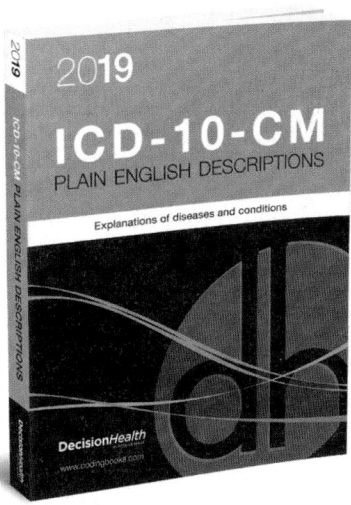

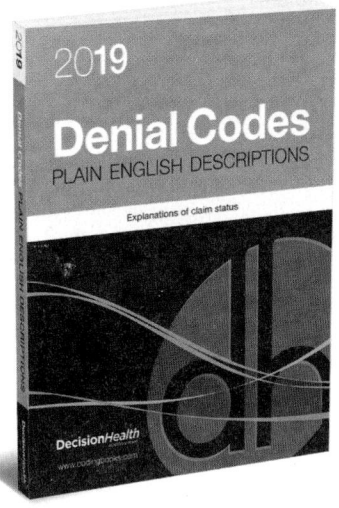

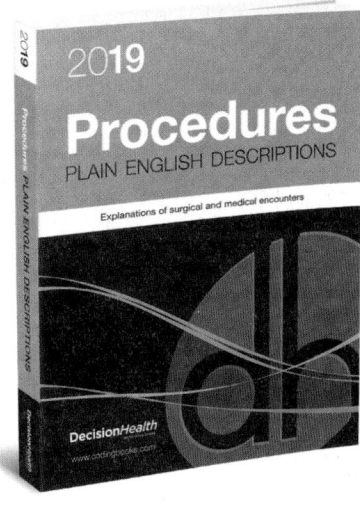

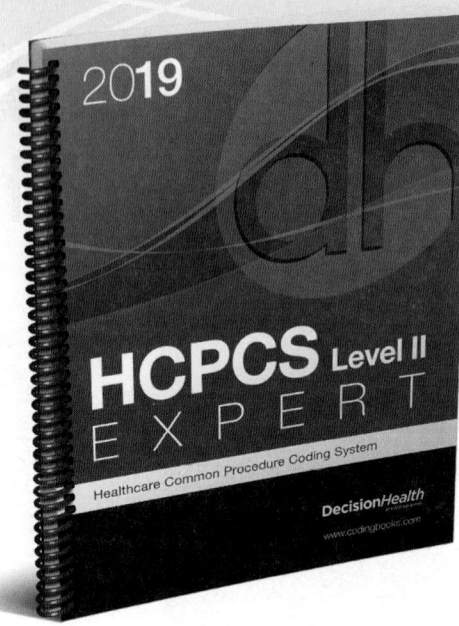

2Ø19

International Classification of Diseases
1Øth Revision Clinical Modification

ICD-1Ø-CM Expert for Physicians

ICD-1Ø-CM Expert for Physicians, 2Ø19

International Classification of Diseases, 1Øth Revision, Clinical Modification

Published by:

DecisionHealth®, an H3.Group division of Simplify Compliance, LLC

100 Winners Circle, Suite 300
Brentwood, TN 37027

Toll-free: 1-855-CALL-DH1 (1-855-225-5341)
http://www.codingbooks.com

Printed in the United States of America

ISBN: 978-1-683Ø8-760-1
Item Number: DHMPBICDPH19

Acknowledgements

Maria Tsigas, *Senior Director, PAC and MP Products*
Renee Dudash, *Senior Director of Operations*
Matt Sharpe, *Senior Production Manager*
AnnMarie Lemoine, *Senior Content Management Specialist*
Karen Long Rayburn, *Content Manager, MP Group*
Lori Becks, RHIA, *Senior Clinical Technical Editor*
Laura Evans, CPC, *Editor*
Susana Lambert, *Publishing Coordinator*
Bradley Clark, *Illustrator*

Table of Contents

Introduction to ICD-10-CM

The World Health Organization (WHO) owns and publishes the *International Statistical Classification of Diseases and Related Health Problems, 10th revision* (ICD-10), and authorized the development of an adaptation of ICD-10 for use in the United States.

ICD-10-Clinical Modification (CM), an expansion of WHO's ICD-10 diagnosis codes, was developed by the National Center for Health Statistics (NCHS), part of the Centers for Disease Control and Prevention (CDC), following a thorough evaluation by a technical advisory panel and additional consultation with physician groups, clinical coders and others to assure clinical accuracy and utility. The first iteration of ICD-10-CM debuted for public comment on the NCHS website in December 1997. However, it took 18 years before the code set was finally used for the classification of morbidity in the U.S.

On Oct. 1, 2015, ICD-10-CM replaced ICD-9-CM as the code set used to classify diagnoses in all U.S. health care settings. Prior to that, ICD-10 codes had been used only to code and classify mortality data for death certificates, beginning Jan. 1, 1999.

The clinical modification represents a significant improvement over ICD-9-CM. Specifically, ICD-10-CM includes the addition of information relevant to ambulatory and managed care encounters; expanded injury codes; the creation of combination diagnosis/symptom codes to reduce the number of codes needed to fully describe a condition; the addition of sixth and seventh characters; the addition of laterality; and greater specificity in code assignment. The new structure allows further expansion than was possible with ICD-9-CM.

In general, ICD-10-CM provides a higher level of detail and the ability to expand to capture new technologies and new advancements in clinical medicine. The code set is designed to allow more accurate reporting of conditions treated, including the ability to track the progression of conditions through treatment.

ICD-10 consists of two parts:

- **ICD-10-CM diagnosis codes,** with consist of three to seven alphanumeric characters and full code titles. These are organized into both an alphabetic index and tabular list.
- **ICD-10 Procedure Coding System (PCS) procedure codes**, developed by the centers for Medicare and Medicaid Services (CMS) for use in U.S. hospital inpatient settings only.

The ICD-10-CM/PCS code sets are maintained and updated by the ICD-10 Coordination and Maintenance Committee, with oversight from CMS and NCHS. The committee meets twice a year to hear proposals for changes to the codes. It then releases its lists of proposed changes to both the CM and PCS code sets in the proposed acute hospital inpatient prospective payment system (IPPS) rule each April and then issues the final version of the code updates in the final hospital rule in July. Separately, the committee releases addenda to the tabular section, updates to the ICD-10-CM Official Guidelines for Coding and Reporting and other information on its website beginning in June. The new codes then take effect Oct. 1 of the same year.

Learn more about the ICD-10-CM/PCS update process on the NCHS website: *https://www.cdc.gov/nchs/icd/icd10cm.htm.*

How to Use the This Manual

Structure of ICD-1Ø-CM

This edition of the ***2019 ICD-10-CM for Physicians Expert*** includes enhancements to assist coders with accurate and efficient selection of the most specific diagnosis code. In addition to the elements of ICD-10-CM maintained by the U.S. Department of Health and Human Services, you'll find icons, illustrations, tips, and definitions throughout the tabular section to help develop a better understanding of the ICD-10-CM codes.

To select a code that corresponds to a diagnosis or reason for the visit documented in the medical record, first locate the term in the Alphabetic Index, and then verify the code in the Tabular List. Make sure to read and adhere to all instructional notations that appear in both the Alphabetic Index and the Tabular List.

ICD-1Ø-CM uses an indented format for both the index and tabular list. The Alphabetical Index contains terms in the ICD-10-CM code set and their corresponding codes. The Tabular List contains categories, subcategories, codes, and descriptors, arranged numerically within the 21 separate chapters. You must use both the Alphabetic Index and Tabular List when locating and assigning a code. Selection of the full code, including laterality and any applicable 7th character, can only be done in the Tabular List.

Alphabetic Index of Diseases and Injuries

The Alphabetic List is divided into two parts: 'Index to Diseases and Injuries' and 'Index to External Causes of Injuries'. Within the index there is a Neoplasm Table.

The Alphabetic Index is an index of diseases, injuries, symptoms and other reasons for a patient encounter.

The main terms are in boldface type and should never be referenced by anatomical site. When using the index, reference the "condition" or other key words to locate potential diagnosis assignment.

Subterms are indented under the main term and indicate the site, type, or etiology for conditions or injuries. More specificity in the condition will be further indented to the right, as needed. Connecting words such as "with," "due to," "in," or "associated with" indicate a relationship between the main term and the subterm.

Table of Drugs and Chemicals

Consult the Table of Drugs and Chemicals when coding a poisoning or adverse effect of a drug. The table, located after the Alphabetic Index to Diseases and Injuries, contains a classification of drugs and other chemical substances associated with poisonings and external causes of adverse effects. The table's rows identify the substance and the columns define the intent: poisoning, accidental (unintentional); poisoning, intentional self-harm; poisoning, assault; poisoning, undetermined; adverse effect; and underdosing. Do not select the final code from the Table of Drugs and Chemicals. Instead, refer back to the tabular section of the manual to ensure correct coding.

In ICD-1Ø, when the drug was correctly prescribed and properly administered and the patient experienced a problem, it is an adverse effect. Assign the code for the nature of the adverse effect followed by the code for the adverse effect of the drug (T36-T5Ø).

Unlike an adverse effect, a poisoning involves a scenario in which the drug was not taken correctly. Poisoning codes have an associated intent: accidental, intentional self-harm, assault, and undetermined. List the poisoning code first, followed by all manifestations of poisonings.

Index to External Cause of Injuries

This section classifies environmental events, circumstances, and conditions as the cause of injury, poisoning and other adverse effects. Located just after the Table of Drugs and Chemicals, the index is organized by main terms that describe the accident, circumstance, event, or specific agent causing the injury or other adverse effect. To locate a code for external causes of an injury or other condition, begin with the Alphabetic Index to External Causes.

Tabular List of Diseases and Injuries

The Tabular List is a numerical listing of the ICD-1Ø codes and their descriptors classified to etiology of conditions or to conditions that affect a specific body system. ICD-1Ø-CM codes contain letters (alpha) and numbers (numeric) and may be 3-7 characters long. Codes with three characters are included as the heading of a category that may be further subdivided by the use of fourth and/or fifth characters and/or sixth characters, which provide greater detail.

A three-character code is to be used only if it is not further subdivided. A code is invalid if it has not been coded to the full number of characters required for that code, including the 7th character, if applicable. The following describes the content of the specific digits:

- First Character – alpha. The only letter not used is the letter 'U', which is reserved for newly discovered diseases of unknown etiology.
- Second Character – numeric
- Third Character – numeric or alpha (not case sensitive)
- Fourth through Seventh Characters – numeric or alpha (not case sensitive). ***Note:*** *For some ICD-1Ø-CM codes, an 'X' is used as a 4th-6th digit character place holder.*

ICD-10-CM Official Guidelines are the Most Authoritative Resource

When there is a question about how to choose or sequence a diagnosis code, the first place to search is also the most authoritative resource - the ICD-10-CM Official Guidelines for Coding and Reporting. These guidelines are updated annually by the ICD-10-CM Coordination and Maintenance Committee and issued each summer at the same time the final ICD-10 code set is released.

Within the ***2019 ICD-10-CM for Physicians Expert*** you will find the most recent version of the guidelines available at press time in the front of the manual. You will also find relevant sections from the guidelines in purple text throughout the tabular code list, located near the codes they impact. That puts the most authoritative coding guidance at your fingertips, with a minimum of page flipping.

For example, under category **E08 Diabetes mellitus due to underlying condition**, you'll find the following paragraph from the official guidelines:

"**Guidelines Section 1.C4.a.6**
Codes under categories E0, Diabetes mellitus due to underlying condition, E09, Drug or chemical induced diabetes mellitus, and E13, Other specified diabetes mellitus, identify complications/manifestations associated with secondary diabetes mellitus. Secondary diabetes is always caused by another condition or event (e.g., cystic fibrosis, malignant neoplasm of pancreas, pancreatectomy, adverse effect of drug, or poisoning)."

Coding Tips Help Fill in the Gaps

In addition to the guidelines, you'll find coding tips in green ink throughout the tabular section. These tips were developed over years of queries to the American Hospital Association Coding Clinic, among other authoritative resources, by DecisionHealth coding editors and subject matter experts. These tips will help you make sense of complicated diagnoses and make the correct code selection when that choice may not be self-evident. For example, under code **E09.36 Drug or chemical induced diabetes mellitus with diabetic cataract**, you'll find the following:

"CODING TIP: Cataracts are more common in diabetic patients. The classification assumes a relationship between cataracts and diabetes, when the patient has diabetes unless the physician specified a different cause."

Definitions Help with Your Understanding of the Scope of a Diagnosis

To assist with coders' understanding of the meaning of certain ICD-10-CM codes, this manual includes brief, plain English descriptions (blue ink). For example, under **F44.1 Dissociative fugue**, you'll find the following:

"DEFINITION: Disorder occurring in response to a severe, recent stressor, in which the patient invents a new personality and becomes unable to remember his/her previous identity, lasting days or months."

Icons and Highlighting Help Quickly Identify Codes, Character Requirements

Make use of the following icons and highlighted codes to quickly identify certain coding elements and how they should be used. Look for a brief key to all of them at the bottom of each page in the tabular section.

Understanding This Manual

The ICD-10-CM Expert contains many icons and highlights that call attention to key indicators and serve as triggers to alert you to instances when you may need additional information to accurately assign a specific code and/or need to take care to understand claims edits impacting a code.

3 4 5 6 7

These icons indicate that an additional digit/character is required to make the code valid.

● ▲

These icons indicate a code addition or change that impacts the code set for the first time this year. The New code icon is used when the code, its descriptor and any instructional notes are first appearing in the code book. The Revised icon is used when an edit is made to the code descriptor or any of its instructional notes. All invalid codes effective in past code years have been removed completely from this manual.

Manifestation

This highlight indicates that these codes are not to be coded on a claim alone. They should be properly sequenced using manifestation coding rules – the etiology, or underlying condition, is sequenced first followed by the manifestation. Codes indicated as manifestations are specified by the Medicare Code Editor (MCE), which detects and reports errors in the coding claims data and is used by most all payers.

Unspecified

This indicator appears on codes that are for use only when the information in the medical record is insufficient to assign a more specific code. For those categories for which an unspecified code is not provided, the "other specified" code may represent both other and unspecified.

A M N P

These icons indicate patient age-related edits used for certain conditions believed to be clinically and virtually impossible in a patient of the stated age. Codes indicated as having an age edit are specified by the Medicare Code Editor (MCE), which detects and reports errors in the coding claims data and is used by most all payers.

♂ ♀

These icons indicate gender-related edits used for certain conditions believed to be clinically and virtually impossible in a patient of the stated sex. Codes indicated as having a sex edit are specified by the Medicare Code Editor (MCE), which detects and reports errors in the coding claims data and is used by most all payers.

HCC

This indicator appears a code if it is designated as a Hierarchical Condition Category under the CMS risk adjustment program. HCCs are used to calculate risk scores to adjust capitated payments made for aged and disabled beneficiaries enrolled in Medicare Advantage plans and certain demonstrations.

HIV

This icon identifies a major HIV-related condition. When the HIV-related condition is coded in combination with an HIV diagnosis, the ICD-10-CM Official Guidelines for Coding and Reporting instruct coders to assign ICD-10-CM code B20 for the HIV as the principal diagnosis or first-listed condition followed by additional codes for the HIV-related conditions.

ICD-10-CM Official Guidelines/Reporting FY 2019 (October 1, 2018 - September 30, 2019)

Narrative changes appear in bold text

Items underlined have been moved within the guidelines since the FY2018 version

***Italics* are used to indicate revisions to heading changes**

The Centers for Medicare and Medicaid Services (CMS) and the National Center for Health Statistics (NCHS), two departments within the U.S. Federal Government's Department of Health and Human Services (DHHS) provide the following guidelines for coding and reporting using the International Classification of Diseases, 10th Revision, Clinical Modification (ICD-10-CM). These guidelines should be used as a companion document to the official version of the ICD-10-CM as published on the NCHS website. The ICD-10-CM is a morbidity classification published by the United States for classifying diagnoses and reason for visits in all health care settings. The ICD-10-CM is based on the ICD-10, the statistical classification of disease published by the World Health Organization (WHO).

These guidelines have been approved by the four organizations that make up the Cooperating Parties for the ICD-10-CM: the American Hospital Association (AHA), the American Health Information Management Association (AHIMA), CMS, and NCHS.

These guidelines are a set of rules that have been developed to accompany and complement the official conventions and instructions provided within the ICD-10-CM itself. The instructions and conventions of the classification take precedence over guidelines. These guidelines are based on the coding and sequencing instructions in the Tabular List and Alphabetic Index of ICD-10-CM, but provide additional instruction. Adherence to these guidelines when assigning ICD-10-CM diagnosis codes is required under the Health Insurance Portability and Accountability Act (HIPAA). The diagnosis codes (Tabular List and Alphabetic Index) have been adopted under HIPAA for all healthcare settings. A joint effort between the healthcare provider and the coder is essential to achieve complete and accurate documentation, code assignment, and reporting of diagnoses and procedures. These guidelines have been developed to assist both the healthcare provider and the coder in identifying those diagnoses that are to be reported. The importance of consistent, complete documentation in the medical record cannot be overemphasized. Without such documentation accurate coding cannot be achieved. The entire record should be reviewed to determine the specific reason for the encounter and the conditions treated.

The term encounter is used for all settings, including hospital admissions. In the context of these guidelines, the term provider is used throughout the guidelines to mean physician or any qualified health care practitioner who is legally accountable for establishing the patient's diagnosis. Only this set of guidelines, approved by the Cooperating Parties, is official.

The guidelines are organized into sections. Section I includes the structure and conventions of the classification and general guidelines that apply to the entire classification, and chapter-specific guidelines that correspond to the chapters as they are arranged in the classification. Section II includes guidelines for selection of principal diagnosis for non-outpatient settings. Section III includes guidelines for reporting additional diagnoses in non-outpatient settings. Section IV is for outpatient coding and reporting. It is necessary to review all sections of the guidelines to fully understand all of the rules and instructions needed to code properly.

Section I. Conventions, general coding guidelines, and chapter specific guidelines

The conventions, general guidelines and chapter-specific guidelines are applicable to all health care settings unless otherwise indicated. The conventions and instructions of the classification take precedence over guidelines.

A. Conventions for the ICD-10-CM

The conventions for the ICD-10-CM are the general rules for use of the classification independent of the guidelines. These conventions are incorporated within the Alphabetic Index and Tabular List of the ICD-10-CM as instructional notes.

1. The Alphabetic Index and Tabular List

The ICD-10-CM is divided into the Alphabetic Index, an alphabetical list of terms and their corresponding code, and the Tabular List, a structured list of codes divided into chapters based on body system or condition. The Alphabetic Index consists of the following parts: the Index of Diseases and Injury, the Index of External Causes of Injury, the Table of Neoplasms and the Table of Drugs and Chemicals.

See Section I.C2. General guidelines

See Section I.C.19. Adverse effects, poisoning, underdosing and toxic effects

2. Format and Structure:

The ICD-10-CM Tabular List contains categories, subcategories and codes. Characters for categories, subcategories and codes may be either a letter or a number. All categories are 3 characters. A three-character category that has no further subdivision is equivalent to a code. Subcategories are either 4 or 5 characters. Codes may be 3, 4, 5, 6 or 7 characters. That is, each level of subdivision after a category is a subcategory. The final level of subdivision is a code. Codes that have applicable 7th characters are still referred to as codes, not subcategories. A code that has an applicable 7th character is considered invalid without the 7th character.

The ICD-10-CM uses an indented format for ease in reference.

3. Use of codes for reporting purposes

For reporting purposes only codes are permissible, not categories or subcategories, and any applicable 7th character is required.

4. Placeholder character

The ICD-10-CM utilizes a placeholder character "X". The "X" is used as a placeholder at certain codes to allow for future expansion. An example of this is at the poisoning, adverse effect and underdosing codes, categories T36-T50.

Where a placeholder exists, the X must be used in order for the code to be considered a valid code.

5. 7th Characters

Certain ICD-10-CM categories have applicable 7th characters. The applicable 7th character is required for all codes within the category, or as the notes in the Tabular List instruct. The 7th character must always be the 7th character in the data field. If a code that requires a 7th character is not 6 characters, a placeholder X must be used to fill in the empty characters.

6. Abbreviations

a. Alphabetic Index abbreviations

NEC "Not elsewhere classifiable"

This abbreviation in the Alphabetic Index represents "other specified". When a specific code is not available for a condition, the Alphabetic Index directs the coder to the "other specified" code in the Tabular List.

NOS "Not otherwise specified"
This abbreviation is the equivalent of unspecified.

b. Tabular List abbreviations

NEC "Not elsewhere classifiable"

This abbreviation in the Tabular List represents "other specified". When a specific code is not available for a condition the Tabular List includes an NEC entry under a code to identify the code as the "other specified" code.

NOS "Not otherwise specified"
This abbreviation is the equivalent of unspecified.

7. Punctuation

[ ] Brackets are used in the Tabular List to enclose synonyms, alternative wording or explanatory phrases. Brackets are used in the Alphabetic Index to identify manifestation codes.

( ) Parentheses are used in both the Alphabetic Index and Tabular List to enclose supplementary words that may be present or absent in the statement of a disease or procedure without affecting the code number to which it is assigned. The terms within the parentheses are referred to as nonessential modifiers. The nonessential modifiers in the Alphabetic Index to Diseases apply to subterms following a main term except when a nonessential modifier and a subentry are mutually exclusive, the subentry takes precedence. For example, in the ICD-10-CM Alphabetic Index under the main term Enteritis, "acute" is a nonessential modifier and "chronic" is a subentry. In this case, the nonessential modifier "acute" does not apply to the subentry "chronic".

: Colons are used in the Tabular List after an incomplete term which needs one or more of the modifiers following the colon to make it assignable to a given category.

8. Use of "and"

See Section I.A.14. Use of the term "And"

9. Other and Unspecified codes

a. "Other" codes

Codes titled "other" or "other specified" are for use when the information in the medical record provides detail for which a specific code does not exist. Alphabetic Index entries with NEC in the line designate "other" codes in the Tabular List. These Alphabetic Index entries represent specific disease entities for which no specific code exists so the term is included within an "other" code.

b. "Unspecified" codes

Codes titled "unspecified" are for use when the information in the medical record is insufficient to assign a more specific code. For those categories for which an unspecified code is not provided, the "other specified" code may represent both other and unspecified.

See Section I.B.18 Use of Signs/Symptom/Unspecified Codes

10. Includes Notes

This note appears immediately under a three character code title to further define, or give examples of, the content of the category.

11. Inclusion terms

List of terms is included under some codes. These terms are the conditions for which that code is to be used. The terms may be synonyms of the code title, or, in the case of "other specified" codes, the terms are a list of the various conditions assigned to that code. The inclusion terms are not necessarily exhaustive. Additional terms found only in the Alphabetic Index may also be assigned to a code.

12. Excludes Notes

The ICD-10-CM has two types of excludes notes. Each type of note has a different definition for use but they are all similar in that they indicate that codes excluded from each other are independent of each other.

a. Excludes1

A type 1 Excludes note is a pure excludes note. It means "NOT CODED HERE!" An Excludes1 note indicates that the code excluded should never be used at the same time as the code above the Excludes1 note. An Excludes1 is used when two conditions cannot occur together, such as a congenital form versus an acquired form of the same condition.

An exception to the Excludes1 definition is the circumstance when the two conditions are unrelated to each other. If it is not clear whether the two conditions involving an Excludes1 note are related or not, query the provider. For example, code F45.8, Other somatoform disorders, has an Excludes1 note for "sleep related teeth grinding (G47.63)," because "teeth grinding" is an inclusion term under F45.8. Only one of these two codes should be assigned for teeth grinding. However psychogenic dysmenorrhea is also an inclusion term under F45.8, and a patient could have both this condition and sleep related teeth grinding. In this case, the two conditions are clearly unrelated to each other, and so it would be appropriate to report F45.8 and G47.63 together.

b. Excludes2

A type 2 excludes note represents "Not included here". An excludes2 note indicates that the condition excluded is not part of the condition represented by the code, but a patient may have both conditions at the same time. When an Excludes2 note appears under a code, it is acceptable to use both the code and the excluded code together, when appropriate.

13. Etiology/manifestation convention ("code first", "use additional code" and "in diseases classified elsewhere" notes)

Certain conditions have both an underlying etiology and multiple body system manifestations due to the underlying etiology. For such conditions, the ICD-10-CM has a coding convention that requires the underlying condition be sequenced first, if applicable, followed by the manifestation. Wherever such a combination exists, there is a "use additional code" note at the etiology code, and a "code first" note at the manifestation code. These instructional notes indicate the proper sequencing order of the codes, etiology followed by manifestation.

In most cases the manifestation codes will have in the code title, "in diseases classified elsewhere." Codes with this title are a component of the etiology/ manifestation convention. The code title indicates that it is a manifestation code. "In diseases classified elsewhere" codes are never permitted to be used as first-listed or principal diagnosis codes. They must be used in conjunction with an underlying condition code and they must be listed following the underlying condition. See category F02, Dementia in other diseases classified elsewhere, for an example of this convention.

There are manifestation codes that do not have "in diseases classified elsewhere" in the title. For such codes, there is a "use additional code" note at the etiology code and a "code first" note at the manifestation code and the rules for sequencing apply.

In addition to the notes in the Tabular List, these conditions also have a specific Alphabetic Index entry structure. In the Alphabetic Index both conditions are listed together with the etiology code first followed by the manifestation codes in brackets. The code in brackets is always to be sequenced second.

An example of the etiology/manifestation convention is dementia in Parkinson's disease. In the Alphabetic Index, code G20 is listed first, followed by code F02.80 or F02.81 in brackets. Code G20 represents the underlying etiology, Parkinson's disease, and must be sequenced first, whereas code F02.80 and F02.81 represent the manifestation of dementia in diseases classified elsewhere, with or without behavioral disturbance.

"Code first" and "Use additional code" notes are also used as sequencing rules in the classification for certain codes that are not part of an etiology/ manifestation combination.

See Section I.B.7. Multiple coding for a single condition.

14. "And"

The word "and" **or "in"** should be interpreted to mean either "and" or "or" when it appears in a title. For example, cases of "tuberculosis of bones", "tuberculosis of joints" and "tuberculosis of bones and joints" are classified to subcategory A18.0, Tuberculosis of bones and joints.

15. "With"

The word "with" should be interpreted to mean "associated with" or "due to" when it appears in a code title, the Alphabetic Index **(either under a main term or subterm),** or an instructional note in the Tabular List. The classification presumes a causal relationship between the two conditions linked by these terms in the Alphabetic Index or Tabular List. These conditions should be coded as related even in the absence of provider documentation explicitly linking them, unless the documentation clearly states the conditions are unrelated or when another guideline exists that specifically requires a documented linkage between two conditions (e.g., sepsis guideline for "acute organ dysfunction that is not clearly associated with the sepsis").

For conditions not specifically linked by these relational terms in the classification or when a guideline requires that a linkage between two conditions be explicitly documented, provider documentation must link the conditions in order to code them as related.

The word "with" in the Alphabetic Index is sequenced immediately following the main term, not in alphabetical order.

16. "See" and "See Also"

The "see" instruction following a main term in the Alphabetic Index indicates that another term should be referenced. It is necessary to go to the main term referenced with the "see" note to locate the correct code.

A "see also" instruction following a main term in the Alphabetic Index instructs that there is another main term that may also be referenced that may provide additional Alphabetic Index entries that may be useful. It is not necessary to follow the "see also" note when the original main term provides the necessary code.

17. "Code also note"

A "code also" note instructs that two codes may be required to fully describe a condition, but this note does not provide sequencing direction. The sequencing depends on the circumstances of the encounter.

18. Default codes

A code listed next to a main term in the ICD-10-CM Alphabetic Index is referred to as a default code. The default code represents that condition that is most commonly associated with the main term, or is the unspecified code for the condition. If a condition is documented in a medical record (for example, appendicitis) without any additional information, such as acute or chronic, the default code should be assigned.

19. Code assignment and Clinical Criteria

The assignment of a diagnosis code is based on the provider's diagnostic statement that the condition exists. The provider's statement that the patient has a particular condition is sufficient. Code assignment is not based on clinical criteria used by the provider to establish the diagnosis.

B. General Coding Guidelines

1. Locating a code in the ICD-10-CM

To select a code in the classification that corresponds to a diagnosis or reason for visit documented in a medical record, first locate the term in the Alphabetic Index, and then verify the code in the Tabular List. Read and be guided by instructional notations that appear in both the Alphabetic Index and the Tabular List.

It is essential to use both the Alphabetic Index and Tabular List when locating and assigning a code. The Alphabetic Index does not always provide the full code. Selection of the full code, including laterality and any applicable 7th character can only be done in the Tabular List. A dash (-) at the end of an Alphabetic Index entry indicates that additional characters are required. Even if a dash is not included at the Alphabetic Index entry, it is necessary to refer to the Tabular List to verify that no 7th character is required.

2. Level of Detail in Coding

Diagnosis codes are to be used and reported at their highest number of characters available.

ICD-10-CM diagnosis codes are composed of codes with 3, 4, 5, 6 or 7 characters. Codes with three characters are included in ICD-10-CM as the heading of a category of codes that may be further subdivided by the use of fourth and/or fifth characters and/or sixth characters, which provide greater detail.

A three-character code is to be used only if it is not further subdivided. A code is invalid if it has not been coded to the full number of characters required for that code, including the 7th character, if applicable.

3. Code or codes from A00.0 through T88.9, Z00-Z99.8

The appropriate code or codes from A00.0 through T88.9, Z00-Z99.8 must be used to identify diagnoses, symptoms, conditions, problems, complaints or other reason(s) for the encounter/visit.

4. Signs and symptoms

Codes that describe symptoms and signs, as opposed to diagnoses, are acceptable for reporting purposes when a related definitive diagnosis has not been established (confirmed) by the provider. Chapter 18 of ICD-10-CM, Symptoms, Signs, and Abnormal Clinical and Laboratory Findings, Not Elsewhere Classified (codes R00.0-R99) contains many, but not all codes for symptoms.

See Section I.B.18 Use of Signs/Symptom/Unspecified Codes

5. Conditions that are an integral part of a disease process

Signs and symptoms that are associated routinely with a disease process should not be assigned as additional codes, unless otherwise instructed by the classification.

6. Conditions that are not an integral part of a disease process

Additional signs and symptoms that may not be associated routinely with a disease process should be coded when present.

7. Multiple coding for a single condition

In addition to the etiology/manifestation convention that requires two codes to fully describe a single condition that affects multiple body systems, there are other single conditions that also require more than one code. "Use additional code" notes are found in the Tabular List at codes that are not part of an etiology/manifestation pair where a secondary code is useful to fully describe a condition. The sequencing rule is the same as the etiology/manifestation pair, "use additional code" indicates that a secondary code should be added, if known.

For example, for bacterial infections that are not included in chapter 1, a secondary code from category B95, Streptococcus, Staphylococcus, and Enterococcus, as the cause of diseases classified elsewhere, or B96,

Other bacterial agents as the cause of diseases classified elsewhere, may be required to identify the bacterial organism causing the infection. A "use additional code" note will normally be found at the infectious disease code, indicating a need for the organism code to be added as a secondary code.

"Code first" notes are also under certain codes that are not specifically manifestation codes but may be due to an underlying cause. When there is a "code first" note and an underlying condition is present, the underlying condition should be sequenced first, if known.

"Code, if applicable, any causal condition first", notes indicate that this code may be assigned as a principal diagnosis when the causal condition is unknown or not applicable. If a causal condition is known, then the code for that condition should be sequenced as the principal or first-listed diagnosis.

Multiple codes may be needed for sequela, complication codes and obstetric codes to more fully describe a condition. See the specific guidelines for these conditions for further instruction.

8. Acute and Chronic Conditions

If the same condition is described as both acute (subacute) and chronic, and separate subentries exist in the Alphabetic Index at the same indentation level, code both and sequence the acute (subacute) code first.

9. Combination Code

A combination code is a single code used to classify:
Two diagnoses, or
A diagnosis with an associated secondary process (manifestation)
A diagnosis with an associated complication

Combination codes are identified by referring to subterm entries in the Alphabetic Index and by reading the inclusion and exclusion notes in the Tabular List.

Assign only the combination code when that code fully identifies the diagnostic conditions involved or when the Alphabetic Index so directs. Multiple coding should not be used when the classification provides a combination code that clearly identifies all of the elements documented in the diagnosis. When the combination code lacks necessary specificity in describing the manifestation or complication, an additional code should be used as a secondary code.

10. Sequela (Late Effects)

A sequela is the residual effect (condition produced) after the acute phase of an illness or injury has terminated. There is no time limit on when a sequela code can be used. The residual may be apparent early, such as in cerebral infarction, or it may occur months or years later, such as that due to a previous injury. Examples of sequela include: scar formation resulting from a burn, deviated septum due to a nasal fracture, and infertility due to tubal occlusion from old tuberculosis. Coding of sequela generally requires two codes sequenced in the following order: the condition or nature of the sequela is sequenced first. The sequela code is sequenced second.

An exception to the above guidelines are those instances where the code for the sequela is followed by a manifestation code identified in the Tabular List and title, or the sequela code has been expanded (at the fourth, fifth or sixth character levels) to include the manifestation(s). The code for the acute phase of an illness or injury that led to the sequela is never used with a code for the late effect.

See Section I.C.9. Sequelae of cerebrovascular disease

See Section I.C.15. Sequelae of complication of pregnancy, childbirth and the puerperium

See Section I.C.19. Application of 7th characters for Chapter 19

11. Impending or Threatened Condition

Code any condition described at the time of discharge as "impending" or "threatened" as follows:

- If it did occur, code as confirmed diagnosis.
- If it did not occur, reference the Alphabetic Index to determine if the condition has a subentry term for "impending" or "threatened" and also reference main term entries for "Impending" and for "Threatened."
- If the subterms are listed, assign the given code.
- If the subterms are not listed, code the existing underlying condition(s) and not the condition described as impending or threatened.

12. Reporting Same Diagnosis Code More than Once

Each unique ICD-10-CM diagnosis code may be reported only once for an encounter. This applies to bilateral conditions when there are no distinct codes identifying laterality or two different conditions classified to the same ICD-10-CM diagnosis code.

13. Laterality

Some ICD-10-CM codes indicate laterality, specifying whether the condition occurs on the left, right or is bilateral. If no bilateral code is provided and the condition is bilateral, assign separate codes for both the left and right side. If the side is not identified in the medical record, assign the code for the unspecified side.

When a patient has a bilateral condition and each side is treated during separate encounters, assign the "bilateral" code (as the condition still exists on both sides), including for the encounter to treat the first side. For the second encounter for treatment after one side has previously been treated and the condition no longer exists on that side, assign the appropriate unilateral code for the side where the condition still exists (e.g., cataract surgery performed on each eye in separate encounters). The bilateral code would not be assigned for the subsequent encounter, as the patient no longer has the condition in the previously-treated site. If the treatment on the first side did not completely resolve the condition, then the bilateral code would still be appropriate.

14. Documentation by Clinicians Other than the Patient's Provider

Code assignment is based on the documentation by patient's provider (i.e., physician or other qualified healthcare practitioner legally accountable for establishing the patient's diagnosis). There are a few exceptions, such as codes for the Body Mass Index (BMI), depth of non-pressure chronic ulcers, pressure ulcer stage, coma scale, and NIH stroke scale (NIHSS) codes, code assignment may be based on medical record documentation from clinicians who are not the patient's provider (i.e., physician or other qualified healthcare practitioner legally accountable for establishing the patient's diagnosis), since this information is typically documented by other clinicians involved in the care of the patient (e.g., a dietitian often documents the BMI and nurses often documents the pressure ulcer stages, and an emergency medical technician often documents the coma scale). However, the associated diagnosis (such as overweight, obesity, acute stroke, or pressure ulcer) must be documented by the patient's provider. If there is conflicting medical record documentation, either from the same clinician or different clinicians, the patient's attending provider should be queried for clarification.

For social determinants of health, such as information found in categories Z55-Z65, Persons with potential health hazards related to socioeconomic and psychosocial circumstances, code assignment may be based on medical record documentation from clinicians involved in the care of the patient who are not the patient's provider since this information represents social information, rather than medical diagnoses.

The BMI, coma scale, and NIHSS codes **and categories Z55-Z65** should only be reported as secondary diagnoses.

15. Syndromes

Follow the Alphabetic Index guidance when coding syndromes. In the absence of Alphabetic Index guidance, assign codes for the documented manifestations of the syndrome. Additional codes for manifestations that are not an integral part of the disease process may also be assigned when the condition does not have a unique code.

16. Documentation of Complications of Care

Codes assignment is based on the provider's documentation of the relationship between the condition and the care or procedure, unless otherwise instructed by the classification. The guideline extends to any complications of care, regardless of the chapter the code is located in. It is important to note that not all conditions that occur during or following medical care or surgery are classified as complications. There must be a cause-and-effect relationship between the care provided and the condition, and an indication in the documentation that it is a complication. Query the provider for clarafication, if the complication is not clearly documented.

17. Borderline Diagnosis

If the provider documents a "borderline" diagnosis at the time of discharge, the diagnosis is coded as confirmed, unless the classification provides a specific entry (e.g., borderline diabetes). If a borderline condition has a specific index entry in ICD-10-CM, it should be coded as such. Since borderline conditions are not uncertain diagnoses, no distinction is made between the care setting (inpatient versus outpatient). Whenever the documentation is unclear regarding a borderline condition, coders are encouraged to query for clarification.

18. Use of Sign/Symptom/ Unspecified Codes

Sign/symptom and "unspecified" codes have acceptable, even necessary, uses. While specific diagnosis codes should be reported when they are supported by the available medical record documentation and clinical knowledge of the patient's health condition, there are instances when signs/symptoms or unspecified codes are the best choices for accurately reflecting the healthcare encounter. Each healthcare encounter should be coded to the level of certainty known for that encounter.

If a definitive diagnosis has not been established by the end of the encounter, it is appropriate to report codes for sign(s) and/or symptom(s) in lieu of a definitive diagnosis. When sufficient clinical information isn't known or available about a particular health condition to assign a more specific code, it is acceptable to report the appropriate "unspecified" code (e.g., a diagnosis of pneumonia has been determined, but not the specific type). Unspecified codes should be reported when they are the codes that most accurately reflect what is known about the patient's condition at the time of that particular encounter. It would be inappropriate to select a specific code that is not supported by the medical record documentation or conduct medically unnecessary diagnostic testing in order to determine a more specific code.

19. Coding for Healthcare Encounters in Hurricane Aftermath

a. Use of External Cause of Morbidity Codes

An external cause of morbidity code should be assigned to identify the cause of the injury(ies) incurred as a result of the hurricane. The use of external cause of morbidity codes is supplemental to the application of ICD-10-CM codes. External cause of morbidity codes are never to be recorded as a principal diagnosis (first-listed in non-inpatient settings). The appropriate injury code should be sequenced before any external cause codes. The external cause of morbidity codes capture how the injury or health condition happened (cause), the intent (unintentional or accidental; or intentional, such as suicide or assault), the place where the event occurred, the activity of the patient at the time of the event, and the person's status (e.g., civilian, military). They should not be assigned for encounters to treat hurricane victims' medical conditions when no injury, adverse effect or poisoning is involved. External cause of morbidity codes should be assigned for each encounter for care and treatment of the injury. External cause of morbidity codes may be assigned in all health care settings. For the purpose of capturing complete and accurate ICD-10-CM data in the aftermath of the hurricane, a healthcare setting should be considered as any location where medical care is provided by licensed healthcare professionals.

b. Sequencing of External Causes of Morbidity Codes

Codes for cataclysmic events, such as a hurricane, take priority over all other external cause codes except child and adult abuse and terrorism and should be sequenced before other external cause of injury codes. Assign as many external cause of morbidity codes as necessary to fully explain each cause. For example, if an injury occurs as a result of a building collapse during the hurricane, external cause codes for both the hurricane and the building collapse should be assigned, with the external causes code for hurricane being sequenced as the first external cause code. For injuries incurred as a direct result of the hurricane, assign the appropriate code(s) for the injuries, followed by the code X37.0-, Hurricane (with the appropriate 7th character), and any other applicable external cause of injury codes. Code X37.0- also should be assigned when an injury is incurred as a result of flooding caused by a levee breaking related to the hurricane. Code X38.-, Flood (with the appropriate 7th character), should be assigned when an injury is from flooding resulting directly from the storm. Code X36.0.-, Collapse of dam or man-made structure, should not be assigned when the cause of the collapse is due to the hurricane. Use of code X36.0- is limited to collapses of man-made structures due to earth surface movements, not due to storm surges directly from a hurricane.

c. Other External Causes of Morbidity Code Issues

For injuries that are not a direct result of the hurricane, such as an evacuee that has incurred an injury as a result of a motor vehicle accident, assign the appropriate external cause of morbidity code(s) to describe the cause of the injury, but do not assign code X37.0-, Hurricane. If it is not clear whether the injury was a direct result of the hurricane, assume the injury is due to the hurricane and assign code X37.0-, Hurricane, as well as any other applicable external cause of morbidity codes. In addition to code X37.0-, Hurricane, other possible applicable external cause of morbidity codes include:

W54.0-, Bitten by dog

X30-, Exposure to excessive natural heat

X31-, Exposure to excessive natural cold

X38-, Flood

d. Use of Z codes

Z codes (other reasons for healthcare encounters) may be assigned as appropriate to further explain the reasons for presenting for healthcare services, including transfers between healthcare facilities. The ICD-10-CM Official Guidelines for Coding and Reporting identify which codes maybe assigned as principal or first-listed diagnosis only, secondary diagnosis only, or principal/first-listed or secondary (depending on the circumstances). Possible applicable Z codes include:

Z59.0, Homelessness

Z59.1, Inadequate housing

Z59.5, Extreme poverty

Z75.1, Person awaiting admission to adequate facility elsewhere

Z75.3, Unavailability and inaccessibility of health-care facilities

Z75.4, Unavailability and inaccessibility of other helping agencies

Z76.2, Encounter for health supervision and care of other healthy infant and child

Z99.12, Encounter for respirator [ventilator] dependence during power failure

The external cause of morbidity codes and the Z codes listed above are not an all-inclusive list. Other codes may be applicable to the encounter based upon the documentation. Assign as many codes as necessary to fully explain each healthcare encounter. Since patient history information may be very limited, use any available documentation to assign the appropriate external cause of morbidity and Z codes.

C. Chapter-Specific Coding Guidelines

In addition to general coding guidelines, there are guidelines for specific diagnoses and/or conditions in the classification. Unless otherwise indicated, these guidelines apply to all health care settings. Please refer to Section II for guidelines on the selection of principal diagnosis.

1. Chapter 1: Certain Infectious and Parasitic Diseases (AØØ-B99)

a. Human Immunodeficiency Virus (HIV) Infections

1) Code only confirmed cases

Code only confirmed cases of HIV infection/illness. This is an exception to the hospital inpatient guideline Section II, H.

In this context, "confirmation" does not require documentation of positive serology or culture for HIV; the provider's diagnostic statement that the patient is HIV positive, or has an HIV-related illness is sufficient.

2) Selection and sequencing of HIV codes

(a) Patient admitted for HIV-related condition

If a patient is admitted for an HIV-related condition, the principal diagnosis should be B20, Human immunodeficiency virus [HIV] disease followed by additional diagnosis codes for all reported HIV-related conditions.

(b) Patient with HIV disease admitted for unrelated condition

If a patient with HIV disease is admitted for an unrelated condition (such as a traumatic injury), the code for the unrelated condition (e.g., the nature of injury code) should be the principal diagnosis. Other diagnoses would be B20 followed by additional diagnosis codes for all reported HIV-related conditions.

(c) Whether the patient is newly diagnosed

Whether the patient is newly diagnosed or has had previous admissions/encounters for HIV conditions is irrelevant to the sequencing decision.

(d) Asymptomatic human immunodeficiency virus

Z21, Asymptomatic human immunodeficiency virus [HIV] infection status, is to be applied when the patient without any documentation of symptoms is listed as being "HIV positive," "known HIV," "HIV test positive," or similar terminology. Do not use this code if the term "AIDS" is used or if the patient is treated for any HIV-related illness or is described as having any condition(s) resulting from his/her HIV positive status; use B20 in these cases.

(e) Patients with inconclusive HIV serology

Patients with inconclusive HIV serology, but no definitive diagnosis or manifestations of the illness, may be assigned code R75, Inconclusive laboratory evidence of human immunodeficiency virus [HIV].

(f) Previously diagnosed HIV-related illness

Patients with any known prior diagnosis of an HIV-related illness should be coded to B20. Once a patient has developed an HIV-related illness, the patient should always be assigned code B20 on every subsequent admission/encounter. Patients previously diagnosed with any HIV illness (B20) should never be assigned to R75 or Z21, Asymptomatic human immunodeficiency virus [HIV] infection status.

(g) HIV Infection in Pregnancy, Childbirth and the Puerperium

During pregnancy, childbirth or the puerperium, a patient admitted (or presenting for a health care encounter) because of an HIV-related illness should receive a principal diagnosis code of O98.7-, Human immunodeficiency [HIV] disease complicating pregnancy, childbirth and the puerperium, followed by B20 and the code(s) for the HIV-related illness(es). Codes from Chapter 15 always take sequencing priority.

Patients with asymptomatic HIV infection status admitted (or presenting for a health care encounter) during pregnancy, childbirth, or the puerperium should receive codes of O98.7- and Z21.

(h) Encounters for testing for HIV

If a patient is being seen to determine his/her HIV status, use code Z11.4, Encounter for screening for human immunodeficiency virus [HIV]. Use additional codes for any associated high risk behavior.

If a patient with signs or symptoms is being seen for HIV testing, code the signs and symptoms. An additional counseling code Z71.7, Human immunodeficiency virus [HIV] counseling, may be used if counseling is provided during the encounter for the test.

When a patient returns to be informed of his/her HIV test results and the test result is negative, use code Z71.7, Human immunodeficiency virus [HIV] counseling.

If the results are positive, see previous guidelines and assign codes as appropriate.

b. Infectious agents as the cause of diseases classified to other chapters

Certain infections are classified in chapters other than Chapter 1 and no organism is identified as part of the infection code. In these instances, it is necessary to use an additional code from Chapter 1 to identify the organism. A code from category B95, Streptococcus, Staphylococcus, and Enterococcus as the cause of diseases classified to other chapters, B96, Other bacterial agents as the cause of diseases classified to other chapters, or B97, Viral agents as the cause of diseases classified to other chapters, is to be used as an additional code to identify the organism. An instructional note will be found at the infection code advising that an additional organism code is required.

c. Infections resistant to antibiotics

Many bacterial infections are resistant to current antibiotics. It is necessary to identify all infections documented as antibiotic resistant. Assign a code from category Z16, Resistance to antimicrobial drugs, following the infection code only if the infection codes does not identify drug resistance.

d. Sepsis, Severe Sepsis, and Septic Shock

1) Coding of Sepsis and Severe Sepsis

(a) Sepsis

For a diagnosis of sepsis, assign the appropriate code for the underlying systemic infection. If the type of infection or causal organism is not further specified, assign code A41.9, Sepsis, unspecified organism.

A code from subcategory R65.2, Severe sepsis, should not be assigned unless severe sepsis or an associated acute organ dysfunction is documented.

(i) Negative or inconclusive blood cultures and sepsis

Negative or inconclusive blood cultures do not preclude a diagnosis of sepsis in patients with clinical evidence of the condition, however, the provider should be queried.

(ii) Urosepsis

The term urosepsis is a nonspecific term. It is not to be considered synonymous with sepsis. It has no default code in the Alphabetic Index. Should a provider use this term, he/she must be queried for clarification.

(iii) Sepsis with organ dysfunction

If a patient has sepsis and associated acute organ dysfunction or multiple organ dysfunction (MOD), follow the instructions for coding severe sepsis.

(iv) Acute organ dysfunction that is not clearly associated with the sepsis

If a patient has sepsis and an acute organ dysfunction, but the medical record documentation indicates that the acute organ dysfunction is related to a medical condition other than the sepsis, do not assign a code from subcategory R65.2, Severe sepsis. An acute organ dysfunction must be associated with the sepsis in order to assign the severe sepsis code. If the documentation is not clear as to whether an acute organ dysfunction is related to the sepsis or another medical condition, query the provider.

(b) Severe sepsis

The coding of severe sepsis requires a minimum of 2 codes: first a code for the underlying systemic infection, followed by a code from subcategory R65.2, Severe sepsis. If the causal organism is not documented, assign code A41.9, Sepsis, unspecified organism, for the infection. Additional code(s) for the associated acute organ dysfunction are also required.

Due to the complex nature of severe sepsis, some cases may require querying the provider prior to assignment of the codes.

2) Septic shock

Septic shock generally refers to circulatory failure associated with severe sepsis, and therefore, it represents a type of acute organ dysfunction.

For cases of septic shock, the code for the systemic infection should be sequenced first, followed by code R65.21, Severe sepsis with septic shock or code T81.12, Postprocedural septic shock. Any additional codes for the other acute organ dysfunctions should also be assigned. As noted in the sequencing instructions in the Tabular List, the code for septic shock cannot be assigned as a principal diagnosis.

3) Sequencing of severe sepsis

If severe sepsis is present on admission, and meets the definition of principal diagnosis, the underlying systemic infection should be assigned as principal diagnosis followed by the appropriate code from subcategory R65.2 as required by the sequencing rules in the Tabular List. A code from subcategory R65.2 can never be assigned as a principal diagnosis.

When severe sepsis develops during an encounter (it was not present on admission) the underlying systemic infection and the appropriate code from subcategory R65.2 should be assigned as secondary diagnoses.

Severe sepsis may be present on admission but the diagnosis may not be confirmed until sometime after admission. If the documentation is not clear whether severe sepsis was present on admission, the provider should be queried.

4) Sepsis and severe sepsis with a localized infection

If the reason for admission is both sepsis or severe sepsis and a localized infection, such as pneumonia or cellulitis, a code(s) for the underlying systemic infection should be assigned first and the code for the localized infection should be assigned as a secondary diagnosis. If the patient has severe sepsis, a code from subcategory R65.2 should also be assigned as a secondary diagnosis. If the patient is admitted with a localized infection, such as pneumonia, and sepsis/severe sepsis doesn't develop until after admission, the localized infection should be assigned first, followed by the appropriate sepsis/severe sepsis codes.

5) Sepsis due to a postprocedural infection

(a) Documentation of causal relationship

As with all postprocedural complications, code assignment is based on the provider's documentation of the relationship between the infection and the procedure.

(b) Sepsis due to a postprocedural infection

For **infections following a procedure, a code from** T81.**40, to T81.43** Infection following a procedure, or **a code from** O86.0**0 to O86.03**, Infection of obstetric surgical wound, **that identifies the site of the infection** should be coded first, **if known. Assign an additional code for sepsis following a procedure (T81.44) or sepsis following an obstetrical procedure (O86.04). Use an additional code to identify the infectious agent.** If the patient has severe sepsis the appropriate code from subcategory R65.2 should also be assigned with the additional code(s) for any acute organ dysfunction.

For infections following infusion, transfusion, therapeutic injection, or immunization, a code from subcategory T80.2, Infections following infusion, transfusion, and therapeutic injection, or code T88.0-, Infection following immunization, should be coded first, followed by the code for the specific infection. If the patient has severe sepsis, the appropriate code from subcategory R65.2 should also be assigned, with the additional codes(s) for any acute organ dysfunction.

(c) Postprocedural infection and postprocedural septic shock

If a postprocedural infection has resulted in postprocedural septic shock, **assign the codes indicated above for sepsis due to a postprocedural infection, followed by code T81.12-, Postprocedural septic shock. Do not assign code R65.21, Severe sepsis with septic shock. Additional code(s) should be assigned for any acute organ dysfunction.**

(c) Postprocedural infection and postprocedural septic shock

In cases where a postprocedural infection has occurred and has resulted in severe sepsis the code for the precipitating complication such as code T81.4, Infection following a procedure, or O86.0, Infection of obstetrical surgical wound should be coded first followed by code R65.20, Severe sepsis without septic shock. A code for the systemic infection should also be assigned.

If a postprocedural infection has resulted in postprocedural septic shock, the code for the precipitating complication such as code T81.4, Infection following a procedure, or O86.0, Infection of obstetrical surgical wound should be coded first followed by code T81.12-, Postprocedural septic shock. A code for the systemic infection should also be assigned.

6) Sepsis and severe sepsis associated with a noninfectious process (condition)

In some cases a noninfectious process (condition), such as trauma, may lead to an infection which can result in sepsis or severe sepsis. If sepsis or severe sepsis is documented as associated with a noninfectious condition, such as a burn or serious injury, and this condition meets the definition for principal diagnosis, the code for the noninfectious condition should be sequenced first, followed by the code for the resulting infection. If severe sepsis, is present a code from subcategory R65.2 should also be assigned with any associated organ dysfunction(s) codes. It is not necessary to assign a code from subcategory R65.1, Systemic inflammatory response syndrome (SIRS) of non-infectious origin, for these cases.

If the infection meets the definition of principal diagnosis it should be sequenced before the non-infectious condition. When both the associated non-infectious condition and the infection meet the definition of principal diagnosis either may be assigned as principal diagnosis.

Only one code from category R65, Symptoms and signs specifically associated with systemic inflammation and infection, should be assigned. Therefore, when a non-infectious condition leads to an infection resulting in severe sepsis, assign the appropriate code from subcategory R65.2, Severe sepsis. Do not additionally assign a code from subcategory R65.1, Systemic inflammatory response syndrome (SIRS) of non-infectious origin.

See Section I.C.18. SIRS due to non-infectious process

7) Sepsis and septic shock complicating abortion, pregnancy, childbirth, and the puerperium

See Section I.C.15. Sepsis and septic shock complicating abortion, pregnancy, childbirth and the puerperium

8) Newborn sepsis

See Section I.C.16. f. *Bacterial sepsis of Newborn*

e. Methicillin Resistant Staphylococcus aureus (MRSA) Conditions

1) Selection and sequencing of MRSA codes

(a) **Combination codes for MRSA infection**

When a patient is diagnosed with an infection that is due to methicillin resistant Staphylococcus aureus (MRSA), and that infection has a combination code that includes the causal organism (e.g., sepsis, pneumonia) assign the appropriate combination code for the condition (e.g., code A41.02, Sepsis due to Methicillin resistant Staphylococcus aureus or code J15.212, Pneumonia due to Methicillin resistant Staphylococcus aureus). Do not assign code B95.62, Methicillin resistant Staphylococcus aureus infection as the cause of diseases classified elsewhere, as an additional code because the combination code includes the type of infection and the MRSA organism. Do not assign a code from subcategory Z16.11, Resistance to penicillins, as an additional diagnosis.

See Section C.1. for instructions on coding and sequencing of sepsis and severe sepsis.

(b) **Other codes for MRSA infection**

When there is documentation of a current infection (e.g., wound infection, stitch abscess, urinary tract infection) due to MRSA, and that infection does not have a combination code that includes the causal organism, assign the appropriate code to identify the condition along with code B95.62, Methicillin resistant Staphylococcus aureus infection as the cause of diseases classified elsewhere for the MRSA infection. Do not assign a code from subcategory Z16.11, Resistance to penicillins.

(c) **Methicillin susceptible Staphylococcus aureus (MSSA) and MRSA colonization**

The condition or state of being colonized or carrying MSSA or MRSA is called colonization or carriage, while an individual person is described as being colonized or being a carrier. Colonization means that MSSA or MSRA is present on or in the body without necessarily causing illness. A positive MRSA colonization test might be documented by the provider as "MRSA screen positive" or "MRSA nasal swab positive".

Assign code Z22.322, Carrier or suspected carrier of Methicillin resistant Staphylococcus aureus, for patients documented as having MRSA colonization. Assign code Z22.321, Carrier or suspected carrier of Methicillin susceptible Staphylococcus aureus, for patient documented as having MSSA colonization. Colonization is not necessarily indicative of a disease process or as the cause of a specific condition the patient may have unless documented as such by the provider

(d) **MRSA colonization and infection**

If a patient is documented as having both MRSA colonization and infection during a hospital admission, code Z22.322, Carrier or suspected carrier of Methicillin resistant Staphylococcus aureus, and a code for the MRSA infection may both be assigned.

f. Zika virus infections

1) Code only confirmed cases

Code only a confirmed diagnosis of Zika virus (A92.5, Zika virus disease) as documented by the provider. This is an exception to the hospital inpatient guideline Section II, H. In this context, "confirmation" does not require documentation of the type of test performed; the physician's diagnostic statement that the condition is confirmed is sufficient. This code should be assigned regardless of the stated mode of transmission.

If the provider documents "suspected", "possible" or "probable" Zika, do not assign code A92.5. Assign a code(s) explaining the reason for encounter (such as fever, rash, or joint pain) or Z20.**821**, Contact with and (suspected) exposure to **Zika virus**.

2. Chapter 2: Neoplasms (CØØ-D49)

General guidelines

Chapter 2 of the ICD-10-CM contains the codes for most benign and all malignant neoplasms. Certain benign neoplasms, such as prostatic adenomas, may be found in the specific body system chapters. To properly code a neoplasm it is necessary to determine from the record if the neoplasm is benign, in-situ, malignant, or of uncertain histologic behavior. If malignant, any secondary (metastatic) sites should also be determined.

Primary malignant neoplasms overlapping site boundaries

A primary malignant neoplasm that overlaps two or more contiguous (next to each other) sites should be classified to the subcategory/code .8 ('overlapping lesion'), unless the combination is specifically indexed elsewhere. For multiple neoplasms of the same site that are not contiguous such as tumors in different quadrants of the same breast, codes for each site should be assigned.

Malignant neoplasm of ectopic tissue

Malignant neoplasms of ectopic tissue are to be coded to the site of origin mentioned, e.g., ectopic pancreatic malignant neoplasms involving the stomach are coded to malignant neoplasm of pancreas, unspecified (C25.9).

The neoplasm table in the Alphabetic Index should be referenced first. However, if the histological term is documented, that term should be referenced first, rather than going immediately to the Neoplasm Table, in order to determine which column in the Neoplasm Table is appropriate. For example, if the documentation indicates "adenoma," refer to the term in the Alphabetic Index to review the entries under this term and the instructional note to "see also neoplasm, by site, benign." The table provides the proper code based on the type of neoplasm and the site. It is important to select the proper column in the table that corresponds to the type of neoplasm. The Tabular List should then be referenced to verify that the correct code has been selected from the table and that a more specific site code does not exist.

See Section I.C.21. Factors influencing health status and contact with health services, Status, for information regarding Z15.0, codes for genetic susceptibility to cancer.

a. Treatment directed at the malignancy

If the treatment is directed at the malignancy, designate the malignancy as the principal diagnosis.

The only exception to this guideline is if a patient admission/encounter is solely for the administration of chemotherapy, immunotherapy or external beam radiation therapy, assign the appropriate Z51.-- code as the first-listed or principal diagnosis, and the diagnosis or problem for which the service is being performed as a secondary diagnosis.

b. Treatment of secondary site

When a patient is admitted because of a primary neoplasm with metastasis and treatment is directed toward the secondary site only, the secondary neoplasm is designated as the principal diagnosis even though the primary malignancy is still present.

c. Coding and sequencing of complications

Coding and sequencing of complications associated with the malignancies or with the therapy thereof are subject to the following guidelines:

1) Anemia associated with malignancy

When admission/encounter is for management of an anemia associated with the malignancy, and the treatment is only for anemia, the appropriate code for the malignancy is sequenced as the principal or first-listed diagnosis followed by the appropriate code for the anemia (such as code D63.0, Anemia in neoplastic disease).

2) Anemia associated with chemotherapy, immunotherapy and radiation therapy

When the admission/encounter is for management of an anemia associated with an adverse effect of the administration of chemotherapy or immunotherapy and the only treatment is for the anemia, the anemia code is sequenced first followed by the appropriate codes for the neoplasm and the adverse effect (T45.1X5-, Adverse effect of antineoplastic and immunosuppressive drugs).

When the admission/encounter is for management of an anemia associated with an adverse effect of radiotherapy, the anemia code should be sequenced first, followed by the appropriate neoplasm code and code Y84.2, Radiological procedure and radiotherapy as the cause of abnormal reaction of the patient, or of later complication, without mention of misadventure at the time of the procedure.

3) Management of dehydration due to the malignancy

When the admission/encounter is for management of dehydration due to the malignancy and only the dehydration is being treated (intravenous rehydration), the dehydration is sequenced first, followed by the code(s) for the malignancy.

4) Treatment of a complication resulting from a surgical procedure

When the admission/encounter is for treatment of a complication resulting from a surgical procedure, designate the complication as the principal or first-listed diagnosis if treatment is directed at resolving the complication.

d. Primary malignancy previously excised

When a primary malignancy has been previously excised or eradicated from its site and there is no further treatment directed to that site and there is no evidence of any existing primary malignancy, a code from category Z85, Personal history of malignant neoplasm, should be used to indicate the former site of the malignancy. Any mention of extension, invasion, or metastasis to another site is coded as a secondary malignant neoplasm to that site. The secondary site may be the principal or first-listed with the Z85 code used as a secondary code.

e. Admissions/Encounters involving chemotherapy, immunotherapy and radiation therapy

1) Episode of care involves surgical removal of neoplasm

When an episode of care involves the surgical removal of a neoplasm, primary or secondary site, followed by adjunct chemotherapy or radiation treatment during the same episode of care, the code for the neoplasm should be assigned as principal or first-listed diagnosis.

2) Patient admission/encounter solely for administration of chemotherapy, immunotherapy and radiation therapy

If a patient admission/encounter is solely for the administration of chemotherapy, immunotherapy or radiation therapy assign code Z51.0, Encounter for antineoplastic external beam radiation therapy, or Z51.11, Encounter for antineoplastic chemotherapy, or Z51.12, Encounter for antineoplastic immunotherapy as the first-listed or principal diagnosis. If a patient receives more than one of these therapies during the same admission more than one of these codes may be assigned, in any sequence.

The malignancy for which the therapy is being administered should be assigned as a secondary diagnosis.

If a patient admission/encounter is for the insertion or implantation of radioactive elements (e.g., brachytherapy) the appropriate code for the malignancy is sequenced as the principal or first-listed diagnosis. Code Z51.0 should not be assigned.

3) Patient admitted for radiation therapy, chemotherapy or immunotherapy and develops complications

When a patient is admitted for the purpose of external beam radiotherapy, immunotherapy or chemotherapy and develops complications such as uncontrolled nausea and vomiting or dehydration, the principal or first-listed diagnosis is Z51.0, Encounter for antineoplastic radiation therapy, or Z51.11, Encounter for antineoplastic chemotherapy, or Z51.12, Encounter for antineoplastic immunotherapy followed by any codes for the complications.

When a patient is admitted for the purpose of insertion or implantation of radioactive elements (e.g., brachytherapy) and develops complications such as uncontrolled nausea and vomiting or dehydration, the principal or first-listed diagnosis is the appropriate code for the malignancy followed by any codes for the complications.

f. Admission/encounter to determine extent of malignancy

When the reason for admission/encounter is to determine the extent of the malignancy, or for a procedure such as paracentesis or thoracentesis, the primary malignancy or appropriate metastatic site is designated as the principal or first-listed diagnosis, even though chemotherapy or radiotherapy is administered.

g. Symptoms, signs, and abnormal findings listed in Chapter 18 associated with neoplasms

Symptoms, signs, and ill-defined conditions listed in Chapter 18 characteristic of, or associated with, an existing primary or secondary site malignancy cannot be used to replace the malignancy as principal or first-listed diagnosis, regardless of the number of admissions or encounters for treatment and care of the neoplasm.

See section I.C.21. Factors influencing health status and contact with health services, Encounter for prophylactic organ removal.

h. Admission/encounter for pain control/management

See Section I.C.6. for information on coding admission/encounter for pain control/management.

i. Malignancy in two or more noncontiguous sites

A patient may have more than one malignant tumor in the same organ. These tumors may represent different primaries or metastatic disease, depending on the site. Should the documentation be unclear, the provider should be queried as to the status of each tumor so that the correct codes can be assigned.

j. Disseminated malignant neoplasm, unspecified

Code C80.0, Disseminated malignant neoplasm, unspecified, is for use only in those cases where the patient has advanced metastatic disease and no known primary or secondary sites are specified. It should not be used in place of assigning codes for the primary site and all known secondary sites.

k. Malignant neoplasm without specification of site

Code C80.1, Malignant (primary) neoplasm, unspecified, equates to Cancer, unspecified. This code should only be used when no determination can be made as to the primary site of a malignancy. This code should rarely be used in the inpatient setting.

l. Sequencing of neoplasm codes

1) Encounter for treatment of primary malignancy

If the reason for the encounter is for treatment of a primary malignancy, assign the malignancy as the principal/first-listed diagnosis. The primary site is to be sequenced first, followed by any metastatic sites.

2) Encounter for treatment of secondary malignancy

When an encounter is for a primary malignancy with metastasis and treatment is directed toward the metastatic (secondary) site(s) only, the metastatic site(s) is designated as the principal/first-listed diagnosis. The primary malignancy is coded as an additional code.

3) Malignant neoplasm in a pregnant patient

When a pregnant woman has a malignant neoplasm, a code from subcategory O9A.1-, Malignant neoplasm complicating pregnancy, childbirth, and the puerperium, should be sequenced first, followed by the appropriate code from Chapter 2 to indicate the type of neoplasm.

4) Encounter for complication associated with a neoplasm

When an encounter is for management of a complication associated with a neoplasm, such as dehydration, and the treatment is only for the complication, the complication is coded first, followed by the appropriate code(s) for the neoplasm.

The exception to this guideline is anemia. When the admission/encounter is for management of an anemia associated with the malignancy, and the treatment is only for anemia, the appropriate code for the malignancy is sequenced as the principal or first-listed diagnosis followed by code D63.0, Anemia in neoplastic disease.

5) Complication from surgical procedure for treatment of a neoplasm

When an encounter is for treatment of a complication resulting from a surgical procedure performed for the treatment of the neoplasm, designate the complication as the principal/first-listed diagnosis. See guideline regarding the coding of a current malignancy versus personal history to determine if the code for the neoplasm should also be assigned.

6) Pathologic fracture due to a neoplasm

When an encounter is for a pathological fracture due to a neoplasm and the focus of treatment is the fracture, a code from subcategory M84.5, Pathological fracture in neoplastic disease, should be sequenced first, followed by the code for the neoplasm.

If the focus of treatment is the neoplasm with an associated pathological fracture, the neoplasm code should be sequenced first, followed by a code from M84.5 for the pathological fracture.

m. Current malignancy versus personal history of malignancy

When a primary malignancy has been excised but further treatment, such as an additional surgery for the malignancy, radiation therapy or chemotherapy is directed to that site, the primary malignancy code should be used until treatment is completed.

When a primary malignancy has been previously excised or eradicated from its site, there is no further treatment (of the malignancy) directed to that site, and there is no evidence of any existing primary malignancy **at that site**, a code from category Z85, Personal history of malignant neoplasm, should be used to indicate the former site of the malignancy.

Subcategories Z85.0 – Z85.7 should only be assigned for the former site of a primary malignancy, not the site of a secondary malignancy. Codes from subcategory Z85.8-, may be assigned for the former site(s) of either a primary or secondary malignancy included in this subcategory.

See Section I.C.21. Factors influencing health status and contact with health services, History (of)

n. Leukemia, Multiple Myeloma, and Malignant Plasma Cell Neoplasms in remission versus personal history

The categories for leukemia, and category C90, Multiple myeloma and malignant plasma cell neoplasms, have codes indicating whether or not the leukemia has achieved remission. There are also codes Z85.6, Personal history of leukemia, and Z85.79, Personal history of other malignant neoplasms of lymphoid, hematopoietic and related tissues. If the documentation is unclear, as to whether the leukemia has achieved remission, the provider should be queried.

See Section I.C.21. Factors influencing health status and contact with health services, History (of)

o. Aftercare following surgery for neoplasm

See Section I.C.21. Factors influencing health status and contact with health services, Aftercare

p. Follow-up care for completed treatment of a malignancy

See Section I.C.21. Factors influencing health status and contact with health services, Follow-up

q. Prophylactic organ removal for prevention of malignancy

See Section I.C. 21, Factors influencing health status and contact with health services, Prophylactic organ removal

r. Malignant neoplasm associated with transplanted organ

A malignant neoplasm of a transplanted organ should be coded as a transplant complication. Assign first the appropriate code from category T86.-, Complications of transplanted organs and tissue, followed by code C80.2, Malignant neoplasm associated with transplanted organ. Use an additional code for the specific malignancy.

3. Chapter 3: Disease of the blood and blood-forming organs and certain disorders involving the immune mechanism (D5Ø-D89)

Reserved for future guideline expansion

4. Chapter 4: Endocrine, Nutritional, and Metabolic Diseases (EØØ-E89)

a. Diabetes mellitus

The diabetes mellitus codes are combination codes that include the type of diabetes mellitus, the body system affected, and the complications affecting that body system. As many codes within a particular category as are necessary to describe all of the complications of the disease may be used. They should be sequenced based on the reason for a particular encounter. Assign as many codes from categories E08 – E13 as needed to identify all of the associated conditions that the patient has.

1) Type of diabetes

The age of a patient is not the sole determining factor, though most type 1 diabetics develop the condition before reaching puberty. For this reason type 1 diabetes mellitus is also referred to as juvenile diabetes.

2) Type of diabetes mellitus not documented

If the type of diabetes mellitus is not documented in the medical record the default is E11.-, Type 2 diabetes mellitus.

3) Diabetes mellitus and the use of insulin and oral hypoglycemics

If the documentation in a medical record does not indicate the type of diabetes but does indicate that the patient uses insulin, code E11-, Type 2 diabetes mellitus, should be assigned. An additional code should be assigned from category Z79 to identify the long-term (current) use of insulin or oral hypoglycemic drugs. If the patient is treated with both oral medications and insulin, only the code for long-term (current) use of insulin should be assigned. Code Z79.4 should not be assigned if insulin is given temporarily to bring a type 2 patient's blood sugar under control during an encounter.

4) Diabetes mellitus in pregnancy and gestational diabetes

See Section I.C.15. Diabetes mellitus in pregnancy.

See Section I.C.15. Gestational (pregnancy induced) diabetes

5) Complications due to insulin pump malfunction

(a) Underdose of insulin due to insulin pump failure

An underdose of insulin due to an insulin pump failure should be assigned to a code from subcategory T85.6, Mechanical complication of other specified internal and external prosthetic devices, implants and grafts, that specifies the type of pump malfunction, as the principal or first-listed code, followed by code T38.3x6-, Underdosing of insulin and oral hypoglycemic [antidiabetic] drugs. Additional codes for the type of diabetes mellitus and any associated complications due to the underdosing should also be assigned.

(b) Overdose of insulin due to insulin pump failure

The principal or first-listed code for an encounter due to an insulin pump malfunction resulting in an overdose of insulin, should also be T85.6-, Mechanical complication of other specified internal and external prosthetic devices, implants and grafts, followed by code T38.3x1-, Poisoning by insulin and oral hypoglycemic [antidiabetic] drugs, accidental (unintentional).

6) Secondary diabetes mellitus

Codes under categories E08, Diabetes mellitus due to underlying condition, and E09, Drug or chemical induced diabetes mellitus, and E13, other specified diabetes mellitus, identify complications/manifestations associated with secondary diabetes mellitus. Secondary diabetes is always caused by another condition or event (e.g., cystic fibrosis, malignant neoplasm of pancreas, pancreatectomy, adverse effect of drug, or poisoning).

(a) Secondary diabetes mellitus and the use of insulin or hypoglycemic drugs *oral*

For patients with secondary diabetes mellitus who routinely use insulin or oral hypoglycemic drugs, an additional code from category Z79 should be assigned to identify the long-term (current) use of insulin or oral hypoglycemic drugs. If the patient is treated with both oral medications and insulin, only the code for long-term (current) use of insulin should be assigned. Code Z79.4 should not be assigned if insulin is given temporarily to bring a type 2 patient's blood sugar under control during an encounter.

(b) Assigning and sequencing secondary diabetes codes and its causes

The sequencing of the secondary diabetes codes in relationship to codes for the cause of the diabetes is based on the Tabular List instructions for categories E08, E09 and E13.

(i) **Secondary diabetes mellitus due to pancreatectomy**

For postpancreatectomy diabetes mellitus (lack of insulin due to the surgical removal of all or part of the pancreas), assign code E89.1, Postprocedural hypoinsulinemia. Assign a code from category E13 and a code from subcategory Z90.41, Acquired absence of pancreas, as additional codes.

(ii) **Secondary diabetes due to drugs**

Secondary diabetes may be caused by an adverse effect of correctly administered medications, poisoning or sequela of poisoning.

See section I.C.19.e for coding of adverse effects and poisoning, and section I.C.20 for external cause code reporting.

5. Chapter 5: Mental, Behavioral and Neurodevelopmental disorders (FØ1 – F99)

a. Pain disorders related to psychological factors

Assign code F45.41, for pain that is exclusively related to psychological disorders. As indicated by the Excludes 1 note under category G89, a code from category G89 should not be assigned with code F45.41

Code F45.42, Pain disorders with related psychological factors, should be used with a code from category G89, Pain, not elsewhere classified, if there is documentation of a psychological component for a patient with acute or chronic pain.

See Section I.C.6. Pain

b. Mental and behavioral disorders due to psychoactive substance use

1) In Remission

Selection of codes for "in remission" for categories F10-F19, Mental and behavioral disorders due to psychoactive substance use (categories F10-F19 with -11, -.21) requires the provider's clinical judgment. The appropriate codes for "in remission" are assigned only on the basis of provider documentation (as defined in the Official Guidelines for Coding and Reporting), unless otherwise instructed by the classification.

Mild substance use disorders in early or sustained remission are classified to the appropriate codes for substance abuse in remission, and moderate or severe substance use disorders in early or sustained remission are classified to the appropriate codes for substance dependence in remission.

2) Psychoactive Substance Use, Abuse And Dependence

When the provider documentation refers to use, abuse and dependence of the same substance (e.g. alcohol, opioid, cannabis, etc.), only one code should be assigned to identify the pattern of use based on the following hierarchy:

- If both use and abuse are documented, assign only the code for abuse
- If both abuse and dependence are documented, assign only the code for dependence
- If use, abuse and dependence are all documented, assign only the code for dependence
- If both use and dependence are documented, assign only the code for dependence.

3) Psychoactive Substance Use *Disorders*

As with all other **unspecified** diagnoses, the codes for **unspecified** psychoactive substance use disorders (F10.9-, F11.9-, F12.9-, F13.9-, F14.9-, F15.9-, F16.9-, **F18.9-, F19.9-**) should only be assigned based on provider documentation and when they meet the definition of a reportable diagnosis (see Section III, Reporting Additional Diagnoses). The codes are to be used only when the psychoactive substance use is associated with a physical, mental or behavioral disorder, and such a relationship is documented by the provider.

c. Factitious Disorder

Factitious disorder imposed on self or Munchausen's syndrome is a disorder in which a person falsely reports or causes his or her own physical or psychological signs or symptoms. For patients with documented factitious disorder on self or Munchausen's syndrome, assign the appropriate code from subcategory F68.1-, Factitious disorder imposed on self.

Munchausen's syndrome by proxy (MSBP) is a disorder in which a caregiver (perpetrator) falsely reports or causes an illness or injury in another person (victim) under his or her care, such as a child, an elderly adult, or a person who has a disability. The condition is also referred to as "factitious disorder imposed on another" or "factitious disorder by proxy." The perpetrator, not the victim, receives this diagnosis. Assign code F68.A, Factitious disorder imposed on another, to the perpetrator's record. For the victim of a patient suffering from MSBP, assign the appropriate code from categories T74, Adult and child abuse, neglect and other maltreatment, confirmed, or T76, Adult and child abuse, neglect and other maltreatment, suspected.

See Section I.C.19.f. Adult and child abuse, neglect and other maltreatment

6. Chapter 6: Diseases of Nervous System and Sense Organs (GØØ-G99)

a. Dominant/nondominant side

Codes from category G81, Hemiplegia and hemiparesis, and subcategories, G83.1, Monoplegia of lower limb, G83.2, Monoplegia of upper limb, and G83.3, Monoplegia, unspecified, identify whether the dominant or nondominant side is affected. Should the affected side be documented, but not specified as dominant or nondominant, and the classification system does not indicate a default, code selection is as follows:

- For ambidextrous patients, the default should be dominant.
- If the left side is affected, the default is non-dominant.
- If the right side is affected, the default is dominant.

b. Pain - Category G89

1) General coding information

Codes in category G89, Pain, not elsewhere classified, may be used in conjunction with codes from other categories and chapters to provide more detail about acute or chronic pain and neoplasm-related pain, unless otherwise indicated below.

If the pain is not specified as acute or chronic, post-thoracotomy, postprocedural, or neoplasm-related, do not assign codes from category G89.

A code from category G89 should not be assigned if the underlying (definitive) diagnosis is known, unless the reason for the encounter is pain control/ management and not management of the underlying condition.

When an admission or encounter is for a procedure aimed at treating the underlying condition (e.g., spinal fusion, kyphoplasty), a code for the underlying condition (e.g., vertebral fracture, spinal stenosis) should be assigned as the principal diagnosis. No code from category G89 should be assigned.

(a) Category G89 Codes as Principal or First-Listed Diagnosis

Category G89 codes are acceptable as principal diagnosis or the first-listed code:

- When pain control or pain management is the reason for the admission/encounter (e.g., a patient with displaced intervertebral disc, nerve impingement and severe back pain presents for injection of steroid into the spinal canal). The underlying cause of the pain should be reported as an additional diagnosis, if known.
- When a patient is admitted for the insertion of a neurostimulator for pain control, assign the appropriate pain code as the principal or first-listed diagnosis. When an admission or encounter is for a procedure aimed at treating the underlying condition and a neurostimulator is inserted for pain control during the same admission/encounter, a code for the underlying condition should be assigned as the principal diagnosis and the appropriate pain code should be assigned as a secondary diagnosis.

(b) Use of Category G89 Codes in Conjunction with Site Specific Pain Codes

(i) **Assigning Category G89 and Site-Specific Pain Codes**

Codes from category G89 may be used in conjunction with codes that identify the site of pain (including codes from chapter 18) if the category G89 code provides additional information. For example, if the code describes the site of the pain, but does not fully describe whether the pain is acute or chronic, then both codes should be assigned.

(ii) **Sequencing of Category G89 Codes with Site-Specific Pain Codes**

The sequencing of category G89 codes with site-specific pain codes (including chapter 18 codes), is dependent on the circumstances of the encounter/admission as follows:

- If the encounter is for pain control or pain management, assign the code from category G89 followed by the code identifying the specific site of pain (e.g., encounter for pain management for acute neck pain from trauma is assigned code G89.11, Acute pain due to trauma, followed by code M54.2, Cervicalgia, to identify the site of pain).
- If the encounter is for any other reason except pain control or pain management, and a related definitive diagnosis has not been established (confirmed) by the provider, assign the code for the specific site of pain first, followed by the appropriate code from category G89.

2) Pain due to devices, implants and grafts

See Section I.C.19. Pain due to medical devices

3) Postoperative Pain

The provider's documentation should be used to guide the coding of postoperative pain, as well as *Section III. Reporting Additional Diagnoses and Section IV. Diagnostic Coding and Reporting in the Outpatient Setting.*

The default for post-thoracotomy and other postoperative pain not specified as acute or chronic is the code for the acute form.

Routine or expected postoperative pain immediately after surgery should not be coded.

(a) **Postoperative pain not associated with specific postoperative complication**

Postoperative pain not associated with a specific postoperative complication is assigned to the appropriate postoperative pain code in category G89.

(b) **Postoperative pain associated with specific postoperative complication**

Postoperative pain associated with a specific postoperative complication (such as painful wire sutures) is assigned to the appropriate code(s) found in Chapter 19, Injury, poisoning, and certain other consequences of external causes. If appropriate, use additional code(s) from category G89 to identify acute or chronic pain (G89.18 or G89.28).

4) Chronic pain

Chronic pain is classified to subcategory G89.2. There is no time frame defining when pain becomes chronic pain. The provider's documentation should be used to guide use of these codes.

5) Neoplasm Related Pain

Code G89.3 is assigned to pain documented as being related, associated or due to cancer, primary or secondary malignancy, or tumor. This code is assigned regardless of whether the pain is acute or chronic.

This code may be assigned as the principal or first-listed code when the stated reason for the admission/encounter is documented as pain control/pain management. The underlying neoplasm should be reported as an additional diagnosis.

When the reason for the admission/encounter is management of the neoplasm and the pain associated with the neoplasm is also documented, code G89.3 may be assigned as an additional diagnosis. It is not necessary to assign an additional code for the site of the pain.

See Section I.C.2 for instructions on the sequencing of neoplasms for all other stated reasons for the admission/encounter (except for pain control/pain management).

6) Chronic pain syndrome

Central pain syndrome (G89.0) and chronic pain syndrome (G89.4) are different than the term "chronic pain," and therefore codes should only be used when the provider has specifically documented this condition.

See Section I.C.5. Pain disorders related to psychological factors

7. Chapter 7: Diseases of Eye and Adnexa (HØØ-H59)

a. Glaucoma

1) Assigning Glaucoma Codes

Assign as many codes from category H40, Glaucoma, as needed to identify the type of glaucoma, the affected eye, and the glaucoma stage.

2) Bilateral glaucoma with same type and stage

When a patient has bilateral glaucoma and both eyes are documented as being the same type and stage, and there is a code for bilateral glaucoma, report only the code for the type of glaucoma, bilateral, with the seventh character for the stage.

When a patient has bilateral glaucoma and both eyes are documented as being the same type and stage, and the classification does not provide a code for bilateral glaucoma (i.e. subcategories H40.10, H40.11 and H40.20) report only one code for the type of glaucoma with the appropriate seventh character for the stage.

3) Bilateral glaucoma stage with different types or stages

When a patient has bilateral glaucoma and each eye is documented as having a different type or stage, and the classification distinguishes laterality, assign the appropriate code for each eye rather than the code for bilateral glaucoma.

When a patient has bilateral glaucoma and each eye is documented as having a different type, and the classification does not distinguish laterality (i.e. subcategories H40.10, H40.11 and H40.20), assign one code for each type of glaucoma with the appropriate seventh character for the stage.

When a patient has bilateral glaucoma and each eye is documented as having the same type, but different stage, and the classification does not distinguish laterality (i.e. subcategories H40.10, H40.11 and H40.20), assign a code for the type of glaucoma for each eye with the seventh character for the specific glaucoma stage documented for each eye.

4) Patient admitted with glaucoma and stage evolves during the admission

If a patient is admitted with glaucoma and the stage progresses during the admission, assign the code for highest stage documented.

5) Indeterminate stage glaucoma

Assignment of the seventh character "4" for "indeterminate stage" should be based on the clinical documentation. The seventh character "4" is used for glaucomas whose stage cannot be clinically determined. This seventh character should not be confused with the seventh character "0", unspecified, which should be assigned when there is no documentation regarding the stage of the glaucoma.

b. Blindness

If "blindness" or "low vision" of both eyes is documented but the visual impairment category is not documented, assign code H54.3, Unqualified visual loss, both eyes. If "blindness" or "low vision" in one eye is documented but the visual impairment category is not documented, assign a code from H54.6-, Unqualified visual loss, one eye. If "blindness" or "visual loss" is documented without any information about whether one or both eyes are affected, assign code H54.7, Unspecified visual loss.

8. Chapter 8: Diseases of Ear and Mastoid Process (H6Ø-H95)

Reserved for future guideline expansion

9. Chapter 9: Diseases of Circulatory System (IØØ-I99)

a. Hypertension

The classification presumes a causal relationship between hypertension and heart involvement and between hypertension and kidney involvement, as the two conditions are linked by the term "with" in the Alphabetic Index. These conditions should be coded as related even in the absence of provider documentation explicitly linking them, unless the documentation clearly states the conditions are unrelated.

For hypertension and conditions not specifically linked by relational terms such as "with," "associated with" or "due to" in the classification, provider documentation must link the conditions in order to code them as related.

1) Hypertension with Heart Disease

Hypertension with heart conditions classified to I50.- or **I51.4-I51.7, I51.89, I51.9**, are assigned to, a code from category I11, Hypertensive heart disease. Use an additional code(s) from category I50, Heart failure, to identify the type(s) of heart failure in those patients with heart failure.

The same heart conditions (I50.-, **I51.4-I51.7, I51.89, I51.9**) with hypertension are coded separately if the provider has **documented they are unrelated to the hypertension**. Sequence according to the circumstances of the admission/encounter.

2) Hypertensive Chronic Kidney Disease

Assign codes from category I12, Hypertensive chronic kidney disease, when both hypertension and a condition classifiable to category N18, Chronic kidney disease (CKD), are present. CKD should not be coded as hypertensive if the **provider indicates the CKD is not related to the hypertension**.

The appropriate code from category N18 should be used as a secondary code with a code from category I12 to identify the stage of chronic kidney disease.

See Section I.C.14. Chronic kidney disease.

If a patient has hypertensive chronic kidney disease and acute renal failure, an additional code for the acute renal failure is required.

3) Hypertensive Heart and Chronic Kidney Disease

Assign codes from combination category I13, Hypertensive heart and chronic kidney disease, when there is hypertension with both heart and kidney involvement. If heart failure is present, assign an additional code from category I50 to identify the type of heart failure.

The appropriate code from category N18, Chronic kidney disease, should be used as a secondary code with a code from category I13 to identify the stage of chronic kidney disease.

See Section I.C.14. Chronic kidney disease.

The codes in category I13, Hypertensive heart and chronic kidney disease, are combination codes that include hypertension, heart disease and chronic kidney disease. The Includes note at I13 specifies that the conditions included at I11 and I12 are included together in I13. If a patient has hypertension, heart disease and chronic kidney disease then a code from I13 should be used, not individual codes for hypertension, heart disease and chronic kidney disease, or codes from I11 or I12.

For patients with both acute renal failure and chronic kidney disease an additional code for acute renal failure is required.

4) Hypertensive Cerebrovascular Disease

For hypertensive cerebrovascular disease, first assign the appropriate code from categories I60-I69, followed by the appropriate hypertension code.

5) Hypertensive Retinopathy

Subcategory H35.0, Background retinopathy and retinal vascular changes, should be used with a code from category I10 – I15, Hypertensive disease to include the systemic hypertension. The sequencing is based on the reason for the encounter.

6) Hypertension, Secondary

Secondary hypertension is due to an underlying condition. Two codes are required: one to identify the underlying etiology and one from category I15 to identify the hypertension. Sequencing of codes is determined by the reason for admission/encounter.

7) Hypertension, Transient

Assign code R03.0, Elevated blood pressure reading without diagnosis of hypertension, unless patient has an established diagnosis of hypertension. Assign code O13.-, Gestational [pregnancy-induced] hypertension without significant proteinuria, or O14.-, Pre-eclampsia, for transient hypertension of pregnancy.

8) Hypertension, Controlled

This diagnostic statement usually refers to an existing state of hypertension under control by therapy. Assign the appropriate code from categories I10-I15, Hypertensive diseases.

9) Hypertension, Uncontrolled

Uncontrolled hypertension may refer to untreated hypertension or hypertension not responding to current therapeutic regimen. In either case, assign the appropriate code from categories I10-I15, Hypertensive diseases.

10) Hypertensive Crisis

Assign a code from category I16, Hypertensive crisis, for documented hypertensive urgency, hypertensive emergency or unspecified hypertensive crisis. Code also any identified hypertensive disease (I10-I15). The sequencing is based on the reason for the encounter.

11) Pulmonary Hypertension

Pulmonary hypertension is classified to category I27, Other pulmonary heart diseases. For secondary pulmonary hypertension (I27.1, I27.2-), code also any associated conditions or adverse effects of drugs or toxins. The sequencing is based on the reason for the encounter**, except for adverse effects of drugs (See Section I.C.19.e.)**

b. Atherosclerotic Coronary Artery Disease and Angina

ICD-10-CM has combination codes for atherosclerotic heart disease with angina pectoris. The subcategories for these codes are I25.11, Atherosclerotic heart disease of native coronary artery with angina pectoris and I25.7, Atherosclerosis of coronary artery bypass graft(s) and coronary artery of transplanted heart with angina pectoris.

When using one of these combination codes it is not necessary to use an additional code for angina pectoris. A causal relationship can be assumed in a patient with both atherosclerosis and angina pectoris, unless the documentation indicates the angina is due to something other than the atherosclerosis.

If a patient with coronary artery disease is admitted due to an acute myocardial infarction (AMI), the AMI should be sequenced before the coronary artery disease.

See Section I.C.9. Acute myocardial infarction (AMI)

c. Intraoperative and Postprocedural Cerebrovascular Accident

Medical record documentation should clearly specify the cause-and-effect relationship between the medical intervention and the cerebrovascular accident in order to assign a code for intraoperative or postprocedural cerebrovascular accident.

Proper code assignment depends on whether it was an infarction or hemorrhage and whether it occurred intraoperatively or postoperatively. If it was a cerebral hemorrhage, code assignment depends on the type of procedure performed.

d. Sequelae of Cerebrovascular Disease

1) Category I69, Sequelae of Cerebrovascular disease

Category I69 is used to indicate conditions classifiable to categories I60-I67 as the causes of sequela (neurologic deficits), themselves classified elsewhere. These "late effects" include neurologic deficits that persist after initial onset of conditions classifiable to categories I60-I67. The neurologic deficits caused by cerebrovascular disease may be present from the onset or may arise at any time after the onset of the condition classifiable to categories I60-I67.

Codes from category I69, Sequelae of cerebrovascular disease, that specify hemiplegia, hemiparesis and monoplegia identify whether the dominant or nondominant side is affected. Should the affected side be documented, but not specified as dominant or nondominant, and the classification system does not indicate a default, code selection is as follows:

- For ambidextrous patients, the default should be dominant.
- If the left side is affected, the default is non-dominant.
- If the right side is affected, the default is dominant.

2) Codes from category I69 with codes from I60-I67

Codes from category I69 may be assigned on a health care record with codes from I60-I67, if the patient has a current cerebrovascular disease and deficits from an old cerebrovascular disease. 3) Codes from category I69 and Personal history of transient ischemic attack (TIA) and cerebral infarction (Z86.73)

Codes from category I69 should not be assigned if the patient does not have neurologic deficits.

See Section I.C.21. 4. History (of) for use of personal history codes

e. Acute myocardial infarction (AMI)

1) Type 1 ST elevation myocardial infarction (STEMI) and non -ST elevation myocardial infarction (NSTEMI)

The ICD-10-CM codes for type 1 acute myocardial infarction (AMI) identify the site, such as anterolateral wall or true posterior wall. Subcategories I21.0-I21.2 and code I21.3 are used for type 1 ST elevation myocardial infarction (STEMI). Code I21.4, Non-ST elevation (NSTEMI) myocardial infarction, is used for type 1 non ST elevation myocardial infarction (NSTEMI) and nontransmural MIs.

If a type 1 NSTEMI evolves to STEMI, assign the STEMI code. If a type 1 STEMI converts to NSTEMI due to thrombolytic therapy, it is still coded as STEMI.

For encounters occurring while the myocardial infarction is equal to, or less than, four weeks old, including transfers to another acute setting or a postacute setting, and myocardial infarction meets the definition for "other diagnoses" (see Section III, Reporting Additional Diagnoses), codes from category I21 may continue to be reported. For encounters after the 4 week time frame and the patient is still receiving care related to the myocardial infarction, the appropriate aftercare code should be assigned, rather than a code from category I21. For old or healed myocardial infarctions not requiring further care, code I25.2, Old myocardial infarction, may be assigned.

2) Acute myocardial infarction, unspecified

Code I21.9, Acute myocardial infarction, unspecified, is the default for the unspecified term acute myocardial infarction or unspecified type. If only type 1 STEMI or transmural MI without the site is documented, query the provider as to the site, or assign code I21.3, ST elevation (STEMI) myocardial infarction of unspecified site.

3) AMI documented as nontransmural or subendocardial but site provided

If an AMI is documented as nontransmural or subendocardial, but the site is provided, it is still coded as a subendocardial AMI.

See Section I.C.21.3 for information on coding status post administration of tPA in a different facility within the last 24 hours.

4) Subsequent acute myocardial infarction

A code from category I22, Subsequent ST elevation (STEMI) and non- ST elevation (NSTEMI) myocardial infarction, is to be used when a patient who has suffered a type 1 or unspecified AMI has a new AMI within the 4 week time frame of the initial AMI. A code from category I22 must be used in conjunction with a code from category I21. The sequencing of the I22 and I21 codes depends on the circumstances of the encounter.

Do not assign code I22 for subsequent myocardial infarctions other than type 1 or unspecified. For subsequent type 2 AMI assign only code I21.A1. For subsequent type 4 or type 5 AMI, assign only code I21.A9.

If a subsequent myocardial infarction of one type occurs within 4 weeks of a myocardial infarction of a different type, assign the appropriate codes from category I21 to identify each type. Do not assign a code from I22. Codes from category I22 should only be assigned if both the initial and subsequent myocardial infarctions are type 1 or unspecified.

5) Other Types of Myocardial Infarction

The ICD-10-CM provides codes for different types of myocardial infarction. Type 1 myocardial infarctions are assigned to codes I21.0-I21.4 **and I21.9.**

Type 2 myocardial infarction, and myocardial infarction due to demand ischemia or secondary to ischemic balance, is assigned to code I21.A1, Myocardial infarction type 2 with a code for the underlying cause. Do not assign code I24.8, Other forms of acute ischemic heart disease for the demand ischemia. Sequencing of type 2 AMI or the underlying cause is dependent on the circumstances of admission. When a type 2 AMI code is described as NSTEMI or STEMI, only assign code I21.A1. Codes I21.01-I21.4 should only be assigned for type 1 AMIs.

Acute myocardial infarctions type 3, 4a, 4b, 4c and 5 are assigned to code I21.A9, Other myocardial infarction type.

The "Code also" and "Code first" notes should be followed related to complications, and for coding of postprocedural myocardial infarctions during or following cardiac surgery.

10. Chapter 10: Diseases of the Respiratory System (J00-J99)

a. Chronic Obstructive Pulmonary Disease [COPD] and Asthma

1) Acute exacerbation of chronic obstructive bronchitis and asthma

The codes in categories J44 and J45 distinguish between uncomplicated cases and those in acute exacerbation. An acute exacerbation is a worsening or a decompensation of a chronic condition. An acute exacerbation is not equivalent to an infection superimposed on a chronic condition, though an exacerbation may be triggered by an infection.

b. Acute Respiratory Failure

1) Acute respiratory failure as principal diagnosis

A code from subcategory J96.0, Acute respiratory failure, or subcategory J96.2, Acute and chronic respiratory failure, may be assigned as a principal diagnosis when it is the condition established after study to be chiefly responsible for occasioning the admission to the hospital, and the selection is supported by the Alphabetic Index and Tabular List. However, chapter-specific coding guidelines (such as obstetrics, poisoning, HIV, newborn) that provide sequencing direction take precedence.

2) Acute respiratory failure as secondary diagnosis

Respiratory failure may be listed as a secondary diagnosis if it occurs after admission, or if it is present on admission, but does not meet the definition of principal diagnosis.

3) Sequencing of acute respiratory failure and another acute condition

When a patient is admitted with respiratory failure and another acute condition, (e.g., myocardial infarction, cerebrovascular accident, aspiration pneumonia), the principal diagnosis will not be the same in every situation. This applies whether the other acute condition is a respiratory or nonrespiratory condition. Selection of the principal diagnosis will be dependent on the circumstances of admission. If both the respiratory failure and the other acute condition are equally responsible for occasioning the admission to the hospital, and there are no chapter-specific sequencing rules, the guideline regarding two or more diagnoses that equally meet the definition for principal diagnosis *(Section II, C.)* may be applied in these situations.

If the documentation is not clear as to whether acute respiratory failure and another condition are equally responsible for occasioning the admission, query the provider for clarification.

c. Influenza due to certain identified influenza influenza viruses

Code only confirmed cases of influenza due to certain identified influenza viruses (category J09), and due to other identified influenza virus (category J10). This is an exception to the hospital inpatient guideline Section II, H. (Uncertain Diagnosis).

In this context, "confirmation" does not require documentation of positive laboratory testing specific for avian or other novel influenza A or other identified influenza virus. However, coding should be based on the provider's diagnostic statement that the patient has avian influenza, or other novel influenza A for category J09, or has another particular identified strain of influenza, such as H1N1 or H3N2, but not identified as novel or variant, for category J10..

If the provider records "suspected" or "possible" or "probable" avian influenza," or novel influenza, or other identified influenza, then the appropriate influenza code from category J11, Influenza due to unidentified influenza virus, should be assigned. A code from category J09, Influenza due to certain identified influenza viruses, should not be assigned nor should a code from category J10, Influenza due to other identified influenza virus.

d. Ventilator associated Pneumonia

1) Documentation of Ventilator associated Pneumonia

As with all procedural or postprocedural complications, code assignment is based on the provider's documentation of the relationship between the condition and the procedure.

Code J95.851, Ventilator associated pneumonia, should be assigned only when the provider has documented ventilator associated pneumonia (VAP). An additional code to identify the organism (e.g., Pseudomonas aeruginosa, code B96.5) should also be assigned. Do not assign an additional code from categories J12-J18 to identify the type of pneumonia.

Code J95.851 should not be assigned for cases where the patient has pneumonia and is on a mechanical ventilator and the provider has not specifically stated that the pneumonia is ventilator-associated pneumonia. If the documentation is unclear as to whether the patient has a pneumonia that is a complication attributable to the mechanical ventilator, query the provider.

2) Ventilator associated Pneumonia Develops after Admission

A patient may be admitted with one type of pneumonia (e.g., code J13, Pneumonia due to Streptococcus pneumonia) and subsequently develop VAP. In this instance, the principal diagnosis would be the appropriate code from categories J12-J18 for the pneumonia diagnosed at the time of admission. Code J95.851, Ventilator associated pneumonia, would be assigned as an additional diagnosis when the provider has also documented the presence of ventilator associated pneumonia.

11. Chapter 11: Diseases of **the** *Digestive System (KØØ-K95)*

Reserved for future guideline expansion

12. Chapter 12: Diseases of **the** *Skin and Subcutaneous Tissue (LØØ-L99)*

a. Pressure ulcer stage codes

1) Pressure ulcer stages

Codes from category L89, Pressure ulcer, are combination codes that identify the site of the pressure ulcer as well as the stage of the ulcer.

The ICD-10-CM classifies pressure ulcer stages based on severity, which is designated by stages 1-4, unspecified stage and unstageable.

Assign as many codes from category L89 as needed to identify all the pressure ulcers the patient has, if applicable.

2) Unstageable pressure ulcers

Assignment of the code for unstageable pressure ulcer (L89.--0) should be based on the clinical documentation. These codes are used for pressure ulcers whose stage cannot be clinically determined (e.g., the ulcer is covered by eschar or has been treated with a skin or muscle graft) and pressure ulcers that are documented as deep tissue injury but not documented as due to trauma. This code should not be confused with the codes for unspecified stage (L89.--9). When there is no documentation regarding the stage of the pressure ulcer, assign the appropriate code for unspecified stage (L89.--9).

3) Documented pressure ulcer stage

Assignment of the pressure ulcer stage code should be guided by clinical documentation of the stage or documentation of the terms found in the Alphabetic Index. For clinical terms describing the stage that are not found in the Alphabetic Index, and there is no documentation of the stage, the provider should be queried.

4) Patients admitted with pressure ulcers documented as healed

No code is assigned if the documentation states that the pressure ulcer is completely healed.

5) Patients admitted with pressure ulcers documented as healing

Pressure ulcers described as healing should be assigned the appropriate pressure ulcer stage code based on the documentation in the medical record. If the documentation does not provide information about the stage of the healing pressure ulcer, assign the appropriate code for unspecified stage.

If the documentation is unclear as to whether the patient has a current (new) pressure ulcer or if the patient is being treated for a healing pressure ulcer, query the provider.

For ulcers that were present on admission but healed at the time of discharge, assign the code for the site and stage of the pressure ulcer at the time of admission.

6) Patient admitted with pressure ulcer evolving into another stage during the admission

If a patient is admitted **to an inpatient hospital** with a pressure ulcer at one stage and it progresses to a higher stage, two separate codes should be assigned: one code for the site and stage of the ulcer on admission and a second code for the same ulcer site and the highest stage reported during the stay.

b. Non-Pressure Chronic Ulcers

1) Patients admitted with non-pressure ulcers documented as healed

No code is assigned if the documentation states that the non-pressure ulcer is completely healed.

2) Patients admitted with non-pressure ulcers documented as healing

Non-pressure ulcers described as healing should be assigned the appropriate non-pressure ulcer code based on the documentation in the medical record. If the documentation does not provide information about the severity of the healing non-pressure ulcer, assign the appropriate code for unspecified severity.

If the documentation is unclear as to whether the patient has a current (new) non-pressure ulcer or if the patient is being treated for a healing non-pressure ulcer, query the provider.

For ulcers that were present on admission but healed at the time of discharge, assign the code for the site and severity of the non-pressure ulcer at the time of admission.

3) Patient admitted with non-pressure ulcer that progresses to another severity level during the admission

If a patient is admitted to an inpatient hospital with a non-pressure ulcer at one severity level and it progresses to a higher severity level, two separate codes should be assigned: one code for the site and severity level of the ulcer on admission and a second code for the same ulcer site and the highest severity level reported during the stay.

See Section I.B.14 for pressure ulcer stage documentation by clinicians other than patient's provider

13. Chapter 13: Diseases of the Musculoskeletal System and Connective Tissue (MØØ-M99)

a. Site and laterality

Most of the codes within Chapter 13 have site and laterality designations. The site represents the bone, joint or the muscle involved. For some conditions where more than one bone, joint or muscle is usually involved, such as osteoarthritis, there is a "multiple sites" code available. For categories where no multiple site code is provided and more than one bone, joint or muscle is involved, multiple codes should be used to indicate the different sites involved.

1) Bone versus joint

For certain conditions, the bone may be affected at the upper or lower end, (e.g., avascular necrosis of bone, M87, Osteoporosis, M80, M81). Though the portion of the bone affected may be at the joint, the site designation will be the bone, not the joint.

b. Acute traumatic versus chronic or recurrent musculoskeletal conditions

Many musculoskeletal conditions are a result of previous injury or trauma to a site, or are recurrent conditions. Bone, joint or muscle conditions that are the result of a healed injury are usually found in chapter 13. Recurrent bone, joint or muscle conditions are also usually found in chapter 13. Any current, acute injury should be coded to the appropriate injury code from chapter 19. Chronic or recurrent conditions should generally be coded with a code from chapter 13. If it is difficult to determine from the documentation in the record which code is best to describe a condition, query the provider.

c. Coding of Pathologic Fractures

7th character A is for use as long as the patient is receiving active treatment for the fracture. While the patient may be seen by a new or different provider over the course of treatment for a pathological fracture, assignment of the 7th character is based on whether the patient is undergoing active treatment and not whether the provider is seeing the patient for the first time.

7th character, D is to be used for encounters after the patient has completed active treatment for the fracture and is receiving routine care for the fracture during the healing or recovery phase. The other 7th characters, listed under each subcategory in the Tabular List, are to be used for subsequent encounters for routine care of fractures during the healing and recovery phase as well as treatment of problems associated with the healing, such as malunions, nonunions, and sequelae.

Care for complications of surgical treatment for fracture repairs during the healing or recovery phase should be coded with the appropriate complication codes.

See Section I.C.19. Coding of traumatic fractures.

d. Osteoporosis

Osteoporosis is a systemic condition, meaning that all bones of the musculoskeletal system are affected. Therefore, site is not a component of the codes under category M81, Osteoporosis without current pathological fracture. The site codes under category M80, Osteoporosis with current pathological fracture, identify the site of the fracture, not the osteoporosis.

1) Osteoporosis without pathological fracture

Category M81, Osteoporosis without current pathological fracture, is for use for patients with osteoporosis who do not currently have a pathologic fracture due to the osteoporosis, even if they have had a fracture in the past. For patients with a history of osteoporosis fractures, status code Z87.310, Personal history of (healed) osteoporosis fracture, should follow the code from M81.

2) Osteoporosis with current pathological fracture

Category M80, Osteoporosis with current pathological fracture, is for patients who have a current pathologic fracture at the time of an encounter. The codes under M80 identify the site of the fracture. A code from category M80, not a traumatic fracture code, should be used for any patient with known osteoporosis who suffers a fracture, even if the patient had a minor fall or trauma, if that fall or trauma would not usually break a normal, healthy bone.

14. Chapter 14: Diseases of Genitourinary System (NØØ-N99)

a. Chronic kidney disease

1) Stages of chronic kidney disease (CKD)

The ICD-10-CM classifies CKD based on severity. The severity of CKD is designated by stages 1-5. Stage 2, code N18.2, equates to mild CKD; stage 3, code N18.3, equates to moderate CKD; and stage 4, code N18.4, equates to severe CKD. Code N18.6, End stage renal disease (ESRD), is assigned when the provider has documented end-stage-renal disease (ESRD).

If both a stage of CKD and ESRD are documented, assign code N18.6 only.

2) Chronic kidney disease and kidney transplant status

Patients who have undergone kidney transplant may still have some form of chronic kidney disease (CKD) because the kidney transplant may not fully restore kidney function. Therefore, the presence of CKD alone does not constitute a transplant complication. Assign the appropriate N18 code for the patient's stage of CKD and code Z94.0, Kidney transplant status. If a transplant complication such as failure or rejection or other transplant complication is documented, see section I.C.19.g for information on coding complications of a kidney transplant. If the documentation is unclear as to whether the patient has a complication of the transplant, query the provider.

3) Chronic kidney disease with other conditions

Patients with CKD may also suffer from other serious conditions, most commonly diabetes mellitus and hypertension. The sequencing of the CKD code in relationship to codes for other contributing conditions is based on the conventions in the Tabular List.

See I.C.9. Hypertensive chronic kidney disease.

See I.C.19. Chronic kidney disease and kidney transplant complications.

15. Chapter 15: Pregnancy, Childbirth, and the Puerperium (OØØ-O9A)

a. General Rules for Obstetric Cases

1) Codes from chapter 15 and sequencing priority

Obstetric cases require codes from chapter 15, codes in the range O00-O9A, Pregnancy, Childbirth, and the Puerperium. Chapter 15 codes have sequencing priority over codes from other chapters. Additional codes from other chapters may be used in conjunction with chapter 15 codes to further specify conditions. Should the provider document that the pregnancy is incidental to the encounter, then code Z33.1, Pregnant state, incidental, should be used in place of any chapter 15 codes. It is the provider's responsibility to state that the condition being treated is not affecting the pregnancy.

2) Chapter 15 codes used only on the maternal record

Chapter 15 codes are to be used only on the maternal record, never on the record of the newborn.

3) Final character for trimester

The majority of codes in Chapter 15 have a final character indicating the trimester of pregnancy. The timeframes for the trimesters are indicated at the beginning of the chapter. If trimester is not a component of a code it is because the condition always occurs in a specific trimester, or the concept of trimester of pregnancy is not applicable. Certain codes have characters for only certain trimesters because the condition does not occur in all trimesters, but it may occur in more than just one.

Assignment of the final character for trimester should be based on the provider's documentation of the trimester (or number of weeks) for the current admission/encounter. This applies to the assignment of trimester for pre-existing conditions as well as those that develop during or are due to the pregnancy. The provider's documentation of the number of weeks may be used to assign the appropriate code identifying the trimester.

Whenever delivery occurs during the current admission, and there is an "in childbirth" option for the obstetric complication being coded, the "in childbirth" code should be assigned.

4) Selection of trimester for inpatient admissions that encompass more than one trimesters

In instances when a patient is admitted to a hospital for complications of pregnancy during one trimester and remains in the hospital into a subsequent trimester, the trimester character for the antepartum complication code should be assigned on the basis of the trimester when the complication developed, not the trimester of the discharge. If the condition developed prior to the current admission/encounter or represents a pre-existing condition, the trimester character for the trimester at the time of the admission/encounter should be assigned.

5) Unspecified trimester

Each category that includes codes for trimester has a code for "unspecified trimester." The "unspecified trimester" code should rarely be used, such as when the documentation in the record is insufficient to determine the trimester and it is not possible to obtain clarification.

6) 7th character for Fetus Identification

Where applicable, a 7th character is to be assigned for certain categories (O31, O32, O33.3 - O33.6, O35, O36, O40, O41, O60.1, O60.2, O64, and O69) to identify the fetus for which the complication code applies.

Assign 7th character "0":

- For single gestations
- When the documentation in the record is insufficient to determine the fetus affected and it is not possible to obtain clarification.
- When it is not possible to clinically determine which fetus is affected.

b. Selection of OB Principal or First-listed Diagnosis

1) Routine outpatient prenatal visits

For routine outpatient prenatal visits when no complications are present, a code from category Z34, Encounter for supervision of normal pregnancy, should be used as the first-listed diagnosis. These codes should not be used in conjunction with chapter 15 codes.

2) Supervision of High-Risk Pregnancy

Codes from category O09, Supervision of high-risk pregnancy, are intended for use only during the prenatal period. For complications during the labor or delivery episode as a result of a high-risk pregnancy, assign the applicable complication codes from Chapter 15. If there are no complications during the labor or delivery episode, assign code O80, Encounter for full-term uncomplicated delivery.

For routine prenatal outpatient visits for patients with high-risk pregnancies, a code from category O09, Supervision of high-risk pregnancy, should be used as the first-listed diagnosis. Secondary chapter 15 codes may be used in conjunction with these codes if appropriate.

3) Episodes when no delivery occurs

In episodes when no delivery occurs, the principal diagnosis should correspond to the principal complication of the pregnancy which necessitated the encounter. Should more than one complication exist, all of which are treated or monitored, any of the complications codes may be sequenced first.

4) When a delivery occurs

When an obstetric patient is admitted and delivers during that admission, the condition that prompted the admission should be sequenced as the principal diagnosis. If multiple conditions prompted the admission, sequence the one most related to the delivery as the principal diagnosis. A code for any complication of the delivery should be assigned as an additional diagnosis. In cases of cesarean delivery, if the patient was admitted with a condition that resulted in the performance of a cesarean procedure, that condition should be selected as the principal diagnosis. If the reason for the admission was unrelated to the condition resulting in the cesarean delivery, the condition related to the reason for the admission should be selected as the principal diagnosis.

5) Outcome of delivery

A code from category Z37, Outcome of delivery, should be included on every maternal record when a delivery has occurred. These codes are not to be used on subsequent records or on the newborn record.

c. Pre-existing conditions versus conditions due to the pregnancy

Certain categories in Chapter 15 distinguish between conditions of the mother that existed prior to pregnancy (pre-existing) and those that are a direct result of pregnancy. When assigning codes from Chapter 15, it is important to assess if a condition was pre-existing prior to pregnancy or developed during or due to the pregnancy in order to assign the correct code.

Categories that do not distinguish between pre-existing and pregnancy-related conditions may be used for either. It is acceptable to use codes specifically for the puerperium with codes complicating pregnancy and childbirth if a condition arises postpartum during the delivery encounter.

d. Pre-existing hypertension in pregnancy

Category O10, Pre-existing hypertension complicating pregnancy, childbirth and the puerperium, includes codes for hypertensive heart and hypertensive chronic kidney disease. When assigning one of the O10 codes that includes hypertensive heart disease or hypertensive chronic kidney disease, it is necessary to add a secondary code from the appropriate hypertension category to specify the type of heart failure or chronic kidney disease.

See Section I.C.9. Hypertension.

e. Fetal Conditions Affecting the Management of the Mother

1) Codes from categories O35 and O36

Codes from categories O35, Maternal care for known or suspected fetal abnormality and damage, and O36, Maternal care for other fetal problems, are assigned only when the fetal condition is actually responsible for modifying the management of the mother, i.e., by requiring diagnostic studies, additional observation, special care, or termination of pregnancy. The fact that the fetal condition exists does not justify assigning a code from this series to the mother's record.

2) In utero surgery

In cases when surgery is performed on the fetus, a diagnosis code from category O35, Maternal care for known or suspected fetal abnormality and damage, should be assigned identifying the fetal condition. Assign the appropriate procedure code for the procedure performed.

No code from Chapter 16, the perinatal codes, should be used on the mother's record to identify fetal conditions. Surgery performed in utero on a fetus is still to be coded as an obstetric encounter.

f. HIV Infection in Pregnancy, Childbirth and the Puerperium

During pregnancy, childbirth or the puerperium, a patient admitted because of an HIV-related illness should receive a principal diagnosis from subcategory O98.7-, Human immunodeficiency [HIV] disease complicating pregnancy, childbirth and the puerperium, followed by the code(s) for the HIV-related illness(es).

Patients with asymptomatic HIV infection status admitted during pregnancy, childbirth, or the puerperium should receive codes of O98.7- and Z21, Asymptomatic human immunodeficiency virus [HIV] infection status.

g. Diabetes mellitus in pregnancy

Diabetes mellitus is a significant complicating factor in pregnancy. Pregnant women who are diabetic should be assigned a code from category O24, Diabetes mellitus in pregnancy, childbirth, and the puerperium, first, followed by the appropriate diabetes code(s) (E08-E13) from Chapter 4.

h. Long term use of insulin and oral hypoglycemics

See section I.C.4.a.3 for information on the long term use of insulin and oral hypoglycemic.

i. Gestational (pregnancy induced) diabetes

Gestational (pregnancy induced) diabetes can occur during the second and third trimester of pregnancy in women who were not diabetic prior to pregnancy. Gestational diabetes can cause complications in the pregnancy similar to those of pre-existing diabetes mellitus. It also puts the woman at greater risk of developing diabetes after the pregnancy. Codes for gestational diabetes are in subcategory O24.4, Gestational diabetes mellitus. No other code from category O24, Diabetes mellitus in pregnancy, childbirth, and the puerperium, should be used with a code from O24.4

The codes under subcategory O24.4 include diet controlled, insulin controlled, and controlled by oral hypoglycemic drugs. If a patient with gestational diabetes is treated with both diet and insulin, only the code for insulin-controlled is required. If a patient with gestational diabetes is treated with both diet and oral hypoglycemic medications, only the code for "controlled by oral hypoglycemic drugs" is required.

Code Z79.4, Long-term (current) use of insulin, or code Z79.84, Long-term (current) use of oral hypoglycemic drugs, should not be assigned with codes from subcategory O24.4.

An abnormal glucose tolerance in pregnancy is assigned a code from subcategory O99.81, Abnormal glucose complicating pregnancy, childbirth, and the puerperium.

j. Sepsis and septic shock complicating abortion, pregnancy, childbirth and the puerperium

When assigning a chapter 15 code for sepsis complicating abortion, pregnancy, childbirth, and the puerperium, a code for the specific type of infection should be assigned as an additional diagnosis. If severe sepsis is present, a code from subcategory R65.2, Severe sepsis, and code(s) for associated organ dysfunction(s) should also be assigned as additional diagnoses.

k. Puerperal sepsis

Code O85, Puerperal sepsis, should be assigned with a secondary code to identify the causal organism (e.g., for a bacterial infection, assign a code from category B95-B96, Bacterial infections in conditions classified elsewhere). A code from category A40, Streptococcal sepsis, or A41, Other sepsis, should not be used for puerperal sepsis. If applicable, use additional codes to identify severe sepsis (R65.2-) and any associated acute organ dysfunction.

l. Alcohol, tobacco *and drug* use during pregnancy, childbirth and the puerperium

1) Alcohol use during pregnancy, childbirth and the puerperium

Codes under subcategory O99.31, Alcohol use complicating pregnancy, childbirth, and the puerperium, should be assigned for any pregnancy case when a mother uses alcohol during the pregnancy or postpartum. A secondary code from category F10, Alcohol related disorders, should also be assigned to identify manifestations of the alcohol use.

2) Tobacco use during pregnancy, childbirth and the puerperium

Codes under subcategory O99.33, Smoking (tobacco) complicating pregnancy, childbirth, and the puerperium, should be assigned for any pregnancy case when a mother uses any type of tobacco product during the pregnancy or postpartum. A secondary code from category F17, Nicotine dependence, or code Z72.0, Tobacco use, should also be assigned to identify the type of nicotine dependence.

3) Drug use during pregnancy, childbirth and the puerperium

Codes under subcategory O99.32, Drug use complicating pregnancy, childbirth, and the puerperium, should be assigned for any pregnancy case when a mother uses drugs during the pregnancy or postpartum. This can involve illegal drugs, or inappropriate use or abuse of prescription drugs. Secondary code(s) from categories F11-F16 and F18-F19 should also be assigned to identify manifestations of the drug use.

m. Poisoning, toxic effects, adverse effects and underdosing in a pregnant patient

A code from subcategory O9A.2, Injury, poisoning and certain other consequences of external causes complicating pregnancy, childbirth, and the puerperium, should be sequenced first, followed by the appropriate injury, poisoning, toxic effect, adverse effect or underdosing code, and then the additional code(s) that specifies the condition caused by the poisoning, toxic effect, adverse effect or underdosing.

See Section I.C.19. Adverse effects, poisoning, underdosing and toxic effects.

n. Normal Delivery, Code O80

1) Encounter for full term uncomplicated delivery

Code O80 should be assigned when a woman is admitted for a full-term normal delivery and delivers a single, healthy infant without any complications antepartum, during the delivery, or postpartum during the delivery episode. Code O80 is always a principal diagnosis. It is not to be used if any other code from chapter 15 is needed to describe a current complication of the antenatal, delivery, or perinatal period. Additional codes from other chapters may be used with code O80 if they are not related to or are in any way complicating the pregnancy.

2) Uncomplicated delivery with resolved antepartum complication

Code O80 may be used if the patient had a complication at some point during the pregnancy, but the complication is not present at the time of the admission for delivery.

3) Outcome of delivery for O80

Z37.0, Single live birth, is the only outcome of delivery code appropriate for use with O80.

o. The Peripartum and Postpartum Periods

1) Peripartum and Postpartum periods

The postpartum period begins immediately after delivery and continues for six weeks following delivery. The peripartum period is defined as the last month of pregnancy to five months postpartum.

2) Peripartum and postpartum complication

A postpartum complication is any complication occurring within the six-week period.

3) Pregnancy-related complications after 6 week period

Chapter 15 codes may also be used to describe pregnancy-related complications after the peripartum or postpartum period if the provider documents that a condition is pregnancy related.

4) Admission for routine postpartum care following delivery outside hospital

When the mother delivers outside the hospital prior to admission and is admitted for routine postpartum care and no complications are noted, code Z39.0, Encounter for care and examination of mother immediately after delivery, should be assigned as the principal diagnosis.

5) Pregnancy associated cardiomyopathy

Pregnancy associated cardiomyopathy, code O90.3, is unique in that it may be diagnosed in the third trimester of pregnancy but may continue to progress months after delivery. For this reason, it is referred to as peripartum cardiomyopathy. Code O90.3 is only for use when the cardiomyopathy develops as a result of pregnancy in a woman who did not have pre-existing heart disease.

p. Code O94, Sequelae of complication of pregnancy, childbirth, and the puerperium

1) Code O94

Code O94, Sequelae of complication of pregnancy, childbirth, and the puerperium, is for use in those cases when an initial complication of a pregnancy develops a sequelae requiring care or treatment at a future date.

2) After the initial postpartum period

This code may be used at any time after the initial postpartum period.

3) Sequencing of Code O94

This code, like all sequela codes, is to be sequenced following the code describing the sequelae of the complication.

q. Termination of Pregnancy and Spontaneous abortions

1) Abortion with Liveborn Fetus

When an attempted termination of pregnancy results in a liveborn fetus, assign code Z33.2, Encounter for elective termination of pregnancy and a code from category Z37, Outcome of Delivery.

2) Retained Products of Conception following an abortion

Subsequent encounters for retained products of conception following a spontaneous abortion or elective termination of pregnancy, without complications are assigned O03.4, Incomplete spontaneous, abortion without complication, or codes O07.4. Failed attempted termination of pregnancy without complication. This advice is appropriate even when the patient was discharged previously with a discharge diagnosis of complete abortion. If the patient has a specific complication associated with the spontaneous abortion or elective termination of pregnancy in addition to retained products of conception, assign the appropriate complication in category O03 or O07 instead of code O03.4 or O07.4.

3) Complications leading to abortion

Codes from Chapter 15 may be used as additional codes to identify any documented complications of the pregnancy in conjunction with codes in categories in O04, O07 and O08.

r. Abuse in a pregnant patient

For suspected or confirmed cases of abuse of a pregnant patient, a code(s) from subcategories O9A.3, Physical abuse complicating pregnancy, childbirth, and the puerperium, O9A.4, Sexual abuse complicating pregnancy, childbirth, and the puerperium, and O9A.5, Psychological abuse complicating pregnancy, childbirth, and the puerperium, should be sequenced first, followed by the appropriate codes (if applicable) to identify any associated current injury due to physical abuse, sexual abuse, and the perpetrator of abuse.

See Section I.C.19.f. Adult and child abuse, neglect and other maltreatment.

16. Chapter 16: Certain Conditions Originating in the Perinatal Period (PØØ-P96)

For coding and reporting purposes the perinatal period is defined as before birth through the 28th day following birth. The following guidelines are provided for reporting purposes

a. General Perinatal Rules

1) Use of Chapter 16 Codes

Codes in this chapter are never for use on the maternal record. Codes from Chapter 15, the obstetric chapter, are never permitted on the newborn record. Chapter 16 codes may be used throughout the life of the patient if the condition is still present.

2) Principal Diagnosis for Birth Record

When coding the birth episode in a newborn record, assign a code from category Z38, Liveborn infants according to place of birth and type of delivery, as the principal diagnosis. A code from category Z38 is assigned only once, to a newborn at the time of birth. If a newborn is transferred to another institution, a code from category Z38 should not be used at the receiving hospital.

A code from category Z38 is used only on the newborn record, not on the mother's record.

3) Use of Codes from other Chapters with Codes from Chapter 16

Codes from other chapters may be used with codes from chapter 16 if the codes from the other chapters provide more specific detail. Codes for signs and symptoms may be assigned when a definitive diagnosis has not been established. If the reason for the encounter is a perinatal condition, the code from chapter 16 should be sequenced first.

4) Use of Chapter 16 Codes after the Perinatal Period

Should a condition originate in the perinatal period, and continue throughout the life of the patient, the perinatal code should continue to be used regardless of the patient's age.

5) Birth process or community acquired conditions

If a newborn has a condition that may be either due to the birth process or community acquired and the documentation does not indicate which it is, the default is due to the birth process and the code from Chapter 16 should be used. If the condition is community-acquired, a code from Chapter 16 should not be assigned.

6) Code all clinically significant conditions

All clinically significant conditions noted on routine newborn examination should be coded. A condition is clinically significant if it requires:

- clinical evaluation; or
- therapeutic treatment; or
- diagnostic procedures; or
- extended length of hospital stay; or
- increased nursing care and/or monitoring; or
- has implications for future health care needs

Note: The perinatal guidelines listed above are the same as the general coding guidelines for "additional diagnoses", except for the final point regarding implications for future health care needs. Codes should be assigned for conditions that have been specified by the provider as having implications for future health care needs.

b. Observation and Evaluation of Newborns for Suspected Conditions not Found

1) Use of Z05 codes

Assign a code from category Z05, Observation and evaluation of newborns and infants for suspected conditions ruled out, to identify those instances when a healthy newborn is evaluated for a suspected condition that is determined after study not to be present. Do not use a code from category Z05 when the patient has identified signs or symptoms of a suspected problem; in such cases code the sign or symptom.

2) *Z05 on Other than the Birth Record*

A code from category Z05 may also be assigned as a principal or first-listed code for readmissions or encounters when the code from category Z38 code no longer applies. Codes from category Z05 are for use only for healthy newborns and infants for which no condition after study is found to be present.

3) Z05 on a birth record

A code from category Z05 is to be used as a secondary code after the code from category Z38, Liveborn infants according to place of birth and type of delivery.

c. Coding Additional Perinatal Diagnoses

1) Assigning codes for conditions that require treatment

Assign codes for conditions that require treatment or further investigation, prolong the length of stay, or require resource utilization.

2) Codes for conditions specified as having implications for future health care needs

Assign codes for conditions that have been specified by the provider as having implications for future health care needs.

Note: This guideline should not be used for adult patients.

d. Prematurity and Fetal Growth Retardation

Providers utilize different criteria in determining prematurity. A code for prematurity should not be assigned unless it is documented. Assignment of codes in categories P05, Disorders of newborn related to slow fetal growth and fetal malnutrition, and P07, Disorders of newborn related to short gestation and low birth weight, not elsewhere classified, should be based on the recorded birth weight and estimated gestational age.

When both birth weight and gestational age are available, two codes from category P07 should be assigned, with the code for birth weight sequenced before the code for gestational age.

e. Low birth weight and immaturity status

Codes from category P07, Disorders of newborn related to short gestation and low birth weight, not elsewhere classified, are for use for a child or adult who was premature or had a low birth weight as a newborn and this is affecting the patient's current health status.

See Section I.C.21. Factors influencing health status and contact with health services, Status.

f. Bacterial Sepsis of Newborn

Category P36, Bacterial sepsis of newborn, includes congenital sepsis. If a perinate is documented as having sepsis without documentation of congenital or community acquired, the default is congenital and a code from category P36 should be assigned. If the P36 code includes the causal organism, an additional code from category B95, Streptococcus, Staphylococcus, and Enterococcus as the cause of diseases classified elsewhere, or B96, Other bacterial agents as the cause of diseases classified elsewhere, should not be assigned. If the P36 code does not include the causal organism, assign an additional code from category B96. If applicable, use additional codes to identify severe sepsis (R65.2-) and any associated acute organ dysfunction.

g. Stillbirth

Code P95, Stillbirth, is only for use in institutions that maintain separate records for stillbirths. No other code should be used with P95. Code P95 should not be used on the mother's record.

17. Chapter 17: Congenital malformations, deformations, and chromosomal abnormalities (Q00-Q99)

Assign an appropriate code(s) from categories Q00-Q99, Congenital malformations, deformations, and chromosomal abnormalities when a malformation/deformation or chromosomal abnormality is documented. A malformation/deformation/or chromosomal abnormality may be the principal/first-listed diagnosis on a record or a secondary diagnosis.

When a malformation/deformation/or chromosomal abnormality does not have a unique code assignment, assign additional code(s) for any manifestations that may be present.

When the code assignment specifically identifies the malformation/deformation/or chromosomal abnormality, manifestations that are an inherent component of the anomaly should not be coded separately. Additional codes should be assigned for manifestations that are not an inherent component.

Codes from Chapter 17 may be used throughout the life of the patient. If a congenital malformation or deformity has been corrected, a personal history code should be used to identify the history of the malformation or deformity. Although present at birth, malformation/deformation/or chromosomal abnormality may not be identified until later in life. Whenever the condition is diagnosed by the physician, it is appropriate to assign a code from codes Q00-Q99. For the birth admission, the appropriate code from category Z38, Liveborn infants, according to place of birth and type of delivery, should be sequenced as the principal diagnosis, followed by any congenital anomaly codes, Q00-Q99.

18. Chapter 18: Symptoms, signs, and abnormal clinical and laboratory findings, not elsewhere classified (RØØ-R99)

Chapter 18 includes symptoms, signs, abnormal results of clinical or other investigative procedures, and ill-defined conditions regarding which no diagnosis classifiable elsewhere is recorded. Signs and symptoms that point to a specific diagnosis have been assigned to a category in other chapters of the classification.

a. Use of symptom codes

Codes that describe symptoms and signs are acceptable for reporting purposes when a related definitive diagnosis has not been established (confirmed) by the provider.

b. Use of a symptom code with a definitive diagnosis code

Codes for signs and symptoms may be reported in addition to a related definitive diagnosis when the sign or symptom is not routinely associated with that diagnosis, such as the various signs and symptoms associated with complex syndromes. The definitive diagnosis code should be sequenced before the symptom code.

Signs or symptoms that are associated routinely with a disease process should not be assigned as additional codes, unless otherwise instructed by the classification.

c. Combination codes that include symptoms

ICD-10-CM contains a number of combination codes that identify both the definitive diagnosis and common symptoms of that diagnosis. When using one of these combination codes, an additional code should not be assigned for the symptom.

d. Repeated falls

Code R29.6, Repeated falls, is for use for encounters when a patient has recently fallen and the reason for the fall is being investigated.

Code Z91.81, History of falling, is for use when a patient has fallen in the past and is at risk for future falls. When appropriate, both codes R29.6 and Z91.81 may be assigned together.

e. Coma scale

The coma scale codes (R40.2-) can be used in conjunction with traumatic brain injury codes, acute cerebrovascular disease or sequelae of cerebrovascular disease codes. These codes are primarily for use by trauma registries, but they may be used in any setting where this information is collected. The coma scale may also be used to assess the status of the central nervous system for other non-trauma conditions, such as monitoring patients in the intensive care unit regardless of medical condition.

The coma scale codes should be sequenced after the diagnosis code(s).

These codes, one from each subcategory, are needed to complete the scale. The 7th character indicates when the scale was recorded. The 7th character should match for all three codes.

At a minimum, report the initial score documented on presentation at your facility. This may be a score from the emergency medicine technician (EMT) or in the emergency department. If desired, a facility may choose to capture multiple Glasgow coma scale scores.

Assign code R40.24, Glasgow coma scale, total score, when only the total score is documented in the medical record and not the individual score(s).

Do not report codes for individual or total Glasgow coma scale scores for a patient with a medically induced coma or a sedated patient.

See Section I.B.14 for coma scale documentation by clinicians other than patient's provider

f. Functional quadriplegia

GUIDELINE HAS BEEN DELETED EFFECTIVE OCTOBER 1, 2017

g. SIRS due to Non-Infectious Process

The systemic inflammatory response syndrome (SIRS) can develop as a result of certain non-infectious disease processes, such as trauma, malignant neoplasm, or pancreatitis. When SIRS is documented with a noninfectious condition, and no subsequent infection is documented, the code for the underlying condition, such as an injury, should be assigned, followed by code R65.10, Systemic inflammatory response syndrome (SIRS) of non-infectious origin without acute organ dysfunction, or code R65.11, Systemic inflammatory response syndrome (SIRS) of non-infectious origin with acute organ dysfunction. If an associated acute organ dysfunction is documented, the appropriate code(s) for the specific type of organ dysfunction(s) should be assigned in addition to code R65.11. If acute organ dysfunction is documented, but it cannot be determined if the acute organ dysfunction is associated with SIRS or due to another condition (e.g., directly due to the trauma), the provider should be queried.

h. Death NOS

Code R99, Ill-defined and unknown cause of mortality, is only for use in the very limited circumstance when a patient who has already died is brought into an emergency department or other healthcare facility and is pronounced dead upon arrival. It does not represent the discharge disposition of death.

i. NIHSS Stroke Scale

The NIH stroke scale (NIHSS) codes (R29.7- -) can be used in conjunction with acute stroke codes (I63) to identify the patient's neurological status and the severity of the stroke. The stroke scale codes should be sequenced after the acute stroke diagnosis code(s).

At a minimum, report the initial score documented. If desired, a facility may choose to capture multiple stroke scale scores.

See Section I.B.14 for NIHSS stroke scale documentation by clinicians other than patient's provider

19. Chapter 19: Injury, poisoning, and certain other consequences of external causes (SØØ-T88)

a. Application of 7th Characters in Chapter 19

Most categories in chapter 19 have a 7th character requirement for each applicable code. Most categories in this chapter have three 7th character values (with the exception of fractures): A, initial encounter, D, subsequent encounter and S, sequela. Categories for traumatic fractures have additional 7th character values. While the patient may be seen by a new or different provider over the course of treatment for an injury, assignment of the 7th character is based on whether the patient is undergoing active treatment and not whether the provider is seeing the patient for the first time.

For complication codes, active treatment refers to treatment for the condition described by the code, even though it may be related to an earlier precipitating problem. For example, code T84.50XA, Infection and inflammatory reaction due to unspecified internal joint prosthesis , initial encounter, is used when active treatment is provided for the infection, even though the condition relates to the prosthetic device, implant or graft that was placed at a previous encounter.

7th character "A", initial encounter is used for each encounter where the patient is receiving active treatment for the condition.

7th character "D" subsequent encounter is used for encounters after the patient has completed active treatment of the condition and is receiving routine care for the condition during the healing or recovery phase.

The aftercare Z codes should not be used for aftercare for conditions such as injuries or poisonings, where 7th characters are provided to identify subsequent care. For example, for aftercare of an injury, assign the acute injury code with the 7th character "D" (subsequent encounter).

7th character "S", sequela, is for use for complications or conditions that arise as a direct result of a condition, such as scar formation after a burn. The scars are sequelae of the burn. When using 7th character "S", it is necessary to use both the injury code that precipitated the sequela and the code for the sequela itself. The "S" is added only to the injury code, not the sequela code. The 7th character "S" identifies the injury responsible for the sequela. The specific type of sequela (e.g. scar) is sequenced first, followed by the injury code.

See Section I.B.10 Sequelae, (Late Effects)

b. Coding of Injuries

When coding injuries, assign separate codes for each injury unless a combination code is provided, in which case the combination code is assigned. **Codes from category** T07, Unspecified multiple injuries should not be assigned in the inpatient setting unless information for a more specific code is not available. Traumatic injury codes (S00-T14.9) are not to be used for normal, healing surgical wounds or to identify complications of surgical wounds.

The code for the most serious injury, as determined by the provider and the focus of treatment, is sequenced first.

1) Superficial injuries

Superficial injuries such as abrasions or contusions are not coded when associated with more severe injuries of the same site.

2) Primary injury with damage to nerves/blood vessels

When a primary injury results in minor damage to peripheral nerves or blood vessels, the primary injury is sequenced first with additional code(s) for injuries to nerves and spinal cord (such as category S04), and/or injury to blood vessels (such as category S15). When the primary injury is to the blood vessels or nerves, that injury should be sequenced first.

c. Coding of Traumatic Fractures

The principles of multiple coding of injuries should be followed in coding fractures. Fractures of specified sites are coded individually by site in accordance with both the provisions within categories S02, S12, S22, S32, S42, S49, S52, S59, S62, S72, S79, S82, S89, S92 and the level of detail furnished by medical record content.

A fracture not indicated as open or closed should be coded to closed. A fracture not indicated whether displaced or not displaced should be coded to displaced.

More specific guidelines are as follows:

1) Initial vs. Subsequent Encounter for Fractures

Traumatic fractures are coded using the appropriate 7th character for initial encounter (A, B, C) for each encounter where the patient is receiving active treatment for the fracture. The appropriate 7th character for initial encounter should also be assigned for a patient who delayed seeking treatment for the fracture or nonunion.

Fractures are coded using the appropriate 7th character for subsequent care for encounters after the patient has completed active treatment of the fracture and is receiving routine care for the fracture during the healing or recovery phase.

Care for complications of surgical treatment for fracture repairs during the healing or recovery phase should be coded with the appropriate complication codes.

Care of complications of fractures, such as malunion and nonunion, should be reported with the appropriate 7th character for subsequent care with nonunion (K, M, N,) or subsequent care with malunion (P, Q, R).

Malunion/nonunion: The appropriate 7th character for initial encounter should also be assigned for a patient who delayed seeking treatment for the fracture or nonunion.

The open fracture designations in the assignment of the 7th character for fractures of the forearm, femur and lower leg, including ankle are based on the Gustilo open fracture classification. When the Gustilo classification type is not specified for an open fracture, the 7th character for open fracture type I or II should be assigned (B, E, H, M, Q).

A code from category M80, not a traumatic fracture code, should be used for any patient with known osteoporosis who suffers a fracture, even if the patient had a minor fall or trauma, if that fall or trauma would not usually break a normal, healthy bone.

See Section I.C.13. Osteoporosis.

The aftercare Z codes should not be used for aftercare for traumatic fractures. For aftercare of a traumatic fracture, assign the acute fracture code with the appropriate 7th character.

2) Multiple fractures sequencing

Multiple fractures are sequenced in accordance with the severity of the fracture.

d. Coding of Burns and Corrosions

The ICD-10-CM makes a distinction between burns and corrosions. The burn codes are for thermal burns, except sunburns, that come from a heat source, such as a fire or hot appliance. The burn codes are also for burns resulting from electricity and radiation. Corrosions are burns due to chemicals. The guidelines are the same for burns and corrosions.

Current burns (T20-T25) are classified by depth, extent and by agent (X code). Burns are classified by depth as first degree (erythema), second degree (blistering), and third degree (full-thickness involvement). Burns of the eye and internal organs (T26-T28) are classified by site, but not by degree.

1) Sequencing of burn and related condition codes

Sequence first the code that reflects the highest degree of burn when more than one burn is present.

a. When the reason for the admission or encounter is for treatment of external multiple burns, sequence first the code that reflects the burn of the highest degree.

b. When a patient has both internal and external burns, the circumstances of admission govern the selection of the principal diagnosis or first-listed diagnosis.

c. When a patient is admitted for burn injuries and other related conditions such as smoke inhalation and/or respiratory failure, the circumstances of admission govern the selection of the principal or first-listed diagnosis.

2) Burns of the same *anatomic* site

Classify burns of the same **anatomic** site **and on the same side** but of different degrees to the subcategory identifying the highest degree recorded in the diagnosis **(e.g., for second and third degree burns of right thigh, assign only code T24.311-)**.

3) Non-healing burns

Non-healing burns are coded as acute burns.

Necrosis of burned skin should be coded as a non-healed burn.

4) Infected Burn

For any documented infected burn site, use an additional code for the infection.

5) Assign separate codes for each burn site

When coding burns, assign separate codes for each burn site. Category T30, Burn and corrosion, body region unspecified is extremely vague and should rarely be used.

Codes for burns of "multiple sites" should only be assigned when the medical record documentation does not specify the individual sites.

6) Burns and Corrosions Classified According to Extent of Body Surface Involved

Assign codes from category T31, Burns classified according to extent of body surface involved, or T32, Corrosions classified according to extent of body surface involved, when the site of the burn is not specified or when there is a need for additional data. It is advisable to use category T31 as additional coding when needed to provide data for evaluating burn mortality, such as that needed by burn units. It is also advisable to use category T31 as an additional code for reporting purposes when there is mention of a third-degree burn involving 20 percent or more of the body surface.

Categories T31 and T32 are based on the classic "rule of nines" in estimating body surface involved: head and neck are assigned nine percent, each arm nine percent, each leg 18 percent, the anterior trunk 18 percent, posterior trunk 18 percent, and genitalia one percent. Providers may change these percentage assignments where necessary to accommodate infants and children who have proportionately larger heads than adults, and patients who have large buttocks, thighs, or abdomen that involve burns.

7) Encounters for treatment of sequela of burns

Encounters for the treatment of the late effects of burns or corrosions (i.e., scars or joint contractures) should be coded with a burn or corrosion code with the 7th character "S" for sequela.

8) Sequelae with a late effect code and current burn

When appropriate, both a code for a current burn or corrosion with 7th character "A" or "D" and a burn or corrosion code with 7th character "S" may be assigned on the same record (when both a current burn and sequelae of an old burn exist). Burns and corrosions do not heal at the same rate and a current healing wound may still exist with sequela of a healed burn or corrosion.

See Section I.B.10 Sequela (Late Effects)

9) Use of an external cause code with burns and corrosions

An external cause code should be used with burns and corrosions to identify the source and intent of the burn, as well as the place where it occurred.

e. Adverse Effects, Poisoning , Underdosing and Toxic Effects

Codes in categories T36-T65 are combination codes that include the substance that was taken as well as the intent. No additional external cause code is required for poisonings, toxic effects, adverse effects and underdosing codes.

1) Do not code directly from the Table of Drugs

Do not code directly from the Table of Drugs and Chemicals. Always refer back to the Tabular List.

2) Use as many codes as necessary to describe

Use as many codes as necessary to describe completely all drugs, medicinal or biological substances.

3) If the same code would describe the causative agent

If the same code would describe the causative agent for more than one adverse reaction, poisoning, toxic effect or underdosing, assign the code only once.

4) If two or more drugs, medicinal or biological substances

If two or more drugs, medicinal or biological substances are reported, code each individually unless a combination code is listed in the Table of Drugs and Chemicals.

5) The occurrence of drug toxicity is classified in ICD-10-CM as follows:

(a) Adverse Effect

When coding an adverse effect of a drug that has been correctly prescribed and properly administered, assign the appropriate code for the nature of the adverse effect followed by the appropriate code for the adverse effect of the drug (T36-T50). The code for the drug should have a 5th or 6th character "5" (for example T36.0X5-) Examples of the nature of an adverse effect are tachycardia, delirium, gastrointestinal hemorrhaging, vomiting, hypokalemia, hepatitis, renal failure, or respiratory failure.

(b) Poisoning

When coding a poisoning or reaction to the improper use of a medication (e.g., overdose, wrong substance given or taken in error, wrong route of administration), first assign the appropriate code from categories T36-T50. The poisoning codes have an associated intent as their 5th or 6th character (accidental, intentional self-harm, assault and undetermined. If the intent of the poisoning is unknown or unspecified, code the intent as accidental intent. The undetermined intent is only for use if the documentation in the record specifies that the intent cannot be determined. Use additional code(s) for all manifestations of poisonings.

If there is also a diagnosis of abuse or dependence of the substance, the abuse or dependence is assigned as an additional code.

Examples of poisoning include:

(i) Error was made in drug prescription

Errors made in drug prescription or in the administration of the drug by provider, nurse, patient, or other person.

(ii) Overdose of a drug intentionally taken

If an overdose of a drug was intentionally taken or administered and resulted in drug toxicity, it would be coded as a poisoning.

(iii) Nonprescribed drug taken with correctly prescribed and properly administered drug

If a nonprescribed drug or medicinal agent was taken in combination with a correctly prescribed and properly administered drug, any drug toxicity or other reaction resulting from the interaction of the two drugs would be classified as a poisoning.

(iv) Interaction of drug(s) and alcohol

When a reaction results from the interaction of a drug(s) and alcohol, this would be classified as poisoning.

See Section I.C.4. if poisoning is the result of insulin pump malfunctions.

(c) **Underdosing**

Underdosing refers to taking less of a medication than is prescribed by a provider or a manufacturer's instruction. **Discontinuing the use of a prescribed medication on the patient's own initiative (not directed by the patient's provider) is also classified as an underdosing.** For underdosing, assign the code from categories T36-T50 (fifth or sixth character "6").

Codes for underdosing should never be assigned as principal or first-listed codes. If a patient has a relapse or exacerbation of the medical condition for which the drug is prescribed because of the reduction in dose, then the medical condition itself should be coded.

Noncompliance (Z91.12-, Z91.13- **and Z91.14-**) or complication of care (Y63.61, Y63.8-Y63.9) codes are to be used with an underdosing code to indicate intent, if known.

(d) Toxic Effects

When a harmful substance is ingested or comes in contact with a person, this is classified as a toxic effect. The toxic effect codes are in categories T51-T65.

Toxic effect codes have an associated intent: accidental, intentional self-harm, assault and undetermined.

f. Adult and child abuse, neglect and other maltreatment

Sequence first the appropriate code from categories T74 (Adult and child abuse, neglect and other maltreatment, confirmed) or T76 (Adult and child abuse, neglect and other maltreatment, suspected) for abuse, neglect and other maltreatment, followed by any accompanying mental health or injury code(s).

If the documentation in the medical record states abuse or neglect it is coded as confirmed (T74.-). It is coded as suspected if it is documented as suspected (T76.-).

For cases of confirmed abuse or neglect an external cause code from the assault section (X92-Y09) should be added to identify the cause of any physical injuries. A perpetrator code (Y07) should be added when the perpetrator of the abuse is known. For suspected cases of abuse or neglect, do not report external cause or perpetrator code.

If a suspected case of abuse, neglect or mistreatment is ruled out during an encounter code Z04.71, Encounter for examination and observation following alleged physical adult abuse, ruled out, or code Z04.72, Encounter for examination and observation following alleged child physical abuse, ruled out, should be used, not a code from T76.

If a suspected case of alleged rape or sexual abuse is ruled out during an encounter code Z04.41, Encounter for examination and observation following alleged adult rape or code Z04.42, Encounter for examination and observation following alleged child rape, should be used, not a code from T76.

If a suspected case of forced sexual exploitation or forced labor exploitation is ruled out during an encounter, code Z04.81, Encounter for examination and observation of victim following forced sexual exploitation, or code Z04.82, Encounter for examination and observation of victim following forced labor exploitation, should be used, not a code from T76.

See Section I.C.15.r Abuse in a pregnant patient.

g. Complications of care

1) General guidelines for complications of care

(a) **Documentation of complications of care**

See Section I.B.16. for information on documentation of complications of care.

2) Pain due to medical devices

Pain associated with devices, implants or grafts left in a surgical site (for example painful hip prosthesis) is assigned to the appropriate code(s) found in Chapter 19, Injury, poisoning, and certain other consequences of external causes. Specific codes for pain due to medical devices are found in the T code section of the ICD-10-CM. Use additional code(s) from category G89 to identify acute or chronic pain due to presence of the device, implant or graft (G89.18 or G89.28).

3) Transplant complications

(a) Transplant complications other than kidney

Codes under category T86, Complications of transplanted organs and tissues, are for use for both complications and rejection of transplanted organs. A transplant complication code is only assigned if the complication affects the function of the transplanted organ. Two codes are required to fully describe a transplant complication: the appropriate code from category T86 and a secondary code that identifies the complication.

Pre-existing conditions or conditions that develop after the transplant are not coded as complications unless they affect the function of the transplanted organs.

See I.C.21.c.3 for transplant organ removal status

See I.C.2.r for malignant neoplasm associated with transplanted organ.

(b) Kidney transplant complications

Patients who have undergone kidney transplant may still have some form of chronic kidney disease (CKD) because the kidney transplant may not fully restore kidney function. Code T86.1- should be assigned for documented complications of a kidney transplant, such as transplant failure or rejection or other transplant complication. Code T86.1- should not be assigned for post kidney transplant patients who have chronic kidney (CKD) unless a transplant complication such as transplant failure or rejection is documented. If the documentation is unclear as to whether the patient has a complication of the transplant, query the provider.

Conditions that affect the function of the transplanted kidney, other than CKD, should be assigned a code from subcategory T86.1, Complications of transplanted organ, Kidney, and a secondary code that identifies the complication.

For patients with CKD following a kidney transplant, but who do not have a complication such as failure or rejection, *see section I.C.14. Chronic kidney disease and kidney transplant status.*

4) Complication codes that include the external cause

As with certain other T codes, some of the complications of care codes have the external cause included in the code. The code includes the nature of the complication as well as the type of procedure that caused the complication. No external cause code indicating the type of procedure is necessary for these codes.

5) Complications of care codes within the body system chapters

Intraoperative and postprocedural complication codes are found within the body system chapters with codes specific to the organs and structures of that body system. These codes should be sequenced first, followed by a code(s) for the specific complication, if applicable.

2Ø. Chapter 2Ø: External Causes of Morbidity (VØØ-Y99)

The external causes of morbidity codes should never be sequenced as the first-listed or principal diagnosis.

External cause codes are intended to provide data for injury research and evaluation of injury prevention strategies. These codes capture how the injury or health condition happened (cause), the intent (unintentional or accidental; or intentional, such as suicide or assault), the place where the event occurred the activity of the patient at the time of the event, and the person's status (e.g., civilian, military).

There is no national requirement for mandatory ICD-10-CM external cause code reporting. Unless a provider is subject to a state-based external cause code reporting mandate or these codes are required by a particular payer, reporting of ICD-10-CM codes in Chapter 20, External Causes of Morbidity, is not required. In the absence of a mandatory reporting requirement, providers are encouraged to voluntarily report external cause codes, as they provide valuable data for injury research and evaluation of injury prevention strategies.

a. General External Cause Coding Guidelines

1) Used with any code in the range of A00.0-T88.9 Z00-Z99

An external cause code may be used with any code in the range of A00.0-T88.9, Z00-Z99, classification that ***represents*** a health condition due to an external cause. Though they are most applicable to injuries, they are also valid for use with such things as infections or diseases due to an external source, and other health conditions, such as a heart attack that occurs during strenuous physical activity.

2) External cause code used for length of treatment

Assign the external cause code, with the appropriate 7th character (initial encounter, subsequent encounter or sequela) for each encounter for which the injury or condition is being treated.

Most categories in this chapter have three 7th character values: A, initial encounter, D, subsequent encounter and S, sequela. While the patient may be seen by a new or different provider over the course of treatment for an injury or condition, assignment of the 7th character for external cause should match the 7th character of the code assigned for the associated injury or condition for the encounter.

3) Use the full range of external cause codes

Use the full range of external cause codes to completely describe the cause, the intent, the place of occurrence, and if applicable, the activity of the patient at the time of the event, and the patient's status, for all injuries, and other health conditions due to an external cause.

4) Assign as many external cause codes as necessary

Assign as many external cause codes as necessary to fully explain each cause. If only one external code can be recorded, assign the code most related to the principal diagnosis.

5) The selection of the appropriate external cause code

The selection of the appropriate external cause code is guided by the Alphabetic Index of External Causes and by Inclusion and Exclusion notes in the Tabular List.

6) External cause code can never be a principal diagnosis

An external cause code can never be a principal (first-listed) diagnosis.

7) Combination external cause codes

Certain of the external cause codes are combination codes that identify sequential events that result in an injury, such as a fall which results in striking against an object. The injury may be due to either event or both. The combination external cause code used should correspond to the sequence of events regardless of which caused the most serious injury.

8) No external cause code needed in certain circumstances

No external cause code from Chapter 20 is needed if the external cause and intent are included in a code from another chapter (e.g. T36.0x1- Poisoning by penicillins, accidental (unintentional)).

b. Place of Occurrence Guideline

Codes from category Y92, Place of occurrence of the external cause, are secondary codes for use after other external cause codes to identify the location of the patient at the time of injury or other condition.

Generally, a place of occurrence code is assigned only once, at the initial encounter for treatment. However, in the rare instance that a new injury occurs during hospitalization, an additional place of occurrence code may be assigned. No 7th characters are used for Y92.

Do not use place of occurrence code Y92.9 if the place is not stated or is not applicable.

c. Activity Code

Assign a code from category Y93, Activity code, to describe the activity of the patient at the time the injury or other health condition occurred.

An activity code is used only once, at the initial encounter for treatment. Only one code from Y93 should be recorded on a medical record. An activity code should be used in conjunction with a place of occurrence code, Y92.

The activity codes are not applicable to poisonings, adverse effects, misadventures or sequela.

Do not assign Y93.9, Unspecified activity, if the activity is not stated.

A code from category Y93 is appropriate for use with external cause and intent codes if identifying the activity provides additional information about the event.

d. Place of Occurrence, Activity, and Status Codes Used with other External Cause Code

When applicable, place of occurrence, activity, and external cause status codes are sequenced after the main external cause code(s). Regardless of the number of external cause codes assigned, there should be only one place of occurrence code, one activity code, and one external cause status code assigned to an encounter.

e. If the Reporting Format Limits the Number of External Cause Codes

If the reporting format limits the number of external cause codes that can be used in reporting clinical data, report the code for the cause/intent most related to the principal diagnosis. If the format permits capture of additional external cause codes, the cause/intent, including medical misadventures, of the additional events should be reported rather than the codes for place, activity, or external status.

f. Multiple External Cause Coding Guidelines

More than one external cause code is required to fully describe the external cause of an illness or injury. The assignment of external cause codes should be sequenced in the following priority:

If two or more events cause separate injuries, an external cause code should be assigned for each cause. The first-listed external cause code will be selected in the following order:

External codes for child and adult abuse take priority over all other external cause codes.

See Section I.C.19., Child and Adult abuse guidelines.

External cause codes for terrorism events take priority over all other external cause codes except child and adult abuse.

External cause codes for cataclysmic events take priority over all other external cause codes except child and adult abuse and terrorism.

External cause codes for transport accidents take priority over all other external cause codes except cataclysmic events, child and adult abuse and terrorism.

Activity and external cause status codes are assigned following all causal (intent) external cause codes.

The first-listed external cause code should correspond to the cause of the most serious diagnosis due to an assault, accident, or self-harm, following the order of hierarchy listed above.

g. Child and Adult Abuse Guideline

Adult and child abuse, neglect and maltreatment are classified as assault. Any of the assault codes may be used to indicate the external cause of any injury resulting from the confirmed abuse.

For confirmed cases of abuse, neglect and maltreatment, when the perpetrator is known, a code from Y07, Perpetrator of maltreatment and neglect, should accompany any other assault codes.

See Section I.C.19. Adult and child abuse, neglect and other maltreatment

h. Unknown or Undetermined Intent Guideline

If the intent (accident, self-harm, assault) of the cause of an injury or other condition is unknown or unspecified, code the intent as accidental intent. All transport accident categories assume accidental intent.

1) Use of undetermined intent

External cause codes for events of undetermined intent are only for use if the documentation in the record specifies that the intent cannot be determined.

i. Sequelae (Late Effects)of External Cause Guidelines

1) Sequelae external cause codes

Sequela are reported using the external cause code with the 7th character "S" for sequela. These codes should be used with any report of a late effect or sequela resulting from a previous injury.

See Section I.B.10 Sequela (Late Effects)

2) Sequela external cause code with a related current injury

A sequela external cause code should never be used with a related current nature of injury code.

3) Use of sequela external cause codes for subsequent visits

Use a late effect external cause code for subsequent visits when a late effect of the initial injury is being treated. Do not use a late effect external cause code for subsequent visits for follow-up care (e.g., to assess healing, to receive rehabilitative therapy) of the injury when no late effect of the injury has been documented.

j. Terrorism Guidelines

1) Cause of injury identified by the Federal Government (FBI) as terrorism

When the cause of an injury is identified by the Federal Government (FBI) as terrorism, the first-listed external cause code should be a code from category Y38, Terrorism. The definition of terrorism employed by the FBI is found at the inclusion note at the beginning of category Y38. Use additional code for place of occurrence (Y92.-). More than one Y38 code may be assigned if the injury is the result of more than one mechanism of terrorism.

2) Cause of an injury is suspected to be the result of terrorism

When the cause of an injury is suspected to be the result of terrorism a code from category Y38 should not be assigned. Suspected cases should be classified as assault.

3) Code Y38.9, Terrorism, secondary effects

Assign code Y38.9, Terrorism, secondary effects, for conditions occurring subsequent to the terrorist event. This code should not be assigned for conditions that are due to the initial terrorist act.

It is acceptable to assign code Y38.9 with another code from Y38 if there is an injury due to the initial terrorist event and an injury that is a subsequent result of the terrorist event.

k. External cause status

A code from category Y99, External cause status, should be assigned whenever any other external cause code is assigned for an encounter, including an Activity code, except for the events noted below. Assign a code from category Y99, External cause status, to indicate the work status of the person at the time the event occurred. The status code indicates whether the event occurred during military activity, whether a non-military person was at work, whether an individual including a student or volunteer was involved in a non-work activity at the time of the causal event.

A code from Y99, External cause status, should be assigned, when applicable, with other external cause codes, such as transport accidents and falls. The external cause status codes are not applicable to poisonings, adverse effects, misadventures or late effects.

Do not assign a code from category Y99 if no other external cause codes (cause, activity) are applicable for the encounter.

An external cause status code is used only once, at the initial encounter for treatment. Only one code from Y99 should be recorded on a medical record.

Do not assign code Y99.9, Unspecified external cause status, if the status is not stated.

21. Chapter 21: Factors influencing health status and contact with health services (Z00-Z99)

Note: The chapter specific guidelines provide additional information about the use of Z codes for specified encounters.

a. Use of Z codes in any healthcare setting

Z codes are for use in any healthcare setting. Z codes may be used as either a first-listed (principal diagnosis code in the inpatient setting) or secondary code, depending on the circumstances of the encounter. Certain Z codes may only be used as first-listed or principal diagnosis.

b. Z Codes indicate a reason for an encounter

Z codes are not procedure codes. A corresponding procedure code must accompany a Z code to describe any procedure performed.

c. Categories of Z Codes

1) Contact/Exposure

Category Z20 indicates contact with, and suspected exposure to, communicable diseases. These codes are for patients who do not show any sign or symptom of a disease but are suspected to have been exposed to it by close personal contact with an infected individual or are in an area where a disease is epidemic.

Category Z77, Other contact with and (suspected) exposures hazardous to health, indicates contact with and suspected exposures hazardous to health.

Contact/exposure codes may be used as a first-listed code to explain an encounter for testing, or, more commonly, as a secondary code to identify a potential risk.

2) Inoculations and vaccinations

Code Z23 is for encounters for inoculations and vaccinations. It indicates that a patient is being seen to receive a prophylactic inoculation against a disease. Procedure codes are required to identify the actual administration of the injection and the type(s) of immunizations given. Code Z23 may be used as a secondary code if the inoculation is given as a routine part of preventive health care, such as a well-baby visit.

3) Status

Status codes indicate that a patient is either a carrier of a disease or has the sequelae or residual of a past disease or condition. This includes such things as the presence of prosthetic or mechanical devices resulting from past treatment. A status code is informative, because the status may affect the course of treatment and its outcome. A status code is distinct from a history code. The history code indicates that the patient no longer has the condition.

A status code should not be used with a diagnosis code from one of the body system chapters, if the diagnosis code includes the information provided by the status code. For example, code Z94.1, Heart transplant status, should not be used with a code from subcategory T86.2, Complications of heart transplant. The status code does not provide additional information. The complication code indicates that the patient is a heart transplant patient.

For encounters for weaning from a mechanical ventilator, assign a code from subcategory J96.1, Chronic respiratory failure, followed by code Z99.11, Dependence on respirator [ventilator] status.

The status Z codes/categories are:

Z14 *Genetic carrier*

Genetic carrier status indicates that a person carries a gene, associated with a particular disease, which may be passed to offspring who may develop that disease. The person does not have the disease and is not at risk of developing the disease.

Z15 *Genetic susceptibility to disease*

Genetic susceptibility indicates that a person has a gene that increases the risk of that person developing the disease.

Codes from category Z15 should not be used as principal or first-listed codes. If the patient has the condition to which he/she is susceptible, and that condition is the reason for the encounter, the code for the current condition should be sequenced first. If the patient is being seen for follow-up after completed treatment for this condition, and the condition no longer exists, a follow-up code should be sequenced first, followed by the appropriate personal history and genetic susceptibility codes. If the purpose of the encounter is genetic counseling associated with procreative management, code Z31.5, Encounter for genetic counseling, should be assigned as the first-listed code, followed by a code from category Z15. Additional codes should be assigned for any applicable family or personal history.

Z16 *Resistance to antimicrobial drugs*
This code indicates that a patient has a condition that is resistant to antimicrobial drug treatment. Sequence the infection code first.

Z17 *Estrogen receptor status*

Z18 *Retained foreign body fragments*

Z19 *Hormone sensitivity malignancy status*

Z21 *Asymptomatic HIV infection status*
This code indicates that a patient has tested positive for HIV but has manifested no signs or symptoms of the disease.

Z22 *Carrier of infectious disease*
Carrier status indicates that a person harbors the specific organisms of a disease without manifest symptoms and is capable of transmitting the infection.

Z28.3 *Underimmunization status*

Z33.1 *Pregnant state, incidental*
This code is a secondary code only for use when the pregnancy is in no way complicating the reason for visit. Otherwise, a code from the obstetric chapter is required.

Z66 *Do not resuscitate*
This code may be used when it is documented by the provider that a patient is on do not resuscitate status at any time during the stay.

Z67 *Blood type*

Z68 *Body mass index (BMI)*
BMI codes should only be assigned when the associated diagnosis (such as overweight or obesity) *meets the definition of a reportable diagnosis (see Section III, Reporting Additional Diagnoses).* ***Do not assign BMI codes during pregnancy. See Section I.B.14 for BMI documentation by clinicians other than the patient's provider.***

Z74.01 *Bed confinement status*

Z76.82 *Awaiting organ transplant status*

Z78 *Other specified health status*
Code Z78.1, Physical restraint status, may be used when it is documented by the provider that a patient has been put in restraints during the current encounter. Please note that this code should not be reported when it is documented by the provider that a patient is temporarily restrained during a procedure.

Z79 Long-term (current) drug therapy
Codes from this category indicate a patient's continuous use of a prescribed drug (including such things as aspirin therapy) for the long-term treatment of a condition or for prophylactic use. It is not for use for patients who have addictions to drugs. This subcategory is not for use of medications for detoxification or maintenance programs to prevent withdrawal symptoms in patients with drug dependence (e.g., methadone maintenance for opiate dependence). Assign the appropriate code for the drug dependence instead.

Assign a code from Z79 if the patient is receiving a medication for an extended period as a prophylactic measure (such as for the prevention of deep vein thrombosis) or as treatment of a chronic condition (such as arthritis) or a disease requiring a lengthy course of treatment (such as cancer). Do not assign a code from category Z79 for medication being administered for a brief period of time to treat an acute illness or injury (such as a course of antibiotics to treat acute bronchitis).

Z88 Allergy status to drugs, medicaments and biological substances
Except: Z88.9, Allergy status to unspecified drugs, medicaments and biological substances status

Z89 Acquired absence of limb

Z90 Acquired absence of organs, not elsewhere classified

Z91.0- Allergy status, other than to drugs and biological substances

Z92.82 Status post administration of tPA (rtPA) in a different facility within the last 24 hours prior to admission to a current facility

Assign code Z92.82, Status post administration of tPA (rtPA) in a different facility within the last 24 hours prior to admission to current facility, as a secondary diagnosis when a patient is received by transfer into a facility and documentation indicates they were administered tissue plasminogen activator (tPA) within the last 24 hours prior to admission to the current facility.

This guideline applies even if the patient is still receiving the tPA at the time they are received into the current facility.

The appropriate code for the condition for which the tPA was administered (such as cerebrovascular disease or myocardial infarction) should be assigned first.

Code Z92.82 is only applicable to the receiving facility record and not to the transferring facility record.

Z93 Artificial opening status

Z94 Transplanted organ and tissue status

Z95 Presence of cardiac and vascular implants and grafts

Z96 Presence of other functional implants

Z97 Presence of other devices

Z98 Other postprocedural states
Assign code Z98.85, Transplanted organ removal status, to indicate that a transplanted organ has been previously removed. This code should not be assigned for the encounter in which the transplanted organ is removed. The complication necessitating removal of the transplant organ should be assigned for that encounter.

See section I.C19. for information on the coding of organ transplant complications.

Z99 Dependence on enabling machines and devices, not elsewhere classified
Note: *Categories Z89-Z90 and Z93-Z99 are for use only if there are no complications or malfunctions of the organ or tissue replaced, the amputation site or the equipment on which the patient is dependent.*

4) History (of)

There are two types of history Z codes, personal and family. Personal history codes explain a patient's past medical condition that no longer exists and is not receiving any treatment, but that has the potential for recurrence, and therefore may require continued monitoring.

Family history codes are for use when a patient has a family member(s) who has had a particular disease that causes the patient to be at higher risk of also contracting the disease.

Personal history codes may be used in conjunction with follow-up codes and family history codes may be used in conjunction with screening codes to explain the need for a test or procedure. History codes are also acceptable on any medical record regardless of the reason for visit. A history of an illness, even if no longer present, is important information that may alter the type of treatment ordered.

The history Z code categories are:

Z80 Family history of primary malignant neoplasm

Z81 Family history of mental and behavioral disorders

Z82 Family history of certain disabilities and chronic diseases (leading to disablement)

Z83 Family history of other specific disorders

Z84 Family history of other conditions

Z85 Personal history of malignant neoplasm

Z86 Personal history of certain other diseases

Z87 Personal history of other diseases and conditions

Z91.4- Personal history of psychological trauma, not elsewhere classified

Z91.5 Personal history of self-harm

Z91.81 History of falling

Z91.82 Personal history of military deployment

Z92 Personal history of medical treatment

Except: Z92.0, Personal history of contraception

Except: Z92.82, Status post administration of tPA (rtPA) in a different facility within the last 24 hours prior to admission to a current facility

5) Screening

Screening is the testing for disease or disease precursors in seemingly well individuals so that early detection and treatment can be provided for those who test positive for the disease (e.g., screening mammogram).

The testing of a person to rule out or confirm a suspected diagnosis because the patient has some sign or symptom is a diagnostic examination, not a screening. In these cases, the sign or symptom is used to explain the reason for the test.

A screening code may be a first-listed code if the reason for the visit is specifically the screening exam. It may also be used as an additional code if the screening is done during an office visit for other health problems. A screening code is not necessary if the screening is inherent to a routine examination, such as a pap smear done during a routine pelvic examination.

Should a condition be discovered during the screening then the code for the condition may be assigned as an additional diagnosis.

The Z code indicates that a screening exam is planned. A procedure code is required to confirm that the screening was performed.

The screening Z codes/categories:

Z11 *Encounter for screening for infectious and parasitic diseases*

Z12 *Encounter for screening for malignant neoplasms*

Z13 *Encounter for screening for other diseases and disorders*

Except: Z13.9, Encounter for screening, unspecified

Z36 *Encounter for antenatal screening for mother*

6) Observation

There are three observation Z code categories. They are for use in very limited circumstances when a person is being observed for a suspected condition that is ruled out. The observation codes are not for use if an injury or illness or any signs or symptoms related to the suspected condition are present. In such cases the diagnosis/symptom code is used with the corresponding external cause code.

The observation codes are to be used as principal diagnosis only. The only exception to this is when the principal diagnosis is required to be a code from category Z38, Liveborn infants according to place of birth and type of delivery. Then a code from category Z05, Encounter for observation and evaluation of newborn for suspected diseases and conditions ruled out, is sequenced after the Z38 code. Additional codes may be used in addition to the observation code but only if they are unrelated to the suspected condition being observed.

Codes from subcategory Z03.7, Encounter for suspected maternal and fetal conditions ruled out, may either be used as a first-listed or as an additional code assignment depending on the case. They are for use in very limited circumstances on a maternal record when an encounter is for a suspected maternal or fetal condition that is ruled out during that encounter (for example, a maternal or fetal condition may be suspected due to an abnormal test result). These codes should not be used when the condition is confirmed. In those cases, the confirmed condition should be coded. In addition, these codes are not for use if an illness or any signs or symptoms related to the suspected condition or problem are present. In such cases the diagnosis/ symptom code is used.

Additional codes may be used in addition to the code from subcategory Z03.7, but only if they are unrelated to the suspected condition being evaluated.

Codes from subcategory Z03.7 may not be used for encounters for antenatal screening of mother. *See Section I.C.21.c.5, Screening.*

For encounters for suspected fetal condition that are inconclusive following testing and evaluation, assign the appropriate code from category O35, O36, O40 or O41.

The observation Z code categories:

Z03 *Encounter for medical observation for suspected diseases and conditions ruled out*

Z04 *Encounter for examination and observation for other reasons*

Except: Z04.9, Encounter for examination and observation for unspecified reason

Z05 *Encounter for observation and evaluation of newborn for suspected diseases and conditions ruled out*

7) Aftercare

Aftercare visit codes cover situations when the initial treatment of a disease has been performed and the patient requires continued care during the healing or recovery phase, or for the long-term consequences of the disease. The aftercare Z code should not be used if treatment is directed at a current, acute disease. The diagnosis code is to be used in these cases. Exceptions to this rule are codes Z51.0, Encounter for antineoplastic radiation therapy, and codes from subcategory Z51.1, Encounter for antineoplastic chemotherapy and immunotherapy. These codes are to be first-listed, followed by the diagnosis code when a patient's encounter is solely to receive radiation therapy, chemotherapy, or immunotherapy for the treatment of a neoplasm. If the reason for the encounter is more than one type of antineoplastic therapy, code Z51.0 and a code from subcategory Z51.1 may be assigned together, in which case one of these codes would be reported as a secondary diagnosis.

The aftercare Z codes should also not be used for aftercare for injuries. For aftercare of an injury, assign the acute injury code with the appropriate 7th character (for subsequent encounter).

The aftercare codes are generally first-listed to explain the specific reason for the encounter. An aftercare code may be used as an additional code when some type of aftercare is provided in addition to the reason for admission and no diagnosis code is applicable. An example of this would be the closure of a colostomy during an encounter for treatment of another condition.

Aftercare codes should be used in conjunction with other aftercare codes or diagnosis codes to provide better detail on the specifics of an aftercare encounter visit, unless otherwise directed by the classification. Should a patient receive multiple types of antineoplastic therapy during the same encounter, code Z51.0, Encounter for antineoplastic radiation therapy, and codes from subcategory Z51.1, Encounter for antineoplastic chemotherapy and immunotherapy, may be used together on a record. The sequencing of multiple aftercare codes depends on the circumstances of the encounter.

Certain aftercare Z code categories need a secondary diagnosis code to describe the resolving condition or sequelae. For others, the condition is included in the code title.

Additional Z code aftercare category terms include fitting and adjustment, and attention to artificial openings.

Status Z codes may be used with aftercare Z codes to indicate the nature of the aftercare. For example code Z95.1, Presence of aortocoronary bypass graft, may be used with code Z48.812, Encounter for surgical aftercare following surgery on the circulatory system, to indicate the surgery for which the aftercare is being performed. A status code should not be used when the aftercare code indicates the type of status, such as using Z43.0, Encounter for attention to tracheostomy, with Z93.0, Tracheostomy status.

The aftercare Z category/codes:

Z42 *Encounter for plastic and reconstructive surgery following medical procedure or healed injury*

Z43 *Encounter for attention to artificial openings*

Z44 *Encounter for fitting and adjustment of external prosthetic device*

Z45 *Encounter for adjustment and management of implanted device*

Z46 *Encounter for fitting and adjustment of other devices*

Z47 *Orthopedic aftercare*

Z48 *Encounter for other postprocedural aftercare*

Z49 *Encounter for care involving renal dialysis*

Z51 *Encounter for other aftercare and medical care*

8) Follow-up

The follow-up codes are used to explain continuing surveillance following completed treatment of a disease, condition, or injury. They imply that the condition has been fully treated and no longer exists. They should not be confused with aftercare codes, or injury codes with a 7th character for subsequent encounter, that explain ongoing care of a healing condition or its sequelae. Follow-up codes may be used in conjunction with history codes to provide the full picture of the healed condition and its treatment. The follow-up code is sequenced first, followed by the history code.

A follow-up code may be used to explain multiple visits. Should a condition be found to have recurred on the follow-up visit, then the diagnosis code for the condition should be assigned in place of the follow-up code.

The follow-up Z code categories:

Z08 *Encounter for follow-up examination after completed treatment for malignant neoplasm*

Z09 *Encounter for follow-up examination after completed treatment for conditions other than malignant neoplasm*

Z39 *Encounter for maternal postpartum care and examination*

9) Donor

Codes in category Z52, Donors of organs and tissues, are used for living individuals who are donating blood or other body tissue. These codes are only for individuals donating for others, not for self-donations. They are not used to identify cadaveric donations.

10) Counseling

Counseling Z codes are used when a patient or family member receives assistance in the aftermath of an illness or injury, or when support is required in coping with family or social problems.

The counseling Z codes/categories:

Z30.0- *Encounter for general counseling and advice on contraception*

Z31.5 *Encounter for procreative genetic counseling*

Z31.6- *Encounter for general counseling and advice on procreation*

Z32.2 *Encounter for childbirth instruction*

Z32.3 *Encounter for childcare instruction*

Z69 *Encounter for mental health services for victim and perpetrator of abuse*

Z70 *Counseling related to sexual attitude, behavior and orientation*

Z71 *Persons encountering health services for other counseling and medical advice, not elsewhere classified*

Z76.81 *Expectant mother prebirth pediatrician visit*

11) Encounters for Obstetrical and Reproductive Services

See Section I.C.15. Pregnancy, Childbirth, and the Puerperium, for further instruction on the use of these codes.

Z codes for pregnancy are for use in those circumstances when none of the problems or complications included in the codes from the Obstetrics chapter exist (a routine prenatal visit or postpartum care). Codes in category Z34, Encounter for supervision of normal pregnancy, are always first-listed and are not to be used with any other code from the OB chapter.

Codes in category Z3A, Weeks of gestation, may be assigned to provide additional information about the pregnancy. Category Z3A codes should not be assigned for pregnancies with abortive outcomes (categories O00-O08), elective termination of pregnancy (code Z33.2), nor for postpartum conditions, as category Z3A is not applicable to these conditions. The date of the admission should be used to determine weeks of gestation for inpatient admissions that encompass more than one gestational week.

The outcome of delivery, category Z37, should be included on all maternal delivery records. It is always a secondary code. Codes in category Z37 should not be used on the newborn record.

Z codes for family planning (contraceptive) or procreative management and counseling should be included on an obstetric record either during the pregnancy or the postpartum stage, if applicable.

Z codes/categories for obstetrical and reproductive services:

Z30 *Encounter for contraceptive management*

Z31 *Encounter for procreative management*

Z32.2 *Encounter for childbirth instruction*

Z32.3 *Encounter for childcare instruction*

Z33 *Pregnant state*

Z34 *Encounter for supervision of normal pregnancy*

Z36 *Encounter for antenatal screening of mother*

Z3A *Weeks of gestation*

Z37 *Outcome of delivery*

Z39 *Encounter for maternal postpartum care and examination*

Z76.81 *Expectant mother prebirth pediatrician visit*

12) Newborns and Infants

See Section I.C.16. Newb*orn (Perinatal) Guidelines, for further instruction on the use of these codes.*

Newborn Z codes/categories:

Z76.1 *Encounter for health supervision and care of foundling*

Z00.1- *Encounter for routine child health examination*

Z38 *Liveborn infants according to place of birth and type of delivery*

13) Routine and administrative examinations

The Z codes allow for the description of encounters for routine examinations, such as, a general check-up, or, examinations for administrative purposes, such as, a pre-employment physical. The codes are not to be used if the examination is for diagnosis of a suspected condition or for treatment purposes. In such cases the diagnosis code is used. During a routine exam, should a diagnosis or condition be discovered, it should be coded as an additional code. Pre-existing and chronic conditions and history codes may also be included as additional codes as long as the examination is for administrative purposes and not focused on any particular condition.

Some of the codes for routine health examinations distinguish between "with" and "without" abnormal findings. Code assignment depends on the information that is known at the time the encounter is being coded. For example, if no abnormal findings were found during the examination, but the encounter is being coded before test results are back, it is acceptable to assign the code for "without abnormal findings." When assigning a code for "with abnormal findings," additional code(s) should be assigned to identify the specific abnormal finding(s).

Pre-operative examination and pre-procedural laboratory examination Z codes are for use only in those situations when a patient is being cleared for a procedure or surgery and no treatment is given.

The Z codes/categories for routine and administrative examinations:

Z00 *Encounter for general examination without complaint, suspected or reported diagnosis*

Z01 *Encounter for other special examination without complaint, suspected or reported diagnosis*

Z02 *Encounter for administrative examination*
Except: Z02.9, Encounter for administrative examinations, unspecified

Z32.0- *Encounter for pregnancy test*

14) Miscellaneous Z codes

The miscellaneous Z codes capture a number of other health care encounters that do not fall into one of the other categories. Certain of these codes identify the reason for the encounter; others are for use as additional codes that provide useful information on circumstances that may affect a patient's care and treatment.

Prophylactic Organ Removal

For encounters specifically for prophylactic removal of an organ (such as prophylactic removal of breasts due to a genetic susceptibility to cancer or a family history of cancer), the principal or first-listed code should be a code from category Z40, Encounter for prophylactic surgery, followed by the appropriate codes to identify the associated risk factor (such as genetic susceptibility or family history).

If the patient has a malignancy of one site and is having prophylactic removal at another site to prevent either a new primary malignancy or metastatic disease, a code for the malignancy should also be assigned in addition to a code from subcategory Z40.0, Encounter for prophylactic surgery for risk factors related to malignant neoplasms. A Z40.0 code should not be assigned if the patient is having organ removal for treatment of a malignancy, such as the removal of the testes for the treatment of prostate cancer.

Miscellaneous Z codes/categories:

Z28 *Immunization not carried out*
Except: Z28.3, Underimmunization status

Z29 *Encounter for other prophylactic measures*

Z40 *Encounter for prophylactic surgery*

Z41 *Encounter for procedures for purposes other than remedying health state*
Except: Z41.9, Encounter for procedure for purposes other than remedying health state, unspecified

Z53 *Persons encountering health services for specific procedures and treatment, not carried out*

Z55 *Problems related to education and literacy*

Z56 *Problems related to employment and unemployment*

Z57 *Occupational exposure to risk factors*

Z58 *Problems related to physical environment*

Z59 *Problems related to housing and economic circumstances*

Z60 *Problems related to social environment*

Z62 *Problems related to upbringing*

Z63 *Other problems related to primary support group, including family circumstances*

Z64 *Problems related to certain psychosocial circumstances*

Z65 *Problems related to other psychosocial circumstances*

Z72 *Problems related to lifestyle*

Note: These codes should be assigned only when the documentation specifies that the patient has an associated problem

Z73 *Problems related to life management difficulty*

Z74 *Problems related to care provider dependency*
Except: Z74.01, Bed confinement status

Z75 *Problems related to medical facilities and other health care*

Z76.0 *Encounter for issue of repeat prescription*

Z76.3 *Healthy person accompanying sick person*

Z76.4 *Other boarder to healthcare facility*

Z76.5 *Malingerer [conscious simulation]*

Z91.1- *Patient's noncompliance with medical treatment and regimen*

Z91.83 *Wandering in diseases classified elsewhere*

Z91.84- *Oral health risk factors*

Z91.89 *Other specified personal risk factors, not elsewhere classified*

See Section I.B.14 for Z55-Z65 Persons with potential health hazards related to socioeconomic and psychosocial circumstances, documentation by clinicians other than the patient's provider

15) Nonspecific Z codes

Certain Z codes are so non-specific, or potentially redundant with other codes in the classification, that there can be little justification for their use in the inpatient setting. Their use in the outpatient setting should be limited to those instances when there is no further documentation to permit more precise coding. Otherwise, any sign or symptom or any other reason for visit that is captured in another code should be used.

Nonspecific Z codes/categories:

Z02.9 *Encounter for administrative examinations, unspecified*

Z04.9 *Encounter for examination and observation for unspecified reason*

Z13.9 *Encounter for screening, unspecified*

Z41.9	*Encounter for procedure for purposes other than remedying health state, unspecified*
Z52.9	*Donor of unspecified organ or tissue*
Z86.59	*Personal history of other mental and behavioral disorders*
Z88.9	*Allergy status to unspecified drugs, medicaments and biological substances status*
Z92.0	*Personal history of contraception*

16) Z Codes That May Only be Principal/First-Listed Diagnosis

The following Z codes/categories may only be reported as the principal/first-listed diagnosis, except when there are multiple encounters on the same day and the medical records for the encounters are combined:

Z00	*Encounter for general examination without complaint, suspected or reported diagnosis* *Except: Z00.6*
Z01	*Encounter for other special examination without complaint, suspected or reported diagnosis*
Z02	*Encounter for administrative examination*
Z03	*Encounter for medical observation for suspected diseases and conditions ruled out*
Z04	*Encounter for examination and observation for other reasons*
Z33.2	*Encounter for elective termination of pregnancy*
Z31.81	*Encounter for male factor infertility in female patient*
Z31.82	*Encounter for Rh incompatibility status*
Z31.83	*Encounter for assisted reproductive fertility procedure cycle*
Z31.84	*Encounter for fertility preservation procedure*
Z34	*Encounter for supervision of normal pregnancy*
Z39	*Encounter for maternal postpartum care and examination*
Z38	*Liveborn infants according to place of birth and type of delivery*
Z40	*Encounter for prophylactic surgery*
Z42	*Encounter for plastic and reconstructive surgery following medical procedure or healed injury*
Z51.0	*Encounter for antineoplastic radiation therapy*
Z51.1-	*Encounter for antineoplastic chemotherapy and immunotherapy*
Z52	*Donors of organs and tissues* *Except: Z52.9, Donor of unspecified organ or tissue*
Z76.1	*Encounter for health supervision and care of foundling*
Z76.2	*Encounter for health supervision and care of other healthy infant and child*
Z99.12	*Encounter for respirator [ventilator] dependence during power failure*

Section II. Selection of Principal Diagnosis

The circumstances of inpatient admission always govern the selection of principal diagnosis. The principal diagnosis is defined in the Uniform Hospital Discharge Data Set (UHDDS) as "that condition established after study to be chiefly responsible for occasioning the admission of the patient to the hospital for care."

The UHDDS definitions are used by hospitals to report inpatient data elements in a standardized manner. These data elements and their definitions can be found in the July 31, 1985, Federal Register (Vol. 50, No, 147), pp. 31038-40.

Since that time the application of the UHDDS definitions has been expanded to include all non-outpatient settings (acute care, short term, long term care and psychiatric hospitals; home health agencies; rehab facilities; nursing homes, etc). The UHDDS definitions also apply to hospice services (all levels of care).

In determining principal diagnosis the coding conventions in the ICD-10-CM, the Tabular List and Alphabetic Index take precedence over these official coding guidelines. (*See Section I.A., Conventions for the ICD-10-CM*)

The importance of consistent, complete documentation in the medical record cannot be overemphasized. Without such documentation the application of all coding guidelines is a difficult, if not impossible, task.

A. Codes for symptoms, signs, and ill-defined conditions

Codes for symptoms, signs, and ill-defined conditions from Chapter 18 are not to be used as principal diagnosis when a related definitive diagnosis has been established.

B. Two or more interrelated conditions, each potentially meeting the definition for principal diagnosis.

When there are two or more interrelated conditions (such as diseases in the same ICD-10-CM chapter or manifestations characteristically associated with a certain disease) potentially meeting the definition of principal diagnosis, either condition may be sequenced first, unless the circumstances of the admission, the therapy provided, the Tabular List, or the Alphabetic Index indicate otherwise.

C. Two or more diagnoses that equally meet the definition for principal diagnosis

In the unusual instance when two or more diagnoses equally meet the criteria for principal diagnosis as determined by the circumstances of admission, diagnostic workup and/or therapy provided, and the Alphabetic Index, Tabular List, or another coding guidelines does not provide sequencing direction, any one of the diagnoses may be sequenced first.

D. Two or more comparative or contrasting conditions.

In those rare instances when two or more contrasting or comparative diagnoses are documented as "either/or" (or similar terminology), they are coded as if the diagnoses were confirmed and the diagnoses are sequenced according to the circumstances of the admission. If no further determination can be made as to which diagnosis should be principal, either diagnosis may be sequenced first.

E. A symptom(s) followed by contrasting/ comparative diagnoses

GUIDELINE HAS BEEN DELETED EFFECTIVE OCTOBER 1, 2014

F. Original treatment plan not carried out

Sequence as the principal diagnosis the condition, which after study occasioned the admission to the hospital, even though treatment may not have been carried out due to unforeseen circumstances.

G. Complications of surgery and other medical care

When the admission is for treatment of a complication resulting from surgery or other medical care, the complication code is sequenced as the principal diagnosis. If the complication is classified to the T80-T88 series and the code lacks the necessary specificity in describing the complication, an additional code for the specific complication should be assigned.

H. Uncertain Diagnosis

If the diagnosis documented at the time of discharge is qualified as "probable", "suspected", "likely", "questionable", "possible", or "still to be ruled out", or other similar terms indicating uncertainty, code the condition as if it existed or was established. The bases for these guidelines are the diagnostic workup, arrangements for further workup or observation, and initial therapeutic approach that correspond most closely with the established diagnosis.

Note: This guideline is applicable only to inpatient admissions to short-term, acute, long-term care and psychiatric hospitals.

I. Admission from Observation Unit

1. Admission Following Medical Observation

When a patient is admitted to an observation unit for a medical condition, which either worsens or does not improve, and is subsequently admitted as an inpatient of the same hospital for this same medical condition, the principal diagnosis would be the medical condition which led to the hospital admission.

2. Admission Following Post-Operative Observation

When a patient is admitted to an observation unit to monitor a condition (or complication) that develops following outpatient surgery, and then is subsequently admitted as an inpatient of the same hospital, hospitals should apply the Uniform Hospital Discharge Data Set (UHDDS) definition of principal diagnosis as "that condition established after study to be chiefly responsible for occasioning the admission of the patient to the hospital for care."

J. Admission from Outpatient Surgery

When a patient receives surgery in the hospital's outpatient surgery department and is subsequently admitted for continuing inpatient care at the same hospital, the following guidelines should be followed in selecting the principal diagnosis for the inpatient admission:

- If the reason for the inpatient admission is a complication, assign the complication as the principal diagnosis.
- If no complication, or other condition, is documented as the reason for the inpatient admission, assign the reason for the outpatient surgery as the principal diagnosis.
- If the reason for the inpatient admission is another condition unrelated to the surgery, assign the unrelated condition as the principal diagnosis.

K. Admissions/Encounters for Rehabilitation

When the purpose for the admission/encounter is rehabilitation, sequence first the code for the condition for which the service is being performed. For example, for an admission/encounter for rehabilitation for right-sided dominant hemiplegia following a cerebrovascular infarction, report code I69.351, Hemiplegia and hemiparesis following cerebral infarction affecting right dominant side, as the first-listed or principal diagnosis.

If the condition for which the rehabilitation service is no longer present, report the appropriate aftercare code as the first-listed or principal diagnosis, unless the rehabilitation service is being provided following an injury. For rehabilitation services following active treatment of an injury, assign the injury code with the appropriate seventh character for subsequent encounter as the first-listed or principal diagnosis. For example, if a patient with severe degenerative osteoarthritis of the hip, underwent hip replacement and the current encounter/admission is for rehabilitation, report code Z47.1, Aftercare following joint replacement surgery, as the first-listed or principal diagnosis. If the patient requires rehabilitation post hip replacement for right intertrochanteric femur fracture, report code S72.141D, Displaced intertrochanteric fracture of right femur, subsequent encounter for closed fracture with routine healing, as the first-listed or principal diagnosis.

See Section I.C.21.c.7, Factors influencing health states and contact with health services, Aftercare.

See Section I.C.19.a for additional information about the use of 7th characters for injury codes.

Section III. Reporting Additional Diagnoses

GENERAL RULES FOR OTHER (ADDITIONAL) DIAGNOSES

For reporting purposes the definition for "other diagnoses" is interpreted as additional conditions that affect patient care in terms of requiring:

- clinical evaluation; or
- therapeutic treatment; or
- diagnostic procedures; or
- extended length of hospital stay; or
- increased nursing care and/or monitoring.

The UHDDS item #11-b defines Other Diagnoses as "all conditions that coexist at the time of admission, that develop subsequently, or that affect the treatment received and/or the length of stay. Diagnoses that relate to an earlier episode which have no bearing on the current hospital stay are to be excluded." UHDDS definitions apply to inpatients in acute care, short-term, long term care and psychiatric hospital setting. The UHDDS definitions are used by acute care short-term hospitals to report inpatient data elements in a standardized manner. These data elements and their definitions can be found in the July 31, 1985, Federal Register (Vol. 50, No, 147), pp. 31038-40.

Since that time the application of the UHDDS definitions has been expanded to include all non-outpatient settings (acute care, short term, long term care and psychiatric hospitals; home health agencies; rehab facilities; nursing homes, etc). The UHDDS definitions also apply to hospice services (all levels of care).

The following guidelines are to be applied in designating "other diagnoses" when neither the Alphabetic Index nor the Tabular List in ICD-10-CM provide direction. The listing of the diagnoses in the patient record is the responsibility of the attending provider.

A. Previous conditions

If the provider has included a diagnosis in the final diagnostic statement, such as the discharge summary or the face sheet, it should ordinarily be coded. Some providers include in the diagnostic statement resolved conditions or diagnoses and status-post procedures from previous admission that have no bearing on the current stay. Such conditions are not to be reported and are coded only if required by hospital policy.

However, history codes (categories Z80-Z87) may be used as secondary codes if the historical condition or family history has an impact on current care or influences treatment.

B. Abnormal findings

Abnormal findings (laboratory, x-ray, pathologic, and other diagnostic results) are not coded and reported unless the provider indicates their clinical significance. If the findings are outside the normal range and the attending provider has ordered other tests to evaluate the condition or prescribed treatment, it is appropriate to ask the provider whether the abnormal finding should be added.

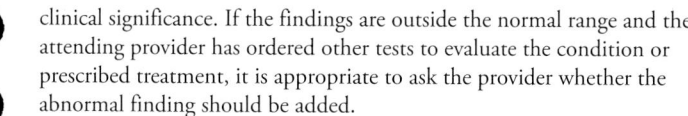

Please note: This differs from the coding practices in the outpatient setting for coding encounters for diagnostic tests that have been interpreted by a provider.

C. Uncertain Diagnosis

If the diagnosis documented at the time of discharge is qualified as "probable", "suspected", "likely", "questionable", "possible", or "still to be ruled out" or other similar terms indicating uncertainty, code the condition as if it existed or was established. The bases for these guidelines are the diagnostic workup, arrangements for further workup or observation, and initial therapeutic approach that correspond most closely with the established diagnosis.

Note: This guideline is applicable only to inpatient admissions to short-term, acute, long-term care and psychiatric hospitals.

Section IV. Diagnostic Coding and Reporting Guidelines for Outpatient Services

These coding guidelines for outpatient diagnoses have been approved for use by hospitals/ providers in coding and reporting hospital-based outpatient services and provider-based office visits. Guidelines in Section I, Conventions, general coding guidelines and chapter-specific guidelines, should also be applied for outpatient services and office visits.

Information about the use of certain abbreviations, punctuation, symbols, and other conventions used in the ICD-10-CM Tabular List (code numbers and titles), can be found in Section IA of these guidelines, under "Conventions Used in the Tabular List." Section I.B. contains general guidelines that apply to the entire classification. Section I.C. contains chapter-specific guidelines that correspond to the chapters as they are arranged in the classification. Information about the correct sequence to use in finding a code is also described in Section I.

The terms encounter and visit are often used interchangeably in describing outpatient service contacts and, therefore, appear together in these guidelines without distinguishing one from the other.

Though the conventions and general guidelines apply to all settings, coding guidelines for outpatient and provider reporting of diagnoses will vary in a number of instances from those for inpatient diagnoses, recognizing that:

The Uniform Hospital Discharge Data Set (UHDDS) definition of principal diagnosis does not apply to hospital-based outpatient services and provider-based office visits.

Coding guidelines for inconclusive diagnoses (probable, suspected, rule out, etc.) were developed for inpatient reporting and do not apply to outpatients.

A. Selection of first-listed condition

In the outpatient setting, the term first-listed diagnosis is used in lieu of principal diagnosis.

In determining the first-listed diagnosis the coding conventions of ICD-10-CM, as well as the general and disease specific guidelines take precedence over the outpatient guidelines.

Diagnoses often are not established at the time of the initial encounter/ visit. It may take two or more visits before the diagnosis is confirmed.

The most critical rule involves beginning the search for the correct code assignment through the Alphabetic Index. Never begin searching initially in the Tabular List as this will lead to coding errors.

1. Outpatient Surgery

When a patient presents for outpatient surgery (same day surgery), code the reason for the surgery as the first-listed diagnosis (reason for the encounter), even if the surgery is not performed due to a contraindication.

2. Observation Stay

When a patient is admitted for observation for a medical condition, assign a code for the medical condition as the first-listed diagnosis.

When a patient presents for outpatient surgery and develops complications requiring admission to observation, code the reason for the surgery as the first reported diagnosis (reason for the encounter), followed by codes for the complications as secondary diagnoses.

B. Codes from A00.0 through T88.9, Z00-Z99

The appropriate code(s) from A00.0 through T88.9, Z00-Z99 must be used to identify diagnoses, symptoms, conditions, problems, complaints, or other reason(s) for the encounter/visit.

C. Accurate reporting of ICD-10-CM diagnosis codes

For accurate reporting of ICD-10-CM diagnosis codes, the documentation should describe the patient's condition, using terminology which includes specific diagnoses as well as symptoms, problems, or reasons for the encounter. There are ICD-10-CM codes to describe all of these.

D. Codes that describe symptoms and signs

Codes that describe symptoms and signs, as opposed to diagnoses, are acceptable for reporting purposes when a diagnosis has not been established (confirmed) by the provider. Chapter 18 of ICD-10-CM, Symptoms, Signs, and Abnormal Clinical and Laboratory Findings Not Elsewhere Classified (codes R00-R99) contain many, but not all codes for symptoms.

E. Encounters for circumstances other than a disease or injury

ICD-10-CM provides codes to deal with encounters for circumstances other than a disease or injury. The Factors Influencing Health Status and Contact with Health Services codes (Z00-Z99) are provided to deal with occasions when circumstances other than a disease or injury are recorded as diagnosis or problems.

See Section I.C.21. Factors influencing health status and contact with health services.

F. Level of Detail in Coding

1. ICD-10-CM codes with 3, 4, 5, 6 or 7 characters

ICD-10-CM is composed of codes with 3, 4, 5, 6 or 7 characters. Codes with three characters are included in ICD-10-CM as the heading of a category of codes that may be further subdivided by the use of fourth, fifth, sixth or seventh characters to provide greater specificity.

2. Use of full number of characters required for a code

A three-character code is to be used only if it is not further subdivided. A code is invalid if it has not been coded to the full number of characters required for that code, including the 7th character, if applicable.

G. ICD-10-CM code for the diagnosis, condition, problem, or other reason for encounter/visit

List first the ICD-10-CM code for the diagnosis, condition, problem, or other reason for encounter/visit shown in the medical record to be chiefly responsible for the services provided. List additional codes that describe any coexisting conditions. In some cases the first-listed diagnosis may be a symptom when a diagnosis has not been established (confirmed) by the physician.

H. Uncertain diagnosis

Do not code diagnoses documented as "probable", "suspected," "questionable," "rule out," or "working diagnosis" or other similar terms indicating uncertainty. Rather, code the condition(s) to the highest degree of certainty for that encounter/visit, such as symptoms, signs, abnormal test results, or other reason for the visit.

Please note: This differs from the coding practices used by short-term, acute care, long-term care and psychiatric hospitals.

I. Chronic diseases

Chronic diseases treated on an ongoing basis may be coded and reported as many times as the patient receives treatment and care for the condition(s)

J. Code all documented conditions that coexist

Code all documented conditions that coexist at the time of the encounter/visit, and require or affect patient care treatment or management. Do not code conditions that were previously treated and no longer exist. However, history codes (categories Z80-Z87) may be used as secondary codes if the historical condition or family history has an impact on current care or influences treatment.

K. Patients receiving diagnostic services only

For patients receiving diagnostic services only during an encounter/visit, sequence first the diagnosis, condition, problem, or other reason for encounter/visit shown in the medical record to be chiefly responsible for the outpatient services provided during the encounter/visit. Codes for other diagnoses (e.g., chronic conditions) may be sequenced as additional diagnoses.

For encounters for routine laboratory/radiology testing in the absence of any signs, symptoms, or associated diagnosis, assign Z01.89, Encounter for other specified special examinations. If routine testing is performed during the same encounter as a test to evaluate a sign, symptom, or diagnosis, it is appropriate to assign both the Z code and the code describing the reason for the non-routine test.

For outpatient encounters for diagnostic tests that have been interpreted by a physician, and the final report is available at the time of coding, code any confirmed or definitive diagnosis(es) documented in the interpretation. Do not code related signs and symptoms as additional diagnoses.

Please note: This differs from the coding practice in the hospital inpatient setting regarding abnormal findings on test results.

L. Patients receiving therapeutic services only

For patients receiving therapeutic services only during an encounter/visit, sequence first the diagnosis, condition, problem, or other reason for encounter/visit shown in the medical record to be chiefly responsible for the outpatient services provided during the encounter/visit. Codes for other diagnoses (e.g., chronic conditions) may be sequenced as additional diagnoses.

The only exception to this rule is that when the primary reason for the admission/encounter is chemotherapy or radiation therapy, the appropriate Z code for the service is listed first, and the diagnosis or problem for which the service is being performed listed second.

M. Patients receiving preoperative evaluations only

For patients receiving preoperative evaluations only, sequence first a code from subcategory Z01.81, Encounter for pre-procedural examinations, to describe the pre-op consultations. Assign a code for the condition to describe the reason for the surgery as an additional diagnosis. Code also any findings related to the pre-op evaluation.

N. Ambulatory surgery

For ambulatory surgery, code the diagnosis for which the surgery was performed. If the postoperative diagnosis is known to be different from the preoperative diagnosis at the time the diagnosis is confirmed, select the postoperative diagnosis for coding, since it is the most definitive.

O. Routine outpatient prenatal visits

See Section I.C.15. Routine outpatient prenatal visits.

P. Encounters for general medical examinations with abnormal findings

The subcategories for encounters for general medical examinations, Z00.0- and encounter for routine child health examination, Z00.12-, provide codes for with and without abnormal findings. Should a general medical examination result in an abnormal finding, the code for general medical examination with abnormal finding should be assigned as the first-listed diagnosis. An examination with abnormal findings refers to a condition/diagnosis that is newly identified or a change in severity of a chronic condition (such as uncontrolled hypertension, or an acute exacerbation of chronic obstructive pulmonary disease) during a routine physical examination. A secondary code for the abnormal finding should also be coded.

Q. Encounters for routine health screenings

See Section I.C.21. Factors influencing health status and contact with health services, Screening

Conversion Table of ICD-1Ø-CM Codes

The National Center for Health Statistics (NCHS) has published an update to the International Classification of Diseases, 10th Revision, Clinical Modification (ICD-10-CM) diagnosis codes, which will become effective October 1, 2018.

The FY 2019 (October 1, 2018-September 30, 2019) Conversion Table for new ICD-10-CM codes is provided to assist users in data retrieval. For each new code the table shows the effective date and its previously assigned code equivalent.

Diagnosis Codes		
Current Code(s) Assignment	Effective October 1	Previous Code(s) Assignment
C43.111	2018	C43.11
C43.112	2018	C43.11
C43.121	2018	C43.12
C43.122	2018	C43.12
C4A.111	2018	C4A.11
C4A.112	2018	C4A.11
C4A.121	2018	C4A.12
C4A.122	2018	C4A.12
C44.1021	2018	C44.102
C44.1022	2018	C44.102
C44.1091	2018	C44.109
C44.1092	2018	C44.109
C44.1121	2018	C44.112
C44.1122	2018	C44.112
C44.1191	2018	C44.119
C44.1192	2018	C44.119
C44.1221	2018	C44.122
C44.1222	2018	C44.122
C44.1291	2018	C44.129
C44.1292	2018	C44.129
C44.131	2018	C44.19
C44.1321	2018	C44.19
C44.1322	2018	C44.19
C44.1391	2018	C44.19
C44.1392	2018	C44.19
C44.1921	2018	C44.192
C44.1922	2018	C44.192
C44.1991	2018	C44.199
C44.1992	2018	C44.199
D03.111	2018	D03.11
D03.112	2018	D03.11
D03.121	2018	D03.12
D03.122	2018	D03.12
D04.111	2018	D04.11
D04.112	2018	D04.11
D04.121	2018	D04.12
D04.122	2018	D04.12
D22.111	2018	D22.11
D22.112	2018	D22.11
D22.121	2018	D22.12
D22.122	2018	D22.12
D23.111	2018	D23.11
D23.112	2018	D23.11
D23.121	2018	D23.12
D23.122	2018	D23.12
E72.81	2018	E72.8
E72.89	2018	E72.8
E75.26	2018	E75.29
E78.41	2018	E78.4
E78.49	2018	E78.4
E88.02	2018	E88.09
F12.23	2018	F12.288
F12.93	2018	F12.988
F53.0	2018	F53
F53.1	2018	F53
F68.A	2018	F68.10
G51.31	2018	G51.3
G51.32	2018	G51.3
G51.33	2018	G51.3
G51.39	2018	G51.3
G71.00	2018	G71.0
G71.01	2018	G71.0
G71.02	2018	G71.0
G71.09	2018	G71.0
H01.00A	2018	H01.001 and H01.002
H01.00B	2018	H01.004 and H01.005
H01.01A	2018	H01.011 and H01.012
H01.01B	2018	H01.014 and H01.015
H01.02A	2018	H01.021 and H01.022
H01.02B	2018	H01.024 and H01.025
H02.151	2018	H02.101-H02.106; H02.109
H02.152	2018	H02.101-H02.106; H02.109
H02.153	2018	H02.101-H02.106; H02.109
H02.154	2018	H02.101-H02.106; H02.109
H02.155	2018	H02.101-H02.106; H02.109
H02.156	2018	H02.101-H02.106; H02.109
H02.159	2018	H02.101-H02.106; H02.109
H02.20A	2018	H02.201 and H02.202

Diagnosis Codes		
Current Code(s) Assignment	Effective October 1	Previous Code(s) Assignment
H02.20B	2018	H02.204 and H02.205
H02.20C	2018	H02.201, H02.202, H02.204 and H02.205
H02.21A	2018	H02.211 and H02.212
H02.21B	2018	H02.214 and H02.215
H02.21C	2018	H02.211, H02.212, H02.214 and H02.215
H02.22A	2018	H02.221 and H02.222
H02.22B	2018	H02.224 and H02.225
H02.22C	2018	H02.221, H02.222, H02.224 and H02.225
H02.23A	2018	H02.231 and H02.232
H02.23B	2018	H02.234 and H02.235
H02.23C	2018	H02.231, H02.232, H02.234 and H02.235
H02.881	2018	H02.89
H02.882	2018	H02.89
H02.883	2018	H02.89
H02.884	2018	H02.89
H02.885	2018	H02.89
H02.886	2018	H02.89
H02.889	2018	H02.89
H02.88A	2018	H02.89
H02.88B	2018	H02.89
H10.821	2018	H10.89
H10.822	2018	H10.89
H10.823	2018	H10.89
H10.829	2018	H10.89
H57.811	2018	H57.8
H57.812	2018	H57.8
H57.813	2018	H57.8
H57.819	2018	H57.8
H57.89	2018	H57.8
I63.81	2018	I63.8
I63.89	2018	I63.8
I67.850	2018	I67.89
I67.858	2018	I67.89
K35.20	2018	K35.2
K35.21	2018	K35.2
K35.30	2018	K35.3
K35.31	2018	K35.3
K35.32	2018	K35.3
K35.33	2018	K35.3
K35.890	2018	K35.89
K35.891	2018	K35.89
K61.31	2018	K61.3
K61.39	2018	K61.3
K61.5	2018	K61.3
K82.A1	2018	K81.0
K82.A2	2018	K82.2 and K81.9

Diagnosis Codes		
Current Code(s) Assignment	Effective October 1	Previous Code(s) Assignment
K83.01	2018	K83.0
K83.09	2018	K83.0
M79.10	2018	M79.1
M79.11	2018	M79.1
M79.12	2018	M79.1
M79.18	2018	M79.1
N35.016	2018	N35.014
N35.116	2018	N35.114
N35.811	2018	N35.8
N35.812	2018	N35.8
N35.813	2018	N35.8
N35.814	2018	N35.8
N35.816	2018	N35.8
N35.819	2018	N35.8
N35.82	2018	N35.8
N35.911	2018	N35.9
N35.912	2018	N35.9
N35.913	2018	N35.9
N35.914	2018	N35.9
N35.916	2018	N35.9
N35.919	2018	N35.9
N35.92	2018	N35.9
N99.116	2018	N99.114
O30.131	2018	O30.101
O30.132	2018	O30.101
O30.133	2018	O30.101
O30.139	2018	O30.101
O30.231	2018	O30.201
O30.232	2018	O30.201
O30.233	2018	O30.201
O30.239	2018	O30.201
O30.831	2018	O30.801
O30.832	2018	O30.801
O30.833	2018	O30.801
O30.839	2018	O30.801
O86.00	2018	O86.0
O86.01	2018	O86.0
O86.02	2018	O86.0
O86.03	2018	O86.0
O86.04	2018	O86.0
O86.09	2018	O86.0
P02.70	2018	P02.7
P02.78	2018	P02.7
P04.11	2018	P04.1
P04.12	2018	P04.1
P04.13	2018	P04.1

Diagnosis Codes		
Current Code(s) Assignment	Effective October 1	Previous Code(s) Assignment
P04.14	2018	P04.1
P04.15	2018	P04.1
P04.16	2018	P04.1
P04.17	2018	P04.1
P04.1A	2018	P04.1
P04.18	2018	P04.1
P04.19	2018	P04.1
P04.40	2018	P04.49
P04.42	2018	P04.49
P04.81	2018	P04.8
P04.89	2018	P04.8
P35.4	2018	P35.8 and A92.5
P74.21	2018	P74.2
P74.22	2018	P74.2
P74.31	2018	P74.3
P74.32	2018	P74.3
P74.41	2018	P74.4
P74.421	2018	P74.4
P74.422	2018	P74.4
P74.49	2018	P74.4
Q51.20	2018	Q51.2
Q51.21	2018	Q51.2
Q51.22	2018	Q51.2
Q51.28	2018	Q51.2
Q93.51	2018	Q93.5
Q93.59	2018	Q93.5
Q93.82	2018	Q93.89
R82.991	2018	R82.99
R82.992	2018	R82.99
R82.993	2018	R82.99
R82.994	2018	R82.99
R82.998	2018	R82.99
R93.811	2018	R93.8
R93.812	2018	R93.8
R93.813	2018	R93.8
R93.819	2018	R93.8
R93.89	2018	R93.8
T43.641A	2018	T43.621A
T43.641D	2018	T43.621D
T43.641S	2018	T43.621S
T43.642A	2018	T43.622A
T43.642D	2018	T43.622D
T43.642S	2018	T43.622S
T43.643A	2018	T43.623A
T43.643D	2018	T43.623D
T43.643S	2018	T43.623S

Diagnosis Codes		
Current Code(s) Assignment	Effective October 1	Previous Code(s) Assignment
T43.644A	2018	T43.624A
T43.644D	2018	T43.624D
T43.644S	2018	T43.624S
T74.51XA	2018	T74.21XA
T74.51XD	2018	T74.21XD
T74.51XS	2018	T74.21XS
T74.52XA	2018	T74.22XA
T74.52XD	2018	T74.22XD
T74.52XS	2018	T74.22XS
T74.61XA	2018	T74.11XA
T74.61XD	2018	T74.11XD
T74.61XS	2018	T74.11XS
T74.62XA	2018	T74.12XA
T74.62XD	2018	T74.12XD
T74.62XS	2018	T74.12XS
T76.51XA	2018	T76.21XA
T76.51XD	2018	T76.21XD
T76.51XS	2018	T76.21XS
T76.52XA	2018	T76.22XA
T76.52XD	2018	T76.22XD
T76.52XS	2018	T76.22XS
T76.61XA	2018	T76.11XA
T76.61XD	2018	T76.11XD
T76.61XS	2018	T76.11XS
T76.62XA	2018	T76.12XA
T76.62XD	2018	T76.12XD
T76.62XS	2018	T76.12XS
T81.40XA	2018	T81.4XXA
T81.40XD	2018	T81.4XXD
T81.40XS	2018	T81.4XXS
T81.41XA	2018	T81.4XXA
T81.41XD	2018	T81.4XXD
T81.41XS	2018	T81.4XXS
T81.42XA	2018	T81.4XXA
T81.42XD	2018	T81.4XXD
T81.42XS	2018	T81.4XXS
T81.43XA	2018	T81.4XXA
T81.43XD	2018	T81.4XXD
T81.43XS	2018	T81.4XXS
T81.44XA	2018	T81.4XXA
T81.44XD	2018	T81.4XXD
T81.44XS	2018	T81.4XXS
T81.49XA	2018	T81.4XXA
T81.49XD	2018	T81.4XXD
T81.49XS	2018	T81.4XXS
Y07.6	2018	Y07.59

Diagnosis Codes		
Current Code(s) Assignment	Effective October 1	Previous Code(s) Assignment
Z04.81	2018	Z04.8
Z04.82	2018	Z04.8
Z04.89	2018	Z04.8
Z13.30	2018	Z13.8
Z13.31	2018	Z13.8
Z13.32	2018	Z13.8
Z13.39	2018	Z13.8
Z13.40	2018	Z13.4
Z13.41	2018	Z13.4

Diagnosis Codes		
Current Code(s) Assignment	Effective October 1	Previous Code(s) Assignment
Z13.42	2018	Z13.4
Z13.49	2018	Z13.4
Z20.821	2018	Z20.828
Z28.83	2018	Z28.89
Z62.813	2018	Z62.810
Z83.430	2018	Z83.49
Z83.438	2018	Z83.49
Z91.42	2018	Z91.410

Source: CMS

A

Aarskog's syndrome Q87.1
Abandonment — *see* Maltreatment
Abasia (-astasia) (hysterical) F44.4
Abderhalden-Kaufmann-Lignac syndrome (cystinosis) E72.04
Abdomen, abdominal — *see also* condition
  acute R10.0
  angina K55.1
  muscle deficiency syndrome Q79.4
Abdominalgia — *see* Pain, abdominal
Abduction contracture, hip or other joint — *see* Contraction, joint
Aberrant (congenital) — *see also* Malposition, congenital
  adrenal gland Q89.1
  artery (peripheral) Q27.8
    basilar NEC Q28.1
    cerebral Q28.3
    coronary Q24.5
    digestive system Q27.8
    eye Q15.8
    lower limb Q27.8
    precerebral Q28.1
    pulmonary Q25.79
    renal Q27.2
    retina Q14.1
    specified site NEC Q27.8
    subclavian Q27.8
    upper limb Q27.8
    vertebral Q28.1
  breast Q83.8
  endocrine gland NEC Q89.2
  hepatic duct Q44.5
  pancreas Q45.3
  parathyroid gland Q89.2
  pituitary gland Q89.2
  sebaceous glands, mucous membrane, mouth, congenital Q38.6
  spleen Q89.09
  subclavian artery Q27.8
  thymus (gland) Q89.2
  thyroid gland Q89.2
  vein (peripheral) NEC Q27.8
    cerebral Q28.3
    digestive system Q27.8
    lower limb Q27.8
    precerebral Q28.1
    specified site NEC Q27.8
    upper limb Q27.8
Aberration
  distantial — *see* Disturbance, visual
  mental F99
Abetalipoproteinemia E78.6
Abiotrophy R68.89
Ablatio, ablation
  retinae — *see* Detachment, retina
Ablepharia, ablepharon Q10.3
Abnormal, abnormality, abnormalities — *see also* Anomaly
  acid-base balance (mixed) E87.4
  albumin R77.0
  alphafetoprotein R77.2
  alveolar ridge K08.9
  anatomical relationship Q89.9
  apertures, congenital, diaphragm Q79.1
  auditory perception H93.29-
    diplacusis — *see* Diplacusis
    hyperacusis — *see* Hyperacusis
    recruitment — *see* Recruitment, auditory
    threshold shift — *see* Shift, auditory threshold
  autosomes Q99.9
    fragile site Q95.5
  basal metabolic rate R94.8
  biosynthesis, testicular androgen E29.1
  bleeding time R79.1
  blood-gas level R79.81
  blood level (of)
    cobalt R79.0
    copper R79.0
    iron R79.0
    lithium R78.89
    magnesium R79.0
    mineral NEC R79.0
    zinc R79.0
  blood pressure
    elevated R03.0
    low reading (nonspecific) R03.1
  blood sugar R73.09
  bowel sounds R19.15
    absent R19.11
    hyperactive R19.12

Abnormal, abnormality, abnormalities - *continued*
  brain scan R94.02
  breathing R06.9
  caloric test R94.138
  cerebrospinal fluid R83.9
    cytology R83.6
    drug level R83.2
    enzyme level R83.0
    hormones R83.1
    immunology R83.4
    microbiology R83.5
    nonmedicinal level R83.3
    specified type NEC R83.8
  chemistry, blood R79.9
    C-reactive protein R79.82
    drugs — *see* Findings, abnormal, in blood
    gas level R79.81
    minerals R79.0
    pancytopenia D61.818
    PTT R79.1
    specified NEC R79.89
    toxins — *see* Findings, abnormal, in blood
  chest sounds (friction) (rales) R09.89
  chromosome, chromosomal Q99.9
    with more than three X chromosomes, female Q97.1
    analysis result R89.8
      bronchial washings R84.8
      cerebrospinal fluid R83.8
      cervix uteri NEC R87.89
      nasal secretions R84.8
      nipple discharge R89.8
      peritoneal fluid R85.89
      pleural fluid R84.8
      prostatic secretions R86.8
      saliva R85.89
      seminal fluid R86.8
      sputum R84.8
      synovial fluid R89.8
      throat scrapings R84.8
      vagina R87.89
      vulva R87.89
      wound secretions R89.8
    dicentric replacement Q93.2
    ring replacement Q93.2
    sex Q99.8
      female phenotype Q97.9
        specified NEC Q97.8
      male phenotype Q98.9
        specified NEC Q98.8
      structural male Q98.6
    specified NEC Q99.8
  clinical findings NEC R68.89
  coagulation D68.9
    newborn, transient P61.6
    profile R79.1
    time R79.1
  communication — *see* Fistula
  conjunctiva, vascular H11.41-
  coronary artery Q24.5
  cortisol-binding globulin E27.8
  course, eustachian tube Q17.8
  creatinine clearance R94.4
  cytology
    anus R85.619
      atypical squamous cells cannot exclude high grade squamous intraepithelial lesion (ASC-H) R85.611
      atypical squamous cells of undetermined significance (ASC-US) R85.610
      cytologic evidence of malignancy R85.614
      high grade squamous intraepithelial lesion (HGSIL) R85.613
      human papillomavirus (HPV) DNA test
        high risk positive R85.81
        low risk postive R85.82
      inadequate smear R85.615
      low grade squamous intraepithelial lesion (LGSIL) R85.612
      satisfactory anal smear but lacking transformation zone R85.616
      specified NEC R85.618
      unsatisfactory smear R85.615
    female genital organs — *see* Abnormal, Papanicolaou (smear)
  dark adaptation curve H53.61
  dentofacial NEC — *see* Anomaly, dentofacial
  development, developmental Q89.9
    central nervous system Q07.9
  diagnostic imaging
    abdomen, abdominal region NEC R93.5
    biliary tract R93.2
    bladder R93.41

Abnormal, abnormality, abnormalities - *continued*
  diagnostic imaging - *continued*
    breast R92.8
    central nervous system NEC R90.89
    cerebrovascular NEC R90.89
    coronary circulation R93.1
    digestive tract NEC R93.3
    gastrointestinal (tract) R93.3
    genitourinary organs R93.89
    head R93.0
    heart R93.1
    intrathoracic organ NEC R93.89
    kidney R93.42-
    limbs R93.6
    liver R93.2
    lung (field) R91.8
    musculoskeletal system NEC R93.7
    renal pelvis R93.41
    retroperitoneum R93.5
    site specified NEC R93.89
    skin and subcutaneous tissue R93.89
    skull R93.0
    testis R93.81-
    urinary organs specified NEC R93.49
    ureter R93.41
  direction, teeth, fully erupted M26.30
  ear ossicles, acquired NEC H74.39-
    ankylosis — *see* Ankylosis, ear ossicles
    discontinuity — *see* Discontinuity, ossicles, ear
    partial loss — *see* Loss, ossicles, ear (partial)
  Ebstein Q22.5
  echocardiogram R93.1
  echoencephalogram R90.81
  echogram — *see* Abnormal, diagnostic imaging
  electrocardiogram [ECG] [EKG] R94.31
  electroencephalogram [EEG] R94.01
  electrolyte — *see* Imbalance, electrolyte
  electromyogram [EMG] R94.131
  electro-oculogram [EOG] R94.110
  electrophysiological intracardiac studies R94.39
  electroretinogram [ERG] R94.111
  erythrocytes
    congenital, with perinatal jaundice D58.9
  feces (color) (contents) (mucus) R19.5
  finding — *see* Findings, abnormal, without diagnosis
  fluid
    amniotic — *see* Abnormal, specimen, specified
    cerebrospinal — *see* Abnormal, cerebrospinal fluid
    peritoneal — *see* Abnormal, specimen, digestive organs
    pleural — *see* Abnormal, specimen, respiratory organs
    synovial — *see* Abnormal, specimen, specified
    thorax (bronchial washings) (pleural fluid) — *see* Abnormal, specimen, respiratory organs
    vaginal — *see* Abnormal, specimen, female genital organs
  form
    teeth K00.2
    uterus — *see* Anomaly, uterus
  function studies
    auditory R94.120
    bladder R94.8
    brain R94.09
    cardiovascular R94.30
    ear R94.128
    endocrine NEC R94.7
    eye NEC R94.118
    kidney R94.4
    liver R94.5
    nervous system
      central NEC R94.09
      peripheral NEC R94.138
    pancreas R94.8
    placenta R94.8
    pulmonary R94.2
    special senses NEC R94.128
    spleen R94.8
    thyroid R94.6
    vestibular R94.121
  gait — *see* Gait
    hysterical F44.4
  gastrin secretion E16.4
  globulin R77.1
    cortisol-binding E27.8
    thyroid-binding E07.89
  glomerular, minor — *see also* N00-N07 with fourth character .0 N05.0
  glucagon secretion E16.3
  glucose tolerance (test) (non-fasting) R73.09
  gravitational (G) forces or states (effect of) T75.81
  hair (color) (shaft) L67.9

Abnormal, abnormality, abnormalities - *continued*
hair (color) (shaft) - *continued*
specified NEC L67.8
hard tissue formation in pulp (dental) K04.3
head movement R25.0
heart
rate R00.9
specified NEC R00.8
shadow R93.1
sounds NEC R01.2
hemoglobin (disease) — *see also* Disease, hemoglobin D58.2
trait — *see* Trait, hemoglobin, abnormal
histology NEC R89.7
immunological findings R89.4
in serum R76.9
specified NEC R76.8
increase in appetite R63.2
involuntary movement — *see* Abnormal, movement, involuntary
jaw closure M26.51
karyotype R89.8
kidney function test R94.4
knee jerk R29.2
leukocyte (cell) (differential) NEC D72.9
liver function test R94.5
loss of
height R29.890
weight R63.4
mammogram NEC R92.8
calcification (calculus) R92.1
microcalcification R92.0
Mantoux test R76.11
movement (disorder) — *see also* Disorder, movement
head R25.0
involuntary R25.9
fasciculation R25.3
of head R25.0
spasm R25.2
specified type NEC R25.8
tremor R25.1
myoglobin (Aberdeen) (Annapolis) R89.7
neonatal screening P09
oculomotor study R94.113
palmar creases Q82.8
Papanicolaou (smear)
anus R85.619
atypical squamous cells cannot exclude high grade squamous intraepithelial lesion (ASC-H) R85.611
atypical squamous cells of undetermined significance (ASC-US) R85.610
cytologic evidence of malignancy R85.614
high grade squamous intraepithelial lesion (HGSIL) R85.613
human papillomavirus (HPV) DNA test
high risk positive R85.81
low risk postive R85.82
inadequate smear R85.615
low grade squamous intraepithelial lesion (LGSIL) R85.612
satisfactory anal smear but lacking transformation zone R85.616
specified NEC R85.618
unsatisfactory smear R85.615
bronchial washings R84.6
cerebrospinal fluid R83.6
cervix R87.619
atypical squamous cells cannot exclude high grade squamous intraepithelial lesion (ASC-H) R87.611
atypical squamous cells of undetermined significance (ASC-US) R87.610
cytologic evidence of malignancy R87.614
high grade squamous intraepithelial lesion (HGSIL) R87.613
inadequate smear R87.615
low grade squamous intraepithelial lesion (LGSIL) R87.612
non-atypical endometrial cells R87.618
satisfactory cervical smear but lacking transformation zone R87.616
specified NEC R87.618
thin preparaton R87.619
unsatisfactory smear R87.615
nasal secretions R84.6
nipple discharge R89.6
peritoneal fluid R85.69
pleural fluid R84.6
prostatic secretions R86.6
saliva R85.69
seminal fluid R86.6

Abnormal, abnormality, abnormalities - *continued*
Papanicolaou (smear) - *continued*
sites NEC R89.6
sputum R84.6
synovial fluid R89.6
throat scrapings R84.6
vagina R87.629
atypical squamous cells cannot exclude high grade squamous intraepithelial lesion (ASC-H) R87.621
atypical squamous cells of undetermined significance (ASC-US) R87.620
cytologic evidence of malignancy R87.624
high grade squamous intraepithelial lesion (HGSIL) R87.623
inadequate smear R87.625
low grade squamous intraepithelial lesion (LGSIL) R87.622
specified NEC R87.628
thin preparation R87.629
unsatisfactory smear R87.625
vulva R87.69
wound secretions R89.6
partial thromboplastin time (PTT) R79.1
pelvis (bony) — *see* Deformity, pelvis
percussion, chest (tympany) R09.89
periods (grossly) — *see* Menstruation
phonocardiogram R94.39
plantar reflex R29.2
plasma
protein R77.9
specified NEC R77.8
viscosity R70.1
pleural (folds) Q34.0
posture R29.3
product of conception O02.9
specified type NEC O02.89
prothrombin time (PT) R79.1
pulmonary
artery, congenital Q25.79
function, newborn P28.89
test results R94.2
pulsations in neck R00.2
pupillary H21.56-
function (reaction) (reflex) — *see* Anomaly, pupil, function
radiological examination — *see* Abnormal, diagnostic imaging
red blood cell (s) (morphology) (volume) R71.8
reflex — *see* Reflex
renal function test R94.4
response to nerve stimulation R94.130
retinal correspondence H53.31
retinal function study R94.111
rhythm, heart — *see also* Arrhythmia
saliva — *see* Abnormal, specimen, digestive organs
scan
kidney R94.4
liver R93.2
thyroid R94.6
secretion
gastrin E16.4
glucagon E16.3
semen, seminal fluid — *see* Abnormal, specimen, male genital organs
serum level (of)
acid phosphatase R74.8
alkaline phosphatase R74.8
amylase R74.8
enzymes R74.9
specified NEC R74.8
lipase R74.8
triacylglycerol lipase R74.8
shape
gravid uterus — *see* Anomaly, uterus
sinus venosus Q21.1
size, tooth, teeth K00.2
spacing, tooth, teeth, fully erupted M26.30
specimen
digestive organs (peritoneal fluid) (saliva) R85.9
cytology R85.69
drug level R85.2
enzyme level R85.0
histology R85.7
hormones R85.1
immunology R85.4
microbiology R85.5
nonmedicinal level R85.3
specified type NEC R85.89
female genital organs (secretions) (smears) R87.9
cytology R87.69
cervix R87.619
human papillomavirus (HPV) DNA test

Abnormal, abnormality, abnormalities - *continued*
specimen - *continued*
female genital organs (secretions) (smears) - *continued*
cytology - *continued*
cervix - *continued*
human papillomavirus (HPV) DNA test - *continued*
high risk positive R87.810
low risk positive R87.820
inadequate (unsatisfactory) smear R87.615
non-atypical endometrial cells R87.618
specified NEC R87.618
vagina R87.629
human papillomavirus (HPV) DNA test
high risk positive R87.811
low risk positive R87.821
inadequate (unsatisfactory) smear R87.625
vulva R87.69
drug level R87.2
enzyme level R87.0
histological R87.7
hormones R87.1
immunology R87.4
microbiology R87.5
nonmedicinal level R87.3
specified type NEC R87.89
male genital organs (prostatic secretions) (semen) R86.9
cytology R86.6
drug level R86.2
enzyme level R86.0
histological R86.7
hormones R86.1
immunology R86.4
microbiology R86.5
nonmedicinal level R86.3
specified type NEC R86.8
nipple discharge — *see* Abnormal, specimen, specified
respiratory organs (bronchial washings) (nasal secretions) (pleural fluid) (sputum) R84.9
cytology R84.6
drug level R84.2
enzyme level R84.0
histology R84.7
hormones R84.1
immunology R84.4
microbiology R84.5
nonmedicinal level R84.3
specified type NEC R84.8
specified organ, system and tissue NOS R89.9
cytology R89.6
drug level R89.2
enzyme level R89.0
histology R89.7
hormones R89.1
immunology R89.4
microbiology R89.5
nonmedicinal level R89.3
specified type NEC R89.8
synovial fluid — *see* Abnormal, specimen, specified
thorax (bronchial washings) (pleural fluids) — *see* Abnormal, specimen, respiratory organs
vagina (secretion) (smear) R87.629
vulva (secretion) (smear) R87.69
wound secretion — *see* Abnormal, specimen, specified
spermatozoa — *see* Abnormal, specimen, male genital organs
sputum (amount) (color) (odor) R09.3
stool (color) (contents) (mucus) R19.5
bloody K92.1
guaiac positive R19.5
synchondrosis Q78.8
thermography — *see also* Abnormal, diagnostic imaging R93.89
thyroid-binding globulin E07.89
tooth, teeth (form) (size) K00.2
toxicology (findings) R78.9
transport protein E88.09
tumor marker NEC R97.8
ultrasound results — *see* Abnormal, diagnostic imaging
umbilical cord complicating delivery O69.9
urination NEC R39.198
urine (constituents) R82.90
bile R82.2
cytological examination R82.8
drugs R82.5
fat R82.0
glucose R81

- **Abrasion** - *continued*
  - lumbar region S30.810
  - malar region S00.81
  - mammary — *see* Abrasion, breast
  - mastoid region S00.81
  - mouth S00.512
  - nail
    - finger — *see* Abrasion, finger
    - toe — *see* Abrasion, toe
  - nape S10.81
  - nasal S00.31
  - neck S10.91
    - specified site NEC S10.81
    - throat S10.11
  - nose S00.31
  - occipital region S00.01
  - oral cavity S00.512
  - orbital region — *see* Abrasion, eyelid
  - palate S00.512
  - palm — *see* Abrasion, hand
  - parietal region S00.01
  - pelvis S30.810
  - penis S30.812
  - perineum
    - female S30.814
    - male S30.810
  - periocular area — *see* Abrasion, eyelid
  - phalanges
    - finger — *see* Abrasion, finger
    - toe — *see* Abrasion, toe
  - pharynx S10.11
  - pinna — *see* Abrasion, ear
  - popliteal space — *see* Abrasion, knee
  - prepuce S30.812
  - pubic region S30.810
  - pudendum
    - female S30.816
    - male S30.815
  - sacral region S30.810
  - scalp S00.01
  - scapular region — *see* Abrasion, shoulder
  - scrotum S30.813
  - shin — *see* Abrasion, leg
  - shoulder S40.21-
  - skin NEC T14.8
  - sternal region S20.319
  - submaxillary region S00.81
  - submental region S00.81
  - subungual
    - finger (s) — *see* Abrasion, finger
    - toe (s) — *see* Abrasion, toe
  - supraclavicular fossa S10.81
  - supraorbital S00.81
  - temple S00.81
  - temporal region S00.81
  - testis S30.813
  - thigh S70.31-
  - thorax, thoracic (wall) S20.91
    - back S20.41-
    - front S20.31-
  - throat S10.11
  - thumb S60.31-
  - toe (s) (lesser) S90.416
    - great S90.41-
  - tongue S00.512
  - tooth, teeth (dentifrice) (habitual) (hard tissues) (occupational) (ritual) (traditional) K03.1
  - trachea S10.11
  - tunica vaginalis S30.813
  - tympanum, tympanic membrane — *see* Abrasion, ear
  - uvula S00.512
  - vagina S30.814
  - vocal cords S10.11
  - vulva S30.814
  - wrist S60.81-
- **Abrism** — *see* Poisoning, food, noxious, plant
- **Abruptio placentae** O45.9-
  - with
    - afibrinogenemia O45.01-
    - coagulation defect O45.00-
      - specified NEC O45.09-
    - disseminated intravascular coagulation O45.02-
    - hypofibrinogenemia O45.01-
  - specified NEC O45.8-
- **Abruption, placenta** — *see* Abruptio placentae
- **Abscess** (connective tissue) (embolic) (fistulous) (infective) (metastatic) (multiple) (pernicious) (pyogenic) (septic) L02.91
  - with
    - diverticular disease (intestine) K57.80
      - with bleeding K57.81
      - large intestine K57.20

- **Abscess** (connective tissue) (embolic) (fistulous) (infective) (metastatic) (multiple) (pernicious) (pyogenic) (septic) - *continued*
  - with - *continued*
    - diverticular disease (intestine) - *continued*
      - large intestine - *continued*
        - with
          - bleeding K57.21
          - small intestine K57.40
            - with bleeding K57.41
      - small intestine K57.00
        - with
          - bleeding K57.01
          - large intestine K57.40
            - with bleeding K57.41
    - lymphangitis - code by site under Abscess
  - abdomen, abdominal
    - cavity K65.1
    - wall L02.211
  - abdominopelvic K65.1
  - accessory sinus — *see* Sinusitis
  - adrenal (capsule) (gland) E27.8
  - alveolar K04.7
    - with sinus K04.6
  - amebic A06.4
    - brain (and liver or lung abscess) A06.6
    - genitourinary tract A06.82
    - liver (without mention of brain or lung abscess) A06.4
    - lung (and liver) (without mention of brain abscess) A06.5
    - specified site NEC A06.89
    - spleen A06.89
  - anerobic A48.0
  - ankle — *see* Abscess, lower limb
  - anorectal K61.2
  - antecubital space — *see* Abscess, upper limb
  - antrum (chronic) (Highmore) — *see* Sinusitis, maxillary
  - anus K61.0
  - apical (tooth) K04.7
    - with sinus (alveolar) K04.6
  - appendix K35.33
  - areola (acute) (chronic) (nonpuerperal) N61.1
    - puerperal, postpartum or gestational — *see* Infection, nipple
  - arm (any part) — *see* Abscess, upper limb
  - artery (wall) I77.89
  - atheromatous I77.2
  - auricle, ear — *see* Abscess, ear, external
  - axilla (region) L02.41-
    - lymph gland or node L04.2
  - back (any part, except buttock) L02.212
  - Bartholin's gland N75.1
    - with
      - abortion — *see* Abortion, by type complicated by, sepsis
      - ectopic or molar pregnancy O08.0
    - following ectopic or molar pregnancy O08.0
  - Bezold's — *see* Mastoiditis, acute
  - bilharziasis B65.1
  - bladder (wall) — *see* Cystitis, specified type NEC
  - bone (subperiosteal) — *see also* Osteomyelitis, specified type NEC
    - accessory sinus (chronic) — *see* Sinusitis
    - chronic or old — *see* Osteomyelitis, chronic
    - jaw (lower) (upper) M27.2
    - mastoid — *see* Mastoiditis, acute, subperiosteal
    - petrous — *see* Petrositis
    - spinal (tuberculous) A18.01
      - nontuberculous — *see* Osteomyelitis, vertebra
  - bowel K63.0
  - brain (any part) (cystic) (otogenic) G06.0
    - amebic (with abscess of any other site) A06.6
    - gonococcal A54.82
    - pheomycotic (chromomycotic) B43.1
    - tuberculous A17.81
  - breast (acute) (chronic) (nonpuerperal) N61.1
    - newborn P39.0
    - puerperal, postpartum, gestational — *see* Mastitis, obstetric, purulent
  - broad ligament N73.2
    - acute N73.0
    - chronic N73.1
  - Brodie's (localized) (chronic) M86.8X-
  - bronchi J98.09
  - buccal cavity K12.2
  - bulbourethral gland N34.0
  - bursa M71.00
    - ankle M71.07-
    - elbow M71.02-
    - foot M71.07-
    - hand M71.04-

- **Abscess** (connective tissue) (embolic) (fistulous) (infective) (metastatic) (multiple) (pernicious) (pyogenic) (septic) - *continued*
  - bursa - *continued*
    - hip M71.05-
    - knee M71.06-
    - multiple sites M71.09
    - pharyngeal J39.1
    - shoulder M71.01-
    - specified site NEC M71.08
    - wrist M71.03-
  - buttock L02.31
  - canthus — *see* Blepharoconjunctivitis
  - cartilage — *see* Disorder, cartilage, specified type NEC
  - cecum K35.33
  - cerebellum, cerebellar G06.0
    - sequelae G09
  - cerebral (embolic) G06.0
    - sequelae G09
  - cervical (meaning neck) L02.11
    - lymph gland or node L04.0
  - cervix (stump) (uteri) — *see* Cervicitis
  - cheek (external) L02.01
    - inner K12.2
  - chest J86.9
    - with fistula J86.0
    - wall L02.213
  - chin L02.01
  - choroid — *see* Inflammation, chorioretinal
  - circumtonsillar J36
  - cold (lung) (tuberculous) — *see also* Tuberculosis, abscess, lung
    - articular — *see* Tuberculosis, joint
  - colon (wall) K63.0
  - colostomy K94.02
  - conjunctiva — *see* Conjunctivitis, acute
  - cornea H16.31-
  - corpus
    - cavernosum N48.21
    - luteum — *see* Oophoritis
  - Cowper's gland N34.0
  - cranium G06.0
  - cul-de-sac (Douglas') (posterior) — *see* Peritonitis, pelvic, female
  - cutaneous — *see* Abscess, by site
  - dental K04.7
    - with sinus (alveolar) K04.6
  - dentoalveolar K04.7
    - with sinus K04.6
  - diaphragm, diaphragmatic K65.1
  - Douglas' cul-de-sac or pouch — *see* Peritonitis, pelvic, female
  - Dubois A50.59
  - ear (middle) — *see also* Otitis, media, suppurative
    - acute — *see* Otitis, media, suppurative, acute
    - external H60.0-
  - entamebic — *see* Abscess, amebic
  - enterostomy K94.12
  - epididymis N45.4
  - epidural G06.2
    - brain G06.0
    - spinal cord G06.1
  - epiglottis J38.7
  - epiploon, epiploic K65.1
  - erysipelatous — *see* Erysipelas
  - esophagus K20.8
  - ethmoid (bone) (chronic) (sinus) J32.2
  - external auditory canal — *see* Abscess, ear, external
  - extradural G06.2
    - brain G06.0
      - sequelae G09
    - spinal cord G06.1
  - extraperitoneal K68.19
  - eye — *see* Endophthalmitis, purulent
  - eyelid H00.03-
  - face (any part, except ear, eye and nose) L02.01
  - fallopian tube — *see* Salpingitis
  - fascia M72.8
  - fauces J39.1
  - fecal K63.0
  - femoral (region) — *see* Abscess, lower limb
  - filaria, filarial — *see* Infestation, filarial
  - finger (any) — *see also* Abscess, hand
    - nail — *see* Cellulitis, finger
  - foot L02.61-
  - forehead L02.01
  - frontal sinus (chronic) J32.1
  - gallbladder K81.0
  - genital organ or tract
    - female (external) N76.4
    - male N49.9
      - multiple sites N49.8

Abscess (connective tissue) (embolic) (fistulous) (infective) (metastatic) (multiple) (pernicious) (pyogenic) (septic) - *continued*

- genital organ or tract - *continued*
  - male - *continued*
    - specified NEC N49.8
- gestational mammary O91.11-
- gestational subareolar O91.11-
- gingival — *see* Peridontitis, localized
- gland, glandular (lymph) (acute) — *see* Lymphadenitis, acute
- gluteal (region) L02.31
- gonorrheal — *see* Gonococcus
- groin L02.214
- gum — *see* Peridontitis, localized
- hand L02.51-
- head NEC L02.811
  - face (any part, except ear, eye and nose) L02.01
- heart — *see* Carditis
- heel — *see* Abscess, foot
- helminthic — *see* Infestation, helminth
- hepatic (cholangitic) (hematogenic) (lymphogenic) (pylephlebitic) K75.0
  - amebic A06.4
- hip (region) — *see* Abscess, lower limb
- horseshoe K61.31
- ileocecal K35.33
- ileostomy (bud) K94.12
- iliac (region) L02.214
  - fossa K35.33
- infraclavicular (fossa) — *see* Abscess, upper limb
- inguinal (region) L02.214
  - lymph gland or node L04.1
- intersphincteric K61.4
- intestine, intestinal NEC K63.0
  - rectal K61.1
- intra-abdominal — *see also* Abscess, peritoneum K65.1
  - following procedure T81.43
    - obstetrical O86.03
  - postprocedural T81.49
    - retroperitoneal K68.11
- intracranial G06.0
- intramammary — *see* Abscess, breast
- intramuscular, following procedure T81.42
  - obstetrical O86.02
- intraorbital — *see* Abscess, orbit
- intraperitoneal K65.1
- intrasphincteric (anus) K61.4
- intraspinal G06.1
- intratonsillar J36
- ischiorectal (fossa) (specified NEC) K61.39
- jaw (bone) (lower) (upper) M27.2
- joint — *see* Arthritis, pyogenic or pyemic
  - spine (tuberculous) A18.01
    - nontuberculous — *see* Spondylopathy, infective
- kidney N15.1
  - with calculus N20.0
    - with hydronephrosis N13.6
  - puerperal (postpartum) O86.21
- knee — *see also* Abscess, lower limb
  - joint M00.9
- labium (majus) (minus) N76.4
- lacrimal
  - caruncle — *see* Inflammation, lacrimal, passages, acute
  - gland — *see* Dacryoadenitis
  - passages (duct) (sac) — *see* Inflammation, lacrimal, passages, acute
- lacunar N34.0
- larynx J38.7
- lateral (alveolar) K04.7
  - with sinus K04.6
- leg (any part) — *see* Abscess, lower limb
- lens H27.8
- lingual K14.0
  - tonsil J36
- lip K13.0
- Littre's gland N34.0
- liver (cholangitic) (hematogenic) (lymphogenic) (pylephlebitic) (pyogenic) K75.0
  - amebic (due to Entamoeba histolytica) (dysenteric) (tropical) A06.4
    - with
      - brain abscess (and liver or lung abscess) A06.6
      - lung abscess A06.5
- loin (region) L02.211
- lower limb L02.41-
- lumbar (tuberculous) A18.01
  - nontuberculous L02.212
- lung (miliary) (putrid) J85.2
  - with pneumonia J85.1

Abscess (connective tissue) (embolic) (fistulous) (infective) (metastatic) (multiple) (pernicious) (pyogenic) (septic) - *continued*

- lung (miliary) (putrid) - *continued*
  - with pneumonia - *continued*
    - due to specified organism (see Pneumonia, in (due to))
  - amebic (with liver abscess) A06.5
    - with
      - brain abscess A06.6
      - pneumonia A06.5
- lymph, lymphatic, gland or node (acute) — *see also* Lymphadenitis, acute
  - mesentery I88.0
- malar M27.2
- mammary gland — *see* Abscess, breast
- marginal, anus K61.0
- mastoid — *see* Mastoiditis, acute
- maxilla, maxillary M27.2
  - molar (tooth) K04.7
    - with sinus K04.6
  - premolar K04.7
  - sinus (chronic) J32.0
- mediastinum J85.3
- meibomian gland — *see* Hordeolum
- meninges G06.2
- mesentery, mesenteric K65.1
- mesosalpinx — *see* Salpingitis
- mons pubis L02.215
- mouth (floor) K12.2
- muscle — *see* Myositis, infective
- myocardium I40.0
- nabothian (follicle) — *see* Cervicitis
- nasal J32.9
- nasopharyngeal J39.1
- navel L02.216
  - newborn P38.9
    - with mild hemorrhage P38.1
    - without hemorrhage P38.9
- neck (region) L02.11
  - lymph gland or node L04.0
- nephritic — *see* Abscess, kidney
- nipple N61.1
  - associated with
    - lactation — *see* Pregnancy, complicated by
    - pregnancy — *see* Pregnancy, complicated by
- nose (external) (fossa) (septum) J34.0
  - sinus (chronic) — *see* Sinusitis
- omentum K65.1
- operative wound T81.49
- orbit, orbital — *see* Cellulitis, orbit
- otogenic G06.0
- ovary, ovarian (corpus luteum) — *see* Oophoritis
- oviduct — *see* Oophoritis
- palate (soft) K12.2
  - hard M27.2
- palmar (space) — *see* Abscess, hand
- pancreas (duct) — *see* Pancreatitis, acute
- parafrenal N48.21
- parametric, parametrium N73.2
  - acute N73.0
  - chronic N73.1
- paranephric N15.1
- parapancreatic — *see* Pancreatitis, acute
- parapharyngeal J39.0
- pararectal K61.1
- parasinus — *see* Sinusitis
- parauterine — *see also* Disease, pelvis, inflammatory N73.2
- paravaginal — *see* Vaginitis
- parietal region (scalp) L02.811
- parodontal — *see* Peridontitis, aggressive, localized
- parotid (duct) (gland) K11.3
  - region K12.2
- pectoral (region) L02.213
- pelvis, pelvic
  - female — *see* Disease, pelvis, inflammatory
  - male, peritoneal K65.1
- penis N48.21
  - gonococcal (accessory gland) (periurethral) A54.1
- perianal K61.0
- periapical K04.7
  - with sinus (alveolar) K04.6
- periappendicular K35.33
- pericardial I30.1
- pericecal K35.33
- pericemental — *see* Peridontitis, aggressive, localized
- pericholecystic — *see* Cholecystitis, acute
- pericoronal — *see* Peridontitis, aggressive, localized
- peridental — *see* Peridontitis, aggressive, localized
- perimetric — *see also* Disease, pelvis, inflammatory N73.2

Abscess (connective tissue) (embolic) (fistulous) (infective) (metastatic) (multiple) (pernicious) (pyogenic) (septic) - *continued*

- perinephric, perinephritic — *see* Abscess, kidney
- perineum, perineal (superficial) L02.215
  - urethra N34.0
- periodontal (parietal) — *see* Peridontitis, aggressive, localized
  - apical K04.7
- periosteum, periosteal — *see also* Osteomyelitis, specified type NEC
  - with osteomyelitis — *see also* Osteomyelitis, specified type NEC
    - acute — *see* Osteomyelitis, acute
    - chronic — *see* Osteomyelitis, chronic
- peripharyngeal J39.0
- peripleuritic J86.9
  - with fistula J86.0
- periprostatic N41.2
- perirectal K61.1
- perirenal (tissue) — *see* Abscess, kidney
- perisinuous (nose) — *see* Sinusitis
- peritoneum, peritoneal (perforated) (ruptured) K65.1
  - with appendicitis — *see also* Appendicitis K35.33
  - pelvic
    - female — *see* Peritonitis, pelvic, female
    - male K65.1
  - postoperative T81.49
  - puerperal, postpartum, childbirth O85
  - tuberculous A18.31
- peritonsillar J36
- perityphlic K35.33
- periureteral N28.89
- periurethral N34.0
  - gonococcal (accessory gland) (periurethral) A54.1
- periuterine — *see also* Disease, pelvis, inflammatory N73.2
- perivesical — *see* Cystitis, specified type NEC
- petrous bone — *see* Petrositis
- phagedenic NOS L02.91
  - chancroid A57
- pharynx, pharyngeal (lateral) J39.1
- pilonidal L05.01
- pituitary (gland) E23.6
- pleura J86.9
  - with fistula J86.0
- popliteal — *see* Abscess, lower limb
- postcecal K35.33
- postlaryngeal J38.7
- postnasal J34.0
- postoperative (any site) — *see also* Infection, postoperative wound T81.49
  - retroperitoneal K68.11
- postpharyngeal J39.0
- posttonsillar J36
- post-typhoid A01.09
- pouch of Douglas — *see* Peritonitis, pelvic, female
- premammary — *see* Abscess, breast
- prepatellar — *see* Abscess, lower limb
- prostate N41.2
  - gonococcal (acute) (chronic) A54.22
- psoas muscle K68.12
- puerperal - code by site under Puerperal, abscess
- pulmonary — *see* Abscess, lung
- pulp, pulpal (dental) K04.01
  - irreversible K04.02
  - reversible K04.01
- rectovaginal septum K63.0
- rectovesical — *see* Cystitis, specified type NEC
- rectum K61.1
- renal — *see* Abscess, kidney
- retina — *see* Inflammation, chorioretinal
- retrobulbar — *see* Abscess, orbit
- retrocecal K65.1
- retrolaryngeal J38.7
- retromammary — *see* Abscess, breast
- retroperitoneal NEC K68.19
  - postprocedural K68.11
- retropharyngeal J39.0
- retrouterine — *see* Peritonitis, pelvic, female
- retrovesical — *see* Cystitis, specified type NEC
- root, tooth K04.7
  - with sinus (alveolar) K04.6
- round ligament — *see also* Disease, pelvis, inflammatory N73.2
- rupture (spontaneous) NOS L02.91
- sacrum (tuberculous) A18.01
  - nontuberculous M46.28
- salivary (duct) (gland) K11.3
- scalp (any part) L02.811
- scapular — *see* Osteomyelitis, specified type NEC
- sclera — *see* Scleritis
- scrofulous (tuberculous) A18.2

Abscess (connective tissue) (embolic) (fistulous) (infective) (metastatic) (multiple) (pernicious) (pyogenic) (septic) - *continued*
- scrotum N49.2
- seminal vesicle N49.0
- septal, dental K04.7
  - with sinus (alveolar) K04.6
- serous — *see* Periostitis
- shoulder (region) — *see* Abscess, upper limb
- sigmoid K63.0
- sinus (accessory) (chronic) (nasal) — *see also* Sinusitis
  - intracranial venous (any) G06.0
- Skene's duct or gland N34.0
- skin — *see* Abscess, by site
- specified site NEC L02.818
- spermatic cord N49.1
- sphenoidal (sinus) (chronic) J32.3
- spinal cord (any part) (staphylococcal) G06.1
  - tuberculous A17.81
- spine (column) (tuberculous) A18.01
  - epidural G06.1
  - nontuberculous — *see* Osteomyelitis, vertebra
- spleen D73.3
  - amebic A06.89
- stitch T81.41
  - following an obstetrical procedure O86.01
- subarachnoid G06.2
  - brain G06.0
  - spinal cord G06.1
- subareolar — *see* Abscess, breast
- subcecal K35.33
- subcutaneous — *see also* Abscess, by site
  - following procedure T81.41
    - obstetrical O86.01
  - pheomycotic (chromomycotic) B43.2
- subdiaphragmatic K65.1
- subdural G06.2
  - brain G06.0
    - sequelae G09
  - spinal cord G06.1
- sub-fascial, following an obstetrical procedure O86.02
- subgaleal L02.811
- subhepatic K65.1
- sublingual K12.2
  - gland K11.3
- submammary — *see* Abscess, breast
- submandibular (region) (space) (triangle) K12.2
  - gland K11.3
- submaxillary (region) L02.01
  - gland K11.3
- submental L02.01
  - gland K11.3
- subperiosteal — *see* Osteomyelitis, specified type NEC
- subphrenic K65.1
  - following an obstetrical procedure O86.03
  - postoperative T81.43
- suburethral N34.0
- sudoriparous L75.8
- supraclavicular (fossa) — *see* Abscess, upper limb
- supralevator K61.5
- suprapelvic, acute N73.0
- suprarenal (capsule) (gland) E27.8
- sweat gland L74.8
- tear duct — *see* Inflammation, lacrimal, passages, acute
- temple L02.01
- temporal region L02.01
- temporosphenoidal G06.0
- tendon (sheath) M65.00
  - ankle M65.07-
  - foot M65.07-
  - forearm M65.03-
  - hand M65.04-
  - lower leg M65.06-
  - pelvic region M65.05-
  - shoulder region M65.01-
  - specified site NEC M65.08
  - thigh M65.05-
  - upper arm M65.02-
- testis N45.4
- thigh — *see* Abscess, lower limb
- thorax J86.9
  - with fistula J86.0
- throat J39.1
- thumb — *see also* Abscess, hand
  - nail — *see* Cellulitis, finger
- thymus (gland) E32.1
- thyroid (gland) E06.0
- toe (any) — *see also* Abscess, foot
  - nail — *see* Cellulitis, toe

Abscess (connective tissue) (embolic) (fistulous) (infective) (metastatic) (multiple) (pernicious) (pyogenic) (septic) - *continued*
- tongue (staphylococcal) K14.0
- tonsil (s) (lingual) J36
- tonsillopharyngeal J36
- tooth, teeth (root) K04.7
  - with sinus (alveolar) K04.6
  - supporting structures NEC — *see* Peridontitis, aggressive, localized
- trachea J39.8
- trunk L02.219
  - abdominal wall L02.211
  - back L02.212
  - chest wall L02.213
  - groin L02.214
  - perineum L02.215
  - umbilicus L02.216
- tubal — *see* Salpingitis
- tuberculous — *see* Tuberculosis, abscess
- tubo-ovarian — *see* Salpingo-oophoritis
- tunica vaginalis N49.1
- umbilicus L02.216
- upper
  - limb L02.41-
  - respiratory J39.8
- urethral (gland) N34.0
- urinary N34.0
- uterus, uterine (wall) — *see also* Endometritis
  - ligament — *see also* Disease, pelvis, inflammatory N73.2
  - neck — *see* Cervicitis
- uvula K12.2
- vagina (wall) — *see* Vaginitis
- vaginorectal — *see* Vaginitis
- vas deferens N49.1
- vermiform appendix K35.33
- vertebra (column) (tuberculous) A18.01
  - nontuberculous — *see* Osteomyelitis, vertebra
- vesical — *see* Cystitis, specified type NEC
- vesico-uterine pouch — *see* Peritonitis, pelvic, female
- vitreous (humor) — *see* Endophthalmitis, purulent
- vocal cord J38.3
- von Bezold's — *see* Mastoiditis, acute
- vulva N76.4
- vulvovaginal gland N75.1
- web space — *see* Abscess, hand
- wound T81.49
- wrist — *see* Abscess, upper limb

Absence (of) (organ or part) (complete or partial)
- adrenal (gland) (congenital) Q89.1
  - acquired E89.6
- albumin in blood E88.09
- alimentary tract (congenital) Q45.8
  - upper Q40.8
- alveolar process (acquired) — *see* Anomaly, alveolar
- ankle (acquired) Z89.44-
- anus (congenital) Q42.3
  - with fistula Q42.2
- aorta (congenital) Q25.41
- appendix, congenital Q42.8
- arm (acquired) Z89.20-
  - above elbow Z89.22-
    - congenital (with hand present) — *see* Agenesis, arm, with hand present
    - and hand — *see* Agenesis, forearm, and hand
  - below elbow Z89.21-
    - congenital (with hand present) — *see* Agenesis, arm, with hand present
    - and hand — *see* Agenesis, forearm, and hand
  - congenital — *see* Defect, reduction, upper limb
  - shoulder (following explantation of shoulder joint prosthesis) (joint) (with or without presence of antibiotic-impregnated cement spacer) Z89.23-
    - congenital (with hand present) — *see* Agenesis, arm, with hand present
- artery (congenital) (peripheral) Q27.8
  - brain Q28.3
  - coronary Q24.5
  - pulmonary Q25.79
  - specified NEC Q27.8
  - umbilical Q27.0
- atrial septum (congenital) Q21.1
- auditory canal (congenital) (external) Q16.1
- auricle (ear) , congenital Q16.0
- bile, biliary duct, congenital Q44.5
- bladder (acquired) Z90.6
  - congenital Q64.5
- bowel sounds R19.11
- brain Q00.0
  - part of Q04.3
- breast (s) (and nipple (s)) (acquired) Z90.1-

Absence (of) (organ or part) (complete or partial) - *continued*
- breast (s) (and nipple (s)) (acquired) - *continued*
  - congenital Q83.8
- broad ligament Q50.6
- bronchus (congenital) Q32.4
- canaliculus lacrimalis, congenital Q10.4
- cerebellum (vermis) Q04.3
- cervix (acquired) (with uterus) Z90.710
  - with remaining uterus Z90.712
  - congenital Q51.5
- chin, congenital Q18.8
- cilia (congenital) Q10.3
  - acquired — *see* Madarosis
- clitoris (congenital) Q52.6
- coccyx, congenital Q76.49
- cold sense R20.8
- congenital
  - lumen — *see* Atresia
  - organ or site NEC — *see* Agenesis
  - septum — *see* Imperfect, closure
- corpus callosum Q04.0
- cricoid cartilage, congenital Q31.8
- diaphragm (with hernia) , congenital Q79.1
- digestive organ (s) or tract, congenital Q45.8
  - acquired NEC Z90.49
  - upper Q40.8
- ductus arteriosus Q28.8
- duodenum (acquired) Z90.49
  - congenital Q41.0
- ear, congenital Q16.9
  - acquired H93.8-
  - auricle Q16.0
  - external Q16.0
  - inner Q16.5
  - lobe, lobule Q17.8
  - middle, except ossicles Q16.4
    - ossicles Q16.3
  - ossicles Q16.3
- ejaculatory duct (congenital) Q55.4
- endocrine gland (congenital) NEC Q89.2
  - acquired E89.89
- epididymis (congenital) Q55.4
  - acquired Z90.79
- epiglottis, congenital Q31.8
- esophagus (congenital) Q39.8
  - acquired (partial) Z90.49
- eustachian tube (congenital) Q16.2
- extremity (acquired) Z89.9
  - congenital Q73.0
  - knee (following explantation of knee joint prosthesis) (joint) (with or without presence of antibiotic-impregnated cement spacer) Z89.52-
  - lower (above knee) Z89.619
    - below knee Z89.51-
  - upper — *see* Absence, arm
- eye (acquired) Z90.01
  - congenital Q11.1
  - muscle (congenital) Q10.3
- eyeball (acquired) Z90.01
- eyelid (fold) (congenital) Q10.3
  - acquired Z90.01
- face, specified part NEC Q18.8
- fallopian tube (s) (acquired) Z90.79
  - congenital Q50.6
- family member (causing problem in home) NEC — *see also* Disruption, family Z63.32
- femur, congenital — *see* Defect, reduction, lower limb, longitudinal, femur
- fibrinogen (congenital) D68.2
  - acquired D65
- finger (s) (acquired) Z89.02-
  - congenital — *see* Agenesis, hand
- foot (acquired) Z89.43-
  - congenital — *see* Agenesis, foot
- forearm (acquired) — *see* Absence, arm, below elbow
- gallbladder (acquired) Z90.49
  - congenital Q44.0
- gamma globulin in blood D80.1
  - hereditary D80.0
- genital organs
  - acquired (female) (male) Z90.79
  - female, congenital Q52.8
    - external Q52.71
    - internal NEC Q52.8
  - male, congenital Q55.8
- genitourinary organs, congenital NEC
  - female Q52.8
  - male Q55.8
- globe (acquired) Z90.01
  - congenital Q11.1
- glottis, congenital Q31.8

- **Absence** (of) (organ or part) (complete or partial) - *continued*
  - hand and wrist (acquired) Z89.11-
    - congenital — *see* Agenesis, hand
  - head, part (acquired) NEC Z90.09
  - heat sense R20.8
  - hip (following explantation of hip joint prosthesis) (joint) (with or without presence of antibiotic-impregnated cement spacer) Z89.62-
  - hymen (congenital) Q52.4
  - ileum (acquired) Z90.49
    - congenital Q41.2
  - immunoglobulin, isolated NEC D80.3
    - IgA D80.2
    - IgG D80.3
    - IgM D80.4
  - incus (acquired) — *see* Loss, ossicles, ear
    - congenital Q16.3
  - inner ear, congenital Q16.5
  - intestine (acquired) (small) Z90.49
    - congenital Q41.9
      - specified NEC Q41.8
    - large Z90.49
      - congenital Q42.9
        - specified NEC Q42.8
  - iris, congenital Q13.1
  - jejunum (acquired) Z90.49
    - congenital Q41.1
  - joint
    - acquired
      - hip (following explantation of hip joint prosthesis) (with or without presence of antibiotic-impregnated cement spacer) Z89.62-
      - knee (following explantation of knee joint prosthesis) (with or without presence of antibiotic-impregnated cement spacer) Z89.52-
      - shoulder (following explantation of shoulder joint prosthesis) (with or without presence of antibiotic-impregnated cement spacer) Z89.23-
    - congenital NEC Q74.8
  - kidney (s) (acquired) Z90.5
    - congenital Q60.2
      - bilateral Q60.1
      - unilateral Q60.0
  - knee (following explantation of knee joint prosthesis) (joint) (with or without presence of antibiotic-impregnated cement spacer) Z89.52-
  - labyrinth, membranous Q16.5
  - larynx (congenital) Q31.8
    - acquired Z90.02
  - leg (acquired) (above knee) Z89.61-
    - below knee (acquired) Z89.51-
    - congenital — *see* Defect, reduction, lower limb
  - lens (acquired) — *see also* Aphakia
    - congenital Q12.3
    - post cataract extraction Z98.4-
  - limb (acquired) — *see* Absence, extremity
  - lip Q38.6
  - liver (congenital) Q44.7
  - lung (fissure) (lobe) (bilateral) (unilateral) (congenital) Q33.3
    - acquired (any part) Z90.2
  - menstruation — *see* Amenorrhea
  - muscle (congenital) (pectoral) Q79.8
    - ocular Q10.3
  - neck, part Q18.8
  - neutrophil — *see* Agranulocytosis
  - nipple (s) (with breast (s)) (acquired) Z90.1
    - congenital Q83.2
  - nose (congenital) Q30.1
    - acquired Z90.09
  - organ
    - of Corti, congenital Q16.5
    - or site, congenital NEC Q89.8
      - acquired NEC Z90.89
  - osseous meatus (ear) Q16.4
  - ovary (acquired)
    - bilateral Z90.722
    - congenital
      - bilateral Q50.02
      - unilateral Q50.01
    - unilateral Z90.721
  - oviduct (acquired)
    - bilateral Z90.722
    - congenital Q50.6
    - unilateral Z90.721
  - pancreas (congenital) Q45.0
    - acquired Z90.410
      - complete Z90.410
      - partial Z90.411
      - total Z90.410
  - parathyroid gland (acquired) E89.2
    - congenital Q89.2

- **Absence** (of) (organ or part) (complete or partial) - *continued*
  - patella, congenital Q74.1
  - penis (congenital) Q55.5
    - acquired Z90.79
  - pericardium (congenital) Q24.8
  - pituitary gland (congenital) Q89.2
    - acquired E89.3
  - prostate (acquired) Z90.79
    - congenital Q55.4
  - pulmonary valve Q22.0
  - punctum lacrimale (congenital) Q10.4
  - radius, congenital — *see* Defect, reduction, upper limb, longitudinal, radius
  - rectum (congenital) Q42.1
    - with fistula Q42.0
    - acquired Z90.49
  - respiratory organ NOS Q34.9
  - rib (acquired) Z90.89
    - congenital Q76.6
  - sacrum, congenital Q76.49
  - salivary gland (s) , congenital Q38.4
  - scrotum, congenital Q55.29
  - seminal vesicles (congenital) Q55.4
    - acquired Z90.79
  - septum
    - atrial (congenital) Q21.1
    - between aorta and pulmonary artery Q21.4
    - ventricular (congenital) Q20.4
  - sex chromosome
    - female phenotype Q97.8
    - male phenotype Q98.8
  - skull bone (congenital) Q75.8
    - with
      - anencephaly Q00.0
      - encephalocele — *see* Encephalocele
      - hydrocephalus Q03.9
        - with spina bifida — *see* Spina bifida, by site, with hydrocephalus
      - microcephaly Q02
  - spermatic cord, congenital Q55.4
  - spine, congenital Q76.49
  - spleen (congenital) Q89.01
    - acquired Z90.81
  - sternum, congenital Q76.7
  - stomach (acquired) (partial) Z90.3
    - congenital Q40.2
  - superior vena cava, congenital Q26.8
  - teeth, tooth (congenital) K00.0
    - acquired (complete) K08.109
      - class I K08.101
      - class II K08.102
      - class III K08.103
      - class IV K08.104
      - due to
        - caries K08.139
          - class I K08.131
          - class II K08.132
          - class III K08.133
          - class IV K08.134
        - periodontal disease K08.129
          - class I K08.121
          - class II K08.122
          - class III K08.123
          - class IV K08.124
        - specified NEC K08.199
          - class I K08.191
          - class II K08.192
          - class III K08.193
          - class IV K08.194
        - trauma K08.119
          - class I K08.111
          - class II K08.112
          - class III K08.113
          - class IV K08.114
      - partial K08.409
        - class I K08.401
        - class II K08.402
        - class III K08.403
        - class IV K08.404
        - due to
          - caries K08.439
            - class I K08.431
            - class II K08.432
            - class III K08.433
            - class IV K08.434
          - periodontal disease K08.429
            - class I K08.421
            - class II K08.422
            - class III K08.423
            - class IV K08.424
          - specified NEC K08.499
            - class I K08.491

- **Absence** (of) (organ or part) (complete or partial) - *continued*
  - teeth, tooth (congenital) - *continued*
    - acquired (complete) - *continued*
      - partial - *continued*
        - due to - *continued*
          - specified NEC - *continued*
            - class II K08.492
            - class III K08.493
            - class IV K08.494
          - trauma K08.419
            - class I K08.411
            - class II K08.412
            - class III K08.413
            - class IV K08.414
  - tendon (congenital) Q79.8
  - testis (congenital) Q55.0
    - acquired Z90.79
  - thumb (acquired) Z89.01-
    - congenital — *see* Agenesis, hand
  - thymus gland Q89.2
  - thyroid (gland) (acquired) E89.0
    - cartilage, congenital Q31.8
    - congenital E03.1
  - toe (s) (acquired) Z89.42-
    - with foot — *see* Absence, foot and ankle
    - congenital — *see* Agenesis, foot
    - great Z89.41-
  - tongue, congenital Q38.3
  - trachea (cartilage) , congenital Q32.1
  - transverse aortic arch, congenital Q25.49
  - tricuspid valve Q22.4
  - umbilical artery, congenital Q27.0
  - upper arm and forearm with hand present, congenital — *see* Agenesis, arm, with hand present
  - ureter (congenital) Q62.4
    - acquired Z90.6
  - urethra, congenital Q64.5
  - uterus (acquired) Z90.710
    - with cervix Z90.710
    - with remaining cervical stump Z90.711
    - congenital Q51.0
  - uvula, congenital Q38.5
  - vagina, congenital Q52.0
  - vas deferens (congenital) Q55.4
    - acquired Z90.79
  - vein (peripheral) congenital NEC Q27.8
    - cerebral Q28.3
    - digestive system Q27.8
    - great Q26.8
    - lower limb Q27.8
    - portal Q26.5
    - precerebral Q28.1
    - specified site NEC Q27.8
    - upper limb Q27.8
  - vena cava (inferior) (superior) , congenital Q26.8
  - ventricular septum Q20.4
  - vertebra, congenital Q76.49
  - vulva, congenital Q52.71
  - wrist (acquired) Z89.12-
- **Absorbent system disease** I87.8
- **Absorption**
  - carbohydrate, disturbance K90.49
  - chemical — *see* Table of Drugs and Chemicals
    - through placenta (newborn) P04.9
      - environmental substance P04.6
      - nutritional substance P04.5
      - obstetric anesthetic or analgesic drug P04.0
  - drug NEC — *see* Table of Drugs and Chemicals
    - addictive
      - through placenta (newborn) — *see also* Newborn, affected by, maternal, use of P04.40
        - cocaine P04.41
        - hallucinogens P04.42
        - specified drug NEC P04.49
    - medicinal
      - through placenta (newborn) P04.19
    - through placenta (newborn) P04.19
      - obstetric anesthetic or analgesic drug P04.0
  - fat, disturbance K90.49
    - pancreatic K90.3
  - noxious substance — *see* Table of Drugs and Chemicals
  - protein, disturbance K90.49
  - starch, disturbance K90.49
  - toxic substance — *see* Table of Drugs and Chemicals
  - uremic — *see* Uremia
- **Abstinence symptoms, syndrome**
  - alcohol F10.239
    - with delirium F10.231
  - cocaine F14.23
  - neonatal P96.1

Abstinence symptoms, syndrome - *continued*
  nicotine — *see* Dependence, drug, nicotine, with, withdrawal
  opioid F11.93
    with dependence F11.23
  psychoactive NEC F19.939
    with
      delirium F19.931
      dependence F19.239
        with
          delirium F19.231
          perceptual disturbance F19.232
        uncomplicated F19.230
      perceptual disturbance F19.932
    uncomplicated F19.930
  sedative F13.939
    with
      delirium F13.931
      dependence F13.239
        with
          delirium F13.231
          perceptual disturbance F13.232
        uncomplicated F13.230
      perceptual disturbance F13.932
    uncomplicated F13.930
  stimulant NEC F15.93
    with dependence F15.23
Abulia R68.89
Abulomania F60.7
Abuse
  adult — *see* Maltreatment, adult
    as reason for
      couple seeking advice (including offender) Z63.0
  alcohol (non-dependent) F10.10
    with
      anxiety disorder F10.180
      intoxication F10.129
        with delirium F10.121
        uncomplicated F10.120
      mood disorder F10.14
      other specified disorder F10.188
      psychosis F10.159
        delusions F10.150
        hallucinations F10.151
      sexual dysfunction F10.181
      sleep disorder F10.182
      unspecified disorder F10.19
    counseling and surveillance Z71.41
    in remission (early) (sustained) F10.11
  amphetamine (or related substance) — *see* Abuse, drug, stimulant NEC
  analgesics (non-prescribed) (over the counter) F55.8
  antacids F55.0
  antidepressants — *see* Abuse, drug, psychoactive NEC
  anxiolytic — *see* Abuse, drug, sedative
  barbiturates — *see* Abuse, drug, sedative
  caffeine — *see* Abuse, drug, stimulant NEC
  cannabis, cannabinoids — *see* Abuse, drug, cannabis
  child — *see* Maltreatment, child
  cocaine — *see* Abuse, drug, cocaine
  drug NEC (non-dependent) F19.10
    with sleep disorder F19.182
    amphetamine type — *see* Abuse, drug, stimulant NEC
    analgesics (non-prescribed) (over the counter) F55.8
    antacids F55.0
    antidepressants — *see* Abuse, drug, psychoactive NEC
    anxiolytics — *see* Abuse, drug, sedative
    barbiturates — *see* Abuse, drug, sedative
    caffeine — *see* Abuse, drug, stimulant NEC
    cannabis F12.10
      with
        anxiety disorder F12.180
        intoxication F12.129
          with
            delirium F12.121
            perceptual disturbance F12.122
          uncomplicated F12.120
        other specified disorder F12.188
        psychosis F12.159
          delusions F12.150
          hallucinations F12.151
        unspecified disorder F12.19
      in remission (early) (sustained) F12.11
    cocaine F14.10
      with
        anxiety disorder F14.180
        intoxication F14.129
          with
            delirium F14.121

Abuse - *continued*
  drug NEC (non-dependent) - *continued*
    cocaine - *continued*
      with - *continued*
        intoxication - *continued*
          with - *continued*
            perceptual disturbance F14.122
          uncomplicated F14.120
        mood disorder F14.14
        other specified disorder F14.188
        psychosis F14.159
          delusions F14.150
          hallucinations F14.151
        sexual dysfunction F14.181
        sleep disorder F14.182
        unspecified disorder F14.19
      in remission (early) (sustained) F14.11
    counseling and surveillance Z71.51
    hallucinogen F16.10
      with
        anxiety disorder F16.180
        flashbacks F16.183
        intoxication F16.129
          with
            delirium F16.121
            perceptual disturbance F16.122
          uncomplicated F16.120
        mood disorder F16.14
        other specified disorder F16.188
        perception disorder, persisting F16.183
        psychosis F16.159
          delusions F16.150
          hallucinations F16.151
        unspecified disorder F16.19
      in remission (early) (sustained) F16.11
    hashish — *see* Abuse, drug, cannabis
    herbal or folk remedies F55.1
    hormones F55.3
    hypnotics — *see* Abuse, drug, sedative
    inhalant F18.10
      with
        anxiety disorder F18.180
        dementia, persisting F18.17
        intoxication F18.129
          with delirium F18.121
          uncomplicated F18.120
        mood disorder F18.14
        other specified disorder F18.188
        psychosis F18.159
          delusions F18.150
          hallucinations F18.151
        unspecified disorder F18.19
      in remission (early) (sustained) F18.11
    in remission (early) (sustained) F19.11
    laxatives F55.2
    LSD — *see* Abuse, drug, hallucinogen
    marihuana — *see* Abuse, drug, cannabis
    morphine type (opioids) — *see* Abuse, drug, opioid
    opioid F11.10
      with
        intoxication F11.129
          with
            delirium F11.121
            perceptual disturbance F11.122
          uncomplicated F11.120
        mood disorder F11.14
        other specified disorder F11.188
        psychosis F11.159
          delusions F11.150
          hallucinations F11.151
        sexual dysfunction F11.181
        sleep disorder F11.182
        unspecified disorder F11.19
      in remission (early) (sustained) F11.11
    PCP (phencyclidine) (or related substance) — *see* Abuse, drug, hallucinogen
    psychoactive NEC F19.10
      with
        amnestic disorder F19.16
        anxiety disorder F19.180
        dementia F19.17
        intoxication F19.129
          with
            delirium F19.121
            perceptual disturbance F19.122
          uncomplicated F19.120
        mood disorder F19.14
        other specified disorder F19.188
        psychosis F19.159
          delusions F19.150
          hallucinations F19.151
        sexual dysfunction F19.181
        sleep disorder F19.182

Abuse - *continued*
  drug NEC (non-dependent) - *continued*
    psychoactive NEC - *continued*
      with - *continued*
        unspecified disorder F19.19
    sedative, hypnotic or anxiolytic F13.10
      with
        anxiety disorder F13.180
        intoxication F13.129
          with delirium F13.121
          uncomplicated F13.120
        mood disorder F13.14
        other specified disorder F13.188
        psychosis F13.159
          delusions F13.150
          hallucinations F13.151
        sexual dysfunction F13.181
        sleep disorder F13.182
        unspecified disorder F13.19
      in remission (early) (sustained) F13.11
    solvent — *see* Abuse, drug, inhalant
    steroids F55.3
    stimulant NEC F15.10
      with
        anxiety disorder F15.180
        intoxication F15.129
          with
            delirium F15.121
            perceptual disturbance F15.122
          uncomplicated F15.120
        mood disorder F15.14
        other specified disorder F15.188
        psychosis F15.159
          delusions F15.150
          hallucinations F15.151
        sexual dysfunction F15.181
        sleep disorder F15.182
        unspecified disorder F15.19
      in remission (early) (sustained) F15.11
    tranquilizers — *see* Abuse, drug, sedative
    vitamins F55.4
  hallucinogens — *see* Abuse, drug, hallucinogen
  hashish — *see* Abuse, drug, cannabis
  herbal or folk remedies F55.1
  hormones F55.3
  hypnotic — *see* Abuse, drug, sedative
  inhalant — *see* Abuse, drug, inhalant
  laxatives F55.2
  LSD — *see* Abuse, drug, hallucinogen
  marihuana — *see* Abuse, drug, cannabis
  morphine type (opioids) — *see* Abuse, drug, opioid
  non-psychoactive substance NEC F55.8
    antacids F55.0
    folk remedies F55.1
    herbal remedies F55.1
    hormones F55.3
    laxatives F55.2
    steroids F55.3
    vitamins F55.4
  opioids — *see* Abuse, drug, opioid
  PCP (phencyclidine) (or related substance) — *see* Abuse, drug, hallucinogen
  physical (adult) (child) — *see* Maltreatment
  psychoactive substance — *see* Abuse, drug, psychoactive NEC
  psychological (adult) (child) — *see* Maltreatment
  sedative — *see* Abuse, drug, sedative
  sexual — *see* Maltreatment
  solvent — *see* Abuse, drug, inhalant
  steroids F55.3
  vitamins F55.4
Acalculia R48.8
  developmental F81.2
Acanthamebiasis (with) B60.10
  conjunctiva B60.12
  keratoconjunctivitis B60.13
  meningoencephalitis B60.11
  other specified B60.19
Acanthocephaliasis B83.8
Acanthocheilonemiasis B74.4
Acanthocytosis E78.6
Acantholysis L11.9
Acanthosis (acquired) (nigricans) L83
  benign Q82.8
  congenital Q82.8
  seborrheic L82.1
    inflamed L82.0
  tongue K14.3
Acapnia E87.3
Acarbia E87.2
Acardia, acardius Q89.8
Acardiacus amorphus Q89.8
Acardiotrophia I51.4

- **Acariasis** B88.0
  - scabies B86
- **Acarodermatitis** (urticarioides) B88.0
- **Acarophobia** F40.218
- **Acatalasemia, acatalasia** E80.3
- **Acathisia** (drug induced) G25.71
- **Accelerated atrioventricular conduction** I45.6
- **Accentuation of personality traits** (type A) Z73.1
- **Accessory** (congenital)
  - adrenal gland Q89.1
  - anus Q43.4
  - appendix Q43.4
  - atrioventricular conduction I45.6
  - auditory ossicles Q16.3
  - auricle (ear) Q17.0
  - biliary duct or passage Q44.5
  - bladder Q64.79
  - blood vessels NEC Q27.9
    - coronary Q24.5
  - bone NEC Q79.8
  - breast tissue, axilla Q83.1
  - carpal bones Q74.0
  - cecum Q43.4
  - chromosome (s) NEC (nonsex) Q92.9
    - with complex rearrangements NEC Q92.5
      - seen only at prometaphase Q92.8
    - partial Q92.9
    - sex
      - female phenotype Q97.8
    - 13 — *see* Trisomy, 13
    - 18 — *see* Trisomy, 18
    - 21 — *see* Trisomy, 21
  - coronary artery Q24.5
  - cusp (s) , heart valve NEC Q24.8
    - pulmonary Q22.3
  - cystic duct Q44.5
  - digit (s) Q69.9
  - ear (auricle) (lobe) Q17.0
  - endocrine gland NEC Q89.2
  - eye muscle Q10.3
  - eyelid Q10.3
  - face bone (s) Q75.8
  - fallopian tube (fimbria) (ostium) Q50.6
  - finger (s) Q69.0
  - foreskin N47.8
  - frontonasal process Q75.8
  - gallbladder Q44.1
  - genital organ (s)
    - female Q52.8
      - external Q52.79
      - internal NEC Q52.8
    - male Q55.8
  - genitourinary organs NEC Q89.8
    - female Q52.8
    - male Q55.8
  - hallux Q69.2
  - heart Q24.8
    - valve NEC Q24.8
      - pulmonary Q22.3
  - hepatic ducts Q44.5
  - hymen Q52.4
  - intestine (large) (small) Q43.4
  - kidney Q63.0
  - lacrimal canal Q10.6
  - leaflet, heart valve NEC Q24.8
  - ligament, broad Q50.6
  - liver Q44.7
    - duct Q44.5
  - lobule (ear) Q17.0
  - lung (lobe) Q33.1
  - muscle Q79.8
  - navicular of carpus Q74.0
  - nervous system, part NEC Q07.8
  - nipple Q83.3
  - nose Q30.8
  - organ or site not listed — *see* Anomaly, by site
  - ovary Q50.31
  - oviduct Q50.6
  - pancreas Q45.3
  - parathyroid gland Q89.2
  - parotid gland (and duct) Q38.4
  - pituitary gland Q89.2
  - preauricular appendage Q17.0
  - prepuce N47.8
  - renal arteries (multiple) Q27.2
  - rib Q76.6
    - cervical Q76.5
  - roots (teeth) K00.2
  - salivary gland Q38.4
  - sesamoid bones Q74.8
    - foot Q74.2
    - hand Q74.0
  - skin tags Q82.8

- **Accessory** (congenital) - *continued*
  - spleen Q89.09
  - sternum Q76.7
  - submaxillary gland Q38.4
  - tarsal bones Q74.2
  - teeth, tooth K00.1
  - tendon Q79.8
  - thumb Q69.1
  - thymus gland Q89.2
  - thyroid gland Q89.2
  - toes Q69.2
  - tongue Q38.3
  - tooth, teeth K00.1
  - tragus Q17.0
  - ureter Q62.5
  - urethra Q64.79
  - urinary organ or tract NEC Q64.8
  - uterus Q51.28
  - vagina Q52.10
  - valve, heart NEC Q24.8
    - pulmonary Q22.3
  - vertebra Q76.49
  - vocal cords Q31.8
  - vulva Q52.79
- **Accident**
  - birth — *see* Birth, injury
  - cardiac — *see* Infarct, myocardium
  - cerebral I63.9
  - cerebrovascular (embolic) (ischemic) (thrombotic) I63.9
    - aborted I63.9
    - hemorrhagic — *see* Hemorrhage, intracranial, intracerebral
    - old (without sequelae) Z86.73
      - with sequelae (of) — *see* Sequelae, infarction, cerebral
  - coronary — *see* Infarct, myocardium
  - craniovascular I63.9
  - vascular, brain I63.9
- **Accidental** — *see* condition
- **Accommodation** (disorder) — *see also* condition
  - hysterical paralysis of F44.89
  - insufficiency of H52.4
  - paresis — *see* Paresis, of accommodation
  - spasm — *see* Spasm, of accommodation
- **Accouchement** — *see* Delivery
- **Accreta placenta** O43.21-
- **Accretio cordis** (nonrheumatic) I31.0
- **Accretions, tooth, teeth** K03.6
- **Acculturation difficulty** Z60.3
- **Accumulation secretion, prostate** N42.89
- **Acephalia, acephalism, acephalus, acephaly** Q00.0
- **Acephalobrachia monster** Q89.8
- **Acephalochirus monster** Q89.8
- **Acephalogaster** Q89.8
- **Acephalostomus monster** Q89.8
- **Acephalothorax** Q89.8
- **Acerophobia** F40.298
- **Acetonemia** R79.89
  - in Type 1 diabetes E10.10
    - with coma E10.11
- **Acetonuria** R82.4
- **Achalasia** (cardia) (esophagus) K22.0
  - congenital Q39.5
  - pylorus Q40.0
  - sphincteral NEC K59.8
- **Ache** (s) — *see* Pain
- **Acheilia** Q38.6
- **Achillobursitis** — *see* Tendinitis, Achilles
- **Achillodynia** — *see* Tendinitis, Achilles
- **Achlorhydria, achlorhydric** (neurogenic) K31.83
  - anemia D50.8
  - diarrhea K31.83
  - psychogenic F45.8
  - secondary to vagotomy K91.1
- **Achluophobia** F40.228
- **Acholia** K82.8
- **Acholuric jaundice** (familial) (splenomegalic) — *see also* Spherocytosis
  - acquired D59.8
- **Achondrogenesis** Q77.0
- **Achondroplasia** (osteosclerosis congenita) Q77.4
- **Achroma, cutis** L80
- **Achromat** (ism) **, achromatopsia** (acquired) (congenital) H53.51
- **Achromia parasitica** B36.0
- **Achromia, congenital** — *see* Albinism
- **Achylia gastrica** K31.89
  - psychogenic F45.8
- **Acid**
  - burn — *see* Corrosion
  - deficiency
    - amide nicotinic E52

- **Acid** - *continued*
  - deficiency - *continued*
    - ascorbic E54
    - folic E53.8
    - nicotinic E52
    - pantothenic E53.8
  - intoxication E87.2
  - peptic disease K30
  - phosphatase deficiency E83.39
  - stomach K30
    - psychogenic F45.8
- **Acidemia** E87.2
  - argininosuccinic E72.22
  - isovaleric E71.110
  - metabolic (newborn) P19.9
    - first noted before onset of labor P19.0
    - first noted during labor P19.1
    - noted at birth P19.2
  - methylmalonic E71.120
  - pipecolic E72.3
  - propionic E71.121
- **Acidity, gastric** (high) K30
  - psychogenic F45.8
- **Acidocytopenia** — *see* Agranulocytosis
- **Acidocytosis** D72.1
- **Acidopenia** — *see* Agranulocytosis
- **Acidosis** (lactic) (respiratory) E87.2
  - in Type 1 diabetes E10.10
    - with coma E10.11
  - kidney, tubular N25.89
  - lactic E87.2
  - metabolic NEC E87.2
    - with respiratory acidosis E87.4
    - hyperchloremic, of newborn P74.421
    - late, of newborn P74.0
  - mixed metabolic and respiratory, newborn P84
  - newborn P84
  - renal (hyperchloremic) (tubular) N25.89
  - respiratory E87.2
    - complicated by
      - metabolic
        - acidosis E87.4
        - alkalosis E87.4
- **Aciduria**
  - 4-hydroxybutyric E72.81
  - argininosuccinic E72.22
  - gamma-hydroxybutyric E72.81
  - glutaric (type I) E72.3
    - type II E71.313
    - type III E71.5-
  - orotic (congenital) (hereditary) (pyrimidine deficiency) E79.8
    - anemia D53.0
- **Acladiosis** (skin) B36.0
- **Aclasis, diaphyseal** Q78.6
- **Acleistocardia** Q21.1
- **Aclusion** — *see* Anomaly, dentofacial, malocclusion
- **Acne** L70.9
  - artificialis L70.8
  - atrophica L70.2
  - cachecticorum (Hebra) L70.8
  - conglobata L70.1
  - cystic L70.0
  - decalvans L66.2
  - excoriée (des jeunes filles) L70.5
  - frontalis L70.2
  - indurata L70.0
  - infantile L70.4
  - keloid L73.0
  - lupoid L70.2
  - necrotic, necrotica (miliaris) L70.2
  - neonatal L70.4
  - nodular L70.0
  - occupational L70.8
  - picker's L70.5
  - pustular L70.0
  - rodens L70.2
  - rosacea L71.9
  - specified NEC L70.8
  - tropica L70.3
  - varioliformis L70.2
  - vulgaris L70.0
- **Acnitis** (primary) A18.4
- **Acosta's disease** T70.29
- **Acoustic** — *see* condition
- **Acousticophobia** F40.298
- **Acquired** — *see also* condition
  - immunodeficiency syndrome (AIDS) B20
- **Acrania** Q00.0
- **Acroangiodermatitis** I78.9
- **Acroasphyxia, chronic** I73.89
- **Acrobystitis** N47.7
- **Acrocephalopolysyndactyly** Q87.0

- **Acrocephalosyndactyly** Q87.0
- **Acrocephaly** Q75.0
- **Acrochondrohyperplasia** — *see* Syndrome, Marfan's
- **Acrocyanosis** I73.8
  - newborn P28.2
    - meaning transient blue hands and feet - omit code
- **Acrodermatitis** L30.8
  - atrophicans (chronica) L90.4
  - continua (Hallopeau) L40.2
  - enteropathica (hereditary) E83.2
  - Hallopeau's L40.2
  - infantile papular L44.4
  - perstans L40.2
  - pustulosa continua L40.2
  - recalcitrant pustular L40.2
- **Acrodynia** — *see* Poisoning, mercury
- **Acromegaly, acromegalia** E22.0
- **Acromelalgia** I73.81
- **Acromicria, acromikria** Q79.8
- **Acronyx** L60.0
- **Acropachy, thyroid** — *see* Thyrotoxicosis
- **Acroparesthesia** (simple) (vasomotor) I73.89
- **Acropathy, thyroid** — *see* Thyrotoxicosis
- **Acrophobia** F40.241
- **Acroposthitis** N47.7
- **Acroscleriasis, acroscleroderma, acrosclerosis** — *see* Sclerosis, systemic
- **Acrosphacelus** I96
- **Acrospiroma, eccrine** — *see* Neoplasm, skin, benign
- **Acrostealgia** — *see* Osteochondropathy
- **Acrotrophodynia** — *see* Immersion
- **ACTH ectopic syndrome** E24.3
- **Actinic** — *see* condition
- **Actinobacillosis, actinobacillus** A28.8
  - mallei A24.0
  - muris A25.1
- **Actinomyces israelii** (infection) — *see* Actinomycosis
- **Actinomycetoma** (foot) B47.1
- **Actinomycosis, actinomycotic** A42.9
  - with pneumonia A42.0
  - abdominal A42.1
  - cervicofacial A42.2
  - cutaneous A42.89
  - gastrointestinal A42.1
  - pulmonary A42.0
  - sepsis A42.7
  - specified site NEC A42.89
- **Actinoneuritis** G62.82
- **Action, heart**
  - disorder I49.9
  - irregular I49.9
    - psychogenic F45.8
- **Activated protein C resistance** D68.51
- **Activation**
  - mast cell (disorder) (syndrome) D89.40
    - idiopathic D89.42
    - monoclonal D89.41
    - secondary D89.43
    - specified type NEC D89.49
- **Active** — *see* condition
- **Acute** — *see also* condition
  - abdomen R10.0
  - gallbladder — *see* Cholecystitis, acute
- **Acyanotic heart disease** (congenital) Q24.9
- **Acystia** Q64.5
- **Adair-Dighton syndrome** (brittle bones and blue sclera, deafness) Q78.0
- **Adamantinoblastoma** — *see* Ameloblastoma
- **Adamantinoma** — *see also* Cyst, calcifying odontogenic
  - long bones C40.90
    - lower limb C40.2-
    - upper limb C40.0-
  - malignant C41.1
    - jaw (bone) (lower) C41.1
      - upper C41.0
  - tibial C40.2-
- **Adamantoblastoma** — *see* Ameloblastoma
- **Adams-Stokes** (-Morgagni) **disease or syndrome** I45.9
- **Adaption reaction** — *see* Disorder, adjustment
- **Addiction** — *see also* Dependence F19.20
  - alcohol, alcoholic (ethyl) (methyl) (wood) (without remission) F10.20
    - with remission F10.21
  - drug — *see* Dependence, drug
  - ethyl alcohol (without remission) F10.20
    - with remission F10.21
  - heroin — *see* Dependence, drug, opioid
  - methyl alcohol (without remission) F10.20
    - with remission F10.21
  - methylated spirit (without remission) F10.20

Addiction - *continued*

  - methylated spirit (without remission) - *continued*
    - with remission F10.21
  - morphine (-like substances) — *see* Dependence, drug, opioid
  - nicotine — *see* Dependence, drug, nicotine
  - opium and opioids — *see* Dependence, drug, opioid
  - tobacco — *see* Dependence, drug, nicotine
- **Addison-Biermer anemia** (pernicious) D51.0
- **Addisonian crisis** E27.2
- **Addison's**
  - anemia (pernicious) D51.0
  - disease (bronze) or syndrome E27.1
    - tuberculous A18.7
  - keloid L94.0
- **Addison-Schilder complex** E71.528
- **Additional** — *see also* Accessory
  - chromosome (s) Q99.8
    - sex — *see* Abnormal, chromosome, sex
    - 21 — *see* Trisomy, 21
- **Adduction contracture, hip or other joint** — *see* Contraction, joint
- **Adenitis** — *see also* Lymphadenitis
  - acute, unspecified site L04.9
  - axillary I88.9
    - acute L04.2
    - chronic or subacute I88.1
  - Bartholin's gland N75.8
  - bulbourethral gland — *see* Urethritis
  - cervical I88.9
    - acute L04.0
    - chronic or subacute I88.1
  - chancroid (Hemophilus ducreyi) A57
  - chronic, unspecified site I88.1
  - Cowper's gland — *see* Urethritis
  - due to Pasteurella multocida (P. septica) A28.0
  - epidemic, acute B27.09
  - gangrenous L04.9
  - gonorrheal NEC A54.89
  - groin I88.9
    - acute L04.1
    - chronic or subacute I88.1
  - infectious (acute) (epidemic) B27.09
  - inguinal I88.9
    - acute L04.1
    - chronic or subacute I88.1
  - lymph gland or node, except mesenteric I88.9
    - acute — *see* Lymphadenitis, acute
    - chronic or subacute I88.1
  - mesenteric (acute) (chronic) (nonspecific) (subacute) I88.0
  - parotid gland (suppurative) — *see* Sialoadenitis
  - salivary gland (any) (suppurative) — *see* Sialoadenitis
  - scrofulous (tuberculous) A18.2
  - Skene's duct or gland — *see* Urethritis
  - strumous, tuberculous A18.2
  - subacute, unspecified site I88.1
  - sublingual gland (suppurative) — *see* Sialoadenitis
  - submandibular gland (suppurative) — *see* Sialoadenitis
  - submaxillary gland (suppurative) — *see* Sialoadenitis
  - tuberculous — *see* Tuberculosis, lymph gland
  - urethral gland — *see* Urethritis
  - Wharton's duct (suppurative) — *see* Sialoadenitis
- **Adenoacanthoma** — *see* Neoplasm, malignant, by site
- **Adenoameloblastoma** — *see* Cyst, calcifying odontogenic
- **Adenocarcinoid** (tumor) — *see* Neoplasm, malignant, by site
- **Adenocarcinoma** — *see also* Neoplasm, malignant, by site
  - acidophil
    - specified site — *see* Neoplasm, malignant, by site
    - unspecified site C75.1
  - adrenal cortical C74.0-
  - alveolar — *see* Neoplasm, lung, malignant
  - apocrine
    - breast — *see* Neoplasm, breast, malignant
    - in situ
      - breast D05.8-
      - specified site NEC — *see* Neoplasm, skin, in situ
      - unspecified site D04.9
    - specified site NEC — *see* Neoplasm, skin, malignant
    - unspecified site C44.99
  - basal cell
    - specified site — *see* Neoplasm, skin, malignant
    - unspecified site C08.9
  - basophil
    - specified site — *see* Neoplasm, malignant, by site

Adenocarcinoma - *continued*

  - basophil - *continued*
    - unspecified site C75.1
  - bile duct type C22.1
    - liver C22.1
    - specified site NEC — *see* Neoplasm, malignant, by site
    - unspecified site C22.1
  - bronchiolar — *see* Neoplasm, lung, malignant
  - bronchioloalveolar — *see* Neoplasm, lung, malignant
  - ceruminous C44.29-
  - cervix, in situ — *see also* Carcinoma, cervix uteri, in situ D06.9
  - chromophobe
    - specified site — *see* Neoplasm, malignant, by site
    - unspecified site C75.1
  - diffuse type
    - specified site — *see* Neoplasm, malignant, by site
    - unspecified site C16.9
  - duct
    - infiltrating
      - with Paget's disease — *see* Neoplasm, breast, malignant
      - specified site — *see* Neoplasm, malignant, by site
      - unspecified site (female) C50.91-
        - male C50.92-
    - specified site — *see* Neoplasm, malignant, by site
    - unspecified site
      - female C56.9
      - male C61
  - eosinophil
    - specified site — *see* Neoplasm, malignant, by site
    - unspecified site C75.1
  - follicular
    - with papillary C73
    - moderately differentiated C73
    - specified site — *see* Neoplasm, malignant, by site
    - trabecular C73
    - unspecified site C73
    - well differentiated C73
  - Hurthle cell C73
  - in
    - adenomatous
      - polyposis coli C18.9
  - infiltrating duct
    - with Paget's disease — *see* Neoplasm, breast, malignant
    - specified site — *see* Neoplasm, by site, malignant
    - unspecified site (female) C50.91-
      - male C50.92-
  - inflammatory
    - specified site — *see* Neoplasm, by site, malignant
    - unspecified site (female) C50.91-
      - male C50.92-
  - intestinal type
    - specified site — *see* Neoplasm, by site, malignant
    - unspecified site C16.9
  - intracystic papillary
  - intraductal
    - breast D05.1-
    - noninfiltrating
      - breast D05.1-
      - papillary
        - with invasion
          - specified site — *see* Neoplasm, by site, malignant
          - unspecified site (female) C50.91-
            - male C50.92-
        - breast D05.1-
        - specified site NEC — *see* Neoplasm, in situ, by site
        - unspecified site D05.1-
      - specified site NEC — *see* Neoplasm, in situ, by site
      - unspecified site D05.1-
    - papillary
      - with invasion
        - specified site — *see* Neoplasm, malignant, by site
        - unspecified site (female) C50.91-
          - male C50.92-
      - breast D05.1-
      - specified site — *see* Neoplasm, in situ, by site
      - unspecified site D05.1-
    - specified site NEC — *see* Neoplasm, in situ, by site
    - unspecified site D05.1-
  - islet cell
    - with exocrine, mixed
      - specified site — *see* Neoplasm, malignant, by site
      - unspecified site C25.9
    - pancreas C25.4

Adenocarcinoma - *continued*
- islet cell - *continued*
  - specified site NEC — *see* Neoplasm, malignant, by site
  - unspecified site C25.4
- lobular
  - in situ
    - breast D05.0-
    - specified site NEC — *see* Neoplasm, in situ, by site
    - unspecified site D05.0-
  - specified site — *see* Neoplasm, malignant, by site
  - unspecified site (female) C50.91-
    - male C50.92-
- mucoid — *see also* Neoplasm, malignant, by site
  - cell
    - specified site — *see* Neoplasm, malignant, by site
    - unspecified site C75.1
- nonencapsulated sclerosing C73
- papillary
  - with follicular C73
  - follicular variant C73
  - intraductal (noninfiltrating)
    - with invasion
      - specified site — *see* Neoplasm, malignant, by site
      - unspecified site (female) C50.91-
        - male C50.92-
    - breast D05.1-
    - specified site NEC — *see* Neoplasm, in situ, by site
    - unspecified site D05.1-
  - serous
    - specified site — *see* Neoplasm, malignant, by site
    - unspecified site C56.9
- papillocystic
  - specified site — *see* Neoplasm, malignant, by site
  - unspecified site C56.9
- pseudomucinous
  - specified site — *see* Neoplasm, malignant, by site
  - unspecified site C56.9
- renal cell C64-
- sebaceous — *see* Neoplasm, skin, malignant
- serous — *see also* Neoplasm, malignant, by site
  - papillary
    - specified site — *see* Neoplasm, malignant, by site
    - unspecified site C56.9
- sweat gland — *see* Neoplasm, skin, malignant
- water-clear cell C75.0

Adenocarcinoma-in-situ — *see also* Neoplasm, in situ, by site
- breast D05.9-

Adenofibroma
- clear cell — *see* Neoplasm, benign, by site
- endometrioid D27.9
  - borderline malignancy D39.10
  - malignant C56-
- mucinous
  - specified site — *see* Neoplasm, benign, by site
  - unspecified site D27.9
- papillary
  - specified site — *see* Neoplasm, benign, by site
  - unspecified site D27.9
- prostate — *see* Enlargement, enlarged, prostate
- serous
  - specified site — *see* Neoplasm, benign, by site
  - unspecified site D27.9
- specified site — *see* Neoplasm, benign, by site
- unspecified site D27.9

Adenofibrosis
- breast — *see* Fibroadenosis, breast
- endometrioid N80.0

Adenoiditis (chronic) J35.02
- with tonsillitis J35.03
- acute J03.90
  - recurrent J03.91
  - specified organism NEC J03.80
    - recurrent J03.81
  - staphylococcal J03.80
    - recurrent J03.81
  - streptococcal J03.00
    - recurrent J03.01

Adenoids — *see* condition

Adenolipoma — *see* Neoplasm, benign, by site

Adenolipomatosis, Launois-Bensaude E88.89

Adenolymphoma
- specified site — *see* Neoplasm, benign, by site
- unspecified site D11.9

Adenoma — *see also* Neoplasm, benign, by site
- acidophil
  - specified site — *see* Neoplasm, benign, by site
  - unspecified site D35.2
- acidophil-basophil, mixed

Adenoma - *continued*
- acidophil-basophil, mixed - *continued*
  - specified site — *see* Neoplasm, benign, by site
  - unspecified site D35.2
- adrenal (cortical) D35.00
  - clear cell D35.00
  - compact cell D35.00
  - glomerulosa cell D35.00
  - heavily pigmented variant D35.00
  - mixed cell D35.00
- alpha-cell
  - pancreas D13.7
  - specified site NEC — *see* Neoplasm, benign, by site
  - unspecified site D13.7
- alveolar D14.30
- apocrine
  - breast D24-
  - specified site NEC — *see* Neoplasm, skin, benign, by site
  - unspecified site D23.9
- basal cell D11.9
- basophil
  - specified site — *see* Neoplasm, benign, by site
  - unspecified site D35.2
- basophil-acidophil, mixed
  - specified site — *see* Neoplasm, benign, by site
  - unspecified site D35.2
- beta-cell
  - pancreas D13.7
  - specified site NEC — *see* Neoplasm, benign, by site
  - unspecified site D13.7
- bile duct D13.4
  - common D13.5
  - extrahepatic D13.5
  - intrahepatic D13.4
  - specified site NEC — *see* Neoplasm, benign, by site
  - unspecified site D13.4
- black D35.00
- bronchial D38.1
  - cylindroid type — *see* Neoplasm, lung, malignant
- ceruminous D23.2-
- chief cell D35.1
- chromophobe
  - specified site — *see* Neoplasm, benign, by site
  - unspecified site D35.2
- colloid
  - specified site — *see* Neoplasm, benign, by site
  - unspecified site D34
- duct
- eccrine, papillary — *see* Neoplasm, skin, benign
- endocrine, multiple
  - single specified site — *see* Neoplasm, uncertain behavior, by site
  - two or more specified sites D44-
  - unspecified site D44.9
- endometrioid — *see also* Neoplasm, benign
  - borderline malignancy — *see* Neoplasm, uncertain behavior, by site
- eosinophil
  - specified site — *see* Neoplasm, benign, by site
  - unspecified site D35.2
- fetal
  - specified site — *see* Neoplasm, benign, by site
  - unspecified site D34
- follicular
  - specified site — *see* Neoplasm, benign, by site
  - unspecified site D34
- hepatocellular D13.4
- Hurthle cell D34
- islet cell
  - pancreas D13.7
  - specified site NEC — *see* Neoplasm, benign, by site
  - unspecified site D13.7
- liver cell D13.4
- macrofollicular
  - specified site — *see* Neoplasm, benign, by site
  - unspecified site D34
- malignant, malignum — *see* Neoplasm, malignant, by site
- microcystic
  - pancreas D13.6
  - specified site NEC — *see* Neoplasm, benign, by site
  - unspecified site D13.6
- microfollicular
  - specified site — *see* Neoplasm, benign, by site
  - unspecified site D34
- mucoid cell
  - specified site — *see* Neoplasm, benign, by site

Adenoma - *continued*
- mucoid cell - *continued*
  - unspecified site D35.2
- multiple endocrine
  - single specified site — *see* Neoplasm, uncertain behavior, by site
  - two or more specified sites D44-
  - unspecified site D44.9
- nipple D24-
- papillary — *see also* Neoplasm, benign, by site
  - eccrine — *see* Neoplasm, skin, benign, by site
- Pick's tubular
  - specified site — *see* Neoplasm, benign, by site
  - unspecified site
    - female D27.9
    - male D29.20
- pleomorphic
  - carcinoma in — *see* Neoplasm, salivary gland, malignant
    - specified site — *see* Neoplasm, malignant, by site
    - unspecified site C08.9
- polypoid — *see also* Neoplasm, benign
  - adenocarcinoma in — *see* Neoplasm, malignant, by site
  - adenocarcinoma in situ — *see* Neoplasm, in situ, by site
- prostate — *see* Neoplasm, benign, prostate
- rete cell D29.20
- sebaceous — *see* Neoplasm, skin, benign
- Sertoli cell
  - specified site — *see* Neoplasm, benign, by site
  - unspecified site
    - female D27.9
    - male D29.20
- skin appendage — *see* Neoplasm, skin, benign
- sudoriferous gland — *see* Neoplasm, skin, benign
- sweat gland — *see* Neoplasm, skin, benign
- testicular
  - specified site — *see* Neoplasm, benign, by site
  - unspecified site
    - female D27.9
    - male D29.20
- tubular — *see also* Neoplasm, benign, by site
  - adenocarcinoma in — *see* Neoplasm, malignant, by site
  - adenocarcinoma in situ — *see* Neoplasm, in situ, by site
  - Pick's
    - specified site — *see* Neoplasm, benign, by site
    - unspecified site
      - female D27.9
      - male D29.20
- tubulovillous — *see also* Neoplasm, benign, by site
  - adenocarcinoma in — *see* Neoplasm, malignant, by site
  - adenocarcinoma in situ — *see* Neoplasm, in situ, by site
- villous — *see* Neoplasm, uncertain behavior, by site
  - adenocarcinoma in — *see* Neoplasm, malignant, by site
  - adenocarcinoma in situ — *see* Neoplasm, in situ, by site
- water-clear cell D35.1

Adenomatosis
- endocrine (multiple) E31.20
  - single specified site — *see* Neoplasm, uncertain behavior, by site
- erosive of nipple D24-
- pluriendocrine — *see* Adenomatosis, endocrine
- pulmonary D38.1
  - malignant — *see* Neoplasm, lung, malignant
- specified site — *see* Neoplasm, benign, by site
- unspecified site D12.6

Adenomatous
- goiter (nontoxic) E04.9
  - with hyperthyroidism — *see* Hyperthyroidism, with, goiter, nodular
  - toxic — *see* Hyperthyroidism, with, goiter, nodular

Adenomyoma — *see also* Neoplasm, benign, by site
- prostate — *see* Enlarged, prostate

Adenomyometritis N80.0

Adenomyosis N80.0

Adenopathy (lymph gland) R59.9
- generalized R59.1
- inguinal R59.0
- localized R59.0
- mediastinal R59.0
- mesentery R59.0
- syphilitic (secondary) A51.49
- tracheobronchial R59.0
  - tuberculous A15.4
    - primary (progressive) A15.7
- tuberculous — *see also* Tuberculosis, lymph gland

Adenopathy (lymph gland) - *continued*
  tuberculous - *continued*
    tracheobronchial A15.4
      primary (progressive) A15.7
Adenosalpingitis — *see* Salpingitis
Adenosarcoma — *see* Neoplasm, malignant, by site
Adenosclerosis I88.8
Adenosis (sclerosing) **breast** — *see* Fibroadenosis, breast
Adenovirus, as cause of disease classified elsewhere B97.0
Adentia (complete) (partial) — *see* Absence, teeth
Adherent — *see also* Adhesions
  labia (minora) N90.89
  pericardium (nonrheumatic) I31.0
    rheumatic I09.2
  placenta (with hemorrhage) O72.0
    without hemorrhage O73.0
  prepuce, newborn N47.0
  scar (skin) L90.5
  tendon in scar L90.5
Adhesions, adhesive (postinfective) K66.0
  with intestinal obstruction K56.50
    complete K56.52
    incomplete K56.51
    partial K56.51
  abdominal (wall) — *see* Adhesions, peritoneum
  appendix K38.8
  bile duct (common) (hepatic) K83.8
  bladder (sphincter) N32.89
  bowel — *see* Adhesions, peritoneum
  cardiac I31.0
    rheumatic I09.2
  cecum — *see* Adhesions, peritoneum
  cervicovaginal N88.1
    congenital Q52.8
    postpartal O90.89
      old N88.1
  cervix N88.1
  ciliary body NEC — *see* Adhesions, iris
  clitoris N90.89
  colon — *see* Adhesions, peritoneum
  common duct K83.8
  congenital — *see also* Anomaly, by site
    fingers — *see* Syndactylism, complex, fingers
    omental, anomalous Q43.3
    peritoneal Q43.3
    tongue (to gum or roof of mouth) Q38.3
  conjunctiva (acquired) H11.21-
    congenital Q15.8
  cystic duct K82.8
  diaphragm — *see* Adhesions, peritoneum
  due to foreign body — *see* Foreign body
  duodenum — *see* Adhesions, peritoneum
  ear
    middle H74.1-
  epididymis N50.89
  epidural — *see* Adhesions, meninges
  epiglottis J38.7
  eyelid H02.59
  female pelvis N73.6
  gallbladder K82.8
  globe H44.89
  heart I31.0
    rheumatic I09.2
  ileocecal (coil) — *see* Adhesions, peritoneum
  ileum — *see* Adhesions, peritoneum
  intestine — *see also* Adhesions, peritoneum
    with obstruction K56.50
      complete K56.52
      incomplete K56.51
      partial K56.51
  intra-abdominal — *see* Adhesions, peritoneum
  iris H21.50-
    anterior H21.51-
    goniosynechiae H21.52-
    posterior H21.54-
    to corneal graft T85.898
  joint — *see* Ankylosis
    knee M23.8X
    temporomandibular M26.61-
  labium (majus) (minus) , congenital Q52.5
  liver — *see* Adhesions, peritoneum
  lung J98.4
  mediastinum J98.59
  meninges (cerebral) (spinal) G96.12
    congenital Q07.8
    tuberculous (cerebral) (spinal) A17.0
  mesenteric — *see* Adhesions, peritoneum
  nasal (septum) (to turbinates) J34.89
  ocular muscle — *see* Strabismus, mechanical
  omentum — *see* Adhesions, peritoneum
  ovary N73.6

Adhesions, adhesive (postinfective) - *continued*
  ovary - *continued*
    congenital (to cecum, kidney or omentum) Q50.39
  paraovarian N73.6
  pelvic (peritoneal)
    female N73.6
      postprocedural N99.4
    male — *see* Adhesions, peritoneum
    postpartal (old) N73.6
    tuberculous A18.17
  penis to scrotum (congenital) Q55.8
  periappendiceal — *see also* Adhesions, peritoneum
  pericardium (nonrheumatic) I31.0
    focal I31.8
    rheumatic I09.2
    tuberculous A18.84
  pericholecystic K82.8
  perigastric — *see* Adhesions, peritoneum
  periovarian N73.6
  periprostatic N42.89
  perirectal — *see* Adhesions, peritoneum
  perirenal N28.89
  peritoneum, peritoneal (postinfective)
    with obstruction (intestinal) K56.50
      complete K56.52
      incomplete K56.51
      partial K56.51
    congenital Q43.3
    pelvic, female N73.6
      postprocedural N99.4
    postpartal, pelvic N73.6
    postprocedural K66.0
    to uterus N73.6
  peritubal N73.6
  periureteral N28.89
  periuterine N73.6
  perivesical N32.89
  perivesicular (seminal vesicle) N50.89
  pleura, pleuritic J94.8
    tuberculous NEC A15.6
  pleuropericardial J94.8
  postoperative (gastrointestinal tract) K66.0
    with obstruction — *see also* Obstruction, intestine, postoperative K91.30
    due to foreign body accidentally left in wound — *see* Foreign body, accidentally left during a procedure
    pelvic peritoneal N99.4
    urethra — *see* Stricture, urethra, postprocedural
    vagina N99.2
  postpartal, old (vulva or perineum) N90.89
  preputial, prepuce N47.5
  pulmonary J98.4
  pylorus — *see* Adhesions, peritoneum
  sciatic nerve — *see* Lesion, nerve, sciatic
  seminal vesicle N50.89
  shoulder (joint) — *see* Capsulitis, adhesive
  sigmoid flexure — *see* Adhesions, peritoneum
  spermatic cord (acquired) N50.89
    congenital Q55.4
  spinal canal G96.12
  stomach — *see* Adhesions, peritoneum
  subscapular — *see* Capsulitis, adhesive
  temporomandibular M26.61-
  tendinitis — *see also* Tenosynovitis, specified type NEC
    shoulder — *see* Capsulitis, adhesive
  testis N44.8
  tongue, congenital (to gum or roof of mouth) Q38.3
    acquired K14.8
  trachea J39.8
  tubo-ovarian N73.6
  tunica vaginalis N44.8
  uterus N73.6
    internal N85.6
    to abdominal wall N73.6
  vagina (chronic) N89.5
    postoperative N99.2
  vitreomacular H43.82-
  vitreous H43.89
  vulva N90.89
Adiaspiromycosis B48.8
Adie (-Holmes) **pupil or syndrome** — *see* Anomaly, pupil, function, tonic pupil
Adiponecrosis neonatorum P83.88
Adiposis — *see also* Obesity
  cerebralis E23.6
  dolorosa E88.2
Adiposity — *see also* Obesity
  heart — *see* Degeneration, myocardial
  localized E65
Adiposogenital dystrophy E23.6

Adjustment
  disorder — *see* Disorder, adjustment
  implanted device — *see* Encounter (for), adjustment (of)
  prosthesis, external — *see* Fitting
  reaction — *see* Disorder, adjustment
Administration of tPA (rtPA)
  in a different facility within the last 24 hours prior to admission to current facility Z92.82
Admission (for) — *see also* Encounter (for)
  adjustment (of)
    artificial
      arm Z44.00-
        complete Z44.01-
        partial Z44.02-
      eye Z44.2
      leg Z44.10-
        complete Z44.11-
        partial Z44.12-
    brain neuropacemaker Z46.2
      implanted Z45.42
    breast
      implant Z45.81
      prosthesis (external) Z44.3
    colostomy belt Z46.89
    contact lenses Z46.0
    cystostomy device Z46.6
    dental prosthesis Z46.3
    device NEC
      abdominal Z46.89
      implanted Z45.89
        cardiac Z45.09
          defibrillator (with synchronous cardiace pacemaker) Z45.02
          pacemaker (cardiac resynchronization therapy (CRT-P)) Z45.018
            pulse generator Z45.010
          resynchronization therapy defibrillator (CRT-D) Z45.02
        hearing device Z45.328
          bone conduction Z45.320
          cochlear Z45.321
        infusion pump Z45.1
        nervous system Z45.49
          CSF drainage Z45.41
          hearing device — *see* Admission, adjustment, device, implanted, hearing device
          neuropacemaker Z45.42
          visual substitution Z45.31
        specified NEC Z45.89
        vascular access Z45.2
        visual substitution Z45.31
      nervous system Z46.2
        implanted — *see* Admission, adjustment, device, implanted, nervous system
      orthodontic Z46.4
      prosthetic Z44.9
        arm — *see* Admission, adjustment, artificial, arm
        breast Z44.3
        dental Z46.3
        eye Z44.2
        leg — *see* Admission, adjustment, artificial, leg
        specified type NEC Z44.8
      substitution
        auditory Z46.2
          implanted — *see* Admission, adjustment, device, implanted, hearing device
        nervous system Z46.2
          implanted — *see* Admission, adjustment, device, implanted, nervous system
        visual Z46.2
          implanted Z45.31
      urinary Z46.6
    hearing aid Z46.1
      implanted — *see* Admission, adjustment, device, implanted, hearing device
    ileostomy device Z46.89
    intestinal appliance or device NEC Z46.89
    neuropacemaker (brain) (peripheral nerve) (spinal cord) Z46.2
      implanted Z45.42
    orthodontic device Z46.4
    orthopedic (brace) (cast) (device) (shoes) Z46.89
    pacemaker (cardiac resynchronization therapy (CRT-P))
      cardiac Z45.018
        pulse generator Z45.010
      nervous system Z46.2
        implanted Z45.42
    portacath (port-a-cath) Z45.2
    prosthesis Z44.9
      arm — *see* Admission, adjustment, artificial, arm

Aftercare - *continued*
- following surgery (for) (on) - *continued*
  - organ transplant - *continued*
    - heart-lung Z48.280
    - kidney Z48.22
    - liver Z48.23
    - lung Z48.24
    - multiple organs NEC Z48.288
    - specified NEC Z48.298
  - orthopedic NEC Z47.89
  - planned wound closure Z48.1
  - removal of internal fixation device Z47.2
  - respiratory system Z48.813
  - scoliosis Z47.82
  - sense organs Z48.810
  - skin and subcutaneous tissue Z48.817
  - specified body system
    - circulatory Z48.812
    - digestive Z48.815
    - genitourinary Z48.816
    - nervous Z48.811
    - oral cavity Z48.814
    - respiratory Z48.813
    - sense organs Z48.810
    - skin and subcutaneous tissue Z48.817
    - teeth Z48.814
  - specified NEC Z48.89
  - spinal Z47.89
  - teeth Z48.814
- fracture - code to fracture with seventh character D
- involving
  - removal of
    - drains Z48.03
    - dressings (nonsurgical) Z48.00
    - staples Z48.02
    - surgical dressings Z48.01
    - sutures Z48.02
- neuropacemaker (brain) (peripheral nerve) (spinal cord) Z46.2
  - implanted Z45.42
- orthopedic NEC Z47.89
- postprocedural — *see* Aftercare, following surgery

After-cataract — *see* Cataract, secondary

Agalactia (primary) O92.3
- elective, secondary or therapeutic O92.5

Agammaglobulinemia (acquired (secondary)) (nonfamilial) (nonfamilial) D80.1
- with
  - immunoglobulin-bearing B-lymphocytes D80.1
  - lymphopenia D81.9
- autosomal recessive (Swiss type) D80.0
- Bruton's X-linked D80.0
- common variable (CVAgamma) D80.1
- congenital sex-linked D80.0
- hereditary D80.0
- lymphopenic D81.9
- Swiss type (autosomal recessive) D80.0
- X-linked (with growth hormone deficiency) (Bruton) D80.0

Aganglionosis (bowel) (colon) Q43.1

Age (old) — *see* Senility

Agenesis
- adrenal (gland) Q89.1
- alimentary tract (complete) (partial) NEC Q45.8
  - upper Q40.8
- anus, anal (canal) Q42.3
  - with fistula Q42.2
- aorta Q25.41
- appendix Q42.8
- arm (complete) Q71.0-
  - with hand present Q71.1-
- artery (peripheral) Q27.9
  - brain Q28.3
  - coronary Q24.5
  - pulmonary Q25.79
  - specified NEC Q27.8
  - umbilical Q27.0
- auditory (canal) (external) Q16.1
- auricle (ear) Q16.0
- bile duct or passage Q44.5
- bladder Q64.5
- bone Q79.9
- brain Q00.0
  - part of Q04.3
- breast (with nipple present) Q83.8
  - with absent nipple Q83.0
- bronchus Q32.4
- canaliculus lacrimalis Q10.4
- carpus — *see* Agenesis, hand
- cartilage Q79.9
- cecum Q42.8
- cerebellum Q04.3
- cervix Q51.5

Agenesis - *continued*
- chin Q18.8
- cilia Q10.3
- circulatory system, part NOS Q28.9
- clavicle Q74.0
- clitoris Q52.6
- coccyx Q76.49
- colon Q42.9
  - specified NEC Q42.8
- corpus callosum Q04.0
- cricoid cartilage Q31.8
- diaphragm (with hernia) Q79.1
- digestive organ (s) or tract (complete) (partial) NEC Q45.8
  - upper Q40.8
- ductus arteriosus Q28.8
- duodenum Q41.0
- ear Q16.9
  - auricle Q16.0
  - lobe Q17.8
- ejaculatory duct Q55.4
- endocrine (gland) NEC Q89.2
- epiglottis Q31.8
- esophagus Q39.8
- eustachian tube Q16.2
- eye Q11.1
  - adnexa Q15.8
- eyelid (fold) Q10.3
- face
  - bones NEC Q75.8
  - specified part NEC Q18.8
- fallopian tube Q50.6
- femur — *see* Defect, reduction, lower limb, longitudinal, femur
- fibula — *see* Defect, reduction, lower limb, longitudinal, fibula
- finger (complete) (partial) — *see* Agenesis, hand
- foot (and toes) (complete) (partial) Q72.3-
- forearm (with hand present) — *see* Agenesis, arm, with hand present
  - and hand Q71.2-
- gallbladder Q44.0
- gastric Q40.2
- genitalia, genital (organ (s))
  - female Q52.8
    - external Q52.71
    - internal NEC Q52.8
  - male Q55.8
- glottis Q31.8
- hair Q84.0
- hand (and fingers) (complete) (partial) Q71.3-
- heart Q24.8
  - valve NEC Q24.8
    - pulmonary Q22.0
- hepatic Q44.7
- humerus — *see* Defect, reduction, upper limb
- hymen Q52.4
- ileum Q41.2
- incus Q16.3
- intestine (small) Q41.9
  - large Q42.9
    - specified NEC Q42.8
- iris (dilator fibers) Q13.1
- jaw M26.09
- jejunum Q41.1
- kidney (s) (partial) Q60.2
  - bilateral Q60.1
  - unilateral Q60.0
- labium (majus) (minus) Q52.71
- labyrinth, membranous Q16.5
- lacrimal apparatus Q10.4
- larynx Q31.8
- leg (complete) Q72.0-
  - with foot present Q72.1-
  - lower leg (with foot present) — *see* Agenesis, leg, with foot present
    - and foot Q72.2-
- lens Q12.3
- limb (complete) Q73.0
  - lower — *see* Agenesis, leg
  - upper — *see* Agenesis, arm
- lip Q38.0
- liver Q44.7
- lung (fissure) (lobe) (bilateral) (unilateral) Q33.3
- mandible, maxilla M26.09
- metacarpus — *see* Agenesis, hand
- metatarsus — *see* Agenesis, foot
- muscle Q79.8
  - eyelid Q10.3
  - ocular Q15.8
- musculoskeletal system NEC Q79.8
- nail (s) Q84.3
- neck, part Q18.8

Agenesis - *continued*
- nerve Q07.8
- nervous system, part NEC Q07.8
- nipple Q83.2
- nose Q30.1
- nuclear Q07.8
- organ
  - of Corti Q16.5
  - or site not listed — *see* Anomaly, by site
- osseous meatus (ear) Q16.1
- ovary
  - bilateral Q50.02
  - unilateral Q50.01
- oviduct Q50.6
- pancreas Q45.0
- parathyroid (gland) Q89.2
- parotid gland (s) Q38.4
- patella Q74.1
- pelvic girdle (complete) (partial) Q74.2
- penis Q55.5
- pericardium Q24.8
- pituitary (gland) Q89.2
- prostate Q55.4
- punctum lacrimale Q10.4
- radioulnar — *see* Defect, reduction, upper limb
- radius — *see* Defect, reduction, upper limb, longitudinal, radius
- rectum Q42.1
  - with fistula Q42.0
- renal Q60.2
  - bilateral Q60.1
  - unilateral Q60.0
- respiratory organ NEC Q34.8
- rib Q76.6
- roof of orbit Q75.8
- round ligament Q52.8
- sacrum Q76.49
- salivary gland Q38.4
- scapula Q74.0
- scrotum Q55.29
- seminal vesicles Q55.4
- septum
  - atrial Q21.1
  - between aorta and pulmonary artery Q21.4
  - ventricular Q20.4
- shoulder girdle (complete) (partial) Q74.0
- skull (bone) Q75.8
  - with
    - anencephaly Q00.0
    - encephalocele — *see* Encephalocele
    - hydrocephalus Q03.9
      - with spina bifida — *see* Spina bifida, by site, with hydrocephalus
    - microcephaly Q02
- spermatic cord Q55.4
- spinal cord Q06.0
- spine Q76.49
- spleen Q89.01
- sternum Q76.7
- stomach Q40.2
- submaxillary gland (s) (congenital) Q38.4
- tarsus — *see* Agenesis, foot
- tendon Q79.8
- testicle Q55.0
- thymus (gland) Q89.2
- thyroid (gland) E03.1
  - cartilage Q31.8
- tibia — *see* Defect, reduction, lower limb, longitudinal, tibia
- tibiofibular — *see* Defect, reduction, lower limb, specified type NEC
- toe (and foot) (complete) (partial) — *see* Agenesis, foot
- tongue Q38.3
- trachea (cartilage) Q32.1
- ulna — *see* Defect, reduction, upper limb, longitudinal, ulna
- upper limb — *see* Agenesis, arm
- ureter Q62.4
- urethra Q64.5
- urinary tract NEC Q64.8
- uterus Q51.0
- uvula Q38.5
- vagina Q52.0
- vas deferens Q55.4
- vein (s) (peripheral) Q27.9
  - brain Q28.3
  - great NEC Q26.8
  - portal Q26.5
- vena cava (inferior) (superior) Q26.8
- vermis of cerebellum Q04.3
- vertebra Q76.49
- vulva Q52.71

Ageusia R43.2
Agitated — *see* condition
Agitation R45.1
Aglossia (congenital) Q38.3
Aglossia-adactylia syndrome Q87.0
Aglycogenosis E74.00
Agnosia (body image) (other senses) (tactile) R48.1
  developmental F88
  verbal R48.1
    auditory R48.1
      developmental F80.2
    developmental F80.2
  visual (object) R48.3
Agoraphobia F40.00
  with panic disorder F40.01
  without panic disorder F40.02
Agrammatism R48.8
Agranulocytopenia — *see* Agranulocytosis
Agranulocytosis (chronic) (cyclical) (genetic) (infantile) (periodic) (pernicious) — *see also* Neutropenia D70.9
  congenital D70.0
  cytoreductive cancer chemotherapy sequela D70.1
  drug-induced D70.2
    due to cytoreductive cancer chemotherapy D70.1
  due to infection D70.3
  secondary D70.4
    drug-induced D70.2
      due to cytoreductive cancer chemotherapy D70.1
Agraphia (absolute) R48.8
  with alexia R48.0
  developmental F81.81
Ague (dumb) — *see* Malaria
Agyria Q04.3
Ahumada-del Castillo syndrome E23.0
Aichomophobia F40.298
AIDS (related complex) B20
Ailment heart — *see* Disease, heart
Ailurophobia F40.218
AIN — *see* Neoplasia, intraepithelial, anal
Ainhum (disease) L94.6
AIPHI
  (acute idiopathic pulmonary hemorrhage in infants (over 28 days old) **)** R04.81
Air
  anterior mediastinum J98.2
  compressed, disease T70.3
  conditioner lung or pneumonitis J67.7
  embolism (artery) (cerebral) (any site) T79.0
    with ectopic or molar pregnancy O08.2
    due to implanted device NEC — *see* Complications, by site and type, specified NEC
    following
      abortion — *see* Abortion by type, complicated by, embolism
      ectopic or molar pregnancy O08.2
      infusion, therapeutic injection or transfusion T80.0
    in pregnancy, childbirth or puerperium — *see* Embolism, obstetric
    traumatic T79.0
  hunger, psychogenic F45.8
  rarefied, effects of — *see* Effect, adverse, high altitude
  sickness T75.3
Airplane sickness T75.3
Akathisia (drug-induced) (treatment-induced) G25.71
  neuroleptic induced (acute) G25.71
  tardive G25.71
Akinesia R29.898
Akinetic mutism R41.89
Akureyri's disease G93.3
Alactasia, congenital E73.0
Alagille's syndrome Q44.7
Alastrim B03
Albers-Schönberg syndrome Q78.2
Albert's syndrome — *see* Tendinitis, Achilles
Albinism, albino E70.30
  with hematologic abnormality E70.339
    Chédiak-Higashi syndrome E70.330
    Hermansky-Pudlak syndrome E70.331
    other specified E70.338
  I E70.320
  II E70.321
  ocular E70.319
    autosomal recessive E70.311
    other specified E70.318
    X-linked E70.310
  oculocutaneous E70.329
    other specified E70.328
    tyrosinase (ty) negative E70.320
    tyrosinase (ty) positive E70.321
  other specified E70.39
Albinismus E70.30
Albright (-McCune) (-Sternberg) **syndrome** Q78.1
Albuminous — *see* condition
Albuminuria, albuminuric (acute) (chronic) (subacute) — *see also* Proteinuria R80.9
  complicating pregnancy — *see* Proteinuria, gestational
    with
      gestational hypertension — *see* Pre-eclampsia
      pre-existing hypertension — *see* Hypertension, complicating pregnancy, pre-existing, with, pre-eclampsia
  gestational — *see* Proteinuria, gestational
    with
      gestational hypertension — *see* Pre-eclampsia
      pre-existing hypertension — *see* Hypertension, complicating pregnancy, pre-existing, with, pre-eclampsia
  orthostatic R80.2
  postural R80.2
  pre-eclamptic — *see* Pre-eclampsia
  scarlatinal A38.8
Albuminurophobia F40.298
Alcaptonuria E70.29
Alcohol, alcoholic, alcohol-induced
  addiction (without remission) F10.20
    with remission F10.21
  amnestic disorder, persisting F10.96
    with dependence F10.26
  anxiety disorder F10.980
  bipolar and related disorder F10.94
  depressive disorder F10.94
  major neurocognitive disorder, amnestic-confabulatory type F10.96
  major neurocognitive disorder, nonamnestic-confabulatory type F10.97
  mild neurocognitive disorder F10.988
  psychotic disorder F10.959
  sexual dysfunction F10.981
  sleep disorder F10.982
  brain syndrome, chronic F10.97
    with dependence F10.27
  cardiopathy I42.6
  counseling and surveillance Z71.41
    family member Z71.42
  delirium (acute) (tremens) (withdrawal) F10.231
    with intoxication F10.921
      in
        abuse F10.121
        dependence F10.221
  dementia F10.97
    with dependence F10.27
  deterioration F10.97
    with dependence F10.27
  hallucinosis (acute) F10.951
    in
      abuse F10.151
      dependence F10.251
  insanity F10.959
  intoxication (acute) (without dependence) F10.129
    with
      delirium F10.121
      dependence F10.229
        with delirium F10.221
        uncomplicated F10.220
    uncomplicated F10.120
  jealousy F10.988
  Korsakoff's, Korsakov's, Korsakow's F10.26
  liver K70.9
    acute — *see* Disease, liver, alcoholic, hepatitis
  mania (acute) (chronic) F10.959
  paranoia, paranoid (type) psychosis F10.950
  pellagra E52
  poisoning, accidental (acute) NEC — *see* Table of Drugs and Chemicals, alcohol, poisoning
  psychosis — *see* Psychosis, alcoholic
  withdrawal (without convulsions) F10.239
    with delirium F10.231
Alcoholism (chronic) (without remission) F10.20
  with
    psychosis — *see* Psychosis, alcoholic
    remission F10.21
  Korsakov's F10.96
    with dependence F10.26
Alder (-Reilly) **anomaly or syndrome** (leukocyte granulation) D72.0
Aldosteronism E26.9
  familial (type I) E26.02
  glucocorticoid-remediable E26.02
  primary (due to (bilateral) adrenal hyperplasia) E26.09
  primary NEC E26.09
  secondary E26.1
Aldosteronism - *continued*
  specified NEC E26.89
Aldosteronoma D44.10
Aldrich (-Wiskott) **syndrome** (eczema-thrombocytopenia) D82.0
Alektorophobia F40.218
Aleppo boil B55.1
Aleukemic — *see* condition
Aleukia
  congenital D70.0
  hemorrhagica D61.9
    congenital D61.09
  splenica D73.1
Alexia R48.0
  developmental F81.0
  secondary to organic lesion R48.0
Algoneurodystrophy M89.00
  ankle M89.07-
  foot M89.07-
  forearm M89.03-
  hand M89.04-
  lower leg M89.06-
  multiple sites M89.0-
  shoulder M89.01-
  specified site NEC M89.08
  thigh M89.05-
  upper arm M89.02-
Algophobia F40.298
Alienation, mental — *see* Psychosis
Alkalemia E87.3
Alkalosis E87.3
  metabolic E87.3
    with respiratory acidosis E87.4
    of newborn P74.41
  respiratory E87.3
Alkaptonuria E70.29
Allen-Masters syndrome N83.8
Allergy, allergic (reaction) (to) T78.40
  air-borne substance NEC (rhinitis) J30.89
  alveolitis (extrinsic) J67.9
    due to
      Aspergillus clavatus J67.4
      Cryptostroma corticale J67.6
      organisms (fungal, thermophilic actinomycete) growing in ventilation (air conditioning) systems J67.7
    specified type NEC J67.8
  anaphylactic reaction or shock T78.2
  angioneurotic edema T78.3
  animal (dander) (epidermal) (hair) (rhinitis) J30.81
  bee sting (anaphylactic shock) — *see* Toxicity, venom, arthropod, bee
  biological — *see* Allergy, drug
  colitis — *see also* Colitis, allergic K52.29
  dander (animal) (rhinitis) J30.81
  dandruff (rhinitis) J30.81
  dental restorative material (existing) K08.55
  dermatitis — *see* Dermatitis, contact, allergic
  diathesis — *see* History, allergy
  drug, medicament & biological (any) (external) (internal) T78.40
    correct substance properly administered — *see* Table of Drugs and Chemicals, by drug, adverse effect
    wrong substance given or taken NEC (by accident) — *see* Table of Drugs and Chemicals, by drug, poisoning
  due to pollen J30.1
  dust (house) (stock) (rhinitis) J30.89
    with asthma — *see* Asthma, allergic extrinsic
  eczema — *see* Dermatitis, contact, allergic
  epidermal (animal) (rhinitis) J30.81
  feathers (rhinitis) J30.89
  food (any) (ingested) NEC T78.1
    anaphylactic shock — *see* Shock, anaphylactic, due to food
    dermatitis — *see* Dermatitis, due to, food
    dietary counseling and surveillance Z71.3
    in contact with skin L23.6
    rhinitis J30.5
    status (without reaction) Z91.018
      eggs Z91.012
      milk products Z91.011
      peanuts Z91.010
      seafood Z91.013
      specified NEC Z91.018
  gastrointestinal — *see also* specific type of allergic reaction
    meaning colitis — *see also* Colitis, allergic K52.29
    meaning gastroenteritis — *see also* Gastroenteritis, allergic K52.29
    meaning other adverse food reaction not elsewhere classified T78.1

Allergy, allergic (reaction) (to) - *continued*
  grain J30.1
  grass (hay fever) (pollen) J30.1
    asthma — *see* Asthma, allergic extrinsic
  hair (animal) (rhinitis) J30.81
  history (of) — *see* History, allergy
  horse serum — *see* Allergy, serum
  inhalant (rhinitis) J30.89
    pollen J30.1
  kapok (rhinitis) J30.89
  medicine — *see* Allergy, drug
  milk protein — *see also* Allergy, food Z91.011
    anaphylactic reaction T78.07
    dermatitis L27.2
    enterocolitis syndrome K52.21
    enteropathy K52.22
    gastroenteritis K52.29
    gastroesophageal reflux — *see also* Reaction, adverse, food K21.9
      with esophagitis K21.0
    proctocolitis K52.82
  nasal, seasonal due to pollen J30.1
  pneumonia J82
  pollen (any) (hay fever) J30.1
    asthma — *see* Asthma, allergic extrinsic
  primrose J30.1
  primula J30.1
  proctocolitis K52.82
  purpura D69.0
  ragweed (hay fever) (pollen) J30.1
    asthma — *see* Asthma, allergic extrinsic
  rose (pollen) J30.1
  seasonal NEC J30.2
  Senecio jacobae (pollen) J30.1
  serum — *see also* Reaction, serum T80.69
    anaphylactic shock T80.59
  shock (anaphylactic) T78.2
    due to
      administration of blood and blood products T80.51
      adverse effect of correct medicinal substance properly administered T88.6
      immunization T80.52
      serum NEC T80.59
      vaccination T80.52
  specific NEC T78.49
  tree (any) (hay fever) (pollen) J30.1
    asthma — *see* Asthma, allergic extrinsic
  upper respiratory J30.9
  urticaria L50.0
  vaccine — *see* Allergy, serum
  wheat — *see* Allergy, food
Allescheriasis B48.2
Alligator skin disease Q80.9
Allocheiria, allochiria R20.8
Almeida's disease — *see* Paracoccidioidomycosis
Alopecia (hereditaria) (seborrheica) L65.9
  androgenic L64.9
    drug-induced L64.0
    specified NEC L64.8
  areata L63.9
    ophiasis L63.2
    specified NEC L63.8
    totalis L63.0
    universalis L63.1
  cicatricial L66.9
    specified NEC L66.8
  circumscripta L63.9
  congenital, congenitalis Q84.0
  due to cytotoxic drugs NEC L65.8
  mucinosa L65.2
  postinfective NEC L65.8
  postpartum L65.0
  premature L64.8
  specific (syphilitic) A51.32
  specified NEC L65.8
  syphilitic (secondary) A51.32
  totalis (capitis) L63.0
  universalis (entire body) L63.1
  X-ray L58.1
Alpers' disease G31.81
Alpine sickness T70.29
Alport syndrome Q87.81
ALTE (apparent life threatening event)
  in newborn and infant R68.13
Alteration (of) **, Altered**
  awareness
    transient R40.4
    unintended under general anesthesia, during procedureT88.53
  mental status R41.82
  pattern of family relationships affecting child Z62.898

Alteration (of) **, Altered** - *continued*
  sensation
    following
      cerebrovascular disease I69.998
        cerebral infarction I69.398
        intracerebral hemorrhage I69.198
        nontraumatic intracranial hemorrhage NEC I69.298
        specified disease NEC I69.898
        subarachnoid hemorrhage I69.098
Alternating — *see* condition
Altitude, high (effects) — *see* Effect, adverse, high altitude
Aluminosis (of lung) J63.0
Alveolitis
  allergic (extrinsic) — *see* Pneumonitis, hypersensitivity
  due to
    Aspergillus clavatus J67.4
    Cryptostroma corticale J67.6
  fibrosing (cryptogenic) (idiopathic) J84.112
  jaw M27.3
  sicca dolorosa M27.3
Alveolus, alveolar — *see* condition
Alymphocytosis D72.810
  thymic (with immunodeficiency) D82.1
Alymphoplasia, thymic D82.1
Alzheimer's disease or sclerosis — *see* Disease, Alzheimer's
Amastia (with nipple present) Q83.8
  with absent nipple Q83.0
Amathophobia F40.228
Amaurosis (acquired) (congenital) — *see also* Blindness
  fugax G45.3
  hysterical F44.6
  Leber's congenital H35.50
  uremic — *see* Uremia
Amaurotic idiocy (infantile) (juvenile) (late) E75.4
Amaxophobia F40.248
Ambiguous genitalia Q56.4
Amblyopia (congenital) (ex anopsia) (partial) (suppression) H53.00-
  anisometropic — *see* Amblyopia, refractive
  deprivation H53.01-
  hysterical F44.6
  nocturnal — *see also* Blindness, night
    vitamin A deficiency E50.5
  refractive H53.02-
  strabismic H53.03-
  suspect H53.04-
  tobacco H53.8
  toxic NEC H53.8
  uremic — *see* Uremia
Ameba, amebic (histolytica) — *see also* Amebiasis
  abscess (liver) A06.4
Amebiasis A06.9
  with abscess — *see* Abscess, amebic
  acute A06.0
  chronic (intestine) A06.1
    with abscess — *see* Abscess, amebic
  cutaneous A06.7
  cutis A06.7
  cystitis A06.81
  genitourinary tract NEC A06.82
  hepatic — *see* Abscess, liver, amebic
  intestine A06.0
  nondysenteric colitis A06.2
  skin A06.7
  specified site NEC A06.89
Ameboma (of intestine) A06.3
Amelia Q73.0
  lower limb — *see* Agenesis, leg
  upper limb — *see* Agenesis, arm
Ameloblastoma — *see also* Cyst, calcifying odontogenic
  long bones C40.9-
    lower limb C40.2-
    upper limb C40.0-
  malignant C41.1
    jaw (bone) (lower) C41.1
      upper C41.0
  tibial C40.2-
Amelogenesis imperfecta K00.5
  nonhereditaria (segmentalis) K00.4
Amenorrhea N91.2
  hyperhormonal E28.8
  primary N91.0
  secondary N91.1
Amentia — *see* Disability, intellectual
  Meynert's (nonalcoholic) F04
American
  leishmaniasis B55.2

American - *continued*
  mountain tick fever A93.2
Ametropia — *see* Disorder, refraction
AMH (asymptomatic microscopic hematuria) R31.21
Amianthosis J61
Amimia R48.8
Amino-acid disorder E72.9
  anemia D53.0
Aminoacidopathy E72.9
Aminoaciduria E72.9
Amnes (t) **ic syndrome** (post-traumatic) F04
  induced by
    alcohol F10.96
      with dependence F10.26
    psychoactive NEC F19.96
      with
        abuse F19.16
        dependence F19.26
    sedative F13.96
      with dependence F13.26
Amnesia R41.3
  anterograde R41.1
  auditory R48.8
  dissociative F44.0
    with dissociative fugue F44.1
  hysterical F44.0
  postictal in epilepsy — *see* Epilepsy
  psychogenic F44.0
  retrograde R41.2
  transient global G45.4
Amnion, amniotic — *see* condition
Amnionitis — *see* Pregnancy, complicated by
Amok F68.8
Amoral traits F60.89
Amphetamine (or other stimulant) **-induced**
  anxiety disorder F15.980
  bipolar and related disorder F15.94
  delirium F15.921
  depressive disorder F15.94
  obsessive-compulsive and related disorder F15.988
  psychotic disorder F15.959
  sexual dysfunction F15.981
  sleep disorder F15.982
  stimulant withdrawal F15.23
Ampulla
  lower esophagus K22.8
  phrenic K22.8
Amputation — *see also* Absence, by site, acquired
  neuroma (postoperative) (traumatic) — *see* Complications, amputation stump, neuroma
  stump (surgical)
    abnormal, painful, or with complication (late) — *see* Complications, amputation stump
    healed or old NOS Z89.9
  traumatic (complete) (partial)
    arm (upper) (complete) S48.91-
      at
        elbow S58.01-
          partial S58.02-
        shoulder joint (complete) S48.01-
          partial S48.02-
      between
        elbow and wrist (complete) S58.11-
          partial S58.12-
        shoulder and elbow (complete) S48.11-
          partial S48.12-
      partial S48.92-
    breast (complete) S28.21-
      partial S28.22-
    clitoris (complete) S38.211
      partial S38.212
    ear (complete) S08.11-
      partial S08.12-
    finger (complete) (metacarpophalangeal) S68.11-
      index S68.11-
      little S68.11-
      middle S68.11-
      partial S68.12-
        index S68.12-
        little S68.12-
        middle S68.12-
        ring S68.12-
      ring S68.11-
      thumb — *see* Amputation, traumatic, thumb
      transphalangeal (complete) S68.61-
        index S68.61-
        little S68.61-
        middle S68.61-
        partial S68.62-
          index S68.62-
          little S68.62-
          middle S68.62-
          ring S68.62-

Amputation - *continued*
  traumatic (complete) (partial) - *continued*
    finger (complete) (metacarpophalangeal) - *continued*
      transphalangeal (complete) - *continued*
        ring S68.61-
    foot (complete) S98.91-
      at ankle level S98.01-
        partial S98.02-
      midfoot S98.31-
        partial S98.32-
      partial S98.92-
    forearm (complete) S58.91-
      at elbow level (complete) S58.01-
        partial S58.02-
      between elbow and wrist (complete) S58.11-
        partial S58.12-
      partial S58.92-
    genital organ (s) (external)
      female (complete) S38.211
        partial S38.212
      male
        penis (complete) S38.221
          partial S38.222
        scrotum (complete) S38.231
          partial S38.232
        testes (complete) S38.231
          partial S38.232
    hand (complete) (wrist level) S68.41-
      finger (s) alone — *see* Amputation, traumatic, finger
      partial S68.42-
      thumb alone — *see* Amputation, traumatic, thumb
      transmetacarpal (complete) S68.71-
        partial S68.72-
    head
      ear — *see* Amputation, traumatic, ear
      nose (partial) S08.812
        complete S08.811
      part S08.89
        scalp S08.0
    hip (and thigh) (complete) S78.91-
      at hip joint (complete) S78.01-
        partial S78.02-
      between hip and knee (complete) S78.11-
        partial S78.12-
      partial S78.92-
    labium (majus) (minus) (complete) S38.21-
      partial S38.21-
    leg (lower) S88.91-
      at knee level S88.01-
        partial S88.02-
      between knee and ankle S88.11-
        partial S88.12-
      partial S88.92-
    nose (partial) S08.812
      complete S08.811
    penis (complete) S38.221
      partial S38.222
    scrotum (complete) S38.231
      partial S38.232
    shoulder — *see* Amputation, traumatic, arm
      at shoulder joint — *see* Amputation, traumatic, arm, at shoulder joint
    testes (complete) S38.231
      partial S38.232
    thigh — *see* Amputation, traumatic, hip
    thorax, part of S28.1
      breast — *see* Amputation, traumatic, breast
    thumb (complete) (metacarpophalangeal) S68.01-
      partial S68.02-
      transphalangeal (complete) S68.51-
        partial S68.52-
    toe (lesser) S98.13-
      great S98.11-
        partial S98.12-
      more than one S98.21-
        partial S98.22-
      partial S98.14-
    vulva (complete) S38.211
      partial S38.212
Amputee (bilateral) (old) Z89.9
Amsterdam dwarfism Q87.1
Amusia R48.8
  developmental F80.89
Amyelencephalus, amyelencephaly Q00.0
Amyelia Q06.0
Amygdalitis — *see* Tonsillitis
Amygdalolith J35.8
Amyloid heart (disease) E85.4 *[I43]*
Amyloidosis (generalized) (primary) E85.9
  with lung involvement E85.4 *[J99]*
Amyloidosis (generalized) (primary) - *continued*
  familial E85.2
  genetic E85.2
  heart E85.4 *[I43]*
  hemodialysis-associated E85.3
  light chain (AL) E85.81
  liver E85.4 *[K77]*
  localized E85.4
  neuropathic heredofamilial E85.1
  non-neuropathic heredofamilial E85.0
  organ limited E85.4
  Portuguese E85.1
  pulmonary E85.4 *[J99]*
  secondary systemic E85.3
  senile systemic (SSA) E85.82
  skin (lichen) (macular) E85.4 *[L99]*
  specified NEC E85.89
  subglottic E85.4 *[J99]*
  wild-type transthyretin-related (ATTR) E85.82
Amylopectinosis (brancher enzyme deficiency) E74.03
Amylophagia — *see* Pica
Amyoplasia congenita Q79.8
Amyotonia M62.89
  congenita G70.2
Amyotrophia, amyotrophy, amyotrophic G71.8
  congenita Q79.8
  diabetic — *see* Diabetes, amyotrophy
  lateral sclerosis G12.21
  neuralgic G54.5
  spinal progressive G12.25
Anacidity, gastric K31.83
  psychogenic F45.8
Anaerosis of newborn P28.89
Analbuminemia E88.09
Analgesia — *see* Anesthesia
Analphalipoproteinemia E78.6
Anaphylactic
  purpura D69.0
  shock or reaction — *see* Shock, anaphylactic
Anaphylactoid shock or reaction — *see* Shock, anaphylactic
Anaphylactoid syndrome of pregnancy O88.01-
Anaphylaxis — *see* Shock, anaphylactic
Anaplasia cervix — *see also* Dysplasia, cervix N87.9
Anaplasmosis, human A77.49
Anarthria R47.1
Anasarca R60.1
  cardiac — *see* Failure, heart, congestive
  lung J18.2
  newborn P83.2
  nutritional E43
  pulmonary J18.2
  renal N04.9
Anastomosis
  aneurysmal — *see* Aneurysm
  arteriovenous ruptured brain I60.8
  intestinal K63.89
    complicated NEC K91.89
      involving urinary tract N99.89
  retinal and choroidal vessels (congenital) Q14.8
Anatomical narrow angle H40.03-
Ancylostoma, ancylostomiasis (braziliense) (caninum) (ceylanicum) (duodenale) B76.0
  Necator americanus B76.1
Andersen's disease (glycogen storage) E74.09
Anderson-Fabry disease E75.21
Andes disease T70.29
Andrews' disease (bacterid) L08.89
Androblastoma
  benign
    specified site — *see* Neoplasm, benign, by site
    unspecified site
      female D27.9
      male D29.20
  malignant
    specified site — *see* Neoplasm, malignant, by site
    unspecified site
      female C56.9
      male C62.90
  specified site — *see* Neoplasm, uncertain behavior, by site
  tubular
    with lipid storage
      specified site — *see* Neoplasm, benign, by site
      unspecified site
        female D27.9
        male D29.20
    specified site — *see* Neoplasm, benign, by site
    unspecified site
      female D27.9
      male D29.20
  unspecified site
Androblastoma - *continued*
  unspecified site - *continued*
    female D39.10
    male D40.10
Androgen insensitivity syndrome — *see also* Syndrome, androgen insensitivity E34.50
Androgen resistance syndrome — *see also* Syndrome, androgen insensitivity E34.50
Android pelvis Q74.2
  with disproportion (fetopelvic) O33.3
    causing obstructed labor O65.3
Androphobia F40.290
Anectasis, pulmonary (newborn) — *see* Atelectasis
Anemia (essential) (general) (hemoglobin deficiency) (infantile) (primary) (profound) D64.9
  with (due to) (in)
    disorder of
      anaerobic glycolysis D55.2
      pentose phosphate pathway D55.1
    koilonychia D50.9
  achlorhydric D50.8
  achrestic D53.1
  Addison (-Biermer) (pernicious) D51.0
  agranulocytic — *see* Agranulocytosis
  amino-acid-deficiency D53.0
  aplastic D61.9
    congenital D61.09
    drug-induced D61.1
    due to
      drugs D61.1
      external agents NEC D61.2
      infection D61.2
      radiation D61.2
    idiopathic D61.3
    red cell (pure) D60.9
      chronic D60.0
      congenital D61.01
      specified type NEC D60.8
      transient D60.1
    specified type NEC D61.89
    toxic D61.2
  aregenerative
    congenital D61.09
  asiderotic D50.9
  atypical (primary) D64.9
  Baghdad spring D55.0
  Balantidium coli A07.0
  Biermer's (pernicious) D51.0
  blood loss (chronic) D50.0
    acute D62
  bothriocephalus B70.0 *[D63.8]*
  brickmaker's B76.9 *[D63.8]*
  cerebral I67.89
  childhood D58.9
  chlorotic D50.8
  chronic
    blood loss D50.0
    hemolytic D58.9
      idiopathic D59.9
    simple D53.9
  chronica congenita aregenerativa D61.09
  combined system disease NEC D51.0 *[G32.0]*
    due to dietary vitamin B12 deficiency D51.3 *[G32.0]*
  complicating pregnancy, childbirth or puerperium — *see* Pregnancy, complicated by (management affected by), anemia
  congenital P61.4
    aplastic D61.09
    due to isoimmunization NOS P55.9
    dyserythropoietic, dyshematopoietic D64.4
    following fetal blood loss P61.3
    Heinz body D58.2
    hereditary hemolytic NOS D58.9
    pernicious D51.0
    spherocytic D58.0
  Cooley's (erythroblastic) D56.1
  cytogenic D51.0
  deficiency D53.9
    2, 3 diphosphoglycurate mutase D55.2
    2, 3 PG D55.2
    6 phosphogluconate dehydrogenase D55.1
    6-PGD D55.1
    amino-acid D53.0
    combined B12 and folate D53.1
    enzyme D55.9
      drug-induced (hemolytic) D59.2
      glucose-6-phosphate dehydrogenase (G6PD) D55.0
      glycolytic D55.2
      nucleotide metabolism D55.3
      related to hexose monophosphate (HMP) shunt pathway NEC D55.1

- **Anemia** (essential) (general) (hemoglobin deficiency) (infantile) (primary) (profound) - *continued*
  - deficiency - *continued*
    - enzyme - *continued*
      - specified type NEC D55.8
    - erythrocytic glutathione D55.1
    - folate D52.9
      - dietary D52.0
      - drug-induced D52.1
    - folic acid D52.9
      - dietary D52.0
      - drug-induced D52.1
    - G SH D55.1
    - GGS-R D55.1
    - glucose-6-phosphate dehydrogenase D55.0
    - glutathione reductase D55.1
    - glyceraldehyde phosphate dehydrogenase D55.2
    - G6PD D55.0
    - hexokinase D55.2
    - iron D50.9
      - secondary to blood loss (chronic) D50.0
    - nutritional D53.9
      - with
        - poor iron absorption D50.8
        - specified deficiency NEC D53.8
    - phosphofructo-aldolase D55.2
    - phosphoglycerate kinase D55.2
    - PK D55.2
    - protein D53.0
    - pyruvate kinase D55.2
    - transcobalamin II D51.2
    - triose-phosphate isomerase D55.2
    - vitamin B12 NOS D51.9
      - dietary D51.3
      - due to
        - intrinsic factor deficiency D51.0
        - selective vitamin B12 malabsorption with proteinuria D51.1
      - pernicious D51.0
      - specified type NEC D51.8
  - Diamond-Blackfan (congenital hypoplastic) D61.01
  - dibothriocephalus B70.0 *[D63.8]*
  - dimorphic D53.1
  - diphasic D53.1
  - Diphyllobothrium (Dibothriocephalus) B70.0 *[D63.8]*
  - due to (in) (with)
    - antineoplastic chemotherapy D64.81
    - blood loss (chronic) D50.0
      - acute D62
    - chemotherapy, antineoplastic D64.81
    - chronic disease classified elsewhere NEC D63.8
    - chronic kidney disease D63.1
    - deficiency
      - amino-acid D53.0
      - copper D53.8
      - folate (folic acid) D52.9
        - dietary D52.0
        - drug-induced D52.1
      - molybdenum D53.8
      - protein D53.0
      - zinc D53.8
    - dietary vitamin B12 deficiency D51.3
    - disorder of
      - glutathione metabolism D55.1
      - nucleotide metabolism D55.3
    - drug — *see* Anemia, by type — *see also* Table of Drugs and Chemicals
    - end stage renal disease D63.1
    - enzyme disorder D55.9
    - fetal blood loss P61.3
    - fish tapeworm (D.latum) infestation B70.0 *[D63.8]*
    - hemorrhage (chronic) D50.0
      - acute D62
    - impaired absorption D50.9
    - loss of blood (chronic) D50.0
      - acute D62
    - myxedema E03.9 *[D63.8]*
    - Necator americanus B76.1 *[D63.8]*
    - prematurity P61.2
    - selective vitamin B12 malabsorption with proteinuria D51.1
    - transcobalamin II deficiency D51.2
  - Dyke-Young type (secondary) (symptomatic) D59.1
  - dyserythropoietic (congenital) D64.4
  - dyshematopoietic (congenital) D64.4
  - Egyptian B76.9 *[D63.8]*
  - elliptocytosis — *see* Elliptocytosis
  - enzyme-deficiency, drug-induced D59.2
  - epidemic — *see also* Ancylostomiasis B76.9 *[D63.8]*
  - erythroblastic
    - familial D56.1

- **Anemia** (essential) (general) (hemoglobin deficiency) (infantile) (primary) (profound) - *continued*
  - erythroblastic - *continued*
    - newborn — *see also* Disease, hemolytic P55.9
    - of childhood D56.1
  - erythrocytic glutathione deficiency D55.1
  - erythropoietin-resistant anemia (EPO resistant anemia) D63.1
  - Faber's (achlorhydric anemia) D50.9
  - factitious (self-induced blood letting) D50.0
  - familial erythroblastic D56.1
  - Fanconi's (congenital pancytopenia) D61.09
  - favism D55.0
  - fish tapeworm (D. latum) infestation B70.0 *[D63.8]*
  - folate (folic acid) deficiency D52.9
  - glucose-6-phosphate dehydrogenase (G6PD) deficiency D55.0
  - glutathione-reductase deficiency D55.1
  - goat's milk D52.0
  - granulocytic — *see* Agranulocytosis
  - Heinz body, congenital D58.2
  - hemolytic D58.9
    - acquired D59.9
      - with hemoglobinuria NEC D59.6
      - autoimmune NEC D59.1
      - infectious D59.4
      - specified type NEC D59.8
      - toxic D59.4
    - acute D59.9
      - due to enzyme deficiency specified type NEC D55.8
      - Lederer's D59.1
    - autoimmune D59.1
      - drug-induced D59.0
    - chronic D58.9
      - idiopathic D59.9
    - cold type (secondary) (symptomatic) D59.1
    - congenital (spherocytic) — *see* Spherocytosis
    - due to
      - cardiac conditions D59.4
      - drugs (nonautoimmune) D59.2
        - autoimmune D59.0
      - enzyme disorder D55.9
        - drug-induced D59.2
      - presence of shunt or other internal prosthetic device D59.4
    - familial D58.9
    - hereditary D58.9
      - due to enzyme disorder D55.9
        - specified type NEC D55.8
      - specified type NEC D58.8
    - idiopathic (chronic) D59.9
    - mechanical D59.4
    - microangiopathic D59.4
    - nonautoimmune D59.4
      - drug-induced D59.2
    - nonspherocytic
      - congenital or hereditary NEC D55.8
        - glucose-6-phosphate dehydrogenase deficiency D55.0
        - pyruvate kinase deficiency D55.2
        - type
          - I D55.1
          - II D55.2
      - type
        - I D55.1
        - II D55.2
    - secondary D59.4
      - autoimmune D59.1
    - specified (hereditary) type NEC D58.8
    - Stransky-Regala type — *see also* Hemoglobinopathy D58.8
    - symptomatic D59.4
      - autoimmune D59.1
    - toxic D59.4
    - warm type (secondary) (symptomatic) D59.1
  - hemorrhagic (chronic) D50.0
    - acute D62
  - Herrick's D57.1
  - hexokinase deficiency D55.2
  - hookworm B76.9 *[D63.8]*
  - hypochromic (idiopathic) (microcytic) (normoblastic) D50.9
    - due to blood loss (chronic) D50.0
      - acute D62
    - familial sex-linked D64.0
    - pyridoxine-responsive D64.3
    - sideroblastic, sex-linked D64.0
  - hypoplasia, red blood cells D61.9
    - congenital or familial D61.01
  - hypoplastic (idiopathic) D61.9
    - congenital or familial (of childhood) D61.01
  - hypoproliferative (refractive) D61.9

- **Anemia** (essential) (general) (hemoglobin deficiency) (infantile) (primary) (profound) - *continued*
  - idiopathic D64.9
    - aplastic D61.3
    - hemolytic, chronic D59.9
  - in (due to) (with)
    - chronic kidney disease D63.1
    - end stage renal disease D63.1
    - failure, kidney (renal) D63.1
    - neoplastic disease — *see also* Neoplasm D63.0
  - intertropical — *see also* Ancylostomiasis D63.8
  - iron deficiency D50.9
    - secondary to blood loss (chronic) D50.0
      - acute D62
    - specified type NEC D50.8
  - Joseph-Diamond-Blackfan (congenital hypoplastic) D61.01
  - Lederer's (hemolytic) D59.1
  - leukoerythroblastic D61.82
  - macrocytic D53.9
    - nutritional D52.0
    - tropical D52.8
  - malarial — *see also* Malaria B54 *[D63.8]*
  - malignant (progressive) D51.0
  - malnutrition D53.9
  - marsh — *see also* Malaria B54 *[D63.8]*
  - Mediterranean (with other hemoglobinopathy) D56.9
  - megaloblastic D53.1
    - combined B12 and folate deficiency D53.1
    - hereditary D51.1
    - nutritional D52.0
    - orotic aciduria D53.0
    - refractory D53.1
    - specified type NEC D53.1
  - megalocytic D53.1
  - microcytic (hypochromic) D50.9
    - due to blood loss (chronic) D50.0
      - acute D62
    - familial D56.8
  - microdrepanocytosis D57.40
  - microelliptopoikilocytic (Rietti-Greppi-Micheli) D56.9
  - miner's B76.9 *[D63.8]*
  - myelodysplastic D46.9
  - myelofibrosis D75.81
  - myelogenous D64.89
  - myelopathic D64.89
  - myelophthisic D61.82
  - myeloproliferative D47.Z9
  - newborn P61.4
    - due to
      - ABO (antibodies, isoimmunization, maternal/fetal incompatibility) P55.1
      - Rh (antibodies, isoimmunization, maternal/fetal incompatibility) P55.0
    - following fetal blood loss P61.3
    - posthemorrhagic (fetal) P61.3
  - nonspherocytic hemolytic — *see* Anemia, hemolytic, nonspherocytic
  - normocytic (infectional) D64.9
    - due to blood loss (chronic) D50.0
      - acute D62
    - myelophthisic D61.82
  - nutritional (deficiency) D53.9
    - with
      - poor iron absorption D50.8
      - specified deficiency NEC D53.8
    - megaloblastic D52.0
  - of prematurity P61.2
  - orotaciduric (congenital) (hereditary) D53.0
  - osteosclerotic D64.89
  - ovalocytosis (hereditary) — *see* Elliptocytosis
  - paludal — *see also* Malaria B54 *[D63.8]*
  - pernicious (congenital) (malignant) (progressive) D51.0
  - pleochromic D64.89
    - of sprue D52.8
  - posthemorrhagic (chronic) D50.0
    - acute D62
    - newborn P61.3
  - postoperative (postprocedural)
    - due to (acute) blood loss D62
      - chronic blood loss D50.0
    - specified NEC D64.9
  - postpartum O90.81
  - pressure D64.89
  - progressive D64.9
    - malignant D51.0
    - pernicious D51.0
  - protein-deficiency D53.0
  - pseudoleukemica infantum D64.89
  - pure red cell D60.9

Anemia (essential) (general) (hemoglobin deficiency) (infantile) (primary) (profound) - *continued*
  pure red cell - *continued*
    congenital D61.01
  pyridoxine-responsive D64.3
  pyruvate kinase deficiency D55.2
  refractory D46.4
    with
      excess of blasts D46.20
        1 (RAEB 1) D46.21
        2 (RAEB 2) D46.22
        in transformation (RAEB T) — *see* Leukemia, acute myeloblastic
      hemochromatosis D46.1
      sideroblasts (ring) (RARS) D46.1
    megaloblastic D53.1
    sideroblastic D46.1
    sideropenic D50.9
    without ring sideroblasts, so stated D46.0
    without sideroblasts without excess of blasts D46.0
  Rietti-Greppi-Micheli D56.9
  scorbutic D53.2
  secondary to
    blood loss (chronic) D50.0
      acute D62
    hemorrhage (chronic) D50.0
      acute D62
  semiplastic D61.89
  sickle-cell — *see* Disease, sickle-cell
  sideroblastic D64.3
    hereditary D64.0
    hypochromic, sex-linked D64.0
    pyridoxine-responsive NEC D64.3
    refractory D46.1
    secondary (due to)
      disease D64.1
      drugs and toxins D64.2
    specified type NEC D64.3
  sideropenic (refractory) D50.9
    due to blood loss (chronic) D50.0
      acute D62
  simple chronic D53.9
  specified type NEC D64.89
  spherocytic (hereditary) — *see* Spherocytosis
  splenic D64.89
  splenomegalic D64.89
  stomatocytosis D58.8
  syphilitic (acquired) (late) A52.79 *[D63.8]*
  target cell D64.89
  thalassemia D56.9
  thrombocytopenic — *see* Thrombocytopenia
  toxic D61.2
  tropical B76.9 *[D63.8]*
    macrocytic D52.8
  tuberculous A18.89 *[D63.8]*
  vegan D51.3
  vitamin
    B6-responsive D64.3
    B12 deficiency (dietary) pernicious D51.0
  von Jaksch's D64.89
  Witts' (achlorhydric anemia) D50.8
Anemophobia F40.228
Anencephalus, anencephaly Q00.0
Anergasia — *see* Psychosis, organic
Anesthesia, anesthetic R20.0
  complication or reaction NEC — *see also* Complications, anesthesia T88.59
  due to
    correct substance properly administered — *see* Table of Drugs and Chemicals, by drug, adverse effect
    overdose or wrong substance given — *see* Table of Drugs and Chemicals, by drug, poisoning
    unintended awareness under general anesthesia during procedure T88.53
    personal history of Z92.84
  cornea H18.81-
  dissociative F44.6
  functional (hysterical) F44.6
  hyperesthetic, thalamic G89.0
  hysterical F44.6
  local skin lesion R20.0
  sexual (psychogenic) F52.1
  shock (due to) T88.2
  skin R20.0
  testicular N50.9
Anetoderma (maculosum) (of) L90.8
  Jadassohn-Pellizzari L90.2
  Schweniger-Buzzi L90.1
Aneurin deficiency E51.9
Aneurysm (anastomotic) (artery) (cirsoid) (diffuse) (false) (fusiform) (multiple) (saccular) I72.9
  abdominal (aorta) I71.4

Aneurysm (anastomotic) (artery) (cirsoid) (diffuse) (false) (fusiform) (multiple) (saccular) - *continued*
  abdominal (aorta) - *continued*
    ruptured I71.3
    syphilitic A52.01
  aorta, aortic (nonsyphilitic) I71.9
    abdominal I71.4
      ruptured I71.3
    arch I71.2
      ruptured I71.1
    arteriosclerotic I71.9
      ruptured I71.8
    ascending I71.2
      ruptured I71.1
    congenital Q25.43
    descending I71.9
      abdominal I71.4
        ruptured I71.3
      ruptured I71.8
      thoracic I71.2
        ruptured I71.1
    root Q25.43
    ruptured I71.8
    sinus, congenital Q25.43
    syphilitic A52.01
    thoracic I71.2
      ruptured I71.1
    thoracoabdominal I71.6
      ruptured I71.5
    thorax, thoracic (arch) I71.2
      ruptured I71.1
    transverse I71.2
      ruptured I71.1
    valve (heart) — *see also* Endocarditis, aortic I35.8
  arteriosclerotic I72.9
    cerebral I67.1
      ruptured — *see* Hemorrhage, intracranial, subarachnoid
  arteriovenous (congenital) — *see also* Malformation, arteriovenous
    acquired I77.0
      brain I67.1
      coronary I25.41
      pulmonary I28.0
    brain Q28.2
      ruptured I60.8
    peripheral — *see* Malformation, arteriovenous, peripheral
    precerebral vessels Q28.0
    specified site NEC — *see also* Malformation, arteriovenous
      acquired I77.0
  basal — *see* Aneurysm, brain
  basilar (trunk) I72.5
  berry (congenital) (nonruptured) I67.1
    ruptured I60.7
  brain I67.1
    arteriosclerotic I67.1
      ruptured — *see* Hemorrhage, intracranial, subarachnoid
    arteriovenous (congenital) (nonruptured) Q28.2
      acquired I67.1
        ruptured I60.8
      ruptured I60.8
    berry (congenital) (nonruptured) I67.1
      ruptured — *see also* Hemorrhage, intracranial, subarachnoid I60.7
    congenital Q28.3
      ruptured I60.7
    meninges I67.1
      ruptured I60.8
    miliary (congenital) (nonruptured) I67.1
      ruptured — *see also* Hemorrhage, intracranial, subarachnoid I60.7
    mycotic I33.0
    ruptured — *see* Hemorrhage, intracranial, subarachnoid
    syphilitic (hemorrhage) A52.05
  cardiac (false) — *see also* Aneurysm, heart I25.3
  carotid artery (common) (external) I72.0
    internal (intracranial) I67.1
      extracranial portion I72.0
    ruptured into brain I60.0-
    syphilitic A52.09
      intracranial A52.05
  cavernous sinus I67.1
    arteriovenous (congenital) (nonruptured) Q28.3
      ruptured I60.8
  celiac I72.8
  central nervous system, syphilitic A52.05
  cerebral — *see* Aneurysm, brain
  chest — *see* Aneurysm, thorax
  circle of Willis I67.1

Aneurysm (anastomotic) (artery) (cirsoid) (diffuse) (false) (fusiform) (multiple) (saccular) - *continued*
  circle of Willis - *continued*
    congenital Q28.3
      ruptured I60.6
    ruptured I60.6
  common iliac artery I72.3
  congenital (peripheral) Q27.8
    aorta (root) (sinus) Q25.43
    brain Q28.3
      ruptured I60.7
    coronary Q24.5
    digestive system Q27.8
    lower limb Q27.8
    pulmonary Q25.79
    retina Q14.1
    specified site NEC Q27.8
    upper limb Q27.8
  conjunctiva — *see* Abnormality, conjunctiva, vascular
  conus arteriosus — *see* Aneurysm, heart
  coronary (arteriosclerotic) (artery) I25.41
    arteriovenous, congenital Q24.5
    congenital Q24.5
    ruptured — *see* Infarct, myocardium
    syphilitic A52.06
    vein I25.89
  cylindroid (aorta) I71.9
    ruptured I71.8
    syphilitic A52.01
  ductus arteriosus Q25.0
  endocardial, infective (any valve) I33.0
  femoral (artery) (ruptured) I72.4
  gastroduodenal I72.8
  gastroepiploic I72.8
  heart (wall) (chronic or with a stated duration of over 4 weeks) I25.3
    valve — *see* Endocarditis
  hepatic I72.8
  iliac (common) (artery) (ruptured) I72.3
  infective I72.9
    endocardial (any valve) I33.0
  innominate (nonsyphilitic) I72.8
    syphilitic A52.09
  interauricular septum — *see* Aneurysm, heart
  interventricular septum — *see* Aneurysm, heart
  intrathoracic (nonsyphilitic) I71.2
    ruptured I71.1
    syphilitic A52.01
  lower limb I72.4
  lung (pulmonary artery) I28.1
  mediastinal (nonsyphilitic) I72.8
    syphilitic A52.09
  miliary (congenital) I67.1
    ruptured — *see* Hemorrhage, intracerebral, subarachnoid, intracranial
  mitral (heart) (valve) I34.8
  mural — *see* Aneurysm, heart
  mycotic I72.9
    endocardial (any valve) I33.0
    ruptured, brain — *see* Hemorrhage, intracerebral, subarachnoid
  myocardium — *see* Aneurysm, heart
  neck I72.0
  pancreaticoduodenal I72.8
  patent ductus arteriosus Q25.0
  peripheral NEC I72.8
    congenital Q27.8
      digestive system Q27.8
      lower limb Q27.8
      specified site NEC Q27.8
      upper limb Q27.8
  popliteal (artery) (ruptured) I72.4
  precerebral
    congenital (nonruptured) Q28.1
    specified site, NEC I72.5
  pulmonary I28.1
    arteriovenous Q25.72
      acquired I28.0
    syphilitic A52.09
    valve (heart) — *see* Endocarditis, pulmonary
  racemose (peripheral) I72.9
    congenital — *see* Aneurysm, congenital
  radial I72.1
  Rasmussen NEC A15.0
  renal (artery) I72.2
  retina — *see also* Disorder, retina, microaneurysms
    congenital Q14.1
    diabetic — *see* Diabetes, microaneurysms, retinal
  sinus of Valsalva Q25.49
  specified NEC I72.8
  spinal (cord) I72.8
    syphilitic (hemorrhage) A52.09

- **Aneurysm** (anastomotic) (artery) (cirsoid) (diffuse) (false) (fusiform) (multiple) (saccular) - *continued*
  - splenic I72.8
  - subclavian (artery) (ruptured) I72.8
    - syphilitic A52.09
  - superior mesenteric I72.8
  - syphilitic (aorta) A52.01
    - central nervous system A52.05
    - congenital (late) A50.54 *[I79.0]*
    - spine, spinal A52.09
  - thoracoabdominal (aorta) I71.6
    - ruptured I71.5
    - syphilitic A52.01
  - thorax, thoracic (aorta) (arch) (nonsyphilitic) I71.2
    - ruptured I71.1
    - syphilitic A52.01
  - traumatic (complication) (early) , specified site — *see* Injury, blood vessel
  - tricuspid (heart) (valve) I07.8
  - ulnar I72.1
  - upper limb (ruptured) I72.1
  - valve, valvular — *see* Endocarditis
  - venous — *see also* Varix I86.8
    - congenital Q27.8
      - digestive system Q27.8
      - lower limb Q27.8
      - specified site NEC Q27.8
      - upper limb Q27.8
  - ventricle — *see* Aneurysm, heart
  - vertebral artery I72.6
  - visceral NEC I72.8
- **Angelman syndrome** Q93.51
- **Anger** R45.4
- **Angiectasis, angiectopia** I99.8
- **Angiitis** I77.6
  - allergic granulomatous M30.1
  - hypersensitivity M31.0
  - necrotizing M31.9
    - specified NEC M31.8
  - nervous system, granulomatous I67.7
- **Angina** (attack) (cardiac) (chest) (heart) (pectoris) (syndrome) (vasomotor) I20.9
  - with
    - atherosclerotic heart disease — *see* Arteriosclerosis, coronary (artery),
    - documented spasm I20.1
  - abdominal K55.1
  - accelerated — *see* Angina, unstable
  - agranulocytic — *see* Agranulocytosis
  - angiospastic — *see* Angina, with documented spasm
  - aphthous B08.5
  - crescendo — *see* Angina, unstable
  - croupous J05.0
  - cruris I73.9
  - de novo effort — *see* Angina, unstable
  - diphtheritic, membranous A36.0
  - equivalent I20.8
  - exudative, chronic J37.0
  - following acute myocardial infarction I23.7
  - gangrenous diphtheritic A36.0
  - intestinal K55.1
  - Ludovici K12.2
  - Ludwig's K12.2
  - malignant diphtheritic A36.0
  - membranous J05.0
    - diphtheritic A36.0
    - Vincent's A69.1
  - mesenteric K55.1
  - monocytic — *see* Mononucleosis, infectious
  - of effort — *see* Angina, specified NEC
  - phlegmonous J36
    - diphtheritic A36.0
  - post-infarctional I23.7
  - pre-infarctional — *see* Angina, unstable
  - Prinzmetal — *see* Angina, with documented spasm
  - progressive — *see* Angina, unstable
  - pseudomembranous A69.1
  - pultaceous, diphtheritic A36.0
  - spasm-induced — *see* Angina, with documented spasm
  - specified NEC I20.8
  - stable I20.8
  - stenocardia — *see* Angina, specified NEC
  - stridulous, diphtheritic A36.2
  - tonsil J36
  - trachealis J05.0
  - unstable I20.0
  - variant — *see* Angina, with documented spasm
  - Vincent's A69.1
  - worsening effort — *see* Angina, unstable
- **Angioblastoma** — *see* Neoplasm, connective tissue, uncertain behavior
- **Angiocholecystitis** — *see* Cholecystitis, acute
- **Angiocholitis** — *see also* Cholecystitis, acute K83.09
- **Angiodysgenesis spinalis** G95.19
- **Angiodysplasia** (cecum) (colon) K55.20
  - with bleeding K55.21
  - duodenum (and stomach) K31.819
    - with bleeding K31.811
  - stomach (and duodenum) K31.819
    - with bleeding K31.811
- **Angioedema** (allergic) (any site) (with urticaria) T78.3
  - hereditary D84.1
- **Angioendothelioma** — *see* Neoplasm, uncertain behavior, by site
  - benign D18.00
    - intra-abdominal D18.03
    - intracranial D18.02
    - skin D18.01
    - specified site NEC D18.09
  - bone — *see* Neoplasm, bone, malignant
  - Ewing's — *see* Neoplasm, bone, malignant
- **Angioendotheliomatosis** C85.8-
- **Angiofibroma** — *see also* Neoplasm, benign, by site
  - juvenile
    - specified site — *see* Neoplasm, benign, by site
    - unspecified site D10.6
- **Angiohemophilia** (A) (B) D68.0
- **Angioid streaks** (choroid) (macula) (retina) H35.33
- **Angiokeratoma** — *see* Neoplasm, skin, benign
  - corporis diffusum E75.21
- **Angioleiomyoma** — *see* Neoplasm, connective tissue, benign
- **Angiolipoma** — *see also* Lipoma
  - infiltrating — *see* Lipoma
- **Angioma** — *see also* Hemangioma, by site
  - capillary I78.1
  - hemorrhagicum hereditaria I78.0
  - intra-abdominal D18.03
  - intracranial D18.02
  - malignant — *see* Neoplasm, connective tissue, malignant
  - plexiform D18.00
    - intra-abdominal D18.03
    - intracranial D18.02
    - skin D18.01
    - specified site NEC D18.09
  - senile I78.1
  - serpiginosum L81.7
  - skin D18.01
  - specified site NEC D18.09
  - spider I78.1
  - stellate I78.1
  - venous Q28.3
- **Angiomatosis** Q82.8
  - bacillary A79.89
  - encephalotrigeminal Q85.8
  - hemorrhagic familial I78.0
  - hereditary familial I78.0
  - liver K76.4
- **Angiomyolipoma** — *see* Lipoma
- **Angiomyoliposarcoma** — *see* Neoplasm, connective tissue, malignant
- **Angiomyoma** — *see* Neoplasm, connective tissue, benign
- **Angiomyosarcoma** — *see* Neoplasm, connective tissue, malignant
- **Angiomyxoma** — *see* Neoplasm, connective tissue, uncertain behavior
- **Angioneurosis** F45.8
- **Angioneurotic edema** (allergic) (any site) (with urticaria) T78.3
  - hereditary D84.1
- **Angiopathia, angiopathy** I99.9
  - cerebral I67.9
    - amyloid E85.4 *[I68.0]*
  - diabetic (peripheral) — *see* Diabetes, angiopathy
  - peripheral I73.9
    - diabetic — *see* Diabetes, angiopathy
    - specified type NEC I73.89
  - retinae syphilitica A52.05
  - retinalis (juvenilis)
    - diabetic — *see* Diabetes, retinopathy
    - proliferative — *see* Retinopathy, proliferative
- **Angiosarcoma** — *see also* Neoplasm, connective tissue, malignant
  - liver C22.3
- **Angiosclerosis** — *see* Arteriosclerosis
- **Angiospasm** (peripheral) (traumatic) (vessel) I73.9
  - brachial plexus G54.0
  - cerebral G45.9
  - cervical plexus G54.2
  - nerve
    - arm — *see* Mononeuropathy, upper limb
      - axillary G54.0
- **Angiospasm** (peripheral) (traumatic) (vessel) - *continued*
  - nerve - *continued*
    - arm - *continued*
      - median — *see* Lesion, nerve, median
      - ulnar — *see* Lesion, nerve, ulnar
    - axillary G54.0
    - leg — *see* Mononeuropathy, lower limb
    - median — *see* Lesion, nerve, median
    - plantar — *see* Lesion, nerve, plantar
    - ulnar — *see* Lesion, nerve, ulnar
- **Angiospastic disease or edema** I73.9
- **Angiostrongyliasis**
  - due to
    - Parastrongylus
      - cantonensis B83.2
      - costaricensis B81.3
  - intestinal B81.3
- **Anguillulosis** — *see* Strongyloidiasis
- **Angulation**
  - cecum — *see* Obstruction, intestine
  - coccyx (acquired) (*see also* subcategory M43.8)
    - congenital NEC Q76.49
  - femur (acquired) — *see also* Deformity, limb, specified type NEC, thigh
    - congenital Q74.2
  - intestine (large) (small) — *see* Obstruction, intestine
  - sacrum (acquired) (*see also* subcategory M43.8)
    - congenital NEC Q76.49
  - sigmoid (flexure) — *see* Obstruction, intestine
  - spine — *see* Dorsopathy, deforming, specified NEC
  - tibia (acquired) — *see also* Deformity, limb, specified type NEC, lower leg
    - congenital Q74.2
  - ureter N13.5
    - with infection N13.6
  - wrist (acquired) — *see also* Deformity, limb, specified type NEC, forearm
    - congenital Q74.0
- **Angulus infectiosus** (lips) K13.0
- **Anhedonia** R45.84
  - sexual F52.0
- **Anhidrosis** L74.4
- **Anhydration** E86.0
- **Anhydremia** E86.0
- **Anidrosis** L74.4
- **Aniridia** (congenital) Q13.1
- **Anisakiasis** (infection) (infestation) B81.0
- **Anisakis larvae infestation** B81.0
- **Aniseikonia** H52.32
- **Anisocoria** (pupil) H57.02
  - congenital Q13.2
- **Anisocytosis** R71.8
- **Anisometropia** (congenital) H52.31
- **Ankle** — *see* condition
- **Ankyloblepharon** (eyelid) (acquired) — *see also* Blepharophimosis
  - filiforme (adnatum) (congenital) Q10.3
  - total Q10.3
- **Ankyloglossia** Q38.1
- **Ankylosis** (fibrous) (osseous) (joint) M24.60
  - ankle M24.67-
  - arthrodesis status Z98.1
  - cricoarytenoid (cartilage) (joint) (larynx) J38.7
  - dental K03.5
  - ear ossicles H74.31-
  - elbow M24.62-
  - foot M24.67-
  - hand M24.64-
  - hip M24.65-
  - incostapedial joint (infectional) — *see* Ankylosis, ear ossicles
  - jaw (temporomandibular) M26.61-
  - knee M24.66-
  - lumbosacral (joint) M43.27
  - postoperative (status) Z98.1
  - produced by surgical fusion, status Z98.1
  - sacro-iliac (joint) M43.28
  - shoulder M24.61-
  - spine (joint) — *see also* Fusion, spine
    - spondylitic — *see* Spondylitis, ankylosing
  - surgical Z98.1
  - temporomandibular M26.61-
  - tooth, teeth (hard tissues) K03.5
  - wrist M24.63-
- **Ankylostoma** — *see* Ancylostoma
- **Ankylostomiasis** — *see* Ancylostomiasis
- **Ankylurethria** — *see* Stricture, urethra
- **Annular** — *see also* condition
  - detachment, cervix N88.8
  - organ or site, congenital NEC — *see* Distortion
  - pancreas (congenital) Q45.1

Anomaly, anomalous (congenital) (unspecified type) - *continued*
  sigmoid (flexure) Q43.9
  simian crease Q82.8
  sinus of Valsalva Q25.49
  skeleton generalized Q78.9
  skin (appendage) Q82.9
  skull Q75.9
    with
      anencephaly Q00.0
      encephalocele — *see* Encephalocele
      hydrocephalus Q03.9
        with spina bifida — *see* Spina bifida, by site, with hydrocephalus
      microcephaly Q02
  specified organ or site NEC Q89.8
  spermatic cord Q55.4
  spine, spinal NEC Q76.49
    column NEC Q76.49
      kyphosis — *see* Kyphosis, congenital
      lordosis — *see* Lordosis, congenital
    cord Q06.9
    nerve root Q07.8
  spleen Q89.09
    agenesis Q89.01
  stenonian duct Q38.4
  sternum NEC Q76.7
  stomach Q40.3
  submaxillary gland Q38.4
  tarsus NEC Q74.2
  tendon Q79.9
  testis — *see* Malformation, testis and scrotum
  thigh NEC Q74.2
  thorax (wall) Q67.8
    bony Q76.9
  throat Q38.8
  thumb Q74.0
  thymus gland Q89.2
  thyroid (gland) Q89.2
    cartilage Q31.8
  tibia NEC Q74.2
    saber A50.56
  toe Q74.2
  tongue Q38.3
  tooth, teeth K00.9
    eruption K00.6
    position, fully erupted M26.30
    spacing, fully erupted M26.30
  trachea (cartilage) Q32.1
  tragus Q17.9
  tricuspid (leaflet) (valve) Q22.9
    atresia or stenosis Q22.4
    Ebstein's Q22.5
  Uhl's (hypoplasia of myocardium, right ventricle) Q24.8
  ulna Q74.0
  umbilical artery Q27.0
  union
    cricoid cartilage and thyroid cartilage Q31.8
    thyroid cartilage and hyoid bone Q31.8
    trachea with larynx Q31.8
  upper limb Q74.0
  urachus Q64.4
  ureter Q62.8
    obstructive NEC Q62.39
      cecoureterocele Q62.32
      orthotopic ureterocele Q62.31
  urethra Q64.70
    absence Q64.5
    double Q64.74
    fistula to rectum Q64.73
    obstructive Q64.39
      stricture Q64.32
    prolapse Q64.71
    specified type NEC Q64.79
  urinary tract Q64.9
  uterus Q51.9
    with only one functioning horn Q51.4
  uvula Q38.5
  vagina Q52.4
  valleculae Q31.8
  valve (heart) NEC Q24.8
    coronary sinus Q24.5
    inferior vena cava Q24.8
    pulmonary Q22.3
    sinus coronario Q24.5
    venae cavae inferioris Q24.8
  vas deferens Q55.4
  vascular Q27.9
    brain Q28.3
    ring Q25.45
  vein (s) (peripheral) Q27.9
    brain Q28.3

Anomaly, anomalous (congenital) (unspecified type) - *continued*
  vein (s) (peripheral) - *continued*
    cerebral Q28.3
    coronary Q24.5
    developmental Q28.3
    great Q26.9
      specified NEC Q26.8
  vena cava (inferior) (superior) Q26.9
  venous — *see* Anomaly, vein(s)
  venous return Q26.8
  ventricular
    bands or folds Q24.8
    septa Q21.0
  vertebra Q76.49
    kyphosis — *see* Kyphosis, congenital
    lordosis — *see* Lordosis, congenital
  vesicourethral orifice Q64.79
  vessel (s) Q27.9
    optic papilla Q14.2
    precerebral Q28.1
  vitelline duct Q43.0
  vitreous body or humor Q14.0
  vulva Q52.70
  wrist (joint) Q74.0
Anomia R48.8
Anonychia (congenital) Q84.3
  acquired L60.8
Anophthalmos, anophthalmus (congenital) (globe) Q11.1
  acquired Z90.01
Anopia, anopsia H53.46-
  quadrant H53.46-
Anorchia, anorchism, anorchidism Q55.0
Anorexia R63.0
  hysterical F44.89
  nervosa F50.00
    atypical F50.9
    binge-eating type F50.2
      with purging F50.02
    restricting type F50.01
Anorgasmy, psychogenic (female) F52.31
  male F52.32
Anosmia R43.0
  hysterical F44.6
  postinfectional J39.8
Anosognosia R41.89
Anosteoplasia Q78.9
Anovulatory cycle N97.0
Anoxemia R09.02
  newborn P84
Anoxia (pathological) R09.02
  altitude T70.29
  cerebral G93.1
    complicating
      anesthesia (general) (local) or other sedation T88.59
        in labor and delivery O74.3
        in pregnancy O29.21-
        postpartum, puerperal O89.2
      delivery (cesarean) (instrumental) O75.4
    during a procedure G97.81
    newborn P84
    resulting from a procedure G97.82
  due to
    drowning T75.1
    high altitude T70.29
  heart — *see* Insufficiency, coronary
  intrauterine P84
  myocardial — *see* Insufficiency, coronary
  newborn P84
  spinal cord G95.11
  systemic (by suffocation) (low content in atmosphere) — *see* Asphyxia, traumatic
Anteflexion — *see* Anteversion
Antenatal
  care (normal pregnancy) Z34.90
  screening (encounter for) of mother — *see also* Encounter, antenatal screening Z36.9
Antepartum — *see* condition
Anterior — *see* condition
Antero-occlusion M26.220
Anteversion
  cervix — *see* Anteversion, uterus
  femur (neck) , congenital Q65.89
  uterus, uterine (cervix) (postinfectional) (postpartal, old) N85.4
    congenital Q51.818
    in pregnancy or childbirth — *see* Pregnancy, complicated by
Anthophobia F40.228
Anthracosilicosis J60

Anthracosis (lung) (occupational) J60
  lingua K14.3
Anthrax A22.9
  with pneumonia A22.1
  cerebral A22.8
  colitis A22.2
  cutaneous A22.0
  gastrointestinal A22.2
  inhalation A22.1
  intestinal A22.2
  meningitis A22.8
  pulmonary A22.1
  respiratory A22.1
  sepsis A22.7
  specified manifestation NEC A22.8
Anthropoid pelvis Q74.2
  with disproportion (fetopelvic) O33.0
Anthropophobia F40.10
  generalized F40.11
Antibodies, maternal (blood group) — *see* Isoimmunization, affecting management of pregnancy
  anti-D — *see* Isoimmunization, affecting management of pregnancy, Rh
    newborn P55.0
Antibody
  anticardiolipin R76.0
    with
      hemorrhagic disorder D68.312
      hypercoagulable state D68.61
  antiphosphatidylglycerol R76.0
    with
      hemorrhagic disorder D68.312
      hypercoagulable state D68.61
  antiphosphatidylinositol R76.0
    with
      hemorrhagic disorder D68.312
      hypercoagulable state D68.61
  antiphosphatidylserine R76.0
    with
      hemorrhagic disorder D68.312
      hypercoagulable state D68.61
  antiphospholipid R76.0
    with
      hemorrhagic disorder D68.312
      hypercoagulable state D68.61
Anticardiolipin syndrome D68.61
Anticoagulant, circulating (intrinsic) — *see also* - Disorder, hemorrhagic D68.318
  drug-induced (extrinsic) — *see also* - Disorder, hemorrhagic D68.32
  iatrogenic D68.32
Antidiuretic hormone syndrome E22.2
Antimonial cholera — *see* Poisoning, antimony
Antiphospholipid
  antibody
    with hemorrhagic disorder D68.312
    syndrome D68.61
Antisocial personality F60.2
Antithrombinemia — *see* Circulating anticoagulants
Antithromboplastinemia D68.318
Antithromboplastinogenemia D68.318
Antitoxin complication or reaction — *see* Complications, vaccination
Antlophobia F40.228
Antritis J32.0
  maxilla J32.0
    acute J01.00
      recurrent J01.01
  stomach K29.60
    with bleeding K29.61
Antrum, antral — *see* condition
Anuria R34
  calculous (impacted) (recurrent) — *see also* Calculus, urinary N20.9
  following
    abortion — *see* Abortion by type complicated by, renal failure
    ectopic or molar pregnancy O08.4
  newborn P96.0
  postprocedural N99.0
  postrenal N13.8
  traumatic (following crushing) T79.5
Anus, anal — *see* condition
Anusitis K62.89
Anxiety F41.9
  depression F41.8
  episodic paroxysmal F41.0
  generalized F41.1
  hysteria F41.8
  neurosis F41.1
  panic type F41.0
  reaction F41.1

Anxiety - *continued*
separation, abnormal (of childhood) F93.0
specified NEC F41.8
state F41.1
Aorta, aortic — *see* condition
Aortectasia — *see* Ectasia, aorta
with aneurysm — *see* Aneurysm, aorta
Aortitis (nonsyphilitic) (calcific) I77.6
arteriosclerotic I70.0
Doehle-Heller A52.02
luetic A52.02
rheumatic — *see* Endocarditis, acute, rheumatic
specific (syphilitic) A52.02
syphilitic A52.02
congenital A50.54 *[I79.1]*
Apathetic thyroid storm — *see* Thyrotoxicosis
Apathy R45.3
Apeirophobia F40.228
Apepsia K30
psychogenic F45.8
Aperistalsis, esophagus K22.0
Apertognathia M26.29
Apert's syndrome Q87.0
Aphagia R13.0
psychogenic F50.9
Aphakia (acquired) (postoperative) H27.0-
congenital Q12.3
Aphasia (amnestic) (global) (nominal) (semantic) (syntactic) R47.01
acquired, with epilepsy (Landau-Kleffner syndrome) — *see* Epilepsy, specified NEC
auditory (developmental) F80.2
developmental (receptive type) F80.2
expressive type F80.1
Wernicke's F80.2
following
cerebrovascular disease I69.920
cerebral infarction I69.320
intracerebral hemorrhage I69.120
nontraumatic intracranial hemorrhage NEC I69.220
specified disease NEC I69.820
subarachnoid hemorrhage I69.020
primary progressive G31.01 *[F02.80]*
with behavioral disturbance G31.01 *[F02.81]*
progressive isolated G31.01 *[F02.80]*
with behavioral disturbance G31.01 *[F02.81]*
sensory F80.2
syphilis, tertiary A52.19
Wernicke's (developmental) F80.2
Aphonia (organic) R49.1
hysterical F44.4
psychogenic F44.4
Aphthae, aphthous — *see also* condition
Bednar's K12.0
cachectic K14.0
epizootic B08.8
fever B08.8
oral (recurrent) K12.0
stomatitis (major) (minor) K12.0
thrush B37.0
ulcer (oral) (recurrent) K12.0
genital organ (s) NEC
female N76.6
male N50.89
larynx J38.7
Apical — *see* condition
Apiphobia F40.218
Aplasia — *see also* Agenesis
abdominal muscle syndrome Q79.4
alveolar process (acquired) — *see* Anomaly, alveolar
congenital Q38.6
aorta (congenital) Q25.41
axialis extracorticalis (congenita) E75.29
bone marrow (myeloid) D61.9
congenital D61.01
brain Q00.0
part of Q04.3
bronchus Q32.4
cementum K00.4
cerebellum Q04.3
cervix (congenital) Q51.5
congenital pure red cell D61.01
corpus callosum Q04.0
cutis congenita Q84.8
erythrocyte congenital D61.01
extracortical axial E75.29
eye Q11.1
fovea centralis (congenital) Q14.1
gallbladder, congenital Q44.0
iris Q13.1
labyrinth, membranous Q16.5
limb (congenital) Q73.8

Aplasia - *continued*
limb (congenital) - *continued*
lower — *see* Defect, reduction, lower limb
upper — *see* Agenesis, arm
lung, congenital (bilateral) (unilateral) Q33.3
pancreas Q45.0
parathyroid-thymic D82.1
Pelizaeus-Merzbacher E75.29
penis Q55.5
prostate Q55.4
red cell (with thymoma) D60.9
acquired D60.9
due to drugs D60.9
adult D60.9
chronic D60.0
congenital D61.01
constitutional D61.01
due to drugs D60.9
hereditary D61.01
of infants D61.01
primary D61.01
pure D61.01
due to drugs D60.9
specified type NEC D60.8
transient D60.1
round ligament Q52.8
skin Q84.8
spermatic cord Q55.4
spleen Q89.01
testicle Q55.0
thymic, with immunodeficiency D82.1
thyroid (congenital) (with myxedema) E03.1
uterus Q51.0
ventral horn cell Q06.1
Apnea, apneic (of) (spells) R06.81
newborn NEC P28.4
obstructive P28.4
sleep (central) (obstructive) (primary) P28.3
prematurity P28.4
sleep G47.30
central (primary) G47.31
idiopathic G47.31
in conditions classified elsewhere G47.37
obstructive (adult) (pediatric) G47.33
hypopnea G47.33
primary central G47.31
specified NEC G47.39
Apneumatosis, newborn P28.0
Apocrine metaplasia (breast) — *see* Dysplasia, mammary, specified type NEC
Apophysitis (bone) — *see also* Osteochondropathy
calcaneus M92.8
juvenile M92.9
Apoplectiform convulsions (cerebral ischemia) I67.82
Apoplexia, apoplexy, apoplectic
adrenal A39.1
heart (auricle) (ventricle) — *see* Infarct, myocardium
heat T67.0
hemorrhagic (stroke) — *see* Hemorrhage, intracranial
meninges, hemorrhagic — *see* Hemorrhage, intracranial, subarachnoid
uremic N18.9 *[I68.8]*
Appearance
bizarre R46.1
specified NEC R46.89
very low level of personal hygiene R46.0
Appendage
epididymal (organ of Morgagni) Q55.4
intestine (epiploic) Q43.8
preauricular Q17.0
testicular (organ of Morgagni) Q55.29
Appendicitis (pneumococcal) (retrocecal) K37
with
gangrene K35.891
perforation NOS K35.32
peritoneal abscess K35.33
peritonitis NEC K35.33
generalized (with perforation or rupture) K35.20
with abscess K35.21
localized K35.30
with
gangrene K35.31
perforation K35.32
and abscess K35.33
rupture (with localized peritonitis) K35.32
acute (catarrhal) (fulminating) (gangrenous) (obstructive) (retrocecal) (suppurative) K35.80
with
gangrene K35.891
peritoneal abscess K35.33

Appendicitis (pneumococcal) (retrocecal) - *continued*
acute (catarrhal) (fulminating) (gangrenous) (obstructive) (retrocecal) (suppurative) - *continued*
with - *continued*
peritonitis NEC K35.33
generalized (with perforation or rupture) K35.20
with abscess K35.21
localized K35.30
with
gangrene K35.31
perforation K35.32
and abscess K35.33
specified NEC K35.890
with gangrene K35.891
amebic A06.89
chronic (recurrent) K36
exacerbation — *see* Appendicitis, acute
gangrenous — *see* Appendicitis, acute
healed (obliterative) K36
interval K36
neurogenic K36
obstructive K36
recurrent K36
relapsing K36
ruptured NOS (with localized peritonitis) K35.32
subacute (adhesive) K36
subsiding K36
suppurative — *see* Appendicitis, acute
tuberculous A18.32
Appendicopathia oxyurica B80
Appendix, appendicular — *see also* condition
epididymis Q55.4
Morgagni
female Q50.5
male (epididymal) Q55.4
testicular Q55.29
testis Q55.29
Appetite
depraved — *see* Pica
excessive R63.2
lack or loss — *see also* Anorexia R63.0
nonorganic origin F50.89
psychogenic F50.89
perverted (hysterical) — *see* Pica
Apple peel syndrome Q41.1
Apprehension state F41.1
Apprehensiveness, abnormal F41.9
Approximal wear K03.0
Apraxia (classic) (ideational) (ideokinetic) (ideomotor) (motor) (verbal) R48.2
following
cerebrovascular disease I69.990
cerebral infarction I69.390
intracerebral hemorrhage I69.190
nontraumatic intracranial hemorrhage NEC I69.290
specified disease NEC I69.890
subarachnoid hemorrhage I69.090
oculomotor, congenital H51.8
Aptyalism K11.7
Apudoma — *see* Neoplasm, uncertain behavior, by site
Aqueous misdirection H40.83-
Arabicum elephantiasis — *see* Infestation, filarial
Arachnitis — *see* Meningitis
Arachnodactyly — *see* Syndrome, Marfan's
Arachnoiditis (acute) (adhesive) (basal) (brain) (cerebrospinal) — *see* Meningitis
Arachnophobia F40.210
Arboencephalitis, Australian A83.4
Arborization block (heart) I45.5
ARC (AIDS-related complex) B20
Arch
aortic Q25.49
bovine Q25.49
Arches — *see* condition
Arcuate uterus Q51.810
Arcuatus uterus Q51.810
Arcus (cornea) **senilis** — *see* Degeneration, cornea, senile
Arc-welder's lung J63.4
Areflexia R29.2
Areola — *see* condition
Argentaffinoma — *see also* Neoplasm, uncertain behavior, by site
malignant — *see* Neoplasm, malignant, by site
syndrome E34.0
Argininemia E72.21
Arginosuccinic aciduria E72.22
Argyll Robertson phenomenon, pupil or syndrome (syphilitic) A52.19
atypical H57.09
nonsyphilitic H57.09

Argyria, argyriasis
- conjunctival H11.13-
- from drug or medicament — *see* Table of Drugs and Chemicals, by substance

Argyrosis, conjunctival H11.13-
Arhinencephaly Q04.1
Ariboflavinosis E53.0
Arm — *see* condition
Arnold-Chiari disease, obstruction or syndrome (type II) Q07.00
- with
  - hydrocephalus Q07.02
    - with spina bifida Q07.03
  - spina bifida Q07.01
    - with hydrocephalus Q07.03
- type III — *see* Encephalocele
- type IV Q04.8

Aromatic amino-acid metabolism disorder E70.9
- specified NEC E70.8

Arousals, confusional G47.51
Arrest, arrested
- cardiac I46.9
  - complicating
    - abortion — *see* Abortion, by type, complicated by, cardiac arrest
    - anesthesia (general) (local) or other sedation — *see* Table of Drugs and Chemicals, by drug,
      - in labor and delivery O74.2
      - in pregnancy O29.11-
      - postpartum, puerperal O89.1
    - delivery (cesarean) (instrumental) O75.4
  - due to
    - cardiac condition I46.2
    - specified condition NEC I46.8
  - intraoperative I97.71-
  - newborn P29.81
  - personal history, successfully resuscitated Z86.74
  - postprocedural I97.12-
    - obstetric procedure O75.4
- cardiorespiratory — *see* Arrest, cardiac
- circulatory — *see* Arrest, cardiac
- deep transverse O64.0
- development or growth
  - bone — *see* Disorder, bone, development or growth
  - child R62.50
  - tracheal rings Q32.1
- epiphyseal
  - complete
    - femur M89.15-
    - humerus M89.12-
    - tibia M89.16-
    - ulna M89.13-
  - forearm M89.13-
    - specified NEC M89.13-
    - ulna — *see* Arrest, epiphyseal, by type, ulna
  - lower leg M89.16-
    - specified NEC M89.168
    - tibia — *see* Arrest, epiphyseal, by type, tibia
  - partial
    - femur M89.15-
    - humerus M89.12-
    - tibia M89.16-
    - ulna M89.13-
  - specified NEC M89.18
- granulopoiesis — *see* Agranulocytosis
- growth plate — *see* Arrest, epiphyseal
- heart — *see* Arrest, cardiac
- legal, anxiety concerning Z65.3
- physeal — *see* Arrest, epiphyseal
- respiratory R09.2
  - newborn P28.81
- sinus I45.5
- spermatogenesis (complete) — *see* Azoospermia
  - incomplete — *see* Oligospermia
- transverse (deep) O64.0

Arrhenoblastoma
- benign
  - specified site — *see* Neoplasm, benign, by site
  - unspecified site
    - female D27.9
    - male D29.20
- malignant
  - specified site — *see* Neoplasm, malignant, by site
  - unspecified site
    - female C56.9
    - male C62.90
- specified site — *see* Neoplasm, uncertain behavior, by site
- unspecified site
  - female D39.10
  - male D40.10

Arrhythmia (auricle) (cardiac) (juvenile) (nodal) (reflex) (sinus) (supraventricular) (transitory) (ventricle) I49.9
- block I45.9
- extrasystolic I49.49
- newborn
  - bradycardia P29.12
  - occurring before birth P03.819
    - before onset of labor P03.810
    - during labor P03.811
  - tachycardia P29.11
- psychogenic F45.8
- specified NEC I49.8
- vagal R55
- ventricular re-entry I47.0

Arrillaga-Ayerza syndrome (pulmonary sclerosis with pulmonary hypertension) I27.0
Arsenical pigmentation L81.8
- from drug or medicament — *see* Table of Drugs and Chemicals

Arsenism — *see* Poisoning, arsenic
Arterial — *see* condition
Arteriofibrosis — *see* Arteriosclerosis
Arteriolar sclerosis — *see* Arteriosclerosis
Arteriolith — *see* Arteriosclerosis
Arteriolitis I77.6
- necrotizing, kidney I77.5
- renal — *see* Hypertension, kidney

Arteriolosclerosis — *see* Arteriosclerosis
Arterionephrosclerosis — *see* Hypertension, kidney
Arteriopathy I77.9
- cerebral autosomal dominant, with subcortical infarcts and leukoencephalopathy (CADASIL) I67.850

Arteriosclerosis, arteriosclerotic (diffuse) (obliterans) (of) (senile) (with calcification) I70.90
- aorta I70.0
- arteries of extremities — *see* Arteriosclerosis, extremities
- brain I67.2
- bypass graft
  - coronary — *see* Arteriosclerosis, coronary, bypass graft
  - extremities — *see* Arteriosclerosis, extremities, bypass graft
- cardiac — *see* Disease, heart, ischemic, atherosclerotic
- cardiopathy — *see* Disease, heart, ischemic, atherosclerotic
- cardiorenal — *see* Hypertension, cardiorenal
- cardiovascular — *see* Disease, heart, ischemic, atherosclerotic
- carotid — *see also* Occlusion, artery, carotid I65.2-
- central nervous system I67.2
- cerebral I67.2
- cerebrovascular I67.2
- coronary (artery) I25.10
  - due to
    - calcified coronary lesion (severely) I25.84
    - lipid rich plaque I25.83
  - bypass graft I25.810
    - with
      - angina pectoris I25.709
        - with documented spasm I25.701
        - specified type NEC I25.708
        - unstable I25.700
      - ischemic chest pain I25.709
    - autologous artery I25.810
      - with
        - angina pectoris I25.729
          - with documented spasm I25.721
          - specified type I25.728
          - unstable I25.720
        - ischemic chest pain I25.729
    - autologous vein I25.810
      - with
        - angina pectoris I25.719
          - with documented spasm I25.711
          - specified type I25.718
          - unstable I25.710
        - ischemic chest pain I25.719
    - nonautologous biological I25.810
      - with
        - angina pectoris I25.739
          - with documented spasm I25.731
          - specified type I25.738
          - unstable I25.730
        - ischemic chest pain I25.739
    - specified type NEC I25.810
      - with
        - angina pectoris I25.799
          - with documented spasm I25.791

Arteriosclerosis, arteriosclerotic (diffuse) (obliterans) (of) (senile) (with calcification) - *continued*
- coronary (artery) - *continued*
  - bypass graft - *continued*
    - specified type NEC - *continued*
      - with - *continued*
        - angina pectoris - *continued*
          - specified type I25.798
          - unstable I25.790
        - ischemic chest pain I25.799
  - native vessel
    - with
      - angina pectoris I25.119
        - with documented spasm I25.111
        - specified type NEC I25.118
        - unstable I25.110
      - ischemic chest pain I25.119
  - transplanted heart I25.811
    - bypass graft I25.812
      - with
        - angina pectoris I25.769
          - with documented spasm I25.761
          - specified type I25.768
          - unstable I25.760
        - ischemic chest pain I25.769
    - native coronary artery I25.811
      - with
        - angina pectoris I25.759
          - with documented spasm I25.751
          - specified type I25.758
          - unstable I25.750
        - ischemic chest pain I25.759
- extremities (native arteries) I70.209
  - bypass graft I70.309
    - autologous vein graft I70.409
      - leg I70.409
        - with
          - gangrene (and intermittent claudication, rest pain and ulcer) I70.469
          - intermittent claudication I70.419
          - rest pain (and intermittent claudication) I70.429
        - bilateral I70.403
          - with
            - gangrene (and intermittent claudication, rest pain and ulcer) I70.463
            - intermittent claudication I70.413
            - rest pain (and intermittent claudication) I70.423
          - specified type NEC I70.493
        - left I70.402
          - with
            - gangrene (and intermittent claudication, rest pain and ulcer) I70.462
            - intermittent claudication I70.412
            - rest pain (and intermittent claudication) I70.422
            - ulceration (and intermittent claudication and rest pain) I70.449
              - ankle I70.443
              - calf I70.442
              - foot site NEC I70.445
              - heel I70.444
              - lower leg NEC I70.448
              - midfoot I70.444
              - thigh I70.441
          - specified type NEC I70.492
        - right I70.401
          - with
            - gangrene (and intermittent claudication, rest pain and ulcer) I70.461
            - intermittent claudication I70.411
            - rest pain (and intermittent claudication) I70.421
            - ulceration (and intermittent claudication and rest pain) I70.439
              - ankle I70.433
              - calf I70.432
              - foot site NEC I70.435
              - heel I70.434
              - lower leg NEC I70.438
              - midfoot I70.434
              - thigh I70.431
          - specified type NEC I70.491
        - specified type NEC I70.499
      - specified NEC I70.408
        - with
          - gangrene (and intermittent claudication, rest pain and ulcer) I70.468
          - intermittent claudication I70.418
          - rest pain (and intermittent claudication) I70.428

Arteriosclerosis, arteriosclerotic (diffuse) (obliterans) (of) (senile) (with calcification) - *continued*
- extremities (native arteries) - *continued*
  - bypass graft - *continued*
    - autologous vein graft - *continued*
      - specified NEC - *continued*
        - with - *continued*
          - ulceration (and intermittent claudication and rest pain) I70.45
        - specified type NEC I70.498
    - leg I70.309
      - with
        - gangrene (and intermittent claudication, rest pain and ulcer) I70.369
        - intermittent claudication I70.319
        - rest pain (and intermittent claudication) I70.329
      - bilateral I70.303
        - with
          - gangrene (and intermittent claudication, rest pain and ulcer) I70.363
          - intermittent claudication I70.313
          - rest pain (and intermittent claudication) I70.323
        - specified type NEC I70.393
      - left I70.302
        - with
          - gangrene (and intermittent claudication, rest pain and ulcer) I70.362
          - intermittent claudication I70.312
          - rest pain (and intermittent claudication) I70.322
          - ulceration (and intermittent claudication and rest pain) I70.349
            - ankle I70.343
            - calf I70.342
            - foot site NEC I70.345
            - heel I70.344
            - lower leg NEC I70.348
            - midfoot I70.344
            - thigh I70.341
        - specified type NEC I70.392
      - right I70.301
        - with
          - gangrene (and intermittent claudication, rest pain and ulcer) I70.361
          - intermittent claudication I70.311
          - rest pain (and intermittent claudication) I70.321
          - ulceration (and intermittent claudication and rest pain) I70.339
            - ankle I70.333
            - calf I70.332
            - foot site NEC I70.335
            - heel I70.334
            - lower leg NEC I70.338
            - midfoot I70.334
            - thigh I70.331
        - specified type NEC I70.391
      - specified type NEC I70.399
    - nonautologous biological graft I70.509
      - leg I70.509
        - with
          - gangrene (and intermittent claudication, rest pain and ulcer) I70.569
          - intermittent claudication I70.519
          - rest pain (and intermittent claudication) I70.529
        - bilateral I70.503
          - with
            - gangrene (and intermittent claudication, rest pain and ulcer) I70.563
            - intermittent claudication I70.513
            - rest pain (and intermittent claudication) I70.523
          - specified type NEC I70.593
        - left I70.502
          - with
            - gangrene (and intermittent claudication, rest pain and ulcer) I70.562
            - intermittent claudication I70.512
            - rest pain (and intermittent claudication) I70.522
            - ulceration (and intermittent claudication and rest pain) I70.549
              - ankle I70.543
              - calf I70.542
              - foot site NEC I70.545
              - heel I70.544
              - lower leg NEC I70.548
              - midfoot I70.544
              - thigh I70.541

Arteriosclerosis, arteriosclerotic (diffuse) (obliterans) (of) (senile) (with calcification) - *continued*
- extremities (native arteries) - *continued*
  - bypass graft - *continued*
    - nonautologous biological graft - *continued*
      - leg - *continued*
        - left - *continued*
          - specified type NEC I70.592
        - right I70.501
          - with
            - gangrene (and intermittent claudication, rest pain and ulcer) I70.561
            - intermittent claudication I70.511
            - rest pain (and intermittent claudication) I70.521
            - ulceration (and intermittent claudication and rest pain) I70.539
              - ankle I70.533
              - calf I70.532
              - foot site NEC I70.535
              - heel I70.534
              - lower leg NEC I70.538
              - midfoot I70.534
              - thigh I70.531
          - specified type NEC I70.591
        - specified type NEC I70.599
      - specified NEC I70.508
        - with
          - gangrene (and intermittent claudication, rest pain and ulcer) I70.568
          - intermittent claudication I70.518
          - rest pain (and intermittent claudication) I70.528
          - ulceration (and intermittent claudication and rest pain) I70.55
        - specified type NEC I70.598
    - nonbiological graft I70.609
      - leg I70.609
        - with
          - gangrene (and intermittent claudication, rest pain and ulcer) I70.669
          - intermittent claudication I70.619
          - rest pain (and intermittent claudication) I70.629
        - bilateral I70.603
          - with
            - gangrene (and intermittent claudication, rest pain and ulcer) I70.663
            - intermittent claudication I70.613
            - rest pain (and intermittent claudication) I70.623
          - specified type NEC I70.693
        - left I70.602
          - with
            - gangrene (and intermittent claudication, rest pain and ulcer) I70.662
            - intermittent claudication I70.612
            - rest pain (and intermittent claudication) I70.622
            - ulceration (and intermittent claudication and rest pain) I70.649
              - ankle I70.643
              - calf I70.642
              - foot site NEC I70.645
              - heel I70.644
              - lower leg NEC I70.648
              - midfoot I70.644
              - thigh I70.641
          - specified type NEC I70.692
        - right I70.601
          - with
            - gangrene (and intermittent claudication, rest pain and ulcer) I70.661
            - intermittent claudication I70.611
            - rest pain (and intermittent claudication) I70.621
            - ulceration (and intermittent claudication and rest pain) I70.639
              - ankle I70.633
              - calf I70.632
              - foot site NEC I70.635
              - heel I70.634
              - lower leg NEC I70.638
              - midfoot I70.634
              - thigh I70.631
          - specified type NEC I70.691
        - specified type NEC I70.699
      - specified NEC I70.608
        - with
          - gangrene (and intermittent claudication, rest pain and ulcer) I70.668
          - intermittent claudication I70.618

Arteriosclerosis, arteriosclerotic (diffuse) (obliterans) (of) (senile) (with calcification) - *continued*
- extremities (native arteries) - *continued*
  - bypass graft - *continued*
    - nonbiological graft - *continued*
      - specified NEC - *continued*
        - with - *continued*
          - rest pain (and intermittent claudication) I70.628
          - ulceration (and intermittent claudication and rest pain) I70.65
        - specified type NEC I70.698
    - specified graft NEC I70.709
      - leg I70.709
        - with
          - gangrene (and intermittent claudication, rest pain and ulcer) I70.769
          - intermittent claudication I70.719
          - rest pain (and intermittent claudication) I70.729
        - bilateral I70.703
          - with
            - gangrene (and intermittent claudication, rest pain and ulcer) I70.763
            - intermittent claudication I70.713
            - rest pain (and intermittent claudication) I70.723
          - specified type NEC I70.793
        - left I70.702
          - with
            - gangrene (and intermittent claudication, rest pain and ulcer) I70.762
            - intermittent claudication I70.712
            - rest pain (and intermittent claudication) I70.722
            - ulceration (and intermittent claudication and rest pain) I70.749
              - ankle I70.743
              - calf I70.742
              - foot site NEC I70.745
              - heel I70.744
              - lower leg NEC I70.748
              - midfoot I70.744
              - thigh I70.741
          - specified type NEC I70.792
        - right I70.701
          - with
            - gangrene (and intermittent claudication, rest pain and ulcer) I70.761
            - intermittent claudication I70.711
            - rest pain (and intermittent claudication) I70.721
            - ulceration (and intermittent claudication and rest pain) I70.739
              - ankle I70.733
              - calf I70.732
              - foot site NEC I70.735
              - heel I70.734
              - lower leg NEC I70.738
              - midfoot I70.734
              - thigh I70.731
          - specified type NEC I70.791
        - specified type NEC I70.799
      - specified NEC I70.708
        - with
          - gangrene (and intermittent claudication, rest pain and ulcer) I70.768
          - intermittent claudication I70.718
          - rest pain (and intermittent claudication) I70.728
          - ulceration (and intermittent claudication and rest pain) I70.75
        - specified type NEC I70.798
    - specified NEC I70.308
      - with
        - gangrene (and intermittent claudication, rest pain and ulcer) I70.368
        - intermittent claudication I70.318
        - rest pain (and intermittent claudication) I70.328
        - ulceration (and intermittent claudication and rest pain) I70.35
      - specified type NEC I70.398
  - leg I70.209
    - with
      - gangrene (and intermittent claudication, rest pain and ulcer) I70.269
      - intermittent claudication I70.219
      - rest pain (and intermittent claudication) I70.229
    - bilateral I70.203
      - with

Arteriosclerosis, arteriosclerotic (diffuse) (obliterans) (of) (senile) (with calcification) - *continued*
extremities (native arteries) - *continued*
leg - *continued*
bilateral - *continued*
with - *continued*
gangrene (and intermittent claudication, rest pain and ulcer) I70.263
intermittent claudication I70.213
rest pain (and intermittent claudication) I70.223
specified type NEC I70.293
left I70.202
with
gangrene (and intermittent claudication, rest pain and ulcer) I70.262
intermittent claudication I70.212
rest pain (and intermittent claudication) I70.222
ulceration (and intermittent claudication and rest pain) I70.249
ankle I70.243
calf I70.242
foot site NEC I70.245
heel I70.244
lower leg NEC I70.248
midfoot I70.244
thigh I70.241
specified type NEC I70.292
right I70.201
with
gangrene (and intermittent claudication, rest pain and ulcer) I70.261
intermittent claudication I70.211
rest pain (and intermittent claudication) I70.221
ulceration (and intermittent claudication and rest pain) I70.239
ankle I70.233
calf I70.232
foot site NEC I70.235
heel I70.234
lower leg NEC I70.238
midfoot I70.234
thigh I70.231
specified type NEC I70.291
specified type NEC I70.299
specified site NEC I70.208
with
gangrene (and intermittent claudication, rest pain and ulcer) I70.268
intermittent claudication I70.218
rest pain (and intermittent claudication) I70.228
ulceration (and intermittent claudication and rest pain) I70.25
specified type NEC I70.298
generalized I70.91
heart (disease) — *see* Arteriosclerosis, coronary (artery),
kidney — *see* Hypertension, kidney
medial — *see* Arteriosclerosis, extremities
mesenteric (artery) K55.1
Mönckeberg's — *see* Arteriosclerosis, extremities
myocarditis I51.4
peripheral (of extremities) — *see* Arteriosclerosis, extremities
pulmonary (idiopathic) I27.0
renal (arterioles) — *see also* Hypertension, kidney
artery I70.1
retina (vascular) I70.8 *[H35.0-]*
specified artery NEC I70.8
spinal (cord) G95.19
vertebral (artery) I67.2
Arteriospasm I73.9
Arteriovenous — *see* condition
Arteritis I77.6
allergic M31.0
aorta (nonsyphilitic) I77.6
syphilitic A52.02
aortic arch M31.4
brachiocephalic M31.4
brain I67.7
syphilitic A52.04
cerebral I67.7
in
diseases classified elsewhere I68.2
systemic lupus erythematosus M32.19
listerial A32.89
syphilitic A52.04
tuberculous A18.89
coronary (artery) I25.89
rheumatic I01.8

Arteritis - *continued*
coronary (artery) - *continued*
rheumatic - *continued*
chronic I09.89
syphilitic A52.06
cranial (left) (right) , giant cell M31.6
deformans — *see* Arteriosclerosis
giant cell NEC M31.6
with polymyalgia rheumatica M31.5
necrosing or necrotizing M31.9
specified NEC M31.8
nodosa M30.0
obliterans — *see* Arteriosclerosis
pulmonary I28.8
rheumatic — *see* Fever, rheumatic
senile — *see* Arteriosclerosis
suppurative I77.2
syphilitic (general) A52.09
brain A52.04
coronary A52.06
spinal A52.09
temporal, giant cell M31.6
young female aortic arch syndrome M31.4
Artery, arterial — *see also* condition
abscess I77.89
single umbilical Q27.0
Arthralgia (allergic) — *see also* Pain, joint
in caisson disease T70.3
temporomandibular M26.62-
Arthritis, arthritic (acute) (chronic) (nonpyogenic) (subacute) M19.90
allergic — *see* Arthritis, specified form NEC
ankylosing (crippling) (spine) — *see also* Spondylitis, ankylosing
sites other than spine — *see* Arthritis, specified form NEC
atrophic — *see* Osteoarthritis
spine — *see* Spondylitis, ankylosing
back — *see* Spondylopathy, inflammatory
blennorrhagic (gonococcal) A54.42
Charcot's — *see* Arthropathy, neuropathic
diabetic — *see* Diabetes, arthropathy, neuropathic
syringomyelic G95.0
chylous (filarial) (*see also* category M01) B74.9
climacteric (any site) NEC — *see* Arthritis, specified form NEC
crystal (-induced) — *see* Arthritis, in, crystals
deformans — *see* Osteoarthritis
degenerative — *see* Osteoarthritis
due to or associated with
acromegaly E22.0
brucellosis — *see* Brucellosis
caisson disease T70.3
diabetes — *see* Diabetes, arthropathy
dracontiasis (*see also* category M01) B72
enteritis NEC
regional — *see* Enteritis, regional
erysipelas (*see also* category M01) A46
erythema
epidemic A25.1
nodosum L52
filariasis NOS B74.9
glanders A24.0
helminthiasis (*see also* category M01) B83.9
hemophilia D66 *[M36.2]*
Henoch- (Schönlein) purpura D69.0 *[M36.4]*
human parvovirus (*see also* category M01) B97.6
infectious disease NEC — *see* category M01
leprosy (see also category M01) — *see also* Leprosy A30.9
Lyme disease A69.23
mycobacteria (*see also* category M01) A31.8
parasitic disease NEC (*see also* category M01) B89
paratyphoid fever (see also category M01) — *see also* Fever, paratyphoid A01.4
rat bite fever (*see also* category M01) A25.1
regional enteritis — *see* Enteritis, regional
respiratory disorder NOS J98.9
serum sickness — *see also* Reaction, serum T80.69
syringomyelia G95.0
typhoid fever A01.04
epidemic erythema A25.1
febrile — *see* Fever, rheumatic
gonococcal A54.42
gouty (acute) — *see* Gout
in (due to)
acromegaly (*see also* subcategory M14.8-) E22.0
amyloidosis (*see also* subcategory M14.8-) E85.4
bacterial disease (*see also* subcategory M01) A49.9
Behçet's syndrome M35.2
caisson disease (*see also* subcategory M14.8-) T70.3

Arthritis, arthritic (acute) (chronic) (nonpyogenic) (subacute) - *continued*
in (due to) - *continued*
coliform bacilli (Escherichia coli) — *see* Arthritis, in, pyogenic organism NEC
crystals M11.9
dicalcium phosphate — *see* Arthritis, in, crystals, specified type NEC
hydroxyapatite M11.0-
pyrophosphate — *see* Arthritis, in, crystals, specified type NEC
specified type NEC M11.80
ankle M11.87-
elbow M11.82-
foot joint M11.87-
hand joint M11.84-
hip M11.85-
knee M11.86-
multiple sites M11.8-
shoulder M11.81-
vertebrae M11.88
wrist M11.83-
dermatoarthritis, lipoid E78.81
dracontiasis (dracunculiasis) (*see also* category M01) B72
endocrine disorder NEC (*see also* subcategory M14.8-) E34.9
enteritis, infectious NEC (*see also* category M01) A09
specified organism NEC (*see also* category M01) A08.8
erythema
multiforme (*see also* subcategory M14.8-) L51.9
nodosum (*see also* subcategory M14.8-) L52
gout — *see* Gout
helminthiasis NEC (*see also* category M01) B83.9
hemochromatosis (*see also* subcategory M14.8-) E83.118
hemoglobinopathy NEC D58.2 *[M36.3]*
hemophilia NEC D66 *[M36.2]*
Hemophilus influenzae M00.8- *[B96.3]*
Henoch (-Schönlein) purpura D69.0 *[M36.4]*
hyperparathyroidism NEC (*see also* subcategory M14.8-) E21.3
hypersensitivity reaction NEC T78.49 *[M36.4]*
hypogammaglobulinemia (*see also* subcategory M14.8-) D80.1
hypothyroidism NEC (*see also* subcategory M14.8-) E03.9
infection — *see* Arthritis, pyogenic or pyemic
spine — *see* Spondylopathy, infective
infectious disease NEC — *see* category M01
leprosy (*see also* category M01) A30.9
leukemia NEC C95.9- *[M36.1]*
lipoid dermatoarthritis E78.81
Lyme disease A69.23
Mediterranean fever, familial (*see also* subcategory M14.8-) M04.1
Meningococcus A39.83
metabolic disorder NEC (*see also* subcategory M14.8-) E88.9
multiple myelomatosis C90.0- *[M36.1]*
mumps B26.85
mycosis NEC (*see also* category M01) B49
myelomatosis (multiple) C90.0- *[M36.1]*
neurological disorder NEC G98.0
ochronosis (*see also* subcategory M14.8-) E70.29
O'nyong-nyong (*see also* category M01) A92.1
parasitic disease NEC (*see also* category M01) B89
paratyphoid fever (*see also* category M01) A01.4
Pseudomonas — *see* Arthritis, pyogenic, bacterial NEC
psoriasis L40.50
pyogenic organism NEC — *see* Arthritis, pyogenic, bacterial NEC
Reiter's disease — *see* Reiter's disease
respiratory disorder NEC (*see also* subcategory M14.8-) J98.9
reticulosis, malignant (*see also* subcategory M14.8-) C86.0
rubella B06.82
Salmonella (arizonae) (cholerae-suis) (enteritidis) (typhimurium) A02.23
sarcoidosis D86.86
specified bacteria NEC — *see* Arthritis, pyogenic, bacterial NEC
sporotrichosis B42.82
syringomyelia G95.0
thalassemia NEC D56.9 *[M36.3]*
tuberculosis — *see* Tuberculosis, arthritis
typhoid fever A01.04
urethritis, Reiter's — *see* Reiter's disease
viral disease NEC (*see also* category M01) B34.9

Arthritis, arthritic (acute) (chronic) (nonpyogenic) (subacute) - *continued*
  infectious or infective — *see also* Arthritis, pyogenic or pyemic
    spine — *see* Spondylopathy, infective
  juvenile M08.90
    with systemic onset — *see* Still's disease
    ankle M08.97-
    elbow M08.92-
    foot joint M08.97-
    hand joint M08.94-
    hip M08.95-
    knee M08.96-
    multiple site M08.99
    pauciarticular M08.40
      ankle M08.47-
      elbow M08.42-
      foot joint M08.47-
      hand joint M08.44-
      hip M08.45-
      knee M08.46-
      shoulder M08.41-
      vertebrae M08.48
      wrist M08.43-
    psoriatic L40.54
    rheumatoid — *see* Arthritis, rheumatoid, juvenile
    shoulder M08.91-
    vertebra M08.98
    specified type NEC M08.80
      ankle M08.87-
      elbow M08.82-
      foot joint M08.87-
      hand joint M08.84-
      hip M08.85-
      knee M08.86-
      multiple site M08.89
      shoulder M08.81-
      specified joint NEC M08.88
      vertebrae M08.88
      wrist M08.83-
    wrist M08.93-
  meaning osteoarthritis — *see* Osteoarthritis
  meningococcal A39.83
  menopausal (any site) NEC — *see* Arthritis, specified form NEC
  mutilans (psoriatic) L40.52
  mycotic NEC (*see also* category M01) B49
  neuropathic (Charcot) — *see* Arthropathy, neuropathic
    diabetic — *see* Diabetes, arthropathy, neuropathic
    nonsyphilitic NEC G98.0
    syringomyelic G95.0
  ochronotic (*see also* subcategory M14.8-) E70.29
  palindromic (any site) — *see* Rheumatism, palindromic
  pneumococcal M00.10
    ankle M00.17-
    elbow M00.12-
    foot joint — *see* Arthritis, pneumococcal, ankle
    hand joint M00.14-
    hip M00.15-
    knee M00.16-
    multiple site M00.19
    shoulder M00.11-
    vertebra M00.18
    wrist M00.13-
  postdysenteric — *see* Arthropathy, postdysenteric
  postmeningococcal A39.84
  postrheumatic, chronic — *see* Arthropathy, postrheumatic, chronic
  primary progressive — *see also* Arthritis, specified form NEC
    spine — *see* Spondylitis, ankylosing
  psoriatic L40.50
  purulent (any site except spine) — *see* Arthritis, pyogenic or pyemic
    spine — *see* Spondylopathy, infective
  pyogenic or pyemic (any site except spine) M00.9
    bacterial NEC M00.80
      ankle M00.87-
      elbow M00.82-
      foot joint — *see* Arthritis, pyogenic, bacterial NEC, ankle
      hand joint M00.84-
      hip M00.85-
      knee M00.86-
      multiple site M00.89
      shoulder M00.81-
      vertebra M00.88
      wrist M00.83-
    pneumococcal — *see* Arthritis, pneumococcal
    spine — *see* Spondylopathy, infective
    staphylococcal — *see* Arthritis, staphylococcal

Arthritis, arthritic (acute) (chronic) (nonpyogenic) (subacute) - *continued*
  pyogenic or pyemic (any site except spine) - *continued*
    streptococcal — *see* Arthritis, streptococcal NEC
      pneumococcal — *see* Arthritis, pneumococcal
  reactive — *see* Reiter's disease
  rheumatic — *see also* Arthritis, rheumatoid
    acute or subacute — *see* Fever, rheumatic
  rheumatoid M06.9
    with
      carditis — *see* Rheumatoid, carditis
      endocarditis — *see* Rheumatoid, carditis
      heart involvement NEC — *see* Rheumatoid, carditis
      lung involvement — *see* Rheumatoid, lung
      myocarditis — *see* Rheumatoid, carditis
      myopathy — *see* Rheumatoid, myopathy
      pericarditis — *see* Rheumatoid, carditis
      polyneuropathy — *see* Rheumatoid, polyneuropathy
      rheumatoid factor — *see* Arthritis, rheumatoid, seropositive
      splenoadenomegaly and leukopenia — *see* Felty's syndrome
      vasculitis — *see* Rheumatoid, vasculitis
      visceral involvement NEC — *see* Rheumatoid, arthritis, with involvement of organs NEC
    juvenile (with or without rheumatoid factor) M08.00
      ankle M08.07-
      elbow M08.02-
      foot joint M08.07-
      hand joint M08.04-
      hip M08.05-
      knee M08.06-
      multiple site M08.09
      shoulder M08.01-
      vertebra M08.08
      wrist M08.03-
    seronegative M06.00
      ankle M06.07-
      elbow M06.02-
      foot joint M06.07-
      hand joint M06.04-
      hip M06.05-
      knee M06.06-
      multiple site M06.09
      shoulder M06.01-
      vertebra M06.08
      wrist M06.03-
    seropositive M05.9
      specified NEC M05.80
        ankle M05.87-
        elbow M05.82-
        foot joint M05.87-
        hand joint M05.84-
        hip M05.85-
        knee M05.86-
        multiple sites M05.89
        shoulder M05.81-
        vertebra — *see* Spondylitis, ankylosing
        wrist M05.83-
      without organ involvement M05.70
        ankle M05.77-
        elbow M05.72-
        foot joint M05.77-
        hand joint M05.74-
        hip M05.75-
        knee M05.76-
        multiple sites M05.79
        shoulder M05.71-
        vertebra — *see* Spondylitis, ankylosing
        wrist M05.73-
    specified type NEC M06.80
      ankle M06.87-
      elbow M06.82-
      foot joint M06.87-
      hand joint M06.84-
      hip M06.85-
      knee M06.86-
      multiple site M06.89
      shoulder M06.81-
      vertebra M06.88
      wrist M06.83-
    spine — *see* Spondylitis, ankylosing
  rubella B06.82
  scorbutic (*see also* subcategory M14.8-) E54
  senile or senescent — *see* Osteoarthritis
  septic (any site except spine) — *see* Arthritis, pyogenic or pyemic
    spine — *see* Spondylopathy, infective

Arthritis, arthritic (acute) (chronic) (nonpyogenic) (subacute) - *continued*
  serum (nontherapeutic) (therapeutic) — *see* Arthropathy, postimmunization
  specified form NEC M13.80
    ankle M13.87-
    elbow M13.82-
    foot joint M13.87-
    hand joint M13.84-
    hip M13.85-
    knee M13.86-
    multiple site M13.89
    shoulder M13.81-
    specified joint NEC M13.88
    wrist M13.83-
  spine — *see also* Spondylopathy, inflammatory
    infectious or infective NEC — *see* Spondylopathy, infective
    Marie-Strümpell — *see* Spondylitis, ankylosing
    pyogenic — *see* Spondylopathy, infective
    rheumatoid — *see* Spondylitis, ankylosing
    traumatic (old) — *see* Spondylopathy, traumatic
    tuberculous A18.01
  staphylococcal M00.00
    ankle M00.07-
    elbow M00.02-
    foot joint — *see* Arthritis, staphylococcal, ankle
    hand joint M00.04-
    hip M00.05-
    knee M00.06-
    multiple site M00.09
    shoulder M00.01-
    vertebra M00.08
    wrist M00.03-
  streptococcal NEC M00.20
    ankle M00.27-
    elbow M00.22-
    foot joint — *see* Arthritis, streptococcal, ankle
    hand joint M00.24-
    hip M00.25-
    knee M00.26-
    multiple site M00.29
    shoulder M00.21-
    vertebra M00.28
    wrist M00.23-
  suppurative — *see* Arthritis, pyogenic or pyemic
  syphilitic (late) A52.16
    congenital A50.55 *[M12.80]*
  syphilitica deformans (Charcot) A52.16
  temporomandibular M26.69
  toxic of menopause (any site) — *see* Arthritis, specified form NEC
  transient — *see* Arthropathy, specified form NEC
  traumatic (chronic) — *see* Arthropathy, traumatic
  tuberculous A18.02
    spine A18.01
  uratic — *see* Gout
  urethritica (Reiter's) — *see* Reiter's disease
  vertebral — *see* Spondylopathy, inflammatory
  villous (any site) — *see* Arthropathy, specified form NEC
Arthrocele — *see* Effusion, joint
Arthrodesis status Z98.1
Arthrodynia — *see also* Pain, joint
Arthrodysplasia Q74.9
Arthrofibrosis, joint — *see* Ankylosis
Arthrogryposis (congenital) Q68.8
  multiplex congenita Q74.3
Arthrokatadysis M24.7
Arthropathy — *see also* Arthritis M12.9
  Charcot's — *see* Arthropathy, neuropathic
    diabetic — *see* Diabetes, arthropathy, neuropathic
    syringomyelic G95.0
  cricoarytenoid J38.7
  crystal (-induced) — *see* Arthritis, in, crystals
  diabetic NEC — *see* Diabetes, arthropathy
  distal interphalangeal, psoriatic L40.51
  enteropathic M07.60
    ankle M07.67-
    elbow M07.62-
    foot joint M07.67-
    hand joint M07.64-
    hip M07.65-
    knee M07.66-
    multiple site M07.69
    shoulder M07.61-
    vertebra M07.68
    wrist M07.63-
  following intestinal bypass M02.00
    ankle M02.07-
    elbow M02.02-
    foot joint M02.07-
    hand joint M02.04-

Arthropathy - *continued*
following intestinal bypass - *continued*
hip M02.05-
knee M02.06-
multiple site M02.09
shoulder M02.01-
vertebra M02.08
wrist M02.03-
gouty — *see also* Gout
in (due to)
Lesch-Nyhan syndrome E79.1 *[M14.8-]*
sickle-cell disorders D57- *[M14.8-]*
hemophilic NEC D66 *[M36.2]*
in (due to)
hyperparathyroidism NEC E21.3 *[M14.8-]*
metabolic disease NOS E88.9 *[M14.8-]*
in (due to)
acromegaly E22.0 *[M14.8-]*
amyloidosis E85.4 *[M14.8-]*
blood disorder NOS D75.9 *[M36.3]*
diabetes — *see* Diabetes, arthropathy
endocrine disease NOS E34.9 *[M14.8-]*
erythema
multiforme L51.9 *[M14.8-]*
nodosum L52 *[M14.8-]*
hemochromatosis E83.118 *[M14.8-]*
hemoglobinopathy NEC D58.2 *[M36.3]*
hemophilia NEC D66 *[M36.2]*
Henoch-Schönlein purpura D69.0 *[M36.4]*
hyperthyroidism E05.90 *[M14.8-]*
hypothyroidism E03.9 *[M14.8-]*
infective endocarditis I33.0 *[M12.80]*
leukemia NEC C95.9- *[M36.1]*
malignant histiocytosis C96.A *[M36.1]*
metabolic disease NOS E88.9 *[M14.8-]*
multiple myeloma C90.0- *[M36.1]*
neoplastic disease NOS (see also
Neoplasm) D49.9 *[M36.1]*
nutritional deficiency
(*see also* subcategory M14.8-) E63.9
psoriasis NOS L40.50
sarcoidosis D86.86
syphilis (late) A52.77
congenital A50.55 *[M12.80]*
thyrotoxicosis (*see also*
subcategory M14.8-) E05.90
ulcerative colitis K51.90 *[M07.60]*
viral hepatitis (postinfectious)
NEC B19.9 *[M12.80]*
Whipple's disease (*see also*
subcategory M14.8-) K90.81
Jaccoud — *see* Arthropathy, postrheumatic, chronic
juvenile — *see* Arthritis, juvenile
psoriatic L40.54
mutilans (psoriatic) L40.52
neuropathic (Charcot) M14.60
ankle M14.67-
diabetic — *see* Diabetes, arthropathy, neuropathic
elbow M14.62-
foot joint M14.67-
hand joint M14.64-
hip M14.65-
knee M14.66-
multiple site M14.69
nonsyphilitic NEC G98.0
shoulder M14.61-
syringomyelic G95.0
vertebra M14.68
wrist M14.63-
osteopulmonary — *see* Osteoarthropathy,
hypertrophic, specified NEC
postdysenteric M02.10
ankle M02.17-
elbow M02.12-
foot joint M02.17-
hand joint M02.14-
hip M02.15-
knee M02.16-
multiple site M02.19
shoulder M02.11-
vertebra M02.18
wrist M02.13-
postimmunization M02.20
ankle M02.27-
elbow M02.22-
foot joint M02.27-
hand joint M02.24-
hip M02.25-
knee M02.26-
multiple site M02.29
shoulder M02.21-
vertebra M02.28
wrist M02.23-

Arthropathy - *continued*
postinfectious NEC B99 *[M12.80]*
in (due to)
enteritis due to Yersinia
enterocolitica A04.6 *[M12.80]*
syphilis A52.77
viral hepatitis NEC B19.9 *[M12.80]*
postrheumatic, chronic (Jaccoud) M12.00
ankle M12.07-
elbow M12.02-
foot joint M12.07-
hand joint M12.04-
hip M12.05-
knee M12.06-
multiple site M12.09
shoulder M12.01-
specified joint NEC M12.08
vertebrae M12.08
wrist M12.03-
psoriatic NEC L40.59
interphalangeal, distal L40.51
reactive M02.9
in (due to)
infective endocarditis I33.0 *[M02.9]*
specified type NEC M02.80
ankle M02.87-
elbow M02.82-
foot joint M02.87-
hand joint M02.84-
hip M02.85-
knee M02.86-
multiple site M02.89
shoulder M02.81-
vertebra M02.88
wrist M02.83-
specified form NEC M12.80
ankle M12.87-
elbow M12.82-
foot joint M12.87-
hand joint M12.84-
hip M12.85-
knee M12.86-
multiple site M12.89
shoulder M12.81-
specified joint NEC M12.88
vertebrae M12.88
wrist M12.83-
syringomyelic G95.0
tabes dorsalis A52.16
tabetic A52.16
transient — *see* Arthropathy, specified form NEC
traumatic M12.50
ankle M12.57-
elbow M12.52-
foot joint M12.57-
hand joint M12.54-
hip M12.55-
knee M12.56-
multiple site M12.59
shoulder M12.51-
specified joint NEC M12.58
vertebrae M12.58
wrist M12.53-
Arthropyosis — *see* Arthritis, pyogenic or pyemic
Arthrosis (deformans) (degenerative)
(localized) — *see also* Osteoarthritis M19.90
spine — *see* Spondylosis
Arthus' phenomenon or reaction T78.41
due to
drug — *see* Table of Drugs and Chemicals, by drug
Articular — *see* condition
Articulation, reverse (teeth) M26.24
Artificial
insemination complication — *see* Complications,
artificial, fertilization
opening status (functioning) (without
complication) Z93.9
anus (colostomy) Z93.3
colostomy Z93.3
cystostomy Z93.50
appendico-vesicostomy Z93.52
cutaneous Z93.51
specified NEC Z93.59
enterostomy Z93.4
gastrostomy Z93.1
ileostomy Z93.2
intestinal tract NEC Z93.4
jejunostomy Z93.4
nephrostomy Z93.6
specified site NEC Z93.8
tracheostomy Z93.0
ureterostomy Z93.6
urethrostomy Z93.6

Artificial - *continued*
opening status (functioning) (without complication)
- *continued*
urinary tract NEC Z93.6
vagina Z93.8
vagina status Z93.8
Arytenoid — *see* condition
Asbestosis (occupational) J61
Ascariasis B77.9
with
complications NEC B77.89
intestinal complications B77.0
pneumonia, pneumonitis B77.81
Ascaridosis, ascaridiasis — *see* Ascariasis
Ascaris (infection) (infestation) (lumbricoides) — *see*
Ascariasis
Ascending — *see* condition
ASC-H
(atypical squamous cells cannot exclude high grade
squamous intraepithelial lesion on cytologic smear)
anus R85.611
cervix R87.611
vagina R87.621
Aschoff's bodies — *see* Myocarditis, rheumatic
Ascites (abdominal) R18.8
cardiac — *see also* Failure, heart, right I50.810
chylous (nonfilarial) I89.8
filarial — *see* Infestation, filarial
due to
cirrhosis, alcoholic K70.31
hepatitis
alcoholic K70.11
chronic active K71.51
S. japonicum B65.2
heart — *see also* Failure, heart, right I50.810
malignant R18.0
pseudochylous R18.8
syphilitic A52.74
tuberculous A18.31
ASC-US
(atypical squamous cells of undetermined
significance on cytologic smear)
anus R85.610
cervix R87.610
vagina R87.620
Aseptic — *see* condition
Asherman's syndrome N85.6
Asialia K11.7
Asiatic cholera — *see* Cholera
Asimultagnosia (simultanagnosia) R48.3
Askin's tumor — *see* Neoplasm, connective tissue,
malignant
Asocial personality F60.2
Asomatognosia R41.4
Aspartylglucosaminuria E77.1
Asperger's disease or syndrome F84.5
Aspergilloma — *see* Aspergillosis
Aspergillosis (with pneumonia) B44.9
bronchopulmonary, allergic B44.81
disseminated B44.7
generalized B44.7
pulmonary NEC B44.1
allergic B44.81
invasive B44.0
specified NEC B44.89
tonsillar B44.2
Aspergillus (flavus) (fumigatus) (infection)
(terreus) — *see* Aspergillosis
Aspermatogenesis — *see* Azoospermia
Aspermia (testis) — *see* Azoospermia
Asphyxia, asphyxiation (by) R09.01
antenatal P84
birth P84
bunny bag — *see* Asphyxia, due to, mechanical
threat to breathing, trapped in bed clothes
crushing S28.0
drowning T75.1
gas, fumes, or vapor — *see* Table of Drugs and
Chemicals
inhalation — *see* Inhalation
intrauterine P84
local I73.00
with gangrene I73.01
mucus — *see also* Foreign body, respiratory tract,
causing asphyxia
newborn P84
pathological R09.01
postnatal P84
mechanical — *see* Asphyxia, due to, mechanical
threat to breathing
prenatal P84
reticularis R23.1

Asphyxia, asphyxiation (by) - *continued*
strangulation — *see* Asphyxia, due to, mechanical threat to breathing
submersion T75.1
traumatic T71.9
due to
crushed chest S28.0
foreign body (in) — *see* Foreign body, respiratory tract, causing asphyxia
low oxygen content of ambient air T71.20
due to
being trapped in
low oxygen environment T71.29
in car trunk T71.221
circumstances undetermined T71.224
done with intent to harm by
another person T71.223
self T71.222
in refrigerator T71.231
circumstances undetermined T71.234
done with intent to harm by
another person T71.233
self T71.232
cave-in T71.21
mechanical threat to breathing (accidental) T71.191
circumstances undetermined T71.194
done with intent to harm by
another person T71.193
self T71.192
hanging T71.161
circumstances undetermined T71.164
done with intent to harm by
another person T71.163
self T71.162
plastic bag T71.121
circumstances undetermined T71.124
done with intent to harm by
another person T71.123
self T71.122
smothering
in furniture T71.151
circumstances undetermined T71.154
done with intent to harm by
another person T71.153
self T71.152
under
another person's body T71.141
circumstances undetermined T71.144
done with intent to harm T71.143
pillow T71.111
circumstances undetermined T71.114
done with intent to harm by
another person T71.113
self T71.112
trapped in bed clothes T71.131
circumstances undetermined T71.134
done with intent to harm by
another person T71.133
self T71.132
vomiting, vomitus — *see* Foreign body, respiratory tract, causing asphyxia

Aspiration
amniotic (clear) fluid (newborn) P24.10
with
pneumonia (pneumonitis) P24.11
respiratory symptoms P24.11
blood
newborn (without respiratory symptoms) P24.20
with
pneumonia (pneumonitis) P24.21
respiratory symptoms P24.21
specified age NEC — *see* Foreign body, respiratory tract
bronchitis J69.0
food or foreign body (with asphyxiation) — *see* Asphyxia, food
liquor (amnii) (newborn) P24.10
with
pneumonia (pneumonitis) P24.11
respiratory symptoms P24.11
meconium (newborn) (without respiratory symptoms) P24.00
with
pneumonitis (pneumonitis) P24.01
respiratory symptoms P24.01
milk (newborn) (without respiratory symptoms) P24.30
with
pneumonia (pneumonitis) P24.31
respiratory symptoms P24.31
specified age NEC — *see* Foreign body, respiratory tract

Aspiration - *continued*
mucus — *see also* Foreign body, by site, causing asphyxia
newborn P24.10
with
pneumonia (pneumonitis) P24.11
respiratory symptoms P24.11
neonatal P24.9
specific NEC (without respiratory symptoms) P24.80
with
pneumonia (pneumonitis) P24.81
respiratory symptoms P24.81
newborn P24.9
specific NEC (without respiratory symptoms) P24.80
with
pneumonia (pneumonitis) P24.81
respiratory symptoms P24.81
pneumonia J69.0
pneumonitis J69.0
syndrome of newborn — *see* Aspiration, by substance, with pneumonia
vernix caseosa (newborn) P24.80
with
pneumonia (pneumonitis) P24.81
respiratory symptoms P24.81
vomitus — *see also* Foreign body, respiratory tract
newborn (without respiratory symptoms) P24.30
with
pneumonia (pneumonitis) P24.31
respiratory symptoms P24.31

Asplenia (congenital) Q89.01
postsurgical Z90.81
Assam fever B55.0
Assault, sexual — *see* Maltreatment
Assmann's focus NEC A15.0
Astasia (-abasia) (hysterical) F44.4
Asteatosis cutis L85.3
Astereognosia, astereognosis R48.1
Asterixis R27.8
in liver disease K71.3
Asteroid hyalitis — *see* Deposit, crystalline
Asthenia, asthenic R53.1
cardiac — *see also* Failure, heart I50.9
psychogenic F45.8
cardiovascular — *see also* Failure, heart I50.9
psychogenic F45.8
heart — *see also* Failure, heart I50.9
psychogenic F45.8
hysterical F44.4
myocardial — *see also* Failure, heart I50.9
psychogenic F45.8
nervous F48.8
neurocirculatory F45.8
neurotic F48.8
psychogenic F48.8
psychoneurotic F48.8
psychophysiologic F48.8
reaction (psychophysiologic) F48.8
senile R54
Asthenopia — *see also* Discomfort, visual
hysterical F44.6
psychogenic F44.6
Asthenospermia — *see* Abnormal, specimen, male genital organs
Asthma, asthmatic (bronchial) (catarrh) (spasmodic) J45.909
with
chronic obstructive bronchitis J44.9
with
acute lower respiratory infection J44.0
exacerbation (acute) J44.1
chronic obstructive pulmonary disease J44.9
with
acute lower respiratory infection J44.0
exacerbation (acute) J44.1
exacerbation (acute) J45.901
hay fever — *see* Asthma, allergic extrinsic
rhinitis, allergic — *see* Asthma, allergic extrinsic
status asthmaticus J45.902
allergic extrinsic J45.909
with
exacerbation (acute) J45.901
status asthmaticus J45.902
atopic — *see* Asthma, allergic extrinsic
cardiac — *see* Failure, ventricular, left
cardiobronchial I50.1
childhood J45.909
with
exacerbation (acute) J45.901
status asthmaticus J45.902
chronic obstructive J44.9

Asthma, asthmatic (bronchial) (catarrh) (spasmodic) - *continued*
chronic obstructive - *continued*
with
acute lower respiratory infection J44.0
exacerbation (acute) J44.1
collier's J60
cough variant J45.991
detergent J69.8
due to
detergent J69.8
inhalation of fumes J68.3
eosinophilic J82
extrinsic, allergic — *see* Asthma, allergic extrinsic
grinder's J62.8
hay — *see* Asthma, allergic extrinsic
heart I50.1
idiosyncratic — *see* Asthma, nonallergic
intermittent (mild) J45.20
with
exacerbation (acute) J45.21
status asthmaticus J45.22
intrinsic, nonallergic — *see* Asthma, nonallergic
Kopp's E32.8
late-onset J45.909
with
exacerbation (acute) J45.901
status asthmaticus J45.902
mild intermittent J45.20
with
exacerbation (acute) J45.21
status asthmaticus J45.22
mild persistent J45.30
with
exacerbation (acute) J45.31
status asthmaticus J45.32
Millar's (laryngismus stridulus) J38.5
miner's J60
mixed J45.909
with
exacerbation (acute) J45.901
status asthmaticus J45.902
moderate persistent J45.40
with
exacerbation (acute) J45.41
status asthmaticus J45.42
nervous — *see* Asthma, nonallergic
nonallergic (intrinsic) J45.909
with
exacerbation (acute) J45.901
status asthmaticus J45.902
persistent
mild J45.30
with
exacerbation (acute) J45.31
status asthmaticus J45.32
moderate J45.40
with
exacerbation (acute) J45.41
status asthmaticus J45.42
severe J45.50
with
exacerbation (acute) J45.51
status asthmaticus J45.52
platinum J45.998
pneumoconiotic NEC J64
potter's J62.8
predominantly allergic J45.909
psychogenic F54
pulmonary eosinophilic J82
red cedar J67.8
Rostan's I50.1
sandblaster's J62.8
sequoiosis J67.8
severe persistent J45.50
with
exacerbation (acute) J45.51
status asthmaticus J45.52
specified NEC J45.998
stonemason's J62.8
thymic E32.8
tuberculous — *see* Tuberculosis, pulmonary
Wichmann's (laryngismus stridulus) J38.5
wood J67.8
Astigmatism (compound) (congenital) H52.20-
irregular H52.21-
regular H52.22-
Astraphobia F40.220
Astroblastoma
specified site — *see* Neoplasm, malignant, by site
unspecified site C71.9
Astrocytoma (cystic)
anaplastic

Astrocytoma (cystic) - *continued*
anaplastic - *continued*
specified site — *see* Neoplasm, malignant, by site
unspecified site C71.9
fibrillary
specified site — *see* Neoplasm, malignant, by site
unspecified site C71.9
fibrous
specified site — *see* Neoplasm, malignant, by site
unspecified site C71.9
gemistocytic
specified site — *see* Neoplasm, malignant, by site
unspecified site C71.9
juvenile
specified site — *see* Neoplasm, malignant, by site
unspecified site C71.9
pilocytic
specified site — *see* Neoplasm, malignant, by site
unspecified site C71.9
piloid
specified site — *see* Neoplasm, malignant, by site
unspecified site C71.9
protoplasmic
specified site — *see* Neoplasm, malignant, by site
unspecified site C71.9
specified site NEC — *see* Neoplasm, malignant, by site
subependymal D43.2
giant cell
specified site — *see* Neoplasm, uncertain behavior, by site
unspecified site D43.2
specified site — *see* Neoplasm, uncertain behavior, by site
unspecified site D43.2
unspecified site C71.9
Astroglioma
specified site — *see* Neoplasm, malignant, by site
unspecified site C71.9
Asymbolia R48.8
Asymmetry — *see also* Distortion
between native and reconstructed breast N65.1
face Q67.0
jaw (lower) — *see* Anomaly, dentofacial, jaw-cranial base relationship, asymmetry
Asynergia, asynergy R27.8
ventricular I51.89
Asystole (heart) — *see* Arrest, cardiac
At risk
for
dental caries Z91.849
high Z91.843
low Z91.841
moderate Z91.842
falling Z91.81
Ataxia, ataxy, ataxic R27.0
acute R27.8
brain (hereditary) G11.9
cerebellar (hereditary) G11.9
with defective DNA repair G11.3
alcoholic G31.2
early-onset G11.1
in
alcoholism G31.2
myxedema E03.9 *[G13.2]*
neoplastic disease — *see also* Neoplasm D49.9 *[G32.81]*
specified disease NEC G32.81
late-onset (Marie's) G11.2
cerebral (hereditary) G11.9
congenital nonprogressive G11.0
family, familial — *see* Ataxia, hereditary
following
cerebrovascular disease I69.993
cerebral infarction I69.393
intracerebral hemorrhage I69.193
nontraumatic intracranial hemorrhage NEC I69.293
specified disease NEC I69.893
subarachnoid hemorrhage I69.093
Friedreich's (heredofamilial) (cerebellar) (spinal) G11.1
gait R26.0
hysterical F44.4
general R27.8
gluten M35.9 *[G32.81]*
with celiac disease K90.0 *[G32.81]*
hereditary G11.9
with neuropathy G60.2
cerebellar — *see* Ataxia, cerebellar
spastic G11.4
specified NEC G11.8
spinal (Friedreich's) G11.1

Ataxia, ataxy, ataxic - *continued*
heredofamilial — *see* Ataxia, hereditary
Hunt's G11.1
hysterical F44.4
locomotor (progressive) (syphilitic) (partial) (spastic) A52.11
diabetic — *see* Diabetes, ataxia
Marie's (cerebellar) (heredofamilial) (late-onset) G11.2
nonorganic origin F44.4
nonprogressive, congenital G11.0
psychogenic F44.4
Roussy-Lévy G60.0
Sanger-Brown's (hereditary) G11.2
spastic hereditary G11.4
spinal
hereditary (Friedreich's) G11.1
progressive (syphilitic) A52.11
spinocerebellar, X-linked recessive G11.1
telangiectasia (Louis-Bar) G11.3
Ataxia-telangiectasia (Louis-Bar) G11.3
Atelectasis (massive) (partial) (pressure) (pulmonary) J98.11
newborn P28.10
due to resorption P28.11
partial P28.19
primary P28.0
secondary P28.19
primary (newborn) P28.0
tuberculous — *see* Tuberculosis, pulmonary
Atelocardia Q24.9
Atelomyelia Q06.1
Atheroembolism
of
extremities
lower I75.02-
upper I75.01-
kidney I75.81
specified NEC I75.89
Atheroma, atheromatous — *see also* Arteriosclerosis I70.90
aorta, aortic I70.0
valve — *see also* Endocarditis, aortic I35.8
aorto-iliac I70.0
artery — *see* Arteriosclerosis
basilar (artery) I67.2
carotid (artery) (common) (internal) I67.2
cerebral (arteries) I67.2
coronary (artery) I25.10
with angina pectoris — *see* Arteriosclerosis, coronary (artery),
degeneration — *see* Arteriosclerosis
heart, cardiac — *see* Disease, heart, ischemic, atherosclerotic
mitral (valve) I34.8
myocardium, myocardial — *see* Disease, heart, ischemic, atherosclerotic
pulmonary valve (heart) — *see also* Endocarditis, pulmonary I37.8
tricuspid (heart) (valve) I36.8
valve, valvular — *see* Endocarditis
vertebral (artery) I67.2
Atheromatosis — *see* Arteriosclerosis
Atherosclerosis — *see also* Arteriosclerosis
coronary
artery I25.10
with angina pectoris — *see* Arteriosclerosis, coronary (artery),
due to
calcified coronary lesion (severely) I25.84
lipid rich plaque I25.83
transplanted heart I25.811
bypass graft I25.812
with angina pectoris — *see* Arteriosclerosis, coronary (artery),
native coronary artery I25.811
with angina pectoris — *see* Arteriosclerosis, coronary (artery),
Athetosis (acquired) R25.8
bilateral (congenital) G80.3
congenital (bilateral) (double) G80.3
double (congenital) G80.3
unilateral R25.8
Athlete's
foot B35.3
heart I51.7
Athrepsia E41
Athyrea (acquired) — *see also* Hypothyroidism
congenital E03.1
Atonia, atony, atonic
bladder (sphincter) (neurogenic) N31.2
capillary I78.8
cecum K59.8

Atonia, atony, atonic - *continued*
cecum - *continued*
psychogenic F45.8
colon — *see* Atony, intestine
congenital P94.2
esophagus K22.8
intestine K59.8
psychogenic F45.8
stomach K31.89
neurotic or psychogenic F45.8
uterus (during labor) O62.2
with hemorrhage (postpartum) O72.1
postpartum (with hemorrhage) O72.1
without hemorrhage O75.89
Atopy — *see* History, allergy
Atransferrinemia, congenital E88.09
Atresia, atretic
alimentary organ or tract NEC Q45.8
upper Q40.8
ani, anus, anal (canal) Q42.3
with fistula Q42.2
aorta (ring) Q25.29
aortic (orifice) (valve) Q23.0
arch Q25.21
congenital with hypoplasia of ascending aorta and defective development of left ventricle (with mitral stenosis) Q23.4
in hypoplastic left heart syndrome Q23.4
aqueduct of Sylvius Q03.0
with spina bifida — *see* Spina bifida, with hydrocephalus
artery NEC Q27.8
cerebral Q28.3
coronary Q24.5
digestive system Q27.8
eye Q15.8
lower limb Q27.8
pulmonary Q25.5
specified site NEC Q27.8
umbilical Q27.0
upper limb Q27.8
auditory canal (external) Q16.1
bile duct (common) (congenital) (hepatic) Q44.2
acquired — *see* Obstruction, bile duct
bladder (neck) Q64.39
obstruction Q64.31
bronchus Q32.4
cecum Q42.8
cervix (acquired) N88.2
congenital Q51.828
in pregnancy or childbirth — *see* Anomaly, cervix, in pregnancy or childbirth
causing obstructed labor O65.5
choana Q30.0
colon Q42.9
specified NEC Q42.8
common duct Q44.2
cricoid cartilage Q31.8
cystic duct Q44.2
acquired K82.8
with obstruction K82.0
digestive organs NEC Q45.8
duodenum Q41.0
ear canal Q16.1
ejaculatory duct Q55.4
epiglottis Q31.8
esophagus Q39.0
with tracheoesophageal fistula Q39.1
eustachian tube Q17.8
fallopian tube (congenital) Q50.6
acquired N97.1
follicular cyst N83.0-
foramen of
Luschka Q03.1
with spina bifida — *see* Spina bifida, with hydrocephalus
Magendie Q03.1
with spina bifida — *see* Spina bifida, with hydrocephalus
gallbladder Q44.1
genital organ
external
female Q52.79
male Q55.8
internal
female Q52.8
male Q55.8
glottis Q31.8
gullet Q39.0
with tracheoesophageal fistula Q39.1
heart valve NEC Q24.8
pulmonary Q22.0
tricuspid Q22.4

Atresia, atretic - *continued*
  hymen Q52.3
    acquired (postinfective) N89.6
  ileum Q41.2
  intestine (small) Q41.9
    large Q42.9
      specified NEC Q42.8
  iris, filtration angle Q15.0
  jejunum Q41.1
  lacrimal apparatus Q10.4
  larynx Q31.8
  meatus urinarius Q64.33
  mitral valve Q23.2
    in hypoplastic left heart syndrome Q23.4
  nares (anterior) (posterior) Q30.0
  nasopharynx Q34.8
  nose, nostril Q30.0
    acquired J34.89
  organ or site NEC Q89.8
  osseous meatus (ear) Q16.1
  oviduct (congenital) Q50.6
    acquired N97.1
  parotid duct Q38.4
    acquired K11.8
  pulmonary (artery) Q25.5
    valve Q22.0
  pulmonic Q22.0
  pupil Q13.2
  rectum Q42.1
    with fistula Q42.0
  salivary duct Q38.4
    acquired K11.8
  sublingual duct Q38.4
    acquired K11.8
  submandibular duct Q38.4
    acquired K11.8
  submaxillary duct Q38.4
    acquired K11.8
  thyroid cartilage Q31.8
  trachea Q32.1
  tricuspid valve Q22.4
  ureter Q62.10
    pelvic junction Q62.11
    vesical orifice Q62.12
  ureteropelvic junction Q62.11
  ureterovesical orifice Q62.12
  urethra (valvular) Q64.39
    stricture Q64.32
  urinary tract NEC Q64.8
  uterus Q51.818
    acquired N85.8
  vagina (congenital) Q52.4
    acquired (postinfectional) (senile) N89.5
  vas deferens Q55.3
  vascular NEC Q27.8
    cerebral Q28.3
    digestive system Q27.8
    lower limb Q27.8
    specified site NEC Q27.8
    upper limb Q27.8
  vein NEC Q27.8
    digestive system Q27.8
    great Q26.8
    lower limb Q27.8
    portal Q26.5
    pulmonary Q26.4
      partial Q26.3
      total Q26.2
    specified site NEC Q27.8
    upper limb Q27.8
  vena cava (inferior) (superior) Q26.8
  vesicourethral orifice Q64.31
  vulva Q52.79
    acquired N90.5
Atrichia, atrichosis — *see* Alopecia
Atrophia — *see also* Atrophy
  cutis senilis L90.8
    due to radiation L57.8
  gyrata of choroid and retina H31.23
  senilis R54
    dermatological L90.8
      due to radiation (nonionizing) (solar) L57.8
  unguium L60.3
    congenita Q84.6
Atrophie blanche (en plaque) (de Milian) L95.0
Atrophoderma, atrophodermia (of) L90.9
  diffusum (idiopathic) L90.4
  maculatum L90.8
    et striatum L90.8
      due to syphilis A52.79
    syphilitic A51.39
  neuriticum L90.8
  Pasini and Pierini L90.3

Atrophoderma, atrophodermia (of) - *continued*
  pigmentosum Q82.1
  reticulatum symmetricum faciei L66.4
  senile L90.8
    due to radiation (nonionizing) (solar) L57.8
  vermiculata (cheeks) L66.4
Atrophy, atrophic (of)
  adrenal (capsule) (gland) E27.49
    primary (autoimmune) E27.1
  alveolar process or ridge (edentulous) K08.20
  anal sphincter (disuse) N81.84
  appendix K38.8
  arteriosclerotic — *see* Arteriosclerosis
  bile duct (common) (hepatic) K83.8
  bladder N32.89
    neurogenic N31.8
  blanche (en plaque) (of Milian) L95.0
  bone (senile) NEC — *see also* Disorder, bone, specified type NEC
    due to
      tabes dorsalis (neurogenic) A52.11
  brain (cortex) (progressive) G31.9
    frontotemporal circumscribed G31.01 *[F02.80]*
      with behavioral disturbance G31.01 *[F02.81]*
    senile NEC G31.1
  breast N64.2
    obstetric — *see* Disorder, breast, specified type NEC
  buccal cavity K13.79
  cardiac — *see* Degeneration, myocardial
  cartilage (infectional) (joint) — *see* Disorder, cartilage, specified NEC
  cerebellar — *see* Atrophy, brain
  cerebral — *see* Atrophy, brain
  cervix (mucosa) (senile) (uteri) N88.8
    menopausal N95.8
  Charcot-Marie-Tooth G60.0
  choroid (central) (macular) (myopic) (retina) H31.10-
    diffuse secondary H31.12-
    gyrate H31.23
    senile H31.11-
  ciliary body — *see* Atrophy, iris
  conjunctiva (senile) H11.89
  corpus cavernosum N48.89
  cortical — *see* Atrophy, brain
  cystic duct K82.8
  Déjérine-Thomas G23.8
  disuse NEC — *see* Atrophy, muscle
  Duchenne-Aran G12.21
  ear H93.8-
  edentulous alveolar ridge K08.20
  endometrium (senile) N85.8
    cervix N88.8
  enteric K63.89
  epididymis N50.89
  eyeball — *see* Disorder, globe, degenerated condition, atrophy
  eyelid (senile) — *see* Disorder, eyelid, degenerative
  facial (skin) L90.9
  fallopian tube (senile) N83.32-
    with ovary N83.33-
  fascioscapulohumeral (Landouzy- Déjérine) G71.02
  fatty, thymus (gland) E32.8
  gallbladder K82.8
  gastric K29.40
    with bleeding K29.41
  gastrointestinal K63.89
  glandular I89.8
  globe H44.52-
  gum — *see* Recession, gingival
  hair L67.8
  heart (brown) — *see* Degeneration, myocardial
  hemifacial Q67.4
    Romberg G51.8
  infantile E41
    paralysis, acute — *see* Poliomyelitis, paralytic
  intestine K63.89
  iris (essential) (progressive) H21.26-
    specified NEC H21.29
  kidney (senile) (terminal) — *see also* Sclerosis, renal N26.1
    congenital or infantile Q60.5
      bilateral Q60.4
      unilateral Q60.3
    hydronephrotic — *see* Hydronephrosis
  lacrimal gland (primary) H04.14-
    secondary H04.15-
  Landouzy-Déjérine G71.02
  laryngitis, infective J37.0
  larynx J38.7
  Leber's optic (hereditary) H47.22
  lip K13.0

Atrophy, atrophic (of) - *continued*
  liver (yellow) K72.90
    with coma K72.91
    acute, subacute K72.00
      with coma K72.01
    chronic K72.10
      with coma K72.11
  lung (senile) J98.4
  macular (dermatological) L90.8
    syphilitic, skin A51.39
      striated A52.79
  mandible (edentulous) K08.20
    minimal K08.21
    moderate K08.22
    severe K08.23
  maxilla K08.20
    minimal K08.24
    moderate K08.25
    severe K08.26
  muscle, muscular (diffuse) (general) (idiopathic) (primary) M62.50
    ankle M62.57-
    Duchenne-Aran G12.21
    foot M62.57-
    forearm M62.53-
    hand M62.54-
    infantile spinal G12.0
    lower leg M62.56-
    multiple sites M62.59
    myelopathic — *see* Atrophy, muscle, spinal
    myotonic G71.11
    neuritic G58.9
    neuropathic (peroneal) (progressive) G60.0
    pelvic (disuse) N81.84
    peroneal G60.0
    progressive (bulbar) G12.21
      adult G12.1
      infantile (spinal) G12.0
      spinal G12.25
        adult G12.1
        infantile G12.0
    pseudohypertrophic G71.02
    shoulder region M62.51-
    specified site NEC M62.58
    spinal G12.9
      adult form G12.1
      Aran-Duchenne G12.21
      childhood form, type II G12.1
      distal G12.1
      hereditary NEC G12.1
      infantile, type I (Werdnig-Hoffmann) G12.0
      juvenile form, type III (Kugelberg-Welander) G12.1
      progressive G12.25
      scapuloperoneal form G12.1
      specified NEC G12.8
    syphilitic A52.78
    thigh M62.55-
    upper arm M62.52-
  myocardium — *see* Degeneration, myocardial
  myometrium (senile) N85.8
    cervix N88.8
  myopathic NEC — *see* Atrophy, muscle
  myotonia G71.11
  nail L60.3
  nasopharynx J31.1
  nerve — *see also* Disorder, nerve
    abducens — *see* Strabismus, paralytic, sixth nerve
    accessory G52.8
    acoustic or auditory — *see* subcategory H93.3
    cranial G52.9
      eighth (auditory) — *see* subcategory H93.3
      eleventh (accessory) G52.8
      fifth (trigeminal) G50.8
      first (olfactory) G52.0
      fourth (trochlear) — *see* Strabismus, paralytic, fourth nerve
      second (optic) H47.20
      sixth (abducens) — *see* Strabismus, paralytic, sixth nerve
      tenth (pneumogastric) (vagus) G52.2
      third (oculomotor) — *see* Strabismus, paralytic, third nerve
      twelfth (hypoglossal) G52.3
    hypoglossal G52.3
    oculomotor — *see* Strabismus, paralytic, third nerve
    olfactory G52.0
    optic (papillomacular bundle)
      syphilitic (late) A52.15
        congenital A50.44
    pneumogastric G52.2
    trigeminal G50.8

Axonotmesis — *see* Injury, nerve
Ayerza's disease or syndrome (pulmonary artery sclerosis with pulmonary hypertension) I27.0
Azoospermia (organic) N46.01
 due to
  drug therapy N46.021
  efferent duct obstruction N46.023
  infection N46.022
  radiation N46.024
  specified cause NEC N46.029
  systemic disease N46.025
Azotemia R79.89
 meaning uremia N19
Aztec ear Q17.3
Azygos
 continuation inferior vena cava Q26.8
 lobe (lung) Q33.1

B

Baastrup's disease — *see* Kissing spine
Babesiosis B60.0
Babington's disease (familial hemorrhagic telangiectasia) I78.0
Babinski's syndrome A52.79
Baby
 crying constantly R68.11
 floppy (syndrome) P94.2
Bacillary — *see* condition
Bacilluria R82.71
Bacillus — *see also* Infection, bacillus
 abortus infection A23.1
 anthracis infection A22.9
 coli infection — *see also* Escherichia coli B96.20
 Flexner's A03.1
 mallei infection A24.0
 Shiga's A03.0
 suipestifer infection — *see* Infection, salmonella
Back — *see* condition
Backache (postural) M54.9
 sacroiliac M53.3
 specified NEC M54.89
Backflow — *see* Reflux
Backward reading (dyslexia) F81.0
Bacteremia R78.81
 with sepsis — *see* Sepsis
Bactericholia — *see* Cholecystitis, acute
Bacterid, bacteride (pustular) L40.3
Bacterium, bacteria, bacterial
 agent NEC, as cause of disease classified elsewhere B96.89
 in blood — *see* Bacteremia
 in urine — *see* Bacteriuria
Bacteriuria, bacteruria R82.71
 asymptomatic R82.71
Bacteroides
 fragilis, as cause of disease classified elsewhere B96.6
Bad
 heart — *see* Disease, heart
 trip
  due to drug abuse — *see* Abuse, drug, hallucinogen
  due to drug dependence — *see* Dependence, drug, hallucinogen
Baelz's disease (cheilitis glandularis apostematosa) K13.0
Baerensprung's disease (eczema marginatum) B35.6
Bagasse disease or pneumonitis J67.1
Bagassosis J67.1
Baker's cyst — *see* Cyst, Baker's
Bakwin-Krida syndrome (metaphyseal dysplasia) Q78.5
Balancing side interference M26.56
Balanitis (circinata) (erosiva) (gangrenosa) (phagedenic) (vulgaris) N48.1
 amebic A06.82
 candidal B37.42
 due to Haemophilus ducreyi A57
 gonococcal (acute) (chronic) A54.23
 xerotica obliterans N48.0
Balanoposthitis N47.6
 gonococcal (acute) (chronic) A54.23
 ulcerative (specific) A63.8
Balanorrhagia — *see* Balanitis
Balantidiasis, balantidiosis A07.0
Bald tongue K14.4
Baldness — *see also* Alopecia
 male-pattern — *see* Alopecia, androgenic
Balkan grippe A78
Balloon disease — *see* Effect, adverse, high altitude
Balo's disease (concentric sclerosis) G37.5
Bamberger-Marie disease — *see* Osteoarthropathy, hypertrophic, specified type NEC
Bancroft's filariasis B74.0
Band (s)
 adhesive — *see* Adhesions, peritoneum
 anomalous or congenital — *see also* Anomaly, by site
  heart (atrial) (ventricular) Q24.8
  intestine Q43.3
  omentum Q43.3
 cervix N88.1
 constricting, congenital Q79.8
 gallbladder (congenital) Q44.1
 intestinal (adhesive) — *see* Adhesions, peritoneum
 obstructive
  intestine K56.50
   complete K56.52
   incomplete K56.51
   partial K56.51
  peritoneum K56.50
   complete K56.52
   incomplete K56.51
   partial K56.51
 periappendiceal, congenital Q43.3
 peritoneal (adhesive) — *see* Adhesions, peritoneum
 uterus N73.6
  internal N85.6
 vagina N89.5
Bandemia D72.825
Bandl's ring (contraction) **, complicating delivery** O62.4
Bangkok hemorrhagic fever A91
Bang's disease (brucella abortus) A23.1
Bankruptcy, anxiety concerning Z59.8
Bannister's disease T78.3
 hereditary D84.1
Banti's disease or syndrome (with cirrhosis) (with portal hypertension) K76.6
Bar, median, prostate — *see* Enlargement, enlarged, prostate
Barcoo disease or rot — *see* Ulcer, skin
Barlow's disease E54
Barodontalgia T70.29
Baron Münchausen syndrome — *see* Disorder, factitious
Barosinusitis T70.1
Barotitis T70.0
Barotrauma T70.29
 odontalgia T70.29
 otitic T70.0
 sinus T70.1
Barraquer (-Simons) **disease or syndrome** (progressive lipodystrophy) E88.1
Barré-Guillain disease or syndrome G61.0
Barrel chest M95.4
Barré-Liéou syndrome (posterior cervical sympathetic) M53.0
Barrett's
 disease — *see* Barrett's, esophagus
 esophagus K22.70
  with dysplasia K22.719
   high grade K22.711
   low grade K22.710
  without dysplasia K22.70
 syndrome — *see* Barrett's, esophagus
 ulcer K22.10
  with bleeding K22.11
  without bleeding K22.10
Bársony (-Polgár) (-Teschendorf) **syndrome** (corkscrew esophagus) K22.4
Barth syndrome E78.71
Bartholinitis (suppurating) N75.8
 gonococcal (acute) (chronic) (with abscess) A54.1
Bartonellosis A44.9
 cutaneous A44.1
 mucocutaneous A44.1
 specified NEC A44.8
 systemic A44.0
Barton's fracture S52.56-
Bartter's syndrome E26.81
Basal — *see* condition
Basan's (hidrotic) **ectodermal dysplasia** Q82.4
Baseball finger — *see* Dislocation, finger
Basedow's disease (exophthalmic goiter) — *see* Hyperthyroidism, with, goiter
Basic — *see* condition
Basilar — *see* condition
Bason's (hidrotic) **ectodermal dysplasia** Q82.4
Basopenia — *see* Agranulocytosis
Basophilia D72.824
Basophilism (cortico-adrenal) (Cushing's) (pituitary) E24.0
Bassen-Kornzweig disease or syndrome E78.6
Bat ear Q17.5
Bateman's
 disease B08.1
 purpura (senile) D69.2
Bathing cramp T75.1
Bathophobia F40.248
Batten (-Mayou) **disease** E75.4
 retina E75.4 *[H36]*
Batten-Steinert syndrome G71.11
Battered — *see* Maltreatment
Battey Mycobacterium infection A31.0
Battle exhaustion F43.0
Battledore placenta O43.19-
Baumgarten-Cruveilhier cirrhosis, disease or syndrome K74.69
Bauxite fibrosis (of lung) J63.1
Bayle's disease (general paresis) A52.17
Bazin's disease (primary) (tuberculous) A18.4
Beach ear — *see* Swimmer's, ear
Beaded hair (congenital) Q84.1
Béal conjunctivitis or syndrome B30.2
Beard's disease (neurasthenia) F48.8
Beat (s)
 atrial, premature I49.1
 ectopic I49.49
 elbow — *see* Bursitis, elbow
 escaped, heart I49.49
 hand — *see* Bursitis, hand
 knee — *see* Bursitis, knee
 premature I49.40
  atrial I49.1
  auricular I49.1
  supraventricular I49.1
Beau's
 disease or syndrome — *see* Degeneration, myocardial
 lines (transverse furrows on fingernails) L60.4
Bechterev's syndrome — *see* Spondylitis, ankylosing
Becker's
 cardiomyopathy I42.8
 disease
  idiopathic mural endomyocardial disease I42.3
  myotonia congenita, recessive form G71.12
 dystrophy G71.01
 pigmented hairy nevus D22.5
Beck's syndrome (anterior spinal artery occlusion) I65.8
Beckwith-Wiedemann syndrome Q87.3
Bed confinement status Z74.01
Bed sore — *see* Ulcer, pressure, by site
Bedbug bite (s) — *see* Bite(s), by site, superficial, insect
Bedclothes, asphyxiation or suffocation by — *see* Asphyxia, traumatic, due to, mechanical, trapped
Bednar's
 aphthae K12.0
 tumor — *see* Neoplasm, malignant, by site
Bedridden Z74.01
Bedsore — *see* Ulcer, pressure, by site
Bedwetting — *see* Enuresis
Bee sting (with allergic or anaphylactic shock) — *see* Toxicity, venom, arthropod, bee
Beer drinker's heart (disease) I42.6
Begbie's disease (exophthalmic goiter) — *see* Hyperthyroidism, with, goiter
Behavior
 antisocial
  adult Z72.811
  child or adolescent Z72.810
 disorder, disturbance — *see* Disorder, conduct
 disruptive — *see* Disorder, conduct
 drug seeking Z76.5
 inexplicable R46.2
 marked evasiveness R46.5
 obsessive-compulsive R46.81
 overactivity R46.3
 poor responsiveness R46.4
 self-damaging (life-style) Z72.89
 sleep-incompatible Z72.821
 slowness R46.4
 specified NEC R46.89
 strange (and inexplicable) R46.2
 suspiciousness R46.5
 type A pattern Z73.1
 undue concern or preoccupation with stressful events R46.6
 verbosity and circumstantial detail obscuring reason for contact R46.7
Behçet's disease or syndrome M35.2
Behr's disease — *see* Degeneration, macula
Beigel's disease or morbus (white piedra) B36.2
Bejel A65

Bekhterev's syndrome — *see* Spondylitis, ankylosing
Belching — *see* Eructation
Bell's
mania F30.8
palsy, paralysis G51.0
infant or newborn P11.3
spasm G51.3-
Bence Jones albuminuria or proteinuria NEC R80.3
Bends T70.3
Benedikt's paralysis or syndrome G46.3
Benign — *see also* condition
prostatic hyperplasia — *see* Hyperplasia, prostate
Bennett's fracture (displaced) S62.21-
Benson's disease — *see* Deposit, crystalline
Bent
back (hysterical) F44.4
nose M95.0
congenital Q67.4
Bereavement (uncomplicated) Z63.4
Bergeron's disease (hysterical chorea) F44.4
Berger's disease — *see* Nephropathy, IgA
Beriberi (dry) E51.11
heart (disease) E51.12
polyneuropathy E51.11
wet E51.12
involving circulatory system E51.11
Berlin's disease or edema (traumatic) S05.8X-
Berlock (berloque) **dermatitis** L56.2
Bernard-Horner syndrome G90.2
Bernard-Soulier disease or thrombopathia D69.1
Bernhardt (-Roth) **disease** — *see* Mononeuropathy, lower limb, meralgia paresthetica
Bernheim's syndrome — *see* Failure, heart, right
Bertielliasis B71.8
Berylliosis (lung) J63.2
Besnier-Boeck (-Schaumann) **disease** — *see* Sarcoidosis
Besnier's
lupus pernio D86.3
prurigo L20.0
Bestiality F65.89
Best's disease H35.50
Betalipoproteinemia, broad or floating E78.2
Beta-mercaptolactate-cysteine disulfiduria E72.09
Betting and gambling Z72.6
pathological (compulsive) F63.0
Bezoar T18.9
intestine T18.3
stomach T18.2
Bezold's abscess — *see* Mastoiditis, acute
Bianchi's syndrome R48.8
Bicornate or bicornis uterus Q51.3
in pregnancy or childbirth O34.00
causing obstructed labor O65.5
Bicuspid aortic valve Q23.1
Biedl-Bardet syndrome Q87.89
Bielschowsky (-Jansky) **disease** E75.4
Biermer's (pernicious) **anemia or disease** D51.0
Biett's disease L93.0
Bifid (congenital)
apex, heart Q24.8
clitoris Q52.6
kidney Q63.8
nose Q30.2
patella Q74.1
scrotum Q55.29
toe NEC Q74.2
tongue Q38.3
ureter Q62.8
uterus Q51.3
uvula Q35.7
Biforis uterus (suprasimplex) Q51.3
Bifurcation (congenital)
gallbladder Q44.1
kidney pelvis Q63.8
renal pelvis Q63.8
rib Q76.6
tongue, congenital Q38.3
trachea Q32.1
ureter Q62.8
urethra Q64.74
vertebra Q76.49
Big spleen syndrome D73.1
Bigeminal pulse R00.8
Bilateral — *see* condition
Bile
duct — *see* condition
pigments in urine R82.2
Bilharziasis — *see also* Schistosomiasis
chyluria B65.0
cutaneous B65.3

Bilharziasis - *continued*
galacturia B65.0
hematochyluria B65.0
intestinal B65.1
lipemia B65.9
lipuria B65.0
oriental B65.2
piarhemia B65.9
pulmonary NOS B65.9 *[J99]*
pneumonia B65.9 *[J17]*
tropical hematuria B65.0
vesical B65.0
Biliary — *see* condition
Bilirubin metabolism disorder E80.7
specified NEC E80.6
Bilirubinemia, familial nonhemolytic E80.4
Bilirubinuria R82.2
Biliuria R82.2
Bilocular stomach K31.2
Binswanger's disease I67.3
Biparta, bipartite
carpal scaphoid Q74.0
patella Q74.1
vagina Q52.10
Bird
face Q75.8
fancier's disease or lung J67.2
Birth
complications in mother — *see* Delivery, complicated
compression during NOS P15.9
defect — *see* Anomaly
immature (less than 37 completed weeks) — *see* Preterm, newborn
extremely (less than 28 completed weeks) — *see* Immaturity, extreme
inattention, at or after — *see* Maltreatment, child, neglect
injury NOS P15.9
basal ganglia P11.1
brachial plexus NEC P14.3
brain (compression) (pressure) P11.2
central nervous system NOS P11.9
cerebellum P11.1
cerebral hemorrhage P10.1
external genitalia P15.5
eye P15.3
face P15.4
fracture
bone P13.9
specified NEC P13.8
clavicle P13.4
femur P13.2
humerus P13.3
long bone, except femur P13.3
radius and ulna P13.3
skull P13.0
spine P11.5
tibia and fibula P13.3
intracranial P11.2
laceration or hemorrhage P10.9
specified NEC P10.8
intraventricular hemorrhage P10.2
laceration
brain P10.1
by scalpel P15.8
peripheral nerve P14.9
liver P15.0
meninges
brain P11.1
spinal cord P11.5
nerve
brachial plexus P14.3
cranial NEC (except facial) P11.4
facial P11.3
peripheral P14.9
phrenic (paralysis) P14.2
paralysis
facial nerve P11.3
spinal P11.5
penis P15.5
rupture
spinal cord P11.5
scalp P12.9
scalpel wound P15.8
scrotum P15.5
skull NEC P13.1
fracture P13.0
specified type NEC P15.8
spinal cord P11.5
spine P11.5
spleen P15.1
sternomastoid (hematoma) P15.2

Birth - *continued*
injury NOS - *continued*
subarachnoid hemorrhage P10.3
subcutaneous fat necrosis P15.6
subdural hemorrhage P10.0
tentorial tear P10.4
testes P15.5
vulva P15.5
lack of care, at or after — *see* Maltreatment, child, neglect
neglect, at or after — *see* Maltreatment, child, neglect
palsy or paralysis, newborn, NOS (birth injury) P14.9
premature (infant) — *see* Preterm, newborn
shock, newborn P96.89
trauma — *see* Birth, injury
weight
low (2499 grams or less) — *see* Low, birthweight
extremely (999 grams or less) — *see* Low, birthweight, extreme
4000 grams to 4499 grams P08.1
4500 grams or more P08.0
Birthmark Q82.5
Birt-Hogg-Dube syndrome Q87.89
Bisalbuminemia E88.09
Biskra's button B55.1
Bite (s) (animal) (human)
abdomen, abdominal
wall S31.159
with penetration into peritoneal cavity S31.659
epigastric region S31.152
with penetration into peritoneal cavity S31.652
left
lower quadrant S31.154
with penetration into peritoneal cavity S31.654
upper quadrant S31.151
with penetration into peritoneal cavity S31.651
periumbilic region S31.155
with penetration into peritoneal cavity S31.655
right
lower quadrant S31.153
with penetration into peritoneal cavity S31.653
upper quadrant S31.150
with penetration into peritoneal cavity S31.650
superficial NEC S30.871
insect S30.861
alveolar (process) — *see* Bite, oral cavity
amphibian (venomous) — *see* Venom, bite, amphibian
animal — *see also* Bite, by site
venomous — *see* Venom
ankle S91.05-
superficial NEC S90.57-
insect S90.56-
antecubital space — *see* Bite, elbow
anus S31.835
superficial NEC S30.877
insect S30.867
arm (upper) S41.15-
lower — *see* Bite, forearm
superficial NEC S40.87-
insect S40.86-
arthropod NEC — *see* Venom, bite, arthropod
auditory canal (external) (meatus) — *see* Bite, ear
auricle, ear — *see* Bite, ear
axilla — *see* Bite, arm
back — *see also* Bite, thorax, back
lower S31.050
with penetration into retroperitoneal space S31.051
superficial NEC S30.870
insect S30.860
bedbug — *see* Bite(s), by site, superficial, insect
breast S21.05-
superficial NEC S20.17-
insect S20.16-
brow — *see* Bite, head, specified site NEC
buttock S31.805
left S31.825
right S31.815
superficial NEC S30.870
insect S30.860
calf — *see* Bite, leg
canaliculus lacrimalis — *see* Bite, eyelid
canthus, eye — *see* Bite, eyelid
centipede — *see* Toxicity, venom, arthropod, centipede
cheek (external) S01.45-
superficial NEC S00.87
insect S00.86
internal — *see* Bite, oral cavity
chest wall — *see* Bite, thorax

Bite (s) (animal) (human) - *continued*
  chigger B88.0
  chin — *see* Bite, head, specified site NEC
  clitoris — *see* Bite, vulva
  costal region — *see* Bite, thorax
  digit (s)
    hand — *see* Bite, finger
    toe — *see* Bite, toe
  ear (canal) (external) S01.35-
    superficial NEC S00.47-
      insect S00.46-
  elbow S51.05-
    superficial NEC S50.37-
      insect S50.36-
  epididymis — *see* Bite, testis
  epigastric region — *see* Bite, abdomen
  epiglottis — *see* Bite, neck, specified site NEC
  esophagus, cervical S11.25
    superficial NEC S10.17
      insect S10.16
  eyebrow — *see* Bite, eyelid
  eyelid S01.15-
    superficial NEC S00.27-
      insect S00.26-
  face NEC — *see* Bite, head, specified site NEC
  finger (s) S61.259
    with
      damage to nail S61.359
    index S61.258
      with
        damage to nail S61.358
      left S61.251
        with
          damage to nail S61.351
      right S61.250
        with
          damage to nail S61.350
      superficial NEC S60.478
        insect S60.46-
    little S61.25-
      with
        damage to nail S61.35-
      superficial NEC S60.47-
        insect S60.46-
    middle S61.25-
      with
        damage to nail S61.35-
      superficial NEC S60.47-
        insect S60.46-
    ring S61.25-
      with
        damage to nail S61.35-
      superficial NEC S60.47-
        insect S60.46-
    superficial NEC S60.479
      insect S60.469
    thumb — *see* Bite, thumb
  flank — *see* Bite, abdomen, wall
  flea — *see* Bite, by site, superficial, insect
  foot (except toe (s) alone) S91.35-
    superficial NEC S90.87-
      insect S90.86-
    toe — *see* Bite, toe
  forearm S51.85-
    elbow only — *see* Bite, elbow
    superficial NEC S50.87-
      insect S50.86-
  forehead — *see* Bite, head, specified site NEC
  genital organs, external
    female S31.552
      superficial NEC S30.876
        insect S30.866
      vagina and vulva — *see* Bite, vulva
    male S31.551
      penis — *see* Bite, penis
      scrotum — *see* Bite, scrotum
      superficial NEC S30.875
        insect S30.865
      testes — *see* Bite, testis
  groin — *see* Bite, abdomen, wall
  gum — *see* Bite, oral cavity
  hand S61.45-
    finger — *see* Bite, finger
    superficial NEC S60.57-
      insect S60.56-
    thumb — *see* Bite, thumb
  head S01.95
    cheek — *see* Bite, cheek
    ear — *see* Bite, ear
    eyelid — *see* Bite, eyelid
    lip — *see* Bite, lip
    nose — *see* Bite, nose
    oral cavity — *see* Bite, oral cavity

Bite (s) (animal) (human) - *continued*
  head - *continued*
    scalp — *see* Bite, scalp
    specified site NEC S01.85
      superficial NEC S00.87
        insect S00.86
    superficial NEC S00.97
      insect S00.96
    temporomandibular area — *see* Bite, cheek
  heel — *see* Bite, foot
  hip S71.05-
    superficial NEC S70.27-
      insect S70.26-
  hymen S31.45
  hypochondrium — *see* Bite, abdomen, wall
  hypogastric region — *see* Bite, abdomen, wall
  inguinal region — *see* Bite, abdomen, wall
  insect — *see* Bite, by site, superficial, insect
  instep — *see* Bite, foot
  interscapular region — *see* Bite, thorax, back
  jaw — *see* Bite, head, specified site NEC
  knee S81.05-
    superficial NEC S80.27-
      insect S80.26-
  labium (majus) (minus) — *see* Bite, vulva
  lacrimal duct — *see* Bite, eyelid
  larynx S11.015
    superficial NEC S10.17
      insect S10.16
  leg (lower) S81.85-
    ankle — *see* Bite, ankle
    foot — *see* Bite, foot
    knee — *see* Bite, knee
    superficial NEC S80.87-
      insect S80.86-
    toe — *see* Bite, toe
    upper — *see* Bite, thigh
  lip S01.551
    superficial NEC S00.571
      insect S00.561
  lizard (venomous) — *see* Venom, bite, reptile
  loin — *see* Bite, abdomen, wall
  lower back — *see* Bite, back, lower
  lumbar region — *see* Bite, back, lower
  malar region — *see* Bite, head, specified site NEC
  mammary — *see* Bite, breast
  marine animals (venomous) — *see* Toxicity, venom, marine animal
  mastoid region — *see* Bite, head, specified site NEC
  mouth — *see* Bite, oral cavity
  nail
    finger — *see* Bite, finger
    toe — *see* Bite, toe
  nape — *see* Bite, neck, specified site NEC
  nasal (septum) (sinus) — *see* Bite, nose
  nasopharynx — *see* Bite, head, specified site NEC
  neck S11.95
    involving
      cervical esophagus — *see* Bite, esophagus, cervical
      larynx — *see* Bite, larynx
      pharynx — *see* Bite, pharynx
      thyroid gland S11.15
      trachea — *see* Bite, trachea
    specified site NEC S11.85
      superficial NEC S10.87
        insect S10.86
    superficial NEC S10.97
      insect S10.96
    throat S11.85
      superficial NEC S10.17
        insect S10.16
  nose (septum) (sinus) S01.25
    superficial NEC S00.37
      insect S00.36
  occipital region — *see* Bite, scalp
  oral cavity S01.552
    superficial NEC S00.572
      insect S00.562
  orbital region — *see* Bite, eyelid
  palate — *see* Bite, oral cavity
  palm — *see* Bite, hand
  parietal region — *see* Bite, scalp
  pelvis S31.050
    with penetration into retroperitoneal space S31.051
    superficial NEC S30.870
      insect S30.860
  penis S31.25
    superficial NEC S30.872
      insect S30.862
  perineum
    female — *see* Bite, vulva
    male — *see* Bite, pelvis

Bite (s) (animal) (human) - *continued*
  periocular area (with or without lacrimal passages) — *see* Bite, eyelid
  phalanges
    finger — *see* Bite, finger
    toe — *see* Bite, toe
  pharynx S11.25
    superficial NEC S10.17
      insect S10.16
  pinna — *see* Bite, ear
  poisonous — *see* Venom
  popliteal space — *see* Bite, knee
  prepuce — *see* Bite, penis
  pubic region — *see* Bite, abdomen, wall
  rectovaginal septum — *see* Bite, vulva
  red bug B88.0
  reptile NEC — *see also* Venom, bite, reptile
    nonvenomous — *see* Bite, by site
    snake — *see* Venom, bite, snake
  sacral region — *see* Bite, back, lower
  sacroiliac region — *see* Bite, back, lower
  salivary gland — *see* Bite, oral cavity
  scalp S01.05
    superficial NEC S00.07
      insect S00.06
  scapular region — *see* Bite, shoulder
  scrotum S31.35
    superficial NEC S30.873
      insect S30.863
  sea-snake (venomous) — *see* Toxicity, venom, snake, sea snake
  shin — *see* Bite, leg
  shoulder S41.05-
    superficial NEC S40.27-
      insect S40.26-
  snake — *see also* Venom, bite, snake
    nonvenomous — *see* Bite, by site
  spermatic cord — *see* Bite, testis
  spider (venomous) — *see* Toxicity, venom, spider
    nonvenomous — *see* Bite, by site, superficial, insect
  sternal region — *see* Bite, thorax, front
  submaxillary region — *see* Bite, head, specified site NEC
  submental region — *see* Bite, head, specified site NEC
  subungual
    finger (s) — *see* Bite, finger
    toe — *see* Bite, toe
  superficial — *see* Bite, by site, superficial
  supraclavicular fossa S11.85
  supraorbital — *see* Bite, head, specified site NEC
  temple, temporal region — *see* Bite, head, specified site NEC
  temporomandibular area — *see* Bite, cheek
  testis S31.35
    superficial NEC S30.873
      insect S30.863
  thigh S71.15-
    superficial NEC S70.37-
      insect S70.36-
  thorax, thoracic (wall) S21.95
    back S21.25-
      with penetration into thoracic cavity S21.45-
    breast — *see* Bite, breast
    front S21.15-
      with penetration into thoracic cavity S21.35-
    superficial NEC S20.97
      back S20.47-
      front S20.37-
      insect S20.96
        back S20.46-
        front S20.36-
  throat — *see* Bite, neck, throat
  thumb S61.05-
    with
      damage to nail S61.15-
    superficial NEC S60.37-
      insect S60.36-
  thyroid S11.15
    superficial NEC S10.87
      insect S10.86
  toe (s) S91.15-
    with
      damage to nail S91.25-
    great S91.15-
      with
        damage to nail S91.25-
    lesser S91.15-
      with
        damage to nail S91.25-
    superficial NEC S90.47-
      great S90.47-

Bite (s) (animal) (human) - *continued*
  toe (s) - *continued*
    superficial NEC - *continued*
      insect S90.46-
        great S90.46-
  tongue S01.552
  trachea S11.025
    superficial NEC S10.17
      insect S10.16
  tunica vaginalis — *see* Bite, testis
  tympanum, tympanic membrane — *see* Bite, ear
  umbilical region S31.155
  uvula — *see* Bite, oral cavity
  vagina — *see* Bite, vulva
  venomous — *see* Venom
  vocal cords S11.035
    superficial NEC S10.17
      insect S10.16
  vulva S31.45
    superficial NEC S30.874
      insect S30.864
  wrist S61.55-
    superficial NEC S60.87-
      insect S60.86-
Biting, cheek or lip K13.1
Biventricular failure (heart) I50.82
Björck (-Thorson) **syndrome** (malignant carcinoid) E34.0
Black
  death A20.9
  eye S00.1-
  hairy tongue K14.3
  heel (foot) S90.3-
  lung (disease) J60
  palm (hand) S60.22-
Blackfan-Diamond anemia or syndrome (congenital hypoplastic anemia) D61.01
Blackhead L70.0
Blackout R55
Bladder — *see* condition
Blast (air) (hydraulic) (immersion) (underwater)
  blindness S05.8X-
  injury
    abdomen or thorax — *see* Injury, by site
    ear (acoustic nerve trauma) — *see* Injury, nerve, acoustic, specified type NEC
  syndrome NEC T70.8
Blastoma — *see* Neoplasm, malignant, by site
  pulmonary — *see* Neoplasm, lung, malignant
Blastomycosis, blastomycotic B40.9
  Brazilian — *see* Paracoccidioidomycosis
  cutaneous B40.3
  disseminated B40.7
  European — *see* Cryptococcosis
  generalized B40.7
  keloidal B48.0
  North American B40.9
  primary pulmonary B40.0
  pulmonary B40.2
    acute B40.0
    chronic B40.1
  skin B40.3
  South American — *see* Paracoccidioidomycosis
  specified NEC B40.89
Bleb (s) R23.8
  emphysematous (lung) (solitary) J43.9
  endophthalmitis H59.43
  filtering (vitreous) , after glaucoma surgery Z98.83
  inflammed (infected) , postprocedural H59.40
    stage 1 H59.41
    stage 2 H59.42
    stage 3 H59.43
  lung (ruptured) J43.9
    congenital — *see* Atelectasis
    newborn P25.8
  subpleural (emphysematous) J43.9
Blebitis, postprocedural H59.40
  stage 1 H59.41
  stage 2 H59.42
  stage 3 H59.43
Bleeder (familial) (hereditary) — *see* Hemophilia
Bleeding — *see also* Hemorrhage
  anal K62.5
  anovulatory N97.0
  atonic, following delivery O72.1
  capillary I78.8
    puerperal O72.2
  contact (postcoital) N93.0
  due to uterine subinvolution N85.3
  ear — *see* Otorrhagia
  excessive, associated with menopausal onset N92.4
  familial — *see* Defect, coagulation
  following intercourse N93.0
Bleeding - *continued*
  gastrointestinal K92.2
  hemorrhoids — *see* Hemorrhoids
  intermenstrual (regular) N92.3
    irregular N92.1
  intraoperative — *see* Complication, intraoperative, hemorrhage
  irregular N92.6
  menopausal N92.4
  newborn, intraventricular — *see* Newborn, affected by, hemorrhage, intraventricular
  nipple N64.59
  nose R04.0
  ovulation N92.3
  postclimacteric N95.0
  postcoital N93.0
  postmenopausal N95.0
  postoperative — *see* Complication, postprocedural, hemorrhage
  preclimacteric N92.4
  pre-pubertal vaginal N93.1
  puberty (excessive, with onset of menstrual periods) N92.2
  rectum, rectal K62.5
    newborn P54.2
  tendencies — *see* Defect, coagulation
  throat R04.1
  tooth socket (post-extraction) K91.840
  umbilical stump P51.9
  uterus, uterine NEC N93.9
    climacteric N92.4
    dysfunctional or functional N93.8
    menopausal N92.4
    preclimacteric or premenopausal N92.4
    unrelated to menstrual cycle N93.9
  vagina, vaginal (abnormal) N93.9
    dysfunctional or functional N93.8
    newborn P54.6
    pre-pubertal N93.1
  vicarious N94.89
Blennorrhagia, blennorrhagic — *see* Gonorrhea
Blennorrhea (acute) (chronic) — *see also* Gonorrhea
  inclusion (neonatal) (newborn) P39.1
  lower genitourinary tract (gonococcal) A54.00
  neonatorum (gonococcal ophthalmia) A54.31
Blepharelosis — *see* Entropion
Blepharitis (angularis) (ciliaris) (eyelid) (marginal) (nonulcerative) H01.009
  herpes zoster B02.39
  left H01.006
    lower H01.005
    upper H01.004
    upper and lower H01.00B
  right H01.003
    lower H01.002
    upper H01.001
    upper and lower H01.00A
  squamous H01.029
    left H01.026
      lower H01.025
      upper H01.024
      upper and lower H01.02B
    right H01.023
      lower H01.022
      upper H01.021
      upper and lower H01.02A
  ulcerative H01.019
    left H01.016
      lower H01.015
      upper H01.014
      upper and lower H01.01B
    right H01.013
      lower H01.012
      upper H01.011
      upper and lower H01.01A
Blepharochalasis H02.30
  congenital Q10.0
  left H02.36
    lower H02.35
    upper H02.34
  right H02.33
    lower H02.32
    upper H02.31
Blepharoclonus H02.59
Blepharoconjunctivitis H10.50-
  angular H10.52-
  contact H10.53-
  ligneous H10.51-
Blepharophimosis (eyelid) H02.529
  congenital Q10.3
  left H02.526
    lower H02.525
    upper H02.524
Blepharophimosis (eyelid) - *continued*
  right H02.523
    lower H02.522
    upper H02.521
Blepharoptosis H02.40-
  congenital Q10.0
  mechanical H02.41-
  myogenic H02.42-
  neurogenic H02.43-
  paralytic H02.43-
Blepharopyorrhea, gonococcal A54.39
Blepharospasm G24.5
  drug induced G24.01
Blighted ovum O02.0
Blind — *see also* Blindness
  bronchus (congenital) Q32.4
  loop syndrome K90.2
    congenital Q43.8
  sac, fallopian tube (congenital) Q50.6
  spot, enlarged — *see* Defect, visual field, localized, scotoma, blind spot area
  tract or tube, congenital NEC — *see* Atresia, by site
Blindness (acquired) (congenital) (both eyes) H54.0X
-
  blast S05.8X-
  color — *see* Deficiency, color vision
  concussion S05.8X-
  cortical H47.619
    left brain H47.612
    right brain H47.611
  day H53.11
  due to injury (current episode) S05.9-
    sequelae -- code to injury with seventh character S
  eclipse (total) — *see* Retinopathy, solar
  emotional (hysterical) F44.6
  face H53.16
  hysterical F44.6
  legal (both eyes) (USA definition) H54.8
  mind R48.8
  night H53.60
    abnormal dark adaptation curve H53.61
    acquired H53.62
    congenital H53.63
    specified type NEC H53.69
    vitamin A deficiency E50.5
  one eye (other eye normal) H54.40
    left (normal vision on right) H54.42-
      low vision on right H54.12-
    low vision, other eye H54.10
    right (normal vision on left) H54.41-
      low vision on left H54.11-
  psychic R48.8
  river B73.01
  snow — *see* Photokeratitis
  sun, solar — *see* Retinopathy, solar
  transient — *see* Disturbance, vision, subjective, loss, transient
  traumatic (current episode) S05.9-
  word (developmental) F81.0
    acquired R48.0
    secondary to organic lesion R48.0
Blister (nonthermal)
  abdominal wall S30.821
  alveolar process S00.522
  ankle S90.52-
  antecubital space — *see* Blister, elbow
  anus S30.827
  arm (upper) S40.82-
  auditory canal — *see* Blister, ear
  auricle — *see* Blister, ear
  axilla — *see* Blister, arm
  back, lower S30.820
  beetle dermatitis L24.89
  breast S20.12-
  brow S00.82
  calf — *see* Blister, leg
  canthus — *see* Blister, eyelid
  cheek S00.82
    internal S00.522
  chest wall — *see* Blister, thorax
  chin S00.82
  costal region — *see* Blister, thorax
  digit (s)
    foot — *see* Blister, toe
    hand — *see* Blister, finger
  due to burn — *see* Burn, by site, second degree
  ear S00.42-
  elbow S50.32-
  epiglottis S10.12
  esophagus, cervical S10.12
  eyebrow — *see* Blister, eyelid
  eyelid S00.22-
  face S00.82

Blister (nonthermal) - *continued*
fever B00.1
finger (s) S60.429
index S60.42-
little S60.42-
middle S60.42-
ring S60.42-
foot (except toe (s) alone) S90.82-
toe — *see* Blister, toe
forearm S50.82-
elbow only — *see* Blister, elbow
forehead S00.82
fracture - omit code
genital organ
female S30.826
male S30.825
gum S00.522
hand S60.52-
head S00.92
ear — *see* Blister, ear
eyelid — *see* Blister, eyelid
lip S00.521
nose S00.32
oral cavity S00.522
scalp S00.02
specified site NEC S00.82
heel — *see* Blister, foot
hip S70.22-
interscapular region S20.429
jaw S00.82
knee S80.22-
larynx S10.12
leg (lower) S80.82-
knee — *see* Blister, knee
upper — *see* Blister, thigh
lip S00.521
malar region S00.82
mammary — *see* Blister, breast
mastoid region S00.82
mouth S00.522
multiple, skin, nontraumatic R23.8
nail
finger — *see* Blister, finger
toe — *see* Blister, toe
nasal S00.32
neck S10.92
specified site NEC S10.82
throat S10.12
nose S00.32
occipital region S00.02
oral cavity S00.522
orbital region — *see* Blister, eyelid
palate S00.522
palm — *see* Blister, hand
parietal region S00.02
pelvis S30.820
penis S30.822
periocular area — *see* Blister, eyelid
phalanges
finger — *see* Blister, finger
toe — *see* Blister, toe
pharynx S10.12
pinna — *see* Blister, ear
popliteal space — *see* Blister, knee
scalp S00.02
scapular region — *see* Blister, shoulder
scrotum S30.823
shin — *see* Blister, leg
shoulder S40.22-
sternal region S20.329
submaxillary region S00.82
submental region S00.82
subungual
finger (s) — *see* Blister, finger
toe (s) — *see* Blister, toe
supraclavicular fossa S10.82
supraorbital S00.82
temple S00.82
temporal region S00.82
testis S30.823
thermal — *see* Burn, second degree, by site
thigh S70.32-
thorax, thoracic (wall) S20.92
back S20.42-
front S20.32-
throat S10.12
thumb S60.32-
toe (s) S90.42-
great S90.42-
tongue S00.522
trachea S10.12
tympanum, tympanic membrane — *see* Blister, ear
upper arm — *see* Blister, arm (upper)

Blister (nonthermal) - *continued*
uvula S00.522
vagina S30.824
vocal cords S10.12
vulva S30.824
wrist S60.82-
Bloating R14.0
Bloch-Sulzberger disease or syndrome Q82.3
Block, blocked
alveolocapillary J84.10
arborization (heart) I45.5
arrhythmic I45.9
atrioventricular (incomplete) (partial) I44.30
with atrioventricular dissociation I44.2
complete I44.2
congenital Q24.6
congenital Q24.6
first degree I44.0
second degree (types I and II) I44.1
specified NEC I44.39
third degree I44.2
types I and II I44.1
auriculoventricular — *see* Block, atrioventricular
bifascicular (cardiac) I45.2
bundle-branch (complete) (false) (incomplete) I45.4
bilateral I45.2
left I44.7
with right bundle branch block I45.2
hemiblock I44.60
anterior I44.4
posterior I44.5
incomplete I44.7
with right bundle branch block I45.2
right I45.10
with
left bundle branch block I45.2
left fascicular block I45.2
specified NEC I45.19
Wilson's type I45.19
cardiac I45.9
conduction I45.9
complete I44.2
fascicular (left) I44.60
anterior I44.4
posterior I44.5
right I45.0
specified NEC I44.69
foramen Magendie (acquired) G91.1
congenital Q03.1
with spina bifida — *see* Spina bifida, by site, with hydrocephalus
heart I45.9
bundle branch I45.4
bilateral I45.2
complete (atrioventricular) I44.2
congenital Q24.6
first degree (atrioventricular) I44.0
second degree (atrioventricular) I44.1
specified type NEC I45.5
third degree (atrioventricular) I44.2
hepatic vein I82.0
intraventricular (nonspecific) I45.4
bundle branch
bilateral I45.2
kidney N28.9
postcystoscopic or postprocedural N99.0
Mobitz (types I and II) I44.1
myocardial — *see* Block, heart
nodal I45.5
organ or site, congenital NEC — *see* Atresia, by site
portal (vein) I81
second degree (types I and II) I44.1
sinoatrial I45.5
sinoauricular I45.5
third degree I44.2
trifascicular I45.3
tubal N97.1
vein NOS I82.90
Wenckebach (types I and II) I44.1
Blockage — *see* Obstruction
Blocq's disease F44.4
Blood
constituents, abnormal R78.9
disease D75.9
donor — *see* Donor, blood
dyscrasia D75.9
with
abortion — *see* Abortion, by type, complicated by, hemorrhage
ectopic pregnancy O08.1
molar pregnancy O08.1
following ectopic or molar pregnancy O08.1
newborn P61.9

Blood - *continued*
dyscrasia - *continued*
puerperal, postpartum O72.3
flukes NEC — *see* Schistosomiasis
in
feces K92.1
occult R19.5
urine — *see* Hematuria
mole O02.0
occult in feces R19.5
pressure
decreased, due to shock following injury T79.4
examination only Z01.30
fluctuating I99.8
high — *see* Hypertension
borderline R03.0
incidental reading, without diagnosis of hypertension R03.0
low — *see also* Hypotension
incidental reading, without diagnosis of hypotension R03.1
spitting — *see* Hemoptysis
staining cornea — *see* Pigmentation, cornea, stromal
transfusion
reaction or complication — *see* Complications, transfusion
type
A (Rh positive) Z67.10
Rh negative Z67.11
AB (Rh positive) Z67.30
Rh negative Z67.31
B (Rh positive) Z67.20
Rh negative Z67.21
O (Rh positive) Z67.40
Rh negative Z67.41
Rh (positive) Z67.90
negative Z67.91
vessel rupture — *see* Hemorrhage
vomiting — *see* Hematemesis
Blood-forming organs, disease D75.9
Bloodgood's disease — *see* Mastopathy, cystic
Bloom (-Machacek) (-Torre) **syndrome** Q82.8
Blount's disease or osteochondrosis — *see* Osteochondrosis, juvenile, tibia
Blue
baby Q24.9
diaper syndrome E72.09
dome cyst (breast) — *see* Cyst, breast
dot cataract Q12.0
nevus D22.9
sclera Q13.5
with fragility of bone and deafness Q78.0
toe syndrome I75.02-
Blueness — *see* Cyanosis
Blues, postpartal O90.6
baby O90.6
Blurring, visual H53.8
Blushing (abnormal) (excessive) R23.2
BMI — *see* Body, mass index
Boarder, hospital NEC Z76.4
accompanying sick person Z76.3
healthy infant or child Z76.2
foundling Z76.1
Bockhart's impetigo L01.02
Bodechtel-Guttman disease (subacute sclerosing panencephalitis) A81.1
Boder-Sedgwick syndrome (ataxia -telangiectasia) G11.3
Body, bodies
Aschoff's — *see* Myocarditis, rheumatic
asteroid, vitreous — *see* Deposit, crystalline
cytoid (retina) — *see* Occlusion, artery, retina
drusen (degenerative) (macula) (retinal) — *see also* Degeneration, macula, drusen
optic disc — *see* Drusen, optic disc
foreign — *see* Foreign body
loose
joint, except knee — *see* Loose, body, joint
knee M23.4-
sheath, tendon — *see* Disorder, tendon, specified type NEC
mass index (BMI)
adult
19.9 or less Z68.1
20.0-20.9 Z68.20
21.0-21.9 Z68.21
22.0-22.9 Z68.22
23.0-23.9 Z68.23
24.0-24.9 Z68.24
25.0-25.9 Z68.25
26.0-26.9 Z68.26
27.0-27.9 Z68.27
28.0-28.9 Z68.28

Briquet's disorder or syndrome F45.0
Brissaud's
infantilism or dwarfism E23.0
motor-verbal tic F95.2
Brittle
bones disease Q78.0
nails L60.3
congenital Q84.6
Broad — *see also* condition
beta disease E78.2
ligament laceration syndrome N83.8
Broad- or floating-betalipoproteinemia E78.2
Brock's syndrome
(atelectasis due to enlarged lymph nodes) J98.19
Brocq-Duhring disease (dermatitis herpetiformis) L13.0
Brodie's abscess or disease M86.8X-
Broken
arches — *see also* Deformity, limb, flat foot
arm (meaning upper limb) — *see* Fracture, arm
back — *see* Fracture, vertebra
bone — *see* Fracture
implant or internal device — *see* Complications, by site and type, mechanical
leg (meaning lower limb) — *see* Fracture, leg
nose S02.2
tooth, teeth — *see* Fracture, tooth
Bromhidrosis, bromidrosis L75.0
Bromidism, bromism G92
due to
correct substance properly administered — *see* Table of Drugs and Chemicals, by drug, adverse effect
overdose or wrong substance given or taken — *see* Table of Drugs and Chemicals, by drug, poisoning
chronic (dependence) F13.20
Bromidrosiphobia F40.298
Bronchi, bronchial — *see* condition
Bronchiectasis (cylindrical) (diffuse) (fusiform) (localized) (saccular) J47.9
with
acute
bronchitis J47.0
lower respiratory infection J47.0
exacerbation (acute) J47.1
congenital Q33.4
tuberculous NEC — *see* Tuberculosis, pulmonary
Bronchiolectasis — *see* Bronchiectasis
Bronchiolitis (acute) (infective) (subacute) J21.9
with
bronchospasm or obstruction J21.9
influenza, flu or grippe — *see* Influenza, with, respiratory manifestations NEC
chemical (chronic) J68.4
acute J68.0
chronic (fibrosing) (obliterative) J44.9
due to
external agent — *see* Bronchitis, acute, due to
human metapneumovirus J21.1
respiratory syncytial virus J21.0
specified organism NEC J21.8
fibrosa obliterans J44.9
influenzal — *see* Influenza, with, respiratory manifestations NEC
obliterans J42
with organizing pneumonia (BOOP) J84.89
obliterative (chronic) (subacute) J44.9
due to fumes or vapors J68.4
due to chemicals, gases, fumes or vapors (inhalation) J68.4
respiratory, interstitial lung disease J84.115
Bronchitis (diffuse) (fibrinous) (hypostatic) (infective) (membranous) J40
with
influenza, flu or grippe — *see* Influenza, with, respiratory manifestations NEC
obstruction (airway) (lung) J44.9
tracheitis (15 years of age and above) J40
acute or subacute J20.9
chronic J42
under 15 years of age J20.9
acute or subacute (with bronchospasm or obstruction) J20.9
with
bronchiectasis J47.0
chronic obstructive pulmonary disease J44.0
chemical (due to gases, fumes or vapors) J68.0
due to
fumes or vapors J68.0
Haemophilus influenzae J20.1
Mycoplasma pneumoniae J20.0
radiation J70.0

Bronchitis (diffuse) (fibrinous) (hypostatic) (infective) (membranous) - *continued*
acute or subacute (with bronchospasm or obstruction) - *continued*
due to - *continued*
specified organism NEC J20.8
Streptococcus J20.2
virus
coxsackie J20.3
echovirus J20.7
parainfluenzae J20.4
respiratory syncytial J20.5
rhinovirus J20.6
viral NEC J20.8
allergic (acute) J45.909
with
exacerbation (acute) J45.901
status asthmaticus J45.902
arachidic T17.528
aspiration (due to fumes or vapors) J68.0
asthmatic J45.9
chronic J44.9
with
acute lower respiratory infection J44.0
exacerbation (acute) J44.1
capillary — *see* Pneumonia, broncho
caseous (tuberculous) A15.5
Castellani's A69.8
catarrhal (15 years of age and above) J40
acute — *see* Bronchitis, acute
chronic J41.0
under 15 years of age J20.9
chemical (acute) (subacute) J68.0
chronic J68.4
due to fumes or vapors J68.0
chronic J68.4
chronic J42
with
airways obstruction J44.9
tracheitis (chronic) J42
asthmatic (obstructive) J44.9
catarrhal J41.0
chemical (due to fumes or vapors) J68.4
due to
chemicals, gases, fumes or vapors (inhalation) J68.4
radiation J70.1
tobacco smoking J41.0
emphysematous J44.9
mucopurulent J41.1
non-obstructive J41.0
obliterans J44.9
obstructive J44.9
purulent J41.1
simple J41.0
croupous — *see* Bronchitis, acute
due to gases, fumes or vapors (chemical) J68.0
emphysematous (obstructive) J44.9
exudative — *see* Bronchitis, acute
fetid J41.1
grippal — *see* Influenza, with, respiratory manifestations NEC
in those under 15 years age — *see* Bronchitis, acute
chronic — *see* Bronchitis, chronic
influenzal — *see* Influenza, with, respiratory manifestations NEC
mixed simple and mucopurulent J41.8
moulder's J62.8
mucopurulent (chronic) (recurrent) J41.1
acute or subacute J20.9
simple (mixed) J41.8
obliterans (chronic) J44.9
obstructive (chronic) (diffuse) J44.9
pituitous J41.1
pneumococcal, acute or subacute J20.2
pseudomembranous, acute or subacute — *see* Bronchitis, acute
purulent (chronic) (recurrent) J41.1
acute or subacute — *see* Bronchitis, acute
putrid J41.1
senile (chronic) J42
simple and mucopurulent (mixed) J41.8
smokers' J41.0
spirochetal NEC A69.8
subacute — *see* Bronchitis, acute
suppurative (chronic) J41.1
acute or subacute — *see* Bronchitis, acute
tuberculous A15.5
under 15 years of age — *see* Bronchitis, acute
chronic — *see* Bronchitis, chronic
viral NEC, acute or subacute — *see also* Bronchitis, acute J20.8
Bronchoalveolitis J18.0

Bronchoaspergillosis B44.1
Bronchocele meaning goiter E04.0
Broncholithiasis J98.09
tuberculous NEC A15.5
Bronchomalacia J98.09
congenital Q32.2
Bronchomycosis NOS B49 *[J99]*
candidal B37.1
Bronchopleuropneumonia — *see* Pneumonia, broncho
Bronchopneumonia — *see* Pneumonia, broncho
Bronchopneumonitis — *see* Pneumonia, broncho
Bronchopulmonary — *see* condition
Bronchopulmonitis — *see* Pneumonia, broncho
Bronchorrhagia (see Hemoptysis)
Bronchorrhea J98.09
acute J20.9
chronic (infective) (purulent) J42
Bronchospasm (acute) J98.01
with
bronchiolitis, acute J21.9
bronchitis, acute (conditions in J20) — *see* Bronchitis, acute
due to external agent — *see* condition, respiratory, acute, due to
exercise induced J45.990
Bronchospirochetosis A69.8
Castellani A69.8
Bronchostenosis J98.09
Bronchus — *see* condition
Brontophobia F40.220
Bronze baby syndrome P83.88
Brooke's tumor — *see* Neoplasm, skin, benign
Brown enamel of teeth (hereditary) K00.5
Brown's sheath syndrome H50.61-
Brown-Séquard disease, paralysis or syndrome G83.81
Bruce sepsis A23.0
Brucellosis (infection) A23.9
abortus A23.1
canis A23.3
dermatitis A23.9
melitensis A23.0
mixed A23.8
sepsis A23.9
melitensis A23.0
specified NEC A23.8
suis A23.2
Bruck-de Lange disease Q87.1
Bruck's disease — *see* Deformity, limb
BRUE (brief resolved unexplained event) R68.13
Brugsch's syndrome Q82.8
Bruise (skin surface intact) — *see also* Contusion
with
open wound — *see* Wound, open
internal organ — *see* Injury, by site
newborn P54.5
scalp, due to birth injury, newborn P12.3
umbilical cord O69.5
Bruit (arterial) R09.89
cardiac R01.1
Brush burn — *see* Abrasion, by site
Bruton's X-linked agammaglobulinemia D80.0
Bruxism
psychogenic F45.8
sleep related G47.63
Bubbly lung syndrome P27.0
Bubo I88.8
blennorrhagic (gonococcal) A54.89
chancroidal A57
climatic A55
due to Haemophilus ducreyi A57
gonococcal A54.89
indolent (nonspecific) I88.8
inguinal (nonspecific) I88.8
chancroidal A57
climatic A55
due to H. ducreyi A57
infective I88.8
scrofulous (tuberculous) A18.2
soft chancre A57
suppurating — *see* Lymphadenitis, acute
syphilitic (primary) A51.0
congenital A50.07
tropical A55
virulent (chancroidal) A57
Bubonic plague A20.0
Bubonocele — *see* Hernia, inguinal
Buccal — *see* condition
Buchanan's disease or osteochondrosis M91.0
Buchem's syndrome (hyperostosis corticalis) M85.2
Bucket-handle fracture or tear (semilunar cartilage) — *see* Tear, meniscus

- **Budd-Chiari syndrome** (hepatic vein thrombosis) I82.0
- **Budgerigar fancier's disease or lung** J67.2
- **Buds**
  - breast E30.1
    - in newborn P96.89
- **Buerger's disease** (thromboangiitis obliterans) I73.1
- **Bulbar** — *see* condition
- **Bulbus cordis** (left ventricle) (persistent) Q21.8
- **Bulimia** (nervosa) F50.2
  - atypical F50.9
  - normal weight F50.9
- **Bulky**
  - stools R19.5
  - uterus N85.2
- **Bulla** (e) R23.8
  - lung (emphysematous) (solitary) J43.9
    - newborn P25.8
- **Bullet wound** — *see also* Wound, open
  - fracture - code as Fracture, by site
  - internal organ — *see* Injury, by site
- **Bundle**
  - branch block (complete) (false) (incomplete) — *see* Block, bundle-branch
  - of His — *see* condition
- **Bunion** M21.61-
  - tailor's M21.62-
- **Bunionette** M21.62-
- **Buphthalmia, buphthalmos** (congenital) Q15.0
- **Burdwan fever** B55.0
- **Bürger-Grütz disease or syndrome** E78.3
- **Buried**
  - penis (congenital) Q55.64
    - acquired N48.83
  - roots K08.3
- **Burke's syndrome** K86.89
- **Burkitt**
  - cell leukemia C91.0-
  - lymphoma (malignant) C83.7-
    - small noncleaved, diffuse C83.7-
    - spleen C83.77
    - undifferentiated C83.7-
  - tumor C83.7-
  - type
    - acute lymphoblastic leukemia C91.0-
    - undifferentiated C83.7-
- **Burn** (electricity) (flame) (hot gas, liquid or hot object) (radiation) (steam) (thermal) T30.0
  - abdomen, abdominal (muscle) (wall) T21.02
    - first degree T21.12
    - second degree T21.22
    - third degree T21.32
  - above elbow T22.039
    - first degree T22.139
    - left T22.032
      - first degree T22.132
      - second degree T22.232
      - third degree T22.332
    - right T22.031
      - first degree T22.131
      - second degree T22.231
      - third degree T22.331
    - second degree T22.239
    - third degree T22.339
  - acid (caustic) (external) (internal) — *see* Corrosion, by site
  - alimentary tract NEC T28.2
    - esophagus T28.1
    - mouth T28.0
    - pharynx T28.0
  - alkaline (caustic) (external) (internal) — *see* Corrosion, by site
  - ankle T25.019
    - first degree T25.119
    - left T25.012
      - first degree T25.112
      - second degree T25.212
      - third degree T25.312
      - multiple with foot — *see* Burn, lower, limb, multiple, ankle and foot
    - right T25.011
      - first degree T25.111
      - second degree T25.211
      - third degree T25.311
    - second degree T25.219
    - third degree T25.319
  - anus — *see* Burn, buttock
  - arm (lower) (upper) — *see* Burn, upper, limb
  - axilla T22.049
    - first degree T22.149
    - left T22.042
      - first degree T22.142

- **Burn** (electricity) (flame) (hot gas, liquid or hot object) (radiation) (steam) (thermal) - *continued*
  - axilla - *continued*
    - left - *continued*
      - second degree T22.242
      - third degree T22.342
    - right T22.041
      - first degree T22.141
      - second degree T22.241
      - third degree T22.341
    - second degree T22.249
    - third degree T22.349
  - back (lower) T21.04
    - first degree T21.14
    - second degree T21.24
    - third degree T21.34
    - upper T21.03
      - first degree T21.13
      - second degree T21.23
      - third degree T21.33
  - blisters - code as Burn, second degree, by site
  - breast (s) — *see* Burn, chest wall
  - buttock (s) T21.05
    - first degree T21.15
    - second degree T21.25
    - third degree T21.35
  - calf T24.039
    - first degree T24.139
    - left T24.032
      - first degree T24.132
      - second degree T24.232
      - third degree T24.332
    - right T24.031
      - first degree T24.131
      - second degree T24.231
      - third degree T24.331
    - second degree T24.239
    - third degree T24.339
  - canthus (eye) — *see* Burn, eyelid
  - caustic acid or alkaline — *see* Corrosion, by site
  - cervix T28.3
  - cheek T20.06
    - first degree T20.16
    - second degree T20.26
    - third degree T20.36
  - chemical (acids) (alkalines) (caustics) (external) (internal) — *see* Corrosion, by site
  - chest wall T21.01
    - first degree T21.11
    - second degree T21.21
    - third degree T21.31
  - chin T20.03
    - first degree T20.13
    - second degree T20.23
    - third degree T20.33
  - colon T28.2
  - conjunctiva (and cornea) — *see* Burn, cornea
  - cornea (and conjunctiva) T26.1-
    - chemical — *see* Corrosion, cornea
  - corrosion (external) (internal) — *see* Corrosion, by site
  - deep necrosis of underlying tissue - code as Burn, third degree, by site
  - dorsum of hand T23.069
    - first degree T23.169
    - left T23.062
      - first degree T23.162
      - second degree T23.262
      - third degree T23.362
    - right T23.061
      - first degree T23.161
      - second degree T23.261
      - third degree T23.361
    - second degree T23.269
    - third degree T23.369
  - due to ingested chemical agent — *see* Corrosion, by site
  - ear (auricle) (external) (canal) T20.01
    - first degree T20.11
    - second degree T20.21
    - third degree T20.31
  - elbow T22.029
    - first degree T22.129
    - left T22.022
      - first degree T22.122
      - second degree T22.222
      - third degree T22.322
    - right T22.021
      - first degree T22.121
      - second degree T22.221
      - third degree T22.321
    - second degree T22.229

- **Burn** (electricity) (flame) (hot gas, liquid or hot object) (radiation) (steam) (thermal) - *continued*
  - elbow - *continued*
    - third degree T22.329
  - epidermal loss - code as Burn, second degree, by site
  - erythema, erythematous - code as Burn, first degree, by site
  - esophagus T28.1
  - extent (percentage of body surface)
    - less than 10 percent T31.0
    - 10-19 percent T31.10
      - with 0-9 percent third degree burns T31.10
      - with 10-19 percent third degree burns T31.11
    - 20-29 percent T31.20
      - with 0-9 percent third degree burns T31.20
      - with 10-19 percent third degree burns T31.21
      - with 20-29 percent third degree burns T31.22
    - 30-39 percent T31.30
      - with 0-9 percent third degree burns T31.30
      - with 10-19 percent third degree burns T31.31
      - with 20-29 percent third degree burns T31.32
      - with 30-39 percent third degree burns T31.33
    - 40-49 percent T31.40
      - with 0-9 percent third degree burns T31.40
      - with 10-19 percent third degree burns T31.41
      - with 20-29 percent third degree burns T31.42
      - with 30-39 percent third degree burns T31.43
      - with 40-49 percent third degree burns T31.44
    - 50-59 percent T31.50
      - with 0-9 percent third degree burns T31.50
      - with 10-19 percent third degree burns T31.51
      - with 20-29 percent third degree burns T31.52
      - with 30-39 percent third degree burns T31.53
      - with 40-49 percent third degree burns T31.54
      - with 50-59 percent third degree burns T31.55
    - 60-69 percent T31.60
      - with 0-9 percent third degree burns T31.60
      - with 10-19 percent third degree burns T31.61
      - with 20-29 percent third degree burns T31.62
      - with 30-39 percent third degree burns T31.63
      - with 40-49 percent third degree burns T31.64
      - with 50-59 percent third degree burns T31.65
      - with 60-69 percent third degree burns T31.66
    - 70-79 percent T31.70
      - with 0-9 percent third degree burns T31.70
      - with 10-19 percent third degree burns T31.71
      - with 20-29 percent third degree burns T31.72
      - with 30-39 percent third degree burns T31.73
      - with 40-49 percent third degree burns T31.74
      - with 50-59 percent third degree burns T31.75
      - with 60-69 percent third degree burns T31.76
      - with 70-79 percent third degree burns T31.77
    - 80-89 percent T31.80
      - with 0-9 percent third degree burns T31.80
      - with 10-19 percent third degree burns T31.81
      - with 20-29 percent third degree burns T31.82
      - with 30-39 percent third degree burns T31.83
      - with 40-49 percent third degree burns T31.84
      - with 50-59 percent third degree burns T31.85
      - with 60-69 percent third degree burns T31.86
      - with 70-79 percent third degree burns T31.87
      - with 80-89 percent third degree burns T31.88
    - 90 percent or more T31.90
      - with 0-9 percent third degree burns T31.90
      - with 10-19 percent third degree burns T31.91
      - with 20-29 percent third degree burns T31.92
      - with 30-39 percent third degree burns T31.93
      - with 40-49 percent third degree burns T31.94
      - with 50-59 percent third degree burns T31.95
      - with 60-69 percent third degree burns T31.96
      - with 70-79 percent third degree burns T31.97
      - with 80-89 percent third degree burns T31.98
      - with 90 percent or more third degree burns T31.99
  - extremity — *see* Burn, limb
  - eye (s) and adnexa T26.4-
    - with resulting rupture and destruction of eyeball T26.2-
    - conjunctival sac — *see* Burn, cornea
    - cornea — *see* Burn, cornea
    - lid — *see* Burn, eyelid
    - periocular area — *see* Burn, eyelid
    - specified site NEC T26.3-
  - eyeball — *see* Burn, eye
  - eyelid (s) T26.0-
    - chemical — *see* Corrosion, eyelid
  - face — *see* Burn, head
  - finger T23.029
    - first degree T23.129
    - left T23.022
      - first degree T23.122
      - second degree T23.222
      - third degree T23.322

- **Burn** (electricity) (flame) (hot gas, liquid or hot object) (radiation) (steam) (thermal) - *continued*
  - finger - *continued*
    - multiple sites (without thumb) T23.039
      - with thumb T23.049
        - first degree T23.149
        - left T23.042
          - first degree T23.142
          - second degree T23.242
          - third degree T23.342
        - right T23.041
          - first degree T23.141
          - second degree T23.241
          - third degree T23.341
        - second degree T23.249
        - third degree T23.349
      - first degree T23.139
      - left T23.032
        - first degree T23.132
        - second degree T23.232
        - third degree T23.332
      - right T23.031
        - first degree T23.131
        - second degree T23.231
        - third degree T23.331
      - second degree T23.239
      - third degree T23.339
    - right T23.021
      - first degree T23.121
      - second degree T23.221
      - third degree T23.321
    - second degree T23.229
    - third degree T23.329
  - flank — *see* Burn, abdominal wall
  - foot T25.029
    - first degree T25.129
    - left T25.022
      - first degree T25.122
      - second degree T25.222
      - third degree T25.322
    - multiple with ankle — *see* Burn, lower, limb, multiple, ankle and foot
    - right T25.021
      - first degree T25.121
      - second degree T25.221
      - third degree T25.321
    - second degree T25.229
    - third degree T25.329
  - forearm T22.019
    - first degree T22.119
    - left T22.012
      - first degree T22.112
      - second degree T22.212
      - third degree T22.312
    - right T22.011
      - first degree T22.111
      - second degree T22.211
      - third degree T22.311
    - second degree T22.219
    - third degree T22.319
  - forehead T20.06
    - first degree T20.16
    - second degree T20.26
    - third degree T20.36
  - fourth degree - code as Burn, third degree, by site
  - friction — *see* Burn, by site
  - from swallowing caustic or corrosive substance NEC — *see* Corrosion, by site
  - full thickness skin loss - code as Burn, third degree, by site
  - gastrointestinal tract NEC T28.2
    - from swallowing caustic or corrosive substance T28.7
  - genital organs
    - external
      - female T21.07
        - first degree T21.17
        - second degree T21.27
        - third degree T21.37
      - male T21.06
        - first degree T21.16
        - second degree T21.26
        - third degree T21.36
    - internal T28.3
      - from caustic or corrosive substance T28.8
  - groin — *see* Burn, abdominal wall
  - hand (s) T23.009
    - back — *see* Burn, dorsum of hand
    - finger — *see* Burn, finger
    - first degree T23.109
    - left T23.002
      - first degree T23.102
      - second degree T23.202

- **Burn** (electricity) (flame) (hot gas, liquid or hot object) (radiation) (steam) (thermal) - *continued*
  - hand (s) - *continued*
    - left - *continued*
      - third degree T23.302
    - multiple sites with wrist T23.099
      - first degree T23.199
      - left T23.092
        - first degree T23.192
        - second degree T23.292
        - third degree T23.392
      - right T23.091
        - first degree T23.191
        - second degree T23.291
        - third degree T23.391
      - second degree T23.299
      - third degree T23.399
    - palm — *see* Burn, palm
    - right T23.001
      - first degree T23.101
      - second degree T23.201
      - third degree T23.301
    - second degree T23.209
    - third degree T23.309
    - thumb — *see* Burn, thumb
  - head (and face) (and neck) T20.00
    - cheek — *see* Burn, cheek
    - chin — *see* Burn, chin
    - ear — *see* Burn, ear
    - eye (s) only — *see* Burn, eye
    - first degree T20.10
    - forehead — *see* Burn, forehead
    - lip — *see* Burn, lip
    - multiple sites T20.09
      - first degree T20.19
      - second degree T20.29
      - third degree T20.39
    - neck — *see* Burn, neck
    - nose — *see* Burn, nose
    - scalp — *see* Burn, scalp
    - second degree T20.20
    - third degree T20.30
  - hip (s) — *see* Burn, thigh
  - inhalation — *see* Burn, respiratory tract
    - caustic or corrosive substance (fumes) — *see* Corrosion, respiratory tract
  - internal organ (s) T28.40
    - alimentary tract T28.2
      - esophagus T28.1
    - eardrum T28.41
    - esophagus T28.1
    - from caustic or corrosive substance (swallowing) NEC — *see* Corrosion, by site
    - genitourinary T28.3
    - mouth T28.0
    - pharynx T28.0
    - respiratory tract — *see* Burn, respiratory tract
    - specified organ NEC T28.49
  - interscapular region — *see* Burn, back, upper
  - intestine (large) (small) T28.2
  - knee T24.029
    - first degree T24.129
    - left T24.022
      - first degree T24.122
      - second degree T24.222
      - third degree T24.322
    - right T24.021
      - first degree T24.121
      - second degree T24.221
      - third degree T24.321
    - second degree T24.229
    - third degree T24.329
  - labium (majus) (minus) — *see* Burn, genital organs, external, female
  - lacrimal apparatus, duct, gland or sac — *see* Burn, eye, specified site NEC
  - larynx T27.0
    - with lung T27.1
  - leg (s) (lower) (upper) — *see* Burn, lower, limb
  - lightning — *see* Burn, by site
  - limb (s)
    - lower (except ankle or foot alone) — *see* Burn, lower, limb
    - upper — *see* Burn, upper limb
  - lip (s) T20.02
    - first degree T20.12
    - second degree T20.22
    - third degree T20.32
  - lower
    - back — *see* Burn, back
    - limb T24.009
      - ankle — *see* Burn, ankle
      - calf — *see* Burn, calf

- **Burn** (electricity) (flame) (hot gas, liquid or hot object) (radiation) (steam) (thermal) - *continued*
  - lower - *continued*
    - limb - *continued*
      - first degree T24.109
      - foot — *see* Burn, foot
      - hip — *see* Burn, thigh
      - knee — *see* Burn, knee
      - left T24.002
        - first degree T24.102
        - second degree T24.202
        - third degree T24.302
      - multiple sites, except ankle and foot T24.099
        - ankle and foot T25.099
          - first degree T25.199
          - left T25.092
            - first degree T25.192
            - second degree T25.292
            - third degree T25.392
          - right T25.091
            - first degree T25.191
            - second degree T25.291
            - third degree T25.391
          - second degree T25.299
          - third degree T25.399
        - first degree T24.199
        - left T24.092
          - first degree T24.192
          - second degree T24.292
          - third degree T24.392
        - right T24.091
          - first degree T24.191
          - second degree T24.291
          - third degree T24.391
        - second degree T24.299
        - third degree T24.399
      - right T24.001
        - first degree T24.101
        - second degree T24.201
        - third degree T24.301
      - second degree T24.209
      - thigh — *see* Burn, thigh
      - third degree T24.309
      - toe — *see* Burn, toe
  - lung (with larynx and trachea) T27.1
  - mouth T28.0
  - neck T20.07
    - first degree T20.17
    - second degree T20.27
    - third degree T20.37
  - nose (septum) T20.04
    - first degree T20.14
    - second degree T20.24
    - third degree T20.34
  - ocular adnexa — *see* Burn, eye
  - orbit region — *see* Burn, eyelid
  - palm T23.059
    - first degree T23.159
    - left T23.052
      - first degree T23.152
      - second degree T23.252
      - third degree T23.352
    - right T23.051
      - first degree T23.151
      - second degree T23.251
      - third degree T23.351
    - second degree T23.259
    - third degree T23.359
  - partial thickness - code as Burn, unspecified degree, by site
  - pelvis — *see* Burn, trunk
  - penis — *see* Burn, genital organs, external, male
  - perineum
    - female — *see* Burn, genital organs, external, female
    - male — *see* Burn, genital organs, external, male
  - periocular area — *see* Burn, eyelid
  - pharynx T28.0
  - rectum T28.2
  - respiratory tract T27.3
    - larynx — *see* Burn, larynx
    - specified part NEC T27.2
    - trachea — *see* Burn, trachea
  - sac, lacrimal — *see* Burn, eye, specified site NEC
  - scalp T20.05
    - first degree T20.15
    - second degree T20.25
    - third degree T20.35
  - scapular region T22.069
    - first degree T22.169
    - left T22.062
      - first degree T22.162
      - second degree T22.262

Burn (electricity) (flame) (hot gas, liquid or hot object) (radiation) (steam) (thermal) - *continued*
scapular region - *continued*
left - *continued*
third degree T22.362
right T22.061
first degree T22.161
second degree T22.261
third degree T22.361
second degree T22.269
third degree T22.369
sclera — *see* Burn, eye, specified site NEC
scrotum — *see* Burn, genital organs, external, male
shoulder T22.059
first degree T22.159
left T22.052
first degree T22.152
second degree T22.252
third degree T22.352
right T22.051
first degree T22.151
second degree T22.251
third degree T22.351
second degree T22.259
third degree T22.359
stomach T28.2
temple — *see* Burn, head
testis — *see* Burn, genital organs, external, male
thigh T24.019
first degree T24.119
left T24.012
first degree T24.112
second degree T24.212
third degree T24.312
right T24.011
first degree T24.111
second degree T24.211
third degree T24.311
second degree T24.219
third degree T24.319
thorax (external) — *see* Burn, trunk
throat (meaning pharynx) T28.0
thumb (s) T23.019
first degree T23.119
left T23.012
first degree T23.112
second degree T23.212
third degree T23.312
multiple sites with fingers T23.049
first degree T23.149
left T23.042
first degree T23.142
second degree T23.242
third degree T23.342
right T23.041
first degree T23.141
second degree T23.241
third degree T23.341
second degree T23.249
third degree T23.349
right T23.011
first degree T23.111
second degree T23.211
third degree T23.311
second degree T23.219
third degree T23.319
toe T25.039
first degree T25.139
left T25.032
first degree T25.132
second degree T25.232
third degree T25.332
right T25.031
first degree T25.131
second degree T25.231
third degree T25.331
second degree T25.239
third degree T25.339
tongue T28.0
tonsil (s) T28.0
trachea T27.0
with lung T27.1
trunk T21.00
abdominal wall — *see* Burn, abdominal wall
anus — *see* Burn, buttock
axilla — *see* Burn, upper limb
back — *see* Burn, back
breast — *see* Burn, chest wall
buttock — *see* Burn, buttock
chest wall — *see* Burn, chest wall
first degree T21.10
flank — *see* Burn, abdominal wall
genital

Burn (electricity) (flame) (hot gas, liquid or hot object) (radiation) (steam) (thermal) - *continued*
trunk - *continued*
genital - *continued*
female — *see* Burn, genital organs, external, female
male — *see* Burn, genital organs, external, male
groin — *see* Burn, abdominal wall
interscapular region — *see* Burn, back, upper
labia — *see* Burn, genital organs, external, female
lower back — *see* Burn, back
penis — *see* Burn, genital organs, external, male
perineum
female — *see* Burn, genital organs, external, female
male — *see* Burn, genital organs, external, male
scapula region — *see* Burn, scapular region
scrotum — *see* Burn, genital organs, external, male
second degree T21.20
specified site NEC T21.09
first degree T21.19
second degree T21.29
third degree T21.39
testes — *see* Burn, genital organs, external, male
third degree T21.30
upper back — *see* Burn, back, upper
vulva — *see* Burn, genital organs, external, female
unspecified site with extent of body surface involved specified
less than 10 percent T31.0
10-19 percent (0-9 percent third degree) T31.10
with 10-19 percent third degree T31.11
20-29 percent (0-9 percent third degree) T31.20
with
10-19 percent third degree T31.21
20-29 percent third degree T31.22
30-39 percent (0-9 percent third degree) T31.30
with
10-19 percent third degree T31.31
20-29 percent third degree T31.32
30-39 percent third degree T31.33
40-49 percent (0-9 percent third degree) T31.40
with
10-19 percent third degree T31.41
20-29 percent third degree T31.42
30-39 percent third degree T31.43
40-49 percent third degree T31.44
50-59 percent (0-9 percent third degree) T31.50
with
10-19 percent third degree T31.51
20-29 percent third degree T31.52
30-39 percent third degree T31.53
40-49 percent third degree T31.54
50-59 percent third degree T31.55
60-69 percent (0-9 percent third degree) T31.60
with
10-19 percent third degree T31.61
20-29 percent third degree T31.62
30-39 percent third degree T31.63
40-49 percent third degree T31.64
50-59 percent third degree T31.65
60-69 percent third degree T31.66
70-79 percent (0-9 percent third degree) T31.70
with
10-19 percent third degree T31.71
20-29 percent third degree T31.72
30-39 percent third degree T31.73
40-49 percent third degree T31.74
50-59 percent third degree T31.75
60-69 percent third degree T31.76
70-79 percent third degree T31.77
80-89 percent (0-9 percent third degree) T31.80
with
10-19 percent third degree T31.81
20-29 percent third degree T31.82
30-39 percent third degree T31.83
40-49 percent third degree T31.84
50-59 percent third degree T31.85
60-69 percent third degree T31.86
70-79 percent third degree T31.87
80-89 percent third degree T31.88
90 percent or more (0-9 percent third degree) T31.90
with
10-19 percent third degree T31.91
20-29 percent third degree T31.92
30-39 percent third degree T31.93
40-49 percent third degree T31.94
50-59 percent third degree T31.95
60-69 percent third degree T31.96
70-79 percent third degree T31.97
80-89 percent third degree T31.98
90-99 percent third degree T31.99

Burn (electricity) (flame) (hot gas, liquid or hot object) (radiation) (steam) (thermal) - *continued*
upper limb T22.00
above elbow — *see* Burn, above elbow
axilla — *see* Burn, axilla
elbow — *see* Burn, elbow
first degree T22.10
forearm — *see* Burn, forearm
hand — *see* Burn, hand
interscapular region — *see* Burn, back, upper
multiple sites T22.099
first degree T22.199
left T22.092
first degree T22.192
second degree T22.292
third degree T22.392
right T22.091
first degree T22.191
second degree T22.291
third degree T22.391
second degree T22.299
third degree T22.399
scapular region — *see* Burn, scapular region
second degree T22.20
shoulder — *see* Burn, shoulder
third degree T22.30
wrist — *see* Burn, wrist
uterus T28.3
vagina T28.3
vulva — *see* Burn, genital organs, external, female
wrist T23.079
first degree T23.179
left T23.072
first degree T23.172
second degree T23.272
third degree T23.372
multiple sites with hand T23.099
first degree T23.199
left T23.092
first degree T23.192
second degree T23.292
third degree T23.392
right T23.091
first degree T23.191
second degree T23.291
third degree T23.391
second degree T23.299
third degree T23.399
right T23.071
first degree T23.171
second degree T23.271
third degree T23.371
second degree T23.279
third degree T23.379
Burnett's syndrome E83.52
Burning
feet syndrome E53.9
sensation R20.8
tongue K14.6
Burn-out (state) Z73.0
Burns' disease or osteochondrosis — *see* Osteochondrosis, juvenile, ulna
Bursa — *see* condition
Bursitis M71.9
Achilles — *see* Tendinitis, Achilles
adhesive — *see* Bursitis, specified NEC
ankle — *see* Enthesopathy, lower limb, ankle, specified type NEC
calcaneal — *see* Enthesopathy, foot, specified type NEC
collateral ligament, tibial — *see* Bursitis, tibial collateral
due to use, overuse, pressure — *see also* Disorder, soft tissue, due to use, specified type NEC
specified NEC — *see* Disorder, soft tissue, due to use, specified NEC
Duplay's M75.0
elbow NEC M70.3-
olecranon M70.2-
finger — *see* Disorder, soft tissue, due to use, specified type NEC, hand
foot — *see* Enthesopathy, foot, specified type NEC
gonococcal A54.49
gouty — *see* Gout
hand M70.1-
hip NEC M70.7-
trochanteric M70.6-
infective NEC M71.10
abscess — *see* Abscess, bursa
ankle M71.17-
elbow M71.12-
foot M71.17-
hand M71.14-

Bursitis - *continued*
infective NEC - *continued*
hip M71.15-
knee M71.16-
multiple sites M71.19
shoulder M71.11-
specified site NEC M71.18
wrist M71.13-
ischial — *see* Bursitis, hip
knee NEC M70.5-
prepatellar M70.4-
occupational NEC — *see also* Disorder, soft tissue, due to, use
olecranon — *see* Bursitis, elbow, olecranon
pharyngeal J39.1
popliteal — *see* Bursitis, knee
prepatellar M70.4-
radiohumeral M77.8
rheumatoid M06.20
ankle M06.27-
elbow M06.22-
foot joint M06.27-
hand joint M06.24-
hip M06.25-
knee M06.26-
multiple site M06.29
shoulder M06.21-
vertebra M06.28
wrist M06.23-
scapulohumeral — *see* Bursitis, shoulder
semimembranous muscle (knee) — *see* Bursitis, knee
shoulder M75.5-
adhesive — *see* Capsulitis, adhesive
specified NEC M71.50
ankle M71.57-
due to use, overuse or pressure — *see* Disorder, soft tissue, due to, use
elbow M71.52-
foot M71.57-
hand M71.54-
hip M71.55-
knee M71.56-
shoulder — *see* Bursitis, shoulder
specified site NEC M71.58
tibial collateral M76.4-
wrist M71.53-
subacromial — *see* Bursitis, shoulder
subcoracoid — *see* Bursitis, shoulder
subdeltoid — *see* Bursitis, shoulder
syphilitic A52.78
Thornwaldt, Tornwaldt J39.2
tibial collateral M76.4-
toe — *see* Enthesopathy, foot, specified type NEC
trochanteric (area) — *see* Bursitis, hip, trochanteric
wrist — *see* Bursitis, hand
Bursopathy M71.9
specified type NEC M71.80
ankle M71.87-
elbow M71.82-
foot M71.87-
hand M71.84-
hip M71.85-
knee M71.86-
multiple sites M71.89
shoulder M71.81-
specified site NEC M71.88
wrist M71.83-
Burst stitches or sutures (complication of surgery) T81.31
external operation wound T81.31
internal operation wound T81.32
Buruli ulcer A31.1
Bury's disease L95.1
Buschke's
disease B45.3
scleredema — *see* Sclerosis, systemic
Busse-Buschke disease B45.3
Buttock — *see* condition
Button
Biskra B55.1
Delhi B55.1
oriental B55.1
Buttonhole deformity (finger) — *see* Deformity, finger, boutonniere
Bwamba fever A92.8
Byssinosis J66.0
Bywaters' syndrome T79.5

C

Cachexia R64
cancerous R64
cardiac — *see* Disease, heart

Cachexia - *continued*
dehydration E86.0
due to malnutrition R64
exophthalmic — *see* Hyperthyroidism
heart — *see* Disease, heart
hypophyseal E23.0
hypopituitary E23.0
lead — *see* Poisoning, lead
malignant R64
marsh — *see* Malaria
nervous F48.8
old age R54
paludal — *see* Malaria
pituitary E23.0
renal N28.9
saturnine — *see* Poisoning, lead
senile R54
Simmonds' E23.0
splenica D73.0
strumipriva E03.4
tuberculous NEC — *see* Tuberculosis
CADASIL
(cerebral autosomal dominant arteriopathy with subcortical infarcts and leukoencephalopathy) I67.850
Café, au lait spots L81.3
Caffeine-induced
anxiety disorder F15.980
sleep disorder F15.982
Caffey's syndrome Q78.8
Caisson disease T70.3
Cake kidney Q63.1
Caked breast (puerperal, postpartum) O92.79
Calabar swelling B74.3
Calcaneal spur — *see* Spur, bone, calcaneal
Calcaneo-apophysitis M92.8
Calcareous — *see* condition
Calcicosis J62.8
Calciferol (vitamin D) **deficiency** E55.9
with rickets E55.0
Calcification
adrenal (capsule) (gland) E27.49
tuberculous E35 *[B90.8]*
aorta I70.0
artery (annular) — *see* Arteriosclerosis
auricle (ear) — *see* Disorder, pinna, specified type NEC
basal ganglia G23.8
bladder N32.89
due to Schistosoma hematobium B65.0
brain (cortex) — *see* Calcification, cerebral
bronchus J98.09
bursa M71.40
ankle M71.47-
elbow M71.42-
foot M71.47-
hand M71.44-
hip M71.45-
knee M71.46-
multiple sites M71.49
shoulder M75.3-
specified site NEC M71.48
wrist M71.43-
cardiac — *see* Degeneration, myocardial
cerebral (cortex) G93.89
artery I67.2
cervix (uteri) N88.8
choroid plexus G93.89
conjunctiva — *see* Concretion, conjunctiva
corpora cavernosa (penis) N48.89
cortex (brain) — *see* Calcification, cerebral
dental pulp (nodular) K04.2
dentinal papilla K00.4
fallopian tube N83.8
falx cerebri G96.19
gallbladder K82.8
general E83.59
heart — *see also* Degeneration, myocardial
valve — *see* Endocarditis
idiopathic infantile arterial (IIAC) Q28.8
intervertebral cartilage or disc (postinfective) — *see* Disorder, disc, specified NEC
intracranial — *see* Calcification, cerebral
joint — *see* Disorder, joint, specified type NEC
kidney N28.89
tuberculous N29 *[B90.1]*
larynx (senile) J38.7
lens — *see* Cataract, specified NEC
lung (active) (postinfectional) J98.4
tuberculous B90.9
lymph gland or node (postinfectional) I89.8
tuberculous — *see also* Tuberculosis, lymph gland B90.8

Calcification - *continued*
mammographic R92.1
massive (paraplegic) — *see* Myositis, ossificans, in, quadriplegia
medial — *see* Arteriosclerosis, extremities
meninges (cerebral) (spinal) G96.19
metastatic E83.59
Mönckeberg's — *see* Arteriosclerosis, extremities
muscle M61.9
due to burns — *see* Myositis, ossificans, in, burns
paralytic — *see* Myositis, ossificans, in, quadriplegia
specified type NEC M61.40
ankle M61.47-
foot M61.47-
forearm M61.43-
hand M61.44-
lower leg M61.46-
multiple sites M61.49
pelvic region M61.45-
shoulder region M61.41-
specified site NEC M61.48
thigh M61.45-
upper arm M61.42-
myocardium, myocardial — *see* Degeneration, myocardial
ovary N83.8
pancreas K86.89
penis N48.89
periarticular — *see* Disorder, joint, specified type NEC
pericardium — *see also* Pericarditis I31.1
pineal gland E34.8
pleura J94.8
postinfectional J94.8
tuberculous NEC B90.9
pulpal (dental) (nodular) K04.2
sclera H15.89
spleen D73.89
subcutaneous L94.2
suprarenal (capsule) (gland) E27.49
tendon (sheath) — *see also* Tenosynovitis, specified type NEC
with bursitis, synovitis or tenosynovitis — *see* Tendinitis, calcific
trachea J39.8
ureter N28.89
uterus N85.8
vitreous — *see* Deposit, crystalline
Calcified — *see* Calcification
Calcinosis (interstitial) (tumoral) (universalis) E83.59
with Raynaud's phenomenon, esophageal dysfunction, sclerodactyly, telangiectasia (CREST syndrome) M34.1
circumscripta (skin) L94.2
cutis L94.2
Calciphylaxis — *see also* Calcification, by site E83.59
Calcium
deposits — *see* Calcification, by site
metabolism disorder E83.50
salts or soaps in vitreous — *see* Deposit, crystalline
Calciuria R82.994
Calculi — *see* Calculus
Calculosis, intrahepatic — *see* Calculus, bile duct
Calculus, calculi, calculous
ampulla of Vater — *see* Calculus, bile duct
anuria (impacted) (recurrent) — *see also* Calculus, urinary N20.9
appendix K38.1
bile duct (common) (hepatic) K80.50
with
calculus of gallbladder — *see* Calculus, gallbladder and bile duct
cholangitis K80.30
with
cholecystitis — *see* Calculus, bile duct, with cholecystitis
obstruction K80.31
acute K80.32
with
chronic cholangitis K80.36
with obstruction K80.37
obstruction K80.33
chronic K80.34
with
acute cholangitis K80.36
with obstruction K80.37
obstruction K80.35
cholecystitis (with cholangitis) K80.40
with obstruction K80.41
acute K80.42
with

Carbuncle - *continued*
lacrimal
gland — *see* Dacryoadenitis
passages (duct) (sac) — *see* Inflammation, lacrimal, passages, acute
leg — *see* Carbuncle, lower limb
lower limb L02.43-
malignant A22.0
navel L02.236
neck L02.13
nose (external) (septum) J34.0
orbit, orbital — *see* Abscess, orbit
palmar (space) — *see* Carbuncle, hand
partes posteriores L02.33
pectoral region L02.233
penis N48.21
perineum L02.235
pinna — *see* Abscess, ear, external
popliteal — *see* Carbuncle, lower limb
scalp L02.831
seminal vesicle N49.0
shoulder — *see* Carbuncle, upper limb
specified site NEC L02.838
temple (region) L02.03
thumb — *see* Carbuncle, hand
toe — *see* Carbuncle, foot
trunk L02.239
abdominal wall L02.231
back L02.232
chest wall L02.233
groin L02.234
perineum L02.235
umbilicus L02.236
umbilicus L02.236
upper limb L02.43-
urethra N34.0
vulva N76.4
Carbunculus — *see* Carbuncle
Carcinoid (tumor) — *see* Tumor, carcinoid
Carcinoidosis E34.0
Carcinoma (malignant) — *see also* Neoplasm, by site, malignant
acidophil
specified site — *see* Neoplasm, malignant, by site
unspecified site C75.1
acidophil-basophil, mixed
specified site — *see* Neoplasm, malignant, by site
unspecified site C75.1
adnexal (skin) — *see* Neoplasm, skin, malignant
adrenal cortical C74.0-
alveolar — *see* Neoplasm, lung, malignant
cell — *see* Neoplasm, lung, malignant
ameloblastic C41.1
upper jaw (bone) C41.0
apocrine
breast — *see* Neoplasm, breast, malignant
specified site NEC — *see* Neoplasm, skin, malignant
unspecified site C44.99
basal cell (pigmented) (see also Neoplasm, skin, malignant) C44.91
fibro-epithelial — *see* Neoplasm, skin, malignant
morphea — *see* Neoplasm, skin, malignant
multicentric — *see* Neoplasm, skin, malignant
basaloid
basal-squamous cell, mixed — *see* Neoplasm, skin, malignant
basophil
specified site — *see* Neoplasm, malignant, by site
unspecified site C75.1
basophil-acidophil, mixed
specified site — *see* Neoplasm, malignant, by site
unspecified site C75.1
basosquamous — *see* Neoplasm, skin, malignant
bile duct
with hepatocellular, mixed C22.0
liver C22.1
specified site NEC — *see* Neoplasm, malignant, by site
unspecified site C22.1
branchial or branchiogenic C10.4
bronchial or bronchogenic — *see* Neoplasm, lung, malignant
bronchiolar — *see* Neoplasm, lung, malignant
bronchioloalveolar — *see* Neoplasm, lung, malignant
C cell
specified site — *see* Neoplasm, malignant, by site
unspecified site C73
ceruminous C44.29-
cervix uteri
in situ D06.9
endocervix D06.0

Carcinoma (malignant) - *continued*
cervix uteri - *continued*
in situ - *continued*
exocervix D06.1
specified site NEC D06.7
chorionic
specified site — *see* Neoplasm, malignant, by site
unspecified site
female C58
male C62.90
chromophobe
specified site — *see* Neoplasm, malignant, by site
unspecified site C75.1
cloacogenic
specified site — *see* Neoplasm, malignant, by site
unspecified site C21.2
diffuse type
specified site — *see* Neoplasm, malignant, by site
unspecified site C16.9
duct (cell)
with Paget's disease — *see* Neoplasm, breast, malignant
infiltrating
with lobular carcinoma (in situ)
specified site — *see* Neoplasm, malignant, by site
unspecified site (female) C50.91-
male C50.92-
specified site — *see* Neoplasm, malignant, by site
unspecified site (female) C50.91-
male C50.92-
ductal
with lobular
specified site — *see* Neoplasm, malignant, by site
unspecified site (female) C50.91-
male C50.92-
ductular, infiltrating
specified site — *see* Neoplasm, malignant, by site
unspecified site (female) C50.91-
male C50.92-
embryonal
liver C22.7
endometrioid
specified site — *see* Neoplasm, malignant, by site
unspecified site
female C56.9
male C61
eosinophil
specified site — *see* Neoplasm, malignant, by site
unspecified site C75.1
epidermoid — *see also* Neoplasm, skin malignant
in situ, Bowen's type — *see* Neoplasm, skin, in situ
fibroepithelial, basal cell — *see* Neoplasm, skin, malignant
follicular
with papillary (mixed) C73
moderately differentiated C73
pure follicle C73
specified site — *see* Neoplasm, malignant, by site
trabecular C73
unspecified site C73
well differentiated C73
generalized, with unspecified primary site C80.0
glycogen-rich — *see* Neoplasm, breast, malignant
granulosa cell C56-
hepatic cell C22.0
hepatocellular C22.0
with bile duct, mixed C22.0
fibrolamellar C22.0
hepatocholangiolitic C22.0
Hurthle cell C73
in
adenomatous
polyposis coli C18.9
pleomorphic adenoma — *see* Neoplasm, salivary glands, malignant
situ — *see* Carcinoma-in-situ
infiltrating
duct
with lobular
specified site — *see* Neoplasm, malignant, by site
unspecified site (female) C50.91-
male C50.92-
with Paget's disease — *see* Neoplasm, breast, malignant
specified site — *see* Neoplasm, malignant
unspecified site (female) C50.91-
male C50.92-
ductular
specified site — *see* Neoplasm, malignant
unspecified site (female) C50.91-
male C50.92-

Carcinoma (malignant) - *continued*
infiltrating - *continued*
lobular
specified site — *see* Neoplasm, malignant
unspecified site (female) C50.91-
male C50.92-
inflammatory
specified site — *see* Neoplasm, malignant
unspecified site (female) C50.91-
male C50.92-
intestinal type
specified site — *see* Neoplasm, malignant, by site
unspecified site C16.9
intracystic
noninfiltrating — *see* Neoplasm, in situ, by site
intraductal (noninfiltrating)
with Paget's disease — *see* Neoplasm, breast, malignant
breast D05.1-
papillary
with invasion
specified site — *see* Neoplasm, malignant, by site
unspecified site (female) C50.91-
male C50.92-
breast D05.1-
specified site NEC — *see* Neoplasm, in situ, by site
unspecified site (female) D05.1-
specified site NEC — *see* Neoplasm, in situ, by site
unspecified site (female) D05.1-
intraepidermal — *see* Neoplasm, in situ
squamous cell, Bowen's type — *see* Neoplasm, skin, in situ
intraepithelial — *see* Neoplasm, in situ, by site
squamous cell — *see* Neoplasm, in situ, by site
intraosseous C41.1
upper jaw (bone) C41.0
islet cell
with exocrine, mixed
specified site — *see* Neoplasm, malignant, by site
unspecified site C25.9
pancreas C25.4
specified site NEC — *see* Neoplasm, malignant, by site
unspecified site C25.4
juvenile, breast — *see* Neoplasm, breast, malignant
large cell
small cell
specified site — *see* Neoplasm, malignant, by site
unspecified site C34.90
Leydig cell (testis)
specified site — *see* Neoplasm, malignant, by site
unspecified site
female C56.9
male C62.90
lipid-rich (female) C50.91-
male C50.92-
liver cell C22.0
liver NEC C22.7
lobular (infiltrating)
with intraductal
specified site — *see* Neoplasm, malignant, by site
unspecified site (female) C50.91-
male C50.92-
noninfiltrating
breast D05.0-
specified site NEC — *see* Neoplasm, in situ, by site
unspecified site D05.0-
specified site — *see* Neoplasm, malignant, by site
unspecified site (female) C50.91-
male C50.92-
medullary
with
amyloid stroma
specified site — *see* Neoplasm, malignant, by site
unspecified site C73
lymphoid stroma
specified site — *see* Neoplasm, malignant, by site
unspecified site (female) C50.91-
male C50.92-
Merkel cell C4A.9
anal margin C4A.51
anal skin C4A.51
canthus C4A.1-
ear and external auricular canal C4A.2-
external auricular canal C4A.2-
eyelid, including canthus C4A.1-
face C4A.30

Carcinoma (malignant) - *continued*
Merkel cell - *continued*
face - *continued*
specified NEC C4A.39
hip C4A.7-
lip C4A.0
lower limb, including hip C4A.7-
neck C4A.4
nodal presentation C7B.1
nose C4A.31
overlapping sites C4A.8
perianal skin C4A.51
scalp C4A.4
secondary C7B.1
shoulder C4A.6-
skin of breast C4A.52
trunk NEC C4A.59
upper limb, including shoulder C4A.6-
visceral metastatic C7B.1
metastatic — *see* Neoplasm, secondary, by site
metatypical — *see* Neoplasm, skin, malignant
morphea, basal cell — *see* Neoplasm, skin, malignant
mucoid
cell
specified site — *see* Neoplasm, malignant, by site
unspecified site C75.1
neuroendocrine — *see also* Tumor, neuroendocrine
high grade, any site C7A.1
poorly differentiated, any site C7A.1
nonencapsulated sclerosing C73
noninfiltrating
intracystic — *see* Neoplasm, in situ, by site
intraductal
breast D05.1-
papillary
breast D05.1-
specified site NEC — *see* Neoplasm, in situ, by site
unspecified site D05.1-
specified site — *see* Neoplasm, in situ, by site
unspecified site D05.1-
lobular
breast D05.0-
specified site NEC — *see* Neoplasm, in situ, by site
unspecified site (female) D05.0-
oat cell
specified site — *see* Neoplasm, malignant, by site
unspecified site C34.90
odontogenic C41.1
upper jaw (bone) C41.0
papillary
with follicular (mixed) C73
follicular variant C73
intraductal (noninfiltrating)
with invasion
specified site — *see* Neoplasm, malignant, by site
unspecified site (female) C50.91-
male C50.92-
breast D05.1-
specified site NEC — *see* Neoplasm, in situ, by site
unspecified site D05.1-
serous
specified site — *see* Neoplasm, malignant, by site
surface
specified site — *see* Neoplasm, malignant, by site
unspecified site C56.9
unspecified site C56.9
papillocystic
specified site — *see* Neoplasm, malignant, by site
unspecified site C56.9
parafollicular cell
specified site — *see* Neoplasm, malignant, by site
unspecified site C73
pilomatrix — *see* Neoplasm, skin, malignant
pseudomucinous
specified site — *see* Neoplasm, malignant, by site
unspecified site C56.9
renal cell C64-
Schmincke — *see* Neoplasm, nasopharynx, malignant
Schneiderian
specified site — *see* Neoplasm, malignant, by site
unspecified site C30.0
sebaceous — *see* Neoplasm, skin, malignant
secondary — *see also* Neoplasm, secondary, by site
Merkel cell C7B.1
secretory, breast — *see* Neoplasm, breast, malignant
serous

Carcinoma (malignant) - *continued*
serous - *continued*
papillary
specified site — *see* Neoplasm, malignant, by site
unspecified site C56.9
surface, papillary
specified site — *see* Neoplasm, malignant, by site
unspecified site C56.9
Sertoli cell
specified site — *see* Neoplasm, malignant, by site
unspecified site C62.90
female C56.9
male C62.90
skin appendage — *see* Neoplasm, skin, malignant
small cell
fusiform cell
specified site — *see* Neoplasm, malignant, by site
unspecified site C34.90
intermediate cell
specified site — *see* Neoplasm, malignant, by site
unspecified site C34.90
large cell
specified site — *see* Neoplasm, malignant, by site
unspecified site C34.90
solid
with amyloid stroma
specified site — *see* Neoplasm, malignant, by site
unspecified site C73
microinvasive
specified site — *see* Neoplasm, malignant, by site
unspecified site C53.9
sweat gland — *see* Neoplasm, skin, malignant
theca cell C56.-
thymic C37
unspecified site (primary) C80.1
water-clear cell C75.0
Carcinoma-in-situ — *see also* Neoplasm, in situ, by site
breast NOS D05.9-
specified type NEC D05.8-
epidermoid — *see also* Neoplasm, in situ, by site
with questionable stromal invasion
cervix D06.9
specified site NEC — *see* Neoplasm, in situ, by site
unspecified site D06.9
Bowen's type — *see* Neoplasm, skin, in situ
intraductal
breast D05.1-
specified site NEC — *see* Neoplasm, in situ, by site
unspecified site D05.1-
lobular
with
infiltrating duct
breast (female) C50.91-
male C50.92-
specified site NEC — *see* Neoplasm, malignant
unspecified site (female) C50.91-
male C50.92-
intraductal
breast D05.8-
specified site NEC — *see* Neoplasm, in situ, by site
unspecified site (female) D05.8-
breast D05.0-
specified site NEC — *see* Neoplasm, in situ, by site
unspecified site D05.0-
squamous cell — *see also* Neoplasm, in situ, by site
with questionable stromal invasion
cervix D06.9
specified site NEC — *see* Neoplasm, in situ, by site
unspecified site D06.9
Carcinomaphobia F45.29
Carcinomatosis C80.0
peritonei C78.6
unspecified site (primary) (secondary) C80.0
Carcinosarcoma — *see* Neoplasm, malignant, by site
embryonal — *see* Neoplasm, malignant, by site
Cardia, cardial — *see* condition
Cardiac — *see also* condition
death, sudden — *see* Arrest, cardiac
pacemaker
in situ Z95.0
management or adjustment Z45.018
tamponade I31.4
Cardialgia — *see* Pain, precordial
Cardiectasis — *see* Hypertrophy, cardiac
Cardiochalasia K21.9
Cardiomalacia I51.5
Cardiomegalia glycogenica diffusa E74.02 *[I43]*

Cardiomegaly — *see also* Hypertrophy, cardiac
congenital Q24.8
glycogen E74.02 *[I43]*
idiopathic I51.7
Cardiomyoliposis I51.5
Cardiomyopathy (familial) (idiopathic) I42.9
alcoholic I42.6
amyloid E85.4 *[I43]*
transthyretin-related (ATTR) familial E85.4
arteriosclerotic — *see* Disease, heart, ischemic, atherosclerotic
beriberi E51.12
cobalt-beer I42.6
congenital I42.4
congestive I42.0
constrictive NOS I42.5
dilated I42.0
due to
alcohol I42.6
beriberi E51.12
cardiac glycogenosis E74.02 *[I43]*
drugs I42.7
external agents NEC I42.7
Friedreich's ataxia G11.1
myotonia atrophica G71.11 *[I43]*
progressive muscular dystrophy G71.09 *[I43]*
glycogen storage E74.02 *[I43]*
hypertensive — *see* Hypertension, heart
hypertrophic (nonobstructive) I42.2
obstructive I42.1
congenital Q24.8
in
Chagas' disease (chronic) B57.2
acute B57.0
sarcoidosis D86.85
ischemic I25.5
metabolic E88.9 *[I43]*
thyrotoxic E05.90 *[I43]*
with thyroid storm E05.91 *[I43]*
newborn I42.8
congenital I42.4
nutritional E63.9 *[I43]*
beriberi E51.12
obscure of Africa I42.8
peripartum O90.3
postpartum O90.3
restrictive NEC I42.5
rheumatic I09.0
secondary I42.9
stress induced I51.81
takotsubo I51.81
thyrotoxic E05.90 *[I43]*
with thyroid storm E05.91 *[I43]*
toxic NEC I42.7
transthyretin-related (ATTR) familial amyloid E85.4
tuberculous A18.84
viral B33.24
Cardionephritis — *see* Hypertension, cardiorenal
Cardionephropathy — *see* Hypertension, cardiorenal
Cardionephrosis — *see* Hypertension, cardiorenal
Cardiopathia nigra I27.0
Cardiopathy — *see also* Disease, heart I51.9
idiopathic I42.9
mucopolysaccharidosis E76.3 *[I52]*
Cardiopericarditis — *see* Pericarditis
Cardiophobia F45.29
Cardiorenal — *see* condition
Cardiorrhexis — *see* Infarct, myocardium
Cardiosclerosis — *see* Disease, heart, ischemic, atherosclerotic
Cardiosis — *see* Disease, heart
Cardiospasm (esophagus) (reflex) (stomach) K22.0
congenital Q39.5
with megaesophagus Q39.5
Cardiostenosis — *see* Disease, heart
Cardiosymphysis I31.0
Cardiovascular — *see* condition
Carditis (acute) (bacterial) (chronic) (subacute) I51.89
meningococcal A39.50
rheumatic — *see* Disease, heart, rheumatic
rheumatoid — *see* Rheumatoid, carditis
viral B33.20
Care (of) (for) (following)
child (routine) Z76.2
family member (handicapped) (sick)
creating problem for family Z63.6
provided away from home for holiday relief Z75.5
unavailable, due to
absence (person rendering care) (sufferer) Z74.2
inability (any reason) of person rendering care Z74.2

Care (of) (for) (following) - *continued*
foundling Z76.1
holiday relief Z75.5
improper — *see* Maltreatment
lack of (at or after birth) (infant) — *see* Maltreatment, child, neglect
lactating mother Z39.1
palliative Z51.5
postpartum
immediately after delivery Z39.0
routine follow-up Z39.2
respite Z75.5
unavailable, due to
absence of person rendering care Z74.2
inability (any reason) of person rendering care Z74.2
well-baby Z76.2
Caries
bone NEC A18.03
dental (dentino enamel junction) (early childhood) (of dentine) (pre-eruptive) (recurrent) (to the pulp) K02.9
arrested (coronal) (root) K02.3
chewing surface
limited to enamel K02.51
penetrating into dentin K02.52
penetrating into pulp K02.53
coronal surface
chewing surface
limited to enamel K02.51
penetrating into dentin K02.52
penetrating into pulp K02.53
pit and fissure surface
limited to enamel K02.51
penetrating into dentin K02.52
penetrating into pulp K02.53
smooth surface
limited to enamel K02.61
penetrating into dentin K02.62
penetrating into pulp K02.63
pit and fissure surface
limited to enamel K02.51
penetrating into dentin K02.52
penetrating into pulp K02.53
primary, cervical origin K02.52
root K02.7
smooth surface
limited to enamel K02.61
penetrating into dentin K02.62
penetrating into pulp K02.63
external meatus — *see* Disorder, ear, external, specified type NEC
hip (tuberculous) A18.02
initial (tooth)
chewing surface K02.51
pit and fissure surface K02.51
smooth surface K02.61
knee (tuberculous) A18.02
labyrinth — *see* subcategory H83.8
limb NEC (tuberculous) A18.03
mastoid process (chronic) — *see* Mastoiditis, chronic
tuberculous A18.03
middle ear — *see* subcategory H74.8
nose (tuberculous) A18.03
orbit (tuberculous) A18.03
ossicles, ear — *see* Abnormal, ear ossicles
petrous bone — *see* Petrositis
root (dental) (tooth) K02.7
sacrum (tuberculous) A18.01
spine, spinal (column) (tuberculous) A18.01
syphilitic A52.77
congenital (early) A50.02 *[M90.80]*
tooth, teeth — *see* Caries, dental
tuberculous A18.03
vertebra (column) (tuberculous) A18.01
Carious teeth — *see* Caries, dental
Carneous mole O02.0
Carnitine insufficiency E71.40
Carotenemia (dietary) E67.1
Carotenosis (cutis) (skin) E67.1
Carotid body or sinus syndrome G90.01
Carotidynia G90.01
Carpal tunnel syndrome — *see* Syndrome, carpal tunnel
Carpenter's syndrome Q87.0
Carpopedal spasm — *see* Tetany
Carr-Barr-Plunkett syndrome Q97.1
Carrier (suspected) **of**
amebiasis Z22.1
bacterial disease NEC Z22.39
diphtheria Z22.2
intestinal infectious NEC Z22.1

Carrier (suspected) **of** - *continued*
bacterial disease NEC - *continued*
intestinal infectious NEC - *continued*
typhoid Z22.0
meningococcal Z22.31
sexually transmitted Z22.4
specified NEC Z22.39
staphylococcal (Methicillin susceptible) Z22.321
Methicillin resistant Z22.322
streptococcal Z22.338
group B Z22.330
complicating pregnancy or delivery O99.82-
typhoid Z22.0
cholera Z22.1
diphtheria Z22.2
gastrointestinal pathogens NEC Z22.1
genetic Z14.8
cystic fibrosis Z14.1
hemophilia A (asymptomatic) Z14.01
symptomatic Z14.02
gestational, pregnant Z33.1
gonorrhea Z22.4
HAA (hepatitis Australian-antigen) B18.8
HB (c) (s) -AG B18.1
hepatitis (viral) B18.9
Australia-antigen (HAA) B18.8
B surface antigen (HBsAg) B18.1
with acute delta- (super) infection B17.0
C B18.2
specified NEC B18.8
human T-cell lymphotropic virus type-1 (HTLV-1) infection Z22.6
infectious organism Z22.9
specified NEC Z22.8
meningococci Z22.31
Salmonella typhosa Z22.0
serum hepatitis — *see* Carrier, hepatitis
staphylococci (Methicillin susceptible) Z22.321
Methicillin resistant Z22.322
streptococci Z22.338
group B Z22.330
complicating pregnancy or delivery O99.82-
syphilis Z22.4
typhoid Z22.0
venereal disease NEC Z22.4
Carrion's disease A44.0
Carter's relapsing fever (Asiatic) A68.1
Cartilage — *see* condition
Caruncle (inflamed)
conjunctiva (acute) — *see* Conjunctivitis, acute
labium (majus) (minus) N90.89
lacrimal — *see* Inflammation, lacrimal, passages
myrtiform N89.8
urethral (benign) N36.2
Cascade stomach K31.2
Caseation lymphatic gland (tuberculous) A18.2
Cassidy (-Scholte) **syndrome** (malignant carcinoid) E34.0
Castellani's disease A69.8
Castration, traumatic, male S38.231
Casts in urine R82.998
Cat
cry syndrome Q93.4
ear Q17.3
eye syndrome Q92.8
Catabolism, senile R54
Catalepsy (hysterical) F44.2
schizophrenic F20.2
Cataplexy (idiopathic) — *see* - Narcolepsy
Cataract (cortical) (immature) (incipient) H26.9
with
neovascularization — *see* Cataract, complicated
age-related — *see* Cataract, senile
anterior
and posterior axial embryonal Q12.0
pyramidal Q12.0
associated with
galactosemia E74.21 *[H28]*
myotonic disorders G71.19 *[H28]*
blue Q12.0
central Q12.0
cerulean Q12.0
complicated H26.20
with
neovascularization H26.21-
ocular disorder H26.22-
glaucomatous flecks H26.23-
congenital Q12.0
coraliform Q12.0
coronary Q12.0
crystalline Q12.0
diabetic — *see* Diabetes, cataract
drug-induced H26.3-

Cataract (cortical) (immature) (incipient) - *continued*
due to
ocular disorder — *see* Cataract, complicated
radiation H26.8
electric H26.8
extraction status Z98.4-
glass-blower's H26.8
heat ray H26.8
heterochromic — *see* Cataract, complicated
hypermature — *see* Cataract, senile, morgagnian type
in (due to)
chronic iridocyclitis — *see* Cataract, complicated
diabetes — *see* Diabetes, cataract
endocrine disease E34.9 *[H28]*
eye disease — *see* Cataract, complicated
hypoparathyroidism E20.9 *[H28]*
malnutrition-dehydration E46 *[H28]*
metabolic disease E88.9 *[H28]*
myotonic disorders G71.19 *[H28]*
nutritional disease E63.9 *[H28]*
infantile — *see* Cataract, presenile
irradiational — *see* Cataract, specified NEC
juvenile — *see* Cataract, presenile
malnutrition-dehydration E46 *[H28]*
morgagnian — *see* Cataract, senile, morgagnian type
myotonic G71.19 *[H28]*
myxedema E03.9 *[H28]*
nuclear
embryonal Q12.0
sclerosis — *see* Cataract, senile, nuclear
presenile H26.00-
combined forms H26.06-
cortical H26.01-
lamellar — *see* Cataract, presenile, cortical
nuclear H26.03-
specified NEC H26.09
subcapsular polar (anterior) H26.04-
posterior H26.05-
zonular — *see* Cataract, presenile, cortical
secondary H26.40
Soemmering's ring H26.41-
specified NEC H26.49-
to eye disease — *see* Cataract, complicated
senile H25.9
brunescens — *see* Cataract, senile, nuclear
combined forms H25.81-
coronary — *see* Cataract, senile, incipient
cortical H25.01-
hypermature — *see* Cataract, senile, morgagnian type
incipient (mature) (total) H25.09-
cortical — *see* Cataract, senile, cortical
subcapsular — *see* Cataract, senile, subcapsular
morgagnian type (hypermature) H25.2-
nuclear (sclerosis) H25.1-
polar subcapsular (anterior) (posterior) — *see* Cataract, senile, incipient
punctate — *see* Cataract, senile, incipient
specified NEC H25.89
subcapsular polar (anterior) H25.03-
posterior H25.04-
snowflake — *see* Diabetes, cataract
specified NEC H26.8
toxic — *see* Cataract, drug-induced
traumatic H26.10-
localized H26.11-
partially resolved H26.12-
total H26.13-
zonular (perinuclear) Q12.0
Cataracta — *see also* Cataract
brunescens — *see* Cataract, senile, nuclear
centralis pulverulenta Q12.0
cerulea Q12.0
complicata — *see* Cataract, complicated
congenita Q12.0
coralliformis Q12.0
coronaria Q12.0
diabetic — *see* Diabetes, cataract
membranacea
accreta — *see* Cataract, secondary
congenita Q12.0
nigra — *see* Cataract, senile, nuclear
sunflower — *see* Cataract, complicated
Catarrh, catarrhal (acute) (febrile) (infectious) (inflammation) — *see also* condition J00
bronchial — *see* Bronchitis
chest — *see* Bronchitis
chronic J31.0
due to congenital syphilis A50.03
enteric — *see* Enteritis
eustachian H68.009
fauces — *see* Pharyngitis

Choked
disc or disk — *see* Papilledema
on food, phlegm, or vomitus NOS — *see* Foreign body, by site
while vomiting NOS — *see* Foreign body, by site
Chokes (resulting from bends) T70.3
Choking sensation R09.89
Cholangiectasis K83.8
Cholangiocarcinoma
with hepatocellular carcinoma, combined C22.0
liver C22.1
specified site NEC — *see* Neoplasm, malignant, by site
unspecified site C22.1
Cholangiohepatitis K83.8
due to fluke infestation B66.1
Cholangiohepatoma C22.0
Cholangiolitis (acute) (chronic) (extrahepatic) (gangrenous) (intrahepatic) K83.09
paratyphoidal — *see* Fever, paratyphoid
typhoidal A01.09
Cholangioma D13.4
malignant — *see* Cholangiocarcinoma
Cholangitis (ascending) (recurrent) (secondary) (stenosing) (suppurative) K83.09
with calculus, bile duct — *see* Calculus, bile duct, with cholangitis
chronic nonsuppurative destructive K74.3
primary K83.09
sclerosing K83.01
sclerosing K83.09
Cholecystectasia K82.8
Cholecystitis K81.9
with
calculus, stones in
bile duct (common) (hepatic) — *see* Calculus, bile duct, with cholecystitis
cystic duct — *see* Calculus, gallbladder, with cholecystitis
gallbladder — *see* Calculus, gallbladder, with cholecystitis
choledocholithiasis — *see* Calculus, bile duct, with cholecystitis
cholelithiasis — *see* Calculus, gallbladder, with cholecystitis
gangrene of gallbladder K82.A1
perforation of gallbladder K82.A2
acute (emphysematous) (gangrenous) (suppurative) K81.0
with
calculus, stones in
cystic duct — *see* Calculus, gallbladder, with cholecystitis, acute
gallbladder — *see* Calculus, gallbladder, with cholecystitis, acute
choledocholithiasis — *see* Calculus, bile duct, with cholecystitis, acute
cholelithiasis — *see* Calculus, gallbladder, with cholecystitis, acute
chronic cholecystitis K81.2
with gallbladder calculus K80.12
with obstruction K80.13
chronic K81.1
with acute cholecystitis K81.2
with gallbladder calculus K80.12
with obstruction K80.13
emphysematous (acute) — *see* Cholecystitis, acute
gangrenous — *see* Cholecystitis, acute
paratyphoidal, current A01.4
suppurative — *see* Cholecystitis, acute
typhoidal A01.09
Cholecystolithiasis — *see* Calculus, gallbladder
Choledochitis (suppurative) K83.09
Choledocholith — *see* Calculus, bile duct
Choledocholithiasis (common duct) (hepatic duct) — *see* Calculus, bile duct
cystic — *see* Calculus, gallbladder
typhoidal A01.09
Cholelithiasis (cystic duct) (gallbladder) (impacted) (multiple) — *see* Calculus, gallbladder
bile duct (common) (hepatic) — *see* Calculus, bile duct
hepatic duct — *see* Calculus, bile duct
specified NEC K80.80
with obstruction K80.81
Cholemia — *see also* Jaundice
familial (simple) (congenital) E80.4
Gilbert's E80.4
Choleperitoneum, choleperitonitis K65.3
Cholera (Asiatic) (epidemic) (malignant) A00.9
antimonial — *see* Poisoning, antimony
classical A00.0
due to Vibrio cholerae 01 A00.9

Cholera (Asiatic) (epidemic) (malignant) - *continued*
due to Vibrio cholerae 01 - *continued*
biovar cholerae A00.0
biovar eltor A00.1
el tor A00.1
el tor A00.1
Cholerine — *see* Cholera
Cholestasis NEC K83.1
with hepatocyte injury K71.0
due to total parenteral nutrition (TPN) K76.89
pure K71.0
Cholesteatoma (ear) (middle) (with reaction) H71.9-
attic H71.0-
external ear (canal) H60.4-
mastoid H71.2-
postmastoidectomy cavity (recurrent) — *see* Complications, postmastoidectomy, recurrent cholesteatoma
recurrent (postmastoidectomy) — *see* Complications, postmastoidectomy, recurrent cholesteatoma
tympanum H71.1-
Cholesteatosis, diffuse H71.3-
Cholesteremia E78.00
Cholesterin in vitreous — *see* Deposit, crystalline
Cholesterol
deposit
retina H35.89
vitreous — *see* Deposit, crystalline
elevated (high) E78.00
with elevated (high) triglycerides E78.2
screening for Z13.220
imbibition of gallbladder K82.4
Cholesterolemia (essential) (pure) E78.00
familial E78.01
hereditary E78.01
Cholesterolosis, cholesterosis (gallbladder) K82.4
cerebrotendinous E75.5
Cholocolic fistula K82.3
Choluria R82.2
Chondritis M94.8X9
aurical H61.03-
costal (Tietze's) M94.0
external ear H61.03-
patella, posttraumatic — *see* Chondromalacia, patella
pinna H61.03-
purulent M94.8X-
tuberculous NEC A18.02
intervertebral A18.01
Chondroblastoma — *see also* Neoplasm, bone, benign
malignant — *see* Neoplasm, bone, malignant
Chondrocalcinosis M11.20
ankle M11.27-
elbow M11.22-
familial M11.10
ankle M11.17-
elbow M11.12-
foot joint M11.17-
hand joint M11.14-
hip M11.15-
knee M11.16-
multiple site M11.19
shoulder M11.11-
vertebrae M11.18
wrist M11.13-
foot joint M11.27-
hand joint M11.24-
hip M11.25-
knee M11.26-
multiple site M11.29
shoulder M11.21-
vertebrae M11.28
specified type NEC M11.20
ankle M11.27-
elbow M11.22-
foot joint M11.27-
hand joint M11.24-
hip M11.25-
knee M11.26-
multiple site M11.29
shoulder M11.21-
vertebrae M11.28
wrist M11.23-
wrist M11.23-
Chondrodermatitis nodularis helicis or anthelicis — *see* Perichondritis, ear
Chondrodysplasia Q78.9
with hemangioma Q78.4
calcificans congenita Q77.3
fetalis Q77.4

Chondrodysplasia - *continued*
metaphyseal (Jansen's) (McKusick's) (Schmid's) Q78.8
punctata Q77.3
Chondrodystrophy, chondrodystrophia (familial) (fetalis) (hypoplastic) Q78.9
calcificans congenita Q77.3
myotonic (congenital) G71.13
punctata Q77.3
Chondroectodermal dysplasia Q77.6
Chondrogenesis imperfecta Q77.4
Chondrolysis M94.35-
Chondroma — *see also* Neoplasm, cartilage, benign
juxtacortical — *see* Neoplasm, bone, benign
periosteal — *see* Neoplasm, bone, benign
Chondromalacia (systemic) M94.20
acromioclavicular joint M94.21-
ankle M94.27-
elbow M94.22-
foot joint M94.27-
glenohumeral joint M94.21-
hand joint M94.24-
hip M94.25-
knee M94.26-
patella M22.4-
multiple sites M94.29
patella M22.4-
rib M94.28
sacroiliac joint M94.259
shoulder M94.21-
sternoclavicular joint M94.21-
vertebral joint M94.28
wrist M94.23-
Chondromatosis — *see also* Neoplasm, cartilage, uncertain behavior
internal Q78.4
Chondromyxosarcoma — *see* Neoplasm, cartilage, malignant
Chondro-osteodysplasia (Morquio-Brailsford type) E76.219
Chondro-osteodystrophy E76.29
Chondro-osteoma — *see* Neoplasm, bone, benign
Chondropathia tuberosa M94.0
Chondrosarcoma — *see* Neoplasm, cartilage, malignant
juxtacortical — *see* Neoplasm, bone, malignant
mesenchymal — *see* Neoplasm, connective tissue, malignant
myxoid — *see* Neoplasm, cartilage, malignant
Chordee (nonvenereal) N48.89
congenital Q54.4
gonococcal A54.09
Chorditis (fibrinous) (nodosa) (tuberosa) J38.2
Chordoma — *see* Neoplasm, vertebral (column), malignant
Chorea (chronic) (gravis) (posthemiplegic) (senile) (spasmodic) G25.5
with
heart involvement I02.0
active or acute (conditions in I01-) I02.0
rheumatic I02.9
with valvular disorder I02.0
rheumatic heart disease (chronic) (inactive) (quiescent) - code to rheumatic heart condition involved
drug-induced G25.4
habit F95.8
hereditary G10
Huntington's G10
hysterical F44.4
minor I02.9
with heart involvement I02.0
progressive G25.5
hereditary G10
rheumatic (chronic) I02.9
with heart involvement I02.0
Sydenham's I02.9
with heart involvement — *see* Chorea, with rheumatic heart disease
nonrheumatic G25.5
Choreoathetosis (paroxysmal) G25.5
Chorioadenoma (destruens) D39.2
Chorioamnionitis O41.12-
Chorioangioma D26.7
Choriocarcinoma — *see* Neoplasm, malignant, by site
combined with
embryonal carcinoma — *see* Neoplasm, malignant, by site
other germ cell elements — *see* Neoplasm, malignant, by site
teratoma — *see* Neoplasm, malignant, by site
specified site — *see* Neoplasm, malignant, by site

Choriocarcinoma - *continued*
unspecified site
female C58
male C62.90
Chorioencephalitis (acute) (lymphocytic) (serous) A87.2
Chorioepithelioma — *see* Choriocarcinoma
Choriomeningitis (acute) (lymphocytic) (serous) A87.2
Chorionepithelioma — *see* Choriocarcinoma
Chorioretinitis — *see also* Inflammation, chorioretinal
disseminated — *see also* Inflammation, chorioretinal, disseminated
in neurosyphilis A52.19
Egyptian B76.9 *[D63.8]*
focal — *see also* Inflammation, chorioretinal, focal
histoplasmic B39.9 *[H32]*
in (due to)
histoplasmosis B39.9 *[H32]*
syphilis (secondary) A51.43
late A52.71
toxoplasmosis (acquired) B58.01
congenital (active) P37.1 *[H32]*
tuberculosis A18.53
juxtapapillary, juxtapapillaris — *see* Inflammation, chorioretinal, focal, juxtapapillary
leprous A30.9 *[H32]*
miner's B76.9 *[D63.8]*
progressive myopia (degeneration) — *see also* Myopia, degenerative H44.2-
syphilitic (secondary) A51.43
congenital (early) A50.01 *[H32]*
late A50.32
late A52.71
tuberculous A18.53
Chorioretinopathy, central serous H35.71-
Choroid — *see* condition
Choroideremia H31.21
Choroiditis — *see* Chorioretinitis
Choroidopathy — *see* Disorder, choroid
Choroidoretinitis — *see* Chorioretinitis
Choroidoretinopathy, central serous — *see* Chorioretinopathy, central serous
Christian-Weber disease M35.6
Christmas disease D67
Chromaffinoma — *see also* Neoplasm, benign, by site
malignant — *see* Neoplasm, malignant, by site
Chromatopsia — *see* Deficiency, color vision
Chromhidrosis, chromidrosis L75.1
Chromoblastomycosis — *see* Chromomycosis
Chromoconversion R82.91
Chromomycosis B43.9
brain abscess B43.1
cerebral B43.1
cutaneous B43.0
skin B43.0
specified NEC B43.8
subcutaneous abscess or cyst B43.2
Chromophytosis B36.0
Chromosome — *see* condition by chromosome involved
D (1) — *see* condition, chromosome 13
E (3) — *see* condition, chromosome 18
G — *see* condition, chromosome 21
Chromotrichomycosis B36.8
Chronic — *see* condition
fracture — *see* Fracture, pathological
Churg-Strauss syndrome M30.1
Chyle cyst, mesentery I89.8
Chylocele (nonfilarial) I89.8
filarial — *see also* Infestation, filarial B74.9 *[N51]*
tunica vaginalis N50.89
filarial — *see also* Infestation, filarial B74.9 *[N51]*
Chylomicronemia (fasting) (with hyperprebetalipoproteinemia) E78.3
Chylopericardium I31.3
acute I30.9
Chylothorax (nonfilarial) I89.8
filarial — *see also* Infestation, filarial B74.9 *[J91.8]*
Chylous — *see* condition
Chyluria (nonfilarial) R82.0
due to
bilharziasis B65.0
Brugia (malayi) B74.1
timori B74.2
schistosomiasis (bilharziasis) B65.0
Wuchereria (bancrofti) B74.0
filarial — *see* Infestation, filarial
Cicatricial (deformity) — *see* Cicatrix
Cicatrix (adherent) (contracted) (painful) (vicious) — *see also* Scar L90.5
adenoid (and tonsil) J35.8
alveolar process M26.79
anus K62.89
auricle — *see* Disorder, pinna, specified type NEC
bile duct (common) (hepatic) K83.8
bladder N32.89
bone — *see* Disorder, bone, specified type NEC
brain G93.89
cervix (postoperative) (postpartal) N88.1
common duct K83.8
cornea H17.9
tuberculous A18.59
duodenum (bulb) , obstructive K31.5
esophagus K22.2
eyelid — *see* Disorder, eyelid function
hypopharynx J39.2
lacrimal passages — *see* Obstruction, lacrimal
larynx J38.7
lung J98.4
middle ear — *see* subcategory H74.8
mouth K13.79
muscle M62.89
with contracture — *see* Contraction, muscle NEC
nasopharynx J39.2
palate (soft) K13.79
penis N48.89
pharynx J39.2
prostate N42.89
rectum K62.89
retina — *see* Scar, chorioretinal
semilunar cartilage — *see* Derangement, meniscus
seminal vesicle N50.89
skin L90.5
infected L08.89
postinfective L90.5
tuberculous B90.8
specified site NEC L90.5
throat J39.2
tongue K14.8
tonsil (and adenoid) J35.8
trachea J39.8
tuberculous NEC B90.9
urethra N36.8
uterus N85.8
vagina N89.8
postoperative N99.2
vocal cord J38.3
wrist, constricting (annular) L90.5
CIDP
(chronic inflammatory demyelinating polyneuropathy) G61.81
CIN — *see* Neoplasia, intraepithelial, cervix
CINCA
(chronic infantile neurological, cutaneous and articular syndrome) M04.2
Cinchonism — *see* Deafness, ototoxic
correct substance properly administered — *see* Table of Drugs and Chemicals, by drug, adverse effect
overdose or wrong substance given or taken — *see* Table of Drugs and Chemicals, by drug, poisoning
Circle of Willis — *see* condition
Circular — *see* condition
Circulating anticoagulants — *see also* - Disorder, hemorrhagic D68.318
due to drugs — *see also* - Disorder, hemorrhagic D68.32
following childbirth O72.3
Circulation
collateral, any site I99.8
defective (lower extremity) I99.9
congenital Q28.9
embryonic Q28.9
failure (peripheral) R57.9
newborn P29.89
fetal, persistent P29.38
heart, incomplete Q28.9
Circulatory system — *see* condition
Circulus senilis (cornea) — *see* Degeneration, cornea, senile
Circumcision (in absence of medical indication) (ritual) (routine) Z41.2
Circumscribed — *see* condition
Circumvallate placenta O43.11-
Cirrhosis, cirrhotic (hepatic) (liver) K74.60
alcoholic K70.30
with ascites K70.31
atrophic — *see* Cirrhosis, liver
Baumgarten-Cruveilhier K74.69
biliary (cholangiolitic) (cholangitic) (hypertrophic) (obstructive) (pericholangiolitic) K74.5
due to
Cirrhosis, cirrhotic (hepatic) (liver) - *continued*
biliary (cholangiolitic) (cholangitic) (hypertrophic) (obstructive) (pericholangiolitic) - *continued*
due to - *continued*
Clonorchiasis B66.1
flukes B66.3
primary K74.3
secondary K74.4
cardiac (of liver) K76.1
Charcot's K74.3
cholangiolitic, cholangitic, cholostatic (primary) K74.3
congestive K76.1
Cruveilhier-Baumgarten K74.69
cryptogenic (liver) K74.69
due to
hepatolenticular degeneration E83.01
Wilson's disease E83.01
xanthomatosis E78.2
fatty K76.0
alcoholic K70.0
Hanot's (hypertrophic) K74.3
hepatic — *see* Cirrhosis, liver
hypertrophic K74.3
Indian childhood K74.69
kidney — *see* Sclerosis, renal
Laennec's K70.30
with ascites K70.31
alcoholic K70.30
with ascites K70.31
nonalcoholic K74.69
liver K74.60
alcoholic K70.30
with ascites K70.31
fatty K70.0
congenital P78.81
syphilitic A52.74
lung (chronic) J84.10
macronodular K74.69
alcoholic K70.30
with ascites K70.31
micronodular K74.69
alcoholic K70.30
with ascites K70.31
mixed type K74.69
monolobular K74.3
nephritis — *see* Sclerosis, renal
nutritional K74.69
alcoholic K70.30
with ascites K70.31
obstructive — *see* Cirrhosis, biliary
ovarian N83.8
pancreas (duct) K86.89
pigmentary E83.110
portal K74.69
alcoholic K70.30
with ascites K70.31
postnecrotic K74.69
alcoholic K70.30
with ascites K70.31
pulmonary J84.10
renal — *see* Sclerosis, renal
spleen D73.2
stasis K76.1
Todd's K74.3
unilobar K74.3
xanthomatous (biliary) K74.5
due to xanthomatosis (familial) (metabolic) (primary) E78.2
Cistern, subarachnoid R93.0
Citrullinemia E72.23
Citrullinuria E72.23
Civatte's disease or poikiloderma L57.3
Clam digger's itch B65.3
Clammy skin R23.1
Clap — *see* Gonorrhea
Clarke-Hadfield syndrome (pancreatic infantilism) K86.89
Clark's paralysis G80.9
Clastothrix L67.8
Claude Bernard-Horner syndrome G90.2
traumatic — *see* Injury, nerve, cervical sympathetic
Claude's disease or syndrome G46.3
Claudicatio venosa intermittens I87.8
Claudication (intermittent) I73.9
cerebral (artery) G45.9
spinal cord (arteriosclerotic) G95.19
syphilitic A52.09
venous (axillary) I87.8
Claustrophobia F40.240
Clavus (infected) L84
Clawfoot (congenital) Q66.89
acquired — *see* Deformity, limb, clawfoot

Clawhand (acquired) — *see also* Deformity, limb, clawhand
- congenital Q68.1

Clawtoe (congenital) Q66.89
- acquired — *see* Deformity, toe, specified NEC

Clay eating — *see* Pica

Cleansing of artificial opening — *see* Attention to, artificial, opening

Cleft (congenital) — *see also* Imperfect, closure
- alveolar process M26.79
- branchial (persistent) Q18.2
  - cyst Q18.0
    - fistula Q18.0
    - sinus Q18.0
- cricoid cartilage, posterior Q31.8
- foot Q72.7
- hand Q71.6
- lip (unilateral) Q36.9
  - with cleft palate Q37.9
    - hard Q37.1
      - with soft Q37.5
    - soft Q37.3
      - with hard Q37.5
  - bilateral Q36.0
    - with cleft palate Q37.8
      - hard Q37.0
        - with soft Q37.4
      - soft Q37.2
        - with hard Q37.4
  - median Q36.1
- nose Q30.2
- palate Q35.9
  - with cleft lip (unilateral) Q37.9
    - bilateral Q37.8
  - hard Q35.1
    - with
      - cleft lip (unilateral) Q37.1
        - bilateral Q37.0
      - soft Q35.5
        - with cleft lip (unilateral) Q37.5
          - bilateral Q37.4
  - medial Q35.5
  - soft Q35.3
    - with
      - cleft lip (unilateral) Q37.3
        - bilateral Q37.2
      - hard Q35.5
        - with cleft lip (unilateral) Q37.5
          - bilateral Q37.4
- penis Q55.69
- scrotum Q55.29
- thyroid cartilage Q31.8
- uvula Q35.7

Cleidocranial dysostosis Q74.0

Cleptomania F63.2

Clicking hip (newborn) R29.4

Climacteric (female) — *see also* Menopause
- arthritis (any site) NEC — *see* Arthritis, specified form NEC
- depression (single episode) F32.89
  - recurrent episode F33.8
- melancholia (single episode) F32.89
  - recurrent episode F33.8
- male (symptoms) (syndrome) NEC N50.89
- paranoid state F22
- polyarthritis NEC — *see* Arthritis, specified form NEC
- symptoms (female) N95.1

Clinical research investigation (clinical trial) (control subject) (normal comparison) (participant) Z00.6

Clitoris — *see* condition

Cloaca (persistent) Q43.7

Clonorchiasis, clonorchis infection (liver) B66.1

Clonus R25.8

Closed bite M26.29

Clostridium (C.)
- **perfringens, as cause of disease classified elsewhere** B96.7

Closure
- congenital, nose Q30.0
- cranial sutures, premature Q75.0
- defective or imperfect NEC — *see* Imperfect, closure
- fistula, delayed — *see* Fistula
- foramen ovale, imperfect Q21.1
- hymen N89.6
- interauricular septum, defective Q21.1
- interventricular septum, defective Q21.0
- lacrimal duct — *see also* Stenosis, lacrimal, duct
  - congenital Q10.5
- nose (congenital) Q30.0
  - acquired M95.0

Closure - *continued*
- of artificial opening — *see* Attention to, artificial, opening
- primary angle, without glaucoma damage H40.06-
- vagina N89.5
- valve — *see* Endocarditis
- vulva N90.5

Clot (blood) — *see also* Embolism
- artery (obstruction) (occlusion) — *see* Embolism
- bladder N32.89
- brain (intradural or extradural) — *see* Occlusion, artery, cerebral
- circulation I74.9
- heart — *see also* Infarct, myocardium
  - not resulting in infarction I51.3
- vein — *see* Thrombosis

Clouded state R40.1
- epileptic — *see* Epilepsy, specified NEC
- paroxysmal — *see* Epilepsy, specified NEC

Cloudy antrum, antra J32.0

Clouston's (hidrotic) **ectodermal dysplasia** Q82.4

Clubbed nail pachydermoperiostosis M89.40 *[L62]*

Clubbing of finger (s) (nails) R68.3

Clubfinger R68.3
- congenital Q68.1

Clubfoot (congenital) Q66.89
- acquired — *see* Deformity, limb, clubfoot
- equinovarus Q66.0
- paralytic — *see* Deformity, limb, clubfoot

Clubhand (congenital) (radial) Q71.4-
- acquired — *see* Deformity, limb, clubhand

Clubnail R68.3
- congenital Q84.6

Clump, kidney Q63.1

Clumsiness, clumsy child syndrome F82

Cluttering F80.81

Clutton's joints A50.51 *[M12.80]*

Coagulation, intravascular (diffuse) (disseminated) — *see also* Defibrination syndrome
- complicating abortion — *see* Abortion, by type, complicated by, intravascular coagulation
- following ectopic or molar pregnancy O08.1

Coagulopathy — *see also* Defect, coagulation
- consumption D65
- intravascular D65
  - newborn P60

Coalition
- calcaneo-scaphoid Q66.89
- tarsal Q66.89

Coalminer's
- elbow — *see* Bursitis, elbow, olecranon
- lung or pneumoconiosis J60

Coalworker's lung or pneumoconiosis J60

Coarctation
- aorta (preductal) (postductal) Q25.1
- pulmonary artery Q25.71

Coated tongue K14.3

Coats' disease (exudative retinopathy) — *see* Retinopathy, exudative

Cocaine-induced
- anxiety disorder F14.980
- bipolar and related disorder F14.94
- depressive disorder F14.94
- obsessive-compulsive and related disorder F14.988
- psychotic disorder F14.959
- sleep disorder F14.982
- sexual dysfunction F14.981

Cocainism — *see* Disorder, cocaine use

Coccidioidomycosis B38.9
- cutaneous B38.3
- disseminated B38.7
- generalized B38.7
- meninges B38.4
- prostate B38.81
- pulmonary B38.2
  - acute B38.0
  - chronic B38.1
- skin B38.3
- specified NEC B38.89

Coccidioidosis — *see* Coccidioidomycosis

Coccidiosis (intestinal) A07.3

Coccydynia, coccygodynia M53.3

Coccyx — *see* condition

Cochin-China diarrhea K90.1

Cockayne's syndrome Q87.1

Cocked up toe — *see* Deformity, toe, specified NEC

Cock's peculiar tumor L72.3

Codman's tumor — *see* Neoplasm, bone, benign

Coenurosis B71.8

Coffee-worker's lung J67.8

Cogan's syndrome H16.32-
- oculomotor apraxia H51.8

Coitus, painful (female) N94.10
- male N53.12
- psychogenic F52.6

Cold J00
- with influenza, flu, or grippe — *see* Influenza, with, respiratory manifestations NEC
- agglutinin disease or hemoglobinuria (chronic) D59.1
- bronchial — *see* Bronchitis
- chest — *see* Bronchitis
- common (head) J00
- effects of T69.9
  - specified effect NEC T69.8
- excessive, effects of T69.9
  - specified effect NEC T69.8
- exhaustion from T69.8
- exposure to T69.9
  - specified effect NEC T69.8
- head J00
- injury syndrome (newborn) P80.0
- on lung — *see* Bronchitis
- rose J30.1
- sensitivity, auto-immune D59.1
- symptoms J00
- virus J00

Coldsore B00.1

Colibacillosis A49.8
- as the cause of other disease — *see also* Escherichia coli B96.20
- generalized A41.50

Colic (bilious) (infantile) (intestinal) (recurrent) (spasmodic) R10.83
- abdomen R10.83
  - psychogenic F45.8
- appendix, appendicular K38.8
- bile duct — *see* Calculus, bile duct
- biliary — *see* Calculus, bile duct
- common duct — *see* Calculus, bile duct
- cystic duct — *see* Calculus, gallbladder
- Devonshire NEC — *see* Poisoning, lead
- gallbladder — *see* Calculus, gallbladder
- gallstone — *see* Calculus, gallbladder
  - gallbladder or cystic duct — *see* Calculus, gallbladder
- hepatic (duct) — *see* Calculus, bile duct
- hysterical F45.8
- kidney N23
- lead NEC — *see* Poisoning, lead
- mucous K58.9
  - with diarrhea K58.0
  - psychogenic F54
- nephritic N23
- painter's NEC — *see* Poisoning, lead
- pancreas K86.89
- psychogenic F45.8
- renal N23
- saturnine NEC — *see* Poisoning, lead
- ureter N23
- urethral N36.8
  - due to calculus N21.1
- uterus NEC N94.89
  - menstrual — *see* Dysmenorrhea
- worm NOS B83.9

Colicystitis — *see* Cystitis

Colitis (acute) (catarrhal) (chronic) (noninfective) (hemorrhagic) — *see also* Enteritis K52.9
- allergic K52.29
  - with
    - food protein-induced enterocolitis syndrome K52.21
    - proctocolitis K52.82
- amebic (acute) — *see also* Amebiasis A06.0
  - nondysenteric A06.2
- anthrax A22.2
- bacillary — *see* Infection, Shigella
- balantidial A07.0
- Clostridium difficile
  - not specified as recurrent A04.72
  - recurrent A04.71
- coccidial A07.3
- collagenous K52.831
- cystica superficialis K52.89
- dietary counseling and surveillance (for) Z71.3
- dietetic — *see also* Colitis, allergic K52.29
- drug-induced K52.1
- due to radiation K52.0
- eosinophilic K52.82
- food hypersensitivity — *see also* Colitis, allergic K52.29
- giardial A07.1
- granulomatous — *see* Enteritis, regional, large intestine
- indeterminate, so stated K52.3

Colitis (acute) (catarrhal) (chronic) (noninfective) (hemorrhagic) - *continued*
infectious — *see* Enteritis, infectious
ischemic K55.9
acute (subacute) — *see also* Ischemia, intestine, acute K55.039
chronic K55.1
due to mesenteric artery insufficiency K55.1
fulminant (acute) — *see also* Ischemia, intestine, acute K55.039
left sided K51.50
with
abscess K51.514
complication K51.519
specified NEC K51.518
fistula K51.513
obstruction K51.512
rectal bleeding K51.511
lymphocytic K52.832
membranous
psychogenic F54
microscopic K52.839
specified NEC K52.838
mucous — *see* Syndrome, irritable, bowel
psychogenic F54
noninfective K52.9
specified NEC K52.89
polyposa — *see* Polyp, colon, inflammatory
protozoal A07.9
pseudomembranous
not specified as recurrent A04.72
recurrent A04.71
pseudomucinous — *see* Syndrome, irritable, bowel
regional — *see* Enteritis, regional, large intestine
infectious A09
segmental — *see* Enteritis, regional, large intestine
septic — *see* Enteritis, infectious
spastic K58.9
with diarrhea K58.0
psychogenic F54
staphylococcal A04.8
foodborne A05.0
subacute ischemic — *see also* Ischemia, intestine, acute K55.039
thromboulcerative — *see also* Ischemia, intestine, acute K55.039
toxic NEC K52.1
due to Clostridium difficile
not specified as recurrent A04.72
recurrent A04.71
transmural — *see* Enteritis, regional, large intestine
trichomonal A07.8
tuberculous (ulcerative) A18.32
ulcerative (chronic) K51.90
with
complication K51.919
abscess K51.914
fistula K51.913
obstruction K51.912
rectal bleeding K51.911
specified complication NEC K51.918
enterocolitis — *see* Enterocolitis, ulcerative
ileocolitis — *see* Ileocolitis, ulcerative
mucosal proctocolitis — *see* Proctocolitis, mucosal
proctitis — *see* Proctitis, ulcerative
pseudopolyposis — *see* Polyp, colon, inflammatory
psychogenic F54
rectosigmoiditis — *see* Rectosigmoiditis, ulcerative
specified type NEC K51.80
with
complication K51.819
abscess K51.814
fistula K51.813
obstruction K51.812
rectal bleeding K51.811
specified complication NEC K51.818
Collagenosis, collagen disease (nonvascular) (vascular) M35.9
cardiovascular I42.8
reactive perforating L87.1
specified NEC M35.8
Collapse R55
adrenal E27.2
cardiorespiratory R57.0
cardiovascular R57.0
newborn P29.89
circulatory (peripheral) R57.9
during or after labor and delivery O75.1
following ectopic or molar pregnancy O08.3
newborn P29.89
during or

Collapse - *continued*
during or - *continued*
after labor and delivery O75.1
resulting from a procedure, not elsewhere classified T81.10
external ear canal — *see* Stenosis, external ear canal
general R55
heart — *see* Disease, heart
heat T67.1
hysterical F44.89
labyrinth, membranous (congenital) Q16.5
lung (massive) — *see also* Atelectasis J98.19
pressure due to anesthesia (general) (local) or other sedation T88.2
during labor and delivery O74.1
in pregnancy O29.02-
postpartum, puerperal O89.09
myocardial — *see* Disease, heart
nervous F48.8
neurocirculatory F45.8
nose M95.0
postoperative T81.10
pulmonary — *see also* Atelectasis J98.19
newborn — *see* Atelectasis
trachea J39.8
tracheobronchial J98.09
valvular — *see* Endocarditis
vascular (peripheral) R57.9
during or after labor and delivery O75.1
following ectopic or molar pregnancy O08.3
newborn P29.89
vertebra M48.50-
cervical region M48.52-
cervicothoracic region M48.53-
in (due to)
metastasis — *see* Collapse, vertebra, in, specified disease NEC
osteoporosis — *see also* Osteoporosis M80.88
cervical region M80.88
cervicothoracic region M80.88
lumbar region M80.88
lumbosacral region M80.88
multiple sites M80.88
occipito-atlanto-axial region M80.88
sacrococcygeal region M80.88
thoracic region M80.88
thoracolumbar region M80.88
specified disease NEC M48.50-
cervical region M48.52-
cervicothoracic region M48.53-
lumbar region M48.56-
lumbosacral region M48.57-
occipito-atlanto-axial region M48.51-
sacrococcygeal region M48.58-
thoracic region M48.54-
thoracolumbar region M48.55-
lumbar region M48.56-
lumbosacral region M48.57-
occipito-atlanto-axial region M48.51-
sacrococcygeal region M48.58-
thoracic region M48.54-
thoracolumbar region M48.55-
Collateral — *see also* condition
circulation (venous) I87.8
dilation, veins I87.8
Colles' fracture S52.53-
Collet (-Sicard) **syndrome** G52.7
Collier's asthma or lung J60
Collodion baby Q80.2
Colloid nodule (of thyroid) (cystic) E04.1
Coloboma (iris) Q13.0
eyelid Q10.3
fundus Q14.8
lens Q12.2
optic disc (congenital) Q14.2
acquired H47.31-
Coloenteritis — *see* Enteritis
Colon — *see* condition
Colonization
MRSA (Methicillin resistant Staphylococcus aureus) Z22.322
MSSA (Methicillin susceptible Staphylococcus aureus) Z22.321
status — *see* Carrier (suspected) of
Coloptosis K63.4
Color blindness — *see* Deficiency, color vision
Colostomy
attention to Z43.3
fitting or adjustment Z46.89
malfunctioning K94.03
status Z93.3
Colpitis (acute) — *see* Vaginitis
Colpocele N81.5

Colpocystitis — *see* Vaginitis
Colpospasm N94.2
Column, spinal, vertebral — *see* condition
Coma R40.20
with
motor response (none) R40.231
abnormal R40.233
abnormal extensor posturing to pain or noxious stimuli (< 2 years of age) R40.232
abnormal flexure posturing to pain or noxious stimuli (0-5 years of age) R40.233
extension R40.232
extensor posturing to pain or noxious stimuli (2-5 years of age) R40.232
flexion/decorticate posturing (< 2 years of age) R40.233
flexion withdrawal R40.234
localizes pain (2-5 years of age) R40.235
normal or spontaneous movement (< 2 years of age) R40.236
obeys commands (2-5 years of age) R40.236
score of
1 R40.231
2 R40.232
3 R40.233
4 R40.234
5 R40.235
6 R40.236
withdraws from pain or noxious stimuli (0-5 years of age) R40.234
withdraws to touch (< 2 years of age) R40.235
opening of eyes (never) R40.211
in response to
pain R40.212
sound R40.213
score of
1 R40.211
2 R40.212
3 R40.213
4 R40.214
spontaneous R40.214
verbal response (none) R40.221
confused conversation R40.224
cooing or babbling or crying appropriately (< 2 years of age) R40.225
inappropriate crying or screaming (< 2 years of age) R40.223
inappropriate words R40.223
inappropriate words (2-5 years of age) R40.224
incomprehensible sounds (2-5 years of age) R40.222
incomprehensible words R40.222
irritable cries (< 2 years of age) R40.224
moans/grunts to pain; restless (< 2 years old) R40.222
oriented R40.225
score of
1 R40.221
2 R40.222
3 R40.223
4 R40.224
5 R40.225
screaming (2-5 years of age) R40.223
uses appropriate words (2- 5 years of age) R40.225
eclamptic — *see* Eclampsia
epileptic — *see* Epilepsy
Glasgow, scale score — *see* Glasgow coma scale
hepatic — *see* Failure, hepatic, by type, with coma
hyperglycemic (diabetic) — *see* Diabetes, by type, with hyperosmolarity, with coma
hyperosmolar (diabetic) — *see* Diabetes, by type, with hyperosmolarity, with coma
hypoglycemic (diabetic) — *see* Diabetes, by type, with hypoglycemia, with coma
nondiabetic E15
in diabetes — *see* Diabetes, coma
insulin-induced — *see* Coma, hypoglycemic
ketoacidotic (diabetic) — *see* Diabetes, by type, with ketoacidosis, with coma
myxedematous E03.5
newborn P91.5
persistent vegetative state R40.3
specified NEC, without documented Glasgow coma scale score, or with partial Glasgow coma scale score reported R40.244
Comatose — *see* Coma
Combat fatigue F43.0
Combined — *see* condition
Comedo, comedones (giant) L70.0
Comedocarcinoma — *see also* Neoplasm, breast, malignant
noninfiltrating

Comedocarcinoma - *continued*
- noninfiltrating - *continued*
  - breast D05.8-
  - specified site — *see* Neoplasm, in situ, by site
  - unspecified site D05.8-

Comedomastitis — *see* Ectasia, mammary duct

Comminuted fracture - code as Fracture, closed

Common
- arterial trunk Q20.0
- atrioventricular canal Q21.2
- atrium Q21.1
- cold (head) J00
- truncus (arteriosus) Q20.0
- variable immunodeficiency — *see* Immunodeficiency, common variable
- ventricle Q20.4

Commotio, commotion (current)
- brain — *see* Injury, intracranial, concussion
- cerebri — *see* Injury, intracranial, concussion
- retinae S05.8X-
- spinal cord — *see* Injury, spinal cord, by region
- spinalis — *see* Injury, spinal cord, by region

Communication
- between
  - base of aorta and pulmonary artery Q21.4
  - left ventricle and right atrium Q20.5
  - pericardial sac and pleural sac Q34.8
  - pulmonary artery and pulmonary vein, congenital Q25.72
- congenital between uterus and digestive or urinary tract Q51.7

Compartment syndrome (deep) (posterior) (traumatic) T79.A0
- abdomen T79.A3
- lower extremity (hip, buttock, thigh, leg, foot, toes) T79.A2
- nontraumatic
  - abdomen M79.A3
  - lower extremity (hip, buttock, thigh, leg, foot, toes) M79.A2-
  - specified site NEC M79.A9
  - upper extremity (shoulder, arm, forearm, wrist, hand, fingers) M79.A1-
- specified site NEC T79.A9
- upper extremity (shoulder, arm, forearm, wrist, hand, fingers) T79.A1

Compensation
- failure — *see* Disease, heart
- neurosis, psychoneurosis — *see* Disorder, factitious

Complaint — *see also* Disease
- bowel, functional K59.9
  - psychogenic F45.8
- intestine, functional K59.9
  - psychogenic F45.8
- kidney — *see* Disease, renal
- miners' J60

Complete — *see* condition

Complex
- Addison-Schilder E71.528
- cardiorenal — *see* Hypertension, cardiorenal
- Costen's M26.69
- disseminated mycobacterium avium- intracellulare (DMAC) A31.2
- Eisenmenger's (ventricular septal defect) I27.83
- hypersexual F52.8
- jumped process, spine — *see* Dislocation, vertebra
- primary, tuberculous A15.7
- Schilder-Addison E71.528
- subluxation (vertebral) M99.19
  - abdomen M99.19
  - acromioclavicular M99.17
  - cervical region M99.11
  - cervicothoracic M99.11
  - costochondral M99.18
  - costovertebral M99.18
  - head region M99.10
  - hip M99.15
  - lower extremity M99.16
  - lumbar region M99.13
  - lumbosacral M99.13
  - occipitocervical M99.10
  - pelvic region M99.15
  - pubic M99.15
  - rib cage M99.18
  - sacral region M99.14
  - sacrococcygeal M99.14
  - sacroiliac M99.14
  - specified NEC M99.19
  - sternochondral M99.18
  - sternoclavicular M99.17
  - thoracic region M99.12
  - thoracolumbar M99.12
  - upper extremity M99.17

Complex - *continued*
- Taussig-Bing (transposition, aorta and overriding pulmonary artery) Q20.1

Complication (s) (from) (of)
- accidental puncture or laceration during a procedure (of) — *see* Complications, intraoperative (intraprocedural), puncture or laceration
- amputation stump (surgical) (late) NEC T87.9
  - dehiscence T87.81
  - infection or inflammation T87.40
    - lower limb T87.4-
    - upper limb T87.4-
  - necrosis T87.50
    - lower limb T87.5-
    - upper limb T87.5-
  - neuroma T87.30
    - lower limb T87.3-
    - upper limb T87.3-
  - specified type NEC T87.89
- anastomosis (and bypass) — *see also* Complications, prosthetic device or implant
  - intestinal (internal) NEC K91.89
    - involving urinary tract N99.89
  - urinary tract (involving intestinal tract) N99.89
  - vascular — *see* Complications, cardiovascular device or implant
- anesthesia, anesthetic — *see also* Anesthesia, complication T88.59
  - brain, postpartum, puerperal O89.2
  - cardiac
    - in
      - labor and delivery O74.2
      - pregnancy O29.19-
    - postpartum, puerperal O89.1
  - central nervous system
    - in
      - labor and delivery O74.3
      - pregnancy O29.29-
    - postpartum, puerperal O89.2
  - difficult or failed intubation T88.4
    - in pregnancy O29.6-
  - failed sedation (conscious) (moderate) during procedure T88.52
  - general, unintended awareness during procedure T88.53
  - hyperthermia, malignant T88.3
  - hypothermia T88.51
  - intubation failure T88.4
  - malignant hyperthermia T88.3
  - pulmonary
    - in
      - labor and delivery O74.1
      - pregnancy NEC O29.09-
    - postpartum, puerperal O89.09
  - shock T88.2
  - spinal and epidural
    - in
      - labor and delivery NEC O74.6
        - headache O74.5
      - pregnancy NEC O29.5X-
    - postpartum, puerperal NEC O89.5
      - headache O89.4
  - unintended awareness under general anesthesia during procedure T88.53
- anti-reflux device — *see* Complications, esophageal anti-reflux device
- aortic (bifurcation) graft — *see* Complications, graft, vascular
- aortocoronary (bypass) graft — *see* Complications, coronary artery (bypass) graft
- aortofemoral (bypass) graft — *see* Complications, extremity artery (bypass) graft
- arteriovenous
  - fistula, surgically created T82.9
    - embolism T82.818
    - fibrosis T82.828
    - hemorrhage T82.838
    - infection or inflammation T82.7
    - mechanical
      - breakdown T82.510
      - displacement T82.520
      - leakage T82.530
      - malposition T82.520
      - obstruction T82.590
      - perforation T82.590
      - protrusion T82.590
    - pain T82.848
    - specified type NEC T82.898
    - stenosis T82.858
    - thrombosis T82.868
  - shunt, surgically created T82.9
    - embolism T82.818
    - fibrosis T82.828

Complication (s) (from) (of) - *continued*
- arteriovenous - *continued*
  - shunt, surgically created - *continued*
    - hemorrhage T82.838
    - infection or inflammation T82.7
    - mechanical
      - breakdown T82.511
      - displacement T82.521
      - leakage T82.531
      - malposition T82.521
      - obstruction T82.591
      - perforation T82.591
      - protrusion T82.591
    - pain T82.848
    - specified type NEC T82.898
    - stenosis T82.858
    - thrombosis T82.868
- arthroplasty — *see* Complications, joint prosthesis
- artificial
  - fertilization or insemination N98.9
    - attempted introduction (of)
      - embryo in embryo transfer N98.3
      - ovum following in vitro fertilization N98.2
    - hyperstimulation of ovaries N98.1
    - infection N98.0
    - specified NEC N98.8
  - heart T82.9
    - embolism T82.817
    - fibrosis T82.827
    - hemorrhage T82.837
    - infection or inflammation T82.7
    - mechanical
      - breakdown T82.512
      - displacement T82.522
      - leakage T82.532
      - malposition T82.522
      - obstruction T82.592
      - perforation T82.592
      - protrusion T82.592
    - pain T82.847
    - specified type NEC T82.897
    - stenosis T82.857
    - thrombosis T82.867
  - opening
    - cecostomy — *see* Complications, colostomy
    - colostomy — *see* Complications, colostomy
    - cystostomy — *see* Complications, cystostomy
    - enterostomy — *see* Complications, enterostomy
    - gastrostomy — *see* Complications, gastrostomy
    - ileostomy — *see* Complications, enterostomy
    - jejunostomy — *see* Complications, enterostomy
    - nephrostomy — *see* Complications, stoma, urinary tract
    - tracheostomy — *see* Complications, tracheostomy
    - ureterostomy — *see* Complications, stoma, urinary tract
    - urethrostomy — *see* Complications, stoma, urinary tract
- balloon implant or device
  - gastrointestinal T85.9
    - embolism T85.818
    - fibrosis T85.828
    - hemorrhage T85.838
    - infection and inflammation T85.79
    - pain T85.848
    - specified type NEC T85.898
    - stenosis T85.858
    - thrombosis T85.868
  - vascular (counterpulsation) T82.9
    - embolism T82.818
    - fibrosis T82.828
    - hemorrhage T82.838
    - infection or inflammation T82.7
    - mechanical
      - breakdown T82.513
      - displacement T82.523
      - leakage T82.533
      - malposition T82.523
      - obstruction T82.593
      - perforation T82.593
      - protrusion T82.593
    - pain T82.848
    - specified type NEC T82.898
    - stenosis T82.858
    - thrombosis T82.868
- bariatric procedure
  - gastric band procedure K95.09
    - infection K95.01
  - specified procedure NEC K95.89
    - infection K95.81
- bile duct implant (prosthetic) T85.9
  - embolism T85.818

Complication (s) (from) (of) - *continued*
bile duct implant (prosthetic) - *continued*
fibrosis T85.828
hemorrhage T85.838
infection and inflammation T85.79
mechanical
breakdown T85.510
displacement T85.520
malfunction T85.510
malposition T85.520
obstruction T85.590
perforation T85.590
protrusion T85.590
specified NEC T85.590
pain T85.848
specified type NEC T85.898
stenosis T85.858
thrombosis T85.868
bladder device (auxiliary) — *see* Complications, genitourinary, device or implant, urinary system
bleeding (postoperative) — *see* Complication, postoperative, hemorrhage
intraoperative — *see* Complication, intraoperative, hemorrhage
blood vessel graft — *see* Complications, graft, vascular
bone
device NEC T84.9
embolism T84.81
fibrosis T84.82
hemorrhage T84.83
infection or inflammation T84.7
mechanical
breakdown T84.318
displacement T84.328
malposition T84.328
obstruction T84.398
perforation T84.398
protrusion T84.398
pain T84.84
specified type NEC T84.89
stenosis T84.85
thrombosis T84.86
graft — *see* Complications, graft, bone
growth stimulator (electrode) — *see* Complications, electronic stimulator device, bone
marrow transplant — *see* Complications, transplant, bone, marrow
brain neurostimulator (electrode) — *see* Complications, electronic stimulator device, brain
breast implant (prosthetic) T85.9
capsular contracture T85.44
embolism T85.818
fibrosis T85.828
hemorrhage T85.838
infection and inflammation T85.79
mechanical
breakdown T85.41
displacement T85.42
leakage T85.43
malposition T85.42
obstruction T85.49
perforation T85.49
protrusion T85.49
specified NEC T85.49
pain T85.848
specified type NEC T85.898
stenosis T85.858
thrombosis T85.868
bypass — *see also* Complications, prosthetic device or implant
aortocoronary — *see* Complications, coronary artery (bypass) graft
arterial — *see also* Complications, graft, vascular
extremity — *see* Complications, extremity artery (bypass) graft
cardiac — *see also* Disease, heart
device, implant or graft T82.9
embolism T82.817
fibrosis T82.827
hemorrhage T82.837
infection or inflammation T82.7
valve prosthesis T82.6
mechanical
breakdown T82.519
specified device NEC T82.518
displacement T82.529
specified device NEC T82.528
leakage T82.539
specified device NEC T82.538
malposition T82.529
specified device NEC T82.528
obstruction T82.599

Complication (s) (from) (of) - *continued*
cardiac - *continued*
device, implant or graft - *continued*
mechanical - *continued*
obstruction - *continued*
specified device NEC T82.598
perforation T82.599
specified device NEC T82.598
protrusion T82.599
specified device NEC T82.598
pain T82.847
specified type NEC T82.897
stenosis T82.857
thrombosis T82.867
cardiovascular device, graft or implant T82.9
aortic graft — *see* Complications, graft, vascular
arteriovenous
fistula, artificial — *see* Complication, arteriovenous, fistula, surgically created
shunt — *see* Complication, arteriovenous, shunt, surgically created
artificial heart — *see* Complication, artificial, heart
balloon (counterpulsation) device — *see* Complication, balloon implant, vascular
carotid artery graft — *see* Complications, graft, vascular
coronary bypass graft — *see* Complication, coronary artery (bypass) graft
dialysis catheter (vascular) — *see* Complication, catheter, dialysis
electronic T82.9
electrode T82.9
embolism T82.817
fibrosis T82.827
hemorrhage T82.837
infection T82.7
mechanical
breakdown T82.110
displacement T82.120
leakage T82.190
obstruction T82.190
perforation T82.190
protrusion T82.190
specified type NEC T82.190
pain T82.847
specified NEC T82.897
stenosis T82.857
thrombosis T82.867
embolism T82.817
fibrosis T82.827
hemorrhage T82.837
infection T82.7
mechanical
breakdown T82.119
displacement T82.129
leakage T82.199
obstruction T82.199
perforation T82.199
protrusion T82.199
specified type NEC T82.199
pain T82.847
pulse generator T82.9
embolism T82.817
fibrosis T82.827
hemorrhage T82.837
infection T82.7
mechanical
breakdown T82.111
displacement T82.121
leakage T82.191
obstruction T82.191
perforation T82.191
protrusion T82.191
specified type NEC T82.191
pain T82.847
specified NEC T82.897
stenosis T82.857
thrombosis T82.867
specified condition NEC T82.897
specified device NEC T82.9
embolism T82.817
fibrosis T82.827
hemorrhage T82.837
infection T82.7
mechanical
breakdown T82.118
displacement T82.128
leakage T82.198
obstruction T82.198
perforation T82.198
protrusion T82.198
specified type NEC T82.198
pain T82.847

Complication (s) (from) (of) - *continued*
cardiovascular device, graft or implant - *continued*
electronic - *continued*
specified device NEC - *continued*
specified NEC T82.897
stenosis T82.857
thrombosis T82.867
stenosis T82.857
thrombosis T82.867
extremity artery graft — *see* Complication, extremity artery (bypass) graft
femoral artery graft — *see* Complication, extremity artery (bypass) graft
heart-lung transplant — *see* Complication, transplant, heart, with lung
heart
transplant — *see* Complication, transplant, heart
valve — *see* Complication, prosthetic device, heart valve
graft — *see* Complication, heart, valve, graft
infection or inflammation T82.7
umbrella device — *see* Complication, umbrella device, vascular
vascular graft (or anastomosis) — *see* Complication, graft, vascular
carotid artery (bypass) graft — *see* Complications, graft, vascular
catheter (device) NEC — *see also* Complications, prosthetic device or implant
cranial infusion
infection and inflammation T85.735
mechanical
breakdown T85.610
displacement T85.620
leakage T85.630
malfunction T85.690
malposition T85.620
obstruction T85.690
perforation T85.690
protrusion T85.690
specified NEC T85.690
cystostomy T83.9
embolism T83.81
fibrosis T83.82
hemorrhage T83.83
infection and inflammation T83.510
mechanical
breakdown T83.010
displacement T83.020
leakage T83.030
malposition T83.020
obstruction T83.090
perforation T83.090
protrusion T83.090
specified NEC T83.090
pain T83.84
specified type NEC T83.89
stenosis T83.85
thrombosis T83.86
dialysis (vascular) T82.9
embolism T82.818
fibrosis T82.828
hemorrhage T82.838
infection and inflammation T82.7
intraperitoneal — *see* Complications, catheter, intraperitoneal
mechanical
breakdown T82.41
displacement T82.42
leakage T82.43
malposition T82.42
obstruction T82.49
perforation T82.49
protrusion T82.49
pain T82.848
specified type NEC T82.898
stenosis T82.858
thrombosis T82.868
epidural infusion T85.9
embolism T85.810
fibrosis T85.820
hemorrhage T85.830
infection and inflammation T85.735
mechanical
breakdown T85.610
displacement T85.620
leakage T85.630
malfunction T85.610
malposition T85.620
obstruction T85.690
perforation T85.690
protrusion T85.690
specified NEC T85.690

- **Complication** (s) (from) (of) - *continued*
  - catheter (device) NEC - *continued*
    - epidural infusion - *continued*
      - pain T85.840
      - specified type NEC T85.890
      - stenosis T85.850
      - thrombosis T85.860
    - intraperitoneal dialysis T85.9
      - embolism T85.818
      - fibrosis T85.828
      - hemorrhage T85.838
      - infection and inflammation T85.71
      - mechanical
        - breakdown T85.611
        - displacement T85.621
        - leakage T85.631
        - malfunction T85.611
        - malposition T85.621
        - obstruction T85.691
        - perforation T85.691
        - protrusion T85.691
        - specified NEC T85.691
      - pain T85.848
      - specified type NEC T85.898
      - stenosis T85.858
      - thrombosis T85.868
    - intrathecal infusion
      - infection and inflammation T85.735
      - mechanical
        - breakdown T85.610
        - displacement T85.620
        - leakage T85.630
        - malfunction T85.690
        - malposition T85.620
        - obstruction T85.690
        - perforation T85.690
        - protrusion T85.690
        - specified NEC T85.690
    - intravenous infusion T82.9
      - embolism T82.818
      - fibrosis T82.828
      - hemorrhage T82.838
      - infection or inflammation T82.7
      - mechanical
        - breakdown T82.514
        - displacement T82.524
        - leakage T82.534
        - malposition T82.524
        - obstruction T82.594
        - perforation T82.594
        - protrusion T82.594
      - pain T82.848
      - specified type NEC T82.898
      - stenosis T82.858
      - thrombosis T82.868
    - spinal infusion
      - infection and inflammation T85.735
      - mechanical
        - breakdown T85.610
        - displacement T85.620
        - leakage T85.630
        - malfunction T85.690
        - malposition T85.620
        - obstruction T85.690
        - perforation T85.690
        - protrusion T85.690
        - specified NEC T85.690
    - subarachnoid infusion
      - infection and inflammation T85.735
      - mechanical
        - breakdown T85.610
        - displacement T85.620
        - leakage T85.630
        - malfunction T85.690
        - malposition T85.620
        - obstruction T85.690
        - perforation T85.690
        - protrusion T85.690
        - specified NEC T85.690
    - subdural infusion T85.9
      - embolism T85.810
      - fibrosis T85.820
      - hemorrhage T85.830
      - infection and inflammation T85.735
      - mechanical
        - breakdown T85.610
        - displacement T85.620
        - leakage T85.630
        - malfunction T85.610
        - malposition T85.620
        - obstruction T85.690
        - perforation T85.690
        - protrusion T85.690

- **Complication** (s) (from) (of) - *continued*
  - catheter (device) NEC - *continued*
    - subdural infusion - *continued*
      - mechanical - *continued*
        - specified NEC T85.690
      - pain T85.840
      - specified type NEC T85.890
      - stenosis T85.850
      - thrombosis T85.860
    - urethral T83.9
      - displacement T83.028
      - embolism T83.81
      - fibrosis T83.82
      - hemorrhage T83.83
      - indwelling
        - breakdown T83.011
        - displacement T83.021
        - infection and inflammation T83.511
        - leakage T83.031
        - specified complication NEC T83.091
      - infection and inflammation T83.511
      - leakage T83.038
      - malposition T83.028
      - mechanical
        - breakdown T83.011
      - obstruction (mechanical) T83.091
      - pain T83.84
      - perforation T83.091
      - protrusion T83.091
      - specified type NEC T83.091
      - stenosis T83.85
      - thrombosis T83.86
    - urinary NEC
      - breakdown T83.018
      - displacement T83.028
      - infection and inflammation T83.518
      - leakage T83.038
      - specified complication NEC T83.098
  - cecostomy (stoma) — *see* Complications, colostomy
  - cesarean delivery wound NEC O90.89
    - disruption O90.0
    - hematoma O90.2
    - infection (following delivery) O86.00
  - chemotherapy (antineoplastic) NEC T88.7
  - chin implant (prosthetic) — *see* Complication, prosthetic device or implant, specified NEC
  - circulatory system I99.8
    - intraoperative I97.88
    - postprocedural I97.89
      - following cardiac surgery — *see also* Infarct, myocardium, associated with revascularization procedure I97.19-
        - postcardiotomy syndrome I97.0
      - hypertension I97.3
      - lymphedema after mastectomy I97.2
      - postcardiotomy syndrome I97.0
      - specified NEC I97.89
  - colostomy (stoma) K94.00
    - hemorrhage K94.01
    - infection K94.02
    - malfunction K94.03
    - mechanical K94.03
    - specified complication NEC K94.09
  - contraceptive device, intrauterine — *see* Complications, intrauterine, contraceptive device
  - cord (umbilical) — *see* Complications, umbilical cord
  - corneal graft — *see* Complications, graft, cornea
  - coronary artery (bypass) graft T82.9
    - atherosclerosis — *see* Arteriosclerosis, coronary (artery),
    - embolism T82.818
    - fibrosis T82.828
    - hemorrhage T82.838
    - infection and inflammation T82.7
    - mechanical
      - breakdown T82.211
      - displacement T82.212
      - leakage T82.213
      - malposition T82.212
      - obstruction T82.218
      - perforation T82.218
      - protrusion T82.218
      - specified NEC T82.218
    - pain T82.848
    - specified type NEC T82.898
    - stenosis T82.858
    - thrombosis T82.868
  - counterpulsation device (balloon) , intra-aortic — *see* Complications, balloon implant, vascular
  - cystostomy (stoma) N99.518

- **Complication** (s) (from) (of) - *continued*
  - cystostomy (stoma) - *continued*
    - catheter — *see* Complications, catheter, cystostomy
    - hemorrhage N99.510
    - infection N99.511
    - malfunction N99.512
    - specified type NEC N99.518
  - delivery — *see also* Complications, obstetric O75.9
    - procedure (instrumental) (manual) (surgical) O75.4
    - specified NEC O75.89
  - dialysis (peritoneal) (renal) — *see also* Complications, infusion
    - catheter (vascular) — *see* Complication, catheter, dialysis
    - peritoneal, intraperitoneal — *see* Complications, catheter, intraperitoneal
  - dorsal column (spinal) neurostimulator — *see* Complications, electronic stimulator device, spinal cord
  - drug NEC T88.7
  - ear procedure — *see also* Disorder, ear
    - intraoperative H95.88
      - hematoma — *see* Complications, intraoperative, hemorrhage (hematoma) (of), ear
      - hemorrhage — *see* Complications, intraoperative, hemorrhage (hematoma) (of), ear
      - laceration — *see* Complications, intraoperative, puncture or laceration..., ear
      - specified NEC H95.88
    - postoperative H95.89
      - external ear canal stenosis H95.81-
      - hematoma — *see* Complications, postprocedural, hematoma (of), ear
      - hemorrhage — *see* Complications, postprocedural, hemorrhage (of), ear
      - postmastoidectomy — *see* Complications, postmastoidectomy
      - seroma — *see* Complications, postprocedural, seroma (of), mastoid process
      - specified NEC H95.89
  - ectopic pregnancy O08.9
    - damage to pelvic organs O08.6
    - embolism O08.2
    - genital infection O08.0
    - hemorrhage (delayed) (excessive) O08.1
    - metabolic disorder O08.5
    - renal failure O08.4
    - shock O08.3
    - specified type NEC O08.0
    - venous complication NEC O08.7
  - electronic stimulator device
    - bladder (urinary) — *see* Complications, electronic stimulator device, urinary
    - bone T84.9
      - breakdown T84.310
      - displacement T84.320
      - embolism T84.81
      - fibrosis T84.82
      - hemorrhage T84.83
      - infection or inflammation T84.7
      - malfunction T84.310
      - malposition T84.320
      - mechanical NEC T84.390
      - obstruction T84.390
      - pain T84.84
      - perforation T84.390
      - protrusion T84.390
      - specified type NEC T84.89
      - stenosis T84.85
      - thrombosis T84.86
    - brain T85.9
      - embolism T85.810
      - fibrosis T85.820
      - hemorrhage T85.830
      - infection and inflammation T85.731
      - mechanical
        - breakdown T85.110
        - displacement T85.120
        - leakage T85.190
        - malposition T85.120
        - obstruction T85.190
        - perforation T85.190
        - protrusion T85.190
        - specified NEC T85.190
      - pain T85.840
      - specified type NEC T85.890
      - stenosis T85.850
      - thrombosis T85.860
    - cardiac (defibrillator) (pacemaker) — *see* Complications, cardiovascular device or implant, electronic

- **Complication** (s) (from) (of) - *continued*
  - fixation device, internal (orthopedic) - *continued*
    - mechanical - *continued*
      - specified type NEC - *continued*
        - limb - *continued*
          - metatarsal T84.293
          - phalanx
            - foot T84.293
            - hand T84.290
          - radius T84.19-
          - tarsal T84.293
          - tibia T84.19-
          - ulna T84.19-
        - specified bone NEC T84.298
        - vertebra T84.296
    - specified type NEC T84.89
      - embolism T84.81
      - fibrosis T84.82
      - hemorrhage T84.83
      - pain T84.84
      - specified complication NEC T84.89
      - stenosis T84.85
      - thrombosis T84.86
  - following
    - acute myocardial infarction NEC I23.8
      - aneurysm (false) (of cardiac wall) (of heart wall) (ruptured) I23.3
      - angina I23.7
      - atrial
        - septal defect I23.1
        - thrombosis I23.6
      - cardiac wall rupture I23.3
      - chordae tendinae rupture I23.4
      - defect
        - septal
          - atrial (heart) I23.1
          - ventricular (heart) I23.2
      - hemopericardium I23.0
      - papillary muscle rupture I23.5
      - rupture
        - cardiac wall I23.3
          - with hemopericardium I23.0
        - chordae tendineae I23.4
        - papillary muscle I23.5
      - specified NEC I23.8
      - thrombosis
        - atrium I23.6
        - auricular appendage I23.6
        - ventricle (heart) I23.6
      - ventricular
        - septal defect I23.2
        - thrombosis I23.6
    - ectopic or molar pregnancy O08.9
      - cardiac arrest O08.81
      - sepsis O08.82
      - specified type NEC O08.89
      - urinary tract infection O08.83
    - termination of pregnancy — *see* Abortion
  - gastrointestinal K92.9
    - bile duct prosthesis — *see* Complications, bile duct implant
    - esophageal anti-reflux device — *see* Complications, esophageal anti-reflux device
    - postoperative
      - colostomy — *see* Complications, colostomy
      - dumping syndrome K91.1
      - enterostomy — *see* Complications, enterostomy
      - gastrostomy — *see* Complications, gastrostomy
      - malabsorption NEC K91.2
      - obstruction — *see also* Obstruction, intestine, postoperative K91.30
      - postcholecystectomy syndrome K91.5
      - specified NEC K91.89
      - vomiting after GI surgery K91.0
    - prosthetic device or implant
      - bile duct prosthesis — *see* Complications, bile duct implant
      - esophageal anti-reflux device — *see* Complications, esophageal anti-reflux device
      - specified type NEC
        - embolism T85.818
        - fibrosis T85.828
        - hemorrhage T85.838
        - mechanical
          - breakdown T85.518
          - displacement T85.528
          - malfunction T85.518
          - malposition T85.528
          - obstruction T85.598
          - perforation T85.598
          - protrusion T85.598
          - specified NEC T85.598
        - pain T85.848

- **Complication** (s) (from) (of) - *continued*
  - gastrointestinal - *continued*
    - prosthetic device or implant - *continued*
      - specified type NEC - *continued*
        - specified complication NEC T85.898
        - stenosis T85.858
        - thrombosis T85.868
  - gastrostomy (stoma) K94.20
    - hemorrhage K94.21
    - infection K94.22
    - malfunction K94.23
    - mechanical K94.23
    - specified complication NEC K94.29
  - genitourinary
    - device or implant T83.9
      - genital tract T83.9
        - infection or inflammation T83.69
        - intrauterine contraceptive device — *see* Complications, intrauterine, contraceptive device
        - mechanical — *see* Complications, by device, mechanical
        - mesh — *see* Complications, mesh
        - penile prosthesis — *see* Complications, prosthetic device, penile
        - specified type NEC T83.89
          - embolism T83.81
          - fibrosis T83.82
          - hemorrhage T83.83
          - pain T83.84
          - specified complication NEC T83.89
          - stenosis T83.85
          - thrombosis T83.86
        - vaginal mesh — *see* Complications, mesh
      - urinary system T83.9
        - cystostomy catheter — *see* Complication, catheter, cystostomy
        - electronic stimulator — *see* Complications, electronic stimulator device, urinary
        - indwelling urethral catheter — *see* Complications, catheter, urethral, indwelling
        - infection or inflammation T83.598
          - indwelling urethral catheter T83.511
        - kidney transplant — *see* Complication, transplant, kidney
        - organ graft — *see* Complication, graft, urinary organ
        - specified type NEC T83.89
          - embolism T83.81
          - fibrosis T83.82
          - hemorrhage T83.83
          - mechanical T83.198
            - breakdown T83.118
            - displacement T83.128
            - malfunction T83.118
            - malposition T83.128
            - obstruction T83.198
            - perforation T83.198
            - protrusion T83.198
            - specified NEC T83.198
        - sphincter, implanted T83.191
        - stent (ileal conduit) (nephroureteral) T83.193
          - ureteral indwelling T83.192
          - pain T83.84
          - specified complication NEC T83.89
          - stenosis T83.85
          - thrombosis T83.86
        - sphincter implant — *see* Complications, implant, urinary sphincter
    - postprocedural
      - pelvic peritoneal adhesions N99.4
      - renal failure N99.0
      - specified NEC N99.89
      - stoma — *see* Complications, stoma, urinary tract
      - urethral stricture — *see* Stricture, urethra, postprocedural
      - vaginal
        - adhesions N99.2
        - vault prolapse N99.3
  - graft (bypass) (patch) — *see also* Complications, prosthetic device or implant
    - aorta — *see* Complications, graft, vascular
    - arterial — *see* Complication, graft, vascular
    - bone T86.839
      - failure T86.831
      - infection T86.832
      - mechanical T84.318
        - breakdown T84.318
        - displacement T84.328
        - protrusion T84.398
        - specified type NEC T84.398
      - rejection T86.830
      - specified type NEC T86.838

- **Complication** (s) (from) (of) - *continued*
  - graft (bypass) (patch) - *continued*
    - carotid artery — *see* Complications, graft, vascular
    - cornea T86.849
      - failure T86.841
      - infection T86.842
      - mechanical T85.398
        - breakdown T85.318
        - displacement T85.328
        - protrusion T85.398
        - specified type NEC T85.398
      - rejection T86.840
      - retroprosthetic membrane T85.398
      - specified type NEC T86.848
    - femoral artery (bypass) — *see* Complication, extremity artery (bypass) graft
    - genital organ or tract — *see* Complications, genitourinary, device or implant, genital tract
    - muscle T84.9
      - breakdown T84.410
      - displacement T84.420
      - embolism T84.81
      - fibrosis T84.82
      - hemorrhage T84.83
      - infection and inflammation T84.7
      - mechanical NEC T84.490
      - pain T84.84
      - specified type NEC T84.89
      - stenosis T84.85
      - thrombosis T84.86
    - nerve — *see* Complication, prosthetic device or implant, specified NEC
    - skin — *see* Complications, prosthetic device or implant, skin graft
    - tendon T84.9
      - breakdown T84.410
      - displacement T84.420
      - embolism T84.81
      - fibrosis T84.82
      - hemorrhage T84.83
      - infection and inflammation T84.7
      - mechanical NEC T84.490
      - pain T84.84
      - specified type NEC T84.89
      - stenosis T84.85
      - thrombosis T84.86
    - urinary organ T83.9
      - embolism T83.81
      - fibrosis T83.82
      - hemorrhage T83.83
      - infection and inflammation T83.598
        - indwelling urethral catheter T83.511
      - mechanical
        - breakdown T83.21
        - displacement T83.22
        - erosion T83.24
        - exposure T83.25
        - leakage T83.23
        - malposition T83.22
        - obstruction T83.29
        - perforation T83.29
        - protrusion T83.29
        - specified NEC T83.29
      - pain T83.84
      - specified type NEC T83.89
      - stenosis T83.85
      - thrombosis T83.86
    - vascular T82.9
      - embolism T82.818
      - femoral artery — *see* Complication, extremity artery (bypass) graft
      - fibrosis T82.828
      - hemorrhage T82.838
      - mechanical
        - breakdown T82.319
          - aorta (bifurcation) T82.310
          - carotid artery T82.311
          - specified vessel NEC T82.318
        - displacement T82.329
          - aorta (bifurcation) T82.320
          - carotid artery T82.321
          - specified vessel NEC T82.328
        - leakage T82.339
          - aorta (bifurcation) T82.330
          - carotid artery T82.331
          - specified vessel NEC T82.338
        - malposition T82.329
          - aorta (bifurcation) T82.320
          - carotid artery T82.321
          - specified vessel NEC T82.328
        - obstruction T82.399
          - aorta (bifurcation) T82.390
          - carotid artery T82.391

Complication (s) (from) (of) - *continued*
graft (bypass) (patch) - *continued*
vascular - *continued*
mechanical - *continued*
obstruction - *continued*
specified vessel NEC T82.398
perforation T82.399
aorta (bifurcation) T82.390
carotid artery T82.391
specified vessel NEC T82.398
protrusion T82.399
aorta (bifurcation) T82.390
carotid artery T82.391
specified vessel NEC T82.398
pain T82.848
specified complication NEC T82.898
stenosis T82.858
thrombosis T82.868
heart I51.9
assist device
infection and inflammation T82.7
following acute myocardial infarction — *see* Complications, following, acute myocardial infarction
postoperative — *see* Complications, circulatory system
transplant — *see* Complication, transplant, heart
and lung (s) — *see* Complications, transplant, heart, with lung
valve
graft (biological) T82.9
embolism T82.817
fibrosis T82.827
hemorrhage T82.837
infection and inflammation T82.7
mechanical T82.228
breakdown T82.221
displacement T82.222
leakage T82.223
malposition T82.222
obstruction T82.228
perforation T82.228
protrusion T82.228
pain T82.847
specified type NEC T82.897
stenosis T82.857
thrombosis T82.867
prosthesis T82.9
embolism T82.817
fibrosis T82.827
hemorrhage T82.837
infection or inflammation T82.6
mechanical T82.09
breakdown T82.01
displacement T82.02
leakage T82.03
malposition T82.02
obstruction T82.09
perforation T82.09
protrusion T82.09
pain T82.847
specified type NEC T82.897
mechanical T82.09
stenosis T82.857
thrombosis T82.867
hematoma
intraoperative — *see* Complication, intraoperative, hemorrhage
postprocedural — *see* Complication, postprocedural, hematoma
hemodialysis — *see* Complications, dialysis
hemorrhage
intraoperative — *see* Complication, intraoperative, hemorrhage
postprocedural — *see* Complication, postprocedural, hemorrhage
ileostomy (stoma) — *see* Complications, enterostomy
immunization (procedure) — *see* Complications, vaccination
implant — *see also* Complications, by site and type
urinary sphincter T83.9
embolism T83.81
fibrosis T83.82
hemorrhage T83.83
infection and inflammation T83.591
mechanical
breakdown T83.111
displacement T83.121
leakage T83.191
malposition T83.121
obstruction T83.191
perforation T83.191

Complication (s) (from) (of) - *continued*
implant - *continued*
urinary sphincter - *continued*
mechanical - *continued*
protrusion T83.191
specified NEC T83.191
pain T83.84
specified type NEC T83.89
stenosis T83.85
thrombosis T83.86
infusion (procedure) T80.90
air embolism T80.0
blood — *see* Complications, transfusion
catheter — *see* Complications, catheter
infection T80.29
pump — *see* Complications, cardiovascular, device or implant
sepsis T80.29
serum reaction — *see also* Reaction, serum T80.69
anaphylactic shock — *see also* Shock, anaphylactic T80.59
specified type NEC T80.89
inhalation therapy NEC T81.81
injection (procedure) T80.90
drug reaction — *see* Reaction, drug
infection T80.29
sepsis T80.29
serum (prophylactic) (therapeutic) — *see* Complications, vaccination
specified type NEC T80.89
vaccine (any) — *see* Complications, vaccination
inoculation (any) — *see* Complications, vaccination
insulin pump
infection and inflammation T85.72
mechanical
breakdown T85.614
displacement T85.624
leakage T85.633
malposition T85.624
obstruction T85.694
perforation T85.694
protrusion T85.694
specified NEC T85.694
intestinal pouch NEC K91.858
intraocular lens (prosthetic) T85.9
embolism T85.818
fibrosis T85.828
hemorrhage T85.838
infection and inflammation T85.79
mechanical
breakdown T85.21
displacement T85.22
malposition T85.22
obstruction T85.29
perforation T85.29
protrusion T85.29
specified NEC T85.29
pain T85.848
specified type NEC T85.898
stenosis T85.858
thrombosis T85.868
intraoperative (intraprocedural)
cardiac arrest — *see also* Infarct, myocardium, associated with revascularization procedure
during cardiac surgery I97.710
during other surgery I97.711
cardiac functional disturbance NEC — *see also* Infarct, myocardium, associated with revascularization procedure
during cardiac surgery I97.790
during other surgery I97.791
hemorrhage (hematoma) (of)
circulatory system organ or structure
during cardiac bypass I97.411
during cardiac catheterization I97.410
during other circulatory system procedure I97.418
during other procedure I97.42
digestive system organ
during procedure on digestive system K91.61
during procedure on other organ K91.62
ear
during procedure on ear and mastoid process H95.21
during procedure on other organ H95.22
endocrine system organ or structure
during procedure on endocrine system organ or structure E36.01
during procedure on other organ E36.02
eye and adnexa
during ophthalmic procedure H59.11-
during other procedure H59.12-
genitourinary organ or structure

Complication (s) (from) (of) - *continued*
intraoperative (intraprocedural) - *continued*
hemorrhage (hematoma) (of) - *continued*
genitourinary organ or structure - *continued*
during procedure on genitourinary organ or structure N99.61
during procedure on other organ N99.62
mastoid process
during procedure on ear and mastoid process H95.21
during procedure on other organ H95.22
musculoskeletal structure
during musculoskeletal surgery M96.810
during non-orthopedic surgery M96.811
during orthopedic surgery M96.810
nervous system
during a nervous system procedure G97.31
during other procedure G97.32
respiratory system
during other procedure J95.62
during procedure on respiratory system organ or structure J95.61
skin and subcutaneous tissue
during a dermatologic procedure L76.01
during a procedure on other organ L76.02
spleen
during a procedure on other organ D78.02
during a procedure on the spleen D78.01
puncture or laceration (accidental) (unintentional) (of)
brain
during a nervous system procedure G97.48
during other procedure G97.49
circulatory system organ or structure
during circulatory system procedure I97.51
during other procedure I97.52
digestive system
during procedure on digestive system K91.71
during procedure on other organ K91.72
ear
during procedure on ear and mastoid process H95.31
during procedure on other organ H95.32
endocrine system organ or structure
during procedure on endocrine system organ or structure E36.11
during procedure on other organ E36.12
eye and adnexa
during ophthalmic procedure H59.21-
during other procedure H59.22-
genitourinary organ or structure
during procedure on genitourinary organ or structure N99.71
during procedure on other organ N99.72
mastoid process
during procedure on ear and mastoid process H95.31
during procedure on other organ H95.32
musculoskeletal structure
during musculoskeletal surgery M96.820
during non-orthopedic surgery M96.821
during orthopedic surgery M96.820
nervous system
during a nervous system procedure G97.48
during other procedure G97.49
respiratory system
during other procedure J95.72
during procedure on respiratory system organ or structure J95.71
skin and subcutaneous tissue
during a dermatologic procedure L76.11
during a procedure on other organ L76.12
spleen
during a procedure on other organ D78.12
during a procedure on the spleen D78.11
specified NEC
circulatory system I97.88
digestive system K91.81
ear H95.88
endocrine system E36.8
eye and adnexa H59.88
genitourinary system N99.81
mastoid process H95.88
musculoskeletal structure M96.89
nervous system G97.81
respiratory system J95.88
skin and subcutaneous tissue L76.81
spleen D78.81
intraperitoneal catheter (dialysis) (infusion) — *see* Complications, catheter, intraperitoneal
intrathecal infusion pump
infection and inflammation T85.738
mechanical

Complication (s) (from) (of) - *continued*
intrathecal infusion pump - *continued*
mechanical - *continued*
breakdown T85.615
displacement T85.625
leakage T85.635
malfunction T85.695
malposition T85.625
obstruction T85.695
perforation T85.695
protrusion T85.695
specified NEC T85.695
intrauterine
contraceptive device
embolism T83.81
fibrosis T83.82
hemorrhage T83.83
infection and inflammation T83.69
mechanical
breakdown T83.31
displacement T83.32
malposition T83.32
obstruction T83.39
perforation T83.39
protrusion T83.39
specified NEC T83.39
pain T83.84
specified type NEC T83.89
stenosis T83.85
thrombosis T83.86
procedure (fetal) , to newborn P96.5
jejunostomy (stoma) — *see* Complications, enterostomy
joint prosthesis, internal T84.9
breakage (fracture) T84.01-
dislocation T84.02-
fracture T84.01-
infection or inflammation T84.50
hip T84.5-
knee T84.5-
specified joint NEC T84.59
instability T84.02-
malposition — *see* Complications, joint prosthesis, mechanical, displacement
mechanical
breakage, broken T84.01-
dislocation T84.02-
fracture T84.01-
instability T84.02-
leakage — *see* Complications, joint prosthesis, mechanical, specified NEC
loosening T84.039
hip T84.03-
knee T84.03-
specified joint NEC T84.038
obstruction — *see* Complications, joint prosthesis, mechanical, specified NEC
perforation — *see* Complications, joint prosthesis, mechanical, specified NEC
osteolysis T84.059
hip T84.05-
knee T84.05-
other specified joint T84.058
protrusion — *see* Complications, joint prosthesis, mechanical, specified NEC
specified complication NEC T84.099
hip T84.09-
knee T84.09-
other specified joint T84.098
subluxation T84.02-
wear of articular bearing surface T84.069
hip T84.06-
knee T84.06-
other specified joint T84.068
specified joint NEC T84.89
embolism T84.81
fibrosis T84.82
hemorrhage T84.83
pain T84.84
specified complication NEC T84.89
stenosis T84.85
thrombosis T84.86
subluxation T84.02-
kidney transplant — *see* Complications, transplant, kidney
labor O75.9
specified NEC O75.89
liver transplant (immune or nonimmune) — *see* Complications, transplant, liver
lumbar puncture G97.1
cerebrospinal fluid leak G97.0
headache or reaction G97.1

Complication (s) (from) (of) - *continued*
lung transplant — *see* Complications, transplant, lung
and heart — *see* Complications, transplant, lung, with heart
male genital N50.9
device, implant or graft — *see* Complications, genitourinary, device or implant, genital tract
postprocedural or postoperative — *see* Complications, genitourinary, postprocedural
specified NEC N99.89
mastoid (process) procedure
intraoperative H95.88
hematoma — *see* Complications, intraoperative, hemorrhage (hematoma) (of), mastoid process
hemorrhage — *see* Complications, intraoperative, hemorrhage (hematoma) (of), mastoid process
laceration — *see* Complications, intraoperative, puncture or laceration..., mastoid process
specified NEC H95.88
postmastoidectomy — *see* Complications, postmastoidectomy
postoperative H95.89
external ear canal stenosis H95.81-
hematoma — *see* Complications..., postprocedural, hematoma (of), mastoid process
hemorrhage — *see* Complications..., postprocedural, hemorrhage (of), mastoid process
postmastoidectomy — *see* Complications, postmastoidectomy
seroma — *see* Complications, postprocedural, seroma (of), mastoid process
specified NEC H95.89
mastoidectomy cavity — *see* Complications, postmastoidectomy
mechanical — *see* Complications, by site and type, mechanical
medical procedures — *see also* Complication(s), intraoperative T88.9
metabolic E88.9
postoperative E89.89
specified NEC E89.89
molar pregnancy NOS O08.9
damage to pelvic organs O08.6
embolism O08.2
genital infection O08.0
hemorrhage (delayed) (excessive) O08.1
metabolic disorder O08.5
renal failure O08.4
shock O08.3
specified type NEC O08.0
venous complication NEC O08.7
musculoskeletal system — *see also* Complication, intraoperative (intraprocedural), by site
device, implant or graft NEC — *see* Complications, orthopedic, device or implant
internal fixation (nail) (plate) (rod) — *see* Complications, fixation device, internal
joint prosthesis — *see* Complications, joint prosthesis
postoperative (postprocedural) M96.89
with osteoporosis — *see* Osteoporosis
fracture following insertion of device — *see* Fracture, following insertion of orthopedic implant, joint prosthesis or bone plate
joint instability after prosthesis removal M96.89
lordosis M96.4
postlaminectomy syndrome NEC M96.1
kyphosis M96.3
pseudarthrosis M96.0
specified complication NEC M96.89
post radiation M96.89
kyphosis M96.2
scoliosis M96.5
specified complication NEC M96.89
nephrostomy (stoma) — *see* Complications, stoma, urinary tract, external NEC
nervous system G98.8
central G96.9
device, implant or graft — *see also* Complication, prosthetic device or implant, specified NEC
electronic stimulator (electrode (s)) — *see* Complications, electronic stimulator device
specified NEC
infection and inflammation T85.738
mechanical T85.695
breakdown T85.615
displacement T85.625
leakage T85.635
malfunction T85.695
malposition T85.625
obstruction T85.695

Complication (s) (from) (of) - *continued*
nervous system - *continued*
device, implant or graft - *continued*
specified NEC - *continued*
mechanical - *continued*
perforation T85.695
protrusion T85.695
specified NEC T85.695
ventricular shunt — *see* Complications, ventricular shunt
electronic stimulator (electrode (s)) — *see* Complications, electronic stimulator device
postprocedural G97.82
intracranial hypotension G97.2
specified NEC G97.82
spinal fluid leak G97.0
newborn, due to intrauterine (fetal) procedure P96.5
nonabsorbable (permanent) sutures — *see* Complication, sutures, permanent
obstetric O75.9
procedure (instrumental) (manual) (surgical) specified NEC O75.4
specified NEC O75.89
surgical wound NEC O90.89
hematoma O90.2
infection O86.00
ocular lens implant — *see* Complications, intraocular lens
ophthalmologic
postprocedural bleb — *see* Blebitis
orbital prosthesis T85.9
embolism T85.818
fibrosis T85.828
hemorrhage T85.838
infection and inflammation T85.79
mechanical
breakdown T85.31-
displacement T85.32-
malposition T85.32-
obstruction T85.39-
perforation T85.39-
protrusion T85.39-
specified NEC T85.39-
pain T85.848
specified type NEC T85.898
stenosis T85.858
thrombosis T85.868
organ or tissue transplant (partial) (total) — *see* Complications, transplant
orthopedic — *see also* Disorder, soft tissue
device or implant T84.9
bone
device or implant — *see* Complication, bone, device NEC
graft — *see* Complication, graft, bone
breakdown T84.418
displacement T84.428
electronic bone stimulator — *see* Complications, electronic stimulator device, bone
embolism T84.81
fibrosis T84.82
fixation device — *see* Complication, fixation device, internal
hemorrhage T84.83
infection or inflammation T84.7
joint prosthesis — *see* Complication, joint prosthesis, internal
malfunction T84.418
malposition T84.428
mechanical NEC T84.498
muscle graft — *see* Complications, graft, muscle
obstruction T84.498
pain T84.84
perforation T84.498
protrusion T84.498
specified complication NEC T84.89
stenosis T84.85
tendon graft — *see* Complications, graft, tendon
thrombosis T84.86
fracture (following insertion of device) — *see* Fracture, following insertion of orthopedic implant, joint prosthesis or bone plate
postprocedural M96.89
fracture — *see* Fracture, following insertion of orthopedic implant, joint prosthesis or bone plate
postlaminectomy syndrome NEC M96.1
kyphosis M96.3
lordosis M96.4
postradiation
kyphosis M96.2
scoliosis M96.5
pseudarthrosis post-fusion M96.0

Complication (s) (from) (of) - *continued*
orthopedic - *continued*
postprocedural - *continued*
specified type NEC M96.89
pacemaker (cardiac) — *see* Complications, cardiovascular device or implant, electronic
pancreas transplant — *see* Complications, transplant, pancreas
penile prosthesis (implant) — *see* Complications, prosthetic device, penile
perfusion NEC T80.90
perineal repair (obstetrical) NEC O90.89
disruption O90.1
hematoma O90.2
infection (following delivery) O86.09
phototherapy T88.9
specified NEC T88.8
postmastoidectomy NEC H95.19-
cyst, mucosal H95.13-
granulation H95.12-
inflammation, chronic H95.11-
recurrent cholesteatoma H95.0-
postoperative — *see* Complications, postprocedural
circulatory — *see* Complications, circulatory system
ear — *see* Complications, ear
endocrine — *see* Complications, endocrine
eye — *see* Complications, eye
lumbar puncture G97.1
cerebrospinal fluid leak G97.0
nervous system (central) (peripheral) — *see* Complications, nervous system
respiratory system — *see* Complications, respiratory system
postprocedural — *see also* Complications, surgical procedure
cardiac arrest — *see also* Infarct, myocardium, associated with revascularization procedure
following cardiac surgery I97.120
following other surgery I97.121
cardiac functional disturbance NEC — *see also* Infarct, myocardium, associated with revascularization procedure
following cardiac surgery I97.190
following other surgery I97.191
cardiac insufficiency
following cardiac surgery I97.110
following other surgery I97.111
chorioretinal scars following retinal surgery H59.81-
following cataract surgery
cataract (lens) fragments H59.02-
cystoid macular edema H59.03-
specified NEC H59.09-
vitreous (touch) syndrome H59.01-
heart failure
following cardiac surgery I97.130
following other surgery I97.131
hematoma (of)
circulatory system organ or structure
following cardiac bypass I97.631
following cardiac catheterization I97.630
following other circulatory system procedure I97.638
following other procedure I97.621
digestive system
following procedure on digestive system K91.870
following procedure on other organ K91.871
ear
following other procedure H95.52
following procedure on ear and mastoid process H95.51
endocrine system
following endocrine system procedure E89.820
following other procedure E89.821
eye and adnexa
following ophthalmic procedure H59.33-
following other procedure H59.34-
genitourinary organ or structure
following procedure on genitourinary organ or structure N99.840
following procedure on other organ N99.841
mastoid process
following other procedure H95.52
following procedure on ear and mastoid process H95.51
musculoskeletal structure
following musculoskeletal surgery M96.840
following non-orthopedic surgery M96.841
following orthopedic surgery M96.840
nervous system
following nervous system procedure G97.61

Complication (s) (from) (of) - *continued*
postprocedural - *continued*
hematoma (of) - *continued*
nervous system - *continued*
following other procedure G97.62
respiratory system
following other procedure J95.861
following procedure on respiratory system organ or structure J95.860
skin and subcutaneous tissue
following dermatologic procedure L76.31
following procedure on other organ L76.32
spleen
following procedure on other organ D78.32
following procedure on the spleen D78.31
hemorrhage (of)
circulatory system organ or structure
following cardiac bypass I97.611
following cardiac catheterization I97.610
following other circulatory system procedure I97.618
following other procedure I97.620
digestive system
following procedure on digestive system K91.840
following procedure on other organ K91.841
ear
following other procedure H95.42
following procedure on ear and mastoid process H95.41
endocrine system
following endocrine system procedure E89.810
following other procedure E89.811
eye and adnexa
following ophthalmic procedure H59.31-
following other procedure H59.32-
genitourinary organ or structure
following procedure on genitourinary organ or structure N99.820
following procedure on other organ N99.821
mastoid process
following other procedure H95.42
following procedure on ear and mastoid process H95.41
musculoskeletal structure
following musculoskeletal surgery M96.830
following non-orthopedic surgery M96.831
following orthopedic surgery M96.830
nervous system
following nervous system procedure G97.51
following other procedure G97.52
respiratory system
following other procedure J95.831
following procedure on respiratory system organ or structure J95.830
skin and subcutaneous tissue
following dermatologic procedure L76.21
following a procedure on other organ L76.22
spleen
following procedure on other organ D78.22
following procedure on the spleen D78.21
seroma (of)
circulatory system organ or structure
following cardiac bypass I97.641
following cardiac catheterization I97.640
following other circulatory system procedure I97.648
following other procedure I97.622
digestive system
following procedure on digestive system K91.872
following procedure on other organ K91.873
ear
following other procedure H95.54
following procedure on ear and mastoid process H95.53
endocrine system
following endocrine system procedure E89.822
following other procedure E89.823
eye and adnexa
following ophthalmic procedure H59.35-
following other procedure H59.36-
genitourinary organ or structure
following procedure on genitourinary organ or structure N99.842
following procedure on other organ N99.843
mastoid process
following other procedure H95.54
following procedure on ear and mastoid process H95.53
musculoskeletal structure
following musculoskeletal surgery M96.842
following non-orthopedic surgery M96.843

Complication (s) (from) (of) - *continued*
postprocedural - *continued*
seroma (of) - *continued*
musculoskeletal structure - *continued*
following orthopedic surgery M96.842
nervous system
following nervous system procedure G97.63
following other procedure G97.64
respiratory system
following other procedure J95.863
following procedure on respiratory system organ or structure J95.862
skin and subcutaneous tissue
following dermatologic procedure L76.33
following procedure on other organ L76.34
spleen
following procedure on other organ D78.34
following procedure on the spleen D78.33
specified NEC
circulatory system I97.89
digestive K91.89
ear H95.89
endocrine E89.89
eye and adnexa H59.89
genitourinary N99.89
mastoid process H95.89
metabolic E89.89
musculoskeletal structure M96.89
nervous system G97.82
respiratory system J95.89
skin and subcutaneous tissue L76.82
spleen D78.89
pregnancy NEC — *see* Pregnancy, complicated by
prosthetic device or implant T85.9
bile duct — *see* Complications, bile duct implant
breast — *see* Complications, breast implant
bulking agent
ureteral
erosion T83.714
exposure T83.724
urethral
erosion T83.713
exposure T83.723
cardiac and vascular NEC — *see* Complications, cardiovascular device or implant
corneal transplant — *see* Complications, graft, cornea
electronic nervous system stimulator — *see* Complications, electronic stimulator device
epidural infusion catheter — *see* Complications, catheter, epidural
esophageal anti-reflux device — *see* Complications, esophageal anti-reflux device
genital organ or tract — *see* Complications, genitourinary, device or implant, genital tract
specified NEC T83.79
heart valve — *see* Complications, heart, valve, prosthesis
infection or inflammation T85.79
intestine transplant T86.892
liver transplant T86.43
lung transplant T86.812
pancreas transplant T86.892
skin graft T86.822
intraocular lens — *see* Complications, intraocular lens
intraperitoneal (dialysis) catheter — *see* Complications, catheter, intraperitoneal
joint — *see* Complications, joint prosthesis, internal
mechanical NEC T85.698
dialysis catheter (vascular) — *see also* Complication, catheter, dialysis, mechanical
peritoneal — *see* Complication, catheter, intraperitoneal, mechanical
gastrointestinal device T85.598
ocular device T85.398
subdural (infusion) catheter T85.690
suture, permanent T85.692
that for bone repair — *see* Complications, fixation device, internal (orthopedic), mechanical
ventricular shunt
breakdown T85.01
displacement T85.02
leakage T85.03
malposition T85.02
obstruction T85.09
perforation T85.09
protrusion T85.09
specified NEC T85.09
mesh

Complication (s) (from) (of) - *continued*
prosthetic device or implant - *continued*
mesh - *continued*
erosion (to surrounding organ or tissue) T83.718
urethral (into pelvic floor muscles) T83.712
vaginal (into pelvic floor muscles) T83.711
exposure (into surrounding organ or tissue) T83.728
urethral (through urethral wall) T83.722
vaginal (into vagina) (through vaginal wall) T83.721
orbital — *see* Complications, orbital prosthesis
penile T83.9
embolism T83.81
fibrosis T83.82
hemorrhage T83.83
infection and inflammation T83.61
mechanical
breakdown T83.410
displacement T83.420
leakage T83.490
malposition T83.420
obstruction T83.490
perforation T83.490
protrusion T83.490
specified NEC T83.490
pain T83.84
specified type NEC T83.89
stenosis T83.85
thrombosis T83.86
prosthetic materials NEC
erosion (to surrounding organ or tissue) T83.718
exposure (into surrounding organ or tissue) T83.728
skin graft T86.829
artificial skin or decellularized allodermis
embolism T85.818
fibrosis T85.828
hemorrhage T85.838
infection and inflammation T85.79
mechanical
breakdown T85.613
displacement T85.623
malfunction T85.613
malposition T85.623
obstruction T85.693
perforation T85.693
protrusion T85.693
specified NEC T85.693
pain T85.848
specified type NEC T85.898
stenosis T85.858
thrombosis T85.868
failure T86.821
infection T86.822
rejection T86.820
specified NEC T86.828
sling
urethral (female) (male)
erosion T83.712
exposure T83.722
specified NEC T85.9
embolism T85.818
fibrosis T85.828
hemorrhage T85.838
infection and inflammation T85.79
mechanical
breakdown T85.618
displacement T85.628
leakage T85.638
malfunction T85.618
malposition T85.628
obstruction T85.698
perforation T85.698
protrusion T85.698
specified NEC T85.698
pain T85.848
specified type NEC T85.898
stenosis T85.858
thrombosis T85.868
subdural infusion catheter — *see* Complications, catheter, subdural
sutures — *see* Complications, sutures
urinary organ or tract NEC — *see* Complications, genitourinary, device or implant, urinary system
vascular — *see* Complications, cardiovascular device or implant
ventricular shunt — *see* Complications, ventricular shunt (device)
puerperium — *see* Puerperal
puncture, spinal G97.1
cerebrospinal fluid leak G97.0
headache or reaction G97.1

Complication (s) (from) (of) - *continued*
pyelogram N99.89
radiation
kyphosis M96.2
scoliosis M96.5
reattached
extremity (infection) (rejection)
lower T87.1X-
upper T87.0X-
specified body part NEC T87.2
reconstructed breast
asymmetry between native and reconstructed breast N65.1
deformity N65.0
disproportion between native and reconstructed breast N65.1
excess tissue N65.0
misshappen N65.0
reimplant NEC — *see also* Complications, prosthetic device or implant
limb (infection) (rejection) — *see* Complications, reattached, extremity
organ (partial) (total) — *see* Complications, transplant
prosthetic device NEC — *see* Complications, prosthetic device
renal N28.9
allograft — *see* Complications, transplant, kidney
dialysis — *see* Complications, dialysis
respirator
mechancial J95.850
specified NEC J95.859
respiratory system J98.9
device, implant or graft — *see* Complication, prosthetic device or implant, specified NEC
lung transplant — *see* Complications, prosthetic device or implant, lung transplant
postoperative J95.89
air leak J95.812
Mendelson's syndrome (chemical pneumonitis) J95.4
pneumothorax J95.811
pulmonary insufficiency (acute) (after nonthoracic surgery) J95.2
chronic J95.3
following thoracic surgery J95.1
respiratory failure (acute) J95.821
acute and chronic J95.822
specified NEC J95.89
subglottic stenosis J95.5
tracheostomy complication — *see* Complications, tracheostomy
therapy T81.89
sedation during labor and delivery O74.9
cardiac O74.2
central nervous system O74.3
pulmonary NEC O74.1
shunt — *see also* Complications, prosthetic device or implant
arteriovenous — *see* Complications, arteriovenous, shunt
ventricular (communicating) — *see* Complications, ventricular shunt
skin
graft T86.829
failure T86.821
infection T86.822
rejection T86.820
specified type NEC T86.828
spinal
anesthesia — *see* Complications, anesthesia, spinal
catheter (epidural) (subdural) — *see* Complications, catheter
puncture or tap G97.1
cerebrospinal fluid leak G97.0
headache or reaction G97.1
stent
bile duct — *see* Complications, bile duct prosthesis
ureteral indwelling
breakdown T83.112
displacement T83.122
leakage T83.192
malposition T83.122
obstruction T83.192
perforation T83.192
protrusion T83.192
specified NEC T83.192
urinary NEC (ileal conduit) (nephroureteral) T83.193
embolism T83.81
fibrosis T83.82
hemorrhage T83.83
infection and inflammation T83.593

Complication (s) (from) (of) - *continued*
stent - *continued*
urinary NEC (ileal conduit) (nephroureteral) - *continued*
mechanical
breakdown T83.113
displacement T83.123
leakage T83.193
malposition T83.123
obstruction T83.193
perforation T83.193
protrusion T83.193
specified NEC T83.193
pain T83.84
specified type NEC T83.89
stenosis T83.85
thrombosis T83.86
vascular
end stent stenosis — *see* Restenosis, stent
in stent stenosis — *see* Restenosis, stent
stoma
digestive tract
colostomy — *see* Complications, colostomy
enterostomy — *see* Complications, enterostomy
esophagostomy — *see* Complications, esophagostomy
gastrostomy — *see* Complications, gastrostomy
urinary tract N99.528
continent N99.538
hemorrhage N99.530
herniation N99.533
infection N99.531
malfunction N99.532
specified type NEC N99.538
stenosis N99.534
cystostomy — *see* Complications, cystostomy
external NOS N99.528
hemorrhage N99.520
herniation N99.523
incontinent N99.528
hemorrhage N99.520
herniation N99.523
infection N99.521
malfunction N99.522
specified type NEC N99.528
stenosis N99.524
infection N99.521
malfunction N99.522
specified type NEC N99.528
stenosis N99.524
stomach banding — *see* Complication(s), bariatric procedure
stomach stapling — *see* Complication(s), bariatric procedure
surgical material, nonabsorbable — *see* Complication, suture, permanent
surgical procedure (on) T81.9
amputation stump (late) — *see* Complications, amputation stump
cardiac — *see* Complications, circulatory system
cholesteatoma, recurrent — *see* Complications, postmastoidectomy, recurrent cholesteatoma
circulatory (early) — *see* Complications, circulatory system
digestive system — *see* Complications, gastrointestinal
dumping syndrome (postgastrectomy) K91.1
ear — *see* Complications, ear
elephantiasis or lymphedema I97.89
postmastectomy I97.2
emphysema (surgical) T81.82
endocrine — *see* Complications, endocrine
eye — *see* Complications, eye
fistula (persistent postoperative) T81.83
foreign body inadvertently left in wound (sponge) (suture) (swab) — *see* Foreign body, accidentally left during a procedure
gastrointestinal — *see* Complications, gastrointestinal
genitourinary NEC N99.89
hematoma
intraoperative — *see* Complication, intraoperative, hemorrhage
postprocedural — *see* Complication, postprocedural, hematoma
hemorrhage
intraoperative — *see* Complication, intraoperative, hemorrhage
postprocedural — *see* Complication, postprocedural, hemorrhage
hepatic failure K91.82
hyperglycemia (postpancreatectomy) E89.1
hypoinsulinemia (postpancreatectomy) E89.1

Complication (s) (from) (of) - *continued*
surgical procedure (on) - *continued*
hypoparathyroidism
(postparathyroidectomy) E89.2
hypopituitarism (posthypophysectomy) E89.3
hypothyroidism (post-thyroidectomy) E89.0
intestinal obstruction — *see also* Obstruction, intestine, postoperative K91.30
intracranial hypotension following ventricular shunting (ventriculostomy) G97.2
lymphedema I97.89
postmastectomy I97.2
malabsorption (postsurgical) NEC K91.2
osteoporosis — *see* Osteoporosis, postsurgical malabsorption
mastoidectomy cavity NEC — *see* Complications, postmastoidectomy
metabolic E89.89
specified NEC E89.89
musculoskeletal — *see* Complications, musculoskeletal system
nervous system (central) (peripheral) — *see* Complications, nervous system
ovarian failure E89.40
asymptomatic E89.40
symptomatic E89.41
peripheral vascular — *see* Complications, surgical procedure, vascular
postcardiotomy syndrome I97.0
postcholecystectomy syndrome K91.5
postcommissurotomy syndrome I97.0
postgastrectomy dumping syndrome K91.1
postlaminectomy syndrome NEC M96.1
kyphosis M96.3
postmastectomy lymphedema syndrome I97.2
postmastoidectomy cholesteatoma — *see* Complications, postmastoidectomy, recurrent cholesteatoma
postvagotomy syndrome K91.1
postvalvulotomy syndrome I97.0
pulmonary insufficiency (acute) J95.2
chronic J95.3
following thoracic surgery J95.1
reattached body part — *see* Complications, reattached
respiratory — *see* Complications, respiratory system
shock (hypovolemic) T81.19
spleen (postoperative) D78.89
intraoperative D78.81
stitch abscess T81.41
subglottic stenosis (postsurgical) J95.5
testicular hypofunction E89.5
transplant — *see* Complications, organ or tissue transplant
urinary NEC N99.89
vaginal vault prolapse (posthysterectomy) N99.3
vascular (peripheral)
artery T81.719
mesenteric T81.710
renal T81.711
specified NEC T81.718
vein T81.72
wound infection T81.49
suture, permanent (wire) NEC T85.9
with repair of bone — *see* Complications, fixation device, internal
embolism T85.818
fibrosis T85.828
hemorrhage T85.838
infection and inflammation T85.79
mechanical
breakdown T85.612
displacement T85.622
malfunction T85.612
malposition T85.622
obstruction T85.692
perforation T85.692
protrusion T85.692
specified NEC T85.692
pain T85.848
specified type NEC T85.898
stenosis T85.858
thrombosis T85.868
tracheostomy J95.00
granuloma J95.09
hemorrhage J95.01
infection J95.02
malfunction J95.03
mechanical J95.03
obstruction J95.03
specified type NEC J95.09
tracheo-esophageal fistula J95.04

Complication (s) (from) (of) - *continued*
transfusion (blood) (lymphocytes) (plasma) T80.92
air emblism T80.0
circulatory overload E87.71
febrile nonhemolytic transfusion reaction R50.84
hemolysis T80.89
hemochromatosis E83.111
hemolytic reaction (antigen unspecified) T80.919
incompatibility reaction (antigen unspecified) T80.919
ABO T80.30
delayed serologic (DSTR) T80.39
hemolytic transfusion reaction (HTR) (unspecified time after transfusion) T80.319
acute (AHTR) (less than 24 hours after transfusion) T80.310
delayed (DHTR) (24 hours or more after transfusion) T80.311
specified NEC T80.39
acute (antigen unspecified) T80.910
delayed (antigen unspecified) T80.911
delayed serologic (DSTR) T80.89
Non-ABO (minor antigens (Duffy) (K) (Kell) (Kidd) (Lewis) (M) (N) (P) (S)) T80.A0
delayed serologic (DSTR) T80.A9
hemolytic transfusion reaction (HTR) (unspecified time after transfusion) T80.A19
acute (AHTR) (less than 24 hours after transfusion) T80.A10
delayed (DHTR) (24 hours or more after transfusion) T80.A11
specified NEC T80.A9
Rh (antigens (C) (c) (D) (E) (e)) (factor) T80.40
delayed serologic (DSTR) T80.49
hemolytic transfusion reaction (HTR) (unspecified time after transfusion) T80.419
acute (AHTR) (less than 24 hours after transfusion) T80.410
delayed (DHTR) (24 hours or more after transfusion) T80.411
specified NEC T80.49
infection T80.29
acute T80.22
reaction NEC T80.89
sepsis T80.29
shock T80.89
transplant T86.90
bone T86.839
failure T86.831
infection T86.832
rejection T86.830
specified type NEC T86.838
bone marrow T86.00
failure T86.02
infection T86.03
rejection T86.01
specified type NEC T86.09
cornea T86.849
failure T86.841
infection T86.842
rejection T86.840
specified type NEC T86.848
failure T86.92
heart T86.20
with lung T86.30
cardiac allograft vasculopathy T86.290
failure T86.32
infection T86.33
rejection T86.31
specified type NEC T86.39
failure T86.22
infection T86.23
rejection T86.21
specified type NEC T86.298
infection T86.93
intestine T86.859
failure T86.851
infection T86.852
rejection T86.850
specified type NEC T86.858
kidney T86.10
failure T86.12
infection T86.13
rejection T86.11
specified type NEC T86.19
liver T86.40
failure T86.42
infection T86.43
rejection T86.41
specified type NEC T86.49
lung T86.819
with heart T86.30
failure T86.32

Complication (s) (from) (of) - *continued*
transplant - *continued*
lung - *continued*
with heart - *continued*
infection T86.33
rejection T86.31
specified type NEC T86.39
failure T86.811
infection T86.812
rejection T86.810
specified type NEC T86.818
malignant neoplasm C80.2
pancreas T86.899
failure T86.891
infection T86.892
rejection T86.890
specified type NEC T86.898
peripheral blood stem cells T86.5
post-transplant lymphoproliferative disorder (PTLD) D47.Z1
rejection T86.91
skin T86.829
failure T86.821
infection T86.822
rejection T86.820
specified type NEC T86.828
specified
tissue T86.899
failure T86.891
infection T86.892
rejection T86.890
specified type NEC T86.898
type NEC T86.99
stem cell (from peripheral blood) (from umbilical cord) T86.5
umbilical cord stem cells T86.5
trauma (early) T79.9
specified NEC T79.8
ultrasound therapy NEC T88.9
umbilical cord NEC
complicating delivery O69.9
specified NEC O69.89
umbrella device, vascular T82.9
embolism T82.818
fibrosis T82.828
hemorrhage T82.838
infection or inflammation T82.7
mechanical
breakdown T82.515
displacement T82.525
leakage T82.535
malposition T82.525
obstruction T82.595
perforation T82.595
protrusion T82.595
pain T82.848
specified type NEC T82.898
stenosis T82.858
thrombosis T82.868
urethral catheter — *see* Complications, catheter, urethral, indwelling
vaccination T88.1
anaphylaxis NEC T80.52
arthropathy — *see* Arthropathy, postimmunization
cellulitis T88.0
encephalitis or encephalomyelitis G04.02
infection (general) (local) NEC T88.0
meningitis G03.8
myelitis G04.02
protein sickness T80.62
rash T88.1
reaction (allergic) T88.1
serum T80.62
sepsis T88.0
serum intoxication, sickness, rash, or other serum reaction NEC T80.62
anaphylactic shock T80.52
shock (allergic) (anaphylactic) T80.52
vaccinia (generalized) (localized) T88.1
vas deferens device or implant — *see* Complications, genitourinary, device or implant, genital tract
vascular I99.9
device or implant T82.9
embolism T82.818
fibrosis T82.828
hemorrhage T82.838
infection or inflammation T82.7
mechanical
breakdown T82.519
specified device NEC T82.518
displacement T82.529
specified device NEC T82.528

- **Complication** (s) (from) (of) - *continued*
  - vascular - *continued*
    - device or implant - *continued*
      - mechanical - *continued*
        - leakage T82.539
          - specified device NEC T82.538
        - malposition T82.529
          - specified device NEC T82.528
        - obstruction T82.599
          - specified device NEC T82.598
        - perforation T82.599
          - specified device NEC T82.598
        - protrusion T82.599
          - specified device NEC T82.598
      - pain T82.848
      - specified type NEC T82.898
      - stenosis T82.858
      - thrombosis T82.868
    - dialysis catheter — *see* Complication, catheter, dialysis
    - following infusion, therapeutic injection or transfusion T80.1
    - graft T82.9
      - embolism T82.818
      - fibrosis T82.828
      - hemorrhage T82.838
      - mechanical
        - breakdown T82.319
          - aorta (bifurcation) T82.310
          - carotid artery T82.311
          - specified vessel NEC T82.318
        - displacement T82.329
          - aorta (bifurcation) T82.320
          - carotid artery T82.321
          - specified vessel NEC T82.328
        - leakage T82.339
          - aorta (bifurcation) T82.330
          - carotid artery T82.331
          - specified vessel NEC T82.338
        - malposition T82.329
          - aorta (bifurcation) T82.320
          - carotid artery T82.321
          - specified vessel NEC T82.328
        - obstruction T82.399
          - aorta (bifurcation) T82.390
          - carotid artery T82.391
          - specified vessel NEC T82.398
        - perforation T82.399
          - aorta (bifurcation) T82.390
          - carotid artery T82.391
          - specified vessel NEC T82.398
        - protrusion T82.399
          - aorta (bifurcation) T82.390
          - carotid artery T82.391
          - specified vessel NEC T82.398
      - pain T82.848
      - specified complication NEC T82.898
      - stenosis T82.858
      - thrombosis T82.868
    - postoperative — *see* Complications, postoperative, circulatory
  - vena cava device (filter) (sieve) (umbrella) — *see* Complications, umbrella device, vascular
  - ventilation therapy NEC T81.81
  - ventilator
    - mechanical J95.850
    - specified NEC J95.859
  - ventricular (communicating) shunt (device) T85.9
    - embolism T85.810
    - fibrosis T85.820
    - hemorrhage T85.830
    - infection and inflammation T85.730
    - mechanical
      - breakdown T85.01
      - displacement T85.02
      - leakage T85.03
      - malposition T85.02
      - obstruction T85.09
      - perforation T85.09
      - protrusion T85.09
      - specified NEC T85.09
    - pain T85.840
    - specified type NEC T85.890
    - stenosis T85.850
    - thrombosis T85.860
  - wire suture, permanent (implanted) — *see* Complications, suture, permanent
- **Compressed air disease** T70.3
- **Compression**
  - with injury - code by Nature of injury
  - artery I77.1
    - celiac, syndrome I77.4
  - brachial plexus G54.0
- **Compression** - *continued*
  - brain (stem) G93.5
    - due to
      - contusion (diffuse) — *see* Injury, intracranial, diffuse
        - focal — *see* Injury, intracranial, focal
      - injury NEC — *see* Injury, intracranial, diffuse
    - traumatic — *see* Injury, intracranial, diffuse
  - bronchus J98.09
  - cauda equina G83.4
  - celiac (artery) (axis) I77.4
  - cerebral — *see* Compression, brain
  - cervical plexus G54.2
  - cord
    - spinal — *see* Compression, spinal
    - umbilical — *see* Compression, umbilical cord
  - cranial nerve G52.9
    - eighth — *see* subcategory H93.3
    - eleventh G52.8
    - fifth G50.8
    - first G52.0
    - fourth — *see* Strabismus, paralytic, fourth nerve
    - ninth G52.1
    - second — *see* Disorder, nerve, optic
    - seventh G51.8
    - sixth — *see* Strabismus, paralytic, sixth nerve
    - tenth G52.2
    - third — *see* Strabismus, paralytic, third nerve
    - twelfth G52.3
  - diver's squeeze T70.3
  - during birth (newborn) P15.9
  - esophagus K22.2
  - eustachian tube — *see* Obstruction, eustachian tube, cartilaginous
  - facies Q67.1
  - fracture
    - nontraumatic NOS — *see* Collapse, vertebra
    - pathological — *see* Fracture, pathological
    - traumatic — *see* Fracture, traumatic
  - heart — *see* Disease, heart
  - intestine — *see* Obstruction, intestine
  - laryngeal nerve, recurrent G52.2
    - with paralysis of vocal cords and larynx J38.00
      - bilateral J38.02
      - unilateral J38.01
  - lumbosacral plexus G54.1
  - lung J98.4
  - lymphatic vessel I89.0
  - medulla — *see* Compression, brain
  - nerve — *see also* Disorder, nerve G58.9
    - arm NEC — *see* Mononeuropathy, upper limb
    - axillary G54.0
    - cranial — *see* Compression, cranial nerve
    - leg NEC — *see* Mononeuropathy, lower limb
    - median (in carpal tunnel) — *see* Syndrome, carpal tunnel
    - optic — *see* Disorder, nerve, optic
    - plantar — *see* Lesion, nerve, plantar
    - posterior tibial (in tarsal tunnel) — *see* Syndrome, tarsal tunnel
    - root or plexus NOS (in) G54.9
      - intervertebral disc disorder NEC — *see* Disorder, disc, with, radiculopathy
        - with myelopathy — *see* Disorder, disc, with, myelopathy
      - neoplastic disease — *see also* Neoplasm D49.9 *[G55]*
      - spondylosis — *see* Spondylosis, with radiculopathy
    - sciatic (acute) — *see* Lesion, nerve, sciatic
    - sympathetic G90.8
    - traumatic — *see* Injury, nerve
    - ulnar — *see* Lesion, nerve, ulnar
    - upper extremity NEC — *see* Mononeuropathy, upper limb
  - spinal (cord) G95.20
    - by displacement of intervertebral disc NEC — *see also* Disorder, disc, with, myelopathy
    - nerve root NOS G54.9
      - due to displacement of intervertebral disc NEC — *see* Disorder, disc, with, radiculopathy
        - with myelopathy — *see* Disorder, disc, with, myelopathy
    - specified NEC G95.29
    - spondylogenic (cervical) (lumbar, lumbosacral) (thoracic) — *see* Spondylosis, with myelopathy NEC
      - anterior — *see* Syndrome, anterior, spinal artery, compression
    - traumatic — *see* Injury, spinal cord, by region
  - subcostal nerve (syndrome) — *see* Mononeuropathy, upper limb, specified NEC
  - sympathetic nerve NEC G90.8
- **Compression** - *continued*
  - syndrome T79.5
  - trachea J39.8
  - ulnar nerve (by scar tissue) — *see* Lesion, nerve, ulnar
  - umbilical cord
    - complicating delivery O69.2
      - cord around neck O69.1
      - prolapse O69.0
      - specified NEC O69.2
  - ureter N13.5
  - vein I87.1
  - vena cava (inferior) (superior) I87.1
- **Compulsion, compulsive**
  - gambling F63.0
  - neurosis F42.8
  - personality F60.5
  - states F42.8
  - swearing F42.8
    - in Gilles de la Tourette's syndrome F95.2
  - tics and spasms F95.9
- **Concato's disease** (pericardial polyserositis) A19.9
  - nontubercular I31.1
  - pleural — *see* Pleurisy, with effusion
- **Concavity chest wall** M95.4
- **Concealed penis** Q55.64
- **Concern** (normal) **about sick person in family** Z63.6
- **Concrescence** (teeth) K00.2
- **Concretio cordis** I31.1
  - rheumatic I09.2
- **Concretion** — *see also* Calculus
  - appendicular K38.1
  - canaliculus — *see* Dacryolith
  - clitoris N90.89
  - conjunctiva H11.12-
  - eyelid — *see* Disorder, eyelid, specified type NEC
  - lacrimal passages — *see* Dacryolith
  - prepuce (male) N47.8
  - salivary gland (any) K11.5
  - seminal vesicle N50.89
  - tonsil J35.8
- **Concussion** (brain) (cerebral) (current) S06.0X9
  - with
    - loss of consciousness of 30 minutes or less S06.0X1
    - loss of consciousness of unspecified durationS06.0X9
  - blast (air) (hydraulic) (immersion) (underwater)
    - abdomen or thorax — *see* Injury, blast, by site
    - ear with acoustic nerve injury — *see* Injury, nerve, acoustic, specified type NEC
  - cauda equina S34.3
  - conus medullaris S34.02
  - ocular S05.8X-
  - spinal (cord)
    - cervical S14.0
    - lumbar S34.01
    - sacral S34.02
    - thoracic S24.0
  - syndrome F07.81
- **Condition** — *see* Disease
- **Conditions arising in the perinatal period** — *see* Newborn, affected by
- **Conduct disorder** — *see* Disorder, conduct
- **Condyloma** A63.0
  - acuminatum A63.0
  - gonorrheal A54.09
  - latum A51.31
  - syphilitic A51.31
    - congenital A50.07
  - venereal, syphilitic A51.31
- **Conflagration** — *see also* Burn
  - asphyxia (by inhalation of gases, fumes or vapors) — *see also* Table of Drugs and Chemicals T59.9-
- **Conflict** (with) — *see also* Discord
  - family Z73.9
  - marital Z63.0
    - involving divorce or estrangement Z63.5
  - parent-child Z62.820
    - parent-adopted child Z62.821
    - parent-biological child Z62.820
    - parent-foster child Z62.822
  - social role NEC Z73.5
- **Confluent** — *see* condition
- **Confusion, confused** R41.0
  - epileptic F05
  - mental state (psychogenic) F44.89
  - psychogenic F44.89
  - reactive (from emotional stress, psychological trauma) F44.89
- **Confusional arousals** G47.51
- **Congelation** T69.9

Constriction - *continued*
external - *continued*
parietal region S00.04
pelvis S30.840
penis S30.842
perineum
female S30.844
male S30.840
periocular area — *see* Constriction, external, eyelid
phalanges
finger — *see* Constriction, external, finger
toe — *see* Constriction, external, toe
pharynx S10.14
pinna — *see* Constriction, external, ear
popliteal space — *see* Constriction, external, knee
prepuce S30.842
pubic region S30.840
pudendum
female S30.846
male S30.845
sacral region S30.840
scalp S00.04
scapular region — *see* Constriction, external, shoulder
scrotum S30.843
shin — *see* Constriction, external, leg
shoulder S40.24-
sternal region S20.349
submaxillary region S00.84
submental region S00.84
subungual
finger (s) — *see* Constriction, external, finger
toe (s) — *see* Constriction, external, toe
supraclavicular fossa S10.84
supraorbital S00.84
temple S00.84
temporal region S00.84
testis S30.843
thigh S70.34-
thorax, thoracic (wall) S20.94
back S20.44-
front S20.34-
throat S10.14
thumb S60.34-
toe (s) (lesser) S90.44-
great S90.44-
tongue S00.542
trachea S10.14
tunica vaginalis S30.843
uvula S00.542
vagina S30.844
vulva S30.844
wrist S60.84-
gallbladder — *see* Obstruction, gallbladder
intestine — *see* Obstruction, intestine
larynx J38.6
congenital Q31.8
specified NEC Q31.8
subglottic Q31.1
organ or site, congenital NEC — *see* Atresia, by site
prepuce (acquired) (congenital) N47.1
pylorus (adult hypertrophic) K31.1
congenital or infantile Q40.0
newborn Q40.0
ring dystocia (uterus) O62.4
spastic — *see also* Spasm
ureter N13.5
ureter N13.5
with infection N13.6
urethra — *see* Stricture, urethra
visual field (peripheral) (functional) — *see* Defect, visual field
Constrictive — *see* condition
Consultation
medical — *see* Counseling, medical
religious Z71.81
specified reason NEC Z71.89
spiritual Z71.81
without complaint or sickness Z71.9
feared complaint unfounded Z71.1
specified reason NEC Z71.89
Consumption — *see* Tuberculosis
Contact (with) — *see also* Exposure (to)
acariasis Z20.7
AIDS virus Z20.6
air pollution Z77.110
algae and algae toxins Z77.121
algae bloom Z77.121
anthrax Z20.810
aromatic amines Z77.020
aromatic (hazardous) compounds NEC Z77.028
aromatic dyes NOS Z77.028
arsenic Z77.010

Contact (with) - *continued*
asbestos Z77.090
bacterial disease NEC Z20.818
benzene Z77.021
blue-green algae bloom Z77.121
body fluids (potentially hazardous) Z77.21
brown tide Z77.121
chemicals (chiefly nonmedicinal) (hazardous) NEC Z77.098
cholera Z20.09
chromium compounds Z77.018
communicable disease Z20.9
bacterial NEC Z20.818
specified NEC Z20.89
viral NEC Z20.828
Zika virus Z20.821
cyanobacteria bloom Z77.121
dyes Z77.098
Escherichia coli (E. coli) Z20.01
fiberglass — *see* Table of Drugs and Chemicals, fiberglass
German measles Z20.4
gonorrhea Z20.2
hazardous metals NEC Z77.018
hazardous substances NEC Z77.29
hazards in the physical environment NEC Z77.128
hazards to health NEC Z77.9
HIV Z20.6
HTLV-III/LAV Z20.6
human immunodeficiency virus (HIV) Z20.6
infection Z20.9
specified NEC Z20.89
infestation (parasitic) NEC Z20.7
intestinal infectious disease NEC Z20.09
Escherichia coli (E. coli) Z20.01
lead Z77.011
meningococcus Z20.811
mold (toxic) Z77.120
nickel dust Z77.018
noise Z77.122
parasitic disease Z20.7
pediculosis Z20.7
pfiesteria piscicida Z77.121
poliomyelitis Z20.89
pollution
air Z77.110
environmental NEC Z77.118
soil Z77.112
water Z77.111
polycyclic aromatic hydrocarbons Z77.028
rabies Z20.3
radiation, naturally occurring NEC Z77.123
radon Z77.123
red tide (Florida) Z77.121
rubella Z20.4
sexually-transmitted disease Z20.2
smallpox (laboratory) Z20.89
syphilis Z20.2
tuberculosis Z20.1
uranium Z77.012
varicella Z20.820
venereal disease Z20.2
viral disease NEC Z20.828
viral hepatitis Z20.5
water pollution Z77.111
Zika virus Z20.821
Contamination, food — *see* Intoxication, foodborne
Contraception, contraceptive
advice Z30.09
counseling Z30.09
device (intrauterine) (in situ) Z97.5
causing menorrhagia T83.83
checking Z30.431
complications — *see* Complications, intrauterine, contraceptive device
in place Z97.5
initial prescription Z30.014
reinsertion Z30.433
removal Z30.432
replacement Z30.433
emergency (postcoital) Z30.012
initial prescription Z30.019
barrier Z30.018
diaphragm Z30.018
injectable Z30.013
intrauterine device Z30.014
pills Z30.011
postcoital (emergency) Z30.012
specified type NEC Z30.018
subdermal implantable Z30.017
transdermal patch hormonal Z30.016
vaginal ring hormonal Z30.015
maintenance Z30.40

Contraception, contraceptive - *continued*
maintenance - *continued*
barrier Z30.49
diaphragm Z30.49
examination Z30.8
injectable Z30.42
intrauterine device Z30.431
pills Z30.41
specified type NEC Z30.49
subdermal implantable Z30.46
transdermal patch hormonal Z30.45
vaginal ring hormonal Z30.44
management Z30.9
specified NEC Z30.8
postcoital (emergency) Z30.012
prescription Z30.019
repeat Z30.40
sterilization Z30.2
surveillance (drug) — *see* Contraception, maintenance
Contraction (s) , contracture, contracted
Achilles tendon — *see also* Short, tendon, Achilles
congenital Q66.89
amputation stump (surgical) (flexion) (late) (next proximal joint) T87.89
anus K59.8
bile duct (common) (hepatic) K83.8
bladder N32.89
neck or sphincter N32.0
bowel, cecum, colon or intestine, any part — *see* Obstruction, intestine
Braxton Hicks — *see* False, labor
breast implant, capsular T85.44
bronchial J98.09
burn (old) — *see* Cicatrix
cervix — *see* Stricture, cervix
cicatricial — *see* Cicatrix
conjunctiva, trachomatous, active A71.1
sequelae (late effect) B94.0
Dupuytren's M72.0
eyelid — *see* Disorder, eyelid function
fascia (lata) (postural) M72.8
Dupuytren's M72.0
palmar M72.0
plantar M72.2
finger NEC — *see also* Deformity, finger
congenital Q68.1
joint — *see* Contraction, joint, hand
flaccid — *see* Contraction, paralytic
gallbladder K82.0
heart valve — *see* Endocarditis
hip — *see* Contraction, joint, hip
hourglass
bladder N32.89
congenital Q64.79
gallbladder K82.0
congenital Q44.1
stomach K31.89
congenital Q40.2
psychogenic F45.8
uterus (complicating delivery) O62.4
hysterical F44.4
internal os — *see* Stricture, cervix
joint (abduction) (acquired) (adduction) (flexion) (rotation) M24.50
ankle M24.57-
congenital NEC Q68.8
hip Q65.89
elbow M24.52-
foot joint M24.57-
hand joint M24.54-
hip M24.55-
congenital Q65.89
hysterical F44.4
knee M24.56-
shoulder M24.51-
wrist M24.53-
kidney (granular) (secondary) N26.9
congenital Q63.8
hydronephritic — *see* Hydronephrosis
Page N26.2
pyelonephritic — *see* Pyelitis, chronic
tuberculous A18.11
ligament — *see also* Disorder, ligament
congenital Q79.8
muscle (postinfective) (postural) NEC M62.40
with contracture of joint — *see* Contraction, joint
ankle M62.47-
congenital Q79.8
sternocleidomastoid Q68.0
extraocular — *see* Strabismus
eye (extrinsic) — *see* Strabismus
foot M62.47-

Contraction (s) **, contracture, contracted** - *continued*
  muscle (postinfective) (postural) NEC - *continued*
    forearm M62.43-
    hand M62.44-
    hysterical F44.4
    ischemic (Volkmann's) T79.6
    lower leg M62.46-
    multiple sites M62.49
    pelvic region M62.45-
    posttraumatic — *see* Strabismus, paralytic
    psychogenic F45.8
      conversion reaction F44.4
    shoulder region M62.41-
    specified site NEC M62.48
    thigh M62.45-
    upper arm M62.42-
  neck — *see* Torticollis
  ocular muscle — *see* Strabismus
  organ or site, congenital NEC — *see* Atresia, by site
  outlet (pelvis) — *see* Contraction, pelvis
  palmar fascia M72.0
  paralytic
    joint — *see* Contraction, joint
    muscle — *see also* Contraction, muscle NEC
      ocular — *see* Strabismus, paralytic
  pelvis (acquired) (general) M95.5
    with disproportion (fetopelvic) O33.1
      causing obstructed labor O65.1
      inlet O33.2
      mid-cavity O33.3
      outlet O33.3
  plantar fascia M72.2
  premature
    atrium I49.1
    auriculoventricular I49.49
    heart I49.49
    junctional I49.2
    supraventricular I49.1
    ventricular I49.3
  prostate N42.89
  pylorus NEC — *see also* Pylorospasm
    psychogenic F45.8
  rectum, rectal (sphincter) K59.8
  ring (Bandl's) (complicating delivery) O62.4
  scar — *see* Cicatrix
  spine — *see* Dorsopathy, deforming
  sternocleidomastoid (muscle) , congenital Q68.0
  stomach K31.89
    hourglass K31.89
      congenital Q40.2
      psychogenic F45.8
    psychogenic F45.8
  tendon (sheath) M62.40
    with contracture of joint — *see* Contraction, joint
    Achilles — *see* Short, tendon, Achilles
    ankle M62.47-
      Achilles — *see* Short, tendon, Achilles
    foot M62.47-
    forearm M62.43-
    hand M62.44-
    lower leg M62.46-
    multiple sites M62.49
    neck M62.48
    pelvic region M62.45-
    shoulder region M62.41-
    specified site NEC M62.48
    thigh M62.45-
    thorax M62.48
    trunk M62.48
    upper arm M62.42-
  toe — *see* Deformity, toe, specified NEC
  ureterovesical orifice (postinfectional) N13.5
    with infection N13.6
  urethra — *see also* Stricture, urethra
    orifice N32.0
  uterus N85.8
    abnormal NEC O62.9
    clonic (complicating delivery) O62.4
    dyscoordinate (complicating delivery) O62.4
    hourglass (complicating delivery) O62.4
    hypertonic O62.4
    hypotonic NEC O62.2
    inadequate
      primary O62.0
      secondary O62.1
    incoordinate (complicating delivery) O62.4
    poor O62.2
    tetanic (complicating delivery) O62.4
  vagina (outlet) N89.5
  vesical N32.89
    neck or urethral orifice N32.0
  visual field — *see* Defect, visual field, generalized

Contraction (s) **, contracture, contracted** - *continued*
  Volkmann's (ischemic) T79.6

Contusion (skin surface intact) T14.8
  abdomen, abdominal (muscle) (wall) S30.1
  adnexa, eye NEC S05.8X-
  adrenal gland S37.812
  alveolar process S00.532
  ankle S90.0-
  antecubital space — *see* Contusion, forearm
  anus S30.3
  arm (upper) S40.02-
    lower (with elbow) — *see* Contusion, forearm
  auditory canal — *see* Contusion, ear
  auricle — *see* Contusion, ear
  axilla — *see* Contusion, arm, upper
  back — *see also* Contusion, thorax, back
    lower S30.0
  bile duct S36.13
  bladder S37.22
  bone NEC T14.8
  brain (diffuse) — *see* Injury, intracranial, diffuse
    focal — *see* Injury, intracranial, focal
  brainstem S06.38-
  breast S20.0-
  broad ligament S37.892
  brow S00.83
  buttock S30.0
  canthus, eye S00.1-
  cauda equina S34.3
  cerebellar, traumatic S06.37-
  cerebral S06.33-
    left side S06.32-
    right side S06.31-
  cheek S00.83
    internal S00.532
  chest (wall) — *see* Contusion, thorax
  chin S00.83
  clitoris S30.23
  colon — *see* Injury, intestine, large, contusion
  common bile duct S36.13
  conjunctiva S05.1-
    with foreign body (in conjunctival sac) — *see* Foreign body, conjunctival sac
  conus medullaris (spine) S34.139
  cornea — *see* Contusion, eyeball
    with foreign body — *see* Foreign body, cornea
  corpus cavernosum S30.21
  cortex (brain) (cerebral) — *see* Injury, intracranial, diffuse
    focal — *see* Injury, intracranial, focal
  costal region — *see* Contusion, thorax
  cystic duct S36.13
  diaphragm S27.802
  duodenum S36.420
  ear S00.43-
  elbow S50.0-
    with forearm — *see* Contusion, forearm
  epididymis S30.22
  epigastric region S30.1
  epiglottis S10.0
  esophagus (thoracic) S27.812
    cervical S10.0
  eyeball S05.1-
  eyebrow S00.1-
  eyelid (and periocular area) S00.1-
  face NEC S00.83
  fallopian tube S37.529
    bilateral S37.522
    unilateral S37.521
  femoral triangle S30.1
  finger (s) S60.00
    with damage to nail (matrix) S60.10
    index S60.02-
      with damage to nail S60.12-
    little S60.05-
      with damage to nail S60.15-
    middle S60.03-
      with damage to nail S60.13-
    ring S60.04-
      with damage to nail S60.14-
    thumb — *see* Contusion, thumb
  flank S30.1
  foot (except toe (s) alone) S90.3-
    toe — *see* Contusion, toe
  forearm S50.1-
    elbow only — *see* Contusion, elbow
  forehead S00.83
  gallbladder S36.122
  genital organs, external
    female S30.202
    male S30.201
  globe (eye) — *see* Contusion, eyeball

Contusion (skin surface intact) - *continued*
  groin S30.1
  gum S00.532
  hand S60.22-
    finger (s) — *see* Contusion, finger
    wrist — *see* Contusion, wrist
  head S00.93
    ear — *see* Contusion, ear
    eyelid — *see* Contusion, eyelid
    lip S00.531
    nose S00.33
    oral cavity S00.532
    scalp S00.03
    specified part NEC S00.83
  heart — *see also* Injury, heart S26.91
  heel — *see* Contusion, foot
  hepatic duct S36.13
  hip S70.0-
  ileum S36.428
  iliac region S30.1
  inguinal region S30.1
  interscapular region S20.229
  intra-abdominal organ S36.92
    colon — *see* Injury, intestine, large, contusion
    liver S36.112
    pancreas — *see* Contusion, pancreas
    rectum S36.62
    small intestine — *see* Injury, intestine, small, contusion
    specified organ NEC S36.892
    spleen — *see* Contusion, spleen
    stomach S36.32
  iris (eye) — *see* Contusion, eyeball
  jaw S00.83
  jejunum S36.428
  kidney S37.01-
    major (greater than 2 cm) S37.02-
    minor (less than 2 cm) S37.01-
  knee S80.0-
  labium (majus) (minus) S30.23
  lacrimal apparatus, gland or sac S05.8X-
  larynx S10.0
  leg (lower) S80.1-
    knee — *see* Contusion, knee
  lens — *see* Contusion, eyeball
  lip S00.531
  liver S36.112
  lower back S30.0
  lumbar region S30.0
  lung S27.329
    bilateral S27.322
    unilateral S27.321
  malar region S00.83
  mastoid region S00.83
  membrane, brain — *see* Injury, intracranial, diffuse
    focal — *see* Injury, intracranial, focal
  mesentery S36.892
  mesosalpinx S37.892
  mouth S00.532
  muscle — *see* Contusion, by site
  nail
    finger — *see* Contusion, finger, with damage to nail
    toe — *see* Contusion, toe, with damage to nail
  nasal S00.33
  neck S10.93
    specified site NEC S10.83
    throat S10.0
  nerve — *see* Injury, nerve
  newborn P54.5
  nose S00.33
  occipital
    lobe (brain) — *see* Injury, intracranial, diffuse
      focal — *see* Injury, intracranial, focal
    region (scalp) S00.03
  orbit (region) (tissues) S05.1-
  ovary S37.429
    bilateral S37.422
    unilateral S37.421
  palate S00.532
  pancreas S36.229
    body S36.221
    head S36.220
    tail S36.222
  parietal
    lobe (brain) — *see* Injury, intracranial, diffuse
      focal — *see* Injury, intracranial, focal
    region (scalp) S00.03
  pelvic organ S37.92
    adrenal gland S37.812
    bladder S37.22
    fallopian tube — *see* Contusion, fallopian tube
    kidney — *see* Contusion, kidney

Contusion (skin surface intact) - *continued*
  pelvic organ - *continued*
    ovary — *see* Contusion, ovary
    prostate S37.822
    specified organ NEC S37.892
    ureter S37.12
    urethra S37.32
    uterus S37.62
  pelvis S30.0
  penis S30.21
  perineum
    female S30.23
    male S30.0
  periocular area S00.1-
  peritoneum S36.81
  periurethral tissue — *see* Contusion, urethra
  pharynx S10.0
  pinna — *see* Contusion, ear
  popliteal space — *see* Contusion, knee
  prepuce S30.21
  prostate S37.822
  pubic region S30.1
  pudendum
    female S30.202
    male S30.201
  quadriceps femoris — *see* Contusion, thigh
  rectum S36.62
  retroperitoneum S36.892
  round ligament S37.892
  sacral region S30.0
  scalp S00.03
    due to birth injury P12.3
  scapular region — *see* Contusion, shoulder
  sclera — *see* Contusion, eyeball
  scrotum S30.22
  seminal vesicle S37.892
  shoulder S40.01-
  skin NEC T14.8
  small intestine — *see* Injury, intestine, small, contusion
  spermatic cord S30.22
  spinal cord — *see* Injury, spinal cord, by region
    cauda equina S34.3
    conus medullaris S34.139
  spleen S36.029
    major S36.021
    minor S36.020
  sternal region S20.219
  stomach S36.32
  subconjunctival S05.1-
  subcutaneous NEC T14.8
  submaxillary region S00.83
  submental region S00.83
  subperiosteal NEC T14.8
  subungual
    finger — *see* Contusion, finger, with damage to nail
    toe — *see* Contusion, toe, with damage to nail
  supraclavicular fossa S10.83
  supraorbital S00.83
  suprarenal gland S37.812
  temple (region) S00.83
  temporal
    lobe (brain) — *see* Injury, intracranial, diffuse
      focal — *see* Injury, intracranial, focal
    region S00.83
  testis S30.22
  thigh S70.1-
  thorax (wall) S20.20
    back S20.22-
    front S20.21-
  throat S10.0
  thumb S60.01-
    with damage to nail S60.11-
  toe (s) (lesser) S90.12-
    with damage to nail S90.22-
    great S90.11-
      with damage to nail S90.21-
  tongue S00.532
  trachea (cervical) S10.0
    thoracic S27.52
  tunica vaginalis S30.22
  tympanum, tympanic membrane — *see* Contusion, ear
  ureter S37.12
  urethra S37.32
  urinary organ NEC S37.892
  uterus S37.62
  uvula S00.532
  vagina S30.23
  vas deferens S37.892
  vesical S37.22
  vocal cord (s) S10.0

Contusion (skin surface intact) - *continued*
  vulva S30.23
  wrist S60.21-
Conus (congenital) (any type) Q14.8
  cornea — *see* Keratoconus
  medullaris syndrome G95.81
Conversion hysteria, neurosis or reaction F44.9
Converter, tuberculosis (test reaction) R76.11
Conviction (legal) **, anxiety concerning** Z65.0
  with imprisonment Z65.1
Convulsions (idiopathic) — *see also* Seizure(s) R56.9
  apoplectiform (cerebral ischemia) I67.82
  dissociative F44.5
  epileptic — *see* Epilepsy
  epileptiform, epileptoid — *see* Seizure, epileptiform
  ether (anesthetic) — *see* Table of Drugs and Chemicals, by drug
  febrile R56.00
    with status epilepticus G40.901
    complex R56.01
      with status epilepticus G40.901
    simple R56.00
  hysterical F44.5
  infantile P90
    epilepsy — *see* Epilepsy
  jacksonian — *see* Epilepsy, localization-related, symptomatic, with simple partial seizures
  myoclonic G25.3
  newborn P90
  obstetrical (nephritic) (uremic) — *see* Eclampsia
  paretic A52.17
  post traumatic R56.1
  psychomotor — *see* Epilepsy, localization-related, symptomatic, with complex partial seizures
  recurrent R56.9
  reflex R25.8
  scarlatinal A38.8
  tetanus, tetanic — *see* Tetanus
  thymic E32.8
Convulsive — *see also* Convulsions
Cooley's anemia D56.1
Coolie itch B76.9
Cooper's
  disease — *see* Mastopathy, cystic
  hernia — *see* Hernia, abdomen, specified site NEC
Copra itch B88.0
Coprophagy F50.89
Coprophobia F40.298
Coproporphyria, hereditary E80.29
Cor
  biloculare Q20.8
  bovis, bovinum — *see* Hypertrophy, cardiac
  pulmonale (chronic) I27.81
    acute I26.09
  triatriatum, triatrium Q24.2
  triloculare Q20.8
    biatrium Q20.4
    biventriculare Q21.1
Corbus' disease (gangrenous balanitis) N48.1
Cord — *see also* condition
  around neck
    complicating delivery O69.81
      with compression O69.1
  bladder G95.89
    tabetic A52.19
Cordis ectopia Q24.8
Corditis (spermatic) N49.1
Corectopia Q13.2
Cori's disease (glycogen storage) E74.03
Corkhandler's disease or lung J67.3
Corkscrew esophagus K22.4
Corkworker's disease or lung J67.3
Corn (infected) L84
Cornea — *see also* condition
  donor Z52.5
  plana Q13.4
Cornelia de Lange syndrome Q87.1
Cornu cutaneum L85.8
Cornual gestation or pregnancy O00.80
  with intrauterine pregnancy O00.81
Coronary (artery) — *see* condition
Coronavirus, as cause of disease classified elsewhere B97.29
  SARS-associated B97.21
Corpora — *see also* condition
  amylacea, prostate N42.89
  cavernosa — *see* condition
Corpulence — *see* Obesity
Corpus — *see* condition
Corrected transposition Q20.5
Corrosion (injury) (acid) (caustic) (chemical) (lime) (external) (internal) T30.4
  abdomen, abdominal (muscle) (wall) T21.42

Corrosion (injury) (acid) (caustic) (chemical) (lime) (external) (internal) - *continued*
  abdomen, abdominal (muscle) (wall) - *continued*
    first degree T21.52
    second degree T21.62
    third degree T21.72
  above elbow T22.439
    first degree T22.539
    left T22.432
      first degree T22.532
      second degree T22.632
      third degree T22.732
    right T22.431
      first degree T22.531
      second degree T22.631
      third degree T22.731
    second degree T22.639
    third degree T22.739
  alimentary tract NEC T28.7
  ankle T25.419
    first degree T25.519
    left T25.412
      first degree T25.512
      second degree T25.612
      third degree T25.712
    multiple with foot — *see* Corrosion, lower, limb, multiple, ankle and foot
    right T25.411
      first degree T25.511
      second degree T25.611
      third degree T25.711
    second degree T25.619
    third degree T25.719
  anus — *see* Corrosion, buttock
  arm (s) (meaning upper limb (s)) — *see* Corrosion, upper limb
  axilla T22.449
    first degree T22.549
    left T22.442
      first degree T22.542
      second degree T22.642
      third degree T22.742
    right T22.441
      first degree T22.541
      second degree T22.641
      third degree T22.741
    second degree T22.649
    third degree T22.749
  back (lower) T21.44
    first degree T21.54
    second degree T21.64
    third degree T21.74
    upper T21.43
      first degree T21.53
      second degree T21.63
      third degree T21.73
  blisters - code as Corrosion, second degree, by site
  breast (s) — *see* Corrosion, chest wall
  buttock (s) T21.45
    first degree T21.55
    second degree T21.65
    third degree T21.75
  calf T24.439
    first degree T24.539
    left T24.432
      first degree T24.532
      second degree T24.632
      third degree T24.732
    right T24.431
      first degree T24.531
      second degree T24.631
      third degree T24.731
    second degree T24.639
    third degree T24.739
  canthus (eye) — *see* Corrosion, eyelid
  cervix T28.8
  cheek T20.46
    first degree T20.56
    second degree T20.66
    third degree T20.76
  chest wall T21.41
    first degree T21.51
    second degree T21.61
    third degree T21.71
  chin T20.43
    first degree T20.53
    second degree T20.63
    third degree T20.73
  colon T28.7
  conjunctiva (and cornea) — *see* Corrosion, cornea
  cornea (and conjunctiva) T26.6-
  deep necrosis of underlying tissue - code as Corrosion, third degree, by site

- **Corrosion** (injury) (acid) (caustic) (chemical) (lime) (external) (internal) - *continued*
  - dorsum of hand T23.469
    - first degree T23.569
    - left T23.462
      - first degree T23.562
      - second degree T23.662
      - third degree T23.762
    - right T23.461
      - first degree T23.561
      - second degree T23.661
      - third degree T23.761
    - second degree T23.669
    - third degree T23.769
  - ear (auricle) (external) (canal) T20.41
    - drum T28.91
    - first degree T20.51
    - second degree T20.61
    - third degree T20.71
  - elbow T22.429
    - first degree T22.529
    - left T22.422
      - first degree T22.522
      - second degree T22.622
      - third degree T22.722
    - right T22.421
      - first degree T22.521
      - second degree T22.621
      - third degree T22.721
    - second degree T22.629
    - third degree T22.729
  - entire body — *see* Corrosion, multiple body regions
  - epidermal loss - code as Corrosion, second degree, by site
  - epiglottis T27.4
  - erythema, erythematous - code as Corrosion, first degree, by site
  - esophagus T28.6
  - extent (percentage of body surface)
    - less than 10 percent T32.0
    - 10-19 percent (0-9 percent third degree) T32.10
      - with 10-19 percent third degree T32.11
    - 20-29 percent (0-9 percent third degree) T32.20
      - with
        - 10-19 percent third degree T32.21
        - 20-29 percent third degree T32.22
    - 30-39 percent (0-9 percent third degree) T32.30
      - with
        - 10-19 percent third degree T32.31
        - 20-29 percent third degree T32.32
        - 30-39 percent third degree T32.33
    - 40-49 percent (0-9 percent third degree) T32.40
      - with
        - 10-19 percent third degree T32.41
        - 20-29 percent third degree T32.42
        - 30-39 percent third degree T32.43
        - 40-49 percent third degree T32.44
    - 50-59 percent (0-9 percent third degree) T32.50
      - with
        - 10-19 percent third degree T32.51
        - 20-29 percent third degree T32.52
        - 30-39 percent third degree T32.53
        - 40-49 percent third degree T32.54
        - 50-59 percent third degree T32.55
    - 60-69 percent (0-9 percent third degree) T32.60
      - with
        - 10-19 percent third degree T32.61
        - 20-29 percent third degree T32.62
        - 30-39 percent third degree T32.63
        - 40-49 percent third degree T32.64
        - 50-59 percent third degree T32.65
        - 60-69 percent third degree T32.66
    - 70-79 percent (0-9 percent third degree) T32.70
      - with
        - 10-19 percent third degree T32.71
        - 20-29 percent third degree T32.72
        - 30-39 percent third degree T32.73
        - 40-49 percent third degree T32.74
        - 50-59 percent third degree T32.75
        - 60-69 percent third degree T32.76
        - 70-79 percent third degree T32.77
    - 80-89 percent (0-9 percent third degree) T32.80
      - with
        - 10-19 percent third degree T32.81
        - 20-29 percent third degree T32.82
        - 30-39 percent third degree T32.83
        - 40-49 percent third degree T32.84
        - 50-59 percent third degree T32.85
        - 60-69 percent third degree T32.86
        - 70-79 percent third degree T32.87
        - 80-89 percent third degree T32.88
    - 90 percent or more (0-9 percent third degree) T32.90

- **Corrosion** (injury) (acid) (caustic) (chemical) (lime) (external) (internal) - *continued*
  - extent (percentage of body surface) - *continued*
    - 90 percent or more (0-9 percent third degree) - *continued*
      - with
        - 10-19 percent third degree T32.91
        - 20-29 percent third degree T32.92
        - 30-39 percent third degree T32.93
        - 40-49 percent third degree T32.94
        - 50-59 percent third degree T32.95
        - 60-69 percent third degree T32.96
        - 70-79 percent third degree T32.97
        - 80-89 percent third degree T32.98
        - 90-99 percent third degree T32.99
  - extremity — *see* Corrosion, limb
  - eye (s) and adnexa T26.9-
    - with resulting rupture and destruction of eyeball T26.7-
    - conjunctival sac — *see* Corrosion, cornea
    - cornea — *see* Corrosion, cornea
    - lid — *see* Corrosion, eyelid
    - periocular area — *see* Corrosion eyelid
    - specified site NEC T26.8-
  - eyeball — *see* Corrosion, eye
  - eyelid (s) T26.5-
  - face — *see* Corrosion, head
  - finger T23.429
    - first degree T23.529
    - left T23.422
      - first degree T23.522
      - second degree T23.622
      - third degree T23.722
    - multiple sites (without thumb) T23.439
      - with thumb T23.449
        - first degree T23.549
        - left T23.442
          - first degree T23.542
          - second degree T23.642
          - third degree T23.742
        - right T23.441
          - first degree T23.541
          - second degree T23.641
          - third degree T23.741
        - second degree T23.649
        - third degree T23.749
      - first degree T23.539
      - left T23.432
        - first degree T23.532
        - second degree T23.632
        - third degree T23.732
      - right T23.431
        - first degree T23.531
        - second degree T23.631
        - third degree T23.731
      - second degree T23.639
      - third degree T23.739
    - right T23.421
      - first degree T23.521
      - second degree T23.621
      - third degree T23.721
    - second degree T23.629
    - third degree T23.729
  - flank — *see* Corrosion, abdomen
  - foot T25.429
    - first degree T25.529
    - left T25.422
      - first degree T25.522
      - second degree T25.622
      - third degree T25.722
    - multiple with ankle — *see* Corrosion, lower, limb, multiple, ankle and foot
    - right T25.421
      - first degree T25.521
      - second degree T25.621
      - third degree T25.721
    - second degree T25.629
    - third degree T25.729
  - forearm T22.419
    - first degree T22.519
    - left T22.412
      - first degree T22.512
      - second degree T22.612
      - third degree T22.712
    - right T22.411
      - first degree T22.511
      - second degree T22.611
      - third degree T22.711
    - second degree T22.619
    - third degree T22.719
  - forehead T20.46
    - first degree T20.56
    - second degree T20.66

- **Corrosion** (injury) (acid) (caustic) (chemical) (lime) (external) (internal) - *continued*
  - forehead - *continued*
    - third degree T20.76
  - fourth degree - code as Corrosion, third degree, by site
  - full thickness skin loss - code as Corrosion, third degree, by site
  - gastrointestinal tract NEC T28.7
  - genital organs
    - external
      - female T21.47
        - first degree T21.57
        - second degree T21.67
        - third degree T21.77
      - male T21.46
        - first degree T21.56
        - second degree T21.66
        - third degree T21.76
    - internal T28.8
  - groin — *see* Corrosion, abdominal wall
  - hand (s) T23.409
    - back — *see* Corrosion, dorsum of hand
    - finger — *see* Corrosion, finger
    - first degree T23.509
    - left T23.402
      - first degree T23.502
      - second degree T23.602
      - third degree T23.702
    - multiple sites with wrist T23.499
      - first degree T23.599
      - left T23.492
        - first degree T23.592
        - second degree T23.692
        - third degree T23.792
      - right T23.491
        - first degree T23.591
        - second degree T23.691
        - third degree T23.791
      - second degree T23.699
      - third degree T23.799
    - palm — *see* Corrosion, palm
    - right T23.401
      - first degree T23.501
      - second degree T23.601
      - third degree T23.701
    - second degree T23.609
    - third degree T23.709
    - thumb — *see* Corrosion, thumb
  - head (and face) (and neck) T20.40
    - cheek — *see* Corrosion, cheek
    - chin — *see* Corrosion, chin
    - ear — *see* Corrosion, ear
    - eye (s) only — *see* Corrosion, eye
    - first degree T20.50
    - forehead — *see* Corrosion, forehead
    - lip — *see* Corrosion, lip
    - multiple sites T20.49
      - first degree T20.59
      - second degree T20.69
      - third degree T20.79
    - neck — *see* Corrosion, neck
    - nose — *see* Corrosion, nose
    - scalp — *see* Corrosion, scalp
    - second degree T20.60
    - third degree T20.70
  - hip (s) — *see* Corrosion, lower, limb
  - inhalation — *see* Corrosion, respiratory tract
  - internal organ (s) — *see also* Corrosion, by site T28.90
    - alimentary tract T28.7
      - esophagus T28.6
    - esophagus T28.6
    - genitourinary T28.8
    - mouth T28.5
    - pharynx T28.5
    - specified organ NEC T28.99
  - interscapular region — *see* Corrosion, back, upper
  - intestine (large) (small) T28.7
  - knee T24.429
    - first degree T24.529
    - left T24.422
      - first degree T24.522
      - second degree T24.622
      - third degree T24.722
    - right T24.421
      - first degree T24.521
      - second degree T24.621
      - third degree T24.721
    - second degree T24.629
    - third degree T24.729
  - labium (majus) (minus) — *see* Corrosion, genital organs, external, female

Corrosion (injury) (acid) (caustic) (chemical) (lime) (external) (internal) - *continued*
- lacrimal apparatus, duct, gland or sac — *see* Corrosion, eye, specified site NEC
- larynx T27.4
  - with lung T27.5
- leg (s) (meaning lower limb (s)) — *see* Corrosion, lower limb
- limb (s)
  - lower — *see* Corrosion, lower, limb
  - upper — *see* Corrosion, upper limb
- lip (s) T20.42
  - first degree T20.52
  - second degree T20.62
  - third degree T20.72
- lower
  - back — *see* Corrosion, back
  - limb T24.409
    - ankle — *see* Corrosion, ankle
    - calf — *see* Corrosion, calf
    - first degree T24.509
    - foot — *see* Corrosion, foot
    - knee — *see* Corrosion, knee
    - left T24.402
      - first degree T24.502
      - second degree T24.602
      - third degree T24.702
    - multiple sites, except ankle and foot T24.499
      - ankle and foot T25.499
        - first degree T25.599
        - left T25.492
          - first degree T25.592
          - second degree T25.692
          - third degree T25.792
        - right T25.491
          - first degree T25.591
          - second degree T25.691
          - third degree T25.791
        - second degree T25.699
        - third degree T25.799
      - first degree T24.599
      - left T24.492
        - first degree T24.592
        - second degree T24.692
        - third degree T24.792
      - right T24.491
        - first degree T24.591
        - second degree T24.691
        - third degree T24.791
      - second degree T24.699
      - third degree T24.799
    - right T24.401
      - first degree T24.501
      - second degree T24.601
      - third degree T24.701
    - second degree T24.609
    - hip — *see* Corrosion, thigh
    - thigh — *see* Corrosion, thigh
    - third degree T24.709
- lung (with larynx and trachea) T27.5
- mouth T28.5
- neck T20.47
  - first degree T20.57
  - second degree T20.67
  - third degree T20.77
- nose (septum) T20.44
  - first degree T20.54
  - second degree T20.64
  - third degree T20.74
- ocular adnexa — *see* Corrosion, eye
- orbit region — *see* Corrosion, eyelid
- palm T23.459
  - first degree T23.559
  - left T23.452
    - first degree T23.552
    - second degree T23.652
    - third degree T23.752
  - right T23.451
    - first degree T23.551
    - second degree T23.651
    - third degree T23.751
  - second degree T23.659
  - third degree T23.759
- partial thickness - code as Corrosion, unspecified degree, by site
- pelvis — *see* Corrosion, trunk
- penis — *see* Corrosion, genital organs, external, male
- perineum
  - female — *see* Corrosion, genital organs, external, female
  - male — *see* Corrosion, genital organs, external, male

Corrosion (injury) (acid) (caustic) (chemical) (lime) (external) (internal) - *continued*
- periocular area — *see* Corrosion, eyelid
- pharynx T28.5
- rectum T28.7
- respiratory tract T27.7
  - larynx — *see* Corrosion, larynx
  - specified part NEC T27.6
  - trachea — *see* Corrosion, larynx
- sac, lacrimal — *see* Corrosion, eye, specified site NEC
- scalp T20.45
  - first degree T20.55
  - second degree T20.65
  - third degree T20.75
- scapular region T22.469
  - first degree T22.569
  - left T22.462
    - first degree T22.562
    - second degree T22.662
    - third degree T22.762
  - right T22.461
    - first degree T22.561
    - second degree T22.661
    - third degree T22.761
  - second degree T22.669
  - third degree T22.769
- sclera — *see* Corrosion, eye, specified site NEC
- scrotum — *see* Corrosion, genital organs, external, male
- shoulder T22.459
  - first degree T22.559
  - left T22.452
    - first degree T22.552
    - second degree T22.652
    - third degree T22.752
  - right T22.451
    - first degree T22.551
    - second degree T22.651
    - third degree T22.751
  - second degree T22.659
  - third degree T22.759
- stomach T28.7
- temple — *see* Corrosion, head
- testis — *see* Corrosion, genital organs, external, male
- thigh T24.419
  - first degree T24.519
  - left T24.412
    - first degree T24.512
    - second degree T24.612
    - third degree T24.712
  - right T24.411
    - first degree T24.511
    - second degree T24.611
    - third degree T24.711
  - second degree T24.619
  - third degree T24.719
- thorax (external) — *see* Corrosion, trunk
- throat (meaning pharynx) T28.5
- thumb (s) T23.419
  - first degree T23.519
  - left T23.412
    - first degree T23.512
    - second degree T23.612
    - third degree T23.712
  - multiple sites with fingers T23.449
    - first degree T23.549
    - left T23.442
      - first degree T23.542
      - second degree T23.642
      - third degree T23.742
    - right T23.441
      - first degree T23.541
      - second degree T23.641
      - third degree T23.741
    - second degree T23.649
    - third degree T23.749
  - right T23.411
    - first degree T23.511
    - second degree T23.611
    - third degree T23.711
  - second degree T23.619
  - third degree T23.719
- toe T25.439
  - first degree T25.539
  - left T25.432
    - first degree T25.532
    - second degree T25.632
    - third degree T25.732
  - right T25.431
    - first degree T25.531
    - second degree T25.631

Corrosion (injury) (acid) (caustic) (chemical) (lime) (external) (internal) - *continued*
- toe - *continued*
  - right - *continued*
    - third degree T25.731
  - second degree T25.639
  - third degree T25.739
- tongue T28.5
- tonsil (s) T28.5
- total body — *see* Corrosion, multiple body regions
- trachea T27.4
  - with lung T27.5
- trunk T21.40
  - abdominal wall — *see* Corrosion, abdominal wall
  - anus — *see* Corrosion, buttock
  - axilla — *see* Corrosion, upper limb
  - back — *see* Corrosion, back
  - breast — *see* Corrosion, chest wall
  - buttock — *see* Corrosion, buttock
  - chest wall — *see* Corrosion, chest wall
  - first degree T21.50
  - flank — *see* Corrosion, abdominal wall
  - genital
    - female — *see* Corrosion, genital organs, external, female
    - male — *see* Corrosion, genital organs, external, male
  - groin — *see* Corrosion, abdominal wall
  - interscapular region — *see* Corrosion, back, upper
  - labia — *see* Corrosion, genital organs, external, female
  - lower back — *see* Corrosion, back
  - penis — *see* Corrosion, genital organs, external, male
  - perineum
    - female — *see* Corrosion, genital organs, external, female
    - male — *see* Corrosion, genital organs, external, male
  - scapular region — *see* Corrosion, upper limb
  - scrotum — *see* Corrosion, genital organs, external, male
  - second degree T21.60
  - shoulder — *see* Corrosion, upper limb
  - specified site NEC T21.49
    - first degree T21.59
    - second degree T21.69
    - third degree T21.79
  - testes — *see* Corrosion, genital organs, external, male
  - third degree T21.70
  - upper back — *see* Corrosion, back, upper
  - vagina T28.8
  - vulva — *see* Corrosion, genital organs, external, female
- unspecified site with extent of body surface involved specified
  - less than 10 percent T32.0
  - 10-19 percent (0-9 percent third degree) T32.10
    - with 10-19 percent third degree T32.11
  - 20-29 percent (0-9 percent third degree) T32.20
    - with
      - 10-19 percent third degree T32.21
      - 20-29 percent third degree T32.22
  - 30-39 percent (0-9 percent third degree) T32.30
    - with
      - 10-19 percent third degree T32.31
      - 20-29 percent third degree T32.32
      - 30-39 percent third degree T32.33
  - 40-49 percent (0-9 percent third degree) T32.40
    - with
      - 10-19 percent third degree T32.41
      - 20-29 percent third degree T32.42
      - 30-39 percent third degree T32.43
      - 40-49 percent third degree T32.44
  - 50-59 percent (0-9 percent third degree) T32.50
    - with
      - 10-19 percent third degree T32.51
      - 20-29 percent third degree T32.52
      - 30-39 percent third degree T32.53
      - 40-49 percent third degree T32.54
      - 50-59 percent third degree T32.55
  - 60-69 percent (0-9 percent third degree) T32.60
    - with
      - 10-19 percent third degree T32.61
      - 20-29 percent third degree T32.62
      - 30-39 percent third degree T32.63
      - 40-49 percent third degree T32.64
      - 50-59 percent third degree T32.65
      - 60-69 percent third degree T32.66
  - 70-79 percent (0-9 percent third degree) T32.70
    - with
      - 10-19 percent third degree T32.71

Corrosion (injury) (acid) (caustic) (chemical) (lime) (external) (internal) - *continued*
unspecified site with extent of body surface involved specified - *continued*
70-79 percent (0-9 percent third degree) - *continued*
with - *continued*
20-29 percent third degree T32.72
30-39 percent third degree T32.73
40-49 percent third degree T32.74
50-59 percent third degree T32.75
60-69 percent third degree T32.76
70-79 percent third degree T32.77
80-89 percent (0-9 percent third degree) T32.80
with
10-19 percent third degree T32.81
20-29 percent third degree T32.82
30-39 percent third degree T32.83
40-49 percent third degree T32.84
50-59 percent third degree T32.85
60-69 percent third degree T32.86
70-79 percent third degree T32.87
80-89 percent third degree T32.88
90 percent or more (0-9 percent third degree) T32.90
with
10-19 percent third degree T32.91
20-29 percent third degree T32.92
30-39 percent third degree T32.93
40-49 percent third degree T32.94
50-59 percent third degree T32.95
60-69 percent third degree T32.96
70-79 percent third degree T32.97
80-89 percent third degree T32.98
90-99 percent third degree T32.99
upper limb (axilla) (scapular region) T22.40
above elbow — *see* Corrosion, above elbow
axilla — *see* Corrosion, axilla
elbow — *see* Corrosion, elbow
first degree T22.50
forearm — *see* Corrosion, forearm
hand — *see* Corrosion, hand
interscapular region — *see* Corrosion, back, upper
multiple sites T22.499
first degree T22.599
left T22.492
first degree T22.592
second degree T22.692
third degree T22.792
right T22.491
first degree T22.591
second degree T22.691
third degree T22.791
second degree T22.699
third degree T22.799
scapular region — *see* Corrosion, scapular region
second degree T22.60
shoulder — *see* Corrosion, shoulder
third degree T22.70
wrist — *see* Corrosion, hand
uterus T28.8
vagina T28.8
vulva — *see* Corrosion, genital organs, external, female
wrist T23.479
first degree T23.579
left T23.472
first degree T23.572
second degree T23.672
third degree T23.772
multiple sites with hand T23.499
first degree T23.599
left T23.492
first degree T23.592
second degree T23.692
third degree T23.792
right T23.491
first degree T23.591
second degree T23.691
third degree T23.791
second degree T23.699
third degree T23.799
right T23.471
first degree T23.571
second degree T23.671
third degree T23.771
second degree T23.679
third degree T23.779
Corrosive burn — *see* Corrosion
Corsican fever — *see* Malaria
Cortical — *see* condition
Cortico-adrenal — *see* condition

Coryza (acute) J00
with grippe or influenza — *see* Influenza, with, respiratory manifestations NEC
syphilitic
congenital (chronic) A50.05
Costen's syndrome or complex M26.69
Costiveness — *see* Constipation
Costochondritis M94.0
Cot death R99
Cotard's syndrome F22
Cotia virus B08.8
Cotton wool spots (retinal) H35.81
Cotungo's disease — *see* Sciatica
Cough (affected) (chronic) (epidemic) (nervous) R05
with hemorrhage — *see* Hemoptysis
bronchial R05
with grippe or influenza — *see* Influenza, with, respiratory manifestations NEC
functional F45.8
hysterical F45.8
laryngeal, spasmodic R05
psychogenic F45.8
smokers' J41.0
tea taster's B49
Counseling (for) Z71.9
abuse NEC
perpetrator Z69.82
victim Z69.81
alcohol abuser Z71.41
family Z71.42
child abuse
nonparental
perpetrator Z69.021
victim Z69.020
parental
perpetrator Z69.011
victim Z69.010
consanguinity Z71.89
contraceptive Z30.09
dietary Z71.3
drug abuser Z71.51
family member Z71.52
exercise Z71.82
family Z71.89
fertility preservation (prior to cancer therapy) (prior to removal of gonads) Z31.62
for non-attending third party Z71.0
related to sexual behavior or orientation Z70.2
genetic
nonprocreative Z71.83
procreative NEC Z31.5
gestational carrier Z31.7
health (advice) (education) (instruction) — *see* Counseling, medical
human immunodeficiency virus (HIV) Z71.7
impotence Z70.1
insulin pump use Z46.81
medical (for) Z71.9
boarding school resident Z59.3
consanguinity Z71.89
feared complaint and no disease found Z71.1
human immunodeficiency virus (HIV) Z71.7
institutional resident Z59.3
on behalf of another Z71.0
related to sexual behavior or orientation Z70.2
person living alone Z60.2
specified reason NEC Z71.89
natural family planning
procreative Z31.61
to avoid pregnancy Z30.02
perpetrator (of)
abuse NEC Z69.82
child abuse
non-parental Z69.021
parental Z69.011
rape NEC Z69.82
spousal abuse Z69.12
procreative NEC Z31.69
fertility preservation (prior to cancer therapy) (prior to removal of gonads) Z31.62
using natural family planning Z31.61
promiscuity Z70.1
rape victim Z69.81
religious Z71.81
sex, sexual (related to) Z70.9
attitude (s) Z70.0
behavior or orientation Z70.1
combined concerns Z70.3
non-responsiveness Z70.1
on behalf of third party Z70.2
specified reason NEC Z70.8
specified reason NEC Z71.89
spiritual Z71.81

Counseling (for) - *continued*
spousal abuse (perpetrator) Z69.12
victim Z69.11
substance abuse Z71.89
alcohol Z71.41
drug Z71.51
tobacco Z71.6
tobacco use Z71.6
use (of)
insulin pump Z46.81
victim (of)
abuse Z69.81
child abuse
by parent Z69.010
non-parental Z69.020
rape NEC Z69.81
Coupled rhythm R00.8
Couvelaire syndrome or uterus (complicating delivery) O45.8X-
Cowperitis — *see* Urethritis
Cowper's gland — *see* condition
Cowpox B08.010
due to vaccination T88.1
Coxa
magna M91.4-
plana M91.2-
valga (acquired) — *see also* Deformity, limb, specified type NEC, thigh
congenital Q65.81
sequelae (late effect) of rickets E64.3
vara (acquired) — *see also* Deformity, limb, specified type NEC, thigh
congenital Q65.82
sequelae (late effect) of rickets E64.3
Coxalgia, coxalgic (nontuberculous) — *see also* Pain, joint, hip
tuberculous A18.02
Coxitis — *see* Monoarthritis, hip
Coxsackie (virus) (infection) B34.1
as cause of disease classified elsewhere B97.11
carditis B33.20
central nervous system NEC A88.8
endocarditis B33.21
enteritis A08.39
meningitis (aseptic) A87.0
myocarditis B33.22
pericarditis B33.23
pharyngitis B08.5
pleurodynia B33.0
specific disease NEC B33.8
Crabs, meaning pubic lice B85.3
Crack baby P04.41
Cracked nipple N64.0
associated with
lactation O92.13
pregnancy O92.11-
puerperium O92.12
Cracked tooth K03.81
Cradle cap L21.0
Craft neurosis F48.8
Cramp (s) R25.2
abdominal — *see* Pain, abdominal
bathing T75.1
colic R10.83
psychogenic F45.8
due to immersion T75.1
fireman T67.2
heat T67.2
immersion T75.1
intestinal — *see* Pain, abdominal
psychogenic F45.8
leg, sleep related G47.62
limb (lower) (upper) NEC R25.2
sleep related G47.62
linotypist's F48.8
organic G25.89
muscle (limb) (general) R25.2
due to immersion T75.1
psychogenic F45.8
occupational (hand) F48.8
organic G25.89
salt-depletion E87.1
sleep related, leg G47.62
stoker's T67.2
swimmer's T75.1
telegrapher's F48.8
organic G25.89
typist's F48.8
organic G25.89
uterus N94.89
menstrual — *see* Dysmenorrhea
writer's F48.8
organic G25.89

Cranial — *see* condition
Craniocleidodysostosis Q74.0
Craniofenestria (skull) Q75.8
Craniolacunia (skull) Q75.8
Craniopagus Q89.4
Craniopathy, metabolic M85.2
Craniopharyngeal — *see* condition
Craniopharyngioma D44.4
Craniorachischisis (totalis) Q00.1
Cranioschisis Q75.8
Craniostenosis Q75.0
Craniosynostosis Q75.0
Craniotabes (cause unknown) M83.8
  neonatal P96.3
  rachitic E64.3
  syphilitic A50.56
Cranium — *see* condition
Craw-craw — *see* Onchocerciasis
Creaking joint — *see* Derangement, joint, specified type NEC
Creeping
  eruption B76.9
  palsy or paralysis G12.22
Crenated tongue K14.8
Creotoxism A05.9
Crepitus
  caput Q75.8
  joint — *see* Derangement, joint, specified type NEC
Crescent or conus choroid, congenital Q14.3
CREST syndrome M34.1
Cretin, cretinism (congenital) (endemic) (nongoitrous) (sporadic) E00.9
  pelvis
    with disproportion (fetopelvic) O33.0
      causing obstructed labor O65.0
  type
    hypothyroid E00.1
    mixed E00.2
    myxedematous E00.1
    neurological E00.0
Creutzfeldt-Jakob disease or syndrome (with dementia) A81.00
  familial A81.09
  iatrogenic A81.09
  specified NEC A81.09
  sporadic A81.09
  variant (vCJD) A81.01
Crib death R99
Cribriform hymen Q52.3
Cri-du-chat syndrome Q93.4
Crigler-Najjar disease or syndrome E80.5
Crime, victim of Z65.4
Crimean hemorrhagic fever A98.0
Criminalism F60.2
Crisis
  abdomen R10.0
  acute reaction F43.0
  addisonian E27.2
  adrenal (cortical) E27.2
  celiac K90.0
  Dietl's N13.8
  emotional — *see also* Disorder, adjustment
    acute reaction to stress F43.0
    specific to childhood and adolescence F93.8
  glaucomatocyclitic — *see* Glaucoma, secondary, inflammation
  heart — *see* Failure, heart
  nitritoid I95.2
    correct substance properly administered — *see* Table of Drugs and Chemicals, by drug, adverse effect
    overdose or wrong substance given or taken — *see* Table of Drugs and Chemicals, by drug, poisoning
  oculogyric H51.8
    psychogenic F45.8
  Pel's (tabetic) A52.11
  psychosexual identity F64.2
  renal N28.0
  sickle-cell D57.00
    with
      acute chest syndrome D57.01
      splenic sequestration D57.02
  state (acute reaction) F43.0
  tabetic A52.11
  thyroid — *see* Thyrotoxicosis with thyroid storm
  thyrotoxic — *see* Thyrotoxicosis with thyroid storm
Crocq's disease (acrocyanosis) I73.89
Crohn's disease — *see* Enteritis, regional
Crooked septum, nasal J34.2
Cross syndrome E70.328
Crossbite (anterior) (posterior) M26.24
Cross-eye — *see* Strabismus, convergent concomitant
Croup, croupous (catarrhal) (infectious) (inflammatory) (nondiphtheritic) J05.0
  bronchial J20.9
  diphtheritic A36.2
  false J38.5
  spasmodic J38.5
    diphtheritic A36.2
  stridulous J38.5
    diphtheritic A36.2
Crouzon's disease Q75.1
Crowding, tooth, teeth, fully erupted M26.31
CRST syndrome M34.1
Cruchet's disease A85.8
Cruelty in children — *see also* Disorder, conduct
Crural ulcer — *see* Ulcer, lower limb
Crush, crushed, crushing T14.8
  abdomen S38.1
  ankle S97.0-
  arm (upper) (and shoulder) S47.-
  axilla — *see* Crush, arm
  back, lower S38.1
  buttock S38.1
  cheek S07.0
  chest S28.0
  cranium S07.1
  ear S07.0
  elbow S57.0-
  extremity
    lower
      ankle — *see* Crush, ankle
      below knee — *see* Crush, leg
      foot — *see* Crush, foot
      hip — *see* Crush, hip
      knee — *see* Crush, knee
      thigh — *see* Crush, thigh
      toe — *see* Crush, toe
    upper
      below elbow S67.9-
      elbow — *see* Crush, elbow
      finger — *see* Crush, finger
      forearm — *see* Crush, forearm
      hand — *see* Crush, hand
      thumb — *see* Crush, thumb
      upper arm — *see* Crush, arm
      wrist — *see* Crush, wrist
  face S07.0
  finger (s) S67.1-
    with hand (and wrist) — *see* Crush, hand, specified site NEC
    index S67.19-
    little S67.19-
    middle S67.19-
    ring S67.19-
    thumb — *see* Crush, thumb
  foot S97.8-
    toe — *see* Crush, toe
  forearm S57.8-
  genitalia, external
    female S38.002
      vagina S38.03
      vulva S38.03
    male S38.001
      penis S38.01
      scrotum S38.02
      testis S38.02
  hand (except fingers alone) S67.2-
    with wrist S67.4-
  head S07.9
    specified NEC S07.8
  heel — *see* Crush, foot
  hip S77.0-
    with thigh S77.2-
  internal organ (abdomen, chest, or pelvis) NEC T14.8
  knee S87.0-
  labium (majus) (minus) S38.03
  larynx S17.0
  leg (lower) S87.8-
    knee — *see* Crush, knee
  lip S07.0
  lower
    back S38.1
    leg — *see* Crush, leg
  neck S17.9
  nerve — *see* Injury, nerve
  nose S07.0
  pelvis S38.1
  penis S38.01
  scalp S07.8
  scapular region — *see* Crush, arm
  scrotum S38.02
  severe, unspecified site T14.8
  shoulder (and upper arm) — *see* Crush, arm
Crush, crushed, crushing - *continued*
  skull S07.1
  syndrome (complication of trauma) T79.5
  testis S38.02
  thigh S77.1-
    with hip S77.2-
  throat S17.8
  thumb S67.0-
    with hand (and wrist) — *see* Crush, hand, specified site NEC
  toe (s) S97.10-
    great S97.11-
    lesser S97.12-
  trachea S17.0
  vagina S38.03
  vulva S38.03
  wrist S67.3-
    with hand S67.4-
Crusta lactea L21.0
Crusts R23.4
Crutch paralysis — *see* Injury, brachial plexus
Cruveilhier-Baumgarten cirrhosis, disease or syndrome K74.69
Cruveilhier's atrophy or disease G12.8
Crying (constant) (continuous) (excessive)
  child, adolescent, or adult R45.83
  infant (baby) (newborn) R68.11
Cryofibrinogenemia D89.2
Cryoglobulinemia (essential) (idiopathic) (mixed) (primary) (purpura) (secondary) (vasculitis) D89.1
  with lung involvement D89.1 *[J99]*
Cryptitis (anal) (rectal) K62.89
Cryptococcosis, cryptococcus (infection) (neoformans) B45.9
  bone B45.3
  cerebral B45.1
  cutaneous B45.2
  disseminated B45.7
  generalized B45.7
  meningitis B45.1
  meningocerebralis B45.1
  osseous B45.3
  pulmonary B45.0
  skin B45.2
  specified NEC B45.8
Cryptopapillitis (anus) K62.89
Cryptophthalmos Q11.2
  syndrome Q87.0
Cryptorchid, cryptorchism, cryptorchidism Q53.9
  bilateral Q53.20
    abdominal Q53.211
    perineal Q53.22
  unilateral Q53.10
    abdominal Q53.111
    perineal Q53.12
Cryptosporidiosis A07.2
  hepatobiliary B88.8
  respiratory B88.8
Cryptostromosis J67.6
Crystalluria R82.998
Cubitus
  congenital Q68.8
  valgus (acquired) M21.0-
    congenital Q68.8
    sequelae (late effect) of rickets E64.3
  varus (acquired) M21.1-
    congenital Q68.8
    sequelae (late effect) of rickets E64.3
Cultural deprivation or shock Z60.3
Curling esophagus K22.4
Curling's ulcer — *see* Ulcer, peptic, acute
Curschmann (-Batten) (-Steinert) **disease or syndrome** G71.11
Curse, Ondine's — *see* Apnea, sleep
Curvature
  organ or site, congenital NEC — *see* Distortion
  penis (lateral) Q55.61
  Pott's (spinal) A18.01
  radius, idiopathic, progressive (congenital) Q74.0
  spine (acquired) (angular) (idiopathic) (incorrect) (postural) — *see* Dorsopathy, deforming
    congenital Q67.5
    due to or associated with
      Charcot-Marie-Tooth disease (*see also*subcategory M49.8) G60.0
      osteitis
        deformans M88.88
        fibrosa cystica (*see also* subcategory M49.8) E21.0
      tuberculosis (Pott's curvature) A18.01
    sequelae (late effect) of rickets E64.3
    tuberculous A18.01

Cyst (colloid) (mucous) (simple) (retention) - *continued*
endometrium, endometrial (uterus) N85.8
ectopic — *see* Endometriosis
enterogenous Q43.8
epidermal, epidermoid (inclusion) (see also Cyst, skin) L72.0
mouth K09.8
oral soft tissue K09.8
epididymis N50.3
epiglottis J38.7
epiphysis cerebri E34.8
epithelial (inclusion) L72.0
epoophoron Q50.5
eruption K09.0
esophagus K22.8
ethmoid sinus J34.1
external female genital organs NEC N90.7
eye NEC H57.89
congenital Q15.8
eyelid (sebaceous) H02.829
infected — *see* Hordeolum
left H02.826
lower H02.825
upper H02.824
right H02.823
lower H02.822
upper H02.821
fallopian tube N83.8
congenital Q50.4
fimbrial (twisted) Q50.4
fissural (oral region) K09.1
follicle (graafian) (hemorrhagic) N83.0-
nabothian N88.8
follicular (atretic) (hemorrhagic) (ovarian) N83.0-
dentigerous K09.0
odontogenic K09.0
skin L72.9
specified NEC L72.8
frontal sinus J34.1
gallbladder K82.8
ganglion — *see* Ganglion
Gartner's duct Q52.4
gingiva K09.0
gland of Moll — *see* Cyst, eyelid
globulomaxillary K09.1
graafian follicle (hemorrhagic) N83.0-
granulosal lutein (hemorrhagic) N83.1-
hemangiomatous D18.00
intra-abdominal D18.03
intracranial D18.02
skin D18.01
specified site NEC D18.09
hemorrhagic M27.49
hydatid — *see also* Echinococcus B67.90
brain B67.99 *[G94]*
liver — *see also* Cyst, liver, hydatid B67.8
lung NEC B67.99 *[J99]*
Morgagni
female Q50.5
male (epididymal) Q55.4
testicular Q55.29
specified site NEC B67.99
hymen N89.8
embryonic Q52.4
hypopharynx J39.2
hypophysis, hypophyseal (duct) (recurrent) E23.6
cerebri E23.6
implantation (dermoid)
external area or site (skin) NEC L72.0
iris — *see* Cyst, iris, implantation
vagina N89.8
vulva N90.7
incisive canal K09.1
inclusion (epidermal) (epithelial) (epidermoid) (squamous) L72.0
not of skin - code under Cyst, by site
intestine (large) (small) K63.89
intracranial — *see* Cyst, brain
intraligamentous — *see also* Disorder, ligament
knee — *see* Derangement, knee
intrasellar E23.6
iris H21.309
exudative H21.31-
idiopathic H21.30-
implantation H21.32-
parasitic H21.33-
pars plana (primary) H21.34-
exudative H21.35-
jaw (bone) M27.40
aneurysmal M27.49
hemorrhagic M27.49
traumatic M27.49

Cyst (colloid) (mucous) (simple) (retention) - *continued*
jaw (bone) - *continued*
developmental (odontogenic) K09.0
fissural K09.1
joint NEC — *see* Disorder, joint, specified type NEC
kidney (acquired) N28.1
calyceal — *see* Hydronephrosis
congenital Q61.00
more than one (multiple) Q61.02
specified as polycystic Q61.3
adult type (autosomal dominant) Q61.2
infantile type (autosomal recessive) NEC Q61.19
collecting duct dilation Q61.11
pyelogenic — *see* Hydronephrosis
simple N28.1
solitary (single) Q61.01
acquired N28.1
labium (majus) (minus) N90.7
sebaceous N90.7
lacrimal — *see also* Disorder, lacrimal system, specified NEC
gland H04.13-
passages or sac — *see* Disorder, lacrimal system, specified NEC
larynx J38.7
lateral periodontal K09.0
lens H27.8
congenital Q12.8
lip (gland) K13.0
liver (idiopathic) (simple) K76.89
congenital Q44.6
hydatid B67.8
granulosus B67.0
multilocularis B67.5
lung J98.4
congenital Q33.0
giant bullous J43.9
lutein N83.1-
lymphangiomatous D18.1
lymphoepithelial, oral soft tissue K09.8
macula — *see* Degeneration, macula, hole
malignant — *see* Neoplasm, malignant, by site
mammary gland — *see* Cyst, breast
mandible M27.40
dentigerous K09.0
radicular K04.8
maxilla M27.40
dentigerous K09.0
radicular K04.8
medial, face and neck Q18.8
median
anterior maxillary K09.1
palatal K09.1
mediastinum, congenital Q34.1
meibomian (gland) — *see* Chalazion
infected — *see* Hordeolum
membrane, brain G93.0
meninges (cerebral) G93.0
spinal G96.19
meniscus, knee — *see* Derangement, knee, meniscus, cystic
mesentery, mesenteric K66.8
chyle I89.8
mesonephric duct
female Q50.5
male Q55.4
milk N64.89
Morgagni (hydatid)
female Q50.5
male (epididymal) Q55.4
testicular Q55.29
mouth K09.8
Müllerian duct Q50.4
appendix testis Q55.29
cervix Q51.6
fallopian tube Q50.4
female Q50.4
male Q55.29
prostatic utricle Q55.4
vagina (embryonal) Q52.4
multilocular (ovary) D39.10
benign — *see* Neoplasm, benign, by site
myometrium N85.8
nabothian (follicle) (ruptured) N88.8
nasoalveolar K09.1
nasolabial K09.1
nasopalatine (anterior) (duct) K09.1
nasopharynx J39.2
neoplastic — *see* Neoplasm, uncertain behavior, by site
benign — *see* Neoplasm, benign, by site

Cyst (colloid) (mucous) (simple) (retention) - *continued*
nervous system NEC G96.8
neuroenteric (congenital) Q06.8
nipple — *see* Cyst, breast
nose (turbinates) J34.1
sinus J34.1
odontogenic, developmental K09.0
omentum (lesser) K66.8
congenital Q45.8
ora serrata — *see* Cyst, retina, ora serrata
oral
region K09.9
developmental (nonodontogenic) K09.1
specified NEC K09.8
soft tissue K09.9
specified NEC K09.8
orbit H05.81-
ovary, ovarian (twisted) N83.20-
adherent N83.20-
chocolate N80.1
corpus
albicans N83.29-
luteum (hemorrhagic) N83.1-
dermoid D27.9
developmental Q50.1
due to failure of involution NEC N83.20-
endometrial N80.1
follicular (graafian) (hemorrhagic) N83.0-
hemorrhagic N83.20-
in pregnancy or childbirth O34.8-
with obstructed labor O65.5
multilocular D39.10
pseudomucinous D27.9
retention N83.29-
serous N83.20-
specified NEC N83.29-
theca lutein (hemorrhagic) N83.1-
tuberculous A18.18
oviduct N83.8
palate (median) (fissural) K09.1
palatine papilla (jaw) K09.1
pancreas, pancreatic (hemorrhagic) (true) K86.2
congenital Q45.2
false K86.3
paralabral
hip M24.85-
shoulder S43.43-
paramesonephric duct Q50.4
female Q50.4
male Q55.29
paranephric N28.1
paraphysis, cerebri, congenital Q04.6
parasitic B89
parathyroid (gland) E21.4
paratubal N83.8
paraurethral duct N36.8
paroophoron Q50.5
parotid gland K11.6
parovarian Q50.5
pelvis, female N94.89
in pregnancy or childbirth O34.8-
causing obstructed labor O65.5
penis (sebaceous) N48.89
periapical K04.8
pericardial (congenital) Q24.8
acquired (secondary) I31.8
pericoronal K09.0
periodontal K04.8
lateral K09.0
peripelvic (lymphatic) N28.1
peritoneum K66.8
chylous I89.8
periventricular, acquired, newborn P91.1
pharynx (wall) J39.2
pilar L72.11
pilonidal (infected) (rectum) L05.91
with abscess L05.01
malignant C44.59-
pituitary (duct) (gland) E23.6
placenta O43.19-
pleura J94.8
popliteal — *see* Cyst, Baker's
porencephalic Q04.6
acquired G93.0
postanal (infected) — *see* Cyst, pilonidal
postmastoidectomy cavity (mucosal) — *see* Complications, postmastoidectomy, cyst
preauricular Q18.1
prepuce N47.4
congenital Q55.69
primordial (jaw) K09.0
prostate N42.83

Cyst (colloid) (mucous) (simple) (retention) - *continued*
- pseudomucinous (ovary) D27.9
- pupillary, miotic H21.27-
- radicular (residual) K04.8
- radiculodental K04.8
- ranular K11.8
- Rathke's pouch E23.6
- rectum (epithelium) (mucous) K62.89
- renal — *see* Cyst, kidney
- residual (radicular) K04.8
- retention (ovary) N83.29-
  - salivary gland K11.6
- retina H33.19-
  - ora serrata H33.11-
  - parasitic H33.12-
- retroperitoneal K68.9
- sacrococcygeal (dermoid) — *see* Cyst, pilonidal
- salivary gland or duct (mucous extravasation or retention) K11.6
- Sampson's N80.1
- sclera H15.89
- scrotum L72.9
  - sebaceous L72.3
- sebaceous (duct) (gland) L72.3
  - breast — *see* Dysplasia, mammary, specified type NEC
  - eyelid — *see* Cyst, eyelid
  - genital organ NEC
    - female N94.89
    - male N50.89
  - scrotum L72.3
- semilunar cartilage (knee) (multiple) — *see* Derangement, knee, meniscus, cystic
- seminal vesicle N50.89
- serous (ovary) N83.20-
- sinus (accessory) (nasal) J34.1
- Skene's gland N36.8
- skin L72.9
  - breast — *see* Dysplasia, mammary, specified type NEC
  - epidermal, epidermoid L72.0
  - epithelial L72.0
  - eyelid — *see* Cyst, eyelid
  - genital organ NEC
    - female N90.7
    - male N50.89
  - inclusion L72.0
  - scrotum L72.9
  - sebaceous L72.3
  - sweat gland or duct L74.8
- solitary
  - bone — *see* Cyst, bone, solitary
  - jaw M27.40
  - kidney N28.1
- spermatic cord N50.89
- sphenoid sinus J34.1
- spinal meninges G96.19
- spleen NEC D73.4
  - congenital Q89.09
  - hydatid — *see also* Echinococcus B67.99 *[D77]*
- Stafne's M27.0
- subarachnoid intrasellar R93.0
- subcutaneous, pheomycotic (chromomycotic) B43.2
- subdural (cerebral) G93.0
  - spinal cord G96.19
- sublingual gland K11.6
- submandibular gland K11.6
- submaxillary gland K11.6
- suburethral N36.8
- suprarenal gland E27.8
- suprasellar — *see* Cyst, brain
- sweat gland or duct L74.8
- synovial — *see also* Cyst, bursa
  - ruptured — *see* Rupture, synovium
- tarsal — *see* Chalazion
- tendon (sheath) — *see* Disorder, tendon, specified type NEC
- testis N44.2
  - tunica albuginea N44.1
- theca lutein (ovary) N83.1-
- Thornwaldt's J39.2
- thymus (gland) E32.8
- thyroglossal duct (infected) (persistent) Q89.2
- thyrolingual duct (infected) (persistent) Q89.2
- thyroid (gland) E04.1
- tongue K14.8
- tonsil J35.8
- tooth — *see* Cyst, dental
- Tornwaldt's J39.2
- trichilemmal (proliferating) L72.12
- trichodermal L72.12
- tubal (fallopian) N83.8

Cyst (colloid) (mucous) (simple) (retention) - *continued*
- tubal (fallopian) - *continued*
  - inflammatory — *see* Salpingitis, chronic
- tubo-ovarian N83.8
  - inflammatory N70.13
- tunica
  - albuginea testis N44.1
  - vaginalis N50.89
- turbinate (nose) J34.1
- Tyson's gland N48.89
- urachus, congenital Q64.4
- ureter N28.89
- ureterovesical orifice N28.89
- urethra, urethral (gland) N36.8
- uterine ligament N83.8
- uterus (body) (corpus) (recurrent) N85.8
  - embryonic Q51.818
    - cervix Q51.6
- vagina, vaginal (implantation) (inclusion) (squamous cell) (wall) N89.8
  - embryonic Q52.4
- vallecula, vallecular (epiglottis) J38.7
- vesical (orifice) N32.89
- vitreous body H43.89
- vulva (implantation) (inclusion) N90.7
  - congenital Q52.79
  - sebaceous gland N90.7
- vulvovaginal gland N90.7
- wolffian
  - female Q50.5
  - male Q55.4

Cystadenocarcinoma — *see* Neoplasm, malignant, by site
- bile duct C22.1
- endometrioid — *see* Neoplasm, malignant, by site
  - specified site — *see* Neoplasm, malignant, by site
  - unspecified site
    - female C56.9
    - male C61
- mucinous
  - papillary
    - specified site — *see* Neoplasm, malignant, by site
    - unspecified site C56.9
  - specified site — *see* Neoplasm, malignant, by site
  - unspecified site C56.9
- papillary
  - mucinous
    - specified site — *see* Neoplasm, malignant, by site
    - unspecified site C56.9
  - pseudomucinous
    - specified site — *see* Neoplasm, malignant, by site
    - unspecified site C56.9
  - serous
    - specified site — *see* Neoplasm, malignant, by site
    - unspecified site C56.9
  - specified site — *see* Neoplasm, malignant, by site
  - unspecified site C56.9
- pseudomucinous
  - papillary
    - specified site — *see* Neoplasm, malignant, by site
    - unspecified site C56.9
  - specified site — *see* Neoplasm, malignant, by site
  - unspecified site C56.9
- serous
  - papillary
    - specified site — *see* Neoplasm, malignant, by site
    - unspecified site C56.9
  - specified site — *see* Neoplasm, malignant, by site
  - unspecified site C56.9

Cystadenofibroma
- clear cell — *see* Neoplasm, benign, by site
- endometrioid D27.9
  - borderline malignancy D39.1-
  - malignant C56.-
- mucinous
  - specified site — *see* Neoplasm, benign, by site
  - unspecified site D27.9
- serous
  - specified site — *see* Neoplasm, benign, by site
  - unspecified site D27.9
- specified site — *see* Neoplasm, benign, by site
- unspecified site D27.9

Cystadenoma — *see also* Neoplasm, benign, by site
- bile duct D13.4
- endometrioid — *see* Neoplasm, benign, by site
  - borderline malignancy — *see* Neoplasm, uncertain behavior, by site
- malignant — *see* Neoplasm, malignant, by site
- mucinous
  - borderline malignancy
    - ovary C56.-

Cystadenoma - *continued*
- mucinous - *continued*
  - borderline malignancy - *continued*
    - specified site NEC — *see* Neoplasm, uncertain behavior, by site
    - unspecified site C56.9
  - papillary
    - borderline malignancy
      - ovary C56.-
      - specified site NEC — *see* Neoplasm, uncertain behavior, by site
      - unspecified site C56.9
    - specified site — *see* Neoplasm, benign, by site
    - unspecified site D27.9
  - specified site — *see* Neoplasm, benign, by site
  - unspecified site D27.9
- papillary
  - borderline malignancy
    - ovary C56.-
    - specified site NEC — *see* Neoplasm, uncertain behavior, by site
    - unspecified site C56.9
  - lymphomatosum
    - specified site — *see* Neoplasm, benign, by site
    - unspecified site D11.9
  - mucinous
    - borderline malignancy
      - ovary C56.-
      - specified site NEC — *see* Neoplasm, uncertain behavior, by site
      - unspecified site C56.9
    - specified site — *see* Neoplasm, benign, by site
    - unspecified site D27.9
  - pseudomucinous
    - borderline malignancy
      - ovary C56.-
      - specified site NEC — *see* Neoplasm, uncertain behavior, by site
      - unspecified site C56.9
    - specified site — *see* Neoplasm, benign, by site
    - unspecified site D27.9
  - serous
    - borderline malignancy
      - ovary C56.-
      - specified site NEC — *see* Neoplasm, uncertain behavior, by site
      - unspecified site C56.9
    - specified site — *see* Neoplasm, benign, by site
    - unspecified site D27.9
  - specified site — *see* Neoplasm, benign, by site
  - unspecified site D27.9
- pseudomucinous
  - borderline malignancy
    - ovary C56.-
    - specified site NEC — *see* Neoplasm, uncertain behavior, by site
    - unspecified site C56.9
  - papillary
    - borderline malignancy
      - ovary C56.-
      - specified site NEC — *see* Neoplasm, uncertain behavior, by site
      - unspecified site C56.9
    - specified site — *see* Neoplasm, benign, by site
    - unspecified site D27.9
  - specified site — *see* Neoplasm, benign, by site
  - unspecified site D27.9
- serous
  - borderline malignancy
    - ovary C56.-
    - specified site NEC — *see* Neoplasm, uncertain behavior, by site
    - unspecified site C56.9
  - papillary
    - borderline malignancy
      - ovary C56.-
      - specified site NEC — *see* Neoplasm, uncertain behavior, by site
      - unspecified site C56.9
    - specified site — *see* Neoplasm, benign, by site
    - unspecified site D27.9
  - specified site — *see* Neoplasm, benign, by site
  - unspecified site D27.9

Cystathionine synthase deficiency E72.11

Cystathioninemia E72.19

Cystathioninuria E72.19

Cystic — *see also* condition
- breast (chronic) — *see* Mastopathy, cystic
- corpora lutea (hemorrhagic) N83.1-
- duct — *see* condition
- eyeball (congenital) Q11.0
- fibrosis — *see* Fibrosis, cystic
- kidney (congenital) Q61.9

- **Cystic** - *continued*
  - kidney (congenital) - *continued*
    - adult type Q61.2
    - infantile type NEC Q61.19
      - collecting duct dilatation Q61.11
    - medullary Q61.5
  - liver, congenital Q44.6
  - lung disease J98.4
    - congenital Q33.0
  - mastitis, chronic — *see* Mastopathy, cystic
  - medullary, kidney Q61.5
  - meniscus — *see* Derangement, knee, meniscus, cystic
  - ovary N83.20-
- **Cysticercosis, cysticerciasis** B69.9
  - with
    - epileptiform fits B69.0
    - myositis B69.81
  - brain B69.0
  - central nervous system B69.0
  - cerebral B69.0
  - ocular B69.1
  - specified NEC B69.89
- **Cysticercus cellulose infestation** — *see* Cysticercosis
- **Cystinosis** (malignant) E72.04
- **Cystinuria** E72.01
- **Cystitis** (exudative) (hemorrhagic) (septic) (suppurative) N30.90
  - with
    - fibrosis — *see* Cystitis, chronic, interstitial
    - hematuria N30.91
    - leukoplakia — *see* Cystitis, chronic, interstitial
    - malakoplakia — *see* Cystitis, chronic, interstitial
    - metaplasia — *see* Cystitis, chronic, interstitial
    - prostatitis N41.3
  - acute N30.00
    - with hematuria N30.01
    - of trigone N30.30
      - with hematuria N30.31
  - allergic — *see* Cystitis, specified type NEC
  - amebic A06.81
  - bilharzial B65.9 *[N33]*
  - blennorrhagic (gonococcal) A54.01
  - bullous — *see* Cystitis, specified type NEC
  - calculous N21.0
  - chlamydial A56.01
  - chronic N30.20
    - with hematuria N30.21
    - interstitial N30.10
      - with hematuria N30.11
    - of trigone N30.30
      - with hematuria N30.31
    - specified NEC N30.20
      - with hematuria N30.21
  - cystic (a) — *see* Cystitis, specified type NEC
  - diphtheritic A36.85
  - echinococcal
    - granulosus B67.39
    - multilocularis B67.69
  - emphysematous — *see* Cystitis, specified type NEC
  - encysted — *see* Cystitis, specified type NEC
  - eosinophilic — *see* Cystitis, specified type NEC
  - follicular — *see* Cystitis, of trigone
  - gangrenous — *see* Cystitis, specified type NEC
  - glandularis — *see* Cystitis, specified type NEC
  - gonococcal A54.01
  - incrusted — *see* Cystitis, specified type NEC
  - interstitial (chronic) — *see* Cystitis, chronic, interstitial
  - irradiation N30.40
    - with hematuria N30.41
  - irritation — *see* Cystitis, specified type NEC
  - malignant — *see* Cystitis, specified type NEC
  - of trigone N30.30
    - with hematuria N30.31
  - panmural — *see* Cystitis, chronic, interstitial
  - polyposa — *see* Cystitis, specified type NEC
  - prostatic N41.3
  - puerperal (postpartum) O86.22
  - radiation — *see* Cystitis, irradiation
  - specified type NEC N30.80
    - with hematuria N30.81
  - subacute — *see* Cystitis, chronic
  - submucous — *see* Cystitis, chronic, interstitial
  - syphilitic (late) A52.76
  - trichomonal A59.03
  - tuberculous A18.12
  - ulcerative — *see* Cystitis, chronic, interstitial
- **Cystocele** (-urethrocele)
  - female N81.10
    - with prolapse of uterus — *see* Prolapse, uterus
    - lateral N81.12
- **Cystocele** (-urethrocele) - *continued*
  - female - *continued*
    - midline N81.11
    - paravaginal N81.12
  - in pregnancy or childbirth O34.8-
    - causing obstructed labor O65.5
  - male N32.89
- **Cystolithiasis** N21.0
- **Cystoma** — *see also* Neoplasm, benign, by site
  - endometrial, ovary N80.1
  - mucinous
    - specified site — *see* Neoplasm, benign, by site
    - unspecified site D27.9
  - serous
    - specified site — *see* Neoplasm, benign, by site
    - unspecified site D27.9
  - simple (ovary) N83.29-
- **Cystoplegia** N31.2
- **Cystoptosis** N32.89
- **Cystopyelitis** — *see* Pyelonephritis
- **Cystorrhagia** N32.89
- **Cystosarcoma phyllodes** D48.6-
  - benign D24-
  - malignant — *see* Neoplasm, breast, malignant
- **Cystostomy**
  - attention to Z43.5
  - complication — *see* Complications, cystostomy
  - status Z93.50
    - appendico-vesicostomy Z93.52
    - cutaneous Z93.51
    - specified NEC Z93.59
- **Cystourethritis** — *see* Urethritis
- **Cystourethrocele** — *see also* Cystocele
  - female N81.10
    - with uterine prolapse — *see* Prolapse, uterus
    - lateral N81.12
    - midline N81.11
    - paravaginal N81.12
  - male N32.89
- **Cytomegalic inclusion disease**
  - congenital P35.1
- **Cytomegalovirus infection** B25.9
- **Cytomycosis** (reticuloendothelial) B39.4
- **Cytopenia** D75.9
  - refractory
    - with multilineage dysplasia D46.A
      - and ring sideroblasts (RCMD RS) D46.B
- **Czerny's disease** (periodic hydrarthrosis of the knee) — *see* Effusion, joint, knee

D

- **Da Costa's syndrome** F45.8
- **Daae** (-Finsen) **disease** (epidemic pleurodynia) B33.0
- **Dabney's grip** B33.0
- **Dacryoadenitis, dacryadenitis** H04.00-
  - acute H04.01-
  - chronic H04.02-
- **Dacryocystitis** H04.30-
  - acute H04.32-
  - chronic H04.41-
  - neonatal P39.1
  - phlegmonous H04.31-
  - syphilitic A52.71
    - congenital (early) A50.01
  - trachomatous, active A71.1
    - sequelae (late effect) B94.0
- **Dacryocystoblenorrhea** — *see* Inflammation, lacrimal, passages, chronic
- **Dacryocystocele** — *see* Disorder, lacrimal system, changes
- **Dacryolith, dacryolithiasis** H04.51-
- **Dacryoma** — *see* Disorder, lacrimal system, changes
- **Dacryopericystitis** — *see* Dacryocystitis
- **Dacryops** H04.11-
- **Dacryostenosis** — *see also* Stenosis, lacrimal
  - congenital Q10.5
- **Dactylitis**
  - bone — *see* Osteomyelitis
  - sickle-cell D57.00
    - Hb C D57.219
    - Hb SS D57.00
    - specified NEC D57.819
  - skin L08.9
  - syphilitic A52.77
  - tuberculous A18.03
- **Dactylolysis spontanea** (ainhum) L94.6
- **Dactylosymphysis** Q70.9
  - fingers — *see* Syndactylism, complex, fingers
  - toes — *see* Syndactylism, complex, toes
- **Damage**
  - arteriosclerotic — *see* Arteriosclerosis
  - brain (nontraumatic) G93.9
    - anoxic, hypoxic G93.1
- **Damage** - *continued*
  - brain (nontraumatic) - *continued*
    - anoxic, hypoxic - *continued*
      - resulting from a procedure G97.82
    - child NEC G80.9
    - due to birth injury P11.2
  - cardiorenal (vascular) — *see* Hypertension, cardiorenal
  - cerebral NEC — *see* Damage, brain
  - coccyx, complicating delivery O71.6
  - coronary — *see* Disease, heart, ischemic
  - eye, birth injury P15.3
  - liver (nontraumatic) K76.9
    - alcoholic K70.9
    - due to drugs — *see* Disease, liver, toxic
    - toxic — *see* Disease, liver, toxic
  - medication T88.7
  - pelvic
    - joint or ligament, during delivery O71.6
    - organ NEC
      - during delivery O71.5
      - following ectopic or molar pregnancy O08.6
  - renal — *see* Disease, renal
  - subendocardium, subendocardial — *see* Degeneration, myocardial
  - vascular I99.9
- **Dana-Putnam syndrome** (subacute combined sclerosis with pernicious anemia) — *see* Degeneration, combined
- **Danbolt** (-Cross) **syndrome** (acrodermatitis enteropathica) E83.2
- **Dandruff** L21.0
- **Dandy-Walker syndrome** Q03.1
  - with spina bifida — *see* Spina bifida
- **Danlos' syndrome** Q79.6
- **Darier** (-White) **disease** (congenital) Q82.8
  - meaning erythema annulare centrifugum L53.1
- **Darier-Roussy sarcoid** D86.3
- **Darling's disease or histoplasmosis** B39.4
- **Darwin's tubercle** Q17.8
- **Dawson's** (inclusion body) **encephalitis** A81.1
- **De Beurmann** (-Gougerot) **disease** B42.1
- **De la Tourette's syndrome** F95.2
- **De Lange's syndrome** Q87.1
- **De Morgan's spots** (senile angiomas) I78.1
- **De Quervain's**
  - disease (tendon sheath) M65.4
  - syndrome E34.51
  - thyroiditis (subacute granulomatous thyroiditis) E06.1
- **De Toni-Fanconi** (-Debré) **syndrome** E72.09
  - with cystinosis E72.04
- **Dead**
  - fetus, retained (mother) O36.4
    - early pregnancy O02.1
  - labyrinth — *see* subcategory H83.2
  - ovum, retained O02.0
- **Deaf nonspeaking NEC** H91.3
- **Deafmutism** (acquired) (congenital) **NEC** H91.3
  - hysterical F44.6
  - syphilitic, congenital (*see also* subcategory H94.8) A50.09
- **Deafness** (acquired) (complete) (hereditary) (partial) H91.9-
  - with blue sclera and fragility of bone Q78.0
  - auditory fatigue — *see* Deafness, specified type NEC
  - aviation T70.0
    - nerve injury — *see* Injury, nerve, acoustic, specified type NEC
  - boilermaker's — *see* subcategory H83.3
  - central — *see* Deafness, sensorineural
  - conductive H90.2
    - and sensorineural
      - mixed H90.8
        - bilateral H90.6
    - bilateral H90.0
    - unilateral H90.1-
      - with restricted hearing on the contralateral side H90.A-
  - congenital H90.5
    - with blue sclera and fragility of bone Q78.0
  - due to toxic agents — *see* Deafness, ototoxic
  - emotional (hysterical) F44.6
  - functional (hysterical) F44.6
  - high frequency H91.9-
  - hysterical F44.6
  - low frequency H91.9-
  - mental R48.8
  - mixed conductive and sensorineural H90.8
    - bilateral H90.6
    - unilateral H90.7-
  - nerve — *see* Deafness, sensorineural

Deafness (acquired) (complete) (hereditary) (partial) - *continued*
- neural — *see* Deafness, sensorineural
- noise-induced (*see also* subcategory H83.3)
  - nerve injury — *see* Injury, nerve, acoustic, specified type NEC
- nonspeaking H91.3
- ototoxic — *see* subcategory H91.0
- perceptive — *see* Deafness, sensorineural
- psychogenic (hysterical) F44.6
- sensorineural H90.5
  - and conductive
    - mixed H90.8
      - bilateral H90.6
    - bilateral H90.3
    - unilateral H90.4-
      - with restricted hearing on the contralateral side H90.A-
- sensory — *see* Deafness, sensorineural
- specified type NEC — *see* subcategory H91.8
- sudden (idiopathic) H91.2-
- syphilitic A52.15
- transient ischemic H93.01-
- traumatic — *see* Injury, nerve, acoustic, specified type NEC
- word (developmental) H93.25

Death (cause unknown) (of) (unexplained) (unspecified cause) R99
- brain G93.82
- cardiac (sudden) (with successful resuscitation) - code to underlying disease
  - family history of Z82.41
  - personal history of Z86.74
- family member (assumed) Z63.4

Debility (chronic) (general) (nervous) R53.81
- congenital or neonatal NOS P96.9
- nervous R53.81
- old age R54
- senile R54

Débove's disease (splenomegaly) R16.1

Decalcification
- bone — *see* Osteoporosis
- teeth K03.89

Decapsulation, kidney N28.89

Decay
- dental — *see* Caries, dental
- senile R54
- tooth, teeth — *see* Caries, dental

Deciduitis (acute)
- following ectopic or molar pregnancy O08.0

Decline (general) — *see* Debility
- cognitive, age-associated R41.81

Decompensation
- cardiac (acute) (chronic) — *see* Disease, heart
- cardiovascular — *see* Disease, cardiovascular
- heart — *see* Disease, heart
- hepatic — *see* Failure, hepatic
- myocardial (acute) (chronic) — *see* Disease, heart
- respiratory J98.8

Decompression sickness T70.3

Decrease (d)
- absolute neutrophile count — *see* Neutropenia
- blood
  - platelets — *see* Thrombocytopenia
  - pressure R03.1
    - due to shock following
      - injury T79.4
      - operation T81.19
- estrogen E28.39
  - postablative E89.40
    - asymptomatic E89.40
    - symptomatic E89.41
- fragility of erythrocytes D58.8
- function
  - lipase (pancreatic) K90.3
  - ovary in hypopituitarism E23.0
  - parenchyma of pancreas K86.89
  - pituitary (gland) (anterior) (lobe) E23.0
    - posterior (lobe) E23.0
- functional activity R68.89
- glucose R73.09
- hematocrit R71.0
- hemoglobin R71.0
- leukocytes D72.819
  - specified NEC D72.818
- libido R68.82
- lymphocytes D72.810
- platelets D69.6
- respiration, due to shock following injury T79.4
- sexual desire R68.82
- tear secretion NEC — *see* Syndrome, dry eye
- tolerance
  - fat K90.49

Decrease (d) - *continued*
- tolerance - *continued*
  - glucose R73.09
  - pancreatic K90.3
  - salt and water E87.8
- vision NEC H54.7
- white blood cell count D72.819
  - specified NEC D72.818

Decubitus (ulcer) — *see* Ulcer, pressure, by site
- cervix N86

Deepening acetabulum — *see* Derangement, joint, specified type NEC, hip

Defect, defective Q89.9
- 3-beta-hydroxysteroid dehydrogenase E25.0
- 11-hydroxylase E25.0
- 21-hydroxylase E25.0
- abdominal wall, congenital Q79.59
- antibody immunodeficiency D80.9
- aorticopulmonary septum Q21.4
- atrial septal (ostium secundum type) Q21.1
  - following acute myocardial infarction (current complication) I23.1
  - ostium primum type Q21.2
- atrioventricular
  - canal Q21.2
  - septum Q21.2
- auricular septal Q21.1
- bilirubin excretion NEC E80.6
- biosynthesis, androgen (testicular) E29.1
- bulbar septum Q21.0
- catalase E80.3
- cell membrane receptor complex (CR3) D71
- circulation I99.9
  - congenital Q28.9
  - newborn Q28.9
- coagulation (factor) — *see also* Deficiency, factor D68.9
  - with
    - ectopic pregnancy O08.1
    - molar pregnancy O08.1
  - acquired D68.4
  - antepartum with hemorrhage — *see* Hemorrhage, antepartum, with coagulation defect
  - due to
    - liver disease D68.4
    - vitamin K deficiency D68.4
  - hereditary NEC D68.2
  - intrapartum O67.0
  - newborn, transient P61.6
  - postpartum O99.13
    - with hemorrhage O72.3
  - specified type NEC D68.8
- complement system D84.1
- conduction (heart) I45.9
  - bone — *see* Deafness, conductive
- congenital, organ or site not listed — *see* Anomaly, by site
- coronary sinus Q21.1
- cushion, endocardial Q21.2
- degradation, glycoprotein E77.1
- dental bridge, crown, fillings — *see* Defect, dental restoration
- dental restoration K08.50
  - specified NEC K08.59
- dentin (hereditary) K00.5
- Descemet's membrane, congenital Q13.89
- developmental — *see also* Anomaly
  - cauda equina Q06.3
- diaphragm
  - with elevation, eventration or hernia — *see* Hernia, diaphragm
  - congenital Q79.1
    - with hernia Q79.0
    - gross (with hernia) Q79.0
- ectodermal, congenital Q82.9
- Eisenmenger's Q21.8
- enzyme
  - catalase E80.3
  - peroxidase E80.3
- esophagus, congenital Q39.9
- extensor retinaculum M62.89
- fibrin polymerization D68.2
- filling
  - bladder R93.41
  - kidney R93.42-
  - renal pelvis R93.41
  - stomach R93.3
  - ureter R93.41
  - urinary organs, specified NEC R93.49
- GABA (gamma aminobutyric acid)
  - metabolic E72.81
- Gerbode Q21.0
- glycoprotein degradation E77.1

Defect, defective - *continued*
- Hageman (factor) D68.2
- hearing — *see* Deafness
- high grade F70
- interatrial septal Q21.1
- interauricular septal Q21.1
- interventricular septal Q21.0
  - with dextroposition of aorta, pulmonary stenosis and hypertrophy of right ventricle Q21.3
  - in tetralogy of Fallot Q21.3
- learning (specific) — *see* Disorder, learning
- lymphocyte function antigen-1 (LFA-1) D84.0
- lysosomal enzyme, post-translational modification E77.0
- major osseous M89.70
  - ankle M89.77-
  - carpus M89.74-
  - clavicle M89.71-
  - femur M89.75-
  - fibula M89.76-
  - fingers M89.74-
  - foot M89.77-
  - forearm M89.73-
  - hand M89.74-
  - humerus M89.72-
  - lower leg M89.76-
  - metacarpus M89.74-
  - metatarsus M89.77-
  - multiple sites M89.79
  - pelvic region M89.75-
  - pelvis M89.75-
  - radius M89.73-
  - scapula M89.71-
  - shoulder region M89.71-
  - specified NEC M89.78
  - tarsus M89.77-
  - thigh M89.75-
  - tibia M89.76-
  - toes M89.77-
  - ulna M89.73-
- mental — *see* Disability, intellectual
- modification, lysosomal enzymes, post-translational E77.0
- obstructive, congenital
  - renal pelvis Q62.39
  - ureter Q62.39
    - atresia — *see* Atresia, ureter
    - cecoureterocele Q62.32
    - megaureter Q62.2
    - orthotopic ureterocele Q62.31
- osseous, major M89.70
  - ankle M89.77-
  - carpus M89.74-
  - clavicle M89.71-
  - femur M89.75-
  - fibula M89.76-
  - fingers M89.74-
  - foot M89.77-
  - forearm M89.73-
  - hand M89.74-
  - humerus M89.72-
  - lower leg M89.76-
  - metacarpus M89.74-
  - metatarsus M89.77-
  - multiple sites M89.9
  - pelvic region M89.75-
  - pelvis M89.75-
  - radius M89.73-
  - scapula M89.71-
  - shoulder region M89.71-
  - specified NEC M89.78
  - tarsus M89.77-
  - thigh M89.75-
  - tibia M89.76-
  - toes M89.77-
  - ulna M89.73-
- osteochondral NEC — *see also* Deformity M95.8
- ostium
  - primum Q21.2
  - secundum Q21.1
- peroxidase E80.3
- placental blood supply — *see* Insufficiency, placental
- platelets, qualitative D69.1
  - constitutional D68.0
- postural NEC, spine — *see* Dorsopathy, deforming
- reduction
  - limb Q73.8
    - lower Q72.9-
      - absence — *see* Agenesis, leg
      - foot — *see* Agenesis, foot
      - longitudinal
        - femur Q72.4-

Defect, defective - *continued*
reduction - *continued*
limb - *continued*
lower - *continued*
longitudinal - *continued*
fibula Q72.6-
tibia Q72.5-
specified type NEC Q72.89-
split foot Q72.7-
specified type NEC Q73.8
upper Q71.9-
absence — *see* Agenesis, arm
forearm — *see* Agenesis, forearm
hand — *see* Agenesis, hand
lobster-claw hand Q71.6-
longitudinal
radius Q71.4-
ulna Q71.5-
specified type NEC Q71.89-
renal pelvis Q63.8
obstructive Q62.39
respiratory system, congenital Q34.9
restoration, dental K08.50
specified NEC K08.59
retinal nerve bundle fibers H35.89
septal (heart) NOS Q21.9
acquired (atrial) (auricular) (ventricular) (old) I51.0
atrial Q21.1
concurrent with acute myocardial infarction — *see* Infarct, myocardium
following acute myocardial infarction (current complication) I23.1
ventricular — *see also* Defect, ventricular septal Q21.0
sinus venosus Q21.1
speech R47.9
developmental F80.9
specified NEC R47.89
Taussig-Bing (aortic transposition and overriding pulmonary artery) Q20.1
teeth, wedge K03.1
vascular (local) I99.9
congenital Q27.9
ventricular septal Q21.0
concurrent with acute myocardial infarction — *see* Infarct, myocardium
following acute myocardial infarction (current complication) I23.2
in tetralogy of Fallot Q21.3
vision NEC H54.7
visual field H53.40
bilateral
heteronymous H53.47
homonymous H53.46-
generalized contraction H53.48-
localized
arcuate H53.43-
scotoma (central area) H53.41-
blind spot area H53.42-
sector H53.43-
specified type NEC H53.45-
voice R49.9
specified NEC R49.8
wedge, tooth, teeth (abrasion) K03.1
Deferentitis N49.1
gonorrheal (acute) (chronic) A54.23
Defibrination (syndrome) D65
antepartum — *see* Hemorrhage, antepartum, with coagulation defect, disseminated intravascular coagulation
following ectopic or molar pregnancy O08.1
intrapartum O67.0
newborn P60
postpartum O72.3
Deficiency, deficient
3-beta hydroxysteroid dehydrogenase E25.0
5-alpha reductase (with male pseudohermaphroditism) E29.1
11-hydroxylase E25.0
21-hydroxylase E25.0
abdominal muscle syndrome Q79.4
accelerator globulin (Ac G) (blood) D68.2
AC globulin (congenital) (hereditary) D68.2
acquired D68.4
acid phosphatase E83.39
activating factor (blood) D68.2
adenosine deaminase (ADA) D81.3
aldolase (hereditary) E74.19
alpha-1-antitrypsin E88.01
amino-acids E72.9
anemia — *see* Anemia
aneurin E51.9

Deficiency, deficient - *continued*
antibody with
hyperimmunoglobulinemia D80.6
near-normal immunoglobins D80.6
antidiuretic hormone E23.2
anti-hemophilic
factor (A) D66
B D67
C D68.1
globulin (AHG) NEC D66
antithrombin (antithrombin III) D68.59
ascorbic acid E54
attention (disorder) (syndrome) F98.8
with hyperactivity — *see* Disorder, attention-deficit hyperactivity
autoprothrombin
I D68.2
II D67
C D68.2
beta-glucuronidase E76.29
biotin E53.8
biotin-dependent carboxylase D81.819
biotinidase D81.810
brancher enzyme (amylopectinosis) E74.03
calciferol E55.9
with
adult osteomalacia M83.8
rickets — *see* Rickets
calcium (dietary) E58
calorie, severe E43
with marasmus E41
and kwashiorkor E42
cardiac — *see* Insufficiency, myocardial
carnitine E71.40
due to
hemodialysis E71.43
inborn errors of metabolism E71.42
Valproic acid therapy E71.43
iatrogenic E71.43
muscle palmityltransferase E71.314
primary E71.41
secondary E71.448
carotene E50.9
central nervous system G96.8
ceruloplasmin (Wilson) E83.01
choline E53.8
Christmas factor D67
chromium E61.4
clotting (blood) — *see also* Deficiency, coagulation factor D68.9
clotting factor NEC (hereditary) — *see also* Deficiency, factor D68.2
coagulation NOS D68.9
with
ectopic pregnancy O08.1
molar pregnancy O08.1
acquired (any) D68.4
antepartum hemorrhage — *see* Hemorrhage, antepartum, with coagulation defect
clotting factor NEC — *see also* Deficiency, factor D68.2
due to
hyperprothrombinemia D68.4
liver disease D68.4
vitamin K deficiency D68.4
newborn, transient P61.6
postpartum O72.3
specified NEC D68.8
cognitive F09
color vision H53.50
achromatopsia H53.51
acquired H53.52
deuteranomaly H53.53
protanomaly H53.54
specified type NEC H53.59
tritanomaly H53.55
combined glucocorticoid and mineralocorticoid E27.49
contact factor D68.2
copper (nutritional) E61.0
corticoadrenal E27.40
primary E27.1
craniofacial axis Q75.0
cyanocobalamin E53.8
C1 esterase inhibitor (C1-INH) D84.1
debrancher enzyme (limit dextrinosis) E74.03
dehydrogenase
long chain/very long chain acyl CoA E71.310
medium chain acyl CoA E71.311
short chain acyl CoA E71.312
diet E63.9
dihydropyrimidine dehydrogenase (DPD) E88.89
disaccharidase E73.9

Deficiency, deficient - *continued*
edema — *see* Malnutrition, severe
endocrine E34.9
energy-supply — *see* Malnutrition
enzymes, circulating NEC E88.09
ergosterol E55.9
with
adult osteomalacia M83.8
rickets — *see* Rickets
essential fatty acid (EFA) E63.0
factor — *see also* Deficiency, coagulation
Hageman D68.2
I (congenital) (hereditary) D68.2
II (congenital) (hereditary) D68.2
IX (congenital) (functional) (hereditary) (with functional defect) D67
multiple (congenital) D68.8
acquired D68.4
V (congenital) (hereditary) D68.2
VII (congenital) (hereditary) D68.2
VIII (congenital) (functional) (hereditary) (with functional defect) D66
with vascular defect D68.0
X (congenital) (hereditary) D68.2
XI (congenital) (hereditary) D68.1
XII (congenital) (hereditary) D68.2
XIII (congenital) (hereditary) D68.2
femoral, proximal focal (congenital) — *see* Defect, reduction, lower limb, longitudinal, femur
fibrin-stabilizing factor (congenital) (hereditary) D68.2
acquired D68.4
fibrinase D68.2
fibrinogen (congenital) (hereditary) D68.2
acquired D65
folate E53.8
folic acid E53.8
foreskin N47.3
fructokinase E74.11
fructose 1,6-diphosphatase E74.19
fructose-1-phosphate aldolase E74.19
GABA (gamma aminobutyric acid) transaminase E72.81
GABA-T (gamma aminobutyric acid transaminase) E72.81
galactokinase E74.29
galactose-1-phosphate uridyl transferase E74.29
gammaglobulin in blood D80.1
hereditary D80.0
glass factor D68.2
glucocorticoid E27.49
mineralocorticoid E27.49
glucose-6-phosphatase E74.01
glucose-6-phosphate dehydrogenase anemia D55.0
glucuronyl transferase E80.5
glycogen synthetase E74.09
gonadotropin (isolated) E23.0
growth hormone (idiopathic) (isolated) E23.0
Hageman factor D68.2
hemoglobin D64.9
hepatophosphorylase E74.09
homogentisate 1,2-dioxygenase E70.29
hormone
anterior pituitary (partial) NEC E23.0
growth E23.0
growth (isolated) E23.0
pituitary E23.0
testicular E29.1
hypoxanthine- (guanine) -phosphoribosyltransferase (HG- PRT) (total H-PRT) E79.1
immunity D84.9
cell-mediated D84.8
with thrombocytopenia and eczema D82.0
combined D81.9
humoral D80.9
IgA (secretory) D80.2
IgG D80.3
IgM D80.4
immuno — *see* Immunodeficiency
immunoglobulin, selective
A (IgA) D80.2
G (IgG) (subclasses) D80.3
M (IgM) D80.4
inositol (B complex) E53.8
intrinsic
factor (congenital) D51.0
sphincter N36.42
with urethral hypermobility N36.43
iodine E61.8
congenital syndrome — *see* Syndrome, iodine-deficiency, congenital
iron E61.1
anemia D50.9

Deficiency, deficient - *continued*
- kalium E87.6
- kappa-light chain D80.8
- labile factor (congenital) (hereditary) D68.2
  - acquired D68.4
- lacrimal fluid (acquired) — *see also* Syndrome, dry eye
  - congenital Q10.6
- lactase
  - congenital E73.0
  - secondary E73.1
- Laki-Lorand factor D68.2
- lecithin cholesterol acyltransferase E78.6
- lipocaic K86.89
- lipoprotein (familial) (high density) E78.6
- liver phosphorylase E74.09
- lysosomal alpha-1, 4 glucosidase E74.02
- magnesium E61.2
- major histocompatibility complex
  - class I D81.6
  - class II D81.7
- manganese E61.3
- menadione (vitamin K) E56.1
  - newborn P53
- mental (familial) (hereditary) — *see* Disability, intellectual
- methylenetetrahydrofolate reductase (MTHFR) E72.12
- mevalonate kinase M04.1
- mineral NEC E61.8
- mineralocorticoid E27.49
  - with glucocorticoid E27.49
- molybdenum (nutritional) E61.5
- moral F60.2
- multiple nutrient elements E61.7
- multiple sulfatase (MSD) E75.26
- muscle
  - carnitine (palmityltransferase) E71.314
  - phosphofructokinase E74.09
- myoadenylate deaminase E79.2
- myocardial — *see* Insufficiency, myocardial
- myophosphorylase E74.04
- NADH diaphorase or reductase (congenital) D74.0
- NADH-methemoglobin reductase (congenital) D74.0
- natrium E87.1
- niacin (amide) (-tryptophan) E52
- nicotinamide E52
- nicotinic acid E52
- number of teeth — *see* Anodontia
- nutrient element E61.9
  - multiple E61.7
  - specified NEC E61.8
- nutrition, nutritional E63.9
  - sequelae — *see* Sequelae, nutritional deficiency
  - specified NEC E63.8
- of interleukin 1 receptor antagonist [DIRA] M04.8
- ornithine transcarbamylase E72.4
- ovarian E28.39
- oxygen — *see* Anoxia
- pantothenic acid E53.8
- parathyroid (gland) E20.9
- perineum (female) N81.89
- phenylalanine hydroxylase E70.1
- phosphoenolpyruvate carboxykinase E74.4
- phosphofructokinase E74.19
- phosphomannomutuse E74.8
- phosphomannose isomerase E74.8
- phosphomannosyl mutase E74.8
- phosphorylase kinase, liver E74.09
- pituitary hormone (isolated) E23.0
- plasma thromboplastin
  - antecedent (PTA) D68.1
  - component (PTC) D67
- plasminogen (type 1) (type 2) E88.02
- platelet NEC D69.1
  - constitutional D68.0
- polyglandular E31.8
  - autoimmune E31.0
- potassium (K) E87.6
- prepuce N47.3
- proaccelerin (congenital) (hereditary) D68.2
  - acquired D68.4
- proconvertin factor (congenital) (hereditary) D68.2
  - acquired D68.4
- protein — *see also* Malnutrition E46
  - anemia D53.0
  - C D68.59
  - S D68.59
- prothrombin (congenital) (heredItary) D68.2
  - acquired D68.4
- Prower factor D68.2
- pseudocholinesterase E88.09

Deficiency, deficient - *continued*
- PTA (plasma thromboplastin antecedent) D68.1
- PTC (plasma thromboplastin component) D67
- purine nucleoside phosphorylase (PNP) D81.5
- pyracin (alpha) (beta) E53.1
- pyridoxal E53.1
- pyridoxamine E53.1
- pyridoxine (derivatives) E53.1
- pyruvate
  - carboxylase E74.4
  - dehydrogenase E74.4
- riboflavin (vitamin B2) E53.0
- salt E87.1
- secretion
  - ovary E28.39
  - salivary gland (any) K11.7
  - urine R34
- selenium (dietary) E59
- serum antitrypsin, familial E88.01
- short stature homeobox gene (SHOX)
  - with
    - dyschondrosteosis Q78.8
    - short stature (idiopathic) E34.3
    - Turner's syndrome Q96.9
- sodium (Na) E87.1
- SPCA (factor VII) D68.2
- sphincter, intrinsic N36.42
  - with urethral hypermobility N36.43
- stable factor (congenital) (hereditary) D68.2
  - acquired D68.4
- Stuart-Prower (factor X) D68.2
- succinic semialdehyde dehydrogenase E72.81
- sucrase E74.39
- sulfatase E75.26
- sulfite oxidase E72.19
- thiamin, thiaminic (chloride) E51.9
  - beriberi (dry) E51.11
    - wet E51.12
- thrombokinase D68.2
  - newborn P53
- thyroid (gland) — *see* Hypothyroidism
- tocopherol E56.0
- tooth bud K00.0
- transcobalamine II (anemia) D51.2
- vanadium E61.6
- vascular I99.9
- vasopressin E23.2
- vertical ridge K06.8
- viosterol — *see* Deficiency, calciferol
- vitamin (multiple) NOS E56.9
  - A E50.9
    - with
      - Bitot's spot (corneal) E50.1
      - follicular keratosis E50.8
      - keratomalacia E50.4
      - manifestations NEC E50.8
      - night blindness E50.5
      - scar of cornea, xerophthalmic E50.6
      - xeroderma E50.8
      - xerophthalmia E50.7
      - xerosis
        - conjunctival E50.0
          - and Bitot's spot E50.1
        - cornea E50.2
          - and ulceration E50.3
    - sequelae E64.1
  - B (complex) NOS E53.9
    - with
      - beriberi (dry) E51.11
        - wet E51.12
      - pellagra E52
  - B1 NOS E51.9
    - beriberi (dry) E51.11
      - with circulatory system manifestations E51.11
      - wet E51.12
  - B12 E53.8
  - B2 (riboflavin) E53.0
  - B6 E53.1
  - C E54
    - sequelae E64.2
  - D E55.9
    - with
      - adult osteomalacia M83.8
      - rickets — *see* Rickets
    - 25-hydroxylase E83.32
  - E E56.0
  - folic acid E53.8
  - G E53.0
  - group B E53.9
    - specified NEC E53.8
  - H (biotin) E53.8
  - K E56.1
    - of newborn P53

Deficiency, deficient - *continued*
- vitamin (multiple) NOS - *continued*
  - nicotinic E52
  - P E56.8
  - PP (pellagra-preventing) E52
  - specified NEC E56.8
  - thiamin E51.9
    - beriberi — *see* Beriberi
- zinc, dietary E60

Deficit — *see also* Deficiency
- attention and concentration R41.840
  - following
    - cerebral infarction I69.310
    - cerebrovascular disease I69.910
      - specified disease NEC I69.810
    - nontraumatic
      - intracerebral hemorrhage I69.110
      - specified intracranial hemorrhage NEC I69.210
      - subarachnoid hemorrhage I69.010
  - disorder — *see* Attention, deficit
- cognitive
  - communication R41.841
  - emotional
    - following
      - cerebral infarction I69.315
      - cerebrovascular disease I69.915
        - specified disease NEC I69.815
      - nontraumatic
        - intracerebral hemorrhage I69.115
        - specified intracranial hemorrhage NEC I69.215
        - subarachnoid hemorrhage I69.015
  - following
    - cerebral infarction I69.319
    - cerebrovascular disease I69.919
      - specified disease NEC I69.819
    - nontraumatic
      - intracerebral hemorrhage I69.119
      - specified intracranial hemorrhage NEC I69.219
      - subarachnoid hemorrhage I69.019
  - social
    - following
      - cerebral infarction I69.315
      - cerebrovascular disease I69.915
        - specified disease NEC I69.815
      - nontraumatic
        - intracerebral hemorrhage I69.115
        - specified intracranial hemorrhage NEC I69.215
        - subarachnoid hemorrhage I69.015
- cognitive NEC R41.89
  - following
    - cerebral infarction I69.318
    - cerebrovascular disease I69.918
      - specified disease NEC I69.818
    - nontraumatic
      - intracerebral hemorrhage I69.118
      - specified intracranial hemorrhage NEC I69.218
      - subarachnoid hemorrhage I69.018
- concentration R41.840
- executive function R41.844
  - following
    - cerebral infarction I69.314
    - cerebrovascular disease I69.914
      - specified disease NEC I69.814
    - nontraumatic
      - intracerebral hemorrhage I69.114
      - specified intracranial hemorrhage NEC I69.214
      - subarachnoid hemorrhage I69.014
- frontal lobe R41.844
  - following
    - cerebral infarction I69.314
    - cerebrovascular disease I69.914
      - specified disease NEC I69.814
    - nontraumatic
      - intracerebral hemorrhage I69.114
      - specified intracranial hemorrhage NEC I69.214
      - subarachnoid hemorrhage I69.014
- memory
  - following
    - cerebral infarction I69.311
    - cerebrovascular disease I69.911
      - specified disease NEC I69.811
    - nontraumatic
      - intracerebral hemorrhage I69.111
      - specified intracranial hemorrhage NEC I69.211
      - subarachnoid hemorrhage I69.011
- neurologic NEC R29.818
  - ischemic
    - reversible (RIND) I63.9
      - prolonged (PRIND) I63.9
- oxygen R09.02

Deficit - *continued*
- prolonged reversible ischemic neurologic (PRIND) I63.9
- psychomotor R41.843
  - following
    - cerebral infarction I69.313
    - cerebrovascular disease I69.913
      - specified disease NEC I69.813
    - nontraumatic
      - intracerebral hemorrhage I69.113
      - specified intracranial hemorrhage NEC I69.213
      - subarachnoid hemorrhage I69.013
- visuospatial R41.842
  - following
    - cerebral infarction I69.312
    - cerebrovascular disease I69.912
      - specified disease NEC I69.812
    - nontraumatic
      - intracerebral hemorrhage I69.112
      - specified intracranial hemorrhage NEC I69.212
      - subarachnoid hemorrhage I69.012

Deflection
- radius — *see* Deformity, limb, specified type NEC, forearm
- septum (acquired) (nasal) (nose) J34.2
- spine — *see* Curvature, spine
- turbinate (nose) J34.2

Defluvium
- capillorum — *see* Alopecia
- ciliorum — *see* Madarosis
- unguium L60.8

Deformity Q89.9
- abdomen, congenital Q89.9
- abdominal wall
  - acquired M95.8
  - congenital Q79.59
- acquired (unspecified site) M95.9
- adrenal gland Q89.1
- alimentary tract, congenital Q45.9
  - upper Q40.9
- ankle (joint) (acquired) — *see also* Deformity, limb, lower leg
  - abduction — *see* Contraction, joint, ankle
  - congenital Q68.8
  - contraction — *see* Contraction, joint, ankle
  - specified type NEC — *see* Deformity, limb, foot, specified NEC
- anus (acquired) K62.89
  - congenital Q43.9
- aorta (arch) (congenital) Q25.40
  - acquired I77.89
- aortic
  - arch, acquired I77.89
  - cusp or valve (congenital) Q23.8
    - acquired — *see also* Endocarditis, aortic I35.8
- arm (acquired) (upper) — *see also* Deformity, limb, upper arm
  - congenital Q68.8
  - forearm — *see* Deformity, limb, forearm
- artery (congenital) (peripheral) NOS Q27.9
  - acquired I77.89
  - coronary (acquired) I25.9
    - congenital Q24.5
  - umbilical Q27.0
- atrial septal Q21.1
- auditory canal (external) (congenital) — *see also* Malformation, ear, external
  - acquired — *see* Disorder, ear, external, specified type NEC
- auricle
  - ear (congenital) — *see also* Malformation, ear, external
    - acquired — *see* Disorder, pinna, deformity
- back — *see* Dorsopathy, deforming
- bile duct (common) (congenital) (hepatic) Q44.5
  - acquired K83.8
- biliary duct or passage (congenital) Q44.5
  - acquired K83.8
- bladder (neck) (trigone) (sphincter) (acquired) N32.89
  - congenital Q64.79
- bone (acquired) NOS M95.9
  - congenital Q79.9
  - turbinate M95.0
- brain (congenital) Q04.9
  - acquired G93.89
  - reduction Q04.3
- breast (acquired) N64.89
  - congenital Q83.9
  - reconstructed N65.0
- bronchus (congenital) Q32.4
  - acquired NEC J98.09
- bursa, congenital Q79.9

Deformity - *continued*
- canaliculi (lacrimalis) (acquired) — *see also* Disorder, lacrimal system, changes
  - congenital Q10.6
- canthus, acquired — *see* Disorder, eyelid, specified type NEC
- capillary (acquired) I78.8
- cardiovascular system, congenital Q28.9
- caruncle, lacrimal (acquired) — *see also* Disorder, lacrimal system, changes
  - congenital Q10.6
- cascade, stomach K31.2
- cecum (congenital) Q43.9
  - acquired K63.89
- cerebral, acquired G93.89
  - congenital Q04.9
- cervix (uterus) (acquired) NEC N88.8
  - congenital Q51.9
- cheek (acquired) M95.2
  - congenital Q18.9
- chest (acquired) (wall) M95.4
  - congenital Q67.8
  - sequelae (late effect) of rickets E64.3
- chin (acquired) M95.2
  - congenital Q18.9
- choroid (congenital) Q14.3
  - acquired H31.8
  - plexus Q07.8
    - acquired G96.19
- cicatricial — *see* Cicatrix
- cilia, acquired — *see* Disorder, eyelid, specified type NEC
- clavicle (acquired) M95.8
  - congenital Q68.8
- clitoris (congenital) Q52.6
  - acquired N90.89
- clubfoot — *see* Clubfoot
- coccyx (acquired) — *see* subcategory M43.8
- colon (congenital) Q43.9
  - acquired K63.89
- concha (ear) , congenital — *see also* Malformation, ear, external
  - acquired — *see* Disorder, pinna, deformity
- cornea (acquired) H18.70
  - congenital Q13.4
  - descemetocele — *see* Descemetocele
  - ectasia — *see* Ectasia, cornea
  - specified NEC H18.79-
  - staphyloma — *see* Staphyloma, cornea
- coronary artery (acquired) I25.9
  - congenital Q24.5
- cranium (acquired) — *see* Deformity, skull
- cricoid cartilage (congenital) Q31.8
  - acquired J38.7
- cystic duct (congenital) Q44.5
  - acquired K82.8
- Dandy-Walker Q03.1
  - with spina bifida — *see* Spina bifida
- diaphragm (congenital) Q79.1
  - acquired J98.6
- digestive organ NOS Q45.9
- ductus arteriosus Q25.0
- duodenal bulb K31.89
- duodenum (congenital) Q43.9
  - acquired K31.89
- dura — *see* Deformity, meninges
- ear (acquired) — *see also* Disorder, pinna, deformity
  - congenital (external) Q17.9
    - internal Q16.5
    - middle Q16.4
      - ossicles Q16.3
    - ossicles Q16.3
- ectodermal (congenital) NEC Q84.9
- ejaculatory duct (congenital) Q55.4
  - acquired N50.89
- elbow (joint) (acquired) — *see also* Deformity, limb, upper arm
  - congenital Q68.8
  - contraction — *see* Contraction, joint, elbow
- endocrine gland NEC Q89.2
- epididymis (congenital) Q55.4
  - acquired N50.89
- epiglottis (congenital) Q31.8
  - acquired J38.7
- esophagus (congenital) Q39.9
  - acquired K22.8
- eustachian tube (congenital) NEC Q17.8
- eye, congenital Q15.9
- eyebrow (congenital) Q18.8
- eyelid (acquired) — *see also* Disorder, eyelid, specified type NEC
  - congenital Q10.3
- face (acquired) M95.2

Deformity - *continued*
- face (acquired) - *continued*
  - congenital Q18.9
- fallopian tube, acquired N83.8
- femur (acquired) — *see* Deformity, limb, specified type NEC, thigh
- fetal
  - with fetopelvic disproportion O33.7
  - causing obstructed labor O66.3
- finger (acquired) M20.00-
  - boutonniere M20.02-
  - congenital Q68.1
  - flexion contracture — *see* Contraction, joint, hand
  - mallet finger M20.01-
  - specified NEC M20.09-
  - swan-neck M20.03-
- flexion (joint) (acquired) — *see also* Deformity, limb, flexion M21.20
  - congenital NOS Q74.9
    - hip Q65.89
- foot (acquired) — *see also* Deformity, limb, lower leg
  - cavovarus (congenital) Q66.1
  - congenital NOS Q66.9
    - specified type NEC Q66.89
  - specified type NEC — *see* Deformity, limb, foot, specified NEC
  - valgus (congenital) Q66.6
    - acquired — *see* Deformity, valgus, ankle
  - varus (congenital) NEC Q66.3
    - acquired — *see* Deformity, varus, ankle
- forearm (acquired) — *see also* Deformity, limb, forearm
  - congenital Q68.8
- forehead (acquired) M95.2
  - congenital Q75.8
- frontal bone (acquired) M95.2
  - congenital Q75.8
- gallbladder (congenital) Q44.1
  - acquired K82.8
- gastrointestinal tract (congenital) NOS Q45.9
  - acquired K63.89
- genitalia, genital organ (s) or system NEC
  - female (congenital) Q52.9
    - acquired N94.89
    - external Q52.70
  - male (congenital) Q55.9
    - acquired N50.89
- globe (eye) (congenital) Q15.8
  - acquired H44.89
- gum, acquired NEC K06.8
- hand (acquired) — *see* Deformity, limb, hand
  - congenital Q68.1
- head (acquired) M95.2
  - congenital Q75.8
- heart (congenital) Q24.9
  - septum Q21.9
    - auricular Q21.1
    - ventricular Q21.0
  - valve (congenital) NEC Q24.8
    - acquired — *see* Endocarditis
- heel (acquired) — *see* Deformity, foot
- hepatic duct (congenital) Q44.5
  - acquired K83.8
- hip (joint) (acquired) — *see also* Deformity, limb, thigh
  - congenital Q65.9
  - due to (previous) juvenile osteochondrosis — *see* Coxa, plana
  - flexion — *see* Contraction, joint, hip
- hourglass — *see* Contraction, hourglass
- humerus (acquired) M21.82-
  - congenital Q74.0
- hypophyseal (congenital) Q89.2
- ileocecal (coil) (valve) (acquired) K63.89
  - congenital Q43.9
- ileum (congenital) Q43.9
  - acquired K63.89
- ilium (acquired) M95.5
  - congenital Q74.2
- integument (congenital) Q84.9
- intervertebral cartilage or disc (acquired) — *see* Disorder, disc, specified NEC
- intestine (large) (small) (congenital) NOS Q43.9
  - acquired K63.89
- intrinsic minus or plus (hand) — *see* Deformity, limb, specified type NEC, forearm
- iris (acquired) H21.89
  - congenital Q13.2
- ischium (acquired) M95.5
  - congenital Q74.2
- jaw (acquired) (congenital) M26.9
- joint (acquired) NEC M21.90

Deformity - *continued*
joint (acquired) NEC - *continued*
congenital Q68.8
elbow M21.92-
hand M21.94-
hip M21.95-
knee M21.96-
shoulder M21.92-
wrist M21.93-
kidney (s) (calyx) (pelvis) (congenital) Q63.9
acquired N28.89
artery (congenital) Q27.2
acquired I77.89
Klippel-Feil (brevicollis) Q76.1
knee (acquired) NEC — *see also* Deformity, limb, lower leg
congenital Q68.2
labium (majus) (minus) (congenital) Q52.79
acquired N90.89
lacrimal passages or duct (congenital) NEC Q10.6
acquired — *see* Disorder, lacrimal system, changes
larynx (muscle) (congenital) Q31.8
acquired J38.7
web (glottic) Q31.0
leg (upper) (acquired) NEC — *see also* Deformity, limb, thigh
congenital Q68.8
lower leg — *see* Deformity, limb, lower leg
lens (acquired) H27.8
congenital Q12.9
lid (fold) (acquired) — *see also* Disorder, eyelid, specified type NEC
congenital Q10.3
ligament (acquired) — *see* Disorder, ligament
congenital Q79.9
limb (acquired) M21.90
clawfoot M21.53-
clawhand M21.51-
clubfoot M21.54-
clubhand M21.52-
congenital, except reduction deformity Q74.9
flat foot M21.4-
flexion M21.20
ankle M21.27-
elbow M21.22-
finger M21.24-
hip M21.25-
knee M21.26-
shoulder M21.21-
toe M21.27-
wrist M21.23-
foot
claw — *see* Deformity, limb, clawfoot
club — *see* Deformity, limb, clubfoot
drop M21.37-
flat — *see* Deformity, limb, flat foot
specified NEC M21.6X-
forearm M21.93-
hand M21.94-
lower leg M21.96-
specified type NEC M21.80
forearm M21.83-
lower leg M21.86-
thigh M21.85-
upper arm M21.82-
thigh M21.95-
unequal length M21.70
short site is
femur M21.75-
fibula M21.76-
humerus M21.72-
radius M21.73-
tibia M21.76-
ulna M21.73-
upper arm M21.92-
valgus — *see* Deformity, valgus
varus — *see* Deformity, varus
wrist drop M21.33-
lip (acquired) NEC K13.0
congenital Q38.0
liver (congenital) Q44.7
acquired K76.89
lumbosacral (congenital) (joint) (region) Q76.49
acquired — *see* subcategory M43.8
kyphosis — *see* Kyphosis, congenital
lordosis — *see* Lordosis, congenital
lung (congenital) Q33.9
acquired J98.4
lymphatic system, congenital Q89.9
Madelung's (radius) Q74.0
mandible (acquired) (congenital) M26.9
maxilla (acquired) (congenital) M26.9
meninges or membrane (congenital) Q07.9

Deformity - *continued*
meninges or membrane (congenital) - *continued*
cerebral Q04.8
acquired G96.19
spinal cord (congenital) G96.19
acquired G96.19
metacarpus (acquired) — *see* Deformity, limb, forearm
congenital Q74.0
metatarsus (acquired) — *see* Deformity, foot
congenital Q66.9
middle ear (congenital) Q16.4
ossicles Q16.3
mitral (leaflets) (valve) I05.8
parachute Q23.2
stenosis, congenital Q23.2
mouth (acquired) K13.79
congenital Q38.6
multiple, congenital NEC Q89.7
muscle (acquired) M62.89
congenital Q79.9
sternocleidomastoid Q68.0
musculoskeletal system (acquired) M95.9
congenital Q79.9
specified NEC M95.8
nail (acquired) L60.8
congenital Q84.6
nasal — *see* Deformity, nose
neck (acquired) M95.3
congenital Q18.9
sternocleidomastoid Q68.0
nervous system (congenital) Q07.9
nipple (congenital) Q83.9
acquired N64.89
nose (acquired) (cartilage) M95.0
bone (turbinate) M95.0
congenital Q30.9
bent or squashed Q67.4
saddle M95.0
syphilitic A50.57
septum (acquired) J34.2
congenital Q30.8
sinus (wall) (congenital) Q30.8
acquired M95.0
syphilitic (congenital) A50.57
late A52.73
ocular muscle (congenital) Q10.3
acquired — *see* Strabismus, mechanical
opticociliary vessels (congenital) Q13.2
orbit (eye) (acquired) H05.30
atrophy — *see* Atrophy, orbit
congenital Q10.7
due to
bone disease NEC H05.32-
trauma or surgery H05.33-
enlargement — *see* Enlargement, orbit
exostosis — *see* Exostosis, orbit
organ of Corti (congenital) Q16.5
ovary (congenital) Q50.39
acquired N83.8
oviduct, acquired N83.8
palate (congenital) Q38.5
acquired M27.8
cleft (congenital) — *see* Cleft, palate
pancreas (congenital) Q45.3
acquired K86.89
parathyroid (gland) Q89.2
parotid (gland) (congenital) Q38.4
acquired K11.8
patella (acquired) — *see* Disorder, patella, specified NEC
pelvis, pelvic (acquired) (bony) M95.5
with disproportion (fetopelvic) O33.0
causing obstructed labor O65.0
congenital Q74.2
rachitic sequelae (late effect) E64.3
penis (glans) (congenital) Q55.69
acquired N48.89
pericardium (congenital) Q24.8
acquired — *see* Pericarditis
pharynx (congenital) Q38.8
acquired J39.2
pinna, acquired — *see also* Disorder, pinna, deformity
congenital Q17.9
pituitary (congenital) Q89.2
posture — *see* Dorsopathy, deforming
prepuce (congenital) Q55.69
acquired N47.8
prostate (congenital) Q55.4
acquired N42.89
pupil (congenital) Q13.2
acquired — *see* Abnormality, pupillary

Deformity - *continued*
pylorus (congenital) Q40.3
acquired K31.89
rachitic (acquired) , old or healed E64.3
radius (acquired) — *see also* Deformity, limb, forearm
congenital Q68.8
rectum (congenital) Q43.9
acquired K62.89
reduction (extremity) (limb) , congenital — *see also* condition and site Q73.8
brain Q04.3
lower — *see* Defect, reduction, lower limb
upper — *see* Defect, reduction, upper limb
renal — *see* Deformity, kidney
respiratory system (congenital) Q34.9
rib (acquired) M95.4
congenital Q76.6
cervical Q76.5
rotation (joint) (acquired) — *see* Deformity, limb, specified site NEC
congenital Q74.9
hip — *see* Deformity, limb, specified type NEC, thigh
congenital Q65.89
sacroiliac joint (congenital) Q74.2
acquired — *see* subcategory M43.8
sacrum (acquired) — *see* subcategory M43.8
saddle
back — *see* Lordosis
nose M95.0
syphilitic A50.57
salivary gland or duct (congenital) Q38.4
acquired K11.8
scapula (acquired) M95.8
congenital Q68.8
scrotum (congenital) — *see also* Malformation, testis and scrotum
acquired N50.89
seminal vesicles (congenital) Q55.4
acquired N50.89
septum, nasal (acquired) J34.2
shoulder (joint) (acquired) — *see* Deformity, limb, upper arm
congenital Q74.0
contraction — *see* Contraction, joint, shoulder
sigmoid (flexure) (congenital) Q43.9
acquired K63.89
skin (congenital) Q82.9
skull (acquired) M95.2
congenital Q75.8
with
anencephaly Q00.0
encephalocele — *see* Encephalocele
hydrocephalus Q03.9
with spina bifida — *see* Spina bifida, by site, with hydrocephalus
microcephaly Q02
soft parts, organs or tissues (of pelvis)
in pregnancy or childbirth NEC O34.8-
causing obstructed labor O65.5
spermatic cord (congenital) Q55.4
acquired N50.89
torsion — *see* Torsion, spermatic cord
spinal — *see* Dorsopathy, deforming
column (acquired) — *see* Dorsopathy, deforming
congenital Q67.5
cord (congenital) Q06.9
acquired G95.89
nerve root (congenital) Q07.9
spine (acquired) — *see also* Dorsopathy, deforming
congenital Q67.5
rachitic E64.3
specified NEC — *see* Dorsopathy, deforming, specified NEC
spleen
acquired D73.89
congenital Q89.09
Sprengel's (congenital) Q74.0
sternocleidomastoid (muscle) , congenital Q68.0
sternum (acquired) M95.4
congenital NEC Q76.7
stomach (congenital) Q40.3
acquired K31.89
submandibular gland (congenital) Q38.4
submaxillary gland (congenital) Q38.4
acquired K11.8
talipes — *see* Talipes
testis (congenital) — *see also* Malformation, testis and scrotum
acquired N44.8
torsion — *see* Torsion, testis
thigh (acquired) — *see also* Deformity, limb, thigh

Deformity - *continued*
thigh (acquired) - *continued*
congenital NEC Q68.8
thorax (acquired) (wall) M95.4
congenital Q67.8
sequelae of rickets E64.3
thumb (acquired) — *see also* Deformity, finger
congenital NEC Q68.1
thymus (tissue) (congenital) Q89.2
thyroid (gland) (congenital) Q89.2
cartilage Q31.8
acquired J38.7
tibia (acquired) — *see also* Deformity, limb, specified type NEC, lower leg
congenital NEC Q68.8
saber (syphilitic) A50.56
toe (acquired) M20.6-
congenital Q66.9
hallux rigidus M20.2-
hallux valgus M20.1-
hallux varus M20.3-
hammer toe M20.4-
specified NEC M20.5X-
tongue (congenital) Q38.3
acquired K14.8
tooth, teeth K00.2
trachea (rings) (congenital) Q32.1
acquired J39.8
transverse aortic arch (congenital) Q25.49
tricuspid (leaflets) (valve) I07.8
atresia or stenosis Q22.4
Ebstein's Q22.5
trunk (acquired) M95.8
congenital Q89.9
ulna (acquired) — *see also* Deformity, limb, forearm
congenital NEC Q68.8
urachus, congenital Q64.4
ureter (opening) (congenital) Q62.8
acquired N28.89
urethra (congenital) Q64.79
acquired N36.8
urinary tract (congenital) Q64.9
urachus Q64.4
uterus (congenital) Q51.9
acquired N85.8
uvula (congenital) Q38.5
vagina (acquired) N89.8
congenital Q52.4
valgus NEC M21.00
ankle M21.07-
elbow M21.02-
hip M21.05-
knee M21.06-
valve, valvular (congenital) (heart) Q24.8
acquired — *see* Endocarditis
varus NEC M21.10
ankle M21.17-
elbow M21.12-
hip M21.15
knee M21.16-
tibia — *see* Osteochondrosis, juvenile, tibia
vas deferens (congenital) Q55.4
acquired N50.89
vein (congenital) Q27.9
great Q26.9
vertebra — *see* Dorsopathy, deforming
vertical talus (congenital) Q66.80
left foot Q66.82
right foot Q66.81
vesicourethral orifice (acquired) N32.89
congenital NEC Q64.79
vessels of optic papilla (congenital) Q14.2
visual field (contraction) — *see* Defect, visual field
vitreous body, acquired H43.89
vulva (congenital) Q52.79
acquired N90.89
wrist (joint) (acquired) — *see also* Deformity, limb, forearm
congenital Q68.8
contraction — *see* Contraction, joint, wrist

Degeneration, degenerative
adrenal (capsule) (fatty) (gland) (hyaline) (infectional) E27.8
amyloid — *see also* Amyloidosis E85.9
anterior cornua, spinal cord G12.29
anterior labral S43.49-
aorta, aortic I70.0
fatty I77.89
aortic valve (heart) — *see* Endocarditis, aortic
arteriovascular — *see* Arteriosclerosis
artery, arterial (atheromatous) (calcareous) — *see also* Arteriosclerosis
cerebral, amyloid E85.4 *[I68.0]*

Degeneration, degenerative - *continued*
artery, arterial (atheromatous) (calcareous) - *continued*
medial — *see* Arteriosclerosis, extremities
articular cartilage NEC — *see* Derangement, joint, articular cartilage, by site
atheromatous — *see* Arteriosclerosis
basal nuclei or ganglia G23.9
specified NEC G23.8
bone NEC — *see* Disorder, bone, specified type NEC
brachial plexus G54.0
brain (cortical) (progressive) G31.9
alcoholic G31.2
arteriosclerotic I67.2
childhood G31.9
specified NEC G31.89
cystic G31.89
congenital Q04.6
in
alcoholism G31.2
beriberi E51.2
cerebrovascular disease I67.9
congenital hydrocephalus Q03.9
with spina bifida — *see also* Spina bifida
Fabry-Anderson disease E75.21
Gaucher's disease E75.22
Hunter's syndrome E76.1
lipidosis
cerebral E75.4
generalized E75.6
mucopolysaccharidosis — *see* Mucopolysaccharidosis
myxedema E03.9 *[G32.89]*
neoplastic disease — *see also* Neoplasm D49.6 *[G32.89]*
Niemann-Pick disease E75.249 *[G32.89]*
sphingolipidosis E75.3 *[G32.89]*
vitamin B12 deficiency E53.8 *[G32.89]*
senile NEC G31.1
breast N64.89
Bruch's membrane — *see* Degeneration, choroid
capillaries (fatty) I78.8
amyloid E85.89 *[I79.8]*
cardiac — *see also* Degeneration, myocardial
valve, valvular — *see* Endocarditis
cardiorenal — *see* Hypertension, cardiorenal
cardiovascular — *see also* Disease, cardiovascular
renal — *see* Hypertension, cardiorenal
cerebellar NOS G31.9
alcoholic G31.2
primary (hereditary) (sporadic) G11.9
cerebral — *see* Degeneration, brain
cerebrovascular I67.9
due to hypertension I67.4
cervical plexus G54.2
cervix N88.8
due to radiation (intended effect) N88.8
adverse effect or misadventure N99.89
chamber angle H21.21-
changes, spine or vertebra — *see* Spondylosis
chorioretinal — *see also* Degeneration, choroid
hereditary H31.20
choroid (colloid) (drusen) H31.10-
atrophy — *see* Atrophy, choroidal
hereditary — *see* Dystrophy, choroidal, hereditary
ciliary body H21.22-
cochlear — *see* subcategory H83.8
combined (spinal cord) (subacute) E53.8 *[G32.0]*
with anemia (pernicious) D51.0 *[G32.0]*
due to dietary vitamin B12 deficiency D51.3 *[G32.0]*
in (due to)
vitamin B12 deficiency E53.8 *[G32.0]*
anemia D51.9 *[G32.0]*
conjunctiva H11.10
concretions — *see* Concretion, conjunctiva
deposits — *see* Deposit, conjunctiva
pigmentations — *see* Pigmentation, conjunctiva
pinguecula — *see* Pinguecula
xerosis — *see* Xerosis, conjunctiva
cornea H18.40
calcerous H18.43
band keratopathy H18.42-
familial, hereditary — *see* Dystrophy, cornea
hyaline (of old scars) H18.49
keratomalacia — *see* Keratomalacia
nodular H18.45-
peripheral H18.46-
senile H18.41-
specified type NEC H18.49
cortical (cerebellar) (parenchymatous) G31.89
alcoholic G31.2

Degeneration, degenerative - *continued*
cortical (cerebellar) (parenchymatous) - *continued*
diffuse, due to arteriopathy I67.2
corticobasal G31.85
cutis L98.8
amyloid E85.4 *[L99]*
dental pulp K04.2
disc disease — *see* Degeneration, intervertebral disc NEC
dorsolateral (spinal cord) — *see* Degeneration, combined
extrapyramidal G25.9
eye, macular — *see also* Degeneration, macula
congenital or hereditary — *see* Dystrophy, retina
facet joints — *see* Spondylosis
fatty
liver NEC K76.0
alcoholic K70.0
grey matter (brain) (Alpers') G31.81
heart — *see also* Degeneration, myocardial
amyloid E85.4 *[I43]*
atheromatous — *see* Disease, heart, ischemic, atherosclerotic
ischemic — *see* Disease, heart, ischemic
hepatolenticular (Wilson's) E83.01
hepatorenal K76.7
hyaline (diffuse) (generalized)
localized — *see* Degeneration, by site
infrapatellar fat pad M79.4
intervertebral disc NOS
with
myelopathy — *see* Disorder, disc, with, myelopathy
radiculitis or radiculopathy — *see* Disorder, disc, with, radiculopathy
cervical, cervicothoracic — *see* Disorder, disc, cervical, degeneration
with
myelopathy — *see* Disorder, disc, cervical, with myelopathy
neuritis, radiculitis or radiculopathy — *see* Disorder, disc, cervical, with neuritis
lumbar region M51.36
with
myelopathy M51.06
neuritis, radiculitis, radiculopathy or sciatica M51.16
lumbosacral region M51.37
with
neuritis, radiculitis, radiculopathy or sciatica M51.17
sacrococcygeal region M53.3
thoracic region M51.34
with
myelopathy M51.04
neuritis, radiculitis, radiculopathy M51.14
thoracolumbar region M51.35
with
myelopathy M51.05
neuritis, radiculitis, radiculopathy M51.15
intestine, amyloid E85.4
iris (pigmentary) H21.23-
ischemic — *see* Ischemia
joint disease — *see* Osteoarthritis
kidney N28.89
amyloid E85.4 *[N29]*
cystic, congenital Q61.9
fatty N28.89
polycystic Q61.3
adult type (autosomal dominant) Q61.2
infantile type (autosomal recessive) NEC Q61.19
collecting duct dilatation Q61.11
Kuhnt-Junius — *see also* Degeneration, macula H35.32-
lens — *see* Cataract
lenticular (familial) (progressive) (Wilson's) (with cirrhosis of liver) E83.01
liver (diffuse) NEC K76.89
amyloid E85.4 *[K77]*
cystic K76.89
congenital Q44.6
fatty NEC K76.0
alcoholic K70.0
hypertrophic K76.89
parenchymatous, acute or subacute K72.00
with coma K72.01
pigmentary K76.89
toxic (acute) K71.9
lung J98.4
lymph gland I89.8
hyaline I89.8
macula, macular (acquired) (age-related) (senile) H35.30

Degeneration, degenerative - *continued*
macula, macular (acquired) (age-related) (senile) - *continued*
angioid streaks H35.33
atrophic age-related H35.31-
congenital or hereditary — *see* Dystrophy, retina
cystoid H35.35-
drusen H35.36-
dry age-related H35.31-
exudative H35.32-
hole H35.34-
nonexudative H35.31-
puckering H35.37-
toxic H35.38-
wet age-related H35.32-
membranous labyrinth, congenital (causing impairment of hearing) Q16.5
meniscus — *see* Derangement, meniscus
mitral — *see* Insufficiency, mitral
Mönckeberg's — *see* Arteriosclerosis, extremities
motor centers, senile G31.1
multi-system G90.3
mural — *see* Degeneration, myocardial
muscle (fatty) (fibrous) (hyaline) (progressive) M62.89
heart — *see* Degeneration, myocardial
myelin, central nervous system G37.9
myocardial, myocardium (fatty) (hyaline) (senile) I51.5
with rheumatic fever (conditions in I00) I09.0
active, acute or subacute I01.2
with chorea I02.0
inactive or quiescent (with chorea) I09.0
hypertensive — *see* Hypertension, heart
rheumatic — *see* Degeneration, myocardial, with rheumatic fever
syphilitic A52.06
nasal sinus (mucosa) J32.9
frontal J32.1
maxillary J32.0
nerve — *see* Disorder, nerve
nervous system G31.9
alcoholic G31.2
amyloid E85.4 *[G99.8]*
autonomic G90.9
fatty G31.89
specified NEC G31.89
nipple N64.89
olivopontocerebellar (hereditary) (familial) G23.8
osseous labyrinth — *see* subcategory H83.8
ovary N83.8
cystic N83.20-
microcystic N83.20-
pallidal pigmentary (progressive) G23.0
pancreas K86.89
tuberculous A18.83
penis N48.89
pigmentary (diffuse) (general)
localized — *see* Degeneration, by site
pallidal (progressive) G23.0
pineal gland E34.8
pituitary (gland) E23.6
popliteal fat pad M79.4
posterolateral (spinal cord) — *see* Degeneration, combined
pulmonary valve (heart) I37.8
pulp (tooth) K04.2
pupillary margin H21.24-
renal — *see* Degeneration, kidney
retina H35.9
hereditary (cerebroretinal) (congenital) (juvenile) (macula) (peripheral) (pigmentary) — *see* Dystrophy, retina
Kuhnt-Junius — *see also* Degeneration, macula H35.32-
macula (cystic) (exudative) (hole) (nonexudative) (pseudohole) (senile) (toxic) — *see* Degeneration, macula
peripheral H35.40
lattice H35.41-
microcystoid H35.42-
paving stone H35.43-
secondary
pigmentary H35.45-
vitreoretinal H35.46-
senile reticular H35.44-
pigmentary (primary) — *see also* Dystrophy, retina
secondary — *see* Degeneration, retina, peripheral, secondary
posterior pole — *see* Degeneration, macula
saccule, congenital (causing impairment of hearing) Q16.5
senile R54

Degeneration, degenerative - *continued*
senile - *continued*
brain G31.1
cardiac, heart or myocardium — *see* Degeneration, myocardial
motor centers G31.1
vascular — *see* Arteriosclerosis
sinus (cystic) — *see also* Sinusitis
polypoid J33.1
skin L98.8
amyloid E85.4 *[L99]*
colloid L98.8
spinal (cord) G31.89
amyloid E85.4 *[G32.89]*
combined (subacute) — *see* Degeneration, combined
dorsolateral — *see* Degeneration, combined
familial NEC G31.89
fatty G31.89
funicular — *see* Degeneration, combined
posterolateral — *see* Degeneration, combined
subacute combined — *see* Degeneration, combined
tuberculous A17.81
spleen D73.0
amyloid E85.4 *[D77]*
stomach K31.89
striatonigral G23.2
suprarenal (capsule) (gland) E27.8
synovial membrane (pulpy) — *see* Disorder, synovium, specified type NEC
tapetoretinal — *see* Dystrophy, retina
thymus (gland) E32.8
fatty E32.8
thyroid (gland) E07.89
tricuspid (heart) (valve) I07.9
tuberculous NEC — *see* Tuberculosis
turbinate J34.89
uterus (cystic) N85.8
vascular (senile) — *see* Arteriosclerosis
hypertensive — *see* Hypertension
vitreoretinal, secondary — *see* Degeneration, retina, peripheral, secondary, vitreoretinal
vitreous (body) H43.81-
Wallerian — *see* Disorder, nerve
Wilson's hepatolenticular E83.01
Deglutition
paralysis R13.0
hysterical F44.4
pneumonia J69.0
Degos' disease I77.89
Dehiscence (of)
amputation stump T87.81
cesarean wound O90.0
closure of
cornea T81.31
craniotomy T81.32
fascia (muscular) (superficial) T81.32
internal organ or tissue T81.32
laceration (external) (internal) T81.33
ligament T81.32
mucosa T81.31
muscle or muscle flap T81.32
ribs or rib cage T81.32
skin and subcutaneous tissue (full-thickness) (superficial) T81.31
skull T81.32
sternum (sternotomy) T81.32
tendon T81.32
traumatic laceration (external) (internal) T81.33
episiotomy O90.1
operation wound NEC T81.31
external operation wound (superficial) T81.31
internal operation wound (deep) T81.32
perineal wound (postpartum) O90.1
traumatic injury wound repair T81.33
wound T81.30
traumatic repair T81.33
Dehydration E86.0
newborn P74.1
Déjérine-Roussy syndrome G89.0
Déjérine-Sottas disease or neuropathy (hypertrophic) G60.0
Déjérine-Thomas atrophy G23.8
Delay, delayed
any plane in pelvis
complicating delivery O66.9
birth or delivery NOS O63.9
closure, ductus arteriosus (Botalli) P29.38
coagulation — *see* Defect, coagulation
conduction (cardiac) (ventricular) I45.9
delivery, second twin, triplet, etc O63.2
development R62.50
global F88

Delay, delayed - *continued*
development - *continued*
intellectual (specific) F81.9
language F80.9
due to hearing loss F80.4
learning F81.9
pervasive F84.9
physiological R62.50
specified stage NEC R62.0
reading F81.0
sexual E30.0
speech F80.9
due to hearing loss F80.4
spelling F81.81
ejaculation F52.32
gastric emptying K30
menarche E30.0
menstruation (cause unknown) N91.0
milestone R62.0
passage of meconium (newborn) P76.0
primary respiration P28.9
puberty (constitutional) E30.0
separation of umbilical cord P96.82
sexual maturation, female E30.0
sleep phase syndrome G47.21
union, fracture — *see* Fracture, by site
vaccination Z28.9
Deletion (s)
autosome Q93.9
identified by fluorescence in situ hybridization (FISH) Q93.89
identified by in situ hybridization (ISH) Q93.89
chromosome
with complex rearrangements NEC Q93.7
part of NEC Q93.59
seen only at prometaphase Q93.89
short arm
4 Q93.3
5p Q93.4
22q11.2 Q93.81
specified NEC Q93.89
long arm chromosome 18 or 21 Q93.89
with complex rearrangements NEC Q93.7
microdeletions NEC Q93.88
Delhi boil or button B55.1
Delinquency (juvenile) (neurotic) F91.8
group Z72.810
Delinquent immunization status Z28.3
Delirium, delirious (acute or subacute) (not alcohol-or drug-induced) (with dementia) R41.0
alcoholic (acute) (tremens) (withdrawal) F10.921
with intoxication F10.921
in
abuse F10.121
dependence F10.221
due to (secondary to)
alcohol
intoxication F10.921
in
abuse F10.121
dependence F10.221
withdrawal F10.231
amphetamine intoxication F15.921
in
abuse F15.121
dependence F15.221
anxiolytic
intoxication F13.921
in
abuse F13.121
dependence F13.221
withdrawal F13.231
cannabis intoxication (acute) F12.921
in
abuse F12.121
dependence F12.221
cocaine intoxication (acute) F14.921
in
abuse F14.121
dependence F14.221
general medical condition F05
hallucinogen intoxication F16.921
in
abuse F16.121
dependence F16.221
hypnotic
intoxication F13.921
in
abuse F13.121
dependence F13.221
withdrawal F13.231
inhalant intoxication (acute) F18.921
in

Delirium, delirious (acute or subacute) (not alcohol-or drug-induced) (with dementia) - *continued*
due to (secondary to) - *continued*
inhalant intoxication (acute) - *continued*
in - *continued*
abuse F18.121
dependence F18.221
multiple etiologies F05
opioid intoxication (acute) F11.921
in
abuse F11.121
dependence F11.221
other (or unknown) substance F19.921
phencyclidine intoxication (acute) F16.921
in
abuse F16.121
dependence F16.221
psychoactive substance NEC intoxication (acute) F19.921
in
abuse F19.121
dependence F19.221
sedative
intoxication F13.921
in
abuse F13.121
dependence F13.221
withdrawal F13.231
unknown etiology F05
exhaustion F43.0
hysterical F44.89
postprocedural (postoperative) F05
puerperal F05
thyroid — *see* Thyrotoxicosis with thyroid storm
traumatic — *see* Injury, intracranial
tremens (alcohol-induced) F10.231
sedative-induced F13.231
Delivery (childbirth) (labor)
arrested active phase O62.1
cesarean (for)
abnormal
pelvis (bony) (deformity) (major) NEC with disproportion (fetopelvic) O33.0
with obstructed labor O65.0
presentation or position O32.9
abruptio placentae — *see also* Abruptio placentae O45.9-
acromion presentation O32.2
atony, uterus O62.2
breech presentation O32.1
incomplete O32.8
brow presentation O32.3
cephalopelvic disproportion O33.9
cerclage O34.3-
chin presentation O32.3
cicatrix of cervix O34.4-
contracted pelvis (general)
inlet O33.2
outlet O33.3
cord presentation or prolapse O69.0
cystocele O34.8-
deformity (acquired) (congenital)
pelvic organs or tissues NEC O34.8-
pelvis (bony) NEC O33.0
disproportion NOS O33.9
eclampsia — *see* Eclampsia
face presentation O32.3
failed
forceps O66.5
induction of labor O61.9
instrumental O61.1
mechanical O61.1
medical O61.0
specified NEC O61.8
surgical O61.1
trial of labor NOS O66.40
following previous cesarean delivery O66.41
vacuum extraction O66.5
ventouse O66.5
fetal-maternal hemorrhage O43.01-
hemorrhage (intrapartum) O67.9
with coagulation defect O67.0
specified cause NEC O67.8
high head at term O32.4
hydrocephalic fetus O33.6
incarceration of uterus O34.51-
incoordinate uterine action O62.4
increased size, fetus O33.5
inertia, uterus O62.2
primary O62.0
secondary O62.1
lateroversion, uterus O34.59-

Delivery (childbirth) (labor) - *continued*
cesarean (for) - *continued*
mal lie O32.9
malposition
fetus O32.9
pelvic organs or tissues NEC O34.8-
uterus NEC O34.59-
malpresentation NOS O32.9
oblique presentation O32.2
occurring after 37 completed weeks of gestation but before 39 completed weeks gestation due to (spontaneous) onset of labor O75.82
oversize fetus O33.5
pelvic tumor NEC O34.8-
placenta previa O44.0-
complete O44.0-
with hemorrhage O44.1-
placental insufficiency O36.51-
planned, occurring after 37 completed weeks of gestation but before 39 completed weeks gestation due to (spontaneous) onset of labor O75.82
polyp, cervix O34.4-
causing obstructed labor O65.5
poor dilatation, cervix O62.0
pre-eclampsia O14.94
mild O14.04
moderate O14.04
severe O14.14
with hemolysis, elevated liver enzymes and low platelet count (HELLP) O14.24
previous
cesarean delivery O34.219
classical (vertical) scar O34.212
low transverse scar O34.211
surgery (to)
cervix O34.4-
gynecological NEC O34.8-
rectum O34.7-
uterus O34.29
vagina O34.6-
prolapse
arm or hand O32.2
uterus O34.52-
prolonged labor NOS O63.9
rectocele O34.8-
retroversion
uterus O34.53-
rigid
cervix O34.4-
pelvic floor O34.8-
perineum O34.7-
vagina O34.6-
vulva O34.7-
sacculation, pregnant uterus O34.59-
scar (s)
cervix O34.4-
cesarean delivery O34.219
classical (vertical) O34.212
low transverse O34.211
transmural uterine O34.29
uterus O34.29
Shirodkar suture in situ O34.3-
shoulder presentation O32.2
stenosis or stricture, cervix O34.4-
streptococcus group B (GBS) carrier state O99.824
transmural uterine scar O34.29
transverse presentation or lie O32.2
tumor, pelvic organs or tissues NEC O34.8-
cervix O34.4-
umbilical cord presentation or prolapse O69.0
without indication O82
completely normal case O80
complicated O75.9
by
abnormal, abnormality (of)
forces of labor O62.9
specified type NEC O62.8
glucose O99.814
uterine contractions NOS O62.9
abruptio placentae — *see also* Abruptio placentae O45.9-
abuse
physical O9A.32
psychological O9A.52
sexual O9A.42
adherent placenta O72.0
without hemorrhage O73.0
alcohol use O99.314
anemia (pre-existing) O99.02
anesthetic death O74.8
annular detachment of cervix O71.3
atony, uterus O62.2

Delivery (childbirth) (labor) - *continued*
complicated - *continued*
by - *continued*
attempted vacuum extraction and forceps O66.5
Bandl's ring O62.4
bariatric surgery status O99.844
biliary tract disorder O26.62
bleeding — *see* Delivery, complicated by, hemorrhage
blood disorder NEC O99.12
cervical dystocia (hypotonic) O62.2
primary O62.0
secondary O62.1
circulatory system disorder O99.42
compression of cord (umbilical) NEC O69.2
condition NEC O99.89
contraction, contracted ring O62.4
cord (umbilical)
around neck
with compression O69.1
without compression O69.81
bruising O69.5
complication O69.9
specified NEC O69.89
compression NEC O69.2
entanglement O69.2
without compression O69.82
hematoma O69.5
presentation O69.0
prolapse O69.0
short O69.3
thrombosis (vessels) O69.5
vascular lesion O69.5
Couvelaire uterus O45.8X-
damage to (injury to) NEC
perineum O71.82
periurethral tissue O71.82
vulva O71.82
delay following rupture of membranes (spontaneous) — *see* Pregnancy, complicated by, premature rupture of membranes
depressed fetal heart tones O76
diabetes O24.92
gestational O24.429
diet controlled O24.420
insulin controlled O24.424
oral drug controlled (antidiabetic) (hypoglycemic) O24.425
pre-existing O24.32
specified NEC O24.82
type 1 O24.02
type 2 O24.12
diastasis recti (abdominis) O71.89
dilatation
bladder O66.8
cervix incomplete, poor or slow O62.0
disease NEC O99.89
disruptio uteri — *see* Delivery, complicated by, rupture, uterus
drug use O99.324
dysfunction, uterus NOS O62.9
hypertonic O62.4
hypotonic O62.2
primary O62.0
secondary O62.1
incoordinate O62.4
eclampsia O15.1
embolism (pulmonary) — *see* Embolism, obstetric
endocrine, nutritional or metabolic disease NEC O99.284
failed
attempted vaginal birth after previous cesarean delivery O66.41
induction of labor O61.9
instrumental O61.1
mechanical O61.1
medical O61.0
specified NEC O61.8
surgical O61.1
trial of labor O66.40
female genital mutilation O65.5
fetal
abnormal acid-base balance O68
acidemia O68
acidosis O68
alkalosis O68
death, early O02.1
deformity O66.3
heart rate or rhythm (abnormal) (non-reassuring) O76
hypoxia O77.8
stress O77.9

Delivery (childbirth) (labor) - *continued*
complicated - *continued*
by - *continued*
fetal - *continued*
stress - *continued*
due to drug administration O77.1
electrocardiographic evidence of O77.8
specified NEC O77.8
ultrasound evidence of O77.8
fever during labor O75.2
gastric banding status O99.844
gastric bypass status O99.844
gastrointestinal disease NEC O99.62
gestational
diabetes O24.429
diet controlled O24.420
insulin (and diet) controlled O24.424
oral drug controlled (antidiabetic) (hypoglycemic) O24.425
edema O12.04
with proteinuria O12.24
proteinuria O12.14
gonorrhea O98.22
hematoma O71.7
ischial spine O71.7
pelvic O71.7
vagina O71.7
vulva or perineum O71.7
hemorrhage (uterine) O67.9
associated with
afibrinogenemia O67.0
coagulation defect O67.0
hyperfibrinolysis O67.0
hypofibrinogenemia O67.0
due to
low implantation of placenta O44.5-
low lying placenta O44.5-
placenta previa O44.1-
marginal O44.3-
partial O44.3-
premature separation of placenta (normally implanted) — *see also* Abruptio placentae O45.9-
retained placenta O72.0
uterine leiomyoma O67.8
placenta NEC O67.8
postpartum NEC (atonic) (immediate) O72.1
with retained or trapped placenta O72.0
delayed O72.2
secondary O72.2
third stage O72.0
hourglass contraction, uterus O62.4
hypertension, hypertensive (pre-existing) — *see* Hypertension, complicated by, childbirth (labor)
hypotension O26.5-
incomplete dilatation (cervix) O62.0
incoordinate uterus contractions O62.4
inertia, uterus O62.2
during latent phase of labor O62.0
primary O62.0
secondary O62.1
infection (maternal) O98.92
carrier state NEC O99.834
gonorrhea O98.22
human immunodeficiency virus (HIV) O98.72
sexually transmitted NEC O98.32
specified NEC O98.82
syphilis O98.12
tuberculosis O98.02
viral hepatitis O98.42
viral NEC O98.52
injury (to mother) — *see also* Delivery, complicated, by, damage to O71.9
nonobstetric O9A.22
caused by abuse — *see* Delivery, complicated by, abuse
intrauterine fetal death, early O02.1
inversion, uterus O71.2
laceration (perineal) O70.9
anus (sphincter) O70.4
with third degree laceration — *see also* Delivery, complicated, by, laceration, perineum, third degree O70.20
with mucosa O70.3
without third degree laceration O70.4
bladder (urinary) O71.5
bowel O71.5
cervix (uteri) O71.3
fourchette O70.0
hymen O70.0
labia O70.0
pelvic
floor O70.1

Delivery (childbirth) (labor) - *continued*
complicated - *continued*
by - *continued*
laceration (perineal) - *continued*
pelvic - *continued*
organ NEC O71.5
perineum, perineal O70.9
first degree O70.0
fourth degree O70.3
muscles O70.1
second degree O70.1
skin O70.0
slight O70.0
third degree O70.20
with
both external anal sphincter (EAS) and internal anal sphincter (IAS) torn (IIIc) O70.23
less than 50% of external anal sphincter (EAS) thickness torn (IIIa) O70.21
more than 50% external anal sphincter (EAS) thickness torn (IIIb) O70.22
IIIa O70.21
IIIb O70.22
IIIc O70.23
peritoneum (pelvic) O71.5
rectovaginal (septum) (without perineal laceration) O71.4
with perineum — *see also* Delivery, complicated, by, laceration, perineum, third degree O70.20
with anal or rectal mucosa O70.3
specified NEC O71.89
sphincter ani — *see* Delivery, complicated, by, laceration, anus (sphincter)
urethra O71.5
uterus O71.81
before labor O71.81
vagina, vaginal (deep) (high) (without perineal laceration) O71.4
with perineum O70.0
muscles, with perineum O70.1
vulva O70.0
liver disorder O26.62
malignancy O9A.12
malnutrition O25.2
malposition, malpresentation
placenta O44.0-
with hemorrhage O44.1-
uterus or cervix O65.5
without obstruction — *see also* Delivery, complicated by, obstruction O32.9
breech O32.1
compound O32.6
face (brow) (chin) O32.3
footling O32.8
high head O32.4
oblique O32.2
specified NEC O32.8
transverse O32.2
unstable lie O32.0
meconium in amniotic fluid O77.0
mental disorder NEC O99.344
metrorrhexis — *see* Delivery, complicated by, rupture, uterus
nervous system disorder O99.354
obesity (pre-existing) O99.214
obesity surgery status O99.844
obstetric trauma O71.9
specified NEC O71.89
obstructed labor
due to
breech (complete) (frank) presentation O64.1
incomplete O64.8
brow presenation O64.3
buttock presentation O64.1
chin presentation O64.2
compound presentation O64.5
contracted pelvis O65.1
deep transverse arrest O64.0
deformed pelvis O65.0
dystocia (fetal) O66.9
due to
conjoined twins O66.3
fetal
abnormality NEC O66.3
ascites O66.3
hydrops O66.3
meningomyelocele O66.3
sacral teratoma O66.3
tumor O66.3
hydrocephalic fetus O66.3
shoulder O66.0

Delivery (childbirth) (labor) - *continued*
complicated - *continued*
by - *continued*
obstructed labor - *continued*
due to - *continued*
face presentation O64.2
fetopelvic disproportion O65.4
footling presentation O64.8
impacted shoulders O66.0
incomplete rotation of fetal head O64.0
large fetus O66.2
locked twins O66.1
malposition O64.9
specified NEC O64.8
malpresentation O64.9
specified NEC O64.8
multiple fetuses NEC O66.6
pelvic
abnormality (maternal) O65.9
organ O65.5
specified NEC O65.8
contraction
inlet O65.2
mid-cavity O65.3
outlet O65.3
persistent (position)
occipitoiliac O64.0
occipitoposterior O64.0
occipitosacral O64.0
occipitotransverse O64.0
prolapsed arm O64.4
shoulder presentation O64.4
specified NEC O66.8
pathological retraction ring, uterus O62.4
penetration, pregnant uterus by instrument O71.1
perforation — *see* Delivery, complicated by, laceration
placenta, placental
ablatio — *see also* Abruptio placentae O45.9-
abnormality O43.9-
specified NEC O43.89-
abruptio — *see also* Abruptio placentae O45.9-
accreta O43.21-
adherent (with hemorrhage) O72.0
without hemorrhage O73.0
detachment (premature) — *see also* Abruptio placentae O45.9-
disorder O43.9-
specified NEC O43.89-
hemorrhage NEC O67.8
increta O43.22-
low (implantation) (lying) O44.4-
with hemorrhage O44.5-
malformation O43.10-
malposition O44.0-
without hemorrhage O44.1-
percreta O43.23-
previa (central) (complete) (lateral) (total) O44.0-
with hemorrhage O44.1-
marginal O44.2-
with hemorrhage O44.3-
partial O44.2-
with hemorrhage O44.3-
retained (with hemorrhage) O72.0
without hemorrhage O73.0
separation (premature) O45.9-
specified NEC O45.8X-
vicious insertion O44.1-
precipitate labor O62.3
premature rupture, membranes — *see also* Pregnancy, complicated by, premature rupture of membranes O42.90
prolapse
arm or hand O32.2
cord (umbilical) O69.0
foot or leg O32.8
uterus O34.52-
prolonged labor O63.9
first stage O63.0
second stage O63.1
protozoal disease (maternal) O98.62
respiratory disease NEC O99.52
retained membranes or portions of placenta O72.2
without hemorrhage O73.1
retarded birth O63.9
retention of secundines (with hemorrhage) O72.0
without hemorrhage O73.0
partial O72.2
without hemorrhage O73.1
rupture
bladder (urinary) O71.5

Delivery (childbirth) (labor) - *continued*
complicated - *continued*
by - *continued*
rupture - *continued*
cervix O71.3
pelvic organ NEC O71.5
urethra O71.5
uterus (during or after labor) O71.1
before labor O71.0-
separation, pubic bone (symphysis pubis) O71.6
shock O75.1
shoulder presentation O64.4
skin disorder NEC O99.72
spasm, cervix O62.4
stenosis or stricture, cervix O65.5
streptococcus group B (GBS) carrier state O99.824
subluxation of symphysis (pubis) O26.72
syphilis (maternal) O98.12
tear — *see* Delivery, complicated by, laceration
tetanic uterus O62.4
trauma (obstetrical) — *see also* Delivery, complicated, by, damage to O71.9
non-obstetric O9A.22
periurethral O71.82
specified NEC O71.89
tuberculosis (maternal) O98.02
tumor, pelvic organs or tissues NEC O65.5
umbilical cord around neck
with compression O69.1
without compression O69.81
uterine inertia O62.2
during latent phase of labor O62.0
primary O62.0
secondary O62.1
vasa previa O69.4
velamentous insertion of cord O43.12-
specified complication NEC O75.89
delayed NOS O63.9
following rupture of membranes
artificial O75.5
second twin, triplet, etc. O63.2
forceps, low following failed vacuum extraction O66.5
missed (at or near term) O36.4
normal O80
obstructed — *see* Delivery, complicated by, obstructed labor
precipitate O62.3
preterm — *see also* Pregnancy, complicated by, preterm labor O60.10
spontaneous O80
term pregnancy NOS O80
uncomplicated O80
vaginal, following previous cesarean delivery O34.219
classical (vertical) scar O34.212
low transverse scar O34.211
Delusions (paranoid) — *see* Disorder, delusional
Dementia (degenerative (primary)) (old age) (old age) (persisting) F03.90
with
aggressive behavior F03.91
behavioral disturbance F03.91
combative behavior F03.91
Lewy bodies G31.83 *[F02.80]*
with behavioral disturbance G31.83 *[F02.81]*
Parkinsonism G31.83 *[F02.80]*
with behavioral disturbance G31.83 *[F02.81]*
Parkinson's disease G20 *[F02.80]*
with behavioral disturbance G20 *[F02.81]*
violent behavior F03.91
alcoholic F10.97
with dependence F10.27
Alzheimer's type — *see* Disease, Alzheimer's
arteriosclerotic — *see* Dementia, vascular
atypical, Alzheimer's type — *see* Disease, Alzheimer's, specified NEC
congenital — *see* Disability, intellectual
frontal (lobe) G31.09 *[F02.80]*
with behavioral disturbance G31.09 *[F02.81]*
frontotemporal G31.09 *[F02.80]*
with behavioral disturbance G31.09 *[F02.81]*
specified NEC G31.09 *[F02.80]*
with behavioral disturbance G31.09 *[F02.81]*
in (due to)
alcohol F10.97
with dependence F10.27
Alzheimer's disease — *see* Disease, Alzheimer's
arteriosclerotic brain disease — *see* Dementia, vascular
cerebral lipidoses E75.- *[F02.80]*
with behavioral disturbance E75.- *[F02.81]*

Dementia (degenerative (primary)) (old age) (old age) (persisting) - *continued*
in (due to) - *continued*
Creutzfeldt-Jakob disease — *see also* Creutzfeldt-Jakob disease or syndrome (with dementia) A81.00
epilepsy G40.- *[F02.80]*
with behavioral disturbance G40.- *[F02.81]*
hepatolenticular degeneration E83.01 *[F02.80]*
with behavioral disturbance E83.01 *[F02.81]*
human immunodeficiency virus (HIV) disease B20 *[F02.80]*
with behavioral disturbance B20 *[F02.81]*
Huntington's disease or chorea G10 *[F02.80]*
with behavioral disturbance G10 *[F02.81]*
hypercalcemia E83.52 *[F02.80]*
with behavioral disturbance E83.52 *[F02.81]*
hypothyroidism, acquired E03.9 *[F02.80]*
with behavioral disturbance E03.9 *[F02.81]*
due to iodine deficiency E01.8 *[F02.80]*
with behavioral disturbance E01.8 *[F02.81]*
inhalants F18.97
with dependence F18.27
multiple
etiologies F03
sclerosis G35 *[F02.80]*
with behavioral disturbance G35 *[F02.81]*
neurosyphilis A52.17 *[F02.80]*
with behavioral disturbance A52.17 *[F02.81]*
juvenile A50.49 *[F02.80]*
with behavioral disturbance A50.49 *[F02.81]*
niacin deficiency E52 *[F02.80]*
with behavioral disturbance E52 *[F02.81]*
paralysis agitans G20 *[F02.80]*
with behavioral disturbance G20 *[F02.81]*
Parkinson's disease G20 *[F02.80]*
pellagra E52 *[F02.80]*
with behavioral disturbance E52 *[F02.81]*
Pick's G31.01 *[F02.80]*
with behavioral disturbance G31.01 *[F02.81]*
polyarteritis nodosa M30.0 *[F02.80]*
with behavioral disturbance M30.0 *[F02.81]*
psychoactive drug F19.97
with dependence F19.27
inhalants F18.97
with dependence F18.27
sedatives, hypnotics or anxiolytics F13.97
with dependence F13.27
sedatives, hypnotics or anxiolytics F13.97
with dependence F13.27
systemic lupus erythematosus M32.- *[F02.80]*
with behavioral disturbance M32.- *[F02.81]*
trypanosomiasis
African B56.9 *[F02.80]*
with behavioral disturbance B56.9 *[F02.81]*
unknown etiology F03
vitamin B12 deficiency E53.8 *[F02.80]*
with behavioral disturbance E53.8 *[F02.81]*
volatile solvents F18.97
with dependence F18.27
with behavioral disturbance G31.83 *[F02.81]*
infantile, infantilis F84.3
Lewy body G31.83 *[F02.80]*
with behavioral disturbance G31.83 *[F02.81]*
multi-infarct — *see* Dementia, vascular
paralytica, paralytic (syphilitic) A52.17 *[F02.80]*
with behavioral disturbance A52.17 *[F02.81]*
juvenilis A50.45
paretic A52.17
praecox — *see* Schizophrenia
presenile F03
Alzheimer's type — *see* Disease, Alzheimer's, early onset
primary degenerative F03
progressive, syphilitic A52.17
senile F03
with acute confusional state F05
Alzheimer's type — *see* Disease, Alzheimer's, late onset
depressed or paranoid type F03
vascular (acute onset) (mixed) (multi-infarct) (subcortical) F01.50
with behavioral disturbance F01.51
Demineralization, bone — *see* Osteoporosis
Demodex folliculorum (infestation) B88.0
Demophobia F40.248
Demoralization R45.3
Demyelination, demyelinization
central nervous system G37.9
specified NEC G37.8
corpus callosum (central) G37.1
disseminated, acute G36.9
specified NEC G36.8

Demyelination, demyelinization - *continued*
global G35
in optic neuritis G36.0
Dengue (classical) (fever) A90
hemorrhagic A91
sandfly A93.1
Dennie-Marfan syphilitic syndrome A50.45
Dens evaginatus, in dente or invaginatus K00.2
Dense breasts R92.2
Density
increased, bone (disseminated) (generalized) (spotted) — *see* Disorder, bone, density and structure, specified type NEC
lung (nodular) J98.4
Dental — *see also* condition
examination Z01.20
with abnormal findings Z01.21
restoration
aesthetically inadequate or displeasing K08.56
defective K08.50
specified NEC K08.59
failure of marginal integrity K08.51
failure of periodontal anatomical integrity K08.54
Dentia praecox K00.6
Denticles (pulp) K04.2
Dentigerous cyst K09.0
Dentin
irregular (in pulp) K04.3
opalescent K00.5
secondary (in pulp) K04.3
sensitive K03.89
Dentinogenesis imperfecta K00.5
Dentinoma — *see* Cyst, calcifying odontogenic
Dentition (syndrome) K00.7
delayed K00.6
difficult K00.7
precocious K00.6
premature K00.6
retarded K00.6
Dependence (on) (syndrome) F19.20
with remission F19.21
alcohol (ethyl) (methyl) (without remission) F10.20
with
amnestic disorder, persisting F10.26
anxiety disorder F10.280
dementia, persisting F10.27
intoxication F10.229
with delirium F10.221
uncomplicated F10.220
mood disorder F10.24
psychotic disorder F10.259
with
delusions F10.250
hallucinations F10.251
remission F10.21
sexual dysfunction F10.281
sleep disorder F10.282
specified disorder NEC F10.288
withdrawal F10.239
with
delirium F10.231
perceptual disturbance F10.232
uncomplicated F10.230
counseling and surveillance Z71.41
amobarbital — *see* Dependence, drug, sedative
amphetamine (s) (type) — *see* Dependence, drug, stimulant NEC
amytal (sodium) — *see* Dependence, drug, sedative
analgesic NEC F55.8
anesthetic (agent) (gas) (general) (local) NEC — *see* Dependence, drug, psychoactive NEC
anxiolytic NEC — *see* Dependence, drug, sedative
barbital (s) — *see* Dependence, drug, sedative
barbiturate (s) (compounds) (drugs classifiable to T42) — *see* Dependence, drug, sedative
benzedrine — *see* Dependence, drug, stimulant NEC
bhang — *see* Dependence, drug, cannabis
bromide (s) NEC — *see* Dependence, drug, sedative
caffeine — *see* Dependence, drug, stimulant NEC
cannabis (sativa) (indica) (resin) (derivatives) (type) — *see* Dependence, drug, cannabis
chloral (betaine) (hydrate) — *see* Dependence, drug, sedative
chlordiazepoxide — *see* Dependence, drug, sedative
coca (leaf) (derivatives) — *see* Dependence, drug, cocaine
cocaine — *see* Dependence, drug, cocaine
codeine — *see* Dependence, drug, opioid
combinations of drugs F19.20
dagga — *see* Dependence, drug, cannabis
demerol — *see* Dependence, drug, opioid
dexamphetamine — *see* Dependence, drug, stimulant NEC

Dependence (on) (syndrome) - *continued*
dexedrine — *see* Dependence, drug, stimulant NEC
dextromethorphan — *see* Dependence, drug, opioid
dextromoramide — *see* Dependence, drug, opioid
dextro-nor-pseudo-ephedrine — *see* Dependence, drug, stimulant NEC
dextrorphan — *see* Dependence, drug, opioid
diazepam — *see* Dependence, drug, sedative
dilaudid — *see* Dependence, drug, opioid
D-lysergic acid diethylamide — *see* Dependence, drug, hallucinogen
drug NEC F19.20
with sleep disorder F19.282
cannabis F12.20
with
anxiety disorder F12.280
intoxication F12.229
with
delirium F12.221
perceptual disturbance F12.222
uncomplicated F12.220
other specified disorder F12.288
psychosis F12.259
delusions F12.250
hallucinations F12.251
unspecified disorder F12.29
withdrawal F12.23
in remission F12.21
cocaine F14.20
with
anxiety disorder F14.280
intoxication F14.229
with
delirium F14.221
perceptual disturbance F14.222
uncomplicated F14.220
mood disorder F14.24
other specified disorder F14.288
psychosis F14.259
delusions F14.250
hallucinations F14.251
sexual dysfunction F14.281
sleep disorder F14.282
unspecified disorder F14.29
withdrawal F14.23
in remission F14.21
withdrawal symptoms in newborn P96.1
counseling and surveillance Z71.51
hallucinogen F16.20
with
anxiety disorder F16.280
flashbacks F16.283
intoxication F16.229
with delirium F16.221
uncomplicated F16.220
mood disorder F16.24
other specified disorder F16.288
perception disorder, persisting F16.283
psychosis F16.259
delusions F16.250
hallucinations F16.251
unspecified disorder F16.29
in remission F16.21
in remission F19.21
inhalant F18.20
with
anxiety disorder F18.280
dementia, persisting F18.27
intoxication F18.229
with delirium F18.221
uncomplicated F18.220
mood disorder F18.24
other specified disorder F18.288
psychosis F18.259
delusions F18.250
hallucinations F18.251
unspecified disorder F18.29
in remission F18.21
nicotine F17.200
with disorder F17.209
in remission F17.201
specified disorder NEC F17.208
withdrawal F17.203
chewing tobacco F17.220
with disorder F17.229
in remission F17.221
specified disorder NEC F17.228
withdrawal F17.223
cigarettes F17.210
with disorder F17.219
in remission F17.211
specified disorder NEC F17.218
withdrawal F17.213

Dependence (on) (syndrome) - *continued*
drug NEC - *continued*
nicotine - *continued*
specified product NEC F17.290
with disorder F17.299
remission F17.291
specified disorder NEC F17.298
withdrawal F17.293
opioid F11.20
with
intoxication F11.229
with
delirium F11.221
perceptual disturbance F11.222
uncomplicated F11.220
mood disorder F11.24
other specified disorder F11.288
psychosis F11.259
delusions F11.250
hallucinations F11.251
sexual dysfunction F11.281
sleep disorder F11.282
unspecified disorder F11.29
withdrawal F11.23
in remission F11.21
psychoactive NEC F19.20
with
amnestic disorder F19.26
anxiety disorder F19.280
dementia F19.27
intoxication F19.229
with
delirium F19.221
perceptual disturbance F19.222
uncomplicated F19.220
mood disorder F19.24
other specified disorder F19.288
psychosis F19.259
delusions F19.250
hallucinations F19.251
sexual dysfunction F19.281
sleep disorder F19.282
unspecified disorder F19.29
withdrawal F19.239
with
delirium F19.231
perceptual disturbance F19.232
uncomplicated F19.230
sedative, hypnotic or anxiolytic F13.20
with
amnestic disorder F13.26
anxiety disorder F13.280
dementia, persisting F13.27
intoxication F13.229
with delirium F13.221
uncomplicated F13.220
mood disorder F13.24
other specified disorder F13.288
psychosis F13.259
delusions F13.250
hallucinations F13.251
sexual dysfunction F13.281
sleep disorder F13.282
unspecified disorder F13.29
withdrawal F13.239
with
delirium F13.231
perceptual disturbance F13.232
uncomplicated F13.230
in remission F13.21
stimulant NEC F15.20
with
anxiety disorder F15.280
intoxication F15.229
with
delirium F15.221
perceptual disturbance F15.222
uncomplicated F15.220
mood disorder F15.24
other specified disorder F15.288
psychosis F15.259
delusions F15.250
hallucinations F15.251
sexual dysfunction F15.281
sleep disorder F15.282
unspecified disorder F15.29
withdrawal F15.23
in remission F15.21
ethyl
alcohol (without remission) F10.20
with remission F10.21
bromide — *see* Dependence, drug, sedative
carbamate F19.20

Dependence (on) (syndrome) - *continued*
ethyl - *continued*
chloride F19.20
morphine — *see* Dependence, drug, opioid
ganja — *see* Dependence, drug, cannabis
glue (airplane) (sniffing) — *see* Dependence, drug, inhalant
glutethimide — *see* Dependence, drug, sedative
hallucinogenics — *see* Dependence, drug, hallucinogen
hashish — *see* Dependence, drug, cannabis
hemp — *see* Dependence, drug, cannabis
heroin (salt) (any) — *see* Dependence, drug, opioid
hypnotic NEC — *see* Dependence, drug, sedative
Indian hemp — *see* Dependence, drug, cannabis
inhalants — *see* Dependence, drug, inhalant
khat — *see* Dependence, drug, stimulant NEC
laudanum — *see* Dependence, drug, opioid
LSD (-25) (derivatives) — *see* Dependence, drug, hallucinogen
luminal — *see* Dependence, drug, sedative
lysergic acid — *see* Dependence, drug, hallucinogen
maconha — *see* Dependence, drug, cannabis
marihuana — *see* Dependence, drug, cannabis
meprobamate — *see* Dependence, drug, sedative
mescaline — *see* Dependence, drug, hallucinogen
methadone — *see* Dependence, drug, opioid
methamphetamine (s) — *see* Dependence, drug, stimulant NEC
methaqualone — *see* Dependence, drug, sedative
methyl
alcohol (without remission) F10.20
with remission F10.21
bromide — *see* Dependence, drug, sedative
morphine — *see* Dependence, drug, opioid
phenidate — *see* Dependence, drug, stimulant NEC
sulfonal — *see* Dependence, drug, sedative
morphine (sulfate) (sulfite) (type) — *see* Dependence, drug, opioid
narcotic (drug) NEC — *see* Dependence, drug, opioid
nembutal — *see* Dependence, drug, sedative
neraval — *see* Dependence, drug, sedative
neravan — *see* Dependence, drug, sedative
neurobarb — *see* Dependence, drug, sedative
nicotine — *see* Dependence, drug, nicotine
nitrous oxide F19.20
nonbarbiturate sedatives and tranquilizers with similar effect — *see* Dependence, drug, sedative
on
artificial heart (fully implantable) (mechanical) Z95.812
aspirator Z99.0
care provider (because of) Z74.9
impaired mobility Z74.09
need for
assistance with personal care Z74.1
continuous supervision Z74.3
no other household member able to render care Z74.2
specified reason NEC Z74.8
machine Z99.89
enabling NEC Z99.89
specified type NEC Z99.89
renal dialysis (hemodialysis) (peritoneal) Z99.2
respirator Z99.11
ventilator Z99.11
wheelchair Z99.3
opiate — *see* Dependence, drug, opioid
opioids — *see* Dependence, drug, opioid
opium (alkaloids) (derivatives) (tincture) — *see* Dependence, drug, opioid
oxygen (long-term) (supplemental) Z99.81
paraldehyde — *see* Dependence, drug, sedative
paregoric — *see* Dependence, drug, opioid
PCP (phencyclidine) (or related substance) — *see* Dependence, drug, hallucinogen
pentobarbital — *see* Dependence, drug, sedative
pentobarbitone (sodium) — *see* Dependence, drug, sedative
pentothal — *see* Dependence, drug, sedative
peyote — *see* Dependence, drug, hallucinogen
phencyclidine (PCP) (or related substance) — *see* Dependence, drug, hallucinogen
phenmetrazine — *see* Dependence, drug, stimulant NEC
phenobarbital — *see* Dependence, drug, sedative
polysubstance F19.20
psilocibin, psilocin, psilocyn, psilocyline — *see* Dependence, drug, hallucinogen
psychostimulant NEC — *see* Dependence, drug, stimulant NEC

- **Dependence** (on) (syndrome) - *continued*
  - secobarbital — *see* Dependence, drug, sedative
  - seconal — *see* Dependence, drug, sedative
  - sedative NEC — *see* Dependence, drug, sedative
  - specified drug NEC — *see* Dependence, drug
  - stimulant NEC — *see* Dependence, drug, stimulant NEC
  - substance NEC — *see* Dependence, drug
  - supplemental oxygen Z99.81
  - tobacco — *see* Dependence, drug, nicotine
    - counseling and surveillance Z71.6
  - tranquilizer NEC — *see* Dependence, drug, sedative
  - vitamin B6 E53.1
  - volatile solvents — *see* Dependence, drug, inhalant
- **Dependency**
  - care-provider Z74.9
  - passive F60.7
  - reactions (persistent) F60.7
- **Depersonalization** (in neurotic state) (neurotic) (syndrome) F48.1
- **Depletion**
  - extracellular fluid E86.9
  - plasma E86.1
  - potassium E87.6
    - nephropathy N25.89
  - salt or sodium E87.1
    - causing heat exhaustion or prostration T67.4
    - nephropathy N28.9
  - volume NOS E86.9
- **Deployment** (current) (military) **status** Z56.82
  - in theater or in support of military war, peacekeeping and humanitarian operations Z56.82
  - personal history of Z91.82
    - military war, peacekeeping and humanitarian deployment (current or past conflict) Z91.82
  - returned from Z91.82
- **Depolarization, premature** I49.40
  - atrial I49.1
  - junctional I49.2
  - specified NEC I49.49
  - ventricular I49.3
- **Deposit**
  - bone in Boeck's sarcoid D86.89
  - calcareous, calcium — *see* Calcification
  - cholesterol
    - retina H35.89
    - vitreous (body) (humor) — *see* Deposit, crystalline
  - conjunctiva H11.11-
  - cornea H18.00-
    - argentous H18.02-
    - due to metabolic disorder H18.03-
    - Kayser-Fleischer ring H18.04-
    - pigmentation — *see* Pigmentation, cornea
  - crystalline, vitreous (body) (humor) H43.2-
  - hemosiderin in old scars of cornea — *see* Pigmentation, cornea, stromal
  - metallic in lens — *see* Cataract, specified NEC
  - skin R23.8
  - tooth, teeth (betel) (black) (green) (materia alba) (orange) (tobacco) K03.6
  - urate, kidney — *see* Calculus, kidney
- **Depraved appetite** — *see* Pica
- **Depressed**
  - HDL cholesterol E78.6
- **Depression** (acute) (mental) F32.9
  - agitated (single episode) F32.2
  - anaclitic — *see* Disorder, adjustment
  - anxiety F41.8
    - persistent F34.1
  - arches — *see also* Deformity, limb, flat foot
  - atypical (single episode) F32.89
    - recurrent episode F33.8
  - basal metabolic rate R94.8
  - bone marrow D75.89
  - central nervous system R09.2
  - cerebral R29.818
    - newborn P91.4
  - cerebrovascular I67.9
  - chest wall M95.4
  - climacteric (single episode) F32.89
    - recurrent episode F33.8
  - endogenous (without psychotic symptoms) F33.2
    - with psychotic symptoms F33.3
  - functional activity R68.89
  - hysterical F44.89
  - involutional (single episode) F32.89
    - recurrent episode F33.8
  - major F32.9
    - with psychotic symptoms F32.3
    - recurrent — *see* Disorder, depressive, recurrent
  - manic-depressive — *see* Disorder, depressive, recurrent
  - masked (single episode) F32.89
- **Depression** (acute) (mental) - *continued*
  - medullary G93.89
  - menopausal (single episode) F32.89
    - recurrent episode F33.8
  - metatarsus — *see* Depression, arches
  - monopolar F33.9
  - nervous F34.1
  - neurotic F34.1
  - nose M95.0
  - postnatal (NOS) F53.0
  - postpartum (NOS) F53.0
  - post-psychotic of schizophrenia F32.89
  - post-schizophrenic F32.89
  - psychogenic (reactive) (single episode) F32.9
  - psychoneurotic F34.1
  - psychotic (single episode) F32.3
    - recurrent F33.3
  - reactive (psychogenic) (single episode) F32.9
    - psychotic (single episode) F32.3
  - recurrent — *see* Disorder, depressive, recurrent
  - respiratory center G93.89
  - seasonal — *see* Disorder, depressive, recurrent
  - senile F03
  - severe, single episode F32.2
  - situational F43.21
  - skull Q67.4
  - specified NEC (single episode) F32.89
  - sternum M95.4
  - visual field — *see* Defect, visual field
  - vital (recurrent) (without psychotic symptoms) F33.2
    - with psychotic symptoms F33.3
    - single episode F32.2
- **Deprivation**
  - cultural Z60.3
  - effects NOS T73.9
    - specified NEC T73.8
  - emotional NEC Z65.8
    - affecting infant or child — *see* Maltreatment, child, psychological
  - food T73.0
  - protein — *see* Malnutrition
  - sleep Z72.820
  - social Z60.4
    - affecting infant or child — *see* Maltreatment, child, psychological
  - specified NEC T73.8
  - vitamins — *see* Deficiency, vitamin
  - water T73.1
- **Derangement**
  - ankle (internal) — *see* Derangement, joint, ankle
  - cartilage (articular) NEC — *see* Derangement, joint, articular cartilage, by site
    - recurrent — *see* Dislocation, recurrent
  - cruciate ligament, anterior, current injury — *see* Sprain, knee, cruciate, anterior
  - elbow (internal) — *see* Derangement, joint, elbow
  - hip (joint) (internal) (old) — *see* Derangement, joint, hip
  - joint (internal) M24.9
    - ankylosis — *see* Ankylosis
    - articular cartilage M24.10
      - ankle M24.17-
      - elbow M24.12-
      - foot M24.17-
      - hand M24.14-
      - hip M24.15-
      - knee NEC M23.9-
      - loose body — *see* Loose, body
      - shoulder M24.11-
      - wrist M24.13-
    - contracture — *see* Contraction, joint
    - current injury — *see also* Dislocation
      - knee, meniscus or cartilage — *see* Tear, meniscus
    - dislocation
      - pathological — *see* Dislocation, pathological
      - recurrent — *see* Dislocation, recurrent
    - knee — *see* Derangement, knee
    - ligament — *see* Disorder, ligament
    - loose body — *see* Loose, body
    - recurrent — *see* Dislocation, recurrent
    - specified type NEC M24.80
      - ankle M24.87-
      - elbow M24.82-
      - foot joint M24.87-
      - hand joint M24.84-
      - hip M24.85-
      - shoulder M24.81-
      - wrist M24.83-
    - temporomandibular M26.69
  - knee (recurrent) M23.9-
    - ligament disruption, spontaneous M23.60-
      - anterior cruciate M23.61-
- **Derangement** - *continued*
  - knee (recurrent) - *continued*
    - ligament disruption, spontaneous - *continued*
      - capsular M23.67-
      - instability, chronic M23.5-
      - lateral collateral M23.64-
      - medial collateral M23.63-
      - posterior cruciate M23.62-
    - loose body M23.4-
    - meniscus M23.30-
      - cystic M23.00-
        - lateral M23.002
          - anterior horn M23.04-
          - posterior horn M23.05-
          - specified NEC M23.06-
        - medial M23.005
          - anterior horn M23.01-
          - posterior horn M23.02-
          - specified NEC M23.03-
      - degenerate — *see* Derangement, knee, meniscus, specified NEC
      - detached — *see* Derangement, knee, meniscus, specified NEC
      - due to old tear or injury M23.20-
        - lateral M23.20-
          - anterior horn M23.24-
          - posterior horn M23.25-
          - specified NEC M23.26-
        - medial M23.20-
          - anterior horn M23.21-
          - posterior horn M23.22-
          - specified NEC M23.23-
      - retained — *see* Derangement, knee, meniscus, specified NEC
      - specified NEC M23.30-
        - lateral M23.30-
          - anterior horn M23.34-
          - posterior horn M23.35-
          - specified NEC M23.36-
        - medial M23.30-
          - anterior horn M23.31-
          - posterior horn M23.32-
          - specified NEC M23.33-
    - old M23.8X-
    - specified NEC — *see* subcategory M23.8
  - low back NEC — *see* Dorsopathy, specified NEC
  - meniscus — *see* Derangement, knee, meniscus
  - mental — *see* Psychosis
  - patella, specified NEC — *see* Disorder, patella, derangement NEC
  - semilunar cartilage (knee) — *see* Derangement, knee, meniscus, specified NEC
  - shoulder (internal) — *see* Derangement, joint, shoulder
- **Dercum's disease** E88.2
- **Derealization** (neurotic) F48.1
- **Dermal** — *see* condition
- **Dermaphytid** — *see* Dermatophytosis
- **Dermatitis** (eczematous) L30.9
  - ab igne L59.0
  - acarine B88.0
  - actinic (due to sun) L57.8
    - other than from sun L59.8
  - allergic — *see* Dermatitis, contact, allergic
  - ambustionis, due to burn or scald — *see* Burn
  - amebic A06.7
  - ammonia L22
  - arsenical (ingested) L27.8
  - artefacta L98.1
    - psychogenic F54
  - atopic L20.9
    - psychogenic F54
    - specified NEC L20.89
  - autoimmune progesterone L30.8
  - berlock, berloque L56.2
  - blastomycotic B40.3
  - blister beetle L24.89
  - bullous, bullosa L13.9
    - mucosynechial, atrophic L12.1
    - seasonal L30.8
    - specified NEC L13.8
  - calorica L59.0
    - due to burn or scald — *see* Burn
  - caterpillar L24.89
  - cercarial B65.3
  - combustionis L59.0
    - due to burn or scald — *see* Burn
  - congelationis T69.1
  - contact (occupational) L25.9
    - allergic L23.9
      - due to
        - adhesives L23.1
        - cement L23.5

Dermatitis (eczematous) - *continued*
  contact (occupational) - *continued*
    allergic - *continued*
      due to - *continued*
        chemical products NEC L23.5
        chromium L23.0
        cosmetics L23.2
        dander (cat) (dog) L23.81
        drugs in contact with skin L23.3
        dyes L23.4
        food in contact with skin L23.6
        hair (cat) (dog) L23.81
        insecticide L23.5
        metals L23.0
        nickel L23.0
        plants, non-food L23.7
        plastic L23.5
        rubber L23.5
        specified agent NEC L23.89
    due to
      cement L25.3
      chemical products NEC L25.3
      cosmetics L25.0
      dander (cat) (dog) L23.81
      drugs in contact with skin L25.1
      dyes L25.2
      food in contact with skin L25.4
      hair (cat) (dog) L23.81
      plants, non-food L25.5
      specified agent NEC L25.8
    irritant L24.9
      due to
        cement L24.5
        chemical products NEC L24.5
        cosmetics L24.3
        detergents L24.0
        drugs in contact with skin L24.4
        food in contact with skin L24.6
        oils and greases L24.1
        plants, non-food L24.7
        solvents L24.2
        specified agent NEC L24.89
  contusiformis L52
  diabetic — *see* E08-E13 with .620
  diaper L22
  diphtheritica A36.3
  dry skin L85.3
  due to
    acetone (contact) (irritant) L24.2
    acids (contact) (irritant) L24.5
    adhesive (s) (allergic) (contact) (plaster) L23.1
      irritant L24.5
    alcohol (irritant) (skin contact) (substances in category T51) L24.2
      taken internally L27.8
    alkalis (contact) (irritant) L24.5
    arsenic (ingested) L27.8
    carbon disulfide (contact) (irritant) L24.2
    caustics (contact) (irritant) L24.5
    cement (contact) L25.3
    cereal (ingested) L27.2
    chemical (s) NEC L25.3
      taken internally L27.8
    chlorocompounds L24.2
    chromium (contact) (irritant) L24.81
    coffee (ingested) L27.2
    cold weather L30.8
    cosmetics (contact) L25.0
      allergic L23.2
      irritant L24.3
    cyclohexanes L24.2
    dander (cat) (dog) L23.81
    Demodex species B88.0
    Dermanyssus gallinae B88.0
    detergents (contact) (irritant) L24.0
    dichromate L24.81
    drugs and medicaments (generalized) (internal use) L27.0
      external — *see* Dermatitis, due to, drugs, in contact with skin
      in contact with skin L25.1
        allergic L23.3
        irritant L24.4
      localized skin eruption L27.1
      specified substance — *see* Table of Drugs and Chemicals
    dyes (contact) L25.2
      allergic L23.4
      irritant L24.89
    epidermophytosis — *see* Dermatophytosis
    esters L24.2
    external irritant NEC L24.9
    fish (ingested) L27.2

Dermatitis (eczematous) - *continued*
  due to - *continued*
    flour (ingested) L27.2
    food (ingested) L27.2
      in contact with skin L25.4
    fruit (ingested) L27.2
    furs (allergic) (contact) L23.81
    glues — *see* Dermatitis, due to, adhesives
    glycols L24.2
    greases NEC (contact) (irritant) L24.1
    hair (cat) (dog) L23.81
    hot
      objects and materials — *see* Burn
      weather or places L59.0
    hydrocarbons L24.2
    infrared rays L59.8
    ingestion, ingested substance L27.9
      chemical NEC L27.8
      drugs and medicaments — *see* Dermatitis, due to, drugs
      food L27.2
      specified NEC L27.8
    insecticide in contact with skin L24.5
    internal agent L27.9
      drugs and medicaments (generalized) — *see* Dermatitis, due to, drugs
      food L27.2
    irradiation — *see* Dermatitis, due to, radioactive substance
    ketones L24.2
    lacquer tree (allergic) (contact) L23.7
    light (sun) NEC L57.8
      acute L56.8
      other L59.8
    Liponyssoides sanguineus B88.0
    low temperature L30.8
    meat (ingested) L27.2
    metals, metal salts (contact) (irritant) L24.81
    milk (ingested) L27.2
    nickel (contact) (irritant) L24.81
    nylon (contact) (irritant) L24.5
    oils NEC (contact) (irritant) L24.1
    paint solvent (contact) (irritant) L24.2
    petroleum products (contact) (irritant) (substances in T52.0) L24.2
    plants NEC (contact) L25.5
      allergic L23.7
      irritant L24.7
    plasters (adhesive) (any) (allergic) (contact) L23.1
      irritant L24.5
    plastic (contact) L25.3
    preservatives (contact) — *see* Dermatitis, due to, chemical, in contact with skin
    primrose (allergic) (contact) L23.7
    primula (allergic) (contact) L23.7
    radiation L59.8
      nonionizing (chronic exposure) L57.8
      sun NEC L57.8
        acute L56.8
    radioactive substance L58.9
      acute L58.0
      chronic L58.1
    radium L58.9
      acute L58.0
      chronic L58.1
    ragweed (allergic) (contact) L23.7
    Rhus (allergic) (contact) (diversiloba) (radicans) (toxicodendron) (venenata) (verniciflua) L23.7
    rubber (contact) L24.5
    Senecio jacobaea (allergic) (contact) L23.7
    solvents (contact) (irritant) (substances in categories T52) L24.2
    specified agent NEC (contact) L25.8
      allergic L23.89
      irritant L24.89
    sunshine NEC L57.8
      acute L56.8
    tetrachlorethylene (contact) (irritant) L24.2
    toluene (contact) (irritant) L24.2
    turpentine (contact) L24.2
    ultraviolet rays (sun NEC) (chronic exposure) L57.8
      acute L56.8
    vaccine or vaccination L27.0
      specified substance — *see* Table of Drugs and Chemicals
    varicose veins — *see* Varix, leg, with, inflammation
    X-rays L58.9
      acute L58.0
      chronic L58.1
  dyshydrotic L30.1
  dysmenorrheica N94.6

Dermatitis (eczematous) - *continued*
  escharotica — *see* Burn
  exfoliative, exfoliativa (generalized) L26
    neonatorum L00
  eyelid — *see also* Dermatosis, eyelid
    allergic H01.119
      left H01.116
        lower H01.115
        upper H01.114
      right H01.113
        lower H01.112
        upper H01.111
    contact — *see* Dermatitis, eyelid, allergic
    due to
      Demodex species B88.0
      herpes (zoster) B02.39
        simplex B00.59
    eczematous H01.139
      left H01.136
        lower H01.135
        upper H01.134
      right H01.133
        lower H01.132
        upper H01.131
  facta, factitia, factitial L98.1
    psychogenic F54
  flexural NEC L20.82
  friction L30.4
  fungus B36.9
    specified type NEC B36.8
  gangrenosa, gangrenous infantum L08.0
  harvest mite B88.0
  heat L59.0
  herpesviral, vesicular (ear) (lip) B00.1
  herpetiformis (bullous) (erythematous) (pustular) (vesicular) L13.0
    juvenile L12.2
    senile L12.0
  hiemalis L30.8
  hypostatic, hypostatica — *see* Varix, leg, with, inflammation
  infectious eczematoid L30.3
  infective L30.3
  irritant — *see* Dermatitis, contact, irritant
  Jacquet's (diaper dermatitis) L22
  Leptus B88.0
  lichenified NEC L28.0
  medicamentosa (generalized) (internal use) — *see* Dermatitis, due to drugs
  mite B88.0
  multiformis L13.0
    juvenile L12.2
  napkin L22
  neurotica L13.0
  nummular L30.0
  papillaris capillitii L73.0
  pellagrous E52
  perioral L71.0
  photocontact L56.2
  polymorpha dolorosa L13.0
  pruriginosa L13.0
  pruritic NEC L30.8
  psychogenic F54
  purulent L08.0
  pustular
    contagious B08.02
    subcorneal L13.1
  pyococcal L08.0
  pyogenica L08.0
  repens L40.2
  Ritter's (exfoliativa) L00
  Schamberg's L81.7
  schistosome B65.3
  seasonal bullous L30.8
  seborrheic L21.9
    infantile L21.1
    specified NEC L21.8
  sensitization NOS L23.9
  septic L08.0
  solare L57.8
  specified NEC L30.8
  stasis I87.2
    with
      varicose ulcer — *see* Varix, leg, with ulcer, with inflammation
      varicose veins — *see* Varix, leg, with, inflammation
    due to postthrombotic syndrome — *see* Syndrome, postthrombotic
  suppurative L08.0
  traumatic NEC L30.4
  trophoneurotica L13.0
  ultraviolet (sun) (chronic exposure) L57.8

Dermatitis (eczematous) - *continued*
ultraviolet (sun) (chronic exposure) - *continued*
acute L56.8
varicose — *see* Varix, leg, with, inflammation
vegetans L10.1
verrucosa B43.0
vesicular, herpesviral B00.1
Dermatoarthritis, lipoid E78.81
Dermatochalasis, eyelid H02.839
left H02.836
lower H02.835
upper H02.834
right H02.833
lower H02.832
upper H02.831
Dermatofibroma (lenticulare) — *see* Neoplasm, skin, benign
protuberans — *see* Neoplasm, skin, uncertain behavior
Dermatofibrosarcoma (pigmented) (protuberans) — *see* Neoplasm, skin, malignant
Dermatographia L50.3
Dermatolysis (exfoliativa) (congenital) Q82.8
acquired L57.4
eyelids — *see* Blepharochalasis
palpebrarum — *see* Blepharochalasis
senile L57.4
Dermatomegaly NEC Q82.8
Dermatomucosomyositis M33.10
with
myopathy M33.12
respiratory involvement M33.11
specified organ involvement NEC M33.19
Dermatomycosis B36.9
furfuracea B36.0
specified type NEC B36.8
Dermatomyositis (acute) (chronic) — *see* also Dermatopolymyositis
adult — *see also* Dermatomyositis, specified NEC M33.10
in (due to) neoplastic disease — *see also* Neoplasm D49.9 *[M36.0]*
juvenile M33.00
with
myopathy M33.02
respiratory involvement M33.01
specified organ involvement NEC M33.09
without myopathy M33.03
specified NEC M33.10
with
myopathy M33.12
respiratory involvement M33.11
specified organ involvement NEC M33.19
without myopathy M33.13
Dermatoneuritis of children — *see* Poisoning, mercury
Dermatophilosis A48.8
Dermatophytid L30.2
Dermatophytide — *see* Dermatophytosis
Dermatophytosis (epidermophyton) (infection) (Microsporum) (tinea) (Trichophyton) B35.9
beard B35.0
body B35.4
capitis B35.0
corporis B35.4
deep-seated B35.8
disseminated B35.8
foot B35.3
granulomatous B35.8
groin B35.6
hand B35.2
nail B35.1
perianal (area) B35.6
scalp B35.0
specified NEC B35.8
Dermatopolymyositis M33.90
with
myopathy M33.92
respiratory involvement M33.91
specified organ involvement NEC M33.99
in neoplastic disease — *see also* Neoplasm D49.9 *[M36.0]*
juvenile M33.00
with
myopathy M33.02
respiratory involvement M33.01
specified organ involvement NEC M33.09
specified NEC M33.10
myopathy M33.12
respiratory involvement M33.11
specified organ involvement NEC M33.19
without myopathy M33.93
Dermatopolyneuritis — *see* Poisoning, mercury
Dermatorrhexis Q79.6
acquired L57.4
Dermatosclerosis — *see also* Scleroderma
localized L94.0
Dermatosis L98.9
Andrews' L08.89
Bowen's — *see* Neoplasm, skin, in situ
bullous L13.9
specified NEC L13.8
exfoliativa L26
eyelid (noninfectious)
dermatitis — *see* Dermatitis, eyelid
discoid lupus erythematosus — *see* Lupus, erythematosus, eyelid
xeroderma — *see* Xeroderma, acquired, eyelid
factitial L98.1
febrile neutrophilic L98.2
gonococcal A54.89
herpetiformis L13.0
juvenile L12.2
linear IgA L13.8
menstrual NEC L98.8
neutrophilic, febrile L98.2
occupational — *see* Dermatitis, contact
papulosa nigra L82.1
pigmentary L81.9
progressive L81.7
Schamberg's L81.7
psychogenic F54
purpuric, pigmented L81.7
pustular, subcorneal L13.1
transient acantholytic L11.1
Dermographia, dermographism L50.3
Dermoid (cyst) — *see also* Neoplasm, benign, by site
with malignant transformation C56-
due to radiation (nonionizing) L57.8
Dermopathy
infiltrative with thyrotoxicosis — *see* Thyrotoxicosis
nephrogenic fibrosing L90.8
Dermophytosis — *see* Dermatophytosis
Descemetocele H18.73-
Descemet's membrane — *see* condition
Descending — *see* condition
Descensus uteri — *see* Prolapse, uterus
Desert
rheumatism B38.0
sore — *see* Ulcer, skin
Desertion (newborn) — *see* Maltreatment
Desmoid (extra-abdominal) (tumor) — *see* Neoplasm, connective tissue, uncertain behavior
abdominal D48.1
Despondency F32.9
Desquamation, skin R23.4
Destruction, destructive — *see also* Damage
articular facet — *see also* Derangement, joint, specified type NEC
knee M23.8X-
vertebra — *see* Spondylosis
bone — *see also* Disorder, bone, specified type NEC
syphilitic A52.77
joint — *see also* Derangement, joint, specified type NEC
sacroiliac M53.3
rectal sphincter K62.89
septum (nasal) J34.89
tuberculous NEC — *see* Tuberculosis
tympanum, tympanic membrane (nontraumatic) — *see* Disorder, tympanic membrane, specified NEC
vertebral disc — *see* Degeneration, intervertebral disc
Destructiveness — *see also* Disorder, conduct
adjustment reaction — *see* Disorder, adjustment
Desultory labor O62.2
Detachment
cartilage — *see* Sprain
cervix, annular N88.8
complicating delivery O71.3
choroid (old) (postinfectional) (simple) (spontaneous) H31.40-
hemorrhagic H31.41-
serous H31.42-
ligament — *see* Sprain
meniscus (knee) — *see also* Derangement, knee, meniscus, specified NEC
current injury — *see* Tear, meniscus
due to old tear or injury — *see* Derangement, knee, meniscus, due to old tear
retina (without retinal break) (serous) H33.2-
with retinal:
break H33.00-
giant H33.03-
multiple H33.02-
Detachment - *continued*
retina (without retinal break) (serous) - *continued*
with retinal: - *continued*
break - *continued*
single H33.01-
dialysis H33.04-
pigment epithelium — *see* Degeneration, retina, separation of layers, pigment epithelium detachment
rhegmatogenous — *see* Detachment, retina, with retinal, break
specified NEC H33.8
total H33.05-
traction H33.4-
vitreous (body) H43.81
Detergent asthma J69.8
Deterioration
epileptic F06.8
general physical R53.81
heart, cardiac — *see* Degeneration, myocardial
mental — *see* Psychosis
myocardial, myocardium — *see* Degeneration, myocardial
senile (simple) R54
Deuteranomaly (anomalous trichromat) H53.53
Deuteranopia (complete) (incomplete) H53.53
Development
abnormal, bone Q79.9
arrested R62.50
bone — *see* Arrest, development or growth, bone
child R62.50
due to malnutrition E45
defective, congenital — *see also* Anomaly, by site
cauda equina Q06.3
left ventricle Q24.8
in hypoplastic left heart syndrome Q23.4
valve Q24.8
pulmonary Q22.3
delayed — *see also* Delay, development R62.50
arithmetical skills F81.2
language (skills) (expressive) F80.1
learning skill F81.9
mixed skills F88
motor coordination F82
reading F81.0
specified learning skill NEC F81.89
speech F80.9
spelling F81.81
written expression F81.81
imperfect, congenital — *see also* Anomaly, by site
heart Q24.9
lungs Q33.6
incomplete
bronchial tree Q32.4
organ or site not listed — *see* Hypoplasia, by site
respiratory system Q34.9
sexual, precocious NEC E30.1
tardy, mental — *see also* Disability, intellectual F79
Developmental — *see* condition
testing, infant or child — *see* Examination, child
Devergie's disease (pityriasis rubra pilaris) L44.0
Deviation (in)
conjugate palsy (eye) (spastic) H51.0
esophagus (acquired) K22.8
eye, skew H51.8
midline (jaw) (teeth) (dental arch) M26.29
specified site NEC — *see* Malposition
nasal septum J34.2
congenital Q67.4
opening and closing of the mandible M26.53
organ or site, congenital NEC — *see* Malposition, congenital
septum (nasal) (acquired) J34.2
congenital Q67.4
sexual F65.9
bestiality F65.89
erotomania F52.8
exhibitionism F65.2
fetishism, fetishistic F65.0
transvestism F65.1
frotteurism F65.81
masochism F65.51
multiple F65.89
necrophilia F65.89
nymphomania F52.8
pederosis F65.4
pedophilia F65.4
sadism, sadomasochism F65.52
satyriasis F52.8
specified type NEC F65.89
transvestism F64.1
voyeurism F65.3
teeth, midline M26.29

Deviation (in) - *continued*
- trachea J39.8
- ureter, congenital Q62.61

Device
- cerebral ventricle (communicating) in situ Z98.2
- contraceptive — *see* Contraceptive, device
- drainage, cerebrospinal fluid, in situ Z98.2

Devic's disease G36.0

Devil's
- grip B33.0
- pinches (purpura simplex) D69.2

Devitalized tooth K04.99

Devonshire colic — *see* Poisoning, lead

Dextraposition, aorta Q20.3
- in tetralogy of Fallot Q21.3

Dextrinosis, limit (debrancher enzyme deficiency) E74.03

Dextrocardia (true) Q24.0
- with
  - complete transposition of viscera Q89.3
  - situs inversus Q89.3

Dextrotransposition, aorta Q20.3

d-glycericacidemia E72.59

Dhat syndrome F48.8

Dhobi itch B35.6

Di George's syndrome D82.1

Di Guglielmo's disease C94.0-

Diabetes, diabetic (mellitus) (sugar) E11.9
- with
  - amyotrophy E11.44
  - arthropathy NEC E11.618
  - autonomic (poly) neuropathy E11.43
  - cataract E11.36
  - Charcot's joints E11.610
  - chronic kidney disease E11.22
  - circulatory complication NEC E11.59
  - complication E11.8
    - specified NEC E11.69
  - dermatitis E11.620
  - foot ulcer E11.621
  - gangrene E11.52
  - gastroparalysis E11.43
  - gastroparesis E11.43
  - glomerulonephrosis, intracapillary E11.21
  - glomerulosclerosis, intercapillary E11.21
  - hyperglycemia E11.65
  - hyperosmolarity E11.00
    - with coma E11.01
  - hypoglycemia E11.649
    - with coma E11.641
  - ketoacidosis E11.10
    - with coma E11.11
  - kidney complications NEC E11.29
  - Kimmelstiel-Wilson disease E11.21
  - loss of protective sensation (LOPS) — *see* Diabetes, by type, with neuropathy
  - mononeuropathy E11.41
  - myasthenia E11.44
  - necrobiosis lipoidica E11.620
  - nephropathy E11.21
  - neuralgia E11.42
  - neurologic complication NEC E11.49
  - neuropathic arthropathy E11.610
  - neuropathy E11.40
  - ophthalmic complication NEC E11.39
  - oral complication NEC E11.638
  - osteomyelitis E11.69
  - periodontal disease E11.630
  - peripheral angiopathy E11.51
    - with gangrene E11.52
  - polyneuropathy E11.42
  - renal complication NEC E11.29
  - renal tubular degeneration E11.29
  - retinopathy E11.319
    - with macular edema E11.311
      - resolved following treatment E11.37
    - nonproliferative E11.329
      - with macular edema E11.321
      - mild E11.329
        - with macular edema E11.321
      - moderate E11.339
        - with macular edema E11.331
      - severe E11.349
        - with macular edema E11.341
    - proliferative E11.359
      - with
        - combined traction retinal detachment and rhegmatogenous retinal detachment E11.354
        - macular edema E11.351
        - stable proliferative diabetic retinopathy E11.355
        - traction retinal detachment involving the macula E11.352

Diabetes, diabetic (mellitus) (sugar) - *continued*
- with - *continued*
  - retinopathy - *continued*
    - proliferative - *continued*
      - with - *continued*
        - traction retinal detachment not involving the macula E11.353
  - skin complication NEC E11.628
  - skin ulcer NEC E11.622
- brittle — *see* Diabetes, type 1
- bronzed E83.110
- complicating pregnancy — *see* Pregnancy, complicated by, diabetes
- dietary counseling and surveillance Z71.3
- due to
  - autoimmune process — *see* Diabetes, type 1
  - immune mediated pancreatic islet beta-cell destruction — *see* Diabetes, type 1
- due to drug or chemical E09.9
  - with
    - amyotrophy E09.44
    - arthropathy NEC E09.618
    - autonomic (poly) neuropathy E09.43
    - cataract E09.36
    - Charcot's joints E09.610
    - chronic kidney disease E09.22
    - circulatory complication NEC E09.59
    - complication E09.8
      - specified NEC E09.69
    - dermatitis E09.620
    - foot ulcer E09.621
    - gangrene E09.52
    - gastroparalysis E09.43
    - gastroparesis E09.43
    - glomerulonephrosis, intracapillary E09.21
    - glomerulosclerosis, intercapillary E09.21
    - hyperglycemia E09.65
    - hyperosmolarity E09.00
      - with coma E09.01
    - hypoglycemia E09.649
      - with coma E09.641
    - ketoacidosis E09.10
      - with coma E09.11
    - kidney complications NEC E09.29
    - Kimmelstiel-Wilson disease E09.21
    - mononeuropathy E09.41
    - myasthenia E09.44
    - necrobiosis lipoidica E09.620
    - nephropathy E09.21
    - neuralgia E09.42
    - neurologic complication NEC E09.49
    - neuropathic arthropathy E09.610
    - neuropathy E09.40
    - ophthalmic complication NEC E09.39
    - oral complication NEC E09.638
    - periodontal disease E09.630
    - peripheral angiopathy E09.51
      - with gangrene E09.52
    - polyneuropathy E09.42
    - renal complication NEC E09.29
    - renal tubular degeneration E09.29
    - retinopathy E09.319
      - with macular edema E09.311
      - resolved following treatment E09.37
      - nonproliferative E09.329
        - with macular edema E09.321
        - mild E09.329
          - with macular edema E09.321
        - moderate E09.339
          - with macular edema E09.331
        - severe E09.349
          - with macular edema E09.341
      - proliferative E09.359
        - with
          - combined traction retinal detachment and rhegmatogenous retinal detachment E09.354
          - macular edema E09.351
          - stable proliferative diabetic retinopathy E09.355
          - traction retinal detachment involving the macula E09.352
          - traction retinal detachment not involving the macula E09.353
    - skin complication NEC E09.628
    - skin ulcer NEC E09.622
- due to underlying condition E08.9
  - with
    - amyotrophy E08.44
    - arthropathy NEC E08.618
    - autonomic (poly) neuropathy E08.43
    - cataract E08.36
    - Charcot's joints E08.610

Diabetes, diabetic (mellitus) (sugar) - *continued*
- due to underlying condition - *continued*
  - with - *continued*
    - chronic kidney disease E08.22
    - circulatory complication NEC E08.59
    - complication E08.8
      - specified NEC E08.69
    - dermatitis E08.620
    - foot ulcer E08.621
    - gangrene E08.52
    - gastroparalysis E08.43
    - gastroparesis E08.43
    - glomerulonephrosis, intracapillary E08.21
    - glomerulosclerosis, intercapillary E08.21
    - hyperglycemia E08.65
    - hyperosmolarity E08.00
      - with coma E08.01
    - hypoglycemia E08.649
      - with coma E08.641
    - ketoacidosis E08.10
      - with coma E08.11
    - kidney complications NEC E08.29
    - Kimmelstiel-WIlson disease E08.21
    - mononeuropathy E08.41
    - myasthenia E08.44
    - necrobiosis lipoidica E08.620
    - nephropathy E08.21
    - neuralgia E08.42
    - neurologic complication NEC E08.49
    - neuropathic arthropathy E08.610
    - neuropathy E08.40
    - ophthalmic complication NEC E08.39
    - oral complication NEC E08.638
    - periodontal disease E08.630
    - peripheral angiopathy E08.51
      - with gangrene E08.52
    - polyneuropathy E08.42
    - renal complication NEC E08.29
    - renal tubular degeneration E08.29
    - retinopathy E08.319
      - with macular edema E08.311
      - resolved following treatment E08.37
      - nonproliferative E08.329
        - with macular edema E08.321
        - mild E08.329
          - with macular edema E08.321
        - moderate E08.339
          - with macular edema E08.331
        - severe E08.349
          - with macular edema E08.341
      - proliferative E08.359
        - with
          - combined traction retinal detachment and rhegmatogenous retinal detachment E08.354
          - macular edema E08.351
          - stable proliferative diabetic retinopathy E08.355
          - traction retinal detachment involving the macula E08.352
          - traction retinal detachment not involving the macula E08.353
    - skin complication NEC E08.628
    - skin ulcer NEC E08.622
- gestational (in pregnancy) O24.419
  - affecting newborn P70.0
  - diet controlled O24.410
  - in childbirth O24.429
    - diet controlled O24.420
    - insulin (and diet) controlled O24.424
    - oral drug controlled (antidiabetic) (hypoglycemic) O24.425
  - insulin (and diet) controlled O24.414
  - oral drug controlled (antidiabetic) (hypoglycemic) O24.415
  - puerperal O24.439
    - diet controlled O24.430
    - insulin (and diet) controlled O24.434
    - oral drug controlled (antidiabetic) (hypoglycemic) O24.435
- hepatogenous E13.9
- idiopathic — *see* Diabetes, type 1
- inadequately controlled - code to Diabetes, by type, with hyperglycemia
- insipidus E23.2
  - nephrogenic N25.1
  - pituitary E23.2
  - vasopressin resistant N25.1
- insulin dependent - code to type of diabetes
- juvenile-onset — *see* Diabetes, type 1
- ketosis-prone — *see* Diabetes, type 1
- latent R73.03
- neonatal (transient) P70.2

Diabetes, diabetic (mellitus) (sugar) - *continued*
  non-insulin dependent - code to type of diabetes
  out of control - code to Diabetes, by type, with hyperglycemia
  phosphate E83.39
  poorly controlled - code to Diabetes, by type, with hyperglycemia
  postpancreatectomy — *see* Diabetes, specified type NEC
  postprocedural — *see* Diabetes, specified type NEC
  secondary diabetes mellitus NEC — *see* Diabetes, specified type NEC
  specified type NEC E13.9
    with
      amyotrophy E13.44
      arthropathy NEC E13.618
      autonomic (poly) neuropathy E13.43
      cataract E13.36
      Charcot's joints E13.610
      chronic kidney disease E13.22
      circulatory complication NEC E13.59
      complication E13.8
        specified NEC E13.69
      dermatitis E13.620
      foot ulcer E13.621
      gangrene E13.52
      gastroparalysis E13.43
      gastroparesis E13.43
      glomerulonephrosis, intracapillary E13.21
      glomerulosclerosis, intercapillary E13.21
      hyperglycemia E13.65
      hyperosmolarity E13.00
        with coma E13.01
      hypoglycemia E13.649
        with coma E13.641
      ketoacidosis E13.10
        with coma E13.11
      kidney complications NEC E13.29
      Kimmelsteil-Wilson disease E13.21
      mononeuropathy E13.41
      myasthenia E13.44
      necrobiosis lipoidica E13.620
      nephropathy E13.21
      neuralgia E13.42
      neurologic complication NEC E13.49
      neuropathic arthropathy E13.610
      neuropathy E13.40
      ophthalmic complication NEC E13.39
      oral complication NEC E13.638
      periodontal disease E13.630
      peripheral angiopathy E13.51
        with gangrene E13.52
      polyneuropathy E13.42
      renal complication NEC E13.29
      renal tubular degeneration E13.29
      retinopathy E13.319
        with macular edema E13.311
        resolved following treatment E13.37
        nonproliferative E13.329
          with macular edema E13.321
          mild E13.329
            with macular edema E13.321
          moderate E13.339
            with macular edema E13.331
          severe E13.349
            with macular edema E13.341
        proliferative E13.359
          with
            combined traction retinal detachment and rhegmatogenous retinal detachment E13.354
            macular edema E13.351
            stable proliferative diabetic retinopathy E13.355
            traction retinal detachment involving the macula E13.352
            traction retinal detachment not involving the macula E13.353
      skin complication NEC E13.628
      skin ulcer NEC E13.622
  steroid-induced — *see* Diabetes, due to, drug or chemical
  type 1 E10.9
    with
      amyotrophy E10.44
      arthropathy NEC E10.618
      autonomic (poly) neuropathy E10.43
      cataract E10.36
      Charcot's joints E10.610
      chronic kidney disease E10.22
      circulatory complication NEC E10.59
      complication E10.8
        specified NEC E10.69

Diabetes, diabetic (mellitus) (sugar) - *continued*
  type 1 - *continued*
    with - *continued*
      dermatitis E10.620
      foot ulcer E10.621
      gangrene E10.52
      gastroparalysis E10.43
      gastroparesis E10.43
      glomerulonephrosis, intracapillary E10.21
      glomerulosclerosis, intercapillary E10.21
      hyperglycemia E10.65
      hypoglycemia E10.649
        with coma E10.641
      ketoacidosis E10.10
        with coma E10.11
      kidney complications NEC E10.29
      Kimmelsteil-Wilson disease E10.21
      mononeuropathy E10.41
      myasthenia E10.44
      necrobiosis lipoidica E10.620
      nephropathy E10.21
      neuralgia E10.42
      neurologic complication NEC E10.49
      neuropathic arthropathy E10.610
      neuropathy E10.40
      ophthalmic complication NEC E10.39
      oral complication NEC E10.638
      osteomyelitis E10.69
      periodontal disease E10.630
      peripheral angiopathy E10.51
        with gangrene E10.52
      polyneuropathy E10.42
      renal complication NEC E10.29
      renal tubular degeneration E10.29
      retinopathy E10.319
        with macular edema E10.311
        resolved following treatment E10.37
        nonproliferative E10.329
          with macular edema E10.321
          mild E10.329
            with macular edema E10.321
          moderate E10.339
            with macular edema E10.331
          severe E10.349
            with macular edema E10.341
        proliferative E10.359
          with
            combined traction retinal detachment and rhegmatogenous retinal detachment E10.354
            macular edema E10.351
            stable proliferative diabetic retinopathy E10.355
            traction retinal detachment involving the macula E10.352
            traction retinal detachment not involving the macula E10.353
      skin complication NEC E10.628
      skin ulcer NEC E10.622
  type 2 E11.9
    with
      amyotrophy E11.44
      arthropathy NEC E11.618
      autonomic (poly) neuropathy E11.43
      cataract E11.36
      Charcot's joints E11.610
      chronic kidney disease E11.22
      circulatory complication NEC E11.59
      complication E11.8
        specified NEC E11.69
      dermatitis E11.620
      foot ulcer E11.621
      gangrene E11.52
      gastroparalysis E11.43
      gastroparesis E11.43
      glomerulonephrosis, intracapillary E11.21
      glomerulosclerosis, intercapillary E11.21
      hyperglycemia E11.65
      hyperosmolarity E11.00
        with coma E11.01
      hypoglycemia E11.649
        with coma E11.641
      ketoacidosis E11.10
        with coma E11.11
      kidney complications NEC E11.29
      Kimmelsteil-Wilson disease E11.21
      mononeuropathy E11.41
      myasthenia E11.44
      necrobiosis lipoidica E11.620
      nephropathy E11.21
      neuralgia E11.42
      neurologic complication NEC E11.49
      neuropathic arthropathy E11.610

Diabetes, diabetic (mellitus) (sugar) - *continued*
  type 2 - *continued*
    with - *continued*
      neuropathy E11.40
      ophthalmic complication NEC E11.39
      oral complication NEC E11.638
      osteomyelitis E11.69
      periodontal disease E11.630
      peripheral angiopathy E11.51
        with gangrene E11.52
      polyneuropathy E11.42
      renal complication NEC E11.29
      renal tubular degeneration E11.29
      retinopathy E11.319
        with macular edema E11.311
        resolved following treatment E11.37
        nonproliferative E11.329
          with macular edema E11.321
          mild E11.329
            with macular edema E11.321
          moderate E11.339
            with macular edema E11.331
          severe E11.349
            with macular edema E11.341
        proliferative E11.359
          with
            combined traction retinal detachment and rhegmatogenous retinal detachment E11.354
            macular edema E11.351
            stable proliferative diabetic retinopathy E11.355
            traction retinal detachment involving the macula E11.352
            traction retinal detachment not involving the macula E11.353
      skin complication NEC E11.628
      skin ulcer NEC E11.622
  uncontrolled
    meaning
      hyperglycemia — *see* Diabetes, by type, with, hyperglycemia
      hypoglycemia — *see* Diabetes, by type, with, hypoglycemia

Diacyclothrombopathia D69.1

Diagnosis deferred R69

Dialysis (intermittent) (treatment)
  noncompliance (with) Z91.15
  renal (hemodialysis) (peritoneal) , status Z99.2
  retina, retinal — *see* Detachment, retina, with retinal, dialysis

Diamond-Blackfan anemia (congenital hypoplastic) D61.01

Diamond-Gardener syndrome (autoerythrocyte sensitization) D69.2

Diaper rash L22

Diaphoresis (excessive) R61

Diaphragm — *see* condition

Diaphragmalgia R07.1

Diaphragmatitis, diaphragmitis J98.6

Diaphysial aclasis Q78.6

Diaphysitis — *see* Osteomyelitis, specified type NEC

Diarrhea, diarrheal (disease) (infantile) (inflammatory) R19.7
  achlorhydric K31.83
  allergic K52.29
    due to
      colitis — *see* Colitis, allergic
      enteritis — *see* Enteritis, allergic
  amebic — *see also* Amebiasis A06.0
    with abscess — *see* Abscess, amebic
    acute A06.0
    chronic A06.1
    nondysenteric A06.2
  bacillary — *see* Dysentery, bacillary
  balantidial A07.0
  cachectic NEC K52.89
  Chilomastix A07.8
  choleriformis A00.1
  chronic (noninfectious) K52.9
  coccidial A07.3
  Cochin-China K90.1
    strongyloidiasis B78.0
  Dientamoeba A07.8
  dietetic — *see also* Diarrhea, allergic K52.29
  drug-induced K52.1
  due to
    bacteria A04.9
      specified NEC A04.8
    Campylobacter A04.5
    Capillaria philippinensis B81.1
    Clostridium difficile
      not specified as recurrent A04.72

Diarrhea, diarrheal (disease) (infantile) (inflammatory) - *continued*
due to - *continued*
Clostridium difficile - *continued*
recurrent A04.71
Clostridium perfringens (C) (F) A04.8
Cryptosporidium A07.2
drugs K52.1
Escherichia coli A04.4
enteroaggregative A04.4
enterohemorrhagic A04.3
enteroinvasive A04.2
enteropathogenic A04.0
enterotoxigenic A04.1
specified NEC A04.4
food hypersensitivity — *see also* Diarrhea, allergic K52.29
Necator americanus B76.1
S. japonicum B65.2
specified organism NEC A08.8
bacterial A04.8
viral A08.39
Staphylococcus A04.8
Trichuris trichiuria B79
virus — *see* Enteritis, viral
Yersinia enterocolitica A04.6
dysenteric A09
endemic A09
epidemic A09
flagellate A07.9
Flexner's (ulcerative) A03.1
functional K59.1
following gastrointestinal surgery K91.89
psychogenic F45.8
Giardia lamblia A07.1
giardial A07.1
hill K90.1
infectious A09
malarial — *see* Malaria
mite B88.0
mycotic NEC B49
neonatal (noninfectious) P78.3
nervous F45.8
neurogenic K59.1
noninfectious K52.9
postgastrectomy K91.1
postvagotomy K91.1
protozoal A07.9
specified NEC A07.8
psychogenic F45.8
specified
bacterium NEC A04.8
virus NEC A08.39
strongyloidiasis B78.0
toxic K52.1
trichomonal A07.8
tropical K90.1
tuberculous A18.32
viral — *see* Enteritis, viral
Diastasis
cranial bones M84.88
congenital NEC Q75.8
joint (traumatic) — *see* Dislocation
muscle M62.00
ankle M62.07-
congenital Q79.8
foot M62.07-
forearm M62.03-
hand M62.04-
lower leg M62.06-
pelvic region M62.05-
shoulder region M62.01-
specified site NEC M62.08
thigh M62.05-
upper arm M62.02-
recti (abdomen)
complicating delivery O71.89
congenital Q79.59
Diastema, tooth, teeth, fully erupted M26.32
Diastematomyelia Q06.2
Diataxia, cerebral G80.4
Diathesis
allergic — *see* History, allergy
bleeding (familial) D69.9
cystine (familial) E72.00
gouty — *see* Gout
hemorrhagic (familial) D69.9
newborn NEC P53
spasmophilic R29.0
Diaz's disease or osteochondrosis (juvenile) (talus) — *see* Osteochondrosis, juvenile, tarsus
Dibothriocephalus, dibothriocephaliasis (latus) (infection) (infestation) B70.0
larval B70.1
Dicephalus, dicephaly Q89.4
Dichotomy, teeth K00.2
Dichromat, dichromatopsia (congenital) — *see* Deficiency, color vision
Dichuchwa A65
Dicroceliasis B66.2
Didelphia, didelphys — *see* Double uterus
Didymytis N45.1
with orchitis N45.3
Dietary
inadequacy or deficiency E63.9
surveillance and counseling Z71.3
Dietl's crisis N13.8
Dieulafoy lesion (hemorrhagic)
duodenum K31.82
esophagus K22.8
intestine (colon) K63.81
stomach K31.82
Difficult, difficulty (in)
acculturation Z60.3
feeding R63.3
newborn P92.9
breast P92.5
specified NEC P92.8
nonorganic (infant or child) F98.29
intubation, in anesthesia T88.4
mechanical, gastroduodenal stoma K91.89
causing obstruction — *see also* Obstruction, intestine, postoperative K91.30
micturition
need to immediately re-void R39.191
position dependent R39.192
specified NEC R39.198
reading (developmental) F81.0
secondary to emotional disorders F93.9
spelling (specific) F81.81
with reading disorder F81.89
due to inadequate teaching Z55.8
swallowing — *see* Dysphagia
walking R26.2
work
conditions NEC Z56.5
schedule Z56.3
Diffuse — *see* condition
DiGeorge's syndrome (thymic hypoplasia) D82.1
Digestive — *see* condition
Dihydropyrimidine dehydrogenase disease (DPD) E88.89
Diktyoma — *see* Neoplasm, malignant, by site
Dilaceration, tooth K00.4
Dilatation
anus K59.8
venule — *see* Hemorrhoids
aorta (focal) (general) — *see* Ectasia, aorta
with aneuysm — *see* Aneurysm, aorta
congenital Q25.44
artery — *see* Aneurysm
bladder (sphincter) N32.89
congenital Q64.79
blood vessel I99.8
bronchial J47.9
with
exacerbation (acute) J47.1
lower respiratory infection J47.0
calyx (due to obstruction) — *see* Hydronephrosis
capillaries I78.8
cardiac (acute) (chronic) — *see also* Hypertrophy, cardiac
congenital Q24.8
valve NEC Q24.8
pulmonary Q22.3
valve — *see* Endocarditis
cavum septi pellucidi Q06.8
cervix (uteri) — *see also* Incompetency, cervix
incomplete, poor, slow complicating delivery O62.0
colon K59.39
congenital Q43.1
psychogenic F45.8
toxic K59.31
common duct (acquired) K83.8
congenital Q44.5
cystic duct (acquired) K82.8
congenital Q44.5
duct, mammary — *see* Ectasia, mammary duct
duodenum K59.8
esophagus K22.8
congenital Q39.5
due to achalasia K22.0
eustachian tube, congenital Q17.8
Dilatation - *continued*
gallbladder K82.8
gastric — *see* Dilatation, stomach
heart (acute) (chronic) — *see also* Hypertrophy, cardiac
congenital Q24.8
valve — *see* Endocarditis
ileum K59.8
psychogenic F45.8
jejunum K59.8
psychogenic F45.8
kidney (calyx) (collecting structures) (cystic) (parenchyma) (pelvis) (idiopathic) N28.89
lacrimal passages or duct — *see* Disorder, lacrimal system, changes
lymphatic vessel I89.0
mammary duct — *see* Ectasia, mammary duct
Meckel's diverticulum (congenital) Q43.0
malignant — *see* Table of Neoplasms, small intestine, malignant
myocardium (acute) (chronic) — *see* Hypertrophy, cardiac
organ or site, congenital NEC — *see* Distortion
pancreatic duct K86.89
pericardium — *see* Pericarditis
pharynx J39.2
prostate N42.89
pulmonary
artery (idiopathic) I28.8
valve, congenital Q22.3
pupil H57.04
rectum K59.39
saccule, congenital Q16.5
salivary gland (duct) K11.8
sphincter ani K62.89
stomach K31.89
acute K31.0
psychogenic F45.8
submaxillary duct K11.8
trachea, congenital Q32.1
ureter (idiopathic) N28.82
congenital Q62.2
due to obstruction N13.4
urethra (acquired) N36.8
vasomotor I73.9
vein I86.8
ventricular, ventricle (acute) (chronic) — *see also* Hypertrophy, cardiac
cerebral, congenital Q04.8
venule NEC I86.8
vesical orifice N32.89
Dilated, dilation — *see* Dilatation
Diminished, diminution
hearing (acuity) — *see* Deafness
sense or sensation (cold) (heat) (tactile) (vibratory) R20.8
vision NEC H54.7
vital capacity R94.2
Diminuta taenia B71.0
Dimitri-Sturge-Weber disease Q85.8
Dimple
congenital sacral Q82.6
parasacral Q82.6
pilonidal or postanal — *see* Cyst, pilonidal
Dioctophyme renalis (infection) (infestation) B83.8
Dipetalonemiasis B74.4
Diphallus Q55.69
Diphtheria, diphtheritic (gangrenous) (hemorrhagic) A36.9
carrier (suspected) Z22.2
cutaneous A36.3
faucial A36.0
infection of wound A36.3
laryngeal A36.2
myocarditis A36.81
nasal, anterior A36.89
nasopharyngeal A36.1
neurological complication A36.89
pharyngeal A36.0
specified site NEC A36.89
tonsillar A36.0
Diphyllobothriasis (intestine) B70.0
larval B70.1
Diplacusis H93.22-
Diplegia (upper limbs) G83.0
congenital (cerebral) G80.8
facial G51.0
lower limbs G82.20
spastic G80.1
Diplococcus, diplococcal — *see* condition
Diplopia H53.2
Dipsomania F10.20
with

Dipsomania - *continued*
  with - *continued*
    psychosis — *see* Psychosis, alcoholic
    remission F10.21
Dipylidiasis B71.1
DIRA
  (deficiency of interleukin 1 receptor antagonist) M04.8
Direction, teeth, abnormal, fully erupted M26.30
Dirofilariasis B74.8
Dirt-eating child F98.3
Disability, disabilities
  heart — *see* Disease, heart
  intellectual F79
    with
      autistic features F84.9
    mild (I.Q.50-69) F70
    moderate (I.Q.35-49) F71
    profound (I.Q. under 20) F73
    severe (I.Q.20-34) F72
    specified level NEC F78
  knowledge acquisition F81.9
  learning F81.9
  limiting activities Z73.6
  spelling, specific F81.81
Disappearance of family member Z63.4
Disarticulation — *see* Amputation
  meaning traumatic amputation — *see* Amputation, traumatic
Discharge (from)
  abnormal finding in — *see* Abnormal, specimen
  breast (female) (male) N64.52
  diencephalic autonomic idiopathic — *see* Epilepsy, specified NEC
  ear — *see also* Otorrhea
    blood — *see* Otorrhagia
  excessive urine R35.8
  nipple N64.52
  penile R36.9
  postnasal R09.82
  prison, anxiety concerning Z65.2
  urethral R36.9
    without blood R36.0
    hematospermia R36.1
  vaginal N89.8
Discitis, diskitis M46.40
  cervical region M46.42
  cervicothoracic region M46.43
  lumbar region M46.46
  lumbosacral region M46.47
  multiple sites M46.49
  occipito-atlanto-axial region M46.41
  pyogenic — *see* Infection, intervertebral disc, pyogenic
  sacrococcygeal region M46.48
  thoracic region M46.44
  thoracolumbar region M46.45
Discoid
  meniscus (congenital) Q68.6
  semilunar cartilage (congenital) — *see* Derangement, knee, meniscus, specified NEC
Discoloration
  nails L60.8
  teeth (posteruptive) K03.7
    during formation K00.8
Discomfort
  chest R07.89
  visual H53.14-
Discontinuity, ossicles, ear H74.2-
Discord (with)
  boss Z56.4
  classmates Z55.4
  counselor Z64.4
  employer Z56.4
  family Z63.8
  fellow employees Z56.4
  in-laws Z63.1
  landlord Z59.2
  lodgers Z59.2
  neighbors Z59.2
  probation officer Z64.4
  social worker Z64.4
  teachers Z55.4
  workmates Z56.4
Discordant connection
  atrioventricular (congenital) Q20.5
  ventriculoarterial Q20.3
Discrepancy
  centric occlusion maximum intercuspation M26.55
  leg length (acquired) — *see* Deformity, limb, unequal length
    congenital — *see* Defect, reduction, lower limb
  uterine size date O26.84-
Discrimination
  ethnic Z60.5
  political Z60.5
  racial Z60.5
  religious Z60.5
  sex Z60.5
Disease, diseased — *see also* Syndrome
  absorbent system I87.8
  acid-peptic K30
  Acosta's T70.29
  Adams-Stokes (-Morgagni) (syncope with heart block) I45.9
  Addison's anemia (pernicious) D51.0
  adenoids (and tonsils) J35.9
  adrenal (capsule) (cortex) (gland) (medullary) E27.9
    hyperfunction E27.0
    specified NEC E27.8
  ainhum L94.6
  airway
    obstructive, chronic J44.9
      due to
        cotton dust J66.0
        specific organic dusts NEC J66.8
    reactive — *see* Asthma
  akamushi (scrub typhus) A75.3
  Albers-Schönberg (marble bones) Q78.2
  Albert's — *see* Tendinitis, Achilles
  alimentary canal K63.9
  alligator-skin Q80.9
    acquired L85.0
  alpha heavy chain C88.3
  alpine T70.29
  altitude T70.20
  alveolar ridge
    edentulous K06.9
      specified NEC K06.8
  alveoli, teeth K08.9
  Alzheimer's G30.9 *[F02.80]*
    with behavioral disturbance G30.9 *[F02.81]*
    early onset G30.0 *[F02.80]*
      with behavioral disturbance G30.0 *[F02.81]*
    late onset G30.1 *[F02.80]*
      with behavioral disturbance G30.1 *[F02.81]*
    specified NEC G30.8 *[F02.80]*
      with behavioral disturbance G30.8 *[F02.81]*
  amyloid — *see* Amyloidosis
  Andersen's (glycogenosis IV) E74.09
  Andes T70.29
  Andrews' (bacterid) L08.89
  angiospastic I73.9
    cerebral G45.9
    vein I87.8
  anterior
    chamber H21.9
    horn cell G12.29
  antiglomerular basement membrane (anti- GBM)
    antibody M31.0
    tubulo-interstitial nephritis N12
  antral — *see* Sinusitis, maxillary
  anus K62.9
    specified NEC K62.89
  aorta (nonsyphilitic) I77.9
    syphilitic NEC A52.02
  aortic (heart) (valve) I35.9
    rheumatic I06.9
  Apollo B30.3
  aponeuroses — *see* Enthesopathy
  appendix K38.9
    specified NEC K38.8
  aqueous (chamber) H21.9
  Arnold-Chiari — *see* Arnold-Chiari disease
  arterial I77.9
    occlusive — *see* Occlusion, by site
      due to stricture or stenosis I77.1
  arteriocardiorenal — *see* Hypertension, cardiorenal
  arteriolar (generalized) (obliterative) I77.9
  arteriorenal — *see* Hypertension, kidney
  arteriosclerotic — *see also* Arteriosclerosis
    cardiovascular — *see* Disease, heart, ischemic, atherosclerotic
    coronary (artery) — *see* Disease, heart, ischemic, atherosclerotic
    heart — *see* Disease, heart, ischemic, atherosclerotic
  artery I77.9
    cerebral I67.9
    coronary I25.10
      with angina pectoris — *see* Arteriosclerosis, coronary (artery),
  arthropod-borne NOS (viral) A94
    specified type NEC A93.8
  atticoantral, chronic H66.20
    left H66.22

Disease, diseased - *continued*
  atticoantral, chronic - *continued*
    left - *continued*
      with right H66.23
    right H66.21
      with left H66.23
  auditory canal — *see* Disorder, ear, external
  auricle, ear NEC — *see* Disorder, pinna
  Australian X A83.4
  autoimmune (systemic) NOS M35.9
    hemolytic (cold type) (warm type) D59.1
      drug-induced D59.0
    thyroid E06.3
  autoinflammatory M04.9
    NOD2-associated M04.8
    specified type NEC M04.8
  aviator's — *see* Effect, adverse, high altitude
  Ayerza's (pulmonary artery sclerosis with pulmonary hypertension) I27.0
  Babington's (familial hemorrhagic telangiectasia) I78.0
  bacterial A49.9
    specified NEC A48.8
    zoonotic A28.9
      specified type NEC A28.8
  Baelz's (cheilitis glandularis apostematosa) K13.0
  bagasse J67.1
  balloon — *see* Effect, adverse, high altitude
  Bang's (brucella abortus) A23.1
  Bannister's T78.3
  barometer makers' — *see* Poisoning, mercury
  Barraquer (-Simons') (progressive lipodystrophy) E88.1
  Barrett's — *see* Barrett's, esophagus
  Bartholin's gland N75.9
  basal ganglia G25.9
    degenerative G23.9
      specified NEC G23.8
    specified NEC G25.89
  Basedow's (exophthalmic goiter) — *see* Hyperthyroidism, with, goiter (diffuse)
  Bateman's B08.1
  Batten-Steinert G71.11
  Battey A31.0
  Beard's (neurasthenia) F48.8
  Becker
    idiopathic mural endomyocardial I42.3
    myotonia congenita G71.12
  Begbie's (exophthalmic goiter) — *see* Hyperthyroidism, with, goiter (diffuse)
  behavioral, organic F07.9
  Beigel's (white piedra) B36.2
  Benson's — *see* Deposit, crystalline
  Bernard-Soulier (thrombopathy) D69.1
  Bernhardt (-Roth) — *see* Mononeuropathy, lower limb, meralgia paresthetica
  Biermer's (pernicious anemia) D51.0
  bile duct (common) (hepatic) K83.9
    with calculus, stones — *see* Calculus, bile duct
    specified NEC K83.8
  biliary (tract) K83.9
    specified NEC K83.8
  Billroth's — *see* Spina bifida
  bird fancier's J67.2
  black lung J60
  bladder N32.9
    in (due to)
      schistosomiasis (bilharziasis) B65.0 *[N33]*
    specified NEC N32.89
  bleeder's D66
  blood D75.9
    forming organs D75.9
    vessel I99.9
  Bloodgood's — *see* Mastopathy, cystic
  Bodechtel-Guttmann (subacute sclerosing panencephalitis) A81.1
  bone — *see also* Disorder, bone
    aluminum M83.4
    fibrocystic NEC
      jaw M27.49
  bone-marrow D75.9
  Borna A83.9
  Bornholm (epidemic pleurodynia) B33.0
  Bouchard's (myopathic dilatation of the stomach) K31.0
  Bouillaud's (rheumatic heart disease) I01.9
  Bourneville (-Brissaud) (tuberous sclerosis) Q85.1
  Bouveret (-Hoffmann) (paroxysmal tachycardia) I47.9
  bowel K63.9
    functional K59.9
      psychogenic F45.8
  brain G93.9

- **Disease, diseased** - *continued*
  - brain - *continued*
    - arterial, artery I67.9
    - arteriosclerotic I67.2
    - congenital Q04.9
    - degenerative — *see* Degeneration, brain
    - inflammatory — *see* Encephalitis
    - organic G93.9
      - arteriosclerotic I67.2
    - parasitic NEC B71.9 *[G94]*
    - senile NEC G31.1
    - specified NEC G93.89
  - breast — *see also* Disorder, breast N64.9
    - cystic (chronic) — *see* Mastopathy, cystic
    - fibrocystic — *see* Mastopathy, cystic
    - Paget's
      - female, unspecified side C50.91-
      - male, unspecified side C50.92-
    - specified NEC N64.89
  - Breda's — *see* Yaws
  - Bretonneau's (diphtheritic malignant angina) A36.0
  - Bright's — *see* Nephritis
    - arteriosclerotic — *see* Hypertension, kidney
  - Brill's (recrudescent typhus) A75.1
  - Brill-Zinsser (recrudescent typhus) A75.1
  - Brion-Kayser — *see* Fever, paratyphoid
  - broad
    - beta E78.2
    - ligament (noninflammatory) N83.9
      - inflammatory — *see* Disease, pelvis, inflammatory
      - specified NEC N83.8
  - Brocq-Duhring (dermatitis herpetiformis) L13.0
  - Brocq's
    - meaning
      - dermatitis herpetiformis L13.0
      - prurigo L28.2
  - bronchopulmonary J98.4
  - bronchus NEC J98.09
  - bronze Addison's E27.1
    - tuberculous A18.7
  - budgerigar fancier's J67.2
  - bullous L13.9
    - chronic of childhood L12.2
    - specified NEC L13.8
  - Buerger's (thromboangiitis obliterans) I73.1
  - Bürger-Grütz (essential familial hyperlipemia) E78.3
  - bursa — *see* Bursopathy
  - caisson T70.3
  - California — *see* Coccidioidomycosis
  - capillaries I78.9
    - specified NEC I78.8
  - Carapata A68.0
  - cardiac — *see* Disease, heart
  - cardiopulmonary, chronic I27.9
  - cardiorenal (hepatic) (hypertensive) (vascular) — *see* Hypertension, cardiorenal
  - cardiovascular (atherosclerotic) I25.10
    - with angina pectoris — *see* Arteriosclerosis, coronary (artery),
    - congenital Q28.9
    - newborn P29.9
      - specified NEC P29.89
    - hypertensive — *see* Hypertension, heart
    - renal (hypertensive) — *see* Hypertension, cardiorenal
    - syphilitic (asymptomatic) A52.00
  - cartilage — *see* Disorder, cartilage
  - Castellani's A69.8
  - Castleman (unicentric) (multicentric) D47.Z2
    - HHV-8-associated — *see also* Herpesvirus, human, 8 D47.Z2
  - cat-scratch A28.1
  - Cavare's (familial periodic paralysis) G72.3
  - cecum K63.9
  - celiac (adult) (infantile) (with steatorrhea) K90.0
  - cellular tissue L98.9
  - central core G71.2
  - cerebellar, cerebellum — *see* Disease, brain
  - cerebral — *see also* Disease, brain
    - degenerative — *see* Degeneration, brain
  - cerebrospinal G96.9
  - cerebrovascular I67.9
    - acute I67.89
      - embolic I63.4-
      - thrombotic I63.3-
    - arteriosclerotic I67.2
    - hereditary NEC I67.858
    - specified NEC I67.89
  - cervix (uteri) (noninflammatory) N88.9
    - inflammatory — *see* Cervicitis
    - specified NEC N88.8
  - Chabert's A22.9

- **Disease, diseased** - *continued*
  - Chandler's (osteochondritis dissecans, hip) — *see* Osteochondritis, dissecans, hip
  - Charlouis — *see* Yaws
  - Chédiak-Steinbrinck (-Higashi) (congenital gigantism of peroxidase granules) E70.330
  - chest J98.9
  - Chiari's (hepatic vein thrombosis) I82.0
  - Chicago B40.9
  - Chignon B36.8
  - chigo, chigoe B88.1
  - childhood granulomatous D71
  - Chinese liver fluke B66.1
  - chlamydial A74.9
    - specified NEC A74.89
  - cholecystic K82.9
  - choroid H31.9
    - specified NEC H31.8
  - Christmas D67
  - chronic bullous of childhood L12.2
  - chylomicron retention E78.3
  - ciliary body H21.9
    - specified NEC H21.89
  - circulatory (system) NEC I99.8
    - newborn P29.9
    - syphilitic A52.00
      - congenital A50.54
  - coagulation factor deficiency (congenital) — *see* Defect, coagulation
  - coccidioidal — *see* Coccidioidomycosis
  - cold
    - agglutinin or hemoglobinuria D59.1
      - paroxysmal D59.6
    - hemagglutinin (chronic) D59.1
  - collagen NOS (nonvascular) (vascular) M35.9
    - specified NEC M35.8
  - colon K63.9
    - functional K59.9
      - congenital Q43.2
    - ischemic — *see also* Ischemia, intestine, acute K55.039
  - colonic inflammatory bowel, unclassified (IBDU) K52.3
  - combined system — *see* Degeneration, combined
  - compressed air T70.3
  - Concato's (pericardial polyserositis) A19.9
    - nontubercular I31.1
    - pleural — *see* Pleurisy, with effusion
  - conjunctiva H11.9
    - chlamydial A74.0
    - specified NEC H11.89
    - viral B30.9
      - specified NEC B30.8
  - connective tissue, systemic (diffuse) M35.9
    - in (due to)
      - hypogammaglobulinemia D80.1 *[M36.8]*
      - ochronosis E70.29 *[M36.8]*
    - specified NEC M35.8
  - Conor and Bruch's (boutonneuse fever) A77.1
  - Cooper's — *see* Mastopathy, cystic
  - Cori's (glycogenosis III) E74.03
  - corkhandler's or corkworker's J67.3
  - cornea H18.9
    - specified NEC H18.89-
  - coronary (artery) — *see* Disease, heart, ischemic, atherosclerotic
    - congenital Q24.5
    - ostial, syphilitic (aortic) (mitral) (pulmonary) A52.03
  - corpus cavernosum N48.9
    - specified NEC N48.89
  - Cotugno's — *see* Sciatica
  - coxsackie (virus) NEC B34.1
  - cranial nerve NOS G52.9
  - Creutzfeldt-Jakob — *see* Creutzfeldt-Jakob disease or syndrome
  - Crocq's (acrocyanosis) I73.89
  - Crohn's — *see* Enteritis, regional
  - Curschmann G71.11
  - cystic
    - breast (chronic) — *see* Mastopathy, cystic
    - kidney, congenital Q61.9
    - liver, congenital Q44.6
    - lung J98.4
      - congenital Q33.0
  - cytomegalic inclusion (generalized) B25.9
    - with pneumonia B25.0
    - congenital P35.1
  - cytomegaloviral B25.9
    - specified NEC B25.8
  - Czerny's (periodic hydrarthrosis of the knee) — *see* Effusion, joint, knee
  - Daae (-Finsen) (epidemic pleurodynia) B33.0

- **Disease, diseased** - *continued*
  - Darling's — *see* Histoplasmosis capsulati
  - Débove's (splenomegaly) R16.1
  - deer fly — *see* Tularemia
  - Degos' I77.89
  - demyelinating, demyelinizating (nervous system) G37.9
    - multiple sclerosis G35
    - specified NEC G37.8
  - dense deposit — *see also* N00-N07 with fourth character .6 N05.6
  - deposition, hydroxyapatite — *see* Disease, hydroxyapatite deposition
  - de Quervain's (tendon sheath) M65.4
    - thyroid (subacute granulomatous thyroiditis) E06.1
  - Devergie's (pityriasis rubra pilaris) L44.0
  - Devic's G36.0
  - diaphorase deficiency D74.0
  - diaphragm J98.6
  - diarrheal, infectious NEC A09
  - digestive system K92.9
    - specified NEC K92.89
  - disc, degenerative — *see* Degeneration, intervertebral disc
  - discogenic — *see also* Displacement, intervertebral disc NEC
    - with myelopathy — *see* Disorder, disc, with, myelopathy
  - diverticular — *see* Diverticula
  - Dubois (thymus) A50.59 *[E35]*
  - Duchenne-Griesinger G71.01
  - Duchenne's
    - muscular dystrophy G71.01
    - pseudohypertrophy, muscles G71.01
  - ductless glands E34.9
  - Duhring's (dermatitis herpetiformis) L13.0
  - duodenum K31.9
    - specified NEC K31.89
  - Dupré's (meningism) R29.1
  - Dupuytren's (muscle contracture) M72.0
  - Durand-Nicholas-Favre (climatic bubo) A55
  - Duroziez's (congenital mitral stenosis) Q23.2
  - ear — *see* Disorder, ear
  - Eberth's — *see* Fever, typhoid
  - Ebola (virus) A98.4
  - Ebstein's heart Q22.5
  - Echinococcus — *see* Echinococcus
  - echovirus NEC B34.1
  - Eddowes' (brittle bones and blue sclera) Q78.0
  - edentulous (alveolar) ridge K06.9
    - specified NEC K06.8
  - Edsall's T67.2
  - Eichstedt's (pityriasis versicolor) B36.0
  - Eisenmenger's (irreversible) I27.83
  - Ellis-van Creveld (chondroectodermal dysplasia) Q77.6
  - end stage renal (ESRD) N18.6
    - due to hypertension I12.0
  - endocrine glands or system NEC E34.9
  - endomyocardial (eosinophilic) I42.3
  - English (rickets) E55.0
  - enteroviral, enterovirus NEC B34.1
    - central nervous system NEC A88.8
  - epidemic B99.9
    - specified NEC B99.8
  - epididymis N50.9
  - Erb (-Landouzy) G71.02
  - Erdheim-Chester (ECD) E88.89
  - esophagus K22.9
    - functional K22.4
    - psychogenic F45.8
    - specified NEC K22.8
  - Eulenburg's (congenital paramyotonia) G71.19
  - eustachian tube — *see* Disorder, eustachian tube
  - external
    - auditory canal — *see* Disorder, ear, external
    - ear — *see* Disorder, ear, external
  - extrapyramidal G25.9
    - specified NEC G25.89
  - eye H57.9
    - anterior chamber H21.9
    - inflammatory NEC H57.89
    - muscle (external) — *see* Strabismus
    - specified NEC H57.89
    - syphilitic — *see* Oculopathy, syphilitic
  - eyeball H44.9
    - specified NEC H44.89
  - eyelid — *see* Disorder, eyelid
    - specified NEC — *see* Disorder, eyelid, specified type NEC
  - eyeworm of Africa B74.3
  - facial nerve (seventh) G51.9
    - newborn (birth injury) P11.3

Disease, diseased - *continued*

- Fahr (of brain) G23.8
- Fahr Volhard (of kidney) I12.-
- fallopian tube (noninflammatory) N83.9
  - inflammatory — *see* Salpingo-oophoritis
  - specified NEC N83.8
- familial periodic paralysis G72.3
- Fanconi's (congenital pancytopenia) D61.09
- fascia NEC — *see also* Disorder, muscle
  - inflammatory — *see* Myositis
  - specified NEC M62.89
- Fauchard's (periodontitis) — *see* Periodontitis
- Favre-Durand-Nicolas (climatic bubo) A55
- Fede's K14.0
- Feer's — *see* Poisoning, mercury
- female pelvic inflammatory — *see also* Disease, pelvis, inflammatory N73.9
  - syphilitic (secondary) A51.42
  - tuberculous A18.17
- Fernels' (aortic aneurysm) I71.9
- fibrocaseous of lung — *see* Tuberculosis, pulmonary
- fibrocystic — *see* Fibrocystic disease
- Fiedler's (leptospiral jaundice) A27.0
- fifth B08.3
- file-cutter's — *see* Poisoning, lead
- fish-skin Q80.9
  - acquired L85.0
- Flajani (-Basedow) (exophthalmic goiter) — *see* Hyperthyroidism, with, goiter (diffuse)
- flax-dresser's J66.1
- fluke — *see* Infestation, fluke
- foot and mouth B08.8
- foot process N04.9
- Forbes' (glycogenosis III) E74.03
- Fordyce-Fox (apocrine miliaria) L75.2
- Fordyce's (ectopic sebaceous glands) (mouth) Q38.6
- Forestier's (rhizomelic pseudopolyarthritis) M35.3
  - meaning ankylosing hyperostosis — *see* Hyperostosis, ankylosing
- Fothergill's
  - neuralgia — *see* Neuralgia, trigeminal
  - scarlatina anginosa A38.9
- Fournier (gangrene) N49.3
  - female N76.89
- fourth B08.8
- Fox (-Fordyce) (apocrine miliaria) L75.2
- Francis' — *see* Tularemia
- Franklin C88.2
- Frei's (climatic bubo) A55
- Friedreich's
  - combined systemic or ataxia G11.1
  - myoclonia G25.3
- frontal sinus — *see* Sinusitis, frontal
- fungus NEC B49
- Gaisböck's (polycythemia hypertonica) D75.1
- gallbladder K82.9
  - calculus — *see* Calculus, gallbladder
  - cholecystitis — *see* Cholecystitis
  - cholesterolosis K82.4
  - fistula — *see* Fistula, gallbladder
  - hydrops K82.1
  - obstruction — *see* Obstruction, gallbladder
  - perforation K82.2
  - specified NEC K82.8
- gamma heavy chain C88.2
- Gamna's (siderotic splenomegaly) D73.2
- Gamstorp's (adynamia episodica hereditaria) G72.3
- Gandy-Nanta (siderotic splenomegaly) D73.2
- ganister J62.8
- gastric — *see* Disease, stomach
- gastroesophageal reflux (GERD) K21.9
  - with esophagitis K21.0
- gastrointestinal (tract) K92.9
  - amyloid E85.4
  - functional K59.9
    - psychogenic F45.8
  - specified NEC K92.89
- Gee (-Herter) (-Heubner) (-Thaysen) (nontropical sprue) K90.0
- genital organs
  - female N94.9
  - male N50.9
- Gerhardt's (erythromelalgia) I73.81
- Gibert's (pityriasis rosea) L42
- Gierke's (glycogenosis I) E74.01
- Gilles de la Tourette's (motor-verbal tic) F95.2
- gingiva K06.9
  - plaque induced K05.00
  - specified NEC K06.8
- gland (lymph) I89.9
- Glanzmann's (hereditary hemorrhagic thrombasthenia) D69.1

Disease, diseased - *continued*

- glass-blower's (cataract) — *see* Cataract, specified NEC
  - salivary gland hypertrophy K11.1
- Glisson's — *see* Rickets
- globe H44.9
  - specified NEC H44.89
- glomerular — *see also* Glomerulonephritis
  - with edema — *see* Nephrosis
  - acute — *see* Nephritis, acute
  - chronic — *see* Nephritis, chronic
  - minimal change N05.0
  - rapidly progressive N01.9
- glycogen storage E74.00
  - Andersen's E74.09
  - Cori's E74.03
  - Forbes' E74.03
  - generalized E74.00
  - glucose-6-phosphatase deficiency E74.01
  - heart E74.02 *[I43]*
  - hepatorenal E74.09
  - Hers' E74.09
  - liver and kidney E74.09
  - McArdle's E74.04
  - muscle phosphofructokinase E74.09
  - myocardium E74.02 *[I43]*
  - Pompe's E74.02
  - Tauri's E74.09
  - type 0 E74.09
  - type I E74.01
  - type II E74.02
  - type III E74.03
  - type IV E74.09
  - type V E74.04
  - type VI-XI E74.09
  - Von Gierke's E74.01
- Goldstein's (familial hemorrhagic telangiectasia) I78.0
- gonococcal NOS A54.9
- graft-versus-host (GVH) D89.813
  - acute D89.810
  - acute on chronic D89.812
  - chronic D89.811
- grainhandler's J67.8
- granulomatous (childhood) (chronic) D71
- Graves' (exophthalmic goiter) — *see* Hyperthyroidism, with, goiter (diffuse)
- Griesinger's — *see* Ancylostomiasis
- Grisel's M43.6
- Gruby's (tinea tonsurans) B35.0
- Guillain-Barré G61.0
- Guinon's (motor-verbal tic) F95.2
- gum K06.9
- gynecological N94.9
- H (Hartnup's) E72.02
- Haff — *see* Poisoning, mercury
- Hageman (congenital factor XII deficiency) D68.2
- hair (color) (shaft) L67.9
  - follicles L73.9
    - specified NEC L73.8
- Hamman's (spontaneous mediastinal emphysema) J98.2
- hand, foot and mouth B08.4
- Hansen's — *see* Leprosy
- Hantavirus, with pulmonary manifestations B33.4
  - with renal manifestations A98.5
- Harada's H30.81-
- Hartnup (pellagra-cerebellar ataxia-renal aminoaciduria) E72.02
- Hart's (pellagra-cerebellar ataxia-renal aminoaciduria) E72.02
- Hashimoto's (struma lymphomatosa) E06.3
- Hb — *see* Disease, hemoglobin
- heart (organic) I51.9
  - with
    - pulmonary edema (acute) — *see also* Failure, ventricular, left I50.1
    - rheumatic fever (conditions in I00)
      - active I01.9
        - with chorea I02.0
        - specified NEC I01.8
      - inactive or quiescent (with chorea) I09.9
        - specified NEC I09.89
  - amyloid E85.4 *[I43]*
  - aortic (valve) I35.9
  - arteriosclerotic or sclerotic (senile) — *see* Disease, heart, ischemic, atherosclerotic
  - artery, arterial — *see* Disease, heart, ischemic, atherosclerotic
  - beer drinkers' I42.6
  - beriberi (wet) E51.12
  - black I27.0
  - congenital Q24.9

Disease, diseased - *continued*

- heart (organic) - *continued*
  - congenital - *continued*
    - cyanotic Q24.9
    - specified NEC Q24.8
  - coronary — *see* Disease, heart, ischemic
  - cryptogenic I51.9
  - fibroid — *see* Myocarditis
  - functional I51.89
    - psychogenic F45.8
  - glycogen storage E74.02 *[I43]*
  - gonococcal A54.83
  - hypertensive — *see* Hypertension, heart
  - hyperthyroid — *see also* Hyperthyroidism E05.90 *[I43]*
    - with thyroid storm E05.91 *[I43]*
  - ischemic (chronic or with a stated duration of over 4 weeks) I25.9
    - atherosclerotic (of) I25.10
      - with angina pectoris — *see* Arteriosclerosis, coronary (artery)
      - coronary artery bypass graft — *see* Arteriosclerosis, coronary (artery),
    - cardiomyopathy I25.5
    - diagnosed on ECG or other special investigation, but currently presenting no symptoms I25.6
    - silent I25.6
    - specified form NEC I25.89
  - kyphoscoliotic I27.1
  - meningococcal A39.50
    - endocarditis A39.51
    - myocarditis A39.52
    - pericarditis A39.53
  - mitral I05.9
    - specified NEC I05.8
  - muscular — *see* Degeneration, myocardial
  - psychogenic (functional) F45.8
  - pulmonary (chronic) I27.9
    - in schistosomiasis B65.9 *[I52]*
    - specified NEC I27.89
  - rheumatic (chronic) (inactive) (old) (quiescent) (with chorea) I09.9
    - active or acute I01.9
      - with chorea (acute) (rheumatic) (Sydenham's) I02.0
    - specified NEC I09.89
  - senile — *see* Myocarditis
  - syphilitic A52.06
    - aortic A52.03
      - aneurysm A52.01
    - congenital A50.54 *[I52]*
  - thyrotoxic — *see also* Thyrotoxicosis E05.90 *[I43]*
    - with thyroid storm E05.91 *[I43]*
  - valve, valvular (obstructive) (regurgitant) — *see also* Endocarditis
    - congenital NEC Q24.8
      - pulmonary Q22.3
  - vascular — *see* Disease, cardiovascular
- heavy chain NEC C88.2
  - alpha C88.3
  - gamma C88.2
  - mu C88.2
- Hebra's
  - pityriasis
    - maculata et circinata L42
    - rubra pilaris L44.0
  - prurigo L28.2
- hematopoietic organs D75.9
- hemoglobin or Hb
  - abnormal (mixed) NEC D58.2
    - with thalassemia D56.9
  - AS genotype D57.3
  - Bart's D56.0
  - C (Hb-C) D58.2
    - with other abnormal hemoglobin NEC D58.2
    - elliptocytosis D58.1
    - Hb-S D57.2-
    - sickle-cell D57.2-
    - thalassemia D56.8
  - Constant Spring D58.2
  - D (Hb-D) D58.2
  - E (Hb-E) D58.2
  - E-beta thalassemia D56.5
  - elliptocytosis D58.1
  - H (Hb-H) (thalassemia) D56.0
    - with other abnormal hemoglobin NEC D56.9
    - Constant Spring D56.0
  - I thalassemia D56.9
  - M D74.0
  - S or SS D57.1
  - SC D57.2-
  - SD D57.8-
  - SE D57.8-

Disease, diseased - *continued*
hemoglobin or Hb - *continued*
spherocytosis D58.0
unstable, hemolytic D58.2
hemolytic (newborn) P55.9
autoimmune (cold type) (warm type) D59.1
drug-induced D59.0
due to or with
incompatibility
ABO (blood group) P55.1
blood (group) (Duffy) (K) (Kell) (Kidd) (Lewis) (M) (S) NEC P55.8
Rh (blood group) (factor) P55.0
Rh negative mother P55.0
specified type NEC P55.8
unstable hemoglobin D58.2
hemorrhagic D69.9
newborn P53
Henoch (-Schönlein) (purpura nervosa) D69.0
hepatic — *see* Disease, liver
hepatobiliary K83.9
toxic K71.9
hepatolenticular E83.01
heredodegenerative NEC
spinal cord G95.89
herpesviral, disseminated B00.7
Hers' (glycogenosis VI) E74.09
Herter (-Gee) (-Heubner) (nontropical sprue) K90.0
Heubner-Herter (nontropical sprue) K90.0
high fetal gene or hemoglobin thalassemia D56.9
Hildenbrand's — *see* Typhus
hip (joint) M25.9
congenital Q65.89
suppurative M00.9
tuberculous A18.02
His (-Werner) (trench fever) A79.0
Hodgson's I71.2
ruptured I71.1
Holla — *see* Spherocytosis
hookworm B76.9
specified NEC B76.8
host-versus-graft D89.813
acute D89.810
acute on chronic D89.812
chronic D89.811
human immunodeficiency virus (HIV) B20
Huntington's G10
with dementia G10 *[F02.80]*
Hutchinson's (cheiropompholyx) — *see* Hutchinson's disease
hyaline (diffuse) (generalized)
membrane (lung) (newborn) P22.0
adult J80
hydatid — *see* Echinococcus
hydroxyapatite deposition M11.00
ankle M11.07-
elbow M11.02-
foot joint M11.07-
hand joint M11.04-
hip M11.05-
knee M11.06-
multiple site M11.09
shoulder M11.01-
vertebra M11.08
wrist M11.03-
hyperkinetic — *see* Hyperkinesia
hypertensive — *see* Hypertension
hypophysis E23.7
Iceland G93.3
I-cell E77.0
immune D89.9
immunoproliferative (malignant) C88.9
small intestinal C88.3
specified NEC C88.8
inclusion B25.9
salivary gland B25.9
infectious, infective B99.9
congenital P37.9
specified NEC P37.8
viral P35.9
specified type NEC P35.8
specified NEC B99.8
inflammatory
penis N48.29
abscess N48.21
cellulitis N48.22
prepuce N47.7
balanoposthitis N47.6
tubo-ovarian — *see* Salpingo-oophoritis
intervertebral disc — *see also* Disorder, disc
with myelopathy — *see* Disorder, disc, with, myelopathy

Disease, diseased - *continued*
intervertebral disc - *continued*
cervical, cervicothoracic — *see* Disorder, disc, cervical
with
myelopathy — *see* Disorder, disc, cervical, with myelopathy
neuritis, radiculitis or radiculopathy — *see* Disorder, disc, cervical, with neuritis
specified NEC — *see* Disorder, disc, cervical, specified type NEC
lumbar (with)
myelopathy M51.06
neuritis, radiculitis, radiculopathy or sciatica M51.16
specified NEC M51.86
lumbosacral (with)
neuritis, radiculitis, radiculopathy or sciatica M51.17
specified NEC M51.87
specified NEC — *see* Disorder, disc, specified NEC
thoracic (with)
myelopathy M51.04
neuritis, radiculitis or radiculopathy M51.14
specified NEC M51.84
thoracolumbar (with)
myelopathy M51.05
neuritis, radiculitis or radiculopathy M51.15
specified NEC M51.85
intestine K63.9
functional K59.9
psychogenic F45.8
specified NEC K59.8
organic K63.9
protozoal A07.9
specified NEC K63.89
iris H21.9
specified NEC H21.89
iron metabolism or storage E83.10
island (scrub typhus) A75.3
itai-itai — *see* Poisoning, cadmium
Jakob-Creutzfeldt — *see* Creutzfeldt-Jakob disease or syndrome
jaw M27.9
fibrocystic M27.49
specified NEC M27.8
jigger B88.1
joint — *see also* Disorder, joint
Charcot's — *see* Arthropathy, neuropathic (Charcot)
degenerative — *see* Osteoarthritis
multiple M15.9
spine — *see* Spondylosis
hypertrophic — *see* Osteoarthritis
sacroiliac M53.3
specified NEC — *see* Disorder, joint, specified type NEC
spine NEC — *see* Dorsopathy
suppurative — *see* Arthritis, pyogenic or pyemic
Jourdain's (acute gingivitis) K05.00
nonplaque induced K05.01
plaque induced K05.00
Kaschin-Beck (endemic polyarthritis) M12.10
ankle M12.17-
elbow M12.12-
foot joint M12.17-
hand joint M12.14-
hip M12.15-
knee M12.16-
multiple site M12.19
shoulder M12.11-
vertebra M12.18
wrist M12.13-
Katayama B65.2
Kedani (scrub typhus) A75.3
Keshan E59
kidney (functional) (pelvis) N28.9
chronic N18.9
hypertensive — *see* Hypertension, kidney
stage 1 N18.1
stage 2 (mild) N18.2
stage 3 (moderate) N18.3
stage 4 (severe) N18.4
stage 5 N18.5
complicating pregnancy — *see* Pregnancy, complicated by, renal disease
cystic (congenital) Q61.9
diabetic — *see* E08-E13 with .22
fibrocystic (congenital) Q61.8
hypertensive — *see* Hypertension, kidney
in (due to)
schistosomiasis (bilharziasis) B65.9 *[N29]*

Disease, diseased - *continued*
kidney (functional) (pelvis) - *continued*
multicystic Q61.4
polycystic Q61.3
adult type Q61.2
childhood type NEC Q61.19
collecting duct dilatation Q61.11
Kimmelstiel (-Wilson) (intercapillary polycystic (congenital) glomerulosclerosis) — *see* E08-E13 with .21
Kimura D21.9
specified site (see Neoplasm, connective tissue benign)
Kinnier Wilson's (hepatolenticular degeneration) E83.01
kissing — *see* Mononucleosis, infectious
Klebs' — *see also* Glomerulonephritis N05.-
Klippel-Feil (brevicollis) Q76.1
Köhler-Pellegrini-Stieda (calcification, knee joint) — *see* Bursitis, tibial collateral
Kok Q89.8
König's (osteochondritis dissecans) — *see* Osteochondritis, dissecans
Korsakoff's (nonalcoholic) F04
alcoholic F10.96
with dependence F10.26
Kostmann's (infantile genetic agranulocytosis) D70.0
kuru A81.81
Kyasanur Forest A98.2
labyrinth, ear — *see* Disorder, ear, inner
lacrimal system — *see* Disorder, lacrimal system
Lafora's — *see* Epilepsy, generalized, idiopathic
Lancereaux-Mathieu (leptospiral jaundice) A27.0
Landry's G61.0
Larrey-Weil (leptospiral jaundice) A27.0
larynx J38.7
legionnaires' A48.1
nonpneumonic A48.2
Lenegre's I44.2
lens H27.9
specified NEC H27.8
Lev's (acquired complete heart block) I44.2
Lewy body (dementia) G31.83 *[F02.80]*
with behavioral disturbance G31.83 *[F02.81]*
Lichtheim's (subacute combined sclerosis with pernicious anemia) D51.0
Lightwood's (renal tubular acidosis) N25.89
Lignac's (cystinosis) E72.04
lip K13.0
lipid-storage E75.6
specified NEC E75.5
Lipschütz's N76.6
liver (chronic) (organic) K76.9
alcoholic (chronic) K70.9
acute — *see* Disease, liver, alcoholic, hepatitis
cirrhosis K70.30
with ascites K70.31
failure K70.40
with coma K70.41
fatty liver K70.0
fibrosis K70.2
hepatitis K70.10
with ascites K70.11
sclerosis K70.2
cystic, congenital Q44.6
drug-induced (idiosyncratic) (toxic) (predictable) (unpredictable) — *see* Disease, liver, toxic
end stage K72.90
due to hepatitis — *see* Hepatitis
fatty, nonalcoholic (NAFLD) K76.0
alcoholic K70.0
fibrocystic (congenital) Q44.6
fluke
Chinese B66.1
oriental B66.1
sheep B66.3
gestational alloimmune (GALD) P78.84
glycogen storage E74.09 *[K77]*
in (due to)
schistosomiasis (bilharziasis) B65.9 *[K77]*
inflammatory K75.9
alcoholic K70.1
specified NEC K75.89
polycystic (congenital) Q44.6
toxic K71.9
with
cholestasis K71.0
cirrhosis (liver) K71.7
fibrosis (liver) K71.7
focal nodular hyperplasia K71.8
hepatic granuloma K71.8
hepatic necrosis K71.10

Disease, diseased - *continued*
liver (chronic) (organic) - *continued*
toxic - *continued*
with - *continued*
hepatic necrosis - *continued*
with coma K71.11
hepatitis NEC K71.6
acute K71.2
chronic
active K71.50
with ascites K71.51
lobular K71.4
persistent K71.3
lupoid K71.50
with ascites K71.51
peliosis hepatis K71.8
veno-occlusive disease (VOD) of liver K71.8
veno-occlusive K76.5
Lobo's (keloid blastomycosis) B48.0
Lobstein's (brittle bones and blue sclera) Q78.0
Ludwig's (submaxillary cellulitis) K12.2
lumbosacral region M53.87
lung J98.4
black J60
congenital Q33.9
cystic J98.4
congenital Q33.0
fibroid (chronic) — *see* Fibrosis, lung
fluke B66.4
oriental B66.4
in
amyloidosis E85.4 *[J99]*
sarcoidosis D86.0
Sjögren's syndrome M35.02
systemic
lupus erythematosus M32.13
sclerosis M34.81
interstitial J84.9
of childhood, specified NEC J84.848
respiratory bronchiolitis J84.115
specified NEC J84.89
obstructive (chronic) J44.9
with
acute
bronchitis J44.0
exacerbation NEC J44.1
lower respiratory infection J44.0
alveolitis, allergic J67.9
asthma J44.9
bronchiectasis J47.9
with
exacerbation (acute) J47.1
lower respiratory infection J47.0
bronchitis J44.9
with
exacerbation (acute) J44.1
lower respiratory infection J44.0
emphysema J43.9
hypersensitivity pneumonitis J67.9
decompensated J44.1
with
exacerbation (acute) J44.1
polycystic J98.4
congenital Q33.0
rheumatoid (diffuse) (interstitial) — *see* Rheumatoid, lung
Lutembacher's (atrial septal defect with mitral stenosis) Q21.1
Lyme A69.20
lymphatic (gland) (system) (channel) (vessel) I89.9
lymphoproliferative D47.9
specified NEC D47.Z9
T-gamma D47.Z9
X-linked D82.3
Magitot's M27.2
malarial — *see* Malaria
malignant — *see also* Neoplasm, malignant, by site
Manson's B65.1
maple bark J67.6
maple-syrup-urine E71.0
Marburg (virus) A98.3
Marion's (bladder neck obstruction) N32.0
Marsh's (exophthalmic goiter) — *see* Hyperthyroidism, with, goiter (diffuse)
mastoid (process) — *see* Disorder, ear, middle
Mathieu's (leptospiral jaundice) A27.0
Maxcy's A75.2
McArdle (-Schmid-Pearson) (glycogenosis V) E74.04
mediastinum J98.59
medullary center (idiopathic) (respiratory) G93.89
Meige's (chronic hereditary edema) Q82.0
meningococcal — *see* Infection, meningococcal

Disease, diseased - *continued*
mental F99
organic F09
mesenchymal M35.9
mesenteric embolic — *see also* Ischemia, intestine, acute K55.039
metabolic, metabolism E88.9
bilirubin E80.7
metal-polisher's J62.8
metastatic — *see also* Neoplasm, secondary, by site C79.9
microvascular - code to condition
microvillus
atrophy Q43.8
inclusion (MVD) Q43.8
middle ear — *see* Disorder, ear, middle
Mikulicz' (dryness of mouth, absent or decreased lacrimation) K11.8
Milroy's (chronic hereditary edema) Q82.0
Minamata — *see* Poisoning, mercury
minicore G71.2
Minor's G95.19
Minot's (hemorrhagic disease, newborn) P53
Minot-von Willebrand-Jürgens (angiohemophilia) D68.0
Mitchell's (erythromelalgia) I73.81
mitral (valve) I05.9
nonrheumatic I34.9
mixed connective tissue M35.1
moldy hay J67.0
Monge's T70.29
Morgagni-Adams-Stokes (syncope with heart block) I45.9
Morgagni's (syndrome) (hyperostosis frontalis interna) M85.2
Morton's (with metatarsalgia) — *see* Lesion, nerve, plantar
Morvan's G60.8
motor neuron (bulbar) (mixed type) (spinal) G12.20
amyotrophic lateral sclerosis G12.21
familial G12.24
progressive bulbar palsy G12.22
specified NEC G12.29
moyamoya I67.5
mu heavy chain disease C88.2
multicore G71.2
muscle — *see also* Disorder, muscle
inflammatory — *see* Myositis
ocular (external) — *see* Strabismus
musculoskeletal system, soft tissue — *see* also Disorder, soft tissue
specified NEC — *see* Disorder, soft tissue, specified type NEC
mushroom workers' J67.5
mycotic B49
myelodysplastic, not classified C94.6
myeloproliferative, not classified C94.6
chronic D47.1
myocardium, myocardial — *see also* Degeneration, myocardial I51.5
primary (idiopathic) I42.9
myoneural G70.9
Naegeli's D69.1
nails L60.9
specified NEC L60.8
Nairobi (sheep virus) A93.8
nasal J34.9
nemaline body G71.2
nerve — *see* Disorder, nerve
nervous system G98.8
autonomic G90.9
central G96.9
specified NEC G96.8
congenital Q07.9
parasympathetic G90.9
specified NEC G98.8
sympathetic G90.9
vegetative G90.9
neuromuscular system G70.9
Newcastle B30.8
Nicolas (-Durand) -Favre (climatic bubo) A55
nipple N64.9
Paget's C50.01-
female C50.01-
male C50.02-
Nishimoto (-Takeuchi) I67.5
nonarthropod-borne NOS (viral) B34.9
enterovirus NEC B34.1
nonautoimmune hemolytic D59.4
drug-induced D59.2
Nonne-Milroy-Meige (chronic hereditary edema) Q82.0
nose J34.9

Disease, diseased - *continued*
nucleus pulposus — *see* Disorder, disc
nutritional E63.9
oast-house-urine E72.19
ocular
herpesviral B00.50
zoster B02.30
obliterative vascular I77.1
Ohara's — *see* Tularemia
Opitz's (congestive splenomegaly) D73.2
Oppenheim-Urbach (necrobiosis lipoidica diabeticorum) — *see* E08-E13 with .620
optic nerve NEC — *see* Disorder, nerve, optic
orbit — *see* Disorder, orbit
Oriental liver fluke B66.1
Oriental lung fluke B66.4
Ormond's N13.5
Oropouche virus A93.0
Osler-Rendu (familial hemorrhagic telangiectasia) I78.0
osteofibrocystic E21.0
Otto's M24.7
outer ear — *see* Disorder, ear, external
ovary (noninflammatory) N83.9
cystic N83.20-
inflammatory — *see* Salpingo-oophoritis
polycystic E28.2
specified NEC N83.8
Owren's (congenital) — *see* Defect, coagulation
pancreas K86.9
cystic K86.2
fibrocystic E84.9
specified NEC K86.89
panvalvular I08.9
specified NEC I08.8
parametrium (noninflammatory) N83.9
parasitic B89
cerebral NEC B71.9 *[G94]*
intestinal NOS B82.9
mouth B37.0
skin NOS B88.9
specified type — *see* Infestation
tongue B37.0
parathyroid (gland) E21.5
specified NEC E21.4
Parkinson's G20
parodontal K05.6
Parrot's (syphilitic osteochondritis) A50.02
Parry's (exophthalmic goiter) — *see* Hyperthyroidism, with, goiter (diffuse)
Parson's (exophthalmic goiter) — *see* Hyperthyroidism, with, goiter (diffuse)
Paxton's (white piedra) B36.2
pearl-worker's — *see* Osteomyelitis, specified type NEC
Pellegrini-Stieda (calcification, knee joint) — *see* Bursitis, tibial collateral
pelvis, pelvic
female NOS N94.9
specified NEC N94.89
gonococcal (acute) (chronic) A54.24
inflammatory (female) N73.9
acute N73.0
chlamydial A56.11
chronic N73.1
specified NEC N73.8
syphilitic (secondary) A51.42
late A52.76
tuberculous A18.17
organ, female N94.9
peritoneum, female NEC N94.89
penis N48.9
inflammatory N48.29
abscess N48.21
cellulitis N48.22
specified NEC N48.89
periapical tissues NOS K04.90
periodontal K05.6
specified NEC K05.5
periosteum — *see* Disorder, bone, specified type NEC
peripheral
arterial I73.9
autonomic nervous system G90.9
nerves — *see* Polyneuropathy
vascular NOS I73.9
peritoneum K66.9
pelvic, female NEC N94.89
specified NEC K66.8
persistent mucosal (middle ear) H66.20
left H66.22
with right H66.23
right H66.21

Disease, diseased - *continued*
persistent mucosal (middle ear) - *continued*
right - *continued*
with left H66.23
Petit's — *see* Hernia, abdomen, specified site NEC
pharynx J39.2
specified NEC J39.2
Phocas' — *see* Mastopathy, cystic
photochromogenic (acid-fast bacilli) (pulmonary) A31.0
nonpulmonary A31.9
Pick's G31.01 *[F02.80]*
with behavioral disturbance G31.01 *[F02.81]*
brain G31.01 *[F02.80]*
with behavioral disturbance G31.01 *[F02.81]*
of pericardium (pericardial pseudocirrhosis of liver) I31.1
pigeon fancier's J67.2
pineal gland E34.8
pink — *see* Poisoning, mercury
Pinkus' (lichen nitidus) L44.1
pinworm B80
Piry virus A93.8
pituitary (gland) E23.7
pituitary-snuff-taker's J67.8
pleura (cavity) J94.9
specified NEC J94.8
pneumatic drill (hammer) T75.21
Pollitzer's (hidradenitis suppurativa) L73.2
polycystic
kidney or renal Q61.3
adult type Q61.2
childhood type NEC Q61.19
collecting duct dilatation Q61.11
liver or hepatic Q44.6
lung or pulmonary J98.4
congenital Q33.0
ovary, ovaries E28.2
spleen Q89.09
polyethylene T84.05-
Pompe's (glycogenosis II) E74.02
Posadas-Wernicke B38.9
Potain's (pulmonary edema) — *see* Edema, lung
prepuce N47.8
inflammatory N47.7
balanoposthitis N47.6
Pringle's (tuberous sclerosis) Q85.1
prion, central nervous system A81.9
specified NEC A81.89
prostate N42.9
specified NEC N42.89
protozoal B64
acanthamebiasis — *see* Acanthamebiasis
African trypanosomiasis — *see* African trypanosomiasis
babesiosis B60.0
Chagas disease — *see* Chagas disease
intestine, intestinal A07.9
leishmaniasis — *see* Leishmaniasis
malaria — *see* Malaria
naegleriasis B60.2
pneumocystosis B59
specified organism NEC B60.8
toxoplasmosis — *see* Toxoplasmosis
pseudo-Hurler's E77.0
psychiatric F99
psychotic — *see* Psychosis
Puente's (simple glandular cheilitis) K13.0
puerperal — *see also* Puerperal O90.89
pulmonary — *see also* Disease, lung
artery I28.9
chronic obstructive J44.9
with
acute bronchitis J44.0
exacerbation (acute) J44.1
lower respiratory infection (acute) J44.0
decompensated J44.1
with
exacerbation (acute) J44.1
heart I27.9
specified NEC I27.89
hypertensive (vascular) — *see also* Hypertension, pulmonary I27.20
primary (idiopathic) I27.0
valve I37.9
rheumatic I09.89
pulp (dental) NOS K04.90
pulseless M31.4
Putnam's (subacute combined sclerosis with pernicious anemia) D51.0
Pyle (-Cohn) (metaphyseal dysplasia) Q78.5
ragpicker's or ragsorter's A22.1
Raynaud's — *see* Raynaud's disease

Disease, diseased - *continued*
reactive airway — *see* Asthma
Reclus' (cystic) — *see* Mastopathy, cystic
rectum K62.9
specified NEC K62.89
Refsum's (heredopathia atactica polyneuritiformis) G60.1
renal (functional) (pelvis) — *see also* Disease, kidney N28.9
with
edema — *see* Nephrosis
glomerular lesion — *see* Glomerulonephritis
with edema — *see* Nephrosis
interstitial nephritis N12
acute N28.9
chronic — *see also* Disease, kidney, chronic N18.9
cystic, congenital Q61.9
diabetic — *see* E08-E13 with .22
end-stage (failure) N18.6
due to hypertension I12.0
fibrocystic (congenital) Q61.8
hypertensive — *see* Hypertension, kidney
lupus M32.14
phosphate-losing (tubular) N25.0
polycystic (congenital) Q61.3
adult type Q61.2
childhood type NEC Q61.19
collecting duct dilatation Q61.11
rapidly progressive N01.9
subacute N01.9
Rendu-Osler-Weber (familial hemorrhagic telangiectasia) I78.0
renovascular (arteriosclerotic) — *see* Hypertension, kidney
respiratory (tract) J98.9
acute or subacute NOS J06.9
due to
chemicals, gases, fumes or vapors (inhalation) J68.3
external agent J70.9
specified NEC J70.8
radiation J70.0
smoke inhalation J70.5
noninfectious J39.8
chronic NOS J98.9
due to
chemicals, gases, fumes or vapors J68.4
external agent J70.9
specified NEC J70.8
radiation J70.1
newborn P27.9
specified NEC P27.8
due to
chemicals, gases, fumes or vapors J68.9
acute or subacute NEC J68.3
chronic J68.4
external agent J70.9
specified NEC J70.8
newborn P28.9
specified type NEC P28.89
upper J39.9
acute or subacute J06.9
noninfectious NEC J39.8
specified NEC J39.8
streptococcal J06.9
retina, retinal H35.9
Batten's or Batten-Mayou E75.4 *[H36]*
specified NEC H35.89
rheumatoid — *see* Arthritis, rheumatoid
rickettsial NOS A79.9
specified type NEC A79.89
Riga (-Fede) (cachectic aphthae) K14.0
Riggs' (compound periodontitis) — *see* Periodontitis
Ritter's L00
Rivalta's (cervicofacial actinomycosis) A42.2
Robles' (onchocerciasis) B73.01
Roger's (congenital interventricular septal defect) Q21.0
Rosenthal's (factor XI deficiency) D68.1
Rossbach's (hyperchlorhydria) K30
Ross River B33.1
Rotes Quérol — *see* Hyperostosis, ankylosing
Roth (-Bernhardt) — *see* Mononeuropathy, lower limb, meralgia paresthetica
Runeberg's (progressive pernicious anemia) D51.0
sacroiliac NEC M53.3
salivary gland or duct K11.9
inclusion B25.9
specified NEC K11.8
virus B25.9
sandworm B76.9
Schimmelbusch's — *see* Mastopathy, cystic
Schmorl's — *see* Schmorl's disease or nodes

Disease, diseased - *continued*
Schönlein (-Henoch) (purpura rheumatica) D69.0
Schottmüller's — *see* Fever, paratyphoid
Schultz's (agranulocytosis) — *see* Agranulocytosis
Schwalbe-Ziehen-Oppenheim G24.1
Schwartz-Jampel G71.13
sclera H15.9
specified NEC H15.89
scrofulous (tuberculous) A18.2
scrotum N50.9
sebaceous glands L73.9
semilunar cartilage, cystic — *see also* Derangement, knee, meniscus, cystic
seminal vesicle N50.9
serum NEC — *see also* Reaction, serum T80.69
sexually transmitted A64
anogenital
herpesviral infection — *see* Herpes, anogenital
warts A63.0
chancroid A57
chlamydial infection — *see* Chlamydia
gonorrhea — *see* Gonorrhea
granuloma inguinale A58
specified organism NEC A63.8
syphilis — *see* Syphilis
trichomoniasis — *see* Trichomoniasis
Sézary C84.1-
shimamushi (scrub typhus) A75.3
shipyard B30.0
sickle-cell D57.1
with crisis (vasoocclusive pain) D57.00
with
acute chest syndrome D57.01
splenic sequestration D57.02
elliptocytosis D57.8-
Hb-C D57.20
with crisis (vasoocclusive pain) D57.219
with
acute chest syndrome D57.211
splenic sequestration D57.212
without crisis D57.20
Hb-SD D57.80
with crisis D57.819
with
acute chest syndrome D57.811
splenic sequestration D57.812
Hb-SE D57.80
with crisis D57.819
with
acute chest syndrome D57.811
splenic sequestration D57.812
specified NEC D57.80
with crisis D57.819
with
acute chest syndrome D57.811
splenic sequestration D57.812
spherocytosis D57.80
with crisis D57.819
with
acute chest syndrome D57.811
splenic sequestration D57.812
thalassemia D57.40
with crisis (vasoocclusive pain) D57.419
with
acute chest syndrome D57.411
splenic sequestration D57.412
without crisis D57.40
silo-filler's J68.8
bronchitis J68.0
pneumonitis J68.0
pulmonary edema J68.1
simian B B00.4
Simons' (progressive lipodystrophy) E88.1
sin nombre virus B33.4
sinus — *see* Sinusitis
Sirkari's B55.0
sixth B08.20
due to human herpesvirus 6 B08.21
due to human herpesvirus 7 B08.22
skin L98.9
due to metabolic disorder NEC E88.9 *[L99]*
specified NEC L98.8
slim (HIV) B20
small vessel I73.9
Sneddon-Wilkinson (subcorneal pustular dermatosis) L13.1
South African creeping B88.0
spinal (cord) G95.9
congenital Q06.9
specified NEC G95.89
spine — *see also* Spondylopathy
joint — *see* Dorsopathy
tuberculous A18.01

Dislocation (articular) - *continued*
- fibula
  - distal end — *see* Dislocation, ankle
  - proximal end — *see* Dislocation, knee
- finger S63.25-
  - index S63.25-
  - interphalangeal S63.27-
    - distal S63.29-
      - index S63.29-
      - little S63.29-
      - middle S63.29-
      - ring S63.29-
    - index S63.27-
    - little S63.27-
    - middle S63.27-
    - proximal S63.28-
      - index S63.28-
      - little S63.28-
      - middle S63.28-
      - ring S63.28-
    - ring S63.27-
  - little S63.25-
  - metacarpophalangeal S63.26-
    - index S63.26-
    - little S63.26-
    - middle S63.26-
    - ring S63.26-
  - middle S63.25-
  - recurrent — *see* Dislocation, recurrent, finger
  - ring S63.25-
  - thumb — *see* Dislocation, thumb
- foot S93.30-
  - recurrent — *see* Dislocation, recurrent, foot
  - specified site NEC S93.33-
  - tarsal joint S93.31-
  - tarsometatarsal joint S93.32-
  - toe — *see* Dislocation, toe
- fracture — *see* Fracture
- glenohumeral (joint) — *see* Dislocation, shoulder
- glenoid — *see* Dislocation, shoulder
- habitual — *see* Dislocation, recurrent
- hip S73.00-
  - anterior S73.03-
    - obturator S73.02-
  - central S73.04-
  - congenital (total) Q65.2
    - bilateral Q65.1
    - partial Q65.5
      - bilateral Q65.4
      - unilateral Q65.3-
    - unilateral Q65.0-
  - developmental M24.85-
  - pathological — *see* Dislocation, pathological NEC, hip
  - posterior S73.01-
  - recurrent — *see* Dislocation, recurrent, hip
- humerus, proximal end — *see* Dislocation, shoulder
- incomplete — *see* Subluxation, by site
- incus — *see* Discontinuity, ossicles, ear
- infracoracoid — *see* Dislocation, shoulder
- innominate (pubic junction) (sacral junction) S33.39
  - acetabulum — *see* Dislocation, hip
- interphalangeal (joint (s))
  - finger S63.279
    - distal S63.29-
      - index S63.29-
      - little S63.29-
      - middle S63.29-
      - ring S63.29-
    - index S63.27-
    - little S63.27-
    - middle S63.27-
    - proximal S63.28-
      - index S63.28-
      - little S63.28-
      - middle S63.28-
      - ring S63.28-
    - ring S63.27-
  - foot or toe — *see* Dislocation, toe
  - thumb S63.12-
- jaw (cartilage) (meniscus) S03.0-
- joint prosthesis — *see* Complications, joint prosthesis, mechanical, displacement, by site
- knee S83.106
  - cap — *see* Dislocation, patella
  - congenital Q68.2
  - old M23.8X-
  - patella — *see* Dislocation, patella
  - pathological — *see* Dislocation, pathological NEC, knee
  - proximal tibia
    - anteriorly S83.11-
    - laterally S83.14-

Dislocation (articular) - *continued*
- knee - *continued*
  - proximal tibia - *continued*
    - medially S83.13-
    - posteriorly S83.12-
  - recurrent — *see also* Derangement, knee, specified NEC
  - specified type NEC S83.19-
- lacrimal gland H04.16-
- lens (complete) H27.10
  - anterior H27.12-
  - congenital Q12.1
  - ocular implant — *see* Complications, intraocular lens
  - partial H27.11-
  - posterior H27.13-
  - traumatic S05.8X-
- ligament - code by site under Dislocation
- lumbar (vertebra) — *see* Dislocation, vertebra, lumbar
- lumbosacral (vertebra) — *see also* Dislocation, vertebra, lumbar
  - congenital Q76.49
- mandible S03.0-
- meniscus (knee) — *see* Tear, meniscus
  - other sites - code by site under Dislocation
- metacarpal (bone)
  - distal end — *see* Dislocation, finger
  - proximal end S63.06-
- metacarpophalangeal (joint)
  - finger S63.26-
    - index S63.26-
    - little S63.26-
    - middle S63.26-
    - ring S63.26-
  - thumb S63.11-
- metatarsal (bone) — *see* Dislocation, foot
- metatarsophalangeal (joint (s)) — *see* Dislocation, toe
- midcarpal (joint) S63.03-
- midtarsal (joint) — *see* Dislocation, foot
- neck S13.20
  - specified site NEC S13.29
  - vertebra — *see* Dislocation, vertebra, cervical
- nose (septal cartilage) S03.1
- occipitoatloid S13.111
- old — *see* Derangement, joint, specified type NEC
- ossicles, ear — *see* Discontinuity, ossicles, ear
- partial — *see* Subluxation, by site
- patella S83.006
  - congenital Q74.1
  - lateral S83.01-
  - recurrent (nontraumatic) M22.0-
    - incomplete M22.1-
  - specified type NEC S83.09-
- pathological NEC M24.30
  - ankle M24.37-
  - elbow M24.32-
  - foot joint M24.37-
  - hand joint M24.34-
  - hip M24.35-
  - knee M24.36-
  - lumbosacral joint — *see* subcategory M53.2
  - pelvic region — *see* Dislocation, pathological, hip
  - sacroiliac — *see* subcategory M53.2
  - shoulder M24.31-
  - wrist M24.33-
- pelvis NEC S33.30
  - specified NEC S33.39
- phalanx
  - finger or hand — *see* Dislocation, finger
  - foot or toe — *see* Dislocation, toe
- prosthesis, internal — *see* Complications, prosthetic device, by site, mechanical
- radial head S53.006
  - anterior S53.01-
  - posterior S53.02-
  - specified type NEC S53.09-
- radiocarpal (joint) S63.02-
- radiohumeral (joint) — *see* Dislocation, radial head
- radioulnar (joint)
  - distal S63.01-
  - proximal — *see* Dislocation, elbow
- radius
  - distal end — *see* Dislocation, wrist
  - proximal end — *see* Dislocation, radial head
- recurrent M24.40
  - ankle M24.47-
  - elbow M24.42-
  - finger M24.44-
  - foot joint M24.47-
  - hand joint M24.44-
  - hip M24.45-

Dislocation (articular) - *continued*
- recurrent - *continued*
  - knee M24.46-
    - patella — *see* Dislocation, patella, recurrent
  - patella — *see* Dislocation, patella, recurrent
  - sacroiliac — *see* subcategory M53.2
  - shoulder M24.41-
  - toe M24.47-
  - vertebra (*see also* subcategory M43.5)
    - atlantoaxial M43.4
      - with myelopathy M43.3
  - wrist M24.43-
- rib (cartilage) S23.29
- sacrococcygeal S33.2
- sacroiliac (joint) (ligament) S33.2
  - congenital Q74.2
  - recurrent — *see* subcategory M53.2
- sacrum S33.2
- scaphoid (bone) (hand) (wrist) — *see* Dislocation, wrist
  - foot — *see* Dislocation, foot
- scapula — *see* Dislocation, shoulder, girdle, scapula
- semilunar cartilage, knee — *see* Tear, meniscus
- septal cartilage (nose) S03.1
- septum (nasal) (old) J34.2
- sesamoid bone - code by site under Dislocation
- shoulder (blade) (ligament) (joint) (traumatic) S43.006
  - acromioclavicular — *see* Dislocation, acromioclavicular
  - chronic — *see* Dislocation, recurrent, shoulder
  - congenital Q68.8
  - girdle S43.30-
    - scapula S43.31-
    - specified site NEC S43.39-
  - humerus S43.00-
    - anterior S43.01-
    - inferior S43.03-
    - posterior S43.02-
  - pathological — *see* Dislocation, pathological NEC, shoulder
  - recurrent — *see* Dislocation, recurrent, shoulder
  - specified type NEC S43.08-
- spine
  - cervical — *see* Dislocation, vertebra, cervical
  - congenital Q76.49
  - due to birth trauma P11.5
  - lumbar — *see* Dislocation, vertebra, lumbar
  - thoracic — *see* Dislocation, vertebra, thoracic
- spontaneous — *see* Dislocation, pathological
- sternoclavicular (joint) S43.206
  - anterior S43.21-
  - posterior S43.22-
- sternum S23.29
- subglenoid — *see* Dislocation, shoulder
- symphysis pubis S33.4
- talus — *see* Dislocation, ankle
- tarsal (bone (s)) (joint (s)) — *see* Dislocation, foot
- tarsometatarsal (joint (s)) — *see* Dislocation, foot
- temporomandibular (joint) S03.0-
- thigh, proximal end — *see* Dislocation, hip
- thorax S23.20
  - specified site NEC S23.29
  - vertebra — *see* Dislocation, vertebra
- thumb S63.10-
  - interphalangeal joint — *see* Dislocation, interphalangeal (joint), thumb
  - metacarpophalangeal joint — *see* Dislocation, metacarpophalangeal (joint), thumb
- thyroid cartilage S13.29
- tibia
  - distal end — *see* Dislocation, ankle
  - proximal end — *see* Dislocation, knee
- tibiofibular (joint)
  - distal — *see* Dislocation, ankle
  - superior — *see* Dislocation, knee
- toe (s) S93.106
  - great S93.10-
    - interphalangeal joint S93.11-
    - metatarsophalangeal joint S93.12-
  - interphalangeal joint S93.119
  - lesser S93.106
    - interphalangeal joint S93.11-
    - metatarsophalangeal joint S93.12-
  - metatarsophalangeal joint S93.12-
- tooth S03.2
- trachea S23.29
- ulna
  - distal end S63.07-
  - proximal end — *see* Dislocation, elbow
- ulnohumeral (joint) — *see* Dislocation, elbow
- vertebra (articular process) (body) (traumatic)
  - cervical S13.101

Dislocation (articular) - *continued*
vertebra (articular process) (body) (traumatic) - *continued*
cervical - *continued*
atlantoaxial joint S13.121
atlantooccipital joint S13.111
atloidooccipital joint S13.111
joint between
C0 and C1 S13.111
C1 and C2 S13.121
C2 and C3 S13.131
C3 and C4 S13.141
C4 and C5 S13.151
C5and C6 S13.161
C6and C7 S13.171
C7and T1 S13.181
occipitoatloid joint S13.111
congenital Q76.49
lumbar S33.101
joint between
L1and L2 S33.111
L2and L3 S33.121
L3 and L4 S33.131
L4and L5 S33.141
nontraumatic — *see* Displacement, intervertebral disc
partial — *see* Subluxation, by site
recurrent NEC — *see* subcategory M43.5
thoracic S23.101
joint between
T1 and T2 S23.111
T2 and T3 S23.121
T3 and T4 S23.123
T4 and T5 S23.131
T5 and T6 S23.133
T6 and T7 S23.141
T7 and T8 S23.143
T8 and T9 S23.151
T9 and T10 S23.153
T10 and T11 S23.161
T11 and T12 S23.163
T12 and L1 S23.171
wrist (carpal bone) S63.006
carpometacarpal joint — *see* Dislocation, carpometacarpal (joint)
distal radioulnar joint — *see* Dislocation, radioulnar (joint), distal
metacarpal bone, proximal — *see* Dislocation, metacarpal (bone), proximal end
midcarpal — *see* Dislocation, midcarpal (joint)
radiocarpal joint — *see* Dislocation, radiocarpal (joint)
recurrent — *see* Dislocation, recurrent, wrist
specified site NEC S63.09-
ulna — *see* Dislocation, ulna, distal end
xiphoid cartilage S23.29
Disorder (of) — *see also* Disease
acantholytic L11.9
specified NEC L11.8
acute
psychotic — *see* Psychosis, acute
stress F43.0
adjustment (grief) F43.20
with
anxiety F43.22
with depressed mood F43.23
conduct disturbance F43.24
with emotional disturbance F43.25
depressed mood F43.21
with anxiety F43.23
other specified symptom F43.29
adrenal (capsule) (gland) (medullary) E27.9
specified NEC E27.8
adrenogenital E25.9
drug-induced E25.8
iatrogenic E25.8
idiopathic E25.8
adult personality (and behavior) F69
specified NEC F68.8
affective (mood) — *see* Disorder, mood
aggressive, unsocialized F91.1
alcohol-related F10.99
with
amnestic disorder, persisting F10.96
anxiety disorder F10.980
dementia, persisting F10.97
intoxication F10.929
with delirium F10.921
uncomplicated F10.920
mood disorder F10.94
other specified F10.988
psychotic disorder F10.959
with

Disorder (of) - *continued*
alcohol-related - *continued*
with - *continued*
psychotic disorder - *continued*
with - *continued*
delusions F10.950
hallucinations F10.951
sexual dysfunction F10.981
sleep disorder F10.982
alcohol use
mild F10.10
with
alcohol-induced
anxiety disorder F10.180
bipolar and related disorder F10.14
depressive disorder F10.14
psychotic disorder F10.159
sexual dysfunction F10.181
sleep disorder F10.182
alcohol intoxication F10.129
delirium F10.121
in remission (early) (sustained) F10.11
moderate or severe F10.20
with
alcohol-induced
anxiety disorder F10.280
bipolar and related disorder F10.24
depressive disorder F10.24
major neurocognitive disorder, amnestic-confabulatory type F10.26
major neurocognitive disorder, nonamnestic-confabulatory type F10.27
mild neurocognitive disorder F10.288
psychotic disorder F10.259
sexual dysfunction F10.281
sleep disorder F10.282
alcohol intoxication F10.229
delirium F10.221
in remission (early) (sustained) F10.21
allergic — *see* Allergy
alveolar NEC J84.09
amino-acid
cystathioninuria E72.19
cystinosis E72.04
cystinuria E72.01
glycinuria E72.09
homocystinuria E72.11
metabolism — *see* Disturbance, metabolism, amino-acid
specified NEC E72.89
neonatal, transitory P74.8
renal transport NEC E72.09
transport NEC E72.09
amnesic, amnestic
alcohol-induced F10.96
with dependence F10.26
due to (secondary to) general medical condition F04
psychoactive NEC-induced F19.96
with
abuse F19.16
dependence F19.26
sedative, hypnotic or anxiolytic-induced F13.96
with dependence F13.26
amphetamine-type substance use
mild F15.10
in remission (early) (sustained) F15.11
moderate F15.20
in remission (early) (sustained) F15.21
severe F15.20
in remission (early) (sustained) F15.21
amphetamine (or other stimulant) use
mild
with
amphetamine (or other stimulant) -induced
anxiety disorder F15.180
bipolar and related disorder F15.14
depressive disorder F15.14
obsessive-compulsive and related disorder F15.188
psychotic disorder F15.159
sexual dysfunction F15.181
amphetamine, cocaine, or other stimulant intoxication
with perceptual disturbances F15.122
without perceptual disturbances F15.129
intoxication delirium F15.121
moderate or severe
with
amphetamine (or other stimulant) -induced
anxiety disorder F15.280
obsessive-compulsive and related disorder F15.288

Disorder (of) - *continued*
amphetamine (or other stimulant) use - *continued*
moderate or severe - *continued*
with - *continued*
amphetamine (or other stimulant) -induced - *continued*
sexual dysfunction F15.281
bipolar and related disorder F15.24
depressive disorder F15.24
psychotic disorder F15.259
amphetamine, cocaine, or other stimulant intoxication
with perceptual disturbances F15.222
without perceptual disturbances F15.229
intoxication delirium F15.221
anaerobic glycolysis with anemia D55.2
anxiety F41.9
due to (secondary to)
alcohol F10.980
in
abuse F10.180
dependence F10.280
amphetamine F15.980
in
abuse F15.180
dependence F15.280
anxiolytic F13.980
in
abuse F13.180
dependence F13.280
caffeine F15.980
in
abuse F15.180
dependence F15.280
cannabis F12.980
in
abuse F12.180
dependence F12.280
cocaine F14.980
in
abuse F14.180
dependence F14.180
general medical condition F06.4
hallucinogen F16.980
in
abuse F16.180
dependence F16.280
hypnotic F13.980
in
abuse F13.180
dependence F13.280
inhalant F18.980
in
abuse F18.180
dependence F18.280
phencyclidine F16.980
in
abuse F16.180
dependence F16.280
psychoactive substance NEC F19.980
in
abuse F19.180
dependence F19.280
sedative F13.980
in
abuse F13.180
dependence F13.280
volatile solvents F18.980
in
abuse F18.180
dependence F18.280
generalized F41.1
illness F45.21
mixed
with depression (mild) F41.8
specified NEC F41.3
organic F06.4
phobic F40.9
of childhood F40.8
specified NEC F41.8
aortic valve — *see* Endocarditis, aortic
aromatic amino-acid metabolism E70.9
specified NEC E70.8
arteriole NEC I77.89
artery NEC I77.89
articulation — *see* Disorder, joint
attachment (childhood)
disinhibited F94.2
reactive F94.1
attention-deficit hyperactivity (adolescent) (adult) (child) F90.9
combined
presentation F90.2

Disorder (of) - *continued*
attention-deficit hyperactivity (adolescent) (adult) (child) - *continued*
combined - *continued*
type F90.2
hyperactive
impulsive presentation F90.1
type F90.1
inattentive
presentation F90.0
type F90.0
specified type NEC F90.8
attention-deficit without hyperactivity (adolescent) (adult) (child) F98.8
auditory processing (central) H93.25
autistic F84.0
autism spectrum F84.0
autoimmune D89.89
autonomic nervous system G90.9
specified NEC G90.8
avoidant
child or adolescent F40.10
restrictive food intake F50.82
balance
acid-base E87.8
mixed E87.4
electrolyte E87.8
fluid NEC E87.8
behavioral (disruptive) — *see* Disorder, conduct
beta-amino-acid metabolism E72.89
bile acid and cholesterol metabolism E78.70
Barth syndrome E78.71
other specified E78.79
Smith-Lemli-Opitz syndrome E78.72
bilirubin excretion E80.6
binge eating F50.81
binocular
movement H51.9
convergence
excess H51.12
insufficiency H51.11
internuclear ophthalmoplegia — *see* Ophthalmoplegia, internuclear
palsy of conjugate gaze H51.0
specified type NEC H51.8
vision NEC — *see* Disorder, vision, binocular
bipolar (I) (type 1) F31.9
and related due to a known physiological condition
with
manic features F06.33
manic- or hypomanic-like episodes F06.33
mixed features F06.34
current (or most recent) episode
depressed F31.9
with psychotic features F31.5
without psychotic features F31.30
mild F31.31
moderate F31.32
severe (without psychotic features) F31.4
with psychotic features F31.5
hypomanic F31.0
manic F31.9
with psychotic features F31.2
without psychotic features F31.10
mild F31.11
moderate F31.12
severe (without psychotic features) F31.13
with psychotic features F31.2
mixed F31.60
mild F31.61
moderate F31.62
severe (without psychotic features) F31.63
with psychotic features F31.64
severe depression (without psychotic features) F31.4
with psychotic features F31.5
in remission (currently) F31.70
in full remission
most recent episode
depressed F31.76
hypomanic F31.72
manic F31.74
mixed F31.78
in partial remission
most recent episode
depressed F31.75
hypomanic F31.71
manic F31.73
mixed F31.77
specified NEC F31.89
II (type 2) F31.81
organic F06.30
single manic episode F30.9

Disorder (of) - *continued*
bipolar (I) (type 1) - *continued*
single manic episode - *continued*
mild F30.11
moderate F30.12
severe (without psychotic symptoms) F30.13
with psychotic symptoms F30.2
bladder N32.9
functional NEC N31.9
in schistosomiasis B65.0 *[N33]*
specified NEC N32.89
bleeding D68.9
blood D75.9
in congenital early syphilis A50.09 *[D77]*
body dysmorphic F45.22
bone M89.9
continuity M84.9
specified type NEC M84.80
ankle M84.87-
fibula M84.86-
foot M84.87-
hand M84.84-
humerus M84.82-
neck M84.88
pelvis M84.859
radius M84.83-
rib M84.88
shoulder M84.81-
skull M84.88
thigh M84.85-
tibia M84.86-
ulna M84.83-
vertebra M84.88
density and structure M85.9
cyst — *see also* Cyst, bone, specified type NEC
aneurysmal — *see* Cyst, bone, aneurysmal
solitary — *see* Cyst, bone, solitary
diffuse idiopathic skeletal hyperostosis — *see* Hyperostosis, ankylosing
fibrous dysplasia (monostotic) — *see* Dysplasia, fibrous, bone
fluorosis — *see* Fluorosis, skeletal
hyperostosis of skull M85.2
osteitis condensans — *see* Osteitis, condensans
specified type NEC M85.8-
ankle M85.87-
foot M85.87-
forearm M85.83-
hand M85.84-
lower leg M85.86-
multiple sites M85.89
neck M85.88
rib M85.88
shoulder M85.81-
skull M85.88
thigh M85.85-
upper arm M85.82-
vertebra M85.88
development and growth NEC M89.20
carpus M89.24-
clavicle M89.21-
femur M89.25-
fibula M89.26-
finger M89.24-
humerus M89.22-
ilium M89.259
ischium M89.259
metacarpus M89.24-
metatarsus M89.27-
multiple sites M89.29
neck M89.28
radius M89.23-
rib M89.28
scapula M89.21-
skull M89.28
tarsus M89.27-
tibia M89.26-
toe M89.27-
ulna M89.23-
vertebra M89.28
specified type NEC M89.8X-
brachial plexus G54.0
branched-chain amino-acid metabolism E71.2
specified NEC E71.19
breast N64.9
agalactia — *see* Agalactia
associated with
lactation O92.70
specified NEC O92.79
pregnancy O92.20
specified NEC O92.29
puerperium O92.20
specified NEC O92.29

Disorder (of) - *continued*
breast - *continued*
cracked nipple — *see* Cracked nipple
galactorrhea — *see* Galactorrhea
hypogalactia O92.4
lactation disorder NEC O92.79
mastitis — *see* Mastitis
nipple infection — *see* Infection, nipple
retracted nipple — *see* Retraction, nipple
specified type NEC N64.89
Briquet's F45.0
bullous, in diseases classified elsewhere L14
caffeine use
mild
with
caffeine-induced
anxiety disorder F15.180
sleep disorder F15.182
moderate or severe
with
caffeine-induced
anxiety disorder F15.280
sleep disorder F15.282
cannabis use
mild F12.10
with
cannabis-induced
anxiety disorder F12.180
psychotic disorder F12.159
sleep disorder F12.188
cannabis intoxication delirium F12.121
with perceptual disturbances F12.122
without perceptual disturbances F12.129
in remission (early) (sustained) F12.11
moderate or severe F12.20
with
cannabis-induced
anxiety disorder F12.280
psychotic disorder F12.259
sleep disorder F12.288
cannabis intoxication
with perceptual disturbances F12.222
without perceptual disturbances F12.229
delirium F12.221
in remission (early) (sustained) F12.21
carbohydrate
absorption, intestinal NEC E74.39
metabolism (congenital) E74.9
specified NEC E74.8
cardiac, functional I51.89
carnitine metabolism E71.40
cartilage M94.9
articular NEC — *see* Derangement, joint, articular cartilage
chondrocalcinosis — *see* Chondrocalcinosis
specified type NEC M94.8X-
articular — *see* Derangement, joint, articular cartilage
multiple sites M94.8X0
catatonia (due to known physiological condition) (with another mental disorder) F06.1
catatonic
due to (secondary to) known physiological condition F06.1
organic F06.1
central auditory processing H93.25
cervical
region NEC M53.82
root (nerve) NEC G54.2
character NOS F60.9
childhood disintegrative NEC F84.3
cholesterol and bile acid metabolism E78.70
Barth syndrome E78.71
other specified E78.79
Smith-Lemli-Opitz syndrome E78.72
choroid H31.9
atrophy — *see* Atrophy, choroid
degeneration — *see* Degeneration, choroid
detachment — *see* Detachment, choroid
dystrophy — *see* Dystrophy, choroid
hemorrhage — *see* Hemorrhage, choroid
rupture — *see* Rupture, choroid
scar — *see* Scar, chorioretinal
solar retinopathy — *see* Retinopathy, solar
specified type NEC H31.8
ciliary body — *see* Disorder, iris
degeneration — *see* Degeneration, ciliary body
coagulation (factor) — *see also* Defect, coagulation D68.9
newborn, transient P61.6
cocaine use
mild F14.10
with

Disorder (of) - *continued*
cocaine use - *continued*
mild - *continued*
with - *continued*
amphetamine, cocaine, or other stimulant intoxication
with perceptual disturbances F14.122
without perceptual disturbances F14.129
cocaine-induced
anxiety disorder F14.180
bipolar and related disorder F14.14
depressive disorder F14.14
obsessive-compulsive and related disorder F14.188
psychotic disorder F14.159
sexual dysfunction F14.181
sleep disorder F14.182
cocaine intoxication delirium F14.121
in remission (early) (sustained) F14.11
moderate or severe F14.20
with
amphetamine, cocaine, or other stimulant intoxication
with perceptual disturbances F14.222
without perceptual disturbances F14.229
cocaine-induced
anxiety disorder F14.280
bipolar and related disorder F14.24
depressive disorder F14.24
obsessive-compulsive and related disorder F14.288
psychotic disorder F14.259
sexual dysfunction F14.281
sleep disorder F14.282
cocaine intoxication delirium F14.221
in remission (early) (sustained) F14.21
coccyx NEC M53.3
cognitive F09
due to (secondary to) general medical condition F09
persisting R41.89
due to
alcohol F10.97
with dependence F10.27
anxiolytics F13.97
with dependence F13.27
hypnotics F13.97
with dependence F13.27
sedatives F13.97
with dependence F13.27
specified substance NEC F19.97
with
abuse F19.17
dependence F19.27
communication F80.9
social pragmatic F80.82
conduct (childhood) F91.9
adjustment reaction — *see* Disorder, adjustment
adolescent onset type F91.2
childhood onset type F91.1
compulsive F63.9
confined to family context F91.0
depressive F91.8
group type F91.2
hyperkinetic — *see* Disorder, attention-deficit hyperactivity
oppositional defiance F91.3
socialized F91.2
solitary aggressive type F91.1
specified NEC F91.8
unsocialized (aggressive) F91.1
conduction, heart I45.9
congenital glycosylation (CDG) E74.8
conjunctiva H11.9
infection — *see* Conjunctivitis
connective tissue, localized L94.9
specified NEC L94.8
conversion (functional neurological symptom disorder)
with
abnormal movement F44.4
anesthesia or sensory loss F44.6
attacks or seizures F44.5
mixed symptoms F44.7
special sensory symptoms F44.6
speech symptoms F44.4
swallowing symptoms F44.4
weakness or paralysis F44.4
convulsive (secondary) — *see* Convulsions
cornea H18.9
deformity — *see* Deformity, cornea
degeneration — *see* Degeneration, cornea
deposits — *see* Deposit, cornea

Disorder (of) - *continued*
cornea - *continued*
due to contact lens H18.82-
specified as edema — *see* Edema, cornea
edema — *see* Edema, cornea
keratitis — *see* Keratitis
keratoconjunctivitis — *see* Keratoconjunctivitis
membrane change — *see* Change, corneal membrane
neovascularization — *see* Neovascularization, cornea
scar — *see* Opacity, cornea
specified type NEC H18.89-
ulcer — *see* Ulcer, cornea
corpus cavernosum N48.9
cranial nerve — *see* Disorder, nerve, cranial
cyclothymic F34.0
defiant oppositional F91.3
delusional (persistent) (systematized) F22
induced F24
depersonalization F48.1
depressive F32.9
due to known physiological condition
with
depressive features F06.31
major depressive-like episode F06.32
mixed features F06.34
major F32.9
with psychotic symptoms F32.3
in remission (full) F32.5
partial F32.4
recurrent F33.9
with psychotic features F33.3
single episode F32.9
mild F32.0
moderate F32.1
severe (without psychotic symptoms) F32.2
with psychotic symptoms F32.3
organic F06.31
persistent F34.1
recurrent F33.9
current episode
mild F33.0
moderate F33.1
severe (without psychotic symptoms) F33.2
with psychotic symptoms F33.3
in remission F33.40
full F33.42
partial F33.41
specified NEC F33.8
single episode — *see* Episode, depressive
specified NEC F32.89
developmental F89
arithmetical skills F81.2
coordination (motor) F82
expressive writing F81.81
language F80.9
expressive F80.1
mixed receptive and expressive F80.2
receptive type F80.2
specified NEC F80.89
learning F81.9
arithmetical F81.2
reading F81.0
mixed F88
motor coordination or function F82
pervasive F84.9
specified NEC F84.8
phonological F80.0
reading F81.0
scholastic skills — *see also* Disorder, learning
mixed F81.89
specified NEC F88
speech F80.9
articulation F80.0
specified NEC F80.89
written expression F81.81
diaphragm J98.6
digestive (system) K92.9
newborn P78.9
specified NEC P78.89
postprocedural — *see* Complication, gastrointestinal
psychogenic F45.8
disc (intervertebral) M51.9
with
myelopathy
cervical region M50.00
cervicothoracic region M50.03
high cervical region M50.01
lumbar region M51.06
mid-cervical region M50.020
sacrococcygeal region M53.3

Disorder (of) - *continued*
disc (intervertebral) - *continued*
with - *continued*
myelopathy - *continued*
thoracic region M51.04
thoracolumbar region M51.05
radiculopathy
cervical region M50.10
cervicothoracic region M50.13
high cervical region M50.11
lumbar region M51.16
lumbosacral region M51.17
mid-cervical region M50.120
sacrococcygeal region M53.3
thoracic region M51.14
thoracolumbar region M51.15
cervical M50.90
with
myelopathy M50.00
C2-C3 M50.01
C3-C4 M50.01
C4-C5 M50.021
C5-C6 M50.022
C6-C7 M50.023
C7-T1 M50.03
cervicothoracic region M50.03
high cervical region M50.01
mid-cervical region M50.020
neuritis, radiculitis or radiculopathy M50.10
C2-C3 M50.11
C3-C4 M50.11
C4-C5 M50.121
C5-C6 M50.122
C6-C7 M50.123
C7-T1 M50.13
cervicothoracic region M50.13
high cervical region M50.11
mid-cervical region M50.120
C2-C3 M50.91
C3-C4 M50.91
C4-C5 M50.921
C5-C6 M50.922
C6-C7 M50.923
C7-T1 M50.93
cervicothoracic region M50.93
degeneration M50.30
C2-C3 M50.31
C3-C4 M50.31
C4-C5 M50.321
C5-C6 M50.322
C6-C7 M50.323
C7-T1 M50.33
cervicothoracic region M50.33
high cervical region M50.31
mid-cervical region M50.320
displacement M50.20
C2-C3 M50.21
C3-C4 M50.21
C4-C5 M50.221
C5-C6 M50.222
C6-C7 M50.223
C7-T1 M50.23
cervicothoracic region M50.23
high cervical region M50.21
mid-cervical region M50.220
high cervical region M50.91
mid-cervical region M50.920
specified type NEC M50.80
C2-C3 M50.81
C3-C4 M50.81
C4-C5 M50.821
C5-C6 M50.822
C6-C7 M50.823
C7-T1 M50.83
cervicothoracic region M50.83
high cervical region M50.81
mid-cervical region M50.820
specified NEC
lumbar region M51.86
lumbosacral region M51.87
sacrococcygeal region M53.3
thoracic region M51.84
thoracolumbar region M51.85
disinhibited attachment (childhood) F94.2
disintegrative, childhood NEC F84.3
disruptive F91.9
mood dysregulation F34.81
specified NEC F91.8
disruptive behavior — *see* Disorder, conduct
dissocial personality F60.2
dissociative F44.9
affecting
motor function F44.4

Disorder (of) - *continued*
  dissociative - *continued*
    affecting - *continued*
      motor function - *continued*
        and sensation F44.7
      sensation F44.6
        and motor function F44.7
    brief reactive F43.0
    due to (secondary to) general medical condition F06.8
    mixed F44.7
    organic F06.8
    other specified NEC F44.89
  double heterozygous sickling — *see* Disease, sickle-cell
  dream anxiety F51.5
  drug induced hemorrhagic D68.32
  drug related F19.99
    abuse — *see* Abuse, drug
    dependence — *see* Dependence, drug
  dysmorphic body F45.22
  dysthymic F34.1
  ear H93.9-
    bleeding — *see* Otorrhagia
    deafness — *see* Deafness
    degenerative H93.09-
    discharge — *see* Otorrhea
    external H61.9-
      auditory canal stenosis — *see* Stenosis, external ear canal
      exostosis — *see* Exostosis, external ear canal
      impacted cerumen — *see* Impaction, cerumen
      otitis — *see* Otitis, externa
      perichondritis — *see* Perichondritis, ear
      pinna — *see* Disorder, pinna
      specified type NEC H61.89-
        in diseases classified elsewhere H62.8X-
    inner H83.9-
      vestibular dysfunction — *see* Disorder, vestibular function
    middle H74.9-
      adhesive H74.1-
      ossicle — *see* Abnormal, ear ossicles
      polyp — *see* Polyp, ear (middle)
      specified NEC, in diseases classified elsewhere H75.8-
    postprocedural — *see* Complications, ear, procedure
    specified NEC, in diseases classified elsewhere H94.8-
  eating (adult) (psychogenic) F50.9
    anorexia — *see* Anorexia
    binge F50.81
    bulimia F50.2
    child F98.29
      pica F98.3
      rumination disorder F98.21
    pica F50.89
      childhood F98.3
  electrolyte (balance) NEC E87.8
    with
      abortion — *see* Abortion by type complicated by specified condition NEC
      ectopic pregnancy O08.5
      molar pregnancy O08.5
    acidosis (metabolic) (respiratory) E87.2
    alkalosis (metabolic) (respiratory) E87.3
  elimination, transepidermal L87.9
    specified NEC L87.8
  emotional (persistent) F34.9
    of childhood F93.9
      specified NEC F93.8
  endocrine E34.9
    postprocedural E89.89
      specified NEC E89.89
  erectile (male) (organic) — *see also* Dysfunction, sexual, male, erectile N52.9
    nonorganic F52.21
  erythematous — *see* Erythema
  esophagus K22.9
    functional K22.4
    psychogenic F45.8
  eustachian tube H69.9-
    infection — *see* Salpingitis, eustachian
    obstruction — *see* Obstruction, eustachian tube
    patulous — *see* Patulous, eustachian tube
    specified NEC H69.8-
  exhibitionistic F65.2
  extrapyramidal G25.9
    in diseases classified elsewhere — *see* category G26
    specified type NEC G25.89
  eye H57.9

Disorder (of) - *continued*
  eye - *continued*
    postprocedural — *see* Complication, postprocedural, eye
  eyelid H02.9
    cyst — *see* Cyst, eyelid
    degenerative H02.70
      chloasma — *see* Chloasma, eyelid
      madarosis — *see* Madarosis
      specified type NEC H02.79
      vitiligo — *see* Vitiligo, eyelid
      xanthelasma — *see* Xanthelasma
    dermatochalasis — *see* Dermatochalasis
    edema — *see* Edema, eyelid
    elephantiasis — *see* Elephantiasis, eyelid
    foreign body, retained — *see* Foreign body, retained, eyelid
    function H02.59
      abnormal innervation syndrome — *see* Syndrome, abnormal innervation
      blepharochalasis — *see* Blepharochalasis
      blepharoclonus — *see* Blepharoclonus
      blepharophimosis — *see* Blepharophimosis
      blepharoptosis — *see* Blepharoptosis
      lagophthalmos — *see* Lagophthalmos
      lid retraction — *see* Retraction, lid
    hypertrichosis — *see* Hypertrichosis, eyelid
    specified type NEC H02.89
    vascular H02.879
      left H02.876
        lower H02.875
        upper H02.874
      right H02.873
        lower H02.872
        upper H02.871
  factitious
    by proxy F68.A
    imposed on another F68.A
    imposed on self F68.10
      with predominantly
        psychological symptoms F68.11
          with physical symptoms F68.13
        physical symptoms F68.12
          with psychological symptoms F68.13
  factor, coagulation — *see* Defect, coagulation
  fatty acid
    metabolism E71.30
      specified NEC E71.39
    oxidation
      LCAD E71.310
      MCAD E71.311
      SCAD E71.312
      specified deficiency NEC E71.318
  feeding (infant or child) — *see also* Disorder, eating R63.3
    or eating disorder F50.9
    specified NEC F50.9
  feigned (with obvious motivation) Z76.5
    without obvious motivation — *see* Disorder, factitious
  female
    hypoactive sexual desire F52.0
    orgasmic F52.31
    sexual interest/arousal F52.22
  fetishistic F65.0
  fibroblastic M72.9
    specified NEC M72.8
  fluency
    adult onset F98.5
    childhood onset F80.81
    following
      cerebral infarction I69.323
      cerebrovascular disease I69.923
        specified disease NEC I69.823
      intracerebral hemorrhage I69.123
      nontraumatic intracranial hemorrhage NEC I69.223
      subarachnoid hemorrhage I69.023
    in conditions classified elsewhere R47.82
  fluid balance E87.8
  follicular (skin) L73.9
    specified NEC L73.8
  frotteuristic F65.81
  fructose metabolism E74.10
    essential fructosuria E74.11
    fructokinase deficiency E74.11
    fructose-1, 6-diphosphatase deficiency E74.19
    hereditary fructose intolerance E74.12
    other specified E74.19
  functional polymorphonuclear neutrophils D71
  gallbladder, biliary tract and pancreas in diseases classified elsewhere K87
  gambling F63.0

Disorder (of) - *continued*
  gamma aminobutyric acid (GABA) metabolism E72.81
  gamma-glutamyl cycle E72.89
  gastric (functional) K31.9
    motility K30
    psychogenic F45.8
    secretion K30
  gastrointestinal (functional) NOS K92.9
    newborn P78.9
    psychogenic F45.8
  gender-identity or -role F64.9
    childhood F64.2
    effect on relationship F66
    of adolescence or adulthood F64.0
      nontranssexual F64.8
    specified NEC F64.8
    uncertainty F66
  genito-pelvic pain penetration F52.6
  genitourinary system
    female N94.9
    male N50.9
    psychogenic F45.8
  globe H44.9
    degenerated condition H44.50
      absolute glaucoma H44.51-
      atrophy H44.52-
      leucocoria H44.53-
    degenerative H44.30
      chalcosis H44.31-
      myopia — *see also* Myopia, degenerative H44.2-
      siderosis H44.32-
      specified type NEC H44.39-
    endophthalmitis — *see* Endophthalmitis
    foreign body, retained — *see* Foreign body, intraocular, old, retained
    hemophthalmos — *see* Hemophthalmos
    hypotony H44.40
      due to
        ocular fistula H44.42-
        specified disorder NEC H44.43-
      flat anterior chamber H44.41-
      primary H44.44-
    luxation — *see* Luxation, globe
    specified type NEC H44.89
  glomerular (in) N05.9
    amyloidosis E85.4 *[N08]*
    cryoglobulinemia D89.1 *[N08]*
    disseminated intravascular coagulation D65 *[N08]*
    Fabry's disease E75.21 *[N08]*
    familial lecithin cholesterol acyltransferase deficiency E78.6 *[N08]*
    Goodpasture's syndrome M31.0
    hemolytic-uremic syndrome D59.3
    Henoch (-Schönlein) purpura D69.0 *[N08]*
    malariae malaria B52.0
    microscopic polyangiitis M31.7 *[N08]*
    multiple myeloma C90.0- *[N08]*
    mumps B26.83
    schistosomiasis B65.9 *[N08]*
    sepsis NEC A41.- *[N08]*
      streptococcal A40.- *[N08]*
    sickle-cell disorders D57.- *[N08]*
    strongyloidiasis B78.9 *[N08]*
    subacute bacterial endocarditis I33.0 *[N08]*
    syphilis A52.75
    systemic lupus erythematosus M32.14
    thrombotic thrombocytopenic purpura M31.1 *[N08]*
    Waldenström macroglobulinemia C88.0 *[N08]*
    Wegener's granulomatosis M31.31
  gluconeogenesis E74.4
  glucosaminoglycan metabolism — *see* Disorder, metabolism, glucosaminoglycan
  glycine metabolism E72.50
    d-glycericacidemia E72.59
    hyperhydroxyprolinemia E72.59
    hyperoxaluria R82.992
      primary E72.53
    hyperprolinemia E72.59
    non-ketotic hyperglycinemia E72.51
    oxalosis E72.53
    oxaluria E72.53
    sarcosinemia E72.59
    trimethylaminuria E72.52
  glycoprotein metabolism E77.9
    specified NEC E77.8
  habit (and impulse) F63.9
    involving sexual behavior NEC F65.9
    specified NEC F63.89
  hallucinogen use
    mild F16.10
      with

Disorder (of) - *continued*
hallucinogen use - *continued*
mild - *continued*
with - *continued*
hallucinogen-induced
anxiety disorder F16.180
bipolar and related disorder F16.14
depressive disorder F16.14
psychotic disorder F16.159
hallucinogen intoxication delirium F16.121
other hallucinogen intoxication F16.129
in remission (early) (sustained) F16.11
moderate or severe F16.20
with
hallucinogen-induced
anxiety disorder F16.280
bipolar and related disorder F16.24
depressive disorder F16.24
psychotic disorder F16.259
hallucinogen intoxication delirium F16.221
other hallucinogen intoxication F16.229
in remission (early) (sustained) F16.21
heart action I49.9
hematological D75.9
newborn (transient) P61.9
specified NEC P61.8
hematopoietic organs D75.9
hemorrhagic NEC D69.9
drug-induced D68.32
due to
extrinsic circulating anticoagulants D68.32
increase in
anti-IIa D68.32
anti-Xa D68.32
intrinsic
circulating anticoagulants D68.318
increase in
antithrombin D68.318
anti-VIIIa D68.318
anti-IXa D68.318
anti-XIa D68.318
following childbirth O72.3
hemostasis — *see* Defect, coagulation
histidine metabolism E70.40
histidinemia E70.41
other specified E70.49
hoarding F42.3
hyperkinetic — *see* Disorder, attention-deficit hyperactivity
hyperleucine-isoleucinemia E71.19
hypervalinemia E71.19
hypoactive sexual desire F52.0
hypochondriacal F45.20
body dysmorphic F45.22
neurosis F45.21
other specified F45.29
identity
dissociative F44.81
of childhood F93.8
illness anxiety F45.21
immune mechanism (immunity) D89.9
specified type NEC D89.89
impaired renal tubular function N25.9
specified NEC N25.89
impulse (control) F63.9
inflammatory
pelvic, in diseases classified elsewhere — *see* category N74
penis N48.29
abscess N48.21
cellulitis N48.22
inhalant use
mild F18.10
with
inhalant-induced
anxiety disorder F18.180
depressive disorder F18.14
major neurocognitive disorder F18.17
mild neurocognitive disorder F18.188
psychotic disorder F18.159
inhalant intoxication F18.129
inhalant intoxication delirium F18.121
in remission (early) (sustained) F18.11
moderate or severe F18.20
with
inhalant-induced
anxiety disorder F18.280
depressive disorder F18.24
major neurocognitive disorder F18.27
mild neurocognitive disorder F18.288
psychotic disorder F18.259
inhalant intoxication F18.229
inhalant intoxication delirium F18.221

Disorder (of) - *continued*
inhalant use - *continued*
moderate or severe - *continued*
in remission (early) (sustained) F18.21
integument, newborn P83.9
specified NEC P83.88
intermittent explosive F63.81
internal secretion pancreas — *see* Increased, secretion, pancreas, endocrine
intestine, intestinal
carbohydrate absorption NEC E74.39
postoperative K91.2
functional NEC K59.9
postoperative K91.89
psychogenic F45.8
vascular K55.9
chronic K55.1
specified NEC K55.8
intraoperative (intraprocedural) — *see* Complications, intraoperative
involuntary emotional expression (IEED) F48.2
iris H21.9
adhesions — *see* Adhesions, iris
atrophy — *see* Atrophy, iris
chamber angle recession — *see* Recession, chamber angle
cyst — *see* Cyst, iris
degeneration — *see* Degeneration, iris
in diseases classified elsewhere H22
iridodialysis — *see* Iridodialysis
iridoschisis — *see* Iridoschisis
miotic pupillary cyst — *see* Cyst, pupillary
pupillary
abnormality — *see* Abnormality, pupillary
membrane — *see* Membrane, pupillary
specified type NEC H21.89
vascular NEC H21.1X-
iron metabolism E83.10
specified NEC E83.19
isovaleric acidemia E71.110
jaw, developmental M27.0
temporomandibular — *see also* Anomaly, dentofacial, temporomandibular joint M26.60-
joint M25.9
derangement — *see* Derangement, joint
effusion — *see* Effusion, joint
fistula — *see* Fistula, joint
hemarthrosis — *see* Hemarthrosis
instability — *see* Instability, joint
osteophyte — *see* Osteophyte
pain — *see* Pain, joint
psychogenic F45.8
specified type NEC M25.80
ankle M25.87-
elbow M25.82-
foot joint M25.87-
hand joint M25.84-
hip M25.85-
knee M25.86-
shoulder M25.81-
wrist M25.83-
stiffness — *see* Stiffness, joint
ketone metabolism E71.32
kidney N28.9
functional (tubular) N25.9
in
schistosomiasis B65.9 *[N29]*
tubular function N25.9
specified NEC N25.89
lacrimal system H04.9
changes H04.69
fistula — *see* Fistula, lacrimal
gland H04.19
atrophy — *see* Atrophy, lacrimal gland
cyst — *see* Cyst, lacrimal, gland
dacryops — *see* Dacryops
dislocation — *see* Dislocation, lacrimal gland
dry eye syndrome — *see* Syndrome, dry eye
infection — *see* Dacryoadenitis
granuloma — *see* Granuloma, lacrimal
inflammation — *see* Inflammation, lacrimal
obstruction — *see* Obstruction, lacrimal
specified NEC H04.89
lactation NEC O92.79
language (developmental) F80.9
expressive F80.1
mixed receptive and expressive F80.2
receptive F80.2
late luteal phase dysphoric N94.89
learning (specific) F81.9
acalculia R48.8
alexia R48.0
mathematics F81.2

Disorder (of) - *continued*
learning (specific) - *continued*
reading F81.0
specified
with impairment in
mathematics F81.2
reading F81.0
written expression F81.81
specified NEC F81.89
spelling F81.81
written expression F81.81
lens H27.9
aphakia — *see* Aphakia
cataract — *see* Cataract
dislocation — *see* Dislocation, lens
specified type NEC H27.8
ligament M24.20
ankle M24.27-
attachment, spine — *see* Enthesopathy, spinal
elbow M24.22-
foot joint M24.27-
hand joint M24.24-
hip M24.25-
knee — *see* Derangement, knee, specified NEC
shoulder M24.21-
vertebra M24.28
wrist M24.23-
ligamentous attachments — *see also* Enthesopathy
spine — *see* Enthesopathy, spinal
lipid
metabolism, congenital E78.9
storage E75.6
specified NEC E75.5
lipoprotein
deficiency (familial) E78.6
metabolism E78.9
specified NEC E78.89
liver K76.9
malarial B54 *[K77]*
low back — *see also* Dorsopathy, specified NEC
lumbosacral
plexus G54.1
root (nerve) NEC G54.4
lung, interstitial, drug-induced J70.4
acute J70.2
chronic J70.3
lymphoproliferative, post-transplant (PTLD) D47.Z1
lysine and hydroxylysine metabolism E72.3
major neurocognitive — *see* Dementia, in (due to)
male
erectile (organic) — *see also* Dysfunction, sexual, male, erectile N52.9
nonorganic F52.21
hypoactive sexual desire F52.0
orgasmic F52.32
manic F30.9
organic F06.33
mast cell activation — *see* Activation, mast cell
mastoid — *see also* Disorder, ear, middle
postprocedural — *see* Complications, ear, procedure
meniscus — *see* Derangement, knee, meniscus
menopausal N95.9
specified NEC N95.8
menstrual N92.6
psychogenic F45.8
specified NEC N92.5
mental (or behavioral) (nonpsychotic) F99
due to (secondary to)
amphetamine
due to drug abuse — *see* Abuse, drug, stimulant
due to drug dependence — *see* Dependence, drug, stimulant
brain disease, damage and dysfunction F09
caffeine use
due to drug abuse — *see* Abuse, drug, stimulant
due to drug dependence — *see* Dependence, drug, stimulant
cannabis use
due to drug abuse — *see* Abuse, drug, cannabis
due to drug dependence — *see* Dependence, drug, cannabis
general medical condition F09
sedative or hypnotic use
due to drug abuse — *see* Abuse, drug, sedative
due to drug dependence — *see* Dependence, drug, sedative
tobacco (nicotine) use — *see* Dependence, drug, nicotine
following organic brain damage F07.9
frontal lobe syndrome F07.0
personality change F07.0
postconcussional syndrome F07.81

Disorder (of) - *continued*
mental (or behavioral) (nonpsychotic) - *continued*
following organic brain damage - *continued*
specified NEC F07.89
infancy, childhood or adolescence F98.9
neurotic — *see* Neurosis
organic or symptomatic F09
presenile, psychotic F03
problem NEC
psychoneurotic — *see* Neurosis
psychotic — *see* Psychosis
puerperal F53.0
senile, psychotic NEC F03
metabolic, amino acid, transitory, newborn P74.8
metabolism NOS E88.9
amino-acid E72.9
aromatic E70.9
albinism — *see* Albinism
histidine E70.40
histidinemia E70.41
other specified E70.49
hyperphenylalaninemia E70.1
classical phenylketonuria E70.0
other specified E70.8
tryptophan E70.5
tyrosine E70.20
hypertyrosinemia E70.21
other specified E70.29
branched chain E71.2
3-methylglutaconic aciduria E71.111
hyperleucine-isoleucinemia E71.19
hypervalinemia E71.19
isovaleric acidemia E71.110
maple syrup urine disease E71.0
methylmalonic acidemia E71.120
organic aciduria NEC E71.118
other specified E71.19
proprionate NEC E71.128
proprionic acidemia E71.121
glycine E72.50
d-glycericacidemia E72.59
hyperhydroxyprolinemia E72.59
hyperoxaluria R82.992
primary E72.53
hyperprolinemia E72.59
non-ketotic hyperglycinemia E72.51
other specified E72.59
sarcosinemia E72.59
trimethylaminuria E72.52
hydroxylysine E72.3
lysine E72.3
ornithine E72.4
other specified E72.89
beta-amino acid E72.89
gamma-glutamyl cycle E72.89
straight-chain E72.89
sulfur-bearing E72.10
homocystinuria E72.11
methylenetetrahydrofolate reductase deficiency E72.12
other specified E72.19
bile acid and cholesterol metabolism E78.70
bilirubin E80.7
specified NEC E80.6
calcium E83.50
hypercalcemia E83.52
hypocalcemia E83.51
other specified E83.59
carbohydrate E74.9
specified NEC E74.8
cholesterol and bile acid metabolism E78.70
congenital E88.9
copper E83.00
Wilson's disease E83.01
specified type NEC E83.09
cystinuria E72.01
fructose E74.10
galactose E74.20
glucosaminoglycan E76.9
mucopolysaccharidosis — *see* Mucopolysaccharidosis
specified NEC E76.8
glutamine E72.89
glycine E72.50
glycogen storage (hepatorenal) E74.09
glycoprotein E77.9
specified NEC E77.8
glycosaminoglycan E76.9
specified NEC E76.8
in labor and delivery O75.89
iron E83.10
isoleucine E71.19
leucine E71.19

Disorder (of) - *continued*
metabolism NOS - *continued*
lipoid E78.9
lipoprotein E78.9
specified NEC E78.89
magnesium E83.40
hypermagnesemia E83.41
hypomagnesemia E83.42
other specified E83.49
mineral E83.9
specified NEC E83.89
mitochondrial E88.40
MELAS syndrome E88.41
MERRF syndrome (myoclonic epilepsy associated with ragged-red fibers) E88.42
other specified E88.49
ornithine E72.4
phosphatases E83.30
phosphorus E83.30
acid phosphatase deficiency E83.39
hypophosphatasia E83.39
hypophosphatemia E83.39
familial E83.31
other specified E83.39
pseudovitamin D deficiency E83.32
plasma protein NEC E88.09
porphyrin — *see* Porphyria
postprocedural E89.89
specified NEC E89.89
purine E79.9
specified NEC E79.8
pyrimidine E79.9
specified NEC E79.8
pyruvate E74.4
serine E72.89
sodium E87.8
specified NEC E88.89
threonine E72.89
valine E71.19
zinc E83.2
methylmalonic acidemia E71.120
micturition NEC — *see also* Difficulty, micturition R39.198
feeling of incomplete emptying R39.14
hesitancy R39.11
poor stream R39.12
psychogenic F45.8
split stream R39.13
straining R39.16
urgency R39.15
mild neurocognitive G31.84
mitochondrial metabolism E88.40
mitral (valve) — *see* Endocarditis, mitral
mixed
anxiety and depressive F41.8
of scholastic skills (developmental) F81.89
receptive expressive language F80.2
mood F39
bipolar — *see* Disorder, bipolar
depressive — *see* Disorder, depressive
due to (secondary to)
alcohol F10.94
amphetamine F15.94
in
abuse F15.14
dependence F15.24
anxiolytic F13.94
in
abuse F13.14
dependence F13.24
cocaine F14.94
in
abuse F14.14
dependence F14.24
general medical condition F06.30
hallucinogen F16.94
in
abuse F16.14
dependence F16.24
hypnotic F13.94
in
abuse F13.14
dependence F13.24
inhalant F18.94
in
abuse F18.14
dependence F18.24
opioid F11.94
in
abuse F11.14
dependence F11.24
phencyclidine (PCP) F16.94
in

Disorder (of) - *continued*
mood - *continued*
due to (secondary to) - *continued*
phencyclidine (PCP) - *continued*
in - *continued*
abuse F16.14
dependence F16.24
physiological condition F06.30
with
depressive features F06.31
major depressive-like episode F06.32
manic features F06.33
mixed features F06.34
psychoactive substance NEC F19.94
in
abuse F19.14
dependence F19.24
sedative F13.94
in
abuse F13.14
dependence F13.24
volatile solvents F18.94
in
abuse F18.14
dependence F18.24
manic episode F30.9
with psychotic symptoms F30.2
in remission (full) F30.4
partial F30.3
specified type NEC F30.8
without psychotic symptoms F30.10
mild F30.11
moderate F30.12
severe F30.13
organic F06.30
right hemisphere F07.89
persistent F34.9
cyclothymia F34.0
dysthymia F34.1
specified type NEC F34.89
recurrent F39
right hemisphere organic F07.89
movement G25.9
drug-induced G25.70
akathisia G25.71
specified NEC G25.79
hysterical F44.4
in diseases classified elsewhere — *see* category G26
periodic limb G47.61
sleep related G47.61
specified NEC G25.89
sleep related NEC G47.69
stereotyped F98.4
treatment-induced G25.9
multiple personality F44.81
muscle M62.9
attachment, spine — *see* Enthesopathy, spinal
in trichinellosis — *see* Trichinellosis, with muscle disorder
psychogenic F45.8
specified type NEC M62.89
tone, newborn P94.9
specified NEC P94.8
muscular
attachments — *see also* Enthesopathy
spine — *see* Enthesopathy, spinal
urethra N36.44
musculoskeletal system, soft tissue — *see* Disorder, soft tissue
postprocedural M96.89
psychogenic F45.8
myoneural G70.9
due to lead G70.1
specified NEC G70.89
toxic G70.1
myotonic NEC G71.19
nail, in diseases classified elsewhere L62
neck region NEC — *see* Dorsopathy, specified NEC
neonatal onset multisystemic inflammatory (NOMID) M04.2
nerve G58.9
abducent NEC — *see* Strabismus, paralytic, sixth nerve
accessory G52.8
acoustic — *see* subcategory H93.3
auditory — *see* subcategory H93.3
auriculotemporal G50.8
axillary G54.0
cerebral — *see* Disorder, nerve, cranial
cranial G52.9
eighth — *see* subcategory H93.3
eleventh G52.8

Disorder (of) - *continued*
personality - *continued*
negativistic F60.89
obsessional F60.5
obsessive (-compulsive) F60.5
organic F07.9
overconscientious F60.5
paranoid F60.0
passive (-dependent) F60.7
passive-aggressive F60.89
pathological NEC F60.9
pseudosocial F60.2
psychopathic F60.2
schizoid F60.1
schizotypal F21
self-defeating F60.7
specified NEC F60.89
type A F60.5
unstable (emotional) F60.3
pervasive, developmental F84.9
phencyclidine use
mild F16.10
with
phencyclidine-induced
anxiety disorder F16.180
bipolar and related disorder F16.14
depressive disorder F16.14
psychotic disorder F16.159
phencyclidine intoxication F16.129
phencyclidine intoxication delirium F16.121
in remission (early) (sustained) F16.11
moderate or severe F16.20
with
phencyclidine-induced
anxiety disorder F16.280
bipolar and related disorder F16.24
depressive disorder F16.24
psychotic disorder F16.259
phencyclidine intoxication F16.229
phencyclidine intoxication delirium F16.221
in remission (early) (sustained) F16.21
phobic anxiety, childhood F40.8
phosphate-losing tubular N25.0
pigmentation L81.9
choroid, congenital Q14.3
diminished melanin formation L81.6
iron L81.8
specified NEC L81.8
pinna (noninfective) H61.10-
deformity, acquired H61.11-
hematoma H61.12-
perichondritis — *see* Perichondritis, ear
specified type NEC H61.19-
pituitary gland E23.7
iatrogenic (postprocedural) E89.3
specified NEC E23.6
platelets D69.1
plexus G54.9
specified NEC G54.8
polymorphonuclear neutrophils D71
porphyrin metabolism — *see* Porphyria
postconcussional F07.81
posthallucinogen perception F16.983
in
abuse F16.183
dependence F16.283
postmenopausal N95.9
specified NEC N95.8
postprocedural (postoperative) — *see* Complications, postprocedural
post-transplant lymphoproliferative D47.Z1
post-traumatic stress (PTSD) F43.10
acute F43.11
chronic F43.12
premenstrual dysphoric (PMDD) F32.81
prepuce N47.8
propionic acidemia E71.121
prostate N42.9
specified NEC N42.89
psychogenic NOS — *see also* condition F45.9
anxiety F41.8
appetite F50.9
asthenic F48.8
cardiovascular (system) F45.8
compulsive F42.8
cutaneous F54
depressive F32.9
digestive (system) F45.8
dysmenorrheic F45.8
dyspneic F45.8
endocrine (system) F54
eye NEC F45.8
feeding — *see* Disorder, eating

Disorder (of) - *continued*
psychogenic NOS - *continued*
functional NEC F45.8
gastric F45.8
gastrointestinal (system) F45.8
genitourinary (system) F45.8
heart (function) (rhythm) F45.8
hyperventilatory F45.8
hypochondriacal — *see* Disorder, hypochondriacal
intestinal F45.8
joint F45.8
learning F81.9
limb F45.8
lymphatic (system) F45.8
menstrual F45.8
micturition F45.8
monoplegic NEC F44.4
motor F44.4
muscle F45.8
musculoskeletal F45.8
neurocirculatory F45.8
obsessive F42.8
occupational F48.8
organ or part of body NEC F45.8
paralytic NEC F44.4
phobic F40.9
physical NEC F45.8
rectal F45.8
respiratory (system) F45.8
rheumatic F45.8
sexual (function) F52.9
skin (allergic) (eczematous) F54
sleep F51.9
specified part of body NEC F45.8
stomach F45.8
psychological F99
associated with
disease classified elsewhere F54
sexual
development F66
relationship F66
uncertainty about gender identity F64.9
psychomotor NEC F44.4
hysterical F44.4
psychoneurotic — *see also* Neurosis
mixed NEC F48.8
psychophysiologic — *see* Disorder, somatoform
psychosexual F65.9
development F66
identity of childhood F64.2
psychosomatic NOS — *see* Disorder, somatoform
multiple F45.0
undifferentiated F45.1
psychotic — *see* Psychosis
transient (acute) F23
puberty E30.9
specified NEC E30.8
pulmonary (valve) — *see* Endocarditis, pulmonary
purine metabolism E79.9
pyrimidine metabolism E79.9
pyruvate metabolism E74.4
reactive attachment (childhood) F94.1
reading R48.0
developmental (specific) F81.0
receptive language F80.2
receptor, hormonal, peripheral — *see also* Syndrome, androgen insensitivity E34.50
recurrent brief depressive F33.8
reflex R29.2
refraction H52.7
aniseikonia H52.32
anisometropia H52.31
astigmatism — *see* Astigmatism
hypermetropia — *see* Hypermetropia
myopia — *see* Myopia
presbyopia H52.4
specified NEC H52.6
relationship F68.8
due to sexual orientation F66
REM sleep behavior G47.52
renal function, impaired (tubular) N25.9
resonance R49.9
specified NEC R49.8
respiratory function, impaired — *see also* Failure, respiration
postprocedural — *see* Complication, postoperative, respiratory system
psychogenic F45.8
retina H35.9
angioid streaks H35.33
changes in vascular appearance H35.01-
degeneration — *see* Degeneration, retina
dystrophy (hereditary) — *see* Dystrophy, retina

Disorder (of) - *continued*
retina - *continued*
edema H35.81
hemorrhage — *see* Hemorrhage, retina
ischemia H35.82
macular degeneration — *see* Degeneration, macula
microaneurysms H35.04-
microvascular abnormality NEC H35.09
neovascularization — *see* Neovascularization, retina
retinopathy — *see* Retinopathy
separation of layers H35.70
central serous chorioretinopathy H35.71-
pigment epithelium detachment (serous) H35.72-
hemorrhagic H35.73-
specified type NEC H35.89
telangiectasis — *see* Telangiectasis, retina
vasculitis — *see* Vasculitis, retina
retroperitoneal K68.9
right hemisphere organic affective F07.89
rumination (infant or child) F98.21
sacrum, sacrococcygeal NEC M53.3
schizoaffective F25.9
bipolar type F25.0
depressive type F25.1
manic type F25.0
mixed type F25.0
specified NEC F25.8
schizoid of childhood F84.5
schizophrenia spectrum and other psychotic disorder F29
specified NEC F28
schizophreniform F20.81
brief F23
schizotypal (personality) F21
secretion, thyrocalcitonin E07.0
sedative, hypnotic, or anxiolytic use
mild F13.10
with
sedative, hypnotic, or anxiolytic-induced
anxiety disorder F13.180
bipolar and related disorder F13.14
depressive disorder F13.14
psychotic disorder F13.159
sexual dysfunction F13.181
sedative, hypnotic, or anxiolytic intoxication F13.129
sedative, hypnotic, or anxiolytic intoxication delirium F13.121
in remission (early) (sustained) F13.11
moderate or severe F13.20
with
sedative, hypnotic, or anxiolytic-induced
anxiety disorder F13.280
bipolar and related disorder F13.24
depressive disorder F13.24
major neurocognitive disorder F13.27
mild neurocognitive disorder F13.288
psychotic disorder F13.259
sexual dysfunction F13.281
sedative, hypnotic, or anxiolytic intoxication F13.229
sedative, hypnotic, or anxiolytic intoxication delirium F13.221
in remission (early) (sustained) F13.21
seizure — *see also* Epilepsy G40.909
intractable G40.919
with status epilepticus G40.911
semantic pragmatic F80.89
with autism F84.0
sense of smell R43.1
psychogenic F45.8
separation anxiety, of childhood F93.0
sexual
arousal, female F52.22
aversion F52.1
function, psychogenic F52.9
interest/arousal, female F52.22
masochism F65.51
maturation F66
nonorganic F52.9
preference — *see also* Deviation, sexual F65.9
fetishistic transvestism F65.1
relationship F66
sadism F65.52
shyness, of childhood and adolescence F40.10
sibling rivalry F93.8
sickle-cell (sickling) (homozygous) — *see* Disease, sickle-cell
heterozygous D57.3
specified type NEC D57.8-
trait D57.3
sinus (nasal) J34.9

- **Disorder** (of) - *continued*
  - sinus (nasal) - *continued*
    - specified NEC J34.89
  - skin L98.9
    - atrophic L90.9
      - specified NEC L90.8
    - granulomatous L92.9
      - specified NEC L92.8
    - hypertrophic L91.9
      - specified NEC L91.8
    - infiltrative NEC L98.6
    - newborn P83.9
      - specified NEC P83.88
    - picking F42.4
    - psychogenic (allergic) (eczematous) F54
  - sleep G47.9
    - breathing-related — *see* Apnea, sleep
    - circadian rhythm G47.20
      - advance sleep phase type G47.22
      - delayed sleep phase type G47.21
      - due to
        - alcohol
          - abuse F10.182
          - dependence F10.282
          - use F10.982
        - amphetamines
          - abuse F15.182
          - dependence F15.282
          - use F15.982
        - caffeine
          - abuse F15.182
          - dependence F15.282
          - use F15.982
        - cocaine
          - abuse F14.182
          - dependence F14.282
          - use F14.982
        - drug NEC
          - abuse F19.182
          - dependence F19.282
          - use F19.982
        - opioid
          - abuse F11.182
          - dependence F11.282
          - use F11.982
        - psychoactive substance NEC
          - abuse F19.182
          - dependence F19.282
          - use F19.982
        - sedative, hypnotic, or anxiolytic
          - abuse F13.182
          - dependence F13.282
          - use F13.982
        - stimulant NEC
          - abuse F15.182
          - dependence F15.282
          - use F15.982
      - free running type G47.24
      - in conditions classified elsewhere G47.27
      - irregular sleep wake type G47.23
      - jet lag type G47.25
      - non-24-hour sleep-wake type G47.24
      - shift work type G47.26
      - specified NEC G47.29
    - due to
      - alcohol
        - abuse F10.182
        - dependence F10.282
        - use F10.982
      - amphetamine
        - abuse F15.182
        - dependence F15.282
        - use F15.982
      - anxiolytic
        - abuse F13.182
        - dependence F13.282
        - use F13.982
      - caffeine
        - abuse F15.182
        - dependence F15.282
        - use F15.982
      - cocaine
        - abuse F14.182
        - dependence F14.282
        - use F14.982
      - drug NEC
        - abuse F19.182
        - dependence F19.282
        - use F19.982
      - hypnotic
        - abuse F13.182
        - dependence F13.282
        - use F13.982

- **Disorder** (of) - *continued*
  - sleep - *continued*
    - due to - *continued*
      - opioid
        - abuse F11.182
        - dependence F11.282
        - use F11.982
      - psychoactive substance NEC
        - abuse F19.182
        - dependence F19.282
        - use F19.982
      - sedative
        - abuse F13.182
        - dependence F13.282
        - use F13.982
      - stimulant NEC
        - abuse F15.182
        - dependence F15.282
        - use F15.982
    - emotional F51.9
    - excessive somnolence — *see* Hypersomnia
    - hypersomnia type — *see* Hypersomnia
    - initiating or maintaining — *see* Insomnia
    - nightmares F51.5
    - nonorganic F51.9
      - specified NEC F51.8
    - parasomnia type G47.50
    - specified NEC G47.8
    - terrors F51.4
    - walking F51.3
  - sleep-wake pattern or schedule — *see also* Disorder, sleep, circadian rhythm G47.9
    - specified NEC G47.8
  - social
    - anxiety (of childhood) F40.10
      - generalized F40.11
    - functioning in childhood F94.9
      - specified NEC F94.8
    - pragmatic F80.82
  - soft tissue M79.9
    - ankle M79.9
    - due to use, overuse and pressure M70.90
      - ankle M70.97-
      - bursitis — *see* Bursitis
      - foot M70.97-
      - forearm M70.93-
      - hand M70.94-
      - lower leg M70.96-
      - multiple sites M70.99
      - pelvic region M70.95-
      - shoulder region M70.91-
      - specified site NEC M70.98
      - specified type NEC M70.80
        - ankle M70.87-
        - foot M70.87-
        - forearm M70.83-
        - hand M70.84-
        - lower leg M70.86-
        - multiple sites M70.89
        - pelvic region M70.85-
        - shoulder region M70.81-
        - specified site NEC M70.88
        - thigh M70.85-
        - upper arm M70.82-
      - thigh M70.95-
      - upper arm M70.92-
    - foot M79.9
    - forearm M79.9
    - hand M79.9
    - lower leg M79.9
    - multiple sites M79.9
    - occupational — *see* Disorder, soft tissue, due to use, overuse and pressure
    - pelvic region M79.9
    - shoulder region M79.9
    - specified type NEC M79.89
    - thigh M79.9
    - upper arm M79.9
  - somatic symptom F45.1
  - somatization F45.0
  - somatoform F45.9
    - pain (persistent) F45.41
    - somatization (multiple) (long-lasting) F45.0
    - specified NEC F45.8
    - undifferentiated F45.1
  - somnolence, excessive — *see* Hypersomnia
  - specific
    - arithmetical F81.2
    - developmental, of motor F82
    - reading F81.0
    - speech and language F80.9
    - spelling F81.81
    - written expression F81.81

- **Disorder** (of) - *continued*
  - speech R47.9
    - articulation (functional) (specific) F80.0
    - developmental F80.9
    - specified NEC R47.89
  - speech-sound F80.0
  - spelling (specific) F81.81
  - spine — *see also* Dorsopathy
    - ligamentous or muscular attachments, peripheral — *see* Enthesopathy, spinal
    - specified NEC — *see* Dorsopathy, specified NEC
  - stereotyped, habit or movement F98.4
  - stimulant use (other) (unspecified)
    - mild F15.10
      - in remission (early) (sustained) F15.11
    - moderate or severe F15.20
      - in remission (early) (sustained) F15.21
  - stomach (functional) — *see* Disorder, gastric
  - stress F43.9
    - acute F43.0
    - post-traumatic F43.10
      - acute F43.11
      - chronic F43.12
  - substance use (other) (unknown)
    - mild F19.10
      - with substance-induced
        - anxiety disorder F19.180
        - bipolar and related disorder F19.14
        - depressive disorder F19.14
        - major neurocognitive disorder F19.17
        - mild neurocognitive disorder F19.188
        - obsessive-compulsive and related disorder F19.188
        - sexual dysfunction F19.181
      - substance intoxication F19.129
      - substance intoxication delirium F19.121
    - moderate or severe F19.20
      - with substance-induced
        - anxiety disorder F19.280
        - bipolar and related disorder F19.24
        - depressive disorder F19.24
        - major neurocognitive disorder F19.27
        - mild neurocognitive disorder F19.288
        - obsessive-compulsive and related disorder F19.288
        - sexual dysfunction F19.281
      - in remission (early) (sustained) F19.21
      - substance intoxication F19.229
      - substance intoxication delirium F19.221
  - sulfur-bearing amino-acid metabolism E72.10
  - sweat gland (eccrine) L74.9
    - apocrine L75.9
      - specified NEC L75.8
    - specified NEC L74.8
  - synovium M67.90
    - acromioclavicular M67.91-
    - ankle M67.97-
    - elbow M67.92-
    - foot M67.97-
    - forearm M67.93-
    - hand M67.94-
    - hip M67.95-
    - knee M67.96-
    - multiple sites M67.99
    - rupture — *see* Rupture, synovium
    - shoulder M67.91-
    - specified type NEC M67.80
      - acromioclavicular M67.81-
      - ankle M67.87-
      - elbow M67.82-
      - foot M67.87-
      - hand M67.84-
      - hip M67.85-
      - knee M67.86-
      - multiple sites M67.89
      - wrist M67.83-
    - synovitis — *see* Synovitis
    - upper arm M67.92-
    - wrist M67.93-
  - temperature regulation, newborn P81.9
    - specified NEC P81.8
  - temporomandibular joint M26.60-
  - tendon M67.90
    - acromioclavicular M67.91-
    - ankle M67.97-
    - contracture — *see* Contracture, tendon
    - elbow M67.92-
    - foot M67.97-
    - forearm M67.93-
    - hand M67.94-
    - hip M67.95-
    - knee M67.96-
    - multiple sites M67.99

- **Disorder** (of) - *continued*
  - tendon - *continued*
    - rupture — *see* Rupture, tendon
    - shoulder M67.91-
    - specified type NEC M67.80
      - acromioclavicular M67.81-
      - ankle M67.87-
      - elbow M67.82-
      - foot M67.87-
      - hand M67.84-
      - hip M67.85-
      - knee M67.86-
      - multiple sites M67.89
      - trunk M67.88
      - wrist M67.83-
    - synovitis — *see* Synovitis
    - tendinitis — *see* Tendinitis
    - tenosynovitis — *see* Tenosynovitis
    - trunk M67.98
    - upper arm M67.92-
    - wrist M67.93-
  - thoracic root (nerve) NEC G54.3
  - thyrocalcitonin hypersecretion E07.0
  - thyroid (gland) E07.9
    - function NEC, neonatal, transitory P72.2
    - iodine-deficiency related E01.8
    - specified NEC E07.89
  - tic — *see* Tic
  - tobacco use
    - chewing tobacco (mild) (moderate) (severe)
      - in remission (early) (sustained) F17.221
    - cigarettes (mild) (moderate) (severe)
      - in remission (early) (sustained) F17.211
    - mild Z72.0
      - in remission (early) (sustained) F17.201
    - moderate F17.200
      - in remission (early) (sustained) F17.201
    - severe F17.200
      - in remission (early) (sustained) F17.201
    - specified product NEC (mild) (moderate) (severe)
      - in remission (early) (sustained) F17.291
  - tooth K08.9
    - development K00.9
      - specified NEC K00.8
    - eruption K00.6
  - Tourette's F95.2
  - trance and possession F44.89
  - transvestic F65.1
  - trauma and stressor-related F43.9
    - other specified F43.8
  - tricuspid (valve) — *see* Endocarditis, tricuspid
  - tryptophan metabolism E70.5
  - tubular, phosphate-losing N25.0
  - tubulo-interstitial (in)
    - brucellosis A23.9 *[N16]*
    - cystinosis E72.04
    - diphtheria A36.84
    - glycogen storage disease E74.00 *[N16]*
    - leukemia NEC C95.9- *[N16]*
    - lymphoma NEC C85.9- *[N16]*
    - mixed cryoglobulinemia D89.1 *[N16]*
    - multiple myeloma C90.0- *[N16]*
    - Salmonella infection A02.25
    - sarcoidosis D86.84
    - sepsis A41.9 *[N16]*
      - streptococcal A40.9 *[N16]*
    - systemic lupus erythematosus M32.15
    - toxoplasmosis B58.83
    - transplant rejection T86.91 *[N16]*
    - Wilson's disease E83.01 *[N16]*
  - tubulo-renal function, impaired N25.9
    - specified NEC N25.89
  - tympanic membrane H73.9-
    - atrophy — *see* Atrophy, tympanic membrane
    - infection — *see* Myringitis
    - perforation — *see* Perforation, tympanum
    - specified NEC H73.89-
  - unsocialized aggressive F91.1
  - urea cycle metabolism E72.20
    - argininemia E72.21
    - arginosuccinic aciduria E72.22
    - citrullinemia E72.23
    - ornithine transcarbamylase deficiency E72.4
    - other specified E72.29
  - ureter (in) N28.9
    - schistosomiasis B65.0 *[N29]*
    - tuberculosis A18.11
  - urethra N36.9
    - specified NEC N36.8
  - urinary system N39.9
    - specified NEC N39.8
  - valve, heart
    - aortic — *see* Endocarditis, aortic

- **Disorder** (of) - *continued*
  - valve, heart - *continued*
    - mitral — *see* Endocarditis, mitral
    - pulmonary — *see* Endocarditis, pulmonary
    - rheumatic
      - aortic — *see* Endocarditis, aortic, rheumatic
      - mitral — *see* Endocarditis, mitral
      - pulmonary — *see* Endocarditis, pulmonary, rheumatic
      - tricuspid — *see* Endocarditis, tricuspid
    - tricuspid — *see* Endocarditis, tricuspid
  - vestibular function H81.9-
    - specified NEC — *see* subcategory H81.8
      - in diseases classified elsewhere H82.-
    - vertigo — *see* Vertigo
  - vision, binocular H53.30
    - abnormal retinal correspondence H53.31
    - diplopia H53.2
    - fusion with defective stereopsis H53.32
    - simultaneous perception H53.33
    - suppression H53.34
  - visual
    - cortex
      - blindness H47.619
        - left brain H47.612
        - right brain H47.611
      - due to
        - inflammatory disorder H47.629
          - left brain H47.622
          - right brain H47.621
        - neoplasm H47.639
          - left brain H47.632
          - right brain H47.631
        - vascular disorder H47.649
          - left brain H47.642
          - right brain H47.641
    - pathway H47.9
      - due to
        - inflammatory disorder H47.51-
        - neoplasm H47.52-
        - vascular disorder H47.53-
      - optic chiasm — *see* Disorder, optic, chiasm
  - vitreous body H43.9
    - crystalline deposits — *see* Deposit, crystalline
    - degeneration — *see* Degeneration, vitreous
    - hemorrhage — *see* Hemorrhage, vitreous
    - opacities — *see* Opacity, vitreous
    - prolapse — *see* Prolapse, vitreous
    - specified type NEC H43.89
  - voice R49.9
    - specified type NEC R49.8
  - volatile solvent use
    - due to drug abuse — *see* Abuse, drug, inhalant
    - due to drug dependence — *see* Dependence, drug, inhalant
  - voyeuristic F65.3
  - white blood cells D72.9
    - specified NEC D72.89
  - withdrawing, child or adolescent F40.10
- **Disorientation** R41.0
- **Displacement, displaced**
  - acquired traumatic of bone, cartilage, joint, tendon NEC — *see* Dislocation
  - adrenal gland (congenital) Q89.1
  - appendix, retrocecal (congenital) Q43.8
  - auricle (congenital) Q17.4
  - bladder (acquired) N32.89
    - congenital Q64.19
  - brachial plexus (congenital) Q07.8
  - brain stem, caudal (congenital) Q04.8
  - canaliculus (lacrimalis) , congenital Q10.6
  - cardia through esophageal hiatus (congenital) Q40.1
  - cerebellum, caudal (congenital) Q04.8
  - cervix — *see* Malposition, uterus
  - colon (congenital) Q43.3
  - device, implant or graft — *see also* Complications, by site and type, mechanical T85.628
    - arterial graft NEC — *see* Complication, cardiovascular device, mechanical, vascular
    - breast (implant) T85.42
    - catheter NEC T85.628
      - dialysis (renal) T82.42
        - intraperitoneal T85.621
      - infusion NEC T82.524
        - spinal (epidural) (subdural) T85.620
      - urinary
        - cystostomy T83.020
        - Hopkins T83.028
        - ileostomy T83.028
        - indwelling T83.021
        - nephrostomy T83.022
        - specified NEC T83.028
        - urostomy T83.028

- **Displacement, displaced** - *continued*
  - device, implant or graft - *continued*
    - electronic (electrode) (pulse generator) (stimulator) — *see* Complication, electronic stimulator
    - fixation, internal (orthopedic) NEC — *see* Complication, fixation device, mechanical
    - gastrointestinal — *see* Complications, prosthetic device, mechanical, gastrointestinal device
    - genital NEC T83.428
      - intrauterine contraceptive device (string) T83.32
      - penile prosthesis (cylinder) (implanted) (pump) (resevoir) T83.420
      - testicular prosthesis T83.421
    - heart NEC — *see* Complication, cardiovascular device, mechanical
    - joint prosthesis — *see* Complications, joint prosthesis, mechanical
    - ocular — *see* Complications, prosthetic device, mechanical, ocular device
    - orthopedic NEC — *see* Complication, orthopedic, device or graft, mechanical
    - specified NEC T85.628
    - urinary NEC T83.128
      - graft T83.22
      - sphincter, implanted T83.121
      - stent (ileal conduit) (nephroureteral) T83.123
        - ureteral indwelling T83.122
    - vascular NEC — *see* Complication, cardiovascular device, mechanical
    - ventricular intracranial shunt T85.02
  - electronic stimulator
    - bone T84.320
    - cardiac — *see* Complications, cardiac device, electronic
    - nervous system — *see* Complication, prosthetic device, mechanical, electronic nervous system stimulator
    - urinary — *see* Complications, electronic stimulator, urinary
  - esophageal mucosa into cardia of stomach, congenital Q39.8
  - esophagus (acquired) K22.8
    - congenital Q39.8
  - eyeball (acquired) (lateral) (old) — *see* Displacement, globe
    - congenital Q15.8
    - current — *see* Avulsion, eye
  - fallopian tube (acquired) N83.4-
    - congenital Q50.6
    - opening (congenital) Q50.6
  - gallbladder (congenital) Q44.1
  - gastric mucosa (congenital) Q40.2
  - globe (acquired) (old) (lateral) H05.21-
    - current — *see* Avulsion, eye
  - heart (congenital) Q24.8
    - acquired I51.89
  - hymen (upward) (congenital) Q52.4
  - intervertebral disc NEC
    - with myelopathy — *see* Disorder, disc, with, myelopathy
    - cervical, cervicothoracic (with) M50.20
      - myelopathy — *see* Disorder, disc, cervical, with myelopathy
      - neuritis, radiculitis or radiculopathy — *see* Disorder, disc, cervical, with neuritis
    - due to trauma — *see* Dislocation, vertebra
    - lumbar region M51.26
      - with
        - myelopathy M51.06
        - neuritis, radiculitis, radiculopathy or sciatica M51.16
    - lumbosacral region M51.27
      - with
        - neuritis, radiculitis, radiculopathy or sciatica M51.17
    - sacrococcygeal region M53.3
    - thoracic region M51.24
      - with
        - myelopathy M51.04
        - neuritis, radiculitis, radiculopathy M51.14
    - thoracolumbar region M51.25
      - with
        - myelopathy M51.05
        - neuritis, radiculitis, radiculopathy M51.15
  - intrauterine device (string) T83.32
  - kidney (acquired) N28.83
    - congenital Q63.2
  - lachrymal, lacrimal apparatus or duct (congenital) Q10.6
  - lens, congenital Q12.1
  - macula (congenital) Q14.1
  - Meckel's diverticulum Q43.0

Displacement, displaced - *continued*
- Meckel's diverticulum - *continued*
  - malignant — *see* Table of Neoplasms, small intestine, malignant
- nail (congenital) Q84.6
  - acquired L60.8
- opening of Wharton's duct in mouth Q38.4
- organ or site, congenital NEC — *see* Malposition, congenital
- ovary (acquired) N83.4-
  - congenital Q50.39
  - free in peritoneal cavity (congenital) Q50.39
  - into hernial sac N83.4-
- oviduct (acquired) N83.4-
  - congenital Q50.6
- parathyroid (gland) E21.4
- parotid gland (congenital) Q38.4
- punctum lacrimale (congenital) Q10.6
- sacro-iliac (joint) (congenital) Q74.2
  - current injury S33.2
  - old — *see* subcategory M53.2
- salivary gland (any) (congenital) Q38.4
- spleen (congenital) Q89.09
- stomach, congenital Q40.2
- sublingual duct Q38.4
- tongue (downward) (congenital) Q38.3
- tooth, teeth, fully erupted M26.30
  - horizontal M26.33
  - vertical M26.34
- trachea (congenital) Q32.1
- ureter or ureteric opening or orifice (congenital) Q62.62
- uterine opening of oviducts or fallopian tubes Q50.6
- uterus, uterine — *see* Malposition, uterus
- ventricular septum Q21.0
  - with rudimentary ventricle Q20.4

Disproportion
- between native and reconstructed breast N65.1
- fiber-type G71.2

Disruptio uteri — *see* Rupture, uterus

Disruption (of)
- ciliary body NEC H21.89
- closure of
  - cornea T81.31
  - craniotomy T81.32
  - fascia (muscular) (superficial) T81.32
  - internal organ or tissue T81.32
  - laceration (external) (internal) T81.33
  - ligament T81.32
  - mucosa T81.31
  - muscle or muscle flap T81.32
  - ribs or rib cage T81.32
  - skin and subcutaneous tissue (full-thickness) (superficial) T81.31
  - skull T81.32
  - sternum (sternotomy) T81.32
  - tendon T81.32
  - traumatic laceration (external) (internal) T81.33
- family Z63.8
  - due to
    - absence of family member due to military deployment Z63.31
    - absence of family member NEC Z63.32
    - alcoholism and drug addiction in family Z63.72
    - bereavement Z63.4
    - death (assumed) or disappearance of family member Z63.4
    - divorce or separation Z63.5
    - drug addiction in family Z63.72
    - return of family member from military deployment (current or past conflict) Z63.71
    - stressful life events NEC Z63.79
- iris NEC H21.89
- ligament (s) — *see also* Sprain
  - knee
    - current injury — *see* Dislocation, knee
    - old (chronic) — *see* Derangement, knee, ligament, instability, chronic
    - spontaneous NEC — *see* Derangement, knee, disruption ligament
- ossicular chain — *see* Discontinuity, ossicles, ear
- pelvic ring (stable) S32.810
  - unstable S32.811
- wound T81.30
  - episiotomy O90.1
  - operation T81.31
    - cesarean O90.0
    - external operation wound (superficial) T81.31
    - internal operation wound (deep) T81.32
  - perineal (obstetric) O90.1
  - traumatic injury repair T81.33
- traumatic injury wound repair T81.33

Dissatisfaction with
- employment Z56.9
- school environment Z55.4

Dissecting — *see* condition

Dissection
- aorta I71.00
  - abdominal I71.02
  - thoracic I71.01
  - thoracoabdominal I71.03
- artery I77.70
  - basilar (trunk) I77.75
  - carotid I77.71
  - cerebral (nonruptured) I67.0
    - ruptured — *see* Hemorrhage, intracranial, subarachnoid
  - coronary I25.42
  - extremity
    - lower I77.77
    - upper I77.76
  - iliac I77.72
  - precerebral
    - congenital (nonruptured) Q28.1
    - specified site NEC I77.75
  - renal I77.73
  - specified NEC I77.79
  - vertebral I77.74
- precerebral artery, congenital (nonruptured) Q28.1
  - Heartland A93.8
- traumatic — *see* Wound, open, by site
- vascular I99.8
- wound — *see* Wound, open

Disseminated — *see* condition

Dissociation
- auriculoventricular or atrioventricular (AV) (any degree) (isorhythmic) I45.89
  - with heart block I44.2
- interference I45.89

Dissociative reaction, state F44.9

Dissolution, vertebra — *see* Osteoporosis

Distension, distention
- abdomen R14.0
- bladder N32.89
- cecum K63.89
- colon K63.89
- gallbladder K82.8
- intestine K63.89
- kidney N28.89
- liver K76.89
- seminal vesicle N50.89
- stomach K31.89
  - acute K31.0
  - psychogenic F45.8
- ureter — *see* Dilatation, ureter
- uterus N85.8

Distoma hepaticum infestation B66.3

Distomiasis B66.9
- bile passages B66.3
- hemic B65.9
- hepatic B66.3
  - due to Clonorchis sinensis B66.1
- intestinal B66.5
- liver B66.3
  - due to Clonorchis sinensis B66.1
- lung B66.4
- pulmonary B66.4

Distomolar (fourth molar) K00.1

Disto-occlusion (Division I) (Division II) M26.212

Distortion (s) (congenital)
- adrenal (gland) Q89.1
- arm NEC Q68.8
- bile duct or passage Q44.5
- bladder Q64.79
- brain Q04.9
- cervix (uteri) Q51.9
- chest (wall) Q67.8
  - bones Q76.8
- clavicle Q74.0
- clitoris Q52.6
- coccyx Q76.49
- common duct Q44.5
- coronary Q24.5
- cystic duct Q44.5
- ear (auricle) (external) Q17.3
  - inner Q16.5
  - middle Q16.4
    - ossicles Q16.3
- endocrine NEC Q89.2
- eustachian tube Q17.8
- eye (adnexa) Q15.8
- face bone (s) NEC Q75.8
- fallopian tube Q50.6
- femur NEC Q68.8
- fibula NEC Q68.8

Distortion (s) (congenital) - *continued*
- finger (s) Q68.1
- foot Q66.9
- genitalia, genital organ (s)
  - female Q52.8
    - external Q52.79
    - internal NEC Q52.8
- gyri Q04.8
- hand bone (s) Q68.1
- heart (auricle) (ventricle) Q24.8
  - valve (cusp) Q24.8
- hepatic duct Q44.5
- humerus NEC Q68.8
- hymen Q52.4
- intrafamilial communications Z63.8
- jaw NEC M26.89
- labium (majus) (minus) Q52.79
- leg NEC Q68.8
- lens Q12.8
- liver Q44.7
- lumbar spine Q76.49
  - with disproportion O33.8
    - causing obstructed labor O65.0
- lumbosacral (joint) (region) Q76.49
  - kyphosis — *see* Kyphosis, congenital
  - lordosis — *see* Lordosis, congenital
- nerve Q07.8
- nose Q30.8
- organ
  - of Corti Q16.5
  - or site not listed — *see* Anomaly, by site
- ossicles, ear Q16.3
- oviduct Q50.6
- pancreas Q45.3
- parathyroid (gland) Q89.2
- pituitary (gland) Q89.2
- radius NEC Q68.8
- sacroiliac joint Q74.2
- sacrum Q76.49
- scapula Q74.0
- shoulder girdle Q74.0
- skull bone (s) NEC Q75.8
  - with
    - anencephalus Q00.0
    - encephalocele — *see* Encephalocele
    - hydrocephalus Q03.9
      - with spina bifida — *see* Spina bifida, with hydrocephalus
    - microcephaly Q02
- spinal cord Q06.8
- spine Q76.49
  - kyphosis — *see* Kyphosis, congenital
  - lordosis — *see* Lordosis, congenital
- spleen Q89.09
- sternum NEC Q76.7
- thorax (wall) Q67.8
  - bony Q76.8
- thymus (gland) Q89.2
- thyroid (gland) Q89.2
- tibia NEC Q68.8
- toe (s) Q66.9
- tongue Q38.3
- trachea (cartilage) Q32.1
- ulna NEC Q68.8
- ureter Q62.8
- urethra Q64.79
  - causing obstruction Q64.39
- uterus Q51.9
- vagina Q52.4
- vertebra Q76.49
  - kyphosis — *see* Kyphosis, congenital
  - lordosis — *see* Lordosis, congenital
- visual — *see also* Disturbance, vision
  - shape and size H53.15
- vulva Q52.79
- wrist (bones) (joint) Q68.8

Distress
- abdomen — *see* Pain, abdominal
- acute respiratory R06.03
  - syndrome (adult) (child) J80
- epigastric R10.13
- fetal P84
  - complicating pregnancy — *see* Stress, fetal
- gastrointestinal (functional) K30
  - psychogenic F45.8
- intestinal (functional) NOS K59.9
  - psychogenic F45.8
- maternal, during labor and delivery O75.0
- relationship, with spouse or intimate partner Z63.0
- respiratory (adult) (child) R06.03
  - newborn P22.9
    - specified NEC P22.8
  - orthopnea R06.01

- **Distress** - *continued*
  - respiratory (adult) (child) - *continued*
    - psychogenic F45.8
    - shortness of breath R06.02
    - specified type NEC R06.09
- **Distribution vessel, atypical** Q27.9
  - coronary artery Q24.5
  - precerebral Q28.1
- **Districhiasis** L68.8
- **Disturbance** (s) — *see also* Disease
  - absorption K90.9
    - calcium E58
    - carbohydrate K90.49
    - fat K90.49
      - pancreatic K90.3
    - protein K90.49
    - starch K90.49
    - vitamin — *see* Deficiency, vitamin
  - acid-base equilibrium E87.8
    - mixed E87.4
  - activity and attention (with hyperkinesis) — *see* Disorder, attention-deficit hyperactivity
  - amino acid transport E72.00
  - assimilation, food K90.9
  - auditory nerve, except deafness — *see* subcategory H93.3
  - behavior — *see* Disorder, conduct
  - blood clotting (mechanism) — *see also* Defect, coagulation D68.9
  - cerebral
    - nerve — *see* Disorder, nerve, cranial
    - status, newborn P91.9
      - specified NEC P91.88
  - circulatory I99.9
  - conduct — *see also* Disorder, conduct F91.9
    - adjustment reaction — *see* Disorder, adjustment
    - compulsive F63.9
    - disruptive F91.9
    - hyperkinetic — *see* Disorder, attention-deficit hyperactivity
    - socialized F91.2
    - specified NEC F91.8
    - unsocialized F91.1
  - coordination R27.8
  - cranial nerve — *see* Disorder, nerve, cranial
  - deep sensibility — *see* Disturbance, sensation
  - digestive K30
    - psychogenic F45.8
  - electrolyte — *see also* Imbalance, electrolyte
    - newborn, transitory P74.49
      - hyperammonemia P74.6
      - hyperchloremia P74.421
      - hyperchloremic metabolic acidosis P74.421
      - hypochloremia P74.422
      - potassium balance
        - hyperkalemia P74.31
        - hypokalemia P74.32
      - sodium balance
        - hypernatremia P74.21
        - hyponatremia P74.22
      - specified type NEC P74.49
  - emotions specific to childhood and adolescence F93.9
    - with
      - anxiety and fearfulness NEC F93.8
      - elective mutism F94.0
      - oppositional disorder F91.3
      - sensitivity (withdrawal) F40.10
      - shyness F40.10
      - social withdrawal F40.10
    - involving relationship problems F93.8
    - mixed F93.8
    - specified NEC F93.8
  - endocrine (gland) E34.9
    - neonatal, transitory P72.9
      - specified NEC P72.8
  - equilibrium R42
  - fructose metabolism E74.10
  - gait — *see* Gait
    - hysterical F44.4
    - psychogenic F44.4
  - gastrointestinal (functional) K30
    - psychogenic F45.8
  - habit, child F98.9
  - hearing, except deafness and tinnitus — *see* Abnormal, auditory perception
  - heart, functional (conditions in I44-I50)
    - due to presence of (cardiac) prosthesis I97.19-
    - postoperative I97.89
      - cardiac surgery — *see also* Infarct, myocardium, associated with revascularization procedure I97.19-
  - hormones E34.9

- **Disturbance** (s) - *continued*
  - innervation uterus (parasympathetic) (sympathetic) N85.8
  - keratinization NEC
    - gingiva K05.10
      - nonplaque induced K05.11
      - plaque induced K05.10
    - lip K13.0
    - oral (mucosa) (soft tissue) K13.29
    - tongue K13.29
  - learning (specific) — *see* Disorder, learning
  - memory — *see* Amnesia
    - mild, following organic brain damage F06.8
  - mental F99
    - associated with diseases classified elsewhere F54
  - metabolism E88.9
    - with
      - abortion — *see* Abortion, by type with other specified complication
      - ectopic pregnancy O08.5
      - molar pregnancy O08.5
    - amino-acid E72.9
      - aromatic E70.9
      - branched-chain E71.2
      - straight-chain E72.89
      - sulfur-bearing E72.10
    - ammonia E72.20
    - arginine E72.21
    - arginosuccinic acid E72.22
    - carbohydrate E74.9
    - cholesterol E78.9
    - citrulline E72.23
    - cystathionine E72.19
    - general E88.9
    - glutamine E72.89
    - histidine E70.40
    - homocystine E72.19
    - hydroxylysine E72.3
    - in labor or delivery O75.89
    - iron E83.10
    - lipoid E78.9
    - lysine E72.3
    - methionine E72.19
    - neonatal, transitory P74.9
      - calcium and magnesium P71.9
        - specified type NEC P71.8
      - carbohydrate metabolism P70.9
        - specified type NEC P70.8
      - specified NEC P74.8
    - ornithine E72.4
    - phosphate E83.39
    - sodium NEC E87.8
    - threonine E72.89
    - tryptophan E70.5
    - tyrosine E70.20
    - urea cycle E72.20
  - motor R29.2
  - nervous, functional R45.0
  - neuromuscular mechanism (eye) , due to syphilis A52.15
  - nutritional E63.9
    - nail L60.3
  - ocular motion H51.9
    - psychogenic F45.8
  - oculogyric H51.8
    - psychogenic F45.8
  - oculomotor H51.9
    - psychogenic F45.8
  - olfactory nerve R43.1
  - optic nerve NEC — *see* Disorder, nerve, optic
  - oral epithelium, including tongue NEC K13.29
  - perceptual due to
    - alcohol withdrawal F10.232
    - amphetamine intoxication F15.922
      - in
        - abuse F15.122
        - dependence F15.222
    - anxiolytic withdrawal F13.232
    - cannabis intoxication (acute) F12.922
      - in
        - abuse F12.122
        - dependence F12.222
    - cocaine intoxication (acute) F14.922
      - in
        - abuse F14.122
        - dependence F14.222
    - hypnotic withdrawal F13.232
    - opioid intoxication (acute) F11.922
      - in
        - abuse F11.122
        - dependence F11.222
    - phencyclidine intoxication (acute) F16.122
    - sedative withdrawal F13.232

- **Disturbance** (s) - *continued*
  - personality (pattern) (trait) — *see also* Disorder, personality F60.9
    - following organic brain damage F07.9
  - polyglandular E31.9
    - specified NEC E31.8
  - potassium balance, newborn
    - hyperkalemia P74.31
    - hypokalemia P74.32
  - psychogenic F45.9
  - psychomotor F44.4
  - psychophysical visual H53.16
  - pupillary — *see* Anomaly, pupil, function
  - reflex R29.2
  - rhythm, heart I49.9
  - salivary secretion K11.7
  - sensation (cold) (heat) (localization) (tactile discrimination) (texture) (vibratory) NEC R20.9
    - hysterical F44.6
    - skin R20.9
      - anesthesia R20.0
      - hyperesthesia R20.3
      - hypoesthesia R20.1
      - paresthesia R20.2
      - specified type NEC R20.8
    - smell R43.9
      - and taste (mixed) R43.8
      - anosmia R43.0
      - parosmia R43.1
      - specified NEC R43.8
    - taste R43.9
      - and smell (mixed) R43.8
      - parageusia R43.2
      - specified NEC R43.8
  - sensory — *see* Disturbance, sensation
  - situational (transient) — *see also* Disorder, adjustment
    - acute F43.0
  - sleep G47.9
    - nonorganic origin F51.9
  - smell — *see* Disturbance, sensation, smell
  - sociopathic F60.2
  - sodium balance, newborn
    - hypernatremia P74.21
    - hyponatremia P74.22
  - speech R47.9
    - developmental F80.9
    - specified NEC R47.89
  - stomach (functional) K31.9
  - sympathetic (nerve) G90.9
  - taste — *see* Disturbance, sensation, taste
  - temperature
    - regulation, newborn P81.9
      - specified NEC P81.8
    - sense R20.8
      - hysterical F44.6
  - tooth
    - eruption K00.6
    - formation K00.4
    - structure, hereditary NEC K00.5
  - touch — *see* Disturbance, sensation
  - vascular I99.9
    - arteriosclerotic — *see* Arteriosclerosis
  - vasomotor I73.9
  - vasospastic I73.9
  - vision, visual H53.9
    - following
      - cerebral infarction I69.398
      - cerebrovascular disease I69.998
        - specified NEC I69.898
      - intracerebral hemorrhage I69.198
      - nontraumatic intracranial hemorrhage NEC I69.298
      - specified disease NEC I69.898
      - subarachnoid hemorrhage I69.098
    - psychophysical H53.16
    - specified NEC H53.8
    - subjective H53.10
      - day blindness H53.11
      - discomfort H53.14-
      - distortions of shape and size H53.15
      - loss
        - sudden H53.13-
        - transient H53.12-
      - specified type NEC H53.19
  - voice R49.9
    - psychogenic F44.4
    - specified NEC R49.8
- **Diuresis** R35.8
- **Diver's palsy, paralysis or squeeze** T70.3
- **Diverticulitis** (acute) K57.92
  - bladder — *see* Cystitis
  - ileum — *see* Diverticulitis, intestine, small

Diverticulitis (acute) - *continued*
- intestine K57.92
  - with
    - abscess, perforation or peritonitis K57.80
      - with bleeding K57.81
    - bleeding K57.93
  - congenital Q43.8
  - large K57.32
    - with
      - abscess, perforation or peritonitis K57.20
        - with bleeding K57.21
      - bleeding K57.33
      - small intestine K57.52
        - with
          - abscess, perforation or peritonitis K57.40
            - with bleeding K57.41
          - bleeding K57.53
  - small K57.12
    - with
      - abscess, perforation or peritonitis K57.00
        - with bleeding K57.01
      - bleeding K57.13
      - large intestine K57.52
        - with
          - abscess, perforation or peritonitis K57.40
            - with bleeding K57.41
          - bleeding K57.53

Diverticulosis K57.90
- with bleeding K57.91
- large intestine K57.30
  - with
    - bleeding K57.31
    - small intestine K57.50
      - with bleeding K57.51
- small intestine K57.10
  - with
    - bleeding K57.11
    - large intestine K57.50
      - with bleeding K57.51

Diverticulum, diverticula (multiple) K57.90
- appendix (noninflammatory) K38.2
- bladder (sphincter) N32.3
  - congenital Q64.6
- bronchus (congenital) Q32.4
  - acquired J98.09
- calyx, calyceal (kidney) N28.89
- cardia (stomach) K31.4
- cecum — *see* Diverticulosis, intestine, large
  - congenital Q43.8
- colon — *see* Diverticulosis, intestine, large
  - congenital Q43.8
- duodenum — *see* Diverticulosis, intestine, small
  - congenital Q43.8
- epiphrenic (esophagus) K22.5
- esophagus (congenital) Q39.6
  - acquired (epiphrenic) (pulsion) (traction) K22.5
- eustachian tube — *see* Disorder, eustachian tube, specified NEC
- fallopian tube N83.8
- gastric K31.4
- heart (congenital) Q24.8
- ileum — *see* Diverticulosis, intestine, small
- jejunum — *see* Diverticulosis, intestine, small
- kidney (pelvis) (calyces) N28.89
  - with calculus — *see* Calculus, kidney
- Meckel's (displaced) (hypertrophic) Q43.0
  - malignant — *see* Table of Neoplasms, small intestine, malignant
- midthoracic K22.5
- organ or site, congenital NEC — *see* Distortion
- pericardium (congenital) (cyst) Q24.8
  - acquired I31.8
- pharyngoesophageal (congenital) Q39.6
  - acquired K22.5
- pharynx (congenital) Q38.7
- rectosigmoid — *see* Diverticulosis, intestine, large
  - congenital Q43.8
- rectum — *see* Diverticulosis, intestine, large
- Rokitansky's K22.5
- seminal vesicle N50.89
- sigmoid — *see* Diverticulosis, intestine, large
  - congenital Q43.8
- stomach (acquired) K31.4
  - congenital Q40.2
- trachea (acquired) J39.8
- ureter (acquired) N28.89
  - congenital Q62.8
- ureterovesical orifice N28.89
- urethra (acquired) N36.1
  - congenital Q64.79
- ventricle, left (congenital) Q24.8
- vesical N32.3
  - congenital Q64.6

Diverticulum, diverticula (multiple) - *continued*
- Zenker's (esophagus) K22.5

Division
- cervix uteri (acquired) N88.8
- glans penis Q55.69
- labia minora (congenital) Q52.79
- ligament (partial or complete) (current) — *see also* Sprain
  - with open wound — *see* Wound, open
- muscle (partial or complete) (current) — *see also* Injury, muscle
  - with open wound — *see* Wound, open
- nerve (traumatic) — *see* Injury, nerve
- spinal cord — *see* Injury, spinal cord, by region
- vein I87.8

Divorce, causing family disruption Z63.5

Dix-Hallpike neurolabyrinthitis — *see* Neuronitis, vestibular

Dizziness R42
- hysterical F44.89
- psychogenic F45.8

DMAC (disseminated mycobacterium avium-intracellulare complex) A31.2

DNR (do not resuscitate) Z66

Doan-Wiseman syndrome (primary splenic neutropenia) — *see* Agranulocytosis

Doehle-Heller aortitis A52.02

Dog bite — *see* Bite

Dohle body panmyelopathic syndrome D72.0

Dolichocephaly Q67.2

Dolichocolon Q43.8

Dolichostenomelia — *see* Syndrome, Marfan's

Donohue's syndrome E34.8

Donor (organ or tissue) Z52.9
- blood (whole) Z52.000
  - autologous Z52.010
  - specified component (lymphocytes) (platelets) NEC Z52.008
    - autologous Z52.018
    - specified donor NEC Z52.098
  - specified donor NEC Z52.090
  - stem cells Z52.001
    - autologous Z52.011
    - specified donor NEC Z52.091
- bone Z52.20
  - autologous Z52.21
  - marrow Z52.3
  - specified type NEC Z52.29
- cornea Z52.5
- egg (Oocyte) Z52.819
  - age 35 and over Z52.812
    - anonymous recipient Z52.812
    - designated recipient Z52.813
  - under age 35 Z52.810
    - anonymous recipient Z52.810
    - designated recipient Z52.811
- kidney Z52.4
- liver Z52.6
- lung Z52.89
- lymphocyte — *see* Donor, blood, specified components NEC
- Oocyte — *see* Donor, egg
- platelets Z52.008
- potential, examination of Z00.5
- semen Z52.89
- skin Z52.10
  - autologous Z52.11
  - specified type NEC Z52.19
- specified organ or tissue NEC Z52.89
- sperm Z52.89

Donovanosis A58

Dorsalgia M54.9
- psychogenic F45.41
- specified NEC M54.89

Dorsopathy M53.9
- deforming M43.9
  - specified NEC — *see* subcategory M43.8
- specified NEC M53.80
  - cervical region M53.82
  - cervicothoracic region M53.83
  - lumbar region M53.86
  - lumbosacral region M53.87
  - occipito-atlanto-axial region M53.81
  - sacrococcygeal region M53.88
  - thoracic region M53.84
  - thoracolumbar region M53.85

Double
- albumin E88.09
- aortic arch Q25.45
- auditory canal Q17.8
- auricle (heart) Q20.8

Double - *continued*
- bladder Q64.79
- cervix Q51.820
  - with doubling of uterus (and vagina) Q51.10
    - with obstruction Q51.11
- inlet ventricle Q20.4
- kidney with double pelvis (renal) Q63.0
- meatus urinarius Q64.75
- monster Q89.4
- outlet
  - left ventricle Q20.2
  - right ventricle Q20.1
- pelvis (renal) with double ureter Q62.5
- tongue Q38.3
- ureter (one or both sides) Q62.5
  - with double pelvis (renal) Q62.5
- urethra Q64.74
- urinary meatus Q64.75
- uterus Q51.20
  - with
    - doubling of cervix (and vagina) Q51.10
      - with obstruction Q51.11
  - complete Q51.21
  - in pregnancy or childbirth O34.59-
    - causing obstructed labor O65.5
  - partial Q51.22
  - specified NEC Q51.28
- vagina Q52.10
  - with doubling of uterus (and cervix) Q51.10
    - with obstruction Q51.11
- vision H53.2
- vulva Q52.79

Douglas' pouch, cul-de-sac — *see* condition

Down syndrome Q90.9
- meiotic nondisjunction Q90.0
- mitotic nondisjunction Q90.1
- mosaicism Q90.1
- translocation Q90.2

DPD (dihydropyrimidine dehydrogenase deficiency) E88.89

Dracontiasis B72

Dracunculiasis, dracunculosis B72

Dream state, hysterical F44.89

Drepanocytic anemia — *see* Disease, sickle-cell

Dresbach's syndrome (elliptocytosis) D58.1

Dreschlera (hawaiiensis) (infection) B43.8

Dressler's syndrome I24.1

Drift, ulnar — *see* Deformity, limb, specified type NEC, forearm

Drinking (alcohol)
- excessive, to excess NEC (without dependence) F10.10
  - habitual (continual) (without remission) F10.20
    - with remission F10.21

Drip, postnasal (chronic) R09.82
- due to
  - allergic rhinitis — *see* Rhinitis, allergic
  - common cold J00
  - gastroesophageal reflux — *see* Reflux, gastroesophageal
  - nasopharyngitis — *see* Nasopharyngitis
  - other know condition - code to condition
  - sinusitis — *see* Sinusitis

Droop
- facial R29.810
  - cerebrovascular disease I69.992
    - cerebral infarction I69.392
    - intracerebral hemorrhage I69.192
    - nontraumatic intracranial hemorrhage NEC I69.292
    - specified disease NEC I69.892
    - subarachnoid hemorrhage I69.092

Drop (in)
- attack NEC R55
- finger — *see* Deformity, finger
- foot — *see* Deformity, limb, foot, drop
- hematocrit (precipitous) R71.0
- hemoglobin R71.0
- toe — *see* Deformity, toe, specified NEC
- wrist — *see* Deformity, limb, wrist drop

Dropped heart beats I45.9

Dropsy, dropsical — *see also* Hydrops
- abdomen R18.8
- brain — *see* Hydrocephalus
- cardiac, heart — *see* Failure, heart, congestive
- gangrenous — *see* Gangrene
- heart — *see* Failure, heart, congestive
- kidney — *see* Nephrosis
- lung — *see* Edema, lung
- newborn due to isoimmunization P56.0
- pericardium — *see* Pericarditis

Drowned, drowning (near) T75.1

Drowsiness R40.0

- **Dysphagia** R13.10
  - cervical R13.19
  - following
    - cerebral infarction I69.391
    - cerebrovascular disease I69.991
      - specified NEC I69.891
    - intracerebral hemorrhage I69.191
    - nontraumatic intracranial hemorrhage NEC I69.291
    - specified disease NEC I69.891
    - subarachnoid hemorrhage I69.091
  - functional (hysterical) F45.8
  - hysterical F45.8
  - nervous (hysterical) F45.8
  - neurogenic R13.19
  - oral phase R13.11
  - oropharyngeal phase R13.12
  - pharyngeal phase R13.13
  - pharyngoesophageal phase R13.14
  - psychogenic F45.8
  - sideropenic D50.1
  - spastica K22.4
  - specified NEC R13.19
- **Dysphagocytosis, congenital** D71
- **Dysphasia** R47.02
  - developmental
    - expressive type F80.1
    - receptive type F80.2
  - following
    - cerebrovascular disease I69.921
      - cerebral infarction I69.321
      - intracerebral hemorrhage I69.121
      - nontraumatic intracranial hemorrhage NEC I69.221
      - specified disease NEC I69.821
      - subarachnoid hemorrhage I69.021
- **Dysphonia** R49.0
  - functional F44.4
  - hysterical F44.4
  - psychogenic F44.4
  - spastica J38.3
- **Dysphoria**
  - gender F64.9
    - in
      - adolescence and adulthood F64.0
      - children F64.2
    - specified NEC F64.8
  - postpartal O90.6
- **Dyspituitarism** E23.3
- **Dysplasia** — *see also* Anomaly
  - acetabular, congenital Q65.89
  - alveolar capillary, with vein misalignment J84.843
  - anus (histologically confirmed) (mild) (moderate) K62.82
    - severe D01.3
  - arrhythmogenic right ventricular I42.8
  - arterial, fibromuscular I77.3
  - asphyxiating thoracic (congenital) Q77.2
  - brain Q07.9
  - bronchopulmonary, perinatal P27.1
  - cervix (uteri) N87.9
    - mild N87.0
    - moderate N87.1
    - severe D06.9
  - chondroectodermal Q77.6
  - colon D12.6
  - craniometaphyseal Q78.8
  - dentinal K00.5
  - diaphyseal, progressive Q78.3
  - dystrophic Q77.5
  - ectodermal (anhidrotic) (congenital) (hereditary) Q82.4
    - hydrotic Q82.8
  - epithelial, uterine cervix — *see* Dysplasia, cervix
  - eye (congenital) Q11.2
  - fibrous
    - bone NEC (monostotic) M85.00
      - ankle M85.07-
      - foot M85.07-
      - forearm M85.03-
      - hand M85.04-
      - lower leg M85.06-
      - multiple site M85.09
      - neck M85.08
      - rib M85.08
      - shoulder M85.01-
      - skull M85.08
      - specified site NEC M85.08
      - thigh M85.05-
      - toe M85.07-
      - upper arm M85.02-
      - vertebra M85.08
    - diaphyseal, progressive Q78.3

- **Dysplasia** - *continued*
  - fibrous - *continued*
    - jaw M27.8
    - polyostotic Q78.1
  - florid osseous — *see also* Cyst, calcifying odontogenic
  - high grade, focal D12.6
  - hip, congenital Q65.89
  - joint, congenital Q74.8
  - kidney Q61.4
    - multicystic Q61.4
  - leg Q74.2
  - lung, congenital (not associated with short gestation) Q33.6
  - mammary (gland) (benign) N60.9-
    - cyst (solitary) — *see* Cyst, breast
    - cystic — *see* Mastopathy, cystic
    - duct ectasia — *see* Ectasia, mammary duct
    - fibroadenosis — *see* Fibroadenosis, breast
    - fibrosclerosis — *see* Fibrosclerosis, breast
    - specified type NEC N60.8-
  - metaphyseal Q78.5
  - muscle Q79.8
  - oculodentodigital Q87.0
  - periapical (cemental) (cemento-osseous) — *see* Cyst, calcifying odontogenic
  - periosteum — *see* Disorder, bone, specified type NEC
  - polyostotic fibrous Q78.1
  - prostate — *see also* Neoplasia, intraepithelial, prostate N42.30
    - severe D07.5
    - specified NEC N42.39
  - renal Q61.4
    - multicystic Q61.4
  - retinal, congenital Q14.1
  - right ventricular, arrhythmogenic I42.8
  - septo-optic Q04.4
  - skin L98.8
  - spinal cord Q06.1
  - spondyloepiphyseal Q77.7
  - thymic, with immunodeficiency D82.1
  - vagina N89.3
    - mild N89.0
    - moderate N89.1
    - severe NEC D07.2
  - vulva N90.3
    - mild N90.0
    - moderate N90.1
    - severe NEC D07.1
- **Dysplasminogenemia** E88.02
- **Dyspnea** (nocturnal) (paroxysmal) R06.00
  - asthmatic (bronchial) J45.909
    - with
      - exacerbation (acute) J45.901
      - bronchitis J45.909
        - with
          - exacerbation (acute) J45.901
          - status asthmaticus J45.902
        - chronic J44.9
      - status asthmaticus J45.902
    - cardiac — *see* Failure, ventricular, left
  - cardiac — *see* Failure, ventricular, left
  - functional F45.8
  - hyperventilation R06.4
  - hysterical F45.8
  - newborn P28.89
  - orthopnea R06.01
  - psychogenic F45.8
  - shortness of breath R06.02
  - specified type NEC R06.09
- **Dyspraxia** R27.8
  - developmental (syndrome) F82
- **Dysproteinemia** E88.09
- **Dysreflexia, autonomic** G90.4
- **Dysrhythmia**
  - cardiac I49.9
    - newborn
      - bradycardia P29.12
      - occurring before birth P03.819
        - before onset of labor P03.810
        - during labor P03.811
      - tachycardia P29.11
    - postoperative I97.89
  - cerebral or cortical — *see* Epilepsy
- **Dyssomnia** — *see* Disorder, sleep
- **Dyssynergia**
  - biliary K83.8
  - bladder sphincter N36.44
  - cerebellaris myoclonica (Hunt's ataxia) G11.1
- **Dysthymia** F34.1
- **Dysthyroidism** E07.9

- **Dystocia** O66.9
  - affecting newborn P03.1
  - cervical (hypotonic) O62.2
    - affecting newborn P03.6
    - primary O62.0
    - secondary O62.1
  - contraction ring O62.4
  - fetal O66.9
    - abnormality NEC O66.3
    - conjoined twins O66.3
    - oversize O66.2
  - maternal O66.9
  - positional O64.9
  - shoulder (girdle) O66.0
    - causing obstructed labor O66.0
  - uterine NEC O62.4
- **Dystonia** G24.9
  - cervical G24.3
  - deformans progressiva G24.1
  - drug induced NEC G24.09
    - acute G24.02
    - specified NEC G24.09
  - familial G24.1
  - idiopathic G24.1
    - familial G24.1
    - nonfamilial G24.2
    - orofacial G24.4
  - lenticularis G24.8
  - musculorum deformans G24.1
  - neuroleptic induced (acute) G24.02
  - orofacial (idiopathic) G24.4
  - oromandibular G24.4
    - due to drug G24.01
  - specified NEC G24.8
  - torsion (familial) (idiopathic) G24.1
    - acquired G24.8
    - genetic G24.1
    - symptomatic (nonfamilial) G24.2
- **Dystonic movements** R25.8
- **Dystrophy, dystrophia**
  - adiposogenital E23.6
  - autosomal recessive, childhood type, muscular dystrophy resembling Duchenne or Becker G71.01
  - Becker's type G71.01
  - cervical sympathetic G90.2
  - choroid (hereditary) H31.20
    - central areolar H31.22
    - choroideremia H31.21
    - gyrate atrophy H31.23
    - specified type NEC H31.29
  - cornea (hereditary) H18.50
    - endothelial H18.51
    - epithelial H18.52
    - granular H18.53
    - lattice H18.54
    - macular H18.55
    - specified type NEC H18.59
  - Duchenne's type G71.01
  - due to malnutrition E45
  - Erb's G71.02
  - Fuchs' H18.51
  - Gower's muscular G71.01
  - hair L67.8
  - infantile neuraxonal G31.89
  - Landouzy-Déjérine G71.02
  - Leyden-Möbius G71.09
  - muscular G71.00
    - autosomal recessive, childhood type, muscular dystrophy resembling Duchenne or Becker G71.01
    - benign (Becker type) G71.01
      - scapuloperoneal with early contractures [Emery-Dreifuss] G71.09
    - congenital (hereditary) (progressive) (with specific morphological abnormalities of the muscle fiber) G71.09
      - myotonic G71.11
    - distal G71.09
    - Duchenne type G71.01
    - Emery-Dreifuss G71.09
    - Erb type G71.02
    - facioscapulohumeral G71.02
    - Gower's G71.01
    - hereditary (progressive) G71.09
    - Landouzy-Déjérine type G71.02
    - limb-girdle G71.09
    - myotonic G71.11
    - progressive (hereditary) G71.09
      - Charcot-Marie (-Tooth) type G60.0
    - pseudohypertrophic (infantile) G71.01
    - scapulohumeral G71.02
    - scapuloperoneal G71.09
    - severe (Duchenne type) G71.01

Dystrophy, dystrophia - *continued*
muscular - *continued*
specified type NEC G71.09
myocardium, myocardial — *see* Degeneration, myocardial
myotonic, myotonica G71.11
nail L60.3
congenital Q84.6
nutritional E45
ocular G71.09
oculocerebrorenal E72.03
oculopharyngeal G71.09
ovarian N83.8
polyglandular E31.8
reflex (neuromuscular) (sympathetic) — *see* Syndrome, pain, complex regional I
retinal (hereditary) H35.50
in
lipid storage disorders E75.6 *[H36]*
systemic lipidoses E75.6 *[H36]*
involving
pigment epithelium H35.54
sensory area H35.53
pigmentary H35.52
vitreoretinal H35.51
Salzmann's nodular — *see* Degeneration, cornea, nodular
scapuloperoneal G71.09
skin NEC L98.8
sympathetic (reflex) — *see* Syndrome, pain, complex regional I
cervical G90.2
tapetoretinal H35.54
thoracic, asphyxiating Q77.2
unguium L60.3
congenital Q84.6
vitreoretinal H35.51
vulva N90.4
yellow (liver) — *see* Failure, hepatic
Dysuria R30.0
psychogenic F45.8

E

Eales' disease H35.06-
Ear — *see also* condition
piercing Z41.3
tropical NEC B36.9 *[H62.40]*
in
aspergillosis B44.89
candidiasis B37.84
moniliasis B37.84
wax (impacted) H61.20
left H61.22
with right H61.23
right H61.21
with left H61.23
Earache — *see* subcategory H92.0
Early satiety R68.81
Eaton-Lambert syndrome — *see* Syndrome, Lambert-Eaton
Eberth's disease (typhoid fever) A01.00
Ebola virus disease A98.4
Ebstein's anomaly or syndrome (heart) Q22.5
Eccentro-osteochondrodysplasia E76.29
Ecchondroma — *see* Neoplasm, bone, benign
Ecchondrosis D48.0
Ecchymosis R58
conjunctiva — *see* Hemorrhage, conjunctiva
eye (traumatic) — *see* Contusion, eyeball
eyelid (traumatic) — *see* Contusion, eyelid
newborn P54.5
spontaneous R23.3
traumatic — *see* Contusion
Echinococciasis — *see* Echinococcus
Echinococcosis — *see* Echinococcus
Echinococcus (infection) B67.90
granulosus B67.4
bone B67.2
liver B67.0
lung B67.1
multiple sites B67.32
specified site NEC B67.39
thyroid B67.31
liver NOS B67.8
granulosus B67.0
multilocularis B67.5
lung NEC B67.99
granulosus B67.1
multilocularis B67.69
multilocularis B67.7
liver B67.5
multiple sites B67.61
specified site NEC B67.69

Echinococcus (infection) - *continued*
specified site NEC B67.99
granulosus B67.39
multilocularis B67.69
thyroid NEC B67.99
granulosus B67.31
multilocularis B67.69 *[E35]*
Echinorhynchiasis B83.8
Echinostomiasis B66.8
Echolalia R48.8
Echovirus, as cause of disease classified elsewhere B97.12
Eclampsia, eclamptic (coma) (convulsions) (delirium) (with hypertension) **NEC** O15.9
complicating
labor and delivery O15.1
postpartum O15.2
pregnancy O15.0-
puerperium O15.2
Economic circumstances affecting care Z59.9
Economo's disease A85.8
Ectasia, ectasis
annuloaortic I35.8
aorta I77.819
with aneurysm — *see* Aneurysm, aorta
abdominal I77.811
thoracic I77.810
thoracoabdominal I77.812
breast — *see* Ectasia, mammary duct
capillary I78.8
cornea H18.71-
gastric antral vascular (GAVE) K31.819
with hemorrhage K31.811
without hemorrhage K31.819
mammary duct N60.4-
salivary gland (duct) K11.8
sclera — *see* Sclerectasia
Ecthyma L08.0
contagiosum B08.02
gangrenosum L08.0
infectiosum B08.02
Ectocardia Q24.8
Ectodermal dysplasia (anhidrotic) Q82.4
Ectodermosis erosiva pluriorificialis L51.1
Ectopic, ectopia (congenital)
abdominal viscera Q45.8
due to defect in anterior abdominal wall Q79.59
ACTH syndrome E24.3
adrenal gland Q89.1
anus Q43.5
atrial beats I49.1
beats I49.49
atrial I49.1
ventricular I49.3
bladder Q64.10
bone and cartilage in lung Q33.5
brain Q04.8
breast tissue Q83.8
cardiac Q24.8
cerebral Q04.8
cordis Q24.8
endometrium — *see* Endometriosis
gastric mucosa Q40.2
gestation — *see* Pregnancy, by site
heart Q24.8
hormone secretion NEC E34.2
kidney (crossed) (pelvis) Q63.2
lens, lentis Q12.1
mole — *see* Pregnancy, by site
organ or site NEC — *see* Malposition, congenital
pancreas Q45.3
pregnancy — *see* Pregnancy, ectopic
pupil — *see* Abnormality, pupillary
renal Q63.2
sebaceous glands of mouth Q38.6
spleen Q89.09
testis Q53.00
bilateral Q53.02
unilateral Q53.01
thyroid Q89.2
tissue in lung Q33.5
ureter Q62.63
ventricular beats I49.3
vesicae Q64.10
Ectromelia Q73.8
lower limb — *see* Defect, reduction, limb, lower, specified type NEC
upper limb — *see* Defect, reduction, limb, upper, specified type NEC
Ectropion H02.109
cervix N86
with cervicitis N72
congenital Q10.1

Ectropion - *continued*
eyelid H02.109
cicatricial H02.119
left H02.116
lower H02.115
upper H02.114
right H02.113
lower H02.112
upper H02.111
congenital Q10.1
left H02.106
lower H02.105
upper H02.104
mechanical H02.129
left H02.126
lower H02.125
upper H02.124
right H02.123
lower H02.122
upper H02.121
paralytic H02.159
left H02.156
lower H02.155
upper H02.154
right H02.153
lower H02.152
upper H02.151
right H02.103
lower H02.102
upper H02.101
senile H02.139
left H02.136
lower H02.135
upper H02.134
right H02.133
lower H02.132
upper H02.131
spastic H02.149
left H02.146
lower H02.145
upper H02.144
right H02.143
lower H02.142
upper H02.141
iris H21.89
lip (acquired) K13.0
congenital Q38.0
urethra N36.8
uvea H21.89
Eczema (acute) (chronic) (erythematous) (fissum) (rubrum) (squamous) — *see also* Dermatitis L30.9
contact — *see* Dermatitis, contact
dyshydrotic L30.1
external ear — *see* Otitis, externa, acute, eczematoid
flexural L20.82
herpeticum B00.0
hypertrophicum L28.0
hypostatic — *see* Varix, leg, with, inflammation
impetiginous L01.1
infantile (due to any substance) L20.83
intertriginous L21.1
seborrheic L21.1
intertriginous NEC L30.4
infantile L21.1
intrinsic (allergic) L20.84
lichenified NEC L28.0
marginatum (hebrae) B35.6
pustular L30.3
stasis I87.2
with varicose veins — *see* Varix, leg, with, inflammation
vaccination, vaccinatum T88.1
varicose — *see* Varix, leg, with, inflammation
Eczematid L30.2
Eddowes (-Spurway) **syndrome** Q78.0
Edema, edematous (infectious) (pitting) (toxic) R60.9
with nephritis — *see* Nephrosis
allergic T78.3
amputation stump (surgical) (sequelae (late effect)) T87.89
angioneurotic (allergic) (any site) (with urticaria) T78.3
hereditary D84.1
angiospastic I73.9
Berlin's (traumatic) S05.8X-
brain (cytotoxic) (vasogenic) G93.6
due to birth injury P11.0
newborn (anoxia or hypoxia) P52.4
birth injury P11.0
traumatic — *see* Injury, intracranial, cerebral edema
cardiac — *see* Failure, heart, congestive

- **Edema, edematous** (infectious) (pitting) (toxic) - *continued*
  - cardiovascular — *see* Failure, heart, congestive
  - cerebral — *see* Edema, brain
  - cerebrospinal — *see* Edema, brain
  - cervix (uteri) (acute) N88.8
    - puerperal, postpartum O90.89
  - chronic hereditary Q82.0
  - circumscribed, acute T78.3
    - hereditary D84.1
  - conjunctiva H11.42-
  - cornea H18.2-
    - idiopathic H18.22-
    - secondary H18.23-
      - due to contact lens H18.21-
  - due to
    - lymphatic obstruction I89.0
    - salt retention E87.0
  - epiglottis — *see* Edema, glottis
  - essential, acute T78.3
    - hereditary D84.1
  - extremities, lower — *see* Edema, legs
  - eyelid NEC H02.849
    - left H02.846
      - lower H02.845
      - upper H02.844
    - right H02.843
      - lower H02.842
      - upper H02.841
  - familial, hereditary Q82.0
  - famine — *see* Malnutrition, severe
  - generalized R60.1
  - glottis, glottic, glottidis (obstructive) (passive) J38.4
    - allergic T78.3
      - hereditary D84.1
  - heart — *see* Failure, heart, congestive
  - heat T67.7
  - hereditary Q82.0
  - inanition — *see* Malnutrition, severe
  - intracranial G93.6
  - iris H21.89
  - joint — *see* Effusion, joint
  - larynx — *see* Edema, glottis
  - legs R60.0
    - due to venous obstruction I87.1
    - hereditary Q82.0
  - localized R60.0
    - due to venous obstruction I87.1
  - lower limbs — *see* Edema, legs
  - lung J81.1
    - with heart condition or failure — *see* Failure, ventricular, left
    - acute J81.0
    - chemical (acute) J68.1
      - chronic J68.1
    - chronic J81.1
      - due to
        - chemicals, gases, fumes or vapors (inhalation) J68.1
        - external agent J70.9
          - specified NEC J70.8
        - radiation J70.1
    - due to
      - chemicals, fumes or vapors (inhalation) J68.1
      - external agent J70.9
        - specified NEC J70.8
      - high altitude T70.29
      - near drowning T75.1
      - radiation J70.0
    - meaning failure, left ventricle I50.1
  - lymphatic I89.0
    - due to mastectomy I97.2
  - macula H35.81
    - cystoid, following cataract surgery — *see* Complications, postprocedural, following cataract surgery
    - diabetic — *see* Diabetes, by type, with, retinopathy, with macular edema
  - malignant — *see* Gangrene, gas
  - Milroy's Q82.0
  - nasopharynx J39.2
  - newborn P83.30
    - hydrops fetalis — *see* Hydrops, fetalis
    - specified NEC P83.39
  - nutritional — *see also* Malnutrition, severe
    - with dyspigmentation, skin and hair E40
  - optic disc or nerve — *see* Papilledema
  - orbit H05.22-
  - pancreas K86.89
  - papilla, optic — *see* Papilledema
  - penis N48.89
  - periodic T78.3
    - hereditary D84.1
- **Edema, edematous** (infectious) (pitting) (toxic) - *continued*
  - pharynx J39.2
  - pulmonary — *see* Edema, lung
  - Quincke's T78.3
    - hereditary D84.1
  - renal — *see* Nephrosis
  - retina H35.81
    - diabetic — *see* Diabetes, by type, with, retinopathy, with macular edema
  - salt E87.0
  - scrotum N50.89
  - seminal vesicle N50.89
  - spermatic cord N50.89
  - spinal (cord) (vascular) (nontraumatic) G95.19
  - starvation — *see* Malnutrition, severe
  - stasis — *see* Hypertension, venous, (chronic)
  - subglottic — *see* Edema, glottis
  - supraglottic — *see* Edema, glottis
  - testis N44.8
  - tunica vaginalis N50.89
  - vas deferens N50.89
  - vulva (acute) N90.89
- **Edentulism** — *see* Absence, teeth, acquired
- **Edsall's disease** T67.2
- **Educational handicap** Z55.9
  - specified NEC Z55.8
- **Edward's syndrome** — *see* Trisomy, 18
- **Effect** (s) (of) (from) — *see* Effect, adverse NEC
- **Effect, adverse**
  - abnormal gravitational (G) forces or states T75.81
  - abuse — *see* Maltreatment
  - air pressure T70.9
    - specified NEC T70.8
  - altitude (high) — *see* Effect, adverse, high altitude
  - anesthesia — *see also* Anesthesia T88.59
    - in labor and delivery O74.9
    - local, toxic
      - in labor and delivery O74.4
      - in pregnancy NEC O29.3-
      - postpartum, puerperal O89.3
    - postpartum, puerperal O89.9
    - specified NEC T88.59
      - in labor and delivery O74.8
      - postpartum, puerperal O89.8
    - spinal and epidural T88.59
      - headache T88.59
        - in labor and delivery O74.5
        - postpartum, puerperal O89.4
      - specified NEC
        - in labor and delivery O74.6
        - postpartum, puerperal O89.5
  - antitoxin — *see* Complications, vaccination
  - atmospheric pressure T70.9
    - due to explosion T70.8
    - high T70.3
    - low — *see* Effect, adverse, high altitude
    - specified effect NEC T70.8
  - biological, correct substance properly administered — *see* Effect, adverse, drug
  - blood (derivatives) (serum) (transfusion) — *see* Complications, transfusion
  - chemical substance — *see* Table of Drugs and Chemicals
  - cold (temperature) (weather) T69.9
    - chilblains T69.1
    - frostbite — *see* Frostbite
    - specified effect NEC T69.8
  - drugs and medicaments T88.7
    - specified drug — *see* Table of Drugs and Chemicals, by drug, adverse effect
    - specified effect - code to condition
  - electric current, electricity (shock) T75.4
    - burn — *see* Burn
  - exertion (excessive) T73.3
  - exposure — *see* Exposure
  - external cause NEC T75.89
  - foodstuffs T78.1
    - allergic reaction — *see* Allergy, food
      - causing anaphylaxis — *see* Shock, anaphylactic, due to food
    - noxious — *see* Poisoning, food, noxious
  - gases, fumes, or vapors T59.9-
    - specified agent — *see* Table of Drugs and Chemicals
  - glue (airplane) sniffing
    - due to drug abuse — *see* Abuse, drug, inhalant
    - due to drug dependence — *see* Dependence, drug, inhalant
  - heat — *see* Heat
  - high altitude NEC T70.29
    - anoxia T70.29
    - on
- **Effect, adverse** - *continued*
  - high altitude NEC - *continued*
    - on - *continued*
      - ears T70.0
      - sinuses T70.1
    - polycythemia D75.1
  - high pressure fluids T70.4
  - hot weather — *see* Heat
  - hunger T73.0
  - immersion, foot — *see* Immersion
  - immunization — *see* Complications, vaccination
  - immunological agents — *see* Complications, vaccination
  - infrared (radiation) (rays) NOS T66
    - dermatitis or eczema L59.8
  - infusion — *see* Complications, infusion
  - lack of care of infants — *see* Maltreatment, child
  - lightning — *see* Lightning
  - medical care T88.9
    - specified NEC T88.8
  - medicinal substance, correct, properly administered — *see* Effect, adverse, drug
  - motion T75.3
  - noise, on inner ear — *see* subcategory H83.3
  - overheated places — *see* Heat
  - psychosocial, of work environment Z56.5
  - radiation (diagnostic) (infrared) (natural source) (therapeutic) (ultraviolet) (X-ray) NOS T66
    - dermatitis or eczema — *see* Dermatitis, due to, radiation
    - fibrosis of lung J70.1
    - pneumonitis J70.0
    - pulmonary manifestations
      - acute J70.0
      - chronic J70.1
    - skin L59.9
  - radioactive substance NOS
    - dermatitis or eczema — *see* Radiodermatitis
  - reduced temperature T69.9
    - immersion foot or hand — *see* Immersion
    - specified effect NEC T69.8
  - serum NEC — *see also* Reaction, serum T80.69
  - specified NEC T78.8
    - external cause NEC T75.89
  - strangulation — *see* Asphyxia, traumatic
  - submersion T75.1
  - thirst T73.1
  - toxic — *see* Toxicity
  - transfusion — *see* Complications, transfusion
  - ultraviolet (radiation) (rays) NOS T66
    - burn — *see* Burn
    - dermatitis or eczema — *see* Dermatitis, due to, ultraviolet rays
      - acute L56.8
  - vaccine (any) — *see* Complications, vaccination
  - vibration — *see* Vibration, adverse effects
  - water pressure NEC T70.9
    - specified NEC T70.8
  - weightlessness T75.82
  - whole blood — *see* Complications, transfusion
  - work environment Z56.5
- **Effects, late** — *see* Sequelae
- **Effluvium**
  - anagen L65.1
  - telogen L65.0
- **Effort syndrome** (psychogenic) F45.8
- **Effusion**
  - amniotic fluid — *see* Pregnancy, complicated by, prematue rupture of membranes
  - brain (serous) G93.6
  - bronchial — *see* Bronchitis
  - cerebral G93.6
  - cerebrospinal — *see also* Meningitis
    - vessel G93.6
  - chest — *see* Effusion, pleura
  - chylous, chyliform (pleura) J94.0
  - intracranial G93.6
  - joint M25.40
    - ankle M25.47-
    - elbow M25.42-
    - foot joint M25.47-
    - hand joint M25.44-
    - hip M25.45-
    - knee M25.46-
    - shoulder M25.41-
    - specified joint NEC M25.48
    - wrist M25.43-
  - malignant pleural J91.0
  - meninges — *see* Meningitis
  - pericardium, pericardial (noninflammatory) I31.3
    - acute — *see* Pericarditis, acute
  - peritoneal (chronic) R18.8
  - pleura, pleurisy, pleuritic, pleuropericardial J90

Effusion - *continued*
pleura, pleurisy, pleuritic, pleuropericardial - *continued*
chylous, chyliform J94.0
due to systemic lupus erythematosis M32.13
in conditions classified elsewhere J91.8
influenzal — *see* Influenza, with, respiratory manifestations NEC
malignant J91.0
newborn P28.89
tuberculous NEC A15.6
primary (progressive) A15.7
spinal — *see* Meningitis
thorax, thoracic — *see* Effusion, pleura
Egg shell nails L60.3
congenital Q84.6
Egyptian splenomegaly B65.1
Ehlers-Danlos syndrome Q79.6
Ehrlichiosis A77.40
due to
E. chafeensis A77.41
E. sennetsu A79.81
specified organism NEC A77.49
Eichstedt's disease B36.0
Eisenmenger's
complex or syndrome I27.83
defect Q21.8
Ejaculation
delayed F52.32
painful N53.12
premature F52.4
retarded N53.11
retrograde N53.14
semen, painful N53.12
psychogenic F52.6
Ekbom's syndrome (restless legs) G25.81
Ekman's syndrome (brittle bones and blue sclera) Q78.0
Elastic skin Q82.8
acquired L57.4
Elastofibroma — *see* Neoplasm, connective tissue, benign
Elastoma (juvenile) Q82.8
Miescher's L87.2
Elastomyofibrosis I42.4
Elastosis
actinic, solar L57.8
atrophicans (senile) L57.4
perforans serpiginosa L87.2
senilis L57.4
Elbow — *see* condition
Electric current, electricity, effects (concussion) (fatal) (nonfatal) (shock) T75.4
burn — *see* Burn
Electric feet syndrome E53.8
Electrocution T75.4
from electroshock gun (taser) T75.4
Electrolyte imbalance E87.8
with
abortion — *see* Abortion by type, complicated by, electrolyte imbalance
ectopic pregnancy O08.5
molar pregnancy O08.5
Elephantiasis (nonfilarial) I89.0
arabicum — *see* Infestation, filarial
bancroftian B74.0
congenital (any site) (hereditary) Q82.0
due to
Brugia (malayi) B74.1
timori B74.2
mastectomy I97.2
Wuchereria (bancrofti) B74.0
eyelid H02.859
left H02.856
lower H02.855
upper H02.854
right H02.853
lower H02.852
upper H02.851
filarial, filariensis — *see* Infestation, filarial
glandular I89.0
graecorum A30.9
lymphangiectatic I89.0
lymphatic vessel I89.0
due to mastectomy I97.2
scrotum (nonfilarial) I89.0
streptococcal I89.0
surgical I97.89
postmastectomy I97.2
telangiectodes I89.0
vulva (nonfilarial) N90.89
Elevated, elevation
antibody titer R76.0

Elevated, elevation - *continued*
basal metabolic rate R94.8
blood pressure — *see also* Hypertension
reading (incidental) (isolated) (nonspecific) , no diagnosis of hypertension R03.0
blood sugar R73.9
body temperature (of unknown origin) R50.9
C-reactive protein (CRP) R79.82
cancer antigen 125 [CA 125] R97.1
carcinoembryonic antigen [CEA] R97.0
cholesterol E78.00
with high triglycerides E78.2
conjugate, eye H51.0
diaphragm, congenital Q79.1
erythrocyte sedimentation rate R70.0
fasting glucose R73.01
fasting triglycerides E78.1
finding on laboratory examination — *see* Findings, abnormal, inconclusive, without diagnosis, by type of exam
GFR (glomerular filtration rate) — *see* Findings, abnormal, inconclusive, without diagnosis, by type of exam
glucose tolerance (oral) R73.02
immunoglobulin level R76.8
indoleacetic acid R82.5
lactic acid dehydrogenase (LDH) level R74.0
leukocytes D72.829
lipoprotein a (Lp (a)) level E78.41
liver function
study R94.5
test R79.89
alkaline phosphatase R74.8
aminotransferase R74.0
bilirubin R17
hepatic enzyme R74.8
lactate dehydrogenase R74.0
Lp (a) (lipoprotein (a)) E78.41
lymphocytes D72.820
prostate specific antigen [PSA] R97.20
Rh titer — *see* Complication(s), transfusion, incompatibility reaction, Rh (factor)
scapula, congenital Q74.0
sedimentation rate R70.0
SGOT R74.0
SGPT R74.0
transaminase level R74.0
triglycerides E78.1
with high cholesterol E78.2
tumor associated antigens [TAA] NEC R97.8
tumor specific antigens [TSA] NEC R97.8
urine level of
catecholamine R82.5
indoleacetic acid R82.5
17-ketosteroids R82.5
steroids R82.5
vanillylmandelic acid (VMA) R82.5
venous pressure I87.8
white blood cell count D72.829
specified NEC D72.828
Elliptocytosis (congenital) (hereditary) D58.1
Hb C (disease) D58.1
hemoglobin disease D58.1
sickle-cell (disease) D57.8-
trait D57.3
Ellison-Zollinger syndrome E16.4
Ellis van Creveld syndrome (chondroectodermal dysplasia) Q77.6
Elongated, elongation (congenital) — *see also* Distortion
bone Q79.9
cervix (uteri) Q51.828
acquired N88.4
hypertrophic N88.4
colon Q43.8
common bile duct Q44.5
cystic duct Q44.5
frenulum, penis Q55.69
labia minora (acquired) N90.69
ligamentum patellae Q74.1
petiolus (epiglottidis) Q31.8
tooth, teeth K00.2
uvula Q38.6
Eltor cholera A00.1
Emaciation (due to malnutrition) E41
Embadomoniasis A07.8
Embedded tooth, teeth K01.0
root only K08.3
Embolic — *see* condition
Embolism (multiple) (paradoxical) I74.9
air (any site) (traumatic) T79.0
following

Embolism (multiple) (paradoxical) - *continued*
air (any site) (traumatic) - *continued*
following - *continued*
abortion — *see* Abortion by type complicated by embolism
ectopic pregnancy O08.2
infusion, therapeutic injection or transfusion T80.0
molar pregnancy O08.2
procedure NEC
artery T81.719
mesenteric T81.710
renal T81.711
specified NEC T81.718
vein T81.72
in pregnancy, childbirth or puerperium — *see* Embolism, obstetric
amniotic fluid (pulmonary) — *see also* Embolism, obstetric
following
abortion — *see* Abortion by type complicated by embolism
ectopic pregnancy O08.2
molar pregnancy O08.2
aorta, aortic I74.10
abdominal I74.09
saddle I74.01
bifurcation I74.09
saddle I74.01
thoracic I74.11
artery I74.9
auditory, internal I65.8
basilar — *see* Occlusion, artery, basilar
carotid (common) (internal) — *see* Occlusion, artery, carotid
cerebellar (anterior inferior) (posterior inferior) (superior) I66.3
cerebral — *see* Occlusion, artery, cerebral
choroidal (anterior) I65.8
communicating posterior I65.8
coronary — *see also* Infarct, myocardium
not resulting in infarction I24.0
extremity I74.4
lower I74.3
upper I74.2
hypophyseal I65.8
iliac I74.5
limb I74.4
lower I74.3
upper I74.2
mesenteric (with gangrene) — *see also* Ischemia, intestine, acute K55.059
ophthalmic — *see* Occlusion, artery, retina
peripheral I74.4
pontine I65.8
precerebral — *see* Occlusion, artery, precerebral
pulmonary — *see* Embolism, pulmonary
renal N28.0
retinal — *see* Occlusion, artery, retina
septic I76
specified NEC I74.8
vertebral — *see* Occlusion, artery, vertebral
basilar (artery) I65.1
blood clot
following
abortion — *see* Abortion by type complicated by embolism
ectopic or molar pregnancy O08.2
in pregnancy, childbirth or puerperium — *see* Embolism, obstetric
brain — *see also* Occlusion, artery, cerebral
following
abortion — *see* Abortion by type complicated by embolism
ectopic or molar pregnancy O08.2
puerperal, postpartum, childbirth — *see* Embolism, obstetric
capillary I78.8
cardiac — *see also* Infarct, myocardium
not resulting in infarction I51.3
carotid (artery) (common) (internal) — *see* Occlusion, artery, carotid
cavernous sinus (venous) — *see* Embolism, intracranial venous sinus
cerebral — *see* Occlusion, artery, cerebral
cholesterol — *see* Atheroembolism
coronary (artery or vein) (systemic) — *see* Occlusion, coronary
due to device, implant or graft — *see also* Complications, by site and type, specified NEC
arterial graft NEC T82.818
breast (implant) T85.818

Embolism (multiple) (paradoxical) - *continued*
  due to device, implant or graft - *continued*
    catheter NEC T85.818
      dialysis (renal) T82.818
        intraperitoneal T85.818
      infusion NEC T82.818
        spinal (epidural) (subdural) T85.810
      urinary (indwelling) T83.81
    electronic (electrode) (pulse generator) (stimulator)
      bone T84.81
      cardiac T82.817
      nervous system (brain) (peripheral nerve) (spinal) T85.810
      urinary T83.81
    fixation, internal (orthopedic) NEC T84.81
    gastrointestinal (bile duct) (esophagus) T85.818
    genital NEC T83.81
    heart (graft) (valve) T82.817
    joint prosthesis T84.81
    ocular (corneal graft) (orbital implant) T85.818
    orthopedic (bone graft) NEC T86.838
    specified NEC T85.818
    urinary (graft) NEC T83.81
    vascular NEC T82.818
    ventricular intracranial shunt T85.810
  extremities
    lower — *see* Embolism, vein, lower extremity
      arterial I74.3
    upper I74.2
  eye H34.9
  fat (cerebral) (pulmonary) (systemic) T79.1
    following
      abortion — *see* Abortion by type complicated by embolism
      ectopic or molar pregnancy O08.2
    complicating delivery — *see* Embolism, obstetric
  following
    abortion — *see* Abortion by type complicated by embolism
    ectopic or molar pregnancy O08.2
    infusion, therapeutic injection or transfusion
      air T80.0
  heart (fatty) — *see also* Infarct, myocardium
    not resulting in infarction I51.3
  hepatic (vein) I82.0
  in pregnancy, childbirth or puerperium — *see* Embolism, obstetric
  intestine (artery) (vein) (with gangrene) — *see also* Ischemia, intestine, acute K55.039
  intracranial — *see also* Occlusion, artery, cerebral
    venous sinus (any) G08
      nonpyogenic I67.6
  intraspinal venous sinuses or veins G08
    nonpyogenic G95.19
  kidney (artery) N28.0
  lateral sinus (venous) — *see* Embolism, intracranial, venous sinus
  leg — *see* Embolism, vein, lower extremity
    arterial I74.3
  longitudinal sinus (venous) — *see* Embolism, intracranial, venous sinus
  lung (massive) — *see* Embolism, pulmonary
  meninges I66.8
  mesenteric (artery) (vein) (with gangrene) — *see also* Ischemia, intestine, acute K55.059
  obstetric (in) (pulmonary)
    childbirth O88.22
      air O88.02
      amniotic fluid O88.12
      blood clot O88.22
      fat O88.82
      pyemic O88.32
      septic O88.32
      specified type NEC O88.82
    pregnancy O88.21-
      air O88.01-
      amniotic fluid O88.11-
      blood clot O88.21-
      fat O88.81-
      pyemic O88.31-
      septic O88.31-
      specified type NEC O88.81-
    puerperal O88.23
      air O88.03
      amniotic fluid O88.13
      blood clot O88.23
      fat O88.83
      pyemic O88.33
      septic O88.33
      specified type NEC O88.83
  ophthalmic — *see* Occlusion, artery, retina
  penis N48.81
  peripheral artery NOS I74.4

Embolism (multiple) (paradoxical) - *continued*
  pituitary E23.6
  popliteal (artery) I74.3
  portal (vein) I81
  postoperative, postrpocedural
    artery T81.719
      mesenteric T81.710
      renal T81.711
      specified NEC T81.718
    vein T81.72
  precerebral artery — *see* Occlusion, artery, precerebral
  puerperal — *see* Embolism, obstetric
  pulmonary (acute) (artery) (vein) I26.99
    with acute cor pulmonale I26.09
    chronic I27.82
    following
      abortion — *see* Abortion by type complicated by embolism
      ectopic or molar pregnancy O08.2
    healed or old Z86.711
    in pregnancy, childbirth or puerperium — *see* Embolism, obstetric
    personal history of Z86.711
    saddle I26.92
      with acute cor pulmonale I26.02
    septic I26.90
      with acute cor pulmonale I26.01
  pyemic (multiple) I76
    following
      abortion — *see* Abortion by type complicated by embolism
      ectopic or molar pregnancy O08.2
    Hemophilus influenzae A41.3
    pneumococcal A40.3
      with pneumonia J13
    puerperal, postpartum, childbirth (any organism) — *see* Embolism, obstetric
    specified organism NEC A41.89
    staphylococcal A41.2
    streptococcal A40.9
  renal (artery) N28.0
    vein I82.3
  retina, retinal — *see* Occlusion, artery, retina
  saddle
    abdominal aorta I74.01
    pulmonary artery I26.92
      with acute cor pulmonale I26.02
  septic (arterial) I76
    complicating abortion — *see* Abortion, by type, complicated by, embolism
  sinus — *see* Embolism, intracranial, venous sinus
  soap complicating abortion — *see* Abortion, by type, complicated by, embolism
  spinal cord G95.19
    pyogenic origin G06.1
  spleen, splenic (artery) I74.8
  upper extremity I74.2
  vein (acute) I82.90
    antecubital I82.61-
      chronic I82.71-
    axillary I82.A1-
      chronic I82.A2-
    basilic I82.61-
      chronic I82.71-
    brachial I82.62-
      chronic I82.72-
    brachiocephalic (innominate) I82.290
      chronic I82.291
    cephalic I82.61-
      chronic I82.71-
    chronic I82.91
    deep (DVT) I82.40-
      calf I82.4Z-
        chronic I82.5Z-
      lower leg I82.4Z-
        chronic I82.5Z-
      thigh I82.4Y-
        chronic I82.5Y-
      upper leg I82.4Y
        chronic I82.5y--
    femoral I82.41-
      chronic I82.51-
    iliac (iliofemoral) I82.42-
      chronic I82.52-
    innominate I82.290
      chronic I82.291
    internal jugular I82.C1-
      chronic I82.C2-
    lower extremity
      deep I82.40-
        chronic I82.50-
        specified NEC I82.49-

Embolism (multiple) (paradoxical) - *continued*
  vein (acute) - *continued*
    lower extremity - *continued*
      deep - *continued*
        specified NEC - *continued*
          chronic NEC I82.59-
      distal
        deep I82.4Z-
      proximal
        deep I82.4Y-
          chronic I82.5Y-
      superficial I82.81-
    popliteal I82.43-
      chronic I82.53-
    radial I82.62-
      chronic I82.72-
    renal I82.3
    saphenous (greater) (lesser) I82.81-
    specified NEC I82.890
      chronic NEC I82.891
    subclavian I82.B1-
      chronic I82.B2-
    thoracic NEC I82.290
      chronic I82.291
    tibial I82.44-
      chronic I82.54-
    ulnar I82.62-
      chronic I82.72-
    upper extremity I82.60-
      chronic I82.70-
      deep I82.62-
        chronic I82.72-
      superficial I82.61-
        chronic I82.71-
  vena cava
    inferior (acute) I82.220
      chronic I82.221
    superior (acute) I82.210
      chronic I82.211
  venous sinus G08
  vessels of brain — *see* Occlusion, artery, cerebral
Embolus — *see* Embolism
Embryoma — *see also* Neoplasm, uncertain behavior, by site
  benign — *see* Neoplasm, benign, by site
  kidney C64.-
  liver C22.0
  malignant — *see also* Neoplasm, malignant, by site
    kidney C64.-
    liver C22.0
    testis C62.9-
      descended (scrotal) C62.1-
      undescended C62.0-
  testis C62.9-
    descended (scrotal) C62.1-
    undescended C62.0-
Embryonic
  circulation Q28.9
  heart Q28.9
  vas deferens Q55.4
Embryopathia NOS Q89.9
Embryotoxon Q13.4
Emesis — *see* Vomiting
Emotional lability R45.86
Emotionality, pathological F60.3
Emotogenic disease — *see* Disorder, psychogenic
Emphysema (atrophic) (bullous) (chronic) (interlobular) (lung) (obstructive) (pulmonary) (senile) (vesicular) J43.9
  cellular tissue (traumatic) T79.7
    surgical T81.82
  centrilobular J43.2
  compensatory J98.3
  congenital (interstitial) P25.0
  conjunctiva H11.89
  connective tissue (traumatic) T79.7
    surgical T81.82
  due to chemicals, gases, fumes or vapors J68.4
  eyelid (s) — *see* Disorder, eyelid, specified type NEC
    surgical T81.82
    traumatic T79.7
  interstitial J98.2
    congenital P25.0
    perinatal period P25.0
  laminated tissue T79.7
    surgical T81.82
  mediastinal J98.2
    newborn P25.2
  orbit, orbital — *see* Disorder, orbit, specified type NEC
  panacinar J43.1
  panlobular J43.1

Emphysema (atrophic) (bullous) (chronic) (interlobular) (lung) (obstructive) (pulmonary) (senile) (vesicular) - *continued*
specified NEC J43.8
subcutaneous (traumatic) T79.7
nontraumatic J98.2
postprocedural T81.82
surgical T81.82
surgical T81.82
thymus (gland) (congenital) E32.8
traumatic (subcutaneous) T79.7
unilateral J43.0
Empty nest syndrome Z60.0
Empyema (acute) (chest) (double) (pleura) (supradiaphragmatic) (thorax) J86.9
with fistula J86.0
accessory sinus (chronic) — *see* Sinusitis
antrum (chronic) — *see* Sinusitis, maxillary
brain (any part) — *see* Abscess, brain
ethmoidal (chronic) (sinus) — *see* Sinusitis, ethmoidal
extradural — *see* Abscess, extradural
frontal (chronic) (sinus) — *see* Sinusitis, frontal
gallbladder K81.0
mastoid (process) (acute) — *see* Mastoiditis, acute
maxilla, maxillary M27.2
sinus (chronic) — *see* Sinusitis, maxillary
nasal sinus (chronic) — *see* Sinusitis
sinus (accessory) (chronic) (nasal) — *see* Sinusitis
sphenoidal (sinus) (chronic) — *see* Sinusitis, sphenoidal
subarachnoid — *see* Abscess, extradural
subdural — *see* Abscess, subdural
tuberculous A15.6
ureter — *see* Ureteritis
ventricular — *see* Abscess, brain
En coup de sabre lesion L94.1
Enamel pearls K00.2
Enameloma K00.2
Enanthema, viral B09
Encephalitis (chronic) (hemorrhagic) (idiopathic) (nonepidemic) (spurious) (subacute) G04.90
acute — *see also* Encephalitis, viral A86
disseminated G04.00
infectious G04.01
noninfectious G04.81
postimmunization (postvaccination) G04.02
postinfectious G04.01
inclusion body A85.8
necrotizing hemorrhagic G04.30
postimmunization G04.32
postinfectious G04.31
specified NEC G04.39
arboviral, arbovirus NEC A85.2
arthropod-borne NEC (viral) A85.2
Australian A83.4
California (virus) A83.5
Central European (tick-borne) A84.1
Czechoslovakian A84.1
Dawson's (inclusion body) A81.1
diffuse sclerosing A81.1
disseminated, acute G04.00
due to
cat scratch disease A28.1
human immunodeficiency virus (HIV) disease B20 *[G05.3]*
malaria — *see* Malaria
rickettsiosis — *see* Rickettsiosis
smallpox inoculation G04.02
typhus — *see* Typhus
Eastern equine A83.2
endemic (viral) A86
epidemic NEC (viral) A86
equine (acute) (infectious) (viral) A83.9
Eastern A83.2
Venezuelan A92.2
Western A83.1
Far Eastern (tick-borne) A84.0
following vaccination or other immunization procedure G04.02
herpes zoster B02.0
herpesviral B00.4
due to herpesvirus 6 B10.01
due to herpesvirus 7 B10.09
specified NEC B10.09
Ilheus (virus) A83.8
inclusion body A81.1
in (due to)
actinomycosis A42.82
adenovirus A85.1
African trypanosomiasis B56.9 *[G05.3]*
Chagas' disease (chronic) B57.42
cytomegalovirus B25.8

Encephalitis (chronic) (hemorrhagic) (idiopathic) (nonepidemic) (spurious) (subacute) - *continued*
in (due to) - *continued*
enterovirus A85.0
herpes (simplex) virus B00.4
due to herpesvirus 6 B10.01
due to herpesvirus 7 B10.09
specified NEC B10.09
infectious disease NEC B99 *[G05.3]*
influenza — *see* Influenza, with, encephalopathy
listeriosis A32.12
measles B05.0
mumps B26.2
naegleriasis B60.2
parasitic disease NEC B89 *[G05.3]*
poliovirus A80.9 *[G05.3]*
rubella B06.01
syphilis
congenital A50.42
late A52.14
systemic lupus erythematosus M32.19
toxoplasmosis (acquired) B58.2
congenital P37.1
tuberculosis A17.82
zoster B02.0
infectious (acute) (virus) NEC A86
Japanese (B type) A83.0
La Crosse A83.5
lead — *see* Poisoning, lead
lethargica (acute) (infectious) A85.8
louping ill A84.8
lupus erythematosus, systemic M32.19
lymphatica A87.2
Mengo A85.8
meningococcal A39.81
Murray Valley A83.4
otitic NEC H66.40 *[G05.3]*
parasitic NOS B71.9
periaxial G37.0
periaxialis (concentrica) (diffuse) G37.5
postchickenpox B01.11
postexanthematous NEC B09
postimmunization G04.02
postinfectious NEC G04.01
postmeasles B05.0
postvaccinal G04.02
postvaricella B01.11
postviral NEC A86
Powassan A84.8
Rasmussen G04.81
Rio Bravo A85.8
Russian
autumnal A83.0
spring-summer (taiga) A84.0
saturnine — *see* Poisoning, lead
specified NEC G04.81
St. Louis A83.3
subacute sclerosing A81.1
summer A83.0
suppurative G04.81
tick-borne A84.9
Torula, torular (cryptococcal) B45.1
toxic NEC G92
trichinosis B75 *[G05.3]*
type
B A83.0
C A83.3
van Bogaert's A81.1
Venezuelan equine A92.2
Vienna A85.8
viral, virus A86
arthropod-borne NEC A85.2
mosquito-borne A83.9
Australian X disease A83.4
California virus A83.5
Eastern equine A83.2
Japanese (B type) A83.0
Murray Valley A83.4
specified NEC A83.8
St. Louis A83.3
type B A83.0
type C A83.3
Western equine A83.1
tick-borne A84.9
biundulant A84.1
central European A84.1
Czechoslovakian A84.1
diphasic meningoencephalitis A84.1
Far Eastern A84.0
Russian spring-summer (taiga) A84.0
specified NEC A84.8
specified type NEC A85.8
Western equine A83.1

Encephalocele Q01.9
frontal Q01.0
nasofrontal Q01.1
occipital Q01.2
specified NEC Q01.8
Encephalocystocele — *see* Encephalocele
Encephaloduroarteriomyosynangiosis (EDAMS) I67.5
Encephalomalacia (brain) (cerebellar) (cerebral) — *see* Softening, brain
Encephalomeningitis — *see* Meningoencephalitis
Encephalomeningocele — *see* Encephalocele
Encephalomeningomyelitis — *see* Meningoencephalitis
Encephalomyelitis — *see also* Encephalitis G04.90
acute disseminated G04.00
infectious G04.01
noninfectious G04.81
postimmunization G04.02
postinfectious G04.01
acute necrotizing hemorrhagic G04.30
postimmunization G04.32
postinfectious G04.31
specified NEC G04.39
benign myalgic G93.3
equine A83.9
Eastern A83.2
Venezuelan A92.2
Western A83.1
in diseases classified elsewhere G05.3
myalgic, benign G93.3
postchickenpox B01.11
postinfectious NEC G04.01
postmeasles B05.0
postvaccinal G04.02
postvaricella B01.11
rubella B06.01
specified NEC G04.81
Venezuelan equine A92.2
Encephalomyelocele — *see* Encephalocele
Encephalomyelomeningitis — *see* Meningoencephalitis
Encephalomyelopathy G96.9
Encephalomyeloradiculitis (acute) G61.0
Encephalomyeloradiculoneuritis (acute) (Guillain-Barré) G61.0
Encephalomyeloradiculopathy G96.9
Encephalopathia hyperbilirubinemica, newborn P57.9
due to isoimmunization (conditions in P55) P57.0
Encephalopathy (acute) G93.40
acute necrotizing hemorrhagic G04.30
postimmunization G04.32
postinfectious G04.31
specified NEC G04.39
alcoholic G31.2
anoxic — *see* Damage, brain, anoxic
arteriosclerotic I67.2
centrolobar progressive (Schilder) G37.0
congenital Q07.9
degenerative, in specified disease NEC G32.89
demyelinating callosal G37.1
due to
drugs - — *see also* Table of Drugs and Chemicals G92
hepatic — *see* Failure, hepatic
hyperbilirubinemic, newborn P57.9
due to isoimmunization (conditions in P55) P57.0
hypertensive I67.4
hypoglycemic E16.2
hypoxic — *see* Damage, brain, anoxic
hypoxic ischemic P91.60
mild P91.61
moderate P91.62
severe P91.63
in (due to) (with)
birth injury P11.1
hyperinsulinism E16.1 *[G94]*
influenza — *see* Influenza, with, encephalopathy
lack of vitamin — *see also* Deficiency, vitamin E56.9 *[G32.89]*
neoplastic disease (see also Neoplasm) D49.9 *[G13.1]*
serum — *see also* Reaction, serum T80.69
syphilis A52.17
trauma (postconcussional) F07.81
current injury — *see* Injury, intracranial
vaccination G04.02
lead — *see* Poisoning, lead
metabolic G93.41
drug induced G92
toxic G92

Encephalopathy (acute) - *continued*
myoclonic, early, symptomatic — *see* Epilepsy, generalized, specified NEC
necrotizing, subacute (Leigh) G31.82
neonatal P91.819
in diseases classified elsewhere P91.811
pellagrous E52 *[G32.89]*
portosystemic — *see* Failure, hepatic
postcontusional F07.81
current injury — *see* Injury, intracranial, diffuse
posthypoglycemic (coma) E16.1 *[G94]*
postradiation G93.89
saturnine — *see* Poisoning, lead
septic G93.41
specified NEC G93.49
spongioform, subacute (viral) A81.09
toxic G92
metabolic G92
traumatic (postconcussional) F07.81
current injury — *see* Injury, intracranial
vitamin B deficiency NEC E53.9 *[G32.89]*
vitamin B1 E51.2
Wernicke's E51.2
Encephalorrhagia — *see* Hemorrhage, intracranial, intracerebral
Encephalosis, posttraumatic F07.81
Enchondroma — *see also* Neoplasm, bone, benign
Enchondromatosis (cartilaginous) (multiple) Q78.4
Encopresis R15.9
functional F98.1
nonorganic origin F98.1
psychogenic F98.1
Encounter (with health service) (for) Z76.89
adjustment and management (of)
breast implant Z45.81
implanted device NEC Z45.89
myringotomy device (stent) (tube) Z45.82
administrative purpose only Z02.9
examination for
adoption Z02.82
armed forces Z02.3
disability determination Z02.71
driving license Z02.4
employment Z02.1
insurance Z02.6
medical certificate NEC Z02.79
paternity testing Z02.81
residential institution admission Z02.2
school admission Z02.0
sports Z02.5
specified reason NEC Z02.89
aftercare — *see* Aftercare
antenatal screening Z36.9
cervical length Z36.86
chromosomal anomalies Z36.0
congenital cardiac abnormalities Z36.83
elevated maternal serum alphafetoprotein level Z36.1
fetal growth retardation Z36.4
fetal lung maturity Z36.84
fetal macrosomia Z36.88
hydrops fetalis Z36.81
intrauterine growth restriction (IUGR) /small-for-dates Z36.4
isoimmunization Z36.5
large-for-dates Z36.88
malformations Z36.3
non-visualized anatomy on a previous scan Z36.2
nuchal translucency Z36.82
raised alphafetoprotein level Z36.1
risk of pre-term labor Z36.86
specified type NEC Z36.89
specified follow-up NEC Z36.2
specified genetic defects NEC Z36.8A
Streptococcus B Z36.85
suspected anomaly Z36.3
uncertain dates Z36.87
assisted reproductive fertility procedure cycle Z31.83
blood typing Z01.83
Rh typing Z01.83
breast augmentation or reduction Z41.1
breast implant exchange (different material) (different size) Z45.81
breast reconstruction following mastectomy Z42.1
check-up — *see* Examination
chemotherapy for neoplasm Z51.11
colonoscopy, screening Z12.11
counseling — *see* Counseling
delivery, full-term, uncomplicated O80
cesarean, without indication O82
desensitization to allergens Z51.6
ear piercing Z41.3

Encounter (with health service) (for) - *continued*
examination — *see* Examination
expectant parent (s) (adoptive) pre-birth pediatrician visit Z76.81
fertility preservation procedure (prior to cancer therapy) (prior to removal of gonads) Z31.84
fitting (of) — *see* Fitting (and adjustment) (of)
genetic
counseling
nonprocreative Z71.83
procreative Z31.5
testing — *see* Test, genetic
hearing conservation and treatment Z01.12
immunotherapy for neoplasm Z51.12
in vitro fertilization cycle Z31.83
instruction (in)
childbirth Z32.2
child care (postpartal) (prenatal) Z32.3
natural family planning
procreative Z31.61
to avoid pregnancy Z30.02
insulin pump titration Z46.81
joint prosthesis insertion following prior explantation of joint prosthesis (staged procedure)
hip Z47.32
knee Z47.33
shoulder Z47.31
laboratory (as part of a general medical examination) Z00.00
with abnormal findings Z00.01
mental health services (for)
abuse NEC
perpetrator Z69.82
victim Z69.81
child abuse
nonparental
perpetrator Z69.021
victim Z69.020
parental
perpetrator Z69.011
victim Z69.010
child neglect
nonparental
perpetrator Z69.021
victim Z69.020
parental
perpetrator Z69.011
victim Z69.010
child psychological abuse
nonparental
perpetrator Z69.021
victim Z69.020
parental
perpetrator Z69.011
victim Z69.010
child sexual abuse
nonparental
perpetrator Z69.021
victim Z69.020
parental
perpetrator Z69.011
victim Z69.010
non-spousal adult abuse (perpetrator) (victim) Z69.81
spousal or partner
abuse
perpetrator Z69.12
victim Z69.11
neglect
perpetrator Z69.12
victim Z69.11
psychological abuse
perpetrator Z69.12
victim Z69.11
violence
perpetrator (physical) (sexual) Z69.12
victim (physical) Z69.11
sexual Z69.81
observation (for) (ruled out)
exposure to (suspected)
anthrax Z03.810
biological agent NEC Z03.818
pediatrician visit, by expectant parent (s) (adoptive) Z76.81
placental sample (taken vaginally) — *see also* Encounter, antenatal screening Z36.9
plastic and reconstructive surgery following medical procedure or healed injury NEC Z42.8
pregnancy
supervision of — *see* Pregnancy, supervision of
test Z32.00
result negative Z32.02
result positive Z32.01

Encounter (with health service) (for) - *continued*
procreative management and counseling for gestational carrier Z31.7
prophylactic measures Z29.9
antivenin Z29.12
fluoride administration Z29.3
immunotherapy for respiratory syncytial virus (RSV) Z29.11
rabies immune globin Z29.14
Rho (D) immune globulin Z29.13
specified NEC Z29.8
radiation therapy (antineoplastic) Z51.0
radiological (as part of a general medical examination) Z00.00
with abnormal findings Z00.01
reconstructive surgery following medical procedure or healed injury NEC Z42.8
removal (of) — *see also* Removal
artificial
arm Z44.00-
complete Z44.01-
partial Z44.02-
eye Z44.2-
leg Z44.10-
complete Z44.11-
partial Z44.12-
breast implant Z45.81
tissue expander (without synchronous insertion of permanent implant) Z45.81
device Z46.9
specified NEC Z46.89
external
fixation device - code to fracture with seventh character D
prosthesis, prosthetic device Z44.9
breast Z44.3-
specified NEC Z44.8
implanted device NEC Z45.89
insulin pump Z46.81
internal fixation device Z47.2
myringotomy device (stent) (tube) Z45.82
nervous system device NEC Z46.2
brain neuropacemaker Z46.2
visual substitution device Z46.2
implanted Z45.31
non-vascular catheter Z46.82
orthodontic device Z46.4
stent
ureteral Z46.6
urinary device Z46.6
repeat cervical smear to confirm findings of recent normal smear following initial abnormal smear Z01.42
respirator [ventilator] use during power failure Z99.12
Rh typing Z01.83
screening — *see* Screening
specified NEC Z76.89
sterilization Z30.2
suspected condition, ruled out
amniotic cavity and membrane Z03.71
cervical shortening Z03.75
fetal anomaly Z03.73
fetal growth Z03.74
maternal and fetal conditions NEC Z03.79
oligohydramnios Z03.71
placental problem Z03.72
polyhydramnios Z03.71
suspected exposure (to) , ruled out
anthrax Z03.810
biological agents NEC Z03.818
termination of pregnancy, elective Z33.2
testing — *see* Test
therapeutic drug level monitoring Z51.81
titration, insulin pump Z46.81
to determine fetal viability of pregnancy O36.80
training
insulin pump Z46.81
X-ray of chest (as part of a general medical examination) Z00.00
with abnormal findings Z00.01
Encystment — *see* Cyst
Endarteritis (bacterial, subacute) (infective) I77.6
brain I67.7
cerebral or cerebrospinal I67.7
deformans — *see* Arteriosclerosis
embolic — *see* Embolism
obliterans — *see also* Arteriosclerosis
pulmonary I28.8
pulmonary I28.8
retina — *see* Vasculitis, retina
senile — *see* Arteriosclerosis
syphilitic A52.09

Endarteritis (bacterial, subacute) (infective) - *continued*
syphilitic - *continued*
brain or cerebral A52.04
congenital A50.54 *[I79.8]*
tuberculous A18.89
Endemic — *see* condition
Endocarditis (chronic) (marantic) (nonbacterial) (thrombotic) (valvular) I38
with rheumatic fever (conditions in I00)
active — *see* Endocarditis, acute, rheumatic
inactive or quiescent (with chorea) I09.1
acute or subacute I33.9
infective I33.0
rheumatic (aortic) (mitral) (pulmonary) (tricuspid) I01.1
with chorea (acute) (rheumatic) (Sydenham's) I02.0
aortic (heart) (nonrheumatic) (valve) I35.8
with
mitral disease I08.0
with tricuspid (valve) disease I08.3
active or acute I01.1
with chorea (acute) (rheumatic) (Sydenham's) I02.0
rheumatic fever (conditions in I00)
active — *see* Endocarditis, acute, rheumatic
inactive or quiescent (with chorea) I06.9
tricuspid (valve) disease I08.2
with mitral (valve) disease I08.3
acute or subacute I33.9
arteriosclerotic I35.8
rheumatic I06.9
with mitral disease I08.0
with tricuspid (valve) disease I08.3
active or acute I01.1
with chorea (acute) (rheumatic) (Sydenham's) I02.0
active or acute I01.1
with chorea (acute) (rheumatic) (Sydenham's) I02.0
specified NEC I06.8
specified cause NEC I35.8
syphilitic A52.03
arteriosclerotic I38
atypical verrucous (Libman-Sacks) M32.11
bacterial (acute) (any valve) (subacute) I33.0
candidal B37.6
congenital Q24.8
constrictive I33.0
Coxiella burnetii A78 *[I39]*
Coxsackie B33.21
due to
prosthetic cardiac valve T82.6
Q fever A78 *[I39]*
Serratia marcescens I33.0
typhoid (fever) A01.02
gonococcal A54.83
infectious or infective (acute) (any valve) (subacute) I33.0
lenta (acute) (any valve) (subacute) I33.0
Libman-Sacks M32.11
listerial A32.82
Löffler's I42.3
malignant (acute) (any valve) (subacute) I33.0
meningococcal A39.51
mitral (chronic) (double) (fibroid) (heart) (inactive) (valve) (with chorea) I05.9
with
aortic (valve) disease I08.0
with tricuspid (valve) disease I08.3
active or acute I01.1
with chorea (acute) (rheumatic) (Sydenham's) I02.0
rheumatic fever (conditions in I00)
active — *see* Endocarditis, acute, rheumatic
inactive or quiescent (with chorea) I05.9
tricuspid (valve) disease I08.1
with aortic (valve) disease I08.3
active or acute I01.1
with chorea (acute) (rheumatic) (Sydenham's) I02.0
bacterial I33.0
arteriosclerotic I34.8
nonrheumatic I34.8
acute or subacute I33.9
specified NEC I05.8
monilial B37.6
multiple valves I08.9
specified disorders I08.8
mycotic (acute) (any valve) (subacute) I33.0
pneumococcal (acute) (any valve) (subacute) I33.0
pulmonary (chronic) (heart) (valve) I37.8

Endocarditis (chronic) (marantic) (nonbacterial) (thrombotic) (valvular) - *continued*
pulmonary (chronic) (heart) (valve) - *continued*
with rheumatic fever (conditions in I00)
active — *see* Endocarditis, acute, rheumatic
inactive or quiescent (with chorea) I09.89
with aortic, mitral or tricuspid disease I08.8
acute or subacute I33.9
rheumatic I01.1
with chorea (acute) (rheumatic) (Sydenham's) I02.0
arteriosclerotic I37.8
congenital Q22.2
rheumatic (chronic) (inactive) (with chorea) I09.89
active or acute I01.1
with chorea (acute) (rheumatic) (Sydenham's) I02.0
syphilitic A52.03
purulent (acute) (any valve) (subacute) I33.0
Q fever A78 *[I39]*
rheumatic (chronic) (inactive) (with chorea) I09.1
active or acute (aortic) (mitral) (pulmonary) (tricuspid) I01.1
with chorea (acute) (rheumatic) (Sydenham's) I02.0
rheumatoid — *see* Rheumatoid, carditis
septic (acute) (any valve) (subacute) I33.0
streptococcal (acute) (any valve) (subacute) I33.0
subacute — *see* Endocarditis, acute
suppurative (acute) (any valve) (subacute) I33.0
syphilitic A52.03
toxic I33.9
tricuspid (chronic) (heart) (inactive) (rheumatic) (valve) (with chorea) I07.9
with
aortic (valve) disease I08.2
mitral (valve) disease I08.3
mitral (valve) disease I08.1
aortic (valve) disease I08.3
rheumatic fever (conditions in I00)
active — *see* Endocarditis, acute, rheumatic
inactive or quiescent (with chorea) I07.8
active or acute I01.1
with chorea (acute) (rheumatic) (Sydenham's) I02.0
arteriosclerotic I36.8
nonrheumatic I36.8
acute or subacute I33.9
specified cause, except rheumatic I36.8
tuberculous — *see* Tuberculosis, endocarditis
typhoid A01.02
ulcerative (acute) (any valve) (subacute) I33.0
vegetative (acute) (any valve) (subacute) I33.0
verrucous (atypical) (nonbacterial) (nonrheumatic) M32.11
Endocardium, endocardial — *see also* condition
cushion defect Q21.2
Endocervicitis — *see also* Cervicitis
due to intrauterine (contraceptive) device T83.69
hyperplastic N72
Endocrine — *see* condition
Endocrinopathy, pluriglandular E31.9
Endodontic
overfill M27.52
underfill M27.53
Endodontitis K04.01
irreversible K04.02
reversible K04.01
Endomastoiditis — *see* Mastoiditis
Endometrioma N80.9
Endometriosis N80.9
appendix N80.5
bladder N80.8
bowel N80.5
broad ligament N80.3
cervix N80.0
colon N80.5
cul-de-sac (Douglas') N80.3
exocervix N80.0
fallopian tube N80.2
female genital organ NEC N80.8
gallbladder N80.8
in scar of skin N80.6
internal N80.0
intestine N80.5
lung N80.8
myometrium N80.0
ovary N80.1
parametrium N80.3
pelvic peritoneum N80.3
peritoneal (pelvic) N80.3
rectovaginal septum N80.4
rectum N80.5

Endometriosis - *continued*
round ligament N80.3
skin (scar) N80.6
specified site NEC N80.8
stromal D39.0
thorax N80.8
umbilicus N80.8
uterus (internal) N80.0
vagina N80.4
vulva N80.8
Endometritis (decidual) (nonspecific) (purulent) (senile) (atrophic) (suppurative) N71.9
with ectopic pregnancy O08.0
acute N71.0
blenorrhagic (gonococcal) (acute) (chronic) A54.24
cervix, cervical (with erosion or ectropion) — *see also* Cervicitis
hyperplastic N72
chlamydial A56.11
chronic N71.1
following
abortion — *see* Abortion by type complicated by genital infection
ectopic or molar pregnancy O08.0
gonococcal, gonorrheal (acute) (chronic) A54.24
hyperplastic — *see also* Hyperplasia, endometrial N85.00-
cervix N72
puerperal, postpartum, childbirth O86.12
subacute N71.0
tuberculous A18.17
Endometrium — *see* condition
Endomyocardiopathy, South African I42.3
Endomyocarditis — *see* Endocarditis
Endomyofibrosis I42.3
Endomyometritis — *see* Endometritis
Endopericarditis — *see* Endocarditis
Endoperineuritis — *see* Disorder, nerve
Endophlebitis — *see* Phlebitis
Endophthalmia — *see* Endophthalmitis, purulent
Endophthalmitis (acute) (infective) (metastatic) (subacute) H44.009
bleb associated H59.4 — *see* also Bleb, inflammed (infected), postprocedural
gonorrheal A54.39
in (due to)
cysticercosis B69.1
onchocerciasis B73.01
toxocariasis B83.0
panuveitis — *see* Panuveitis
parasitic H44.12-
purulent H44.00-
panophthalmitis — *see* Panophthalmitis
vitreous abscess H44.02-
specified NEC H44.19
sympathetic — *see* Uveitis, sympathetic
Endosalpingioma D28.2
Endosalpingiosis N94.89
Endosteitis — *see* Osteomyelitis
Endothelioma, bone — *see* Neoplasm, bone, malignant
Endotheliosis (hemorrhagic infectional) D69.8
Endotoxemia - code to condition
Endotrachelitis — *see* Cervicitis
Engelmann (-Camurati) **syndrome** Q78.3
English disease — *see* Rickets
Engman's disease L30.3
Engorgement
breast N64.59
newborn P83.4
puerperal, postpartum O92.79
lung (passive) — *see* Edema, lung
pulmonary (passive) — *see* Edema, lung
stomach K31.89
venous, retina — *see* Occlusion, retina, vein, engorgement
Enlargement, enlarged — *see also* Hypertrophy
adenoids J35.2
with tonsils J35.3
alveolar ridge K08.89
congenital — *see* Anomaly, alveolar
apertures of diaphragm (congenital) Q79.1
gingival K06.1
heart, cardiac — *see* Hypertrophy, cardiac
labium majus, childhood asymmetric (CALME) N90.61
lacrimal gland, chronic H04.03-
liver — *see* Hypertrophy, liver
lymph gland or node R59.9
generalized R59.1
localized R59.0
orbit H05.34-

Enlargement, enlarged - *continued*
- organ or site, congenital NEC — *see* Anomaly, by site
- parathyroid (gland) E21.0
- pituitary fossa R93.0
- prostate N40.0
  - with lower urinary tract symptoms (LUTS) N40.1
  - without lower urinary tract symtpoms (LUTS) N40.0
- sella turcica R93.0
- spleen — *see* Splenomegaly
- thymus (gland) (congenital) E32.0
- thyroid (gland) — *see* Goiter
- tongue K14.8
- tonsils J35.1
  - with adenoids J35.3
- uterus N85.2
- vestibular aqueduct Q16.5

Enophthalmos H05.40-
- due to
  - orbital tissue atrophy H05.41-
  - trauma or surgery H05.42-

Enostosis M27.8

Entamebic, entamebiasis — *see* Amebiasis

Entanglement
- umbilical cord (s) O69.82
  - with compression O69.2
  - around neck (with compression) O69.81
    - with compression O69.1
    - without compression O69.81
  - of twins in monoamniotic sac O69.2
  - without compression O69.82

Enteralgia — *see* Pain, abdominal

Enteric — *see* condition

Enteritis (acute) (diarrheal) (hemorrhagic) (noninfective) K52.9
- adenovirus A08.2
- aertrycke infection A02.0
- allergic K52.29
  - with
    - eosinophilic gastritis or gastroenteritis K52.81
    - food protein-induced enterocolitis syndrome K52.21
    - food protein-induced enteropathy K52.22
    - FPIES K52.21
- amebic (acute) A06.0
  - with abscess — *see* Abscess, amebic
  - chronic A06.1
    - with abscess — *see* Abscess, amebic
    - nondysenteric A06.2
  - nondysenteric A06.2
- astrovirus A08.32
- bacillary NOS A03.9
- bacterial A04.9
  - specified NEC A04.8
- calicivirus A08.31
- candidal B37.82
- Chilomastix A07.8
- choleriformis A00.1
- chronic (noninfectious) K52.9
  - ulcerative — *see* Colitis, ulcerative
- cicatrizing (chronic) — *see* Enteritis, regional, small intestine
- Clostridium
  - botulinum (food poisoning) A05.1
  - difficile
    - not specified as recurrent A04.72
    - recurrent A04.71
- coccidial A07.3
- coxsackie virus A08.39
- dietetic — *see also* Enteritis, allergic K52.29
- drug-induced K52.1
- due to
  - astrovirus A08.32
  - calicivirus A08.31
  - coxsackie virus A08.39
  - drugs K52.1
  - echovirus A08.39
  - enterovirus NEC A08.39
  - food hypersensitivity — *see also* Enteritis, allergic K52.29
  - infectious organism (bacterial) (viral) — *see* Enteritis, infectious
  - torovirus A08.39
  - Yersinia enterocolitica A04.6
- echovirus A08.39
- eltor A00.1
- enterovirus NEC A08.39
- eosinophilic K52.81
- epidemic (infectious) A09
- fulminant — *see also* Ischemia, intestine, acute K55.019
- gangrenous — *see* Enteritis, infectious

Enteritis (acute) (diarrheal) (hemorrhagic) (noninfective) - *continued*
- giardial A07.1
- infectious NOS A09
  - due to
    - adenovirus A08.2
    - Aerobacter aerogenes A04.8
    - Arizona (bacillus) A02.0
    - bacteria NOS A04.9
      - specified NEC A04.8
    - Campylobacter A04.5
    - Clostridium difficile
      - not specified as recurrent A04.72
      - recurrent A04.71
    - Clostridium perfringens A04.8
    - Enterobacter aerogenes A04.8
    - enterovirus A08.39
    - Escherichia coli A04.4
      - enteroaggregative A04.4
      - enterohemorrhagic A04.3
      - enteroinvasive A04.2
      - enteropathogenic A04.0
      - enterotoxigenic A04.1
      - specified NEC A04.4
    - specified
      - bacteria NEC A04.8
      - virus NEC A08.39
    - Staphylococcus A04.8
    - virus NEC A08.4
      - specified type NEC A08.39
    - Yersinia enterocolitica A04.6
  - specified organism NEC A08.8
- influenzal — *see* Influenza, with, digestive manifestations
- ischemic K55.9
  - acute — *see also* Ischemia, intestine, acute K55.019
  - chronic K55.1
- microsporidial A07.8
- mucomembranous, myxomembranous — *see* Syndrome, irritable bowel
- mucous — *see* Syndrome, irritable bowel
- necroticans A05.2
- necrotizing of newborn — *see* Enterocolitis, necrotizing, in newborn
- neurogenic — *see* Syndrome, irritable bowel
- newborn necrotizing — *see* Enterocolitis, necrotizing, in newborn
- noninfectious K52.9
- norovirus A08.11
- parasitic NEC B82.9
- paratyphoid (fever) — *see* Fever, paratyphoid
- protozoal A07.9
  - specified NEC A07.8
- radiation K52.0
- regional (of) K50.90
  - with
    - complication K50.919
      - abscess K50.914
      - fistula K50.913
      - intestinal obstruction K50.912
      - rectal bleeding K50.911
      - specified complication NEC K50.918
  - colon — *see* Enteritis, regional, large intestine
  - duodenum — *see* Enteritis, regional, small intestine
  - ileum — *see* Enteritis, regional, small intestine
  - jejunum — *see* Enteritis, regional, small intestine
  - large bowel — *see* Enteritis, regional, large intestine
  - large intestine (colon) (rectum) K50.10
    - with
      - complication K50.119
        - abscess K50.114
        - fistula K50.113
        - intestinal obstruction K50.112
        - rectal bleeding K50.111
        - small intestine (duodenum) (ileum) (jejunum) involvement K50.80
          - with
            - complication K50.819
              - abscess K50.814
              - fistula K50.813
              - intestinal obstruction K50.812
              - rectal bleeding K50.811
              - specified complication NEC K50.818
        - specified complication NEC K50.118
  - rectum — *see* Enteritis, regional, large intestine
  - small intestine (duodenum) (ileum) (jejunum) K50.00
    - with
      - complication K50.019
        - abscess K50.014

Enteritis (acute) (diarrheal) (hemorrhagic) (noninfective) - *continued*
- regional (of) - *continued*
  - small intestine (duodenum) (ileum) (jejunum) - *continued*
    - with - *continued*
      - complication - *continued*
        - fistula K50.013
        - intestinal obstruction K50.012
        - large intestine (colon) (rectum) involvement K50.80
          - with
            - complication K50.819
              - abscess K50.814
              - fistula K50.813
              - intestinal obstruction K50.812
              - rectal bleeding K50.811
              - specified complication NEC K50.818
        - rectal bleeding K50.011
        - specified complication NEC K50.018
- rotaviral A08.0
- Salmonella, salmonellosis (arizonae) (cholerae-suis) (enteritidis) (typhimurium) A02.0
- segmental — *see* Enteritis, regional
- septic A09
- Shigella — *see* Infection, Shigella
- small round structured NEC A08.19
- spasmodic, spastic — *see* Syndrome, irritable bowel
- staphylococcal A04.8
  - due to food A05.0
- torovirus A08.39
- toxic NEC K52.1
  - due to Clostridium difficile
    - not specified as recurrent A04.72
    - recurrent A04.71
- trichomonal A07.8
- tuberculous A18.32
- typhosa A01.00
- ulcerative (chronic) — *see* Colitis, ulcerative
- viral A08.4
  - adenovirus A08.2
  - enterovirus A08.39
  - Rotavirus A08.0
  - small round structured NEC A08.19
  - specified NEC A08.39
  - virus specified NEC A08.39

Enterobiasis B80

Enterobius vermicularis (infection) (infestation) B80

Enterocele — *see also* Hernia, abdomen
- pelvic, pelvis (acquired) (congenital) N81.5
- vagina, vaginal (acquired) (congenital) NEC N81.5

Enterocolitis — *see also* Enteritis K52.9
- due to Clostridium difficile
  - not specified as recurrent A04.72
  - recurrent A04.71
- fulminant ischemic — *see also* Ischemia, intestine, acute K55.059
- granulomatous — *see* Enteritis, regional
- hemorrhagic (acute) — *see also* Ischemia, intestine, acute K55.059
  - chronic K55.1
- infectious NEC A09
- ischemic K55.9
- necrotizing K55.30
  - with
    - perforation K55.33
    - pneumatosis K55.32
      - and perforation K55.33
  - due to Clostridium difficile
    - not specified as recurrent A04.72
    - recurrent A04.71
  - in non-newborn K55.30
    - stage 1 (without pneumatosis, without perforation) K55.31
    - stage 2 (with pneumatosis, without perforation) K55.32
    - stage 3 (with pneumatosis, with perforation) K55.33
  - in newborn P77.9
    - stage 1 (without pneumatosis, without perforation) P77.1
    - stage 2 (with pneumatosis, without perforation) P77.2
    - stage 3 (with pneumatosis, with perforation) P77.3
  - without pneumatosis or perforation K55.31
- noninfectious K52.9
  - newborn — *see* Enterocolitis, necrotizing, in newborn
- pseudomembranous (newborn)
  - not specified as recurrent A04.72
  - recurrent A04.71

Enterocolitis - *continued*
radiation K52.0
newborn — *see* Enterocolitis, necrotizing, in newborn
ulcerative (chronic) — *see* Pancolitis, ulcerative (chronic)
Enterogastritis — *see* Enteritis
Enteropathy K63.9
food protein-induced enterocolitis (FPIES) K52.22
celiac-gluten-sensitive K90.0
non-celiac K90.41
hemorrhagic, terminal — *see also* Ischemia, intestine, acute K55.059
protein-losing K90.49
Enteroperitonitis — *see* Peritonitis
Enteroptosis K63.4
Enterorrhagia K92.2
Enterospasm — *see also* Syndrome, irritable, bowel
psychogenic F45.8
Enterostenosis — *see also* Obstruction, intestine, specified NEC K56.699
Enterostomy
complication — *see* Complication, enterostomy
status Z93.4
Enterovirus, as cause of disease classified elsewhere B97.10
coxsackievirus B97.11
echovirus B97.12
other specified B97.19
Enthesopathy (peripheral) M77.9
Achilles tendinitis — *see* Tendinitis, Achilles
ankle and tarsus M77.9
specified type NEC — *see* Enthesopathy, foot, specified type NEC
anterior tibial syndrome M76.81-
calcaneal spur — *see* Spur, bone, calcaneal
elbow region M77.8
lateral epicondylitis — *see* Epicondylitis, lateral
medial epicondylitis — *see* Epicondylitis, medial
foot NEC M77.9
metatarsalgia — *see* Metatarsalgia
specified type NEC M77.5-
forearm M77.9
gluteal tendinitis — *see* Tendinitis, gluteal
hand M77.9
hip — *see* Enthesopathy, lower limb, specified type NEC
iliac crest spur — *see* Spur, bone, iliac crest
iliotibial band syndrome — *see* Syndrome, iliotibial band
knee — *see* Enthesopathy, lower limb, lower leg, specified type NEC
lateral epicondylitis — *see* Epicondylitis, lateral
lower limb (excluding foot) M76.9
Achilles tendinitis — *see* Tendinitis, Achilles
anterior tibial syndrome M76.81-
gluteal tendinitis — *see* Tendinitis, gluteal
iliac crest spur — *see* Spur, bone, iliac crest
iliotibial band syndrome — *see* Syndrome, iliotibial band
patellar tendinitis — *see* Tendinitis, patellar
pelvic region — *see* Enthesopathy, lower limb, specified type NEC
peroneal tendinitis — *see* Tendinitis, peroneal
posterior tibial syndrome M76.82-
psoas tendinitis — *see* Tendinitis, psoas
shoulder M77.9
specified type NEC M76.89-
tibial collateral bursitis — *see* Bursitis, tibial collateral
medial epicondylitis — *see* Epicondylitis, medial
metatarsalgia — *see* Metatarsalgia
multiple sites M77.9
patellar tendinitis — *see* Tendinitis, patellar
pelvis M77.9
periarthritis of wrist — *see* Periarthritis, wrist
peroneal tendinitis — *see* Tendinitis, peroneal
posterior tibial syndrome M76.82-
psoas tendinitis — *see* Tendinitis, psoas
shoulder region — *see* Lesion, shoulder
specified site NEC M77.9
specified type NEC M77.8
spinal M46.00
cervical region M46.02
cervicothoracic region M46.03
lumbar region M46.06
lumbosacral region M46.07
multiple sites M46.09
occipito-atlanto-axial region M46.01
sacrococcygeal region M46.08
thoracic region M46.04
thoracolumbar region M46.05

Enthesopathy (peripheral) - *continued*
tibial collateral bursitis — *see* Bursitis, tibial collateral
upper arm M77.9
wrist and carpus NEC M77.8
calcaneal spur — *see* Spur, bone, calcaneal
periarthritis of wrist — *see* Periarthritis, wrist
Entomophobia F40.218
Entomophthoromycosis B46.8
Entrance, air into vein — *see* Embolism, air
Entrapment, nerve — *see* Neuropathy, entrapment
Entropion (eyelid) (paralytic) H02.009
cicatricial H02.019
left H02.016
lower H02.015
upper H02.014
right H02.013
lower H02.012
upper H02.011
congenital Q10.2
left H02.006
lower H02.005
upper H02.004
mechanical H02.029
left H02.026
lower H02.025
upper H02.024
right H02.023
lower H02.022
upper H02.021
right H02.003
lower H02.002
upper H02.001
senile H02.039
left H02.036
lower H02.035
upper H02.034
right H02.033
lower H02.032
upper H02.031
spastic H02.049
left H02.046
lower H02.045
upper H02.044
right H02.043
lower H02.042
upper H02.041
Enucleated eye (traumatic, current) S05.7-
Enuresis R32
functional F98.0
habit disturbance F98.0
nocturnal N39.44
psychogenic F98.0
nonorganic origin F98.0
psychogenic F98.0
Eosinopenia — *see* Agranulocytosis
Eosinophilia (allergic) (hereditary) (idiopathic) (secondary) D72.1
with
angiolymphoid hyperplasia (ALHE) D18.01
infiltrative J82
Löffler's J82
peritoneal — *see* Peritonitis, eosinophilic
pulmonary NEC J82
tropical (pulmonary) J82
Eosinophilia-myalgia syndrome M35.8
Ependymitis (acute) (cerebral) (chronic) (granular) — *see* Encephalomyelitis
Ependymoblastoma
specified site — *see* Neoplasm, malignant, by site
unspecified site C71.9
Ependymoma (epithelial) (malignant)
anaplastic
specified site — *see* Neoplasm, malignant, by site
unspecified site C71.9
benign
specified site — *see* Neoplasm, benign, by site
unspecified site D33.2
myxopapillary D43.2
specified site — *see* Neoplasm, uncertain behavior, by site
unspecified site D43.2
papillary D43.2
specified site — *see* Neoplasm, uncertain behavior, by site
unspecified site D43.2
specified site — *see* Neoplasm, malignant, by site
unspecified site C71.9
Ependymopathy G93.89
Ephelis, ephelides L81.2
Epiblepharon (congenital) Q10.3
Epicanthus, epicanthic fold (eyelid) (congenital) Q10.3

Epicondylitis (elbow)
lateral M77.1-
medial M77.0-
Epicystitis — *see* Cystitis
Epidemic — *see* condition
Epidermidalization, cervix — *see* Dysplasia, cervix
Epidermis, epidermal — *see* condition
Epidermodysplasia verruciformis B07.8
Epidermolysis
bullosa (congenital) Q81.9
acquired L12.30
drug-induced L12.31
specified cause NEC L12.35
dystrophica Q81.2
letalis Q81.1
simplex Q81.0
specified NEC Q81.8
necroticans combustiformis L51.2
due to drug — *see* Table of Drugs and Chemicals, by drug
Epidermophytid — *see* Dermatophytosis
Epidermophytosis (infected) — *see* Dermatophytosis
Epididymis — *see* condition
Epididymitis (acute) (nonvenereal) (recurrent) (residual) N45.1
with orchitis N45.3
blennorrhagic (gonococcal) A54.23
caseous (tuberculous) A18.15
chlamydial A56.19
filarial — *see also* Infestation, filarial B74.9 *[N51]*
gonococcal A54.23
syphilitic A52.76
tuberculous A18.15
Epididymo-orchitis — *see also* Epididymitis N45.3
Epidural — *see* condition
Epigastrium, epigastric — *see* condition
Epigastrocele — *see* Hernia, ventral
Epiglottis — *see* condition
Epiglottitis, epiglottiditis (acute) J05.10
with obstruction J05.11
chronic J37.0
Epignathus Q89.4
Epilepsia partialis continua — *see also* Kozhevnikof's epilepsy G40.1-
Epilepsy, epileptic, epilepsia (attack) (cerebral) (convulsion) (fit) (seizure) G40.909
Note: the following terms are to be considered equivalent to intractable: pharmacoresistant (pharmacologically resistant) , treatment resistant, refractory (medically) and poorly controlled
with
complex partial seizures — *see* Epilepsy, localization-related, symptomatic, with complex partial seizures
grand mal seizures on awakening — *see* Epilepsy, generalized, specified NEC
myoclonic absences — *see* Epilepsy, generalized, specified NEC
myoclonic-astatic seizures — *see* Epilepsy, generalized, specified NEC
simple partial seizures — *see* Epilepsy, localization-related, symptomatic, with simple partial seizures
akinetic — *see* Epilepsy, generalized, specified NEC
benign childhood with centrotemporal EEG spikes — *see* Epilepsy, localization-related, idiopathic
benign myoclonic in infancy G40.80-
Bravais-jacksonian — *see* Epilepsy, localization-related, symptomatic, with simple partial seizures
childhood
with occipital EEG paroxysms — *see* Epilepsy, localization-related, idiopathic
absence G40.A09
intractable G40.A19
with status epilepticus G40.A11
without status epilepticus G40.A19
not intractable G40.A09
with status epilepticus G40.A01
without status epilepticus G40.A09
climacteric — *see* Epilepsy, specified NEC
cysticercosis B69.0
deterioration (mental) F06.8
due to syphilis A52.19
focal — *see* Epilepsy, localization-related, symptomatic, with simple partial seizures
generalized
idiopathic G40.309
intractable G40.319
with status epilepticus G40.311
without status epilepticus G40.319
not intractable G40.309
with status epilepticus G40.301

Epilepsy, epileptic, epilepsia (attack) (cerebral) (convulsion) (fit) (seizure) - *continued*
generalized - *continued*
idiopathic - *continued*
not intractable - *continued*
without status epilepticus G40.309
specified NEC G40.409
intractable G40.419
with status epilepticus G40.411
without status epilepticus G40.419
not intractable G40.409
with status epilepticus G40.401
without status epilepticus G40.409
impulsive petit mal — *see* Epilepsy, juvenile myoclonic
intractable G40.919
with status epilepticus G40.911
without status epilepticus G40.919
juvenile absence G40.A09
intractable G40.A19
with status epilepticus G40.A11
without status epilepticus G40.A19
not intractable G40.A09
with status epilepticus G40.A01
without status epilepticus G40.A09
juvenile myoclonic G40.B09
intractable G40.B19
with status epilepticus G40.B11
without status epilepticus G40.B19
not intractable G40.B09
with status epilepticus G40.B01
without status epilepticus G40.B09
localization-related (focal) (partial)
idiopathic G40.009
with seizures of localized onset G40.009
intractable G40.019
with status epilepticus G40.011
without status epilepticus G40.019
not intractable G40.009
with status epilepticus G40.001
without status epilepticus G40.009
symptomatic
with complex partial seizures G40.209
intractable G40.219
with status epilepticus G40.211
without status epilepticus G40.219
not intractable G40.209
with status epilepticus G40.201
without status epilepticus G40.209
with simple partial seizures G40.109
intractable G40.119
with status epilepticus G40.111
without status epilepticus G40.119
not intractable G40.109
with status epilepticus G40.101
without status epilepticus G40.109
myoclonus, myoclonic — *see* Epilepsy, generalized, specified NEC
progressive — *see* Epilepsy, generalized, idiopathic
not intractable G40.909
with status epilepticus G40.901
without status epilepticus G40.909
on awakening — *see* Epilepsy, generalized, specified NEC
parasitic NOS B71.9 *[G94]*
partialis continua — *see also* Kozhevnikof's epilepsy G40.1-
peripheral — *see* Epilepsy, specified NEC
procursiva — *see* Epilepsy, localization-related, symptomatic, with simple partial seizures
progressive (familial) myoclonic — *see* Epilepsy, generalized, idiopathic
reflex — *see* Epilepsy, specified NEC
related to
alcohol G40.509
not intractable G40.509
with status epilepticus G40.501
without status epliepticus G40.509
drugs G40.509
not intractable G40.509
with status epilepticus G40.501
without status epliepticus G40.509
external causes G40.509
not intractable G40.509
with status epilepticus G40.501
without status epliepticus G40.509
hormonal changes G40.509
not intractable G40.509
with status epilepticus G40.501
without status epliepticus G40.509
sleep deprivation G40.509
not intractable G40.509

Epilepsy, epileptic, epilepsia (attack) (cerebral) (convulsion) (fit) (seizure) - *continued*
related to - *continued*
sleep deprivation - *continued*
not intractable - *continued*
with status epilepticus G40.501
without status epliepticus G40.509
stress G40.509
not intractable G40.509
with status epilepticus G40.501
without status epliepticus G40.509
somatomotor — *see* Epilepsy, localization-related, symptomatic, with simple partial seizures
somatosensory — *see* Epilepsy, localization-related, symptomatic, with simple partial seizures
spasms G40.822
intractable G40.824
with status epilepticus G40.823
without status epilepticus G40.824
not intractable G40.822
with status epilepticus G40.821
without status epilepticus G40.822
specified NEC G40.802
intractable G40.804
with status epilepticus G40.803
without status epilepticus G40.804
not intractable G40.802
with status epilepticus G40.801
without status epilepticus G40.802
syndromes
generalized
idiopathic G40.309
intractable G40.319
with status epilepticus G40.311
without status epilepticus G40.319
not intractable G40.309
with status epilepticus G40.301
without status epilepticus G40.309
specified NEC G40.409
intractable G40.419
with status epilepticus G40.411
without status epilepticus G40.419
not intractable G40.409
with status epilepticus G40.401
without status epilepticus G40.409
localization-related (focal) (partial)
idiopathic G40.009
with seizures of localized onset G40.009
intractable G40.019
with status epilepticus G40.011
without status epilepticus G40.019
not intractable G40.009
with status epilepticus G40.001
without status epilepticus G40.009
symptomatic
with complex partial seizures G40.209
intractable G40.219
with status epilepticus G40.211
without status epilepticus G40.219
not intractable G40.209
with status epilepticus G40.201
without status epilepticus G40.209
with simple partial seizures G40.109
intractable G40.119
with status epilepticus G40.111
without status epilepticus G40.119
not intractable G40.109
with status epilepticus G40.101
without status epilepticus G40.109
specified NEC G40.802
intractable G40.804
with status epilepticus G40.803
without status epilepticus G40.804
not intractable G40.802
with status epilepticus G40.801
without status epilepticus G40.802
tonic (-clonic) — *see* Epilepsy, generalized, specified NEC
twilight F05
uncinate (gyrus) — *see* Epilepsy, localization-related, symptomatic, with complex partial seizures
Unverricht (-Lundborg) (familial myoclonic) — *see* Epilepsy, generalized, idiopathic
visceral — *see* Epilepsy, specified NEC
visual — *see* Epilepsy, specified NEC
Epiloia Q85.1
Epimenorrhea N92.0
Epipharyngitis — *see* Nasopharyngitis
Epiphora H04.20-
due to
excess lacrimation H04.21-
insufficient drainage H04.22-
Epiphyseal arrest — *see* Arrest, epiphyseal

Epiphyseolysis, epiphysiolysis — *see* Osteochondropathy
Epiphysitis — *see also* Osteochondropathy
juvenile M92.9
syphilitic (congenital) A50.02
Epiplocele — *see* Hernia, abdomen
Epiploitis — *see* Peritonitis
Epiplosarcomphalocele — *see* Hernia, umbilicus
Episcleritis (suppurative) H15.10-
in (due to)
syphilis A52.71
tuberculosis A18.51
nodular H15.12-
periodica fugax H15.11-
angioneurotic — *see* Edema, angioneurotic
syphilitic (late) A52.71
tuberculous A18.51
Episode
affective, mixed F39
depersonalization (in neurotic state) F48.1
depressive F32.9
major F32.9
mild F32.0
moderate F32.1
severe (without psychotic symptoms) F32.2
with psychotic symptoms F32.3
recurrent F33.9
brief F33.8
specified NEC F32.89
hypomanic F30.8
manic F30.9
with
psychotic symptoms F30.2
remission (full) F30.4
partial F30.3
other specified F30.8
recurrent F31.89
without psychotic symptoms F30.10
mild F30.11
moderate F30.12
severe (without psychotic symptoms) F30.13
with psychotic symptoms F30.2
psychotic F23
organic F06.8
schizophrenic (acute) NEC, brief F23
Epispadias (female) (male) Q64.0
Episplenitis D73.89
Epistaxis (multiple) R04.0
hereditary I78.0
vicarious menstruation N94.89
Epithelioma (malignant) — *see* also Neoplasm, malignant, by site
adenoides cysticum — *see* Neoplasm, skin, benign
basal cell — *see* Neoplasm, skin, malignant
benign — *see* Neoplasm, benign, by site
Bowen's — *see* Neoplasm, skin, in situ
calcifying, of Malherbe — *see* Neoplasm, skin, benign
external site — *see* Neoplasm, skin, malignant
intraepidermal, Jadassohn — *see* Neoplasm, skin, benign
squamous cell — *see* Neoplasm, malignant, by site
Epitheliomatosis pigmented Q82.1
Epitheliopathy, multifocal placoid pigment H30.14-
Epithelium, epithelial — *see* condition
Epituberculosis (with atelectasis) (allergic) A15.7
Eponychia Q84.6
Epstein's
nephrosis or syndrome — *see* Nephrosis
pearl K09.8
Epulis (gingiva) (fibrous) (giant cell) K06.8
Equinia A24.0
Equinovarus (congenital) (talipes) Q66.0
acquired — *see* Deformity, limb, clubfoot
Equivalent
convulsive (abdominal) — *see* Epilepsy, specified NEC
epileptic (psychic) — *see* Epilepsy, localization-related, symptomatic, with complex partial seizures
Erb (-Duchenne) **paralysis** (birth injury) (newborn) P14.0
Erb-Goldflam disease or syndrome G70.00
with exacerbation (acute) G70.01
in crisis G70.01
Erb's
disease G71.02
palsy, paralysis (brachial) (birth) (newborn) P14.0
spinal (spastic) syphilitic A52.17
pseudohypertrophic muscular dystrophy G71.02
Erdheim's syndrome (acromegalic macrospondylitis) E22.0
Erection, painful (persistent) — *see* Priapism

Ergosterol deficiency (vitamin D) E55.9
 with
  adult osteomalacia M83.8
  rickets — *see* Rickets
Ergotism — *see also* Poisoning, food, noxious, plant
 from ergot used as drug (migraine therapy) — *see* Table of Drugs and Chemicals
Erosio interdigitalis blastomycetica B37.2
Erosion
 artery I77.2
  without rupture I77.89
 bone — *see* Disorder, bone, density and structure, specified NEC
 bronchus J98.09
 cartilage (joint) — *see* Disorder, cartilage, specified type NEC
 cervix (uteri) (acquired) (chronic) (congenital) N86
  with cervicitis N72
 cornea (nontraumatic) — *see* Ulcer, cornea
  recurrent H18.83-
  traumatic — *see* Abrasion, cornea
 dental (idiopathic) (occupational) (due to diet, drugs or vomiting) K03.2
 duodenum, postpyloric — *see* Ulcer, duodenum
 esophagus K22.10
  with bleeding K22.11
 gastric — *see* Ulcer, stomach
 gastrojejunal — *see* Ulcer, gastrojejunal
 implanted mesh — *see* Complications, mesh
 intestine K63.3
 lymphatic vessel I89.8
 pylorus, pyloric (ulcer) — *see* Ulcer, stomach
 spine, aneurysmal A52.09
 stomach — *see* Ulcer, stomach
 subcutaneous device pocket
  nervous system prosthetic device, implant, or graft T85.890
  other internal prosthetic device, implant, or graft T85.898
 teeth (idiopathic) (occupational) (due to diet, drugs or vomiting) K03.2
 urethra N36.8
 uterus N85.8
Erotomania F52.8
Error
 metabolism, inborn -- se Disorder, metabolism
 refractive — *see* Disorder, refraction
Eructation R14.2
 nervous or psychogenic F45.8
Eruption
 creeping B76.9
 drug (generalized) (taken internally) L27.0
  fixed L27.1
  in contact with skin — *see* Dermatitis, due to drugs
  localized L27.1
 Hutchinson, summer L56.4
 Kaposi's varicelliform B00.0
 napkin L22
 polymorphous light (sun) L56.4
 recalcitrant pustular L13.8
 ringed R23.8
 skin (nonspecific) R21
  creeping (meaning hookworm) B76.9
  due to inoculation/vaccination (generalized) — *see also* Dermatitis, due to, vaccine L27.0
   localized L27.1
  erysipeloid A26.0
  feigned L98.1
  Kaposi's varicelliform B00.0
  lichenoid L28.0
  meaning dermatitis — *see* Dermatitis
  toxic NEC L53.0
 tooth, teeth, abnormal (incomplete) (late) (premature) (sequence) K00.6
 vesicular R23.8
Erysipelas (gangrenous) (infantile) (newborn) (phlegmonous) (suppurative) A46
 external ear A46 *[H62.40]*
 puerperal, postpartum O86.89
Erysipeloid A26.9
 cutaneous (Rosenbach's) A26.0
 disseminated A26.8
 sepsis A26.7
 specified NEC A26.8
Erythema, erythematous (infectional) (inflammation) L53.9
 ab igne L59.0
 annulare (centrifugum) (rheumaticum) L53.1
 arthriticum epidemicum A25.1
 brucellum — *see* Brucellosis
 chronic figurate NEC L53.3
 chronicum migrans (Borrelia burgdorferi) A69.20
 diaper L22

Erythema, erythematous (infectional) (inflammation) - *continued*
 due to
  chemical NEC L53.0
   in contact with skin L24.5
  drug (internal use) — *see* Dermatitis, due to, drugs
 elevatum diutinum L95.1
 endemic E52
 epidemic, arthritic A25.1
 figuratum perstans L53.3
 gluteal L22
 heat - code by site under Burn, first degree
 ichthyosiforme congenitum bullous Q80.3
 in diseases classified elsewhere L54
 induratum (nontuberculous) L52
  tuberculous A18.4
 infectiosum B08.3
 intertrigo L30.4
 iris L51.9
 marginatum L53.2
  in (due to) acute rheumatic fever I00
 medicamentosum — *see* Dermatitis, due to, drugs
 migrans A26.0
  chronicum A69.20
  tongue K14.1
 multiforme (major) (minor) L51.9
  bullous, bullosum L51.1
  conjunctiva L51.1
  nonbullous L51.0
  pemphigoides L12.0
  specified NEC L51.8
 napkin L22
 neonatorum P83.88
  toxic P83.1
 nodosum L52
  tuberculous A18.4
 palmar L53.8
 pernio T69.1
 rash, newborn P83.88
 scarlatiniform (recurrent) (exfoliative) L53.8
 solare L55.0
 specified NEC L53.8
 toxic, toxicum NEC L53.0
  newborn P83.1
 tuberculous (primary) A18.4
Erythematous, erythematosus — *see* condition
Erythermalgia (primary) I73.81
Erythralgia I73.81
Erythrasma L08.1
Erythredema (polyneuropathy) — *see* Poisoning, mercury
Erythremia (acute) C94.0-
 chronic D45
 secondary D75.1
Erythroblastopenia — *see also* Aplasia, red cell D60.9
 congenital D61.01
Erythroblastophthisis D61.09
Erythroblastosis (fetalis) (newborn) P55.9
 due to
  ABO (antibodies) (incompatibility) (isoimmunization) P55.1
  Rh (antibodies) (incompatibility) (isoimmunization) P55.0
Erythrocyanosis (crurum) I73.89
Erythrocythemia — *see* Erythremia
Erythrocytosis (megalosplenic) (secondary) D75.1
 familial D75.0
 oval, hereditary — *see* Elliptocytosis
 secondary D75.1
 stress D75.1
Erythroderma (secondary) — *see also* Erythema L53.9
 bullous ichthyosiform, congenital Q80.3
 desquamativum L21.1
 ichthyosiform, congenital (bullous) Q80.3
 neonatorum P83.88
 psoriaticum L40.8
Erythrodysesthesia, palmar plantar (PPE) L27.1
Erythrogenesis imperfecta D61.09
Erythroleukemia C94.0-
Erythromelalgia I73.81
Erythrophagocytosis D75.89
Erythrophobia F40.298
Erythroplakia, oral epithelium, and tongue K13.29
Erythroplasia (Queyrat) D07.4
 specified site — *see* Neoplasm, skin, in situ
 unspecified site D07.4
Escherichia coli (E. coli)
 , as cause of disease classified elsewhere B96.20
 non-O157 Shiga toxin-producing (with known O group) B96.22
 non-Shiga toxin-producing B96.29

Escherichia coli (E. coli)
, as cause of disease classified elsewhere - *continued*
 O157 with confirmation of Shiga toxin when H antigen is unknown, or is not H7 B96.21
 O157:H- (nonmotile) with confirmation of Shiga toxin B96.21
 O157:H7 with or without confirmation of Shiga toxin-production B96.21
 Shiga toxin-producing (with unspecified O group) (STEC) B96.23
 O157 B96.21
 O157:H7 with or without confirmation of Shiga toxin-production B96.21
  specified NEC B96.22
 specified NEC B96.29
Esophagismus K22.4
Esophagitis (acute) (alkaline) (chemical) (chronic) (infectional) (necrotic) (peptic) (postoperative) K20.9
 candidal B37.81
 due to gastrointestinal reflux disease K21.0
 eosinophilic K20.0
 reflux K21.0
 specified NEC K20.8
 tuberculous A18.83
 ulcerative K22.10
  with bleeding K22.11
Esophagocele K22.5
Esophagomalacia K22.8
Esophagospasm K22.4
Esophagostenosis K22.2
Esophagostomiasis B81.8
Esophagotracheal — *see* condition
Esophagus — *see* condition
Esophoria H50.51
 convergence, excess H51.12
 divergence, insufficiency H51.8
Esotropia — *see* Strabismus, convergent concomitant
Espundia B55.2
Essential — *see* condition
Esthesioneuroblastoma C30.0
Esthesioneurocytoma C30.0
Esthesioneuroepithelioma C30.0
Esthiomene A55
Estivo-autumnal malaria (fever) B50.9
Estrangement (marital) Z63.5
 parent-child NEC Z62.890
Estriasis — *see* Myiasis
Ethanolism — *see* Alcoholism
Etherism — *see* Dependence, drug, inhalant
Ethmoid, ethmoidal — *see* condition
Ethmoiditis (chronic) (nonpurulent) (purulent) — *see also* Sinusitis, ethmoidal
 influenzal — *see* Influenza, with, respiratory manifestations NEC
 Woakes' J33.1
Ethylism — *see* Alcoholism
Eulenburg's disease (congenital paramyotonia) G71.19
Eumycetoma B47.0
Eunuchoidism E29.1
 hypogonadotropic E23.0
European blastomycosis — *see* Cryptococcosis
Eustachian — *see* condition
Evaluation (for) (of)
 development state
  adolescent Z00.3
  period of
   delayed growth in childhood Z00.70
    with abnormal findings Z00.71
   rapid growth in childhood Z00.2
  puberty Z00.3
 growth and developmental state (period of rapid growth) Z00.2
  delayed growth Z00.70
   with abnormal findings Z00.71
 mental health (status) Z00.8
  requested by authority Z04.6
 period of
  delayed growth in childhood Z00.70
   with abnormal findings Z00.71
  rapid growth in childhood Z00.2
 suspected condition — *see* Observation
Evans syndrome D69.41
Event
 apparent life threatening in newborn and infant (ALTE) R68.13
 brief resolved unexplained event (BRUE) R68.13
Eventration — *see also* Hernia, ventral
 colon into chest — *see* Hernia, diaphragm
 diaphragm (congenital) Q79.1
Eversion
 bladder N32.89

- **Eversion** - *continued*
  - cervix (uteri) N86
    - with cervicitis N72
  - foot NEC — *see also* Deformity, valgus, ankle
    - congenital Q66.6
  - punctum lacrimale (postinfectional) (senile) H04.52-
  - ureter (meatus) N28.89
  - urethra (meatus) N36.8
  - uterus N81.4
- **Evidence**
  - cytologic
    - of malignancy on anal smear R85.614
    - of malignancy on cervical smear R87.614
    - of malignancy on vaginal smear R87.624
- **Evisceration**
  - birth injury P15.8
  - traumatic NEC
    - eye — *see* Enucleated eye
- **Evulsion** — *see* Avulsion
- **Ewing's sarcoma or tumor** — *see* Neoplasm, bone, malignant
- **Examination** (for) (following) (general) (of) (routine) Z00.00
  - with abnormal findings Z00.01
  - abuse, physical (alleged) , ruled out
    - adult Z04.71
    - child Z04.72
  - adolescent (development state) Z00.3
  - alleged rape or sexual assault (victim) , ruled out
    - adult Z04.41
    - child Z04.42
  - allergy Z01.82
  - annual (adult) (periodic) (physical) Z00.00
    - with abnormal findings Z00.01
    - gynecological Z01.419
      - with abnormal findings Z01.411
  - antibody response Z01.84
  - blood — *see* Examination, laboratory
  - blood pressure Z01.30
    - with abnormal findings Z01.31
  - cancer staging — *see* Neoplasm, malignant, by site
  - cervical Papanicolaou smear Z12.4
    - as part of routine gynecological examination Z01.419
      - with abnormal findings Z01.411
  - child (over 28 days old) Z00.129
    - with abnormal findings Z00.121
    - under 28 days old — *see* Newborn, examination
  - clinical research control or normal comparison (control) (participant) Z00.6
  - contraceptive (drug) maintenance (routine) Z30.8
    - device (intrauterine) Z30.431
  - dental Z01.20
    - with abnormal findings Z01.21
  - developmental — *see* Examination, child
  - donor (potential) Z00.5
  - ear Z01.10
    - with abnormal findings NEC Z01.118
  - eye Z01.00
    - with abnormal findings Z01.01
  - following
    - accident NEC Z04.3
      - transport Z04.1
      - work Z04.2
    - assault, alleged, ruled out
      - adult Z04.71
      - child Z04.72
    - motor vehicle accident Z04.1
    - treatment (for) Z09
      - combined NEC Z09
        - fracture Z09
        - malignant neoplasm Z08
      - malignant neoplasm Z08
      - mental disorder Z09
      - specified condition NEC Z09
  - follow-up (routine) (following) Z09
    - chemotherapy NEC Z09
      - malignant neoplasm Z08
    - fracture Z09
    - malignant neoplasm Z08
    - postpartum Z39.2
    - psychotherapy Z09
    - radiotherapy NEC Z09
      - malignant neoplasm Z08
    - surgery NEC Z09
      - malignant neoplasm Z08
  - forced sexual exploitation Z04.81
  - forced labor exploitation Z04.82
  - gynecological Z01.419
    - with abnormal findings Z01.411
    - for contraceptive maintenance Z30.8
  - health — *see* Examination, medical
  - hearing Z01.10
- **Examination** (for) (following) (general) (of) (routine) - *continued*
  - hearing - *continued*
    - with abnormal findings NEC Z01.118
    - infant or child (over 28 days old) Z00.129
      - with abnormal findings Z00.121
    - following failed hearing screening Z01.110
  - immunity status testing Z01.84
  - laboratory (as part of a general medical examination) Z00.00
    - with abnormal findings Z00.01
    - preprocedural Z01.812
  - lactating mother Z39.1
  - medical (adult) (for) (of) Z00.00
    - with abnormal findings Z00.01
    - administrative purpose only Z02.9
      - specified NEC Z02.89
    - admission to
      - armed forces Z02.3
      - old age home Z02.2
      - prison Z02.89
      - residential institution Z02.2
      - school Z02.0
        - following illness or medical treatment Z02.0
      - summer camp Z02.89
    - adoption Z02.82
    - blood alcohol or drug level Z02.83
    - camp (summer) Z02.89
    - clinical research, normal subject (control) (participant) Z00.6
    - control subject in clinical research (normal comparison) (participant) Z00.6
    - donor (potential) Z00.5
    - driving license Z02.4
    - general (adult) Z00.00
      - with abnormal findings Z00.01
    - immigration Z02.89
    - insurance purposes Z02.6
    - marriage Z02.89
    - medicolegal reasons NEC Z04.89
    - naturalization Z02.89
    - participation in sport Z02.5
    - paternity testing Z02.81
    - population survey Z00.8
    - pre-employment Z02.1
    - pre-operative — *see* Examination, pre-procedural
    - pre-procedural
      - cardiovascular Z01.810
      - respiratory Z01.811
      - specified NEC Z01.818
    - preschool children
      - for admission to school Z02.0
    - prisoners
      - for entrance into prison Z02.89
    - recruitment for armed forces Z02.3
    - specified NEC Z00.8
    - sport competition Z02.5
  - medicolegal reason NEC Z04.89
    - following
      - forced sexual exploitation Z04.81
      - forced labor exploitation Z04.82
  - newborn — *see* Newborn, examination
  - pelvic (annual) (periodic) Z01.419
    - with abnormal findings Z01.411
  - period of rapid growth in childhood Z00.2
  - periodic (adult) (annual) (routine) Z00.00
    - with abnormal findings Z00.01
  - physical (adult) — *see also* Examination, medical Z00.00
    - sports Z02.5
  - postpartum
    - immediately after delivery Z39.0
    - routine follow-up Z39.2
  - prenatal (normal pregnancy) — *see also* Pregnancy, normal Z34.9-
  - pre-chemotherapy (antineoplastic) Z01.818
  - pre-procedural (pre-operative)
    - cardiovascular Z01.810
    - laboratory Z01.812
    - respiratory Z01.811
    - specified NEC Z01.818
  - prior to chemotherapy (antineoplastic) Z01.818
  - psychiatric NEC Z00.8
    - follow-up not needing further care Z09
    - requested by authority Z04.6
  - radiological (as part of a general medical examination) Z00.00
    - with abnormal findings Z00.01
  - repeat cervical smear to confirm findings of recent normal smear following initial abnormal smear Z01.42
  - skin (hypersensitivity) Z01.82
  - special — *see also* Examination, by type Z01.89
- **Examination** (for) (following) (general) (of) (routine) - *continued*
  - special - *continued*
    - specified type NEC Z01.89
  - specified type or reason NEC Z04.89
  - teeth Z01.20
    - with abnormal findings Z01.21
  - urine — *see* Examination, laboratory
  - vision Z01.00
    - with abnormal findings Z01.01
    - infant or child (over 28 days old) Z00.129
      - with abnormal findings Z00.121
- **Exanthem, exanthema** — *see also* Rash
  - with enteroviral vesicular stomatitis B08.4
  - Boston A88.0
  - epidemic with meningitis A88.0 *[G02]*
  - subitum B08.20
    - due to human herpesvirus 6 B08.21
    - due to human herpesvirus 7 B08.22
  - viral, virus B09
    - specified type NEC B08.8
- **Excess, excessive, excessively**
  - alcohol level in blood R78.0
  - androgen (ovarian) E28.1
  - attrition, tooth, teeth K03.0
  - carotene, carotin (dietary) E67.1
  - cold, effects of T69.9
    - specified effect NEC T69.8
  - convergence H51.12
  - crying
    - in child, adolescent, or adult R45.83
    - in infant R68.11
  - development, breast N62
  - divergence H51.8
  - drinking (alcohol) NEC (without dependence) F10.10
    - habitual (continual) (without remission) F10.20
  - eating R63.2
  - estrogen E28.0
  - fat — *see also* Obesity
    - in heart — *see* Degeneration, myocardial
    - localized E65
  - foreskin N47.8
  - gas R14.0
  - glucagon E16.3
  - heat — *see* Heat
  - intermaxillary vertical dimension of fully erupted teeth M26.37
  - interocclusal distance of fully erupted teeth M26.37
  - kalium E87.5
  - large
    - colon K59.39
      - congenital Q43.8
    - infant P08.0
    - organ or site, congenital NEC — *see* Anomaly, by site
  - long
    - organ or site, congenital NEC — *see* Anomaly, by site
  - menstruation (with regular cycle) N92.0
    - with irregular cycle N92.1
  - napping Z72.821
  - natrium E87.0
  - number of teeth K00.1
  - nutrient (dietary) NEC R63.2
  - potassium (K) E87.5
  - salivation K11.7
  - secretion — *see also* Hypersecretion
    - milk O92.6
    - sputum R09.3
    - sweat R61
  - sexual drive F52.8
  - short
    - organ or site, congenital NEC — *see* Anomaly, by site
    - umbilical cord in labor or delivery O69.3
  - skin L98.7
    - and subcutaneous tissue L98.7
    - eyelid (acquired) — *see* Blepharochalasis
      - congenital Q10.3
  - sodium (Na) E87.0
  - spacing of fully erupted teeth M26.32
  - sputum R09.3
  - sweating R61
  - thirst R63.1
    - due to deprivation of water T73.1
  - tuberosity of jaw M26.07
  - vitamin
    - A (dietary) E67.0
      - administered as drug (prolonged intake) — *see* Table of Drugs and Chemicals, vitamins, adverse effect

Excess, excessive, excessively - *continued*
vitamin - *continued*
A (dietary) - *continued*
overdose or wrong substance given or taken — *see* Table of Drugs and Chemicals, vitamins, poisoning
D (dietary) E67.3
administered as drug (prolonged intake) — *see* Table of Drugs and Chemicals, vitamins, adverse effect
overdose or wrong substance given or taken — *see* Table of Drugs and Chemicals, vitamins, poisoning
weight
gain R63.5
loss R63.4
Excitability, abnormal, under minor stress (personality disorder) F60.3
Excitation
anomalous atrioventricular I45.6
psychogenic F30.8
reactive (from emotional stress, psychological trauma) F30.8
Excitement
hypomanic F30.8
manic F30.9
mental, reactive (from emotional stress, psychological trauma) F30.8
state, reactive (from emotional stress, psychological trauma) F30.8
Excoriation (traumatic) — *see also* Abrasion
neurotic L98.1
skin picking disorder F42.4
Exfoliation
due to erythematous conditions according to extent of body surface involved L49.0
10-19 percent of body surface L49.1
20-29 percent of body surface L49.2
30-39 percent of body surface L49.3
40-49 percent of body surface L49.4
50-59 percent of body surface L49.5
60-69 percent of body surface L49.6
70-79 percent of body surface L49.7
80-89 percent of body surface L49.8
90-99 percent of body surface L49.9
less than 10 percent of body surface L49.0
teeth, due to systemic causes K08.0
Exfoliative — *see* condition
Exhaustion, exhaustive (physical NEC) R53.83
battle F43.0
cardiac — *see* Failure, heart
delirium F43.0
due to
cold T69.8
excessive exertion T73.3
exposure T73.2
neurasthenia F48.8
heart — *see* Failure, heart
heat — *see also* Heat, exhaustion T67.5
due to
salt depletion T67.4
water depletion T67.3
maternal, complicating delivery O75.81
mental F48.8
myocardium, myocardial — *see* Failure, heart
nervous F48.8
old age R54
psychogenic F48.8
psychosis F43.0
senile R54
vital NEC Z73.0
Exhibitionism F65.2
Exocervicitis — *see* Cervicitis
Exomphalos Q79.2
meaning hernia — *see* Hernia, umbilicus
Exophoria H50.52
convergence, insufficiency H51.11
divergence, excess H51.8
Exophthalmos H05.2-
congenital Q15.8
constant NEC H05.24-
displacement, globe — *see* Displacement, globe
due to thyrotoxicosis (hyperthyroidism) — *see* Hyperthyroidism, with, goiter (diffuse)
dysthyroid — *see* Hyperthyroidism, with, goiter (diffuse)
goiter — *see* Hyperthyroidism, with, goiter (diffuse)
intermittent NEC H05.25-
malignant — *see* Hyperthyroidism, with, goiter (diffuse)
orbital
edema — *see* Edema, orbit
hemorrhage — *see* Hemorrhage, orbit

Exophthalmos - *continued*
pulsating NEC H05.26-
thyrotoxic, thyrotropic — *see* Hyperthyroidism, with, goiter (diffuse)
Exostosis — *see also* Disorder, bone
cartilaginous — *see* Neoplasm, bone, benign
congenital (multiple) Q78.6
external ear canal H61.81-
gonococcal A54.49
jaw (bone) M27.8
multiple, congenital Q78.6
orbit H05.35-
osteocartilaginous — *see* Neoplasm, bone, benign
syphilitic A52.77
Exotropia — *see* Strabismus, divergent concomitant
Explanation of
investigation finding Z71.2
medication Z71.89
Exposure (to) — *see also* Contact, with T75.89
acariasis Z20.7
AIDS virus Z20.6
air pollution Z77.110
algae and algae toxins Z77.121
algae bloom Z77.121
anthrax Z20.810
aromatic amines Z77.020
aromatic (hazardous) compounds NEC Z77.028
aromatic dyes NOS Z77.028
arsenic Z77.010
asbestos Z77.090
bacterial disease NEC Z20.818
benzene Z77.021
blue-green algae bloom Z77.121
body fluids (potentially hazardous) Z77.21
brown tide Z77.121
chemicals (chiefly nonmedicinal) (hazardous) NEC Z77.098
cholera Z20.09
chromium compounds Z77.018
cold, effects of T69.9
specified effect NEC T69.8
communicable disease Z20.9
bacterial NEC Z20.818
specified NEC Z20.89
viral NEC Z20.828
Zika virus Z20.821
cyanobacteria bloom Z77.121
disaster Z65.5
discrimination Z60.5
dyes Z77.098
effects of T73.9
environmental tobacco smoke (acute) (chronic) Z77.22
Escherichia coli (E. coli) Z20.01
exhaustion due to T73.2
fiberglass — *see* Table of Drugs and Chemicals, fiberglass
German measles Z20.4
gonorrhea Z20.2
hazardous metals NEC Z77.018
hazardous substances NEC Z77.29
hazards in the physical environment NEC Z77.128
hazards to health NEC Z77.9
human immunodeficiency virus (HIV) Z20.6
human T-lymphotropic virus type-1 (HTLV-1) Z20.89
implanted
mesh — *see* Complications, mesh
prosthetic materials NEC — *see* Complications, prosthetic materials NEC
infestation (parasitic) NEC Z20.7
intestinal infectious disease NEC Z20.09
Escherichia coli (E. coli) Z20.01
lead Z77.011
meningococcus Z20.811
mold (toxic) Z77.120
nickel dust Z77.018
noise Z77.122
occupational
air contaminants NEC Z57.39
dust Z57.2
environmental tobacco smoke Z57.31
extreme temperature Z57.6
noise Z57.0
radiation Z57.1
risk factors Z57.9
specified NEC Z57.8
toxic agents (gases) (liquids) (solids) (vapors) in agriculture Z57.4
toxic agents (gases) (liquids) (solids) (vapors) in industry NEC Z57.5
vibration Z57.7
parasitic disease NEC Z20.7

Exposure (to) - *continued*
pediculosis Z20.7
persecution Z60.5
pfiesteria piscicida Z77.121
poliomyelitis Z20.89
polycyclic aromatic hydrocarbons Z77.028
pollution
air Z77.110
environmental NEC Z77.118
soil Z77.112
water Z77.111
prenatal (drugs) (toxic chemicals) — *see* Newborn, affected by, noxious substances transmitted via placenta or breast milk
rabies Z20.3
radiation, naturally occurring NEC Z77.123
radon Z77.123
red tide (Florida) Z77.121
rubella Z20.4
second hand tobacco smoke (acute) (chronic) Z77.22
in the perinatal period P96.81
sexually-transmitted disease Z20.2
smallpox (laboratory) Z20.89
syphilis Z20.2
terrorism Z65.4
torture Z65.4
tuberculosis Z20.1
uranium Z77.012
varicella Z20.820
venereal disease Z20.2
viral disease NEC Z20.828
war Z65.5
water pollution Z77.111
Zika virus Z20.821
Exsanguination — *see* Hemorrhage
Exstrophy
abdominal contents Q45.8
bladder Q64.10
cloacal Q64.12
specified type NEC Q64.19
supravesical fissure Q64.11
Extensive — *see* condition
Extra — *see also* Accessory
marker chromosomes (normal individual) Q92.61
in abnormal individual Q92.62
rib Q76.6
cervical Q76.5
Extrasystoles (supraventricular) I49.49
atrial I49.1
auricular I49.1
junctional I49.2
ventricular I49.3
Extrauterine gestation or pregnancy — *see* Pregnancy, by site
Extravasation
blood R58
chyle into mesentery I89.8
pelvicalyceal N13.8
pyelosinus N13.8
urine (from ureter) R39.0
vesicant agent
antineoplastic chemotherapy T80.810
other agent NEC T80.818
Extremity — *see* condition, limb
Extrophy — *see* Exstrophy
Extroversion
bladder Q64.19
uterus N81.4
complicating delivery O71.2
postpartal (old) N81.4
Extruded tooth (teeth) M26.34
Extrusion
breast implant (prosthetic) T85.42
eye implant (globe) (ball) T85.328
intervertebral disc — *see* Displacement, intervertebral disc
ocular lens implant (prosthetic) — *see* Complications, intraocular lens
vitreous — *see* Prolapse, vitreous
Exudate
pleural — *see* Effusion, pleura
retina H35.89
Exudative — *see* condition
Eye, eyeball, eyelid — *see* condition
Eyestrain — *see* Disturbance, vision, subjective
Eyeworm disease of Africa B74.3

F

Faber's syndrome (achlorhydric anemia) D50.9
Fabry (-Anderson) **disease** E75.21
Faciocephalalgia, autonomic — *see also* Neuropathy, peripheral, autonomic G90.09

Alphabetic Index to Diseases
Excess, excessive, excessively — Faciocephalalgia, autonomic

Factor (s)
- psychic, associated with diseases classified elsewhere F54
- psychological
  - affecting physical conditions F54
  - or behavioral
    - affecting general medical condition F54
    - associated with disorders or diseases classified elsewhere F54

Fahr disease (of brain) G23.8

Fahr Volhard disease (of kidney) I12.-

Failure, failed
- abortion — *see* Abortion, attempted
- aortic (valve) I35.8
  - rheumatic I06.8
- attempted abortion — *see* Abortion, attempted
- biventricular I50.82
  - due to left heart failure I50.814
- bone marrow — *see* Anemia, aplastic
- cardiac — *see* Failure, heart
- cardiorenal (chronic) — *see also* Failure, renal, and Failure, heart I50.9
  - hypertensive I13.2
- cardiorespiratory — *see also* Failure, heart R09.2
- cardiovascular (chronic) — *see* Failure, heart
- cerebrovascular I67.9
- cervical dilatation in labor O62.0
- circulation, circulatory (peripheral) R57.9
  - newborn P29.89
- compensation — *see* Disease, heart
- compliance with medical treatment or regimen — *see* Noncompliance
- congestive — *see* Failure, heart, congestive
- dental implant (endosseous) M27.69
  - due to
    - failure of dental prosthesis M27.63
    - lack of attached gingiva M27.62
    - occlusal trauma (poor prosthetic design) M27.62
    - parafunctional habits M27.62
    - periodontal infection (peri-implantitis) M27.62
    - poor oral hygiene M27.62
  - osseointegration M27.61
    - due to
      - complications of systemic disease M27.61
      - poor bone quality M27.61
    - iatrogenic M27.61
  - post-osseointegration
    - biological M27.62
    - due to complications of systemic disease M27.62
    - iatrogenic M27.62
    - mechanical M27.63
  - pre-integration M27.61
  - pre-osseointegration M27.61
  - specified NEC M27.69
- descent of head (at term) of pregnancy (mother) O32.4
- endosseous dental implant — *see* Failure, dental implant
- engagement of head (term of pregnancy) (mother) O32.4
- erection (penile) — *see also* Dysfunction, sexual, male, erectile N52.9
  - nonorganic F52.21
- examination (s) , anxiety concerning Z55.2
- expansion terminal respiratory units (newborn) (primary) P28.0
- forceps NOS (with subsequent cesarean delivery) O66.5
- gain weight (child over 28 days old) R62.51
  - adult R62.7
  - newborn P92.6
- genital response (male) F52.21
  - female F52.22
- heart (acute) (senile) (sudden) I50.9
  - with
    - acute pulmonary edema — *see* Failure, ventricular, left
    - decompensation — *see also* Failure, heart, by type as diastolic or systolic, acute and chronic I50.9
    - dilatation — *see* Disease, heart
    - normal ejection fraction — *see* Failure, heart, diastolic
    - preserved ejection fraction — *see* Failure, heart, diastolic
    - reduced ejection fraction — *see* Failure, heart, systolic
  - arteriosclerotic I70.90
  - biventricular I50.82
    - due to left heart failure I50.814
  - combined left-right sided I50.82
    - due to left heart failure I50.814

Failure, failed - *continued*
- heart (acute) (senile) (sudden) - *continued*
  - compensated — *see also* Failure, heart, by type as diastolic or systolic, chronic I50.9
  - complicating
    - anesthesia (general) (local) or other sedation
      - in labor and delivery O74.2
      - in pregnancy O29.12-
      - postpartum, puerperal O89.1
    - delivery (cesarean) (instrumental) O75.4
  - congestive I50.9
    - with rheumatic fever (conditions in I00)
      - active I01.8
      - inactive or quiescent (with chorea) I09.81
    - newborn P29.0
    - rheumatic (chronic) (inactive) (with chorea) I09.81
      - active or acute I01.8
        - with chorea I02.0
  - decompensated — *see also* Failure, heart, by type as diastolic or systolic, acute and chronic I50.9
  - degenerative — *see* Degeneration, myocardial
  - diastolic (congestive) (left ventricular) I50.30
    - acute (congestive) I50.31
      - and (on) chronic (congestive) I50.33
    - chronic (congestive) I50.32
      - and (on) acute (congestive) I50.33
    - combined with systolic (congestive) I50.40
      - acute (congestive) I50.41
        - and (on) chronic (congestive) I50.43
      - chronic (congestive) I50.42
        - and (on) acute (congestive) I50.43
  - due to presence of cardiac prosthesis I97.13-
  - end stage — *see also* Failure, heart, by type as diastolic or systolic, chronic I50.84
  - following cardiac surgery I97.13-
  - high output NOS I50.83
  - hypertensive — *see* Hypertension, heart
  - left (ventricular) — *see also* Failure, ventricular, left
    - combined diastolic and systolic — *see* Failure, heart, diastolic, combined with systolic
    - diastolic — *see* Failure, heart, diastolic
    - systolic — *see* Failure, heart, systolic
  - low output (syndrome) NOS I50.9
  - newborn P29.0
  - organic — *see* Disease, heart
  - peripartum O90.3
  - postprocedural I97.13-
  - rheumatic (chronic) (inactive) I09.9
  - right (isolated) (ventricular) I50.810
    - acute I50.811
      - and (on) chronic I50.813
    - chronic I50.812
      - and acute I50.813
    - secondary to left heart failure I50.814
  - specified NEC I50.89

  Note: heart failure stages A, B, C, and D are based on the American College of Cardiology and American Heart Association stages of heart failure, which complement and should not be confused with the New York Heart Association Classification of Heart Failure, into Class I, Class II, Class III, and Class IV

  - stage A Z91.89
  - stage B — *see also* Failure, heart, by type as diastolic or systolic I50.9
  - stage C — *see also* Failure, heart, by type as diastolic or systolic I50.9
  - stage D — *see also* Failure, heart, by type as diastolic or systolic, chronic I50.84
  - systolic (congestive) (left ventricular) I50.20
    - acute (congestive) I50.21
      - and (on) chronic (congestive) I50.23
    - chronic (congestive) I50.22
      - and (on) acute (congestive) I50.23
    - combined with diastolic (congestive) I50.40
      - acute (congestive) I50.41
        - and (on) chronic (congestive) I50.43
      - chronic (congestive) I50.42
        - and (on) acute (congestive) I50.43
  - thyrotoxic — *see also* Thyrotoxicosis E05.90 *[I43]*
    - with
      - high output — *see also* Thyrotoxicosis I50.83
      - thyroid storm E05.91 *[I43]*
        - high output — *see also* Thyrotoxicosis I50.83
  - valvular — *see* Endocarditis
- hepatic K72.90
  - with coma K72.91
  - acute or subacute K72.00
    - with coma K72.01
    - due to drugs K71.10
      - with coma K71.11

Failure, failed - *continued*
- hepatic - *continued*
  - alcoholic (acute) (chronic) (subacute) K70.40
    - with coma K70.41
  - chronic K72.10
    - with coma K72.11
    - due to drugs (acute) (subacute) (chronic) K71.10
      - with coma K71.11
  - due to drugs (acute) (subacute) (chronic) K71.10
    - with coma K71.11
  - postprocedural K91.82
- hepatorenal K76.7
- induction (of labor) O61.9
  - abortion — *see* Abortion, attempted
  - by
    - oxytocic drugs O61.0
    - prostaglandins O61.0
  - instrumental O61.1
  - mechanical O61.1
  - medical O61.0
  - specified NEC O61.8
  - surgical O61.1
- intubation during anesthesia T88.4
  - in pregnancy O29.6-
  - labor and delivery O74.7
  - postpartum, puerperal O89.6
- involution, thymus (gland) E32.0
- kidney — *see also* Disease, kidney, chronic N19
  - acute — *see also* Failure, renal, acute N17.9-
  - diabetic — *see* E08-E13 with .22
- lactation (complete) O92.3
  - partial O92.4
- Leydig's cell, adult E29.1
- liver — *see* Failure, hepatic
- menstruation at puberty N91.0
- mitral I05.8
- myocardial, myocardium — *see also* Failure, heart I50.9
  - chronic — *see also* Failure, heart, congestive I50.9
  - congestive — *see also* Failure, heart, congestive I50.9
- orgasm (female) (psychogenic) F52.31
  - male F52.32
- ovarian (primary) E28.39
  - iatrogenic E89.40
    - asymptomatic E89.40
    - symptomatic E89.41
  - postprocedural (postablative) (postirradiation) (postsurgical) E89.40
    - asymptomatic E89.40
    - symptomatic E89.41
- ovulation causing infertility N97.0
- polyglandular, autoimmune E31.0
- prosthetic joint implant — *see* Complications, joint prosthesis, mechanical, breakdown, by site
- renal N19
  - with
    - tubular necrosis (acute) N17.0
  - acute N17.9
    - with
      - cortical necrosis N17.1
      - medullary necrosis N17.2
      - tubular necrosis N17.0
    - specified NEC N17.8
  - chronic N18.9
    - hypertensive — *see* Hypertension, kidney
  - congenital P96.0
  - end stage (chronic) N18.6
    - due to hypertension I12.0
  - following
    - abortion — *see* Abortion by type complicated by specified condition NEC
    - crushing T79.5
    - ectopic or molar pregnancy O08.4
    - labor and delivery (acute) O90.4
  - hypertensive — *see* Hypertension, kidney
  - postprocedural N99.0
- respiration, respiratory J96.90
  - with
    - hypercapnia J96.92
    - hypercarbia J96.02
    - hypoxia J96.91
  - acute J96.00
    - with
      - hypercapnia J96.02
      - hypercarbia J96.02
      - hypoxia J96.01
  - center G93.89
  - acute and (on) chronic J96.20
    - with
      - hypercapnia J96.22
      - hypercarbia J96.22
      - hypoxia J96.21

Fever (inanition) (of unknown origin) (persistent) (with chills) (with rigor) - *continued*
  Cameroon — *see* Malaria
  Canton A75.9
  catarrhal (acute) J00
    chronic J31.0
  cat-scratch A28.1
  Central Asian hemorrhagic A98.0
  cerebral — *see* Encephalitis
  cerebrospinal meningococcal A39.0
  Chagres B50.9
  Chandipura A92.8
  Changuinola A93.1
  Charcot's (biliary) (hepatic) (intermittent) — *see* Calculus, bile duct
  Chikungunya (viral) (hemorrhagic) A92.0
  Chitral A93.1
  Colombo — *see* Fever, paratyphoid
  Colorado tick (virus) A93.2
  congestive (remittent) — *see* Malaria
  Congo virus A98.0
  continued malarial B50.9
  Corsican — *see* Malaria
  Crimean-Congo hemorrhagic A98.0
  Cyprus — *see* Brucellosis
  dandy A90
  deer fly — *see* Tularemia
  dengue (virus) A90
    hemorrhagic A91
    sandfly A93.1
  desert B38.0
  drug induced R50.2
  due to
    conditions classified elsewhere R50.81
    heat T67.0
  enteric A01.00
  enteroviral exanthematous (Boston exanthem) A88.0
  ephemeral (of unknown origin) R50.9
  epidemic hemorrhagic A98.5
  erysipelatous — *see* Erysipelas
  estivo-autumnal (malarial) B50.9
  famine A75.0
  five day A79.0
  following delivery O86.4
  Fort Bragg A27.89
  gastroenteric A01.00
  gastromalarial — *see* Malaria
  Gibraltar — *see* Brucellosis
  glandular — *see* Mononucleosis, infectious
  Guama (viral) A92.8
  Haverhill A25.1
  hay (allergic) J30.1
    with asthma (bronchial) J45.909
      with
        exacerbation (acute) J45.901
        status asthmaticus J45.902
    due to
      allergen other than pollen J30.89
      pollen, any plant or tree J30.1
  heat (effects) T67.0
  hematuric, bilious B50.8
  hemoglobinuric (malarial) (bilious) B50.8
  hemorrhagic (arthropod-borne) NOS A94
    with renal syndrome A98.5
    arenaviral A96.9
      specified NEC A96.8
    Argentinian A96.0
    Bangkok A91
    Bolivian A96.1
    Central Asian A98.0
    Chikungunya A92.0
    Crimean-Congo A98.0
    dengue (virus) A91
    epidemic A98.5
    Junin (virus) A96.0
    Korean A98.5
    Kyasanur forest A98.2
    Machupo (virus) A96.1
    mite-borne A93.8
    mosquito-borne A92.8
    Omsk A98.1
    Philippine A91
    Russian A98.5
    Singapore A91
    Southeast Asia A91
    Thailand A91
    tick-borne NEC A93.8
    viral A99
      specified NEC A98.8
  hepatic — *see* Cholecystitis
  herpetic — *see* Herpes
  icterohemorrhagic A27.0
  Indiana A93.8

Fever (inanition) (of unknown origin) (persistent) (with chills) (with rigor) - *continued*
  infective B99.9
    specified NEC B99.8
  intermittent (bilious) — *see also* Malaria
    of unknown origin R50.9
    pernicious B50.9
  iodide R50.2
  Japanese river A75.3
  jungle — *see also* Malaria
    yellow A95.0
  Junin (virus) hemorrhagic A96.0
  Katayama B65.2
  kedani A75.3
  Kenya (tick) A77.1
  Kew Garden A79.1
  Korean hemorrhagic A98.5
  Lassa A96.2
  Lone Star A77.0
  Machupo (virus) hemorrhagic A96.1
  malaria, malarial — *see* Malaria
  Malta A23.9
  Marseilles A77.1
  marsh — *see* Malaria
  Mayaro (viral) A92.8
  Mediterranean — *see also* Brucellosis A23.9
    familial M04.1
    tick A77.1
  meningeal — *see* Meningitis
  Meuse A79.0
  Mexican A75.2
  mianeh A68.1
  miasmatic — *see* Malaria
  mosquito-borne (viral) A92.9
    hemorrhagic A92.8
  mountain — *see also* Brucellosis
    meaning Rocky Mountain spotted fever A77.0
    tick (American) (Colorado) (viral) A93.2
  Mucambo (viral) A92.8
  mud A27.9
  Neapolitan — *see* Brucellosis
  neutropenic D70.9
  newborn P81.9
    environmental P81.0
  Nine-Mile A78
  non-exanthematous tick A93.2
  North Asian tick-borne A77.2
  Omsk hemorrhagic A98.1
  O'nyong-nyong (viral) A92.1
  Oropouche (viral) A93.0
  Oroya A44.0
  paludal — *see* Malaria
  Panama (malarial) B50.9
  Pappataci A93.1
  paratyphoid A01.4
    A A01.1
    B A01.2
    C A01.3
  parrot A70
  periodic (Mediterranean) M04.1
  persistent (of unknown origin) R50.9
  petechial A39.0
  pharyngoconjunctival B30.2
  Philippine hemorrhagic A91
  phlebotomus A93.1
  Piry (virus) A93.8
  Pixuna (viral) A92.8
  Plasmodium ovale B53.0
  polioviral (nonparalytic) A80.4
  Pontiac A48.2
  postimmunization R50.83
  postoperative R50.82
    due to infection T81.40
  posttransfusion R50.84
  postvaccination R50.83
  presenting with conditions classified elsewhere R50.81
  pretibial A27.89
  puerperal O86.4
  Q A78
  quadrilateral A78
  quartan (malaria) B52.9
  Queensland (coastal) (tick) A77.3
  quintan A79.0
  rabbit — *see* Tularemia
  rat-bite A25.9
    due to
      Spirillum A25.0
      Streptobacillus moniliformis A25.1
  recurrent — *see* Fever, relapsing
  relapsing (Borrelia) A68.9
    Carter's (Asiatic) A68.1
    Dutton's (West African) A68.1

Fever (inanition) (of unknown origin) (persistent) (with chills) (with rigor) - *continued*
  relapsing (Borrelia) - *continued*
    Koch's A68.9
    louse-borne A68.0
    Novy's
      louse-borne A68.0
      tick-borne A68.1
    Obermeyer's (European) A68.0
    tick-borne A68.1
  remittent (bilious) (congestive) (gastric) — *see* Malaria
  rheumatic (active) (acute) (chronic) (subacute) I00
    with central nervous system involvement I02.9
    active with heart involvement — *see* category I01
    inactive or quiescent with
      cardiac hypertrophy I09.89
      carditis I09.9
      endocarditis I09.1
        aortic (valve) I06.9
          with mitral (valve) disease I08.0
        mitral (valve) I05.9
          with aortic (valve) disease I08.0
        pulmonary (valve) I09.89
        tricuspid (valve) I07.8
      heart disease NEC I09.89
      heart failure (congestive) (conditions in category I50.) I09.81
      left ventricular failure (conditions in I50.1- I50.4-) I09.81
      myocarditis, myocardial degeneration (conditions in I51.4) I09.0
      pancarditis I09.9
      pericarditis I09.2
  Rift Valley (viral) A92.4
  Rocky Mountain spotted A77.0
  rose J30.1
  Ross River B33.1
  Russian hemorrhagic A98.5
  San Joaquin (Valley) B38.0
  sandfly A93.1
  Sao Paulo A77.0
  scarlet A38.9
  seven day (leptospirosis) (autumnal) (Japanese) A27.89
    dengue A90
  shin-bone A79.0
  Singapore hemorrhagic A91
  solar A90
  Songo A98.5
  sore B00.1
  South African tick-bite A68.1
  Southeast Asia hemorrhagic A91
  spinal — *see* Meningitis
  spirillary A25.0
  splenic — *see* Anthrax
  spotted A77.9
    American A77.0
    Brazilian A77.0
    cerebrospinal meningitis A39.0
    Colombian A77.0
    due to Rickettsia
      australis A77.3
      conorii A77.1
      rickettsii A77.0
      sibirica A77.2
      specified type NEC A77.8
    Ehrlichiosis A77.40
      due to
        E. chafeensis A77.41
        specified organism NEC A77.49
    Rocky Mountain A77.0
  steroid R50.2
  streptobacillary A25.1
  subtertian B50.9
  Sumatran mite A75.3
  sun A90
  swamp A27.9
  swine A02.8
  sylvatic, yellow A95.0
  Tahyna B33.8
  tertian — *see* Malaria, tertian
  Thailand hemorrhagic A91
  thermic T67.0
  three-day A93.1
  tick
    American mountain A93.2
    Colorado A93.2
    Kemerovo A93.8
    Mediterranean A77.1
    mountain A93.2
    nonexanthematous A93.2
    Quaranfil A93.8

- **Fever** (inanition) (of unknown origin) (persistent) (with chills) (with rigor) - *continued*
  - tick-bite NEC A93.8
  - tick-borne (hemorrhagic) NEC A93.8
  - trench A79.0
  - tsutsugamushi A75.3
  - typhogastric A01.00
  - typhoid (abortive) (hemorrhagic) (intermittent) (malignant) A01.00
    - complicated by
      - arthritis A01.04
      - heart involvement A01.02
      - meningitis A01.01
      - osteomyelitis A01.05
      - pneumonia A01.03
      - specified NEC A01.09
  - typhomalarial — *see* Malaria
  - typhus — *see* Typhus (fever)
  - undulant — *see* Brucellosis
  - unknown origin R50.9
  - uveoparotid D86.89
  - valley B38.0
  - Venezuelan equine A92.2
  - vesicular stomatitis A93.8
  - viral hemorrhagic — *see* Fever, hemorrhagic, by type of virus
  - Volhynian A79.0
  - Wesselsbron (viral) A92.8
  - West
    - African B50.8
    - Nile (viral) A92.30
      - with
        - complications NEC A92.39
        - cranial nerve disorders A92.32
        - encephalitis A92.31
        - encephalomyelitis A92.31
        - neurologic manifestation NEC A92.32
        - optic neuritis A92.32
        - polyradiculitis A92.32
  - Whitmore's — *see* Melioidosis
  - Wolhynian A79.0
  - worm B83.9
  - yellow A95.9
    - jungle A95.0
    - sylvatic A95.0
    - urban A95.1
  - Zika virus A92.5
- **Fibrillation**
  - atrial or auricular (established) I48.91
    - chronic I48.2
    - paroxysmal I48.0
    - permanent I48.2
    - persistent I48.1
  - cardiac I49.8
  - heart I49.8
  - muscular M62.89
  - ventricular I49.01
- **Fibrin**
  - ball or bodies, pleural (sac) J94.1
  - chamber, anterior (eye) (gelatinous exudate) — *see* Iridocyclitis, acute
- **Fibrinogenolysis** — *see* Fibrinolysis
- **Fibrinogenopenia** D68.8
  - acquired D65
  - congenital D68.2
- **Fibrinolysis** (hemorrhagic) (acquired) D65
  - antepartum hemorrhage — *see* Hemorrhage, antepartum, with coagulation defect
  - following
    - abortion — *see* Abortion by type complicated by hemorrhage
    - ectopic or molar pregnancy O08.1
  - intrapartum O67.0
  - newborn, transient P60
  - postpartum O72.3
- **Fibrinopenia** (hereditary) D68.2
  - acquired D68.4
- **Fibrinopurulent** — *see* condition
- **Fibrinous** — *see* condition
- **Fibroadenoma**
  - cellular intracanalicular D24-
  - giant D24-
  - intracanalicular
    - cellular D24-
    - giant D24-
    - specified site — *see* Neoplasm, benign, by site
    - unspecified site D24-
  - juvenile D24-
  - pericanalicular
    - specified site — *see* Neoplasm, benign, by site
    - unspecified site D24-
  - phyllodes D24-
  - prostate D29.1
- **Fibroadenoma** - *continued*
  - specified site NEC — *see* Neoplasm, benign, by site
  - unspecified site D24-
- **Fibroadenosis, breast** (chronic) (cystic) (diffuse) (periodic) (segmental) N60.2-
- **Fibroangioma** — *see also* Neoplasm, benign, by site
  - juvenile
    - specified site — *see* Neoplasm, benign, by site
    - unspecified site D10.6
- **Fibrochondrosarcoma** — *see* Neoplasm, cartilage, malignant
- **Fibrocystic**
  - disease — *see also* Fibrosis, cystic
    - breast — *see* Mastopathy, cystic
    - jaw M27.49
    - kidney (congenital) Q61.8
    - liver Q44.6
    - pancreas E84.9
  - kidney (congenital) Q61.8
- **Fibrodysplasia ossificans progressiva** — *see* Myositis, ossificans, progressiva
- **Fibroelastosis** (cordis) (endocardial) (endomyocardial) I42.4
- **Fibroid** (tumor) — *see also* Neoplasm, connective tissue, benign
  - disease, lung (chronic) — *see* Fibrosis, lung
  - heart (disease) — *see* Myocarditis
  - in pregnancy or childbirth O34.1-
    - causing obstructed labor O65.5
  - induration, lung (chronic) — *see* Fibrosis, lung
  - lung — *see* Fibrosis, lung
  - pneumonia (chronic) — *see* Fibrosis, lung
  - uterus — *see also* Leiomyoma, uterus D25.9
- **Fibrolipoma** — *see* Lipoma
- **Fibroliposarcoma** — *see* Neoplasm, connective tissue, malignant
- **Fibroma** — *see also* Neoplasm, connective tissue, benign
  - ameloblastic — *see* Cyst, calcifying odontogenic
  - bone (nonossifying) — *see* Disorder, bone, specified type NEC
    - ossifying — *see* Neoplasm, bone, benign
  - cementifying — *see* Neoplasm, bone, benign
  - chondromyxoid — *see* Neoplasm, bone, benign
  - desmoplastic — *see* Neoplasm, connective tissue, uncertain behavior
  - durum — *see* Neoplasm, connective tissue, benign
  - fascial — *see* Neoplasm, connective tissue, benign
  - invasive — *see* Neoplasm, connective tissue, uncertain behavior
  - molle — *see* Lipoma
  - myxoid — *see* Neoplasm, connective tissue, benign
  - nasopharynx, nasopharyngeal (juvenile) D10.6
  - nonosteogenic (nonossifying) — *see* Dysplasia, fibrous
  - odontogenic (central) — *see* Cyst, calcifying odontogenic
  - ossifying — *see* Neoplasm, bone, benign
  - periosteal — *see* Neoplasm, bone, benign
  - soft — *see* Lipoma
- **Fibromatosis** M72.9
  - abdominal — *see* Neoplasm, connective tissue, uncertain behavior
  - aggressive — *see* Neoplasm, connective tissue, uncertain behavior
  - congenital generalized — *see* Neoplasm, connective tissue, uncertain behavior
  - Dupuytren's M72.0
  - gingival K06.1
  - palmar (fascial) M72.0
  - plantar (fascial) M72.2
  - pseudosarcomatous (proliferative) (subcutaneous) M72.4
  - retroperitoneal D48.3
  - specified NEC M72.8
- **Fibromyalgia** M79.7
- **Fibromyoma** — *see also* Neoplasm, connective tissue, benign
  - uterus (corpus) — *see also* Leiomyoma, uterus
    - in pregnancy or childbirth — *see* Fibroid, in pregnancy or childbirth
      - causing obstructed labor O65.5
- **Fibromyositis** M79.7
- **Fibromyxolipoma** D17.9
- **Fibromyxoma** — *see* Neoplasm, connective tissue, benign
- **Fibromyxosarcoma** — *see* Neoplasm, connective tissue, malignant
- **Fibro-odontoma, ameloblastic** — *see* Cyst, calcifying odontogenic
- **Fibro-osteoma** — *see* Neoplasm, bone, benign
- **Fibroplasia, retrolental** H35.17-
- **Fibropurulent** — *see* condition
- **Fibrosarcoma** — *see also* Neoplasm, connective tissue, malignant
  - ameloblastic C41.1
    - upper jaw (bone) C41.0
  - congenital — *see* Neoplasm, connective tissue, malignant
  - fascial — *see* Neoplasm, connective tissue, malignant
  - infantile — *see* Neoplasm, connective tissue, malignant
  - odontogenic C41.1
    - upper jaw (bone) C41.0
  - periosteal — *see* Neoplasm, bone, malignant
- **Fibrosclerosis**
  - breast N60.3-
  - multifocal M35.5
  - penis (corpora cavernosa) N48.6
- **Fibrosis, fibrotic**
  - adrenal (gland) E27.8
  - amnion O41.8X-
  - anal papillae K62.89
  - arteriocapillary — *see* Arteriosclerosis
  - bladder N32.89
    - interstitial — *see* Cystitis, chronic, interstitial
    - localized submucosal — *see* Cystitis, chronic, interstitial
    - panmural — *see* Cystitis, chronic, interstitial
  - breast — *see* Fibrosclerosis, breast
  - capillary — *see also* Arteriosclerosis I70.90
    - lung (chronic) — *see* Fibrosis, lung
  - cardiac — *see* Myocarditis
  - cervix N88.8
  - chorion O41.8X-
  - corpus cavernosum (sclerosing) N48.6
  - cystic (of pancreas) E84.9
    - with
      - distal intestinal obstruction syndrome E84.19
      - fecal impaction E84.19
      - intestinal manifestations NEC E84.19
      - pulmonary manifestations E84.0
      - specified manifestations NEC E84.8
  - due to device, implant or graft — *see also* Complications, by site and type, specified NEC T85.828
    - arterial graft NEC T82.828
    - breast (implant) T85.828
    - catheter NEC T85.828
      - dialysis (renal) T82.828
        - intraperitoneal T85.828
      - infusion NEC T82.828
        - spinal (epidural) (subdural) T85.820
      - urinary (indwelling) T83.82
    - electronic (electrode) (pulse generator) (stimulator)
      - bone T84.82
      - cardiac T82.827
      - nervous system (brain) (peripheral nerve) (spinal) T85.820
      - urinary T83.82
    - fixation, internal (orthopedic) NEC T84.82
    - gastrointestinal (bile duct) (esophagus) T85.828
    - genital NEC T83.82
    - heart NEC T82.827
    - joint prosthesis T84.82
    - ocular (corneal graft) (orbital implant) NEC T85.828
    - orthopedic NEC T84.82
    - specified NEC T85.828
    - urinary NEC T83.82
    - vascular NEC T82.828
    - ventricular intracranial shunt T85.820
  - ejaculatory duct N50.89
  - endocardium — *see* Endocarditis
  - endomyocardial (tropical) I42.3
  - epididymis N50.89
  - eye muscle — *see* Strabismus, mechanical
  - heart — *see* Myocarditis
  - hepatic — *see* Fibrosis, liver
  - hepatolienal (portal hypertension) K76.6
  - hepatosplenic (portal hypertension) K76.6
  - infrapatellar fat pad M79.4
  - intrascrotal N50.89
  - kidney N26.9
  - liver K74.0
    - with sclerosis K74.2
    - alcoholic K70.2
  - lung (atrophic) (chronic) (confluent) (massive) (perialveolar) (peribronchial) J84.10
    - with
      - anthracosilicosis J60
      - anthracosis J60
      - asbestosis J61
      - bagassosis J67.1
      - bauxite J63.1

- **Fire, Saint Anthony's** — *see* Erysipelas
- **Fire-setting**
  - pathological (compulsive) F63.1
- **Fish hook stomach** K31.89
- **Fishmeal-worker's lung** J67.8
- **Fissure, fissured**
  - anus, anal K60.2
    - acute K60.0
    - chronic K60.1
    - congenital Q43.8
  - ear, lobule, congenital Q17.8
  - epiglottis (congenital) Q31.8
  - larynx J38.7
    - congenital Q31.8
  - lip K13.0
    - congenital — *see* Cleft, lip
  - nipple N64.0
    - associated with
      - lactation O92.13
      - pregnancy O92.11-
      - puerperium O92.12
  - nose Q30.2
  - palate (congenital) — *see* Cleft, palate
  - skin R23.4
  - spine (congenital) — *see also* Spina bifida
    - with hydrocephalus — *see* Spina bifida, by site, with hydrocephalus
  - tongue (acquired) K14.5
    - congenital Q38.3
- **Fistula** (cutaneous) L98.8
  - abdomen (wall) K63.2
    - bladder N32.2
    - intestine NEC K63.2
    - ureter N28.89
    - uterus N82.5
  - abdominorectal K63.2
  - abdominosigmoidal K63.2
  - abdominothoracic J86.0
  - abdominouterine N82.5
    - congenital Q51.7
  - abdominovesical N32.2
  - accessory sinuses — *see* Sinusitis
  - actinomycotic — *see* Actinomycosis
  - alveolar antrum — *see* Sinusitis, maxillary
  - alveolar process K04.6
  - anorectal K60.5
  - antrobuccal — *see* Sinusitis, maxillary
  - antrum — *see* Sinusitis, maxillary
  - anus, anal (recurrent) (infectional) K60.3
    - congenital Q43.6
      - with absence, atresia and stenosis Q42.2
    - tuberculous A18.32
  - aorta-duodenal I77.2
  - appendix, appendicular K38.3
  - arteriovenous (acquired) (nonruptured) I77.0
    - brain I67.1
      - congenital Q28.2
        - ruptured I60.8
      - ruptured I60.8
    - cerebral — *see* Fistula, arteriovenous, brain
    - congenital (peripheral) — *see also* Malformation, arteriovenous
      - brain Q28.2
        - ruptured I60.8
      - coronary Q24.5
      - pulmonary Q25.72
    - coronary I25.41
      - congenital Q24.5
    - pulmonary I28.0
      - congenital Q25.72
    - surgically created (for dialysis) Z99.2
      - complication — *see* Complication, arteriovenous, fistula, surgically created
    - traumatic — *see* Injury, blood vessel
  - artery I77.2
  - aural (mastoid) — *see* Mastoiditis, chronic
  - auricle — *see also* Disorder, pinna, specified type NEC
    - congenital Q18.1
  - Bartholin's gland N82.8
  - bile duct (common) (hepatic) K83.3
    - with calculus, stones — *see* Calculus, bile duct
  - biliary (tract) — *see* Fistula, bile duct
  - bladder (sphincter) NEC — *see also* Fistula, vesico- N32.2
    - into seminal vesicle N32.2
  - bone — *see also* Disorder, bone, specified type NEC
    - with osteomyelitis, chronic — *see* Osteomyelitis, chronic, with draining sinus
  - brain G93.89
    - arteriovenous (acquired) I67.1
      - congenital Q28.2
  - branchial (cleft) Q18.0

Fistula (cutaneous) - *continued*

  - branchiogenous Q18.0
  - breast N61.0
    - puerperal, postpartum or gestational, due to mastitis (purulent) — *see* Mastitis, obstetric, purulent
  - bronchial J86.0
  - bronchocutaneous, bronchomediastinal, bronchopleural, bronchopleuromediastinal (infective) J86.0
    - tuberculous NEC A15.5
  - bronchoesophageal J86.0
    - congenital Q39.2
      - with atresia of esophagus Q39.1
  - bronchovisceral J86.0
  - buccal cavity (infective) K12.2
  - cecosigmoidal K63.2
  - cecum K63.2
  - cerebrospinal (fluid) G96.0
  - cervical, lateral Q18.1
  - cervicoaural Q18.1
  - cervicosigmoidal N82.4
  - cervicovesical N82.1
  - cervix N82.8
  - chest (wall) J86.0
  - cholecystenteric — *see* Fistula, gallbladder
  - cholecystocolic — *see* Fistula, gallbladder
  - cholecystocolonic — *see* Fistula, gallbladder
  - cholecystoduodenal — *see* Fistula, gallbladder
  - cholecystogastric — *see* Fistula, gallbladder
  - cholecystointestinal — *see* Fistula, gallbladder
  - choledochoduodenal — *see* Fistula, bile duct
  - cholocolic K82.3
  - coccyx — *see* Sinus, pilonidal
  - colon K63.2
  - colostomy K94.09
  - common duct — *see* Fistula, bile duct
  - congenital, site not listed — *see* Anomaly, by site
  - coronary, arteriovenous I25.41
    - congenital Q24.5
  - costal region J86.0
  - cul-de-sac, Douglas' N82.8
  - cystic duct — *see also* Fistula, gallbladder
    - congenital Q44.5
  - dental K04.6
  - diaphragm J86.0
  - duodenum K31.6
  - ear (external) (canal) — *see* Disorder, ear, external, specified type NEC
  - enterocolic K63.2
  - enterocutaneous K63.2
  - enterouterine N82.4
    - congenital Q51.7
  - enterovaginal N82.4
    - congenital Q52.2
    - large intestine N82.3
    - small intestine N82.2
  - enterovesical N32.1
  - epididymis N50.89
    - tuberculous A18.15
  - esophagobronchial J86.0
    - congenital Q39.2
      - with atresia of esophagus Q39.1
  - esophagocutaneous K22.8
  - esophagopleural-cutaneous J86.0
  - esophagotracheal J86.0
    - congenital Q39.2
      - with atresia of esophagus Q39.1
  - esophagus K22.8
    - congenital Q39.2
      - with atresia of esophagus Q39.1
  - ethmoid — *see* Sinusitis, ethmoidal
  - eyeball (cornea) (sclera) — *see* Disorder, globe, hypotony
  - eyelid H01.8
  - fallopian tube, external N82.5
  - fecal K63.2
    - congenital Q43.6
  - from periapical abscess K04.6
  - frontal sinus — *see* Sinusitis, frontal
  - gallbladder K82.3
    - with calculus, cholelithiasis, stones — *see* Calculus, gallbladder
  - gastric K31.6
  - gastrocolic K31.6
    - congenital Q40.2
    - tuberculous A18.32
  - gastroenterocolic K31.6
  - gastroesophageal K31.6
  - gastrojejunal K31.6
  - gastrojejunocolic K31.6
  - genital tract (female) N82.9
    - specified NEC N82.8

Fistula (cutaneous) - *continued*

  - genital tract (female) - *continued*
    - to intestine NEC N82.4
    - to skin N82.5
  - hepatic artery-portal vein, congenital Q26.6
  - hepatopleural J86.0
  - hepatopulmonary J86.0
  - ileorectal or ileosigmoidal K63.2
  - ileovaginal N82.2
  - ileovesical N32.1
  - ileum K63.2
  - in ano K60.3
    - tuberculous A18.32
  - inner ear (labyrinth) — *see* subcategory H83.1
  - intestine NEC K63.2
  - intestinocolonic (abdominal) K63.2
  - intestinoureteral N28.89
  - intestinouterine N82.4
  - intestinovaginal N82.4
    - large intestine N82.3
    - small intestine N82.2
  - intestinovesical N32.1
  - ischiorectal (fossa) K61.39
  - jejunum K63.2
  - joint M25.10
    - ankle M25.17-
    - elbow M25.12-
    - foot joint M25.17-
    - hand joint M25.14-
    - hip M25.15-
    - knee M25.16-
    - shoulder M25.11-
    - specified joint NEC M25.18
    - tuberculous — *see* Tuberculosis, joint
    - vertebrae M25.18
    - wrist M25.13-
  - kidney N28.89
  - labium (majus) (minus) N82.8
  - labyrinth — *see* subcategory H83.1
  - lacrimal (gland) (sac) H04.61-
  - lacrimonasal duct — *see* Fistula, lacrimal
  - laryngotracheal, congenital Q34.8
  - larynx J38.7
  - lip K13.0
    - congenital Q38.0
  - lumbar, tuberculous A18.01
  - lung J86.0
  - lymphatic I89.8
  - mammary (gland) N61.0
  - mastoid (process) (region) — *see* Mastoiditis, chronic
  - maxillary J32.0
  - medial, face and neck Q18.8
  - mediastinal J86.0
  - mediastinobronchial J86.0
  - mediastinocutaneous J86.0
  - middle ear — *see* subcategory H74.8
  - mouth K12.2
  - nasal J34.89
    - sinus — *see* Sinusitis
  - nasopharynx J39.2
  - nipple N64.0
  - nose J34.89
  - oral (cutaneous) K12.2
    - maxillary J32.0
    - nasal (with cleft palate) — *see* Cleft, palate
  - orbit, orbital — *see* Disorder, orbit, specified type NEC
  - oroantral J32.0
  - oviduct, external N82.5
  - palate (hard) M27.8
  - pancreatic K86.89
  - pancreaticoduodenal K86.89
  - parotid (gland) K11.4
    - region K12.2
  - penis N48.89
  - perianal K60.3
  - pericardium (pleura) (sac) — *see* Pericarditis
  - pericecal K63.2
  - perineorectal K60.4
  - perineosigmoidal K63.2
  - perineum, perineal (with urethral involvement) NEC N36.0
    - tuberculous A18.13
    - ureter N28.89
  - perirectal K60.4
    - tuberculous A18.32
  - peritoneum K65.9
  - pharyngoesophageal J39.2
  - pharynx J39.2
    - branchial cleft (congenital) Q18.0
  - pilonidal (infected) (rectum) — *see* Sinus, pilonidal

Fistula (cutaneous) - *continued*
pleura, pleural, pleurocutaneous, pleuroperitoneal J86.0
tuberculous NEC A15.6
pleuropericardial I31.8
portal vein-hepatic artery, congenital Q26.6
postauricular H70.81-
postoperative, persistent T81.83
specified site — *see* Fistula, by site
preauricular (congenital) Q18.1
prostate N42.89
pulmonary J86.0
arteriovenous I28.0
congenital Q25.72
tuberculous — *see* Tuberculosis, pulmonary
pulmonoperitoneal J86.0
rectolabial N82.4
rectosigmoid (intercommunicating) K63.2
rectoureteral N28.89
rectourethral N36.0
congenital Q64.73
rectouterine N82.4
congenital Q51.7
rectovaginal N82.3
congenital Q52.2
tuberculous A18.18
rectovesical N32.1
congenital Q64.79
rectovesicovaginal N82.3
rectovulval N82.4
congenital Q52.79
rectum (to skin) K60.4
congenital Q43.6
with absence, atresia and stenosis Q42.0
tuberculous A18.32
renal N28.89
retroauricular — *see* Fistula, postauricular
salivary duct or gland (any) K11.4
congenital Q38.4
scrotum (urinary) N50.89
tuberculous A18.15
semicircular canals — *see* subcategory H83.1
sigmoid K63.2
to bladder N32.1
sinus — *see* Sinusitis
skin L98.8
to genital tract (female) N82.5
splenocolic D73.89
stercoral K63.2
stomach K31.6
sublingual gland K11.4
submandibular gland K11.4
submaxillary (gland) K11.4
region K12.2
thoracic J86.0
duct I89.8
thoracoabdominal J86.0
thoracogastric J86.0
thoracointestinal J86.0
thorax J86.0
thyroglossal duct Q89.2
thyroid E07.89
trachea, congenital (external) (internal) Q32.1
tracheoesophageal J86.0
congenital Q39.2
with atresia of esophagus Q39.1
following tracheostomy J95.04
traumatic arteriovenous — *see* Injury, blood vessel, by site
tuberculous - code by site under Tuberculosis
typhoid A01.09
umbilicourinary Q64.8
urachus, congenital Q64.4
ureter (persistent) N28.89
ureteroabdominal N28.89
ureterorectal N28.89
ureterosigmoido-abdominal N28.89
ureterovaginal N82.1
ureterovesical N32.2
urethra N36.0
congenital Q64.79
tuberculous A18.13
urethroperineal N36.0
urethroperineovesical N32.2
urethrorectal N36.0
congenital Q64.73
urethroscrotal N50.89
urethrovaginal N82.1
urethrovesical N32.2
urinary (tract) (persistent) (recurrent) N36.0
uteroabdominal N82.5
congenital Q51.7
uteroenteric, uterointestinal N82.4

Fistula (cutaneous) - *continued*
uteroenteric, uterointestinal - *continued*
congenital Q51.7
uterorectal N82.4
congenital Q51.7
uteroureteric N82.1
uterourethral Q51.7
uterovaginal N82.8
uterovesical N82.1
congenital Q51.7
uterus N82.8
vagina (postpartal) (wall) N82.8
vaginocutaneous (postpartal) N82.5
vaginointestinal NEC N82.4
large intestine N82.3
small intestine N82.2
vaginoperineal N82.5
vasocutaneous, congenital Q55.7
vesical NEC N32.2
vesicoabdominal N32.2
vesicocervicovaginal N82.1
vesicocolic N32.1
vesicocutaneous N32.2
vesicoenteric N32.1
vesicointestinal N32.1
vesicometrorectal N82.4
vesicoperineal N32.2
vesicorectal N32.1
congenital Q64.79
vesicosigmoidal N32.1
vesicosigmoidovaginal N82.3
vesicoureteral N32.2
vesicoureterovaginal N82.1
vesicourethral N32.2
vesicourethrorectal N32.1
vesicouterine N82.1
congenital Q51.7
vesicovaginal N82.0
vulvorectal N82.4
congenital Q52.79
Fit R56.9
epileptic — *see* Epilepsy
fainting R55
hysterical F44.5
newborn P90
Fitting (and adjustment) (of)
artificial
arm — *see* Admission, adjustment, artificial, arm
breast Z44.3
eye Z44.2
leg — *see* Admission, adjustment, artificial, leg
automatic implantable cardiac defibrillator (with synchronous cardiac pacemaker) Z45.02
brain neuropacemaker Z46.2
implanted Z45.42
cardiac defibrillator — *see* Fitting (and adjustment) (of), automatic implantable cardiac defibrillator
catheter, non-vascular Z46.82
colostomy belt Z46.89
contact lenses Z46.0
CRT-D (resynchronization therapy defibrillator) Z45.02
CRT-P (cardiac resynchronization therapy pacemaker) Z45.018
pulse generator Z45.010
cystostomy device Z46.6
defibrillator, cardiac — *see* Fitting (and adjustment) (of), automatic implantable cardiac defibrillator
dentures Z46.3
device NOS Z46.9
abdominal Z46.89
gastrointestinal NEC Z46.59
implanted NEC Z45.89
nervous system Z46.2
implanted — *see* Admission, adjustment, device, implanted, nervous system
orthodontic Z46.4
orthoptic Z46.0
orthotic Z46.89
prosthetic (external) Z44.9
breast Z44.3
dental Z46.3
eye Z44.2
specified NEC Z44.8
specified NEC Z46.89
substitution
auditory Z46.2
implanted — *see* Admission, adjustment, device, implanted, hearing device
nervous system Z46.2
implanted — *see* Admission, adjustment, device, implanted, nervous system
visual Z46.2

Fitting (and adjustment) (of) - *continued*
device NOS - *continued*
substitution - *continued*
visual - *continued*
implanted Z45.31
urinary Z46.6
gastric lap band Z46.51
gastrointestinal appliance NEC Z46.59
glasses (reading) Z46.0
hearing aid Z46.1
ileostomy device Z46.89
insulin pump Z46.81
intestinal appliance NEC Z46.89
myringotomy device (stent) (tube) Z45.82
neuropacemaker Z46.2
implanted Z45.42
non-vascular catheter Z46.82
orthodontic device Z46.4
orthopedic device (brace) (cast) (corset) (shoes) Z46.89
pacemaker (cardiac) (cardiac resynchronization therapy (CRT-P)) Z45.018
nervous system (brain) (peripheral nerve) (spinal cord) Z46.2
implanted Z45.42
pulse generator Z45.010
portacath (port-a-cath) Z45.2
prosthesis (external) Z44.9
arm — *see* Admission, adjustment, artificial, arm
breast Z44.3
dental Z46.3
eye Z44.2
leg — *see* Admission, adjustment, artificial, leg
specified NEC Z44.8
spectacles Z46.0
wheelchair Z46.89
Fitzhugh-Curtis syndrome
due to
Chlamydia trachomatis A74.81
Neisseria gonorrhorea (gonococcal peritonitis) A54.85
Fitz's syndrome (acute hemorrhagic pancreatitis) — *see also* Pancreatitis, acute K85.80
Fixation
joint — *see* Ankylosis
larynx J38.7
stapes — *see* Ankylosis, ear ossicles
deafness — *see* Deafness, conductive
uterus (acquired) — *see* Malposition, uterus
vocal cord J38.3
Flabby ridge K06.8
Flaccid — *see also* condition
palate, congenital Q38.5
Flail
chest S22.5
newborn (birth injury) P13.8
joint (paralytic) M25.20
ankle M25.27-
elbow M25.22-
foot joint M25.27-
hand joint M25.24-
hip M25.25-
knee M25.26-
shoulder M25.21-
specified joint NEC M25.28
wrist M25.23-
Flajani's disease — *see* Hyperthyroidism, with, goiter (diffuse)
Flap, liver K71.3
Flashbacks (residual to hallucinogen use) F16.283
Flat
chamber (eye) — *see* Disorder, globe, hypotony, flat anterior chamber
chest, congenital Q67.8
foot (acquired) (fixed type) (painful) (postural) — *see also* Deformity, limb, flat foot
congenital (rigid) (spastic (everted)) Q66.5-
rachitic sequelae (late effect) E64.3
organ or site, congenital NEC — *see* Anomaly, by site
pelvis M95.5
with disproportion (fetopelvic) O33.0
causing obstructed labor O65.0
congenital Q74.2
Flatau-Schilder disease G37.0
Flatback syndrome M40.30
lumbar region M40.36
lumbosacral region M40.37
thoracolumbar region M40.35
Flattening
head, femur M89.8X5
hip — *see* Coxa, plana
lip (congenital) Q18.8

Flattening - *continued*
nose (congenital) Q67.4
acquired M95.0
Flatulence R14.3
psychogenic F45.8
Flatus R14.3
vaginalis N89.8
Flax-dresser's disease J66.1
Flea bite — *see* Injury, bite, by site, superficial, insect
Flecks, glaucomatous (subcapsular) — *see* Cataract, complicated
Fleischer (-Kayser) **ring** (cornea) H18.04-
Fleshy mole O02.0
Flexibilitas cerea — *see* Catalepsy
Flexion
amputation stump (surgical) T87.89
cervix — *see* Malposition, uterus
contracture, joint — *see* Contraction, joint
deformity, joint — *see also* Deformity, limb, flexion M21.20
hip, congenital Q65.89
uterus — *see also* Malposition, uterus
lateral — *see* Lateroversion, uterus
Flexner-Boyd dysentery A03.2
Flexner's dysentery A03.1
Flexure — *see* Flexion
Flint murmur (aortic insufficiency) I35.1
Floater, vitreous — *see* Opacity, vitreous
Floating
cartilage (joint) — *see also* Loose, body, joint
knee — *see* Derangement, knee, loose body
gallbladder, congenital Q44.1
kidney N28.89
congenital Q63.8
spleen D73.89
Flooding N92.0
Floor — *see* condition
Floppy
baby syndrome (nonspecific) P94.2
iris syndrome (intraoperative) (IFIS) H21.81
nonrheumatic mitral valve syndrome I34.1
Flu — *see also* Influenza
avian — *see also* Influenza, due to, identified novel influenza A virus J09.X2
bird — *see also* Influenza, due to, identified novel influenza A virus J09.X2
intestinal NEC A08.4
swine (viruses that normally cause infections in pigs) — *see also* Influenza, due to, identified novel influenza A virus J09.X2
Fluctuating blood pressure I99.8
Fluid
abdomen R18.8
chest J94.8
heart — *see* Failure, heart, congestive
joint — *see* Effusion, joint
loss (acute) E86.9
lung — *see* Edema, lung
overload E87.70
specified NEC E87.79
peritoneal cavity R18.8
pleural cavity J94.8
retention R60.9
Flukes NEC — *see also* Infestation, fluke
blood NEC — *see* Schistosomiasis
liver B66.3
Fluor (vaginalis) N89.8
trichomonal or due to Trichomonas (vaginalis) A59.00
Fluorosis
dental K00.3
skeletal M85.10
ankle M85.17-
foot M85.17-
forearm M85.13-
hand M85.14-
lower leg M85.16-
multiple site M85.19
neck M85.18
rib M85.18
shoulder M85.11-
skull M85.18
specified site NEC M85.18
thigh M85.15-
toe M85.17-
upper arm M85.12-
vertebra M85.18
Flush syndrome E34.0
Flushing R23.2
menopausal N95.1
Flutter
atrial or auricular I48.92
atypical I48.4

Flutter - *continued*
atrial or auricular - *continued*
type I I48.3
type II I48.4
typical I48.3
heart I49.8
atrial or auricular I48.92
atypical I48.4
type I I48.3
type II I48.4
typical I48.3
ventricular I49.02
ventricular I49.02
FNHTR (febrile nonhemolytic transfusion reaction) R50.84
Fochier's abscess - code by site under Abscess
Focus, Assmann's — *see* Tuberculosis, pulmonary
Fogo selvagem L10.3
Foix-Alajouanine syndrome G95.19
Fold, folds (anomalous) — *see also* Anomaly, by site
Descemet's membrane — *see* Change, corneal membrane, Descemet's, fold
epicanthic Q10.3
heart Q24.8
Folie à deux F24
Follicle
cervix (nabothian) (ruptured) N88.8
graafian, ruptured, with hemorrhage N83.0-
nabothian N88.8
Follicular — *see* condition
Folliculitis (superficial) L73.9
abscedens et suffodiens L66.3
cyst N83.0-
decalvans L66.2
deep — *see* Furuncle, by site
gonococcal (acute) (chronic) A54.01
keloid, keloidalis L73.0
pustular L01.02
ulerythematosa reticulata L66.4
Folliculome lipidique
specified site — *see* Neoplasm, benign, by site
unspecified site
female D27.9
male D29.20
Følling's disease E70.0
Follow-up — *see* Examination, follow-up
Fong's syndrome (hereditary osteo -onychodysplasia) Q87.2
Food
allergy L27.2
asphyxia (from aspiration or inhalation) — *see* Foreign body, by site
choked on — *see* Foreign body, by site
deprivation T73.0
specified kind of food NEC E63.8
intoxication — *see* Poisoning, food
lack of T73.0
poisoning — *see* Poisoning, food
rejection NEC — *see* Disorder, eating
strangulation or suffocation — *see* Foreign body, by site
toxemia — *see* Poisoning, food
Foot — *see* condition
Foramen ovale (nonclosure) (patent) (persistent) Q21.1
Forbes' glycogen storage disease E74.03
Fordyce-Fox disease L75.2
Fordyce's disease (mouth) Q38.6
Forearm — *see* condition
Foreign body
with
laceration — *see* Laceration, by site, with foreign body
puncture wound — *see* Puncture, by site, with foreign body
accidentally left following a procedure T81.509
aspiration T81.506
resulting in
adhesions T81.516
obstruction T81.526
perforation T81.536
specified complication NEC T81.596
cardiac catheterization T81.505
resulting in
acute reaction T81.60
aseptic peritonitis T81.61
specified NEC T81.69
adhesions T81.515
obstruction T81.525
perforation T81.535
specified complication NEC T81.595
causing
acute reaction T81.60

Foreign body - *continued*
accidentally left following a procedure - *continued*
causing - *continued*
acute reaction - *continued*
aseptic peritonitis T81.61
specified complication NEC T81.69
adhesions T81.519
aseptic peritonitis T81.61
obstruction T81.529
perforation T81.539
specified complication NEC T81.599
endoscopy T81.504
resulting in
adhesions T81.514
obstruction T81.524
perforation T81.534
specified complication NEC T81.594
immunization T81.503
resulting in
adhesions T81.513
obstruction T81.523
perforation T81.533
specified complication NEC T81.593
infusion T81.501
resulting in
adhesions T81.511
obstruction T81.521
perforation T81.531
specified complication NEC T81.591
injection T81.503
resulting in
adhesions T81.513
obstruction T81.523
perforation T81.533
specified complication NEC T81.593
kidney dialysis T81.502
resulting in
adhesions T81.512
obstruction T81.522
perforation T81.532
specified complication NEC T81.592
packing removal T81.507
resulting in
acute reaction T81.60
aseptic peritonitis T81.61
specified NEC T81.69
adhesions T81.517
obstruction T81.527
perforation T81.537
specified complication NEC T81.597
puncture T81.506
resulting in
adhesions T81.516
obstruction T81.526
perforation T81.536
specified complication NEC T81.596
specified procedure NEC T81.508
resulting in
acute reaction T81.60
aseptic peritonitis T81.61
specified NEC T81.69
adhesions T81.518
obstruction T81.528
perforation T81.538
specified complication NEC T81.598
surgical operation T81.500
resulting in
acute reaction T81.60
aseptic peritonitis T81.61
specified NEC T81.69
adhesions T81.510
obstruction T81.520
perforation T81.530
specified complication NEC T81.590
transfusion T81.501
resulting in
adhesions T81.511
obstruction T81.521
perforation T81.531
specified complication NEC T81.591
alimentary tract T18.9
anus T18.5
colon T18.4
esophagus — *see* Foreign body, esophagus
mouth T18.0
multiple sites T18.8
rectosigmoid (junction) T18.5
rectum T18.5
small intestine T18.3
specified site NEC T18.8
stomach T18.2
anterior chamber (eye) S05.5-

Foreign body - *continued*
  retained (old) (nonmagnetic) (in) - *continued*
    lens - *continued*
      magnetic — *see* Foreign body, intraocular, old, retained, magnetic, lens
    muscle — *see* Foreign body, retained, soft tissue
    orbit — *see* Foreign body, orbit, old
    posterior wall of globe — *see* Foreign body, intraocular, old, retained, posterior wall
      magnetic — *see* Foreign body, intraocular, old, retained, magnetic, posterior wall
    retrobulbar — *see* Foreign body, orbit, old, retrobulbar
    soft tissue M79.5
    vitreous — *see* Foreign body, intraocular, old, retained, vitreous body
      magnetic — *see* Foreign body, intraocular, old, retained, magnetic, vitreous body
  retina S05.5-
  superficial, without open wound
    abdomen, abdominal (wall) S30.851
    alveolar process S00.552
    ankle S90.55-
    antecubital space — *see* Foreign body, superficial, forearm
    anus S30.857
    arm (upper) S40.85-
    auditory canal — *see* Foreign body, superficial, ear
    auricle — *see* Foreign body, superficial, ear
    axilla — *see* Foreign body, superficial, arm
    back, lower S30.850
    breast S20.15-
    brow S00.85
    buttock S30.850
    calf — *see* Foreign body, superficial, leg
    canthus — *see* Foreign body, superficial, eyelid
    cheek S00.85
      internal S00.552
    chest wall — *see* Foreign body, superficial, thorax
    chin S00.85
    clitoris S30.854
    costal region — *see* Foreign body, superficial, thorax
    digit (s)
      hand — *see* Foreign body, superficial, finger
      foot — *see* Foreign body, superficial, toe
    ear S00.45-
    elbow S50.35-
    epididymis S30.853
    epigastric region S30.851
    epiglottis S10.15
    esophagus, cervical S10.15
    eyebrow — *see* Foreign body, superficial, eyelid
    eyelid S00.25-
    face S00.85
    finger (s) S60.459
      index S60.45-
      little S60.45-
      middle S60.45-
      ring S60.45-
    flank S30.851
    foot (except toe (s) alone) S90.85-
      toe — *see* Foreign body, superficial, toe
    forearm S50.85-
      elbow only — *see* Foreign body, superficial, elbow
    forehead S00.85
    genital organs, external
      female S30.856
      male S30.855
    groin S30.851
    gum S00.552
    hand S60.55-
    head S00.95
      ear — *see* Foreign body, superficial, ear
      eyelid — *see* Foreign body, superficial, eyelid
      lip S00.551
      nose S00.35
      oral cavity S00.552
      scalp S00.05
      specified site NEC S00.85
    heel — *see* Foreign body, superficial, foot
    hip S70.25-
    inguinal region S30.851
    interscapular region S20.459
    jaw S00.85
    knee S80.25-
    labium (majus) (minus) S30.854
    larynx S10.15
    leg (lower) S80.85-
      knee — *see* Foreign body, superficial, knee
      upper — *see* Foreign body, superficial, thigh
    lip S00.551

Foreign body - *continued*
  superficial, without open wound - *continued*
    lower back S30.850
    lumbar region S30.850
    malar region S00.85
    mammary — *see* Foreign body, superficial, breast
    mastoid region S00.85
    mouth S00.552
    nail
      finger — *see* Foreign body, superficial, finger
      toe — *see* Foreign body, superficial, toe
    nape S10.85
    nasal S00.35
    neck S10.95
      specified site NEC S10.85
      throat S10.15
    nose S00.35
    occipital region S00.05
    oral cavity S00.552
    orbital region — *see* Foreign body, superficial, eyelid
    palate S00.552
    palm — *see* Foreign body, superficial, hand
    parietal region S00.05
    pelvis S30.850
    penis S30.852
    perineum
      female S30.854
      male S30.850
    periocular area — *see* Foreign body, superficial, eyelid
    phalanges
      finger — *see* Foreign body, superficial, finger
      toe — *see* Foreign body, superficial, toe
    pharynx S10.15
    pinna — *see* Foreign body, superficial, ear
    popliteal space — *see* Foreign body, superficial, knee
    prepuce S30.852
    pubic region S30.850
    pudendum
      female S30.856
      male S30.855
    sacral region S30.850
    scalp S00.05
    scapular region — *see* Foreign body, superficial, shoulder
    scrotum S30.853
    shin — *see* Foreign body, superficial, leg
    shoulder S40.25-
    sternal region S20.359
    submaxillary region S00.85
    submental region S00.85
    subungual
      finger (s) — *see* Foreign body, superficial, finger
      toe (s) — *see* Foreign body, superficial, toe
    supraclavicular fossa S10.85
    supraorbital S00.85
    temple S00.85
    temporal region S00.85
    testis S30.853
    thigh S70.35-
    thorax, thoracic (wall) S20.95
      back S20.45-
      front S20.35-
    throat S10.15
    thumb S60.35-
    toe (s) (lesser) S90.456
      great S90.45-
    tongue S00.552
    trachea S10.15
    tunica vaginalis S30.853
    tympanum, tympanic membrane — *see* Foreign body, superficial, ear
    uvula S00.552
    vagina S30.854
    vocal cords S10.15
    vulva S30.854
    wrist S60.85-
  swallowed T18.9
  trachea T17.408
    causing
      asphyxiation T17.400
        food (bone) (seed) T17.420
        gastric contents (vomitus) T17.410
        specified type NEC T17.490
      injury NEC T17.408
        food (bone) (seed) T17.428
        gastric contents (vomitus) T17.418
        specified type NEC T17.498
  type of fragment — *see* Retained, foreign body fragments (type of)
  vitreous (humor) S05.5-

Forestier's disease (rhizomelic pseudopolyarthritis) M35.3
  meaning ankylosing hyperostosis — *see* Hyperostosis, ankylosing
Formation
  hyalin in cornea — *see* Degeneration, cornea
  sequestrum in bone (due to infection) — *see* Osteomyelitis, chronic
  valve
    colon, congenital Q43.8
    ureter (congenital) Q62.39
Formication R20.2
Fort Bragg fever A27.89
Fossa — *see also* condition
  pyriform — *see* condition
Foster-Kennedy syndrome H47.14-
Fothergill's
  disease (trigeminal neuralgia) — *see also* Neuralgia, trigeminal
    scarlatina anginosa A38.9
Foul breath R19.6
Foundling Z76.1
Fournier disease or gangrene N49.3
  female N76.89
Fourth
  cranial nerve — *see* condition
  molar K00.1
Foville's (peduncular) **disease or syndrome** G46.3
Fox (-Fordyce) **disease** (apocrine miliaria) L75.2
FPIES (food protein-induced enteropathy syndrome) K52.21
Fracture, burst — *see* Fracture, traumatic, by site
Fracture, chronic — *see* Fracture, pathological, by site
Fracture, insufficiency — *see* Fracture, pathological, by site
Fracture, nontraumatic, NEC
  atypical
    femur M84.750-
      complete
        oblique M84.759
          left side M84.758
          right side M84.757
        transverse M84.756
          left side M84.755
          right side M84.754
      incomplete M84.753
        left side M84.752
        right side M84.751
Fracture, pathological (pathologic) — *see also* Fracture, traumatic M84.40
  ankle M84.47-
  carpus M84.44-
  clavicle M84.41-
  compression (not due to trauma) — *see also* Collapse, vertebra M48.50-
  dental implant M27.63
  dental restorative material K08.539
    with loss of material K08.531
    without loss of material K08.530
  due to
    neoplastic disease NEC — *see also* Neoplasm M84.50
      ankle M84.57-
      carpus M84.54-
      clavicle M84.51-
      femur M84.55
      fibula M84.56-
      finger M84.54-
      hip M84.559
      humerus M84.52-
      ilium M84.550
      ischium M84.550
      metacarpus M84.54-
      metatarsus M84.57-
      neck M84.58
      pelvis M84.550
      radius M84.53-
      rib M84.58
      scapula M84.51-
      skull M84.58
      specified site NEC M84.58
      tarsus M84.57-
      tibia M84.56-
      toe M84.57-
      ulna M84.53-
      vertebra M84.58
    osteoporosis M80.00
      disuse — *see* Osteoporosis, specified type NEC, with pathological fracture
      drug-induced — *see* Osteoporosis, drug induced, with pathological fracture

Fracture, pathological (pathologic) - *continued*
due to - *continued*
osteoporosis - *continued*
idiopathic — *see* Osteoporosis, specified type NEC, with pathological fracture
postmenopausal — *see* Osteoporosis, postmenopausal, with pathological fracture
postoophorectomy — *see* Osteoporosis, postoophorectomy, with pathological fracture
postsurgical malabsorption — *see* Osteoporosis, specified type NEC, with pathological fracture
specified cause NEC — *see* Osteoporosis, specified type NEC, with pathological fracture
specified disease NEC M84.60
ankle M84.67-
carpus M84.64-
clavicle M84.61-
femur M84.65-
fibula M84.66-
finger M84.64-
hip M84.65-
humerus M84.62-
ilium M84.650
ischium M84.650
metacarpus M84.64-
metatarsus M84.67-
neck M84.68
radius M84.63-
rib M84.68
scapula M84.61-
skull M84.68
tarsus M84.67-
tibia M84.66-
toe M84.67-
ulna M84.63-
vertebra M84.68
femur M84.45-
fibula M84.46-
finger M84.44-
hip M84.459
humerus M84.42-
ilium M84.454
ischium M84.454
joint prosthesis — *see* Complications, joint prosthesis, mechanical, breakdown, by site
periprosthetic — *see* Fracture, pathological, periprosthetic
metacarpus M84.44-
metatarsus M84.47-
neck M84.48
pelvis M84.454
periprosthetic M97.9
ankle M97.2-
elbow M97.4-
finger M97.8
hip M97.0-
knee M97.1-
other specified joint M97.8
shoulder M97.3-
spinal joint M97.8
toe joint M97.8
wrist joint M97.8
radius M84.43-
restorative material (dental) K08.539
with loss of material K08.531
without loss of material K08.530
rib M84.48
scapula M84.41-
skull M84.48
tarsus M84.47-
tibia M84.46-
toe M84.47-
ulna M84.43-
vertebra M84.48

Fracture, traumatic (abduction) (adduction) (separation) — *see also* Fracture, pathological T14.8
acetabulum S32.40-
column
anterior (displaced) (iliopubic) S32.43-
nondisplaced S32.436
posterior (displaced) (ilioischial) S32.443
nondisplaced S32.44-
dome (displaced) S32.48-
nondisplaced S32.48
specified NEC S32.49-
transverse (displaced) S32.45-
with associated posterior wall fracture (displaced) S32.46-
nondisplaced S32.46-
nondisplaced S32.45-
wall
anterior (displaced) S32.41-
nondisplaced S32.41-

Fracture, traumatic (abduction) (adduction) (separation) - *continued*
acetabulum - *continued*
wall - *continued*
medial (displaced) S32.47-
nondisplaced S32.47-
posterior (displaced) S32.42-
with associated transverse fracture (displaced) S32.46-
nondisplaced S32.46-
nondisplaced S32.42-
acromion — *see* Fracture, scapula, acromial process
ankle S82.899
bimalleolar (displaced) S82.84-
nondisplaced S82.84-
lateral malleolus only (displaced) S82.6-
nondisplaced S82.6-
medial malleolus (displaced) S82.5-
associated with Maisonneuve's fracture — *see* Fracture, Maisonneuve's
nondisplaced S82.5-
talus — *see* Fracture, tarsal, talus
trimalleolar (displaced) S82.85-
nondisplaced S82.85-
arm (upper) — *see also* Fracture, humerus, shaft
humerus — *see* Fracture, humerus
radius — *see* Fracture, radius
ulna — *see* Fracture, ulna
astragalus — *see* Fracture, tarsal, talus
atlas — *see* Fracture, neck, cervical vertebra, first
axis — *see* Fracture, neck, cervical vertebra, second
back — *see* Fracture, vertebra
Barton's — *see* Barton's fracture
base of skull — *see* Fracture, skull, base
basicervical (basal) (femoral) S72.0
Bennett's — *see* Bennett's fracture
bimalleolar — *see* Fracture, ankle, bimalleolar
blow-out S02.3-
bone NEC T14.8
birth injury P13.9
following insertion of orthopedic implant, joint prosthesis or bone plate — *see* Fracture, following insertion of orthopedic implant, joint prosthesis or bone plate
in (due to) neoplastic disease NEC — *see* Fracture, pathological, due to, neoplastic disease
pathological (cause unknown) — *see* Fracture, pathological
breast bone — *see* Fracture, sternum
bucket handle (semilunar cartilage) — *see* Tear, meniscus
burst — *see* Fracture, traumatic, by site
calcaneus — *see* Fracture, tarsal, calcaneus
carpal bone (s) S62.10-
capitate (displaced) S62.13-
nondisplaced S62.13-
cuneiform — *see* Fracture, carpal bone, triquetrum
hamate (body) (displaced) S62.143
hook process (displaced) S62.15-
nondisplaced S62.15-
nondisplaced S62.14-
larger multangular — *see* Fracture, carpal bones, trapezium
lunate (displaced) S62.12-
nondisplaced S62.12-
navicular S62.00-
distal pole (displaced) S62.01-
nondisplaced S62.01-
middle third (displaced) S62.02-
nondisplaced S62.02-
proximal third (displaced) S62.03-
nondisplaced S62.03-
volar tuberosity — *see* Fracture, carpal bones, navicular, distal pole
os magnum — *see* Fracture, carpal bones, capitate
pisiform (displaced) S62.16-
nondisplaced S62.16-
semilunar — *see* Fracture, carpal bones, lunate
smaller multangular — *see* Fracture, carpal bones, trapezoid
trapezium (displaced) S62.17-
nondisplaced S62.17-
trapezoid (displaced) S62.18-
nondisplaced S62.18-
triquetrum (displaced) S62.11-
nondisplaced S62.11-
unciform — *see* Fracture, carpal bones, hamate
cervical — *see* Fracture, vertebra, cervical
clavicle S42.00-
acromial end (displaced) S42.03-
nondisplaced S42.03-
birth injury P13.4
lateral end — *see* Fracture, clavicle, acromial end

Fracture, traumatic (abduction) (adduction) (separation) - *continued*
clavicle - *continued*
shaft (displaced) S42.02-
nondisplaced S42.02-
sternal end (anterior) (displaced) S42.01-
nondisplaced S42.01-
posterior S42.01-
coccyx S32.2
collapsed — *see* Collapse, vertebra
collar bone — *see* Fracture, clavicle
Colles' — *see* Colles' fracture
coronoid process — *see* Fracture, ulna, upper end, coronoid process
corpus cavernosum penis S39.840
costochondral cartilage S23.41
costochondral, costosternal junction — *see* Fracture, rib
cranium — *see* Fracture, skull
cricoid cartilage S12.8
cuboid (ankle) — *see* Fracture, tarsal, cuboid
cuneiform
foot — *see* Fracture, tarsal, cuneiform
wrist — *see* Fracture, carpal, triquetrum
delayed union — *see* Delay, union, fracture
dental restorative material K08.539
with loss of material K08.531
without loss of material K08.530
due to
birth injury — *see* Birth, injury, fracture
osteoporosis — *see* Osteoporosis, with fracture
Dupuytren's — *see* Fracture, ankle, lateral malleolus
elbow S42.40-
ethmoid (bone) (sinus) — *see* Fracture, skull, base
face bone S02.92
fatigue — *see also* Fracture, stress
vertebra M48.40
cervical region M48.42
cervicothoracic region M48.43
lumbar region M48.46
lumbosacral region M48.47
occipito-atlanto-axial region M48.41
sacrococcygeal region M48.48
thoracic region M48.44
thoracolumbar region M48.45
femur, femoral S72.9-
basicervical (basal) S72.0
birth injury P13.2
capital epiphyseal S79.01-
condyles, epicondyles — *see* Fracture, femur, lower end
distal end — *see* Fracture, femur, lower end
epiphysis
head — *see* Fracture, femur, upper end, epiphysis
lower — *see* Fracture, femur, lower end, epiphysis
upper — *see* Fracture, femur, upper end, epiphysis
following insertion of implant, prosthesis or plate M96.66-
head — *see* Fracture, femur, upper end, head
intertrochanteric — *see* Fracture, femur, trochanteric
intratrochanteric — *see* Fracture, femur, trochanteric
lower end S72.40-
condyle (displaced) S72.41-
lateral (displaced) S72.42-
nondisplaced S72.42-
medial (displaced) S72.43-
nondisplaced S72.43-
nondisplaced S72.41-
epiphysis (displaced) S72.44-
nondisplaced S72.44-
physeal S79.10-
Salter-Harris
Type I S79.11-
Type II S79.12-
Type III S79.13-
Type IV S79.14-
specified NEC S79.19-
specified NEC S72.49-
supracondylar (displaced) S72.45-
with intracondylar extension (displaced) S72.46 -
nondisplaced S72.46-
nondisplaced S72.45-
torus S72.47-
neck — *see* Fracture, femur, upper end, neck
pertrochanteric — *see* Fracture, femur, trochanteric
shaft (lower third) (middle third) (upper third) S72.30-
comminuted (displaced) S72.35-

Fracture, traumatic (abduction) (adduction) (separation) - *continued*
femur, femoral - *continued*
shaft (lower third) (middle third) (upper third) - *continued*
comminuted (displaced) - *continued*
nondisplaced S72.35-
oblique (displaced) S72.33-
nondisplaced S72.33-
segmental (displaced) S72.36-
nondisplaced S72.36-
specified NEC S72.39-
spiral (displaced) S72.34-
nondisplaced S72.34-
transverse (displaced) S72.32-
nondisplaced S72.32-
specified site NEC — *see* subcategory S72.8
subcapital (displaced) S72.01-
subtrochanteric (region) (section) (displaced) S72.2-
nondisplaced S72.2-
transcervical — *see* Fracture, femur, upper end, neck
transtrochanteric — *see* Fracture, femur, trochanteric
trochanteric S72.10-
apophyseal (displaced) S72.13-
nondisplaced S72.13-
greater trochanter (displaced) S72.11-
nondisplaced S72.11-
intertrochanteric (displaced) S72.14-
nondisplaced S72.14-
lesser trochanter (displaced) S72.12-
nondisplaced S72.12-
upper end S72.00-
apophyseal (displaced) S72.13-
nondisplaced S72.13-
cervicotrochanteric — *see* Fracture, femur, upper end, neck, base
epiphysis (displaced) S72.02-
nondisplaced S72.02-
head S72.05-
articular (displaced) S72.06-
nondisplaced S72.06-
specified NEC S72.09-
intertrochanteric (displaced) S72.14-
nondisplaced S72.14-
intracapsular S72.01-
midcervical (displaced) S72.03-
nondisplaced S72.03-
neck S72.00-
base (displaced) S72.04-
nondisplaced S72.04-
specified NEC S72.09-
pertrochanteric — *see* Fracture, femur, upper end, trochanteric
physeal S79.00-
Salter-Harris type I S79.01-
specified NEC S79.09-
subcapital (displaced) S72.01-
subtrochanteric (displaced) S72.2-
nondisplaced S72.2-
transcervical — *see* Fracture, femur, upper end, midcervical
trochanteric S72.10-
greater (displaced) S72.11-
nondisplaced S72.11-
lesser (displaced) S72.12-
nondisplaced S72.12-
fibula (shaft) (styloid) S82.40-
comminuted (displaced) S82.45-
nondisplaced S82.45-
following insertion of implant, prosthesis or plate M96.67-
involving ankle or malleolus — *see* Fracture, fibula, lateral malleolus
lateral malleolus (displaced) S82.6-
nondisplaced S82.6-
lower end
physeal S89.30-
Salter-Harris
Type I S89.31-
Type II S89.32-
specified NEC S89.39-
specified NEC S82.83-
torus S82.82-
oblique (displaced) S82.43-
nondisplaced S82.43-
segmental (displaced) S82.46-
nondisplaced S82.46-
specified NEC S82.49-
spiral (displaced) S82.44-
nondisplaced S82.44-

Fracture, traumatic (abduction) (adduction) (separation) - *continued*
fibula (shaft) (styloid) - *continued*
transverse (displaced) S82.42-
nondisplaced S82.42-
upper end
physeal S89.20-
Salter-Harris
Type I S89.21-
Type II S89.22-
specified NEC S89.29-
specified NEC S82.83-
torus S82.81-
finger (except thumb) S62.60-
distal phalanx (displaced) S62.63-
nondisplaced S62.66-
index S62.60-
distal phalanx (displaced) S62.63-
nondisplaced S62.66-
middle phalanx (displaced) S62.62-
nondisplaced S62.65-
proximal phalanx (displaced) S62.61-
nondisplaced S62.64-
little S62.60-
distal phalanx (displaced) S62.63-
nondisplaced S62.66-
middle phalanx (displaced) S62.62-
nondisplaced S62.65-
proximal phalanx (displaced) S62.61-
nondisplaced S62.64-
middle phalanx (displaced) S62.62-
nondisplaced S62.65-
middle S62.60-
distal phalanx (displaced) S62.63-
nondisplaced S62.66-
middle phalanx (displaced) S62.62-
nondisplaced S62.65-
proximal phalanx (displaced) S62.61-
nondisplaced S62.64-
proximal phalanx (displaced) S62.61-
nondisplaced S62.64-
ring S62.60-
distal phalanx (displaced) S62.63-
nondisplaced S62.66-
middle phalanx (displaced) S62.62-
nondisplaced S62.65-
proximal phalanx (displaced) S62.61-
nondisplaced S62.64-
thumb — *see* Fracture, thumb
following insertion (intraoperative) (postoperative) of orthopedic implant, joint prosthesis or bone plate M96.69
femur M96.66-
fibula M96.67-
humerus M96.62-
pelvis M96.65
radius M96.63-
specified bone NEC M96.69
tibia M96.67-
ulna M96.63-
foot S92.90-
astragalus — *see* Fracture, tarsal, talus
calcaneus — *see* Fracture, tarsal, calcaneus
cuboid — *see* Fracture, tarsal, cuboid
cuneiform — *see* Fracture, tarsal, cuneiform
metatarsal — *see* Fracture, metatarsal
navicular — *see* Fracture, tarsal, navicular
sesamoid S92.81-
specified NEC S92.81-
talus — *see* Fracture, tarsal, talus
tarsal — *see* Fracture, tarsal
toe — *see* Fracture, toe
forearm S52.9-
radius — *see* Fracture, radius
ulna — *see* Fracture, ulna
fossa (anterior) (middle) (posterior) S02.19
frontal (bone) (skull) S02.0
sinus S02.19
glenoid (cavity) (scapula) — *see* Fracture, scapula, glenoid cavity
greenstick — *see* Fracture, by site
hallux — *see* Fracture, toe, great
hand S62.9-
carpal — *see* Fracture, carpal bone
finger (except thumb) — *see* Fracture, finger
metacarpal — *see* Fracture, metacarpal
navicular (scaphoid) (hand) — *see* Fracture, carpal bone, navicular
thumb — *see* Fracture, thumb
healed or old
with complications - code by Nature of the complication
heel bone — *see* Fracture, tarsal, calcaneus

Fracture, traumatic (abduction) (adduction) (separation) - *continued*
Hill-Sachs S42.29-
hip — *see* Fracture, femur, neck
humerus S42.30-
anatomical neck — *see* Fracture, humerus, upper end
articular process — *see* Fracture, humerus, lower end
capitellum — *see* Fracture, humerus, lower end, condyle, lateral
distal end — *see* Fracture, humerus, lower end
epiphysis
lower — *see* Fracture, humerus, lower end, physeal
upper — *see* Fracture, humerus, upper end, physeal
external condyle — *see* Fracture, humerus, lower end, condyle, lateral
following insertion of implant, prosthesis or plate M96.62-
great tuberosity — *see* Fracture, humerus, upper end, greater tuberosity
intercondylar — *see* Fracture, humerus, lower end
internal epicondyle — *see* Fracture, humerus, lower end, epicondyle, medial
lesser tuberosity — *see* Fracture, humerus, upper end, lesser tuberosity
lower end S42.40-
condyle
lateral (displaced) S42.45-
nondisplaced S42.45-
medial (displaced) S42.46-
nondisplaced S42.46-
epicondyle
lateral (displaced) S42.43-
nondisplaced S42.43-
medial (displaced) S42.44-
incarcerated S42.44-
nondisplaced S42.44-
physeal S49.10-
Salter-Harris
Type I S49.11-
Type II S49.12-
Type III S49.13-
Type IV S49.14-
specified NEC S49.19-
specified NEC (displaced) S42.49-
nondisplaced S42.49-
supracondylar (simple) (displaced) S42.41-
with intercondylar fracture — *see* Fracture, humerus, lower end
comminuted (displaced) S42.42-
nondisplaced S42.42-
nondisplaced S42.41-
torus S42.48-
transcondylar (displaced) S42.47-
nondisplaced S42.47-
proximal end — *see* Fracture, humerus, upper end
shaft S42.30-
comminuted (displaced) S42.35-
nondisplaced S42.35-
greenstick S42.31-
oblique (displaced) S42.33-
nondisplaced S42.33-
segmental (displaced) S42.36-
nondisplaced S42.36-
specified NEC S42.39-
spiral (displaced) S42.34-
nondisplaced S42.34-
transverse (displaced) S42.32-
nondisplaced S42.32-
supracondylar — *see* Fracture, humerus, lower end
surgical neck — *see* Fracture, humerus, upper end, surgical neck
trochlea — *see* Fracture, humerus, lower end, condyle, medial
tuberosity — *see* Fracture, humerus, upper end
upper end S42.20-
anatomical neck — *see* Fracture, humerus, upper end, specified NEC
articular head — *see* Fracture, humerus, upper end, specified NEC
epiphysis — *see* Fracture, humerus, upper end, physeal
greater tuberosity (displaced) S42.25-
nondisplaced S42.25-
lesser tuberosity (displaced) S42.26-
nondisplaced S42.26-
physeal S49.00-
Salter-Harris
Type I S49.01-
Type II S49.02-

Fracture, traumatic (abduction) (adduction) (separation) - *continued*
humerus - *continued*
upper end - *continued*
physeal - *continued*
Salter-Harris - *continued*
Type III S49.03-
Type IV S49.04-
specified NEC S49.09-
specified NEC (displaced) S42.29-
nondisplaced S42.29-
surgical neck (displaced) S42.21-
four-part S42.24-
nondisplaced S42.21-
three-part S42.23-
two-part (displaced) S42.22-
nondisplaced S42.22-
torus S42.27-
transepiphyseal — *see* Fracture, humerus, upper end, physeal
hyoid bone S12.8
ilium S32.30-
with disruption of pelvic ring — *see* Disruption, pelvic ring
avulsion (displaced) S32.31-
nondisplaced S32.31-
specified NEC S32.39-
impaction, impacted - code as Fracture, by site
innominate bone — *see* Fracture, ilium
instep — *see* Fracture, foot
ischium S32.60-
with disruption of pelvic ring — *see* Disruption, pelvic ring
avulsion (displaced) S32.61-
nondisplaced S32.61-
specified NEC S32.69-
jaw (bone) (lower) — *see* Fracture, mandible
upper — *see* Fracture, maxilla
joint prosthesis — *see* Complications, joint prosthesis, mechanical, breakdown, by site
periprosthetic — *see* Fracture, traumatic, periprosthetic
knee cap — *see* Fracture, patella
larynx S12.8
late effects — *see* Sequelae, fracture
leg (lower) S82.9-
ankle — *see* Fracture, ankle
femur — *see* Fracture, femur
fibula — *see* Fracture, fibula
malleolus — *see* Fracture, ankle
patella — *see* Fracture, patella
specified site NEC S82.89-
tibia — *see* Fracture, tibia
lumbar spine — *see* Fracture, vertebra, lumbar
lumbosacral spine S32.9
Maisonneuve's (displaced) S82.86-
nondisplaced S82.86-
malar bone — *see also* Fracture, maxilla S02.400
left side S02.40B
right side S02.40A
malleolus — *see* Fracture, ankle
malunion — *see* Fracture, by site
mandible (lower jaw (bone)) S02.609
alveolus S02.67-
angle (of jaw) S02.65-
body, unspecified S02.600
left side S02.602
right side S02.601
condylar process S02.61-
coronoid process S02.63-
ramus, unspecified S02.64-
specified site NEC S02.69
subcondylar process S02.62-
symphysis S02.66
manubrium (sterni) S22.21
dissociation from sternum S22.23
march — *see* Fracture, traumatic, stress, by site
maxilla, maxillary (bone) (sinus) (superior) (upper jaw) S02.401
alveolus S02.42
inferior — *see* Fracture, mandible
LeFort I S02.411
LeFort II S02.412
LeFort III S02.413
left side S02.40D
right side S02.40C
metacarpal S62.309
base (displaced) S62.319
nondisplaced S62.349
fifth S62.30-
base (displaced) S62.31-
nondisplaced S62.34-
neck (displaced) S62.33-

Fracture, traumatic (abduction) (adduction) (separation) - *continued*
metacarpal - *continued*
fifth - *continued*
neck (displaced) - *continued*
nondisplaced S62.36-
shaft (displaced) S62.32-
nondisplaced S62.35-
specified NEC S62.398
first S62.20-
base NEC (displaced) S62.23-
nondisplaced S62.23-
Bennett's — *see* Bennett's fracture
neck (displaced) S62.25-
nondisplaced S62.25-
shaft (displaced) S62.24-
nondisplaced S62.24-
specified NEC S62.29-
fourth S62.30-
base (displaced) S62.31-
nondisplaced S62.34-
neck (displaced) S62.33-
nondisplaced S62.36-
shaft (displaced) S62.32-
nondisplaced S62.35-
specified NEC S62.39-
neck (displaced) S62.33-
nondisplaced S62.36-
Rolando's — *see* Rolando's fracture
second S62.30-
base (displaced) S62.31-
nondisplaced S62.34-
neck (displaced) S62.33-
nondisplaced S62.36-
shaft (displaced) S62.32-
nondisplaced S62.35-
specified NEC S62.39-
shaft (displaced) S62.32-
nondisplaced S62.35-
third S62.30-
base (displaced) S62.31-
nondisplaced S62.34-
neck (displaced) S62.33-
nondisplaced S62.36-
shaft (displaced) S62.32-
nondisplaced S62.35-
specified NEC S62.39-
specified NEC S62.399
metastatic — *see* Fracture, pathological, due to, neoplastic disease — *see also* Neoplasm
metatarsal bone S92.30-
fifth (displaced) S92.35-
nondisplaced S92.35-
first (displaced) S92.31-
nondisplaced S92.31-
fourth (displaced) S92.34-
nondisplaced S92.34-
physeal S99.10-
Salter-Harris
Type I S99.11-
Type II S99.12-
Type III S99.13-
Type IV S99.14-
specified NEC S99.19-
second (displaced) S92.32-
nondisplaced S92.32-
third (displaced) S92.33-
nondisplaced S92.33-
Monteggia's — *see* Monteggia's fracture
multiple
hand (and wrist) NEC — *see* Fracture, by site
ribs — *see* Fracture, rib, multiple
nasal (bone (s)) S02.2
navicular (scaphoid) (foot) — *see also* Fracture, tarsal, navicular
hand — *see* Fracture, carpal, navicular
neck S12.9
cervical vertebra S12.9
fifth (displaced) S12.400
nondisplaced S12.401
specified type NEC (displaced) S12.490
nondisplaced S12.491
first (displaced) S12.000
burst (stable) S12.01
unstable S12.02
lateral mass (displaced) S12.040
nondisplaced S12.041
nondisplaced S12.001
posterior arch (displaced) S12.030
nondisplaced S12.031
specified type NEC (displaced) S12.090
nondisplaced S12.091
fourth (displaced) S12.300

Fracture, traumatic (abduction) (adduction) (separation) - *continued*
neck - *continued*
cervical vertebra - *continued*
fourth (displaced) - *continued*
nondisplaced S12.301
specified type NEC (displaced) S12.390
nondisplaced S12.391
second (displaced) S12.100
nondisplaced S12.101
dens (anterior) (displaced) (type II) S12.110
nondisplaced S12.112
posterior S12.111
specified type NEC (displaced) S12.120
nondisplaced S12.121
specified type NEC (displaced) S12.190
nondisplaced S12.191
seventh (displaced) S12.600
nondisplaced S12.601
specified type NEC (displaced) S12.690
nondisplaced S12.691
sixth (displaced) S12.500
nondisplaced S12.501
specified type NEC (displaced) S12.590
nondisplaced S12.591
third (displaced) S12.200
nondisplaced S12.201
specified type NEC (displaced) S12.290
nondisplaced S12.291
hyoid bone S12.8
larynx S12.8
specified site NEC S12.8
thyroid cartilage S12.8
trachea S12.8
neoplastic NEC — *see* Fracture, pathological, due to, neoplastic disease
neural arch — *see* Fracture, vertebra
newborn — *see* Birth, injury, fracture
nontraumatic — *see* Fracture, pathological
nonunion — *see* Nonunion, fracture
nose, nasal (bone) (septum) S02.2
occiput — *see* Fracture, skull, base, occiput
odontoid process — *see* Fracture, neck, cervical vertebra, second
olecranon (process) (ulna) — *see* Fracture, ulna, upper end, olecranon process
orbit, orbital (bone) (region) S02.8-
floor (blow-out) S02.3-
roof S02.19
os
calcis — *see* Fracture, tarsal, calcaneus
magnum — *see* Fracture, carpal, capitate
pubis — *see* Fracture, pubis
palate S02.8-
parietal bone (skull) S02.0
patella S82.00-
comminuted (displaced) S82.04-
nondisplaced S82.04-
longitudinal (displaced) S82.02-
nondisplaced S82.02-
osteochondral (displaced) S82.01-
nondisplaced S82.01-
specified NEC S82.09-
transverse (displaced) S82.03-
nondisplaced S82.03-
pedicle (of vertebral arch) — *see* Fracture, vertebra
pelvis, pelvic (bone) S32.9
acetabulum — *see* Fracture, acetabulum
circle — *see* Disruption, pelvic ring
following insertion of implant, prosthesis or plate M96.65
ilium — *see* Fracture, ilium
ischium — *see* Fracture, ischium
multiple
with disruption of pelvic ring (circle) — *see* Disruption, pelvic ring
without disruption of pelvic ring (circle) S32.82
pubis — *see* Fracture, pubis
specified site NEC S32.89
sacrum — *see* Fracture, sacrum
periprosthetic, around internal prosthetic joint M97.9
ankle M97.2-
elbow M97.4-
finger M97.8
hip M97.0-
knee M97.1--
shoulder M97.3-
specified joint NEC M97.8
spine M97.8
toe M97.8
wrist M97.8
phalanx
foot — *see* Fracture, toe

Fracture, traumatic (abduction) (adduction) (separation) - *continued*
 phalanx - *continued*
  hand — *see* Fracture, finger
 pisiform — *see* Fracture, carpal, pisiform
 pond — *see* Fracture, skull
 prosthetic device, internal — *see* Complications, prosthetic device, by site, mechanical
 pubis S32.50-
  with disruption of pelvic ring — *see* Disruption, pelvic ring
  specified site NEC S32.59-
  superior rim S32.51-
 radius S52.9-
  distal end — *see* Fracture, radius, lower end
  following insertion of implant, prosthesis or plate M96.63-
  head — *see* Fracture, radius, upper end, head
  lower end S52.50-
   Barton's — *see* Barton's fracture
   Colles' — *see* Colles' fracture
   extraarticular NEC S52.55-
   intraarticular NEC S52.57-
   physeal S59.20-
    Salter-Harris
     Type I S59.21-
     Type II S59.22-
     Type III S59.23-
     Type IV S59.24-
    specified NEC S59.29-
   Smith's — *see* Smith's fracture
   specified NEC S52.59-
   styloid process (displaced) S52.51-
    nondisplaced S52.51-
   torus S52.52-
  neck — *see* Fracture, radius, upper end
  proximal end — *see* Fracture, radius, upper end
  shaft S52.30-
   bent bone S52.38-
   comminuted (displaced) S52.35-
    nondisplaced S52.35-
   Galeazzi's — *see* Galeazzi's fracture
   greenstick S52.31-
   oblique (displaced) S52.33-
    nondisplaced S52.33-
   segmental (displaced) S52.36-
    nondisplaced S52.36-
   specified NEC S52.39-
   spiral (displaced) S52.34-
    nondisplaced S52.34-
   transverse (displaced) S52.32-
    nondisplaced S52.32-
  upper end S52.10-
   head (displaced) S52.12-
    nondisplaced S52.12-
   neck (displaced) S52.13-
    nondisplaced S52.13-
   specified NEC S52.18-
   physeal S59.10-
    Salter-Harris
     Type I S59.11-
     Type II S59.12-
     Type III S59.13-
     Type IV S59.14-
    specified NEC S59.19-
   torus S52.11-
 ramus
  inferior or superior, pubis — *see* Fracture, pubis
  mandible — *see* Fracture, mandible
 restorative material (dental) K08.539
  with loss of material K08.531
  without loss of material K08.530
 rib S22.3-
  with flail chest — *see* Flail, chest
  multiple S22.4-
   with flail chest — *see* Flail, chest
 root, tooth — *see* Fracture, tooth
 sacrum S32.10
  specified NEC S32.19
  Type
   1 S32.14
   2 S32.15
   3 S32.16
   4 S32.17
  Zone
   I S32.119
    displaced (minimally) S32.111
     severely S32.112
    nondisplaced S32.110
   II S32.129
    displaced (minimally) S32.121
     severely S32.122
    nondisplaced S32.120

Fracture, traumatic (abduction) (adduction) (separation) - *continued*
 sacrum - *continued*
  Zone - *continued*
   III S32.139
    displaced (minimally) S32.131
     severely S32.132
    nondisplaced S32.130
 scaphoid (hand) — *see also* Fracture, carpal, navicular
  foot — *see* Fracture, tarsal, navicular
 scapula S42.10-
  acromial process (displaced) S42.12-
   nondisplaced S42.12-
  body (displaced) S42.11-
   nondisplaced S42.11-
  coracoid process (displaced) S42.13-
   nondisplaced S42.13-
  glenoid cavity (displaced) S42.14-
   nondisplaced S42.14-
  neck (displaced) S42.15-
   nondisplaced S42.15-
  specified NEC S42.19-
 semilunar bone, wrist — *see* Fracture, carpal, lunate
 sequelae — *see* Sequelae, fracture
 sesamoid bone
  foot S92.81-
  hand — *see* Fracture, carpal
  other — *see* Fracture, traumatic, by site
 shepherd's — *see* Fracture, tarsal, talus
 shoulder (girdle) S42.9-
  blade — *see* Fracture, scapula
 sinus (ethmoid) (frontal) S02.19
 skull S02.91
  base S02.10-
   occiput S02.119
    condyle S02.113
     type I S02.110
      left side S02.11B
      right side S02.11A
     type II S02.111
      left side S02.11D
      right side S02.11C
     type III S02.112
      left side S02.11F
      right side S02.11E
     specified NEC S02.118
      left side S02.11H
      right side S02.11G
   specified NEC S02.19
  birth injury P13.0
  frontal bone S02.0
  parietal bone S02.0
  specified site NEC S02.8-
  temporal bone S02.19
  vault S02.0
 Smith's — *see* Smith's fracture
 sphenoid (bone) (sinus) S02.19
 spine — *see* Fracture, vertebra
 spinous process — *see* Fracture, vertebra
 spontaneous (cause unknown) — *see* Fracture, pathological
 stave (of thumb) — *see* Fracture, metacarpal, first
 sternum S22.20
  with flail chest — *see* Flail, chest
  body S22.22
  manubrium S22.21
  xiphoid (process) S22.24
 stress M84.30
  ankle M84.37-
  carpus M84.34-
  clavicle M84.31-
  femoral neck M84.359
  femur M84.35-
  fibula M84.36-
  finger M84.34-
  hip M84.359
  humerus M84.32-
  ilium M84.350
  ischium M84.350
  metacarpus M84.34-
  metatarsus M84.37-
  neck — *see* Fracture, fatigue, vertebra
  pelvis M84.350
  radius M84.33-
  rib M84.38
  scapula M84.31-
  skull M84.38
  tarsus M84.37-
  tibia M84.36-
  toe M84.37-
  ulna M84.33-
  vertebra — *see* Fracture, fatigue, vertebra

Fracture, traumatic (abduction) (adduction) (separation) - *continued*
 supracondylar, elbow — *see* Fracture, humerus, lower end, supracondylar
 symphysis pubis — *see* Fracture, pubis
 talus (ankle bone) — *see* Fracture, tarsal, talus
 tarsal bone (s) S92.20-
  astragalus — *see* Fracture, tarsal, talus
  calcaneus S92.00-
   anterior process (displaced) S92.02-
    nondisplaced S92.02-
   body (displaced) S92.01-
    nondisplaced S92.01-
   extraarticular NEC (displaced) S92.05-
    nondisplaced S92.05-
   intraarticular (displaced) S92.06-
    nondisplaced S92.06-
   physeal S99.00-
    Salter-Harris
     Type I S99.01-
     Type II S99.02-
     Type III S99.03-
     Type IV S99.04-
    specified NEC S99.09-
   tuberosity (displaced) S92.04-
    avulsion (displaced) S92.03-
     nondisplaced S92.03-
    nondisplaced S92.04-
  cuboid (displaced) S92.21-
   nondisplaced S92.21-
  cuneiform
   intermediate (displaced) S92.23-
    nondisplaced S92.23-
   lateral (displaced) S92.22-
    nondisplaced S92.22-
   medial (displaced) S92.24-
    nondisplaced S92.24-
  navicular (displaced) S92.25-
   nondisplaced S92.25-
  scaphoid — *see* Fracture, tarsal, navicular
  talus S92.10-
   avulsion (displaced) S92.15-
    nondisplaced S92.15-
   body (displaced) S92.12-
    nondisplaced S92.12-
   dome (displaced) S92.14-
    nondisplaced S92.14-
   head (displaced) S92.12-
    nondisplaced S92.12-
   lateral process (displaced) S92.14-
    nondisplaced S92.14-
   neck (displaced) S92.11-
    nondisplaced S92.11-
   posterior process (displaced) S92.13-
    nondisplaced S92.13-
   specified NEC S92.19-
 temporal bone (styloid) S02.19
 thorax (bony) S22.9
  with flail chest — *see* Flail, chest
  rib S22.3-
   multiple S22.4-
    with flail chest — *see* Flail, chest
  sternum S22.20
   body S22.22
   manubrium S22.21
   xiphoid process S22.24
  vertebra (displaced) S22.009
   burst (stable) S22.001
    unstable S22.002
   eighth S22.069
    burst (stable) S22.061
     unstable S22.062
    specified type NEC S22.068
    wedge compression S22.060
   eleventh S22.089
    burst (stable) S22.081
     unstable S22.082
    specified type NEC S22.088
    wedge compression S22.080
   fifth S22.059
    burst (stable) S22.051
     unstable S22.052
    specified type NEC S22.058
    wedge compression S22.050
   first S22.019
    burst (stable) S22.011
     unstable S22.012
    specified type NEC S22.018
    wedge compression S22.010
   fourth S22.049
    burst (stable) S22.041
     unstable S22.042
    specified type NEC S22.048

- **Fracture, traumatic** (abduction) (adduction) (separation) - *continued*
  - thorax (bony) - *continued*
    - vertebra (displaced) - *continued*
      - fourth - *continued*
        - wedge compression S22.040
      - ninth S22.079
        - burst (stable) S22.071
          - unstable S22.072
        - specified type NEC S22.078
        - wedge compression S22.070
      - nondisplaced S22.001
      - second S22.029
        - burst (stable) S22.021
          - unstable S22.022
        - specified type NEC S22.028
        - wedge compression S22.020
      - seventh S22.069
        - burst (stable) S22.061
          - unstable S22.062
        - specified type NEC S22.068
        - wedge compression S22.060
      - sixth S22.059
        - burst (stable) S22.051
          - unstable S22.052
        - specified type NEC S22.058
        - wedge compression S22.050
      - specified type NEC S22.008
      - tenth S22.079
        - burst (stable) S22.071
          - unstable S22.072
        - specified type NEC S22.078
        - wedge compression S22.070
      - third S22.039
        - burst (stable) S22.031
          - unstable S22.032
        - specified type NEC S22.038
        - wedge compression S22.030
      - twelfth S22.089
        - burst (stable) S22.081
          - unstable S22.082
        - specified type NEC S22.088
        - wedge compression S22.080
      - wedge compression S22.000
  - thumb S62.50-
    - distal phalanx (displaced) S62.52-
      - nondisplaced S62.52-
    - proximal phalanx (displaced) S62.51-
      - nondisplaced S62.51-
  - thyroid cartilage S12.8
  - tibia (shaft) S82.20-
    - comminuted (displaced) S82.25-
      - nondisplaced S82.25-
    - condyles — *see* Fracture, tibia, upper end
    - distal end — *see* Fracture, tibia, lower end
    - epiphysis
      - lower — *see* Fracture, tibia, lower end
      - upper — *see* Fracture, tibia, upper end
    - following insertion of implant, prosthesis or plate M96.67-
    - head (involving knee joint) — *see* Fracture, tibia, upper end
    - intercondyloid eminence — *see* Fracture, tibia, upper end
    - involving ankle or malleolus — *see* Fracture, ankle, medial malleolus
    - lower end S82.30-
      - physeal S89.10-
        - Salter-Harris
          - Type I S89.11-
          - Type II S89.12-
          - Type III S89.13-
          - Type IV S89.14-
        - specified NEC S89.19-
      - pilon (displaced) S82.87-
        - nondisplaced S82.87-
      - specified NEC S82.39-
      - torus S82.31-
    - malleolus — *see* Fracture, ankle, medial malleolus
    - oblique (displaced) S82.23-
      - nondisplaced S82.23-
    - pilon — *see* Fracture, tibia, lower end, pilon
    - proximal end — *see* Fracture, tibia, upper end
    - segmental (displaced) S82.26-
      - nondisplaced S82.26-
    - specified NEC S82.29-
    - spine — *see* Fracture, tibia, upper end, spine
    - spiral (displaced) S82.24-
      - nondisplaced S82.24-
    - transverse (displaced) S82.22-
      - nondisplaced S82.22-
    - tuberosity — *see* Fracture, tibia, upper end, tuberosity

- **Fracture, traumatic** (abduction) (adduction) (separation) - *continued*
  - tibia (shaft) - *continued*
    - upper end S82.10-
      - bicondylar (displaced) S82.14-
        - nondisplaced S82.14-
      - lateral condyle (displaced) S82.12-
        - nondisplaced S82.12-
      - medial condyle (displaced) S82.13-
        - nondisplaced S82.13-
      - physeal S89.00-
        - Salter-Harris
          - Type I S89.01-
          - Type II S89.02-
          - Type III S89.03-
          - Type IV S89.04-
        - specified NEC S89.09-
      - plateau — *see* Fracture, tibia, upper end, bicondylar
      - spine (displaced) S82.11-
        - nondisplaced S82.11-
      - torus S82.16-
      - specified NEC S82.19-
      - tuberosity (displaced) S82.15-
        - nondisplaced S82.15-
  - toe S92.91-
    - great (displaced) S92.40-
      - distal phalanx (displaced) S92.42-
        - nondisplaced S92.42-
      - nondisplaced S92.40-
      - proximal phalanx (displaced) S92.41-
        - nondisplaced S92.41-
      - specified NEC S92.49-
    - lesser (displaced) S92.50-
      - distal phalanx (displaced) S92.53-
        - nondisplaced S92.53-
      - medial phalanx (displaced) S92.52-
        - nondisplaced S92.52-
      - nondisplaced S92.50-
      - proximal phalanx (displaced) S92.51-
        - nondisplaced S92.51-
      - specified NEC S92.59-
    - physeal
      - phalanx S99.20-
        - Salter-Harris
          - Type I S99.21-
          - Type II S99.22-
          - Type III S99.23-
          - Type IV S99.24-
        - specified NEC S99.29-
  - tooth (root) S02.5
  - trachea (cartilage) S12.8
  - transverse process — *see* Fracture, vertebra
  - trapezium or trapezoid bone — *see* Fracture, carpal
  - trimalleolar — *see* Fracture, ankle, trimalleolar
  - triquetrum (cuneiform of carpus) — *see* Fracture, carpal, triquetrum
  - trochanter — *see* Fracture, femur, trochanteric
  - tuberosity (external) — *see* Fracture, traumatic, by site
  - ulna (shaft) S52.20-
    - bent bone S52.28-
    - coronoid process — *see* Fracture, ulna, upper end, coronoid process
    - distal end — *see* Fracture, ulna, lower end
    - following insertion of implant, prosthesis or plate M96.63-
    - head S52.60-
    - lower end S52.60-
      - physeal S59.00-
        - Salter-Harris
          - Type I S59.01-
          - Type II S59.02-
          - Type III S59.03-
          - Type IV S59.04-
        - specified NEC S59.09-
      - specified NEC S52.69-
      - styloid process (displaced) S52.61-
        - nondisplaced S52.61-
      - torus S52.62-
    - proximal end — *see* Fracture, ulna, upper end
    - shaft S52.20-
      - comminuted (displaced) S52.25-
        - nondisplaced S52.25-
      - greenstick S52.21-
      - Monteggia's — *see* Monteggia's fracture
      - oblique (displaced) S52.23-
        - nondisplaced S52.23-
      - segmental (displaced) S52.26-
        - nondisplaced S52.26-
      - specified NEC S52.29-
      - spiral (displaced) S52.24-
        - nondisplaced S52.24-

- **Fracture, traumatic** (abduction) (adduction) (separation) - *continued*
  - ulna (shaft) - *continued*
    - shaft - *continued*
      - transverse (displaced) S52.22-
        - nondisplaced S52.22-
    - upper end S52.00-
      - coronoid process (displaced) S52.04-
        - nondisplaced S52.04-
      - olecranon process (displaced) S52.02-
        - with intraarticular extension S52.03-
        - nondisplaced S52.02-
          - with intraarticular extension S52.03-
      - specified NEC S52.09-
      - torus S52.01-
  - unciform — *see* Fracture, carpal, hamate
  - vault of skull S02.0
  - vertebra, vertebral (arch) (body) (column) (neural arch) (pedicle) (spinous process) (transverse process)
    - atlas — *see* Fracture, neck, cervical vertebra, first
    - axis — *see* Fracture, neck, cervical vertebra, second
    - cervical (teardrop) S12.9
      - axis — *see* Fracture, neck, cervical vertebra, second
      - first (atlas) — *see* Fracture, neck, cervical vertebra, first
      - second (axis) — *see* Fracture, neck, cervical vertebra, second
    - chronic M84.48
    - coccyx S32.2
    - dorsal — *see* Fracture, thorax, vertebra
    - lumbar S32.009
      - burst (stable) S32.001
        - unstable S32.002
      - fifth S32.059
        - burst (stable) S32.051
          - unstable S32.052
        - specified type NEC S32.058
        - wedge compression S32.050
      - first S32.019
        - burst (stable) S32.011
          - unstable S32.012
        - specified type NEC S32.018
        - wedge compression S32.010
      - fourth S32.049
        - burst (stable) S32.041
          - unstable S32.042
        - specified type NEC S32.048
        - wedge compression S32.040
      - second S32.029
        - burst (stable) S32.021
          - unstable S32.022
        - specified type NEC S32.028
        - wedge compression S32.020
      - specified type NEC S32.008
      - third S32.039
        - burst (stable) S32.031
          - unstable S32.032
        - specified type NEC S32.038
        - wedge compression S32.030
      - wedge compression S32.000
    - metastatic — *see* Collapse, vertebra, in, specified disease NEC — *see also* Neoplasm
    - newborn (birth injury) P11.5
    - sacrum S32.10
      - specified NEC S32.19
      - Type
        - 1 S32.14
        - 2 S32.15
        - 3 S32.16
        - 4 S32.17
      - Zone
        - I S32.119
          - displaced (minimally) S32.111
            - severely S32.112
          - nondisplaced S32.110
        - II S32.129
          - displaced (minimally) S32.121
            - severely S32.122
          - nondisplaced S32.120
        - III S32.139
          - displaced (minimally) S32.131
            - severely S32.132
          - nondisplaced S32.130
    - thoracic — *see* Fracture, thorax, vertebra
  - vertex S02.0
  - vomer (bone) S02.2
  - wrist S62.10-
    - carpal — *see* Fracture, carpal bone
    - navicular (scaphoid) (hand) — *see* Fracture, carpal, navicular

Fracture, traumatic (abduction) (adduction) (separation) - *continued*
- xiphisternum, xiphoid (process) S22.24
- zygoma S02.402
  - left side S02.40F
  - right side S02.40E

Fragile, fragility
- autosomal site Q95.5
- bone, congenital (with blue sclera) Q78.0
- capillary (hereditary) D69.8
- hair L67.8
- nails L60.3
- non-sex chromosome site Q95.5
- X chromosome Q99.2

Fragilitas
- crinium L67.8
- ossium (with blue sclerae) (hereditary) Q78.0
- unguium L60.3
  - congenital Q84.6

Fragments, cataract (lens)
- **, following cataract surgery** H59.02-
- retained foreign body — *see* Retained, foreign body fragments (type of)

Frailty (frail) R54
- mental R41.81

Frambesia, frambesial (tropica) — *see also* Yaws
- initial lesion or ulcer A66.0
- primary A66.0

Frambeside
- gummatous A66.4
- of early yaws A66.2

Frambesioma A66.1

Franceschetti-Klein (-Wildervanck) **disease or syndrome** Q75.4

Francis' disease — *see* Tularemia

Franklin disease C88.2

Frank's essential thrombocytopenia D69.3

Fraser's syndrome Q87.0

Freckle (s) L81.2
- malignant melanoma in — *see* Melanoma
- melanotic (Hutchinson's) — *see* Melanoma, in situ
- retinal D49.81

Frederickson's hyperlipoproteinemia, type
- I and V E78.3
- IIA E78.00
- IIB and III E78.2
- IV E78.1

Freeman Sheldon syndrome Q87.0

Freezing — *see also* Effect, adverse, cold T69.9

Freiberg's disease
- (infraction of metatarsal head or osteochondrosis) — *see* Osteochondrosis, juvenile, metatarsus

Frei's disease A55

Fremitus, friction, cardiac R01.2

Frenum, frenulum
- external os Q51.828
- tongue (shortening) (congenital) Q38.1

Frequency micturition (nocturnal) R35.0
- psychogenic F45.8

Frey's syndrome
- auriculotemporal G50.8
- hyperhidrosis L74.52

Friction
- burn — *see* Burn, by site
- fremitus, cardiac R01.2
- precordial R01.2
- sounds, chest R09.89

Friderichsen-Waterhouse syndrome or disease A39.1

Friedländer's B (bacillus) **NEC** — *see also* condition A49.8

Friedreich's
- ataxia G11.1
- combined systemic disease G11.1
- facial hemihypertrophy Q67.4
- sclerosis (cerebellum) (spinal cord) G11.1

Frigidity F52.22

Fröhlich's syndrome E23.6

Frontal — *see also* condition
- lobe syndrome F07.0

Frostbite (superficial) T33.90
- with
  - partial thickness skin loss — *see* Frostbite (superficial), by site
  - tissue necrosis T34.90
- abdominal wall T33.3
  - with tissue necrosis T34.3
- ankle T33.81-
  - with tissue necrosis T34.81-
- arm T33.4-
  - with tissue necrosis T34.4-
  - finger (s) — *see* Frostbite, finger

Frostbite (superficial) - *continued*
- arm - *continued*
  - hand — *see* Frostbite, hand
  - wrist — *see* Frostbite, wrist
- ear T33.01-
  - with tissue necrosis T34.01-
- face T33.09
  - with tissue necrosis T34.09
- finger T33.53-
  - with tissue necrosis T34.53-
- foot T33.82-
  - with tissue necrosis T34.82-
- hand T33.52-
  - with tissue necrosis T34.52-
- head T33.09
  - with tissue necrosis T34.09
  - ear — *see* Frostbite, ear
  - nose — *see* Frostbite, nose
- hip (and thigh) T33.6-
  - with tissue necrosis T34.6-
- knee T33.7-
  - with tissue necrosis T34.7-
- leg T33.9-
  - with tissue necrosis T34.9-
  - ankle — *see* Frostbite, ankle
  - foot — *see* Frostbite, foot
  - knee — *see* Frostbite, knee
  - lower T33.7-
    - with tissue necrosis T34.7-
  - thigh — *see* Frostbite, hip
  - toe — *see* Frostbite, toe
- limb
  - lower T33.99
    - with tissue necrosis T34.99
  - upper — *see* Frostbite, arm
- neck T33.1
  - with tissue necrosis T34.1
- nose T33.02
  - with tissue necrosis T34.02
- pelvis T33.3
  - with tissue necrosis T34.3
- specified site NEC T33.99
  - with tissue necrosis T34.99
- thigh — *see* Frostbite, hip
- thorax T33.2
  - with tissue necrosis T34.2
- toes T33.83-
  - with tissue necrosis T34.83-
- trunk T33.99
  - with tissue necrosis T34.99
- wrist T33.51-
  - with tissue necrosis T34.51-

Frotteurism F65.81

Frozen — *see also* Effect, adverse, cold T69.9
- pelvis (female) N94.89
  - male K66.8
- shoulder — *see* Capsulitis, adhesive

Fructokinase deficiency E74.11

Fructose 1,6 diphosphatase deficiency E74.19

Fructosemia (benign) (essential) E74.12

Fructosuria (benign) (essential) E74.11

Fuchs'
- black spot (myopic) — *see also* Myopia, degenerative H44.2-
- dystrophy (corneal endothelium) H18.51
- heterochromic cyclitis — *see* Cyclitis, Fuchs' heterochromic

Fucosidosis E77.1

Fugue R68.89
- dissociative F44.1
- hysterical (dissociative) F44.1
- postictal in epilepsy — *see* Epilepsy
- reaction to exceptional stress (transient) F43.0

Fulminant, fulminating — *see* condition

Functional — *see also* condition
- bleeding (uterus) N93.8

Functioning, intellectual, borderline R41.83

Fundus — *see* condition

Fungemia NOS B49

Fungus, fungous
- cerebral G93.89
- disease NOS B49
- infection — *see* Infection, fungus

Funiculitis (acute) (chronic) (endemic) N49.1
- gonococcal (acute) (chronic) A54.23
- tuberculous A18.15

Funnel
- breast (acquired) M95.4
  - congenital Q67.6
  - sequelae (late effect) of rickets E64.3
- chest (acquired) M95.4
  - congenital Q67.6
  - sequelae (late effect) of rickets E64.3

Funnel - *continued*
- pelvis (acquired) M95.5
  - with disproportion (fetopelvic) O33.3
    - causing obstructed labor O65.3
  - congenital Q74.2

FUO (fever of unknown origin) R50.9

Furfur L21.0
- microsporon B36.0

Furrier's lung J67.8

Furrowed K14.5
- nail (s) (transverse) L60.4
  - congenital Q84.6
- tongue K14.5
  - congenital Q38.3

Furuncle L02.92
- abdominal wall L02.221
- ankle — *see* Furuncle, lower limb
- anus K61.0
- antecubital space — *see* Furuncle, upper limb
- arm — *see* Furuncle, upper limb
- auditory canal, external — *see* Abscess, ear, external
- auricle (ear) — *see* Abscess, ear, external
- axilla (region) L02.42-
- back (any part) L02.222
- breast N61.1
- buttock L02.32
- cheek (external) L02.02
- chest wall L02.223
- chin L02.02
- corpus cavernosum N48.21
- ear, external — *see* Abscess, ear, external
- external auditory canal — *see* Abscess, ear, external
- eyelid — *see* Abscess, eyelid
- face L02.02
- femoral (region) — *see* Furuncle, lower limb
- finger — *see* Furuncle, hand
- flank L02.221
- foot L02.62-
- forehead L02.02
- gluteal (region) L02.32
- groin L02.224
- hand L02.52-
- head L02.821
  - face L02.02
- hip — *see* Furuncle, lower limb
- kidney — *see* Abscess, kidney
- knee — *see* Furuncle, lower limb
- labium (majus) (minus) N76.4
- lacrimal
  - gland — *see* Dacryoadenitis
  - passages (duct) (sac) — *see* Inflammation, lacrimal, passages, acute
- leg (any part) — *see* Furuncle, lower limb
- lower limb L02.42-
- malignant A22.0
- mouth K12.2
- navel L02.226
- neck L02.12
- nose J34.0
- orbit, orbital — *see* Abscess, orbit
- palmar (space) — *see* Furuncle, hand
- partes posteriores L02.32
- pectoral region L02.223
- penis N48.21
- perineum L02.225
- pinna — *see* Abscess, ear, external
- popliteal — *see* Furuncle, lower limb
- prepatellar — *see* Furuncle, lower limb
- scalp L02.821
- seminal vesicle N49.0
- shoulder — *see* Furuncle, upper limb
- specified site NEC L02.828
- submandibular K12.2
- temple (region) L02.02
- thumb — *see* Furuncle, hand
- toe — *see* Furuncle, foot
- trunk L02.229
  - abdominal wall L02.221
  - back L02.222
  - chest wall L02.223
  - groin L02.224
  - perineum L02.225
  - umbilicus L02.226
- umbilicus L02.226
- upper limb L02.42-
- vulva N76.4

Furunculosis — *see* Furuncle

Fused — *see* Fusion, fused

Fusion, fused (congenital)
- astragaloscaphoid Q74.2
- atria Q21.1
- auditory canal Q16.1
- auricles, heart Q21.1

- **Fusion, fused** (congenital) - *continued*
  - binocular with defective stereopsis H53.32
  - bone Q79.8
  - cervical spine M43.22
  - choanal Q30.0
  - commissure, mitral valve Q23.2
  - cusps, heart valve NEC Q24.8
    - mitral Q23.2
    - pulmonary Q22.1
    - tricuspid Q22.4
  - ear ossicles Q16.3
  - fingers Q70.0-
  - hymen Q52.3
  - joint (acquired) — *see also* Ankylosis
    - congenital Q74.8
  - kidneys (incomplete) Q63.1
  - labium (majus) (minus) Q52.5
  - larynx and trachea Q34.8
  - limb, congenital Q74.8
    - lower Q74.2
    - upper Q74.0
  - lobes, lung Q33.8
  - lumbosacral (acquired) M43.27
    - arthrodesis status Z98.1
    - congenital Q76.49
    - postprocedural status Z98.1
  - nares, nose, nasal, nostril (s) Q30.0
  - organ or site not listed — *see* Anomaly, by site
  - ossicles Q79.9
    - auditory Q16.3
  - pulmonic cusps Q22.1
  - ribs Q76.6
  - sacroiliac (joint) (acquired) M43.28
    - arthrodesis status Z98.1
    - congenital Q74.2
    - postprocedural status Z98.1
  - spine (acquired) NEC M43.20
    - arthrodesis status Z98.1
    - cervical region M43.22
    - cervicothoracic region M43.23
    - congenital Q76.49
    - lumbar M43.26
    - lumbosacral region M43.27
    - occipito-atlanto-axial region M43.21
    - postoperative status Z98.1
    - sacrococcygeal region M43.28
    - thoracic region M43.24
    - thoracolumbar region M43.25
  - sublingual duct with submaxillary duct at opening in mouth Q38.4
  - testes Q55.1
  - toes Q70.2-
  - tooth, teeth K00.2
  - trachea and esophagus Q39.8
  - twins Q89.4
  - vagina Q52.4
  - ventricles, heart Q21.0
  - vertebra (arch) — *see* Fusion, spine
  - vulva Q52.5
- **Fusospirillosis** (mouth) (tongue) (tonsil) A69.1
- **Fussy baby** R68.12

G

- **Gain in weight** (abnormal) (excessive) — *see also* Weight, gain
- **Gaisböck's disease** (polycythemia hypertonica) D75.1
- **Gait abnormality** R26.9
  - ataxic R26.0
  - falling R29.6
  - hysterical (ataxic) (staggering) F44.4
  - paralytic R26.1
  - spastic R26.1
  - specified type NEC R26.89
  - staggering R26.0
  - unsteadiness R26.81
  - walking difficulty NEC R26.2
- **Galactocele** (breast) N64.89
  - puerperal, postpartum O92.79
- **Galactokinase deficiency** E74.29
- **Galactophoritis** N61.0
  - gestational, puerperal, postpartum O91.2-
- **Galactorrhea** O92.6
  - not associated with childbirth N64.3
- **Galactosemia** (classic) (congenital) E74.21
- **Galactosuria** E74.29
- **Galacturia** R82.0
  - schistosomiasis (bilharziasis) B65.0
- **GALD** (gestational alloimmune liver disease) P78.84
- **Galeazzi's fracture** S52.37-
- **Galen's vein** — *see* condition
- **Galeophobia** F40.218
- **Gall duct** — *see* condition
- **Gallbladder** — *see also* condition
  - acute K81.0
- **Gallop rhythm** R00.8
- **Gallstone** (colic) (cystic duct) (gallbladder) (impacted) (multiple) — *see also* Calculus, gallbladder
  - with
    - cholecystitis — *see* Calculus, gallbladder, with cholecystitis
  - bile duct (common) (hepatic) — *see* Calculus, bile duct
  - causing intestinal obstruction K56.3
  - specified NEC K80.80
    - with obstruction K80.81
- **Gambling** Z72.6
  - pathological (compulsive) F63.0
- **Gammopathy** (of undetermined significance [MGUS]) D47.2
  - associated with lymphoplasmacytic dyscrasia D47.2
  - monoclonal D47.2
  - polyclonal D89.0
- **Gamna's disease** (siderotic splenomegaly) D73.1
- **Gamophobia** F40.298
- **Gampsodactylia** (congenital) Q66.7
- **Gamstorp's disease** (adynamia episodica hereditaria) G72.3
- **Gandy-Nanta disease** (siderotic splenomegaly) D73.1
- **Gang**
  - membership offenses Z72.810
- **Gangliocytoma** D36.10
- **Ganglioglioma** — *see* Neoplasm, uncertain behavior, by site
- **Ganglion** (compound) (diffuse) (joint) (tendon (sheath)) M67.40
  - ankle M67.47-
  - foot M67.47-
  - forearm M67.43-
  - hand M67.44-
  - lower leg M67.46-
  - multiple sites M67.49
  - of yaws (early) (late) A66.6
  - pelvic region M67.45-
  - periosteal — *see* Periostitis
  - shoulder region M67.41-
  - specified site NEC M67.48
  - thigh region M67.45-
  - tuberculous A18.09
  - upper arm M67.42-
  - wrist M67.43-
- **Ganglioneuroblastoma** — *see* Neoplasm, nerve, malignant
- **Ganglioneuroma** D36.10
  - malignant — *see* Neoplasm, nerve, malignant
- **Ganglioneuromatosis** D36.10
- **Ganglionitis**
  - fifth nerve — *see* Neuralgia, trigeminal
  - gasserian (postherpetic) (postzoster) B02.21
  - geniculate G51.1
    - newborn (birth injury) P11.3
    - postherpetic, postzoster B02.21
  - herpes zoster B02.21
  - postherpetic geniculate B02.21
- **Gangliosidosis** E75.10
  - GM1 E75.19
  - GM2 E75.00
    - other specified E75.09
    - Sandhoff disease E75.01
    - Tay-Sachs disease E75.02
  - GM3 E75.19
  - mucolipidosis IV E75.11
- **Gangosa** A66.5
- **Gangrene, gangrenous** (connective tissue) (dropsical) (dry) (moist) (skin) (ulcer) — *see also* Necrosis I96
  - with diabetes (mellitus) — *see* Diabetes, gangrene
  - abdomen (wall) I96
  - alveolar M27.3
  - appendix K35.80
    - with
      - peritonitis, localized — *see also* Appendicitis K35.31
  - arteriosclerotic (general) (senile) — *see* Arteriosclerosis, extremities, with, gangrene
  - auricle I96
  - Bacillus welchii A48.0
  - bladder (infectious) — *see* Cystitis, specified type NEC
  - bowel, cecum, or colon — *see* Gangrene, intestine
  - Clostridium perfringens or welchii A48.0
  - cornea H18.89-
  - corpora cavernosa N48.29
    - noninfective N48.89
- **Gangrene, gangrenous** (connective tissue) (dropsical) (dry) (moist) (skin) (ulcer) - *continued*
  - cutaneous, spreading I96
  - decubital — *see* Ulcer, pressure, by site
  - diabetic (any site) — *see* Diabetes, gangrene
  - epidemic — *see* Poisoning, food, noxious, plant
  - epididymis (infectional) N45.1
  - erysipelas — *see* Erysipelas
  - emphysematous — *see* Gangrene, gas
  - extremity (lower) (upper) I96
  - Fournier N49.3
    - female N76.89
  - fusospirochetal A69.0
  - gallbladder — *see* Cholecystitis, acute
  - gas (bacillus) A48.0
    - following
      - abortion — *see* Abortion by type complicated by infection
      - ectopic or molar pregnancy O08.0
  - glossitis K14.0
  - hernia — *see* Hernia, by site, with gangrene
  - intestine, intestinal (hemorrhagic) (massive) — *see also* Infarct, intestine K55.069
    - with
      - mesenteric embolism — *see also* Infarct, intestine K55.069
      - obstruction — *see* Obstruction, intestine
  - laryngitis J04.0
  - limb (lower) (upper) I96
  - lung J85.0
    - spirochetal A69.8
  - lymphangitis I89.1
  - Meleney's (synergistic) — *see* Ulcer, skin
  - mesentery — *see also* Infarct, intestine K55.069
    - with
      - embolism — *see also* Infarct, intestine K55.069
      - intestinal obstruction — *see* Obstruction, intestine
  - mouth A69.0
  - ovary — *see* Oophoritis
  - pancreas — *see* Pancreatitis, acute
  - penis N48.29
    - noninfective N48.89
  - perineum I96
  - pharynx — *see also* Pharyngitis
    - Vincent's A69.1
  - presenile I73.1
  - progressive synergistic — *see* Ulcer, skin
  - pulmonary J85.0
  - pulpal (dental) K04.1
  - quinsy J36
  - Raynaud's (symmetric gangrene) I73.01
  - retropharyngeal J39.2
  - scrotum N49.3
    - noninfective N50.89
  - senile (atherosclerotic) — *see* Arteriosclerosis, extremities, with, gangrene
  - spermatic cord N49.1
    - noninfective N50.89
  - spine I96
  - spirochetal NEC A69.8
  - spreading cutaneous I96
  - stomatitis A69.0
  - symmetrical I73.01
  - testis (infectional) N45.2
    - noninfective N44.8
  - throat — *see also* Pharyngitis
    - diphtheritic A36.0
    - Vincent's A69.1
  - thyroid (gland) E07.89
  - tooth (pulp) K04.1
  - tuberculous NEC — *see* Tuberculosis
  - tunica vaginalis N49.1
    - noninfective N50.89
  - umbilicus I96
  - uterus — *see* Endometritis
  - uvulitis K12.2
  - vas deferens N49.1
    - noninfective N50.89
  - vulva N76.89
- **Ganister disease** J62.8
- **Ganser's syndrome** (hysterical) F44.89
- **Gardner-Diamond syndrome** (autoerythrocyte sensitization) D69.2
- **Gargoylism** E76.01
- **Garré's disease, osteitis** (sclerosing) , **osteomyelitis** — *see* Osteomyelitis, specified type NEC
- **Garrod's pad, knuckle** M72.1
- **Gartner's duct**
  - cyst Q52.4
  - persistent Q50.6

- **Gas** R14.3
  - asphyxiation, inhalation, poisoning, suffocation NEC — *see* Table of Drugs and Chemicals
  - excessive R14.0
  - gangrene A48.0
    - following
      - abortion — *see* Abortion by type complicated by infection
      - ectopic or molar pregnancy O08.0
  - on stomach R14.0
  - pains R14.1
- **Gastralgia** — *see also* Pain, abdominal
- **Gastrectasis** K31.0
  - psychogenic F45.8
- **Gastric** — *see* condition
- **Gastrinoma**
  - malignant
    - pancreas C25.4
    - specified site NEC — *see* Neoplasm, malignant, by site
    - unspecified site C25.4
  - specified site — *see* Neoplasm, uncertain behavior
  - unspecified site D37.9
- **Gastritis** (simple) K29.70
  - with bleeding K29.71
  - acute (erosive) K29.00
    - with bleeding K29.01
  - alcoholic K29.20
    - with bleeding K29.21
  - allergic K29.60
    - with bleeding K29.61
  - atrophic (chronic) K29.40
    - with bleeding K29.41
  - chronic (antral) (fundal) K29.50
    - with bleeding K29.51
    - atrophic K29.40
      - with bleeding K29.41
    - superficial K29.30
      - with bleeding K29.31
  - dietary counseling and surveillance Z71.3
  - due to diet deficiency E63.9
  - eosinophilic K52.81
  - giant hypertrophic K29.60
    - with bleeding K29.61
  - granulomatous K29.60
    - with bleeding K29.61
  - hypertrophic (mucosa) K29.60
    - with bleeding K29.61
  - nervous F54
  - spastic K29.60
    - with bleeding K29.61
  - specified NEC K29.60
    - with bleeding K29.61
  - superficial chronic K29.30
    - with bleeding K29.31
  - tuberculous A18.83
  - viral NEC A08.4
- **Gastrocarcinoma** — *see* Neoplasm, malignant, stomach
- **Gastrocolic** — *see* condition
- **Gastrodisciasis, gastrodiscoidiasis** B66.8
- **Gastroduodenitis** K29.90
  - with bleeding K29.91
  - virus, viral A08.4
    - specified type NEC A08.39
- **Gastrodynia** — *see* Pain, abdominal
- **Gastroenteritis** (acute) (chronic) (noninfectious) — *see also* Enteritis K52.9
  - allergic K52.29
    - with
      - eosinophilic gastritis or gastroenteritis K52.81
      - food protein-induced enterocolitis syndrome K52.21
      - food protein-induced enteropathy K52.22
  - dietetic — *see also* Gastroenteritis, allergic K52.29
  - drug-induced K52.1
  - due to
    - Cryptosporidium A07.2
    - drugs K52.1
    - food poisoning — *see* Intoxication, foodborne
    - radiation K52.0
  - eosinophilic K52.81
  - epidemic (infectious) A09
  - food hypersensitivity — *see also* Gastroenteritis, allergic K52.29
  - infectious — *see* Enteritis, infectious
  - influenzal — *see* Influenza, with gastroenteritis
  - noninfectious K52.9
    - specified NEC K52.89
  - rotaviral A08.0
  - Salmonella A02.0
  - toxic K52.1
  - viral NEC A08.4

Gastroenteritis (acute) (chronic) (noninfectious) - *continued*

  - viral NEC - *continued*
    - acute infectious A08.39
      - type Norwalk A08.11
    - infantile (acute) A08.39
    - Norwalk agent A08.11
    - rotaviral A08.0
    - severe of infants A08.39
    - specified type NEC A08.39
- **Gastroenteropathy** — *see also* Gastroenteritis K52.9
  - acute, due to Norwalk agent A08.11
  - acute, due to Norovirus A08.11
  - infectious A09
- **Gastroenteroptosis** K63.4
- **Gastroesophageal laceration- hemorrhage syndrome** K22.6
- **Gastrointestinal** — *see* condition
- **Gastrojejunal** — *see* condition
- **Gastrojejunitis** — *see also* Enteritis K52.9
- **Gastrojejunocolic** — *see* condition
- **Gastroliths** K31.89
- **Gastromalacia** K31.89
- **Gastroparalysis** K31.84
  - diabetic — *see* Diabetes, gastroparalysis
- **Gastroparesis** K31.84
  - diabetic — *see* Diabetes, by type, with gastroparesis
- **Gastropathy** K31.9
  - congestive portal K31.89
  - erythematous K29.70
  - exudative K90.89
  - portal hypertensive K31.89
- **Gastroptosis** K31.89
- **Gastrorrhagia** K92.2
  - psychogenic F45.8
- **Gastroschisis** (congenital) Q79.3
- **Gastrospasm** (neurogenic) (reflex) K31.89
  - neurotic F45.8
  - psychogenic F45.8
- **Gastrostaxis** — *see* Gastritis, with bleeding
- **Gastrostenosis** K31.89
- **Gastrostomy**
  - attention to Z43.1
  - status Z93.1
- **Gastrosuccorrhea** (continuous) (intermittent) K31.89
  - neurotic F45.8
  - psychogenic F45.8
- **Gatophobia** F40.218
- **Gaucher's disease or splenomegaly** (adult) (infantile) E75.22
- **Gee** (-Herter) (-Thaysen) **disease** (nontropical sprue) K90.0
- **Gélineau's syndrome** G47.419
  - with cataplexy G47.411
- **Gemination, tooth, teeth** K00.2
- **Gemistocytoma**
  - specified site — *see* Neoplasm, malignant, by site
  - unspecified site C71.9
- **General, generalized** — *see* condition
- **Genetic**
  - carrier (status)
    - cystic fibrosis Z14.1
    - hemophilia A (asymptomatic) Z14.01
      - symptomatic Z14.02
    - specified NEC Z14.8
  - susceptibility to disease NEC Z15.89
    - malignant neoplasm Z15.09
      - breast Z15.01
      - endometrium Z15.04
      - ovary Z15.02
      - prostate Z15.03
      - specified NEC Z15.09
    - multiple endocrine neoplasia Z15.81
- **Genital** — *see* condition
- **Genito-anorectal syndrome** A55
- **Genitourinary system** — *see* condition
- **Genu**
  - congenital Q74.1
  - extrorsum (acquired) — *see also* Deformity, varus, knee
    - congenital Q74.1
    - sequelae (late effect) of rickets E64.3
  - introrsum (acquired) — *see also* Deformity, valgus, knee
    - congenital Q74.1
    - sequelae (late effect) of rickets E64.3
  - rachitic (old) E64.3
  - recurvatum (acquired) — *see also* Deformity, limb, specified type NEC, lower leg
    - congenital Q68.2
    - sequelae (late effect) of rickets E64.3
  - valgum (acquired) (knock-knee) M21.06-
    - congenital Q74.1

Genu - *continued*

  - valgum (acquired) (knock-knee) - *continued*
    - sequelae (late effect) of rickets E64.3
  - varum (acquired) (bowleg) M21.16-
    - congenital Q74.1
    - sequelae (late effect) of rickets E64.3
- **Geographic tongue** K14.1
- **Geophagia** — *see* Pica
- **Geotrichosis** B48.3
  - stomatitis B48.3
- **Gephyrophobia** F40.242
- **Gerbode defect** Q21.0
- **GERD** (gastroesophageal reflux disease) K21.9
- **Gerhardt's**
  - disease (erythromelalgia) I73.81
  - syndrome (vocal cord paralysis) J38.00
    - bilateral J38.02
    - unilateral J38.01
- **German measles** — *see also* Rubella
  - exposure to Z20.4
- **Germinoblastoma** (diffuse) C85.9-
  - follicular C82.9-
- **Germinoma** — *see* Neoplasm, malignant, by site
- **Gerontoxon** — *see* Degeneration, cornea, senile
- **Gerstmann's syndrome** R48.8
  - developmental F81.2
- **Gerstmann-Sträussler-Scheinker syndrome** (GSS) A81.82
- **Gestation** (period) — *see also* Pregnancy
  - ectopic — *see* Pregnancy, by site
  - multiple O30.9-
    - greater than quadruplets — *see* Pregnancy, multiple (gestation), specified NEC
    - specified NEC — *see* Pregnancy, multiple (gestation), specified NEC
- **Gestational**
  - mammary abscess O91.11-
  - purulent mastitis O91.11-
  - subareolar abscess O91.11-
- **Ghon tubercle, primary infection** A15.7
- **Ghost**
  - teeth K00.4
  - vessels (cornea) H16.41-
- **Ghoul hand** A66.3
- **Gianotti-Crosti disease** L44.4
- **Giant**
  - cell
    - epulis K06.8
    - peripheral granuloma K06.8
  - esophagus, congenital Q39.5
  - kidney, congenital Q63.3
  - urticaria T78.3
    - hereditary D84.1
- **Giardiasis** A07.1
- **Gibert's disease or pityriasis** L42
- **Giddiness** R42
  - hysterical F44.89
  - psychogenic F45.8
- **Gierke's disease** (glycogenosis I) E74.01
- **Gigantism** (cerebral) (hypophyseal) (pituitary) E22.0
  - constitutional E34.4
- **Gilbert's disease or syndrome** E80.4
- **Gilchrist's disease** B40.9
- **Gilford-Hutchinson disease** E34.8
- **Gilles de la Tourette's disease or syndrome** (motor-verbal tic) F95.2
- **Gingivitis** K05.10
  - acute (catarrhal) K05.00
    - necrotizing A69.1
    - nonplaque induced K05.01
    - plaque induced K05.00
  - chronic (desquamative) (hyperplastic) (simple marginal) (pregnancy associated) (ulcerative) K05.10
    - nonplaque induced K05.11
    - plaque induced K05.10
  - expulsiva — *see* Periodontitis
  - necrotizing ulcerative (acute) A69.1
  - pellagrous E52
    - acute necrotizing A69.1
  - Vincent's A69.1
- **Gingivoglossitis** K14.0
- **Gingivopericementitis** — *see* Periodontitis
- **Gingivosis** — *see* Gingivitis, chronic
- **Gingivostomatitis** K05.10
  - herpesviral B00.2
  - necrotizing ulcerative (acute) A69.1
- **Gland, glandular** — *see* condition
- **Glanders** A24.0
- **Glanzmann** (-Naegeli) **disease or thrombasthenia** D69.1
- **Glasgow coma scale**
  - total score

Glasgow coma scale - *continued*
- total score - *continued*
  - 3-8 R40.243
  - 9-12 R40.242
  - 13-15 R40.241

Glass-blower's disease (cataract) — *see* Cataract, specified NEC

Glaucoma H40.9
- with
  - increased episcleral venous pressure H40.81-
  - pseudoexfoliation of lens — *see* Glaucoma, open angle, primary, capsular
- absolute H44.51-
- angle-closure (primary) H40.20-
  - acute (attack) (crisis) H40.21-
  - chronic H40.22-
  - intermittent H40.23-
  - residual stage H40.24-
- borderline H40.00-
- capsular (with pseudoexfoliation of lens) — *see* Glaucoma, open angle, primary, capsular
- childhood Q15.0
- closed angle — *see* Glaucoma, angle-closure
- congenital Q15.0
- corticosteroid-induced — *see* Glaucoma, secondary, drugs
- hypersecretion H40.82-
- in (due to)
  - amyloidosis E85.4 *[H42]*
  - aniridia Q13.1 *[H42]*
  - concussion of globe — *see* Glaucoma, secondary, trauma
  - dislocation of lens — *see* Glaucoma, secondary
  - disorder of lens NEC — *see* Glaucoma, secondary
  - drugs — *see* Glaucoma, secondary, drugs
  - endocrine disease NOS E34.9 *[H42]*
  - eye
    - inflammation — *see* Glaucoma, secondary, inflammation
    - trauma — *see* Glaucoma, secondary, trauma
  - hypermature cataract — *see* Glaucoma, secondary
  - iridocyclitis — *see* Glaucoma, secondary, inflammation
  - lens disorder — *see* Glaucoma, secondary,
  - Lowe's syndrome E72.03 *[H42]*
  - metabolic disease NOS E88.9 *[H42]*
  - ocular disorders NEC — *see* Glaucoma, secondary
  - onchocerciasis B73.02
  - pupillary block — *see* Glaucoma, secondary
  - retinal vein occlusion — *see* Glaucoma, secondary
  - Rieger's anomaly Q13.81 *[H42]*
  - rubeosis of iris — *see* Glaucoma, secondary
  - tumor of globe — *see* Glaucoma, secondary
- infantile Q15.0
- low tension — *see* Glaucoma, open angle, primary, low-tension
- malignant H40.83-
- narrow angle — *see* Glaucoma, angle-closure
- newborn Q15.0
- noncongestive (chronic) — *see* Glaucoma, open angle
- nonobstructive — *see* Glaucoma, open angle
- obstructive — *see also* Glaucoma, angle-closure
  - due to lens changes — *see* Glaucoma, secondary
- open angle H40.10-
  - primary H40.11-
    - capsular (with pseudoexfoliation of lens) H40.14-
    - low-tension H40.12-
    - pigmentary H40.13-
    - residual stage H40.15-
- phacolytic — *see* Glaucoma, secondary
- pigmentary — *see* Glaucoma, open angle, primary, pigmentary
- postinfectious — *see* Glaucoma, secondary, inflammation
- secondary (to) H40.5-
  - drugs H40.6-
  - inflammation H40.4-
  - trauma H40.3-
- simple (chronic) H40.11-
- simplex H40.11-
- specified type NEC H40.89
- suspect H40.00-
- syphilitic A52.71
- traumatic — *see also* Glaucoma, secondary, trauma
  - newborn (birth injury) P15.3
- tuberculous A18.59

Glaucomatous flecks (subcapsular) — *see* Cataract, complicated

Glazed tongue K14.4

Gleet (gonococcal) A54.01

Glénard's disease K63.4

Glioblastoma (multiforme)
- with sarcomatous component
  - specified site — *see* Neoplasm, malignant, by site
  - unspecified site C71.9
- giant cell
  - specified site — *see* Neoplasm, malignant, by site
  - unspecified site C71.9
- specified site — *see* Neoplasm, malignant, by site
- unspecified site C71.9

Glioma (malignant)
- astrocytic
  - specified site — *see* Neoplasm, malignant, by site
  - unspecified site C71.9
- mixed
  - specified site — *see* Neoplasm, malignant, by site
  - unspecified site C71.9
- nose Q30.8
- specified site NEC — *see* Neoplasm, malignant, by site
- subependymal D43.2
  - specified site — *see* Neoplasm, uncertain behavior, by site
  - unspecified site D43.2
- unspecified site C71.9

Gliomatosis cerebri C71.0

Glioneuroma — *see* Neoplasm, uncertain behavior, by site

Gliosarcoma
- specified site — *see* Neoplasm, malignant, by site
- unspecified site C71.9

Gliosis (cerebral) G93.89
- spinal G95.89

Glisson's disease — *see* Rickets

Globinuria R82.3

Globus (hystericus) F45.8

Glomangioma D18.00
- intra-abdominal D18.03
- intracranial D18.02
- skin D18.01
- specified site NEC D18.09

Glomangiomyoma D18.00
- intra-abdominal D18.03
- intracranial D18.02
- skin D18.01
- specified site NEC D18.09

Glomangiosarcoma — *see* Neoplasm, connective tissue, malignant

Glomerular
- disease in syphilis A52.75
- nephritis — *see* Glomerulonephritis

Glomerulitis — *see* Glomerulonephritis

Glomerulonephritis — *see also* Nephritis N05.9
- with
  - edema — *see* Nephrosis
  - minimal change N05.0
  - minor glomerular abnormality N05.0
- acute N00.9
- chronic N03.9
- crescentic (diffuse) NEC — *see also* N00-N07 with fourth character .7 N05.7
- dense deposit — *see also* N00-N07 with fourth character .6 N05.6
- diffuse
  - crescentic — *see also* N00-N07 with fourth character .7 N05.7
  - endocapillary proliferative — *see also* N00-N07 with fourth character .4 N05.4
  - membranous — *see also* N00-N07 with fourth character .2 N05.2
  - mesangial proliferative — *see also* N00-N07 with fourth character .3 N05.3
  - mesangiocapillary — *see also* N00-N07 with fourth character .5 N05.5
  - sclerosing N18.9
- endocapillary proliferative (diffuse) NEC — *see also* N00-N07 with fourth character .4 N05.4
- extracapillary NEC — *see also* N00-N07 with fourth character .7 N05.7
- focal (and segmental) — *see also* N00-N07 with fourth character .1 N05.1
- hypocomplementemic — *see* Glomerulonephritis, membranoproliferative
- IgA — *see* Nephropathy, IgA
- immune complex (circulating) NEC N05.8
- in (due to)
  - amyloidosis E85.4 *[N08]*
  - bilharziasis B65.9 *[N08]*
  - cryoglobulinemia D89.1 *[N08]*
  - defibrination syndrome D65 *[N08]*
  - diabetes mellitus — *see* Diabetes, glomerulosclerosis
  - disseminated intravascular coagulation D65 *[N08]*
  - Fabry (-Anderson) disease E75.21 *[N08]*

Glomerulonephritis - *continued*
- in (due to) - *continued*
  - Goodpasture's syndrome M31.0
  - hemolytic-uremic syndrome D59.3
  - Henoch (-Schönlein) purpura D69.0 *[N08]*
  - lecithin cholesterol acyltransferase deficiency E78.6 *[N08]*
  - microscopic polyangiitis M31.7 *[N08]*
  - multiple myeloma C90.0- *[N08]*
  - Plasmodium malariae B52.0
  - schistosomiasis B65.9 *[N08]*
  - sepsis A41.9 *[N08]*
    - streptococcal A40- *[N08]*
  - sickle-cell disorders D57.- *[N08]*
  - strongyloidiasis B78.9 *[N08]*
  - subacute bacterial endocarditis I33.0 *[N08]*
  - syphilis (late) congenital A50.59 *[N08]*
  - systemic lupus erythematosus M32.14
  - thrombotic thrombocytopenic purpura M31.1 *[N08]*
  - typhoid fever A01.09
  - Waldenström macroglobulinemia C88.0 *[N08]*
  - Wegener's granulomatosis M31.31
- latent or quiescent N03.9
- lobular, lobulonodular — *see* Glomerulonephritis, membranoproliferative
- membranoproliferative (diffuse) (type 1 or 3) — *see also* N00-N07 with fourth character .5 N05.5
  - dense deposit (type 2) NEC — *see also* N00-N07 with fourth character .6 N05.6
- membranous (diffuse) NEC — *see also* N00-N07 with fourth character .2 N05.2
- mesangial
  - IgA/IgG — *see* Nephropathy, IgA
  - proliferative (diffuse) NEC — *see also* N00-N07 with fourth character .3 N05.3
- mesangiocapillary (diffuse) NEC — *see also* N00-N07 with fourth character .5 N05.5
- necrotic, necrotizing NEC — *see also* N00-N07 with fourth character .8 N05.8
- nodular — *see* Glomerulonephritis, membranoproliferative
- poststreptococcal NEC N05.9
  - acute N00.9
  - chronic N03.9
  - rapidly progressive N01.9
- proliferative NEC — *see also* N00-N07 with fourth character .8 N05.8
  - diffuse (lupus) M32.14
- rapidly progressive N01.9
- sclerosing, diffuse N18.9
- specified pathology NEC — *see also* N00-N07 with fourth character .8 N05.8
- subacute N01.9

Glomerulopathy — *see* Glomerulonephritis

Glomerulosclerosis — *see also* Sclerosis, renal
- intercapillary (nodular) (with diabetes) — *see* Diabetes, glomerulosclerosis
- intracapillary — *see* Diabetes, glomerulosclerosis

Glossagra K14.6

Glossalgia K14.6

Glossitis (chronic superficial) (gangrenous) (Moeller's) K14.0
- areata exfoliativa K14.1
- atrophic K14.4
- benign migratory K14.1
- cortical superficial, sclerotic K14.0
- Hunter's D51.0
- interstitial, sclerous K14.0
- median rhomboid K14.2
- pellagrous E52
- superficial, chronic K14.0

Glossocele K14.8

Glossodynia K14.6
- exfoliativa K14.4

Glossoncus K14.8

Glossopathy K14.9

Glossophytia K14.3

Glossoplegia K14.8

Glossoptosis K14.8

Glossopyrosis K14.6

Glossotrichia K14.3

Glossy skin L90.8

Glottis — *see* condition

Glottitis — *see also* Laryngitis J04.0

Glucagonoma
- pancreas
  - benign D13.7
  - malignant C25.4
  - uncertain behavior D37.8
- specified site NEC
  - benign — *see* Neoplasm, benign, by site
  - malignant — *see* Neoplasm, malignant, by site

Glucagonoma - *continued*
  specified site NEC - *continued*
    uncertain behavior — *see* Neoplasm, uncertain behavior, by site
  unspecified site
    benign D13.7
    malignant C25.4
    uncertain behavior D37.8
Glucoglycinuria E72.51
Glucose-galactose malabsorption E74.39
Glue
  ear — *see* Otitis, media, nonsuppurative, chronic, mucoid
  sniffing (airplane) — *see* Abuse, drug, inhalant
    dependence — *see* Dependence, drug, inhalant
Glutaric aciduria E72.3
Glycinemia E72.51
Glycinuria (renal) (with ketosis) E72.09
Glycogen
  infiltration — *see* Disease, glycogen storage
  storage disease — *see* Disease, glycogen storage
Glycogenosis (diffuse) (generalized) — *see also* Disease, glycogen storage
  cardiac E74.02 *[I43]*
  diabetic, secondary — *see* Diabetes, glycogenosis, secondary
  pulmonary interstitial J84.842
Glycopenia E16.2
Glycosuria R81
  renal E74.8
Gnathostoma spinigerum (infection) (infestation) **, gnathostomiasis** (wandering swelling) B83.1
Goiter (plunging) (substernal) E04.9
  with
    hyperthyroidism (recurrent) — *see* Hyperthyroidism, with, goiter
    thyrotoxicosis — *see* Hyperthyroidism, with, goiter
  adenomatous — *see* Goiter, nodular
  cancerous C73
  congenital (nontoxic) E03.0
    diffuse E03.0
    parenchymatous E03.0
    transitory, with normal functioning P72.0
  cystic E04.2
    due to iodine-deficiency E01.1
  due to
    enzyme defect in synthesis of thyroid hormone E07.1
    iodine-deficiency (endemic) E01.2
  dyshormonogenetic (familial) E07.1
  endemic (iodine-deficiency) E01.2
    diffuse E01.0
    multinodular E01.1
  exophthalmic — *see* Hyperthyroidism, with, goiter
  iodine-deficiency (endemic) E01.2
    diffuse E01.0
    multinodular E01.1
    nodular E01.1
  lingual Q89.2
  lymphadenoid E06.3
  malignant C73
  multinodular (cystic) (nontoxic) E04.2
    toxic or with hyperthyroidism E05.20
      with thyroid storm E05.21
  neonatal NEC P72.0
  nodular (nontoxic) (due to) E04.9
    with
      hyperthyroidism E05.20
        with thyroid storm E05.21
      thyrotoxicosis E05.20
        with thyroid storm E05.21
    endemic E01.1
    iodine-deficiency E01.1
    sporadic E04.9
    toxic E05.20
      with thyroid storm E05.21
  nontoxic E04.9
    diffuse (colloid) E04.0
    multinodular E04.2
    simple E04.0
    specified NEC E04.8
    uninodular E04.1
  simple E04.0
  toxic — *see* Hyperthyroidism, with, goiter
  uninodular (nontoxic) E04.1
    toxic or with hyperthyroidism E05.10
      with thyroid storm E05.11
Goiter-deafness syndrome E07.1
Goldberg syndrome Q89.8
Goldberg-Maxwell syndrome E34.51
Goldblatt's hypertension or kidney I70.1
Goldenhar (-Gorlin) **syndrome** Q87.0
Goldflam-Erb disease or syndrome G70.00
  with exacerbation (acute) G70.01
  in crisis G70.01
Goldscheider's disease Q81.8
Goldstein's disease
  (familial hemorrhagic telangiectasia) I78.0
Golfer's elbow — *see* Epicondylitis, medial
Gonadoblastoma
  specified site — *see* Neoplasm, uncertain behavior, by site
  unspecified site
    female D39.10
    male D40.10
Gonecystitis — *see* Vesiculitis
Gongylonemiasis B83.8
Goniosynechiae — *see* Adhesions, iris, goniosynechiae
Gonococcemia A54.86
Gonococcus, gonococcal (disease) (infection) — *see also* condition A54.9
  anus A54.6
  bursa, bursitis A54.49
  conjunctiva, conjunctivitis (neonatorum) A54.31
  endocardium A54.83
  eye A54.30
    conjunctivitis A54.31
    iridocyclitis A54.32
    keratitis A54.33
    newborn A54.31
    other specified A54.39
  fallopian tubes (acute) (chronic) A54.24
  genitourinary (organ) (system) (tract) (acute)
    lower A54.00
      with abscess (accessory gland) (periurethral) A54.1
    upper — *see also* condition A54.29
  heart A54.83
  iridocyclitis A54.32
  joint A54.42
  lymphatic (gland) (node) A54.89
  meninges, meningitis A54.81
  musculoskeletal A54.40
    arthritis A54.42
    osteomyelitis A54.43
    other specified A54.49
    spondylopathy A54.41
  pelviperitonitis A54.24
  pelvis (acute) (chronic) A54.24
  pharynx A54.5
  proctitis A54.6
  pyosalpinx (acute) (chronic) A54.24
  rectum A54.6
  skin A54.89
  specified site NEC A54.89
  tendon sheath A54.49
  throat A54.5
  urethra (acute) (chronic) A54.01
    with abscess (accessory gland) (periurethral) A54.1
  vulva (acute) (chronic) A54.02
Gonocytoma
  specified site — *see* Neoplasm, uncertain behavior, by site
  unspecified site
    female D39.10
    male D40.10
Gonorrhea (acute) (chronic) A54.9
  Bartholin's gland (acute) (chronic) (purulent) A54.02
    with abscess (accessory gland) (periurethral) A54.1
  bladder A54.01
  cervix A54.03
  conjunctiva, conjunctivitis (neonatorum) A54.31
  contact Z20.2
  Cowper's gland (with abscess) A54.1
  exposure to Z20.2
  fallopian tube (acute) (chronic) A54.24
  kidney (acute) (chronic) A54.21
  lower genitourinary tract A54.00
    with abscess (accessory gland) (periurethral) A54.1
  ovary (acute) (chronic) A54.24
  pelvis (acute) (chronic) A54.24
    female pelvic inflammatory disease A54.24
  penis A54.09
  prostate (acute) (chronic) A54.22
  seminal vesicle (acute) (chronic) A54.23
  specified site not listed — *see also* Gonococcus A54.89
  spermatic cord (acute) (chronic) A54.23
  urethra A54.01
    with abscess (accessory gland) (periurethral) A54.1
  vagina A54.02
  vas deferens (acute) (chronic) A54.23
  vulva A54.02
Goodall's disease A08.19
Goodpasture's syndrome M31.0
Gopalan's syndrome (burning feet) E53.0
Gorlin-Chaudry-Moss syndrome Q87.0
Gottron's papules L94.4
Gougerot-Blum syndrome
  (pigmented purpuric lichenoid dermatitis) L81.7
Gougerot-Carteaud disease or syndrome
  (confluent reticulate papillomatosis) L83
Gougerot's syndrome (trisymptomatic) L81.7
Gouley's syndrome (constrictive pericarditis) I31.1
Goundou A66.6
Gout, chronic — *see also* Gout, gouty M1A.9
  drug-induced M1A.20
    ankle M1A.27-
    elbow M1A.22-
    foot joint M1A.27-
    hand joint M1A.24-
    hip M1A.25-
    knee M1A.26-
    multiple site M1A.29-
    shoulder M1A.21-
    vertebrae M1A.28
    wrist M1A.23-
  idiopathic M1A.00
    ankle M1A.07-
    elbow M1A.02-
    foot joint M1A.07-
    hand joint M1A.04-
    hip M1A.05-
    knee M1A.06-
    multiple site M1A.09
    shoulder M1A.01-
    vertebrae M1A.08
    wrist M1A.03-
  in (due to) renal impairment M1A.30
    ankle M1A.37-
    elbow M1A.32-
    foot joint M1A.37-
    hand joint M1A.34-
    hip M1A.35-
    knee M1A.36-
    multiple site M1A.39
    shoulder M1A.31-
    vertebrae M1A.38
    wrist M1A.33-
  lead-induced M1A.10
    ankle M1A.17-
    elbow M1A.12-
    foot joint M1A.17-
    hand joint M1A.14-
    hip M1A.15-
    knee M1A.16-
    multiple site M1A.19
    shoulder M1A.11-
    vertebrae M1A.18
    wrist M1A.13-
  primary — *see* Gout, chronic, idiopathic
  saturnine — *see* Gout, chronic, lead-induced
  secondary NEC M1A.40
    ankle M1A.47-
    elbow M1A.42-
    foot joint M1A.47-
    hand joint M1A.44-
    hip M1A.45-
    knee M1A.46-
    multiple site M1A.49
    shoulder M1A.41-
    vertebrae M1A.48
    wrist M1A.43-
  syphilitic (*see also* subcategory M14.8-) A52.77
  tophi M1A.9
Gout, gouty (acute) (attack) (flare) — *see also* Gout, chronic M10.9
  drug-induced M10.20
    ankle M10.27-
    elbow M10.22-
    foot joint M10.27-
    hand joint M10.24-
    hip M10.25-
    knee M10.26-
    multiple site M10.29
    shoulder M10.21-
    vertebrae M10.28
    wrist M10.23-
  idiopathic M10.00
    ankle M10.07-
    elbow M10.02-
    foot joint M10.07-
    hand joint M10.04-
    hip M10.05-
    knee M10.06-
    multiple site M10.09
    shoulder M10.01-

Headache - *continued*
primary - *continued*
exertional G44.84
stabbing G44.85
thunderclap G44.53
rebound G44.40
intractable G44.41
not intractable G44.40
short lasting unilateral neuralgiform, with conjunctival injection and tearing (SUNCT) G44.059
intractable G44.051
not intractable G44.059
specified syndrome NEC G44.89
spinal and epidural anesthesia - induced T88.59
in labor and delivery O74.5
in pregnancy O29.4-
postpartum, puerperal O89.4
spinal fluid loss (from puncture) G97.1
stabbing (primary) G44.85
tension (-type) G44.209
chronic G44.229
intractable G44.221
not intractable G44.229
episodic G44.219
intractable G44.211
not intractable G44.219
intractable G44.201
not intractable G44.209
thunderclap (primary) G44.53
vascular NEC G44.1
Healthy
infant
accompanying sick mother Z76.3
receiving care Z76.2
person accompanying sick person Z76.3
Hearing examination Z01.10
with abnormal findings NEC Z01.118
infant or child (over 28 days old) Z00.129
with abnormal findings Z00.121
following failed hearing screening Z01.110
for hearing conservation and treatment Z01.12
Heart — *see* condition
Heart beat
abnormality R00.9
specified NEC R00.8
awareness R00.2
rapid R00.0
slow R00.1
Heartburn R12
psychogenic F45.8
Heartland virus disease A93.8
Heat (effects) T67.9
apoplexy T67.0
burn — *see also* Burn L55.9
collapse T67.1
cramps T67.2
dermatitis or eczema L59.0
edema T67.7
erythema - code by site under Burn, first degree
excessive T67.9
specified effect NEC T67.8
exhaustion T67.5
anhydrotic T67.3
due to
salt (and water) depletion T67.4
water depletion T67.3
with salt depletion T67.4
fatigue (transient) T67.6
fever T67.0
hyperpyrexia T67.0
prickly L74.0
prostration — *see* Heat, exhaustion
pyrexia T67.0
rash L74.0
specified effect NEC T67.8
stroke T67.0
sunburn — *see* Sunburn
syncope T67.1
Heavy-for-dates NEC (infant) (4000g to 4499g) P08.1
exceptionally (4500g or more) P08.0
Hebephrenia, hebephrenic (schizophrenia) F20.1
Heberden's disease or nodes (with arthropathy) M15.1
Hebra's
pityriasis L26
prurigo L28.2
Heel — *see* condition
Heerfordt's disease D86.89
Hegglin's anomaly or syndrome D72.0
Heilmeyer-Schoner disease D45
Heine-Medin disease A80.9
Heinz body anemia, congenital D58.2
Heliophobia F40.228
Heller's disease or syndrome F84.3
HELLP syndrome
(hemolysis, elevated liver enzymes and low platelet count) O14.2-
complicating
childbirth O14.24
puerperium O14.25
Helminthiasis — *see also* Infestation, helminth
Ancylostoma B76.0
intestinal B82.0
mixed types (types classifiable to more than one of the titles B65.0-B81.3 and B81.8) B81.4
specified type NEC B81.8
mixed types (intestinal) (types classifiable to more than one of the titles B65.0-B81.3 and B81.8) B81.4
Necator (americanus) B76.1
specified type NEC B83.8
Heloma L84
Hemangioblastoma — *see* Neoplasm, connective tissue, uncertain behavior
malignant — *see* Neoplasm, connective tissue, malignant
Hemangioendothelioma — *see also* Neoplasm, uncertain behavior, by site
benign D18.00
intra-abdominal D18.03
intracranial D18.02
skin D18.01
specified site NEC D18.09
bone (diffuse) — *see* Neoplasm, bone, malignant
epithelioid — *see also* Neoplasm, uncertain behavior, by site
malignant — *see* Neoplasm, malignant, by site
malignant — *see* Neoplasm, connective tissue, malignant
Hemangiofibroma — *see* Neoplasm, benign, by site
Hemangiolipoma — *see* Lipoma
Hemangioma D18.00
arteriovenous D18.00
intra-abdominal D18.03
intracranial D18.02
skin D18.01
specified site NEC D18.09
capillary D18.00
intra-abdominal D18.03
intracranial D18.02
skin D18.01
specified site NEC D18.09
cavernous D18.00
intra-abdominal D18.03
intracranial D18.02
skin D18.01
specified site NEC D18.09
epithelioid D18.00
intra-abdominal D18.03
intracranial D18.02
skin D18.01
specified site NEC D18.09
histiocytoid D18.00
intra-abdominal D18.03
intracranial D18.02
skin D18.01
specified site NEC D18.09
infantile D18.00
intra-abdominal D18.03
intracranial D18.02
skin D18.01
specified site NEC D18.09
intra-abdominal D18.03
intracranial D18.02
intramuscular D18.00
intra-abdominal D18.03
intracranial D18.02
skin D18.01
specified site NEC D18.09
intrathoracic structures D18.09
juvenile D18.00
malignant — *see* Neoplasm,connective tissue, malignant
plexiform D18.00
intra-abdominal D18.03
intracranial D18.02
skin D18.01
specified site NEC D18.09
racemose D18.00
intra-abdominal D18.03
intracranial D18.02
skin D18.01
specified site NEC D18.09
sclerosing — *see* Neoplasm,skin, benign
Hemangioma - *continued*
simplex D18.00
intra-abdominal D18.03
intracranial D18.02
skin D18.01
specified site NEC D18.09
skin D18.01
specified site NEC D18.09
venous D18.00
intra-abdominal D18.03
intracranial D18.02
skin D18.01
specified site NEC D18.09
verrucous keratotic D18.00
intra-abdominal D18.03
intracranial D18.02
skin D18.01
specified site NEC D18.09
Hemangiomatosis (systemic) I78.8
involving single site — *see* Hemangioma
Hemangiopericytoma — *see also* Neoplasm, connective tissue, uncertain behavior
benign — *see* Neoplasm, connective tissue, benign
malignant — *see* Neoplasm, connective tissue, malignant
Hemangiosarcoma — *see* Neoplasm, connective tissue, malignant
Hemarthrosis (nontraumatic) M25.00
ankle M25.07-
elbow M25.02-
foot joint M25.07-
hand joint M25.04-
hip M25.05-
in hemophilic arthropathy — *see* Arthropathy, hemophilic
knee M25.06-
shoulder M25.01-
specified joint NEC M25.08
traumatic — *see* Sprain, by site
vertebrae M25.08
wrist M25.03-
Hematemesis K92.0
with ulcer - code by site under Ulcer, with hemorrhage K27.4
newborn, neonatal P54.0
due to swallowed maternal blood P78.2
Hematidrosis L74.8
Hematinuria — *see also* Hemoglobinuria
malarial B50.8
Hematobilia K83.8
Hematocele
female NEC N94.89
with ectopic pregnancy O00.90
with intrauterine pregnancy O00.91
ovary N83.8
male N50.1
Hematochezia — *see also* Melena K92.1
Hematochyluria — *see also* Infestation, filarial
schistosomiasis (bilharziasis) B65.0
Hematocolpos (with hematometra or hematosalpinx) N89.7
Hematocornea — *see* Pigmentation, cornea, stromal
Hematogenous — *see* condition
Hematoma (traumatic) (skin surface intact) — *see also* Contusion
with
injury of internal organs — *see* Injury, by site
open wound — *see* Wound, open
amputation stump (surgical) (late) T87.89
aorta, dissecting I71.00
abdominal I71.02
thoracic I71.01
thoracoabdominal I71.03
aortic intramural — *see* Dissection, aorta
arterial (complicating trauma) — *see* Injury, blood vessel, by site
auricle — *see* Contusion, ear
nontraumatic — *see* Disorder, pinna, hematoma
birth injury NEC P15.8
brain (traumatic)
with
cerebral laceration or contusion (diffuse) — *see* Injury, intracranial, diffuse
focal — *see* Injury, intracranial, focal
cerebellar, traumatic S06.37-
newborn NEC P52.4
birth injury P10.1
intracerebral, traumatic — *see* Injury, intracranial, intracerebral hemorrhage
nontraumatic — *see* Hemorrhage, intracranial
subarachnoid, arachnoid, traumatic — *see* Injury, intracranial, subarachnoid hemorrhage

Hematoma (traumatic) (skin surface intact) - *continued*
brain (traumatic) - *continued*
subdural, traumatic — *see* Injury, intracranial, subdural hemorrhage
breast (nontraumatic) N64.89
broad ligament (nontraumatic) N83.7
traumatic S37.892
cerebellar, traumatic S06.37-
cerebral — *see* Hematoma, brain
cerebrum S06.36-
left S06.35-
right S06.34-
cesarean delivery wound O90.2
complicating delivery (perineal) (pelvic) (vagina) (vulva) O71.7
corpus cavernosum (nontraumatic) N48.89
epididymis (nontraumatic) N50.1
epidural (traumatic) — *see* Injury, intracranial, epidural hemorrhage
spinal — *see* Injury, spinal cord, by region
episiotomy O90.2
face, birth injury P15.4
genital organ NEC (nontraumatic)
female (nonobstetric) N94.89
traumatic S30.202
male N50.1
traumatic S30.201
internal organs — *see* Injury, by site
intracerebral, traumatic — *see* Injury, intracranial, intracerebral hemorrhage
intraoperative — *see* Complications, intraoperative, hemorrhage
labia (nontraumatic) (nonobstetric) N90.89
liver (subcapsular) (nontraumatic) K76.89
birth injury P15.0
mediastinum — *see* Injury, intrathoracic
mesosalpinx (nontraumatic) N83.7
traumatic S37.898
muscle - code by site under Contusion
nontraumatic
muscle M79.81
soft tissue M79.81
obstetrical surgical wound O90.2
orbit, orbital (nontraumatic) — *see also* Hemorrhage, orbit
traumatic — *see* Contusion, orbit
pelvis (female) (nontraumatic) (nonobstetric) N94.89
obstetric O71.7
traumatic — *see* Injury, by site
penis (nontraumatic) N48.89
birth injury P15.5
perianal (nontraumatic) K64.5
perineal S30.23
complicating delivery O71.7
perirenal — *see* Injury, kidney
pinna — *see* Contusion, ear
nontraumatic — *see* Disorder, pinna, hematoma
placenta O43.89-
postoperative (postprocedural) — *see* Complication, postprocedural, hematoma
retroperitoneal (nontraumatic) K66.1
traumatic S36.892
scrotum, superficial S30.22
birth injury P15.5
seminal vesicle (nontraumatic) N50.1
traumatic S37.892
spermatic cord (traumatic) S37.892
nontraumatic N50.1
spinal (cord) (meninges) — *see also* Injury, spinal cord, by region
newborn (birth injury) P11.5
spleen D73.5
intraoperative — *see* Complications, intraoperative, hemorrhage, spleen
postprocedural (postoperative) — *see* Complications, postprocedural, hemorrhage, spleen
sternocleidomastoid, birth injury P15.2
sternomastoid, birth injury P15.2
subarachnoid (traumatic) — *see* Injury, intracranial, subarachnoid hemorrhage
newborn (nontraumatic) P52.5
due to birth injury P10.3
nontraumatic — *see* Hemorrhage, intracranial, subarachnoid
subdural (traumatic) — *see* Injury, intracranial, subdural hemorrhage
newborn (localized) P52.8
birth injury P10.0
nontraumatic — *see* Hemorrhage, intracranial, subdural

Hematoma (traumatic) (skin surface intact) - *continued*
superficial, newborn P54.5
testis (nontraumatic) N50.1
birth injury P15.5
tunica vaginalis (nontraumatic) N50.1
umbilical cord, complicating delivery O69.5
uterine ligament (broad) (nontraumatic) N83.7
traumatic S37.892
vagina (ruptured) (nontraumatic) N89.8
complicating delivery O71.7
vas deferens (nontraumatic) N50.1
traumatic S37.892
vitreous — *see* Hemorrhage, vitreous
vulva (nontraumatic) (nonobstetric) N90.89
complicating delivery O71.7
newborn (birth injury) P15.5
Hematometra N85.7
with hematocolpos N89.7
Hematomyelia (central) G95.19
newborn (birth injury) P11.5
traumatic T14.8
Hematomyelitis G04.90
Hematoperitoneum — *see* Hemoperitoneum
Hematophobia F40.230
Hematopneumothorax (see Hemothorax)
Hematopoiesis, cyclic D70.4
Hematoporphyria — *see* Porphyria
Hematorachis, hematorrhachis G95.19
newborn (birth injury) P11.5
Hematosalpinx N83.6
with
hematocolpos N89.7
hematometra N85.7
with hematocolpos N89.7
infectional — *see* Salpingitis
Hematospermia R36.1
Hematothorax (see Hemothorax)
Hematuria R31.9
due to sulphonamide, sulfonamide — *see* Table of Drugs and Chemicals, by drug
benign (familial) (of childhood) — *see also* Hematuria, idiopathic
essential microscopic R31.1
endemic — *see also* Schistosomiasis B65.0
gross R31.0
idiopathic N02.9
with glomerular lesion
crescentic (diffuse) glomerulonephritis N02.7
dense deposit disease N02.6
endocapillary proliferative glomerulonephritis N02.4
focal and segmental hyalinosis or sclerosis N02.1
membranoproliferative (diffuse) N02.5
membranous (diffuse) N02.2
mesangial proliferative (diffuse) N02.3
mesangiocapillary (diffuse) N02.5
minor abnormality N02.0
proliferative NEC N02.8
specified pathology NEC N02.8
intermittent — *see* Hematuria, idiopathic
malarial B50.8
microscopic NEC (with symptoms) R31.29
asymptomatic R31.21
benign essential R31.1
paroxysmal — *see also* Hematuria, idiopathic
nocturnal D59.5
persistent — *see* Hematuria, idiopathic
recurrent — *see* Hematuria, idiopathic
tropical — *see also* Schistosomiasis B65.0
tuberculous A18.13
Hemeralopia (day blindness) H53.11
vitamin A deficiency E50.5
Hemi-akinesia R41.4
Hemianalgesia R20.0
Hemianencephaly Q00.0
Hemianesthesia R20.0
Hemianopia, hemianopsia (heteronymous) H53.47
homonymous H53.46-
syphilitic A52.71
Hemiathetosis R25.8
Hemiatrophy R68.89
cerebellar G31.9
face, facial, progressive (Romberg) G51.8
tongue K14.8
Hemiballism (us) G25.5
Hemicardia Q24.8
Hemicephalus, hemicephaly Q00.0
Hemichorea G25.5
Hemicolitis, left — *see* Colitis, left sided
Hemicrania
congenital malformation Q00.0
continua G44.51

Hemicrania - *continued*
meaning migraine — *see also* Migraine G43.909
paroxysmal G44.039
chronic G44.049
intractable G44.041
not intractable G44.049
episodic G44.039
intractable G44.031
not intractable G44.039
intractable G44.031
not intractable G44.039
Hemidystrophy — *see* Hemiatrophy
Hemiectromelia Q73.8
Hemihypalgesia R20.8
Hemihypesthesia R20.1
Hemi-inattention R41.4
Hemimelia Q73.8
lower limb — *see* Defect, reduction, lower limb, specified type NEC
upper limb — *see* Defect, reduction, upper limb, specified type NEC
Hemiparalysis — *see* Hemiplegia
Hemiparesis — *see* Hemiplegia
Hemiparesthesia R20.2
Hemiparkinsonism G20
Hemiplegia G81.9-
alternans facialis G83.89
ascending NEC G81.90
spinal G95.89
congenital (cerebral) G80.8
spastic G80.2
embolic (current episode) I63.4-
flaccid G81.0-
following
cerebrovascular disease I69.959
cerebral infarction I69.35-
intracerebral hemorrhage I69.15-
nontraumatic intracranial hemorrhage NEC I69.25-
specified disease NEC I69.85-
stroke NOS I69.35-
subarachnoid hemorrhage I69.05-
hysterical F44.4
newborn NEC P91.88
birth injury P11.9
spastic G81.1-
congenital G80.2
thrombotic (current episode) I63.3-
Hemisection, spinal cord — *see* Injury, spinal cord, by region
Hemispasm (facial) R25.2
Hemisporosis B48.8
Hemitremor R25.1
Hemivertebra Q76.49
failure of segmentation with scoliosis Q76.3
fusion with scoliosis Q76.3
Hemochromatosis E83.119
with refractory anemia D46.1
due to repeated red blood cell transfusion E83.111
hereditary (primary) E83.110
neonatal P78.84
primary E83.110
specified NEC E83.118
Hemoglobin — *see also* condition
abnormal (disease) — *see* Disease, hemoglobin
AS genotype D57.3
Constant Spring D58.2
E-beta thalassemia D56.5
fetal, hereditary persistence (HPFH) D56.4
H Constant Spring D56.0
low NOS D64.9
S (Hb S) , heterozygous D57.3
Hemoglobinemia D59.9
due to blood transfusion T80.89
paroxysmal D59.6
nocturnal D59.5
Hemoglobinopathy (mixed) D58.2
with thalassemia D56.8
sickle-cell D57.1
with thalassemia D57.40
with crisis (vasoocclusive pain) D57.419
with
acute chest syndrome D57.411
splenic sequestration D57.412
without crisis D57.40
Hemoglobinuria R82.3
with anemia, hemolytic, acquired (chronic) NEC D59.6
cold (agglutinin) (paroxysmal) (with Raynaud's syndrome) D59.6
due to exertion or hemolysis NEC D59.6
intermittent D59.6
malarial B50.8

- **Hemoglobinuria** - *continued*
  - march D59.6
  - nocturnal (paroxysmal) D59.5
  - paroxysmal (cold) D59.6
    - nocturnal D59.5
- **Hemolymphangioma** D18.1
- **Hemolysis**
  - intravascular
    - with
      - abortion — *see* Abortion, by type, complicated by, hemorrhage
      - ectopic or molar pregnancy O08.1
      - hemorrhage
        - antepartum — *see* Hemorrhage, antepartum, with coagulation defect
        - intrapartum — *see also* Hemorrhage, complicating, delivery O67.0
    - postpartum O72.3
  - neonatal (excessive) P58.9
    - specified NEC P58.8
- **Hemolytic** — *see* condition
- **Hemopericardium** I31.2
  - following acute myocardial infarction (current complication) I23.0
  - newborn P54.8
  - traumatic — *see* Injury, heart, with hemopericardium
- **Hemoperitoneum** K66.1
  - infectional K65.9
  - traumatic S36.899
    - with open wound — *see* Wound, open, with penetration into peritoneal cavity
- **Hemophilia** (classical) (familial) (hereditary) D66
  - A D66
  - B D67
  - C D68.1
  - acquired D68.311
  - autoimmune D68.311
  - calcipriva — *see also* Defect, coagulation D68.4
  - nonfamilial — *see also* Defect, coagulation D68.4
  - secondary D68.311
  - vascular D68.0
- **Hemophthalmos** H44.81-
- **Hemopneumothorax** — *see also* Hemothorax
  - traumatic S27.2
- **Hemoptysis** R04.2
  - newborn P26.9
  - tuberculous — *see* Tuberculosis, pulmonary
- **Hemorrhage, hemorrhagic** (concealed) R58
  - abdomen R58
  - accidental antepartum — *see* Hemorrhage, antepartum
  - acute idiopathic pulmonary, in infants R04.81
  - adenoid J35.8
  - adrenal (capsule) (gland) E27.49
    - medulla E27.8
    - newborn P54.4
  - after delivery — *see* Hemorrhage, postpartum
  - alveolar
    - lung, newborn P26.8
    - process K08.89
  - alveolus K08.89
  - amputation stump (surgical) T87.89
  - anemia (chronic) D50.0
    - acute D62
  - antepartum (with) O46.90
    - with coagulation defect O46.00-
      - afibrinogenemia O46.01-
      - disseminated intravascular coagulation O46.02-
      - hypofibrinogenemia O46.01-
      - specified defect NEC O46.09-
    - before 20 weeks gestation O20.9
      - specified type NEC O20.8
      - threatened abortion O20.0
    - due to
      - abruptio placenta — *see also* Abruptio placentae O45.9-
      - leiomyoma, uterus — *see* Hemorrhage, antepartum, specified cause NEC
      - placenta previa O44.1-
    - specified cause NEC — *see* subcategory O46.8X-
  - anus (sphincter) K62.5
  - apoplexy (stroke) — *see* Hemorrhage, intracranial, intracerebral
  - arachnoid — *see* Hemorrhage, intracranial, subarachnoid
  - artery R58
    - brain — *see* Hemorrhage, intracranial, intracerebral
  - basilar (ganglion) I61.0
  - bladder N32.89
  - bowel K92.2
    - newborn P54.3

- **Hemorrhage, hemorrhagic** (concealed) - *continued*
  - brain (miliary) (nontraumatic) — *see* Hemorrhage, intracranial, intracerebral
    - due to
      - birth injury P10.1
      - syphilis A52.05
    - epidural or extradural (traumatic) — *see* Injury, intracranial, epidural hemorrhage
    - newborn P52.4
      - birth injury P10.1
    - subarachnoid — *see* Hemorrhage, intracranial, subarachnoid
    - subdural — *see* Hemorrhage, intracranial, subdural
  - brainstem (nontraumatic) I61.3
    - traumatic S06.38-
  - breast N64.59
  - bronchial tube — *see* Hemorrhage, lung
  - bronchopulmonary — *see* Hemorrhage, lung
  - bronchus — *see* Hemorrhage, lung
  - bulbar I61.5
  - capillary I78.8
    - primary D69.8
  - cecum K92.2
  - cerebellar, cerebellum (nontraumatic) I61.4
    - newborn P52.6
    - traumatic S06.37-
  - cerebral, cerebrum — *see also* Hemorrhage, intracranial, intracerebral
    - newborn (anoxic) P52.4
      - birth injury P10.1
    - lobe I61.1
  - cerebromeningeal I61.8
  - cerebrospinal — *see* Hemorrhage, intracranial, intracerebral
  - cervix (uteri) (stump) NEC N88.8
  - chamber, anterior (eye) — *see* Hyphema
  - childbirth — *see* Hemorrhage, complicating, delivery
  - choroid H31.30-
    - expulsive H31.31-
  - ciliary body — *see* Hyphema
  - cochlea — *see* subcategory H83.8
  - colon K92.2
  - complicating
    - abortion — *see* Abortion, by type, complicated by, hemorrhage
    - delivery O67.9
      - associated with coagulation defect (afibrinogenemia) (DIC) (hyperfibrinolysis) O67.0
      - specified cause NEC O67.8
    - surgical procedure — *see* Hemorrhage, intraoperative
  - conjunctiva H11.3-
    - newborn P54.8
  - cord, newborn (stump) P51.9
  - corpus luteum (ruptured) cyst N83.1-
  - cortical (brain) I61.1
  - cranial — *see* Hemorrhage, intracranial
  - cutaneous R23.3
    - due to autosensitivity, erythrocyte D69.2
    - newborn P54.5
  - delayed
    - following ectopic or molar pregnancy O08.1
    - postpartum O72.2
  - diathesis (familial) D69.9
  - disease D69.9
    - newborn P53
    - specified type NEC D69.8
  - due to or associated with
    - afibrinogenemia or other coagulation defect (conditions in categories D65-D69)
      - antepartum — *see* Hemorrhage, antepartum, with coagulation defect
      - intrapartum O67.0
    - dental implant M27.61
    - device, implant or graft — *see also* Complications, by site and type, specified NEC T85.838
      - arterial graft NEC T82.838
      - breast T85.838
      - catheter NEC T85.838
        - dialysis (renal) T82.838
          - intraperitoneal T85.838
        - infusion NEC T82.838
          - spinal (epidural) (subdural) T85.830
        - urinary (indwelling) T83.83
      - electronic (electrode) (pulse generator) (stimulator)
        - bone T84.83
        - cardiac T82.837
        - nervous system (brain) (peripheral nerve) (spinal) T85.830
        - urinary T83.83

- **Hemorrhage, hemorrhagic** (concealed) - *continued*
  - due to or associated with - *continued*
    - device, implant or graft - *continued*
      - fixation, internal (orthopedic) NEC T84.83
      - gastrointestinal (bile duct) (esophagus) T85.838
      - genital NEC T83.83
      - heart NEC T82.837
      - joint prosthesis T84.83
      - ocular (corneal graft) (orbital implant) NEC T85.838
      - orthopedic NEC T84.83
        - bone graft T86.838
      - specified NEC T85.838
      - urinary NEC T83.83
      - vascular NEC T82.838
      - ventricular intracranial shunt T85.830
  - duodenum, duodenal K92.2
    - ulcer — *see* Ulcer, duodenum, with hemorrhage
  - dura mater — *see* Hemorrhage, intracranial, subdural
  - endotracheal — *see* Hemorrhage, lung
  - epicranial subaponeurotic (massive) , birth injury P12.2
  - epidural (traumatic) — *see also* Injury, intracranial, epidural hemorrhage
    - nontraumatic I62.1
  - esophagus K22.8
    - varix I85.01
      - secondary I85.11
  - excessive, following ectopic gestation (subsequent episode) O08.1
  - extradural (traumatic) — *see* Injury, intracranial, epidural hemorrhage
    - birth injury P10.8
    - newborn (anoxic) (nontraumatic) P52.8
    - nontraumatic I62.1
  - eye NEC H57.89
    - fundus — *see* Hemorrhage, retina
    - lid — *see* Disorder, eyelid, specified type NEC
  - fallopian tube N83.6
  - fibrinogenolysis — *see* Fibrinolysis
  - fibrinolytic (acquired) — *see* Fibrinolysis
  - from
    - ear (nontraumatic) — *see* Otorrhagia
    - tracheostomy stoma J95.01
  - fundus, eye — *see* Hemorrhage, retina
  - funis — *see* Hemorrhage, umbilicus, cord
  - gastric — *see* Hemorrhage, stomach
  - gastroenteric K92.2
    - newborn P54.3
  - gastrointestinal (tract) K92.2
    - newborn P54.3
  - genital organ, male N50.1
  - genitourinary (tract) NOS R31.9
  - gingiva K06.8
  - globe (eye) — *see* Hemophthalmos
  - graafian follicle cyst (ruptured) N83.0-
  - gum K06.8
  - heart I51.89
  - hypopharyngeal (throat) R04.1
  - intermenstrual (regular) N92.3
    - irregular N92.1
  - internal (organs) NEC R58
    - capsule I61.0
    - ear — *see* subcategory H83.8
    - newborn P54.8
  - intestine K92.2
    - newborn P54.3
  - intra-abdominal R58
  - intra-alveolar (lung) , newborn P26.8
  - intracerebral (nontraumatic) — *see* Hemorrhage, intracranial, intracerebral
  - intracranial (nontraumatic) I62.9
    - birth injury P10.9
    - epidural, nontraumatic I62.1
    - extradural, nontraumatic I62.1
    - newborn P52.9
      - specified NEC P52.8
    - intracerebral (nontraumatic) (in) I61.9
      - brain stem I61.3
      - cerebellum I61.4
      - newborn P52.4
        - birth injury P10.1
      - hemisphere I61.2
        - cortical (superficial) I61.1
        - subcortical (deep) I61.0
      - intraoperative
        - during a nervous system procedure G97.31
        - during other procedure G97.32
      - intraventricular I61.5
      - multiple localized I61.6
      - postprocedural
        - following a nervous system procedure G97.51

Hemorrhoids (bleeding) (without mention of degree) - *continued*
skin tags - *continued*
anus K64.4
residual K64.4
specified NEC K64.8
strangulated — *see also* Hemorrhoids, by degree K64.8
thrombosed — *see also* Hemorrhoids, by degree K64.5
ulcerated — *see also* Hemorrhoids, by degree K64.8
Hemosalpinx N83.6
with
hematocolpos N89.7
hematometra N85.7
with hematocolpos N89.7
Hemosiderosis (dietary) E83.19
pulmonary, idiopathic E83.1- *[J84.03]*
transfusion T80.89
Hemothorax (bacterial) (nontuberculous) J94.2
newborn P54.8
traumatic S27.1
with pneumothorax S27.2
tuberculous NEC A15.6
Henoch (-Schönlein) **disease or syndrome** (purpura) D69.0
Henpue, henpuye A66.6
Hepar lobatum (syphilitic) A52.74
Hepatalgia K76.89
Hepatitis K75.9
acute B17.9
with coma K72.01
with hepatic failure — *see* Failure, hepatic
alcoholic — *see* Hepatitis, alcoholic
infectious B17.9
non-viral K72.0
viral B17.9
alcoholic (acute) (chronic) K70.10
with ascites K70.11
amebic — *see* Abscess, liver, amebic
anicteric, (viral) — *see* Hepatitis, viral
antigen-associated (HAA) — *see* Hepatitis, B
Australia-antigen (positive) — *see* Hepatitis, B
autoimmune K75.4
B B19.10
with hepatic coma B19.11
acute B16.9
with
delta-agent (coinfection) (without hepatic coma) B16.1
with hepatic coma B16.0
hepatic coma (without delta-agent coinfection) B16.2
chronic B18.1
with delta-agent B18.0
bacterial NEC K75.89
C (viral) B19.20
with hepatic coma B19.21
acute B17.10
with hepatic coma B17.11
chronic B18.2
catarrhal (acute) B15.9
with hepatic coma B15.0
cholangiolitic K75.89
cholestatic K75.89
chronic K73.9
active NEC K73.2
lobular NEC K73.1
persistent NEC K73.0
specified NEC K73.8
cytomegaloviral B25.1
due to ethanol (acute) (chronic) — *see* Hepatitis, alcoholic
epidemic B15.9
with hepatic coma B15.0
fulminant NEC (viral) — *see* Hepatitis, viral
neonatal giant cell P59.29
granulomatous NEC K75.3
herpesviral B00.81
history of
B Z86.19
C Z86.19
homologous serum — *see* Hepatitis, viral, type B
in (due to)
mumps B26.81
toxoplasmosis (acquired) B58.1
congenital (active) P37.1 *[K77]*
infectious, infective B15.9
acute (subacute) B17.9
chronic B18.9
inoculation — *see* Hepatitis, viral, type B
interstitial (chronic) K74.69
lupoid NEC K75.4

Hepatitis - *continued*
malignant NEC (with hepatic failure) K72.90
with coma K72.91
neonatal (idiopathic) (toxic) P59.29
newborn P59.29
postimmunization — *see* Hepatitis, viral, type B
post-transfusion — *see* Hepatitis, viral, type B
reactive, nonspecific K75.2
serum — *see* Hepatitis, viral, type B
specified type NEC
with hepatic failure — *see* Failure, hepatic
syphilitic (late) A52.74
congenital (early) A50.08 *[K77]*
late A50.59 *[K77]*
secondary A51.45
toxic — *see also* Disease, liver, toxic K71.6
tuberculous A18.83
viral, virus B19.9
with hepatic coma B19.0
acute B17.9
chronic B18.9
specified NEC B18.8
type
B B18.1
with delta-agent B18.0
C B18.2
congenital P35.3
coxsackie B33.8 *[K77]*
cytomegalic inclusion B25.1
in remission, any type - code to Hepatitis, chronic, by type
non-A, non-B B17.8
specified type NEC (with or without coma) B17.8
type
A B15.9
with hepatic coma B15.0
B B19.10
with hepatic coma B19.11
acute B16.9
with
delta-agent (coinfection) (without hepatic coma) B16.1
with hepatic coma B16.0
hepatic coma (without delta-agent coinfection) B16.2
chronic B18.1
with delta-agent B18.0
C B19.20
with hepatic coma B19.21
acute B17.10
with hepatic coma B17.11
chronic B18.2
E B17.2
non-A, non-B B17.8
Hepatization lung (acute) — *see* Pneumonia, lobar
Hepatoblastoma C22.2
Hepatocarcinoma C22.0
Hepatocholangiocarcinoma C22.0
Hepatocholangioma, benign D13.4
Hepatocholangitis K75.89
Hepatolenticular degeneration E83.01
Hepatoma (malignant) C22.0
benign D13.4
embryonal C22.0
Hepatomegaly — *see also* Hypertrophy, liver
with splenomegaly R16.2
congenital Q44.7
in mononucleosis
gammaherpesviral B27.09
infectious specified NEC B27.89
Hepatoptosis K76.89
Hepatorenal syndrome following labor and delivery O90.4
Hepatosis K76.89
Hepatosplenomegaly R16.2
hyperlipemic (Bürger-Grütz type) E78.3 *[K77]*
Hereditary — *see* condition
Heredodegeneration, macular — *see* Dystrophy, retina
Heredopathia atactica polyneuritiformis G60.1
Heredosyphilis — *see* Syphilis, congenital
Herlitz' syndrome Q81.1
Hermansky-Pudlak syndrome E70.331
Hermaphrodite, hermaphroditism (true) Q56.0
46,XX with streak gonads Q99.1
46,XX/46,XY Q99.0
46,XY with streak gonads Q99.1
chimera 46,XX/46,XY Q99.0
Hernia, hernial (acquired) (recurrent) K46.9
with
gangrene — *see* Hernia, by site, with, gangrene
incarceration — *see* Hernia, by site, with, obstruction

Hernia, hernial (acquired) (recurrent) - *continued*
with - *continued*
irreducible — *see* Hernia, by site, with, obstruction
obstruction — *see* Hernia, by site, with, obstruction
strangulation — *see* Hernia, by site, with, obstruction
abdomen, abdominal K46.9
with
gangrene (and obstruction) K46.1
obstruction K46.0
femoral — *see* Hernia, femoral
incisional — *see* Hernia, incisional
inguinal — *see* Hernia, inguinal
specified site NEC K45.8
with
gangrene (and obstruction) K45.1
obstruction K45.0
umbilical — *see* Hernia, umbilical
wall — *see* Hernia, ventral
appendix — *see* Hernia, abdomen
bladder (mucosa) (sphincter)
congenital (female) (male) Q79.51
female — *see* Cystocele
male N32.89
brain, congenital — *see* Encephalocele
cartilage, vertebra — *see* Displacement, intervertebral disc
cerebral, congenital — *see also* Encephalocele
endaural Q01.8
ciliary body (traumatic) S05.2-
colon — *see* Hernia, abdomen
Cooper's — *see* Hernia, abdomen, specified site NEC
crural — *see* Hernia, femoral
diaphragm, diaphragmatic K44.9
with
gangrene (and obstruction) K44.1
obstruction K44.0
congenital Q79.0
direct (inguinal) — *see* Hernia, inguinal
diverticulum, intestine — *see* Hernia, abdomen
double (inguinal) — *see* Hernia, inguinal, bilateral
due to adhesions (with obstruction) K56.50
epigastric — *see also* Hernia, ventral K43.9
esophageal hiatus — *see* Hernia, hiatal
external (inguinal) — *see* Hernia, inguinal
fallopian tube N83.4-
fascia M62.89
femoral K41.90
with
gangrene (and obstruction) K41.40
not specified as recurrent K41.40
recurrent K41.41
obstruction K41.30
not specified as recurrent K41.30
recurrent K41.31
bilateral K41.20
with
gangrene (and obstruction) K41.10
not specified as recurrent K41.10
recurrent K41.11
obstruction K41.00
not specified as recurrent K41.00
recurrent K41.01
not specified as recurrent K41.20
recurrent K41.21
unilateral K41.90
with
gangrene (and obstruction) K41.40
not specified as recurrent K41.40
recurrent K41.41
obstruction K41.30
not specified as recurrent K41.30
recurrent K41.31
not specified as recurrent K41.90
recurrent K41.91
not specified as recurrent K41.90
recurrent K41.91
foramen magnum G93.5
congenital Q01.8
funicular (umbilical) — *see also* Hernia, umbilicus
spermatic (cord) — *see* Hernia, inguinal
gastrointestinal tract — *see* Hernia, abdomen
Hesselbach's — *see* Hernia, femoral, specified site NEC
hiatal (esophageal) (sliding) K44.9
with
gangrene (and obstruction) K44.1
obstruction K44.0
congenital Q40.1
hypogastric — *see* Hernia, ventral

Hernia, hernial (acquired) (recurrent) - *continued*
incarcerated — *see also* Hernia, by site, with obstruction
with gangrene — *see* Hernia, by site, with gangrene
incisional K43.2
with
gangrene (and obstruction) K43.1
obstruction K43.0
indirect (inguinal) — *see* Hernia, inguinal
inguinal (direct) (external) (funicular) (indirect) (internal) (oblique) (scrotal) (sliding) K40.90
with
gangrene (and obstruction) K40.40
not specified as recurrent K40.40
recurrent K40.41
obstruction K40.30
not specified as recurrent K40.30
recurrent K40.31
not specified as recurrent K40.90
recurrent K40.91
bilateral K40.20
with
gangrene (and obstruction) K40.10
not specified as recurrent K40.10
recurrent K40.11
obstruction K40.00
not specified as recurrent K40.00
recurrent K40.01
not specified as recurrent K40.20
recurrent K40.21
unilateral K40.90
with
gangrene (and obstruction) K40.40
not specified as recurrent K40.40
recurrent K40.41
obstruction K40.30
not specified as recurrent K40.30
recurrent K40.31
not specified as recurrent K40.90
recurrent K40.91
internal — *see also* Hernia, abdomen
inguinal — *see* Hernia, inguinal
interstitial — *see* Hernia, abdomen
intervertebral cartilage or disc — *see* Displacement, intervertebral disc
intestine, intestinal — *see* Hernia, by site
intra-abdominal — *see* Hernia, abdomen
iris (traumatic) S05.2-
irreducible — *see also* Hernia, by site, with obstruction
with gangrene — *see* Hernia, by site, with gangrene
ischiatic — *see* Hernia, abdomen, specified site NEC
ischiorectal — *see* Hernia, abdomen, specified site NEC
lens (traumatic) S05.2-
linea (alba) (semilunaris) — *see* Hernia, ventral
Littre's — *see* Hernia, abdomen
lumbar — *see* Hernia, abdomen, specified site NEC
lung (subcutaneous) J98.4
mediastinum J98.59
mesenteric (internal) — *see* Hernia, abdomen
midline — *see* Hernia, ventral
muscle (sheath) M62.89
nucleus pulposus — *see* Displacement, intervertebral disc
oblique (inguinal) — *see* Hernia, inguinal
obstructive — *see also* Hernia, by site, with obstruction
with gangrene — *see* Hernia, by site, with gangrene
obturator — *see* Hernia, abdomen, specified site NEC
omental — *see* Hernia, abdomen
ovary N83.4-
oviduct N83.4-
paraesophageal — *see also* Hernia, diaphragm
congenital Q40.1
parastomal K43.5
with
gangrene (and obstruction) K43.4
obstruction K43.3
paraumbilical — *see* Hernia, umbilicus
perineal — *see* Hernia, abdomen, specified site NEC
Petit's — *see* Hernia, abdomen, specified site NEC
postoperative — *see* Hernia, incisional
pregnant uterus — *see* Abnormal, uterus in pregnancy or childbirth
prevesical N32.89
properitoneal — *see* Hernia, abdomen, specified site NEC

Hernia, hernial (acquired) (recurrent) - *continued*
pudendal — *see* Hernia, abdomen, specified site NEC
rectovaginal N81.6
retroperitoneal — *see* Hernia, abdomen, specified site NEC
Richter's — *see* Hernia, abdomen, with obstruction
Rieux's, Riex's — *see* Hernia, abdomen, specified site NEC
sac condition (adhesion) (dropsy) (inflammation) (laceration) (suppuration) - code by site under Hernia
sciatic — *see* Hernia, abdomen, specified site NEC
scrotum, scrotal — *see* Hernia, inguinal
sliding (inguinal) — *see also* Hernia, inguinal
hiatus — *see* Hernia, hiatal
spigelian — *see* Hernia, ventral
spinal — *see* Spina bifida
strangulated — *see also* Hernia, by site, with obstruction
with gangrene — *see* Hernia, by site, with gangrene
subxiphoid — *see* Hernia, ventral
supra-umbilicus — *see* Hernia, ventral
tendon — *see* Disorder, tendon, specified type NEC
Treitz's (fossa) — *see* Hernia, abdomen, specified site NEC
tunica vaginalis Q55.29
umbilicus, umbilical K42.9
with
gangrene (and obstruction) K42.1
obstruction K42.0
ureter N28.89
urethra, congenital Q64.79
urinary meatus, congenital Q64.79
uterus N81.4
pregnant — *see* Abnormal, uterus in pregnancy or childbirth
vaginal (anterior) (wall) — *see* Cystocele
Velpeau's — *see* Hernia, femoral
ventral K43.9
with
gangrene (and obstruction) K43.7
obstruction K43.6
recurrent — *see* Hernia, incisional
incisional K43.2
with
gangrene (and obstruction) K43.1
obstruction K43.0
specified NEC K43.9
with
gangrene (and obstruction) K43.7
obstruction K43.6
vesical
congenital (female) (male) Q79.51
female — *see* Cystocele
male N32.89
vitreous (into wound) S05.2-
into anterior chamber — *see* Prolapse, vitreous
Herniation — *see also* Hernia
brain (stem) G93.5
cerebral G93.5
mediastinum J98.59
nucleus pulposus — *see* Displacement, intervertebral disc
Herpangina B08.5
Herpes, herpesvirus, herpetic B00.9
anogenital A60.9
perianal skin A60.1
rectum A60.1
urogenital tract A60.00
cervix A60.03
male genital organ NEC A60.02
penis A60.01
specified site NEC A60.09
vagina A60.04
vulva A60.04
blepharitis (zoster) B02.39
simplex B00.59
circinatus B35.4
bullosus L12.0
conjunctivitis (simplex) B00.53
zoster B02.31
cornea B02.33
encephalitis B00.4
due to herpesvirus 6 B10.01
due to herpesvirus 7 B10.09
specified NEC B10.09
eye (zoster) B02.30
simplex B00.50
eyelid (zoster) B02.39
simplex B00.59
facialis B00.1

Herpes, herpesvirus, herpetic - *continued*
febrilis B00.1
geniculate ganglionitis B02.21
genital, genitalis A60.00
female A60.09
male A60.02
gestational, gestationis O26.4-
gingivostomatitis B00.2
human B00.9
1 — *see* Herpes, simplex
2 — *see* Herpes, simplex
3 — *see* Varicella
4 — *see* Mononucleosis, Epstein-Barr (virus)
5 — *see* Disease, cytomegalic inclusion (generalized)
6
encephalitis B10.01
specified NEC B10.81
7
encephalitis B10.09
specified NEC B10.82
8 B10.89
infection NEC B10.89
Kaposi's sarcoma associated B10.89
iridocyclitis (simplex) B00.51
zoster B02.32
iris (vesicular erythema multiforme) L51.9
iritis (simplex) B00.51
Kaposi's sarcoma associated B10.89
keratitis (simplex) (dendritic) (disciform) (interstitial) B00.52
zoster (interstitial) B02.33
keratoconjunctivitis (simplex) B00.52
zoster B02.33
labialis B00.1
lip B00.1
meningitis (simplex) B00.3
zoster B02.1
ophthalmicus (zoster) NEC B02.30
simplex B00.50
penis A60.01
perianal skin A60.1
pharyngitis, pharyngotonsillitis B00.2
rectum A60.1
scrotum A60.02
sepsis B00.7
simplex B00.9
complicated NEC B00.89
congenital P35.2
conjunctivitis B00.53
external ear B00.1
eyelid B00.59
hepatitis B00.81
keratitis (interstitial) B00.52
myleitis B00.82
specified complication NEC B00.89
visceral B00.89
stomatitis B00.2
tonsurans B35.0
visceral B00.89
vulva A60.04
whitlow B00.89
zoster — *see also* condition B02.9
auricularis B02.21
complicated NEC B02.8
conjunctivitis B02.31
disseminated B02.7
encephalitis B02.0
eye (lid) B02.39
geniculate ganglionitis B02.21
keratitis (interstitial) B02.33
meningitis B02.1
myelitis B02.24
neuritis, neuralgia B02.29
ophthalmicus NEC B02.30
oticus B02.21
polyneuropathy B02.23
specified complication NEC B02.8
trigeminal neuralgia B02.22
Herpesvirus (human) — *see* Herpes
Herpetophobia F40.218
Herrick's anemia — *see* Disease, sickle-cell
Hers' disease E74.09
Herter-Gee syndrome K90.0
Herxheimer's reaction R68.89
Hesitancy
of micturition R39.11
urinary R39.11
Hesselbach's hernia — *see* Hernia, femoral, specified site NEC
Heterochromia (congenital) Q13.2
cataract — *see* Cataract, complicated

Heterochromia (congenital) - *continued*
cyclitis (Fuchs) — *see* Cyclitis, Fuchs' heterochromic
hair L67.1
iritis — *see* Cyclitis, Fuchs' heterochromic
retained metallic foreign body (nonmagnetic) — *see* Foreign body, intraocular, old, retained
magnetic — *see* Foreign body, intraocular, old, retained, magnetic
uveitis — *see* Cyclitis, Fuchs' heterochromic
Heterophoria — *see* Strabismus, heterophoria
Heterophyes, heterophyiasis (small intestine) B66.8
Heterotopia, heterotopic — *see also* Malposition, congenital
cerebralis Q04.8
Heterotropia — *see* Strabismus
Heubner-Herter disease K90.0
Hexadactylism Q69.9
HGSIL (cytology finding)
(high grade squamous intraepithelial lesion on cytologic smear) (Pap smear finding)
anus R85.613
cervix R87.613
biopsy (histology) finding — *see* Neoplasia, intraepithelial, cervix, grade II or grade III
vagina R87.623
biopsy (histology) finding — *see* Neoplasia, intraepithelial, vagina, grade II or grade III
Hibernoma — *see* Lipoma
Hiccup, hiccough R06.6
epidemic B33.0
psychogenic F45.8
Hidden penis (congenital) Q55.64
acquired N48.83
Hidradenitis (axillaris) (suppurative) L73.2
Hidradenoma (nodular) — *see also* Neoplasm, skin, benign
clear cell — *see* Neoplasm, skin, benign
papillary — *see* Neoplasm, skin, benign
Hidrocystoma — *see* Neoplasm, skin, benign
High
altitude effects T70.20
anoxia T70.29
on
ears T70.0
sinuses T70.1
polycythemia D75.1
arch
foot Q66.7
palate, congenital Q38.5
arterial tension — *see* Hypertension
basal metabolic rate R94.8
blood pressure — *see also* Hypertension
borderline R03.0
reading (incidental) (isolated) (nonspecific) , without diagnosis of hypertension R03.0
cholesterol E78.00
with high triglycerides E78.2
diaphragm (congenital) Q79.1
expressed emotional level within family Z63.8
head at term O32.4
palate, congenital Q38.5
risk
infant NEC Z76.2
sexual behavior (heterosexual) Z72.51
bisexual Z72.53
homosexual Z72.52
scrotal testis, testes
bilateral Q53.23
unilateral Q53.13
temperature (of unknown origin) R50.9
thoracic rib Q76.6
triglycerides E78.1
with high cholesterol E78.2
Hildenbrand's disease A75.0
Hilum — *see* condition
Hip — *see* condition
Hippel's disease Q85.8
Hippophobia F40.218
Hippus H57.09
Hirschsprung's disease or megacolon Q43.1
Hirsutism, hirsuties L68.0
Hirudiniasis
external B88.3
internal B83.4
Hiss-Russell dysentery A03.1
Histidinemia, histidinuria E70.41
Histiocytoma — *see also* Neoplasm, skin, benign
fibrous — *see also* Neoplasm, skin, benign
atypical — *see* Neoplasm, connective tissue, uncertain behavior
malignant — *see* Neoplasm, connective tissue, malignant

Histiocytosis D76.3
acute differentiated progressive C96.0
Langerhans' cell NEC C96.6
multifocal X
multisystemic (disseminated) C96.0
unisystemic C96.5
pulmonary, adult (adult PLCH) J84.82
unifocal (X) C96.6
lipid, lipoid D76.3
essential E75.29
malignant C96.A
mononuclear phagocytes NEC D76.1
Langerhans' cells C96.6
non-Langerhans cell D76.3
polyostotic sclerosing D76.3
sinus, with massive lymphadenopathy D76.3
syndrome NEC D76.3
X NEC C96.6
acute (progressive) C96.0
chronic C96.6
multifocal C96.5
multisystemic C96.0
unifocal C96.6
Histoplasmosis B39.9
with pneumonia NEC B39.2
African B39.5
American — *see* Histoplasmosis, capsulati
capsulati B39.4
disseminated B39.3
generalized B39.3
pulmonary B39.2
acute B39.0
chronic B39.1
Darling's B39.4
duboisii B39.5
lung NEC B39.2
History
family (of) — *see also* History, personal (of)
alcohol abuse Z81.1
allergy NEC Z84.89
anemia Z83.2
arthritis Z82.61
asthma Z82.5
blindness Z82.1
cardiac death (sudden) Z82.41
carrier of genetic disease Z84.81
chromosomal anomaly Z82.79
chronic
disabling disease NEC Z82.8
lower respiratory disease Z82.5
colonic polyps Z83.71
congenital malformations and deformations Z82.79
polycystic kidney Z82.71
consanguinity Z84.3
deafness Z82.2
diabetes mellitus Z83.3
disability NEC Z82.8
disease or disorder (of)
allergic NEC Z84.89
behavioral NEC Z81.8
blood and blood-forming organs Z83.2
cardiovascular NEC Z82.49
chronic disabling NEC Z82.8
digestive Z83.79
ear NEC Z83.52
endocrine NEC Z83.49
elevated lipoprotein (a) (Lp (a)) Z83.430
eye NEC Z83.518
glaucoma Z83.511
familial hypercholesterolemia Z83.42
genitourinary NEC Z84.2
glaucoma Z83.511
hematological Z83.2
immune mechanism Z83.2
infectious NEC Z83.1
ischemic heart Z82.49
kidney Z84.1
lipoprotein metabolism Z83.438
mental NEC Z81.8
metabolic Z83.49
musculoskeletal NEC Z82.69
neurological NEC Z82.0
nutritional Z83.49
parasitic NEC Z83.1
psychiatric NEC Z81.8
respiratory NEC Z83.6
skin and subcutaneous tissue NEC Z84.0
specified NEC Z84.89
drug abuse NEC Z81.3
elevated lipoprotein (a) (Lp (a)) Z83.430
epilepsy Z82.0
familial hypercholesterolemia Z83.42
genetic disease carrier Z84.81

History - *continued*
family (of) - *continued*
glaucoma Z83.511
hearing loss Z82.2
human immunodeficiency virus (HIV) infection Z83.0
Huntington's chorea Z82.0
hyperlipidemia, familial combined Z83.438
intellectual disability Z81.0
leukemia Z80.6
lipidemia NEC Z83.438
malignant neoplasm (of) NOS Z80.9
bladder Z80.52
breast Z80.3
bronchus Z80.1
digestive organ Z80.0
gastrointestinal tract Z80.0
genital organ Z80.49
ovary Z80.41
prostate Z80.42
specified organ NEC Z80.49
testis Z80.43
hematopoietic NEC Z80.7
intrathoracic organ NEC Z80.2
kidney Z80.51
lung Z80.1
lymphatic NEC Z80.7
ovary Z80.41
prostate Z80.42
respiratory organ NEC Z80.2
specified site NEC Z80.8
testis Z80.43
trachea Z80.1
urinary organ or tract Z80.59
bladder Z80.52
kidney Z80.51
mental
disorder NEC Z81.8
multiple endocrine neoplasia (MEN) syndrome Z83.41
osteoporosis Z82.62
polycystic kidney Z82.71
polyps (colon) Z83.71
psychiatric disorder Z81.8
psychoactive substance abuse NEC Z81.3
respiratory condition NEC Z83.6
asthma and other lower respiratory conditions Z82.5
self-harmful behavior Z81.8
SIDS (sudden infant death syndrome) Z84.82
skin condition Z84.0
specified condition NEC Z84.89
stroke (cerebrovascular) Z82.3
substance abuse NEC Z81.4
alcohol Z81.1
drug NEC Z81.3
psychoactive NEC Z81.3
tobacco Z81.2
sudden
cardiac death Z82.41
infant death syndrome (SIDS) Z84.82
tobacco abuse Z81.2
violence, violent behavior Z81.8
visual loss Z82.1
personal (of) — *see also* History, family (of)
abuse
childhood Z62.819
forced labor or sexual exploitation in childhood Z62.813
physical Z62.810
psychological Z62.811
sexual Z62.810
adult Z91.419
forced labor or sexual exploitation Z91.42
physical and sexual Z91.410
psychological Z91.411
alcohol dependence F10.21
allergy (to) Z88.9
analgesic agent NEC Z88.6
anesthetic Z88.4
antibiotic agent NEC Z88.1
anti-infective agent NEC Z88.3
contrast media Z91.041
drugs, medicaments and biological substances Z88.9
specified NEC Z88.8
food Z91.018
additives Z91.02
eggs Z91.012
milk products Z91.011
peanuts Z91.010
seafood Z91.013
specified food NEC Z91.018

History - *continued*
  personal (of) - *continued*
    obstetric complications Z87.59
      childbirth Z87.59
      pregnancy Z87.59
      pre-term labor Z87.51
      puerperium Z87.59
    osteoporosis fractures Z87.31
    parasuicide (attempt) Z91.5
    physical trauma NEC Z87.828
      self-harm or suicide attempt Z91.5
    poisoning NEC Z91.89
      self-harm or suicide attempt Z91.5
    poor personal hygiene Z91.89
    pneumonia (recurrent) Z87.01
    preterm labor Z87.51
    prolonged reversible ischemic neurologic deficit (PRIND) Z86.73
    procedure during pregnancy Z98.870
    procedure while a fetus Z98.871
    prostatic dysplasia Z87.430
    psychological
      abuse
        adult Z91.411
        child Z62.811
      trauma, specified NEC Z91.49
    radiation therapy Z92.3
    removal
      implant
        breast Z98.86
    renal calculi Z87.442
    respiratory condition NEC Z87.09
    retained foreign body fully removed Z87.821
    risk factors NEC Z91.89
    self-harm Z91.5
    self-poisoning attempt Z91.5
    sex reassignment Z87.890
    sleep-wake cycle problem Z72.821
    specified NEC Z87.898
    steroid therapy (systemic) Z92.241
      inhaled Z92.240
    stroke without residual deficits Z86.73
    substance abuse NEC F10-F19
    sudden cardiac arrest Z86.74
    sudden cardiac death successfully resuscitated Z86.74
    suicide attempt Z91.5
    surgery NEC Z98.890
      with uterine scar Z98.891
      sex reassignment Z87.890
      transplant — *see* Transplant
    thrombophlebitis Z86.72
    thrombosis (venous) Z86.718
      pulmonary Z86.711
    tobacco dependence Z87.891
    transient ischemic attack (TIA) without residual deficits Z86.73
    trauma (physical) NEC Z87.828
      psychological NEC Z91.49
      self-harm Z91.5
    traumatic brain injury Z87.820
    unhealthy sleep-wake cycle Z72.821
    unintended awareness under general anesthesia Z92.84
    urinary calculi Z87.442
    urinary (recurrent) (tract) infection (s) Z87.440
    uterine scar from previous surgery Z98.891
    vaginal dysplasia Z87.411
    venous thrombosis or embolism Z86.718
      pulmonary Z86.711
    vulvar dysplasia Z87.412
His-Werner disease A79.0
HIV — *see also* Human, immunodeficiency
  virus B20
  laboratory evidence (nonconclusive) R75
  positive, seropositive Z21
  nonconclusive test (in infants) R75
Hives (bold) — *see* Urticaria
Hoarseness R49.0
Hobo Z59.0
Hodgkin disease — *see* Lymphoma, Hodgkin
Hodgson's disease I71.2
  ruptured I71.1
Hoffa-Kastert disease E88.89
Hoffa's disease E88.89
Hoffmann-Bouveret syndrome I47.9
Hoffmann's syndrome E03.9 *[G73.7]*
Hole (round)
  macula H35.34-
  retina (without detachment) — *see* Break, retina, round hole
    with detachment — *see* Detachment, retina, with retinal, break
Holiday relief care Z75.5
Hollenhorst's plaque — *see* Occlusion, artery, retina
Hollow foot (congenital) Q66.7
  acquired — *see* Deformity, limb, foot, specified NEC
Holoprosencephaly Q04.2
Holt-Oram syndrome Q87.2
Homelessness Z59.0
Homesickness — *see* Disorder, adjustment
Homocystinemia, homocystinuria E72.11
Homogentisate 1,2-dioxygenase deficiency E70.29
Homologous serum hepatitis (prophylactic) (therapeutic) — *see* Hepatitis, viral, type B
Honeycomb lung J98.4
  congenital Q33.0
Hooded
  clitoris Q52.6
  penis Q55.69
Hookworm (anemia) (disease) (infection) (infestation) B76.9
  specified NEC B76.8
Hordeolum (eyelid) (externum) (recurrent) H00.019
  internum H00.029
    left H00.026
      lower H00.025
      upper H00.024
    right H00.023
      lower H00.022
      upper H00.021
  left H00.016
    lower H00.015
    upper H00.014
  right H00.013
    lower H00.012
    upper H00.011
Horn
  cutaneous L85.8
  nail L60.2
    congenital Q84.6
Horner (-Claude Bernard) **syndrome** G90.2
  traumatic — *see* Injury, nerve, cervical sympathetic
Horseshoe kidney (congenital) Q63.1
Horton's headache or neuralgia G44.099
  intractable G44.091
  not intractable G44.099
Hospital hopper syndrome — *see* Disorder, factitious
Hospitalism in children — *see* Disorder, adjustment
Hostility R45.5
  towards child Z62.3
Hot flashes
  menopausal N95.1
Hourglass (contracture) — *see also* Contraction, hourglass
  stomach K31.89
    congenital Q40.2
    stricture K31.2
Household, housing circumstance affecting care Z59.9
  specified NEC Z59.8
Housemaid's knee — *see* Bursitis, prepatellar
Hudson (-Stähli) **line** (cornea) — *see* Pigmentation, cornea, anterior
Human
  bite (open wound) — *see also* Bite
    intact skin surface — *see* Bite, superficial
  herpesvirus — *see* Herpes
  immunodeficiency virus (HIV) disease (infection) B20
    asymptomatic status Z21
    contact Z20.6
    counseling Z71.7
    dementia B20 *[F02.80]*
      with behavioral disturbance B20 *[F02.81]*
    exposure to Z20.6
    laboratory evidence R75
    type-2 (HIV 2) as cause of disease classified elsewhere B97.35
  papillomavirus (HPV)
    DNA test positive
      high risk
        cervix R87.810
        vagina R87.811
      low risk
        cervix R87.820
        vagina R87.821
    screening for Z11.51
  T-cell lymphotropic virus
    type-1 (HTLV-I) infection B33.3
      as cause of disease classified elsewhere B97.33
      carrier Z22.6
    type-2 (HTLV-II) as cause of disease classified elsewhere B97.34
Humidifier lung or pneumonitis J67.7
Humiliation (experience) **in childhood** Z62.898
Humpback (acquired) — *see* Kyphosis
Hunchback (acquired) — *see* Kyphosis
Hunger T73.0
  air, psychogenic F45.8
Hungry bone syndrome E83.81
Hunner's ulcer — *see* Cystitis, chronic, interstitial
Hunter's
  glossitis D51.0
  syndrome E76.1
Huntington's disease or chorea G10
  with dementia G10 *[F02.80]*
    with behavioral disturbance G10 *[F02.81]*
Hunt's
  disease or syndrome (herpetic geniculate ganglionitis) B02.21
    dyssynergia cerebellaris myoclonica G11.1
  neuralgia B02.21
Hurler (-Scheie) **disease or syndrome** E76.02
Hurst's disease G36.1
Hurthle cell
  adenocarcinoma C73
  adenoma D34
  carcinoma C73
  tumor D34
Hutchinson-Boeck disease or syndrome — *see* Sarcoidosis
Hutchinson-Gilford disease or syndrome E34.8
Hutchinson's
  disease, meaning
    angioma serpiginosum L81.7
    pompholyx (cheiropompholyx) L30.1
    prurigo estivalis L56.4
    summer eruption or summer prurigo L56.4
  melanotic freckle — *see* Melanoma, in situ
    malignant melanoma in — *see* Melanoma
  teeth or incisors (congenital syphilis) A50.52
  triad (congenital syphilis) A50.53
Hyalin plaque, sclera, senile H15.89
Hyaline membrane (disease) (lung) (pulmonary) (newborn) P22.0
Hyalinosis
  cutis (et mucosae) E78.89
  focal and segmental (glomerular) — *see also* N00-N07 with fourth character .1 N05.1
Hyalitis, hyalosis, asteroid — *see also* Deposit, crystalline
  syphilitic (late) A52.71
Hydatid
  cyst or tumor — *see* Echinococcus
  mole — *see* Hydatidiform mole
  Morgagni
    female Q50.5
    male (epididymal) Q55.4
      testicular Q55.29
Hydatidiform mole (benign) (complicating pregnancy) (delivered) (undelivered) O01.9
  classical O01.0
  complete O01.0
  incomplete O01.1
  invasive D39.2
  malignant D39.2
  partial O01.1
Hydatidosis — *see* Echinococcus
Hydradenitis (axillaris) (suppurative) L73.2
Hydradenoma — *see* Hidradenoma
Hydramnios O40.-
Hydrancephaly, hydranencephaly Q04.3
  with spina bifida — *see* Spina bifida, with hydrocephalus
Hydrargyrism NEC — *see* Poisoning, mercury
Hydrarthrosis — *see also* Effusion, joint
  gonococcal A54.42
  intermittent M12.40
    ankle M12.47-
    elbow M12.42-
    foot joint M12.47-
    hand joint M12.44-
    hip M12.45-
    knee M12.46-
    multiple site M12.49
    shoulder M12.41-
    specified joint NEC M12.48
    wrist M12.43-
  of yaws (early) (late) (*see also* subcategory M14.8-) A66.6
  syphilitic (late) A52.77
    congenital A50.55 *[M12.80]*
Hydremia D64.89
Hydrencephalocele (congenital) — *see* Encephalocele

- **Hydrencephalomeningocele** (congenital) — *see* Encephalocele
- **Hydroa** R23.8
  - aestivale L56.4
  - vacciniforme L56.4
- **Hydroadenitis** (axillaris) (suppurative) L73.2
- **Hydrocalycosis** — *see* Hydronephrosis
- **Hydrocele** (spermatic cord) (testis) (tunica vaginalis) N43.3
  - canal of Nuck N94.89
  - communicating N43.2
    - congenital P83.5
  - congenital P83.5
  - encysted N43.0
  - female NEC N94.89
  - infected N43.1
  - newborn P83.5
  - round ligament N94.89
  - specified NEC N43.2
  - spinalis — *see* Spina bifida
  - vulva N90.89
- **Hydrocephalus** (acquired) (external) (internal) (malignant) (recurrent) G91.9
  - aqueduct Sylvius stricture Q03.0
  - causing disproportion O33.6
    - with obstructed labor O66.3
  - communicating G91.0
  - congenital (external) (internal) Q03.9
    - with spina bifida Q05.4
      - cervical Q05.0
      - dorsal Q05.1
      - lumbar Q05.2
      - lumbosacral Q05.2
      - sacral Q05.3
      - thoracic Q05.1
      - thoracolumbar Q05.1
    - specified NEC Q03.8
  - due to toxoplasmosis (congenital) P37.1
  - foramen Magendie block (acquired) G91.1
    - congenital — *see also* Hydrocephalus, congenital Q03.1
  - in (due to)
    - infectious disease NEC B89 *[G91.4]*
    - neoplastic disease NEC (see also Neoplasm) G91.4
    - parasitic disease B89 *[G91.4]*
  - newborn Q03.9
    - with spina bifida — *see* Spina bifida, with hydrocephalus
  - noncommunicating G91.1
  - normal pressure G91.2
    - secondary G91.0
  - obstructive G91.1
  - otitic G93.2
  - post-traumatic NEC G91.3
  - secondary G91.4
    - post-traumatic G91.3
  - specified NEC G91.8
  - syphilitic, congenital A50.49
- **Hydrocolpos** (congenital) N89.8
- **Hydrocystoma** — *see* Neoplasm, skin, benign
- **Hydroencephalocele** (congenital) — *see* Encephalocele
- **Hydroencephalomeningocele** (congenital) — *see* Encephalocele
- **Hydrohematopneumothorax** — *see* Hemothorax
- **Hydromeningitis** — *see* Meningitis
- **Hydromeningocele** (spinal) — *see also* Spina bifida
  - cranial — *see* Encephalocele
- **Hydrometra** N85.8
- **Hydrometrocolpos** N89.8
- **Hydromicrocephaly** Q02
- **Hydromphalos** (since birth) Q45.8
- **Hydromyelia** Q06.4
- **Hydromyelocele** — *see* Spina bifida
- **Hydronephrosis** (atrophic) (early) (functionless) (intermittent) (primary) (secondary) **NEC** N13.30
  - with
    - infection N13.6
    - obstruction (by) (of)
      - renal calculus N13.2
        - with infection N13.6
      - ureteral NEC N13.1
        - with infection N13.6
        - calculus N13.2
          - with infection N13.6
      - ureteropelvic junction (congenital) Q62.11
        - acquired N13.0
          - with infection N13.6
    - ureteral stricture NEC N13.1
      - with infection N13.6
  - congenital Q62.0
    - due to acquired occlusion of ureteropelvic junction N13.0
- **Hydronephrosis** (atrophic) (early) (functionless) (intermittent) (primary) (secondary) **NEC** - *continued*
  - specified type NEC N13.39
  - tuberculous A18.11
- **Hydropericarditis** — *see* Pericarditis
- **Hydropericardium** — *see* Pericarditis
- **Hydroperitoneum** R18.8
- **Hydrophobia** — *see* Rabies
- **Hydrophthalmos** Q15.0
- **Hydropneumohemothorax** — *see* Hemothorax
- **Hydropneumopericarditis** — *see* Pericarditis
- **Hydropneumopericardium** — *see* Pericarditis
- **Hydropneumothorax** J94.8
  - traumatic — *see* Injury, intrathoracic, lung
  - tuberculous NEC A15.6
- **Hydrops** R60.9
  - abdominis R18.8
  - articulorum intermittens — *see* Hydrarthrosis, intermittent
  - cardiac — *see* Failure, heart, congestive
  - causing obstructed labor (mother) O66.3
  - endolymphatic H81.0-
  - fetal — *see* Pregnancy, complicated by, hydrops, fetalis
  - fetalis P83.2
    - due to
      - ABO isoimmunization P56.0
      - alpha thalassemia D56.0
      - hemolytic disease P56.90
        - specified NEC P56.99
      - isoimmunization (ABO) (Rh) P56.0
      - other specified nonhemolytic disease NEC P83.2
      - Rh incompatibility P56.0
    - during pregnancy — *see* Pregnancy, complicated by, hydrops, fetalis
  - gallbladder K82.1
  - joint — *see* Effusion, joint
  - labyrinth H81.0-
  - newborn (idiopathic) P83.2
    - due to
      - ABO isoimmunization P56.0
      - alpha thalassemia D56.0
      - hemolytic disease P56.90
        - specified NEC P56.99
      - isoimmunization (ABO) (Rh) P56.0
      - Rh incompatibility P56.0
  - nutritional — *see* Malnutrition, severe
  - pericardium — *see* Pericarditis
  - pleura — *see* Hydrothorax
  - spermatic cord — *see* Hydrocele
- **Hydropyonephrosis** N13.6
- **Hydrorachis** Q06.4
- **Hydrorrhea** (nasal) J34.89
  - pregnancy — *see* Rupture, membranes, premature
- **Hydrosadenitis** (axillaris) (suppurative) L73.2
- **Hydrosalpinx** (fallopian tube) (follicularis) N70.11
- **Hydrothorax** (double) (pleura) J94.8
  - chylous (nonfilarial) I89.8
    - filarial — *see also* Infestation, filarial B74.9 *[J91.8]*
  - traumatic — *see* Injury, intrathoracic
  - tuberculous NEC (non primary) A15.6
- **Hydroureter** — *see also* Hydronephrosis N13.4
  - with infection N13.6
  - congenital Q62.39
- **Hydroureteronephrosis** — *see* Hydronephrosis
- **Hydrourethra** N36.8
- **Hydroxykynureninuria** E70.8
- **Hydroxylysinemia** E72.3
- **Hydroxyprolinemia** E72.59
- **Hygiene, sleep**
  - abuse Z72.821
  - inadequate Z72.821
  - poor Z72.821
- **Hygroma** (congenital) (cystic) D18.1
  - praepatellare, prepatellar — *see* Bursitis, prepatellar
- **Hymen** — *see* condition
- **Hymenolepis, hymenolepiasis** (diminuta) (infection) (infestation) (nana) B71.0
- **Hypalgesia** R20.8
- **Hyperacidity** (gastric) K31.89
  - psychogenic F45.8
- **Hyperactive, hyperactivity** F90.9
  - basal cell, uterine cervix — *see* Dysplasia, cervix
  - bowel sounds R19.12
  - cervix epithelial (basal) — *see* Dysplasia, cervix
  - child F90.9
    - attention deficit — *see* Disorder, attention-deficit hyperactivity
  - detrusor muscle N32.81
  - gastrointestinal K31.89
    - psychogenic F45.8
  - nasal mucous membrane J34.3
- **Hyperactive, hyperactivity** - *continued*
  - stomach K31.89
  - thyroid (gland) — *see* Hyperthyroidism
- **Hyperacusis** H93.23-
- **Hyperadrenalism** E27.5
- **Hyperadrenocorticism** E24.9
  - congenital E25.0
  - iatrogenic E24.2
    - correct substance properly administered — *see* Table of Drugs and Chemicals, by drug, adverse effect
    - overdose or wrong substance given or taken — *see* Table of Drugs and Chemicals, by drug, poisoning
  - not associated with Cushing's syndrome E27.0
  - pituitary-dependent E24.0
- **Hyperaldosteronism** E26.9
  - familial (type I) E26.02
  - glucocorticoid-remediable E26.02
  - primary (due to (bilateral) adrenal hyperplasia) E26.09
  - primary NEC E26.09
  - secondary E26.1
  - specified NEC E26.89
- **Hyperalgesia** R20.8
- **Hyperalimentation** R63.2
  - carotene, carotin E67.1
  - specified NEC E67.8
  - vitamin
    - A E67.0
    - D E67.3
- **Hyperaminoaciduria**
  - arginine E72.21
  - cystine E72.01
  - lysine E72.3
  - ornithine E72.4
- **Hyperammonemia** (congenital) E72.20
- **Hyperazotemia** — *see* Uremia
- **Hyperbetalipoproteinemia** (familial) E78.00
  - with prebetalipoproteinemia E78.2
- **Hyperbicarbonatemia** P74.41
- **Hyperbilirubinemia**
  - constitutional E80.6
  - familial conjugated E80.6
  - neonatal (transient) — *see* Jaundice, newborn
- **Hypercalcemia, hypocalciuric, familial** E83.52
- **Hypercalciuria, idiopathic** R82.994
- **Hypercapnia** R06.89
  - newborn P84
- **Hypercarotenemia** (dietary) E67.1
- **Hypercementosis** K03.4
- **Hyperchloremia** E87.8
- **Hyperchlorhydria** K31.89
  - neurotic F45.8
  - psychogenic F45.8
- **Hypercholesterinemia** — *see* Hypercholesterolemia
- **Hypercholesterolemia** (essential) (primary) (pure) E78.00
  - with hyperglyceridemia, endogenous E78.2
  - dietary counseling and surveillance Z71.3
  - familial E78.01
  - hereditary E78.01
- **Hyperchylia gastrica, psychogenic** F45.8
- **Hyperchylomicronemia** (familial) (primary) E78.3
  - with hyperbetalipoproteinemia E78.3
- **Hypercoagulable** (state) D68.59
  - activated protein C resistance D68.51
  - antithrombin (III) deficiency D68.59
  - factor V Leiden mutation D68.51
  - primary NEC D68.59
  - protein C deficiency D68.59
  - protein S deficiency D68.59
  - prothrombin gene mutation D68.52
  - secondary D68.69
  - specified NEC D68.69
- **Hypercoagulation** (state) D68.59
- **Hypercorticalism, pituitary-dependent** E24.0
- **Hypercorticosolism** — *see* Cushing's, syndrome
- **Hypercorticosteronism** E24.2
  - correct substance properly administered — *see* Table of Drugs and Chemicals, by drug, adverse effect
  - overdose or wrong substance given or taken — *see* Table of Drugs and Chemicals, by drug, poisoning
- **Hypercortisonism** E24.2
  - correct substance properly administered — *see* Table of Drugs and Chemicals, by drug, adverse effect
  - overdose or wrong substance given or taken — *see* Table of Drugs and Chemicals, by drug, poisoning
- **Hyperekplexia** Q89.8
- **Hyperelectrolytemia** E87.8
- **Hyperemesis** R11.10
  - with nausea R11.2
  - gravidarum (mild) O21.0

Hyperemesis - *continued*
  gravidarum (mild) - *continued*
    with
      carbohydrate depletion O21.1
      dehydration O21.1
      electrolyte imbalance O21.1
      metabolic disturbance O21.1
    severe (with metabolic disturbance) O21.1
  projectile R11.12
  psychogenic F45.8
Hyperemia (acute) (passive) R68.89
  anal mucosa K62.89
  bladder N32.89
  cerebral I67.89
  conjunctiva H11.43-
  ear internal, acute — *see* subcategory H83.0
  enteric K59.8
  eye — *see* Hyperemia, conjunctiva
  eyelid (active) (passive) — *see* Disorder, eyelid, specified type NEC
  intestine K59.8
  iris — *see* Disorder, iris, vascular
  kidney N28.89
  labyrinth — *see* subcategory H83.0
  liver (active) K76.89
  lung (passive) — *see* Edema, lung
  pulmonary (passive) — *see* Edema, lung
  renal N28.89
  retina H35.89
  stomach K31.89
Hyperesthesia (body surface) R20.3
  larynx (reflex) J38.7
    hysterical F44.89
  pharynx (reflex) J39.2
    hysterical F44.89
Hyperestrogenism (drug-induced) (iatrogenic) E28.0
Hyperexplexia Q89.8
Hyperfibrinolysis — *see* Fibrinolysis
Hyperfructosemia E74.19
Hyperfunction
  adrenal cortex, not associated with Cushing's syndrome E27.0
    medulla E27.5
      adrenomedullary E27.5
    virilism E25.9
      congenital E25.0
  ovarian E28.8
  pancreas K86.89
  parathyroid (gland) E21.3
  pituitary (gland) (anterior) E22.9
    specified NEC E22.8
  polyglandular E31.1
  testicular E29.0
Hypergammaglobulinemia D89.2
  polyclonal D89.0
  Waldenström D89.0
Hypergastrinemia E16.4
Hyperglobulinemia R77.1
Hyperglycemia, hyperglycemic (transient) R73.9
  coma — *see* Diabetes, by type, with coma
  postpancreatectomy E89.1
Hyperglyceridemia (endogenous) (essential) (familial) (hereditary) (pure) E78.1
  mixed E78.3
Hyperglycinemia (non-ketotic) E72.51
Hypergonadism
  ovarian E28.8
  testicular (primary) (infantile) E29.0
Hyperheparinemia D68.32
Hyperhidrosis, hyperidrosis R61
  focal
    primary L74.519
      axilla L74.510
      face L74.511
      palms L74.512
      soles L74.513
    secondary L74.52
  generalized R61
  localized
    primary L74.519
      axilla L74.510
      face L74.511
      palms L74.512
      soles L74.513
    secondary L74.52
  psychogenic F45.8
  secondary R61
    focal L74.52
Hyperhistidinemia E70.41
Hyperhomocysteinemia E72.11
Hyperhydroxyprolinemia E72.59
Hyperinsulinism (functional) E16.1
  with
Hyperinsulinism (functional) - *continued*
  with - *continued*
    coma (hypoglycemic) E15
    encephalopathy E16.1 *[G94]*
  ectopic E16.1
  therapeutic misadventure (from administration of insulin) — *see* subcategory T38.3
Hyperkalemia E87.5
Hyperkeratosis — *see also* Keratosis L85.9
  cervix N88.0
  due to yaws (early) (late) (palmar or plantar) A66.3
  follicularis Q82.8
    penetrans (in cutem) L87.0
  palmoplantaris climacterica L85.1
  pinta A67.1
  senile (with pruritus) L57.0
  universalis congenita Q80.8
  vocal cord J38.3
  vulva N90.4
Hyperkinesia, hyperkinetic (disease) (reaction) (syndrome) (childhood) (adolescence) — *see also* Disorder, attention-deficit hyperactivity
  heart I51.89
Hyperleucine-isoleucinemia E71.19
Hyperlipemia, hyperlipidemia E78.5
  combined E78.2
    familial E78.49
  group
    A E78.00
    B E78.1
    C E78.2
    D E78.3
  mixed E78.2
  specified NEC E78.49
Hyperlipidosis E75.6
  hereditary NEC E75.5
Hyperlipoproteinemia E78.5
  Fredrickson's type
    I E78.3
    IIa E78.00
    IIb E78.2
    III E78.2
    IV E78.1
    V E78.3
  low-density-lipoprotein-type (LDL) E78.00
  very-low-density-lipoprotein-type (VLDL) E78.1
Hyperlucent lung, unilateral J43.0
Hyperlysinemia E72.3
Hypermagnesemia E83.41
  neonatal P71.8
Hypermenorrhea N92.0
Hypermethioninemia E72.19
Hypermetropia (congenital) H52.0-
Hypermobility, hypermotility
  cecum — *see* Syndrome, irritable bowel
  coccyx — *see* subcategory M53.2
  colon — *see* Syndrome, irritable bowel
    psychogenic F45.8
  ileum K58.9
  intestine — *see also* Syndrome, irritable bowel K58.9
    psychogenic F45.8
  meniscus (knee) — *see* Derangement, knee, meniscus
  scapula — *see* Instability, joint, shoulder
  stomach K31.89
    psychogenic F45.8
  syndrome M35.7
  urethra N36.41
    with intrinsic sphincter deficiency N36.43
Hypernasality R49.21
Hypernatremia E87.0
Hypernephroma C64.-
Hyperopia — *see* Hypermetropia
Hyperorexia nervosa F50.2
Hyperornithinemia E72.4
Hyperosmia R43.1
Hyperosmolality E87.0
Hyperostosis (monomelic) — *see also* Disorder, bone, density and structure, specified NEC
  ankylosing (spine) M48.10
    cervical region M48.12
    cervicothoracic region M48.13
    lumbar region M48.16
    lumbosacral region M48.17
    multiple sites M48.19
    occipito-atlanto-axial region M48.11
    sacrococcygeal region M48.18
    thoracic region M48.14
    thoracolumbar region M48.15
  cortical (skull) M85.2
    infantile M89.8X-
  frontal, internal of skull M85.2
Hyperostosis (monomelic) - *continued*
  interna frontalis M85.2
  skeletal, diffuse idiopathic — *see* Hyperostosis, ankylosing
  skull M85.2
    congenital Q75.8
  vertebral, ankylosing — *see* Hyperostosis, ankylosing
Hyperovarism E28.8
Hyperoxaluria R82.992
  primary E72.53
Hyperparathyroidism E21.3
  primary E21.0
  secondary (renal) N25.81
    non-renal E21.1
  specified NEC E21.2
  tertiary E21.2
Hyperpathia R20.8
Hyperperistalsis R19.2
  psychogenic F45.8
Hyperpermeability, capillary I78.8
Hyperphagia R63.2
Hyperphenylalaninemia NEC E70.1
Hyperphoria (alternating) H50.53
Hyperphosphatemia E83.39
Hyperpiesis, hyperpiesia — *see* Hypertension
Hyperpigmentation — *see also* Pigmentation
  melanin NEC L81.4
  postinflammatory L81.0
Hyperpinealism E34.8
Hyperpituitarism E22.9
Hyperplasia, hyperplastic
  adenoids J35.2
  adrenal (capsule) (cortex) (gland) E27.8
    with
      sexual precocity (male) E25.9
        congenital E25.0
      virilism, adrenal E25.9
        congenital E25.0
      virilization (female) E25.9
        congenital E25.0
    congenital E25.0
      salt-losing E25.0
  adrenomedullary E27.5
  angiolymphoid, eosinophilia (ALHE) D18.01
  appendix (lymphoid) K38.0
  artery, fibromuscular I77.3
  bone — *see also* Hypertrophy, bone
    marrow D75.89
  breast — *see also* Hypertrophy, breast
    ductal (atypical) N60.9-
  C-cell, thyroid E07.0
  cementation (tooth) (teeth) K03.4
  cervical gland R59.0
  cervix (uteri) (basal cell) (endometrium) (polypoid) — *see also* Dysplasia, cervix
    congenital Q51.828
  clitoris, congenital Q52.6
  denture K06.2
  endocervicitis N72
  endometrium, endometrial (adenomatous) (benign) (cystic) (glandular) (glandular-cystic) (polypoid) N85.00
    with atypia N85.02
    cervix — *see* Dysplasia, cervix
    complex (without atypia) N85.01
    simple (without atypia) N85.01
  epithelial L85.9
    focal, oral, including tongue K13.29
    nipple N62
    skin L85.9
    tongue K13.29
    vaginal wall N89.3
  erythroid D75.89
  fibromuscular of artery (carotid) (renal) I77.3
  genital
    female NEC N94.89
    male N50.89
  gingiva K06.1
  glandularis cystica uteri (interstitialis) — *see also* Hyperplasia, endometrial N85.00-
  gum K06.1
  hymen, congenital Q52.4
  irritative, edentulous (alveolar) K06.2
  jaw M26.09
    alveolar M26.79
    lower M26.03
      alveolar M26.72
    upper M26.01
      alveolar M26.71
  kidney (congenital) Q63.3
  labia N90.69
    epithelial N90.3

Hyperplasia, hyperplastic - *continued*
  liver (congenital) Q44.7
    nodular, focal K76.89
  lymph gland or node R59.9
  mandible, mandibular M26.03
    alveolar M26.72
    unilateral condylar M27.8
  maxilla, maxillary M26.01
    alveolar M26.71
  myometrium, myometrial N85.2
  neuroendocrine cell, of infancy J84.841
  nose
    lymphoid J34.89
    polypoid J33.9
  oral mucosa (irritative) K13.6
  organ or site, congenital NEC — *see* Anomaly, by site
  ovary N83.8
  palate, papillary (irritative) K13.6
  pancreatic islet cells E16.9
    alpha E16.8
      with excess
        gastrin E16.4
        glucagon E16.3
    beta E16.1
  parathyroid (gland) E21.0
  pharynx (lymphoid) J39.2
  prostate (adenofibromatous) (nodular) N40.0
    with lower urinary tract symptoms (LUTS) N40.1
    without lower urinary tract symtpoms (LUTS) N40.0
  renal artery I77.89
  reticulo-endothelial (cell) D75.89
  salivary gland (any) K11.1
  Schimmelbusch's — *see* Mastopathy, cystic
  suprarenal capsule (gland) E27.8
  thymus (gland) (persistent) E32.0
  thyroid (gland) — *see* Goiter
  tonsils (faucial) (infective) (lingual) (lymphoid) J35.1
    with adenoids J35.3
  unilateral condylar M27.8
  uterus, uterine N85.2
    endometrium (glandular) — *see also* Hyperplasia, endometrial N85.00-
  vulva N90.69
    epithelial N90.3
Hyperpnea — *see* Hyperventilation
Hyperpotassemia E87.5
Hyperprebetalipoproteinemia (familial) E78.1
Hyperprolactinemia E22.1
Hyperprolinemia (type I) (type II) E72.59
Hyperproteinemia E88.09
Hyperprothrombinemia, causing coagulation factor deficiency D68.4
Hyperpyrexia R50.9
  heat (effects) T67.0
  malignant, due to anesthetic T88.3
  rheumatic — *see* Fever, rheumatic
  unknown origin R50.9
Hyper-reflexia R29.2
Hypersalivation K11.7
Hypersecretion
  ACTH (not associated with Cushing's syndrome) E27.0
    pituitary E24.0
  adrenaline E27.5
  adrenomedullary E27.5
  androgen (testicular) E29.0
    ovarian (drug-induced) (iatrogenic) E28.1
  calcitonin E07.0
  catecholamine E27.5
  corticoadrenal E24.9
  cortisol E24.9
  epinephrine E27.5
  estrogen E28.0
  gastric K31.89
    psychogenic F45.8
  gastrin E16.4
  glucagon E16.3
  hormone (s)
    ACTH (not associated with Cushing's syndrome) E27.0
      pituitary E24.0
    antidiuretic E22.2
    growth E22.0
    intestinal NEC E34.1
    ovarian androgen E28.1
    pituitary E22.9
    testicular E29.0
    thyroid stimulating E05.80
      with thyroid storm E05.81
  insulin — *see* Hyperinsulinism

Hypersecretion - *continued*
  lacrimal glands — *see* Epiphora
  medulloadrenal E27.5
  milk O92.6
  ovarian androgens E28.1
  salivary gland (any) K11.7
  thyrocalcitonin E07.0
  upper respiratory J39.8
Hypersegmentation, leukocytic, hereditary D72.0
Hypersensitive, hypersensitiveness, hypersensitivity — *see also* Allergy
  carotid sinus G90.01
  colon — *see* Irritable, colon
  drug T88.7
  gastrointestinal K52.29
    immediate K52.29
    psychogenic F45.8
  labyrinth — *see* subcategory H83.2
  pain R20.8
  pneumonitis — *see* Pneumonitis, allergic
  reaction T78.40
    upper respiratory tract NEC J39.3
Hypersomnia (organic) G47.10
  due to
    alcohol
      abuse F10.182
      dependence F10.282
      use F10.982
    amphetamines
      abuse F15.182
      dependence F15.282
      use F15.982
    caffeine
      abuse F15.182
      dependence F15.282
      use F15.982
    cocaine
      abuse F14.182
      dependence F14.282
      use F14.982
    drug NEC
      abuse F19.182
      dependence F19.282
      use F19.982
    medical condition G47.14
    mental disorder F51.13
    opioid
      abuse F11.182
      dependence F11.282
      use F11.982
    psychoactive substance NEC
      abuse F19.182
      dependence F19.282
      use F19.982
    sedative, hypnotic, or anxiolytic
      abuse F13.182
      dependence F13.282
      use F13.982
    stimulant NEC
      abuse F15.182
      dependence F15.282
      use F15.982
  idiopathic G47.11
    with long sleep time G47.11
    without long sleep time G47.12
  menstrual related G47.13
  nonorganic origin F51.11
    specified NEC F51.19
  not due to a substance or known physiological condition F51.11
    specified NEC F51.19
  primary F51.11
  recurrent G47.13
  specified NEC G47.19
Hyperspleniа, hypersplenism D73.1
Hyperstimulation, ovaries
  (associated with induced ovulation) N98.1
Hypersusceptibility — *see* Allergy
Hypertelorism (ocular) (orbital) Q75.2
Hypertension, hypertensive (accelerated) (benign) (essential) (idiopathic) (malignant) (systemic) I10
  with
    heart failure (congestive) I11.0
    heart involvement (conditions in I50.-, I51.4- I51.9 due to hypertension) — *see* Hypertension, heart
    kidney involvement — *see* Hypertension, kidney
  benign, intracranial G93.2
  borderline R03.0
  cardiorenal (disease) I13.10
    with heart failure I13.0
      with stage 1 through stage 4 chronic kidney disease I13.0
      with stage 5 or end stage renal disease I13.2

Hypertension, hypertensive (accelerated) (benign) (essential) (idiopathic) (malignant) (systemic) - *continued*
  cardiorenal (disease) - *continued*
    without heart failure I13.10
      with stage 1 through stage 4 chronic kidney disease I13.10
      with stage 5 or end stage renal disease I13.11
  cardiovascular
    disease (arteriosclerotic) (sclerotic) — *see* Hypertension, heart
    renal (disease) — *see* Hypertension, cardiorenal
  chronic venous — *see* Hypertension, venous (chronic)
  complicating
    childbirth (labor) O16.4
      pre-existing O10.92
        with
          heart disease O10.12
            with renal disease O10.32
          pre-eclampsia O11.4
          renal disease O10.22
            with heart disease O10.32
        essential O10.02
        secondary O10.42
    pregnancy O16.-
      with edema — *see also* Pre-eclampsia O14.9-
      gestational (pregnancy induced) (without proteinuria) O13.-
        with proteinuria O14.9-
          mild pre-eclampsia O14.0-
          moderate pre-eclampsia O14.0-
          severe pre-eclampsia O14.1-
            with hemolysis, elevated liver enzymes and low platelet count (HELLP) O14.2-
      pre-existing O10.91-
        with
          heart disease O10.11-
            with renal disease O10.31-
          pre-eclampsia — *see* category O11
          renal disease O10.21-
            with heart disease O10.31-
        essential O10.01-
        secondary O10.41-
      transient O13.-
    puerperium, pre-existing O16.5
      pre-existing
        with
          heart disease O10.13
            with renal disease O10.33
          pre-eclampsia O11.5
          renal disease O10.23
            with heart disease O10.33
        essential O10.03
      pregnancy-induced O13.9
      secondary O10.43
  crisis I16.9
  due to
    endocrine disorders I15.2
    pheochromocytoma I15.2
    renal disorders NEC I15.1
      arterial I15.0
    renovascular disorders I15.0
    specified disease NEC I15.8
  emergency I16.1
  encephalopathy I67.4
  gestational (without significant proteinuria) (pregnancy-induced) (transient) O13.-
    with significant proteinuria — *see* Pre-eclampsia
    complicating
      delivery O13.4
      puerperium O13.5
  Goldblatt's I70.1
  heart (disease) (conditions in I51.4-I51.9 due to hypertension) I11.9
    with
      heart failure (congestive) I11.0
      kidney disease (chronic) — *see* Hypertension, cardiorenal
  intracranial (benign) G93.2
  kidney I12.9
    with
      heart disease — *see* Hypertension, cardiorenal
      stage 5 chronic kidney disease (CKD) or end stage renal disease (ESRD) I12.0
      stage 1 through stage 4 chronic kidney disease I12.9
  lesser circulation I27.0
  maternal O16.-
  newborn P29.2
    pulmonary (persistent) P29.30
  ocular H40.05-
  pancreatic duct - code to underlying condition

Hypotrichosis — *see* Alopecia
Hypotropia H50.2-
Hypoventilation R06.89
congenital central alveolar G47.35
sleep related
idiopathic nonobstructive alveolar G47.34
in conditions classified elsewhere G47.36
Hypovitaminosis — *see* Deficiency, vitamin
Hypovolemia E86.1
surgical shock T81.19
traumatic (shock) T79.4
Hypoxemia R09.02
newborn P84
sleep related, in conditions classified elsewhere G47.36
Hypoxia — *see also* Anoxia R09.02
cerebral, during a procedure NEC G97.81
postprocedural NEC G97.82
intrauterine P84
myocardial — *see* Insufficiency, coronary
newborn P84
sleep-related G47.34
Hypsarhythmia — *see* Epilepsy, generalized, specified NEC
Hysteralgia, pregnant uterus O26.89-
Hysteria, hysterical (conversion) (dissociative state) F44.9
anxiety F41.8
convulsions F44.5
psychosis, acute F44.9
Hysteroepilepsy F44.5

I

I.Q.
under 20 F73
20-34 F72
35-49 F71
50-69 F70
IBDU
(colonic inflammatory bowel dissease unclassified) K52.3
Ichthyoparasitism due to Vandellia cirrhosa B88.8
Ichthyosis (congenital) Q80.9
acquired L85.0
fetalis Q80.4
hystrix Q80.8
lamellar Q80.2
lingual K13.29
palmaris and plantaris Q82.8
simplex Q80.0
vera Q80.8
vulgaris Q80.0
X-linked Q80.1
Ichthyotoxism — *see* Poisoning, fish
bacterial — *see* Intoxication, foodborne
Icteroanemia, hemolytic (acquired) D59.9
congenital — *see* Spherocytosis
Icterus — *see also* Jaundice
conjunctiva R17
newborn P59.9
gravis, newborn P55.0
hematogenous (acquired) D59.9
hemolytic (acquired) D59.9
congenital — *see* Spherocytosis
hemorrhagic (acute) (leptospiral) (spirochetal) A27.0
newborn P53
infectious B15.9
with hepatic coma B15.0
leptospiral A27.0
spirochetal A27.0
neonatorum — *see* Jaundice, newborn
spirochetal A27.0
Ictus solaris, solis T67.0
Id reaction (due to bacteria) L30.2
Ideation
homicidal R45.850
suicidal R45.851
Identity disorder (child) F64.9
gender role F64.2
psychosexual F64.2
Idioglossia F80.0
Idiopathic — *see* condition
Idiot, idiocy (congenital) F73
amaurotic (Bielschowsky (-Jansky)) (family) (infantile (late)) (juvenile (late)) (Vogt-Spielmeyer) E75.4
microcephalic Q02
IgE asthma J45.909
IIAC (idiopathic infantile arterial calcification) Q28.8
Ileitis (chronic) (noninfectious) — *see also* Enteritis K52.9
backwash — *see* Pancolitis, ulcerative (chronic)
infectious A09

Ileitis (chronic) (noninfectious) - *continued*
regional (ulcerative) — *see* Enteritis, regional, small intestine
segmental — *see* Enteritis, regional
terminal (ulcerative) — *see* Enteritis, regional, small intestine
Ileocolitis — *see also* Enteritis K52.9
infectious A09
regional — *see* Enteritis, regional
ulcerative K51.0-
Ileostomy
attention to Z43.2
malfunctioning K94.13
status Z93.2
with complication — *see* Complications, enterostomy
Ileotyphus — *see* Typhoid
Ileum — *see* condition
Ileus (bowel) (colon) (inhibitory) (intestine) K56.7
adynamic K56.0
due to gallstone (in intestine) K56.3
duodenal (chronic) K31.5
gallstone K56.3
mechanical NEC — *see also* Obstruction, intestine, specified NEC K56.699
meconium P76.0
in cystic fibrosis E84.11
meaning meconium plug (without cystic fibrosis) P76.0
myxedema K59.8
neurogenic K56.0
Hirschsprung's disease or megacolon Q43.1
newborn
due to meconium P76.0
in cystic fibrosis E84.11
meaning meconium plug (without cystic fibrosis) P76.0
transitory P76.1
obstructive — *see also* Obstruction, intestine, specified NEC K56.699
paralytic K56.0
postoperative K91.89
Iliac — *see* condition
Iliotibial band syndrome M76.3-
Illiteracy Z55.0
Illness — *see also* Disease R69
manic-depressive — *see* Disorder, bipolar
Imbalance R26.89
autonomic G90.8
constituents of food intake E63.1
electrolyte E87.8
with
abortion — *see* Abortion by type, complicated by, electrolyte imbalance
molar pregnancy O08.5
due to hyperemesis gravidarum O21.1
following ectopic or molar pregnancy O08.5
neonatal, transitory NEC P74.49
potassium
hyperkalemia P74.31
hypokalemia P74.32
sodium
hypernatremia P74.21
hyponatremia P74.22
endocrine E34.9
eye muscle NOS H50.9
hormone E34.9
hysterical F44.4
labyrinth — *see* subcategory H83.2
posture R29.3
protein-energy — *see* Malnutrition
sympathetic G90.8
Imbecile, imbecility (I.Q.35-49) F71
Imbedding, intrauterine device T83.39
Imbibition, cholesterol (gallbladder) K82.4
Imbrication, teeth,, fully erupted M26.30
Imerslund (-Gräsbeck) **syndrome** D51.1
Immature — *see also* Immaturity
birth (less than 37 completed weeks) — *see* Preterm, newborn
extremely (less than 28 completed weeks) — *see* Immaturity, extreme
personality F60.89
Immaturity (less than 37 completed weeks) — *see also* Preterm, newborn
extreme of newborn (less than 28 completed weeks of gestation) (less than 196 completed days of gestation) (unspecified weeks of gestation) P07.20
gestational age
23 completed weeks (23 weeks, 0 days through 23 weeks, 6 days) P07.22
24 completed weeks (24 weeks, 0 days through 24 weeks, 6 days) P07.23

Immaturity (less than 37 completed weeks) - *continued*
extreme of newborn (less than 28 completed weeks of gestation) (less than 196 completed days of gestation) (unspecified weeks of gestation) - *continued*
gestational age - *continued*
25 completed weeks (25 weeks, 0 days through 25 weeks, 6 days) P07.24
26 completed weeks (26 weeks, 0 days through 26 weeks, 6 days) P07.25
27 completed weeks (27 weeks, 0 days through 27 weeks, 6 days) P07.26
less than 23 completed weeks P07.21
fetus or infant light-for-dates — *see* Light-for-dates
lung, newborn P28.0
organ or site NEC — *see* Hypoplasia
pulmonary, newborn P28.0
reaction F60.89
sexual (female) (male) , after puberty E30.0
Immersion T75.1
hand T69.01-
foot T69.02-
Immobile, immobility
complete, due to severe physical disability or frailty R53.2
intestine K59.8
syndrome (paraplegic) M62.3
Immune reconstitution (inflammatory) **syndrome [IRIS]** D89.3
Immunization — *see also* Vaccination
ABO — *see* Incompatibility, ABO
in newborn P55.1
appropriate for age
child (over 28 days old) Z00.129
with abnormal findings Z00.121
complication — *see* Complications, vaccination
encounter for Z23
not done (not carried out) Z28.9
because (of)
acute illness of patient Z28.01
allergy to vaccine (or component) Z28.04
caregiver refusal Z28.82
chronic illness of patient Z28.02
contraindication NEC Z28.09
delay in delivery of vaccine Z28.83
group pressure Z28.1
guardian refusal Z28.82
immune compromised state of patient Z28.03
lack of availability of vaccine Z28.83
manufacturer delay of vaccine Z28.83
parent refusal Z28.82
patient's belief Z28.1
patient had disease being vaccinated against Z28.81
patient refusal Z28.21
religious beliefs of patient Z28.1
specified reason NEC Z28.89
of patient Z28.29
unavailability of vaccine Z28.83
unspecified patient reason Z28.20
Rh factor
affecting management of pregnancy NEC O36.09-
anti-D antibody O36.01-
from transfusion — *see* Complication(s), transfusion, incompatibility reaction, Rh (factor)
Immunocytoma C83.0-
Immunodeficiency D84.9
with
adenosine-deaminase deficiency D81.3
antibody defects D80.9
specified type NEC D80.8
hyperimmunoglobulinemia D80.6
increased immunoglobulin M (IgM) D80.5
major defect D82.9
specified type NEC D82.8
partial albinism D82.8
short-limbed stature D82.2
thrombocytopenia and eczema D82.0
antibody with
hyperimmunoglobulinemia D80.6
near-normal immunoglobulins D80.6
autosomal recessive, Swiss type D80.0
combined D81.9
biotin-dependent carboxylase D81.819
biotinidase D81.810
holocarboxylase synthetase D81.818
specified type NEC D81.818
severe (SCID) D81.9
with
low or normal B-cell numbers D81.2
low T- and B-cell numbers D81.1
reticular dysgenesis D81.0

Inadequate, inadequacy - *continued*
intrafamilial communication Z63.8
material resources Z59.9
mental — *see* Disability, intellectual
parental supervision or control of child Z62.0
personality F60.7
pulmonary
function R06.89
newborn P28.5
ventilation, newborn P28.5
sample of cytologic smear
anus R85.615
cervix R87.615
vagina R87.625
social F60.7
insurance Z59.7
skills NEC Z73.4
supervision of child by parent Z62.0
teaching affecting education Z55.8
welfare support Z59.7
Inanition R64
with edema — *see* Malnutrition, severe
due to
deprivation of food T73.0
malnutrition — *see* Malnutrition
fever R50.9
Inappropriate
change in quantitative human chorionic gonadotropin (hCG) in early pregnancy O02.81
diet or eating habits Z72.4
level of quantitative human chorionic gonadotropin (hCG) for gestational age in early pregnancy O02.81
secretion
antidiuretic hormone (ADH) (excessive) E22.2
deficiency E23.2
pituitary (posterior) E22.2
Inattention at or after birth — *see* Neglect
Incarceration, incarcerated
enterocele K46.0
gangrenous K46.1
epiplocele K46.0
gangrenous K46.1
exomphalos K42.0
gangrenous K42.1
hernia — *see also* Hernia, by site, with obstruction
with gangrene — *see* Hernia, by site, with gangrene
iris, in wound — *see* Injury, eye, laceration, with prolapse
lens, in wound — *see* Injury, eye, laceration, with prolapse
omphalocele K42.0
prison, anxiety concerning Z65.1
rupture — *see* Hernia, by site
sarcoepiplocele K46.0
gangrenous K46.1
sarcoepiplomphalocele K42.0
with gangrene K42.1
uterus N85.8
gravid O34.51-
causing obstructed labor O65.5
Incised wound
external — *see* Laceration
internal organs — *see* Injury, by site
Incision, incisional
hernia K43.2
with
gangrene (and obstruction) K43.1
obstruction K43.0
surgical, complication — *see* Complications, surgical procedure
traumatic
external — *see* Laceration
internal organs — *see* Injury, by site
Inclusion
azurophilic leukocytic D72.0
blennorrhea (neonatal) (newborn) P39.1
gallbladder in liver (congenital) Q44.1
Incompatibility
ABO
affecting management of pregnancy O36.11-
anti-A sensitization O36.11-
anti-B sensitization O36.19-
specified NEC O36.19-
infusion or transfusion reaction — *see* Complication(s), transfusion, incompatibility reaction, ABO
newborn P55.1
blood (group) (Duffy) (K) (Kell) (Kidd) (Lewis) (M) (S) NEC
affecting management of pregnancy O36.11-
anti-A sensitization O36.11-

Incompatibility - *continued*
blood (group) (Duffy) (K) (Kell) (Kidd) (Lewis) (M) (S) NEC - *continued*
affecting management of pregnancy - *continued*
anti-B sensitization O36.19-
infusion or transfusion reaction T80.89
newborn P55.8
divorce or estrangement Z63.5
Rh (blood group) (factor) Z31.82
affecting management of pregnancy NEC O36.09-
anti-D antibody O36.01-
infusion or transfusion reaction — *see* Complication(s), transfusion, incompatibility reaction, Rh (factor)
newborn P55.0
rhesus — *see* Incompatibility, Rh
Incompetency, incompetent, incompetence
annular
aortic (valve) — *see* Insufficiency, aortic
mitral (valve) I34.0
pulmonary valve (heart) I37.1
aortic (valve) — *see* Insufficiency, aortic
cardiac valve — *see* Endocarditis
cervix, cervical (os) N88.3
in pregnancy O34.3-
chronotropic I45.89
with
autonomic dysfunction G90.8
ischemic heart disease I25.89
left ventricular dysfunction I51.89
sinus node dysfunction I49.8
esophagogastric (junction) (sphincter) K22.0
mitral (valve) — *see* Insufficiency, mitral
pelvic fundus N81.89
pubocervical tissue N81.82
pulmonary valve (heart) I37.1
congenital Q22.3
rectovaginal tissue N81.83
tricuspid (annular) (valve) — *see* Insufficiency, tricuspid
valvular — *see* Endocarditis
congenital Q24.8
vein, venous (saphenous) (varicose) — *see* Varix, leg
Incomplete — *see also* condition
bladder, emptying R33.9
defecation R15.0
expansion lungs (newborn) NEC — *see* Atelectasis
rotation, intestine Q43.3
Inconclusive
diagnostic imaging due to excess body fat of patient R93.9
findings on diagnostic imaging of breast NEC R92.8
mammogram (due to dense breasts) R92.2
Incontinence R32
anal sphincter R15.9
coital N39.491
feces R15.9
nonorganic origin F98.1
insensible (urinary) N39.42
overflow N39.490
postural (urinary) N39.492
psychogenic F45.8
rectal R15.9
reflex N39.498
stress (female) (male) N39.3
and urge N39.46
urethral sphincter R32
urge N39.41
and stress (female) (male) N39.46
urine (urinary) R32
continuous N39.45
due to cognitive impairment, or severe physical disability or immobility R39.81
functional R39.81
insensible N39.42
mixed (stress and urge) N39.46
nocturnal N39.44
nonorganic origin F98.0
overflow N39.490
post dribbling N39.43
postural N39.492
reflex N39.498
specified NEC N39.498
stress (female) (male) N39.3
and urge N39.46
total N39.498
unaware N39.42
urge N39.41
and stress (female) (male) N39.46
Incontinentia pigmenti Q82.3
Incoordinate, incoordination
esophageal-pharyngeal (newborn) — *see* Dysphagia

Incoordinate, incoordination - *continued*
muscular R27.8
uterus (action) (contractions) (complicating delivery) O62.4
Increase, increased
abnormal, in development R63.8
androgens (ovarian) E28.1
anticoagulants (antithrombin) (anti-VIIIa) (anti-IXa) (anti-Xa) (anti-XIa) — *see* Circulating anticoagulants
cold sense R20.8
estrogen E28.0
function
adrenal
cortex — *see* Cushing's, syndrome
medulla E27.5
pituitary (gland) (anterior) (lobe) E22.9
posterior E22.2
heat sense R20.8
intracranial pressure (benign) G93.2
permeability, capillaries I78.8
pressure, intracranial G93.2
secretion
gastrin E16.4
glucagon E16.3
pancreas, endocrine E16.9
growth hormone-releasing hormone E16.8
pancreatic polypeptide E16.8
somatostatin E16.8
vasoactive-intestinal polypeptide E16.8
sphericity, lens Q12.4
splenic activity D73.1
venous pressure I87.8
portal K76.6
Increta placenta O43.22-
Incrustation, cornea, foreign body (lead) (zinc) — *see* Foreign body, cornea
Incyclophoria H50.54
Incyclotropia — *see* Cyclotropia
Indeterminate sex Q56.4
India rubber skin Q82.8
Indigestion (acid) (bilious) (functional) K30
catarrhal K31.89
due to decomposed food NOS A05.9
nervous F45.8
psychogenic F45.8
Indirect — *see* condition
Induratio penis plastica N48.6
Induration, indurated
brain G93.89
breast (fibrous) N64.51
puerperal, postpartum O92.29
broad ligament N83.8
chancre
anus A51.1
congenital A50.07
extragenital NEC A51.2
corpora cavernosa (penis) (plastic) N48.6
liver (chronic) K76.89
lung (black) (chronic) (fibroid) — *see also* Fibrosis, lung J84.10
essential brown J84.03
penile (plastic) N48.6
phlebitic — *see* Phlebitis
skin R23.4
Inebriety (without dependence) — *see* Alcohol, intoxication
Inefficiency, kidney N28.9
Inelasticity, skin R23.4
Inequality, leg (length) (acquired) — *see also* Deformity, limb, unequal length
congenital — *see* Defect, reduction, lower limb
lower leg — *see* Deformity, limb, unequal length
Inertia
bladder (neurogenic) N31.2
stomach K31.89
psychogenic F45.8
uterus, uterine during labor O62.2
during latent phase of labor O62.0
primary O62.0
secondary O62.1
vesical (neurogenic) N31.2
Infancy, infantile, infantilism — *see also* condition
celiac K90.0
genitalia, genitals (after puberty) E30.0
Herter's (nontropical sprue) K90.0
intestinal K90.0
Lorain E23.0
pancreatic K86.89
pelvis M95.5
with disproportion (fetopelvic) O33.1
causing obstructed labor O65.1
pituitary E23.0

Infancy, infantile, infantilism - *continued*
renal N25.0
uterus — *see* Infantile, genitalia
Infant (s) — *see also* Infancy
excessive crying R68.11
irritable child R68.12
lack of care — *see* Neglect
liveborn (singleton) Z38.2
born in hospital Z38.00
by cesarean Z38.01
born outside hospital Z38.1
multiple NEC Z38.8
born in hospital Z38.68
by cesarean Z38.69
born outside hospital Z38.7
quadruplet Z38.8
born in hospital Z38.63
by cesarean Z38.64
born outside hospital Z38.7
quintuplet Z38.8
born in hospital Z38.65
by cesarean Z38.66
born outside hospital Z38.7
triplet Z38.8
born in hospital Z38.61
by cesarean Z38.62
born outside hospital Z38.7
twin Z38.5
born in hospital Z38.30
by cesarean Z38.31
born outside hospital Z38.4
of diabetic mother (syndrome of) P70.1
gestational diabetes P70.0
Infantile — *see also* condition
genitalia, genitals E30.0
os, uterine E30.0
penis E30.0
testis E29.1
uterus E30.0
Infantilism — *see* Infancy
Infarct, infarction
adrenal (capsule) (gland) E27.49
appendices epiploicae — *see also* Infarct, intestine K55.069
bowel — *see also* Infarct, intestine K55.069
brain (stem) — *see* Infarct, cerebral
breast N64.89
brewer's (kidney) N28.0
cardiac — *see* Infarct, myocardium
cerebellar — *see* Infarct, cerebral
cerebral — *see also* Occlusion, artery cerebral or precerebral, with infarction I63.9-
aborted I63.9
cortical I63.9
due to
cerebral venous thrombosis, nonpyogenic I63.6
embolism
cerebral arteries I63.4-
precerebral arteries I63.1-
occlusion NEC
cerebral arteries I63.5-
precerebral arteries I63.2-
small artery I63.81
stenosis NEC
cerebral arteries I63.5-
precerebral arteries I63.2-
small artery I63.81
thrombosis
cerebral artery I63.3-
precerebral artery I63.0-
intraoperative
during cardiac surgery I97.810
during other surgery I97.811
postprocedural
following cardiac surgery I97.820
following other surgery I97.821
specified NEC I63.89
colon (acute) (agnogenic) (embolic) (hemorrhagic) (nonocclusive) (nonthrombotic) (occlusive) (segmental) (thrombotic) (with gangrene) — *see also* Infarct, intestine K55.049
coronary artery — *see* Infarct, myocardium
embolic — *see* Embolism
fallopian tube N83.8
gallbladder K82.8
heart — *see* Infarct, myocardium
hepatic K76.3
hypophysis (anterior lobe) E23.6
impending (myocardium) I20.0
intestine (acute) (agnogenic) (embolic) (hemorrhagic) (nonocclusive) (nonthrombotic) (occlusive) (thrombotic) (with gangrene) K55.069
diffuse K55.062

Infarct, infarction - *continued*
intestine (acute) (agnogenic) (embolic) (hemorrhagic) (nonocclusive) (nonthrombotic) (occlusive) (thrombotic) (with gangrene) - *continued*
focal K55.061
large K55.049
diffuse K55.042
focal K55.041
small K55.029
diffuse K55.022
focal K55.021
kidney N28.0
lacunar I63.81
liver K76.3
lung (embolic) (thrombotic) — *see* Embolism, pulmonary
lymph node I89.8
mesentery, mesenteric (embolic) (thrombotic) (with gangrene) — *see also* Infarct, intestine K55.069
muscle (ischemic) M62.20
ankle M62.27-
foot M62.27-
forearm M62.23-
hand M62.24-
lower leg M62.26-
pelvic region M62.25-
shoulder region M62.21-
specified site NEC M62.28
thigh M62.25-
upper arm M62.22-
myocardium, myocardial (acute) (with stated duration of 4 weeks or less) I21.9
associated with revascularization procedure I21.A9
diagnosed on ECG, but presenting no symptoms I25.2
due to
demand ischemia I21.A1
ischemic imbalance I21.A1
healed or old I25.2
intraoperative — *see also* Infarct, myocardium, associated with revascularization procedure
during cardiac surgery I97.790
during other surgery I97.791
non-Q wave I21.4
non-ST elevation (NSTEMI) I21.4
subsequent I22.2
nontransmural I21.4
past (diagnosed on ECG or other investigation, but currently presenting no symptoms) I25.2
postprocedural — *see also* Infarct, myocardium, associated with revascularization procedure
following cardiac surgery surgery — *see also* Infarct, myocardium, type 4 or type 5 I97.190
following other surgery I97.191
Q wave (see also, Infarct, myocardium, by site) I21.3
secondary to
demand ischemia I21.A1
ischemic imbalance I21.A1
ST elevation (STEMI) I21.3
anterior (anteroapical) (anterolateral) (anteroseptal) (Q wave) (wall) I21.09
subsequent I22.0
inferior (diaphragmatic) (inferolateral) (inferoposterior) (wall) NEC I21.19
subsequent I22.1
inferoposterior transmural (Q wave) I21.11
involving
coronary artery of anterior wall NEC I21.09
coronary artery of inferior wall NEC I21.19
diagonal coronary artery I21.02
left anterior descending coronary artery I21.02
left circumflex coronary artery I21.21
left main coronary artery I21.01
oblique marginal coronary artery I21.21
right coronary artery I21.11
lateral (apical-lateral) (basal-lateral) (high) I21.29
subsequent I22.8
posterior (posterobasal) (posterolateral) (posteroseptal) (true) I21.29
subsequent I22.8
septal I21.29
subsequent I22.8
specified NEC I21.29
subsequent I22.8
subsequent I22.9
subsequent (recurrent) (reinfarction) I22.9
anterior (anteroapical) (anterolateral) (anteroseptal) (wall) I22.0
diaphragmatic (wall) I22.1
inferior (diaphragmatic) (inferolateral) (inferoposterior) (wall) I22.1

Infarct, infarction - *continued*
myocardium, myocardial (acute) (with stated duration of 4 weeks or less) - *continued*
subsequent (recurrent) (reinfarction) - *continued*
lateral (apical-lateral) (basal-lateral) (high) I22.8
non-ST elevation (NSTEMI) I22.2
posterior (posterobasal) (posterolateral) (posteroseptal) (true) I22.8
septal I22.8
specified NEC I22.8
ST elevation I22.9
anterior (anteroapical) (anterolateral) (anteroseptal) (wall) I22.0
inferior (diaphragmatic) (inferolateral) (inferoposterior) (wall) I22.1
specified NEC I22.8
subendocardial I22.2
transmural I22.9
anterior (anteroapical) (anterolateral) (anteroseptal) (wall) I22.0
diaphragmatic (wall) I22.1
inferior (diaphragmatic) (inferolateral) (inferoposterior) (wall) I22.1
lateral (apical-lateral) (basal-lateral) (high) I22.8
posterior (posterobasal) (posterolateral) (posteroseptal) (true) I22.8
specified NEC I22.8
type 1 — *see also* Infarction, myocardial, subsequent, by site, or by ST elevation or non-ST elevation I22.9
type 2 I21.A1
type 3 I21.A9
type 4 I21.A9
type 5 I21.A9
syphilitic A52.06
transmural I21.9
anterior (anteroapical) (anterolateral) (anteroseptal) (Q wave) (wall) NEC I21.09
inferior (diaphragmatic) (inferolateral) (inferoposterior) (Q wave) (wall) NEC I21.19
inferoposterior (Q wave) I21.11
lateral (apical-lateral) (basal-lateral) (high) NEC I21.29
posterior (posterobasal) (posterolateral) (posteroseptal) (true) NEC I21.29
septal NEC I21.29
specified NEC I21.29
type 1 — *see also* Infarction, myocardial, by site, or by ST elevation or non-ST elevation I21.9
type 2 I21.A1
type 3 I21.A9
type 4 (a) (b) (c) I21.A9
type 5 I21.A9
nontransmural I21.4
omentum — *see also* Infarct, intestine K55.069
ovary N83.8
pancreas K86.89
papillary muscle — *see* Infarct, myocardium
parathyroid gland E21.4
pituitary (gland) E23.6
placenta O43.81-
prostate N42.89
pulmonary (artery) (vein) (hemorrhagic) — *see* Embolism, pulmonary
renal (embolic) (thrombotic) N28.0
retina, retinal (artery) — *see* Occlusion, artery, retina
spinal (cord) (acute) (embolic) (nonembolic) G95.11
spleen D73.5
embolic or thrombotic I74.8
subendocardial (acute) (nontransmural) I21.4
suprarenal (capsule) (gland) E27.49
testis N50.1
thrombotic — *see also* Thrombosis
artery, arterial — *see* Embolism
thyroid (gland) E07.89
ventricle (heart) — *see* Infarct, myocardium
Infecting — *see* condition
Infection, infected, infective (opportunistic) B99.9
with
drug resistant organism — *see* Resistance (to), drug — *see also* specific organism
lymphangitis — *see* Lymphangitis
organ dysfunction (acute) R65.20
with septic shock R65.21
abscess (skin) - code by site under Abscess
Absidia — *see* Mucormycosis
Acanthamoeba — *see* Acanthamebiasis
Acanthocheilonema (perstans) (streptocerca) B74.4
accessory sinus (chronic) — *see* Sinusitis
achorion — *see* Dermatophytosis
Acremonium falciforme B47.0
acromioclavicular M00.9

Infection, infected, infective (opportunistic) - *continued*
  Actinobacillus (actinomycetem-comitans) A28.8
    mallei A24.0
    muris A25.1
  Actinomadura B47.1
  Actinomyces (israelii) — *see also* Actinomycosis A42.9
  Actinomycetales — *see* Actinomycosis
  actinomycotic NOS — *see* Actinomycosis
  adenoid (and tonsil) J03.90
    chronic J35.02
  adenovirus NEC
    as cause of disease classified elsewhere B97.0
    unspecified nature or site B34.0
  aerogenes capsulatus A48.0
  aertrycke — *see* Infection, salmonella
  alimentary canal NOS — *see* Enteritis, infectious
  Allescheria boydii B48.2
  Alternaria B48.8
  alveolus, alveolar (process) K04.7
  Ameba, amebic (histolytica) — *see* Amebiasis
  amniotic fluid, sac or cavity O41.10-
    chorioamnionitis O41.12-
    placentitis O41.14-
  amputation stump (surgical) — *see* Complication, amputation stump, infection
  Ancylostoma (duodenalis) B76.0
  Anisakiasis, Anisakis larvae B81.0
  anthrax — *see* Anthrax
  antrum (chronic) — *see* Sinusitis, maxillary
  anus, anal (papillae) (sphincter) K62.89
  arbovirus (arbor virus) A94
    specified type NEC A93.8
  artificial insemination N98.0
  Ascaris lumbricoides — *see* Ascariasis
  Ascomycetes B47.0
  Aspergillus (flavus) (fumigatus) (terreus) — *see* Aspergillosis
  atypical
    acid-fast (bacilli) — *see* Mycobacterium, atypical
    mycobacteria — *see* Mycobacterium, atypical
    virus A81.9
      specified type NEC A81.89
  auditory meatus (external) — *see* Otitis, externa, infective
  auricle (ear) — *see* Otitis, externa, infective
  axillary gland (lymph) L04.2
  Bacillus A49.9
    abortus A23.1
    anthracis — *see* Anthrax
    Ducrey's (any location) A57
    Flexner's A03.1
    Friedländer's NEC A49.8
    gas (gangrene) A48.0
    mallei A24.0
    melitensis A23.0
    paratyphoid, paratyphosus A01.4
      A A01.1
      B A01.2
      C A01.3
    Shiga (-Kruse) A03.0
    suipestifer — *see* Infection, salmonella
    swimming pool A31.1
    typhosa A01.00
    welchii — *see* Gangrene, gas
  bacterial NOS A49.9
    as cause of disease classified elsewhere B96.89
      Clostridium perfringens [C. perfringens] B96.7
      Bacteroides fragilis [B. fragilis] B96.6
      Enterobacter sakazakii B96.89
      Enterococcus B95.2
      Escherichia coli [E. coli] — *see also* Escherichia coli B96.20
      Helicobacter pylori [H.pylori] B96.81
      Hemophilus influenzae [H. influenzae] B96.3
      Klebsiella pneumoniae [K. pneumoniae] B96.1
      Mycoplasma pneumoniae [M. pneumoniae] B96.0
      Proteus (mirabilis) (morganii) B96.4
      Pseudomonas (aeruginosa) (mallei) (pseudomallei) B96.5
      Staphylococcus B95.8
        aureus (methicillin susceptible) (MSSA) B95.61
          methicillin resistant (MRSA) B95.62
        specified NEC B95.7
      Streptococcus B95.5
        group A B95.0
        group B B95.1
        pneumoniae B95.3
        specified NEC B95.4
      Vibrio vulnificus B96.82
    specified NEC A48.8

Infection, infected, infective (opportunistic) - *continued*
  Bacterium
    paratyphosum A01.4
      A A01.1
      B A01.2
      C A01.3
    typhosum A01.00
  Bacteroides NEC A49.8
    fragilis, as cause of disease classified elsewhere B96.6
  Balantidium coli A07.0
  Bartholin's gland N75.8
  Basidiobolus B46.8
  bile duct (common) (hepatic) — *see* Cholangitis
  bladder — *see* Cystitis
  Blastomyces, blastomycotic — *see also* Blastomycosis
    brasiliensis — *see* Paracoccidioidomycosis
    dermatitidis — *see* Blastomycosis
    European — *see* Cryptococcosis
    Loboi B48.0
    North American B40.9
    South American — *see* Paracoccidioidomycosis
  bleb, postprocedure — *see* Blebitis
  bone — *see* Osteomyelitis
  Bordetella — *see* Whooping cough
  Borrelia bergdorfi A69.20
  brain — *see also* Encephalitis G04.90
    membranes — *see* Meningitis
    septic G06.0
      meninges — *see* Meningitis, bacterial
  branchial cyst Q18.0
  breast — *see* Mastitis
  bronchus — *see* Bronchitis
  Brucella A23.9
    abortus A23.1
    canis A23.3
    melitensis A23.0
    mixed A23.8
    specified NEC A23.8
    suis A23.2
  Brugia (malayi) B74.1
    timori B74.2
  bursa — *see* Bursitis, infective
  buttocks (skin) L08.9
  Campylobacter, intestinal A04.5
    as cause of disease classified elsewhere B96.81
  Candida (albicans) (tropicalis) — *see* Candidiasis
  candiru B88.8
  Capillaria (intestinal) B81.1
    hepatica B83.8
    philippinensis B81.1
  cartilage — *see* Disorder, cartilage, specified type NEC
  catheter-related bloodstream (CRBSI) T80.211
  cat liver fluke B66.0
  cellulitis - code by site under Cellulitis
  central line-associated T80.219
    bloodstream (CLABSI) T80.211
    specified NEC T80.218
  Cephalosporium falciforme B47.0
  cerebrospinal — *see* Meningitis
  cervical gland (lymph) L04.0
  cervix — *see* Cervicitis
  cesarean delivery wound (puerperal) O86.00
  cestodes — *see* Infestation, cestodes
  chest J22
  Chilomastix (intestinal) A07.8
  Chlamydia, chlamydial A74.9
    anus A56.3
    genitourinary tract A56.2
      lower A56.00
      specified NEC A56.19
    lymphogranuloma A55
    pharynx A56.4
    psittaci A70
    rectum A56.3
    sexually transmitted NEC A56.8
  cholera — *see* Cholera
  Cladosporium
    bantianum (brain abscess) B43.1
    carrionii B43.0
    castellanii B36.1
    trichoides (brain abscess) B43.1
    werneckii B36.1
  Clonorchis (sinensis) (liver) B66.1
  Clostridium NEC
    bifermentans A48.0
    botulinum (food poisoning) A05.1
      infant A48.51
      wound A48.52
    difficile

Infection, infected, infective (opportunistic) - *continued*
  Clostridium NEC - *continued*
    difficile - *continued*
      as cause of disease classified elsewhere B96.89
      foodborne (disease)
        not specified as recurrent A04.72
        recurrent A04.71
      gas gangrene A48.0
      necrotizing enterocolitis
        not specified as recurrent A04.72
        recurrent A04.71
      sepsis A41.4
    gas-forming NEC A48.0
    histolyticum A48.0
    novyi, causing gas gangrene A48.0
    oedematiens A48.0
    perfringens
      as cause of disease classified elsewhere B96.7
      due to food A05.2
      foodborne (disease) A05.2
      gas gangrene A48.0
      sepsis A41.4
    septicum, causing gas gangrene A48.0
    sordellii, causing gas gangrene A48.0
    welchii
      as cause of disease classified elsewhere B96.7
      foodborne (disease) A05.2
      gas gangrene A48.0
      necrotizing enteritis A05.2
      sepsis A41.4
  Coccidioides (immitis) — *see* Coccidioidomycosis
  colon — *see* Enteritis, infectious
  colostomy K94.02
  common duct — *see* Cholangitis
  congenital P39.9
    Candida (albicans) P37.5
    cytomegalovirus P35.1
    hepatitis, viral P35.3
    herpes simplex P35.2
    infectious or parasitic disease P37.9
      specified NEC P37.8
    listeriosis (disseminated) P37.2
    malaria NEC P37.4
      falciparum P37.3
    Plasmodium falciparum P37.3
    poliomyelitis P35.8
    rubella P35.0
    skin P39.4
    toxoplasmosis (acute) (subacute) (chronic) P37.1
    tuberculosis P37.0
    urinary (tract) P39.3
    vaccinia P35.8
    virus P35.9
      specified type NEC P35.8
  Conidiobolus B46.8
  coronavirus NEC B34.2
    as cause of disease classified elsewhere B97.29
    severe acute respiratory syndrome (SARS associated) B97.21
  corpus luteum — *see* Salpingo-oophoritis
  Corynebacterium diphtheriae — *see* Diphtheria
  cotia virus B08.8
  Coxiella burnetii A78
  coxsackie — *see* Coxsackie
  Cryptococcus neoformans — *see* Cryptococcosis
  Cryptosporidium A07.2
  Cunninghamella — *see* Mucormycosis
  cyst — *see* Cyst
  cystic duct — *see also* Cholecystitis K81.9
  Cysticercus cellulosae — *see* Cysticercosis
  cytomegalovirus, cytomegaloviral B25.9
    congenital P35.1
    maternal, maternal care for (suspected) damage to fetus O35.3
    mononucleosis B27.10
      with
        complication NEC B27.19
        meningitis B27.12
        polyneuropathy B27.11
  delta-agent (acute) , in hepatitis B carrier B17.0
  dental (pulpal origin) K04.7
  Deuteromycetes B47.0
  Dicrocoelium dendriticum B66.2
  Dipetalonema (perstans) (streptocerca) B74.4
  diphtherial — *see* Diphtheria
  Diphyllobothrium (adult) (latum) (pacificum) B70.0
    larval B70.1
  Diplogonoporus (grandis) B71.8
  Dipylidium caninum B67.4
  Dirofilaria B74.8
  Dracunculus medinensis B72
  Drechslera (hawaiiensis) B43.8

Infection, infected, infective (opportunistic) - *continued*
  Ducrey Haemophilus (any location) A57
  due to or resulting from
    artificial insemination N98.0
    central venous catheter T80.219
      bloodstream T80.211
      exit or insertion site T80.212
      localized T80.212
      port or reservoir T80.212
      specified NEC T80.218
      tunnel T80.212
    device, implant or graft — *see also* Complications, by site and type, infection or inflammation T85.79
      arterial graft NEC T82.7
      breast (implant) T85.79
      catheter NEC T85.79
        dialysis (renal) T82.7
          intraperitoneal T85.71
        infusion NEC T82.7
          cranial T85.735
          intrathecal T85.735
          spinal (epidural) (subdural) T85.735
          subarachnoid T85.735
        urinary T83.518
          cystostomy T83.510
          Hopkins T83.518
          ileostomy T83.518
          nephrostomy T83.512
          specified NEC T83.518
          urethral indwelling T83.511
          urostomy T83.518
      electronic (electrode) (pulse generator) (stimulator)
        bone T84.7
        cardiac T82.7
        nervous system T85.738
          brain T85.731
          cranial nerve T85.732
          gastric nerve T85.732
          generator pocket T85.734
          neurostimulator generator T85.734
          peripheral nerve T85.732
          sacral nerve T85.732
          spinal cord T85.733
          vagal nerve T85.732
        urinary T83.590
      fixation, internal (orthopedic) NEC — *see* Complication, fixation device, infection
      gastrointestinal (bile duct) (esophagus) T85.79
        neurostimulator electrode (lead) T85.732
      genital NEC T83.69
      heart NEC T82.7
        valve (prosthesis) T82.6
          graft T82.7
      joint prosthesis — *see* Complication, joint prosthesis, infection
      ocular (corneal graft) (orbital implant) NEC T85.79
      orthopedic NEC T84.7
      penile (cylinder) (pump) (resevoir) T83.61
      specified NEC T85.79
      testicular T83.62
      urinary NEC T83.598
        ileal conduit stent T83.593
        implanted neurostimulation T83.590
        implanted sphincter T83.591
        indwelling ureteral stent T83.592
        nephroureteral stent T83.593
        specified stent NEC T83.593
      vascular NEC T82.7
      ventricular intracranial (communicating) shunt T85.730
    Hickman catheter T80.219
      bloodstream T80.211
      localized T80.212
      specified NEC T80.218
    immunization or vaccination T88.0
    infusion, injection or transfusion NEC T80.29
      acute T80.22
    injury NEC - code by site under Wound, open
    peripherally inserted central catheter (PICC) T80.219
      bloodstream T80.211
      localized T80.212
      specified NEC T80.218
    portacath (port-a-cath) T80.219
      bloodstream T80.211
      localized T80.212
      specified NEC T80.218
    pulmonary artery catheter — *see* Infection, due to or resulting from, central venous catheter

Infection, infected, infective (opportunistic) - *continued*
  due to or resulting from - *continued*
    surgery T81.40
    Swan Ganz catheter — *see* Infection, due to or resulting from, central venous catheter
    triple lumen catheter T80.219
      bloodstream T80.211
      localized T80.212
      specified NEC T80.218
    umbilical venous catheter T80.219
      bloodstream T80.211
      localized T80.212
      specified NEC T80.218
  during labor NEC O75.3
  ear (middle) — *see also* Otitis media
    external — *see* Otitis, externa, infective
    inner — *see* subcategory H83.0
  Eberthella typhosa A01.00
  Echinococcus — *see* Echinococcus
  echovirus
    as cause of disease classified elsewhere B97.12
    unspecified nature or site B34.1
  endocardium I33.0
  endocervix — *see* Cervicitis
  Entamoeba — *see* Amebiasis
  enteric — *see* Enteritis, infectious
  Enterobacter sakazakii B96.89
  Enterobius vermicularis B80
  enterostomy K94.12
  enterovirus B34.1
    as cause of disease classified elsewhere B97.10
      coxsackievirus B97.11
      echovirus B97.12
      specified NEC B97.19
  Entomophthora B46.8
  Epidermophyton — *see* Dermatophytosis
  epididymis — *see* Epididymitis
  episiotomy (puerperal) O86.09
  Erysipelothrix (insidiosa) (rhusiopathiae) — *see* Erysipeloid
  erythema infectiosum B08.3
  Escherichia (E.) coli NEC A49.8
    as cause of disease classified elsewhere — *see also* Escherichia coli B96.20
    congenital P39.8
      sepsis P36.4
    generalized A41.51
    intestinal — *see* Enteritis, infectious, due to, Escherichia coli
  ethmoidal (chronic) (sinus) — *see* Sinusitis, ethmoidal
  eustachian tube (ear) — *see* Salpingitis, eustachian
  external auditory canal (meatus) NEC — *see* Otitis, externa, infective
  eye (purulent) — *see* Endophthalmitis, purulent
  eyelid — *see* Inflammation, eyelid
  fallopian tube — *see* Salpingo-oophoritis
  Fasciola (gigantica) (hepatica) (indica) B66.3
  Fasciolopsis (buski) B66.5
  filarial — *see* Infestation, filarial
  finger (skin) L08.9
    nail L03.01-
      fungus B35.1
  fish tapeworm B70.0
    larval B70.1
  flagellate, intestinal A07.9
  fluke — *see* Infestation, fluke
  focal
    teeth (pulpal origin) K04.7
    tonsils J35.01
  Fonsecaea (compactum) (pedrosoi) B43.0
  food — *see* Intoxication, foodborne
  foot (skin) L08.9
    dermatophytic fungus B35.3
  Francisella tularensis — *see* Tularemia
  frontal (sinus) (chronic) — *see* Sinusitis, frontal
  fungus NOS B49
    beard B35.0
    dermatophytic — *see* Dermatophytosis
    foot B35.3
    groin B35.6
    hand B35.2
    nail B35.1
    pathogenic to compromised host only B48.8
    perianal (area) B35.6
    scalp B35.0
    skin B36.9
      foot B35.3
      hand B35.2
      toenails B35.1
  Fusarium B48.8
  gallbladder — *see* Cholecystitis

Infection, infected, infective (opportunistic) - *continued*
  gas bacillus — *see* Gangrene, gas
  gastrointestinal — *see* Enteritis, infectious
  generalized NEC — *see* Sepsis
  generator pocket, implanted electronic neurostimulator T85.734
  genital organ or tract
    female — *see* Disease, pelvis, inflammatory
    male N49.9
      multiple sites N49.8
      specified NEC N49.8
  Ghon tubercle, primary A15.7
  Giardia lamblia A07.1
  gingiva (chronic) K05.10
    acute K05.00
      nonplaque induced K05.01
      plaque induced K05.00
    nonplaque induced K05.11
    plaque induced K05.10
  glanders A24.0
  glenosporopsis B48.0
  Gnathostoma (spinigerum) B83.1
  Gongylonema B83.8
  gonococcal — *see* Gonococcus
  gram-negative bacilli NOS A49.9
  guinea worm B72
  gum (chronic) K05.10
    acute K05.00
      nonplaque induced K05.01
      plaque induced K05.00
    nonplaque induced K05.11
    plaque induced K05.10
  Haemophilus — *see* Infection, Hemophilus
  heart — *see* Carditis
  Helicobacter pylori A04.8
    as cause of disease classified elsewhere B96.81
  helminths B83.9
    intestinal B82.0
      mixed (types classifiable to more than one of the titles B65.0-B81.3 and B81.8) B81.4
      specified type NEC B81.8
    specified type NEC B83.8
  Hemophilus
    aegyptius, systemic A48.4
    ducrey (any location) A57
    influenzae NEC A49.2
      as cause of disease classified elsewhere B96.3
    generalized A41.3
  herpes (simplex) — *see also* Herpes
    congenital P35.2
    disseminated B00.7
    zoster B02.9
  herpesvirus, herpesviral — *see* Herpes
  hip (joint) NEC M00.9
    due to internal joint prosthesis
      left T84.52
      right T84.51
    skin NEC L08.9
  Heterophyes (heterophyes) B66.8
  Histoplasma — *see* Histoplasmosis
    American B39.4
    capsulatum B39.4
  hookworm B76.9
  human
    papilloma virus A63.0
    T-cell lymphotropic virus type-1 (HTLV-1) B33.3
  hydrocele N43.0
  Hymenolepis B71.0
  hypopharynx — *see* Pharyngitis
  inguinal (lymph) glands L04.1
    due to soft chancre A57
  intervertebral disc, pyogenic M46.30
    cervical region M46.32
    cervicothoracic region M46.33
    lumbar region M46.36
    lumbosacral region M46.37
    multiple sites M46.39
    occipito-atlanto-axial region M46.31
    sacrococcygeal region M46.38
    thoracic region M46.34
    thoracolumbar region M46.35
  intestine, intestinal — *see* Enteritis, infectious
    specified NEC A08.8
  intra-amniotic affecting newborn NEC P39.2
  Isospora belli or hominis A07.3
  Japanese B encephalitis A83.0
  jaw (bone) (lower) (upper) M27.2
  joint NEC M00.9
    due to internal joint prosthesis T84.50
  kidney (cortex) (hematogenous) N15.9
    with calculus N20.0
      with hydronephrosis N13.6

Infection, infected, infective (opportunistic) - *continued*
kidney (cortex) (hematogenous) - *continued*
following ectopic gestation O08.83
pelvis and ureter (cystic) N28.85
puerperal (postpartum) O86.21
specified NEC N15.8
Klebsiella (K.) pneumoniae NEC A49.8
as cause of disease classified elsewhere B96.1
knee (joint) NEC M00.9
joint M00.9
due to internal joint prosthesis
left T84.54
right T84.53
skin L08.9
Koch's — *see* Tuberculosis
labia (majora) (minora) (acute) — *see* Vulvitis
lacrimal
gland — *see* Dacryoadenitis
passages (duct) (sac) — *see* Inflammation, lacrimal, passages
lancet fluke B66.2
larynx NEC J38.7
leg (skin) NOS L08.9
Legionella pneumophila A48.1
nonpneumonic A48.2
Leishmania — *see also* Leishmaniasis
aethiopica B55.1
braziliensis B55.2
chagasi B55.0
donovani B55.0
infantum B55.0
major B55.1
mexicana B55.1
tropica B55.1
lentivirus, as cause of disease classified elsewhere B97.31
Leptosphaeria senegalensis B47.0
Leptospira interrogans A27.9
autumnalis A27.89
canicola A27.89
hebdomadis A27.89
icterohaemorrhagiae A27.0
pomona A27.89
specified type NEC A27.89
leptospirochetal NEC — *see* Leptospirosis
Listeria monocytogenes — *see also* Listeriosis
congenital P37.2
Loa loa B74.3
with conjunctival infestation B74.3
eyelid B74.3
Loboa loboi B48.0
local, skin (staphylococcal) (streptococcal) L08.9
abscess - code by site under Abscess
cellulitis - code by site under Cellulitis
specified NEC L08.89
ulcer — *see* Ulcer, skin
Loefflerella mallei A24.0
lung — *see also* Pneumonia J18.9
atypical Mycobacterium A31.0
spirochetal A69.8
tuberculous — *see* Tuberculosis, pulmonary
virus — *see* Pneumonia, viral
lymph gland — *see also* Lymphadenitis, acute
mesenteric I88.0
lymphoid tissue, base of tongue or posterior pharynx, NEC (chronic) J35.03
Madurella (grisea) (mycetomii) B47.0
major
following ectopic or molar pregnancy O08.0
puerperal, postpartum, childbirth O85
Malassezia furfur B36.0
Malleomyces
mallei A24.0
pseudomallei (whitmori) — *see* Melioidosis
mammary gland N61.0
Mansonella (ozzardi) (perstans) (streptocerca) B74.4
mastoid — *see* Mastoiditis
maxilla, maxillary M27.2
sinus (chronic) — *see* Sinusitis, maxillary
mediastinum J98.51
Medina (worm) B72
meibomian cyst or gland — *see* Hordeolum
meninges — *see* Meningitis, bacterial
meningococcal — *see also* condition A39.9
adrenals A39.1
brain A39.81
cerebrospinal A39.0
conjunctiva A39.89
endocardium A39.51
heart A39.50
endocardium A39.51
myocardium A39.52

Infection, infected, infective (opportunistic) - *continued*
meningococcal - *continued*
heart - *continued*
pericardium A39.53
joint A39.83
meninges A39.0
meningococcemia A39.4
acute A39.2
chronic A39.3
myocardium A39.52
pericardium A39.53
retrobulbar neuritis A39.82
specified site NEC A39.89
mesenteric lymph nodes or glands NEC I88.0
Metagonimus B66.8
metatarsophalangeal M00.9
methicillin
resistant Staphylococcus aureus (MRSA) A49.02
susceptible Staphylococcus aureus (MSSA) A49.01
Microsporum, microsporic — *see* Dermatophytosis
mixed flora (bacterial) NEC A49.8
Monilia — *see* Candidiasis
Monosporium apiospermum B48.2
mouth, parasitic B37.0
Mucor — *see* Mucormycosis
muscle NEC — *see* Myositis, infective
mycelium NOS B49
mycetoma B47.9
actinomycotic NEC B47.1
mycotic NEC B47.0
Mycobacterium, mycobacterial — *see* Mycobacterium
Mycoplasma NEC A49.3
pneumoniae, as cause of disease classified elsewhere B96.0
mycotic NOS B49
pathogenic to compromised host only B48.8
skin NOS B36.9
myocardium NEC I40.0
nail (chronic)
with lymphangitis — *see* Lymphangitis, acute, digit
finger L03.01-
fungus B35.1
ingrowing L60.0
toe L03.03-
fungus B35.1
nasal sinus (chronic) — *see* Sinusitis
nasopharynx — *see* Nasopharyngitis
navel L08.82
Necator americanus B76.1
Neisseria — *see* Gonococcus
Neotestudina rosatii B47.0
newborn P39.9
intra-amniotic NEC P39.2
skin P39.4
specified type NEC P39.8
nipple N61.0
associated with
lactation O91.03
pregnancy O91.01-
puerperium O91.02
Nocardia — *see* Nocardiosis
obstetrical surgical wound (puerperal) O86.00
incisional site
deep O86.02
superficial O86.01
organ and space site O86.03
surgical site specified NEC O86.09
Oesophagostomum (apiostomum) B81.8
Oestrus ovis — *see* Myiasis
Oidium albicans B37.9
Onchocerca (volvulus) — *see* Onchocerciasis
oncovirus, as cause of disease classified elsewhere B97.32
operation wound T81.49
Opisthorchis (felineus) (viverrini) B66.0
orbit, orbital — *see* Inflammation, orbit
orthopoxvirus NEC B08.09
ovary — *see* Salpingo-oophoritis
Oxyuris vermicularis B80
pancreas (acute) — *see* Pancreatitis, acute
abscess — *see* Pancreatitis, acute
specified NEC — *see also* Pancreatitis, acute K85.80
papillomavirus, as cause of disease classified elsewhere B97.7
papovavirus NEC B34.4
Paracoccidioides brasiliensis — *see* Paracoccidioidomycosis
Paragonimus (westermani) B66.4
parainfluenza virus B34.8

Infection, infected, infective (opportunistic) - *continued*
parameningococcus NOS A39.9
parapoxvirus B08.60
specified NEC B08.69
parasitic B89
Parastrongylus
cantonensis B83.2
costaricensis B81.3
paratyphoid A01.4
Type A A01.1
Type B A01.2
Type C A01.3
paraurethral ducts N34.2
parotid gland — *see* Sialoadenitis
parvovirus NEC B34.3
as cause of disease classified elsewhere B97.6
Pasteurella NEC A28.0
multocida A28.0
pestis — *see* Plague
pseudotuberculosis A28.0
septica (cat bite) (dog bite) A28.0
tularensis — *see* Tularemia
pelvic, female — *see* Disease, pelvis, inflammatory
Penicillium (marneffei) B48.4
penis (glans) (retention) NEC N48.29
periapical K04.5
peridental, periodontal K05.20
generalized — *see* Peridontitis, aggressive, generalized
localized — *see* Peridontitis, aggressive, localized
perinatal period P39.9
specified type NEC P39.8
perineal repair (puerperal) O86.09
periorbital — *see* Inflammation, orbit
perirectal K62.89
perirenal — *see* Infection, kidney
peritoneal — *see* Peritonitis
periureteral N28.89
Petriellidium boydii B48.2
pharynx — *see also* Pharyngitis
coxsackievirus B08.5
posterior, lymphoid (chronic) J35.03
Phialophora
gougerotii (subcutaneous abscess or cyst) B43.2
jeanselmei (subcutaneous abscess or cyst) B43.2
verrucosa (skin) B43.0
Piedraia hortae B36.3
pinta A67.9
intermediate A67.1
late A67.2
mixed A67.3
primary A67.0
pinworm B80
pityrosporum furfur B36.0
pleuro-pneumonia-like organism (PPLO)
NEC A49.3
as cause of disease classified elsewhere B96.0
pneumococcus, pneumococcal NEC A49.1
as cause of disease classified elsewhere B95.3
generalized (purulent) A40.3
with pneumonia J13
Pneumocystis carinii (pneumonia) B59
Pneumocystis jiroveci (pneumonia) B59
port or reservoir T80.212
postoperative T81.40
postoperative wound T81.49
surgical site
deep incisional T81.42
organ and space T81.43
specified NEC T81.49
superficial incisional T81.41
postprocedural T81.40
postvaccinal T88.0
prepuce NEC N47.7
with penile inflammation N47.6
prion — *see* Disease, prion, central nervous system
prostate (capsule) — *see* Prostatitis
Proteus (mirabilis) (morganii) (vulgaris) NEC A49.8
as cause of disease classified elsewhere B96.4
protozoal NEC B64
intestinal A07.9
specified NEC A07.8
specified NEC B60.8
Pseudoallescheria boydii B48.2
Pseudomonas NEC A49.8
as cause of disease classified elsewhere B96.5
mallei A24.0
pneumonia J15.1
pseudomallei — *see* Melioidosis
puerperal O86.4
genitourinary tract NEC O86.89
major or generalized O85

Infection, infected, infective (opportunistic) - *continued*
puerperal - *continued*
minor O86.4
specified NEC O86.89
pulmonary — *see* Infection, lung
purulent — *see* Abscess
Pyrenochaeta romeroi B47.0
Q fever A78
rectum (sphincter) K62.89
renal — *see also* Infection, kidney
pelvis and ureter (cystic) N28.85
reovirus, as cause of disease classified elsewhere B97.5
respiratory (tract) NEC J98.8
acute J22
chronic J98.8
influenzal (upper) (acute) — *see* Influenza, with, respiratory manifestations NEC
lower (acute) J22
chronic — *see* Bronchitis, chronic
rhinovirus J00
syncytial virus, as cause of disease classified elsewhere B97.4
upper (acute) NOS J06.9
chronic J39.8
streptococcal J06.9
viral NOS J06.9
resulting from
presence of internal prosthesis, implant, graft — *see* Complications, by site and type, infection
retortamoniasis A07.8
retroperitoneal NEC K68.9
retrovirus B33.3
as cause of disease classified elsewhere B97.30
human
immunodeficiency, type 2 (HIV 2) B97.35
T-cell lymphotropic
type I (HTLV-I) B97.33
type II (HTLV-II) B97.34
lentivirus B97.31
oncovirus B97.32
specified NEC B97.39
Rhinosporidium (seeberi) B48.1
rhinovirus
as cause of disease classified elsewhere B97.89
unspecified nature or site B34.8
Rhizopus — *see* Mucormycosis
rickettsial NOS A79.9
roundworm (large) NEC B82.0
Ascariasis — *see also* Ascariasis B77.9
rubella — *see* Rubella
Saccharomyces — *see* Candidiasis
salivary duct or gland (any) — *see* Sialoadenitis
Salmonella (aertrycke) (arizonae) (callinarum) (cholerae-suis) (enteritidis) (suipestifer) (typhimurium) A02.9
with
(gastro) enteritis A02.0
sepsis A02.1
specified manifestation NEC A02.8
due to food (poisoning) A02.9
hirschfeldii A01.3
localized A02.20
arthritis A02.23
meningitis A02.21
osteomyelitis A02.24
pneumonia A02.22
pyelonephritis A02.25
specified NEC A02.29
paratyphi A01.4
A A01.1
B A01.2
C A01.3
schottmuelleri A01.2
typhi, typhosa — *see* Typhoid
Sarcocystis A07.8
scabies B86
Schistosoma — *see* Infestation, Schistosoma
scrotum (acute) NEC N49.2
seminal vesicle — *see* Vesiculitis
septic
localized, skin — *see* Abscess
sheep liver fluke B66.3
Shigella A03.9
boydii A03.2
dysenteriae A03.0
flexneri A03.1
group
A A03.0
B A03.1
C A03.2

Infection, infected, infective (opportunistic) - *continued*
Shigella - *continued*
group - *continued*
D A03.3
Schmitz (-Stutzer) A03.0
schmitzii A03.0
shigae A03.0
sonnei A03.3
specified NEC A03.8
shoulder (joint) NEC M00.9
due to internal joint prosthesis T84.59
skin NEC L08.9
sinus (accessory) (chronic) (nasal) — *see also* Sinusitis
pilonidal — *see* Sinus, pilonidal
skin NEC L08.89
Skene's duct or gland — *see* Urethritis
skin (local) (staphylococcal) (streptococcal) L08.9
abscess - code by site under Abscess
cellulitis - code by site under Cellulitis
due to fungus B36.9
specified type NEC B36.8
mycotic B36.9
specified type NEC B36.8
newborn P39.4
ulcer — *see* Ulcer, skin
slow virus A81.9
specified NEC A81.89
Sparganum (mansoni) (proliferum) (baxteri) B70.1
specific — *see also* Syphilis
to perinatal period — *see* Infection, congenital
specified NEC B99.8
spermatic cord NEC N49.1
sphenoidal (sinus) — *see* Sinusitis, sphenoidal
spinal cord NOS — *see also* Myelitis G04.91
abscess G06.1
meninges — *see* Meningitis
streptococcal G04.89
Spirillum A25.0
spirochetal NOS A69.9
lung A69.8
specified NEC A69.8
Spirometra larvae B70.1
spleen D73.89
Sporotrichum, Sporothrix (schenckii) — *see* Sporotrichosis
staphylococcal, unspecified site
aureus (methicillin susceptible) (MSSA) A49.01
methicillin resistant (MRSA) A49.02
as cause of disease classified elsewhere B95.8
aureus (methicillin susceptible) (MSSA) B95.61
methicillin resistant (MRSA) B95.62
specified NEC B95.7
food poisoning A05.0
generalized (purulent) A41.2
pneumonia — *see* Pneumonia, staphylococcal
Stellantchasmus falcatus B66.8
streptobacillus moniliformis A25.1
streptococcal NEC A49.1
as cause of disease classified elsewhere B95.5
B genitourinary complicating
childbirth O98.82
pregnancy O98.81-
puerperium O98.83
congenital
sepsis P36.10
group B P36.0
specified NEC P36.19
generalized (purulent) A40.9
Streptomyces B47.1
Strongyloides (stercoralis) — *see* Strongyloidiasis
stump (amputation) (surgical) — *see* Complication, amputation stump, infection
subcutaneous tissue, local L08.9
suipestifer — *see* Infection, salmonella
swimming pool bacillus A31.1
Taenia — *see* Infestation, Taenia
Taeniarhynchus saginatus B68.1
tapeworm — *see* Infestation, tapeworm
tendon (sheath) — *see* Tenosynovitis, infective NEC
Ternidens diminutus B81.8
testis — *see* Orchitis
threadworm B80
throat — *see* Pharyngitis
thyroglossal duct K14.8
toe (skin) L08.9
cellulitis L03.03-
fungus B35.1
nail L03.03-
fungus B35.1
tongue NEC K14.0
parasitic B37.0

Infection, infected, infective (opportunistic) - *continued*
tonsil (and adenoid) (faucial) (lingual) (pharyngeal) — *see* Tonsillitis
tooth, teeth K04.7
periapical K04.7
peridental, periodontal K05.20
generalized — *see* Peridontitis, aggressive, generalized
localized — *see* Peridontitis, aggressive, localized
pulp K04.01
irreversible K04.02
reversible K04.01
socket M27.3
TORCH — *see* Infection, congenital
without active infection P00.2
Torula histolytica — *see* Cryptococcosis
Toxocara (canis) (cati) (felis) B83.0
Toxoplasma gondii — *see* Toxoplasma
trachea, chronic J42
trematode NEC — *see* Infestation, fluke
trench fever A79.0
Treponema pallidum — *see* Syphilis
Trichinella (spiralis) B75
Trichomonas A59.9
cervix A59.09
intestine A07.8
prostate A59.02
specified site NEC A59.8
urethra A59.03
urogenitalis A59.00
vagina A59.01
vulva A59.01
Trichophyton, trichophytic — *see* Dermatophytosis
Trichosporon (beigelii) cutaneum B36.2
Trichostrongylus B81.2
Trichuris (trichiura) B79
Trombicula (irritans) B88.0
Trypanosoma
brucei
gambiense B56.0
rhodesiense B56.1
cruzi — *see* Chagas' disease
tubal — *see* Salpingo-oophoritis
tuberculous NEC — *see* Tuberculosis
tubo-ovarian — *see* Salpingo-oophoritis
tunnel T80.212
tunica vaginalis N49.1
tympanic membrane NEC — *see* Myringitis
typhoid (abortive) (ambulant) (bacillus) — *see* Typhoid
typhus A75.9
flea-borne A75.2
mite-borne A75.3
recrudescent A75.1
tick-borne A77.9
African A77.1
North Asian A77.2
umbilicus L08.82
ureter N28.86
urethra — *see* Urethritis
urinary (tract) N39.0
bladder — *see* Cystitis
complicating
pregnancy O23.4-
specified type NEC O23.3-
kidney — *see* Infection, kidney
newborn P39.3
puerperal (postpartum) O86.20
tuberculous A18.13
urethra — *see* Urethritis
uterus, uterine — *see* Endometritis
vaccination T88.0
vaccinia not from vaccination B08.011
vagina (acute) — *see* Vaginitis
varicella B01.9
varicose veins — *see* Varix
vas deferens NEC N49.1
vesical — *see* Cystitis
Vibrio
cholerae A00.0
El Tor A00.1
parahaemolyticus (food poisoning) A05.3
vulnificus
as cause of disease classified elsewhere B96.82
foodborne intoxication A05.5
Vincent's (gum) (mouth) (tonsil) A69.1
virus, viral NOS B34.9
adenovirus
as cause of disease classified elsewhere B97.0
unspecified nature or site B34.0
arborvirus, arbovirus arthropod-borne A94

Infection, infected, infective (opportunistic) - *continued*
  virus, viral NOS - *continued*
    as cause of disease classified elsewhere B97.89
      adenovirus B97.0
      coronavirus B97.29
        SARS-associated B97.21
      coxsackievirus B97.11
      echovirus B97.12
      enterovirus B97.10
        coxsackievirus B97.11
        echovirus B97.12
        specified NEC B97.19
      human
        immunodeficiency, type 2 (HIV 2) B97.35
        T-cell lymphotropic,
          type I (HTLV-I) B97.33
          type II (HTLV-II) B97.34
        metapneumovirus B97.81
      papillomavirus B97.7
      parvovirus B97.6
      reovirus B97.5
      respiratory syncytial B97.4
      retrovirus B97.30
        human
          immunodeficiency, type 2 (HIV 2) B97.35
          T-cell lymphotropic,
            type I (HTLV-I) B97.33
            type II (HTLV-II) B97.34
        lentivirus B97.31
        oncovirus B97.32
        specified NEC B97.39
      specified NEC B97.89
    central nervous system A89
      atypical A81.9
        specified NEC A81.89
      enterovirus NEC A88.8
        meningitis A87.0
      slow virus A81.9
        specified NEC A81.89
      specified NEC A88.8
    chest J98.8
    cotia B08.8
    coxsackie — *see also* Infection, coxsackie B34.1
      as cause of disease classified elsewhere B97.11
    ECHO
      as cause of disease classified elsewhere B97.12
      unspecified nature or site B34.1
    encephalitis, tick-borne A84.9
    enterovirus, as cause of disease classified elsewhere B97.10
      coxsackievirus B97.11
      echovirus B97.12
      specified NEC B97.19
    exanthem NOS B09
    human papilloma as cause of disease classified elsewhere B97.7
    human metapneumovirus as cause of disease classified elsewhere B97.81
    intestine — *see* Enteritis, viral
    respiratory syncytial
      as cause of disease classified elsewhere B97.4
      bronchopneumonia J12.1
      common cold syndrome J00
      nasopharyngitis (acute) J00
    rhinovirus
      as cause of disease classified elsewhere B97.89
      unspecified nature or site B34.8
    slow A81.9
      specified NEC A81.89
    specified type NEC B33.8
      as cause of disease classified elsewhere B97.89
      unspecified nature or site B34.8
    unspecified nature or site B34.9
    West Nile — *see* Virus, West Nile
  vulva (acute) — *see* Vulvitis
  West Nile — *see* Virus, West Nile
  whipworm B79
  worms B83.9
    specified type NEC B83.8
  Wuchereria (bancrofti) B74.0
    malayi B74.1
  yatapoxvirus B08.70
    specified NEC B08.79
  yeast — *see also* Candidiasis B37.9
  yellow fever — *see* Fever, yellow
  Yersinia
    enterocolitica (intestinal) A04.6
    pestis — *see* Plague
    pseudotuberculosis A28.2
  Zeis' gland — *see* Hordeolum
  Zika virus A92.5
    congenital P35.4

Infection, infected, infective (opportunistic) - *continued*
  zoonotic bacterial NOS A28.9
  Zopfia senegalensis B47.0
Infective, infectious — *see* condition
Infertility
  female N97.9
    age-related N97.8
    associated with
      anovulation N97.0
      cervical (mucus) disease or anomaly N88.3
      congenital anomaly
        cervix N88.3
        fallopian tube N97.1
        uterus N97.2
        vagina N97.8
      dysmucorrhea N88.3
      fallopian tube disease or anomaly N97.1
      pituitary-hypothalamic origin E23.0
      specified origin NEC N97.8
      Stein-Leventhal syndrome E28.2
      uterine disease or anomaly N97.2
      vaginal disease or anomaly N97.8
    due to
      cervical anomaly N88.3
      fallopian tube anomaly N97.1
      ovarian failure E28.39
      Stein-Leventhal syndrome E28.2
      uterine anomaly N97.2
      vaginal anomaly N97.8
    nonimplantation N97.2
    origin
      cervical N88.3
      tubal (block) (occlusion) (stenosis) N97.1
      uterine N97.2
      vaginal N97.8
  male N46.9
    azoospermia N46.01
      extratesticular cause N46.029
        drug therapy N46.021
        efferent duct obstruction N46.023
        infection N46.022
        radiation N46.024
        specified cause NEC N46.029
        systemic disease N46.025
    oligospermia N46.11
      extratesticular cause N46.129
        drug therapy N46.121
        efferent duct obstruction N46.123
        infection N46.122
        radiation N46.124
        specified cause NEC N46.129
        systemic disease N46.125
    specified type NEC N46.8
Infestation B88.9
  Acanthocheilonema (perstans) (streptocerca) B74.4
  Acariasis B88.0
    demodex folliculorum B88.0
    sarcoptes scabiei B86
    trombiculae B88.0
  Agamofilaria streptocerca B74.4
  Ancylostoma, ankylostoma (braziliense) (caninum) (ceylanicum) (duodenale) B76.0
    americanum B76.1
    new world B76.1
  Anisakis larvae, anisakiasis B81.0
  arthropod NEC B88.2
  Ascaris lumbricoides — *see* Ascariasis
  Balantidium coli A07.0
  beef tapeworm B68.1
  Bothriocephalus (latus) B70.0
    larval B70.1
  broad tapeworm B70.0
    larval B70.1
  Brugia (malayi) B74.1
    timori B74.2
  candiru B88.8
  Capillaria
    hepatica B83.8
    philippinensis B81.1
  cat liver fluke B66.0
  cestodes B71.9
    diphyllobothrium — *see* Infestation, diphyllobothrium
    dipylidiasis B71.1
    hymenolepiasis B71.0
    specified type NEC B71.8
  chigger B88.0
  chigo, chigoe B88.1
  Clonorchis (sinensis) (liver) B66.1
  coccidial A07.3
  crab-lice B85.3
  Cysticercus cellulosae — *see* Cysticercosis

Infestation - *continued*
  Demodex (folliculorum) B88.0
  Dermanyssus gallinae B88.0
  Dermatobia (hominis) — *see* Myiasis
  Dibothriocephalus (latus) B70.0
    larval B70.1
  Dicrocoelium dendriticum B66.2
  Diphyllobothrium (adult) (latum) (intestinal) (pacificum) B70.0
    larval B70.1
  Diplogonoporus (grandis) B71.8
  Dipylidium caninum B67.4
  Distoma hepaticum B66.3
  dog tapeworm B67.4
  Dracunculus medinensis B72
  dragon worm B72
  dwarf tapeworm B71.0
  Echinococcus — *see* Echinococcus
  Echinostomum ilocanum B66.8
  Entamoeba (histolytica) — *see* Infection, Ameba
  Enterobius vermicularis B80
  eyelid
    in (due to)
      leishmaniasis B55.1
      loiasis B74.3
      onchocerciasis B73.09
      phthiriasis B85.3
    parasitic NOS B89
  eyeworm B74.3
  Fasciola (gigantica) (hepatica) (indica) B66.3
  Fasciolopsis (buski) (intestine) B66.5
  filarial B74.9
    bancroftian B74.0
    conjunctiva B74.9
    due to
      Acanthocheilonema (perstans) (streptocerca) B74.4
      Brugia (malayi) B74.1
        timori B74.2
      Dracunculus medinensis B72
      guinea worm B72
      loa loa B74.3
      Mansonella (ozzardi) (perstans) (streptocerca) B74.4
      Onchocerca volvulus B73.00
        eye B73.00
        eyelid B73.09
      Wuchereria (bancrofti) B74.0
    Malayan B74.1
    ozzardi B74.4
    specified type NEC B74.8
  fish tapeworm B70.0
    larval B70.1
  fluke B66.9
    blood NOS — *see* Schistosomiasis
    cat liver B66.0
    intestinal B66.5
    liver (sheep) B66.3
      cat B66.0
      Chinese B66.1
      due to clonorchiasis B66.1
      oriental B66.1
    lancet B66.2
    lung (oriental) B66.4
    sheep liver B66.3
    specified type NEC B66.8
  fly larvae — *see* Myiasis
  Gasterophilus (intestinalis) — *see* Myiasis
  Gastrodiscoides hominis B66.8
  Giardia lamblia A07.1
  Gnathostoma (spinigerum) B83.1
  Gongylonema B83.8
  guinea worm B72
  helminth B83.9
    angiostrongyliasis B83.2
      intestinal B81.3
    gnathostomiasis B83.1
    hirudiniasis, internal B83.4
    intestinal B82.0
      angiostrongyliasis B81.3
      anisakiasis B81.0
      ascariasis — *see* Ascariasis
      capillariasis B81.1
      cysticercosis — *see* Cysticercosis
      diphyllobothriasis — *see* Infestation, diphyllobothriasis
      dracunculiasis B72
      echinococcus — *see* Echinococcosis
      enterobiasis B80
      filariasis - — *see* Infestation, filarial
      fluke — *see* Infestation, fluke
      hookworm — *see* Infestation, hookworm

Inflammation, inflamed, inflammatory (with exudation) - *continued*
due to device, implant or graft - *continued*
catheter - *continued*
urinary - *continued*
Hopkins T83.518
ileostomy T83.518
nephrostomy T83.512
specified NEC T83.518
urethral indwelling T83.511
urostomy T83.518
electronic (electrode) (pulse generator) (stimulator)
bone T84.7
cardiac T82.7
nervous system T85.738
brain T85.731
cranial nerve T85.732
gastric nerve T85.732
neurostimulator generator T85.734
peripheral nerve T85.732
sacral nerve T85.732
spinal cord T85.733
vagal nerve T85.732
urinary T83.590
fixation, internal (orthopedic) NEC — *see* Complication, fixation device, infection
gastrointestinal (bile duct) (esophagus) T85.79
neurostimulator electrode (lead) T85.732
genital NEC T83.69
heart NEC T82.7
valve (prosthesis) T82.6
graft T82.7
joint prosthesis — *see* Complication, joint prosthesis, infection
ocular (corneal graft) (orbital implant) NEC T85.79
orthopedic NEC T84.7
penile (cylinder) (pump) (resevoir) T83.61
specified NEC T85.79
testicular T83.62
urinary NEC T83.598
ileal conduit stent T83.593
implanted neurostimulation T83.590
implanted sphincter T83.591
indwelling ureteral stent T83.592
nephroureteral stent T83.593
specified stent NEC T83.593
vascular NEC T82.7
ventricular intracranial (communicating) shunt T85.730
duodenum K29.80
with bleeding K29.81
dura mater — *see* Meningitis
ear (middle) — *see also* Otitis, media
external — *see* Otitis, externa
inner — *see* subcategory H83.0
epididymis — *see* Epididymitis
esophagus K20.9
ethmoidal (sinus) (chronic) — *see* Sinusitis, ethmoidal
eustachian tube (catarrhal) — *see* Salpingitis, eustachian
eyelid H01.9
abscess — *see* Abscess, eyelid
blepharitis — *see* Blepharitis
chalazion — *see* Chalazion
dermatosis (noninfectious) — *see* Dermatosis, eyelid
hordeolum — *see* Hordeolum
specified NEC H01.8
fallopian tube — *see* Salpingo-oophoritis
fascia — *see* Myositis
follicular, pharynx J31.2
frontal (sinus) (chronic) — *see* Sinusitis, frontal
gallbladder — *see* Cholecystitis
gastric — *see* Gastritis
gastrointestinal — *see* Enteritis
genital organ (internal) (diffuse)
female — *see* Disease, pelvis, inflammatory
male N49.9
multiple sites N49.8
specified NEC N49.8
gland (lymph) — *see* Lymphadenitis
glottis — *see* Laryngitis
granular, pharynx J31.2
gum K05.10
nonplaque induced K05.11
plaque induced K05.10
heart — *see* Carditis
hepatic duct — *see* Cholangitis
ileoanal (internal) pouch K91.850
ileum — *see also* Enteritis
regional or terminal — *see* Enteritis, regional

Inflammation, inflamed, inflammatory (with exudation) - *continued*
intestine (any part) — *see* Enteritis
intestinal pouch K91.850
jaw (acute) (bone) (chronic) (lower) (suppurative) (upper) M27.2
joint NEC — *see* Arthritis
sacroiliac M46.1
kidney — *see* Nephritis
knee (joint) M13.169
tuberculous A18.02
labium (majus) (minus) — *see* Vulvitis
lacrimal
gland — *see* Dacryoadenitis
passages (duct) (sac) — *see also* Dacryocystitis
canaliculitis — *see* Canaliculitis, lacrimal
larynx — *see* Laryngitis
leg NOS L08.9
lip K13.0
liver (capsule) — *see also* Hepatitis
chronic K73.9
suppurative K75.0
lung (acute) — *see also* Pneumonia
chronic J98.4
lymph gland or node — *see* Lymphadenitis
lymphatic vessel — *see* Lymphangitis
maxilla, maxillary M27.2
sinus (chronic) — *see* Sinusitis, maxillary
membranes of brain or spinal cord — *see* Meningitis
meninges — *see* Meningitis
mouth K12.1
muscle — *see* Myositis
myocardium — *see* Myocarditis
nasal sinus (chronic) — *see* Sinusitis
nasopharynx — *see* Nasopharyngitis
navel L08.82
nerve NEC — *see* Neuralgia
nipple N61.0
puerperal, postpartum or gestational — *see* Infection, nipple
nose — *see* Rhinitis
oculomotor (nerve) — *see* Strabismus, paralytic, third nerve
optic nerve — *see* Neuritis, optic
orbit (chronic) H05.10
acute H05.00
abscess — *see* Abscess, orbit
cellulitis — *see* Cellulitis, orbit
osteomyelitis — *see* Osteomyelitis, orbit
periostitis — *see* Periostitis, orbital
tenonitis — *see* Tenonitis, eye
granuloma — *see* Granuloma, orbit
myositis — *see* Myositis, orbital
ovary — *see* Salpingo-oophoritis
oviduct — *see* Salpingo-oophoritis
pancreas (acute) — *see* Pancreatitis
parametrium N73.0
parotid region L08.9
pelvis, female — *see* Disease, pelvis, inflammatory
penis (corpora cavernosa) N48.29
perianal K62.89
pericardium — *see* Pericarditis
perineum (female) (male) L08.9
perirectal K62.89
peritoneum — *see* Peritonitis
periuterine — *see* Disease, pelvis, inflammatory
perivesical — *see* Cystitis
petrous bone (acute) (chronic) — *see* Petrositis
pharynx (acute) — *see* Pharyngitis
pia mater — *see* Meningitis
pleura — *see* Pleurisy
polyp, colon — *see also* Polyp, colon, inflammatory K51.40
prostate — *see also* Prostatitis
specified type NEC N41.8
rectosigmoid — *see* Rectosigmoiditis
rectum — *see also* Proctitis K62.89
respiratory, upper — *see also* Infection, respiratory, upper J06.9
acute, due to radiation J70.0
chronic, due to external agent — *see* condition, respiratory, chronic, due to
due to
chemicals, gases, fumes or vapors (inhalation) J68.2
radiation J70.1
retina — *see* Chorioretinitis
retrocecal — *see* Appendicitis
retroperitoneal — *see* Peritonitis
salivary duct or gland (any) (suppurative) — *see* Sialoadenitis
scorbutic, alveoli, teeth E54
scrotum N49.2

Inflammation, inflamed, inflammatory (with exudation) - *continued*
seminal vesicle — *see* Vesiculitis
sigmoid — *see* Enteritis
sinus — *see* Sinusitis
Skene's duct or gland — *see* Urethritis
skin L08.9
spermatic cord N49.1
sphenoidal (sinus) — *see* Sinusitis, sphenoidal
spinal
cord — *see* Encephalitis
membrane — *see* Meningitis
nerve — *see* Disorder, nerve
spine — *see* Spondylopathy, inflammatory
spleen (capsule) D73.89
stomach — *see* Gastritis
subcutaneous tissue L08.9
suprarenal (gland) E27.8
synovial — *see* Tenosynovitis
tendon (sheath) NEC — *see* Tenosynovitis
testis — *see* Orchitis
throat (acute) — *see* Pharyngitis
thymus (gland) E32.8
thyroid (gland) — *see* Thyroiditis
tongue K14.0
tonsil — *see* Tonsillitis
trachea — *see* Tracheitis
trochlear (nerve) — *see* Strabismus, paralytic, fourth nerve
tubal — *see* Salpingo-oophoritis
tuberculous NEC — *see* Tuberculosis
tubo-ovarian — *see* Salpingo-oophoritis
tunica vaginalis N49.1
tympanic membrane — *see* Tympanitis
umbilicus, umbilical L08.82
uterine ligament — *see* Disease, pelvis, inflammatory
uterus (catarrhal) — *see* Endometritis
uveal tract (anterior) NOS — *see also* Iridocyclitis
posterior — *see* Chorioretinitis
vagina — *see* Vaginitis
vas deferens N49.1
vein — *see also* Phlebitis
intracranial or intraspinal (septic) G08
thrombotic I80.9
leg — *see* Phlebitis, leg
lower extremity — *see* Phlebitis, leg
vocal cord J38.3
vulva — *see* Vulvitis
Wharton's duct (suppurative) — *see* Sialoadenitis
Inflation, lung, imperfect (newborn) — *see* Atelectasis
Influenza (bronchial) (epidemic) (respiratory (upper)) (unidentified influenza virus) (unidentified influenza virus) J11.1
with
digestive manifestations J11.2
encephalopathy J11.81
enteritis J11.2
gastroenteritis J11.2
gastrointestinal manifestations J11.2
laryngitis J11.1
myocarditis J11.82
otitis media J11.83
pharyngitis J11.1
pneumonia J11.00
specified type J11.08
respiratory manifestations NEC J11.1
specified manifestation NEC J11.89
A/H5N1 — *see also* Influenza, due to, identified novel influenza A virus J09.X2
avian — *see also* Influenza, due to, identified novel influenza A virus J09.X2
bird — *see also* Influenza, due to, identified novel influenza A virus J09.X2
novel (2009) H1N1 influenza — *see also* Influenza, due to, identified influenza virus NEC J10.1
novel influenza A/H1N1 — *see also* Influenza, due to, identified influenza virus NEC J10.1
due to
avian — *see also* Influenza, due to, identified novel influenza A virus J09.X2
identified influenza virus NEC J10.1
with
digestive manifestations J10.2
encephalopathy J10.81
enteritis J10.2
gastroenteritis J10.2
gastrointestinal manifestations J10.2
laryngitis J10.1
myocarditis J10.82
otitis media J10.83
pharyngitis J10.1

Influenza (bronchial) (epidemic) (respiratory (upper)) (unidentified influenza virus) (unidentified influenza virus) - *continued*
- due to - *continued*
  - identified influenza virus NEC - *continued*
    - with - *continued*
      - pneumonia (unspecified type) J10.00
        - with same identified influenza virus J10.01
        - specified type NEC J10.08
      - respiratory manifestations NEC J10.1
      - specified manifestation NEC J10.89
  - identified novel influenza A virus J09.X2
    - with
      - digestive manifestations J09.X3
      - encephalopathy J09.X9
      - enteritis J09.X3
      - gastroenteritis J09.X3
      - gastrointestinal manifestations J09.X3
      - laryngitis J09.X2
      - myocarditis J09.X9
      - otitis media J09.X9
      - pharyngitis J09.X2
      - pneumonia J09.X1
      - respiratory manifestations NEC J09.X2
      - specified manifestation NEC J09.X9
      - upper respiratory symptoms J09.X2
- of other animal origin, not bird or swine — *see also* Influenza, due to, identified novel influenza A virus J09.X2
- swine (viruses that normally cause infections in pigs) — *see also* Influenza, due to, identified novel influenza A virus J09.X2

Influenzal — *see* Influenza

Influenza-like disease — *see* Influenza

Infraction, Freiberg's (metatarsal head) — *see* Osteochondrosis, juvenile, metatarsus

Infraeruption of tooth (teeth) M26.34

Infusion complication, misadventure, or reaction — *see* Complications, infusion

Ingestion
- chemical — *see* Table of Drugs and Chemicals, by substance, poisoning
- drug or medicament
  - correct substance properly administered — *see* Table of Drugs and Chemicals, by drug, adverse effect
  - overdose or wrong substance given or taken — *see* Table of Drugs and Chemicals, by drug, poisoning
- foreign body — *see* Foreign body, alimentary tract
- tularemia A21.3

Ingrowing
- hair (beard) L73.1
- nail (finger) (toe) L60.0

Inguinal — *see also* condition
- testicle Q53.9
  - bilateral Q53.212
  - unilateral Q53.112

Inhalant-induced
- anxiety disorder F18.980
- depressive disorder F18.94
- major neurocognitive disorder F18.97
- mild neurocognitive disorder F18.988
- psychotic disorder F18.959

Inhalation
- anthrax A22.1
- flame T27.3
- food or foreign body — *see* Foreign body, by site
- gases, fumes, or vapors NEC T59.9-
  - specified agent — *see* Table of Drugs and Chemicals, by substance
- liquid or vomitus — *see* Asphyxia
- meconium (newborn) P24.00
  - with
    - pneumonia (pneumonitis) P24.01
    - with respiratory symptoms P24.01
- mucus — *see* Asphyxia, mucus
- oil or gasoline (causing suffocation) — *see* Foreign body, by site
- smoke J70.5
  - due to chemicals, gases, fumes and vapors J68.9
- steam — *see* Toxicity, vapors
- stomach contents or secretions — *see* Foreign body, by site
  - due to anesthesia (general) (local) or other sedation T88.59
    - in labor and delivery O74.0
    - in pregnancy O29.01-
    - postpartum, puerperal O89.01

Inhibition, orgasm
- female F52.31
- male F52.32

Inhibitor, systemic lupus erythematosus (presence of) D68.62

Iniencephalus, iniencephaly Q00.2

Injection, traumatic jet (air) (industrial) (water) (paint or dye) T70.4

Injury — *see also* specified injury type T14.90
- abdomen, abdominal S39.91
  - blood vessel — *see* Injury, blood vessel, abdomen
  - cavity — *see* Injury, intra-abdominal
  - contusion S30.1
  - internal — *see* Injury, intra-abdominal
  - intra-abdominal organ — *see* Injury, intra-abdominal
  - nerve — *see* Injury, nerve, abdomen
  - open — *see* Wound, open, abdomen
  - specified NEC S39.81
  - superficial — *see* Injury, superficial, abdomen
- Achilles tendon S86.00-
  - laceration S86.02-
  - specified type NEC S86.09-
  - strain S86.01-
- acoustic, resulting in deafness — *see* Injury, nerve, acoustic
- adrenal (gland) S37.819
  - contusion S37.812
  - laceration S37.813
  - specified type NEC S37.818
- alveolar (process) S09.93
- ankle S99.91-
  - contusion — *see* Contusion, ankle
  - dislocation — *see* Dislocation, ankle
  - fracture — *see* Fracture, ankle
  - nerve — *see* Injury, nerve, ankle
  - open — *see* Wound, open, ankle
  - specified type NEC S99.81-
  - sprain — *see* Sprain, ankle
  - superficial — *see* Injury, superficial, ankle
- anterior chamber, eye — *see* Injury, eye, specified site NEC
- anus — *see* Injury, abdomen
- aorta (thoracic) S25.00
  - abdominal S35.00
    - laceration (minor) (superficial) S35.01
      - major S35.02
    - specified type NEC S35.09
  - laceration (minor) (superficial) S25.01
    - major S25.02
  - specified type NEC S25.09
- arm (upper) S49.9-
  - blood vessel — *see* Injury, blood vessel, arm
  - contusion — *see* Contusion, arm, upper
  - fracture — *see* Fracture, humerus
  - lower — *see* Injury, forearm
  - muscle — *see* Injury, muscle, shoulder
  - nerve — *see* Injury, nerve, arm
  - open — *see* Wound, open, arm
  - specified type NEC S49.8-
  - superficial — *see* Injury, superficial, arm
- artery (complicating trauma) — *see also* Injury, blood vessel, by site
  - cerebral or meningeal — *see* Injury, intracranial
- auditory canal (external) (meatus) S09.91
- auricle, auris, ear S09.91
- axilla — *see* Injury, shoulder
- back — *see* Injury, back, lower
- bile duct S36.13
- birth — *see also* Birth, injury P15.9
- bladder (sphincter) S37.20
  - at delivery O71.5
  - contusion S37.22
  - laceration S37.23
  - obstetrical trauma O71.5
  - specified type NEC S37.29
- blast (air) (hydraulic) (immersion) (underwater) NEC T14.8
  - acoustic nerve trauma — *see* Injury, nerve, acoustic
  - bladder — *see* Injury, bladder
  - brain — *see* Concussion
  - colon — *see* Injury, intestine, large, blast injury
  - ear (primary) S09.31-
    - secondary S09.39-
  - generalized T70.8
  - lung — *see* Injury, intrathoracic, lung, blast injury
  - multiple body organs T70.8
  - peritoneum S36.81
  - rectum S36.61
  - retroperitoneum S36.898
  - small intestine S36.419
    - duodenum S36.410
    - specified site NEC S36.418
  - specified
    - intra-abdominal organ NEC S36.898

Injury - *continued*
- blast (air) (hydraulic) (immersion) (underwater) NEC - *continued*
  - specified - *continued*
    - pelvic organ NEC S37.899
- blood vessel NEC T14.8
  - abdomen S35.9-
    - aorta — *see* Injury, aorta, abdominal
    - celiac artery — *see* Injury, blood vessel, celiac artery
    - iliac vessel — *see* Injury, blood vessel, iliac
    - laceration S35.91
    - mesenteric vessel — *see* Injury, mesenteric
    - portal vein — *see* Injury, blood vessel, portal vein
    - renal vessel — *see* Injury, blood vessel, renal
    - specified vessel NEC S35.8X-
    - splenic vessel — *see* Injury, blood vessel, splenic
    - vena cava — *see* Injury, vena cava, inferior
  - ankle — *see* Injury, blood vessel, foot
  - aorta (abdominal) (thoracic) — *see* Injury, aorta
  - arm (upper) NEC S45.90-
    - forearm — *see* Injury, blood vessel, forearm
    - laceration S45.91-
    - specified
      - site NEC S45.80-
        - laceration S45.81-
        - specified type NEC S45.89-
      - type NEC S45.99-
    - superficial vein S45.30-
      - laceration S45.31-
      - specified type NEC S45.39-
  - axillary
    - artery S45.00-
      - laceration S45.01-
      - specified type NEC S45.09-
    - vein S45.20-
      - laceration S45.21-
      - specified type NEC S45.29-
  - azygos vein — *see* Injury, blood vessel, thoracic, specified site NEC
  - brachial
    - artery S45.10-
      - laceration S45.11-
      - specified type NEC S45.19-
    - vein S45.20-
      - laceration S45.219
      - specified type NEC S45.29-
  - carotid artery (common) (external) (internal, extracranial) S15.00-
    - internal, intracranial S06.8-
    - laceration (minor) (superficial) S15.01-
      - major S15.02-
    - specified type NEC S15.09-
  - celiac artery S35.219
    - branch S35.299
      - laceration (minor) (superficial) S35.291
        - major S35.292
      - specified NEC S35.298
    - laceration (minor) (superficial) S35.211
      - major S35.212
    - specified type NEC S35.218
  - cerebral — *see* Injury, intracranial
  - deep plantar — *see* Injury, blood vessel, plantar artery
  - digital (hand) — *see* Injury, blood vessel, finger
  - dorsal
    - artery (foot) S95.00-
      - laceration S95.01-
      - specified type NEC S95.09-
    - vein (foot) S95.20-
      - laceration S95.21-
      - specified type NEC S95.29-
  - due to accidental laceration during procedure — *see* Laceration, accidental complicating surgery
  - extremity — *see* Injury, blood vessel, limb
  - femoral
    - artery (common) (superficial) S75.00-
      - laceration (minor) (superficial) S75.01-
        - major S75.02-
      - specified type NEC S75.09-
    - vein (hip level) (thigh level) S75.10-
      - laceration (minor) (superficial) S75.11-
        - major S75.12-
      - specified type NEC S75.19-
  - finger S65.50-
    - index S65.50-
      - laceration S65.51-
      - specified type NEC S65.59-
    - laceration S65.51-
    - little S65.50-
      - laceration S65.51-
      - specified type NEC S65.59-

- **Injury** - *continued*
  - blood vessel NEC - *continued*
    - finger - *continued*
      - middle S65.50-
        - laceration S65.51-
        - specified type NEC S65.59-
      - specified type NEC S65.59-
      - thumb — *see* Injury, blood vessel, thumb
    - foot S95.90-
      - dorsal
        - artery — *see* Injury, blood vessel, dorsal, artery
        - vein — *see* Injury, blood vessel, dorsal, vein
      - laceration S95.91-
      - plantar artery — *see* Injury, blood vessel, plantar artery
      - specified
        - site NEC S95.80-
          - laceration S95.81-
          - specified type NEC S95.89-
        - specified type NEC S95.99-
    - forearm S55.90-
      - laceration S55.91-
      - radial artery — *see* Injury, blood vessel, radial artery
      - specified
        - site NEC S55.80-
          - laceration S55.81-
          - specified type NEC S55.89-
        - type NEC S55.99-
      - ulnar artery — *see* Injury, blood vessel, ulnar artery
      - vein S55.20-
        - laceration S55.21-
        - specified type NEC S55.29-
    - gastric
      - artery — *see* Injury, mesenteric, artery, branch
      - vein — *see* Injury, blood vessel, abdomen
    - gastroduodenal artery — *see* Injury, mesenteric, artery, branch
    - greater saphenous vein (lower leg level) S85.30-
      - hip (and thigh) level S75.20-
        - laceration (minor) (superficial) S75.21-
          - major S75.22-
        - specified type NEC S75.29-
      - laceration S85.31-
      - specified type NEC S85.39-
    - hand (level) S65.90-
      - finger — *see* Injury, blood vessel, finger
      - laceration S65.91-
      - palmar arch — *see* Injury, blood vessel, palmar arch
      - radial artery — *see* Injury, blood vessel, radial artery, hand
      - specified
        - site NEC S65.80-
          - laceration S65.81-
          - specified type NEC S65.89-
        - type NEC S65.99-
      - thumb — *see* Injury, blood vessel, thumb
      - ulnar artery — *see* Injury, blood vessel, ulnar artery, hand
    - head S09.0
      - intracranial — *see* Injury, intracranial
      - multiple S09.0
    - hepatic
      - artery — *see* Injury, mesenteric, artery
      - vein — *see* Injury, vena cava, inferior
    - hip S75.90-
      - femoral artery — *see* Injury, blood vessel, femoral, artery
      - femoral vein — *see* Injury, blood vessel, femoral, vein
      - greater saphenous vein — *see* Injury, blood vessel, greater saphenous, hip level
      - laceration S75.91-
      - specified
        - site NEC S75.80-
          - laceration S75.81-
          - specified type NEC S75.89-
        - type NEC S75.99-
    - hypogastric (artery) (vein) — *see* Injury, blood vessel, iliac
    - iliac S35.5-
      - artery S35.51-
      - specified vessel NEC S35.5-
      - uterine vessel — *see* Injury, blood vessel, uterine
      - vein S35.51-
    - innominate — *see* Injury, blood vessel, thoracic, innominate
    - intercostal (artery) (vein) — *see* Injury, blood vessel, thoracic, intercostal
    - jugular vein (external) S15.20-
      - internal S15.30-

- **Injury** - *continued*
  - blood vessel NEC - *continued*
    - jugular vein (external) - *continued*
      - internal - *continued*
        - laceration (minor) (superficial) S15.31-
          - major S15.32-
        - specified type NEC S15.39-
      - laceration (minor) (superficial) S15.21-
        - major S15.22-
      - specified type NEC S15.29-
    - leg (level) (lower) S85.90-
      - greater saphenous — *see* Injury, blood vessel, greater saphenous
      - laceration S85.91-
      - lesser saphenous — *see* Injury, blood vessel, lesser saphenous
      - peroneal artery — *see* Injury, blood vessel, peroneal artery
      - popliteal
        - artery — *see* Injury, blood vessel, popliteal, artery
        - vein — *see* Injury, blood vessel, popliteal, vein
      - specified
        - site NEC S85.80-
          - laceration S85.81-
          - specified type NEC S85.89-
        - type NEC S85.99-
      - thigh — *see* Injury, blood vessel, hip
      - tibial artery — *see* Injury, blood vessel, tibial artery
    - lesser saphenous vein (lower leg level) S85.40-
      - laceration S85.41-
      - specified type NEC S85.49-
    - limb
      - lower — *see* Injury, blood vessel, leg
      - upper — *see* Injury, blood vessel, arm
    - lower back — *see* Injury, blood vessel, abdomen
      - specified NEC — *see* Injury, blood vessel, abdomen, specified, site NEC
    - mammary (artery) (vein) — *see* Injury, blood vessel, thoracic, specified site NEC
    - mesenteric (inferior) (superior)
      - artery — *see* Injury, mesenteric, artery
      - vein — *see* Injury, mesenteric, vein
    - neck S15.9
      - specified site NEC S15.8
    - ovarian (artery) (vein) — *see* subcategory S35.8
    - palmar arch (superficial) S65.20-
      - deep S65.30-
        - laceration S65.31-
        - specified type NEC S65.39-
      - laceration S65.21-
      - specified type NEC S65.29-
    - pelvis — *see* Injury, blood vessel, abdomen
      - specified NEC — *see* Injury, blood vessel, abdomen, specified, site NEC
    - peroneal artery S85.20-
      - laceration S85.21-
      - specified type NEC S85.29-
    - plantar artery (deep) (foot) S95.10-
      - laceration S95.11-
      - specified type NEC S95.19-
    - popliteal
      - artery S85.00-
        - laceration S85.01-
        - specified type NEC S85.09-
      - vein S85.50-
        - laceration S85.51-
        - specified type NEC S85.59-
    - portal vein S35.319
      - laceration S35.311
      - specified type NEC S35.318
    - precerebral — *see* Injury, blood vessel, neck
    - pulmonary (artery) (vein) — *see* Injury, blood vessel, thoracic, pulmonary
    - radial artery (forearm level) S55.10-
      - hand and wrist (level) S65.10-
        - laceration S65.11-
        - specified type NEC S65.19-
      - laceration S55.11-
      - specified type NEC S55.19-
    - renal
      - artery S35.40-
        - laceration S35.41-
        - specified NEC S35.49-
      - vein S35.40-
        - laceration S35.41-
        - specified NEC S35.49-
    - saphenous vein (greater) (lower leg level) — *see* Injury, blood vessel, greater saphenous
      - hip and thigh level — *see* Injury, blood vessel, greater saphenous, hip level

- **Injury** - *continued*
  - blood vessel NEC - *continued*
    - saphenous vein (greater) (lower leg level) - *continued*
      - lesser — *see* Injury, blood vessel, lesser saphenous
    - shoulder
      - specified NEC — *see* Injury, blood vessel, arm, specified site NEC
      - superficial vein — *see* Injury, blood vessel, arm, superficial vein
    - specified NEC T14.8
    - splenic
      - artery — *see* Injury, blood vessel, celiac artery, branch
      - vein S35.329
        - laceration S35.321
        - specified NEC S35.328
    - subclavian — *see* Injury, blood vessel, thoracic, innominate
    - thigh — *see* Injury, blood vessel, hip
    - thoracic S25.90
      - aorta S25.00
        - laceration (minor) (superficial) S25.01
          - major S25.02
        - specified type NEC S25.09
      - azygos vein — *see* Injury, blood vessel, thoracic, specified, site NEC
      - innominate
        - artery S25.10-
          - laceration (minor) (superficial) S25.11-
            - major S25.12-
          - specified type NEC S25.19-
        - vein S25.30-
          - laceration (minor) (superficial) S25.31-
            - major S25.32-
          - specified type NEC S25.39-
      - intercostal S25.50-
        - laceration S25.51-
        - specified type NEC S25.59-
      - laceration S25.91
      - mammary vessel — *see* Injury, blood vessel, thoracic, specified, site NEC
      - pulmonary S25.40-
        - laceration (minor) (superficial) S25.41-
          - major S25.42-
        - specified type NEC S25.49-
      - specified
        - site NEC S25.80-
          - laceration S25.81-
          - specified type NEC S25.89-
        - type NEC S25.99
      - subclavian — *see* Injury, blood vessel, thoracic, innominate
      - vena cava (superior) S25.20
        - laceration (minor) (superficial) S25.21
          - major S25.22
        - specified type NEC S25.29
    - thumb S65.40-
      - laceration S65.41-
      - specified type NEC S65.49-
    - tibial artery S85.10-
      - anterior S85.13-
        - laceration S85.14-
        - specified injury NEC S85.15-
      - laceration S85.11-
      - posterior S85.16-
        - laceration S85.17-
        - specified injury NEC S85.18-
      - specified injury NEC S85.12-
    - ulnar artery (forearm level) S55.00-
      - hand and wrist (level) S65.00-
        - laceration S65.01-
        - specified type NEC S65.09-
      - laceration S55.01-
      - specified type NEC S55.09-
    - upper arm (level) — *see* Injury, blood vessel, arm
      - superficial vein — *see* Injury, blood vessel, arm, superficial vein
    - uterine S35.5-
      - artery S35.53-
      - vein S35.53-
    - vena cava — *see* Injury, vena cava
    - vertebral artery S15.10-
      - laceration (minor) (superficial) S15.11-
        - major S15.12-
      - specified type NEC S15.19-
    - wrist (level) — *see* Injury, blood vessel, hand
  - brachial plexus S14.3
    - newborn P14.3
  - brain (traumatic) S06.9-
    - diffuse (axonal) S06.2X-
    - focal S06.30-

Injury - *continued*
 hip - *continued*
 open — *see* Wound, open, hip
 sprain — *see* Sprain, hip
 superficial — *see* Injury, superficial, hip
 specified NEC S79.81-
 hymen S39.94
 hypogastric
 blood vessel — *see* Injury, blood vessel, iliac
 plexus — *see* Injury, nerve, lumbosacral,
 sympathetic
 ileum — *see* Injury, intestine, small
 iliac region S39.91
 instrumental (during surgery) — *see* Laceration,
 accidental complicating surgery
 birth injury — *see* Birth, injury
 nonsurgical — *see* Injury, by site
 obstetrical O71.9
 bladder O71.5
 cervix O71.3
 high vaginal O71.4
 perineal NOS O70.9
 urethra O71.5
 uterus O71.5
 with rupture or perforation O71.1
 internal T14.8
 aorta — *see* Injury, aorta
 bladder (sphincter) — *see* Injury, bladder
 with
 ectopic or molar pregnancy O08.6
 following ectopic or molar pregnancy O08.6
 obstetrical trauma O71.5
 bronchus, bronchi — *see* Injury, intrathoracic,
 bronchus
 cecum — *see* Injury, intestine, large
 cervix (uteri) — *see also* Injury, uterus
 with ectopic or molar pregnancy O08.6
 following ectopic or molar pregnancy O08.6
 obstetrical trauma O71.3
 chest — *see* Injury, intrathoracic
 gastrointestinal tract — *see* Injury, intra-abdominal
 heart — *see* Injury, heart
 intestine NEC — *see* Injury, intestine
 intrauterine — *see* Injury, uterus
 mesentery — *see* Injury, intra-abdominal,
 specified, site NEC
 pelvis, pelvic (organ) S37.90
 following ectopic or molar pregnancy
 (subsequent episode) O08.6
 obstetrical trauma NEC O71.5
 rupture or perforation O71.1
 specified NEC S39.83
 rectum — *see* Injury, intestine, large, rectum
 stomach — *see* Injury, stomach
 ureter — *see* Injury, ureter
 urethra (sphincter) following ectopic or molar
 pregnancy O08.6
 uterus — *see* Injury, uterus
 interscapular area — *see* Injury, thorax
 intestine
 large S36.509
 ascending (right) S36.500
 blast injury (primary) S36.510
 secondary S36.590
 contusion S36.520
 laceration S36.530
 specified type NEC S36.590
 blast injury (primary) S36.519
 ascending (right) S36.510
 descending (left) S36.512
 rectum S36.61
 sigmoid S36.513
 specified site NEC S36.518
 transverse S36.511
 contusion S36.529
 ascending (right) S36.520
 descending (left) S36.522
 rectum S36.62
 sigmoid S36.523
 specified site NEC S36.528
 transverse S36.521
 descending (left) S36.502
 blast injury (primary) S36.512
 secondary S36.592
 contusion S36.522
 laceration S36.532
 specified type NEC S36.592
 laceration S36.539
 ascending (right) S36.530
 descending (left) S36.532
 rectum S36.63
 sigmoid S36.533
 specified site NEC S36.538

Injury - *continued*
rectum S36.60
 blast injury (primary) S36.61
 secondary S36.69
 contusion S36.62
 laceration S36.63
 specified type NEC S36.69
 sigmoid S36.503
 blast injury (primary) S36.513
 secondary S36.593
 contusion S36.523
 laceration S36.533
 specified type NEC S36.593
 specified
 site NEC S36.508
 blast injury (primary) S36.518
 secondary S36.598
 contusion S36.528
 laceration S36.538
 specified type NEC S36.598
 type NEC S36.599
 ascending (right) S36.590
 descending (left) S36.592
 rectum S36.69
 sigmoid S36.593
 specified site NEC S36.598
 transverse S36.591
 transverse S36.501
 blast injury (primary) S36.511
 secondary S36.591
 contusion S36.521
 laceration S36.531
 specified type NEC S36.591
 small S36.409
 blast injury (primary) S36.419
 duodenum S36.410
 secondary S36.499
 duodenum S36.490
 specified site NEC S36.498
 specified site NEC S36.418
 contusion S36.429
 duodenum S36.420
 specified site NEC S36.428
 duodenum S36.400
 blast injury (primary) S36.410
 secondary S36.490
 contusion S36.420
 laceration S36.430
 specified NEC S36.490
 laceration S36.439
 duodenum S36.430
 specified site NEC S36.438
 specified
 type NEC S36.499
 duodenum S36.490
 specified site NEC S36.498
 site NEC S36.408
 intra-abdominal S36.90
 adrenal gland — *see* Injury, adrenal gland
 bladder — *see* Injury, bladder
 colon — *see* Injury, intestine, large
 contusion S36.92
 fallopian tube — *see* Injury, fallopian tube
 gallbladder — *see* Injury, gallbladder
 intestine — *see* Injury, intestine
 laceration S36.93
 liver — *see* Injury, liver
 kidney — *see* Injury, kidney
 ovary — *see* Injury, ovary
 pancreas — *see* Injury, pancreas
 pelvic NOS S37.90
 peritoneum — *see* Injury, intra-abdominal,
 specified, site NEC
 prostate — *see* Injury, prostate
 rectum — *see* Injury, intestine, large, rectum
 retroperitoneum — *see* Injury, intra-abdominal,
 specified, site NEC
 seminal vesicle — *see* Injury, pelvis, organ,
 specified site NEC
 small intestine — *see* Injury, intestine, small
 specified
 site NEC S36.899
 contusion S36.892
 laceration S36.893
 specified type NEC S36.898
 type NEC S36.99
 pelvic S37.90
type NEC S37.99
 spleen — *see* Injury, spleen
 stomach — *see* Injury, stomach
 ureter — *see* Injury, ureter
 urethra — *see* Injury, urethra
 uterus — *see* Injury, uterus
 vas deferens — *see* Injury, pelvis, organ, specified
intracranial, focal
 cerebral edema, traumatic S06.1X-
 diffuse S06.1X-
 focal S06.1X-
 diffuse (axonal) S06.2X-
 epidural hemorrhage (traumatic) S06.4X-
 focal brain injury S06.30-
left side S06.35-
 right side S06.34-
 subarachnoid hemorrhage, traumatic S06.6X-
intrathoracic S27.9
 bronchus S27.409
 bilateral S27.402
 blast injury (primary) S27.419
 bilateral S27.412
 secondary — *see* Injury, intrathoracic, bronchus,
 specified type NEC
 unilateral S27.411
 contusion S27.429
 bilateral S27.422
 unilateral S27.421
 laceration S27.439
 bilateral S27.432
 unilateral S27.431
 specified type NEC S27.499
 bilateral S27.492
 unilateral S27.491
 unilateral S27.401
 diaphragm S27.809
 contusion S27.802
 laceration S27.803
 specified type NEC S27.808
 esophagus (thoracic) S27.819
 contusion S27.812
 laceration S27.813
 specified type NEC S27.818
 heart — *see* Injury, heart
 hemopneumothorax S27.2
 hemothorax S27.1
 lung S27.309
 aspiration J69.0
 bilateral S27.302
 blast injury (primary) S27.319
 bilateral S27.312
 secondary — *see* Injury, intrathoracic, lung,
 specified type NEC
 unilateral S27.311
 contusion S27.329
 bilateral S27.322
 unilateral S27.321
 laceration S27.339
 bilateral S27.332
 unilateral S27.331
 specified type NEC S27.399
 bilateral S27.392
 unilateral S27.391
 unilateral S27.301
 pleura S27.60
 laceration S27.63
 specified type NEC S27.69
 pneumothorax S27.0
 specified organ NEC S27.899
 contusion S27.892
 laceration S27.893
 specified type NEC S27.898

Injury - *continued*
intrathoracic - *continued*
trachea, thoracic - *continued*
contusion S27.52
laceration S27.53
specified type NEC S27.59
iris — *see* Injury, eye, specified site NEC
penetrating — *see* Injury, eyeball, penetrating
jaw S09.93
jejunum — *see* Injury, intestine, small
joint NOS T14.8
old or residual — *see* Disorder, joint, specified type NEC
kidney S37.00-
acute (nontraumatic) N17.9
contusion — *see* Contusion, kidney
laceration — *see* Laceration, kidney
specified NEC S37.09-
knee S89.9-
contusion — *see* Contusion, knee
dislocation — *see* Dislocation, knee
meniscus (lateral) (medial) — *see* Sprain, knee, specified site NEC
old injury or tear — *see* Derangement, knee, meniscus, due to old injury
open — *see* Wound, open, knee
specified NEC S89.8-
sprain — *see* Sprain, knee
superficial — *see* Injury, superficial, knee
labium (majus) (minus) S39.94
labyrinth, ear S09.30-
lacrimal apparatus, duct, gland, or sac — *see* Injury, eye, specified site NEC
larynx NEC S19.81
leg (lower) S89.9-
blood vessel — *see* Injury, blood vessel, leg
contusion — *see* Contusion, leg
fracture — *see* Fracture, leg
muscle — *see* Injury, muscle, leg
nerve — *see* Injury, nerve, leg
open — *see* Wound, open, leg
specified NEC S89.8-
superficial — *see* Injury, superficial, leg
lens, eye — *see* Injury, eye, specified site NEC
penetrating — *see* Injury, eyeball, penetrating
limb NEC T14.8
lip S09.93
liver S36.119
contusion S36.112
laceration S36.113
major (stellate) S36.116
minor S36.114
moderate S36.115
specified NEC S36.118
lower back S39.92
specified NEC S39.82
lumbar, lumbosacral (region) S39.92
plexus — *see* Injury, lumbosacral plexus
lumbosacral plexus S34.4
lung — *see also* Injury, intrathoracic, lung
aspiration J69.0
transfusion-related (TRALI) J95.84
lymphatic thoracic duct — *see* Injury, intrathoracic, specified organ NEC
malar region S09.93
mastoid region S09.90
maxilla S09.93
mediastinum — *see* Injury, intrathoracic, specified organ NEC
membrane, brain — *see* Injury, intracranial
meningeal artery — *see* Injury, intracranial, subdural hemorrhage
meninges (cerebral) — *see* Injury, intracranial
mesenteric
artery
branch S35.299
laceration (minor) (superficial) S35.291
major S35.292
specified NEC S35.298
inferior S35.239
laceration (minor) (superficial) S35.231
major S35.232
specified NEC S35.238
superior S35.229
laceration (minor) (superficial) S35.221
major S35.222
specified NEC S35.228
plexus (inferior) (superior) — *see* Injury, nerve, lumbosacral, sympathetic
vein
inferior S35.349
laceration S35.341
specified NEC S35.348

Injury - *continued*
mesenteric - *continued*
vein - *continued*
superior S35.339
laceration S35.331
specified NEC S35.338
mesentery — *see* Injury, intra-abdominal, specified site NEC
mesosalpinx — *see* Injury, pelvic organ, specified site NEC
middle ear S09.30-
midthoracic region NOS S29.9
mouth S09.93
multiple NOS T07
muscle (and fascia) (and tendon)
abdomen S39.001
laceration S39.021
specified type NEC S39.091
strain S39.011
abductor
thumb, forearm level — *see* Injury, muscle, thumb, abductor
adductor
thigh S76.20-
laceration S76.22-
specified type NEC S76.29-
strain S76.21-
ankle — *see* Injury, muscle, foot
anterior muscle group, at leg level (lower) S86.20-
laceration S86.22-
specified type NEC S86.29-
strain S86.21-
arm (upper) — *see* Injury, muscle, shoulder
biceps (parts NEC) S46.20-
laceration S46.22-
long head S46.10-
laceration S46.12-
strain S46.11-
specified type NEC S46.19-
specified type NEC S46.29-
strain S46.21-
extensor
finger (s) (other than thumb) — *see* Injury, muscle, finger by site, extensor
forearm level, specified NEC — *see* Injury, muscle, forearm, extensor
thumb — *see* Injury, muscle, thumb, extensor
toe (large) (ankle level) (foot level) — *see* Injury, muscle, toe, extensor
finger
extensor (forearm level) S56.40-
hand level S66.309
laceration S66.329
specified type NEC S66.399
strain S66.319
laceration S56.429
specified type NEC S56.499
strain S56.419
flexor (forearm level) S56.10-
hand level S66.109
laceration S66.129
specified type NEC S66.199
strain S66.119
laceration S56.129
specified type NEC S56.199
strain S56.119
intrinsic S66.509
laceration S66.529
specified type NEC S66.599
strain S66.519
index
extensor (forearm level)
hand level S66.308
laceration S66.32-
specified type NEC S66.39-
strain S66.31-
specified type NEC S56.492-
flexor (forearm level)
hand level S66.108
laceration S66.12-
specified type NEC S66.19-
strain S66.11-
specified type NEC S56.19-
strain S56.11-
intrinsic S66.50-
laceration S66.52-
specified type NEC S66.59-
strain S66.51-
little
extensor (forearm level)
hand level S66.30-
laceration S66.32-
specified type NEC S66.39-

Injury - *continued*
muscle (and fascia) (and tendon) - *continued*
finger - *continued*
little - *continued*
extensor (forearm level) - *continued*
hand level - *continued*
strain S66.31-
laceration S56.42-
specified type NEC S56.49-
strain S56.41-
flexor (forearm level)
hand level S66.10-
laceration S66.12-
specified type NEC S66.19-
strain S66.11-
laceration S56.12-
specified type NEC S56.19-
strain S56.11-
intrinsic S66.50-
laceration S66.52-
specified type NEC S66.59-
strain S66.51-
middle
extensor (forearm level)
hand level S66.30-
laceration S66.32-
specified type NEC S66.39-
strain S66.31-
laceration S56.42-
specified type NEC S56.49-
strain S56.41-
flexor (forearm level)
hand level S66.10-
laceration S66.12-
specified type NEC S66.19-
strain S66.11-
laceration S56.12-
specified type NEC S56.19-
strain S56.11-
intrinsic S66.50-
laceration S66.52-
specified type NEC S66.59-
strain S66.51-
ring
extensor (forearm level)
hand level S66.30-
laceration S66.32-
specified type NEC S66.39-
strain S66.31-
laceration S56.42-
specified type NEC S56.49-
strain S56.41-
flexor (forearm level)
hand level S66.10-
laceration S66.12-
specified type NEC S66.19-
strain S66.11-
laceration S56.12-
specified type NEC S56.19-
strain S56.11-
intrinsic S66.50-
laceration S66.52-
specified type NEC S66.59-
strain S66.51-
flexor
finger (s) (other than thumb) — *see* Injury, muscle, finger
forearm level, specified NEC — *see* Injury, muscle, forearm, flexor
thumb — *see* Injury, muscle, thumb, flexor
toe (long) (ankle level) (foot level) — *see* Injury, muscle, toe, flexor
foot S96.90-
intrinsic S96.20-
laceration S96.22-
specified type NEC S96.29-
strain S96.21-
laceration S96.92-
long extensor, toe — *see* Injury, muscle, toe, extensor
long flexor, toe — *see* Injury, muscle, toe, flexor
specified
site NEC S96.80-
laceration S96.82-
specified type NEC S96.89-
strain S96.81-
type NEC S96.99-
strain S96.91-
forearm (level) S56.90-
extensor S56.50-
laceration S56.52-
specified type NEC S56.59-
strain S56.51-

Injury - *continued*
muscle (and fascia) (and tendon) - *continued*
forearm (level) - *continued*
flexor S56.20-
laceration S56.22-
specified type NEC S56.29-
strain S56.21-
laceration S56.92-
specified S56.99-
site NEC S56.80-
laceration S56.82-
strain S56.81-
type NEC S56.89-
strain S56.91-
hand (level) S66.90-
laceration S66.92-
specified
site NEC S66.80-
laceration S66.82-
specified type NEC S66.89-
strain S66.81-
type NEC S66.99-
strain S66.91-
head S09.10
laceration S09.12
specified type NEC S09.19
strain S09.11
hip NEC S76.00-
laceration S76.02-
specified type NEC S76.09-
strain S76.01-
intrinsic
ankle and foot level — *see* Injury, muscle, foot, intrinsic
finger (other than thumb) — *see* Injury, muscle, finger by site, intrinsic
foot (level) — *see* Injury, muscle, foot, intrinsic
thumb — *see* Injury, muscle, thumb, intrinsic
leg (level) (lower) S86.90-
Achilles tendon — *see* Injury, Achilles tendon
anterior muscle group — *see* Injury, muscle, anterior muscle group
laceration S86.92-
peroneal muscle group — *see* Injury, muscle, peroneal muscle group
posterior muscle group — *see* Injury, muscle, posterior muscle group, leg level
specified
site NEC S86.80-
laceration S86.82-
specified type NEC S86.89-
strain S86.81-
type NEC S86.99-
strain S86.91-
long
extensor toe, at ankle and foot level — *see* Injury, muscle, toe, extensor
flexor, toe, at ankle and foot level — *see* Injury, muscle, toe, flexor
head, biceps — *see* Injury, muscle, biceps, long head
lower back S39.002
laceration S39.022
specified type NEC S39.092
strain S39.012
neck (level) S16.9
laceration S16.2
specified type NEC S16.8
strain S16.1
pelvis S39.003
laceration S39.023
specified type NEC S39.093
strain S39.013
peroneal muscle group, at leg level (lower) S86.30-
laceration S86.32-
specified type NEC S86.39-
strain S86.31-
posterior muscle (group)
leg level (lower) S86.10-
laceration S86.12-
specified type NEC S86.19-
strain S86.11-
thigh level S76.30-
laceration S76.32-
specified type NEC S76.39-
strain S76.31-
quadriceps (thigh) S76.10-
laceration S76.12-
specified type NEC S76.19-
strain S76.11-
shoulder S46.90-
laceration S46.92-
rotator cuff — *see* Injury, rotator cuff

Injury - *continued*
muscle (and fascia) (and tendon) - *continued*
shoulder - *continued*
specified site NEC S46.80-
laceration S46.82-
strain S46.81-
specified type NEC S46.89-
strain S46.91-
specified type NEC S46.99-
thigh NEC (level) S76.90-
adductor — *see* Injury, muscle, adductor, thigh
laceration S76.92-
posterior muscle (group) — *see* Injury, muscle, posterior muscle, thigh level
quadriceps — *see* Injury, muscle, quadriceps
specified
site NEC S76.80-
laceration S76.82-
specified type NEC S76.89-
strain S76.81-
type NEC S76.99-
strain S76.91-
thorax (level) S29.009
back wall S29.002
front wall S29.001
laceration S29.029
back wall S29.022
front wall S29.021
specified type NEC S29.099
back wall S29.092
front wall S29.091
strain S29.019
back wall S29.012
front wall S29.011
thumb
abductor (forearm level) S56.30-
laceration S56.32-
specified type NEC S56.39-
strain S56.31-
extensor (forearm level) S56.30-
hand level S66.20-
laceration S66.22-
specified type NEC S66.29-
strain S66.21-
laceration S56.32-
specified type NEC S56.39-
strain S56.31-
flexor (forearm level) S56.00-
hand level S66.00-
laceration S66.02-
specified type NEC S66.09-
strain S66.01-
laceration S56.02-
specified type NEC S56.09-
strain S56.01-
wrist level — *see* Injury, muscle, thumb, flexor, hand level
intrinsic S66.40-
laceration S66.42-
specified type NEC S66.49-
strain S66.41-
toe — *see also* Injury, muscle, foot
extensor, long S96.10-
laceration S96.12-
specified type NEC S96.19-
strain S96.11-
flexor, long S96.00-
laceration S96.02-
specified type NEC S96.09-
strain S96.01-
triceps S46.30-
laceration S46.32-
specified type NEC S46.39-
strain S46.31-
wrist (and hand) level — *see* Injury, muscle, hand
musculocutaneous nerve — *see* Injury, nerve, musculocutaneous
myocardium — *see* Injury, heart
nape — *see* Injury, neck
nasal (septum) (sinus) S09.92
nasopharynx S09.92
neck S19.9
specified NEC S19.80
specified site NEC S19.89
nerve NEC T14.8
abdomen S34.9
peripheral S34.6
specified site NEC S34.8
abducens S04.4-
contusion S04.4-
laceration S04.4-
specified type NEC S04.4-
abducent — *see* Injury, nerve, abducens

Injury - *continued*
nerve NEC - *continued*
accessory S04.7-
contusion S04.7-
laceration S04.7-
specified type NEC S04.7-
acoustic S04.6-
contusion S04.6-
laceration S04.6-
specified type NEC S04.6-
ankle S94.9-
cutaneous sensory S94.3-
specified site NEC — *see* subcategory S94.8
anterior crural, femoral — *see* Injury, nerve, femoral
arm (upper) S44.9-
axillary — *see* Injury, nerve, axillary
cutaneous — *see* Injury, nerve, cutaneous, arm
median — *see* Injury, nerve, median, upper arm
musculocutaneous — *see* Injury, nerve, musculocutaneous
radial — *see* Injury, nerve, radial, upper arm
specified site NEC — *see* subcategory S44.8
ulnar — *see* Injury, nerve, ulnar, arm
auditory — *see* Injury, nerve, acoustic
axillary S44.3-
brachial plexus — *see* Injury, brachial plexus
cervical sympathetic S14.5
cranial S04.9
contusion S04.9
eighth (acoustic or auditory) — *see* Injury, nerve, acoustic
eleventh (accessory) — *see* Injury, nerve, accessory
fifth (trigeminal) — *see* Injury, nerve, trigeminal
first (olfactory) — *see* Injury, nerve, olfactory
fourth (trochlear) — *see* Injury, nerve, trochlear
laceration S04.9
ninth (glossopharyngeal) — *see* Injury, nerve, glossopharyngeal
second (optic) — *see* Injury, nerve, optic
seventh (facial) — *see* Injury, nerve, facial
sixth (abducent) — *see* Injury, nerve, abducens
specified
nerve NEC S04.89-
contusion S04.89-
laceration S04.89-
specified type NEC S04.89-
type NEC S04.9
tenth (pneumogastric or vagus) — *see* Injury, nerve, vagus
third (oculomotor) — *see* Injury, nerve, oculomotor
twelfth (hypoglossal) — *see* Injury, nerve, hypoglossal
cutaneous sensory
ankle (level) S94.3-
arm (upper) (level) S44.5-
foot (level) — *see* Injury, nerve, cutaneous sensory, ankle
forearm (level) S54.3-
hip (level) S74.2-
leg (lower level) S84.2-
shoulder (level) — *see* Injury, nerve, cutaneous sensory, arm
thigh (level) — *see* Injury, nerve, cutaneous sensory, hip
deep peroneal — *see* Injury, nerve, peroneal, foot
digital
finger S64.4-
index S64.49-
little S64.49-
middle S64.49-
ring S64.49-
thumb S64.3-
toe — *see* Injury, nerve, ankle, specified site NEC
eighth cranial (acoustic or auditory) — *see* Injury, nerve, acoustic
eleventh cranial (accessory) — *see* Injury, nerve, accessory
facial S04.5-
contusion S04.5-
laceration S04.5-
newborn P11.3
specified type NEC S04.5-
femoral (hip level) (thigh level) S74.1-
fifth cranial (trigeminal) — *see* Injury, nerve, trigeminal
finger (digital) — *see* Injury, nerve, digital, finger
first cranial (olfactory) — *see* Injury, nerve, olfactory
foot S94.9-
cutaneous sensory S94.3-

Injury - *continued*
  nerve NEC - *continued*
    foot - *continued*
      deep peroneal S94.2-
      lateral plantar S94.0-
      medial plantar S94.1-
      specified site NEC — *see* subcategory S94.8
    forearm (level) S54.9-
      cutaneous sensory — *see* Injury, nerve, cutaneous sensory, forearm
      median — *see* Injury, nerve, median
      radial — *see* Injury, nerve, radial
      specified site NEC — *see* subcategory S54.8
      ulnar — *see* Injury, nerve, ulnar
    fourth cranial (trochlear) — *see* Injury, nerve, trochlear
    glossopharyngeal S04.89-
      specified type NEC S04.89-
    hand S64.9-
      median — *see* Injury, nerve, median, hand
      radial — *see* Injury, nerve, radial, hand
      specified NEC — *see* subcategory S64.8
      ulnar — *see* Injury, nerve, ulnar, hand
    hip (level) S74.9-
      cutaneous sensory — *see* Injury, nerve, cutaneous sensory, hip
      femoral — *see* Injury, nerve, femoral
      sciatic — *see* Injury, nerve, sciatic
      specified site NEC — *see* subcategory S74.8
    hypoglossal S04.89-
      specified type NEC S04.89-
    lateral plantar S94.0-
    leg (lower) S84.9-
      cutaneous sensory — *see* Injury, nerve, cutaneous sensory, leg
      peroneal — *see* Injury, nerve, peroneal
      specified site NEC — *see* subcategory S84.8
      tibial — *see* Injury, nerve, tibial
      upper — *see* Injury, nerve, thigh
    lower
      back — *see* Injury, nerve, abdomen, specified site NEC
        peripheral — *see* Injury, nerve, abdomen, peripheral
      limb — *see* Injury, nerve, leg
    lumbar spinal — *see* Injury, nerve, spinal, lumbar
    lumbar plexus — *see* Injury, nerve, lumbosacral, sympathetic
    lumbosacral
      plexus — *see* Injury, nerve, lumbosacral, sympathetic
      sympathetic S34.5
    medial plantar S94.1-
    median (forearm level) S54.1-
      hand (level) S64.1-
      upper arm (level) S44.1-
      wrist (level) — *see* Injury, nerve, median, hand
    musculocutaneous S44.4-
    musculospiral (upper arm level) — *see* Injury, nerve, radial, upper arm
    neck S14.9
      peripheral S14.4
      specified site NEC S14.8
      sympathetic S14.5
    ninth cranial (glossopharyngeal) — *see* Injury, nerve, glossopharyngeal
    oculomotor S04.1-
      contusion S04.1-
      laceration S04.1-
      specified type NEC S04.1-
    olfactory S04.81-
      specified type NEC S04.81-
    optic S04.01-
      contusion S04.01-
      laceration S04.01-
      specified type NEC S04.01-
    pelvic girdle — *see* Injury, nerve, hip
    pelvis — *see* Injury, nerve, abdomen, specified site NEC
      peripheral — *see* Injury, nerve, abdomen, peripheral
    peripheral NEC T14.8
      abdomen — *see* Injury, nerve, abdomen, peripheral
      lower back — *see* Injury, nerve, abdomen, peripheral
      neck — *see* Injury, nerve, neck, peripheral
      pelvis — *see* Injury, nerve, abdomen, peripheral
      specified NEC T14.8
    peroneal (lower leg level) S84.1-
      foot S94.2-
    plexus
      brachial — *see* Injury, brachial plexus

Injury - *continued*
  nerve NEC - *continued*
    plexus - *continued*
      celiac, coeliac — *see* Injury, nerve, lumbosacral, sympathetic
      mesenteric, inferior — *see* Injury, nerve, lumbosacral, sympathetic
      sacral — *see* Injury, lumbosacral plexus
      spinal
        brachial — *see* Injury, brachial plexus
        lumbosacral — *see* Injury, lumbosacral plexus
    pneumogastric — *see* Injury, nerve, vagus
    radial (forearm level) S54.2-
      hand (level) S64.2-
      upper arm (level) S44.2-
      wrist (level) — *see* Injury, nerve, radial, hand
    root — *see* Injury, nerve, spinal, root
    sacral plexus — *see* Injury, lumbosacral plexus
    sacral spinal — *see* Injury, nerve, spinal, sacral
    sciatic (hip level) (thigh level) S74.0-
    second cranial (optic) — *see* Injury, nerve, optic
    seventh cranial (facial) — *see* Injury, nerve, facial
    shoulder — *see* Injury, nerve, arm
    sixth cranial (abducent) — *see* Injury, nerve, abducens
    spinal
      plexus — *see* Injury, nerve, plexus, spinal
      root
        cervical S14.2
        dorsal S24.2
        lumbar S34.21
        sacral S34.22
        thoracic — *see* Injury, nerve, spinal, root, dorsal
    splanchnic — *see* Injury, nerve, lumbosacral, sympathetic
    sympathetic NEC — *see* Injury, nerve, lumbosacral, sympathetic
      cervical — *see* Injury, nerve, cervical sympathetic
    tenth cranial (pneumogastric or vagus) — *see* Injury, nerve, vagus
    thigh (level) — *see* Injury, nerve, hip
      cutaneous sensory — *see* Injury, nerve, cutaneous sensory, hip
      femoral — *see* Injury, nerve, femoral
      sciatic — *see* Injury, nerve, sciatic
      specified NEC — *see* Injury, nerve, hip
    third cranial (oculomotor) — *see* Injury, nerve, oculomotor
    thorax S24.9
      peripheral S24.3
      specified site NEC S24.8
      sympathetic S24.4
    thumb, digital — *see* Injury, nerve, digital, thumb
    tibial (lower leg level) (posterior) S84.0-
    toe — *see* Injury, nerve, ankle
    trigeminal S04.3-
      contusion S04.3-
      laceration S04.3-
      specified type NEC S04.3-
    trochlear S04.2-
      contusion S04.2-
      laceration S04.2-
      specified type NEC S04.2-
    twelfth cranial (hypoglossal) — *see* Injury, nerve, hypoglossal
    ulnar (forearm level) S54.0-
      arm (upper) (level) S44.0-
      hand (level) S64.0-
      wrist (level) — *see* Injury, nerve, ulnar, hand
    vagus S04.89-
      specified type NEC S04.89-
    wrist (level) — *see* Injury, nerve, hand
  ninth cranial nerve (glossopharyngeal) — *see* Injury, nerve, glossopharyngeal
  nose (septum) S09.92
  obstetrical O71.9
    specified NEC O71.89
  occipital (region) (scalp) S09.90
    lobe — *see* Injury, intracranial
  optic chiasm S04.02
  optic radiation S04.03-
  optic tract and pathways S04.03-
  orbit, orbital (region) — *see* Injury, eye
    penetrating (with foreign body) — *see* Injury, eye, orbit, penetrating
    specified NEC — *see* Injury, eye, specified site NEC
  ovary, ovarian S37.409
    bilateral S37.402
      contusion S37.422
      laceration S37.432
      specified type NEC S37.492
    blood vessel — *see* Injury, blood vessel, ovarian

Injury - *continued*
  ovary, ovarian - *continued*
    contusion S37.429
      bilateral S37.422
      unilateral S37.421
    laceration S37.439
      bilateral S37.432
      unilateral S37.431
    specified type NEC S37.499
      bilateral S37.492
      unilateral S37.491
    unilateral S37.401
      contusion S37.421
      laceration S37.431
      specified type NEC S37.491
  palate (hard) (soft) S09.93
  pancreas S36.209
    body S36.201
      contusion S36.221
      laceration S36.231
        major S36.261
        minor S36.241
        moderate S36.251
      specified type NEC S36.291
    contusion S36.229
    head S36.200
      contusion S36.220
      laceration S36.230
        major S36.260
        minor S36.240
        moderate S36.250
      specified type NEC S36.290
    laceration S36.239
      major S36.269
      minor S36.249
      moderate S36.259
    specified type NEC S36.299
    tail S36.202
      contusion S36.222
      laceration S36.232
        major S36.262
        minor S36.242
        moderate S36.252
      specified type NEC S36.292
  parietal (region) (scalp) S09.90
    lobe — *see* Injury, intracranial
  patellar ligament (tendon) S76.10-
    laceration S76.12-
    specified NEC S76.19-
    strain S76.11-
  pelvis, pelvic (floor) S39.93
    complicating delivery O70.1
    joint or ligament, complicating delivery O71.6
    organ S37.90
      with ectopic or molar pregnancy O08.6
      complication of abortion — *see* Abortion
      contusion S37.92
      following ectopic or molar pregnancy O08.6
      laceration S37.93
      obstetrical trauma NEC O71.5
      specified
        site NEC S37.899
          contusion S37.892
          laceration S37.893
          specified type NEC S37.898
        type NEC S37.99
    specified NEC S39.83
  penis S39.94
  perineum S39.94
  peritoneum S36.81
    laceration S36.893
  periurethral tissue — *see* Injury, urethra
    complicating delivery O71.82
  phalanges
    foot — *see* Injury, foot
    hand — *see* Injury, hand
  pharynx NEC S19.85
  pleura — *see* Injury, intrathoracic, pleura
  plexus
    brachial — *see* Injury, brachial plexus
    cardiac — *see* Injury, nerve, thorax, sympathetic
    celiac, coeliac — *see* Injury, nerve, lumbosacral, sympathetic
    esophageal — *see* Injury, nerve, thorax, sympathetic
    hypogastric — *see* Injury, nerve, lumbosacral, sympathetic
    lumbar, lumbosacral — *see* Injury, lumbosacral plexus
    mesenteric — *see* Injury, nerve, lumbosacral, sympathetic
    pulmonary — *see* Injury, nerve, thorax, sympathetic

Injury - *continued*
  postcardiac surgery (syndrome) I97.0
  prepuce S39.94
  prostate S37.829
    contusion S37.822
    laceration S37.823
    specified type NEC S37.828
  pubic region S39.94
  pudendum S39.94
  pulmonary plexus — *see* Injury, nerve, thorax, sympathetic
  rectovaginal septum NEC S39.83
  rectum — *see* Injury, intestine, large, rectum
  retina — *see* Injury, eye, specified site NEC
    penetrating — *see* Injury, eyeball, penetrating
  retroperitoneal — *see* Injury, intra-abdominal, specified site NEC
  rotator cuff (muscle (s)) (tendon (s)) S46.00-
    laceration S46.02-
    specified type NEC S46.09-
    strain S46.01-
  round ligament — *see* Injury, pelvic organ, specified site NEC
  sacral plexus — *see* Injury, lumbosacral plexus
  salivary duct or gland S09.93
  scalp S09.90
    newborn (birth injury) P12.9
      due to monitoring (electrode) (sampling incision) P12.4
      specified NEC P12.89
        caput succedaneum P12.81
  scapular region — *see* Injury, shoulder
  sclera — *see* Injury, eye, specified site NEC
    penetrating — *see* Injury, eyeball, penetrating
  scrotum S39.94
  second cranial nerve (optic) — *see* Injury, nerve, optic
  seminal vesicle — *see* Injury, pelvic organ, specified site NEC
  seventh cranial nerve (facial) — *see* Injury, nerve, facial
  shoulder S49.9-
    blood vessel — *see* Injury, blood vessel, arm
    contusion — *see* Contusion, shoulder
    dislocation — *see* Dislocation, shoulder
    fracture — *see* Fracture, shoulder
    muscle — *see* Injury, muscle, shoulder
    nerve — *see* Injury, nerve, shoulder
    open — *see* Wound, open, shoulder
    specified type NEC S49.8-
    sprain — *see* Sprain, shoulder girdle
    superficial — *see* Injury, superficial, shoulder
  sinus
    cavernous — *see* Injury, intracranial
    nasal S09.92
  sixth cranial nerve (abducent) — *see* Injury, nerve, abducens
  skeleton, birth injury P13.9
    specified part NEC P13.8
  skin NEC T14.8
    surface intact — *see* Injury, superficial
  skull NEC S09.90
  specified NEC T14.8
  spermatic cord (pelvic region) S37.898
    scrotal region S39.848
  spinal (cord)
    cervical (neck) S14.109
      anterior cord syndrome S14.139
        C1 level S14.131
        C2 level S14.132
        C3 level S14.133
        C4 level S14.134
        C5 level S14.135
        C6 level S14.136
        C7 level S14.137
        C8 level S14.138
      Brown-Séquard syndrome S14.149
        C1 level S14.141
        C2 level S14.142
        C3 level S14.143
        C4 level S14.144
        C5 level S14.145
        C6 level S14.146
        C7 level S14.147
        C8 level S14.148
      C1 level S14.101
      C2 level S14.102
      C3 level S14.103
      C4 level S14.104
      C5 level S14.105
      C6 level S14.106
      C7 level S14.107
      C8 level S14.108

Injury - *continued*
  spinal (cord) - *continued*
    cervical (neck) - *continued*
      central cord syndrome S14.129
        C1 level S14.121
        C2 level S14.122
        C3 level S14.123
        C4 level S14.124
        C5 level S14.125
        C6 level S14.126
        C7 level S14.127
        C8 level S14.128
      complete lesion S14.119
        C1 level S14.111
        C2 level S14.112
        C3 level S14.113
        C4 level S14.114
        C5 level S14.115
        C6 level S14.116
        C7 level S14.117
        C8 level S14.118
      concussion S14.0
      edema S14.0
      incomplete lesion specified NEC S14.159
        C1 level S14.151
        C2 level S14.152
        C3 level S14.153
        C4 level S14.154
        C5 level S14.155
        C6 level S14.156
        C7 level S14.157
        C8 level S14.158
      posterior cord syndrome S14.159
        C1 level S14.151
        C2 level S14.152
        C3 level S14.153
        C4 level S14.154
        C5 level S14.155
        C6 level S14.156
        C7 level S14.157
        C8 level S14.158
    dorsal — *see* Injury, spinal, thoracic
    lumbar S34.109
      complete lesion S34.119
        L1 level S34.111
        L2 level S34.112
        L3 level S34.113
        L4 level S34.114
        L5 level S34.115
      concussion S34.01
      edema S34.01
      incomplete lesion S34.129
        L1 level S34.121
        L2 level S34.122
        L3 level S34.123
        L4 level S34.124
        L5 level S34.125
      L1 level S34.101
      L2 level S34.102
      L3 level S34.103
      L4 level S34.104
      L5 level S34.105
    nerve root NEC
      cervical — *see* Injury, nerve, spinal, root, cervical
      dorsal — *see* Injury, nerve, spinal, root, dorsal
      lumbar S34.21
      sacral S34.22
      thoracic — *see* Injury, nerve, spinal, root, dorsal
    plexus
      brachial — *see* Injury, brachial plexus
      lumbosacral — *see* Injury, lumbosacral plexus
    sacral S34.139
      complete lesion S34.131
      incomplete lesion S34.132
    thoracic S24.109
      anterior cord syndrome S24.139
        T1 level S24.131
        T2-T6 level S24.132
        T7-T10 level S24.133
        T11-T12 level S24.134
      Brown-Séquard syndrome S24.149
        T1 level S24.141
        T2-T6 level S24.142
        T7-T10 level S24.143
        T11-T12 level S24.144
      complete lesion S24.119
        T1 level S24.111
        T2-T6 level S24.112
        T7-T10 level S24.113
        T11-T12 level S24.114
      concussion S24.0
      edema S24.0
      incomplete lesion specified NEC S24.159

Injury - *continued*
  spinal (cord) - *continued*
    thoracic - *continued*
      incomplete lesion specified NEC - *continued*
        T1 level S24.151
        T2-T6 level S24.152
        T7-T10 level S24.153
        T11-T12 level S24.154
      posterior cord syndrome S24.159
        T1 level S24.151
        T2-T6 level S24.152
        T7-T10 level S24.153
        T11-T12 level S24.154
      T1 level S24.101
      T2-T6 level S24.102
      T7-T10 level S24.103
      T11-T12 level S24.104
  splanchnic nerve — *see* Injury, nerve, lumbosacral, sympathetic
  spleen S36.00
    contusion S36.029
      major S36.021
      minor S36.020
    laceration S36.039
      major (massive) (stellate) S36.032
      moderate S36.031
      superficial (capsular) (minor) S36.030
    specified type NEC S36.09
  splenic artery — *see* Injury, blood vessel, celiac artery, branch
  stellate ganglion — *see* Injury, nerve, thorax, sympathetic
  sternal region S29.9
  stomach S36.30
    contusion S36.32
    laceration S36.33
    specified type NEC S36.39
  subconjunctival — *see* Injury, eye, conjunctiva
  subcutaneous NEC T14.8
  submaxillary region S09.93
  submental region S09.93
  subungual
    fingers — *see* Injury, hand
    toes — *see* Injury, foot
  superficial NEC T14.8
    abdomen, abdominal (wall) S30.92
      abrasion S30.811
      bite S30.871
        insect S30.861
      contusion S30.1
      external constriction S30.841
      foreign body S30.851
    abrasion — *see* Abrasion, by site
    adnexa, eye NEC — *see* Injury, eye, specified site NEC
    alveolar process — *see* Injury, superficial, oral cavity
    ankle S90.91-
      abrasion — *see* Abrasion, ankle
      blister — *see* Blister, ankle
      bite — *see* Bite, ankle
      contusion — *see* Contusion, ankle
      external constriction — *see* Constriction, external, ankle
      foreign body — *see* Foreign body, superficial, ankle
    anus S30.98
    arm (upper) S40.92-
      abrasion — *see* Abrasion, arm
      bite — *see* Bite, superficial, arm
      blister — *see* Blister, arm (upper)
      contusion — *see* Contusion, arm
      external constriction — *see* Constriction, external, arm
      foreign body — *see* Foreign body, superficial, arm
    auditory canal (external) (meatus) — *see* Injury, superficial, ear
    auricle — *see* Injury, superficial, ear
    axilla — *see* Injury, superficial, arm
    back — *see also* Injury, superficial, thorax, back
      lower S30.91
        abrasion S30.810
        contusion S30.0
        external constriction S30.840
        superficial
          bite NEC S30.870
            insect S30.860
          foreign body S30.850
    bite NEC — *see* Bite, superficial NEC, by site
    blister — *see* Blister, by site
    breast S20.10-
      abrasion — *see* Abrasion, breast

- **Injury** - *continued*
  - superficial NEC - *continued*
    - breast - *continued*
      - bite — *see* Bite, superficial, breast
      - contusion — *see* Contusion, breast
      - external constriction — *see* Constriction, external, breast
      - foreign body — *see* Foreign body, superficial, breast
    - brow — *see* Injury, superficial, head, specified NEC
    - buttock S30.91
    - calf — *see* Injury, superficial, leg
    - canthus, eye — *see* Injury, superficial, periocular area
    - cheek (external) — *see* Injury, superficial, head, specified NEC
      - internal — *see* Injury, superficial, oral cavity
    - chest wall — *see* Injury, superficial, thorax
    - chin — *see* Injury, superficial, head NEC
    - clitoris S30.95
    - conjunctiva — *see* Injury, eye, conjunctiva
      - with foreign body (in conjunctival sac) — *see* Foreign body, conjunctival sac
    - contusion — *see* Contusion, by site
    - costal region — *see* Injury, superficial, thorax
    - digit (s)
      - hand — *see* Injury, superficial, finger
    - ear (auricle) (canal) (external) S00.40-
      - abrasion — *see* Abrasion, ear
      - bite — *see* Bite, superficial, ear
      - contusion — *see* Contusion, ear
      - external constriction — *see* Constriction, external, ear
      - foreign body — *see* Foreign body, superficial, ear
    - elbow S50.90-
      - abrasion — *see* Abrasion, elbow
      - bite — *see* Bite, superficial, elbow
      - blister — *see* Blister, elbow
      - contusion — *see* Contusion, elbow
      - external constriction — *see* Constriction, external, elbow
      - foreign body — *see* Foreign body, superficial, elbow
    - epididymis S30.94
    - epigastric region S30.92
    - epiglottis — *see* Injury, superficial, throat
    - esophagus
      - cervical — *see* Injury, superficial, throat
    - external constriction — *see* Constriction, external, by site
    - extremity NEC T14.8
    - eyeball NEC — *see* Injury, eye, specified site NEC
    - eyebrow — *see* Injury, superficial, periocular area
    - eyelid S00.20-
      - abrasion — *see* Abrasion, eyelid
      - bite — *see* Bite, superficial, eyelid
      - contusion — *see* Contusion, eyelid
      - external constriction — *see* Constriction, external, eyelid
      - foreign body — *see* Foreign body, superficial, eyelid
    - face NEC — *see* Injury, superficial, head, specified NEC
    - finger (s) S60.949
      - abrasion — *see* Abrasion, finger
      - bite — *see* Bite, superficial, finger
      - blister — *see* Blister, finger
      - contusion — *see* Contusion, finger
      - external constriction — *see* Constriction, external, finger
      - foreign body — *see* Foreign body, superficial, finger
      - insect bite — *see* Bite, by site, superficial, insect
      - index S60.94-
      - little S60.94-
      - middle S60.94-
      - ring S60.94-
    - flank S30.92
    - foot S90.92-
      - abrasion — *see* Abrasion, foot
      - bite — *see* Bite, foot
      - blister — *see* Blister, foot
      - contusion — *see* Contusion, foot
      - external constriction — *see* Constriction, external, foot
      - foreign body — *see* Foreign body, superficial, foot
    - forearm S50.91-
      - abrasion — *see* Abrasion, forearm
      - bite — *see* Bite, forearm, superficial
      - blister — *see* Blister, forearm
      - contusion — *see* Contusion, forearm

- **Injury** - *continued*
  - superficial NEC - *continued*
    - forearm - *continued*
      - elbow only — *see* Injury, superficial, elbow
      - external constriction — *see* Constriction, external, forearm
      - foreign body — *see* Foreign body, superficial, forearm
    - forehead — *see* Injury, superficial, head NEC
    - foreign body — *see* Foreign body, superficial
    - genital organs, external
      - female S30.97
      - male S30.96
    - globe (eye) — *see* Injury, eye, specified site NEC
    - groin S30.92
    - gum — *see* Injury, superficial, oral cavity
    - hand S60.92-
      - abrasion — *see* Abrasion, hand
      - bite — *see* Bite, superficial, hand
      - contusion — *see* Contusion, hand
      - external constriction — *see* Constriction, external, hand
      - foreign body — *see* Foreign body, superficial, hand
    - head S00.90
      - ear — *see* Injury, superficial, ear
      - eyelid — *see* Injury, superficial, eyelid
      - nose S00.30
      - oral cavity S00.502
      - scalp S00.00
      - specified site NEC S00.80
    - heel — *see* Injury, superficial, foot
    - hip S70.91-
      - abrasion — *see* Abrasion, hip
      - bite — *see* Bite, superficial, hip
      - blister — *see* Blister, hip
      - contusion — *see* Contusion, hip
      - external constriction — *see* Constriction, external, hip
      - foreign body — *see* Foreign body, superficial, hip
    - iliac region — *see* Injury, superficial, abdomen
    - inguinal region — *see* Injury, superficial, abdomen
    - insect bite — *see* Bite, by site, superficial, insect
    - interscapular region — *see* Injury, superficial, thorax, back
    - jaw — *see* Injury, superficial, head, specified NEC
    - knee S80.91-
      - abrasion — *see* Abrasion, knee
      - bite — *see* Bite, superficial, knee
      - blister — *see* Blister, knee
      - contusion — *see* Contusion, knee
      - external constriction — *see* Constriction, external, knee
      - foreign body — *see* Foreign body, superficial, knee
    - labium (majus) (minus) S30.95
    - lacrimal (apparatus) (gland) (sac) — *see* Injury, eye, specified site NEC
    - larynx — *see* Injury, superficial, throat
    - leg (lower) S80.92-
      - abrasion — *see* Abrasion, leg
      - bite — *see* Bite, superficial, leg
      - contusion — *see* Contusion, leg
      - external constriction — *see* Constriction, external, leg
      - foreign body — *see* Foreign body, superficial, leg
      - knee — *see* Injury, superficial, knee
    - limb NEC T14.8
    - lip S00.501
    - lower back S30.91
    - lumbar region S30.91
    - malar region — *see* Injury, superficial, head, specified NEC
    - mammary — *see* Injury, superficial, breast
    - mastoid region — *see* Injury, superficial, head, specified NEC
    - mouth — *see* Injury, superficial, oral cavity
    - muscle NEC T14.8
    - nail NEC T14.8
      - finger — *see* Injury, superficial, finger
      - toe — *see* Injury, superficial, toe
    - nasal (septum) — *see* Injury, superficial, nose
    - neck S10.90
      - specified site NEC S10.80
    - nose (septum) S00.30
    - occipital region — *see* Injury, superficial, scalp
    - oral cavity S00.502
    - orbital region — *see* Injury, superficial, periocular area
    - palate — *see* Injury, superficial, oral cavity
    - palm — *see* Injury, superficial, hand
    - parietal region — *see* Injury, superficial, scalp
    - pelvis S30.91

- **Injury** - *continued*
  - superficial NEC - *continued*
    - pelvis - *continued*
      - girdle — *see* Injury, superficial, hip
    - penis S30.93
    - perineum
      - female S30.95
      - male S30.91
    - periocular area S00.20-
      - abrasion — *see* Abrasion, eyelid
      - bite — *see* Bite, superficial, eyelid
      - contusion — *see* Contusion, eyelid
      - external constriction — *see* Constriction, external, eyelid
      - foreign body — *see* Foreign body, superficial, eyelid
    - phalanges
      - finger — *see* Injury, superficial, finger
      - toe — *see* Injury, superficial, toe
    - pharynx — *see* Injury, superficial, throat
    - pinna — *see* Injury, superficial, ear
    - popliteal space — *see* Injury, superficial, knee
    - prepuce S30.93
    - pubic region S30.91
    - pudendum
      - female S30.97
      - male S30.96
    - sacral region S30.91
    - scalp S00.00
    - scapular region — *see* Injury, superficial, shoulder
    - sclera — *see* Injury, eye, specified site NEC
    - scrotum S30.94
    - shin — *see* Injury, superficial, leg
    - shoulder S40.91-
      - abrasion — *see* Abrasion, shoulder
      - bite — *see* Bite, superficial, shoulder
      - blister — *see* Blister, shoulder
      - contusion — *see* Contusion, shoulder
      - external constriction — *see* Constriction, external, shoulder
      - foreign body — *see* Foreign body, superficial, shoulder
    - skin NEC T14.8
    - sternal region — *see* Injury, superficial, thorax, front
    - subconjunctival — *see* Injury, eye, specified site NEC
    - subcutaneous NEC T14.8
    - submaxillary region — *see* Injury, superficial, head, specified NEC
    - submental region — *see* Injury, superficial, head, specified NEC
    - subungual
      - finger (s) — *see* Injury, superficial, finger
      - toe (s) — *see* Injury, superficial, toe
    - supraclavicular fossa — *see* Injury, superficial, neck
    - supraorbital — *see* Injury, superficial, head, specified NEC
    - temple — *see* Injury, superficial, head, specified NEC
    - temporal region — *see* Injury, superficial, head, specified NEC
    - testis S30.94
    - thigh S70.92-
      - abrasion — *see* Abrasion, thigh
      - bite — *see* Bite, superficial, thigh
      - blister — *see* Blister, thigh
      - contusion — *see* Contusion, thigh
      - external constriction — *see* Constriction, external, thigh
      - foreign body — *see* Foreign body, superficial, thigh
    - thorax, thoracic (wall) S20.90
      - abrasion — *see* Abrasion, thorax
      - back S20.40-
      - bite — *see* Bite, thorax, superficial
      - blister — *see* Blister, thorax
      - contusion — *see* Contusion, thorax
      - external constriction — *see* Constriction, external, thorax
      - foreign body — *see* Foreign body, superficial, thorax
      - front S20.30-
    - throat S10.10
      - abrasion S10.11
      - bite S10.17
        - insect S10.16
      - blister S10.12
      - contusion S10.0
      - external constriction S10.14
      - foreign body S10.15
    - thumb S60.93-

Insomnia (organic) - *continued*
  due to - *continued*
    stimulant NEC - *continued*
      abuse F15.182
      dependence F15.282
      use F15.982
  fatal familial (FFI) A81.83
  idiopathic F51.01
  learned F51.3
  nonorganic origin F51.01
  not due to a substance or known physiological condition F51.01
    specified NEC F51.09
  paradoxical F51.03
  primary F51.01
  psychiatric F51.05
  psychophysiologic F51.04
  related to psychopathology F51.05
  short-term F51.02
  specified NEC G47.09
  stress-related F51.02
  transient F51.02
  without objective findings F51.02
Inspiration
  food or foreign body — *see* Foreign body, by site
  mucus — *see* Asphyxia, mucus
Inspissated bile syndrome (newborn) P59.1
Instability
  emotional (excessive) F60.3
  joint (post-traumatic) M25.30
    ankle M25.37-
    due to old ligament injury — *see* Disorder, ligament
    elbow M25.32-
    flail — *see* Flail, joint
    foot M25.37-
    hand M25.34-
    hip M25.35-
    knee M25.36-
    lumbosacral — *see* subcategory M53.2
    prosthesis — *see* Complications, joint prosthesis, mechanical, displacement, by site
    sacroiliac — *see* subcategory M53.2
    secondary to
      old ligament injury — *see* Disorder, ligament
      removal of joint prosthesis M96.89
    shoulder (region) M25.31-
    spine — *see* subcategory M53.2
    wrist M25.33-
  knee (chronic) M23.5-
  lumbosacral — *see* subcategory M53.2
  nervous F48.8
  personality (emotional) F60.3
  spine — *see* Instability, joint, spine
  vasomotor R55
Institutional syndrome (childhood) F94.2
Institutionalization, affecting child Z62.22
  disinhibited attachment F94.2
Insufficiency, insufficient
  accommodation, old age H52.4
  adrenal (gland) E27.40
    primary E27.1
  adrenocortical E27.40
    drug-induced E27.3
    iatrogenic E27.3
    primary E27.1
  anatomic crown height K08.89
  anterior (occlusal) guidance M26.54
  anus K62.89
  aortic (valve) I35.1
    with
      mitral (valve) disease I08.0
        with tricuspid (valve) disease I08.3
      stenosis I35.2
      tricuspid (valve) disease I08.2
        with mitral (valve) disease I08.3
    congenital Q23.1
    rheumatic I06.1
      with
        mitral (valve) disease I08.0
          with tricuspid (valve) disease I08.3
        stenosis I06.2
          with mitral (valve) disease I08.0
            with tricuspid (valve) disease I08.3
        tricuspid (valve) disease I08.2
          with mitral (valve) disease I08.3
    specified cause NEC I35.1
    syphilitic A52.03
  arterial I77.1
    basilar G45.0
    carotid (hemispheric) G45.1
    cerebral I67.81
    coronary (acute or subacute) I24.8

Insufficiency, insufficient - *continued*
  arterial - *continued*
    mesenteric K55.1
    peripheral I73.9
    precerebral (multiple) (bilateral) G45.2
    vertebral G45.0
  arteriovenous I99.8
  biliary K83.8
  cardiac — *see also* Insufficiency, myocardial
    due to presence of (cardiac) prosthesis I97.11-
    postprocedural I97.11-
  cardiorenal, hypertensive I13.2
  cardiovascular — *see* Disease, cardiovascular
  cerebrovascular (acute) I67.81
    with transient focal neurological signs and symptoms G45.8
  circulatory NEC I99.8
    newborn P29.89
  clinical crown length K08.89
  convergence H51.11
  coronary (acute or subacute) I24.8
    chronic or with a stated duration of over 4 weeks I25.89
  corticoadrenal E27.40
    primary E27.1
  dietary E63.9
  divergence H51.8
  food T73.0
  gastroesophageal K22.8
  gonadal
    ovary E28.39
    testis E29.1
  heart — *see also* Insufficiency, myocardial
    newborn P29.0
    valve — *see* Endocarditis
  hepatic — *see* Failure, hepatic
  idiopathic autonomic G90.09
  interocclusal distance of fully erupted teeth (ridge) M26.36
  kidney N28.9
    acute N28.9
    chronic N18.9
  lacrimal (secretion) H04.12-
    passages — *see* Stenosis, lacrimal
  liver — *see* Failure, hepatic
  lung — *see* Insufficiency, pulmonary
  mental (congenital) — *see* Disability, intellectual
  mesenteric K55.1
  mitral (valve) I34.0
    with
      aortic valve disease I08.0
        with tricuspid (valve) disease I08.3
      obstruction or stenosis I05.2
        with aortic valve disease I08.0
      tricuspid (valve) disease I08.1
        with aortic (valve) disease I08.3
    congenital Q23.3
    rheumatic I05.1
      with
        aortic valve disease I08.0
          with tricuspid (valve) disease I08.3
        obstruction or stenosis I05.2
          with aortic valve disease I08.0
            with tricuspid (valve) disease I08.3
        tricuspid (valve) disease I08.1
          with aortic (valve) disease I08.3
      active or acute I01.1
        with chorea, rheumatic (Sydenham's) I02.0
    specified cause, except rheumatic I34.0
  muscle — *see also* Disease, muscle
    heart — *see* Insufficiency, myocardial
    ocular NEC H50.9
  myocardial, myocardium (with arteriosclerosis) — *see also* Failure, heart I50.9
    with
      rheumatic fever (conditions in I00) I09.0
        active, acute or subacute I01.2
          with chorea I02.0
        inactive or quiescent (with chorea) I09.0
    congenital Q24.8
    hypertensive — *see* Hypertension, heart
    newborn P29.0
    rheumatic I09.0
      active, acute, or subacute I01.2
    syphilitic A52.06
  nourishment T73.0
  pancreatic K86.89
    exocrine K86.81
  parathyroid (gland) E20.9
  peripheral vascular (arterial) I73.9
  pituitary E23.0
  placental (mother) O36.51-
  platelets D69.6

Insufficiency, insufficient - *continued*
  prenatal care affecting management of pregnancy O09.3-
  progressive pluriglandular E31.0
  pulmonary J98.4
    acute, following surgery (nonthoracic) J95.2
      thoracic J95.1
    chronic, following surgery J95.3
    following
      shock J98.4
      trauma J98.4
    newborn P28.5
    valve I37.1
      with stenosis I37.2
      congenital Q22.2
      rheumatic I09.89
        with aortic, mitral or tricuspid (valve) disease I08.8
  pyloric K31.89
  renal (acute) N28.9
    chronic N18.9
  respiratory R06.89
    newborn P28.5
  rotation — *see* Malrotation
  sleep syndrome F51.12
  social insurance Z59.7
  suprarenal E27.40
    primary E27.1
  tarso-orbital fascia, congenital Q10.3
  testis E29.1
  thyroid (gland) (acquired) E03.9
    congenital E03.1
  tricuspid (valve) (rheumatic) I07.1
    with
      aortic (valve) disease I08.2
        with mitral (valve) disease I08.3
      mitral (valve) disease I08.1
        with aortic (valve) disease I08.3
      obstruction or stenosis I07.2
        with aortic (valve) disease I08.2
          with mitral (valve) disease I08.3
    congenital Q22.8
    nonrheumatic I36.1
      with stenosis I36.2
  urethral sphincter R32
  valve, valvular (heart) I38
    aortic — *see* Insufficiency, aortic (valve)
    mitral — *see* Insufficiency, mitral (valve)
    pulmonary — *see* Insufficiency, pulmonary, valve
    tricuspid — *see* Insufficiency, tricuspid (valve)
    congenital Q24.8
  vascular I99.8
    intestine K55.9
      acute — *see also* Ischemia, intestine, acute K55.059
    mesenteric K55.1
    peripheral I73.9
    renal — *see* Hypertension, kidney
  velopharyngeal
    acquired K13.79
    congenital Q38.8
  venous (chronic) (peripheral) I87.2
  ventricular — *see* Insufficiency, myocardial
  welfare support Z59.7
Insufflation, fallopian Z31.41
Insular — *see* condition
Insulinoma
  pancreas
    benign D13.7
    malignant C25.4
    uncertain behavior D37.8
  specified site
    benign — *see* Neoplasm, by site, benign
    malignant — *see* Neoplasm, by site, malignant
    uncertain behavior — *see* Neoplasm, by site, uncertain behavior
  unspecified site
    benign D13.7
    malignant C25.4
    uncertain behavior D37.8
Insuloma — *see* Insulinoma
Interference
  balancing side M26.56
  non-working side M26.56
Intermenstrual — *see* condition
Intermittent — *see* condition
Internal — *see* condition
Interrogation
  cardiac defibrillator (automatic) (implantable) Z45.02
  cardiac pacemaker Z45.018
  cardiac (event) (loop) recorder Z45.09
  infusion pump (implanted) (intrathecal) Z45.1

Interrogation - *continued*
neurostimulator Z46.2
Interruption
aortic arch Q25.21
bundle of His I44.30
phase-shift, sleep cycle — *see* Disorder, sleep, circadian rhythm
sleep phase-shift, or 24 hour sleep-wake cycle — *see* Disorder, sleep, circadian rhythm
Interstitial — *see* condition
Intertrigo L30.4
labialis K13.0
Intervertebral disc — *see* condition
Intestine, intestinal — *see* condition
Intolerance
carbohydrate K90.49
disaccharide, hereditary E73.0
fat NEC K90.49
pancreatic K90.3
food K90.49
dietary counseling and surveillance Z71.3
fructose E74.10
hereditary E74.12
glucose (-galactose) E74.39
gluten K90.41
lactose E73.9
specified NEC E73.8
lysine E72.3
milk NEC K90.49
lactose E73.9
protein K90.49
starch NEC K90.49
sucrose (-isomaltose) E74.31
Intoxicated NEC (without dependence) — *see* Alcohol, intoxication
Intoxication
acid E87.2
alcoholic (acute) (without dependence) — *see* Alcohol, intoxication
alimentary canal K52.1
amphetamine (without dependence) — *see* Abuse, drug, stimulant, with intoxication
with dependence — *see* Dependence, drug, stimulant, with intoxication
anxiolytic (acute) (without dependence) — *see* Abuse, drug, sedative, with intoxication
with dependence — *see* Dependence, drug, sedative, with intoxication
caffeine F15.929
with dependence — *see* Dependence, drug, stimulant, with intoxication
cannabinoids (acute) (without dependence) — *see* Use, cannabis, with intoxication
with
abuse — *see* Abuse, drug, cannabis, with intoxication
dependence — *see* Dependence, drug, cannabis, with intoxication
chemical — *see* Table of Drugs and Chemicals
via placenta or breast milk — *see* - Absorption, chemical, through placenta
cocaine (acute) (without dependence) — *see* Abuse, drug, cocaine, with intoxication
with dependence — *see* Dependence, drug, cocaine, with intoxication
drug
acute (without dependence) — *see* Abuse, drug, by type with intoxication
with dependence — *see* Dependence, drug, by type with intoxication
addictive
via placenta or breast milk — *see* Absorption, drug, addictive, through placenta
newborn P93.8
gray baby syndrome P93.0
overdose or wrong substance given or taken — *see* Table of Drugs and Chemicals, by drug, poisoning
enteric K52.1
foodborne A05.9
bacterial A05.9
classical (Clostridium botulinum) A05.1
due to
Bacillus cereus A05.4
bacterium A05.9
specified NEC A05.8
Clostridium
botulinum A05.1
perfringens A05.2
welchii A05.2
Salmonella A02.9
with
(gastro) enteritis A02.0

Intoxication - *continued*
foodborne - *continued*
due to - *continued*
Salmonella - *continued*
with - *continued*
localized infection (s) A02.20
arthritis A02.23
meningitis A02.21
osteomyelitis A02.24
pneumonia A02.22
pyelonephritis A02.25
specified NEC A02.29
sepsis A02.1
specified manifestation NEC A02.8
Staphylococcus A05.0
Vibrio
parahaemolyticus A05.3
vulnificus A05.5
enterotoxin, staphylococcal A05.0
noxious — *see* Poisoning, food, noxious
gastrointestinal K52.1
hallucinogenic (without dependence) — *see* Abuse, drug, hallucinogen, with intoxication
with dependence — *see* Dependence, drug, hallucinogen, with intoxication
hypnotic (acute) (without dependence) — *see* Abuse, drug, sedative, with intoxication
with dependence — *see* Dependence, drug, sedative, with intoxication
inhalant (acute) (without dependence) — *see* Abuse, drug, inhalant, with intoxication
with dependence — *see* Dependence, drug, inhalant, with intoxication
meaning
inebriation — *see* category F10
poisoning — *see* Table of Drugs and Chemicals
methyl alcohol (acute) (without dependence) — *see* Alcohol, intoxication
opioid (acute) (without dependence) — *see* Abuse, drug, opioid, with intoxication
with dependence — *see* Dependence, drug, opioid, with intoxication
pathologic NEC (without dependence) — *see* Alcohol, intoxication
phencyclidine (without dependence) — *see* Abuse, drug, hallucinogen, with intoxication
with dependence - — *see* Dependence, drug, hallucinogen, with intoxication
potassium (K) E87.5
psychoactive substance NEC (without dependence) — *see* Abuse, drug, psychoactive NEC, with intoxication
with dependence — *see* Dependence, drug, psychoactive NEC, with intoxication
sedative (acute) (without dependence) — *see* Abuse, drug, sedative, with intoxication
with dependence — *see* Dependence, drug, sedative, with intoxication
serum — *see also* Reaction, serum T80.69
uremic — *see* Uremia
volatile solvents (acute) (without dependence) — *see* Abuse, drug, inhalant, with intoxication
with dependence — *see* Dependence, drug, inhalant, with intoxication
water E87.79
Intraabdominal testis, testes
bilateral Q53.211
unilateral Q53.111
Intracranial — *see* condition
Intrahepatic gallbladder Q44.1
Intraligamentous — *see* condition
Intrathoracic — *see also* condition
kidney Q63.2
Intrauterine contraceptive device
checking Z30.431
insertion Z30.430
immediately following removal Z30.433
in situ Z97.5
management Z30.431
reinsertion Z30.433
removal Z30.432
replacement Z30.433
retention in pregnancy O26.3-
Intraventricular — *see* condition
Intrinsic deformity — *see* Deformity
Intubation, difficult or failed T88.4
Intumescence, lens (eye) (cataract) — *see* Cataract
Intussusception (bowel) (colon) (enteric) (ileocecal) (ileocolic) (intestine) (rectum) K56.1
appendix K38.8
congenital Q43.8
ureter (with obstruction) N13.5

Invagination (bowel, colon, intestine or rectum) K56.1
Inversion
albumin-globulin (A-G) ratio E88.09
bladder N32.89
cecum — *see* Intussusception
cervix N88.8
chromosome in normal individual Q95.1
circadian rhythm — *see* Disorder, sleep, circadian rhythm
nipple N64.59
congenital Q83.8
gestational — *see* Retraction, nipple
puerperal, postpartum — *see* Retraction, nipple
nyctohemeral rhythm — *see* Disorder, sleep, circadian rhythm
optic papilla Q14.2
organ or site, congenital NEC — *see* Anomaly, by site
sleep rhythm — *see* Disorder, sleep, circadian rhythm
testis (congenital) Q55.29
uterus (chronic) (postinfectional) (postpartal, old) N85.5
postpartum O71.2
vagina (posthysterectomy) N99.3
ventricular Q20.5
Investigation — *see also* Examination Z04.9
clinical research subject (control) (normal comparison) (participant) Z00.6
Involuntary movement, abnormal R25.9
Involution, involutional — *see also* condition
breast, cystic — *see* Dysplasia, mammary, specified type NEC
depression (single episode) F32.89
recurrent episode F33.9
melancholia (single episode) F32.89
recurrent episode F33.8
ovary, senile — *see* Atrophy, ovary
thymus failure E32.8
IRDS (type I) P22.0
type II P22.1
Irideremia Q13.1
Iridis rubeosis — *see* Disorder, iris, vascular
Iridochoroiditis (panuveitis) — *see* Panuveitis
Iridocyclitis H20.9
acute H20.0-
hypopyon H20.05-
primary H20.01-
recurrent H20.02-
secondary (noninfectious) H20.04-
infectious H20.03-
chronic H20.1-
due to allergy — *see* Iridocyclitis, acute, secondary
endogenous — *see* Iridocyclitis, acute, primary
Fuchs' — *see* Cyclitis, Fuchs' heterochromic
gonococcal A54.32
granulomatous — *see* Iridocyclitis, chronic
herpes, herpetic (simplex) B00.51
zoster B02.32
hypopyon — *see* Iridocyclitis, acute, hypopyon
in (due to)
ankylosing spondylitis M45.9
gonococcal infection A54.32
herpes (simplex) virus B00.51
zoster B02.32
infectious disease NOS B99
parasitic disease NOS B89 *[H22]*
sarcoidosis D86.83
syphilis A51.43
tuberculosis A18.54
zoster B02.32
lens-induced H20.2-
nongranulomatous — *see* Iridocyclitis, acute
recurrent — *see* Iridocyclitis, acute, recurrent
rheumatic — *see* Iridocyclitis, chronic
subacute — *see* Iridocyclitis, acute
sympathetic — *see* Uveitis, sympathetic
syphilitic (secondary) A51.43
tuberculous (chronic) A18.54
Vogt-Koyanagi H20.82-
Iridocyclochoroiditis (panuveitis) — *see* Panuveitis
Iridodialysis H21.53-
Iridodonesis H21.89
Iridoplegia (complete) (partial) (reflex) H57.09
Iridoschisis H21.25-
Iris — *see also* condition
bombé — *see* Membrane, pupillary
Iritis — *see also* Iridocyclitis
chronic — *see* Iridocyclitis, chronic
diabetic — *see* E08-E13 with .39
due to
herpes simplex B00.51

Iritis - *continued*
due to - *continued*
leprosy A30.9 *[H22]*
gonococcal A54.32
gouty — *see also* Gout, by type M10.9 *[H22]*
granulomatous — *see* Iridocyclitis, chronic
lens induced — *see* Iridocyclitis, lens-induced
papulosa (syphilitic) A52.71
rheumatic — *see* Iridocyclitis, chronic
syphilitic (secondary) A51.43
congenital (early) A50.01
late A52.71
tuberculous A18.54
Iron — *see* condition
Iron-miner's lung J63.4
Irradiated enamel (tooth, teeth) K03.89
Irradiation effects, adverse T66
Irreducible, irreducibility — *see* condition
Irregular, irregularity
action, heart I49.9
alveolar process K08.89
bleeding N92.6
breathing R06.89
contour of cornea (acquired) — *see* Deformity, cornea
congenital Q13.4
contour, reconstructed breast N65.0
dentin (in pulp) K04.3
eye movements H55.89
nystagmus — *see* Nystagmus
saccadic H55.81
labor O62.2
menstruation (cause unknown) N92.6
periods N92.6
prostate N42.9
pupil — *see* Abnormality, pupillary
reconstructed breast N65.0
respiratory R06.89
septum (nasal) J34.2
shape, organ or site, congenital NEC — *see* Distortion
sleep-wake pattern (rhythm) G47.23
Irritable, irritability R45.4
bladder N32.89
bowel (syndrome) K58.9
with
constipation K58.1
diarrhea K58.0
mixed K58.2
psychogenic F45.8
specified NEC K58.8
bronchial — *see* Bronchitis
cerebral, in newborn P91.3
colon — *see also* Irritable, bowel K58.9
with diarrhea K58.0
psychogenic F45.8
duodenum K59.8
heart (psychogenic) F45.8
hip — *see* Derangement, joint, specified type NEC, hip
ileum K59.8
infant R68.12
jejunum K59.8
rectum K59.8
stomach K31.89
psychogenic F45.8
sympathetic G90.8
urethra N36.8
Irritation
anus K62.89
axillary nerve G54.0
bladder N32.89
brachial plexus G54.0
bronchial — *see* Bronchitis
cervical plexus G54.2
cervix — *see* Cervicitis
choroid, sympathetic — *see* Endophthalmitis
cranial nerve — *see* Disorder, nerve, cranial
gastric K31.89
psychogenic F45.8
globe, sympathetic — *see* Uveitis, sympathetic
labyrinth — *see* subcategory H83.2
lumbosacral plexus G54.1
meninges (traumatic) — *see* Injury, intracranial
nontraumatic — *see* Meningismus
nerve — *see* Disorder, nerve
nervous R45.0
penis N48.89
perineum NEC L29.3
peripheral autonomic nervous system G90.8
peritoneum — *see* Peritonitis
pharynx J39.2
plantar nerve — *see* Lesion, nerve, plantar

Irritation - *continued*
spinal (cord) (traumatic) — *see also* Injury, spinal cord, by region
nerve G58.9
root NEC — *see* Radiculopathy
nontraumatic — *see* Myelopathy
stomach K31.89
psychogenic F45.8
sympathetic nerve NEC G90.8
ulnar nerve — *see* Lesion, nerve, ulnar
vagina N89.8
Ischemia, ischemic I99.8
brain — *see* Ischemia, cerebral
bowel (transient)
acute — *see also* Ischemia, intestine, acute K55.059
chronic K55.1
due to mesenteric artery insufficiency K55.1
cardiac (see Disease, heart, ischemic)
cardiomyopathy I25.5
cerebral (chronic) (generalized) I67.82
arteriosclerotic I67.2
intermittent G45.9
newborn P91.0
recurrent focal G45.8
transient G45.9
colon chronic (due to mesenteric artery insufficiency) K55.1
coronary — *see* Disease, heart, ischemic
demand (coronary) — *see also* Angina I24.8
with myocardial infarction I21.A1
resulting in myocardial infarction I21.A1
heart (chronic or with a stated duration of over 4 weeks) I25.9
acute or with a stated duration of 4 weeks or less I24.9
subacute I24.9
infarction, muscle — *see* Infarct, muscle
intestine (large) (small) (transient) K55.9
acute K55.059
diffuse K55.052
focal K55.051
large K55.039
diffuse K55.032
focal K55.031
small K55.019
diffuse K55.012
focal K55.011
chronic K55.1
due to mesenteric artery insufficiency K55.1
kidney N28.0
mesenteric, acute — *see also* Ischemia, intestine, acute K55.059
muscle, traumatic T79.6
myocardium, myocardial (chronic or with a stated duration of over 4 weeks) I25.9
acute, without myocardial infarction I51.3
silent (asymptomatic) I25.6
transient of newborn P29.4
renal N28.0
retina, retinal — *see* Occlusion, artery, retina
small bowel
acute K55.019
diffuse K55.012
focal K55.011
chronic K55.1
due to mesenteric artery insufficiency K55.1
spinal cord G95.11
subendocardial — *see* Insufficiency, coronary
supply (coronary) — *see also* Angina I25.9
due to vasospasm I20.1
Ischial spine — *see* condition
Ischialgia — *see* Sciatica
Ischiopagus Q89.4
Ischium, ischial — *see* condition
Ischuria R34
Iselin's disease or osteochondrosis — *see* Osteochondrosis, juvenile, metatarsus
Islands of
parotid tissue in
lymph nodes Q38.6
neck structures Q38.6
submaxillary glands in
fascia Q38.6
lymph nodes Q38.6
neck muscles Q38.6
Islet cell tumor, pancreas D13.7
Isoimmunization NEC — *see also* Incompatibility
affecting management of pregnancy (ABO) (with hydrops fetalis) O36.11-
anti-A sensitization O36.11-
anti-B sensitization O36.19-
anti-c sensitization O36.09-

Isoimmunization NEC - *continued*
affecting management of pregnancy (ABO) (with hydrops fetalis) - *continued*
anti-C sensitization O36.09-
anti-e sensitization O36.09-
anti-E sensitization O36.09-
Rh NEC O36.09-
anti-D antibody O36.01-
specified NEC O36.19-
newborn P55.9
with
hydrops fetalis P56.0
kernicterus P57.0
ABO (blood groups) P55.1
Rhesus (Rh) factor P55.0
specified type NEC P55.8
Isolation, isolated
dwelling Z59.8
family Z63.79
social Z60.4
Isoleucinosis E71.19
Isomerism atrial appendages
(with asplenia or polysplenia) Q20.6
Isosporiasis, isosporosis A07.3
Isovaleric acidemia E71.110
Issue of
medical certificate Z02.79
for disability determination Z02.71
repeat prescription (appliance) (glasses) (medicinal substance, medicament, medicine) Z76.0
contraception — *see* Contraception
Itch, itching — *see also* Pruritus
baker's L23.6
barber's B35.0
bricklayer's L24.5
cheese B88.0
clam digger's B65.3
coolie B76.9
copra B88.0
dew B76.9
dhobi B35.6
filarial — *see* Infestation, filarial
grain B88.0
grocer's B88.0
ground B76.9
harvest B88.0
jock B35.6
Malabar B35.5
beard B35.0
foot B35.3
scalp B35.0
meaning scabies B86
Norwegian B86
perianal L29.0
poultrymen's B88.0
sarcoptic B86
scabies B86
scrub B88.0
straw B88.0
swimmer's B65.3
water B76.9
winter L29.8
Ivemark's syndrome
(asplenia with congenital heart disease) Q89.01
Ivory bones Q78.2
Ixodiasis NEC B88.8

J

Jaccoud's syndrome — *see* Arthropathy, postrheumatic, chronic
Jackson's
membrane Q43.3
paralysis or syndrome G83.89
veil Q43.3
Jacquet's dermatitis (diaper dermatitis) L22
Jadassohn-Pellizari's disease or anetoderma L90.2
Jadassohn's
blue nevus — *see* Nevus
intraepidermal epithelioma — *see* Neoplasm, skin, benign
Jaffe-Lichtenstein (-Uehlinger) **syndrome** — *see* Dysplasia, fibrous, bone NEC
Jakob-Creutzfeldt disease or syndrome — *see* Creutzfeldt-Jakob disease or syndrome
Jaksch-Luzet disease D64.89
Jamaican
neuropathy G92
paraplegic tropical ataxic-spastic syndrome G92
Janet's disease F48.8
Janiceps Q89.4
Jansky-Bielschowsky amaurotic idiocy E75.4
Japanese
B-type encephalitis A83.0

Keratoconjunctivitis - *continued*
  shipyard B30.0
  sicca (Sjogren's) M35.0-
    not Sjogren's H16.22-
  specified type NEC H16.29-
  tuberculous (phlyctenular) A18.52
  vernal H16.26-
Keratoconus H18.60-
  congenital Q13.4
  stable H18.61-
  unstable H18.62-
Keratocyst (dental) (odontogenic) — *see* Cyst, calcifying odontogenic
Keratoderma, keratodermia (congenital) (palmaris et plantaris) (symmetrical) Q82.8
  acquired L85.1
    in diseases classified elsewhere L86
  climactericum L85.1
  gonococcal A54.89
  gonorrheal A54.89
  punctata L85.2
  Reiter's — *see* Reiter's disease
Keratodermatocele — *see* Descemetocele
Keratoglobus H18.79
  congenital Q15.8
    with glaucoma Q15.0
Keratohemia — *see* Pigmentation, cornea, stromal
Keratoiritis — *see also* Iridocyclitis
  syphilitic A50.39
  tuberculous A18.54
Keratoma L57.0
  palmaris and plantaris hereditarium Q82.8
  senile L57.0
Keratomalacia H18.44-
  vitamin A deficiency E50.4
Keratomegaly Q13.4
Keratomycosis B49
  nigrans, nigricans (palmaris) B36.1
Keratopathy H18.9
  band H18.42-
  bullous H18.1-
  bullous (aphakic) , following cataract surgery H59.01-
Keratoscleritis, tuberculous A18.52
Keratosis L57.0
  actinic L57.0
  arsenical L85.8
  congenital, specified NEC Q80.8
  female genital NEC N94.89
  follicularis Q82.8
    acquired L11.0
    congenita Q82.8
    et parafollicularis in cutem penetrans L87.0
    spinulosa (decalvans) Q82.8
    vitamin A deficiency E50.8
  gonococcal A54.89
  male genital (external) N50.89
  nigricans L83
  obturans, external ear (canal) — *see* Cholesteatoma, external ear
  palmaris et plantaris (inherited) (symmetrical) Q82.8
    acquired L85.1
  penile N48.89
  pharynx J39.2
  pilaris, acquired L85.8
  punctata (palmaris et plantaris) L85.2
  scrotal N50.89
  seborrheic L82.1
    inflamed L82.0
  senile L57.0
  solar L57.0
  tonsillaris J35.8
  vagina N89.4
  vegetans Q82.8
  vitamin A deficiency E50.8
  vocal cord J38.3
Kerato-uveitis — *see* Iridocyclitis
Kerion (celsi) B35.0
Kernicterus of newborn
  (not due to isoimmunization) P57.9
  due to isoimmunization (conditions in P55.0-P55.9) P57.0
  specified type NEC P57.8
Kerunoparalysis T75.09
Keshan disease E59
Ketoacidosis E87.2
  diabetic — *see* Diabetes, by type, with ketoacidosis
Ketonuria R82.4
Ketosis NEC E88.89
  diabetic — *see* Diabetes, by type, with with ketoacidosis
Kew Garden fever A79.1
Kidney — *see* condition
Kienböck's disease — *see also* Osteochondrosis, juvenile, hand, carpal lunate
  adult M93.1
Kimmelstiel (-Wilson) **disease** — *see* Diabetes, Kimmelstiel (-Wilson) disease
Kimura disease D21.9
  specified site (see Neoplasm, connective tissue benign)
Kink, kinking
  artery I77.1
  hair (acquired) L67.8
  ileum or intestine — *see* Obstruction, intestine
  Lane's — *see* Obstruction, intestine
  organ or site, congenital NEC — *see* Anomaly, by site
  ureter (pelvic junction) N13.5
    with
      hydronephrosis N13.1
        with infection N13.6
      pyelonephritis (chronic) N11.1
    congenital Q62.39
  vein (s) I87.8
    caval I87.1
    peripheral I87.1
Kinnier Wilson's disease (hepatolenticular degeneration) E83.01
Kissing spine M48.20
  cervical region M48.22
  cervicothoracic region M48.23
  lumbar region M48.26
  lumbosacral region M48.27
  occipito-atlanto-axial region M48.21
  thoracic region M48.24
  thoracolumbar region M48.25
Klatskin's tumor C24.0
Klauder's disease A26.8
Klebs' disease — *see also* Glomerulonephritis N05.-
Klebsiella (K.)
  pneumoniae, as cause of disease classified elsewhere B96.1
Klein (e) **-Levin syndrome** G47.13
Kleptomania F63.2
Klinefelter's syndrome Q98.4
  karyotype 47,XXY Q98.0
  male with more than two X chromosomes Q98.1
Klippel-Feil deficiency, disease, or syndrome (brevicollis) Q76.1
Klippel's disease I67.2
Klippel-Trenaunay (-Weber) **syndrome** Q87.2
Klumpke (-Déjerine) **palsy, paralysis** (birth) (newborn) P14.1
Knee — *see* condition
Knock knee (acquired) M21.06-
  congenital Q74.1
Knot (s)
  intestinal, syndrome (volvulus) K56.2
  surfer S89.8-
  umbilical cord (true) O69.2
Knotting (of)
  hair L67.8
  intestine K56.2
Knuckle pad (Garrod's) M72.1
Koch's
  infection — *see* Tuberculosis
  relapsing fever A68.9
Koch-Weeks' conjunctivitis — *see* Conjunctivitis, acute, mucopurulent
Köebner's syndrome Q81.8
Köenig's disease (osteochondritis dissecans) — *see* Osteochondritis, dissecans
Köhler-Pellegrini-Steida disease or syndrome (calcification, knee joint) — *see* Bursitis, tibial collateral
Köhler's disease
  patellar — *see* Osteochondrosis, juvenile, patella
  tarsal navicular — *see* Osteochondrosis, juvenile, tarsus
Koilonychia L60.3
  congenital Q84.6
Kojevnikov's, epilepsy — *see* Kozhevnikof's epilepsy
Koplik's spots B05.9
Kopp's asthma E32.8
Korsakoff's (Wernicke)
  disease, psychosis or syndrome (alcoholic) F10.96
  with dependence F10.26
  drug-induced
    due to drug abuse — *see* Abuse, drug, by type, with amnestic disorder
    due to drug dependence — *see* Dependence, drug, by type, with amnestic disorder
  nonalcoholic F04
Korsakov's disease, psychosis or syndrome — *see* Korsakoff's disease
Korsakow's disease, psychosis or syndrome — *see* Korsakoff's disease
Kostmann's disease or syndrome (infantile genetic agranulocytosis) — *see* Agranulocytosis
Kozhevnikof's epilepsy G40.109
  intractable G40.119
    with status epilepticus G40.111
    without status epilepticus G40.119
  not intractable G40.109
    with status epilepticus G40.101
    without status epilepticus G40.109
Krabbe's
  disease E75.23
  syndrome, congenital muscle hypoplasia Q79.8
Kraepelin-Morel disease — *see* Schizophrenia
Kraft-Weber-Dimitri disease Q85.8
Kraurosis
  ani K62.89
  penis N48.0
  vagina N89.8
  vulva N90.4
Kreotoxism A05.9
Krukenberg's
  spindle — *see* Pigmentation, cornea, posterior
  tumor C79.6-
Kufs' disease E75.4
Kugelberg-Welander disease G12.1
Kuhnt-Junius degeneration — *see also* Degeneration, macula H35.32-
Kümmell's disease or spondylitis — *see* Spondylopathy, traumatic
Kupffer cell sarcoma C22.3
Kuru A81.81
Kussmaul's
  disease M30.0
  respiration E87.2
    in diabetic acidosis — *see* Diabetes, by type, with ketoacidosis
Kwashiorkor E40
  marasmic, marasmus type E42
Kyasanur Forest disease A98.2
Kyphoscoliosis, kyphoscoliotic (acquired) — *see also* Scoliosis M41.9
  congenital Q67.5
  heart (disease) I27.1
  sequelae of rickets E64.3
  tuberculous A18.01
Kyphosis, kyphotic (acquired) M40.209
  cervical region M40.202
  cervicothoracic region M40.203
  congenital Q76.419
    cervical region Q76.412
    cervicothoracic region Q76.413
    occipito-atlanto-axial region Q76.411
    thoracic region Q76.414
    thoracolumbar region Q76.415
  Morquio-Brailsford type (spinal) (*see also*subcategory M49.8) E76.219
  postlaminectomy M96.3
  postradiation therapy M96.2
  postural (adolescent) M40.00
    cervicothoracic region M40.03
    thoracic region M40.04
    thoracolumbar region M40.05
  secondary NEC M40.10
    cervical region M40.12
    cervicothoracic region M40.13
    thoracic region M40.14
    thoracolumbar region M40.15
  sequelae of rickets E64.3
  specified type NEC M40.299
    cervical region M40.292
    cervicothoracic region M40.293
    thoracic region M40.294
    thoracolumbar region M40.295
  syphilitic, congenital A50.56
  thoracic region M40.204
  thoracolumbar region M40.205
  tuberculous A18.01
Kyrle disease L87.0

L

Labia, labium — *see* condition
Labile
  blood pressure R09.89
  vasomotor system I73.9
Labioglossal paralysis G12.29
Labium leporinum — *see* Cleft, lip
Labor — *see* Delivery
Labored breathing — *see* Hyperventilation

Labyrinthitis (circumscribed) (destructive) (diffuse) (inner ear) (latent) (purulent) (suppurative) (*see also*subcategory H83.0)
  syphilitic A52.79
Laceration
  with abortion — *see* Abortion, by type, complicated by laceration of pelvic organs
  abdomen, abdominal
    wall S31.119
      with
        foreign body S31.129
        penetration into peritoneal cavity S31.619
          with foreign body S31.629
      epigastric region S31.112
        with
          foreign body S31.122
          penetration into peritoneal cavity S31.612
            with foreign body S31.622
      left
        lower quadrant S31.114
          with
            foreign body S31.124
            penetration into peritoneal cavity S31.614
              with foreign body S31.624
        upper quadrant S31.111
          with
            foreign body S31.121
            penetration into peritoneal cavity S31.611
              with foreign body S31.621
      periumbilic region S31.115
        with
          foreign body S31.125
          penetration into peritoneal cavity S31.615
            with foreign body S31.625
      right
        lower quadrant S31.113
          with
            foreign body S31.123
            penetration into peritoneal cavity S31.613
              with foreign body S31.623
        upper quadrant S31.110
          with
            foreign body S31.120
            penetration into peritoneal cavity S31.610
              with foreign body S31.620
  accidental, complicating surgery — *see* Complications, surgical, accidental puncture or laceration
  Achilles tendon S86.02-
  adrenal gland S37.813
  alveolar (process) — *see* Laceration, oral cavity
  ankle S91.01-
    with
      foreign body S91.02-
  antecubital space — *see* Laceration, elbow
  anus (sphincter) S31.831
    with
      ectopic or molar pregnancy O08.6
      foreign body S31.832
    complicating delivery — *see* Delivery, complicated, by, laceration, anus (sphincter)
    following ectopic or molar pregnancy O08.6
    nontraumatic, nonpuerperal — *see* Fissure, anus
  arm (upper) S41.11-
    with foreign body S41.12-
    lower — *see* Laceration, forearm
  auditory canal (external) (meatus) — *see* Laceration, ear
  auricle, ear — *see* Laceration, ear
  axilla — *see* Laceration, arm
  back — *see also* Laceration, thorax, back
    lower S31.010
      with
        foreign body S31.020
          with penetration into retroperitoneal space S31.021
        penetration into retroperitoneal space S31.011
  bile duct S36.13
  bladder S37.23
    with ectopic or molar pregnancy O08.6
    following ectopic or molar pregnancy O08.6
    obstetrical trauma O71.5
  blood vessel — *see* Injury, blood vessel
  bowel — *see also* Laceration, intestine
    with ectopic or molar pregnancy O08.6
    complicating abortion — *see* Abortion, by type, complicated by, specified condition NEC
    following ectopic or molar pregnancy O08.6
    obstetrical trauma O71.5
  brain (any part) (cortex) (diffuse) (membrane) — *see also* Injury, intracranial, diffuse
    during birth P10.8
      with hemorrhage P10.1

Laceration - *continued*
  brain (any part) (cortex) (diffuse) (membrane) - *continued*
    focal — *see* Injury, intracranial, focal brain injury
  brainstem S06.38-
  breast S21.01-
    with foreign body S21.02-
  broad ligament S37.893
    with ectopic or molar pregnancy O08.6
    following ectopic or molar pregnancy O08.6
    laceration syndrome N83.8
    obstetrical trauma O71.6
    syndrome (laceration) N83.8
  buttock S31.801
    with foreign body S31.802
    left S31.821
      with foreign body S31.822
    right S31.811
      with foreign body S31.812
  calf — *see* Laceration, leg
  canaliculus lacrimalis — *see* Laceration, eyelid
  canthus, eye — *see* Laceration, eyelid
  capsule, joint — *see* Sprain
  causing eversion of cervix uteri (old) N86
  central (perineal) , complicating delivery O70.9
  cerebellum, traumatic S06.37-
  cerebral S06.33-
    left side S06.32-
    during birth P10.8
      with hemorrhage P10.1
    right side S06.31-
  cervix (uteri)
    with ectopic or molar pregnancy O08.6
    following ectopic or molar pregnancy O08.6
    nonpuerperal, nontraumatic N88.1
    obstetrical trauma (current) O71.3
    old (postpartal) N88.1
    traumatic S37.63
  cheek (external) S01.41-
    with foreign body S01.42-
    internal — *see* Laceration, oral cavity
  chest wall — *see* Laceration, thorax
  chin — *see* Laceration, head, specified site NEC
  chordae tendinae NEC I51.1
    concurrent with acute myocardial infarction — *see* Infarct, myocardium
    following acute myocardial infarction (current complication) I23.4
  clitoris — *see* Laceration, vulva
  colon — *see* Laceration, intestine, large, colon
  common bile duct S36.13
  cortex (cerebral) — *see* Injury, intracranial, diffuse
  costal region — *see* Laceration, thorax
  cystic duct S36.13
  diaphragm S27.803
  digit (s)
    hand — *see* Laceration, finger
    foot — *see* Laceration, toe
  duodenum S36.430
  ear (canal) (external) S01.31-
    with foreign body S01.32-
    drum S09.2-
  elbow S51.01-
    with
      foreign body S51.02-
  epididymis — *see* Laceration, testis
  epigastric region — *see* Laceration, abdomen, wall, epigastric region
  esophagus K22.8
    traumatic
      cervical S11.21
        with foreign body S11.22
      thoracic S27.813
  eye (ball) S05.3-
    with prolapse or loss of intraocular tissue S05.2-
    penetrating S05.6-
  eyebrow — *see* Laceration, eyelid
  eyelid S01.11-
    with foreign body S01.12-
  face NEC — *see* Laceration, head, specified site NEC
  fallopian tube S37.539
    bilateral S37.532
    unilateral S37.531
  finger (s) S61.219
    with
      damage to nail S61.319
        with
          foreign body S61.329
      foreign body S61.229
    index S61.218
      with
        damage to nail S61.318

Laceration - *continued*
  finger (s) - *continued*
    index - *continued*
      with - *continued*
        damage to nail - *continued*
          with
            foreign body S61.328
        foreign body S61.228
      left S61.211
        with
          damage to nail S61.311
            with
              foreign body S61.321
          foreign body S61.221
      right S61.210
        with
          damage to nail S61.310
            with
              foreign body S61.320
          foreign body S61.220
    little S61.218
      with
        damage to nail S61.318
          with
            foreign body S61.328
        foreign body S61.228
      left S61.217
        with
          damage to nail S61.317
            with
              foreign body S61.327
          foreign body S61.227
      right S61.216
        with
          damage to nail S61.316
            with
              foreign body S61.326
          foreign body S61.226
    middle S61.218
      with
        damage to nail S61.318
          with
            foreign body S61.328
        foreign body S61.228
      left S61.213
        with
          damage to nail S61.313
            with
              foreign body S61.323
          foreign body S61.223
      right S61.212
        with
          damage to nail S61.312
            with
              foreign body S61.322
          foreign body S61.222
    ring S61.218
      with
        damage to nail S61.318
          with
            foreign body S61.328
        foreign body S61.228
      left S61.215
        with
          damage to nail S61.315
            with
              foreign body S61.325
          foreign body S61.225
      right S61.214
        with
          damage to nail S61.314
            with
              foreign body S61.324
          foreign body S61.224
  flank S31.119
    with foreign body S31.129
  foot (except toe (s) alone) S91.319
    with foreign body S91.329
    left S91.312
      with foreign body S91.322
    right S91.311
      with foreign body S91.321
    toe — *see* Laceration, toe
  forearm S51.819
    with
      foreign body S51.829
    elbow only — *see* Laceration, elbow
    left S51.812
      with
        foreign body S51.822
    right S51.811
      with
        foreign body S51.821

- **Laceration** - *continued*
  - forehead S01.81
    - with foreign body S01.82
  - fourchette O70.0
    - with ectopic or molar pregnancy O08.6
    - complicating delivery O70.0
    - following ectopic or molar pregnancy O08.6
  - gallbladder S36.123
  - genital organs, external
    - female S31.512
      - with foreign body S31.522
      - vagina — *see* Laceration, vagina
      - vulva — *see* Laceration, vulva
    - male S31.511
      - with foreign body S31.521
      - penis — *see* Laceration, penis
      - scrotum — *see* Laceration, scrotum
      - testis — *see* Laceration, testis
  - groin — *see* Laceration, abdomen, wall
  - gum — *see* Laceration, oral cavity
  - hand S61.419
    - with
      - foreign body S61.429
    - finger — *see* Laceration, finger
    - left S61.412
      - with
        - foreign body S61.422
    - right S61.411
      - with
        - foreign body S61.421
    - thumb — *see* Laceration, thumb
  - head S01.91
    - with foreign body S01.92
    - cheek — *see* Laceration, cheek
    - ear — *see* Laceration, ear
    - eyelid — *see* Laceration, eyelid
    - lip — *see* Laceration, lip
    - nose — *see* Laceration, nose
    - oral cavity — *see* Laceration, oral cavity
    - scalp S01.01
      - with foreign body S01.02
    - specified site NEC S01.81
      - with foreign body S01.82
    - temporomandibular area — *see* Laceration, cheek
  - heart — *see* Injury, heart, laceration
  - heel — *see* Laceration, foot
  - hepatic duct S36.13
  - hip S71.019
    - with foreign body S71.029
    - left S71.012
      - with foreign body S71.022
    - right S71.011
      - with foreign body S71.021
  - hymen — *see* Laceration, vagina
  - hypochondrium — *see* Laceration, abdomen, wall
  - hypogastric region — *see* Laceration, abdomen, wall
  - ileum S36.438
  - inguinal region — *see* Laceration, abdomen, wall
  - instep — *see* Laceration, foot
  - internal organ — *see* Injury, by site
  - interscapular region — *see* Laceration, thorax, back
  - intestine
    - large
      - colon S36.539
        - ascending S36.530
        - descending S36.532
        - sigmoid S36.533
        - specified site NEC S36.538
      - rectum S36.63
        - transverse S36.531
    - small S36.439
      - duodenum S36.430
      - specified site NEC S36.438
  - intra-abdominal organ S36.93
    - intestine — *see* Laceration, intestine
    - liver — *see* Laceration, liver
    - pancreas — *see* Laceration, pancreas
    - peritoneum S36.81
    - specified site NEC S36.893
    - spleen — *see* Laceration, spleen
    - stomach — *see* Laceration, stomach
  - intracranial NEC — *see also* Injury, intracranial, diffuse
    - birth injury P10.9
  - jaw — *see* Laceration, head, specified site NEC
  - jejunum S36.438
  - joint capsule — *see* Sprain, by site
  - kidney S37.03-
    - major (greater than 3 cm) (massive) (stellate) S37.06-
    - minor (less than 1 cm) S37.04-
    - moderate (1 to 3 cm) S37.05-
      - multiple S37.06-

- **Laceration** - *continued*
  - knee S81.01-
    - with foreign body S81.02-
  - labium (majus) (minus) — *see* Laceration, vulva
  - lacrimal duct — *see* Laceration, eyelid
  - large intestine — *see* Laceration, intestine, large
  - larynx S11.011
    - with foreign body S11.012
  - leg (lower) S81.819
    - with foreign body S81.829
    - foot — *see* Laceration, foot
    - knee — *see* Laceration, knee
    - left S81.812
      - with foreign body S81.822
    - right S81.811
      - with foreign body S81.821
    - upper — *see* Laceration, thigh
  - ligament — *see* Sprain
  - lip S01.511
    - with foreign body S01.521
  - liver S36.113
    - major (stellate) S36.116
    - minor S36.114
    - moderate S36.115
  - loin — *see* Laceration, abdomen, wall
  - lower back — *see* Laceration, back, lower
  - lumbar region — *see* Laceration, back, lower
  - lung S27.339
    - bilateral S27.332
    - unilateral S27.331
  - malar region — *see* Laceration, head, specified site NEC
  - mammary — *see* Laceration, breast
  - mastoid region — *see* Laceration, head, specified site NEC
  - meninges — *see* Injury, intracranial, diffuse
  - meniscus — *see* Tear, meniscus
  - mesentery S36.893
  - mesosalpinx S37.893
  - mouth — *see* Laceration, oral cavity
  - muscle — *see* Injury, muscle, by site, laceration
  - nail
    - finger — *see* Laceration, finger, with damage to nail
    - toe — *see* Laceration, toe, with damage to nail
  - nasal (septum) (sinus) — *see* Laceration, nose
  - nasopharynx — *see* Laceration, head, specified site NEC
  - neck S11.91
    - with foreign body S11.92
    - involving
      - cervical esophagus S11.21
        - with foreign body S11.22
      - larynx — *see* Laceration, larynx
      - pharynx — *see* Laceration, pharynx
      - thyroid gland — *see* Laceration, thyroid gland
      - trachea — *see* Laceration, trachea
    - specified site NEC S11.81
      - with foreign body S11.82
  - nerve — *see* Injury, nerve
  - nose (septum) (sinus) S01.21
    - with foreign body S01.22
  - ocular NOS S05.3-
    - adnexa NOS S01.11-
  - oral cavity S01.512
    - with foreign body S01.522
  - orbit (eye) — *see* Wound, open, ocular, orbit
  - ovary S37.439
    - bilateral S37.432
    - unilateral S37.431
  - palate — *see* Laceration, oral cavity
  - palm — *see* Laceration, hand
  - pancreas S36.239
    - body S36.231
      - major S36.261
      - minor S36.241
      - moderate S36.251
    - head S36.230
      - major S36.260
      - minor S36.240
      - moderate S36.250
    - major S36.269
    - minor S36.249
    - moderate S36.259
    - tail S36.232
      - major S36.262
      - minor S36.242
      - moderate S36.252
  - pelvic S31.010
    - with
      - foreign body S31.020
        - penetration into retroperitoneal cavity S31.021
      - penetration into retroperitoneal cavity S31.011

- **Laceration** - *continued*
  - pelvic - *continued*
    - floor — *see also* Laceration, back, lower
      - with ectopic or molar pregnancy O08.6
      - complicating delivery O70.1
      - following ectopic or molar pregnancy O08.6
      - old (postpartal) N81.89
    - organ S37.93
      - with ectopic or molar pregnancy O08.6
      - adrenal gland S37.813
      - bladder S37.23
      - fallopian tube — *see* Laceration, fallopian tube
      - following ectopic or molar pregnancy O08.6
      - kidney — *see* Laceration, kidney
      - obstetrical trauma O71.5
      - ovary — *see* Laceration, ovary
      - prostate S37.823
      - specified site NEC S37.893
      - ureter S37.13
      - urethra S37.33
      - uterus S37.63
  - penis S31.21
    - with foreign body S31.22
  - perineum
    - female S31.41
      - with
        - ectopic or molar pregnancy O08.6
        - foreign body S31.42
      - during delivery O70.9
        - first degree O70.0
        - fourth degree O70.3
        - second degree O70.1
        - third degree — *see also* Delivery, complicated, by, laceration, perineum, third degree O70.20
      - old (postpartal) N81.89
      - postpartal N81.89
      - secondary (postpartal) O90.1
    - male S31.119
      - with foreign body S31.129
  - periocular area (with or without lacrimal passages) — *see* Laceration, eyelid
  - peritoneum S36.893
  - periumbilic region — *see* Laceration, abdomen, wall, periumbilic
  - periurethral tissue — *see* Laceration, urethra
  - phalanges
    - finger — *see* Laceration, finger
    - toe — *see* Laceration, toe
  - pharynx S11.21
    - with foreign body S11.22
  - pinna — *see* Laceration, ear
  - popliteal space — *see* Laceration, knee
  - prepuce — *see* Laceration, penis
  - prostate S37.823
  - pubic region S31.119
    - with foreign body S31.129
  - pudendum — *see* Laceration, genital organs, external
  - rectovaginal septum — *see* Laceration, vagina
  - rectum S36.63
  - retroperitoneum S36.893
  - round ligament S37.893
  - sacral region — *see* Laceration, back, lower
  - sacroiliac region — *see* Laceration, back, lower
  - salivary gland — *see* Laceration, oral cavity
  - scalp S01.01
    - with foreign body S01.02
  - scapular region — *see* Laceration, shoulder
  - scrotum S31.31
    - with foreign body S31.32
  - seminal vesicle S37.893
  - shin — *see* Laceration, leg
  - shoulder S41.019
    - with foreign body S41.029
    - left S41.012
      - with foreign body S41.022
    - right S41.011
      - with foreign body S41.021
  - small intestine — *see* Laceration, intestine, small
  - spermatic cord — *see* Laceration, testis
  - spinal cord (meninges) — *see also* Injury, spinal cord, by region
    - due to injury at birth P11.5
    - newborn (birth injury) P11.5
  - spleen S36.039
    - major (massive) (stellate) S36.032
    - moderate S36.031
    - superficial (minor) S36.030
  - sternal region — *see* Laceration, thorax, front
  - stomach S36.33
  - submaxillary region — *see* Laceration, head, specified site NEC

- **Landouzy's disease** (icterohemorrhagic leptospirosis) A27.0
- **Landry-Guillain-Barré, syndrome or paralysis** G61.0
- **Landry's disease or paralysis** G61.0
- **Lane's**
  - band Q43.3
  - kink — *see* Obstruction, intestine
  - syndrome K90.2
- **Langdon Down syndrome** — *see* Trisomy, 21
- **Lapsed immunization schedule status** Z28.3
- **Large**
  - baby (regardless of gestational age) (4000g to 4499g) P08.1
  - ear, congenital Q17.1
  - physiological cup Q14.2
  - stature R68.89
- **Large-for-dates NEC** (infant) (4000g to 4499g) P08.1
  - affecting management of pregnancy O36.6-
  - exceptionally (4500g or more) P08.0
- **Larsen-Johansson disease orosteochondrosis** — *see* Osteochondrosis, juvenile, patella
- **Larsen's syndrome** (flattened facies and multiple congenital dislocations) Q74.8
- **Larva migrans**
  - cutaneous B76.9
    - Ancylostoma B76.0
  - visceral B83.0
- **Laryngeal** — *see* condition
- **Laryngismus** (stridulus) J38.5
  - congenital P28.89
  - diphtheritic A36.2
- **Laryngitis** (acute) (edematous) (fibrinous) (infective) (infiltrative) (malignant) (membranous) (phlegmonous) (pneumococcal) (pseudomembranous) (septic) (subglottic) (suppurative) (ulcerative) J04.0
  - with
    - influenza, flu, or grippe — *see* Influenza, with, laryngitis
    - tracheitis (acute) — *see* Laryngotracheitis
  - atrophic J37.0
  - catarrhal J37.0
  - chronic J37.0
    - with tracheitis (chronic) J37.1
  - diphtheritic A36.2
  - due to external agent — *see* Inflammation, respiratory, upper, due to
  - Hemophilus influenzae J04.0
  - H. influenzae J04.0
  - hypertrophic J37.0
  - influenzal — *see* Influenza, with, respiratory manifestations NEC
  - obstructive J05.0
  - sicca J37.0
  - spasmodic J05.0
    - acute J04.0
  - streptococcal J04.0
  - stridulous J05.0
  - syphilitic (late) A52.73
    - congenital A50.59 *[J99]*
      - early A50.03 *[J99]*
  - tuberculous A15.5
  - Vincent's A69.1
- **Laryngocele** (congenital) (ventricular) Q31.3
- **Laryngofissure** J38.7
  - congenital Q31.8
- **Laryngomalacia** (congenital) Q31.5
- **Laryngopharyngitis** (acute) J06.0
  - chronic J37.0
  - due to external agent — *see* Inflammation, respiratory, upper, due to
- **Laryngoplegia** J38.00
  - bilateral J38.02
  - unilateral J38.01
- **Laryngoptosis** J38.7
- **Laryngospasm** J38.5
- **Laryngostenosis** J38.6
- **Laryngotracheitis** (acute) (Infectional) (infective) (viral) J04.2
  - atrophic J37.1
  - catarrhal J37.1
  - chronic J37.1
  - diphtheritic A36.2
  - due to external agent — *see* Inflammation, respiratory, upper, due to
  - Hemophilus influenzae J04.2
  - hypertrophic J37.1
  - influenzal — *see* Influenza, with, respiratory manifestations NEC
  - pachydermic J38.7

- **Laryngotracheitis** (acute) (Infectional) (infective) (viral) - *continued*
  - sicca J37.1
  - spasmodic J38.5
    - acute J05.0
  - streptococcal J04.2
  - stridulous J38.5
  - syphilitic (late) A52.73
    - congenital A50.59 *[J99]*
      - early A50.03 *[J99]*
  - tuberculous A15.5
  - Vincent's A69.1
- **Laryngotracheobronchitis** — *see* Bronchitis
- **Larynx, laryngeal** — *see* condition
- **Lassa fever** A96.2
- **Lassitude** — *see* Weakness
- **Late**
  - talker R62.0
  - walker R62.0
- **Late effect** (s) — *see* Sequelae
- **Latent** — *see* condition
- **Laterocession** — *see* Lateroversion
- **Lateroflexion** — *see* Lateroversion
- **Lateroversion**
  - cervix — *see* Lateroversion, uterus
  - uterus, uterine (cervix) (postinfectional) (postpartal, old) N85.4
    - congenital Q51.818
    - in pregnancy or childbirth O34.59-
- **Lathyrism** — *see* Poisoning, food, noxious, plant
- **Launois' syndrome** (pituitary gigantism) E22.0
- **Launois-Bensaude adenolipomatosis** E88.89
- **Laurence-Moon** (-Bardet) **-Biedl syndrome** Q87.89
- **Lax, laxity** — *see also* Relaxation
  - ligament (ous) — *see also* Disorder, ligament
    - familial M35.7
    - knee — *see* Derangement, knee
  - skin (acquired) L57.4
    - congenital Q82.8
- **Laxative habit** F55.2
- **Lazy leukocyte syndrome** D70.8
- **Lead miner's lung** J63.6
- **Leak, leakage**
  - air NEC J93.82
    - postprocedural J95.812
  - amniotic fluid — *see* Rupture, membranes, premature
  - blood (microscopic) , fetal, into maternal circulation
    - affecting management of pregnancy — *see* Pregnancy, complicated by
  - cerebrospinal fluid G96.0
    - from spinal (lumbar) puncture G97.0
  - device, implant or graft — *see also* Complications, by site and type, mechanical
    - arterial graft NEC — *see* Complication, cardiovascular device, mechanical, vascular
    - breast (implant) T85.43
    - catheter NEC T85.638
      - urinary T83.038
        - cystostomy T83.030
        - Hopkins T83.038
        - ileostomy T83.038
        - indwelling T83.031
        - nephrostomy T83.032
        - specified NEC T83.038
        - urostomy T83.038
      - dialysis (renal) T82.43
        - intraperitoneal T85.631
      - infusion NEC T82.534
        - spinal (epidural) (subdural) T85.630
    - gastrointestinal — *see* Complications, prosthetic device, mechanical, gastrointestinal device
    - genital NEC T83.498
      - penile prosthesis (cylinder) (implanted) (pump) (resevoir) T83.490
      - testicular prosthesis T83.491
    - heart NEC — *see* Complication, cardiovascular device, mechanical
    - joint prosthesis — *see* Complications, joint prosthesis, mechanical, specified NEC, by site
    - ocular NEC — *see* Complications, prosthetic device, mechanical, ocular device
    - orthopedic NEC — *see* Complication, orthopedic, device, mechanical
    - persistent air J93.82
    - specified NEC T85.638
    - urinary NEC — *see also* Complication, genitourinary, device, urinary, mechanical
      - graft T83.23
    - vascular NEC — *see* Complication, cardiovascular device, mechanical
    - ventricular intracranial shunt T85.03
  - urine — *see* Incontinence

- **Leaky heart** — *see* Endocarditis
- **Learning defect** (specific) F81.9
- **Leather bottle stomach** C16.9
- **Leber's**
  - congenital amaurosis H35.50
  - optic atrophy (hereditary) H47.22
- **Lederer's anemia** D59.1
- **Leeches** (external) — *see* Hirudiniasis
- **Leg** — *see* condition
- **Legg** (-Calvé)
  - **-Perthes disease, syndrome or osteochondrosis** M91.1-
- **Legionellosis** A48.1
  - nonpneumonic A48.2
- **Legionnaires'**
  - disease A48.1
    - nonpneumonic A48.2
  - pneumonia A48.1
- **Leigh's disease** G31.82
- **Leiner's disease** L21.1
- **Leiofibromyoma** — *see* Leiomyoma
- **Leiomyoblastoma** — *see* Neoplasm, connective tissue, benign
- **Leiomyofibroma** — *see also* Neoplasm, connective tissue, benign
  - uterus (cervix) (corpus) D25.9
- **Leiomyoma** — *see also* Neoplasm, connective tissue, benign
  - bizarre — *see* Neoplasm, connective tissue, benign
  - cellular — *see* Neoplasm, connective tissue, benign
  - epithelioid — *see* Neoplasm, connective tissue, benign
  - uterus (cervix) (corpus) D25.9
    - intramural D25.1
    - submucous D25.0
    - subserosal D25.2
  - vascular — *see* Neoplasm, connective tissue, benign
- **Leiomyoma, leiomyomatosis** (intravascular) — *see* Neoplasm, connective tissue, uncertain behavior
- **Leiomyosarcoma** — *see also* Neoplasm, connective tissue, malignant
  - epithelioid — *see* Neoplasm, connective tissue, malignant
  - myxoid — *see* Neoplasm, connective tissue, malignant
- **Leishmaniasis** B55.9
  - American (mucocutaneous) B55.2
    - cutaneous B55.1
  - Asian Desert B55.1
  - Brazilian B55.2
  - cutaneous (any type) B55.1
  - dermal — *see also* Leishmaniasis, cutaneous
    - post-kala-azar B55.0
  - eyelid B55.1
  - infantile B55.0
  - Mediterranean B55.0
  - mucocutaneous (American) (New World) B55.2
  - naso-oral B55.2
  - nasopharyngeal B55.2
  - old world B55.1
  - tegumentaria diffusa B55.1
  - visceral B55.0
- **Leishmanoid, dermal** — *see also* Leishmaniasis, cutaneous
  - post-kala-azar B55.0
- **Lenegre's disease** I44.2
- **Lengthening, leg** — *see* Deformity, limb, unequal length
- **Lennert's lymphoma** — *see* Lymphoma, Lennert's
- **Lennox-Gastaut syndrome** G40.812
  - intractable G40.814
    - with status epilepticus G40.813
    - without status epilepticus G40.814
  - not intractable G40.812
    - with status epilepticus G40.811
    - without status epilepticus G40.812
- **Lens** — *see* condition
- **Lenticonus** (anterior) (posterior) (congenital) Q12.8
- **Lenticular degeneration, progressive** E83.01
- **Lentiglobus** (posterior) (congenital) Q12.8
- **Lentigo** (congenital) L81.4
  - maligna — *see also* Melanoma, in situ
    - melanoma — *see* Melanoma
- **Lentivirus, as cause of disease classified elsewhere** B97.31
- **Leontiasis**
  - ossium M85.2
  - syphilitic (late) A52.78
    - congenital A50.59
- **Lepothrix** A48.8
- **Lepra** — *see* Leprosy
- **Leprechaunism** E34.8

- **Leprosy** A30.-
  - with muscle disorder A30.9 *[M63.80]*
    - ankle A30.9 *[M63.87-]*
    - foot A30.9 *[M63.87-]*
    - forearm A30.9 *[M63.83-]*
    - hand A30.9 *[M63.84-]*
    - lower leg A30.9 *[M63.86-]*
    - multiple sites A30.9 *[M63.89]*
    - pelvic region A30.9 *[M63.85-]*
    - shoulder region A30.9 *[M63.81-]*
    - specified site NEC A30.9 *[M63.88]*
    - thigh A30.9 *[M63.85-]*
    - upper arm A30.9 *[M63.82-]*
  - anesthetic A30.9
  - BB A30.3
  - BL A30.4
  - borderline (infiltrated) (neuritic) A30.3
    - lepromatous A30.4
    - tuberculoid A30.2
  - BT A30.2
  - dimorphous (infiltrated) (neuritic) A30.3
  - I A30.0
  - indeterminate (macular) (neuritic) A30.0
  - lepromatous (diffuse) (infiltrated) (macular) (neuritic) (nodular) A30.5
  - LL A30.5
  - macular (early) (neuritic) (simple) A30.9
  - maculoanesthetic A30.9
  - mixed A30.3
  - neural A30.9
  - nodular A30.5
  - primary neuritic A30.3
  - specified type NEC A30.8
  - TT A30.1
  - tuberculoid (major) (minor) A30.1
- **Leptocytosis, hereditary** D56.9
- **Leptomeningitis** (chronic) (circumscribed) (hemorrhagic) (nonsuppurative) — *see* Meningitis
- **Leptomeningopathy** G96.19
- **Leptospiral** — *see* condition
- **Leptospirochetal** — *see* condition
- **Leptospirosis** A27.9
  - canicola A27.89
  - due to Leptospira interrogans serovar icterohaemorrhagiae A27.0
  - icterohemorrhagica A27.0
  - pomona A27.89
  - Weil's disease A27.0
- **Leptus dermatitis** B88.0
- **Leriche's syndrome** (aortic bifurcation occlusion) I74.09
- **Leri's pleonosteosis** Q78.8
- **Leri-Weill syndrome** Q77.8
- **Lermoyez' syndrome** — *see* Vertigo, peripheral NEC
- **Lesch-Nyhan syndrome** E79.1
- **Leser-Trélat disease** L82.1
  - inflamed L82.0
- **Lesion** (s) (nontraumatic)
  - abducens nerve — *see* Strabismus, paralytic, sixth nerve
  - alveolar process K08.9
  - angiocentric immunoproliferative D47.Z9
  - anorectal K62.9
  - aortic (valve) I35.9
  - auditory nerve — *see* subcategory H93.3
  - basal ganglion G25.9
  - bile duct — *see* Disease, bile duct
  - biomechanical M99.9
    - specified type NEC M99.89
      - abdomen M99.89
      - acromioclavicular M99.87
      - cervical region M99.81
      - cervicothoracic M99.81
      - costochondral M99.88
      - costovertebral M99.88
      - head region M99.80
      - hip M99.85
      - lower extremity M99.86
      - lumbar region M99.83
      - lumbosacral M99.83
      - occipitocervical M99.80
      - pelvic region M99.85
      - pubic M99.85
      - rib cage M99.88
      - sacral region M99.84
      - sacrococcygeal M99.84
      - sacroiliac M99.84
      - specified NEC M99.89
      - sternochondral M99.88
      - sternoclavicular M99.87
      - thoracic region M99.82
      - thoracolumbar M99.82
      - upper extremity M99.87

- **Lesion** (s) (nontraumatic) - *continued*
  - bladder N32.9
  - bone — *see* Disorder, bone
  - brachial plexus G54.0
  - brain G93.9
    - congenital Q04.9
    - vascular I67.9
      - degenerative I67.9
      - hypertensive I67.4
  - buccal cavity K13.79
  - calcified — *see* Calcification
  - canthus — *see* Disorder, eyelid
  - carate — *see* Pinta, lesions
  - cardia K31.9
  - cardiac — *see also* Disease, heart I51.9
    - congenital Q24.9
    - valvular — *see* Endocarditis
  - cauda equina G83.4
  - cecum K63.9
  - cerebral — *see* Lesion, brain
  - cerebrovascular I67.9
    - degenerative I67.9
    - hypertensive I67.4
  - cervical (nerve) root NEC G54.2
  - chiasmal — *see* Disorder, optic, chiasm
  - chorda tympani G51.8
  - coin, lung R91.1
  - colon K63.9
  - combined periodontic - endodontic K05.5
  - congenital — *see* Anomaly, by site
  - conjunctiva H11.9
  - conus medullaris — *see* Injury, conus medullaris
  - coronary artery — *see* Ischemia, heart
  - cranial nerve G52.9
    - eighth — *see* Disorder, ear
    - eleventh G52.9
    - fifth G50.9
    - first G52.0
    - fourth — *see* Strabismus, paralytic, fourth nerve
    - seventh G51.9
    - sixth — *see* Strabismus, paralytic, sixth nerve
    - tenth G52.2
    - twelfth G52.3
  - cystic — *see* Cyst
  - degenerative — *see* Degeneration
  - duodenum K31.9
  - edentulous (alveolar) ridge, associated with trauma, due to traumatic occlusion K06.2
  - en coup de sabre L94.1
  - eyelid — *see* Disorder, eyelid
  - gasserian ganglion G50.8
  - gastric K31.9
  - gastroduodenal K31.9
  - gastrointestinal K63.9
  - gingiva, associated with trauma K06.2
  - glomerular
    - focal and segmental — *see also* N00-N07 with fourth character .1 N05.1
    - minimal change — *see also* N00-N07 with fourth character .0 N05.0
  - heart (organic) — *see* Disease, heart
  - hyperchromic, due to pinta (carate) A67.1
  - hyperkeratotic — *see* Hyperkeratosis
  - hypothalamic E23.7
  - ileocecal K63.9
  - ileum K63.9
  - iliohypogastric nerve G57.8-
  - inflammatory — *see* Inflammation
  - intestine K63.9
  - intracerebral — *see* Lesion, brain
  - intrachiasmal (optic) — *see* Disorder, optic, chiasm
  - intracranial, space-occupying R90.0
  - joint — *see* Disorder, joint
    - sacroiliac (old) M53.3
  - keratotic — *see* Keratosis
  - kidney — *see* Disease, renal
  - laryngeal nerve (recurrent) G52.2
  - lip K13.0
  - liver K76.9
  - lumbosacral
    - plexus G54.1
    - root (nerve) NEC G54.4
  - lung (coin) R91.1
  - maxillary sinus J32.0
  - mitral I05.9
  - Morel-Lavallée — *see* Hematoma, by site
  - motor cortex NEC G93.89
  - mouth K13.79
  - nerve G58.9
    - femoral G57.2-
    - median G56.1-
      - carpal tunnel syndrome — *see* Syndrome, carpal tunnel

- **Lesion** (s) (nontraumatic) - *continued*
  - nerve - *continued*
    - plantar G57.6-
    - popliteal (lateral) G57.3-
      - medial G57.4-
    - radial G56.3-
    - sciatic G57.0-
    - spinal — *see* Injury, nerve, spinal
    - ulnar G56.2-
  - nervous system, congenital Q07.9
  - nonallopathic — *see* Lesion, biomechanical
  - nose (internal) J34.89
  - obstructive — *see* Obstruction
  - obturator nerve G57.8-
  - oral mucosa K13.70
  - organ or site NEC — *see* Disease, by site
  - osteolytic — *see* Osteolysis
  - peptic K27.9
  - periodontal, due to traumatic occlusion K05.5
  - pharynx J39.2
  - pigment, pigmented (skin) L81.9
  - pinta — *see* Pinta, lesions
  - polypoid — *see* Polyp
  - prechiasmal (optic) — *see* Disorder, optic, chiasm
  - primary — *see also* Syphilis, primary A51.0
    - carate A67.0
    - pinta A67.0
    - yaws A66.0
  - pulmonary J98.4
    - valve I37.9
  - pylorus K31.9
  - rectosigmoid K63.9
  - retina, retinal H35.9
  - sacroiliac (joint) (old) M53.3
  - salivary gland K11.9
    - benign lymphoepithelial K11.8
  - saphenous nerve G57.8-
  - sciatic nerve G57.0-
  - secondary — *see* Syphilis, secondary
  - shoulder (region) M75.9-
    - specified NEC M75.8-
  - sigmoid K63.9
  - sinus (accessory) (nasal) J34.89
  - skin L98.9
    - suppurative L08.0
  - SLAP S43.43-
  - spinal cord G95.9
    - congenital Q06.9
  - spleen D73.89
  - stomach K31.9
  - superior glenoid labrum S43.43-
  - syphilitic — *see* Syphilis
  - tertiary — *see* Syphilis, tertiary
  - thoracic root (nerve) NEC G54.3
  - tonsillar fossa J35.9
  - tooth, teeth K08.9
    - white spot
      - chewing surface K02.51
      - pit and fissure surface K02.51
      - smooth surface K02.61
  - traumatic — *see* specific type of injury by site
  - tricuspid (valve) I07.9
    - nonrheumatic I36.9
  - trigeminal nerve G50.9
  - ulcerated or ulcerative — *see* Ulcer, skin
  - uterus N85.9
  - vagina N89.8
  - vulva N90.89
  - vagus nerve G52.2
  - valvular — *see* Endocarditis
  - vascular I99.9
    - affecting central nervous system I67.9
    - following trauma NEC T14.8
    - umbilical cord, complicating delivery O69.5
  - warty — *see* Verruca
  - white spot (tooth)
    - chewing surface K02.51
    - pit and fissure surface K02.51
    - smooth surface K02.61
- **Lethargic** — *see* condition
- **Lethargy** R53.83
- **Letterer-Siwe's disease** C96.0
- **Leukemia, leukemic** C95.9-
  - acute basophilic C94.8-
  - acute bilineal C95.0-
  - acute erythroid C94.0-
  - acute lymphoblastic C91.0-
  - acute megakaryoblastic C94.2-
  - acute megakaryocytic C94.2-
  - acute mixed lineage C95.0-
  - acute monoblastic (monoblastic/monocytic) C93.0-
  - acute monocytic (monoblastic/monocytic) C93.0-

Leukemia, leukemic - *continued*
acute myeloblastic (minimal differentiation) (with maturation) C92.0-
acute myeloid, NOS C92.0-
with
11q23-abnormality C92.6-
dysplasia of remaining hematopoesis and/or myelodysplastic disease in its history C92.A-
multilineage dysplasia C92.A-
variation of MLL-gene C92.6-
M6 (a) (b) C94.0-
M7 C94.2-
acute myelomonocytic C92.5-
acute promyelocytic C92.4-
adult T-cell (HTLV-1-associated) (acute variant) (chronic variant) (lymphomatoid variant) (smouldering variant) C91.5-
aggressive NK-cell C94.8-
AML (1/ETO) (M0) (M1) (M2) (without a FAB classification) C92.0-
AML M3 C92.4-
AML M4 (Eo with inv (16) or t (16;16)) C92.5-
AML M5 C93.0-
AML M5a C93.0-
AML M5b C93.0-
AML Me with t (15;17) and variants C92.4-
atypical chronic myeloid, BCR/ABL-negative C92.2 -
biphenotypic acute C95.0-
blast cell C95.0-
Burkitt-type, mature B-cell C91.A-
chronic lymphocytic, of B-cell type C91.1-
chronic monocytic C93.1-
chronic myelogenous (Philadelphia chromosome (Ph1) positive) (t (9;22)) (q34;q11) (with crisis of blast cells) C92.1-
chronic myeloid, BCR/ABL-positive C92.1-
atypical, BCR/ABL-negative C92.2-
chronic myelomonocytic C93.1-
chronic neutrophilic D47.1
CMML (-1) (-2) (with eosinophilia) C93.1-
granulocytic (*see also* Category C92) C92.9-
hairy cell C91.4-
juvenile myelomonocytic C93.3-
lymphoid C91.9-
specified NEC C91.Z-
mast cell C94.3-
mature B-cell, Burkitt-type C91.A-
monocytic (subacute) C93.9-
specified NEC C93.Z-
myelogenous (*see also* Category C92) C92.9-
myeloid C92.9-
acute C92.0-
specified NEC C92.Z-
plasma cell C90.1-
plasmacytic C90.1-
prolymphocytic
of B-cell type C91.3-
of T-cell type C91.6-
specified NEC C94.8-
stem cell, of unclear lineage C95.0-
subacute lymphocytic C91.9-
T-cell large granular lymphocytic C91.Z-
unspecified cell type C95.9-
acute C95.0-
chronic C95.1-
Leukemoid reaction — *see also* Reaction, leukemoid D72.823-
Leukoaraiosis (hypertensive) I67.81
Leukoariosis — *see* Leukoaraiosis
Leukocoria — *see* Disorder, globe, degenerated condition, leucocoria
Leukocytopenia D72.819
Leukocytosis D72.829
eosinophilic D72.1
Leukoderma, leukodermia NEC L81.5
syphilitic A51.39
late A52.79
Leukodystrophy E75.29
Leukoedema, oral epithelium K13.29
Leukoencephalitis G04.81
acute (subacute) hemorrhagic G36.1
postimmunization or postvaccinal G04.02
postinfectious G04.01
subacute sclerosing A81.1
van Bogaert's (sclerosing) A81.1
Leukoencephalopathy — *see also* Encephalopathy G93.49
Binswanger's I67.3
heroin vapor G92
metachromatic E75.25
multifocal (progressive) A81.2
postimmunization and postvaccinal G04.02

Leukoencephalopathy - *continued*
progressive multifocal A81.2
reversible, posterior G93.6
van Bogaert's (sclerosing) A81.1
vascular, progressive I67.3
Leukoerythroblastosis D75.9
Leukokeratosis — *see also* Leukoplakia
mouth K13.21
nicotina palati K13.24
oral mucosa K13.21
tongue K13.21
vocal cord J38.3
Leukokraurosis vulva (e) N90.4
Leukoma (cornea) — *see also* Opacity, cornea
adherent H17.0-
interfering with central vision — *see* Opacity, cornea, central
Leukomalacia, cerebral, newborn P91.2
periventricular P91.2
Leukomelanopathy, hereditary D72.0
Leukonychia (punctata) (striata) L60.8
congenital Q84.4
Leukopathia unguium L60.8
congenital Q84.4
Leukopenia D72.819
basophilic D72.818
chemotherapy (cancer) induced D70.1
congenital D70.0
cyclic D70.0
drug induced NEC D70.2
due to cytoreductive cancer chemotherapy D70.1
eosinophilic D72.818
familial D70.0
infantile genetic D70.0
malignant D70.9
periodic D70.0
transitory neonatal P61.5
Leukopenic — *see* condition
Leukoplakia
anus K62.89
bladder (postinfectional) N32.89
buccal K13.21
cervix (uteri) N88.0
esophagus K22.8
gingiva K13.21
hairy (oral mucosa) (tongue) K13.3
kidney (pelvis) N28.89
larynx J38.7
lip K13.21
mouth K13.21
oral epithelium, including tongue (mucosa) K13.21
palate K13.21
pelvis (kidney) N28.89
penis (infectional) N48.0
rectum K62.89
syphilitic (late) A52.79
tongue K13.21
ureter (postinfectional) N28.89
urethra (postinfectional) N36.8
uterus N85.8
vagina N89.4
vocal cord J38.3
vulva N90.4
Leukorrhea N89.8
due to Trichomonas (vaginalis) A59.00
trichomonal A59.00
Leukosarcoma C85.9-
Levocardia (isolated) Q24.1
with situs inversus Q89.3
Levotransposition Q20.5
Lev's disease or syndrome
(acquired complete heart block) I44.2
Levulosuria — *see* Fructosuria
Levurid L30.2
Lewy body (ies) (dementia) (disease) G31.83
Leyden-Moebius dystrophy G71.09
Leydig cell
carcinoma
specified site — *see* Neoplasm, malignant, by site
unspecified site
female C56.9
male C62.9-
tumor
benign
specified site — *see* Neoplasm, benign, by site
unspecified site
female D27.-
male D29.2-
malignant
specified site — *see* Neoplasm, malignant, by site
unspecified site
female C56.-
male C62.9-

Leydig cell - *continued*
tumor - *continued*
specified site — *see* Neoplasm, uncertain behavior, by site
unspecified site
female D39.1-
male D40.1-
Leydig-Sertoli cell tumor
specified site — *see* Neoplasm, benign, by site
unspecified site
female D27.-
male D29.2-
LGSIL
(Low grade squamous intraepithelial lesion on cytologic smear of)
anus R85.612
cervix R87.612
vagina R87.622
Liar, pathologic F60.2
Libido
decreased R68.82
Libman-Sacks disease M32.11
Lice (infestation) B85.2
body (Pediculus corporis) B85.1
crab B85.3
head (Pediculus capitis) B85.0
mixed (classifiable to more than one of the titles B85.0-B85.3) B85.4
pubic (Phthirus pubis) B85.3
Lichen L28.0
albus L90.0
penis N48.0
vulva N90.4
amyloidosis E85.4 *[L99]*
atrophicus L90.0
penis N48.0
vulva N90.4
congenital Q82.8
myxedematosus L98.5
nitidus L44.1
pilaris Q82.8
acquired L85.8
planopilaris L66.1
planus (chronicus) L43.9
annularis L43.8
bullous L43.1
follicular L66.1
hypertrophic L43.0
moniliformis L44.3
of Wilson L43.9
specified NEC L43.8
subacute (active) L43.3
tropicus L43.3
ruber
acuminatus L44.0
moniliformis L44.3
planus L43.9
sclerosus (et atrophicus) L90.0
penis N48.0
vulva N90.4
scrofulosus (primary) (tuberculous) A18.4
simplex (chronicus) (circumscriptus) L28.0
striatus L44.2
urticatus L28.2
Lichenification L28.0
Lichenoides tuberculosis (primary) A18.4
Lichtheim's disease or syndrome — *see* Degeneration, combined
Lien migrans D73.89
Ligament — *see* condition
Light
for gestational age — *see* Light for dates
headedness R42
Light-for-dates (infant) P05.00
with weight of
499 grams or less P05.01
500-749 grams P05.02
750-999 grams P05.03
1000-1249 grams P05.04
1250-1499 grams P05.05
1500-1749 grams P05.06
1750-1999 grams P05.07
2000-2499 grams P05.08
2500 grams and over P05.09
specified NEC P05.09
and small-for-dates — *see* Small for dates
affecting management of pregnancy O36.59-
Lightning (effects) (stroke) (struck by) T75.00
burn — *see* Burn
foot E53.8
shock T75.01
specified effect NEC T75.09
Lightwood-Albright syndrome N25.89

Lightwood's disease or syndrome
(renal tubular acidosis) N25.89
Lignac (-de Toni) (-Fanconi) (-Debré)
disease or syndrome E72.09
with cystinosis E72.04
Ligneous thyroiditis E06.5
Likoff's syndrome I20.8
Limb — *see* condition
Limbic epilepsy personality syndrome F07.0
Limitation, limited
activities due to disability Z73.6
cardiac reserve — *see* Disease, heart
eye muscle duction, traumatic — *see* Strabismus, mechanical
mandibular range of motion M26.52
Lindau (-von Hippel) **disease** Q85.8
Line (s)
Beau's L60.4
Harris' — *see* Arrest, epiphyseal
Hudson's (cornea) — *see* Pigmentation, cornea, anterior
Stähli's (cornea) — *see* Pigmentation, cornea, anterior
Linea corneae senilis — *see* Change, cornea, senile
Lingua
geographica K14.1
nigra (villosa) K14.3
plicata K14.5
tylosis K13.29
Lingual — *see* condition
Linguatulosis B88.8
Linitis (gastric) **plasticaC16.9**
Lip — *see* condition
Lipedema — *see* Edema
Lipemia — *see also* Hyperlipidemia
retina, retinalis E78.3
Lipidosis E75.6
cerebral (infantile) (juvenile) (late) E75.4
cerebroretinal E75.4
cerebroside E75.22
cholesterol (cerebral) E75.5
glycolipid E75.21
hepatosplenomegalic E78.3
sphingomyelin — *see* Niemann-Pick disease or syndrome
sulfatide E75.29
Lipoadenoma — *see* Neoplasm, benign, by site
Lipoblastoma — *see* Lipoma
Lipoblastomatosis — *see* Lipoma
Lipochondrodystrophy E76.01
Lipochrome histiocytosis (familial) D71
Lipodermatosclerosis — *see* Varix, leg, with, inflammation
ulcerated — *see* Varix, leg, with, ulcer, with inflammation by site
Lipodystrophia progressiva E88.1
Lipodystrophy (progressive) E88.1
insulin E88.1
intestinal K90.81
mesenteric K65.4
Lipofibroma — *see* Lipoma
Lipofuscinosis, neuronal (with ceroidosis) E75.4
Lipogranuloma, sclerosing L92.8
Lipogranulomatosis E78.89
Lipoid — *see also* condition
histiocytosis D76.3
essential E75.29
nephrosis N04.9
proteinosis of Urbach E78.89
Lipoidemia — *see* Hyperlipidemia
Lipoidosis — *see* Lipidosis
Lipoma D17.9
fetal D17.9
fat cell D17.9
infiltrating D17.9
intramuscular D17.9
pleomorphic D17.9
site classification
arms (skin) (subcutaneous) D17.2-
connective tissue D17.30
intra-abdominal D17.5
intrathoracic D17.4
peritoneum D17.79
retroperitoneum D17.79
specified site NEC D17.39
spermatic cord D17.6
face (skin) (subcutaneous) D17.0
genitourinary organ NEC D17.72
head (skin) (subcutaneous) D17.0
intra-abdominal D17.5
intrathoracic D17.4
kidney D17.71
legs (skin) (subcutaneous) D17.2-

Lipoma - *continued*
site classification - *continued*
neck (skin) (subcutaneous) D17.0
peritoneum D17.79
retroperitoneum D17.79
skin D17.30
specified site NEC D17.39
specified site NEC D17.79
spermatic cord D17.6
subcutaneous D17.30
specified site NEC D17.39
trunk (skin) (subcutaneous) D17.1
unspecified D17.9
spindle cell D17.9
Lipomatosis E88.2
dolorosa (Dercum) E88.2
fetal — *see* Lipoma
Launois-Bensaude E88.89
Lipomyoma — *see* Lipoma
Lipomyxoma — *see* Lipoma
Lipomyxosarcoma — *see* Neoplasm, connective tissue, malignant
Lipoprotein metabolism disorder E78.9
Lipoproteinemia E78.5
broad-beta E78.2
floating-beta E78.2
hyper-pre-beta E78.1
Liposarcoma — *see also* Neoplasm, connective tissue, malignant
dedifferentiated — *see* Neoplasm, connective tissue, malignant
differentiated type — *see* Neoplasm, connective tissue, malignant
embryonal — *see* Neoplasm, connective tissue, malignant
mixed type — *see* Neoplasm, connective tissue, malignant
myxoid — *see* Neoplasm, connective tissue, malignant
pleomorphic — *see* Neoplasm, connective tissue, malignant
round cell — *see* Neoplasm, connective tissue, malignant
well differentiated type — *see* Neoplasm, connective tissue, malignant
Liposynovitis prepatellaris E88.89
Lipping, cervix N86
Lipschütz disease or ulcer N76.6
Lipuria R82.0
schistosomiasis (bilharziasis) B65.0
Lisping F80.0
Lissauer's paralysis A52.17
Lissencephalia, lissencephaly Q04.3
Listeriosis, listerellosis A32.9
congenital (disseminated) P37.2
cutaneous A32.0
neonatal, newborn (disseminated) P37.2
oculoglandular A32.81
specified NEC A32.89
Lithemia E79.0
Lithiasis — *see* Calculus
Lithosis J62.8
Lithuria R82.998
Litigation, anxiety concerning Z65.3
Little leaguer's elbow — *see* Epicondylitis, medial
Little's disease G80.9
Littre's
gland — *see* condition
hernia — *see* Hernia, abdomen
Littritis — *see* Urethritis
Livedo (annularis) (racemosa) (reticularis) R23.1
Liver — *see* condition
Living alone (problems with) Z60.2
with handicapped person Z74.2
Lloyd's syndrome — *see* Adenomatosis, endocrine
Loa loa, loaiasis, loasis B74.3
Lobar — *see* condition
Lobomycosis B48.0
Lobo's disease B48.0
Lobotomy syndrome F07.0
Lobstein (-Ekman) **disease or syndrome** Q78.0
Lobster-claw hand Q71.6-
Lobulation (congenital) — *see also* Anomaly, by site
kidney, Q63.1
liver, abnormal Q44.7
spleen Q89.09
Lobule, lobular — *see* condition
Local, localized — *see* condition
Locked twins causing obstructed labor O66.1
Locked-in state G83.5
Locking
joint — *see* Derangement, joint, specified type NEC
knee — *see* Derangement, knee

Lockjaw — *see* Tetanus
Löffler's
endocarditis I42.3
eosinophilia J82
pneumonia J82
syndrome (eosinophilic pneumonitis) J82
Loiasis (with conjunctival infestation) (eyelid) B74.3
Lone Star fever A77.0
Long
labor O63.9
first stage O63.0
second stage O63.1
QT syndrome I45.81
Longitudinal stripes or grooves, nails L60.8
congenital Q84.6
Long-term (current) (prophylactic) **drug therapy** (use of)
agents affecting estrogen receptors and estrogen levels NEC Z79.818
anastrozole (Arimidex) Z79.811
antibiotics Z79.2
short-term use - omit code
anticoagulants Z79.01
anti-inflammatory, non-steroidal (NSAID) Z79.1
antiplatelet Z79.02
antithrombotics Z79.02
aromatase inhibitors Z79.811
aspirin Z79.82
birth control pill or patch Z79.3
bisphosphonates Z79.83
contraceptive, oral Z79.3
drug, specified NEC Z79.899
estrogen receptor downregulators Z79.818
Evista Z79.810
exemestane (Aromasin) Z79.811
Fareston Z79.810
fulvestrant (Faslodex) Z79.818
gonadotropin-releasing hormone (GnRH) agonist Z79.818
goserelin acetate (Zoladex) Z79.818
hormone replacement Z79.890
insulin Z79.4
letrozole (Femara) Z79.811
leuprolide acetate (leuprorelin) (Lupron) Z79.818
megestrol acetate (Megace) Z79.818
methadone for pain management Z79.891
Nolvadex Z79.810
non-steroidal anti-inflammatories (NSAID) Z79.1
opiate analgesic Z79.891
oral
antidiabetic Z79.84
contraceptive Z79.3
hypoglycemic Z79.84
raloxifene (Evista) Z79.810
selective estrogen receptor modulators (SERMs) Z79.810
steroids
inhaled Z79.51
systemic Z79.52
tamoxifen (Nolvadex) Z79.810
toremifene (Fareston) Z79.810
Loop
intestine — *see* Volvulus
vascular on papilla (optic) Q14.2
Loose — *see also* condition
body
joint M24.00
ankle M24.07-
elbow M24.02-
hand M24.04-
hip M24.05-
knee M23.4-
shoulder (region) M24.01-
specified site NEC M24.08
vertebra M24.08
toe M24.07-
wrist M24.03-
knee M23.4-
sheath, tendon — *see* Disorder, tendon, specified type NEC
cartilage — *see* Loose, body, joint
skin and subcutaneous tissue (following bariatric surgery weight loss) (following dietary weight loss) L98.7
tooth, teeth K08.89
Loosening
aseptic
joint prosthesis — *see* Complications, joint prosthesis, mechanical, loosening, by site
epiphysis — *see* Osteochondropathy
mechanical
joint prosthesis — *see* Complications, joint prosthesis, mechanical, loosening, by site

- **Looser-Milkman** (-Debray) **syndrome** M83.8
- **Lop ear** (deformity) Q17.3
- **Lorain** (-Levi) **short stature syndrome** E23.0
- **Lordosis** M40.50
  - acquired — *see* Lordosis, specified type NEC
  - congenital Q76.429
    - lumbar region Q76.426
    - lumbosacral region Q76.427
    - sacral region Q76.428
    - sacrococcygeal region Q76.428
    - thoracolumbar region Q76.425
  - lumbar region M40.56
  - lumbosacral region M40.57
  - postsurgical M96.4
  - postural — *see* Lordosis, specified type NEC
  - rachitic (late effect) (sequelae) E64.3
  - sequelae of rickets E64.3
  - specified type NEC M40.40
    - lumbar region M40.46
    - lumbosacral region M40.47
    - thoracolumbar region M40.45
  - thoracolumbar region M40.55
  - tuberculous A18.01
- **Loss** (of)
  - appetite (see Anorexia) R63.0
    - hysterical F50.89
    - nonorganic origin F50.89
    - psychogenic F50.89
  - blood — *see* Hemorrhage
  - bone — *see* Loss, substance of, bone
  - control, sphincter, rectum R15.9
    - nonorganic origin F98.1
  - consciousness, transient R55
    - traumatic — *see* Injury, intracranial
  - elasticity, skin R23.4
  - family (member) in childhood Z62.898
  - fluid (acute) E86.9
  - function of labyrinth — *see* subcategory H83.2
  - hair, nonscarring — *see* Alopecia
  - hearing — *see also* Deafness
    - central NOS H90.5
    - conductive H90.2
      - bilateral H90.0
      - unilateral
        - with
          - restricted hearing on the contralateral side H90.A1-
          - unrestricted hearing on the contralateral side H90.1-
    - mixed conductive and sensorineural hearing loss H90.8
      - bilateral H90.6
      - unilateral
        - with
          - restricted hearing on the contralateral side H90.A3-
          - unrestricted hearing on the contralateral side H90.7-
    - neural NOS H90.5
    - perceptive NOS H90.5
    - sensorineural NOS H90.5
      - bilateral H90.3
      - unilateral
        - with
          - restricted hearing on the contralateral side H90.A2-
          - unrestricted hearing on the contralateral side H90.4-
    - sensory NOS H90.5
  - height R29.890
  - limb or member, traumatic, current — *see* Amputation, traumatic
  - love relationship in childhood Z62.898
  - memory — *see also* Amnesia
    - mild, following organic brain damage F06.8
  - mind — *see* Psychosis
  - occlusal vertical dimension of fully erupted teeth M26.37
  - organ or part — *see* Absence, by site, acquired
  - ossicles, ear (partial) H74.32-
  - parent in childhood Z63.4
  - pregnancy, recurrent N96
    - care in current pregnancy O26.2-
    - without current pregnancy N96
  - recurrent pregnancy — *see* Loss, pregnancy, recurrent
  - self-esteem, in childhood Z62.898
  - sense of
    - smell — *see* Disturbance, sensation, smell
    - taste — *see* Disturbance, sensation, taste
    - touch R20.8
  - sensory R44.9
    - dissociative F44.6

- **Loss** (of) - *continued*
  - sexual desire F52.0
  - sight (acquired) (complete) (congenital) — *see* Blindness
  - substance of
    - bone — *see* Disorder, bone, density and structure, specified NEC
      - horizontal alveolar K06.3
    - cartilage — *see* Disorder, cartilage, specified type NEC
      - auricle (ear) — *see* Disorder, pinna, specified type NEC
    - vitreous (humor) H15.89
  - tooth, teeth — *see* Absence, teeth, acquired
  - vision, visual H54.7
    - both eyes H54.3
    - one eye H54.60
      - left (normal vision on right) H54.62
      - right (normal vision on left) H54.61
    - specified as blindness — *see* Blindness
    - subjective
      - sudden H53.13-
      - transient H53.12-
  - vitreous — *see* Prolapse, vitreous
  - voice — *see* Aphonia
  - weight (abnormal) (cause unknown) R63.4
- **Louis-Bar syndrome** (ataxia-telangiectasia) G11.3
- **Louping ill** (encephalitis) A84.8
- **Louse, lousiness** — *see* Lice
- **Low**
  - achiever, school Z55.3
  - back syndrome M54.5
  - basal metabolic rate R94.8
  - birthweight (2499 grams or less) P07.10
    - with weight of
      - 1000-1249 grams P07.14
      - 1250-1499 grams P07.15
      - 1500-1749 grams P07.16
      - 1750-1999 grams P07.17
      - 2000-2499 grams P07.18
    - extreme (999 grams or less) P07.00
      - with weight of
        - 499 grams or less P07.01
        - 500-749 grams P07.02
        - 750-999 grams P07.03
    - for gestational age — *see* Light for dates
  - blood pressure — *see also* Hypotension
    - reading (incidental) (isolated) (nonspecific) R03.1
  - cardiac reserve — *see* Disease, heart
  - function — *see also* Hypofunction
    - kidney N28.9
  - hematocrit D64.9
  - hemoglobin D64.9
  - income Z59.6
  - level of literacy Z55.0
  - lying
    - kidney N28.89
    - organ or site, congenital — *see* Malposition, congenital
  - output syndrome (cardiac) — *see* Failure, heart
  - platelets (blood) — *see* Thrombocytopenia
  - reserve, kidney N28.89
  - salt syndrome E87.1
  - self esteem R45.81
  - set ears Q17.4
  - vision H54.2X-
    - one eye (other eye normal) H54.50
      - left (normal vision on right) H54.52A-
      - other eye blind — *see* Blindness
      - right (normal vision on left) H54.511-
- **Low-density-lipoprotein-type** (LDL) **hyperlipoproteinemia** E78.00
- **Lowe's syndrome** E72.03
- **Lown-Ganong-Levine syndrome** I45.6
- **LSD reaction** (acute) (without dependence) F16.90
  - with dependence F16.20
- **L-shaped kidney** Q63.8
- **Ludwig's angina or disease** K12.2
- **Lues** (venerea) **, luetic** — *see* Syphilis
- **Luetscher's syndrome** (dehydration) E86.0
- **Lumbago, lumbalgia** M54.5
  - with sciatica M54.4-
    - due to intervertebral disc disorder M51.17
  - due to displacement, intervertebral disc M51.27
    - with sciatica M51.17
- **Lumbar** — *see* condition
- **Lumbarization, vertebra, congenital** Q76.49
- **Lumbermen's itch** B88.0
- **Lump** — *see also* Mass
  - breast N63.0
    - axillary tail
      - left N63.32
      - right N63.31

- **Lump** - *continued*
  - breast - *continued*
    - left
      - lower inner quadrant N63.24
      - lower outer quadrant N63.23
      - unspecified quadrant N63.20
      - upper inner quadrant N63.22
      - upper outer quadrant N63.21
    - right
      - lower inner quadrant N63.14
      - lower outer quadrant N63.13
      - unspecified quadrant N63.10
      - upper inner quadrant N63.12
      - upper outer quadrant N63.11
    - subareolar
      - left N63.42
      - right N63.41
- **Lunacy** — *see* Psychosis
- **Lung** — *see* condition
- **Lupoid** (miliary) **of Boeck** D86.3
- **Lupus**
  - anticoagulant D68.62
    - with
      - hemorrhagic disorder D68.312
      - hypercoagulable state D68.62
    - finding without diagnosis R76.0
  - discoid (local) L93.0
  - erythematosus (discoid) (local) L93.0
    - disseminated — *see* Lupus, erythematosus, systemic
    - eyelid H01.129
      - left H01.126
        - lower H01.125
        - upper H01.124
      - right H01.123
        - lower H01.122
        - upper H01.121
    - profundus L93.2
    - specified NEC L93.2
    - subacute cutaneous L93.1
    - systemic M32.9
      - with organ or system involvement M32.10
        - endocarditis M32.11
        - lung M32.13
        - pericarditis M32.12
        - renal (glomerular) M32.14
          - tubulo-interstitial M32.15
        - specified organ or system NEC M32.19
      - drug-induced M32.0
      - inhibitor (presence of) D68.62
        - with
          - hemorrhagic disorder D68.312
          - hypercoagulable state D68.62
        - finding without diagnosis R76.0
      - specified NEC M32.8
  - exedens A18.4
  - hydralazine M32.0
    - correct substance properly administered — *see* Table of Drugs and Chemicals, by drug, adverse effect
    - overdose or wrong substance given or taken — *see* Table of Drugs and Chemicals, by drug, poisoning
  - nephritis (chronic) M32.14
  - nontuberculous, not disseminated L93.0
  - panniculitis L93.2
  - pernio (Besnier) D86.3
  - systemic — *see* Lupus, erythematosus, systemic
  - tuberculous A18.4
    - eyelid A18.4
  - vulgaris A18.4
    - eyelid A18.4
- **Luteinoma** D27.-
- **Lutembacher's disease or syndrome** (atrial septal defect with mitral stenosis) Q21.1
- **Luteoma** D27.-
- **Lutz** (-Splendore-de Almeida) **disease** — *see* Paracoccidioidomycosis
- **Luxation** — *see also* Dislocation
  - eyeball (nontraumatic) — *see* Luxation, globe
    - birth injury P15.3
  - globe, nontraumatic H44.82-
  - lacrimal gland — *see* Dislocation, lacrimal gland
  - lens (old) (partial) (spontaneous)
    - congenital Q12.1
    - syphilitic A50.39
- **Lycanthropy** F22
- **Lyell's syndrome** L51.2
  - due to drug L51.2
    - correct substance properly administered — *see* Table of Drugs and Chemicals, by drug, adverse effect

Lyell's syndrome - *continued*
  due to drug - *continued*
    overdose or wrong substance given or taken — *see* Table of Drugs and Chemicals, by drug, poisoning
Lyme disease A69.20
Lymph
  gland or node — *see* condition
  scrotum — *see* Infestation, filarial
Lymphadenitis I88.9
  with ectopic or molar pregnancy O08.0
  acute L04.9
    axilla L04.2
    face L04.0
    head L04.0
    hip L04.3
    limb
      lower L04.3
      upper L04.2
    neck L04.0
    shoulder L04.2
    specified site NEC L04.8
    trunk L04.1
  anthracosis (occupational) J60
  any site, except mesenteric I88.9
    chronic I88.1
    subacute I88.1
  breast
    gestational — *see* Mastitis, obstetric
    puerperal, postpartum (nonpurulent) O91.22
  chancroidal (congenital) A57
  chronic I88.1
    mesenteric I88.0
  due to
    Brugia (malayi) B74.1
      timori B74.2
    chlamydial lymphogranuloma A55
    diphtheria (toxin) A36.89
    lymphogranuloma venereum A55
    Wuchereria bancrofti B74.0
  following ectopic or molar pregnancy O08.0
  gonorrheal A54.89
  infective — *see* Lymphadenitis, acute
  mesenteric (acute) (chronic) (nonspecific) (subacute) I88.0
    due to Salmonella typhi A01.09
    tuberculous A18.39
  mycobacterial A31.8
  purulent — *see* Lymphadenitis, acute
  pyogenic — *see* Lymphadenitis, acute
  regional, nonbacterial I88.8
  septic — *see* Lymphadenitis, acute
  subacute, unspecified site I88.1
  suppurative — *see* Lymphadenitis, acute
  syphilitic (early) (secondary) A51.49
    late A52.79
  tuberculous — *see* Tuberculosis, lymph gland
  venereal (chlamydial) A55
Lymphadenoid goiter E06.3
Lymphadenopathy (generalized) R59.1
  angioimmunoblastic, with dysproteinemia (AILD) C86.5
  due to toxoplasmosis (acquired) B58.89
    congenital (acute) (subacute) (chronic) P37.1
  localized R59.0
  syphilitic (early) (secondary) A51.49
Lymphadenosis R59.1
Lymphangiectasis I89.0
  conjunctiva H11.89
  postinfectional I89.0
  scrotum I89.0
Lymphangiectatic elephantiasis, nonfilarial I89.0
Lymphangioendothelioma D18.1
  malignant — *see* Neoplasm, connective tissue, malignant
Lymphangioleiomyomatosis J84.81
Lymphangioma D18.1
  capillary D18.1
  cavernous D18.1
  cystic D18.1
  malignant — *see* Neoplasm, connective tissue, malignant
Lymphangiomyoma D18.1
Lymphangiomyomatosis J84.81
Lymphangiosarcoma — *see* Neoplasm, connective tissue, malignant
Lymphangitis I89.1
  with
    abscess - code by site under Abscess
    cellulitis - code by site under Cellulitis
    ectopic or molar pregnancy O08.0
  acute L03.91
    abdominal wall L03.321

Lymphangitis - *continued*
  acute - *continued*
    ankle — *see* Lymphangitis, acute, lower limb
    arm — *see* Lymphangitis, acute, upper limb
    auricle (ear) — *see* Lymphangitis, acute, ear
    axilla L03.12-
    back (any part) L03.322
    buttock L03.327
    cervical (meaning neck) L03.222
    cheek (external) L03.212
    chest wall L03.323
    digit
      finger — *see* Lymphangitis, acute, finger
      toe — *see* Lymphangitis, acute, toe
    ear (external) H60.1-
    external auditory canal — *see* Lymphangitis, acute, ear
    eyelid — *see* Abscess, eyelid
    face NEC L03.212
    finger (intrathecal) (periosteal) (subcutaneous) (subcuticular) L03.02-
    foot — *see* Lymphangitis, acute, lower limb
    gluteal (region) L03.327
    groin L03.324
    hand — *see* Lymphangitis, acute, upper limb
    head NEC L03.891
      face (any part, except ear, eye and nose) L03.212
    heel — *see* Lymphangitis, acute, lower limb
    hip — *see* Lymphangitis, acute, lower limb
    jaw (region) L03.212
    knee — *see* Lymphangitis, acute, lower limb
    leg — *see* Lymphangitis, acute, lower limb
    lower limb L03.12-
      toe — *see* Lymphangitis, acute, toe
    navel L03.326
    neck (region) L03.222
    orbit, orbital — *see* Cellulitis, orbit
    pectoral (region) L03.323
    perineal, perineum L03.325
    scalp (any part) L03.891
    shoulder — *see* Lymphangitis, acute, upper limb
    specified site NEC L03.898
    thigh — *see* Lymphangitis, acute, lower limb
    thumb (intrathecal) (periosteal) (subcutaneous) (subcuticular) — *see* Lymphangitis, acute, finger
    toe (intrathecal) (periosteal) (subcutaneous) (subcuticular) L03.04-
    trunk L03.329
      abdominal wall L03.321
      back (any part) L03.322
      buttock L03.327
      chest wall L03.323
      groin L03.324
      perineal, perineum L03.325
      umbilicus L03.326
    umbilicus L03.326
    upper limb L03.12-
      axilla — *see* Lymphangitis, acute, axilla
      finger — *see* Lymphangitis, acute, finger
      thumb — *see* Lymphangitis, acute, finger
    wrist — *see* Lymphangitis, acute, upper limb
  breast
    gestational — *see* Mastitis, obstetric
  chancroidal A57
  chronic (any site) I89.1
  due to
    Brugia (malayi) B74.1
      timori B74.2
    Wuchereria bancrofti B74.0
  following ectopic or molar pregnancy O08.89
  penis
    acute N48.29
    gonococcal (acute) (chronic) A54.09
  puerperal, postpartum, childbirth O86.89
  strumous, tuberculous A18.2
  subacute (any site) I89.1
  tuberculous — *see* Tuberculosis, lymph gland
Lymphatic (vessel) — *see* condition
Lymphatism E32.8
Lymphectasia I89.0
Lymphedema (acquired) — *see also* Elephantiasis
  congenital Q82.0
  hereditary (chronic) (idiopathic) Q82.0
  postmastectomy I97.2
  praecox I89.0
  secondary I89.0
  surgical NEC I97.89
    postmastectomy (syndrome) I97.2
Lymphoblastic — *see* condition
Lymphoblastoma (diffuse) — *see* Lymphoma, lymphoblastic (diffuse)
  giant follicular — *see* Lymphoma, lymphoblastic (diffuse)

Lymphoblastoma (diffuse) - *continued*
  macrofollicular — *see* Lymphoma, lymphoblastic (diffuse)
Lymphocele I89.8
Lymphocytic
  chorioencephalitis (acute) (serous) A87.2
  choriomeningitis (acute) (serous) A87.2
  meningoencephalitis A87.2
Lymphocytoma, benign cutis L98.8
Lymphocytopenia D72.810
Lymphocytosis (symptomatic) D72.820
  infectious (acute) B33.8
Lymphoepithelioma — *see* Neoplasm, malignant, by site
Lymphogranuloma (malignant) — *see also* Lymphoma, Hodgkin
  chlamydial A55
  inguinale A55
  venereum (any site) (chlamydial) (with stricture of rectum) A55
Lymphogranulomatosis (malignant) — *see also* Lymphoma, Hodgkin
  benign (Boeck's sarcoid) (Schaumann's) D86.1
Lymphohistiocytosis, hemophagocytic (familial) D76.1
Lymphoid — *see* condition
Lymphoma (of) (malignant) C85.90
  adult T-cell (HTLV-1-associated) (acute variant) (chronic variant) (lymphomatoid variant) (smouldering variant) C91.5-
  anaplastic large cell
    ALK-negative C84.7-
    ALK-positive C84.6-
    CD30-positive C84.6-
    primary cutaneous C86.6
  angioimmunoblastic T-cell C86.5
  BALT C88.4
  B-cell C85.1-
  B-precursor C83.5-
  blastic NK-cell C86.4
  blastic plasmacytoid dendritic cell neoplasm (BPDCN) C86.4
  bronchial-associated lymphoid tissue [BALT-lymphoma] C88.4
  Burkitt (atypical) C83.7-
  Burkitt-like C83.7-
  centrocytic C83.1-
  cutaneous follicle center C82.6-
  cutaneous T-cell C84.A-
  diffuse follicle center C82.5-
  diffuse large cell C83.3-
    anaplastic C83.3-
    B-cell C83.3-
    CD30-positive C83.3-
    centroblastic C83.3-
    immunoblastic C83.3-
    plasmablastic C83.3-
    subtype not specified C83.3-
    T-cell rich C83.3-
  enteropathy-type (associated) (intestinal) T-cell C86.2
  extranodal NK/T-cell, nasal type C86.0
  extranodal marginal zone B-cell lymphoma of mucosa-associated lymphoid tissue [MALT-lymphoma] C88.4
  follicular C82.9-
    grade
      I C82.0-
      II C82.1-
      III C82.2-
      IIIa C82.3-
      IIIb C82.4-
    specified NEC C82.8-
  hepatosplenic T-cell (alpha-beta) (gamma-delta) C86.1
  histiocytic C85.9-
    true C96.A
  Hodgkin C81.9
    lymphocyte-rich (classical) C81.4-
    lymphocyte depleted (classical) C81.3-
    mixed cellularity (classical) C81.2-
    nodular sclerosis (classical) C81.1-
    specified NEC (classical) C81.7-
    lymphocyte-rich classical C81.4-
    lymphocyte depleted classical C81.3-
    mixed cellularity classical C81.2-
    nodular
      lymphocyte predominant C81.0-
      sclerosis (classical) C81.1-
  intravascular large B-cell C83.8-
  Lennert's C84.4-
  lymphoblastic B-cell C83.5-
  lymphoblastic (diffuse) C83.5-

Lymphoma (of) (malignant) - *continued*
  lymphoblastic T-cell C83.5-
  lymphoepithelioid C84.4-
  lymphoplasmacytic C83.0-
    with IgM-production C88.0
  MALT C88.4
  mantle cell C83.1-
  mature T-cell NEC C84.4-
  mature T/NK-cell C84.9-
    specified NEC C84.Z-
  mediastinal (thymic) large B-cell C85.2-
  Mediterranean C88.3
  mucosa-associated lymphoid tissue [MALT-lymphoma] C88.4
  NK/T cell C84.9-
  nodal marginal zone C83.0-
  non-follicular (diffuse) C83.9-
    specified NEC C83.8-
  non-Hodgkin — *see also* Lymphoma, by type C85.9-
    specified NEC C85.8-
  non-leukemic variant of B-CLL C83.0-
  peripheral T-cell, not classified C84.4-
  primary cutaneous
    anaplastic large cell C86.6
    CD30-positive large T-cell C86.6
  primary effusion B-cell C83.8-
  SALT C88.4
  skin-associated lymphoid tissue [SALT-lymphoma] C88.4
  small cell B-cell C83.0-
  splenic marginal zone C83.0-
  subcutaneous panniculitis-like T-cell C86.3
  T-precursor C83.5-
  true histiocytic C96.A
Lymphomatosis — *see* Lymphoma
Lymphopathia venereum, veneris A55
Lymphopenia D72.810
Lymphoplasmacytic leukemia — *see* Leukemia, chronic lymphocytic, B-cell type
Lymphoproliferation, X-linked disease D82.3
Lymphoreticulosis, benign (of inoculation) A28.1
Lymphorrhea I89.8
Lymphosarcoma (diffuse) — *see also* Lymphoma C85.9-
Lymphostasis I89.8
Lypemania — *see* Melancholia
Lysine and hydroxylysine metabolism disorder E72.3
Lyssa — *see* Rabies

M

Macacus ear Q17.3
Maceration, wet feet, tropical (syndrome) T69.02-
MacLeod's syndrome J43.0
Macrocephalia, macrocephaly Q75.3
Macrocheilia, macrochilia (congenital) Q18.6
Macrocolon — *see also* Megacolon Q43.1
Macrocornea Q15.8
  with glaucoma Q15.0
Macrocytic — *see* condition
Macrocytosis D75.89
Macrodactylia, macrodactylism (fingers) (thumbs) Q74.0
  toes Q74.2
Macrodontia K00.2
Macrogenia M26.05
Macrogenitosomia (adrenal) (male) (praecox) E25.9
  congenital E25.0
Macroglobulinemia (idiopathic) (primary) C88.0
  monoclonal (essential) D47.2
  Waldenström C88.0
Macroglossia (congenital) Q38.2
  acquired K14.8
Macrognathia, macrognathism (congenital) (mandibular) (maxillary) M26.09
Macrogyria (congenital) Q04.8
Macrohydrocephalus — *see* Hydrocephalus
Macromastia — *see* Hypertrophy, breast
Macrophthalmos Q11.3
  in congenital glaucoma Q15.0
Macropsia H53.15
Macrosigmoid K59.39
  congenital Q43.2
Macrospondylitis , acromegalic E22.0
Macrostomia (congenital) Q18.4
Macrotia (external ear) (congenital) Q17.1
Macula
  cornea, corneal — *see* Opacity, cornea
  degeneration (atrophic) (exudative) (senile) — *see also* Degeneration, macula
    hereditary — *see* Dystrophy, retina
Maculae ceruleae -- B85.1
Maculopathy, toxic — *see* Degeneration, macula, toxic
Madarosis (eyelid) H02.729
  left H02.726
    lower H02.725
    upper H02.724
  right H02.723
    lower H02.722
    upper H02.721
Madelung's
  deformity (radius) Q74.0
  disease
    radial deformity Q74.0
    symmetrical lipomas, neck E88.89
Madness — *see* Psychosis
Madura
  foot B47.9
    actinomycotic B47.1
    mycotic B47.0
Maduromycosis B47.0
Maffucci's syndrome Q78.4
Magnesium metabolism disorder — *see* Disorder, metabolism, magnesium
Main en griffe (acquired) — *see also* Deformity, limb, clawhand
  congenital Q74.0
Maintenance (encounter for)
  antineoplastic chemotherapy Z51.11
  antineoplastic radiation therapy Z51.0
  methadone F11.20
Majocchi's
  disease L81.7
  granuloma B35.8
Major — *see* condition
Mal de los pintos — *see* Pinta
Mal de mer T75.3
Malabar itch (any site) B35.5
Malabsorption K90.9
  calcium K90.89
  carbohydrate K90.49
  disaccharide E73.9
  fat K90.49
  galactose E74.20
  glucose (-galactose) E74.39
  intestinal K90.9
    specified NEC K90.89
  isomaltose E74.31
  lactose E73.9
  methionine E72.19
  monosaccharide E74.39
  postgastrectomy K91.2
  postsurgical K91.2
  protein K90.49
  starch K90.49
  sucrose E74.39
  syndrome K90.9
    postsurgical K91.2
Malacia, bone (adult) M83.9
  juvenile — *see* Rickets
Malacoplakia
  bladder N32.89
  pelvis (kidney) N28.89
  ureter N28.89
  urethra N36.8
Malacosteon, juvenile — *see* Rickets
Maladaptation — *see* Maladjustment
Maladie de Roger Q21.0
Maladjustment
  conjugal Z63.0
    involving divorce or estrangement Z63.5
  educational Z55.4
  family Z63.9
  marital Z63.0
    involving divorce or estrangement Z63.5
  occupational NEC Z56.89
  simple, adult — *see* Disorder, adjustment
  situational — *see* Disorder, adjustment
  social Z60.9
    due to
      acculturation difficulty Z60.3
      discrimination and persecution (perceived) Z60.5
      exclusion and isolation Z60.4
      life-cycle (phase of life) transition Z60.0
      rejection Z60.4
      specified reason NEC Z60.8
Malaise R53.81
Malakoplakia — *see* Malacoplakia
Malaria, malarial (fever) B54
  with
    blackwater fever B50.8
      hemoglobinuric (bilious) B50.8
    hemoglobinuria B50.8
Malaria, malarial (fever) - *continued*
  accidentally induced (therapeutically) - code by type under Malaria
  algid B50.9
  cerebral B50.0 *[G94]*
  clinically diagnosed (without parasitological confirmation) B54
  congenital NEC P37.4
    falciparum P37.3
  congestion, congestive B54
  continued (fever) B50.9
  estivo-autumnal B50.9
  falciparum B50.9
    with complications NEC B50.8
      cerebral B50.0 *[G94]*
    severe B50.8
  hemorrhagic B54
  malariae B52.9
    with
      complications NEC B52.8
      glomerular disorder B52.0
  malignant (tertian) — *see* Malaria, falciparum
  mixed infections - code to first listed type in B50-B53
  ovale B53.0
  parasitologically confirmed NEC B53.8
  pernicious, acute — *see* Malaria, falciparum
  Plasmodium (P.)
    falciparum NEC — *see* Malaria, falciparum
    malariae NEC B52.9
      with Plasmodium
        falciparum (and or vivax) — *see* Malaria, falciparum
        vivax — *see also* Malaria, vivax
          and falciparum — *see* Malaria, falciparum
    ovale B53.0
      with Plasmodium malariae — *see also* Malaria, malariae
        and vivax — *see also* Malaria, vivax
          and falciparum — *see* Malaria, falciparum
    simian B53.1
      with Plasmodium malariae — *see also* Malaria, malariae
        and vivax — *see also* Malaria, vivax
          and falciparum — *see* Malaria, falciparum
    vivax NEC B51.9
      with Plasmodium falciparum — *see* Malaria, falciparum
  quartan — *see* Malaria, malariae
  quotidian — *see* Malaria, falciparum
  recurrent B54
  remittent B54
  specified type NEC (parasitologically confirmed) B53.8
  spleen B54
  subtertian (fever) — *see* Malaria, falciparum
  tertian (benign) — *see also* Malaria, vivax
    malignant B50.9
  tropical B50.9
  typhoid B54
  vivax B51.9
    with
      complications NEC B51.8
      ruptured spleen B51.0
Malassez's disease (cystic) N50.89
Malassimilation K90.9
Maldescent, testis Q53.9
  bilateral Q53.20
    abdominal Q53.211
    perineal Q53.22
  unilateral Q53.10
    abdominal Q53.111
    perineal Q53.12
Maldevelopment — *see also* Anomaly
  brain Q07.9
  colon Q43.9
  hip Q74.2
    congenital dislocation Q65.2
      bilateral Q65.1
      unilateral Q65.0-
  mastoid process Q75.8
  middle ear Q16.4
    except ossicles Q16.4
    ossicles Q16.3
  ossicles Q16.3
  spine Q76.49
  toe Q74.2
Male type pelvis Q74.2
  with disproportion (fetopelvic) O33.3
    causing obstructed labor O65.3
Malformation (congenital) — *see also* Anomaly
  adrenal gland Q89.1

Malfunction - *continued*
cystostomy (stoma) - *continued*
catheter T83.010
enteric stoma K94.13
enterostomy K94.13
esophagostomy K94.33
gastroenteric K31.89
gastrostomy K94.23
ileostomy K94.13
valve K94.13
intrathecal infusion pump T85.615
jejunostomy K94.13
nervous system device, implant or graft, specified NEC T85.615
pacemaker — *see* Malfunction, cardiac electronic device
prosthetic device, internal — *see* Complications, prosthetic device, by site, mechanical
tracheostomy J95.03
urinary device NEC — *see* Complication, genitourinary, device, urinary, mechanical
valve
colostomy K94.03
heart T82.09
ileostomy K94.13
vascular graft or shunt NEC — *see* Complication, cardiovascular device, mechanical, vascular
ventricular (communicating shunt) T85.01
Malherbe's tumor — *see* Neoplasm, skin, benign
Malibu disease L98.8
Malignancy — *see also* Neoplasm, malignant, by site
unspecified site (primary) C80.1
Malignant — *see* condition
Malingerer, malingering Z76.5
Mallet finger (acquired) — *see* Deformity, finger, mallet finger
congenital Q74.0
sequelae of rickets E64.3
Malleus A24.0
Mallory's bodies R89.7
Mallory-Weiss syndrome K22.6
Malnutrition E46
degree
first E44.1
mild (protein) E44.1
moderate (protein) E44.0
second E44.0
severe (protein-energy) E43
intermediate form E42
with
kwashiorkor (and marasmus) E42
marasmus E41
third E43
following gastrointestinal surgery K91.2
intrauterine
light-for-dates — *see* Light for dates
small-for-dates — *see* Small for dates
lack of care, or neglect (child) (infant) T76.02
confirmed T74.02
malignant E40
protein E46
calorie E46
mild E44.1
moderate E44.0
severe E43
intermediate form E42
with
kwashiorkor (and marasmus) E42
marasmus E41
energy E46
mild E44.1
moderate E44.0
severe E43
intermediate form E42
with
kwashiorkor (and marasmus) E42
marasmus E41
severe (protein-energy) E43
with
kwashiorkor (and marasmus) E42
marasmus E41
Malocclusion (teeth) M26.4
Angle's M26.219
class I M26.211
class II M26.212
class III M26.213
due to
abnormal swallowing M26.59
mouth breathing M26.59
tongue, lip or finger habits M26.59
temporomandibular (joint) M26.69
Malposition
cervix — *see* Malposition, uterus

Malposition - *continued*
congenital
adrenal (gland) Q89.1
alimentary tract Q45.8
lower Q43.8
upper Q40.8
aorta Q25.49
appendix Q43.8
arterial trunk Q20.0
artery (peripheral) Q27.8
coronary Q24.5
digestive system Q27.8
lower limb Q27.8
pulmonary Q25.79
specified site NEC Q27.8
upper limb Q27.8
auditory canal Q17.8
causing impairment of hearing Q16.9
auricle (ear) Q17.4
causing impairment of hearing Q16.9
cervical Q18.2
biliary duct or passage Q44.5
bladder (mucosa) — *see* Exstrophy, bladder
brachial plexus Q07.8
brain tissue Q04.8
breast Q83.8
bronchus Q32.4
cecum Q43.8
clavicle Q74.0
colon Q43.8
digestive organ or tract NEC Q45.8
lower Q43.8
upper Q40.8
ear (auricle) (external) Q17.4
ossicles Q16.3
endocrine (gland) NEC Q89.2
epiglottis Q31.8
eustachian tube Q17.8
eye Q15.8
facial features Q18.8
fallopian tube Q50.6
finger (s) Q68.1
supernumerary Q69.0
foot Q66.9
gallbladder Q44.1
gastrointestinal tract Q45.8
genitalia, genital organ (s) or tract
female Q52.8
external Q52.79
internal NEC Q52.8
male Q55.8
glottis Q31.8
hand Q68.1
heart Q24.8
dextrocardia Q24.0
with complete transposition of viscera Q89.3
hepatic duct Q44.5
hip (joint) Q65.89
intestine (large) (small) Q43.8
with anomalous adhesions, fixation or malrotation Q43.3
joint NEC Q68.8
kidney Q63.2
larynx Q31.8
limb Q68.8
lower Q68.8
upper Q68.8
liver Q44.7
lung (lobe) Q33.8
nail (s) Q84.6
nerve Q07.8
nervous system NEC Q07.8
nose, nasal (septum) Q30.8
organ or site not listed — *see* Anomaly, by site
ovary Q50.39
pancreas Q45.3
parathyroid (gland) Q89.2
patella Q74.1
peripheral vascular system Q27.8
pituitary (gland) Q89.2
respiratory organ or system NEC Q34.8
rib (cage) Q76.6
supernumerary in cervical region Q76.5
scapula Q74.0
shoulder Q74.0
spinal cord Q06.8
spleen Q89.09
sternum NEC Q76.7
stomach Q40.2
symphysis pubis Q74.2
thymus (gland) Q89.2
thyroid (gland) (tissue) Q89.2
cartilage Q31.8

Malposition - *continued*
congenital - *continued*
toe (s) Q66.9
supernumerary Q69.2
tongue Q38.3
trachea Q32.1
ureter Q62.60
deviation Q62.61
displacement Q62.62
ectopia Q62.63
specified type NEC Q62.69
uterus Q51.818
vein (s) (peripheral) Q27.8
great Q26.8
vena cava (inferior) (superior) Q26.8
device, implant or graft — *see also* Complications, by site and type, mechanical T85.628
arterial graft NEC — *see* Complication, cardiovascular device, mechanical, vascular
breast (implant) T85.42
catheter NEC T85.628
cystostomy T83.020
dialysis (renal) T82.42
intraperitoneal T85.621
infusion NEC T82.524
spinal (epidural) (subdural) T85.620
urinary — *see also* Displacement, device, catheter, urinary T83.028
electronic (electrode) (pulse generator) (stimulator)
bone T84.320
cardiac T82.129
electrode T82.120
pulse generator T82.121
specified type NEC T82.128
nervous system — *see* Complication, prosthetic device, mechanical, electronic nervous system stimulator
urinary — *see* Complication, genitourinary, device, urinary, mechanical
fixation, internal (orthopedic) NEC — *see* Complication, fixation device, mechanical
gastrointestinal — *see* Complications, prosthetic device, mechanical, gastrointestinal device
genital NEC T83.428
intrauterine contraceptive device (string) T83.32
penile prosthesis (cylinder) (implanted) (pump) (resevoir) T83.420
testicular prosthesis T83.421
heart NEC — *see* Complication, cardiovascular device, mechanical
joint prosthesis — *see* Complication, joint prosthesis, mechanical
ocular NEC — *see* Complications, prosthetic device, mechanical, ocular device
orthopedic NEC — *see* Complication, orthopedic, device, mechanical
specified NEC T85.628
urinary NEC — *see also* Complication, genitourinary, device, urinary, mechanical
graft T83.22
vascular NEC — *see* Complication, cardiovascular device, mechanical
ventricular intracranial shunt T85.02
fetus — *see* Pregnancy, complicated by (management affected by), presentation, fetal
gallbladder K82.8
gastrointestinal tract, congenital Q45.8
heart, congenital NEC Q24.8
joint prosthesis — *see* Complications, joint prosthesis, mechanical, displacement, by site
stomach K31.89
congenital Q40.2
tooth, teeth, fully erupted M26.30
uterus (acute) (acquired) (adherent) (asymptomatic) (postinfectional) (postpartal, old) N85.4
anteflexion or anteversion N85.4
congenital Q51.818
flexion N85.4
lateral — *see* Lateroversion, uterus
inversion N85.5
lateral (flexion) (version) — *see* Lateroversion, uterus
in pregnancy or childbirth — *see* subcategory O34.5
retroflexion or retroversion — *see* Retroversion, uterus
Malposture R29.3
Malrotation
cecum Q43.3
colon Q43.3
intestine Q43.3
kidney Q63.2
Malta fever — *see* Brucellosis

Melanoma (malignant) - *continued*
skin - *continued*
anus, anal (skin) C43.51
arm C43.6-
auditory canal (external) C43.2-
auricle (ear) C43.2-
auricular canal (external) C43.2-
axilla, axillary fold C43.59
back C43.59
breast (female) (male) C43.52
brow C43.39
buttock C43.59
canthus (eye) C43.1-
cheek (external) C43.39
chest wall C43.59
chin C43.39
ear (external) C43.2-
elbow C43.6-
external meatus (ear) C43.2-
eyebrow C43.39
eyelid (lower) (upper) C43.1-
face C43.30
specified NEC C43.39
female genital organ (external) NEC C51.9
finger C43.6-
flank C43.59
foot C43.7-
forearm C43.6-
forehead C43.39
foreskin C60.0
glabella C43.39
gluteal region C43.59
groin C43.59
hand C43.6-
heel C43.7-
helix C43.2-
hip C43.7-
interscapular region C43.59
jaw (external) C43.39
knee C43.7-
labium C51.9
majus C51.0
minus C51.1
leg C43.7-
lip (lower) (upper) C43.0
lower limb NEC C43.7-
male genital organ (external) NEC C63.9
nail
finger C43.6-
toe C43.7-
nasolabial groove C43.39
nates C43.59
neck C43.4
nose (external) C43.31
overlapping site C43.8
palpebra C43.1-
penis C60.9
perianal skin C43.51
perineum C43.51
pinna C43.2-
popliteal fossa or space C43.7-
prepuce C60.0
pudendum C51.9
scalp C43.4
scrotum C63.2
shoulder C43.6-
skin NEC C43.9
submammary fold C43.52
temple C43.39
thigh C43.7-
toe C43.7-
trunk NEC C43.59
umbilicus C43.59
upper limb NEC C43.6-
vulva C51.9
overlapping sites C51.8
spindle cell
with epithelioid, mixed — *see* Melanoma, skin, by site
type A C69.4-
type B C69.4-
superficial spreading — *see* Melanoma, skin, by site
Melanosarcoma — *see also* Melanoma
epithelioid cell — *see* Melanoma
Melanosis L81.4
addisonian E27.1
tuberculous A18.7
adrenal E27.1
colon K63.89
conjunctiva — *see* Pigmentation, conjunctiva
congenital Q13.89
cornea (presenile) (senile) — *see also* Pigmentation, cornea

Melanosis - *continued*
cornea (presenile) (senile) - *continued*
congenital Q13.4
eye NEC H57.89
congenital Q15.8
lenticularis progressiva Q82.1
liver K76.89
precancerous — *see also* Melanoma, in situ
malignant melanoma in — *see* Melanoma
Riehl's L81.4
sclera H15.89
congenital Q13.89
suprarenal E27.1
tar L81.4
toxic L81.4
Melanuria R82.998
MELAS syndrome E88.41
Melasma L81.1
adrenal (gland) E27.1
suprarenal (gland) E27.1
Melena K92.1
with ulcer - code by site under Ulcer, with hemorrhage K27.4
due to swallowed maternal blood P78.2
newborn, neonatal P54.1
due to swallowed maternal blood P78.2
Meleney's
gangrene (cutaneous) — *see* Ulcer, skin
ulcer (chronic undermining) — *see* Ulcer, skin
Melioidosis A24.9
acute A24.1
chronic A24.2
fulminating A24.1
pneumonia A24.1
pulmonary (chronic) A24.2
acute A24.1
subacute A24.2
sepsis A24.1
specified NEC A24.3
subacute A24.2
Melitensis, febris A23.0
Melkersson (-Rosenthal) **syndrome** G51.2
Mellitus, diabetes — *see* Diabetes
Melorheostosis (bone) — *see* Disorder, bone, density and structure, specified NEC
Meloschisis Q18.4
Melotia Q17.4
Membrana
capsularis lentis posterior Q13.89
epipapillaris Q14.2
Membranacea placenta O43.19-
Membranaceous uterus N85.8
Membrane (s) **, membranous** — *see also* condition
cyclitic — *see* Membrane, pupillary
folds, congenital — *see* Web
Jackson's Q43.3
over face of newborn P28.9
premature rupture — *see* Rupture, membranes, premature
pupillary H21.4-
persistent Q13.89
retained (with hemorrhage) (complicating delivery) O72.2
without hemorrhage O73.1
secondary cataract — *see* Cataract, secondary
unruptured (causing asphyxia) — *see* Asphyxia, newborn
vitreous — *see* Opacity, vitreous, membranes and strands
Membranitis — *see* Chorioamnionitis
Memory disturbance, lack or loss — *see also* Amnesia
mild, following organic brain damage F06.8
Menadione deficiency E56.1
Menarche
delayed E30.0
precocious E30.1
Mendacity, pathologic F60.2
Mendelson's syndrome (due to anesthesia) J95.4
in labor and delivery O74.0
in pregnancy O29.01-
obstetric O74.0
postpartum, puerperal O89.01
Ménétrier's disease or syndrome K29.60
with bleeding K29.61
Ménière's disease, syndrome or vertigo H81.0-
Meninges, meningeal — *see* condition
Meningioma — *see also* Neoplasm, meninges, benign
angioblastic — *see* Neoplasm, meninges, benign
angiomatous — *see* Neoplasm, meninges, benign
endotheliomatous — *see* Neoplasm, meninges, benign

Meningioma - *continued*
fibroblastic — *see* Neoplasm, meninges, benign
fibrous — *see* Neoplasm, meninges, benign
hemangioblastic — *see* Neoplasm, meninges, benign
hemangiopericytic — *see* Neoplasm, meninges, benign
malignant — *see* Neoplasm, meninges, malignant
meningiothelial — *see* Neoplasm, meninges, benign
meningotheliomatous — *see* Neoplasm, meninges, benign
mixed — *see* Neoplasm, meninges, benign
multiple — *see* Neoplasm, meninges, uncertain behavior
papillary — *see* Neoplasm, meninges, uncertain behavior
psammomatous — *see* Neoplasm, meninges, benign
syncytial — *see* Neoplasm, meninges, benign
transitional — *see* Neoplasm, meninges, benign
Meningiomatosis (diffuse) — *see* Neoplasm, meninges, uncertain behavior
Meningism — *see* Meningismus
Meningismus (infectional) (pneumococcal) R29.1
due to serum or vaccine R29.1
influenzal — *see* Influenza, with, manifestations NEC
Meningitis (basal) (basic) (brain) (cerebral) (cervical) (congestive) (diffuse) (hemorrhagic) (infantile) (membranous) (metastatic) (nonspecific) (pontine) (progressive) (simple) (spinal) (subacute) (sympathetic) (toxic) G03.9
abacterial G03.0
actinomycotic A42.81
adenoviral A87.1
arbovirus A87.8
aseptic (acute) G03.0
bacterial G00.9
Escherichia coli (E. coli) G00.8
Friedländer (bacillus) G00.8
gram-negative G00.9
H. influenzae G00.0
Klebsiella G00.8
pneumococcal G00.1
specified organism NEC G00.8
staphylococcal G00.3
streptococcal (acute) G00.2
benign recurrent (Mollaret) G03.2
candidal B37.5
caseous (tuberculous) A17.0
cerebrospinal A39.0
chronic NEC G03.1
clear cerebrospinal fluid NEC G03.0
coxsackievirus A87.0
cryptococcal B45.1
diplococcal (gram positive) A39.0
echovirus A87.0
enteroviral A87.0
eosinophilic B83.2
epidemic NEC A39.0
Escherichia coli (E. coli) G00.8
fibrinopurulent G00.9
specified organism NEC G00.8
Friedländer (bacillus) G00.8
gonococcal A54.81
gram-negative cocci G00.9
gram-positive cocci G00.9
Haemophilus (influenzae) G00.0
H. influenzae G00.0
in (due to)
adenovirus A87.1
African trypanosomiasis B56.9 *[G02]*
anthrax A22.8
bacterial disease NEC A48.8 *[G01]*
Chagas' disease (chronic) B57.41
chickenpox B01.0
coccidioidomycosis B38.4
Diplococcus pneumoniae G00.1
enterovirus A87.0
herpes (simplex) virus B00.3
zoster B02.1
infectious mononucleosis B27.92
leptospirosis A27.81
Listeria monocytogenes A32.11
Lyme disease A69.21
measles B05.1
mumps (virus) B26.1
neurosyphilis (late) A52.13
parasitic disease NEC B89 *[G02]*
poliovirus A80.9 *[G02]*
preventive immunization, inoculation or vaccination G03.8
rubella B06.02
Salmonella infection A02.21
specified cause NEC G03.8

Meningitis (basal) (basic) (brain) (cerebral) (cervical) (congestive) (diffuse) (hemorrhagic) (infantile) (membranous) (metastatic) (nonspecific) (pontine) (progressive) (simple) (spinal) (subacute) (sympathetic) (toxic) - *continued*
in (due to) - *continued*
Streptococcal pneumoniae G00.1
typhoid fever A01.01
varicella B01.0
viral disease NEC A87.8
whooping cough A37.90
zoster B02.1
infectious G00.9
influenzal (H. influenzae) G00.0
Klebsiella G00.8
leptospiral (aseptic) A27.81
lymphocytic (acute) (benign) (serous) A87.2
meningococcal A39.0
Mima polymorpha G00.8
Mollaret (benign recurrent) G03.2
monilial B37.5
mycotic NEC B49 *[G02]*
Neisseria A39.0
nonbacterial G03.0
nonpyogenic NEC G03.0
ossificans G96.19
pneumococcal streptococcus pneumoniae G00.1
poliovirus A80.9 *[G02]*
postmeasles B05.1
purulent G00.9
specified organism NEC G00.8
pyogenic G00.9
specified organism NEC G00.8
Salmonella (arizonae) (Cholerae-Suis) (enteritidis) (typhimurium) A02.21
septic G00.9
specified organism NEC G00.8
serosa circumscripta NEC G03.0
serous NEC G93.2
specified organism NEC G00.8
sporotrichosis B42.81
staphylococcal G00.3
sterile G03.0
Streptococcal (acute) G00.2
pneumoniae G00.1
suppurative G00.9
specified organism NEC G00.8
syphilitic (late) (tertiary) A52.13
acute A51.41
congenital A50.41
secondary A51.41
Torula histolytica (cryptococcal) B45.1
traumatic (complication of injury) T79.8
tuberculous A17.0
typhoid A01.01
viral NEC A87.9
Yersinia pestis A20.3
Meningocele (spinal) — *see also* Spina bifida
with hydrocephalus — *see* Spina bifida, by site, with hydrocephalus
acquired (traumatic) G96.19
cerebral — *see* Encephalocele
Meningocerebritis — *see* Meningoencephalitis
Meningococcemia A39.4
acute A39.2
chronic A39.3
Meningococcus, meningococcal — *see also* condition A39.9
adrenalitis, hemorrhagic A39.1
carrier (suspected) of Z22.31
meningitis (cerebrospinal) A39.0
Meningoencephalitis — *see also* Encephalitis G04.90
acute NEC — *see also* Encephalitis, viral A86
bacterial NEC G04.2
California A83.5
diphasic A84.1
eosinophilic B83.2
epidemic A39.81
herpesviral, herpetic B00.4
due to herpesvirus 6 B10.01
due to herpesvirus 7 B10.09
specified NEC B10.09
in (due to)
blastomycosis NEC B40.81
diseases classified elsewhere G05.3
free-living amebae B60.2
Hemophilus influenzae (H .influenzae) G00.0
herpes B00.4
due to herpesvirus 6 B10.01
due to herpesvirus 7 B10.09
specified NEC B10.09
H. influenzae G00.0

Meningoencephalitis - *continued*
in (due to) - *continued*
Lyme disease A69.22
mercury — *see* subcategory T56.1
mumps B26.2
Naegleria (amebae) (organisms) (fowleri) B60.2
Parastrongylus cantonensis B83.2
toxoplasmosis (acquired) B58.2
congenital P37.1
infectious (acute) (viral) A86
influenzal (H. influenzae) G00.0
Listeria monocytogenes A32.12
lymphocytic (serous) A87.2
mumps B26.2
parasitic NEC B89 *[G05.3]*
pneumococcal G04.2
primary amebic B60.2
specific (syphilitic) A52.14
specified organism NEC G04.81
staphylococcal G04.2
streptococcal G04.2
syphilitic A52.14
toxic NEC G92
due to mercury — *see* subcategory T56.1
tuberculous A17.82
virus NEC A86
Meningoencephalocele — *see also* Encephalocele
syphilitic A52.19
congenital A50.49
Meningoencephalomyelitis — *see also* Meningoencephalitis
acute NEC (viral) A86
disseminated G04.00
postimmunization or postvaccination G04.02
postinfectious G04.01
due to
actinomycosis A42.82
Torula B45.1
Toxoplasma or toxoplasmosis (acquired) B58.2
congenital P37.1
postimmunization or postvaccination G04.02
Meningoencephalomyelopathy G96.9
Meningoencephalopathy G96.9
Meningomyelitis — *see also* Meningoencephalitis
bacterial NEC G04.2
blastomycotic NEC B40.81
cryptococcal B45.1
in diseases classified elsewhere G05.4
meningococcal A39.81
syphilitic A52.14
tuberculous A17.82
Meningomyelocele — *see also* Spina bifida
syphilitic A52.19
Meningomyeloneuritis — *see* Meningoencephalitis
Meningoradiculitis — *see* Meningitis
Meningovascular — *see* condition
Menkes' disease or syndrome E83.09
meaning maple-syrup-urine disease E71.0
Menometrorrhagia N92.1
Menopause, menopausal (asymptomatic) (state) Z78.0
arthritis (any site) NEC — *see* Arthritis, specified form NEC
bleeding N92.4
depression (single episode) F32.89
agitated (single episode) F32.2
recurrent episode F33.9
psychotic (single episode) F32.89
recurrent episode F33.9
recurrent episode F33.8
melancholia (single episode) F32.89
recurrent episode F33.8
paranoid state F22
premature E28.319
asymptomatic E28.319
postirradiation E89.40
postsurgical E89.40
symptomatic E28.310
postirradiation E89.41
postsurgical E89.41
psychosis NEC F28
symptomatic N95.1
toxic polyarthritis NEC — *see* Arthritis, specified form NEC
Menorrhagia (primary) N92.0
climacteric N92.4
menopausal N92.4
menopausal N92.4
postclimacteric N95.0
postmenopausal N95.0
preclimacteric or premenopausal N92.4
pubertal (menses retained) N92.2
Menostaxis N92.0

Menses, retention N94.89
Menstrual — *see* Menstruation
Menstruation
absent — *see* Amenorrhea
anovulatory N97.0
cycle, irregular N92.6
delayed N91.0
disorder N93.9
psychogenic F45.8
during pregnancy O20.8
excessive (with regular cycle) N92.0
with irregular cycle N92.1
at puberty N92.2
frequent N92.0
infrequent — *see* Oligomenorrhea
irregular N92.6
specified NEC N92.5
latent N92.5
membranous N92.5
painful — *see also* Dysmenorrhea N94.6
primary N94.4
psychogenic F45.8
secondary N94.5
passage of clots N92.0
precocious E30.1
protracted N92.5
rare — *see* Oligomenorrhea
retained N94.89
retrograde N92.5
scanty — *see* Oligomenorrhea
suppression N94.89
vicarious (nasal) N94.89
Mental — *see also* condition
deficiency — *see* Disability, intellectual
deterioration — *see* Psychosis
disorder — *see* Disorder, mental
exhaustion F48.8
insufficiency (congenital) — *see* Disability, intellectual
observation without need for further medical care Z03.89
retardation — *see* Disability, intellectual
subnormality — *see* Disability, intellectuall
upset — *see* Disorder, mental
Meralgia paresthetica G57.1-
Mercurial — *see* condition
Mercurialism — *see* subcategory T56.1
Merkel cell tumor — *see* Carcinoma, Merkel cell
Merocele — *see* Hernia, femoral
Meromelia
lower limb — *see* Defect, reduction, lower limb
intercalary
femur — *see* Defect, reduction, lower limb, specified type NEC
tibiofibular (complete) (incomplete) — *see* Defect, reduction, lower limb
upper limb — *see* Defect, reduction, upper limb
intercalary, humeral, radioulnar — *see* Agenesis, arm, with hand present
MERRF syndrome
(myoclonic epilepsy associated with ragged-red fiber) E88.42
Merzbacher-Pelizaeus disease E75.29
Mesaortitis — *see* Aortitis
Mesarteritis — *see* Arteritis
Mesencephalitis — *see* Encephalitis
Mesenchymoma — *see also* Neoplasm, connective tissue, uncertain behavior
benign — *see* Neoplasm, connective tissue, benign
malignant — *see* Neoplasm, connective tissue, malignant
Mesenteritis
retractile K65.4
sclerosing K65.4
Mesentery, mesenteric — *see* condition
Mesiodens, mesiodentes K00.1
Mesio-occlusion M26.213
Mesocolon — *see* condition
Mesonephroma (malignant) — *see* Neoplasm, malignant, by site
benign — *see* Neoplasm, benign, by site
Mesophlebitis — *see* Phlebitis
Mesostromal dysgenesia Q13.89
Mesothelioma (malignant) C45.9
benign
mesentery D19.1
mesocolon D19.1
omentum D19.1
peritoneum D19.1
pleura D19.0
specified site NEC D19.7
unspecified site D19.9
biphasic C45.9

Mesothelioma (malignant) - *continued*
  biphasic - *continued*
    benign
      mesentery D19.1
      mesocolon D19.1
      omentum D19.1
      peritoneum D19.1
      pleura D19.0
      specified site NEC D19.7
      unspecified site D19.9
  cystic D48.4
  epithelioid C45.9
    benign
      mesentery D19.1
      mesocolon D19.1
      omentum D19.1
      peritoneum D19.1
      pleura D19.0
      specified site NEC D19.7
      unspecified site D19.9
  fibrous C45.9
    benign
      mesentery D19.1
      mesocolon D19.1
      omentum D19.1
      peritoneum D19.1
      pleura D19.0
      specified site NEC D19.7
      unspecified site D19.9
  site classification
    liver C45.7
    lung C45.7
    mediastinum C45.7
    mesentery C45.1
    mesocolon C45.1
    omentum C45.1
    pericardium C45.2
    peritoneum C45.1
    pleura C45.0
      parietal C45.0
    retroperitoneum C45.7
    specified site NEC C45.7
    unspecified C45.9
Metabolic syndrome E88.81
Metagonimiasis B66.8
Metagonimus infestation (intestine) B66.8
Metal
  pigmentation L81.8
  polisher's disease J62.8
Metamorphopsia H53.15
Metaplasia
  apocrine (breast) — *see* Dysplasia, mammary, specified type NEC
  cervix (squamous) — *see* Dysplasia, cervix
  endometrium (squamous) (uterus) N85.8
  esophagus K22.7-
  kidney (pelvis) (squamous) N28.89
  myelogenous D73.1
  myeloid (agnogenic) (megakaryocytic) D73.1
  spleen D73.1
  squamous cell, bladder N32.89
Metastasis, metastatic
  abscess — *see* Abscess
  calcification E83.59
  cancer
    from specified site — *see* Neoplasm, malignant, by site
    to specified site — *see* Neoplasm, secondary, by site
  deposits (in) — *see* Neoplasm, secondary, by site
  disease — *see also* Neoplasm, secondary, by site C79.9
  spread (to) — *see* Neoplasm, secondary, by site
Metastrongyliasis B83.8
Metatarsalgia M77.4-
  anterior G57.6-
  Morton's G57.6-
Metatarsus, metatarsal — *see also* condition
  adductus, congenital Q66.22
  valgus (abductus) , congenital Q66.6
  varus (congenital) Q66.22
    primus Q66.21
Methadone use — *see* Use, opioid
Methemoglobinemia D74.9
  acquired (with sulfhemoglobinemia) D74.8
  congenital D74.0
  enzymatic (congenital) D74.0
  Hb M disease D74.0
  hereditary D74.0
  toxic D74.8
Methemoglobinuria — *see* Hemoglobinuria
Methioninemia E72.19
Methylmalonic acidemia E71.120
Metritis (catarrhal) (hemorrhagic) (septic) (suppurative) — *see also* Endometritis
  cervical — *see* Cervicitis
Metropathia hemorrhagica N93.8
Metroperitonitis — *see* Peritonitis, pelvic, female
Metrorrhagia N92.1
  climacteric N92.4
  menopausal N92.4
  postpartum NEC (atonic) (following delivery of placenta) O72.1
    delayed or secondary O72.2
  preclimacteric or premenopausal N92.4
  psychogenic F45.8
Metrorrhexis — *see* Rupture, uterus
Metrosalpingitis N70.91
Metrostaxis N93.8
Metrovaginitis — *see* Endometritis
Meyer-Schwickerath and Weyers syndrome Q87.0
Meynert's amentia (nonalcoholic) F04
  alcoholic F10.96
    with dependence F10.26
Mibelli's disease (porokeratosis) Q82.8
Mice, joint — *see* Loose, body, joint
  knee M23.4-
Micrencephalon, micrencephaly Q02
Microalbuminuria R80.9
Microaneurysm, retinal — *see also* Disorder, retina, microaneurysms
  diabetic — *see* E08-E13 with .31
Microangiopathy (peripheral) I73.9
  thrombotic M31.1
Microcalcifications, breast R92.0
Microcephalus, microcephalic, microcephaly Q02
  due to toxoplasmosis (congenital) P37.1
Microcheilia Q18.7
Microcolon (congenital) Q43.8
Microcornea (congenital) Q13.4
Microcytic — *see* condition
Microdeletions NEC Q93.88
Microdontia K00.2
Microdrepanocytosis D57.40
  with crisis (vasoocclusive pain) D57.419
    with
      acute chest syndrome D57.411
      splenic sequestration D57.412
Microembolism
  atherothrombotic — *see* Atheroembolism
  retinal — *see* Occlusion, artery, retina
Microencephalon Q02
Microfilaria streptocerca infestation — *see* Onchocerciasis
Microgastria (congenital) Q40.2
Microgenia M26.06
Microgenitalia, congenital
  female Q52.8
  male Q55.8
Microglioma — *see* Lymphoma, non-Hodgkin, specified NEC
Microglossia (congenital) Q38.3
Micrognathia, micrognathism (congenital) (mandibular) (maxillary) M26.09
Microgyria (congenital) Q04.3
Microinfarct of heart — *see* Insufficiency, coronary
Microlentia (congenital) Q12.8
Microlithiasis, alveolar, pulmonary J84.02
Micromastia N64.82
Micromyelia (congenital) Q06.8
Micropenis Q55.62
Microphakia (congenital) Q12.8
Microphthalmos, microphthalmia (congenital) Q11.2
  due to toxoplasmosis P37.1
Micropsia H53.15
Microscopic polyangiitis (polyarteritis) M31.7
Microsporidiosis B60.8
  intestinal A07.8
Microsporon furfur infestation B36.0
Microsporosis — *see also* Dermatophytosis
  nigra B36.1
Microstomia (congenital) Q18.5
Microtia (congenital) (external ear) Q17.2
Microtropia H50.40
Microvillus inclusion disease (MVD) (MVID) Q43.8
Micturition
  disorder NEC — *see also* Difficulty, micturition R39.198
    psychogenic F45.8
  frequency R35.0
    psychogenic F45.8
  hesitancy R39.11
  incomplete emptying R39.14
  nocturnal R35.1
  painful R30.9
Micturition - *continued*
  painful - *continued*
    dysuria R30.0
    psychogenic F45.8
    tenesmus R30.1
  poor stream R39.12
  position dependent R39.192
  split stream R39.13
  straining R39.16
  urgency R39.15
Mid plane — *see* condition
Middle
  ear — *see* condition
  lobe (right) syndrome J98.19
Miescher's elastoma L87.2
Mietens' syndrome Q87.2
Migraine (idiopathic) G43.909
  with refractory migraine G43.919
    with status migrainosus G43.911
    without status migrainosus G43.919
  with aura (acute-onset) (prolonged) (typical) (without headache) G43.109
    with refractory migraine G43.119
      with status migrainosus G43.111
      without status migrainosus G43.119
    intractable G43.119
      with status migrainosus G43.111
      without status migrainosus G43.119
    not intractable G43.109
      with status migrainosus G43.101
      without status migrainosus G43.109
    persistent G43.509
      with cerebral infarction G43.609
        with refractory migraine G43.619
          with status migrainosus G43.611
          without status migrainosus G43.619
        intractable G43.619
          with status migrainosus G43.611
          without status migrainosus G43.619
        not intractable G43.609
          with status migrainosus G43.601
          without status migrainosus G43.609
        without refractory migraine G43.609
          with status migrainosus G43.601
          without status migrainosus G43.609
      without cerebral infarction G43.509
        with refractory migraine G43.519
          with status migrainosus G43.511
          without status migrainosus G43.519
        intractable G43.519
          with status migrainosus G43.511
          without status migrainosus G43.519
        not intractable G43.509
          with status migrainosus G43.501
          without status migrainosus G43.509
        without refractory migraine G43.509
          with status migrainosus G43.501
          without status migrainosus G43.509
    without mention of refractory migraine G43.109
      with status migrainosus G43.101
      without status migrainosus G43.109
  abdominal G43.D0
    with refractory migraine G43.D1
    intractable G43.D1
    not intractable G43.D0
    without refractory migraine G43.D0
  basilar — *see* Migraine, with aura
  classical — *see* Migraine, with aura
  common — *see* Migraine, without aura
  complicated G43.109
  equivalents — *see* Migraine, with aura
  familiar — *see* Migraine, hemiplegic
  hemiplegic G43.409
    with refractory migraine G43.419
      with status migrainosus G43.411
      without status migrainosus G43.419
    intractable G43.419
      with status migrainosus G43.411
      without status migrainosus G43.419
    not intractable G43.409
      with status migrainosus G43.401
      without status migrainosus G43.409
    without refractory migraine G43.409
      with status migrainosus G43.401
      without status migrainosus G43.409
  intractable G43.919
    with status migrainosus G43.911
    without status migrainosus G43.919
  menstrual G43.829
    with refractory migraine G43.839
      with status migrainosus G43.831
      without status migrainosus G43.839
    intractable G43.839

Migraine (idiopathic) - *continued*
  menstrual - *continued*
    intractable - *continued*
      with status migrainosus G43.831
      without status migrainosus G43.839
    not intractable 4G43.829
      with status migrainosus G43.821
      without status migrainosus G43.829
    without refractory migraine G43.829
      with status migrainosus G43.821
      without status migrainosus G43.829
  menstrually related — *see* Migraine, menstrual
  not intractable G43.909
    with status migrainosus G43.901
    without status migrainosus G43.919
  ophthalmoplegic G43.B0
    with refractory migraine G43.B1
    intractable G43.B1
    not intractable G43.B0
    without refractory migraine G43.B0
  persistent aura (with, without) cerebral infarction — *see* Migraine, with aura, persistent
  preceded or accompanied by transient focal neurological phenomena — *see* Migraine, with aura
  pre-menstrual — *see* Migraine, menstrual
  pure menstrual — *see* Migraine, menstrual
  retinal — *see* Migraine, with aura
  specified NEC G43.809
    intractable G43.819
      with status migrainosus G43.811
      without status migrainosus G43.819
    not intractable G43.809
      with status migrainosus G43.801
      without status migrainosus G43.809
  sporadic — *see* Migraine, hemiplegic
  transformed — *see* Migraine, without aura, chronic
  triggered seizures — *see* Migraine, with aura
  without aura G43.009
    with refractory migraine G43.019
      with status migrainosus G43.011
      without status migrainosus G43.019
    chronic G43.709
      with refractory migraine G43.719
        with status migrainosus G43.711
        without status migrainosus G43.719
      intractable
        with status migrainosus G43.711
        without status migrainosus G43.719
      not intractable
        with status migrainosus G43.701
        without status migrainosus G43.709
      without refractory migraine G43.709
        with status migrainosus G43.701
        without status migrainosus G43.709
    intractable
      with status migrainosus G43.011
      without status migrainosus G43.019
    not intractable
      with status migrainosus G43.001
      without status migrainosus G43.009
    without mention of refractory migraine G43.009
      with status migrainosus G43.001
      without status migrainosus G43.009
  without refractory migraineG43.909
    with status migrainosus G43.901
    without status migrainosus G43.919
Migrant, social Z59.0
Migration, anxiety concerning Z60.3
Migratory, migrating — *see also* condition
  person Z59.0
  testis Q55.29
Mikity-Wilson disease or syndrome P27.0
Mikulicz' disease or syndrome K11.8
Miliaria L74.3
  alba L74.1
  apocrine L75.2
  crystallina L74.1
  profunda L74.2
  rubra L74.0
  tropicalis L74.2
Miliary — *see* condition
Milium L72.0
  colloid L57.8
Milk
  crust L21.0
  excessive secretion O92.6
  poisoning — *see* Poisoning, food, noxious
  retention O92.79
  sickness — *see* Poisoning, food, noxious
  spots I31.0
Milk-alkali disease or syndrome E83.52
Milk-leg (deep vessels) (nonpuerperal) — *see* Embolism, vein, lower extremity
  complicating pregnancy O22.3-
  puerperal, postpartum, childbirth O87.1
Milkman's disease or syndrome M83.8
Milky urine — *see* Chyluria
Millard-Gubler (-Foville) **paralysis or syndrome** G46.3
Millar's asthma J38.5
Miller Fisher syndrome G61.0
Mills' disease — *see* Hemiplegia
Millstone maker's pneumoconiosis J62.8
Milroy's disease (chronic hereditary edema) Q82.0
Minamata disease T56.1
Miners' asthma or lung J60
Minkowski-Chauffard syndrome — *see* Spherocytosis
Minor — *see* condition
Minor's disease (hematomyelia) G95.19
Minot's disease (hemorrhagic disease) **, newborn** P53
Minot-von Willebrand-Jurgens disease or syndrome (angiohemophilia) D68.0
Minus (and plus) **hand** (intrinsic) — *see* Deformity, limb, specified type NEC, forearm
Miosis (pupil) H57.03
Mirizzi's syndrome (hepatic duct stenosis) K83.1
Mirror writing F81.0
Misadventure (of) (prophylactic) (therapeutic) — *see also* Complications T88.9
  administration of insulin (by accident) — *see* subcategory T38.3
  infusion — *see* Complications, infusion
  local applications (of fomentations, plasters, etc.) T88.9
    burn or scald — *see* Burn
    specified NEC T88.8
  medical care (early) (late) T88.9
    adverse effect of drugs or chemicals — *see* Table of Drugs and Chemicals
  medical care (early) (late)
    burn or scald — *see* Burn
    specified NEC T88.8
  specified NEC T88.8
  surgical procedure (early) (late) — *see* Complications, surgical procedure
  transfusion — *see* Complications, transfusion
  vaccination or other immunological procedure — *see* Complications, vaccination
Miscarriage O03.9
Misdirection, aqueous H40.83-
Misperception, sleep state F51.02
Misplaced, misplacement
  ear Q17.4
  kidney (acquired) N28.89
    congenital Q63.2
  organ or site, congenital NEC — *see* Malposition, congenital
Missed
  abortion O02.1
  delivery O36.4
Missing — *see also* Absence
  string of intrauterine contraceptive device T83.32
Misuse of drugs F19.99
Mitchell's disease (erythromelalgia) I73.81
Mite (s) (infestation) B88.9
  diarrhea B88.0
  grain (itch) B88.0
  hair follicle (itch) B88.0
  in sputum B88.0
Mitral — *see* condition
Mittelschmerz N94.0
Mixed — *see* condition
MMN (multifocal motor neuropathy) G61.82
MNGIE
  (Mitochondrial Neurogastrointestinal Encephalopathy) **syndrome** E88.49
Mobile, mobility
  cecum Q43.3
  excessive — *see* Hypermobility
  gallbladder, congenital Q44.1
  kidney N28.89
  organ or site, congenital NEC — *see* Malposition, congenital
Mobitz heart block (atrioventricular) I44.1
Moebius, Möbius
  disease (ophthalmoplegic migraine) — *see* Migraine, ophthalmoplegic
  syndrome Q87.0
    congenital oculofacial paralysis (with other anomalies) Q87.0
    ophthalmoplegic migraine — *see* Migraine, ophthalmoplegic
Moeller's glossitis K14.0
Mohr's syndrome (Types I and II) Q87.0
Mola destruens D39.2
Molar pregnancy O02.0
Molarization of premolars K00.2
Molding, head (during birth) **- omit code**
Mole (pigmented) — *see also* Nevus
  blood O02.0
  Breus' O02.0
  cancerous — *see* Melanoma
  carneous O02.0
  destructive D39.2
  fleshy O02.0
  hydatid, hydatidiform (benign) (complicating pregnancy) (delivered) (undelivered) O01.9
    classical O01.0
    complete O01.0
    incomplete O01.1
    invasive D39.2
    malignant D39.2
    partial O01.1
  intrauterine O02.0
  invasive (hydatidiform) D39.2
  malignant
    meaning
      malignant hydatidiform mole D39.2
      melanoma — *see* Melanoma
  nonhydatidiform O02.0
  nonpigmented — *see* Nevus
  pregnancy NEC O02.0
  skin — *see* Nevus
  tubal O00.10-
    with intrauterine pregnancy O00.11-
  vesicular — *see* Mole, hydatidiform
Molimen, molimina (menstrual) N94.3
Molluscum contagiosum (epitheliale) B08.1
Mönckeberg's arteriosclerosis, disease, or sclerosis — *see* Arteriosclerosis, extremities
Mondini's malformation (cochlea) Q16.5
Mondor's disease I80.8
Monge's disease T70.29
Monilethrix (congenital) Q84.1
Moniliasis — *see also* Candidiasis B37.9
  neonatal P37.5
Monitoring (encounter for)
  therapeutic drug level Z51.81
Monkey malaria B53.1
Monkeypox B04
Monoarthritis M13.10
  ankle M13.17-
  elbow M13.12-
  foot joint M13.17-
  hand joint M13.14-
  hip M13.15-
  knee M13.16-
  shoulder M13.11-
  wrist M13.13-
Monoblastic — *see* condition
Monochromat (ism) **, monochromatopsia** (acquired) (congenital) H53.51
Monocytic — *see* condition
Monocytopenia D72.818
Monocytosis (symptomatic) D72.821
Monomania — *see* Psychosis
Mononeuritis G58.9
  cranial nerve — *see* Disorder, nerve, cranial
  femoral nerve G57.2-
  lateral
    cutaneous nerve of thigh G57.1-
    popliteal nerve G57.3-
  lower limb G57.9-
    specified nerve NEC G57.8-
  medial popliteal nerve G57.4-
  median nerve G56.1-
  multiplex G58.7
  plantar nerve G57.6-
  posterior tibial nerve G57.5-
  radial nerve G56.3-
  sciatic nerve G57.0-
  specified NEC G58.8
  tibial nerve G57.4-
  ulnar nerve G56.2-
  upper limb G56.9-
    specified nerve NEC G56.8-
  vestibular — *see* subcategory H93.3
Mononeuropathy G58.9
  carpal tunnel syndrome — *see* Syndrome, carpal tunnel
  diabetic NEC — *see* E08-E13 with .41
  femoral nerve — *see* Lesion, nerve, femoral
  ilioinguinal nerve G57.8-
  in diseases classified elsewhere — *see* category G59
  intercostal G58.0

Mononeuropathy - *continued*
lower limb G57.9-
causalgia — *see* Causalgia, lower limb
femoral nerve — *see* Lesion, nerve, femoral
meralgia paresthetica G57.1-
plantar nerve — *see* Lesion, nerve, plantar
popliteal nerve — *see* Lesion, nerve, popliteal
sciatic nerve — *see* Lesion, nerve, sciatic
specified NEC G57.8-
tarsal tunnel syndrome — *see* Syndrome, tarsal tunnel
median nerve — *see* Lesion, nerve, median
multiplex G58.7
obturator nerve G57.8-
popliteal nerve — *see* Lesion, nerve, popliteal
radial nerve — *see* Lesion, nerve, radial
saphenous nerve G57.8-
specified NEC G58.8
tarsal tunnel syndrome — *see* Syndrome, tarsal tunnel
tuberculous A17.83
ulnar nerve — *see* Lesion, nerve, ulnar
upper limb G56.9-
carpal tunnel syndrome — *see* Syndrome, carpal tunnel
causalgia — *see* Causalgia
median nerve — *see* Lesion, nerve, median
radial nerve — *see* Lesion, nerve, radial
specified site NEC G56.8-
ulnar nerve — *see* Lesion, nerve, ulnar
Mononucleosis, infectious B27.90
with
complication NEC B27.99
meningitis B27.92
polyneuropathy B27.91
cytomegaloviral B27.10
with
complication NEC B27.19
meningitis B27.12
polyneuropathy B27.11
Epstein-Barr (virus) B27.00
with
complication NEC B27.09
meningitis B27.02
polyneuropathy B27.01
gammaherpesviral B27.00
with
complication NEC B27.09
meningitis B27.02
polyneuropathy B27.01
specified NEC B27.80
with
complication NEC B27.89
meningitis B27.82
polyneuropathy B27.81
Monoplegia G83.3-
congenital (cerebral) G80.8
spastic G80.1
embolic (current episode) I63.4-
following
cerebrovascular disease
cerebral infarction
lower limb I69.34-
upper limb I69.33-
intracerebral hemorrhage
lower limb I69.14-
upper limb I69.13-
lower limb I69.94-
nontraumatic intracranial hemorrhage NEC
lower limb I69.24-
upper limb I69.23-
specified disease NEC
lower limb I69.84-
upper limb I69.83-
stroke NOS
lower limb I69.34-
upper limb I69.33-
subarachnoid hemorrhage
lower limb I69.04-
upper limb I69.03-
upper limb I69.93-
hysterical (transient) F44.4
lower limb G83.1-
psychogenic (conversion reaction) F44.4
thrombotic (current episode) I63.3-
transient R29.818
upper limb G83.2-
Monorchism, monorchidism Q55.0
Monosomy — *see also* Deletion, chromosome Q93.9
specified NEC Q93.89
whole chromosome
meiotic nondisjunction Q93.0
mitotic nondisjunction Q93.1

Monosomy - *continued*
whole chromosome - *continued*
mosaicism Q93.1
X Q96.9
Monster, monstrosity (single) Q89.7
acephalic Q00.0
twin Q89.4
Monteggia's fracture (-dislocation) S52.27-
Mooren's ulcer (cornea) — *see* Ulcer, cornea, Mooren's
Moore's syndrome — *see* Epilepsy, specified NEC
Mooser-Neill reaction A75.2
Mooser's bodies A75.2
Morbidity not stated or unknown R69
Morbilli — *see* Measles
Morbus — *see also* Disease
angelicus, anglorum E55.0
Beigel B36.2
caducus — *see* Epilepsy
celiacus K90.0
comitialis — *see* Epilepsy
cordis — *see also* Disease, heart I51.9
valvulorum — *see* Endocarditis
coxae senilis M16.9
tuberculous A18.02
hemorrhagicus neonatorum P53
maculosus neonatorum P54.5
Morel (-Stewart) (-Morgagni) **syndrome** M85.2
Morel-Kraepelin disease — *see* Schizophrenia
Morel-Moore syndrome M85.2
Morgagni's
cyst, organ, hydatid, or appendage
female Q50.5
male (epididymal) Q55.4
testicular Q55.29
syndrome M85.2
Morgagni-Stewart-Morel syndrome M85.2
Morgagni-Stokes-Adams syndrome I45.9
Morgagni-Turner (-Albright) **syndrome** Q96.9
Moria F07.0
Moron (I.Q.50-69) F70
Morphea L94.0
Morphinism (without remission) F11.20
with remission F11.21
Morphinomania (without remission) F11.20
with remission F11.21
Morquio (-Ullrich) (-Brailsford)
disease or syndrome — *see* Mucopolysaccharidosis
Mortification (dry) (moist) — *see* Gangrene
Morton's metatarsalgia (neuralgia) (neuroma) (syndrome) G57.6-
Morvan's disease or syndrome G60.8
Mosaicism, mosaic (autosomal) (chromosomal)
45,X/other cell lines NEC with abnormal sex chromosome Q96.4
45,X/46,XX Q96.3
sex chromosome
female Q97.8
lines with various numbers of X chromosomes Q97.2
male Q98.7
XY Q96.3
Moschowitz' disease M31.1
Mother yaw A66.0
Motion sickness (from travel, any vehicle) (from roundabouts or swings) T75.3
Mottled, mottling, teeth (enamel) (endemic) (nonendemic) K00.3
Mounier-Kuhn syndrome Q32.4
with bronchiectasis J47.9
exacerbation (acute) J47.1
lower respiratory infection J47.0
acquired J98.09
with bronchiectasis J47.9
with
exacerbation (acute) J47.1
lower respiratory infection J47.0
Mountain
sickness T70.29
with polycythemia , acquired (acute) D75.1
tick fever A93.2
Mouse, joint — *see* Loose, body, joint
knee M23.4-
Mouth — *see* condition
Movable
coccyx — *see* subcategory M53.2
kidney N28.89
congenital Q63.8
spleen D73.89
Movements, dystonic R25.8
Moyamoya disease I67.5
MRSA (Methicillin resistant Staphylococcus aureus)
infection A49.02

MRSA (Methicillin resistant Staphylococcus aureus) - *continued*
infection - *continued*
as the cause of diseases classified elsewhere B95.62
sepsis A41.02
MSD (multiple sulfatase deficiency) E75.26
MSSA
(Methicillin susceptible Staphylococcus aureus)
infection A49.01
as the cause of diseases classified elsewhere B95.61
sepsis A41.01
Mucha-Habermann disease L41.0
Mucinosis (cutaneous) (focal) (papular) (reticular erythematous) (skin) L98.5
oral K13.79
Mucocele
appendix K38.8
buccal cavity K13.79
gallbladder K82.1
lacrimal sac, chronic H04.43-
nasal sinus J34.1
nose J34.1
salivary gland (any) K11.6
sinus (accessory) (nasal) J34.1
turbinate (bone) (middle) (nasal) J34.1
uterus N85.8
Mucolipidosis
I E77.1
II, III E77.0
IV E75.11
Mucopolysaccharidosis E76.3
beta-gluduronidase deficiency E76.29
cardiopathy E76.3 *[I52]*
Hunter's syndrome E76.1
Hurler's syndrome E76.01
Hurler-Scheie syndrome E76.02
Maroteaux-Lamy syndrome E76.29
Morquio syndrome E76.219
A E76.210
B E76.211
classic E76.210
Sanfilippo syndrome E76.22
Scheie's syndrome E76.03
specified NEC E76.29
type
I
Hurler's syndrome E76.01
Hurler-Scheie syndrome E76.02
Scheie's syndrome E76.03
II E76.1
III E76.22
IV E76.219
IVA E76.210
IVB E76.211
VI E76.29
VII E76.29
Mucormycosis B46.5
cutaneous B46.3
disseminated B46.4
gastrointestinal B46.2
generalized B46.4
pulmonary B46.0
rhinocerebral B46.1
skin B46.3
subcutaneous B46.3
Mucositis (ulcerative) K12.30
due to drugs NEC K12.32
gastrointestinal K92.81
mouth (oral) (oropharyngeal) K12.30
due to antineoplastic therapy K12.31
due to drugs NEC K12.32
due to radiation K12.33
specified NEC K12.39
viral K12.39
nasal J34.81
oral cavity — *see* Mucositis, mouth
oral soft tissues — *see* Mucositis, mouth
vagina and vulva N76.81
Mucositis necroticans agranulocytica — *see* Agranulocytosis
Mucous — *see also* condition
patches (syphilitic) A51.39
congenital A50.07
Mucoviscidosis E84.9
with meconium obstruction E84.11
Mucus
asphyxia or suffocation — *see* Asphyxia, mucus
in stool R19.5
plug — *see* Asphyxia, mucus
Muguet B37.0
Mulberry molars (congenital syphilis) A50.52

Myositis - *continued*
infective - *continued*
upper limb - *continued*
upper arm M60.02-
interstitial M60.10
ankle M60.17-
foot M60.17-
forearm M60.13-
hand M60.14-
lower leg M60.16-
multiple sites M60.19
shoulder region M60.11-
specified site NEC M60.18
thigh M60.15-
upper arm M60.12-
mycotic B49 *[M63.8-]*
orbital, chronic H05.12-
ossificans or ossifying (circumscripta) — *see also* Ossification, muscle, specified NEC
in (due to)
burns M61.30
ankle M61.37-
foot M61.37-
forearm M61.33-
hand M61.34-
lower leg M61.36-
multiple sites M61.39
pelvic region M61.35-
shoulder region M61.31-
specified site NEC M61.38
thigh M61.35-
upper arm M61.32-
quadriplegia or paraplegia M61.20
ankle M61.27-
foot M61.27-
forearm M61.23-
hand M61.24-
lower leg M61.26-
multiple sites M61.29
pelvic region M61.25-
shoulder region M61.21-
specified site NEC M61.28
thigh M61.25-
upper arm M61.22-
progressiva M61.10
ankle M61.17-
finger M61.14-
foot M61.17-
forearm M61.13-
hand M61.14-
lower leg M61.16-
multiple sites M61.19
pelvic region M61.15-
shoulder region M61.11-
specified site NEC M61.18
thigh M61.15-
toe M61.17-
upper arm M61.12-
traumatica M61.00
ankle M61.07-
foot M61.07-
forearm M61.03-
hand M61.04-
lower leg M61.06-
multiple sites M61.09
pelvic region M61.05-
shoulder region M61.01-
specified site NEC M61.08
thigh M61.05-
upper arm M61.02-
purulent — *see* Myositis, infective
specified type NEC M60.80
ankle M60.87-
foot M60.87-
forearm M60.83-
hand M60.84-
lower leg M60.86-
multiple sites M60.89
pelvic region M60.85-
shoulder region M60.81-
specified site NEC M60.88
thigh M60.85-
upper arm M60.82-
suppurative — *see* Myositis, infective
traumatic (old) — *see* Myositis, specified type NEC
Myospasia impulsiva F95.2
Myotonia (acquisita) (intermittens) M62.89
atrophica G71.11
chondrodystrophic G71.13
congenita (acetazolamide responsive) (dominant) (recessive) G71.12
drug-induced G71.14
dystrophica G71.11
Myotonia (acquisita) (intermittens) - *continued*
fluctuans G71.19
levior G71.12
permanens G71.19
symptomatic G71.19
Myotonic pupil — *see* Anomaly, pupil, function, tonic pupil
Myriapodiasis B88.2
Myringitis H73.2-
with otitis media — *see* Otitis, media
acute H73.00-
bullous H73.01-
specified NEC H73.09-
bullous — *see* Myringitis, acute, bullous
chronic H73.1-
Mysophobia F40.228
Mytilotoxism — *see* Poisoning, fish
Myxadenitis labialis K13.0
Myxedema (adult) (idiocy) (infantile) (juvenile) — *see also* Hypothyroidism E03.9
circumscribed E05.90
with storm E05.91
coma E03.5
congenital E00.1
cutis L98.5
localized (pretibial) E05.90
with storm E05.91
papular L98.5
Myxochondrosarcoma — *see* Neoplasm, cartilage, malignant
Myxofibroma — *see* Neoplasm, connective tissue, benign
odontogenic — *see* Cyst, calcifying odontogenic
Myxofibrosarcoma — *see* Neoplasm, connective tissue, malignant
Myxolipoma D17.9
Myxoliposarcoma — *see* Neoplasm, connective tissue, malignant
Myxoma — *see also* Neoplasm, connective tissue, benign
nerve sheath — *see* Neoplasm, nerve, benign
odontogenic — *see* Cyst, calcifying odontogenic
Myxosarcoma — *see* Neoplasm, connective tissue, malignant

N

Naegeli's
disease Q82.8
leukemia, monocytic C93.1-
Naegleriasis (with meningoencephalitis) B60.2
Naffziger's syndrome G54.0
Naga sore — *see* Ulcer, skin
Nägele's pelvis M95.5
with disproportion (fetopelvic) O33.0
causing obstructed labor O65.0
Nail — *see also* condition
biting F98.8
patella syndrome Q87.2
Nanism, nanosomia — *see* Dwarfism
Nanophyetiasis B66.8
Nanukayami A27.89
Napkin rash L22
Narcolepsy G47.419
with cataplexy G47.411
in conditions classified elsewhere G47.429
with cataplexy G47.421
Narcosis R06.89
Narcotism — *see* Dependence
NARP (Neuropathy, Ataxia and Retinitis pigmentosa) **syndrome** E88.49
Narrow
anterior chamber angle H40.03-
gingival width (of periodontal soft tissue) K05.5
pelvis — *see* Contraction, pelvis
Narrowing — *see also* Stenosis
artery I77.1
auditory, internal I65.8
basilar — *see* Occlusion, artery, basilar
carotid — *see* Occlusion, artery, carotid
cerebellar — *see* Occlusion, artery, cerebellar
cerebral — *see* Occlusion artery, cerebral
choroidal — *see* Occlusion, artery, cerebral, specified NEC
communicating posterior — *see* Occlusion, artery, cerebral, specified NEC
coronary — *see also* Disease, heart, ischemic, atherosclerotic
congenital Q24.5
syphilitic A50.54 *[I52]*
due to syphilis NEC A52.06
hypophyseal — *see* Occlusion, artery, cerebral, specified NEC
Narrowing - *continued*
artery - *continued*
pontine — *see* Occlusion, artery, cerebral, specified NEC
precerebral — *see* Occlusion, artery, precerebral
vertebral — *see* Occlusion, artery, vertebral
auditory canal (external) — *see* Stenosis, external ear canal
eustachian tube — *see* Obstruction, eustachian tube
eyelid — *see* Disorder, eyelid function
larynx J38.6
mesenteric artery — *see also* Ischemia, intestine, acute K55.059
palate M26.89
palpebral fissure — *see* Disorder, eyelid function
ureter N13.5
with infection N13.6
urethra — *see* Stricture, urethra
Narrowness, abnormal, eyelid Q10.3
Nasal — *see* condition
Nasolachrymal, nasolacrimal — *see* condition
Nasopharyngeal — *see also* condition
pituitary gland Q89.2
torticollis M43.6
Nasopharyngitis (acute) (infective) (streptococcal) (subacute) J00
chronic (suppurative) (ulcerative) J31.1
Nasopharynx, nasopharyngeal — *see* condition
Natal tooth, teeth K00.6
Nausea (without vomiting) R11.0
with vomiting R11.2
gravidarum — *see* Hyperemesis, gravidarum
marina T75.3
navalis T75.3
Navel — *see* condition
Neapolitan fever — *see* Brucellosis
Near drowning T75.1
Nearsightedness — *see* Myopia
Near-syncope R55
Nebula, cornea — *see* Opacity, cornea
Necator americanus infestation B76.1
Necatoriasis B76.1
Neck — *see* condition
Necrobiosis R68.89
lipoidica NEC L92.1
with diabetes — *see* E08-E13 with .620
Necrolysis, toxic epidermal L51.2
due to drug
correct substance properly administered — *see* Table of Drugs and Chemicals, by drug, adverse effect
overdose or wrong substance given or taken — *see* Table of Drugs and Chemicals, by drug, poisoning
Necrophilia F65.89
Necrosis, necrotic (ischemic) — *see also* Gangrene
adrenal (capsule) (gland) E27.49
amputation stump (surgical) (late) T87.50
arm T87.5-
leg T87.5-
antrum J32.0
aorta (hyaline) — *see also* Aneurysm, aorta
cystic medial — *see* Dissection, aorta
artery I77.5
bladder (aseptic) (sphincter) N32.89
bone — *see also* Osteonecrosis M87.9
aseptic or avascular — *see* Osteonecrosis
idiopathic M87.00
ethmoid J32.2
jaw M27.2
tuberculous — *see* Tuberculosis, bone
brain I67.89
breast (aseptic) (fat) (segmental) N64.1
bronchus J98.09
central nervous system NEC I67.89
cerebellar I67.89
cerebral I67.89
colon — *see also* Infarct, intestine K55.049
cornea H18.89-
cortical (acute) (renal) N17.1
cystic medial (aorta) — *see* Dissection, aorta
dental pulp K04.1
esophagus K22.8
ethmoid (bone) J32.2
eyelid — *see* Disorder, eyelid, degenerative
fat, fatty (generalized) — *see also* Disorder, soft tissue, specified type NEC
abdominal wall K65.4
breast (aseptic) (segmental) N64.1
localized — *see* Degeneration, by site, fatty
mesentery K65.4
omentum K65.4
pancreas K86.89

Necrosis, necrotic (ischemic) - *continued*
fat, fatty (generalized) - *continued*
peritoneum K65.4
skin (subcutaneous) , newborn P83.0
subcutaneous, due to birth injury P15.6
gallbladder — *see* Cholecystitis, acute
heart — *see* Infarct, myocardium
hip, aseptic or avascular — *see* Osteonecrosis, by type, femur
intestine (acute) (hemorrhagic) (massive) — *see also* Infarct, intestine K55.069
jaw M27.2
kidney (bilateral) N28.0
acute N17.9
cortical (acute) (bilateral) N17.1
with ectopic or molar pregnancy O08.4
medullary (bilateral) (in acute renal failure) (papillary) N17.2
papillary (bilateral) (in acute renal failure) N17.2
tubular N17.0
with ectopic or molar pregnancy O08.4
complicating
abortion — *see* Abortion, by type, complicated by, tubular necrosis
ectopic or molar pregnancy O08.4
pregnancy — *see* Pregnancy, complicated by, diseases of, specified type or system NEC
following ectopic or molar pregnancy O08.4
traumatic T79.5
larynx J38.7
liver (with hepatic failure) (cell) — *see* Failure, hepatic
hemorrhagic, central K76.2
lung J85.0
lymphatic gland — *see* Lymphadenitis, acute
mammary gland (fat) (segmental) N64.1
mastoid (chronic) — *see* Mastoiditis, chronic
medullary (acute) (renal) N17.2
mesentery — *see also* Infarct, intestine K55.069
fat K65.4
mitral valve — *see* Insufficiency, mitral
myocardium, myocardial — *see* Infarct, myocardium
nose J34.0
omentum (with mesenteric infarction) — *see also* Infarct, intestine K55.069
fat K65.4
orbit, orbital — *see* Osteomyelitis, orbit
ossicles, ear — *see* Abnormal, ear ossicles
ovary N70.92
pancreas (aseptic) (duct) (fat) K86.89
acute (infective) — *see* Pancreatitis, acute
infective — *see* Pancreatitis, acute
papillary (acute) (renal) N17.2
perineum N90.89
peritoneum (with mesenteric infarction) — *see also* Infarct, intestine K55.069
fat K65.4
pharynx J02.9
in granulocytopenia — *see* Neutropenia
Vincent's A69.1
phosphorus — *see* subcategory T54.2
pituitary (gland) E23.0
postpartum O99.285
Sheehan O99.285
pressure — *see* Ulcer, pressure, by site
pulmonary J85.0
pulp (dental) K04.1
radiation — *see* Necrosis, by site
radium — *see* Necrosis, by site
renal — *see* Necrosis, kidney
sclera H15.89
scrotum N50.89
skin or subcutaneous tissue NEC I96
spine, spinal (column) — *see also* Osteonecrosis, by type, vertebra
cord G95.19
spleen D73.5
stomach K31.89
stomatitis (ulcerative) A69.0
subcutaneous fat, newborn P83.88
subendocardial (acute) I21.4
chronic I25.89
suprarenal (capsule) (gland) E27.49
testis N50.89
thymus (gland) E32.8
tonsil J35.8
trachea J39.8
tuberculous NEC — *see* Tuberculosis
tubular (acute) (anoxic) (renal) (toxic) N17.0
postprocedural N99.0
vagina N89.8
vertebra — *see also* Osteonecrosis, by type, vertebra

Necrosis, necrotic (ischemic) - *continued*
vertebra - *continued*
tuberculous A18.01
vulva N90.89
X-ray — *see* Necrosis, by site
Necrospermia — *see* Infertility, male
Need (for)
care provider because (of)
assistance with personal care Z74.1
continuous supervision required Z74.3
impaired mobility Z74.09
no other household member able to render care Z74.2
specified reason NEC Z74.8
immunization — *see* Vaccination
vaccination — *see* Vaccination
Neglect
adult
confirmed T74.01
history of Z91.412
suspected T76.01
child (childhood)
confirmed T74.02
history of Z62.812
suspected T76.02
emotional, in childhood Z62.898
hemispatial R41.4
left-sided R41.4
sensory R41.4
visuospatial R41.4
Neisserian infection NEC — *see* Gonococcus
Nelaton's syndrome G60.8
Nelson's syndrome E24.1
Nematodiasis (intestinal) B82.0
Ancylostoma B76.0
Neonatal — *see also* Newborn
acne L70.4
bradycardia P29.12
tachycardia P29.11
screening, abnormal findings on P09
tooth, teeth K00.6
Neonatorum — *see* condition
Neoplasia
endocrine, multiple (MEN) E31.20
type I E31.21
type IIA E31.22
type IIB E31.23
intraepithelial (histologically confirmed)
anal (AIN) (histologically confirmed) K62.82
grade I K62.82
grade II K62.82
severe D01.3
cervical glandular (histologically confirmed) D06.9
cervix (uteri) (CIN) (histologically confirmed) N87.9
glandular D06.9
grade I N87.0
grade II N87.1
grade III (severe dysplasia) — *see also* Carcinoma, cervix uteri, in situ D06.9
prostate (histologically confirmed) (PIN) N42.31
grade I N42.31
grade II N42.31
grade III (severe dysplasia) D07.5
vagina (histologically confirmed) (VAIN) N89.3
grade I N89.0
grade II N89.1
grade III (severe dysplasia) D07.2
vulva (histologically confirmed) (VIN) N90.3
grade I N90.0
grade II N90.1
grade III (severe dysplasia) D07.1
Neoplasm, neoplastic — *see also* Table of Neoplasms
lipomatous, benign — *see* Lipoma
malignant mast cell C96.20
specified type NEC C96.29
mast cell, of uncertain behavior NEC D47.09

Notes:

The list below gives the code numbers for neoplasms by anatomical site. For each site there are six possible code numbers according to whether the neoplasm in question is malignant, benign, in situ, of uncertain behavior, or of unspecified nature. The description of the neoplasm will often indicate which of the six columns is appropriate; e.g., malignant melanoma of skin, benign fibroadenoma of breast, carcinoma in situ of cervix uteri. Where such descriptors are not present, the remainder of the Index should be consulted where guidance is given to the appropriate column for each morphological (histological) variety listed; e.g., Mesonephroma -- see Neoplasm, malignant; Embryoma -- see also Neoplasm, uncertain behavior; Disease, Bowen's -- see Neoplasm, skin, in situ. However, the guidance in the Index can be overridden if one of the descriptors mentioned above is present; e.g., malignant adenoma of colon to C18.9 and not to D12.6 as the adjective "malignant" overrides the Index entry "Adenoma - see also Neoplasm, benign."

Codes listed with a dash -, following the code have a required additional character for laterality. The tabular must be reviewed for the complete code.

Neoplasm, neoplastic	Malignant Primary	Malignant Secondary	Ca in situ	Benign	Uncertain Behavior	Unspecified Behavior
Neoplasm, neoplastic	C80.1	C79.9	D09.9	D36.9	D48.9	D49.9
abdomen, abdominal	C76.2	C79.8-	D09.8	D36.7	D48.7	D49.89
cavity	C76.2	C79.8-	D09.8	D36.7	D48.7	D49.89
organ	C76.2	C79.8-	D09.8	D36.7	D48.7	D49.89
viscera	C76.2	C79.8-	D09.8	D36.7	D48.7	D49.89
wall — *see also* Neoplasm, abdomen, wall, skin	C44.509	C79.2-	D04.5	D23.5	D48.5	D49.2
connective tissue	C49.4	C79.8-	-	D21.4	D48.1	D49.2
skin	C44.509					
basal cell carcinoma	C44.519	-	-	-	-	-
specified type NEC	C44.599	-	-	-	-	-
squamous cell carcinoma	C44.529	-	-	-	-	-
abdominopelvic	C76.8	C79.8-	-	D36.7	D48.7	D49.89
accessory sinus — *see* Neoplasm, sinus						
acoustic nerve	C72.4-	C79.49	-	D33.3	D43.3	D49.7
adenoid (pharynx) (tissue)	C11.1	C79.89	D00.08	D10.6	D37.05	D49.0
adipose tissue — *see also* Neoplasm, connective tissue	C49.4	C79.89	-	D21.9	D48.1	D49.2
adnexa (uterine)	C57.4	C79.89	D07.39	D28.7	D39.8	D49.59
adrenal	C74.9-	C79.7-	D09.3	D35.0-	D44.1-	D49.7
capsule	C74.9-	C79.7-	D09.3	D35.0-	D44.1-	D49.7
cortex	C74.0-	C79.7-	D09.3	D35.0-	D44.1-	D49.7
gland	C74.9-	C79.7-	D09.3	D35.0-	D44.1-	D49.7
medulla	C74.1-	C79.7-	D09.3	D35.0-	D44.1-	D49.7
ala nasi (external) — *see also* Neoplasm, skin, nose	C44.301	C79.2	D04.39	D23.39	D48.5	D49.2
alimentary canal or tract NEC	C26.9	C78.80	D01.9	D13.9	D37.9	D49.0
alveolar	C03.9	C79.89	D00.03	D10.39	D37.09	D49.0
mucosa	C03.9	C79.89	D00.03	D10.39	D37.09	D49.0
lower	C03.1	C79.89	D00.03	D10.39	D37.09	D49.0
upper	C03.0	C79.89	D00.03	D10.39	D37.09	D49.0
ridge or process	C41.1	C79.51	-	D16.5-	D48.0	D49.2
carcinoma	C03.9	C79.8-	-	-	-	-
lower	C03.1	C79.8-	-	-	-	-
upper	C03.0	C79.8-	-	-	-	-
lower	C41.1	C79.51	-	D16.5-	D48.0	D49.2
mucosa	C03.9	C79.89	D00.03	D10.39	D37.09	D49.0
lower	C03.1	C79.89	D00.03	D10.39	D37.09	D49.0
upper	C03.0	C79.89	D00.03	D10.39	D37.09	D49.0
upper	C41.0	C79.51	-	D16.4-	D48.0	D49.2
sulcus	C06.1	C79.89	D00.02	D10.39	D37.09	D49.0
alveolus	C03.9	C79.89	D00.03	D10.39	D37.09	D49.0
lower	C03.1	C79.89	D00.03	D10.39	D37.09	D49.0
upper	C03.0	C79.89	D00.03	D10.39	D37.09	D49.0
ampulla of Vater	C24.1	C78.89	D01.5	D13.5	D37.6	D49.0
ankle NEC	C76.5-	C79.89	D04.7-	D36.7	D48.7	D49.89
anorectum, anorectal (junction)	C21.8	C78.5	D01.3	D12.9	D37.8	D49.0
antecubital fossa or space	C76.4-	C79.89	D04.6-	D36.7	D48.7	D49.89
antrum (Highmore) (maxillary)	C31.0	C78.39	D02.3	D14.0	D38.5	D49.1
pyloric	C16.3	C78.89	D00.2	D13.1	D37.1	D49.0
tympanicum	C30.1	C78.39	D02.3	D14.0	D38.5	D49.1
anus, anal	C21.0	C78.5	D01.3	D12.9	D37.8	D49.0
canal	C21.1	C78.5	D01.3	D12.9	D37.8	D49.0
cloacogenic zone	C21.2	C78.5	D01.3	D12.9	D37.8	D49.0
margin — *see also* Neoplasm, anus, skin	C44.500	C79.2	D04.5	D23.5	D48.5	D49.2
overlapping lesion with rectosigmoid junction or rectum	C21.8	-	-	-	-	-
skin	C44.500	C79.2	D04.5	D23.5	D48.5	D49.2
basal cell carcinoma	C44.510	-	-	-	-	-
specified type NEC	C44.590	-	-	-	-	-
squamous cell carcinoma	C44.520	-	-	-	-	-
sphincter	C21.1	C78.5	D01.3	D12.9	D37.8	D49.0
aorta (thoracic)	C49.3	C79.89	-	D21.3	D48.1	D49.2
abdominal	C49.4	C79.89	-	D21.4	D48.1	D49.2
aortic body	C75.5	C79.89	-	D35.6	D44.7	D49.7
aponeurosis	C49.9	C79.89	-	D21.9	D48.1	D49.2
palmar	C49.1-	C79.89	-	D21.1-	D48.1	D49.2
plantar	C49.2-	C79.89	-	D21.2-	D48.1	D49.2
appendix	C18.1	C78.5	D01.0	D12.1	D37.3	D49.0
arachnoid	C70.9	C79.49	-	D32.9	D42.9	D49.7
cerebral	C70.0	C79.32	-	D32.0	D42.0	D49.7
spinal	C70.1	C79.49	-	D32.1	D42.1	D49.7
areola	C50.0-	C79.81	D05.-	D24.-	D48.6-	D49.3
arm NEC	C76.4-	C79.89	D04.6-	D36.7	D48.7	D49.89
artery — *see* Neoplasm, connective tissue						
aryepiglottic fold	C13.1	C79.89	D00.08	D10.7	D37.05	D49.0
hypopharyngeal aspect	C13.1	C79.89	D00.08	D10.7	D37.05	D49.0
laryngeal aspect	C32.1	C78.39	D02.0	D14.1	D38.0	D49.1
marginal zone	C13.1	C79.89	D00.08	D10.7	D37.05	D49.0
arytenoid (cartilage)	C32.3	C78.39	D02.0	D14.1	D38.0	D49.1
fold — *see* Neoplasm, aryepiglottic						
associated with transplanted organ	C80.2	-	-	-	-	-
atlas	C41.2	C79.51	-	D16.6	D48.0	D49.2
atrium, cardiac	C38.0	C79.89	-	D15.1	D48.7	D49.89
auditory						
canal (external) (skin)	C44.20-	C79.2	D04.2-	D23.2-	D48.5	D49.2
internal	C30.1	C78.39	D02.3	D14.0	D38.5	D49.1
nerve	C72.4-	C79.49	-	D33.3	D43.3	D49.7
tube	C30.1	C78.39	D02.3	D14.0	D38.5	D49.1
opening	C11.2	C79.89	D00.08	D10.6	D37.05	D49.0
auricle, ear — *see also* Neoplasm, skin, ear	C44.20-	C79.2	D04.2-	D23.2-	D48.5	D49.2
auricular canal (external) — *see also* Neoplasm, skin, ear	C44.20-	C79.2	D04.2-	D23.2-	D48.5	D49.2
internal	C30.1	C78.39	D02.3	D14.0	D38.5	D49.2
autonomic nerve or nervous system NEC (see Neoplasm, nerve, peripheral)						
axilla, axillary	C76.1	C79.89	D09.8	D36.7	D48.7	D49.89
fold — *see also* Neoplasm, skin, trunk	C44.509	C79.2	D04.5	D23.5	D48.5	D49.2
back NEC	C76.8	C79.89	D04.5	D36.7	D48.7	D49.89
Bartholin's gland	C51.0	C79.82	D07.1	D28.0	D39.8	D49.59
basal ganglia	C71.0	C79.31	-	D33.0	D43.0	D49.6
basis pedunculi	C71.7	C79.31	-	D33.1	D43.1	D49.6
bile or biliary (tract)	C24.9	C78.89	D01.5	D13.5	D37.6	D49.0
canaliculi (biliferi) (intrahepatic)	C22.1	C78.7	D01.5	D13.4	D37.6	D49.0
canals, interlobular	C22.1	C78.89	D01.5	D13.4	D37.6	D49.0
duct or passage (common) (cystic) (extrahepatic)	C24.0	C78.89	D01.5	D13.5	D37.6	D49.0
interlobular	C22.1	C78.89	D01.5	D13.4	D37.6	D49.0
intrahepatic	C22.1	C78.7	D01.5	D13.4	D37.6	D49.0
and extrahepatic	C24.8	C78.89	D01.5	D13.5	D37.6	D49.0
bladder (urinary)	C67.9	C79.11	D09.0	D30.3	D41.4	D49.4
dome	C67.1	C79.11	D09.0	D30.3	D41.4	D49.4
neck	C67.5	C79.11	D09.0	D30.3	D41.4	D49.4
orifice	C67.9	C79.11	D09.0	D30.3	D41.4	D49.4
ureteric	C67.6	C79.11	D09.0	D30.3	D41.4	D49.4
urethral	C67.5	C79.11	D09.0	D30.3	D41.4	D49.4
overlapping lesion	C67.8	-	-	-	-	-
sphincter	C67.8	C79.11	D09.0	D30.3	D41.4	D49.4
trigone	C67.0	C79.11	D09.0	D30.3	D41.4	D49.4
urachus	C67.7	C79.11	D09.0	D30.3	D41.4	D49.4
wall	C67.9	C79.11	D09.0	D30.3	D41.4	D49.4
anterior	C67.3	C79.11	D09.0	D30.3	D41.4	D49.4
lateral	C67.2	C79.11	D09.0	D30.3	D41.4	D49.4
posterior	C67.4	C79.11	D09.0	D30.3	D41.4	D49.4
blood vessel — *see* Neoplasm, connective tissue						
bone (periosteum)	C41.9	C79.51	-	D16.9-	D48.0	D49.2
acetabulum	C41.4	C79.51	-	D16.8-	D48.0	D49.2
ankle	C40.3-	C79.51	-	D16.3-	-	-
arm NEC	C40.0-	C79.51	-	D16.0-	-	-
astragalus	C40.3-	C79.51	-	D16.3-	-	-
atlas	C41.2	C79.51	-	D16.6-	D48.0	D49.2
axis	C41.2	C79.51	-	D16.6-	D48.0	D49.2
back NEC	C41.2	C79.51	-	D16.6-	D48.0	D49.2
calcaneus	C40.3-	C79.51	-	D16.3-	-	-
calvarium	C41.0	C79.51	-	D16.4-	D48.0	D49.2
carpus (any)	C40.1-	C79.51	-	D16.1-	-	-

Neoplasm, neoplastic	Malignant Primary	Malignant Secondary	Ca in situ	Benign	Uncertain Behavior	Unspecified Behavior
bone - *continued*						
cartilage NEC	C41.9	C79.51	-	D16.9-	D48.0	D49.2
clavicle	C41.3	C79.51	-	D16.7-	D48.0	D49.2
clivus	C41.0	C79.51	-	D16.4-	D48.0	D49.2
coccygeal vertebra	C41.4	C79.51	-	D16.8-	D48.0	D49.2
coccyx	C41.4	C79.51	-	D16.8-	D48.0	D49.2
costal cartilage	C41.3	C79.51	-	D16.7-	D48.0	D49.2
costovertebral joint	C41.3	C79.51	-	D16.7-	D48.0	D49.2
cranial	C41.0	C79.51	-	D16.4-	D48.0	D49.2
cuboid	C40.3-	C79.51	-	D16.3-	-	-
cuneiform	C41.9	C79.51	-	D16.9-	D48.0	D49.2
elbow	C40.0-	C79.51	-	D16.0-	-	-
ethmoid (labyrinth)	C41.0	C79.51	-	D16.4-	D48.0	D49.2
face	C41.0	C79.51	-	D16.4-	D48.0	D49.2
femur (any part)	C40.2-	C79.51	-	D16.2-	-	-
fibula (any part)	C40.2-	C79.51	-	D16.2-	-	-
finger (any)	C40.1-	C79.51	-	D16.1-	-	-
foot	C40.3-	C79.51	-	D16.3-	-	-
forearm	C40.0-	C79.51	-	D16.0-	-	-
frontal	C41.0	C79.51	-	D16.4-	D48.0	D49.2
hand	C40.1-	C79.51	-	D16.1-	-	-
heel	C40.3-	C79.51	-	D16.3-	-	-
hip	C41.4	C79.51	-	D16.8-	D48.0	D49.2
humerus (any part)	C40.0-	C79.51	-	D16.0-	-	-
hyoid	C41.0	C79.51	-	D16.4-	D48.0	D49.2
ilium	C41.4	C79.51	-	D16.8-	D48.0	D49.2
innominate	C41.4	C79.51	-	D16.8-	D48.0	D49.2
intervertebral cartilage or disc	C41.2	C79.51	-	D16.6-	D48.0	D49.2
ischium	C41.4	C79.51	-	D16.8-	D48.0	D49.2
jaw (lower)	C41.1	C79.51	-	D16.5-	D48.0	D49.2
knee	C40.2-	C79.51	-	D16.2-	-	-
leg NEC	C40.2-	C79.51	-	D16.2-	-	-
limb NEC	C40.9-	C79.51	-	D16.9-	-	-
lower (long bones)	C40.2-	C79.51	-	D16.2-	-	-
short bones	C40.3-	C79.51	-	D16.3-	-	-
upper (long bones)	C40.0-	C79.51	-	D16.0-	-	-
short bones	C40.1-	C79.51	-	D16.1-	-	-
malar	C41.0	C79.51	-	D16.4-	D48.0	D49.2
mandible	C41.1	C79.51	-	D16.5-	D48.0	D49.2
marrow NEC (any bone)	C96.9	C79.52	-	-	D47.9	D49.89
mastoid	C41.0	C79.51	-	D16.4-	D48.0	D49.2
maxilla, maxillary (superior)	C41.0	C79.51	-	D16.4-	D48.0	D49.2
inferior	C41.1	C79.51	-	D16.5-	D48.0	D49.2
metacarpus (any)	C40.1-	C79.51	-	D16.1-	-	-
metatarsus (any)	C40.3-	C79.51	-	D16.3-	-	-
overlapping sites	C40.8-	-	-	-	-	-
navicular						
ankle	C40.3-	C79.51	-	-	-	-
hand	C40.1-	C79.51	-	-	-	-
nose, nasal	C41.0	C79.51	-	D16.4-	D48.0	D49.2
occipital	C41.0	C79.51	-	D16.4-	D48.0	D49.2
orbit	C41.0	C79.51	-	D16.4-	D48.0	D49.2
parietal	C41.0	C79.51	-	D16.4-	D48.0	D49.2
patella	C40.2-	C79.51	-	-	-	-
pelvic	C41.4	C79.51	-	D16.8	D48.0	D49.2
phalanges						
foot	C40.3-	C79.51	-	-	-	-
hand	C40.1-	C79.51	-	-	-	-
pubic	C41.4	C79.51	-	D16.8	D48.0	D49.2
radius (any part)	C40.0-	C79.51	-	D16.0-	-	-
rib	C41.3	C79.51	-	D16.7	D48.0	D49.2
sacral vertebra	C41.4	C79.51	-	D16.8	D48.0	D49.2
sacrum	C41.4	C79.51	-	D16.8	D48.0	D49.2
scaphoid						
of ankle	C40.3-	C79.51	-	-	-	-
of hand	C40.1-	C79.51	-	-	-	-
scapula (any part)	C40.0-	C79.51	-	D16.0-	-	-
sella turcica	C41.0	C79.51	-	D16.4-	D48.0	D49.2
shoulder	C40.0-	C79.51	-	D16.0-	-	-
skull	C41.0	C79.51	-	D16.4-	D48.0	D49.2
sphenoid	C41.0	C79.51	-	D16.4-	D48.0	D49.2
spine, spinal (column)	C41.2	C79.51	-	D16.6	D48.0	D49.2
coccyx	C41.4	C79.51	-	D16.8	D48.0	D49.2
sacrum	C41.4	C79.51	-	D16.8	D48.0	D49.2
sternum	C41.3	C79.51	-	D16.7	D48.0	D49.2
tarsus (any)	C40.3-	C79.51	-	-	-	-
temporal	C41.0	C79.51	-	D16.4-	D48.0	D49.2
thumb	C40.1-	C79.51	-	-	-	-
tibia (any part)	C40.2-	C79.51	-	-	-	-

Neoplasm, neoplastic	Malignant Primary	Malignant Secondary	Ca in situ	Benign	Uncertain Behavior	Unspecified Behavior
bone - *continued*						
toe (any)	C40.3-	C79.51	-	-	-	-
trapezium	C40.1-	C79.51	-	-	-	-
trapezoid	C40.1-	C79.51	-	-	-	-
turbinate	C41.0	C79.51	-	D16.4-	D48.0	D49.2
ulna (any part)	C40.0-	C79.51	-	D16.0-	-	-
unciform	C40.1-	C79.51	-	-	-	-
vertebra (column)	C41.2	C79.51	-	D16.6	D48.0	D49.2
coccyx	C41.4	C79.51	-	D16.8	D48.0	D49.2
sacrum	C41.4	C79.51	-	D16.8	D48.0	D49.2
vomer	C41.0	C79.51	-	D16.4-	D48.0	D49.2
wrist	C40.1-	C79.51	-	-	-	-
xiphoid process	C41.3	C79.51	-	D16.7	D48.0	D49.2
zygomatic	C41.0	C79.51	-	D16.4-	D48.0	D49.2
book-leaf (mouth)	C06.89	C79.89	D00.00	D10.39	D37.09	D49.0
bowel — *see* Neoplasm, intestine						
brachial plexus	C47.1-	C79.89	-	D36.12	D48.2	D49.2
brain NEC	C71.9	C79.31	-	D33.2	D43.2	D49.6
basal ganglia	C71.0	C79.31	-	D33.0	D43.0	D49.6
cerebellopontine angle	C71.6	C79.31	-	D33.1	D43.1	D49.6
cerebellum NOS	C71.6	C79.31	-	D33.1	D43.1	D49.6
cerebrum	C71.0	C79.31	-	D33.0	D43.0	D49.6
choroid plexus	C71.7	C79.31	-	D33.1	D43.1	D49.6
corpus callosum	C71.8	C79.31	-	D33.2	D43.2	D49.6
corpus striatum	C71.0	C79.31	-	D33.0	D43.0	D49.6
cortex (cerebral)	C71.0	C79.31	-	D33.0	D43.0	D49.6
frontal lobe	C71.1	C79.31	-	D33.0	D43.0	D49.6
globus pallidus	C71.0	C79.31	-	D33.0	D43.0	D49.6
hippocampus	C71.2	C79.31	-	D33.0	D43.0	D49.6
hypothalamus	C71.0	C79.31	-	D33.0	D43.0	D49.6
internal capsule	C71.0	C79.31	-	D33.0	D43.0	D49.6
medulla oblongata	C71.7	C79.31	-	D33.1	D43.1	D49.6
meninges	C70.0	C79.32	-	D32.0	D42.0	D49.7
midbrain	C71.7	C79.31	-	D33.1	D43.1	D49.6
occipital lobe	C71.4	C79.31	-	D33.0	D43.0	D49.6
overlapping lesion	C71.8	C79.31	-	-	-	-
parietal lobe	C71.3	C79.31	-	D33.0	D43.0	D49.6
peduncle	C71.7	C79.31	-	D33.1	D43.1	D49.6
pons	C71.7	C79.31	-	D33.1	D43.1	D49.6
stem	C71.7	C79.31	-	D33.1	D43.1	D49.6
tapetum	C71.8	C79.31	-	D33.2	D43.2	D49.6
temporal lobe	C71.2	C79.31	-	D33.0	D43.0	D49.6
thalamus	C71.0	C79.31	-	D33.0	D43.0	D49.6
uncus	C71.2	C79.31	-	D33.0	D43.0	D49.6
ventricle (floor)	C71.5	C79.31	-	D33.0	D43.0	D49.6
fourth	C71.7	C79.31	-	D33.1	D43.1	D49.6
branchial (cleft) (cyst) (vestiges)	C10.4	C79.89	D00.08	D10.5	D37.05	D49.0
breast (connective tissue) (glandular tissue) (soft parts)	C50.9-	C79.81	D05.-	D24.-	D48.6-	D49.3
areola	C50.0-	C79.81	D05.-	D24.-	D48.6-	D49.3
axillary tail	C50.6-	C79.81	D05.-	D24.-	D48.6-	D49.3
central portion	C50.1-	C79.81	D05.-	D24.-	D48.6-	D49.3
inner	C50.8-	C79.81	D05.-	D24.-	D48.6-	D49.3
lower	C50.8-	C79.81	D05.-	D24.-	D48.6-	D49.3
lower-inner quadrant	C50.3-	C79.81	D05.-	D24.-	D48.6-	D49.3
lower-outer quadrant	C50.5-	C79.81	D05.-	D24.-	D48.6-	D49.3
mastectomy site (skin) — *see also* Neoplasm, breast, skin	C44.501	C79.2	-	-	-	-
specified as breast tissue	C50.8-	C79.81	-	-	-	-
midline	C50.8-	C79.81	D05.-	D24.-	D48.6-	D49.3
nipple	C50.0-	C79.81	D05.-	D24.-	D48.6-	D49.3
outer	C50.8-	C79.81	D05.-	D24.-	D48.6-	D49.3
overlapping lesion	C50.8-	-	-	-	-	-
skin	C44.501	C79.2	D04.5	D23.5	D48.5	D49.2
basal cell carcinoma	C44.511	-	-	-	-	-
specified type NEC	C44.591	-	-	-	-	-
squamous cell carcinoma	C44.521	-	-	-	-	-
tail (axillary)	C50.6-	C79.81	D05.-	D24.-	D48.6-	D49.3
upper	C50.8-	C79.81	D05.-	D24.-	D48.6-	D49.3
upper-inner quadrant	C50.2-	C79.81	D05.-	D24.-	D48.6-	D49.3
upper-outer quadrant	C50.4-	C79.81	D05.-	D24.-	D48.6-	D49.3
broad ligament	C57.1	C79.82	D07.39	D28.2	D39.8	D49.59
bronchiogenic, bronchogenic (lung)	C34.9-	C78.0-	D02.2-	D14.3-	D38.1	D49.1
bronchiole	C34.9-	C78.0-	D02.2-	D14.3-	D38.1	D49.1
bronchus	C34.9-	C78.0-	D02.2-	D14.3-	D38.1	D49.1
carina	C34.0-	C78.0-	D02.2-	D14.3-	D38.1	D49.1
lower lobe of lung	C34.3-	C78.0-	D02.2-	D14.3-	D38.1	D49.1
main	C34.0-	C78.0-	D02.2-	D14.3-	D38.1	D49.1
middle lobe of lung	C34.2	C78.0-	D02.21	D14.31	D38.1	D49.1

Neoplasm, neoplastic	Malignant Primary	Malignant Secondary	Ca in situ	Benign	Uncertain Behavior	Unspecified Behavior
bronchus - *continued*						
overlapping lesion	C34.8-	-	-	-	-	-
upper lobe of lung	C34.1-	C78.0-	D02.2-	D14.3-	D38.1	D49.1
brow	C44.309	C79.2	D04.39	D23.39	D48.5	D49.2
basal cell carcinoma	C44.319	-	-	-	-	-
specified type NEC	C44.399	-	-	-	-	-
squamous cell carcinoma	C44.329	-	-	-	-	-
buccal (cavity)	C06.9	C79.89	D00.00	D10.39	D37.09	D49.0
commissure	C06.0	C79.89	D00.02	D10.39	D37.09	D49.0
groove (lower) (upper)	C06.1	C79.89	D00.02	D10.39	D37.09	D49.0
mucosa	C06.0	C79.89	D00.02	D10.39	D37.09	D49.0
sulcus (lower) (upper)	C06.1	C79.89	D00.02	D10.39	D37.09	D49.0
bulbourethral gland	C68.0	C79.19	D09.19	D30.4	D41.3	D49.59
bursa — *see* Neoplasm, connective tissue						
buttock NEC	C76.3	C79.89	D04.5	D36.7	D48.7	D49.89
calf	C76.5-	C79.89	D04.7-	D36.7	D48.7	D49.89
calvarium	C41.0	C79.51	-	D16.4-	D48.0	D49.2
calyx, renal	C65.-	C79.0-	D09.19	D30.1-	D41.1-	D49.51-
canal						
anal	C21.1	C78.5	D01.3	D12.9	D37.8	D49.0
auditory (external) — *see also* Neoplasm, skin, ear	C44.20-	C79.2	D04.2-	D23.2-	D48.5	D49.2
auricular (external) — *see also* Neoplasm, skin, ear	C44.20-	C79.2	D04.2-	D23.2-	D48.5	D49.2
canaliculi, biliary (biliferi) (intrahepatic)	C22.1	C78.7	D01.5	D13.4	D37.6	D49.0
canthus (eye) (inner) (outer)	C44.10-	C79.2	D04.1-	D23.1-	D48.5	D49.2
basal cell carcinoma	C44.11-	-	-	-	-	-
sebaceous cell	C44.13-	-	-	-	-	-
specified type NEC	C44.19-	-	-	-	-	-
squamous cell carcinoma	C44.12-	-	-	-	-	-
capillary — *see* Neoplasm, connective tissue						
caput coli	C18.0	C78.5	D01.0	D12.0	D37.4	D49.0
carcinoid — *see* Tumor, carcinoid						
cardia (gastric)	C16.0	C78.89	D00.2	D13.1	D37.1	D49.0
cardiac orifice (stomach)	C16.0	C78.89	D00.2	D13.1	D37.1	D49.0
cardio-esophageal junction	C16.0	C78.89	D00.2	D13.1	D37.1	D49.0
cardio-esophagus	C16.0	C78.89	D00.2	D13.1	D37.1	D49.0
carina (bronchus)	C34.0-	C78.0-	D02.2-	D14.3-	D38.1	D49.1
carotid (artery)	C49.0	C79.89	-	D21.0	D48.1	D49.2
body	C75.4	C79.89	-	D35.5	D44.6	D49.7
carpus (any bone)	C40.1-	C79.51	-	D16.1-	-	-
cartilage (articular) (joint) NEC — *see also* Neoplasm, bone	C41.9	C79.51	-	D16.9-	D48.0	D49.2
arytenoid	C32.3	C78.39	D02.0	D14.1	D38.0	D49.1
auricular	C49.0	C79.89	-	D21.0	D48.1	D49.2
bronchi	C34.0-	C78.39	-	D14.3-	D38.1	D49.1
costal	C41.3	C79.51	-	D16.7	D48.0	D49.2
cricoid	C32.3	C78.39	D02.0	D14.1	D38.0	D49.1
cuneiform	C32.3	C78.39	D02.0	D14.1	D38.0	D49.1
ear (external)	C49.0	C79.89	-	D21.0	D48.1	D49.2
ensiform	C41.3	C79.51	-	D16.7	D48.0	D49.2
epiglottis	C32.1	C78.39	D02.0	D14.1	D38.0	D49.1
anterior surface	C10.1	C79.89	D00.08	D10.5	D37.05	D49.0
eyelid	C49.0	C79.89	-	D21.0	D48.1	D49.2
intervertebral	C41.2	C79.51	-	D16.6	D48.0	D49.2
larynx, laryngeal	C32.3	C78.39	D02.0	D14.1	D38.0	D49.1
nose, nasal	C30.0	C78.39	D02.3	D14.0	D38.5	D49.1
pinna	C49.0	C79.89	-	D21.0	D48.1	D49.2
rib	C41.3	C79.51	-	D16.7	D48.0	D49.2
semilunar (knee)	C40.2-	C79.51	-	D16.2-	D48.0	D49.2
thyroid	C32.3	C78.39	D02.0	D14.1	D38.0	D49.1
trachea	C33	C78.39	D02.1	D14.2	D38.1	D49.1
cauda equina	C72.1	C79.49	-	D33.4	D43.4	D49.7
cavity						
buccal	C06.9	C79.89	D00.00	D10.30	D37.09	D49.0
nasal	C30.0	C78.39	D02.3	D14.0	D38.5	D49.1
oral	C06.9	C79.89	D00.00	D10.30	D37.09	D49.0
peritoneal	C48.2	C78.6	-	D20.1	D48.4	D49.0
tympanic	C30.1	C78.39	D02.3	D14.0	D38.5	D49.1
cecum	C18.0	C78.5	D01.0	D12.0	D37.4	D49.0
central nervous system	C72.9	C79.40	-	-	-	-
cerebellopontine (angle)	C71.6	C79.31	-	D33.1	D43.1	D49.6
cerebellum, cerebellar	C71.6	C79.31	-	D33.1	D43.1	D49.6
cerebrum, cerebral (cortex) (hemisphere) (white matter)	C71.0	C79.31	-	D33.0	D43.0	D49.6
meninges	C70.0	C79.32	-	D32.0	D42.0	D49.7

Neoplasm, neoplastic	Malignant Primary	Malignant Secondary	Ca in situ	Benign	Uncertain Behavior	Unspecified Behavior
cerebrum, cerebral - *continued*						
peduncle	C71.7	C79.31	-	D33.1	D43.1	D49.6
ventricle	C71.5	C79.31	-	D33.0	D43.0	D49.6
fourth	C71.7	C79.31	-	D33.1	D43.1	D49.6
cervical region	C76.0	C79.89	D09.8	D36.7	D48.7	D49.89
cervix (cervical) (uteri) (uterus)	C53.9	C79.82	D06.9	D26.0	D39.0	D49.59
canal	C53.0	C79.82	D06.0	D26.0	D39.0	D49.59
endocervix (canal) (gland)	C53.0	C79.82	D06.0	D26.0	D39.0	D49.59
exocervix	C53.1	C79.82	D06.1	D26.0	D39.0	D49.59
external os	C53.1	C79.82	D06.1	D26.0	D39.0	D49.59
internal os	C53.0	C79.82	D06.0	D26.0	D39.0	D49.59
nabothian gland	C53.0	C79.82	D06.0	D26.0	D39.0	D49.59
overlapping lesion	C53.8	-	-	-	-	-
squamocolumnar junction	C53.8	C79.82	D06.7	D26.0	D39.0	D49.59
stump	C53.8	C79.82	D06.7	D26.0	D39.0	D49.59
cheek	C76.0	C79.89	D09.8	D36.7	D48.7	D49.89
external	C44.309	C79.2	D04.39	D23.39	D48.5	D49.2
basal cell carcinoma	C44.319	-	-	-	-	-
specified type NEC	C44.399	-	-	-	-	-
squamous cell carcinoma	C44.329	-	-	-	-	-
inner aspect	C06.0	C79.89	D00.02	D10.39	D37.09	D49.0
internal	C06.0	C79.89	D00.02	D10.39	D37.09	D49.0
mucosa	C06.0	C79.89	D00.02	D10.39	D37.09	D49.0
chest (wall) NEC	C76.1	C79.89	D09.8	D36.7	D48.7	D49.89
chiasma opticum	C72.3-	C79.49	-	D33.3	D43.3	D49.7
chin	C44.309	C79.2	D04.39	D23.39	D48.5	D49.2
basal cell carcinoma	C44.319	-	-	-	-	-
specified type NEC	C44.399	-	-	-	-	-
squamous cell carcinoma	C44.329	-	-	-	-	-
choana	C11.3	C79.89	D00.08	D10.6	D37.05	D49.0
cholangiole	C22.1	C78.89	D01.5	D13.4	D37.6	D49.0
choledochal duct	C24.0	C78.89	D01.5	D13.5	D37.6	D49.0
choroid	C69.3-	C79.49	D09.2-	D31.3-	D48.7	D49.81
plexus	C71.5	C79.31	-	D33.0	D43.0	D49.6
ciliary body	C69.4-	C79.49	D09.2-	D31.4-	D48.7	D49.89
clavicle	C41.3	C79.51	-	D16.7	D48.0	D49.2
clitoris	C51.2	C79.82	D07.1	D28.0	D39.8	D49.59
clivus	C41.0	C79.51	-	D16.4-	D48.0	D49.2
cloacogenic zone	C21.2	C78.5	D01.3	D12.9	D37.8	D49.0
coccygeal						
body or glomus	C49.5	C79.89	-	D21.5	D48.1	D49.2
vertebra	C41.4	C79.51	-	D16.8	D48.0	D49.2
coccyx	C41.4	C79.51	-	D16.8	D48.0	D49.2
colon — *see also* Neoplasm, intestine, large	C18.9	C78.5	-	-	-	-
with rectum	C19	C78.5	D01.1	D12.7	D37.5	D49.0
column, spinal — *see* Neoplasm, spine						
columnella — *see also* Neoplasm, skin, face	C44.390	C79.2	D04.39	D23.39	D48.5	D49.2
commissure						
labial, lip	C00.6	C79.89	D00.01	D10.39	D37.01	D49.0
laryngeal	C32.0	C78.39	D02.0	D14.1	D38.0	D49.1
common (bile) duct	C24.0	C78.89	D01.5	D13.5	D37.6	D49.0
concha — *see also* Neoplasm, skin, ear	C44.20-	C79.2	D04.2-	D23.2-	D48.5	D49.2
nose	C30.0	C78.39	D02.3	D14.0	D38.5	D49.1
conjunctiva	C69.0-	C79.49	D09.2-	D31.0-	D48.7	D49.89
connective tissue NEC	C49.9	C79.89	-	D21.9	D48.1	D49.2
Note: For neoplasms of connective tissue (blood vessel, bursa, fascia, ligament, muscle, peripheral nerves, sympathetic and parasympathetic nerves and ganglia, synovia, tendon, etc.) or of morphological types that indicate connective tissue, code according to the list under "Neoplasm, connective tissue". For sites that do not appear in this list, code to neoplasm of that site; e.g., fibrosarcoma, pancreas (C25.9)						
Note: Morphological types that indicate connective tissue appear in their proper place in the alphabetic index with the instruction "see Neoplasm, connective tissue ...."						
abdomen	C49.4	C79.89	-	D21.4	D48.1	D49.2

Neoplasm, neoplastic	Malignant Primary	Malignant Secondary	Ca in situ	Benign	Uncertain Behavior	Unspecified Behavior
connective tissue NEC - *continued*						
abdominal wall	C49.4	C79.89	-	D21.4	D48.1	D49.2
ankle	C49.2-	C79.89	-	D21.2-	D48.1	D49.2
antecubital fossa or space	C49.1-	C79.89	-	D21.1-	D48.1	D49.2
arm	C49.1-	C79.89	-	D21.1-	D48.1	D49.2
auricle (ear)	C49.0	C79.89	-	D21.0	D48.1	D49.2
axilla	C49.3	C79.89	-	D21.3	D48.1	D49.2
back	C49.6	C79.89	-	D21.6	D48.1	D49.2
breast — *see* Neoplasm, breast						
buttock	C49.5	C79.89	-	D21.5	D48.1	D49.2
calf	C49.2-	C79.89	-	D21.2-	D48.1	D49.2
cervical region	C49.0	C79.89	-	D21.0	D48.1	D49.2
cheek	C49.0	C79.89	-	D21.0	D48.1	D49.2
chest (wall)	C49.3	C79.89	-	D21.3	D48.1	D49.2
chin	C49.0	C79.89	-	D21.0	D48.1	D49.2
diaphragm	C49.3	C79.89	-	D21.3	D48.1	D49.2
ear (external)	C49.0	C79.89	-	D21.0	D48.1	D49.2
elbow	C49.1-	C79.89	-	D21.1-	D48.1	D49.2
extrarectal	C49.5	C79.89	-	D21.5	D48.1	D49.2
extremity	C49.9	C79.89	-	D21.9	D48.1	D49.2
lower	C49.2-	C79.89	-	D21.2-	D48.1	D49.2
upper	C49.1-	C79.89	-	D21.1-	D48.1	D49.2
eyelid	C49.0	C79.89	-	D21.0	D48.1	D49.2
face	C49.0	C79.89	-	D21.0	D48.1	D49.2
finger	C49.1-	C79.89	-	D21.1-	D48.1	D49.2
flank	C49.6	C79.89	-	D21.6	D48.1	D49.2
foot	C49.2-	C79.89	-	D21.2-	D48.1	D49.2
forearm	C49.1-	C79.89	-	D21.1-	D48.1	D49.2
forehead	C49.0	C79.89	-	D21.0	D48.1	D49.2
gastric	C49.4	C79.89	-	D21.4	D48.1	D49.2
gastrointestinal	C49.4	C79.89	-	D21.4	D48.1	D49.2
gluteal region	C49.5	C79.89	-	D21.5	D48.1	D49.2
great vessels NEC	C49.3	C79.89	-	D21.3	D48.1	D49.2
groin	C49.5	C79.89	-	D21.5	D48.1	D49.2
hand	C49.1-	C79.89	-	D21.1-	D48.1	D49.2
head	C49.0	C79.89	-	D21.0	D48.1	D49.2
heel	C49.2-	C79.89	-	D21.2-	D48.1	D49.2
hip	C49.2-	C79.89	-	D21.2-	D48.1	D49.2
hypochondrium	C49.4	C79.89	-	D21.4	D48.1	D49.2
iliopsoas muscle	C49.5	C79.89	-	D21.5	D48.1	D49.2
infraclavicular region	C49.3	C79.89	-	D21.3	D48.1	D49.2
inguinal (canal) (region)	C49.5	C79.89	-	D21.5	D48.1	D49.2
intestinal	C49.4	C79.89	-	D21.4	D48.1	D49.2
intrathoracic	C49.3	C79.89	-	D21.3	D48.1	D49.2
ischiorectal fossa	C49.5	C79.89	-	D21.5	D48.1	D49.2
jaw	C03.9	C79.89	D00.03	D10.39	D48.1	D49.0
knee	C49.2-	C79.89	-	D21.2-	D48.1	D49.2
leg	C49.2-	C79.89	-	D21.2-	D48.1	D49.2
limb NEC	C49.9	C79.89	-	D21.9	D48.1	D49.2
lower	C49.2-	C79.89	-	D21.2-	D48.1	D49.2
upper	C49.1-	C79.89	-	D21.1-	D48.1	D49.2
nates	C49.5	C79.89	-	D21.5	D48.1	D49.2
neck	C49.0	C79.89	-	D21.0	D48.1	D49.2
orbit	C69.6-	C79.49	D09.2-	D31.6-	D48.1	D49.89
overlapping lesion	C49.8	-	-	-	-	-
pararectal	C49.5	C79.89	-	D21.5	D48.1	D49.2
para-urethral	C49.5	C79.89	-	D21.5	D48.1	D49.2
paravaginal	C49.5	C79.89	-	D21.5	D48.1	D49.2
pelvis (floor)	C49.5	C79.89	-	D21.5	D48.1	D49.2
pelvo-abdominal	C49.8	C79.89	-	D21.6	D48.1	D49.2
perineum	C49.5	C79.89	-	D21.5	D48.1	D49.2
perirectal (tissue)	C49.5	C79.89	-	D21.5	D48.1	D49.2
periurethral (tissue)	C49.5	C79.89	-	D21.5	D48.1	D49.2
popliteal fossa or space	C49.2-	C79.89	-	D21.2-	D48.1	D49.2
presacral	C49.5	C79.89	-	D21.5	D48.1	D49.2
psoas muscle	C49.4	C79.89	-	D21.4	D48.1	D49.2
pterygoid fossa	C49.0	C79.89	-	D21.0	D48.1	D49.2
rectovaginal septum or wall	C49.5	C79.89	-	D21.5	D48.1	D49.2
rectovesical	C49.5	C79.89	-	D21.5	D48.1	D49.2
retroperitoneum	C48.0	C78.6	-	D20.0	D48.3	D49.0
sacrococcygeal region	C49.5	C79.89	-	D21.5	D48.1	D49.2
scalp	C49.0	C79.89	-	D21.0	D48.1	D49.2
scapular region	C49.3	C79.89	-	D21.3	D48.1	D49.2
shoulder	C49.1-	C79.89	-	D21.1-	D48.1	D49.2
skin (dermis) NEC — *see also* Neoplasm, skin, by site	C44.90	C79.2	D04.9	D23.9	D48.5	D49.2
stomach	C49.4	C79.89	-	D21.4	D48.1	D49.2
submental	C49.0	C79.89	-	D21.0	D48.1	D49.2
supraclavicular region	C49.0	C79.89	-	D21.0	D48.1	D49.2
connective tissue NEC - *continued*						
temple	C49.0	C79.89	-	D21.0	D48.1	D49.2
temporal region	C49.0	C79.89	-	D21.0	D48.1	D49.2
thigh	C49.2-	C79.89	-	D21.2-	D48.1	D49.2
thoracic (duct) (wall)	C49.3	C79.89	-	D21.3	D48.1	D49.2
thorax	C49.3	C79.89	-	D21.3	D48.1	D49.2
thumb	C49.1-	C79.89	-	D21.1-	D48.1	D49.2
toe	C49.2-	C79.89	-	D21.2-	D48.1	D49.2
trunk	C49.6	C79.89	-	D21.6	D48.1	D49.2
umbilicus	C49.4	C79.89	-	D21.4	D48.1	D49.2
vesicorectal	C49.5	C79.89	-	D21.5	D48.1	D49.2
wrist	C49.1-	C79.89	-	D21.1-	D48.1	D49.2
conus medullaris	C72.0	C79.49	-	D33.4	D43.4	D49.7
cord (true) (vocal)	C32.0	C78.39	D02.0	D14.1	D38.0	D49.1
false	C32.1	C78.39	D02.0	D14.1	D38.0	D49.1
spermatic	C63.1-	C79.82	D07.69	D29.8	D40.8	D49.59
spinal (cervical) (lumbar) (thoracic)	C72.0	C79.49	-	D33.4	D43.4	D49.7
cornea (limbus)	C69.1-	C79.49	D09.2-	D31.1-	D48.7	D49.89
corpus						
albicans	C56.-	C79.6-	D07.39	D27.-	D39.1-	D49.59
callosum, brain	C71.0	C79.31	-	D33.2	D43.2	D49.6
cavernosum	C60.2	C79.82	D07.4	D29.0	D40.8	D49.59
gastric	C16.2	C78.89	D00.2	D13.1	D37.1	D49.0
overlapping sites	C54.8	-	-	-	-	-
penis	C60.2	C79.82	D07.4	D29.0	D40.8	D49.59
striatum, cerebrum	C71.0	C79.31	-	D33.0	D43.0	D49.6
uteri	C54.9	C79.82	D07.0	D26.1	D39.0	D49.59
isthmus	C54.0	C79.82	D07.0	D26.1	D39.0	D49.59
cortex						
adrenal	C74.0-	C79.7-	D09.3	D35.0-	D44.1-	D49.7
cerebral	C71.0	C79.31	-	D33.0	D43.0	D49.6
costal cartilage	C41.3	C79.51	-	D16.7	D48.0	D49.2
costovertebral joint	C41.3	C79.51	-	D16.7	D48.0	D49.2
Cowper's gland	C68.0	C79.19	D09.19	D30.4	D41.3	D49.59
cranial (fossa, any)	C71.9	C79.31	-	D33.2	D43.2	D49.6
meninges	C70.0	C79.32	-	D32.0	D42.0	D49.7
nerve	C72.50	C79.49	-	D33.3	D43.3	D49.7
specified NEC	C72.59	C79.49	-	D33.3	D43.3	D49.7
craniobuccal pouch	C75.2	C79.89	D09.3	D35.2	D44.3	D49.7
craniopharyngeal (duct) (pouch)	C75.2	C79.89	D09.3	D35.3	D44.4	D49.7
cricoid	C13.0	C79.89	D00.08	D10.7	D37.05	D49.0
cartilage	C32.3	C78.39	D02.0	D14.1	D38.0	D49.1
cricopharynx	C13.0	C79.89	D00.08	D10.7	D37.05	D49.0
crypt of Morgagni	C21.8	C78.5	D01.3	D12.9	D37.8	D49.0
crystalline lens	C69.4-	C79.49	D09.2-	D31.4-	D48.7	D49.89
cul-de-sac (Douglas')	C48.1	C78.6	-	D20.1	D48.4	D49.0
cuneiform cartilage	C32.3	C78.39	D02.0	D14.1	D38.0	D49.1
cutaneous — *see* Neoplasm, skin						
cutis — *see* Neoplasm, skin						
cystic (bile) duct (common)	C24.0	C78.89	D01.5	D13.5	D37.6	D49.0
dermis — *see* Neoplasm, skin						
diaphragm	C49.3	C79.89	-	D21.3	D48.1	D49.2
digestive organs, system, tube, or tract NEC	C26.9	C78.89	D01.9	D13.9	D37.9	D49.0
disc, intervertebral	C41.2	C79.51	-	D16.6	D48.0	D49.2
disease, generalized	C80.0	-	-	-	-	-
disseminated	C80.0	-	-	-	-	-
Douglas' cul-de-sac or pouch	C48.1	C78.6	-	D20.1	D48.4	D49.0
duodenojejunal junction	C17.8	C78.4	D01.49	D13.39	D37.2	D49.0
duodenum	C17.0	C78.4	D01.49	D13.2	D37.2	D49.0
dura (cranial) (mater)	C70.9	C79.49	-	D32.9	D42.9	D49.7
cerebral	C70.0	C79.32	-	D32.0	D42.0	D49.7
spinal	C70.1	C79.49	-	D32.1	D42.1	D49.7
ear (external) — *see also* Neoplasm, skin, ear	C44.20-	C79.2	D04.2-	D23.2-	D48.5	D49.2
auricle or auris — *see also* Neoplasm, skin, ear	C44.20-	C79.2	D04.2-	D23.2-	D48.5	D49.2
canal, external — *see also* Neoplasm, skin, ear	C44.20-	C79.2	D04.2-	D23.2-	D48.5	D49.2
cartilage	C49.0	C79.89	-	D21.0	D48.1	D49.2
external meatus — *see also* Neoplasm, skin, ear	C44.20-	C79.2	D04.2-	D23.2-	D48.5	D49.2
inner	C30.1	C78.39	D02.3	D14.0	D38.5	D49.1
lobule — *see also* Neoplasm, skin, ear	C44.20-	C79.2	D04.2-	D23.2-	D48.5	D49.2
middle	C30.1	C78.39	D02.3	D14.0	D38.5	D49.1
overlapping lesion with accessory sinuses	C31.8	-	-	-	-	-

Neoplasm, neoplastic	Malignant Primary	Malignant Secondary	Ca in situ	Benign	Uncertain Behavior	Unspecified Behavior
ear - *continued*						
skin	C44.20-	C79.2	D04.2-	D23.2-	D48.5	D49.2
basal cell carcinoma	C44.21-	-	-	-	-	-
specified type NEC	C44.29-	-	-	-	-	-
squamous cell carcinoma	C44.22-	-	-	-	-	-
earlobe	C44.20-	C79.2	D04.2-	D23.2-	D48.5	D49.2
basal cell carcinoma	C44.21-	-	-	-	-	-
specified type NEC	C44.29-	-	-	-	-	-
squamous cell carcinoma	C44.22-	-	-	-	-	-
ejaculatory duct	C63.7	C79.82	D07.69	D29.8	D40.8	D49.59
elbow NEC	C76.4-	C79.89	D04.6-	D36.7	D48.7	D49.89
endocardium	C38.0	C79.89	-	D15.1	D48.7	D49.89
endocervix (canal) (gland)	C53.0	C79.82	D06.0	D26.0	D39.0	D49.59
endocrine gland NEC	C75.9	C79.89	D09.3	D35.9	D44.9	D49.7
pluriglandular	C75.8	C79.89	D09.3	D35.7	D44.9	D49.7
endometrium (gland) (stroma)	C54.1	C79.82	D07.0	D26.1	D39.0	D49.59
ensiform cartilage	C41.3	C79.51	-	D16.7	D48.0	D49.2
enteric — *see* Neoplasm, intestine						
ependyma (brain)	C71.5	C79.31	-	D33.0	D43.0	D49.6
fourth ventricle	C71.7	C79.31	-	D33.1	D43.1	D49.6
epicardium	C38.0	C79.89	-	D15.1	D48.7	D49.89
epididymis	C63.0-	C79.82	D07.69	D29.3-	D40.8	D49.59
epidural	C72.9	C79.49	-	D33.9	D43.9	D49.7
epiglottis	C32.1	C78.39	D02.0	D14.1	D38.0	D49.1
anterior aspect or surface	C10.1	C79.89	D00.08	D10.5	D37.05	D49.0
cartilage	C32.3	C78.39	D02.0	D14.1	D38.0	D49.1
free border (margin)	C10.1	C79.89	D00.08	D10.5	D37.05	D49.0
junctional region	C10.8	C79.89	D00.08	D10.5	D37.05	D49.0
posterior (laryngeal) surface	C32.1	C78.39	D02.0	D14.1	D38.0	D49.1
suprahyoid portion	C32.1	C78.39	D02.0	D14.1	D38.0	D49.1
esophagogastric junction	C16.0	C78.89	D00.2	D13.1	D37.1	D49.0
esophagus	C15.9	C78.89	D00.1	D13.0	D37.8	D49.0
abdominal	C15.5	C78.89	D00.1	D13.0	D37.8	D49.0
cervical	C15.3	C78.89	D00.1	D13.0	D37.8	D49.0
distal (third)	C15.5	C78.89	D00.1	D13.0	D37.8	D49.0
lower (third)	C15.5	C78.89	D00.1	D13.0	D37.8	D49.0
middle (third)	C15.4	C78.89	D00.1	D13.0	D37.8	D49.0
overlapping lesion	C15.8	-	-	-	-	-
proximal (third)	C15.3	C78.89	D00.1	D13.0	D37.8	D49.0
thoracic	C15.4	C78.89	D00.1	D13.0	D37.8	D49.0
upper (third)	C15.3	C78.89	D00.1	D13.0	D37.8	D49.0
ethmoid (sinus)	C31.1	C78.39	D02.3	D14.0	D38.5	D49.1
bone or labyrinth	C41.0	C79.51	-	D16.4-	D48.0	D49.2
eustachian tube	C30.1	C78.39	D02.3	D14.0	D38.5	D49.1
exocervix	C53.1	C79.82	D06.1	D26.0	D39.0	D49.59
external						
meatus (ear) — *see also* Neoplasm, skin, ear	C44.20-	C79.2	D04.2-	D23.2-	D48.5	D49.2
os, cervix uteri	C53.1	C79.82	D06.1	D26.0	D39.0	D49.59
extradural	C72.9	C79.49	-	D33.9	D43.9	D49.7
extrahepatic (bile) duct	C24.0	C78.89	D01.5	D13.5	D37.6	D49.0
overlapping lesion with gallbladder	C24.8	-	-	-	-	-
extraocular muscle	C69.6-	C79.49	D09.2-	D31.6-	D48.7	D49.89
extrarectal	C76.3	C79.89	D09.8	D36.7	D48.7	D49.89
extremity	C76.8	C79.89	D04.8	D36.7	D48.7	D49.89
lower	C76.5-	C79.89	D04.7-	D36.7	D48.7	D49.89
upper	C76.4-	C79.89	D04.6-	D36.7	D48.7	D49.89
eye NEC	C69.9-	C79.49	D09.2	D31.9	D48.7	D49.89
overlapping sites	C69.8	-	-	-	-	-
eyeball	C69.9-	C79.49	D09.2-	D31.9-	D48.7	D49.89
eyebrow	C44.309	C79.2	D04.39	D23.39	D48.5	D49.2
basal cell carcinoma	C44.319	-	-	-	-	-
specified type NEC	C44.399	-	-	-	-	-
squamous cell carcinoma	C44.329	-	-	-	-	-
eyelid (lower) (skin) (upper)	C44.10-	-	-	-	-	-
basal cell carcinoma	C44.11-	-	-	-	-	-
sebaceous cell	C44.13-	-	-	-	-	-
specified type NEC	C44.19-	-	-	-	-	-
squamous cell carcinoma	C44.12-	-	-	-	-	-
cartilage	C49.0	C79.89	-	D21.0	D48.1	D49.2
face NEC	C76.0	C79.89	D04.39	D36.7	D48.7	D49.89
fallopian tube (accessory)	C57.0-	C79.82	D07.39	D28.2	D39.8	D49.59
falx (cerebella) (cerebri)	C70.0	C79.32	-	D32.0	D42.0	D49.7
fascia — *see also* Neoplasm, connective tissue						
palmar	C49.1-	C79.89	-	D21.1-	D48.1	D49.2
plantar	C49.2-	C79.89	-	D21.2-	D48.1	D49.2
fatty tissue — *see* Neoplasm, connective tissue						

Neoplasm, neoplastic	Malignant Primary	Malignant Secondary	Ca in situ	Benign	Uncertain Behavior	Unspecified Behavior
fauces, faucial NEC	C10.9	C79.89	D00.08	D10.5	D37.05	D49.0
pillars	C09.1	C79.89	D00.08	D10.5	D37.05	D49.0
tonsil	C09.9	C79.89	D00.08	D10.4	D37.05	D49.0
femur (any part)	C40.2-	-	-	D16.2-	-	-
fetal membrane	C58	C79.82	D07.0	D26.7	D39.2	D49.59
fibrous tissue — *see* Neoplasm, connective tissue						
fibula (any part)	C40.2-	C79.51	-	D16.2-	-	-
filum terminale	C72.0	C79.49	-	D33.4	D43.4	D49.7
finger NEC	C76.4-	C79.89	D04.6-	D36.7	D48.7	D49.89
flank NEC	C76.8	C79.89	D04.5	D36.7	D48.7	D49.89
follicle, nabothian	C53.0	C79.82	D06.0	D26.0	D39.0	D49.59
foot NEC	C76.5-	C79.89	D04.7-	D36.7	D48.7	D49.89
forearm NEC	C76.4-	C79.89	D04.6-	D36.7	D48.7	D49.89
forehead (skin)	C44.309	C79.2	D04.39	D23.39	D48.5	D49.2
basal cell carcinoma	C44.319	-	-	-	-	-
specified type NEC	C44.399	-	-	-	-	-
squamous cell carcinoma	C44.329	-	-	-	-	-
foreskin	C60.0	C79.82	D07.4	D29.0	D40.8	D49.59
fornix						
pharyngeal	C11.3	C79.89	D00.08	D10.6	D37.05	D49.0
vagina	C52	C79.82	D07.2	D28.1	D39.8	D49.59
fossa (of)						
anterior (cranial)	C71.9	C79.31	-	D33.2	D43.2	D49.6
cranial	C71.9	C79.31	-	D33.2	D43.2	D49.6
ischiorectal	C76.3	C79.89	D09.8	D36.7	D48.7	D49.89
middle (cranial)	C71.9	C79.31	-	D33.2	D43.2	D49.6
piriform	C12	C79.89	D00.08	D10.7	D37.05	D49.0
pituitary	C75.1	C79.89	D09.3	D35.2	D44.3	D49.7
posterior (cranial)	C71.9	C79.31	-	D33.2	D43.2	D49.6
pterygoid	C49.0	C79.89	-	D21.0	D48.1	D49.2
pyriform	C12	C79.89	D00.08	D10.7	D37.05	D49.0
Rosenmuller	C11.2	C79.89	D00.08	D10.6	D37.05	D49.0
tonsillar	C09.0	C79.89	D00.08	D10.5	D37.05	D49.0
fourchette	C51.9	C79.82	D07.1	D28.0	D39.8	D49.59
frenulum						
labii — *see* Neoplasm, lip, internal						
linguae	C02.2	C79.89	D00.07	D10.1	D37.02	D49.0
frontal						
bone	C41.0	C79.51	-	D16.4-	D48.0	D49.2
lobe, brain	C71.1	C79.31	-	D33.0	D43.0	D49.6
pole	C71.1	C79.31	-	D33.0	D43.0	D49.6
sinus	C31.2	C78.39	D02.3	D14.0	D38.5	D49.1
fundus						
stomach	C16.1	C78.89	D00.2	D13.1	D37.1	D49.0
uterus	C54.3	C79.82	D07.0	D26.1	D39.0	D49.59
gall duct (extrahepatic)	C24.0	C78.89	D01.5	D13.5	D37.6	D49.0
intrahepatic	C22.1	C78.7	D01.5	D13.4	D37.6	D49.0
gallbladder	C23	C78.89	D01.5	D13.5	D37.6	D49.0
overlapping lesion with extrahepatic bile ducts	C24.8	-	-	-	-	-
ganglia — *see also* Neoplasm, nerve, peripheral	C47.9	C79.89	-	D36.10	D48.2	D49.2
basal	C71.0	C79.31	-	D33.0	D43.0	D49.6
cranial nerve	C72.50	C79.49	-	D33.3	D43.3	D49.7
Gartner's duct	C52	C79.82	D07.2	D28.1	D39.8	D49.59
gastric — *see* Neoplasm, stomach						
gastrocolic	C26.9	C78.89	D01.9	D13.9	D37.9	D49.0
gastroesophageal junction	C16.0	C78.89	D00.2	D13.1	D37.1	D49.0
gastrointestinal (tract) NEC	C26.9	C78.89	D01.9	D13.9	D37.9	D49.0
generalized	C80.0	-	-	-	-	-
genital organ or tract						
female NEC	C57.9	C79.82	D07.30	D28.9	D39.9	D49.59
overlapping lesion	C57.8	-	-	-	-	-
specified site NEC	C57.7	C79.82	D07.39	D28.7	D39.8	D49.59
male NEC	C63.9	C79.82	D07.60	D29.9	D40.9	D49.59
overlapping lesion	C63.8	-	-	-	-	-
specified site NEC	C63.7	C79.82	D07.69	D29.8	D40.8	D49.59
genitourinary tract						
female	C57.9	C79.82	D07.30	D28.9	D39.9	D49.59
male	C63.9	C79.82	D07.60	D29.9	D40.9	D49.59
gingiva (alveolar) (marginal)	C03.9	C79.89	D00.03	D10.39	D37.09	D49.0
lower	C03.1	C79.89	D00.03	D10.39	D37.09	D49.0
mandibular	C03.1	C79.89	D00.03	D10.39	D37.09	D49.0
maxillary	C03.0	C79.89	D00.03	D10.39	D37.09	D49.0
upper	C03.0	C79.89	D00.03	D10.39	D37.09	D49.0
gland, glandular (lymphatic) (system) — *see also* Neoplasm, lymph gland						

Neoplasm, neoplastic	Malignant Primary	Malignant Secondary	Ca in situ	Benign	Uncertain Behavior	Unspecified Behavior
gland, glandular - *continued*						
endocrine NEC	C75.9	C79.89	D09.3	D35.9	D44.9	D49.7
salivary — *see* Neoplasm, salivary gland						
glans penis	C60.1	C79.82	D07.4	D29.0	D40.8	D49.59
globus pallidus	C71.0	C79.31	-	D33.0	D43.0	D49.6
glomus						
coccygeal	C49.5	C79.89	-	D21.5	D48.1	D49.2
jugularis	C75.5	C79.89	-	D35.6	D44.7	D49.7
glosso-epiglottic fold (s)	C10.1	C79.89	D00.08	D10.5	D37.05	D49.0
glossopalatine fold	C09.1	C79.89	D00.08	D10.5	D37.05	D49.0
glossopharyngeal sulcus	C09.0	C79.89	D00.08	D10.5	D37.05	D49.0
glottis	C32.0	C78.39	D02.0	D14.1	D38.0	D49.1
gluteal region	C76.3	C79.89	D04.5	D36.7	D48.7	D49.89
great vessels NEC	C49.3	C79.89	-	D21.3	D48.1	D49.2
groin NEC	C76.3	C79.89	D04.5	D36.7	D48.7	D49.89
gum	C03.9	C79.89	D00.03	D10.39	D37.09	D49.0
lower	C03.1	C79.89	D00.03	D10.39	D37.09	D49.0
upper	C03.0	C79.89	D00.03	D10.39	D37.09	D49.0
hand NEC	C76.4-	C79.89	D04.6-	D36.7	D48.7	D49.89
head NEC	C76.0	C79.89	D04.4	D36.7	D48.7	D49.89
heart	C38.0	C79.89	-	D15.1	D48.7	D49.89
heel NEC	C76.5-	C79.89	D04.7-	D36.7	D48.7	D49.89
helix — *see also* Neoplasm, skin, ear	C44.20-	C79.2	D04.2-	D23.2-	D48.5	D49.2
hematopoietic, hemopoietic tissue NEC	C96.9	-	-	-	-	-
specified NEC	C96.Z	-	-	-	-	-
hemisphere, cerebral	C71.0	C79.31	-	D33.0	D43.0	D49.6
hemorrhoidal zone	C21.1	C78.5	D01.3	D12.9	D37.8	D49.0
hepatic — *see also* Index to disease, by histology	C22.9	C78.7	D01.5	D13.4	D37.6	D49.0
duct (bile)	C24.0	C78.89	D01.5	D13.5	D37.6	D49.0
flexure (colon)	C18.3	C78.5	D01.0	D12.3	D37.4	D49.0
primary	C22.8	C78.7	D01.5	D13.4	D37.6	D49.0
hepatobiliary	C24.9	C78.89	D01.5	D13.5	D37.6	D49.0
hepatoblastoma	C22.2	C78.7	D01.5	D13.4	D37.6	D49.0
hepatoma	C22.0	C78.7	D01.5	D13.4	D37.6	D49.0
hilus of lung	C34.0-	C78.0-	D02.2-	D14.3-	D38.1	D49.1
hip NEC	C76.5-	C79.89	D04.7-	D36.7	D48.7	D49.89
hippocampus, brain	C71.2	C79.31	-	D33.0	D43.0	D49.6
humerus (any part)	C40.0-	C79.51	-	D16.0-	-	-
hymen	C52	C79.82	D07.2	D28.1	D39.8	D49.59
hypopharynx, hypopharyngeal NEC	C13.9	C79.89	D00.08	D10.7	D37.05	D49.0
overlapping lesion	C13.8	-	-	-	-	-
postcricoid region	C13.0	C79.89	D00.08	D10.7	D37.05	D49.0
posterior wall	C13.2	C79.89	D00.08	D10.7	D37.05	D49.0
pyriform fossa (sinus)	C12	C79.89	D00.08	D10.7	D37.05	D49.0
hypophysis	C75.1	C79.89	D09.3	D35.2	D44.3	D49.7
hypothalamus	C71.0	C79.31	-	D33.0	D43.0	D49.6
ileocecum, ileocecal (coil) (junction) (valve)	C18.0	C78.5	D01.0	D12.0	D37.4	D49.0
ileum	C17.2	C78.4	D01.49	D13.39	D37.2	D49.0
ilium	C41.4	C79.51	-	D16.8	D48.0	D49.2
immunoproliferative NEC	C88.9	-	-	-	-	-
infraclavicular (region)	C76.1	C79.89	D04.5	D36.7	D48.7	D49.89
inguinal (region)	C76.3	C79.89	D04.5	D36.7	D48.7	D49.89
insula	C71.0	C79.31	-	D33.0	D43.0	D49.6
insular tissue (pancreas)	C25.4	C78.89	D01.7	D13.7	D37.8	D49.0
brain	C71.0	C79.31	-	D33.0	D43.0	D49.6
interarytenoid fold	C13.1	C79.89	D00.08	D10.7	D37.05	D49.0
hypopharyngeal aspect	C13.1	C79.89	D00.08	D10.7	D37.05	D49.0
laryngeal aspect	C32.1	C78.39	D02.0	D14.1	D38.0	D49.1
marginal zone	C13.1	C79.89	D00.08	D10.7	D37.05	D49.0
interdental papillae	C03.9	C79.89	D00.03	D10.39	D37.09	D49.0
lower	C03.1	C79.89	D00.03	D10.39	D37.09	D49.0
upper	C03.0	C79.89	D00.03	D10.39	D37.09	D49.0
internal						
capsule	C71.0	C79.31	-	D33.0	D43.0	D49.6
os (cervix)	C53.0	C79.82	D06.0	D26.0	D39.0	D49.59
intervertebral cartilage or disc	C41.2	C79.51	-	D16.6	D48.0	D49.2
intestine, intestinal	C26.0	C78.80	D01.40	D13.9	D37.8	D49.0
large	C18.9	C78.5	D01.0	D12.6	D37.4	D49.0
appendix	C18.1	C78.5	D01.0	D12.1	D37.3	D49.0
caput coli	C18.0	C78.5	D01.0	D12.0	D37.4	D49.0
cecum	C18.0	C78.5	D01.0	D12.0	D37.4	D49.0
colon	C18.9	C78.5	D01.0	D12.6	D37.4	D49.0
and rectum	C19	C78.5	D01.1	D12.7	D37.5	D49.0
ascending	C18.2	C78.5	D01.0	D12.2	D37.4	D49.0

Neoplasm, neoplastic	Malignant Primary	Malignant Secondary	Ca in situ	Benign	Uncertain Behavior	Unspecified Behavior
intestine, intestinal - *continued*						
caput	C18.0	C78.5	D01.0	D12.0	D37.4	D49.0
descending	C18.6	C78.5	D01.0	D12.4	D37.4	D49.0
distal	C18.6	C78.5	D01.0	D12.4	D37.4	D49.0
left	C18.6	C78.5	D01.0	D12.4	D37.4	D49.0
overlapping lesion	C18.8	-	-	-	-	-
pelvic	C18.7	C78.5	D01.0	D12.5	D37.4	D49.0
right	C18.2	C78.5	D01.0	D12.2	D37.4	D49.0
sigmoid (flexure)	C18.7	C78.5	D01.0	D12.5	D37.4	D49.0
transverse	C18.4	C78.5	D01.0	D12.3	D37.4	D49.0
hepatic flexure	C18.3	C78.5	D01.0	D12.3	D37.4	D49.0
ileocecum, ileocecal (coil) (valve)	C18.0	C78.5	D01.0	D12.0	D37.4	D49.0
overlapping lesion	C18.8	-	-	-	-	-
sigmoid flexure (lower) (upper)	C18.7	C78.5	D01.0	D12.5	D37.4	D49.0
splenic flexure	C18.5	C78.5	D01.0	D12.3	D37.4	D49.0
small	C17.9	C78.4	D01.40	D13.30	D37.2	D49.0
duodenum	C17.0	C78.4	D01.49	D13.2	D37.2	D49.0
ileum	C17.2	C78.4	D01.49	D13.39	D37.2	D49.0
jejunum	C17.1	C78.4	D01.49	D13.39	D37.2	D49.0
overlapping lesion	C17.8	-	-	-	-	-
tract NEC	C26.0	C78.89	D01.40	D13.9	D37.8	D49.0
intra-abdominal	C76.2	C79.89	D09.8	D36.7	D48.7	D49.89
intracranial NEC	C71.9	C79.31	-	D33.2	D43.2	D49.6
intrahepatic (bile) duct	C22.1	C78.7	D01.5	D13.4	D37.6	D49.0
intraocular	C69.9-	C79.49	D09.2-	D31.9-	D48.7	D49.89
intraorbital	C69.6-	C79.49	D09.2-	D31.6-	D48.7	D49.89
intrasellar	C75.1	C79.89	D09.3	D35.2	D44.3	D49.7
intrathoracic (cavity) (organs)	C76.1	C79.89	D09.8	D15.9	D48.7	D49.89
specified NEC	C76.1	C79.89	D09.8	D15.7	-	-
iris	C69.4-	C79.49	D09.2-	D31.4-	D48.7	D49.89
ischiorectal (fossa)	C76.3	C79.89	D09.8	D36.7	D48.7	D49.89
ischium	C41.4	C79.51	-	D16.8	D48.0	D49.2
island of Reil	C71.0	C79.31	-	D33.0	D43.0	D49.6
islands or islets of Langerhans	C25.4	C78.89	D01.7	D13.7	D37.8	D49.0
isthmus uteri	C54.0	C79.82	D07.0	D26.1	D39.0	D49.59
jaw	C76.0	C79.89	D09.8	D36.7	D48.7	D49.89
bone	C41.1	C79.51	-	D16.5-	D48.0	D49.2
lower	C41.1	C79.51	-	D16.5-	-	-
upper	C41.0	C79.51	-	D16.4-	-	-
carcinoma (any type) (lower) (upper)	C76.0	C79.89	-	-	-	-
skin — *see also* Neoplasm, skin, face	C44.309	C79.2	D04.39	D23.39	D48.5	D49.2
soft tissues	C03.9	C79.89	D00.03	D10.39	D37.09	D49.0
lower	C03.1	C79.89	D00.03	D10.39	D37.09	D49.0
upper	C03.0	C79.89	D00.03	D10.39	D37.09	D49.0
jejunum	C17.1	C78.4	D01.49	D13.39	D37.2	D49.0
joint NEC — *see also* Neoplasm, bone	C41.9	C79.51	-	D16.9-	D48.0	D49.2
acromioclavicular	C40.0-	C79.51	-	D16.0-	-	-
bursa or synovial membrane — *see* Neoplasm, connective tissue						
costovertebral	C41.3	C79.51	-	D16.7	D48.0	D49.2
sternocostal	C41.3	C79.51	-	D16.7	D48.0	D49.2
temporomandibular	C41.1	C79.51	-	D16.5-	D48.0	D49.2
junction						
anorectal	C21.8	C78.5	D01.3	D12.9	D37.8	D49.0
cardioesophageal	C16.0	C78.89	D00.2	D13.1	D37.1	D49.0
esophagogastric	C16.0	C78.89	D00.2	D13.1	D37.1	D49.0
gastroesophageal	C16.0	C78.89	D00.2	D13.1	D37.1	D49.0
hard and soft palate	C05.9	C79.89	D00.00	D10.39	D37.09	D49.0
ileocecal	C18.0	C78.5	D01.0	D12.0	D37.4	D49.0
pelvirectal	C19	C78.5	D01.1	D12.7	D37.5	D49.0
pelviureteric	C65.-	C79.0-	D09.19	D30.1-	D41.1-	D49.59
rectosigmoid	C19	C78.5	D01.1	D12.7	D37.5	D49.0
squamocolumnar, of cervix	C53.8	C79.82	D06.7	D26.0	D39.0	D49.59
Kaposi's sarcoma — *see* Kaposi's, sarcoma						
kidney (parenchymal)	C64.-	C79.0-	D09.19	D30.0-	D41.0-	D49.51-
calyx	C65.-	C79.0-	D09.19	D30.1-	D41.1-	D49.51-
hilus	C65.-	C79.0-	D09.19	D30.1-	D41.1-	D49.51-
pelvis	C65.-	C79.0-	D09.19	D30.1-	D41.1-	D49.51-
knee NEC	C76.5-	C79.89	D04.7-	D36.7	D48.7	D49.89
labia (skin)	C51.9	C79.82	D07.1	D28.0	D39.8	D49.59
majora	C51.0	C79.82	D07.1	D28.0	D39.8	D49.59
minora	C51.1	C79.82	D07.1	D28.0	D39.8	D49.59
labial — *see also* Neoplasm, lip	C00.9	C79.89	D00.01	D10.0	D37.01	D49.0
sulcus (lower) (upper)	C06.1	C79.89	D00.02	D10.39	D37.09	D49.0

Neoplasm, neoplastic	Malignant Primary	Malignant Secondary	Ca in situ	Benign	Uncertain Behavior	Unspecified Behavior
labium (skin)	C51.9	C79.82	D07.1	D28.0	D39.8	D49.59
majus	C51.0	C79.82	D07.1	D28.0	D39.8	D49.59
minus	C51.1	C79.82	D07.1	D28.0	D39.8	D49.59
lacrimal						
canaliculi	C69.5-	C79.49	D09.2-	D31.5-	D48.7	D49.89
duct (nasal)	C69.5-	C79.49	D09.2-	D31.5-	D48.7	D49.89
gland	C69.5-	C79.49	D09.2-	D31.5-	D48.7	D49.89
punctum	C69.5-	C79.49	D09.2-	D31.5-	D48.7	D49.89
sac	C69.5-	C79.49	D09.2-	D31.5-	D48.7	D49.89
Langerhans, islands or islets	C25.4	C78.89	D01.7	D13.7	D37.8	D49.0
laryngopharynx	C13.9	C79.89	D00.08	D10.7	D37.05	D49.0
larynx, laryngeal NEC	C32.9	C78.39	D02.0	D14.1	D38.0	D49.1
aryepiglottic fold	C32.1	C78.39	D02.0	D14.1	D38.0	D49.1
cartilage (arytenoid) (cricoid) (cuneiform) (thyroid)	C32.3	C78.39	D02.0	D14.1	D38.0	D49.1
commissure (anterior) (posterior)	C32.0	C78.39	D02.0	D14.1	D38.0	D49.1
extrinsic NEC	C32.1	C78.39	D02.0	D14.1	D38.0	D49.1
meaning hypopharynx	C13.9	C79.89	D00.08	D10.7	D37.05	D49.0
interarytenoid fold	C32.1	C78.39	D02.0	D14.1	D38.0	D49.1
intrinsic	C32.0	C78.39	D02.0	D14.1	D38.0	D49.1
overlapping lesion	C32.8	-	-	-	-	-
ventricular band	C32.1	C78.39	D02.0	D14.1	D38.0	D49.1
leg NEC	C76.5-	C79.89	D04.7-	D36.7	D48.7	D49.89
lens, crystalline	C69.4-	C79.49	D09.2-	D31.4-	D48.7	D49.89
lid (lower) (upper)	C44.10-	C79.2	D04.1-	D23.1-	D48.5	D49.2
basal cell carcinoma	C44.11-	-	-	-	-	-
sebaceous cell	C44.13-	-	-	-	-	-
specified type NEC	C44.19-	-	-	-	-	-
squamous cell carcinoma	C44.12-	-	-	-	-	-
ligament — *see also* Neoplasm, connective tissue						
broad	C57.1	C79.82	D07.39	D28.2	D39.8	D49.59
Mackenrodt's	C57.7	C79.82	D07.39	D28.7	D39.8	D49.59
non-uterine — *see* Neoplasm, connective tissue						
round	C57.2	C79.82	-	D28.2	D39.8	D49.59
sacro-uterine	C57.3	C79.82	-	D28.2	D39.8	D49.59
uterine	C57.3	C79.82	-	D28.2	D39.8	D49.59
utero-ovarian	C57.7	C79.82	D07.39	D28.2	D39.8	D49.59
uterosacral	C57.3	C79.82	-	D28.2	D39.8	D49.59
limb	C76.8	C79.89	D04.8	D36.7	D48.7	D49.89
lower	C76.5-	C79.89	D04.7-	D36.7	D48.7	D49.89
upper	C76.4-	C79.89	D04.6-	D36.7	D48.7	D49.89
limbus of cornea	C69.1-	C79.49	D09.2-	D31.1-	D48.7	D49.89
lingual NEC — *see also* Neoplasm, tongue	C02.9	C79.89	D00.07	D10.1	D37.02	D49.0
lingula, lung	C34.1-	C78.0-	D02.2-	D14.3-	D38.1	D49.1
lip	C00.9	C79.89	D00.01	D10.0	D37.01	D49.0
buccal aspect — *see* Neoplasm, lip, internal						
commissure	C00.6	C79.89	D00.01	D10.0	D37.01	D49.0
external	C00.2	C79.89	D00.01	D10.0	D37.01	D49.0
lower	C00.1	C79.89	D00.01	D10.0	D37.01	D49.0
upper	C00.0	C79.89	D00.01	D10.0	D37.01	D49.0
frenulum — *see* Neoplasm, lip, internal						
inner aspect — *see* Neoplasm, lip, internal						
internal	C00.5	C79.89	D00.01	D10.0	D37.01	D49.0
lower	C00.4	C79.89	D00.01	D10.0	D37.01	D49.0
upper	C00.3	C79.89	D00.01	D10.0	D37.01	D49.0
lipstick area	C00.2	C79.89	D00.01	D10.0	D37.01	D49.0
lower	C00.1	C79.89	D00.01	D10.0	D37.01	D49.0
upper	C00.0	C79.89	D00.01	D10.0	D37.01	D49.0
lower	C00.1	C79.89	D00.01	D10.0	D37.01	D49.0
internal	C00.4	C79.89	D00.01	D10.0	D37.01	D49.0
mucosa — *see* Neoplasm, lip, internal						
oral aspect — *see* Neoplasm, lip, internal						
overlapping lesion	C00.8	-	-	-	-	-
with oral cavity or pharynx	C14.8	-	-	-	-	-
skin (commissure) (lower) (upper)	C44.00	C79.2	D04.0	D23.0	D48.5	D49.2
basal cell carcinoma	C44.01	-	-	-	-	-
specified type NEC	C44.09	-	-	-	-	-
squamous cell carcinoma	C44.02	-	-	-	-	-
upper	C00.0	C79.89	D00.01	D10.0	D37.01	D49.0
internal	C00.3	C79.89	D00.01	D10.0	D37.01	D49.0
vermilion border	C00.2	C79.89	D00.01	D10.0	D37.01	D49.0

Neoplasm, neoplastic	Malignant Primary	Malignant Secondary	Ca in situ	Benign	Uncertain Behavior	Unspecified Behavior
lip - *continued*						
lower	C00.1	C79.89	D00.01	D10.0	D37.01	D49.0
upper	C00.0	C79.89	D00.01	D10.0	D37.01	D49.0
lipomatous — *see* Lipoma, by site						
liver — *see also* Index to disease, by histology	C22.9	C78.7	D01.5	D13.4	D37.6	D49.0
primary	C22.8	C78.7	D01.5	D13.4	D37.6	D49.0
lumbosacral plexus	C47.5	C79.89	-	D36.16	D48.2	D49.2
lung	C34.9-	C78.0-	D02.2-	D14.3-	D38.1	D49.1
azygos lobe	C34.1-	C78.0-	D02.2-	D14.3-	D38.1	D49.1
carina	C34.0-	C78.0-	D02.2-	D14.3-	D38.1	D49.1
hilus	C34.0-	C78.0-	D02.2-	D14.3-	D38.1	D49.1
linqula	C34.1-	C78.0-	D02.2-	D14.3-	D38.1	D49.1
lobe NEC	C34.9-	C78.0-	D02.2-	D14.3-	D38.1	D49.1
lower lobe	C34.3-	C78.0-	D02.2-	D14.3-	D38.1	D49.1
main bronchus	C34.0-	C78.0-	D02.2-	D14.3-	D38.1	D49.1
mesothelioma — *see* Mesothelioma						
middle lobe	C34.2	C78.0-	D02.21	D14.31	D38.1	D49.1
overlapping lesion	C34.8-	-	-	-	-	-
upper lobe	C34.1-	C78.0-	D02.2-	D14.3-	D38.1	D49.1
lymph, lymphatic channel NEC	C49.9	C79.89	-	D21.9	D48.1	D49.2
gland (secondary)	-	C77.9	-	D36.0	D48.7	D49.89
abdominal	-	C77.2	-	D36.0	D48.7	D49.89
aortic	-	C77.2	-	D36.0	D48.7	D49.89
arm	-	C77.3	-	D36.0	D48.7	D49.89
auricular (anterior) (posterior)	-	C77.0	-	D36.0	D48.7	D49.89
axilla, axillary	-	C77.3	-	D36.0	D48.7	D49.89
brachial	-	C77.3	-	D36.0	D48.7	D49.89
bronchial	-	C77.1	-	D36.0	D48.7	D49.89
bronchopulmonary	-	C77.1	-	D36.0	D48.7	D49.89
celiac	-	C77.2	-	D36.0	D48.7	D49.89
cervical	-	C77.0	-	D36.0	D48.7	D49.89
cervicofacial	-	C77.0	-	D36.0	D48.7	D49.89
Cloquet	-	C77.4	-	D36.0	D48.7	D49.89
colic	-	C77.2	-	D36.0	D48.7	D49.89
common duct	-	C77.2	-	D36.0	D48.7	D49.89
cubital	-	C77.3	-	D36.0	D48.7	D49.89
diaphragmatic	-	C77.1	-	D36.0	D48.7	D49.89
epigastric, inferior	-	C77.1	-	D36.0	D48.7	D49.89
epitrochlear	-	C77.3	-	D36.0	D48.7	D49.89
esophageal	-	C77.1	-	D36.0	D48.7	D49.89
face	-	C77.0	-	D36.0	D48.7	D49.89
femoral	-	C77.4	-	D36.0	D48.7	D49.89
gastric	-	C77.2	-	D36.0	D48.7	D49.89
groin	-	C77.4	-	D36.0	D48.7	D49.89
head	-	C77.0	-	D36.0	D48.7	D49.89
hepatic	-	C77.2	-	D36.0	D48.7	D49.89
hilar (pulmonary)	-	C77.1	-	D36.0	D48.7	D49.89
splenic	-	C77.2	-	D36.0	D48.7	D49.89
hypogastric	-	C77.5	-	D36.0	D48.7	D49.89
ileocolic	-	C77.2	-	D36.0	D48.7	D49.89
iliac	-	C77.5	-	D36.0	D48.7	D49.89
infraclavicular	-	C77.3	-	D36.0	D48.7	D49.89
inguina, inguinal	-	C77.4	-	D36.0	D48.7	D49.89
innominate	-	C77.1	-	D36.0	D48.7	D49.89
intercostal	-	C77.1	-	D36.0	D48.7	D49.89
intestinal	-	C77.2	-	D36.0	D48.7	D49.89
intrabdominal	-	C77.2	-	D36.0	D48.7	D49.89
intrapelvic	-	C77.5	-	D36.0	D48.7	D49.89
intrathoracic	-	C77.1	-	D36.0	D48.7	D49.89
jugular	-	C77.0	-	D36.0	D48.7	D49.89
leg	-	C77.4	-	D36.0	D48.7	D49.89
limb						
lower	-	C77.4	-	D36.0	D48.7	D49.89
upper	-	C77.3	-	D36.0	D48.7	D49.89
lower limb	-	C77.4	-	D36.0	D48.7	D49.89
lumbar	-	C77.2	-	D36.0	D48.7	D49.89
mandibular	-	C77.0	-	D36.0	D48.7	D49.89
mediastinal	-	C77.1	-	D36.0	D48.7	D49.89
mesenteric (inferior) (superior)	-	C77.2	-	D36.0	D48.7	D49.89
midcolic	-	C77.2	-	D36.0	D48.7	D49.89
multiple sites in categories C77.0 - C77.5	-	C77.8	-	D36.0	D48.7	D49.89
neck	-	C77.0	-	D36.0	D48.7	D49.89
obturator	-	C77.5	-	D36.0	D48.7	D49.89
occipital	-	C77.0	-	D36.0	D48.7	D49.89
pancreatic	-	C77.2	-	D36.0	D48.7	D49.89
para-aortic	-	C77.2	-	D36.0	D48.7	D49.89

Neoplasm, neoplastic	Malignant Primary	Malignant Secondary	Ca in situ	Benign	Uncertain Behavior	Unspecified Behavior
lymph, lymphatic channel NEC - *continued*						
paracervical	-	C77.5	-	D36.0	D48.7	D49.89
parametrial	-	C77.5	-	D36.0	D48.7	D49.89
parasternal	-	C77.1	-	D36.0	D48.7	D49.89
parotid	-	C77.0	-	D36.0	D48.7	D49.89
pectoral	-	C77.3	-	D36.0	D48.7	D49.89
pelvic	-	C77.5	-	D36.0	D48.7	D49.89
peri-aortic	-	C77.2	-	D36.0	D48.7	D49.89
peripancreatic	-	C77.2	-	D36.0	D48.7	D49.89
popliteal	-	C77.4	-	D36.0	D48.7	D49.89
porta hepatis	-	C77.2	-	D36.0	D48.7	D49.89
portal	-	C77.2	-	D36.0	D48.7	D49.89
preauricular	-	C77.0	-	D36.0	D48.7	D49.89
prelaryngeal	-	C77.0	-	D36.0	D48.7	D49.89
presymphysial	-	C77.5	-	D36.0	D48.7	D49.89
pretracheal	-	C77.0	-	D36.0	D48.7	D49.89
primary (any site) NEC	C96.9	-	-	-	-	-
pulmonary (hiler)	-	C77.1	-	D36.0	D48.7	D49.89
pyloric	-	C77.2	-	D36.0	D48.7	D49.89
retroperitoneal	-	C77.2	-	D36.0	D48.7	D49.89
retropharyngeal	-	C77.0	-	D36.0	D48.7	D49.89
Rosenmuller's	-	C77.4	-	D36.0	D48.7	D49.89
sacral	-	C77.5	-	D36.0	D48.7	D49.89
scalene	-	C77.0	-	D36.0	D48.7	D49.89
site NEC	-	C77.9	-	D36.0	D48.7	D49.89
splenic (hilar)	-	C77.2	-	D36.0	D48.7	D49.89
subclavicular	-	C77.3	-	D36.0	D48.7	D49.89
subinguinal	-	C77.4	-	D36.0	D48.7	D49.89
sublingual	-	C77.0	-	D36.0	D48.7	D49.89
submandibular	-	C77.0	-	D36.0	D48.7	D49.89
submaxillary	-	C77.0	-	D36.0	D48.7	D49.89
submental	-	C77.0	-	D36.0	D48.7	D49.89
subscapular	-	C77.3	-	D36.0	D48.7	D49.89
supraclavicular	-	C77.0	-	D36.0	D48.7	D49.89
thoracic	-	C77.1	-	D36.0	D48.7	D49.89
tibial	-	C77.4	-	D36.0	D48.7	D49.89
tracheal	-	C77.1	-	D36.0	D48.7	D49.89
tracheobronchial	-	C77.1	-	D36.0	D48.7	D49.89
upper limb	-	C77.3	-	D36.0	D48.7	D49.89
Virchow's	-	C77.0	-	D36.0	D48.7	D49.89
node — *see also* Neoplasm, lymph gland						
primary NEC	C96.9	-	-	-	-	-
vessel — *see also* Neoplasm, connective tissue	C49.9	C79.89	-	D21.9	D48.1	D49.2
Mackenrodt's ligament	C57.7	C79.82	D07.39	D28.7	D39.8	D49.59
malar	C41.0	C79.51	-	D16.4-	D48.0	D49.2
region — *see* Neoplasm, cheek						
mammary gland — *see* Neoplasm, breast						
mandible	C41.1	C79.51	-	D16.5-	D48.0	D49.2
alveolar						
mucosa (carcinoma)	C03.1	C79.89	D00.03	D10.39	D37.09	D49.0
ridge or process	C41.1	C79.51	-	D16.5-	D48.0	D49.2
marrow (bone) NEC	C96.9	C79.52	-	-	D47.9	D49.89
mastectomy site (skin) — *see also* Neoplasm, breast, skin	C44.501	C79.2	-	-	-	-
specified as breast tissue	C50.8-	C79.81	-	-	-	-
mastoid (air cells) (antrum) (cavity)	C30.1	C78.39	D02.3	D14.0	D38.5	D49.1
bone or process	C41.0	C79.51	-	D16.4-	D48.0	D49.2
maxilla, maxillary (superior)	C41.0	C79.51	-	D16.4-	D48.0	D49.2
alveolar						
mucosa	C03.0	C79.89	D00.03	D10.39	D37.09	D49.0
ridge or process (carcinoma)	C41.0	C79.51	-	D16.4-	D48.0	D49.2
antrum	C31.0	C78.39	D02.3	D14.0	D38.5	D49.1
carcinoma	C03.0	C79.51	-	-	-	-
inferior — *see* Neoplasm, mandible						
sinus	C31.0	C78.39	D02.3	D14.0	D38.5	D49.1
meatus external (ear) — *see also* Neoplasm, skin, ear	C44.20-	C79.2	D04.2-	D23.2-	D48.5	D49.2
Meckel diverticulum, malignant	C17.3	C78.4	D01.49	D13.39	D37.2	D49.0
mediastinum, mediastinal	C38.3	C78.1	-	D15.2	D38.3	D49.89
anterior	C38.1	C78.1	-	D15.2	D38.3	D49.89
posterior	C38.2	C78.1	-	D15.2	D38.3	D49.89
medulla						
adrenal	C74.1-	C79.7-	D09.3	D35.0-	D44.1-	D49.7
oblongata	C71.7	C79.31	-	D33.1	D43.1	D49.6

Neoplasm, neoplastic	Malignant Primary	Malignant Secondary	Ca in situ	Benign	Uncertain Behavior	Unspecified Behavior
meibomian gland	C44.10-	C79.2	D04.1-	D23.1-	D48.5	D49.2
basal cell carcinoma	C44.11-	-	-	-	-	-
sebaceous cell	C44.13-	-	-	-	-	-
specified type NEC	C44.19-	-	-	-	-	-
squamous cell carcinoma	C44.12-	-	-	-	-	-
melanoma — *see* Melanoma						
meninges	C70.9	C79.49	-	D32.9	D42.9	D49.7
brain	C70.0	C79.32	-	D32.0	D42.0	D49.7
cerebral	C70.0	C79.32	-	D32.0	D42.0	D49.7
crainial	C70.0	C79.32	-	D32.0	D42.0	D49.7
intracranial	C70.0	C79.32	-	D32.0	D42.0	D49.7
spinal (cord)	C70.1	C79.49	-	D32.1	D42.1	D49.7
meniscus, knee joint (lateral) (medial)	C40.2-	C79.51	-	D16.2-	D48.0	D49.2
Merkel cell — *see* Carcinoma, Merkel cell						
mesentery, mesenteric	C48.1	C78.6	-	D20.1	D48.4	D49.0
mesoappendix	C48.1	C78.6	-	D20.1	D48.4	D49.0
mesocolon	C48.1	C78.6	-	D20.1	D48.4	D49.0
mesopharynx — *see* Neoplasm, oropharynx						
mesosalpinx	C57.1	C79.82	D07.39	D28.2	D39.8	D49.59
mesothelial tissue — *see* Mesothelioma						
mesothelioma — *see* Mesothelioma						
mesovarium	C57.1	C79.82	D07.39	D28.2	D39.8	D49.59
metacarpus (any bone)	C40.1-	C79.51	-	D16.1-	-	-
metastatic NEC — *see also* Neoplasm, by site, secondary	-	C79.9	-	-	-	-
metatarsus (any bone)	C40.3-	C79.51	-	D16.3-	-	-
midbrain	C71.7	C79.31	-	D33.1	D43.1	D49.6
milk duct — *see* Neoplasm, breast						
mons						
pubis	C51.9	C79.82	D07.1	D28.0	D39.8	D49.59
veneris	C51.9	C79.82	D07.1	D28.0	D39.8	D49.59
motor tract	C72.9	C79.49	-	D33.9	D43.9	D49.7
brain	C71.9	C79.31	-	D33.2	D43.2	D49.6
cauda equina	C72.1	C79.49	-	D33.4	D43.4	D49.7
spinal	C72.0	C79.49	-	D33.4	D43.4	D49.7
mouth	C06.9	C79.89	D00.00	D10.30	D37.09	D49.0
book-leaf	C06.89	C79.89	-	-	-	-
floor	C04.9	C79.89	D00.06	D10.2	D37.09	D49.0
anterior portion	C04.0	C79.89	D00.06	D10.2	D37.09	D49.0
lateral portion	C04.1	C79.89	D00.06	D10.2	D37.09	D49.0
overlapping lesion	C04.8	-	-	-	-	-
overlapping NEC	C06.80	-	-	-	-	-
roof	C05.9	C79.89	D00.00	D10.39	D37.09	D49.0
specified part NEC	C06.89	C79.89	D00.00	D10.39	D37.09	D49.0
vestibule	C06.1	C79.89	D00.00	D10.39	D37.09	D49.0
mucosa						
alveolar (ridge or process)	C03.9	C79.89	D00.03	D10.39	D37.09	D49.0
lower	C03.1	C79.89	D00.03	D10.39	D37.09	D49.0
upper	C03.0	C79.89	D00.03	D10.39	D37.09	D49.0
buccal	C06.0	C79.89	D00.02	D10.39	D37.09	D49.0
cheek	C06.0	C79.89	D00.02	D10.39	D37.09	D49.0
lip — *see* Neoplasm, lip, internal						
nasal	C30.0	C78.39	D02.3	D14.0	D38.5	D49.1
oral	C06.0	C79.89	D00.02	D10.39	D37.09	D49.0
Mullerian duct						
female	C57.7	C79.82	D07.39	D28.7	D39.8	D49.59
male	C63.7	C79.82	D07.69	D29.8	D40.8	D49.59
muscle — *see also* Neoplasm, connective tissue						
extraocular	C69.6-	C79.49	D09.2-	D31.6-	D48.7	D49.89
myocardium	C38.0	C79.89	-	D15.1	D48.7	D49.89
myometrium	C54.2	C79.82	D07.0	D26.1	D39.0	D49.59
myopericardium	C38.0	C79.89	-	D15.1	D48.7	D49.89
nabothian gland (follicle)	C53.0	C79.82	D06.0	D26.0	D39.0	D49.59
nail — *see also* Neoplasm, skin, limb	C44.90	C79.2	D04.9	D23.9	D48.5	D49.2
finger — *see also* Neoplasm, skin, limb, upper	C44.60-	C79.2	D04.6-	D23.6-	D48.5	D49.2
toe — *see also* Neoplasm, skin, limb, lower	C44.70-	C79.2	D04.7-	D23.7-	D48.5	D49.2
nares, naris (anterior) (posterior)	C30.0	C78.39	D02.3	D14.0	D38.5	D49.1
nasal — *see* Neoplasm, nose						
nasolabial groove — *see also* Neoplasm, skin, face	C44.309	C79.2	D04.39	D23.39	D48.5	D49.2
nasolacrimal duct	C69.5-	C79.49	D09.2-	D31.5-	D48.7	D49.89

Neoplasm, neoplastic	Malignant Primary	Malignant Secondary	Ca in situ	Benign	Uncertain Behavior	Unspecified Behavior
nasopharynx, nasopharyngeal	C11.9	C79.89	D00.08	D10.6	D37.05	D49.0
- floor	C11.3	C79.89	D00.08	D10.6	D37.05	D49.0
- overlapping lesion	C11.8	-	-	-	-	-
- roof	C11.0	C79.89	D00.08	D10.6	D37.05	D49.0
- wall	C11.9	C79.89	D00.08	D10.6	D37.05	D49.0
- - anterior	C11.3	C79.89	D00.08	D10.6	D37.05	D49.0
- - lateral	C11.2	C79.89	D00.08	D10.6	D37.05	D49.0
- - posterior	C11.1	C79.89	D00.08	D10.6	D37.05	D49.0
- - superior	C11.0	C79.89	D00.08	D10.6	D37.05	D49.0
nates — *see also* Neoplasm, skin, trunk	C44.509	C79.2	D04.5	D23.5	D48.5	D49.2
neck NEC	C76.0	C79.89	D09.8	D36.7	D48.7	D49.89
- skin	C44.40	-	-	-	-	-
- - basal cell carcinoma	C44.41	-	-	-	-	-
- - specified type NEC	C44.49	-	-	-	-	-
- - squamous cell carcinoma	C44.42	-	-	-	-	-
nerve (ganglion)	C47.9	C79.89	-	D36.10	D48.2	D49.2
- abducens	C72.59	C79.49	-	D33.3	D43.3	D49.7
- accessory (spinal)	C72.59	C79.49	-	D33.3	D43.3	D49.7
- acoustic	C72.4-	C79.49	-	D33.3	D43.3	D49.7
- auditory	C72.4-	C79.49	-	D33.3	D43.3	D49.7
- autonomic NEC — *see also* Neoplasm, nerve, peripheral	C47.9	C79.89	-	D36.10	D48.2	D49.2
- brachial	C47.1-	C79.89	-	D36.12	D48.2	D49.2
- cranial	C72.50	C79.49	-	D33.3	D43.3	D49.7
- - specified NEC	C72.59	C79.49	-	D33.3	D43.3	D49.7
- facial	C72.59	C79.49	-	D33.3	D43.3	D49.7
- femoral	C47.2-	C79.89	-	D36.13	D48.2	D49.2
- ganglion NEC — *see also* Neoplasm, nerve, peripheral	C47.9	C79.89	-	D36.10	D48.2	D49.2
- glossopharyngeal	C72.59	C79.49	-	D33.3	D43.3	D49.7
- hypoglossal	C72.59	C79.49	-	D33.3	D43.3	D49.7
- intercostal	C47.3	C79.89	-	D36.14	D48.2	D49.2
- lumbar	C47.6	C79.89	-	D36.17	D48.2	D49.2
- median	C47.1-	C79.89	-	D36.12	D48.2	D49.2
- obturator	C47.2-	C79.89	-	D36.13	D48.2	D49.2
- oculomotor	C72.59	C79.49	-	D33.3	D43.3	D49.7
- olfactory	C47.2-	C79.49	-	D33.3	D43.3	D49.7
- optic	C72.3-	C79.49	-	D33.3	D43.3	D49.7
- parasympathetic NEC	C47.9	C79.89	-	D36.10	D48.2	D49.2
- peripheral NEC	C47.9	C79.89	-	D36.10	D48.2	D49.2
- - abdomen	C47.4	C79.89	-	D36.15	D48.2	D49.2
- - abdominal wall	C47.4	C79.89	-	D36.15	D48.2	D49.2
- - ankle	C47.2-	C79.89	-	D36.13	D48.2	D49.2
- - antecubital fossa or space	C47.1-	C79.89	-	D36.12	D48.2	D49.2
- - arm	C47.1-	C79.89	-	D36.12	D48.2	D49.2
- - auricle (ear)	C47.0	C79.89	-	D36.11	D48.2	D49.2
- - axilla	C47.3	C79.89	-	D36.12	D48.2	D49.2
- - back	C47.6	C79.89	-	D36.17	D48.2	D49.2
- - buttock	C47.5	C79.89	-	D36.16	D48.2	D49.2
- - calf	C47.2-	C79.89	-	D36.13	D48.2	D49.2
- - cervical region	C47.0	C79.89	-	D36.11	D48.2	D49.2
- - cheek	C47.0	C79.89	-	D36.11	D48.2	D49.2
- - chest (wall)	C47.3	C79.89	-	D36.14	D48.2	D49.2
- - chin	C47.0	C79.89	-	D36.11	D48.2	D49.2
- - ear (external)	C47.0	C79.89	-	D36.11	D48.2	D49.2
- - elbow	C47.1-	C79.89	-	D36.12	D48.2	D49.2
- - extrarectal	C47.5	C79.89	-	D36.16	D48.2	D49.2
- - extremity	C47.9	C79.89	-	D36.10	D48.2	D49.2
- - - lower	C47.2-	C79.89	-	D36.13	D48.2	D49.2
- - - upper	C47.1-	C79.89	-	D36.12	D48.2	D49.2
- - eyelid	C47.0	C79.89	-	D36.11	D48.2	D49.2
- - face	C47.0	C79.89	-	D36.11	D48.2	D49.2
- - finger	C47.1-	C79.89	-	D36.12	D48.2	D49.2
- - flank	C47.6	C79.89	-	D36.17	D48.2	D49.2
- - foot	C47.2-	C79.89	-	D36.13	D48.2	D49.2
- - forearm	C47.1-	C79.89	-	D36.12	D48.2	D49.2
- - forehead	C47.0	C79.89	-	D36.11	D48.2	D49.2
- - gluteal region	C47.5	C79.89	-	D36.16	D48.2	D49.2
- - groin	C47.5	C79.89	-	D36.16	D48.2	D49.2
- - hand	C47.1-	C79.89	-	D36.12	D48.2	D49.2
- - head	C47.0	C79.89	-	D36.11	D48.2	D49.2
- - heel	C47.2-	C79.89	-	D36.13	D48.2	D49.2
- - hip	C47.2-	C79.89	-	D36.13	D48.2	D49.2
- - infraclavicular region	C47.3	C79.89	-	D36.14	D48.2	D49.2
- - inguinal (canal) (region)	C47.5	C79.89	-	D36.16	D48.2	D49.2
- - intrathoracic	C47.3	C79.89	-	D36.14	D48.2	D49.2
- - ischiorectal fossa	C47.5	C79.89	-	D36.16	D48.2	D49.2
- - knee	C47.2-	C79.89	-	D36.13	D48.2	D49.2

Neoplasm, neoplastic	Malignant Primary	Malignant Secondary	Ca in situ	Benign	Uncertain Behavior	Unspecified Behavior
nerve - *continued*						
- - leg	C47.2-	C79.89	-	D36.13	D48.2	D49.2
- - limb NEC	C47.9	C79.89	-	D36.10	D48.2	D49.2
- - - lower	C47.2-	C79.89	-	D36.13	D48.2	D49.2
- - - upper	C47.1-	C79.89	-	D36.12	D48.2	D49.2
- - nates	C47.5	C79.89	-	D36.16	D48.2	D49.2
- - neck	C47.0	C79.89	-	D36.11	D48.2	D49.2
- - orbit	C69.6-	C79.49	-	D31.6-	D48.7	D49.2
- - pararectal	C47.5	C79.89	-	D36.16	D48.2	D49.2
- - paraurethral	C47.5	C79.89	-	D36.16	D48.2	D49.2
- - paravaginal	C47.5	C79.89	-	D36.16	D48.2	D49.2
- - pelvis (floor)	C47.5	C79.89	-	D36.16	D48.2	D49.2
- - pelvoabdominal	C47.8	C79.89	-	D36.17	D48.2	D49.2
- - perineum	C47.5	C79.89	-	D36.16	D48.2	D49.2
- - perirectal (tissue)	C47.5	C79.89	-	D36.16	D48.2	D49.2
- - periurethral (tissue)	C47.5	C79.89	-	D36.16	D48.2	D49.2
- - popliteal fossa or space	C47.2-	C79.89	-	D36.13	D48.2	D49.2
- - presacral	C47.5	C79.89	-	D36.16	D48.2	D49.2
- - pterygoid fossa	C47.0	C79.89	-	D36.11	D48.2	D49.2
- - rectovaginal septum or wall	C47.5	C79.89	-	D36.16	D48.2	D49.2
- - rectovesical	C47.5	C79.89	-	D36.16	D48.2	D49.2
- - sacrococcygeal region	C47.5	C79.89	-	D36.16	D48.2	D49.2
- - scalp	C47.0	C79.89	-	D36.11	D48.2	D49.2
- - scapular region	C47.3	C79.89	-	D36.14	D48.2	D49.2
- - shoulder	C47.1-	C79.89	-	D36.12	D48.2	D49.2
- - submental	C47.0	C79.89	-	D36.11	D48.2	D49.2
- - supraclavicular region	C47.0	C79.89	-	D36.11	D48.2	D49.2
- - temple	C47.0	C79.89	-	D36.11	D48.2	D49.2
- - temporal region	C47.0	C79.89	-	D36.11	D48.2	D49.2
- - thigh	C47.2-	C79.89	-	D36.13	D48.2	D49.2
- - thoracic (duct) (wall)	C47.3	C79.89	-	D36.14	D48.2	D49.2
- - thorax	C47.3	C79.89	-	D36.14	D48.2	D49.2
- - thumb	C47.1-	C79.89	-	D36.12	D48.2	D49.2
- - toe	C47.2-	C79.89	-	D36.13	D48.2	D49.2
- - trunk	C47.6	C79.89	-	D36.17	D48.2	D49.2
- - umbilicus	C47.4	C79.89	-	D36.15	D48.2	D49.2
- - vesicorectal	C47.5	C79.89	-	D36.16	D48.2	D49.2
- - wrist	C47.1-	C79.89	-	D36.12	D48.2	D49.2
- radial	C47.1-	C79.89	-	D36.12	D48.2	D49.2
- sacral	C47.5	C79.89	-	D36.16	D48.2	D49.2
- sciatic	C47.2-	C79.89	-	D36.13	D48.2	D49.2
- spinal NEC	C47.9	C79.89	-	D36.10	D48.2	D49.2
- - accessory	C72.59	C79.49	-	D33.3	D43.3	D49.7
- sympathetic NEC — *see also* Neoplasm, nerve, peripheral	C47.9	C79.89	-	D36.10	D48.2	D49.2
- trigeminal	C72.59	C79.49	-	D33.3	D43.3	D49.7
- trochlear	C72.59	C79.49	-	D33.3	D43.3	D49.7
- ulnar	C47.1-	C79.89	-	D36.12	D48.2	D49.2
- vagus	C72.59	C79.49	-	D33.3	D43.3	D49.7
nervous system (central)	C72.9	C79.40	-	D33.9	D43.9	D49.7
- autonomic — *see* Neoplasm, nerve, peripheral						
- parasympathetic — *see* Neoplasm, nerve, peripheral						
- specified site NEC	-	C79.49	-	D33.7	D43.8	-
- sympathetic — *see* Neoplasm, nerve, peripheral						
nevus — *see* Nevus						
nipple	C50.0-	C79.81	D05.-	D24.-	-	-
nose, nasal	C76.0	C79.89	D09.8	D36.7	D48.7	D49.89
- ala (external) (nasi) — *see also* Neoplasm, nose, skin	C44.301	C79.2	D04.39	D23.39	D48.5	D49.2
- bone	C41.0	C79.51	-	D16.4-	D48.0	D49.2
- cartilage	C30.0	C78.39	D02.3	D14.0	D38.5	D49.1
- cavity	C30.0	C78.39	D02.3	D14.0	D38.5	D49.1
- choana	C11.3	C79.89	D00.08	D10.6	D37.05	D49.0
- external (skin) — *see also* Neoplasm, nose, skin	C44.301	C79.2	D04.39	D23.39	D48.5	D49.2
- fossa	C30.0	C78.39	D02.3	D14.0	D38.5	D49.1
- internal	C30.0	C78.39	D02.3	D14.0	D38.5	D49.1
- mucosa	C30.0	C78.39	D02.3	D14.0	D38.5	D49.1
- septum	C30.0	C78.39	D02.3	D14.0	D38.5	D49.1
- - posterior margin	C11.3	C79.89	D00.08	D10.6	D37.05	D49.0
- sinus — *see* Neoplasm, sinus						
- skin	C44.301	C79.2	D04.39	D23.39	D48.5	D49.2
- - basal cell carcinoma	C44.311	-	-	-	-	-
- - specified type NEC	C44.391	-	-	-	-	-
- - squamous cell carcinoma	C44.321	-	-	-	-	-
- turbinate (mucosa)	C30.0	C78.39	D02.3	D14.0	D38.5	D49.1

Neoplasm, neoplastic	Malignant Primary	Malignant Secondary	Ca in situ	Benign	Uncertain Behavior	Unspecified Behavior
nose, nasal - *continued*						
bone	C41.0	C79.51	-	D16.4-	D48.0	D49.2
vestibule	C30.0	C78.39	D02.3	D14.0	D38.5	D49.1
nostril	C30.0	C78.39	D02.3	D14.0	D38.5	D49.1
nucleus pulposus	C41.2	C79.51	-	D16.6	D48.0	D49.2
occipital						
bone	C41.0	C79.51	-	D16.4-	D48.0	D49.2
lobe or pole, brain	C71.4	C79.31	-	D33.0	D43.0	D49.6
odontogenic — *see* Neoplasm, jaw bone						
olfactory nerve or bulb	C72.2-	C79.49	-	D33.3	D43.3	D49.7
olive (brain)	C71.7	C79.31	-	D33.1	D43.1	D49.6
omentum	C48.1	C78.6	-	D20.1	D48.4	D49.0
operculum (brain)	C71.0	C79.31	-	D33.0	D43.0	D49.6
optic nerve, chiasm, or tract	C72.3-	C79.49	-	D33.3	D43.3	D49.7
oral (cavity)	C06.9	C79.89	D00.00	D10.30	D37.09	D49.0
ill-defined	C14.8	C79.89	D00.00	D10.30	D37.09	D49.0
mucosa	C06.0	C79.89	D00.02	D10.39	D37.09	D49.0
orbit	C69.6-	C79.49	D09.2-	D31.6-	D48.7	D49.89
autonomic nerve	C69.6-	C79.49	-	D31.6-	D48.7	D49.2
bone	C41.0	C79.51	-	D16.4-	D48.0	D49.2
eye	C69.6-	C79.49	D09.2-	D31.6-	D48.7	D49.89
peripheral nerves	C69.6-	C79.49	-	D31.6-	D48.7	D49.2
soft parts	C69.6-	C79.49	D09.2-	D31.6-	D48.7	D49.89
organ of Zuckerkandl	C75.5	C79.89	-	D35.6	D44.7	D49.7
oropharynx	C10.9	C79.89	D00.08	D10.5	D37.05	D49.0
branchial cleft (vestige)	C10.4	C79.89	D00.08	D10.5	D37.05	D49.0
junctional region	C10.8	C79.89	D00.08	D10.5	D37.05	D49.0
lateral wall	C10.2	C79.89	D00.08	D10.5	D37.05	D49.0
overlapping lesion	C10.8	-	-	-	-	-
pillars or fauces	C09.1	C79.89	D00.08	D10.5	D37.05	D49.0
posterior wall	C10.3	C79.89	D00.08	D10.5	D37.05	D49.0
vallecula	C10.0	C79.89	D00.08	D10.5	D37.05	D49.0
os						
external	C53.1	C79.82	D06.1	D26.0	D39.0	D49.59
internal	C53.0	C79.82	D06.0	D26.0	D39.0	D49.59
ovary	C56.-	C79.6-	D07.39	D27.-	D39.1-	D49.59
oviduct	C57.0-	C79.82	D07.39	D28.2	D39.8	D49.59
palate	C05.9	C79.89	D00.00	D10.39	D37.09	D49.0
hard	C05.0	C79.89	D00.05	D10.39	D37.09	D49.0
junction of hard and soft palate	C05.9	C79.89	D00.00	D10.39	D37.09	D49.0
overlapping lesions	C05.8	-	-	-	-	-
soft	C05.1	C79.89	D00.04	D10.39	D37.09	D49.0
nasopharyngeal surface	C11.3	C79.89	D00.08	D10.6	D37.05	D49.0
posterior surface	C11.3	C79.89	D00.08	D10.6	D37.05	D49.0
superior surface	C11.3	C79.89	D00.08	D10.6	D37.05	D49.0
palatoglossal arch	C09.1	C79.89	D00.00	D10.5	D37.09	D49.0
palatopharyngeal arch	C09.1	C79.89	D00.00	D10.5	D37.09	D49.0
pallium	C71.0	C79.31	-	D33.0	D43.0	D49.6
palpebra	C44.10-	C79.2	D04.1-	D23.1-	D48.5	D49.2
basal cell carcinoma	C44.11-	-	-	-	-	-
sebaceous cell	C44.13-	-	-	-	-	-
specified type NEC	C44.19-	-	-	-	-	-
squamous cell carcinoma	C44.12-	-	-	-	-	-
pancreas	C25.9	C78.89	D01.7	D13.6	D37.8	D49.0
body	C25.1	C78.89	D01.7	D13.6	D37.8	D49.0
duct (of Santorini) (of Wirsung)	C25.3	C78.89	D01.7	D13.6	D37.8	D49.0
ectopic tissue	C25.7	C78.89	-	D13.6	D37.8	D49.0
head	C25.0	C78.89	D01.7	D13.6	D37.8	D49.0
islet cells	C25.4	C78.89	D01.7	D13.7	D37.8	D49.0
neck	C25.7	C78.89	D01.7	D13.6	D37.8	D49.0
overlapping lesion	C25.8	-	-	-	-	-
tail	C25.2	C78.89	D01.7	D13.6	D37.8	D49.0
para-aortic body	C75.5	C79.89	-	D35.6	D44.7	D49.7
paraganglion NEC	C75.5	C79.89	-	D35.6	D44.7	D49.7
parametrium	C57.3	C79.82	-	D28.2	D39.8	D49.59
paranephric	C48.0	C78.6	-	D20.0	D48.3	D49.0
pararectal	C76.3	C79.89	-	D36.7	D48.7	D49.89
parasagittal (region)	C76.0	C79.89	D09.8	D36.7	D48.7	D49.89
parasellar	C72.9	C79.49	-	D33.9	D43.8	D49.7
parathyroid (gland)	C75.0	C79.89	D09.3	D35.1	D44.2	D49.7
paraurethral	C76.3	C79.89	-	D36.7	D48.7	D49.89
gland	C68.1	C79.19	D09.19	D30.8	D41.8	D49.59
paravaginal	C76.3	C79.89	-	D36.7	D48.7	D49.89
parenchyma, kidney	C64.-	C79.0-	D09.19	D30.0-	D41.0-	D49.51-
parietal						
bone	C41.0	C79.51	-	D16.4-	D48.0	D49.2
lobe, brain	C71.3	C79.31	-	D33.0	D43.0	D49.6
paroophoron	C57.1	C79.82	D07.39	D28.2	D39.8	D49.59

Neoplasm, neoplastic	Malignant Primary	Malignant Secondary	Ca in situ	Benign	Uncertain Behavior	Unspecified Behavior
parotid (duct) (gland)	C07	C79.89	D00.00	D11.0	D37.030	D49.0
parovarium	C57.1	C79.82	D07.39	D28.2	D39.8	D49.59
patella	C40.20	C79.51	-	-	-	-
peduncle, cerebral	C71.7	C79.31	-	D33.1	D43.1	D49.6
pelvirectal junction	C19	C78.5	D01.1	D12.7	D37.5	D49.0
pelvis, pelvic	C76.3	C79.89	D09.8	D36.7	D48.7	D49.89
bone	C41.4	C79.51	-	D16.8	D48.0	D49.2
floor	C76.3	C79.89	D09.8	D36.7	D48.7	D49.89
renal	C65.-	C79.0-	D09.19	D30.1-	D41.1-	D49.51-
viscera	C76.3	C79.89	D09.8	D36.7	D48.7	D49.89
wall	C76.3	C79.89	D09.8	D36.7	D48.7	D49.89
pelvo-abdominal	C76.8	C79.89	D09.8	D36.7	D48.7	D49.89
penis	C60.9	C79.82	D07.4	D29.0	D40.8	D49.59
body	C60.2	C79.82	D07.4	D29.0	D40.8	D49.59
corpus (cavernosum)	C60.2	C79.82	D07.4	D29.0	D40.8	D49.59
glans	C60.1	C79.82	D07.4	D29.0	D40.8	D49.59
overlapping sites	C60.8	-	-	-	-	-
skin NEC	C60.9	C79.82	D07.4	D29.0	D40.8	D49.59
periadrenal (tissue)	C48.0	C78.6	-	D20.0	D48.3	D49.0
perianal (skin) — *see also* Neoplasm, anus, skin	C44.500	C79.2	D04.5	D23.5	D48.5	D49.2
pericardium	C38.0	C79.89	-	D15.1	D48.7	D49.89
perinephric	C48.0	C78.6	-	D20.0	D48.3	D49.0
perineum	C76.3	C79.89	D09.8	D36.7	D48.7	D49.89
periodontal tissue NEC	C03.9	C79.89	D00.03	D10.39	D37.09	D49.0
periosteum — *see* Neoplasm, bone						
peripancreatic	C48.0	C78.6	-	D20.0	D48.3	D49.0
peripheral nerve NEC	C47.9	C79.89	-	D36.10	D48.2	D49.2
perirectal (tissue)	C76.3	C79.89	-	D36.7	D48.7	D49.89
perirenal (tissue)	C48.0	C78.6	-	D20.0	D48.3	D49.0
peritoneum, peritoneal (cavity)	C48.2	C78.6	-	D20.1	D48.4	D49.0
benign mesothelial tissue — *see* Mesothelioma, benign						
overlapping lesion	C48.8	-	-	-	-	-
with digestive organs	C26.9	-	-	-	-	-
parietal	C48.1	C78.6	-	D20.1	D48.4	D49.0
pelvic	C48.1	C78.6	-	D20.1	D48.4	D49.0
specified part NEC	C48.1	C78.6	-	D20.1	D48.4	D49.0
peritonsillar (tissue)	C76.0	C79.89	D09.8	D36.7	D48.7	D49.89
periurethral tissue	C76.3	C79.89	-	D36.7	D48.7	D49.89
phalanges						
foot	C40.3-	C79.51	-	D16.3-	-	-
hand	C40.1-	C79.51	-	D16.1-	-	-
pharynx, pharyngeal	C14.0	C79.89	D00.08	D10.9	D37.05	D49.0
bursa	C11.1	C79.89	D00.08	D10.6	D37.05	D49.0
fornix	C11.3	C79.89	D00.08	D10.6	D37.05	D49.0
recess	C11.2	C79.89	D00.08	D10.6	D37.05	D49.0
region	C14.0	C79.89	D00.08	D10.9	D37.05	D49.0
tonsil	C11.1	C79.89	D00.08	D10.6	D37.05	D49.0
wall (lateral) (posterior)	C14.0	C79.89	D00.08	D10.9	D37.05	D49.0
pia mater	C70.9	C79.40	-	D32.9	D42.9	D49.7
cerebral	C70.0	C79.32	-	D32.0	D42.0	D49.7
cranial	C70.0	C79.32	-	D32.0	D42.0	D49.7
spinal	C70.1	C79.49	-	D32.1	D42.1	D49.7
pillars of fauces	C09.1	C79.89	D00.08	D10.5	D37.05	D49.0
pineal (body) (gland)	C75.3	C79.89	D09.3	D35.4	D44.5	D49.7
pinna (ear) NEC — *see also* Neoplasm, skin, ear	C44.20-	C79.2	D04.2-	D23.2-	D48.5	D49.2
piriform fossa or sinus	C12	C79.89	D00.08	D10.7	D37.05	D49.0
pituitary (body) (fossa) (gland) (lobe)	C75.1	C79.89	D09.3	D35.2	D44.3	D49.7
placenta	C58	C79.82	D07.0	D26.7	D39.2	D49.59
pleura, pleural (cavity)	C38.4	C78.2	-	D19.0	D38.2	D49.1
overlapping lesion with heart or mediastinum	C38.8	-	-	-	-	-
parietal	C38.4	C78.2	-	D19.0	D38.2	D49.1
visceral	C38.4	C78.2	-	D19.0	D38.2	D49.1
plexus						
brachial	C47.1-	C79.89	-	D36.12	D48.2	D49.2
cervical	C47.0	C79.89	-	D36.11	D48.2	D49.2
choroid	C71.5	C79.31	-	D33.0	D43.0	D49.6
lumbosacral	C47.5	C79.89	-	D36.16	D48.2	D49.2
sacral	C47.5	C79.89	-	D36.16	D48.2	D49.2
pluriendocrine	C75.8	C79.89	D09.3	D35.7	D44.9	D49.7
pole						
frontal	C71.1	C79.31	-	D33.0	D43.0	D49.6
occipital	C71.4	C79.31	-	D33.0	D43.0	D49.6
pons (varolii)	C71.7	C79.31	-	D33.1	D43.1	D49.6
popliteal fossa or space	C76.5-	C79.89	D04.7-	D36.7	D48.7	D49.89

Neoplasm, neoplastic	Malignant Primary	Malignant Secondary	Ca in situ	Benign	Uncertain Behavior	Unspecified Behavior
postcricoid (region)	C13.0	C79.89	D00.08	D10.7	D37.05	D49.0
posterior fossa (cranial)	C71.9	C79.31	-	D33.2	D43.2	D49.6
postnasal space	C11.9	C79.89	D00.08	D10.6	D37.05	D49.0
prepuce	C60.0	C79.82	D07.4	D29.0	D40.8	D49.59
prepylorus	C16.4	C78.89	D00.2	D13.1	D37.1	D49.0
presacral (region)	C76.3	C79.89	-	D36.7	D48.7	D49.89
prostate (gland)	C61	C79.82	D07.5	D29.1	D40.0	D49.59
utricle	C68.0	C79.19	D09.19	D30.4	D41.3	D49.59
pterygoid fossa	C49.0	C79.89	-	D21.0	D48.1	D49.2
pubic bone	C41.4	C79.51	-	D16.8	D48.0	D49.2
pudenda, pudendum (female)	C51.9	C79.82	D07.1	D28.0	D39.8	D49.59
pulmonary — *see also* Neoplasm, lung	C34.9-	C78.0-	D02.2-	D14.3-	D38.1	D49.1
putamen	C71.0	C79.31	-	D33.0	D43.0	D49.6
pyloric						
antrum	C16.3	C78.89	D00.2	D13.1	D37.1	D49.0
canal	C16.4	C78.89	D00.2	D13.1	D37.1	D49.0
pylorus	C16.4	C78.89	D00.2	D13.1	D37.1	D49.0
pyramid (brain)	C71.7	C79.31	-	D33.1	D43.1	D49.6
pyriform fossa or sinus	C12	C79.89	D00.08	D10.7	D37.05	D49.0
radius (any part)	C40.0-	C79.51	-	D16.0-	-	-
Rathke's pouch	C75.1	C79.89	D09.3	D35.2	D44.3	D49.7
rectosigmoid (junction)	C19	C78.5	D01.1	D12.7	D37.5	D49.0
overlapping lesion with anus or rectum	C21.8	-	-	-	-	-
rectouterine pouch	C48.1	C78.6	-	D20.1	D48.4	D49.0
rectovaginal septum or wall	C76.3	C79.89	D09.8	D36.7	D48.7	D49.89
rectovesical septum	C76.3	C79.89	D09.8	D36.7	D48.7	D49.89
rectum (ampulla)	C20	C78.5	D01.2	D12.8	D37.5	D49.0
and colon	C19	C78.5	D01.1	D12.7	D37.5	D49.0
overlapping lesion with anus or rectosigmoid junction	C21.8	-	-	-	-	-
renal	C64.-	C79.0-	D09.19	D30.0-	D41.0-	D49.51-
calyx	C65.-	C79.0-	D09.19	D30.1-	D41.1-	D49.51-
hilus	C65.-	C79.0-	D09.19	D30.1-	D41.1-	D49.51-
parenchyma	C64.-	C79.0-	D09.19	D30.0-	D41.0-	D49.51-
pelvis	C65.-	C79.0-	D09.19	D30.1-	D41.1-	D49.51-
respiratory						
organs or system NEC	C39.9	C78.30	D02.4	D14.4	D38.6	D49.1
tract NEC	C39.9	C78.30	D02.4	D14.4	D38.5	D49.1
upper	C39.0	C78.30	D02.4	D14.4	D38.5	D49.1
retina	C69.2-	C79.49	D09.2-	D31.2-	D48.7	D49.81
retrobulbar	C69.6-	C79.49	-	D31.6-	D48.7	D49.89
retrocecal	C48.0	C78.6	-	D20.0	D48.3	D49.0
retromolar (area) (triangle) (trigone)	C06.2	C79.89	D00.00	D10.39	D37.09	D49.0
retro-orbital	C76.0	C79.89	D09.8	D36.7	D48.7	D49.89
retroperitoneal (space) (tissue)	C48.0	C78.6	-	D20.0	D48.3	D49.0
retroperitoneum	C48.0	C78.6	-	D20.0	D48.3	D49.0
retropharyngeal	C14.0	C79.89	D00.08	D10.9	D37.05	D49.0
retrovesical (septum)	C76.3	C79.89	D09.8	D36.7	D48.7	D49.89
rhinencephalon	C71.0	C79.31	-	D33.0	D43.0	D49.6
rib	C41.3	C79.51	-	D16.7	D48.0	D49.2
Rosenmuller's fossa	C11.2	C79.89	D00.08	D10.6	D37.05	D49.0
round ligament	C57.2	C79.82	-	D28.2	D39.8	D49.59
sacrococcyx, sacrococcygeal	C41.4	C79.51		D16.8	D48.0	D49.2
region	C76.3	C79.89	D09.8	D36.7	D48.7	D49.89
sacrouterine ligament	C57.3	C79.82	-	D28.2	D39.8	D49.59
sacrum, sacral (vertebra)	C41.4	C79.51	-	D16.8	D48.0	D49.2
salivary gland or duct (major)	C08.9	C79.89	D00.00	D11.9	D37.039	D49.0
minor NEC	C06.9	C79.89	D00.00	D10.39	D37.04	D49.0
overlapping lesion	C08.9	-	-	-	-	-
parotid	C07	C79.89	D00.00	D11.0	D37.030	D49.0
pluriglandular	C08.9	C79.89	D00.00	D11.9	D37.039	D49.0
sublingual	C08.1	C79.89	D00.00	D11.7	D37.031	D49.0
submandibular	C08.0	C79.89	D00.00	D11.7	D37.032	D49.0
submaxillary	C08.0	C79.89	D00.00	D11.7	D37.032	D49.0
salpinx (uterine)	C57.0-	C79.82	D07.39	D28.2	D39.8	D49.59
Santorini's duct	C25.3	C78.89	D01.7	D13.6	D37.8	D49.0
scalp	C44.40	C79.2	D04.4	D23.4	D48.5	D49.2
basal cell carcinoma	C44.41	-	-	-	-	-
specified type NEC	C44.49	-	-	-	-	-
squamous cell carcinoma	C44.42	-	-	-	-	-
scapula (any part)	C40.0-	C79.51	-	D16.0-	-	-
scapular region	C76.1	C79.89	D09.8	D36.7	D48.7	D49.89
scar NEC — *see also* Neoplasm, skin, by site	C44.90	C79.2	D04.9	D23.9	D48.5	D49.2
sciatic nerve	C47.2-	C79.89	-	D36.13	D48.2	D49.2
sclera	C69.4-	C79.49	D09.2-	D31.4-	D48.7	D49.89
scrotum (skin)	C63.2	C79.82	D07.61	D29.4	D40.8	D49.59
sebaceous gland — *see* Neoplasm, skin						
sella turcica	C75.1	C79.89	D09.3	D35.2	D44.3	D49.7
bone	C41.0	C79.51	-	D16.4-	D48.0	D49.2
semilunar cartilage (knee)	C40.2-	C79.51	-	D16.2-	D48.0	D49.2
seminal vesicle	C63.7	C79.82	D07.69	D29.8	D40.8	D49.59
septum						
nasal	C30.0	C78.39	D02.3	D14.0	D38.5	D49.1
posterior margin	C11.3	C79.89	D00.08	D10.6	D37.05	D49.0
rectovaginal	C76.3	C79.89	D09.8	D36.7	D48.7	D49.89
rectovesical	C76.3	C79.89	D09.8	D36.7	D48.7	D49.89
urethrovaginal	C57.9	C79.82	D07.30	D28.9	D39.9	D49.59
vesicovaginal	C57.9	C79.82	D07.30	D28.9	D39.9	D49.59
shoulder NEC	C76.4-	C79.89	D04.6-	D36.7	D48.7	D49.89
sigmoid flexure (lower) (upper)	C18.7	C78.5	D01.0	D12.5	D37.4	D49.0
sinus (accessory)	C31.9	C78.39	D02.3	D14.0	D38.5	D49.1
bone (any)	C41.0	C79.51	-	D16.4-	D48.0	D49.2
ethmoidal	C31.1	C78.39	D02.3	D14.0	D38.5	D49.1
frontal	C31.2	C78.39	D02.3	D14.0	D38.5	D49.1
maxillary	C31.0	C78.39	D02.3	D14.0	D38.5	D49.1
nasal, paranasal NEC	C31.9	C78.39	D02.3	D14.0	D38.5	D49.1
overlapping lesion	C31.8	-	-	-	-	-
pyriform	C12	C79.89	D00.08	D10.7	D37.05	D49.0
sphenoid	C31.3	C78.39	D02.3	D14.0	D38.5	D49.1
skeleton, skeletal NEC	C41.9	C79.51	-	D16.9-	D48.0	D49.2
Skene's gland	C68.1	C79.19	D09.19	D30.8	D41.8	D49.59
skin NOS	C44.90	C79.2	D04.9	D23.9	D48.5	D49.2
abdominal wall	C44.509	C79.2	D04.5	D23.5	D48.5	D49.2
basal cell carcinoma	C44.519	-	-	-	-	-
specified type NEC	C44.599	-	-	-	-	-
squamous cell carcinoma	C44.529	-	-	-	-	-
ala nasi — *see also* Neoplasm, nose, skin	C44.301	C79.2	D04.39	D23.39	D48.5	D49.2
ankle — *see also* Neoplasm, skin, limb, lower	C44.70-	C79.2	D04.7-	D23.7-	D48.5	D49.2
antecubital space — *see also* Neoplasm, skin, limb, upper	C44.60-	C79.2	D04.6-	D23.6-	D48.5	D49.2
anus	C44.500	C79.2	D04.5	D23.5	D48.5	D49.2
basal cell carcinoma	C44.510	-	-	-	-	-
specified type NEC	C44.590	-	-	-	-	-
squamous cell carcinoma	C44.520	-	-	-	-	-
arm — *see also* Neoplasm, skin, limb, upper	C44.60-	C79.2	D04.6-	D23.6-	D48.5	D49.2
auditory canal (external) — *see also* Neoplasm, skin, ear	C44.20-	C79.2	D04.2-	D23.2-	D48.5	D49.2
auricle (ear) — *see also* Neoplasm, skin, ear	C44.20-	C79.2	D04.2-	D23.2-	D48.5	D49.2
auricular canal (external) — *see also* Neoplasm, skin, ear	C44.20-	C79.2	D04.2-	D23.2-	D48.5	D49.2
axilla, axillary fold — *see also* Neoplasm, skin, trunk	C44.509	C79.2	D04.5	D23.5	D48.5	D49.2
back — *see also* Neoplasm, skin, trunk	C44.509	C79.2	D04.5	D23.5	D48.5	D49.2
basal cell carcinoma	C44.91					
breast	C44.501	C79.2	D04.5	D23.5	D48.5	D49.2
basal cell carcinoma	C44.511	-	-	-	-	-
specified type NEC	C44.591	-	-	-	-	-
squamous cell carcinoma	C44.521	-	-	-	-	-
brow — *see also* Neoplasm, skin, face	C44.309	C79.2	D04.39	D23.39	D48.5	D49.2
buttock — *see also* Neoplasm, skin, trunk	C44.509	C79.2	D04.5	D23.5	D48.5	D49.2
calf — *see also* Neoplasm, skin, limb, lower	C44.70-	C79.2	D04.7-	D23.7-	D48.5	D49.2
canthus (eye) (inner) (outer)	C44.10-	C79.2	D04.1-	D23.1-	D48.5	D49.2
basal cell carcinoma	C44.11-	-	-	-	-	-
sebaceous cell	C44.13-	-	-	-	-	-
specified type NEC	C44.19-	-	-	-	-	-
squamous cell carcinoma	C44.12-	-	-	-	-	-
cervical region — *see also* Neoplasm, skin, neck	C44.40	C79.2	D04.4	D23.4	D48.5	D49.2
cheek (external) — *see also* Neoplasm, skin, face	C44.309	C79.2	D04.39	D23.39	D48.5	D49.2
chest (wall) — *see also* Neoplasm, skin, trunk	C44.509	C79.2	D04.5	D23.5	D48.5	D49.2
chin — *see also* Neoplasm, skin, face	C44.309	C79.2	D04.39	D23.39	D48.5	D49.2
clavicular area — *see also* Neoplasm, skin, trunk	C44.509	C79.2	D04.5	D23.5	D48.5	D49.2

Neoplasm, neoplastic	Malignant Primary	Malignant Secondary	Ca in situ	Benign	Uncertain Behavior	Unspecified Behavior
skin NOS - *continued*						
clitoris	C51.2	C79.82	D07.1	D28.0	D39.8	D49.59
columnella — *see also* Neoplasm, skin, face	C44.309	C79.2	D04.39	D23.39	D48.5	D49.2
concha — *see also* Neoplasm, skin, ear	C44.20-	C79.2	D04.2-	D23.2-	D48.5	D49.2
ear (external)	C44.20-	C79.2	D04.2-	D23.2-	D48.5	D49.2
basal cell carcinoma	C44.21-	-	-	-	-	-
specified type NEC	C44.29-	-	-	-	-	-
squamous cell carcinoma	C44.22-	-	-	-	-	-
elbow — *see also* Neoplasm, skin, limb, upper	C44.60-	C79.2	D04.6-	D23.6-	D48.5	D49.2
eyebrow — *see also* Neoplasm, skin, face	C44.309	C79.2	D04.39	D23.39	D48.5	D49.2
eyelid	C44.10-	C79.2	D04.1-	D23.1-	D48.5	D49.2
basal cell carcinoma	C44.11-	-	-	-	-	-
sebaceous cell	C44.13-	-	-	-	-	-
specified type NEC	C44.19-	-	-	-	-	-
squamous cell carcinoma	C44.12-	-	-	-	-	-
face NOS	C44.300	C79.2	D04.30	D23.30	D48.5	D49.2
basal cell carcinoma	C44.310	-	-	-	-	-
specified type NEC	C44.390	-	-	-	-	-
squamous cell carcinoma	C44.320	-	-	-	-	-
female genital organs (external)	C51.9	C79.82	D07.1	D28.0	D39.8	D49.59
clitoris	C51.2	C79.82	D07.1	D28.0	D39.8	D49.59
labium NEC	C51.9	C79.82	D07.1	D28.0	D39.8	D49.59
majus	C51.0	C79.82	D07.1	D28.0	D39.8	D49.59
minus	C51.1	C79.82	D07.1	D28.0	D39.8	D49.59
pudendum	C51.9	C79.82	D07.1	D28.0	D39.8	D49.59
vulva	C51.9	C79.82	D07.1	D28.0	D39.8	D49.59
finger — *see also* Neoplasm, skin, limb, upper	C44.60-	C79.2	D04.6-	D23.6-	D48.5	D49.2
flank — *see also* Neoplasm, skin, trunk	C44.509	C79.2	D04.5	D23.5	D48.5	D49.2
foot — *see also* Neoplasm, skin, limb, lower	C44.70-	C79.2	D04.7-	D23.7-	D48.5	D49.2
forearm — *see also* Neoplasm, skin, limb, upper	C44.60-	C79.2	D04.6-	D23.6-	D48.5	D49.2
forehead — *see also* Neoplasm, skin, face	C44.309	C79.2	D04.39	D23.39	D48.5	D49.2
glabella — *see also* Neoplasm, skin, face	C44.309	C79.2	D04.39	D23.39	D48.5	D49.2
gluteal region — *see also* Neoplasm, skin, trunk	C44.509	C79.2	D04.5	D23.5	D48.5	D49.2
groin — *see also* Neoplasm, skin, trunk	C44.509	C79.2	D04.5	D23.5	D48.5	D49.2
hand — *see also* Neoplasm, skin, limb, upper	C44.60-	C79.2	D04.6-	D23.6-	D48.5	D49.2
head NEC — *see also* Neoplasm, skin, scalp	C44.40	C79.2	D04.4	D23.4	D48.5	D49.2
heel — *see also* Neoplasm, skin, limb, lower	C44.70-	C79.2	D04.7-	D23.7-	D48.5	D49.2
helix — *see also* Neoplasm, skin, ear	C44.20-	C79.2	D04.2-	D23.2-	D48.5	D49.2
hip — *see also* Neoplasm, skin, limb, lower	C44.70-	C79.2	D04.7-	D23.7-	D48.5	D49.2
infraclavicular region — *see also* Neoplasm, skin, trunk	C44.509	C79.2	D04.5	D23.5	D48.5	D49.2
inguinal region — *see also* Neoplasm, skin, trunk	C44.509	C79.2	D04.5	D23.5	D48.5	D49.2
jaw — *see also* Neoplasm, skin, face	C44.309	C79.2	D04.39	D23.39	D48.5	D49.2
Kaposi's sarcoma — *see* Kaposi's, sarcoma, skin						
knee — *see also* Neoplasm, skin, limb, lower	C44.70-	C79.2	D04.7-	D23.7-	D48.5	D49.2
labia						
majora	C51.0	C79.82	D07.1	D28.0	D39.8	D49.59
minora	C51.1	C79.82	D07.1	D28.0	D39.8	D49.59
leg — *see also* Neoplasm, skin, limb, lower	C44.70-	C79.2	D04.7-	D23.7-	D48.5	D49.2
lid (lower) (upper)	C44.10-	C79.2	D04.1-	D23.1-	D48.5	D49.2
basal cell carcinoma	C44.11-	-	-	-	-	-
sebaceous cell	C44.13-	-	-	-	-	-
specified type NEC	C44.19-	-	-	-	-	-
squamous cell carcinoma	C44.12-	-	-	-	-	-
limb NEC	C44.90	C79.2	D04.9	D23.9	D48.5	D49.2
basal cell carcinoma	C44.91					
lower	C44.70-	C79.2	D04.7-	D23.7-	D48.5	D49.2
basal cell carcinoma	C44.71-	-	-	-	-	-
specified type NEC	C44.79-	-	-	-	-	-
squamous cell carcinoma	C44.72-	-	-	-	-	-
upper	C44.60-	C79.2	D04.6-	D23.6-	D48.5	D49.2
basal cell carcinoma	C44.61-	-	-	-	-	-
specified type NEC	C44.69-	-	-	-	-	-
squamous cell carcinoma	C44.62-	-	-	-	-	-
lip (lower) (upper)	C44.00	C79.2	D04.0	D23.0	D48.5	D49.2
basal cell carcinoma	C44.01	-	-	-	-	-
specified type NEC	C44.09	-	-	-	-	-
squamous cell carcinoma	C44.02	-	-	-	-	-
male genital organs	C63.9	C79.82	D07.60	D29.9	D40.8	D49.59
penis	C60.9	C79.82	D07.4	D29.0	D40.8	D49.59
prepuce	C60.0	C79.82	D07.4	D29.0	D40.8	D49.59
scrotum	C63.2	C79.82	D07.61	D29.4	D40.8	D49.59
mastectomy site (skin) — *see also* Neoplasm, skin, breast	C44.501	C79.2	-	-	-	-
specified as breast tissue	C50.8-	C79.81	-	-	-	-
meatus, acoustic (external) — *see also* Neoplasm, skin, ear	C44.20-	C79.2	D04.2-	D23.2-	D48.5	D49.2
melanotic — *see* Melanoma						
Merkel cell — *see* Carcinoma, Merkel cell						
nates — *see also* Neoplasm, skin, trunk	C44.509	C79.2	D04.5	D23.5	D48.5	D49.2
neck	C44.40	C79.2	D04.4	D23.4	D48.5	D49.2
basal cell carcinoma	C44.41	-	-	-	-	-
specified type NEC	C44.49	-	-	-	-	-
squamous cell carcinoma	C44.42	-	-	-	-	-
nevus — *see* Nevus, skin						
nose (external) — *see also* Neoplasm, nose, skin	C44.301	C79.2	D04.39	D23.39	D48.5	D49.2
overlapping lesion	C44.80	-	-	-	-	-
basal cell carcinoma	C44.81	-	-	-	-	-
specified type NEC	C44.89	-	-	-	-	-
squamous cell carcinoma	C44.82	-	-	-	-	-
palm — *see also* Neoplasm, skin, limb, upper	C44.60-	C79.2	D04.6-	D23.6-	D48.5	D49.2
palpebra	C44.10-	C79.2	D04.1-	D23.1-	D48.5	D49.2
basal cell carcinoma	C44.11-	-	-	-	-	-
sebaceous cell	C44.13-	-	-	-	-	-
specified type NEC	C44.19-	-	-	-	-	-
squamous cell carcinoma	C44.12-	-	-	-	-	-
penis NEC	C60.9	C79.82	D07.4	D29.0	D40.8	D49.59
perianal — *see also* Neoplasm, skin, anus	C44.500	C79.2	D04.5	D23.5	D48.5	D49.2
perineum — *see also* Neoplasm, skin, anus	C44.500	C79.2	D04.5	D23.5	D48.5	D49.2
pinna — *see also* Neoplasm, skin, ear	C44.20-	C79.2	D04.2-	D23.2-	D48.5	D49.2
plantar — *see also* Neoplasm, skin, limb, lower	C44.70-	C79.2	D04.7-	D23.7-	D48.5	D49.2
popliteal fossa or space — *see also* Neoplasm, skin, limb, lower	C44.70-	C79.2	D04.7-	D23.7-	D48.5	D49.2
prepuce	C60.0	C79.82	D07.4	D29.0	D40.8	D49.59
pubes — *see also* Neoplasm, skin, trunk	C44.509	C79.2	D04.5	D23.5	D48.5	D49.2
sacrococcygeal region — *see also* Neoplasm, skin, trunk	C44.509	C79.2	D04.5	D23.5	D48.5	D49.2
scalp	C44.40	C79.2	D04.4	D23.4	D48.5	D49.2
basal cell carcinoma	C44.41	-	-	-	-	-
specified type NEC	C44.49	-	-	-	-	-
squamous cell carcinoma	C44.42	-	-	-	-	-
scapular region — *see also* Neoplasm, skin, trunk	C44.509	C79.2	D04.5	D23.5	D48.5	D49.2
scrotum	C63.2	C79.82	D07.61	D29.4	D40.8	D49.59
shoulder — *see also* Neoplasm, skin, limb, upper	C44.60-	C79.2	D04.6-	D23.6-	D48.5	D49.2
sole (foot) — *see also* Neoplasm, skin, limb, lower	C44.70-	C79.2	D04.7-	D23.7-	D48.5	D49.2
specified sites NEC	C44.80	C79.2	D04.8	D23.9	D48.5	D49.2
basal cell carcinoma	C44.81	-	-	-	-	-
specified type NEC	C44.89	-	-	-	-	-
squamous cell carcinoma	C44.82	-	-	-	-	-
specified type NEC	C44.99	-	-	-	-	-
squamous cell carcinoma	C44.92	-	-	-	-	-
submammary fold — *see also* Neoplasm, skin, trunk	C44.509	C79.2	D04.5	D23.5	D48.5	D49.2

Neoplasm, neoplastic	Malignant Primary	Malignant Secondary	Ca in situ	Benign	Uncertain Behavior	Unspecified Behavior
skin NOS - *continued*						
supraclavicular region — *see also* Neoplasm, skin, neck	C44.40	C79.2	D04.4	D23.4	D48.5	D49.2
temple — *see also* Neoplasm, skin, face	C44.309	C79.2	D04.39	D23.39	D48.5	D49.2
thigh — *see also* Neoplasm, skin, limb, lower	C44.70-	C79.2	D04.7-	D23.7-	D48.5	D49.2
thoracic wall — *see also* Neoplasm, skin, trunk	C44.509	C79.2	D04.5	D23.5	D48.5	D49.2
thumb — *see also* Neoplasm, skin, limb, upper	C44.60-	C79.2	D04.6-	D23.6-	D48.5	D49.2
toe — *see also* Neoplasm, skin, limb, lower	C44.70-	C79.2	D04.7-	D23.7-	D48.5	D49.2
tragus — *see also* Neoplasm, skin, ear	C44.20-	C79.2	D04.2-	D23.2-	D48.5	D49.2
trunk	C44.509	C79.2	D04.5	D23.5	D48.5	D49.2
basal cell carcinoma	C44.519	-	-	-	-	-
specified type NEC	C44.599	-	-	-	-	-
squamous cell carcinoma	C44.529	-	-	-	-	-
umbilicus — *see also* Neoplasm, skin, trunk	C44.509	C79.2	D04.5	D23.5	D48.5	D49.2
vulva	C51.9	C79.82	D07.1	D28.0	D39.8	D49.59
overlapping lesion	C51.8	-	-	-	-	-
wrist — *see also* Neoplasm, skin, limb, upper	C44.60-	C79.2	D04.6-	D23.6-	D48.5	D49.2
skull	C41.0	C79.51	-	D16.4-	D48.0	D49.2
soft parts or tissues — *see* Neoplasm, connective tissue						
specified site NEC	C76.8	C79.89	D09.8	D36.7	D48.7	D49.89
spermatic cord	C63.1-	C79.82	D07.69	D29.8	D40.8	D49.59
sphenoid	C31.3	C78.39	D02.3	D14.0	D38.5	D49.1
bone	C41.0	C79.51	-	D16.4-	D48.0	D49.2
sinus	C31.3	C78.39	D02.3	D14.0	D38.5	D49.1
sphincter						
anal	C21.1	C78.5	D01.3	D12.9	D37.8	D49.0
of Oddi	C24.0	C78.89	D01.5	D13.5	D37.6	D49.0
spine, spinal (column)	C41.2	C79.51	-	D16.6	D48.0	D49.2
bulb	C71.7	C79.31	-	D33.1	D43.1	D49.6
coccyx	C41.4	C79.51	-	D16.8	D48.0	D49.2
cord (cervical) (lumbar) (sacral) (thoracic)	C72.0	C79.49	-	D33.4	D43.4	D49.7
dura mater	C70.1	C79.49	-	D32.1	D42.1	D49.7
lumbosacral	C41.2	C79.51	-	D16.6	D48.0	D49.2
marrow NEC	C96.9	C79.52	-	-	D47.9	D49.89
membrane	C70.1	C79.49	-	D32.1	D42.1	D49.7
meninges	C70.1	C79.49	-	D32.1	D42.1	D49.7
nerve (root)	C47.9	C79.89	-	D36.10	D48.2	D49.2
pia mater	C70.1	C79.49	-	D32.1	D42.1	D49.7
root	C47.9	C79.89	-	D36.10	D48.2	D49.2
sacrum	C41.4	C79.51	-	D16.8	D48.0	D49.2
spleen, splenic NEC	C26.1	C78.89	D01.7	D13.9	D37.8	D49.0
flexure (colon)	C18.5	C78.5	D01.0	D12.3	D37.4	D49.0
stem, brain	C71.7	C79.31	-	D33.1	D43.1	D49.6
Stensen's duct	C07	C79.89	D00.00	D11.0	D37.030	D49.0
sternum	C41.3	C79.51	-	D16.7	D48.0	D49.2
stomach	C16.9	C78.89	D00.2	D13.1	D37.1	D49.0
antrum (pyloric)	C16.3	C78.89	D00.2	D13.1	D37.1	D49.0
body	C16.2	C78.89	D00.2	D13.1	D37.1	D49.0
cardia	C16.0	C78.89	D00.2	D13.1	D37.1	D49.0
cardiac orifice	C16.0	C78.89	D00.2	D13.1	D37.1	D49.0
corpus	C16.2	C78.89	D00.2	D13.1	D37.1	D49.0
fundus	C16.1	C78.89	D00.2	D13.1	D37.1	D49.0
greater curvature NEC	C16.6	C78.89	D00.2	D13.1	D37.1	D49.0
lesser curvature NEC	C16.5	C78.89	D00.2	D13.1	D37.1	D49.0
overlapping lesion	C16.8	-	-	-	-	-
prepylorus	C16.4	C78.89	D00.2	D13.1	D37.1	D49.0
pylorus	C16.4	C78.89	D00.2	D13.1	D37.1	D49.0
wall NEC	C16.9	C78.89	D00.2	D13.1	D37.1	D49.0
anterior NEC	C16.8	C78.89	D00.2	D13.1	D37.1	D49.0
posterior NEC	C16.8	C78.89	D00.2	D13.1	D37.1	D49.0
stroma, endometrial	C54.1	C79.82	D07.0	D26.1	D39.0	D49.59
stump, cervical	C53.8	C79.82	D06.7	D26.0	D39.0	D49.59
subcutaneous (nodule) (tissue) NEC — *see* Neoplasm, connective tissue						
subdural	C70.9	C79.32	-	D32.9	D42.9	D49.7
subglottis, subglottic	C32.2	C78.39	D02.0	D14.1	D38.0	D49.1
sublingual	C04.9	C79.89	D00.06	D10.2	D37.09	D49.0
gland or duct	C08.1	C79.89	D00.00	D11.7	D37.031	D49.0
submandibular gland	C08.0	C79.89	D00.00	D11.7	D37.032	D49.0
submaxillary gland or duct	C08.0	C79.89	D00.00	D11.7	D37.032	D49.0
submental	C76.0	C79.89	D09.8	D36.7	D48.7	D49.89
subpleural	C34.9-	C78.0-	D02.2-	D14.3-	D38.1	D49.1
substernal	C38.1	C78.1	-	D15.2	D38.3	D49.89
sudoriferous, sudoriparous gland, site unspecified	C44.90	C79.2	D04.9	D23.9	D48.5	D49.2
specified site — *see* Neoplasm, skin						
supraclavicular region	C76.0	C79.89	D09.8	D36.7	D48.7	D49.89
supraglottis	C32.1	C78.39	D02.0	D14.1	D38.0	D49.1
suprarenal	C74.9-	C79.7-	D09.3	D35.0-	D44.1-	D49.7
capsule	C74.9-	C79.7-	D09.3	D35.0-	D44.1-	D49.7
cortex	C74.0-	C79.7-	D09.3	D35.0-	D44.1-	D49.7
gland	C74.9-	C79.7-	D09.3	D35.0-	D44.1-	D49.7
medulla	C74.1-	C79.7-	D09.3	D35.0-	D44.1-	D49.7
suprasellar (region)	C71.9	C79.31	-	D33.2	D43.2	D49.6
supratentorial (brain) NEC	C71.0	C79.31	-	D33.0	D43.0	D49.6
sweat gland (apocrine) (eccrine) , site unspecified	C44.90	C79.2	D04.9	D23.9	D48.5	D49.2
specified site — *see* Neoplasm, skin						
sympathetic nerve or nervous system NEC	C47.9	C79.89	-	D36.10	D48.2	D49.2
symphysis pubis	C41.4	C79.51	-	D16.8	D48.0	D49.2
synovial membrane — *see* Neoplasm, connective tissue						
tapetum, brain	C71.8	C79.31	-	D33.2	D43.2	D49.6
tarsus (any bone)	C40.3-	C79.51	-	D16.3-	-	-
temple (skin) — *see also* Neoplasm, skin, face	C44.309	C79.2	D04.39	D23.39	D48.5	D49.2
temporal						
bone	C41.0	C79.51	-	D16.4-	D48.0	D49.2
lobe or pole	C71.2	C79.31	-	D33.0	D43.0	D49.6
region	C76.0	C79.89	D09.8	D36.7	D48.7	D49.89
skin — *see also* Neoplasm, skin, face	C44.309	C79.2	D04.39	D23.39	D48.5	D49.2
tendon (sheath) — *see* Neoplasm, connective tissue						
tentorium (cerebelli)	C70.0	C79.32	-	D32.0	D42.0	D49.7
testis, testes	C62.9-	C79.82	D07.69	D29.2-	D40.1-	D49.59
descended	C62.1-	C79.82	D07.69	D29.2-	D40.1-	D49.59
ectopic	C62.0-	C79.82	D07.69	D29.2-	D40.1-	D49.59
retained	C62.0-	C79.82	D07.69	D29.2-	D40.1-	D49.59
scrotal	C62.1-	C79.82	D07.69	D29.2-	D40.1-	D49.59
undescended	C62.0-	C79.82	D07.69	D29.2-	D40.1-	D49.59
unspecified whether descended or undescended	C62.9-	C79.82	D07.69	D29.2-	D40.1-	D49.59
thalamus	C71.0	C79.31	-	D33.0	D43.0	D49.6
thigh NEC	C76.5-	C79.89	D04.7-	D36.7	D48.7	D49.89
thorax, thoracic (cavity) (organs NEC)	C76.1	C79.89	D09.8	D36.7	D48.7	D49.89
duct	C49.3	C79.89	-	D21.3	D48.1	D49.2
wall NEC	C76.1	C79.89	D09.8	D36.7	D48.7	D49.89
throat	C14.0	C79.89	D00.08	D10.9	D37.05	D49.0
thumb NEC	C76.4-	C79.89	D04.6-	D36.7	D48.7	D49.89
thymus (gland)	C37	C79.89	D09.3	D15.0	D38.4	D49.89
thyroglossal duct	C73	C79.89	D09.3	D34	D44.0	D49.7
thyroid (gland)	C73	C79.89	D09.3	D34	D44.0	D49.7
cartilage	C32.3	C78.39	D02.0	D14.1	D38.0	D49.1
tibia (any part)	C40.2-	C79.51	-	D16.2-	-	-
toe NEC	C76.5-	C79.89	D04.7-	D36.7	D48.7	D49.89
tongue	C02.9	C79.89	D00.07	D10.1	D37.02	D49.0
anterior (two-thirds) NEC	C02.3	C79.89	D00.07	D10.1	D37.02	D49.0
dorsal surface	C02.0	C79.89	D00.07	D10.1	D37.02	D49.0
ventral surface	C02.2	C79.89	D00.07	D10.1	D37.02	D49.0
base (dorsal surface)	C01	C79.89	D00.07	D10.1	D37.02	D49.0
border (lateral)	C02.1	C79.89	D00.07	D10.1	D37.02	D49.0
dorsal surface NEC	C02.0	C79.89	D00.07	D10.1	D37.02	D49.0
fixed part NEC	C01	C79.89	D00.07	D10.1	D37.02	D49.0
foreamen cecum	C02.0	C79.89	D00.07	D10.1	D37.02	D49.0
frenulum linguae	C02.2	C79.89	D00.07	D10.1	D37.02	D49.0
junctional zone	C02.8	C79.89	D00.07	D10.1	D37.02	D49.0
margin (lateral)	C02.1	C79.89	D00.07	D10.1	D37.02	D49.0
midline NEC	C02.0	C79.89	D00.07	D10.1	D37.02	D49.0
mobile part NEC	C02.3	C79.89	D00.07	D10.1	D37.02	D49.0
overlapping lesion	C02.8	-	-	-	-	-
posterior (third)	C01	C79.89	D00.07	D10.1	D37.02	D49.0
root	C01	C79.89	D00.07	D10.1	D37.02	D49.0
surface (dorsal)	C02.0	C79.89	D00.07	D10.1	D37.02	D49.0

Neoplasm, neoplastic	Malignant Primary	Malignant Secondary	Ca in situ	Benign	Uncertain Behavior	Unspecified Behavior
tongue - *continued*						
base	C01	C79.89	D00.07	D10.1	D37.02	D49.0
ventral	C02.2	C79.89	D00.07	D10.1	D37.02	D49.0
tip	C02.1	C79.89	D00.07	D10.1	D37.02	D49.0
tonsil	C02.4	C79.89	D00.07	D10.1	D37.02	D49.0
tonsil	C09.9	C79.89	D00.08	D10.4	D37.05	D49.0
fauces, faucial	C09.9	C79.89	D00.08	D10.4	D37.05	D49.0
lingual	C02.4	C79.89	D00.07	D10.1	D37.02	D49.0
overlapping sites	C09.8	-	-	-	-	-
palatine	C09.9	C79.89	D00.08	D10.4	D37.05	D49.0
pharyngeal	C11.1	C79.89	D00.08	D10.6	D37.05	D49.0
pillar (anterior) (posterior)	C09.1	C79.89	D00.08	D10.5	D37.05	D49.0
tonsillar fossa	C09.0	C79.89	D00.08	D10.5	D37.05	D49.0
tooth socket NEC	C03.9	C79.89	D00.03	D10.39	D37.09	D49.0
trachea (cartilage) (mucosa)	C33	C78.39	D02.1	D14.2	D38.1	D49.1
overlapping lesion with bronchus or lung	C34.8-	-	-	-	-	-
tracheobronchial	C34.8-	C78.39	D02.1	D14.2	D38.1	D49.1
overlapping lesion with lung	C34.8-	-	-	-	-	-
tragus — *see also* Neoplasm, skin, ear	C44.20-	C79.2	D04.2-	D23.2-	D48.5	D49.2
trunk NEC	C76.8	C79.89	D04.5	D36.7	D48.7	D49.89
tubo-ovarian	C57.8	C79.82	D07.39	D28.7	D39.8	D49.59
tunica vaginalis	C63.7	C79.82	D07.69	D29.8	D40.8	D49.59
turbinate (bone)	C41.0	C79.51	-	D16.4-	D48.0	D49.2
nasal	C30.0	C78.39	D02.3	D14.0	D38.5	D49.1
tympanic cavity	C30.1	C78.39	D02.3	D14.0	D38.5	D49.1
ulna (any part)	C40.0-	C79.51	-	D16.0-	-	-
umbilicus, umbilical — *see also* Neoplasm, skin, trunk	C44.509	C79.2	D04.5	D23.5	D48.5	D49.2
uncus, brain	C71.2	C79.31	-	D33.0	D43.0	D49.6
unknown site or unspecified	C80.1	C79.9	D09.9	D36.9	D48.9	D49.9
urachus	C67.7	C79.11	D09.0	D30.3	D41.4	D49.4
ureter, ureteral	C66.-	C79.19	D09.19	D30.2-	D41.2-	D49.59
orifice (bladder)	C67.6	C79.11	D09.0	D30.3	D41.4	D49.4
ureter-bladder (junction)	C67.6	C79.11	D09.0	D30.3	D41.4	D49.4
urethra, urethral (gland)	C68.0	C79.19	D09.19	D30.4	D41.3	D49.59
orifice, internal	C67.5	C79.11	D09.0	D30.3	D41.4	D49.4
urethrovaginal (septum)	C57.9	C79.82	D07.30	D28.9	D39.8	D49.59
urinary organ or system	C68.9	C79.10	D09.10	D30.9	D41.9	D49.59
bladder — *see* Neoplasm, bladder						
overlapping lesion	C68.8	-	-	-	-	-
specified sites NEC	C68.8	C79.19	D09.19	D30.8	D41.8	D49.59
utero-ovarian	C57.8	C79.82	D07.39	D28.7	D39.8	D49.59
ligament	C57.1	C79.82	D07.39	D28.2	D39.8	D49.59
uterosacral ligament	C57.3	C79.82	-	D28.2	D39.8	D49.59
uterus, uteri, uterine	C55	C79.82	D07.0	D26.9	D39.0	D49.59
adnexa NEC	C57.4	C79.82	D07.39	D28.7	D39.8	D49.59
body	C54.9	C79.82	D07.0	D26.1	D39.0	D49.59
cervix	C53.9	C79.82	D06.9	D26.0	D39.0	D49.59
cornu	C54.9	C79.82	D07.0	D26.1	D39.0	D49.59
corpus	C54.9	C79.82	D07.0	D26.1	D39.0	D49.59
endocervix (canal) (gland)	C53.0	C79.82	D06.0	D26.0	D39.0	D49.59
endometrium	C54.1	C79.82	D07.0	D26.1	D39.0	D49.59
exocervix	C53.1	C79.82	D06.1	D26.0	D39.0	D49.59
external os	C53.1	C79.82	D06.1	D26.0	D39.0	D49.59
fundus	C54.3	C79.82	D07.0	D26.1	D39.0	D49.59
internal os	C53.0	C79.82	D06.0	D26.0	D39.0	D49.59
isthmus	C54.0	C79.82	D07.0	D26.1	D39.0	D49.59
ligament	C57.3	C79.82	-	D28.2	D39.8	D49.59
broad	C57.1	C79.82	D07.39	D28.2	D39.8	D49.59
round	C57.2	C79.82	-	D28.2	D39.8	D49.59
lower segment	C54.0	C79.82	D07.0	D26.1	D39.0	D49.59
myometrium	C54.2	C79.82	D07.0	D26.1	D39.0	D49.59
overlapping sites	C54.8	-	-	-	-	-
squamocolumnar junction	C53.8	C79.82	D06.7	D26.0	D39.0	D49.59
tube	C57.0-	C79.82	D07.39	D28.2	D39.8	D49.59
utricle, prostatic	C68.0	C79.19	D09.19	D30.4	D41.3	D49.59
uveal tract	C69.4-	C79.49	D09.2-	D31.4-	D48.7	D49.89
uvula	C05.2	C79.89	D00.04	D10.39	D37.09	D49.0
vagina, vaginal (fornix) (vault) (wall)	C52	C79.82	D07.2	D28.1	D39.8	D49.59
vaginovesical	C57.9	C79.82	D07.30	D28.9	D39.9	D49.59
septum	C57.9	C79.82	D07.30	D28.9	D39.9	D49.59
vallecula (epiglottis)	C10.0	C79.89	D00.08	D10.5	D37.05	D49.0
vas deferens	C63.1-	C79.82	D07.69	D29.8	D40.8	D49.59
vascular — *see* Neoplasm, connective tissue						
Vater's ampulla	C24.1	C78.89	D01.5	D13.5	D37.6	D49.0

Neoplasm, neoplastic	Malignant Primary	Malignant Secondary	Ca in situ	Benign	Uncertain Behavior	Unspecified Behavior
vein, venous — *see* Neoplasm, connective tissue						
vena cava (abdominal) (inferior)	C49.4	C79.89	-	D21.4	D48.1	D49.2
superior	C49.3	C79.89	-	D21.3	D48.1	D49.2
ventricle (cerebral) (floor) (lateral) (third)	C71.5	C79.31	-	D33.0	D43.0	D49.6
cardiac (left) (right)	C38.0	C79.89	-	D15.1	D48.7	D49.89
fourth	C71.7	C79.31	-	D33.1	D43.1	D49.6
ventricular band of larynx	C32.1	C78.39	D02.0	D14.1	D38.0	D49.1
ventriculus — *see* Neoplasm, stomach						
vermillion border — *see* Neoplasm, lip						
vermis, cerebellum	C71.6	C79.31	-	D33.1	D43.1	D49.6
vertebra (column)	C41.2	C79.51	-	D16.6	D48.0	D49.2
coccyx	C41.4	C79.51	-	D16.8-	D48.0	D49.2
marrow NEC	C96.9	C79.52	-	-	D47.9	D49.89
sacrum	C41.4	C79.51	-	D16.8-	D48.0	D49.2
vesical — *see* Neoplasm, bladder						
vesicle, seminal	C63.7	C79.82	D07.69	D29.8	D40.8	D49.59
vesicocervical tissue	C57.9	C79.82	D07.30	D28.9	D39.9	D49.59
vesicorectal	C76.3	C79.82	D09.8	D36.7	D48.7	D49.89
vesicovaginal	C57.9	C79.82	D07.30	D28.9	D39.9	D49.59
septum	C57.9	C79.82	D07.30	D28.9	D39.8	D49.59
vessel (blood) — *see* Neoplasm, connective tissue						
vestibular gland, greater	C51.0	C79.82	D07.1	D28.0	D39.8	D49.59
vestibule						
mouth	C06.1	C79.89	D00.00	D10.39	D37.09	D49.0
nose	C30.0	C78.39	D02.3	D14.0	D38.5	D49.1
Virchow's gland	C77.0	C77.0	-	D36.0	D48.7	D49.89
viscera NEC	C76.8	C79.89	D09.8	D36.7	D48.7	D49.89
vocal cords (true)	C32.0	C78.39	D02.0	D14.1	D38.0	D49.1
false	C32.1	C78.39	D02.0	D14.1	D38.0	D49.1
vomer	C41.0	C79.51	-	D16.4-	D48.0	D49.2
vulva	C51.9	C79.82	D07.1	D28.0	D39.8	D49.59
vulvovaginal gland	C51.0	C79.82	D07.1	D28.0	D39.8	D49.59
Waldeyer's ring	C14.2	C79.89	D00.08	D10.9	D37.05	D49.0
Wharton's duct	C08.0	C79.89	D00.00	D11.7	D37.032	D49.0
white matter (central) (cerebral)	C71.0	C79.31	-	D33.0	D43.0	D49.6
windpipe	C33	C78.39	D02.1	D14.2	D38.1	D49.1
Wirsung's duct	C25.3	C78.89	D01.7	D13.6	D37.8	D49.0
wolffian (body) (duct)						
female	C57.7	C79.82	D07.39	D28.7	D39.8	D49.59
male	C63.7	C79.82	D07.69	D29.8	D40.8	D49.59
womb — *see* Neoplasm, uterus						
wrist NEC	C76.4-	C79.89	D04.6-	D36.7	D48.7	D49.89
xiphoid process	C41.3	C79.51	-	D16.7	D48.0	D49.2
Zuckerkandl organ	C75.5	C79.89	-	D35.6	D44.7	D49.7

Neovascularization
  ciliary body — *see* Disorder, iris, vascular
  cornea H16.40-
    deep H16.44-
    ghost vessels — *see* Ghost, vessels
    localized H16.43-
    pannus — *see* Pannus
  iris — *see* Disorder, iris, vascular
  retina H35.05-
Nephralgia N23
Nephritis, nephritic (albuminuric) (azotemic) (congenital) (disseminated) (epithelial) (familial) (focal) (granulomatous) (hemorrhagic) (infantile) (nonsuppurative, excretory) (uremic) N05.9
  with
    dense deposit disease N05.6
    diffuse
      crescentic glomerulonephritis N05.7
      endocapillary proliferative glomerulonephritis N05.4
      membranous glomerulonephritis N05.2
      mesangial proliferative glomerulonephritis N05.3
      mesangiocapillary glomerulonephritis N05.5
    edema — *see* Nephrosis
    focal and segmental glomerular lesions N05.1
    foot process disease N04.9
    glomerular lesion
      diffuse sclerosing N05.8
      hypocomplementemic — *see* Nephritis, membranoproliferative
      IgA — *see* Nephropathy, IgA
      lobular, lobulonodular — *see* Nephritis, membranoproliferative
      nodular — *see* Nephritis, membranoproliferative
    lesion of
      glomerulonephritis, proliferative N05.8
      renal necrosis N05.9
    minor glomerular abnormality N05.0
    specified morphological changes NEC N05.8
  acute N00.9
    with
      dense deposit disease N00.6
      diffuse
        crescentic glomerulonephritis N00.7
        endocapillary proliferative glomerulonephritis N00.4
        membranous glomerulonephritis N00.2
        mesangial proliferative glomerulonephritis N00.3
        mesangiocapillary glomerulonephritis N00.5
      focal and segmental glomerular lesions N00.1
      minor glomerular abnormality N00.0
      specified morphological changes NEC N00.8
  amyloid E85.4 *[N08]*
  antiglomerular basement membrane (anti-GBM) antibody NEC
    in Goodpasture's syndrome M31.0
  antitubular basement membrane (tubulo-interstitial) NEC N12
    toxic — *see* Nephropathy, toxic
  arteriolar — *see* Hypertension, kidney
  arteriosclerotic — *see* Hypertension, kidney
  ascending — *see* Nephritis, tubulo-interstitial
  atrophic N03.9
  Balkan (endemic) N15.0
  calculous, calculus — *see* Calculus, kidney
  cardiac — *see* Hypertension, kidney
  cardiovascular — *see* Hypertension, kidney
  chronic N03.9
    with
      dense deposit disease N03.6
      diffuse
        crescentic glomerulonephritis N03.7
        endocapillary proliferative glomerulonephritis N03.4
        membranous glomerulonephritis N03.2
        mesangial proliferative glomerulonephritis N03.3
        mesangiocapillary glomerulonephritis N03.5
      focal and segmental glomerular lesions N03.1
      minor glomerular abnormality N03.0
      specified morphological changes NEC N03.8
    arteriosclerotic — *see* Hypertension, kidney
  cirrhotic N26.9
  complicating pregnancy O26.83-
  croupous N00.9
  degenerative — *see* Nephrosis
  diffuse sclerosing N05.8
  due to
    diabetes mellitus — *see* E08-E13 with .21
    subacute bacterial endocarditis I33.0
    systemic lupus erythematosus (chronic) M32.14
    typhoid fever A01.09

Nephritis, nephritic (albuminuric) (azotemic) (congenital) (disseminated) (epithelial) (familial) (focal) (granulomatous) (hemorrhagic) (infantile) (nonsuppurative, excretory) (uremic) - *continued*
  gonococcal (acute) (chronic) A54.21
  hypocomplementemic — *see* Nephritis, membranoproliferative
  IgA — *see* Nephropathy, IgA
  immune complex (circulating) NEC N05.8
  infective — *see* Nephritis, tubulo-interstitial
  interstitial — *see* Nephritis, tubulo-interstitial
  lead N14.3
  membranoproliferative (diffuse) (type 1 or 3) — *see also* N00-N07 with fourth character .5 N05.5
    type 2 — *see also* N00-N07 with fourth character .6 N05.6
  minimal change N05.0
  necrotic, necrotizing NEC — *see also* N00-N07 with fourth character .8 N05.8
  nephrotic — *see* Nephrosis
  nodular — *see* Nephritis, membranoproliferative
  polycystic Q61.3
    adult type Q61.2
    autosomal
      dominant Q61.2
      recessive NEC Q61.19
    childhood type NEC Q61.19
    infantile type NEC Q61.19
  poststreptococcal N05.9
    acute N00.9
    chronic N03.9
    rapidly progressive N01.9
  proliferative NEC — *see also* N00-N07 with fourth character .8 N05.8
  purulent — *see* Nephritis, tubulo-interstitial
  rapidly progressive N01.9
    with
      dense deposit disease N01.6
      diffuse
        crescentic glomerulonephritis N01.7
        endocapillary proliferative glomerulonephritis N01.4
        membranous glomerulonephritis N01.2
        mesangial proliferative glomerulonephritis N01.3
        mesangiocapillary glomerulonephritis N01.5
      focal and segmental glomerular lesions N01.1
      minor glomerular abnormality N01.0
      specified morphological changes NEC N01.8
  salt losing or wasting NEC N28.89
  saturnine N14.3
  sclerosing, diffuse N05.8
  septic — *see* Nephritis, tubulo-interstitial
  specified pathology NEC — *see also* N00-N07 with fourth character .8 N05.8
  subacute N01.9
  suppurative — *see* Nephritis, tubulo-interstitial
  syphilitic (late) A52.75
    congenital A50.59 *[N08]*
    early (secondary) A51.44
  toxic — *see* Nephropathy, toxic
  tubal, tubular — *see* Nephritis, tubulo-interstitial
  tuberculous A18.11
  tubulo-interstitial (in) N12
    acute (infectious) N10
    chronic (infectious) N11.9
      nonobstructive N11.8
        reflux-associated N11.0
      obstructive N11.1
      specified NEC N11.8
    due to
      brucellosis A23.9 *[N16]*
      cryoglobulinemia D89.1 *[N16]*
      glycogen storage disease E74.00 *[N16]*
    Sjögren's syndrome M35.04
  vascular — *see* Hypertension, kidney
  war N00.9
Nephroblastoma (epithelial) (mesenchymal) C64-
Nephrocalcinosis E83.59 *[N29]*
Nephrocystitis, pustular — *see* Nephritis, tubulo-interstitial
Nephrolithiasis (congenital) (pelvis) (recurrent) — *see also* Calculus, kidney
Nephroma C64-
  mesoblastic D41.0-
Nephronephritis — *see* Nephrosis
Nephronophthisis Q61.5
Nephropathia epidemica A98.5
Nephropathy — *see also* Nephritis N28.9
  with
    edema — *see* Nephrosis
    glomerular lesion — *see* Glomerulonephritis
  amyloid, hereditary E85.0

Nephropathy - *continued*
  analgesic N14.0
    with medullary necrosis, acute N17.2
  Balkan (endemic) N15.0
  chemical — *see* Nephropathy, toxic
  diabetic — *see* E08-E13 with .21
  drug-induced N14.2
    specified NEC N14.1
  focal and segmental hyalinosis or sclerosis N02.1
  heavy metal-induced N14.3
  hereditary NEC N07.9
    with
      dense deposit disease N07.6
      diffuse
        crescentic glomerulonephritis N07.7
        endocapillary proliferative glomerulonephritis N07.4
        membranous glomerulonephritis N07.2
        mesangial proliferative glomerulonephritis N07.3
        mesangiocapillary glomerulonephritis N07.5
      focal and segmental glomerular lesions N07.1
      minor glomerular abnormality N07.0
      specified morphological changes NEC N07.8
  hypercalcemic N25.89
  hypertensive — *see* Hypertension, kidney
  hypokalemic (vacuolar) N25.89
  IgA N02.8
    with glomerular lesion N02.9
      focal and segmental hyalinosis or sclerosis N02.1
      membranoproliferative (diffuse) N02.5
      membranous (diffuse) N02.2
      mesangial proliferative (diffuse) N02.3
      mesangiocapillary (diffuse) N02.5
      proliferative NEC N02.8
      specified pathology NEC N02.8
  lead N14.3
  membranoproliferative (diffuse) N02.5
  membranous (diffuse) N02.2
  mesangial (IgA/IgG) — *see* Nephropathy, IgA
    proliferative (diffuse) N02.3
  mesangiocapillary (diffuse) N02.5
  obstructive N13.8
  phenacetin N17.2
  phosphate-losing N25.0
  potassium depletion N25.89
  pregnancy-related O26.83-
  proliferative NEC — *see also* N00-N07 with fourth character .8 N05.8
  protein-losing N25.89
  saturnine N14.3
  sickle-cell D57.- *[N08]*
  toxic NEC N14.4
    due to
      drugs N14.2
        analgesic N14.0
        specified NEC N14.1
      heavy metals N14.3
  vasomotor N17.0
  water-losing N25.89
Nephroptosis N28.83
Nephropyosis — *see* Abscess, kidney
Nephrorrhagia N28.89
Nephrosclerosis (arteriolar) (arteriosclerotic) (chronic) (hyaline) — *see also* Hypertension, kidney
  hyperplastic — *see* Hypertension, kidney
  senile N26.9
Nephrosis, nephrotic (Epstein's) (syndrome) (congenital) N04.9
  with
    foot process disease N04.9
    glomerular lesion N04.1
    hypocomplementemic N04.5
  acute N04.9
  anoxic — *see* Nephrosis, tubular
  chemical — *see* Nephrosis, tubular
  cholemic K76.7
  diabetic — *see* E08-E13 with .21
  Finnish type (congenital) Q89.8
  hemoglobin N10
  hemoglobinuric — *see* Nephrosis, tubular
  in
    amyloidosis E85.4 *[N08]*
    diabetes mellitus — *see* E08-E13 with .21
    epidemic hemorrhagic fever A98.5
    malaria (malariae) B52.0
  ischemic — *see* Nephrosis, tubular
  lipoid N04.9
  lower nephron — *see* Nephrosis, tubular
  malarial (malariae) B52.0
  minimal change N04.0
  myoglobin N10
  necrotizing — *see* Nephrosis, tubular

Neuropathy, neuropathic - *continued*
bladder N31.9
atonic (motor) (sensory) N31.2
autonomous N31.2
flaccid N31.2
nonreflex N31.2
reflex N31.1
uninhibited N31.0
brachial plexus G54.0
cervical plexus G54.2
chronic
progressive segmentally demyelinating G62.89
relapsing demyelinating G62.89
Déjérine-Sottas G60.0
diabetic — *see* E08-E13 with .40
mononeuropathy — *see* E08-E13 with .41
polyneuropathy — *see* E08-E13 with .42
entrapment G58.9
iliohypogastric nerve G57.8-
ilioinguinal nerve G57.8-
lateral cutaneous nerve of thigh G57.1-
median nerve G56.0-
obturator nerve G57.8-
peroneal nerve G57.3-
posterior tibial nerve G57.5-
saphenous nerve G57.8-
ulnar nerve G56.2-
facial nerve G51.9
hereditary G60.9
motor and sensory (types I-IV) G60.0
sensory G60.8
specified NEC G60.8
hypertrophic G60.0
Charcot-Marie-Tooth G60.0
Déjérine-Sottas G60.0
interstitial progressive G60.0
of infancy G60.0
Refsum G60.1
idiopathic G60.9
progressive G60.3
specified NEC G60.8
in association with hereditary ataxia G60.2
intercostal G58.0
ischemic — *see* Disorder, nerve
Jamaica (ginger) G62.2
leg NEC G57.9-
lower extremity G57.9-
lumbar plexus G54.1
median nerve G56.1-
motor and sensory — *see also* Polyneuropathy
hereditary (types I-IV) G60.0
multifocal motor (MMN) G61.82
multiple (acute) (chronic) — *see* Polyneuropathy
optic (nerve) — *see also* Neuritis, optic
ischemic H47.01-
paraneoplastic (sensorial) (Denny Brown) D49.9 *[G13.0]*
peripheral (nerve) — *see also* Polyneuropathy G62.9
autonomic G90.9
idiopathic G90.09
in (due to)
amyloidosis E85.4 *[G99.0]*
diabetes mellitus — *see* E08-E13 with .43
endocrine disease NEC E34.9 *[G99.0]*
gout M10.00 *[G99.0]*
hyperthyroidism E05.90 *[G99.0]*
with thyroid storm E05.91 *[G99.0]*
metabolic disease NEC E88.9 *[G99.0]*
idiopathic G60.9
progressive G60.3
in (due to)
antitetanus serum G62.0
arsenic G62.2
drugs NEC G62.0
lead G62.2
organophosphate compounds G62.2
toxic agent NEC G62.2
plantar nerves G57.6-
progressive
hypertrophic interstitial G60.0
inflammatory G62.81
radicular NEC — *see* Radiculopathy
sacral plexus G54.1
sciatic G57.0-
serum G61.1
toxic NEC G62.2
trigeminal sensory G50.8
ulnar nerve G56.2-
uremic N18.9 *[G63]*
vitamin B12 E53.8 *[G63]*
with anemia (pernicious) D51.0 *[G63]*
due to dietary deficiency D51.3 *[G63]*

Neurophthisis — *see also* Disorder, nerve
peripheral, diabetic — *see* E08-E13 with .42
Neuroretinitis — *see* Chorioretinitis
Neuroretinopathy, hereditary optic H47.22
Neurosarcoma — *see* Neoplasm, nerve, malignant
Neurosclerosis — *see* Disorder, nerve
Neurosis, neurotic F48.9
anankastic F42.8
anxiety (state) F41.1
panic type F41.0
asthenic F48.8
bladder F45.8
cardiac (reflex) F45.8
cardiovascular F45.8
character F60.9
colon F45.8
compensation F68.10
compulsive, compulsion F42.8
conversion F44.9
craft F48.8
cutaneous F45.8
depersonalization F48.1
depressive (reaction) (type) F34.1
environmental F48.8
excoriation L98.1
fatigue F48.8
functional — *see* Disorder, somatoform
gastric F45.8
gastrointestinal F45.8
heart F45.8
hypochondriacal F45.21
hysterical F44.9
incoordination F45.8
larynx F45.8
vocal cord F45.8
intestine F45.8
larynx (sensory) F45.8
hysterical F44.4
mixed NEC F48.8
musculoskeletal F45.8
obsessional F42.8
obsessive-compulsive F42.8
occupational F48.8
ocular NEC F45.8
organ — *see* Disorder, somatoform
pharynx F45.8
phobic F40.9
posttraumatic (situational) F43.10
acute F43.11
chronic F43.12
psychasthenic (type) F48.8
railroad F48.8
rectum F45.8
respiratory F45.8
rumination F45.8
sexual F65.9
situational F48.8
social F40.10
generalized F40.11
specified type NEC F48.8
state F48.9
with depersonalization episode F48.1
stomach F45.8
traumatic F43.10
acute F43.11
chronic F43.12
vasomotor F45.8
visceral F45.8
war F48.8
Neurospongioblastosis diffusa Q85.1
Neurosyphilis (arrested) (early) (gumma) (late) (latent) (recurrent) (relapse) A52.3
with ataxia (cerebellar) (locomotor) (spastic) (spinal) A52.19
aneurysm (cerebral) A52.05
arachnoid (adhesive) A52.13
arteritis (any artery) (cerebral) A52.04
asymptomatic A52.2
congenital A50.40
dura (mater) A52.13
general paresis A52.17
hemorrhagic A52.05
juvenile (asymptomatic) (meningeal) A50.40
leptomeninges (aseptic) A52.13
meningeal, meninges (adhesive) A52.13
meningitis A52.13
meningovascular (diffuse) A52.13
optic atrophy A52.15
parenchymatous (degenerative) A52.19
paresis, paretic A52.17
juvenile A50.45
remission in (sustained) A52.3
serological (without symptoms) A52.2

Neurosyphilis (arrested) (early) (gumma) (late) (latent) (recurrent) (relapse) - *continued*
specified nature or site NEC A52.19
tabes, tabetic (dorsalis) A52.11
juvenile A50.45
taboparesis A52.17
juvenile A50.45
thrombosis (cerebral) A52.05
vascular (cerebral) NEC A52.05
Neurothekeoma — *see* Neoplasm, nerve, benign
Neurotic — *see* Neurosis
Neurotoxemia — *see* Toxemia
Neutroclusion M26.211
Neutropenia, neutropenic (chronic) (genetic) (idiopathic) (immune) (infantile) (malignant) (pernicious) (splenic) D70.9
congenital (primary) D70.0
cyclic D70.4
cytoreductive cancer chemotherapy sequela D70.1
drug-induced D70.2
due to cytoreductive cancer chemotherapy D70.1
due to infection D70.3
fever D70.9
neonatal, transitory (isoimmune) (maternal transfer) P61.5
periodic D70.4
secondary (cyclic) (periodic) (splenic) D70.4
drug-induced D70.2
due to cytoreductive cancer chemotherapy D70.1
toxic D70.8
Neutrophilia, hereditary giant D72.0
Nevocarcinoma — *see* Melanoma
Nevus D22.9
achromic — *see* Neoplasm, skin, benign
amelanotic — *see* Neoplasm, skin, benign
angiomatousD18.00
intra-abdominal D18.03
intracranial D18.02
skin D18.01
specified site NEC D18.09
araneus I78.1
balloon cell — *see* Neoplasm, skin, benign
bathing trunk D48.5
blue — *see* Neoplasm, skin, benign
cellular — *see* Neoplasm, skin, benign
giant — *see* Neoplasm, skin, benign
Jadassohn's — *see* Neoplasm, skin, benign
malignant — *see* Melanoma
capillary D18.00
intra-abdominal D18.03
intracranial D18.02
skin D18.01
specified site NEC D18.09
cavernous D18.00
intra-abdominal D18.03
intracranial D18.02
skin D18.01
specified site NEC D18.09
cellular — *see* Neoplasm, skin, benign
blue — *see* Neoplasm, skin, benign
choroid D31.3-
comedonicus Q82.5
conjunctiva D31.0-
dermal — *see* Neoplasm, skin, benign
with epidermal nevus — *see* Neoplasm, skin, benign
dysplastic — *see* Neoplasm, skin, benign
eye D31.9-
flammeus Q82.5
hemangiomatous D18.00
intra-abdominal D18.03
intracranial D18.02
skin D18.01
specified site NEC D18.09
iris D31.4-
lacrimal gland D31.5-
lymphatic D18.1
magnocellular
specified site — *see* Neoplasm, benign, by site
unspecified site D31.40
malignant — *see* Melanoma
meaning hemangioma D18.00
intra-abdominal D18.03
intracranial D18.02
skin D18.01
specified site NEC D18.09
mouth (mucosa) D10.30
specified site NEC D10.39
white sponge Q38.6
multiplex Q85.1
non-neoplastic I78.1
oral mucosa D10.30
specified site NEC D10.39

- **Nevus** - *continued*
  - oral mucosa - *continued*
    - white sponge Q38.6
  - orbit D31.6-
  - pigmented
    - giant — *see also* Neoplasm, skin, uncertain behavior D48.5
      - malignant melanoma in — *see* Melanoma
  - portwine Q82.5
  - retina D31.2-
  - retrobulbar D31.6-
  - sanguineous Q82.5
  - senile I78.1
  - skin D22.9
    - abdominal wall D22.5
    - ala nasi D22.39
    - ankle D22.7-
    - anus, anal D22.5
    - arm D22.6-
    - auditory canal (external) D22.2-
    - auricle (ear) D22.2-
    - auricular canal (external) D22.2-
    - axilla, axillary fold D22.5
    - back D22.5
    - breast D22.5
    - brow D22.39
    - buttock D22.5
    - canthus (eye) D22.1-
    - cheek (external) D22.39
    - chest wall D22.5
    - chin D22.39
    - ear (external) D22.2-
    - external meatus (ear) D22.2-
    - eyebrow D22.39
    - eyelid (lower) (upper) D22.1-
    - face D22.30
      - specified NEC D22.39
    - female genital organ (external) NEC D28.0
    - finger D22.6-
    - flank D22.5
    - foot D22.7-
    - forearm D22.6-
    - forehead D22.39
    - foreskin D29.0
    - genital organ (external) NEC
      - female D28.0
      - male D29.9
    - gluteal region D22.5
    - groin D22.5
    - hand D22.6-
    - heel D22.7-
    - helix D22.2-
    - hip D22.7-
    - interscapular region D22.5
    - jaw D22.39
    - knee D22.7-
    - labium (majus) (minus) D28.0
    - leg D22.7-
    - lip (lower) (upper) D22.0
    - lower limb D22.7-
    - male genital organ (external) D29.9
    - nail D22.9
      - finger D22.6-
      - toe D22.7-
    - nasolabial groove D22.39
    - nates D22.5
    - neck D22.4
    - nose (external) D22.39
    - palpebra D22.1-
    - penis D29.0
    - perianal skin D22.5
    - perineum D22.5
    - pinna D22.2-
    - popliteal fossa or space D22.7-
    - prepuce D29.0
    - pudendum D28.0
    - scalp D22.4
    - scrotum D29.4
    - shoulder D22.6-
    - submammary fold D22.5
    - temple D22.39
    - thigh D22.7-
    - toe D22.7-
    - trunk NEC D22.5
    - umbilicus D22.5
    - upper limb D22.6-
    - vulva D28.0
  - specified site NEC — *see* Neoplasm, by site, benign
  - spider I78.1
  - stellar I78.1
  - strawberry Q82.5
  - Sutton's benign D22.9
  - unius lateris Q82.5

- **Nevus** - *continued*
  - Unna's Q82.5
  - vascular Q82.5
  - verrucous Q82.5
- **Newborn** (infant) (liveborn) (singleton) Z38.2
  - acne L70.4
  - abstinence syndrome P96.1
  - affected by
    - abnormalities of membranes P02.9
      - specified NEC P02.8
    - abruptio placenta P02.1
    - amino-acid metabolic disorder, transitory P74.8
    - amniocentesis (while in utero) P00.6
    - amnionitis P02.78
    - apparent life threatening event (ALTE) R68.13
    - bleeding (into)
      - cerebral cortex P52.22
      - germinal matrix P52.0
      - ventricles P52.1
    - breech delivery P03.0
    - cardiac arrest P29.81
    - cardiomyopathy I42.8
      - congenital I42.4
    - cerebral ischemia P91.0
    - Cesarean delivery P03.4
    - chemotherapy agents P04.11
    - chorioamnionitis P02.78
    - cocaine (crack) P04.41
    - complications of labor and delivery P03.9
      - specified NEC P03.89
    - compression of umbilical cord NEC P02.5
    - contracted pelvis P03.1
    - delivery P03.9
      - Cesarean P03.4
      - forceps P03.2
      - vacuum extractor P03.3
    - drugs of addiction P04.40
      - cocaine P04.41
      - hallucinogens P04.42
      - specified drug NEC P04.49
    - environmental chemicals P04.6
    - entanglement (knot) in umbilical cord P02.5
    - fetal (intrauterine)
      - growth retardation P05.9
      - inflammatory response syndrome (FIRS) P02.70
      - malnutrition not light or small for gestational age P05.2
    - FIRS (fetal inflammatory response syndrome) P02.70
    - forceps delivery P03.2
    - heart rate abnormalities
      - bradycardia P29.12
      - intrauterine P03.819
        - before onset of labor P03.810
        - during labor P03.811
      - tachycardia P29.11
    - hemorrhage (antepartum) P02.1
      - cerebellar (nontraumatic) P52.6
      - intracerebral (nontraumatic) P52.4
      - intracranial (nontraumatic) P52.9
        - specified NEC P52.8
      - intraventricular (nontraumatic) P52.3
        - grade 1 P52.0
        - grade 2 P52.1
        - grade 3 P52.21
        - grade 4 P52.22
      - posterior fossa (nontraumatic) P52.6
      - subarachnoid (nontraumatic) P52.5
      - subependymal P52.0
        - with intracerebral extension P52.22
        - with intraventricular extension P52.1
          - with enlargment of ventricles P52.21
        - without intraventricular extension P52.0
    - hypoxic ischemic encephalopathy [HIE] P91.60
      - mild P91.61
      - moderate P91.62
      - severe P91.63
    - induction of labor P03.89
    - intestinal perforation P78.0
    - intrauterine (fetal) blood loss P50.9
      - due to (from)
        - cut end of co-twin cord P50.5
        - hemorrhage into
          - co-twin P50.3
          - maternal circulation P50.4
        - placenta P50.2
        - ruptured cord blood P50.1
        - vasa previa P50.0
      - specified NEC P50.8
    - intrauterine (fetal) hemorrhage P50.9
    - intrauterine (in utero) procedure P96.5
    - malpresentation (malposition) NEC P03.1
    - maternal (complication of) (use of)

- **Newborn** (infant) (liveborn) (singleton) - *continued*
  - affected by - *continued*
    - maternal (complication of) (use of) - *continued*
      - alcohol P04.3
      - amphetamines P04.16
      - analgesia (maternal) P04.0
      - anesthesia (maternal) P04.0
      - anticonvulsants P04.13
      - antidepressants P04.15
      - antineoplastic chemotherapy P04.11
      - anxiolytics P04.1A
      - blood loss P02.1
      - cannabis P04.81
      - circulatory disease P00.3
      - condition P00.9
        - specified NEC P00.89
      - cytotoxic drugs P04.12
      - delivery P03.9
        - Cesarean P03.4
        - forceps P03.2
        - vacuum extractor P03.3
      - diabetes mellitus (pre-existing) P70.1
      - disorder P00.9
        - specified NEC P00.89
      - drugs (addictive) (illegal) NEC P04.49
      - ectopic pregnancy P01.4
      - gestational diabetes P70.0
      - hemorrhage P02.1
      - hypertensive disorder P00.0
      - incompetent cervix P01.0
      - infectious disease P00.2
      - injury P00.5
      - labor and delivery P03.9
      - malpresentation before labor P01.7
      - maternal death P01.6
      - medical procedure P00.7
      - medication P04.19
        - specified type NEC P04.18
      - multiple pregnancy P01.5
      - nutritional disorder P00.4
      - oligohydramnios P01.2
      - opiates P04.14
        - administered for procedures during pregnancy or labor and delivery P04.0
      - parasitic disease P00.2
      - periodontal disease P00.81
      - placenta previa P02.0
      - polyhydramnios P01.3
      - precipitate delivery P03.5
      - pregnancy P01.9
        - specified P01.8
      - premature rupture of membranes P01.1
      - renal disease P00.1
      - respiratory disease P00.3
      - sedative-hypnotics P04.17
      - surgical procedure P00.6
      - tranquilizers administered for procedures during pregnancy or labor and delivery P04.0
      - urinary tract disease P00.1
      - uterine contraction (abnormal) P03.6
    - meconium peritonitis P78.0
    - medication (legal) (maternal use) (prescribed) P04.19
    - membrane abnormalities P02.9
      - specified NEC P02.8
    - membranitis P02.78
    - methamphetamine (s) P04.49
    - mixed metabolic and respiratory acidosis P84
    - neonatal abstinence syndrome P96.1
    - noxious substances transmitted via placenta or breast milk P04.9
      - cannabis P04.81
      - specified NEC P04.89
    - nutritional supplements P04.5
    - placenta previa P02.0
    - placental
      - abnormality (functional) (morphological) P02.20
        - specified NEC P02.29
      - dysfunction P02.29
      - infarction P02.29
      - insufficiency P02.29
      - separation NEC P02.1
      - transfusion syndromes P02.3
    - placentitis P02.78
    - precipitate delivery P03.5
    - prolapsed cord P02.4
    - respiratory arrest P28.81
    - slow intrauterine growth P05.9
    - tobacco P04.2
    - twin to twin transplacental transfusion P02.3
    - umbilical cord (tightly) around neck P02.5
    - umbilical cord condition P02.60
      - short cord P02.69

Newborn (infant) (liveborn) (singleton) - *continued*
affected by - *continued*
umbilical cord condition - *continued*
specified NEC P02.69
uterine contractions (abnormal) P03.6
vasa previa P02.69
from intrauterine blood loss P50.0
apnea P28.4
primary P28.3
obstructive P28.4
sleep (central) (obstructive) (primary) P28.3
born in hospital Z38.00
by cesarean Z38.01
born outside hospital Z38.1
breast buds P96.89
breast engorgement P83.4
check-up — *see* Newborn, examination
convulsion P90
dehydration P74.1
examination
8 to 28 days old Z00.111
under 8 days old Z00.110
fever P81.9
environmentally-induced P81.0
hyperbilirubinemia P59.9
of prematurity P59.0
hypernatremia P74.21
hyponatremia P74.22
infection P39.9
candidal P37.5
specified NEC P39.8
urinary tract P39.3
jaundice P59.9
due to
breast milk inhibitor P59.3
hepatocellular damage P59.20
specified NEC P59.29
preterm delivery P59.0
of prematurity P59.0
specified NEC P59.8
late metabolic acidosis P74.0
mastitis P39.0
infective P39.0
noninfective P83.4
multiple born NEC Z38.8
born in hospital Z38.68
by cesarean Z38.69
born outside hospital Z38.7
omphalitis P38.9
with mild hemorrhage P38.1
without hemorrhage P38.9
post-term P08.21
prolonged gestation (over 42 completed weeks) P08.22
quadruplet Z38.8
born in hospital Z38.63
by cesarean Z38.64
born outside hospital Z38.7
quintuplet Z38.8
born in hospital Z38.65
by cesarean Z38.66
born outside hospital Z38.7
seizure P90
sepsis (congenital) P36.9
due to
anaerobes NEC P36.5
Escherichia coli P36.4
Staphylococcus P36.30
aureus P36.2
specified NEC P36.39
Streptococcus P36.10
group B P36.0
specified NEC P36.19
specified NEC P36.8
triplet Z38.8
born in hospital Z38.61
by cesarean Z38.62
born outside hospital Z38.7
twin Z38.5
born in hospital Z38.30
by cesarean Z38.31
born outside hospital Z38.4
vomiting P92.09
bilious P92.01
weight check Z00.111
Newcastle conjunctivitis or disease B30.8
Nezelof's syndrome (pure alymphocytosis) D81.4
Niacin (amide) **deficiency** E52
Nicolas (-Durand) **-Favre disease** A55
Nicotine — *see* Tobacco
Nicotinic acid deficiency E52
Niemann-Pick disease or syndrome E75.249
specified NEC E75.248
Niemann-Pick disease or syndrome - *continued*
type
A E75.240
B E75.241
C E75.242
D E75.243
Night
blindness — *see* Blindness, night
sweats R61
terrors (child) F51.4
Nightmares (REM sleep type) F51.5
NIHSS (National Institutes of Health Stroke Scale) **score** R29.7-
Nipple — *see* condition
Nisbet's chancre A57
Nishimoto (-Takeuchi) **disease** I67.5
Nitritoid crisis or reaction — *see* Crisis, nitritoid
Nitrosohemoglobinemia D74.8
Njovera A65
Nocardiosis, nocardiasis A43.9
cutaneous A43.1
lung A43.0
pneumonia A43.0
pulmonary A43.0
specified site NEC A43.8
Nocturia R35.1
psychogenic F45.8
Nocturnal — *see* condition
Nodal rhythm I49.8
Node (s) — *see also* Nodule
Bouchard's (with arthropathy) M15.2
Haygarth's M15.8
Heberden's (with arthropathy) M15.1
larynx J38.7
lymph — *see* condition
milker's B08.03
Osler's I33.0
Schmorl's — *see* Schmorl's disease
singer's J38.2
teacher's J38.2
tuberculous — *see* Tuberculosis, lymph gland
vocal cord J38.2
Nodule (s) **, nodular**
actinomycotic — *see* Actinomycosis
breast NEC — *see also* Lump, breast N63.0
colloid (cystic) , thyroid E04.1
cutaneous — *see* Swelling, localized
endometrial (stromal) D26.1
Haygarth's M15.8
inflammatory — *see* Inflammation
juxta-articular
syphilitic A52.77
yaws A66.7
larynx J38.7
lung, solitary (subsegmental branch of the bronchial tree) R91.1
multiple R91.8
milker's B08.03
prostate N40.2
with lower urinary tract symptoms (LUTS) N40.3
without lower urinary tract symtpoms (LUTS) N40.2
pulmonary, solitary (subsegmental branch of the bronchial tree) R91.1
retrocardiac R09.89
rheumatoid M06.30
ankle M06.37-
elbow M06.32-
foot joint M06.37-
hand joint M06.34-
hip M06.35-
knee M06.36-
multiple site M06.39
shoulder M06.31-
vertebra M06.38
wrist M06.33-
scrotum (inflammatory) N49.2
singer's J38.2
solitary, lung (subsegmental branch of the bronchial tree) R91.1
multiple R91.8
subcutaneous — *see* Swelling, localized
teacher's J38.2
thyroid (cold) (gland) (nontoxic) E04.1
with thyrotoxicosis E05.20
with thyroid storm E05.21
toxic or with hyperthyroidism E05.20
with thyroid storm E05.21
vocal cord J38.2
Noma (gangrenous) (hospital) (infective) A69.0
auricle I96
mouth A69.0
pudendi N76.89
Noma (gangrenous) (hospital) (infective) - *continued*
vulvae N76.89
Nomad, nomadism Z59.0
NOMID
(neonatal onset multisystemic inflammatory disorder) M04.2
Nonadherence to medical treatment Z91.19
Nonautoimmune hemolytic anemia D59.4
drug-induced D59.2
Nonclosure — *see also* Imperfect, closure
ductus arteriosus (Botallo's) Q25.0
foramen
botalli Q21.1
ovale Q21.1
Noncompliance Z91.19
with
dietary regimen Z91.11
dialysis Z91.15
medical treatment Z91.19
medication regimen NEC Z91.14
underdosing — *see also* Table of Drugs and Chemicals, categories T36-T50, with final character 6 Z91.14
intentional NEC Z91.128
due to financial hardship of patient Z91.120
unintentional NEC Z91.138
due to patient's age related debility Z91.130
renal dialysis Z91.15
Nondescent (congenital) — *see also* Malposition, congenital
cecum Q43.3
colon Q43.3
testicle Q53.9
bilateral Q53.20
abdominal Q53.211
perineal Q53.22
unilateral Q53.10
abdominal Q53.111
perineal Q53.12
Nondevelopment
brain Q02
part of Q04.3
heart Q24.8
organ or site, congenital NEC — *see* Hypoplasia
Nonengagement
head NEC O32.4
in labor, causing obstructed labor O64.8
Nonexanthematous tick fever A93.2
Nonexpansion, lung (newborn) P28.0
Nonfunctioning
cystic duct — *see also* Disease, gallbladder K82.8
gallbladder — *see also* Disease, gallbladder K82.8
kidney N28.9
labyrinth — *see* subcategory H83.2
Non-Hodgkin lymphoma NEC — *see* Lymphoma, non-Hodgkin
Nonimplantation, ovum N97.2
Noninsufflation, fallopian tube N97.1
Non-ketotic hyperglycinemia E72.51
Nonne-Milroy syndrome Q82.0
Nonovulation N97.0
Non-palpable testicle (s)
bilateral R39.84
unilateral R39.83
Nonpatent fallopian tube N97.1
Nonpneumatization, lung NEC P28.0
Nonrotation — *see* Malrotation
Nonsecretion, urine — *see* Anuria
Nonunion
fracture — *see* Fracture, by site
joint, following fusion or arthrodesis M96.0
organ or site, congenital NEC — *see* Imperfect, closure
symphysis pubis, congenital Q74.2
Nonvisualization, gallbladder R93.2
Nonvital, nonvitalized tooth K04.99
Non-working side interference M26.56
Noonan's syndrome Q87.1
Normocytic anemia (infectional) **due to blood loss** (chronic) D50.0
acute D62
Norrie's disease (congenital) Q15.8
North American blastomycosis B40.9
Norwegian itch B86
Nose, nasal — *see* condition
Nosebleed R04.0
Nose-picking F98.8
Nosomania F45.21
Nosophobia F45.22
Nostalgia F43.20
Notch of iris Q13.2
Notching nose, congenital (tip) Q30.2

Nothnagel's
- syndrome — *see* Strabismus, paralytic, third nerve
- vasomotor acroparesthesia I73.89

Novy's relapsing fever A68.9
- louse-borne A68.0
- tick-borne A68.1

Noxious
- foodstuffs, poisoning by — *see* Poisoning, food, noxious, plant
- substances transmitted through placenta or breast milk P04.9

Nucleus pulposus — *see* condition
Numbness R20.0
Nuns' knee — *see* Bursitis, prepatellar
Nursemaid's elbow S53.03-
Nutcracker esophagus K22.4
Nutmeg liver K76.1
Nutrient element deficiency E61.9
- specified NEC E61.8

Nutrition deficient or insufficient — *see also* Malnutrition E46
- due to
  - insufficient food T73.0
  - lack of
    - care (child) T76.02
      - adult T76.01
    - food T73.0

Nutritional stunting E45
Nyctalopia (night blindness) — *see* Blindness, night
Nycturia R35.1
- psychogenic F45.8

Nymphomania F52.8
Nystagmus H55.00
- benign paroxysmal — *see* Vertigo, benign paroxysmal
- central positional H81.4-
- congenital H55.01
- dissociated H55.04
- latent H55.02
- miners' H55.09
- positional
  - benign paroxysmal H81.4-
  - central H81.4-
- specified form NEC H55.09
- visual deprivation H55.03

O

Obermeyer's relapsing fever (European) A68.0
Obesity E66.9
- with alveolar hypoventilation E66.2
- adrenal E27.8
- complicating
  - childbirth O99.214
  - pregnancy O99.21-
  - puerperium O99.215
- constitutional E66.8
- dietary counseling and surveillance Z71.3
- drug-induced E66.1
- due to
  - drug E66.1
  - excess calories E66.09
    - morbid E66.01
    - severe E66.01
- endocrine E66.8
- endogenous E66.8
- exogenous E66.09
- familial E66.8
- glandular E66.8
- hypothyroid — *see* Hypothyroidism
- hypoventilation syndrome (OHS) E66.2
- morbid E66.01
  - with
    - alveolar hypoventilation E66.2
    - obesity hypoventilation syndrome (OHS) E66.2
  - due to excess calories E66.01
- nutritional E66.09
- pituitary E23.6
- severe E66.01
- specified type NEC E66.8

Oblique — *see* condition
Obliteration
- appendix (lumen) K38.8
- artery I77.1
- bile duct (noncalculous) K83.1
- common duct (noncalculous) K83.1
- cystic duct — *see* Obstruction, gallbladder
- disease, arteriolar I77.1
- endometrium N85.8
- eye, anterior chamber — *see* Disorder, globe, hypotony
- fallopian tube N97.1
- lymphatic vessel I89.0
  - due to mastectomy I97.2

Obliteration - *continued*
- organ or site, congenital NEC — *see* Atresia, by site
- ureter N13.5
  - with infection N13.6
- urethra — *see* Stricture, urethra
- vein I87.8
- vestibule (oral) K08.89

Observation (following) (for)
- (without need for further medical care) Z04.9
- accident NEC Z04.3
  - at work Z04.2
  - transport Z04.1
- adverse effect of drug Z03.6
- alleged rape or sexual assault (victim) , ruled out
  - adult Z04.41
  - child Z04.42
- criminal assault Z04.89
- development state
  - adolescent Z00.3
  - period of rapid growth in childhood Z00.2
  - puberty Z00.3
- disease, specified NEC Z03.89
- following work accident Z04.2
- forced sexual exploitation Z04.81
- forced labor exploitation Z04.82
- growth and development state — *see* Observation, development state
- injuries (accidental) NEC — *see also* Observation, accident
- newborn (for)
  - suspected condition, related to exposure from the mother or birth process — *see* - Newborn, affected by, maternal
    - ruled out Z05.9
      - cardiac Z05.0
      - connective tissue Z05.73
      - gastrointestinal Z05.5
      - genetic Z05.41
      - genitourinary Z05.6
      - immunologic Z05.43
      - infectious Z05.1
      - metabolic Z05.42
      - musculoskeletal Z05.72
      - neurological Z05.2
      - respiratory Z05.3
      - skin and subcutaneous tissue Z05.71
      - specified condition NEC Z05.8
- postpartum
  - immediately after delivery Z39.0
  - routine follow-up Z39.2
- pregnancy (normal) (without complication) Z34.9-
  - high risk O09.9-
- suicide attempt, alleged NEC Z03.89
  - self-poisoning Z03.6
- suspected, ruled out — *see also* Suspected condition, ruled out
  - abuse, physical
    - adult Z04.71
    - child Z04.72
  - accident at work Z04.2
  - adult battering victim Z04.71
  - child battering victim Z04.72
  - condition NEC Z03.89
    - newborn — *see also* Observation, newborn (for), suspected condition, ruled out Z05.9
  - drug poisoning or adverse effect Z03.6
  - exposure (to)
    - anthrax Z03.810
    - biological agent NEC Z03.818
  - inflicted injury NEC Z04.89
  - suicide attempt, alleged Z03.89
    - self-poisoning Z03.6
  - toxic effects from ingested substance (drug) (poison) Z03.6
- toxic effects from ingested substance (drug) (poison) Z03.6

Obsession, obsessional state F42.8
- mixed thoughts and acts F42.2

Obsessive-compulsive neurosis or reaction F42.8
Obstetric embolism, septic — *see* Embolism, obstetric, septic
Obstetrical trauma (complicating delivery) O71.9
- with or following ectopic or molar pregnancy O08.6
- specified type NEC O71.89

Obstipation — *see* Constipation
Obstruction, obstructed, obstructive
- airway J98.8
  - with
    - allergic alveolitis J67.9
    - asthma J45.909
      - with
        - exacerbation (acute) J45.901
        - status asthmaticus J45.902

Obstruction, obstructed, obstructive - *continued*
- airway - *continued*
  - with - *continued*
    - bronchiectasis J47.9
      - with
        - exacerbation (acute) J47.1
        - lower respiratory infection J47.0
    - bronchitis (chronic) J44.9
    - emphysema J43.9
  - chronic J44.9
    - with
      - allergic alveolitis — *see* Pneumonitis, hypersensitivity
      - bronchiectasis J47.9
        - with
          - exacerbation (acute) J47.1
          - lower respiratory infection J47.0
  - due to
    - foreign body — *see* Foreign body, by site, causing asphyxia
    - inhalation of fumes or vapors J68.9
    - laryngospasm J38.5
- ampulla of Vater K83.1
- aortic (heart) (valve) — *see* Stenosis, aortic
- aortoiliac I74.09
- aqueduct of Sylvius G91.1
  - congenital Q03.0
    - with spina bifida — *see* Spina bifida, by site, with hydrocephalus
- Arnold-Chiari — *see* Arnold-Chiari disease
- artery — *see also* Atherosclerosis, artery I70.9
  - stent — *see* Restenosis, stent
  - basilar (complete) (partial) — *see* Occlusion, artery, basilar
  - carotid (complete) (partial) — *see* Occlusion, artery, carotid
  - cerebellar — *see* Occlusion, artery, cerebellar
  - cerebral (anterior) (middle) (posterior) — *see* Occlusion, artery, cerebral
  - precerebral — *see* Occlusion, artery, precerebral
  - renal N28.0
  - retinal NEC — *see* Occlusion, artery, retina
  - vertebral (complete) (partial) — *see* Occlusion, artery, vertebral
- band (intestinal) — *see also* Obstruction, intestine, specified NEC K56.699
- bile duct or passage (common) (hepatic) (noncalculous) K83.1
  - with calculus K80.51
  - congenital (causing jaundice) Q44.3
- biliary (duct) (tract) K83.1
  - gallbladder K82.0
- bladder-neck (acquired) N32.0
  - congenital Q64.31
  - due to hyperplasia (hypertrophy) of prostate — *see* Hyperplasia, prostate
- bowel — *see* Obstruction, intestine
- bronchus J98.09
- canal, ear — *see* Stenosis, external ear canal
- cardia K22.2
- caval veins (inferior) (superior) I87.1
- cecum — *see* Obstruction, intestine
- circulatory I99.8
- colon — *see* Obstruction, intestine
- common duct (noncalculous) K83.1
- coronary (artery) — *see* Occlusion, coronary
- cystic duct — *see also* Obstruction, gallbladder
  - with calculus K80.21
- device, implant or graft — *see also* Complications, by site and type, mechanical T85.698
  - arterial graft NEC — *see* Complication, cardiovascular device, mechanical, vascular
  - catheter NEC T85.628
    - cystostomy T83.090
    - dialysis (renal) T82.49
      - intraperitoneal T85.691
    - Hopkins T83.098
    - ileostomy T83.098
    - infusion NEC T82.594
      - spinal (epidural) (subdural) T85.690
    - nephrostomy T83.092
    - urethral indwelling T83.091
    - urinary T83.098
    - urostomy T83.098
  - due to infection T85.79
  - gastrointestinal — *see* Complications, prosthetic device, mechanical, gastrointestinal device
  - genital NEC T83.498
    - intrauterine contraceptive device T83.39
    - penile prosthesis (cylinder) (implanted) (pump) (resevoir) T83.490
    - testicular prosthesis T83.491

Obstruction, obstructed, obstructive - *continued*
device, implant or graft - *continued*
heart NEC — *see* Complication, cardiovascular device, mechanical
joint prosthesis — *see* Complications, joint prosthesis, mechanical, specified NEC, by site
orthopedic NEC — *see* Complication, orthopedic, device, mechanical
specified NEC T85.628
urinary NEC — *see also* Complication, genitourinary, device, urinary, mechanical
graft T83.29
vascular NEC — *see* Complication, cardiovascular device, mechanical
ventricular intracranial shunt T85.09
due to foreign body accidentally left in operative wound T81.529
duodenum K31.5
ejaculatory duct N50.89
esophagus K22.2
eustachian tube (complete) (partial) H68.10-
cartilagenous (extrinsic) H68.13-
intrinsic H68.12-
osseous H68.11-
fallopian tube (bilateral) N97.1
fecal K56.41
with hernia — *see* Hernia, by site, with obstruction
foramen of Monro (congenital) Q03.8
with spina bifida — *see* Spina bifida, by site, with hydrocephalus
foreign body — *see* Foreign body
gallbladder K82.0
with calculus, stones K80.21
congenital Q44.1
gastric outlet K31.1
gastrointestinal — *see* Obstruction, intestine
hepatic K76.89
duct (noncalculous) K83.1
hepatobiliary K83.1
ileum — *see* Obstruction, intestine
iliofemoral (artery) I74.5
intestine K56.609
complete K56.601
incomplete K56.600
partial K56.600
with
adhesions (intestinal) (peritoneal) K56.50
complete K56.52
incomplete K56.51
partial K56.51
adynamic K56.0
by gallstone K56.3
congenital (small) Q41.9
large Q42.9
specified part NEC Q42.8
neurogenic K56.0
Hirschsprung's disease or megacolon Q43.1
newborn P76.9
due to
fecaliths P76.8
inspissated milk P76.2
meconium (plug) P76.0
in mucoviscidosis E84.11
specified NEC P76.8
postoperative K91.30
complete K91.32
incomplete K91.31
partial K91.31
reflex K56.0
specified NEC K56.699
complete K56.691
incomplete K56.690
partial K56.690
volvulus K56.2
intracardiac ball valve prosthesis T82.09
jejunum — *see* Obstruction, intestine
joint prosthesis — *see* Complications, joint prosthesis, mechanical, specified NEC, by site
kidney (calices) N28.89
labor — *see* Delivery
lacrimal (passages) (duct)
by
dacryolith — *see* Dacryolith
stenosis — *see* Stenosis, lacrimal
congenital Q10.5
neonatal H04.53-
lacrimonasal duct — *see* Obstruction, lacrimal
lacteal, with steatorrhea K90.2
laryngitis — *see* Laryngitis
larynx NEC J38.6
congenital Q31.8
lung J98.4
disease, chronic J44.9

Obstruction, obstructed, obstructive - *continued*
lymphatic I89.0
meconium (plug)
newborn P76.0
due to fecaliths P76.0
in mucoviscidosis E84.11
mitral — *see* Stenosis, mitral
nasal J34.89
nasolacrimal duct — *see also* Obstruction, lacrimal
congenital Q10.5
nasopharynx J39.2
nose J34.89
organ or site, congenital NEC — *see* Atresia, by site
pancreatic duct K86.89
parotid duct or gland K11.8
pelviureteral junction N13.5
with hydronephrosis N13.0
congenital Q62.39
pharynx J39.2
portal (circulation) (vein) I81
prostate — *see also* Hyperplasia, prostate
valve (urinary) N32.0
pulmonary valve (heart) I37.0
pyelonephritis (chronic) N11.1
pylorus
adult K31.1
congenital or infantile Q40.0
rectosigmoid — *see* Obstruction, intestine
rectum K62.4
renal N28.89
outflow N13.8
pelvis, congenital Q62.39
respiratory J98.8
chronic J44.9
retinal (vessels) H34.9
salivary duct (any) K11.8
with calculus K11.5
sigmoid — *see* Obstruction, intestine
sinus (accessory) (nasal) J34.89
Stensen's duct K11.8
stomach NEC K31.89
acute K31.0
congenital Q40.2
due to pylorospasm K31.3
submandibular duct K11.8
submaxillary gland K11.8
with calculus K11.5
thoracic duct I89.0
thrombotic — *see* Thrombosis
trachea J39.8
tracheostomy airway J95.03
tricuspid (valve) — *see* Stenosis, tricuspid
upper respiratory, congenital Q34.8
ureter (functional) (pelvic junction) NEC N13.5
with
hydronephrosis N13.1
with infection N13.6
pyelonephritis (chronic) N11.1
congenital Q62.39
due to calculus — *see* Calculus, ureter
urethra NEC N36.8
congenital Q64.39
urinary (moderate) N13.9
due to hyperplasia (hypertrophy) of prostate — *see* Hyperplasia, prostate
organ or tract (lower) N13.9
prostatic valve N32.0
specified NEC N13.8
uropathy N13.9
uterus N85.8
vagina N89.5
valvular — *see* Endocarditis
vein, venous I87.1
caval (inferior) (superior) I87.1
thrombotic — *see* Thrombosis
vena cava (inferior) (superior) I87.1
vesical NEC N32.0
vesicourethral orifice N32.0
congenital Q64.31
vessel NEC I99.8
stent — *see* Restenosis, stent

Obturator — *see* condition

Occlusal wear, teeth K03.0

Occlusio pupillae — *see* Membrane, pupillary

Occlusion, occluded
anus K62.4
congenital Q42.3
with fistula Q42.2
aortoiliac (chronic) I74.09
aqueduct of Sylvius G91.1
congenital Q03.0
with spina bifida — *see* Spina bifida, by site, with hydrocephalus

Occlusion, occluded - *continued*
artery — *see also* Atherosclerosis, artery I70.9
auditory, internal I65.8
basilar I65.1
with
infarction I63.22
due to
embolism I63.12
thrombosis I63.02
brain or cerebral I66.9
with infarction (due to) I63.5-
embolism I63.4-
thrombosis I63.3-
carotid I65.2-
with
infarction I63.23-
due to
embolism I63.13-
thrombosis I63.03-
cerebellar (anterior inferior) (posterior inferior) (superior) I66.3
with infarction I63.54-
due to
embolism I63.44-
thrombosis I63.34-
cerebral I66.9
with infarction I63.50
due to
embolism I63.40
specified NEC I63.49
thrombosis I63.30
specified NEC I63.39
anterior I66.1-
with infarction I63.52-
due to
embolism I63.42-
thrombosis I63.32-
middle I66.0-
with infarction I63.51-
due to
embolism I63.41-
thrombosis I63.31-
posterior I66.2-
with infarction I63.53-
due to
embolism I63.43-
thrombosis I63.33-
specified NEC I66.8
with infarction I63.59
due to
embolism I63.4-
thrombosis I63.3-
choroidal (anterior) — *see* Occlusion, artery, precerebral, specified NEC
communicating posterior — *see* Occlusion, artery, precerebral, specified NEC
complete
coronary I25.82
extremities I70.92
coronary (acute) (thrombotic) (without myocardial infarction) I24.0
with myocardial infarction — *see* Infarction, myocardium
chronic total I25.82
complete I25.82
healed or old I25.2
total (chronic) I25.82
hypophyseal — *see* Occlusion, artery, precerebral, specified NEC
iliac I74.5
lower extremities due to stenosis or stricture I77.1
mesenteric (embolic) (thrombotic) — *see also* Infarct, intestine K55.069
perforating — *see* Occlusion, artery, cerebral, specified NEC
peripheral I77.9
thrombotic or embolic I74.4
pontine — *see* Occlusion, artery, precerebral, specified NEC
precerebral I65.9
with infarction I63.20
specified NEC I63.29
due to
embolism I63.10
specified NEC I63.19
thrombosis I63.00
specified NEC I63.09
basilar — *see* Occlusion, artery, basilar
carotid — *see* Occlusion, artery, carotid
puerperal O88.23
specified NEC I65.8
with infarction I63.29
due to

Occlusion, occluded - *continued*
- artery - *continued*
  - precerebral - *continued*
    - specified NEC - *continued*
      - with infarction - *continued*
        - due to - *continued*
          - embolism I63.19
          - thrombosis I63.09
    - vertebral — *see* Occlusion, artery, vertebral
  - renal N28.0
  - retinal
    - central H34.1-
    - partial H34.21-
    - branch H34.23-
    - transient H34.0-
  - spinal — *see* Occlusion, artery, precerebral, vertebral
  - total (chronic)
    - coronary I25.82
    - extremities I70.92
  - vertebral I65.0-
    - with
      - infarction I63.21-
        - due to
          - embolism I63.11-
          - thrombosis I63.01-
- basilar artery — *see* Occlusion, artery, basilar
- bile duct (common) (hepatic) (noncalculous) K83.1
- bowel — *see* Obstruction, intestine
- carotid (artery) (common) (internal) — *see* Occlusion, artery, carotid
- centric (of teeth) M26.59
  - maximum intercuspation discrepancy M26.55
- cerebellar (artery) — *see* Occlusion, artery, cerebellar
- cerebral (artery) — *see* Occlusion, artery, cerebral
- cerebrovascular — *see also* Occlusion, artery, cerebral
  - with infarction I63.5-
- cervical canal — *see* Stricture, cervix
- cervix (uteri) — *see* Stricture, cervix
- choanal Q30.0
- choroidal (artery) — *see* Occlusion, artery, precerebral, specified NEC
- colon — *see* Obstruction, intestine
- communicating posterior artery — *see* Occlusion, artery, precerebral, specified NEC
- coronary (artery) (vein) (thrombotic) — *see also* Infarct, myocardium
  - chronic total I25.82
  - healed or old I25.2
  - not resulting in infarction I24.0
  - total (chronic) I25.82
- cystic duct — *see* Obstruction, gallbladder
- embolic — *see* Embolism
- fallopian tube N97.1
  - congenital Q50.6
- gallbladder — *see also* Obstruction, gallbladder
  - congenital (causing jaundice) Q44.1
- gingiva, traumatic K06.2
- hymen N89.6
  - congenital Q52.3
- hypophyseal (artery) — *see* Occlusion, artery, precerebral, specified NEC
- iliac artery I74.5
- intestine — *see* Obstruction, intestine
- lacrimal passages — *see* Obstruction, lacrimal
- lung J98.4
- lymph or lymphatic channel I89.0
- mammary duct N64.89
- mesenteric artery (embolic) (thrombotic) — *see also* Infarct, intestine K55.069
- nose J34.89
  - congenital Q30.0
- organ or site, congenital NEC — *see* Atresia, by site
- oviduct N97.1
  - congenital Q50.6
- peripheral arteries
  - due to stricture or stenosis I77.1
  - upper extremity I74.2
- pontine (artery) — *see* Occlusion, artery, precerebral, specified NEC
- posterior lingual, of mandibular teeth M26.29
- precerebral artery — *see* Occlusion, artery, precerebral
- punctum lacrimale — *see* Obstruction, lacrimal
- pupil — *see* Membrane, pupillary
- pylorus, adult — *see also* Stricture, pylorus K31.1
- renal artery N28.0
- retina, retinal
  - artery — *see* Occlusion, artery, retinal
  - vein (central) H34.81-
    - engorgement H34.82-

Occlusion, occluded - *continued*
- retina, retinal - *continued*
  - vein (central) - *continued*
    - tributary H34.83-
  - vessels H34.9
- spinal artery — *see* Occlusion, artery, precerebral, vertebral
- teeth (mandibular) (posterior lingual) M26.29
- thoracic duct I89.0
- thrombotic — *see* Thrombosis, artery
- traumatic
  - edentulous (alveolar) ridge K06.2
  - gingiva K06.2
  - periodontal K05.5
- tubal N97.1
- ureter (complete) (partial) N13.5
  - congenital Q62.10
- ureteropelvic junction N13.5
  - congenital Q62.11
- ureterovesical orifice N13.5
  - congenital Q62.12
- urethra — *see* Stricture, urethra
- uterus N85.8
- vagina N89.5
- vascular NEC I99.8
- vein — *see* Thrombosis
  - retinal — *see* Occlusion, retinal, vein
- vena cava (inferior) (superior) — *see* Embolism, vena cava
- ventricle (brain) NEC G91.1
- vertebral (artery) — *see* Occlusion, artery, vertebral
- vessel (blood) I99.8
- vulva N90.5

Occult
- blood in feces (stools) R19.5

Occupational
- problems NEC Z56.89

Ochlophobia — *see* Agoraphobia

Ochronosis (endogenous) E70.29

Ocular muscle — *see* condition

Oculogyric crisis or disturbance H51.8
- psychogenic F45.8

Oculomotor syndrome H51.9

Oculopathy
- syphilitic NEC A52.71
  - congenital
    - early A50.01
    - late A50.30
  - early (secondary) A51.43
  - late A52.71

Oddi's sphincter spasm K83.4

Odontalgia K08.89

Odontoameloblastoma — *see* Cyst, calcifying odontogenic

Odontoclasia K03.89

Odontodysplasia, regional K00.4

Odontogenesis imperfecta K00.5

Odontoma (ameloblastic) (complex) (compound) (fibroameloblastic) — *see* Cyst, calcifying odontogenic

Odontomyelitis (closed) (open) K04.01
- irreversible K04.02
- reversible K04.01

Odontorrhagia K08.89

Odontosarcoma, ameloblastic C41.1
- upper jaw (bone) C41.0

Oestriasis — *see* Myiasis

Oguchi's disease H53.63

Ohara's disease — *see* Tularemia

OHS (obesity hypoventilation syndrome) E66.2

Oidiomycosis — *see* Candidiasis

Oidium albicans infection — *see* Candidiasis

Old age (without mention of debility) R54
- dementia F03

Old (previous) **myocardial infarction** I25.2

Olfactory — *see* condition

Oligemia — *see* Anemia

Oligoastrocytoma
- specified site — *see* Neoplasm, malignant, by site
- unspecified site C71.9

Oligocythemia D64.9

Oligodendroblastoma
- specified site — *see* Neoplasm, malignant
- unspecified site C71.9

Oligodendroglioma
- anaplastic type
  - specified site — *see* Neoplasm, malignant, by site
  - unspecified site C71.9
- specified site — *see* Neoplasm, malignant, by site
- unspecified site C71.9

Oligodontia — *see* Anodontia

Oligoencephalon Q02

Oligohidrosis L74.4

Oligohydramnios O41.0-

Oligohydrosis L74.4

Oligomenorrhea N91.5
- primary N91.3
- secondary N91.4

Oligophrenia — *see also* Disability, intellectual
- phenylpyruvic E70.0

Oligospermia N46.11
- due to
  - drug therapy N46.121
  - efferent duct obstruction N46.123
  - infection N46.122
  - radiation N46.124
  - specified cause NEC N46.129
  - systemic disease N46.125

Oligotrichia — *see* Alopecia

Oliguria R34
- with, complicating or following ectopic or molar pregnancy O08.4
- postprocedural N99.0

Ollier's disease Q78.4

Omenotocele — *see* Hernia, abdomen, specified site NEC

Omentitis — *see* Peritonitis

Omentum, omental — *see* condition

Omphalitis (congenital) (newborn) P38.9
- with mild hemorrhage P38.1
- without hemorrhage P38.9
- not of newborn L08.82
- tetanus A33

Omphalocele Q79.2

Omphalomesenteric duct, persistent Q43.0

Omphalorrhagia, newborn P51.9

Omsk hemorrhagic fever A98.1

Onanism (excessive) F98.8

Onchocerciasis, onchocercosis B73.1
- with
  - eye disease B73.00
    - endophthalmitis B73.01
    - eyelid B73.09
    - glaucoma B73.02
    - specified NEC B73.09
- eye NEC B73.00
- eyelid B73.09

Oncocytoma — *see* Neoplasm, benign, by site

Oncovirus, as cause of disease classified elsewhere B97.32

Ondine's curse — *see* Apnea, sleep

Oneirophrenia F23

Onychauxis L60.2
- congenital Q84.5

Onychia — *see also* Cellulitis, digit
- with lymphangitis — *see* Lymphangitis, acute, digit
- candidal B37.2
- dermatophytic B35.1

Onychitis — *see also* Cellulitis, digit
- with lymphangitis — *see* Lymphangitis, acute, digit

Onychocryptosis L60.0

Onychodystrophy L60.3
- congenital Q84.6

Onychogryphosis, onychogryposis L60.2

Onycholysis L60.1

Onychomadesis L60.8

Onychomalacia L60.3

Onychomycosis (finger) (toe) B35.1

Onycho-osteodysplasia Q87.2

Onychophagia F98.8

Onychophosis L60.8

Onychoptosis L60.8

Onychorrhexis L60.3
- congenital Q84.6

Onychoschizia L60.3

Onyxis (finger) (toe) L60.0

Onyxitis — *see also* Cellulitis, digit
- with lymphangitis — *see* Lymphangitis, acute, digit

Oophoritis (cystic) (infectional) (interstitial) N70.92
- with salpingitis N70.93
- acute N70.02
  - with salpingitis N70.03
- chronic N70.12
  - with salpingitis N70.13
- complicating abortion — *see* Abortion, by type, complicated by, oophoritis

Oophorocele N83.4-

Opacity, opacities
- cornea H17.-
  - central H17.1-
  - congenital Q13.3
  - degenerative — *see* Degeneration, cornea
  - hereditary — *see* Dystrophy, cornea
  - inflammatory — *see* Keratitis
  - minor H17.81-
  - peripheral H17.82-

- **Opacity, opacities** - *continued*
  - cornea - *continued*
    - sequelae of trachoma (healed) B94.0
    - specified NEC H17.89
  - enamel (teeth) (fluoride) (nonfluoride) K00.3
  - lens — *see* Cataract
  - snowball — *see* Deposit, crystalline
  - vitreous (humor) NEC H43.39-
    - congenital Q14.0
    - membranes and strands H43.31-
- **Opalescent dentin** (hereditary) K00.5
- **Open, opening**
  - abnormal, organ or site, congenital — *see* Imperfect, closure
  - angle with
    - borderline
      - findings
        - high risk H40.02-
        - low risk H40.01-
      - intraocular pressure H40.00-
    - cupping of discs H40.01-
    - glaucoma (primary) — *see* Glaucoma, open angle
  - bite
    - anterior M26.220
    - posterior M26.221
  - false — *see* Imperfect, closure
  - margin on tooth restoration K08.51
  - restoration margins of tooth K08.51
  - wound — *see* Wound, open
- **Operational fatigue** F48.8
- **Operative** — *see* condition
- **Operculitis** — *see* Periodontitis
- **Operculum** — *see* Break, retina
- **Ophiasis** L63.2
- **Ophthalmia** — *see also* Conjunctivitis H10.9
  - actinic rays — *see* Photokeratitis
  - allergic (acute) — *see* Conjunctivitis, acute, atopic
  - blennorrhagic (gonococcal) (neonatorum) A54.31
  - diphtheritic A36.86
  - Egyptian A71.1
  - electrica — *see* Photokeratitis
  - gonococcal (neonatorum) A54.31
  - metastatic — *see* Endophthalmitis, purulent
  - migraine — *see* Migraine, ophthalmoplegic
  - neonatorum, newborn P39.1
    - gonococcal A54.31
  - nodosa H16.24-
  - purulent — *see* Conjunctivitis, acute, mucopurulent
  - spring — *see* Conjunctivitis, acute, atopic
  - sympathetic — *see* Uveitis, sympathetic
- **Ophthalmitis** — *see* Ophthalmia
- **Ophthalmocele** (congenital) Q15.8
- **Ophthalmoneuromyelitis** G36.0
- **Ophthalmoplegia** — *see also* Strabismus, paralytic
  - anterior internuclear — *see* Ophthalmoplegia, internuclear
  - ataxia-areflexia G61.0
  - diabetic — *see* E08-E13 with .39
  - exophthalmic E05.00
    - with thyroid storm E05.01
  - external H49.88-
    - progressive H49.4-
      - with pigmentary retinopathy — *see* Kearns-Sayre syndrome
    - total H49.3-
  - internal (complete) (total) H52.51-
  - internuclear H51.2-
  - migraine — *see* Migraine, ophthalmoplegic
  - Parinaud's H49.88-
  - progressive external — *see* Ophthalmoplegia, external, progressive
  - supranuclear, progressive G23.1
  - total (external) — *see* Ophthalmoplegia, external, total
- **Opioid** (s)
  - abuse — *see* Abuse, drug, opioids
  - dependence — *see* Dependence, drug, opioids
  - induced, without use disorder
    - anxiety disorder F11.988
    - delirium F11.921
    - depressive disorder F11.94
    - sexual dysfunction F11.981
    - sleep disorder F11.982
- **Opisthognathism** M26.09
- **Opisthorchiasis** (felineus) (viverrini) B66.0
- **Opitz' disease** D73.2
- **Opiumism** — *see* Dependence, drug, opioid
- **Oppenheim's disease** G70.2
- **Oppenheim-Urbach disease** (necrobiosis lipoidica diabeticorum) — *see* E08-E13 with .620
- **Optic nerve** — *see* condition
- **Orbit** — *see* condition
- **Orchioblastoma** C62.9-
- **Orchitis** (gangrenous) (nonspecific) (septic) (suppurative) N45.2
  - blennorrhagic (gonococcal) (acute) (chronic) A54.23
  - chlamydial A56.19
  - filarial — *see also* Infestation, filarial B74.9 *[N51]*
  - gonococcal (acute) (chronic) A54.23
  - mumps B26.0
  - syphilitic A52.76
  - tuberculous A18.15
- **Orf** (virus disease) B08.02
- **Organic** — *see also* condition
  - brain syndrome F09
  - heart — *see* Disease, heart
  - mental disorder F09
  - psychosis F09
- **Orgasm**
  - anejaculatory N53.13
- **Oriental**
  - bilharziasis B65.2
  - schistosomiasis B65.2
- **Orifice** — *see* condition
- **Origin of both great vessels from right ventricle** Q20.1
- **Ormond's disease** (with ureteral obstruction) N13.5
  - with infection N13.6
- **Ornithine metabolism disorder** E72.4
- **Ornithinemia** (Type I) (Type II) E72.4
- **Ornithosis** A70
- **Orotaciduria, oroticaciduria** (congenital) (hereditary) (pyrimidine deficiency) E79.8
  - anemia D53.0
- **Orthodontics**
  - adjustment Z46.4
  - fitting Z46.4
- **Orthopnea** R06.01
- **Orthopoxvirus** B08.09
  - specified NEC B08.09
- **Os, uterus** — *see* condition
- **Osgood-Schlatter disease or osteochondrosis** — *see* Osteochondrosis, juvenile, tibia
- **Osler** (-Weber) **-Rendu disease** I78.0
- **Osler's nodes** I33.0
- **Osmidrosis** L75.0
- **Osseous** — *see* condition
- **Ossification**
  - artery — *see* Arteriosclerosis
  - auricle (ear) — *see* Disorder, pinna, specified type NEC
  - bronchial J98.09
  - cardiac — *see* Degeneration, myocardial
  - cartilage (senile) — *see* Disorder, cartilage, specified type NEC
  - coronary (artery) — *see* Disease, heart, ischemic, atherosclerotic
  - diaphragm J98.6
  - ear, middle — *see* Otosclerosis
  - falx cerebri G96.19
  - fontanel, premature Q75.0
  - heart — *see also* Degeneration, myocardial
    - valve — *see* Endocarditis
  - larynx J38.7
  - ligament — *see* Disorder, tendon, specified type NEC
    - posterior longitudinal — *see* Spondylopathy, specified NEC
  - meninges (cerebral) (spinal) G96.19
  - multiple, eccentric centers — *see* Disorder, bone, development or growth
  - muscle — *see also* Calcification, muscle
    - due to burns — *see* Myositis, ossificans, in, burns
    - paralytic — *see* Myositis, ossificans, in, quadriplegia
    - progressive — *see* Myositis, ossificans, progressiva
    - specified NEC M61.50
      - ankle M61.57-
      - foot M61.57-
      - forearm M61.53-
      - hand M61.54-
      - lower leg M61.56-
      - multiple sites M61.59
      - pelvic region M61.55-
      - shoulder region M61.51-
      - specified site NEC M61.58
      - thigh M61.55-
      - upper arm M61.52-
    - traumatic — *see* Myositis, ossificans, traumatica
  - myocardium, myocardial — *see* Degeneration, myocardial
  - penis N48.89
  - periarticular — *see* Disorder, joint, specified type NEC
- **Ossification** - *continued*
  - pinna — *see* Disorder, pinna, specified type NEC
  - rider's bone — *see* Ossification, muscle, specified NEC
  - sclera H15.89
  - subperiosteal, post-traumatic M89.8X-
  - tendon — *see* Disorder, tendon, specified type NEC
  - trachea J39.8
  - tympanic membrane — *see* Disorder, tympanic membrane, specified NEC
  - vitreous (humor) — *see* Deposit, crystalline
- **Osteitis** — *see also* Osteomyelitis
  - alveolar M27.3
  - condensans M85.30
    - ankle M85.37-
    - foot M85.37-
    - forearm M85.33-
    - hand M85.34-
    - lower leg M85.36-
    - multiple site M85.39
    - neck M85.38
    - rib M85.38
    - shoulder M85.31-
    - skull M85.38
    - specified site NEC M85.38
    - thigh M85.35-
    - toe M85.37-
    - upper arm M85.32-
    - vertebra M85.38
  - deformans M88.9
    - in (due to)
      - malignant neoplasm of bone C41.9 *[M90.60]*
      - neoplastic disease — *see also* Neoplasm D49.9 *[M90.60]*
        - carpus D49.9 *[M90.64-]*
        - clavicle D49.9 *[M90.61-]*
        - femur D49.9 *[M90.65-]*
        - fibula D49.9 *[M90.66-]*
        - finger D49.9 *[M90.64-]*
        - humerus D49.9 *[M90.62-]*
        - ilium D49.9 *[M90.65-]*
        - ischium D49.9 *[M90.65-]*
        - metacarpus D49.9 *[M90.64-]*
        - metatarsus D49.9 *[M90.67-]*
        - multiple sites D49.9 *[M90.69]*
        - neck D49.9 *[M90.68]*
        - radius D49.9 *[M90.63-]*
        - rib D49.9 *[M90.68]*
        - scapula D49.9 *[M90.61-]*
        - skull D49.9 *[M90.68]*
        - tarsus D49.9 *[M90.67-]*
        - tibia D49.9 *[M90.66-]*
        - toe D49.9 *[M90.67-]*
        - ulna D49.9 *[M90.63-]*
        - vertebra D49.9 *[M90.68]*
    - skull M88.0
    - specified NEC — *see* Paget's disease, bone, by site
    - vertebra M88.1
  - due to yaws A66.6
  - fibrosa NEC — *see* Cyst, bone, by site
    - circumscripta — *see* Dysplasia, fibrous, bone NEC
    - cystica (generalisata) E21.0
    - disseminata Q78.1
    - osteoplastica E21.0
  - fragilitans Q78.0
  - Garr's (sclerosing) — *see* Osteomyelitis, specified type NEC
  - jaw (acute) (chronic) (lower) (suppurative) (upper) M27.2
  - parathyroid E21.0
  - petrous bone (acute) (chronic) — *see* Petrositis
  - sclerotic, nonsuppurative — *see* Osteomyelitis, specified type NEC
  - tuberculosa A18.09
    - cystica D86.89
    - multiplex cystoides D86.89
- **Osteoarthritis** M19.90
  - ankle M19.07-
  - elbow M19.02-
  - foot joint M19.07-
  - generalized M15.9
    - erosive M15.4
    - primary M15.0
    - specified NEC M15.8
  - hand joint M19.04-
    - first carpometacarpal joint M18.9
  - hip M16.1-
    - bilateral M16.0
    - due to hip dysplasia (unilateral) M16.3-
      - bilateral M16.2
  - interphalangeal
    - distal (Heberden) M15.1
    - proximal (Bouchard) M15.2

Osteoarthritis - *continued*
knee M17.1-
bilateral M17.0
shoulder M19.01-
spine — *see* Spondylosis
wrist M19.03-
post-traumatic NEC M19.92
ankle M19.17-
elbow M19.12-
foot joint M19.17-
hand joint M19.14-
first carpometacarpal joint M18.3-
bilateral M18.2
hip M16.5-
bilateral M16.4
knee M17.3-
bilateral M17.2
shoulder M19.11-
wrist M19.13-
primary M19.91
ankle M19.07-
elbow M19.02-
foot joint M19.07-
hand joint M19.04-
first carpometacarpal joint M18.1-
bilateral M18.0
hip M16.1-
bilateral M16.0
knee M17.1-
bilateral M17.0
shoulder M19.01-
spine — *see* Spondylosis
wrist M19.03-
secondary M19.93
ankle M19.27-
elbow M19.22-
foot joint M19.27-
hand joint M19.24-
first carpometacarpal joint M18.5-
bilateral M18.4
hip M16.7
bilateral M16.6
knee M17.5
bilateral M17.4
multiple M15.3
shoulder M19.21-
spine — *see* Spondylosis
wrist M19.23-
Osteoarthropathy (hypertrophic) M19.90
ankle — *see* Osteoarthritis, primary, ankle
elbow — *see* Osteoarthritis, primary, elbow
foot joint — *see* Osteoarthritis, primary, foot
hand joint — *see* Osteoarthritis, primary, hand joint
knee joint — *see* Osteoarthritis, primary, knee
multiple site — *see* Osteoarthritis, primary, multiple joint
pulmonary — *see also* Osteoarthropathy, specified type NEC
hypertrophic — *see* Osteoarthropathy, hypertrophic, specified type NEC
secondary hypertrophic — *see* Osteoarthropathy, specified type NEC
shoulder — *see* Osteoarthritis, primary, shoulder
specified joint NEC — *see* Osteoarthritis, primary, specified joint NEC
specified type NEC M89.40
carpus M89.44-
clavicle M89.41-
femur M89.45-
fibula M89.46-
finger M89.44-
humerus M89.42-
ilium M89.459
ischium M89.459
metacarpus M89.44-
metatarsus M89.47-
multiple sites M89.49
neck M89.48
radius M89.43-
rib M89.48
scapula M89.41-
skull M89.48
tarsus M89.47-
tibia M89.46-
toe M89.47-
ulna M89.43-
vertebra M89.48
secondary — *see* Osteoarthropathy, specified type NEC
spine — *see* Spondylosis
wrist — *see* Osteoarthritis, primary, wrist
Osteoarthrosis (degenerative) (hypertrophic) (joint) — *see also* Osteoarthritis
deformans alkaptonurica E70.29 *[M36.8]*
erosive M15.4
generalized M15.9
primary M15.0
polyarticular M15.9
spine — *see* Spondylosis
Osteoblastoma — *see* Neoplasm, bone, benign
aggressive — *see* Neoplasm, bone, uncertain behavior
Osteochondritis — *see also* Osteochondropathy, by site
Brailsford's — *see* Osteochondrosis, juvenile, radius
dissecans M93.20
ankle M93.27-
elbow M93.22-
foot M93.27-
hand M93.24-
hip M93.25-
knee M93.26-
multiple sites M93.29
shoulder joint M93.21-
specified site NEC M93.28
wrist M93.23-
juvenile M92.9
patellar — *see* Osteochondrosis, juvenile, patella
syphilitic (congenital) (early) A50.02 *[M90.80]*
ankle A50.02 *[M90.87-]*
elbow A50.02 *[M90.82-]*
foot A50.02 *[M90.87-]*
forearm A50.02 *[M90.83-]*
hand A50.02 *[M90.84-]*
hip A50.02 *[M90.85-]*
knee A50.02 *[M90.86-]*
multiple sites A50.02 *[M90.89]*
shoulder joint A50.02 *[M90.81-]*
specified site NEC A50.02 *[M90.88]*
Osteochondroarthrosis deformans endemica — *see* Disease, Kaschin-Beck
Osteochondrodysplasia Q78.9
with defects of growth of tubular bones and spine Q77.9
specified NEC Q77.8
specified NEC Q78.8
Osteochondrodystrophy E78.9
Osteochondrolysis — *see* Osteochondritis, dissecans
Osteochondroma — *see* Neoplasm, bone, benign
Osteochondromatosis D48.0
syndrome Q78.4
Osteochondromyxosarcoma — *see* Neoplasm, bone, malignant
Osteochondropathy M93.90
ankle M93.97-
elbow M93.92-
foot M93.97-
hand M93.94-
hip M93.95-
Kienböck's disease of adults M93.1
knee M93.96-
multiple joints M93.99
osteochondritis dissecans — *see* Osteochondritis, dissecans
osteochondrosis — *see* Osteochondrosis
shoulder region M93.91-
slipped upper femoral epiphysis — *see* Slipped, epiphysis, upper femoral
specified joint NEC M93.98
specified type NEC M93.80
ankle M93.87-
elbow M93.82-
foot M93.87-
hand M93.84-
hip M93.85-
knee M93.86-
multiple joints M93.89
shoulder region M93.81-
specified joint NEC M93.88
wrist M93.83-
syphilitic, congenital
early A50.02 *[M90.80]*
late A50.56 *[M90.80]*
wrist M93.93-
Osteochondrosarcoma — *see* Neoplasm, bone, malignant
Osteochondrosis — *see also* Osteochondropathy, by site
acetabulum (juvenile) M91.0
adult — *see* Osteochondropathy, specified type NEC, by site
astragalus (juvenile) — *see* Osteochondrosis, juvenile, tarsus
Blount's — *see* Osteochondrosis, juvenile, tibia
Osteochondrosis - *continued*
Buchanan's M91.0
Burns' — *see* Osteochondrosis, juvenile, ulna
calcaneus (juvenile) — *see* Osteochondrosis, juvenile, tarsus
capitular epiphysis (femur) (juvenile) — *see* Legg-Calvé-Perthes disease
carpal (juvenile) (lunate) (scaphoid) — *see* Osteochondrosis, juvenile, hand, carpal lunate
adult M93.1
coxae juvenilis — *see* Legg-Calvé-Perthes disease
deformans juvenilis, coxae — *see* Legg-Calvé-Perthes disease
Diaz's — *see* Osteochondrosis, juvenile, tarsus
dissecans (knee) (shoulder) — *see* Osteochondritis, dissecans
femoral capital epiphysis (juvenile) — *see* Legg-Calvé-Perthes disease
femur (head) , juvenile — *see* Legg-Calvé-Perthes disease
fibula (juvenile) — *see* Osteochondrosis, juvenile, fibula
foot NEC (juvenile) M92.8
Freiberg's — *see* Osteochondrosis, juvenile, metatarsus
Haas' (juvenile) — *see* Osteochondrosis, juvenile, humerus
Haglund's — *see* Osteochondrosis, juvenile, tarsus
hip (juvenile) — *see* Legg-Calvé-Perthes disease
humerus (capitulum) (head) (juvenile) — *see* Osteochondrosis, juvenile, humerus
ilium, iliac crest (juvenile) M91.0
ischiopubic synchondrosis M91.0
Iselin's — *see* Osteochondrosis, juvenile, metatarsus
juvenile, juvenilis M92.9
after congenital dislocation of hip reduction — *see* Osteochondrosis, juvenile, hip, specified NEC
arm — *see* Osteochondrosis, juvenile, upper limb NEC
capitular epiphysis (femur) — *see* Legg-Calvé-Perthes disease
clavicle, sternal epiphysis — *see* Osteochondrosis, juvenile, upper limb NEC
coxae — *see* Legg-Calvé-Perthes disease
deformans M92.9
fibula M92.5-
foot NEC M92.8
hand M92.20-
carpal lunate M92.21-
metacarpal head M92.22-
specified site NEC M92.29-
head of femur — *see* Legg-Calvé-Perthes disease
hip and pelvis M91.9-
coxa plana — *see* Coxa, plana
femoral head — *see* Legg-Calvé-Perthes disease
pelvis M91.0
pseudocoxalgia — *see* Pseudocoxalgia
specified NEC M91.8-
humerus M92.0-
limb
lower NEC M92.8
upper NEC — *see* Osteochondrosis, juvenile, upper limb NEC
medial cuneiform bone — *see* Osteochondrosis, juvenile, tarsus
metatarsus M92.7-
patella M92.4-
radius M92.1-
specified site NEC M92.8
spine M42.00
cervical region M42.02
cervicothoracic region M42.03
lumbar region M42.06
lumbosacral region M42.07
multiple sites M42.09
occipito-atlanto-axial region M42.01
sacrococcygeal region M42.08
thoracic region M42.04
thoracolumbar region M42.05
tarsus M92.6-
tibia M92.5-
ulna M92.1-
upper limb NEC M92.3-
vertebra (body) (epiphyseal plates) (Calvé's) (Scheuermann's) — *see* Osteochondrosis, juvenile, spine
Kienböck's — *see* Osteochondrosis, juvenile, hand, carpal lunate
adult M93.1
Köhler's
patellar — *see* Osteochondrosis, juvenile, patella
tarsal navicular — *see* Osteochondrosis, juvenile, tarsus

Osteochondrosis - *continued*
  Legg-Perthes (-Calvé) (-Waldenström) — *see* Legg-Calvé-Perthes disease
  limb
    lower NEC (juvenile) M92.8
    upper NEC (juvenile) — *see* Osteochondrosis, juvenile, upper limb NEC
  lunate bone (carpal) (juvenile) — *see also* Osteochondrosis, juvenile, hand, carpal lunate
    adult M93.1
  Mauclaire's — *see* Osteochondrosis, juvenile, hand, metacarpal
  metacarpal (head) (juvenile) — *see* Osteochondrosis, juvenile, hand, metacarpal
  metatarsus (fifth) (head) (juvenile) (second) — *see* Osteochondrosis, juvenile, metatarsus
  navicular (juvenile) — *see* Osteochondrosis, juvenile, tarsus
  os
    calcis (juvenile) — *see* Osteochondrosis, juvenile, tarsus
    tibiale externum (juvenile) — *see* Osteochondrosis, juvenile, tarsus
  Osgood-Schlatter — *see* Osteochondrosis, juvenile, tibia
  Panner's — *see* Osteochondrosis, juvenile, humerus
  patellar center (juvenile) (primary) (secondary) — *see* Osteochondrosis, juvenile, patella
  pelvis (juvenile) M91.0
  Pierson's M91.0
  radius (head) (juvenile) — *see* Osteochondrosis, juvenile, radius
  Scheuermann's — *see* Osteochondrosis, juvenile, spine
  Sever's — *see* Osteochondrosis, juvenile, tarsus
  Sinding-Larsen — *see* Osteochondrosis, juvenile, patella
  spine M42.9
    adult M42.10
      cervical region M42.12
      cervicothoracic region M42.13
      lumbar region M42.16
      lumbosacral region M42.17
      multiple sites M42.19
      occipito-atlanto-axial region M42.11
      sacrococcygeal region M42.18
      thoracic region M42.14
      thoracolumbar region M42.15
    juvenile — *see* Osteochondrosis, juvenile, spine
  symphysis pubis (juvenile) M91.0
  syphilitic (congenital) A50.02
  talus (juvenile) — *see* Osteochondrosis, juvenile, tarsus
  tarsus (navicular) (juvenile) — *see* Osteochondrosis, juvenile, tarsus
  tibia (proximal) (tubercle) (juvenile) — *see* Osteochondrosis, juvenile, tibia
  tuberculous — *see* Tuberculosis, bone
  ulna (lower) (juvenile) — *see* Osteochondrosis, juvenile, ulna
  van Neck's M91.0
  vertebral — *see* Osteochondrosis, spine
Osteoclastoma D48.0
  malignant — *see* Neoplasm, bone, malignant
Osteodynia — *see* Disorder, bone, specified type NEC
Osteodystrophy Q78.9
  azotemic N25.0
  congenital Q78.9
  parathyroid, secondary E21.1
  renal N25.0
Osteofibroma — *see* Neoplasm, bone, benign
Osteofibrosarcoma — *see* Neoplasm, bone, malignant
Osteogenesis imperfecta Q78.0
Osteogenic — *see* condition
Osteolysis M89.50
  carpus M89.54-
  clavicle M89.51-
  femur M89.55-
  fibula M89.56-
  finger M89.54-
  humerus M89.52-
  ilium M89.559
  ischium M89.559
  joint prosthesis (periprosthetic) — *see* Complications, joint prosthesis, mechanical, periprosthetic, osteolysis, by site
  metacarpus M89.54-
  metatarsus M89.57-
  multiple sites M89.59
  neck M89.58

Osteolysis - *continued*
  periprosthetic — *see* Complications, joint prosthesis, mechanical, periprosthetic, osteolysis, by site
  radius M89.53-
  rib M89.58
  scapula M89.51-
  skull M89.58
  tarsus M89.57-
  tibia M89.56-
  toe M89.57-
  ulna M89.53-
  vertebra M89.58
Osteoma — *see also* Neoplasm, bone, benign
  osteoid — *see also* Neoplasm, bone, benign
    giant — *see* Neoplasm, bone, benign
Osteomalacia M83.9
  adult M83.9
    drug-induced NEC M83.5
    due to
      malabsorption (postsurgical) M83.2
      malnutrition M83.3
    specified NEC M83.8
  aluminium-induced M83.4
  infantile — *see* Rickets
  juvenile — *see* Rickets
  oncogenic E83.89
  pelvis M83.8
  puerperal M83.0
  senile M83.1
  vitamin-D-resistant in adults E83.31 *[M90.8-]*
    carpus E83.31 *[M90.84-]*
    clavicle E83.31 *[M90.81-]*
    femur E83.31 *[M90.85-]*
    fibula E83.31 *[M90.86-]*
    finger E83.31 *[M90.84-]*
    humerus E83.31 *[M90.82-]*
    ilium E83.31 *[M90.859]*
    ischium E83.31 *[M90.859]*
    metacarpus E83.31 *[M90.84-]*
    metatarsus E83.31 *[M90.87-]*
    multiple sites E83.31 *[M90.89]*
    neck E83.31 *[M90.88]*
    radius E83.31 *[M90.83-]*
    rib E83.31 *[M90.88]*
    scapula E83.31 *[M90.819]*
    skull E83.31 *[M90.88]*
    tarsus E83.31 *[M90.879]*
    tibia E83.31 *[M90.869]*
    toe E83.31 *[M90.879]*
    ulna E83.31 *[M90.839]*
    vertebra E83.31 *[M90.88]*
Osteomyelitis (general) (infective) (localized) (neonatal) (purulent) (septic) (staphylococcal) (streptococcal) (suppurative) (with periostitis) M86.9
  acute M86.10
    carpus M86.14-
    clavicle M86.11-
    femur M86.15-
    fibula M86.16-
    finger M86.14-
    hematogenous M86.00
      carpus M86.04-
      clavicle M86.01-
      femur M86.05-
      fibula M86.06-
      finger M86.04-
      humerus M86.02-
      ilium M86.059
      ischium M86.059
      mandible M27.2
      metacarpus M86.04-
      metatarsus M86.07-
      multiple sites M86.09
      neck M86.08
      orbit H05.02-
      petrous bone — *see* Petrositis
      radius M86.03-
      rib M86.08
      scapula M86.01-
      skull M86.08
      tarsus M86.07-
      tibia M86.06-
      toe M86.07-
      ulna M86.03-
      vertebra — *see* Osteomyelitis, vertebra
    humerus M86.12-
    ilium M86.159
    ischium M86.159
    mandible M27.2
    metacarpus M86.14-
    metatarsus M86.17-
    multiple sites M86.19

Osteomyelitis (general) (infective) (localized) (neonatal) (purulent) (septic) (staphylococcal) (streptococcal) (suppurative) (with periostitis) - *continued*
  acute - *continued*
    neck M86.18
    orbit H05.02-
    petrous bone — *see* Petrositis
    radius M86.13-
    rib M86.18
    scapula M86.11-
    skull M86.18
    tarsus M86.17-
    tibia M86.16-
    toe M86.17-
    ulna M86.13-
    vertebra — *see* Osteomyelitis, vertebra
  chronic (or old) M86.60
    with draining sinus M86.40
      carpus M86.44-
      clavicle M86.41-
      femur M86.45-
      fibula M86.46-
      finger M86.44-
      humerus M86.42-
      ilium M86.459
      ischium M86.459
      mandible M27.2
      metacarpus M86.44-
      metatarsus M86.47-
      multiple sites M86.49
      neck M86.48
      orbit H05.02-
      petrous bone — *see* Petrositis
      radius M86.43-
      rib M86.48
      scapula M86.41-
      skull M86.48
      tarsus M86.47-
      tibia M86.46-
      toe M86.47-
      ulna M86.43-
      vertebra — *see* Osteomyelitis, vertebra
    carpus M86.64-
    clavicle M86.61-
    femur M86.65-
    fibula M86.66-
    finger M86.64-
    hematogenous NEC M86.50
      carpus M86.54-
      clavicle M86.51-
      femur M86.55-
      fibula M86.56-
      finger M86.54-
      humerus M86.52-
      ilium M86.559
      ischium M86.559
      mandible M27.2
      metacarpus M86.54-
      metatarsus M86.57-
      multifocal M86.30
        carpus M86.34-
        clavicle M86.31-
        femur M86.35-
        fibula M86.36-
        finger M86.34-
        humerus M86.32-
        ilium M86.359
        ischium M86.359
        metacarpus M86.34-
        metatarsus M86.37-
        multiple sites M86.39
        neck M86.38
        radius M86.33-
        rib M86.38
        scapula M86.31-
        skull M86.38
        tarsus M86.37-
        tibia M86.36-
        toe M86.37-
        ulna M86.33-
        vertebra — *see* Osteomyelitis, vertebra
      multiple sites M86.59
      neck M86.58
      orbit H05.02-
      petrous bone — *see* Petrositis
      radius M86.53-
      rib M86.58
      scapula M86.51-
      skull M86.58
      tarsus M86.57-
      tibia M86.56-
      toe M86.57-

Osteomyelitis (general) (infective) (localized) (neonatal) (purulent) (septic) (staphylococcal) (streptococcal) (suppurative) (with periostitis) - *continued*
  chronic (or old) - *continued*
    hematogenous NEC - *continued*
      ulna M86.53-
      vertebra — *see* Osteomyelitis, vertebra
    humerus M86.62-
    ilium M86.659
    ischium M86.659
    mandible M27.2
    metacarpus M86.64-
    metatarsus M86.67-
    multifocal — *see* Osteomyelitis, chronic, hematogenous, multifocal
    multiple sites M86.69
    neck M86.68
    orbit H05.02-
    petrous bone — *see* Petrositis
    radius M86.63-
    rib M86.68
    scapula M86.61-
    skull M86.68
    tarsus M86.67-
    tibia M86.66-
    toe M86.67-
    ulna M86.63-
    vertebra — *see* Osteomyelitis, vertebra
  echinococcal B67.2
  Garr's — *see* Osteomyelitis, specified type NEC
  in diabetes mellitus — *see* E08-E13 with .69
  jaw (acute) (chronic) (lower) (neonatal) (suppurative) (upper) M27.2
  nonsuppurating — *see* Osteomyelitis, specified type NEC
  orbit H05.02-
  petrous bone — *see* Petrositis
  Salmonella (arizonae) (cholerae-suis) (enteritidis) (typhimurium) A02.24
  sclerosing, nonsuppurative — *see* Osteomyelitis, specified type NEC
  specified type NEC (*see also* subcategory M86.8X-)
    mandible M27.2
    orbit H05.02-
    petrous bone — *see* Petrositis
    vertebra — *see* Osteomyelitis, vertebra
  subacute M86.20
    carpus M86.24-
    clavicle M86.21-
    femur M86.25-
    fibula M86.26-
    finger M86.24-
    humerus M86.22-
    mandible M27.2
    metacarpus M86.24-
    metatarsus M86.27-
    multiple sites M86.29
    neck M86.28
    orbit H05.02-
    petrous bone — *see* Petrositis
    radius M86.23-
    rib M86.28
    scapula M86.21-
    skull M86.28
    tarsus M86.27-
    tibia M86.26-
    toe M86.27-
    ulna M86.23-
    vertebra — *see* Osteomyelitis, vertebra
  syphilitic A52.77
    congenital (early) A50.02 *[M90.80]*
  tuberculous — *see* Tuberculosis, bone
  typhoid A01.05
  vertebra M46.20
    cervical region M46.22
    cervicothoracic region M46.23
    lumbar region M46.26
    lumbosacral region M46.27
    occipito-atlanto-axial region M46.21
    sacrococcygeal region M46.28
    thoracic region M46.24
    thoracolumbar region M46.25
Osteomyelofibrosis D47.4
Osteomyelosclerosis D75.89
Osteonecrosis M87.9
  due to
    drugs — *see* Osteonecrosis, secondary, due to, drugs
    trauma — *see* Osteonecrosis, secondary, due to, trauma
  idiopathic aseptic M87.00
    ankle M87.07-

Osteonecrosis - *continued*
  idiopathic aseptic - *continued*
    carpus M87.03-
    clavicle M87.01-
    femur M87.05-
    fibula M87.06-
    finger M87.04-
    humerus M87.02-
    ilium M87.050
    ischium M87.050
    metacarpus M87.04-
    metatarsus M87.07-
    multiple sites M87.09
    neck M87.08
    pelvis M87.050
    radius M87.03-
    rib M87.08
    scapula M87.01-
    skull M87.08
    tarsus M87.07-
    tibia M87.06-
    toe M87.07-
    ulna M87.03-
    vertebra M87.08
  secondary NEC M87.30
    carpus M87.33-
    clavicle M87.31-
    due to
      drugs M87.10
        carpus M87.13-
        clavicle M87.11-
        femur M87.15-
        fibula M87.16-
        finger M87.14-
        humerus M87.12-
        ilium M87.159
        ischium M87.159
        jaw M87.180
        metacarpus M87.14-
        metatarsus M87.17-
        multiple sites M87.19
        neck M87.18
        radius M87.13-
        rib M87.18
        scapula M87.11-
        skull M87.18
        tarsus M87.17-
        tibia M87.16-
        toe M87.17-
        ulna M87.13-
        vertebra M87.18
      hemoglobinopathy NEC D58.2 *[M90.50]*
        carpus D58.2 *[M90.54-]*
        clavicle D58.2 *[M90.51-]*
        femur D58.2 *[M90.55-]*
        fibula D58.2 *[M90.56-]*
        finger D58.2 *[M90.54-]*
        humerus D58.2 *[M90.52-]*
        ilium D58.2 *[M90.55-]*
        ischium D58.2 *[M90.55-]*
        metacarpus D58.2 *[M90.54-]*
        metatarsus D58.2 *[M90.57-]*
        multiple sites D58.2 *[M90.58]*
        neck D58.2 *[M90.58]*
        radius D58.2 *[M90.53-]*
        rib D58.2 *[M90.58]*
        scapula D58.2 *[M90.51-]*
        skull D58.2 *[M90.58]*
        tarsus D58.2 *[M90.57-]*
        tibia D58.2 *[M90.56-]*
        toe D58.2 *[M90.57-]*
        ulna D58.2 *[M90.53-]*
        vertebra D58.2 *[M90.58]*
      trauma (previous) M87.20
        carpus M87.23-
        clavicle M87.21-
        femur M87.25-
        fibula M87.26-
        finger M87.24-
        humerus M87.22-
        ilium M87.25-
        ischium M87.25-
        metacarpus M87.24-
        metatarsus M87.27-
        multiple sites M87.29
        neck M87.28
        radius M87.23-
        rib M87.28
        scapula M87.21-
        skull M87.28
        tarsus M87.27-
        tibia M87.26-
        toe M87.27-

Osteonecrosis - *continued*
  secondary NEC - *continued*
    due to - *continued*
      trauma (previous) - *continued*
        ulna M87.23-
        vertebra M87.28
    femur M87.35-
    fibula M87.36-
    finger M87.34-
    humerus M87.32-
    ilium M87.350
    in
      caisson disease T70.3 *[M90.50]*
        carpus T70.3 *[M90.54-]*
        clavicle T70.3 *[M90.51-]*
        femur T70.3 *[M90.55-]*
        fibula T70.3 *[M90.56-]*
        finger T70.3 *[M90.54-]*
        humerus T70.3 *[M90.52-]*
        ilium T70.3 *[M90.55-]*
        ischium T70.3 *[M90.55-]*
        metacarpus T70.3 *[M90.54-]*
        metatarsus T70.3 *[M90.57-]*
        multiple sites T70.3 *[M90.59]*
        neck T70.3 *[M90.58]*
        radius T70.3 *[M90.53-]*
        rib T70.3 *[M90.58]*
        scapula T70.3 *[M90.51-]*
        skull T70.3 *[M90.58]*
        tarsus T70.3 *[M90.57-]*
        tibia T70.3 *[M90.56-]*
        toe T70.3 *[M90.57-]*
        ulna T70.3 *[M90.53-]*
        vertebra T70.3 *[M90.58]*
    ischium M87.350
    metacarpus M87.34-
    metatarsus M87.37-
    multiple site M87.39
    neck M87.38
    radius M87.33-
    rib M87.38
    scapula M87.319
    skull M87.38
    tarsus M87.379
    tibia M87.366
    toe M87.379
    ulna M87.33-
    vertebra M87.38
  specified type NEC M87.80
    carpus M87.83-
    clavicle M87.81-
    femur M87.85-
    fibula M87.86-
    finger M87.84-
    humerus M87.82-
    ilium M87.85-
    ischium M87.85-
    metacarpus M87.84-
    metatarsus M87.87-
    multiple sites M87.89
    neck M87.88
    radius M87.83-
    rib M87.88
    scapula M87.81-
    skull M87.88
    tarsus M87.87-
    tibia M87.86-
    toe M87.87-
    ulna M87.83-
    vertebra M87.88
Osteo-onycho-arthro-dysplasia Q87.2
Osteo-onychodysplasia, hereditary Q87.2
Osteopathia condensans disseminata Q78.8
Osteopathy — *see also* Osteomyelitis, Osteonecrosis, Osteoporosis
  after poliomyelitis M89.60
    carpus M89.64-
    clavicle M89.61-
    femur M89.65-
    fibula M89.66-
    finger M89.64-
    humerus M89.62-
    ilium M89.659
    ischium M89.659
    metacarpus M89.64-
    metatarsus M89.67-
    multiple sites M89.69
    neck M89.68
    radius M89.63-
    rib M89.68
    scapula M89.61-
    skull M89.68
    tarsus M89.67-

Osteopathy - *continued*
after poliomyelitis - *continued*
tibia M89.66-
toe M89.67-
ulna M89.63-
vertebra M89.68
in (due to)
renal osteodystrophy N25.0
specified diseases classified elsewhere — *see* subcategory M90.8
Osteopenia M85.8-
borderline M85.8-
Osteoperiostitis — *see* Osteomyelitis, specified type NEC
Osteopetrosis (familial) Q78.2
Osteophyte M25.70
ankle M25.77-
elbow M25.72-
foot joint M25.77-
hand joint M25.74-
hip M25.75-
knee M25.76-
shoulder M25.71-
spine M25.78
vertebrae M25.78
wrist M25.73-
Osteopoikilosis Q78.8
Osteoporosis (female) (male) M81.0
with current pathological fracture M80.00
age-related M81.0
with current pathologic fracture M80.00
carpus M80.04-
clavicle M80.01-
fibula M80.06-
finger M80.04-
humerus M80.02-
ilium M80.05-
ischium M80.05-
metacarpus M80.04-
metatarsus M80.07-
pelvis M80.05-
radius M80.03-
scapula M80.01-
tarsus M80.07-
tibia M80.06-
toe M80.07-
ulna M80.03-
vertebra M80.08
disuse M81.8
with current pathological fracture M80.80
carpus M80.84-
clavicle M80.81-
fibula M80.86-
finger M80.84-
humerus M80.82-
ilium M80.85-
ischium M80.85-
metacarpus M80.84-
metatarsus M80.87-
pelvis M80.85-
radius M80.83-
scapula M80.81-
tarsus M80.87-
tibia M80.86-
toe M80.87-
ulna M80.83-
vertebra M80.88
drug-induced — *see* Osteoporosis, specified type NEC
idiopathic — *see* Osteoporosis, specified type NEC
involutional — *see* Osteoporosis, age-related
Lequesne M81.6
localized M81.6
postmenopausal M81.0
with pathological fracture M80.00
carpus M80.04-
clavicle M80.01-
fibula M80.06-
finger M80.04-
humerus M80.02-
ilium M80.05-
ischium M80.05-
metacarpus M80.04-
metatarsus M80.07-
pelvis M80.05-
radius M80.03-
scapula M80.01-
tarsus M80.07-
tibia M80.06-
toe M80.07-
ulna M80.03-
vertebra M80.08

Osteoporosis (female) (male) - *continued*
postoophorectomy — *see* Osteoporosis, specified type NEC
postsurgical malabsorption — *see* Osteoporosis, specified type NEC
post-traumatic — *see* Osteoporosis, specified type NEC
senile — *see* Osteoporosis, age-related
specified type NEC M81.8
with pathological fracture M80.80
carpus M80.84-
clavicle M80.81-
fibula M80.86-
finger M80.84-
humerus M80.82-
ilium M80.85-
ischium M80.85-
metacarpus M80.84-
metatarsus M80.87-
pelvis M80.85-
radius M80.83-
scapula M80.81-
tarsus M80.87-
tibia M80.86-
toe M80.87-
ulna M80.83-
vertebra M80.88
Osteopsathyrosis (idiopathica) Q78.0
Osteoradionecrosis, jaw (acute) (chronic) (lower) (suppurative) (upper) M27.2
Osteosarcoma (any form) — *see* Neoplasm, bone, malignant
Osteosclerosis Q78.2
acquired M85.8-
congenita Q77.4
fragilitas (generalisata) Q78.2
myelofibrosis D75.81
Osteosclerotic anemia D64.89
Osteosis
cutis L94.2
renal fibrocystic N25.0
Österreicher-Turner syndrome Q87.2
Ostium
atrioventriculare commune Q21.2
primum (arteriosum) (defect) (persistent) Q21.2
secundum (arteriosum) (defect) (patent) (persistent) Q21.1
Ostrum-Furst syndrome Q75.8
Otalgia — *see* subcategory H92.0
Otitis (acute) H66.90
with effusion — *see also* Otitis, media, nonsuppurative
purulent — *see* Otitis, media, suppurative
adhesive — *see* subcategory H74.1
chronic — *see also* Otitis, media, chronic
with effusion — *see also* Otitis, media, nonsuppurative, chronic
externa H60.9-
abscess — *see* Abscess, ear, external
acute (noninfective) H60.50-
actinic H60.51-
chemical H60.52-
contact H60.53-
eczematoid H60.54-
infective — *see* Otitis, externa, infective
reactive H60.55-
specified NEC H60.59-
cellulitis — *see* Cellulitis, ear
chronic H60.6-
diffuse — *see* Otitis, externa, infective, diffuse
hemorrhagic — *see* Otitis, externa, infective, hemorrhagic
in (due to)
aspergillosis B44.89
candidiasis B37.84
erysipelas A46 *[H62.40]*
herpes (simplex) virus infection B00.1
zoster B02.8
impetigo L01.00 *[H62.40]*
infectious disease NEC B99 *[H62.4-]*
mycosis NEC B36.9 *[H62.40]*
parasitic disease NEC B89 *[H62.40]*
viral disease NEC B34.9 *[H62.40]*
zoster B02.8
infective NEC H60.39-
abscess — *see* Abscess, ear, external
cellulitis — *see* Cellulitis, ear
diffuse H60.31-
hemorrhagic H60.32-
swimmer's ear — *see* Swimmer's, ear
malignant H60.2-
mycotic NEC B36.9 *[H62.40]*
in

Otitis (acute) - *continued*
externa - *continued*
mycotic NEC - *continued*
in - *continued*
aspergillosis B44.89
candidiasis B37.84
moniliasis B37.84
necrotizing — *see* Otitis, externa, malignant
Pseudomonas aeruginosa — *see* Otitis, externa, malignant
reactive — *see* Otitis, externa, acute, reactive
specified NEC — *see* subcategory H60.8
tropical NEC B36.9 *[H62.40]*
in
aspergillosis B44.89
candidiasis B37.84
moniliasis B37.84
insidiosa — *see* Otosclerosis
interna — *see* subcategory H83.0
media (hemorrhagic) (staphylococcal) (streptococcal) H66.9-
with effusion (nonpurulent) — *see* Otitis, media, nonsuppurative
acute, subacute H66.90
allergic — *see* Otitis, media, nonsuppurative, acute, allergic
exudative — *see* Otitis, media, suppurative, acute
mucoid — *see* Otitis, media, nonsuppurative, acute
necrotizing — *see also* Otitis, media, suppurative, acute
in
measles B05.3
scarlet fever A38.0
nonsuppurative NEC — *see* Otitis, media, nonsuppurative, acute
purulent — *see* Otitis, media, suppurative, acute
sanguinous — *see* Otitis, media, nonsuppurative, acute
secretory — *see* Otitis, media, nonsuppurative, acute, serous
seromucinous — *see* Otitis, media, nonsuppurative, acute
serous — *see* Otitis, media, nonsuppurative, acute, serous
suppurative — *see* Otitis, media, suppurative, acute
allergic — *see* Otitis, media, nonsuppurative
catarrhal — *see* Otitis, media, nonsuppurative
chronic H66.90
with effusion (nonpurulent) — *see* Otitis, media, nonsuppurative, chronic
allergic — *see* Otitis, media, nonsuppurative, chronic, allergic
benign suppurative — *see* Otitis, media, suppurative, chronic, tubotympanic
catarrhal — *see* Otitis, media, nonsuppurative, chronic, serous
exudative — *see* Otitis, media, nonsuppurative, chronic
mucinous — *see* Otitis, media, nonsuppurative, chronic, mucoid
mucoid — *see* Otitis, media, nonsuppurative, chronic, mucoid
nonsuppurative NEC — *see* Otitis, media, nonsuppurative, chronic
purulent — *see* Otitis, media, suppurative, chronic
secretory — *see* Otitis, media, nonsuppurative, chronic, mucoid
seromucinous — *see* Otitis, media, nonsuppurative, chronic
serous — *see* Otitis, media, nonsuppurative, chronic, serous
suppurative — *see* Otitis, media, suppurative, chronic
transudative — *see* Otitis, media, nonsuppurative, chronic, mucoid
exudative — *see* Otitis, media, suppurative
in (due to) (with)
influenza — *see* Influenza, with, otitis media
measles B05.3
scarlet fever A38.0
tuberculosis A18.6
viral disease NEC B34.- *[H67.-]*
mucoid — *see* Otitis, media, nonsuppurative
nonsuppurative H65.9-
acute or subacute NEC H65.19-
allergic H65.11-
recurrent H65.11-
recurrent H65.19-
secretory — *see* Otitis, media, nonsuppurative, serous

P

Pain (s) - *continued*
- chronic - *continued*
  - associated with significant psychosocial dysfunction G89.4
  - due to trauma G89.21
  - neoplasm related G89.3
  - postoperative NEC G89.28
  - postprocedural NEC G89.28
  - post-thoracotomy G89.22
  - specified NEC G89.29
- coccyx M53.3
- colon — *see* Pain, abdominal
- coronary — *see* Angina
- costochondral R07.1
- diaphragm R07.1
- due to cancer G89.3
- due to device, implant or graft — *see also* Complications, by site and type, specified NEC T85.848
  - arterial graft NEC T82.848
  - breast (implant) T85.848
  - catheter NEC T85.848
    - dialysis (renal) T82.848
      - intraperitoneal T85.848
    - infusion NEC T82.848
      - spinal (epidural) (subdural) T85.840
    - urinary (indwelling) T83.84
  - electronic (electrode) (pulse generator) (stimulator)
    - bone T84.84
    - cardiac T82.847
    - nervous system (brain) (peripheral nerve) (spinal) T85.840
    - urinary T83.84
  - fixation, internal (orthopedic) NEC T84.84
  - gastrointestinal (bile duct) (esophagus) T85.848
  - genital NEC T83.84
  - heart NEC T82.847
  - infusion NEC T85.848
  - joint prosthesis T84.84
  - ocular (corneal graft) (orbital implant) NEC T85.848
  - orthopedic NEC T84.84
  - specified NEC T85.848
  - urinary NEC T83.84
  - vascular NEC T82.848
  - ventricular intracranial shunt T85.840
- due to malignancy (primary) (secondary) G89.3
- ear — *see* subcategory H92.0
- epigastric, epigastrium R10.13
- eye — *see* Pain, ocular
- face, facial R51
  - atypical G50.1
- female genital organs NEC N94.89
- finger — *see* Pain, limb, upper
- flank — *see* Pain, abdominal
- foot — *see* Pain, limb, lower
- gallbladder K82.9
- gas (intestinal) R14.1
- gastric — *see* Pain, abdominal
- generalized NOS R52
- genital organ
  - female N94.89
  - male N50.89
- groin — *see* Pain, abdominal, lower
- hand — *see* Pain, limb, upper
- head — *see* Headache
- heart — *see* Pain, precordial
- infra-orbital — *see* Neuralgia, trigeminal
- intercostal R07.82
- intermenstrual N94.0
- jaw R68.84
- joint M25.50
  - ankle M25.57-
  - elbow M25.52-
  - finger M25.54-
  - foot M25.57-
  - hand M25.54-
  - hip M25.55-
  - knee M25.56-
  - shoulder M25.51-
  - toe M25.57-
  - wrist M25.53-
- kidney N23
- laryngeal R07.0
- leg — *see* Pain, limb, lower
- limb M79.609
  - lower M79.60-
    - foot M79.67-
    - lower leg M79.66-
    - thigh M79.65-
    - toe M79.67-
  - upper M79.60-
    - axilla M79.62-

Pain (s) - *continued*
- limb - *continued*
  - upper - *continued*
    - finger M79.64-
    - forearm M79.63-
    - hand M79.64-
    - upper arm M79.62-
- loin M54.5
- low back M54.5
- lumbar region M54.5
- mandibular R68.84
- mastoid — *see* subcategory H92.0
- maxilla R68.84
- menstrual — *see also* Dysmenorrhea N94.6
- metacarpophalangeal (joint) — *see* Pain, joint, hand
- metatarsophalangeal (joint) — *see* Pain, joint, foot
- mouth K13.79
- muscle — *see* Myalgia
- musculoskeletal — *see also* Pain, by site M79.18
- myofascial M79.18
- nasal J34.89
- nasopharynx J39.2
- neck NEC M54.2
- nerve NEC — *see* Neuralgia
- neuromuscular — *see* Neuralgia
- nose J34.89
- ocular H57.1-
- ophthalmic — *see* Pain, ocular
- orbital region — *see* Pain, ocular
- ovary N94.89
- over heart — *see* Pain, precordial
- ovulation N94.0
- pelvic (female) R10.2
- penis N48.89
- pericardial — *see* Pain, precordial
- perineal, perineum R10.2
- pharynx J39.2
- pleura, pleural, pleuritic R07.81
- postoperative NOS G89.18
- postprocedural NOS G89.18
- post-thoracotomy G89.12
- precordial (region) R07.2
- premenstrual N94.3
- psychogenic (persistent) (any site) F45.41
- radicular (spinal) — *see* Radiculopathy
- rectum K62.89
- respiration R07.1
- retrosternal R07.2
- rheumatoid, muscular — *see* Myalgia
- rib R07.81
- root (spinal) — *see* Radiculopathy
- round ligament (stretch) R10.2
- sacroiliac M53.3
- sciatic — *see* Sciatica
- scrotum N50.82
- seminal vesicle N50.89
- shoulder M25.51-
- spermatic cord N50.89
- spinal root — *see* Radiculopathy
- spine M54.9
  - cervical M54.2
  - low back M54.5
    - with sciatica M54.4-
  - thoracic M54.6
- stomach — *see* Pain, abdominal
- substernal R07.2
- temporomandibular (joint) M26.62-
- testis N50.81-
- thoracic spine M54.6
  - with radicular and visceral pain M54.14
- throat R07.0
- tibia — *see* Pain, limb, lower
- toe — *see* Pain, limb, lower
- tongue K14.6
- tooth K08.89
- trigeminal — *see* Neuralgia, trigeminal
- tumor associated G89.3
- ureter N23
- urinary (organ) (system) N23
- uterus NEC N94.89
- vagina R10.2
- vertebrogenic (syndrome) M54.89
- vesical R39.89
  - associated with micturition — *see* Micturition, painful
- vulva R10.2

Painful — *see also* Pain
- coitus
  - female N94.10
  - male N53.12
  - psychogenic F52.6
- ejaculation (semen) N53.12
  - psychogenic F52.6

Painful - *continued*
- erection — *see* Priapism
- feet syndrome E53.8
- joint replacement (hip) (knee) T84.84
- menstruation — *see* Dysmenorrhea
  - psychogenic F45.8
- micturition — *see* Micturition, painful
- respiration R07.1
- scar NEC L90.5
- wire sutures T81.89

Painter's colic — *see* subcategory T56.0

Palate — *see* condition

Palatoplegia K13.79

Palatoschisis — *see* Cleft, palate

Palilalia R48.8

Palliative care Z51.5

Pallor R23.1
- optic disc, temporal — *see* Atrophy, optic

Palmar — *see also* condition
- fascia — *see* condition

Palpable
- cecum K63.89
- kidney N28.89
- ovary N83.8
- prostate N42.9
- spleen — *see* Splenomegaly

Palpitations (heart) R00.2
- psychogenic F45.8

Palsy — *see also* Paralysis G83.9
- atrophic diffuse (progressive) G12.22
- Bell's — *see also* Palsy, facial
  - newborn P11.3
- brachial plexus NEC G54.0
  - newborn (birth injury) P14.3
- brain — *see* Palsy, cerebral
- bulbar (progressive) (chronic) G12.22
  - of childhood (Fazio-Londe) G12.1
  - pseudo NEC G12.29
  - supranuclear (progressive) G23.1
- cerebral (congenital) G80.9
  - ataxic G80.4
  - athetoid G80.3
  - choreathetoid G80.3
  - diplegic G80.8
    - spastic G80.1
  - dyskinetic G80.3
    - athetoid G80.3
    - choreathetoid G80.3
    - distonic G80.3
  - dystonic G80.3
  - hemiplegic G80.8
    - spastic G80.2
  - mixed G80.8
  - monoplegic G80.8
    - spastic G80.1
  - paraplegic G80.8
    - spastic G80.1
  - quadriplegic G80.8
    - spastic G80.0
  - spastic G80.1
    - diplegic G80.1
    - hemiplegic G80.2
    - monoplegic G80.1
    - quadriplegic G80.0
    - specified NEC G80.1
    - tetrapelgic G80.0
  - specified NEC G80.8
  - syphilitic A52.12
    - congenital A50.49
  - tetraplegic G80.8
    - spastic G80.0
- cranial nerve — *see also* Disorder, nerve, cranial
  - multiple G52.7
    - in
      - infectious disease B99 *[G53]*
      - neoplastic disease — *see also* Neoplasm D49.9 *[G53]*
      - parasitic disease B89 *[G53]*
      - sarcoidosis D86.82
- creeping G12.22
- diver's T70.3
- Erb's P14.0
- facial G51.0
  - newborn (birth injury) P11.3
- glossopharyngeal G52.1
- Klumpke (-Déjérine) P14.1
- lead — *see* subcategory T56.0
- median nerve (tardy) G56.1-
- nerve G58.9
  - specified NEC G58.8
- peroneal nerve (acute) (tardy) G57.3-
- progressive supranuclear G23.1
- pseudobulbar NEC G12.29

Palsy - *continued*
  radial nerve (acute) G56.3-
  seventh nerve — *see also* Palsy, facial
    newborn P11.3
  shaking — *see* Parkinsonism
  spastic (cerebral) (spinal) G80.1
  ulnar nerve (tardy) G56.2-
  wasting G12.29
Paludism — *see* Malaria
Panangiitis M30.0
Panaris, panaritium — *see also* Cellulitis, digit
  with lymphangitis — *see* Lymphangitis, acute, digit
Panarteritis nodosa M30.0
  brain or cerebral I67.7
Pancake heart R93.1
  with cor pulmonale (chronic) I27.81
Pancarditis (acute) (chronic) I51.89
  rheumatic I09.89
    active or acute I01.8
Pancoast's syndrome or tumor C34.1-
Pancolitis, ulcerative (chronic) K51.00
  with
    complication K51.019
    abscess K51.014
    fistula K51.013
    obstruction K51.012
    rectal bleeding K51.011
    specified complication NEC K51.018
Pancreas, pancreatic — *see* condition
Pancreatitis (annular) (apoplectic) (calcareous) (edematous) (hemorrhagic) (malignant) (recurrent) (subacute) (suppurative) K85.90
  with necrosis (uninfected) K85.91
    infected K85.92
  acute (without necrosis or infection) K85.90
    with necrosis (uninfected) K85.91
      infected K85.92
    alcohol induced (without necrosis or infection) K85.20
      with necrosis (uninfected) K85.21
        infected K85.22
    biliary (without necrosis or infection) K85.10
      with necrosis (uninfected) K85.11
        infected K85.12
    drug induced (without necrosis or infection) K85.30
      with necrosis (uninfected) K85.31
        infected K85.32
    gallstone (without necrosis or infection) K85.10
      with necrosis (uninfected) K85.11
        infected K85.12
    idiopathic (without necrosis or infection) K85.00
      with necrosis (uninfected) K85.01
        infected K85.02
    specified NEC (without necrosis or infection) K85.80
      with necrosis (uninfected) K85.81
        infected K85.82
  chronic (infectious) K86.1
    alcohol-induced K86.0
    recurrent K86.1
    relapsing K86.1
  cystic (chronic) K86.1
  cytomegaloviral B25.2
  fibrous (chronic) K86.1
  gangrenous — *see* Pancreatitis, acute
  gallstone (without necrosis or infection) K85.10
    with necrosis (uninfected) K85.11
      infected K85.12
  interstitial (chronic) K86.1
    acute — *see also* Pancreatitis, acute K85.80
  mumps B26.3
  recurrent (chronic) K86.1
  relapsing, chronic K86.1
  syphilitic A52.74
Pancreatoblastoma — *see* Neoplasm, pancreas, malignant
Pancreolithiasis K86.89
Pancytolysis D75.89
Pancytopenia (acquired) D61.818
  with
    malformations D61.09
    myelodysplastic syndrome — *see* Syndrome, myelodysplastic
  antineoplastic chemotherapy induced D61.810
  congenital D61.09
  drug-induced NEC D61.811
PANDAS
  (pediatric autoimmune neuropsychiatric disorders associated with streptococcal infections syndrome) D89.89
Panencephalitis, subacute, sclerosing A81.1
Panhematopenia D61.9
  congenital D61.09
  constitutional D61.09
  splenic, primary D73.1
Panhemocytopenia D61.9
  congenital D61.09
  constitutional D61.09
Panhypogonadism E29.1
Panhypopituitarism E23.0
  prepubertal E23.0
Panic (attack) (state) F41.0
  reaction to exceptional stress (transient) F43.0
Panmyelopathy, familial, constitutional D61.09
Panmyelophthisis D61.82
  congenital D61.09
Panmyelosis (acute) (with myelofibrosis) C94.4-
Panner's disease — *see* Osteochondrosis, juvenile, humerus
Panneuritis endemica E51.11
Panniculitis (nodular) (nonsuppurative) M79.3
  back M54.00
    cervical region M54.02
    cervicothoracic region M54.03
    lumbar region M54.06
    lumbosacral region M54.07
    multiple sites M54.09
    occipito-atlanto-axial region M54.01
    sacrococcygeal region M54.08
    thoracic region M54.04
    thoracolumbar region M54.05
  lupus L93.2
  mesenteric K65.4
  neck M54.02
    cervicothoracic region M54.03
    occipito-atlanto-axial region M54.01
  relapsing M35.6
Panniculus adiposus (abdominal) E65
Pannus (allergic) (cornea) (degenerativus) (keratic) H16.42-
  abdominal (symptomatic) E65
  trachomatosus, trachomatous (active) A71.1
Panophthalmitis H44.01-
Pansinusitis (chronic) (hyperplastic) (nonpurulent) (purulent) J32.4
  acute J01.40
    recurrent J01.41
  tuberculous A15.8
Panuveitis (sympathetic) H44.11-
Panvalvular disease I08.9
  specified NEC I08.8
PAPA
  (pyogenic arthritis, pyoderma gangrenosum, and acne syndrome) M04.8
Papanicolaou smear, cervix Z12.4
  as part of routine gynecological examination Z01.419
    with abnormal findings Z01.411
  for suspected neoplasm Z12.4
  nonspecific abnormal finding R87.619
  routine Z01.419
    with abnormal findings Z01.411
Papilledema (choked disc) H47.10
  associated with
    decreased ocular pressure H47.12
    increased intracranial pressure H47.11
    retinal disorder H47.13
  Foster-Kennedy syndrome H47.14-
Papillitis H46.00
  anus K62.89
  chronic lingual K14.4
  necrotizing, kidney N17.2
  optic H46.0-
  rectum K62.89
  renal, necrotizing N17.2
  tongue K14.0
Papilloma — *see also* Neoplasm, benign, by site
  acuminatum (female) (male) (anogenital) A63.0
  basal cell L82.1
    inflamed L82.0
  benign pinta (primary) A67.0
  bladder (urinary) (transitional cell) D41.4
  choroid plexus (lateral ventricle) (third ventricle) D33.0
    anaplastic C71.5
    fourth ventricle D33.1
    malignant C71.5
  renal pelvis (transitional cell) D41.1-
    benign D30.1-
  Schneiderian
    specified site — *see* Neoplasm, benign, by site
    unspecified site D14.0
  serous surface
    borderline malignancy
Papilloma - *continued*
  serous surface - *continued*
    borderline malignancy - *continued*
      specified site — *see* Neoplasm, uncertain behavior, by site
      unspecified site D39.10
    specified site — *see* Neoplasm, benign, by site
    unspecified site D27.9
  transitional (cell)
    bladder (urinary) D41.4
    inverted type — *see* Neoplasm, uncertain behavior, by site
    renal pelvis D41.1-
    ureter D41.2-
  ureter (transitional cell) D41.2-
    benign D30.2-
  urothelial — *see* Neoplasm, uncertain behavior, by site
  villous — *see* Neoplasm, uncertain behavior, by site
    adenocarcinoma in — *see* Neoplasm, malignant, by site
      in situ — *see* Neoplasm, in situ
  yaws, plantar or palmar A66.1
Papillomata, multiple, of yaws A66.1
Papillomatosis — *see also* Neoplasm, benign, by site
  confluent and reticulated L83
  cystic, breast — *see* Mastopathy, cystic
  ductal, breast — *see* Mastopathy, cystic
  intraductal (diffuse) — *see* Neoplasm, benign, by site
  subareolar duct D24-
Papillomavirus, as cause of disease classified elsewhere B97.7
Papillon-Léage and Psaume syndrome Q87.0
Papule (s) R23.8
  carate (primary) A67.0
  fibrous, of nose D22.39
  Gottron's L94.4
  pinta (primary) A67.0
Papulosis
  lymphomatoid C86.6
  malignant I77.89
Papyraceous fetus O31.0-
Para-albuminemia E88.09
Paracephalus Q89.7
Parachute mitral valve Q23.2
Paracoccidioidomycosis B41.9
  disseminated B41.7
  generalized B41.7
  mucocutaneous-lymphangitic B41.8
  pulmonary B41.0
  specified NEC B41.8
  visceral B41.8
Paradentosis K05.4
Paraffinoma T88.8
Paraganglioma D44.7
  adrenal D35.0-
    malignant C74.1-
  aortic body D44.7
    malignant C75.5
  carotid body D44.6
    malignant C75.4
  chromaffin — *see also* Neoplasm, benign, by site
    malignant — *see* Neoplasm, malignant, by site
  extra-adrenal D44.7
    malignant C75.5
      specified site — *see* Neoplasm, malignant, by site
      unspecified site C75.5
    specified site — *see* Neoplasm, uncertain behavior, by site
    unspecified site D44.7
  gangliocytic D13.2
    specified site — *see* Neoplasm, benign, by site
    unspecified site D13.2
  glomus jugulare D44.7
    malignant C75.5
  jugular D44.7
  malignant C75.5
    specified site — *see* Neoplasm, malignant, by site
    unspecified site C75.5
  nonchromaffin D44.7
    malignant C75.5
      specified site — *see* Neoplasm, malignant, by site
      unspecified site C75.5
    specified site — *see* Neoplasm, uncertain behavior, by site
    unspecified site D44.7
  parasympathetic D44.7
    specified site — *see* Neoplasm, uncertain behavior, by site
    unspecified site D44.7
  specified site — *see* Neoplasm, uncertain behavior, by site

- **Paraganglioma** - *continued*
  - sympathetic D44.7
    - specified site — *see* Neoplasm, uncertain behavior, by site
    - unspecified site D44.7
  - unspecified site D44.7
- **Parageusia** R43.2
  - psychogenic F45.8
- **Paragonimiasis** B66.4
- **Paragranuloma, Hodgkin** — *see* Lymphoma, Hodgkin, specified NEC
- **Parahemophilia** — *see also* Defect, coagulation D68.2
- **Parakeratosis** R23.4
  - variegata L41.0
- **Paralysis, paralytic** (complete) (incomplete) G83.9
  - with
    - syphilis A52.17
  - abducens, abducent (nerve) — *see* Strabismus, paralytic, sixth nerve
  - abductor, lower extremity G57.9-
  - accessory nerve G52.8
  - accommodation — *see also* Paresis, of accommodation
    - hysterical F44.89
  - acoustic nerve (except Deafness) — *see* subcategory H93.3
  - agitans — *see also* Parkinsonism G20
    - arteriosclerotic G21.4
  - alternating (oculomotor) G83.89
  - amyotrophic G12.21
  - ankle G57.9-
  - anus (sphincter) K62.89
  - arm — *see* Monoplegia, upper limb
  - ascending (spinal) , acute G61.0
  - association G12.29
  - asthenic bulbar G70.00
    - with exacerbation (acute) G70.01
    - in crisis G70.01
  - ataxic (hereditary) G11.9
    - general (syphilitic) A52.17
  - atrophic G58.9
    - infantile, acute — *see* Poliomyelitis, paralytic
    - progressive G12.22
    - spinal (acute) — *see* Poliomyelitis, paralytic
  - axillary G54.0
  - Babinski-Nageotte's G83.89
  - Bell's G51.0
    - newborn P11.3
  - Benedikt's G46.3
  - birth injury P14.9
    - spinal cord P11.5
  - bladder (neurogenic) (sphincter) N31.2
  - bowel, colon or intestine K56.0
  - brachial plexus G54.0
    - birth injury P14.3
    - newborn (birth injury) P14.3
  - brain G83.9
    - diplegia G83.0
    - triplegia G83.89
  - bronchial J98.09
  - Brown-Séquard G83.81
  - bulbar (chronic) (progressive) G12.22
    - infantile — *see* Poliomyelitis, paralytic
    - poliomyelitic — *see* Poliomyelitis, paralytic
    - pseudo G12.29
  - bulbospinal G70.00
    - with exacerbation (acute) G70.01
    - in crisis G70.01
  - cardiac — *see also* Failure, heart I50.9
  - cerebrocerebellar, diplegic G80.1
  - cervical
    - plexus G54.2
    - sympathetic G90.09
  - Céstan-Chenais G46.3
  - Charcot-Marie-Tooth type G60.0
  - Clark's G80.9
  - colon K56.0
  - compressed air T70.3
  - compression
    - arm G56.9-
    - leg G57.9-
    - lower extremity G57.9-
    - upper extremity G56.9-
  - congenital (cerebral) — *see* Palsy, cerebral
  - conjugate movement (gaze) (of eye) H51.0
    - cortical (nuclear) (supranuclear) H51.0
  - cordis — *see* Failure, heart
  - cranial or cerebral nerve G52.9
  - creeping G12.22
  - crossed leg G83.89
  - crutch — *see* Injury, brachial plexus
  - deglutition R13.0

- **Paralysis, paralytic** (complete) (incomplete) - *continued*
  - deglutition - *continued*
    - hysterical F44.4
  - dementia A52.17
  - descending (spinal) NEC G12.29
  - diaphragm (flaccid) J98.6
    - due to accidental dissection of phrenic nerve during procedure — *see* Puncture, accidental complicating surgery
  - digestive organs NEC K59.8
  - diplegic — *see* Diplegia
  - divergence (nuclear) H51.8
  - diver's T70.3
  - Duchenne's
    - birth injury P14.0
    - due to or associated with
      - motor neuron disease G12.22
      - muscular dystrophy G71.01
  - due to intracranial or spinal birth injury — *see* Palsy, cerebral
  - embolic (current episode) I63.4-
  - Erb (-Duchenne) (birth) (newborn) P14.0
  - Erb's syphilitic spastic spinal A52.17
  - esophagus K22.8
  - eye muscle (extrinsic) H49.9
    - intrinsic — *see also* Paresis, of accommodation
  - facial (nerve) G51.0
    - birth injury P11.3
    - congenital P11.3
    - following operation NEC — *see* Puncture, accidental complicating surgery
    - newborn (birth injury) P11.3
  - familial (recurrent) (periodic) G72.3
    - spastic G11.4
  - fauces J39.2
  - finger G56.9-
  - gait R26.1
  - gastric nerve (nondiabetic) G52.2
  - gaze, conjugate H51.0
  - general (progressive) (syphilitic) A52.17
    - juvenile A50.45
  - glottis J38.00
    - bilateral J38.02
    - unilateral J38.01
  - gluteal G54.1
  - Gubler (-Millard) G46.3
  - hand — *see* Monoplegia, upper limb
  - heart — *see* Arrest, cardiac
  - hemiplegic — *see* Hemiplegia
  - hyperkalemic periodic (familial) G72.3
  - hypoglossal (nerve) G52.3
  - hypokalemic periodic G72.3
  - hysterical F44.4
  - ileus K56.0
  - infantile — *see also* Poliomyelitis, paralytic A80.30
    - bulbar — *see* Poliomyelitis, paralytic
    - cerebral — *see* Palsy, cerebral
    - spastic — *see* Palsy, cerebral, spastic
  - infective — *see* Poliomyelitis, paralytic
  - inferior nuclear G83.9
  - internuclear — *see* Ophthalmoplegia, internuclear
  - intestine K56.0
  - iris H57.09
    - due to diphtheria (toxin) A36.89
  - ischemic, Volkmann's (complicating trauma) T79.6
  - Jackson's G83.89
  - jake — *see* Poisoning, food, noxious, plant
  - Jamaica ginger (jake) G62.2
  - juvenile general A50.45
  - Klumpke (-Déjérine) (birth) (newborn) P14.1
  - labioglossal (laryngeal) (pharyngeal) G12.29
  - Landry's G61.0
  - laryngeal nerve (recurrent) (superior) (unilateral) J38.00
    - bilateral J38.02
    - unilateral J38.01
  - larynx J38.00
    - bilateral J38.02
    - due to diphtheria (toxin) A36.2
    - unilateral J38.01
  - lateral G12.23
  - lead — *see* subcategory T56.0
  - left side — *see* Hemiplegia
  - leg G83.1-
    - both — *see* Paraplegia
    - crossed G83.89
    - hysterical F44.4
    - psychogenic F44.4
    - transient or transitory R29.818
      - traumatic NEC — *see* Injury, nerve, leg
  - levator palpebrae superioris — *see* Blepharoptosis, paralytic

- **Paralysis, paralytic** (complete) (incomplete) - *continued*
  - limb — *see* Monoplegia
  - lip K13.0
  - Lissauer's A52.17
  - lower limb — *see* Monoplegia, lower limb
    - both — *see* Paraplegia
  - lung J98.4
  - median nerve G56.1-
  - medullary (tegmental) G83.89
  - mesencephalic NEC G83.89
    - tegmental G83.89
  - middle alternating G83.89
  - Millard-Gubler-Foville G46.3
  - monoplegic — *see* Monoplegia
  - motor G83.9
  - muscle, muscular NEC G72.89
    - due to nerve lesion G58.9
    - eye (extrinsic) H49.9
      - intrinsic — *see* Paresis, of accommodation
      - oblique — *see* Strabismus, paralytic, fourth nerve
    - iris sphincter H21.9
    - ischemic (Volkmann's) (complicating trauma) T79.6
    - progressive G12.21
    - pseudohypertrophic G71.02
  - musculocutaneous nerve G56.9-
  - musculospiral G56.9-
  - nerve — *see also* Disorder, nerve
    - abducent — *see* Strabismus, paralytic, sixth nerve
    - accessory G52.8
    - auditory (except Deafness) — *see* subcategory H93.3
    - birth injury P14.9
    - cranial or cerebral G52.9
    - facial G51.0
      - birth injury P11.3
      - congenital P11.3
      - newborn (birth injury) P11.3
    - fourth or trochlear — *see* Strabismus, paralytic, fourth nerve
    - newborn (birth injury) P14.9
    - oculomotor — *see* Strabismus, paralytic, third nerve
    - phrenic (birth injury) P14.2
    - radial G56.3-
    - seventh or facial G51.0
      - newborn (birth injury) P11.3
    - sixth or abducent — *see* Strabismus, paralytic, sixth nerve
    - syphilitic A52.15
    - third or oculomotor — *see* Strabismus, paralytic, third nerve
    - trigeminal G50.9
    - trochlear — *see* Strabismus, paralytic, fourth nerve
    - ulnar G56.2-
  - normokalemic periodic G72.3
  - ocular H49.9
    - alternating G83.89
  - oculofacial, congenital (Moebius) Q87.0
  - oculomotor (external bilateral) (nerve) — *see* Strabismus, paralytic, third nerve
  - palate (soft) K13.79
  - paratrigeminal G50.9
  - periodic (familial) (hyperkalemic) (hypokalemic) (myotonic) (normokalemic) (potassium sensitive) (secondary) G72.3
  - peripheral autonomic nervous system — *see* Neuropathy, peripheral, autonomic
  - peroneal (nerve) G57.3-
  - pharynx J39.2
  - phrenic nerve G56.8-
  - plantar nerve (s) G57.6-
  - pneumogastric nerve G52.2
  - poliomyelitis (current) — *see* Poliomyelitis, paralytic
  - popliteal nerve G57.3-
  - postepileptic transitory G83.84
  - progressive (atrophic) (bulbar) (spinal) G12.22
    - general A52.17
    - infantile acute — *see* Poliomyelitis, paralytic
    - supranuclear G23.1
  - pseudobulbar G12.29
  - pseudohypertrophic (muscle) G71.09
  - psychogenic F44.4
  - quadriceps G57.9-
  - quadriplegic — *see* Tetraplegia
  - radial nerve G56.3-
  - rectus muscle (eye) H49.9
  - recurrent isolated sleep G47.53
  - respiratory (muscle) (system) (tract) R06.81
    - center NEC G93.89
    - congenital P28.89

Paralysis, paralytic (complete) (incomplete) - *continued*
respiratory (muscle) (system) (tract) - *continued*
newborn P28.89
right side — *see* Hemiplegia
saturnine — *see* subcategory T56.0
sciatic nerve G57.0-
senile G83.9
shaking — *see* Parkinsonism
shoulder G56.9-
sleep, recurrent isolated G47.53
spastic G83.9
cerebral — *see* Palsy, cerebral, spastic
congenital (cerebral) — *see* Palsy, cerebral, spastic
familial G11.4
hereditary G11.4
quadriplegic G80.0
syphilitic (spinal) A52.17
sphincter, bladder — *see* Paralysis, bladder
spinal (cord) G83.9
accessory nerve G52.8
acute — *see* Poliomyelitis, paralytic
ascending acute G61.0
atrophic (acute) — *see also* Poliomyelitis, paralytic
spastic, syphilitic A52.17
congenital NEC — *see* Palsy, cerebral
infantile — *see* Poliomyelitis, paralytic
hereditary G95.89
progressive G12.21
sequelae NEC G83.89
sternomastoid G52.8
stomach K31.84
diabetic — *see* Diabetes, by type, with gastroparesis
nerve G52.2
diabetic — *see* Diabetes, by type, with gastroparesis
stroke — *see* Infarct, brain
subcapsularis G56.8-
supranuclear (progressive) G23.1
sympathetic G90.8
cervical G90.09
nervous system — *see* Neuropathy, peripheral, autonomic
syndrome G83.9
specified NEC G83.89
syphilitic spastic spinal (Erb's) A52.17
thigh G57.9-
throat J39.2
diphtheritic A36.0
muscle J39.2
thrombotic (current episode) I63.3-
thumb G56.9-
tick — *see* Toxicity, venom, arthropod, specified NEC
Todd's (postepileptic transitory paralysis) G83.84
toe G57.6-
tongue K14.8
transient R29.5
arm or leg NEC R29.818
traumatic NEC — *see* Injury, nerve
trapezius G52.8
traumatic, transient NEC — *see* Injury, nerve
trembling — *see* Parkinsonism
triceps brachii G56.9-
trigeminal nerve G50.9
trochlear (nerve) — *see* Strabismus, paralytic, fourth nerve
ulnar nerve G56.2-
upper limb — *see* Monoplegia, upper limb
uremic N18.9 *[G99.8]*
uveoparotitic D86.89
uvula K13.79
postdiphtheritic A36.0
vagus nerve G52.2
vasomotor NEC G90.8
velum palati K13.79
vesical — *see* Paralysis, bladder
vestibular nerve (except Vertigo) — *see* subcategory H93.3
vocal cords J38.00
bilateral J38.02
unilateral J38.01
Volkmann's (complicating trauma) T79.6
wasting G12.29
Weber's G46.3
wrist G56.9-
Paramedial urethrovesical orifice Q64.79
Paramenia N92.6
Parametritis — *see also* Disease, pelvis, inflammatory N73.2
acute N73.0
Parametritis - *continued*
complicating abortion — *see* Abortion, by type, complicated by, parametritis
Parametrium, parametric — *see* condition
Paramnesia — *see* Amnesia
Paramolar K00.1
Paramyloidosis E85.89
Paramyoclonus multiplex G25.3
Paramyotonia (congenita) G71.19
Parangi — *see* Yaws
Paranoia (querulans) F22
senile F03
Paranoid
dementia (senile) F03
praecox — *see* Schizophrenia
personality F60.0
psychosis (climacteric) (involutional) (menopausal) F22
psychogenic (acute) F23
senile F03
reaction (acute) F23
chronic F22
schizophrenia F20.0
state (climacteric) (involutional) (menopausal) (simple) F22
senile F03
tendencies F60.0
traits F60.0
trends F60.0
type, psychopathic personality F60.0
Paraparesis — *see* Paraplegia
Paraphasia R47.02
Paraphilia F65.9
Paraphimosis (congenital) N47.2
chancroidal A57
Paraphrenia, paraphrenic (late) F22
schizophrenia F20.0
Paraplegia (lower) G82.20
ataxic — *see* Degeneration, combined, spinal cord
complete G82.21
congenital (cerebral) G80.8
spastic G80.1
familial spastic G11.4
functional (hysterical) F44.4
hereditary, spastic G11.4
hysterical F44.4
incomplete G82.22
Pott's A18.01
psychogenic F44.4
spastic
Erb's spinal, syphilitic A52.17
hereditary G11.4
tropical G04.1
syphilitic (spastic) A52.17
traumatic
current injury - code to injury with seventh character A
sequela of previous injury - code to injury with seventh character S
tropical spastic G04.1
Parapoxvirus B08.60
specified NEC B08.69
Paraproteinemia D89.2
benign (familial) D89.2
monoclonal D47.2
secondary to malignant disease D47.2
Parapsoriasis L41.9
en plaques L41.4
guttata L41.1
large plaque L41.4
retiform, retiformis L41.5
small plaque L41.3
specified NEC L41.8
varioliformis (acuta) L41.0
Parasitic — *see also* condition
disease NEC B89
stomatitis B37.0
sycosis (beard) (scalp) B35.0
twin Q89.4
Parasitism B89
intestinal B82.9
skin B88.9
specified — *see* Infestation
Parasitophobia F40.218
Parasomnia G47.50
due to
alcohol
abuse F10.182
dependence F10.282
use F10.982
amphetamines
abuse F15.182
dependence F15.282
Parasomnia - *continued*
due to - *continued*
amphetamines - *continued*
use F15.982
caffeine
abuse F15.182
dependence F15.282
use F15.982
cocaine
abuse F14.182
dependence F14.282
use F14.982
drug NEC
abuse F19.182
dependence F19.282
use F19.982
opioid
abuse F11.182
dependence F11.282
use F11.982
psychoactive substance NEC
abuse F19.182
dependence F19.282
use F19.982
sedative, hypnotic, or anxiolytic
abuse F13.182
dependence F13.282
use F13.982
stimulant NEC
abuse F15.182
dependence F15.282
use F15.982
in conditions classified elsewhere G47.54
nonorganic origin F51.8
organic G47.50
specified NEC G47.59
Paraspadias Q54.9
Paraspasmus facialis G51.8
Parasuicide (attempt)
history of (personal) Z91.5
in family Z81.8
Parathyroid gland — *see* condition
Parathyroid tetany E20.9
Paratrachoma A74.0
Paratyphilitis — *see* Appendicitis
Paratyphoid (fever) — *see* Fever, paratyphoid
Paratyphus — *see* Fever, paratyphoid
Paraurethral duct Q64.79
nonorganic origin F51.5
Paraurethritis — *see also* Urethritis
gonococcal (acute) (chronic) (with abscess) A54.1
Paravaccinia NEC B08.04
Paravaginitis — *see* Vaginitis
Parencephalitis — *see also* Encephalitis
sequelae G09
Parent-child conflict — *see* Conflict, parent-child
estrangement NEC Z62.890
Paresis — *see also* Paralysis
accommodation — *see* Paresis, of accommodation
Bernhardt's G57.1-
bladder (sphincter) — *see also* Paralysis, bladder
tabetic A52.17
bowel, colon or intestine K56.0
extrinsic muscle, eye H49.9
general (progressive) (syphilitic) A52.17
juvenile A50.45
heart — *see* Failure, heart
insane (syphilitic) A52.17
juvenile (general) A50.45
of accommodation H52.52-
peripheral progressive (idiopathic) G60.3
pseudohypertrophic G71.09
senile G83.9
syphilitic (general) A52.17
congenital A50.45
vesical NEC N31.2
Paresthesia — *see also* Disturbance, sensation, skin R20.2
Bernhardt G57.1-
Paretic — *see* condition
Parinaud's
conjunctivitis H10.89
oculoglandular syndrome H10.89
ophthalmoplegia H49.88-
Parkinsonism (idiopathic) (primary) G20
with neurogenic orthostatic hypotension (symptomatic) G90.3
arteriosclerotic G21.4
dementia G31.83 *[F02.80]*
with behavioral disturbance G31.83 *[F02.81]*
due to
drugs NEC G21.19
neuroleptic G21.11

Parkinsonism (idiopathic) (primary) - *continued*
- medication-induced NEC G21.19
- neuroleptic induced G21.11
- postencephalitic G21.3
- secondary G21.9
  - due to
    - arteriosclerosis G21.4
    - drugs NEC G21.19
      - neuroleptic G21.11
    - encephalitis G21.3
    - external agents NEC G21.2
    - syphilis A52.19
  - specified NEC G21.8
- syphilitic A52.19
- treatment-induced NEC G21.19
- vascular G21.4

Parkinson's disease, syndrome or tremor — *see* Parkinsonism
Parodontitis — *see* Periodontitis
Parodontosis K05.4
Paronychia — *see also* Cellulitis, digit
- with lymphangitis — *see* Lymphangitis, acute, digit
- candidal (chronic) B37.2
- tuberculous (primary) A18.4

Parorexia (psychogenic) F50.89
Parosmia R43.1
- psychogenic F45.8

Parotid gland — *see* condition
Parotitis, parotiditis (allergic) (nonspecific toxic) (purulent) (septic) (suppurative) — *see also* Sialoadenitis
- epidemic — *see* Mumps
- infectious — *see* Mumps
- postoperative K91.89
- surgical K91.89

Parrot fever A70
Parrot's disease
- (early congenital syphilitic pseudoparalysis) A50.02

Parry-Romberg syndrome G51.8
Parry's disease or syndrome E05.00
- with thyroid storm E05.01

Pars planitis — *see* Cyclitis
Parsonage (-Aldren) **-Turner syndrome** G54.5
Parson's disease (exophthalmic goiter) E05.00
- with thyroid storm E05.01

Particolored infant Q82.8
Parturition — *see* Delivery
Parulis K04.7
- with sinus K04.6

Parvovirus, as cause of disease classified elsewhere B97.6
Pasini and Pierini's atrophoderma L90.3
Passage
- false, urethra N36.5
- meconium (newborn) during delivery P03.82
- of sounds or bougies — *see* Attention to, artificial, opening

Passive — *see* condition
- smoking Z77.22

Pasteurella septica A28.0
Pasteurellosis — *see* Infection, Pasteurella
PAT (paroxysmal atrial tachycardia) I47.1
Patau's syndrome — *see* Trisomy, 13
Patches
- mucous (syphilitic) A51.39
  - congenital A50.07
- smokers' (mouth) K13.24

Patellar — *see* condition
Patent — *see also* Imperfect, closure
- canal of Nuck Q52.4
- cervix N88.3
- ductus arteriosus or Botallo's Q25.0
- foramen
  - botalli Q21.1
  - ovale Q21.1
- interauricular septum Q21.1
- interventricular septum Q21.0
- omphalomesenteric duct Q43.0
- os (uteri) — *see* Patent, cervix
- ostium secundum Q21.1
- urachus Q64.4
- vitelline duct Q43.0

Paterson (-Brown) (-Kelly) **syndrome or web** D50.1
Pathologic, pathological — *see also* condition
- asphyxia R09.01
- fire-setting F63.1
- gambling F63.0
- ovum O02.0
- resorption, tooth K03.3
- stealing F63.2

Pathology (of) — *see* Disease
- periradicular, associated with previous endodontic treatment NEC M27.59

Pattern, sleep-wake, irregular G47.23
Patulous — *see also* Imperfect, closure (congenital)
- alimentary tract Q45.8
  - lower Q43.8
  - upper Q40.8
- eustachian tube H69.0-

Pause, sinoatrial I49.5
Paxton's disease B36.2
Pearl (s)
- enamel K00.2
- Epstein's K09.8

Pearl-worker's disease — *see* Osteomyelitis, specified type NEC
Pectenosis K62.4
Pectoral — *see* condition
Pectus
- carinatum (congenital) Q67.7
  - acquired M95.4
  - rachitic sequelae (late effect) E64.3
- excavatum (congenital) Q67.6
  - acquired M95.4
  - rachitic sequelae (late effect) E64.3
- recurvatum (congenital) Q67.6

Pedatrophia E41
Pederosis F65.4
Pediculosis (infestation) B85.2
- capitis (head-louse) (any site) B85.0
- corporis (body-louse) (any site) B85.1
- eyelid B85.0
- mixed (classifiable to more than one of the titles B85.0-B85.3) B85.4
- pubis (pubic louse) (any site) B85.3
- vestimenti B85.1
- vulvae B85.3

Pediculus (infestation) — *see* Pediculosis
Pedophilia F65.4
Peg-shaped teeth K00.2
Pelade — *see* Alopecia, areata
Pelger-Huët anomaly or syndrome D72.0
Peliosis (rheumatica) D69.0
- hepatis K76.4
  - with toxic liver disease K71.8

Pelizaeus-Merzbacher disease E75.29
Pellagra (alcoholic) (with polyneuropathy) E52
Pellagra-cerebellar-ataxia-renal aminoaciduria syndrome E72.02
Pellegrini (-Stieda) **disease or syndrome** — *see* Bursitis, tibial collateral
Pellizzi's syndrome E34.8
Pel's crisis A52.11
Pelvic — *see also* condition
- examination (periodic) (routine) Z01.419
  - with abnormal findings Z01.411
- kidney, congenital Q63.2

Pelviolithiasis — *see* Calculus, kidney
Pelviperitonitis — *see also* Peritonitis, pelvic
- gonococcal A54.24
- puerperal O85

Pelvis — *see* condition or type
Pemphigoid L12.9
- benign, mucous membrane L12.1
- bullous L12.0
- cicatricial L12.1
- juvenile L12.2
- ocular L12.1
- specified NEC L12.8

Pemphigus L10.9
- benign familial (chronic) Q82.8
- Brazilian L10.3
- circinatus L13.0
- conjunctiva L12.1
- drug-induced L10.5
- erythematosus L10.4
- foliaceous L10.2
- gangrenous — *see* Gangrene
- neonatorum L01.03
- ocular L12.1
- paraneoplastic L10.81
- specified NEC L10.89
- syphilitic (congenital) A50.06
- vegetans L10.1
- vulgaris L10.0
- wildfire L10.3

Pendred's syndrome E07.1
Pendulous
- abdomen, in pregnancy — *see* Pregnancy, complicated by, abnormal, pelvic organs or tissues NEC
- breast N64.89

Penetrating wound — *see also* Puncture
- with internal injury — *see* Injury, by site
- eyeball — *see* Puncture, eyeball

Penetrating wound - *continued*
- orbit (with or without foreign body) — *see* Puncture, orbit
- uterus by instrument with or following ectopic or molar pregnancy O08.6

Penicillosis B48.4
Penis — *see* condition
Penitis N48.29
Pentalogy of Fallot Q21.8
Pentasomy X syndrome Q97.1
Pentosuria (essential) E74.8
Percreta placenta O43.23-
Peregrinating patient — *see* Disorder, factitious
Perforation, perforated (nontraumatic) (of)
- accidental during procedure (blood vessel) (nerve) (organ) — *see* Complication, accidental puncture or laceration
- antrum — *see* Sinusitis, maxillary
- appendix K35.32
  - with localized peritonitis K35.32
- atrial septum, multiple Q21.1
- attic, ear — *see* Perforation, tympanum, attic
- bile duct (common) (hepatic) K83.2
  - cystic K82.2
- bladder (urinary)
  - with or following ectopic or molar pregnancy O08.6
  - obstetrical trauma O71.5
  - traumatic S37.29
    - at delivery O71.5
- bowel K63.1
  - with or following ectopic or molar pregnancy O08.6
  - newborn P78.0
  - obstetrical trauma O71.5
  - traumatic — *see* Laceration, intestine
- broad ligament N83.8
  - with or following ectopic or molar pregnancy O08.6
  - obstetrical trauma O71.6
- by
  - device, implant or graft — *see also* Complications, by site and type, mechanical T85.628
    - arterial graft NEC — *see* Complication, cardiovascular device, mechanical, vascular
    - breast (implant) T85.49
    - catheter NEC T85.698
      - cystostomy T83.090
      - dialysis (renal) T82.49
        - intraperitoneal T85.691
      - infusion NEC T82.594
        - spinal (epidural) (subdural) T85.690
      - urinary — *see also* Complications, catheter, urinary T83.098
    - electronic (electrode) (pulse generator) (stimulator)
      - bone T84.390
      - cardiac T82.199
        - electrode T82.190
        - pulse generator T82.191
        - specified type NEC T82.198
      - nervous system — *see* Complication, prosthetic device, mechanical, electronic nervous system stimulator
      - urinary — *see* Complication, genitourinary, device, urinary, mechanical
    - fixation, internal (orthopedic) NEC — *see* Complication, fixation device, mechanical
    - gastrointestinal — *see* Complications, prosthetic device, mechanical, gastrointestinal device
    - genital NEC T83.498
      - intrauterine contraceptive device T83.39
      - penile prosthesis T83.490
    - heart NEC — *see* Complication, cardiovascular device, mechanical
    - joint prosthesis — *see* Complications, joint prosthesis, mechanical, specified NEC, by site
    - ocular NEC — *see* Complications, prosthetic device, mechanical, ocular device
    - orthopedic NEC — *see* Complication, orthopedic, device, mechanical
    - specified NEC T85.628
    - urinary NEC — *see also* Complication, genitourinary, device, urinary, mechanical
      - graft T83.29
    - vascular NEC — *see* Complication, cardiovascular device, mechanical
    - ventricular intracranial shunt T85.09
  - foreign body left accidentally in operative wound T81.539
  - instrument (any) during a procedure, accidental — *see* Puncture, accidental complicating surgery

Perforation, perforated (nontraumatic) (of) - *continued*
cecum K35.32
with localized peritonitis K35.32
cervix (uteri) N88.8
with or following ectopic or molar pregnancy O08.6
obstetrical trauma O71.3
colon K63.1
newborn P78.0
obstetrical trauma O71.5
traumatic — *see* Laceration, intestine, large
common duct (bile) K83.2
cornea (due to ulceration) — *see* Ulcer, cornea, perforated
cystic duct K82.2
diverticulum (intestine) K57.80
with bleeding K57.81
large intestine K57.20
with
bleeding K57.21
small intestine K57.40
with bleeding K57.41
small intestine K57.00
with
bleeding K57.01
large intestine K57.40
with bleeding K57.41
ear drum — *see* Perforation, tympanum
esophagus K22.3
ethmoidal sinus — *see* Sinusitis, ethmoidal
frontal sinus — *see* Sinusitis, frontal
gallbladder K82.2
heart valve — *see* Endocarditis
ileum K63.1
newborn P78.0
obstetrical trauma O71.5
traumatic — *see* Laceration, intestine, small
instrumental, surgical (accidental) (blood vessel) (nerve) (organ) — *see* Puncture, accidental complicating surgery
intestine NEC K63.1
with ectopic or molar pregnancy O08.6
newborn P78.0
obstetrical trauma O71.5
traumatic — *see* Laceration, intestine
ulcerative NEC K63.1
newborn P78.0
jejunum, jejunal K63.1
obstetrical trauma O71.5
traumatic — *see* Laceration, intestine, small
ulcer — *see* Ulcer, gastrojejunal, with perforation
joint prosthesis — *see* Complications, joint prosthesis, mechanical, specified NEC, by site
mastoid (antrum) (cell) — *see* Disorder, mastoid, specified NEC
maxillary sinus — *see* Sinusitis, maxillary
membrana tympani — *see* Perforation, tympanum
nasal
septum J34.89
congenital Q30.3
syphilitic A52.73
sinus J34.89
congenital Q30.8
due to sinusitis — *see* Sinusitis
palate — *see also* Cleft, palate Q35.9
syphilitic A52.79
palatine vault — *see also* Cleft, palate, hard Q35.1
syphilitic A52.79
congenital A50.59
pars flaccida (ear drum) — *see* Perforation, tympanum, attic
pelvic
floor S31.030
with
ectopic or molar pregnancy O08.6
penetration into retroperitoneal space S31.031
retained foreign body S31.040
with penetration into retroperitoneal space S31.041
following ectopic or molar pregnancy O08.6
obstetrical trauma O70.1
organ S37.99
adrenal gland S37.818
bladder — *see* Perforation, bladder
fallopian tube S37.599
bilateral S37.592
unilateral S37.591
kidney S37.09-
obstetrical trauma O71.5
ovary S37.499
bilateral S37.492
unilateral S37.491

Perforation, perforated (nontraumatic) (of) - *continued*
pelvic - *continued*
organ - *continued*
prostate S37.828
specified organ NEC S37.898
ureter — *see* Perforation, ureter
urethra — *see* Perforation, urethra
uterus — *see* Perforation, uterus
perineum — *see* Laceration, perineum
pharynx J39.2
rectum K63.1
newborn P78.0
obstetrical trauma O71.5
traumatic S36.63
root canal space due to endodontic treatment M27.51
sigmoid K63.1
newborn P78.0
obstetrical trauma O71.5
traumatic S36.533
sinus (accessory) (chronic) (nasal) J34.89
sphenoidal sinus — *see* Sinusitis, sphenoidal
surgical (accidental) (by instrument) (blood vessel) (nerve) (organ) — *see* Puncture, accidental complicating surgery
traumatic
external — *see* Puncture
eye — *see* Puncture, eyeball
internal organ — *see* Injury, by site
tympanum, tympanic (membrane) (persistent post-traumatic) (postinflammatory) H72.9-
attic H72.1-
multiple — *see* Perforation, tympanum, multiple
total — *see* Perforation, tympanum, total
central H72.0-
multiple — *see* Perforation, tympanum, multiple
total — *see* Perforation, tympanum, total
marginal NEC — *see* subcategory H72.2
multiple H72.81-
pars flaccida — *see* Perforation, tympanum, attic
total H72.82-
traumatic, current episode S09.2-
typhoid, gastrointestinal — *see* Typhoid
ulcer — *see* Ulcer, by site, with perforation
ureter N28.89
traumatic S37.19
urethra N36.8
with ectopic or molar pregnancy O08.6
following ectopic or molar pregnancy O08.6
obstetrical trauma O71.5
traumatic S37.39
at delivery O71.5
uterus
with ectopic or molar pregnancy O08.6
by intrauterine contraceptive device T83.39
following ectopic or molar pregnancy O08.6
obstetrical trauma O71.1
traumatic S37.69
obstetric O71.1
uvula K13.79
syphilitic A52.79
vagina
obstetrical trauma O71.4
other trauma — *see* Puncture, vagina
Periadenitis mucosa necrotica recurrens K12.0
Periappendicitis (acute) — *see* Appendicitis
Periarteritis nodosa (disseminated) (infectious) (necrotizing) M30.0
Periarthritis (joint) — *see also* Enthesopathy
Duplay's M75.0-
gonococcal A54.42
humeroscapularis — *see* Capsulitis, adhesive
scapulohumeral — *see* Capsulitis, adhesive
shoulder — *see* Capsulitis, adhesive
wrist M77.2-
Periarthrosis (angioneural) — *see* Enthesopathy
Pericapsulitis, adhesive (shoulder) — *see* Capsulitis, adhesive
Pericarditis (with decompensation) (with effusion) I31.9
with rheumatic fever (conditions in I00)
active — *see* Pericarditis, rheumatic
inactive or quiescent I09.2
acute (hemorrhagic) (nonrheumatic) (Sicca) I30.9
with chorea (acute) (rheumatic) (Sydenham's) I02.0
benign I30.8
nonspecific I30.0
rheumatic I01.0
with chorea (acute) (Sydenham's) I02.0
adhesive or adherent (chronic) (external) (internal) I31.0

Pericarditis (with decompensation) (with effusion) - *continued*
adhesive or adherent (chronic) (external) (internal) - *continued*
acute — *see* Pericarditis, acute
rheumatic I09.2
bacterial (acute) (subacute) (with serous or seropurulent effusion) I30.1
calcareous I31.1
cholesterol (chronic) I31.8
acute I30.9
chronic (nonrheumatic) I31.9
rheumatic I09.2
constrictive (chronic) I31.1
coxsackie B33.23
fibrinocaseous (tuberculous) A18.84
fibrinopurulent I30.1
fibrinous I30.8
fibrous I31.0
gonococcal A54.83
idiopathic I30.0
in systemic lupus erythematosus M32.12
infective I30.1
meningococcal A39.53
neoplastic (chronic) I31.8
acute I30.9
obliterans, obliterating I31.0
plastic I31.0
pneumococcal I30.1
postinfarction I24.1
purulent I30.1
rheumatic (active) (acute) (with effusion) (with pneumonia) I01.0
with chorea (acute) (rheumatic) (Sydenham's) I02.0
chronic or inactive (with chorea) I09.2
rheumatoid — *see* Rheumatoid, carditis
septic I30.1
serofibrinous I30.8
staphylococcal I30.1
streptococcal I30.1
suppurative I30.1
syphilitic A52.06
tuberculous A18.84
uremic N18.9 *[I32]*
viral I30.1
Pericardium, pericardial — *see* condition
Pericellulitis — *see* Cellulitis
Pericementitis (chronic) (suppurative) — *see also* Periodontitis
acute K05.20
generalized — *see* Peridontitis, aggressive, generalized
localized — *see* Peridontitis, aggressive, localized
Perichondritis
auricle — *see* Perichondritis, ear
bronchus J98.09
ear (external) H61.00-
acute H61.01-
chronic H61.02-
external auditory canal — *see* Perichondritis, ear
larynx J38.7
syphilitic A52.73
typhoid A01.09
nose J34.89
pinna — *see* Perichondritis, ear
trachea J39.8
Periclasia K05.4
Pericoronitis — *see* Periodontitis
Pericystitis N30.90
with hematuria N30.91
Peridiverticulitis (intestine) K57.92
cecum — *see* Diverticulitis, intestine, large
colon — *see* Diverticulitis, intestine, large
duodenum — *see* Diverticulitis, intestine, small
intestine — *see* Diverticulitis, intestine
jejunum — *see* Diverticulitis, intestine, small
rectosigmoid — *see* Diverticulitis, intestine, large
rectum — *see* Diverticulitis, intestine, large
sigmoid — *see* Diverticulitis, intestine, large
Periendocarditis — *see* Endocarditis
Periepididymitis N45.1
Perifolliculitis L01.02
abscedens, caput, scalp L66.3
capitis, abscedens (et suffodiens) L66.3
superficial pustular L01.02
Perihepatitis K65.8
Perilabyrinthitis (acute) — *see* subcategory H83.0
Perimeningitis — *see* Meningitis
Perimetritis — *see* Endometritis
Perimetrosalpingitis — *see* Salpingo-oophoritis
Perineocele N81.81
Perinephric, perinephritic — *see* condition

Perinephritis — *see also* Infection, kidney
purulent — *see* Abscess, kidney
Perineum, perineal — *see* condition
Perineuritis NEC — *see* Neuralgia
Periodic — *see* condition
Periodontitis (chronic) (complex) (compound) (local) (simplex) K05.30
acute K05.20
generalized K05.229
moderate K05.222
severe K05.223
slight K05.221
localized K05.219
moderate K05.212
severe K05.213
slight K05.211
apical K04.5
acute (pulpal origin) K04.4
generalized K05.329
moderate K05.322
severe K05.323
slight K05.321
localized K05.319
moderate K05.312
severe K05.313
slight K05.311
Periodontoclasia K05.4
Periodontosis (juvenile) K05.4
Periods — *see also* Menstruation
heavy N92.0
irregular N92.6
shortened intervals (irregular) N92.1
Perionychia — *see also* Cellulitis, digit
with lymphangitis — *see* Lymphangitis, acute, digit
Perioophoritis — *see* Salpingo-oophoritis
Periorchitis N45.2
Periosteum, periosteal — *see* condition
Periostitis (albuminosa) (circumscribed) (diffuse) (infective) (monomelic) — *see also* Osteomyelitis
alveolar M27.3
alveolodental M27.3
dental M27.3
gonorrheal A54.43
jaw (lower) (upper) M27.2
orbit H05.03-
syphilitic A52.77
congenital (early) A50.02 *[M90.80]*
secondary A51.46
tuberculous — *see* Tuberculosis, bone
yaws (hypertrophic) (early) (late) A66.6 *[M90.80]*
Periostosis (hyperplastic) — *see also* Disorder, bone, specified type NEC
with osteomyelitis — *see* Osteomyelitis, specified type NEC
Peripartum
cardiomyopathy O90.3
Periphlebitis — *see* Phlebitis
Periproctitis K62.89
Periprostatitis — *see* Prostatitis
Perirectal — *see* condition
Perirenal — *see* condition
Perisalpingitis — *see* Salpingo-oophoritis
Perisplenitis (infectional) D73.89
Peristalsis, visible or reversed R19.2
Peritendinitis — *see* Enthesopathy
Peritoneum, peritoneal — *see* condition
Peritonitis (adhesive) (bacterial) (fibrinous) (hemorrhagic) (idiopathic) (localized) (perforative) (primary) (with adhesions) (with effusion) K65.9
with or following
abscess K65.1
appendicitis
with perforation or rupture K35.32
generalized — *see also* Appendicitis K35.20
localized — *see also* Appendicitis K35.30
diverticular disease (intestine) K57.80
with bleeding K57.81
large intestine K57.20
with
bleeding K57.21
small intestine K57.40
with bleeding K57.41
small intestine K57.00
with
bleeding K57.01
large intestine K57.40
with bleeding K57.41
ectopic or molar pregnancy O08.0
acute (generalized) K65.0
aseptic T81.61
bile, biliary K65.3
chemical T81.61
chlamydial A74.81

Peritonitis (adhesive) (bacterial) (fibrinous) (hemorrhagic) (idiopathic) (localized) (perforative) (primary) (with adhesions) (with effusion) - *continued*
complicating abortion — *see* Abortion, by type, complicated by, pelvic peritonitis
congenital P78.1
chronic proliferative K65.8
diaphragmatic K65.0
diffuse K65.0
diphtheritic A36.89
disseminated K65.0
due to
bile K65.3
foreign
body or object accidentally left during a procedure (instrument) (sponge) (swab) T81.599
substance accidentally left during a procedure (chemical) (powder) (talc) T81.61
talc T81.61
urine K65.8
eosinophilic K65.8
acute K65.0
fibrocaseous (tuberculous) A18.31
fibropurulent K65.0
following ectopic or molar pregnancy O08.0
general (ized) K65.0
gonococcal A54.85
meconium (newborn) P78.0
neonatal P78.1
meconium P78.0
pancreatic K65.0
paroxysmal, familial E85.0
benign E85.0
pelvic
female N73.5
acute N73.3
chronic N73.4
with adhesions N73.6
male K65.0
periodic, familial E85.0
proliferative, chronic K65.8
puerperal, postpartum, childbirth O85
purulent K65.0
septic K65.0
specified NEC K65.8
spontaneous bacterial K65.2
subdiaphragmatic K65.0
subphrenic K65.0
suppurative K65.0
syphilitic A52.74
congenital (early) A50.08 *[K67]*
talc T81.61
tuberculous A18.31
urine K65.8
Peritonsillar — *see* condition
Peritonsillitis J36
Perityphlitis K37
Periureteritis N28.89
Periurethral — *see* condition
Periurethritis (gangrenous) — *see* Urethritis
Periuterine — *see* condition
Perivaginitis — *see* Vaginitis
Perivasculitis, retinal H35.06-
Perivasitis (chronic) N49.1
Perivesiculitis (seminal) — *see* Vesiculitis
Perlèche NEC K13.0
due to
candidiasis B37.83
moniliasis B37.83
riboflavin deficiency E53.0
vitamin B2 (riboflavin) deficiency E53.0
Pernicious — *see* condition
Pernio, perniosis T69.1
Perpetrator (of abuse) — *see* Index to External Causes of Injury, Perpetrator
Persecution
delusion F22
social Z60.5
Perseveration (tonic) R48.8
Persistence, persistent (congenital)
anal membrane Q42.3
with fistula Q42.2
arteria stapedia Q16.3
atrioventricular canal Q21.2
branchial cleft NOS Q18.2
cyst Q18.0
fistula Q18.0
sinus Q18.0
bulbus cordis in left ventricle Q21.8
canal of Cloquet Q14.0
capsule (opaque) Q12.8
cilioretinal artery or vein Q14.8

Persistence, persistent (congenital) - *continued*
cloaca Q43.7
communication — *see* Fistula, congenital
convolutions
aortic arch Q25.46
fallopian tube Q50.6
oviduct Q50.6
uterine tube Q50.6
double aortic arch Q25.45
ductus arteriosus (Botalli) Q25.0
fetal
circulation P29.38
form of cervix (uteri) Q51.828
hemoglobin, hereditary (HPFH) D56.4
foramen
Botalli Q21.1
ovale Q21.1
Gartner's duct Q52.4
hemoglobin, fetal (hereditary) (HPFH) D56.4
hyaloid
artery (generally incomplete) Q14.0
system Q14.8
hymen, in pregnancy or childbirth — *see* Pregnancy, complicated by, abnormal, vulva
lanugo Q84.2
left
posterior cardinal vein Q26.8
root with right arch of aorta Q25.49
superior vena cava Q26.1
Meckel's diverticulum Q43.0
malignant — *see* Table of Neoplasms, small intestine, malignant
mucosal disease (middle ear) — *see* Otitis, media, suppurative, chronic, tubotympanic
nail (s) , anomalous Q84.6
omphalomesenteric duct Q43.0
organ or site not listed — *see* Anomaly, by site
ostium
atrioventriculare commune Q21.2
primum Q21.2
secundum Q21.1
ovarian rests in fallopian tube Q50.6
pancreatic tissue in intestinal tract Q43.8
primary (deciduous)
teeth K00.6
vitreous hyperplasia Q14.0
pupillary membrane Q13.89
right aortic arch Q25.47
rhesus (Rh) titer — *see* Complication(s), transfusion, incompatibility reaction, Rh (factor)
sinus
urogenitalis
female Q52.8
male Q55.8
venosus with imperfect incorporation in right auricle Q26.8
thymus (gland) (hyperplasia) E32.0
thyroglossal duct Q89.2
thyrolingual duct Q89.2
truncus arteriosus or communis Q20.0
tunica vasculosa lentis Q12.2
umbilical sinus Q64.4
urachus Q64.4
vitelline duct Q43.0
Person (with)
admitted for clinical research, as a control subject (normal comparison) (participant) Z00.6
awaiting admission to adequate facility elsewhere Z75.1
concern (normal) about sick person in family Z63.6
consulting on behalf of another Z71.0
feigning illness Z76.5
living (in)
alone Z60.2
boarding school Z59.3
residential institution Z59.3
without
adequate housing (heating) (space) Z59.1
housing (permanent) (temporary) Z59.0
person able to render necessary care Z74.2
shelter Z59.0
on waiting list Z75.1
sick or handicapped in family Z63.6
Personality (disorder) F60.9
accentuation of traits (type A pattern) Z73.1
affective F34.0
aggressive F60.3
amoral F60.2
anacastic, anankastic F60.5
antisocial F60.2
anxious F60.6
asocial F60.2
asthenic F60.7

Personality (disorder) - *continued*
  avoidant F60.6
  borderline F60.3
  change due to organic condition (enduring) F07.0
  compulsive F60.5
  cycloid F34.0
  cyclothymic F34.0
  dependent F60.7
  depressive F34.1
  dissocial F60.2
  dual F44.81
  eccentric F60.89
  emotionally unstable F60.3
  expansive paranoid F60.0
  explosive F60.3
  fanatic F60.0
  haltlose type F60.89
  histrionic F60.4
  hyperthymic F34.0
  hypothymic F34.1
  hysterical F60.4
  immature F60.89
  inadequate F60.7
  labile (emotional) F60.3
  mixed (nonspecific) F60.89
  morally defective F60.2
  multiple F44.81
  narcissistic F60.81
  obsessional F60.5
  obsessive (-compulsive) F60.5
  organic F07.0
  overconscientious F60.5
  paranoid F60.0
  passive (-dependent) F60.7
  passive-aggressive F60.89
  pathologic F60.9
  pattern defect or disturbance F60.9
  pseudopsychopathic (organic) F07.0
  pseudoretarded (organic) F07.0
  psychoinfantile F60.4
  psychoneurotic NEC F60.89
  psychopathic F60.2
  querulant F60.0
  sadistic F60.89
  schizoid F60.1
  self-defeating F60.7
  sensitive paranoid F60.0
  sociopathic (amoral) (antisocial) (asocial) (dissocial) F60.2
  specified NEC F60.89
  type A Z73.1
  unstable (emotional) F60.3
Perthes' disease — *see* Legg-Calvé-Perthes disease
Pertussis — *see also* Whooping cough A37.90
Perversion, perverted
  appetite F50.89
    psychogenic F50.89
  function
    pituitary gland E23.2
      posterior lobe E22.2
  sense of smell and taste R43.8
    psychogenic F45.8
  sexual — *see* Deviation, sexual
Pervious, congenital — *see also* Imperfect, closure
  ductus arteriosus Q25.0
Pes (congenital) — *see also* Talipes
  acquired — *see also* Deformity, limb, foot, specified NEC
    planus — *see* Deformity, limb, flat foot
  adductus Q66.89
  cavus Q66.7
  deformity NEC, acquired — *see* Deformity, limb, foot, specified NEC
  planus (acquired) (any degree) — *see also* Deformity, limb, flat foot
    rachitic sequelae (late effect) E64.3
  valgus Q66.6
Pest, pestis — *see* Plague
Petechia, petechiae R23.3
  newborn P54.5
Petechial typhus A75.9
Peter's anomaly Q13.4
Petit mal seizure — *see* Epilepsy, generalized, specified NEC
Petit's hernia — *see* Hernia, abdomen, specified site NEC
Petrellidosis B48.2
Petrositis H70.20-
  acute H70.21-
  chronic H70.22-
Peutz-Jeghers disease or syndrome Q85.8
Peyronie's disease N48.6
PFAPA
  (periodic fever, aphthous stomatitis, pharyngitis, and adenopathy syndrome) M04.8
Pfeiffer's disease — *see* Mononucleosis, infectious
Phagedena (dry) (moist) (sloughing) — *see also* Gangrene
  geometric L88
  penis N48.29
  tropical — *see* Ulcer, skin
  vulva N76.6
Phagedenic — *see* condition
Phakoma H35.89
Phakomatosis — *see also* specific eponymous syndromes Q85.9
  Bourneville's Q85.1
  specified NEC Q85.8
Phantom limb syndrome (without pain) G54.7
  with pain G54.6
Pharyngeal pouch syndrome D82.1
Pharyngitis (acute) (catarrhal) (gangrenous) (infective) (malignant) (membranous) (phlegmonous) (pseudomembranous) (simple) (subacute) (suppurative) (ulcerative) (viral) J02.9
  with influenza, flu, or grippe — *see* Influenza, with, pharyngitis
  aphthous B08.5
  atrophic J31.2
  chlamydial A56.4
  chronic (atrophic) (granular) (hypertrophic) J31.2
  coxsackievirus B08.5
  diphtheritic A36.0
  enteroviral vesicular B08.5
  follicular (chronic) J31.2
  fusospirochetal A69.1
  gonococcal A54.5
  granular (chronic) J31.2
  herpesviral B00.2
  hypertrophic J31.2
  infectional, chronic J31.2
  influenzal — *see* Influenza, with, respiratory manifestations NEC
  lymphonodular, acute (enteroviral) B08.8
  pneumococcal J02.8
  purulent J02.9
  putrid J02.9
  septic J02.0
  sicca J31.2
  specified organism NEC J02.8
  staphylococcal J02.8
  streptococcal J02.0
  syphilitic, congenital (early) A50.03
  tuberculous A15.8
  vesicular, enteroviral B08.5
  viral NEC J02.8
Pharyngoconjunctivitis, viral B30.2
Pharyngolaryngitis (acute) J06.0
  chronic J37.0
Pharyngoplegia J39.2
Pharyngotonsillitis, herpesviral B00.2
Pharyngotracheitis, chronic J42
Pharynx, pharyngeal — *see* condition
Phencyclidine-induced
  anxiety disorder F16.980
  bipolar and related disorder F16.94
  depressive disorder F16.94
  psychotic disorder F16.959
Phenomenon
  Arthus' — *see* Arthus' phenomenon
  jaw-winking Q07.8
  lupus erythematosus (LE) cell M32.9
  Raynaud's (secondary) I73.00
    with gangrene I73.01
  vasomotor R55
  vasospastic I73.9
  vasovagal R55
  Wenckebach's I44.1
Phenylketonuria E70.1
  classical E70.0
  maternal E70.1
Pheochromoblastoma
  specified site — *see* Neoplasm, malignant, by site
  unspecified site C74.10
Pheochromocytoma
  malignant
    specified site — *see* Neoplasm, malignant, by site
    unspecified site C74.10
  specified site — *see* Neoplasm, benign, by site
  unspecified site D35.00
Pheohyphomycosis — *see* Chromomycosis
Pheomycosis — *see* Chromomycosis
Phimosis (congenital) (due to infection) N47.1
  chancroidal A57
Phlebectasia — *see also* Varix
  congenital Q27.4
Phlebitis (infective) (pyemic) (septic) (suppurative) I80.9
  antepartum — *see* Thrombophlebitis, antepartum
  blue — *see* Phlebitis, leg, deep
  breast, superficial I80.8
  cavernous (venous) sinus — *see* Phlebitis, intracranial (venous) sinus
  cerebral (venous) sinus — *see* Phlebitis, intracranial (venous) sinus
  chest wall, superficial I80.8
  cranial (venous) sinus — *see* Phlebitis, intracranial (venous) sinus
  deep (vessels) — *see* Phlebitis, leg, deep
  due to implanted device — *see* Complications, by site and type, specified NEC
  during or resulting from a procedure T81.72
  femoral vein (superficial) I80.1-
  femoropopliteal vein I80.0-
  gestational — *see* Phlebopathy, gestational
  hepatic veins I80.8
  iliofemoral — *see* Phlebitis, femoral vein
  intracranial (venous) sinus (any) G08
    nonpyogenic I67.6
  intraspinal venous sinuses and veins G08
    nonpyogenic G95.19
  lateral (venous) sinus — *see* Phlebitis, intracranial (venous) sinus
  leg I80.3
    antepartum — *see* Thrombophlebitis, antepartum
    deep (vessels) NEC I80.20-
      iliac I80.21-
      popliteal vein I80.22-
      specified vessel NEC I80.29-
      tibial vein I80.23-
    femoral vein (superficial) I80.1-
    superficial (vessels) I80.0-
  longitudinal sinus — *see* Phlebitis, intracranial (venous) sinus
  lower limb — *see* Phlebitis, leg
  migrans, migrating (superficial) I82.1
  pelvic
    with ectopic or molar pregnancy O08.0
    following ectopic or molar pregnancy O08.0
    puerperal, postpartum O87.1
  popliteal vein — *see* Phlebitis, leg, deep, popliteal
  portal (vein) K75.1
  postoperative T81.72
  pregnancy — *see* Thrombophlebitis, antepartum
  puerperal, postpartum, childbirth O87.0
    deep O87.1
    pelvic O87.1
    superficial O87.0
  retina — *see* Vasculitis, retina
  saphenous (accessory) (great) (long) (small) — *see* Phlebitis, leg, superficial
  sinus (meninges) — *see* Phlebitis, intracranial (venous) sinus
  specified site NEC I80.8
  syphilitic A52.09
  tibial vein — *see* Phlebitis, leg, deep, tibial
  ulcerative I80.9
    leg — *see* Phlebitis, leg
  umbilicus I80.8
  uterus (septic) — *see* Endometritis
  varicose (leg) (lower limb) — *see* Varix, leg, with, inflammation
Phlebofibrosis I87.8
Phleboliths I87.8
Phlebopathy,
  gestational O22.9-
  puerperal O87.9
Phlebosclerosis I87.8
Phlebothrombosis — *see also* Thrombosis
  antepartum — *see* Thrombophlebitis, antepartum
  pregnancy — *see* Thrombophlebitis, antepartum
  puerperal — *see* Thrombophlebitis, puerperal
Phlebotomus fever A93.1
Phlegmasia
  alba dolens O87.1
    nonpuerperal — *see* Phlebitis, femoral vein
  cerulea dolens — *see* Phlebitis, leg, deep
Phlegmon — *see* Abscess
Phlegmonous — *see* condition
Phlyctenulosis (allergic) (keratoconjunctivitis) (nontuberculous) — *see also* Keratoconjunctivitis
  cornea — *see* Keratoconjunctivitis
  tuberculous A18.52
Phobia, phobic F40.9
  animal F40.218
    spiders F40.210
  examination F40.298

Phobia, phobic - *continued*
reaction F40.9
simple F40.298
social F40.10
generalized F40.11
specific (isolated) F40.298
animal F40.218
spiders F40.210
blood F40.230
injection F40.231
injury F40.233
men F40.290
natural environment F40.228
thunderstorms F40.220
situational F40.248
bridges F40.242
closed in spaces F40.240
flying F40.243
heights F40.241
specified focus NEC F40.298
transfusion F40.231
women F40.291
specified NEC F40.8
medical care NEC F40.232
state F40.9
Phocas' disease — *see* Mastopathy, cystic
Phocomelia Q73.1
lower limb — *see* Agenesis, leg, with foot present
upper limb — *see* Agenesis, arm, with hand present
Phoria H50.50
Phosphate-losing tubular disorder N25.0
Phosphatemia E83.39
Phosphaturia E83.39
Photodermatitis (sun) L56.8
chronic L57.8
due to drug L56.8
light other than sun L59.8
Photokeratitis H16.13-
Photophobia H53.14-
Photophthalmia — *see* Photokeratitis
Photopsia H53.19
Photoretinitis — *see* Retinopathy, solar
Photosensitivity, photosensitization (sun)
skin L56.8
light other than sun L59.8
Phrenitis — *see* Encephalitis
Phrynoderma (vitamin A deficiency) E50.8
Phthiriasis (pubis) B85.3
with any infestation classifiable to B85.0-B85.2 B85.4
Phthirus infestation — *see* Phthiriasis
Phthisis — *see also* Tuberculosis
bulbi (infectional) — *see* Disorder, globe, degenerated condition, atrophy
eyeball (due to infection) — *see* Disorder, globe, degenerated condition, atrophy
Phycomycosis — *see* Zygomycosis
Physalopteriasis B81.8
Physical restraint status Z78.1
Phytobezoar T18.9
intestine T18.3
stomach T18.2
Pian — *see* Yaws
Pianoma A66.1
Pica F50.89
in adults F50.89
infant or child F98.3
Picking, nose F98.8
Pick-Niemann disease — *see* Niemann-Pick disease or syndrome
Pick's
cerebral atrophy G31.01 *[F02.80]*
with behavioral disturbance G31.01 *[F02.81]*
disease or syndrome (brain) G31.01 *[F02.80]*
with behavioral disturbance G31.01 *[F02.81]*
brain G31.01 *[F02.80]*
with behavioral disturbance G31.01 *[F02.81]*
pericardium (pericardial pseudocirrhosis of liver) I31.1
syndrome
brain G31.01 *[F02.80]*
with behavioral disturbance G31.01 *[F02.81]*
of heart (pericardial pseudocirrhosis of liver) I31.1
Pickwickian syndrome E66.2
Piebaldism E70.39
Piedra (beard) (scalp) B36.8
black B36.3
white B36.2
Pierre Robin deformity or syndrome Q87.0
Pierson's disease or osteochondrosis M91.0
Pig-bel A05.2
Pigeon
breast or chest (acquired) M95.4

Pigeon - *continued*
breast or chest (acquired) - *continued*
congenital Q67.7
rachitic sequelae (late effect) E64.3
breeder's disease or lung J67.2
fancier's disease or lung J67.2
toe — *see* Deformity, toe, specified NEC
Pigmentation (abnormal) (anomaly) L81.9
conjunctiva H11.13-
cornea (anterior) H18.01-
posterior H18.05-
stromal H18.06-
diminished melanin formation NEC L81.6
iron L81.8
lids, congenital Q82.8
limbus corneae — *see* Pigmentation, cornea
metals L81.8
optic papilla, congenital Q14.2
retina, congenital (grouped) (nevoid) Q14.1
scrotum, congenital Q82.8
tattoo L81.8
Piles — *see also* Hemorrhoids K64.9
Pili
annulati or torti (congenital) Q84.1
incarnati L73.1
Pill roller hand (intrinsic) — *see* Parkinsonism
Pilomatrixoma — *see* Neoplasm, skin, benign
malignant — *see* Neoplasm, skin, malignant
Pilonidal — *see* condition
Pimple R23.8
PIN — *see* Neoplasia, intraepithelial, prostate
Pinched nerve — *see* Neuropathy, entrapment
Pindborg tumor — *see* Cyst, calcifying odontogenic
Pineal body or gland — *see* condition
Pinealoblastoma C75.3
Pinealoma D44.5
malignant C75.3
Pineoblastoma C75.3
Pineocytoma D44.5
Pinguecula H11.15-
Pingueculitis H10.81-
Pinhole meatus — *see also* Stricture, urethra N35.919
Pink
disease — *see* subcategory T56.1
eye — *see* Conjunctivitis, acute, mucopurulent
Pinkus' disease (lichen nitidus) L44.1
Pinpoint
meatus — *see* Stricture, urethra
os (uteri) — *see* Stricture, cervix
Pins and needles R20.2
Pinta A67.9
cardiovascular lesions A67.2
chancre (primary) A67.0
erythematous plaques A67.1
hyperchromic lesions A67.1
hyperkeratosis A67.1
lesions A67.9
cardiovascular A67.2
hyperchromic A67.1
intermediate A67.1
late A67.2
mixed A67.3
primary A67.0
skin (achromic) (cicatricial) (dyschromic) A67.2
hyperchromic A67.1
mixed (achromic and hyperchromic) A67.3
papule (primary) A67.0
skin lesions (achromic) (cicatricial) (dyschromic) A67.2
hyperchromic A67.1
mixed (achromic and hyperchromic) A67.3
vitiligo A67.2
Pintids A67.1
Pinworm (disease) (infection) (infestation) B80
Piroplasmosis B60.0
Pistol wound — *see* Gunshot wound
Pitchers' elbow — *see* Derangement, joint, specified type NEC, elbow
Pithecoid pelvis Q74.2
with disproportion (fetopelvic) O33.0
causing obstructed labor O65.0
Pithiatism F48.8
Pitted — *see* Pitting
Pitting — *see also* Edema R60.9
lip R60.0
nail L60.8
teeth K00.4
Pituitary gland — *see* condition
Pituitary-snuff-taker's disease J67.8
Pityriasis (capitis) L21.0
alba L30.5
circinata (et maculata) L42

Pityriasis (capitis) - *continued*
furfuracea L21.0
Hebra's L26
lichenoides L41.0
chronica L41.1
et varioliformis (acuta) L41.0
maculata (et circinata) L30.5
nigra B36.1
pilaris, Hebra's L44.0
rosea L42
rotunda L44.8
rubra (Hebra) pilaris L44.0
simplex L30.5
specified type NEC L30.5
streptogenes L30.5
versicolor (scrotal) B36.0
Placenta, placental — *see* Pregnancy, complicated by (care of) (management affected by), specified condition
Placentitis O41.14-
Plagiocephaly Q67.3
Plague A20.9
abortive A20.8
ambulatory A20.8
asymptomatic A20.8
bubonic A20.0
cellulocutaneous A20.1
cutaneobubonic A20.1
lymphatic gland A20.0
meningitis A20.3
pharyngeal A20.8
pneumonic (primary) (secondary) A20.2
pulmonary, pulmonic A20.2
septicemic A20.7
tonsillar A20.8
septicemic A20.7
Planning, family
contraception Z30.9
procreation Z31.69
Plaque (s)
artery, arterial — *see* Arteriosclerosis
calcareous — *see* Calcification
coronary, lipid rich I25.83
epicardial I31.8
erythematous, of pinta A67.1
Hollenhorst's — *see* Occlusion, artery, retina
lipid rich, coronary I25.83
pleural (without asbestos) J92.9
with asbestos J92.0
tongue K13.29
Plasmacytoma C90.3-
extramedullary C90.2-
medullary C90.0-
solitary C90.3-
Plasmacytopenia D72.818
Plasmacytosis D72.822
Plaster ulcer — *see* Ulcer, pressure, by site
Plateau iris syndrome (post-iridectomy) (postprocedural) (without glaucoma) H21.82
with glaucoma H40.22-
Platybasia Q75.8
Platyonychia (congenital) Q84.6
acquired L60.8
Platypelloid pelvis M95.5
with disproportion (fetopelvic) O33.0
causing obstructed labor O65.0
congenital Q74.2
Platyspondylisis Q76.49
Plaut (-Vincent) **disease** — *see also* Vincent's A69.1
Plethora R23.2
newborn P61.1
Pleura, pleural — *see* condition
Pleuralgia R07.81
Pleurisy (acute) (adhesive) (chronic) (costal) (diaphragmatic) (double) (dry) (fibrinous) (fibrous) (interlobar) (latent) (plastic) (primary) (residual) (sicca) (sterile) (subacute) (unresolved) R09.1
with
adherent pleura J86.0
effusion J90
chylous, chyliform J94.0
tuberculous (non primary) A15.6
primary (progressive) A15.7
tuberculosis — *see* Pleurisy, tuberculous (non primary)
encysted — *see* Pleurisy, with effusion
exudative — *see* Pleurisy, with effusion
fibrinopurulent, fibropurulent — *see* Pyothorax
hemorrhagic — *see* Hemothorax
pneumococcal J90
purulent — *see* Pyothorax
septic — *see* Pyothorax
serofibrinous — *see* Pleurisy, with effusion

Pleurisy (acute) (adhesive) (chronic) (costal) (diaphragmatic) (double) (dry) (fibrinous) (fibrous) (interlobar) (latent) (plastic) (primary) (residual) (sicca) (sterile) (subacute) (unresolved) - *continued*
seropurulent — *see* Pyothorax
serous — *see* Pleurisy, with effusion
staphylococcal J86.9
streptococcal J90
suppurative — *see* Pyothorax
traumatic (post) (current) — *see* Injury, intrathoracic, pleura
tuberculous (with effusion) (non primary) A15.6
primary (progressive) A15.7
Pleuritis sicca — *see* Pleurisy
Pleurobronchopneumonia — *see* Pneumonia, broncho-
Pleurodynia R07.81
epidemic B33.0
viral B33.0
Pleuropericarditis — *see also* Pericarditis
acute I30.9
Pleuropneumonia (acute) (bilateral) (double) (septic) — *see also* Pneumonia J18.8
chronic — *see* Fibrosis, lung
Pleuro-pneumonia-like-organism (PPLO) **, as cause of disease classified elsewhere** B96.0
Pleurorrhea — *see* Pleurisy, with effusion
Plexitis, brachial G54.0
Plica
polonica B85.0
syndrome, knee M67.5-
tonsil J35.8
Plicated tongue K14.5
Plug
bronchus NEC J98.09
meconium (newborn) NEC syndrome P76.0
mucus — *see* Asphyxia, mucus
Plumbism — *see* subcategory T56.0
Plummer's disease E05.20
with thyroid storm E05.21
Plummer-Vinson syndrome D50.1
Pluricarential syndrome of infancy E40
Plus (and minus) **hand** (intrinsic) — *see* Deformity, limb, specified type NEC, forearm
Pneumathemia — *see* Air, embolism
Pneumatic hammer (drill) **syndrome** T75.21
Pneumatocele (lung) J98.4
intracranial G93.89
tension J44.9
Pneumatosis
cystoides intestinalis K63.89
intestinalis K63.89
peritonei K66.8
Pneumaturia R39.89
Pneumoblastoma — *see* Neoplasm, lung, malignant
Pneumocephalus G93.89
Pneumococcemia A40.3
Pneumococcus, pneumococcal — *see* condition
Pneumoconiosis (due to) (inhalation of) J64
with tuberculosis (any type in A15) J65
aluminum J63.0
asbestos J61
bagasse, bagassosis J67.1
bauxite J63.1
beryllium J63.2
coal miners' (simple) J60
coalworkers' (simple) J60
collier's J60
cotton dust J66.0
diatomite (diatomaceous earth) J62.8
dust
inorganic NEC J63.6
lime J62.8
marble J62.8
organic NEC J66.8
fumes or vapors (from silo) J68.9
graphite J63.3
grinder's J62.8
kaolin J62.8
mica J62.8
millstone maker's J62.8
mineral fibers NEC J61
miner's J60
moldy hay J67.0
potter's J62.8
rheumatoid — *see* Rheumatoid, lung
sandblaster's J62.8
silica, silicate NEC J62.8
with carbon J60
stonemason's J62.8
talc (dust) J62.0
Pneumocystis carinii pneumonia B59
Pneumocystis jiroveci (pneumonia) B59
Pneumocystosis (with pneumonia) B59
Pneumohemopericardium I31.2
Pneumohemothorax J94.2
traumatic S27.2
Pneumohydropericardium — *see* Pericarditis
Pneumohydrothorax — *see* Hydrothorax
Pneumomediastinum J98.2
congenital or perinatal P25.2
Pneumomycosis B49 *[J99]*
Pneumonia (acute) (double) (migratory) (purulent) (septic) (unresolved) J18.9
with
lung abscess J85.1
due to specified organism — *see* Pneumonia, in (due to)
influenza — *see* Influenza, with, pneumonia
adenoviral J12.0
adynamic J18.2
alba A50.04
allergic (eosinophilic) J82
alveolar — *see* Pneumonia, lobar
anaerobes J15.8
anthrax A22.1
apex, apical — *see* Pneumonia, lobar
Ascaris B77.81
aspiration J69.0
due to
aspiration of microorganisms
bacterial J15.9
viral J12.9
food (regurgitated) J69.0
gastric secretions J69.0
milk (regurgitated) J69.0
oils, essences J69.1
solids, liquids NEC J69.8
vomitus J69.0
newborn P24.81
amniotic fluid (clear) P24.11
blood P24.21
liquor (amnii) P24.11
meconium P24.01
milk P24.31
mucus P24.11
food (regurgitated) P24.31
specified NEC P24.81
stomach contents P24.31
postprocedural J95.4
atypical NEC J18.9
bacillus J15.9
specified NEC J15.8
bacterial J15.9
specified NEC J15.8
Bacteroides (fragilis) (oralis) (melaninogenicus) J15.8
basal, basic, basilar — *see* Pneumonia, by type
bronchiolitis obliterans organized (BOOP) J84.89
broncho-, bronchial (confluent) (croupous) (diffuse) (disseminated) (hemorrhagic) (involving lobes) (lobar) (terminal) J18.0
allergic (eosinophilic) J82
aspiration — *see* Pneumonia, aspiration
bacterial J15.9
specified NEC J15.8
chronic — *see* Fibrosis, lung
diplococcal J13
Eaton's agent J15.7
Escherichia coli (E. coli) J15.5
Friedländer's bacillus J15.0
Hemophilus influenzae J14
hypostatic J18.2
inhalation — *see also* Pneumonia, aspiration
due to fumes or vapors (chemical) J68.0
of oils or essences J69.1
Klebsiella (pneumoniae) J15.0
lipid, lipoid J69.1
endogenous J84.89
Mycoplasma (pneumoniae) J15.7
pleuro-pneumonia-like-organisms (PPLO) J15.7
pneumococcal J13
Proteus J15.6
Pseudomonas J15.1
Serratia marcescens J15.6
specified organism NEC J16.8
staphylococcal — *see* Pneumonia, staphylococcal
streptococcal NEC J15.4
group B J15.3
pneumoniae J13
viral, virus — *see* Pneumonia, viral
Butyrivibrio (fibriosolvens) J15.8
Candida B37.1
caseous — *see* Tuberculosis, pulmonary
catarrhal — *see* Pneumonia, broncho
chlamydial J16.0
Pneumonia (acute) (double) (migratory) (purulent) (septic) (unresolved) - *continued*
chlamydial - *continued*
congenital P23.1
cholesterol J84.89
cirrhotic (chronic) — *see* Fibrosis, lung
Clostridium (haemolyticum) (novyi) J15.8
confluent — *see* Pneumonia, broncho
congenital (infective) P23.9
due to
bacterium NEC P23.6
Chlamydia P23.1
Escherichia coli P23.4
Haemophilus influenzae P23.6
infective organism NEC P23.8
Klebsiella pneumoniae P23.6
Mycoplasma P23.6
Pseudomonas P23.5
Staphylococcus P23.2
Streptococcus (except group B) P23.6
group B P23.3
viral agent P23.0
specified NEC P23.8
croupous — *see* Pneumonia, lobar
cryptogenic organizing J84.116
cytomegalic inclusion B25.0
cytomegaloviral B25.0
deglutition — *see* Pneumonia, aspiration
desquamative interstitial J84.117
diffuse — *see* Pneumonia, broncho
diplococcal, diplococcus (broncho-) (lobar) J13
disseminated (focal) — *see* Pneumonia, broncho
Eaton's agent J15.7
embolic, embolism — *see* Embolism, pulmonary
Enterobacter J15.6
eosinophilic J82
Escherichia coli (E. coli) J15.5
Eubacterium J15.8
fibrinous — *see* Pneumonia, lobar
fibroid, fibrous (chronic) — *see* Fibrosis, lung
Friedländer's bacillus J15.0
Fusobacterium (nucleatum) J15.8
gangrenous J85.0
giant cell (measles) B05.2
gonococcal A54.84
gram-negative bacteria NEC J15.6
anaerobic J15.8
Hemophilus influenzae (broncho) (lobar) J14
human metapneumovirus J12.3
hypostatic (broncho) (lobar) J18.2
in (due to)
actinomycosis A42.0
adenovirus J12.0
anthrax A22.1
ascariasis B77.81
aspergillosis B44.9
Bacillus anthracis A22.1
Bacterium anitratum J15.6
candidiasis B37.1
chickenpox B01.2
Chlamydia J16.0
neonatal P23.1
coccidioidomycosis B38.2
acute B38.0
chronic B38.1
cytomegalovirus disease B25.0
Diplococcus (pneumoniae) J13
Eaton's agent J15.7
Enterobacter J15.6
Escherichia coli (E. coli) J15.5
Friedländer's bacillus J15.0
fumes and vapors (chemical) (inhalation) J68.0
gonorrhea A54.84
Hemophilus influenzae (H. influenzae) J14
Herellea J15.6
histoplasmosis B39.2
acute B39.0
chronic B39.1
human metapneumovirus J12.3
Klebsiella (pneumoniae) J15.0
measles B05.2
Mycoplasma (pneumoniae) J15.7
nocardiosis, nocardiasis A43.0
ornithosis A70
parainfluenza virus J12.2
pleuro-pneumonia-like-organism (PPLO) J15.7
pneumococcus J13
pneumocystosis (Pneumocystis carinii) (Pneumocystis jiroveci) B59
Proteus J15.6
Pseudomonas NEC J15.1
pseudomallei A24.1
psittacosis A70

Pneumothorax NOS - *continued*
spontaneous NOS - *continued*
primary J93.11
secondary J93.12
tension J93.0
tense valvular, infectional J93.0
tension (spontaneous) J93.0
traumatic S27.0
with hemothorax S27.2
tuberculous — *see* Tuberculosis, pulmonary
Podagra — *see also* Gout M10.9
Podencephalus Q01.9
Poikilocytosis R71.8
Poikiloderma L81.6
Civatte's L57.3
congenital Q82.8
vasculare atrophicans L94.5
Poikilodermatomyositis M33.10
with
myopathy M33.12
respiratory involvement M33.11
specified organ involvement NEC M33.19
Pointed ear (congenital) Q17.3
Poison ivy, oak, sumac or other plant dermatitis (allergic) (contact) L23.7
Poisoning (acute) — *see also* Table of Drugs and Chemicals
algae and toxins T65.82-
Bacillus B (aertrycke) (cholerae (suis)) (paratyphosus) (suipestifer) A02.9
botulinus A05.1
bacterial toxins A05.9
berries, noxious — *see* Poisoning, food, noxious, berries
botulism A05.1
ciguatera fish T61.0-
Clostridium botulinum A05.1
death-cap (Amanita phalloides) (Amanita verna) — *see* Poisoning, food, noxious, mushrooms
drug — *see* Table of Drugs and Chemicals, by drug, poisoning
epidemic, fish (noxious) — *see* Poisoning, seafood
bacterial A05.9
fava bean D55.0
fish (noxious) T61.9-
bacterial — *see* Intoxication, foodborne, by agent
ciguatera fish — *see* Poisoning, ciguatera fish
scombroid fish — *see* Poisoning, scombroid fish
specified type NEC T61.77-
food (acute) (diseased) (infected) (noxious) NEC T62.9-
bacterial — *see* Intoxication, foodborne, by agent
due to
Bacillus (aertrycke) (choleraesuis) (paratyphosus) (suipestifer) A02.9
botulinus A05.1
Clostridium (perfringens) (Welchii) A05.2
salmonella (aertrycke) (callinarum) (choleraesuis) (enteritidis) (paratyphi) (suipestifer) A02.9
with
gastroenteritis A02.0
sepsis A02.1
staphylococcus A05.0
Vibrio
parahaemolyticus A05.3
vulnificus A05.5
noxious or naturally toxic T62.9-
berries — *see* subcategory T62.1-
fish — *see* Poisoning, seafood
mushrooms — *see* subcategory T62.0X-
plants NEC — *see* subcategory T62.2X-
seafood — *see* Poisoning, seafood
specified NEC — *see* subcategory T62.8X-
ichthyotoxism — *see* Poisoning, seafood
kreotoxism, food A05.9
latex T65.81-
lead T56.0-
mushroom — *see* Poisoning, food, noxious, mushroom
mussels — *see also* Poisoning, shellfish
bacterial — *see* Intoxication, foodborne, by agent
nicotine (tobacco) T65.2-
noxious foodstuffs — *see* Poisoning, food, noxious
plants, noxious — *see* Poisoning, food, noxious, plants NEC
ptomaine — *see* Poisoning, food
radiation J70.0
Salmonella (arizonae) (cholerae-suis) (enteritidis) (typhimurium) A02.9
scombroid fish T61.1-
seafood (noxious) T61.9-
bacterial — *see* Intoxication, foodborne, by agent

Poisoning (acute) - *continued*
seafood (noxious) - *continued*
fish — *see* Poisoning, fish
shellfish — *see* Poisoning, shellfish
specified NEC — *see* subcategory T61.8X-
shellfish (amnesic) (azaspiracid) (diarrheic) (neurotoxic) (noxious) (paralytic) T61.78-
bacterial — *see* Intoxication, foodborne, by agent
ciguatera mollusk — *see* Poisoning, ciguatera fish
specified substance NEC T65.891
Staphylococcus, food A05.0
tobacco (nicotine) T65.2-
water E87.79
Poker spine — *see* Spondylitis, ankylosing
Poland syndrome Q79.8
Polioencephalitis (acute) (bulbar) A80.9
inferior G12.22
influenzal — *see* Influenza, with, encephalopathy
superior hemorrhagic (acute) (Wernicke's) E51.2
Wernicke's E51.2
Polioencephalomyelitis (acute) (anterior) A80.9
with beriberi E51.2
Polioencephalopathy, superior hemorrhagic E51.2
with
beriberi E51.11
pellagra E52
Poliomeningoencephalitis — *see* Meningoencephalitis
Poliomyelitis (acute) (anterior) (epidemic) A80.9
with paralysis (bulbar) — *see* Poliomyelitis, paralytic
abortive A80.4
ascending (progressive) — *see* Poliomyelitis, paralytic
bulbar (paralytic) — *see* Poliomyelitis, paralytic
congenital P35.8
nonepidemic A80.9
nonparalytic A80.4
paralytic A80.30
specified NEC A80.39
vaccine-associated A80.0
wild virus
imported A80.1
indigenous A80.2
spinal, acute A80.9
Poliosis (eyebrow) (eyelashes) L67.1
circumscripta, acquired L67.1
Pollakiuria R35.0
psychogenic F45.8
Pollinosis J30.1
Pollitzer's disease L73.2
Polyadenitis — *see also* Lymphadenitis
malignant A20.0
Polyalgia M79.89
Polyangiitis M30.0
microscopic M31.7
overlap syndrome M30.8
Polyarteritis
microscopic M31.7
nodosa M30.0
with lung involvement M30.1
juvenile M30.2
related condition NEC M30.8
Polyarthralgia — *see* Pain, joint
Polyarthritis, polyarthropathy — *see also* Arthritis M13.0
due to or associated with other specified conditions — *see* Arthritis
epidemic (Australian) (with exanthema) B33.1
infective — *see* Arthritis, pyogenic or pyemic
inflammatory M06.4
juvenile (chronic) (seronegative) M08.3
migratory — *see* Fever, rheumatic
rheumatic, acute — *see* Fever, rheumatic
Polyarthrosis M15.9
post-traumatic M15.3
primary M15.0
specified NEC M15.8
Polycarential syndrome of infancy E40
Polychondritis (atrophic) (chronic) — *see also* Disorder, cartilage, specified type NEC
relapsing M94.1
Polycoria Q13.2
Polycystic (disease)
degeneration, kidney Q61.3
autosomal dominant (adult type) Q61.2
autosomal recessive (infantile type) NEC Q61.19
kidney Q61.3
autosomal
dominant Q61.2
recessive NEC Q61.19
autosomal dominant (adult type) Q61.2
autosomal recessive (childhood type) NEC Q61.19

Polycystic (disease) - *continued*
kidney - *continued*
infantile type NEC Q61.19
liver Q44.6
lung J98.4
congenital Q33.0
ovary, ovaries E28.2
spleen Q89.09
Polycythemia (secondary) D75.1
acquired D75.1
benign (familial) D75.0
due to
donor twin P61.1
erythropoietin D75.1
fall in plasma volume D75.1
high altitude D75.1
maternal-fetal transfusion P61.1
stress D75.1
emotional D75.1
erythropoietin D75.1
familial (benign) D75.0
Gaisböck's (hypertonica) D75.1
high altitude D75.1
hypertonica D75.1
hypoxemic D75.1
neonatorum P61.1
nephrogenous D75.1
relative D75.1
secondary D75.1
spurious D75.1
stress D75.1
vera D45
Polycytosis cryptogenica D75.1
Polydactylism, polydactyly Q69.9
toes Q69.2
Polydipsia R63.1
Polydystrophy, pseudo-Hurler E77.0
Polyembryoma — *see* Neoplasm, malignant, by site
Polyglandular
deficiency E31.0
dyscrasia E31.9
dysfunction E31.9
syndrome E31.8
Polyhydramnios O40.-
Polymastia Q83.1
Polymenorrhea N92.0
Polymyalgia M35.3
arteritica, giant cell M31.5
rheumatica M35.3
with giant cell arteritis M31.5
Polymyositis (acute) (chronic) (hemorrhagic) M33.20
with
myopathy M33.22
respiratory involvement M33.21
skin involvement — *see* Dermatopolymyositis
specified organ involvement NEC M33.29
ossificans (generalisata) (progressiva) — *see* Myositis, ossificans, progressiva
Polyneuritis, polyneuritic — *see also* Polyneuropathy
acute (post-) infective G61.0
alcoholic G62.1
cranialis G52.7
demyelinating, chronic inflammatory (CIDP) G61.81
diabetic — *see* Diabetes, polyneuropathy
diphtheritic A36.83
due to lack of vitamin NEC E56.9 *[G63]*
endemic E51.11
erythredema — *see* subcategory T56.1
febrile, acute G61.0
hereditary ataxic G60.1
idiopathic, acute G61.0
infective (acute) G61.0
inflammatory, chronic demyelinating (CIDP) G61.81
nutritional E63.9 *[G63]*
postinfective (acute) G61.0
specified NEC G62.89
Polyneuropathy (peripheral) G62.9
alcoholic G62.1
amyloid (Portuguese) E85.1 *[G63]*
transthyretin-related (ATTR) familial E85.1
arsenical G62.2
critical illness G62.81
demyelinating, chronic inflammatory (CIDP) G61.81
diabetic — *see* Diabetes, polyneuropathy
drug-induced G62.0
hereditary G60.9
specified NEC G60.8
idiopathic G60.9
progressive G60.3

Polyneuropathy (peripheral) - *continued*
- in (due to)
  - alcohol G62.1
    - sequelae G65.2
  - amyloidosis, familial (Portuguese) E85.1 *[G63]*
  - antitetanus serum G61.1
  - arsenic G62.2
    - sequelae G65.2
  - avitaminosis NEC E56.9 *[G63]*
  - beriberi E51.11
  - collagen vascular disease NEC M35.9 *[G63]*
  - deficiency (of)
    - B (-complex) vitamins E53.9 *[G63]*
    - vitamin B6 E53.1 *[G63]*
  - diabetes — *see* Diabetes, polyneuropathy
  - diphtheria A36.83
  - drug or medicament G62.0
    - correct substance properly administered — *see* Table of Drugs and Chemicals, by drug, adverse effect
    - overdose or wrong substance given or taken — *see* Table of Drugs and Chemicals, by drug, poisoning
  - endocrine disease NEC E34.9 *[G63]*
  - herpes zoster B02.23
  - hypoglycemia E16.2 *[G63]*
  - infectious
    - disease NEC B99 *[G63]*
    - mononucleosis B27.91
  - lack of vitamin NEC E56.9 *[G63]*
  - lead G62.2
    - sequelae G65.2
  - leprosy A30.9 *[G63]*
  - Lyme disease A69.22
  - metabolic disease NEC E88.9 *[G63]*
  - microscopic polyangiitis M31.7 *[G63]*
  - mumps B26.84
  - neoplastic disease — *see also* Neoplasm D49.9 *[G63]*
  - nutritional deficiency NEC E63.9 *[G63]*
  - organophosphate compounds G62.2
    - sequelae G65.2
  - parasitic disease NEC B89 *[G63]*
  - pellagra E52 *[G63]*
  - polyarteritis nodosa M30.0
  - porphyria E80.20 *[G63]*
  - radiation G62.82
  - rheumatoid arthritis — *see* Rheumatoid, polyneuropathy
  - sarcoidosis D86.89
  - serum G61.1
  - syphilis (late) A52.15
    - congenital A50.43
  - systemic
    - connective tissue disorder M35.9 *[G63]*
    - lupus erythematosus M32.19
  - toxic agent NEC G62.2
    - sequelae G65.2
- transthyretin-related (ATTR) familial amyloid E85.1
  - triorthocresyl phosphate G62.2
    - sequelae G65.2
  - tuberculosis A17.89
  - uremia N18.9 *[G63]*
  - vitamin B12 deficiency E53.8 *[G63]*
    - with anemia (pernicious) D51.0 *[G63]*
      - due to dietary deficiency D51.3 *[G63]*
  - zoster B02.23
- inflammatory G61.9
  - chronic demyelinating (CIDP) G61.81
  - sequelae G65.1
  - specified NEC G61.89
- lead G62.2
  - sequelae G65.2
- nutritional NEC E63.9 *[G63]*
- postherpetic (zoster) B02.23
- progressive G60.3
- radiation-induced G62.82
- sensory (hereditary) (idiopathic) G60.8
- specified NEC G62.89
- syphilitic (late) A52.15
  - congenital A50.43

Polyopia H53.8

Polyorchism, polyorchidism Q55.21

Polyosteoarthritis — *see also* Osteoarthritis, generalized M15.9-
- post-traumatic M15.3
- specified NEC M15.8

Polyostotic fibrous dysplasia Q78.1

Polyotia Q17.0

Polyp, polypus
- accessory sinus J33.8
- adenocarcinoma in — *see* Neoplasm, malignant, by site
- adenocarcinoma in situ in — *see* Neoplasm, in situ, by site
- adenoid tissue J33.0
- adenomatous — *see also* Neoplasm, benign, by site
  - adenocarcinoma in — *see* Neoplasm, malignant, by site
  - adenocarcinoma in situ in — *see* Neoplasm, in situ, by site
  - carcinoma in — *see* Neoplasm, malignant, by site
  - carcinoma in situ in — *see* Neoplasm, in situ, by site
  - multiple — *see* Neoplasm, benign
    - adenocarcinoma in — *see* Neoplasm, malignant, by site
    - adenocarcinoma in situ in — *see* Neoplasm, in situ, by site
- antrum J33.8
- anus, anal (canal) K62.0
- Bartholin's gland N84.3
- bladder D41.4
- carcinoma in — *see* Neoplasm, malignant, by site
- carcinoma in situ in — *see* Neoplasm, in situ, by site
- cecum D12.0
- cervix (uteri) N84.1
  - in pregnancy or childbirth — *see* Pregnancy, complicated by, abnormal, cervix
  - mucous N84.1
  - nonneoplastic N84.1
- choanal J33.0
- cholesterol K82.4
- clitoris N84.3
- colon K63.5
  - adenomatous D12.6
  - ascending D12.2
  - cecum D12.0
  - descending D12.4
  - inflammatory K51.40
    - with
      - abscess K51.414
      - complication K51.419
        - specified NEC K51.418
      - fistula K51.413
      - intestinal obstruction K51.412
      - rectal bleeding K51.411
  - sigmoid D12.5
  - transverse D12.3
- corpus uteri N84.0
- dental K04.01
  - irreversible K04.02
  - reversible K04.01
- duodenum K31.7
- ear (middle) H74.4-
- endometrium N84.0
- ethmoidal (sinus) J33.8
- fallopian tube N84.8
- female genital tract N84.9
  - specified NEC N84.8
- frontal (sinus) J33.8
- gallbladder K82.4
- gingiva, gum K06.8
- labia, labium (majus) (minus) N84.3
- larynx (mucous) J38.1
  - adenomatous D14.1
- malignant — *see* Neoplasm, malignant, by site
- maxillary (sinus) J33.8
- middle ear — *see* Polyp, ear (middle)
- myometrium N84.0
- nares
  - anterior J33.9
  - posterior J33.0
- nasal (mucous) J33.9
  - cavity J33.0
  - septum J33.0
- nasopharyngeal J33.0
- nose (mucous) J33.9
- oviduct N84.8
- pharynx J39.2
- placenta O90.89
- prostate — *see* Enlargement, enlarged, prostate
- pudenda, pudendum N84.3
- pulpal (dental) K04.01
  - irreversible K04.02
  - reversible K04.01
- rectum (nonadenomatous) K62.1
  - adenomatous — *see* Polyp, adenomatous
- septum (nasal) J33.0
- sinus (accessory) (ethmoidal) (frontal) (maxillary) (sphenoidal) J33.8
- sphenoidal (sinus) J33.8
- stomach K31.7
  - adenomatous D13.1
- tube, fallopian N84.8
- turbinate, mucous membrane J33.8
- umbilical, newborn P83.6
- ureter N28.89
- urethra N36.2
- uterus (body) (corpus) (mucous) N84.0
  - cervix N84.1
  - in pregnancy or childbirth — *see* Pregnancy, complicated by, tumor, uterus
- vagina N84.2
- vocal cord (mucous) J38.1
- vulva N84.3

Polyphagia R63.2

Polyploidy Q92.7

Polypoid — *see* condition

Polyposis — *see also* Polyp
- coli (adenomatous) D12.6
  - adenocarcinoma in C18.9
  - adenocarcinoma in situ in — *see* Neoplasm, in situ, by site
  - carcinoma in C18.9
- colon (adenomatous) D12.6
- familial D12.6
  - adenocarcinoma in situ in — *see* Neoplasm, in situ, by site
- intestinal (adenomatous) D12.6
- malignant lymphomatous C83.1-
- multiple, adenomatous — *see also* Neoplasm, benign D36.9

Polyradiculitis — *see* Polyneuropathy

Polyradiculoneuropathy (acute) (postinfective) (segmentally demyelinating) G61.0

Polyserositis
- due to pericarditis I31.1
- pericardial I31.1
- periodic, familial E85.0
- tuberculous A19.9
  - acute A19.1
  - chronic A19.8

Polysplenia syndrome Q89.09

Polysyndactyly — *see also* Syndactylism, syndactyly Q70.4

Polytrichia L68.3

Polyunguia Q84.6

Polyuria R35.8
- nocturnal R35.1
- psychogenic F45.8

Pompe's disease (glycogen storage) E74.02

Pompholyx L30.1

Poncet's disease (tuberculous rheumatism) A18.09

Pond fracture — *see* Fracture, skull

Ponos B55.0

Pons, pontine — *see* condition

Poor
- aesthetic of existing restoration of tooth K08.56
- contractions, labor O62.2
- gingival margin to tooth restoration K08.51
- personal hygiene R46.0
- prenatal care, affecting management of pregnancy — *see* Pregnancy, complicated by, insufficient, prenatal care
- sucking reflex (newborn) R29.2
- urinary stream R39.12
- vision NEC H54.7

Poradenitis, nostras inguinalis or venerea A55

Porencephaly (congenital) (developmental) (true) Q04.6
- acquired G93.0
- nondevelopmental G93.0
- traumatic (post) F07.89

Porocephaliasis B88.8

Porokeratosis Q82.8

Poroma, eccrine — *see* Neoplasm, skin, benign

Porphyria (South African) E80.20
- acquired E80.20
- acute intermittent (hepatic) (Swedish) E80.21
- cutanea tarda (hereditary) (symptomatic) E80.1
- due to drugs E80.20
  - correct substance properly administered — *see* Table of Drugs and Chemicals, by drug, adverse effect
  - overdose or wrong substance given or taken — *see* Table of Drugs and Chemicals, by drug, poisoning
- erythropoietic (congenital) (hereditary) E80.0
- hepatocutaneous type E80.1
- secondary E80.20
- toxic NEC E80.20
- variegata E80.20

Porphyrinuria — *see* Porphyria

Porphyruria — *see* Porphyria

Port wine nevus, mark, or stain Q82.5

Portal — *see* condition

Posadas-Wernicke disease B38.9
Positive
culture (nonspecific)
blood R78.81
bronchial washings R84.5
cerebrospinal fluid R83.5
cervix uteri R87.5
nasal secretions R84.5
nipple discharge R89.5
nose R84.5
staphylococcus (Methicillin susceptible) Z22.321
Methicillin resistant Z22.322
peritoneal fluid R85.5
pleural fluid R84.5
prostatic secretions R86.5
saliva R85.5
seminal fluid R86.5
sputum R84.5
synovial fluid R89.5
throat scrapings R84.5
urine R82.79
vagina R87.5
vulva R87.5
wound secretions R89.5
PPD (skin test) R76.11
serology for syphilis A53.0
false R76.8
with signs or symptoms - code as Syphilis, by site and stage
skin test, tuberculin (without active tuberculosis) R76.11
test, human immunodeficiency virus (HIV) R75
VDRL A53.0
with signs or symptoms - code by site and stage under Syphilis A53.9
Wassermann reaction A53.0
Postcardiotomy syndrome I97.0
Postcaval ureter Q62.62
Postcholecystectomy syndrome K91.5
Postclimacteric bleeding N95.0
Postcommissurotomy syndrome I97.0
Postconcussional syndrome F07.81
Postcontusional syndrome F07.81
Postcricoid region — *see* condition
Post-dates (40-42 weeks) (pregnancy) (mother) O48.0
more than 42 weeks gestation O48.1
Postencephalitic syndrome F07.89
Posterior — *see* condition
Posterolateral sclerosis (spinal cord) — *see* Degeneration, combined
Postexanthematous — *see* condition
Postfebrile — *see* condition
Postgastrectomy dumping syndrome K91.1
Posthemiplegic chorea — *see* Monoplegia
Posthemorrhagic anemia (chronic) D50.0
acute D62
newborn P61.3
Postherpetic neuralgia (zoster) B02.29
trigeminal B02.22
Posthitis N47.7
Postimmunization complication or reaction — *see* Complications, vaccination
Postinfectious — *see* condition
Postlaminectomy syndrome NEC M96.1
Postleukotomy syndrome F07.0
Postmastectomy lymphedema (syndrome) I97.2
Postmaturity, postmature (over 42 weeks)
maternal (over 42 weeks gestation) O48.1
newborn P08.22
Postmeasles complication NEC — *see also* condition B05.89
Postmenopausal
endometrium (atrophic) N95.8
suppurative — *see also* Endometritis N71.9
osteoporosis — *see* Osteoporosis, postmenopausal
Postnasal drip R09.82
due to
allergic rhinitis — *see* Rhinitis, allergic
common cold J00
gastroesophageal reflux — *see* Reflux, gastroesophageal
nasopharyngitis — *see* Nasopharyngitis
other know condition - code to condition
sinusitis — *see* Sinusitis
Postnatal — *see* condition
Postoperative (postprocedural) — *see* Complication, postoperative
pneumothorax, therapeutic Z98.3
state NEC Z98.890
Postpancreatectomy hyperglycemia E89.1
Postpartum — *see* Puerperal
Postphlebitic syndrome — *see* Syndrome, postthrombotic
Postpolio (myelitic) **syndrome** G14
Postpoliomyelitic — *see also* condition
osteopathy — *see* Osteopathy, after poliomyelitis
Postprocedural — *see also* Postoperative
hypoinsulinemia E89.1
Postschizophrenic depression F32.89
Postsurgery status — *see also* Status (post)
pneumothorax, therapeutic Z98.3
Post-term (40-42 weeks) (pregnancy) (mother) O48.0
infant P08.21
more than 42 weeks gestation (mother) O48.1
Post-traumatic brain syndrome, nonpsychotic F07.81
Post-typhoid abscess A01.09
Postures, hysterical F44.2
Postvaccinal reaction or complication — *see* Complications, vaccination
Postvalvulotomy syndrome I97.0
Potain's
disease (pulmonary edema) — *see* Edema, lung
syndrome (gastrectasis with dyspepsia) K31.0
Potter's
asthma J62.8
facies Q60.6
lung J62.8
syndrome (with renal agenesis) Q60.6
Pott's
curvature (spinal) A18.01
disease or paraplegia A18.01
spinal curvature A18.01
tumor, puffy — *see* Osteomyelitis, specified type NEC
Pouch
bronchus Q32.4
Douglas' — *see* condition
esophagus, esophageal, congenital Q39.6
acquired K22.5
gastric K31.4
Hartmann's K82.8
pharynx, pharyngeal (congenital) Q38.7
Pouchitis K91.850
Poultrymen's itch B88.0
Poverty NEC Z59.6
extreme Z59.5
Poxvirus NEC B08.8
Prader-Willi syndrome Q87.1
Preauricular appendage or tag Q17.0
Prebetalipoproteinemia (acquired) (essential) (familial) (hereditary) (primary) (secondary) E78.1
with chylomicronemia E78.3
Precipitate labor or delivery O62.3
Preclimacteric bleeding (menorrhagia) N92.4
Precocious
adrenarche E30.1
menarche E30.1
menstruation E30.1
pubarche E30.1
puberty E30.1
central E22.8
sexual development NEC E30.1
thelarche E30.8
Precocity, sexual (constitutional) (cryptogenic) (female) (idiopathic) (male) E30.1
with adrenal hyperplasia E25.9
congenital E25.0
Precordial pain R07.2
Predeciduous teeth K00.2
Prediabetes, prediabetic R73.03
complicating
pregnancy — *see* Pregnancy, complicated by, diseases of, specified type or system NEC
puerperium O99.89
Predislocation status of hip at birth Q65.6
Pre-eclampsia O14.9-
with pre-existing hypertension — *see* Hypertension, complicating pregnancy, pre-existing, with, pre-eclampsia
complicating
childbirth O14.94
puerperium O14.95
mild O14.0-
complicating
childbirth O14.04
puerperium O14.05
moderate O14.0-
complicating
childbirth O14.04
puerperium O14.05
severe O14.1-
with hemolysis, elevated liver enzymes and low platelet count (HELLP) O14.2-
Pre-eclampsia - *continued*
severe - *continued*
with hemolysis, elevated liver enzymes and low platelet count (HELLP) - *continued*
complicating
childbirth O14.24
puerperium O14.25
complicating
childbirth O14.14
puerperium O14.15
Pre-eruptive color change, teeth, tooth K00.8
Pre-excitation atrioventricular conduction I45.6
Preglaucoma H40.00-
Pregnancy (single) (uterine) — *see also* Delivery and Puerperal
Note: The Tabular must be reviewed for assignment of the appropriate character indicating the trimester of the pregnancy
Note: The Tabular must be reviewed for assignment of appropriate seventh character for multiple gestation codes in Chapter 15
abdominal (ectopic) O00.00
with intrauterine pregnancy O00.01
with viable fetus O36.7-
ampullar O00.10-
with intrauterine pregnancy O00.11-
biochemical O02.81
broad ligament O00.80
with intrauterine pregnancy O00.81
cervical O00.80
with intrauterine pregnancy O00.81
chemical O02.81
complicated NOS O26.9-
complicated by (care of) (management affected by)
abnormal, abnormality
cervix O34.4-
causing obstructed labor O65.5
cord (umbilical) O69.9
fetal heart rate or rhythm O36.83-
findings on antenatal screening of mother O28.9
biochemical O28.1
cytological O28.2
chromosomal O28.5
genetic O28.5
hematological O28.0
radiological O28.4
specified NEC O28.8
ultrasonic O28.3
glucose (tolerance) NEC O99.810
pelvic organs O34.9-
specified NEC O34.8-
causing obstructed labor O65.5
pelvis (bony) (major) NEC O33.0
perineum O34.7-
position
placenta O44.0-
with hemorrhage O44.1-
uterus O34.59-
uterus O34.59-
causing obstructed labor O65.5
congenital O34.0-
vagina O34.6-
causing obstructed labor O65.5
vulva O34.7-
causing obstructed labor O65.5
abruptio placentae — *see* Abruptio placentae
abscess or cellulitis
bladder O23.1-
breast O91.11-
genital organ or tract O23.9-
abuse
physical O9A.31-
psychological O9A.51-
sexual O9A.41-
adverse effect anesthesia O29.9-
aspiration pneumonitis O29.01-
cardiac arrest O29.11-
cardiac complication NEC O29.19-
cardiac failure O29.12-
central nervous system complication NEC O29.29-
cerebral anoxia O29.21-
failed or difficult intubation O29.6-
inhalation of stomach contents or secretions NOS O29.01-
local, toxic reaction O29.3X
Mendelson's syndrome O29.01-
pressure collapse of lung O29.02-
pulmonary complications NEC O29.09-
specified NEC O29.8X-
spinal and epidural type NEC O29.5X
induced headache O29.4-

Pregnancy (single) (uterine) - *continued*
- complicated by (care of) (management affected by) - *continued*
  - albuminuria — *see also* Proteinuria, gestational O12.1-
  - alcohol use O99.31-
  - amnionitis O41.12-
  - anaphylactoid syndrome of pregnancy O88.01-
  - anemia (conditions in D50-D64) (pre-existing) O99.01-
    - complicating the puerperium O99.03
  - antepartum hemorrhage O46.9-
    - with coagulation defect — *see* Hemorrhage, antepartum, with coagulation defect
    - specified NEC O46.8X-
  - appendicitis O99.61-
  - atrophy (yellow) (acute) liver (subacute) O26.61-
  - bariatric surgery status O99.84-
  - bicornis or bicornuate uterus O34.0-
  - biliary tract problems O26.61-
  - breech presentation O32.1
  - cardiovascular diseases (conditions in I00-I09, I20-I52, I70-I99) O99.41-
  - cerebrovascular disorders (conditions in I60-I69) O99.41-
  - cervical shortening O26.87-
  - cervicitis O23.51-
  - chloasma (gravidarum) O26.89-
  - cholestasis (intrahepatic) O26.61-
  - cholecystitis O99.61-
  - chorioamnionitis O41.12-
  - circulatory system disorder (conditions in I00-I09, I20-I99, O99.41-)
  - compound presentation O32.6
  - conjoined twins O30.02-
  - connective system disorders (conditions in M00-M99) O99.89
  - contracted pelvis (general) O33.1
    - inlet O33.2
    - outlet O33.3
  - convulsions (eclamptic) (uremic) — *see also* Eclampsia O15.9-
  - cracked nipple O92.11-
  - cystitis O23.1-
  - cystocele O34.8-
  - death of fetus (near term) O36.4
    - early pregnancy O02.1
    - of one fetus or more in multiple gestation O31.2-
  - deciduitis O41.14-
  - decreased fetal movement O36.81-
  - dental problems O99.61-
  - diabetes (mellitus) O24.91-
    - gestational (pregnancy induced) — *see* Diabetes, gestational
    - pre-existing O24.31-
      - specified NEC O24.81-
      - type 1 O24.01-
      - type 2 O24.11-
  - digestive system disorders (conditions in K00-K93) O99.61-
  - diseases of — *see* Pregnancy, complicated by, specified body system disease
    - biliary tract O26.61-
    - blood NEC (conditions in D65-D77) O99.11-
    - liver O26.61-
    - specified NEC O99.89
  - disorders of — *see* Pregnancy, complicated by, specified body system disorder
    - amniotic fluid and membranes O41.9-
      - specified NEC O41.8X-
    - biliary tract O26.61-
    - ear and mastoid process (conditions in H60-H95) O99.89
    - eye and adnexa (conditions in H00-H59) O99.89
    - liver O26.61-
    - skin (conditions in L00-L99) O99.71-
    - specified NEC O99.89
  - displacement, uterus NEC O34.59-
    - causing obstructed labor O65.5
  - disproportion (due to) O33.9
    - fetal (ascites) (hydrops) (meningomyelocele) (sacral teratoma) (tumor) deformities NEC O33.7
    - generally contracted pelvis O33.1
    - hydrocephalic fetus O33.6
    - inlet contraction of pelvis O33.2
    - mixed maternal and fetal origin O33.4
    - specified NEC O33.8
  - double uterus O34.0-
    - causing obstructed labor O65.5
  - drug use (conditions in F11-F19) O99.32-

Pregnancy (single) (uterine) - *continued*
- complicated by (care of) (management affected by) - *continued*
  - eclampsia, eclamptic (coma) (convulsions) (delirium) (nephritis) (uremia) — *see also* Eclampsia O15.-
  - ectopic pregnancy — *see* Pregnancy, ectopic
  - edema O12.0-
    - with
      - gestational hypertension, mild — *see also* Pre-eclampsia O14.0-
    - proteinuria O12.2-
  - effusion, amniotic fluid — *see* Pregnancy, complicated by, premature rupture of membranes
  - elderly
    - multigravida O09.52-
    - primigravida O09.51-
  - embolism — *see also* Embolism, obstetric, pregnancy O88.-
  - endocrine diseases NEC O99.28-
  - endometritis O86.12
  - excessive weight gain O26.0-
  - exhaustion O26.81-
    - during labor and delivery O75.81
  - face presentation O32.3
  - failed induction of labor O61.9
    - instrumental O61.1
    - mechanical O61.1
    - medical O61.0
    - specified NEC O61.8
    - surgical O61.1
  - failed or difficult intubation for anesthesia O29.6-
  - false labor (pains) O47.9
    - at or after 37 completed weeks of pregnancy O47.1
    - before 37 completed weeks of pregnancy O47.0-
  - fatigue O26.81-
    - during labor and delivery O75.81
  - fatty metamorphosis of liver O26.61-
  - female genital mutilation O34.8- *[N90.81-]*
  - fetal (maternal care for)
    - abnormality or damage O35.9
      - acid-base balance O68
      - specified type NEC O35.8
    - acidemia O68
    - acidosis O68
    - alkalosis O68
    - anemia and thrombocytopenia O36.82-
    - anencephaly O35.0
    - chromosomal abnormality (conditions in Q90-Q99) O35.1
    - conjoined twins O30.02-
    - damage from
      - amniocentesis O35.7
      - biopsy procedures O35.7
      - drug addiction O35.5
      - hematological investigation O35.7
      - intrauterine contraceptive device O35.7
      - maternal
        - alcohol addiction O35.4
        - cytomegalovirus infection O35.3
        - disease NEC O35.8
        - drug addiction O35.5
        - listeriosis O35.8
        - rubella O35.3
        - toxoplasmosis O35.8
        - viral infection O35.3
      - medical procedure NEC O35.7
      - radiation O35.6
    - death (near term) O36.4
      - early pregnancy O02.1
    - decreased movement O36.81-
    - disproportion due to deformity (fetal) O33.7
    - excessive growth (large for dates) O36.6-
    - growth retardation O36.59-
      - light for dates O36.59-
      - small for dates O36.59-
    - heart rate irregularity (bradycardia) (decelerations) (tachycardia) O76
    - hereditary disease O35.2
    - hydrocephalus O35.0
    - intrauterine death O36.4
    - poor growth O36.59-
      - light for dates O36.59-
      - small for dates O36.59-
    - problem O36.9-
      - specified NEC O36.89-
    - reduction (elective) O31.3-
    - selective termination O31.3-
    - spina bifida O35.0
    - thrombocytopenia O36.82-
  - fibroid (tumor) (uterus) O34.1-
  - fissure of nipple O92.11-

Pregnancy (single) (uterine) - *continued*
- complicated by (care of) (management affected by) - *continued*
  - gallstones O99.61-
  - gastric banding status O99.84-
  - gastric bypass status O99.84-
  - genital herpes (asymptomatic) (history of) (inactive) O98.3-
  - genital tract infection O23.9-
  - glomerular diseases (conditions in N00-N07) O26.83-
    - with hypertension, pre-existing — *see* Hypertension, complicating, pregnancy, pre-existing, with, renal disease
  - gonorrhea O98.21-
  - grand multiparity O09.4
  - habitual aborter — *see* Pregnancy, complicated by, recurrent pregnancy loss
  - HELLP syndrome (hemolysis, elevated liver enzymes and low platelet count) O14.2-
  - hemorrhage
    - antepartum — *see* Hemorrhage, antepartum
    - before 20 completed weeks gestation O20.9
      - specified NEC O20.8
    - due to premature separation, placenta — *see also* Abruptio placentae O45.9-
    - early O20.9
      - specified NEC O20.8
    - threatened abortion O20.0
  - hemorrhoids O22.4-
  - hepatitis (viral) O98.41-
  - herniation of uterus O34.59-
  - high
    - head at term O32.4
    - risk — *see* Supervision (of) (for), high-risk
  - history of in utero procedure during previous pregnancy O09.82-
  - HIV O98.71-
  - human immunodeficiency virus (HIV) disease O98.71-
  - hydatidiform mole — *see also* Mole, hydatidiform O01.9-
  - hydramnios O40.-
  - hydrocephalic fetus (disproportion) O33.6
  - hydrops
    - amnii O40.-
    - fetalis O36.2-
      - associated with isoimmunization — *see also* Pregnancy, complicated by, isoimmunization O36.11-
  - hydrorrhea O42.90
  - hyperemesis (gravidarum) (mild) — *see also* Hyperemesis, gravidarum O21.0-
  - hypertension — *see* Hypertension, complicating pregnancy
  - hypertensive
    - heart and renal disease, pre-existing — *see* Hypertension, complicating, pregnancy, pre-existing, with, heart disease, with renal disease
    - heart disease, pre-existing — *see* Hypertension, complicating, pregnancy, pre-existing, with, heart disease
    - renal disease, pre-existing — *see* Hypertension, complicating, pregnancy, pre-existing, with, renal disease
  - hypotension O26.5-
  - immune disorders NEC (conditions in D80-D89) O99.11-
  - incarceration, uterus O34.51-
  - incompetent cervix O34.3-
  - inconclusive fetal viability O36.80
  - infection (s) O98.91-
    - amniotic fluid or sac O41.10-
    - bladder O23.1-
    - carrier state NEC O99.830
      - streptococcus B O99.820
    - genital organ or tract O23.9-
      - specified NEC O23.59-
    - genitourinary tract O23.9-
    - gonorrhea O98.21-
    - hepatitis (viral) O98.41-
    - HIV O98.71-
    - human immunodeficiency virus (HIV) O98.71-
    - kidney O23.0-
    - nipple O91.01-
    - parasitic disease O98.91-
      - specified NEC O98.81-
    - protozoal disease O98.61-
    - sexually transmitted NEC O98.31-
    - specified type NEC O98.81-
    - syphilis O98.11-
    - tuberculosis O98.01-
    - urethra O23.2-

Pregnancy (single) (uterine) - *continued*
complicated by (care of) (management affected by) - *continued*
infection (s) - *continued*
urinary (tract) O23.4-
specified NEC O23.3-
viral disease O98.51-
injury or poisoning (conditions in S00-T88) O9A.21-
due to abuse
physical O9A.31-
psychological O9A.51-
sexual O9A.41-
insufficient
prenatal care O09.3-
weight gain O26.1-
insulin resistance O26.89
intrauterine fetal death (near term) O36.4
early pregnancy O02.1
multiple gestation (one fetus or more) O31.2-
isoimmunization O36.11-
anti-A sensitization O36.11-
anti-B sensitization O36.19-
Rh O36.09-
anti-D antibody O36.01-
specified NEC O36.19-
laceration of uterus NEC O71.81
malformation
placenta, placental (vessel) O43.10-
specified NEC O43.19-
uterus (congenital) O34.0-
malnutrition (conditions in E40-E46) O25.1-
maternal hypotension syndrome O26.5-
mental disorders (conditions in F01-F09, F20-F99) O99.34-
alcohol use O99.31-
drug use O99.32-
smoking O99.33-
mentum presentation O32.3
metabolic disorders O99.28-
missed
abortion O02.1
delivery O36.4
multiple gestations O30.9-
conjoined twins O30.02-
specified number of multiples NEC — *see* Pregnancy, multiple (gestation), specified NEC
quadruplet — *see* Pregnancy, quadruplet
specified complication NEC O31.8X-
triplet — *see* Pregnancy, triplet
twin — *see* Pregnancy, twin
musculoskeletal condition (conditions is M00-M99) O99.89
necrosis, liver (conditions in K72) O26.61-
neoplasm
benign
cervix O34.4-
corpus uteri O34.1-
uterus O34.1-
malignant O9A.11-
nephropathy NEC O26.83-
nervous system condition (conditions in G00-G99) O99.35-
nutritional diseases NEC O99.28-
obesity (pre-existing) O99.21-
obesity surgery status O99.84-
oblique lie or presentation O32.2
older mother — *see* Pregnancy, complicated by, elderly
oligohydramnios O41.0-
with premature rupture of membranes — *see also* Pregnancy, complicated by, premature rupture of membranes O42.-
onset (spontaneous) of labor after 37 completed weeks of gestation but before 39 completed weeks gestation, with delivery by (planned) cesarean section O75.82
oophoritis O23.52-
overdose, drug — *see also* Table of Drugs and Chemicals, by drug, poisoning O9A.21-
oversize fetus O33.5
papyraceous fetus O31.0-
pelvic inflammatory disease O99.89
periodontal disease O99.61-
peripheral neuritis O26.82-
peritoneal (pelvic) adhesions O99.89
phlebitis O22.9-
phlebopathy O22.9-
phlebothrombosis (superficial) O22.2-
deep O22.3-
placenta accreta O43.21-
placenta increta O43.22-
placenta percreta O43.23-

Pregnancy (single) (uterine) - *continued*
complicated by (care of) (management affected by) - *continued*
placenta previa O44.0-
complete O44.0-
with hemorrhage O44.1-
marginal O44.2-
with hemorrhage O44.3-
partial O44.2-
with hemorrhage O44.3-
placental disorder O43.9-
specified NEC O43.89-
placental dysfunction O43.89-
placental infarction O43.81-
placental insufficiency O36.51-
placental transfusion syndromes
fetomaternal O43.01-
fetus to fetus O43.02-
maternofetal O43.01-
placentitis O41.14-
pneumonia O99.51-
poisoning — *see also* Table of Drugs and Chemicals O9A.21-
polyhydramnios O40-
polymorphic eruption of pregnancy O26.86
poor obstetric history NEC O09.29-
postmaturity (post-term) (40 to 42 weeks) O48.0
more than 42 completed weeks gestation (prolonged) O48.1
pre-eclampsia O14.9-
mild O14.0-
moderate O14.0-
severe O14.1-
with hemolysis, elevated liver enzymes and low platelet count (HELLP) O14.2-
premature labor — *see* Pregnancy, complicated by, preterm labor
premature rupture of membranes O42.90
full-term, unspecified as to length of time between rupture and onset of labor O42.92
with onset of labor
within 24 hours O42.00
at or after 37 weeks gestation, onset of labor within 24 hours of rupture O42.02
pre-term (before 37 completed weeks of gestation) O42.01-
after 24 hours O42.10
at or after 37 weeks gestation, onset of labor more than 24 hours following rupture O42.12
pre-term (before 37 completed weeks of gestation) O42.11-
at or after 37 weeks gestation, unspecified as to length of time between rupture and onset of labor O42.92
pre-term (before 37 completed weeks of gestation) O42.91-
premature separation of placenta — *see also* Abruptio placentae O45.9-
presentation, fetal — *see* Delivery, complicated by, malposition
preterm delivery O60.10
preterm labor
with delivery O60.10
preterm O60.10
term O60.20
second trimester
with term delivery O60.22
without delivery O60.02
with preterm delivery
second trimester O60.12
third trimester O60.13
third trimester
with term delivery O60.23
without delivery O60.03
with third trimester preterm delivery O60.14
without delivery O60.00
second trimester O60.02
third trimester O60.03
previous history of — *see* Pregnancy, supervision of, high-risk
prolapse, uterus O34.52-
proteinuria (gestational) — *see also* Proteinuria, gestational O12.1-
with edema O12.2-
pruritic urticarial papules and plaques of pregnancy (PUPPP) O26.86
pruritus (neurogenic) O26.89-
psychosis or psychoneurosis (puerperal) F53.1
ptyalism O26.89-
PUPPP (pruritic urticarial papules and plaques of pregnancy) O26.86
pyelitis O23.0-
recurrent pregnancy loss O26.2-

Pregnancy (single) (uterine) - *continued*
complicated by (care of) (management affected by) - *continued*
renal disease or failure NEC O26.83-
with secondary hypertension, pre-existing — *see* Hypertension, complicating, pregnancy, pre-existing, secondary
hypertensive, pre-existing — *see* Hypertension, complicating, pregnancy, pre-existing, with, renal disease
respiratory condition (conditions in J00-J99) O99.51-
retained, retention
dead ovum O02.0
intrauterine contraceptive device O26.3-
retroversion, uterus O34.53-
Rh immunization, incompatibility or sensitization NEC O36.09-
anti-D antibody O36.01-
rupture
amnion (premature) — *see also* Pregnancy, complicated by, premature rupture of membranes O42-
membranes (premature) — *see also* Pregnancy, complicated by, premature rupture of membranes O42-
uterus (during labor) O71.1
before onset of labor O71.0-
salivation (excessive) O26.89-
salpingitis O23.52-
salpingo-oophoritis O23.52-
sepsis (conditions in A40, A41) O98.81-
size date discrepancy (uterine) O26.84-
skin condition (conditions in L00-L99) O99.71-
smoking (tobacco) O99.33-
social problem O09.7-
specified condition NEC O26.89-
spotting O26.85-
streptococcus group B (GBS) carrier state O99.820
subluxation of symphysis (pubis) O26.71-
syphilis (conditions in A50-A53) O98.11-
threatened
abortion O20.0
labor O47.9
at or after 37 completed weeks of gestation O47.1
before 37 completed weeks of gestation O47.0-
thrombophlebitis (superficial) O22.2-
thrombosis O22.9-
cerebral venous O22.5-
cerebrovenous sinus O22.5-
deep O22.3-
tobacco use disorder (smoking) O99.33-
torsion of uterus O34.59-
toxemia O14.9-
transverse lie or presentation O32.2
tuberculosis (conditions in A15-A19) O98.01-
tumor (benign)
cervix O34.4-
malignant O9A.11-
uterus O34.1-
unstable lie O32.0
upper respiratory infection O99.51-
urethritis O23.2-
uterine size date discrepancy O26.84-
vaginitis or vulvitis O23.59-
varicose veins (lower extremities) O22.0-
genitals O22.1-
legs O22.0-
perineal O22.1-
vaginal or vulval O22.1-
venereal disease NEC (conditions in A63.8) O98.31-
venous disorders O22.9-
specified NEC O22.8X-
viral diseases (conditions in A80-B09, B25-B34) O98.51-
very young mother — *see* Pregnancy, complicated by, young mother
vomiting O21.9
due to diseases classified elsewhere O21.8
hyperemesis gravidarum (mild) — *see also* Hyperemesis, gravidarum O21.0-
late (occurring after 20 weeks of gestation) O21.2
young mother
multigravida O09.62-
primigravida O09.61-
concealed O09.3-
continuing following
elective fetal reduction of one or more fetus O31.3-
intrauterine death of one or more fetus O31.2-
spontaneous abortion of one or more fetus O31.1-
cornual O00.80

Pregnancy (single) (uterine) - *continued*
cornual - *continued*
with intrauterine pregnancy O00.81
ectopic (ruptured) O00.90
with intrauterine pregnancy O00.91
abdominal O00.00
with
intrauterine pregnancy O00.01
viable fetus O36.7-
cervical O00.80
with intrauterine pregnancy O00.81
complicated (by) O08.9
afibrinogenemia O08.1
cardiac arrest O08.81
chemical damage of pelvic organ (s) O08.6
circulatory collapse O08.3
defibrination syndrome O08.1
electrolyte imbalance O08.5
embolism (amniotic fluid) (blood clot) (pulmonary) (septic) O08.2
endometritis O08.0
genital tract and pelvic infection O08.0
hemorrhage (delayed) (excessive) O08.1
infection
genital tract or pelvic O08.0
kidney O08.83
urinary tract O08.83
intravascular coagulation O08.1
laceration of pelvic organ (s) O08.6
metabolic disorder O08.5
oliguria O08.4
oophoritis O08.0
parametritis O08.0
pelvic peritonitis O08.0
perforation of pelvic organ (s) O08.6
renal failure or shutdown O08.4
salpingitis or salpingo-oophoritis O08.0
sepsis O08.82
shock O08.83
septic O08.82
specified condition NEC O08.89
tubular necrosis (renal) O08.4
uremia O08.4
urinary infection O08.83
venous complication NEC O08.7
embolism O08.2
cornual O00.80
with intrauterine pregnancy O00.81
intraligamentous O00.80
with intrauterine pregnancy O00.81
mural O00.80
with intrauterine pregnancy O00.81
ovarian O00.20-
with intrauterine pregnancy O00.21-
specified site NEC O00.80
with intrauterine pregnancy O00.81
tubal (ruptured) O00.10-
with intrauterine pregnancy O00.11-
examination (normal) Z34.9-
high-risk — *see* Pregnancy, supervision of, high-risk
first Z34.0-
specified Z34.8-
extrauterine — *see* Pregnancy, ectopic
fallopian O00.10-
with intrauterine pregnancy O00.11-
false F45.8
gestational carrier Z33.3
heptachorionic, hepta-amniotic (septuplets) O30.83-
hexachorionic, hexa-amniotic (sextuplets) O30.83-
hidden O09.3-
high-risk — *see* Pregnancy, supervision of, high-risk
incidental finding Z33.1
interstitial O00.80
with intrauterine pregnancy O00.81
intraligamentous O00.80
with intrauterine pregnancy O00.81
intramural O00.80
with intrauterine pregnancy O00.81
intraperitoneal O00.00
with intrauterine pregnancy O00.01
isthmian O00.10-
with intrauterine pregnancy O00.11-
mesometric (mural) O00.80
with intrauterine pregnancy O00.81
molar NEC O02.0
complicated (by) O08.9
afibrinogenemia O08.1
cardiac arrest O08.81
chemical damage of pelvic organ (s) O08.6
circulatory collapse O08.3
defibrination syndrome O08.1
electrolyte imbalance O08.5

Pregnancy (single) (uterine) - *continued*
molar NEC - *continued*
complicated (by) - *continued*
embolism (amniotic fluid) (blood clot) (pulmonary) (septic) O08.2
endometritis O08.0
genital tract and pelvic infection O08.0
hemorrhage (delayed) (excessive) O08.1
infection
genital tract or pelvic O08.0
kidney O08.83
urinary tract O08.83
intravascular coagulation O08.1
laceration of pelvic organ (s) O08.6
metabolic disorder O08.5
oliguria O08.4
oophoritis O08.0
parametritis O08.0
pelvic peritonitis O08.0
perforation of pelvic organ (s) O08.6
renal failure or shutdown O08.4
salpingitis or salpingo-oophoritis O08.0
sepsis O08.82
shock O08.3
septic O08.82
specified condition NEC O08.89
tubular necrosis (renal) O08.4
uremia O08.4
urinary infection O08.83
venous complication NEC O08.7
embolism O08.2
hydatidiform — *see also* Mole, hydatidiform O01.9-
multiple (gestation) O30.9-
greater than quadruplets — *see* Pregnancy, multiple (gestation), specified NEC
specified NEC O30.80-
with
two or more monoamniotic fetuses O30.82-
two or more monochorionic fetuses O30.81-
number of chorions and amnions are both equal to the number of fetuses O30.83-
two or more monoamniotic fetuses O30.82-
two or more monochorionic fetuses O30.81-
unable to determine number of placenta and number of amniotic sacs O30.89-
unspecified number of placenta and unspecified number of amniotic sacs O30.80-
mural O00.80
with intrauterine pregnancy O00.81
normal (supervision of) Z34.9-
high-risk — *see* Pregnancy, supervision of, high-risk
first Z34.0-
specified Z34.8-
ovarian O00.20-
with intrauterine pregnancy O00.21-
pentachorionic, penta-amniotic (quintuplets) O30.83-
postmature (40 to 42 weeks) O48.0
more than 42 weeks gestation O48.1
post-term (40 to 42 weeks) O48.0
prenatal care only Z34.9-
high-risk — *see* Pregnancy, supervision of, high-risk
first Z34.0-
specified Z34.8-
prolonged (more than 42 weeks gestation) O48.1
quadruplet O30.20-
with
two or more monoamniotic fetuses O30.22-
two or more monochorionic fetuses O30.21-
quadrachorionic/quadra-amniotic O30.23-
two or more monoamniotic fetuses O30.22-
two or more monochorionic fetuses O30.21-
unable to determine number of placenta and number of amniotic sacs O30.29-
unspecified number of placenta and unspecified number of amniotic sacs O30.20-
quintuplet — *see* Pregnancy, multiple (gestation), specified NEC
sextuplet — *see* Pregnancy, multiple (gestation), specified NEC
supervision of
concealed pregnancy O09.3-
elderly mother
multigravida O09.52-
primigravida O09.51-
hidden pregnancy O09.3-
high-risk O09.9-
due to (history of)
ectopic pregnancy O09.1-

Pregnancy (single) (uterine) - *continued*
supervision of - *continued*
high-risk - *continued*
due to (history of) - *continued*
elderly — *see* Pregnancy, supervision, elderly mother
grand multiparity O09.4
infertility O09.0-
insufficient prenatal care O09.3-
in utero procedure during previous pregnancy O09.82-
in vitro fertilization O09.81-
molar pregnancy O09.A-
multiple previous pregnancies O09.4-
older mother — *see* Pregnancy, supervision of, elderly mother
poor reproductive or obstetric history NEC O09.29-
pre-term labor O09.21-
previous
neonatal death O09.29-
social problems O09.7-
specified NEC O09.89-
very young mother — *see* Pregnancy, supervision, young mother
resulting from in vitro fertilization O09.81-
normal Z34.9-
first Z34.0-
specified NEC Z34.8-
young mother
multigravida O09.62-
primigravida O09.61-
triplet O30.10-
with
two or more monoamniotic fetuses O30.12-
two or more monochorionic fetuses O30.11-
trichorionic/triamniotic O30.13-
two or more monoamniotic fetuses O30.12-
two or more monochorionic fetuses O30.11-
unable to determine number of placenta and number of amniotic sacs O30.19-
unspecified number of placenta and unspecified number of amniotic sacs O30.10-
tubal (with abortion) (with rupture) O00.10-
with intrauterine pregnancy O00.11-
twin O30.00-
conjoined O30.02-
dichorionic/diamniotic (two placenta, two amniotic sacs) O30.04-
monochorionic/diamniotic (one placenta, two amniotic sacs) O30.03-
monochorionic/monoamniotic (one placenta, one amniotic sac) O30.01-
unable to determine number of placenta and number of amniotic sacs O30.09-
unspecified number of placenta and unspecified number of amniotic sacs O30.00-
unwanted Z64.0
weeks of gestation
8 weeks Z3A.08
9 weeks Z3A.09
10 weeks Z3A.10
11 weeks Z3A.11
12 weeks Z3A.12
13 weeks Z3A.13
14 weeks Z3A.14
15 weeks Z3A.15
16 weeks Z3A.16
17 weeks Z3A.17
18 weeks Z3A.18
19 weeks Z3A.19
20 weeks Z3A.20
21 weeks Z3A.21
22 weeks Z3A.22
23 weeks Z3A.23
24 weeks Z3A.24
25 weeks Z3A.25
26 weeks Z3A.26
27 weeks Z3A.27
28 weeks Z3A.28
29 weeks Z3A.29
30 weeks Z3A.30
31 weeks Z3A.31
32 weeks Z3A.32
33 weeks Z3A.33
34 weeks Z3A.34
35 weeks Z3A.35
36 weeks Z3A.36
37 weeks Z3A.37
38 weeks Z3A.38
39 weeks Z3A.39
40 weeks Z3A.40
41 weeks Z3A.41

Pregnancy (single) (uterine) - *continued*
  weeks of gestation - *continued*
    42 weeks Z3A.42
    greater than 42 weeks Z3A.49
    less than 8 weeks Z3A.01
    not specified Z3A.00
Preiser's disease — *see* Osteonecrosis, secondary, due to, trauma, metacarpus
Pre-kwashiorkor — *see* Malnutrition, severe
Preleukemia (syndrome) D46.9
Preluxation, hip, congenital Q65.6
Premature — *see also* condition
  adrenarche E27.0
  aging E34.8
  beats I49.40
    atrial I49.1
    auricular I49.1
    supraventricular I49.1
  birth NEC — *see* Preterm, newborn
  closure, foramen ovale Q21.8
  contraction
    atrial I49.1
    atrioventricular I49.2
    auricular I49.1
    auriculoventricular I49.49
    heart (extrasystole) I49.49
    junctional I49.2
    ventricular I49.3
  delivery — *see also* Pregnancy, complicated by, preterm labor O60.10
  ejaculation F52.4
  infant NEC — *see* Preterm, newborn
    light-for-dates — *see* Light for dates
  labor — *see* Pregnancy, complicated by, preterm labor
  lungs P28.0
  menopause E28.319
    asymptomatic E28.319
    symptomatic E28.310
  newborn
    extreme (less than 28 completed weeks) — *see* Immaturity, extreme
    less than 37 completed weeks — *see* Preterm, newborn
  puberty E30.1
  rupture membranes or amnion — *see* Pregnancy, complicated by, premature rupture of membranes
  senility E34.8
  thelarche E30.8
  ventricular systole I49.3
Prematurity NEC (less than 37 completed weeks) — *see* Preterm, newborn
  extreme (less than 28 completed weeks) — *see* Immaturity, extreme
Premenstrual
  dysphoric disorder (PMDD) F32.81
  tension (syndrome) N94.3
Premolarization, cuspids K00.2
Prenatal
  care, normal pregnancy — *see* Pregnancy, normal
  screening of mother — *see also* Encounter, antenatal screening Z36.9
  teeth K00.6
Preparatory care for subsequent treatment NEC
  for dialysis Z49.01
    peritoneal Z49.02
Prepartum — *see* condition
Preponderance, left or right ventricular I51.7
Prepuce — *see* condition
PRES
  (posterior reversible encephalopathy syndrome) I67.83
Presbycardia R54
Presbycusis, presbyacusia H91.1-
Presbyesophagus K22.8
Presbyophrenia F03
Presbyopia H52.4
Prescription of contraceptives (initial) Z30.019
  barrier Z30.018
  diaphragm Z30.018
  emergency (postcoital) Z30.012
  implantable subdermal Z30.017
  injectable Z30.013
  intrauterine contraceptive device Z30.014
  pills Z30.011
  postcoital (emergency) Z30.012
  repeat Z30.40
    barrier Z30.49
    diaphragm Z30.49
    implantable subdermal Z30.46
    injectable Z30.42
    pills Z30.41
    specified type NEC Z30.49

Prescription of contraceptives (initial) - *continued*
  repeat - *continued*
    transdermal patch hormonal Z30.45
    vaginal ring hormonal Z30.44
  specified type NEC Z30.018
    transdermal patch hormonal Z30.016
    vaginal ring hormonal Z30.015
Presence (of)
  ankle-joint implant (functional) (prosthesis) Z96.66-
  aortocoronary (bypass) graft Z95.1
  arterial-venous shunt (dialysis) Z99.2
  artificial
    eye (globe) Z97.0
    heart (fully implantable) (mechanical) Z95.812
      valve Z95.2
    larynx Z96.3
    lens (intraocular) Z96.1
    limb (complete) (partial) Z97.1-
      arm Z97.1-
        bilateral Z97.15
      leg Z97.1-
        bilateral Z97.16
  audiological implant (functional) Z96.29
  bladder implant (functional) Z96.0
  bone
    conduction hearing device Z96.29
    implant (functional) NEC Z96.7
    joint (prosthesis) — *see* Presence, joint implant
  cardiac
    defibrillator (functional) (with synchronous cardiac pacemaker) Z95.810
    implant or graft Z95.9
      specified type NEC Z95.818
    pacemaker Z95.0
    resynchronization therapy
      defibrillator Z95.810
      pacemaker Z95.0
  cerebrospinal fluid drainage device Z98.2
  cochlear implant (functional) Z96.21
  contact lens (es) Z97.3
  coronary artery graft or prosthesis Z95.5
  CRT-D (cardiac resynchronization therapy defibrillator) Z95.810
  CRT-P (cardiac resynchronization therapy pacemaker) Z95.0
  cardioverter-defibrillator (ICD) Z95.810
  CSF shunt Z98.2
  dental prosthesis device Z97.2
  dentures Z97.2
  device (external) NEC Z97.8
    cardiac NEC Z95.818
    heart assist Z95.811
    implanted (functional) Z96.9
      specified NEC Z96.89
    prosthetic Z97.8
  ear implant Z96.20
    cochlear implant Z96.21
    myringotomy tube Z96.22
    specified type NEC Z96.29
  elbow-joint implant (functional) (prosthesis) Z96.62-
  endocrine implant (functional) NEC Z96.49
  eustachian tube stent or device (functional) Z96.29
  external hearing-aid or device Z97.4
  finger-joint implant (functional) (prosthetic) Z96.69-
  functional implant Z96.9
    specified NEC Z96.89
  graft
    cardiac NEC Z95.818
    vascular NEC Z95.828
  hearing-aid or device (external) Z97.4
    implant (bone) (cochlear) (functional) Z96.21
  heart assist device Z95.811
  heart valve implant (functional) Z95.2
    prosthetic Z95.2
    specified type NEC Z95.4
    xenogenic Z95.3
  hip-joint implant (functional) (prosthesis) Z96.64-
  ICD (cardioverter-defibrillator) Z95.810
  implanted device (artificial) (functional) (prosthetic) Z96.9
    automatic cardiac defibrillator (with synchronous cardiac pacemaker) Z95.810
    cardiac pacemaker Z95.0
    cochlear Z96.21
    dental Z96.5
    heart Z95.812
    heart valve Z95.2
      prosthetic Z95.2
      specified NEC Z95.4
      xenogenic Z95.3
    insulin pump Z96.41
    intraocular lens Z96.1
    joint Z96.60

Presence (of) - *continued*
  implanted device (artificial) (functional) (prosthetic) - *continued*
    joint - *continued*
      ankle Z96.66-
      elbow Z96.62-
      finger Z96.69-
      hip Z96.64-
      knee Z96.65-
      shoulder Z96.61-
      specified NEC Z96.698
      wrist Z96.63-
    larynx Z96.3
    myringotomy tube Z96.22
    otological Z96.20
      cochlear Z96.21
      eustachian stent Z96.29
      myringotomy Z96.22
      specified NEC Z96.29
      stapes Z96.29
    skin Z96.81
    skull plate Z96.7
    specified NEC Z96.89
    urogenital Z96.0
  insulin pump (functional) Z96.41
  intestinal bypass or anastomosis Z98.0
  intraocular lens (functional) Z96.1
  intrauterine contraceptive device (IUD) Z97.5
  intravascular implant (functional) (prosthetic) NEC Z95.9
    coronary artery Z95.5
    defibrillator (with synchronous cardiac pacemaker) Z95.810
    peripheral vessel (with angioplasty) Z95.820
  joint implant (prosthetic) (any) Z96.60
    ankle — *see* Presence, ankle joint implant
    elbow — *see* Presence, elbow joint implant
    finger — *see* Presence, finger joint implant
    hip — *see* Presence, hip joint implant
    knee — *see* Presence, knee joint implant
    shoulder — *see* Presence, shoulder joint implant
    specified joint NEC Z96.698
    wrist — *see* Presence, wrist joint implant
  knee-joint implant (functional) (prosthesis) Z96.65-
  laryngeal implant (functional) Z96.3
  mandibular implant (dental) Z96.5
  myringotomy tube (s) Z96.22
  orthopedic-joint implant (prosthetic) (any) — *see* Presence, joint implant
  otological implant (functional) Z96.29
  shoulder-joint implant (functional) (prosthesis) Z96.61-
  skull-plate implant Z96.7
  spectacles Z97.3
  stapes implant (functional) Z96.29
  systemic lupus erythematosus [SLE] inhibitor D68.62
  tendon implant (functional) (graft) Z96.7
  tooth root (s) implant Z96.5
  ureteral stent Z96.0
  urethral stent Z96.0
  urogenital implant (functional) Z96.0
  vascular implant or device Z95.9
    access port device Z95.828
    specified type NEC Z95.828
  wrist-joint implant (functional) (prosthesis) Z96.63-
Presenile — *see also* condition
  dementia F03
  premature aging E34.8
Presentation, fetal — *see* Delivery , complicated by, malposition
Prespondylolisthesis (congenital) Q76.2
Pressure
  area, skin — *see* Ulcer, pressure, by site
  brachial plexus G54.0
  brain G93.5
    injury at birth NEC P11.1
  cerebral — *see* Pressure, brain
  chest R07.89
  cone, tentorial G93.5
  hyposystolic — *see also* Hypotension
    incidental reading, without diagnosis of hypotension R03.1
  increased
    intracranial (benign) G93.2
      injury at birth P11.0
    intraocular H40.05-
  lumbosacral plexus G54.1
  mediastinum J98.59
  necrosis (chronic) — *see* Ulcer, pressure, by site
  parental, inappropriate (excessive) Z62.6
  sore (chronic) — *see* Ulcer, pressure, by site
  spinal cord G95.20

Pressure - *continued*
ulcer (chronic) — *see* Ulcer, pressure, by site
venous, increased I87.8
Pre-syncope R55
Preterm
delivery — *see also* Pregnancy, complicated by, preterm labor O60.10
labor — *see* Pregnancy, complicated by, preterm labor
newborn (infant) P07.30
gestational age
28 completed weeks (28 weeks, 0 days through 28 weeks, 6 days) P07.31
29 completed weeks (29 weeks, 0 days through 29 weeks, 6 days) P07.32
30 completed weeks (30 weeks, 0 days through 30 weeks, 6 days) P07.33
31 completed weeks (31 weeks, 0 days through 31 weeks, 6 days) P07.34
32 completed weeks (32 weeks, 0 days through 32 weeks, 6 days) P07.35
33 completed weeks (33 weeks, 0 days through 33 weeks, 6 days) P07.36
34 completed weeks (34 weeks, 0 days through 34 weeks, 6 days) P07.37
35 completed weeks (35 weeks, 0 days through 35 weeks, 6 days) P07.38
36 completed weeks (36 weeks, 0 days through 36 weeks, 6 days) P07.39
Previa
placenta (total) (without hemorrhage) O44.0-
with hemorrhage O44.1-
complete O44.0-
with hemorrhage O44.1-
low — *see also* Delivery, complicated, by, placenta, low O44.4-
with hemorrhage O44.5-
marginal O44.2-
with hemorrhage O44.3-
partial O44.2-
with hemorrhage O44.3-
vasa O69.4
Priapism N48.30
due to
disease classified elsewhere N48.32
drug N48.33
specified cause NEC N48.39
trauma N48.31
Prickling sensation (skin) R20.2
Prickly heat L74.0
Primary — *see* condition
Primigravida
elderly, affecting management of pregnancy, labor and delivery (supervision only) — *see* Pregnancy, complicated by, elderly, primigravida
older, affecting management of pregnancy, labor and delivery (supervision only) — *see* Pregnancy, complicated by, elderly, primigravida
very young, affecting management of pregnancy, labor and delivery (supervision only) — *see* Pregnancy, complicated by, young mother, primigravida
Primipara
elderly, affecting management of pregnancy, labor and delivery (supervision only) — *see* Pregnancy, complicated by, elderly, primigravida
older, affecting management of pregnancy, labor and delivery (supervision only) — *see* Pregnancy, complicated by, elderly, primigravida
very young, affecting management of pregnancy, labor and delivery (supervision only) — *see* Pregnancy, complicated by, young mother, primigravida
Primus varus (bilateral) Q66.2
PRIND
(Prolonged reversible ischemic neurologic deficit) I63.9
Pringle's disease (tuberous sclerosis) Q85.1
Prinzmetal angina I20.1
Prizefighter ear — *see* Cauliflower ear
Problem (with) (related to)
academic Z55.8
acculturation Z60.3
adjustment (to)
change of job Z56.1
life-cycle transition Z60.0
pension Z60.0
retirement Z60.0
adopted child Z62.821
alcoholism in family Z63.72
atypical parenting situation Z62.9
bankruptcy Z59.8
behavioral (adult) F69

Problem (with) (related to) - *continued*
behavioral (adult) - *continued*
drug seeking Z76.5
birth of sibling affecting child Z62.898
care (of)
provider dependency Z74.9
specified NEC Z74.8
sick or handicapped person in family or household Z63.6
child
abuse (affecting the child) — *see* Maltreatment, child
custody or support proceedings Z65.3
in welfare custody Z62.21
in care of non-parental family member Z62.21
in foster care Z62.21
living in orphanage or group home Z62.22
child-rearing Z62.9
specified NEC Z62.898
communication (developmental) F80.9
conflict or discord (with)
boss Z56.4
classmates Z55.4
counselor Z64.4
employer Z56.4
family Z63.9
specified NEC Z63.8
probation officer Z64.4
social worker Z64.4
teachers Z55.4
workmates Z56.4
conviction in legal proceedings Z65.0
with imprisonment Z65.1
counselor Z64.4
creditors Z59.8
digestive K92.9
drug addict in family Z63.72
ear — *see* Disorder, ear
economic Z59.9
affecting care Z59.9
specified NEC Z59.8
education Z55.9
specified NEC Z55.8
employment Z56.9
change of job Z56.1
discord Z56.4
environment Z56.5
sexual harassment Z56.81
specified NEC Z56.89
stress NEC Z56.6
stressful schedule Z56.3
threat of job loss Z56.2
unemployment Z56.0
enuresis, child F98.0
eye H57.9
failed examinations (school) Z55.2
falling Z91.81
family — *see also* Disruption, family Z63.9-
specified NEC Z63.8
feeding (elderly) (infant) R63.3
newborn P92.9
breast P92.5
overfeeding P92.4
slow P92.2
specified NEC P92.8
underfeeding P92.3
nonorganic F50.89
finance Z59.9
specified NEC Z59.8
foreclosure on loan Z59.8
foster child Z62.822
frightening experience (s) in childhood Z62.898
genital NEC
female N94.9
male N50.9
health care Z75.9
specified NEC Z75.8
hearing — *see* Deafness
homelessness Z59.0
housing Z59.9
inadequate Z59.1
isolated Z59.8
specified NEC Z59.8
identity (of childhood) F93.8
illegitimate pregnancy (unwanted) Z64.0
illiteracy Z55.0
impaired mobility Z74.09
imprisonment or incarceration Z65.1
inadequate teaching affecting education Z55.8
inappropriate (excessive) parental pressure Z62.6
influencing health status NEC Z78.9
in-law Z63.1
institutionalization, affecting child Z62.22

Problem (with) (related to) - *continued*
intrafamilial communication Z63.8
jealousy, child F93.8
landlord Z59.2
language (developmental) F80.9
learning (developmental) F81.9
legal Z65.3
conviction without imprisonment Z65.0
imprisonment Z65.1
release from prison Z65.2
life-management Z73.9
specified NEC Z73.89
life-style Z72.9
gambling Z72.6
high-risk sexual behavior (heterosexual) Z72.51
bisexual Z72.53
homosexual Z72.52
inappropriate eating habits Z72.4
self-damaging behavior NEC Z72.89
specified NEC Z72.89
tobacco use Z72.0
literacy Z55.9
low level Z55.0
specified NEC Z55.8
living alone Z60.2
lodgers Z59.2
loss of love relationship in childhood Z62.898
marital Z63.0
involving
divorce Z63.5
estrangement Z63.5
gender identity F66
mastication K08.89
medical
care, within family Z63.6
facilities Z75.9
specified NEC Z75.8
mental F48.9
multiparity Z64.1
negative life events in childhood Z62.9
altered pattern of family relationships Z62.898
frightening experience Z62.898
loss of
love relationship Z62.898
self-esteem Z62.898
physical abuse (alleged) — *see* Maltreatment, child
removal from home Z62.29
specified event NEC Z62.898
neighbor Z59.2
neurological NEC R29.818
new step-parent affecting child Z62.898
none (feared complaint unfounded) Z71.1
occupational NEC Z56.89
parent-child — *see* Conflict, parent-child
personal hygiene Z91.89
personality F69
phase-of-life transition, adjustment Z60.0
presence of sick or disabled person in family or household Z63.79
needing care Z63.6
primary support group (family) Z63.9
specified NEC Z63.8
probation officer Z64.4
psychiatric F99
psychosexual (development) F66
psychosocial Z65.9
religious or spiritual Z65.8
specified NEC Z65.8
relationship Z63.9
childhood F93.8
release from prison Z65.2
religious or spiritual Z65.8
removal from home affecting child Z62.29
seeking and accepting known hazardous and harmful behavioral or psychological interventions Z65.8
chemical, nutritional or physical interventions Z65.8
sexual function (nonorganic) F52.9
sight H54.7
sleep disorder, child F51.9
smell — *see* Disturbance, sensation, smell
social
environment Z60.9
specified NEC Z60.8
exclusion and rejection Z60.4
worker Z64.4
speech R47.9
developmental F80.9
specified NEC R47.89
swallowing — *see* Dysphagia
taste — *see* Disturbance, sensation, taste
tic, child F95.0
underachievement in school Z55.3

Problem (with) (related to) - *continued*
unemployment Z56.0
threatened Z56.2
unwanted pregnancy Z64.0
upbringing Z62.9
specified NEC Z62.898
urinary N39.9
voice production R47.89
work schedule (stressful) Z56.3
Procedure (surgical)
converted
arthroscopic to open Z53.33
laparoscopic to open Z53.31
specified procedure NEC to open Z53.39
thoracoscopic to open Z53.32
for purpose other than remedying health state Z41.9
specified NEC Z41.8
not done Z53.9
because of
administrative reasons Z53.8
contraindication Z53.09
smoking Z53.01
patient's decision Z53.20
for reasons of belief or group pressure Z53.1
left against medical advice (AMA) Z53.21
specified reason NEC Z53.29
specified reason NEC Z53.8
Procidentia (uteri) N81.3
Proctalgia K62.89
fugax K59.4
spasmodic K59.4
Proctitis K62.89
amebic (acute) A06.0
chlamydial A56.3
gonococcal A54.6
granulomatous — *see* Enteritis, regional, large intestine
herpetic A60.1
radiation K62.7
tuberculous A18.32
ulcerative (chronic) K51.20
with
complication K51.219
abscess K51.214
fistula K51.213
obstruction K51.212
rectal bleeding K51.211
specified NEC K51.218
Proctocele
female (without uterine prolapse) N81.6
with uterine prolapse N81.2
complete N81.3
male K62.3
Proctocolitis
food-induced eosinophilic K52.82
food protein-induced K52.82
milk protein-induced K52.82
mucosal — *see* Rectosigmoiditis, ulcerative
Proctoptosis K62.3
Proctorrhagia K62.5
Proctosigmoiditis K63.89
ulcerative (chronic) — *see* Rectosigmoiditis, ulcerative
Proctospasm K59.4
psychogenic F45.8
Profichet's disease — *see* Disorder, soft tissue, specified type NEC
Progeria E34.8
Prognathism (mandibular) (maxillary) M26.19
Progonoma (melanotic) — *see* Neoplasm, benign, by site
Progressive — *see* condition
Prolactinoma
specified site — *see* Neoplasm, benign, by site
unspecified site D35.2
Prolapse, prolapsed
anus, anal (canal) (sphincter) K62.2
arm or hand O32.2
causing obstructed labor O64.4
bladder (mucosa) (sphincter) (acquired)
congenital Q79.4
female — *see* Cystocele
male N32.89
breast implant (prosthetic) T85.49
cecostomy K94.09
cecum K63.4
cervix, cervical (hypertrophied) N81.2
anterior lip, obstructing labor O65.5
congenital Q51.828
postpartal, old N81.2
stump N81.85
ciliary body (traumatic) — *see* Laceration, eye(ball), with prolapse or loss of interocular tissue

Prolapse, prolapsed - *continued*
colon (pedunculated) K63.4
colostomy K94.09
disc (intervertebral) — *see* Displacement, intervertebral disc
eye implant (orbital) T85.398
lens (ocular) — *see* Complications, intraocular lens
fallopian tube N83.4-
gastric (mucosa) K31.89
genital, female N81.9
specified NEC N81.89
globe, nontraumatic — *see* Luxation, globe
ileostomy bud K94.19
intervertebral disc — *see* Displacement, intervertebral disc
intestine (small) K63.4
iris (traumatic) — *see* Laceration, eye(ball), with prolapse or loss of interocular tissue
nontraumatic H21.89
kidney N28.83
congenital Q63.2
laryngeal muscles or ventricle J38.7
liver K76.89
meatus urinarius N36.8
mitral (valve) I34.1
ocular lens implant — *see* Complications, intraocular lens
organ or site, congenital NEC — *see* Malposition, congenital
ovary N83.4-
pelvic floor, female N81.89
perineum, female N81.89
rectum (mucosa) (sphincter) K62.3
due to trichuris trichuria B79
spleen D73.89
stomach K31.89
umbilical cord
complicating delivery O69.0
urachus, congenital Q64.4
ureter N28.89
with obstruction N13.5
with infection N13.6
ureterovesical orifice N28.89
urethra (acquired) (infected) (mucosa) N36.8
congenital Q64.71
urinary meatus N36.8
congenital Q64.72
uterovaginal N81.4
complete N81.3
incomplete N81.2
uterus (with prolapse of vagina) N81.4
complete N81.3
congenital Q51.818
first degree N81.2
in pregnancy or childbirth — *see* Pregnancy, complicated by, abnormal, uterus
incomplete N81.2
postpartal (old) N81.4
second degree N81.2
third degree N81.3
uveal (traumatic) — *see* Laceration, eye(ball), with prolapse or loss of interocular tissue
vagina (anterior) (wall) — *see* Cystocele
with prolapse of uterus N81.4
complete N81.3
incomplete N81.2
posterior wall N81.6
posthysterectomy N99.3
vitreous (humor) H43.0-
in wound — *see* Laceration, eye(ball), with prolapse or loss of interocular tissue
womb — *see* Prolapse, uterus
Prolapsus, female N81.9
specified NEC N81.89
Proliferation (s)
prostate, atypical small acinar N42.32
primary cutaneous CD30-positive large T-cell C86.6
Proliferative — *see* condition
Prolonged, prolongation (of)
bleeding (time) (idiopathic) R79.1
coagulation (time) R79.1
gestation (over 42 completed weeks)
mother O48.1
newborn P08.22
interval I44.0
labor O63.9
first stage O63.0
second stage O63.1
partial thromboplastin time (PTT) R79.1
pregnancy (more than 42 weeks gestation) O48.1
prothrombin time R79.1
QT interval I45.81
uterine contractions in labor O62.4

Prominence, prominent
auricle (congenital) (ear) Q17.5
ischial spine or sacral promontory
with disproportion (fetopelvic) O33.0
causing obstructed labor O65.0
nose (congenital) acquired M95.0
Promiscuity — *see* High, risk, sexual behavior
Pronation
ankle — *see* Deformity, limb, foot, specified NEC
foot — *see also* Deformity, limb, foot, specified NEC
congenital Q74.2
Prophylactic
administration of
antibiotics, long-term Z79.2
short-term use - omit code
drug — *see also* Long-term (current) drug therapy (use of) Z79.899-
medication Z79.899
organ removal (for neoplasia management) Z40.00
breast Z40.01
fallopian tube (s) Z40.03
with ovary (s) Z40.02
ovary (s) Z40.02
specified site NEC Z40.09
surgery Z40.9
for risk factors related to malignant neoplasm — *see* Prophylactic, organ removal
specified NEC Z40.8
vaccination Z23
Propionic acidemia E71.121
Proptosis (ocular) — *see also* Exophthalmos
thyroid — *see* Hyperthyroidism, with goiter
Prosecution, anxiety concerning Z65.3
Prosopagnosia R48.3
Prostadynia N42.81
Prostate, prostatic — *see* condition
Prostatism — *see* Hyperplasia, prostate
Prostatitis (congestive) (suppurative) (with cystitis) N41.9
acute N41.0
cavitary N41.8
chronic N41.1
diverticular N41.8
due to Trichomonas (vaginalis) A59.02
fibrous N41.1
gonococcal (acute) (chronic) A54.22
granulomatous N41.4
hypertrophic N41.1
subacute N41.1
trichomonal A59.02
tuberculous A18.14
Prostatocystitis N41.3
Prostatorrhea N42.89
Prostatosis N42.82
Prostration R53.83
heat — *see also* Heat, exhaustion
anhydrotic T67.3
due to
salt (and water) depletion T67.4
water depletion T67.3
nervous F48.8
senile R54
Protanomaly (anomalous trichromat) H53.54
Protanopia (complete) (incomplete) H53.54
Protection (against) (from) — *see* Prophylactic
Protein
deficiency NEC — *see* Malnutrition
malnutrition — *see* Malnutrition
sickness — *see also* Reaction, serum T80.69
Proteinemia R77.9
Proteinosis
alveolar (pulmonary) J84.01
lipid or lipoid (of Urbach) E78.89
Proteinuria R80.9
Bence Jones R80.3
complicating pregnancy — *see* Proteinuria, gestational
gestational
complicating
childbirth O12.14
pregnancy O12.1-
with edema O12.2-
puerperium O12.15
idiopathic R80.0
isolated R80.0
with glomerular lesion N06.9
dense deposit disease N06.6
diffuse
crescentic glomerulonephritis N06.7
endocapillary proliferative glomerulonephritis N06.4
mesangiocapillary glomerulonephritis N06.5

Proteinuria - *continued*
isolated - *continued*
with glomerular lesion - *continued*
focal and segmental hyalinosis or sclerosis N06.1
membranous (diffuse) N06.2
mesangial proliferative (diffuse) N06.3
minimal change N06.0
specified pathology NEC N06.8
orthostatic R80.2
with glomerular lesion — *see* Proteinuria, isolated, with glomerular lesion
persistent R80.1
with glomerular lesion — *see* Proteinuria, isolated, with glomerular lesion
postural R80.2
with glomerular lesion — *see* Proteinuria, isolated, with glomerular lesion
pre-eclamptic — *see* Pre-eclampsia
puerperal O12.15
specified type NEC R80.8
Proteolysis, pathologic D65
Proteus (mirabilis) (morganii)
, as cause of disease classified elsewhere B96.4
Prothrombin gene mutation D68.52
Protoporphyria, erythropoietic E80.0
Protozoal — *see also* condition
disease B64
specified NEC B60.8
Protrusion, protrusio
acetabuli M24.7
acetabulum (into pelvis) M24.7
device, implant or graft — *see also* Complications, by site and type, mechanical T85.698
arterial graft NEC — *see* Complication, cardiovascular device, mechanical, vascular
breast (implant) T85.49
catheter NEC T85.698
cystostomy T83.090
dialysis (renal) T82.49
intraperitoneal T85.691
infusion NEC T82.594
spinal (epidural) (subdural) T85.690
urinary — *see also* Complications, catheter, urinary T83.098
electronic (electrode) (pulse generator) (stimulator)
bone T84.390
nervous system — *see* Complication, prosthetic device, mechanical, electronic nervous system stimulator
fixation, internal (orthopedic) NEC — *see* Complication, fixation device, mechanical
gastrointestinal — *see* Complications, prosthetic device, mechanical, gastrointestinal device
genital NEC T83.498
intrauterine contraceptive device T83.39
penile prosthesis (cylinder) (implanted) (pump) (resevoir) T83.490
testicular prosthesis T83.491
heart NEC — *see* Complication, cardiovascular device, mechanical
joint prosthesis — *see* Complications, joint prosthesis, mechanical, specified NEC, by site
ocular NEC — *see* Complications, prosthetic device, mechanical, ocular device
orthopedic NEC — *see* Complication, orthopedic, device, mechanical
specified NEC T85.628
urinary NEC — *see also* Complication, genitourinary, device, urinary, mechanical graft T83.29
vascular NEC — *see* Complication, cardiovascular device, mechanical
ventricular intracranial shunt T85.09
intervertebral disc — *see* Displacement, intervertebral disc
joint prosthesis — *see* Complications, joint prosthesis, mechanical, specified NEC, by site
nucleus pulposus — *see* Displacement, intervertebral disc
Prune belly (syndrome) Q79.4
Prurigo (ferox) (gravis) (Hebrae) (Hebra's) (mitis) (simplex) L28.2
Besnier's L20.0
estivalis L56.4
nodularis L28.1
psychogenic F45.8
Pruritus, pruritic (essential) L29.9
ani, anus L29.0
psychogenic F45.8
anogenital L29.3
psychogenic F45.8
due to onchocerca volvulus B73.1

Pruritus, pruritic (essential) - *continued*
gravidarum — *see* Pregnancy, complicated by, specified pregnancy-related condition NEC
hiemalis L29.8
neurogenic (any site) F45.8
perianal L29.0
psychogenic (any site) F45.8
scroti, scrotum L29.1
psychogenic F45.8
senile, senilis L29.8
specified NEC L29.8
psychogenic F45.8
Trichomonas A59.9
vulva, vulvae L29.2
psychogenic F45.8
Pseudarthrosis, pseudoarthrosis (bone) — *see* Nonunion, fracture
clavicle, congenital Q74.0
joint, following fusion or arthrodesis M96.0
Pseudoaneurysm — *see* Aneurysm
Pseudoangina (pectoris) — *see* Angina
Pseudoangioma I81
Pseudoarteriosus Q28.8
Pseudoarthrosis — *see* Pseudarthrosis
Pseudobulbar affect (PBA) F48.2
Pseudochromhidrosis L67.8
Pseudocirrhosis, liver, pericardial I31.1
Pseudocowpox B08.03
Pseudocoxalgia M91.3-
Pseudocroup J38.5
Pseudo-Cushing's syndrome, alcohol -induced E24.4
Pseudocyesis F45.8
Pseudocyst
lung J98.4
pancreas K86.3
retina — *see* Cyst, retina
Pseudoelephantiasis neuroarthritica Q82.0
Pseudoexfoliation, capsule (lens) — *see* Cataract, specified NEC
Pseudofolliculitis barbae L73.1
Pseudoglioma H44.89
Pseudohemophilia (Bernuth's) (hereditary) (type B) D68.0
Type A D69.8
vascular D69.8
Pseudohermaphroditism Q56.3
adrenal E25.8
female Q56.2
with adrenocortical disorder E25.8
without adrenocortical disorder Q56.2
adrenal (congenital) E25.0
unspecified E25.9
male Q56.1
with
adrenocortical disorder E25.8
androgen resistance E34.51
cleft scrotum Q56.1
feminizing testis E34.51
5-alpha-reductase deficiency E29.1
without gonadal disorder Q56.1
adrenal E25.8
unspecified E25.9
Pseudo-Hurler's polydystrophy E77.0
Pseudohydrocephalus G93.2
Pseudohypertrophic muscular dystrophy (Erb's) G71.02
Pseudohypertrophy, muscle G71.09
Pseudohypoparathyroidism E20.1
Pseudoinsomnia F51.03
Pseudoleukemia, infantile D64.89
Pseudomembranous — *see* condition
Pseudomeningocele (cerebral) (infective) (post-traumatic) G96.19
postprocedural (spinal) G97.82
Pseudomenses (newborn) P54.6
Pseudomenstruation (newborn) P54.6
Pseudomonas
aeruginosa, as cause of disease classified elsewhere B96.5
mallei infection A24.0
as cause of disease classified elsewhere B96.5
pseudomallei, as cause of disease classified elsewhere B96.5
Pseudomyotonia G71.19
Pseudomyxoma peritonei C78.6
Pseudoneuritis, optic (nerve) (disc) (papilla)
, congenital Q14.2
Pseudo-obstruction intestine (acute) (chronic) (idiopathic) (intermittent secondary) (primary) K59.8
Pseudopapilledema H47.33-
congenital Q14.2

Pseudoparalysis
arm or leg R29.818
atonic, congenital P94.2
Pseudopelade L66.0
Pseudophakia Z96.1
Pseudopolyarthritis, rhizomelic M35.3
Pseudopolycythemia D75.1
Pseudopseudohypoparathyroidism E20.1
Pseudopterygium H11.81-
Pseudoptosis (eyelid) — *see* Blepharochalasis
Pseudopuberty, precocious
female heterosexual E25.8
male isosexual E25.8
Pseudorickets (renal) N25.0
Pseudorubella B08.20
Pseudosclerema, newborn P83.88
Pseudosclerosis (brain)
of Westphal (Strümpell) E83.01
Jakob's — *see* Creutzfeldt-Jakob disease or syndrome
spastic — *see* Creutzfeldt-Jakob disease or syndrome
Pseudotetanus — *see* Convulsions
Pseudotetany R29.0
hysterical F44.5
Pseudotruncus arteriosus Q25.49
Pseudotuberculosis A28.2
enterocolitis A04.8
pasteurella (infection) A28.0
Pseudotumor
cerebri G93.2
orbital H05.11-
Pseudoxanthoma elasticum Q82.8
Psilosis (sprue) (tropical) K90.1
nontropical K90.0
Psittacosis A70
Psoitis M60.88
Psoriasis L40.9
arthropathic L40.50
arthritis mutilans L40.52
distal interphalangeal L40.51
juvenile L40.54
other specified L40.59
spondylitis L40.53
buccal K13.29
flexural L40.8
guttate L40.4
mouth K13.29
nummular L40.0
plaque L40.0
psychogenic F54
pustular (generalized) L40.1
palmaris et plantaris L40.3
specified NEC L40.8
vulgaris L40.0
Psychasthenia F48.8
Psychiatric disorder or problem F99
Psychogenic — *see also* condition
factors associated with physical conditions F54
Psychological and behavioral factors affecting medical condition F59
Psychoneurosis, psychoneurotic — *see also* Neurosis
anxiety (state) F41.1
depersonalization F48.1
hypochondriacal F45.21
hysteria F44.9
neurasthenic F48.8
personality NEC F60.89
Psychopathy, psychopathic
affectionless F94.2
autistic F84.5
constitution, post-traumatic F07.81
personality — *see* Disorder, personality
sexual — *see* Deviation, sexual
state F60.2
Psychosexual identity disorder of childhood F64.2
Psychosis, psychotic F29
acute (transient) F23
hysterical F44.9
affective — *see* Disorder, mood
alcoholic F10.959
with
abuse F10.159
anxiety disorder F10.980
with
abuse F10.180
dependence F10.280
delirium tremens F10.231
delusions F10.950
with
abuse F10.150
dependence F10.250

Puerperal, puerperium
(complicated by, complications) - *continued*
  diabetes O24.93
    gestational — *see* Puerperal, gestational diabetes
    pre-existing O24.33
      specified NEC O24.83
      type 1 O24.03
      type 2 O24.13
  digestive system disorder O99.63
  disease O90.9
    breast NEC O92.29
    cerebrovascular (acute) O99.43
    nonobstetric NEC O99.89
    tubo-ovarian O86.19
    Valsuani's O99.03
  disorder O90.9
    biliary tract O26.63
    lactation O92.70
    liver O26.63
    nonobstetric NEC O99.89
  disruption
    cesarean wound O90.0
    episiotomy wound O90.1
    perineal laceration wound O90.1
  drug use O99.325
  eclampsia (with pre-existing hypertension) O15.2
  embolism (pulmonary) (blood clot) — *see*
    Embolism, obstetric, puerperal
  endocrine, nutritional or metabolic disease
    NEC O99.285
  endophlebitis — *see* Puerperal, phlebitis
  endotrachelitis O86.11
  failure
    lactation (complete) O92.3
      partial O92.4
    renal, acute O90.4
  fever (of unknown origin) O86.4
    septic O85
  fissure, nipple O92.12
    associated with lactation O92.13
  fistula
    breast (due to mastitis) O91.12
      associated with lactation O91.13
    nipple O91.02
      associated with lactation O91.03
  galactophoritis O91.22
    associated with lactation O91.23
  galactorrhea O92.6
  gastric banding status O99.845
  gastric bypass status O99.845
  gastrointestinal disease NEC O99.63
  gestational
    diabetes O24.439
      diet controlled O24.430
      insulin (and diet) controlled O24.434
      oral drug controlled (antidiabetic)
        (hypoglycemic) O24.435
    edema O12.05
      with proteinuria O12.25
    proteinuria O12.15
  gonorrhea O98.23
  hematoma, subdural O99.43
  hemiplegia, cerebral O99.355
    due to cerbrovascular disorder O99.43
  hemorrhage O72.1
    brain O99.43
    bulbar O99.43
    cerebellar O99.43
    cerebral O99.43
    cortical O99.43
    delayed or secondary O72.2
    extradural O99.43
    internal capsule O99.43
    intracranial O99.43
    intrapontine O99.43
    meningeal O99.43
    pontine O99.43
    retained placenta O72.0
    subarachnoid O99.43
    subcortical O99.43
    subdural O99.43
    third stage O72.0
    uterine, delayed O72.2
    ventricular O99.43
  hemorrhoids O87.2
  hepatorenal syndrome O90.4
  hypertension — *see* Hypertension, complicating,
    puerperium
  hypertrophy, breast O92.29
  induration breast (fibrous) O92.29
  infection O86.4
    cervix O86.11
    generalized O85

Puerperal, puerperium (complicated by,
complications) - *continued*
  infection - *continued*
    genital tract NEC O86.19
      obstetric surgical wound O86.09
    kidney (bacillus coli) O86.21
    maternal O98.93
      carrier state NEC O99.835
      gonorrhea O98.23
      human immunodeficiency virus (HIV) O98.73
      protozoal O98.63
      sexually transmitted NEC O98.33
      specified NEC O98.83
      streptococcus group B (GBS) carrier
        state O99.825
      syphilis O98.13
      tuberculosis O98.03
      viral hepatitis O98.43
      viral NEC O98.53
    nipple O91.02
      associated with lactation O91.03
    peritoneum O85
    renal O86.21
    specified NEC O86.89
    urinary (asymptomatic) (tract) NEC O86.20
      bladder O86.22
      kidney O86.21
      specified site NEC O86.29
      urethra O86.22
    vagina O86.13
    vein — *see* Puerperal, phlebitis
  ischemia, cerebral O99.43
  lymphangitis O86.89
    breast O91.22
      associated with lactation O91.23
  malignancy O9A.13
  malnutrition O25.3
  mammillitis O91.02
    associated with lactation O91.03
  mammitis O91.22
    associated with lactation O91.23
  mania F30.8
  mastitis O91.22
    associated with lactation O91.23
    purulent O91.12
      associated with lactation O91.13
  melancholia — *see* Disorder, depressive
  mental disorder NEC O99.345
  metroperitonitis O85
  metrorrhagia — *see* Hemorrhage, postpartum
  metrosalpingitis O86.19
  metrovaginitis O86.13
  milk leg O87.1
  monoplegia, cerebral O99.43
  mood disturbance O90.6
  necrosis, liver (acute) (subacute) (conditions in
    subcategory K72.0) O26.63
    with renal failure O90.4
  nervous system disorder O99.355
  neuritis O90.89
  obesity (pre-existing prior to pregnancy) O99.215
  obesity surgery status O99.845
  occlusion, precerebral artery O99.43
  paralysis
    bladder (sphincter) O90.89
    cerebral O99.43
  paralytic stroke O99.43
  parametritis O85
  paravaginitis O86.13
  pelviperitonitis O85
  perimetritis O86.12
  perimetrosalpingitis O86.19
  perinephritis O86.21
  periphlebitis — *see* Puerperal phlebitis
  peritoneal infection O85
  peritonitis (pelvic) O85
  perivaginitis O86.13
  phlebitis O87.0
    deep O87.1
    pelvic O87.1
    superficial O87.0
  phlebothrombosis, deep O87.1
  phlegmasia alba dolens O87.1
  placental polyp O90.89
  pneumonia, embolic — *see* Embolism, obstetric,
    puerperal
  pre-eclampsia — *see* Pre-eclampsia
  psychosis (NOS) F53.1
  pyelitis O86.21
  pyelocystitis O86.29
  pyelonephritis O86.21
  pyelonephrosis O86.21
  pyemia O85

Puerperal, puerperium (complicated by,
complications) - *continued*
  pyocystitis O86.29
  pyohemia O85
  pyometra O86.12
  pyonephritis O86.21
  pyosalpingitis O86.19
  pyrexia (of unknown origin) O86.4
  renal
    disease NEC O90.89
    failure O90.4
  respiratory disease NEC O99.53
  retention
    decidua — *see* Retention, decidua
    placenta O72.0
    secundines — *see* Retention, secundines
  retrated nipple O92.02
  salpingo-ovaritis O86.19
  salpingoperitonitis O85
  secondary perineal tear O90.1
  sepsis (pelvic) O85
  sepsis O85
  septic thrombophlebitis O86.81
  skin disorder NEC O99.73
  specified condition NEC O99.89
  stroke O99.43
  subinvolution (uterus) O90.89
  subluxation of symphysis (pubis) O26.73
  suppuration — *see* Puerperal, abscess
  tetanus A34
  thelitis O91.02
    associated with lactation O91.03
  thrombocytopenia O72.3
  thrombophlebitis (superficial) O87.0
    deep O87.1
    pelvic O87.1
    septic O86.81
  thrombosis (venous) — *see* Thrombosis, puerperal
  thyroiditis O90.5
  toxemia (eclamptic) (pre-eclamptic) (with
    convulsions) O15.2
  trauma, non-obstetric O9A.23
    caused by abuse (physical) (suspected) O9A.33
      confirmed O9A.33
      psychological (suspected) O9A.53
        confirmed O9A.53
      sexual (suspected) O9A.43
        confirmed O9A.43
  uremia (due to renal failure) O90.4
  urethritis O86.22
  vaginitis O86.13
  varicose veins (legs) O87.4
    vulva or perineum O87.8
  venous O87.9
  vulvitis O86.19
  vulvovaginitis O86.13
  white leg O87.1
Puerperium — *see* Puerperal
Pulmolithiasis J98.4
Pulmonary — *see* condition
Pulpitis (acute) (anachoretic) (chronic) (hyperplastic)
  (putrescent) (suppurative) (ulcerative) K04.01
  irreversible K04.02
  reversible K04.01
Pulpless tooth K04.99
Pulse
  alternating R00.8
  bigeminal R00.8
  fast R00.0
  feeble, rapid due to shock following injury T79.4
  rapid R00.0
  weak R09.89
Pulsus alternans or trigeminus R00.8
Punch drunk F07.81
Punctum lacrimale occlusion — *see* Obstruction,
  lacrimal
Puncture
  abdomen, abdominal
    wall S31.139
      with
        foreign body S31.149
        penetration into peritoneal cavity S31.639
          with foreign body S31.649
      epigastric region S31.132
        with
          foreign body S31.142
          penetration into peritoneal cavity S31.632
            with foreign body S31.642
      left
        lower quadrant S31.134
          with
            foreign body S31.144
            penetration into peritoneal cavity S31.634

- **Puncture** - *continued*
  - abdomen, abdominal - *continued*
    - wall - *continued*
      - left - *continued*
        - lower quadrant - *continued*
          - with - *continued*
            - penetration into peritoneal cavity - *continued*
              - with foreign body S31.644
        - upper quadrant S31.131
          - with
            - foreign body S31.141
            - penetration into peritoneal cavity S31.631
              - with foreign body S31.641
      - periumbilic region S31.135
        - with
          - foreign body S31.145
          - penetration into peritoneal cavity S31.635
            - with foreign body S31.645
      - right
        - lower quadrant S31.133
          - with
            - foreign body S31.143
            - penetration into peritoneal cavity S31.633
              - with foreign body S31.643
        - upper quadrant S31.130
          - with
            - foreign body S31.140
            - penetration into peritoneal cavity S31.630
              - with foreign body S31.640
  - accidental, complicating surgery — *see* Complication, accidental puncture or laceration
  - alveolar (process) — *see* Puncture, oral cavity
  - ankle S91.039
    - with
      - foreign body S91.049
    - left S91.032
      - with
        - foreign body S91.042
    - right S91.031
      - with
        - foreign body S91.041
  - anus S31.833
    - with foreign body S31.834
  - arm (upper) S41.139
    - with foreign body S41.149
    - left S41.132
      - with foreign body S41.142
    - lower — *see* Puncture, forearm
    - right S41.131
      - with foreign body S41.141
  - auditory canal (external) (meatus) — *see* Puncture, ear
  - auricle, ear — *see* Puncture, ear
  - axilla — *see* Puncture, arm
  - back — *see also* Puncture, thorax, back
    - lower S31.030
      - with
        - foreign body S31.040
          - with penetration into retroperitoneal space S31.041
        - penetration into retroperitoneal space S31.031
  - bladder (traumatic) S37.29
    - nontraumatic N32.89
  - breast S21.039
    - with foreign body S21.049
    - left S21.032
      - with foreign body S21.042
    - right S21.031
      - with foreign body S21.041
  - buttock S31.803
    - with foreign body S31.804
    - left S31.823
      - with foreign body S31.824
    - right S31.813
      - with foreign body S31.814
  - by
    - device, implant or graft — *see* Complications, by site and type, mechanical
    - foreign body left accidentally in operative wound T81.539
    - instrument (any) during a procedure, accidental — *see* Puncture, accidental complicating surgery
  - calf — *see* Puncture, leg
  - canaliculus lacrimalis — *see* Puncture, eyelid
  - canthus, eye — *see* Puncture, eyelid
  - cervical esophagus S11.23
    - with foreign body S11.24
  - cheek (external) S01.439
    - with foreign body S01.449
    - left S01.432
      - with foreign body S01.442
    - right S01.431

- **Puncture** - *continued*
  - cheek (external) - *continued*
    - right - *continued*
      - with foreign body S01.441
    - internal — *see* Puncture, oral cavity
  - chest wall — *see* Puncture, thorax
  - chin — *see* Puncture, head, specified site NEC
  - clitoris — *see* Puncture, vulva
  - costal region — *see* Puncture, thorax
  - digit (s)
    - hand — *see* Puncture, finger
    - foot — *see* Puncture, toe
  - ear (canal) (external) S01.339
    - with foreign body S01.349
    - left S01.332
      - with foreign body S01.342
    - right S01.331
      - with foreign body S01.341
    - drum S09.2-
  - elbow S51.039
    - with
      - foreign body S51.049
    - left S51.032
      - with
        - foreign body S51.042
    - right S51.031
      - with
        - foreign body S51.041
  - epididymis — *see* Puncture, testis
  - epigastric region — *see* Puncture, abdomen, wall, epigastric
  - epiglottis S11.83
    - with foreign body S11.84
  - esophagus
    - cervical S11.23
      - with foreign body S11.24
    - thoracic S27.818
  - eyeball S05.6-
    - with foreign body S05.5-
  - eyebrow — *see* Puncture, eyelid
  - eyelid S01.13-
    - with foreign body S01.14-
    - left S01.132
      - with foreign body S01.142
    - right S01.131
      - with foreign body S01.141
  - face NEC — *see* Puncture, head, specified site NEC
  - finger (s) S61.239
    - with
      - damage to nail S61.339
        - with
          - foreign body S61.349
      - foreign body S61.249
    - index S61.238
      - with
        - damage to nail S61.338
          - with
            - foreign body S61.348
        - foreign body S61.248
      - left S61.231
        - with
          - damage to nail S61.331
            - with
              - foreign body S61.341
          - foreign body S61.241
      - right S61.230
        - with
          - damage to nail S61.330
            - with
              - foreign body S61.340
          - foreign body S61.240
    - little S61.238
      - with
        - damage to nail S61.338
          - with
            - foreign body S61.348
        - foreign body S61.248
      - left S61.237
        - with
          - damage to nail S61.337
            - with
              - foreign body S61.347
          - foreign body S61.247
      - right S61.236
        - with
          - damage to nail S61.336
            - with
              - foreign body S61.346
          - foreign body S61.246
    - middle S61.238
      - with
        - damage to nail S61.338
          - with

- **Puncture** - *continued*
  - finger (s) - *continued*
    - middle - *continued*
      - with - *continued*
        - damage to nail - *continued*
          - with - *continued*
            - foreign body S61.348
        - foreign body S61.248
      - left S61.233
        - with
          - damage to nail S61.333
            - with
              - foreign body S61.343
          - foreign body S61.243
      - right S61.232
        - with
          - damage to nail S61.332
            - with
              - foreign body S61.342
          - foreign body S61.242
    - ring S61.238
      - with
        - damage to nail S61.338
          - with
            - foreign body S61.348
        - foreign body S61.248
      - left S61.235
        - with
          - damage to nail S61.335
            - with
              - foreign body S61.345
          - foreign body S61.245
      - right S61.234
        - with
          - damage to nail S61.334
            - with
              - foreign body S61.344
          - foreign body S61.244
  - flank S31.139
    - with foreign body S31.149
  - foot (except toe (s) alone) S91.339
    - with foreign body S91.349
    - left S91.332
      - with foreign body S91.342
    - right S91.331
      - with foreign body S91.341
    - toe — *see* Puncture, toe
  - forearm S51.839
    - with
      - foreign body S51.849
    - elbow only — *see* Puncture, elbow
    - left S51.832
      - with
        - foreign body S51.842
    - right S51.831
      - with
        - foreign body S51.841
  - forehead — *see* Puncture, head, specified site NEC
  - genital organs, external
    - female S31.532
      - with foreign body S31.542
      - vagina — *see* Puncture, vagina
      - vulva — *see* Puncture, vulva
    - male S31.531
      - with foreign body S31.541
      - penis — *see* Puncture, penis
      - scrotum — *see* Puncture, scrotum
      - testis — *see* Puncture, testis
  - groin — *see* Puncture, abdomen, wall
  - gum — *see* Puncture, oral cavity
  - hand S61.439
    - with
      - foreign body S61.449
    - finger — *see* Puncture, finger
    - left S61.432
      - with
        - foreign body S61.442
    - right S61.431
      - with
        - foreign body S61.441
    - thumb — *see* Puncture, thumb
  - head S01.93
    - with foreign body S01.94
    - cheek — *see* Puncture, cheek
    - ear — *see* Puncture, ear
    - eyelid — *see* Puncture, eyelid
    - lip — *see* Puncture, oral cavity
    - nose — *see* Puncture, nose
    - oral cavity — *see* Puncture, oral cavity
    - scalp S01.03
      - with foreign body S01.04
    - specified site NEC S01.83
      - with foreign body S01.84

Puncture - *continued*
head - *continued*
temporomandibular area — *see* Puncture, cheek
heart S26.99
with hemopericardium S26.09
without hemopericardium S26.19
heel — *see* Puncture, foot
hip S71.039
with foreign body S71.049
left S71.032
with foreign body S71.042
right S71.031
with foreign body S71.041
hymen — *see* Puncture, vagina
hypochondrium — *see* Puncture, abdomen, wall
hypogastric region — *see* Puncture, abdomen, wall
inguinal region — *see* Puncture, abdomen, wall
instep — *see* Puncture, foot
internal organs — *see* Injury, by site
interscapular region — *see* Puncture, thorax, back
intestine
large
colon S36.599
ascending S36.590
descending S36.592
sigmoid S36.593
specified site NEC S36.598
transverse S36.591
rectum S36.69
small S36.499
duodenum S36.490
specified site NEC S36.498
intra-abdominal organ S36.99
gallbladder S36.128
intestine — *see* Puncture, intestine
liver S36.118
pancreas — *see* Puncture, pancreas
peritoneum S36.81
specified site NEC S36.898
spleen S36.09
stomach S36.39
jaw — *see* Puncture, head, specified site NEC
knee S81.039
with foreign body S81.049
left S81.032
with foreign body S81.042
right S81.031
with foreign body S81.041
labium (majus) (minus) — *see* Puncture, vulva
lacrimal duct — *see* Puncture, eyelid
larynx S11.013
with foreign body S11.014
leg (lower) S81.839
with foreign body S81.849
foot — *see* Puncture, foot
knee — *see* Puncture, knee
left S81.832
with foreign body S81.842
right S81.831
with foreign body S81.841
upper — *see* Puncture, thigh
lip S01.531
with foreign body S01.541
loin — *see* Puncture, abdomen, wall
lower back — *see* Puncture, back, lower
lumbar region — *see* Puncture, back, lower
malar region — *see* Puncture, head, specified site NEC
mammary — *see* Puncture, breast
mastoid region — *see* Puncture, head, specified site NEC
mouth — *see* Puncture, oral cavity
nail
finger — *see* Puncture, finger, with damage to nail
toe — *see* Puncture, toe, with damage to nail
nasal (septum) (sinus) — *see* Puncture, nose
nasopharynx — *see* Puncture, head, specified site NEC
neck S11.93
with foreign body S11.94
involving
cervical esophagus — *see* Puncture, cervical esophagus
larynx — *see* Puncture, larynx
pharynx — *see* Puncture, pharynx
thyroid gland — *see* Puncture, thyroid gland
trachea — *see* Puncture, trachea
specified site NEC S11.83
with foreign body S11.84
nose (septum) (sinus) S01.23
with foreign body S01.24
ocular — *see* Puncture, eyeball
oral cavity S01.532

Puncture - *continued*
oral cavity - *continued*
with foreign body S01.542
orbit S05.4-
palate — *see* Puncture, oral cavity
palm — *see* Puncture, hand
pancreas S36.299
body S36.291
head S36.290
tail S36.292
pelvis — *see* Puncture, back, lower
penis S31.23
with foreign body S31.24
perineum
female S31.43
with foreign body S31.44
male S31.139
with foreign body S31.149
periocular area (with or without lacrimal passages) — *see* Puncture, eyelid
phalanges
finger — *see* Puncture, finger
toe — *see* Puncture, toe
pharynx S11.23
with foreign body S11.24
pinna — *see* Puncture, ear
popliteal space — *see* Puncture, knee
prepuce — *see* Puncture, penis
pubic region S31.139
with foreign body S31.149
pudendum — *see* Puncture, genital organs, external
rectovaginal septum — *see* Puncture, vagina
sacral region — *see* Puncture, back, lower
sacroiliac region — *see* Puncture, back, lower
salivary gland — *see* Puncture, oral cavity
scalp S01.03
with foreign body S01.04
scapular region — *see* Puncture, shoulder
scrotum S31.33
with foreign body S31.34
shin — *see* Puncture, leg
shoulder S41.039
with foreign body S41.049
left S41.032
with foreign body S41.042
right S41.031
with foreign body S41.041
spermatic cord — *see* Puncture, testis
sternal region — *see* Puncture, thorax, front
submaxillary region — *see* Puncture, head, specified site NEC
submental region — *see* Puncture, head, specified site NEC
subungual
finger (s) — *see* Puncture, finger, with damage to nail
toe — *see* Puncture, toe, with damage to nail
supraclavicular fossa — *see* Puncture, neck, specified site NEC
temple, temporal region — *see* Puncture, head, specified site NEC
temporomandibular area — *see* Puncture, cheek
testis S31.33
with foreign body S31.34
thigh S71.139
with foreign body S71.149
left S71.132
with foreign body S71.142
right S71.131
with foreign body S71.141
thorax, thoracic (wall) S21.93
with foreign body S21.94
back S21.23-
with
foreign body S21.24-
with penetration S21.44
penetration S21.43
breast — *see* Puncture, breast
front S21.13-
with
foreign body S21.14-
with penetration S21.34
penetration S21.33
throat — *see* Puncture, neck
thumb S61.039
with
damage to nail S61.139
with
foreign body S61.149
foreign body S61.049
left S61.032
with
damage to nail S61.132

Puncture - *continued*
thumb - *continued*
left - *continued*
with - *continued*
damage to nail - *continued*
with
foreign body S61.142
foreign body S61.042
right S61.031
with
damage to nail S61.131
with
foreign body S61.141
foreign body S61.041
thyroid gland S11.13
with foreign body S11.14
toe (s) S91.139
with
damage to nail S91.239
with
foreign body S91.249
foreign body S91.149
great S91.133
with
damage to nail S91.233
with
foreign body S91.243
foreign body S91.143
left S91.132
with
damage to nail S91.232
with
foreign body S91.242
foreign body S91.142
right S91.131
with
damage to nail S91.231
with
foreign body S91.241
foreign body S91.141
lesser S91.136
with
damage to nail S91.236
with
foreign body S91.246
foreign body S91.146
left S91.135
with
damage to nail S91.235
with
foreign body S91.245
foreign body S91.145
right S91.134
with
damage to nail S91.234
with
foreign body S91.244
foreign body S91.144
tongue — *see* Puncture, oral cavity
trachea S11.023
with foreign body S11.024
tunica vaginalis — *see* Puncture, testis
tympanum, tympanic membrane S09.2-
umbilical region S31.135
with foreign body S31.145
uvula — *see* Puncture, oral cavity
vagina S31.43
with foreign body S31.44
vocal cords S11.033
with foreign body S11.034
vulva S31.43
with foreign body S31.44
wrist S61.539
with
foreign body S61.549
left S61.532
with
foreign body S61.542
right S61.531
with
foreign body S61.541
PUO (pyrexia of unknown origin) R50.9
Pupillary membrane (persistent) Q13.89
Pupillotonia — *see* Anomaly, pupil, function, tonic pupil
Purpura D69.2
abdominal D69.0
allergic D69.0
anaphylactoid D69.0
annularis telangiectodes L81.7
arthritic D69.0
autoerythrocyte sensitization D69.2
autoimmune D69.0

- **Radiculomyelitis** — *see also* Encephalitis
  - toxic, due to
    - Clostridium tetani A35
    - Corynebacterium diphtheriae A36.82
- **Radiculopathy** M54.10
  - cervical region M54.12
  - cervicothoracic region M54.13
  - due to
    - disc disorder
      - C3 M50.11
      - C4 M50.11
      - C5 M50.121
      - C6 M50.122
      - C7 M50.123
      - C8 M50.13
    - displacement of intervertebral disc — *see* Disorder, disc, with, radiculopathy
  - leg M54.1-
  - lumbar region M54.16
  - lumbosacral region M54.17
  - occipito-atlanto-axial region M54.11
  - postherpetic B02.29
  - sacrococcygeal region M54.18
  - syphilitic A52.11
  - thoracic region (with visceral pain) M54.14
  - thoracolumbar region M54.15
- **Radiodermal burns** (acute, chronic, or occupational) — *see* Burn
- **Radiodermatitis** L58.9
  - acute L58.0
  - chronic L58.1
- **Radiotherapy session** Z51.0
- **RAEB** (refractory anemia with excess blasts) D46.2-
- **Rage, meaning rabies** — *see* Rabies
- **Ragpicker's disease** A22.1
- **Ragsorter's disease** A22.1
- **Raillietiniasis** B71.8
- **Railroad neurosis** F48.8
- **Railway spine** F48.8
- **Raised** — *see also* Elevated
  - antibody titer R76.0
- **Rake teeth, tooth** M26.39
- **Rales** R09.89
- **Ramifying renal pelvis** Q63.8
- **Ramsay-Hunt disease or syndrome** — *see also* Hunt's disease B02.21
  - meaning dyssynergia cerebellaris myoclonica G11.1
- **Ranula** K11.6
  - congenital Q38.4
- **Rape**
  - adult
    - confirmed T74.21
    - suspected T76.21
  - alleged, observation or examination, ruled out
    - adult Z04.41
    - child Z04.42
  - child
    - confirmed T74.22
    - suspected T76.22
- **Rapid**
  - feeble pulse, due to shock, following injury T79.4
  - heart (beat) R00.0
    - psychogenic F45.8
  - second stage (delivery) O62.3
  - time-zone change syndrome G47.25
- **Rarefaction, bone** — *see* Disorder, bone, density and structure, specified NEC
- **Rash** (toxic) R21
  - canker A38.9
  - diaper L22
  - drug (internal use) L27.0
    - contact — *see also* Dermatitis, due to, drugs, external L25.1
  - following immunization T88.1
  - food — *see* Dermatitis, due to, food
  - heat L74.0
  - napkin (psoriasiform) L22
  - nettle — *see* Urticaria
  - pustular L08.0
  - rose R21
    - epidemic B06.9
  - scarlet A38.9
  - serum — *see also* Reaction, serum T80.69
  - wandering tongue K14.1
- **Rasmussen aneurysm** — *see* Tuberculosis, pulmonary
- **Rasmussen encephalitis** G04.81
- **Rat-bite fever** A25.9
  - due to Streptobacillus moniliformis A25.1
  - spirochetal (morsus muris) A25.0
- **Rathke's pouch tumor** D44.3
- **Raymond** (-Céstan) **syndrome** I65.8
- **Raynaud's disease, phenomenon or syndrome** (secondary) I73.00
  - with gangrene (symmetric) I73.01
- **RDS** (newborn) (type I) P22.0
  - type II P22.1
- **Reaction** — *see also* Disorder
  - adaptation — *see* Disorder, adjustment
  - adjustment (anxiety) (conduct disorder) (depressiveness) (distress) — *see* Disorder, adjustment
    - with
      - mutism, elective (child) (adolescent) F94.0
  - adverse
    - food (any) (ingested) NEC T78.1
      - anaphylactic — *see* Shock, anaphylactic, due to food
  - affective — *see* Disorder, mood
  - allergic — *see* Allergy
  - anaphylactic — *see* Shock, anaphylactic
  - anaphylactoid — *see* Shock, anaphylactic
  - anesthesia — *see* Anesthesia, complication
  - antitoxin (prophylactic) (therapeutic) — *see* Complications, vaccination
  - anxiety F41.1
  - Arthus — *see* Arthus' phenomenon
  - asthenic F48.8
  - combat and operational stress F43.0
  - compulsive F42.8
  - conversion F44.9
  - crisis, acute F43.0
  - deoxyribonuclease (DNA) (DNase) hypersensitivity D69.2
  - depressive (single episode) F32.9
    - affective (single episode) F31.4
      - recurrent episode F33.9
    - neurotic F34.1
    - psychoneurotic F34.1
    - psychotic F32.3
    - recurrent — *see* Disorder, depressive, recurrent
  - dissociative F44.9
  - drug NEC T88.7
    - addictive — *see* Dependence, drug
      - transmitted via placenta or breast milk — *see* Absorption, drug, addictive, through placenta
    - allergic — *see* Allergy, drug
    - lichenoid L43.2
    - newborn P93.8
      - gray baby syndrome P93.0
    - overdose or poisoning (by accident) — *see* Table of Drugs and Chemicals, by drug, poisoning
    - photoallergic L56.1
    - phototoxic L56.0
    - withdrawal — *see* Dependence, by drug, with, withdrawal
      - infant of dependent mother P96.1
      - newborn P96.1
    - wrong substance given or taken (by accident) — *see* Table of Drugs and Chemicals, by drug, poisoning
  - fear F40.9
    - child (abnormal) F93.8
  - febrile nonhemolytic transfusion (FNHTR) R50.84
  - fluid loss, cerebrospinal G97.1
  - foreign
    - body NEC — *see* Granuloma, foreign body
      - in operative wound (inadvertently left) — *see* Foreign body, accidentally left during a procedure
    - substance accidentally left during a procedure (chemical) (powder) (talc) T81.60
      - aseptic peritonitis T81.61
      - body or object (instrument) (sponge) (swab) — *see* Foreign body, accidentally left during a procedure
      - specified reaction NEC T81.69
  - grief — *see* Disorder, adjustment
  - Herxheimer's R68.89
  - hyperkinetic — *see* Hyperkinesia
  - hypochondriacal F45.20
  - hypoglycemic, due to insulin E16.0
    - with coma (diabetic) — *see* Diabetes, coma
      - nondiabetic E15
    - therapeutic misadventure — *see* subcategory T38.3
  - hypomanic F30.8
  - hysterical F44.9
  - immunization — *see* Complications, vaccination
  - incompatibility
    - ABO blood group (infusion) (transfusion) — *see* Complication(s), transfusion, incompatibility reaction, ABO
      - delayed serologic T80.39
    - minor blood group (Duffy) (E) (K) (Kell) (Kidd) (Lewis) (M) (N) (P) (S) T80.89

Reaction - *continued*

  - incompatibility - *continued*
    - Rh (factor) (infusion) (transfusion) — *see* Complication(s), transfusion, incompatibility reaction, Rh (factor)
  - inflammatory — *see* Infection
  - infusion — *see* Complications, infusion
  - inoculation (immune serum) — *see* Complications, vaccination
  - insulin T38.3-
  - involutional psychotic — *see* Disorder, depressive
  - leukemoid D72.823
    - basophilic D72.823
    - lymphocytic D72.823
    - monocytic D72.823
    - myelocytic D72.823
    - neutrophilic D72.823
  - LSD (acute)
    - due to drug abuse — *see* Abuse, drug, hallucinogen
    - due to drug dependence — *see* Dependence, drug, hallucinogen
  - lumbar puncture G97.1
  - manic-depressive — *see* Disorder, bipolar
  - neurasthenic F48.8
  - neurogenic — *see* Neurosis
  - neurotic F48.9
  - neurotic-depressive F34.1
  - nitritoid — *see* Crisis, nitritoid
  - nonspecific
    - to
      - cell mediated immunity measurement of gamma interferon antigen response without active tuberculosis R76.12
      - QuantiFERON-TB test (QFT) without active tuberculosis R76.12
      - tuberculin test — *see also* Reaction, tuberculin skin test R76.11
  - obsessive-compulsive F42.8
  - organic, acute or subacute — *see* Delirium
  - paranoid (acute) F23
    - chronic F22
    - senile F03
  - passive dependency F60.7
  - phobic F40.9
  - post-traumatic stress, uncomplicated Z73.3
  - psychogenic F99
  - psychoneurotic — *see also* Neurosis
    - compulsive F42.8
    - depersonalization F48.1
    - depressive F34.1
    - hypochondriacal F45.20
    - neurasthenic F48.8
    - obsessive F42.8
  - psychophysiologic — *see* Disorder, somatoform
  - psychosomatic — *see* Disorder, somatoform
  - psychotic — *see* Psychosis
  - scarlet fever toxin — *see* Complications, vaccination
  - schizophrenic F23
    - acute (brief) (undifferentiated) F23
    - latent F21
    - undifferentiated (acute) (brief) F23
  - serological for syphilis — *see* Serology for syphilis
  - serum T80.69
    - anaphylactic (immediate) — *see also* Shock, anaphylactic T80.59
    - specified reaction NEC
      - due to
        - administration of blood and blood products T80.61
        - immunization T80.62
        - serum specified NEC T80.69
        - vaccination T80.62
  - situational — *see* Disorder, adjustment
  - somatization — *see* Disorder, somatoform
  - spinal puncture G97.1
  - stress (severe) F43.9
    - acute (agitation) ("daze") (disorientation) (disturbance of consciousness) (flight reaction) (fugue) F43.0
    - specified NEC F43.8
  - surgical procedure — *see* Complications, surgical procedure
  - tetanus antitoxin — *see* Complications, vaccination
  - toxic, to local anesthesia T88.59
    - in labor and delivery O74.4
    - in pregnancy O29.3X-
    - postpartum, puerperal O89.3
  - toxin-antitoxin — *see* Complications, vaccination
  - transfusion (blood) (bone marrow) (lymphocytes) (allergic) — *see* Complications, transfusion
  - tuberculin skin test, abnormal R76.11
  - vaccination (any) — *see* Complications, vaccination

Reaction - *continued*
withdrawing, child or adolescent F93.8
Reactive airway disease — *see* Asthma
Reactive depression — *see* Reaction, depressive
Rearrangement
chromosomal
balanced (in) Q95.9
abnormal individual (autosomal) Q95.2
non-sex (autosomal) chromosomes Q95.2
sex/non-sex chromosomes Q95.3
specified NEC Q95.8
Recalcitrant patient — *see* Noncompliance
Recanalization, thrombus — *see* Thrombosis
Recession, receding
chamber angle (eye) H21.55-
chin M26.09
gingival (postinfective) (postoperative)
generalized K06.020
minimal K06.021
moderate K06.022
severe K06.023
localized K06.010
minimal K06.011
moderate K06.012
severe K06.013
Recklinghausen disease Q85.01
bones E21.0
Reclus' disease (cystic) — *see* Mastopathy, cystic
Recrudescent typhus (fever) A75.1
Recruitment, auditory H93.21-
Rectalgia K62.89
Rectitis K62.89
Rectocele
female (without uterine prolapse) N81.6
with uterine prolapse N81.4
incomplete N81.2
in pregnancy — *see* Pregnancy, complicated by, abnormal, pelvic organs or tissues NEC
male K62.3
Rectosigmoid junction — *see* condition
Rectosigmoiditis K63.89
ulcerative (chronic) K51.30
with
complication K51.319
abscess K51.314
fistula K51.313
obstruction K51.312
rectal bleeding K51.311
specified NEC K51.318
Rectourethral — *see* condition
Rectovaginal — *see* condition
Rectovesical — *see* condition
Rectum, rectal — *see* condition
Recurrent — *see* condition
pregnancy loss — *see* Loss (of), pregnancy, recurrent
Red bugs B88.0
Red tide — *see also* Table of Drugs and Chemicals T65.82-
Red-cedar lung or pneumonitis J67.8
Reduced
mobility Z74.09
ventilatory or vital capacity R94.2
Redundant, redundancy
anus (congenital) Q43.8
clitoris N90.89
colon (congenital) Q43.8
foreskin (congenital) N47.8
intestine (congenital) Q43.8
labia N90.69
organ or site, congenital NEC — *see* Accessory
panniculus (abdominal) E65
prepuce (congenital) N47.8
pylorus K31.89
rectum (congenital) Q43.8
scrotum N50.89
sigmoid (congenital) Q43.8
skin L98.7
and subcutaneous tissue L98.7
of face L57.4
eyelids — *see* Blepharochalasis
stomach K31.89
Reduplication — *see* Duplication
Reflex R29.2
hyperactive gag J39.2
pupillary, abnormal — *see* Anomaly, pupil, function
vasoconstriction I73.9
vasovagal R55
Reflux K21.9
acid K21.9
esophageal K21.9
with esophagitis K21.0
newborn P78.83

Reflux - *continued*
gastroesophageal K21.9
with esophagitis K21.0
mitral — *see* Insufficiency, mitral
ureteral — *see* Reflux, vesicoureteral
vesicoureteral (with scarring) N13.70
with
nephropathy N13.729
with hydroureter N13.739
bilateral N13.732
unilateral N13.731
bilateral N13.722
unilateral N13.721
without hydroureter N13.729
bilateral N13.722
unilateral N13.721
pyelonephritis (chronic) N11.0
congenital Q62.7
without nephropathy N13.71
Reforming, artificial openings — *see* Attention to, artificial, opening
Refractive error — *see* Disorder, refraction
Refsum's disease or syndrome G60.1
Refusal of
food, psychogenic F50.89
treatment (because of) Z53.20
left against medical advice (AMA) Z53.21
patient's decision NEC Z53.29
reasons of belief or group pressure Z53.1
Regional — *see* condition
Regurgitation R11.10
aortic (valve) — *see* Insufficiency, aortic
food — *see also* Vomiting
with reswallowing — *see* Rumination
newborn P92.1
gastric contents — *see* Vomiting
heart — *see* Endocarditis
mitral (valve) — *see* Insufficiency, mitral
congenital Q23.3
myocardial — *see* Endocarditis
pulmonary (valve) (heart) I37.1
congenital Q22.2
syphilitic A52.03
tricuspid — *see* Insufficiency, tricuspid
valve, valvular — *see* Endocarditis
congenital Q24.8
vesicoureteral — *see* Reflux, vesicoureteral
Reichmann's disease or syndrome K31.89
Reifenstein syndrome E34.52
Reinsertion
implantable subdermal contraceptive Z30.46
intrauterine contraceptive device Z30.433
Reiter's disease, syndrome, or urethritis M02.30
ankle M02.37-
elbow M02.32-
foot joint M02.37-
hand joint M02.34-
hip M02.35-
knee M02.36-
multiple site M02.39
shoulder M02.31-
vertebra M02.38
wrist M02.33-
Rejection
food, psychogenic F50.89
transplant T86.91
bone T86.830
marrow T86.01
cornea T86.840
heart T86.21
with lung (s) T86.31
intestine T86.850
kidney T86.11
liver T86.41
lung (s) T86.810
with heart T86.31
organ (immune or nonimmune cause) T86.91
pancreas T86.890
skin (allograft) (autograft) T86.820
specified NEC T86.890
stem cell (peripheral blood) (umbilical cord) T86.5
Relapsing fever A68.9
Carter's (Asiatic) A68.1
Dutton's (West African) A68.1
Koch's A68.9
louse-borne (epidemic) A68.0
Novy's (American) A68.1
Obermeyers's (European) A68.0
Spirillum A68.9
tick-borne (endemic) A68.1
Relationship
occlusal
open anterior M26.220

Relationship - *continued*
occlusal - *continued*
open posterior M26.221
Relaxation
anus (sphincter) K62.89
psychogenic F45.8
arch (foot) — *see also* Deformity, limb, flat foot
back ligaments — *see* Instability, joint, spine
bladder (sphincter) N31.2
cardioesophageal K21.9
cervix — *see* Incompetency, cervix
diaphragm J98.6
joint (capsule) (ligament) (paralytic) — *see* Flail, joint
congenital NEC Q74.8
lumbosacral (joint) — *see* subcategory M53.2
pelvic floor N81.89
perineum N81.89
posture R29.3
rectum (sphincter) K62.89
sacroiliac (joint) — *see* subcategory M53.2
scrotum N50.89
urethra (sphincter) N36.44
vesical N31.2
Release from prison, anxiety concerning Z65.2
Remains
canal of Cloquet Q14.0
capsule (opaque) Q14.8
Remittent fever (malarial) B54
Remnant
canal of Cloquet Q14.0
capsule (opaque) Q14.8
cervix, cervical stump (acquired) (postoperative) N88.8
cystic duct, postcholecystectomy K91.5
fingernail L60.8
congenital Q84.6
meniscus, knee — *see* Derangement, knee, meniscus, specified NEC
thyroglossal duct Q89.2
tonsil J35.8
infected (chronic) J35.01
urachus Q64.4
Removal (from) (of)
artificial
arm Z44.00-
complete Z44.01-
partial Z44.02-
eye Z44.2-
leg Z44.10-
complete Z44.11-
partial Z44.12-
breast implant Z45.81
cardiac pulse generator (battery) (end-of-life) Z45.010
catheter (urinary) (indwelling) Z46.6
from artificial opening — *see* Attention to, artificial, opening
non-vascular Z46.82
vascular NEC Z45.2
drains Z48.03
device Z46.9
contraceptive Z30.432
implantable subdermal Z30.46
implanted NEC Z45.89
specified NEC Z46.89
dressing (nonsurgical) Z48.00
surgical Z48.01
external
fixation device - code to fracture with seventh character D
prosthesis, prosthetic device Z44.9
breast Z44.3-
specified NEC Z44.8
home in childhood (to foster home or institution) Z62.29
ileostomy Z43.2
insulin pump Z46.81
myringotomy device (stent) (tube) Z45.82
nervous system device NEC Z46.2
brain neuropacemaker Z46.2
visual substitution device Z46.2
implanted Z45.31
non-vascular catheter Z46.82
orthodontic device Z46.4
organ, prophylactic (for neoplasia management) — *see* Prophylactic, organ removal
staples Z48.02
stent
ureteral Z46.6
suture Z48.02
urinary device Z46.6
vascular access device or catheter Z45.2

Ren
  arcuatus Q63.1
  mobile, mobilis N28.89
    congenital Q63.8
  unguliformis Q63.1
Renal — *see* condition
Rendu-Osler-Weber disease or syndrome I78.0
Reninoma D41.0-
Renon-Delille syndrome E23.3
Reovirus, as cause of disease classified elsewhere B97.5
Repeated falls NEC R29.6
Replaced chromosome by dicentric ring Q93.2
Replacement by artificial or mechanical device or prosthesis of
  bladder Z96.0
  blood vessel NEC Z95.828
  bone NEC Z96.7
  cochlea Z96.21
  coronary artery Z95.5
  eustachian tube Z96.29
  eye globe Z97.0
  heart Z95.812
    valve Z95.2
      prosthetic Z95.2
      specified NEC Z95.4
      xenogenic Z95.3
  intestine Z96.89
  joint Z96.60
    hip — *see* Presence, hip joint implant
    knee — *see* Presence, knee joint implant
    specified site NEC Z96.698
  larynx Z96.3
  lens Z96.1
  limb (s) — *see* Presence, artificial, limb
  mandible NEC (for tooth root implant (s)) Z96.5
  organ NEC Z96.89
  peripheral vessel NEC Z95.828
  stapes Z96.29
  teeth Z97.2
  tendon Z96.7
  tissue NEC Z96.89
  tooth root (s) Z96.5
  vessel NEC Z95.828
    coronary (artery) Z95.5
Request for expert evidence Z04.89
Reserve, decreased or low
  cardiac — *see* Disease, heart
  kidney N28.89
Residual — *see also* condition
  ovary syndrome N99.83
  state, schizophrenic F20.5
  urine R39.198
Resistance, resistant (to)
  activated protein C D68.51
  complicating pregnancy O26.89
  insulin E88.81
  organism (s)
    to
      drug Z16.30
        aminoglycosides Z16.29
        amoxicillin Z16.11
        ampicillin Z16.11
        antibiotic (s) Z16.20
          multiple Z16.24
          specified NEC Z16.29
        antifungal Z16.32
        antimicrobial (single) Z16.30
          multiple Z16.35
          specified NEC Z16.39
        antimycobacterial (single) Z16.341
          multiple Z16.342
        antiparasitic Z16.31
        antiviral Z16.33
        beta lactam antibiotics Z16.10
          specified NEC Z16.19
        cephalosporins Z16.19
        extended beta lactamase (ESBL) Z16.12
        fluoroquinolones Z16.23
        macrolides Z16.29
        methicillin — *see* MRSA
        multiple drugs (MDRO)
          antibiotics Z16.24
          antimicrobial Z16.35
          antimycobacterials Z16.342
        penicillins Z16.11
        quinine (and related compounds) Z16.31
        quinolones Z16.23
        sulfonamides Z16.29
        tetracyclines Z16.29
        tuberculostatics (single) Z16.341
          multiple Z16.342
        vancomycin Z16.21

Resistance, resistant (to) - *continued*
  organism (s) - *continued*
    to - *continued*
      drug - *continued*
        vancomycin - *continued*
          related antibiotics Z16.22
  thyroid hormone E07.89
Resorption
  dental (roots) K03.3
    alveoli M26.79
  teeth (external) (internal) (pathological) (roots) K03.3
Respiration
  Cheyne-Stokes R06.3
  decreased due to shock, following injury T79.4
  disorder of, psychogenic F45.8
  insufficient, or poor R06.89
    newborn P28.5
  painful R07.1
  sighing, psychogenic F45.8
Respiratory — *see also* condition
  distress syndrome (newborn) (type I) P22.0
    type II P22.1
  syncytial virus, as cause of disease classified elsewhere B97.4
Respite care Z75.5
Response (drug)
  photoallergic L56.1
  phototoxic L56.0
Restenosis
  stent
    vascular
      end stent
        adjacent to stent — *see* Arteriosclerosis
        within the stent
          coronary T82.855
          peripheral T82.856
      in stent
        coronary vessel T82.855
        peripheral vessel T82.856
Restless legs (syndrome) G25.81
Restlessness R45.1
Restoration (of)
  dental
    aesthetically inadequate or displeasing K08.56
    defective K08.50
      specified NEC K08.59
    failure of marginal integrity K08.51
    failure of periodontal anatomical intergrity K08.54
  organ continuity from previous sterilization (tuboplasty) (vasoplasty) Z31.0
    aftercare Z31.42
  tooth (existing)
    contours biologically incompatible with oral health K08.54
    open margins K08.51
    overhanging K08.52
    poor aesthetic K08.56
    poor gingival margins K08.51
  unsatisfactory, of tooth K08.50
    specified NEC K08.59
Restorative material (dental)
  allergy to K08.55
  fractured K08.539
    with loss of material K08.531
    without loss of material K08.530
  unrepairable overhanging of K08.52
Restriction of housing space Z59.1
Rests, ovarian, in fallopian tube Q50.6
Restzustand (schizophrenic) F20.5
Retained — *see also* Retention
  cholelithiasis following cholecystectomy K91.86
  foreign body fragments (type of) Z18.9
    acrylics Z18.2
    animal quill (s) or spines Z18.31
    cement Z18.83
    concrete Z18.83
    crystalline Z18.83
    depleted isotope Z18.09
    depleted uranium Z18.01
    diethylhexyl phthalates Z18.2
    glass Z18.81
    isocyanate Z18.2
    magnetic metal Z18.11
    metal Z18.10
    nonmagnectic metal Z18.12
    nontherapeutic radioactive Z18.09
    organic NEC Z18.39
    plastic Z18.2
    quill (s) (animal) Z18.31
    radioactive (nontherapeutic) NEC Z18.09
    specified NEC Z18.89
    spine (s) (animal) Z18.31

Retained - *continued*
  foreign body fragments (type of) - *continued*
    stone Z18.83
    tooth (teeth) Z18.32
    wood Z18.33
  fragments (type of) Z18.9
    acrylics Z18.2
    animal quill (s) or spines Z18.31
    cement Z18.83
    concrete Z18.83
    crystalline Z18.83
    depleted isotope Z18.09
    depleted uranium Z18.01
    diethylhexyl phthalates Z18.2
    glass Z18.81
    isocyanate Z18.2
    magnetic metal Z18.11
    metal Z18.10
    nonmagnectic metal Z18.12
    nontherapeutic radioactive Z18.09
    organic NEC Z18.39
    plastic Z18.2
    quill (s) (animal) Z18.31
    radioactive (nontherapeutic) NEC Z18.09
    specified NEC Z18.89
    spine (s) (animal) Z18.31
    stone Z18.83
    tooth (teeth) Z18.32
    wood Z18.33
  gallstones, following cholecystectomy K91.86
Retardation
  development, developmental, specific — *see* Disorder, developmental
  endochondral bone growth — *see* Disorder, bone, development or growth
  growth R62.50
    due to malnutrition E45
  mental — *see* Disability, intellectual
  motor function, specific F82
  physical (child) R62.52
    due to malnutrition E45
  reading (specific) F81.0
  spelling (specific) (without reading disorder) F81.81
Retching — *see* Vomiting
Retention — *see also* Retained
  bladder — *see* Retention, urine
  carbon dioxide E87.2
  cholelithiasis following cholecystectomy K91.86
  cyst — *see* Cyst
  dead
    fetus (at or near term) (mother) O36.4
      early fetal death O02.1
    ovum O02.0
  decidua (fragments) (following delivery) (with hemorrhage) O72.2
    without hemorrhage O73.1
  deciduous tooth K00.6
  dental root K08.3
  fecal — *see* Constipation
  fetus
    dead O36.4
      early O02.1
  fluid R60.9
  foreign body — *see also* Foreign body, retained
    current trauma - code as Foreign body, by site or type
  gallstones, following cholecystectomy K91.86
  gastric K31.89
  intrauterine contraceptive device, in pregnancy — *see* Pregnancy, complicated by, retention, intrauterine device
  membranes (complicating delivery) (with hemorrhage) O72.2
    with abortion — *see* Abortion, by type
    without hemorrhage O73.1
  meniscus — *see* Derangement, meniscus
  menses N94.89
  milk (puerperal, postpartum) O92.79
  nitrogen, extrarenal R39.2
  ovary syndrome N99.83
  placenta (total) (with hemorrhage) O72.0
    without hemorrhage O73.0
    portions or fragments (with hemorrhage) O72.2
      without hemorrhage O73.1
  products of conception
    early pregnancy (dead fetus) O02.1
    following
      delivery (with hemorrhage) O72.2
        without hemorrhage O73.1
  secundines (following delivery) (with hemorrhage) O72.0
    without hemorrhage O73.0

Rheumatoid - *continued*
myopathy - *continued*
shoulder M05.41-
vertebra — *see* Spondylitis, ankylosing
wrist M05.43-
pericarditis — *see* Rheumatoid, carditis
polyarthritis — *see* Arthritis, rheumatoid
polyneuropathy M05.50
ankle M05.57-
elbow M05.52-
foot joint M05.57-
hand joint M05.54-
hip M05.55-
knee M05.56-
multiple site M05.59
shoulder M05.51-
vertebra — *see* Spondylitis, ankylosing
wrist M05.53-
vasculitis M05.20
ankle M05.27-
elbow M05.22-
foot joint M05.27-
hand joint M05.24-
hip M05.25-
knee M05.26-
multiple site M05.29
shoulder M05.21-
vertebra — *see* Spondylitis, ankylosing
wrist M05.23-
Rhinitis (atrophic) (catarrhal) (chronic) (croupous) (fibrinous) (granulomatous) (hyperplastic) (hypertrophic) (membranous) (obstructive) (purulent) (suppurative) (ulcerative) J31.0
with
sore throat — *see* Nasopharyngitis
acute J00
allergic J30.9
with asthma J45.909
with
exacerbation (acute) J45.901
status asthmaticus J45.902
due to
food J30.5
pollen J30.1
nonseasonal J30.89
perennial J30.89
seasonal NEC J30.2
specified NEC J30.89
infective J00
pneumococcal J00
syphilitic A52.73
congenital A50.05 *[J99]*
tuberculous A15.8
vasomotor J30.0
Rhinoantritis (chronic) — *see* Sinusitis, maxillary
Rhinodacryolith — *see* Dacryolith
Rhinolith (nasal sinus) J34.89
Rhinomegaly J34.89
Rhinopharyngitis (acute) (subacute) — *see also* Nasopharyngitis
chronic J31.1
destructive ulcerating A66.5
mutilans A66.5
Rhinophyma L71.1
Rhinorrhea J34.89
cerebrospinal (fluid) G96.0
paroxysmal — *see* Rhinitis, allergic
spasmodic — *see* Rhinitis, allergic
Rhinosalpingitis — *see* Salpingitis, eustachian
Rhinoscleroma A48.8
Rhinosporidiosis B48.1
Rhinovirus infection NEC B34.8
Rhizomelic chondrodysplasia punctata E71.540
Rhythm
atrioventricular nodal I49.8
disorder I49.9
coronary sinus I49.8
ectopic I49.8
nodal I49.8
escape I49.9
heart, abnormal I49.9
idioventricular I44.2
nodal I49.8
sleep, inversion G47.2-
nonorganic origin — *see* Disorder, sleep, circadian rhythm, psychogenic
Rhytidosis facialis L98.8
Rib — *see also* condition
cervical Q76.5
Riboflavin deficiency E53.0
Rice bodies — *see also* Loose, body, joint
knee M23.4-
Richter syndrome — *see* Leukemia, chronic lymphocytic, B-cell type
Richter's hernia — *see* Hernia, abdomen, with obstruction
Ricinism — *see* Poisoning, food, noxious, plant
Rickets (active) (acute) (adolescent) (chest wall) (congenital) (current) (infantile) (intestinal) E55.0
adult — *see* Osteomalacia
celiac K90.0
hypophosphatemic with nephrotic-glycosuric dwarfism E72.09
inactive E64.3
kidney N25.0
renal N25.0
sequelae, any E64.3
vitamin-D-resistant E83.31 *[M90.80]*
Rickettsial disease A79.9
specified type NEC A79.89
Rickettsialpox (Rickettsia akari) A79.1
Rickettsiosis A79.9
due to
Ehrlichia sennetsu A79.81
Rickettsia akari (rickettsialpox) A79.1
specified type NEC A79.89
tick-borne A77.9
vesicular A79.1
Rider's bone — *see* Ossification, muscle, specified NEC
Ridge, alveolus — *see also* condition
flabby K06.8
Ridged ear, congenital Q17.3
Riedel's
lobe, liver Q44.7
struma, thyroiditis or disease E06.5
Rieger's anomaly or syndrome Q13.81
Riehl's melanosis L81.4
Rietti-Greppi-Micheli anemia D56.9
Rieux's hernia — *see* Hernia, abdomen, specified site NEC
Riga (-Fede) **disease** K14.0
Riggs' disease — *see* Periodontitis
Right aortic arch Q25.47
Right middle lobe syndrome J98.11
Rigid, rigidity — *see also* condition
abdominal R19.30
with severe abdominal pain R10.0
epigastric R19.36
generalized R19.37
left lower quadrant R19.34
left upper quadrant R19.32
periumbilic R19.35
right lower quadrant R19.33
right upper quadrant R19.31
articular, multiple, congenital Q68.8
cervix (uteri) in pregnancy — *see* Pregnancy, complicated by, abnormal, cervix
hymen (acquired) (congenital) N89.6
nuchal R29.1
pelvic floor in pregnancy — *see* Pregnancy, complicated by, abnormal, pelvic organs or tissues NEC
perineum or vulva in pregnancy — *see* Pregnancy, complicated by, abnormal, vulva
spine — *see* Dorsopathy, specified NEC
vagina in pregnancy — *see* Pregnancy, complicated by, abnormal, vagina
Rigors R68.89
with fever R50.9
Riley-Day syndrome G90.1
RIND (reversible ischemic neurologic deficit) I63.9
Ring (s)
aorta (vascular) Q25.45
Bandl's O62.4
contraction, complicating delivery O62.4
esophageal, lower (muscular) K22.2
Fleischer's (cornea) H18.04-
hymenal, tight (acquired) (congenital) N89.6
Kayser-Fleischer (cornea) H18.04-
retraction, uterus, pathological O62.4
Schatzki's (esophagus) (lower) K22.2
congenital Q39.3
Soemmerring's — *see* Cataract, secondary
vascular (congenital) Q25.8
aorta Q25.45
Ringed hair (congenital) Q84.1
Ringworm B35.9
beard B35.0
black dot B35.0
body B35.4
Burmese B35.5
corporeal B35.4
foot B35.3
groin B35.6
Ringworm - *continued*
hand B35.2
honeycomb B35.0
nails B35.1
perianal (area) B35.6
scalp B35.0
specified NEC B35.8
Tokelau B35.5
Rise, venous pressure I87.8
Rising, PSA following treatment for malignant neoplasm of prostate R97.21
Risk
for
dental caries Z91.849
high Z91.843
low Z91.841
moderate Z91.842
suicidal
meaning personal history of attempted suicide Z91.5
meaning suicidal ideation — *see* Ideation, suicidal
Ritter's disease L00
Rivalry, sibling Z62.891
Rivalta's disease A42.2
River blindness B73.01
Robert's pelvis Q74.2
with disproportion (fetopelvic) O33.0
causing obstructed labor O65.0
Robin (-Pierre) **syndrome** Q87.0
Robinow-Silvermann-Smith syndrome Q87.1
Robinson's (hidrotic)
ectodermal dysplasia or syndrome Q82.4
Robles' disease B73.01
Rocky Mountain (spotted) **fever** A77.0
Roetheln — *see* Rubella
Roger's disease Q21.0
Rokitansky-Aschoff sinuses (gallbladder) K82.8
Rolando's fracture (displaced) S62.22-
nondisplaced S62.22-
Romano-Ward (prolonged QT interval) **syndrome** I45.81
Romberg's disease or syndrome G51.8
Roof, mouth — *see* condition
Rosacea L71.9
acne L71.9
keratitis L71.8
specified NEC L71.8
Rosary, rachitic E55.0
Rose
cold J30.1
fever J30.1
rash R21
epidemic B06.9
Rosenbach's erysipeloid A26.0
Rosenthal's disease or syndrome D68.1
Roseola B09
infantum B08.20
due to human herpesvirus 6 B08.21
due to human herpesvirus 7 B08.22
Ross River disease or fever B33.1
Rossbach's disease K31.89
psychogenic F45.8
Rostan's asthma (cardiac) — *see* Failure, ventricular, left
Rotation
anomalous, incomplete or insufficient, intestine Q43.3
cecum (congenital) Q43.3
colon (congenital) Q43.3
spine, incomplete or insufficient — *see* Dorsopathy, deforming, specified NEC
tooth, teeth, fully erupted M26.35
vertebra, incomplete or insufficient — *see* Dorsopathy, deforming, specified NEC
Rotes Quérol disease or syndrome — *see* Hyperostosis, ankylosing
Roth (-Bernhardt) **disease or syndrome** — *see* Meralgia paraesthetica
Rothmund (-Thomson) **syndrome** Q82.8
Rotor's disease or syndrome E80.6
Round
back (with wedging of vertebrae) — *see* Kyphosis
sequelae (late effect) of rickets E64.3
worms (large) (infestation) NEC B82.0
Ascariasis — *see also* Ascariasis B77.9
Roussy-Lévy syndrome G60.0
Rubella (German measles) B06.9
complication NEC B06.09
neurological B06.00
congenital P35.0
contact Z20.4
exposure to Z20.4
maternal

Rubella (German measles) - *continued*
maternal - *continued*
manifest rubella in infant P35.0
care for (suspected) damage to fetus O35.3
suspected damage to fetus affecting management of pregnancy O35.3
specified complications NEC B06.89
Rubeola (meaning measles) — *see* Measles
meaning rubella — *see* Rubella
Rubeosis, iris — *see* Disorder, iris, vascular
Rubinstein-Taybi syndrome Q87.2
Rudimentary (congenital) — *see also* Agenesis
arm — *see* Defect, reduction, upper limb
bone Q79.9
cervix uteri Q51.828
eye Q11.2
lobule of ear Q17.3
patella Q74.1
respiratory organs in thoracopagus Q89.4
tracheal bronchus Q32.4
uterus Q51.818
in male Q56.1
vagina Q52.0
Ruled out condition — *see* Observation, suspected
Rumination R11.10
with nausea R11.2
disorder of infancy F98.21
neurotic F42.8
newborn P92.1
obsessional F42.8
psychogenic F42.8
Runeberg's disease D51.0
Runny nose R09.89
Rupia (syphilitic) A51.39
congenital A50.06
tertiary A52.79
Rupture, ruptured
abscess (spontaneous) - code by site under Abscess
aneurysm — *see* Aneurysm
anus (sphincter) — *see* Laceration, anus
aorta, aortic I71.8
abdominal I71.3
arch I71.1
ascending I71.1
descending I71.8
abdominal I71.3
thoracic I71.1
syphilitic A52.01
thoracoabdominal I71.5
thorax, thoracic I71.1
transverse I71.1
traumatic — *see* Injury, aorta, laceration, major
valve or cusp — *see also* Endocarditis, aortic I35.8
appendix (with peritonitis) — *see also* Appendicitis K35.32
with localized peritonitis — *see also* Appendicitis K35.32
arteriovenous fistula, brain I60.8
artery I77.2
brain — *see* Hemorrhage, intracranial, intracerebral
coronary — *see* Infarct, myocardium
heart — *see* Infarct, myocardium
pulmonary I28.8
traumatic (complication) — *see* Injury, blood vessel
bile duct (common) (hepatic) K83.2
cystic K82.2
bladder (sphincter) (nontraumatic) (spontaneous) N32.89
following ectopic or molar pregnancy O08.6
obstetrical trauma O71.5
traumatic S37.29
blood vessel — *see also* Hemorrhage
brain — *see* Hemorrhage, intracranial, intracerebral
heart — *see* Infarct, myocardium
traumatic (complication) — *see* Injury, blood vessel, laceration, major, by site
bone — *see* Fracture
bowel (nontraumatic) K63.1
brain
aneurysm (congenital) — *see also* Hemorrhage, intracranial, subarachnoid
syphilitic A52.05
hemorrhagic — *see* Hemorrhage, intracranial, intracerebral
capillaries I78.8
cardiac (auricle) (ventricle) (wall) I23.3
with hemopericardium I23.0
infectional I40.9
traumatic — *see* Injury, heart
cartilage (articular) (current) — *see also* Sprain

Rupture, ruptured - *continued*
cartilage (articular) (current) - *continued*
knee S83.3-
semilunar — *see* Tear, meniscus
cecum (with peritonitis) K65.0
with peritoneal abscess K35.33
traumatic S36.598
celiac artery, traumatic — *see* Injury, blood vessel, celiac artery, laceration, major
cerebral aneurysm (congenital) (see Hemorrhage, intracranial, subarachnoid)
cervix (uteri)
with ectopic or molar pregnancy O08.6
following ectopic or molar pregnancy O08.6
obstetrical trauma O71.3
traumatic S37.69
chordae tendineae NEC I51.1
concurrent with acute myocardial infarction — *see* Infarct, myocardium
following acute myocardial infarction (current complication) I23.4
choroid (direct) (indirect) (traumatic) H31.32-
circle of Willis I60.6
colon (nontraumatic) K63.1
traumatic — *see* Injury, intestine, large
cornea (traumatic) — *see* Injury, eye, laceration
coronary (artery) (thrombotic) — *see* Infarct, myocardium
corpus luteum (infected) (ovary) N83.1-
cyst — *see* Cyst
cystic duct K82.2
Descemet's membrane — *see* Change, corneal membrane, Descemet's, rupture
traumatic — *see* Injury, eye, laceration
diaphragm, traumatic — *see* Injury, intrathoracic, diaphragm
disc — *see* Rupture, intervertebral disc
diverticulum (intestine) K57.80
with bleeding K57.81
bladder N32.3
large intestine K57.20
with
bleeding K57.21
small intestine K57.40
with bleeding K57.41
small intestine K57.00
with
bleeding K57.01
large intestine K57.40
with bleeding K57.41
duodenal stump K31.89
ear drum (nontraumatic) — *see also* Perforation, tympanum
traumatic S09.2-
due to blast injury — *see* Injury, blast, ear
esophagus K22.3
eye (without prolapse or loss of intraocular tissue) — *see* Injury, eye, laceration
fallopian tube NEC (nonobstetric) (nontraumatic) N83.8
due to pregnancy O00.10-
with intrauterine pregnancy O00.11-
fontanel P13.1
gallbladder K82.2
traumatic S36.128
gastric — *see also* Rupture, stomach
vessel K92.2
globe (eye) (traumatic) — *see* Injury, eye, laceration
graafian follicle (hematoma) N83.0-
heart — *see* Rupture, cardiac
hymen (nontraumatic) (nonintentional) N89.8
internal organ, traumatic — *see* Injury, by site
intervertebral disc — *see* Displacement, intervertebral disc
traumatic — *see* Rupture, traumatic, intervertebral disc
intestine NEC (nontraumatic) K63.1
traumatic — *see* Injury, intestine
iris — *see also* Abnormality, pupillary
traumatic — *see* Injury, eye, laceration
joint capsule, traumatic — *see* Sprain
kidney (traumatic) S37.06-
birth injury P15.8
nontraumatic N28.89
lacrimal duct (traumatic) — *see* Injury, eye, specified site NEC
lens (cataract) (traumatic) — *see* Cataract, traumatic
ligament, traumatic — *see* Rupture, traumatic, ligament, by site
liver S36.116
birth injury P15.0
lymphatic vessel I89.8

Rupture, ruptured - *continued*
marginal sinus (placental) (with hemorrhage) — *see* Hemorrhage, antepartum, specified cause NEC
membrana tympani (nontraumatic) — *see* Perforation, tympanum
membranes (spontaneous)
artificial
delayed delivery following O75.5
delayed delivery following — *see* Pregnancy, complicated by, premature rupture of membranes
meningeal artery I60.8
meniscus (knee) — *see also* Tear, meniscus
old — *see* Derangement, meniscus
site other than knee - code as Sprain
mesenteric artery, traumatic — *see* Injury, mesenteric, artery, laceration, major
mesentery (nontraumatic) K66.8
traumatic — *see* Injury, intra-abdominal, specified, site NEC
mitral (valve) I34.8
muscle (traumatic) — *see also* Strain
diastasis — *see* Diastasis, muscle
nontraumatic M62.10
ankle M62.17-
foot M62.17-
forearm M62.13-
hand M62.14-
lower leg M62.16-
pelvic region M62.15-
shoulder region M62.11-
specified site NEC M62.18
thigh M62.15-
upper arm M62.12-
traumatic — *see* Strain, by site
musculotendinous junction NEC, nontraumatic — *see* Rupture, tendon, spontaneous
mycotic aneurysm causing cerebral hemorrhage — *see* Hemorrhage, intracranial, subarachnoid
myocardium, myocardial — *see* Rupture, cardiac
traumatic — *see* Injury, heart
nontraumatic, meaning hernia — *see* Hernia
obstructed — *see* Hernia, by site, obstructed
operation wound — *see* Disruption, wound, operation
ovary, ovarian N83.8
corpus luteum cyst N83.1-
follicle (graafian) N83.0-
oviduct (nonobstetric) (nontraumatic) N83.8
due to pregnancy O00.10-
with intrauterine pregnancy O00.11-
pancreas (nontraumatic) K86.89
traumatic S36.299
papillary muscle NEC I51.2
following acute myocardial infarction (current complication) I23.5
pelvic
floor, complicating delivery O70.1
organ NEC, obstetrical trauma O71.5
perineum (nonobstetric) (nontraumatic) N90.89
complicating delivery — *see* Delivery, complicated, by, laceration, anus (sphincter)
postoperative wound — *see* Disruption, wound, operation
prostate (traumatic) S37.828
pulmonary
artery I28.8
valve (heart) I37.8
vein I28.8
vessel I28.8
pus tube — *see* Salpingitis
pyosalpinx — *see* Salpingitis
rectum (nontraumatic) K63.1
traumatic S36.69
retina, retinal (traumatic) (without detachment) — *see also* Break, retina
with detachment — *see* Detachment, retina, with retinal, break
rotator cuff (nontraumatic) M75.10-
complete M75.12-
incomplete M75.11-
sclera — *see* Injury, eye, laceration
sigmoid (nontraumatic) K63.1
traumatic S36.593
spinal cord — *see also* Injury, spinal cord, by region
due to injury at birth P11.5
newborn (birth injury) P11.5
spleen (traumatic) S36.09
birth injury P15.1
congenital (birth injury) P15.1
due to P. vivax malaria B51.0
nontraumatic D73.5
spontaneous D73.5

Rupture, ruptured - *continued*
splenic vein R58
traumatic — *see* Injury, blood vessel, splenic vein
stomach (nontraumatic) (spontaneous) K31.89
traumatic S36.39
supraspinatus (complete) (incomplete) (nontraumatic) — *see* Tear, rotator cuff
symphysis pubis
obstetric O71.6
traumatic S33.4
synovium (cyst) M66.10
ankle M66.17-
elbow M66.12-
finger M66.14-
foot M66.17-
forearm M66.13-
hand M66.14-
pelvic region M66.15-
shoulder region M66.11-
specified site NEC M66.18
thigh M66.15-
toe M66.17-
upper arm M66.12-
wrist M66.13-
tendon (traumatic) — *see* Strain
nontraumatic (spontaneous) M66.9
ankle M66.87-
extensor M66.20
ankle M66.27-
foot M66.27-
forearm M66.23-
hand M66.24-
lower leg M66.26-
multiple sites M66.29
pelvic region M66.25-
shoulder region M66.21-
specified site NEC M66.28
thigh M66.25-
upper arm M66.22-
flexor M66.30
ankle M66.37-
foot M66.37-
forearm M66.33-
hand M66.34-
lower leg M66.36-
multiple sites M66.39
pelvic region M66.35-
shoulder region M66.31-
specified site NEC M66.38
thigh M66.35-
upper arm M66.32-
foot M66.87-
forearm M66.83-
hand M66.84-
lower leg M66.86-
multiple sites M66.89
pelvic region M66.85-
shoulder region M66.81-
specified
site NEC M66.88
tendon M66.80
thigh M66.85-
upper arm M66.82-
thoracic duct I89.8
tonsil J35.8
traumatic
aorta — *see* Injury, aorta, laceration, major
diaphragm — *see* Injury, intrathoracic, diaphragm
external site — *see* Wound, open, by site
eye — *see* Injury, eye, laceration
internal organ — *see* Injury, by site
intervertebral disc
cervical S13.0
lumbar S33.0
thoracic S23.0
kidney S37.06-
ligament — *see also* Sprain
ankle — *see* Sprain, ankle
carpus — *see* Rupture, traumatic, ligament, wrist
collateral (hand) — *see* Rupture, traumatic, ligament, finger, collateral
finger (metacarpophalangeal) (interphalangeal) S63.40-
collateral S63.41-
index S63.41-
little S63.41-
middle S63.41-
ring S63.41-
index S63.40-
little S63.40-
middle S63.40-
palmar S63.42-
index S63.42-

Rupture, ruptured - *continued*
traumatic - *continued*
ligament - *continued*
finger (metacarpophalangeal) (interphalangeal) - *continued*
palmar - *continued*
little S63.42-
middle S63.42-
ring S63.42-
ring S63.40-
specified site NEC S63.499
index S63.49-
little S63.49-
middle S63.49-
ring S63.49-
volar plate S63.43-
index S63.43-
little S63.43-
middle S63.43-
ring S63.43-
foot — *see* Sprain, foot
radial collateral S53.2-
radiocarpal — *see* Rupture, traumatic, ligament, wrist, radiocarpal
ulnar collateral S53.3-
ulnocarpal — *see* Rupture, traumatic, ligament, wrist, ulnocarpal
wrist S63.30-
collateral S63.31-
radiocarpal S63.32-
specified site NEC S63.39-
ulnocarpal (palmar) S63.33-
liver S36.116
membrana tympani — *see* Rupture, ear drum, traumatic
muscle or tendon — *see* Strain
myocardium — *see* Injury, heart
pancreas S36.299
rectum S36.69
sigmoid S36.593
spleen S36.09
stomach S36.39
symphysis pubis S33.4
tympanum, tympanic (membrane) — *see* Rupture, ear drum, traumatic
ureter S37.19
uterus S37.69
vagina — *see* Injury, vagina
vena cava — *see* Injury, vena cava, laceration, major
tricuspid (heart) (valve) I07.8
tube, tubal (nonobstetric) (nontraumatic) N83.8
abscess — *see* Salpingitis
due to pregnancy O00.10-
with intrauterine pregnancy O00.11-
tympanum, tympanic (membrane) (nontraumatic) — *see also* Perforation, tympanic membrane H72.9-
traumatic — *see* Rupture, ear drum, traumatic
umbilical cord, complicating delivery O69.89
ureter (traumatic) S37.19
nontraumatic N28.89
urethra (nontraumatic) N36.8
with ectopic or molar pregnancy O08.6
following ectopic or molar pregnancy O08.6
obstetrical trauma O71.5
traumatic S37.39
uterosacral ligament (nonobstetric) (nontraumatic) N83.8
uterus (traumatic) S37.69
before labor O71.0-
during or after labor O71.1
nonpuerperal, nontraumatic N85.8
pregnant (during labor) O71.1
before labor O71.0-
vagina — *see* Injury, vagina
valve, valvular (heart) — *see* Endocarditis
varicose vein — *see* Varix
varix — *see* Varix
vena cava R58
traumatic — *see* Injury, vena cava, laceration, major
vesical (urinary) N32.89
vessel (blood) R58
pulmonary I28.8
traumatic — *see* Injury, blood vessel
viscus R19.8
vulva complicating delivery O70.0
Russell-Silver syndrome Q87.1
Russian spring-summer type encephalitis A84.0
Rust's disease (tuberculous cervical spondylitis) A18.01
Ruvalcaba-Myhre-Smith syndrome E71.440
Rytand-Lipsitch syndrome I44.2

S

Saber, sabre shin or tibia (syphilitic) A50.56 *[M90.8-]*
Sac lacrimal — *see* condition
Saccharomyces infection B37.9
Saccharopinuria E72.3
Saccular — *see* condition
Sacculation
aorta (nonsyphilitic) — *see* Aneurysm, aorta
bladder N32.3
intralaryngeal (congenital) (ventricular) Q31.3
larynx (congenital) (ventricular) Q31.3
organ or site, congenital — *see* Distortion
pregnant uterus — *see* Pregnancy, complicated by, abnormal, uterus
ureter N28.89
urethra N36.1
vesical N32.3
Sachs' amaurotic familial idiocy or disease E75.02
Sachs-Tay disease E75.02
Sacks-Libman disease M32.11
Sacralgia M53.3
Sacralization Q76.49
Sacrodynia M53.3
Sacroiliac joint — *see* condition
Sacroiliitis NEC M46.1
Sacrum — *see* condition
Saddle
back — *see* Lordosis
embolus
abdominal aorta I74.01
pulmonary artery I26.92
with acute cor pulmonale I26.02
injury - code to condition
nose M95.0
due to syphilis A50.57
Sadism (sexual) F65.52
Sadness, postpartal O90.6
Sadomasochism F65.50
Saemisch's ulcer (cornea) — *see* Ulcer, cornea, central
Sagging
skin and subcutaneous tissue (following bariatric surgery weight loss) (following dietary weight loss) L98.7
Sahib disease B55.0
Sailors' skin L57.8
Saint
Anthony's fire — *see* Erysipelas
triad — *see* Hernia, diaphragm
Vitus' dance — *see* Chorea, Sydenham's
Salaam
attack (s) — *see* Epilepsy, spasms
tic R25.8
Salicylism
abuse F55.8
overdose or wrong substance given — *see* Table of Drugs and Chemicals, by drug, poisoning
Salivary duct or gland — *see* condition
Salivation, excessive K11.7
Salmonella — *see* Infection, Salmonella
Salmonellosis A02.0
Salpingitis (catarrhal) (fallopian tube) (nodular) (pseudofollicular) (purulent) (septic) N70.91
with oophoritis N70.93
acute N70.01
with oophoritis N70.03
chlamydial A56.11
chronic N70.11
with oophoritis N70.13
complicating abortion — *see* Abortion, by type, complicated by, salpingitis
ear — *see* Salpingitis, eustachian
eustachian (tube) H68.00-
acute H68.01-
chronic H68.02-
follicularis N70.11
with oophoritis N70.13
gonococcal (acute) (chronic) A54.24
interstitial, chronic N70.11
with oophoritis N70.13
isthmica nodosa N70.11
with oophoritis N70.13
specific (gonococcal) (acute) (chronic) A54.24
tuberculous (acute) (chronic) A18.17
venereal (gonococcal) (acute) (chronic) A54.24
Salpingocele N83.4-
Salpingo-oophoritis (catarrhal) (purulent) (ruptured) (septic) (suppurative) N70.93
acute N70.03
with ectopic or molar pregnancy O08.0

Schistosomiasis - *continued*
bladder B65.0
chestermani B65.8
colon B65.1
cutaneous B65.3
due to
S. haematobium B65.0
S. japonicum B65.2
S. mansoni B65.1
S. mattheii B65.8
Eastern B65.2
genitourinary tract B65.0
intestinal B65.1
lung NEC B65.9 *[J99]*
pneumonia B65.9 *[J17]*
Manson's (intestinal) B65.1
oriental B65.2
pulmonary NEC B65.9 *[J99]*
pneumonia B65.9
Schistosoma
haematobium B65.0
japonicum B65.2
mansoni B65.1
specified type NEC B65.8
urinary B65.0
vesical B65.0
Schizencephaly Q04.6
Schizoaffective psychosis F25.9
Schizodontia K00.2
Schizoid personality F60.1
Schizophrenia, schizophrenic F20.9
acute (brief) (undifferentiated) F23
atypical (form) F20.3
borderline F21
catalepsy F20.2
catatonic (type) (excited) (withdrawn) F20.2
cenesthopathic, cenesthesiopathic F20.89
childhood type F84.5
chronic undifferentiated F20.5
cyclic F25.0
disorganized (type) F20.1
flexibilitas cerea F20.2
hebephrenic (type) F20.1
incipient F21
latent F21
negative type F20.5
paranoid (type) F20.0
paraphrenic F20.0
post-psychotic depression F32.89
prepsychotic F21
prodromal F21
pseudoneurotic F21
pseudopsychopathic F21
reaction F23
residual (state) (type) F20.5
restzustand F20.5
schizoaffective (type) — *see* Psychosis, schizoaffective
simple (type) F20.89
simplex F20.89
specified type NEC F20.89
spectrum and other psychotic disorder F29
specified NEC F28
stupor F20.2
syndrome of childhood F84.5
undifferentiated (type) F20.3
chronic F20.5
Schizothymia (persistent) F60.1
Schlatter-Osgood disease or osteochondrosis — *see* Osteochondrosis, juvenile, tibia
Schlatter's tibia — *see* Osteochondrosis, juvenile, tibia
Schmidt's syndrome (polyglandular, autoimmune) E31.0
Schmincke's carcinoma or tumor — *see* Neoplasm, nasopharynx, malignant
Schmitz (-Stutzer) **dysentery** A03.0
Schmorl's disease or nodes
lumbar region M51.46
lumbosacral region M51.47
sacrococcygeal region M53.3
thoracic region M51.44
thoracolumbar region M51.45
Schneiderian
papilloma — *see* Neoplasm, nasopharynx, benign
specified site — *see* Neoplasm, benign, by site
unspecified site D14.0
specified site — *see* Neoplasm, malignant, by site
unspecified site C30.0
Scholte's syndrome (malignant carcinoid) E34.0
Scholz (-Bielchowsky-Henneberg) **disease or syndrome** E75.25
Schönlein (-Henoch) **disease or purpura** (primary) (rheumatic) D69.0
Schottmuller's disease A01.4
Schroeder's syndrome (endocrine hypertensive) E27.0
Schüller-Christian disease or syndrome C96.5
Schultze's type acroparesthesia, simple I73.89
Schultz's disease or syndrome — *see* Agranulocytosis
Schwalbe-Ziehen-Oppenheim disease G24.1
Schwannoma — *see also* Neoplasm, nerve, benign
malignant — *see also* Neoplasm, nerve, malignant
with rhabdomyoblastic differentiation — *see* Neoplasm, nerve, malignant
melanocytic — *see* Neoplasm, nerve, benign
pigmented — *see* Neoplasm, nerve, benign
Schwannomatosis Q85.03
Schwartz (-Jampel) **syndrome** G71.13
Schwartz-Bartter syndrome E22.2
Schweniger-Buzzi anetoderma L90.1
Sciatic — *see* condition
Sciatica (infective)
with lumbago M54.4-
due to intervertebral disc disorder — *see* Disorder, disc, with, radiculopathy
due to displacement of intervertebral disc (with lumbago) — *see* Disorder, disc, with, radiculopathy
wallet M54.3-
Scimitar syndrome Q26.8
Sclera — *see* condition
Sclerectasia H15.84-
Scleredema
adultorum — *see* Sclerosis, systemic
Buschke's — *see* Sclerosis, systemic
newborn P83.0
Sclerema (adiposum) (edematosum) (neonatorum) (newborn) P83.0
adultorum — *see* Sclerosis, systemic
Scleriasis — *see* Scleroderma
Scleritis H15.00-
with corneal involvement H15.04-
anterior H15.01-
brawny H15.02-
in (due to) zoster B02.34
posterior H15.03-
specified type NEC H15.09-
syphilitic A52.71
tuberculous (nodular) A18.51
Sclerochoroiditis H31.8
Scleroconjunctivitis — *see* Scleritis
Sclerocystic ovary syndrome E28.2
Sclerodactyly, sclerodactylia L94.3
Scleroderma, sclerodermia (acrosclerotic) (diffuse) (generalized) (progressive) (pulmonary) — *see also* Sclerosis, systemic M34.9-
circumscribed L94.0
linear L94.1
localized L94.0
newborn P83.88
systemic M34.9
Sclerokeratitis H16.8
tuberculous A18.52
Scleroma nasi A48.8
Scleromalacia (perforans) H15.05-
Scleromyxedema L98.5
Sclérose en plaques G35
Sclerosis, sclerotic
adrenal (gland) E27.8
Alzheimer's — *see* Disease, Alzheimer's
amyotrophic (lateral) G12.21
aorta, aortic I70.0
valve — *see* Endocarditis, aortic
artery, arterial, arteriolar, arteriovascular — *see* Arteriosclerosis
ascending multiple G35
brain (generalized) (lobular) G37.9
artery, arterial I67.2
diffuse G37.0
disseminated G35
insular G35
Krabbe's E75.23
miliary G35
multiple G35
presenile (Alzheimer's) — *see* Disease, Alzheimer's, early onset
senile (arteriosclerotic) I67.2
stem, multiple G35
tuberous Q85.1
bulbar, multiple G35
bundle of His I44.39
cardiac — *see* Disease, heart, ischemic, atherosclerotic

Sclerosis, sclerotic - *continued*
cardiorenal — *see* Hypertension, cardiorenal
cardiovascular — *see also* Disease, cardiovascular
renal — *see* Hypertension, cardiorenal
cerebellar — *see* Sclerosis, brain
cerebral — *see* Sclerosis, brain
cerebrospinal (disseminated) (multiple) G35
cerebrovascular I67.2
choroid — *see* Degeneration, choroid
combined (spinal cord) — *see also* Degeneration, combined
multiple G35
concentric (Balo) G37.5
cornea — *see* Opacity, cornea
coronary (artery) I25.10
with angina pectoris — *see* Arteriosclerosis, coronary (artery),
corpus cavernosum
female N90.89
male N48.6
diffuse (brain) (spinal cord) G37.0
disseminated G35
dorsal G35
dorsolateral (spinal cord) — *see* Degeneration, combined
endometrium N85.5
extrapyramidal G25.9
eye, nuclear (senile) — *see* Cataract, senile, nuclear
focal and segmental (glomerular) — *see also* N00-N07 with fourth character .1 N05.1
Friedreich's (spinal cord) G11.1
funicular (spermatic cord) N50.89
general (vascular) — *see* Arteriosclerosis
gland (lymphatic) I89.8
hepatic K74.1
alcoholic K70.2
hereditary
cerebellar G11.9
spinal (Friedreich's ataxia) G11.1
hippocampal G93.81
insular G35
kidney — *see* Sclerosis, renal
larynx J38.7
lateral (amyotrophic) (descending) (spinal) G12.21
primary G12.23
lens, senile nuclear — *see* Cataract, senile, nuclear
liver K74.1
with fibrosis K74.2
alcoholic K70.2
alcoholic K70.2
cardiac K76.1
lung — *see* Fibrosis, lung
mastoid — *see* Mastoiditis, chronic
mesial temporal G93.81
mitral I05.8
Mönckeberg's (medial) — *see* Arteriosclerosis, extremities
multiple (brain stem) (cerebral) (generalized) (spinal cord) G35
myocardium, myocardial — *see* Disease, heart, ischemic, atherosclerotic
nuclear (senile) , eye — *see* Cataract, senile, nuclear
ovary N83.8
pancreas K86.89
penis N48.6
peripheral arteries — *see* Arteriosclerosis, extremities
plaques G35
pluriglandular E31.8
polyglandular E31.8
posterolateral (spinal cord) — *see* Degeneration, combined
presenile (Alzheimer's) — *see* Disease, Alzheimer's, early onset
primary, lateral G12.23
progressive, systemic M34.0
pulmonary — *see* Fibrosis, lung
artery I27.0
valve (heart) — *see* Endocarditis, pulmonary
renal N26.9
with
cystine storage disease E72.09
hypertensive heart disease (conditions in I11) — *see* Hypertension, cardiorenal
arteriolar (hyaline) (hyperplastic) — *see* Hypertension, kidney
retina (senile) (vascular) H35.00
senile (vascular) — *see* Arteriosclerosis
spinal (cord) (progressive) G95.89
ascending G61.0
combined — *see also* Degeneration, combined
multiple G35
syphilitic A52.11

- **Screening** (for) - *continued*
  - neoplasm (malignant) (of) - *continued*
    - breast Z12.39
      - routine mammogram Z12.31
    - cervix Z12.4
    - colon Z12.11
    - genitourinary organs NEC Z12.79
      - bladder Z12.6
      - cervix Z12.4
      - ovary Z12.73
      - prostate Z12.5
      - testis Z12.71
      - vagina Z12.72
    - hematopoietic system Z12.89
    - intestinal tract Z12.10
      - colon Z12.11
      - rectum Z12.12
      - small intestine Z12.13
    - lung Z12.2
    - lymph (glands) Z12.89
    - nervous system Z12.82
    - oral cavity Z12.81
    - prostate Z12.5
    - rectum Z12.12
    - respiratory organs Z12.2
    - skin Z12.83
    - small intestine Z12.13
    - specified site NEC Z12.89
    - stomach Z12.0
  - nephropathy Z13.89
  - nervous system disorders NEC Z13.858
  - neurological condition Z13.89
  - osteoporosis Z13.820
  - parasitic infestation Z11.9
    - specified NEC Z11.8
  - phenylketonuria Z13.228
  - plague Z11.2
  - poisoning (chemical) (heavy metal) Z13.88
  - poliomyelitis Z11.59
  - postnatal, chromosomal abnormalities Z13.89
  - prenatal, of mother — *see also* Encounter, antenatal screening Z36.9
  - protozoal disease Z11.6
    - intestinal Z11.0
  - pulmonary tuberculosis Z11.1
  - radiation exposure Z13.88
  - respiratory condition Z13.83
  - respiratory tuberculosis Z11.1
  - rheumatoid arthritis Z13.828
  - rubella Z11.59
  - schistosomiasis Z11.6
  - sexually-transmitted disease NEC Z11.3
    - human immunodeficiency virus (HIV) Z11.4
  - sickle-cell disease or trait Z13.0
  - skin condition Z13.89
  - sleeping sickness Z11.6
  - special Z13.9
    - specified NEC Z13.89
  - syphilis Z11.3
  - tetanus Z11.2
  - trachoma Z11.8
  - traumatic brain injury Z13.850
  - trypanosomiasis Z11.6
  - tuberculosis, respiratory Z11.1
  - venereal disease Z11.3
  - viral encephalitis (mosquito- or tick-borne) Z11.59
  - whooping cough Z11.2
  - worms, intestinal Z11.6
  - yaws Z11.8
  - yellow fever Z11.59
- **Scrofula, scrofulosis** (tuberculosis of cervical lymph glands) A18.2
- **Scrofulide** (primary) (tuberculous) A18.4
- **Scrofuloderma, scrofulodermia** (any site) (primary) A18.4
- **Scrofulosus lichen** (primary) (tuberculous) A18.4
- **Scrofulous** — *see* condition
- **Scrotal tongue** K14.5
- **Scrotum** — *see* condition
- **Scurvy, scorbutic** E54
  - anemia D53.2
  - gum E54
  - infantile E54
  - rickets E55.0 *[M90.80]*
- **Sealpox** B08.62
- **Seasickness** T75.3
- **Seatworm** (infection) (infestation) B80
- **Sebaceous** — *see also* condition
  - cyst — *see* Cyst, sebaceous
- **Seborrhea, seborrheic** L21.9
  - capillitii R23.8
  - capitis L21.0
  - dermatitis L21.9
- **Seborrhea, seborrheic** - *continued*
  - dermatitis - *continued*
    - infantile L21.1
  - eczema L21.9
    - infantile L21.1
  - sicca L21.0
- **Seckel's syndrome** Q87.1
- **Seclusion, pupil** — *see* Membrane, pupillary
- **Second hand tobacco smoke exposure** (acute) (chronic) Z77.22
  - in the perinatal period P96.81
- **Secondary**
  - dentin (in pulp) K04.3
  - neoplasm, secondaries — *see* Table of Neoplasms, secondary
- **Secretion**
  - antidiuretic hormone, inappropriate E22.2
  - catecholamine, by pheochromocytoma E27.5
  - hormone
    - antidiuretic, inappropriate (syndrome) E22.2
    - by
      - carcinoid tumor E34.0
      - pheochromocytoma E27.5
    - ectopic NEC E34.2
  - urinary
    - excessive R35.8
    - suppression R34
- **Section**
  - nerve, traumatic — *see* Injury, nerve
- **Sedative, hypnotic, or anxiolytic-induced**
  - anxiety disorder F13.980
  - bipolar and related disorder F13.94
  - delirium F13.921
  - depressive disorder F13.94
  - major neurocognitive disorder F13.97
  - mild neurocognitive disorder F13.988
  - psychotic disorder F13.959
  - sexual dysfunction F13.981
  - sleep disorder F13.982
- **Segmentation, incomplete** (congenital) — *see also* Fusion
  - bone NEC Q78.8
  - lumbosacral (joint) (vertebra) Q76.49
- **Seitelberger's syndrome** (infantile neuraxonal dystrophy) G31.89
- **Seizure** (s) — *see also* Convulsions R56.9
  - akinetic — *see* Epilepsy, generalized, specified NEC
  - atonic — *see* Epilepsy, generalized, specified NEC
  - autonomic (hysterical) F44.5
  - convulsive — *see* Convulsions
  - cortical (focal) (motor) — *see* Epilepsy, localization-related, symptomatic, with simple partial seizures
  - disorder — *see also* Epilepsy G40.909
  - due to stroke — *see* Sequelae (of), disease, cerebrovascular, by type, specified NEC
  - epileptic — *see* Epilepsy
  - febrile (simple) R56.00
    - with status epilepticus G40.901
    - complex (atypical) (complicated) R56.01
      - with status epilepticus G40.901
  - grand mal G40.409
    - intractable G40.419
      - with status epilepticus G40.411
      - without status epilepticus G40.419
    - not intractable G40.409
      - with status epilepticus G40.401
      - without status epilepticus G40.409
  - heart — *see* Disease, heart
  - hysterical F44.5
  - intractable G40.919
    - with status epilepticus G40.911
  - Jacksonian (focal) (motor type) (sensory type) — *see* Epilepsy, localization-related, symptomatic, with simple partial seizures
  - newborn P90
  - nonspecific epileptic
    - atonic — *see* Epilepsy, generalized, specified NEC
    - clonic — *see* Epilepsy, generalized, specified NEC
    - myoclonic — *see* Epilepsy, generalized, specified NEC
    - tonic — *see* Epilepsy, generalized, specified NEC
    - tonic-clonic — *see* Epilepsy, generalized, specified NEC
  - partial, developing into secondarily generalized seizures
    - complex — *see* Epilepsy, localization-related, symptomatic, with complex partial seizures
    - simple — *see* Epilepsy, localization-related, symptomatic, with simple partial seizures
  - petit mal G40.409
    - intractable G40.419
      - with status epilepticus G40.411
      - without status epilepticus G40.419
- **Seizure** (s) - *continued*
  - petit mal - *continued*
    - not intractable G40.409
      - with status epilepticus G40.401
      - without status epilepticus G40.409
  - post traumatic R56.1
  - recurrent G40.909
  - specified NEC G40.89
  - uncinate — *see* Epilepsy, localization-related, symptomatic, with complex partial seizures
- **Selenium deficiency, dietary** E59
- **Self-damaging behavior** (life-style) Z72.89
- **Self-harm** (attempted)
  - history (personal) Z91.5
    - in family Z81.8
- **Self-mutilation** (attempted)
  - history (personal) Z91.5
    - in family Z81.8
- **Self-poisoning**
  - history (personal) Z91.5
    - in family Z81.8
  - observation following (alleged) attempt Z03.6
- **Semicoma** R40.1
- **Seminal vesiculitis** N49.0
- **Seminoma** C62.9-
  - specified site — *see* Neoplasm, malignant, by site
- **Senear-Usher disease or syndrome** L10.4
- **Senectus** R54
- **Senescence** (without mention of psychosis) R54
- **Senile, senility** — *see also* condition R41.81
  - with
    - acute confusional state F05
    - mental changes NOS F03
    - psychosis NEC — *see* Psychosis, senile
  - asthenia R54
  - cervix (atrophic) N88.8
  - debility R54
  - endometrium (atrophic) N85.8
  - fallopian tube (atrophic) — *see* Atrophy, fallopian tube
  - heart (failure) R54
  - ovary (atrophic) — *see* Atrophy, ovary
  - premature E34.8
  - vagina, vaginitis (atrophic) N95.2
  - wart L82.1
- **Sensation**
  - burning (skin) R20.8
    - tongue K14.6
  - loss of R20.8
  - prickling (skin) R20.2
  - tingling (skin) R20.2
- **Sense loss**
  - smell — *see* Disturbance, sensation, smell
  - taste — *see* Disturbance, sensation, taste
  - touch R20.8
- **Sensibility disturbance** (cortical) (deep) (vibratory) R20.9
- **Sensitive, sensitivity** — *see also* Allergy
  - carotid sinus G90.01
  - child (excessive) F93.8
  - cold, autoimmune D59.1
  - dentin K03.89
  - gluten (non-celiac) K90.41
  - latex Z91.040
  - methemoglobin D74.8
  - tuberculin, without clinical or radiological symptoms R76.11
  - visual
    - glare H53.71
    - impaired contrast H53.72
- **Sensitiver Beziehungswahn** F22
- **Sensitization, auto-erythrocytic** D69.2
- **Separation**
  - anxiety, abnormal (of childhood) F93.0
  - apophysis, traumatic - code as Fracture, by site
  - choroid — *see* Detachment, choroid
  - epiphysis, epiphyseal
    - nontraumatic — *see also* Osteochondropathy, specified type NEC
      - upper femoral — *see* Slipped, epiphysis, upper femoral
    - traumatic - code as Fracture, by site
  - fracture — *see* Fracture
  - infundibulum cardiac from right ventricle by a partition Q24.3
  - joint (traumatic) (current) - code by site under Dislocation
  - pubic bone, obstetrical trauma O71.6
  - retina, retinal — *see* Detachment, retina
  - symphysis pubis, obstetrical trauma O71.6
  - tracheal ring, incomplete, congenital Q32.1
- **Sepsis** (generalized) (unspecified organism) A41.9
  - with

Sepsis (generalized) (unspecified organism) - *continued*
- with - *continued*
  - organ dysfunction (acute) (multiple) R65.20
    - with septic shock R65.21
- actinomycotic A42.7
- adrenal hemorrhage syndrome (meningococcal) A39.1
- anaerobic A41.4
- Bacillus anthracis A22.7
- Brucella — *see also* Brucellosis A23.9
- candidal B37.7
- cryptogenic A41.9
- due to device, implant or graft T85.79
  - arterial graft NEC T82.7
  - breast (implant) T85.79
  - catheter NEC T85.79
    - dialysis (renal) T82.7
      - intraperitoneal T85.71
    - infusion NEC T82.7
      - spinal (cranial) (epidural) (intrathecal) (spinal) (subarachnoid) (subdural) T85.735
    - urethral indwelling T83.511
    - urinary T83.518
  - ectopic or molar pregnancy O08.82
  - electronic (electrode) (pulse generator) (stimulator)
    - bone T84.7
    - cardiac T82.7
    - nervous system T85.738
      - brain T85.731
      - neurostimulator generator T85.734
      - peripheral nerve T85.732
      - spinal cord T85.733
    - urinary T83.590
  - fixation, internal (orthopedic) — *see* Complication, fixation device, infection
  - gastrointestinal (bile duct) (esophagus) T85.79
    - neurostimulator electrode (lead) T85.732
  - genital T83.69
  - heart NEC T82.7
    - valve (prosthesis) T82.6
      - graft T82.7
  - joint prosthesis — *see* Complication, joint prosthesis, infection
  - ocular (corneal graft) (orbital implant) T85.79
  - orthopedic NEC T84.7
    - fixation device, internal — *see* Complication, fixation device, infection
  - specified NEC T85.79
  - vascular T82.7
  - ventricular intracranial (communicating) shunt T85.730
- during labor O75.3
- Enterococcus A41.81
- Erysipelothrix (rhusiopathiae) (erysipeloid) A26.7
- Escherichia coli (E. coli) A41.5
- extraintestinal yersiniosis A28.2
- following
  - abortion (subsequent episode) O08.0
    - current episode — *see* Abortion
  - ectopic or molar pregnancy O08.82
  - immunization T88.0
  - infusion, therapeutic injection or transfusion NEC T80.29
  - obstetrical procedure O86.04
- gangrenous A41.9
- gonococcal A54.86
- Gram-negative (organism) A41.5
  - anaerobic A41.4
- Haemophilus influenzae A41.3
- herpesviral B00.7
- intra-abdominal K65.1
- intraocular — *see* Endophthalmitis, purulent
- Listeria monocytogenes A32.7
- localized - code to specific localized infection
  - in operation wound T81.49
  - skin — *see* Abscess
- malleus A24.0
- melioidosis A24.1
- meningeal — *see* Meningitis
- meningococcal A39.4
  - acute A39.2
  - chronic A39.3
- MSSA (Methicillin susceptible Staphylococcus aureus) A41.01
- newborn P36.9
  - due to
    - anaerobes NEC P36.5
    - Escherichia coli P36.4
    - Staphylococcus P36.30
      - aureus P36.2
      - specified NEC P36.39
    - Streptococcus P36.10

Sepsis (generalized) (unspecified organism) - *continued*
- newborn - *continued*
  - due to - *continued*
    - Streptococcus - *continued*
      - group B P36.0
      - specified NEC P36.19
  - specified NEC P36.8
- Pasteurella multocida A28.0
- pelvic, puerperal, postpartum, childbirth O85
- postprocedural T81.44
- pneumococcal A40.3
- puerperal, postpartum, childbirth (pelvic) O85
- Salmonella (arizonae) (cholerae-suis) (enteritidis) (typhimurium) A02.1
- severe R65.20
  - with septic shock R65.21
- skin, localized — *see* Abscess
- Shigella — *see also* Dysentery, bacillary A03.9
- specified organism NEC A41.89
- Staphylococcus, staphylococcal A41.2
  - aureus (methicillin susceptible) (MSSA) A41.01
    - methicillin resistant (MRSA) A41.02
  - coagulase-negative A41.1
  - specified NEC A41.1
- Streptococcus, streptococcal A40.9
  - agalactiae A40.1
  - group
    - A A40.0
    - B A40.1
    - D A41.81
  - neonatal P36.10
    - group B P36.0
    - specified NEC P36.19
  - pneumoniae A40.3
  - pyogenes A40.0
  - specified NEC A40.8
- tracheostomy stoma J95.02
- tularemic A21.7
- umbilical, umbilical cord (newborn) — *see* Sepsis, newborn
- Yersinia pestis A20.7

Septate — *see* Septum

Septic — *see* condition
- arm — *see* Cellulitis, upper limb
  - with lymphangitis — *see* Lymphangitis, acute, upper limb
- embolus — *see* Embolism
- finger — *see* Cellulitis, digit
  - with lymphangitis — *see* Lymphangitis, acute, digit
- foot — *see* Cellulitis, lower limb
  - with lymphangitis — *see* Lymphangitis, acute, lower limb
- gallbladder (acute) K81.0
- hand — *see* Cellulitis, upper limb
  - with lymphangitis — *see* Lymphangitis, acute, upper limb
- joint — *see* Arthritis, pyogenic or pyemic
- leg — *see* Cellulitis, lower limb
  - with lymphangitis — *see* Lymphangitis, acute, lower limb
- nail — *see also* Cellulitis, digit
  - with lymphangitis — *see* Lymphangitis, acute, digit
- sore — *see also* Abscess
  - throat J02.0
    - streptococcal J02.0
- spleen (acute) D73.89
- teeth, tooth (pulpal origin) K04.4
- throat — *see* Pharyngitis
- thrombus — *see* Thrombosis
- toe — *see* Cellulitis, digit
  - with lymphangitis — *see* Lymphangitis, acute, digit
- tonsils, chronic J35.01
  - with adenoiditis J35.03
- uterus — *see* Endometritis

Septicemia A41.9
- meaning sepsis — *see* Sepsis

Septum, septate (congenital) — *see also* Anomaly, by site
- anal Q42.3
  - with fistula Q42.2
- aqueduct of Sylvius Q03.0
  - with spina bifida — *see* Spina bifida, by site, with hydrocephalus
- uterus Q51.20
  - complete Q51.21
  - partial Q51.22
  - specified NEC Q51.28
- vagina Q52.10

Septum, septate (congenital) - *continued*
- vagina - *continued*
  - in pregnancy — *see* Pregnancy, complicated by, abnormal vagina
    - causing obstructed labor O65.5
  - longitudinal Q52.129
    - microperforate
      - left side Q52.124
      - right side Q52.123
    - nonobstruction Q52.120
    - obstructing Q52.129
      - left side Q52.122
      - right side Q52.121
  - transverse Q52.11

Sequelae (of) — *see also* condition
- abscess, intracranial or intraspinal (conditions in G06) G09
- amputation -- code to injury with seventh character S
- burn and corrosion -- code to injury with seventh character S
- calcium deficiency E64.8
- cerebrovascular disease — *see* Sequelae, disease, cerebrovascular
- childbirth O94
- contusion -- code to injury with seventh character S
- corrosion — *see* Sequelae, burn and corrosion
- crushing injury -- code to injury with seventh character S
- disease
  - cerebrovascular I69.90
    - alteration of sensation I69.998
    - aphasia I69.920
    - apraxia I69.990
    - ataxia I69.993
    - cognitive deficits I69.91
    - disturbance of vision I69.998
    - dysarthria I69.922
    - dysphagia I69.991
    - dysphasia I69.921
    - facial droop I69.992
    - facial weakness I69.992
    - fluency disorder I69.923
    - hemiplegia I69.95-
    - hemorrhage
      - intracerebral — *see* Sequelae, hemorrhage, intracerebral
      - intracranial, nontraumatic NEC — *see* Sequelae, hemorrhage, intracranial, nontraumatic
      - subarachnoid — *see* Sequelae, hemorrhage, subarachnoid
    - language deficit I69.928
    - monoplegia
      - lower limb I69.94-
      - upper limb I69.93-
    - paralytic syndrome I69.96-
    - specified effect NEC I69.998
    - specified type NEC I69.80
      - alteration of sensation I69.898
      - aphasia I69.820
      - apraxia I69.890
      - ataxia I69.893
      - cognitive deficits I69.81
      - disturbance of vision I69.898
      - dysarthria I69.822
      - dysphagia I69.891
      - dysphasia I69.821
      - facial droop I69.892
      - facial weakness I69.892
      - fluency disorder I69.823
      - hemiplegia I69.85-
      - language deficit I69.828
      - monoplegia
        - lower limb I69.84-
        - upper limb I69.83-
      - paralytic syndrome I69.86-
      - specified effect NEC I69.898
    - speech deficit I69.928
      - speech deficit I69.828
    - stroke NOS — *see* Sequelae, stroke NOS
- dislocation -- code to injury with seventh character S
- encephalitis or encephalomyelitis (conditions in G04) G09
  - in infectious disease NEC B94.8
  - viral B94.1
- external cause -- code to injury with seventh character S
- foreign body entering natural orifice -- code to injury with seventh character S
- fracture -- code to injury with seventh character S
- frostbite -- code to injury with seventh character S
- Hansen's disease B92

- **Sequelae** (of) - *continued*
  - hemorrhage
    - intracerebral I69.10
      - alteration of sensation I69.198
      - aphasia I69.120
      - apraxia I69.190
      - ataxia I69.193
      - cognitive deficits I69.11
      - disturbance of vision I69.198
      - dysarthria I69.122
      - dysphagia I69.191
      - dysphasia I69.121
      - facial droop I69.192
      - facial weakness I69.192
      - fluency disorder I69.123
      - hemiplegia I69.15-
      - language deficit NEC I69.128
      - monoplegia
        - lower limb I69.14-
        - upper limb I69.13-
      - paralytic syndrome I69.16-
      - specified effect NEC I69.198
      - speech deficit NEC I69.128
    - intracranial, nontraumatic NEC I69.20
      - alteration of sensation I69.298
      - aphasia I69.220
      - apraxia I69.290
      - ataxia I69.293
      - cognitive deficits I69.21
      - disturbance of vision I69.298
      - dysarthria I69.222
      - dysphagia I69.291
      - dysphasia I69.221
      - facial droop I69.292
      - facial weakness I69.292
      - fluency disorder I69.223
      - hemiplegia I69.25-
      - language deficit NEC I69.228
      - monoplegia
        - lower limb I69.24-
        - upper limb I69.23-
      - paralytic syndrome I69.26-
      - specified effect NEC I69.298
      - speech deficit NEC I69.228
    - subarachnoid I69.00
      - alteration of sensation I69.098
      - aphasia I69.020
      - apraxia I69.090
      - ataxia I69.093
      - cognitive deficits — *see* subcategory I69.01-
      - disturbance of vision I69.098
      - dysarthria I69.022
      - dysphagia I69.091
      - dysphasia I69.021
      - facial droop I69.092
      - facial weakness I69.092
      - fluency disorder I69.023
      - hemiplegia I69.05-
      - language deficit NEC I69.028
      - monoplegia
        - lower limb I69.04-
        - upper limb I69.03-
      - paralytic syndrome I69.06-
      - specified effect NEC I69.098
      - speech deficit NEC I69.028
  - hepatitis, viral B94.2
  - hyperalimentation E68
  - infarction
    - cerebral I69.30
      - alteration of sensation I69.398
      - aphasia I69.320
      - apraxia I69.390
      - ataxia I69.393
      - cognitive deficits I69.31
      - disturbance of vision I69.398
      - dysarthria I69.322
      - dysphagia I69.391
      - dysphasia I69.321
      - facial droop I69.392
      - facial weakness I69.392
      - fluency disorder I69.323
      - hemiplegia I69.35-
      - language deficit NEC I69.328
      - monoplegia
        - lower limb I69.34-
        - upper limb I69.33-
      - paralytic syndrome I69.36-
      - specified effect NEC I69.398
      - speech deficit NEC I69.328
  - infection, pyogenic, intracranial or intraspinal G09
  - infectious disease B94.9
    - specified NEC B94.8
  - injury -- code to injury with seventh character S

- **Sequelae** (of) - *continued*
  - leprosy B92
  - meningitis
    - bacterial (conditions in G00) G09
    - other or unspecified cause (conditions in G03) G09
  - muscle (and tendon) injury -- code to injury with seventh character S
  - myelitis — *see* Sequelae, encephalitis
  - niacin deficiency E64.8
  - nutritional deficiency E64.9
    - specified NEC E64.8
  - obstetrical condition O94
  - parasitic disease B94.9
  - phlebitis or thrombophlebitis of intracranial or intraspinal venous sinuses and veins (conditions in G08) G09
  - poisoning -- code to poisoning with seventh character S
    - nonmedicinal substance — *see* Sequelae, toxic effect, nonmedicinal substance
  - poliomyelitis (acute) B91
  - pregnancy O94
  - protein-energy malnutrition E64.0
  - puerperium O94
  - rickets E64.3
  - selenium deficiency E64.8
  - sprain and strain -- code to injury with seventh character S
  - stroke NOS I69.30
    - alteration in sensation I69.398
    - aphasia I69.320
    - apraxia I69.390
    - ataxia I69.393
    - cognitive deficits I69.31
    - disturbance of vision I69.398
    - dysarthria I69.322
    - dysphagia I69.391
    - dysphasia I69.321
    - facial droop I69.392
    - facial weakness I69.392
    - hemiplegia I69.35-
    - language deficit NEC I69.328
    - monoplegia
      - lower limb I69.34-
      - upper limb I69.33-
    - paralytic syndrome I69.36-
    - specified effect NEC I69.398
    - speech deficit NEC I69.328
  - tendon and muscle injury -- code to injury with seventh character S
  - thiamine deficiency E64.8
  - trachoma B94.0
  - tuberculosis B90.9
    - bones and joints B90.2
    - central nervous system B90.0
    - genitourinary B90.1
    - pulmonary (respiratory) B90.9
    - specified organs NEC B90.8
  - viral
    - encephalitis B94.1
    - hepatitis B94.2
  - vitamin deficiency NEC E64.8
    - A E64.1
    - B E64.8
    - C E64.2
  - wound, open -- code to injury with seventh character S
- **Sequestration** — *see also* Sequestrum
  - disk — *see* Displacement, intervertebral disk
  - lung, congenital Q33.2
- **Sequestrum**
  - bone — *see* Osteomyelitis, chronic
  - dental M27.2
  - jaw bone M27.2
  - orbit — *see* Osteomyelitis, orbit
  - sinus (accessory) (nasal) — *see* Sinusitis
- **Sequoiosis lung or pneumonitis** J67.8
- **Serology for syphilis**
  - doubtful
    - with signs or symptoms - code by site and stage under Syphilis
    - follow-up of latent syphilis — *see* Syphilis, latent
  - negative, with signs or symptoms - code by site and stage under Syphilis
  - positive A53.0
    - with signs or symptoms - code by site and stage under Syphilis
  - reactivated A53.0
- **Seroma** — *see also* Hematoma
  - postprocedural — *see* Complication, postprocedural, seroma
  - traumatic, secondary and recurrent T79.2
- **Seropurulent** — *see* condition
- **Serositis, multiple** K65.8
  - pericardial I31.1
  - peritoneal K65.8
- **Serous** — *see* condition
- **Sertoli cell**
  - adenoma
    - specified site — *see* Neoplasm, benign, by site
    - unspecified site
      - female D27.9
      - male D29.20
  - carcinoma
    - specified site — *see* Neoplasm, malignant, by site
    - unspecified site (male) C62.9-
      - female C56.9
  - tumor
    - with lipid storage
      - specified site — *see* Neoplasm, benign, by site
      - unspecified site
        - female D27.9
        - male D29.20
    - specified site — *see* Neoplasm, benign, by site
    - unspecified site
      - female D27.9
      - male D29.20
- **Sertoli-Leydig cell tumor** — *see* Neoplasm, benign, by site
  - specified site — *see* Neoplasm, benign, by site
  - unspecified site
    - female D27.9
    - male D29.20
- **Serum**
  - allergy, allergic reaction — *see also* Reaction, serum T80.69
    - shock — *see also* Shock, anaphylactic T80.59
  - arthritis — *see also* Reaction, serum T80.69
  - complication or reaction NEC — *see also* Reaction, serum T80.69
  - disease NEC — *see also* Reaction, serum T80.69
  - hepatitis — *see also* Hepatitis, viral, type B
    - carrier (suspected) of B18.1
  - intoxication — *see also* Reaction, serum T80.69
  - neuritis — *see also* Reaction, serum T80.69
  - neuropathy G61.1
  - poisoning NEC — *see also* Reaction, serum T80.69
  - rash NEC — *see also* Reaction, serum T80.69
  - reaction NEC — *see also* Reaction, serum T80.69
  - sickness NEC — *see also* Reaction, serum T80.69
  - urticaria — *see also* Reaction, serum T80.69
- **Sesamoiditis** M25.8-
- **Severe sepsis** R65.20
  - with septic shock R65.21
- **Sever's disease or osteochondrosis** — *see* Osteochondrosis, juvenile, tarsus
- **Sex**
  - chromosome mosaics Q97.8
    - lines with various numbers of X chromosomes Q97.2
  - education Z70.8
  - reassignment surgery status Z87.890
- **Sextuplet pregnancy** — *see* Pregnancy, sextuplet
- **Sexual**
  - function, disorder of (psychogenic) F52.9
  - immaturity (female) (male) E30.0
  - impotence (psychogenic) organic origin NEC — *see* Dysfunction, sexual, male
  - precocity (constitutional) (cryptogenic) (female) (idiopathic) (male) E30.1
- **Sexuality, pathologic** — *see* Deviation, sexual
- **Sézary disease** C84.1-
- **Shadow, lung** R91.8
- **Shaking palsy or paralysis** — *see* Parkinsonism
- **Shallowness, acetabulum** — *see* Derangement, joint, specified type NEC, hip
- **Shaver's disease** J63.1
- **Sheath** (tendon) — *see* condition
- **Sheathing, retinal vessels** H35.01-
- **Shedding**
  - nail L60.8
  - premature, primary (deciduous) teeth K00.6
- **Sheehan's disease or syndrome** E23.0
- **Shelf, rectal** K62.89
- **Shell teeth** K00.5
- **Shellshock** (current) F43.0
  - lasting state — *see* Disorder, post-traumatic stress
- **Shield kidney** Q63.1
- **Shift**
  - auditory threshold (temporary) H93.24-
  - mediastinal R93.89
- **Shifting sleep-work schedule** (affecting sleep) G47.26
- **Shiga** (-Kruse) **dysentery** A03.0
- **Shiga's bacillus** A03.0
- **Shigella** (dysentery) — *see* Dysentery, bacillary

Sigmoiditis — *see also* Enteritis K52.9
  infectious A09
  noninfectious K52.9
Silfverskföld's syndrome Q78.9
Silicosiderosis J62.8
Silicosis, silicotic (simple) (complicated) J62.8
  with tuberculosis J65
Silicotuberculosis J65
Silo-fillers' disease J68.8
  bronchitis J68.0
  pneumonitis J68.0
  pulmonary edema J68.1
Silver's syndrome Q87.1
Simian malaria B53.1
Simmonds' cachexia or disease E23.0
Simons' disease or syndrome
  (progressive lipodystrophy) E88.1
Simple, simplex — *see* condition
Simulation, conscious (of illness) Z76.5
Simultanagnosia (asimultagnosia) R48.3
Sin Nombre virus disease (Hantavirus) (cardio)
  -pulmonary syndrome) B33.4
Sinding-Larsen disease or osteochondrosis — *see*
  Osteochondrosis, juvenile, patella
Singapore hemorrhagic fever A91
Singer's node or nodule J38.2
Single
  atrium Q21.2
  coronary artery Q24.5
  umbilical artery Q27.0
  ventricle Q20.4
Singultus R06.6
  epidemicus B33.0
Sinus — *see also* Fistula
  abdominal K63.89
  arrest I45.5
  arrhythmia I49.8
  bradycardia R00.1
  branchial cleft (internal) (external) Q18.0
  coccygeal — *see* Sinus, pilonidal
  dental K04.6
  dermal (congenital) Q06.8
    with abscess Q06.8
    coccygeal, pilonidal — *see* Sinus, coccygeal
  infected, skin NEC L08.89
  marginal, ruptured or bleeding — *see* Hemorrhage,
    antepartum, specified cause NEC
  medial, face and neck Q18.8
  pause I45.5
  pericranii Q01.9
  pilonidal (infected) (rectum) L05.92
    with abscess L05.02
  preauricular Q18.1
  rectovaginal N82.3
  Rokitansky-Aschoff (gallbladder) K82.8
  sacrococcygeal (dermoid) (infected) — *see* Sinus,
    pilonidal
  tachycardia R00.0
    paroxysmal I47.1
  tarsi syndrome M25.57-
  testis N50.89
  tract (postinfective) — *see* Fistula
  urachus Q64.4
Sinusitis (accessory) (chronic) (hyperplastic) (nasal)
  (nonpurulent) (purulent) J32.9
  acute J01.90
    ethmoidal J01.20
      recurrent J01.21
    frontal J01.10
      recurrent J01.11
    involving more than one sinus, other than
      pansinusitis J01.80
      recurrent J01.81
    maxillary J01.00
      recurrent J01.01
    pansinusitis J01.40
      recurrent J01.41
    recurrent J01.91
    specified NEC J01.80
      recurrent J01.81
    sphenoidal J01.30
      recurrent J01.31
  allergic — *see* Rhinitis, allergic
  due to high altitude T70.1
  ethmoidal J32.2
    acute J01.20
      recurrent J01.21
  frontal J32.1
    acute J01.10
      recurrent J01.11
  influenzal — *see* Influenza, with, respiratory
    manifestations NEC

Sinusitis (accessory) (chronic) (hyperplastic) (nasal)
(nonpurulent) (purulent) - *continued*
  involving more than one sinus but not
    pansinusitis J32.8
    acute J01.80
      recurrent J01.81
  maxillary J32.0
    acute J01.00
      recurrent J01.01
  sphenoidal J32.3
    acute J01.30
      recurrent J01.31
  tuberculous, any sinus A15.8
Sinusitis-bronchiectasis-situs inversus (syndrome)
  (triad) Q89.3
Sipple's syndrome E31.22
Sirenomelia (syndrome) Q87.2
Siriasis T67.0
Sirkari's disease B55.0
Siti A65
Situation, psychiatric F99
Situational
  disturbance (transient) — *see* Disorder, adjustment
    acute F43.0
  maladjustment — *see* Disorder, adjustment
  reaction — *see* Disorder, adjustment
    acute F43.0
Situs inversus or transversus (abdominalis)
  (thoracis) Q89.3
Sixth disease B08.20
  due to human herpesvirus 6 B08.21
  due to human herpesvirus 7 B08.22
Sjögren-Larsson syndrome Q87.1
Sjögren's syndrome or disease — *see* Sicca
  syndrome
Skeletal — *see* condition
Skene's gland — *see* condition
Skenitis — *see* Urethritis
Skerljevo A65
Skevas-Zerfus disease — *see* Toxicity, venom,
  marine animal, sea anemone
Skin — *see also* condition
  clammy R23.1
  donor — *see* Donor, skin
  hidebound M35.9
Slate-dressers' or slate-miners' lung J62.8
Sleep
  apnea — *see* Apnea, sleep
  deprivation Z72.820
  disorder or disturbance G47.9
    child F51.9
    nonorganic origin F51.9
    specified NEC G47.8
  disturbance G47.9
    nonorganic origin F51.9
  drunkenness F51.9
  rhythm inversion G47.2-
  terrors F51.4
  walking F51.3
    hysterical F44.89
Sleep hygiene
  abuse Z72.821
  inadequate Z72.821
  poor Z72.821
Sleeping sickness — *see* Sickness, sleeping
Sleeplessness — *see* Insomnia
  menopausal N95.1
Sleep-wake schedule disorder G47.20
Slim disease (in HIV infection) B20
Slipped, slipping
  epiphysis (traumatic) — *see*
    also Osteochondropathy, specified type NEC
    capital femoral (traumatic)
      acute (on chronic) S79.01-
    current traumatic - code as Fracture, by site
    upper femoral (nontraumatic) M93.00-
      acute M93.01-
        on chronic M93.03-
      chronic M93.02-
  intervertebral disc — *see* Displacement,
    intervertebral disc
  ligature, umbilical P51.8
  patella — *see* Disorder, patella, derangement NEC
  rib M89.8X8
  sacroiliac joint — *see* subcategory M53.2
  tendon — *see* Disorder, tendon
  ulnar nerve, nontraumatic — *see* Lesion, nerve,
    ulnar
  vertebra NEC — *see* Spondylolisthesis
Slocumb's syndrome E27.0
Sloughing (multiple) (phagedena) (skin) — *see*
  also Gangrene
  abscess — *see* Abscess

Sloughing (multiple) (phagedena) (skin) - *continued*
  appendix K38.8
  fascia — *see* Disorder, soft tissue, specified type
    NEC
  scrotum N50.89
  tendon — *see* Disorder, tendon
  transplanted organ — *see* Rejection, transplant
  ulcer — *see* Ulcer, skin
Slow
  feeding, newborn P92.2
  flow syndrome, coronary I20.8
  heart (beat) R00.1
Slowing, urinary stream R39.198
Sluder's neuralgia (syndrome) G44.89
Slurred, slurring speech R47.81
Small (ness)
  for gestational age — *see* Small for dates
  introitus, vagina N89.6
  kidney (unknown cause) N27.9
    bilateral N27.1
    unilateral N27.0
  ovary (congenital) Q50.39
  pelvis
    with disproportion (fetopelvic) O33.1
      causing obstructed labor O65.1
  uterus N85.8
  white kidney N03.9
Small-and-light-for-dates — *see* Small for dates
Small-for-dates (infant) P05.10
  with weight of
    499 grams or less P05.11
    500-749 grams P05.12
    750-999 grams P05.13
    1000-1249 grams P05.14
    1250-1499 grams P05.15
    1500-1749 grams P05.16
    1750-1999 grams P05.17
    2000-2499 grams P05.18
    2500 grams and over P05.19
  specified NEC P05.19
Smallpox B03
Smearing, fecal R15.1
Smith-Lemli-Opitz syndrome E78.72
Smith's fracture S52.54-
Smoker — *see* Dependence, drug, nicotine
Smoker's
  bronchitis J41.0
  cough J41.0
  palate K13.24
  throat J31.2
  tongue K13.24
Smoking
  passive Z77.22
Smothering spells R06.81
Snaggle teeth, tooth M26.39
Snapping
  finger — *see* Trigger finger
  hip — *see* Derangement, joint, specified type NEC,
    hip
    involving the iliotiblial band M76.3-
  knee — *see* Derangement, knee
    involving the iliotiblial band M76.3-
Sneddon-Wilkinson disease or syndrome
  (sub-corneal pustular dermatosis) L13.1
Sneezing (intractable) R06.7
Sniffing
  cocaine
    abuse — *see* Abuse, drug, cocaine
    dependence — *see* Dependence, drug, cocaine
  gasoline
    abuse — *see* Abuse, drug, inhalant
    dependence — *see* Dependence, drug, inhalant
  glue (airplane)
    abuse — *see* Abuse, drug, inhalant
    drug dependence — *see* Dependence, drug,
      inhalant
Sniffles
  newborn P28.89
Snoring R06.83
Snow blindness — *see* Photokeratitis
Snuffles (non-syphilitic) R06.5
  newborn P28.89
  syphilitic (infant) A50.05 *[J99]*
Social
  exclusion Z60.4
    due to discrimination or persecution
      (perceived) Z60.5
  migrant Z59.0
    acculturation difficulty Z60.3
  rejection Z60.4
    due to discrimination or persecution Z60.5
  role conflict NEC Z73.5
  skills inadequacy NEC Z73.4

Social - *continued*
transplantation Z60.3
Sodoku A25.0
Soemmerring's ring — *see* Cataract, secondary
Soft — *see also* condition
nails L60.3
Softening
bone — *see* Osteomalacia
brain (necrotic) (progressive) G93.89
congenital Q04.8
embolic I63.4-
hemorrhagic — *see* Hemorrhage, intracranial, intracerebral
occlusive I63.5-
thrombotic I63.3-
cartilage M94.2-
patella M22.4-
cerebellar — *see* Softening, brain
cerebral — *see* Softening, brain
cerebrospinal — *see* Softening, brain
myocardial, heart — *see* Degeneration, myocardial
spinal cord G95.89
stomach K31.89
Soldier's
heart F45.8
patches I31.0
Solitary
cyst, kidney N28.1
kidney, congenital Q60.0
Solvent abuse — *see* Abuse, drug, inhalant
dependence — *see* Dependence, drug, inhalant
Somatization reaction, somatic reaction — *see* Disorder, somatoform
Somnambulism F51.3
hysterical F44.89
Somnolence R40.0
nonorganic origin F51.11
Sonne dysentery A03.3
Soor B37.0
Sore
bed — *see* Ulcer, pressure, by site
chiclero B55.1
Delhi B55.1
desert — *see* Ulcer, skin
eye H57.1-
Lahore B55.1
mouth K13.79
canker K12.0
muscle M79.10
Naga — *see* Ulcer, skin
of skin — *see* Ulcer, skin
oriental B55.1
pressure — *see* Ulcer, pressure, by site
skin L98.9
soft A57
throat (acute) — *see also* Pharyngitis
with influenza, flu, or grippe — *see* Influenza, with, respiratory manifestations NEC
chronic J31.2
coxsackie (virus) B08.5
diphtheritic A36.0
herpesviral B00.2
influenzal — *see* Influenza, with, respiratory manifestations NEC
septic J02.0
streptococcal (ulcerative) J02.0
viral NEC J02.8
coxsackie B08.5
tropical — *see* Ulcer, skin
veldt — *see* Ulcer, skin
Soto's syndrome (cerebral gigantism) Q87.3
South African cardiomyopathy syndrome I42.8
Southeast Asian hemorrhagic fever A91
Spacing
abnormal, tooth, teeth, fully erupted M26.30
excessive, tooth, fully erupted M26.32
Spade-like hand (congenital) Q68.1
Spading nail L60.8
congenital Q84.6
Spanish collar N47.1
Sparganosis B70.1
Spasm (s) , spastic, spasticity — *see also* condition R25.2
accommodation — *see* Spasm, of accommodation
ampulla of Vater K83.4
anus, ani (sphincter) (reflex) K59.4
psychogenic F45.8
artery I73.9
cerebral G45.9
Bell's G51.3-
bladder (sphincter, external or internal) N32.89
psychogenic F45.8
bronchus, bronchiole J98.01

Spasm (s) , spastic, spasticity - *continued*
cardia K22.0
cardiac I20.1
carpopedal — *see* Tetany
cerebral (arteries) (vascular) G45.9
cervix, complicating delivery O62.4
ciliary body (of accommodation) — *see* Spasm, of accommodation
colon — *see also* Irritable, bowel K58.9
with diarrhea K58.0
psychogenic F45.8
common duct K83.8
compulsive — *see* Tic
conjugate H51.8
coronary (artery) I20.1
diaphragm (reflex) R06.6
epidemic B33.0
psychogenic F45.8
duodenum K59.8
epidemic diaphragmatic (transient) B33.0
esophagus (diffuse) K22.4
psychogenic F45.8
facial G51.3-
fallopian tube N83.8
gastrointestinal (tract) K31.89
psychogenic F45.8
glottis J38.5
hysterical F44.4
psychogenic F45.8
conversion reaction F44.4
reflex through recurrent laryngeal nerve J38.5
habit — *see* Tic
heart I20.1
hemifacial (clonic) G51.3-
hourglass — *see* Contraction, hourglass
hysterical F44.4
infantile — *see* Epilepsy, spasms
inferior oblique, eye H51.8
intestinal — *see also* Syndrome, irritable bowel K58.9
psychogenic F45.8
larynx, laryngeal J38.5
hysterical F44.4
psychogenic F45.8
conversion reaction F44.4
levator palpebrae superioris — *see* Disorder, eyelid function
muscle NEC M62.838
back M62.830
nerve, trigeminal G51.0
nervous F45.8
nodding F98.4
occupational F48.8
oculogyric H51.8
psychogenic F45.8
of accommodation H52.53-
ophthalmic artery — *see* Occlusion, artery, retina
perineal, female N94.89
peroneo-extensor — *see also* Deformity, limb, flat foot
pharynx (reflex) J39.2
hysterical F45.8
psychogenic F45.8
psychogenic F45.8
pylorus NEC K31.3
adult hypertrophic K31.89
congenital or infantile Q40.0
psychogenic F45.8
rectum (sphincter) K59.4
psychogenic F45.8
retinal (artery) — *see* Occlusion, artery, retina
sigmoid — *see also* Syndrome, irritable bowel K58.9
psychogenic F45.8
sphincter of Oddi K83.4
stomach K31.89
neurotic F45.8
throat J39.2
hysterical F45.8
psychogenic F45.8
tic F95.9
chronic F95.1
transient of childhood F95.0
tongue K14.8
torsion (progressive) G24.1
trigeminal nerve — *see* Neuralgia, trigeminal
ureter N13.5
urethra (sphincter) N35.919
uterus N85.8
complicating labor O62.4
vagina N94.2
psychogenic F52.5
vascular I73.9

Spasm (s) , spastic, spasticity - *continued*
vasomotor I73.9
vein NEC I87.8
viscera — *see* Pain, abdominal
Spasmodic — *see* condition
Spasmophilia — *see* Tetany
Spasmus nutans F98.4
Spastic, spasticity — *see also* Spasm
child (cerebral) (congenital) (paralysis) G80.1
Speaker's throat R49.8
Specific, specified — *see* condition
Speech
defect, disorder, disturbance, impediment R47.9
psychogenic, in childhood and adolescence F98.8
slurring R47.81
specified NEC R47.89
Spencer's disease A08.19
Spens' syndrome (syncope with heart block) I45.9
Sperm counts (fertility testing) Z31.41
postvasectomy Z30.8
reversal Z31.42
Spermatic cord — *see* condition
Spermatocele N43.40
congenital Q55.4
multiple N43.42
single N43.41
Spermatocystitis N49.0
Spermatocytoma C62.9-
specified site — *see* Neoplasm, malignant, by site
Spermatorrhea N50.89
Sphacelus — *see* Gangrene
Sphenoidal — *see* condition
Sphenoiditis (chronic) — *see* Sinusitis, sphenoidal
Sphenopalatine ganglion neuralgia G90.09
Sphericity, increased, lens (congenital) Q12.4
Spherocytosis (congenital) (familial) (hereditary) D58.0
hemoglobin disease D58.0
sickle-cell (disease) D57.8-
Spherophakia Q12.4
Sphincter — *see* condition
Sphincteritis, sphincter of Oddi — *see* Cholangitis
Sphingolipidosis E75.3
specified NEC E75.29
Sphingomyelinosis E75.3
Spicule tooth K00.2
Spider
bite — *see* Toxicity, venom, spider
fingers — *see* Syndrome, Marfan's
nevus I78.1
toes — *see* Syndrome, Marfan's
vascular I78.1
Spiegler-Fendt
benign lymphocytoma L98.8
sarcoid L08.89
Spielmeyer-Vogt disease E75.4
Spina bifida (aperta) Q05.9
with hydrocephalus NEC Q05.4
cervical Q05.5
with hydrocephalus Q05.0
dorsal Q05.6
with hydrocephalus Q05.1
lumbar Q05.7
with hydrocephalus Q05.2
lumbosacral Q05.7
with hydrocephalus Q05.2
occulta Q76.0
sacral Q05.8
with hydrocephalus Q05.3
thoracic Q05.6
with hydrocephalus Q05.1
thoracolumbar Q05.6
with hydrocephalus Q05.1
Spindle, Krukenberg's — *see* Pigmentation, cornea, posterior
Spine, spinal — *see* condition
Spiradenoma (eccrine) — *see* Neoplasm, skin, benign
Spirillosis A25.0
Spirillum
minus A25.0
obermeieri infection A68.0
Spirochetal — *see* condition
Spirochetosis A69.9
arthritic, arthritica A69.9
bronchopulmonary A69.8
icterohemorrhagic A27.0
lung A69.8
Spirometrosis B70.1
Spitting blood — *see* Hemoptysis
Splanchnoptosis K63.4
Spleen, splenic — *see* condition
Splenectasis — *see* Splenomegaly

Status (post) - *continued*
organ replacement - *continued*
by organ transplant (heterologous) (homologous) — *see* Transplant
pacemaker
brain Z96.89
cardiac Z95.0
specified NEC Z96.89
pancreatectomy Z90.410
complete Z90.410
partial Z90.411
total Z90.410
physical restraint Z78.1
pneumonectomy (complete) (partial) Z90.2
pneumothorax, therapeutic Z98.3
postcommotio cerebri F07.81
postoperative (postprocedural) NEC Z98.890
breast implant Z98.82
dental Z98.818
crown Z98.811
fillings Z98.811
restoration Z98.811
sealant Z98.810
specified NEC Z98.818
uterine scar Z98.891
pneumothorax, therapeutic Z98.3
postpartum (routine follow-up) Z39.2
care immediately after delivery Z39.0
postsurgical (postprocedural) NEC Z98.890
pneumothorax, therapeutic Z98.3
pregnancy, incidental Z33.1
prosthesis coronary angioplasty Z95.5
pseudophakia Z96.1
renal dialysis (hemodialysis) (peritoneal) Z99.2
retained foreign body — *see* Retained, foreign body fragments (type of)
reversed jejunal transposition (for bypass) Z98.0
salpingo-oophorectomy
bilateral Z90.722
unilateral Z90.721
sex reassignment surgery status Z87.890
shunt
arteriovenous (for dialysis) Z99.2
cerebrospinal fluid Z98.2
ventricular (communicating) (for drainage) Z98.2
splenectomy Z90.81
thymicolymphaticus E32.8
thymicus E32.8
thymolymphaticus E32.8
thyroidectomy (hypothyroidism) E89.0
tooth (teeth) extraction — *see also* Absence, teeth, acquired K08.409
tPA (rtPA) administration in a different facility within the last 24 hours prior to admission to current facility Z92.82
tracheostomy Z93.0
transplant — *see* Transplant
organ removed Z98.85
tubal ligation Z98.51
underimmunization Z28.3
ureterostomy Z93.6
urethrostomy Z93.6
vagina, artificial Z93.8
vasectomy Z98.52
wheelchair confinement Z99.3
Stealing
child problem F91.8
in company with others Z72.810
pathological (compulsive) F63.2
Steam burn — *see* Burn
Steatocystoma multiplex L72.2
Steatohepatitis (nonalcoholic) (NASH) K75.81
Steatoma L72.3
eyelid (cystic) — *see* Dermatosis, eyelid
infected — *see* Hordeolum
Steatorrhea (chronic) K90.9
with lacteal obstruction K90.2
idiopathic (adult) (infantile) K90.9
pancreatic K90.3
primary K90.0
tropical K90.1
Steatosis E88.89
heart — *see* Degeneration, myocardial
kidney N28.89
liver NEC K76.0
Steele-Richardson-Olszewski disease or syndrome G23.1
Steinbrocker's syndrome G90.8
Steinert's disease G71.11
Stein-Leventhal syndrome E28.2
Stein's syndrome E28.2
STEMI — *see also* - Infarct, myocardium, ST elevation I21.3
Stenocardia I20.8
Stenocephaly Q75.8
Stenosis, stenotic (cicatricial) — *see also* Stricture
ampulla of Vater K83.1
anus, anal (canal) (sphincter) K62.4
and rectum K62.4
congenital Q42.3
with fistula Q42.2
aorta (ascending) (supraventricular) (congenital) Q25.1
arteriosclerotic I70.0
calcified I70.0
supravalvular Q25.3
aortic (valve) I35.0
with insufficiency I35.2
congenital Q23.0
rheumatic I06.0
with
incompetency, insufficiency or regurgitation I06.2
with mitral (valve) disease I08.0
with tricuspid (valve) disease I08.3
mitral (valve) disease I08.0
with tricuspid (valve) disease I08.3
tricuspid (valve) disease I08.2
with mitral (valve) disease I08.3
specified cause NEC I35.0
syphilitic A52.03
aqueduct of Sylvius (congenital) Q03.0
with spina bifida — *see* Spina bifida, by site, with hydrocephalus
acquired G91.1
artery NEC — *see also* Arteriosclerosis I77.1
celiac I77.4
cerebral — *see* Occlusion, artery, cerebral
extremities — *see* Arteriosclerosis, extremities
precerebral — *see* Occlusion, artery, precerebral
pulmonary (congenital) Q25.6
acquired I28.8
renal I70.1
stent
coronary T82.855
peripheral T82.856
bile duct (common) (hepatic) K83.1
congenital Q44.3
bladder-neck (acquired) N32.0
congenital Q64.31
brain G93.89
bronchus J98.09
congenital Q32.3
syphilitic A52.72
cardia (stomach) K22.2
congenital Q39.3
cardiovascular — *see* Disease, cardiovascular
caudal M48.08
cervix, cervical (canal) N88.2
congenital Q51.828
in pregnancy or childbirth — *see* Pregnancy, complicated by, abnormal cervix
colon — *see also* Obstruction, intestine
congenital Q42.9
specified NEC Q42.8
colostomy K94.03
common (bile) duct K83.1
congenital Q44.3
coronary (artery) — *see* Disease, heart, ischemic, atherosclerotic
cystic duct — *see* Obstruction, gallbladder
due to presence of device, implant or graft — *see also* Complications, by site and type, specified NEC T85.858
arterial graft NEC T82.858
breast (implant) T85.858
catheter T85.858
dialysis (renal) T82.858
intraperitoneal T85.858
infusion NEC T82.858
spinal (epidural) (subdural) T85.850
urinary (indwelling) T83.85
fixation, internal (orthopedic) NEC T84.85
gastrointestinal (bile duct) (esophagus) T85.858
genital NEC T83.85
heart NEC T82.857
joint prosthesis T84.85
ocular (corneal graft) (orbital implant) NEC T85.858
orthopedic NEC T84.85
specified NEC T85.858
urinary NEC T83.85
vascular NEC T82.858
ventricular intracranial shunt T85.850
duodenum K31.5
congenital Q41.0
Stenosis, stenotic (cicatricial) - *continued*
ejaculatory duct NEC N50.89
endocervical os — *see* Stenosis, cervix
enterostomy K94.13
esophagus K22.2
congenital Q39.3
syphilitic A52.79
congenital A50.59 *[K23]*
eustachian tube — *see* Obstruction, eustachian tube
external ear canal (acquired) H61.30-
congenital Q16.1
due to
inflammation H61.32-
trauma H61.31-
postprocedural H95.81-
specified cause NEC H61.39-
gallbladder — *see* Obstruction, gallbladder
glottis J38.6
heart valve (congenital) Q24.8
aortic Q23.0
mitral Q23.2
pulmonary Q22.1
tricuspid Q22.4
hepatic duct K83.1
hymen N89.6
hypertrophic subaortic (idiopathic) I42.1
ileum — *see also* Obstruction, intestine, specified NEC K56.699
congenital Q41.2
infundibulum cardia Q24.3
intervertebral foramina — *see also* Lesion, biomechanical, specified NEC
connective tissue M99.79
abdomen M99.79
cervical region M99.71
cervicothoracic M99.71
head region M99.70
lumbar region M99.73
lumbosacral M99.73
occipitocervical M99.70
sacral region M99.74
sacrococcygeal M99.74
sacroiliac M99.74
specified NEC M99.79
thoracic region M99.72
thoracolumbar M99.72
disc M99.79
abdomen M99.79
cervical region M99.71
cervicothoracic M99.71
head region M99.70
lower extremity M99.76
lumbar region M99.73
lumbosacral M99.73
occipitocervical M99.70
pelvic M99.75
rib cage M99.78
sacral region M99.74
sacrococcygeal M99.74
sacroiliac M99.74
specified NEC M99.79
thoracic region M99.72
thoracolumbar M99.72
upper extremity M99.77
osseous M99.69
abdomen M99.69
cervical region M99.61
cervicothoracic M99.61
head region M99.60
lower extremity M99.66
lumbar region M99.63
lumbosacral M99.63
occipitocervical M99.60
pelvic M99.65
rib cage M99.68
sacral region M99.64
sacrococcygeal M99.64
sacroiliac M99.64
specified NEC M99.69
thoracic region M99.62
thoracolumbar M99.62
upper extremity M99.67
subluxation — *see* Stenosis, intervertebral foramina, osseous
intestine — *see also* Obstruction, intestine
congenital (small) Q41.9
large Q42.9
specified NEC Q42.8
specified NEC Q41.8
jejunum — *see also* Obstruction, intestine, specified NEC K56.699
congenital Q41.1
lacrimal (passage)

Stenosis, stenotic (cicatricial) - *continued*
lacrimal (passage) - *continued*
canaliculi H04.54-
congenital Q10.5
duct H04.55-
punctum H04.56-
sac H04.57-
lacrimonasal duct — *see* Stenosis, lacrimal, duct
congenital Q10.5
larynx J38.6
congenital NEC Q31.8
subglottic Q31.1
syphilitic A52.73
congenital A50.59 *[J99]*
mitral (chronic) (inactive) (valve) I05.0
with
aortic valve disease I08.0
incompetency, insufficiency or regurgitation I05.2
active or acute I01.1
with rheumatic or Sydenham's chorea I02.0
congenital Q23.2
specified cause, except rheumatic I34.2
syphilitic A52.03
myocardium, myocardial — *see also* Degeneration, myocardial
hypertrophic subaortic (idiopathic) I42.1
nares (anterior) (posterior) J34.89
congenital Q30.0
nasal duct — *see also* Stenosis, lacrimal, duct
congenital Q10.5
nasolacrimal duct — *see also* Stenosis, lacrimal, duct
congenital Q10.5
neural canal — *see also* Lesion, biomechanical, specified NEC
connective tissue M99.49
abdomen M99.49
cervical region M99.41
cervicothoracic M99.41
head region M99.40
lower extremity M99.46
lumbar region M99.43
lumbosacral M99.43
occipitocervical M99.40
pelvic M99.45
rib cage M99.48
sacral region M99.44
sacrococcygeal M99.44
sacroiliac M99.44
specified NEC M99.49
thoracic region M99.42
thoracolumbar M99.42
upper extremity M99.47
intervertebral disc M99.59
abdomen M99.59
cervical region M99.51
cervicothoracic M99.51
head region M99.50
lower extremity M99.56
lumbar region M99.53
lumbosacral M99.53
occipitocervical M99.50
pelvic M99.55
rib cage M99.58
sacral region M99.54
sacrococcygeal M99.54
sacroiliac M99.54
specified NEC M99.59
thoracic region M99.52
thoracolumbar M99.52
upper extremity M99.57
osseous M99.39
abdomen M99.39
cervical region M99.31
cervicothoracic M99.31
head region M99.30
lower extremity M99.36
lumbar region M99.33
lumbosacral M99.33
pelvic M99.35
rib cage M99.38
occipitocervical M99.30
sacral region M99.34
sacrococcygeal M99.34
sacroiliac M99.34
specified NEC M99.39
thoracic region M99.32
thoracolumbar M99.32
upper extremity M99.37
subluxation M99.29
cervical region M99.21
cervicothoracic M99.21

Stenosis, stenotic (cicatricial) - *continued*
neural canal - *continued*
subluxation - *continued*
head region M99.20
lower extremity M99.26
lumbar region M99.23
lumbosacral M99.23
occipitocervical M99.20
pelvic M99.25
rib cage M99.28
sacral region M99.24
sacrococcygeal M99.24
sacroiliac M99.24
specified NEC M99.29
thoracic region M99.22
thoracolumbar M99.22
upper extremity M99.27
organ or site, congenital NEC — *see* Atresia, by site
papilla of Vater K83.1
pulmonary (artery) (congenital) Q25.6
with ventricular septal defect, transposition of aorta, and hypertrophy of right ventricle Q21.3
acquired I28.8
in tetralogy of Fallot Q21.3
infundibular Q24.3
subvalvular Q24.3
supravalvular Q25.6
valve I37.0
with insufficiency I37.2
congenital Q22.1
rheumatic I09.89
with aortic, mitral or tricuspid (valve) disease I08.8
vein, acquired I28.8
vessel NEC I28.8
pulmonic (congenital) Q22.1
infundibular Q24.3
subvalvular Q24.3
pylorus (hypertrophic) (acquired) K31.1
adult K31.1
congenital Q40.0
infantile Q40.0
rectum (sphincter) — *see* Stricture, rectum
renal artery I70.1
congenital Q27.1
salivary duct (any) K11.8
sphincter of Oddi K83.1
spinal M48.00
cervical region M48.02
cervicothoracic region M48.03
lumbar region (NOS) (without neurogenic claudication) M48.061
with neurogenic claudication M48.062
lumbosacral region M48.07
occipito-atlanto-axial region M48.01
sacrococcygeal region M48.08
thoracic region M48.04
thoracolumbar region M48.05
stent
vascular
end stent
adjacent to stent — *see* Arteriosclerosis
within the stent
coronary T82.855
peripheral T82.856
in stent
coronary vessel T82.855
peripheral vessel T82.856
stomach, hourglass K31.2
subaortic (congenital) Q24.4
hypertrophic (idiopathic) I42.1
subglottic J38.6
congenital Q31.1
postprocedural J95.5
trachea J39.8
congenital Q32.1
syphilitic A52.73
tuberculous NEC A15.5
tracheostomy J95.03
tricuspid (valve) I07.0
with
aortic (valve) disease I08.2
incompetency, insufficiency or regurgitation I07.2
with aortic (valve) disease I08.2
with mitral (valve) disease I08.3
mitral (valve) disease I08.1
with aortic (valve) disease I08.3
congenital Q22.4
nonrheumatic I36.0
with insufficiency I36.2
tubal N97.1
ureter — *see* Atresia, ureter

Stenosis, stenotic (cicatricial) - *continued*
ureteropelvic junction, congenital Q62.11
ureterovesical orifice, congenital Q62.12
urethra (valve) — *see also* Stricture, urethra
congenital Q64.32
urinary meatus, congenital Q64.33
vagina N89.5
congenital Q52.4
in pregnancy — *see* Pregnancy, complicated by, abnormal vagina
causing obstructed labor O65.5
valve (cardiac) (heart) — *see also* Endocarditis I38
congenital Q24.8
aortic Q23.0
mitral Q23.2
pulmonary Q22.1
tricuspid Q22.4
vena cava (inferior) (superior) I87.1
congenital Q26.0
vesicourethral orifice Q64.31
vulva N90.5
Stent jail T82.897
Stercolith (impaction) K56.41
appendix K38.1
Stercoraceous, stercoral ulcer K63.3
anus or rectum K62.6
Stereotypies NEC F98.4
Sterility — *see* Infertility
Sterilization — *see* Encounter (for), sterilization
Sternalgia — *see* Angina
Sternopagus Q89.4
Sternum bifidum Q76.7
Steroid
effects (adverse) (adrenocortical) (iatrogenic)
cushingoid E24.2
correct substance properly administered — *see* Table of Drugs and Chemicals, by drug, adverse effect
overdose or wrong substance given or taken — *see* Table of Drugs and Chemicals, by drug, poisoning
diabetes — *see* category E09
correct substance properly administered — *see* Table of Drugs and Chemicals, by drug, adverse effect
overdose or wrong substance given or taken — *see* Table of Drugs and Chemicals, by drug, poisoning
fever R50.2
insufficiency E27.3
correct substance properly administered — *see* Table of Drugs and Chemicals, by drug, adverse effect
overdose or wrong substance given or taken — *see* Table of Drugs and Chemicals, by drug, poisoning
responder H40.04-
Stevens-Johnson disease or syndrome L51.1
toxic epidermal necrolysis overlap L51.3
Stewart-Morel syndrome M85.2
Sticker's disease B08.3
Sticky eye — *see* Conjunctivitis, acute, mucopurulent
Stieda's disease — *see* Bursitis, tibial collateral
Stiff neck — *see* Torticollis
Stiff-man syndrome G25.82
Stiffness, joint NEC M25.60-
ankle M25.67-
ankylosis — *see* Ankylosis, joint
contracture — *see* Contraction, joint
elbow M25.62-
foot M25.67-
hand M25.64-
hip M25.65-
knee M25.66-
shoulder M25.61-
wrist M25.63-
Stigmata congenital syphilis A50.59
Stillbirth P95
Still-Felty syndrome — *see* Felty's syndrome
Still's disease or syndrome (juvenile) M08.20
adult-onset M06.1
ankle M08.27-
elbow M08.22-
foot joint M08.27-
hand joint M08.24-
hip M08.25-
knee M08.26-
multiple site M08.29
shoulder M08.21-
vertebra M08.28
wrist M08.23-
Stimulation, ovary E28.1

- **Sting** (venomous)
  - (with allergic or anaphylactic shock) — *see* Table of Drugs and Chemicals, by animal or substance, poisoning
- **Stippled epiphyses** Q78.8
- **Stitch**
  - abscess T81.41
  - burst (in operation wound) — *see* Disruption, wound, operation
- **Stokes' disease** E05.00
  - with thyroid storm E05.01
- **Stokes-Adams disease or syndrome** I45.9
- **Stokvis** (-Talma) **disease** D74.8
- **Stoma malfunction**
  - colostomy K94.03
  - enterostomy K94.13
  - gastrostomy K94.23
  - ileostomy K94.13
  - tracheostomy J95.03
- **Stomach** — *see* condition
- **Stomatitis** (denture) (ulcerative) K12.1
  - angular K13.0
    - due to dietary or vitamin deficiency E53.0
  - aphthous K12.0
  - bovine B08.61
  - candidal B37.0
  - catarrhal K12.1
  - diphtheritic A36.89
  - due to
    - dietary deficiency E53.0
    - thrush B37.0
    - vitamin deficiency
      - B group NEC E53.9
      - B2 (riboflavin) E53.0
  - epidemic B08.8
  - epizootic B08.8
  - follicular K12.1
  - gangrenous A69.0
  - Geotrichum B48.3
  - herpesviral, herpetic B00.2
  - herpetiformis K12.0
  - malignant K12.1
  - membranous acute K12.1
  - monilial B37.0
  - mycotic B37.0
  - necrotizing ulcerative A69.0
  - parasitic B37.0
  - septic K12.1
  - spirochetal A69.1
  - suppurative (acute) K12.2
  - ulceromembranous A69.1
  - vesicular K12.1
    - with exanthem (enteroviral) B08.4
    - virus disease A93.8
  - Vincent's A69.1
- **Stomatocytosis** D58.8
- **Stomatomycosis** B37.0
- **Stomatorrhagia** K13.79
- **Stone** (s) — *see also* Calculus
  - bladder (diverticulum) N21.0
  - cystine E72.09
  - heart syndrome I50.1
  - kidney N20.0
  - prostate N42.0
  - pulpal (dental) K04.2
  - renal N20.0
  - salivary gland or duct (any) K11.5
  - urethra (impacted) N21.1
  - urinary (duct) (impacted) (passage) N20.9
    - bladder (diverticulum) N21.0
    - lower tract N21.9
    - specified NEC N21.8
  - xanthine E79.8 *[N22]*
- **Stonecutter's lung** J62.8
- **Stonemason's asthma, disease, lung or pneumoconiosis** J62.8
- **Stoppage**
  - heart — *see* Arrest, cardiac
  - urine — *see* Retention, urine
- **Storm, thyroid** — *see* Thyrotoxicosis
- **Strabismus** (congenital) (nonparalytic) H50.9
  - concomitant H50.40
    - convergent — *see* Strabismus, convergent concomitant
    - divergent — *see* Strabismus, divergent concomitant
  - convergent concomitant H50.00
    - accommodative component H50.43
    - alternating H50.05
      - with
        - A pattern H50.06
        - specified nonconcomitances NEC H50.08
        - V pattern H50.07

- **Strabismus** (congenital) (nonparalytic) - *continued*
  - convergent concomitant - *continued*
    - monocular H50.01-
      - with
        - A pattern H50.02-
        - specified nonconcomitances NEC H50.04-
        - V pattern H50.03-
    - intermittent H50.31-
      - alternating H50.32
  - cyclotropia H50.41
  - divergent concomitant H50.10
    - alternating H50.15
      - with
        - A pattern H50.16
        - specified noncomitances NEC H50.18
        - V pattern H50.17
    - monocular H50.11-
      - with
        - A pattern H50.12-
        - specified noncomitances NEC H50.14-
        - V pattern H50.13-
    - intermittent H50.33
      - alternating H50.34
  - Duane's syndrome H50.81-
  - due to adhesions, scars H50.69
  - heterophoria H50.50
    - alternating H50.55
    - cyclophoria H50.54
    - esophoria H50.51
    - exophoria H50.52
    - vertical H50.53
  - heterotropia H50.40
    - intermittent H50.30
  - hypertropia H50.2-
  - hypotropia — *see* Hypertropia
  - latent H50.50
  - mechanical H50.60
    - Brown's sheath syndrome H50.61-
    - specified type NEC H50.69
  - monofixation syndrome H50.42
  - paralytic H49.9
    - abducens nerve H49.2-
    - fourth nerve H49.1-
    - Kearns-Sayre syndrome H49.81-
    - ophthalmoplegia (external)
      - progressive H49.4-
        - with pigmentary retinopathy H49.81-
      - total H49.3-
    - sixth nerve H49.2-
    - specified type NEC H49.88-
    - third nerve H49.0-
    - trochlear nerve H49.1-
  - specified type NEC H50.89
  - vertical H50.2-
- **Strain**
  - back S39.012
  - cervical S16.1
  - eye NEC — *see* Disturbance, vision, subjective
  - heart — *see* Disease, heart
  - low back S39.012
  - mental NOS Z73.3
    - work-related Z56.6
  - muscle (tendon) — *see* Injury, muscle, by site, strain
  - neck S16.1
  - postural — *see also* Disorder, soft tissue, due to use
  - physical NOS Z73.3
    - work-related Z56.6
  - psychological NEC Z73.3
  - tendon — *see* Injury, muscle, by site, strain
- **Straining, on urination** R39.16
- **Strand, vitreous** — *see* Opacity, vitreous, membranes and strands
- **Strangulation, strangulated** — *see also* Asphyxia, traumatic
  - appendix K38.8
  - bladder-neck N32.0
  - bowel or colon K56.2
  - food or foreign body — *see* Foreign body, by site
  - hemorrhoids — *see* Hemorrhoids, with complication
  - hernia — *see also* Hernia, by site, with obstruction
    - with gangrene — *see* Hernia, by site, with gangrene
  - intestine (large) (small) K56.2
    - with hernia — *see also* Hernia, by site, with obstruction
      - with gangrene — *see* Hernia, by site, with gangrene
  - mesentery K56.2
  - mucus — *see* Asphyxia, mucus
  - omentum K56.2
  - organ or site, congenital NEC — *see* Atresia, by site
  - ovary — *see* Torsion, ovary
  - penis N48.89

- **Strangulation, strangulated** - *continued*
  - penis - *continued*
    - foreign body T19.4
  - rupture — *see* Hernia, by site, with obstruction
  - stomach due to hernia — *see also* Hernia, by site, with obstruction
    - with gangrene — *see* Hernia, by site, with gangrene
  - vesicourethral orifice N32.0
- **Strangury** R30.0
- **Straw itch** B88.0
- **Strawberry**
  - gallbladder K82.4
  - mark Q82.5
  - tongue (red) (white) K14.3
- **Streak** (s)
  - macula, angioid H35.33
  - ovarian Q50.32
- **Strephosymbolia** F81.0
  - secondary to organic lesion R48.8
- **Streptobacillary fever** A25.1
- **Streptobacillosis** A25.1
- **Streptobacillus moniliformis** A25.1
- **Streptococcus, streptococcal** — *see also* condition
  - as cause of disease classified elsewhere B95.5
  - group
    - A, as cause of disease classified elsewhere B95.0
    - B, as cause of disease classified elsewhere B95.1
    - D, as cause of disease classified elsewhere B95.2
  - pneumoniae, as cause of disease classified elsewhere B95.3
  - specified NEC, as cause of disease classified elsewhere B95.4
- **Streptomycosis** B47.1
- **Streptotrichosis** A48.8
- **Stress** F43.9
  - family — *see* Disruption, family
  - fetal P84
    - complicating pregnancy O77.9
      - due to drug administration O77.1
  - mental NEC Z73.3
    - work-related Z56.6
  - physical NEC Z73.3
    - work-related Z56.6
  - polycythemia D75.1
  - reaction — *see also* Reaction, stress F43.9
  - work schedule Z56.3
- **Stretching, nerve** — *see* Injury, nerve
- **Striae albicantes, atrophicae or distensae** (cutis) L90.6
- **Stricture** — *see also* Stenosis
  - ampulla of Vater K83.1
  - anus (sphincter) K62.4
    - congenital Q42.3
      - with fistula Q42.2
    - infantile Q42.3
      - with fistula Q42.2
  - aorta (ascending) (congenital) Q25.1
    - arteriosclerotic I70.0
    - calcified I70.0
    - supravalvular, congenital Q25.3
  - aortic (valve) — *see* Stenosis, aortic
  - aqueduct of Sylvius (congenital) Q03.0
    - with spina bifida — *see* Spina bifida, by site, with hydrocephalus
    - acquired G91.1
  - artery I77.1
    - basilar — *see* Occlusion, artery, basilar
    - carotid — *see* Occlusion, artery, carotid
    - celiac I77.4
    - congenital (peripheral) Q27.8
      - cerebral Q28.3
      - coronary Q24.5
      - digestive system Q27.8
      - lower limb Q27.8
      - retinal Q14.1
      - specified site NEC Q27.8
      - umbilical Q27.0
      - upper limb Q27.8
    - coronary — *see* Disease, heart, ischemic, atherosclerotic
      - congenital Q24.5
    - precerebral — *see* Occlusion, artery, precerebral
    - pulmonary (congenital) Q25.6
      - acquired I28.8
    - renal I70.1
    - vertebral — *see* Occlusion, artery, vertebral
  - auditory canal (external) (congenital)
    - acquired — *see* Stenosis, external ear canal
  - bile duct (common) (hepatic) K83.1
    - congenital Q44.3
    - postoperative K91.89
  - bladder N32.89

Stricture - *continued*
bladder - *continued*
neck N32.0
bowel — *see* Obstruction, intestine
brain G93.89
bronchus J98.09
congenital Q32.3
syphilitic A52.72
cardia (stomach) K22.2
congenital Q39.3
cardiac — *see also* Disease, heart
orifice (stomach) K22.2
cecum — *see* Obstruction, intestine
cervix, cervical (canal) N88.2
congenital Q51.828
in pregnancy — *see* Pregnancy, complicated by, abnormal cervix
causing obstructed labor O65.5
colon — *see also* Obstruction, intestine
congenital Q42.9
specified NEC Q42.8
colostomy K94.03
common (bile) duct K83.1
coronary (artery) — *see* Disease, heart, ischemic, atherosclerotic
cystic duct — *see* Obstruction, gallbladder
digestive organs NEC, congenital Q45.8
duodenum K31.5
congenital Q41.0
ear canal (external) (congenital) Q16.1
acquired — *see* Stricture, auditory canal, acquired
ejaculatory duct N50.89
enterostomy K94.13
esophagus K22.2
congenital Q39.3
syphilitic A52.79
congenital A50.59 *[K23]*
eustachian tube — *see also* Obstruction, eustachian tube
congenital Q17.8
fallopian tube N97.1
gonococcal A54.24
tuberculous A18.17
gallbladder — *see* Obstruction, gallbladder
glottis J38.6
heart — *see also* Disease, heart
valve — *see also* Endocarditis I38
aortic Q23.0
mitral Q23.2
pulmonary Q22.1
tricuspid Q22.4
hepatic duct K83.1
hourglass, of stomach K31.2
hymen N89.6
hypopharynx J39.2
ileum — *see also* Obstruction, intestine, specified NEC K56.699
congenital Q41.2
intestine — *see also* Obstruction, intestine
congenital (small) Q41.9
large Q42.9
specified NEC Q42.8
specified NEC Q41.8
ischemic K55.1
jejunum — *see also* Obstruction, intestine, specified NEC K56.699
congenital Q41.1
lacrimal passages — *see also* Stenosis, lacrimal
congenital Q10.5
larynx J38.6
congenital NEC Q31.8
subglottic Q31.1
syphilitic A52.73
congenital A50.59 *[J99]*
meatus
ear (congenital) Q16.1
acquired — *see* Stricture, auditory canal, acquired
osseous (ear) (congenital) Q16.1
acquired — *see* Stricture, auditory canal, acquired
urinarius — *see also* Stricture, urethra
congenital Q64.33
mitral (valve) — *see* Stenosis, mitral
myocardium, myocardial I51.5
hypertrophic subaortic (idiopathic) I42.1
nares (anterior) (posterior) J34.89
congenital Q30.0
nasal duct — *see also* Stenosis, lacrimal, duct
congenital Q10.5
nasolacrimal duct — *see also* Stenosis, lacrimal, duct
congenital Q10.5
nasopharynx J39.2
syphilitic A52.73

Stricture - *continued*
nose J34.89
congenital Q30.0
nostril (anterior) (posterior) J34.89
congenital Q30.0
syphilitic A52.73
congenital A50.59 *[J99]*
organ or site, congenital NEC — *see* Atresia, by site
os uteri — *see* Stricture, cervix
osseous meatus (ear) (congenital) Q16.1
acquired — *see* Stricture, auditory canal, acquired
oviduct — *see* Stricture, fallopian tube
pelviureteric junction (congenital) Q62.11
acquired, with hydronephrosis N13.0
penis, by foreign body T19.4
pharynx J39.2
prostate N42.89
pulmonary, pulmonic
artery (congenital) Q25.6
acquired I28.8
noncongenital I28.8
infundibulum (congenital) Q24.3
valve I37.0
congenital Q22.1
vein, acquired I28.8
vessel NEC I28.8
punctum lacrimale — *see also* Stenosis, lacrimal, punctum
congenital Q10.5
pylorus (hypertrophic) K31.1
adult K31.1
congenital Q40.0
infantile Q40.0
rectosigmoid — *see also* Obstruction, intestine, specified NEC K56.699
rectum (sphincter) K62.4
congenital Q42.1
with fistula Q42.0
due to
chlamydial lymphogranuloma A55
irradiation K91.89
lymphogranuloma venereum A55
gonococcal A54.6
inflammatory (chlamydial) A55
syphilitic A52.74
tuberculous A18.32
renal artery I70.1
congenital Q27.1
salivary duct or gland (any) K11.8
sigmoid (flexure) — *see* Obstruction, intestine
spermatic cord N50.89
stoma (following) (of)
colostomy K94.03
enterostomy K94.13
gastrostomy K94.23
ileostomy K94.13
tracheostomy J95.03
stomach K31.89
congenital Q40.2
hourglass K31.2
subaortic Q24.4
hypertrophic (acquired) (idiopathic) I42.1
subglottic J38.6
syphilitic NEC A52.79
trachea J39.8
congenital Q32.1
syphilitic A52.73
tuberculous NEC A15.5
tracheostomy J95.03
tricuspid (valve) — *see* Stenosis, tricuspid
tunica vaginalis N50.89
ureter (postoperative) N13.5
with
hydronephrosis N13.1
with infection N13.6
pyelonephritis (chronic) N11.1
congenital — *see* Atresia, ureter
tuberculous A18.11
ureteropelvic junction (congenital) Q62.11
acquired, with hydronephrosis N13.0
ureterovesical orifice N13.5
with infection N13.6
urethra (organic) (spasmodic) — *see also* Stricture, urethra, male N35.919
associated with schistosomiasis B65.0 *[N37]*
congenital Q64.39
valvular (posterior) Q64.2
due to
infection — *see* Stricture, urethra, postinfective
trauma — *see* Stricture, urethra, post-traumatic
female N35.92
gonococcal, gonorrheal A54.01

Stricture - *continued*
urethra (organic) (spasmodic) - *continued*
infective NEC — *see* Stricture, urethra, postinfective
late effect (sequelae) of injury — *see* Stricture, urethra, post-traumatic
male N35.919
anterior urethra N35.914
bulbous urethra N35.912
meatal N35.911
membranous urethra N35.913
overlapping sites N35.916
postcatheterization — *see* Stricture, urethra, postprocedural
postinfective NEC
female N35.12
male N35.119
anterior urethra N35.114
bulbous urethra N35.112
meatal N35.111
membranous urethra N35.113
overlapping sites N35.116
postobstetric N35.021
postoperative — *see* Stricture, urethra, postprocedural
postprocedural
female N99.12
male N99.114
anterior bulbous urethra N99.113
bulbous urethra N99.111
fossa navicularis N99.115
meatal N99.110
membranous urethra N99.112
overlapping sites N99.116
post-traumatic
female N35.028
due to childbirth N35.021
male N35.014
anterior urethra N35.013
bulbous urethra N35.011
meatal N35.010
membranous urethra N35.012
overlapping sites N35.016
sequela (late effect) of
childbirth N35.021
injury — *see* Stricture, urethra, post-traumatic
specified cause NEC
female N35.82
male N35.819
anterior urethra N35.814
bulbous urethra N35.812
meatal N35.811
membranous urethra N35.813
overlapping sites N35.816
syphilitic A52.76
traumatic — *see* Stricture, urethra, post-traumatic
valvular (posterior) , congenital Q64.2
urinary meatus — *see* Stricture, urethra
uterus, uterine (synechiae) N85.6
os (external) (internal) — *see* Stricture, cervix
vagina (outlet) — *see* Stenosis, vagina
valve (cardiac) (heart) — *see also* Endocarditis
congenital
aortic Q23.0
mitral Q23.2
pulmonary Q22.1
tricuspid Q22.4
vas deferens N50.89
congenital Q55.4
vein I87.1
vena cava (inferior) (superior) NEC I87.1
congenital Q26.0
vesicourethral orifice N32.0
congenital Q64.31
vulva (acquired) N90.5
Stridor R06.1
congenital (larynx) P28.89
Stridulous — *see* condition
Stroke (apoplectic) (brain) (embolic) (ischemic) (paralytic) (thrombotic) I63.9
cryptogenic — *see also* infarction, cerebral I63.9
epileptic — *see* Epilepsy
heat T67.0
in evolution I63.9
intraoperative
during cardiac surgery I97.810
during other surgery I97.811
lightning — *see* Lightning
meaning
cerebral hemorrhage - code to Hemorrhage, intracranial
cerebral infarction - code to Infarction, cerebral
postprocedural

Stroke (apoplectic) (brain) (embolic) (ischemic) (paralytic) (thrombotic) - *continued*
postprocedural - *continued*
following cardiac surgery I97.820
following other surgery I97.821
unspecified (NOS) I63.9
Stromatosis, endometrial D39.0
Strongyloidiasis, strongyloidosis B78.9
cutaneous B78.1
disseminated B78.7
intestinal B78.0
Strophulus pruriginosus L28.2
Struck by lightning — *see* Lightning
Struma — *see also* Goiter
Hashimoto E06.3
lymphomatosa E06.3
nodosa (simplex) E04.9
endemic E01.2
multinodular E01.1
multinodular E04.2
iodine-deficiency related E01.1
toxic or with hyperthyroidism E05.20
with thyroid storm E05.21
multinodular E05.20
with thyroid storm E05.21
uninodular E05.10
with thyroid storm E05.11
toxicosa E05.20
with thyroid storm E05.21
multinodular E05.20
with thyroid storm E05.21
uninodular E05.10
with thyroid storm E05.11
uninodular E04.1
ovarii D27.-
Riedel's E06.5
Strumipriva cachexia E03.4
Strümpell-Marie spine — *see* Spondylitis, ankylosing
Strümpell-Westphal pseudosclerosis E83.01
Stuart deficiency disease (factor X) D68.2
Stuart-Prower factor deficiency (factor X) D68.2
Student's elbow — *see* Bursitis, elbow, olecranon
Stump — *see* Amputation
Stunting, nutritional E45
Stupor (catatonic) R40.1
depressive (single episode) F32.89
recurrent episode F33.8
dissociative F44.2
manic F30.2
manic-depressive F31.89
psychogenic (anergic) F44.2
reaction to exceptional stress (transient) F43.0
Sturge (-Weber) (-Dimitri) (-Kalischer) **disease or syndrome** Q85.8
Stuttering F80.81
adult onset F98.5
childhood onset F80.81
following cerebrovascular disease — *see* Disorder, fluency. following cerebrovascular disease
in conditions classified elsewhere R47.82
Sty, stye (external) (internal) (meibomian) (zeisian) — *see* Hordeolum
Subacidity, gastric K31.89
psychogenic F45.8
Subacute — *see* condition
Subarachnoid — *see* condition
Subcortical — *see* condition
Subcostal syndrome, nerve compression — *see* Mononeuropathy, upper limb, specified site NEC
Subcutaneous, subcuticular — *see* condition
Subdural — *see* condition
Subendocardium — *see* condition
Subependymoma
specified site — *see* Neoplasm, uncertain behavior, by site
unspecified site D43.2
Suberosis J67.3
Subglossitis — *see* Glossitis
Subhemophilia D66
Subinvolution
breast (postlactational) (postpuerperal) N64.89
puerperal O90.89
uterus (chronic) (nonpuerperal) N85.3
puerperal O90.89
Sublingual — *see* condition
Sublinguitis — *see* Sialoadenitis
Subluxatable hip Q65.6
Subluxation — *see also* Dislocation
acromioclavicular S43.11-
ankle S93.0-
atlantoaxial, recurrent M43.4
with myelopathy M43.3

Subluxation - *continued*
carpometacarpal (joint) NEC S63.05-
thumb S63.04-
complex, vertebral — *see* Complex, subluxation
congenital — *see also* Malposition, congenital
hip — *see* Dislocation, hip, congenital, partial
joint (excluding hip)
lower limb Q68.8
shoulder Q68.8
upper limb Q68.8
elbow (traumatic) S53.10-
anterior S53.11-
lateral S53.14-
medial S53.13-
posterior S53.12-
specified type NEC S53.19-
finger S63.20-
index S63.20-
interphalangeal S63.22-
distal S63.24-
index S63.24-
little S63.24-
middle S63.24-
ring S63.24-
index S63.22-
little S63.22-
middle S63.22-
proximal S63.23-
index S63.23-
little S63.23-
middle S63.23-
ring S63.23-
ring S63.22-
little S63.20-
metacarpophalangeal S63.21-
index S63.21-
little S63.21-
middle S63.21-
ring S63.21-
middle S63.20-
ring S63.20-
foot S93.30-
specified site NEC S93.33-
tarsal joint S93.31-
tarsometatarsal joint S93.32-
toe — *see* Subluxation, toe
hip S73.00-
anterior S73.03-
obturator S73.02-
central S73.04-
posterior S73.01-
interphalangeal (joint)
finger S63.22-
distal joint S63.24-
index S63.24-
little S63.24-
middle S63.24-
ring S63.24-
index S63.22-
little S63.22-
middle S63.22-
proximal joint S63.23-
index S63.23-
little S63.23-
middle S63.23-
ring S63.23-
ring S63.22-
thumb S63.12-
toe S93.13-
great S93.13-
lesser S93.13-
joint prosthesis — *see* Complications, joint prosthesis, mechanical, displacement, by site
knee S83.10-
cap — *see* Subluxation, patella
patella — *see* Subluxation, patella
proximal tibia
anteriorly S83.11-
laterally S83.14-
medially S83.13-
posteriorly S83.12-
specified type NEC S83.19-
lens — *see* Dislocation, lens, partial
ligament, traumatic — *see* Sprain, by site
metacarpal (bone)
proximal end S63.06-
metacarpophalangeal (joint)
finger S63.21-
index S63.21-
little S63.21-
middle S63.21-
ring S63.21-
thumb S63.11-

Subluxation - *continued*
metatarsophalangeal joint S93.14-
great toe S93.14-
lesser toe S93.14-
midcarpal (joint) S63.03-
patella S83.00-
lateral S83.01-
recurrent (nontraumatic) — *see* Dislocation, patella, recurrent, incomplete
specified type NEC S83.09-
pathological — *see* Dislocation, pathological
radial head S53.00-
anterior S53.01-
nursemaid's elbow S53.03-
posterior S53.02-
specified type NEC S53.09-
radiocarpal (joint) S63.02-
radioulnar (joint)
distal S63.01-
proximal — *see* Subluxation, elbow
shoulder
congenital Q68.8
girdle S43.30-
scapula S43.31-
specified site NEC S43.39-
traumatic S43.00-
anterior S43.01-
inferior S43.03-
posterior S43.02-
specified type NEC S43.08-
sternoclavicular (joint) S43.20-
anterior S43.21-
posterior S43.22-
symphysis (pubis)
thumb S63.103
interphalangeal joint — *see* Subluxation, interphalangeal (joint), thumb
metacarpophalangeal joint — *see* Subluxation, metacarpophalangeal (joint), thumb
toe (s) S93.10-
great S93.10-
interphalangeal joint S93.13-
metatarsophalangeal joint S93.14-
interphalangeal joint S93.13-
lesser S93.10-
interphalangeal joint S93.13-
metatarsophalangeal joint S93.14-
metatarsophalangeal joint S93.149
ulnohumeral joint — *see* Subluxation, elbow
vertebral
recurrent NEC — *see* subcategory M43.5
traumatic
cervical S13.100
atlantoaxial joint S13.120
atlantooccipital joint S13.110
atloidooccipital joint S13.110
joint between
C0 and C1 S13.110
C1 and C2 S13.120
C2 and C3 S13.130
C3 and C4 S13.140
C4 and C5 S13.150
C5and C6 S13.160
C6and C7 S13.170
C7and T1 S13.180
occipitoatloid joint S13.110
lumbar S33.100
joint between
L1and L2 S33.110
L2and L3 S33.120
L3 and L4 S33.130
L4and L5 S33.140
thoracic S23.100
joint between
T1and T2 S23.110
T2and T3 S23.120
T3 and T4 S23.122
T4 and T5 S23.130
T5 and T6 S23.132
T6 and T7 S23.140
T7 and T8 S23.142
T8 and T9 S23.150
T9 and T10 S23.152
T10 and T11 S23.160
T11 and T12 S23.162
T12 and L1 S23.170
ulna
distal end S63.07-
proximal end — *see* Subluxation, elbow
wrist (carpal bone) S63.00-
carpometacarpal joint — *see* Subluxation, carpometacarpal (joint)

Swelling (of) - *continued*
arm - *continued*
forearm M79.89
breast — *see also* Lump, breast N63.0
Calabar B74.3
cervical gland R59.0
chest, localized R22.2
ear H93.8-
extremity (lower) (upper) — *see* Disorder, soft tissue, specified type NEC
finger M79.89
foot M79.89
glands R59.9
generalized R59.1
localized R59.0
hand M79.89
head (localized) R22.0
inflammatory — *see* Inflammation
intra-abdominal — *see* Mass, abdominal
joint — *see* Effusion, joint
leg M79.89
lower M79.89
limb — *see* Disorder, soft tissue, specified type NEC
localized (skin) R22.9
chest R22.2
head R22.0
limb
lower — *see* Mass, localized, limb, lower
upper — *see* Mass, localized, limb, upper
neck R22.1
trunk R22.2
neck (localized) R22.1
pelvic — *see* Mass, abdominal
scrotum N50.89
splenic — *see* Splenomegaly
testis N50.89
toe M79.89
umbilical R19.09
wandering, due to Gnathostoma (spinigerum) B83.1
white — *see* Tuberculosis, arthritis
Swift (-Feer) **disease**
overdose or wrong substance given or taken — *see* Table of Drugs and Chemicals, by drug, poisoning
Swimmer's
cramp T75.1
ear H60.33-
itch B65.3
Swimming in the head R42
Swollen — *see* Swelling
Swyer syndrome Q99.1
Sycosis L73.8
barbae (not parasitic) L73.8
contagiosa (mycotic) B35.0
lupoides L73.8
mycotic B35.0
parasitic B35.0
vulgaris L73.8
Sydenham's chorea — *see* Chorea, Sydenham's
Sylvatic yellow fever A95.0
Sylvest's disease B33.0
Symblepharon H11.23-
congenital Q10.3
Symond's syndrome G93.2
Sympathetic — *see* condition
Sympatheticotonia G90.8
Sympathicoblastoma
specified site — *see* Neoplasm, malignant, by site
unspecified site C74.90
Sympathogonioma — *see* Sympathicoblastoma
Symphalangy (fingers) (toes) Q70.9
Symptoms NEC R68.89
breast NEC N64.59
cold J00
development NEC R63.8
factitious, self-induced — *see* Disorder, factitious
genital organs, female R10.2
involving
abdomen NEC R19.8
appearance NEC R46.89
awareness R41.9
altered mental status R41.82
amnesia — *see* Amnesia
borderline intellectual functioning R41.83
coma — *see* Coma
disorientation R41.0
neurologic neglect syndrome R41.4
senile cognitive decline R41.81
specified symptom NEC R41.89
behavior NEC R46.89
cardiovascular system NEC R09.89
chest NEC R09.89
circulatory system NEC R09.89
cognitive functions R41.9

Symptoms NEC - *continued*
involving - *continued*
cognitive functions - *continued*
altered mental status R41.82
amnesia — *see* Amnesia
borderline intellectual functioning R41.83
coma — *see* Coma
disorientation R41.0
neurologic neglect syndrome R41.4
senile cognitive decline R41.81
specified symptom NEC R41.89
development NEC R62.50
digestive system NEC R19.8
emotional state NEC R45.89
emotional lability R45.86
food and fluid intake R63.8
general perceptions and sensations R44.9
specified NEC R44.8
musculoskeletal system R29.91
specified NEC R29.898
nervous system R29.90
specified NEC R29.818
pelvis NEC R19.8
respiratory system NEC R09.89
skin and integument R23.9
urinary system R39.9
menopausal N95.1
metabolism NEC R63.8
neurotic F48.8
of infancy R68.19
pelvis NEC, female R10.2
skin and integument NEC R23.9
subcutaneous tissue NEC R23.9
viral cold J00
Sympus Q74.2
Syncephalus Q89.4
Synchondrosis
abnormal (congenital) Q78.8
ischiopubic M91.0
Synchysis (scintillans) (senile) (vitreous body) H43.89
Syncope (near) (pre-) R55
anginosa I20.8
bradycardia R00.1
cardiac R55
carotid sinus G90.01
due to spinal (lumbar) puncture G97.1
heart R55
heat T67.1
laryngeal R05
psychogenic F48.8
tussive R05
vasoconstriction R55
vasodepressor R55
vasomotor R55
vasovagal R55
Syndactylism, syndactyly Q70.9
complex (with synostosis)
fingers Q70.0-
toes Q70.2-
simple (without synostosis)
fingers Q70.1-
toes Q70.3-
Syndrome — *see also* Disease
5q minus NOS D46.C
48,XXXX Q97.1
49,XXXXX Q97.1
abdominal
acute R10.0
muscle deficiency Q79.4
abnormal innervation H02.519
left H02.516
lower H02.515
upper H02.514
right H02.513
lower H02.512
upper H02.511
abstinence, neonatal P96.1
acid pulmonary aspiration, obstetric O74.0
acquired immunodeficiency — *see* Human, immunodeficiency virus (HIV) disease
acute abdominal R10.0
acute respiratory distress (adult) (child) J80
idiopathic J84.114
Adair-Dighton Q78.0
Adams-Stokes (-Morgagni) I45.9
adiposogenital E23.6
adrenal
hemorrhage (meningococcal) A39.1
meningococcic A39.1
adrenocortical — *see* Cushing's, syndrome
adrenogenital E25.9

Syndrome - *continued*
adrenogenital - *continued*
congenital, associated with enzyme deficiency E25.0
afferent loop NEC K91.89
Alagille's Q44.7
alcohol withdrawal (without convulsions) — *see* Dependence, alcohol, with, withdrawal
Alder's D72.0
Aldrich (-Wiskott) D82.0
alien hand R41.4
Alport Q87.81
alveolar hypoventilation E66.2
alveolocapillary block J84.10
amnesic, amnestic (confabulatory) (due to) — *see* Disorder, amnesic
amyostatic (Wilson's disease) E83.01
androgen insensitivity E34.50
complete E34.51
partial E34.52
androgen resistance — *see also* Syndrome, androgen insensitivity E34.50
Angelman Q93.51
anginal — *see* Angina
ankyloglossia superior Q38.1
anterior
chest wall R07.89
cord G83.82
spinal artery G95.19
compression M47.019
cervical region M47.012
cervicothoracic region M47.013
lumbar region M47.016
occipito-atlanto-axial region M47.011
thoracic region M47.014
thoracolumbar region M47.015
tibial M76.81-
antibody deficiency D80.9
agammaglobulinemic D80.1
hereditary D80.0
congenital D80.0
hypogammaglobulinemic D80.1
hereditary D80.0
anticardiolipin (-antibody) D68.61
antidepressant discontinuation T43.205
antiphospholipid (-antibody) D68.61
aortic
arch M31.4
bifurcation I74.09
aortomesenteric duodenum occlusion K31.5
apical ballooning (transient left ventricular) I51.81
arcuate ligament I77.4
argentaffin, argintaffinoma E34.0
Arnold-Chiari — *see* Arnold-Chiari disease
Arrillaga-Ayerza I27.0
arterial tortuosity Q87.82
arteriovenous steal T82.898-
Asherman's N85.6
aspiration, of newborn — *see* Aspiration, by substance, with pneumonia
meconium P24.01
ataxia-telangiectasia G11.3
auriculotemporal G50.8
autoerythrocyte sensitization (Gardner-Diamond) D69.2
autoimmune polyglandular E31.0
autoimmune lymphoproliferative [ALPS] D89.82
autoinflammatory M04.9
specified type NEC M04.8
autosomal — *see* Abnormal, autosomes
Avellis' G46.8
Ayerza (-Arrillaga) I27.0
Babinski-Nageotte G83.89
Bakwin-Krida Q78.5
bare lymphocyte D81.6
Barré-Guillain G61.0
Barré-Liéou M53.0
Barrett's — *see* Barrett's, esophagus
Barsony-Polgar K22.4
Barsony-Teschendorf K22.4
Barth E78.71
Bartter's E26.81
basal cell nevus Q87.89
Basedow's E05.00
with thyroid storm E05.01
basilar artery G45.0
Batten-Steinert G71.11
battered
baby or child — *see* Maltreatment, child, physical abuse
spouse — *see* Maltreatment, adult, physical abuse
Beals Q87.40
Beau's I51.5

- **Syndrome** - *continued*
  - Beck's I65.8
  - Benedikt's G46.3
  - Béquez César (-Steinbrinck-Chédiak-Higashi) E70.330
  - Bernhardt-Roth — *see* Meralgia paresthetica
  - Bernheim's — *see* Failure, heart, right
  - big spleen D73.1
  - bilateral polycystic ovarian E28.2
  - Bing-Horton's — *see* Horton's headache
  - Birt-Hogg-Dube syndrome Q87.89
  - Björck (-Thorsen) E34.0
  - black
    - lung J60
    - widow spider bite — *see* Toxicity, venom, spider, black widow
  - Blackfan-Diamond D61.01
  - Blau M04.8
  - blind loop K90.2
    - congenital Q43.8
    - postsurgical K91.2
  - blue sclera Q78.0
  - blue toe I75.02-
  - Boder-Sedgewick G11.3
  - Boerhaave's K22.3
  - Borjeson Forssman Lehmann Q89.8
  - Bouillaud's I01.9
  - Bourneville (-Pringle) Q85.1
  - Bouveret (-Hoffman) I47.9
  - brachial plexus G54.0
  - bradycardia-tachycardia I49.5
  - brain (nonpsychotic) F09
    - with psychosis, psychotic reaction F09
    - acute or subacute — *see* Delirium
    - congenital — *see* Disability, intellectual
    - organic F09
      - post-traumatic (nonpsychotic) F07.81
        - psychotic F09
    - personality change F07.0
    - postcontusional F07.81
    - post-traumatic, nonpsychotic F07.81
    - psycho-organic F09
    - psychotic F06.8
  - brain stem stroke G46.3
  - Brandt's (acrodermatitis enteropathica) E83.2
  - broad ligament laceration N83.8
  - Brock's J98.11
  - bronze baby P83.88
  - Brown-Sequard G83.81
  - Brugada I49.8
  - bubbly lung P27.0
  - Buchem's M85.2
  - Budd-Chiari I82.0
  - bulbar (progressive) G12.22
  - Bürger-Grütz E78.3
  - Burke's K86.89
  - Burnett's (milk-alkali) E83.52
  - burning feet E53.9
  - Bywaters' T79.5
  - Call-Fleming I67.841
  - carbohydrate-deficient glycoprotein (CDGS) E77.8
  - carcinogenic thrombophlebitis I82.1
  - carcinoid E34.0
  - cardiac asthma I50.1
  - cardiacos negros I27.0
  - cardiofaciocutaneous Q87.89
  - cardiopulmonary-obesity E66.2
  - cardiorenal — *see* Hypertension, cardiorenal
  - cardiorespiratory distress (idiopathic) , newborn P22.0
  - cardiovascular renal — *see* Hypertension, cardiorenal
  - carotid
    - artery (hemispheric) (internal) G45.1
    - body G90.01
    - sinus G90.01
  - carpal tunnel G56.0-
  - Cassidy (-Scholte) E34.0
  - cat cry Q93.4
  - cat eye Q92.8
  - cauda equina G83.4
  - causalgia — *see* Causalgia
  - celiac K90.0
    - artery compression I77.4
    - axis I77.4
  - central pain G89.0
  - cerebellar
    - hereditary G11.9
    - stroke G46.4
  - cerebellomedullary malformation — *see* Spina bifida
  - cerebral
    - artery

- **Syndrome** - *continued*
  - cerebral - *continued*
    - artery - *continued*
      - anterior G46.1
      - middle G46.0
      - posterior G46.2
    - gigantism E22.0
  - cervical (root) M53.1
    - disc — *see* Disorder, disc, cervical, with neuritis
    - fusion Q76.1
    - posterior, sympathicus M53.0
    - rib Q76.5
    - sympathetic paralysis G90.2
  - cervicobrachial (diffuse) M53.1
  - cervicocranial M53.0
  - cervicodorsal outlet G54.2
  - cervicothoracic outlet G54.0
  - Céstan (-Raymond) I65.8
  - Charcot's (angina cruris) (intermittent claudication) I73.9
  - Charcot-Weiss-Baker G90.09
  - CHARGE Q89.8
  - Chédiak-Higashi (-Steinbrinck) E70.330
  - chest wall R07.1
  - Chiari's (hepatic vein thrombosis) I82.0
  - Chilaiditi's Q43.3
  - child maltreatment — *see* Maltreatment, child
  - chondrocostal junction M94.0
  - chondroectodermal dysplasia Q77.6
  - chromosome 4 short arm deletion Q93.3
  - chromosome 5 short arm deletion Q93.4
  - chronic
    - infantile neurological, cutaneous and articular (CINCA) M04.2
    - pain G89.4
      - personality F68.8
  - Clarke-Hadfield K86.89
  - Clerambault's automatism G93.89
  - Clouston's (hidrotic ectodermal dysplasia) Q82.4
  - clumsiness, clumsy child F82
  - cluster headache G44.009
    - intractable G44.001
    - not intractable G44.009
  - Coffin-Lowry Q89.8
  - cold injury (newborn) P80.0
  - combined immunity deficiency D81.9
  - compartment (deep) (posterior) (traumatic) T79.A0
    - abdomen T79.A3
    - lower extremity (hip, buttock, thigh, leg, foot, toes) T79.A2
    - nontraumatic
      - abdomen M79.A3
      - lower extremity (hip, buttock, thigh, leg, foot, toes) M79.A2-
      - specified site NEC M79.A9
      - upper extremity (shoulder, arm, forearm, wrist, hand, fingers) M79.A1-
    - postprocedural — *see* Syndrome, compartment, nontraumatic
    - specified site NEC T79.A9
    - upper extremity (shoulder, arm, forearm, wrist, hand, fingers) T79.A1
  - complex regional pain — *see* Syndrome, pain, complex regional
  - compression T79.5
    - anterior spinal — *see* Syndrome, anterior, spinal artery, compression
    - cauda equina G83.4
    - celiac artery I77.4
    - vertebral artery M47.029
      - occipito-atlanto-axial region M47.021
      - cervical region M47.022
  - concussion F07.81
  - congenital
    - affecting multiple systems NEC Q87.89
    - central alveolar hypoventilation G47.35
    - facial diplegia Q87.0
    - muscular hypertrophy-cerebral Q87.89
    - oculo-auriculovertebral Q87.0
    - oculofacial diplegia (Moebius) Q87.0
    - rubella (manifest) P35.0
  - congestion-fibrosis (pelvic) , female N94.89
  - congestive dysmenorrhea N94.6
  - Conn's E26.01
  - connective tissue M35.9
    - overlap NEC M35.1
  - conus medullaris G95.81
  - cord
    - anterior G83.82
    - posterior G83.83
  - coronary
    - acute NEC I24.9
    - insufficiency or intermediate I20.0

- **Syndrome** - *continued*
  - coronary - *continued*
    - slow flow I20.8
  - Costen's (complex) M26.69
  - costochondral junction M94.0
  - costoclavicular G54.0
  - costovertebral E22.0
  - Cowden Q85.8
  - craniovertebral M53.0
  - Creutzfeldt-Jakob — *see* Creutzfeldt-Jakob disease or syndrome
  - cri-du-chat Q93.4
  - crib death R99
  - cricopharyngeal — *see* Dysphagia
  - croup J05.0
  - CRPS I — *see* Syndrome, pain, complex regional I
  - crush T79.5
  - cubital tunnel — *see* Lesion, nerve, ulnar
  - Curschmann (-Batten) (-Steinert) G71.11
  - Cushing's E24.9
    - alcohol-induced E24.4
    - due to
      - alcohol
      - drugs E24.2
      - ectopic ACTH E24.3
      - overproduction of pituitary ACTH E24.0
    - drug-induced E24.2
    - overdose or wrong substance given or taken — *see* Table of Drugs and Chemicals, by drug, poisoning
    - pituitary-dependent E24.0
    - specified type NEC E24.8
  - cryopyrin-associated periodic M04.2
  - cryptophthalmos Q87.0
  - cystic duct stump K91.5
  - Dana-Putnam D51.0
  - Danbolt (-Cross) (acrodermatitis enteropathica) E83.2
  - Dandy-Walker Q03.1
    - with spina bifida Q07.01
  - Danlos' Q79.6
  - defibrination — *see also* Fibrinolysis
    - with
      - antepartum hemorrhage — *see* Hemorrhage, antepartum, with coagulation defect
      - intrapartum hemorrhage — *see* Hemorrhage, complicating, delivery
    - newborn P60
    - postpartum O72.3
  - Degos' I77.89
  - Déjérine-Roussy G89.0
  - delayed sleep phase G47.21
  - demyelinating G37.9
  - dependence — *see* F10-F19 with fourth character .2
  - depersonalization (-derealization) F48.1
  - De Quervain E34.51
  - de Toni-Fanconi (-Debré) E72.09
    - with cystinosis E72.04
  - diabetes mellitus-hypertension-nephrosis — *see* Diabetes, nephrosis
  - diabetes mellitus in newborn infant P70.2
  - diabetes-nephrosis — *see* Diabetes, nephrosis
  - diabetic amyotrophy — *see* Diabetes, amyotrophy
  - dialysis associated steal T82.898-
  - Diamond-Blackfan D61.01
  - Diamond-Gardener D69.2
  - DIC (diffuse or disseminated intravascular coagulopathy) D65
  - di George's D82.1
  - Dighton's Q78.0
  - disequilibrium E87.8
  - Döhle body-panmyelopathic D72.0
  - dorsolateral medullary G46.4
  - double athetosis G80.3
  - Down — *see also* Down syndrome Q90.9
  - Dresbach's (elliptocytosis) D58.1
  - Dressler's (postmyocardial infarction) I24.1
    - postcardiotomy I97.0
  - drug withdrawal, infant of dependent mother P96.1
  - dry eye H04.12-
  - due to abnormality
    - chromosomal Q99.9
      - sex
        - female phenotype Q97.9
        - male phenotype Q98.9
      - specified NEC Q99.8
  - dumping (postgastrectomy) K91.1
    - nonsurgical K31.89
  - Dupré's (meningism) R29.1
  - dysmetabolic X E88.81
  - dyspraxia, developmental F82
  - Eagle-Barrett Q79.4
  - Eaton-Lambert — *see* Syndrome, Lambert-Eaton

Syndrome - *continued*
- trisomy - *continued*
  - 21 - *continued*
    - meiotic nondisjunction Q90.0
    - mitotic nondisjunction Q90.1
    - mosaicism Q90.1
    - translocation Q90.2
  - 22 Q92.8
- tropical wet feet T69.0-
- Trousseau's I82.1
- tumor lysis (following antineoplastic chemotherapy) (spontaneous) NEC E88.3
- tumor necrosis factor receptor associated periodic (TRAPS) M04.1
- Twiddler's (due to)
  - automatic implantable defibrillator T82.198
  - cardiac pacemaker T82.198
- Unverricht (-Lundborg) — *see* Epilepsy, generalized, idiopathic
- upward gaze H51.8
- uremia, chronic — *see also* Disease, kidney, chronic N18.9
- urethral N34.3
- urethro-oculo-articular — *see* Reiter's disease
- urohepatic K76.7
- vago-hypoglossal G52.7
- vascular NEC in cerebrovascular disease G46.8
- vasoconstriction, reversible cerebrovascular I67.841
- vasomotor I73.9
- vasospastic (traumatic) T75.22
- vasovagal R55
- van Buchem's M85.2
- van der Hoeve's Q78.0
- VATER Q87.2
- velo-cardio-facial Q93.81
- vena cava (inferior) (superior) (obstruction) I87.1
- vertebral
  - artery G45.0
    - compression — *see* Syndrome, anterior, spinal artery, compression
  - steal G45.0
- vertebro-basilar artery G45.0
- vertebrogenic (pain) M54.89
- vertiginous — *see* Disorder, vestibular function
- Vinson-Plummer D50.1
- virus B34.9
- visceral larva migrans B83.0
- visual disorientation H53.8
- vitamin B6 deficiency E53.1
- vitreal corneal H59.01-
- vitreous (touch) H59.01-
- Vogt-Koyanagi H20.82-
- Volkmann's T79.6
- von Schroetter's I82.890
- von Willebrand (-Jürgen) D68.0
- Waldenström-Kjellberg D50.1
- Wallenberg's G46.3
- water retention E87.79
- Waterhouse (-Friderichsen) A39.1
- Weber-Gubler G46.3
- Weber-Leyden G46.3
- Weber's G46.3
- Wegener's M31.30
  - with
    - kidney involvement M31.31
    - lung involvement M31.30
      - with kidney involvement M31.31
- Weingarten's (tropical eosinophilia) J82
- Weiss-Baker G90.09
- Werdnig-Hoffman G12.0
- Wermer's E31.21
- Werner's E34.8
- Wernicke-Korsakoff (nonalcoholic) F04
  - alcoholic F10.26
- West's — *see* Epilepsy, spasms
- Westphal-Strümpell E83.01
- wet
  - feet (maceration) (tropical) T69.0-
  - lung, newborn P22.1
- whiplash S13.4
- whistling face Q87.0
- Wilkie's K55.1
- Wilkinson-Sneddon L13.1
- Williams Q93.82
- Willebrand (-Jürgens) D68.0
- Wilson's (hepatolenticular degeneration) E83.01
- Wiskott-Aldrich D82.0
- withdrawal — *see* Withdrawal, state
  - drug
    - infant of dependent mother P96.1
    - therapeutic use, newborn P96.2
- Woakes' (ethmoiditis) J33.1
- Wright's (hyperabduction) G54.0

Syndrome - *continued*
- X I20.9
- XXXX Q97.1
- XXXXX Q97.1
- XXXXY Q98.1
- XXY Q98.0
- Yao M04.8
- yellow nail L60.5
- Zahorsky's B08.5
- Zellweger syndrome E71.510
- Zellweger-like syndrome E71.541

Synechia (anterior) (iris) (posterior) (pupil) — *see also* Adhesions, iris
- intra-uterine (traumatic) N85.6

Synesthesia R20.8

Syngamiasis, syngamosis B83.3

Synodontia K00.2

Synorchidism, synorchism Q55.1

Synostosis (congenital) Q78.8
- astragalo-scaphoid Q74.2
- radioulnar Q74.0

Synovial sarcoma — *see* Neoplasm, connective tissue, malignant

Synovioma (malignant) — *see also* Neoplasm, connective tissue, malignant
- benign — *see* Neoplasm, connective tissue, benign

Synoviosarcoma — *see* Neoplasm, connective tissue, malignant

Synovitis — *see also* Tenosynovitis M65.9
- crepitant
  - hand M70.0-
  - wrist M70.03-
- gonococcal A54.49
- gouty — *see* Gout
- in (due to)
  - crystals M65.8-
  - gonorrhea A54.49
  - syphilis (late) A52.78
  - use, overuse, pressure — *see* Disorder, soft tissue, due to use
- infective NEC — *see* Tenosynovitis, infective NEC
- specified NEC — *see* Tenosynovitis, specified type NEC
- syphilitic A52.78
  - congenital (early) A50.02
- toxic — *see* Synovitis, transient
- transient M67.3-
  - ankle M67.37-
  - elbow M67.32-
  - foot joint M67.37-
  - hand joint M67.34-
  - hip M67.35-
  - knee M67.36-
  - multiple site M67.39
  - pelvic region M67.35-
  - shoulder M67.31-
  - specified joint NEC M67.38
  - wrist M67.33-
- traumatic, current — *see* Sprain
- tuberculous — *see* Tuberculosis, synovitis
- villonodular (pigmented) M12.2-
  - ankle M12.27-
  - elbow M12.22-
  - foot joint M12.27-
  - hand joint M12.24-
  - hip M12.25-
  - knee M12.26-
  - multiple site M12.29
  - pelvic region M12.25-
  - shoulder M12.21-
  - specified joint NEC M12.28
  - vertebrae M12.28
  - wrist M12.23-

Syphilid A51.39
- congenital A50.06
- newborn A50.06
- tubercular (late) A52.79

Syphilis, syphilitic (acquired) A53.9
- abdomen (late) A52.79
- acoustic nerve A52.15
- adenopathy (secondary) A51.49
- adrenal (gland) (with cortical hypofunction) A52.79
- age under 2 years NOS — *see also* Syphilis, congenital, early
  - acquired A51.9
- alopecia (secondary) A51.32
- anemia (late) A52.79 *[D63.8]*
- aneurysm (aorta) (ruptured) A52.01
  - central nervous system A52.05
  - congenital A50.54 *[I79.0]*
- anus (late) A52.74
  - primary A51.1
  - secondary A51.39

Syphilis, syphilitic (acquired) - *continued*
- aorta (arch) (abdominal) (thoracic) A52.02
  - aneurysm A52.01
- aortic (insufficiency) (regurgitation) (stenosis) A52.03
  - aneurysm A52.01
- arachnoid (adhesive) (cerebral) (spinal) A52.13
- asymptomatic — *see* Syphilis, latent
- ataxia (locomotor) A52.11
- atrophoderma maculatum A51.39
- auricular fibrillation A52.06
- bladder (late) A52.76
- bone A52.77
  - secondary A51.46
- brain A52.17
- breast (late) A52.79
- bronchus (late) A52.72
- bubo (primary) A51.0
- bulbar palsy A52.19
- bursa (late) A52.78
- cardiac decompensation A52.06
- cardiovascular A52.00
- central nervous system (late) (recurrent) (relapse) (tertiary) A52.3
  - with
    - ataxia A52.11
    - general paralysis A52.17
      - juvenile A50.45
    - paresis (general) A52.17
      - juvenile A50.45
    - tabes (dorsalis) A52.11
      - juvenile A50.45
    - taboparesis A52.17
      - juvenile A50.45
  - aneurysm A52.05
  - congenital A50.40
  - juvenile A50.40
  - remission in (sustained) A52.3
  - serology doubtful, negative, or positive A52.3
  - specified nature or site NEC A52.19
  - vascular A52.05
- cerebral A52.17
  - meningovascular A52.13
  - nerves (multiple palsies) A52.15
  - sclerosis A52.17
  - thrombosis A52.05
- cerebrospinal (tabetic type) A52.12
- cerebrovascular A52.05
- cervix (late) A52.76
- chancre (multiple) A51.0
  - extragenital A51.2
  - Rollet's A51.0
- Charcot's joint A52.16
- chorioretinitis A51.43
  - congenital A50.01
  - late A52.71
  - prenatal A50.01
- choroiditis — *see* Syphilitic chorioretinitis
- choroidoretinitis — *see* Syphilitic chorioretinitis
- ciliary body (secondary) A51.43
  - late A52.71
- colon (late) A52.74
- combined spinal sclerosis A52.11
- condyloma (latum) A51.31
- congenital A50.9
  - with
    - paresis (general) A50.45
    - tabes (dorsalis) A50.45
    - taboparesis A50.45
  - chorioretinitis, choroiditis A50.01 *[H32]*
  - early, or less than 2 years after birth NEC A50.2
    - with manifestations — *see* Syphilis, congenital, early, symptomatic
    - latent (without manifestations) A50.1
      - negative spinal fluid test A50.1
      - serology positive A50.1
    - symptomatic A50.09
      - cutaneous A50.06
      - mucocutaneous A50.07
      - oculopathy A50.01
      - osteochondropathy A50.02
      - pharyngitis A50.03
      - pneumonia A50.04
      - rhinitis A50.05
      - visceral A50.08
  - interstitial keratitis A50.31
  - juvenile neurosyphilis A50.45
  - late, or 2 years or more after birth NEC A50.7
    - chorioretinitis, choroiditis A50.32
    - interstitial keratitis A50.31
    - juvenile neurosyphilis A50.45
    - latent (without manifestations) A50.6
      - negative spinal fluid test A50.6

Syphilis, syphilitic (acquired) - *continued*
seropositive
with signs or symptoms - code by site and stage under Syphilis
follow-up of latent syphilis — *see* Syphilis, latent
only finding — *see* Syphilis, latent
seventh nerve (paralysis) A52.15
sinus, sinusitis (late) A52.73
skeletal system A52.77
skin (with ulceration) (early) (secondary) A51.39
late or tertiary A52.79
small intestine A52.74
spastic spinal paralysis A52.17
spermatic cord (late) A52.76
spinal (cord) A52.12
spleen A52.79
splenomegaly A52.79
spondylitis A52.77
staphyloma A52.71
stigmata (congenital) A50.59
stomach A52.74
synovium A52.78
tabes dorsalis (late) A52.11
juvenile A50.45
tabetic type A52.11
juvenile A50.45
taboparesis A52.17
juvenile A50.45
tachycardia A52.06
tendon (late) A52.78
tertiary A52.9
with symptoms NEC A52.79
cardiovascular A52.00
central nervous system A52.3
multiple NEC A52.79
specified site NEC A52.79
testis A52.76
thorax A52.73
throat A52.73
thymus (gland) (late) A52.79
thyroid (late) A52.79
tongue (late) A52.79
tonsil (lingual) (late) A52.73
primary A51.2
secondary A51.39
trachea (late) A52.73
tunica vaginalis (late) A52.76
ulcer (any site) (early) (secondary) A51.39
late A52.79
perforating A52.79
foot A52.11
urethra (late) A52.76
urogenital (late) A52.76
uterus (late) A52.76
uveal tract (secondary) A51.43
late A52.71
uveitis (secondary) A51.43
late A52.71
uvula (late) (perforated) A52.79
vagina A51.0
late A52.76
valvulitis NEC A52.03
vascular A52.00
brain (cerebral) A52.05
ventriculi A52.74
vesicae urinariae (late) A52.76
viscera (abdominal) (late) A52.74
secondary A51.49
vitreous (opacities) (late) A52.71
hemorrhage A52.71
vulva A51.0
late A52.76
secondary A51.39
Syphiloma A52.79
cardiovascular system A52.00
central nervous system A52.3
circulatory system A52.00
congenital A50.59
Syphilophobia F45.29
Syringadenoma — *see also* Neoplasm, skin, benign
papillary — *see* Neoplasm, skin, benign
Syringobulbia G95.0
Syringocystadenoma — *see* Neoplasm, skin, benign
papillary — *see* Neoplasm, skin, benign
Syringoma — *see also* Neoplasm, skin, benign
chondroid — *see* Neoplasm, skin, benign
Syringomyelia G95.0
Syringomyelitis — *see* Encephalitis
Syringomyelocele — *see* Spina bifida
Syringopontia G95.0
System, systemic — *see also* condition
disease, combined — *see* Degeneration, combined

System, systemic - *continued*
inflammatory response syndrome (SIRS) of non-infectious origin (without organ dysfunction) R65.10
with acute organ dysfunction R65.11
lupus erythematosus M32.9
inhibitor present D68.62

T

Tabacism, tabacosis, tabagism — *see also* Poisoning, tobacco
meaning dependence (without remission) F17.200
with
disorder F17.299
in remission F17.211
specified disorder NEC F17.298
withdrawal F17.203
Tabardillo A75.9
flea-borne A75.2
louse-borne A75.0
Tabes, tabetic A52.10
with
central nervous system syphilis A52.10
Charcot's joint A52.16
cord bladder A52.19
crisis, viscera (any) A52.19
paralysis, general A52.17
paresis (general) A52.17
perforating ulcer (foot) A52.19
arthropathy (Charcot) A52.16
bladder A52.19
bone A52.11
cerebrospinal A52.12
congenital A50.45
conjugal A52.10
dorsalis A52.11
juvenile A50.49
juvenile A50.49
latent A52.19
mesenterica A18.39
paralysis, insane, general A52.17
spasmodic A52.17
syphilis (cerebrospinal) A52.12
Taboparalysis A52.17
Taboparesis (remission) A52.17
juvenile A50.45
TAC (trigeminal autonomic cephalgia) **NEC** G44.099
intractable G44.091
not intractable G44.099
Tache noir S60.22-
Tachyalimentation K91.2
Tachyarrhythmia, tachyrhythmia — *see* Tachycardia
Tachycardia R00.0
atrial (paroxysmal) I47.1
auricular I47.1
AV nodal re-entry (re-entrant) I47.1
junctional (paroxysmal) I47.1
newborn P29.11
nodal (paroxysmal) I47.1
non-paroxysmal AV nodal I45.89
paroxysmal (sustained) (nonsustained) I47.9
with sinus bradycardia I49.5
atrial (PAT) I47.1
atrioventricular (AV) (re-entrant) I47.1
psychogenic F54
junctional I47.1
ectopic I47.1
nodal I47.1
psychogenic (atrial) (supraventricular) (ventricular) F54
supraventricular (sustained) I47.1
psychogenic F54
ventricular I47.2
psychogenic F54
psychogenic F45.8
sick sinus I49.5
sinoauricular NOS R00.0
paroxysmal I47.1
sinus [sinusal] NOS R00.0
paroxysmal I47.1
supraventricular I47.1
ventricular (paroxysmal) (sustained) I47.2
psychogenic F54
Tachygastria K31.89
Tachypnea R06.82
hysterical F45.8
newborn (idiopathic) (transitory) P22.1
psychogenic F45.8
transitory, of newborn P22.1
TACO (transfusion associated circulatory overload) E87.71

Taenia (infection) (infestation) B68.9
diminuta B71.0
echinococcal infestation B67.90
mediocanellata B68.1
nana B71.0
saginata B68.1
solium (intestinal form) B68.0
larval form — *see* Cysticercosis
Taeniasis (intestine) — *see* Taenia
Tag (hypertrophied skin) (infected) L91.8
adenoid J35.8
anus K64.4
hemorrhoidal K64.4
hymen N89.8
perineal N90.89
preauricular Q17.0
sentinel K64.4
skin L91.8
accessory (congenital) Q82.8
anus K64.4
congenital Q82.8
preauricular Q17.0
tonsil J35.8
urethra, urethral N36.8
vulva N90.89
Tahyna fever B33.8
Takahara's disease E80.3
Takayasu's disease or syndrome M31.4
Talcosis (pulmonary) J62.0
Talipes (congenital) Q66.89
acquired, planus — *see* Deformity, limb, flat foot
asymmetric Q66.89
calcaneovalgus Q66.4
calcaneovarus Q66.1
calcaneus Q66.89
cavus Q66.7
equinovalgus Q66.6
equinovarus Q66.0
equinus Q66.89
percavus Q66.7
planovalgus Q66.6
planus (acquired) (any degree) — *see also* Deformity, limb, flat foot
congenital Q66.5-
due to rickets (sequelae) E64.3
valgus Q66.6
varus Q66.3
Tall stature, constitutional E34.4
Talma's disease M62.89
Talon noir S90.3-
hand S60.22-
heel S90.3-
toe S90.1-
Tamponade, heart I31.4
Tanapox (virus disease) B08.71
Tangier disease E78.6
Tantrum, child problem F91.8
Tapeworm (infection) (infestation) — *see* Infestation, tapeworm
Tapia's syndrome G52.7
TAR (thrombocytopenia with absent radius) **syndrome** Q87.2
Tarral-Besnier disease L44.0
Tarsal tunnel syndrome — *see* Syndrome, tarsal tunnel
Tarsalgia — *see* Pain, limb, lower
Tarsitis (eyelid) H01.8
syphilitic A52.71
tuberculous A18.4
Tartar (teeth) (dental calculus) K03.6
Tattoo (mark) L81.8
Tauri's disease E74.09
Taurodontism K00.2
Taussig-Bing syndrome Q20.1
Taybi's syndrome Q87.2
Tay-Sachs amaurotic familial idiocy or disease E75.02
TBI (traumatic brain injury) S06.9
Teacher's node or nodule J38.2
Tear, torn (traumatic) — *see also* Laceration
with abortion — *see* Abortion
annular fibrosis M51.35
anus, anal (sphincter) S31.831
complicating delivery
with third degree perineal laceration — *see also* Delivery, complicated, by, laceration, perineum, third degree O70.20
with mucosa O70.3
without third degree perineal laceration O70.4
nontraumatic (healed) (old) K62.81
articular cartilage, old — *see* Derangement, joint, articular cartilage, by site
bladder

Tear, torn (traumatic) - *continued*
bladder - *continued*
with ectopic or molar pregnancy O08.6
following ectopic or molar pregnancy O08.6
obstetrical O71.5
traumatic — *see* Injury, bladder
bowel
with ectopic or molar pregnancy O08.6
following ectopic or molar pregnancy O08.6
obstetrical trauma O71.5
broad ligament
with ectopic or molar pregnancy O08.6
following ectopic or molar pregnancy O08.6
obstetrical trauma O71.6
bucket handle (knee) (meniscus) — *see* Tear, meniscus
capsule, joint — *see* Sprain
cartilage — *see also* Sprain
articular, old — *see* Derangement, joint, articular cartilage, by site
cervix
with ectopic or molar pregnancy O08.6
following ectopic or molar pregnancy O08.6
obstetrical trauma (current) O71.3
old N88.1
traumatic — *see* Injury, uterus
dural G97.41
nontraumatic G96.11
internal organ — *see* Injury, by site
knee cartilage
articular (current) S83.3-
old — *see* Derangement, knee, meniscus, due to old tear
ligament — *see* Sprain
meniscus (knee) (current injury) S83.209
bucket-handle S83.20-
lateral
bucket-handle S83.25-
complex S83.27-
peripheral S83.26-
specified type NEC S83.28-
medial
bucket-handle S83.21-
complex S83.23-
peripheral S83.22-
specified type NEC S83.24-
old — *see* Derangement, knee, meniscus, due to old tear
site other than knee - code as Sprain
specified type NEC S83.20-
muscle — *see* Strain
pelvic
floor, complicating delivery O70.1
organ NEC, obstetrical trauma O71.5
with ectopic or molar pregnancy O08.6
following ectopic or molar pregnancy O08.6
perineal, secondary O90.1
periurethral tissue, obstetrical trauma O71.82
with ectopic or molar pregnancy O08.6
following ectopic or molar pregnancy O08.6
rectovaginal septum — *see* Laceration, vagina
retina, retinal (without detachment) (horseshoe) — *see also* Break, retina, horseshoe
with detachment — *see* Detachment, retina, with retinal, break
rotator cuff (nontraumatic) M75.10-
complete M75.12-
incomplete M75.11-
traumatic S46.01-
capsule S43.42-
semilunar cartilage, knee — *see* Tear, meniscus
supraspinatus (complete) (incomplete) (nontraumatic) — *see also* Tear, rotator cuff M75.10-
tendon — *see* Strain
tentorial, at birth P10.4
umbilical cord
complicating delivery O69.89
urethra
with ectopic or molar pregnancy O08.6
following ectopic or molar pregnancy O08.6
obstetrical trauma O71.5
uterus — *see* Injury, uterus
vagina — *see* Laceration, vagina
vessel, from catheter — *see* Puncture, accidental complicating surgery
vulva, complicating delivery O70.0
Tear-stone — *see* Dacryolith
Teeth — *see also* condition
grinding
psychogenic F45.8
sleep related G47.63
Teething (syndrome) K00.7
Telangiectasia, telangiectasis (verrucous) I78.1
ataxic (cerebellar) (Louis-Bar) G11.3
familial I78.0
hemorrhagic, hereditary (congenital) (senile) I78.0
hereditary, hemorrhagic (congenital) (senile) I78.0
juxtafoveal H35.07-
macular H35.07-
macularis eruptiva perstans D47.01
parafoveal H35.07-
retinal (idiopathic) (juxtafoveal) (macular) (parafoveal) H35.07-
spider I78.1
Telephone scatologia F65.89
Telescoped bowel or intestine K56.1
congenital Q43.8
Temperature
body, high (of unknown origin) R50.9
cold, trauma from T69.9
newborn P80.0
specified effect NEC T69.8
Temple — *see* condition
Temporal — *see* condition
Temporomandibular joint pain-dysfunction syndrome M26.62-
Temporosphenoidal — *see* condition
Tendency
bleeding — *see* Defect, coagulation
suicide
meaning personal history of attempted suicide Z91.5
meaning suicidal ideation — *see* Ideation, suicidal
to fall R29.6
Tenderness, abdominal R10.819
epigastric R10.816
generalized R10.817
left lower quadrant R10.814
left upper quadrant R10.812
periumbilic R10.815
right lower quadrant R10.813
right upper quadrant R10.811
rebound R10.829
epigastric R10.826
generalized R10.827
left lower quadrant R10.824
left upper quadrant R10.822
periumbilic R10.825
right lower quadrant R10.823
right upper quadrant R10.821
Tendinitis, tendonitis — *see also* Enthesopathy
Achilles M76.6-
adhesive — *see* Tenosynovitis, specified type NEC
shoulder — *see* Capsulitis, adhesive
bicipital M75.2-
calcific M65.2-
ankle M65.27-
foot M65.27-
forearm M65.23-
hand M65.24-
lower leg M65.26-
multiple sites M65.29
pelvic region M65.25-
shoulder M75.3-
specified site NEC M65.28
thigh M65.25-
upper arm M65.22-
due to use, overuse, pressure — *see also* Disorder, soft tissue, due to use
specified NEC — *see* Disorder, soft tissue, due to use, specified NEC
gluteal M76.0-
patellar M76.5-
peroneal M76.7-
psoas M76.1-
tibial (posterior) M76.82-
anterior M76.81-
trochanteric — *see* Bursitis, hip, trochanteric
Tendon — *see* condition
Tendosynovitis — *see* Tenosynovitis
Tenesmus (rectal) R19.8
vesical R30.1
Tennis elbow — *see* Epicondylitis, lateral
Tenonitis — *see also* Tenosynovitis
eye (capsule) H05.04-
Tenontosynovitis — *see* Tenosynovitis
Tenontothecitis — *see* Tenosynovitis
Tenophyte — *see* Disorder, synovium, specified type NEC
Tenosynovitis — *see also* Synovitis M65.9
adhesive — *see* Tenosynovitis, specified type NEC
shoulder — *see* Capsulitis, adhesive
bicipital (calcifying) — *see* Tendinitis, bicipital
gonococcal A54.49
in (due to)
Tenosynovitis - *continued*
in (due to) - *continued*
crystals M65.8-
gonorrhea A54.49
syphilis (late) A52.78
use, overuse, pressure — *see also* Disorder, soft tissue, due to use
specified NEC — *see* Disorder, soft tissue, due to use, specified NEC
infective NEC M65.1-
ankle M65.17-
foot M65.17-
forearm M65.13-
hand M65.14-
lower leg M65.16-
multiple sites M65.19
pelvic region M65.15-
shoulder region M65.11-
specified site NEC M65.18
thigh M65.15-
upper arm M65.12-
radial styloid M65.4
shoulder region M65.81-
adhesive — *see* Capsulitis, adhesive
specified type NEC M65.88
ankle M65.87-
foot M65.87-
forearm M65.83-
hand M65.84-
lower leg M65.86-
multiple sites M65.89
pelvic region M65.85-
shoulder region M65.81-
specified site NEC M65.88
thigh M65.85-
upper arm M65.82-
tuberculous — *see* Tuberculosis, tenosynovitis
Tenovaginitis — *see* Tenosynovitis
Tension
arterial, high — *see also* Hypertension
without diagnosis of hypertension R03.0
headache G44.209
intractable G44.201
not intractable G44.209
nervous R45.0
pneumothorax J93.0
premenstrual N94.3
state (mental) F48.9
Tentorium — *see* condition
Teratencephalus Q89.8
Teratism Q89.7
Teratoblastoma (malignant) — *see* Neoplasm, malignant, by site
Teratocarcinoma — *see also* Neoplasm, malignant, by site
liver C22.7
Teratoma (solid) — *see also* Neoplasm, uncertain behavior, by site
with embryonal carcinoma, mixed — *see* Neoplasm, malignant, by site
with malignant transformation — *see* Neoplasm, malignant, by site
adult (cystic) — *see* Neoplasm, benign, by site
benign — *see* Neoplasm, benign, by site
combined with choriocarcinoma — *see* Neoplasm, malignant, by site
cystic (adult) — *see* Neoplasm, benign, by site
differentiated — *see* Neoplasm, benign, by site
embryonal — *see also* Neoplasm, malignant, by site
liver C22.7
immature — *see* Neoplasm, malignant, by site
liver C22.7
adult, benign, cystic, differentiated type or mature D13.4
malignant — *see also* Neoplasm, malignant, by site
anaplastic — *see* Neoplasm, malignant, by site
intermediate — *see* Neoplasm, malignant, by site
specified site — *see* Neoplasm, malignant, by site
unspecified site C62.90
undifferentiated — *see* Neoplasm, malignant, by site
mature — *see* Neoplasm, uncertain behavior, by site
malignant — *see* Neoplasm, by site, malignant, by site
ovary D27.-
embryonal, immature or malignant C56-
solid — *see* Neoplasm, uncertain behavior, by site
testis C62.9-
adult, benign, cystic, differentiated type or mature D29.2-
scrotal C62.1-
undescended C62.0-

Termination
- anomalous — *see also* Malposition, congenital
  - right pulmonary vein Q26.3
- pregnancy, elective Z33.2

Ternidens diminutus infestation B81.8
Ternidensiasis B81.8
Terror (s) **night** (child) F51.4
Terrorism, victim of Z65.4
Terry's syndrome — *see also* Myopia, degenerative H44.2-
Tertiary — *see* condition
Test, tests, testing (for)
- adequacy (for dialysis)
  - hemodialysis Z49.31
  - peritoneal Z49.32
- blood pressure Z01.30
  - abnormal reading — *see* Blood, pressure
- blood-alcohol Z04.89
  - positive — *see* Findings, abnormal, in blood
- blood-drug Z04.89
  - positive — *see* Findings, abnormal, in blood
- blood typing Z01.83
  - Rh typing Z01.83
- cardiac pulse generator (battery) Z45.010
- fertility Z31.41
- genetic
  - disease carrier status for procreative management
    - female Z31.430
    - male Z31.440
  - male partner of patient with recurrent pregnancy loss Z31.441
  - procreative management NEC
    - female Z31.438
    - male Z31.448
- hearing Z01.10
  - with abnormal findings NEC Z01.118
  - infant or child (over 28 days old) Z00.129
    - with abnormal findings Z00.121
- HIV (human immunodeficiency virus)
  - nonconclusive (in infants) R75
  - positive Z21
  - seropositive Z21
- immunity status Z01.84
- intelligence NEC Z01.89
- laboratory (as part of a general medical examination) Z00.00
  - with abnormal finding Z00.01
  - for medicolegal reason NEC Z04.89
- male partner of patient with recurrent pregnancy loss Z31.441
- Mantoux (for tuberculosis) Z11.1
  - abnormal result R76.11
- pregnancy, positive first pregnancy — *see* Pregnancy, normal, first
- procreative Z31.49
  - fertility Z31.41
- skin, diagnostic
  - allergy Z01.82
    - special screening examination — *see* Screening, by name of disease
  - Mantoux Z11.1
  - tuberculin Z11.1
- specified NEC Z01.89
- tuberculin Z11.1
  - abnormal result R76.11
- vision Z01.00
  - with abnormal findings Z01.01
  - infant or child (over 28 days old) Z00.129
    - with abnormal findings Z00.121
- Wassermann Z11.3
  - positive — *see* Serology for syphilis, positive

Testicle, testicular, testis — *see also* condition
- feminization syndrome — *see also* Syndrome, androgen insensitivity E34.51
- migrans Q55.29

Tetanus, tetanic (cephalic) (convulsions) A35
- with
  - abortion A34
  - ectopic or molar pregnancy O08.0
- following ectopic or molar pregnancy O08.0
- inoculation reaction (due to serum) — *see* Complications, vaccination
- neonatorum A33
- obstetrical A34
- puerperal, postpartum, childbirth A34

Tetany (due to) R29.0
- alkalosis E87.3
- associated with rickets E55.0
- convulsions R29.0
  - hysterical F44.5
- functional (hysterical) F44.5
- hyperkinetic R29.0
  - hysterical F44.5

Tetany (due to) - *continued*
- hyperpnea R06.4
  - hysterical F44.5
  - psychogenic F45.8
- hyperventilation — *see also* Hyperventilation R06.4
  - hysterical F44.5
- neonatal (without calcium or magnesium deficiency) P71.3
- parathyroid (gland) E20.9
- parathyroprival E89.2
- post- (para) thyroidectomy E89.2
- postoperative E89.2
- pseudotetany R29.0
- psychogenic (conversion reaction) F44.5

Tetralogy of Fallot Q21.3
Tetraplegia (chronic) — *see also* Quadriplegia G82.50
Thailand hemorrhagic fever A91
Thalassanemia — *see* Thalassemia
Thalassemia (anemia) (disease) D56.9
- with other hemoglobinopathy D56.8
- alpha (major) (severe) (triple gene defect) D56.0
  - minor D56.3
  - silent carrier D56.3
  - trait D56.3
- beta (severe) D56.1
  - homozygous D56.1
  - major D56.1
  - minor D56.3
  - trait D56.3
- delta-beta (homozygous) D56.2
  - minor D56.3
  - trait D56.3
- dominant D56.8
- hemoglobin
  - C D56.8
  - E-beta D56.5
- intermedia D56.1
- major D56.1
- minor D56.3
- mixed D56.8
- sickle-cell — *see* Disease, sickle-cell, thalassemia
- specified type NEC D56.8
- trait D56.3
- variants D56.8

Thanatophoric dwarfism or short stature Q77.1
Thaysen-Gee disease (nontropical sprue) K90.0
Thaysen's disease K90.0
Thecoma D27-
- luteinized D27-
- malignant C56-

Thelarche, premature E30.8
Thelaziasis B83.8
Thelitis N61.0
- puerperal, postpartum or gestational — *see* Infection, nipple

Therapeutic — *see* condition
Therapy
- drug, long-term (current) (prophylactic)
  - agents affecting estrogen receptors and estrogen levels NEC Z79.818
  - anastrozole (Arimidex) Z79.811
  - antibiotics Z79.2
    - short-term use - omit code
  - anticoagulants Z79.01
  - anti-inflammatory Z79.1
  - antiplatelet Z79.02
  - antithrombotics Z79.02
  - aromatase inhibitors Z79.811
  - aspirin Z79.82
  - birth control pill or patch Z79.3
  - bisphosphonates Z79.83
  - contraceptive, oral Z79.3
  - drug, specified NEC Z79.899
  - estrogen receptor downregulators Z79.818
  - Evista Z79.810
  - exemestane (Aromasin) Z79.811
  - Fareston Z79.810
  - fulvestrant (Faslodex) Z79.818
  - gonadotropin-releasing hormone (GnRH) agonist Z79.818
  - goserelin acetate (Zoladex) Z79.818
  - hormone replacement Z79.890
  - insulin Z79.4
  - letrozole (Femara) Z79.811
  - leuprolide acetate (leuprorelin) (Lupron) Z79.818
  - megestrol acetate (Megace) Z79.818
  - methadone
    - for pain management Z79.891
    - maintenance therapy F11.20
  - Nolvadex Z79.810
  - opiate analgesic Z79.891
  - oral contraceptive Z79.3

Therapy - *continued*
- drug, long-term (current) (prophylactic) - *continued*
  - raloxifene (Evista) Z79.810
  - selective estrogen receptor modulators (SERMs) Z79.810
  - short term - omit code
  - steroids
    - inhaled Z79.51
    - systemic Z79.52
  - tamoxifen (Nolvadex) Z79.810
  - toremifene (Fareston) Z79.810

Thermic — *see* condition
Thermography (abnormal) — *see also* Abnormal, diagnostic imaging R93.89
- breast R92.8

Thermoplegia T67.0
Thesaurismosis, glycogen — *see* Disease, glycogen storage
Thiamin deficiency E51.9
- specified NEC E51.8

Thiaminic deficiency with beriberi E51.11
Thibierge-Weissenbach syndrome — *see* Sclerosis, systemic
Thickening
- bone — *see* Hypertrophy, bone
- breast N64.59
- endometrium R93.89
- epidermal L85.9
  - specified NEC L85.8
- hymen N89.6
- larynx J38.7
- nail L60.2
  - congenital Q84.5
- periosteal — *see* Hypertrophy, bone
- pleura J92.9
  - with asbestos J92.0
- skin R23.4
- subepiglottic J38.7
- tongue K14.8
- valve, heart — *see* Endocarditis

Thigh — *see* condition
Thinning vertebra — *see* Spondylopathy, specified NEC
Thirst, excessive R63.1
- due to deprivation of water T73.1

Thomsen disease G71.12
Thoracic — *see also* condition
- kidney Q63.2
- outlet syndrome G54.0

Thoracogastroschisis (congenital) Q79.8
Thoracopagus Q89.4
Thorax — *see* condition
Thorn's syndrome N28.89
Thorson-Björck syndrome E34.0
Threadworm (infection) (infestation) B80
Threatened
- abortion O20.0
  - with subsequent abortion O03.9
- job loss, anxiety concerning Z56.2
- labor (without delivery) O47.9
  - at or after 37 completed weeks of gestation O47.1
  - before 37 completed weeks of gestation O47.0-
- loss of job, anxiety concerning Z56.2
- miscarriage O20.0
- unemployment, anxiety concerning Z56.2

Three-day fever A93.1
Threshers' lung J67.0
Thrix annulata (congenital) Q84.1
Throat — *see* condition
Thrombasthenia (Glanzmann) (hemorrhagic) (hereditary) D69.1
Thromboangiitis I73.1
- obliterans (general) I73.1
  - cerebral I67.89
  - vessels
    - brain I67.89
    - spinal cord I67.89

Thromboarteritis — *see* Arteritis
Thromboasthenia (Glanzmann) (hemorrhagic) (hereditary) D69.1
Thrombocytasthenia (Glanzmann) D69.1
Thrombocythemia (essential) (hemorrhagic) (idiopathic) (primary) D47.3
Thrombocytopathy (dystrophic) (granulopenic) D69.1
Thrombocytopenia, thrombocytopenic D69.6
- with absent radius (TAR) Q87.2
- congenital D69.42
- dilutional D69.59
- due to
  - drugs D69.59
  - extracorporeal circulation of blood D69.59
  - (massive) blood transfusion D69.59

Thrombocytopenia, thrombocytopenic - *continued*
  due to - *continued*
    platelet alloimmunization D69.59
  essential D69.3
  heparin induced (HIT) D75.82
  hereditary D69.42
  idiopathic D69.3
  neonatal, transitory P61.0
    due to
      exchange transfusion P61.0
      idiopathic maternal thrombocytopenia P61.0
      isoimmunization P61.0
  primary NEC D69.49
    idiopathic D69.3
  puerperal, postpartum O72.3
  secondary D69.59
  transient neonatal P61.0
Thrombocytosis, essential D47.3
  primary D47.3
Thromboembolism — *see* Embolism
Thrombopathy (Bernard-Soulier) D69.1
  constitutional D68.0
  Willebrand-Jurgens D68.0
Thrombopenia — *see* Thrombocytopenia
Thrombophilia D68.59
  primary NEC D68.59
  secondary NEC D68.69
  specified NEC D68.69
Thrombophlebitis I80.9
  antepartum O22.2-
    deep O22.3-
    superficial O22.2-
  cavernous (venous) sinus G08
    complicating pregnancy O22.5-
    nonpyogenic I67.6
  cerebral (sinus) (vein) G08
    nonpyogenic I67.6
    sequelae G09
  due to implanted device — *see* Complications, by site and type, specified NEC
  during or resulting from a procedure NEC T81.72
  femoral vein (superficial) I80.1-
  femoropopliteal vein I80.0-
  hepatic (vein) I80.8
  idiopathic, recurrent I82.1
  iliofemoral I80.1-
  intracranial venous sinus (any) G08
    nonpyogenic I67.6
    sequelae G09
  intraspinal venous sinuses and veins G08
    nonpyogenic G95.19
  lateral (venous) sinus G08
    nonpyogenic I67.6
  leg I80.3
    superficial I80.0-
  longitudinal (venous) sinus G08
    nonpyogenic I67.6
  lower extremity I80.299
  migrans, migrating I82.1
  pelvic
    with ectopic or molar pregnancy O08.0
    following ectopic or molar pregnancy O08.0
    puerperal O87.1
  popliteal vein — *see* Phlebitis, leg, deep, popliteal
  portal (vein) K75.1
  postoperative T81.72
  pregnancy — *see* Thrombophlebitis, antepartum
  puerperal, postpartum, childbirth O87.0
    deep O87.1
    pelvic O87.1
    septic O86.81
    superficial O87.0
  saphenous (greater) (lesser) I80.0-
  sinus (intracranial) G08
    nonpyogenic I67.6
  specified site NEC I80.8
  tibial vein I80.23-
Thrombosis, thrombotic (bland) (multiple) (progressive) (silent) (vessel) I82.90
  anal K64.5
  antepartum — *see* Thrombophlebitis, antepartum
  aorta, aortic I74.10
    abdominal I74.09
      saddle I74.01
    bifurcation I74.09
    saddle I74.01
    specified site NEC I74.19
    terminal I74.09
    thoracic I74.11
    valve — *see* Endocarditis, aortic
  apoplexy I63.3-
  artery, arteries (postinfectional) I74.9

Thrombosis, thrombotic (bland) (multiple) (progressive) (silent) (vessel) - *continued*
  artery, arteries (postinfectional) - *continued*
    auditory, internal — *see* Occlusion, artery, precerebral, specified NEC
    basilar — *see* Occlusion, artery, basilar
    carotid (common) (internal) — *see* Occlusion, artery, carotid
    cerebellar (anterior inferior) (posterior inferior) (superior) — *see* Occlusion, artery, cerebellar
    cerebral — *see* Occlusion, artery, cerebral
    choroidal (anterior) — *see* Occlusion, artery, precerebral, specified NEC
    communicating, posterior — *see* Occlusion, artery, precerebral, specified NEC
    coronary — *see also* Infarct, myocardium
      not resulting in infarction I24.0
    hepatic I74.8
    hypophyseal — *see* Occlusion, artery, precerebral, specified NEC
    iliac I74.5
    limb I74.4
      lower I74.3
      upper I74.2
    meningeal, anterior or posterior — *see* Occlusion, artery, cerebral, specified NEC
    mesenteric (with gangrene) — *see also* Infarct, intestine K55.069
    ophthalmic — *see* Occlusion, artery, retina
    pontine — *see* Occlusion, artery, precerebral, specified NEC
    precerebral — *see* Occlusion, artery, precerebral
    pulmonary (iatrogenic) — *see* Embolism, pulmonary
    renal N28.0
    retinal — *see* Occlusion, artery, retina
    spinal, anterior or posterior G95.11
    traumatic NEC T14.8
    vertebral — *see* Occlusion, artery, vertebral
  atrium, auricular — *see also* Infarct, myocardium
    following acute myocardial infarction (current complication) I23.6
    not resulting in infarction I51.3
    old I51.3
  basilar (artery) — *see* Occlusion, artery, basilar
  brain (artery) (stem) — *see also* Occlusion, artery, cerebral
    due to syphilis A52.05
    puerperal O99.43
    sinus — *see* Thrombosis, intracranial venous sinus
  capillary I78.8
  cardiac — *see also* Infarct, myocardium
    not resulting in infarction I51.3
    old I51.3
    valve — *see* Endocarditis
  carotid (artery) (common) (internal) — *see* Occlusion, artery, carotid
  cavernous (venous) sinus — *see* Thrombosis, intracranial venous sinus
  cerebellar artery (anterior inferior) (posterior inferior) (superior) I66.3
  cerebral (artery) — *see* Occlusion, artery, cerebral
  cerebrovenous sinus — *see also* Thrombosis, intracranial venous sinus
    puerperium O87.3
  chronic I82.91
  coronary (artery) (vein) — *see also* Infarct, myocardium
    not resulting in infarction I24.0
  corpus cavernosum N48.89
  cortical I66.9
  deep — *see* Embolism, vein, lower extremity
  due to device, implant or graft — *see also* Complications, by site and type, specified NEC T85.868
    arterial graft NEC T82.868
    breast (implant) T85.868
    catheter NEC T85.868
      dialysis (renal) T82.868
        intraperitoneal T85.868
      infusion NEC T82.868
        spinal (epidural) (subdural) T85.860
      urinary (indwelling) T83.86
    electronic (electrode) (pulse generator) (stimulator)
      bone T84.86
      cardiac T82.867
      nervous system (brain) (peripheral nerve) (spinal) T85.860
      urinary T83.86
    fixation, internal (orthopedic) NEC T84.86
    gastrointestinal (bile duct) (esophagus) T85.868
    genital NEC T83.86
    heart T82.867

Thrombosis, thrombotic (bland) (multiple) (progressive) (silent) (vessel) - *continued*
  due to device, implant or graft - *continued*
    joint prosthesis T84.86
    ocular (corneal graft) (orbital implant) NEC T85.868
    orthopedic NEC T84.86
    specified NEC T85.868
    urinary NEC T83.86
    vascular NEC T82.868
    ventricular intracranial shunt T85.860
  during the puerperium — *see* Thrombosis, puerperal
  endocardial — *see also* Infarct, myocardium
    not resulting in infarction I51.3
  eye — *see* Occlusion, retina
  genital organ
    female NEC N94.89
      pregnancy — *see* Thrombophlebitis, antepartum
    male N50.1
  gestational — *see* Phlebopathy, gestational
  heart (chamber) — *see also* Infarct, myocardium
    not resulting in infarction I51.3
    old I51.3
  hepatic (vein) I82.0
    artery I74.8
  history (of) Z86.718
  intestine (with gangrene) — *see also* Infarct, intestine K55.069
  intracardiac NEC (apical) (atrial) (auricular) (ventricular) (old) I51.3
  intracranial (arterial) I66.9
    venous sinus (any) G08
      nonpyogenic origin I67.6
      puerperium O87.3
  intramural — *see also* Infarct, myocardium
    not resulting in infarction I51.3
    old I51.3
  intraspinal venous sinuses and veins G08
    nonpyogenic G95.19
  kidney (artery) N28.0
  lateral (venous) sinus — *see* Thrombosis, intracranial venous sinus
  leg — *see* Thrombosis, vein, lower extremity
    arterial I74.3
  liver (venous) I82.0
    artery I74.8
    portal vein I81
  longitudinal (venous) sinus — *see* Thrombosis, intracranial venous sinus
  lower limb — *see* Thrombosis, vein, lower extremity
  lung (iatrogenic) (postoperative) — *see* Embolism, pulmonary
  meninges (brain) (arterial) I66.8
  mesenteric (artery) (with gangrene) — *see also* Infarct, intestine K55.069
    vein (inferior) (superior) I81
  mitral I34.8
  mural — *see also* Infarct, myocardium
    due to syphilis A52.06
    not resulting in infarction I51.3
    old I51.3
  omentum (with gangrene) — *see also* Infarct, intestine K55.069
  ophthalmic — *see* Occlusion, retina
  pampiniform plexus (male) N50.1
  parietal — *see also* Infarct, myocardium
    not resulting in infarction I24.0
  penis, superficial vein N48.81
  perianal venous K64.5
  peripheral arteries I74.4
    upper I74.2
  personal history (of) Z86.718
  portal I81
    due to syphilis A52.09
  precerebral artery — *see* Occlusion, artery, precerebral
  puerperal, postpartum O87.0
    brain (artery) O99.43
      venous (sinus) O87.3
    cardiac O99.43
    cerebral (artery) O99.43
      venous (sinus) O87.3
    superficial O87.0
  pulmonary (artery) (iatrogenic) (postoperative) (vein) — *see* Embolism, pulmonary
  renal (artery) N28.0
    vein I82.3
  resulting from presence of device, implant or graft — *see* Complications, by site and type, specified NEC
  retina, retinal — *see* Occlusion, retina
  scrotum N50.1
  seminal vesicle N50.1

Thrombosis, thrombotic (bland) (multiple) (progressive) (silent) (vessel) - *continued*
- sigmoid (venous) sinus — *see* Thrombosis, intracranial venous sinus
- sinus, intracranial (any) — *see* Thrombosis, intracranial venous sinus
- specified site NEC I82.890
  - chronic I82.891
- spermatic cord N50.1
- spinal cord (arterial) G95.11
  - due to syphilis A52.09
  - pyogenic origin G06.1
- spleen, splenic D73.5
  - artery I74.8
- testis N50.1
- tumor — *see* Neoplasm, unspecified behavior, by site
- traumatic NEC T14.8
- tricuspid I07.8
- tunica vaginalis N50.1
- umbilical cord (vessels) , complicating delivery O69.5
- vas deferens N50.1
- vein (acute) I82.90
  - antecubital I82.61-
    - chronic I82.71-
  - axillary I82.A1-
    - chronic I82.A2-
  - basilic I82.61-
    - chronic I82.71-
  - brachial I82.62-
    - chronic I82.72-
  - brachiocephalic (innominate) I82.290
    - chronic I82.291
  - cerebral, nonpyogenic I67.6
  - cephalic I82.61-
    - chronic I82.71-
  - chronic I82.91
  - deep (DVT) I82.40-
    - calf I82.4Z-
      - chronic I82.5Z-
    - lower leg I82.4Z-
      - chronic I82.5Z-
    - thigh I82.4Y-
      - chronic I82.5Y-
    - upper leg I82.4Y
      - chronic I82.5y--
  - femoral I82.41-
    - chronic I82.51-
  - iliac (iliofemoral) I82.42-
    - chronic I82.52-
  - innominate I82.290
    - chronic I82.291
  - internal jugular I82.C1-
    - chronic I82.C2-
  - lower extremity
    - deep I82.40-
      - chronic I82.50-
      - specified NEC I82.49-
        - chronic NEC I82.59-
    - distal
      - deep I82.4Z-
    - proximal
      - deep I82.4Y-
        - chronic I82.5Y-
    - superficial I82.81-
  - perianal K64.5
  - popliteal I82.43-
    - chronic I82.53-
  - radial I82.62-
    - chronic I82.72-
  - renal I82.3
  - saphenous (greater) (lesser) I82.81-
  - specified NEC I82.890
    - chronic NEC I82.891
  - subclavian I82.B1-
    - chronic I82.B2-
  - thoracic NEC I82.290
    - chronic I82.291
  - tibial I82.44-
    - chronic I82.54-
  - ulnar I82.62-
    - chronic I82.72-
  - upper extremity I82.60-
    - chronic I82.70-
    - deep I82.62-
      - chronic I82.72-
    - superficial I82.61-
      - chronic I82.71-
- vena cava
  - inferior I82.220
    - chronic I82.221
  - superior I82.210

Thrombosis, thrombotic (bland) (multiple) (progressive) (silent) (vessel) - *continued*
- vena cava - *continued*
  - superior - *continued*
    - chronic I82.211
- venous, perianal K64.5
- ventricle — *see also* Infarct, myocardium
  - following acute myocardial infarction (current complication) I23.6
  - not resulting in infarction I24.0
  - old I51.3

Thrombus — *see* Thrombosis

Thrush — *see also* Candidiasis
- oral B37.0
- newborn P37.5
- vaginal B37.3

Thumb — *see also* condition
- sucking (child problem) F98.8

Thymitis E32.8

Thymoma (benign) D15.0
- malignant C37

Thymus, thymic (gland) — *see* condition

Thyrocele — *see* Goiter

Thyroglossal — *see also* condition
- cyst Q89.2
- duct, persistent Q89.2

Thyroid (gland) (body) — *see also* condition
- hormone resistance E07.89
- lingual Q89.2
- nodule (cystic) (nontoxic) (single) E04.1

Thyroiditis E06.9
- acute (nonsuppurative) (pyogenic) (suppurative) E06.0
- autoimmune E06.3
- chronic (nonspecific) (sclerosing) E06.5
  - with thyrotoxicosis, transient E06.2
  - fibrous E06.5
  - lymphadenoid E06.3
  - lymphocytic E06.3
  - lymphoid E06.3
- de Quervain's E06.1
- drug-induced E06.4
- fibrous (chronic) E06.5
- giant-cell (follicular) E06.1
- granulomatous (de Quervain) (subacute) E06.1
- Hashimoto's (struma lymphomatosa) E06.3
- iatrogenic E06.4
- ligneous E06.5
- lymphocytic (chronic) E06.3
- lymphoid E06.3
- lymphomatous E06.3
- nonsuppurative E06.1
- postpartum, puerperal O90.5
- pseudotuberculous E06.1
- pyogenic E06.0
- radiation E06.4
- Riedel's E06.5
- subacute (granulomatous) E06.1
- suppurative E06.0
- tuberculous A18.81
- viral E06.1
- woody E06.5

Thyrolingual duct, persistent Q89.2

Thyromegaly E01.0

Thyrotoxic
- crisis — *see* Thyrotoxicosis
- heart disease or failure — *see also* Thyrotoxicosis E05.90 *[I43]*
  - with thyroid storm E05.91 *[I43]*
- storm — *see* Thyrotoxicosis

Thyrotoxicosis (recurrent) E05.90
- with
  - goiter (diffuse) E05.00
    - with thyroid storm E05.01
    - adenomatous uninodular E05.10
      - with thyroid storm E05.11
    - multinodular E05.20
      - with thyroid storm E05.21
    - nodular E05.20
      - with thyroid storm E05.21
    - uninodular E05.10
      - with thyroid storm E05.11
  - infiltrative
    - dermopathy E05.00
      - with thyroid storm E05.01
    - ophthalmopathy E05.00
      - with thyroid storm E05.01
  - single thyroid nodule E05.10
    - with thyroid storm E05.11
  - thyroid storm E05.91
- due to
  - ectopic thyroid nodule or tissue E05.30
    - with thyroid storm E05.31

Thyrotoxicosis (recurrent) - *continued*
- due to - *continued*
  - ingestion of (excessive) thyroid material E05.40
    - with thyroid storm E05.41
  - overproduction of thyroid-stimulating hormone E05.80
    - with thyroid storm E05.81
  - specified cause NEC E05.80
    - with thyroid storm E05.81
- factitia E05.40
  - with thyroid storm E05.41
- heart — *see also* Failure, heart, high -output E05.90 *[I43]*
  - with thyroid storm — *see also* Failure, heart, high-output E05.91 *[I43]*
  - failure — *see also* Failure, heart, high-output E05.90 *[I43]*
- neonatal (transient) P72.1
- transient with chronic thyroiditis E06.2

Tibia vara — *see* Osteochondrosis, juvenile, tibia

Tic (disorder) F95.9
- breathing F95.8
- child problem F95.0
- compulsive F95.1
- de la Tourette F95.2
- degenerative (generalized) (localized) G25.69
  - facial G25.69
- disorder
  - chronic
    - motor F95.1
    - vocal F95.1
  - combined vocal and multiple motor F95.2
  - transient F95.0
- douloureux G50.0
  - atypical G50.1
  - postherpetic, postzoster B02.22
- drug-induced G25.61
- eyelid F95.8
- habit F95.9
  - chronic F95.1
  - transient of childhood F95.0
- lid, transient of childhood F95.0
- motor-verbal F95.2
- occupational F48.8
- orbicularis F95.8
  - transient of childhood F95.0
- organic origin G25.69
- provisional F95.0
- postchoreic G25.69
- psychogenic, compulsive F95.1
- salaam R25.8
- spasm (motor or vocal) F95.9
  - chronic F95.1
  - transient of childhood F95.0
- specified NEC F95.8

Tick-borne — *see* condition

Tietze's disease or syndrome M94.0

Tight, tightness
- anus K62.89
- chest R07.89
- fascia (lata) M62.89
- foreskin (congenital) N47.1
- hymen, hymenal ring N89.6
- introitus (acquired) (congenital) N89.6
- rectal sphincter K62.89
- tendon — *see* Short, tendon
- urethral sphincter N35.919

Tilting vertebra — *see* Dorsopathy, deforming, specified NEC

Timidity, child F93.8

Tinea (intersecta) (tarsi) B35.9
- amiantacea L44.8
- asbestina B35.0
- barbae B35.0
- beard B35.0
- black dot B35.0
- blanca B36.2
- capitis B35.0
- corporis B35.4
- cruris B35.6
- flava B36.0
- foot B35.3
- furfuracea B36.0
- imbricata (Tokelau) B35.5
- kerion B35.0
- manuum B35.2
- microsporic — *see* Dermatophytosis
- nigra B36.1
- nodosa — *see* Piedra
- pedis B35.3
- scalp B35.0
- specified NEC B35.8
- sycosis B35.0

Tinea (intersecta) (tarsi) - *continued*
- tonsurans B35.0
- trichophytic — *see* Dermatophytosis
- unguium B35.1
- versicolor B36.0

Tingling sensation (skin) R20.2
Tin-miner's lung J63.5
Tinnitus NOS H93.1-
- audible H93.1-
- aurium H93.1-
- pulsatile H93.A-
- subjective H93.1-

Tipped tooth (teeth) M26.33
Tipping
- pelvis M95.5
  - with disproportion (fetopelvic) O33.0
    - causing obstructed labor O65.0
- tooth (teeth) , fully erupted M26.33

Tiredness R53.83
Tissue — *see* condition
Tobacco (nicotine)
- abuse — *see* Tobacco, use
- dependence — *see* Dependence, drug, nicotine
- harmful use Z72.0
- heart — *see* Tobacco, toxic effect
- maternal use, affecting newborn P04.2
- toxic effect — *see* Table of Drugs and Chemicals, by substance, poisoning
  - chewing tobacco — *see* Table of Drugs and Chemicals, by substance, poisoning
  - cigarettes — *see* Table of Drugs and Chemicals, by substance, poisoning
- use Z72.0
  - complicating
    - childbirth O99.334
    - pregnancy O99.33-
    - puerperium O99.335
  - counseling and surveillance Z71.6
  - history Z87.891
- withdrawal state — *see also* Dependence, drug, nicotine F17.203

Tocopherol deficiency E56.0
Todd's
- cirrhosis K74.3
- paralysis (postepileptic) (transitory) G83.84

Toe — *see* condition
Toilet, artificial opening — *see* Attention to, artificial, opening
Tokelau (ringworm) B35.5
Tollwut — *see* Rabies
Tommaselli's disease R31.9
- correct substance properly administered — *see* Table of Drugs and Chemicals, by drug, adverse effect
- overdose or wrong substance given or taken — *see* Table of Drugs and Chemicals, by drug, poisoning

Tongue — *see also* condition
- tie Q38.1

Tonic pupil — *see* Anomaly, pupil, function, tonic pupil
Toni-Fanconi syndrome (cystinosis) E72.09
- with cystinosis E72.04

Tonsil — *see* condition
Tonsillitis (acute) (catarrhal) (croupous) (follicular) (gangrenous) (infective) (lacunar) (lingual) (malignant) (membranous) (parenchymatous) (phlegmonous) (pseudomembranous) (purulent) (septic) (subacute) (suppurative) (toxic) (ulcerative) (vesicular) (viral) J03.90
- chronic J35.01
  - with adenoiditis J35.03
- diphtheritic A36.0
- hypertrophic J35.01
  - with adenoiditis J35.03
- recurrent J03.91
- specified organism NEC J03.80
  - recurrent J03.81
- staphylococcal J03.80
  - recurrent J03.81
- streptococcal J03.00
  - recurrent J03.01
- tuberculous A15.8
- Vincent's A69.1

Tooth, teeth — *see* condition
Toothache K08.89
Topagnosis R20.8
Tophi — *see* Gout, chronic
TORCH infection — *see* Infection, congenital
- without active infection P00.2

Torn — *see* Tear
Tornwaldt's cyst or disease J39.2
Torsion
- accessory tube — *see* Torsion, fallopian tube
- adnexa (female) — *see* Torsion, fallopian tube

Torsion - *continued*
- aorta, acquired I77.1
- appendix epididymis N44.04
- appendix testis N44.03
- bile duct (common) (hepatic) K83.8
  - congenital Q44.5
- bowel, colon or intestine K56.2
- cervix — *see* Malposition, uterus
- cystic duct K82.8
- dystonia — *see* Dystonia, torsion
- epididymis (appendix) N44.04
- fallopian tube N83.52-
  - with ovary N83.53
- gallbladder K82.8
  - congenital Q44.1
- hydatid of Morgagni
  - female N83.52-
  - male N44.03
- kidney (pedicle) (leading to infarction) N28.0
- Meckel's diverticulum (congenital) Q43.0
  - malignant — *see* Table of Neoplasms, small intestine, malignant
- mesentery K56.2
- omentum K56.2
- organ or site, congenital NEC — *see* Anomaly, by site
- ovary (pedicle) N83.51-
  - with fallopian tube N83.53
  - congenital Q50.2
- oviduct — *see* Torsion, fallopian tube
- penis (acquired) N48.82
  - congenital Q55.63
- spasm — *see* Dystonia, torsion
- spermatic cord N44.02
  - extravaginal N44.01
  - intravaginal N44.02
- spleen D73.5
- testis, testicle N44.00
  - appendix N44.03
- tibia — *see* Deformity, limb, specified type NEC, lower leg
- uterus — *see* Malposition, uterus

Torticollis (intermittent) (spastic) M43.6
- congenital (sternomastoid) Q68.0
- due to birth injury P15.8
- hysterical F44.4
- ocular R29.891
- psychogenic F45.8
  - conversion reaction F44.4
- rheumatic M43.6
- rheumatoid M06.88
- spasmodic G24.3
- traumatic, current S13.4

Tortipelvis G24.1
Tortuous
- aortic arch Q25.46
- artery I77.1
- organ or site, congenital NEC — *see* Distortion
- retinal vessel, congenital Q14.1
- ureter N13.8
- urethra N36.8
- vein — *see* Varix

Torture, victim of Z65.4
Torula, torular (histolytica) (infection) — *see* Cryptococcosis
Torulosis — *see* Cryptococcosis
Torus (mandibularis) (palatinus) M27.0
- fracture — *see* Fracture, by site, torus

Touraine's syndrome Q79.8
Tourette's syndrome F95.2
Tourniquet syndrome — *see* Constriction, external, by site
Tower skull Q75.0
- with exophthalmos Q87.0

Toxemia R68.89
- bacterial — *see* Sepsis
- burn — *see* Burn
- eclamptic (with pre-existing hypertension) — *see* Eclampsia
- erysipelatous — *see* Erysipelas
- fatigue R68.89
- food — *see* Poisoning, food
- gastrointestinal K52.1
- intestinal K52.1
- kidney — *see* Uremia
- malarial — *see* Malaria
- myocardial — *see* Myocarditis, toxic
- of pregnancy — *see* Pre-eclampsia
- pre-eclamptic — *see* Pre-eclampsia
- small intestine K52.1
- staphylococcal, due to food A05.0
- stasis R68.89
- uremic — *see* Uremia

Toxemia - *continued*
- urinary — *see* Uremia

Toxemica cerebropathia psychica (nonalcoholic) F04
- alcoholic — *see* Alcohol, amnestic disorder

Toxic (poisoning) — *see also* condition T65.91
- effect — *see* Table of Drugs and Chemicals, by substance, poisoning
- shock syndrome A48.3
- thyroid (gland) — *see* Thyrotoxicosis

Toxicemia — *see* Toxemia
Toxicity — *see* Table of Drugs and Chemicals, by substance, poisoning
- fava bean D55.0
- food, noxious — *see* Poisoning, food
- from drug or nonmedicinal substance — *see* Table of Drugs and Chemicals, by drug

Toxicosis — *see also* Toxemia
- capillary, hemorrhagic D69.0

Toxinfection, gastrointestinal K52.1
Toxocariasis B83.0
Toxoplasma, toxoplasmosis (acquired) B58.9
- with
  - hepatitis B58.1
  - meningoencephalitis B58.2
  - ocular involvement B58.00
  - other organ involvement B58.89
  - pneumonia, pneumonitis B58.3
- congenital (acute) (subacute) (chronic) P37.1
- maternal, manifest toxoplasmosis in infant (acute) (subacute) (chronic) P37.1

tPA (rtPA)
- **administation in a different facility within the last 24 hours prior to admission to current facility** Z92.82

Trabeculation, bladder N32.89
Trachea — *see* condition
Tracheitis (catarrhal) (infantile) (membranous) (plastic) (septal) (suppurative) (viral) J04.10
- with
  - bronchitis (15 years of age and above) J40
    - acute or subacute — *see* Bronchitis, acute
    - chronic J42
    - tuberculous NEC A15.5
    - under 15 years of age J20.9
  - laryngitis (acute) J04.2
    - chronic J37.1
    - tuberculous NEC A15.5
- acute J04.10
  - with obstruction J04.11
- chronic J42
  - with
    - bronchitis (chronic) J42
    - laryngitis (chronic) J37.1
- diphtheritic (membranous) A36.89
- due to external agent — *see* Inflammation, respiratory, upper, due to
- syphilitic A52.73
- tuberculous A15.5

Trachelitis (nonvenereal) — *see* Cervicitis
Tracheobronchial — *see* condition
Tracheobronchitis (15 years of age and above) — *see also* Bronchitis
- due to
  - Bordetella bronchiseptica A37.80
    - with pneumonia A37.81
  - Francisella tularensis A21.8

Tracheobronchomegaly Q32.4
- with bronchiectasis J47.9
  - with
    - exacerbation (acute) J47.1
    - lower respiratory infection J47.0
- acquired J98.09
  - with bronchiectasis J47.9
    - with
      - exacerbation (acute) J47.1
      - lower respiratory infection J47.0

Tracheobronchopneumonitis — *see* Pneumonia, broncho-
Tracheocele (external) (internal) J39.8
- congenital Q32.1

Tracheomalacia J39.8
- congenital Q32.0

Tracheopharyngitis (acute) J06.9
- chronic J42
- due to external agent — *see* Inflammation, respiratory, upper, due to

Tracheostenosis J39.8
Tracheostomy
- complication — *see* Complication, tracheostomy
- status Z93.0
  - attention to Z43.0
  - malfunctioning J95.03

- **Trachoma, trachomatous** A71.9
  - active (stage) A71.1
  - contraction of conjunctiva A71.1
  - dubium A71.0
  - initial (stage) A71.0
  - healed or sequelae B94.0
  - pannus A71.1
  - Türck's J37.0
- **Traction, vitreomacular** H43.82-
- **Train sickness** T75.3
- **Trait** (s)
  - Hb-S D57.3
  - hemoglobin
    - abnormal NEC D58.2
      - with thalassemia D56.3
    - C — *see* Disease, hemoglobin C
    - S (Hb-S) D57.3
  - Lepore D56.3
  - personality, accentuated Z73.1
  - sickle-cell D57.3
    - with elliptocytosis or spherocytosis D57.3
  - type A personality Z73.1
- **Tramp** Z59.0
- **Trance** R41.89
  - hysterical F44.89
- **Transaminasemia** R74.0
- **Transection**
  - abdomen (partial) S38.3
  - aorta (incomplete) — *see also* Injury, aorta
    - complete — *see* Injury, aorta, laceration, major
  - carotid artery (incomplete) — *see also* Injury, blood vessel, carotid, laceration
    - complete — *see* Injury, blood vessel, carotid, laceration, major
  - celiac artery (incomplete) S35.211
    - branch (incomplete) S35.291
      - complete S35.292
    - complete S35.212
  - innominate
    - artery (incomplete) — *see also* Injury, blood vessel, thoracic, innominate, artery, laceration
      - complete — *see* Injury, blood vessel, thoracic, innominate, artery, laceration, major
    - vein (incomplete) — *see also* Injury, blood vessel, thoracic, innominate, vein, laceration
      - complete — *see* Injury, blood vessel, thoracic, innominate, vein, laceration, major
  - jugular vein (external) (incomplete) — *see also* Injury, blood vessel, jugular vein, laceration
    - complete — *see* Injury, blood vessel, jugular vein, laceration, major
    - internal (incomplete) — *see also* Injury, blood vessel, jugular vein, internal, laceration
      - complete — *see* Injury, blood vessel, jugular vein, internal, laceration, major
  - mesenteric artery (incomplete) — *see also* Injury, mesenteric, artery, laceration
    - complete — *see* Injury, mesenteric artery, laceration, major
  - pulmonary vessel (incomplete) — *see also* Injury, blood vessel, thoracic, pulmonary, laceration
    - complete — *see* Injury, blood vessel, thoracic, pulmonary, laceration, major
  - subclavian — *see* Transection, innominate
  - vena cava (incomplete) — *see also* Injury, vena cava
    - complete — *see* Injury, vena cava, laceration, major
  - vertebral artery (incomplete) — *see also* Injury, blood vessel, vertebral, laceration
    - complete — *see* Injury, blood vessel, vertebral, laceration, major
- **Transfusion**
  - associated (red blood cell)
    - hemochromatosis E83.111
  - blood
    - ABO incompatible — *see* Complication(s), transfusion, incompatibility reaction, ABO
    - minor blood group (Duffy) (E) (K) (Kell) (Kidd) (Lewis) (M) (N) (P) (S) T80.89
    - reaction or complication — *see* Complications, transfusion
  - fetomaternal (mother) — *see* Pregnancy, complicated by, placenta, transfusion syndrome
  - maternofetal (mother) — *see* Pregnancy, complicated by, placenta, transfusion syndrome
  - placental (syndrome) (mother) — *see* Pregnancy, complicated by, placenta, transfusion syndrome
  - reaction (adverse) — *see* Complications, transfusion
  - related acute lung injury (TRALI) J95.84
  - twin-to-twin — *see* Pregnancy, complicated by, placenta, transfusion syndrome, fetus to fetus
- **Transient** (meaning homeless) — *see also* condition Z59.0
- **Translocation**
  - balanced autosomal Q95.9
    - in normal individual Q95.0
  - chromosomes NEC Q99.8
    - balanced and insertion in normal individual Q95.0
  - Down syndrome Q90.2
  - trisomy
    - 13 Q91.6
    - 18 Q91.2
    - 21 Q90.2
- **Translucency, iris** — *see* Degeneration, iris
- **Transmission of chemical substances through the placenta** — *see* Absorption, chemical, through placenta
- **Transparency, lung, unilateral** J43.0
- **Transplant** (ed) (status) Z94.9
  - awaiting organ Z76.82
  - bone Z94.6
    - marrow Z94.81
  - candidate Z76.82
  - complication — *see* Complication, transplant
  - cornea Z94.7
  - heart Z94.1
    - and lung (s) Z94.3
    - valve Z95.2
      - prosthetic Z95.2
      - specified NEC Z95.4
      - xenogenic Z95.3
  - intestine Z94.82
  - kidney Z94.0
  - liver Z94.4
  - lung (s) Z94.2
    - and heart Z94.3
  - organ (failure) (infection) (rejection) Z94.9
    - removal status Z98.85
  - pancreas Z94.83
  - skin Z94.5
  - social Z60.3
  - specified organ or tissue NEC Z94.89
  - stem cells Z94.84
  - tissue Z94.9
- **Transplants, ovarian, endometrial** N80.1
- **Transposed** — *see* Transposition
- **Transposition** (congenital) — *see also* Malposition, congenital
  - abdominal viscera Q89.3
  - aorta (dextra) Q20.3
  - appendix Q43.8
  - colon Q43.8
  - corrected Q20.5
  - great vessels (complete) (partial) Q20.3
  - heart Q24.0
    - with complete transposition of viscera Q89.3
  - intestine (large) (small) Q43.8
  - reversed jejunal (for bypass) (status) Z98.0
  - scrotum Q55.23
  - stomach Q40.2
    - with general transposition of viscera Q89.3
  - tooth, teeth, fully erupted M26.30
  - vessels, great (complete) (partial) Q20.3
  - viscera (abdominal) (thoracic) Q89.3
- **Transsexualism** F64.0
- **Transverse** — *see also* condition
  - arrest (deep) , in labor O64.0
  - lie (mother) O32.2
    - causing obstructed labor O64.8
- **Transvestism, transvestitism** (dual-role) F64.1
  - fetishistic F65.1
- **Trapped placenta** (with hemorrhage) O72.0
  - without hemorrhage O73.0
- **TRAPS**
  - (tumor necrosis factor receptor associated periodic syndrome) M04.1
- **Trauma, traumatism** — *see also* Injury
  - acoustic — *see* subcategory H83.3
  - birth — *see* Birth, injury
  - complicating ectopic or molar pregnancy O08.6
  - during delivery O71.9
  - following ectopic or molar pregnancy O08.6
  - obstetric O71.9
    - specified NEC O71.89
  - occlusal
    - primary K08.81
    - secondary K08.82
- **Traumatic** — *see also* condition
  - brain injury S06.9
- **Treacher Collins syndrome** Q75.4
- **Treitz's hernia** — *see* Hernia, abdomen, specified site NEC
- **Trematode infestation** — *see* Infestation, fluke
- **Trematodiasis** — *see* Infestation, fluke
- **Trembling paralysis** — *see* Parkinsonism
- **Tremor** (s) R25.1
  - drug induced G25.1
  - essential (benign) G25.0
  - familial G25.0
  - hereditary G25.0
  - hysterical F44.4
  - intention G25.2
  - medication induced postural G25.1
  - mercurial — *see* subcategory T56.1
  - Parkinson's — *see* Parkinsonism
  - psychogenic (conversion reaction) F44.4
  - senilis R54
  - specified type NEC G25.2
- **Trench**
  - fever A79.0
  - foot — *see* Immersion, foot
  - mouth A69.1
- **Treponema pallidum infection** — *see* Syphilis
- **Treponematosis**
  - due to
    - T. pallidum — *see* Syphilis
    - T. pertenue — *see* Yaws
- **Triad**
  - Hutchinson's (congenital syphilis) A50.53
  - Kartagener's Q89.3
  - Saint's — *see* Hernia, diaphragm
- **Trichiasis** (eyelid) H02.059
  - with entropion — *see* Entropion
  - left H02.056
    - lower H02.055
    - upper H02.054
  - right H02.053
    - lower H02.052
    - upper H02.051
- **Trichinella spiralis** (infection) (infestation) B75
- **Trichinellosis, trichiniasis, trichinelliasis, trichinosis** B75
  - with muscle disorder B75 *[M63.80]*
    - ankle B75 *[M63.87-]*
    - foot B75 *[M63.87-]*
    - forearm B75 *[M63.83-]*
    - hand B75 *[M63.84-]*
    - lower leg B75 *[M63.86-]*
    - multiple sites B75 *[M63.89]*
    - pelvic region B75 *[M63.85-]*
    - shoulder region B75 *[M63.81-]*
    - specified site NEC B75 *[M63.88]*
    - thigh B75 *[M63.85-]*
    - upper arm B75 *[M63.82-]*
- **Trichobezoar** T18.9
  - intestine T18.3
  - stomach T18.2
- **Trichocephaliasis, trichocephalosis** B79
- **Trichocephalus infestation** B79
- **Trichoclasis** L67.8
- **Trichoepithelioma** — *see also* Neoplasm, skin, benign
  - malignant — *see* Neoplasm, skin, malignant
- **Trichofolliculoma** — *see* Neoplasm, skin, benign
- **Tricholemmoma** — *see* Neoplasm, skin, benign
- **Trichomoniasis** A59.9
  - bladder A59.03
  - cervix A59.09
  - intestinal A07.8
  - prostate A59.02
  - seminal vesicles A59.09
  - specified site NEC A59.8
  - urethra A59.03
  - urogenitalis A59.00
  - vagina A59.01
  - vulva A59.01
- **Trichomycosis**
  - axillaris A48.8
  - nodosa, nodularis B36.8
- **Trichonodosis** L67.8
- **Trichophytid, trichophyton infection** — *see* Dermatophytosis
- **Trichophytobezoar** T18.9
  - intestine T18.3
  - stomach T18.2
- **Trichophytosis** — *see* Dermatophytosis
- **Trichoptilosis** L67.8
- **Trichorrhexis** (nodosa) (invaginata) L67.0
- **Trichosis axillaris** A48.8
- **Trichosporosis nodosa** B36.2
- **Trichostasis spinulosa** (congenital) Q84.1
- **Trichostrongyliasis, trichostrongylosis** (small intestine) B81.2
- **Trichostrongylus infection** B81.2
- **Trichotillomania** F63.3
- **Trichromat, trichromatopsia, anomalous** (congenital) H53.55
- **Trichuriasis** B79

- **Trichuris trichiura** (infection) (infestation) (any site) B79
- **Tricuspid** (valve) — *see* condition
- **Trifid** — *see also* Accessory
  - kidney (pelvis) Q63.8
  - tongue Q38.3
- **Trigeminal neuralgia** — *see* Neuralgia, trigeminal
- **Trigeminy** R00.8
- **Trigger finger** (acquired) M65.30
  - congenital Q74.0
  - index finger M65.32-
  - little finger M65.35-
  - middle finger M65.33-
  - ring finger M65.34-
  - thumb M65.31-
- **Trigonitis** (bladder) (chronic) (pseudomembranous) N30.30
  - with hematuria N30.31
- **Trigonocephaly** Q75.0
- **Trilocular heart** — *see* Cor triloculare
- **Trimethylaminuria** E72.52
- **Tripartite placenta** O43.19-
- **Triphalangeal thumb** Q74.0
- **Triple** — *see also* Accessory
  - kidneys Q63.0
  - uteri Q51.818
  - X, female Q97.0
- **Triplegia** G83.89
  - congenital G80.8
- **Triplet** (newborn) — *see also* Newborn, triplet
  - complicating pregnancy — *see* Pregnancy, triplet
- **Triplication** — *see* Accessory
- **Triploidy** Q92.7
- **Trismus** R25.2
  - neonatorum A33
  - newborn A33
- **Trisomy** (syndrome) Q92.9
  - autosomes Q92.9
  - chromosome specified NEC Q92.8
    - partial Q92.2
      - due to unbalanced translocation Q92.5
    - whole (nonsex chromosome)
      - meiotic nondisjunction Q92.0
      - mitotic nondisjunction Q92.1
      - mosaicism Q92.1
    - specified NEC Q92.8
  - due to
    - dicentrics — *see* Extra, marker chromosomes
    - extra rings — *see* Extra, marker chromosomes
    - isochromosomes — *see* Extra, marker chromosomes
  - specified NEC Q92.8
  - whole chromosome Q92.9
    - meiotic nondisjunction Q92.0
    - mitotic nondisjunction Q92.1
    - mosaicism Q92.1
    - partial Q92.9
    - specified NEC Q92.8
  - 13 (partial) Q91.7
    - meiotic nondisjunction Q91.4
    - mitotic nondisjunction Q91.5
    - mosaicism Q91.5
    - translocation Q91.6
  - 18 (partial) Q91.3
    - meiotic nondisjunction Q91.0
    - mitotic nondisjunction Q91.1
    - mosaicism Q91.1
    - translocation Q91.2
  - 20 Q92.8
  - 21 (partial) Q90.9
    - meiotic nondisjunction Q90.0
    - mitotic nondisjunction Q90.1
    - mosaicism Q90.1
    - translocation Q90.2
  - 22 Q92.8
- **Tritanomaly, tritanopia** H53.55
- **Trombiculosis, trombiculiasis, trombidiosis** B88.0
- **Trophedema** (congenital) (hereditary) Q82.0
- **Trophoblastic disease** — *see also* Mole, hydatidiform O01.9
- **Tropholymphedema** Q82.0
- **Trophoneurosis NEC** G96.8
  - disseminated M34.9
- **Tropical** — *see* condition
- **Trouble** — *see also* Disease
  - heart — *see* Disease, heart
  - kidney — *see* Disease, renal
  - nervous R45.0
  - sinus — *see* Sinusitis
- **Trousseau's syndrome** (thrombophlebitis migrans) I82.1
- **Truancy, childhood**
  - from school Z72.810
- **Truncus**
  - arteriosus (persistent) Q20.0
  - communis Q20.0
- **Trunk** — *see* condition
- **Trypanosomiasis**
  - African B56.9
    - by Trypanosoma brucei
      - gambiense B56.0
      - rhodesiense B56.1
  - American — *see* Chagas' disease
  - Brazilian — *see* Chagas' disease
  - by Trypanosoma
    - brucei gambiense B56.0
    - brucei rhodesiense B56.1
    - cruzi — *see* Chagas' disease
  - gambiensis, Gambian B56.0
  - rhodesiensis, Rhodesian B56.1
  - South American — *see* Chagas' disease
  - where
    - African trypanosomiasis is prevalent B56.9
    - Chagas' disease is prevalent B57.2
- **T-shaped incisors** K00.2
- **Tsutsugamushi** (disease) (fever) A75.3
- **Tube, tubal, tubular** — *see* condition
- **Tubercle** — *see also* Tuberculosis
  - brain, solitary A17.81
  - Darwin's Q17.8
  - Ghon, primary infection A15.7
- **Tuberculid, tuberculide** (indurating, subcutaneous) (lichenoid) (miliary) (papulonecrotic) (primary) (skin) A18.4
- **Tuberculoma** — *see also* Tuberculosis
  - brain A17.81
  - meninges (cerebral) (spinal) A17.1
  - spinal cord A17.81
- **Tuberculosis, tubercular, tuberculous** (calcification) (calcified) (caseous) (chromogenic acid-fast bacilli) (degeneration) (fibrocaseous) (fistula) (interstitial) (isolated circumscribed lesions) (necrosis) (parenchymatous) (ulcerative) A15.9
  - with pneumoconiosis (any condition in J60-J64) J65
  - abdomen (lymph gland) A18.39
  - abscess (respiratory) A15.9
    - bone A18.03
      - hip A18.02
      - knee A18.02
      - sacrum A18.01
      - specified site NEC A18.03
      - spinal A18.01
      - vertebra A18.01
    - brain A17.81
    - breast A18.89
    - Cowper's gland A18.15
    - dura (mater) (cerebral) (spinal) A17.81
    - epidural (cerebral) (spinal) A17.81
    - female pelvis A18.17
    - frontal sinus A15.8
    - genital organs NEC A18.10
    - genitourinary A18.10
    - gland (lymphatic) — *see* Tuberculosis, lymph gland
    - hip A18.02
    - intestine A18.32
    - ischiorectal A18.32
    - joint NEC A18.02
      - hip A18.02
      - knee A18.02
      - specified NEC A18.02
      - vertebral A18.01
    - kidney A18.11
    - knee A18.02
    - latent R76.11
    - lumbar (spine) A18.01
    - lung — *see* Tuberculosis, pulmonary
    - meninges (cerebral) (spinal) A17.0
    - muscle A18.09
    - perianal (fistula) A18.32
    - perinephritic A18.11
    - perirectal A18.32
    - rectum A18.32
    - retropharyngeal A15.8
    - sacrum A18.01
    - scrofulous A18.2
    - scrotum A18.15
    - skin (primary) A18.4
    - spinal cord A17.81
    - spine or vertebra (column) A18.01
    - subdiaphragmatic A18.31
    - testis A18.15
    - urinary A18.13
    - uterus A18.17
  - accessory sinus — *see* Tuberculosis, sinus
  - Addison's disease A18.7

Tuberculosis, tubercular, tuberculous (calcification) (calcified) (caseous) (chromogenic acid-fast bacilli) (degeneration) (fibrocaseous) (fistula) (interstitial) (isolated circumscribed lesions) (necrosis) (parenchymatous) (ulcerative) - *continued*

  - adenitis — *see* Tuberculosis, lymph gland
  - adenoids A15.8
  - adenopathy — *see* Tuberculosis, lymph gland
  - adherent pericardium A18.84
  - adnexa (uteri) A18.17
  - adrenal (capsule) (gland) A18.7
  - alimentary canal A18.32
  - anemia A18.89
  - ankle (joint) (bone) A18.02
  - anus A18.32
  - apex, apical — *see* Tuberculosis, pulmonary
  - appendicitis, appendix A18.32
  - arachnoid A17.0
  - artery, arteritis A18.89
    - cerebral A18.89
  - arthritis (chronic) (synovial) A18.02
    - spine or vertebra (column) A18.01
  - articular — *see* Tuberculosis, joint
  - ascites A18.31
  - asthma — *see* Tuberculosis, pulmonary
  - axilla, axillary (gland) A18.2
  - bladder A18.12
  - bone A18.03
    - hip A18.02
    - knee A18.02
    - limb NEC A18.03
    - sacrum A18.01
    - spine or vertebral column A18.01
  - bowel (miliary) A18.32
  - brain A17.81
  - breast A18.89
  - broad ligament A18.17
  - bronchi, bronchial, bronchus A15.5
    - ectasia, ectasis (bronchiectasis) — *see* Tuberculosis, pulmonary
    - fistula A15.5
      - primary (progressive) A15.7
    - gland or node A15.4
      - primary (progressive) A15.7
    - lymph gland or node A15.4
      - primary (progressive) A15.7
  - bronchiectasis — *see* Tuberculosis, pulmonary
  - bronchitis A15.5
  - bronchopleural A15.6
  - bronchopneumonia, bronchopneumonic — *see* Tuberculosis, pulmonary
  - bronchorrhagia A15.5
  - bronchotracheal A15.5
  - bronze disease A18.7
  - buccal cavity A18.83
  - bulbourethral gland A18.15
  - bursa A18.09
  - cachexia A15.9
  - cardiomyopathy A18.84
  - caries — *see* Tuberculosis, bone
  - cartilage A18.02
    - intervertebral A18.01
  - catarrhal — *see* Tuberculosis, respiratory
  - cecum A18.32
  - cellulitis (primary) A18.4
  - cerebellum A17.81
  - cerebral, cerebrum A17.81
  - cerebrospinal A17.81
    - meninges A17.0
  - cervical (lymph gland or node) A18.2
  - cervicitis, cervix (uteri) A18.16
  - chest — *see* Tuberculosis, respiratory
  - chorioretinitis A18.53
  - choroid, choroiditis A18.53
  - ciliary body A18.54
  - colitis A18.32
  - collier's J65
  - colliquativa (primary) A18.4
  - colon A18.32
  - complex, primary A15.7
  - congenital P37.0
  - conjunctiva A18.59
  - connective tissue (systemic) A18.89
  - contact Z20.1
  - cornea (ulcer) A18.52
  - Cowper's gland A18.15
  - coxae A18.02
  - coxalgia A18.02
  - cul-de-sac of Douglas A18.17
  - curvature, spine A18.01
  - cutis (colliquativa) (primary) A18.4
  - cyst, ovary A18.18
  - cystitis A18.12

Tuberculosis, tubercular, tuberculous (calcification) (calcified) (caseous) (chromogenic acid-fast bacilli) (degeneration) (fibrocaseous) (fistula) (interstitial) (isolated circumscribed lesions) (necrosis) (parenchymatous) (ulcerative) - *continued*
  dactylitis A18.03
  diarrhea A18.32
  diffuse — *see* Tuberculosis, miliary
  digestive tract A18.32
  disseminated — *see* Tuberculosis, miliary
  duodenum A18.32
  dura (mater) (cerebral) (spinal) A17.0
    abscess (cerebral) (spinal) A17.81
  dysentery A18.32
  ear (inner) (middle) A18.6
    bone A18.03
    external (primary) A18.4
    skin (primary) A18.4
  elbow A18.02
  emphysema — *see* Tuberculosis, pulmonary
  empyema A15.6
  encephalitis A17.82
  endarteritis A18.89
  endocarditis A18.84
    aortic A18.84
    mitral A18.84
    pulmonary A18.84
    tricuspid A18.84
  endocrine glands NEC A18.82
  endometrium A18.17
  enteric, enterica, enteritis A18.32
  enterocolitis A18.32
  epididymis, epididymitis A18.15
  epidural abscess (cerebral) (spinal) A17.81
  epiglottis A15.5
  episcleritis A18.51
  erythema (induratum) (nodosum) (primary) A18.4
  esophagus A18.83
  eustachian tube A18.6
  exposure (to) Z20.1
  exudative — *see* Tuberculosis, pulmonary
  eye A18.50
  eyelid (primary) (lupus) A18.4
  fallopian tube (acute) (chronic) A18.17
  fascia A18.09
  fauces A15.8
  female pelvic inflammatory disease A18.17
  finger A18.03
  first infection A15.7
  gallbladder A18.83
  ganglion A18.09
  gastritis A18.83
  gastrocolic fistula A18.32
  gastroenteritis A18.32
  gastrointestinal tract A18.32
  general, generalized — *see* Tuberculosis, miliary
  genital organs A18.10
  genitourinary A18.10
  genu A18.02
  glandula suprarenalis A18.7
  glandular, general A18.2
  glottis A15.5
  grinder's J65
  gum A18.83
  hand A18.03
  heart A18.84
  hematogenous — *see* Tuberculosis, miliary
  hemoptysis — *see* Tuberculosis, pulmonary
  hemorrhage NEC — *see* Tuberculosis, pulmonary
  hemothorax A15.6
  hepatitis A18.83
  hilar lymph nodes A15.4
    primary (progressive) A15.7
  hip (joint) (disease) (bone) A18.02
  hydropneumothorax A15.6
  hydrothorax A15.6
  hypoadrenalism A18.7
  hypopharynx A15.8
  ileocecal (hyperplastic) A18.32
  ileocolitis A18.32
  ileum A18.32
  iliac spine (superior) A18.03
  immunological findings only A15.7
  indurativa (primary) A18.4
  infantile A15.7
  infection A15.9
    without clinical manifestations A15.7
  infraclavicular gland A18.2
  inguinal gland A18.2
  inguinalis A18.2
  intestine (any part) A18.32
  iridocyclitis A18.54
  iris, iritis A18.54

Tuberculosis, tubercular, tuberculous (calcification) (calcified) (caseous) (chromogenic acid-fast bacilli) (degeneration) (fibrocaseous) (fistula) (interstitial) (isolated circumscribed lesions) (necrosis) (parenchymatous) (ulcerative) - *continued*
  ischiorectal A18.32
  jaw A18.03
  jejunum A18.32
  joint A18.02
    vertebral A18.01
  keratitis (interstitial) A18.52
  keratoconjunctivitis A18.52
  kidney A18.11
  knee (joint) A18.02
  kyphosis, kyphoscoliosis A18.01
  laryngitis A15.5
  larynx A15.5
  latent R76.11
  leptomeninges, leptomeningitis (cerebral) (spinal) A17.0
  lichenoides (primary) A18.4
  linguae A18.83
  lip A18.83
  liver A18.83
  lordosis A18.01
  lung — *see* Tuberculosis, pulmonary
  lupus vulgaris A18.4
  lymph gland or node (peripheral) A18.2
    abdomen A18.39
    bronchial A15.4
      primary (progressive) A15.7
    cervical A18.2
    hilar A15.4
      primary (progressive) A15.7
    intrathoracic A15.4
      primary (progressive) A15.7
    mediastinal A15.4
      primary (progressive) A15.7
    mesenteric A18.39
    retroperitoneal A18.39
    tracheobronchial A15.4
      primary (progressive) A15.7
  lymphadenitis — *see* Tuberculosis, lymph gland
  lymphangitis — *see* Tuberculosis, lymph gland
  lymphatic (gland) (vessel) — *see* Tuberculosis, lymph gland
  mammary gland A18.89
  marasmus A15.9
  mastoiditis A18.03
  mediastinal lymph gland or node A15.4
    primary (progressive) A15.7
  mediastinitis A15.8
    primary (progressive) A15.7
  mediastinum A15.8
    primary (progressive) A15.7
  medulla A17.81
  melanosis, Addisonian A18.7
  meninges, meningitis (basilar) (cerebral) (cerebrospinal) (spinal) A17.0
  meningoencephalitis A17.82
  mesentery, mesenteric (gland or node) A18.39
  miliary A19.9
    acute A19.2
      multiple sites A19.1
      single specified site A19.0
    chronic A19.8
    specified NEC A19.8
  millstone makers' J65
  miner's J65
  molder's J65
  mouth A18.83
  multiple A19.9
    acute A19.1
    chronic A19.8
  muscle A18.09
  myelitis A17.82
  myocardium, myocarditis A18.84
  nasal (passage) (sinus) A15.8
  nasopharynx A15.8
  neck gland A18.2
  nephritis A18.11
  nerve (mononeuropathy) A17.83
  nervous system A17.9
  nose (septum) A15.8
  ocular A18.50
  omentum A18.31
  oophoritis (acute) (chronic) A18.17
  optic (nerve trunk) (papilla) A18.59
  orbit A18.59
  orchitis A18.15
  organ, specified NEC A18.89
  osseous — *see* Tuberculosis, bone
  osteitis — *see* Tuberculosis, bone

Tuberculosis, tubercular, tuberculous (calcification) (calcified) (caseous) (chromogenic acid-fast bacilli) (degeneration) (fibrocaseous) (fistula) (interstitial) (isolated circumscribed lesions) (necrosis) (parenchymatous) (ulcerative) - *continued*
  osteomyelitis — *see* Tuberculosis, bone
  otitis media A18.6
  ovary, ovaritis (acute) (chronic) A18.17
  oviduct (acute) (chronic) A18.17
  pachymeningitis A17.0
  palate (soft) A18.83
  pancreas A18.83
  papulonecrotic (a) (primary) A18.4
  parathyroid glands A18.82
  paronychia (primary) A18.4
  parotid gland or region A18.83
  pelvis (bony) A18.03
  penis A18.15
  peribronchitis A15.5
  pericardium, pericarditis A18.84
  perichondritis, larynx A15.5
  periostitis — *see* Tuberculosis, bone
  perirectal fistula A18.32
  peritoneum NEC A18.31
  peritonitis A18.31
  pharynx, pharyngitis A15.8
  phlyctenulosis (keratoconjunctivitis) A18.52
  phthisis NEC — *see* Tuberculosis, pulmonary
  pituitary gland A18.82
  pleura, pleural, pleurisy, pleuritis (fibrinous) (obliterative) (purulent) (simple plastic) (with effusion) A15.6
    primary (progressive) A15.7
  pneumonia, pneumonic — *see* Tuberculosis, pulmonary
  pneumothorax (spontaneous) (tense valvular) — *see* Tuberculosis, pulmonary
  polyneuropathy A17.89
  polyserositis A19.9
    acute A19.1
    chronic A19.8
  potter's J65
  prepuce A18.15
  primary (complex) A15.7
  proctitis A18.32
  prostate, prostatitis A18.14
  pulmonalis — *see* Tuberculosis, pulmonary
  pulmonary (cavitated) (fibrotic) (infiltrative) (nodular) A15.0
    childhood type or first infection A15.7
    primary (complex) A15.7
  pyelitis A18.11
  pyelonephritis A18.11
  pyemia — *see* Tuberculosis, miliary
  pyonephrosis A18.11
  pyopneumothorax A15.6
  pyothorax A15.6
  rectum (fistula) (with abscess) A18.32
  reinfection stage — *see* Tuberculosis, pulmonary
  renal A18.11
  renis A18.11
  respiratory A15.9
    primary A15.7
    specified site NEC A15.8
  retina, retinitis A18.53
  retroperitoneal (lymph gland or node) A18.39
  rheumatism NEC A18.09
  rhinitis A15.8
  sacroiliac (joint) A18.01
  sacrum A18.01
  salivary gland A18.83
  salpingitis (acute) (chronic) A18.17
  sandblaster's J65
  sclera A18.51
  scoliosis A18.01
  scrofulous A18.2
  scrotum A18.15
  seminal tract or vesicle A18.15
  senile A15.9
  septic — *see* Tuberculosis, miliary
  shoulder (joint) A18.02
    blade A18.03
  sigmoid A18.32
  sinus (any nasal) A15.8
    bone A18.03
    epididymis A18.15
  skeletal NEC A18.03
  skin (any site) (primary) A18.4
  small intestine A18.32
  soft palate A18.83
  spermatic cord A18.15
  spine, spinal (column) A18.01
    cord A17.81

Tuberculosis, tubercular, tuberculous (calcification) (calcified) (caseous) (chromogenic acid-fast bacilli) (degeneration) (fibrocaseous) (fistula) (interstitial) (isolated circumscribed lesions) (necrosis) (parenchymatous) (ulcerative) - *continued*
spine, spinal (column) - *continued*
medulla A17.81
membrane A17.0
meninges A17.0
spleen, splenitis A18.85
spondylitis A18.01
sternoclavicular joint A18.02
stomach A18.83
stonemason's J65
subcutaneous tissue (cellular) (primary) A18.4
subcutis (primary) A18.4
subdeltoid bursa A18.83
submaxillary (region) A18.83
supraclavicular gland A18.2
suprarenal (capsule) (gland) A18.7
swelling, joint (see also category M01) — *see also* Tuberculosis, joint A18.02
symphysis pubis A18.02
synovitis A18.09
articular A18.02
spine or vertebra A18.01
systemic — *see* Tuberculosis, miliary
tarsitis A18.4
tendon (sheath) — *see* Tuberculosis, tenosynovitis
tenosynovitis A18.09
spine or vertebra A18.01
testis A18.15
throat A15.8
thymus gland A18.82
thyroid gland A18.81
tongue A18.83
tonsil, tonsillitis A15.8
trachea, tracheal A15.5
lymph gland or node A15.4
primary (progressive) A15.7
tracheobronchial A15.5
lymph gland or node A15.4
primary (progressive) A15.7
tubal (acute) (chronic) A18.17
tunica vaginalis A18.15
ulcer (skin) (primary) A18.4
bowel or intestine A18.32
specified NEC - code under Tuberculosis, by site
unspecified site A15.9
ureter A18.11
urethra, urethral (gland) A18.13
urinary organ or tract A18.13
uterus A18.17
uveal tract A18.54
uvula A18.83
vagina A18.18
vas deferens A18.15
verruca, verrucosa (cutis) (primary) A18.4
vertebra (column) A18.01
vesiculitis A18.15
vulva A18.18
wrist (joint) A18.02
Tuberculum
Carabelli — *see* Note at K00.2
occlusal — *see* Note at K00.2
paramolare K00.2
Tuberosity, entire maxillary M26.07
Tuberous sclerosis (brain) Q85.1
Tubo-ovarian — *see* condition
Tuboplasty, after previous sterilization Z31.0
aftercare Z31.42
Tubotympanitis, catarrhal (chronic) — *see* Otitis, media, nonsuppurative, chronic, serous
Tularemia A21.9
with
conjunctivitis A21.1
pneumonia A21.2
abdominal A21.3
bronchopneumonic A21.2
conjunctivitis A21.1
cryptogenic A21.3
enteric A21.3
gastrointestinal A21.3
generalized A21.7
ingestion A21.3
intestinal A21.3
oculoglandular A21.1
ophthalmic A21.1
pneumonia (any) , pneumonic A21.2
pulmonary A21.2
sepsis A21.7
specified NEC A21.8
typhoidal A21.7

Tularemia - *continued*
ulceroglandular A21.0
Tularensis conjunctivitis A21.1
Tumefaction — *see also* Swelling
liver — *see* Hypertrophy, liver
Tumor — *see also* Neoplasm, unspecified behavior, by site
acinar cell — *see* Neoplasm, uncertain behavior, by site
acinic cell — *see* Neoplasm, uncertain behavior, by site
adenocarcinoid — *see* Neoplasm, malignant, by site
adenomatoid — *see also* Neoplasm, benign, by site
odontogenic — *see* Cyst, calcifying odontogenic
adnexal (skin) — *see* Neoplasm, skin, benign, by site
adrenal
cortical (benign) D35.0-
malignant C74.0-
rest — *see* Neoplasm, benign, by site
alpha-cell
malignant
pancreas C25.4
specified site NEC — *see* Neoplasm, malignant, by site
unspecified site C25.4
pancreas D13.7
specified site NEC — *see* Neoplasm, benign, by site
unspecified site D13.7
aneurysmal — *see* Aneurysm
aortic body D44.7
malignant C75.5
Askin's — *see* Neoplasm, connective tissue, malignant
basal cell — *see also* Neoplasm, skin, uncertain behavior D48.5
Bednar — *see* Neoplasm, skin, malignant
benign (unclassified) — *see* Neoplasm, benign, by site
beta-cell
malignant
pancreas C25.4
specified site NEC — *see* Neoplasm, malignant, by site
unspecified site C25.4
pancreas D13.7
specified site NEC — *see* Neoplasm, benign, by site
unspecified site D13.7
Brenner D27.9
borderline malignancy D39.1-
malignant C56-
proliferating D39.1-
bronchial alveolar, intravascular D38.1
Brooke's — *see* Neoplasm, skin, benign
brown fat — *see* Lipoma
Burkitt — *see* Lymphoma, Burkitt
calcifying epithelial odontogenic — *see* Cyst, calcifying odontogenic
carcinoid
benign D3A.00
appendix D3A.020
ascending colon D3A.022
bronchus (lung) D3A.090
cecum D3A.021
colon D3A.029
descending colon D3A.024
duodenum D3A.010
foregut NOS D3A.094
hindgut NOS D3A.096
ileum D3A.012
jejunum D3A.011
kidney D3A.093
large intestine D3A.029
lung (bronchus) D3A.090
midgut NOS D3A.095
rectum D3A.026
sigmoid colon D3A.025
small intestine D3A.019
specified NEC D3A.098
stomach D3A.092
thymus D3A.091
transverse colon D3A.023
malignant C7A.00
appendix C7A.020
ascending colon C7A.022
bronchus (lung) C7A.090
cecum C7A.021
colon C7A.029
descending colon C7A.024
duodenum C7A.010
foregut NOS C7A.094

Tumor - *continued*
carcinoid - *continued*
malignant - *continued*
hindgut NOS C7A.096
ileum C7A.012
jejunum C7A.011
kidney C7A.093
large intestine C7A.029
lung (bronchus) C7A.090
midgut NOS C7A.095
rectum C7A.026
sigmoid colon C7A.025
small intestine C7A.019
specified NEC C7A.098
stomach C7A.092
thymus C7A.091
transverse colon C7A.023
mesentary metastasis C7B.04
secondary C7B.00
bone C7B.03
distant lymph nodes C7B.01
liver C7B.02
peritoneum C7B.04
specified NEC C7B.09
carotid body D44.6
malignant C75.4
cells — *see also* Neoplasm, unspecified behavior, by site
benign — *see* Neoplasm, benign, by site
malignant — *see* Neoplasm, malignant, by site
uncertain whether benign or malignant — *see* Neoplasm, uncertain behavior, by site
cervix, in pregnancy or childbirth — *see* Pregnancy, complicated by, tumor, cervix
chondromatous giant cell — *see* Neoplasm, bone, benign
chromaffin — *see also* Neoplasm, benign, by site
malignant — *see* Neoplasm, malignant, by site
Cock's peculiar L72.3
Codman's — *see* Neoplasm, bone, benign
dentigerous, mixed — *see* Cyst, calcifying odontogenic
dermoid — *see* Neoplasm, benign, by site
with malignant transformation C56-
desmoid (extra-abdominal) — *see also* Neoplasm, connective tissue, uncertain behavior
abdominal — *see* Neoplasm, connective tissue, uncertain behavior
embolus — *see* Neoplasm, secondary, by site
embryonal (mixed) — *see also* Neoplasm, uncertain behavior, by site
liver C22.7
endodermal sinus
specified site — *see* Neoplasm, malignant, by site
unspecified site
female C56.-
male C62.90
epithelial
benign — *see* Neoplasm, benign, by site
malignant — *see* Neoplasm, malignant, by site
Ewing's — *see* Neoplasm, bone, malignant, by site
fatty — *see* Lipoma
fibroid — *see* Leiomyoma
G cell
malignant
pancreas C25.4
specified site NEC — *see* Neoplasm, malignant, by site
unspecified site C25.4
specified site — *see* Neoplasm, uncertain behavior, by site
unspecified site D37.8
germ cell — *see also* Neoplasm, malignant, by site
mixed — *see* Neoplasm, malignant, by site
ghost cell, odontogenic — *see* Cyst, calcifying odontogenic
giant cell — *see also* Neoplasm, uncertain behavior, by site
bone D48.0
malignant — *see* Neoplasm, bone, malignant
chondromatous — *see* Neoplasm, bone, benign
malignant — *see* Neoplasm, malignant, by site
soft parts — *see* Neoplasm, connective tissue, uncertain behavior
malignant — *see* Neoplasm, connective tissue, malignant
glomus D18.00
intra-abdominal D18.03
intracranial D18.02
jugulare D44.7
malignant C75.5
skin D18.01
specified site NEC D18.09

Tumor - *continued*
gonadal stromal — *see* Neoplasm, uncertain behavior, by site
granular cell — *see also* Neoplasm, connective tissue, benign
malignant — *see* Neoplasm, connective tissue, malignant
granulosa cell D39.1-
juvenile D39.1-
malignant C56-
granulosa cell-theca cell D39.1-
malignant C56-
Grawitz's C64-
hemorrhoidal — *see* Hemorrhoids
hilar cell D27-
hilus cell D27-
Hurthle cell (benign) D34
malignant C73
hydatid — *see* Echinococcus
hypernephroid — *see also* Neoplasm, uncertain behavior, by site
interstitial cell — *see also* Neoplasm, uncertain behavior, by site
benign — *see* Neoplasm, benign, by site
malignant — *see* Neoplasm, malignant, by site
intravascular bronchial alveolar D38.1
islet cell — *see* Neoplasm, benign, by site
malignant — *see* Neoplasm, malignant, by site
pancreas C25.4
specified site NEC — *see* Neoplasm, malignant, by site
unspecified site C25.4
pancreas D13.7
specified site NEC — *see* Neoplasm, benign, by site
unspecified site D13.7
juxtaglomerular D41.0-
Klatskin's C24.0
Krukenberg's C79.6-
Leydig cell — *see* Neoplasm, uncertain behavior, by site
benign — *see* Neoplasm, benign, by site
specified site — *see* Neoplasm, benign, by site
unspecified site
female D27.9
male D29.20
malignant — *see* Neoplasm, malignant, by site
specified site — *see* Neoplasm, malignant, by site
unspecified site
female C56.9
male C62.90
specified site — *see* Neoplasm, uncertain behavior, by site
unspecified site
female D39.10
male D40.10
lipid cell, ovary D27-
lipoid cell, ovary D27-
malignant — *see also* Neoplasm, malignant, by site C80.1
fusiform cell (type) C80.1
giant cell (type) C80.1
localized, plasma cell — *see* Plasmacytoma, solitary
mixed NEC C80.1
small cell (type) C80.1
spindle cell (type) C80.1
unclassified C80.1
mast cell D47.09
melanotic, neuroectodermal — *see* Neoplasm, benign, by site
Merkel cell — *see* Carcinoma, Merkel cell
mesenchymal
malignant — *see* Neoplasm, connective tissue, malignant
mixed — *see* Neoplasm, connective tissue, uncertain behavior
mesodermal, mixed — *see also* Neoplasm, malignant, by site
liver C22.4
mesonephric — *see also* Neoplasm, uncertain behavior, by site
malignant — *see* Neoplasm, malignant, by site
metastatic
from specified site — *see* Neoplasm, malignant, by site
of specified site — *see* Neoplasm, malignant, by site
to specified site — *see* Neoplasm, secondary, by site
mixed NEC — *see also* Neoplasm, benign, by site
malignant — *see* Neoplasm, malignant, by site
mucinous of low malignant potential

Tumor - *continued*
mucinous of low malignant potential - *continued*
specified site — *see* Neoplasm, malignant, by site
unspecified site C56.9
mucocarcinoid
specified site — *see* Neoplasm, malignant, by site
unspecified site C18.1
mucoepidermoid — *see* Neoplasm, uncertain behavior, by site
Müllerian, mixed
specified site — *see* Neoplasm, malignant, by site
unspecified site C54.9
myoepithelial — *see* Neoplasm, benign, by site
neuroectodermal (peripheral) — *see* Neoplasm, malignant, by site
primitive
specified site — *see* Neoplasm, malignant, by site
unspecified site C71.9
neuroendocrine D3A.8
malignant poorly differentiated C7A.1
secondary NEC C7B.8
specified NEC C7A.8
neurogenic olfactory C30.0
nonencapsulated sclerosing C73
odontogenic (adenomatoid) (benign) (calcifying epithelial) (keratocystic) (squamous) — *see* Cyst, calcifying odontogenic
malignant C41.1
upper jaw (bone) C41.0
ovarian stromal D39.1-
ovary, in pregnancy — *see* Pregnancy, complicated by
pacinian — *see* Neoplasm, skin, benign
Pancoast's — *see* Pancoast's syndrome
papillary — *see also* Papilloma
cystic D37.9
mucinous of low malignant potential C56-
specified site — *see* Neoplasm, malignant, by site
unspecified site C56.9
serous of low malignant potential
specified site — *see* Neoplasm, malignant, by site
unspecified site C56.9
pelvic, in pregnancy or childbirth — *see* Pregnancy, complicated by
phantom F45.8
phyllodes D48.6-
benign D24-
malignant — *see* Neoplasm, breast, malignant
Pindborg — *see* Cyst, calcifying odontogenic
placental site trophoblastic D39.2
plasma cell (malignant) (localized) — *see* Plasmacytoma, solitary
polyvesicular vitelline
specified site — *see* Neoplasm, malignant, by site
unspecified site
female C56.9
male C62.90
Pott's puffy — *see* Osteomyelitis, specified NEC
Rathke's pouch D44.3
retinal anlage — *see* Neoplasm, benign, by site
salivary gland type, mixed — *see* Neoplasm, salivary gland, benign
malignant — *see* Neoplasm, salivary gland, malignant
Sampson's N80.1
Schmincke's — *see* Neoplasm, nasopharynx, malignant
sclerosing stromal D27-
sebaceous — *see* Cyst, sebaceous
secondary — *see* Neoplasm, secondary, by site
carcinoid C7B.00
bone C7B.03
distant lymph nodes C7B.01
liver C7B.02
peritoneum C7B.04
specified NEC C7B.09
neuroendocrine NEC C7B.8
serous of low malignant potential
specified site — *see* Neoplasm, malignant, by site
unspecified site C56.9
Sertoli cell — *see* Neoplasm, benign, by site
with lipid storage
specified site — *see* Neoplasm, benign, by site
unspecified site
female D27.9
male D29.20
specified site — *see* Neoplasm, benign, by site
unspecified site
female D27.9
male D29.20
Sertoli-Leydig cell — *see* Neoplasm, benign, by site
specified site — *see* Neoplasm, benign, by site
unspecified site

Tumor - *continued*
Sertoli-Leydig cell - *continued*
unspecified site - *continued*
female D27.9
male D29.20
sex cord (-stromal) — *see* Neoplasm, uncertain behavior, by site
with annular tubules D39.1-
skin appendage — *see* Neoplasm, skin, benign
smooth muscle — *see* Neoplasm, connective tissue, uncertain behavior
soft tissue
benign — *see* Neoplasm, connective tissue, benign
malignant — *see* Neoplasm, connective tissue, malignant
sternomastoid (congenital) Q68.0
stromal
endometrial D39.0
gastric D48.1
benign D21.4
malignant C16.9
uncertain behavior D48.1
gastrointestinal C49.A-
benign D21.4
esophagus C49.A1
large intestine C49.A4
malignant C49.A0
colon C49.A4
duodenum C49.A3
esophagus C49.A1
ileum C49.A3
jejunum C49.A3
large intestine C49.A4
Meckel diverticulum C49.A3
omentum C49.A9
peritoneum C49.A9
rectum C49.A5
small intestine C49.A3
specified site NEC C49.A9
stomach C49.A2
rectum C49.A5
small intestine C49.A3
specified site NEC C49.A9
stomach C49.A2
uncertain behavior D48.1
intestine
benign D21.4
malignant
large C49.A4
small C49.A3
uncertain behavior D48.1
ovarian D39.1-
stomach C49.A2
benign D21.4
malignant C49.A2
uncertain behavior D48.1
testicular D40.10
sweat gland — *see also* Neoplasm, skin, uncertain behavior
benign — *see* Neoplasm, skin, benign
malignant — *see* Neoplasm, skin, malignant
syphilitic, brain A52.17
testicular stromal D40.1-
theca cell D27.-
theca cell-granulosa cell D39.1-
Triton, malignant — *see* Neoplasm, nerve, malignant
trophoblastic, placental site D39.2
turban D23.4
uterus (body) , in pregnancy or childbirth — *see* Pregnancy, complicated by, tumor, uterus
vagina, in pregnancy or childbirth — *see* Pregnancy, complicated by
varicose — *see* Varix
von Recklinghausen's — *see* Neurofibromatosis
vulva or perineum, in pregnancy or childbirth — *see* Pregnancy, complicated by
causing obstructed labor O65.5
Warthin's — *see* Neoplasm, salivary gland, benign
Wilms' C64-
yolk sac — *see* Neoplasm, malignant, by site
specified site — *see* Neoplasm, malignant, by site
unspecified site
female C56.9
male C62.90

Tumor lysis syndrome (following antineoplastic chemotherapy) (spontaneous) **NEC** E88.3
Tumorlet — *see* Neoplasm, uncertain behavior, by site
Tungiasis B88.1
Tunica vasculosa lentis Q12.2
Turban tumor D23.4

Ulcer, ulcerated, ulcerating, ulceration, ulcerative - *continued*
lower limb (atrophic) (chronic) (neurogenic) (perforating) (pyogenic) (trophic) (tropical) - *continued*
midfoot - *continued*
with - *continued*
bone involvement without evidence of necrosis L97.406
bone necrosis L97.404
exposed fat layer L97.402
muscle involvement without evidence of necrosis L97.405
muscle necrosis L97.403
skin breakdown only L97.401
specified severity NEC L97.408
left L97.429
with
bone involvement without evidence of necrosis L97.426
bone necrosis L97.424
exposed fat layer L97.422
muscle involvement without evidence of necrosis L97.425
muscle necrosis L97.423
skin breakdown only L97.421
specified severity NEC L97.428
right L97.419
with
bone involvement without evidence of necrosis L97.416
bone necrosis L97.414
exposed fat layer L97.412
muscle involvement without evidence of necrosis L97.415
muscle necrosis L97.413
skin breakdown only L97.411
specified severity NEC L97.418
right L97.919
with
bone involvement without evidence of necrosis L97.916
bone necrosis L97.914
exposed fat layer L97.912
muscle involvement without evidence of necrosis L97.915
muscle necrosis L97.913
skin breakdown only L97.911
specified severity NEC L97.918
thigh L97.109
with
bone involvement without evidence of necrosis L97.106
bone necrosis L97.104
muscle involvement without evidence of necrosis L97.105
exposed fat layer L97.102
muscle necrosis L97.103
skin breakdown only L97.101
specified severity NEC L97.108
left L97.129
with
bone involvement without evidence of necrosis L97.126
bone necrosis L97.124
exposed fat layer L97.122
muscle involvement without evidence of necrosis L97.125
muscle necrosis L97.123
skin breakdown only L97.121
specified severity NEC L97.128
right L97.119
with
bone involvement without evidence of necrosis L97.116
bone necrosis L97.114
exposed fat layer L97.112
muscle involvement without evidence of necrosis L97.115
muscle necrosis L97.113
skin breakdown only L97.111
specified severity NEC L97.118
toe L97.509
with
bone involvement without evidence of necrosis L97.506
bone necrosis L97.504
exposed fat layer L97.502
muscle involvement without evidence of necrosis L97.505
muscle necrosis L97.503
skin breakdown only L97.501
specified severity NEC L97.508

Ulcer, ulcerated, ulcerating, ulceration, ulcerative - *continued*
lower limb (atrophic) (chronic) (neurogenic) (perforating) (pyogenic) (trophic) (tropical) - *continued*
toe - *continued*
left L97.529
with
bone involvement without evidence of necrosis L97.526
bone necrosis L97.524
exposed fat layer L97.522
muscle involvement without evidence of necrosis L97.525
muscle necrosis L97.523
skin breakdown only L97.521
specified severity NEC L97.528
right L97.519
with
bone involvement without evidence of necrosis L97.516
bone necrosis L97.514
exposed fat layer L97.512
muscle involvement without evidence of necrosis L97.515
muscle necrosis L97.513
skin breakdown only L97.511
specified severity NEC L97.518
leprous A30.1
syphilitic A52.19
varicose — *see* Varix, leg, with, ulcer
luetic — *see* Ulcer, syphilitic
lung J98.4
tuberculous — *see* Tuberculosis, pulmonary
malignant — *see* Neoplasm, malignant, by site
marginal NEC — *see* Ulcer, gastrojejunal
meatus (urinarius) N34.2
Meckel's diverticulum Q43.0
malignant — *see* Table of Neoplasms, small intestine, malignant
Meleney's (chronic undermining) — *see* Ulcer, skin
Mooren's (cornea) — *see* Ulcer, cornea, Mooren's
mycobacterial (skin) A31.1
nasopharynx J39.2
neck, uterus N86
neurogenic NEC — *see* Ulcer, skin
nose, nasal (passage) (infective) (septum) J34.0
skin — *see* Ulcer, skin
spirochetal A69.8
varicose (bleeding) I86.8
oral mucosa (traumatic) K12.1
palate (soft) K12.1
penis (chronic) N48.5
peptic (site unspecified) K27.9
with
hemorrhage K27.4
and perforation K27.6
perforation K27.5
acute K27.3
with
hemorrhage K27.0
and perforation K27.2
perforation K27.1
chronic K27.7
with
hemorrhage K27.4
and perforation K27.6
perforation K27.5
esophagus K22.10
with bleeding K22.11
newborn P78.82
perforating K27.5
skin — *see* Ulcer, skin
peritonsillar J35.8
phagedenic (tropical) — *see* Ulcer, skin
pharynx J39.2
phlebitis — *see* Phlebitis
plaster — *see* Ulcer, pressure, by site
popliteal space — *see* Ulcer, lower limb
postpyloric — *see* Ulcer, duodenum
prepuce N47.7
prepyloric — *see* Ulcer, stomach
pressure (pressure area) L89.9-
ankle L89.5-
back L89.1-
buttock L89.3-
coccyx L89.15-
contiguous site of back, buttock, hip L89.4-
elbow L89.0-
face L89.81-
head L89.81-
heel L89.6-
hip L89.2-

Ulcer, ulcerated, ulcerating, ulceration, ulcerative - *continued*
pressure (pressure area) - *continued*
sacral region (tailbone) L89.15-
specified site NEC L89.89-
stage 1 (healing) (pre-ulcer skin changes limited to persistent focal edema)
ankle L89.5-
back L89.1-
buttock L89.3-
coccyx L89.15-
contiguous site of back, buttock, hip L89.4-
elbow L89.0-
face L89.81-
head L89.81-
heel L89.6-
hip L89.2-
sacral region (tailbone) L89.15-
specified site NEC L89.89-
stage 2 (healing) (abrasion, blister, partial thickness skin loss involving epidermis and/or dermis)
ankle L89.5-
back L89.1-
buttock L89.3-
coccyx L89.15-
contiguous site of back, buttock, hip L89.4-
elbow L89.0-
face L89.81-
head L89.81-
heel L89.6-
hip L89.2-
sacral region (tailbone) L89.15-
specified site NEC L89.89-
stage 3 (healing) (full thickness skin loss involving damage or necrosis of subcutaneous tissue)
ankle L89.5-
back L89.1-
buttock L89.3-
coccyx L89.15-
contiguous site of back, buttock, hip L89.4-
elbow L89.0-
face L89.81-
head L89.81-
heel L89.6-
hip L89.2-
sacral region (tailbone) L89.15-
specified site NEC L89.89-
stage 4 (healing) (necrosis of soft tissues through to underlying muscle, tendon, or bone)
ankle L89.5-
back L89.1-
buttock L89.3-
coccyx L89.15-
contiguous site of back, buttock, hip L89.4-
elbow L89.0-
face L89.81-
head L89.81-
heel L89.6-
hip L89.2-
sacral region (tailbone) L89.15-
specified site NEC L89.89-
unspecified stage
ankle L89.5-
back L89.1-
buttock L89.3-
coccyx L89.15-
contiguous site of back, buttock, hip L89.4-
elbow L89.0-
face L89.81-
head L89.81-
heel L89.6-
hip L89.2-
sacral region (tailbone) L89.15-
specified site NEC L89.89-
unstageable
ankle L89.5-
back L89.1-
buttock L89.3-
coccyx L89.15-
contiguous site of back, buttock, hip L89.4-
elbow L89.0-
face L89.81-
head L89.81-
heel L89.6-
hip L89.2-
sacral region (tailbone) L89.15-
specified site NEC L89.89-
primary of intestine K63.3
with perforation K63.1
prostate N41.9
pyloric — *see* Ulcer, stomach
rectosigmoid K63.3
with perforation K63.1

Ulcer, ulcerated, ulcerating, ulceration, ulcerative - *continued*
- rectum (sphincter) (solitary) K62.6
  - stercoraceous, stercoral K62.6
- retina — *see* Inflammation, chorioretinal
- rodent — *see also* Neoplasm, skin, malignant
- sclera — *see* Scleritis
- scrofulous (tuberculous) A18.2
- scrotum N50.89
  - tuberculous A18.15
  - varicose I86.1
- seminal vesicle N50.89
- sigmoid — *see* Ulcer, intestine
- skin (atrophic) (chronic) (neurogenic) (non-healing) (perforating) (pyogenic) (trophic) (tropical) L98.499
  - with gangrene — *see* Gangrene
  - amebic A06.7
  - back — *see* Ulcer, back
  - buttock — *see* Ulcer, buttock
  - decubitus — *see* Ulcer, pressure
  - lower limb — *see* Ulcer, lower limb
  - mycobacterial A31.1
  - specified site NEC L98.499
    - with
      - bone involvement without evidence of necrosis L98.496
      - bone necrosis L98.494
      - exposed fat layer L98.492
      - muscle involvement without evidence of necrosis L98.495
      - muscle necrosis L98.493
      - skin breakdown only L98.491
      - specified severity NEC L98.498
  - tuberculous (primary) A18.4
  - varicose — *see* Ulcer, varicose
- sloughing — *see* Ulcer, skin
- solitary, anus or rectum (sphincter) K62.6
- sore throat J02.9
  - streptococcal J02.0
- spermatic cord N50.89
- spine (tuberculous) A18.01
- stasis (venous) — *see* Varix, leg, with, ulcer
  - without varicose veins I87.2
- stercoraceous, stercoral K63.3
  - with perforation K63.1
  - anus or rectum K62.6
- stoma, stomal — *see* Ulcer, gastrojejunal
- stomach (eroded) (peptic) (round) K25.9
  - with
    - hemorrhage K25.4
      - and perforation K25.6
    - perforation K25.5
  - acute K25.3
    - with
      - hemorrhage K25.0
        - and perforation K25.2
      - perforation K25.1
  - chronic K25.7
    - with
      - hemorrhage K25.4
        - and perforation K25.6
      - perforation K25.5
- stomal — *see* Ulcer, gastrojejunal
- stomatitis K12.1
- stress — *see* Ulcer, peptic
- strumous (tuberculous) A18.2
- submucosal, bladder — *see* Cystitis, interstitial
- syphilitic (any site) (early) (secondary) A51.39
  - late A52.79
  - perforating A52.79
    - foot A52.11
- testis N50.89
- thigh — *see* Ulcer, lower limb
- throat J39.2
  - diphtheritic A36.0
- toe — *see* Ulcer, lower limb
- tongue (traumatic) K14.0
- tonsil J35.8
  - diphtheritic A36.0
- trachea J39.8
- trophic — *see* Ulcer, skin
- tropical — *see* Ulcer, skin
- tuberculous — *see* Tuberculosis, ulcer
- tunica vaginalis N50.89
- turbinate J34.89
- typhoid (perforating) — *see* Typhoid
- unspecified site — *see* Ulcer, skin
- urethra (meatus) — *see* Urethritis
- uterus N85.8
  - cervix N86
    - with cervicitis N72
  - neck N86

Ulcer, ulcerated, ulcerating, ulceration, ulcerative - *continued*
- uterus - *continued*
  - neck - *continued*
    - with cervicitis N72
- vagina N76.5
  - in Behçet's disease M35.2 *[N77.0]*
  - pessary N89.8
- valve, heart I33.0
- varicose (lower limb, any part) — *see also* Varix, leg, with, ulcer
  - broad ligament I86.2
  - esophagus — *see* Varix, esophagus
  - inflamed or infected — *see* Varix, leg, with ulcer, with inflammation
  - nasal septum I86.8
  - perineum I86.3
  - scrotum I86.1
  - specified site NEC I86.8
  - sublingual I86.0
  - vulva I86.3
- vas deferens N50.89
- vulva (acute) (infectional) N76.6
  - in (due to)
    - Behçet's disease M35.2 *[N77.0]*
    - herpesviral (herpes simplex) infection A60.04
    - tuberculosis A18.18
- vulvobuccal, recurring N76.6
- X-ray L58.1
- yaws A66.4

Ulcerosa scarlatina A38.8
Ulcus — *see also* Ulcer
- cutis tuberculosum A18.4
- duodeni — *see* Ulcer, duodenum
- durum (syphilitic) A51.0
  - extragenital A51.2
- gastrojejunale — *see* Ulcer, gastrojejunal
- hypostaticum — *see* Ulcer, varicose
- molle (cutis) (skin) A57
- serpens corneae — *see* Ulcer, cornea, central
- ventriculi — *see* Ulcer, stomach

Ulegyria Q04.8
Ulerythema
- ophryogenes, congenital Q84.2
- sycosiforme L73.8

Ullrich (-Bonnevie) (-Turner) **syndrome** — *see also* Turner's syndrome Q87.1
Ullrich-Feichtiger syndrome Q87.0
Ulnar — *see* condition
Ulorrhagia, ulorrhea K06.8
Umbilicus, umbilical — *see* condition
Unacceptable
- contours of tooth K08.54
- morphology of tooth K08.54

Unavailability (of)
- bed at medical facility Z75.1
- health service-related agencies Z75.4
- medical facilities (at) Z75.3
  - due to
    - investigation by social service agency Z75.2
    - lack of services at home Z75.0
    - remoteness from facility Z75.3
    - waiting list Z75.1
  - home Z75.0
  - outpatient clinic Z75.3
- schooling Z55.1
- social service agencies Z75.4

Uncinaria americana infestation B76.1
Uncinariasis B76.9
Uncongenial work Z56.5
Unconscious (ness) — *see* Coma
Under observation — *see* Observation
Underachievement in school Z55.3
Underdevelopment — *see also* Undeveloped
- nose Q30.1
- sexual E30.0

Underdosing — *see also* Table of Drugs and Chemicals, categories T36-T50, with final character 6 Z91.14
- intentional NEC Z91.128
  - due to financial hardship of patient Z91.120
- unintentional NEC Z91.138
  - due to patient's age related debility Z91.130

Underfeeding, newborn P92.3
Underfill, endodontic M27.53
Underimmunization status Z28.3
Undernourishment — *see* Malnutrition
Undernutrition — *see* Malnutrition
Underweight R63.6
- for gestational age — *see* Light for dates

Underwood's disease P83.0
Undescended — *see also* Malposition, congenital
- cecum Q43.3

Undescended - *continued*
- colon Q43.3
- testicle — *see* Cryptorchid

Undeveloped, undevelopment — *see also* Hypoplasia
- brain (congenital) Q02
- cerebral (congenital) Q02
- heart Q24.8
- lung Q33.6
- testis E29.1
- uterus E30.0

Undiagnosed (disease) R69
Undulant fever — *see* Brucellosis
Unemployment, anxiety concerning Z56.0
- threatened Z56.2

Unequal length (acquired) (limb) — *see also* Deformity, limb, unequal length
- leg — *see also* Deformity, limb, unequal length
  - congenital Q72.9-

Unextracted dental root K08.3
Unguis incarnatus L60.0
Unhappiness R45.2
Unicornate uterus Q51.4
- in pregnancy or childbirth O34.00

Unilateral — *see also* condition
- development, breast N64.89
- organ or site, congenital NEC — *see* Agenesis, by site

Unilocular heart Q20.8
Union, abnormal — *see also* Fusion
- larynx and trachea Q34.8

Universal mesentery Q43.3
Unrepairable overhanging of dental restorative materials K08.52
Unsatisfactory
- restoration of tooth K08.50
  - specified NEC K08.59
- sample of cytologic smear
  - anus R85.615
  - cervix R87.615
  - vagina R87.625
- surroundings Z59.1
  - work Z56.5

Unsoundness of mind — *see* Psychosis
Unstable
- back NEC — *see* Instability, joint, spine
- hip (congenital) Q65.6
  - acquired — *see* Derangement, joint, specified type NEC, hip
- joint — *see* Instability, joint
  - secondary to removal of joint prosthesis M96.89
- lie (mother) O32.0
- lumbosacral joint (congenital)
  - acquired — *see* subcategory M53.2
- sacroiliac — *see* subcategory M53.2
- spine NEC — *see* Instability, joint, spine

Unsteadiness on feet R26.81
Untruthfulness, child problem F91.8
Unverricht (-Lundborg) **disease or epilepsy** — *see* Epilepsy, generalized, idiopathic
Unwanted pregnancy Z64.0
Upbringing, institutional Z62.22
- away from parents NEC Z62.29
- in care of non-parental family member Z62.21
- in foster care Z62.21
- in orphanage or group home Z62.22
- in welfare custody Z62.21

Upper respiratory — *see* condition
Upset
- gastric K30
- gastrointestinal K30
  - psychogenic F45.8
- intestinal (large) (small) K59.9
  - psychogenic F45.8
- menstruation N93.9
- mental F48.9
- stomach K30
  - psychogenic F45.8

Urachus — *see also* condition
- patent or persistent Q64.4

Urbach-Oppenheim disease (necrobiosis lipoidica diabeticorum) — *see* E08-E13 with .620
Urbach's lipoid proteinosis E78.89
Urbach-Wiethe disease E78.89
Urban yellow fever A95.1
Urea
- blood, high — *see* Uremia
- cycle metabolism disorder — *see* Disorder, urea cycle metabolism

Uremia, uremic N19
- with
  - ectopic or molar pregnancy O08.4

- **Uremia, uremic** - *continued*
  - with - *continued*
    - polyneuropathy N18.9 *[G63]*
  - chronic NOS — *see also* Disease, kidney, chronic N18.9
    - due to hypertension — *see* Hypertensive, kidney
  - complicating
    - ectopic or molar pregnancy O08.4
  - congenital P96.0
  - extrarenal R39.2
  - following ectopic or molar pregnancy O08.4
  - newborn P96.0
  - prerenal R39.2
- **Ureter, ureteral** — *see* condition
- **Ureteralgia** N23
- **Ureterectasis** — *see* Hydroureter
- **Ureteritis** N28.89
  - cystica N28.86
  - due to calculus N20.1
    - with calculus, kidney N20.2
      - with hydronephrosis N13.2
  - gonococcal (acute) (chronic) A54.21
  - nonspecific N28.89
- **Ureterocele** N28.89
  - congenital (orthotopic) Q62.31
    - ectopic Q62.32
- **Ureterolith, ureterolithiasis** — *see* Calculus, ureter
- **Ureterostomy**
  - attention to Z43.6
  - status Z93.6
- **Urethra, urethral** — *see* condition
- **Urethralgia** R39.89
- **Urethritis** (anterior) (posterior) N34.2
  - calculous N21.1
  - candidal B37.41
  - chlamydial A56.01
  - diplococcal (gonococcal) A54.01
    - with abscess (accessory gland) (periurethral) A54.1
  - gonococcal A54.01
    - with abscess (accessory gland) (periurethral) A54.1
  - nongonococcal N34.1
    - Reiter's — *see* Reiter's disease
  - nonspecific N34.1
  - nonvenereal N34.1
  - postmenopausal N34.2
  - puerperal O86.22
  - Reiter's — *see* Reiter's disease
  - specified NEC N34.2
  - trichomonal or due to Trichomonas (vaginalis) A59.03
- **Urethrocele** N81.0
  - with
    - cystocele — *see* Cystocele
    - prolapse of uterus — *see* Prolapse, uterus
- **Urethrolithiasis** (with colic or infection) N21.1
- **Urethrorectal** — *see* condition
- **Urethrorrhagia** N36.8
- **Urethrorrhea** R36.9
- **Urethrostomy**
  - attention to Z43.6
  - status Z93.6
- **Urethrotrigonitis** — *see* Trigonitis
- **Urethrovaginal** — *see* condition
- **Urgency**
  - fecal R15.2
  - hypertensive — *see* Hypertension
  - urinary R39.15
- **Urhidrosis, uridrosis** L74.8
- **Uric acid in blood** (increased) E79.0
- **Uricacidemia** (asymptomatic) E79.0
- **Uricemia** (asymptomatic) E79.0
- **Uricosuria** R82.998
- **Urinary** — *see* condition
- **Urination**
  - frequent R35.0
  - painful R30.9
- **Urine**
  - blood in — *see* Hematuria
  - discharge, excessive R35.8
  - enuresis, nonorganic origin F98.0
  - extravasation R39.0
  - frequency R35.0
  - incontinence R32
    - nonorganic origin F98.0
  - intermittent stream R39.198
  - pus in N39.0
  - retention or stasis R33.9
    - organic R33.8
      - drug-induced R33.0
    - psychogenic F45.8
  - secretion
    - deficient R34
    - excessive R35.8
- **Urine** - *continued*
  - secretion - *continued*
    - frequency R35.0
  - stream
    - intermittent R39.198
    - slowing R39.198
    - splitting R39.13
    - weak R39.12
- **Urinemia** — *see* Uremia
- **Urinoma, urethra** N36.8
- **Uroarthritis, infectious** (Reiter's) — *see* Reiter's disease
- **Urodialysis** R34
- **Urolithiasis** — *see* Calculus, urinary
- **Uronephrosis** — *see* Hydronephrosis
- **Uropathy** N39.9
  - obstructive N13.9
    - specified NEC N13.8
  - reflux N13.9
    - specified NEC N13.8
  - vesicoureteral reflux-associated — *see* Reflux, vesicoureteral
- **Urosepsis - code to condition**
- **Urticaria** L50.9
  - with angioneurotic edema T78.3
    - hereditary D84.1
  - allergic L50.0
  - cholinergic L50.5
  - chronic L50.8
  - cold, familial L50.2
  - contact L50.6
  - dermatographic L50.3
  - due to
    - cold or heat L50.2
    - drugs L50.0
    - food L50.0
    - inhalants L50.0
    - plants L50.6
    - serum — *see also* Reaction, serum T80.69
  - factitial L50.3
  - familial cold M04.2
  - giant T78.3
    - hereditary D84.1
  - gigantea T78.3
  - idiopathic L50.1
  - larynx T78.3
    - hereditary D84.1
  - neonatorum P83.88
  - nonallergic L50.1
  - papulosa (Hebra) L28.2
  - pigmentosa D47.01
    - congenital Q82.2
    - of neonatal onset Q82.2
    - of newborn onset Q82.2
  - recurrent periodic L50.8
  - serum — *see also* Reaction, serum T80.69
  - solar L56.3
  - specified type NEC L50.8
  - thermal (cold) (heat) L50.2
  - vibratory L50.4
  - xanthelasmoidea — *see* Urticaria pigmentosa
- **Use** (of)
  - alcohol Z72.89
    - with
      - intoxication F10.929
      - sleep disorder F10.982
    - harmful — *see* Abuse, alcohol
  - amphetamines — *see* Use, stimulant NEC
  - caffeine — *see* Use, stimulant NEC
  - cannabis F12.90
    - with
      - anxiety disorder F12.980
      - intoxication F12.929
        - with
          - delirium F12.921
          - perceptual disturbance F12.922
        - uncomplicated F12.920
      - other specified disorder F12.988
      - psychosis F12.959
        - delusions F12.950
        - hallucinations F12.951
      - unspecified disorder F12.99
      - withdrawal F12.93
  - cocaine F14.90
    - with
      - anxiety disorder F14.980
      - intoxication F14.929
        - with
          - delirium F14.921
          - perceptual disturbance F14.922
        - uncomplicated F14.920
      - other specified disorder F14.988
      - psychosis F14.959
- **Use** (of) - *continued*
  - cocaine - *continued*
    - with - *continued*
      - psychosis - *continued*
        - delusions F14.950
        - hallucinations F14.951
      - sexual dysfunction F14.981
      - sleep disorder F14.982
      - unspecified disorder F14.99
    - harmful — *see* Abuse, drug, cocaine
  - drug (s) NEC F19.90
    - with sleep disorder F19.982
    - harmful — *see* Abuse, drug, by type
  - hallucinogen NEC F16.90
    - with
      - anxiety disorder F16.980
      - intoxication F16.929
        - with
          - delirium F16.921
        - uncomplicated F16.920
      - mood disorder F16.94
      - other specified disorder F16.988
      - perception disorder (flashbacks) F16.983
      - psychosis F16.959
        - delusions F16.950
        - hallucinations F16.951
      - unspecified disorder F16.99
    - harmful — *see* Abuse, drug, hallucinogen NEC
  - inhalants F18.90
    - with
      - anxiety disorder F18.980
      - intoxication F18.929
        - with delirium F18.921
        - uncomplicated F18.920
      - mood disorder F18.94
      - other specified disorder F18.988
      - persisting dementia F18.97
      - psychosis F18.959
        - delusions F18.950
        - hallucinations F18.951
      - unspecified disorder F18.99
    - harmful — *see* Abuse, drug, inhalant
  - methadone — *see* Use, opioid
  - nonprescribed drugs F19.90
    - harmful — *see* Abuse, non-psychoactive substance
  - opioid F11.90
    - with
      - disorder F11.99
        - mood F11.94
        - sleep F11.982
        - specified type NEC F11.988
      - intoxication F11.929
        - with
          - delirium F11.921
          - perceptual disturbance F11.922
        - uncomplicated F11.920
      - withdrawal F11.93
    - harmful — *see* Abuse, drug, opioid
  - patent medicines F19.90
    - harmful — *see* Abuse, non-psychoactive substance
  - psychoactive drug NEC F19.90
    - with
      - anxiety disorder F19.980
      - intoxication F19.929
        - with
          - delirium F19.921
          - perceptual disturbance F19.922
        - uncomplicated F19.920
      - mood disorder F19.94
      - other specified disorder F19.988
      - persisting
        - amnestic disorder F19.96
        - dementia F19.97
      - psychosis F19.959
        - delusions F19.950
        - hallucinations F19.951
      - sexual dysfunction F19.981
      - sleep disorder F19.982
      - unspecified disorder F19.99
      - withdrawal F19.939
        - with
          - delirium F19.931
          - perceptual disturbance F19.932
        - uncomplicated F19.930
    - harmful — *see* Abuse, drug NEC, psychoactive NEC
  - sedative, hypnotic, or anxiolytic F13.90
    - with
      - anxiety disorder F13.980
      - intoxication F13.929
        - with
          - delirium F13.921
        - uncomplicated F13.920

Use (of) - *continued*
sedative, hypnotic, or anxiolytic - *continued*
with - *continued*
other specified disorder F13.988
persisting
amnestic disorder F13.96
dementia F13.97
psychosis F13.959
delusions F13.950
hallucinations F13.951
sexual dysfunction F13.981
sleep disorder F13.982
unspecified disorder F13.99
harmful — *see* Abuse, drug, sedative, hypnotic, or anxiolytic
stimulant NEC F15.90
with
anxiety disorder F15.980
intoxication F15.929
with
delirium F15.921
perceptual disturbance F15.922
uncomplicated F15.920
mood disorder F15.94
other specified disorder F15.988
psychosis F15.959
delusions F15.950
hallucinations F15.951
sexual dysfunction F15.981
sleep disorder F15.982
unspecified disorder F15.99
withdrawal F15.93
harmful — *see* Abuse, drug, stimulant NEC
tobacco Z72.0
with dependence — *see* Dependence, drug, nicotine
volatile solvents — *see also* Use, inhalant F18.90
harmful — *see* Abuse, drug, inhalant
Usher-Senear disease or syndrome L10.4
Uta B55.1
Uteromegaly N85.2
Uterovaginal — *see* condition
Uterovesical — *see* condition
Uveal — *see* condition
Uveitis (anterior) — *see also* Iridocyclitis
acute — *see* Iridocyclitis, acute
chronic — *see* Iridocyclitis, chronic
due to toxoplasmosis (acquired) B58.09
congenital P37.1
granulomatous — *see* Iridocyclitis, chronic
heterochromic — *see* Cyclitis, Fuchs' heterochromic
lens-induced — *see* Iridocyclitis, lens-induced
posterior — *see* Chorioretinitis
sympathetic H44.13-
syphilitic (secondary) A51.43
congenital (early) A50.01
late A52.71
tuberculous A18.54
Uveoencephalitis — *see* Inflammation, chorioretinal
Uveokeratitis — *see* Iridocyclitis
Uveoparotitis D86.89
Uvula — *see* condition
Uvulitis (acute) (catarrhal) (chronic) (membranous) (suppurative) (ulcerative) K12.2

V

Vaccination (prophylactic)
complication or reaction — *see* Complications, vaccination
delayed Z28.9
encounter for Z23
not done — *see* Immunization, not done, because (of)
Vaccinia (generalized) (localized) T88.1
congenital P35.8
without vaccination B08.011
Vacuum, in sinus (accessory) (nasal) J34.89
Vagabond, vagabondage Z59.0
Vagabond's disease B85.1
Vagina, vaginal — *see* condition
Vaginalitis (tunica) (testis) N49.1
Vaginismus (reflex) N94.2
functional F52.5
nonorganic F52.5
psychogenic F52.5
secondary N94.2
Vaginitis (acute) (circumscribed) (diffuse) (emphysematous) (nonvenereal) (ulcerative) N76.0
with ectopic or molar pregnancy O08.0
amebic A06.82
atrophic, postmenopausal N95.2
bacterial N76.0
blennorrhagic (gonococcal) A54.02
Vaginitis (acute) (circumscribed) (diffuse) (emphysematous) (nonvenereal) (ulcerative) - *continued*
candidal B37.3
chlamydial A56.02
chronic N76.1
due to Trichomonas (vaginalis) A59.01
following ectopic or molar pregnancy O08.0
gonococcal A54.02
with abscess (accessory gland) (periurethral) A54.1
granuloma A58
in (due to)
candidiasis B37.3
herpesviral (herpes simplex) infection A60.04
pinworm infection B80 *[N77.1]*
monilial B37.3
mycotic (candidal) B37.3
postmenopausal atrophic N95.2
puerperal (postpartum) O86.13
senile (atrophic) N95.2
subacute or chronic N76.1
syphilitic (early) A51.0
late A52.76
trichomonal A59.01
tuberculous A18.18
Vaginosis — *see* Vaginitis
Vagotonia G52.2
Vagrancy Z59.0
VAIN — *see* Neoplasia, intraepithelial, vagina
Vallecula — *see* condition
Valley fever B38.0
Valsuani's disease — *see* Anemia, obstetric
Valve, valvular (formation) — *see also* condition
cerebral ventricle (communicating) in situ Z98.2
cervix, internal os Q51.828
congenital NEC — *see* Atresia, by site
ureter (pelvic junction) (vesical orifice) Q62.39
urethra (congenital) (posterior) Q64.2
Valvulitis (chronic) — *see* Endocarditis
Valvulopathy — *see* Endocarditis
Van Bogaert's leukoencephalopathy (sclerosing) (subacute) A81.1
Van Bogaert-Scherer-Epstein disease or syndrome E75.5
Van Buchem's syndrome M85.2
Van Creveld-von Gierke disease E74.01
Van der Hoeve (-de Kleyn) **syndrome** Q78.0
Van der Woude's syndrome Q38.0
Van Neck's disease or osteochondrosis M91.0
Vanishing lung J44.9
Vapor asphyxia or suffocation T59.9
specified agent — *see* Table of Drugs and Chemicals
Variance, lethal ball, prosthetic heart valve T82.09
Variants, thalassemic D56.8
Variations in hair color L67.1
Varicella B01.9
with
complications NEC B01.89
encephalitis B01.11
encephalomyelitis B01.11
meningitis B01.0
myelitis B01.12
pneumonia B01.2
congenital P35.8
Varices — *see* Varix
Varicocele (scrotum) (thrombosed) I86.1
ovary I86.2
perineum I86.3
spermatic cord (ulcerated) I86.1
Varicose
aneurysm (ruptured) I77.0
dermatitis — *see* Varix, leg, with, inflammation
eczema — *see* Varix, leg, with, inflammation
phlebitis — *see* Varix, with, inflammation
tumor — *see* Varix
ulcer (lower limb, any part) — *see also* Varix, leg, with, ulcer
anus — *see also* Hemorrhoids K64.8
esophagus — *see* Varix, esophagus
inflamed or infected — *see* Varix, leg, with ulcer, with inflammation
nasal septum I86.8
perineum I86.3
scrotum I86.1
specified site NEC I86.8
vein — *see* Varix
vessel — *see* Varix, leg
Varicosis, varicosities, varicosity — *see* Varix
Variola (major) (minor) B03
Varioloid B03
Varix (lower limb) (ruptured) I83.90
with
edema I83.899
Varix (lower limb) (ruptured) - *continued*
with - *continued*
inflammation I83.10
with ulcer (venous) I83.209
pain I83.819
specified complication NEC I83.899
stasis dermatitis I83.10
with ulcer (venous) I83.209
swelling I83.899
ulcer I83.009
with inflammation I83.209
aneurysmal I77.0
asymptomatic I83.9-
bladder I86.2
broad ligament I86.2
complicating
childbirth (lower extremity) O87.4
anus or rectum O87.2
genital (vagina, vulva or perineum) O87.8
pregnancy (lower extremity) O22.0-
anus or rectum O22.4-
genital (vagina, vulva or perineum) O22.1-
puerperium (lower extremity) O87.4
anus or rectum O87.2
genital (vagina, vulva, perineum) O87.8
congenital (any site) Q27.8
esophagus (idiopathic) (primary) (ulcerated) I85.00
bleeding I85.01
congenital Q27.8
in (due to)
alcoholic liver disease I85.10
bleeding I85.11
cirrhosis of liver I85.10
bleeding I85.11
portal hypertension I85.10
bleeding I85.11
schistosomiasis I85.10
bleeding I85.11
toxic liver disease I85.10
bleeding I85.11
secondary I85.10
bleeding I85.11
gastric I86.4
inflamed or infected I83.10
ulcerated I83.209
labia (majora) I86.3
leg (asymptomatic) I83.90
with
edema I83.899
inflammation I83.10
with ulcer — *see* Varix, leg, with, ulcer, with inflammation by site
pain I83.819
specified complication NEC I83.899
swelling I83.899
ulcer I83.009
with inflammation I83.209
ankle I83.003
with inflammation I83.203
calf I83.002
with inflammation I83.202
foot NEC I83.005
with inflammation I83.205
heel I83.004
with inflammation I83.204
lower leg NEC I83.008
with inflammation I83.208
midfoot I83.004
with inflammation I83.204
thigh I83.001
with inflammation I83.201
bilateral (asymptomatic) I83.93
with
edema I83.893
pain I83.813
specified complication NEC I83.893
swelling I83.893
ulcer I83.0-
with inflammation I83.209
left (asymptomatic) I83.92
with
edema I83.892
pain I83.812
specified complication NEC I83.892
swelling I83.892
inflammation I83.12
with ulcer — *see* Varix, leg, with, ulcer, with inflammation by site
ulcer I83.029
with inflammation I83.229
ankle I83.023
with inflammation I83.223
calf I83.022

- **Vision, visual** - *continued*
  - blurred, blurring H53.8
    - hysterical F44.6
  - defect, defective NEC H54.7
  - disorientation (syndrome) H53.8
  - disturbance H53.9
    - hysterical F44.6
  - double H53.2
  - examination Z01.00
    - with abnormal findings Z01.01
  - field, limitation (defect) — *see* Defect, visual field
  - hallucinations R44.1
  - halos H53.19
  - loss — *see* Loss, vision
    - sudden — *see* Disturbance, vision, subjective, loss, sudden
  - low (both eyes) — *see* Low, vision
  - perception, simultaneous without fusion H53.33
- **Vitality, lack or want of** R53.83
  - newborn P96.89
- **Vitamin deficiency** — *see* Deficiency, vitamin
- **Vitelline duct, persistent** Q43.0
- **Vitiligo** L80
  - eyelid H02.739
    - left H02.736
      - lower H02.735
      - upper H02.734
    - right H02.733
      - lower H02.732
      - upper H02.731
  - pinta A67.2
  - vulva N90.89
- **Vitreal corneal syndrome** H59.01-
- **Vitreoretinopathy, proliferative** — *see also* Retinopathy, proliferative
  - with retinal detachment — *see* Detachment, retina, traction
- **Vitreous** — *see also* condition
  - touch syndrome — *see* Complication, postprocedural, following cataract surgery
- **Vocal cord** — *see* condition
- **Vogt-Koyanagi syndrome** H20.82-
- **Vogt's disease or syndrome** G80.3
- **Vogt-Spielmeyer amaurotic idiocy or disease** E75.4
- **Voice**
  - change R49.9
    - specified NEC R49.8
  - loss — *see* Aphonia
- **Volhynian fever** A79.0
- **Volkmann's ischemic contracture or paralysis** (complicating trauma) T79.6
- **Volvulus** (bowel) (colon) (intestine) K56.2
  - with perforation K56.2
  - congenital Q43.8
  - duodenum K31.5
  - fallopian tube — *see* Torsion, fallopian tube
  - oviduct — *see* Torsion, fallopian tube
  - stomach (due to absence of gastrocolic ligament) K31.89
- **Vomiting** R11.10
  - with nausea R11.2
  - asphyxia — *see* Foreign body, by site, causing asphyxia, gastric contents
  - bilious (cause unknown) R11.14
    - in newborn P92.01
    - following gastro-intestinal surgery K91.0
  - blood — *see* Hematemesis
  - causing asphyxia, choking, or suffocation — *see* Foreign body, by site
  - cyclical G43.A0
    - with refractory migraine G43.A1
    - intractable G43.A1
    - not intractable G43.A0
    - psychogenic F50.89
    - without refractory migraine G43.A0
  - fecal mater R11.13
  - following gastrointestinal surgery K91.0
    - psychogenic F50.89
  - functional K31.89
  - hysterical F50.89
  - nervous F50.89
  - neurotic F50.89
  - newborn NEC P92.09
    - bilious P92.01
  - periodic R11.10
    - psychogenic F50.89
  - projectile R11.12
  - psychogenic F50.89
  - uremic — *see* Uremia
  - without nausea R11.11
- **Vomito negro** — *see* Fever, yellow
- **Von Bezold's abscess** — *see* Mastoiditis, acute
- **Von Economo-Cruchet disease** A85.8
- **Von Eulenburg's disease** G71.19
- **Von Gierke's disease** E74.01
- **Von Hippel** (-Lindau) **disease or syndrome** Q85.8
- **Von Jaksch's anemia or disease** D64.89
- **Von Recklinghausen**
  - disease (neurofibromatosis) Q85.01
    - bones E21.0
- **Von Schroetter's syndrome** I82.890
- **Von Willebrand** (-Jurgens) (-Minot) **disease or syndrome** D68.0
- **Von Zumbusch's disease** L40.1
- **Voyeurism** F65.3
- **Vrolik's disease** Q78.0
- **Vulva** — *see* condition
- **Vulvismus** N94.2
- **Vulvitis** (acute) (allergic) (atrophic) (hypertrophic) (intertriginous) (senile) N76.2
  - with ectopic or molar pregnancy O08.0
  - adhesive, congenital Q52.79
  - blennorrhagic (gonococcal) A54.02
  - candidal B37.3
  - chlamydial A56.02
  - due to Haemophilus ducreyi A57
  - following ectopic or molar pregnancy O08.0
  - gonococcal A54.02
    - with abscess (accessory gland) (periurethral) A54.1
  - herpesviral A60.04
  - leukoplakic N90.4
  - monilial B37.3
  - puerperal (postpartum) O86.19
  - subacute or chronic N76.3
  - syphilitic (early) A51.0
    - late A52.76
  - trichomonal A59.01
  - tuberculous A18.18
- **Vulvodynia** N94.819
  - specified NEC N94.818
- **Vulvorectal** — *see* condition
- **Vulvovaginitis** (acute) — *see* Vaginitis

W

- **Waiting list, person on** Z75.1
  - for organ transplant Z76.82
  - undergoing social agency investigation Z75.2
- **Waldenström**
  - hypergammaglobulinemia D89.0
  - syndrome or macroglobulinemia C88.0
- **Waldenström-Kjellberg syndrome** D50.1
- **Walking**
  - difficulty R26.2
    - psychogenic F44.4
  - sleep F51.3
    - hysterical F44.89
- **Wall, abdominal** — *see* condition
- **Wallenberg's disease or syndrome** G46.3
- **Wallgren's disease** I87.8
- **Wandering**
  - gallbladder, congenital Q44.1
  - in diseases classified elsewhere Z91.83
  - kidney, congenital Q63.8
  - organ or site, congenital NEC — *see* Malposition, congenital, by site
  - pacemaker (heart) I49.8
  - spleen D73.89
- **War neurosis** F48.8
- **Wart** (due to HPV) (filiform) (infectious) (viral) B07.9
  - anogenital region (venereal) A63.0
  - common B07.8
  - external genital organs (venereal) A63.0
  - flat B07.8
  - Hassal-Henle's (of cornea) H18.49
  - Peruvian A44.1
  - plantar B07.0
  - prosector (tuberculous) A18.4
  - seborrheic L82.1
    - inflamed L82.0
  - senile (seborrheic) L82.1
    - inflamed L82.0
  - tuberculous A18.4
  - venereal A63.0
- **Warthin's tumor** — *see* Neoplasm, salivary gland, benign
- **Wassilieff's disease** A27.0
- **Wasting**
  - disease R64
    - due to malnutrition E41
  - extreme (due to malnutrition) E41
  - muscle NEC — *see* Atrophy, muscle
- **Water**
  - clefts (senile cataract) — *see* Cataract, senile, incipient
  - deprivation of T73.1
- **Water** - *continued*
  - intoxication E87.79
  - itch B76.9
  - lack of T73.1
  - loading E87.70
  - on
    - brain — *see* Hydrocephalus
    - chest J94.8
  - poisoning E87.79
- **Waterbrash** R12
- **Waterhouse** (-Friderichsen) **syndrome or disease** (meningococcal) A39.1
- **Water-losing nephritis** N25.89
- **Watermelon stomach** K31.819
  - with hemorrhage K31.811
  - without hemorrhage K31.819
- **Watsoniasis** B66.8
- **Wax in ear** — *see* Impaction, cerumen
- **Weak, weakening, weakness** (generalized) R53.1
  - arches (acquired) — *see also* Deformity, limb, flat foot
  - bladder (sphincter) R32
  - facial R29.810
    - following
      - cerebrovascular disease I69.992
        - cerebral infarction I69.392
        - intracerebral hemorrhage I69.192
        - nontraumatic intracranial hemorrhage NEC I69.292
        - specified disease NEC I69.892
        - stroke I69.392
        - subarachnoid hemorrhage I69.092
  - foot (double) — *see* Weak, arches
  - heart, cardiac — *see* Failure, heart
  - mind F70
  - muscle M62.81
  - myocardium — *see* Failure, heart
  - newborn P96.89
  - pelvic fundus N81.89
  - pubocervical tissue N81.82
  - senile R54
  - rectovaginal tissue N81.83
  - urinary stream R39.12
  - valvular — *see* Endocarditis
- **Wear, worn** (with normal or routine use)
  - articular bearing surface of internal joint prosthesis — *see* Complications, joint prosthesis, mechanical, wear of articular bearing surfaces, by site
  - device, implant or graft — *see* Complications, by site, mechanical complication
  - tooth, teeth (approximal) (hard tissues) (interproximal) (occlusal) K03.0
- **Weather, weathered**
  - effects of
    - cold T69.9
      - specified effect NEC T69.8
    - hot — *see* Heat
  - skin L57.8
- **Weaver's syndrome** Q87.3
- **Web, webbed** (congenital)
  - duodenal Q43.8
  - esophagus Q39.4
  - fingers Q70.1-
  - larynx (glottic) (subglottic) Q31.0
  - neck (pterygium colli) Q18.3
  - Paterson-Kelly D50.1
  - popliteal syndrome Q87.89
  - toes Q70.3-
- **Weber-Christian disease** M35.6
- **Weber-Cockayne syndrome** (epidermolysis bullosa) Q81.8
- **Weber-Gubler syndrome** G46.3
- **Weber-Leyden syndrome** G46.3
- **Weber-Osler syndrome** I78.0
- **Weber's paralysis or syndrome** G46.3
- **Wedge-shaped or wedging vertebra** — *see* Collapse, vertebra NEC
- **Wegener's granulomatosis or syndrome** M31.30
  - with
    - kidney involvement M31.31
    - lung involvement M31.30
      - with kidney involvement M31.31
- **Wegner's disease** A50.02
- **Weight**
  - 1000-2499 grams at birth (low) — *see* Low, birthweight
  - 999 grams or less at birth (extremely low) — *see* Low, birthweight, extreme
  - and length below 10th percentile for gestational age P05.1-
  - below but length above 10th percentile for gestational age P05.0-

Weight - *continued*
  gain (abnormal) (excessive) R63.5
    in pregnancy — *see* Pregnancy, complicated by, excessive weight gain
    low — *see* Pregnancy, complicated by, insufficient, weight gain
  loss (abnormal) (cause unknown) R63.4
Weightlessness (effect of) T75.82
Weil (l) -Marchesani syndrome Q87.1
Weil's disease A27.0
Weingarten's syndrome J82
Weir Mitchell's disease I73.81
Weiss-Baker syndrome G90.09
Wells' disease L98.3
Wen — *see* Cyst, sebaceous
Wenckebach's block or phenomenon I44.1
Werdnig-Hoffmann syndrome (muscular atrophy) G12.0
Werlhof's disease D69.3
Wermer's disease or syndrome E31.21
Werner-His disease A79.0
Werner's disease or syndrome E34.8
Wernicke-Korsakoff's syndrome or psychosis (alcoholic) F10.96
  with dependence F10.26
  drug-induced
    due to drug abuse — *see* Abuse, drug, by type, with amnestic disorder
    due to drug dependence — *see* Dependence, drug, by type, with amnestic disorder
  nonalcoholic F04
Wernicke-Posadas disease B38.9
Wernicke's
  developmental aphasia F80.2
  disease or syndrome E51.2
  encephalopathy E51.2
  polioencephalitis, superior E51.2
West African fever B50.8
Westphal-Strümpell syndrome E83.01
West's syndrome — *see* Epilepsy, spasms
Wet
  feet, tropical (maceration) (syndrome) — *see* Immersion, foot
  lung (syndrome) , newborn P22.1
Wharton's duct — *see* condition
Wheal — *see* Urticaria
Wheezing R06.2
Whiplash injury S13.4
Whipple's disease (*see also* subcategory M14.8-) K90.81
Whipworm (disease) (infection) (infestation) B79
Whistling face Q87.0
White — *see also* condition
  kidney, small N03.9
  leg, puerperal, postpartum, childbirth O87.1
  mouth B37.0
  patches of mouth K13.29
  spot lesions, teeth
    chewing surface K02.51
    pit and fissure surface K02.51
    smooth surface K02.61
Whitehead L70.0
Whitlow — *see also* Cellulitis, digit
  with lymphangitis — *see* Lymphangitis, acute, digit
  herpesviral B00.89
Whitmore's disease or fever — *see* Melioidosis
Whooping cough A37.90
  with pneumonia A37.91
    due to Bordetella
      bronchiseptica A37.81
      parapertussis A37.11
      pertussis A37.01
    specified organism NEC A37.81
  due to
    Bordetella
      bronchiseptica A37.80
        with pneumonia A37.81
      parapertussis A37.10
        with pneumonia A37.11
      pertussis A37.00
        with pneumonia A37.01
      specified NEC A37.80
        with pneumonia A37.81
Wichman's asthma J38.5
Wide cranial sutures, newborn P96.3
Widening aorta — *see* Ectasia, aorta
  with aneurysm — *see* Aneurysm, aorta
Wilkie's disease or syndrome K55.1
Wilkinson-Sneddon disease or syndrome L13.1
Willebrand (-Jürgens) **thrombopathy** D68.0
Williams syndrome Q93.82
Willige-Hunt disease or syndrome G23.1
Wilms' tumor C64-
Wilson-Mikity syndrome P27.0
Wilson's
  disease or syndrome E83.01
  hepatolenticular degeneration E83.01
  lichen ruber L43.9
Window — *see also* Imperfect, closure
  aorticopulmonary Q21.4
Winter — *see* condition
Wiskott-Aldrich syndrome D82.0
Withdrawal state — *see also* Dependence, drug by type, with withdrawal
  alcohol
    with perceptual disturbances F10.232
    without perceptual disturbances F10.239
  caffeine F15.93
  cannabis F12.23
  newborn
    correct therapeutic substance properly administered P96.2
    infant of dependent mother P96.1
  therapeutic substance, neonatal P96.2
without loss of consciousness S06.0X0
Witts' anemia D50.8
Witzelsucht F07.0
Woakes' ethmoiditis or syndrome J33.1
Wolff-Hirschorn syndrome Q93.3
Wolff-Parkinson-White syndrome I45.6
Wolhynian fever A79.0
Wolman's disease E75.5
Wood lung or pneumonitis J67.8
Woolly, wooly hair (congenital) (nevus) Q84.1
Woolsorter's disease A22.1
Word
  blindness (congenital) (developmental) F81.0
  deafness (congenital) (developmental) H93.25
Worm (s) (infection) (infestation) — *see also* Infestation, helminth
  guinea B72
  in intestine NEC B82.0
Worm-eaten soles A66.3
Worn out — *see* Exhaustion
  cardiac
    defibrillator (with synchronous cardiace pacemaker) Z45.02
    pacemaker
      battery Z45.010
      lead Z45.018
  device, implant or graft — *see* Complications, by site, mechanical
Worried well Z71.1
Worries R45.82
Wound check Z48.0-
  due to injury - code to Injury, by site, using appropriate seventh character for subsequent encounter
Wound, open T14.8-
  abdomen, abdominal
    wall S31.109
      with penetration into peritoneal cavity S31.609
      bite — *see* Bite, abdomen, wall
      epigastric region S31.102
        with penetration into peritoneal cavity S31.602
        bite — *see* Bite, abdomen, wall, epigastric region
        laceration — *see* Laceration, abdomen, wall, epigastric region
        puncture — *see* Puncture, abdomen, wall, epigastric region
      laceration — *see* Laceration, abdomen, wall
      left
        lower quadrant S31.104
          with penetration into peritoneal cavity S31.604
          bite — *see* Bite, abdomen, wall, left, lower quadrant
          laceration — *see* Laceration, abdomen, wall, left, lower quadrant
          puncture — *see* Puncture, abdomen, wall, left, lower quadrant
        upper quadrant S31.101
          with penetration into peritoneal cavity S31.601
          bite — *see* Bite, abdomen, wall, left, upper quadrant
          laceration — *see* Laceration, abdomen, wall, left, upper quadrant
          puncture — *see* Puncture, abdomen, wall, left, upper quadrant
      periumbilic region S31.105
        with penetration into peritoneal cavity S31.605
        bite — *see* Bite, abdomen, wall, periumbilic region
        laceration — *see* Laceration, abdomen, wall, periumbilic region
Wound, open - *continued*
  abdomen, abdominal - *continued*
    wall - *continued*
      periumbilic region - *continued*
        puncture — *see* Puncture, abdomen, wall, periumbilic region
      puncture — *see* Puncture, abdomen, wall
      right
        lower quadrant S31.103
          with penetration into peritoneal cavity S31.603
          bite — *see* Bite, abdomen, wall, right, lower quadrant
          laceration — *see* Laceration, abdomen, wall, right, lower quadrant
          puncture — *see* Puncture, abdomen, wall, right, lower quadrant
        upper quadrant S31.100
          with penetration into peritoneal cavity S31.600
          bite — *see* Bite, abdomen, wall, right, upper quadrant
          laceration — *see* Laceration, abdomen, wall, right, upper quadrant
          puncture — *see* Puncture, abdomen, wall, right, upper quadrant
  alveolar (process) — *see* Wound, open, oral cavity
  ankle S91.00-
    bite — *see* Bite, ankle
    laceration — *see* Laceration, ankle
    puncture — *see* Puncture, ankle
  antecubital space — *see* Wound, open, elbow
  anterior chamber, eye — *see* Wound, open, ocular
  anus S31.839
    bite S31.835
    laceration — *see* Laceration, anus
    puncture — *see* Puncture, anus
  arm (upper) S41.10-
    with amputation — *see* Amputation, traumatic, arm
    bite — *see* Bite, arm
    forearm — *see* Wound, open, forearm
    laceration — *see* Laceration, arm
    puncture — *see* Puncture, arm
  auditory canal (external) (meatus) — *see* Wound, open, ear
  auricle, ear — *see* Wound, open, ear
  axilla — *see* Wound, open, arm
  back — *see also* Wound, open, thorax, back
    lower S31.000
      with penetration into retroperitoneal space S31.001
      bite — *see* Bite, back, lower
      laceration — *see* Laceration, back, lower
      puncture — *see* Puncture, back, lower
  bite — *see* Bite
  blood vessel — *see* Injury, blood vessel
  breast S21.00-
    with amputation — *see* Amputation, traumatic, breast
    bite — *see* Bite, breast
    laceration — *see* Laceration, breast
    puncture — *see* Puncture, breast
  buttock S31.809
    bite — *see* Bite, buttock
    laceration — *see* Laceration, buttock
    left S31.829
    puncture — *see* Puncture, buttock
    right S31.819
  calf — *see* Wound, open, leg
  canaliculus lacrimalis — *see* Wound, open, eyelid
  canthus, eye — *see* Wound, open, eyelid
  cervical esophagus S11.20
    bite S11.25
    laceration — *see* Laceration, esophagus, traumatic, cervical
    puncture — *see* Puncture, cervical esophagus
  cheek (external) S01.40-
    bite — *see* Bite, cheek
    laceration — *see* Laceration, cheek
    puncture — *see* Puncture, cheek
    internal — *see* Wound, open, oral cavity
  chest wall — *see* Wound, open, thorax
  chin — *see* Wound, open, head, specified site NEC
  choroid — *see* Wound, open, ocular
  ciliary body (eye) — *see* Wound, open, ocular
  clitoris S31.40
    with amputation — *see* Amputation, traumatic, clitoris
    bite S31.45
    laceration — *see* Laceration, vulva
    puncture — *see* Puncture, vulva
  conjunctiva — *see* Wound, open, ocular
  cornea — *see* Wound, open, ocular
  costal region — *see* Wound, open, thorax

Wound, open - *continued*
perineum - *continued*
female S31.502
laceration — *see* Laceration, perineum
male S31.501
puncture — *see* Puncture, perineum
periocular area (with or without lacrimal passages) — *see* Wound, open, eyelid
periumbilic region S31.105
with penetration into peritoneal cavity S31.605
bite — *see* Bite, abdomen, wall, periumbilic region
laceration — *see* Laceration, abdomen, wall, periumbilic region
puncture — *see* Puncture, abdomen, wall, periumbilic region
phalanges
finger — *see* Wound, open, finger
toe — *see* Wound, open, toe
pharynx S11.20
pinna — *see* Wound, open, ear
popliteal space — *see* Wound, open, knee
prepuce — *see* Wound, open, penis
pubic region — *see* Wound, open, back, lower
pudendum — *see* Wound, open, genital organs, external
puncture wound — *see* Puncture
rectovaginal septum — *see* Wound, open, vagina
right
lower quadrant S31.103
with penetration into peritoneal cavity S31.603
bite — *see* Bite, abdomen, wall, right, lower quadrant
laceration — *see* Laceration, abdomen, wall, right, lower quadrant
puncture — *see* Puncture, abdomen, wall, right, lower quadrant
upper quadrant S31.100
with penetration into peritoneal cavity S31.600
bite — *see* Bite, abdomen, wall, right, upper quadrant
laceration — *see* Laceration, abdomen, wall, right, upper quadrant
puncture — *see* Puncture, abdomen, wall, right, upper quadrant
sacral region — *see* Wound, open, back, lower
sacroiliac region — *see* Wound, open, back, lower
salivary gland — *see* Wound, open, oral cavity
scalp S01.00
bite S01.05
laceration — *see* Laceration, scalp
puncture — *see* Puncture, scalp
scalpel, newborn (birth injury) P15.8
scapular region — *see* Wound, open, shoulder
sclera — *see* Wound, open, ocular
scrotum S31.30
with amputation — *see* Amputation, traumatic, scrotum
bite S31.35
laceration — *see* Laceration, scrotum
puncture — *see* Puncture, scrotum
shin — *see* Wound, open, leg
shoulder S41.00-
with amputation — *see* Amputation, traumatic, arm
bite — *see* Bite, shoulder
laceration — *see* Laceration, shoulder
puncture — *see* Puncture, shoulder
skin NOS T14.8
spermatic cord — *see* Wound, open, testis
sternal region — *see* Wound, open, thorax, front wall
submaxillary region — *see* Wound, open, head, specified site NEC
submental region — *see* Wound, open, head, specified site NEC
subungual
finger (s) — *see* Wound, open, finger
toe (s) — *see* Wound, open, toe
supraclavicular region — *see* Wound, open, neck, specified site NEC
temple, temporal region — *see* Wound, open, head, specified site NEC
temporomandibular area — *see* Wound, open, cheek
testis S31.30
with amputation — *see* Amputation, traumatic, testes
bite S31.35
laceration — *see* Laceration, testis
puncture — *see* Puncture, testis
thigh S71.10-
with amputation — *see* Amputation, traumatic, hip
bite — *see* Bite, thigh
laceration — *see* Laceration, thigh

Wound, open - *continued*
thigh - *continued*
puncture — *see* Puncture, thigh
thorax, thoracic (wall) S21.90
back S21.20-
with penetration S21.40
bite — *see* Bite, thorax
breast — *see* Wound, open, breast
front S21.10-
with penetration S21.30
laceration — *see* Laceration, thorax
puncture — *see* Puncture, thorax
throat — *see* Wound, open, neck
thumb S61.009
with
amputation — *see* Amputation, traumatic, thumb
damage to nail S61.109
bite — *see* Bite, thumb
laceration — *see* Laceration, thumb
left S61.002
with
damage to nail S61.102
puncture — *see* Puncture, thumb
right S61.001
with
damage to nail S61.101
thyroid (gland) — *see* Wound, open, neck, thyroid
toe (s) S91.109
with
amputation — *see* Amputation, traumatic, toe
damage to nail S91.209
bite — *see* Bite, toe
great S91.103
with
damage to nail S91.203
left S91.102
with
damage to nail S91.202
right S91.101
with
damage to nail S91.201
laceration — *see* Laceration, toe
lesser S91.106
with
damage to nail S91.206
left S91.105
with
damage to nail S91.205
right S91.104
with
damage to nail S91.204
puncture — *see* Puncture, toe
tongue — *see* Wound, open, oral cavity
trachea (cervical region) — *see* Wound, open, neck, trachea
tunica vaginalis — *see* Wound, open, testis
tympanum, tympanic membrane S09.2-
laceration — *see* Laceration, ear, drum
puncture — *see* Puncture, tympanum
umbilical region — *see* Wound, open, abdomen, wall, periumbilic region
uvula — *see* Wound, open, oral cavity
vagina S31.40
bite S31.45
laceration — *see* Laceration, vagina
puncture — *see* Puncture, vagina
vocal cord S11.039
bite — *see* Bite, vocal cord
laceration S11.031
with foreign body S11.032
puncture S11.033
with foreign body S11.034
vitreous (humor) — *see* Wound, open, ocular
vulva S31.40
with amputation — *see* Amputation, traumatic, vulva
bite S31.45
laceration — *see* Laceration, vulva
puncture — *see* Puncture, vulva
wrist S61.50-
bite — *see* Bite, wrist
laceration — *see* Laceration, wrist
puncture — *see* Puncture, wrist
Wound, superficial — *see* Injury — *see also* specified injury type
Wright's syndrome G54.0
Wrist — *see* condition
Wrong drug (by accident) (given in error) — *see* Table of Drugs and Chemicals, by drug, poisoning
Wry neck — *see* Torticollis
Wuchereria (bancrofti) **infestation** B74.0
Wuchereriasis B74.0
Wuchernde Struma Langhans C73

X

Xanthelasma (eyelid) (palpebrarum) H02.60
left H02.66
lower H02.65
upper H02.64
right H02.63
lower H02.62
upper H02.61
Xanthelasmatosis (essential) E78.2
Xanthinuria, hereditary E79.8
Xanthoastrocytoma
specified site — *see* Neoplasm, malignant, by site
unspecified site C71.9
Xanthofibroma — *see* Neoplasm, connective tissue, benign
Xanthogranuloma D76.3
Xanthoma (s) **, xanthomatosis** (primary) (familial) (hereditary) E75.5
with
hyperlipoproteinemia
Type I E78.3
Type III E78.2
Type IV E78.1
Type V E78.3
bone (generalisata) C96.5
cerebrotendinous E75.5
cutaneotendinous E75.5
disseminatum (skin) E78.2
eruptive E78.2
hypercholesterinemic E78.00
hypercholesterolemic E78.00
hyperlipidemic E78.5
joint E75.5
multiple (skin) E78.2
tendon (sheath) E75.5
tubo-eruptive E78.2
tuberosum E78.2
tuberous E78.2
verrucous, oral mucosa K13.4
Xanthosis R23.8
Xenophobia F40.10
Xeroderma — *see also* Ichthyosis
acquired L85.0
eyelid H01.149
left H01.146
lower H01.145
upper H01.144
right H01.143
lower H01.142
upper H01.141
pigmentosum Q82.1
vitamin A deficiency E50.8
Xerophthalmia (vitamin A deficiency) E50.7
unrelated to vitamin A deficiency — *see* Keratoconjunctivitis
Xerosis
conjunctiva H11.14-
with Bitot's spots — *see also* Pigmentation, conjunctiva
vitamin A deficiency E50.1
vitamin A deficiency E50.0
cornea H18.89-
with ulceration — *see* Ulcer, cornea
vitamin A deficiency E50.3
vitamin A deficiency E50.2
cutis L85.3
skin L85.3
Xerostomia K11.7
Xiphopagus Q89.4
XO syndrome Q96.9
X-ray (of)
abnormal findings — *see* Abnormal, diagnostic imaging
breast (mammogram) (routine) Z12.31
chest
routine (as part of a general medical examination) Z00.00
with abnormal findings Z00.01
routine (as part of a general medical examination) Z00.00
with abnormal findings Z00.01
XXXXY syndrome Q98.1
XXY syndrome Q98.0

Y

Yaba pox (virus disease) B08.72
Yatapoxvirus B08.70
specified NEC B08.79
Yawning R06.89
psychogenic F45.8
Yaws A66.9
bone lesions A66.6
butter A66.1

Yaws - *continued*
chancre A66.0
cutaneous, less than five years after infection A66.2
early (cutaneous) (macular) (maculopapular) (micropapular) (papular) A66.2
frambeside A66.2
skin lesions NEC A66.2
eyelid A66.2
ganglion A66.6
gangosis, gangosa A66.5
gumma, gummata A66.4
bone A66.6
gummatous
frambeside A66.4
osteitis A66.6
periostitis A66.6
hydrarthrosis (*see also* subcategory M14.8-) A66.6
hyperkeratosis (early) (late) A66.3
initial lesions A66.0
joint lesions (*see also* subcategory M14.8-) A66.6
juxta-articular nodules A66.7
late nodular (ulcerated) A66.4
latent (without clinical manifestations) (with positive serology) A66.8
mother A66.0
mucosal A66.7
multiple papillomata A66.1
nodular, late (ulcerated) A66.4
osteitis A66.6
papilloma, plantar or palmar A66.1
periostitis (hypertrophic) A66.6
specified NEC A66.7
ulcers A66.4
wet crab A66.1
Yeast infection — *see also* Candidiasis B37.9
Yellow
atrophy (liver) — *see* Failure, hepatic
fever — *see* Fever, yellow
jack — *see* Fever, yellow
jaundice — *see* Jaundice
nail syndrome L60.5
Yersiniosis — *see also* Infection, Yersinia
extraintestinal A28.2
intestinal A04.6

Z

Zahorsky's syndrome (herpangina) B08.5
Zellweger's syndrome Q87.89
Zenker's diverticulum (esophagus) K22.5
Ziehen-Oppenheim disease G24.1
Zieve's syndrome K70.0
Zika NOS A92.5
congenital P35.4
Zinc
deficiency, dietary E60
metabolism disorder E83.2
Zollinger-Ellison syndrome E16.4
Zona — *see* Herpes, zoster
Zoophobia F40.218
Zoster (herpes) — *see* Herpes, zoster
Zygomycosis B46.9
specified NEC B46.8
Zymotic — *see* condition

Substance	Poisoning Accidental (unintentional)	Poisoning Intentional self-harm	Poisoning Assault	Poisoning Undetermined	Adverse effect	Underdosing
1-propanol	T51.3X1-	T51.3X2-	T51.3X3-	T51.3X4-	-	-
2-propanol	T51.2X1-	T51.2X2-	T51.2X3-	T51.2X4-	-	-
2,4-D (dichlorophen-oxyacetic acid)	T60.3X1-	T60.3X2-	T60.3X3-	T60.3X4-	-	-
2,4-toluene diisocyanate	T65.0X1-	T65.0X2-	T65.0X3-	T65.0X4-	-	-
2,4,5-T (trichloro-phenoxyacetic acid)	T60.1X1-	T60.1X2-	T60.1X3-	T60.1X4-	-	-
3,4-methylenedioxymethamphetamine	T43.641-	T43.642-	T43.643-	T43.644-	-	-
14-hydroxydihydro-morphinone	T40.2X1-	T40.2X2-	T40.2X3-	T40.2X4-	T40.2X5-	T40.2X6-
ABOB	T37.5X1-	T37.5X2-	T37.5X3-	T37.5X4-	T37.5X5-	T37.5X6-
Abrine	T62.2X1-	T62.2X2-	T62.2X3-	T62.2X4-	-	-
Abrus (seed)	T62.2X1-	T62.2X2-	T62.2X3-	T62.2X4-	-	-
Absinthe	T51.0X1-	T51.0X2-	T51.0X3-	T51.0X4-	-	-
beverage	T51.0X1-	T51.0X2-	T51.0X3-	T51.0X4-	-	-
Acaricide	T60.8X1-	T60.8X2-	T60.8X3-	T60.8X4-	-	-
Acebutolol	T44.7X1-	T44.7X2-	T44.7X3-	T44.7X4-	T44.7X5-	T44.7X6-
Acecarbromal	T42.6X1-	T42.6X2-	T42.6X3-	T42.6X4-	T42.6X5-	T42.6X6-
Aceclidine	T44.1X1-	T44.1X2-	T44.1X3-	T44.1X4-	T44.1X5-	T44.1X6-
Acedapsone	T37.0X1-	T37.0X2-	T37.0X3-	T37.0X4-	T37.0X5-	T37.0X6-
Acefylline piperazine	T48.6X1-	T48.6X2-	T48.6X3-	T48.6X4-	T48.6X5-	T48.6X6-
Acemorphan	T40.2X1-	T40.2X2-	T40.2X3-	T40.2X4-	T40.2X5-	T40.2X6-
Acenocoumarin	T45.511-	T45.512-	T45.513-	T45.514-	T45.515-	T45.516-
Acenocoumarol	T45.511-	T45.512-	T45.513-	T45.514-	T45.515-	T45.516-
Acepifylline	T48.6X1-	T48.6X2-	T48.6X3-	T48.6X4-	T48.6X5-	T48.6X6-
Acepromazine	T43.3X1-	T43.3X2-	T43.3X3-	T43.3X4-	T43.3X5-	T43.3X6-
Acesulfamethoxypyridazine	T37.0X1-	T37.0X2-	T37.0X3-	T37.0X4-	T37.0X5-	T37.0X6-
Acetal	T52.8X1-	T52.8X2-	T52.8X3-	T52.8X4-	-	-
Acetaldehyde (vapor)	T52.8X1-	T52.8X2-	T52.8X3-	T52.8X4-	-	-
liquid	T65.891-	T65.892-	T65.893-	T65.894-	-	-
P-Acetamidophenol	T39.1X1-	T39.1X2-	T39.1X3-	T39.1X4-	T39.1X5-	T39.1X6-
Acetaminophen	T39.1X1-	T39.1X2-	T39.1X3-	T39.1X4-	T39.1X5-	T39.1X6-
Acetaminosalol	T39.1X1-	T39.1X2-	T39.1X3-	T39.1X4-	T39.1X5-	T39.1X6-
Acetanilide	T39.1X1-	T39.1X2-	T39.1X3-	T39.1X4-	T39.1X5-	T39.1X6-
Acetarsol	T37.3X1-	T37.3X2-	T37.3X3-	T37.3X4-	T37.3X5-	T37.3X6-
Acetazolamide	T50.2X1-	T50.2X2-	T50.2X3-	T50.2X4-	T50.2X5-	T50.2X6-
Acetiamine	T45.2X1-	T45.2X2-	T45.2X3-	T45.2X4-	T45.2X5-	T45.2X6-
Acetic						
acid	T54.2X1-	T54.2X2-	T54.2X3-	T54.2X4-	-	-
with sodium acetate (ointment)	T49.3X1-	T49.3X2-	T49.3X3-	T49.3X4-	T49.3X5-	T49.3X6-
ester (solvent) (vapor)	T52.8X1-	T52.8X2-	T52.8X3-	T52.8X4-	-	-
irrigating solution	T50.3X1-	T50.3X2-	T50.3X3-	T50.3X4-	T50.3X5-	T50.3X6-
medicinal (lotion)	T49.2X1-	T49.2X2-	T49.2X3-	T49.2X4-	T49.2X5-	T49.2X6-
anhydride	T65.891-	T65.892-	T65.893-	T65.894-	-	-
ether (vapor)	T52.8X1-	T52.8X2-	T52.8X3-	T52.8X4-	-	-
Acetohexamide	T38.3X1-	T38.3X2-	T38.3X3-	T38.3X4-	T38.3X5-	T38.3X6-
Acetohydroxamic acid	T50.991-	T50.992-	T50.993-	T50.994-	T50.995-	T50.996-
Acetomenaphthone	T45.7X1-	T45.7X2-	T45.7X3-	T45.7X4-	T45.7X5-	T45.7X6-
Acetomorphine	T40.1X1-	T40.1X2-	T40.1X3-	T40.1X4-	-	-
Acetone (oils)	T52.4X1-	T52.4X2-	T52.4X3-	T52.4X4-	-	-
chlorinated	T52.4X1-	T52.4X2-	T52.4X3-	T52.4X4-	-	-
vapor	T52.4X1-	T52.4X2-	T52.4X3-	T52.4X4-	-	-
Acetonitrile	T52.8X1-	T52.8X2-	T52.8X3-	T52.8X4-	-	-
Acetophenazine	T43.3X1-	T43.3X2-	T43.3X3-	T43.3X4-	T43.3X5-	T43.3X6-
Acetophenetedin	T39.1X1-	T39.1X2-	T39.1X3-	T39.1X4-	T39.1X5-	T39.1X6-
Acetophenone	T52.4X1-	T52.4X2-	T52.4X3-	T52.4X4-	-	-
Acetorphine	T40.2X1-	T40.2X2-	T40.2X3-	T40.2X4-	-	-
Acetosulfone (sodium)	T37.1X1-	T37.1X2-	T37.1X3-	T37.1X4-	T37.1X5-	T37.1X6-
Acetrizoate (sodium)	T50.8X1-	T50.8X2-	T50.8X3-	T50.8X4-	T50.8X5-	T50.8X6-
Acetrizoic acid	T50.8X1-	T50.8X2-	T50.8X3-	T50.8X4-	T50.8X5-	T50.8X6-
Acetyl						
bromide	T53.6X1-	T53.6X2-	T53.6X3-	T53.6X4-	-	-
chloride	T53.6X1-	T53.6X2-	T53.6X3-	T53.6X4-	-	-
Acetylcarbromal	T42.6X1-	T42.6X2-	T42.6X3-	T42.6X4-	T42.6X5-	T42.6X6-
Acetylcholine						
chloride	T44.1X1-	T44.1X2-	T44.1X3-	T44.1X4-	T44.1X5-	T44.1X6-
derivative	T44.1X1-	T44.1X2-	T44.1X3-	T44.1X4-	T44.1X5-	T44.1X6-
Acetylcysteine	T48.4X1-	T48.4X2-	T48.4X3-	T48.4X4-	T48.4X5-	T48.4X6-
Acetyldigitoxin	T46.0X1-	T46.0X2-	T46.0X3-	T46.0X4-	T46.0X5-	T46.0X6-
Acetyldigoxin	T46.0X1-	T46.0X2-	T46.0X3-	T46.0X4-	T46.0X5-	T46.0X6-
Acetyldihydrocodeine	T40.2X1-	T40.2X2-	T40.2X3-	T40.2X4-	-	-
Acetyldihydrocodeinone	T40.2X1-	T40.2X2-	T40.2X3-	T40.2X4-	-	-
Acetylene (gas)	T59.891-	T59.892-	T59.893-	T59.894-	-	-
dichloride	T53.6X1-	T53.6X2-	T53.6X3-	T53.6X4-	-	-
incomplete combustion of	T58.11X-	T58.12X-	T58.13X-	T58.14X-	-	-
industrial	T59.891-	T59.892-	T59.893-	T59.894-	-	-
Acetylene - *continued*						
tetrachloride	T53.6X1-	T53.6X2-	T53.6X3-	T53.6X4-	-	-
vapor	T53.6X1-	T53.6X2-	T53.6X3-	T53.6X4-	-	-
Acetylpheneturide	T42.6X1-	T42.6X2-	T42.6X3-	T42.6X4-	T42.6X5-	T42.6X6-
Acetylphenylhydrazine	T39.8X1-	T39.8X2-	T39.8X3-	T39.8X4-	T39.8X5-	T39.8X6-
Acetylsalicylic acid (salts)	T39.011-	T39.012-	T39.013-	T39.014-	T39.015-	T39.016-
enteric coated	T39.011-	T39.012-	T39.013-	T39.014-	T39.015-	T39.016-
Acetylsulfamethoxypyridazine	T37.0X1-	T37.0X2-	T37.0X3-	T37.0X4-	T37.0X5-	T37.0X6-
Achromycin	T36.4X1-	T36.4X2-	T36.4X3-	T36.4X4-	T36.4X5-	T36.4X6-
ophthalmic preparation	T49.5X1-	T49.5X2-	T49.5X3-	T49.5X4-	T49.5X5-	T49.5X6-
topical NEC	T49.0X1-	T49.0X2-	T49.0X3-	T49.0X4-	T49.0X5-	T49.0X6-
Aciclovir	T37.5X1-	T37.5X2-	T37.5X3-	T37.5X4-	T37.5X5-	T37.5X6-
Acid (corrosive) **NEC**	T54.2X1-	T54.2X2-	T54.2X3-	T54.2X4-	-	-
Acidifying agent NEC	T50.901-	T50.902-	T50.903-	T50.904-	T50.905-	T50.906-
Acipimox	T46.6X1-	T46.6X2-	T46.6X3-	T46.6X4-	T46.6X5-	T46.6X6-
Acitretin	T50.991-	T50.992-	T50.993-	T50.994-	T50.995-	T50.996-
Aclarubicin	T45.1X1-	T45.1X2-	T45.1X3-	T45.1X4-	T45.1X5-	T45.1X6-
Aclatonium napadisilate	T48.1X1-	T48.1X2-	T48.1X3-	T48.1X4-	T48.1X5-	T48.1X6-
Aconite (wild)	T46.991-	T46.992-	T46.993-	T46.994-	T46.995-	T46.996-
Aconitine	T46.991-	T46.992-	T46.993-	T46.994-	T46.995-	T46.996-
Aconitum ferox	T46.991-	T46.992-	T46.993-	T46.994-	T46.995-	T46.996-
Acridine	T65.6X1-	T65.6X2-	T65.6X3-	T65.6X4-	-	-
vapor	T59.891-	T59.892-	T59.893-	T59.894-	-	-
Acriflavine	T37.91X-	T37.92X-	T37.93X-	T37.94X-	T37.95X-	T37.96X-
Acriflavinium chloride	T49.0X1-	T49.0X2-	T49.0X3-	T49.0X4-	T49.0X5-	T49.0X6-
Acrinol	T49.0X1-	T49.0X2-	T49.0X3-	T49.0X4-	T49.0X5-	T49.0X6-
Acrisorcin	T49.0X1-	T49.0X2-	T49.0X3-	T49.0X4-	T49.0X5-	T49.0X6-
Acrivastine	T45.0X1-	T45.0X2-	T45.0X3-	T45.0X4-	T45.0X5-	T45.0X6-
Acrolein (gas)	T59.891-	T59.892-	T59.893-	T59.894-	-	-
liquid	T54.1X1-	T54.1X2-	T54.1X3-	T54.1X4-	-	-
Acrylamide	T65.891-	T65.892-	T65.893-	T65.894-	-	-
Acrylic resin	T49.3X1-	T49.3X2-	T49.3X3-	T49.3X4-	T49.3X5-	T49.3X6-
Acrylonitrile	T65.891-	T65.892-	T65.893-	T65.894-	-	-
Actaea spicata	T62.2X1-	T62.2X2-	T62.2X3-	T62.2X4-	-	-
berry	T62.1X1-	T62.1X2-	T62.1X3-	T62.1X4-	-	-
Acterol	T37.3X1-	T37.3X2-	T37.3X3-	T37.3X4-	T37.3X5-	T37.3X6-
ACTH	T38.811-	T38.812-	T38.813-	T38.814-	T38.815-	T38.816-
Actinomycin C	T45.1X1-	T45.1X2-	T45.1X3-	T45.1X4-	T45.1X5-	T45.1X6-
Actinomycin D	T45.1X1-	T45.1X2-	T45.1X3-	T45.1X4-	T45.1X5-	T45.1X6-
Activated charcoal — *see also* Charcoal, medicinal	T47.6X1-	T47.6X2-	T47.6X3-	T47.6X4-	T47.6X5-	T47.6X6-
Acyclovir	T37.5X1-	T37.5X2-	T37.5X3-	T37.5X4-	T37.5X5-	T37.5X6-
Adenine	T45.2X1-	T45.2X2-	T45.2X3-	T45.2X4-	T45.2X5-	T45.2X6-
arabinoside	T37.5X1-	T37.5X2-	T37.5X3-	T37.5X4-	T37.5X5-	T37.5X6-
Adenosine (phosphate)	T46.2X1-	T46.2X2-	T46.2X3-	T46.2X4-	T46.2X5-	T46.2X6-
ADH	T38.891-	T38.892-	T38.893-	T38.894-	T38.895-	T38.896-
Adhesive NEC	T65.891-	T65.892-	T65.893-	T65.894-	-	-
Adicillin	T36.0X1-	T36.0X2-	T36.0X3-	T36.0X4-	T36.0X5-	T36.0X6-
Adiphenine	T44.3X1-	T44.3X2-	T44.3X3-	T44.3X4-	T44.3X5-	T44.3X6-
Adipiodone	T50.8X1-	T50.8X2-	T50.8X3-	T50.8X4-	T50.8X5-	T50.8X6-
Adjunct, pharmaceutical	T50.901-	T50.902-	T50.903-	T50.904-	T50.905-	T50.906-
Adrenal (extract, cortex or medulla) (glucocorticoids) (hormones) (mineralocorticoids)	T38.0X1-	T38.0X2-	T38.0X3-	T38.0X4-	T38.0X5-	T38.0X6-
ENT agent	T49.6X1-	T49.6X2-	T49.6X3-	T49.6X4-	T49.6X5-	T49.6X6-
ophthalmic preparation	T49.5X1-	T49.5X2-	T49.5X3-	T49.5X4-	T49.5X5-	T49.5X6-
topical NEC	T49.0X1-	T49.0X2-	T49.0X3-	T49.0X4-	T49.0X5-	T49.0X6-
Adrenaline	T44.5X1-	T44.5X2-	T44.5X3-	T44.5X4-	T44.5X5-	T44.5X6-
Adrenalin — *see* Adrenaline						
Adrenergic NEC	T44.901-	T44.902-	T44.903-	T44.904-	T44.905-	T44.906-
blocking agent NEC	T44.8X1-	T44.8X2-	T44.8X3-	T44.8X4-	T44.8X5-	T44.8X6-
beta, heart	T44.7X1-	T44.7X2-	T44.7X3-	T44.7X4-	T44.7X5-	T44.7X6-
specified NEC	T44.991-	T44.992-	T44.993-	T44.994-	T44.995-	T44.996-
Adrenochrome						
(mono) semicarbazone	T46.991-	T46.992-	T46.993-	T46.994-	T46.995-	T46.996-
derivative	T46.991-	T46.992-	T46.993-	T46.994-	T46.995-	T46.996-
Adrenocorticotrophic hormone	T38.811-	T38.812-	T38.813-	T38.814-	T38.815-	T38.816-
Adrenocorticotrophin	T38.811-	T38.812-	T38.813-	T38.814-	T38.815-	T38.816-
Adriamycin	T45.1X1-	T45.1X2-	T45.1X3-	T45.1X4-	T45.1X5-	T45.1X6-
Aerosol spray NEC	T65.91X-	T65.92X-	T65.93X-	T65.94X-	-	-
Aerosporin	T36.8X1-	T36.8X2-	T36.8X3-	T36.8X4-	T36.8X5-	T36.8X6-
ENT agent	T49.6X1-	T49.6X2-	T49.6X3-	T49.6X4-	T49.6X5-	T49.6X6-
ophthalmic preparation	T49.5X1-	T49.5X2-	T49.5X3-	T49.5X4-	T49.5X5-	T49.5X6-
topical NEC	T49.0X1-	T49.0X2-	T49.0X3-	T49.0X4-	T49.0X5-	T49.0X6-
Aethusa cynapium	T62.2X1-	T62.2X2-	T62.2X3-	T62.2X4-	-	-
Afghanistan black	T40.7X1-	T40.7X2-	T40.7X3-	T40.7X4-	T40.7X5-	T40.7X6-
Aflatoxin	T64.01X-	T64.02X-	T64.03X-	T64.04X-	-	-

Substance	Poisoning Accidental (unintentional)	Poisoning Intentional self-harm	Poisoning Assault	Poisoning Undetermined	Adverse effect	Underdosing
Afloqualone	T42.8X1-	T42.8X2-	T42.8X3-	T42.8X4-	T42.8X5-	T42.8X6-
African boxwood	T62.2X1-	T62.2X2-	T62.2X3-	T62.2X4-	-	-
Agar	T47.4X1-	T47.4X2-	T47.4X3-	T47.4X4-	T47.4X5-	T47.4X6-
Agonist						
predominantly						
alpha-adrenoreceptor	T44.4X1-	T44.4X2-	T44.4X3-	T44.4X4-	T44.4X5-	T44.4X6-
beta-adrenoreceptor	T44.5X1-	T44.5X2-	T44.5X3-	T44.5X4-	T44.5X5-	T44.5X6-
Agricultural agent NEC	T65.91X-	T65.92X-	T65.93X-	T65.94X-	-	-
Agrypnal	T42.3X1-	T42.3X2-	T42.3X3-	T42.3X4-	T42.3X5-	T42.3X6-
AHLG	T50.Z11-	T50.Z12-	T50.Z13-	T50.Z14-	T50.Z15-	T50.Z16-
Air contaminant (s), **source/type NOS**	T65.91X-	T65.92X-	T65.93X-	T65.94X-	-	-
Ajmaline	T46.2X1-	T46.2X2-	T46.2X3-	T46.2X4-	T46.2X5-	T46.2X6-
Akee	T62.1X1-	T62.1X2-	T62.1X3-	T62.1X4-	-	-
Akrinol	T49.0X1-	T49.0X2-	T49.0X3-	T49.0X4-	T49.0X5-	T49.0X6-
Akritoin	T37.8X1-	T37.8X2-	T37.8X3-	T37.8X4-	T37.8X5-	T37.8X6-
Alacepril	T46.4X1-	T46.4X2-	T46.4X3-	T46.4X4-	T46.4X5-	T46.4X6-
Alantolactone	T37.4X1-	T37.4X2-	T37.4X3-	T37.4X4-	T37.4X5-	T37.4X6-
Albamycin	T36.8X1-	T36.8X2-	T36.8X3-	T36.8X4-	T36.8X5-	T36.8X6-
Albendazole	T37.4X1-	T37.4X2-	T37.4X3-	T37.4X4-	T37.4X5-	T37.4X6-
Albumin						
bovine	T45.8X1-	T45.8X2-	T45.8X3-	T45.8X4-	T45.8X5-	T45.8X6-
human serum	T45.8X1-	T45.8X2-	T45.8X3-	T45.8X4-	T45.8X5-	T45.8X6-
salt-poor	T45.8X1-	T45.8X2-	T45.8X3-	T45.8X4-	T45.8X5-	T45.8X6-
normal human serum	T45.8X1-	T45.8X2-	T45.8X3-	T45.8X4-	T45.8X5-	T45.8X6-
Albuterol	T48.6X1-	T48.6X2-	T48.6X3-	T48.6X4-	T48.6X5-	T48.6X6-
Albutoin	T42.0X1-	T42.0X2-	T42.0X3-	T42.0X4-	T42.0X5-	T42.0X6-
Alclometasone	T49.0X1-	T49.0X2-	T49.0X3-	T49.0X4-	T49.0X5-	T49.0X6-
Alcohol	T51.91X-	T51.92X-	T51.93X-	T51.94X-	-	-
absolute	T51.0X1-	T51.0X2-	T51.0X3-	T51.0X4-	-	-
beverage	T51.0X1-	T51.0X2-	T51.0X3-	T51.0X4-	-	-
allyl	T51.8X1-	T51.8X2-	T51.8X3-	T51.8X4-	-	-
amyl	T51.3X1-	T51.3X2-	T51.3X3-	T51.3X4-	-	-
antifreeze	T51.1X1-	T51.1X2-	T51.1X3-	T51.1X4-	-	-
beverage	T51.0X1-	T51.0X2-	T51.0X3-	T51.0X4-	-	-
butyl	T51.3X1-	T51.3X2-	T51.3X3-	T51.3X4-	-	-
dehydrated	T51.0X1-	T51.0X2-	T51.0X3-	T51.0X4-	-	-
beverage	T51.0X1-	T51.0X2-	T51.0X3-	T51.0X4-	-	-
denatured	T51.0X1-	T51.0X2-	T51.0X3-	T51.0X4-	-	-
deterrent NEC	T50.6X1-	T50.6X2-	T50.6X3-	T50.6X4-	T50.6X5-	T50.6X6-
diagnostic (gastric function)	T50.8X1-	T50.8X2-	T50.8X3-	T50.8X4-	T50.8X5-	T50.8X6-
ethyl	T51.0X1-	T51.0X2-	T51.0X3-	T51.0X4-	-	-
beverage	T51.0X1-	T51.0X2-	T51.0X3-	T51.0X4-	-	-
grain	T51.0X1-	T51.0X2-	T51.0X3-	T51.0X4-	-	-
beverage	T51.0X1-	T51.0X2-	T51.0X3-	T51.0X4-	-	-
industrial	T51.0X1-	T51.0X2-	T51.0X3-	T51.0X4-	-	-
isopropyl	T51.2X1-	T51.2X2-	T51.2X3-	T51.2X4-	-	-
methyl	T51.1X1-	T51.1X2-	T51.1X3-	T51.1X4-	-	-
preparation for consumption	T51.0X1-	T51.0X2-	T51.0X3-	T51.0X4-	-	-
propyl	T51.3X1-	T51.3X2-	T51.3X3-	T51.3X4-	-	-
secondary	T51.2X1-	T51.2X2-	T51.2X3-	T51.2X4-	-	-
radiator	T51.1X1-	T51.1X2-	T51.1X3-	T51.1X4-	-	-
rubbing	T51.2X1-	T51.2X2-	T51.2X3-	T51.2X4-	-	-
specified type NEC	T51.8X1-	T51.8X2-	T51.8X3-	T51.8X4-	-	-
surgical	T51.0X1-	T51.0X2-	T51.0X3-	T51.0X4-	-	-
vapor (from any type of Alcohol)	T59.891-	T59.892-	T59.893-	T59.894-	-	-
wood	T51.1X1-	T51.1X2-	T51.1X3-	T51.1X4-	-	-
Alcuronium (chloride)	T48.1X1-	T48.1X2-	T48.1X3-	T48.1X4-	T48.1X5-	T48.1X6-
Aldactone	T50.0X1-	T50.0X2-	T50.0X3-	T50.0X4-	T50.0X5-	T50.0X6-
Aldesulfone sodium	T37.1X1-	T37.1X2-	T37.1X3-	T37.1X4-	T37.1X5-	T37.1X6-
Aldicarb	T60.0X1-	T60.0X2-	T60.0X3-	T60.0X4-	-	-
Aldomet	T46.5X1-	T46.5X2-	T46.5X3-	T46.5X4-	T46.5X5-	T46.5X6-
Aldosterone	T50.0X1-	T50.0X2-	T50.0X3-	T50.0X4-	T50.0X5-	T50.0X6-
Aldrin (dust)	T60.1X1-	T60.1X2-	T60.1X3-	T60.1X4-	-	-
Aleve — *see* Naproxen						
Alexitol sodium	T47.1X1-	T47.1X2-	T47.1X3-	T47.1X4-	T47.1X5-	T47.1X6-
Alfacalcidol	T45.2X1-	T45.2X2-	T45.2X3-	T45.2X4-	T45.2X5-	T45.2X6-
Alfadolone	T41.1X1-	T41.1X2-	T41.1X3-	T41.1X4-	T41.1X5-	T41.1X6-
Alfaxalone	T41.1X1-	T41.1X2-	T41.1X3-	T41.1X4-	T41.1X5-	T41.1X6-
Alfentanil	T40.4X1-	T40.4X2-	T40.4X3-	T40.4X4-	T40.4X5-	T40.4X6-
Alfuzosin (hydrochloride)	T44.8X1-	T44.8X2-	T44.8X3-	T44.8X4-	T44.8X5-	T44.8X6-
Algae (harmful) (toxin)	T65.821-	T65.822-	T65.823-	T65.824-	-	-
Algeldrate	T47.1X1-	T47.1X2-	T47.1X3-	T47.1X4-	T47.1X5-	T47.1X6-
Algin	T47.8X1-	T47.8X2-	T47.8X3-	T47.8X4-	T47.8X5-	T47.8X6-
Alglucerase	T45.3X1-	T45.3X2-	T45.3X3-	T45.3X4-	T45.3X5-	T45.3X6-
Alidase	T45.3X1-	T45.3X2-	T45.3X3-	T45.3X4-	T45.3X5-	T45.3X6-
Alimemazine	T43.3X1-	T43.3X2-	T43.3X3-	T43.3X4-	T43.3X5-	T43.3X6-

Substance	Poisoning Accidental (unintentional)	Poisoning Intentional self-harm	Poisoning Assault	Poisoning Undetermined	Adverse effect	Underdosing
Aliphatic thiocyanates	T65.0X1-	T65.0X2-	T65.0X3-	T65.0X4-	-	-
Alizapride	T45.0X1-	T45.0X2-	T45.0X3-	T45.0X4-	T45.0X5-	T45.0X6-
Alkali (caustic)	T54.3X1-	T54.3X2-	T54.3X3-	T54.3X4-	-	-
Alkaline antiseptic solution (aromatic)	T49.6X1-	T49.6X2-	T49.6X3-	T49.6X4-	T49.6X5-	T49.6X6-
Alkalinizing agents (medicinal)	T50.901-	T50.902-	T50.903-	T50.904-	T50.905-	T50.906-
Alkalizing agent NEC	T50.901-	T50.902-	T50.903-	T50.904-	T50.905-	T50.906-
Alka-seltzer	T39.011-	T39.012-	T39.013-	T39.014-	T39.015-	T39.016-
Alkavervir	T46.5X1-	T46.5X2-	T46.5X3-	T46.5X4-	T46.5X5-	T46.5X6-
Alkonium (bromide)	T49.0X1-	T49.0X2-	T49.0X3-	T49.0X4-	T49.0X5-	T49.0X6-
Alkylating drug NEC	T45.1X1-	T45.1X2-	T45.1X3-	T45.1X4-	T45.1X5-	T45.1X6-
antimyeloproliferative	T45.1X1-	T45.1X2-	T45.1X3-	T45.1X4-	T45.1X5-	T45.1X6-
lymphatic	T45.1X1-	T45.1X2-	T45.1X3-	T45.1X4-	T45.1X5-	T45.1X6-
Alkylisocyanate	T65.0X1-	T65.0X2-	T65.0X3-	T65.0X4-	-	-
Allantoin	T49.4X1-	T49.4X2-	T49.4X3-	T49.4X4-	T49.4X5-	T49.4X6-
Allegron	T43.011-	T43.012-	T43.013-	T43.014-	T43.015-	T43.016-
Allethrin	T49.0X1-	T49.0X2-	T49.0X3-	T49.0X4-	T49.0X5-	T49.0X6-
Allobarbital	T42.3X1-	T42.3X2-	T42.3X3-	T42.3X4-	T42.3X5-	T42.3X6-
Allopurinol	T50.4X1-	T50.4X2-	T50.4X3-	T50.4X4-	T50.4X5-	T50.4X6-
Allyl						
Alcohol	T51.8X1-	T51.8X2-	T51.8X3-	T51.8X4-	-	-
disulfide	T46.6X1-	T46.6X2-	T46.6X3-	T46.6X4-	T46.6X5-	T46.6X6-
Allylestrenol	T38.5X1-	T38.5X2-	T38.5X3-	T38.5X4-	T38.5X5-	T38.5X6-
Allylisopropylacetylurea	T42.6X1-	T42.6X2-	T42.6X3-	T42.6X4-	T42.6X5-	T42.6X6-
Allylisopropylmalonylurea	T42.3X1-	T42.3X2-	T42.3X3-	T42.3X4-	T42.3X5-	T42.3X6-
Allylthiourea	T49.3X1-	T49.3X2-	T49.3X3-	T49.3X4-	T49.3X5-	T49.3X6-
Allyltribromide	T42.6X1-	T42.6X2-	T42.6X3-	T42.6X4-	T42.6X5-	T42.6X6-
Allypropymal	T42.3X1-	T42.3X2-	T42.3X3-	T42.3X4-	T42.3X5-	T42.3X6-
Almagate	T47.1X1-	T47.1X2-	T47.1X3-	T47.1X4-	T47.1X5-	T47.1X6-
Almasilate	T47.1X1-	T47.1X2-	T47.1X3-	T47.1X4-	T47.1X5-	T47.1X6-
Almitrine	T50.7X1-	T50.7X2-	T50.7X3-	T50.7X4-	T50.7X5-	T50.7X6-
Aloes	T47.2X1-	T47.2X2-	T47.2X3-	T47.2X4-	T47.2X5-	T47.2X6-
Aloglutamol	T47.1X1-	T47.1X2-	T47.1X3-	T47.1X4-	T47.1X5-	T47.1X6-
Aloin	T47.2X1-	T47.2X2-	T47.2X3-	T47.2X4-	T47.2X5-	T47.2X6-
Aloxidone	T42.2X1-	T42.2X2-	T42.2X3-	T42.2X4-	T42.2X5-	T42.2X6-
Alpha						
acetyldigoxin	T46.0X1-	T46.0X2-	T46.0X3-	T46.0X4-	T46.0X5-	T46.0X6-
adrenergic blocking drug	T44.6X1-	T44.6X2-	T44.6X3-	T44.6X4-	T44.6X5-	T44.6X6-
amylase	T45.3X1-	T45.3X2-	T45.3X3-	T45.3X4-	T45.3X5-	T45.3X6-
tocoferol (acetate)	T45.2X1-	T45.2X2-	T45.2X3-	T45.2X4-	T45.2X5-	T45.2X6-
tocopherol	T45.2X1-	T45.2X2-	T45.2X3-	T45.2X4-	T45.2X5-	T45.2X6-
Alphadolone	T41.1X1-	T41.1X2-	T41.1X3-	T41.1X4-	T41.1X5-	T41.1X6-
Alphaprodine	T40.4X1-	T40.4X2-	T40.4X3-	T40.4X4-	T40.4X5-	T40.4X6-
Alphaxalone	T41.1X1-	T41.1X2-	T41.1X3-	T41.1X4-	T41.1X5-	T41.1X6-
Alprazolam	T42.4X1-	T42.4X2-	T42.4X3-	T42.4X4-	T42.4X5-	T42.4X6-
Alprenolol	T44.7X1-	T44.7X2-	T44.7X3-	T44.7X4-	T44.7X5-	T44.7X6-
Alprostadil	T46.7X1-	T46.7X2-	T46.7X3-	T46.7X4-	T46.7X5-	T46.7X6-
Alsactide	T38.811-	T38.812-	T38.813-	T38.814-	T38.815-	T38.816-
Alseroxylon	T46.5X1-	T46.5X2-	T46.5X3-	T46.5X4-	T46.5X5-	T46.5X6-
Alteplase	T45.611-	T45.612-	T45.613-	T45.614-	T45.615-	T45.616-
Altizide	T50.2X1-	T50.2X2-	T50.2X3-	T50.2X4-	T50.2X5-	T50.2X6-
Altretamine	T45.1X1-	T45.1X2-	T45.1X3-	T45.1X4-	T45.1X5-	T45.1X6-
Alum (medicinal)	T49.4X1-	T49.4X2-	T49.4X3-	T49.4X4-	T49.4X5-	T49.4X6-
nonmedicinal (ammonium) (potassium)	T56.891-	T56.892-	T56.893-	T56.894-	-	-
Aluminium, aluminum						
acetate	T49.2X1-	T49.2X2-	T49.2X3-	T49.2X4-	T49.2X5-	T49.2X6-
solution	T49.0X1-	T49.0X2-	T49.0X3-	T49.0X4-	T49.0X5-	T49.0X6-
aspirin	T39.011-	T39.012-	T39.013-	T39.014-	T39.015-	T39.016-
bis (acetylsalicylate)	T39.011-	T39.012-	T39.013-	T39.014-	T39.015-	T39.016-
carbonate (gel, basic)	T47.1X1-	T47.1X2-	T47.1X3-	T47.1X4-	T47.1X5-	T47.1X6-
chlorhydroxide-complex	T47.1X1-	T47.1X2-	T47.1X3-	T47.1X4-	T47.1X5-	T47.1X6-
chloride	T49.2X1-	T49.2X2-	T49.2X3-	T49.2X4-	T49.2X5-	T49.2X6-
clofibrate	T46.6X1-	T46.6X2-	T46.6X3-	T46.6X4-	T46.6X5-	T46.6X6-
diacetate	T49.2X1-	T49.2X2-	T49.2X3-	T49.2X4-	T49.2X5-	T49.2X6-
glycinate	T47.1X1-	T47.1X2-	T47.1X3-	T47.1X4-	T47.1X5-	T47.1X6-
hydroxide (gel)	T47.1X1-	T47.1X2-	T47.1X3-	T47.1X4-	T47.1X5-	T47.1X6-
hydroxide-magnesium carb. gel	T47.1X1-	T47.1X2-	T47.1X3-	T47.1X4-	T47.1X5-	T47.1X6-
magnesium silicate	T47.1X1-	T47.1X2-	T47.1X3-	T47.1X4-	T47.1X5-	T47.1X6-
nicotinate	T46.7X1-	T46.7X2-	T46.7X3-	T46.7X4-	T46.7X5-	T46.7X6-
ointment (surgical) (topical)	T49.3X1-	T49.3X2-	T49.3X3-	T49.3X4-	T49.3X5-	T49.3X6-
phosphate	T47.1X1-	T47.1X2-	T47.1X3-	T47.1X4-	T47.1X5-	T47.1X6-
salicylate	T39.091-	T39.092-	T39.093-	T39.094-	T39.095-	T39.096-
silicate	T47.1X1-	T47.1X2-	T47.1X3-	T47.1X4-	T47.1X5-	T47.1X6-
sodium silicate	T47.1X1-	T47.1X2-	T47.1X3-	T47.1X4-	T47.1X5-	T47.1X6-
subacetate	T49.2X1-	T49.2X2-	T49.2X3-	T49.2X4-	T49.2X5-	T49.2X6-
sulfate	T49.0X1-	T49.0X2-	T49.0X3-	T49.0X4-	T49.0X5-	T49.0X6-
tannate	T47.6X1-	T47.6X2-	T47.6X3-	T47.6X4-	T47.6X5-	T47.6X6-

Substance	Poisoning Accidental (unintentional)	Poisoning Intentional self-harm	Poisoning Assault	Poisoning Undetermined	Adverse effect	Underdosing
Aluminium, aluminum - *continued*						
topical NEC	T49.3X1-	T49.3X2-	T49.3X3-	T49.3X4-	T49.3X5-	T49.3X6-
Alurate	T42.3X1-	T42.3X2-	T42.3X3-	T42.3X4-	T42.3X5-	T42.3X6-
Alverine	T44.3X1-	T44.3X2-	T44.3X3-	T44.3X4-	T44.3X5-	T44.3X6-
Alvodine	T40.2X1-	T40.2X2-	T40.2X3-	T40.2X4-	T40.2X5-	T40.2X6-
Amanita phalloides	T62.0X1-	T62.0X2-	T62.0X3-	T62.0X4-	-	-
Amanitine	T62.0X1-	T62.0X2-	T62.0X3-	T62.0X4-	-	-
Amantadine	T42.8X1-	T42.8X2-	T42.8X3-	T42.8X4-	T42.8X5-	T42.8X6-
Ambazone	T49.6X1-	T49.6X2-	T49.6X3-	T49.6X4-	T49.6X5-	T49.6X6-
Ambenonium (chloride)	T44.0X1-	T44.0X2-	T44.0X3-	T44.0X4-	T44.0X5-	T44.0X6-
Ambroxol	T48.4X1-	T48.4X2-	T48.4X3-	T48.4X4-	T48.4X5-	T48.4X6-
Ambuphylline	T48.6X1-	T48.6X2-	T48.6X3-	T48.6X4-	T48.6X5-	T48.6X6-
Ambutonium bromide	T44.3X1-	T44.3X2-	T44.3X3-	T44.3X4-	T44.3X5-	T44.3X6-
Amcinonide	T49.0X1-	T49.0X2-	T49.0X3-	T49.0X4-	T49.0X5-	T49.0X6-
Amdinocilline	T36.0X1-	T36.0X2-	T36.0X3-	T36.0X4-	T36.0X5-	T36.0X6-
Ametazole	T50.8X1-	T50.8X2-	T50.8X3-	T50.8X4-	T50.8X5-	T50.8X6-
Amethocaine	T41.3X1-	T41.3X2-	T41.3X3-	T41.3X4-	T41.3X5-	T41.3X6-
regional	T41.3X1-	T41.3X2-	T41.3X3-	T41.3X4-	T41.3X5-	T41.3X6-
spinal	T41.3X1-	T41.3X2-	T41.3X3-	T41.3X4-	T41.3X5-	T41.3X6-
Amethopterin	T45.1X1-	T45.1X2-	T45.1X3-	T45.1X4-	T45.1X5-	T45.1X6-
Amezinium metilsulfate	T44.991-	T44.992-	T44.993-	T44.994-	T44.995-	T44.996-
Amfebutamone	T43.291-	T43.292-	T43.293-	T43.294-	T43.295-	T43.296-
Amfepramone	T50.5X1-	T50.5X2-	T50.5X3-	T50.5X4-	T50.5X5-	T50.5X6-
Amfetamine	T43.621-	T43.622-	T43.623-	T43.624-	T43.625-	T43.626-
Amfetaminil	T43.621-	T43.622-	T43.623-	T43.624-	T43.625-	T43.626-
Amfomycin	T36.8X1-	T36.8X2-	T36.8X3-	T36.8X4-	T36.8X5-	T36.8X6-
Amidefrine mesilate	T48.5X1-	T48.5X2-	T48.5X3-	T48.5X4-	T48.5X5-	T48.5X6-
Amidone	T40.3X1-	T40.3X2-	T40.3X3-	T40.3X4-	T40.3X5-	T40.3X6-
Amidopyrine	T39.2X1-	T39.2X2-	T39.2X3-	T39.2X4-	T39.2X5-	T39.2X6-
Amidotrizoate	T50.8X1-	T50.8X2-	T50.8X3-	T50.8X4-	T50.8X5-	T50.8X6-
Amiflamine	T43.1X1-	T43.1X2-	T43.1X3-	T43.1X4-	T43.1X5-	T43.1X6-
Amikacin	T36.5X1-	T36.5X2-	T36.5X3-	T36.5X4-	T36.5X5-	T36.5X6-
Amikhelline	T46.3X1-	T46.3X2-	T46.3X3-	T46.3X4-	T46.3X5-	T46.3X6-
Amiloride	T50.2X1-	T50.2X2-	T50.2X3-	T50.2X4-	T50.2X5-	T50.2X6-
Aminacrine	T49.0X1-	T49.0X2-	T49.0X3-	T49.0X4-	T49.0X5-	T49.0X6-
Amineptine	T43.011-	T43.012-	T43.013-	T43.014-	T43.015-	T43.016-
Aminitrozole	T37.3X1-	T37.3X2-	T37.3X3-	T37.3X4-	T37.3X5-	T37.3X6-
Amino acids	T50.3X1-	T50.3X2-	T50.3X3-	T50.3X4-	T50.3X5-	T50.3X6-
Aminoacetic acid (derivatives)	T50.3X1-	T50.3X2-	T50.3X3-	T50.3X4-	T50.3X5-	T50.3X6-
Aminoacridine	T49.0X1-	T49.0X2-	T49.0X3-	T49.0X4-	T49.0X5-	T49.0X6-
Aminobenzoic acid (-p)	T49.3X1-	T49.3X2-	T49.3X3-	T49.3X4-	T49.3X5-	T49.3X6-
4-Aminobutyric acid	T43.8X1-	T43.8X2-	T43.8X3-	T43.8X4-	T43.8X5-	T43.8X6-
Aminocaproic acid	T45.621-	T45.622-	T45.623-	T45.624-	T45.625-	T45.626-
Aminoethylisothiourium	T45.8X1-	T45.8X2-	T45.8X3-	T45.8X4-	T45.8X5-	T45.8X6-
Aminofenazone	T39.2X1-	T39.2X2-	T39.2X3-	T39.2X4-	T39.2X5-	T39.2X6-
Aminoglutethimide	T45.1X1-	T45.1X2-	T45.1X3-	T45.1X4-	T45.1X5-	T45.1X6-
Aminohippuric acid	T50.8X1-	T50.8X2-	T50.8X3-	T50.8X4-	T50.8X5-	T50.8X6-
Aminomethylbenzoic acid	T45.691-	T45.692-	T45.693-	T45.694-	T45.695-	T45.696-
Aminometradine	T50.2X1-	T50.2X2-	T50.2X3-	T50.2X4-	T50.2X5-	T50.2X6-
Aminopentamide	T44.3X1-	T44.3X2-	T44.3X3-	T44.3X4-	T44.3X5-	T44.3X6-
Aminophenazone	T39.2X1-	T39.2X2-	T39.2X3-	T39.2X4-	T39.2X5-	T39.2X6-
Aminophenol	T54.0X1-	T54.0X2-	T54.0X3-	T54.0X4-	-	-
4-Aminophenol derivatives	T39.1X1-	T39.1X2-	T39.1X3-	T39.1X4-	T39.1X5	T39.1X6-
Aminophenylpyridone	T43.591-	T43.592-	T43.593-	T43.594-	T43.595-	T43.596-
Aminophylline	T48.6X1-	T48.6X2-	T48.6X3-	T48.6X4-	T48.6X5-	T48.6X6-
Aminopterin sodium	T45.1X1-	T45.1X2-	T45.1X3-	T45.1X4-	T45.1X5-	T45.1X6-
Aminopyrine	T39.2X1-	T39.2X2-	T39.2X3-	T39.2X4-	T39.2X5-	T39.2X6-
8-Aminoquinoline drugs	T37.2X1-	T37.2X2-	T37.2X3-	T37.2X4-	T37.2X5-	T37.2X6-
Aminorex	T50.5X1-	T50.5X2-	T50.5X3-	T50.5X4-	T50.5X5-	T50.5X6-
Aminosalicylic acid	T37.1X1-	T37.1X2-	T37.1X3-	T37.1X4-	T37.1X5-	T37.1X6-
Aminosalylum	T37.1X1-	T37.1X2-	T37.1X3-	T37.1X4-	T37.1X5-	T37.1X6-
Amiodarone	T46.2X1-	T46.2X2-	T46.2X3-	T46.2X4-	T46.2X5-	T46.2X6-
Amiphenazole	T50.7X1-	T50.7X2-	T50.7X3-	T50.7X4-	T50.7X5-	T50.7X6-
Amiquinsin	T46.5X1-	T46.5X2-	T46.5X3-	T46.5X4-	T46.5X5-	T46.5X6-
Amisometradine	T50.2X1-	T50.2X2-	T50.2X3-	T50.2X4-	T50.2X5-	T50.2X6-
Amisulpride	T43.591-	T43.592-	T43.593-	T43.594-	T43.595-	T43.596-
Amitriptyline	T43.011-	T43.012-	T43.013-	T43.014-	T43.015-	T43.016-
Amitriptylinoxide	T43.011-	T43.012-	T43.013-	T43.014-	T43.015-	T43.016-
Amlexanox	T48.6X1-	T48.6X2-	T48.6X3-	T48.6X4-	T48.6X5-	T48.6X6-
Ammonia (fumes) (gas) (vapor)	T59.891-	T59.892-	T59.893-	T59.894-	-	-
aromatic spirit	T48.991-	T48.992-	T48.993-	T48.994-	T48.995-	T48.996-
liquid (household)	T54.3X1-	T54.3X2-	T54.3X3-	T54.3X4-	-	-
Ammoniated mercury	T49.0X1-	T49.0X2-	T49.0X3-	T49.0X4-	T49.0X5-	T49.0X6-
Ammonium						
acid tartrate	T49.5X1-	T49.5X2-	T49.5X3-	T49.5X4-	T49.5X5-	T49.5X6-
bromide	T42.6X1-	T42.6X2-	T42.6X3-	T42.6X4-	T42.6X5-	T42.6X6-
carbonate	T54.3X1-	T54.3X2-	T54.3X3-	T54.3X4-	-	-

Substance	Poisoning Accidental (unintentional)	Poisoning Intentional self-harm	Poisoning Assault	Poisoning Undetermined	Adverse effect	Underdosing
Ammonium - *continued*						
chloride	T50.991-	T50.992-	T50.993-	T50.994-	T50.995-	T50.996-
expectorant	T48.4X1-	T48.4X2-	T48.4X3-	T48.4X4-	T48.4X5-	T48.4X6-
compounds (household) NEC	T54.3X1-	T54.3X2-	T54.3X3-	T54.3X4-	-	-
fumes (any usage)	T59.891-	T59.892-	T59.893-	T59.894-	-	-
industrial	T54.3X1-	T54.3X2-	T54.3X3-	T54.3X4-	-	-
ichthyosulronate	T49.4X1-	T49.4X2-	T49.4X3-	T49.4X4-	T49.4X5-	T49.4X6-
mandelate	T37.91X-	T37.92X-	T37.93X-	T37.94X-	T37.95X-	T37.96X-
sulfamate	T60.3X1-	T60.3X2-	T60.3X3-	T60.3X4-	-	-
sulfonate resin	T47.8X1-	T47.8X2-	T47.8X3-	T47.8X4-	T47.8X5-	T47.8X6-
Amobarbital (sodium)	T42.3X1-	T42.3X2-	T42.3X3-	T42.3X4-	T42.3X5-	T42.3X6-
Amodiaquine	T37.2X1-	T37.2X2-	T37.2X3-	T37.2X4-	T37.2X5-	T37.2X6-
Amopyroquin (e)	T37.2X1-	T37.2X2-	T37.2X3-	T37.2X4-	T37.2X5-	T37.2X6-
Amoxapine	T43.011-	T43.012-	T43.013-	T43.014-	T43.015-	T43.016-
Amoxicillin	T36.0X1-	T36.0X2-	T36.0X3-	T36.0X4-	T36.0X5-	T36.0X6-
Amperozide	T43.591-	T43.592-	T43.593-	T43.594-	T43.595-	T43.596-
Amphenidone	T43.591-	T43.592-	T43.593-	T43.594-	T43.595-	T43.596-
Amphetamine NEC	T43.621-	T43.622-	T43.623-	T43.624-	T43.625-	T43.626-
Amphomycin	T36.8X1-	T36.8X2-	T36.8X3-	T36.8X4-	T36.8X5-	T36.8X6-
Amphotalide	T37.4X1-	T37.4X2-	T37.4X3-	T37.4X4-	T37.4X5-	T37.4X6-
Amphotericin B	T36.7X1-	T36.7X2-	T36.7X3-	T36.7X4-	T36.7X5-	T36.7X6-
topical	T49.0X1-	T49.0X2-	T49.0X3-	T49.0X4-	T49.0X5-	T49.0X6-
Ampicillin	T36.0X1-	T36.0X2-	T36.0X3-	T36.0X4-	T36.0X5-	T36.0X6-
Amprotropine	T44.3X1-	T44.3X2-	T44.3X3-	T44.3X4-	T44.3X5-	T44.3X6-
Amsacrine	T45.1X1-	T45.1X2-	T45.1X3-	T45.1X4-	T45.1X5-	T45.1X6-
Amygdaline	T62.2X1-	T62.2X2-	T62.2X3-	T62.2X4-	-	-
Amyl						
acetate	T52.8X1-	T52.8X2-	T52.8X3-	T52.8X4-	-	-
vapor	T59.891-	T59.892-	T59.893-	T59.894-	-	-
alcohol	T51.3X1-	T51.3X2-	T51.3X3-	T51.3X4-	-	-
chloride	T53.6X1-	T53.6X2-	T53.6X3-	T53.6X4-	-	-
formate	T52.8X1-	T52.8X2-	T52.8X3-	T52.8X4-	-	-
nitrite	T46.3X1-	T46.3X2-	T46.3X3-	T46.3X4-	T46.3X5-	T46.3X6-
propionate	T65.891-	T65.892-	T65.893-	T65.894-	-	-
Amylase	T47.5X1-	T47.5X2-	T47.5X3-	T47.5X4-	T47.5X5-	T47.5X6-
Amyleine, regional	T41.3X1-	T41.3X2-	T41.3X3-	T41.3X4-	T41.3X5-	T41.3X6-
Amylene						
dichloride	T53.6X1-	T53.6X2-	T53.6X3-	T53.6X4-	-	-
hydrate	T51.3X1-	T51.3X2-	T51.3X3-	T51.3X4-	-	-
Amylmetacresol	T49.6X1-	T49.6X2-	T49.6X3-	T49.6X4-	T49.6X5-	T49.6X6-
Amylobarbitone	T42.3X1-	T42.3X2-	T42.3X3-	T42.3X4-	T42.3X5-	T42.3X6-
Amylocaine, regional	T41.3X1-	T41.3X2-	T41.3X3-	T41.3X4-	T41.3X5-	T41.3X6-
infiltration (subcutaneous)	T41.3X1-	T41.3X2-	T41.3X3-	T41.3X4-	T41.3X5-	T41.3X6-
nerve block (peripheral) (plexus)	T41.3X1-	T41.3X2-	T41.3X3-	T41.3X4-	T41.3X5-	T41.3X6-
spinal	T41.3X1-	T41.3X2-	T41.3X3-	T41.3X4-	T41.3X5-	T41.3X6-
topical (surface)	T41.3X1-	T41.3X2-	T41.3X3-	T41.3X4-	T41.3X5-	T41.3X6-
Amylopectin	T47.6X1-	T47.6X2-	T47.6X3-	T47.6X4-	T47.6X5-	T47.6X6-
Amytal (sodium)	T42.3X1-	T42.3X2-	T42.3X3-	T42.3X4-	T42.3X5-	T42.3X6-
Anabolic steroid	T38.7X1-	T38.7X2-	T38.7X3-	T38.7X4-	T38.7X5-	T38.7X6-
Analeptic NEC	T50.7X1-	T50.7X2-	T50.7X3-	T50.7X4-	T50.7X5-	T50.7X6-
Analgesic	T39.91X-	T39.92X-	T39.93X-	T39.94X-	T39.95X-	T39.96X-
anti-inflammatory NEC	T39.91X-	T39.92X-	T39.93X-	T39.94X-	T39.95X-	T39.96X-
propionic acid derivative	T39.311-	T39.312-	T39.313-	T39.314-	T39.315-	T39.316-
antirheumatic NEC	T39.4X1-	T39.4X2-	T39.4X3	T39.4X4-	T39.4X5-	T39.4X6-
aromatic NEC	T39.1X1-	T39.1X2-	T39.1X3-	T39.1X4-	T39.1X5-	T39.1X6-
narcotic NEC	T40.601-	T40.602-	T40.603-	T40.604-	T40.605-	T40.606-
combination	T40.601-	T40.602-	T40.603-	T40.604-	T40.605-	T40.606-
obstetric	T40.601-	T40.602-	T40.603-	T40.604-	T40.605-	T40.606-
non-narcotic NEC	T39.91X-	T39.92X-	T39.93X-	T39.94X-	T39.95X-	T39.96X-
combination	T39.91X-	T39.92X-	T39.93X-	T39.94X-	T39.95X-	T39.96X-
pyrazole	T39.2X1-	T39.2X2-	T39.2X3-	T39.2X4-	T39.2X5-	T39.2X6-
specified NEC	T39.8X1-	T39.8X2-	T39.8X3-	T39.8X4-	T39.8X5-	T39.8X6-
Analgin	T39.2X1-	T39.2X2-	T39.2X3-	T39.2X4-	T39.2X5-	T39.2X6-
Anamirta cocculus	T62.1X1-	T62.1X2-	T62.1X3-	T62.1X4-	-	-
Ancillin	T36.0X1-	T36.0X2-	T36.0X3-	T36.0X4-	T36.0X5-	T36.0X6-
Ancrod	T45.691-	T45.692-	T45.693-	T45.694-	T45.695-	T45.696-
Androgen	T38.7X1-	T38.7X2-	T38.7X3-	T38.7X4-	T38.7X5-	T38.7X6-
Androgen-estrogen mixture	T38.7X1-	T38.7X2-	T38.7X3-	T38.7X4-	T38.7X5-	T38.7X6-
Androstalone	T38.7X1-	T38.7X2-	T38.7X3-	T38.7X4-	T38.7X5-	T38.7X6-
Androstanolone	T38.7X1-	T38.7X2-	T38.7X3-	T38.7X4-	T38.7X5-	T38.7X6-
Androsterone	T38.7X1-	T38.7X2-	T38.7X3-	T38.7X4-	T38.7X5-	T38.7X6-
Anemone pulsatilla	T62.2X1-	T62.2X2-	T62.2X3-	T62.2X4-	-	-
Anesthesia						
caudal	T41.3X1-	T41.3X2-	T41.3X3-	T41.3X4-	T41.3X5-	T41.3X6-
endotracheal	T41.0X1-	T41.0X2-	T41.0X3-	T41.0X4-	T41.0X5-	T41.0X6-
epidural	T41.3X1-	T41.3X2-	T41.3X3-	T41.3X4-	T41.3X5-	T41.3X6-
inhalation	T41.0X1-	T41.0X2-	T41.0X3-	T41.0X4-	T41.0X5-	T41.0X6-

Substance	Poisoning Accidental (unintentional)	Poisoning Intentional self-harm	Poisoning Assault	Poisoning Undetermined	Adverse effect	Underdosing
Anesthesia - *continued*						
local	T41.3X1-	T41.3X2-	T41.3X3-	T41.3X4-	T41.3X5-	T41.3X6-
mucosal	T41.3X1-	T41.3X2-	T41.3X3-	T41.3X4-	T41.3X5-	T41.3X6-
muscle relaxation	T48.1X1-	T48.1X2-	T48.1X3-	T48.1X4-	T48.1X5-	T48.1X6-
nerve blocking	T41.3X1-	T41.3X2-	T41.3X3-	T41.3X4-	T41.3X5-	T41.3X6-
plexus blocking	T41.3X1-	T41.3X2-	T41.3X3-	T41.3X4-	T41.3X5-	T41.3X6-
potentiated	T41.201-	T41.202-	T41.203-	T41.204-	T41.205-	T41.206-
rectal	T41.201-	T41.202-	T41.203-	T41.204-	T41.205-	T41.206-
general	T41.201-	T41.202-	T41.203-	T41.204-	T41.205-	T41.206-
local	T41.3X1-	T41.3X2-	T41.3X3-	T41.3X4-	T41.3X5-	T41.3X6-
regional	T41.3X1-	T41.3X2-	T41.3X3-	T41.3X4-	T41.3X5-	T41.3X6-
surface	T41.3X1-	T41.3X2-	T41.3X3-	T41.3X4-	T41.3X5-	T41.3X6-
Anesthetic NEC — *see also* Anesthesia	T41.41X-	T41.42X-	T41.43X-	T41.44X-	T41.45X-	T41.46X-
with muscle relaxant	T41.201-	T41.202-	T41.203-	T41.204-	T41.205-	T41.206-
general	T41.201-	T41.202-	T41.203-	T41.204-	T41.205-	T41.206-
local	T41.3X1-	T41.3X2-	T41.3X3-	T41.3X4-	T41.3X5-	T41.3X6-
gaseous NEC	T41.0X1-	T41.0X2-	T41.0X3-	T41.0X4-	T41.0X5-	T41.0X6-
general NEC	T41.201-	T41.202-	T41.203-	T41.204-	T41.205-	T41.206-
halogenated hydrocarbon derivatives NEC	T41.0X1-	T41.0X2-	T41.0X3-	T41.0X4-	T41.0X5-	T41.0X6-
infiltration NEC	T41.3X1-	T41.3X2-	T41.3X3-	T41.3X4-	T41.3X5-	T41.3X6-
intravenous NEC	T41.1X1-	T41.1X2-	T41.1X3-	T41.1X4-	T41.1X5-	T41.1X6-
local NEC	T41.3X1-	T41.3X2-	T41.3X3-	T41.3X4-	T41.3X5-	T41.3X6-
rectal	T41.201-	T41.202-	T41.203-	T41.204-	T41.205-	T41.206-
general	T41.201-	T41.202-	T41.203-	T41.204-	T41.205-	T41.206-
local	T41.3X1-	T41.3X2-	T41.3X3-	T41.3X4-	T41.3X5-	T41.3X6-
regional NEC	T41.3X1-	T41.3X2-	T41.3X3-	T41.3X4-	T41.3X5-	T41.3X6-
spinal NEC	T41.3X1-	T41.3X2-	T41.3X3-	T41.3X4-	T41.3X5-	T41.3X6-
thiobarbiturate	T41.1X1-	T41.1X2-	T41.1X3-	T41.1X4-	T41.1X5-	T41.1X6-
topical	T41.3X1-	T41.3X2-	T41.3X3-	T41.3X4-	T41.3X5-	T41.3X6-
Aneurine	T45.2X1-	T45.2X2-	T45.2X3-	T45.2X4-	T45.2X5-	T45.2X6-
Angio-Conray	T50.8X1-	T50.8X2-	T50.8X3-	T50.8X4-	T50.8X5-	T50.8X6-
Angiotensin	T44.5X1-	T44.5X2-	T44.5X3-	T44.5X4-	T44.5X5-	T44.5X6-
Angiotensinamide	T44.991-	T44.992-	T44.993-	T44.994-	T44.995-	T44.996-
Anhydrohydroxy-progesterone	T38.5X1-	T38.5X2-	T38.5X3-	T38.5X4-	T38.5X5-	T38.5X6-
Anhydron	T50.2X1-	T50.2X2-	T50.2X3-	T50.2X4-	T50.2X5-	T50.2X6-
Anileridine	T40.4X1-	T40.4X2-	T40.4X3-	T40.4X4-	T40.4X5-	T40.4X6-
Aniline (dye) (liquid)	T65.3X1-	T65.3X2-	T65.3X3-	T65.3X4-	-	-
analgesic	T39.1X1-	T39.1X2-	T39.1X3-	T39.1X4-	T39.1X5-	T39.1X6-
derivatives, therapeutic NEC	T39.1X1-	T39.1X2-	T39.1X3-	T39.1X4-	T39.1X5-	T39.1X6-
vapor	T65.3X1-	T65.3X2-	T65.3X3-	T65.3X4-	-	-
Aniscoropine	T44.3X1-	T44.3X2-	T44.3X3-	T44.3X4-	T44.3X5-	T44.3X6-
Anise oil	T47.5X1-	T47.5X2-	T47.5X3-	T47.5X4-	T47.5X5-	T47.5X6-
Anisidine	T65.3X1-	T65.3X2-	T65.3X3-	T65.3X4-	-	-
Anisindione	T45.511-	T45.512-	T45.513-	T45.514-	T45.515-	T45.516-
Anisotropine methyl-bromide	T44.3X1-	T44.3X2-	T44.3X3-	T44.3X4-	T44.3X5-	T44.3X6-
Anistreplase	T45.611-	T45.612-	T45.613-	T45.614-	T45.615-	T45.616-
Anorexiant (central)	T50.5X1-	T50.5X2-	T50.5X3-	T50.5X4-	T50.5X5-	T50.5X6-
Anorexic agents	T50.5X1-	T50.5X2-	T50.5X3-	T50.5X4-	T50.5X5-	T50.5X6-
Ansamycin	T36.6X1-	T36.6X2-	T36.6X3-	T36.6X4-	T36.6X5-	T36.6X6-
Ant (bite) (sting)	T63.421-	T63.422-	T63.423-	T63.424-	-	-
Ant poison — *see* Insecticide						
Antabuse	T50.6X1-	T50.6X2-	T50.6X3-	T50.6X4-	T50.6X5-	T50.6X6-
Antacid NEC	T47.1X1-	T47.1X2-	T47.1X3-	T47.1X4-	T47.1X5-	T47.1X6-
Antagonist						
Aldosterone	T50.0X1-	T50.0X2-	T50.0X3-	T50.0X4-	T50.0X5-	T50.0X6-
alpha-adrenoreceptor	T44.6X1-	T44.6X2-	T44.6X3-	T44.6X4-	T44.6X5-	T44.6X6-
anticoagulant	T45.7X1-	T45.7X2-	T45.7X3-	T45.7X4-	T45.7X5-	T45.7X6-
beta-adrenoreceptor	T44.7X1-	T44.7X2-	T44.7X3-	T44.7X4-	T44.7X5-	T44.7X6-
extrapyramidal NEC	T44.3X1-	T44.3X2-	T44.3X3-	T44.3X4-	T44.3X5-	T44.3X6-
folic acid	T45.1X1-	T45.1X2-	T45.1X3-	T45.1X4-	T45.1X5-	T45.1X6-
H2 receptor	T47.0X1-	T47.0X2-	T47.0X3-	T47.0X4-	T47.0X5-	T47.0X6-
heavy metal	T45.8X1-	T45.8X2-	T45.8X3-	T45.8X4-	T45.8X5-	T45.8X6-
narcotic analgesic	T50.7X1-	T50.7X2-	T50.7X3-	T50.7X4-	T50.7X5-	T50.7X6-
opiate	T50.7X1-	T50.7X2-	T50.7X3-	T50.7X4-	T50.7X5-	T50.7X6-
pyrimidine	T45.1X1-	T45.1X2-	T45.1X3-	T45.1X4-	T45.1X5-	T45.1X6-
serotonin	T46.5X1-	T46.5X2-	T46.5X3-	T46.5X4-	T46.5X5-	T46.5X6-
Antazolin (e)	T45.0X1-	T45.0X2-	T45.0X3-	T45.0X4-	T45.0X5-	T45.0X6-
Anterior pituitary hormone NEC	T38.811-	T38.812-	T38.813-	T38.814-	T38.815-	T38.816-
Anthelmintic NEC	T37.4X1-	T37.4X2-	T37.4X3-	T37.4X4-	T37.4X5-	T37.4X6-
Anthiolimine	T37.4X1-	T37.4X2-	T37.4X3-	T37.4X4-	T37.4X5-	T37.4X6-
Anthralin	T49.4X1-	T49.4X2-	T49.4X3-	T49.4X4-	T49.4X5-	T49.4X6-
Anthramycin	T45.1X1-	T45.1X2-	T45.1X3-	T45.1X4-	T45.1X5-	T45.1X6-
Antiadrenergic NEC	T44.8X1-	T44.8X2-	T44.8X3-	T44.8X4-	T44.8X5-	T44.8X6-
Antiallergic NEC	T45.0X1-	T45.0X2-	T45.0X3-	T45.0X4-	T45.0X5-	T45.0X6-

Substance	Poisoning Accidental (unintentional)	Poisoning Intentional self-harm	Poisoning Assault	Poisoning Undetermined	Adverse effect	Underdosing
Anti-anemic (drug) (preparation)	T45.8X1-	T45.8X2-	T45.8X3-	T45.8X4-	T45.8X5-	T45.8X6-
Antiandrogen NEC	T38.6X1-	T38.6X2-	T38.6X3-	T38.6X4-	T38.6X5-	T38.6X6-
Antianxiety drug NEC	T43.501-	T43.502-	T43.503-	T43.504-	T43.505-	T43.506-
Antiaris toxicaria	T65.891-	T65.892-	T65.893-	T65.894-	-	-
Antiarteriosclerotic drug	T46.6X1-	T46.6X2-	T46.6X3-	T46.6X4-	T46.6X5-	T46.6X6-
Antiasthmatic drug NEC	T48.6X1-	T48.6X2-	T48.6X3-	T48.6X4-	T48.6X5-	T48.6X6-
Antibiotic NEC	T36.91X-	T36.92X-	T36.93X-	T36.94X-	T36.95X-	T36.96X-
aminoglycoside	T36.5X1-	T36.5X2-	T36.5X3-	T36.5X4-	T36.5X5-	T36.5X6-
anticancer	T45.1X1-	T45.1X2-	T45.1X3-	T45.1X4-	T45.1X5-	T45.1X6-
antifungal	T36.7X1-	T36.7X2-	T36.7X3-	T36.7X4-	T36.7X5-	T36.7X6-
antimycobacterial	T36.5X1-	T36.5X2-	T36.5X3-	T36.5X4-	T36.5X5-	T36.5X6-
antineoplastic	T45.1X1-	T45.1X2-	T45.1X3-	T45.1X4-	T45.1X5-	T45.1X6-
cephalosporin (group)	T36.1X1-	T36.1X2-	T36.1X3-	T36.1X4-	T36.1X5-	T36.1X6-
chloramphenicol (group)	T36.2X1-	T36.2X2-	T36.2X3-	T36.2X4-	T36.2X5-	T36.2X6-
ENT	T49.6X1-	T49.6X2-	T49.6X3-	T49.6X4-	T49.6X5-	T49.6X6-
eye	T49.5X1-	T49.5X2-	T49.5X3-	T49.5X4-	T49.5X5-	T49.5X6-
fungicidal (local)	T49.0X1-	T49.0X2-	T49.0X3-	T49.0X4-	T49.0X5-	T49.0X6-
intestinal	T36.8X1-	T36.8X2-	T36.8X3-	T36.8X4-	T36.8X5-	T36.8X6-
b-lactam NEC	T36.1X1-	T36.1X2-	T36.1X3-	T36.1X4-	T36.1X5-	T36.1X6-
local	T49.0X1-	T49.0X2-	T49.0X3-	T49.0X4-	T49.0X5-	T49.0X6-
macrolides	T36.3X1-	T36.3X2-	T36.3X3-	T36.3X4-	T36.3X5-	T36.3X6-
polypeptide	T36.8X1-	T36.8X2-	T36.8X3-	T36.8X4-	T36.8X5-	T36.8X6-
specified NEC	T36.8X1-	T36.8X2-	T36.8X3-	T36.8X4-	T36.8X5-	T36.8X6-
tetracycline (group)	T36.4X1-	T36.4X2-	T36.4X3-	T36.4X4-	T36.4X5-	T36.4X6-
throat	T49.6X1-	T49.6X2-	T49.6X3-	T49.6X4-	T49.6X5-	T49.6X6-
Anticancer agents NEC	T45.1X1-	T45.1X2-	T45.1X3-	T45.1X4-	T45.1X5-	T45.1X6-
Anticholesterolemic drug NEC	T46.6X1-	T46.6X2-	T46.6X3-	T46.6X4-	T46.6X5-	T46.6X6-
Anticholinergic NEC	T44.3X1-	T44.3X2-	T44.3X3-	T44.3X4-	T44.3X5-	T44.3X6-
Anticholinesterase	T44.0X1-	T44.0X2-	T44.0X3-	T44.0X4-	T44.0X5-	T44.0X6-
organophosphorus	T44.0X1-	T44.0X2-	T44.0X3-	T44.0X4-	T44.0X5-	T44.0X6-
insecticide	T60.0X1-	T60.0X2-	T60.0X3-	T60.0X4-	-	-
nerve gas	T59.891-	T59.892-	T59.893-	T59.894-	-	-
reversible	T44.0X1-	T44.0X2-	T44.0X3-	T44.0X4-	T44.0X5-	T44.0X6-
ophthalmological	T49.5X1-	T49.5X2-	T49.5X3-	T49.5X4-	T49.5X5-	T49.5X6-
Anticoagulant NEC	T45.511-	T45.512-	T45.513-	T45.514-	T45.515-	T45.516-
Antagonist	T45.7X1-	T45.7X2-	T45.7X3-	T45.7X4-	T45.7X5-	T45.7X6-
Anti-common-cold drug NEC	T48.5X1-	T48.5X2-	T48.5X3-	T48.5X4-	T48.5X5-	T48.5X6-
Anticonvulsant	T42.71X-	T42.72X-	T42.73X-	T42.74X-	T42.75X-	T42.76X-
barbiturate	T42.3X1-	T42.3X2-	T42.3X3-	T42.3X4-	T42.3X5-	T42.3X6-
combination (with barbiturate)	T42.3X1-	T42.3X2-	T42.3X3-	T42.3X4-	T42.3X5-	T42.3X6-
hydantoin	T42.0X1-	T42.0X2-	T42.0X3-	T42.0X4-	T42.0X5-	T42.0X6-
hypnotic NEC	T42.6X1-	T42.6X2-	T42.6X3-	T42.6X4-	T42.6X5-	T42.6X6-
oxazolidinedione	T42.2X1-	T42.2X2-	T42.2X3-	T42.2X4-	T42.2X5-	T42.2X6-
pyrimidinedione	T42.6X1-	T42.6X2-	T42.6X3-	T42.6X4-	T42.6X5-	T42.6X6-
specified NEC	T42.6X1-	T42.6X2-	T42.6X3-	T42.6X4-	T42.6X5-	T42.6X6-
succinimide	T42.2X1-	T42.2X2-	T42.2X3-	T42.2X4-	T42.2X5-	T42.2X6-
Anti-D immunoglobulin (human)	T50.Z11-	T50.Z12-	T50.Z13-	T50.Z14-	T50.Z15-	T50.Z16-
Antidepressant	T43.201-	T43.202-	T43.203-	T43.204-	T43.205-	T43.206-
monoamine oxidase inhibitor	T43.1X1-	T43.1X2-	T43.1X3-	T43.1X4-	T43.1X5-	T43.1X6-
selective serotonin norepinephrine reuptake inhibitor	T43.211-	T43.212-	T43.213-	T43.214-	T43.215-	T43.216-
selective serotonin reuptake inhibitor	T43.221-	T43.222-	T43.223-	T43.224-	T43.225-	T43.226-
specified NEC	T43.291-	T43.292-	T43.293-	T43.294-	T43.295-	T43.296-
tetracyclic	T43.021-	T43.022-	T43.023-	T43.024-	T43.025-	T43.026-
triazolopyridine	T43.211-	T43.212-	T43.213-	T43.214-	T43.215-	T43.216-
tricyclic	T43.011-	T43.012-	T43.013-	T43.014-	T43.015-	T43.016-
Antidiabetic NEC	T38.3X1-	T38.3X2-	T38.3X3-	T38.3X4-	T38.3X5-	T38.3X6-
biguanide	T38.3X1-	T38.3X2-	T38.3X3-	T38.3X4-	T38.3X5-	T38.3X6-
and sulfonyl combined	T38.3X1-	T38.3X2-	T38.3X3-	T38.3X4-	T38.3X5-	T38.3X6-
combined	T38.3X1-	T38.3X2-	T38.3X3-	T38.3X4-	T38.3X5-	T38.3X6-
sulfonylurea	T38.3X1-	T38.3X2-	T38.3X3-	T38.3X4-	T38.3X5-	T38.3X6-
Antidiarrheal drug NEC	T47.6X1-	T47.6X2-	T47.6X3-	T47.6X4-	T47.6X5-	T47.6X6-
absorbent	T47.6X1-	T47.6X2-	T47.6X3-	T47.6X4-	T47.6X5-	T47.6X6-
Antidiphtheria serum	T50.Z11-	T50.Z12-	T50.Z13-	T50.Z14-	T50.Z15-	T50.Z16-
Antidiuretic hormone	T38.891-	T38.892-	T38.893-	T38.894-	T38.895-	T38.896-
Antidote NEC	T50.6X1-	T50.6X2-	T50.6X3-	T50.6X4-	T50.6X5-	T50.6X6-
heavy metal	T45.8X1-	T45.8X2-	T45.8X3-	T45.8X4-	T45.8X5-	T45.8X6-
Antidysrhythmic NEC	T46.2X1-	T46.2X2-	T46.2X3-	T46.2X4-	T46.2X5-	T46.2X6-
Antiemetic drug	T45.0X1-	T45.0X2-	T45.0X3-	T45.0X4-	T45.0X5-	T45.0X6-
Antiepilepsy agent	T42.71X-	T42.72X-	T42.73X-	T42.74X-	T42.75X-	T42.76X-
combination	T42.5X1-	T42.5X2-	T42.5X3-	T42.5X4-	T42.5X5-	T42.5X6-
mixed	T42.5X1-	T42.5X2-	T42.5X3-	T42.5X4-	T42.5X5-	T42.5X6-
specified, NEC	T42.6X1-	T42.6X2-	T42.6X3-	T42.6X4-	T42.6X5-	T42.6X6-
Antiestrogen NEC	T38.6X1-	T38.6X2-	T38.6X3-	T38.6X4-	T38.6X5-	T38.6X6-
Antifertility pill	T38.4X1-	T38.4X2-	T38.4X3-	T38.4X4-	T38.4X5-	T38.4X6-

Substance	Poisoning Accidental (unintentional)	Poisoning Intentional self-harm	Poisoning Assault	Poisoning Undetermined	Adverse effect	Underdosing
Antifibrinolytic drug	T45.621-	T45.622-	T45.623-	T45.624-	T45.625-	T45.626-
Antifilarial drug	T37.4X1-	T37.4X2-	T37.4X3-	T37.4X4-	T37.4X5-	T37.4X6-
Antiflatulent	T47.5X1-	T47.5X2-	T47.5X3-	T47.5X4-	T47.5X5-	T47.5X6-
Antifreeze	T65.91X-	T65.92X-	T65.93X-	T65.94X-	-	-
alcohol	T51.1X1-	T51.1X2-	T51.1X3-	T51.1X4-	-	-
ethylene glycol	T51.8X1-	T51.8X2-	T51.8X3-	T51.8X4-	-	-
Antifungal						
antibiotic (systemic)	T36.7X1-	T36.7X2-	T36.7X3-	T36.7X4-	T36.7X5-	T36.7X6-
anti-infective NEC	T37.91X-	T37.92X-	T37.93X-	T37.94X-	T37.95X-	T37.96X-
disinfectant, local	T49.0X1-	T49.0X2-	T49.0X3-	T49.0X4-	T49.0X5-	T49.0X6-
nonmedicinal (spray)	T60.3X1-	T60.3X2-	T60.3X3-	T60.3X4-	-	-
topical	T49.0X1-	T49.0X2-	T49.0X3-	T49.0X4-	T49.0X5-	T49.0X6-
Anti-gastric-secretion drug NEC	T47.1X1-	T47.1X2-	T47.1X3-	T47.1X4-	T47.1X5-	T47.1X6-
Antigonadotrophin NEC	T38.6X1-	T38.6X2-	T38.6X3-	T38.6X4-	T38.6X5-	T38.6X6-
Antihallucinogen	T43.501-	T43.502-	T43.503-	T43.504-	T43.505-	T43.506-
Antihelmintics	T37.4X1-	T37.4X2-	T37.4X3-	T37.4X4-	T37.4X5-	T37.4X6-
Antihemophilic						
factor	T45.8X1-	T45.8X2-	T45.8X3-	T45.8X4-	T45.8X5-	T45.8X6-
fraction	T45.8X1-	T45.8X2-	T45.8X3-	T45.8X4-	T45.8X5-	T45.8X6-
globulin concentrate	T45.7X1-	T45.7X2-	T45.7X3-	T45.7X4-	T45.7X5-	T45.7X6-
human plasma	T45.8X1-	T45.8X2-	T45.8X3-	T45.8X4-	T45.8X5-	T45.8X6-
plasma, dried	T45.7X1-	T45.7X2-	T45.7X3-	T45.7X4-	T45.7X5-	T45.7X6-
Antihemorrhoidal preparation	T49.2X1-	T49.2X2-	T49.2X3-	T49.2X4-	T49.2X5-	T49.2X6-
Antiheparin drug	T45.7X1-	T45.7X2-	T45.7X3-	T45.7X4-	T45.7X5-	T45.7X6-
Antihistamine	T45.0X1-	T45.0X2-	T45.0X3-	T45.0X4-	T45.0X5-	T45.0X6-
Antihookworm drug	T37.4X1-	T37.4X2-	T37.4X3-	T37.4X4-	T37.4X5-	T37.4X6-
Anti-human lymphocytic globulin	T50.Z11-	T50.Z12-	T50.Z13-	T50.Z14-	T50.Z15-	T50.Z16-
Antihyperlipidemic drug	T46.6X1-	T46.6X2-	T46.6X3-	T46.6X4-	T46.6X5-	T46.6X6-
Antihypertensive drug NEC	T46.5X1-	T46.5X2-	T46.5X3-	T46.5X4-	T46.5X5-	T46.5X6-
Anti-infective NEC	T37.91X-	T37.92X-	T37.93X-	T37.94X-	T37.95X-	T37.96X-
anthelmintic	T37.4X1-	T37.4X2-	T37.4X3-	T37.4X4-	T37.4X5-	T37.4X6-
antibiotics	T36.91X-	T36.92X-	T36.93X-	T36.94X-	T36.95X-	T36.96X-
specified NEC	T36.8X1-	T36.8X2-	T36.8X3-	T36.8X4-	T36.8X5-	T36.8X6-
antimalarial	T37.2X1-	T37.2X2-	T37.2X3-	T37.2X4-	T37.2X5-	T37.2X6-
antimycobacterial NEC	T37.1X1-	T37.1X2-	T37.1X3-	T37.1X4-	T37.1X5-	T37.1X6-
antibiotics	T36.5X1-	T36.5X2-	T36.5X3-	T36.5X4-	T36.5X5-	T36.5X6-
antiprotozoal NEC	T37.3X1-	T37.3X2-	T37.3X3-	T37.3X4-	T37.3X5-	T37.3X6-
blood	T37.2X1-	T37.2X2-	T37.2X3-	T37.2X4-	T37.2X5-	T37.2X6-
antiviral	T37.5X1-	T37.5X2-	T37.5X3-	T37.5X4-	T37.5X5-	T37.5X6-
arsenical	T37.8X1-	T37.8X2-	T37.8X3-	T37.8X4-	T37.8X5-	T37.8X6-
bismuth, local	T49.0X1-	T49.0X2-	T49.0X3-	T49.0X4-	T49.0X5-	T49.0X6-
ENT	T49.6X1-	T49.6X2-	T49.6X3-	T49.6X4-	T49.6X5-	T49.6X6-
eye NEC	T49.5X1-	T49.5X2-	T49.5X3-	T49.5X4-	T49.5X5-	T49.5X6-
heavy metals NEC	T37.8X1-	T37.8X2-	T37.8X3-	T37.8X4-	T37.8X5-	T37.8X6-
local NEC	T49.0X1-	T49.0X2-	T49.0X3-	T49.0X4-	T49.0X5-	T49.0X6-
specified NEC	T49.0X1-	T49.0X2-	T49.0X3-	T49.0X4-	T49.0X5-	T49.0X6-
mixed	T37.91X-	T37.92X-	T37.93X-	T37.94X-	T37.95X-	T37.96X-
ophthalmic preparation	T49.5X1-	T49.5X2-	T49.5X3-	T49.5X4-	T49.5X5-	T49.5X6-
topical NEC	T49.0X1-	T49.0X2-	T49.0X3-	T49.0X4-	T49.0X5-	T49.0X6-
Anti-inflammatory drug NEC	T39.391-	T39.392-	T39.393-	T39.394-	T39.395-	T39.396-
local	T49.0X1-	T49.0X2-	T49.0X3-	T49.0X4-	T49.0X5-	T49.0X6-
nonsteroidal NEC	T39.391-	T39.392-	T39.393-	T39.394-	T39.395-	T39.396-
propionic acid derivative	T39.311-	T39.312-	T39.313-	T39.314-	T39.315-	T39.316-
specified NEC	T39.391-	T39.392-	T39.393-	T39.394-	T39.395-	T39.396-
Antikaluretic	T50.3X1-	T50.3X2-	T50.3X3-	T50.3X4-	T50.3X5-	T50.3X6-
Antiknock (tetraethyl lead)	T56.0X1-	T56.0X2-	T56.0X3-	T56.0X4-	-	-
Antilipemic drug NEC	T46.6X1-	T46.6X2-	T46.6X3-	T46.6X4-	T46.6X5-	T46.6X6-
Antimalarial	T37.2X1-	T37.2X2-	T37.2X3-	T37.2X4-	T37.2X5-	T37.2X6-
prophylactic NEC	T37.2X1-	T37.2X2-	T37.2X3-	T37.2X4-	T37.2X5-	T37.2X6-
pyrimidine derivative	T37.2X1-	T37.2X2-	T37.2X3-	T37.2X4-	T37.2X5-	T37.2X6-
Antimetabolite	T45.1X1-	T45.1X2-	T45.1X3-	T45.1X4-	T45.1X5-	T45.1X6-
Antimitotic agent	T45.1X1-	T45.1X2-	T45.1X3-	T45.1X4-	T45.1X5-	T45.1X6-
Antimony (compounds) (vapor) **NEC**	T56.891-	T56.892-	T56.893-	T56.894-	-	-
anti-infectives	T37.8X1-	T37.8X2-	T37.8X3-	T37.8X4-	T37.8X5-	T37.8X6-
dimercaptosuccinate	T37.3X1-	T37.3X2-	T37.3X3-	T37.3X4-	T37.3X5-	T37.3X6-
hydride	T56.891-	T56.892-	T56.893-	T56.894-	-	-
pesticide (vapor)	T60.8X1-	T60.8X2-	T60.8X3-	T60.8X4-	-	-
potassium (sodium) tartrate	T37.8X1-	T37.8X2-	T37.8X3-	T37.8X4-	T37.8X5-	T37.8X6-
sodium dimercaptosuccinate	T37.3X1-	T37.3X2-	T37.3X3-	T37.3X4-	T37.3X5-	T37.3X6-
tartrated	T37.8X1-	T37.8X2-	T37.8X3-	T37.8X4-	T37.8X5-	T37.8X6-
Antimuscarinic NEC	T44.3X1-	T44.3X2-	T44.3X3-	T44.3X4-	T44.3X5-	T44.3X6-
Antimycobacterial drug NEC	T37.1X1-	T37.1X2-	T37.1X3-	T37.1X4-	T37.1X5-	T37.1X6-
antibiotics	T36.5X1-	T36.5X2-	T36.5X3-	T36.5X4-	T36.5X5-	T36.5X6-
combination	T37.1X1-	T37.1X2-	T37.1X3-	T37.1X4-	T37.1X5-	T37.1X6-
Antinausea drug	T45.0X1-	T45.0X2-	T45.0X3-	T45.0X4-	T45.0X5-	T45.0X6-
Antinematode drug	T37.4X1-	T37.4X2-	T37.4X3-	T37.4X4-	T37.4X5-	T37.4X6-
Antineoplastic NEC	T45.1X1-	T45.1X2-	T45.1X3-	T45.1X4-	T45.1X5-	T45.1X6-
alkaloidal	T45.1X1-	T45.1X2-	T45.1X3-	T45.1X4-	T45.1X5-	T45.1X6-
antibiotics	T45.1X1-	T45.1X2-	T45.1X3-	T45.1X4-	T45.1X5-	T45.1X6-
combination	T45.1X1-	T45.1X2-	T45.1X3-	T45.1X4-	T45.1X5-	T45.1X6-
estrogen	T38.5X1-	T38.5X2-	T38.5X3-	T38.5X4-	T38.5X5-	T38.5X6-
steroid	T38.7X1-	T38.7X2-	T38.7X3-	T38.7X4-	T38.7X5-	T38.7X6-
Antiparasitic drug (systemic)	T37.91X-	T37.92X-	T37.93X-	T37.94X-	T37.95X-	T37.96X-
local	T49.0X1-	T49.0X2-	T49.0X3-	T49.0X4-	T49.0X5-	T49.0X6-
specified NEC	T37.8X1-	T37.8X2-	T37.8X3-	T37.8X4-	T37.8X5-	T37.8X6-
Antiparkinsonism drug NEC	T42.8X1-	T42.8X2-	T42.8X3-	T42.8X4-	T42.8X5-	T42.8X6-
Antiperspirant NEC	T49.2X1-	T49.2X2-	T49.2X3-	T49.2X4-	T49.2X5-	T49.2X6-
Antiphlogistic NEC	T39.4X1-	T39.4X2-	T39.4X3-	T39.4X4-	T39.4X5-	T39.4X6-
Antiplatyhelmintic drug	T37.4X1-	T37.4X2-	T37.4X3-	T37.4X4-	T37.4X5-	T37.4X6-
Antiprotozoal drug NEC	T37.3X1-	T37.3X2-	T37.3X3-	T37.3X4-	T37.3X5-	T37.3X6-
blood	T37.2X1-	T37.2X2-	T37.2X3-	T37.2X4-	T37.2X5-	T37.2X6-
local	T49.0X1-	T49.0X2-	T49.0X3-	T49.0X4-	T49.0X5-	T49.0X6-
Antipruritic drug NEC	T49.1X1-	T49.1X2-	T49.1X3-	T49.1X4-	T49.1X5-	T49.1X6-
Antipsychotic drug	T43.501-	T43.502-	T43.503-	T43.504-	T43.505-	T43.506-
specified NEC	T43.591-	T43.592-	T43.593-	T43.594-	T43.595-	T43.596-
Antipyretic	T39.91X-	T39.92X-	T39.93X-	T39.94X-	T39.95X-	T39.96X-
specified NEC	T39.8X1-	T39.8X2-	T39.8X3-	T39.8X4-	T39.8X5-	T39.8X6-
Antipyrine	T39.2X1-	T39.2X2-	T39.2X3-	T39.2X4-	T39.2X5-	T39.2X6-
Antirabies hyperimmune serum	T50.Z11-	T50.Z12-	T50.Z13-	T50.Z14-	T50.Z15-	T50.Z16-
Antirheumatic NEC	T39.4X1-	T39.4X2-	T39.4X3-	T39.4X4-	T39.4X5-	T39.4X6-
Antirigidity drug NEC	T42.8X1-	T42.8X2-	T42.8X3-	T42.8X4-	T42.8X5-	T42.8X6-
Antischistosomal drug	T37.4X1-	T37.4X2-	T37.4X3-	T37.4X4-	T37.4X5-	T37.4X6-
Antiscorpion sera	T50.Z11-	T50.Z12-	T50.Z13-	T50.Z14-	T50.Z15-	T50.Z16-
Antiseborrheics	T49.4X1-	T49.4X2-	T49.4X3-	T49.4X4-	T49.4X5-	T49.4X6-
Antiseptics (external) (medicinal)	T49.0X1-	T49.0X2-	T49.0X3-	T49.0X4-	T49.0X5-	T49.0X6-
Antistine	T45.0X1-	T45.0X2-	T45.0X3-	T45.0X4-	T45.0X5-	T45.0X6-
Antitapeworm drug	T37.4X1-	T37.4X2-	T37.4X3-	T37.4X4-	T37.4X5-	T37.4X6-
Antitetanus immunoglobulin	T50.Z11-	T50.Z12-	T50.Z13-	T50.Z14-	T50.Z15-	T50.Z16-
Antithrombotic	T45.521-	T45.522-	T45.523-	T45.524-	T45.525-	T45.526-
Antithyroid drug NEC	T38.2X1-	T38.2X2-	T38.2X3-	T38.2X4-	T38.2X5-	T38.2X6-
Antitoxin	T50.Z11-	T50.Z12-	T50.Z13-	T50.Z14-	T50.Z15-	T50.Z16-
diphtheria	T50.Z11-	T50.Z12-	T50.Z13-	T50.Z14-	T50.Z15-	T50.Z16-
gas gangrene	T50.Z11-	T50.Z12-	T50.Z13-	T50.Z14-	T50.Z15-	T50.Z16-
tetanus	T50.Z11-	T50.Z12-	T50.Z13-	T50.Z14-	T50.Z15-	T50.Z16-
Antitrichomonal drug	T37.3X1-	T37.3X2-	T37.3X3-	T37.3X4-	T37.3X5-	T37.3X6-
Antituberculars	T37.1X1-	T37.1X2-	T37.1X3-	T37.1X4-	T37.1X5-	T37.1X6-
antibiotics	T36.5X1-	T36.5X2-	T36.5X3-	T36.5X4-	T36.5X5-	T36.5X6-
Antitussive NEC	T48.3X1-	T48.3X2-	T48.3X3-	T48.3X4-	T48.3X5-	T48.3X6-
codeine mixture	T40.2X1-	T40.2X2-	T40.2X3-	T40.2X4-	T40.2X5-	T40.2X6-
opiate	T40.2X1-	T40.2X2-	T40.2X3-	T40.2X4-	T40.2X5-	T40.2X6-
Antivaricose drug	T46.8X1-	T46.8X2-	T46.8X3-	T46.8X4-	T46.8X5-	T46.8X6-
Antivenin, antivenom (sera)	T50.Z11-	T50.Z12-	T50.Z13-	T50.Z14-	T50.Z15-	T50.Z16-
crotaline	T50.Z11-	T50.Z12-	T50.Z13-	T50.Z14-	T50.Z15-	T50.Z16-
spider bite	T50.Z11-	T50.Z12-	T50.Z13-	T50.Z14-	T50.Z15-	T50.Z16-
Antivertigo drug	T45.0X1-	T45.0X2-	T45.0X3-	T45.0X4-	T45.0X5-	T45.0X6-
Antiviral drug NEC	T37.5X1-	T37.5X2-	T37.5X3-	T37.5X4-	T37.5X5-	T37.5X6-
eye	T49.5X1-	T49.5X2-	T49.5X3-	T49.5X4-	T49.5X5-	T49.5X6-
Antiwhipworm drug	T37.4X1-	T37.4X2	T37.4X3	T37.4X4-	T37.4X5-	T37.4X6-
Antrol — *see also* by specific chemical substance	T60.91X-	T60.92X-	T60.93X-	T60.94X-	-	-
fungicide	T60.91X-	T60.92X-	T60.93X-	T60.94X-	-	-
ANTU (alpha naphthylthiourea)	T60.4X1-	T60.4X2-	T60.4X3-	T60.4X4-	-	-
Apalcillin	T36.0X1-	T36.0X2-	T36.0X3-	T36.0X4-	T36.0X5-	T36.0X6-
APC	T48.5X1-	T48.5X2-	T48.5X3-	T48.5X4-	T48.5X5-	T48.5X6-
Aplonidine	T44.4X1-	T44.4X2-	T44.4X3-	T44.4X4-	T44.4X5-	T44.4X6-
Apomorphine	T47.7X1-	T47.7X2-	T47.7X3-	T47.7X4-	T47.7X5-	T47.7X6-
Appetite depressants, central	T50.5X1-	T50.5X2-	T50.5X3-	T50.5X4-	T50.5X5-	T50.5X6-
Apraclonidine (hydrochloride)	T44.4X1-	T44.4X2-	T44.4X3-	T44.4X4-	T44.4X5-	T44.4X6-
Apresoline	T46.5X1-	T46.5X2-	T46.5X3-	T46.5X4-	T46.5X5-	T46.5X6-
Aprindine	T46.2X1-	T46.2X2-	T46.2X3-	T46.2X4-	T46.2X5-	T46.2X6-
Aprobarbital	T42.3X1-	T42.3X2-	T42.3X3-	T42.3X4-	T42.3X5-	T42.3X6-
Apronalide	T42.6X1-	T42.6X2-	T42.6X3-	T42.6X4-	T42.6X5-	T42.6X6-
Aprotinin	T45.621-	T45.622-	T45.623-	T45.624-	T45.625-	T45.626-
Aptocaine	T41.3X1-	T41.3X2-	T41.3X3-	T41.3X4-	T41.3X5-	T41.3X6-
Aqua fortis	T54.2X1-	T54.2X2-	T54.2X3-	T54.2X4-	-	-
Ara-A	T37.5X1-	T37.5X2-	T37.5X3-	T37.5X4-	T37.5X5-	T37.5X6-
Ara-C	T45.1X1-	T45.1X2-	T45.1X3-	T45.1X4-	T45.1X5-	T45.1X6-
Arachis oil	T49.3X1-	T49.3X2-	T49.3X3-	T49.3X4-	T49.3X5-	T49.3X6-
cathartic	T47.4X1-	T47.4X2-	T47.4X3-	T47.4X4-	T47.4X5-	T47.4X6-
Aralen	T37.2X1-	T37.2X2-	T37.2X3-	T37.2X4-	T37.2X5-	T37.2X6-
Arecoline	T44.1X1-	T44.1X2-	T44.1X3-	T44.1X4-	T44.1X5-	T44.1X6-

Arginine - Benisone
Table of Drugs and Chemicals

Substance	Poisoning Accidental (unintentional)	Poisoning Intentional self-harm	Poisoning Assault	Poisoning Undetermined	Adverse effect	Underdosing
Arginine	T50.991-	T50.992-	T50.993-	T50.994-	T50.995-	T50.996-
glutamate	T50.991-	T50.992-	T50.993-	T50.994-	T50.995-	T50.996-
Argyrol	T49.0X1-	T49.0X2-	T49.0X3-	T49.0X4-	T49.0X5-	T49.0X6-
ENT agent	T49.6X1-	T49.6X2-	T49.6X3-	T49.6X4-	T49.6X5-	T49.6X6-
ophthalmic preparation	T49.5X1-	T49.5X2-	T49.5X3-	T49.5X4-	T49.5X5-	T49.5X6-
Aristocort	T38.0X1-	T38.0X2-	T38.0X3-	T38.0X4-	T38.0X5-	T38.0X6-
ENT agent	T49.6X1-	T49.6X2-	T49.6X3-	T49.6X4-	T49.6X5-	T49.6X6-
ophthalmic preparation	T49.5X1-	T49.5X2-	T49.5X3-	T49.5X4-	T49.5X5-	T49.5X6-
topical NEC	T49.0X1-	T49.0X2-	T49.0X3-	T49.0X4-	T49.0X5-	T49.0X6-
Aromatics, corrosive	T54.1X1-	T54.1X2-	T54.1X3-	T54.1X4-	-	-
disinfectants	T54.1X1-	T54.1X2-	T54.1X3-	T54.1X4-	-	-
Arsenate of lead	T57.0X1-	T57.0X2-	T57.0X3-	T57.0X4-	-	-
herbicide	T57.0X1-	T57.0X2-	T57.0X3-	T57.0X4-	-	-
Arsenic, arsenicals (compounds) (dust) (vapor) **NEC**	T57.0X1-	T57.0X2-	T57.0X3-	T57.0X4-	-	-
anti-infectives	T37.8X1-	T37.8X2-	T37.8X3-	T37.8X4-	T37.8X5-	T37.8X6-
pesticide (dust) (fumes)	T57.0X1-	T57.0X2-	T57.0X3-	T57.0X4-	-	-
Arsine (gas)	T57.0X1-	T57.0X2-	T57.0X3-	T57.0X4-	-	-
Arsphenamine (silver)	T37.8X1-	T37.8X2-	T37.8X3-	T37.8X4-	T37.8X5-	T37.8X6-
Arsthinol	T37.3X1-	T37.3X2-	T37.3X3-	T37.3X4-	T37.3X5-	T37.3X6-
Artane	T44.3X1-	T44.3X2-	T44.3X3-	T44.3X4-	T44.3X5-	T44.3X6-
Arthropod (venomous) **NEC**	T63.481-	T63.482-	T63.483-	T63.484-	-	-
Articaine	T41.3X1-	T41.3X2-	T41.3X3-	T41.3X4-	T41.3X5-	T41.3X6-
Asbestos	T57.8X1-	T57.8X2-	T57.8X3-	T57.8X4-	-	-
Ascaridole	T37.4X1-	T37.4X2-	T37.4X3-	T37.4X4-	T37.4X5-	T37.4X6-
Ascorbic acid	T45.2X1-	T45.2X2-	T45.2X3-	T45.2X4-	T45.2X5-	T45.2X6-
Asiaticoside	T49.0X1-	T49.0X2-	T49.0X3-	T49.0X4-	T49.0X5-	T49.0X6-
Asparaginase	T45.1X1-	T45.1X2-	T45.1X3-	T45.1X4-	T45.1X5-	T45.1X6-
Aspidium (oleoresin)	T37.4X1-	T37.4X2-	T37.4X3-	T37.4X4-	T37.4X5-	T37.4X6-
Aspirin (aluminum) (soluble)	T39.011-	T39.012-	T39.013-	T39.014-	T39.015-	T39.016-
Aspoxicillin	T36.0X1-	T36.0X2-	T36.0X3-	T36.0X4-	T36.0X5-	T36.0X6-
Astemizole	T45.0X1-	T45.0X2-	T45.0X3-	T45.0X4-	T45.0X5-	T45.0X6-
Astringent (local)	T49.2X1-	T49.2X2-	T49.2X3-	T49.2X4-	T49.2X5-	T49.2X6-
specified NEC	T49.2X1-	T49.2X2-	T49.2X3-	T49.2X4-	T49.2X5-	T49.2X6-
Astromicin	T36.5X1-	T36.5X2-	T36.5X3-	T36.5X4-	T36.5X5-	T36.5X6-
Ataractic drug NEC	T43.501-	T43.502-	T43.503-	T43.504-	T43.505-	T43.506-
Atenolol	T44.7X1-	T44.7X2-	T44.7X3-	T44.7X4-	T44.7X5-	T44.7X6-
Atonia drug, intestinal	T47.4X1-	T47.4X2-	T47.4X3-	T47.4X4-	T47.4X5-	T47.4X6-
Atophan	T50.4X1-	T50.4X2-	T50.4X3-	T50.4X4-	T50.4X5-	T50.4X6-
Atracurium besilate	T48.1X1-	T48.1X2-	T48.1X3-	T48.1X4-	T48.1X5-	T48.1X6-
Atropine	T44.3X1-	T44.3X2-	T44.3X3-	T44.3X4-	T44.3X5-	T44.3X6-
derivative	T44.3X1-	T44.3X2-	T44.3X3-	T44.3X4-	T44.3X5-	T44.3X6-
methonitrate	T44.3X1-	T44.3X2-	T44.3X3-	T44.3X4-	T44.3X5-	T44.3X6-
Attapulgite	T47.6X1-	T47.6X2-	T47.6X3-	T47.6X4-	T47.6X5-	T47.6X6-
Auramine	T65.891-	T65.892-	T65.893-	T65.894-	-	-
dye	T65.6X1-	T65.6X2-	T65.6X3-	T65.6X4-	-	-
fungicide	T60.3X1-	T60.3X2-	T60.3X3-	T60.3X4-	-	-
Auranofin	T39.4X1-	T39.4X2-	T39.4X3-	T39.4X4-	T39.4X5-	T39.4X6-
Aurantiin	T46.991-	T46.992-	T46.993-	T46.994-	T46.995-	T46.996-
Aureomycin	T36.4X1-	T36.4X2-	T36.4X3-	T36.4X4-	T36.4X5-	T36.4X6-
ophthalmic preparation	T49.5X1-	T49.5X2-	T49.5X3-	T49.5X4-	T49.5X5-	T49.5X6-
topical NEC	T49.0X1-	T49.0X2-	T49.0X3-	T49.0X4-	T49.0X5-	T49.0X6-
Aurothioglucose	T39.4X1-	T39.4X2-	T39.4X3-	T39.4X4-	T39.4X5-	T39.4X6-
Aurothioglycanide	T39.4X1-	T39.4X2-	T39.4X3-	T39.4X4-	T39.4X5-	T39.4X6-
Aurothiomalate sodium	T39.4X1-	T39.4X2-	T39.4X3-	T39.4X4-	T39.4X5-	T39.4X6-
Aurotioprol	T39.4X1-	T39.4X2-	T39.4X3-	T39.4X4-	T39.4X5-	T39.4X6-
Automobile fuel	T52.0X1-	T52.0X2-	T52.0X3-	T52.0X4-	-	-
Autonomic nervous system agent NEC	T44.901-	T44.902-	T44.903-	T44.904-	T44.905-	T44.906-
Avlosulfon	T37.1X1-	T37.1X2-	T37.1X3-	T37.1X4-	T37.1X5-	T37.1X6-
Avomine	T42.6X1-	T42.6X2-	T42.6X3-	T42.6X4-	T42.6X5-	T42.6X6-
Axerophthol	T45.2X1-	T45.2X2-	T45.2X3-	T45.2X4-	T45.2X5-	T45.2X6-
Azacitidine	T45.1X1-	T45.1X2-	T45.1X3-	T45.1X4-	T45.1X5-	T45.1X6-
Azacyclonol	T43.591-	T43.592-	T43.593-	T43.594-	T43.595-	T43.596-
Azadirachta	T60.2X1-	T60.2X2-	T60.2X3-	T60.2X4-	-	-
Azanidazole	T37.3X1-	T37.3X2-	T37.3X3-	T37.3X4-	T37.3X5-	T37.3X6-
Azapetine	T46.7X1-	T46.7X2-	T46.7X3-	T46.7X4-	T46.7X5-	T46.7X6-
Azapropazone	T39.2X1-	T39.2X2-	T39.2X3-	T39.2X4-	T39.2X5-	T39.2X6-
Azaribine	T45.1X1-	T45.1X2-	T45.1X3-	T45.1X4-	T45.1X5-	T45.1X6-
Azaserine	T45.1X1-	T45.1X2-	T45.1X3-	T45.1X4-	T45.1X5-	T45.1X6-
Azatadine	T45.0X1-	T45.0X2-	T45.0X3-	T45.0X4-	T45.0X5-	T45.0X6-
Azatepa	T45.1X1-	T45.1X2-	T45.1X3-	T45.1X4-	T45.1X5-	T45.1X6-
Azathioprine	T45.1X1-	T45.1X2-	T45.1X3-	T45.1X4-	T45.1X5-	T45.1X6-
Azelaic acid	T49.0X1-	T49.0X2-	T49.0X3-	T49.0X4-	T49.0X5-	T49.0X6-
Azelastine	T45.0X1-	T45.0X2-	T45.0X3-	T45.0X4-	T45.0X5-	T45.0X6-
Azidocillin	T36.0X1-	T36.0X2-	T36.0X3-	T36.0X4-	T36.0X5-	T36.0X6-
Azidothymidine	T37.5X1-	T37.5X2-	T37.5X3-	T37.5X4-	T37.5X5-	T37.5X6-

Substance	Poisoning Accidental (unintentional)	Poisoning Intentional self-harm	Poisoning Assault	Poisoning Undetermined	Adverse effect	Underdosing
Azinphos (ethyl) (methyl)	T60.0X1-	T60.0X2-	T60.0X3-	T60.0X4-	-	-
Aziridine (chelating)	T54.1X1-	T54.1X2-	T54.1X3-	T54.1X4-	-	-
Azithromycin	T36.3X1-	T36.3X2-	T36.3X3-	T36.3X4-	T36.3X5-	T36.3X6-
Azlocillin	T36.0X1-	T36.0X2-	T36.0X3-	T36.0X4-	T36.0X5-	T36.0X6-
Azobenzene smoke	T65.3X1-	T65.3X2-	T65.3X3-	T65.3X4-	-	-
acaricide	T60.8X1-	T60.8X2-	T60.8X3-	T60.8X4-	-	-
Azosulfamide	T37.0X1-	T37.0X2-	T37.0X3-	T37.0X4-	T37.0X5-	T37.0X6-
AZT	T37.5X1-	T37.5X2-	T37.5X3-	T37.5X4-	T37.5X5-	T37.5X6-
Aztreonam	T36.1X1-	T36.1X2-	T36.1X3-	T36.1X4-	T36.1X5-	T36.1X6-
Azulfidine	T37.0X1-	T37.0X2-	T37.0X3-	T37.0X4-	T37.0X5-	T37.0X6-
Azuresin	T50.8X1-	T50.8X2-	T50.8X3-	T50.8X4-	T50.8X5-	T50.8X6-
Bacampicillin	T36.0X1-	T36.0X2-	T36.0X3-	T36.0X4-	T36.0X5-	T36.0X6-
Bacillus						
lactobacillus	T47.8X1-	T47.8X2-	T47.8X3-	T47.8X4-	T47.8X5-	T47.8X6-
subtilis	T47.6X1-	T47.6X2-	T47.6X3-	T47.6X4-	T47.6X5-	T47.6X6-
Bacimycin	T49.0X1-	T49.0X2-	T49.0X3-	T49.0X4-	T49.0X5-	T49.0X6-
ophthalmic preparation	T49.5X1-	T49.5X2-	T49.5X3-	T49.5X4-	T49.5X5-	T49.5X6-
Bacitracin zinc	T49.0X1-	T49.0X2-	T49.0X3-	T49.0X4-	T49.0X5-	T49.0X6-
with neomycin	T49.0X1-	T49.0X2-	T49.0X3-	T49.0X4-	T49.0X5-	T49.0X6-
ENT agent	T49.6X1-	T49.6X2-	T49.6X3-	T49.6X4-	T49.6X5-	T49.6X6-
ophthalmic preparation	T49.5X1-	T49.5X2-	T49.5X3-	T49.5X4-	T49.5X5-	T49.5X6-
topical NEC	T49.0X1-	T49.0X2-	T49.0X3-	T49.0X4-	T49.0X5-	T49.0X6-
Baclofen	T42.8X1-	T42.8X2-	T42.8X3-	T42.8X4-	T42.8X5-	T42.8X6-
Baking soda	T50.991-	T50.992-	T50.993-	T50.994-	T50.995-	T50.996-
BAL	T45.8X1-	T45.8X2-	T45.8X3-	T45.8X4-	T45.8X5-	T45.8X6-
Bambuterol	T48.6X1-	T48.6X2-	T48.6X3-	T48.6X4-	T48.6X5-	T48.6X6-
Bamethan (sulfate)	T46.7X1-	T46.7X2-	T46.7X3-	T46.7X4-	T46.7X5-	T46.7X6-
Bamifylline	T48.6X1-	T48.6X2-	T48.6X3-	T48.6X4-	T48.6X5-	T48.6X6-
Bamipine	T45.0X1-	T45.0X2-	T45.0X3-	T45.0X4-	T45.0X5-	T45.0X6-
Baneberry — *see* Actaea spicata						
Banewort — *see* Belladonna						
Barbenyl	T42.3X1-	T42.3X2-	T42.3X3-	T42.3X4-	T42.3X5-	T42.3X6-
Barbexaclone	T42.6X1-	T42.6X2-	T42.6X3-	T42.6X4-	T42.6X5-	T42.6X6-
Barbital	T42.3X1-	T42.3X2-	T42.3X3-	T42.3X4-	T42.3X5-	T42.3X6-
sodium	T42.3X1-	T42.3X2-	T42.3X3-	T42.3X4-	T42.3X5-	T42.3X6-
Barbitone	T42.3X1-	T42.3X2-	T42.3X3-	T42.3X4-	T42.3X5-	T42.3X6-
Barbiturate NEC	T42.3X1-	T42.3X2-	T42.3X3-	T42.3X4-	T42.3X5-	T42.3X6-
with tranquilizer	T42.3X1-	T42.3X2-	T42.3X3-	T42.3X4-	T42.3X5-	T42.3X6-
anesthetic (intravenous)	T41.1X1-	T41.1X2-	T41.1X3-	T41.1X4-	T41.1X5-	T41.1X6-
Barium (carbonate) (chloride) (sulfite)	T57.8X1-	T57.8X2-	T57.8X3-	T57.8X4-	-	-
diagnostic agent	T50.8X1-	T50.8X2-	T50.8X3-	T50.8X4-	T50.8X5-	T50.8X6-
pesticide	T60.4X1-	T60.4X2-	T60.4X3-	T60.4X4-	-	-
rodenticide	T60.4X1-	T60.4X2-	T60.4X3-	T60.4X4-	-	-
sulfate (medicinal)	T50.8X1-	T50.8X2-	T50.8X3-	T50.8X4-	T50.8X5-	T50.8X6-
Barrier cream	T49.3X1-	T49.3X2-	T49.3X3-	T49.3X4-	T49.3X5-	T49.3X6-
Basic fuchsin	T49.0X1-	T49.0X2-	T49.0X3-	T49.0X4-	T49.0X5-	T49.0X6-
Battery acid or fluid	T54.2X1-	T54.2X2-	T54.2X3-	T54.2X4-	-	-
Bay rum	T51.8X1-	T51.8X2-	T51.8X3-	T51.8X4-	-	-
BCG (vaccine)	T50.A91-	T50.A92-	T50.A93-	T50.A94-	T50.A95-	T50.A96-
BCNU	T45.1X1-	T45.1X2-	T45.1X3-	T45.1X4-	T45.1X5-	T45.1X6-
Bearsfoot	T62.2X1-	T62.2X2-	T62.2X3-	T62.2X4-	-	-
Beclamide	T42.6X1-	T42.6X2-	T42.6X3-	T42.6X4-	T42.6X5-	T42.6X6-
Beclomethasone	T44.5X1-	T44.5X2-	T44.5X3-	T44.5X4-	T44.5X5-	T44.5X6-
Bee (sting) (venom)	T63.441-	T63.442-	T63.443-	T63.444-	-	-
Befunolol	T49.5X1-	T49.5X2-	T49.5X3-	T49.5X4-	T49.5X5-	T49.5X6-
Bekanamycin	T36.5X1-	T36.5X2-	T36.5X3-	T36.5X4-	T36.5X5-	T36.5X6-
Belladonna — *see also* Nightshade						
alkaloids	T44.3X1-	T44.3X2-	T44.3X3-	T44.3X4-	T44.3X5-	T44.3X6-
extract	T44.3X1-	T44.3X2-	T44.3X3-	T44.3X4-	T44.3X5-	T44.3X6-
herb	T44.3X1-	T44.3X2-	T44.3X3-	T44.3X4-	T44.3X5-	T44.3X6-
Bemegride	T50.7X1-	T50.7X2-	T50.7X3-	T50.7X4-	T50.7X5-	T50.7X6-
Benactyzine	T44.3X1-	T44.3X2-	T44.3X3-	T44.3X4-	T44.3X5-	T44.3X6-
Benadryl	T45.0X1-	T45.0X2-	T45.0X3-	T45.0X4-	T45.0X5-	T45.0X6-
Benaprizine	T44.3X1-	T44.3X2-	T44.3X3-	T44.3X4-	T44.3X5-	T44.3X6-
Benazepril	T46.4X1-	T46.4X2-	T46.4X3-	T46.4X4-	T46.4X5-	T46.4X6-
Bencyclane	T46.7X1-	T46.7X2-	T46.7X3-	T46.7X4-	T46.7X5-	T46.7X6-
Bendazol	T46.3X1-	T46.3X2-	T46.3X3-	T46.3X4-	T46.3X5-	T46.3X6-
Bendrofluazide	T50.2X1-	T50.2X2-	T50.2X3-	T50.2X4-	T50.2X5-	T50.2X6-
Bendroflumethiazide	T50.2X1-	T50.2X2-	T50.2X3-	T50.2X4-	T50.2X5-	T50.2X6-
Benemid	T50.4X1-	T50.4X2-	T50.4X3-	T50.4X4-	T50.4X5-	T50.4X6-
Benethamine penicillin	T36.0X1-	T36.0X2-	T36.0X3-	T36.0X4-	T36.0X5-	T36.0X6-
Benexate	T47.1X1-	T47.1X2-	T47.1X3-	T47.1X4-	T47.1X5-	T47.1X6-
Benfluorex	T46.6X1-	T46.6X2-	T46.6X3-	T46.6X4-	T46.6X5-	T46.6X6-
Benfotiamine	T45.2X1-	T45.2X2-	T45.2X3-	T45.2X4-	T45.2X5-	T45.2X6-
Benisone	T49.0X1-	T49.0X2-	T49.0X3-	T49.0X4-	T49.0X5-	T49.0X6-

Table of Drugs and Chemicals
Arginine — Benisone

Substance	Poisoning Accidental (unintentional)	Poisoning Intentional self-harm	Poisoning Assault	Poisoning Undetermined	Adverse effect	Underdosing
Benomyl	T60.0X1-	T60.0X2-	T60.0X3-	T60.0X4-	-	-
Benoquin	T49.8X1-	T49.8X2-	T49.8X3-	T49.8X4-	T49.8X5-	T49.8X6-
Benoxinate	T41.3X1-	T41.3X2-	T41.3X3-	T41.3X4-	T41.3X5-	T41.3X6-
Benperidol	T43.4X1-	T43.4X2-	T43.4X3-	T43.4X4-	T43.4X5-	T43.4X6-
Benproperine	T48.3X1-	T48.3X2-	T48.3X3-	T48.3X4-	T48.3X5-	T48.3X6-
Benserazide	T42.8X1-	T42.8X2-	T42.8X3-	T42.8X4-	T42.8X5-	T42.8X6-
Bentazepam	T42.4X1-	T42.4X2-	T42.4X3-	T42.4X4-	T42.4X5-	T42.4X6-
Bentiromide	T50.8X1-	T50.8X2-	T50.8X3-	T50.8X4-	T50.8X5-	T50.8X6-
Bentonite	T49.3X1-	T49.3X2-	T49.3X3-	T49.3X4-	T49.3X5-	T49.3X6-
Benzalbutyramide	T46.6X1-	T46.6X2-	T46.6X3-	T46.6X4-	T46.6X5-	T46.6X6-
Benzalkonium (chloride)	T49.0X1-	T49.0X2-	T49.0X3-	T49.0X4-	T49.0X5-	T49.0X6-
ophthalmic preparation	T49.5X1-	T49.5X2-	T49.5X3-	T49.5X4-	T49.5X5-	T49.5X6-
Benzamidosalicylate (calcium)	T37.1X1-	T37.1X2-	T37.1X3-	T37.1X4-	T37.1X5-	T37.1X6-
Benzamine	T41.3X1-	T41.3X2-	T41.3X3-	T41.3X4-	T41.3X5-	T41.3X6-
lactate	T49.1X1-	T49.1X2-	T49.1X3-	T49.1X4-	T49.1X5-	T49.1X6-
Benzamphetamine	T50.5X1-	T50.5X2-	T50.5X3-	T50.5X4-	T50.5X5-	T50.5X6-
Benzapril hydrochloride	T46.5X1-	T46.5X2-	T46.5X3-	T46.5X4-	T46.5X5-	T46.5X6-
Benzathine benzylpenicillin	T36.0X1-	T36.0X2-	T36.0X3-	T36.0X4-	T36.0X5-	T36.0X6-
Benzathine penicillin	T36.0X1-	T36.0X2-	T36.0X3-	T36.0X4-	T36.0X5-	T36.0X6-
Benzatropine	T42.8X1-	T42.8X2-	T42.8X3-	T42.8X4-	T42.8X5-	T42.8X6-
Benzbromarone	T50.4X1-	T50.4X2-	T50.4X3-	T50.4X4-	T50.4X5-	T50.4X6-
Benzcarbimine	T45.1X1-	T45.1X2-	T45.1X3-	T45.1X4-	T45.1X5-	T45.1X6-
Benzedrex	T44.991-	T44.992-	T44.993-	T44.994-	T44.995-	T44.996-
Benzedrine (amphetamine)	T43.621-	T43.622-	T43.623-	T43.624-	T43.625-	T43.626-
Benzenamine	T65.3X1-	T65.3X2-	T65.3X3-	T65.3X4-	-	-
Benzene	T52.1X1-	T52.1X2-	T52.1X3-	T52.1X4-	-	-
homologues (acetyl) (dimethyl) (methyl) (solvent)	T52.2X1-	T52.2X2-	T52.2X3-	T52.2X4-	-	-
Benzethonium (chloride)	T49.0X1-	T49.0X2-	T49.0X3-	T49.0X4-	T49.0X5-	T49.0X6-
Benzfetamine	T50.5X1-	T50.5X2-	T50.5X3-	T50.5X4-	T50.5X5-	T50.5X6-
Benzhexol	T44.3X1-	T44.3X2-	T44.3X3-	T44.3X4-	T44.3X5-	T44.3X6-
Benzhydramine (chloride)	T45.0X1-	T45.0X2-	T45.0X3-	T45.0X4-	T45.0X5-	T45.0X6-
Benzidine	T65.891-	T65.892-	T65.893-	T65.894-	-	-
Benzilonium bromide	T44.3X1-	T44.3X2-	T44.3X3-	T44.3X4-	T44.3X5-	T44.3X6-
Benzimidazole	T60.3X1-	T60.3X2-	T60.3X3-	T60.3X4-	-	-
Benzin (e) — *see* Ligroin						
Benziodarone	T46.3X1-	T46.3X2-	T46.3X3-	T46.3X4-	T46.3X5-	T46.3X6-
Benznidazole	T37.3X1-	T37.3X2-	T37.3X3-	T37.3X4-	T37.3X5-	T37.3X6-
Benzocaine	T41.3X1-	T41.3X2-	T41.3X3-	T41.3X4-	T41.3X5-	T41.3X6-
Benzodiapin	T42.4X1-	T42.4X2-	T42.4X3-	T42.4X4-	T42.4X5-	T42.4X6-
Benzodiazepine NEC	T42.4X1-	T42.4X2-	T42.4X3-	T42.4X4-	T42.4X5-	T42.4X6-
Benzoic acid	T49.0X1-	T49.0X2-	T49.0X3-	T49.0X4-	T49.0X5-	T49.0X6-
with salicylic acid	T49.0X1-	T49.0X2-	T49.0X3-	T49.0X4-	T49.0X5-	T49.0X6-
Benzoin (tincture)	T48.5X1-	T48.5X2-	T48.5X3-	T48.5X4-	T48.5X5-	T48.5X6-
Benzol (benzene)	T52.1X1-	T52.1X2-	T52.1X3-	T52.1X4-	-	-
vapor	T52.0X1-	T52.0X2-	T52.0X3-	T52.0X4-	-	-
Benzomorphan	T40.2X1-	T40.2X2-	T40.2X3-	T40.2X4-	T40.2X5-	T40.2X6-
Benzonatate	T48.3X1-	T48.3X2-	T48.3X3-	T48.3X4-	T48.3X5-	T48.3X6-
Benzophenones	T49.3X1-	T49.3X2-	T49.3X3-	T49.3X4-	T49.3X5-	T49.3X6-
Benzopyrone	T46.991-	T46.992-	T46.993-	T46.994-	T46.995-	T46.996-
Benzothiadiazides	T50.2X1-	T50.2X2-	T50.2X3-	T50.2X4-	T50.2X5-	T50.2X6-
Benzoxonium chloride	T49.0X1-	T49.0X2-	T49.0X3-	T49.0X4-	T49.0X5-	T49.0X6-
Benzoyl peroxide	T49.0X1-	T49.0X2-	T49.0X3-	T49.0X4-	T49.0X5-	T49.0X6-
Benzoylpas calcium	T37.1X1-	T37.1X2-	T37.1X3-	T37.1X4-	T37.1X5-	T37.1X6-
Benzperidin	T43.591-	T43.592-	T43.593-	T43.594-	T43.595-	T43.596-
Benzperidol	T43.591-	T43.592-	T43.593-	T43.594-	T43.595-	T43.596-
Benzphetamine	T50.5X1-	T50.5X2-	T50.5X3-	T50.5X4-	T50.5X5-	T50.5X6-
Benzpyrinium bromide	T44.1X1-	T44.1X2-	T44.1X3-	T44.1X4-	T44.1X5-	T44.1X6-
Benzquinamide	T45.0X1-	T45.0X2-	T45.0X3-	T45.0X4-	T45.0X5-	T45.0X6-
Benzthiazide	T50.2X1-	T50.2X2-	T50.2X3-	T50.2X4-	T50.2X5-	T50.2X6-
Benztropine						
anticholinergic	T44.3X1-	T44.3X2-	T44.3X3-	T44.3X4-	T44.3X5-	T44.3X6-
antiparkinson	T42.8X1-	T42.8X2-	T42.8X3-	T42.8X4-	T42.8X5-	T42.8X6-
Benzydamine	T49.0X1-	T49.0X2-	T49.0X3-	T49.0X4-	T49.0X5-	T49.0X6-
Benzyl						
acetate	T52.8X1-	T52.8X2-	T52.8X3-	T52.8X4-	-	-
alcohol	T49.0X1-	T49.0X2-	T49.0X3-	T49.0X4-	T49.0X5-	T49.0X6-
benzoate	T49.0X1-	T49.0X2-	T49.0X3-	T49.0X4-	T49.0X5-	T49.0X6-
Benzoic acid	T49.0X1-	T49.0X2-	T49.0X3-	T49.0X4-	T49.0X5-	T49.0X6-
morphine	T40.2X1-	T40.2X2-	T40.2X3-	T40.2X4-	-	-
nicotinate	T46.6X1-	T46.6X2-	T46.6X3-	T46.6X4-	T46.6X5-	T46.6X6-
penicillin	T36.0X1-	T36.0X2-	T36.0X3-	T36.0X4-	T36.0X5-	T36.0X6-
Benzylhydrochlorthia-zide	T50.2X1-	T50.2X2-	T50.2X3-	T50.2X4-	T50.2X5-	T50.2X6-
Benzylpenicillin	T36.0X1-	T36.0X2-	T36.0X3-	T36.0X4-	T36.0X5-	T36.0X6-
Benzylthiouracil	T38.2X1-	T38.2X2-	T38.2X3-	T38.2X4-	T38.2X5-	T38.2X6-
Bephenium hydroxy-naphthoate	T37.4X1-	T37.4X2-	T37.4X3-	T37.4X4-	T37.4X5-	T37.4X6-
Bepridil	T46.1X1-	T46.1X2-	T46.1X3-	T46.1X4-	T46.1X5-	T46.1X6-

Substance	Poisoning Accidental (unintentional)	Poisoning Intentional self-harm	Poisoning Assault	Poisoning Undetermined	Adverse effect	Underdosing
Bergamot oil	T65.891-	T65.892-	T65.893-	T65.894-	-	-
Bergapten	T50.991-	T50.992-	T50.993-	T50.994-	T50.995-	T50.996-
Berries, poisonous	T62.1X1-	T62.1X2-	T62.1X3-	T62.1X4-	-	-
Beryllium (compounds)	T56.7X1-	T56.7X2-	T56.7X3-	T56.7X4-	-	-
b-acetyldigoxin	T46.0X1-	T46.0X2-	T46.0X3-	T46.0X4-	T46.0X5-	T46.0X6-
beta adrenergic blocking agent, heart	T44.7X1-	T44.7X2-	T44.7X3-	T44.7X4-	T44.7X5-	T44.7X6-
b-benzalbutyramide	T46.6X1-	T46.6X2-	T46.6X3-	T46.6X4-	T46.6X5-	T46.6X6-
Betacarotene	T45.2X1-	T45.2X2-	T45.2X3-	T45.2X4-	T45.2X5-	T45.2X6-
b-eucaine	T49.1X1-	T49.1X2-	T49.1X3-	T49.1X4-	T49.1X5-	T49.1X6-
Beta-Chlor	T42.6X1-	T42.6X2-	T42.6X3-	T42.6X4-	T42.6X5-	T42.6X6-
b-galactosidase	T47.5X1-	T47.5X2-	T47.5X3-	T47.5X4-	T47.5X5-	T47.5X6-
Betahistine	T46.7X1-	T46.7X2-	T46.7X3-	T46.7X4-	T46.7X5-	T46.7X6-
Betaine	T47.5X1-	T47.5X2-	T47.5X3-	T47.5X4-	T47.5X5-	T47.5X6-
Betamethasone	T49.0X1-	T49.0X2-	T49.0X3-	T49.0X4-	T49.0X5-	T49.0X6-
topical	T49.0X1-	T49.0X2-	T49.0X3-	T49.0X4-	T49.0X5-	T49.0X6-
Betamicin	T36.8X1-	T36.8X2-	T36.8X3-	T36.8X4-	T36.8X5-	T36.8X6-
Betanidine	T46.5X1-	T46.5X2-	T46.5X3-	T46.5X4-	T46.5X5-	T46.5X6-
b-sitosterol (s)	T46.6X1-	T46.6X2-	T46.6X3-	T46.6X4-	T46.6X5-	T46.6X6-
Betaxolol	T44.7X1-	T44.7X2-	T44.7X3-	T44.7X4-	T44.7X5-	T44.7X6-
Betazole	T50.8X1-	T50.8X2-	T50.8X3-	T50.8X4-	T50.8X5-	T50.8X6-
Bethanechol	T44.1X1-	T44.1X2-	T44.1X3-	T44.1X4-	T44.1X5-	T44.1X6-
chloride	T44.1X1-	T44.1X2-	T44.1X3-	T44.1X4-	T44.1X5-	T44.1X6-
Bethanidine	T46.5X1-	T46.5X2-	T46.5X3-	T46.5X4-	T46.5X5-	T46.5X6-
Betoxycaine	T41.3X1-	T41.3X2-	T41.3X3-	T41.3X4-	T41.3X5-	T41.3X6-
Betula oil	T49.3X1-	T49.3X2-	T49.3X3-	T49.3X4-	T49.3X5-	T49.3X6-
Bevantolol	T44.7X1-	T44.7X2-	T44.7X3-	T44.7X4-	T44.7X5-	T44.7X6-
Bevonium metilsulfate	T44.3X1-	T44.3X2-	T44.3X3-	T44.3X4-	T44.3X5-	T44.3X6-
Bezafibrate	T46.6X1-	T46.6X2-	T46.6X3-	T46.6X4-	T46.6X5-	T46.6X6-
Bezitramide	T40.4X1-	T40.4X2-	T40.4X3-	T40.4X4-	T40.4X5-	T40.4X6-
BHA	T50.991-	T50.992-	T50.993-	T50.994-	T50.995-	T50.996-
Bhang	T40.7X1-	T40.7X2-	T40.7X3-	T40.7X4-	T40.7X5-	T40.7X6-
BHC (medicinal)	T49.0X1-	T49.0X2-	T49.0X3-	T49.0X4-	T49.0X5-	T49.0X6-
nonmedicinal (vapor)	T53.6X1-	T53.6X2-	T53.6X3-	T53.6X4-	-	-
Bialamicol	T37.3X1-	T37.3X2-	T37.3X3-	T37.3X4-	T37.3X5-	T37.3X6-
Bibenzonium bromide	T48.3X1-	T48.3X2-	T48.3X3-	T48.3X4-	T48.3X5-	T48.3X6-
Bibrocathol	T49.5X1-	T49.5X2-	T49.5X3-	T49.5X4-	T49.5X5-	T49.5X6-
Bichloride of mercury — *see* Mercury, chloride						
Bichromates (calcium) (potassium) (sodium) (crystals)	T57.8X1-	T57.8X2-	T57.8X3-	T57.8X4-	-	-
fumes	T56.2X1-	T56.2X2-	T56.2X3-	T56.2X4-	-	-
Biclotymol	T49.6X1-	T49.6X2-	T49.6X3-	T49.6X4-	T49.6X5-	T49.6X6-
Bicucculine	T50.7X1-	T50.7X2-	T50.7X3-	T50.7X4-	T50.7X5-	T50.7X6-
Bifemelane	T43.291-	T43.292-	T43.293-	T43.294-	T43.295-	T43.296-
Biguanide derivatives, oral	T38.3X1-	T38.3X2-	T38.3X3-	T38.3X4-	T38.3X5-	T38.3X6-
Bile salts	T47.5X1-	T47.5X2-	T47.5X3-	T47.5X4-	T47.5X5-	T47.5X6-
Biligrafin	T50.8X1-	T50.8X2-	T50.8X3-	T50.8X4-	T50.8X5-	T50.8X6-
Bilopaque	T50.8X1-	T50.8X2-	T50.8X3-	T50.8X4-	T50.8X5-	T50.8X6-
Binifibrate	T46.6X1-	T46.6X2-	T46.6X3-	T46.6X4-	T46.6X5-	T46.6X6-
Binitrobenzol	T65.3X1-	T65.3X2-	T65.3X3-	T65.3X4-	-	-
Bioflavonoid (s)	T46.991-	T46.992-	T46.993-	T46.994-	T46.995-	T46.996-
Biological substance NEC	T50.901-	T50.902-	T50.903-	T50.904-	T50.905-	T50.906-
Biotin	T45.2X1-	T45.2X2-	T45.2X3-	T45.2X4-	T45.2X5-	T45.2X6-
Biperiden	T44.3X1-	T44.3X2-	T44.3X3-	T44.3X4-	T44.3X5-	T44.3X6-
Bisacodyl	T47.2X1-	T47.2X2-	T47.2X3-	T47.2X4-	T47.2X5-	T47.2X6-
Bisbentiamine	T45.2X1-	T45.2X2-	T45.2X3-	T45.2X4-	T45.2X5-	T45.2X6-
Bisbutiamine	T45.2X1-	T45.2X2-	T45.2X3-	T45.2X4-	T45.2X5-	T45.2X6-
Bisdequalinium (salts) (diacetate)	T49.6X1-	T49.6X2-	T49.6X3-	T49.6X4-	T49.6X5-	T49.6X6-
Bishydroxycoumarin	T45.511-	T45.512-	T45.513-	T45.514-	T45.515-	T45.516-
Bismarsen	T37.8X1-	T37.8X2-	T37.8X3-	T37.8X4-	T37.8X5-	T37.8X6-
Bismuth salts	T47.6X1-	T47.6X2-	T47.6X3-	T47.6X4-	T47.6X5-	T47.6X6-
aluminate	T47.1X1-	T47.1X2-	T47.1X3-	T47.1X4-	T47.1X5-	T47.1X6-
anti-infectives	T37.8X1-	T37.8X2-	T37.8X3-	T37.8X4-	T37.8X5-	T37.8X6-
formic iodide	T49.0X1-	T49.0X2-	T49.0X3-	T49.0X4-	T49.0X5-	T49.0X6-
glycolylarsenate	T49.0X1-	T49.0X2-	T49.0X3-	T49.0X4-	T49.0X5-	T49.0X6-
nonmedicinal (compounds) NEC	T65.91X-	T65.92X-	T65.93X-	T65.94X-	-	-
subcarbonate	T47.6X1-	T47.6X2-	T47.6X3-	T47.6X4-	T47.6X5-	T47.6X6-
subsalicylate	T37.8X1-	T37.8X2-	T37.8X3-	T37.8X4-	T37.8X5-	T37.8X6-
sulfarsphenamine	T37.8X1-	T37.8X2-	T37.8X3-	T37.8X4-	T37.8X5-	T37.8X6-
Bisoprolol	T44.7X1-	T44.7X2-	T44.7X3-	T44.7X4-	T44.7X5-	T44.7X6-
Bisoxatin	T47.2X1-	T47.2X2-	T47.2X3-	T47.2X4-	T47.2X5-	T47.2X6-
Bisulepin (hydrochloride)	T45.0X1-	T45.0X2-	T45.0X3-	T45.0X4-	T45.0X5-	T45.0X6-
Bithionol	T37.8X1-	T37.8X2-	T37.8X3-	T37.8X4-	T37.8X5-	T37.8X6-
anthelminthic	T37.4X1-	T37.4X2-	T37.4X3-	T37.4X4-	T37.4X5-	T37.4X6-
Bitolterol	T48.6X1-	T48.6X2-	T48.6X3-	T48.6X4-	T48.6X5-	T48.6X6-

Substance	Poisoning Accidental (unintentional)	Poisoning Intentional self-harm	Poisoning Assault	Poisoning Undetermined	Adverse effect	Underdosing
Bitoscanate	T37.4X1-	T37.4X2-	T37.4X3-	T37.4X4-	T37.4X5-	T37.4X6-
Bitter almond oil	T62.8X1-	T62.8X2-	T62.8X3-	T62.8X4-	-	-
Bittersweet	T62.2X1-	T62.2X2-	T62.2X3-	T62.2X4-	-	-
Black						
flag	T60.91X-	T60.92X-	T60.93X-	T60.94X-	-	-
henbane	T62.2X1-	T62.2X2-	T62.2X3-	T62.2X4-	-	-
leaf (40)	T60.91X-	T60.92X-	T60.93X-	T60.94X-	-	-
widow spider (bite)	T63.311-	T63.312-	T63.313-	T63.314-	-	-
antivenin	T50.Z11-	T50.Z12-	T50.Z13-	T50.Z14-	T50.Z15-	T50.Z16-
Blast furnace gas (carbon monoxide from)	T58.8X1-	T58.8X2-	T58.8X3-	T58.8X4-	-	-
Bleach	T54.91X-	T54.92X-	T54.93X-	T54.94X-	-	-
Bleaching agent (medicinal)	T49.4X1-	T49.4X2-	T49.4X3-	T49.4X4-	T49.4X5-	T49.4X6-
Bleomycin	T45.1X1-	T45.1X2-	T45.1X3-	T45.1X4-	T45.1X5-	T45.1X6-
Blockain	T41.3X1-	T41.3X2-	T41.3X3-	T41.3X4-	T41.3X5-	T41.3X6-
infiltration (subcutaneous)	T41.3X1-	T41.3X2-	T41.3X3-	T41.3X4-	T41.3X5-	T41.3X6-
nerve block (peripheral) (plexus)	T41.3X1-	T41.3X2-	T41.3X3-	T41.3X4-	T41.3X5-	T41.3X6-
topical (surface)	T41.3X1-	T41.3X2-	T41.3X3-	T41.3X4-	T41.3X5-	T41.3X6-
Blockers, calcium channel	T46.1X1-	T46.1X2-	T46.1X3-	T46.1X4-	T46.1X5-	T46.1X6-
Blood (derivatives) (natural) (plasma) (whole)	T45.8X1-	T45.8X2-	T45.8X3-	T45.8X4-	T45.8X5-	T45.8X6-
dried	T45.8X1-	T45.8X2-	T45.8X3-	T45.8X4-	T45.8X5-	T45.8X6-
drug affecting NEC	T45.91X-	T45.92X-	T45.93X-	T45.94X-	T45.95X-	T45.96X-
expander NEC	T45.8X1-	T45.8X2-	T45.8X3-	T45.8X4-	T45.8X5-	T45.8X6-
fraction NEC	T45.8X1-	T45.8X2-	T45.8X3-	T45.8X4-	T45.8X5-	T45.8X6-
substitute (macromolecular)	T45.8X1-	T45.8X2-	T45.8X3-	T45.8X4-	T45.8X5-	T45.8X6-
Blue velvet	T40.2X1-	T40.2X2-	T40.2X3-	T40.2X4-	-	-
Bone meal	T62.8X1-	T62.8X2-	T62.8X3-	T62.8X4-	-	-
Bonine	T45.0X1-	T45.0X2-	T45.0X3-	T45.0X4-	T45.0X5-	T45.0X6-
Bopindolol	T44.7X1-	T44.7X2-	T44.7X3-	T44.7X4-	T44.7X5-	T44.7X6-
Boracic acid	T49.0X1-	T49.0X2-	T49.0X3-	T49.0X4-	T49.0X5-	T49.0X6-
ENT agent	T49.6X1-	T49.6X2-	T49.6X3-	T49.6X4-	T49.6X5-	T49.6X6-
ophthalmic preparation	T49.5X1-	T49.5X2-	T49.5X3-	T49.5X4-	T49.5X5-	T49.5X6-
Borane complex	T57.8X1-	T57.8X2-	T57.8X3-	T57.8X4-	-	-
Borate (s)	T57.8X1-	T57.8X2-	T57.8X3-	T57.8X4-	-	-
buffer	T50.991-	T50.992-	T50.993-	T50.994-	T50.995-	T50.996-
cleanser	T54.91X-	T54.92X-	T54.93X-	T54.94X-	-	-
sodium	T57.8X1-	T57.8X2-	T57.8X3-	T57.8X4-	-	-
Borax (cleanser)	T54.91X-	T54.92X-	T54.93X-	T54.94X-	-	-
Bordeaux mixture	T60.3X1-	T60.3X2-	T60.3X3-	T60.3X4-	-	-
Boric acid	T49.0X1-	T49.0X2-	T49.0X3-	T49.0X4-	T49.0X5-	T49.0X6-
ENT agent	T49.6X1-	T49.6X2-	T49.6X3-	T49.6X4-	T49.6X5-	T49.6X6-
ophthalmic preparation	T49.5X1-	T49.5X2-	T49.5X3-	T49.5X4-	T49.5X5-	T49.5X6-
Bornaprine	T44.3X1-	T44.3X2-	T44.3X3-	T44.3X4-	T44.3X5-	T44.3X6-
Boron	T57.8X1-	T57.8X2-	T57.8X3-	T57.8X4-	-	-
hydride NEC	T57.8X1-	T57.8X2-	T57.8X3-	T57.8X4-	-	-
fumes or gas	T57.8X1-	T57.8X2-	T57.8X3-	T57.8X4-	-	-
trifluoride	T59.891-	T59.892-	T59.893-	T59.894-	-	-
Botox	T48.291-	T48.292-	T48.293-	T48.294-	T48.295-	T48.296-
Botulinus anti-toxin (type A, B)	T50.Z11-	T50.Z12-	T50.Z13-	T50.Z14-	T50.Z15-	T50.Z16-
Brake fluid vapor	T59.891-	T59.892-	T59.893-	T59.894-	-	-
Brallobarbital	T42.3X1-	T42.3X2-	T42.3X3-	T42.3X4-	T42.3X5-	T42.3X6-
Bran (wheat)	T47.4X1-	T47.4X2-	T47.4X3-	T47.4X4-	T47.4X5-	T47.4X6-
Brass (fumes)	T56.891-	T56.892-	T56.893-	T56.894-	-	-
Brasso	T52.0X1-	T52.0X2-	T52.0X3-	T52.0X4-	-	-
Bretylium tosilate	T46.2X1-	T46.2X2-	T46.2X3-	T46.2X4-	T46.2X5-	T46.2X6-
Brevital (sodium)	T41.1X1-	T41.1X2-	T41.1X3-	T41.1X4-	T41.1X5-	T41.1X6-
Brinase	T45.3X1-	T45.3X2-	T45.3X3-	T45.3X4-	T45.3X5-	T45.3X6-
British antilewisite	T45.8X1-	T45.8X2-	T45.8X3-	T45.8X4-	T45.8X5-	T45.8X6-
Brodifacoum	T60.4X1-	T60.4X2-	T60.4X3-	T60.4X4-	-	-
Bromal (hydrate)	T42.6X1-	T42.6X2-	T42.6X3-	T42.6X4-	T42.6X5-	T42.6X6-
Bromazepam	T42.4X1-	T42.4X2-	T42.4X3-	T42.4X4-	T42.4X5-	T42.4X6-
Bromazine	T45.0X1-	T45.0X2-	T45.0X3-	T45.0X4-	T45.0X5-	T45.0X6-
Brombenzylcyanide	T59.3X1-	T59.3X2-	T59.3X3-	T59.3X4-	-	-
Bromelains	T45.3X1-	T45.3X2-	T45.3X3-	T45.3X4-	T45.3X5-	T45.3X6-
Bromethalin	T60.4X1-	T60.4X2-	T60.4X3-	T60.4X4-	-	-
Bromhexine	T48.4X1-	T48.4X2-	T48.4X3-	T48.4X4-	T48.4X5-	T48.4X6-
Bromide salts	T42.6X1-	T42.6X2-	T42.6X3-	T42.6X4-	T42.6X5-	T42.6X6-
Bromindione	T45.511-	T45.512-	T45.513-	T45.514-	T45.515-	T45.516-
Bromine						
compounds (medicinal)	T42.6X1-	T42.6X2-	T42.6X3-	T42.6X4-	T42.6X5-	T42.6X6-
sedative	T42.6X1-	T42.6X2-	T42.6X3-	T42.6X4-	T42.6X5-	T42.6X6-
vapor	T59.891-	T59.892-	T59.893-	T59.894-	-	-
Bromisoval	T42.6X1-	T42.6X2-	T42.6X3-	T42.6X4-	T42.6X5-	T42.6X6-
Bromisovalum	T42.6X1-	T42.6X2-	T42.6X3-	T42.6X4-	T42.6X5-	T42.6X6-
Bromobenzylcyanide	T59.3X1-	T59.3X2-	T59.3X3-	T59.3X4-	-	-
Bromochlorosalicylani-lide	T49.0X1-	T49.0X2-	T49.0X3-	T49.0X4-	T49.0X5-	T49.0X6-

Substance	Poisoning Accidental (unintentional)	Poisoning Intentional self-harm	Poisoning Assault	Poisoning Undetermined	Adverse effect	Underdosing
Bromocriptine	T42.8X1-	T42.8X2-	T42.8X3-	T42.8X4-	T42.8X5-	T42.8X6-
Bromodiphenhydramine	T45.0X1-	T45.0X2-	T45.0X3-	T45.0X4-	T45.0X5-	T45.0X6-
Bromoform	T42.6X1-	T42.6X2-	T42.6X3-	T42.6X4-	T42.6X5-	T42.6X6-
Bromophenol blue reagent	T50.991-	T50.992-	T50.993-	T50.994-	T50.995-	T50.996-
Bromopride	T47.8X1-	T47.8X2-	T47.8X3-	T47.8X4-	T47.8X5-	T47.8X6-
Bromosalicylchloranitide	T49.0X1-	T49.0X2-	T49.0X3-	T49.0X4-	T49.0X5-	T49.0X6-
Bromosalicylhydroxamic acid	T37.1X1-	T37.1X2-	T37.1X3-	T37.1X4-	T37.1X5-	T37.1X6-
Bromo-seltzer	T39.1X1-	T39.1X2-	T39.1X3-	T39.1X4-	T39.1X5-	T39.1X6-
Bromoxynil	T60.3X1-	T60.3X2-	T60.3X3-	T60.3X4-	-	-
Bromperidol	T43.4X1-	T43.4X2-	T43.4X3-	T43.4X4-	T43.4X5-	T43.4X6-
Brompheniramine	T45.0X1-	T45.0X2-	T45.0X3-	T45.0X4-	T45.0X5-	T45.0X6-
Bromsulfophthalein	T50.8X1-	T50.8X2-	T50.8X3-	T50.8X4-	T50.8X5-	T50.8X6-
Bromural	T42.6X1-	T42.6X2-	T42.6X3-	T42.6X4-	T42.6X5-	T42.6X6-
Bromvaletone	T42.6X1-	T42.6X2-	T42.6X3-	T42.6X4-	T42.6X5-	T42.6X6-
Bronchodilator NEC	T48.6X1-	T48.6X2-	T48.6X3-	T48.6X4-	T48.6X5-	T48.6X6-
Brotizolam	T42.4X1-	T42.4X2-	T42.4X3-	T42.4X4-	T42.4X5-	T42.4X6-
Brovincamine	T46.7X1-	T46.7X2-	T46.7X3-	T46.7X4-	T46.7X5-	T46.7X6-
Brown recluse spider (bite) (venom)	T63.331-	T63.332-	T63.333-	T63.334-	-	-
Brown spider (bite) (venom)	T63.391-	T63.392-	T63.393-	T63.394-	-	-
Broxaterol	T48.6X1-	T48.6X2-	T48.6X3-	T48.6X4-	T48.6X5-	T48.6X6-
Broxuridine	T45.1X1-	T45.1X2-	T45.1X3-	T45.1X4-	T45.1X5-	T45.1X6-
Broxyquinoline	T37.8X1-	T37.8X2-	T37.8X3-	T37.8X4-	T37.8X5-	T37.8X6-
Bruceine	T48.291-	T48.292-	T48.293-	T48.294-	T48.295-	T48.296-
Brucia	T62.2X1-	T62.2X2-	T62.2X3-	T62.2X4-	-	-
Brucine	T65.1X1-	T65.1X2-	T65.1X3-	T65.1X4-	-	-
Brunswick green — *see* Copper						
Bruten — *see* Ibuprofen						
Bryonia	T47.2X1-	T47.2X2-	T47.2X3-	T47.2X4-	T47.2X5-	T47.2X6-
Buclizine	T45.0X1-	T45.0X2-	T45.0X3-	T45.0X4-	T45.0X5-	T45.0X6-
Buclosamide	T49.0X1-	T49.0X2-	T49.0X3-	T49.0X4-	T49.0X5-	T49.0X6-
Budesonide	T44.5X1-	T44.5X2-	T44.5X3-	T44.5X4-	T44.5X5-	T44.5X6-
Budralazine	T46.5X1-	T46.5X2-	T46.5X3-	T46.5X4-	T46.5X5-	T46.5X6-
Bufferin	T39.011-	T39.012-	T39.013-	T39.014-	T39.015-	T39.016-
Buflomedil	T46.7X1-	T46.7X2-	T46.7X3-	T46.7X4-	T46.7X5-	T46.7X6-
Buformin	T38.3X1-	T38.3X2-	T38.3X3-	T38.3X4-	T38.3X5-	T38.3X6-
Bufotenine	T40.991-	T40.992-	T40.993-	T40.994-	-	-
Bufrolin	T48.6X1-	T48.6X2-	T48.6X3-	T48.6X4-	T48.6X5-	T48.6X6-
Bufylline	T48.6X1-	T48.6X2-	T48.6X3-	T48.6X4-	T48.6X5-	T48.6X6-
Bulk filler	T50.5X1-	T50.5X2-	T50.5X3-	T50.5X4-	T50.5X5-	T50.5X6-
cathartic	T47.4X1-	T47.4X2-	T47.4X3-	T47.4X4-	T47.4X5-	T47.4X6-
Bumetanide	T50.1X1-	T50.1X2-	T50.1X3-	T50.1X4-	T50.1X5-	T50.1X6-
Bunaftine	T46.2X1-	T46.2X2-	T46.2X3-	T46.2X4-	T46.2X5-	T46.2X6-
Bunamiodyl	T50.8X1-	T50.8X2-	T50.8X3-	T50.8X4-	T50.8X5-	T50.8X6-
Bunazosin	T44.6X1-	T44.6X2-	T44.6X3-	T44.6X4-	T44.6X5-	T44.6X6-
Bunitrolol	T44.7X1-	T44.7X2-	T44.7X3-	T44.7X4-	T44.7X5-	T44.7X6-
Buphenine	T46.7X1-	T46.7X2-	T46.7X3-	T46.7X4-	T46.7X5-	T46.7X6-
Bupivacaine	T41.3X1-	T41.3X2-	T41.3X3-	T41.3X4-	T41.3X5-	T41.3X6-
infiltration (subcutaneous)	T41.3X1-	T41.3X2-	T41.3X3-	T41.3X4-	T41.3X5-	T41.3X6-
nerve block (peripheral) (plexus)	T41.3X1-	T41.3X2-	T41.3X3-	T41.3X4-	T41.3X5-	T41.3X6-
spinal	T41.3X1-	T41.3X2-	T41.3X3-	T41.3X4-	T41.3X5-	T41.3X6-
Bupranolol	T44.7X1-	T44.7X2-	T44.7X3-	T44.7X4-	T44.7X5-	T44.7X6-
Buprenorphine	T40.4X1-	T40.4X2-	T40.4X3-	T40.4X4-	T40.4X5-	T40.4X6-
Bupropion	T43.291-	T43.292-	T43.293-	T43.294-	T43.295-	T43.296-
Burimamide	T47.1X1-	T47.1X2-	T47.1X3-	T47.1X4-	T47.1X5-	T47.1X6-
Buserelin	T38.891-	T38.892-	T38.893-	T38.894-	T38.895-	T38.896-
Buspirone	T43.591-	T43.592-	T43.593-	T43.594-	T43.595-	T43.596-
Busulfan, busulphan	T45.1X1-	T45.1X2-	T45.1X3-	T45.1X4-	T45.1X5-	T45.1X6-
Butabarbital (sodium)	T42.3X1-	T42.3X2-	T42.3X3-	T42.3X4-	T42.3X5-	T42.3X6-
Butabarbitone	T42.3X1-	T42.3X2-	T42.3X3-	T42.3X4-	T42.3X5-	T42.3X6-
Butabarpal	T42.3X1-	T42.3X2-	T42.3X3-	T42.3X4-	T42.3X5-	T42.3X6-
Butacaine	T41.3X1-	T41.3X2-	T41.3X3-	T41.3X4-	T41.3X5-	T41.3X6-
Butalamine	T46.7X1-	T46.7X2-	T46.7X3-	T46.7X4-	T46.7X5-	T46.7X6-
Butalbital	T42.3X1-	T42.3X2-	T42.3X3-	T42.3X4-	T42.3X5-	T42.3X6-
Butallylonal	T42.3X1-	T42.3X2-	T42.3X3-	T42.3X4-	T42.3X5-	T42.3X6-
Butamben	T41.3X1-	T41.3X2-	T41.3X3-	T41.3X4-	T41.3X5-	T41.3X6-
Butamirate	T48.3X1-	T48.3X2-	T48.3X3-	T48.3X4-	T48.3X5-	T48.3X6-
Butane (distributed in mobile container)	T59.891-	T59.892-	T59.893-	T59.894-	-	-
distributed through pipes	T59.891-	T59.892-	T59.893-	T59.894-	-	-
incomplete combustion	T58.11X-	T58.12X-	T58.13X-	T58.14X-	-	-
Butanilicaine	T41.3X1-	T41.3X2-	T41.3X3-	T41.3X4-	T41.3X5-	T41.3X6-
Butanol	T51.3X1-	T51.3X2-	T51.3X3-	T51.3X4-	-	-
Butanone, 2-butanone	T52.4X1-	T52.4X2-	T52.4X3-	T52.4X4-	-	-
Butantrone	T49.4X1-	T49.4X2-	T49.4X3-	T49.4X4-	T49.4X5-	T49.4X6-
Butaperazine	T43.3X1-	T43.3X2-	T43.3X3-	T43.3X4-	T43.3X5-	T43.3X6-
Butazolidin	T39.2X1-	T39.2X2-	T39.2X3-	T39.2X4-	T39.2X5-	T39.2X6-

Substance	Poisoning Accidental (unintentional)	Poisoning Intentional self-harm	Poisoning Assault	Poisoning Undetermined	Adverse effect	Underdosing
Butetamate	T48.6X1-	T48.6X2-	T48.6X3-	T48.6X4-	T48.6X5-	T48.6X6-
Butethal	T42.3X1-	T42.3X2-	T42.3X3-	T42.3X4-	T42.3X5-	T42.3X6-
Butethamate	T44.3X1-	T44.3X2-	T44.3X3-	T44.3X4-	T44.3X5-	T44.3X6-
Buthalitone (sodium)	T41.1X1-	T41.1X2-	T41.1X3-	T41.1X4-	T41.1X5-	T41.1X6-
Butisol (sodium)	T42.3X1-	T42.3X2-	T42.3X3-	T42.3X4-	T42.3X5-	T42.3X6-
Butizide	T50.2X1-	T50.2X2-	T50.2X3-	T50.2X4-	T50.2X5-	T50.2X6-
Butobarbital	T42.3X1-	T42.3X2-	T42.3X3-	T42.3X4-	T42.3X5-	T42.3X6-
sodium	T42.3X1-	T42.3X2-	T42.3X3-	T42.3X4-	T42.3X5-	T42.3X6-
Butobarbitone	T42.3X1-	T42.3X2-	T42.3X3-	T42.3X4-	T42.3X5-	T42.3X6-
Butoconazole (nitrate)	T49.0X1-	T49.0X2-	T49.0X3-	T49.0X4-	T49.0X5-	T49.0X6-
Butorphanol	T40.4X1-	T40.4X2-	T40.4X3-	T40.4X4-	T40.4X5-	T40.4X6-
Butriptyline	T43.011-	T43.012-	T43.013-	T43.014-	T43.015-	T43.016-
Butropium bromide	T44.3X1-	T44.3X2-	T44.3X3-	T44.3X4-	T44.3X5-	T44.3X6-
Butter of antimony — *see* Antimony						
Buttercups	T62.2X1-	T62.2X2-	T62.2X3-	T62.2X4-	-	-
Butyl						
acetate (secondary)	T52.8X1-	T52.8X2-	T52.8X3-	T52.8X4-	-	-
alcohol	T51.3X1-	T51.3X2-	T51.3X3-	T51.3X4-	-	-
aminobenzoate	T41.3X1-	T41.3X2-	T41.3X3-	T41.3X4-	T41.3X5-	T41.3X6-
butyrate	T52.8X1-	T52.8X2-	T52.8X3-	T52.8X4-	-	-
carbinol	T51.3X1-	T51.3X2-	T51.3X3-	T51.3X4-	-	-
carbitol	T52.3X1-	T52.3X2-	T52.3X3-	T52.3X4-	-	-
cellosolve	T52.3X1-	T52.3X2-	T52.3X3-	T52.3X4-	-	-
chloral (hydrate)	T42.6X1-	T42.6X2-	T42.6X3-	T42.6X4-	T42.6X5-	T42.6X6-
formate	T52.8X1-	T52.8X2-	T52.8X3-	T52.8X4-	-	-
lactate	T52.8X1-	T52.8X2-	T52.8X3-	T52.8X4-	-	-
propionate	T52.8X1-	T52.8X2-	T52.8X3-	T52.8X4-	-	-
scopolamine bromide	T44.3X1-	T44.3X2-	T44.3X3-	T44.3X4-	T44.3X5-	T44.3X6-
thiobarbital sodium	T41.1X1-	T41.1X2-	T41.1X3-	T41.1X4-	T41.1X5-	T41.1X6-
Butylated hydroxy-anisole	T50.991-	T50.992-	T50.993-	T50.994-	T50.995-	T50.996-
Butylchloral hydrate	T42.6X1-	T42.6X2-	T42.6X3-	T42.6X4-	T42.6X5-	T42.6X6-
Butyltoluene	T52.2X1-	T52.2X2-	T52.2X3-	T52.2X4-	-	-
Butyn	T41.3X1-	T41.3X2-	T41.3X3-	T41.3X4-	T41.3X5-	T41.3X6-
Butyrophenone (-based tranquilizers)	T43.4X1-	T43.4X2-	T43.4X3-	T43.4X4-	T43.4X5-	T43.4X6-
Cabergoline	T42.8X1-	T42.8X2-	T42.8X3-	T42.8X4-	T42.8X5-	T42.8X6-
Cacodyl, cacodylic acid	T57.0X1-	T57.0X2-	T57.0X3-	T57.0X4-	-	-
Cactinomycin	T45.1X1-	T45.1X2-	T45.1X3-	T45.1X4-	T45.1X5-	T45.1X6-
Cade oil	T49.4X1-	T49.4X2-	T49.4X3-	T49.4X4-	T49.4X5-	T49.4X6-
Cadexomer iodine	T49.0X1-	T49.0X2-	T49.0X3-	T49.0X4-	T49.0X5-	T49.0X6-
Cadmium (chloride) (fumes) (oxide)	T56.3X1-	T56.3X2-	T56.3X3-	T56.3X4-	-	-
sulfide (medicinal) NEC	T49.4X1-	T49.4X2-	T49.4X3-	T49.4X4-	T49.4X5-	T49.4X6-
Cadralazine	T46.5X1-	T46.5X2-	T46.5X3-	T46.5X4-	T46.5X5-	T46.5X6-
Caffeine	T43.611-	T43.612-	T43.613-	T43.614-	T43.615-	T43.616-
Calabar bean	T62.2X1-	T62.2X2-	T62.2X3-	T62.2X4-	-	-
Caladium seguinum	T62.2X1-	T62.2X2-	T62.2X3-	T62.2X4-	-	-
Calamine (lotion)	T49.3X1-	T49.3X2-	T49.3X3-	T49.3X4-	T49.3X5-	T49.3X6-
Calcifediol	T45.2X1-	T45.2X2-	T45.2X3-	T45.2X4-	T45.2X5-	T45.2X6-
Calciferol	T45.2X1-	T45.2X2-	T45.2X3-	T45.2X4-	T45.2X5-	T45.2X6-
Calcitonin	T50.991-	T50.992-	T50.993-	T50.994-	T50.995-	T50.996-
Calcitriol	T45.2X1-	T45.2X2-	T45.2X3-	T45.2X4-	T45.2X5-	T45.2X6-
Calcium	T50.3X1-	T50.3X2-	T50.3X3-	T50.3X4-	T50.3X5-	T50.3X6-
actylsalicylate	T39.011-	T39.012-	T39.013-	T39.014-	T39.015-	T39.016-
benzamidosalicylate	T37.1X1-	T37.1X2-	T37.1X3-	T37.1X4-	T37.1X5-	T37.1X6-
bromide	T42.6X1-	T42.6X2-	T42.6X3-	T42.6X4-	T42.6X5-	T42.6X6-
bromolactobionate	T42.6X1-	T42.6X2-	T42.6X3-	T42.6X4-	T42.6X5-	T42.6X6-
carbaspirin	T39.011-	T39.012-	T39.013-	T39.014-	T39.015-	T39.016-
carbimide	T50.6X1-	T50.6X2-	T50.6X3-	T50.6X4-	T50.6X5-	T50.6X6-
carbonate	T47.1X1-	T47.1X2-	T47.1X3-	T47.1X4-	T47.1X5-	T47.1X6-
chloride	T50.991-	T50.992-	T50.993-	T50.994-	T50.995-	T50.996-
anhydrous	T50.991-	T50.992-	T50.993-	T50.994-	T50.995-	T50.996-
cyanide	T57.8X1-	T57.8X2-	T57.8X3-	T57.8X4-	-	-
dioctyl sulfosuccinate	T47.4X1-	T47.4X2-	T47.4X3-	T47.4X4-	T47.4X5-	T47.4X6-
disodium edathamil	T45.8X1-	T45.8X2-	T45.8X3-	T45.8X4-	T45.8X5-	T45.8X6-
disodium edetate	T45.8X1-	T45.8X2-	T45.8X3-	T45.8X4-	T45.8X5-	T45.8X6-
dobesilate	T46.991-	T46.992-	T46.993-	T46.994-	T46.995-	T46.996-
EDTA	T45.8X1-	T45.8X2-	T45.8X3-	T45.8X4-	T45.8X5-	T45.8X6-
ferrous citrate	T45.4X1-	T45.4X2-	T45.4X3-	T45.4X4-	T45.4X5-	T45.4X6-
folinate	T45.8X1-	T45.8X2-	T45.8X3-	T45.8X4-	T45.8X5-	T45.8X6-
glubionate	T50.3X1-	T50.3X2-	T50.3X3-	T50.3X4-	T50.3X5-	T50.3X6-
gluconate	T50.3X1-	T50.3X2-	T50.3X3-	T50.3X4-	T50.3X5-	T50.3X6-
gluconogalactogluc-onate	T50.3X1-	T50.3X2-	T50.3X3-	T50.3X4-	T50.3X5-	T50.3X6-
hydrate, hydroxide	T54.3X1-	T54.3X2-	T54.3X3-	T54.3X4-	-	-
hypochlorite	T54.3X1-	T54.3X2-	T54.3X3-	T54.3X4-	-	-
iodide	T48.4X1-	T48.4X2-	T48.4X3-	T48.4X4-	T48.4X5-	T48.4X6-
ipodate	T50.8X1-	T50.8X2-	T50.8X3-	T50.8X4-	T50.8X5-	T50.8X6-
Calcium - *continued*						
lactate	T50.3X1-	T50.3X2-	T50.3X3-	T50.3X4-	T50.3X5-	T50.3X6-
leucovorin	T45.8X1-	T45.8X2-	T45.8X3-	T45.8X4-	T45.8X5-	T45.8X6-
mandelate	T37.91X-	T37.92X-	T37.93X-	T37.94X-	T37.95X-	T37.96X-
oxide	T54.3X1-	T54.3X2-	T54.3X3-	T54.3X4-	-	-
pantothenate	T45.2X1-	T45.2X2-	T45.2X3-	T45.2X4-	T45.2X5-	T45.2X6-
phosphate	T50.3X1-	T50.3X2-	T50.3X3-	T50.3X4-	T50.3X5-	T50.3X6-
salicylate	T39.091-	T39.092-	T39.093-	T39.094-	T39.095-	T39.096-
salts	T50.3X1-	T50.3X2-	T50.3X3-	T50.3X4-	T50.3X5-	T50.3X6-
Calculus-dissolving drug	T50.991-	T50.992-	T50.993-	T50.994-	T50.995-	T50.996-
Calomel	T49.0X1-	T49.0X2-	T49.0X3-	T49.0X4-	T49.0X5-	T49.0X6-
Caloric agent	T50.3X1-	T50.3X2-	T50.3X3-	T50.3X4-	T50.3X5-	T50.3X6-
Calusterone	T38.7X1-	T38.7X2-	T38.7X3-	T38.7X4-	T38.7X5-	T38.7X6-
Camazepam	T42.4X1-	T42.4X2-	T42.4X3-	T42.4X4-	T42.4X5-	T42.4X6-
Camomile	T49.0X1-	T49.0X2-	T49.0X3-	T49.0X4-	T49.0X5-	T49.0X6-
Camoquin	T37.2X1-	T37.2X2-	T37.2X3-	T37.2X4-	T37.2X5-	T37.2X6-
Camphor						
insecticide	T60.2X1-	T60.2X2-	T60.2X3-	T60.2X4-	-	-
medicinal	T49.8X1-	T49.8X2-	T49.8X3-	T49.8X4-	T49.8X5-	T49.8X6-
Camylofin	T44.3X1-	T44.3X2-	T44.3X3-	T44.3X4-	T44.3X5-	T44.3X6-
Cancer chemotherapy drug regimen	T45.1X1-	T45.1X2-	T45.1X3-	T45.1X4-	T45.1X5-	T45.1X6-
Candeptin	T49.0X1-	T49.0X2-	T49.0X3-	T49.0X4-	T49.0X5-	T49.0X6-
Candicidin	T49.0X1-	T49.0X2-	T49.0X3-	T49.0X4-	T49.0X5-	T49.0X6-
Cannabinol	T40.7X1-	T40.7X2-	T40.7X3-	T40.7X4-	T40.7X5-	T40.7X6-
Cannabis (derivatives)	T40.7X1-	T40.7X2-	T40.7X3-	T40.7X4-	T40.7X5-	T40.7X6-
Canned heat	T51.1X1-	T51.1X2-	T51.1X3-	T51.1X4-	-	-
Canrenoic acid	T50.0X1-	T50.0X2-	T50.0X3-	T50.0X4-	T50.0X5-	T50.0X6-
Canrenone	T50.0X1-	T50.0X2-	T50.0X3-	T50.0X4-	T50.0X5-	T50.0X6-
Cantharides, cantharidin, cantharis	T49.8X1-	T49.8X2-	T49.8X3-	T49.8X4-	T49.8X5-	T49.8X6-
Canthaxanthin	T50.991-	T50.992-	T50.993-	T50.994-	T50.995-	T50.996-
Capillary-active drug NEC	T46.901-	T46.902-	T46.903-	T46.904-	T46.905-	T46.906-
Capreomycin	T36.8X1-	T36.8X2-	T36.8X3-	T36.8X4-	T36.8X5-	T36.8X6-
Capsicum	T49.4X1-	T49.4X2-	T49.4X3-	T49.4X4-	T49.4X5-	T49.4X6-
Captafol	T60.3X1-	T60.3X2-	T60.3X3-	T60.3X4-	-	-
Captan	T60.3X1-	T60.3X2-	T60.3X3-	T60.3X4-	-	-
Captodiame, captodiamine	T43.591-	T43.592-	T43.593-	T43.594-	T43.595-	T43.596-
Captopril	T46.4X1-	T46.4X2-	T46.4X3-	T46.4X4-	T46.4X5-	T46.4X6-
Caramiphen	T44.3X1-	T44.3X2-	T44.3X3-	T44.3X4-	T44.3X5-	T44.3X6-
Carazolol	T44.7X1-	T44.7X2-	T44.7X3-	T44.7X4-	T44.7X5-	T44.7X6-
Carbachol	T44.1X1-	T44.1X2-	T44.1X3-	T44.1X4-	T44.1X5-	T44.1X6-
Carbacrylamine (resin)	T50.3X1-	T50.3X2-	T50.3X3-	T50.3X4-	T50.3X5-	T50.3X6-
Carbamate (insecticide)	T60.0X1-	T60.0X2-	T60.0X3-	T60.0X4-	-	-
Carbamate (sedative)	T42.6X1-	T42.6X2-	T42.6X3-	T42.6X4-	T42.6X5-	T42.6X6-
herbicide	T60.0X1-	T60.0X2-	T60.0X3-	T60.0X4-	-	-
insecticide	T60.0X1-	T60.0X2-	T60.0X3-	T60.0X4-	-	-
Carbamazepine	T42.1X1-	T42.1X2-	T42.1X3-	T42.1X4-	T42.1X5-	T42.1X6-
Carbamide	T47.3X1-	T47.3X2-	T47.3X3-	T47.3X4-	T47.3X5-	T47.3X6-
peroxide	T49.0X1-	T49.0X2-	T49.0X3-	T49.0X4-	T49.0X5-	T49.0X6-
topical	T49.8X1-	T49.8X2-	T49.8X3-	T49.8X4-	T49.8X5-	T49.8X6-
Carbamylcholine chloride	T44.1X1-	T44.1X2-	T44.1X3-	T44.1X4-	T44.1X5-	T44.1X6-
Carbaril	T60.0X1-	T60.0X2-	T60.0X3-	T60.0X4-	-	-
Carbarsone	T37.3X1-	T37.3X2-	T37.3X3-	T37.3X4-	T37.3X5-	T37.3X6-
Carbaryl	T60.0X1-	T60.0X2-	T60.0X3-	T60.0X4-	-	-
Carbaspirin	T39.011-	T39.012-	T39.013-	T39.014-	T39.015-	T39.016-
Carbazochrome (salicylate) (sodium sulfonate)	T49.4X1-	T49.4X2-	T49.4X3-	T49.4X4-	T49.4X5-	T49.4X6-
Carbenicillin	T36.0X1-	T36.0X2-	T36.0X3-	T36.0X4-	T36.0X5-	T36.0X6-
Carbenoxolone	T47.1X1-	T47.1X2-	T47.1X3-	T47.1X4-	T47.1X5-	T47.1X6-
Carbetapentane	T48.3X1-	T48.3X2-	T48.3X3-	T48.3X4-	T48.3X5-	T48.3X6-
Carbethyl salicylate	T39.091-	T39.092-	T39.093-	T39.094-	T39.095-	T39.096-
Carbidopa (with levodopa)	T42.8X1-	T42.8X2-	T42.8X3-	T42.8X4-	T42.8X5-	T42.8X6-
Carbimazole	T38.2X1-	T38.2X2-	T38.2X3-	T38.2X4-	T38.2X5-	T38.2X6-
Carbinol	T51.1X1-	T51.1X2-	T51.1X3-	T51.1X4-	-	-
Carbinoxamine	T45.0X1-	T45.0X2-	T45.0X3-	T45.0X4-	T45.0X5-	T45.0X6-
Carbiphene	T39.8X1-	T39.8X2-	T39.8X3-	T39.8X4-	T39.8X5-	T39.8X6-
Carbitol	T52.3X1-	T52.3X2-	T52.3X3-	T52.3X4-	-	-
Carbo medicinalis	T47.6X1-	T47.6X2-	T47.6X3-	T47.6X4-	T47.6X5-	T47.6X6-
Carbocaine	T41.3X1-	T41.3X2-	T41.3X3-	T41.3X4-	T41.3X5-	T41.3X6-
infiltration (subcutaneous)	T41.3X1-	T41.3X2-	T41.3X3-	T41.3X4-	T41.3X5-	T41.3X6-
nerve block (peripheral) (plexus)	T41.3X1-	T41.3X2-	T41.3X3-	T41.3X4-	T41.3X5-	T41.3X6-
topical (surface)	T41.3X1-	T41.3X2-	T41.3X3-	T41.3X4-	T41.3X5-	T41.3X6-
Carbocisteine	T48.4X1-	T48.4X2-	T48.4X3-	T48.4X4-	T48.4X5-	T48.4X6-
Carbocromen	T46.3X1-	T46.3X2-	T46.3X3-	T46.3X4-	T46.3X5-	T46.3X6-
Carbol fuchsin	T49.0X1-	T49.0X2-	T49.0X3-	T49.0X4-	T49.0X5-	T49.0X6-
Carbolic acid — *see also* Phenol	T54.0X1-	T54.0X2-	T54.0X3-	T54.0X4-	-	-

Substance	Poisoning Accidental (unintentional)	Poisoning Intentional self-harm	Poisoning Assault	Poisoning Undetermined	Adverse effect	Underdosing
Carbolonium (bromide)	T48.1X1-	T48.1X2-	T48.1X3-	T48.1X4-	T48.1X5-	T48.1X6-
Carbomycin	T36.8X1-	T36.8X2-	T36.8X3-	T36.8X4-	T36.8X5-	T36.8X6-
Carbon						
bisulfide (liquid)	T65.4X1-	T65.4X2-	T65.4X3-	T65.4X4-	-	-
vapor	T65.4X1-	T65.4X2-	T65.4X3-	T65.4X4-	-	-
dioxide (gas)	T59.7X1-	T59.7X2-	T59.7X3-	T59.7X4-	-	-
medicinal	T41.5X1-	T41.5X2-	T41.5X3-	T41.5X4-	T41.5X5-	T41.5X6-
nonmedicinal	T59.7X1-	T59.7X2-	T59.7X3-	T59.7X4-	-	-
snow	T49.4X1-	T49.4X2-	T49.4X3-	T49.4X4-	T49.4X5-	T49.4X6-
disulfide (liquid)	T65.4X1-	T65.4X2-	T65.4X3-	T65.4X4-	-	-
vapor	T65.4X1-	T65.4X2-	T65.4X3-	T65.4X4-	-	-
monoxide (from incomplete combustion)	T58.91X-	T58.92X-	T58.93X-	T58.94X-	-	-
blast furnace gas	T58.8X1-	T58.8X2-	T58.8X3-	T58.8X4-	-	-
butane (distributed in mobile container)	T58.11X-	T58.12X-	T58.13X-	T58.14X-	-	-
distributed through pipes	T58.11X-	T58.12X-	T58.13X-	T58.14X-	-	-
charcoal fumes	T58.2X1-	T58.2X2-	T58.2X3-	T58.2X4-	-	-
coal	T58.2X1-	T58.2X2-	T58.2X3-	T58.2X4-	-	-
coke (in domestic stoves, fireplaces)	T58.2X1-	T58.2X2-	T58.2X3-	T58.2X4-	-	-
gas (piped)	T58.11X-	T58.12X-	T58.13X-	T58.14X-	-	-
solid (in domestic stoves, fireplaces)	T58.2X1-	T58.2X2-	T58.2X3-	T58.2X4-	-	-
exhaust gas (motor) not in transit	T58.01X-	T58.02X-	T58.03X-	T58.04X-	-	-
combustion engine, any not in watercraft	T58.01X-	T58.02X-	T58.03X-	T58.04X-	-	-
farm tractor, not in transit	T58.01X-	T58.02X-	T58.03X-	T58.04X-	-	-
gas engine	T58.01X-	T58.02X-	T58.03X-	T58.04X-	-	-
motor pump	T58.01X-	T58.02X-	T58.03X-	T58.04X-	-	-
motor vehicle, not in transit	T58.01X-	T58.02X-	T58.03X-	T58.04X-	-	-
fuel (in domestic use)	T58.2X1-	T58.2X2-	T58.2X3-	T58.2X4-	-	-
gas (piped)	T58.11X-	T58.12X-	T58.13X-	T58.14X-	-	-
in mobile container	T58.11X-	T58.12X-	T58.13X-	T58.14X-	-	-
piped (natural)	T58.11X-	T58.12X-	T58.13X-	T58.14X-	-	-
utility	T58.11X-	T58.12X-	T58.13X-	T58.14X-	-	-
in mobile container	T58.11X-	T58.12X-	T58.13X-	T58.14X-	-	-
illuminating gas	T58.11X-	T58.12X-	T58.13X-	T58.14X-	-	-
industrial fuels or gases, any	T58.8X1-	T58.8X2-	T58.8X3-	T58.8X4-	-	-
kerosene (in domestic stoves, fireplaces)	T58.2X1-	T58.2X2-	T58.2X3-	T58.2X4-	-	-
kiln gas or vapor	T58.8X1-	T58.8X2-	T58.8X3-	T58.8X4-	-	-
motor exhaust gas, not in transit	T58.01X-	T58.02X-	T58.03X-	T58.04X-	-	-
piped gas (manufactured) (natural)	T58.11X-	T58.12X-	T58.13X-	T58.14X-	-	-
producer gas	T58.8X1-	T58.8X2-	T58.8X3-	T58.8X4-	-	-
propane (distributed in mobile container)	T58.11X-	T58.12X-	T58.13X-	T58.14X-	-	-
distributed through pipes	T58.11X-	T58.12X-	T58.13X-	T58.14X-	-	-
specified source NEC	T58.8X1-	T58.8X2-	T58.8X3-	T58.8X4-	-	-
stove gas	T58.11X-	T58.12X-	T58.13X-	T58.14X-	-	-
piped	T58.11X-	T58.12X-	T58.13X-	T58.14X-	-	-
utility gas	T58.11X-	T58.12X-	T58.13X-	T58.14X-	-	-
piped	T58.11X-	T58.12X-	T58.13X-	T58.14X-	-	-
water gas	T58.11X-	T58.12X-	T58.13X-	T58.14X-	-	-
wood (in domestic stoves, fireplaces)	T58.2X1-	T58.2X2-	T58.2X3-	T58.2X4-	-	-
tetrachloride (vapor) NEC	T53.0X1-	T53.0X2-	T53.0X3-	T53.0X4-	-	-
liquid (cleansing agent) NEC	T53.0X1-	T53.0X2-	T53.0X3-	T53.0X4-	-	-
solvent	T53.0X1-	T53.0X2-	T53.0X3-	T53.0X4-	-	-
Carbonic acid gas	T59.7X1-	T59.7X2-	T59.7X3-	T59.7X4-	-	-
anhydrase inhibitor NEC	T50.2X1-	T50.2X2-	T50.2X3-	T50.2X4-	T50.2X5-	T50.2X6-
Carbophenothion	T60.0X1-	T60.0X2-	T60.0X3-	T60.0X4-	-	-
Carboplatin	T45.1X1-	T45.1X2-	T45.1X3-	T45.1X4-	T45.1X5-	T45.1X6-
Carboprost	T48.0X1-	T48.0X2-	T48.0X3-	T48.0X4-	T48.0X5-	T48.0X6-
Carboquone	T45.1X1-	T45.1X2-	T45.1X3-	T45.1X4-	T45.1X5-	T45.1X6-
Carbowax	T49.3X1-	T49.3X2-	T49.3X3-	T49.3X4-	T49.3X5-	T49.3X6-
Carboxymethyl-cellulose	T47.4X1-	T47.4X2-	T47.4X3-	T47.4X4-	T47.4X5-	T47.4X6-
S-Carboxymethyl-cysteine	T48.4X1-	T48.4X2-	T48.4X3-	T48.4X4-	T48.4X5-	T48.4X6-
Carbrital	T42.3X1-	T42.3X2-	T42.3X3-	T42.3X4-	T42.3X5-	T42.3X6-
Carbromal	T42.6X1-	T42.6X2-	T42.6X3-	T42.6X4-	T42.6X5-	T42.6X6-
Carbutamide	T38.3X1-	T38.3X2-	T38.3X3-	T38.3X4-	T38.3X5-	T38.3X6-
Carbuterol	T48.6X1-	T48.6X2-	T48.6X3-	T48.6X4-	T48.6X5-	T48.6X6-
Cardiac						
depressants	T46.2X1-	T46.2X2-	T46.2X3-	T46.2X4-	T46.2X5-	T46.2X6-
rhythm regulator	T46.2X1-	T46.2X2-	T46.2X3-	T46.2X4-	T46.2X5-	T46.2X6-
specified NEC	T46.2X1-	T46.2X2-	T46.2X3-	T46.2X4-	T46.2X5-	T46.2X6-

Substance	Poisoning Accidental (unintentional)	Poisoning Intentional self-harm	Poisoning Assault	Poisoning Undetermined	Adverse effect	Underdosing
Cardiografin	T50.8X1-	T50.8X2-	T50.8X3-	T50.8X4-	T50.8X5-	T50.8X6-
Cardio-green	T50.8X1-	T50.8X2-	T50.8X3-	T50.8X4-	T50.8X5-	T50.8X6-
Cardiotonic (glycoside) **NEC**	T46.0X1-	T46.0X2-	T46.0X3-	T46.0X4-	T46.0X5-	T46.0X6-
Cardiovascular drug NEC	T46.901-	T46.902-	T46.903-	T46.904-	T46.905-	T46.906-
Cardrase	T50.2X1-	T50.2X2-	T50.2X3-	T50.2X4-	T50.2X5-	T50.2X6-
Carfecillin	T36.0X1-	T36.0X2-	T36.0X3-	T36.0X4-	T36.0X5-	T36.0X6-
Carfenazine	T43.3X1-	T43.3X2-	T43.3X3-	T43.3X4-	T43.3X5-	T43.3X6-
Carfusin	T49.0X1-	T49.0X2-	T49.0X3-	T49.0X4-	T49.0X5-	T49.0X6-
Carindacillin	T36.0X1-	T36.0X2-	T36.0X3-	T36.0X4-	T36.0X5-	T36.0X6-
Carisoprodol	T42.8X1-	T42.8X2-	T42.8X3-	T42.8X4-	T42.8X5-	T42.8X6-
Carmellose	T47.4X1-	T47.4X2-	T47.4X3-	T47.4X4-	T47.4X5-	T47.4X6-
Carminative	T47.5X1-	T47.5X2-	T47.5X3-	T47.5X4-	T47.5X5-	T47.5X6-
Carmofur	T45.1X1-	T45.1X2-	T45.1X3-	T45.1X4-	T45.1X5-	T45.1X6-
Carmustine	T45.1X1-	T45.1X2-	T45.1X3-	T45.1X4-	T45.1X5-	T45.1X6-
Carotene	T45.2X1-	T45.2X2-	T45.2X3-	T45.2X4-	T45.2X5-	T45.2X6-
Carphenazine	T43.3X1-	T43.3X2-	T43.3X3-	T43.3X4-	T43.3X5-	T43.3X6-
Carpipramine	T42.4X1-	T42.4X2-	T42.4X3-	T42.4X4-	T42.4X5-	T42.4X6-
Carprofen	T39.311-	T39.312-	T39.313-	T39.314-	T39.315-	T39.316-
Carpronium chloride	T44.3X1-	T44.3X2-	T44.3X3-	T44.3X4-	T44.3X5-	T44.3X6-
Carrageenan	T47.8X1-	T47.8X2-	T47.8X3-	T47.8X4-	T47.8X5-	T47.8X6-
Carteolol	T44.7X1-	T44.7X2-	T44.7X3-	T44.7X4-	T44.7X5-	T44.7X6-
Carter's Little Pills	T47.2X1-	T47.2X2-	T47.2X3-	T47.2X4-	T47.2X5-	T47.2X6-
Cascara (sagrada)	T47.2X1-	T47.2X2-	T47.2X3-	T47.2X4-	T47.2X5-	T47.2X6-
Cassava	T62.2X1-	T62.2X2-	T62.2X3-	T62.2X4-	-	-
Castellani's paint	T49.0X1-	T49.0X2-	T49.0X3-	T49.0X4-	T49.0X5-	T49.0X6-
Castor						
bean	T62.2X1-	T62.2X2-	T62.2X3-	T62.2X4-	-	-
oil	T47.2X1-	T47.2X2-	T47.2X3-	T47.2X4-	T47.2X5-	T47.2X6-
Catalase	T45.3X1-	T45.3X2-	T45.3X3-	T45.3X4-	T45.3X5-	T45.3X6-
Caterpillar (sting)	T63.431-	T63.432-	T63.433-	T63.434-	-	-
Catha (edulis) (tea)	T43.691-	T43.692-	T43.693-	T43.694-	-	-
Cathartic NEC	T47.4X1-	T47.4X2-	T47.4X3-	T47.4X4-	T47.4X5-	T47.4X6-
anthacene derivative	T47.2X1-	T47.2X2-	T47.2X3-	T47.2X4-	T47.2X5-	T47.2X6-
bulk	T47.4X1-	T47.4X2-	T47.4X3-	T47.4X4-	T47.4X5-	T47.4X6-
contact	T47.2X1-	T47.2X2-	T47.2X3-	T47.2X4-	T47.2X5-	T47.2X6-
emollient NEC	T47.4X1-	T47.4X2-	T47.4X3-	T47.4X4-	T47.4X5-	T47.4X6-
irritant NEC	T47.2X1-	T47.2X2-	T47.2X3-	T47.2X4-	T47.2X5-	T47.2X6-
mucilage	T47.4X1-	T47.4X2-	T47.4X3-	T47.4X4-	T47.4X5-	T47.4X6-
saline	T47.3X1-	T47.3X2-	T47.3X3-	T47.3X4-	T47.3X5-	T47.3X6-
vegetable	T47.2X1-	T47.2X2-	T47.2X3-	T47.2X4-	T47.2X5-	T47.2X6-
Cathine	T50.5X1-	T50.5X2-	T50.5X3-	T50.5X4-	T50.5X5-	T50.5X6-
Cathomycin	T36.8X1-	T36.8X2-	T36.8X3-	T36.8X4-	T36.8X5-	T36.8X6-
Cation exchange resin	T50.3X1-	T50.3X2-	T50.3X3-	T50.3X4-	T50.3X5-	T50.3X6-
Caustic (s) **NEC**	T54.91X-	T54.92X-	T54.93X-	T54.94X-	-	-
alkali	T54.3X1-	T54.3X2-	T54.3X3-	T54.3X4-	-	-
hydroxide	T54.3X1-	T54.3X2-	T54.3X3-	T54.3X4-	-	-
potash	T54.3X1-	T54.3X2-	T54.3X3-	T54.3X4-	-	-
soda	T54.3X1-	T54.3X2-	T54.3X3-	T54.3X4-	-	-
specified NEC	T54.91X-	T54.92X-	T54.93X-	T54.94X-	-	-
Ceepryn	T49.0X1-	T49.0X2-	T49.0X3-	T49.0X4-	T49.0X5-	T49.0X6-
ENT agent	T49.6X1-	T49.6X2-	T49.6X3-	T49.6X4-	T49.6X5-	T49.6X6-
lozenges	T49.6X1-	T49.6X2-	T49.6X3-	T49.6X4-	T49.6X5-	T49.6X6-
Cefacetrile	T36.1X1-	T36.1X2-	T36.1X3-	T36.1X4-	T36.1X5-	T36.1X6-
Cefaclor	T36.1X1-	T36.1X2-	T36.1X3-	T36.1X4-	T36.1X5-	T36.1X6-
Cefadroxil	T36.1X1-	T36.1X2-	T36.1X3-	T36.1X4-	T36.1X5-	T36.1X6-
Cefalexin	T36.1X1-	T36.1X2-	T36.1X3-	T36.1X4-	T36.1X5-	T36.1X6-
Cefaloglycin	T36.1X1-	T36.1X2-	T36.1X3-	T36.1X4-	T36.1X5-	T36.1X6-
Cefaloridine	T36.1X1-	T36.1X2-	T36.1X3-	T36.1X4-	T36.1X5-	T36.1X6-
Cefalosporins	T36.1X1-	T36.1X2-	T36.1X3-	T36.1X4-	T36.1X5-	T36.1X6-
Cefalotin	T36.1X1-	T36.1X2-	T36.1X3-	T36.1X4-	T36.1X5-	T36.1X6-
Cefamandole	T36.1X1-	T36.1X2-	T36.1X3-	T36.1X4-	T36.1X5-	T36.1X6-
Cefamycin antibiotic	T36.1X1-	T36.1X2-	T36.1X3-	T36.1X4-	T36.1X5-	T36.1X6-
Cefapirin	T36.1X1-	T36.1X2-	T36.1X3-	T36.1X4-	T36.1X5-	T36.1X6-
Cefatrizine	T36.1X1-	T36.1X2-	T36.1X3-	T36.1X4-	T36.1X5-	T36.1X6-
Cefazedone	T36.1X1-	T36.1X2-	T36.1X3-	T36.1X4-	T36.1X5-	T36.1X6-
Cefazolin	T36.1X1-	T36.1X2-	T36.1X3-	T36.1X4-	T36.1X5-	T36.1X6-
Cefbuperazone	T36.1X1-	T36.1X2-	T36.1X3-	T36.1X4-	T36.1X5-	T36.1X6-
Cefetamet	T36.1X1-	T36.1X2-	T36.1X3-	T36.1X4-	T36.1X5-	T36.1X6-
Cefixime	T36.1X1-	T36.1X2-	T36.1X3-	T36.1X4-	T36.1X5-	T36.1X6-
Cefmenoxime	T36.1X1-	T36.1X2-	T36.1X3-	T36.1X4-	T36.1X5-	T36.1X6-
Cefmetazole	T36.1X1-	T36.1X2-	T36.1X3-	T36.1X4-	T36.1X5-	T36.1X6-
Cefminox	T36.1X1-	T36.1X2-	T36.1X3-	T36.1X4-	T36.1X5-	T36.1X6-
Cefonicid	T36.1X1-	T36.1X2-	T36.1X3-	T36.1X4-	T36.1X5-	T36.1X6-
Cefoperazone	T36.1X1-	T36.1X2-	T36.1X3-	T36.1X4-	T36.1X5-	T36.1X6-
Ceforanide	T36.1X1-	T36.1X2-	T36.1X3-	T36.1X4-	T36.1X5-	T36.1X6-
Cefotaxime	T36.1X1-	T36.1X2-	T36.1X3-	T36.1X4-	T36.1X5-	T36.1X6-
Cefotetan	T36.1X1-	T36.1X2-	T36.1X3-	T36.1X4-	T36.1X5-	T36.1X6-
Cefotiam	T36.1X1-	T36.1X2-	T36.1X3-	T36.1X4-	T36.1X5-	T36.1X6-

Substance	Poisoning Accidental (unintentional)	Poisoning Intentional self-harm	Poisoning Assault	Poisoning Undetermined	Adverse effect	Underdosing
Cefoxitin	T36.1X1-	T36.1X2-	T36.1X3-	T36.1X4-	T36.1X5-	T36.1X6-
Cefpimizole	T36.1X1-	T36.1X2-	T36.1X3-	T36.1X4-	T36.1X5-	T36.1X6-
Cefpiramide	T36.1X1-	T36.1X2-	T36.1X3-	T36.1X4-	T36.1X5-	T36.1X6-
Cefradine	T36.1X1-	T36.1X2-	T36.1X3-	T36.1X4-	T36.1X5-	T36.1X6-
Cefroxadine	T36.1X1-	T36.1X2-	T36.1X3-	T36.1X4-	T36.1X5-	T36.1X6-
Cefsulodin	T36.1X1-	T36.1X2-	T36.1X3-	T36.1X4-	T36.1X5-	T36.1X6-
Ceftazidime	T36.1X1-	T36.1X2-	T36.1X3-	T36.1X4-	T36.1X5-	T36.1X6-
Cefteram	T36.1X1-	T36.1X2-	T36.1X3-	T36.1X4-	T36.1X5-	T36.1X6-
Ceftezole	T36.1X1-	T36.1X2-	T36.1X3-	T36.1X4-	T36.1X5-	T36.1X6-
Ceftizoxime	T36.1X1-	T36.1X2-	T36.1X3-	T36.1X4-	T36.1X5-	T36.1X6-
Ceftriaxone	T36.1X1-	T36.1X2-	T36.1X3-	T36.1X4-	T36.1X5-	T36.1X6-
Cefuroxime	T36.1X1-	T36.1X2-	T36.1X3-	T36.1X4-	T36.1X5-	T36.1X6-
Cefuzonam	T36.1X1-	T36.1X2-	T36.1X3-	T36.1X4-	T36.1X5-	T36.1X6-
Celestone	T38.0X1-	T38.0X2-	T38.0X3-	T38.0X4-	T38.0X5-	T38.0X6-
topical	T49.0X1-	T49.0X2-	T49.0X3-	T49.0X4-	T49.0X5-	T49.0X6-
Celiprolol	T44.7X1-	T44.7X2-	T44.7X3-	T44.7X4-	T44.7X5-	T44.7X6-
Cell stimulants and proliferants	T49.8X1-	T49.8X2-	T49.8X3-	T49.8X4-	T49.8X5-	T49.8X6-
Cellosolve	T52.91X-	T52.92X-	T52.93X-	T52.94X-	-	-
Cellulose						
cathartic	T47.4X1-	T47.4X2-	T47.4X3-	T47.4X4-	T47.4X5-	T47.4X6-
hydroxyethyl	T47.4X1-	T47.4X2-	T47.4X3-	T47.4X4-	T47.4X5-	T47.4X6-
nitrates (topical)	T49.3X1-	T49.3X2-	T49.3X3-	T49.3X4-	T49.3X5-	T49.3X6-
oxidized	T49.4X1-	T49.4X2-	T49.4X3-	T49.4X4-	T49.4X5-	T49.4X6-
Centipede (bite)	T63.411-	T63.412-	T63.413-	T63.414-	-	-
Central nervous system						
depressants	T42.71X-	T42.72X-	T42.73X-	T42.74X-	T42.75X-	T42.76X-
anesthetic (general) NEC	T41.201-	T41.202-	T41.203-	T41.204-	T41.205-	T41.206-
gases NEC	T41.0X1-	T41.0X2-	T41.0X3-	T41.0X4-	T41.0X5-	T41.0X6-
intravenous	T41.1X1-	T41.1X2-	T41.1X3-	T41.1X4-	T41.1X5-	T41.1X6-
barbiturates	T42.3X1-	T42.3X2-	T42.3X3-	T42.3X4-	T42.3X5-	T42.3X6-
benzodiazepines	T42.4X1-	T42.4X2-	T42.4X3-	T42.4X4-	T42.4X5-	T42.4X6-
bromides	T42.6X1-	T42.6X2-	T42.6X3-	T42.6X4-	T42.6X5-	T42.6X6-
cannabis sativa	T40.7X1-	T40.7X2-	T40.7X3-	T40.7X4-	T40.7X5-	T40.7X6-
chloral hydrate	T42.6X1-	T42.6X2-	T42.6X3-	T42.6X4-	T42.6X5-	T42.6X6-
ethanol	T51.0X1-	T51.0X2-	T51.0X3-	T51.0X4-	-	-
hallucinogenics	T40.901-	T40.902-	T40.903-	T40.904-	T40.905-	T40.906-
hypnotics	T42.71X-	T42.72X-	T42.73X-	T42.74X-	T42.75X-	T42.76X-
specified NEC	T42.6X1-	T42.6X2-	T42.6X3-	T42.6X4-	T42.6X5-	T42.6X6-
muscle relaxants	T42.8X1-	T42.8X2-	T42.8X3-	T42.8X4-	T42.8X5-	T42.8X6-
paraldehyde	T42.6X1-	T42.6X2-	T42.6X3-	T42.6X4-	T42.6X5-	T42.6X6-
sedatives; sedative-hypnotics	T42.71X-	T42.72X-	T42.73X-	T42.74X-	T42.75X-	T42.76X-
mixed NEC	T42.6X1-	T42.6X2-	T42.6X3-	T42.6X4-	T42.6X5-	T42.6X6-
specified NEC	T42.6X1-	T42.6X2-	T42.6X3-	T42.6X4-	T42.6X5-	T42.6X6-
muscle-tone depressants	T42.8X1-	T42.8X2-	T42.8X3-	T42.8X4-	T42.8X5-	T42.8X6-
stimulants	T43.601-	T43.602-	T43.603-	T43.604-	T43.605-	T43.606-
amphetamines	T43.621-	T43.622-	T43.623-	T43.624-	T43.625-	T43.626-
analeptics	T50.7X1-	T50.7X2-	T50.7X3-	T50.7X4-	T50.7X5-	T50.7X6-
antidepressants	T43.201-	T43.202-	T43.203-	T43.204-	T43.205-	T43.206-
opiate antagonists	T50.7X1-	T50.7X2-	T50.7X3-	T50.7X4-	T50.7X5-	T50.7X6-
specified NEC	T43.691-	T43.692-	T43.693-	T43.694-	T43.695-	T43.696-
Cephalexin	T36.1X1-	T36.1X2-	T36.1X3-	T36.1X4-	T36.1X5-	T36.1X6-
Cephaloglycin	T36.1X1-	T36.1X2-	T36.1X3-	T36.1X4-	T36.1X5-	T36.1X6-
Cephaloridine	T36.1X1-	T36.1X2-	T36.1X3-	T36.1X4-	T36.1X5-	T36.1X6-
Cephalosporins	T36.1X1-	T36.1X2-	T36.1X3-	T36.1X4	T36.1X5	T36.1X6
N (adicillin)	T36.0X1-	T36.0X2-	T36.0X3-	T36.0X4-	T36.0X5-	T36.0X6-
Cephalothin	T36.1X1-	T36.1X2-	T36.1X3-	T36.1X4-	T36.1X5-	T36.1X6-
Cephalotin	T36.1X1-	T36.1X2-	T36.1X3-	T36.1X4-	T36.1X5-	T36.1X6-
Cephradine	T36.1X1-	T36.1X2-	T36.1X3-	T36.1X4-	T36.1X5-	T36.1X6-
Cerbera (odallam)	T62.2X1-	T62.2X2-	T62.2X3-	T62.2X4-	-	-
Cerberin	T46.0X1-	T46.0X2-	T46.0X3-	T46.0X4-	T46.0X5-	T46.0X6-
Cerebral stimulants	T43.601-	T43.602-	T43.603-	T43.604-	T43.605-	T43.606-
psychotherapeutic	T43.601-	T43.602-	T43.603-	T43.604-	T43.605-	T43.606-
specified NEC	T43.691-	T43.692-	T43.693-	T43.694-	T43.695-	T43.696-
Cerium oxalate	T45.0X1-	T45.0X2-	T45.0X3-	T45.0X4-	T45.0X5-	T45.0X6-
Cerous oxalate	T45.0X1-	T45.0X2-	T45.0X3-	T45.0X4-	T45.0X5-	T45.0X6-
Ceruletide	T50.8X1-	T50.8X2-	T50.8X3-	T50.8X4-	T50.8X5-	T50.8X6-
Cetalkonium (chloride)	T49.0X1-	T49.0X2-	T49.0X3-	T49.0X4-	T49.0X5-	T49.0X6-
Cethexonium chloride	T49.0X1-	T49.0X2-	T49.0X3-	T49.0X4-	T49.0X5-	T49.0X6-
Cetiedil	T46.7X1-	T46.7X2-	T46.7X3-	T46.7X4-	T46.7X5-	T46.7X6-
Cetirizine	T45.0X1-	T45.0X2-	T45.0X3-	T45.0X4-	T45.0X5-	T45.0X6-
Cetomacrogol	T50.991-	T50.992-	T50.993-	T50.994-	T50.995-	T50.996-
Cetotiamine	T45.2X1-	T45.2X2-	T45.2X3-	T45.2X4-	T45.2X5-	T45.2X6-
Cetoxime	T45.0X1-	T45.0X2-	T45.0X3-	T45.0X4-	T45.0X5-	T45.0X6-
Cetraxate	T47.1X1-	T47.1X2-	T47.1X3-	T47.1X4-	T47.1X5-	T47.1X6-
Cetrimide	T49.0X1-	T49.0X2-	T49.0X3-	T49.0X4-	T49.0X5-	T49.0X6-
Cetrimonium (bromide)	T49.0X1-	T49.0X2-	T49.0X3-	T49.0X4-	T49.0X5-	T49.0X6-

Substance	Poisoning Accidental (unintentional)	Poisoning Intentional self-harm	Poisoning Assault	Poisoning Undetermined	Adverse effect	Underdosing
Cetylpyridinium chloride	T49.0X1-	T49.0X2-	T49.0X3-	T49.0X4-	T49.0X5-	T49.0X6-
ENT agent	T49.6X1-	T49.6X2-	T49.6X3-	T49.6X4-	T49.6X5-	T49.6X6-
lozenges	T49.6X1-	T49.6X2-	T49.6X3-	T49.6X4-	T49.6X5-	T49.6X6-
Cevadilla — *see* Sabadilla						
Cevitamic acid	T45.2X1-	T45.2X2-	T45.2X3-	T45.2X4-	T45.2X5-	T45.2X6-
Chalk, precipitated	T47.1X1-	T47.1X2-	T47.1X3-	T47.1X4-	T47.1X5-	T47.1X6-
Chamomile	T49.0X1-	T49.0X2-	T49.0X3-	T49.0X4-	T49.0X5-	T49.0X6-
Ch'an su	T46.0X1-	T46.0X2-	T46.0X3-	T46.0X4-	T46.0X5-	T46.0X6-
Charcoal	T47.6X1-	T47.6X2-	T47.6X3-	T47.6X4-	T47.6X5-	T47.6X6-
activated — *see also* Charcoal, medicinal	T47.6X1-	T47.6X2-	T47.6X3-	T47.6X4-	T47.6X5-	T47.6X6-
fumes (Carbon monoxide)	T58.2X1-	T58.2X2-	T58.2X3-	T58.2X4-	-	-
industrial	T58.8X1-	T58.8X2-	T58.8X3-	T58.8X4-	-	-
medicinal (activated)	T47.6X1-	T47.6X2-	T47.6X3-	T47.6X4-	T47.6X5-	T47.6X6-
antidiarrheal	T47.6X1-	T47.6X2-	T47.6X3-	T47.6X4-	T47.6X5-	T47.6X6-
poison control	T47.8X1-	T47.8X2-	T47.8X3-	T47.8X4-	T47.8X5-	T47.8X6-
specified use other than for diarrhea	T47.8X1-	T47.8X2-	T47.8X3-	T47.8X4-	T47.8X5-	T47.8X6-
topical	T49.8X1-	T49.8X2-	T49.8X3-	T49.8X4-	T49.8X5-	T49.8X6-
Chaulmosulfone	T37.1X1-	T37.1X2-	T37.1X3-	T37.1X4-	T37.1X5-	T37.1X6-
Chelating agent NEC	T50.6X1-	T50.6X2-	T50.6X3-	T50.6X4-	T50.6X5-	T50.6X6-
Chelidonium majus	T62.2X1-	T62.2X2-	T62.2X3-	T62.2X4-	-	-
Chemical substance NEC	T65.91X-	T65.92X-	T65.93X-	T65.94X-	-	-
Chenodeoxycholic acid	T47.5X1-	T47.5X2-	T47.5X3-	T47.5X4-	T47.5X5-	T47.5X6-
Chenodiol	T47.5X1-	T47.5X2-	T47.5X3-	T47.5X4-	T47.5X5-	T47.5X6-
Chenopodium	T37.4X1-	T37.4X2-	T37.4X3-	T37.4X4-	T37.4X5-	T37.4X6-
Cherry laurel	T62.2X1-	T62.2X2-	T62.2X3-	T62.2X4-	-	-
Chinidin (e)	T46.2X1-	T46.2X2-	T46.2X3-	T46.2X4-	T46.2X5-	T46.2X6-
Chiniofon	T37.8X1-	T37.8X2-	T37.8X3-	T37.8X4-	T37.8X5-	T37.8X6-
Chlophedianol	T48.3X1-	T48.3X2-	T48.3X3-	T48.3X4-	T48.3X5-	T48.3X6-
Chloral	T42.6X1-	T42.6X2-	T42.6X3-	T42.6X4-	T42.6X5-	T42.6X6-
derivative	T42.6X1-	T42.6X2-	T42.6X3-	T42.6X4-	T42.6X5-	T42.6X6-
hydrate	T42.6X1-	T42.6X2-	T42.6X3-	T42.6X4-	T42.6X5-	T42.6X6-
Chloralamide	T42.6X1-	T42.6X2-	T42.6X3-	T42.6X4-	T42.6X5-	T42.6X6-
Chloralodol	T42.6X1-	T42.6X2-	T42.6X3-	T42.6X4-	T42.6X5-	T42.6X6-
Chloralose	T60.4X1-	T60.4X2-	T60.4X3-	T60.4X4-	-	-
Chlorambucil	T45.1X1-	T45.1X2-	T45.1X3-	T45.1X4-	T45.1X5-	T45.1X6-
Chloramine	T57.8X1-	T57.8X2-	T57.8X3-	T57.8X4-	-	-
T	T49.0X1-	T49.0X2-	T49.0X3-	T49.0X4-	T49.0X5-	T49.0X6-
topical	T49.0X1-	T49.0X2-	T49.0X3-	T49.0X4-	T49.0X5-	T49.0X6-
Chloramphenicol	T36.2X1-	T36.2X2-	T36.2X3-	T36.2X4-	T36.2X5-	T36.2X6-
ENT agent	T49.6X1-	T49.6X2-	T49.6X3-	T49.6X4-	T49.6X5-	T49.6X6-
ophthalmic preparation	T49.5X1-	T49.5X2-	T49.5X3-	T49.5X4-	T49.5X5-	T49.5X6-
topical NEC	T49.0X1-	T49.0X2-	T49.0X3-	T49.0X4-	T49.0X5-	T49.0X6-
Chlorate (potassium) (sodium) **NEC**	T60.3X1-	T60.3X2-	T60.3X3-	T60.3X4-	-	-
herbicide	T60.3X1-	T60.3X2-	T60.3X3-	T60.3X4-	-	-
Chlorazanil	T50.2X1-	T50.2X2-	T50.2X3-	T50.2X4-	T50.2X5-	T50.2X6-
Chlorbenzene, chlorbenzol	T53.7X1-	T53.7X2-	T53.7X3-	T53.7X4-	-	-
Chlorbenzoxamine	T44.3X1-	T44.3X2-	T44.3X3-	T44.3X4-	T44.3X5-	T44.3X6-
Chlorbutol	T42.6X1-	T42.6X2-	T42.6X3-	T42.6X4-	T42.6X5-	T42.6X6-
Chlorcyclizine	T45.0X1-	T45.0X2-	T45.0X3-	T45.0X4-	T45.0X5-	T45.0X6-
Chlordan (e) (dust)	T60.1X1-	T60.1X2-	T60.1X3-	T60.1X4-	-	-
Chlordantoin	T49.0X1-	T49.0X2-	T49.0X3-	T49.0X4-	T49.0X5-	T49.0X6-
Chlordiazepoxide	T42.4X1-	T42.4X2-	T42.4X3-	T42.4X4-	T42.4X5-	T42.4X6-
Chlordiethyl benzamide	T49.3X1-	T49.3X2-	T49.3X3-	T49.3X4-	T49.3X5-	T49.3X6-
Chloresium	T49.8X1-	T49.8X2-	T49.8X3-	T49.8X4-	T49.8X5-	T49.8X6-
Chlorethiazol	T42.6X1-	T42.6X2-	T42.6X3-	T42.6X4-	T42.6X5-	T42.6X6-
Chlorethyl — *see* Ethyl chloride						
Chloretone	T42.6X1-	T42.6X2-	T42.6X3-	T42.6X4-	T42.6X5-	T42.6X6-
Chlorex	T53.6X1-	T53.6X2-	T53.6X3-	T53.6X4-	-	-
insecticide	T60.1X1-	T60.1X2-	T60.1X3-	T60.1X4-	-	-
Chlorfenvinphos	T60.0X1-	T60.0X2-	T60.0X3-	T60.0X4-	-	-
Chlorhexadol	T42.6X1-	T42.6X2-	T42.6X3-	T42.6X4-	T42.6X5-	T42.6X6-
Chlorhexamide	T45.1X1-	T45.1X2-	T45.1X3-	T45.1X4-	T45.1X5-	T45.1X6-
Chlorhexidine	T49.0X1-	T49.0X2-	T49.0X3-	T49.0X4-	T49.0X5-	T49.0X6-
Chlorhydroxyquinolin	T49.0X1-	T49.0X2-	T49.0X3-	T49.0X4-	T49.0X5-	T49.0X6-
Chloride of lime (bleach)	T54.3X1-	T54.3X2-	T54.3X3-	T54.3X4-	-	-
Chlorimipramine	T43.011-	T43.012-	T43.013-	T43.014-	T43.015-	T43.016-
Chlorinated						
camphene	T53.6X1-	T53.6X2-	T53.6X3-	T53.6X4-	-	-
diphenyl	T53.7X1-	T53.7X2-	T53.7X3-	T53.7X4-	-	-
hydrocarbons NEC	T53.91X-	T53.92X-	T53.93X-	T53.94X-	-	-
solvents	T53.91X-	T53.92X-	T53.93X-	T53.94X-	-	-
lime (bleach)	T54.3X1-	T54.3X2-	T54.3X3-	T54.3X4-	-	-
and boric acid solution	T49.0X1-	T49.0X2-	T49.0X3-	T49.0X4-	T49.0X5-	T49.0X6-
naphthalene (insecticide)	T60.1X1-	T60.1X2-	T60.1X3-	T60.1X4-	-	-
industrial (non-pesticide)	T53.7X1-	T53.7X2-	T53.7X3-	T53.7X4-	-	-

Substance	Poisoning Accidental (unintentional)	Poisoning Intentional self-harm	Poisoning Assault	Poisoning Undetermined	Adverse effect	Underdosing
Chlorinated *- continued*						
pesticide NEC	T60.8X1-	T60.8X2-	T60.8X3-	T60.8X4-	-	-
soda — *see also* sodium hypochlorite						
solution	T49.0X1-	T49.0X2-	T49.0X3-	T49.0X4-	T49.0X5-	T49.0X6-
Chlorine (fumes) (gas)	T59.4X1-	T59.4X2-	T59.4X3-	T59.4X4-	-	-
bleach	T54.3X1-	T54.3X2-	T54.3X3-	T54.3X4-	-	-
compound gas NEC	T59.4X1-	T59.4X2-	T59.4X3-	T59.4X4-	-	-
disinfectant	T59.4X1-	T59.4X2-	T59.4X3-	T59.4X4-	-	-
releasing agents NEC	T59.4X1-	T59.4X2-	T59.4X3-	T59.4X4-	-	-
Chlorisondamine chloride	T46.991-	T46.992-	T46.993-	T46.994-	T46.995-	T46.996-
Chlormadinone	T38.5X1-	T38.5X2-	T38.5X3-	T38.5X4-	T38.5X5-	T38.5X6-
Chlormephos	T60.0X1-	T60.0X2-	T60.0X3-	T60.0X4-	-	-
Chlormerodrin	T50.2X1-	T50.2X2-	T50.2X3-	T50.2X4-	T50.2X5-	T50.2X6-
Chlormethiazole	T42.6X1-	T42.6X2-	T42.6X3-	T42.6X4-	T42.6X5-	T42.6X6-
Chlormethine	T45.1X1-	T45.1X2-	T45.1X3-	T45.1X4-	T45.1X5-	T45.1X6-
Chlormethylenecycline	T36.4X1-	T36.4X2-	T36.4X3-	T36.4X4-	T36.4X5-	T36.4X6-
Chlormezanone	T42.6X1-	T42.6X2-	T42.6X3-	T42.6X4-	T42.6X5-	T42.6X6-
Chloroacetic acid	T60.3X1-	T60.3X2-	T60.3X3-	T60.3X4-	-	-
Chloroacetone	T59.3X1-	T59.3X2-	T59.3X3-	T59.3X4-	-	-
Chloroacetophenone	T59.3X1-	T59.3X2-	T59.3X3-	T59.3X4-	-	-
Chloroaniline	T53.7X1-	T53.7X2-	T53.7X3-	T53.7X4-	-	-
Chlorobenzene, chlorobenzol	T53.7X1-	T53.7X2-	T53.7X3-	T53.7X4-	-	-
Chlorobromomethane (fire extinguisher)	T53.6X1-	T53.6X2-	T53.6X3-	T53.6X4-	-	-
Chlorobutanol	T49.0X1-	T49.0X2-	T49.0X3-	T49.0X4-	T49.0X5-	T49.0X6-
Chlorocresol	T49.0X1-	T49.0X2-	T49.0X3-	T49.0X4-	T49.0X5-	T49.0X6-
Chlorodehydro-methyltestosterone	T38.7X1-	T38.7X2-	T38.7X3-	T38.7X4-	T38.7X5-	T38.7X6-
Chlorodinitrobenzene	T53.7X1-	T53.7X2-	T53.7X3-	T53.7X4-	-	-
dust or vapor	T53.7X1-	T53.7X2-	T53.7X3-	T53.7X4-	-	-
Chlorodiphenyl	T53.7X1-	T53.7X2-	T53.7X3-	T53.7X4-	-	-
Chloroethane — *see* Ethyl chloride						
Chloroethylene	T53.6X1-	T53.6X2-	T53.6X3-	T53.6X4-	-	-
Chlorofluorocarbons	T53.5X1-	T53.5X2-	T53.5X3-	T53.5X4-	-	-
Chloroform (fumes) (vapor)	T53.1X1-	T53.1X2-	T53.1X3-	T53.1X4-	-	-
anesthetic	T41.0X1-	T41.0X2-	T41.0X3-	T41.0X4-	T41.0X5-	T41.0X6-
solvent	T53.1X1-	T53.1X2-	T53.1X3-	T53.1X4-	-	-
water, concentrated	T41.0X1-	T41.0X2-	T41.0X3-	T41.0X4-	T41.0X5-	T41.0X6-
Chloroguanide	T37.2X1-	T37.2X2-	T37.2X3-	T37.2X4-	T37.2X5-	T37.2X6-
Chloromycetin	T36.2X1-	T36.2X2-	T36.2X3-	T36.2X4-	T36.2X5-	T36.2X6-
ENT agent	T49.6X1-	T49.6X2-	T49.6X3-	T49.6X4-	T49.6X5-	T49.6X6-
ophthalmic preparation	T49.5X1-	T49.5X2-	T49.5X3-	T49.5X4-	T49.5X5-	T49.5X6-
otic solution	T49.6X1-	T49.6X2-	T49.6X3-	T49.6X4-	T49.6X5-	T49.6X6-
topical NEC	T49.0X1-	T49.0X2-	T49.0X3-	T49.0X4-	T49.0X5-	T49.0X6-
Chloronitrobenzene	T53.7X1-	T53.7X2-	T53.7X3-	T53.7X4-	-	-
dust or vapor	T53.7X1-	T53.7X2-	T53.7X3-	T53.7X4-	-	-
Chlorophacinone	T60.4X1-	T60.4X2-	T60.4X3-	T60.4X4-	-	-
Chlorophenol	T53.7X1-	T53.7X2-	T53.7X3-	T53.7X4-	-	-
Chlorophenothane	T60.1X1-	T60.1X2-	T60.1X3-	T60.1X4-	-	-
Chlorophyll	T50.991-	T50.992-	T50.993-	T50.994-	T50.995-	T50.996-
Chloropicrin (fumes)	T53.6X1-	T53.6X2-	T53.6X3-	T53.6X4-	-	-
fumigant	T60.8X1-	T60.8X2-	T60.8X3-	T60.8X4-	-	-
fungicide	T60.3X1-	T60.3X2-	T60.3X3-	T60.3X4-	-	-
pesticide	T60.8X1-	T60.8X2-	T60.8X3-	T60.8X4-	-	-
Chloroprocaine	T41.3X1-	T41.3X2-	T41.3X3-	T41.3X4-	T41.3X5-	T41.3X6-
infiltration (subcutaneous)	T41.3X1-	T41.3X2-	T41.3X3-	T41.3X4-	T41.3X5-	T41.3X6-
nerve block (peripheral) (plexus)	T41.3X1-	T41.3X2-	T41.3X3-	T41.3X4-	T41.3X5-	T41.3X6-
spinal	T41.3X1-	T41.3X2-	T41.3X3-	T41.3X4-	T41.3X5-	T41.3X6-
Chloroptic	T49.5X1-	T49.5X2-	T49.5X3-	T49.5X4-	T49.5X5-	T49.5X6-
Chloropurine	T45.1X1-	T45.1X2-	T45.1X3-	T45.1X4-	T45.1X5-	T45.1X6-
Chloropyramine	T45.0X1-	T45.0X2-	T45.0X3-	T45.0X4-	T45.0X5-	T45.0X6-
Chloropyrifos	T60.0X1-	T60.0X2-	T60.0X3-	T60.0X4-	-	-
Chloropyrilene	T45.0X1-	T45.0X2-	T45.0X3-	T45.0X4-	T45.0X5-	T45.0X6-
Chloroquine	T37.2X1-	T37.2X2-	T37.2X3-	T37.2X4-	T37.2X5-	T37.2X6-
Chlorothalonil	T60.3X1-	T60.3X2-	T60.3X3-	T60.3X4-	-	-
Chlorothen	T45.0X1-	T45.0X2-	T45.0X3-	T45.0X4-	T45.0X5-	T45.0X6-
Chlorothiazide	T50.2X1-	T50.2X2-	T50.2X3-	T50.2X4-	T50.2X5-	T50.2X6-
Chlorothymol	T49.4X1-	T49.4X2-	T49.4X3-	T49.4X4-	T49.4X5-	T49.4X6-
Chlorotrianisene	T38.5X1-	T38.5X2-	T38.5X3-	T38.5X4-	T38.5X5-	T38.5X6-
Chlorovinyldichloro-arsine, not in war	T57.0X1-	T57.0X2-	T57.0X3-	T57.0X4-	-	-
Chloroxine	T49.4X1-	T49.4X2-	T49.4X3-	T49.4X4-	T49.4X5-	T49.4X6-
Chloroxylenol	T49.0X1-	T49.0X2-	T49.0X3-	T49.0X4-	T49.0X5-	T49.0X6-
Chlorphenamine	T45.0X1-	T45.0X2-	T45.0X3-	T45.0X4-	T45.0X5-	T45.0X6-
Chlorphenesin	T42.8X1-	T42.8X2-	T42.8X3-	T42.8X4-	T42.8X5-	T42.8X6-
topical (antifungal)	T49.0X1-	T49.0X2-	T49.0X3-	T49.0X4-	T49.0X5-	T49.0X6-

Substance	Poisoning Accidental (unintentional)	Poisoning Intentional self-harm	Poisoning Assault	Poisoning Undetermined	Adverse effect	Underdosing
Chlorpheniramine	T45.0X1-	T45.0X2-	T45.0X3-	T45.0X4-	T45.0X5-	T45.0X6-
Chlorphenoxamine	T45.0X1-	T45.0X2-	T45.0X3-	T45.0X4-	T45.0X5-	T45.0X6-
Chlorphentermine	T50.5X1-	T50.5X2-	T50.5X3-	T50.5X4-	T50.5X5-	T50.5X6-
Chlorprocaine — *see* Chloroprocaine						
Chlorproguanil	T37.2X1-	T37.2X2-	T37.2X3-	T37.2X4-	T37.2X5-	T37.2X6-
Chlorpromazine	T43.3X1-	T43.3X2-	T43.3X3-	T43.3X4-	T43.3X5-	T43.3X6-
Chlorpropamide	T38.3X1-	T38.3X2-	T38.3X3-	T38.3X4-	T38.3X5-	T38.3X6-
Chlorprothixene	T43.4X1-	T43.4X2-	T43.4X3-	T43.4X4-	T43.4X5-	T43.4X6-
Chlorquinaldol	T49.0X1-	T49.0X2-	T49.0X3-	T49.0X4-	T49.0X5-	T49.0X6-
Chlorquinol	T49.0X1-	T49.0X2-	T49.0X3-	T49.0X4-	T49.0X5-	T49.0X6-
Chlortalidone	T50.2X1-	T50.2X2-	T50.2X3-	T50.2X4-	T50.2X5-	T50.2X6-
Chlortetracycline	T36.4X1-	T36.4X2-	T36.4X3-	T36.4X4-	T36.4X5-	T36.4X6-
Chlorthalidone	T50.2X1-	T50.2X2-	T50.2X3-	T50.2X4-	T50.2X5-	T50.2X6-
Chlorthiophos	T60.0X1-	T60.0X2-	T60.0X3-	T60.0X4-	-	-
Chlortrianisene	T38.5X1-	T38.5X2-	T38.5X3-	T38.5X4-	T38.5X5-	T38.5X6-
Chlor-Trimeton	T45.0X1-	T45.0X2-	T45.0X3-	T45.0X4-	T45.0X5-	T45.0X6-
Chlorthion	T60.0X1-	T60.0X2-	T60.0X3-	T60.0X4-	-	-
Chlorzoxazone	T42.8X1-	T42.8X2-	T42.8X3-	T42.8X4-	T42.8X5-	T42.8X6-
Choke damp	T59.7X1-	T59.7X2-	T59.7X3-	T59.7X4-	-	-
Cholagogues	T47.5X1-	T47.5X2-	T47.5X3-	T47.5X4-	T47.5X5-	T47.5X6-
Cholebrine	T50.8X1-	T50.8X2-	T50.8X3-	T50.8X4-	T50.8X5-	T50.8X6-
Cholecalciferol	T45.2X1-	T45.2X2-	T45.2X3-	T45.2X4-	T45.2X5-	T45.2X6-
Cholecystokinin	T50.8X1-	T50.8X2-	T50.8X3-	T50.8X4-	T50.8X5-	T50.8X6-
Cholera vaccine	T50.A91-	T50.A92-	T50.A93-	T50.A94-	T50.A95-	T50.A96-
Choleretic	T47.5X1-	T47.5X2-	T47.5X3-	T47.5X4-	T47.5X5-	T47.5X6-
Cholesterol-lowering agents	T46.6X1-	T46.6X2-	T46.6X3-	T46.6X4-	T46.6X5-	T46.6X6-
Cholestyramine (resin)	T46.6X1-	T46.6X2-	T46.6X3-	T46.6X4-	T46.6X5-	T46.6X6-
Cholic acid	T47.5X1-	T47.5X2-	T47.5X3-	T47.5X4-	T47.5X5-	T47.5X6-
Choline	T48.6X1-	T48.6X2-	T48.6X3-	T48.6X4-	T48.6X5-	T48.6X6-
chloride	T50.991-	T50.992-	T50.993-	T50.994-	T50.995-	T50.996-
dihydrogen citrate	T50.991-	T50.992-	T50.993-	T50.994-	T50.995-	T50.996-
salicylate	T39.091-	T39.092-	T39.093-	T39.094-	T39.095-	T39.096-
theophyllinate	T48.6X1-	T48.6X2-	T48.6X3-	T48.6X4-	T48.6X5-	T48.6X6-
Cholinergic (drug) **NEC**	T44.1X1-	T44.1X2-	T44.1X3-	T44.1X4-	T44.1X5-	T44.1X6-
muscle tone enhancer	T44.1X1-	T44.1X2-	T44.1X3-	T44.1X4-	T44.1X5-	T44.1X6-
organophosphorus	T44.0X1-	T44.0X2-	T44.0X3-	T44.0X4-	T44.0X5-	T44.0X6-
insecticide	T60.0X1-	T60.0X2-	T60.0X3-	T60.0X4-	-	-
nerve gas	T59.891-	T59.892-	T59.893-	T59.894-	-	-
trimethyl ammonium propanediol	T44.1X1-	T44.1X2-	T44.1X3-	T44.1X4-	T44.1X5-	T44.1X6-
Cholinesterase reactivator	T50.6X1-	T50.6X2-	T50.6X3-	T50.6X4-	T50.6X5-	T50.6X6-
Cholografin	T50.8X1-	T50.8X2-	T50.8X3-	T50.8X4-	T50.8X5-	T50.8X6-
Chorionic gonadotropin	T38.891-	T38.892-	T38.893-	T38.894-	T38.895-	T38.896-
Chromate	T56.2X1-	T56.2X2-	T56.2X3-	T56.2X4-	-	-
dust or mist	T56.2X1-	T56.2X2-	T56.2X3-	T56.2X4-	-	-
lead — *see also* lead	T56.0X1-	T56.0X2-	T56.0X3-	T56.0X4-	-	-
paint	T56.0X1-	T56.0X2-	T56.0X3-	T56.0X4-	-	-
Chromic						
acid	T56.2X1-	T56.2X2-	T56.2X3-	T56.2X4-	-	-
dust or mist	T56.2X1-	T56.2X2-	T56.2X3-	T56.2X4-	-	-
phosphate 32P	T45.1X1-	T45.1X2-	T45.1X3-	T45.1X4-	T45.1X5-	T45.1X6-
Chromium	T56.2X1-	T56.2X2-	T56.2X3-	T56.2X4-	-	-
compounds — *see* Chromate						
sesquioxide	T50.8X1-	T50.8X2-	T50.8X3-	T50.8X4-	T50.8X5-	T50.8X6-
Chromomycin A3	T45.1X1-	T45.1X2-	T45.1X3-	T45.1X4-	T45.1X5-	T45.1X6-
Chromonar	T46.3X1-	T46.3X2-	T46.3X3-	T46.3X4-	T46.3X5-	T46.3X6-
Chromyl chloride	T56.2X1-	T56.2X2-	T56.2X3-	T56.2X4-	-	-
Chrysarobin	T49.4X1-	T49.4X2-	T49.4X3-	T49.4X4-	T49.4X5-	T49.4X6-
Chrysazin	T47.2X1-	T47.2X2-	T47.2X3-	T47.2X4-	T47.2X5-	T47.2X6-
Chymar	T45.3X1-	T45.3X2-	T45.3X3-	T45.3X4-	T45.3X5-	T45.3X6-
ophthalmic preparation	T49.5X1-	T49.5X2-	T49.5X3-	T49.5X4-	T49.5X5-	T49.5X6-
Chymopapain	T45.3X1-	T45.3X2-	T45.3X3-	T45.3X4-	T45.3X5-	T45.3X6-
Chymotrypsin	T45.3X1-	T45.3X2-	T45.3X3-	T45.3X4-	T45.3X5-	T45.3X6-
ophthalmic preparation	T49.5X1-	T49.5X2-	T49.5X3-	T49.5X4-	T49.5X5-	T49.5X6-
Cianidanol	T50.991-	T50.992-	T50.993-	T50.994-	T50.995-	T50.996-
Cianopramine	T43.011-	T43.012-	T43.013-	T43.014-	T43.015-	T43.016-
Cibenzoline	T46.2X1-	T46.2X2-	T46.2X3-	T46.2X4-	T46.2X5-	T46.2X6-
Ciclacillin	T36.0X1-	T36.0X2-	T36.0X3-	T36.0X4-	T36.0X5-	T36.0X6-
Ciclobarbital — *see* Hexobarbital						
Ciclonicate	T46.7X1-	T46.7X2-	T46.7X3-	T46.7X4-	T46.7X5-	T46.7X6-
Ciclopirox (olamine)	T49.0X1-	T49.0X2-	T49.0X3-	T49.0X4-	T49.0X5-	T49.0X6-
Ciclosporin	T45.1X1-	T45.1X2-	T45.1X3-	T45.1X4-	T45.1X5-	T45.1X6-
Cicuta maculata or virosa	T62.2X1-	T62.2X2-	T62.2X3-	T62.2X4-	-	-
Cicutoxin	T62.2X1-	T62.2X2-	T62.2X3-	T62.2X4-	-	-
Cigarette lighter fluid	T52.0X1-	T52.0X2-	T52.0X3-	T52.0X4-	-	-
Cigarettes (tobacco)	T65.221-	T65.222-	T65.223-	T65.224-	-	-

Substance	Poisoning Accidental (unintentional)	Poisoning Intentional self-harm	Poisoning Assault	Poisoning Undetermined	Adverse effect	Underdosing
Ciguatoxin	T61.01X-	T61.02X-	T61.03X-	T61.04X-	-	-
Cilazapril	T46.4X1-	T46.4X2-	T46.4X3-	T46.4X4-	T46.4X5-	T46.4X6-
Cimetidine	T47.0X1-	T47.0X2-	T47.0X3-	T47.0X4-	T47.0X5-	T47.0X6-
Cimetropium bromide	T44.3X1-	T44.3X2-	T44.3X3-	T44.3X4-	T44.3X5-	T44.3X6-
Cinchocaine	T41.3X1-	T41.3X2-	T41.3X3-	T41.3X4-	T41.3X5-	T41.3X6-
topical (surface)	T41.3X1-	T41.3X2-	T41.3X3-	T41.3X4-	T41.3X5-	T41.3X6-
Cinchona	T37.2X1-	T37.2X2-	T37.2X3-	T37.2X4-	T37.2X5-	T37.2X6-
Cinchonine alkaloids	T37.2X1-	T37.2X2-	T37.2X3-	T37.2X4-	T37.2X5-	T37.2X6-
Cinchophen	T50.4X1-	T50.4X2-	T50.4X3-	T50.4X4-	T50.4X5-	T50.4X6-
Cinepazide	T46.7X1-	T46.7X2-	T46.7X3-	T46.7X4-	T46.7X5-	T46.7X6-
Cinnamedrine	T48.5X1-	T48.5X2-	T48.5X3-	T48.5X4-	T48.5X5-	T48.5X6-
Cinnarizine	T45.0X1-	T45.0X2-	T45.0X3-	T45.0X4-	T45.0X5-	T45.0X6-
Cinoxacin	T37.8X1-	T37.8X2-	T37.8X3-	T37.8X4-	T37.8X5-	T37.8X6-
Ciprofibrate	T46.6X1-	T46.6X2-	T46.6X3-	T46.6X4-	T46.6X5-	T46.6X6-
Ciprofloxacin	T36.8X1-	T36.8X2-	T36.8X3-	T36.8X4-	T36.8X5-	T36.8X6-
Cisapride	T47.8X1-	T47.8X2-	T47.8X3-	T47.8X4-	T47.8X5-	T47.8X6-
Cisplatin	T45.1X1-	T45.1X2-	T45.1X3-	T45.1X4-	T45.1X5-	T45.1X6-
Citalopram	T43.221-	T43.222-	T43.223-	T43.224-	T43.225-	T43.226-
Citanest	T41.3X1-	T41.3X2-	T41.3X3-	T41.3X4-	T41.3X5-	T41.3X6-
infiltration (subcutaneous)	T41.3X1-	T41.3X2-	T41.3X3-	T41.3X4-	T41.3X5-	T41.3X6-
nerve block (peripheral) (plexus)	T41.3X1-	T41.3X2-	T41.3X3-	T41.3X4-	T41.3X5-	T41.3X6-
Citric acid	T47.5X1-	T47.5X2-	T47.5X3-	T47.5X4-	T47.5X5-	T47.5X6-
Citrovorum (factor)	T45.8X1-	T45.8X2-	T45.8X3-	T45.8X4-	T45.8X5-	T45.8X6-
Claviceps purpurea	T62.2X1-	T62.2X2-	T62.2X3-	T62.2X4-	-	-
Clavulanic acid	T36.1X1-	T36.1X2-	T36.1X3-	T36.1X4-	T36.1X5-	T36.1X6-
Cleaner, cleansing agent, type not specified	T65.891-	T65.892-	T65.893-	T65.894-	-	-
of paint or varnish	T52.91X-	T52.92X-	T52.93X-	T52.94X-	-	-
specified type NEC	T65.891-	T65.892-	T65.893-	T65.894-	-	-
Clebopride	T47.8X1-	T47.8X2-	T47.8X3-	T47.8X4-	T47.8X5-	T47.8X6-
Clefamide	T37.3X1-	T37.3X2-	T37.3X3-	T37.3X4-	T37.3X5-	T37.3X6-
Clemastine	T45.0X1-	T45.0X2-	T45.0X3-	T45.0X4-	T45.0X5-	T45.0X6-
Clematis vitalba	T62.2X1-	T62.2X2-	T62.2X3-	T62.2X4-	-	-
Clemizole	T45.0X1-	T45.0X2-	T45.0X3-	T45.0X4-	T45.0X5-	T45.0X6-
penicillin	T36.0X1-	T36.0X2-	T36.0X3-	T36.0X4-	T36.0X5-	T36.0X6-
Clenbuterol	T48.6X1-	T48.6X2-	T48.6X3-	T48.6X4-	T48.6X5-	T48.6X6-
Clidinium bromide	T44.3X1-	T44.3X2-	T44.3X3-	T44.3X4-	T44.3X5-	T44.3X6-
Clindamycin	T36.8X1-	T36.8X2-	T36.8X3-	T36.8X4-	T36.8X5-	T36.8X6-
Clinofibrate	T46.6X1-	T46.6X2-	T46.6X3-	T46.6X4-	T46.6X5-	T46.6X6-
Clioquinol	T37.8X1-	T37.8X2-	T37.8X3-	T37.8X4-	T37.8X5-	T37.8X6-
Cliradon	T40.2X1-	T40.2X2-	T40.2X3-	T40.2X4-	-	-
Clobazam	T42.4X1-	T42.4X2-	T42.4X3-	T42.4X4-	T42.4X5-	T42.4X6-
Clobenzorex	T50.5X1-	T50.5X2-	T50.5X3-	T50.5X4-	T50.5X5-	T50.5X6-
Clobetasol	T49.0X1-	T49.0X2-	T49.0X3-	T49.0X4-	T49.0X5-	T49.0X6-
Clobetasone	T49.0X1-	T49.0X2-	T49.0X3-	T49.0X4-	T49.0X5-	T49.0X6-
Clobutinol	T48.3X1-	T48.3X2-	T48.3X3-	T48.3X4-	T48.3X5-	T48.3X6-
Clocortolone	T38.0X1-	T38.0X2-	T38.0X3-	T38.0X4-	T38.0X5-	T38.0X6-
Clodantoin	T49.0X1-	T49.0X2-	T49.0X3-	T49.0X4-	T49.0X5-	T49.0X6-
Clodronic acid	T50.991-	T50.992-	T50.993-	T50.994-	T50.995-	T50.996-
Clofazimine	T37.1X1-	T37.1X2-	T37.1X3-	T37.1X4-	T37.1X5-	T37.1X6-
Clofedanol	T48.3X1-	T48.3X2-	T48.3X3-	T48.3X4-	T48.3X5-	T48.3X6-
Clofenamide	T50.2X1-	T50.2X2-	T50.2X3-	T50.2X4-	T50.2X5-	T50.2X6-
Clofenotane	T49.0X1-	T49.0X2-	T49.0X3-	T49.0X4-	T49.0X5-	T49.0X6-
Clofezone	T39.2X1-	T39.2X2-	T39.2X3-	T39.2X4-	T39.2X5-	T39.2X6-
Clofibrate	T46.6X1-	T46.6X2-	T46.6X3-	T46.6X4-	T46.6X5-	T46.6X6-
Clofibride	T46.6X1-	T46.6X2-	T46.6X3-	T46.6X4-	T46.6X5-	T46.6X6-
Cloforex	T50.5X1-	T50.5X2-	T50.5X3-	T50.5X4-	T50.5X5-	T50.5X6-
Clomethiazole	T42.6X1-	T42.6X2-	T42.6X3-	T42.6X4-	T42.6X5-	T42.6X6-
Clometocillin	T36.0X1-	T36.0X2-	T36.0X3-	T36.0X4-	T36.0X5-	T36.0X6-
Clomifene	T38.5X1-	T38.5X2-	T38.5X3-	T38.5X4-	T38.5X5-	T38.5X6-
Clomiphene	T38.5X1-	T38.5X2-	T38.5X3-	T38.5X4-	T38.5X5-	T38.5X6-
Clomipramine	T43.011-	T43.012-	T43.013-	T43.014-	T43.015-	T43.016-
Clomocycline	T36.4X1-	T36.4X2-	T36.4X3-	T36.4X4-	T36.4X5-	T36.4X6-
Clonazepam	T42.4X1-	T42.4X2-	T42.4X3-	T42.4X4-	T42.4X5-	T42.4X6-
Clonidine	T46.5X1-	T46.5X2-	T46.5X3-	T46.5X4-	T46.5X5-	T46.5X6-
Clonixin	T39.8X1-	T39.8X2-	T39.8X3-	T39.8X4-	T39.8X5-	T39.8X6-
Clopamide	T50.2X1-	T50.2X2-	T50.2X3-	T50.2X4-	T50.2X5-	T50.2X6-
Clopenthixol	T43.4X1-	T43.4X2-	T43.4X3-	T43.4X4-	T43.4X5-	T43.4X6-
Cloperastine	T48.3X1-	T48.3X2-	T48.3X3-	T48.3X4-	T48.3X5-	T48.3X6-
Clophedianol	T48.3X1-	T48.3X2-	T48.3X3-	T48.3X4-	T48.3X5-	T48.3X6-
Cloponone	T36.2X1-	T36.2X2-	T36.2X3-	T36.2X4-	T36.2X5-	T36.2X6-
Cloprednol	T38.0X1-	T38.0X2-	T38.0X3-	T38.0X4-	T38.0X5-	T38.0X6-
Cloral betaine	T42.6X1-	T42.6X2-	T42.6X3-	T42.6X4-	T42.6X5-	T42.6X6-
Cloramfenicol	T36.2X1-	T36.2X2-	T36.2X3-	T36.2X4-	T36.2X5-	T36.2X6-
Clorazepate (dipotassium)	T42.4X1-	T42.4X2-	T42.4X3-	T42.4X4-	T42.4X5-	T42.4X6-
Clorexolone	T50.2X1-	T50.2X2-	T50.2X3-	T50.2X4-	T50.2X5-	T50.2X6-
Clorfenamine	T45.0X1-	T45.0X2-	T45.0X3-	T45.0X4-	T45.0X5-	T45.0X6-

Substance	Poisoning Accidental (unintentional)	Poisoning Intentional self-harm	Poisoning Assault	Poisoning Undetermined	Adverse effect	Underdosing
Clorgiline	T43.1X1-	T43.1X2-	T43.1X3-	T43.1X4-	T43.1X5-	T43.1X6-
Clorotepine	T44.3X1-	T44.3X2-	T44.3X3-	T44.3X4-	T44.3X5-	T44.3X6-
Clorox (bleach)	T54.91X-	T54.92X-	T54.93X-	T54.94X-	-	-
Clorprenaline	T48.6X1-	T48.6X2-	T48.6X3-	T48.6X4-	T48.6X5-	T48.6X6-
Clortermine	T50.5X1-	T50.5X2-	T50.5X3-	T50.5X4-	T50.5X5-	T50.5X6-
Clotiapine	T43.591-	T43.592-	T43.593-	T43.594-	T43.595-	T43.596-
Clotiazepam	T42.4X1-	T42.4X2-	T42.4X3-	T42.4X4-	T42.4X5-	T42.4X6-
Clotibric acid	T46.6X1-	T46.6X2-	T46.6X3-	T46.6X4-	T46.6X5-	T46.6X6-
Clotrimazole	T49.0X1-	T49.0X2-	T49.0X3-	T49.0X4-	T49.0X5-	T49.0X6-
Cloxacillin	T36.0X1-	T36.0X2-	T36.0X3-	T36.0X4-	T36.0X5-	T36.0X6-
Cloxazolam	T42.4X1-	T42.4X2-	T42.4X3-	T42.4X4-	T42.4X5-	T42.4X6-
Cloxiquine	T49.0X1-	T49.0X2-	T49.0X3-	T49.0X4-	T49.0X5-	T49.0X6-
Clozapine	T42.4X1-	T42.4X2-	T42.4X3-	T42.4X4-	T42.4X5-	T42.4X6-
Coagulant NEC	T45.7X1-	T45.7X2-	T45.7X3-	T45.7X4-	T45.7X5-	T45.7X6-
Coal (carbon monoxide from — *see also* Carbon, monoxide, coal)	T58.2X1-	T58.2X2-	T58.2X3-	T58.2X4-	-	-
oil — *see* Kerosene						
tar	T49.1X1-	T49.1X2-	T49.1X3-	T49.1X4-	T49.1X5-	T49.1X6-
fumes	T59.891-	T59.892-	T59.893-	T59.894-	-	-
medicinal (ointment)	T49.4X1-	T49.4X2-	T49.4X3-	T49.4X4-	T49.4X5-	T49.4X6-
analgesics NEC	T39.2X1-	T39.2X2-	T39.2X3-	T39.2X4-	T39.2X5-	T39.2X6-
naphtha (solvent)	T52.0X1-	T52.0X2-	T52.0X3-	T52.0X4-	-	-
Cobalamine	T45.2X1-	T45.2X2-	T45.2X3-	T45.2X4-	T45.2X5-	T45.2X6-
Cobalt (nonmedicinal) (fumes) (industrial)	T56.891-	T56.892-	T56.893-	T56.894-	-	-
medicinal (trace) (chloride)	T45.8X1-	T45.8X2-	T45.8X3-	T45.8X4-	T45.8X5-	T45.8X6-
Cobra (venom)	T63.041-	T63.042-	T63.043-	T63.044-	-	-
Coca (leaf)	T40.5X1-	T40.5X2-	T40.5X3-	T40.5X4-	T40.5X5-	T40.5X6-
Cocaine	T40.5X1-	T40.5X2-	T40.5X3-	T40.5X4-	T40.5X5-	T40.5X6-
topical anesthetic	T41.3X1-	T41.3X2-	T41.3X3-	T41.3X4-	T41.3X5-	T41.3X6-
Cocarboxylase	T45.3X1-	T45.3X2-	T45.3X3-	T45.3X4-	T45.3X5-	T45.3X6-
Coccidioidin	T50.8X1-	T50.8X2-	T50.8X3-	T50.8X4-	T50.8X5-	T50.8X6-
Cocculus indicus	T62.1X1-	T62.1X2-	T62.1X3-	T62.1X4-	-	-
Cochineal	T65.6X1-	T65.6X2-	T65.6X3-	T65.6X4-	-	-
medicinal products	T50.991-	T50.992-	T50.993-	T50.994-	T50.995-	T50.996-
Codeine	T40.2X1-	T40.2X2-	T40.2X3-	T40.2X4-	T40.2X5-	T40.2X6-
Cod-liver oil	T45.2X1-	T45.2X2-	T45.2X3-	T45.2X4-	T45.2X5-	T45.2X6-
Coenzyme A	T50.991-	T50.992-	T50.993-	T50.994-	T50.995-	T50.996-
Coffee	T62.8X1-	T62.8X2-	T62.8X3-	T62.8X4-	-	-
Cogalactoiso-merase	T50.991-	T50.992-	T50.993-	T50.994-	T50.995-	T50.996-
Cogentin	T44.3X1-	T44.3X2-	T44.3X3-	T44.3X4-	T44.3X5-	T44.3X6-
Coke fumes or gas (carbon monoxide)	T58.2X1-	T58.2X2-	T58.2X3-	T58.2X4-	-	-
industrial use	T58.8X1-	T58.8X2-	T58.8X3-	T58.8X4-	-	-
Colace	T47.4X1-	T47.4X2-	T47.4X3-	T47.4X4-	T47.4X5-	T47.4X6-
Colaspase	T45.1X1-	T45.1X2-	T45.1X3-	T45.1X4-	T45.1X5-	T45.1X6-
Colchicine	T50.4X1-	T50.4X2-	T50.4X3-	T50.4X4-	T50.4X5-	T50.4X6-
Colchicum	T62.2X1-	T62.2X2-	T62.2X3-	T62.2X4-	-	-
Cold cream	T49.3X1-	T49.3X2-	T49.3X3-	T49.3X4-	T49.3X5-	T49.3X6-
Colecalciferol	T45.2X1-	T45.2X2-	T45.2X3-	T45.2X4-	T45.2X5-	T45.2X6-
Colestipol	T46.6X1-	T46.6X2-	T46.6X3-	T46.6X4-	T46.6X5-	T46.6X6-
Colestyramine	T46.6X1-	T46.6X2-	T46.6X3-	T46.6X4-	T46.6X5-	T46.6X6-
Colimycin	T36.8X1-	T36.8X2-	T36.8X3-	T36.8X4-	T36.8X5-	T36.8X6-
Colistimethate	T36.8X1-	T36.8X2-	T36.8X3-	T36.8X4-	T36.8X5-	T36.8X6-
Colistin	T36.8X1-	T36.8X2-	T36.8X3-	T36.8X4-	T36.8X5-	T36.8X6-
sulfate (eye preparation)	T49.5X1-	T49.5X2-	T49.5X3-	T49.5X4-	T49.5X5-	T49.5X6-
Collagen	T50.991-	T50.992-	T50.993-	T50.994-	T50.995-	T50.996-
Collagenase	T49.4X1-	T49.4X2-	T49.4X3-	T49.4X4-	T49.4X5-	T49.4X6-
Collodion	T49.3X1-	T49.3X2-	T49.3X3-	T49.3X4-	T49.3X5-	T49.3X6-
Colocynth	T47.2X1-	T47.2X2-	T47.2X3-	T47.2X4-	T47.2X5-	T47.2X6-
Colophony adhesive	T49.3X1-	T49.3X2-	T49.3X3-	T49.3X4-	T49.3X5-	T49.3X6-
Colorant — *see also* Dye	T50.991-	T50.992-	T50.993-	T50.994-	T50.995-	T50.996-
Coloring matter — *see* Dye(s)						
Combustion gas (after combustion) — *see* Carbon, monoxide						
prior to combustion	T59.891-	T59.892-	T59.893-	T59.894-	-	-
Compazine	T43.3X1-	T43.3X2-	T43.3X3-	T43.3X4-	T43.3X5-	T43.3X6-
Compound						
42 (warfarin)	T60.4X1-	T60.4X2-	T60.4X3-	T60.4X4-	-	-
269 (endrin)	T60.1X1-	T60.1X2-	T60.1X3-	T60.1X4-	-	-
497 (dieldrin)	T60.1X1-	T60.1X2-	T60.1X3-	T60.1X4-	-	-
1080 (sodium fluoroacetate)	T60.4X1-	T60.4X2-	T60.4X3-	T60.4X4-	-	-
3422 (parathion)	T60.0X1-	T60.0X2-	T60.0X3-	T60.0X4-	-	-
3911 (phorate)	T60.0X1-	T60.0X2-	T60.0X3-	T60.0X4-	-	-
3956 (toxaphene)	T60.1X1-	T60.1X2-	T60.1X3-	T60.1X4-	-	-
4049 (malathion)	T60.0X1-	T60.0X2-	T60.0X3-	T60.0X4-	-	-
4069 (malathion)	T60.0X1-	T60.0X2-	T60.0X3-	T60.0X4-	-	-

Substance	Poisoning Accidental (unintentional)	Poisoning Intentional self-harm	Poisoning Assault	Poisoning Undetermined	Adverse effect	Underdosing
Compound - *continued*						
4124 (dicapthon)	T60.0X1-	T60.0X2-	T60.0X3-	T60.0X4-	-	-
E (cortisone)	T38.0X1-	T38.0X2-	T38.0X3-	T38.0X4-	T38.0X5-	T38.0X6-
F (hydrocortisone)	T38.0X1-	T38.0X2-	T38.0X3-	T38.0X4-	T38.0X5-	T38.0X6-
Congener, anabolic	T38.7X1-	T38.7X2-	T38.7X3-	T38.7X4-	T38.7X5-	T38.7X6-
Congo red	T50.8X1-	T50.8X2-	T50.8X3-	T50.8X4-	T50.8X5-	T50.8X6-
Coniine, conine	T62.2X1-	T62.2X2-	T62.2X3-	T62.2X4-	-	-
Conium (maculatum)	T62.2X1-	T62.2X2-	T62.2X3-	T62.2X4-	-	-
Conjugated estrogenic substances	T38.5X1-	T38.5X2-	T38.5X3-	T38.5X4-	T38.5X5-	T38.5X6-
Contac	T48.5X1-	T48.5X2-	T48.5X3-	T48.5X4-	T48.5X5-	T48.5X6-
Contact lens solution	T49.5X1-	T49.5X2-	T49.5X3-	T49.5X4-	T49.5X5-	T49.5X6-
Contraceptive (oral)	T38.4X1-	T38.4X2-	T38.4X3-	T38.4X4-	T38.4X5-	T38.4X6-
vaginal	T49.8X1-	T49.8X2-	T49.8X3-	T49.8X4-	T49.8X5-	T49.8X6-
Contrast medium, radiography	T50.8X1-	T50.8X2-	T50.8X3-	T50.8X4-	T50.8X5-	T50.8X6-
Convallaria glycosides	T46.0X1-	T46.0X2-	T46.0X3-	T46.0X4-	T46.0X5-	T46.0X6-
Convallaria majalis	T62.2X1-	T62.2X2-	T62.2X3-	T62.2X4-	-	-
berry	T62.1X1-	T62.1X2-	T62.1X3-	T62.1X4-	-	-
Copper (dust) (fumes) (nonmedicinal) **NEC**	T56.4X1-	T56.4X2-	T56.4X3-	T56.4X4-	-	-
arsenate, arsenite	T57.0X1-	T57.0X2-	T57.0X3-	T57.0X4-	-	-
insecticide	T60.2X1-	T60.2X2-	T60.2X3-	T60.2X4-	-	-
emetic	T47.7X1-	T47.7X2-	T47.7X3-	T47.7X4-	T47.7X5-	T47.7X6-
fungicide	T60.3X1-	T60.3X2-	T60.3X3-	T60.3X4-	-	-
gluconate	T49.0X1-	T49.0X2-	T49.0X3-	T49.0X4-	T49.0X5-	T49.0X6-
insecticide	T60.2X1-	T60.2X2-	T60.2X3-	T60.2X4-	-	-
medicinal (trace)	T45.8X1-	T45.8X2-	T45.8X3-	T45.8X4-	T45.8X5-	T45.8X6-
oleate	T49.0X1-	T49.0X2-	T49.0X3-	T49.0X4-	T49.0X5-	T49.0X6-
sulfate	T56.4X1-	T56.4X2-	T56.4X3-	T56.4X4-	-	-
cupric	T56.4X1-	T56.4X2-	T56.4X3-	T56.4X4-	-	-
fungicide	T60.3X1-	T60.3X2-	T60.3X3-	T60.3X4-	-	-
medicinal						
ear	T49.6X1-	T49.6X2-	T49.6X3-	T49.6X4-	T49.6X5-	T49.6X6-
emetic	T47.7X1-	T47.7X2-	T47.7X3-	T47.7X4-	T47.7X5-	T47.7X6-
eye	T49.5X1-	T49.5X2-	T49.5X3-	T49.5X4-	T49.5X5-	T49.5X6-
cuprous	T56.4X1-	T56.4X2-	T56.4X3-	T56.4X4-	-	-
fungicide	T60.3X1-	T60.3X2-	T60.3X3-	T60.3X4-	-	-
medicinal						
ear	T49.6X1-	T49.6X2-	T49.6X3-	T49.6X4-	T49.6X5-	T49.6X6-
emetic	T47.7X1-	T47.7X2-	T47.7X3-	T47.7X4-	T47.7X5-	T47.7X6-
eye	T49.5X1-	T49.5X2-	T49.5X3-	T49.5X4-	T49.5X5-	T49.5X6-
Copperhead snake (bite) (venom)	T63.061-	T63.062-	T63.063-	T63.064-	-	-
Coral (sting)	T63.691-	T63.692-	T63.693-	T63.694-	-	-
snake (bite) (venom)	T63.021-	T63.022-	T63.023-	T63.024-	-	-
Corbadrine	T49.6X1-	T49.6X2-	T49.6X3-	T49.6X4-	T49.6X5-	T49.6X6-
Cordite	T65.891-	T65.892-	T65.893-	T65.894-	-	-
vapor	T59.891-	T59.892-	T59.893-	T59.894-	-	-
Cordran	T49.0X1-	T49.0X2-	T49.0X3-	T49.0X4-	T49.0X5-	T49.0X6-
Corn cures	T49.4X1-	T49.4X2-	T49.4X3-	T49.4X4-	T49.4X5-	T49.4X6-
Corn starch	T49.3X1-	T49.3X2-	T49.3X3-	T49.3X4-	T49.3X5-	T49.3X6-
Cornhusker's lotion	T49.3X1-	T49.3X2-	T49.3X3-	T49.3X4-	T49.3X5-	T49.3X6-
Coronary vasodilator NEC	T46.3X1-	T46.3X2-	T46.3X3-	T46.3X4-	T46.3X5-	T46.3X6-
Corrosive NEC	T54.91X-	T54.92X-	T54.93X-	T54.94X-	-	-
acid NEC	T54.2X1-	T54.2X2-	T54.2X3-	T54.2X4-	-	-
aromatics	T54.1X1-	T54.1X2-	T54.1X3-	T54.1X4-	-	-
disinfectant	T54.1X1-	T54.1X2-	T54.1X3-	T54.1X4-	-	-
fumes NEC	T54.91X-	T54.92X-	T54.93X-	T54.94X-	-	-
specified NEC	T54.91X-	T54.92X-	T54.93X-	T54.94X-	-	-
sublimate	T56.1X1-	T56.1X2-	T56.1X3-	T56.1X4-	-	-
Cortate	T38.0X1-	T38.0X2-	T38.0X3-	T38.0X4-	T38.0X5-	T38.0X6-
Cort-Dome	T38.0X1-	T38.0X2-	T38.0X3-	T38.0X4-	T38.0X5-	T38.0X6-
ENT agent	T49.6X1-	T49.6X2-	T49.6X3-	T49.6X4-	T49.6X5-	T49.6X6-
ophthalmic preparation	T49.5X1-	T49.5X2-	T49.5X3-	T49.5X4-	T49.5X5-	T49.5X6-
topical NEC	T49.0X1-	T49.0X2-	T49.0X3-	T49.0X4-	T49.0X5-	T49.0X6-
Cortef	T38.0X1-	T38.0X2-	T38.0X3-	T38.0X4-	T38.0X5-	T38.0X6-
ENT agent	T49.6X1-	T49.6X2-	T49.6X3-	T49.6X4-	T49.6X5-	T49.6X6-
ophthalmic preparation	T49.5X1-	T49.5X2-	T49.5X3-	T49.5X4-	T49.5X5-	T49.5X6-
topical NEC	T49.0X1-	T49.0X2-	T49.0X3-	T49.0X4-	T49.0X5-	T49.0X6-
Corticosteroid	T38.0X1-	T38.0X2-	T38.0X3-	T38.0X4-	T38.0X5-	T38.0X6-
ENT agent	T49.6X1-	T49.6X2-	T49.6X3-	T49.6X4-	T49.6X5-	T49.6X6-
mineral	T50.0X1-	T50.0X2-	T50.0X3-	T50.0X4-	T50.0X5-	T50.0X6-
ophthalmic	T49.5X1-	T49.5X2-	T49.5X3-	T49.5X4-	T49.5X5-	T49.5X6-
topical NEC	T49.0X1-	T49.0X2-	T49.0X3-	T49.0X4-	T49.0X5-	T49.0X6-
Corticotropin	T38.811-	T38.812-	T38.813-	T38.814-	T38.815-	T38.816-
Cortisol	T49.0X1-	T49.0X2-	T49.0X3-	T49.0X4-	T49.0X5-	T49.0X6-
ENT agent	T49.6X1-	T49.6X2-	T49.6X3-	T49.6X4-	T49.6X5-	T49.6X6-
ophthalmic preparation	T49.5X1-	T49.5X2-	T49.5X3-	T49.5X4-	T49.5X5-	T49.5X6-
Cortisol - *continued*						
topical NEC	T49.0X1-	T49.0X2-	T49.0X3-	T49.0X4-	T49.0X5-	T49.0X6-
Cortisone (acetate)	T38.0X1-	T38.0X2-	T38.0X3-	T38.0X4-	T38.0X5-	T38.0X6-
ENT agent	T49.6X1-	T49.6X2-	T49.6X3-	T49.6X4-	T49.6X5-	T49.6X6-
ophthalmic preparation	T49.5X1-	T49.5X2-	T49.5X3-	T49.5X4-	T49.5X5-	T49.5X6-
topical NEC	T49.0X1-	T49.0X2-	T49.0X3-	T49.0X4-	T49.0X5-	T49.0X6-
Cortivazol	T38.0X1-	T38.0X2-	T38.0X3-	T38.0X4-	T38.0X5-	T38.0X6-
Cortogen	T38.0X1-	T38.0X2-	T38.0X3-	T38.0X4-	T38.0X5-	T38.0X6-
ENT agent	T49.6X1-	T49.6X2-	T49.6X3-	T49.6X4-	T49.6X5-	T49.6X6-
ophthalmic preparation	T49.5X1-	T49.5X2-	T49.5X3-	T49.5X4-	T49.5X5-	T49.5X6-
Cortone	T38.0X1-	T38.0X2-	T38.0X3-	T38.0X4-	T38.0X5-	T38.0X6-
ENT agent	T49.6X1-	T49.6X2-	T49.6X3-	T49.6X4-	T49.6X5-	T49.6X6-
ophthalmic preparation	T49.5X1-	T49.5X2-	T49.5X3-	T49.5X4-	T49.5X5-	T49.5X6-
Cortril	T38.0X1-	T38.0X2-	T38.0X3-	T38.0X4-	T38.0X5-	T38.0X6-
ENT agent	T49.6X1-	T49.6X2-	T49.6X3-	T49.6X4-	T49.6X5-	T49.6X6-
ophthalmic preparation	T49.5X1-	T49.5X2-	T49.5X3-	T49.5X4-	T49.5X5-	T49.5X6-
topical NEC	T49.0X1-	T49.0X2-	T49.0X3-	T49.0X4-	T49.0X5-	T49.0X6-
Corynebacterium parvum	T45.1X1-	T45.1X2-	T45.1X3-	T45.1X4-	T45.1X5-	T45.1X6-
Cosmetic preparation	T49.8X1-	T49.8X2-	T49.8X3-	T49.8X4-	T49.8X5-	T49.8X6-
Cosmetics	T49.8X1-	T49.8X2-	T49.8X3-	T49.8X4-	T49.8X5-	T49.8X6-
Cosyntropin	T38.811-	T38.812-	T38.813-	T38.814-	T38.815-	T38.816-
Cotarnine	T45.7X1-	T45.7X2-	T45.7X3-	T45.7X4-	T45.7X5-	T45.7X6-
Co-trimoxazole	T36.8X1-	T36.8X2-	T36.8X3-	T36.8X4-	T36.8X5-	T36.8X6-
Cottonseed oil	T49.3X1-	T49.3X2-	T49.3X3-	T49.3X4-	T49.3X5-	T49.3X6-
Cough mixture (syrup)	T48.4X1-	T48.4X2-	T48.4X3-	T48.4X4-	T48.4X5-	T48.4X6-
containing opiates	T40.2X1-	T40.2X2-	T40.2X3-	T40.2X4-	T40.2X5-	T40.2X6-
expectorants	T48.4X1-	T48.4X2-	T48.4X3-	T48.4X4-	T48.4X5-	T48.4X6-
Coumadin	T45.511-	T45.512-	T45.513-	T45.514-	T45.515-	T45.516-
rodenticide	T60.4X1-	T60.4X2-	T60.4X3-	T60.4X4-	-	-
Coumaphos	T60.0X1-	T60.0X2-	T60.0X3-	T60.0X4-	-	-
Coumarin	T45.511-	T45.512-	T45.513-	T45.514-	T45.515-	T45.516-
Coumetarol	T45.511-	T45.512-	T45.513-	T45.514-	T45.515-	T45.516-
Cowbane	T62.2X1-	T62.2X2-	T62.2X3-	T62.2X4-	-	-
Cozyme	T45.2X1-	T45.2X2-	T45.2X3-	T45.2X4-	T45.2X5-	T45.2X6-
Crack	T40.5X1-	T40.5X2-	T40.5X3-	T40.5X4-	-	-
Crataegus extract	T46.0X1-	T46.0X2-	T46.0X3-	T46.0X4-	T46.0X5-	T46.0X6-
Creolin	T54.1X1-	T54.1X2-	T54.1X3-	T54.1X4-	-	-
disinfectant	T54.1X1-	T54.1X2-	T54.1X3-	T54.1X4-	-	-
Creosol (compound)	T49.0X1-	T49.0X2-	T49.0X3-	T49.0X4-	T49.0X5-	T49.0X6-
Creosote (coal tar) (beechwood)	T49.0X1-	T49.0X2-	T49.0X3-	T49.0X4-	T49.0X5-	T49.0X6-
medicinal (expectorant)	T48.4X1-	T48.4X2-	T48.4X3-	T48.4X4-	T48.4X5-	T48.4X6-
syrup	T48.4X1-	T48.4X2-	T48.4X3-	T48.4X4-	T48.4X5-	T48.4X6-
Cresol (s)	T49.0X1-	T49.0X2-	T49.0X3-	T49.0X4-	T49.0X5-	T49.0X6-
and soap solution	T49.0X1-	T49.0X2-	T49.0X3-	T49.0X4-	T49.0X5-	T49.0X6-
Cresyl acetate	T49.0X1-	T49.0X2-	T49.0X3-	T49.0X4-	T49.0X5-	T49.0X6-
Cresylic acid	T49.0X1-	T49.0X2-	T49.0X3-	T49.0X4-	T49.0X5-	T49.0X6-
Crimidine	T60.4X1-	T60.4X2-	T60.4X3-	T60.4X4-	-	-
Croconazole	T37.8X1-	T37.8X2-	T37.8X3-	T37.8X4-	T37.8X5-	T37.8X6-
Cromoglicic acid	T48.6X1-	T48.6X2-	T48.6X3-	T48.6X4-	T48.6X5-	T48.6X6-
Cromolyn	T48.6X1-	T48.6X2-	T48.6X3-	T48.6X4-	T48.6X5-	T48.6X6-
Cromonar	T46.3X1-	T46.3X2-	T46.3X3-	T46.3X4-	T46.3X5-	T46.3X6-
Cropropamide	T39.8X1-	T39.8X2-	T39.8X3-	T39.8X4-	T39.8X5-	T39.8X6-
with crotethamide	T50.7X1-	T50.7X2-	T50.7X3-	T50.7X4-	T50.7X5-	T50.7X6-
Crotamiton	T49.0X1-	T49.0X2-	T49.0X3-	T49.0X4-	T49.0X5-	T49.0X6-
Crotethamide	T39.8X1-	T39.8X2-	T39.8X3-	T39.8X4-	T39.8X5-	T39.8X6-
with cropropamide	T50.7X1-	T50.7X2-	T50.7X3-	T50.7X4-	T50.7X5-	T50.7X6-
Croton (oil)	T47.2X1-	T47.2X2-	T47.2X3-	T47.2X4-	T47.2X5-	T47.2X6-
chloral	T42.6X1-	T42.6X2-	T42.6X3-	T42.6X4-	T42.6X5-	T42.6X6-
Crude oil	T52.0X1-	T52.0X2-	T52.0X3-	T52.0X4-	-	-
Cryogenine	T39.8X1-	T39.8X2-	T39.8X3-	T39.8X4-	T39.8X5-	T39.8X6-
Cryolite (vapor)	T60.1X1-	T60.1X2-	T60.1X3-	T60.1X4-	-	-
insecticide	T60.1X1-	T60.1X2-	T60.1X3-	T60.1X4-	-	-
Cryptenamine (tannates)	T46.5X1-	T46.5X2-	T46.5X3-	T46.5X4-	T46.5X5-	T46.5X6-
Crystal violet	T49.0X1-	T49.0X2-	T49.0X3-	T49.0X4-	T49.0X5-	T49.0X6-
Cuckoopint	T62.2X1-	T62.2X2-	T62.2X3-	T62.2X4-	-	-
Cumetharol	T45.511-	T45.512-	T45.513-	T45.514-	T45.515-	T45.516-
Cupric						
acetate	T60.3X1-	T60.3X2-	T60.3X3-	T60.3X4-	-	-
acetoarsenite	T57.0X1-	T57.0X2-	T57.0X3-	T57.0X4-	-	-
arsenate	T57.0X1-	T57.0X2-	T57.0X3-	T57.0X4-	-	-
gluconate	T49.0X1-	T49.0X2-	T49.0X3-	T49.0X4-	T49.0X5-	T49.0X6-
oleate	T49.0X1-	T49.0X2-	T49.0X3-	T49.0X4-	T49.0X5-	T49.0X6-
sulfate	T56.4X1-	T56.4X2-	T56.4X3-	T56.4X4-	-	-
Cuprous sulfate — *see also* Copper sulfate	T56.4X1-	T56.4X2-	T56.4X3-	T56.4X4-	-	-
Curare, curarine	T48.1X1-	T48.1X2-	T48.1X3-	T48.1X4-	T48.1X5-	T48.1X6-
Cyamemazine	T43.3X1-	T43.3X2-	T43.3X3-	T43.3X4-	T43.3X5-	T43.3X6-

Substance	Poisoning Accidental (unintentional)	Poisoning Intentional self-harm	Poisoning Assault	Poisoning Undetermined	Adverse effect	Underdosing
Cyamopsis tetragono-loba	T46.6X1-	T46.6X2-	T46.6X3-	T46.6X4-	T46.6X5-	T46.6X6-
Cyanacetyl hydrazide	T37.1X1-	T37.1X2-	T37.1X3-	T37.1X4-	T37.1X5-	T37.1X6-
Cyanic acid (gas)	T59.891-	T59.892-	T59.893-	T59.894-	-	-
Cyanide (s) (compounds) (potassium) (sodium) **NEC**	T65.0X1-	T65.0X2-	T65.0X3-	T65.0X4-	-	-
dust or gas (inhalation) NEC	T57.3X1-	T57.3X2-	T57.3X3-	T57.3X4-	-	-
fumigant	T65.0X1-	T65.0X2-	T65.0X3-	T65.0X4-	-	-
hydrogen	T57.3X1-	T57.3X2-	T57.3X3-	T57.3X4-	-	-
mercuric — *see* Mercury						
pesticide (dust) (fumes)	T65.0X1-	T65.0X2-	T65.0X3-	T65.0X4-	-	-
Cyanoacrylate adhesive	T49.3X1-	T49.3X2-	T49.3X3-	T49.3X4-	T49.3X5-	T49.3X6-
Cyanocobalamin	T45.8X1-	T45.8X2-	T45.8X3-	T45.8X4-	T45.8X5-	T45.8X6-
Cyanogen (chloride) (gas) **NEC**	T59.891-	T59.892-	T59.893-	T59.894-	-	-
Cyclacillin	T36.0X1-	T36.0X2-	T36.0X3-	T36.0X4-	T36.0X5-	T36.0X6-
Cyclaine	T41.3X1-	T41.3X2-	T41.3X3-	T41.3X4-	T41.3X5-	T41.3X6-
Cyclamate	T50.991-	T50.992-	T50.993-	T50.994-	T50.995-	T50.996-
Cyclamen europaeum	T62.2X1-	T62.2X2-	T62.2X3-	T62.2X4-	-	-
Cyclandelate	T46.7X1-	T46.7X2-	T46.7X3-	T46.7X4-	T46.7X5-	T46.7X6-
Cyclazocine	T50.7X1-	T50.7X2-	T50.7X3-	T50.7X4-	T50.7X5-	T50.7X6-
Cyclizine	T45.0X1-	T45.0X2-	T45.0X3-	T45.0X4-	T45.0X5-	T45.0X6-
Cyclobarbital	T42.3X1-	T42.3X2-	T42.3X3-	T42.3X4-	T42.3X5-	T42.3X6-
Cyclobarbitone	T42.3X1-	T42.3X2-	T42.3X3-	T42.3X4-	T42.3X5-	T42.3X6-
Cyclobenzaprine	T48.1X1-	T48.1X2-	T48.1X3-	T48.1X4-	T48.1X5-	T48.1X6-
Cyclodrine	T44.3X1-	T44.3X2-	T44.3X3-	T44.3X4-	T44.3X5-	T44.3X6-
Cycloguanil embonate	T37.2X1-	T37.2X2-	T37.2X3-	T37.2X4-	T37.2X5-	T37.2X6-
Cyclohexane	T52.8X1-	T52.8X2-	T52.8X3-	T52.8X4-	-	-
Cyclohexanol	T51.8X1-	T51.8X2-	T51.8X3-	T51.8X4-	-	-
Cyclohexanone	T52.4X1-	T52.4X2-	T52.4X3-	T52.4X4-	-	-
Cycloheximide	T60.3X1-	T60.3X2-	T60.3X3-	T60.3X4-	-	-
Cyclohexyl acetate	T52.8X1-	T52.8X2-	T52.8X3-	T52.8X4-	-	-
Cycloleucin	T45.1X1-	T45.1X2-	T45.1X3-	T45.1X4-	T45.1X5-	T45.1X6-
Cyclomethycaine	T41.3X1-	T41.3X2-	T41.3X3-	T41.3X4-	T41.3X5-	T41.3X6-
Cyclopentamine	T44.4X1-	T44.4X2-	T44.4X3-	T44.4X4-	T44.4X5-	T44.4X6-
Cyclopenthiazide	T50.2X1-	T50.2X2-	T50.2X3-	T50.2X4-	T50.2X5-	T50.2X6-
Cyclopentolate	T44.3X1-	T44.3X2-	T44.3X3-	T44.3X4-	T44.3X5-	T44.3X6-
Cyclophosphamide	T45.1X1-	T45.1X2-	T45.1X3-	T45.1X4-	T45.1X5-	T45.1X6-
Cycloplegic drug	T49.5X1-	T49.5X2-	T49.5X3-	T49.5X4-	T49.5X5-	T49.5X6-
Cyclopropane	T41.291-	T41.292-	T41.293-	T41.294-	T41.295-	T41.296-
Cyclopyrabital	T39.8X1-	T39.8X2-	T39.8X3-	T39.8X4-	T39.8X5-	T39.8X6-
Cycloserine	T37.1X1-	T37.1X2-	T37.1X3-	T37.1X4-	T37.1X5-	T37.1X6-
Cyclosporin	T45.1X1-	T45.1X2-	T45.1X3-	T45.1X4-	T45.1X5-	T45.1X6-
Cyclothiazide	T50.2X1-	T50.2X2-	T50.2X3-	T50.2X4-	T50.2X5-	T50.2X6-
Cycrimine	T44.3X1-	T44.3X2-	T44.3X3-	T44.3X4-	T44.3X5-	T44.3X6-
Cyhalothrin	T60.1X1-	T60.1X2-	T60.1X3-	T60.1X4-	-	-
Cymarin	T46.0X1-	T46.0X2-	T46.0X3-	T46.0X4-	T46.0X5-	T46.0X6-
Cypermethrin	T60.1X1-	T60.1X2-	T60.1X3-	T60.1X4-	-	-
Cyphenothrin	T60.2X1-	T60.2X2-	T60.2X3-	T60.2X4-	-	-
Cyproheptadine	T45.0X1-	T45.0X2-	T45.0X3-	T45.0X4-	T45.0X5-	T45.0X6-
Cyproterone	T38.6X1-	T38.6X2-	T38.6X3-	T38.6X4-	T38.6X5-	T38.6X6-
Cysteamine	T50.6X1-	T50.6X2-	T50.6X3-	T50.6X4-	T50.6X5-	T50.6X6-
Cytarabine	T45.1X1-	T45.1X2-	T45.1X3-	T45.1X4-	T45.1X5-	T45.1X6-
Cytisus						
laburnum	T62.2X1-	T62.2X2-	T62.2X3-	T62.2X4-	-	-
scoparius	T62.2X1-	T62.2X2-	T62.2X3-	T62.2X4-	-	-
Cytochrome C	T47.5X1-	T47.5X2-	T47.5X3-	T47.5X4-	T47.5X5-	T47.5X6-
Cytomel	T38.1X1-	T38.1X2-	T38.1X3-	T38.1X4-	T38.1X5-	T38.1X6-
Cytosine arabinoside	T45.1X1-	T45.1X2-	T45.1X3-	T45.1X4-	T45.1X5-	T45.1X6-
Cytoxan	T45.1X1-	T45.1X2-	T45.1X3-	T45.1X4-	T45.1X5-	T45.1X6-
Cytozyme	T45.7X1-	T45.7X2-	T45.7X3-	T45.7X4-	T45.7X5-	T45.7X6-
2,4-D	T60.3X1-	T60.3X2-	T60.3X3-	T60.3X4-	-	-
Dacarbazine	T45.1X1-	T45.1X2-	T45.1X3-	T45.1X4-	T45.1X5-	T45.1X6-
Dactinomycin	T45.1X1-	T45.1X2-	T45.1X3-	T45.1X4-	T45.1X5-	T45.1X6-
DADPS	T37.1X1-	T37.1X2-	T37.1X3-	T37.1X4-	T37.1X5-	T37.1X6-
Dakin's solution	T49.0X1-	T49.0X2-	T49.0X3-	T49.0X4-	T49.0X5-	T49.0X6-
Dalapon (sodium)	T60.3X1-	T60.3X2-	T60.3X3-	T60.3X4-	-	-
Dalmane	T42.4X1-	T42.4X2-	T42.4X3-	T42.4X4-	T42.4X5-	T42.4X6-
Danazol	T38.6X1-	T38.6X2-	T38.6X3-	T38.6X4-	T38.6X5-	T38.6X6-
Danilone	T45.511-	T45.512-	T45.513-	T45.514-	T45.515-	T45.516-
Danthron	T47.2X1-	T47.2X2-	T47.2X3-	T47.2X4-	T47.2X5-	T47.2X6-
Dantrolene	T42.8X1-	T42.8X2-	T42.8X3-	T42.8X4-	T42.8X5-	T42.8X6-
Dantron	T47.2X1-	T47.2X2-	T47.2X3-	T47.2X4-	T47.2X5-	T47.2X6-
Daphne (gnidium) (mezereum)	T62.2X1-	T62.2X2-	T62.2X3-	T62.2X4-	-	-
berry	T62.1X1-	T62.1X2-	T62.1X3-	T62.1X4-	-	-
Dapsone	T37.1X1-	T37.1X2-	T37.1X3-	T37.1X4-	T37.1X5-	T37.1X6-
Daraprim	T37.2X1-	T37.2X2-	T37.2X3-	T37.2X4-	T37.2X5-	T37.2X6-
Darnel	T62.2X1-	T62.2X2-	T62.2X3-	T62.2X4-	-	-
Darvon	T39.8X1-	T39.8X2-	T39.8X3-	T39.8X4-	T39.8X5-	T39.8X6-
Daunomycin	T45.1X1-	T45.1X2-	T45.1X3-	T45.1X4-	T45.1X5-	T45.1X6-

Substance	Poisoning Accidental (unintentional)	Poisoning Intentional self-harm	Poisoning Assault	Poisoning Undetermined	Adverse effect	Underdosing
Daunorubicin	T45.1X1-	T45.1X2-	T45.1X3-	T45.1X4-	T45.1X5-	T45.1X6-
DBI	T38.3X1-	T38.3X2-	T38.3X3-	T38.3X4-	T38.3X5-	T38.3X6-
D-Con	T60.91X-	T60.92X-	T60.93X-	T60.94X-	-	-
insecticide	T60.2X1-	T60.2X2-	T60.2X3-	T60.2X4-	-	-
rodenticide	T60.4X1-	T60.4X2-	T60.4X3-	T60.4X4-	-	-
DDAVP	T38.891-	T38.892-	T38.893-	T38.894-	T38.895-	T38.896-
DDE (bis (chlorophenyl) **-dichloroethylene)**	T60.2X1-	T60.2X2-	T60.2X3-	T60.2X4-	-	-
DDS	T37.1X1-	T37.1X2-	T37.1X3-	T37.1X4-	T37.1X5-	T37.1X6-
DDT (dust)	T60.1X1-	T60.1X2-	T60.1X3-	T60.1X4-	-	-
Deadly nightshade — *see also* Belladonna	T62.2X1-	T62.2X2-	T62.2X3-	T62.2X4-	-	-
berry	T62.1X1-	T62.1X2-	T62.1X3-	T62.1X4-	-	-
Deamino-D-arginine vasopressin	T38.891-	T38.892-	T38.893-	T38.894-	T38.895-	T38.896-
Deanol (aceglumate)	T50.991-	T50.992-	T50.993-	T50.994-	T50.995-	T50.996-
Debrisoquine	T46.5X1-	T46.5X2-	T46.5X3-	T46.5X4-	T46.5X5-	T46.5X6-
Decaborane	T57.8X1-	T57.8X2-	T57.8X3-	T57.8X4-	-	-
fumes	T59.891-	T59.892-	T59.893-	T59.894-	-	-
Decadron	T38.0X1-	T38.0X2-	T38.0X3-	T38.0X4-	T38.0X5-	T38.0X6-
ENT agent	T49.6X1-	T49.6X2-	T49.6X3-	T49.6X4-	T49.6X5-	T49.6X6-
ophthalmic preparation	T49.5X1-	T49.5X2-	T49.5X3-	T49.5X4-	T49.5X5-	T49.5X6-
topical NEC	T49.0X1-	T49.0X2-	T49.0X3-	T49.0X4-	T49.0X5-	T49.0X6-
Decahydronaphthalene	T52.8X1-	T52.8X2-	T52.8X3-	T52.8X4-	-	-
Decalin	T52.8X1-	T52.8X2-	T52.8X3-	T52.8X4-	-	-
Decamethonium (bromide)	T48.1X1-	T48.1X2-	T48.1X3-	T48.1X4-	T48.1X5-	T48.1X6-
Decholin	T47.5X1-	T47.5X2-	T47.5X3-	T47.5X4-	T47.5X5-	T47.5X6-
Declomycin	T36.4X1-	T36.4X2-	T36.4X3-	T36.4X4-	T36.4X5-	T36.4X6-
Decongestant, nasal (mucosa)	T48.5X1-	T48.5X2-	T48.5X3-	T48.5X4-	T48.5X5-	T48.5X6-
combination	T48.5X1-	T48.5X2-	T48.5X3-	T48.5X4-	T48.5X5-	T48.5X6-
Deet	T60.8X1-	T60.8X2-	T60.8X3-	T60.8X4-	-	-
Deferoxamine	T45.8X1-	T45.8X2-	T45.8X3-	T45.8X4-	T45.8X5-	T45.8X6-
Deflazacort	T38.0X1-	T38.0X2-	T38.0X3-	T38.0X4-	T38.0X5-	T38.0X6-
Deglycyrrhizinized extract of licorice	T48.4X1-	T48.4X2-	T48.4X3-	T48.4X4-	T48.4X5-	T48.4X6-
Dehydrocholic acid	T47.5X1-	T47.5X2-	T47.5X3-	T47.5X4-	T47.5X5-	T47.5X6-
Dehydroemetine	T37.3X1-	T37.3X2-	T37.3X3-	T37.3X4-	T37.3X5-	T37.3X6-
Dekalin	T52.8X1-	T52.8X2-	T52.8X3-	T52.8X4-	-	-
Delalutin	T38.5X1-	T38.5X2-	T38.5X3-	T38.5X4-	T38.5X5-	T38.5X6-
Delorazepam	T42.4X1-	T42.4X2-	T42.4X3-	T42.4X4-	T42.4X5-	T42.4X6-
Delphinium	T62.2X1-	T62.2X2-	T62.2X3-	T62.2X4-	-	-
Deltamethrin	T60.1X1-	T60.1X2-	T60.1X3-	T60.1X4-	-	-
Deltasone	T38.0X1-	T38.0X2-	T38.0X3-	T38.0X4-	T38.0X5-	T38.0X6-
Deltra	T38.0X1-	T38.0X2-	T38.0X3-	T38.0X4-	T38.0X5-	T38.0X6-
Delvinal	T42.3X1-	T42.3X2-	T42.3X3-	T42.3X4-	T42.3X5-	T42.3X6-
Demecarium (bromide)	T49.5X1-	T49.5X2-	T49.5X3-	T49.5X4-	T49.5X5-	T49.5X6-
Demeclocycline	T36.4X1-	T36.4X2-	T36.4X3-	T36.4X4-	T36.4X5-	T36.4X6-
Demecolcine	T45.1X1-	T45.1X2-	T45.1X3-	T45.1X4-	T45.1X5-	T45.1X6-
Demegestone	T38.5X1-	T38.5X2-	T38.5X3-	T38.5X4-	T38.5X5-	T38.5X6-
Demelanizing agents	T49.8X1-	T49.8X2-	T49.8X3-	T49.8X4-	T49.8X5-	T49.8X6-
Demephion -O and -S	T60.0X1-	T60.0X2-	T60.0X3-	T60.0X4-	-	-
Demerol	T40.2X1-	T40.2X2-	T40.2X3-	T40.2X4-	T40.2X5-	T40.2X6-
Demethylchlortetracycline	T36.4X1-	T36.4X2-	T36.4X3-	T36.4X4-	T36.4X5-	T36.4X6-
Demethyltetracycline	T36.4X1-	T36.4X2-	T36.4X3-	T36.4X4-	T36.4X5-	T36.4X6-
Demeton -O and -S	T60.0X1-	T60.0X2-	T60.0X3-	T60.0X4-	-	-
Demulcent (external)	T49.3X1-	T49.3X2-	T49.3X3-	T49.3X4-	T49.3X5-	T49.3X6-
specified NEC	T49.3X1-	T49.3X2-	T49.3X3-	T49.3X4-	T49.3X5-	T49.3X6-
Demulen	T38.4X1-	T38.4X2-	T38.4X3-	T38.4X4-	T38.4X5-	T38.4X6-
Denatured alcohol	T51.0X1-	T51.0X2-	T51.0X3-	T51.0X4-	-	-
Dendrid	T49.5X1-	T49.5X2-	T49.5X3-	T49.5X4-	T49.5X5-	T49.5X6-
Dental drug, topical application NEC	T49.7X1-	T49.7X2-	T49.7X3-	T49.7X4-	T49.7X5-	T49.7X6-
Dentifrice	T49.7X1-	T49.7X2-	T49.7X3-	T49.7X4-	T49.7X5-	T49.7X6-
Deodorant spray (feminine hygiene)	T49.8X1-	T49.8X2-	T49.8X3-	T49.8X4-	T49.8X5-	T49.8X6-
Deoxycortone	T50.0X1-	T50.0X2-	T50.0X3-	T50.0X4-	T50.0X5-	T50.0X6-
2-Deoxy-5-fluorouridine	T45.1X1-	T45.1X2-	T45.1X3-	T45.1X4-	T45.1X5-	T45.1X6-
5-Deoxy-5-fluorouridine	T45.1X1-	T45.1X2-	T45.1X3-	T45.1X4-	T45.1X5-	T45.1X6-
Deoxyribonuclease (pancreatic)	T45.3X1-	T45.3X2-	T45.3X3-	T45.3X4-	T45.3X5-	T45.3X6-
Depilatory	T49.4X1-	T49.4X2-	T49.4X3-	T49.4X4-	T49.4X5-	T49.4X6-
Deprenalin	T42.8X1-	T42.8X2-	T42.8X3-	T42.8X4-	T42.8X5-	T42.8X6-
Deprenyl	T42.8X1-	T42.8X2-	T42.8X3-	T42.8X4-	T42.8X5-	T42.8X6-
Depressant, appetite	T50.5X1-	T50.5X2-	T50.5X3-	T50.5X4-	T50.5X5-	T50.5X6-
Depressant						
appetite (central)	T50.5X1-	T50.5X2-	T50.5X3-	T50.5X4-	T50.5X5-	T50.5X6-
cardiac	T46.2X1-	T46.2X2-	T46.2X3-	T46.2X4-	T46.2X5-	T46.2X6-

Depressant - Diemal

Table of Drugs and Chemicals

Table of Drugs and Chemicals

Depressant — Diemal

Substance	Poisoning Accidental (unintentional)	Poisoning Intentional self-harm	Poisoning Assault	Poisoning Undetermined	Adverse effect	Underdosing
Depressant - *continued*						
central nervous system (anesthetic) — *see also* Central nervous system, depressants	T42.71X-	T42.72X-	T42.73X-	T42.74X-	T42.75X-	T42.76X-
general anesthetic	T41.201-	T41.202-	T41.203-	T41.204-	T41.205-	T41.206-
muscle tone	T42.8X1-	T42.8X2-	T42.8X3-	T42.8X4-	T42.8X5-	T42.8X6-
muscle tone, central	T42.8X1-	T42.8X2-	T42.8X3-	T42.8X4-	T42.8X5-	T42.8X6-
psychotherapeutic	T43.501-	T43.502-	T43.503-	T43.504-	T43.505-	T43.506-
Deptropine	T45.0X1-	T45.0X2-	T45.0X3-	T45.0X4-	T45.0X5-	T45.0X6-
Dequalinium (chloride)	T49.0X1-	T49.0X2-	T49.0X3-	T49.0X4-	T49.0X5-	T49.0X6-
Derris root	T60.2X1-	T60.2X2-	T60.2X3-	T60.2X4-	-	-
Deserpidine	T46.5X1-	T46.5X2-	T46.5X3-	T46.5X4-	T46.5X5-	T46.5X6-
Desferrioxamine	T45.8X1-	T45.8X2-	T45.8X3-	T45.8X4-	T45.8X5-	T45.8X6-
Desipramine	T43.011-	T43.012-	T43.013-	T43.014-	T43.015-	T43.016-
Deslanoside	T46.0X1-	T46.0X2-	T46.0X3-	T46.0X4-	T46.0X5-	T46.0X6-
Desloughing agent	T49.4X1-	T49.4X2-	T49.4X3-	T49.4X4-	T49.4X5-	T49.4X6-
Desmethylimipramine	T43.011-	T43.012-	T43.013-	T43.014-	T43.015-	T43.016-
Desmopressin	T38.891-	T38.892-	T38.893-	T38.894-	T38.895-	T38.896-
Desocodeine	T40.2X1-	T40.2X2-	T40.2X3-	T40.2X4-	T40.2X5-	T40.2X6-
Desogestrel	T38.5X1-	T38.5X2-	T38.5X3-	T38.5X4-	T38.5X5-	T38.5X6-
Desomorphine	T40.2X1-	T40.2X2-	T40.2X3-	T40.2X4-	-	-
Desonide	T49.0X1-	T49.0X2-	T49.0X3-	T49.0X4-	T49.0X5-	T49.0X6-
Desoximetasone	T49.0X1-	T49.0X2-	T49.0X3-	T49.0X4-	T49.0X5-	T49.0X6-
Desoxycorticosteroid	T50.0X1-	T50.0X2-	T50.0X3-	T50.0X4-	T50.0X5-	T50.0X6-
Desoxycortone	T50.0X1-	T50.0X2-	T50.0X3-	T50.0X4-	T50.0X5-	T50.0X6-
Desoxyephedrine	T43.621-	T43.622-	T43.623-	T43.624-	T43.625-	T43.626-
Detaxtran	T46.6X1-	T46.6X2-	T46.6X3-	T46.6X4-	T46.6X5-	T46.6X6-
Detergent	T49.2X1-	T49.2X2-	T49.2X3-	T49.2X4-	T49.2X5-	T49.2X6-
external medication	T49.2X1-	T49.2X2-	T49.2X3-	T49.2X4-	T49.2X5-	T49.2X6-
local	T49.2X1-	T49.2X2-	T49.2X3-	T49.2X4-	T49.2X5-	T49.2X6-
medicinal	T49.2X1-	T49.2X2-	T49.2X3-	T49.2X4-	T49.2X5-	T49.2X6-
nonmedicinal	T55.1X1-	T55.1X2-	T55.1X3-	T55.1X4-	-	-
specified NEC	T55.1X1-	T55.1X2-	T55.1X3-	T55.1X4-	-	-
Deterrent, alcohol	T50.6X1-	T50.6X2-	T50.6X3-	T50.6X4-	T50.6X5-	T50.6X6-
Detoxifying agent	T50.6X1-	T50.6X2-	T50.6X3-	T50.6X4-	T50.6X5-	T50.6X6-
Detrothyronine	T38.1X1-	T38.1X2-	T38.1X3-	T38.1X4-	T38.1X5-	T38.1X6-
Dettol (external medication)	T49.0X1-	T49.0X2-	T49.0X3-	T49.0X4-	T49.0X5-	T49.0X6-
Dexamethasone	T38.0X1-	T38.0X2-	T38.0X3-	T38.0X4-	T38.0X5-	T38.0X6-
ENT agent	T49.6X1-	T49.6X2-	T49.6X3-	T49.6X4-	T49.6X5-	T49.6X6-
ophthalmic preparation	T49.5X1-	T49.5X2-	T49.5X3-	T49.5X4-	T49.5X5-	T49.5X6-
topical NEC	T49.0X1-	T49.0X2-	T49.0X3-	T49.0X4-	T49.0X5-	T49.0X6-
Dexamfetamine	T43.621-	T43.622-	T43.623-	T43.624-	T43.625-	T43.626-
Dexamphetamine	T43.621-	T43.622-	T43.623-	T43.624-	T43.625-	T43.626-
Dexbrompheniramine	T45.0X1-	T45.0X2-	T45.0X3-	T45.0X4-	T45.0X5-	T45.0X6-
Dexchlorpheniramine	T45.0X1-	T45.0X2-	T45.0X3-	T45.0X4-	T45.0X5-	T45.0X6-
Dexedrine	T43.621-	T43.622-	T43.623-	T43.624-	T43.625-	T43.626-
Dexetimide	T44.3X1-	T44.3X2-	T44.3X3-	T44.3X4-	T44.3X5-	T44.3X6-
Dexfenfluramine	T50.5X1-	T50.5X2-	T50.5X3-	T50.5X4-	T50.5X5-	T50.5X6-
Dexpanthenol	T45.2X1-	T45.2X2-	T45.2X3-	T45.2X4-	T45.2X5-	T45.2X6-
Dextran (40) (70) (150)	T45.8X1-	T45.8X2-	T45.8X3-	T45.8X4-	T45.8X5-	T45.8X6-
Dextriferron	T45.4X1-	T45.4X2-	T45.4X3-	T45.4X4-	T45.4X5-	T45.4X6-
Dextro calcium pantothenate	T45.2X1-	T45.2X2-	T45.2X3-	T45.2X4-	T45.2X5-	T45.2X6-
Dextro pantothenyl alcohol	T45.2X1-	T45.2X2-	T45.2X3-	T45.2X4-	T45.2X5-	T45.2X6-
Dextroamphetamine	T43.621-	T43.622-	T43.623-	T43.624-	T43.625-	T43.626-
Dextromethorphan	T48.3X1-	T48.3X2-	T48.3X3-	T48.3X4-	T48.3X5-	T48.3X6-
Dextromoramide	T40.4X1-	T40.4X2-	T40.4X3-	T40.4X4-	-	-
topical	T49.8X1-	T49.8X2-	T49.8X3-	T49.8X4-	T49.8X5-	T49.8X6-
Dextropropoxyphene	T40.4X1-	T40.4X2-	T40.4X3-	T40.4X4-	T40.4X5-	T40.4X6-
Dextrorphan	T40.2X1-	T40.2X2-	T40.2X3-	T40.2X4-	T40.2X5-	T40.2X6-
Dextrose	T50.3X1-	T50.3X2-	T50.3X3-	T50.3X4-	T50.3X5-	T50.3X6-
concentrated solution, intravenous	T46.8X1-	T46.8X2-	T46.8X3-	T46.8X4-	T46.8X5-	T46.8X6-
Dextrothyroxin	T38.1X1-	T38.1X2-	T38.1X3-	T38.1X4-	T38.1X5-	T38.1X6-
Dextrothyroxine sodium	T38.1X1-	T38.1X2-	T38.1X3-	T38.1X4-	T38.1X5-	T38.1X6-
DFP	T44.0X1-	T44.0X2-	T44.0X3-	T44.0X4-	T44.0X5-	T44.0X6-
DHE	T37.3X1-	T37.3X2-	T37.3X3-	T37.3X4-	T37.3X5-	T37.3X6-
45	T46.5X1-	T46.5X2-	T46.5X3-	T46.5X4-	T46.5X5-	T46.5X6-
Diabinese	T38.3X1-	T38.3X2-	T38.3X3-	T38.3X4-	T38.3X5-	T38.3X6-
Diacetone alcohol	T52.4X1-	T52.4X2-	T52.4X3-	T52.4X4-	-	-
Diacetyl monoxime	T50.991-	T50.992-	T50.993-	T50.994-	-	-
Diacetylmorphine	T40.1X1-	T40.1X2-	T40.1X3-	T40.1X4-	-	-
Diachylon plaster	T49.4X1-	T49.4X2-	T49.4X3-	T49.4X4-	T49.4X5-	T49.4X6-
Diaethylstilboestrolum	T38.5X1-	T38.5X2-	T38.5X3-	T38.5X4-	T38.5X5-	T38.5X6-
Diagnostic agent NEC	T50.8X1-	T50.8X2-	T50.8X3-	T50.8X4-	T50.8X5-	T50.8X6-
Dial (soap)	T49.2X1-	T49.2X2-	T49.2X3-	T49.2X4-	T49.2X5-	T49.2X6-
sedative	T42.3X1-	T42.3X2-	T42.3X3-	T42.3X4-	T42.3X5-	T42.3X6-
Dialkyl carbonate	T52.91X-	T52.92X-	T52.93X-	T52.94X-	-	-
Diallylbarbituric acid	T42.3X1-	T42.3X2-	T42.3X3-	T42.3X4-	T42.3X5-	T42.3X6-
Diallymal	T42.3X1-	T42.3X2-	T42.3X3-	T42.3X4-	T42.3X5-	T42.3X6-
Dialysis solution (intraperitoneal)	T50.3X1-	T50.3X2-	T50.3X3-	T50.3X4-	T50.3X5-	T50.3X6-
Diaminodiphenylsulfone	T37.1X1-	T37.1X2-	T37.1X3-	T37.1X4-	T37.1X5-	T37.1X6-
Diamorphine	T40.1X1-	T40.1X2-	T40.1X3-	T40.1X4-	-	-
Diamox	T50.2X1-	T50.2X2-	T50.2X3-	T50.2X4-	T50.2X5-	T50.2X6-
Diamthazole	T49.0X1-	T49.0X2-	T49.0X3-	T49.0X4-	T49.0X5-	T49.0X6-
Dianthone	T47.2X1-	T47.2X2-	T47.2X3-	T47.2X4-	T47.2X5-	T47.2X6-
Diaphenylsulfone	T37.0X1-	T37.0X2-	T37.0X3-	T37.0X4-	T37.0X5-	T37.0X6-
Diasone (sodium)	T37.1X1-	T37.1X2-	T37.1X3-	T37.1X4-	T37.1X5-	T37.1X6-
Diastase	T47.5X1-	T47.5X2-	T47.5X3-	T47.5X4-	T47.5X5-	T47.5X6-
Diatrizoate	T50.8X1-	T50.8X2-	T50.8X3-	T50.8X4-	T50.8X5-	T50.8X6-
Diazepam	T42.4X1-	T42.4X2-	T42.4X3-	T42.4X4-	T42.4X5-	T42.4X6-
Diazinon	T60.0X1-	T60.0X2-	T60.0X3-	T60.0X4-	-	-
Diazomethane (gas)	T59.891-	T59.892-	T59.893-	T59.894-	-	-
Diazoxide	T46.5X1-	T46.5X2-	T46.5X3-	T46.5X4-	T46.5X5-	T46.5X6-
Dibekacin	T36.5X1-	T36.5X2-	T36.5X3-	T36.5X4-	T36.5X5-	T36.5X6-
Dibenamine	T44.6X1-	T44.6X2-	T44.6X3-	T44.6X4-	T44.6X5-	T44.6X6-
Dibenzepin	T43.011-	T43.012-	T43.013-	T43.014-	T43.015-	T43.016-
Dibenzheptropine	T45.0X1-	T45.0X2-	T45.0X3-	T45.0X4-	T45.0X5-	T45.0X6-
Dibenzyline	T44.6X1-	T44.6X2-	T44.6X3-	T44.6X4-	T44.6X5-	T44.6X6-
Diborane (gas)	T59.891-	T59.892-	T59.893-	T59.894-	-	-
Dibromochloropropane	T60.8X1-	T60.8X2-	T60.8X3-	T60.8X4-	-	-
Dibromodulcitol	T45.1X1-	T45.1X2-	T45.1X3-	T45.1X4-	T45.1X5-	T45.1X6-
Dibromoethane	T53.6X1-	T53.6X2-	T53.6X3-	T53.6X4-	-	-
Dibromomannitol	T45.1X1-	T45.1X2-	T45.1X3-	T45.1X4-	T45.1X5-	T45.1X6-
Dibromopropamidine isethionate	T49.0X1-	T49.0X2-	T49.0X3-	T49.0X4-	T49.0X5-	T49.0X6-
Dibrompropamidine	T49.0X1-	T49.0X2-	T49.0X3-	T49.0X4-	T49.0X5-	T49.0X6-
Dibucaine	T41.3X1-	T41.3X2-	T41.3X3-	T41.3X4-	T41.3X5-	T41.3X6-
topical (surface)	T41.3X1-	T41.3X2-	T41.3X3-	T41.3X4-	T41.3X5-	T41.3X6-
Dibunate sodium	T48.3X1-	T48.3X2-	T48.3X3-	T48.3X4-	T48.3X5-	T48.3X6-
Dibutoline sulfate	T44.3X1-	T44.3X2-	T44.3X3-	T44.3X4-	T44.3X5-	T44.3X6-
Dicamba	T60.3X1-	T60.3X2-	T60.3X3-	T60.3X4-	-	-
Dicapthon	T60.0X1-	T60.0X2-	T60.0X3-	T60.0X4-	-	-
Dichlobenil	T60.3X1-	T60.3X2-	T60.3X3-	T60.3X4-	-	-
Dichlone	T60.3X1-	T60.3X2-	T60.3X3-	T60.3X4-	-	-
Dichloralphenozone	T42.6X1-	T42.6X2-	T42.6X3-	T42.6X4-	T42.6X5-	T42.6X6-
Dichlorbenzidine	T65.3X1-	T65.3X2-	T65.3X3-	T65.3X4-	-	-
Dichlorhydrin	T52.8X1-	T52.8X2-	T52.8X3-	T52.8X4-	-	-
Dichlorhydroxyquinoline	T37.8X1-	T37.8X2-	T37.8X3-	T37.8X4-	T37.8X5-	T37.8X6-
Dichlorobenzene	T53.7X1-	T53.7X2-	T53.7X3-	T53.7X4-	-	-
Dichlorobenzyl alcohol	T49.6X1-	T49.6X2-	T49.6X3-	T49.6X4-	T49.6X5-	T49.6X6-
Dichlorodifluoromethane	T53.5X1-	T53.5X2-	T53.5X3-	T53.5X4-	-	-
Dichloroethane	T52.8X1-	T52.8X2-	T52.8X3-	T52.8X4-	-	-
Sym-Dichloroethyl ether	T53.6X1-	T53.6X2-	T53.6X3-	T53.6X4-	-	-
Dichloroethyl sulfide, not in war	T59.891-	T59.892-	T59.893-	T59.894-	-	-
Dichloroethylene	T53.6X1-	T53.6X2-	T53.6X3-	T53.6X4-	-	-
Dichloroformoxine, not in war	T59.891-	T59.892-	T59.893-	T59.894-	-	-
Dichlorohydrin, alpha-dichlorohydrin	T52.8X1-	T52.8X2-	T52.8X3-	T52.8X4-	-	-
Dichloromethane (solvent)	T53.4X1-	T53.4X2-	T53.4X3-	T53.4X4-	-	-
vapor	T53.4X1-	T53.4X2-	T53.4X3-	T53.4X4-	-	-
Dichloronaphthoquinone	T60.3X1-	T60.3X2-	T60.3X3-	T60.3X4-	-	-
Dichlorophen	T37.4X1-	T37.4X2-	T37.4X3-	T37.4X4-	T37.4X5-	T37.4X6-
2,4-Dichlorophenoxyacetic acid	T60.3X1-	T60.3X2-	T60.3X3-	T60.3X4-	-	-
Dichloropropene	T60.3X1-	T60.3X2-	T60.3X3-	T60.3X4-	-	-
Dichloropropionic acid	T60.3X1-	T60.3X2-	T60.3X3-	T60.3X4-	-	-
Dichlorphenamide	T50.2X1-	T50.2X2-	T50.2X3-	T50.2X4-	T50.2X5-	T50.2X6-
Dichlorvos	T60.0X1-	T60.0X2-	T60.0X3-	T60.0X4-	-	-
Diclofenac	T39.391-	T39.392-	T39.393-	T39.394-	T39.395-	T39.396-
Diclofenamide	T50.2X1-	T50.2X2-	T50.2X3-	T50.2X4-	T50.2X5-	T50.2X6-
Diclofensine	T43.291-	T43.292-	T43.293-	T43.294-	T43.295-	T43.296-
Diclonixine	T39.8X1-	T39.8X2-	T39.8X3-	T39.8X4-	T39.8X5-	T39.8X6-
Dicloxacillin	T36.0X1-	T36.0X2-	T36.0X3-	T36.0X4-	T36.0X5-	T36.0X6-
Dicophane	T49.0X1-	T49.0X2-	T49.0X3-	T49.0X4-	T49.0X5-	T49.0X6-
Dicoumarol, dicoumarin, dicumarol	T45.511-	T45.512-	T45.513-	T45.514-	T45.515-	T45.516-
Dicrotophos	T60.0X1-	T60.0X2-	T60.0X3-	T60.0X4-	-	-
Dicyanogen (gas)	T65.0X1-	T65.0X2-	T65.0X3-	T65.0X4-	-	-
Dicyclomine	T44.3X1-	T44.3X2-	T44.3X3-	T44.3X4-	T44.3X5-	T44.3X6-
Dicycloverine	T44.3X1-	T44.3X2-	T44.3X3-	T44.3X4-	T44.3X5-	T44.3X6-
Dideoxycytidine	T37.5X1-	T37.5X2-	T37.5X3-	T37.5X4-	T37.5X5-	T37.5X6-
Dideoxyinosine	T37.5X1-	T37.5X2-	T37.5X3-	T37.5X4-	T37.5X5-	T37.5X6-
Dieldrin (vapor)	T60.1X1-	T60.1X2-	T60.1X3-	T60.1X4-	-	-
Diemal	T42.3X1-	T42.3X2-	T42.3X3-	T42.3X4-	T42.3X5-	T42.3X6-

Substance	Poisoning Accidental (unintentional)	Poisoning Intentional self-harm	Poisoning Assault	Poisoning Undetermined	Adverse effect	Underdosing
Dienestrol	T38.5X1-	T38.5X2-	T38.5X3-	T38.5X4-	T38.5X5-	T38.5X6-
Dienoestrol	T38.5X1-	T38.5X2-	T38.5X3-	T38.5X4-	T38.5X5-	T38.5X6-
Dietetic drug NEC	T50.901-	T50.902-	T50.903-	T50.904-	T50.905-	T50.906-
Diethazine	T42.8X1-	T42.8X2-	T42.8X3-	T42.8X4-	T42.8X5-	T42.8X6-
Diethyl						
barbituric acid	T42.3X1-	T42.3X2-	T42.3X3-	T42.3X4-	T42.3X5-	T42.3X6-
carbamazine	T37.4X1-	T37.4X2-	T37.4X3-	T37.4X4-	T37.4X5-	T37.4X6-
carbinol	T51.3X1-	T51.3X2-	T51.3X3-	T51.3X4-	-	-
carbonate	T52.8X1-	T52.8X2-	T52.8X3-	T52.8X4-	-	-
ether (vapor) — *see also* ether	T41.0X1-	T41.0X2-	T41.0X3-	T41.0X4-	T41.0X5-	T41.0X6-
oxide	T52.8X1-	T52.8X2-	T52.8X3-	T52.8X4-	-	-
propion	T50.5X1-	T50.5X2-	T50.5X3-	T50.5X4-	T50.5X5-	T50.5X6-
stilbestrol	T38.5X1-	T38.5X2-	T38.5X3-	T38.5X4-	T38.5X5-	T38.5X6-
toluamide (nonmedicinal)	T60.8X1-	T60.8X2-	T60.8X3-	T60.8X4-	-	-
medicinal	T49.3X1-	T49.3X2-	T49.3X3-	T49.3X4-	T49.3X5-	T49.3X6-
Diethylcarbamazine	T37.4X1-	T37.4X2-	T37.4X3-	T37.4X4-	T37.4X5-	T37.4X6-
Diethylene						
dioxide	T52.8X1-	T52.8X2-	T52.8X3-	T52.8X4-	-	-
glycol (monoacetate) (monobutyl ether) (monoethyl ether)	T52.3X1-	T52.3X2-	T52.3X3-	T52.3X4-	-	-
Diethylhexylphthalate	T65.891-	T65.892-	T65.893-	T65.894-	-	-
Diethylpropion	T50.5X1-	T50.5X2-	T50.5X3-	T50.5X4-	T50.5X5-	T50.5X6-
Diethylstilbestrol	T38.5X1-	T38.5X2-	T38.5X3-	T38.5X4-	T38.5X5-	T38.5X6-
Diethylstilboestrol	T38.5X1-	T38.5X2-	T38.5X3-	T38.5X4-	T38.5X5-	T38.5X6-
Diethylsulfone-diethylmethane	T42.6X1-	T42.6X2-	T42.6X3-	T42.6X4-	T42.6X5-	T42.6X6-
Diethyltoluamide	T49.0X1-	T49.0X2-	T49.0X3-	T49.0X4-	T49.0X5-	T49.0X6-
Diethyltryptamine (DET)	T40.991-	T40.992-	T40.993-	T40.994-	-	-
Difebarbamate	T42.3X1-	T42.3X2-	T42.3X3-	T42.3X4-	T42.3X5-	T42.3X6-
Difencloxazine	T40.2X1-	T40.2X2-	T40.2X3-	T40.2X4-	T40.2X5-	T40.2X6-
Difenidol	T45.0X1-	T45.0X2-	T45.0X3-	T45.0X4-	T45.0X5-	T45.0X6-
Difenoxin	T47.6X1-	T47.6X2-	T47.6X3-	T47.6X4-	T47.6X5-	T47.6X6-
Difetarsone	T37.3X1-	T37.3X2-	T37.3X3-	T37.3X4-	T37.3X5-	T37.3X6-
Diffusin	T45.3X1-	T45.3X2-	T45.3X3-	T45.3X4-	T45.3X5-	T45.3X6-
Diflorasone	T49.0X1-	T49.0X2-	T49.0X3-	T49.0X4-	T49.0X5-	T49.0X6-
Diflos	T44.0X1-	T44.0X2-	T44.0X3-	T44.0X4-	T44.0X5-	T44.0X6-
Diflubenzuron	T60.1X1-	T60.1X2-	T60.1X3-	T60.1X4-	-	-
Diflucortolone	T49.0X1-	T49.0X2-	T49.0X3-	T49.0X4-	T49.0X5-	T49.0X6-
Diflunisal	T39.091-	T39.092-	T39.093-	T39.094-	T39.095-	T39.096-
Difluoromethyldopa	T42.8X1-	T42.8X2-	T42.8X3-	T42.8X4-	T42.8X5-	T42.8X6-
Difluorophate	T44.0X1-	T44.0X2-	T44.0X3-	T44.0X4-	T44.0X5-	T44.0X6-
Digestant NEC	T47.5X1-	T47.5X2-	T47.5X3-	T47.5X4-	T47.5X5-	T47.5X6-
Digitalin (e)	T46.0X1-	T46.0X2-	T46.0X3-	T46.0X4-	T46.0X5-	T46.0X6-
Digitalis (leaf) (glycoside)	T46.0X1-	T46.0X2-	T46.0X3-	T46.0X4-	T46.0X5-	T46.0X6-
lanata	T46.0X1-	T46.0X2-	T46.0X3-	T46.0X4-	T46.0X5-	T46.0X6-
purpurea	T46.0X1-	T46.0X2-	T46.0X3-	T46.0X4-	T46.0X5-	T46.0X6-
Digitoxin	T46.0X1-	T46.0X2-	T46.0X3-	T46.0X4-	T46.0X5-	T46.0X6-
Digitoxose	T46.0X1-	T46.0X2-	T46.0X3-	T46.0X4-	T46.0X5-	T46.0X6-
Digoxin	T46.0X1-	T46.0X2-	T46.0X3-	T46.0X4-	T46.0X5-	T46.0X6-
Digoxine	T46.0X1-	T46.0X2-	T46.0X3-	T46.0X4-	T46.0X5-	T46.0X6-
Dihydralazine	T46.5X1-	T46.5X2-	T46.5X3-	T46.5X4-	T46.5X5-	T46.5X6-
Dihydrazine	T46.5X1-	T46.5X2-	T46.5X3-	T46.5X4-	T46.5X5-	T46.5X6-
Dihydrocodeine	T40.2X1-	T40.2X2-	T40.2X3-	T40.2X4-	T40.2X5-	T40.2X6-
Dihydrocodeinone	T40.2X1-	T40.2X2-	T40.2X3-	T40.2X4-	T40.2X5-	T40.2X6-
Dihydroergocornine	T46.7X1-	T46.7X2-	T46.7X3-	T46.7X4-	T46.7X5	T46.7X6
Dihydroergocristine (mesilate)	T46.7X1-	T46.7X2-	T46.7X3-	T46.7X4-	T46.7X5-	T46.7X6-
Dihydroergokryptine	T46.7X1-	T46.7X2-	T46.7X3-	T46.7X4-	T46.7X5-	T46.7X6-
Dihydroergotamine	T46.5X1-	T46.5X2-	T46.5X3-	T46.5X4-	T46.5X5-	T46.5X6-
Dihydroergotoxine	T46.7X1-	T46.7X2-	T46.7X3-	T46.7X4-	T46.7X5-	T46.7X6-
mesilate	T46.7X1-	T46.7X2-	T46.7X3-	T46.7X4-	T46.7X5-	T46.7X6-
Dihydrohydroxycodeinone	T40.2X1-	T40.2X2-	T40.2X3-	T40.2X4-	T40.2X5-	T40.2X6-
Dihydrohydroxymorphinone	T40.2X1-	T40.2X2-	T40.2X3-	T40.2X4-	T40.2X5-	T40.2X6-
Dihydroisocodeine	T40.2X1-	T40.2X2-	T40.2X3-	T40.2X4-	T40.2X5-	T40.2X6-
Dihydromorphine	T40.2X1-	T40.2X2-	T40.2X3-	T40.2X4-	-	-
Dihydromorphinone	T40.2X1-	T40.2X2-	T40.2X3-	T40.2X4-	T40.2X5-	T40.2X6-
Dihydrostreptomycin	T36.5X1-	T36.5X2-	T36.5X3-	T36.5X4-	T36.5X5-	T36.5X6-
Dihydrotachysterol	T45.2X1-	T45.2X2-	T45.2X3-	T45.2X4-	T45.2X5-	T45.2X6-
Dihydroxyaluminum aminoacetate	T47.1X1-	T47.1X2-	T47.1X3-	T47.1X4-	T47.1X5-	T47.1X6-
Dihydroxyaluminum sodium carbonate	T47.1X1-	T47.1X2-	T47.1X3-	T47.1X4-	T47.1X5-	T47.1X6-
Dihydroxyanthraquinone	T47.2X1-	T47.2X2-	T47.2X3-	T47.2X4-	T47.2X5-	T47.2X6-
Dihydroxycodeinone	T40.2X1-	T40.2X2-	T40.2X3-	T40.2X4-	T40.2X5-	T40.2X6-
Dihydroxypropyl theophylline	T50.2X1-	T50.2X2-	T50.2X3-	T50.2X4-	T50.2X5-	T50.2X6-
Diiodohydroxyquin	T37.8X1-	T37.8X2-	T37.8X3-	T37.8X4-	T37.8X5-	T37.8X6-
topical	T49.0X1-	T49.0X2-	T49.0X3-	T49.0X4-	T49.0X5-	T49.0X6-
Diiodohydroxyquinoline	T37.8X1-	T37.8X2-	T37.8X3-	T37.8X4-	T37.8X5-	T37.8X6-
Diiodotyrosine	T38.2X1-	T38.2X2-	T38.2X3-	T38.2X4-	T38.2X5-	T38.2X6-

Substance	Poisoning Accidental (unintentional)	Poisoning Intentional self-harm	Poisoning Assault	Poisoning Undetermined	Adverse effect	Underdosing
Diisopromine	T44.3X1-	T44.3X2-	T44.3X3-	T44.3X4-	T44.3X5-	T44.3X6-
Diisopropylamine	T46.3X1-	T46.3X2-	T46.3X3-	T46.3X4-	T46.3X5-	T46.3X6-
Diisopropylfluorophos-phonate	T44.0X1-	T44.0X2-	T44.0X3-	T44.0X4-	T44.0X5-	T44.0X6-
Dilantin	T42.0X1-	T42.0X2-	T42.0X3-	T42.0X4-	T42.0X5-	T42.0X6-
Dilaudid	T40.2X1-	T40.2X2-	T40.2X3-	T40.2X4-	T40.2X5-	T40.2X6-
Dilazep	T46.3X1-	T46.3X2-	T46.3X3-	T46.3X4-	T46.3X5-	T46.3X6-
Dill	T47.5X1-	T47.5X2-	T47.5X3-	T47.5X4-	T47.5X5-	T47.5X6-
Diloxanide	T37.3X1-	T37.3X2-	T37.3X3-	T37.3X4-	T37.3X5-	T37.3X6-
Diltiazem	T46.1X1-	T46.1X2-	T46.1X3-	T46.1X4-	T46.1X5-	T46.1X6-
Dimazole	T49.0X1-	T49.0X2-	T49.0X3-	T49.0X4-	T49.0X5-	T49.0X6-
Dimefline	T50.7X1-	T50.7X2-	T50.7X3-	T50.7X4-	T50.7X5-	T50.7X6-
Dimefox	T60.0X1-	T60.0X2-	T60.0X3-	T60.0X4-	-	-
Dimemorfan	T48.3X1-	T48.3X2-	T48.3X3-	T48.3X4-	T48.3X5-	T48.3X6-
Dimenhydrinate	T45.0X1-	T45.0X2-	T45.0X3-	T45.0X4-	T45.0X5-	T45.0X6-
Dimercaprol (British anti-lewisite)	T45.8X1-	T45.8X2-	T45.8X3-	T45.8X4-	T45.8X5-	T45.8X6-
Dimercaptopropanol	T45.8X1-	T45.8X2-	T45.8X3-	T45.8X4-	T45.8X5-	T45.8X6-
Dimestrol	T38.5X1-	T38.5X2-	T38.5X3-	T38.5X4-	T38.5X5-	T38.5X6-
Dimetane	T45.0X1-	T45.0X2-	T45.0X3-	T45.0X4-	T45.0X5-	T45.0X6-
Dimethicone	T47.1X1-	T47.1X2-	T47.1X3-	T47.1X4-	T47.1X5-	T47.1X6-
Dimethindene	T45.0X1-	T45.0X2-	T45.0X3-	T45.0X4-	T45.0X5-	T45.0X6-
Dimethisoquin	T49.1X1-	T49.1X2-	T49.1X3-	T49.1X4-	T49.1X5-	T49.1X6-
Dimethisterone	T38.5X1-	T38.5X2-	T38.5X3-	T38.5X4-	T38.5X5-	T38.5X6-
Dimethoate	T60.0X1-	T60.0X2-	T60.0X3-	T60.0X4-	-	-
Dimethocaine	T41.3X1-	T41.3X2-	T41.3X3-	T41.3X4-	T41.3X5-	T41.3X6-
Dimethoxanate	T48.3X1-	T48.3X2-	T48.3X3-	T48.3X4-	T48.3X5-	T48.3X6-
Dimethyl						
arsine, arsinic acid	T57.0X1-	T57.0X2-	T57.0X3-	T57.0X4-	-	-
carbinol	T51.2X1-	T51.2X2-	T51.2X3-	T51.2X4-	-	-
carbonate	T52.8X1-	T52.8X2-	T52.8X3-	T52.8X4-	-	-
diguanide	T38.3X1-	T38.3X2-	T38.3X3-	T38.3X4-	T38.3X5-	T38.3X6-
ketone	T52.4X1-	T52.4X2-	T52.4X3-	T52.4X4-	-	-
vapor	T52.4X1-	T52.4X2-	T52.4X3-	T52.4X4-	-	-
meperidine	T40.2X1-	T40.2X2-	T40.2X3-	T40.2X4-	T40.2X5-	T40.2X6-
parathion	T60.0X1-	T60.0X2-	T60.0X3-	T60.0X4-	-	-
phthlate	T49.3X1-	T49.3X2-	T49.3X3-	T49.3X4-	T49.3X5-	T49.3X6-
polysiloxane	T47.8X1-	T47.8X2-	T47.8X3-	T47.8X4-	T47.8X5-	T47.8X6-
sulfate (fumes)	T59.891-	T59.892-	T59.893-	T59.894-	-	-
liquid	T65.891-	T65.892-	T65.893-	T65.894-	-	-
sulfoxide (nonmedicinal)	T52.8X1-	T52.8X2-	T52.8X3-	T52.8X4-	-	-
medicinal	T49.4X1-	T49.4X2-	T49.4X3-	T49.4X4-	T49.4X5-	T49.4X6-
tryptamine	T40.991-	T40.992-	T40.993-	T40.994-	-	-
tubocurarine	T48.1X1-	T48.1X2-	T48.1X3-	T48.1X4-	T48.1X5-	T48.1X6-
Dimethylamine sulfate	T49.4X1-	T49.4X2-	T49.4X3-	T49.4X4-	T49.4X5-	T49.4X6-
Dimethylformamide	T52.8X1-	T52.8X2-	T52.8X3-	T52.8X4-	-	-
Dimethyltubocurarinium chloride	T48.1X1-	T48.1X2-	T48.1X3-	T48.1X4-	T48.1X5-	T48.1X6-
Dimeticone	T47.1X1-	T47.1X2-	T47.1X3-	T47.1X4-	T47.1X5-	T47.1X6-
Dimetilan	T60.0X1-	T60.0X2-	T60.0X3-	T60.0X4-	-	-
Dimetindene	T45.0X1-	T45.0X2-	T45.0X3-	T45.0X4-	T45.0X5-	T45.0X6-
Dimetotiazine	T43.3X1-	T43.3X2-	T43.3X3-	T43.3X4-	T43.3X5-	T43.3X6-
Dimorpholamine	T50.7X1-	T50.7X2-	T50.7X3-	T50.7X4-	T50.7X5-	T50.7X6-
Dimoxyline	T46.3X1-	T46.3X2-	T46.3X3-	T46.3X4-	T46.3X5-	T46.3X6-
Dinitrobenzene	T65.3X1-	T65.3X2-	T65.3X3-	T65.3X4-	-	-
vapor	T59.891-	T59.892-	T59.893-	T59.894-	-	-
Dinitrobenzol	T65.3X1-	T65.3X2-	T65.3X3-	T65.3X4-	-	-
vapor	T59.891-	T59.892-	T59.893-	T59.894-	-	-
Dinitrobutylphenol	T65.3X1-	T65.3X2-	T65.3X3-	T65.3X4-	-	-
Dinitro (-ortho-) **cresol** (pesticide) (spray)	T65.3X1-	T65.3X2-	T65.3X3-	T65.3X4-	-	-
Dinitrocyclohexylphenol	T65.3X1-	T65.3X2-	T65.3X3-	T65.3X4-	-	-
Dinitrophenol	T65.3X1-	T65.3X2-	T65.3X3-	T65.3X4-	-	-
Dinoprost	T48.0X1-	T48.0X2-	T48.0X3-	T48.0X4-	T48.0X5-	T48.0X6-
Dinoprostone	T48.0X1-	T48.0X2-	T48.0X3-	T48.0X4-	T48.0X5-	T48.0X6-
Dinoseb	T60.3X1-	T60.3X2-	T60.3X3-	T60.3X4-	-	-
Dioctyl sulfosuccinate (calcium) (sodium)	T47.4X1-	T47.4X2-	T47.4X3-	T47.4X4-	T47.4X5-	T47.4X6-
Diodone	T50.8X1-	T50.8X2-	T50.8X3-	T50.8X4-	T50.8X5-	T50.8X6-
Diodoquin	T37.8X1-	T37.8X2-	T37.8X3-	T37.8X4-	T37.8X5-	T37.8X6-
Dionin	T40.2X1-	T40.2X2-	T40.2X3-	T40.2X4-	T40.2X5-	T40.2X6-
Diosmin	T46.991-	T46.992-	T46.993-	T46.994-	T46.995-	T46.996-
Dioxane	T52.8X1-	T52.8X2-	T52.8X3-	T52.8X4-	-	-
Dioxathion	T60.0X1-	T60.0X2-	T60.0X3-	T60.0X4-	-	-
Dioxin	T53.7X1-	T53.7X2-	T53.7X3-	T53.7X4-	-	-
Dioxopromethazine	T43.3X1-	T43.3X2-	T43.3X3-	T43.3X4-	T43.3X5-	T43.3X6-
Dioxyline	T46.3X1-	T46.3X2-	T46.3X3-	T46.3X4-	T46.3X5-	T46.3X6-
Dipentene	T52.8X1-	T52.8X2-	T52.8X3-	T52.8X4-	-	-
Diperodon	T41.3X1-	T41.3X2-	T41.3X3-	T41.3X4-	T41.3X5-	T41.3X6-

Diphacinone - Elastase

Table of Drugs and Chemicals

Substance	Poisoning Accidental (unintentional)	Poisoning Intentional self-harm	Poisoning Assault	Poisoning Undetermined	Adverse effect	Underdosing
Diphacinone	T60.4X1-	T60.4X2-	T60.4X3-	T60.4X4-	-	-
Diphemanil	T44.3X1-	T44.3X2-	T44.3X3-	T44.3X4-	T44.3X5-	T44.3X6-
metilsulfate	T44.3X1-	T44.3X2-	T44.3X3-	T44.3X4-	T44.3X5-	T44.3X6-
Diphenadione	T45.511-	T45.512-	T45.513-	T45.514-	T45.515-	T45.516-
rodenticide	T60.4X1-	T60.4X2-	T60.4X3-	T60.4X4-	-	-
Diphenhydramine	T45.0X1-	T45.0X2-	T45.0X3-	T45.0X4-	T45.0X5-	T45.0X6-
Diphenidol	T45.0X1-	T45.0X2-	T45.0X3-	T45.0X4-	T45.0X5-	T45.0X6-
Diphenoxylate	T47.6X1-	T47.6X2-	T47.6X3-	T47.6X4-	T47.6X5-	T47.6X6-
Diphenylamine	T65.3X1-	T65.3X2-	T65.3X3-	T65.3X4-	-	-
Diphenylbutazone	T39.2X1-	T39.2X2-	T39.2X3-	T39.2X4-	T39.2X5-	T39.2X6-
Diphenylchloroarsine, not in war	T57.0X1-	T57.0X2-	T57.0X3-	T57.0X4-	-	-
Diphenylhydantoin	T42.0X1-	T42.0X2-	T42.0X3-	T42.0X4-	T42.0X5-	T42.0X6-
Diphenylmethane dye	T52.1X1-	T52.1X2-	T52.1X3-	T52.1X4-	-	-
Diphenylpyraline	T45.0X1-	T45.0X2-	T45.0X3-	T45.0X4-	T45.0X5-	T45.0X6-
Diphtheria						
antitoxin	T50.Z11-	T50.Z12-	T50.Z13-	T50.Z14-	T50.Z15-	T50.Z16-
toxoid	T50.A91-	T50.A92-	T50.A93-	T50.A94-	T50.A95-	T50.A96-
with tetanus toxoid	T50.A21-	T50.A22-	T50.A23-	T50.A24-	T50.A25-	T50.A26-
with pertussis component	T50.A11-	T50.A12-	T50.A13-	T50.A14-	T50.A15-	T50.A16-
vaccine	T50.A91-	T50.A92-	T50.A93-	T50.A94-	T50.A95-	T50.A96-
combination						
including pertussis	T50.A11-	T50.A12-	T50.A13-	T50.A14-	T50.A15-	T50.A16-
without pertussis	T50.A21-	T50.A22-	T50.A23-	T50.A24-	T50.A25-	T50.A26-
Diphylline	T50.2X1-	T50.2X2-	T50.2X3-	T50.2X4-	T50.2X5-	T50.2X6-
Dipipanone	T40.4X1-	T40.4X2-	T40.4X3-	T40.4X4-	-	-
Dipivefrine	T49.5X1-	T49.5X2-	T49.5X3-	T49.5X4-	T49.5X5-	T49.5X6-
Diplovax	T50.B91-	T50.B92-	T50.B93-	T50.B94-	T50.B95-	T50.B96-
Diprophylline	T50.2X1-	T50.2X2-	T50.2X3-	T50.2X4-	T50.2X5-	T50.2X6-
Dipropyline	T48.291-	T48.292-	T48.293-	T48.294-	T48.295-	T48.296-
Dipyridamole	T46.3X1-	T46.3X2-	T46.3X3-	T46.3X4-	T46.3X5-	T46.3X6-
Dipyrone	T39.2X1-	T39.2X2-	T39.2X3-	T39.2X4-	T39.2X5-	T39.2X6-
Diquat (dibromide)	T60.3X1-	T60.3X2-	T60.3X3-	T60.3X4-	-	-
Disinfectant	T65.891-	T65.892-	T65.893-	T65.894-	-	-
alkaline	T54.3X1-	T54.3X2-	T54.3X3-	T54.3X4-	-	-
aromatic	T54.1X1-	T54.1X2-	T54.1X3-	T54.1X4-	-	-
intestinal	T37.8X1-	T37.8X2-	T37.8X3-	T37.8X4-	T37.8X5-	T37.8X6-
Disipal	T42.8X1-	T42.8X2-	T42.8X3-	T42.8X4-	T42.8X5-	T42.8X6-
Disodium edetate	T50.6X1-	T50.6X2-	T50.6X3-	T50.6X4-	T50.6X5-	T50.6X6-
Disoprofol	T41.291-	T41.292-	T41.293-	T41.294-	T41.295-	T41.296-
Disopyramide	T46.2X1-	T46.2X2-	T46.2X3-	T46.2X4-	T46.2X5-	T46.2X6-
Distigmine (bromide)	T44.0X1-	T44.0X2-	T44.0X3-	T44.0X4-	T44.0X5-	T44.0X6-
Disulfamide	T50.2X1-	T50.2X2-	T50.2X3-	T50.2X4-	T50.2X5-	T50.2X6-
Disulfanilamide	T37.0X1-	T37.0X2-	T37.0X3-	T37.0X4-	T37.0X5-	T37.0X6-
Disulfiram	T50.6X1-	T50.6X2-	T50.6X3-	T50.6X4-	T50.6X5-	T50.6X6-
Disulfoton	T60.0X1-	T60.0X2-	T60.0X3-	T60.0X4-	-	-
Dithiazanine iodide	T37.4X1-	T37.4X2-	T37.4X3-	T37.4X4-	T37.4X5-	T37.4X6-
Dithiocarbamate	T60.0X1-	T60.0X2-	T60.0X3-	T60.0X4-	-	-
Dithranol	T49.4X1-	T49.4X2-	T49.4X3-	T49.4X4-	T49.4X5-	T49.4X6-
Diucardin	T50.2X1-	T50.2X2-	T50.2X3-	T50.2X4-	T50.2X5-	T50.2X6-
Diupres	T50.2X1-	T50.2X2-	T50.2X3-	T50.2X4-	T50.2X5-	T50.2X6-
Diuretic NEC	T50.2X1-	T50.2X2-	T50.2X3-	T50.2X4-	T50.2X5-	T50.2X6-
benzothiadiazine	T50.2X1-	T50.2X2-	T50.2X3-	T50.2X4-	T50.2X5-	T50.2X6-
carbonic acid anhydrase inhibitors	T50.2X1-	T50.2X2-	T50.2X3-	T50.2X4-	T50.2X5-	T50.2X6-
furfuryl NEC	T50.2X1-	T50.2X2-	T50.2X3-	T50.2X4-	T50.2X5-	T50.2X6-
loop (high-ceiling)	T50.1X1-	T50.1X2-	T50.1X3-	T50.1X4-	T50.1X5-	T50.1X6-
mercurial NEC	T50.2X1-	T50.2X2-	T50.2X3-	T50.2X4-	T50.2X5-	T50.2X6-
osmotic	T50.2X1-	T50.2X2-	T50.2X3-	T50.2X4-	T50.2X5-	T50.2X6-
purine NEC	T50.2X1-	T50.2X2-	T50.2X3-	T50.2X4-	T50.2X5-	T50.2X6-
saluretic NEC	T50.2X1-	T50.2X2-	T50.2X3-	T50.2X4-	T50.2X5-	T50.2X6-
sulfonamide	T50.2X1-	T50.2X2-	T50.2X3-	T50.2X4-	T50.2X5-	T50.2X6-
thiazide NEC	T50.2X1-	T50.2X2-	T50.2X3-	T50.2X4-	T50.2X5-	T50.2X6-
xanthine	T50.2X1-	T50.2X2-	T50.2X3-	T50.2X4-	T50.2X5-	T50.2X6-
Diurgin	T50.2X1-	T50.2X2-	T50.2X3-	T50.2X4-	T50.2X5-	T50.2X6-
Diuril	T50.2X1-	T50.2X2-	T50.2X3-	T50.2X4-	T50.2X5-	T50.2X6-
Diuron	T60.3X1-	T60.3X2-	T60.3X3-	T60.3X4-	-	-
Divalproex	T42.6X1-	T42.6X2-	T42.6X3-	T42.6X4-	T42.6X5-	T42.6X6-
Divinyl ether	T41.0X1-	T41.0X2-	T41.0X3-	T41.0X4-	T41.0X5-	T41.0X6-
Dixanthogen	T49.0X1-	T49.0X2-	T49.0X3-	T49.0X4-	T49.0X5-	T49.0X6-
Dixyrazine	T43.3X1-	T43.3X2-	T43.3X3-	T43.3X4-	T43.3X5-	T43.3X6-
D-lysergic acid diethylamide	T40.8X1-	T40.8X2-	T40.8X3-	T40.8X4-	-	-
DMCT	T36.4X1-	T36.4X2-	T36.4X3-	T36.4X4-	T36.4X5-	T36.4X6-
DMSO — *see* Dimethyl sulfoxide						
DNBP	T60.3X1-	T60.3X2-	T60.3X3-	T60.3X4-	-	-
DNOC	T65.3X1-	T65.3X2-	T65.3X3-	T65.3X4-	-	-
Dobutamine	T44.5X1-	T44.5X2-	T44.5X3-	T44.5X4-	T44.5X5-	T44.5X6-
DOCA	T38.0X1-	T38.0X2-	T38.0X3-	T38.0X4-	T38.0X5-	T38.0X6-

Substance	Poisoning Accidental (unintentional)	Poisoning Intentional self-harm	Poisoning Assault	Poisoning Undetermined	Adverse effect	Underdosing
Docusate sodium	T47.4X1-	T47.4X2-	T47.4X3-	T47.4X4-	T47.4X5-	T47.4X6-
Dodicin	T49.0X1-	T49.0X2-	T49.0X3-	T49.0X4-	T49.0X5-	T49.0X6-
Dofamium chloride	T49.0X1-	T49.0X2-	T49.0X3-	T49.0X4-	T49.0X5-	T49.0X6-
Dolophine	T40.3X1-	T40.3X2-	T40.3X3-	T40.3X4-	T40.3X5-	T40.3X6-
Doloxene	T39.8X1-	T39.8X2-	T39.8X3-	T39.8X4-	T39.8X5-	T39.8X6-
Domestic gas (after combustion) — *see* Gas, utility						
prior to combustion	T59.891-	T59.892-	T59.893-	T59.894-	-	-
Domiodol	T48.4X1-	T48.4X2-	T48.4X3-	T48.4X4-	T48.4X5-	T48.4X6-
Domiphen (bromide)	T49.0X1-	T49.0X2-	T49.0X3-	T49.0X4-	T49.0X5-	T49.0X6-
Domperidone	T45.0X1-	T45.0X2-	T45.0X3-	T45.0X4-	T45.0X5-	T45.0X6-
Dopa	T42.8X1-	T42.8X2-	T42.8X3-	T42.8X4-	T42.8X5-	T42.8X6-
Dopamine	T44.991-	T44.992-	T44.993-	T44.994-	T44.995-	T44.996-
Doriden	T42.6X1-	T42.6X2-	T42.6X3-	T42.6X4-	T42.6X5-	T42.6X6-
Dormiral	T42.3X1-	T42.3X2-	T42.3X3-	T42.3X4-	T42.3X5-	T42.3X6-
Dormison	T42.6X1-	T42.6X2-	T42.6X3-	T42.6X4-	T42.6X5-	T42.6X6-
Dornase	T48.4X1-	T48.4X2-	T48.4X3-	T48.4X4-	T48.4X5-	T48.4X6-
Dorsacaine	T41.3X1-	T41.3X2-	T41.3X3-	T41.3X4-	T41.3X5-	T41.3X6-
Dosulepin	T43.011-	T43.012-	T43.013-	T43.014-	T43.015-	T43.016-
Dothiepin	T43.011-	T43.012-	T43.013-	T43.014-	T43.015-	T43.016-
Doxantrazole	T48.6X1-	T48.6X2-	T48.6X3-	T48.6X4-	T48.6X5-	T48.6X6-
Doxapram	T50.7X1-	T50.7X2-	T50.7X3-	T50.7X4-	T50.7X5-	T50.7X6-
Doxazosin	T44.6X1-	T44.6X2-	T44.6X3-	T44.6X4-	T44.6X5-	T44.6X6-
Doxepin	T43.011-	T43.012-	T43.013-	T43.014-	T43.015-	T43.016-
Doxifluridine	T45.1X1-	T45.1X2-	T45.1X3-	T45.1X4-	T45.1X5-	T45.1X6-
Doxorubicin	T45.1X1-	T45.1X2-	T45.1X3-	T45.1X4-	T45.1X5-	T45.1X6-
Doxycycline	T36.4X1-	T36.4X2-	T36.4X3-	T36.4X4-	T36.4X5-	T36.4X6-
Doxylamine	T45.0X1-	T45.0X2-	T45.0X3-	T45.0X4-	T45.0X5-	T45.0X6-
Dramamine	T45.0X1-	T45.0X2-	T45.0X3-	T45.0X4-	T45.0X5-	T45.0X6-
Drano (drain cleaner)	T54.3X1-	T54.3X2-	T54.3X3-	T54.3X4-	-	-
Dressing, live pulp	T49.7X1-	T49.7X2-	T49.7X3-	T49.7X4-	T49.7X5-	T49.7X6-
Drocode	T40.2X1-	T40.2X2-	T40.2X3-	T40.2X4-	T40.2X5-	T40.2X6-
Dromoran	T40.2X1-	T40.2X2-	T40.2X3-	T40.2X4-	T40.2X5-	T40.2X6-
Dromostanolone	T38.7X1-	T38.7X2-	T38.7X3-	T38.7X4-	T38.7X5-	T38.7X6-
Dronabinol	T40.7X1-	T40.7X2-	T40.7X3-	T40.7X4-	T40.7X5-	T40.7X6-
Droperidol	T43.591-	T43.592-	T43.593-	T43.594-	T43.595-	T43.596-
Dropropizine	T48.3X1-	T48.3X2-	T48.3X3-	T48.3X4-	T48.3X5-	T48.3X6-
Drostanolone	T38.7X1-	T38.7X2-	T38.7X3-	T38.7X4-	T38.7X5-	T38.7X6-
Drotaverine	T44.3X1-	T44.3X2-	T44.3X3-	T44.3X4-	T44.3X5-	T44.3X6-
Drotrecogin alfa	T45.511-	T45.512-	T45.513-	T45.514-	T45.515-	T45.516-
Drug NEC	T50.901-	T50.902-	T50.903-	T50.904-	T50.905-	T50.906-
specified NEC	T50.991-	T50.992-	T50.993-	T50.994-	T50.995-	T50.996-
DTIC	T45.1X1-	T45.1X2-	T45.1X3-	T45.1X4-	T45.1X5-	T45.1X6-
Duboisine	T44.3X1-	T44.3X2-	T44.3X3-	T44.3X4-	T44.3X5-	T44.3X6-
Dulcolax	T47.2X1-	T47.2X2-	T47.2X3-	T47.2X4-	T47.2X5-	T47.2X6-
Duponol (C) (EP)	T49.2X1-	T49.2X2-	T49.2X3-	T49.2X4-	T49.2X5-	T49.2X6-
Durabolin	T38.7X1-	T38.7X2-	T38.7X3-	T38.7X4-	T38.7X5-	T38.7X6-
Dyclone	T41.3X1-	T41.3X2-	T41.3X3-	T41.3X4-	T41.3X5-	T41.3X6-
Dyclonine	T41.3X1-	T41.3X2-	T41.3X3-	T41.3X4-	T41.3X5-	T41.3X6-
Dydrogesterone	T38.5X1-	T38.5X2-	T38.5X3-	T38.5X4-	T38.5X5-	T38.5X6-
Dye NEC	T65.6X1-	T65.6X2-	T65.6X3-	T65.6X4-	-	-
antiseptic	T49.0X1-	T49.0X2-	T49.0X3-	T49.0X4-	T49.0X5-	T49.0X6-
diagnostic agents	T50.8X1-	T50.8X2-	T50.8X3-	T50.8X4-	T50.8X5-	T50.8X6-
pharmaceutical NEC	T50.901-	T50.902-	T50.903-	T50.904-	T50.905-	T50.906-
Dyflos	T44.0X1-	T44.0X2-	T44.0X3-	T44.0X4-	T44.0X5-	T44.0X6-
Dymelor	T38.3X1-	T38.3X2-	T38.3X3-	T38.3X4-	T38.3X5-	T38.3X6-
Dynamite	T65.3X1-	T65.3X2-	T65.3X3-	T65.3X4-	-	-
fumes	T59.891-	T59.892-	T59.893-	T59.894-	-	-
Dyphylline	T44.3X1-	T44.3X2-	T44.3X3-	T44.3X4-	T44.3X5-	T44.3X6-
Ear drug NEC	T49.6X1-	T49.6X2-	T49.6X3-	T49.6X4-	T49.6X5-	T49.6X6-
Ear preparations	T49.6X1-	T49.6X2-	T49.6X3-	T49.6X4-	T49.6X5-	T49.6X6-
Echothiophate, echothiopate, ecothiopate	T49.5X1-	T49.5X2-	T49.5X3-	T49.5X4-	T49.5X5-	T49.5X6-
Econazole	T49.0X1-	T49.0X2-	T49.0X3-	T49.0X4-	T49.0X5-	T49.0X6-
Ecothiopate iodide	T49.5X1-	T49.5X2-	T49.5X3-	T49.5X4-	T49.5X5-	T49.5X6-
Ecstasy	T43.641-	T43.642-	T43.643-	T43.644-	-	-
Ectylurea	T42.6X1-	T42.6X2-	T42.6X3-	T42.6X4-	T42.6X5-	T42.6X6-
Edathamil disodium	T45.8X1-	T45.8X2-	T45.8X3-	T45.8X4-	T45.8X5-	T45.8X6-
Edecrin	T50.1X1-	T50.1X2-	T50.1X3-	T50.1X4-	T50.1X5-	T50.1X6-
Edetate, disodium (calcium)	T45.8X1-	T45.8X2-	T45.8X3-	T45.8X4-	T45.8X5-	T45.8X6-
Edoxudine	T49.5X1-	T49.5X2-	T49.5X3-	T49.5X4-	T49.5X5-	T49.5X6-
Edrophonium	T44.0X1-	T44.0X2-	T44.0X3-	T44.0X4-	T44.0X5-	T44.0X6-
chloride	T44.0X1-	T44.0X2-	T44.0X3-	T44.0X4-	T44.0X5-	T44.0X6-
EDTA	T50.6X1-	T50.6X2-	T50.6X3-	T50.6X4-	T50.6X5-	T50.6X6-
Eflornithine	T37.2X1-	T37.2X2-	T37.2X3-	T37.2X4-	T37.2X5-	T37.2X6-
Efloxate	T46.3X1-	T46.3X2-	T46.3X3-	T46.3X4-	T46.3X5-	T46.3X6-
Elase	T49.8X1-	T49.8X2-	T49.8X3-	T49.8X4-	T49.8X5-	T49.8X6-
Elastase	T47.5X1-	T47.5X2-	T47.5X3-	T47.5X4-	T47.5X5-	T47.5X6-

Table of Drugs and Chemicals

Diphacinone — Elastase

Substance	Poisoning Accidental (unintentional)	Poisoning Intentional self-harm	Poisoning Assault	Poisoning Undetermined	Adverse effect	Underdosing
Elaterium	T47.2X1-	T47.2X2-	T47.2X3-	T47.2X4-	T47.2X5-	T47.2X6-
Elcatonin	T50.991-	T50.992-	T50.993-	T50.994-	T50.995-	T50.996-
Elder	T62.2X1-	T62.2X2-	T62.2X3-	T62.2X4-	-	-
berry, (unripe)	T62.1X1-	T62.1X2-	T62.1X3-	T62.1X4-	-	-
Electrolyte balance drug	T50.3X1-	T50.3X2-	T50.3X3-	T50.3X4-	T50.3X5-	T50.3X6-
Electrolytes NEC	T50.3X1-	T50.3X2-	T50.3X3-	T50.3X4-	T50.3X5-	T50.3X6-
Electrolytic agent NEC	T50.3X1-	T50.3X2-	T50.3X3-	T50.3X4-	T50.3X5-	T50.3X6-
Elemental diet	T50.901-	T50.902-	T50.903-	T50.904-	T50.905-	T50.906-
Elliptinium acetate	T45.1X1-	T45.1X2-	T45.1X3-	T45.1X4-	T45.1X5-	T45.1X6-
Embramine	T45.0X1-	T45.0X2-	T45.0X3-	T45.0X4-	T45.0X5-	T45.0X6-
Emepronium (salts)	T44.3X1-	T44.3X2-	T44.3X3-	T44.3X4-	T44.3X5-	T44.3X6-
bromide	T44.3X1-	T44.3X2-	T44.3X3-	T44.3X4-	T44.3X5-	T44.3X6-
Emetic NEC	T47.7X1-	T47.7X2-	T47.7X3-	T47.7X4-	T47.7X5-	T47.7X6-
Emetine	T37.3X1-	T37.3X2-	T37.3X3-	T37.3X4-	T37.3X5-	T37.3X6-
Emollient NEC	T49.3X1-	T49.3X2-	T49.3X3-	T49.3X4-	T49.3X5-	T49.3X6-
Emorfazone	T39.8X1-	T39.8X2-	T39.8X3-	T39.8X4-	T39.8X5-	T39.8X6-
Emylcamate	T43.591-	T43.592-	T43.593-	T43.594-	T43.595-	T43.596-
Enalapril	T46.4X1-	T46.4X2-	T46.4X3-	T46.4X4-	T46.4X5-	T46.4X6-
Enalaprilat	T46.4X1-	T46.4X2-	T46.4X3-	T46.4X4-	T46.4X5-	T46.4X6-
Encainide	T46.2X1-	T46.2X2-	T46.2X3-	T46.2X4-	T46.2X5-	T46.2X6-
Endocaine	T41.3X1-	T41.3X2-	T41.3X3-	T41.3X4-	T41.3X5-	T41.3X6-
Endosulfan	T60.2X1-	T60.2X2-	T60.2X3-	T60.2X4-	-	-
Endothall	T60.3X1-	T60.3X2-	T60.3X3-	T60.3X4-	-	-
Endralazine	T46.5X1-	T46.5X2-	T46.5X3-	T46.5X4-	T46.5X5-	T46.5X6-
Endrin	T60.1X1-	T60.1X2-	T60.1X3-	T60.1X4-	-	-
Enflurane	T41.0X1-	T41.0X2-	T41.0X3-	T41.0X4-	T41.0X5-	T41.0X6-
Enhexymal	T42.3X1-	T42.3X2-	T42.3X3-	T42.3X4-	T42.3X5-	T42.3X6-
Enocitabine	T45.1X1-	T45.1X2-	T45.1X3-	T45.1X4-	T45.1X5-	T45.1X6-
Enovid	T38.4X1-	T38.4X2-	T38.4X3-	T38.4X4-	T38.4X5-	T38.4X6-
Enoxacin	T36.8X1-	T36.8X2-	T36.8X3-	T36.8X4-	T36.8X5-	T36.8X6-
Enoxaparin (sodium)	T45.511-	T45.512-	T45.513-	T45.514-	T45.515-	T45.516-
Enpiprazole	T43.591-	T43.592-	T43.593-	T43.594-	T43.595-	T43.596-
Enprofylline	T48.6X1-	T48.6X2-	T48.6X3-	T48.6X4-	T48.6X5-	T48.6X6-
Enprostil	T47.1X1-	T47.1X2-	T47.1X3-	T47.1X4-	T47.1X5-	T47.1X6-
ENT preparations (anti-infectives)	T49.6X1-	T49.6X2-	T49.6X3-	T49.6X4-	T49.6X5-	T49.6X6-
Enterogastrone	T38.891-	T38.892-	T38.893-	T38.894-	T38.895-	T38.896-
Enviomycin	T36.8X1-	T36.8X2-	T36.8X3-	T36.8X4-	T36.8X5-	T36.8X6-
Enzodase	T45.3X1-	T45.3X2-	T45.3X3-	T45.3X4-	T45.3X5-	T45.3X6-
Enzyme NEC	T45.3X1-	T45.3X2-	T45.3X3-	T45.3X4-	T45.3X5-	T45.3X6-
depolymerizing	T49.8X1-	T49.8X2-	T49.8X3-	T49.8X4-	T49.8X5-	T49.8X6-
fibrolytic	T45.3X1-	T45.3X2-	T45.3X3-	T45.3X4-	T45.3X5-	T45.3X6-
gastric	T47.5X1-	T47.5X2-	T47.5X3-	T47.5X4-	T47.5X5-	T47.5X6-
intestinal	T47.5X1-	T47.5X2-	T47.5X3-	T47.5X4-	T47.5X5-	T47.5X6-
local action	T49.4X1-	T49.4X2-	T49.4X3-	T49.4X4-	T49.4X5-	T49.4X6-
proteolytic	T49.4X1-	T49.4X2-	T49.4X3-	T49.4X4-	T49.4X5-	T49.4X6-
thrombolytic	T45.3X1-	T45.3X2-	T45.3X3-	T45.3X4-	T45.3X5-	T45.3X6-
EPAB	T41.3X1-	T41.3X2-	T41.3X3-	T41.3X4-	T41.3X5-	T41.3X6-
Epanutin	T42.0X1-	T42.0X2-	T42.0X3-	T42.0X4-	T42.0X5-	T42.0X6-
Ephedra	T44.991-	T44.992-	T44.993-	T44.994-	T44.995-	T44.996-
Ephedrine	T44.991-	T44.992-	T44.993-	T44.994-	T44.995-	T44.996-
Epichlorhydrin, epichlorohydrin	T52.8X1-	T52.8X2-	T52.8X3-	T52.8X4-	-	-
Epicillin	T36.0X1-	T36.0X2-	T36.0X3-	T36.0X4-	T36.0X5-	T36.0X6-
Epiestriol	T38.5X1-	T38.5X2-	T38.5X3-	T38.5X4-	T38.5X5-	T38.5X6-
Epilim — *see* Sodium valproate						
Epimestrol	T38.5X1-	T38.5X2-	T38.5X3-	T38.5X4-	T38.5X5-	T38.5X6-
Epinephrine	T44.5X1-	T44.5X2-	T44.5X3-	T44.5X4-	T44.5X5-	T44.5X6-
Epirubicin	T45.1X1-	T45.1X2-	T45.1X3-	T45.1X4-	T45.1X5-	T45.1X6-
Epitiostanol	T38.7X1-	T38.7X2-	T38.7X3-	T38.7X4-	T38.7X5-	T38.7X6-
Epitizide	T50.2X1-	T50.2X2-	T50.2X3-	T50.2X4-	T50.2X5-	T50.2X6-
EPN	T60.0X1-	T60.0X2-	T60.0X3-	T60.0X4-	-	-
EPO	T45.8X1-	T45.8X2-	T45.8X3-	T45.8X4-	T45.8X5-	T45.8X6-
Epoetin alpha	T45.8X1-	T45.8X2-	T45.8X3-	T45.8X4-	T45.8X5-	T45.8X6-
Epomediol	T50.991-	T50.992-	T50.993-	T50.994-	T50.995-	T50.996-
Epoprostenol	T45.521-	T45.522-	T45.523-	T45.524-	T45.525-	T45.526-
Epoxy resin	T65.891-	T65.892-	T65.893-	T65.894-	-	-
Eprazinone	T48.4X1-	T48.4X2-	T48.4X3-	T48.4X4-	T48.4X5-	T48.4X6-
Epsilon amino-caproic acid	T45.621-	T45.622-	T45.623-	T45.624-	T45.625-	T45.626-
Epsom salt	T47.3X1-	T47.3X2-	T47.3X3-	T47.3X4-	T47.3X5-	T47.3X6-
Eptazocine	T40.4X1-	T40.4X2-	T40.4X3-	T40.4X4-	T40.4X5-	T40.4X6-
Equanil	T43.591-	T43.592-	T43.593-	T43.594-	T43.595-	T43.596-
Equisetum	T62.2X1-	T62.2X2-	T62.2X3-	T62.2X4-	-	-
diuretic	T50.2X1-	T50.2X2-	T50.2X3-	T50.2X4-	T50.2X5-	T50.2X6-
Ergobasine	T48.0X1-	T48.0X2-	T48.0X3-	T48.0X4-	T48.0X5-	T48.0X6-
Ergocalciferol	T45.2X1-	T45.2X2-	T45.2X3-	T45.2X4-	T45.2X5-	T45.2X6-
Ergoloid mesylates	T46.7X1-	T46.7X2-	T46.7X3-	T46.7X4-	T46.7X5-	T46.7X6-
Ergometrine	T48.0X1-	T48.0X2-	T48.0X3-	T48.0X4-	T48.0X5-	T48.0X6-
Ergonovine	T48.0X1-	T48.0X2-	T48.0X3-	T48.0X4-	T48.0X5-	T48.0X6-
Ergot NEC	T64.81X-	T64.82X-	T64.83X-	T64.84X-	-	-
derivative	T48.0X1-	T48.0X2-	T48.0X3-	T48.0X4-	T48.0X5-	T48.0X6-
medicinal (alkaloids)	T48.0X1-	T48.0X2-	T48.0X3-	T48.0X4-	T48.0X5-	T48.0X6-
prepared	T48.0X1-	T48.0X2-	T48.0X3-	T48.0X4-	T48.0X5-	T48.0X6-
Ergotamine	T46.5X1-	T46.5X2-	T46.5X3-	T46.5X4-	T46.5X5-	T46.5X6-
Ergotocine	T48.0X1-	T48.0X2-	T48.0X3-	T48.0X4-	T48.0X5-	T48.0X6-
Ergotrate	T48.0X1-	T48.0X2-	T48.0X3-	T48.0X4-	T48.0X5-	T48.0X6-
Eritrityl tetranitrate	T46.3X1-	T46.3X2-	T46.3X3-	T46.3X4-	T46.3X5-	T46.3X6-
Erythrityl tetranitrate	T46.3X1-	T46.3X2-	T46.3X3-	T46.3X4-	T46.3X5-	T46.3X6-
Erythrol tetranitrate	T46.3X1-	T46.3X2-	T46.3X3-	T46.3X4-	T46.3X5-	T46.3X6-
Erythromycin (salts)	T36.3X1-	T36.3X2-	T36.3X3-	T36.3X4-	T36.3X5-	T36.3X6-
ophthalmic preparation	T49.5X1-	T49.5X2-	T49.5X3-	T49.5X4-	T49.5X5-	T49.5X6-
topical NEC	T49.0X1-	T49.0X2-	T49.0X3-	T49.0X4-	T49.0X5-	T49.0X6-
Erythropoietin	T45.8X1-	T45.8X2-	T45.8X3-	T45.8X4-	T45.8X5-	T45.8X6-
human	T45.8X1-	T45.8X2-	T45.8X3-	T45.8X4-	T45.8X5-	T45.8X6-
Escin	T46.991-	T46.992-	T46.993-	T46.994-	T46.995-	T46.996-
Esculin	T45.2X1-	T45.2X2-	T45.2X3-	T45.2X4-	T45.2X5-	T45.2X6-
Esculoside	T45.2X1-	T45.2X2-	T45.2X3-	T45.2X4-	T45.2X5-	T45.2X6-
ESDT (ether-soluble tar distillate)	T49.1X1-	T49.1X2-	T49.1X3-	T49.1X4-	T49.1X5-	T49.1X6-
Eserine	T49.5X1-	T49.5X2-	T49.5X3-	T49.5X4-	T49.5X5-	T49.5X6-
Esflurbiprofen	T39.311-	T39.312-	T39.313-	T39.314-	T39.315-	T39.316-
Eskabarb	T42.3X1-	T42.3X2-	T42.3X3-	T42.3X4-	T42.3X5-	T42.3X6-
Eskalith	T43.8X1-	T43.8X2-	T43.8X3-	T43.8X4-	T43.8X5-	T43.8X6-
Esmolol	T44.7X1-	T44.7X2-	T44.7X3-	T44.7X4-	T44.7X5-	T44.7X6-
Estanozolol	T38.7X1-	T38.7X2-	T38.7X3-	T38.7X4-	T38.7X5-	T38.7X6-
Estazolam	T42.4X1-	T42.4X2-	T42.4X3-	T42.4X4-	T42.4X5-	T42.4X6-
Estradiol	T38.5X1-	T38.5X2-	T38.5X3-	T38.5X4-	T38.5X5-	T38.5X6-
with testosterone	T38.7X1-	T38.7X2-	T38.7X3-	T38.7X4-	T38.7X5-	T38.7X6-
benzoate	T38.5X1-	T38.5X2-	T38.5X3-	T38.5X4-	T38.5X5-	T38.5X6-
Estramustine	T45.1X1-	T45.1X2-	T45.1X3-	T45.1X4-	T45.1X5-	T45.1X6-
Estriol	T38.5X1-	T38.5X2-	T38.5X3-	T38.5X4-	T38.5X5-	T38.5X6-
Estrogen	T38.5X1-	T38.5X2-	T38.5X3-	T38.5X4-	T38.5X5-	T38.5X6-
with progesterone	T38.5X1-	T38.5X2-	T38.5X3-	T38.5X4-	T38.5X5-	T38.5X6-
conjugated	T38.5X1-	T38.5X2-	T38.5X3-	T38.5X4-	T38.5X5-	T38.5X6-
Estrone	T38.5X1-	T38.5X2-	T38.5X3-	T38.5X4-	T38.5X5-	T38.5X6-
Estropipate	T38.5X1-	T38.5X2-	T38.5X3-	T38.5X4-	T38.5X5-	T38.5X6-
Etacrynate sodium	T50.1X1-	T50.1X2-	T50.1X3-	T50.1X4-	T50.1X5-	T50.1X6-
Etacrynic acid	T50.1X1-	T50.1X2-	T50.1X3-	T50.1X4-	T50.1X5-	T50.1X6-
Etafedrine	T48.6X1-	T48.6X2-	T48.6X3-	T48.6X4-	T48.6X5-	T48.6X6-
Etafenone	T46.3X1-	T46.3X2-	T46.3X3-	T46.3X4-	T46.3X5-	T46.3X6-
Etambutol	T37.1X1-	T37.1X2-	T37.1X3-	T37.1X4-	T37.1X5-	T37.1X6-
Etamiphyllin	T48.6X1-	T48.6X2-	T48.6X3-	T48.6X4-	T48.6X5-	T48.6X6-
Etamivan	T50.7X1-	T50.7X2-	T50.7X3-	T50.7X4-	T50.7X5-	T50.7X6-
Etamsylate	T45.7X1-	T45.7X2-	T45.7X3-	T45.7X4-	T45.7X5-	T45.7X6-
Etebenecid	T50.4X1-	T50.4X2-	T50.4X3-	T50.4X4-	T50.4X5-	T50.4X6-
Ethacridine	T49.0X1-	T49.0X2-	T49.0X3-	T49.0X4-	T49.0X5-	T49.0X6-
Ethacrynic acid	T50.1X1-	T50.1X2-	T50.1X3-	T50.1X4-	T50.1X5-	T50.1X6-
Ethadione	T42.2X1-	T42.2X2-	T42.2X3-	T42.2X4-	T42.2X5-	T42.2X6-
Ethambutol	T37.1X1-	T37.1X2-	T37.1X3-	T37.1X4-	T37.1X5-	T37.1X6-
Ethamide	T50.2X1-	T50.2X2-	T50.2X3-	T50.2X4-	T50.2X5-	T50.2X6-
Ethamivan	T50.7X1-	T50.7X2-	T50.7X3-	T50.7X4-	T50.7X5-	T50.7X6-
Ethamsylate	T45.7X1-	T45.7X2-	T45.7X3-	T45.7X4-	T45.7X5-	T45.7X6-
Ethanol	T51.0X1-	T51.0X2-	T51.0X3-	T51.0X4-	-	-
beverage	T51.0X1-	T51.0X2-	T51.0X3-	T51.0X4-	-	-
Ethanolamine oleate	T46.8X1-	T46.8X2-	T46.8X3-	T46.8X4-	T46.8X5-	T46.8X6-
Ethaverine	T44.3X1-	T44.3X2-	T44.3X3-	T44.3X4-	T44.3X5-	T44.3X6-
Ethchlorvynol	T42.6X1-	T42.6X2-	T42.6X3-	T42.6X4-	T42.6X5-	T42.6X6-
Ethebenecid	T50.4X1-	T50.4X2-	T50.4X3-	T50.4X4-	T50.4X5-	T50.4X6-
Ether (vapor)	T41.0X1-	T41.0X2-	T41.0X3-	T41.0X4-	T41.0X5-	T41.0X6-
anesthetic	T41.0X1-	T41.0X2-	T41.0X3-	T41.0X4-	T41.0X5-	T41.0X6-
divinyl	T41.0X1-	T41.0X2-	T41.0X3-	T41.0X4-	T41.0X5-	T41.0X6-
ethyl (medicinal)	T41.0X1-	T41.0X2-	T41.0X3-	T41.0X4-	T41.0X5-	T41.0X6-
nonmedicinal	T52.8X1-	T52.8X2-	T52.8X3-	T52.8X4-	-	-
petroleum — *see* Ligroin						
solvent	T52.8X1-	T52.8X2-	T52.8X3-	T52.8X4-	-	-
Ethiazide	T50.2X1-	T50.2X2-	T50.2X3-	T50.2X4-	T50.2X5-	T50.2X6-
Ethidium chloride (vapor)	T59.891-	T59.892-	T59.893-	T59.894-	-	-
Ethinamate	T42.6X1-	T42.6X2-	T42.6X3-	T42.6X4-	T42.6X5-	T42.6X6-
Ethinylestradiol, ethinyloestradiol	T38.5X1-	T38.5X2-	T38.5X3-	T38.5X4-	T38.5X5-	T38.5X6-
with						
levonorgestrel	T38.4X1-	T38.4X2-	T38.4X3-	T38.4X4-	T38.4X5-	T38.4X6-
norethisterone	T38.4X1-	T38.4X2-	T38.4X3-	T38.4X4-	T38.4X5-	T38.4X6-
Ethiodized oil (131 I)	T50.8X1-	T50.8X2-	T50.8X3-	T50.8X4-	T50.8X5-	T50.8X6-
Ethion	T60.0X1-	T60.0X2-	T60.0X3-	T60.0X4-	-	-
Ethionamide	T37.1X1-	T37.1X2-	T37.1X3-	T37.1X4-	T37.1X5-	T37.1X6-

Substance	Poisoning Accidental (unintentional)	Poisoning Intentional self-harm	Poisoning Assault	Poisoning Undetermined	Adverse effect	Underdosing
Ethioniamide	T37.1X1-	T37.1X2-	T37.1X3-	T37.1X4-	T37.1X5-	T37.1X6-
Ethisterone	T38.5X1-	T38.5X2-	T38.5X3-	T38.5X4-	T38.5X5-	T38.5X6-
Ethobral	T42.3X1-	T42.3X2-	T42.3X3-	T42.3X4-	T42.3X5-	T42.3X6-
Ethocaine (infiltration) (topical)	T41.3X1-	T41.3X2-	T41.3X3-	T41.3X4-	T41.3X5-	T41.3X6-
nerve block (peripheral) (plexus)	T41.3X1-	T41.3X2-	T41.3X3-	T41.3X4-	T41.3X5-	T41.3X6-
spinal	T41.3X1-	T41.3X2-	T41.3X3-	T41.3X4-	T41.3X5-	T41.3X6-
Ethoheptazine	T40.4X1-	T40.4X2-	T40.4X3-	T40.4X4-	T40.4X5-	T40.4X6-
Ethopropazine	T44.3X1-	T44.3X2-	T44.3X3-	T44.3X4-	T44.3X5-	T44.3X6-
Ethosuximide	T42.2X1-	T42.2X2-	T42.2X3-	T42.2X4-	T42.2X5-	T42.2X6-
Ethotoin	T42.0X1-	T42.0X2-	T42.0X3-	T42.0X4-	T42.0X5-	T42.0X6-
Ethoxazene	T37.91X-	T37.92X-	T37.93X-	T37.94X-	T37.95X-	T37.96X-
Ethoxazorutoside	T46.991-	T46.992-	T46.993-	T46.994-	T46.995-	T46.996-
2-Ethoxyethanol	T52.3X1-	T52.3X2-	T52.3X3-	T52.3X4-	-	-
Ethoxzolamide	T50.2X1-	T50.2X2-	T50.2X3-	T50.2X4-	T50.2X5-	T50.2X6-
Ethyl						
acetate	T52.8X1-	T52.8X2-	T52.8X3-	T52.8X4-	-	-
alcohol	T51.0X1-	T51.0X2-	T51.0X3-	T51.0X4-	-	-
beverage	T51.0X1-	T51.0X2-	T51.0X3-	T51.0X4-	-	-
aldehyde (vapor)	T59.891-	T59.892-	T59.893-	T59.894-	-	-
liquid	T52.8X1-	T52.8X2-	T52.8X3-	T52.8X4-	-	-
aminobenzoate	T41.3X1-	T41.3X2-	T41.3X3-	T41.3X4-	T41.3X5-	T41.3X6-
aminophenothiazine	T43.3X1-	T43.3X2-	T43.3X3-	T43.3X4-	T43.3X5-	T43.3X6-
benzoate	T52.8X1-	T52.8X2-	T52.8X3-	T52.8X4-	-	-
biscoumacetate	T45.511-	T45.512-	T45.513-	T45.514-	T45.515-	T45.516-
bromide (anesthetic)	T41.0X1-	T41.0X2-	T41.0X3-	T41.0X4-	T41.0X5-	T41.0X6-
carbamate	T45.1X1-	T45.1X2-	T45.1X3-	T45.1X4-	T45.1X5-	T45.1X6-
carbinol	T51.3X1-	T51.3X2-	T51.3X3-	T51.3X4-	-	-
carbonate	T52.8X1-	T52.8X2-	T52.8X3-	T52.8X4-	-	-
chaulmoograte	T37.1X1-	T37.1X2-	T37.1X3-	T37.1X4-	T37.1X5-	T37.1X6-
chloride (anesthetic)	T41.0X1-	T41.0X2-	T41.0X3-	T41.0X4-	T41.0X5-	T41.0X6-
anesthetic (local)	T41.3X1-	T41.3X2-	T41.3X3-	T41.3X4-	T41.3X5-	T41.3X6-
inhaled	T41.0X1-	T41.0X2-	T41.0X3-	T41.0X4-	T41.0X5-	T41.0X6-
local	T49.4X1-	T49.4X2-	T49.4X3-	T49.4X4-	T49.4X5-	T49.4X6-
solvent	T53.6X1-	T53.6X2-	T53.6X3-	T53.6X4-	-	-
dibunate	T48.3X1-	T48.3X2-	T48.3X3-	T48.3X4-	T48.3X5-	T48.3X6-
dichloroarsine (vapor)	T57.0X1-	T57.0X2-	T57.0X3-	T57.0X4-	-	-
estranol	T38.7X1-	T38.7X2-	T38.7X3-	T38.7X4-	T38.7X5-	T38.7X6-
ether — *see also* ether	T52.8X1-	T52.8X2-	T52.8X3-	T52.8X4-	-	-
formate NEC (solvent)	T52.0X1-	T52.0X2-	T52.0X3-	T52.0X4-	-	-
fumarate	T49.4X1-	T49.4X2-	T49.4X3-	T49.4X4-	T49.4X5-	T49.4X6-
hydroxyisobutyrate NEC (solvent)	T52.8X1-	T52.8X2-	T52.8X3-	T52.8X4-	-	-
iodoacetate	T59.3X1-	T59.3X2-	T59.3X3-	T59.3X4-	-	-
lactate NEC (solvent)	T52.8X1-	T52.8X2-	T52.8X3-	T52.8X4-	-	-
loflazepate	T42.4X1-	T42.4X2-	T42.4X3-	T42.4X4-	T42.4X5-	T42.4X6-
mercuric chloride	T56.1X1-	T56.1X2-	T56.1X3-	T56.1X4-	-	-
methylcarbinol	T51.8X1-	T51.8X2-	T51.8X3-	T51.8X4-	-	-
morphine	T40.2X1-	T40.2X2-	T40.2X3-	T40.2X4-	T40.2X5-	T40.2X6-
noradrenaline	T48.6X1-	T48.6X2-	T48.6X3-	T48.6X4-	T48.6X5-	T48.6X6-
oxybutyrate NEC (solvent)	T52.8X1-	T52.8X2-	T52.8X3-	T52.8X4-	-	-
Ethylene (gas)	T59.891-	T59.892-	T59.893-	T59.894-	-	-
anesthetic (general)	T41.0X1-	T41.0X2-	T41.0X3-	T41.0X4-	T41.0X5-	T41.0X6-
chlorohydrin	T52.8X1-	T52.8X2-	T52.8X3-	T52.8X4-	-	-
vapor	T53.6X1-	T53.6X2-	T53.6X3-	T53.6X4-	-	-
dichloride	T52.8X1-	T52.8X2-	T52.8X3-	T52.8X4-	-	-
vapor	T53.6X1-	T53.6X2-	T53.6X3-	T53.6X4-	-	-
dinitrate	T52.3X1-	T52.3X2-	T52.3X3-	T52.3X4-	-	-
glycol (s)	T52.8X1-	T52.8X2-	T52.8X3-	T52.8X4-	-	-
dinitrate	T52.3X1-	T52.3X2-	T52.3X3-	T52.3X4-	-	-
monobutyl ether	T52.3X1-	T52.3X2-	T52.3X3-	T52.3X4-	-	-
imine	T54.1X1-	T54.1X2-	T54.1X3-	T54.1X4-	-	-
oxide (fumigant) (nonmedicinal)	T59.891-	T59.892-	T59.893-	T59.894-	-	-
medicinal	T49.0X1-	T49.0X2-	T49.0X3-	T49.0X4-	T49.0X5-	T49.0X6-
Ethylenediamine theophylline	T48.6X1-	T48.6X2-	T48.6X3-	T48.6X4-	T48.6X5-	T48.6X6-
Ethylenediaminetetra-acetic acid	T50.6X1-	T50.6X2-	T50.6X3-	T50.6X4-	T50.6X5-	T50.6X6-
Ethylenedinitrilotetra-acetate	T50.6X1-	T50.6X2-	T50.6X3-	T50.6X4-	T50.6X5-	T50.6X6-
Ethylestrenol	T38.7X1-	T38.7X2-	T38.7X3-	T38.7X4-	T38.7X5-	T38.7X6-
Ethylhydroxycellulose	T47.4X1-	T47.4X2-	T47.4X3-	T47.4X4-	T47.4X5-	T47.4X6-
Ethylidene						
chloride NEC	T53.6X1-	T53.6X2-	T53.6X3-	T53.6X4-	-	-
diacetate	T60.3X1-	T60.3X2-	T60.3X3-	T60.3X4-	-	-
dicoumarin	T45.511-	T45.512-	T45.513-	T45.514-	T45.515-	T45.516-
dicoumarol	T45.511-	T45.512-	T45.513-	T45.514-	T45.515-	T45.516-
diethyl ether	T52.0X1-	T52.0X2-	T52.0X3-	T52.0X4-	-	-
Ethylmorphine	T40.2X1-	T40.2X2-	T40.2X3-	T40.2X4-	T40.2X5-	T40.2X6-
Ethylnorepinephrine	T48.6X1-	T48.6X2-	T48.6X3-	T48.6X4-	T48.6X5-	T48.6X6-

Substance	Poisoning Accidental (unintentional)	Poisoning Intentional self-harm	Poisoning Assault	Poisoning Undetermined	Adverse effect	Underdosing
Ethylparachlorophen-oxyisobutyrate	T46.6X1-	T46.6X2-	T46.6X3-	T46.6X4-	T46.6X5-	T46.6X6-
Ethynodiol	T38.4X1-	T38.4X2-	T38.4X3-	T38.4X4-	T38.4X5-	T38.4X6-
with mestranol diacetate	T38.4X1-	T38.4X2-	T38.4X3-	T38.4X4-	T38.4X5-	T38.4X6-
Etidocaine	T41.3X1-	T41.3X2-	T41.3X3-	T41.3X4-	T41.3X5-	T41.3X6-
infiltration (subcutaneous)	T41.3X1-	T41.3X2-	T41.3X3-	T41.3X4-	T41.3X5-	T41.3X6-
nerve (peripheral) (plexus)	T41.3X1-	T41.3X2-	T41.3X3-	T41.3X4-	T41.3X5-	T41.3X6-
Etidronate	T50.991-	T50.992-	T50.993-	T50.994-	T50.995-	T50.996-
Etidronic acid (disodium salt)	T50.991-	T50.992-	T50.993-	T50.994-	T50.995-	T50.996-
Etifoxine	T42.6X1-	T42.6X2-	T42.6X3-	T42.6X4-	T42.6X5-	T42.6X6-
Etilefrine	T44.4X1-	T44.4X2-	T44.4X3-	T44.4X4-	T44.4X5-	T44.4X6-
Etilfen	T42.3X1-	T42.3X2-	T42.3X3-	T42.3X4-	T42.3X5-	T42.3X6-
Etinodiol	T38.4X1-	T38.4X2-	T38.4X3-	T38.4X4-	T38.4X5-	T38.4X6-
Etiroxate	T46.6X1-	T46.6X2-	T46.6X3-	T46.6X4-	T46.6X5-	T46.6X6-
Etizolam	T42.4X1-	T42.4X2-	T42.4X3-	T42.4X4-	T42.4X5-	T42.4X6-
Etodolac	T39.391-	T39.392-	T39.393-	T39.394-	T39.395-	T39.396-
Etofamide	T37.3X1-	T37.3X2-	T37.3X3-	T37.3X4-	T37.3X5-	T37.3X6-
Etofibrate	T46.6X1-	T46.6X2-	T46.6X3-	T46.6X4-	T46.6X5-	T46.6X6-
Etofylline	T46.7X1-	T46.7X2-	T46.7X3-	T46.7X4-	T46.7X5-	T46.7X6-
clofibrate	T46.6X1-	T46.6X2-	T46.6X3-	T46.6X4-	T46.6X5-	T46.6X6-
Etoglucid	T45.1X1-	T45.1X2-	T45.1X3-	T45.1X4-	T45.1X5-	T45.1X6-
Etomidate	T41.1X1-	T41.1X2-	T41.1X3-	T41.1X4-	T41.1X5-	T41.1X6-
Etomide	T39.8X1-	T39.8X2-	T39.8X3-	T39.8X4-	T39.8X5-	T39.8X6-
Etomidoline	T44.3X1-	T44.3X2-	T44.3X3-	T44.3X4-	T44.3X5-	T44.3X6-
Etoposide	T45.1X1-	T45.1X2-	T45.1X3-	T45.1X4-	T45.1X5-	T45.1X6-
Etorphine	T40.2X1-	T40.2X2-	T40.2X3-	T40.2X4-	T40.2X5-	T40.2X6-
Etoval	T42.3X1-	T42.3X2-	T42.3X3-	T42.3X4-	T42.3X5-	T42.3X6-
Etozolin	T50.1X1-	T50.1X2-	T50.1X3-	T50.1X4-	T50.1X5-	T50.1X6-
Etretinate	T50.991-	T50.992-	T50.993-	T50.994-	T50.995-	T50.996-
Etryptamine	T43.691-	T43.692-	T43.693-	T43.694-	T43.695-	T43.696-
Etybenzatropine	T44.3X1-	T44.3X2-	T44.3X3-	T44.3X4-	T44.3X5-	T44.3X6-
Etynodiol	T38.4X1-	T38.4X2-	T38.4X3-	T38.4X4-	T38.4X5-	T38.4X6-
Eucaine	T41.3X1-	T41.3X2-	T41.3X3-	T41.3X4-	T41.3X5-	T41.3X6-
Eucalyptus oil	T49.7X1-	T49.7X2-	T49.7X3-	T49.7X4-	T49.7X5-	T49.7X6-
Eucatropine	T49.5X1-	T49.5X2-	T49.5X3-	T49.5X4-	T49.5X5-	T49.5X6-
Eucodal	T40.2X1-	T40.2X2-	T40.2X3-	T40.2X4-	T40.2X5-	T40.2X6-
Euneryl	T42.3X1-	T42.3X2-	T42.3X3-	T42.3X4-	T42.3X5-	T42.3X6-
Euphthalmine	T44.3X1-	T44.3X2-	T44.3X3-	T44.3X4-	T44.3X5-	T44.3X6-
Eurax	T49.0X1-	T49.0X2-	T49.0X3-	T49.0X4-	T49.0X5-	T49.0X6-
Euresol	T49.4X1-	T49.4X2-	T49.4X3-	T49.4X4-	T49.4X5-	T49.4X6-
Euthroid	T38.1X1-	T38.1X2-	T38.1X3-	T38.1X4-	T38.1X5-	T38.1X6-
Evans blue	T50.8X1-	T50.8X2-	T50.8X3-	T50.8X4-	T50.8X5-	T50.8X6-
Evipal	T42.3X1-	T42.3X2-	T42.3X3-	T42.3X4-	T42.3X5-	T42.3X6-
sodium	T41.1X1-	T41.1X2-	T41.1X3-	T41.1X4-	T41.1X5-	T41.1X6-
Evipan	T42.3X1-	T42.3X2-	T42.3X3-	T42.3X4-	T42.3X5-	T42.3X6-
sodium	T41.1X1-	T41.1X2-	T41.1X3-	T41.1X4-	T41.1X5-	T41.1X6-
Exalamide	T49.0X1-	T49.0X2-	T49.0X3-	T49.0X4-	T49.0X5-	T49.0X6-
Exalgin	T39.1X1-	T39.1X2-	T39.1X3-	T39.1X4-	T39.1X5-	T39.1X6-
Excipients, pharmaceutical	T50.901-	T50.902-	T50.903-	T50.904-	T50.905-	T50.906-
Exhaust gas (engine) (motor vehicle)	T58.01X-	T58.02X-	T58.03X-	T58.04X-	-	-
Ex-Lax (phenolphthalein)	T47.2X1-	T47.2X2-	T47.2X3-	T47.2X4-	T47.2X5-	T47.2X6-
Expectorant NEC	T48.4X1-	T48.4X2-	T48.4X3-	T48.4X4-	T48.4X5-	T48.4X6-
Extended insulin zinc suspension	T38.3X1-	T38.3X2-	T38.3X3-	T38.3X4-	T38.3X5-	T38.3X6-
External medications (skin) (mucous membrane)	T49.91X-	T49.92X-	T49.93X-	T49.94X-	T49.95X-	T49.96X-
dental agent	T49.7X1-	T49.7X2-	T49.7X3-	T49.7X4-	T49.7X5-	T49.7X6-
ENT agent	T49.6X1-	T49.6X2-	T49.6X3-	T49.6X4-	T49.6X5-	T49.6X6-
ophthalmic preparation	T49.5X1-	T49.5X2-	T49.5X3-	T49.5X4-	T49.5X5-	T49.5X6-
specified NEC	T49.8X1-	T49.8X2-	T49.8X3-	T49.8X4-	T49.8X5-	T49.8X6-
Extrapyramidal antagonist NEC	T44.3X1-	T44.3X2-	T44.3X3-	T44.3X4-	T44.3X5-	T44.3X6-
Eye agents (anti-infective)	T49.5X1-	T49.5X2-	T49.5X3-	T49.5X4-	T49.5X5-	T49.5X6-
Eye drug NEC	T49.5X1-	T49.5X2-	T49.5X3-	T49.5X4-	T49.5X5-	T49.5X6-
FAC (fluorouracil + doxorubicin + cyclophosphamide)	T45.1X1-	T45.1X2-	T45.1X3-	T45.1X4-	T45.1X5-	T45.1X6-
Factor						
I (fibrinogen)	T45.8X1-	T45.8X2-	T45.8X3-	T45.8X4-	T45.8X5-	T45.8X6-
III (thromboplastin)	T45.8X1-	T45.8X2-	T45.8X3-	T45.8X4-	T45.8X5-	T45.8X6-
VIII (antihemophilic Factor) (concentrate)	T45.8X1-	T45.8X2-	T45.8X3-	T45.8X4-	T45.8X5-	T45.8X6-
IX complex	T45.7X1-	T45.7X2-	T45.7X3-	T45.7X4-	T45.7X5-	T45.7X6-
human	T45.8X1-	T45.8X2-	T45.8X3-	T45.8X4-	T45.8X5-	T45.8X6-
Famotidine	T47.0X1-	T47.0X2-	T47.0X3-	T47.0X4-	T47.0X5-	T47.0X6-
Fat suspension, intravenous	T50.991-	T50.992-	T50.993-	T50.994-	T50.995-	T50.996-
Fazadinium bromide	T48.1X1-	T48.1X2-	T48.1X3-	T48.1X4-	T48.1X5-	T48.1X6-
Febarbamate	T42.3X1-	T42.3X2-	T42.3X3-	T42.3X4-	T42.3X5-	T42.3X6-
Fecal softener	T47.4X1-	T47.4X2-	T47.4X3-	T47.4X4-	T47.4X5-	T47.4X6-

Substance	Poisoning Accidental (unintentional)	Poisoning Intentional self-harm	Poisoning Assault	Poisoning Undetermined	Adverse effect	Underdosing
Fedrilate	T48.3X1-	T48.3X2-	T48.3X3-	T48.3X4-	T48.3X5-	T48.3X6-
Felodipine	T46.1X1-	T46.1X2-	T46.1X3-	T46.1X4-	T46.1X5-	T46.1X6-
Felypressin	T38.891-	T38.892-	T38.893-	T38.894-	T38.895-	T38.896-
Femoxetine	T43.221-	T43.222-	T43.223-	T43.224-	T43.225-	T43.226-
Fenalcomine	T46.3X1-	T46.3X2-	T46.3X3-	T46.3X4-	T46.3X5-	T46.3X6-
Fenamisal	T37.1X1-	T37.1X2-	T37.1X3-	T37.1X4-	T37.1X5-	T37.1X6-
Fenazone	T39.2X1-	T39.2X2-	T39.2X3-	T39.2X4-	T39.2X5-	T39.2X6-
Fenbendazole	T37.4X1-	T37.4X2-	T37.4X3-	T37.4X4-	T37.4X5-	T37.4X6-
Fenbutrazate	T50.5X1-	T50.5X2-	T50.5X3-	T50.5X4-	T50.5X5-	T50.5X6-
Fencamfamine	T43.691-	T43.692-	T43.693-	T43.694-	T43.695-	T43.696-
Fendiline	T46.1X1-	T46.1X2-	T46.1X3-	T46.1X4-	T46.1X5-	T46.1X6-
Fenetylline	T43.691-	T43.692-	T43.693-	T43.694-	T43.695-	T43.696-
Fenflumizole	T39.391-	T39.392-	T39.393-	T39.394-	T39.395-	T39.396-
Fenfluramine	T50.5X1-	T50.5X2-	T50.5X3-	T50.5X4-	T50.5X5-	T50.5X6-
Fenobarbital	T42.3X1-	T42.3X2-	T42.3X3-	T42.3X4-	T42.3X5-	T42.3X6-
Fenofibrate	T46.6X1-	T46.6X2-	T46.6X3-	T46.6X4-	T46.6X5-	T46.6X6-
Fenoprofen	T39.311-	T39.312-	T39.313-	T39.314-	T39.315-	T39.316-
Fenoterol	T48.6X1-	T48.6X2-	T48.6X3-	T48.6X4-	T48.6X5-	T48.6X6-
Fenoverine	T44.3X1-	T44.3X2-	T44.3X3-	T44.3X4-	T44.3X5-	T44.3X6-
Fenoxazoline	T48.5X1-	T48.5X2-	T48.5X3-	T48.5X4-	T48.5X5-	T48.5X6-
Fenproporex	T50.5X1-	T50.5X2-	T50.5X3-	T50.5X4-	T50.5X5-	T50.5X6-
Fenquizone	T50.2X1-	T50.2X2-	T50.2X3-	T50.2X4-	T50.2X5-	T50.2X6-
Fentanyl	T40.4X1-	T40.4X2-	T40.4X3-	T40.4X4-	T40.4X5-	T40.4X6-
Fentazin	T43.3X1-	T43.3X2-	T43.3X3-	T43.3X4-	T43.3X5-	T43.3X6-
Fenthion	T60.0X1-	T60.0X2-	T60.0X3-	T60.0X4-	-	-
Fenticlor	T49.0X1-	T49.0X2-	T49.0X3-	T49.0X4-	T49.0X5-	T49.0X6-
Fenylbutazone	T39.2X1-	T39.2X2-	T39.2X3-	T39.2X4-	T39.2X5-	T39.2X6-
Feprazone	T39.2X1-	T39.2X2-	T39.2X3-	T39.2X4-	T39.2X5-	T39.2X6-
Fer de lance (bite) (venom)	T63.061-	T63.062-	T63.063-	T63.064-	-	-
Ferric — *see also* Iron						
chloride	T45.4X1-	T45.4X2-	T45.4X3-	T45.4X4-	T45.4X5-	T45.4X6-
citrate	T45.4X1-	T45.4X2-	T45.4X3-	T45.4X4-	T45.4X5-	T45.4X6-
hydroxide						
colloidal	T45.4X1-	T45.4X2-	T45.4X3-	T45.4X4-	T45.4X5-	T45.4X6-
polymaltose	T45.4X1-	T45.4X2-	T45.4X3-	T45.4X4-	T45.4X5-	T45.4X6-
pyrophosphate	T45.4X1-	T45.4X2-	T45.4X3-	T45.4X4-	T45.4X5-	T45.4X6-
Ferritin	T45.4X1-	T45.4X2-	T45.4X3-	T45.4X4-	T45.4X5-	T45.4X6-
Ferrocholinate	T45.4X1-	T45.4X2-	T45.4X3-	T45.4X4-	T45.4X5-	T45.4X6-
Ferrodextrane	T45.4X1-	T45.4X2-	T45.4X3-	T45.4X4-	T45.4X5-	T45.4X6-
Ferropolimaler	T45.4X1-	T45.4X2-	T45.4X3-	T45.4X4-	T45.4X5-	T45.4X6-
Ferrous — *see also* Iron						
phosphate	T45.4X1-	T45.4X2-	T45.4X3-	T45.4X4-	T45.4X5-	T45.4X6-
salt	T45.4X1-	T45.4X2-	T45.4X3-	T45.4X4-	T45.4X5-	T45.4X6-
with folic acid	T45.4X1-	T45.4X2-	T45.4X3-	T45.4X4-	T45.4X5-	T45.4X6-
Ferrous fumerate, gluconate, lactate, salt NEC, sulfate (medicinal)	T45.4X1-	T45.4X2-	T45.4X3-	T45.4X4-	T45.4X5-	T45.4X6-
Ferrovanadium (fumes)	T59.891-	T59.892-	T59.893-	T59.894-	-	-
Ferrum — *see* Iron						
Fertilizers NEC	T65.891-	T65.892-	T65.893-	T65.894-	-	-
with herbicide mixture	T60.3X1-	T60.3X2-	T60.3X3-	T60.3X4-	-	-
Fetoxilate	T47.6X1-	T47.6X2-	T47.6X3-	T47.6X4-	T47.6X5-	T47.6X6-
Fiber, dietary	T47.4X1-	T47.4X2-	T47.4X3-	T47.4X4-	T47.4X5-	T47.4X6-
Fiberglass	T65.831-	T65.832-	T65.833-	T65.834-	-	-
Fibrinogen (human)	T45.8X1-	T45.8X2-	T45.8X3-	T45.8X4-	T45.8X5-	T45.8X6-
Fibrinolysin (human)	T45.691-	T45.692-	T45.693-	T45.694-	T45.695-	T45.696-
Fibrinolysis						
affecting drug	T45.601-	T45.602-	T45.603-	T45.604-	T45.605-	T45.606-
inhibitor NEC	T45.621-	T45.622-	T45.623-	T45.624-	T45.625-	T45.626-
Fibrinolytic drug	T45.611-	T45.612-	T45.613-	T45.614-	T45.615-	T45.616-
Filix mas	T37.4X1-	T37.4X2-	T37.4X3-	T37.4X4-	T37.4X5-	T37.4X6-
Filtering cream	T49.3X1-	T49.3X2-	T49.3X3-	T49.3X4-	T49.3X5-	T49.3X6-
Fiorinal	T39.011-	T39.012-	T39.013-	T39.014-	T39.015-	T39.016-
Firedamp	T59.891-	T59.892-	T59.893-	T59.894-	-	-
Fish, noxious, nonbacterial	T61.91X-	T61.92X-	T61.93X-	T61.94X-	-	-
ciguatera	T61.01X-	T61.02X-	T61.03X-	T61.04X-	-	-
scombroid	T61.11X-	T61.12X-	T61.13X-	T61.14X-	-	-
shell	T61.781-	T61.782-	T61.783-	T61.784-	-	-
specified NEC	T61.771-	T61.772-	T61.773-	T61.774-	-	-
Flagyl	T37.3X1-	T37.3X2-	T37.3X3-	T37.3X4-	T37.3X5-	T37.3X6-
Flavine adenine dinucleotide	T45.2X1-	T45.2X2-	T45.2X3-	T45.2X4-	T45.2X5-	T45.2X6-
Flavodic acid	T46.991-	T46.992-	T46.993-	T46.994-	T46.995-	T46.996-
Flavoxate	T44.3X1-	T44.3X2-	T44.3X3-	T44.3X4-	T44.3X5-	T44.3X6-
Flaxedil	T48.1X1-	T48.1X2-	T48.1X3-	T48.1X4-	T48.1X5-	T48.1X6-
Flaxseed (medicinal)	T49.3X1-	T49.3X2-	T49.3X3-	T49.3X4-	T49.3X5-	T49.3X6-
Flecainide	T46.2X1-	T46.2X2-	T46.2X3-	T46.2X4-	T46.2X5-	T46.2X6-
Fleroxacin	T36.8X1-	T36.8X2-	T36.8X3-	T36.8X4-	T36.8X5-	T36.8X6-
Floctafenine	T39.8X1-	T39.8X2-	T39.8X3-	T39.8X4-	T39.8X5-	T39.8X6-

Substance	Poisoning Accidental (unintentional)	Poisoning Intentional self-harm	Poisoning Assault	Poisoning Undetermined	Adverse effect	Underdosing
Flomax	T44.6X1-	T44.6X2-	T44.6X3-	T44.6X4-	T44.6X5-	T44.6X6-
Flomoxef	T36.1X1-	T36.1X2-	T36.1X3-	T36.1X4-	T36.1X5-	T36.1X6-
Flopropione	T44.3X1-	T44.3X2-	T44.3X3-	T44.3X4-	T44.3X5-	T44.3X6-
Florantyrone	T47.5X1-	T47.5X2-	T47.5X3-	T47.5X4-	T47.5X5-	T47.5X6-
Floraquin	T37.8X1-	T37.8X2-	T37.8X3-	T37.8X4-	T37.8X5-	T37.8X6-
Florinef	T38.0X1-	T38.0X2-	T38.0X3-	T38.0X4-	T38.0X5-	T38.0X6-
ENT agent	T49.6X1-	T49.6X2-	T49.6X3-	T49.6X4-	T49.6X5-	T49.6X6-
ophthalmic preparation	T49.5X1-	T49.5X2-	T49.5X3-	T49.5X4-	T49.5X5-	T49.5X6-
topical NEC	T49.0X1-	T49.0X2-	T49.0X3-	T49.0X4-	T49.0X5-	T49.0X6-
Flowers of sulfur	T49.4X1-	T49.4X2-	T49.4X3-	T49.4X4-	T49.4X5-	T49.4X6-
Floxuridine	T45.1X1-	T45.1X2-	T45.1X3-	T45.1X4-	T45.1X5-	T45.1X6-
Fluanisone	T43.4X1-	T43.4X2-	T43.4X3-	T43.4X4-	T43.4X5-	T43.4X6-
Flubendazole	T37.4X1-	T37.4X2-	T37.4X3-	T37.4X4-	T37.4X5-	T37.4X6-
Fluclorolone acetonide	T49.0X1-	T49.0X2-	T49.0X3-	T49.0X4-	T49.0X5-	T49.0X6-
Flucloxacillin	T36.0X1-	T36.0X2-	T36.0X3-	T36.0X4-	T36.0X5-	T36.0X6-
Fluconazole	T37.8X1-	T37.8X2-	T37.8X3-	T37.8X4-	T37.8X5-	T37.8X6-
Flucytosine	T37.8X1-	T37.8X2-	T37.8X3-	T37.8X4-	T37.8X5-	T37.8X6-
Fludeoxyglucose (18F)	T50.8X1-	T50.8X2-	T50.8X3-	T50.8X4-	T50.8X5-	T50.8X6-
Fludiazepam	T42.4X1-	T42.4X2-	T42.4X3-	T42.4X4-	T42.4X5-	T42.4X6-
Fludrocortisone	T50.0X1-	T50.0X2-	T50.0X3-	T50.0X4-	T50.0X5-	T50.0X6-
ENT agent	T49.6X1-	T49.6X2-	T49.6X3-	T49.6X4-	T49.6X5-	T49.6X6-
ophthalmic preparation	T49.5X1-	T49.5X2-	T49.5X3-	T49.5X4-	T49.5X5-	T49.5X6-
topical NEC	T49.0X1-	T49.0X2-	T49.0X3-	T49.0X4-	T49.0X5-	T49.0X6-
Fludroxycortide	T49.0X1-	T49.0X2-	T49.0X3-	T49.0X4-	T49.0X5-	T49.0X6-
Flufenamic acid	T39.391-	T39.392-	T39.393-	T39.394-	T39.395-	T39.396-
Fluindione	T45.511-	T45.512-	T45.513-	T45.514-	T45.515-	T45.516-
Flumequine	T37.8X1-	T37.8X2-	T37.8X3-	T37.8X4-	T37.8X5-	T37.8X6-
Flumethasone	T49.0X1-	T49.0X2-	T49.0X3-	T49.0X4-	T49.0X5-	T49.0X6-
Flumethiazide	T50.2X1-	T50.2X2-	T50.2X3-	T50.2X4-	T50.2X5-	T50.2X6-
Flumidin	T37.5X1-	T37.5X2-	T37.5X3-	T37.5X4-	T37.5X5-	T37.5X6-
Flunarizine	T46.7X1-	T46.7X2-	T46.7X3-	T46.7X4-	T46.7X5-	T46.7X6-
Flunidazole	T37.8X1-	T37.8X2-	T37.8X3-	T37.8X4-	T37.8X5-	T37.8X6-
Flunisolide	T48.6X1-	T48.6X2-	T48.6X3-	T48.6X4-	T48.6X5-	T48.6X6-
Flunitrazepam	T42.4X1-	T42.4X2-	T42.4X3-	T42.4X4-	T42.4X5-	T42.4X6-
Fluocinolone (acetonide)	T49.0X1-	T49.0X2-	T49.0X3-	T49.0X4-	T49.0X5-	T49.0X6-
Fluocinonide	T49.0X1-	T49.0X2-	T49.0X3-	T49.0X4-	T49.0X5-	T49.0X6-
Fluocortin (butyl)	T49.0X1-	T49.0X2-	T49.0X3-	T49.0X4-	T49.0X5-	T49.0X6-
Fluocortolone	T49.0X1-	T49.0X2-	T49.0X3-	T49.0X4-	T49.0X5-	T49.0X6-
Fluohydrocortisone	T38.0X1-	T38.0X2-	T38.0X3-	T38.0X4-	T38.0X5-	T38.0X6-
ENT agent	T49.6X1-	T49.6X2-	T49.6X3-	T49.6X4-	T49.6X5-	T49.6X6-
ophthalmic preparation	T49.5X1-	T49.5X2-	T49.5X3-	T49.5X4-	T49.5X5-	T49.5X6-
topical NEC	T49.0X1-	T49.0X2-	T49.0X3-	T49.0X4-	T49.0X5-	T49.0X6-
Fluonid	T49.0X1-	T49.0X2-	T49.0X3-	T49.0X4-	T49.0X5-	T49.0X6-
Fluopromazine	T43.3X1-	T43.3X2-	T43.3X3-	T43.3X4-	T43.3X5-	T43.3X6-
Fluoracetate	T60.8X1-	T60.8X2-	T60.8X3-	T60.8X4-	-	-
Fluorescein	T50.8X1-	T50.8X2-	T50.8X3-	T50.8X4-	T50.8X5-	T50.8X6-
Fluorhydrocortisone	T50.0X1-	T50.0X2-	T50.0X3-	T50.0X4-	T50.0X5-	T50.0X6-
Fluoride (nonmedicinal) (pesticide) (sodium) **NEC**	T60.8X1-	T60.8X2-	T60.8X3-	T60.8X4-	-	-
hydrogen — *see* Hydrofluoric acid						
medicinal NEC	T50.991-	T50.992-	T50.993-	T50.994-	T50.995-	T50.996-
dental use	T49.7X1-	T49.7X2-	T49.7X3-	T49.7X4-	T49.7X5-	T49.7X6-
not pesticide NEC	T54.91X-	T54.92X-	T54.93X-	T54.94X-	-	-
stannous	T49.7X1-	T49.7X2-	T49.7X3-	T49.7X4-	T49.7X5-	T49.7X6-
Fluorinated corticosteroids	T38.0X1-	T38.0X2-	T38.0X3-	T38.0X4-	T38.0X5-	T38.0X6-
Fluorine (gas)	T59.5X1-	T59.5X2-	T59.5X3-	T59.5X4-	-	-
salt — *see* Fluoride(s)						
Fluoristan	T49.7X1-	T49.7X2-	T49.7X3-	T49.7X4-	T49.7X5-	T49.7X6-
Fluormetholone	T49.0X1-	T49.0X2-	T49.0X3-	T49.0X4-	T49.0X5-	T49.0X6-
Fluoroacetate	T60.8X1-	T60.8X2-	T60.8X3-	T60.8X4-	-	-
Fluorocarbon monomer	T53.6X1-	T53.6X2-	T53.6X3-	T53.6X4-	-	-
Fluorocytosine	T37.8X1-	T37.8X2-	T37.8X3-	T37.8X4-	T37.8X5-	T37.8X6-
Fluorodeoxyuridine	T45.1X1-	T45.1X2-	T45.1X3-	T45.1X4-	T45.1X5-	T45.1X6-
Fluorometholone	T49.0X1-	T49.0X2-	T49.0X3-	T49.0X4-	T49.0X5-	T49.0X6-
ophthalmic preparation	T49.5X1-	T49.5X2-	T49.5X3-	T49.5X4-	T49.5X5-	T49.5X6-
Fluorophosphate insecticide	T60.0X1-	T60.0X2-	T60.0X3-	T60.0X4-	-	-
Fluorosol	T46.3X1-	T46.3X2-	T46.3X3-	T46.3X4-	T46.3X5-	T46.3X6-
Fluorouracil	T45.1X1-	T45.1X2-	T45.1X3-	T45.1X4-	T45.1X5-	T45.1X6-
Fluorphenylalanine	T49.5X1-	T49.5X2-	T49.5X3-	T49.5X4-	T49.5X5-	T49.5X6-
Fluothane	T41.0X1-	T41.0X2-	T41.0X3-	T41.0X4-	T41.0X5-	T41.0X6-
Fluoxetine	T43.221-	T43.222-	T43.223-	T43.224-	T43.225-	T43.226-
Fluoxymesterone	T38.7X1-	T38.7X2-	T38.7X3-	T38.7X4-	T38.7X5-	T38.7X6-
Flupenthixol	T43.4X1-	T43.4X2-	T43.4X3-	T43.4X4-	T43.4X5-	T43.4X6-
Flupentixol	T43.4X1-	T43.4X2-	T43.4X3-	T43.4X4-	T43.4X5-	T43.4X6-
Fluphenazine	T43.3X1-	T43.3X2-	T43.3X3-	T43.3X4-	T43.3X5-	T43.3X6-
Fluprednidene	T49.0X1-	T49.0X2-	T49.0X3-	T49.0X4-	T49.0X5-	T49.0X6-
Fluprednisolone	T38.0X1-	T38.0X2-	T38.0X3-	T38.0X4-	T38.0X5-	T38.0X6-

Substance	Poisoning Accidental (unintentional)	Poisoning Intentional self-harm	Poisoning Assault	Poisoning Undetermined	Adverse effect	Underdosing
Fluradoline	T39.8X1-	T39.8X2-	T39.8X3-	T39.8X4-	T39.8X5-	T39.8X6-
Flurandrenolide	T49.0X1-	T49.0X2-	T49.0X3-	T49.0X4-	T49.0X5-	T49.0X6-
Flurandrenolone	T49.0X1-	T49.0X2-	T49.0X3-	T49.0X4-	T49.0X5-	T49.0X6-
Flurazepam	T42.4X1-	T42.4X2-	T42.4X3-	T42.4X4-	T42.4X5-	T42.4X6-
Flurbiprofen	T39.311-	T39.312-	T39.313-	T39.314-	T39.315-	T39.316-
Flurobate	T49.0X1-	T49.0X2-	T49.0X3-	T49.0X4-	T49.0X5-	T49.0X6-
Fluroxene	T41.0X1-	T41.0X2-	T41.0X3-	T41.0X4-	T41.0X5-	T41.0X6-
Fluspirilene	T43.591-	T43.592-	T43.593-	T43.594-	T43.595-	T43.596-
Flutamide	T38.6X1-	T38.6X2-	T38.6X3-	T38.6X4-	T38.6X5-	T38.6X6-
Flutazolam	T42.4X1-	T42.4X2-	T42.4X3-	T42.4X4-	T42.4X5-	T42.4X6-
Fluticasone propionate	T38.0X1-	T38.0X2-	T38.0X3-	T38.0X4-	T38.0X5-	T38.0X6-
Flutoprazepam	T42.4X1-	T42.4X2-	T42.4X3-	T42.4X4-	T42.4X5-	T42.4X6-
Flutropium bromide	T48.6X1-	T48.6X2-	T48.6X3-	T48.6X4-	T48.6X5-	T48.6X6-
Fluvoxamine	T43.221-	T43.222-	T43.223-	T43.224-	T43.225-	T43.226-
Folacin	T45.8X1-	T45.8X2-	T45.8X3-	T45.8X4-	T45.8X5-	T45.8X6-
Folic acid	T45.8X1-	T45.8X2-	T45.8X3-	T45.8X4-	T45.8X5-	T45.8X6-
with ferrous salt	T45.2X1-	T45.2X2-	T45.2X3-	T45.2X4-	T45.2X5-	T45.2X6-
antagonist	T45.1X1-	T45.1X2-	T45.1X3-	T45.1X4-	T45.1X5-	T45.1X6-
Folinic acid	T45.8X1-	T45.8X2-	T45.8X3-	T45.8X4-	T45.8X5-	T45.8X6-
Folium stramoniae	T48.6X1-	T48.6X2-	T48.6X3-	T48.6X4-	T48.6X5-	T48.6X6-
Follicle-stimulating hormone, human	T38.811-	T38.812-	T38.813-	T38.814-	T38.815-	T38.816-
Folpet	T60.3X1-	T60.3X2-	T60.3X3-	T60.3X4-	-	-
Fominoben	T48.3X1-	T48.3X2-	T48.3X3-	T48.3X4-	T48.3X5-	T48.3X6-
Food, foodstuffs, noxious, nonbacterial, NEC	T62.91X-	T62.92X-	T62.93X-	T62.94X-	-	-
berries	T62.1X1-	T62.1X2-	T62.1X3-	T62.1X4-	-	-
fish — *see also* Fish	T61.91X-	T61.92X-	T61.93X-	T61.94X-	-	-
mushrooms	T62.0X1-	T62.0X2-	T62.0X3-	T62.0X4-	-	-
plants	T62.2X1-	T62.2X2-	T62.2X3-	T62.2X4-	-	-
seafood	T61.91X-	T61.92X-	T61.93X-	T61.94X-	-	-
specified NEC	T61.8X1-	T61.8X2-	T61.8X3-	T61.8X4-	-	-
seeds	T62.2X1-	T62.2X2-	T62.2X3-	T62.2X4-	-	-
shellfish	T61.781-	T61.782-	T61.783-	T61.784-	-	-
specified NEC	T62.8X1-	T62.8X2-	T62.8X3-	T62.8X4-	-	-
Fool's parsley	T62.2X1-	T62.2X2-	T62.2X3-	T62.2X4-	-	-
Formaldehyde (solution) **, gas or vapor**	T59.2X1-	T59.2X2-	T59.2X3-	T59.2X4-	-	-
fungicide	T60.3X1-	T60.3X2-	T60.3X3-	T60.3X4-	-	-
Formalin	T59.2X1-	T59.2X2-	T59.2X3-	T59.2X4-	-	-
fungicide	T60.3X1-	T60.3X2-	T60.3X3-	T60.3X4-	-	-
vapor	T59.2X1-	T59.2X2-	T59.2X3-	T59.2X4-	-	-
Formic acid	T54.2X1-	T54.2X2-	T54.2X3-	T54.2X4-	-	-
vapor	T59.891-	T59.892-	T59.893-	T59.894-	-	-
Foscarnet sodium	T37.5X1-	T37.5X2-	T37.5X3-	T37.5X4-	T37.5X5-	T37.5X6-
Fosfestrol	T38.5X1-	T38.5X2-	T38.5X3-	T38.5X4-	T38.5X5-	T38.5X6-
Fosfomycin	T36.8X1-	T36.8X2-	T36.8X3-	T36.8X4-	T36.8X5-	T36.8X6-
Fosfonet sodium	T37.5X1-	T37.5X2-	T37.5X3-	T37.5X4-	T37.5X5-	T37.5X6-
Fosinopril	T46.4X1-	T46.4X2-	T46.4X3-	T46.4X4-	T46.4X5-	T46.4X6-
sodium	T46.4X1-	T46.4X2-	T46.4X3-	T46.4X4-	T46.4X5-	T46.4X6-
Fowler's solution	T57.0X1-	T57.0X2-	T57.0X3-	T57.0X4-	-	-
Foxglove	T62.2X1-	T62.2X2-	T62.2X3-	T62.2X4-	-	-
Framycetin	T36.5X1-	T36.5X2-	T36.5X3-	T36.5X4-	T36.5X5-	T36.5X6-
Frangula	T47.2X1-	T47.2X2-	T47.2X3-	T47.2X4-	T47.2X5-	T47.2X6-
extract	T47.2X1-	T47.2X2-	T47.2X3-	T47.2X4-	T47.2X5-	T47.2X6-
Frei antigen	T50.8X1-	T50.8X2-	T50.8X3-	T50.8X4-	T50.8X5-	T50.8X6-
Freon	T53.5X1-	T53.5X2-	T53.5X3-	T53.5X4-	-	-
Fructose	T50.3X1-	T50.3X2-	T50.3X3-	T50.3X4-	T50.3X5-	T50.3X6-
Frusemide	T50.1X1-	T50.1X2-	T50.1X3-	T50.1X4-	T50.1X5-	T50.1X6-
FSH	T38.811-	T38.812-	T38.813-	T38.814-	T38.815-	T38.816-
Ftorafur	T45.1X1-	T45.1X2-	T45.1X3-	T45.1X4-	T45.1X5-	T45.1X6-
Fuel						
automobile	T52.0X1-	T52.0X2-	T52.0X3-	T52.0X4-	-	-
exhaust gas, not in transit	T58.01X-	T58.02X-	T58.03X-	T58.04X-	-	-
vapor NEC	T52.0X1-	T52.0X2-	T52.0X3-	T52.0X4-	-	-
gas (domestic use) — *see also* Carbon, monoxide, fuel, utility	T59.891-	T59.892-	T59.893-	T59.894-	-	-
utility	T59.891-	T59.892-	T59.893-	T59.894-	-	-
in mobile container	T59.891-	T59.892-	T59.893-	T59.894-	-	-
incomplete combustion of — *see* Carbon, monoxide, fuel, utility						
piped (natural)	T59.891-	T59.892-	T59.893-	T59.894-	-	-
industrial, incomplete combustion	T58.8X1-	T58.8X2-	T58.8X3-	T58.8X4-	-	-
Fugillin	T36.8X1-	T36.8X2-	T36.8X3-	T36.8X4-	T36.8X5-	T36.8X6-
Fulminate of mercury	T56.1X1-	T56.1X2-	T56.1X3-	T56.1X4-	-	-
Fulvicin	T36.7X1-	T36.7X2-	T36.7X3-	T36.7X4-	T36.7X5-	T36.7X6-
Fumadil	T36.8X1-	T36.8X2-	T36.8X3-	T36.8X4-	T36.8X5-	T36.8X6-
Fumagillin	T36.8X1-	T36.8X2-	T36.8X3-	T36.8X4-	T36.8X5-	T36.8X6-
Fumaric acid	T49.4X1-	T49.4X2-	T49.4X3-	T49.4X4-	T49.4X5-	T49.4X6-
Fumes (from)	T59.91X-	T59.92X-	T59.93X-	T59.94X-	-	-
carbon monoxide — *see* Carbon, monoxide						
charcoal (domestic use) — *see* Charcoal, fumes						
chloroform — *see* Chloroform						
coke (in domestic stoves, fireplaces) — *see* Coke fumes						
corrosive NEC	T54.91X-	T54.92X-	T54.93X-	T54.94X-	-	-
ether — *see* ether						
freons	T53.5X1-	T53.5X2-	T53.5X3-	T53.5X4-	-	-
hydrocarbons	T59.891-	T59.892-	T59.893-	T59.894-	-	-
petroleum (liquefied)	T59.891-	T59.892-	T59.893-	T59.894-	-	-
distributed through pipes (pure or mixed with air)	T59.891-	T59.892-	T59.893-	T59.894-	-	-
lead — *see* lead						
metal — *see* Metals, or the specified metal						
nitrogen dioxide	T59.0X1-	T59.0X2-	T59.0X3-	T59.0X4-	-	-
pesticides — *see* Pesticides						
petroleum (liquefied)	T59.891-	T59.892-	T59.893-	T59.894-	-	-
distributed through pipes (pure or mixed with air)	T59.891-	T59.892-	T59.893-	T59.894-	-	-
polyester	T59.891-	T59.892-	T59.893-	T59.894-	-	-
specified source NEC — *see also* substance specified	T59.891-	T59.892-	T59.893-	T59.894-	-	-
sulfur dioxide	T59.1X1-	T59.1X2-	T59.1X3-	T59.1X4-	-	-
Fumigant NEC	T60.91X-	T60.92X-	T60.93X-	T60.94X-	-	-
Fungi, noxious, used as food	T62.0X1-	T62.0X2-	T62.0X3-	T62.0X4-	-	-
Fungicide NEC (nonmedicinal)	T60.3X1-	T60.3X2-	T60.3X3-	T60.3X4-	-	-
Fungizone	T36.7X1-	T36.7X2-	T36.7X3-	T36.7X4-	T36.7X5-	T36.7X6-
topical	T49.0X1-	T49.0X2-	T49.0X3-	T49.0X4-	T49.0X5-	T49.0X6-
Furacin	T49.0X1-	T49.0X2-	T49.0X3-	T49.0X4-	T49.0X5-	T49.0X6-
Furadantin	T37.91X-	T37.92X-	T37.93X-	T37.94X-	T37.95X-	T37.96X-
Furazolidone	T37.8X1-	T37.8X2-	T37.8X3-	T37.8X4-	T37.8X5-	T37.8X6-
Furazolium chloride	T49.0X1-	T49.0X2-	T49.0X3-	T49.0X4-	T49.0X5-	T49.0X6-
Furfural	T52.8X1-	T52.8X2-	T52.8X3-	T52.8X4-	-	-
Furnace (coal burning) (domestic) **, gas from**	T58.2X1-	T58.2X2-	T58.2X3-	T58.2X4-	-	-
industrial	T58.8X1-	T58.8X2-	T58.8X3-	T58.8X4-	-	-
Furniture polish	T65.891-	T65.892-	T65.893-	T65.894-	-	-
Furosemide	T50.1X1-	T50.1X2-	T50.1X3-	T50.1X4-	T50.1X5-	T50.1X6-
Furoxone	T37.91X-	T37.92X-	T37.93X-	T37.94X-	T37.95X-	T37.96X-
Fursultiamine	T45.2X1-	T45.2X2-	T45.2X3-	T45.2X4-	T45.2X5-	T45.2X6-
Fusafungine	T36.8X1-	T36.8X2-	T36.8X3-	T36.8X4-	T36.8X5-	T36.8X6-
Fusel oil (any) (amyl) (butyl) (propyl) **, vapor**	T51.3X1-	T51.3X2-	T51.3X3-	T51.3X4-	-	-
Fusidate (ethanolamine) (sodium)	T36.8X1-	T36.8X2-	T36.8X3-	T36.8X4-	T36.8X5-	T36.8X6-
Fusidic acid	T36.8X1-	T36.8X2-	T36.8X3-	T36.8X4-	T36.8X5-	T36.8X6-
Fytic acid, nonasodium	T50.6X1-	T50.6X2-	T50.6X3-	T50.6X4-	T50.6X5-	T50.6X6-
GABA	T43.8X1-	T43.8X2-	T43.8X3-	T43.8X4-	T43.8X5-	T43.8X6-
Gadopentetic acid	T50.8X1-	T50.8X2-	T50.8X3-	T50.8X4-	T50.8X5-	T50.8X6-
Galactose	T50.3X1-	T50.3X2-	T50.3X3-	T50.3X4-	T50.3X5-	T50.3X6-
b-Galactosidase	T47.5X1-	T47.5X2-	T47.5X3-	T47.5X4-	T47.5X5-	T47.5X6-
Galantamine	T44.0X1-	T44.0X2-	T44.0X3-	T44.0X4-	T44.0X5-	T44.0X6-
Gallamine (triethiodide)	T48.1X1-	T48.1X2-	T48.1X3-	T48.1X4-	T48.1X5-	T48.1X6-
Gallium citrate	T50.991-	T50.992-	T50.993-	T50.994-	T50.995-	T50.996-
Gallopamil	T46.1X1-	T46.1X2-	T46.1X3-	T46.1X4-	T46.1X5-	T46.1X6-
Gamboge	T47.2X1-	T47.2X2-	T47.2X3-	T47.2X4-	T47.2X5-	T47.2X6-
Gamimune	T50.Z11-	T50.Z12-	T50.Z13-	T50.Z14-	T50.Z15-	T50.Z16-
Gamma globulin	T50.Z11-	T50.Z12-	T50.Z13-	T50.Z14-	T50.Z15-	T50.Z16-
Gamma-aminobutyric acid	T43.8X1-	T43.8X2-	T43.8X3-	T43.8X4-	T43.8X5-	T43.8X6-
Gamma-benzene hexachloride (medicinal)	T49.0X1-	T49.0X2-	T49.0X3-	T49.0X4-	T49.0X5-	T49.0X6-
nonmedicinal, vapor	T53.6X1-	T53.6X2-	T53.6X3-	T53.6X4-	-	-
Gamma-BHC (medicinal) — *see also* Gamma-benzene hexachloride	T49.0X1-	T49.0X2-	T49.0X3-	T49.0X4-	T49.0X5-	T49.0X6-
Gamulin	T50.Z11-	T50.Z12-	T50.Z13-	T50.Z14-	T50.Z15-	T50.Z16-
Ganciclovir (sodium)	T37.5X1-	T37.5X2-	T37.5X3-	T37.5X4-	T37.5X5-	T37.5X6-
Ganglionic blocking drug NEC	T44.2X1-	T44.2X2-	T44.2X3-	T44.2X4-	T44.2X5-	T44.2X6-
specified NEC	T44.2X1-	T44.2X2-	T44.2X3-	T44.2X4-	T44.2X5-	T44.2X6-
Ganja	T40.7X1-	T40.7X2-	T40.7X3-	T40.7X4-	T40.7X5-	T40.7X6-
Garamycin	T36.5X1-	T36.5X2-	T36.5X3-	T36.5X4-	T36.5X5-	T36.5X6-
ophthalmic preparation	T49.5X1-	T49.5X2-	T49.5X3-	T49.5X4-	T49.5X5-	T49.5X6-
topical NEC	T49.0X1-	T49.0X2-	T49.0X3-	T49.0X4-	T49.0X5-	T49.0X6-

Substance	Poisoning Accidental (unintentional)	Poisoning Intentional self-harm	Poisoning Assault	Poisoning Undetermined	Adverse effect	Underdosing
Gardenal	T42.3X1-	T42.3X2-	T42.3X3-	T42.3X4-	T42.3X5-	T42.3X6-
Gardepanyl	T42.3X1-	T42.3X2-	T42.3X3-	T42.3X4-	T42.3X5-	T42.3X6-
Gas NEC	T59.91X-	T59.92X-	T59.93X-	T59.94X-	-	-
acetylene	T59.891-	T59.892-	T59.893-	T59.894-	-	-
incomplete combustion of	T58.11X-	T58.12X-	T58.13X-	T58.14X-	-	-
air contaminants, source or type not specified	T59.91X-	T59.92X-	T59.93X-	T59.94X-	-	-
anesthetic	T41.0X1-	T41.0X2-	T41.0X3-	T41.0X4-	T41.0X5-	T41.0X6-
blast furnace	T58.8X1-	T58.8X2-	T58.8X3-	T58.8X4-	-	-
butane — *see* butane						
carbon monoxide — *see* Carbon, monoxide						
chlorine	T59.4X1-	T59.4X2-	T59.4X3-	T59.4X4-	-	-
coal	T58.2X1-	T58.2X2-	T58.2X3-	T58.2X4-	-	-
cyanide	T57.3X1-	T57.3X2-	T57.3X3-	T57.3X4-	-	-
dicyanogen	T65.0X1-	T65.0X2-	T65.0X3-	T65.0X4-	-	-
domestic — *see* Domestic gas						
exhaust	T58.01X-	T58.02X-	T58.03X-	T58.04X-	-	-
from utility (for cooking, heating, or lighting) (after combustion) — *see* Carbon, monoxide, fuel, utility						
prior to combustion	T59.891-	T59.892-	T59.893-	T59.894-	-	-
from wood- or coal-burning stove or fireplace	T58.2X1-	T58.2X2-	T58.2X3-	T58.2X4-	-	-
fuel (domestic use) (after combustion) — *see also* Carbon, monoxide, fuel						
industrial use	T58.8X1-	T58.8X2-	T58.8X3-	T58.8X4-	-	-
prior to combustion	T59.891-	T59.892-	T59.893-	T59.894-	-	-
utility	T59.891-	T59.892-	T59.893-	T59.894-	-	-
in mobile container	T59.891-	T59.892-	T59.893-	T59.894-	-	-
incomplete combustion of — *see* Carbon, monoxide, fuel, utility						
piped (natural)	T59.891-	T59.892-	T59.893-	T59.894-	-	-
garage	T58.01X-	T58.02X-	T58.03X-	T58.04X-	-	-
hydrocarbon NEC	T59.891-	T59.892-	T59.893-	T59.894-	-	-
incomplete combustion of — *see* Carbon, monoxide, fuel, utility						
liquefied — *see* butane						
piped	T59.891-	T59.892-	T59.893-	T59.894-	-	-
hydrocyanic acid	T65.0X1-	T65.0X2-	T65.0X3-	T65.0X4-	-	-
illuminating (after combustion)	T58.11X-	T58.12X-	T58.13X-	T58.14X-	-	-
prior to combustion	T59.891-	T59.892-	T59.893-	T59.894-	-	-
incomplete combustion, any — *see* Carbon, monoxide						
kiln	T58.8X1-	T58.8X2-	T58.8X3-	T58.8X4-	-	-
lacrimogenic	T59.3X1-	T59.3X2-	T59.3X3-	T59.3X4-	-	-
liquefied petroleum — *see* butane						
marsh	T59.891-	T59.892-	T59.893-	T59.894-	-	-
motor exhaust, not in transit	T58.01X-	T58.02X-	T58.03X-	T58.04X-	-	-
mustard, not in war	T59.891-	T59.892-	T59.893-	T59.894-	-	-
natural	T60.001	T50.002-	T59.090-	T59.094-	-	-
nerve, not in war	T59.91X-	T59.92X-	T59.93X-	T59.94X-	-	-
oil	T52.0X1-	T52.0X2-	T52.0X3-	T52.0X4-	-	-
petroleum (liquefied) (distributed in mobile containers)	T59.891-	T59.892-	T59.893-	T59.894-	-	-
piped (pure or mixed with air)	T59.891-	T59.892-	T59.893-	T59.894-	-	-
piped (manufactured) (natural) NEC	T59.891-	T59.892-	T59.893-	T59.894-	-	-
producer	T58.8X1-	T58.8X2-	T58.8X3-	T58.8X4-	-	-
propane — *see* propane						
refrigerant (chlorofluoro-carbon)	T53.5X1-	T53.5X2-	T53.5X3-	T53.5X4-	-	-
not chlorofluoro-carbon	T59.891-	T59.892-	T59.893-	T59.894-	-	-
sewer	T59.91X-	T59.92X-	T59.93X-	T59.94X-	-	-
specified source NEC	T59.91X-	T59.92X-	T59.93X-	T59.94X-	-	-
stove (after combustion)	T58.11X-	T58.12X-	T58.13X-	T58.14X-	-	-
prior to combustion	T59.891-	T59.892-	T59.893-	T59.894-	-	-
tear	T59.3X1-	T59.3X2-	T59.3X3-	T59.3X4-	-	-
therapeutic	T41.5X1-	T41.5X2-	T41.5X3-	T41.5X4-	T41.5X5-	T41.5X6-
utility (for cooking, heating, or lighting) (piped) NEC	T59.891-	T59.892-	T59.893-	T59.894-	-	-
in mobile container	T59.891-	T59.892-	T59.893-	T59.894-	-	-

Substance	Poisoning Accidental (unintentional)	Poisoning Intentional self-harm	Poisoning Assault	Poisoning Undetermined	Adverse effect	Underdosing
Gas NEC - *continued* incomplete combustion of — *see* Carbon, monoxide, fuel, utilty						
piped (natural)	T59.891-	T59.892-	T59.893-	T59.894-	-	-
water	T58.11X-	T58.12X-	T58.13X-	T58.14X-	-	-
incomplete combustion of — *see* Carbon, monoxide, fuel, utility						
Gaseous substance — *see* Gas						
Gasoline	T52.0X1-	T52.0X2-	T52.0X3-	T52.0X4-	-	-
vapor	T52.0X1-	T52.0X2-	T52.0X3-	T52.0X4-	-	-
Gastric enzymes	T47.5X1-	T47.5X2-	T47.5X3-	T47.5X4-	T47.5X5-	T47.5X6-
Gastrografin	T50.8X1-	T50.8X2-	T50.8X3-	T50.8X4-	T50.8X5-	T50.8X6-
Gastrointestinal drug	T47.91X-	T47.92X-	T47.93X-	T47.94X-	T47.95X-	T47.96X-
biological	T47.8X1-	T47.8X2-	T47.8X3-	T47.8X4-	T47.8X5-	T47.8X6-
specified NEC	T47.8X1-	T47.8X2-	T47.8X3-	T47.8X4-	T47.8X5-	T47.8X6-
Gaultheria procumbens	T62.2X1-	T62.2X2-	T62.2X3-	T62.2X4-	-	-
Gefarnate	T44.3X1-	T44.3X2-	T44.3X3-	T44.3X4-	T44.3X5-	T44.3X6-
Gelatin (intravenous)	T45.8X1-	T45.8X2-	T45.8X3-	T45.8X4-	T45.8X5-	T45.8X6-
absorbable (sponge)	T45.7X1-	T45.7X2-	T45.7X3-	T45.7X4-	T45.7X5-	T45.7X6-
Gelfilm	T49.8X1-	T49.8X2-	T49.8X3-	T49.8X4-	T49.8X5-	T49.8X6-
Gelfoam	T45.7X1-	T45.7X2-	T45.7X3-	T45.7X4-	T45.7X5-	T45.7X6-
Gelsemine	T50.991-	T50.992-	T50.993-	T50.994-	T50.995-	T50.996-
Gelsemium (sempervirens)	T62.2X1-	T62.2X2-	T62.2X3-	T62.2X4-	-	-
Gemeprost	T48.0X1-	T48.0X2-	T48.0X3-	T48.0X4-	T48.0X5-	T48.0X6-
Gemfibrozil	T46.6X1-	T46.6X2-	T46.6X3-	T46.6X4-	T46.6X5-	T46.6X6-
Gemonil	T42.3X1-	T42.3X2-	T42.3X3-	T42.3X4-	T42.3X5-	T42.3X6-
Gentamicin	T36.5X1-	T36.5X2-	T36.5X3-	T36.5X4-	T36.5X5-	T36.5X6-
ophthalmic preparation	T49.5X1-	T49.5X2-	T49.5X3-	T49.5X4-	T49.5X5-	T49.5X6-
topical NEC	T49.0X1-	T49.0X2-	T49.0X3-	T49.0X4-	T49.0X5-	T49.0X6-
Gentian	T47.5X1-	T47.5X2-	T47.5X3-	T47.5X4-	T47.5X5-	T47.5X6-
violet	T49.0X1-	T49.0X2-	T49.0X3-	T49.0X4-	T49.0X5-	T49.0X6-
Gepefrine	T44.4X1-	T44.4X2-	T44.4X3-	T44.4X4-	T44.4X5-	T44.4X6-
Gestonorone caproate	T38.5X1-	T38.5X2-	T38.5X3-	T38.5X4-	T38.5X5-	T38.5X6-
Gexane	T49.0X1-	T49.0X2-	T49.0X3-	T49.0X4-	T49.0X5-	T49.0X6-
Gila monster (venom)	T63.111-	T63.112-	T63.113-	T63.114-	-	-
Ginger	T47.5X1-	T47.5X2-	T47.5X3-	T47.5X4-	T47.5X5-	T47.5X6-
Jamaica — *see* Jamaica, ginger						
Gitalin	T46.0X1-	T46.0X2-	T46.0X3-	T46.0X4-	T46.0X5-	T46.0X6-
amorphous	T46.0X1-	T46.0X2-	T46.0X3-	T46.0X4-	T46.0X5-	T46.0X6-
Gitaloxin	T46.0X1-	T46.0X2-	T46.0X3-	T46.0X4-	T46.0X5-	T46.0X6-
Gitoxin	T46.0X1-	T46.0X2-	T46.0X3-	T46.0X4-	T46.0X5-	T46.0X6-
Glafenine	T39.8X1-	T39.8X2-	T39.8X3-	T39.8X4-	T39.8X5-	T39.8X6-
Glandular extract (medicinal) **NEC**	T50.Z91-	T50.Z92-	T50.Z93-	T50.Z94-	T50.Z95-	T50.Z96-
Glaucarubin	T37.3X1-	T37.3X2-	T37.3X3-	T37.3X4-	T37.3X5-	T37.3X6-
Glibenclamide	T38.3X1-	T38.3X2-	T38.3X3-	T38.3X4-	T38.3X5-	T38.3X6-
Glibornuride	T38.3X1-	T38.3X2-	T38.3X3-	T38.3X4-	T38.3X5-	T38.3X6-
Gliclazide	T38.3X1-	T38.3X2-	T38.3X3-	T38.3X4-	T38.3X5-	T38.3X6-
Glimidine	T38.3X1-	T38.3X2-	T38.3X3-	T38.3X4-	T38.3X5-	T38.3X6-
Glipizide	T38.3X1-	T38.3X2-	T38.3X3-	T38.3X4-	T38.3X5-	T38.3X6-
Gliquidone	T38.3X1-	T38.3X2-	T38.3X3-	T38.3X4-	T38.3X5-	T38.3X6-
Glisolamide	T38.3X1-	T38.3X2-	T38.3X3-	T38.3X4-	T38.3X5-	T38.3X6-
Glisoxepide	T38.3X1-	T38.3X2-	T38.3X3-	T38.3X4-	T38.3X5-	T38.3X6-
Globin zinc insulin	T38.3X1-	T38.3X2-	T38.3X3-	T38.3X4-	T38.3X5-	T38.3X6-
Globulin						
antilymphocytic	T50.Z11-	T50.Z12-	T50.Z13-	T50.Z14-	T50.Z15-	T50.Z16-
antirhesus	T50.Z11-	T50.Z12-	T50.Z13-	T50.Z14-	T50.Z15-	T50.Z16-
antivenin	T50.Z11-	T50.Z12-	T50.Z13-	T50.Z14-	T50.Z15-	T50.Z16-
antiviral	T50.Z11-	T50.Z12-	T50.Z13-	T50.Z14-	T50.Z15-	T50.Z16-
Glucagon	T38.3X1-	T38.3X2-	T38.3X3-	T38.3X4-	T38.3X5-	T38.3X6-
Glucocorticoids	T38.0X1-	T38.0X2-	T38.0X3-	T38.0X4-	T38.0X5-	T38.0X6-
Glucocorticosteroid	T38.0X1-	T38.0X2-	T38.0X3-	T38.0X4-	T38.0X5-	T38.0X6-
Gluconic acid	T50.991-	T50.992-	T50.993-	T50.994-	T50.995-	T50.996-
Glucosamine sulfate	T39.4X1-	T39.4X2-	T39.4X3-	T39.4X4-	T39.4X5-	T39.4X6-
Glucose	T50.3X1-	T50.3X2-	T50.3X3-	T50.3X4-	T50.3X5-	T50.3X6-
with sodium chloride	T50.3X1-	T50.3X2-	T50.3X3-	T50.3X4-	T50.3X5-	T50.3X6-
Glucosulfone sodium	T37.1X1-	T37.1X2-	T37.1X3-	T37.1X4-	T37.1X5-	T37.1X6-
Glucurolactone	T47.8X1-	T47.8X2-	T47.8X3-	T47.8X4-	T47.8X5-	T47.8X6-
Glue NEC	T52.8X1-	T52.8X2-	T52.8X3-	T52.8X4-	-	-
Glutamic acid	T47.5X1-	T47.5X2-	T47.5X3-	T47.5X4-	T47.5X5-	T47.5X6-
Glutaral (medicinal)	T49.0X1-	T49.0X2-	T49.0X3-	T49.0X4-	T49.0X5-	T49.0X6-
nonmedicinal	T65.891-	T65.892-	T65.893-	T65.894-	-	-
Glutaraldehyde (nonmedicinal)	T65.891-	T65.892-	T65.893-	T65.894-	-	-
medicinal	T49.0X1-	T49.0X2-	T49.0X3-	T49.0X4-	T49.0X5-	T49.0X6-
Glutathione	T50.6X1-	T50.6X2-	T50.6X3-	T50.6X4-	T50.6X5-	T50.6X6-

Substance	Poisoning Accidental (unintentional)	Poisoning Intentional self-harm	Poisoning Assault	Poisoning Undetermined	Adverse effect	Underdosing
Glutethimide	T42.6X1-	T42.6X2-	T42.6X3-	T42.6X4-	T42.6X5-	T42.6X6-
Glyburide	T38.3X1-	T38.3X2-	T38.3X3-	T38.3X4-	T38.3X5-	T38.3X6-
Glycerin	T47.4X1-	T47.4X2-	T47.4X3-	T47.4X4-	T47.4X5-	T47.4X6-
Glycerol	T47.4X1-	T47.4X2-	T47.4X3-	T47.4X4-	T47.4X5-	T47.4X6-
borax	T49.6X1-	T49.6X2-	T49.6X3-	T49.6X4-	T49.6X5-	T49.6X6-
intravenous	T50.3X1-	T50.3X2-	T50.3X3-	T50.3X4-	T50.3X5-	T50.3X6-
iodinated	T48.4X1-	T48.4X2-	T48.4X3-	T48.4X4-	T48.4X5-	T48.4X6-
Glycerophosphate	T50.991-	T50.992-	T50.993-	T50.994-	T50.995-	T50.996-
Glyceryl						
gualacolate	T48.4X1-	T48.4X2-	T48.4X3-	T48.4X4-	T48.4X5-	T48.4X6-
nitrate	T46.3X1-	T46.3X2-	T46.3X3-	T46.3X4-	T46.3X5-	T46.3X6-
triacetate (topical)	T49.0X1-	T49.0X2-	T49.0X3-	T49.0X4-	T49.0X5-	T49.0X6-
trinitrate	T46.3X1-	T46.3X2-	T46.3X3-	T46.3X4-	T46.3X5-	T46.3X6-
Glycine	T50.3X1-	T50.3X2-	T50.3X3-	T50.3X4-	T50.3X5-	T50.3X6-
Glyclopyramide	T38.3X1-	T38.3X2-	T38.3X3-	T38.3X4-	T38.3X5-	T38.3X6-
Glycobiarsol	T37.3X1-	T37.3X2-	T37.3X3-	T37.3X4-	T37.3X5-	T37.3X6-
Glycols (ether)	T52.3X1-	T52.3X2-	T52.3X3-	T52.3X4-	-	-
Glyconiazide	T37.1X1-	T37.1X2-	T37.1X3-	T37.1X4-	T37.1X5-	T37.1X6-
Glycopyrrolate	T44.3X1-	T44.3X2-	T44.3X3-	T44.3X4-	T44.3X5-	T44.3X6-
Glycopyrronium	T44.3X1-	T44.3X2-	T44.3X3-	T44.3X4-	T44.3X5-	T44.3X6-
bromide	T44.3X1-	T44.3X2-	T44.3X3-	T44.3X4-	T44.3X5-	T44.3X6-
Glycoside, cardiac (stimulant)	T46.0X1-	T46.0X2-	T46.0X3-	T46.0X4-	T46.0X5-	T46.0X6-
Glycyclamide	T38.3X1-	T38.3X2-	T38.3X3-	T38.3X4-	T38.3X5-	T38.3X6-
Glycyrrhiza extract	T48.4X1-	T48.4X2-	T48.4X3-	T48.4X4-	T48.4X5-	T48.4X6-
Glycyrrhizic acid	T48.4X1-	T48.4X2-	T48.4X3-	T48.4X4-	T48.4X5-	T48.4X6-
Glycyrrhizinate potassium	T48.4X1-	T48.4X2-	T48.4X3-	T48.4X4-	T48.4X5-	T48.4X6-
Glymidine sodium	T38.3X1-	T38.3X2-	T38.3X3-	T38.3X4-	T38.3X5-	T38.3X6-
Glyphosate	T60.3X1-	T60.3X2-	T60.3X3-	T60.3X4-	-	-
Glyphylline	T48.6X1-	T48.6X2-	T48.6X3-	T48.6X4-	T48.6X5-	T48.6X6-
Gold						
colloidal (I98Au)	T45.1X1-	T45.1X2-	T45.1X3-	T45.1X4-	T45.1X5-	T45.1X6-
salts	T39.4X1-	T39.4X2-	T39.4X3-	T39.4X4-	T39.4X5-	T39.4X6-
Golden sulfide of antimony	T56.891-	T56.892-	T56.893-	T56.894-	-	-
Goldylocks	T62.2X1-	T62.2X2-	T62.2X3-	T62.2X4-	-	-
Gonadal tissue extract	T38.901-	T38.902-	T38.903-	T38.904-	T38.905-	T38.906-
female	T38.5X1-	T38.5X2-	T38.5X3-	T38.5X4-	T38.5X5-	T38.5X6-
male	T38.7X1-	T38.7X2-	T38.7X3-	T38.7X4-	T38.7X5-	T38.7X6-
Gonadorelin	T38.891-	T38.892-	T38.893-	T38.894-	T38.895-	T38.896-
Gonadotropin	T38.891-	T38.892-	T38.893-	T38.894-	T38.895-	T38.896-
chorionic	T38.891-	T38.892-	T38.893-	T38.894-	T38.895-	T38.896-
pituitary	T38.811-	T38.812-	T38.813-	T38.814-	T38.815-	T38.816-
Goserelin	T45.1X1-	T45.1X2-	T45.1X3-	T45.1X4-	T45.1X5-	T45.1X6-
Grain alcohol	T51.0X1-	T51.0X2-	T51.0X3-	T51.0X4-	-	-
Gramicidin	T49.0X1-	T49.0X2-	T49.0X3-	T49.0X4-	T49.0X5-	T49.0X6-
Granisetron	T45.0X1-	T45.0X2-	T45.0X3-	T45.0X4-	T45.0X5-	T45.0X6-
Gratiola officinalis	T62.2X1-	T62.2X2-	T62.2X3-	T62.2X4-	-	-
Grease	T65.891-	T65.892-	T65.893-	T65.894-	-	-
Green hellebore	T62.2X1-	T62.2X2-	T62.2X3-	T62.2X4-	-	-
Green soap	T49.2X1-	T49.2X2-	T49.2X3-	T49.2X4-	T49.2X5-	T49.2X6-
Grifulvin	T36.7X1-	T36.7X2-	T36.7X3-	T36.7X4-	T36.7X5-	T36.7X6-
Griseofulvin	T36.7X1-	T36.7X2-	T36.7X3-	T36.7X4-	T36.7X5-	T36.7X6-
Growth hormone	T38.811-	T38.812-	T38.813-	T38.814-	T38.815-	T38.816-
Guaiac reagent	T50.991-	T50.992-	T50.993-	T50.994-	T50.995-	T50.996-
Guaiacol derivatives	T48.4X1-	T48.4X2-	T48.4X3-	T48.4X4-	T48.4X5-	T48.4X6-
Guaifenesin	T48.4X1-	T48.4X2-	T48.4X3-	T48.4X4-	T48.4X5-	T48.4X6-
Guaimesal	T48.4X1-	T48.4X2-	T48.4X3-	T48.4X4-	T48.4X5-	T48.4X6-
Guaiphenesin	T48.4X1-	T48.4X2-	T48.4X3-	T48.4X4-	T48.4X5-	T48.4X6-
Guamecycline	T36.4X1-	T36.4X2-	T36.4X3-	T36.4X4-	T36.4X5-	T36.4X6-
Guanabenz	T46.5X1-	T46.5X2-	T46.5X3-	T46.5X4-	T46.5X5-	T46.5X6-
Guanacline	T46.5X1-	T46.5X2-	T46.5X3-	T46.5X4-	T46.5X5-	T46.5X6-
Guanadrel	T46.5X1-	T46.5X2-	T46.5X3-	T46.5X4-	T46.5X5-	T46.5X6-
Guanatol	T37.2X1-	T37.2X2-	T37.2X3-	T37.2X4-	T37.2X5-	T37.2X6-
Guanethidine	T46.5X1-	T46.5X2-	T46.5X3-	T46.5X4-	T46.5X5-	T46.5X6-
Guanfacine	T46.5X1-	T46.5X2-	T46.5X3-	T46.5X4-	T46.5X5-	T46.5X6-
Guano	T65.891-	T65.892-	T65.893-	T65.894-	-	-
Guanochlor	T46.5X1-	T46.5X2-	T46.5X3-	T46.5X4-	T46.5X5-	T46.5X6-
Guanoclor	T46.5X1-	T46.5X2-	T46.5X3-	T46.5X4-	T46.5X5-	T46.5X6-
Guanoctine	T46.5X1-	T46.5X2-	T46.5X3-	T46.5X4-	T46.5X5-	T46.5X6-
Guanoxabenz	T46.5X1-	T46.5X2-	T46.5X3-	T46.5X4-	T46.5X5-	T46.5X6-
Guanoxan	T46.5X1-	T46.5X2-	T46.5X3-	T46.5X4-	T46.5X5-	T46.5X6-
Guar gum (medicinal)	T46.6X1-	T46.6X2-	T46.6X3-	T46.6X4-	T46.6X5-	T46.6X6-
Hachimycin	T36.7X1-	T36.7X2-	T36.7X3-	T36.7X4-	T36.7X5-	T36.7X6-
Hair						
dye	T49.4X1-	T49.4X2-	T49.4X3-	T49.4X4-	T49.4X5-	T49.4X6-
preparation NEC	T49.4X1-	T49.4X2-	T49.4X3-	T49.4X4-	T49.4X5-	T49.4X6-
Halazepam	T42.4X1-	T42.4X2-	T42.4X3-	T42.4X4-	T42.4X5-	T42.4X6-
Halcinolone	T49.0X1-	T49.0X2-	T49.0X3-	T49.0X4-	T49.0X5-	T49.0X6-
Halcinonide	T49.0X1-	T49.0X2-	T49.0X3-	T49.0X4-	T49.0X5-	T49.0X6-
Halethazole	T49.0X1-	T49.0X2-	T49.0X3-	T49.0X4-	T49.0X5-	T49.0X6-
Hallucinogen NEC	T40.901-	T40.902-	T40.903-	T40.904-	T40.905-	T40.906-
Halofantrine	T37.2X1-	T37.2X2-	T37.2X3-	T37.2X4-	T37.2X5-	T37.2X6-
Halofenate	T46.6X1-	T46.6X2-	T46.6X3-	T46.6X4-	T46.6X5-	T46.6X6-
Halometasone	T49.0X1-	T49.0X2-	T49.0X3-	T49.0X4-	T49.0X5-	T49.0X6-
Haloperidol	T43.4X1-	T43.4X2-	T43.4X3-	T43.4X4-	T43.4X5-	T43.4X6-
Haloprogin	T49.0X1-	T49.0X2-	T49.0X3-	T49.0X4-	T49.0X5-	T49.0X6-
Halotex	T49.0X1-	T49.0X2-	T49.0X3-	T49.0X4-	T49.0X5-	T49.0X6-
Halothane	T41.0X1-	T41.0X2-	T41.0X3-	T41.0X4-	T41.0X5-	T41.0X6-
Haloxazolam	T42.4X1-	T42.4X2-	T42.4X3-	T42.4X4-	T42.4X5-	T42.4X6-
Halquinols	T49.0X1-	T49.0X2-	T49.0X3-	T49.0X4-	T49.0X5-	T49.0X6-
Hamamelis	T49.2X1-	T49.2X2-	T49.2X3-	T49.2X4-	T49.2X5-	T49.2X6-
Haptendextran	T45.8X1-	T45.8X2-	T45.8X3-	T45.8X4-	T45.8X5-	T45.8X6-
Harmonyl	T46.5X1-	T46.5X2-	T46.5X3-	T46.5X4-	T46.5X5-	T46.5X6-
Hartmann's solution	T50.3X1-	T50.3X2-	T50.3X3-	T50.3X4-	T50.3X5-	T50.3X6-
Hashish	T40.7X1-	T40.7X2-	T40.7X3-	T40.7X4-	T40.7X5-	T40.7X6-
Hawaiian Woodrose seeds	T40.991-	T40.992-	T40.993-	T40.994-	-	-
HCB	T60.3X1-	T60.3X2-	T60.3X3-	T60.3X4-	-	-
HCH	T53.6X1-	T53.6X2-	T53.6X3-	T53.6X4-	-	-
medicinal	T49.0X1-	T49.0X2-	T49.0X3-	T49.0X4-	T49.0X5-	T49.0X6-
HCN	T57.3X1-	T57.3X2-	T57.3X3-	T57.3X4-	-	-
Headache cures, drugs, powders NEC	T50.901-	T50.902-	T50.903-	T50.904-	T50.905-	T50.906-
Heavenly Blue (morning glory)	T40.991-	T40.992-	T40.993-	T40.994-	-	-
Heavy metal antidote	T45.8X1-	T45.8X2-	T45.8X3-	T45.8X4-	T45.8X5-	T45.8X6-
Hedaquinium	T49.0X1-	T49.0X2-	T49.0X3-	T49.0X4-	T49.0X5-	T49.0X6-
Hedge hyssop	T62.2X1-	T62.2X2-	T62.2X3-	T62.2X4-	-	-
Heet	T49.8X1-	T49.8X2-	T49.8X3-	T49.8X4-	T49.8X5-	T49.8X6-
Helenin	T37.4X1-	T37.4X2-	T37.4X3-	T37.4X4-	T37.4X5-	T37.4X6-
Helium (nonmedicinal) **NEC**	T59.891-	T59.892-	T59.893-	T59.894-	-	-
medicinal	T48.991-	T48.992-	T48.993-	T48.994-	T48.995-	T48.996-
Hellebore (black) (green) (white)	T62.2X1-	T62.2X2-	T62.2X3-	T62.2X4-	-	-
Hematin	T45.8X1-	T45.8X2-	T45.8X3-	T45.8X4-	T45.8X5-	T45.8X6-
Hematinic preparation	T45.8X1-	T45.8X2-	T45.8X3-	T45.8X4-	T45.8X5-	T45.8X6-
Hematological agent	T45.91X-	T45.92X-	T45.93X-	T45.94X-	T45.95X-	T45.96X-
specified NEC	T45.8X1-	T45.8X2-	T45.8X3-	T45.8X4-	T45.8X5-	T45.8X6-
Hemlock	T62.2X1-	T62.2X2-	T62.2X3-	T62.2X4-	-	-
Hemostatic	T45.621-	T45.622-	T45.623-	T45.624-	T45.625-	T45.626-
drug, systemic	T45.621-	T45.622-	T45.623-	T45.624-	T45.625-	T45.626-
Hemostyptic	T49.4X1-	T49.4X2-	T49.4X3-	T49.4X4-	T49.4X5-	T49.4X6-
Henbane	T62.2X1-	T62.2X2-	T62.2X3-	T62.2X4-	-	-
Heparin (sodium)	T45.511-	T45.512-	T45.513-	T45.514-	T45.515-	T45.516-
action reverser	T45.7X1-	T45.7X2-	T45.7X3-	T45.7X4-	T45.7X5-	T45.7X6-
Heparin-fraction	T45.511-	T45.512-	T45.513-	T45.514-	T45.515-	T45.516-
Heparinoid (systemic)	T45.511-	T45.512-	T45.513-	T45.514-	T45.515-	T45.516-
Hepatic secretion stimulant	T47.8X1-	T47.8X2-	T47.8X3-	T47.8X4-	T47.8X5-	T47.8X6-
Hepatitis B						
immune globulin	T50.Z11-	T50.Z12-	T50.Z13-	T50.Z14-	T50.Z15-	T50.Z16-
vaccine	T50.B91-	T50.B92-	T50.B93-	T50.B94-	T50.B95-	T50.B96-
Hepronicate	T46.7X1-	T46.7X2-	T46.7X3-	T46.7X4-	T46.7X5-	T46.7X6-
Heptabarb	T42.3X1-	T42.3X2-	T42.3X3-	T42.3X4-	T42.3X5-	T42.3X6-
Heptabarbital	T42.3X1-	T42.3X2-	T42.3X3-	T42.3X4-	T42.3X5-	T42.3X6-
Heptabarbitone	T42.3X1-	T42.3X2-	T42.3X3-	T42.3X4-	T42.3X5-	T42.3X6-
Heptachlor	T60.1X1-	T60.1X2-	T60.1X3-	T60.1X4-	-	-
Heptalgin	T40.2X1-	T40.2X2-	T40.2X3-	T40.2X4-	T40.2X5-	T40.2X6-
Heptaminol	T46.3X1-	T46.3X2-	T46.3X3-	T46.3X4-	T46.3X5-	T46.3X6-
Herbicide NEC	T60.3X1-	T60.3X2-	T60.3X3-	T60.3X4-	-	-
Heroin	T40.1X1-	T40.1X2-	T40.1X3-	T40.1X4-	-	-
Herplex	T49.5X1-	T49.5X2-	T49.5X3-	T49.5X4-	T49.5X5-	T49.5X6-
HES	T45.8X1-	T45.8X2-	T45.8X3-	T45.8X4-	T45.8X5-	T45.8X6-
Hesperidin	T46.991-	T46.992-	T46.993-	T46.994-	T46.995-	T46.996-
Hetacillin	T36.0X1-	T36.0X2-	T36.0X3-	T36.0X4-	T36.0X5-	T36.0X6-
Hetastarch	T45.8X1-	T45.8X2-	T45.8X3-	T45.8X4-	T45.8X5-	T45.8X6-
HETP	T60.0X1-	T60.0X2-	T60.0X3-	T60.0X4-	-	-
Hexachlorobenzene (vapor)	T60.3X1-	T60.3X2-	T60.3X3-	T60.3X4-	-	-
Hexachlorocyclohexane	T53.6X1-	T53.6X2-	T53.6X3-	T53.6X4-	-	-
Hexachlorophene	T49.0X1-	T49.0X2-	T49.0X3-	T49.0X4-	T49.0X5-	T49.0X6-
Hexadiline	T46.3X1-	T46.3X2-	T46.3X3-	T46.3X4-	T46.3X5-	T46.3X6-
Hexadimethrine (bromide)	T45.7X1-	T45.7X2-	T45.7X3-	T45.7X4-	T45.7X5-	T45.7X6-
Hexadylamine	T46.3X1-	T46.3X2-	T46.3X3-	T46.3X4-	T46.3X5-	T46.3X6-
Hexaethyl tetraphos-phate	T60.0X1-	T60.0X2-	T60.0X3-	T60.0X4-	-	-
Hexafluorenium bromide	T48.1X1-	T48.1X2-	T48.1X3-	T48.1X4-	T48.1X5-	T48.1X6-
Hexafluronium (bromide)	T48.1X1-	T48.1X2-	T48.1X3-	T48.1X4-	T48.1X5-	T48.1X6-
Hexa-germ	T49.2X1-	T49.2X2-	T49.2X3-	T49.2X4-	T49.2X5-	T49.2X6-
Hexahydrobenzol	T52.8X1-	T52.8X2-	T52.8X3-	T52.8X4-	-	-
Hexahydrocresol (s)	T51.8X1-	T51.8X2-	T51.8X3-	T51.8X4-	-	-
arsenide	T57.0X1-	T57.0X2-	T57.0X3-	T57.0X4-	-	-

Substance	Poisoning Accidental (unintentional)	Poisoning Intentional self-harm	Poisoning Assault	Poisoning Undetermined	Adverse effect	Underdosing
Hexahydrocresol - *continued*						
arseniurated	T57.0X1-	T57.0X2-	T57.0X3-	T57.0X4-	-	-
cyanide	T57.3X1-	T57.3X2-	T57.3X3-	T57.3X4-	-	-
gas	T59.891-	T59.892-	T59.893-	T59.894-	-	-
Fluoride (liquid)	T57.8X1-	T57.8X2-	T57.8X3-	T57.8X4-	-	-
vapor	T59.891-	T59.892-	T59.893-	T59.894-	-	-
phophorated	T60.0X1-	T60.0X2-	T60.0X3-	T60.0X4-	-	-
sulfate	T57.8X1-	T57.8X2-	T57.8X3-	T57.8X4-	-	-
sulfide (gas)	T59.6X1-	T59.6X2-	T59.6X3-	T59.6X4-	-	-
arseniurated	T57.0X1-	T57.0X2-	T57.0X3-	T57.0X4-	-	-
sulfurated	T57.8X1-	T57.8X2-	T57.8X3-	T57.8X4-	-	-
Hexahydrophenol	T51.8X1-	T51.8X2-	T51.8X3-	T51.8X4-	-	-
Hexalen	T51.8X1-	T51.8X2-	T51.8X3-	T51.8X4-	-	-
Hexamethonium bromide	T44.2X1-	T44.2X2-	T44.2X3-	T44.2X4-	T44.2X5-	T44.2X6-
Hexamethylene	T52.8X1-	T52.8X2-	T52.8X3-	T52.8X4-	-	-
Hexamethylmelamine	T45.1X1-	T45.1X2-	T45.1X3-	T45.1X4-	T45.1X5-	T45.1X6-
Hexamidine	T49.0X1-	T49.0X2-	T49.0X3-	T49.0X4-	T49.0X5-	T49.0X6-
Hexamine (mandelate)	T37.8X1-	T37.8X2-	T37.8X3-	T37.8X4-	T37.8X5-	T37.8X6-
Hexanone, 2-hexanone	T52.4X1-	T52.4X2-	T52.4X3-	T52.4X4-	-	-
Hexanuorenium	T48.1X1-	T48.1X2-	T48.1X3-	T48.1X4-	T48.1X5-	T48.1X6-
Hexapropymate	T42.6X1-	T42.6X2-	T42.6X3-	T42.6X4-	T42.6X5-	T42.6X6-
Hexasonium iodide	T44.3X1-	T44.3X2-	T44.3X3-	T44.3X4-	T44.3X5-	T44.3X6-
Hexcarbacholine bromide	T48.1X1-	T48.1X2-	T48.1X3-	T48.1X4-	T48.1X5-	T48.1X6-
Hexemal	T42.3X1-	T42.3X2-	T42.3X3-	T42.3X4-	T42.3X5-	T42.3X6-
Hexestrol	T38.5X1-	T38.5X2-	T38.5X3-	T38.5X4-	T38.5X5-	T38.5X6-
Hexethal (sodium)	T42.3X1-	T42.3X2-	T42.3X3-	T42.3X4-	T42.3X5-	T42.3X6-
Hexetidine	T37.8X1-	T37.8X2-	T37.8X3-	T37.8X4-	T37.8X5-	T37.8X6-
Hexobarbital	T42.3X1-	T42.3X2-	T42.3X3-	T42.3X4-	T42.3X5-	T42.3X6-
rectal	T41.291-	T41.292-	T41.293-	T41.294-	T41.295-	T41.296-
sodium	T41.1X1-	T41.1X2-	T41.1X3-	T41.1X4-	T41.1X5-	T41.1X6-
Hexobendine	T46.3X1-	T46.3X2-	T46.3X3-	T46.3X4-	T46.3X5-	T46.3X6-
Hexocyclium	T44.3X1-	T44.3X2-	T44.3X3-	T44.3X4-	T44.3X5-	T44.3X6-
metilsulfate	T44.3X1-	T44.3X2-	T44.3X3-	T44.3X4-	T44.3X5-	T44.3X6-
Hexoestrol	T38.5X1-	T38.5X2-	T38.5X3-	T38.5X4-	T38.5X5-	T38.5X6-
Hexone	T52.4X1-	T52.4X2-	T52.4X3-	T52.4X4-	-	-
Hexoprenaline	T48.6X1-	T48.6X2-	T48.6X3-	T48.6X4-	T48.6X5-	T48.6X6-
Hexylcaine	T41.3X1-	T41.3X2-	T41.3X3-	T41.3X4-	T41.3X5-	T41.3X6-
Hexylresorcinol	T52.2X1-	T52.2X2-	T52.2X3-	T52.2X4-	-	-
HGH (human growth hormone)	T38.811-	T38.812-	T38.813-	T38.814-	T38.815-	T38.816-
Hinkle's pills	T47.2X1-	T47.2X2-	T47.2X3-	T47.2X4-	T47.2X5-	T47.2X6-
Histalog	T50.8X1-	T50.8X2-	T50.8X3-	T50.8X4-	T50.8X5-	T50.8X6-
Histamine (phosphate)	T50.8X1-	T50.8X2-	T50.8X3-	T50.8X4-	T50.8X5-	T50.8X6-
Histoplasmin	T50.8X1-	T50.8X2-	T50.8X3-	T50.8X4-	T50.8X5-	T50.8X6-
Holly berries	T62.2X1-	T62.2X2-	T62.2X3-	T62.2X4-	-	-
Homatropine	T44.3X1-	T44.3X2-	T44.3X3-	T44.3X4-	T44.3X5-	T44.3X6-
methylbromide	T44.3X1-	T44.3X2-	T44.3X3-	T44.3X4-	T44.3X5-	T44.3X6-
Homochlorcyclizine	T45.0X1-	T45.0X2-	T45.0X3-	T45.0X4-	T45.0X5-	T45.0X6-
Homosalate	T49.3X1-	T49.3X2-	T49.3X3-	T49.3X4-	T49.3X5-	T49.3X6-
Homo-tet	T50.Z11-	T50.Z12-	T50.Z13-	T50.Z14-	T50.Z15-	T50.Z16-
Hormone	T38.801-	T38.802-	T38.803-	T38.804-	T38.805-	T38.806-
adrenal cortical steroids	T38.0X1-	T38.0X2-	T38.0X3-	T38.0X4-	T38.0X5-	T38.0X6-
androgenic	T38.7X1-	T38.7X2-	T38.7X3-	T38.7X4-	T38.7X5-	T38.7X6-
anterior pituitary NEC	T38.811-	T38.812-	T38.813-	T38.814-	T38.815-	T38.816-
antidiabetic agents	T38.3X1-	T38.3X2-	T38.3X3-	T38.3X4-	T38.3X5-	T38.3X6-
antidiuretic	T38.891-	T38.892-	T38.893-	T38.894-	T38.895-	T38.896-
cancer therapy	T45.1X1-	T45.1X2-	T45.1X3-	T45.1X4-	T45.1X5-	T45.1X6-
follicle stimulating	T38.811-	T38.812-	T38.813-	T38.814-	T38.815-	T38.816-
gonadotropic	T38.891-	T38.892-	T38.893-	T38.894-	T38.895-	T38.896-
pituitary	T38.811-	T38.812-	T38.813-	T38.814-	T38.815-	T38.816-
growth	T38.811-	T38.812-	T38.813-	T38.814-	T38.815-	T38.816-
luteinizing	T38.811-	T38.812-	T38.813-	T38.814-	T38.815-	T38.816-
ovarian	T38.5X1-	T38.5X2-	T38.5X3-	T38.5X4-	T38.5X5-	T38.5X6-
oxytocic	T48.0X1-	T48.0X2-	T48.0X3-	T48.0X4-	T48.0X5-	T48.0X6-
parathyroid (derivatives)	T50.991-	T50.992-	T50.993-	T50.994-	T50.995-	T50.996-
pituitary (posterior) NEC	T38.891-	T38.892-	T38.893-	T38.894-	T38.895-	T38.896-
anterior	T38.811-	T38.812-	T38.813-	T38.814-	T38.815-	T38.816-
specified, NEC	T38.891-	T38.892-	T38.893-	T38.894-	T38.895-	T38.896-
thyroid	T38.1X1-	T38.1X2-	T38.1X3-	T38.1X4-	T38.1X5-	T38.1X6-
Hornet (sting)	T63.451-	T63.452-	T63.453-	T63.454-	-	-
Horse anti-human lymphocytic serum	T50.Z11-	T50.Z12-	T50.Z13-	T50.Z14-	T50.Z15-	T50.Z16-
Horticulture agent NEC	T65.91X-	T65.92X-	T65.93X-	T65.94X-	-	-
with pesticide	T60.91X-	T60.92X-	T60.93X-	T60.94X-	-	-
Human						
albumin	T45.8X1-	T45.8X2-	T45.8X3-	T45.8X4-	T45.8X5-	T45.8X6-
growth hormone (HGH)	T38.811-	T38.812-	T38.813-	T38.814-	T38.815-	T38.816-
immune serum	T50.Z11-	T50.Z12-	T50.Z13-	T50.Z14-	T50.Z15-	T50.Z16-
Hyaluronidase	T45.3X1-	T45.3X2-	T45.3X3-	T45.3X4-	T45.3X5-	T45.3X6-

Substance	Poisoning Accidental (unintentional)	Poisoning Intentional self-harm	Poisoning Assault	Poisoning Undetermined	Adverse effect	Underdosing
Hyazyme	T45.3X1-	T45.3X2-	T45.3X3-	T45.3X4-	T45.3X5-	T45.3X6-
Hycodan	T40.2X1-	T40.2X2-	T40.2X3-	T40.2X4-	T40.2X5-	T40.2X6-
Hydantoin derivative NEC	T42.0X1-	T42.0X2-	T42.0X3-	T42.0X4-	T42.0X5-	T42.0X6-
Hydeltra	T38.0X1-	T38.0X2-	T38.0X3-	T38.0X4-	T38.0X5-	T38.0X6-
Hydergine	T44.6X1-	T44.6X2-	T44.6X3-	T44.6X4-	T44.6X5-	T44.6X6-
Hydrabamine penicillin	T36.0X1-	T36.0X2-	T36.0X3-	T36.0X4-	T36.0X5-	T36.0X6-
Hydralazine	T46.5X1-	T46.5X2-	T46.5X3-	T46.5X4-	T46.5X5-	T46.5X6-
Hydrargaphen	T49.0X1-	T49.0X2-	T49.0X3-	T49.0X4-	T49.0X5-	T49.0X6-
Hydrargyri amino-chloridum	T49.0X1-	T49.0X2-	T49.0X3-	T49.0X4-	T49.0X5-	T49.0X6-
Hydrastine	T48.291-	T48.292-	T48.293-	T48.294-	T48.295-	T48.296-
Hydrazine	T54.1X1-	T54.1X2-	T54.1X3-	T54.1X4-	-	-
monoamine oxidase inhibitors	T43.1X1-	T43.1X2-	T43.1X3-	T43.1X4-	T43.1X5-	T43.1X6-
Hydrazoic acid, azides	T54.2X1-	T54.2X2-	T54.2X3-	T54.2X4-	-	-
Hydriodic acid	T48.4X1-	T48.4X2-	T48.4X3-	T48.4X4-	T48.4X5-	T48.4X6-
Hydrocarbon gas	T59.891-	T59.892-	T59.893-	T59.894-	-	-
incomplete combustion of — *see* Carbon, monoxide, fuel, utility						
liquefied (mobile container)	T59.891-	T59.892-	T59.893-	T59.894-	-	-
piped (natural)	T59.891-	T59.892-	T59.893-	T59.894-	-	-
Hydrochloric acid (liquid)	T54.2X1-	T54.2X2-	T54.2X3-	T54.2X4-	-	-
medicinal (digestant)	T47.5X1-	T47.5X2-	T47.5X3-	T47.5X4-	T47.5X5-	T47.5X6-
vapor	T59.891-	T59.892-	T59.893-	T59.894-	-	-
Hydrochlorothiazide	T50.2X1-	T50.2X2-	T50.2X3-	T50.2X4-	T50.2X5-	T50.2X6-
Hydrocodone	T40.2X1-	T40.2X2-	T40.2X3-	T40.2X4-	T40.2X5-	T40.2X6-
Hydrocortisone (derivatives)	T38.0X1-	T38.0X2-	T38.0X3-	T38.0X4-	T38.0X5-	T38.0X6-
aceponate	T49.0X1-	T49.0X2-	T49.0X3-	T49.0X4-	T49.0X5-	T49.0X6-
ENT agent	T49.6X1-	T49.6X2-	T49.6X3-	T49.6X4-	T49.6X5-	T49.6X6-
ophthalmic preparation	T49.5X1-	T49.5X2-	T49.5X3-	T49.5X4-	T49.5X5-	T49.5X6-
topical NEC	T49.0X1-	T49.0X2-	T49.0X3-	T49.0X4-	T49.0X5-	T49.0X6-
Hydrocortone	T38.0X1-	T38.0X2-	T38.0X3-	T38.0X4-	T38.0X5-	T38.0X6-
ENT agent	T49.6X1-	T49.6X2-	T49.6X3-	T49.6X4-	T49.6X5-	T49.6X6-
ophthalmic preparation	T49.5X1-	T49.5X2-	T49.5X3-	T49.5X4-	T49.5X5-	T49.5X6-
topical NEC	T49.0X1-	T49.0X2-	T49.0X3-	T49.0X4-	T49.0X5-	T49.0X6-
Hydrocyanic acid (liquid)	T57.3X1-	T57.3X2-	T57.3X3-	T57.3X4-	-	-
gas	T65.0X1-	T65.0X2-	T65.0X3-	T65.0X4-	-	-
Hydroflumethiazide	T50.2X1-	T50.2X2-	T50.2X3-	T50.2X4-	T50.2X5-	T50.2X6-
Hydrofluoric acid (liquid)	T54.2X1-	T54.2X2-	T54.2X3-	T54.2X4-	-	-
vapor	T59.891-	T59.892-	T59.893-	T59.894-	-	-
Hydrogen	T59.891-	T59.892-	T59.893-	T59.894-	-	-
arsenide	T57.0X1-	T57.0X2-	T57.0X3-	T57.0X4-	-	-
arseniureted	T57.0X1-	T57.0X2-	T57.0X3-	T57.0X4-	-	-
chloride	T57.8X1-	T57.8X2-	T57.8X3-	T57.8X4-	-	-
cyanide (salts)	T57.3X1-	T57.3X2-	T57.3X3-	T57.3X4-	-	-
gas	T57.3X1-	T57.3X2-	T57.3X3-	T57.3X4-	-	-
Fluoride	T59.5X1-	T59.5X2-	T59.5X3-	T59.5X4-	-	-
vapor	T59.5X1-	T59.5X2-	T59.5X3-	T59.5X4-	-	-
peroxide	T49.0X1-	T49.0X2-	T49.0X3-	T49.0X4-	T49.0X5-	T49.0X6-
phosphureted	T57.1X1-	T57.1X2-	T57.1X3-	T57.1X4-	-	-
sulfide	T59.6X1-	T59.6X2-	T59.6X3-	T59.6X4-	-	-
arseniureted	T57.0X1-	T57.0X2-	T57.0X3-	T57.0X4-	-	-
sulfureted	T59.6X1-	T59.6X2-	T59.6X3-	T59.6X4-	-	-
Hydromethylpyridine	T46.7X1-	T46.7X2-	T46.7X3-	T46.7X4-	T46.7X5-	T46.7X6-
Hydromorphinol	T40.2X1-	T40.2X2-	T40.2X3-	T40.2X4-	-	-
Hydromorphinone	T40.2X1-	T40.2X2-	T40.2X3-	T40.2X4-	T40.2X5-	T40.2X6-
Hydromorphone	T40.2X1-	T40.2X2-	T40.2X3-	T40.2X4-	T40.2X5-	T40.2X6-
Hydromox	T50.2X1-	T50.2X2-	T50.2X3-	T50.2X4-	T50.2X5-	T50.2X6-
Hydrophilic lotion	T49.3X1-	T49.3X2-	T49.3X3-	T49.3X4-	T49.3X5-	T49.3X6-
Hydroquinidine	T46.2X1-	T46.2X2-	T46.2X3-	T46.2X4-	T46.2X5-	T46.2X6-
Hydroquinone	T52.2X1-	T52.2X2-	T52.2X3-	T52.2X4-	-	-
vapor	T59.891-	T59.892-	T59.893-	T59.894-	-	-
Hydrosulfuric acid (gas)	T59.6X1-	T59.6X2-	T59.6X3-	T59.6X4-	-	-
Hydrotalcite	T47.1X1-	T47.1X2-	T47.1X3-	T47.1X4-	T47.1X5-	T47.1X6-
Hydrous wool fat	T49.3X1-	T49.3X2-	T49.3X3-	T49.3X4-	T49.3X5-	T49.3X6-
Hydroxide, caustic	T54.3X1-	T54.3X2-	T54.3X3-	T54.3X4-	-	-
Hydroxocobalamin	T45.8X1-	T45.8X2-	T45.8X3-	T45.8X4-	T45.8X5-	T45.8X6-
Hydroxyamphetamine	T49.5X1-	T49.5X2-	T49.5X3-	T49.5X4-	T49.5X5-	T49.5X6-
Hydroxycarbamide	T45.1X1-	T45.1X2-	T45.1X3-	T45.1X4-	T45.1X5-	T45.1X6-
Hydroxychloroquine	T37.8X1-	T37.8X2-	T37.8X3-	T37.8X4-	T37.8X5-	T37.8X6-
Hydroxydihydrocodeinone	T40.2X1-	T40.2X2-	T40.2X3-	T40.2X4-	T40.2X5-	T40.2X6-
Hydroxyestrone	T38.5X1-	T38.5X2-	T38.5X3-	T38.5X4-	T38.5X5-	T38.5X6-
Hydroxyethyl starch	T45.8X1-	T45.8X2-	T45.8X3-	T45.8X4-	T45.8X5-	T45.8X6-
Hydroxymethylpenta-none	T52.4X1-	T52.4X2-	T52.4X3-	T52.4X4-	-	-
Hydroxyphenamate	T43.591-	T43.592-	T43.593-	T43.594-	T43.595-	T43.596-
Hydroxyphenylbutazone	T39.2X1-	T39.2X2-	T39.2X3-	T39.2X4-	T39.2X5-	T39.2X6-
Hydroxyprogesterone	T38.5X1-	T38.5X2-	T38.5X3-	T38.5X4-	T38.5X5-	T38.5X6-
caproate	T38.5X1-	T38.5X2-	T38.5X3-	T38.5X4-	T38.5X5-	T38.5X6-

Substance	Poisoning Accidental (unintentional)	Poisoning Intentional self-harm	Poisoning Assault	Poisoning Undetermined	Adverse effect	Underdosing
Hydroxyquinoline (derivatives) **NEC**	T37.8X1-	T37.8X2-	T37.8X3-	T37.8X4-	T37.8X5-	T37.8X6-
Hydroxystilbamidine	T37.3X1-	T37.3X2-	T37.3X3-	T37.3X4-	T37.3X5-	T37.3X6-
Hydroxytoluene (nonmedicinal)	T54.0X1-	T54.0X2-	T54.0X3-	T54.0X4-	-	-
medicinal	T49.0X1-	T49.0X2-	T49.0X3-	T49.0X4-	T49.0X5-	T49.0X6-
Hydroxyurea	T45.1X1-	T45.1X2-	T45.1X3-	T45.1X4-	T45.1X5-	T45.1X6-
Hydroxyzine	T43.591-	T43.592-	T43.593-	T43.594-	T43.595-	T43.596-
Hyoscine	T44.3X1-	T44.3X2-	T44.3X3-	T44.3X4-	T44.3X5-	T44.3X6-
Hyoscyamine	T44.3X1-	T44.3X2-	T44.3X3-	T44.3X4-	T44.3X5-	T44.3X6-
Hyoscyamus	T44.3X1-	T44.3X2-	T44.3X3-	T44.3X4-	T44.3X5-	T44.3X6-
dry extract	T44.3X1-	T44.3X2-	T44.3X3-	T44.3X4-	T44.3X5-	T44.3X6-
Hypaque	T50.8X1-	T50.8X2-	T50.8X3-	T50.8X4-	T50.8X5-	T50.8X6-
Hypertussis	T50.Z11-	T50.Z12-	T50.Z13-	T50.Z14-	T50.Z15-	T50.Z16-
Hypnotic	T42.71X-	T42.72X-	T42.73X-	T42.74X-	T42.75X-	T42.76X-
anticonvulsant	T42.71X-	T42.72X-	T42.73X-	T42.74X-	T42.75X-	T42.76X-
specified NEC	T42.6X1-	T42.6X2-	T42.6X3-	T42.6X4-	T42.6X5-	T42.6X6-
Hypochlorite	T49.0X1-	T49.0X2-	T49.0X3-	T49.0X4-	T49.0X5-	T49.0X6-
Hypophysis, posterior	T38.891-	T38.892-	T38.893-	T38.894-	T38.895-	T38.896-
Hypotensive NEC	T46.5X1-	T46.5X2-	T46.5X3-	T46.5X4-	T46.5X5-	T46.5X6-
Hypromellose	T49.5X1-	T49.5X2-	T49.5X3-	T49.5X4-	T49.5X5-	T49.5X6-
Ibacitabine	T37.5X1-	T37.5X2-	T37.5X3-	T37.5X4-	T37.5X5-	T37.5X6-
Ibopamine	T44.991-	T44.992-	T44.993-	T44.994-	T44.995-	T44.996-
Ibufenac	T39.311-	T39.312-	T39.313-	T39.314-	T39.315-	T39.316-
Ibuprofen	T39.311-	T39.312-	T39.313-	T39.314-	T39.315-	T39.316-
Ibuproxam	T39.311-	T39.312-	T39.313-	T39.314-	T39.315-	T39.316-
Ibuterol	T48.6X1-	T48.6X2-	T48.6X3-	T48.6X4-	T48.6X5-	T48.6X6-
Ichthammol	T49.0X1-	T49.0X2-	T49.0X3-	T49.0X4-	T49.0X5-	T49.0X6-
Ichthyol	T49.4X1-	T49.4X2-	T49.4X3-	T49.4X4-	T49.4X5-	T49.4X6-
Idarubicin	T45.1X1-	T45.1X2-	T45.1X3-	T45.1X4-	T45.1X5-	T45.1X6-
Idrocilamide	T42.8X1-	T42.8X2-	T42.8X3-	T42.8X4-	T42.8X5-	T42.8X6-
Ifenprodil	T46.7X1-	T46.7X2-	T46.7X3-	T46.7X4-	T46.7X5-	T46.7X6-
Ifosfamide	T45.1X1-	T45.1X2-	T45.1X3-	T45.1X4-	T45.1X5-	T45.1X6-
Iletin	T38.3X1-	T38.3X2-	T38.3X3-	T38.3X4-	T38.3X5-	T38.3X6-
Ilex	T62.2X1-	T62.2X2-	T62.2X3-	T62.2X4-	-	-
Illuminating gas (after combustion)	T58.11X-	T58.12X-	T58.13X-	T58.14X-	-	-
prior to combustion	T59.891-	T59.892-	T59.893-	T59.894-	-	-
Ilopan	T45.2X1-	T45.2X2-	T45.2X3-	T45.2X4-	T45.2X5-	T45.2X6-
Iloprost	T46.7X1-	T46.7X2-	T46.7X3-	T46.7X4-	T46.7X5-	T46.7X6-
Ilotycin	T36.3X1-	T36.3X2-	T36.3X3-	T36.3X4-	T36.3X5-	T36.3X6-
ophthalmic preparation	T49.5X1-	T49.5X2-	T49.5X3-	T49.5X4-	T49.5X5-	T49.5X6-
topical NEC	T49.0X1-	T49.0X2-	T49.0X3-	T49.0X4-	T49.0X5-	T49.0X6-
Imidazole-4-carboxamide	T45.1X1-	T45.1X2-	T45.1X3-	T45.1X4-	T45.1X5-	T45.1X6-
Imipenem	T36.0X1-	T36.0X2-	T36.0X3-	T36.0X4-	T36.0X5-	T36.0X6-
Imipramine	T43.011-	T43.012-	T43.013-	T43.014-	T43.015-	T43.016-
Iminostilbene	T42.1X1-	T42.1X2-	T42.1X3-	T42.1X4-	T42.1X5-	T42.1X6-
Immu-G	T50.Z11-	T50.Z12-	T50.Z13-	T50.Z14-	T50.Z15-	T50.Z16-
Immuglobin	T50.Z11-	T50.Z12-	T50.Z13-	T50.Z14-	T50.Z15-	T50.Z16-
Immune						
globulin	T50.Z11-	T50.Z12-	T50.Z13-	T50.Z14-	T50.Z15-	T50.Z16-
serum globulin	T50.Z11-	T50.Z12-	T50.Z13-	T50.Z14-	T50.Z15-	T50.Z16-
Immunoglobin human (intravenous) (normal)	T50.Z11-	T50.Z12-	T50.Z13-	T50.Z14-	T50.Z15-	T50.Z16-
unmodified	T50.Z11-	T50.Z12-	T50.Z13-	T50.Z14-	T50.Z15-	T50.Z16-
Immunosuppressive drug	T45.1X1-	T45.1X2-	T45.1X3-	T45.1X4-	T45.1X5-	T45.1X6-
Immu-tetanus	T50.Z11-	T50.Z12-	T50.Z13-	T50.Z14-	T50.Z15-	T50.Z16-
Indalpine	T43.221-	T43.222-	T43.223-	T43.224-	T43.225-	T43.226-
Indanazoline	T48.5X1-	T48.5X2-	T48.5X3-	T48.5X4-	T48.5X5-	T48.5X6-
Indandione (derivatives)	T45.511-	T45.512-	T45.513-	T45.514-	T45.515-	T45.516-
Indapamide	T46.5X1-	T46.5X2-	T46.5X3-	T46.5X4-	T46.5X5-	T46.5X6-
Indendione (derivatives)	T45.511-	T45.512-	T45.513-	T45.514-	T45.515-	T45.516-
Indenolol	T44.7X1-	T44.7X2-	T44.7X3-	T44.7X4-	T44.7X5-	T44.7X6-
Inderal	T44.7X1-	T44.7X2-	T44.7X3-	T44.7X4-	T44.7X5-	T44.7X6-
Indian						
hemp	T40.7X1-	T40.7X2-	T40.7X3-	T40.7X4-	T40.7X5-	T40.7X6-
tobacco	T62.2X1-	T62.2X2-	T62.2X3-	T62.2X4-	-	-
Indigo carmine	T50.8X1-	T50.8X2-	T50.8X3-	T50.8X4-	T50.8X5-	T50.8X6-
Indobufen	T45.521-	T45.522-	T45.523-	T45.524-	T45.525-	T45.526-
Indocin	T39.2X1-	T39.2X2-	T39.2X3-	T39.2X4-	T39.2X5-	T39.2X6-
Indocyanine green	T50.8X1-	T50.8X2-	T50.8X3-	T50.8X4-	T50.8X5-	T50.8X6-
Indometacin	T39.391-	T39.392-	T39.393-	T39.394-	T39.395-	T39.396-
Indomethacin	T39.391-	T39.392-	T39.393-	T39.394-	T39.395-	T39.396-
farnesil	T39.4X1-	T39.4X2-	T39.4X3-	T39.4X4-	T39.4X5-	T39.4X6-
Indoramin	T44.6X1-	T44.6X2-	T44.6X3-	T44.6X4-	T44.6X5-	T44.6X6-
Industrial						
alcohol	T51.0X1-	T51.0X2-	T51.0X3-	T51.0X4-	-	-
fumes	T59.891-	T59.892-	T59.893-	T59.894-	-	-
solvents (fumes) (vapors)	T52.91X-	T52.92X-	T52.93X-	T52.94X-	-	-
Influenza vaccine	T50.B91-	T50.B92-	T50.B93-	T50.B94-	T50.B95-	T50.B96-
Ingested substance NEC	T65.91X-	T65.92X-	T65.93X-	T65.94X-	-	-
INH	T37.1X1-	T37.1X2-	T37.1X3-	T37.1X4-	T37.1X5-	T37.1X6-
Inhalation, gas (noxious) — *see* Gas						
Inhibitor						
angiotensin-converting enzyme	T46.4X1-	T46.4X2-	T46.4X3-	T46.4X4-	T46.4X5-	T46.4X6-
carbonic anhydrase	T50.2X1-	T50.2X2-	T50.2X3-	T50.2X4-	T50.2X5-	T50.2X6-
fibrinolysis	T45.621-	T45.622-	T45.623-	T45.624-	T45.625-	T45.626-
monoamine oxidase NEC	T43.1X1-	T43.1X2-	T43.1X3-	T43.1X4-	T43.1X5-	T43.1X6-
hydrazine	T43.1X1-	T43.1X2-	T43.1X3-	T43.1X4-	T43.1X5-	T43.1X6-
postsynaptic	T43.8X1-	T43.8X2-	T43.8X3-	T43.8X4-	T43.8X5-	T43.8X6-
prothrombin synthesis	T45.511-	T45.512-	T45.513-	T45.514-	T45.515-	T45.516-
Ink	T65.891-	T65.892-	T65.893-	T65.894-	-	-
Inorganic substance NEC	T57.91X-	T57.92X-	T57.93X-	T57.94X-	-	-
Inosine pranobex	T37.5X1-	T37.5X2-	T37.5X3-	T37.5X4-	T37.5X5-	T37.5X6-
Inositol	T50.991-	T50.992-	T50.993-	T50.994-	T50.995-	T50.996-
nicotinate	T46.7X1-	T46.7X2-	T46.7X3-	T46.7X4-	T46.7X5-	T46.7X6-
Inproquone	T45.1X1-	T45.1X2-	T45.1X3-	T45.1X4-	T45.1X5-	T45.1X6-
Insect (sting) **, venomous**	T63.481-	T63.482-	T63.483-	T63.484-	-	-
ant	T63.421-	T63.422-	T63.423-	T63.424-	-	-
bee	T63.441-	T63.442-	T63.443-	T63.444-	-	-
caterpillar	T63.431-	T63.432-	T63.433-	T63.434-	-	-
hornet	T63.451-	T63.452-	T63.453-	T63.454-	-	-
wasp	T63.461-	T63.462-	T63.463-	T63.464-	-	-
Insecticide NEC	T60.91X-	T60.92X-	T60.93X-	T60.94X-	-	-
carbamate	T60.0X1-	T60.0X2-	T60.0X3-	T60.0X4-	-	-
chlorinated	T60.1X1-	T60.1X2-	T60.1X3-	T60.1X4-	-	-
mixed	T60.91X-	T60.92X-	T60.93X-	T60.94X-	-	-
organochlorine	T60.1X1-	T60.1X2-	T60.1X3-	T60.1X4-	-	-
organophosphorus	T60.0X1-	T60.0X2-	T60.0X3-	T60.0X4-	-	-
Insular tissue extract	T38.3X1-	T38.3X2-	T38.3X3-	T38.3X4-	T38.3X5-	T38.3X6-
Insulin (amorphous) (globin) (isophane) (Lente) (NPH) (Semilente) (Ultralente)	T38.3X1-	T38.3X2-	T38.3X3-	T38.3X4-	T38.3X5-	T38.3X6-
defalan	T38.3X1-	T38.3X2-	T38.3X3-	T38.3X4-	T38.3X5-	T38.3X6-
human	T38.3X1-	T38.3X2-	T38.3X3-	T38.3X4-	T38.3X5-	T38.3X6-
injection, soluble	T38.3X1-	T38.3X2-	T38.3X3-	T38.3X4-	T38.3X5-	T38.3X6-
biphasic	T38.3X1-	T38.3X2-	T38.3X3-	T38.3X4-	T38.3X5-	T38.3X6-
intermediate acting	T38.3X1-	T38.3X2-	T38.3X3-	T38.3X4-	T38.3X5-	T38.3X6-
protamine zinc	T38.3X1-	T38.3X2-	T38.3X3-	T38.3X4-	T38.3X5-	T38.3X6-
slow acting	T38.3X1-	T38.3X2-	T38.3X3-	T38.3X4-	T38.3X5-	T38.3X6-
zinc						
protamine injection	T38.3X1-	T38.3X2-	T38.3X3-	T38.3X4-	T38.3X5-	T38.3X6-
suspension (amorphous) (crystalline)	T38.3X1-	T38.3X2-	T38.3X3-	T38.3X4-	T38.3X5-	T38.3X6-
Interferon (alpha) (beta) (gamma)	T37.5X1-	T37.5X2-	T37.5X3-	T37.5X4-	T37.5X5-	T37.5X6-
Intestinal motility control drug	T47.6X1-	T47.6X2-	T47.6X3-	T47.6X4-	T47.6X5-	T47.6X6-
biological	T47.8X1-	T47.8X2-	T47.8X3-	T47.8X4-	T47.8X5-	T47.8X6-
Intranarcon	T41.1X1-	T41.1X2-	T41.1X3-	T41.1X4-	T41.1X5-	T41.1X6-
Intravenous						
amino acids	T50.991-	T50.992-	T50.993-	T50.994-	T50.995-	T50.996-
fat suspension	T50.991-	T50.992-	T50.993-	T50.994-	T50.995-	T50.996-
Inulin	T50.8X1-	T50.8X2-	T50.8X3-	T50.8X4-	T50.8X5-	T50.8X6-
Invert sugar	T50.3X1-	T50.3X2-	T50.3X3-	T50.3X4-	T50.3X5-	T50.3X6-
Inza — *see* Naproxen						
Iobenzamic acid	T50.8X1-	T50.8X2-	T50.8X3-	T50.8X4-	T50.8X5-	T50.8X6-
Iocarmic acid	T50.8X1-	T50.8X2-	T50.8X3-	T50.8X4-	T50.8X5-	T50.8X6-
Iocetamic acid	T50.8X1-	T50.8X2-	T50.8X3-	T50.8X4-	T50.8X5-	T50.8X6-
Iodamide	T50.8X1-	T50.8X2-	T50.8X3-	T50.8X4-	T50.8X5-	T50.8X6-
Iodide NEC — *see also* Iodine	T49.0X1-	T49.0X2-	T49.0X3-	T49.0X4-	T49.0X5-	T49.0X6-
mercury (ointment)	T49.0X1-	T49.0X2-	T49.0X3-	T49.0X4-	T49.0X5-	T49.0X6-
methylate	T49.0X1-	T49.0X2-	T49.0X3-	T49.0X4-	T49.0X5-	T49.0X6-
potassium (expectorant) NEC	T48.4X1-	T48.4X2-	T48.4X3-	T48.4X4-	T48.4X5-	T48.4X6-
Iodinated						
contrast medium	T50.8X1-	T50.8X2-	T50.8X3-	T50.8X4-	T50.8X5-	T50.8X6-
glycerol	T48.4X1-	T48.4X2-	T48.4X3-	T48.4X4-	T48.4X5-	T48.4X6-
human serum albumin (131I)	T50.8X1-	T50.8X2-	T50.8X3-	T50.8X4-	T50.8X5-	T50.8X6-
Iodine (antiseptic, external) (tincture) **NEC**	T49.0X1-	T49.0X2-	T49.0X3-	T49.0X4-	T49.0X5-	T49.0X6-
125 — *see also* Radiation sickness, and Exposure to radioactivce isotopes	T50.8X1-	T50.8X2-	T50.8X3-	T50.8X4-	T50.8X5-	T50.8X6-
therapeutic	T50.991-	T50.992-	T50.993-	T50.994-	T50.995-	T50.996-
131 — *see also* Radiation sickness, and Exposure to radioactivce isotopes	T50.8X1-	T50.8X2-	T50.8X3-	T50.8X4-	T50.8X5-	T50.8X6-
therapeutic	T38.2X1-	T38.2X2-	T38.2X3-	T38.2X4-	T38.2X5-	T38.2X6-

Substance	Poisoning Accidental (unintentional)	Poisoning Intentional self-harm	Poisoning Assault	Poisoning Undetermined	Adverse effect	Underdosing
Iodine NEC - *continued*						
diagnostic	T50.8X1-	T50.8X2-	T50.8X3-	T50.8X4-	T50.8X5-	T50.8X6-
for thyroid conditions (antithyroid)	T38.2X1-	T38.2X2-	T38.2X3-	T38.2X4-	T38.2X5-	T38.2X6-
solution	T49.0X1-	T49.0X2-	T49.0X3-	T49.0X4-	T49.0X5-	T49.0X6-
vapor	T59.891-	T59.892-	T59.893-	T59.894-	-	-
Iodipamide	T50.8X1-	T50.8X2-	T50.8X3-	T50.8X4-	T50.8X5-	T50.8X6-
Iodized (poppy seed) **oil**	T50.8X1-	T50.8X2-	T50.8X3-	T50.8X4-	T50.8X5-	T50.8X6-
Iodobismitol	T37.8X1-	T37.8X2-	T37.8X3-	T37.8X4-	T37.8X5-	T37.8X6-
Iodochlorhydroxyquin	T37.8X1-	T37.8X2-	T37.8X3-	T37.8X4-	T37.8X5-	T37.8X6-
topical	T49.0X1-	T49.0X2-	T49.0X3-	T49.0X4-	T49.0X5-	T49.0X6-
Iodochlorhydroxyquinoline	T37.8X1-	T37.8X2-	T37.8X3-	T37.8X4-	T37.8X5-	T37.8X6-
Iodocholesterol (131I)	T50.8X1-	T50.8X2-	T50.8X3-	T50.8X4-	T50.8X5-	T50.8X6-
Iodoform	T49.0X1-	T49.0X2-	T49.0X3-	T49.0X4-	T49.0X5-	T49.0X6-
Iodohippuric acid	T50.8X1-	T50.8X2-	T50.8X3-	T50.8X4-	T50.8X5-	T50.8X6-
Iodopanoic acid	T50.8X1-	T50.8X2-	T50.8X3-	T50.8X4-	T50.8X5-	T50.8X6-
Iodophthalein (sodium)	T50.8X1-	T50.8X2-	T50.8X3-	T50.8X4-	T50.8X5-	T50.8X6-
Iodopyracet	T50.8X1-	T50.8X2-	T50.8X3-	T50.8X4-	T50.8X5-	T50.8X6-
Iodoquinol	T37.8X1-	T37.8X2-	T37.8X3-	T37.8X4-	T37.8X5-	T37.8X6-
Iodoxamic acid	T50.8X1-	T50.8X2-	T50.8X3-	T50.8X4-	T50.8X5-	T50.8X6-
Iofendylate	T50.8X1-	T50.8X2-	T50.8X3-	T50.8X4-	T50.8X5-	T50.8X6-
Ioglycamic acid	T50.8X1-	T50.8X2-	T50.8X3-	T50.8X4-	T50.8X5-	T50.8X6-
Iohexol	T50.8X1-	T50.8X2-	T50.8X3-	T50.8X4-	T50.8X5-	T50.8X6-
Ion exchange resin						
anion	T47.8X1-	T47.8X2-	T47.8X3-	T47.8X4-	T47.8X5-	T47.8X6-
cation	T50.3X1-	T50.3X2-	T50.3X3-	T50.3X4-	T50.3X5-	T50.3X6-
cholestyramine	T46.6X1-	T46.6X2-	T46.6X3-	T46.6X4-	T46.6X5-	T46.6X6-
intestinal	T47.8X1-	T47.8X2-	T47.8X3-	T47.8X4-	T47.8X5-	T47.8X6-
Iopamidol	T50.8X1-	T50.8X2-	T50.8X3-	T50.8X4-	T50.8X5-	T50.8X6-
Iopanoic acid	T50.8X1-	T50.8X2-	T50.8X3-	T50.8X4-	T50.8X5-	T50.8X6-
Iophenoic acid	T50.8X1-	T50.8X2-	T50.8X3-	T50.8X4-	T50.8X5-	T50.8X6-
Iopodate, sodium	T50.8X1-	T50.8X2-	T50.8X3-	T50.8X4-	T50.8X5-	T50.8X6-
Iopodic acid	T50.8X1-	T50.8X2-	T50.8X3-	T50.8X4-	T50.8X5-	T50.8X6-
Iopromide	T50.8X1-	T50.8X2-	T50.8X3-	T50.8X4-	T50.8X5-	T50.8X6-
Iopydol	T50.8X1-	T50.8X2-	T50.8X3-	T50.8X4-	T50.8X5-	T50.8X6-
Iotalamic acid	T50.8X1-	T50.8X2-	T50.8X3-	T50.8X4-	T50.8X5-	T50.8X6-
Iothalamate	T50.8X1-	T50.8X2-	T50.8X3-	T50.8X4-	T50.8X5-	T50.8X6-
Iothiouracil	T38.2X1-	T38.2X2-	T38.2X3-	T38.2X4-	T38.2X5-	T38.2X6-
Iotrol	T50.8X1-	T50.8X2-	T50.8X3-	T50.8X4-	T50.8X5-	T50.8X6-
Iotrolan	T50.8X1-	T50.8X2-	T50.8X3-	T50.8X4-	T50.8X5-	T50.8X6-
Iotroxate	T50.8X1-	T50.8X2-	T50.8X3-	T50.8X4-	T50.8X5-	T50.8X6-
Iotroxic acid	T50.8X1-	T50.8X2-	T50.8X3-	T50.8X4-	T50.8X5-	T50.8X6-
Ioversol	T50.8X1-	T50.8X2-	T50.8X3-	T50.8X4-	T50.8X5-	T50.8X6-
Ioxaglate	T50.8X1-	T50.8X2-	T50.8X3-	T50.8X4-	T50.8X5-	T50.8X6-
Ioxaglic acid	T50.8X1-	T50.8X2-	T50.8X3-	T50.8X4-	T50.8X5-	T50.8X6-
Ioxitalamic acid	T50.8X1-	T50.8X2-	T50.8X3-	T50.8X4-	T50.8X5-	T50.8X6-
Ipecac	T47.7X1-	T47.7X2-	T47.7X3-	T47.7X4-	T47.7X5-	T47.7X6-
Ipecacuanha	T48.4X1-	T48.4X2-	T48.4X3-	T48.4X4-	T48.4X5-	T48.4X6-
Ipodate, calcium	T50.8X1-	T50.8X2-	T50.8X3-	T50.8X4-	T50.8X5-	T50.8X6-
Ipral	T42.3X1-	T42.3X2-	T42.3X3-	T42.3X4-	T42.3X5-	T42.3X6-
Ipratropium (bromide)	T48.6X1-	T48.6X2-	T48.6X3-	T48.6X4-	T48.6X5-	T48.6X6-
Ipriflavone	T46.3X1-	T46.3X2-	T46.3X3-	T46.3X4-	T46.3X5-	T46.3X6-
Iprindole	T43.011-	T43.012-	T43.013-	T43.014-	T43.015-	T43.016-
Iproclozide	T43.1X1-	T43.1X2-	T43.1X3-	T43.1X4-	T43.1X5-	T43.1X6-
Iprofenin	T50.8X1-	T50.8X2-	T50.8X3-	T50.8X4-	T50.8X5-	T50.8X6-
Iproheptine	T49.2X1-	T49.2X2-	T49.2X3-	T49.2X4-	T49.2X5-	T49.2X6-
Iproniazid	T43.1X1-	T43.1X2-	T43.1X3-	T43.1X4-	T43.1X5-	T43.1X6-
Iproplatin	T45.1X1-	T45.1X2-	T45.1X3-	T45.1X4-	T45.1X5-	T45.1X6-
Iproveratril	T46.1X1-	T46.1X2-	T46.1X3-	T46.1X4-	T46.1X5-	T46.1X6-
Iron (compounds) (medicinal) **NEC**	T45.4X1-	T45.4X2-	T45.4X3-	T45.4X4-	T45.4X5-	T45.4X6-
ammonium	T45.4X1-	T45.4X2-	T45.4X3-	T45.4X4-	T45.4X5-	T45.4X6-
dextran injection	T45.4X1-	T45.4X2-	T45.4X3-	T45.4X4-	T45.4X5-	T45.4X6-
nonmedicinal	T56.891-	T56.892-	T56.893-	T56.894-	-	-
salts	T45.4X1-	T45.4X2-	T45.4X3-	T45.4X4-	T45.4X5-	T45.4X6-
sorbitex	T45.4X1-	T45.4X2-	T45.4X3-	T45.4X4-	T45.4X5-	T45.4X6-
sorbitol citric acid complex	T45.4X1-	T45.4X2-	T45.4X3-	T45.4X4-	T45.4X5-	T45.4X6-
Irrigating fluid (vaginal)	T49.8X1-	T49.8X2-	T49.8X3-	T49.8X4-	T49.8X5-	T49.8X6-
eye	T49.5X1-	T49.5X2-	T49.5X3-	T49.5X4-	T49.5X5-	T49.5X6-
Isepamicin	T36.5X1-	T36.5X2-	T36.5X3-	T36.5X4-	T36.5X5-	T36.5X6-
Isoaminile (citrate)	T48.3X1-	T48.3X2-	T48.3X3-	T48.3X4-	T48.3X5-	T48.3X6-
Isoamyl nitrite	T46.3X1-	T46.3X2-	T46.3X3-	T46.3X4-	T46.3X5-	T46.3X6-
Isobenzan	T60.1X1-	T60.1X2-	T60.1X3-	T60.1X4-	-	-
Isobutyl acetate	T52.8X1-	T52.8X2-	T52.8X3-	T52.8X4-	-	-
Isocarboxazid	T43.1X1-	T43.1X2-	T43.1X3-	T43.1X4-	T43.1X5-	T43.1X6-
Isoconazole	T49.0X1-	T49.0X2-	T49.0X3-	T49.0X4-	T49.0X5-	T49.0X6-
Isocyanate	T65.0X1-	T65.0X2-	T65.0X3-	T65.0X4-	-	-
Isoephedrine	T44.991-	T44.992-	T44.993-	T44.994-	T44.995-	T44.996-
Isoetarine	T48.6X1-	T48.6X2-	T48.6X3-	T48.6X4-	T48.6X5-	T48.6X6-
Isoethadione	T42.2X1-	T42.2X2-	T42.2X3-	T42.2X4-	T42.2X5-	T42.2X6-
Isoetharine	T44.5X1-	T44.5X2-	T44.5X3-	T44.5X4-	T44.5X5-	T44.5X6-
Isoflurane	T41.0X1-	T41.0X2-	T41.0X3-	T41.0X4-	T41.0X5-	T41.0X6-
Isoflurophate	T44.0X1-	T44.0X2-	T44.0X3-	T44.0X4-	T44.0X5-	T44.0X6-
Isomaltose, ferric complex	T45.4X1-	T45.4X2-	T45.4X3-	T45.4X4-	T45.4X5-	T45.4X6-
Isometheptene	T44.3X1-	T44.3X2-	T44.3X3-	T44.3X4-	T44.3X5-	T44.3X6-
Isoniazid	T37.1X1-	T37.1X2-	T37.1X3-	T37.1X4-	T37.1X5-	T37.1X6-
with						
rifampicin	T36.6X1-	T36.6X2-	T36.6X3-	T36.6X4-	T36.6X5-	T36.6X6-
thioacetazone	T37.1X1-	T37.1X2-	T37.1X3-	T37.1X4-	T37.1X5-	T37.1X6-
Isonicotinic acid hydrazide	T37.1X1-	T37.1X2-	T37.1X3-	T37.1X4-	T37.1X5-	T37.1X6-
Isonipecaine	T40.4X1-	T40.4X2-	T40.4X3-	T40.4X4-	T40.4X5-	T40.4X6-
Isopentaquine	T37.2X1-	T37.2X2-	T37.2X3-	T37.2X4-	T37.2X5-	T37.2X6-
Isophane insulin	T38.3X1-	T38.3X2-	T38.3X3-	T38.3X4-	T38.3X5-	T38.3X6-
Isophorone	T65.891-	T65.892-	T65.893-	T65.894-	-	-
Isophosphamide	T45.1X1-	T45.1X2-	T45.1X3-	T45.1X4-	T45.1X5-	T45.1X6-
Isopregnenone	T38.5X1-	T38.5X2-	T38.5X3-	T38.5X4-	T38.5X5-	T38.5X6-
Isoprenaline	T48.6X1-	T48.6X2-	T48.6X3-	T48.6X4-	T48.6X5-	T48.6X6-
Isopromethazine	T43.3X1-	T43.3X2-	T43.3X3-	T43.3X4-	T43.3X5-	T43.3X6-
Isopropamide	T44.3X1-	T44.3X2-	T44.3X3-	T44.3X4-	T44.3X5-	T44.3X6-
iodide	T44.3X1-	T44.3X2-	T44.3X3-	T44.3X4-	T44.3X5-	T44.3X6-
Isopropanol	T51.2X1-	T51.2X2-	T51.2X3-	T51.2X4-	-	-
Isopropyl						
acetate	T52.8X1-	T52.8X2-	T52.8X3-	T52.8X4-	-	-
alcohol	T51.2X1-	T51.2X2-	T51.2X3-	T51.2X4-	-	-
medicinal	T49.4X1-	T49.4X2-	T49.4X3-	T49.4X4-	T49.4X5-	T49.4X6-
ether	T52.8X1-	T52.8X2-	T52.8X3-	T52.8X4-	-	-
Isopropylaminophenazone	T39.2X1-	T39.2X2-	T39.2X3-	T39.2X4-	T39.2X5-	T39.2X6-
Isoproterenol	T48.6X1-	T48.6X2-	T48.6X3-	T48.6X4-	T48.6X5-	T48.6X6-
Isosorbide dinitrate	T46.3X1-	T46.3X2-	T46.3X3-	T46.3X4-	T46.3X5-	T46.3X6-
Isothipendyl	T45.0X1-	T45.0X2-	T45.0X3-	T45.0X4-	T45.0X5-	T45.0X6-
Isotretinoin	T50.991-	T50.992-	T50.993-	T50.994-	T50.995-	T50.996-
Isoxazolyl penicillin	T36.0X1-	T36.0X2-	T36.0X3-	T36.0X4-	T36.0X5-	T36.0X6-
Isoxicam	T39.391-	T39.392-	T39.393-	T39.394-	T39.395-	T39.396-
Isoxsuprine	T46.7X1-	T46.7X2-	T46.7X3-	T46.7X4-	T46.7X5-	T46.7X6-
Ispagula	T47.4X1-	T47.4X2-	T47.4X3-	T47.4X4-	T47.4X5-	T47.4X6-
husk	T47.4X1-	T47.4X2-	T47.4X3-	T47.4X4-	T47.4X5-	T47.4X6-
Isradipine	T46.1X1-	T46.1X2-	T46.1X3-	T46.1X4-	T46.1X5-	T46.1X6-
I-thyroxine sodium	T38.1X1-	T38.1X2-	T38.1X3-	T38.1X4-	T38.1X5-	T38.1X6-
Itraconazole	T37.8X1-	T37.8X2-	T37.8X3-	T37.8X4-	T37.8X5-	T37.8X6-
Itramin tosilate	T46.3X1-	T46.3X2-	T46.3X3-	T46.3X4-	T46.3X5-	T46.3X6-
Ivermectin	T37.4X1-	T37.4X2-	T37.4X3-	T37.4X4-	T37.4X5-	T37.4X6-
Izoniazid	T37.1X1-	T37.1X2-	T37.1X3-	T37.1X4-	T37.1X5-	T37.1X6-
with thioacetazone	T37.1X1-	T37.1X2-	T37.1X3-	T37.1X4-	T37.1X5-	T37.1X6-
Jalap	T47.2X1-	T47.2X2-	T47.2X3-	T47.2X4-	T47.2X5-	T47.2X6-
Jamaica						
dogwood (bark)	T39.8X1-	T39.8X2-	T39.8X3-	T39.8X4-	T39.8X5-	T39.8X6-
ginger	T65.891-	T65.892-	T65.893-	T65.894-	-	-
root	T62.2X1-	T62.2X2-	T62.2X3-	T62.2X4-	-	-
Jatropha	T62.2X1-	T62.2X2-	T62.2X3-	T62.2X4-	-	-
curcas	T62.2X1-	T62.2X2-	T62.2X3-	T62.2X4-	-	-
Jectofer	T45.4X1-	T45.4X2-	T45.4X3-	T45.4X4-	T45.4X5-	T45.4X6-
Jellyfish (sting)	T63.621-	T63.622-	T63.623-	T63.624-	-	-
Jequirity (bean)	T62.2X1-	T62.2X2-	T62.2X3-	T62.2X4-	-	-
Jimson weed (stramonium)	T62.2X1-	T62.2X2-	T62.2X3-	T62.2X4-	-	-
seeds	T62.2X1-	T62.2X2-	T62.2X3-	T62.2X4-	-	-
Josamycin	T36.3X1-	T36.3X2-	T36.3X3-	T36.3X4-	T36.3X5-	T36.3X6-
Juniper tar	T49.1X1-	T49.1X2-	T49.1X3-	T49.1X4-	T49.1X5-	T49.1X6-
Kallidinogenase	T46.7X1-	T46.7X2-	T46.7X3-	T46.7X4-	T46.7X5-	T46.7X6-
Kallikrein	T46.7X1-	T46.7X2-	T46.7X3-	T46.7X4-	T46.7X5-	T46.7X6-
Kanamycin	T36.5X1-	T36.5X2-	T36.5X3-	T36.5X4-	T36.5X5-	T36.5X6-
Kantrex	T36.5X1-	T36.5X2-	T36.5X3-	T36.5X4-	T36.5X5-	T36.5X6-
Kaolin	T47.6X1-	T47.6X2-	T47.6X3-	T47.6X4-	T47.6X5-	T47.6X6-
light	T47.6X1-	T47.6X2-	T47.6X3-	T47.6X4-	T47.6X5-	T47.6X6-
Karaya (gum)	T47.4X1-	T47.4X2-	T47.4X3-	T47.4X4-	T47.4X5-	T47.4X6-
Kebuzone	T39.2X1-	T39.2X2-	T39.2X3-	T39.2X4-	T39.2X5-	T39.2X6-
Kelevan	T60.1X1-	T60.1X2-	T60.1X3-	T60.1X4-	-	-
Kemithal	T41.1X1-	T41.1X2-	T41.1X3-	T41.1X4-	T41.1X5-	T41.1X6-
Kenacort	T38.0X1-	T38.0X2-	T38.0X3-	T38.0X4-	T38.0X5-	T38.0X6-
Keratolytic drug NEC	T49.4X1-	T49.4X2-	T49.4X3-	T49.4X4-	T49.4X5-	T49.4X6-
anthracene	T49.4X1-	T49.4X2-	T49.4X3-	T49.4X4-	T49.4X5-	T49.4X6-
Keratoplastic NEC	T49.4X1-	T49.4X2-	T49.4X3-	T49.4X4-	T49.4X5-	T49.4X6-
Kerosene, kerosine (fuel) (solvent) **NEC**	T52.0X1-	T52.0X2-	T52.0X3-	T52.0X4-	-	-
insecticide	T52.0X1-	T52.0X2-	T52.0X3-	T52.0X4-	-	-
vapor	T52.0X1-	T52.0X2-	T52.0X3-	T52.0X4-	-	-
Ketamine	T41.291-	T41.292-	T41.293-	T41.294-	T41.295-	T41.296-

Substance	Poisoning Accidental (unintentional)	Poisoning Intentional self-harm	Poisoning Assault	Poisoning Undetermined	Adverse effect	Underdosing
Ketazolam	T42.4X1-	T42.4X2-	T42.4X3-	T42.4X4-	T42.4X5-	T42.4X6-
Ketazon	T39.2X1-	T39.2X2-	T39.2X3-	T39.2X4-	T39.2X5-	T39.2X6-
Ketobemidone	T40.4X1-	T40.4X2-	T40.4X3-	T40.4X4-	-	-
Ketoconazole	T49.0X1-	T49.0X2-	T49.0X3-	T49.0X4-	T49.0X5-	T49.0X6-
Ketols	T52.4X1-	T52.4X2-	T52.4X3-	T52.4X4-	-	-
Ketone oils	T52.4X1-	T52.4X2-	T52.4X3-	T52.4X4-	-	-
Ketoprofen	T39.311-	T39.312-	T39.313-	T39.314-	T39.315-	T39.316-
Ketorolac	T39.8X1-	T39.8X2-	T39.8X3-	T39.8X4-	T39.8X5-	T39.8X6-
Ketotifen	T45.0X1-	T45.0X2-	T45.0X3-	T45.0X4-	T45.0X5-	T45.0X6-
Khat	T43.691-	T43.692-	T43.693-	T43.694-	-	-
Khellin	T46.3X1-	T46.3X2-	T46.3X3-	T46.3X4-	T46.3X5-	T46.3X6-
Khelloside	T46.3X1-	T46.3X2-	T46.3X3-	T46.3X4-	T46.3X5-	T46.3X6-
Kiln gas or vapor (carbon monoxide)	T58.8X1-	T58.8X2-	T58.8X3-	T58.8X4-	-	-
Kitasamycin	T36.3X1-	T36.3X2-	T36.3X3-	T36.3X4-	T36.3X5-	T36.3X6-
Konsyl	T47.4X1-	T47.4X2-	T47.4X3-	T47.4X4-	T47.4X5-	T47.4X6-
Kosam seed	T62.2X1-	T62.2X2-	T62.2X3-	T62.2X4-	-	-
Krait (venom)	T63.091-	T63.092-	T63.093-	T63.094-	-	-
Kwell (insecticide)	T60.1X1-	T60.1X2-	T60.1X3-	T60.1X4-	-	-
anti-infective (topical)	T49.0X1-	T49.0X2-	T49.0X3-	T49.0X4-	T49.0X5-	T49.0X6-
Labetalol	T44.8X1-	T44.8X2-	T44.8X3-	T44.8X4-	T44.8X5-	T44.8X6-
Laburnum (seeds)	T62.2X1-	T62.2X2-	T62.2X3-	T62.2X4-	-	-
leaves	T62.2X1-	T62.2X2-	T62.2X3-	T62.2X4-	-	-
Lachesine	T49.5X1-	T49.5X2-	T49.5X3-	T49.5X4-	T49.5X5-	T49.5X6-
Lacidipine	T46.5X1-	T46.5X2-	T46.5X3-	T46.5X4-	T46.5X5-	T46.5X6-
Lacquer	T65.6X1-	T65.6X2-	T65.6X3-	T65.6X4-	-	-
Lacrimogenic gas	T59.3X1-	T59.3X2-	T59.3X3-	T59.3X4-	-	-
Lactated potassic saline	T50.3X1-	T50.3X2-	T50.3X3-	T50.3X4-	T50.3X5-	T50.3X6-
Lactic acid	T49.8X1-	T49.8X2-	T49.8X3-	T49.8X4-	T49.8X5-	T49.8X6-
Lactobacillus						
acidophilus	T47.6X1-	T47.6X2-	T47.6X3-	T47.6X4-	T47.6X5-	T47.6X6-
compound	T47.6X1-	T47.6X2-	T47.6X3-	T47.6X4-	T47.6X5-	T47.6X6-
bifidus, lyophilized	T47.6X1-	T47.6X2-	T47.6X3-	T47.6X4-	T47.6X5-	T47.6X6-
bulgaricus	T47.6X1-	T47.6X2-	T47.6X3-	T47.6X4-	T47.6X5-	T47.6X6-
sporogenes	T47.6X1-	T47.6X2-	T47.6X3-	T47.6X4-	T47.6X5-	T47.6X6-
Lactoflavin	T45.2X1-	T45.2X2-	T45.2X3-	T45.2X4-	T45.2X5-	T45.2X6-
Lactose (as excipient)	T50.901-	T50.902-	T50.903-	T50.904-	T50.905-	T50.906-
Lactuca (virosa) (extract)	T42.6X1-	T42.6X2-	T42.6X3-	T42.6X4-	T42.6X5-	T42.6X6-
Lactucarium	T42.6X1-	T42.6X2-	T42.6X3-	T42.6X4-	T42.6X5-	T42.6X6-
Lactulose	T47.3X1-	T47.3X2-	T47.3X3-	T47.3X4-	T47.3X5-	T47.3X6-
Laevo — *see* Levo-						
Lanatosides	T46.0X1-	T46.0X2-	T46.0X3-	T46.0X4-	T46.0X5-	T46.0X6-
Lanolin	T49.3X1-	T49.3X2-	T49.3X3-	T49.3X4-	T49.3X5-	T49.3X6-
Largactil	T43.3X1-	T43.3X2-	T43.3X3-	T43.3X4-	T43.3X5-	T43.3X6-
Larkspur	T62.2X1-	T62.2X2-	T62.2X3-	T62.2X4-	-	-
Laroxyl	T43.011-	T43.012-	T43.013-	T43.014-	T43.015-	T43.016-
Lasix	T50.1X1-	T50.1X2-	T50.1X3-	T50.1X4-	T50.1X5-	T50.1X6-
Lassar's paste	T49.4X1-	T49.4X2-	T49.4X3-	T49.4X4-	T49.4X5-	T49.4X6-
Latamoxef	T36.1X1-	T36.1X2-	T36.1X3-	T36.1X4-	T36.1X5-	T36.1X6-
Latex	T65.811-	T65.812-	T65.813-	T65.814-	-	-
Lathyrus (seed)	T62.2X1-	T62.2X2-	T62.2X3-	T62.2X4-	-	-
Laudanum	T40.0X1-	T40.0X2-	T40.0X3-	T40.0X4-	T40.0X5-	T40.0X6-
Laudexium	T48.1X1-	T48.1X2-	T48.1X3-	T48.1X4-	T48.1X5-	T48.1X6-
Laughing gas	T41.0X1-	T41.0X2-	T41.0X3-	T41.0X4-	T41.0X5-	T41.0X6-
Laurel, black or cherry	T62.2X1-	T62.2X2-	T62.2X3-	T62.2X4-	-	-
Laurolinium	T49.0X1-	T49.0X2-	T49.0X3-	T49.0X4-	T49.0X5-	T49.0X6-
Lauryl sulfoacetate	T49.2X1-	T49.2X2-	T49.2X3-	T49.2X4-	T49.2X5-	T49.2X6-
Laxative NEC	T47.4X1-	T47.4X2-	T47.4X3-	T47.4X4-	T47.4X5-	T47.4X6-
osmotic	T47.3X1-	T47.3X2-	T47.3X3-	T47.3X4-	T47.3X5-	T47.3X6-
saline	T47.3X1-	T47.3X2-	T47.3X3-	T47.3X4-	T47.3X5-	T47.3X6-
stimulant	T47.2X1-	T47.2X2-	T47.2X3-	T47.2X4-	T47.2X5-	T47.2X6-
L-dopa	T42.8X1-	T42.8X2-	T42.8X3-	T42.8X4-	T42.8X5-	T42.8X6-
Lead (dust) (fumes) (vapor) **NEC**	T56.0X1-	T56.0X2-	T56.0X3-	T56.0X4-	-	-
acetate	T49.2X1-	T49.2X2-	T49.2X3-	T49.2X4-	T49.2X5-	T49.2X6-
alkyl (fuel additive)	T56.0X1-	T56.0X2-	T56.0X3-	T56.0X4-	-	-
anti-infectives	T37.8X1-	T37.8X2-	T37.8X3-	T37.8X4-	T37.8X5-	T37.8X6-
antiknock compound (tetraethyl)	T56.0X1-	T56.0X2-	T56.0X3-	T56.0X4-	-	-
arsenate, arsenite (dust) (herbicide) (insecticide) (vapor)	T57.0X1-	T57.0X2-	T57.0X3-	T57.0X4-	-	-
carbonate	T56.0X1-	T56.0X2-	T56.0X3-	T56.0X4-	-	-
paint	T56.0X1-	T56.0X2-	T56.0X3-	T56.0X4-	-	-
chromate	T56.0X1-	T56.0X2-	T56.0X3-	T56.0X4-	-	-
paint	T56.0X1-	T56.0X2-	T56.0X3-	T56.0X4-	-	-
dioxide	T56.0X1-	T56.0X2-	T56.0X3-	T56.0X4-	-	-
inorganic	T56.0X1-	T56.0X2-	T56.0X3-	T56.0X4-	-	-
iodide	T56.0X1-	T56.0X2-	T56.0X3-	T56.0X4-	-	-

Substance	Poisoning Accidental (unintentional)	Poisoning Intentional self-harm	Poisoning Assault	Poisoning Undetermined	Adverse effect	Underdosing
Lead NEC - *continued*						
pigment (paint)	T56.0X1-	T56.0X2-	T56.0X3-	T56.0X4-	-	-
monoxide (dust)	T56.0X1-	T56.0X2-	T56.0X3-	T56.0X4-	-	-
paint	T56.0X1-	T56.0X2-	T56.0X3-	T56.0X4-	-	-
organic	T56.0X1-	T56.0X2-	T56.0X3-	T56.0X4-	-	-
oxide	T56.0X1-	T56.0X2-	T56.0X3-	T56.0X4-	-	-
paint	T56.0X1-	T56.0X2-	T56.0X3-	T56.0X4-	-	-
paint	T56.0X1-	T56.0X2-	T56.0X3-	T56.0X4-	-	-
salts	T56.0X1-	T56.0X2-	T56.0X3-	T56.0X4-	-	-
specified compound NEC	T56.0X1-	T56.0X2-	T56.0X3-	T56.0X4-	-	-
tetra-ethyl	T56.0X1-	T56.0X2-	T56.0X3-	T56.0X4-	-	-
Lebanese red	T40.7X1-	T40.7X2-	T40.7X3-	T40.7X4-	T40.7X5-	T40.7X6-
Lefetamine	T39.8X1-	T39.8X2-	T39.8X3-	T39.8X4-	T39.8X5-	T39.8X6-
Lenperone	T43.4X1-	T43.4X2-	T43.4X3-	T43.4X4-	T43.4X5-	T43.4X6-
Lente lietin (insulin)	T38.3X1-	T38.3X2-	T38.3X3-	T38.3X4-	T38.3X5-	T38.3X6-
Leptazol	T50.7X1-	T50.7X2-	T50.7X3-	T50.7X4-	T50.7X5-	T50.7X6-
Leptophos	T60.0X1-	T60.0X2-	T60.0X3-	T60.0X4-	-	-
Leritine	T40.2X1-	T40.2X2-	T40.2X3-	T40.2X4-	T40.2X5-	T40.2X6-
Letosteine	T48.4X1-	T48.4X2-	T48.4X3-	T48.4X4-	T48.4X5-	T48.4X6-
Letter	T38.1X1-	T38.1X2-	T38.1X3-	T38.1X4-	T38.1X5-	T38.1X6-
Lettuce opium	T42.6X1-	T42.6X2-	T42.6X3-	T42.6X4-	T42.6X5-	T42.6X6-
Leucinocaine	T41.3X1-	T41.3X2-	T41.3X3-	T41.3X4-	T41.3X5-	T41.3X6-
Leucocianidol	T46.991-	T46.992-	T46.993-	T46.994-	T46.995-	T46.996-
Leucovorin (factor)	T45.8X1-	T45.8X2-	T45.8X3-	T45.8X4-	T45.8X5-	T45.8X6-
Leukeran	T45.1X1-	T45.1X2-	T45.1X3-	T45.1X4-	T45.1X5-	T45.1X6-
Leuprolide	T38.891-	T38.892-	T38.893-	T38.894-	T38.895-	T38.896-
Levalbuterol	T48.6X1-	T48.6X2-	T48.6X3-	T48.6X4-	T48.6X5-	T48.6X6-
Levallorphan	T50.7X1-	T50.7X2-	T50.7X3-	T50.7X4-	T50.7X5-	T50.7X6-
Levamisole	T37.4X1-	T37.4X2-	T37.4X3-	T37.4X4-	T37.4X5-	T37.4X6-
Levanil	T42.6X1-	T42.6X2-	T42.6X3-	T42.6X4-	T42.6X5-	T42.6X6-
Levarterenol	T44.4X1-	T44.4X2-	T44.4X3-	T44.4X4-	T44.4X5-	T44.4X6-
Levdropropizine	T48.3X1-	T48.3X2-	T48.3X3-	T48.3X4-	T48.3X5-	T48.3X6-
Levobunolol	T49.5X1-	T49.5X2-	T49.5X3-	T49.5X4-	T49.5X5-	T49.5X6-
Levocabastine (hydrochloride)	T45.0X1-	T45.0X2-	T45.0X3-	T45.0X4-	T45.0X5-	T45.0X6-
Levocarnitine	T50.991-	T50.992-	T50.993-	T50.994-	T50.995-	T50.996-
Levodopa	T42.8X1-	T42.8X2-	T42.8X3-	T42.8X4-	T42.8X5-	T42.8X6-
with carbidopa	T42.8X1-	T42.8X2-	T42.8X3-	T42.8X4-	T42.8X5-	T42.8X6-
Levo-dromoran	T40.2X1-	T40.2X2-	T40.2X3-	T40.2X4-	T40.2X5-	T40.2X6-
Levoglutamide	T50.991-	T50.992-	T50.993-	T50.994-	T50.995-	T50.996-
Levoid	T38.1X1-	T38.1X2-	T38.1X3-	T38.1X4-	T38.1X5-	T38.1X6-
Levo-iso-methadone	T40.3X1-	T40.3X2-	T40.3X3-	T40.3X4-	T40.3X5-	T40.3X6-
Levomepromazine	T43.3X1-	T43.3X2-	T43.3X3-	T43.3X4-	T43.3X5-	T43.3X6-
Levonordefrin	T49.6X1-	T49.6X2-	T49.6X3-	T49.6X4-	T49.6X5-	T49.6X6-
Levonorgestrel	T38.4X1-	T38.4X2-	T38.4X3-	T38.4X4-	T38.4X5-	T38.4X6-
with ethinylestradiol	T38.5X1-	T38.5X2-	T38.5X3-	T38.5X4-	T38.5X5-	T38.5X6-
Levopromazine	T43.3X1-	T43.3X2-	T43.3X3-	T43.3X4-	T43.3X5-	T43.3X6-
Levoprome	T42.6X1-	T42.6X2-	T42.6X3-	T42.6X4-	T42.6X5-	T42.6X6-
Levopropoxyphene	T40.4X1-	T40.4X2-	T40.4X3-	T40.4X4-	T40.4X5-	T40.4X6-
Levopropylhexedrine	T50.5X1-	T50.5X2-	T50.5X3-	T50.5X4-	T50.5X5-	T50.5X6-
Levoproxyphylline	T48.6X1-	T48.6X2-	T48.6X3-	T48.6X4-	T48.6X5-	T48.6X6-
Levorphanol	T40.4X1-	T40.4X2-	T40.4X3-	T40.4X4-	T40.4X5-	T40.4X6-
Levothyroxine	T38.1X1-	T38.1X2-	T38.1X3-	T38.1X4-	T38.1X5-	T38.1X6-
sodium	T38.1X1-	T38.1X2-	T38.1X3-	T38.1X4-	T38.1X5-	T38.1X6-
Levsin	T44.3X1-	T44.3X2-	T44.3X3-	T44.3X4-	T44.3X5-	T44.3X6-
Levulose	T50.3X1-	T50.3X2-	T50.3X3-	T50.3X4-	T50.3X5-	T50.3X6-
Lewisite (gas) , **not in war**	T57.0X1-	T57.0X2-	T57.0X3-	T57.0X4-	-	-
Librium	T42.4X1-	T42.4X2-	T42.4X3-	T42.4X4-	T42.4X5-	T42.4X6-
Lidex	T49.0X1-	T49.0X2-	T49.0X3-	T49.0X4-	T49.0X5-	T49.0X6-
Lidocaine	T41.3X1-	T41.3X2-	T41.3X3-	T41.3X4-	T41.3X5-	T41.3X6-
regional	T41.3X1-	T41.3X2-	T41.3X3-	T41.3X4-	T41.3X5-	T41.3X6-
spinal	T41.3X1-	T41.3X2-	T41.3X3-	T41.3X4-	T41.3X5-	T41.3X6-
Lidofenin	T50.8X1-	T50.8X2-	T50.8X3-	T50.8X4-	T50.8X5-	T50.8X6-
Lidoflazine	T46.1X1-	T46.1X2-	T46.1X3-	T46.1X4-	T46.1X5-	T46.1X6-
Lighter fluid	T52.0X1-	T52.0X2-	T52.0X3-	T52.0X4-	-	-
Lignin hemicellulose	T47.6X1-	T47.6X2-	T47.6X3-	T47.6X4-	T47.6X5-	T47.6X6-
Lignocaine	T41.3X1-	T41.3X2-	T41.3X3-	T41.3X4-	T41.3X5-	T41.3X6-
regional	T41.3X1-	T41.3X2-	T41.3X3-	T41.3X4-	T41.3X5-	T41.3X6-
spinal	T41.3X1-	T41.3X2-	T41.3X3-	T41.3X4-	T41.3X5-	T41.3X6-
Ligroin (e) (solvent)	T52.0X1-	T52.0X2-	T52.0X3-	T52.0X4-	-	-
vapor	T59.891-	T59.892-	T59.893-	T59.894-	-	-
Ligustrum vulgare	T62.2X1-	T62.2X2-	T62.2X3-	T62.2X4-	-	-
Lily of the valley	T62.2X1-	T62.2X2-	T62.2X3-	T62.2X4-	-	-
Lime (chloride)	T54.3X1-	T54.3X2-	T54.3X3-	T54.3X4-	-	-
Limonene	T52.8X1-	T52.8X2-	T52.8X3-	T52.8X4-	-	-
Lincomycin	T36.8X1-	T36.8X2-	T36.8X3-	T36.8X4-	T36.8X5-	T36.8X6-
Lindane (insecticide) (nonmedicinal) (vapor)	T53.6X1-	T53.6X2-	T53.6X3-	T53.6X4-	-	-
medicinal	T49.0X1-	T49.0X2-	T49.0X3-	T49.0X4-	T49.0X5-	T49.0X6-

Substance	Poisoning Accidental (unintentional)	Poisoning Intentional self-harm	Poisoning Assault	Poisoning Undetermined	Adverse effect	Underdosing
Liniments NEC	T49.91X-	T49.92X-	T49.93X-	T49.94X-	T49.95X-	T49.96X-
Linoleic acid	T46.6X1-	T46.6X2-	T46.6X3-	T46.6X4-	T46.6X5-	T46.6X6-
Linolenic acid	T46.6X1-	T46.6X2-	T46.6X3-	T46.6X4-	T46.6X5-	T46.6X6-
Linseed	T47.4X1-	T47.4X2-	T47.4X3-	T47.4X4-	T47.4X5-	T47.4X6-
Liothyronine	T38.1X1-	T38.1X2-	T38.1X3-	T38.1X4-	T38.1X5-	T38.1X6-
Liotrix	T38.1X1-	T38.1X2-	T38.1X3-	T38.1X4-	T38.1X5-	T38.1X6-
Lipancreatin	T47.5X1-	T47.5X2-	T47.5X3-	T47.5X4-	T47.5X5-	T47.5X6-
Lipo-alprostadil	T46.7X1-	T46.7X2-	T46.7X3-	T46.7X4-	T46.7X5-	T46.7X6-
Lipo-Lutin	T38.5X1-	T38.5X2-	T38.5X3-	T38.5X4-	T38.5X5-	T38.5X6-
Lipotropic drug NEC	T50.901-	T50.902-	T50.903-	T50.904-	T50.905-	T50.906-
Liquefied petroleum gases	T59.891-	T59.892-	T59.893-	T59.894-	-	-
piped (pure or mixed with air)	T59.891-	T59.892-	T59.893-	T59.894-	-	-
Liquid						
paraffin	T47.4X1-	T47.4X2-	T47.4X3-	T47.4X4-	T47.4X5-	T47.4X6-
petrolatum	T47.4X1-	T47.4X2-	T47.4X3-	T47.4X4-	T47.4X5-	T47.4X6-
topical	T49.3X1-	T49.3X2-	T49.3X3-	T49.3X4-	T49.3X5-	T49.3X6-
specified NEC	T65.891-	T65.892-	T65.893-	T65.894-	-	-
substance	T65.91X-	T65.92X-	T65.93X-	T65.94X-	-	-
Liquor creosolis compositus	T65.891-	T65.892-	T65.893-	T65.894-	-	-
Liquorice	T48.4X1-	T48.4X2-	T48.4X3-	T48.4X4-	T48.4X5-	T48.4X6-
extract	T47.8X1-	T47.8X2-	T47.8X3-	T47.8X4-	T47.8X5-	T47.8X6-
Lisinopril	T46.4X1-	T46.4X2-	T46.4X3-	T46.4X4-	T46.4X5-	T46.4X6-
Lisuride	T42.8X1-	T42.8X2-	T42.8X3-	T42.8X4-	T42.8X5-	T42.8X6-
Lithane	T43.8X1-	T43.8X2-	T43.8X3-	T43.8X4-	T43.8X5-	T43.8X6-
Lithium	T56.891-	T56.892-	T56.893-	T56.894-	-	-
gluconate	T43.591-	T43.592-	T43.593-	T43.594-	T43.595-	T43.596-
salts (carbonate)	T43.591-	T43.592-	T43.593-	T43.594-	T43.595-	T43.596-
Lithonate	T43.8X1-	T43.8X2-	T43.8X3-	T43.8X4-	T43.8X5-	T43.8X6-
Liver						
extract	T45.8X1-	T45.8X2-	T45.8X3-	T45.8X4-	T45.8X5-	T45.8X6-
for parenteral use	T45.8X1-	T45.8X2-	T45.8X3-	T45.8X4-	T45.8X5-	T45.8X6-
fraction 1	T45.8X1-	T45.8X2-	T45.8X3-	T45.8X4-	T45.8X5-	T45.8X6-
hydrolysate	T45.8X1-	T45.8X2-	T45.8X3-	T45.8X4-	T45.8X5-	T45.8X6-
Lizard (bite) (venom)	T63.121-	T63.122-	T63.123-	T63.124-	-	-
LMD	T45.8X1-	T45.8X2-	T45.8X3-	T45.8X4-	T45.8X5-	T45.8X6-
Lobelia	T62.2X1-	T62.2X2-	T62.2X3-	T62.2X4-	-	-
Lobeline	T50.7X1-	T50.7X2-	T50.7X3-	T50.7X4-	T50.7X5-	T50.7X6-
Local action drug NEC	T49.8X1-	T49.8X2-	T49.8X3-	T49.8X4-	T49.8X5-	T49.8X6-
Locorten	T49.0X1-	T49.0X2-	T49.0X3-	T49.0X4-	T49.0X5-	T49.0X6-
Lofepramine	T43.011-	T43.012-	T43.013-	T43.014-	T43.015-	T43.016-
Lolium temulentum	T62.2X1-	T62.2X2-	T62.2X3-	T62.2X4-	-	-
Lomotil	T47.6X1-	T47.6X2-	T47.6X3-	T47.6X4-	T47.6X5-	T47.6X6-
Lomustine	T45.1X1-	T45.1X2-	T45.1X3-	T45.1X4-	T45.1X5-	T45.1X6-
Lonidamine	T45.1X1-	T45.1X2-	T45.1X3-	T45.1X4-	T45.1X5-	T45.1X6-
Loperamide	T47.6X1-	T47.6X2-	T47.6X3-	T47.6X4-	T47.6X5-	T47.6X6-
Loprazolam	T42.4X1-	T42.4X2-	T42.4X3-	T42.4X4-	T42.4X5-	T42.4X6-
Lorajmine	T46.2X1-	T46.2X2-	T46.2X3-	T46.2X4-	T46.2X5-	T46.2X6-
Loratidine	T45.0X1-	T45.0X2-	T45.0X3-	T45.0X4-	T45.0X5-	T45.0X6-
Lorazepam	T42.4X1-	T42.4X2-	T42.4X3-	T42.4X4-	T42.4X5-	T42.4X6-
Lorcainide	T46.2X1-	T46.2X2-	T46.2X3-	T46.2X4-	T46.2X5-	T46.2X6-
Lormetazepam	T42.4X1-	T42.4X2-	T42.4X3-	T42.4X4-	T42.4X5-	T42.4X6-
Lotions NEC	T49.91X-	T49.92X-	T49.93X-	T49.94X-	T49.95X-	T49.96X-
Lotusate	T42.3X1-	T42.3X2-	T42.3X3-	T42.3X4-	T42.3X5-	T42.3X6-
Lovastatin	T46.6X1-	T46.6X2-	T46.6X3-	T46.6X4-	T46.6X5-	T46.6X6-
Lowila	T49.2X1-	T49.2X2-	T49.2X3-	T49.2X4-	T49.2X5-	T49.2X6-
Loxapine	T43.591-	T43.592-	T43.593-	T43.594-	T43.595-	T43.596-
Lozenges (throat)	T49.6X1-	T49.6X2-	T49.6X3-	T49.6X4-	T49.6X5-	T49.6X6-
LSD	T40.8X1-	T40.8X2-	T40.8X3-	T40.8X4-	-	-
L-Tryptophan — *see* amino acid						
Lubricant, eye	T49.5X1-	T49.5X2-	T49.5X3-	T49.5X4-	T49.5X5-	T49.5X6-
Lubricating oil NEC	T52.0X1-	T52.0X2-	T52.0X3-	T52.0X4-	-	-
Lucanthone	T37.4X1-	T37.4X2-	T37.4X3-	T37.4X4-	T37.4X5-	T37.4X6-
Luminal	T42.3X1-	T42.3X2-	T42.3X3-	T42.3X4-	T42.3X5-	T42.3X6-
Lung irritant (gas) **NEC**	T59.91X-	T59.92X-	T59.93X-	T59.94X-	-	-
Luteinizing hormone	T38.811-	T38.812-	T38.813-	T38.814-	T38.815-	T38.816-
Lutocylol	T38.5X1-	T38.5X2-	T38.5X3-	T38.5X4-	T38.5X5-	T38.5X6-
Lutromone	T38.5X1-	T38.5X2-	T38.5X3-	T38.5X4-	T38.5X5-	T38.5X6-
Lututrin	T48.291-	T48.292-	T48.293-	T48.294-	T48.295-	T48.296-
Lye (concentrated)	T54.3X1-	T54.3X2-	T54.3X3-	T54.3X4-	-	-
Lygranum (skin test)	T50.8X1-	T50.8X2-	T50.8X3-	T50.8X4-	T50.8X5-	T50.8X6-
Lymecycline	T36.4X1-	T36.4X2-	T36.4X3-	T36.4X4-	T36.4X5-	T36.4X6-
Lymphogranuloma venereum antigen	T50.8X1-	T50.8X2-	T50.8X3-	T50.8X4-	T50.8X5-	T50.8X6-
Lynestrenol	T38.4X1-	T38.4X2-	T38.4X3-	T38.4X4-	T38.4X5-	T38.4X6-
Lyovac Sodium Edecrin	T50.1X1-	T50.1X2-	T50.1X3-	T50.1X4-	T50.1X5-	T50.1X6-
Lypressin	T38.891-	T38.892-	T38.893-	T38.894-	T38.895-	T38.896-
Lysergic acid diethylamide	T40.8X1-	T40.8X2-	T40.8X3-	T40.8X4-	-	-

Substance	Poisoning Accidental (unintentional)	Poisoning Intentional self-harm	Poisoning Assault	Poisoning Undetermined	Adverse effect	Underdosing
Lysergide	T40.8X1-	T40.8X2-	T40.8X3-	T40.8X4-	-	-
Lysine vasopressin	T38.891-	T38.892-	T38.893-	T38.894-	T38.895-	T38.896-
Lysol	T54.1X1-	T54.1X2-	T54.1X3-	T54.1X4-	-	-
Lysozyme	T49.0X1-	T49.0X2-	T49.0X3-	T49.0X4-	T49.0X5-	T49.0X6-
Lytta (vitatta)	T49.8X1-	T49.8X2-	T49.8X3-	T49.8X4-	T49.8X5-	T49.8X6-
Mace	T59.3X1-	T59.3X2-	T59.3X3-	T59.3X4-	-	-
Macrogol	T50.991-	T50.992-	T50.993-	T50.994-	T50.995-	T50.996-
Macrolide						
anabolic drug	T38.7X1-	T38.7X2-	T38.7X3-	T38.7X4-	T38.7X5-	T38.7X6-
antibiotic	T36.3X1-	T36.3X2-	T36.3X3-	T36.3X4-	T36.3X5-	T36.3X6-
Mafenide	T49.0X1-	T49.0X2-	T49.0X3-	T49.0X4-	T49.0X5-	T49.0X6-
Magaldrate	T47.1X1-	T47.1X2-	T47.1X3-	T47.1X4-	T47.1X5-	T47.1X6-
Magic mushroom	T40.991-	T40.992-	T40.993-	T40.994-	-	-
Magnamycin	T36.8X1-	T36.8X2-	T36.8X3-	T36.8X4-	T36.8X5-	T36.8X6-
Magnesia magma	T47.1X1-	T47.1X2-	T47.1X3-	T47.1X4-	T47.1X5-	T47.1X6-
Magnesium NEC	T56.891-	T56.892-	T56.893-	T56.894-	-	-
carbonate	T47.1X1-	T47.1X2-	T47.1X3-	T47.1X4-	T47.1X5-	T47.1X6-
citrate	T47.4X1-	T47.4X2-	T47.4X3-	T47.4X4-	T47.4X5-	T47.4X6-
hydroxide	T47.1X1-	T47.1X2-	T47.1X3-	T47.1X4-	T47.1X5-	T47.1X6-
oxide	T47.1X1-	T47.1X2-	T47.1X3-	T47.1X4-	T47.1X5-	T47.1X6-
peroxide	T49.0X1-	T49.0X2-	T49.0X3-	T49.0X4-	T49.0X5-	T49.0X6-
salicylate	T39.091-	T39.092-	T39.093-	T39.094-	T39.095-	T39.096-
silicofluoride	T50.3X1-	T50.3X2-	T50.3X3-	T50.3X4-	T50.3X5-	T50.3X6-
sulfate	T47.4X1-	T47.4X2-	T47.4X3-	T47.4X4-	T47.4X5-	T47.4X6-
thiosulfate	T45.0X1-	T45.0X2-	T45.0X3-	T45.0X4-	T45.0X5-	T45.0X6-
trisilicate	T47.1X1-	T47.1X2-	T47.1X3-	T47.1X4-	T47.1X5-	T47.1X6-
Malathion (medicinal)	T49.0X1-	T49.0X2-	T49.0X3-	T49.0X4-	T49.0X5-	T49.0X6-
insecticide	T60.0X1-	T60.0X2-	T60.0X3-	T60.0X4-	-	-
Male fern extract	T37.4X1-	T37.4X2-	T37.4X3-	T37.4X4-	T37.4X5-	T37.4X6-
M-AMSA	T45.1X1-	T45.1X2-	T45.1X3-	T45.1X4-	T45.1X5-	T45.1X6-
Mandelic acid	T37.8X1-	T37.8X2-	T37.8X3-	T37.8X4-	T37.8X5-	T37.8X6-
Manganese (dioxide) (salts)	T57.2X1-	T57.2X2-	T57.2X3-	T57.2X4-	-	-
medicinal	T50.991-	T50.992-	T50.993-	T50.994-	T50.995-	T50.996-
Mannitol	T47.3X1-	T47.3X2-	T47.3X3-	T47.3X4-	T47.3X5-	T47.3X6-
hexanitrate	T46.3X1-	T46.3X2-	T46.3X3-	T46.3X4-	T46.3X5-	T46.3X6-
Mannomustine	T45.1X1-	T45.1X2-	T45.1X3-	T45.1X4-	T45.1X5-	T45.1X6-
MAO inhibitors	T43.1X1-	T43.1X2-	T43.1X3-	T43.1X4-	T43.1X5-	T43.1X6-
Mapharsen	T37.8X1-	T37.8X2-	T37.8X3-	T37.8X4-	T37.8X5-	T37.8X6-
Maphenide	T49.0X1-	T49.0X2-	T49.0X3-	T49.0X4-	T49.0X5-	T49.0X6-
Maprotiline	T43.021-	T43.022-	T43.023-	T43.024-	T43.025-	T43.026-
Marcaine	T41.3X1-	T41.3X2-	T41.3X3-	T41.3X4-	T41.3X5-	T41.3X6-
infiltration (subcutaneous)	T41.3X1-	T41.3X2-	T41.3X3-	T41.3X4-	T41.3X5-	T41.3X6-
nerve block (peripheral) (plexus)	T41.3X1-	T41.3X2-	T41.3X3-	T41.3X4-	T41.3X5-	T41.3X6-
Marezine	T45.0X1-	T45.0X2-	T45.0X3-	T45.0X4-	T45.0X5-	T45.0X6-
Marihuana	T40.7X1-	T40.7X2-	T40.7X3-	T40.7X4-	T40.7X5-	T40.7X6-
Marijuana	T40.7X1-	T40.7X2-	T40.7X3-	T40.7X4-	T40.7X5-	T40.7X6-
Marine (sting)	T63.691-	T63.692-	T63.693-	T63.694-	-	-
animals (sting)	T63.691-	T63.692-	T63.693-	T63.694-	-	-
plants (sting)	T63.711-	T63.712-	T63.713-	T63.714-	-	-
Marplan	T43.1X1-	T43.1X2-	T43.1X3-	T43.1X4-	T43.1X5-	T43.1X6-
Marsh gas	T59.891-	T59.892-	T59.893-	T59.894-	-	-
Marsilid	T43.1X1-	T43.1X2-	T43.1X3-	T43.1X4-	T43.1X5-	T43.1X6-
Matulane	T45.1X1-	T45.1X2-	T45.1X3-	T45.1X4-	T45.1X5-	T45.1X6-
Mazindol	T50.5X1-	T50.5X2-	T50.5X3-	T50.5X4-	T50.5X5-	T50.5X6-
MCPA	T60.3X1-	T60.3X2-	T60.3X3-	T60.3X4-	-	-
MDMA	T43.641-	T43.642-	T43.643-	T43.644-	-	-
Meadow saffron	T62.2X1-	T62.2X2-	T62.2X3-	T62.2X4-	-	-
Measles virus vaccine (attenuated)	T50.B91-	T50.B92-	T50.B93-	T50.B94-	T50.B95-	T50.B96-
Meat, noxious	T62.8X1-	T62.8X2-	T62.8X3-	T62.8X4-	-	-
Meballymal	T42.3X1-	T42.3X2-	T42.3X3-	T42.3X4-	T42.3X5-	T42.3X6-
Mebanazine	T43.1X1-	T43.1X2-	T43.1X3-	T43.1X4-	T43.1X5-	T43.1X6-
Mebaral	T42.3X1-	T42.3X2-	T42.3X3-	T42.3X4-	T42.3X5-	T42.3X6-
Mebendazole	T37.4X1-	T37.4X2-	T37.4X3-	T37.4X4-	T37.4X5-	T37.4X6-
Mebeverine	T44.3X1-	T44.3X2-	T44.3X3-	T44.3X4-	T44.3X5-	T44.3X6-
Mebhydrolin	T45.0X1-	T45.0X2-	T45.0X3-	T45.0X4-	T45.0X5-	T45.0X6-
Mebumal	T42.3X1-	T42.3X2-	T42.3X3-	T42.3X4-	T42.3X5-	T42.3X6-
Mebutamate	T43.591-	T43.592-	T43.593-	T43.594-	T43.595-	T43.596-
Mecamylamine	T44.2X1-	T44.2X2-	T44.2X3-	T44.2X4-	T44.2X5-	T44.2X6-
Mechlorethamine	T45.1X1-	T45.1X2-	T45.1X3-	T45.1X4-	T45.1X5-	T45.1X6-
Mecillinam	T36.0X1-	T36.0X2-	T36.0X3-	T36.0X4-	T36.0X5-	T36.0X6-
Meclizine (hydrochloride)	T45.0X1-	T45.0X2-	T45.0X3-	T45.0X4-	T45.0X5-	T45.0X6-
Meclocycline	T36.4X1-	T36.4X2-	T36.4X3-	T36.4X4-	T36.4X5-	T36.4X6-
Meclofenamate	T39.391-	T39.392-	T39.393-	T39.394-	T39.395-	T39.396-
Meclofenamic acid	T39.391-	T39.392-	T39.393-	T39.394-	T39.395-	T39.396-
Meclofenoxate	T43.691-	T43.692-	T43.693-	T43.694-	T43.695-	T43.696-
Meclozine	T45.0X1-	T45.0X2-	T45.0X3-	T45.0X4-	T45.0X5-	T45.0X6-

Substance	Poisoning Accidental (unintentional)	Poisoning Intentional self-harm	Poisoning Assault	Poisoning Undetermined	Adverse effect	Underdosing
Mecobalamin	T45.8X1-	T45.8X2-	T45.8X3-	T45.8X4-	T45.8X5-	T45.8X6-
Mecoprop	T60.3X1-	T60.3X2-	T60.3X3-	T60.3X4-	-	-
Mecrilate	T49.3X1-	T49.3X2-	T49.3X3-	T49.3X4-	T49.3X5-	T49.3X6-
Mecysteine	T48.4X1-	T48.4X2-	T48.4X3-	T48.4X4-	T48.4X5-	T48.4X6-
Medazepam	T42.4X1-	T42.4X2-	T42.4X3-	T42.4X4-	T42.4X5-	T42.4X6-
Medicament NEC	T50.901-	T50.902-	T50.903-	T50.904-	T50.905-	T50.906-
Medinal	T42.3X1-	T42.3X2-	T42.3X3-	T42.3X4-	T42.3X5-	T42.3X6-
Medomin	T42.3X1-	T42.3X2-	T42.3X3-	T42.3X4-	T42.3X5-	T42.3X6-
Medrogestone	T38.5X1-	T38.5X2-	T38.5X3-	T38.5X4-	T38.5X5-	T38.5X6-
Medroxalol	T44.8X1-	T44.8X2-	T44.8X3-	T44.8X4-	T44.8X5-	T44.8X6-
Medroxyprogesterone acetate (depot)	T38.5X1-	T38.5X2-	T38.5X3-	T38.5X4-	T38.5X5-	T38.5X6-
Medrysone	T49.0X1-	T49.0X2-	T49.0X3-	T49.0X4-	T49.0X5-	T49.0X6-
Mefenamic acid	T39.391-	T39.392-	T39.393-	T39.394-	T39.395-	T39.396-
Mefenorex	T50.5X1-	T50.5X2-	T50.5X3-	T50.5X4-	T50.5X5-	T50.5X6-
Mefloquine	T37.2X1-	T37.2X2-	T37.2X3-	T37.2X4-	T37.2X5-	T37.2X6-
Mefruside	T50.2X1-	T50.2X2-	T50.2X3-	T50.2X4-	T50.2X5-	T50.2X6-
Megahallucinogen	T40.901-	T40.902-	T40.903-	T40.904-	T40.905-	T40.906-
Megestrol	T38.5X1-	T38.5X2-	T38.5X3-	T38.5X4-	T38.5X5-	T38.5X6-
Meglumine						
antimoniate	T37.8X1-	T37.8X2-	T37.8X3-	T37.8X4-	T37.8X5-	T37.8X6-
diatrizoate	T50.8X1-	T50.8X2-	T50.8X3-	T50.8X4-	T50.8X5-	T50.8X6-
iodipamide	T50.8X1-	T50.8X2-	T50.8X3-	T50.8X4-	T50.8X5-	T50.8X6-
iotroxate	T50.8X1-	T50.8X2-	T50.8X3-	T50.8X4-	T50.8X5-	T50.8X6-
MEK (methyl ethyl ketone)	T52.4X1-	T52.4X2-	T52.4X3-	T52.4X4-	-	-
Meladinin	T49.3X1-	T49.3X2-	T49.3X3-	T49.3X4-	T49.3X5-	T49.3X6-
Meladrazine	T44.3X1-	T44.3X2-	T44.3X3-	T44.3X4-	T44.3X5-	T44.3X6-
Melaleuca alternifolia oil	T49.0X1-	T49.0X2-	T49.0X3-	T49.0X4-	T49.0X5-	T49.0X6-
Melanizing agents	T49.3X1-	T49.3X2-	T49.3X3-	T49.3X4-	T49.3X5-	T49.3X6-
Melanocyte-stimulating hormone	T38.891-	T38.892-	T38.893-	T38.894-	T38.895-	T38.896-
Melarsonyl potassium	T37.3X1-	T37.3X2-	T37.3X3-	T37.3X4-	T37.3X5-	T37.3X6-
Melarsoprol	T37.3X1-	T37.3X2-	T37.3X3-	T37.3X4-	T37.3X5-	T37.3X6-
Melia azedarach	T62.2X1-	T62.2X2-	T62.2X3-	T62.2X4-	-	-
Melitracen	T43.011-	T43.012-	T43.013-	T43.014-	T43.015-	T43.016-
Mellaril	T43.3X1-	T43.3X2-	T43.3X3-	T43.3X4-	T43.3X5-	T43.3X6-
Meloxine	T49.3X1-	T49.3X2-	T49.3X3-	T49.3X4-	T49.3X5-	T49.3X6-
Melperone	T43.4X1-	T43.4X2-	T43.4X3-	T43.4X4-	T43.4X5-	T43.4X6-
Melphalan	T45.1X1-	T45.1X2-	T45.1X3-	T45.1X4-	T45.1X5-	T45.1X6-
Memantine	T43.8X1-	T43.8X2-	T43.8X3-	T43.8X4-	T43.8X5-	T43.8X6-
Menadiol	T45.7X1-	T45.7X2-	T45.7X3-	T45.7X4-	T45.7X5-	T45.7X6-
sodium sulfate	T45.7X1-	T45.7X2-	T45.7X3-	T45.7X4-	T45.7X5-	T45.7X6-
Menadione	T45.7X1-	T45.7X2-	T45.7X3-	T45.7X4-	T45.7X5-	T45.7X6-
sodium bisulfite	T45.7X1-	T45.7X2-	T45.7X3-	T45.7X4-	T45.7X5-	T45.7X6-
Menaphthone	T45.7X1-	T45.7X2-	T45.7X3-	T45.7X4-	T45.7X5-	T45.7X6-
Menaquinone	T45.7X1-	T45.7X2-	T45.7X3-	T45.7X4-	T45.7X5-	T45.7X6-
Menatetrenone	T45.7X1-	T45.7X2-	T45.7X3-	T45.7X4-	T45.7X5-	T45.7X6-
Meningococcal vaccine	T50.A91-	T50.A92-	T50.A93-	T50.A94-	T50.A95-	T50.A96-
Menningovax (-AC) (-C)	T50.A91-	T50.A92-	T50.A93-	T50.A94-	T50.A95-	T50.A96-
Menotropins	T38.811-	T38.812-	T38.813-	T38.814-	T38.815-	T38.816-
Menthol	T48.5X1-	T48.5X2-	T48.5X3-	T48.5X4-	T48.5X5-	T48.5X6-
Mepacrine	T37.2X1-	T37.2X2-	T37.2X3-	T37.2X4-	T37.2X5-	T37.2X6-
Meparfynol	T42.6X1-	T42.6X2-	T42.6X3-	T42.6X4-	T42.6X5-	T42.6X6-
Mepartricin	T36.7X1-	T36.7X2-	T36.7X3-	T36.7X4-	T36.7X5-	T36.7X6-
Mepazine	T43.3X1-	T43.3X2-	T43.3X3-	T43.3X4-	T43.3X5-	T43.3X6-
Mepenzolate	T44.3X1-	T44.3X2-	T44.3X3-	T44.3X4-	T44.3X5-	T44.3X6-
bromide	T44.3X1-	T44.3X2-	T44.3X3-	T44.3X4-	T44.3X5-	T44.3X6-
Meperidine	T40.4X1-	T40.4X2-	T40.4X3-	T40.4X4-	T40.4X5-	T40.4X6-
Mephebarbital	T42.3X1-	T42.3X2-	T42.3X3-	T42.3X4-	T42.3X5-	T42.3X6-
Mephenamin (e)	T42.8X1-	T42.8X2-	T42.8X3-	T42.8X4-	T42.8X5-	T42.8X6-
Mephenesin	T42.8X1-	T42.8X2-	T42.8X3-	T42.8X4-	T42.8X5-	T42.8X6-
Mephenhydramine	T45.0X1-	T45.0X2-	T45.0X3-	T45.0X4-	T45.0X5-	T45.0X6-
Mephenoxalone	T42.8X1-	T42.8X2-	T42.8X3-	T42.8X4-	T42.8X5-	T42.8X6-
Mephentermine	T44.991-	T44.992-	T44.993-	T44.994-	T44.995-	T44.996-
Mephenytoin	T42.0X1-	T42.0X2-	T42.0X3-	T42.0X4-	T42.0X5-	T42.0X6-
with phenobarbital	T42.3X1-	T42.3X2-	T42.3X3-	T42.3X4-	T42.3X5-	T42.3X6-
Mephobarbital	T42.3X1-	T42.3X2-	T42.3X3-	T42.3X4-	T42.3X5-	T42.3X6-
Mephosfolan	T60.0X1-	T60.0X2-	T60.0X3-	T60.0X4-	-	-
Mepindolol	T44.7X1-	T44.7X2-	T44.7X3-	T44.7X4-	T44.7X5-	T44.7X6-
Mepiperphenidol	T44.3X1-	T44.3X2-	T44.3X3-	T44.3X4-	T44.3X5-	T44.3X6-
Mepitiostane	T38.7X1-	T38.7X2-	T38.7X3-	T38.7X4-	T38.7X5-	T38.7X6-
Mepivacaine	T41.3X1-	T41.3X2-	T41.3X3-	T41.3X4-	T41.3X5-	T41.3X6-
epidural	T41.3X1-	T41.3X2-	T41.3X3-	T41.3X4-	T41.3X5-	T41.3X6-
Meprednisone	T38.0X1-	T38.0X2-	T38.0X3-	T38.0X4-	T38.0X5-	T38.0X6-
Meprobam	T43.591-	T43.592-	T43.593-	T43.594-	T43.595-	T43.596-
Meprobamate	T43.591-	T43.592-	T43.593-	T43.594-	T43.595-	T43.596-
Meproscillarin	T46.0X1-	T46.0X2-	T46.0X3-	T46.0X4-	T46.0X5-	T46.0X6-
Meprylcaine	T41.3X1-	T41.3X2-	T41.3X3-	T41.3X4-	T41.3X5-	T41.3X6-

Substance	Poisoning Accidental (unintentional)	Poisoning Intentional self-harm	Poisoning Assault	Poisoning Undetermined	Adverse effect	Underdosing
Meptazinol	T39.8X1-	T39.8X2-	T39.8X3-	T39.8X4-	T39.8X5-	T39.8X6-
Mepyramine	T45.0X1-	T45.0X2-	T45.0X3-	T45.0X4-	T45.0X5-	T45.0X6-
Mequitazine	T43.3X1-	T43.3X2-	T43.3X3-	T43.3X4-	T43.3X5-	T43.3X6-
Meralluride	T50.2X1-	T50.2X2-	T50.2X3-	T50.2X4-	T50.2X5-	T50.2X6-
Merbaphen	T50.2X1-	T50.2X2-	T50.2X3-	T50.2X4-	T50.2X5-	T50.2X6-
Merbromin	T49.0X1-	T49.0X2-	T49.0X3-	T49.0X4-	T49.0X5-	T49.0X6-
Mercaptobenzothiazole salts	T49.0X1-	T49.0X2-	T49.0X3-	T49.0X4-	T49.0X5-	T49.0X6-
Mercaptomerin	T50.2X1-	T50.2X2-	T50.2X3-	T50.2X4-	T50.2X5-	T50.2X6-
Mercaptopurine	T45.1X1-	T45.1X2-	T45.1X3-	T45.1X4-	T45.1X5-	T45.1X6-
Mercumatilin	T50.2X1-	T50.2X2-	T50.2X3-	T50.2X4-	T50.2X5-	T50.2X6-
Mercuramide	T50.2X1-	T50.2X2-	T50.2X3-	T50.2X4-	T50.2X5-	T50.2X6-
Mercurochrome	T49.0X1-	T49.0X2-	T49.0X3-	T49.0X4-	T49.0X5-	T49.0X6-
Mercurophylline	T50.2X1-	T50.2X2-	T50.2X3-	T50.2X4-	T50.2X5-	T50.2X6-
Mercury, mercurial, mercuric, mercurous (compounds) (cyanide) (fumes) (nonmedicinal) (vapor) **NEC**	T56.1X1-	T56.1X2-	T56.1X3-	T56.1X4-	-	-
ammoniated	T49.0X1-	T49.0X2-	T49.0X3-	T49.0X4-	T49.0X5-	T49.0X6-
anti-infective						
local	T49.0X1-	T49.0X2-	T49.0X3-	T49.0X4-	T49.0X5-	T49.0X6-
systemic	T37.8X1-	T37.8X2-	T37.8X3-	T37.8X4-	T37.8X5-	T37.8X6-
topical	T49.0X1-	T49.0X2-	T49.0X3-	T49.0X4-	T49.0X5-	T49.0X6-
chloride (ammoniated)	T49.0X1-	T49.0X2-	T49.0X3-	T49.0X4-	T49.0X5-	T49.0X6-
fungicide	T56.1X1-	T56.1X2-	T56.1X3-	T56.1X4-	-	-
diuretic NEC	T50.2X1-	T50.2X2-	T50.2X3-	T50.2X4-	T50.2X5-	T50.2X6-
fungicide	T56.1X1-	T56.1X2-	T56.1X3-	T56.1X4-	-	-
organic (fungicide)	T56.1X1-	T56.1X2-	T56.1X3-	T56.1X4-	-	-
oxide, yellow	T49.0X1-	T49.0X2-	T49.0X3-	T49.0X4-	T49.0X5-	T49.0X6-
Mersalyl	T50.2X1-	T50.2X2-	T50.2X3-	T50.2X4-	T50.2X5-	T50.2X6-
Merthiolate	T49.0X1-	T49.0X2-	T49.0X3-	T49.0X4-	T49.0X5-	T49.0X6-
ophthalmic preparation	T49.5X1-	T49.5X2-	T49.5X3-	T49.5X4-	T49.5X5-	T49.5X6-
Meruvax	T50.B91-	T50.B92-	T50.B93-	T50.B94-	T50.B95-	T50.B96-
Mesalazine	T47.8X1-	T47.8X2-	T47.8X3-	T47.8X4-	T47.8X5-	T47.8X6-
Mescal buttons	T40.991-	T40.992-	T40.993-	T40.994-	-	-
Mescaline	T40.991-	T40.992-	T40.993-	T40.994-	-	-
Mesna	T48.4X1-	T48.4X2-	T48.4X3-	T48.4X4-	T48.4X5-	T48.4X6-
Mesoglycan	T46.6X1-	T46.6X2-	T46.6X3-	T46.6X4-	T46.6X5-	T46.6X6-
Mesoridazine	T43.3X1-	T43.3X2-	T43.3X3-	T43.3X4-	T43.3X5-	T43.3X6-
Mestanolone	T38.7X1-	T38.7X2-	T38.7X3-	T38.7X4-	T38.7X5-	T38.7X6-
Mesterolone	T38.7X1-	T38.7X2-	T38.7X3-	T38.7X4-	T38.7X5-	T38.7X6-
Mestranol	T38.5X1-	T38.5X2-	T38.5X3-	T38.5X4-	T38.5X5-	T38.5X6-
Mesulergine	T42.8X1-	T42.8X2-	T42.8X3-	T42.8X4-	T42.8X5-	T42.8X6-
Mesulfen	T49.0X1-	T49.0X2-	T49.0X3-	T49.0X4-	T49.0X5-	T49.0X6-
Mesuximide	T42.2X1-	T42.2X2-	T42.2X3-	T42.2X4-	T42.2X5-	T42.2X6-
Metabutethamine	T41.3X1-	T41.3X2-	T41.3X3-	T41.3X4-	T41.3X5-	T41.3X6-
Metactesylacetate	T49.0X1-	T49.0X2-	T49.0X3-	T49.0X4-	T49.0X5-	T49.0X6-
Metacycline	T36.4X1-	T36.4X2-	T36.4X3-	T36.4X4-	T36.4X5-	T36.4X6-
Metaldehyde (snail killer) **NEC**	T60.8X1-	T60.8X2-	T60.8X3-	T60.8X4-	-	-
Metals (heavy) (nonmedicinal)	T56.91X-	T56.92X-	T56.93X-	T56.94X-	-	-
dust, fumes, or vapor NEC	T56.91X-	T56.92X-	T56.93X-	T56.94X-	-	-
light NEC	T56.91X-	T56.92X-	T56.93X-	T56.94X-	-	-
dust, fumes, or vapor NEC	T56.91X-	T56.92X-	T56.93X-	T56.94X-	-	-
specified NEC	T56.891-	T56.892-	T56.893-	T56.894-	-	-
thallium	T56.811-	T56.812-	T56.813-	T56.814-	-	-
Metamfetamine	T43.621-	T43.622-	T43.623-	T43.624-	T43.625-	T43.626-
Metamizole sodium	T39.2X1-	T39.2X2-	T39.2X3-	T39.2X4-	T39.2X5-	T39.2X6-
Metampicillin	T36.0X1-	T36.0X2-	T36.0X3-	T36.0X4-	T36.0X5-	T36.0X6-
Metamucil	T47.4X1-	T47.4X2-	T47.4X3-	T47.4X4-	T47.4X5-	T47.4X6-
Metandienone	T38.7X1-	T38.7X2-	T38.7X3-	T38.7X4-	T38.7X5-	T38.7X6-
Metandrostenolone	T38.7X1-	T38.7X2-	T38.7X3-	T38.7X4-	T38.7X5-	T38.7X6-
Metaphen	T49.0X1-	T49.0X2-	T49.0X3-	T49.0X4-	T49.0X5-	T49.0X6-
Metaphos	T60.0X1-	T60.0X2-	T60.0X3-	T60.0X4-	-	-
Metapramine	T43.011-	T43.012-	T43.013-	T43.014-	T43.015-	T43.016-
Metaproterenol	T48.291-	T48.292-	T48.293-	T48.294-	T48.295-	T48.296-
Metaraminol	T44.4X1-	T44.4X2-	T44.4X3-	T44.4X4-	T44.4X5-	T44.4X6-
Metaxalone	T42.8X1-	T42.8X2-	T42.8X3-	T42.8X4-	T42.8X5-	T42.8X6-
Metenolone	T38.7X1-	T38.7X2-	T38.7X3-	T38.7X4-	T38.7X5-	T38.7X6-
Metergoline	T42.8X1-	T42.8X2-	T42.8X3-	T42.8X4-	T42.8X5-	T42.8X6-
Metescufylline	T46.991-	T46.992-	T46.993-	T46.994-	T46.995-	T46.996-
Metetoin	T42.0X1-	T42.0X2-	T42.0X3-	T42.0X4-	T42.0X5-	T42.0X6-
Metformin	T38.3X1-	T38.3X2-	T38.3X3-	T38.3X4-	T38.3X5-	T38.3X6-
Methacholine	T44.1X1-	T44.1X2-	T44.1X3-	T44.1X4-	T44.1X5-	T44.1X6-
Methacycline	T36.4X1-	T36.4X2-	T36.4X3-	T36.4X4-	T36.4X5-	T36.4X6-
Methadone	T40.3X1-	T40.3X2-	T40.3X3-	T40.3X4-	T40.3X5-	T40.3X6-
Methallenestril	T38.5X1-	T38.5X2-	T38.5X3-	T38.5X4-	T38.5X5-	T38.5X6-
Methallenoestril	T38.5X1-	T38.5X2-	T38.5X3-	T38.5X4-	T38.5X5-	T38.5X6-
Methamphetamine	T43.621-	T43.622-	T43.623-	T43.624-	T43.625-	T43.626-
Methampyrone	T39.2X1-	T39.2X2-	T39.2X3-	T39.2X4-	T39.2X5-	T39.2X6-

Substance	Poisoning Accidental (unintentional)	Poisoning Intentional self-harm	Poisoning Assault	Poisoning Undetermined	Adverse effect	Underdosing
Methandienone	T38.7X1-	T38.7X2-	T38.7X3-	T38.7X4-	T38.7X5-	T38.7X6-
Methandriol	T38.7X1-	T38.7X2-	T38.7X3-	T38.7X4-	T38.7X5-	T38.7X6-
Methandrostenolone	T38.7X1-	T38.7X2-	T38.7X3-	T38.7X4-	T38.7X5-	T38.7X6-
Methane	T59.891-	T59.892-	T59.893-	T59.894-	-	-
Methanethiol	T59.891-	T59.892-	T59.893-	T59.894-	-	-
Methaniazide	T37.1X1-	T37.1X2-	T37.1X3-	T37.1X4-	T37.1X5-	T37.1X6-
Methanol (vapor)	T51.1X1-	T51.1X2-	T51.1X3-	T51.1X4-	-	-
Methantheline	T44.3X1-	T44.3X2-	T44.3X3-	T44.3X4-	T44.3X5-	T44.3X6-
Methanthelinium bromide	T44.3X1-	T44.3X2-	T44.3X3-	T44.3X4-	T44.3X5-	T44.3X6-
Methaphenilene	T45.0X1-	T45.0X2-	T45.0X3-	T45.0X4-	T45.0X5-	T45.0X6-
Methapyrilene	T45.0X1-	T45.0X2-	T45.0X3-	T45.0X4-	T45.0X5-	T45.0X6-
Methaqualone (compound)	T42.6X1-	T42.6X2-	T42.6X3-	T42.6X4-	T42.6X5-	T42.6X6-
Metharbital	T42.3X1-	T42.3X2-	T42.3X3-	T42.3X4-	T42.3X5-	T42.3X6-
Methazolamide	T50.2X1-	T50.2X2-	T50.2X3-	T50.2X4-	T50.2X5-	T50.2X6-
Methdilazine	T43.3X1-	T43.3X2-	T43.3X3-	T43.3X4-	T43.3X5-	T43.3X6-
Methedrine	T43.621-	T43.622-	T43.623-	T43.624-	T43.625-	T43.626-
Methenamine (mandelate)	T37.8X1-	T37.8X2-	T37.8X3-	T37.8X4-	T37.8X5-	T37.8X6-
Methenolone	T38.7X1-	T38.7X2-	T38.7X3-	T38.7X4-	T38.7X5-	T38.7X6-
Methergine	T48.0X1-	T48.0X2-	T48.0X3-	T48.0X4-	T48.0X5-	T48.0X6-
Methetoin	T42.0X1-	T42.0X2-	T42.0X3-	T42.0X4-	T42.0X5-	T42.0X6-
Methiacil	T38.2X1-	T38.2X2-	T38.2X3-	T38.2X4-	T38.2X5-	T38.2X6-
Methicillin	T36.0X1-	T36.0X2-	T36.0X3-	T36.0X4-	T36.0X5-	T36.0X6-
Methimazole	T38.2X1-	T38.2X2-	T38.2X3-	T38.2X4-	T38.2X5-	T38.2X6-
Methiodal sodium	T50.8X1-	T50.8X2-	T50.8X3-	T50.8X4-	T50.8X5-	T50.8X6-
Methionine	T50.991-	T50.992-	T50.993-	T50.994-	T50.995-	T50.996-
Methisazone	T37.5X1-	T37.5X2-	T37.5X3-	T37.5X4-	T37.5X5-	T37.5X6-
Methisoprinol	T37.5X1-	T37.5X2-	T37.5X3-	T37.5X4-	T37.5X5-	T37.5X6-
Methitural	T42.3X1-	T42.3X2-	T42.3X3-	T42.3X4-	T42.3X5-	T42.3X6-
Methixene	T44.3X1-	T44.3X2-	T44.3X3-	T44.3X4-	T44.3X5-	T44.3X6-
Methobarbital, methobarbitone	T42.3X1-	T42.3X2-	T42.3X3-	T42.3X4-	T42.3X5-	T42.3X6-
Methocarbamol	T42.8X1-	T42.8X2-	T42.8X3-	T42.8X4-	T42.8X5-	T42.8X6-
skeletal muscle relaxant	T48.1X1-	T48.1X2-	T48.1X3-	T48.1X4-	T48.1X5-	T48.1X6-
Methohexital	T41.1X1-	T41.1X2-	T41.1X3-	T41.1X4-	T41.1X5-	T41.1X6-
Methohexitone	T41.1X1-	T41.1X2-	T41.1X3-	T41.1X4-	T41.1X5-	T41.1X6-
Methoin	T42.0X1-	T42.0X2-	T42.0X3-	T42.0X4-	T42.0X5-	T42.0X6-
Methopholine	T39.8X1-	T39.8X2-	T39.8X3-	T39.8X4-	T39.8X5-	T39.8X6-
Methopromazine	T43.3X1-	T43.3X2-	T43.3X3-	T43.3X4-	T43.3X5-	T43.3X6-
Methorate	T48.3X1-	T48.3X2-	T48.3X3-	T48.3X4-	T48.3X5-	T48.3X6-
Methoserpidine	T46.5X1-	T46.5X2-	T46.5X3-	T46.5X4-	T46.5X5-	T46.5X6-
Methotrexate	T45.1X1-	T45.1X2-	T45.1X3-	T45.1X4-	T45.1X5-	T45.1X6-
Methotrimeprazine	T43.3X1-	T43.3X2-	T43.3X3-	T43.3X4-	T43.3X5-	T43.3X6-
Methoxa-Dome	T49.3X1-	T49.3X2-	T49.3X3-	T49.3X4-	T49.3X5-	T49.3X6-
Methoxamine	T44.4X1-	T44.4X2-	T44.4X3-	T44.4X4-	T44.4X5-	T44.4X6-
Methoxsalen	T50.991-	T50.992-	T50.993-	T50.994-	T50.995-	T50.996-
Methoxyaniline	T65.3X1-	T65.3X2-	T65.3X3-	T65.3X4-	-	-
Methoxybenzyl penicillin	T36.0X1-	T36.0X2-	T36.0X3-	T36.0X4-	T36.0X5-	T36.0X6-
Methoxychlor	T53.7X1-	T53.7X2-	T53.7X3-	T53.7X4-	-	-
Methoxy-DDT	T53.7X1-	T53.7X2-	T53.7X3-	T53.7X4-	-	-
2-Methoxyethanol	T52.3X1-	T52.3X2-	T52.3X3-	T52.3X4-	-	-
Methoxyflurane	T41.0X1-	T41.0X2-	T41.0X3-	T41.0X4-	T41.0X5-	T41.0X6-
Methoxyphenamine	T48.6X1-	T48.6X2-	T48.6X3-	T48.6X4-	T48.6X5-	T48.6X6-
Methoxypromazine	T43.3X1-	T43.3X2-	T43.3X3-	T43.3X4-	T43.3X5-	T43.3X6-
5-Methoxypsoralen (5-MOP)	T50.991-	T50.992-	T50.993-	T50.994-	T50.995-	T50.996-
8-Methoxypsoralen (8-MOP)	T50.991-	T50.992-	T50.993-	T50.994-	T50.995-	T50.996-
Methscopolamine bromide	T44.3X1-	T44.3X2-	T44.3X3-	T44.3X4-	T44.3X5-	T44.3X6-
Methsuximide	T42.2X1-	T42.2X2-	T42.2X3-	T42.2X4-	T42.2X5-	T42.2X6-
Methyclothiazide	T50.2X1-	T50.2X2-	T50.2X3-	T50.2X4-	T50.2X5-	T50.2X6-
Methyl						
acetate	T52.4X1-	T52.4X2-	T52.4X3-	T52.4X4-	-	-
acetone	T52.4X1-	T52.4X2-	T52.4X3-	T52.4X4-	-	-
acrylate	T65.891-	T65.892-	T65.893-	T65.894-	-	-
alcohol	T51.1X1-	T51.1X2-	T51.1X3-	T51.1X4-	-	-
aminophenol	T65.3X1-	T65.3X2-	T65.3X3-	T65.3X4-	-	-
amphetamine	T43.621-	T43.622-	T43.623-	T43.624-	T43.625-	T43.626-
androstanolone	T38.7X1-	T38.7X2-	T38.7X3-	T38.7X4-	T38.7X5-	T38.7X6-
atropine	T44.3X1-	T44.3X2-	T44.3X3-	T44.3X4-	T44.3X5-	T44.3X6-
benzene	T52.2X1-	T52.2X2-	T52.2X3-	T52.2X4-	-	-
benzoate	T52.8X1-	T52.8X2-	T52.8X3-	T52.8X4-	-	-
benzol	T52.2X1-	T52.2X2-	T52.2X3-	T52.2X4-	-	-
bromide (gas)	T59.891-	T59.892-	T59.893-	T59.894-	-	-
fumigant	T60.8X1-	T60.8X2-	T60.8X3-	T60.8X4-	-	-
butanol	T51.3X1-	T51.3X2-	T51.3X3-	T51.3X4-	-	-
carbinol	T51.1X1-	T51.1X2-	T51.1X3-	T51.1X4-	-	-
carbonate	T52.8X1-	T52.8X2-	T52.8X3-	T52.8X4-	-	-
CCNU	T45.1X1-	T45.1X2-	T45.1X3-	T45.1X4-	T45.1X5-	T45.1X6-
cellosolve	T52.91X-	T52.92X-	T52.93X-	T52.94X-	-	-
cellulose	T47.4X1-	T47.4X2-	T47.4X3-	T47.4X4-	T47.4X5-	T47.4X6-

Substance	Poisoning Accidental (unintentional)	Poisoning Intentional self-harm	Poisoning Assault	Poisoning Undetermined	Adverse effect	Underdosing
Methyl - *continued*						
chloride (gas)	T59.891-	T59.892-	T59.893-	T59.894-	-	-
chloroformate	T59.3X1-	T59.3X2-	T59.3X3-	T59.3X4-	-	-
cyclohexane	T52.8X1-	T52.8X2-	T52.8X3-	T52.8X4-	-	-
cyclohexanol	T51.8X1-	T51.8X2-	T51.8X3-	T51.8X4-	-	-
cyclohexanone	T52.8X1-	T52.8X2-	T52.8X3-	T52.8X4-	-	-
cyclohexyl acetate	T52.8X1-	T52.8X2-	T52.8X3-	T52.8X4-	-	-
demeton	T60.0X1-	T60.0X2-	T60.0X3-	T60.0X4-	-	-
dihydromorphinone	T40.2X1-	T40.2X2-	T40.2X3-	T40.2X4-	T40.2X5-	T40.2X6-
ergometrine	T48.0X1-	T48.0X2-	T48.0X3-	T48.0X4-	T48.0X5-	T48.0X6-
ergonovine	T48.0X1-	T48.0X2-	T48.0X3-	T48.0X4-	T48.0X5-	T48.0X6-
ethyl ketone	T52.4X1-	T52.4X2-	T52.4X3-	T52.4X4-	-	-
glucamine antimonate	T37.8X1-	T37.8X2-	T37.8X3-	T37.8X4-	T37.8X5-	T37.8X6-
hydrazine	T65.891-	T65.892-	T65.893-	T65.894-	-	-
iodide	T65.891-	T65.892-	T65.893-	T65.894-	-	-
isobutyl ketone	T52.4X1-	T52.4X2-	T52.4X3-	T52.4X4-	-	-
isothiocyanate	T60.3X1-	T60.3X2-	T60.3X3-	T60.3X4-	-	-
mercaptan	T59.891-	T59.892-	T59.893-	T59.894-	-	-
morphine NEC	T40.2X1-	T40.2X2-	T40.2X3-	T40.2X4-	T40.2X5-	T40.2X6-
nicotinate	T49.4X1-	T49.4X2-	T49.4X3-	T49.4X4-	T49.4X5-	T49.4X6-
paraben	T49.0X1-	T49.0X2-	T49.0X3-	T49.0X4-	T49.0X5-	T49.0X6-
parafynol	T42.6X1-	T42.6X2-	T42.6X3-	T42.6X4-	T42.6X5-	T42.6X6-
parathion	T60.0X1-	T60.0X2-	T60.0X3-	T60.0X4-	-	-
peridol	T43.4X1-	T43.4X2-	T43.4X3-	T43.4X4-	T43.4X5-	T43.4X6-
phenidate	T43.631-	T43.632-	T43.633-	T43.634-	T43.635-	T43.636-
prednisolone	T38.0X1-	T38.0X2-	T38.0X3-	T38.0X4-	T38.0X5-	T38.0X6-
ENT agent	T49.6X1-	T49.6X2-	T49.6X3-	T49.6X4-	T49.6X5-	T49.6X6-
ophthalmic preparation	T49.5X1-	T49.5X2-	T49.5X3-	T49.5X4-	T49.5X5-	T49.5X6-
topical NEC	T49.0X1-	T49.0X2-	T49.0X3-	T49.0X4-	T49.0X5-	T49.0X6-
propylcarbinol	T51.3X1-	T51.3X2-	T51.3X3-	T51.3X4-	-	-
rosaniline NEC	T49.0X1-	T49.0X2-	T49.0X3-	T49.0X4-	T49.0X5-	T49.0X6-
salicylate	T49.2X1-	T49.2X2-	T49.2X3-	T49.2X4-	T49.2X5-	T49.2X6-
sulfate (fumes)	T59.891-	T59.892-	T59.893-	T59.894-	-	-
liquid	T52.8X1-	T52.8X2-	T52.8X3-	T52.8X4-	-	-
sulfonal	T42.6X1-	T42.6X2-	T42.6X3-	T42.6X4-	T42.6X5-	T42.6X6-
testosterone	T38.7X1-	T38.7X2-	T38.7X3-	T38.7X4-	T38.7X5-	T38.7X6-
thiouracil	T38.2X1-	T38.2X2-	T38.2X3-	T38.2X4-	T38.2X5-	T38.2X6-
Methylamphetamine	T43.621-	T43.622-	T43.623-	T43.624-	T43.625-	T43.626-
Methylated spirit	T51.1X1-	T51.1X2-	T51.1X3-	T51.1X4-	-	-
Methylatropine nitrate	T44.3X1-	T44.3X2-	T44.3X3-	T44.3X4-	T44.3X5-	T44.3X6-
Methylbenactyzium bromide	T44.3X1-	T44.3X2-	T44.3X3-	T44.3X4-	T44.3X5-	T44.3X6-
Methylbenzethonium chloride	T49.0X1-	T49.0X2-	T49.0X3-	T49.0X4-	T49.0X5-	T49.0X6-
Methylcellulose	T47.4X1-	T47.4X2-	T47.4X3-	T47.4X4-	T47.4X5-	T47.4X6-
laxative	T47.4X1-	T47.4X2-	T47.4X3-	T47.4X4-	T47.4X5-	T47.4X6-
Methylchlorophenoxy-acetic acid	T60.3X1-	T60.3X2-	T60.3X3-	T60.3X4-	-	-
Methyldopa	T46.5X1-	T46.5X2-	T46.5X3-	T46.5X4-	T46.5X5-	T46.5X6-
Methyldopate	T46.5X1-	T46.5X2-	T46.5X3-	T46.5X4-	T46.5X5-	T46.5X6-
Methylene						
blue	T50.6X1-	T50.6X2-	T50.6X3-	T50.6X4-	T50.6X5-	T50.6X6-
chloride or dichloride (solvent) NEC	T53.4X1-	T53.4X2-	T53.4X3-	T53.4X4-	-	-
Methylenedioxyamphetamine	T43.621-	T43.622-	T43.623-	T43.624-	T43.625-	T43.626-
Methylenedioxymethamphetamine	T43.641-	T43.642-	T43.643-	T43.644-	-	-
Methylergometrine	T48.0X1-	T48.0X2-	T48.0X3-	T48.0X4-	T48.0X5-	T48.0X6-
Methylergonovine	T48.0X1-	T48.0X2-	T48.0X3-	T48.0X4-	T48.0X5-	T48.0X6-
Methylestrenolone	T38.5X1-	T38.5X2-	T38.5X3-	T38.5X4-	T38.5X5-	T38.5X6-
Methylethyl cellulose	T50.991-	T50.992-	T50.993-	T50.994-	T50.995-	T50.996-
Methylhexabital	T42.3X1-	T42.3X2-	T42.3X3-	T42.3X4-	T42.3X5-	T42.3X6-
Methylmorphine	T40.2X1-	T40.2X2-	T40.2X3-	T40.2X4-	T40.2X5-	T40.2X6-
Methylparaben (ophthalmic)	T49.5X1-	T49.5X2-	T49.5X3-	T49.5X4-	T49.5X5-	T49.5X6-
Methylparafynol	T42.6X1-	T42.6X2-	T42.6X3-	T42.6X4-	T42.6X5-	T42.6X6-
Methylpentynol, methylpenthynol	T42.6X1-	T42.6X2-	T42.6X3-	T42.6X4-	T42.6X5-	T42.6X6-
Methylphenidate	T43.631-	T43.632-	T43.633-	T43.634-	T43.635-	T43.636-
Methylphenobarbital	T42.3X1-	T42.3X2-	T42.3X3-	T42.3X4-	T42.3X5-	T42.3X6-
Methylpolysiloxane	T47.1X1-	T47.1X2-	T47.1X3-	T47.1X4-	T47.1X5-	T47.1X6-
Methylprednisolone — *see* Methyl, prednisolone						
Methylrosaniline	T49.0X1-	T49.0X2-	T49.0X3-	T49.0X4-	T49.0X5-	T49.0X6-
Methylrosanilinium chloride	T49.0X1-	T49.0X2-	T49.0X3-	T49.0X4-	T49.0X5-	T49.0X6-
Methyltestosterone	T38.7X1-	T38.7X2-	T38.7X3-	T38.7X4-	T38.7X5-	T38.7X6-
Methylthionine chloride	T50.6X1-	T50.6X2-	T50.6X3-	T50.6X4-	T50.6X5-	T50.6X6-
Methylthioninium chloride	T50.6X1-	T50.6X2-	T50.6X3-	T50.6X4-	T50.6X5-	T50.6X6-
Methylthiouracil	T38.2X1-	T38.2X2-	T38.2X3-	T38.2X4-	T38.2X5-	T38.2X6-
Methyprylon	T42.6X1-	T42.6X2-	T42.6X3-	T42.6X4-	T42.6X5-	T42.6X6-
Methysergide	T46.5X1-	T46.5X2-	T46.5X3-	T46.5X4-	T46.5X5-	T46.5X6-
Metiamide	T47.1X1-	T47.1X2-	T47.1X3-	T47.1X4-	T47.1X5-	T47.1X6-

Substance	Poisoning Accidental (unintentional)	Poisoning Intentional self-harm	Poisoning Assault	Poisoning Undetermined	Adverse effect	Underdosing
Meticillin	T36.0X1-	T36.0X2-	T36.0X3-	T36.0X4-	T36.0X5-	T36.0X6-
Meticrane	T50.2X1-	T50.2X2-	T50.2X3-	T50.2X4-	T50.2X5-	T50.2X6-
Metildigoxin	T46.0X1-	T46.0X2-	T46.0X3-	T46.0X4-	T46.0X5-	T46.0X6-
Metipranolol	T49.5X1-	T49.5X2-	T49.5X3-	T49.5X4-	T49.5X5-	T49.5X6-
Metirosine	T46.5X1-	T46.5X2-	T46.5X3-	T46.5X4-	T46.5X5-	T46.5X6-
Metisazone	T37.5X1-	T37.5X2-	T37.5X3-	T37.5X4-	T37.5X5-	T37.5X6-
Metixene	T44.3X1-	T44.3X2-	T44.3X3-	T44.3X4-	T44.3X5-	T44.3X6-
Metizoline	T48.5X1-	T48.5X2-	T48.5X3-	T48.5X4-	T48.5X5-	T48.5X6-
Metoclopramide	T45.0X1-	T45.0X2-	T45.0X3-	T45.0X4-	T45.0X5-	T45.0X6-
Metofenazate	T43.3X1-	T43.3X2-	T43.3X3-	T43.3X4-	T43.3X5-	T43.3X6-
Metofoline	T39.8X1-	T39.8X2-	T39.8X3-	T39.8X4-	T39.8X5-	T39.8X6-
Metolazone	T50.2X1-	T50.2X2-	T50.2X3-	T50.2X4-	T50.2X5-	T50.2X6-
Metopon	T40.2X1-	T40.2X2-	T40.2X3-	T40.2X4-	T40.2X5-	T40.2X6-
Metoprine	T45.1X1-	T45.1X2-	T45.1X3-	T45.1X4-	T45.1X5-	T45.1X6-
Metoprolol	T44.7X1-	T44.7X2-	T44.7X3-	T44.7X4-	T44.7X5-	T44.7X6-
Metrifonate	T60.0X1-	T60.0X2-	T60.0X3-	T60.0X4-	-	-
Metrizamide	T50.8X1-	T50.8X2-	T50.8X3-	T50.8X4-	T50.8X5-	T50.8X6-
Metrizoic acid	T50.8X1-	T50.8X2-	T50.8X3-	T50.8X4-	T50.8X5-	T50.8X6-
Metronidazole	T37.8X1-	T37.8X2-	T37.8X3-	T37.8X4-	T37.8X5-	T37.8X6-
Metycaine	T41.3X1-	T41.3X2-	T41.3X3-	T41.3X4-	T41.3X5-	T41.3X6-
infiltration (subcutaneous)	T41.3X1-	T41.3X2-	T41.3X3-	T41.3X4-	T41.3X5-	T41.3X6-
nerve block (peripheral) (plexus)	T41.3X1-	T41.3X2-	T41.3X3-	T41.3X4-	T41.3X5-	T41.3X6-
topical (surface)	T41.3X1-	T41.3X2-	T41.3X3-	T41.3X4-	T41.3X5-	T41.3X6-
Metyrapone	T50.8X1-	T50.8X2-	T50.8X3-	T50.8X4-	T50.8X5-	T50.8X6-
Mevinphos	T60.0X1-	T60.0X2-	T60.0X3-	T60.0X4-	-	-
Mexazolam	T42.4X1-	T42.4X2-	T42.4X3-	T42.4X4-	T42.4X5-	T42.4X6-
Mexenone	T49.3X1-	T49.3X2-	T49.3X3-	T49.3X4-	T49.3X5-	T49.3X6-
Mexiletine	T46.2X1-	T46.2X2-	T46.2X3-	T46.2X4-	T46.2X5-	T46.2X6-
Mezereon	T62.2X1-	T62.2X2-	T62.2X3-	T62.2X4-	-	-
berries	T62.1X1-	T62.1X2-	T62.1X3-	T62.1X4-	-	-
Mezlocillin	T36.0X1-	T36.0X2-	T36.0X3-	T36.0X4-	T36.0X5-	T36.0X6-
Mianserin	T43.021-	T43.022-	T43.023-	T43.024-	T43.025-	T43.026-
Micatin	T49.0X1-	T49.0X2-	T49.0X3-	T49.0X4-	T49.0X5-	T49.0X6-
Miconazole	T49.0X1-	T49.0X2-	T49.0X3-	T49.0X4-	T49.0X5-	T49.0X6-
Micronomicin	T36.5X1-	T36.5X2-	T36.5X3-	T36.5X4-	T36.5X5-	T36.5X6-
Midazolam	T42.4X1-	T42.4X2-	T42.4X3-	T42.4X4-	T42.4X5-	T42.4X6-
Midecamycin	T36.3X1-	T36.3X2-	T36.3X3-	T36.3X4-	T36.3X5-	T36.3X6-
Mifepristone	T38.6X1-	T38.6X2-	T38.6X3-	T38.6X4-	T38.6X5-	T38.6X6-
Milk of magnesia	T47.1X1-	T47.1X2-	T47.1X3-	T47.1X4-	T47.1X5-	T47.1X6-
Millipede (tropical) (venomous)	T63.411-	T63.412-	T63.413-	T63.414-	-	-
Miltown	T43.591-	T43.592-	T43.593-	T43.594-	T43.595-	T43.596-
Milverine	T44.3X1-	T44.3X2-	T44.3X3-	T44.3X4-	T44.3X5-	T44.3X6-
Minaprine	T43.291-	T43.292-	T43.293-	T43.294-	T43.295-	T43.296-
Minaxolone	T41.291-	T41.292-	T41.293-	T41.294-	T41.295-	T41.296-
Mineral						
acids	T54.2X1-	T54.2X2-	T54.2X3-	T54.2X4-	-	-
oil (laxative) (medicinal)	T47.4X1-	T47.4X2-	T47.4X3-	T47.4X4-	T47.4X5-	T47.4X6-
emulsion	T47.2X1-	T47.2X2-	T47.2X3-	T47.2X4-	T47.2X5-	T47.2X6-
nonmedicinal	T52.0X1-	T52.0X2-	T52.0X3-	T52.0X4-	-	-
topical	T49.3X1-	T49.3X2-	T49.3X3-	T49.3X4-	T49.3X5-	T49.3X6-
salt NEC	T50.3X1-	T50.3X2-	T50.3X3-	T50.3X4-	T50.3X5-	T50.3X6-
spirits	T52.0X1-	T52.0X2-	T52.0X3-	T52.0X4-	-	-
Mineralocorticosteroid	T50.0X1-	T50.0X2-	T50.0X3-	T50.0X4-	T50.0X5-	T50.0X6-
Minocycline	T36.4X1-	T36.4X2-	T36.4X3-	T36.4X4-	T36.4X5-	T36.4X6-
Minoxidil	T46.7X1-	T46.7X2-	T46.7X3-	T46.7X4-	T46.7X5-	T46.7X6-
Miokamycin	T36.3X1-	T36.3X2-	T36.3X3-	T36.3X4-	T36.3X5-	T36.3X6-
Miotic drug	T49.5X1-	T49.5X2-	T49.5X3-	T49.5X4-	T49.5X5-	T49.5X6-
Mipafox	T60.0X1-	T60.0X2-	T60.0X3-	T60.0X4-	-	-
Mirex	T60.1X1-	T60.1X2-	T60.1X3-	T60.1X4-	-	-
Mirtazapine	T43.021-	T43.022-	T43.023-	T43.024-	T43.025-	T43.026-
Misonidazole	T37.3X1-	T37.3X2-	T37.3X3-	T37.3X4-	T37.3X5-	T37.3X6-
Misoprostol	T47.1X1-	T47.1X2-	T47.1X3-	T47.1X4-	T47.1X5-	T47.1X6-
Mithramycin	T45.1X1-	T45.1X2-	T45.1X3-	T45.1X4-	T45.1X5-	T45.1X6-
Mitobronitol	T45.1X1-	T45.1X2-	T45.1X3-	T45.1X4-	T45.1X5-	T45.1X6-
Mitoguazone	T45.1X1-	T45.1X2-	T45.1X3-	T45.1X4-	T45.1X5-	T45.1X6-
Mitolactol	T45.1X1-	T45.1X2-	T45.1X3-	T45.1X4-	T45.1X5-	T45.1X6-
Mitomycin	T45.1X1-	T45.1X2-	T45.1X3-	T45.1X4-	T45.1X5-	T45.1X6-
Mitopodozide	T45.1X1-	T45.1X2-	T45.1X3-	T45.1X4-	T45.1X5-	T45.1X6-
Mitotane	T45.1X1-	T45.1X2-	T45.1X3-	T45.1X4-	T45.1X5-	T45.1X6-
Mitoxantrone	T45.1X1-	T45.1X2-	T45.1X3-	T45.1X4-	T45.1X5-	T45.1X6-
Mivacurium chloride	T48.1X1-	T48.1X2-	T48.1X3-	T48.1X4-	T48.1X5-	T48.1X6-
Miyari bacteria	T47.6X1-	T47.6X2-	T47.6X3-	T47.6X4-	T47.6X5-	T47.6X6-
Moclobemide	T43.1X1-	T43.1X2-	T43.1X3-	T43.1X4-	T43.1X5-	T43.1X6-
Moderil	T46.5X1-	T46.5X2-	T46.5X3-	T46.5X4-	T46.5X5-	T46.5X6-
Mofebutazone	T39.2X1-	T39.2X2-	T39.2X3-	T39.2X4-	T39.2X5-	T39.2X6-
Mogadon — *see* Nitrazepam						
Molindone	T43.591-	T43.592-	T43.593-	T43.594-	T43.595-	T43.596-

Substance	Poisoning Accidental (unintentional)	Poisoning Intentional self-harm	Poisoning Assault	Poisoning Undetermined	Adverse effect	Underdosing
Molsidomine	T46.3X1-	T46.3X2-	T46.3X3-	T46.3X4-	T46.3X5-	T46.3X6-
Mometasone	T49.0X1-	T49.0X2-	T49.0X3-	T49.0X4-	T49.0X5-	T49.0X6-
Monistat	T49.0X1-	T49.0X2-	T49.0X3-	T49.0X4-	T49.0X5-	T49.0X6-
Monkshood	T62.2X1-	T62.2X2-	T62.2X3-	T62.2X4-	-	-
Monoamine oxidase inhibitor NEC	T43.1X1-	T43.1X2-	T43.1X3-	T43.1X4-	T43.1X5-	T43.1X6-
hydrazine	T43.1X1-	T43.1X2-	T43.1X3-	T43.1X4-	T43.1X5-	T43.1X6-
Monobenzone	T49.4X1-	T49.4X2-	T49.4X3-	T49.4X4-	T49.4X5-	T49.4X6-
Monochloroacetic acid	T60.3X1-	T60.3X2-	T60.3X3-	T60.3X4-	-	-
Monochlorobenzene	T53.7X1-	T53.7X2-	T53.7X3-	T53.7X4-	-	-
Monoethanolamine	T46.8X1-	T46.8X2-	T46.8X3-	T46.8X4-	T46.8X5-	T46.8X6-
oleate	T46.8X1-	T46.8X2-	T46.8X3-	T46.8X4-	T46.8X5-	T46.8X6-
Monooctanoin	T50.991-	T50.992-	T50.993-	T50.994-	T50.995-	T50.996-
Monophenylbutazone	T39.2X1-	T39.2X2-	T39.2X3-	T39.2X4-	T39.2X5-	T39.2X6-
Monosodium glutamate	T65.891-	T65.892-	T65.893-	T65.894-	-	-
Monosulfiram	T49.0X1-	T49.0X2-	T49.0X3-	T49.0X4-	T49.0X5-	T49.0X6-
Monoxide, carbon — *see* Carbon, monoxide						
Monoxidine hydrochloride	T46.1X1-	T46.1X2-	T46.1X3-	T46.1X4-	T46.1X5-	T46.1X6-
Monuron	T60.3X1-	T60.3X2-	T60.3X3-	T60.3X4-	-	-
Moperone	T43.4X1-	T43.4X2-	T43.4X3-	T43.4X4-	T43.4X5-	T43.4X6-
Mopidamol	T45.1X1-	T45.1X2-	T45.1X3-	T45.1X4-	T45.1X5-	T45.1X6-
MOPP (mechloreth-amine + vincristine + prednisone + procarba-zine)	T45.1X1-	T45.1X2-	T45.1X3-	T45.1X4-	T45.1X5-	T45.1X6-
Morfin	T40.2X1-	T40.2X2-	T40.2X3-	T40.2X4-	T40.2X5-	T40.2X6-
Morinamide	T37.1X1-	T37.1X2-	T37.1X3-	T37.1X4-	T37.1X5-	T37.1X6-
Morning glory seeds	T40.991-	T40.992-	T40.993-	T40.994-	-	-
Moroxydine	T37.5X1-	T37.5X2-	T37.5X3-	T37.5X4-	T37.5X5-	T37.5X6-
Morphazinamide	T37.1X1-	T37.1X2-	T37.1X3-	T37.1X4-	T37.1X5-	T37.1X6-
Morphine	T40.2X1-	T40.2X2-	T40.2X3-	T40.2X4-	T40.2X5-	T40.2X6-
antagonist	T50.7X1-	T50.7X2-	T50.7X3-	T50.7X4-	T50.7X5-	T50.7X6-
Morpholinylethylmorphine	T40.2X1-	T40.2X2-	T40.2X3-	T40.2X4-	-	-
Morsuximide	T42.2X1-	T42.2X2-	T42.2X3-	T42.2X4-	T42.2X5-	T42.2X6-
Mosapramine	T43.591-	T43.592-	T43.593-	T43.594-	T43.595-	T43.596-
Moth balls — *see also* Pesticides	T60.2X1-	T60.2X2-	T60.2X3-	T60.2X4-	-	-
naphthalene	T60.2X1-	T60.2X2-	T60.2X3-	T60.2X4-	-	-
paradichlorobenzene	T60.1X1-	T60.1X2-	T60.1X3-	T60.1X4-	-	-
Motor exhaust gas	T58.01X-	T58.02X-	T58.03X-	T58.04X-	-	-
Mouthwash (antiseptic) (zinc chloride)	T49.6X1-	T49.6X2-	T49.6X3-	T49.6X4-	T49.6X5-	T49.6X6-
Moxastine	T45.0X1-	T45.0X2-	T45.0X3-	T45.0X4-	T45.0X5-	T45.0X6-
Moxaverine	T44.3X1-	T44.3X2-	T44.3X3-	T44.3X4-	T44.3X5-	T44.3X6-
Moxisylyte	T46.7X1-	T46.7X2-	T46.7X3-	T46.7X4-	T46.7X5-	T46.7X6-
Mucilage, plant	T47.4X1-	T47.4X2-	T47.4X3-	T47.4X4-	T47.4X5-	T47.4X6-
Mucolytic drug	T48.4X1-	T48.4X2-	T48.4X3-	T48.4X4-	T48.4X5-	T48.4X6-
Mucomyst	T48.4X1-	T48.4X2-	T48.4X3-	T48.4X4-	T48.4X5-	T48.4X6-
Mucous membrane agents (external)	T49.91X-	T49.92X-	T49.93X-	T49.94X-	T49.95X-	T49.96X-
specified NEC	T49.8X1-	T49.8X2-	T49.8X3-	T49.8X4-	T49.8X5-	T49.8X6-
Mumps						
immune globulin (human)	T50.Z11-	T50.Z12-	T50.Z13-	T50.Z14-	T50.Z15-	T50.Z16-
skin test antigen	T50.8X1-	T50.8X2-	T50.8X3-	T50.8X4-	T50.8X5-	T50.8X6-
vaccine	T50.B91-	T50.B92-	T50.B93-	T50.B94-	T50.B95-	T50.B96-
Mumpsvax	T50.B91-	T50.B92-	T50.B93-	T50.B94-	T50.B95-	T50.B96-
Mupirocin	T49.0X1-	T49.0X2-	T49.0X3-	T49.0X4-	T49.0X5-	T49.0X6-
Muriatic acid — *see* Hydrochloric acid						
Muromonab-CD3	T45.1X1-	T45.1X2-	T45.1X3-	T45.1X4-	T45.1X5-	T45.1X6-
Muscle-action drug NEC	T48.201-	T48.202-	T48.203-	T48.204-	T48.205-	T48.206-
Muscle affecting agents NEC	T48.201-	T48.202-	T48.203-	T48.204-	T48.205-	T48.206-
oxytocic	T48.0X1-	T48.0X2-	T48.0X3-	T48.0X4-	T48.0X5-	T48.0X6-
relaxants	T48.201-	T48.202-	T48.203-	T48.204-	T48.205-	T48.206-
central nervous system	T42.8X1-	T42.8X2-	T42.8X3-	T42.8X4-	T42.8X5-	T42.8X6-
skeletal	T48.1X1-	T48.1X2-	T48.1X3-	T48.1X4-	T48.1X5-	T48.1X6-
smooth	T44.3X1-	T44.3X2-	T44.3X3-	T44.3X4-	T44.3X5-	T44.3X6-
Muscle relaxant — *see* Relaxant, muscle						
Muscle-tone depressant, central NEC	T42.8X1-	T42.8X2-	T42.8X3-	T42.8X4-	T42.8X5-	T42.8X6-
specified NEC	T42.8X1-	T42.8X2-	T42.8X3-	T42.8X4-	T42.8X5-	T42.8X6-
Mushroom, noxious	T62.0X1-	T62.0X2-	T62.0X3-	T62.0X4-	-	-
Mussel, noxious	T61.781-	T61.782-	T61.783-	T61.784-	-	-
Mustard (emetic)	T47.7X1-	T47.7X2-	T47.7X3-	T47.7X4-	T47.7X5-	T47.7X6-
black	T47.7X1-	T47.7X2-	T47.7X3-	T47.7X4-	T47.7X5-	T47.7X6-
gas, not in war	T59.91X-	T59.92X-	T59.93X-	T59.94X-	-	-
nitrogen	T45.1X1-	T45.1X2-	T45.1X3-	T45.1X4-	T45.1X5-	T45.1X6-
Mustine	T45.1X1-	T45.1X2-	T45.1X3-	T45.1X4-	T45.1X5-	T45.1X6-

Substance	Poisoning Accidental (unintentional)	Poisoning Intentional self-harm	Poisoning Assault	Poisoning Undetermined	Adverse effect	Underdosing
M-vac	T45.1X1-	T45.1X2-	T45.1X3-	T45.1X4-	T45.1X5-	T45.1X6-
Mycifradin	T36.5X1-	T36.5X2-	T36.5X3-	T36.5X4-	T36.5X5-	T36.5X6-
topical	T49.0X1-	T49.0X2-	T49.0X3-	T49.0X4-	T49.0X5-	T49.0X6-
Mycitracin	T36.8X1-	T36.8X2-	T36.8X3-	T36.8X4-	T36.8X5-	T36.8X6-
ophthalmic preparation	T49.5X1-	T49.5X2-	T49.5X3-	T49.5X4-	T49.5X5-	T49.5X6-
Mycostatin	T36.7X1-	T36.7X2-	T36.7X3-	T36.7X4-	T36.7X5-	T36.7X6-
topical	T49.0X1-	T49.0X2-	T49.0X3-	T49.0X4-	T49.0X5-	T49.0X6-
Mycotoxins	T64.81X-	T64.82X-	T64.83X-	T64.84X-	-	-
aflatoxin	T64.01X-	T64.02X-	T64.03X-	T64.04X-	-	-
specified NEC	T64.81X-	T64.82X-	T64.83X-	T64.84X-	-	-
Mydriacyl	T44.3X1-	T44.3X2-	T44.3X3-	T44.3X4-	T44.3X5-	T44.3X6-
Mydriatic drug	T49.5X1-	T49.5X2-	T49.5X3-	T49.5X4-	T49.5X5-	T49.5X6-
Myelobromal	T45.1X1-	T45.1X2-	T45.1X3-	T45.1X4-	T45.1X5-	T45.1X6-
Myleran	T45.1X1-	T45.1X2-	T45.1X3-	T45.1X4-	T45.1X5-	T45.1X6-
Myochrysin (e)	T39.2X1-	T39.2X2-	T39.2X3-	T39.2X4-	T39.2X5-	T39.2X6-
Myoneural blocking agents	T48.1X1-	T48.1X2-	T48.1X3-	T48.1X4-	T48.1X5-	T48.1X6-
Myralact	T49.0X1-	T49.0X2-	T49.0X3-	T49.0X4-	T49.0X5-	T49.0X6-
Myristica fragrans	T62.2X1-	T62.2X2-	T62.2X3-	T62.2X4-	-	-
Myristicin	T65.891-	T65.892-	T65.893-	T65.894-	-	-
Mysoline	T42.3X1-	T42.3X2-	T42.3X3-	T42.3X4-	T42.3X5-	T42.3X6-
Nabilone	T40.7X1-	T40.7X2-	T40.7X3-	T40.7X4-	T40.7X5-	T40.7X6-
Nabumetone	T39.391-	T39.392-	T39.393-	T39.394-	T39.395-	T39.396-
Nadolol	T44.7X1-	T44.7X2-	T44.7X3-	T44.7X4-	T44.7X5-	T44.7X6-
Nafcillin	T36.0X1-	T36.0X2-	T36.0X3-	T36.0X4-	T36.0X5-	T36.0X6-
Nafoxidine	T38.6X1-	T38.6X2-	T38.6X3-	T38.6X4-	T38.6X5-	T38.6X6-
Naftazone	T46.991-	T46.992-	T46.993-	T46.994-	T46.995-	T46.996-
Naftidrofuryl (oxalate)	T46.7X1-	T46.7X2-	T46.7X3-	T46.7X4-	T46.7X5-	T46.7X6-
Naftifine	T49.0X1-	T49.0X2-	T49.0X3-	T49.0X4-	T49.0X5-	T49.0X6-
Nail polish remover	T52.91X-	T52.92X-	T52.93X-	T52.94X-	-	-
Nalbuphine	T40.4X1-	T40.4X2-	T40.4X3-	T40.4X4-	T40.4X5-	T40.4X6-
Naled	T60.0X1-	T60.0X2-	T60.0X3-	T60.0X4-	-	-
Nalidixic acid	T37.8X1-	T37.8X2-	T37.8X3-	T37.8X4-	T37.8X5-	T37.8X6-
Nalorphine	T50.7X1-	T50.7X2-	T50.7X3-	T50.7X4-	T50.7X5-	T50.7X6-
Naloxone	T50.7X1-	T50.7X2-	T50.7X3-	T50.7X4-	T50.7X5-	T50.7X6-
Naltrexone	T50.7X1-	T50.7X2-	T50.7X3-	T50.7X4-	T50.7X5-	T50.7X6-
Namenda	T43.8X1-	T43.8X2-	T43.8X3-	T43.8X4-	T43.8X5-	T43.8X6-
Nandrolone	T38.7X1-	T38.7X2-	T38.7X3-	T38.7X4-	T38.7X5-	T38.7X6-
Naphazoline	T48.5X1-	T48.5X2-	T48.5X3-	T48.5X4-	T48.5X5-	T48.5X6-
Naphtha (painters') (petroleum)	T52.0X1-	T52.0X2-	T52.0X3-	T52.0X4-	-	-
solvent	T52.0X1-	T52.0X2-	T52.0X3-	T52.0X4-	-	-
vapor	T52.0X1-	T52.0X2-	T52.0X3-	T52.0X4-	-	-
Naphthalene (non-chlorinated)	T60.2X1-	T60.2X2-	T60.2X3-	T60.2X4-	-	-
chlorinated	T60.1X1-	T60.1X2-	T60.1X3-	T60.1X4-	-	-
vapor	T60.1X1-	T60.1X2-	T60.1X3-	T60.1X4-	-	-
insecticide or moth repellent	T60.2X1-	T60.2X2-	T60.2X3-	T60.2X4-	-	-
chlorinated	T60.1X1-	T60.1X2-	T60.1X3-	T60.1X4-	-	-
vapor	T60.2X1-	T60.2X2-	T60.2X3-	T60.2X4-	-	-
chlorinated	T60.1X1-	T60.1X2-	T60.1X3-	T60.1X4-	-	-
Naphthol	T65.891-	T65.892-	T65.893-	T65.894-	-	-
Naphthylamine	T65.891-	T65.892-	T65.893-	T65.894-	-	-
Naphthylthiourea (ANTU)	T60.4X1-	T60.4X2-	T60.4X3-	T60.4X4-	-	-
Naprosyn — *see* Naproxen						
Naproxen	T39.311-	T39.312-	T39.313-	T39.314-	T39.315-	T39.316-
Narcotic (drug)	T40.601-	T40.602-	T40.603-	T40.604-	T40.605-	T40.606-
analgesic NEC	T40.601-	T40.602-	T40.603-	T40.604-	T40.605-	T40.606-
antagonist	T50.7X1-	T50.7X2-	T50.7X3-	T50.7X4-	T50.7X5-	T50.7X6-
specified NEC	T40.691-	T40.692-	T40.693-	T40.694-	T40.695-	T40.696-
synthetic	T40.4X1-	T40.4X2-	T40.4X3-	T40.4X4-	T40.4X5-	T40.4X6-
Narcotine	T48.3X1-	T48.3X2-	T48.3X3-	T48.3X4-	T48.3X5-	T48.3X6-
Nardil	T43.1X1-	T43.1X2-	T43.1X3-	T43.1X4-	T43.1X5-	T43.1X6-
Nasal drug NEC	T49.6X1-	T49.6X2-	T49.6X3-	T49.6X4-	T49.6X5-	T49.6X6-
Natamycin	T49.0X1-	T49.0X2-	T49.0X3-	T49.0X4-	T49.0X5-	T49.0X6-
Natrium cyanide — *see* Cyanide(s)						
Natural						
blood (product)	T45.8X1-	T45.8X2-	T45.8X3-	T45.8X4-	T45.8X5-	T45.8X6-
gas (piped)	T59.891-	T59.892-	T59.893-	T59.894-	-	-
incomplete combustion	T58.11X-	T58.12X-	T58.13X-	T58.14X-	-	-
Nealbarbital	T42.3X1-	T42.3X2-	T42.3X3-	T42.3X4-	T42.3X5-	T42.3X6-
Nectadon	T48.3X1-	T48.3X2-	T48.3X3-	T48.3X4-	T48.3X5-	T48.3X6-
Nedocromil	T48.6X1-	T48.6X2-	T48.6X3-	T48.6X4-	T48.6X5-	T48.6X6-
Nefopam	T39.8X1-	T39.8X2-	T39.8X3-	T39.8X4-	T39.8X5-	T39.8X6-
Nematocyst (sting)	T63.691-	T63.692-	T63.693-	T63.694-	-	-
Nembutal	T42.3X1-	T42.3X2-	T42.3X3-	T42.3X4-	T42.3X5-	T42.3X6-
Nemonapride	T43.591-	T43.592-	T43.593-	T43.594-	T43.595-	T43.596-
Neoarsphenamine	T37.8X1-	T37.8X2-	T37.8X3-	T37.8X4-	T37.8X5-	T37.8X6-
Neocinchophen	T50.4X1-	T50.4X2-	T50.4X3-	T50.4X4-	T50.4X5-	T50.4X6-
Neomycin (derivatives)	T36.5X1-	T36.5X2-	T36.5X3-	T36.5X4-	T36.5X5-	T36.5X6-
with						
bacitracin	T49.0X1-	T49.0X2-	T49.0X3-	T49.0X4-	T49.0X5-	T49.0X6-
neostigmine	T44.0X1-	T44.0X2-	T44.0X3-	T44.0X4-	T44.0X5-	T44.0X6-
ENT agent	T49.6X1-	T49.6X2-	T49.6X3-	T49.6X4-	T49.6X5-	T49.6X6-
ophthalmic preparation	T49.5X1-	T49.5X2-	T49.5X3-	T49.5X4-	T49.5X5-	T49.5X6-
topical NEC	T49.0X1-	T49.0X2-	T49.0X3-	T49.0X4-	T49.0X5-	T49.0X6-
Neonal	T42.3X1-	T42.3X2-	T42.3X3-	T42.3X4-	T42.3X5-	T42.3X6-
Neoprontosil	T37.0X1-	T37.0X2-	T37.0X3-	T37.0X4-	T37.0X5-	T37.0X6-
Neosalvarsan	T37.8X1-	T37.8X2-	T37.8X3-	T37.8X4-	T37.8X5-	T37.8X6-
Neosilversalvarsan	T37.8X1-	T37.8X2-	T37.8X3-	T37.8X4-	T37.8X5-	T37.8X6-
Neosporin	T36.8X1-	T36.8X2-	T36.8X3-	T36.8X4-	T36.8X5-	T36.8X6-
ENT agent	T49.6X1-	T49.6X2-	T49.6X3-	T49.6X4-	T49.6X5-	T49.6X6-
opthalmic preparation	T49.5X1-	T49.5X2-	T49.5X3-	T49.5X4-	T49.5X5-	T49.5X6-
topical NEC	T49.0X1-	T49.0X2-	T49.0X3-	T49.0X4-	T49.0X5-	T49.0X6-
Neostigmine bromide	T44.0X1-	T44.0X2-	T44.0X3-	T44.0X4-	T44.0X5-	T44.0X6-
Neraval	T42.3X1-	T42.3X2-	T42.3X3-	T42.3X4-	T42.3X5-	T42.3X6-
Neravan	T42.3X1-	T42.3X2-	T42.3X3-	T42.3X4-	T42.3X5-	T42.3X6-
Nerium oleander	T62.2X1-	T62.2X2-	T62.2X3-	T62.2X4-	-	-
Nerve gas, not in war	T59.91X-	T59.92X-	T59.93X-	T59.94X-	-	-
Nesacaine	T41.3X1-	T41.3X2-	T41.3X3-	T41.3X4-	T41.3X5-	T41.3X6-
infiltration (subcutaneous)	T41.3X1-	T41.3X2-	T41.3X3-	T41.3X4-	T41.3X5-	T41.3X6-
nerve block (peripheral) (plexus)	T41.3X1-	T41.3X2-	T41.3X3-	T41.3X4-	T41.3X5-	T41.3X6-
Netilmicin	T36.5X1-	T36.5X2-	T36.5X3-	T36.5X4-	T36.5X5-	T36.5X6-
Neurobarb	T42.3X1-	T42.3X2-	T42.3X3-	T42.3X4-	T42.3X5-	T42.3X6-
Neuroleptic drug NEC	T43.501-	T43.502-	T43.503-	T43.504-	T43.505-	T43.506-
Neuromuscular blocking drug	T48.1X1-	T48.1X2-	T48.1X3-	T48.1X4-	T48.1X5-	T48.1X6-
Neutral insulin injection	T38.3X1-	T38.3X2-	T38.3X3-	T38.3X4-	T38.3X5-	T38.3X6-
Neutral spirits	T51.0X1-	T51.0X2-	T51.0X3-	T51.0X4-	-	-
beverage	T51.0X1-	T51.0X2-	T51.0X3-	T51.0X4-	-	-
Niacin	T46.7X1-	T46.7X2-	T46.7X3-	T46.7X4-	T46.7X5-	T46.7X6-
Niacinamide	T45.2X1-	T45.2X2-	T45.2X3-	T45.2X4-	T45.2X5-	T45.2X6-
Nialamide	T43.1X1-	T43.1X2-	T43.1X3-	T43.1X4-	T43.1X5-	T43.1X6-
Niaprazine	T42.6X1-	T42.6X2-	T42.6X3-	T42.6X4-	T42.6X5-	T42.6X6-
Nicametate	T46.7X1-	T46.7X2-	T46.7X3-	T46.7X4-	T46.7X5-	T46.7X6-
Nicardipine	T46.1X1-	T46.1X2-	T46.1X3-	T46.1X4-	T46.1X5-	T46.1X6-
Nicergoline	T46.7X1-	T46.7X2-	T46.7X3-	T46.7X4-	T46.7X5-	T46.7X6-
Nickel (carbonyl) (tetra -carbonyl) (fumes) (vapor)	T56.891-	T56.892-	T56.893-	T56.894-	-	-
Nickelocene	T56.891-	T56.892-	T56.893-	T56.894-	-	-
Niclosamide	T37.4X1-	T37.4X2-	T37.4X3-	T37.4X4-	T37.4X5-	T37.4X6-
Nicofuranose	T46.7X1-	T46.7X2-	T46.7X3-	T46.7X4-	T46.7X5-	T46.7X6-
Nicomorphine	T40.2X1-	T40.2X2-	T40.2X3-	T40.2X4-	-	-
Nicorandil	T46.3X1-	T46.3X2-	T46.3X3-	T46.3X4-	T46.3X5-	T46.3X6-
Nicotiana (plant)	T62.2X1-	T62.2X2-	T62.2X3-	T62.2X4-	-	-
Nicotinamide	T45.2X1-	T45.2X2-	T45.2X3-	T45.2X4-	T45.2X5-	T45.2X6-
Nicotine (insecticide) (spray) (sulfate) **NEC**	T60.2X1-	T60.2X2-	T60.2X3-	T60.2X4-	-	-
from tobacco	T65.291-	T65.292-	T65.293-	T65.294-	-	-
cigarettes	T65.221-	T65.222-	T65.223-	T65.224-	-	-
not insecticide	T65.291-	T65.292-	T65.293-	T65.294-	-	-
Nicotinic acid	T46.7X1-	T46.7X2-	T46.7X3-	T46.7X4-	T46.7X5-	T46.7X6-
Nicotinyl alcohol	T46.7X1-	T46.7X2-	T46.7X3-	T46.7X4-	T46.7X5-	T46.7X6-
Nicoumalone	T45.511-	T45.512-	T45.513-	T45.514-	T45.515-	T45.516-
Nifedipine	T46.1X1-	T46.1X2-	T46.1X3-	T46.1X4-	T46.1X5-	T46.1X6-
Nifenazone	T39.2X1-	T39.2X2-	T39.2X3-	T39.2X4-	T39.2X5-	T39.2X6-
Nifuraldezone	T37.91X-	T37.92X-	T37.93X-	T37.94X-	T37.95X-	T37.96X-
Nifuratel	T37.8X1-	T37.8X2-	T37.8X3-	T37.8X4-	T37.8X5-	T37.8X6-
Nifurtimox	T37.3X1-	T37.3X2-	T37.3X3-	T37.3X4-	T37.3X5-	T37.3X6-
Nifurtoinol	T37.8X1-	T37.8X2-	T37.8X3-	T37.8X4-	T37.8X5-	T37.8X6-
Nightshade, deadly (solanum — *see also* Belladonna	T62.2X1-	T62.2X2-	T62.2X3-	T62.2X4-	-	-
berry	T62.1X1-	T62.1X2-	T62.1X3-	T62.1X4-	-	-
Nikethamide	T50.7X1-	T50.7X2-	T50.7X3-	T50.7X4-	T50.7X5-	T50.7X6-
Nilstat	T36.7X1-	T36.7X2-	T36.7X3-	T36.7X4-	T36.7X5-	T36.7X6-
topical	T49.0X1-	T49.0X2-	T49.0X3-	T49.0X4-	T49.0X5-	T49.0X6-
Nilutamide	T38.6X1-	T38.6X2-	T38.6X3-	T38.6X4-	T38.6X5-	T38.6X6-
Nimesulide	T39.391-	T39.392-	T39.393-	T39.394-	T39.395-	T39.396-
Nimetazepam	T42.4X1-	T42.4X2-	T42.4X3-	T42.4X4-	T42.4X5-	T42.4X6-
Nimodipine	T46.1X1-	T46.1X2-	T46.1X3-	T46.1X4-	T46.1X5-	T46.1X6-
Nimorazole	T37.3X1-	T37.3X2-	T37.3X3-	T37.3X4-	T37.3X5-	T37.3X6-
Nimustine	T45.1X1-	T45.1X2-	T45.1X3-	T45.1X4-	T45.1X5-	T45.1X6-
Niridazole	T37.4X1-	T37.4X2-	T37.4X3-	T37.4X4-	T37.4X5-	T37.4X6-
Nisentil	T40.2X1-	T40.2X2-	T40.2X3-	T40.2X4-	T40.2X5-	T40.2X6-
Nisoldipine	T46.1X1-	T46.1X2-	T46.1X3-	T46.1X4-	T46.1X5-	T46.1X6-
Nitramine	T65.3X1-	T65.3X2-	T65.3X3-	T65.3X4-	-	-
Nitrate, organic	T46.3X1-	T46.3X2-	T46.3X3-	T46.3X4-	T46.3X5-	T46.3X6-

Substance	Poisoning Accidental (unintentional)	Poisoning Intentional self-harm	Poisoning Assault	Poisoning Undetermined	Adverse effect	Underdosing
Nitrazepam	T42.4X1-	T42.4X2-	T42.4X3-	T42.4X4-	T42.4X5-	T42.4X6-
Nitrefazole	T50.6X1-	T50.6X2-	T50.6X3-	T50.6X4-	T50.6X5-	T50.6X6-
Nitrendipine	T46.1X1-	T46.1X2-	T46.1X3-	T46.1X4-	T46.1X5-	T46.1X6-
Nitric						
acid (liquid)	T54.2X1-	T54.2X2-	T54.2X3-	T54.2X4-	-	-
vapor	T59.891-	T59.892-	T59.893-	T59.894-	-	-
oxide (gas)	T59.0X1-	T59.0X2-	T59.0X3-	T59.0X4-	-	-
Nitrimidazine	T37.3X1-	T37.3X2-	T37.3X3-	T37.3X4-	T37.3X5-	T37.3X6-
Nitrite, amyl (medicinal) (vapor)	T46.3X1-	T46.3X2-	T46.3X3-	T46.3X4-	T46.3X5-	T46.3X6-
Nitroaniline	T65.3X1-	T65.3X2-	T65.3X3-	T65.3X4-	-	-
vapor	T59.891-	T59.892-	T59.893-	T59.894-	-	-
Nitrobenzene, nitrobenzol	T65.3X1-	T65.3X2-	T65.3X3-	T65.3X4-	-	-
vapor	T65.3X1-	T65.3X2-	T65.3X3-	T65.3X4-	-	-
Nitrocellulose	T65.891-	T65.892-	T65.893-	T65.894-	-	-
lacquer	T65.891-	T65.892-	T65.893-	T65.894-	-	-
Nitrodiphenyl	T65.3X1-	T65.3X2-	T65.3X3-	T65.3X4-	-	-
Nitrofural	T49.0X1-	T49.0X2-	T49.0X3-	T49.0X4-	T49.0X5-	T49.0X6-
Nitrofurantoin	T37.8X1-	T37.8X2-	T37.8X3-	T37.8X4-	T37.8X5-	T37.8X6-
Nitrofurazone	T49.0X1-	T49.0X2-	T49.0X3-	T49.0X4-	T49.0X5-	T49.0X6-
Nitrogen	T59.0X1-	T59.0X2-	T59.0X3-	T59.0X4-	-	-
mustard	T45.1X1-	T45.1X2-	T45.1X3-	T45.1X4-	T45.1X5-	T45.1X6-
Nitroglycerin, nitro-glycerol (medicinal)	T46.3X1-	T46.3X2-	T46.3X3-	T46.3X4-	T46.3X5-	T46.3X6-
nonmedicinal	T65.5X1-	T65.5X2-	T65.5X3-	T65.5X4-	-	-
fumes	T65.5X1-	T65.5X2-	T65.5X3-	T65.5X4-	-	-
Nitroglycol	T52.3X1-	T52.3X2-	T52.3X3-	T52.3X4-	-	-
Nitrohydrochloric acid	T54.2X1-	T54.2X2-	T54.2X3-	T54.2X4-	-	-
Nitromersol	T49.0X1-	T49.0X2-	T49.0X3-	T49.0X4-	T49.0X5-	T49.0X6-
Nitronaphthalene	T65.891-	T65.892-	T65.893-	T65.894-	-	-
Nitrophenol	T54.0X1-	T54.0X2-	T54.0X3-	T54.0X4-	-	-
Nitropropane	T52.8X1-	T52.8X2-	T52.8X3-	T52.8X4-	-	-
Nitroprusside	T46.5X1-	T46.5X2-	T46.5X3-	T46.5X4-	T46.5X5-	T46.5X6-
Nitrosodimethylamine	T65.3X1-	T65.3X2-	T65.3X3-	T65.3X4-	-	-
Nitrothiazol	T37.4X1-	T37.4X2-	T37.4X3-	T37.4X4-	T37.4X5-	T37.4X6-
Nitrotoluene, nitrotoluol	T65.3X1-	T65.3X2-	T65.3X3-	T65.3X4-	-	-
vapor	T65.3X1-	T65.3X2-	T65.3X3-	T65.3X4-	-	-
Nitrous						
acid (liquid)	T54.2X1-	T54.2X2-	T54.2X3-	T54.2X4-	-	-
fumes	T59.891-	T59.892-	T59.893-	T59.894-	-	-
ether spirit	T46.3X1-	T46.3X2-	T46.3X3-	T46.3X4-	T46.3X5-	T46.3X6-
oxide	T41.0X1-	T41.0X2-	T41.0X3-	T41.0X4-	T41.0X5-	T41.0X6-
Nitroxoline	T37.8X1-	T37.8X2-	T37.8X3-	T37.8X4-	T37.8X5-	T37.8X6-
Nitrozone	T49.0X1-	T49.0X2-	T49.0X3-	T49.0X4-	T49.0X5-	T49.0X6-
Nizatidine	T47.0X1-	T47.0X2-	T47.0X3-	T47.0X4-	T47.0X5-	T47.0X6-
Nizofenone	T43.8X1-	T43.8X2-	T43.8X3-	T43.8X4-	T43.8X5-	T43.8X6-
Noctec	T42.6X1-	T42.6X2-	T42.6X3-	T42.6X4-	T42.6X5-	T42.6X6-
Noludar	T42.6X1-	T42.6X2-	T42.6X3-	T42.6X4-	T42.6X5-	T42.6X6-
Nomegestrol	T38.5X1-	T38.5X2-	T38.5X3-	T38.5X4-	T38.5X5-	T38.5X6-
Nomifensine	T43.291-	T43.292-	T43.293-	T43.294-	T43.295-	T43.296-
Nonoxinol	T49.8X1-	T49.8X2-	T49.8X3-	T49.8X4-	T49.8X5-	T49.8X6-
Nonylphenoxy (polyethoxy-ethanol)	T49.8X1-	T49.8X2-	T49.8X3-	T49.8X4-	T49.8X5-	T49.8X6-
Noptil	T42.3X1-	T42.3X2-	T42.3X3-	T42.3X4-	T42.3X5-	T42.3X6-
Noradrenaline	T44.4X1-	T44.4X2-	T44.4X3-	T44.4X4-	T44.4X5-	T44.4X6-
Noramidopyrine	T39.2X1-	T39.2X2-	T39.2X3-	T39.2X4-	T39.2X5-	T39.2X6-
methanesulfonate sodium	T39.2X1-	T39.2X2-	T39.2X3-	T39.2X4-	T39.2X5-	T39.2X6-
Norbormide	T60.4X1-	T60.4X2-	T60.4X3-	T60.4X4-	-	-
Nordazepam	T42.4X1-	T42.4X2-	T42.4X3-	T42.4X4-	T42.4X5-	T42.4X6-
Norepinephrine	T44.4X1-	T44.4X2-	T44.4X3-	T44.4X4-	T44.4X5-	T44.4X6-
Norethandrolone	T38.7X1-	T38.7X2-	T38.7X3-	T38.7X4-	T38.7X5-	T38.7X6-
Norethindrone	T38.4X1-	T38.4X2-	T38.4X3-	T38.4X4-	T38.4X5-	T38.4X6-
Norethisterone (acetate) (enantate)	T38.4X1-	T38.4X2-	T38.4X3-	T38.4X4-	T38.4X5-	T38.4X6-
with ethinylestradiol	T38.5X1-	T38.5X2-	T38.5X3-	T38.5X4-	T38.5X5-	T38.5X6-
Noretynodrel	T38.5X1-	T38.5X2-	T38.5X3-	T38.5X4-	T38.5X5-	T38.5X6-
Norfenefrine	T44.4X1-	T44.4X2-	T44.4X3-	T44.4X4-	T44.4X5-	T44.4X6-
Norfloxacin	T36.8X1-	T36.8X2-	T36.8X3-	T36.8X4-	T36.8X5-	T36.8X6-
Norgestrel	T38.4X1-	T38.4X2-	T38.4X3-	T38.4X4-	T38.4X5-	T38.4X6-
Norgestrienone	T38.4X1-	T38.4X2-	T38.4X3-	T38.4X4-	T38.4X5-	T38.4X6-
Norlestrin	T38.4X1-	T38.4X2-	T38.4X3-	T38.4X4-	T38.4X5-	T38.4X6-
Norlutin	T38.4X1-	T38.4X2-	T38.4X3-	T38.4X4-	T38.4X5-	T38.4X6-
Normal serum albumin (human) **, salt-poor**	T45.8X1-	T45.8X2-	T45.8X3-	T45.8X4-	T45.8X5-	T45.8X6-
Normethandrone	T38.5X1-	T38.5X2-	T38.5X3-	T38.5X4-	T38.5X5-	T38.5X6-
Normison — *see* Benzodiazepines						
Normorphine	T40.2X1-	T40.2X2-	T40.2X3-	T40.2X4-	-	-
Norpseudoephedrine	T50.5X1-	T50.5X2-	T50.5X3-	T50.5X4-	T50.5X5-	T50.5X6-

Substance	Poisoning Accidental (unintentional)	Poisoning Intentional self-harm	Poisoning Assault	Poisoning Undetermined	Adverse effect	Underdosing
Nortestosterone (furanpropionate)	T38.7X1-	T38.7X2-	T38.7X3-	T38.7X4-	T38.7X5-	T38.7X6-
Nortriptyline	T43.011-	T43.012-	T43.013-	T43.014-	T43.015-	T43.016-
Noscapine	T48.3X1-	T48.3X2-	T48.3X3-	T48.3X4-	T48.3X5-	T48.3X6-
Nose preparations	T49.6X1-	T49.6X2-	T49.6X3-	T49.6X4-	T49.6X5-	T49.6X6-
Novobiocin	T36.5X1-	T36.5X2-	T36.5X3-	T36.5X4-	T36.5X5-	T36.5X6-
Novocain (infiltration) (topical)	T41.3X1-	T41.3X2-	T41.3X3-	T41.3X4-	T41.3X5-	T41.3X6-
nerve block (peripheral) (plexus)	T41.3X1-	T41.3X2-	T41.3X3-	T41.3X4-	T41.3X5-	T41.3X6-
spinal	T41.3X1-	T41.3X2-	T41.3X3-	T41.3X4-	T41.3X5-	T41.3X6-
Noxious foodstuff	T62.91X-	T62.92X-	T62.93X-	T62.94X-	-	-
specified NEC	T62.8X1-	T62.8X2-	T62.8X3-	T62.8X4-	-	-
Noxiptiline	T43.011-	T43.012-	T43.013-	T43.014-	T43.015-	T43.016-
Noxytiolin	T49.0X1-	T49.0X2-	T49.0X3-	T49.0X4-	T49.0X5-	T49.0X6-
NPH Iletin (insulin)	T38.3X1-	T38.3X2-	T38.3X3-	T38.3X4-	T38.3X5-	T38.3X6-
Numorphan	T40.2X1-	T40.2X2-	T40.2X3-	T40.2X4-	T40.2X5-	T40.2X6-
Nunol	T42.3X1-	T42.3X2-	T42.3X3-	T42.3X4-	T42.3X5-	T42.3X6-
Nupercaine (spinal anesthetic)	T41.3X1-	T41.3X2-	T41.3X3-	T41.3X4-	T41.3X5-	T41.3X6-
topical (surface)	T41.3X1-	T41.3X2-	T41.3X3-	T41.3X4-	T41.3X5-	T41.3X6-
Nutmeg oil (liniment)	T49.3X1-	T49.3X2-	T49.3X3-	T49.3X4-	T49.3X5-	T49.3X6-
Nutritional supplement	T50.901-	T50.902-	T50.903-	T50.904-	T50.905-	T50.906-
Nux vomica	T65.1X1-	T65.1X2-	T65.1X3-	T65.1X4-	-	-
Nydrazid	T37.1X1-	T37.1X2-	T37.1X3-	T37.1X4-	T37.1X5-	T37.1X6-
Nylidrin	T46.7X1-	T46.7X2-	T46.7X3-	T46.7X4-	T46.7X5-	T46.7X6-
Nystatin	T36.7X1-	T36.7X2-	T36.7X3-	T36.7X4-	T36.7X5-	T36.7X6-
topical	T49.0X1-	T49.0X2-	T49.0X3-	T49.0X4-	T49.0X5-	T49.0X6-
Nytol	T45.0X1-	T45.0X2-	T45.0X3-	T45.0X4-	T45.0X5-	T45.0X6-
Obidoxime chloride	T50.6X1-	T50.6X2-	T50.6X3-	T50.6X4-	T50.6X5-	T50.6X6-
Octafonium (chloride)	T49.3X1-	T49.3X2-	T49.3X3-	T49.3X4-	T49.3X5-	T49.3X6-
Octamethyl pyrophos-phoramide	T60.0X1-	T60.0X2-	T60.0X3-	T60.0X4-	-	-
Octanoin	T50.991-	T50.992-	T50.993-	T50.994-	T50.995-	T50.996-
Octatropine methyl-bromide	T44.3X1-	T44.3X2-	T44.3X3-	T44.3X4-	T44.3X5-	T44.3X6-
Octotiamine	T45.2X1-	T45.2X2-	T45.2X3-	T45.2X4-	T45.2X5-	T45.2X6-
Octoxinol (9)	T49.8X1-	T49.8X2-	T49.8X3-	T49.8X4-	T49.8X5-	T49.8X6-
Octreotide	T38.991-	T38.992-	T38.993-	T38.994-	T38.995-	T38.996-
Octyl nitrite	T46.3X1-	T46.3X2-	T46.3X3-	T46.3X4-	T46.3X5-	T46.3X6-
Oestradiol	T38.5X1-	T38.5X2-	T38.5X3-	T38.5X4-	T38.5X5-	T38.5X6-
Oestriol	T38.5X1-	T38.5X2-	T38.5X3-	T38.5X4-	T38.5X5-	T38.5X6-
Oestrogen	T38.5X1-	T38.5X2-	T38.5X3-	T38.5X4-	T38.5X5-	T38.5X6-
Oestrone	T38.5X1-	T38.5X2-	T38.5X3-	T38.5X4-	T38.5X5-	T38.5X6-
Ofloxacin	T36.8X1-	T36.8X2-	T36.8X3-	T36.8X4-	T36.8X5-	T36.8X6-
Oil (of)	T65.891-	T65.892-	T65.893-	T65.894-	-	-
bitter almond	T62.8X1-	T62.8X2-	T62.8X3-	T62.8X4-	-	-
cloves	T49.7X1-	T49.7X2-	T49.7X3-	T49.7X4-	T49.7X5-	T49.7X6-
colors	T65.6X1-	T65.6X2-	T65.6X3-	T65.6X4-	-	-
fumes	T59.891-	T59.892-	T59.893-	T59.894-	-	-
lubricating	T52.0X1-	T52.0X2-	T52.0X3-	T52.0X4-	-	-
Niobe	T52.8X1-	T52.8X2-	T52.8X3-	T52.8X4-	-	-
vitriol (liquid)	T54.2X1-	T54.2X2-	T54.2X3-	T54.2X4-	-	-
fumes	T54.2X1-	T54.2X2-	T54.2X3-	T54.2X4-	-	-
wintergreen (bitter) NEC	T49.3X1-	T49.3X2-	T49.3X3-	T49.3X4-	T49.3X5-	T49.3X6-
Oily preparation (for skin)	T49.3X1-	T49.3X2-	T49.3X3-	T49.3X4-	T49.3X5-	T49.3X6-
Ointment NEC	T49.3X1-	T49.3X2-	T49.3X3-	T49.3X4-	T49.3X5-	T49.3X6-
Olanzapine	T43.591-	T43.592-	T43.593-	T43.594-	T43.595-	T43.596-
Oleander	T62.2X1-	T62.2X2-	T62.2X3-	T62.2X4-	-	-
Oleandomycin	T36.3X1-	T36.3X2-	T36.3X3-	T36.3X4-	T36.3X5-	T36.3X6-
Oleandrin	T46.0X1-	T46.0X2-	T46.0X3-	T46.0X4-	T46.0X5-	T46.0X6-
Oleic acid	T46.6X1-	T46.6X2-	T46.6X3-	T46.6X4-	T46.6X5-	T46.6X6-
Oleovitamin A	T45.2X1-	T45.2X2-	T45.2X3-	T45.2X4-	T45.2X5-	T45.2X6-
Oleum ricini	T47.2X1-	T47.2X2-	T47.2X3-	T47.2X4-	T47.2X5-	T47.2X6-
Olive oil (medicinal) **NEC**	T47.4X1-	T47.4X2-	T47.4X3-	T47.4X4-	T47.4X5-	T47.4X6-
Olivomycin	T45.1X1-	T45.1X2-	T45.1X3-	T45.1X4-	T45.1X5-	T45.1X6-
Olsalazine	T47.8X1-	T47.8X2-	T47.8X3-	T47.8X4-	T47.8X5-	T47.8X6-
Omeprazole	T47.1X1-	T47.1X2-	T47.1X3-	T47.1X4-	T47.1X5-	T47.1X6-
OMPA	T60.0X1-	T60.0X2-	T60.0X3-	T60.0X4-	-	-
Oncovin	T45.1X1-	T45.1X2-	T45.1X3-	T45.1X4-	T45.1X5-	T45.1X6-
Ondansetron	T45.0X1-	T45.0X2-	T45.0X3-	T45.0X4-	T45.0X5-	T45.0X6-
Ophthaine	T41.3X1-	T41.3X2-	T41.3X3-	T41.3X4-	T41.3X5-	T41.3X6-
Ophthetic	T41.3X1-	T41.3X2-	T41.3X3-	T41.3X4-	T41.3X5-	T41.3X6-
Opiate NEC	T40.601-	T40.602-	T40.603-	T40.604-	T40.605-	T40.606-
antagonists	T50.7X1-	T50.7X2-	T50.7X3-	T50.7X4-	T50.7X5-	T50.7X6-
Opioid NEC	T40.2X1-	T40.2X2-	T40.2X3-	T40.2X4-	T40.2X5-	T40.2X6-
Opipramol	T43.011-	T43.012-	T43.013-	T43.014-	T43.015-	T43.016-
Opium alkaloids (total)	T40.0X1-	T40.0X2-	T40.0X3-	T40.0X4-	T40.0X5-	T40.0X6-
standardized powdered	T40.0X1-	T40.0X2-	T40.0X3-	T40.0X4-	T40.0X5-	T40.0X6-
tincture (camphorated)	T40.0X1-	T40.0X2-	T40.0X3-	T40.0X4-	T40.0X5-	T40.0X6-
Oracon	T38.4X1-	T38.4X2-	T38.4X3-	T38.4X4-	T38.4X5-	T38.4X6-

Substance	Poisoning Accidental (unintentional)	Poisoning Intentional self-harm	Poisoning Assault	Poisoning Undetermined	Adverse effect	Underdosing
Oragrafin	T50.8X1-	T50.8X2-	T50.8X3-	T50.8X4-	T50.8X5-	T50.8X6-
Oral contraceptives	T38.4X1-	T38.4X2-	T38.4X3-	T38.4X4-	T38.4X5-	T38.4X6-
Oral rehydration salts	T50.3X1-	T50.3X2-	T50.3X3-	T50.3X4-	T50.3X5-	T50.3X6-
Orazamide	T50.991-	T50.992-	T50.993-	T50.994-	T50.995-	T50.996-
Orciprenaline	T48.291-	T48.292-	T48.293-	T48.294-	T48.295-	T48.296-
Organidin	T48.4X1-	T48.4X2-	T48.4X3-	T48.4X4-	T48.4X5-	T48.4X6-
Organonitrate NEC	T46.3X1-	T46.3X2-	T46.3X3-	T46.3X4-	T46.3X5-	T46.3X6-
Organophosphates	T60.0X1-	T60.0X2-	T60.0X3-	T60.0X4-	-	-
Orimune	T50.B91-	T50.B92-	T50.B93-	T50.B94-	T50.B95-	T50.B96-
Orinase	T38.3X1-	T38.3X2-	T38.3X3-	T38.3X4-	T38.3X5-	T38.3X6-
Ormeloxifene	T38.6X1-	T38.6X2-	T38.6X3-	T38.6X4-	T38.6X5-	T38.6X6-
Ornidazole	T37.3X1-	T37.3X2-	T37.3X3-	T37.3X4-	T37.3X5-	T37.3X6-
Ornithine aspartate	T50.991-	T50.992-	T50.993-	T50.994-	T50.995-	T50.996-
Ornoprostil	T47.1X1-	T47.1X2-	T47.1X3-	T47.1X4-	T47.1X5-	T47.1X6-
Orphenadrine (hydrochloride)	T42.8X1-	T42.8X2-	T42.8X3-	T42.8X4-	T42.8X5-	T42.8X6-
Ortal (sodium)	T42.3X1-	T42.3X2-	T42.3X3-	T42.3X4-	T42.3X5-	T42.3X6-
Orthoboric acid	T49.0X1-	T49.0X2-	T49.0X3-	T49.0X4-	T49.0X5-	T49.0X6-
ENT agent	T49.6X1-	T49.6X2-	T49.6X3-	T49.6X4-	T49.6X5-	T49.6X6-
ophthalmic preparation	T49.5X1-	T49.5X2-	T49.5X3-	T49.5X4-	T49.5X5-	T49.5X6-
Orthocaine	T41.3X1-	T41.3X2-	T41.3X3-	T41.3X4-	T41.3X5-	T41.3X6-
Orthodichlorobenzene	T53.7X1-	T53.7X2-	T53.7X3-	T53.7X4-	-	-
Ortho-Novum	T38.4X1-	T38.4X2-	T38.4X3-	T38.4X4-	T38.4X5-	T38.4X6-
Orthotolidine (reagent)	T54.2X1-	T54.2X2-	T54.2X3-	T54.2X4-	-	-
Osmic acid (liquid)	T54.2X1-	T54.2X2-	T54.2X3-	T54.2X4-	-	-
fumes	T54.2X1-	T54.2X2-	T54.2X3-	T54.2X4-	-	-
Osmotic diuretics	T50.2X1-	T50.2X2-	T50.2X3-	T50.2X4-	T50.2X5-	T50.2X6-
Otilonium bromide	T44.3X1-	T44.3X2-	T44.3X3-	T44.3X4-	T44.3X5-	T44.3X6-
Otorhinolaryngological drug NEC	T49.6X1-	T49.6X2-	T49.6X3-	T49.6X4-	T49.6X5-	T49.6X6-
Ouabain (e)	T46.0X1-	T46.0X2-	T46.0X3-	T46.0X4-	T46.0X5-	T46.0X6-
Ovarian						
hormone	T38.5X1-	T38.5X2-	T38.5X3-	T38.5X4-	T38.5X5-	T38.5X6-
stimulant	T38.5X1-	T38.5X2-	T38.5X3-	T38.5X4-	T38.5X5-	T38.5X6-
Ovral	T38.4X1-	T38.4X2-	T38.4X3-	T38.4X4-	T38.4X5-	T38.4X6-
Ovulen	T38.4X1-	T38.4X2-	T38.4X3-	T38.4X4-	T38.4X5-	T38.4X6-
Oxacillin	T36.0X1-	T36.0X2-	T36.0X3-	T36.0X4-	T36.0X5-	T36.0X6-
Oxalic acid	T54.2X1-	T54.2X2-	T54.2X3-	T54.2X4-	-	-
ammonium salt	T50.991-	T50.992-	T50.993-	T50.994-	T50.995-	T50.996-
Oxamniquine	T37.4X1-	T37.4X2-	T37.4X3-	T37.4X4-	T37.4X5-	T37.4X6-
Oxanamide	T43.591-	T43.592-	T43.593-	T43.594-	T43.595-	T43.596-
Oxandrolone	T38.7X1-	T38.7X2-	T38.7X3-	T38.7X4-	T38.7X5-	T38.7X6-
Oxantel	T37.4X1-	T37.4X2-	T37.4X3-	T37.4X4-	T37.4X5-	T37.4X6-
Oxapium iodide	T44.3X1-	T44.3X2-	T44.3X3-	T44.3X4-	T44.3X5-	T44.3X6-
Oxaprotiline	T43.021-	T43.022-	T43.023-	T43.024-	T43.025-	T43.026-
Oxaprozin	T39.311-	T39.312-	T39.313-	T39.314-	T39.315-	T39.316-
Oxatomide	T45.0X1-	T45.0X2-	T45.0X3-	T45.0X4-	T45.0X5-	T45.0X6-
Oxazepam	T42.4X1-	T42.4X2-	T42.4X3-	T42.4X4-	T42.4X5-	T42.4X6-
Oxazimedrine	T50.5X1-	T50.5X2-	T50.5X3-	T50.5X4-	T50.5X5-	T50.5X6-
Oxazolam	T42.4X1-	T42.4X2-	T42.4X3-	T42.4X4-	T42.4X5-	T42.4X6-
Oxazolidine derivatives	T42.2X1-	T42.2X2-	T42.2X3-	T42.2X4-	T42.2X5-	T42.2X6-
Oxazolidinedione (derivative)	T42.2X1-	T42.2X2-	T42.2X3-	T42.2X4-	T42.2X5-	T42.2X6-
Ox bile extract	T47.5X1-	T47.5X2-	T47.5X3-	T47.5X4-	T47.5X5-	T47.5X6-
Oxcarbazepine	T42.1X1-	T42.1X2-	T42.1X3-	T42.1X4-	T42.1X5-	T42.1X6-
Oxedrine	T44.4X1-	T44.4X2-	T44.4X3-	T44.4X4-	T44.4X5-	T44.4X6-
Oxeladin (citrate)	T48.3X1-	T48.3X2-	T48.3X3-	T48.3X4-	T48.3X5-	T48.3X6-
Oxendolone	T38.5X1-	T38.5X2-	T38.5X3-	T38.5X4-	T38.5X5-	T38.5X6-
Oxetacaine	T41.3X1-	T41.3X2-	T41.3X3-	T41.3X4-	T41.3X5-	T41.3X6-
Oxethazine	T41.3X1-	T41.3X2-	T41.3X3-	T41.3X4-	T41.3X5-	T41.3X6-
Oxetorone	T39.8X1-	T39.8X2-	T39.8X3-	T39.8X4-	T39.8X5-	T39.8X6-
Oxiconazole	T49.0X1-	T49.0X2-	T49.0X3-	T49.0X4-	T49.0X5-	T49.0X6-
Oxidizing agent NEC	T54.91X-	T54.92X-	T54.93X-	T54.94X-	-	-
Oxipurinol	T50.4X1-	T50.4X2-	T50.4X3-	T50.4X4-	T50.4X5-	T50.4X6-
Oxitriptan	T43.291-	T43.292-	T43.293-	T43.294-	T43.295-	T43.296-
Oxitropium bromide	T48.6X1-	T48.6X2-	T48.6X3-	T48.6X4-	T48.6X5-	T48.6X6-
Oxodipine	T46.1X1-	T46.1X2-	T46.1X3-	T46.1X4-	T46.1X5-	T46.1X6-
Oxolamine	T48.3X1-	T48.3X2-	T48.3X3-	T48.3X4-	T48.3X5-	T48.3X6-
Oxolinic acid	T37.8X1-	T37.8X2-	T37.8X3-	T37.8X4-	T37.8X5-	T37.8X6-
Oxomemazine	T43.3X1-	T43.3X2-	T43.3X3-	T43.3X4-	T43.3X5-	T43.3X6-
Oxophenarsine	T37.3X1-	T37.3X2-	T37.3X3-	T37.3X4-	T37.3X5-	T37.3X6-
Oxprenolol	T44.7X1-	T44.7X2-	T44.7X3-	T44.7X4-	T44.7X5-	T44.7X6-
Oxsoralen	T49.3X1-	T49.3X2-	T49.3X3-	T49.3X4-	T49.3X5-	T49.3X6-
Oxtriphylline	T48.6X1-	T48.6X2-	T48.6X3-	T48.6X4-	T48.6X5-	T48.6X6-
Oxybate sodium	T41.291-	T41.292-	T41.293-	T41.294-	T41.295-	T41.296-
Oxybuprocaine	T41.3X1-	T41.3X2-	T41.3X3-	T41.3X4-	T41.3X5-	T41.3X6-
Oxybutynin	T44.3X1-	T44.3X2-	T44.3X3-	T44.3X4-	T44.3X5-	T44.3X6-
Oxychlorosene	T49.0X1-	T49.0X2-	T49.0X3-	T49.0X4-	T49.0X5-	T49.0X6-
Oxycodone	T40.2X1-	T40.2X2-	T40.2X3-	T40.2X4-	T40.2X5-	T40.2X6-
Oxyfedrine	T46.3X1-	T46.3X2-	T46.3X3-	T46.3X4-	T46.3X5-	T46.3X6-

Substance	Poisoning Accidental (unintentional)	Poisoning Intentional self-harm	Poisoning Assault	Poisoning Undetermined	Adverse effect	Underdosing
Oxygen	T41.5X1-	T41.5X2-	T41.5X3-	T41.5X4-	T41.5X5-	T41.5X6-
Oxylone	T49.0X1-	T49.0X2-	T49.0X3-	T49.0X4-	T49.0X5-	T49.0X6-
ophthalmic preparation	T49.5X1-	T49.5X2-	T49.5X3-	T49.5X4-	T49.5X5-	T49.5X6-
Oxymesterone	T38.7X1-	T38.7X2-	T38.7X3-	T38.7X4-	T38.7X5-	T38.7X6-
Oxymetazoline	T48.5X1-	T48.5X2-	T48.5X3-	T48.5X4-	T48.5X5-	T48.5X6-
Oxymetholone	T38.7X1-	T38.7X2-	T38.7X3-	T38.7X4-	T38.7X5-	T38.7X6-
Oxymorphone	T40.2X1-	T40.2X2-	T40.2X3-	T40.2X4-	T40.2X5-	T40.2X6-
Oxypertine	T43.591-	T43.592-	T43.593-	T43.594-	T43.595-	T43.596-
Oxyphenbutazone	T39.2X1-	T39.2X2-	T39.2X3-	T39.2X4-	T39.2X5-	T39.2X6-
Oxyphencyclimine	T44.3X1-	T44.3X2-	T44.3X3-	T44.3X4-	T44.3X5-	T44.3X6-
Oxyphenisatine	T47.2X1-	T47.2X2-	T47.2X3-	T47.2X4-	T47.2X5-	T47.2X6-
Oxyphenonium bromide	T44.3X1-	T44.3X2-	T44.3X3-	T44.3X4-	T44.3X5-	T44.3X6-
Oxypolygelatin	T45.8X1-	T45.8X2-	T45.8X3-	T45.8X4-	T45.8X5-	T45.8X6-
Oxyquinoline (derivatives)	T37.8X1-	T37.8X2-	T37.8X3-	T37.8X4-	T37.8X5-	T37.8X6-
Oxytetracycline	T36.4X1-	T36.4X2-	T36.4X3-	T36.4X4-	T36.4X5-	T36.4X6-
Oxytocic drug NEC	T48.0X1-	T48.0X2-	T48.0X3-	T48.0X4-	T48.0X5-	T48.0X6-
Oxytocin (synthetic)	T48.0X1-	T48.0X2-	T48.0X3-	T48.0X4-	T48.0X5-	T48.0X6-
Ozone	T59.891-	T59.892-	T59.893-	T59.894-	-	-
PABA	T49.3X1-	T49.3X2-	T49.3X3-	T49.3X4-	T49.3X5-	T49.3X6-
Packed red cells	T45.8X1-	T45.8X2-	T45.8X3-	T45.8X4-	T45.8X5-	T45.8X6-
Padimate	T49.3X1-	T49.3X2-	T49.3X3-	T49.3X4-	T49.3X5-	T49.3X6-
Paint NEC	T65.6X1-	T65.6X2-	T65.6X3-	T65.6X4-	-	-
cleaner	T52.91X-	T52.92X-	T52.93X-	T52.94X-	-	-
fumes NEC	T59.891-	T59.892-	T59.893-	T59.894-	-	-
lead (fumes)	T56.0X1-	T56.0X2-	T56.0X3-	T56.0X4-	-	-
solvent NEC	T52.8X1-	T52.8X2-	T52.8X3-	T52.8X4-	-	-
stripper	T52.8X1-	T52.8X2-	T52.8X3-	T52.8X4-	-	-
Palfium	T40.2X1-	T40.2X2-	T40.2X3-	T40.2X4-	-	-
Palm kernel oil	T50.991-	T50.992-	T50.993-	T50.994-	T50.995-	T50.996-
Paludrine	T37.2X1-	T37.2X2-	T37.2X3-	T37.2X4-	T37.2X5-	T37.2X6-
PAM (pralidoxime)	T50.6X1-	T50.6X2-	T50.6X3-	T50.6X4-	T50.6X5-	T50.6X6-
Pamaquine (naphthoute)	T37.2X1-	T37.2X2-	T37.2X3-	T37.2X4-	T37.2X5-	T37.2X6-
Panadol	T39.1X1-	T39.1X2-	T39.1X3-	T39.1X4-	T39.1X5-	T39.1X6-
Pancreatic						
digestive secretion stimulant	T47.8X1-	T47.8X2-	T47.8X3-	T47.8X4-	T47.8X5-	T47.8X6-
dornase	T45.3X1-	T45.3X2-	T45.3X3-	T45.3X4-	T45.3X5-	T45.3X6-
Pancreatin	T47.5X1-	T47.5X2-	T47.5X3-	T47.5X4-	T47.5X5-	T47.5X6-
Pancrelipase	T47.5X1-	T47.5X2-	T47.5X3-	T47.5X4-	T47.5X5-	T47.5X6-
Pancuronium (bromide)	T48.1X1-	T48.1X2-	T48.1X3-	T48.1X4-	T48.1X5-	T48.1X6-
Pangamic acid	T45.2X1-	T45.2X2-	T45.2X3-	T45.2X4-	T45.2X5-	T45.2X6-
Panthenol	T45.2X1-	T45.2X2-	T45.2X3-	T45.2X4-	T45.2X5-	T45.2X6-
topical	T49.8X1-	T49.8X2-	T49.8X3-	T49.8X4-	T49.8X5-	T49.8X6-
Pantopon	T40.0X1-	T40.0X2-	T40.0X3-	T40.0X4-	T40.0X5-	T40.0X6-
Pantothenic acid	T45.2X1-	T45.2X2-	T45.2X3-	T45.2X4-	T45.2X5-	T45.2X6-
Panwarfin	T45.511-	T45.512-	T45.513-	T45.514-	T45.515-	T45.516-
Papain	T47.5X1-	T47.5X2-	T47.5X3-	T47.5X4-	T47.5X5-	T47.5X6-
digestant	T47.5X1-	T47.5X2-	T47.5X3-	T47.5X4-	T47.5X5-	T47.5X6-
Papaveretum	T40.0X1-	T40.0X2-	T40.0X3-	T40.0X4-	T40.0X5-	T40.0X6-
Papaverine	T44.3X1-	T44.3X2-	T44.3X3-	T44.3X4-	T44.3X5-	T44.3X6-
Para-acetamidophenol	T39.1X1-	T39.1X2-	T39.1X3-	T39.1X4-	T39.1X5-	T39.1X6-
Para-aminobenzoic acid	T49.3X1-	T49.3X2-	T49.3X3-	T49.3X4-	T49.3X5-	T49.3X6-
Para-aminophenol derivatives	T39.1X1-	T39.1X2-	T39.1X3-	T39.1X4-	T39.1X5-	T39.1X6-
Para-aminosalicylic acid	T37.1X1-	T37.1X2-	T37.1X3-	T37.1X4-	T37.1X5-	T37.1X6-
Paracetaldehyde	T42.6X1-	T42.6X2-	T42.6X3-	T42.6X4-	T42.6X5-	T42.6X6-
Paracetamol	T39.1X1-	T39.1X2-	T39.1X3-	T39.1X4-	T39.1X5-	T39.1X6-
Parachlorophenol (camphorated)	T49.0X1-	T49.0X2-	T49.0X3-	T49.0X4-	T49.0X5-	T49.0X6-
Paracodin	T40.2X1-	T40.2X2-	T40.2X3-	T40.2X4-	T40.2X5-	T40.2X6-
Paradione	T42.2X1-	T42.2X2-	T42.2X3-	T42.2X4-	T42.2X5-	T42.2X6-
Paraffin (s) (wax)	T52.0X1-	T52.0X2-	T52.0X3-	T52.0X4-	-	-
liquid (medicinal)	T47.4X1-	T47.4X2-	T47.4X3-	T47.4X4-	T47.4X5-	T47.4X6-
nonmedicinal	T52.0X1-	T52.0X2-	T52.0X3-	T52.0X4-	-	-
Paraformaldehyde	T60.3X1-	T60.3X2-	T60.3X3-	T60.3X4-	-	-
Paraldehyde	T42.6X1-	T42.6X2-	T42.6X3-	T42.6X4-	T42.6X5-	T42.6X6-
Paramethadione	T42.2X1-	T42.2X2-	T42.2X3-	T42.2X4-	T42.2X5-	T42.2X6-
Paramethasone	T38.0X1-	T38.0X2-	T38.0X3-	T38.0X4-	T38.0X5-	T38.0X6-
acetate	T49.0X1-	T49.0X2-	T49.0X3-	T49.0X4-	T49.0X5-	T49.0X6-
Paraoxon	T60.0X1-	T60.0X2-	T60.0X3-	T60.0X4-	-	-
Paraquat	T60.3X1-	T60.3X2-	T60.3X3-	T60.3X4-	-	-
Parasympatholytic NEC	T44.3X1-	T44.3X2-	T44.3X3-	T44.3X4-	T44.3X5-	T44.3X6-
Parasympathomimetic drug NEC	T44.1X1-	T44.1X2-	T44.1X3-	T44.1X4-	T44.1X5-	T44.1X6-
Parathion	T60.0X1-	T60.0X2-	T60.0X3-	T60.0X4-	-	-
Parathormone	T50.991-	T50.992-	T50.993-	T50.994-	T50.995-	T50.996-
Parathyroid extract	T50.991-	T50.992-	T50.993-	T50.994-	T50.995-	T50.996-
Paratyphoid vaccine	T50.A91-	T50.A92-	T50.A93-	T50.A94-	T50.A95-	T50.A96-
Paredrine	T44.4X1-	T44.4X2-	T44.4X3-	T44.4X4-	T44.4X5-	T44.4X6-
Paregoric	T40.0X1-	T40.0X2-	T40.0X3-	T40.0X4-	T40.0X5-	T40.0X6-

Substance	Poisoning Accidental (unintentional)	Poisoning Intentional self-harm	Poisoning Assault	Poisoning Undetermined	Adverse effect	Underdosing
Pargyline	T46.5X1-	T46.5X2-	T46.5X3-	T46.5X4-	T46.5X5-	T46.5X6-
Paris green	T57.0X1-	T57.0X2-	T57.0X3-	T57.0X4-	-	-
insecticide	T57.0X1-	T57.0X2-	T57.0X3-	T57.0X4-	-	-
Parnate	T43.1X1-	T43.1X2-	T43.1X3-	T43.1X4-	T43.1X5-	T43.1X6-
Paromomycin	T36.5X1-	T36.5X2-	T36.5X3-	T36.5X4-	T36.5X5-	T36.5X6-
Paroxypropione	T45.1X1-	T45.1X2-	T45.1X3-	T45.1X4-	T45.1X5-	T45.1X6-
Parzone	T40.2X1-	T40.2X2-	T40.2X3-	T40.2X4-	T40.2X5-	T40.2X6-
PAS	T37.1X1-	T37.1X2-	T37.1X3-	T37.1X4-	T37.1X5-	T37.1X6-
Pasiniazid	T37.1X1-	T37.1X2-	T37.1X3-	T37.1X4-	T37.1X5-	T37.1X6-
PBB (polybrominated biphenyls)	T65.891-	T65.892-	T65.893-	T65.894-	-	-
PCB	T65.891-	T65.892-	T65.893-	T65.894-	-	-
PCP						
meaning pentachlorophenol	T60.1X1-	T60.1X2-	T60.1X3-	T60.1X4-	-	-
fungicide	T60.3X1-	T60.3X2-	T60.3X3-	T60.3X4-	-	-
herbicide	T60.3X1-	T60.3X2-	T60.3X3-	T60.3X4-	-	-
insecticide	T60.1X1-	T60.1X2-	T60.1X3-	T60.1X4-	-	-
meaning phencyclidine	T40.991-	T40.992-	T40.993-	T40.994-	-	-
Peach kernel oil (emulsion)	T47.4X1-	T47.4X2-	T47.4X3-	T47.4X4-	T47.4X5-	T47.4X6-
Peanut oil (emulsion) **NEC**	T47.4X1-	T47.4X2-	T47.4X3-	T47.4X4-	T47.4X5-	T47.4X6-
topical	T49.3X1-	T49.3X2-	T49.3X3-	T49.3X4-	T49.3X5-	T49.3X6-
Pearly Gates (morning glory seeds)	T40.991-	T40.992-	T40.993-	T40.994-	-	-
Pecazine	T43.3X1-	T43.3X2-	T43.3X3-	T43.3X4-	T43.3X5-	T43.3X6-
Pectin	T47.6X1-	T47.6X2-	T47.6X3-	T47.6X4-	T47.6X5-	T47.6X6-
Pefloxacin	T37.8X1-	T37.8X2-	T37.8X3-	T37.8X4-	T37.8X5-	T37.8X6-
Pegademase, bovine	T50.Z91-	T50.Z92-	T50.Z93-	T50.Z94-	T50.Z95-	T50.Z96-
Pelletierine tannate	T37.4X1-	T37.4X2-	T37.4X3-	T37.4X4-	T37.4X5-	T37.4X6-
Pemirolast (potassium)	T48.6X1-	T48.6X2-	T48.6X3-	T48.6X4-	T48.6X5-	T48.6X6-
Pemoline	T50.7X1-	T50.7X2-	T50.7X3-	T50.7X4-	T50.7X5-	T50.7X6-
Pempidine	T44.2X1-	T44.2X2-	T44.2X3-	T44.2X4-	T44.2X5-	T44.2X6-
Penamecillin	T36.0X1-	T36.0X2-	T36.0X3-	T36.0X4-	T36.0X5-	T36.0X6-
Penbutolol	T44.7X1-	T44.7X2-	T44.7X3-	T44.7X4-	T44.7X5-	T44.7X6-
Penethamate	T36.0X1-	T36.0X2-	T36.0X3-	T36.0X4-	T36.0X5-	T36.0X6-
Penfluridol	T43.591-	T43.592-	T43.593-	T43.594-	T43.595-	T43.596-
Penflutizide	T50.2X1-	T50.2X2-	T50.2X3-	T50.2X4-	T50.2X5-	T50.2X6-
Pengitoxin	T46.0X1-	T46.0X2-	T46.0X3-	T46.0X4-	T46.0X5-	T46.0X6-
Penicillamine	T50.6X1-	T50.6X2-	T50.6X3-	T50.6X4-	T50.6X5-	T50.6X6-
Penicillin (any)	T36.0X1-	T36.0X2-	T36.0X3-	T36.0X4-	T36.0X5-	T36.0X6-
Penicillinase	T45.3X1-	T45.3X2-	T45.3X3-	T45.3X4-	T45.3X5-	T45.3X6-
Penicilloyl polylysine	T50.8X1-	T50.8X2-	T50.8X3-	T50.8X4-	T50.8X5-	T50.8X6-
Penimepicycline	T36.4X1-	T36.4X2-	T36.4X3-	T36.4X4-	T36.4X5-	T36.4X6-
Pentachloroethane	T53.6X1-	T53.6X2-	T53.6X3-	T53.6X4-	-	-
Pentachloronaphthalene	T53.7X1-	T53.7X2-	T53.7X3-	T53.7X4-	-	-
Pentachlorophenol (pesticide)	T60.1X1-	T60.1X2-	T60.1X3-	T60.1X4-	-	-
fungicide	T60.3X1-	T60.3X2-	T60.3X3-	T60.3X4-	-	-
herbicide	T60.3X1-	T60.3X2-	T60.3X3-	T60.3X4-	-	-
insecticide	T60.1X1-	T60.1X2-	T60.1X3-	T60.1X4-	-	-
Pentaerythritol	T46.3X1-	T46.3X2-	T46.3X3-	T46.3X4-	T46.3X5-	T46.3X6-
chloral	T42.6X1-	T42.6X2-	T42.6X3-	T42.6X4-	T42.6X5-	T42.6X6-
tetranitrate NEC	T46.3X1-	T46.3X2-	T46.3X3-	T46.3X4-	T46.3X5-	T46.3X6-
Pentaerythrityl tetranitrate	T46.3X1-	T46.3X2-	T46.3X3-	T46.3X4-	T46.3X5-	T46.3X6-
Pentagastrin	T50.8X1-	T50.8X2-	T50.8X3-	T50.8X4-	T50.8X5-	T50.8X6-
Pentalin	T53.6X1-	T53.6X2-	T53.6X3-	T53.6X4-	-	-
Pentamethonium bromide	T44.2X1-	T44.2X2-	T44.2X3-	T44.2X4-	T44.2X5-	T44.2X6-
Pentamidine	T37.3X1-	T37.3X2-	T37.3X3-	T37.3X4-	T37.3X5-	T37.3X6-
Pentanol	T51.3X1-	T51.3X2-	T51.3X3-	T51.3X4-	-	-
Pentapyrrolinium (bitartrate)	T44.2X1-	T44.2X2-	T44.2X3-	T44.2X4-	T44.2X5-	T44.2X6-
Pentaquine	T37.2X1-	T37.2X2-	T37.2X3-	T37.2X4-	T37.2X5-	T37.2X6-
Pentazocine	T40.4X1-	T40.4X2-	T40.4X3-	T40.4X4-	T40.4X5-	T40.4X6-
Pentetrazole	T50.7X1-	T50.7X2-	T50.7X3-	T50.7X4-	T50.7X5-	T50.7X6-
Penthienate bromide	T44.3X1-	T44.3X2-	T44.3X3-	T44.3X4-	T44.3X5-	T44.3X6-
Pentifylline	T46.7X1-	T46.7X2-	T46.7X3-	T46.7X4-	T46.7X5-	T46.7X6-
Pentobarbital	T42.3X1-	T42.3X2-	T42.3X3-	T42.3X4-	T42.3X5-	T42.3X6-
sodium	T42.3X1-	T42.3X2-	T42.3X3-	T42.3X4-	T42.3X5-	T42.3X6-
Pentobarbitone	T42.3X1-	T42.3X2-	T42.3X3-	T42.3X4-	T42.3X5-	T42.3X6-
Pentolonium tartrate	T44.2X1-	T44.2X2-	T44.2X3-	T44.2X4-	T44.2X5-	T44.2X6-
Pentosan polysulfate (sodium)	T39.8X1-	T39.8X2-	T39.8X3-	T39.8X4-	T39.8X5-	T39.8X6-
Pentostatin	T45.1X1-	T45.1X2-	T45.1X3-	T45.1X4-	T45.1X5-	T45.1X6-
Pentothal	T41.1X1-	T41.1X2-	T41.1X3-	T41.1X4-	T41.1X5-	T41.1X6-
Pentoxifylline	T46.7X1-	T46.7X2-	T46.7X3-	T46.7X4-	T46.7X5-	T46.7X6-
Pentoxyverine	T48.3X1-	T48.3X2-	T48.3X3-	T48.3X4-	T48.3X5-	T48.3X6-
Pentrinat	T46.3X1-	T46.3X2-	T46.3X3-	T46.3X4-	T46.3X5-	T46.3X6-
Pentylenetetrazole	T50.7X1-	T50.7X2-	T50.7X3-	T50.7X4-	T50.7X5-	T50.7X6-
Pentylsalicylamide	T37.1X1-	T37.1X2-	T37.1X3-	T37.1X4-	T37.1X5-	T37.1X6-
Pentymal	T42.3X1-	T42.3X2-	T42.3X3-	T42.3X4-	T42.3X5-	T42.3X6-
Peplomycin	T45.1X1-	T45.1X2-	T45.1X3-	T45.1X4-	T45.1X5-	T45.1X6-
Peppermint (oil)	T47.5X1-	T47.5X2-	T47.5X3-	T47.5X4-	T47.5X5-	T47.5X6-

Substance	Poisoning Accidental (unintentional)	Poisoning Intentional self-harm	Poisoning Assault	Poisoning Undetermined	Adverse effect	Underdosing
Pepsin	T47.5X1-	T47.5X2-	T47.5X3-	T47.5X4-	T47.5X5-	T47.5X6-
digestant	T47.5X1-	T47.5X2-	T47.5X3-	T47.5X4-	T47.5X5-	T47.5X6-
Pepstatin	T47.1X1-	T47.1X2-	T47.1X3-	T47.1X4-	T47.1X5-	T47.1X6-
Peptavlon	T50.8X1-	T50.8X2-	T50.8X3-	T50.8X4-	T50.8X5-	T50.8X6-
Perazine	T43.3X1-	T43.3X2-	T43.3X3-	T43.3X4-	T43.3X5-	T43.3X6-
Percaine (spinal)	T41.3X1-	T41.3X2-	T41.3X3-	T41.3X4-	T41.3X5-	T41.3X6-
topical (surface)	T41.3X1-	T41.3X2-	T41.3X3-	T41.3X4-	T41.3X5-	T41.3X6-
Perchloroethylene	T53.3X1-	T53.3X2-	T53.3X3-	T53.3X4-	-	-
medicinal	T37.4X1-	T37.4X2-	T37.4X3-	T37.4X4-	T37.4X5-	T37.4X6-
vapor	T53.3X1-	T53.3X2-	T53.3X3-	T53.3X4-	-	-
Percodan	T40.2X1-	T40.2X2-	T40.2X3-	T40.2X4-	T40.2X5-	T40.2X6-
Percogesic — *see also* acetaminophen	T45.0X1-	T45.0X2-	T45.0X3-	T45.0X4-	T45.0X5-	T45.0X6-
Percorten	T38.0X1-	T38.0X2-	T38.0X3-	T38.0X4-	T38.0X5-	T38.0X6-
Pergolide	T42.8X1-	T42.8X2-	T42.8X3-	T42.8X4-	T42.8X5-	T42.8X6-
Pergonal	T38.811-	T38.812-	T38.813-	T38.814-	T38.815-	T38.816-
Perhexilene	T46.3X1-	T46.3X2-	T46.3X3-	T46.3X4-	T46.3X5-	T46.3X6-
Perhexiline (maleate)	T46.3X1-	T46.3X2-	T46.3X3-	T46.3X4-	T46.3X5-	T46.3X6-
Periactin	T45.0X1-	T45.0X2-	T45.0X3-	T45.0X4-	T45.0X5-	T45.0X6-
Periciazine	T43.3X1-	T43.3X2-	T43.3X3-	T43.3X4-	T43.3X5-	T43.3X6-
Periclor	T42.6X1-	T42.6X2-	T42.6X3-	T42.6X4-	T42.6X5-	T42.6X6-
Perindopril	T46.4X1-	T46.4X2-	T46.4X3-	T46.4X4-	T46.4X5-	T46.4X6-
Perisoxal	T39.8X1-	T39.8X2-	T39.8X3-	T39.8X4-	T39.8X5-	T39.8X6-
Peritoneal dialysis solution	T50.3X1-	T50.3X2-	T50.3X3-	T50.3X4-	T50.3X5-	T50.3X6-
Peritrate	T46.3X1-	T46.3X2-	T46.3X3-	T46.3X4-	T46.3X5-	T46.3X6-
Perlapine	T42.4X1-	T42.4X2-	T42.4X3-	T42.4X4-	T42.4X5-	T42.4X6-
Permanganate	T65.891-	T65.892-	T65.893-	T65.894-	-	-
Permethrin	T60.1X1-	T60.1X2-	T60.1X3-	T60.1X4-	-	-
Pernocton	T42.3X1-	T42.3X2-	T42.3X3-	T42.3X4-	T42.3X5-	T42.3X6-
Pernoston	T42.3X1-	T42.3X2-	T42.3X3-	T42.3X4-	T42.3X5-	T42.3X6-
Peronine	T40.2X1-	T40.2X2-	T40.2X3-	T40.2X4-	-	-
Perphenazine	T43.3X1-	T43.3X2-	T43.3X3-	T43.3X4-	T43.3X5-	T43.3X6-
Pertofrane	T43.011-	T43.012-	T43.013-	T43.014-	T43.015-	T43.016-
Pertussis						
immune serum (human)	T50.Z11-	T50.Z12-	T50.Z13-	T50.Z14-	T50.Z15-	T50.Z16-
vaccine (with diphtheria toxoid) (with tetanus toxoid)	T50.A11-	T50.A12-	T50.A13-	T50.A14-	T50.A15-	T50.A16-
Peruvian balsam	T49.0X1-	T49.0X2-	T49.0X3-	T49.0X4-	T49.0X5-	T49.0X6-
Peruvoside	T46.0X1-	T46.0X2-	T46.0X3-	T46.0X4-	T46.0X5-	T46.0X6-
Pesticide (dust) (fumes) (vapor) **NEC**	T60.91X-	T60.92X-	T60.93X-	T60.94X-	-	-
arsenic	T57.0X1-	T57.0X2-	T57.0X3-	T57.0X4-	-	-
chlorinated	T60.1X1-	T60.1X2-	T60.1X3-	T60.1X4-	-	-
cyanide	T65.0X1-	T65.0X2-	T65.0X3-	T65.0X4-	-	-
kerosene	T52.0X1-	T52.0X2-	T52.0X3-	T52.0X4-	-	-
mixture (of compounds)	T60.91X-	T60.92X-	T60.93X-	T60.94X-	-	-
naphthalene	T60.2X1-	T60.2X2-	T60.2X3-	T60.2X4-	-	-
organochlorine (compounds)	T60.1X1-	T60.1X2-	T60.1X3-	T60.1X4-	-	-
petroleum (distillate) (products) NEC	T60.8X1-	T60.8X2-	T60.8X3-	T60.8X4-	-	-
specified ingredient NEC	T60.8X1-	T60.8X2-	T60.8X3-	T60.8X4-	-	-
strychnine	T65.1X1-	T65.1X2-	T65.1X3-	T65.1X4-	-	-
thallium	T60.4X1-	T60.4X2-	T60.4X3-	T60.4X4-	-	-
Pethidine	T40.4X1-	T40.4X2-	T40.4X3-	T40.4X4-	T40.4X5-	T40.4X6-
Petrichloral	T42.6X1-	T42.6X2-	T42.6X3-	T42.6X4-	T42.6X5-	T42.6X6-
Petrol	T52.0X1-	T52.0X2-	T52.0X3-	T52.0X4-	-	-
vapor	T52.0X1-	T52.0X2-	T52.0X3-	T52.0X4-	-	-
Petrolatum	T49.3X1-	T49.3X2-	T49.3X3-	T49.3X4-	T49.3X5-	T49.3X6-
hydrophilic	T49.3X1-	T49.3X2-	T49.3X3-	T49.3X4-	T49.3X5-	T49.3X6-
liquid	T47.4X1-	T47.4X2-	T47.4X3-	T47.4X4-	T47.4X5-	T47.4X6-
topical	T49.3X1-	T49.3X2-	T49.3X3-	T49.3X4-	T49.3X5-	T49.3X6-
nonmedicinal	T52.0X1-	T52.0X2-	T52.0X3-	T52.0X4-	-	-
red veterinary	T49.3X1-	T49.3X2-	T49.3X3-	T49.3X4-	T49.3X5-	T49.3X6-
white	T49.3X1-	T49.3X2-	T49.3X3-	T49.3X4-	T49.3X5-	T49.3X6-
Petroleum (products) **NEC**	T52.0X1-	T52.0X2-	T52.0X3-	T52.0X4-	-	-
benzine (s) — *see* Ligroin						
ether — *see* Ligroin						
jelly — *see* Petrolatum						
naphtha — *see* Ligroin						
pesticide	T60.8X1-	T60.8X2-	T60.8X3-	T60.8X4-	-	-
solids	T52.0X1-	T52.0X2-	T52.0X3-	T52.0X4-	-	-
solvents	T52.0X1-	T52.0X2-	T52.0X3-	T52.0X4-	-	-
vapor	T52.0X1-	T52.0X2-	T52.0X3-	T52.0X4-	-	-
Peyote	T40.991-	T40.992-	T40.993-	T40.994-	-	-
Phanodorm, phanodorn	T42.3X1-	T42.3X2-	T42.3X3-	T42.3X4-	T42.3X5-	T42.3X6-
Phanquinone	T37.3X1-	T37.3X2-	T37.3X3-	T37.3X4-	T37.3X5-	T37.3X6-
Phanquone	T37.3X1-	T37.3X2-	T37.3X3-	T37.3X4-	T37.3X5-	T37.3X6-

Substance	Poisoning Accidental (unintentional)	Poisoning Intentional self-harm	Poisoning Assault	Poisoning Undetermined	Adverse effect	Underdosing
Pharmaceutical						
adjunct NEC	T50.901-	T50.902-	T50.903-	T50.904-	T50.905-	T50.906-
excipient NEC	T50.901-	T50.902-	T50.903-	T50.904-	T50.905-	T50.906-
sweetener	T50.901-	T50.902-	T50.903-	T50.904-	T50.905-	T50.906-
viscous agent	T50.901-	T50.902-	T50.903-	T50.904-	T50.905-	T50.906-
Phemitone	T42.3X1-	T42.3X2-	T42.3X3-	T42.3X4-	T42.3X5-	T42.3X6-
Phenacaine	T41.3X1-	T41.3X2-	T41.3X3-	T41.3X4-	T41.3X5-	T41.3X6-
Phenacemide	T42.6X1-	T42.6X2-	T42.6X3-	T42.6X4-	T42.6X5-	T42.6X6-
Phenacetin	T39.1X1-	T39.1X2-	T39.1X3-	T39.1X4-	T39.1X5-	T39.1X6-
Phenadoxone	T40.2X1-	T40.2X2-	T40.2X3-	T40.2X4-	-	-
Phenaglycodol	T43.591-	T43.592-	T43.593-	T43.594-	T43.595-	T43.596-
Phenantoin	T42.0X1-	T42.0X2-	T42.0X3-	T42.0X4-	T42.0X5-	T42.0X6-
Phenaphthazine reagent	T50.991-	T50.992-	T50.993-	T50.994-	T50.995-	T50.996-
Phenazocine	T40.4X1-	T40.4X2-	T40.4X3-	T40.4X4-	T40.4X5-	T40.4X6-
Phenazone	T39.2X1-	T39.2X2-	T39.2X3-	T39.2X4-	T39.2X5-	T39.2X6-
Phenazopyridine	T39.8X1-	T39.8X2-	T39.8X3-	T39.8X4-	T39.8X5-	T39.8X6-
Phenbenicillin	T36.0X1-	T36.0X2-	T36.0X3-	T36.0X4-	T36.0X5-	T36.0X6-
Phenbutrazate	T50.5X1-	T50.5X2-	T50.5X3-	T50.5X4-	T50.5X5-	T50.5X6-
Phencyclidine	T40.991-	T40.992-	T40.993-	T40.994-	T40.995-	T40.996-
Phendimetrazine	T50.5X1-	T50.5X2-	T50.5X3-	T50.5X4-	T50.5X5-	T50.5X6-
Phenelzine	T43.1X1-	T43.1X2-	T43.1X3-	T43.1X4-	T43.1X5-	T43.1X6-
Phenemal	T42.3X1-	T42.3X2-	T42.3X3-	T42.3X4-	T42.3X5-	T42.3X6-
Phenergan	T42.6X1-	T42.6X2-	T42.6X3-	T42.6X4-	T42.6X5-	T42.6X6-
Pheneticillin	T36.0X1-	T36.0X2-	T36.0X3-	T36.0X4-	T36.0X5-	T36.0X6-
Pheneturide	T42.6X1-	T42.6X2-	T42.6X3-	T42.6X4-	T42.6X5-	T42.6X6-
Phenformin	T38.3X1-	T38.3X2-	T38.3X3-	T38.3X4-	T38.3X5-	T38.3X6-
Phenglutarimide	T44.3X1-	T44.3X2-	T44.3X3-	T44.3X4-	T44.3X5-	T44.3X6-
Phenicarbazide	T39.8X1-	T39.8X2-	T39.8X3-	T39.8X4-	T39.8X5-	T39.8X6-
Phenindamine	T45.0X1-	T45.0X2-	T45.0X3-	T45.0X4-	T45.0X5-	T45.0X6-
Phenindione	T45.511-	T45.512-	T45.513-	T45.514-	T45.515-	T45.516-
Pheniprazine	T43.1X1-	T43.1X2-	T43.1X3-	T43.1X4-	T43.1X5-	T43.1X6-
Pheniramine	T45.0X1-	T45.0X2-	T45.0X3-	T45.0X4-	T45.0X5-	T45.0X6-
Phenisatin	T47.2X1-	T47.2X2-	T47.2X3-	T47.2X4-	T47.2X5-	T47.2X6-
Phenmetrazine	T50.5X1-	T50.5X2-	T50.5X3-	T50.5X4-	T50.5X5-	T50.5X6-
Phenobal	T42.3X1-	T42.3X2-	T42.3X3-	T42.3X4-	T42.3X5-	T42.3X6-
Phenobarbital	T42.3X1-	T42.3X2-	T42.3X3-	T42.3X4-	T42.3X5-	T42.3X6-
with						
mephenytoin	T42.3X1-	T42.3X2-	T42.3X3-	T42.3X4-	T42.3X5-	T42.3X6-
phenytoin	T42.3X1-	T42.3X2-	T42.3X3-	T42.3X4-	T42.3X5-	T42.3X6-
sodium	T42.3X1-	T42.3X2-	T42.3X3-	T42.3X4-	T42.3X5-	T42.3X6-
Phenobarbitone	T42.3X1-	T42.3X2-	T42.3X3-	T42.3X4-	T42.3X5-	T42.3X6-
Phenobutiodil	T50.8X1-	T50.8X2-	T50.8X3-	T50.8X4-	T50.8X5-	T50.8X6-
Phenoctide	T49.0X1-	T49.0X2-	T49.0X3-	T49.0X4-	T49.0X5-	T49.0X6-
Phenol	T49.0X1-	T49.0X2-	T49.0X3-	T49.0X4-	T49.0X5-	T49.0X6-
disinfectant	T54.0X1-	T54.0X2-	T54.0X3-	T54.0X4-	-	-
in oil injection	T46.8X1-	T46.8X2-	T46.8X3-	T46.8X4-	T46.8X5-	T46.8X6-
medicinal	T49.1X1-	T49.1X2-	T49.1X3-	T49.1X4-	T49.1X5-	T49.1X6-
nonmedicinal NEC	T54.0X1-	T54.0X2-	T54.0X3-	T54.0X4-	-	-
pesticide	T60.8X1-	T60.8X2-	T60.8X3-	T60.8X4-	-	-
red	T50.8X1-	T50.8X2-	T50.8X3-	T50.8X4-	T50.8X5-	T50.8X6-
Phenolic preparation	T49.1X1-	T49.1X2-	T49.1X3-	T49.1X4-	T49.1X5-	T49.1X6-
Phenolphthalein	T47.2X1-	T47.2X2-	T47.2X3-	T47.2X4-	T47.2X5-	T47.2X6-
Phenolsulfonphthalein	T50.8X1-	T50.8X2-	T50.8X3-	T50.8X4-	T50.8X5-	T50.8X6-
Phenomorphan	T40.2X1-	T40.2X2-	T40.2X3-	T40.2X4-	-	-
Phenonyl	T42.3X1-	T42.3X2-	T42.3X3-	T42.3X4-	T42.3X5-	T42.3X6-
Phenoperidine	T40.4X1-	T40.4X2-	T40.4X3-	T40.4X4-	-	-
Phenopyrazone	T46.991-	T46.992-	T46.993-	T46.994-	T46.995-	T46.996-
Phenoquin	T50.4X1-	T50.4X2-	T50.4X3-	T50.4X4-	T50.4X5-	T50.4X6-
Phenothiazine (psychotropic) **NEC**	T43.3X1-	T43.3X2-	T43.3X3-	T43.3X4-	T43.3X5-	T43.3X6-
insecticide	T60.2X1-	T60.2X2-	T60.2X3-	T60.2X4-	-	-
Phenothrin	T49.0X1-	T49.0X2-	T49.0X3-	T49.0X4-	T49.0X5-	T49.0X6-
Phenoxybenzamine	T46.7X1-	T46.7X2-	T46.7X3-	T46.7X4-	T46.7X5-	T46.7X6-
Phenoxyethanol	T49.0X1-	T49.0X2-	T49.0X3-	T49.0X4-	T49.0X5-	T49.0X6-
Phenoxymethyl penicillin	T36.0X1-	T36.0X2-	T36.0X3-	T36.0X4-	T36.0X5-	T36.0X6-
Phenprobamate	T42.8X1-	T42.8X2-	T42.8X3-	T42.8X4-	T42.8X5-	T42.8X6-
Phenprocoumon	T45.511-	T45.512-	T45.513-	T45.514-	T45.515-	T45.516-
Phensuximide	T42.2X1-	T42.2X2-	T42.2X3-	T42.2X4-	T42.2X5-	T42.2X6-
Phentermine	T50.5X1-	T50.5X2-	T50.5X3-	T50.5X4-	T50.5X5-	T50.5X6-
Phenthicillin	T36.0X1-	T36.0X2-	T36.0X3-	T36.0X4-	T36.0X5-	T36.0X6-
Phentolamine	T46.7X1-	T46.7X2-	T46.7X3-	T46.7X4-	T46.7X5-	T46.7X6-
Phenyl						
butazone	T39.2X1-	T39.2X2-	T39.2X3-	T39.2X4-	T39.2X5-	T39.2X6-
enediamine	T65.3X1-	T65.3X2-	T65.3X3-	T65.3X4-	-	-
hydrazine	T65.3X1-	T65.3X2-	T65.3X3-	T65.3X4-	-	-
antineoplastic	T45.1X1-	T45.1X2-	T45.1X3-	T45.1X4-	T45.1X5-	T45.1X6-
mercuric compounds — *see* Mercury						
Phenyl - *continued*						
salicylate	T49.3X1-	T49.3X2-	T49.3X3-	T49.3X4-	T49.3X5-	T49.3X6-
Phenylalanine mustard	T45.1X1-	T45.1X2-	T45.1X3-	T45.1X4-	T45.1X5-	T45.1X6-
Phenylbutazone	T39.2X1-	T39.2X2-	T39.2X3-	T39.2X4-	T39.2X5-	T39.2X6-
Phenylenediamine	T65.3X1-	T65.3X2-	T65.3X3-	T65.3X4-	-	-
Phenylephrine	T44.4X1-	T44.4X2-	T44.4X3-	T44.4X4-	T44.4X5-	T44.4X6-
Phenylethylbiguanide	T38.3X1-	T38.3X2-	T38.3X3-	T38.3X4-	T38.3X5-	T38.3X6-
Phenylmercuric						
acetate	T49.0X1-	T49.0X2-	T49.0X3-	T49.0X4-	T49.0X5-	T49.0X6-
borate	T49.0X1-	T49.0X2-	T49.0X3-	T49.0X4-	T49.0X5-	T49.0X6-
nitrate	T49.0X1-	T49.0X2-	T49.0X3-	T49.0X4-	T49.0X5-	T49.0X6-
Phenylmethylbarbitone	T42.3X1-	T42.3X2-	T42.3X3-	T42.3X4-	T42.3X5-	T42.3X6-
Phenylpropanol	T47.5X1-	T47.5X2-	T47.5X3-	T47.5X4-	T47.5X5-	T47.5X6-
Phenylpropanolamine	T44.991-	T44.992-	T44.993-	T44.994-	T44.995-	T44.996-
Phenylsulfthion	T60.0X1-	T60.0X2-	T60.0X3-	T60.0X4-	-	-
Phenyltoloxamine	T45.0X1-	T45.0X2-	T45.0X3-	T45.0X4-	T45.0X5-	T45.0X6-
Phenyramidol, phenyramidon	T39.8X1-	T39.8X2-	T39.8X3-	T39.8X4-	T39.8X5-	T39.8X6-
Phenytoin	T42.0X1-	T42.0X2-	T42.0X3-	T42.0X4-	T42.0X5-	T42.0X6-
with Phenobarbital	T42.3X1-	T42.3X2-	T42.3X3-	T42.3X4-	T42.3X5-	T42.3X6-
pHisoHex	T49.2X1-	T49.2X2-	T49.2X3-	T49.2X4-	T49.2X5-	T49.2X6-
Pholcodine	T48.3X1-	T48.3X2-	T48.3X3-	T48.3X4-	T48.3X5-	T48.3X6-
Pholedrine	T46.991-	T46.992-	T46.993-	T46.994-	T46.995-	T46.996-
Phorate	T60.0X1-	T60.0X2-	T60.0X3-	T60.0X4-	-	-
Phosdrin	T60.0X1-	T60.0X2-	T60.0X3-	T60.0X4-	-	-
Phosfolan	T60.0X1-	T60.0X2-	T60.0X3-	T60.0X4-	-	-
Phosgene (gas)	T59.891-	T59.892-	T59.893-	T59.894-	-	-
Phosphamidon	T60.0X1-	T60.0X2-	T60.0X3-	T60.0X4-	-	-
Phosphate	T65.891-	T65.892-	T65.893-	T65.894-	-	-
laxative	T47.4X1-	T47.4X2-	T47.4X3-	T47.4X4-	T47.4X5-	T47.4X6-
organic	T60.0X1-	T60.0X2-	T60.0X3-	T60.0X4-	-	-
solvent	T52.91X-	T52.92X-	T52.93X-	T52.94X-	-	-
tricresyl	T65.891-	T65.892-	T65.893-	T65.894-	-	-
Phosphine	T57.1X1-	T57.1X2-	T57.1X3-	T57.1X4-	-	-
fumigant	T57.1X1-	T57.1X2-	T57.1X3-	T57.1X4-	-	-
Phospholine	T49.5X1-	T49.5X2-	T49.5X3-	T49.5X4-	T49.5X5-	T49.5X6-
Phosphoric acid	T54.2X1-	T54.2X2-	T54.2X3-	T54.2X4-	-	-
Phosphorus (compound) **NEC**	T57.1X1-	T57.1X2-	T57.1X3-	T57.1X4-	-	-
pesticide	T60.0X1-	T60.0X2-	T60.0X3-	T60.0X4-	-	-
Phthalates	T65.891-	T65.892-	T65.893-	T65.894-	-	-
Phthalic anhydride	T65.891-	T65.892-	T65.893-	T65.894-	-	-
Phthalimidoglutarimide	T42.6X1-	T42.6X2-	T42.6X3-	T42.6X4-	T42.6X5-	T42.6X6-
Phthalylsulfathiazole	T37.0X1-	T37.0X2-	T37.0X3-	T37.0X4-	T37.0X5-	T37.0X6-
Phylloquinone	T45.7X1-	T45.7X2-	T45.7X3-	T45.7X4-	T45.7X5-	T45.7X6-
Physeptone	T40.3X1-	T40.3X2-	T40.3X3-	T40.3X4-	T40.3X5-	T40.3X6-
Physostigma venenosum	T62.2X1-	T62.2X2-	T62.2X3-	T62.2X4-	-	-
Physostigmine	T49.5X1-	T49.5X2-	T49.5X3-	T49.5X4-	T49.5X5-	T49.5X6-
Phytolacca decandra	T62.2X1-	T62.2X2-	T62.2X3-	T62.2X4-	-	-
berries	T62.1X1-	T62.1X2-	T62.1X3-	T62.1X4-	-	-
Phytomenadione	T45.7X1-	T45.7X2-	T45.7X3-	T45.7X4-	T45.7X5-	T45.7X6-
Phytonadione	T45.7X1-	T45.7X2-	T45.7X3-	T45.7X4-	T45.7X5-	T45.7X6-
Picoperine	T48.3X1-	T48.3X2-	T48.3X3-	T48.3X4-	T48.3X5-	T48.3X6-
Picosulfate (sodium)	T47.2X1-	T47.2X2-	T47.2X3-	T47.2X4-	T47.2X5-	T47.2X6-
Picric (acid)	T54.2X1-	T54.2X2-	T54.2X3-	T54.2X4-	-	-
Picrotoxin	T50.7X1-	T50.7X2-	T50.7X3-	T50.7X4-	T50.7X5-	T50.7X6-
Piketoprofen	T49.0X1-	T49.0X2-	T49.0X3-	T49.0X4-	T49.0X5-	T49.0X6-
Pilocarpine	T44.1X1-	T44.1X2-	T44.1X3-	T44.1X4-	T44.1X5-	T44.1X6-
Pilocarpus (jaborandi) **extract**	T44.1X1-	T44.1X2-	T44.1X3-	T44.1X4-	T44.1X5-	T44.1X6-
Pilsicainide (hydrochloride)	T46.2X1-	T46.2X2-	T46.2X3-	T46.2X4-	T46.2X5-	T46.2X6-
Pimaricin	T36.7X1-	T36.7X2-	T36.7X3-	T36.7X4-	T36.7X5-	T36.7X6-
Pimeclone	T50.7X1-	T50.7X2-	T50.7X3-	T50.7X4-	T50.7X5-	T50.7X6-
Pimelic ketone	T52.8X1-	T52.8X2-	T52.8X3-	T52.8X4-	-	-
Pimethixene	T45.0X1-	T45.0X2-	T45.0X3-	T45.0X4-	T45.0X5-	T45.0X6-
Piminodine	T40.2X1-	T40.2X2-	T40.2X3-	T40.2X4-	T40.2X5-	T40.2X6-
Pimozide	T43.591-	T43.592-	T43.593-	T43.594-	T43.595-	T43.596-
Pinacidil	T46.5X1-	T46.5X2-	T46.5X3-	T46.5X4-	T46.5X5-	T46.5X6-
Pinaverium bromide	T44.3X1-	T44.3X2-	T44.3X3-	T44.3X4-	T44.3X5-	T44.3X6-
Pinazepam	T42.4X1-	T42.4X2-	T42.4X3-	T42.4X4-	T42.4X5-	T42.4X6-
Pindolol	T44.7X1-	T44.7X2-	T44.7X3-	T44.7X4-	T44.7X5-	T44.7X6-
Pindone	T60.4X1-	T60.4X2-	T60.4X3-	T60.4X4-	-	-
Pine oil (disinfectant)	T65.891-	T65.892-	T65.893-	T65.894-	-	-
Pinkroot	T37.4X1-	T37.4X2-	T37.4X3-	T37.4X4-	T37.4X5-	T37.4X6-
Pipadone	T40.2X1-	T40.2X2-	T40.2X3-	T40.2X4-	-	-
Pipamazine	T45.0X1-	T45.0X2-	T45.0X3-	T45.0X4-	T45.0X5-	T45.0X6-
Pipamperone	T43.4X1-	T43.4X2-	T43.4X3-	T43.4X4-	T43.4X5-	T43.4X6-
Pipazetate	T48.3X1-	T48.3X2-	T48.3X3-	T48.3X4-	T48.3X5-	T48.3X6-
Pipemidic acid	T37.8X1-	T37.8X2-	T37.8X3-	T37.8X4-	T37.8X5-	T37.8X6-
Pipenzolate bromide	T44.3X1-	T44.3X2-	T44.3X3-	T44.3X4-	T44.3X5-	T44.3X6-
Piperacetazine	T43.3X1-	T43.3X2-	T43.3X3-	T43.3X4-	T43.3X5-	T43.3X6-

Piperacillin - Pravastatin
Table of Drugs and Chemicals
Table of Drugs and Chemicals

Substance	Poisoning Accidental (unintentional)	Poisoning Intentional self-harm	Poisoning Assault	Poisoning Undetermined	Adverse effect	Underdosing
Piperacillin	T36.0X1-	T36.0X2-	T36.0X3-	T36.0X4-	T36.0X5-	T36.0X6-
Piperazine	T37.4X1-	T37.4X2-	T37.4X3-	T37.4X4-	T37.4X5-	T37.4X6-
estrone sulfate	T38.5X1-	T38.5X2-	T38.5X3-	T38.5X4-	T38.5X5-	T38.5X6-
Piper cubeba	T62.2X1-	T62.2X2-	T62.2X3-	T62.2X4-	-	-
Piperidione	T48.3X1-	T48.3X2-	T48.3X3-	T48.3X4-	T48.3X5-	T48.3X6-
Piperidolate	T44.3X1-	T44.3X2-	T44.3X3-	T44.3X4-	T44.3X5-	T44.3X6-
Piperocaine	T41.3X1-	T41.3X2-	T41.3X3-	T41.3X4-	T41.3X5-	T41.3X6-
infiltration (subcutaneous)	T41.3X1-	T41.3X2-	T41.3X3-	T41.3X4-	T41.3X5-	T41.3X6-
nerve block (peripheral) (plexus)	T41.3X1-	T41.3X2-	T41.3X3-	T41.3X4-	T41.3X5-	T41.3X6-
topical (surface)	T41.3X1-	T41.3X2-	T41.3X3-	T41.3X4-	T41.3X5-	T41.3X6-
Piperonyl butoxide	T60.8X1-	T60.8X2-	T60.8X3-	T60.8X4-	-	-
Pipethanate	T44.3X1-	T44.3X2-	T44.3X3-	T44.3X4-	T44.3X5-	T44.3X6-
Pipobroman	T45.1X1-	T45.1X2-	T45.1X3-	T45.1X4-	T45.1X5-	T45.1X6-
Pipotiazine	T43.3X1-	T43.3X2-	T43.3X3-	T43.3X4-	T43.3X5-	T43.3X6-
Pipoxizine	T45.0X1-	T45.0X2-	T45.0X3-	T45.0X4-	T45.0X5-	T45.0X6-
Pipradrol	T43.691-	T43.692-	T43.693-	T43.694-	T43.695-	T43.696-
Piprinhydrinate	T45.0X1-	T45.0X2-	T45.0X3-	T45.0X4-	T45.0X5-	T45.0X6-
Pirarubicin	T45.1X1-	T45.1X2-	T45.1X3-	T45.1X4-	T45.1X5-	T45.1X6-
Pirazinamide	T37.1X1-	T37.1X2-	T37.1X3-	T37.1X4-	T37.1X5-	T37.1X6-
Pirbuterol	T48.6X1-	T48.6X2-	T48.6X3-	T48.6X4-	T48.6X5-	T48.6X6-
Pirenzepine	T47.1X1-	T47.1X2-	T47.1X3-	T47.1X4-	T47.1X5-	T47.1X6-
Piretanide	T50.1X1-	T50.1X2-	T50.1X3-	T50.1X4-	T50.1X5-	T50.1X6-
Piribedil	T42.8X1-	T42.8X2-	T42.8X3-	T42.8X4-	T42.8X5-	T42.8X6-
Piridoxilate	T46.3X1-	T46.3X2-	T46.3X3-	T46.3X4-	T46.3X5-	T46.3X6-
Piritramide	T40.4X1-	T40.4X2-	T40.4X3-	T40.4X4-	-	-
Piromidic acid	T37.8X1-	T37.8X2-	T37.8X3-	T37.8X4-	T37.8X5-	T37.8X6-
Piroxicam	T39.391-	T39.392-	T39.393-	T39.394-	T39.395-	T39.396-
beta-cyclodextrin complex	T39.8X1-	T39.8X2-	T39.8X3-	T39.8X4-	T39.8X5-	T39.8X6-
Pirozadil	T46.6X1-	T46.6X2-	T46.6X3-	T46.6X4-	T46.6X5-	T46.6X6-
Piscidia (bark) (erythrina)	T39.8X1-	T39.8X2-	T39.8X3-	T39.8X4-	T39.8X5-	T39.8X6-
Pitch	T65.891-	T65.892-	T65.893-	T65.894-	-	-
Pitkin's solution	T41.3X1-	T41.3X2-	T41.3X3-	T41.3X4-	T41.3X5-	T41.3X6-
Pitocin	T48.0X1-	T48.0X2-	T48.0X3-	T48.0X4-	T48.0X5-	T48.0X6-
Pitressin (tannate)	T38.891-	T38.892-	T38.893-	T38.894-	T38.895-	T38.896-
Pituitary extracts (posterior)	T38.891-	T38.892-	T38.893-	T38.894-	T38.895-	T38.896-
anterior	T38.811-	T38.812-	T38.813-	T38.814-	T38.815-	T38.816-
Pituitrin	T38.891-	T38.892-	T38.893-	T38.894-	T38.895-	T38.896-
Pivampicillin	T36.0X1-	T36.0X2-	T36.0X3-	T36.0X4-	T36.0X5-	T36.0X6-
Pivmecillinam	T36.0X1-	T36.0X2-	T36.0X3-	T36.0X4-	T36.0X5-	T36.0X6-
Placental hormone	T38.891-	T38.892-	T38.893-	T38.894-	T38.895-	T38.896-
Placidyl	T42.6X1-	T42.6X2-	T42.6X3-	T42.6X4-	T42.6X5-	T42.6X6-
Plague vaccine	T50.A91-	T50.A92-	T50.A93-	T50.A94-	T50.A95-	T50.A96-
Plant						
food or fertilizer NEC	T65.891-	T65.892-	T65.893-	T65.894-	-	-
containing herbicide	T60.3X1-	T60.3X2-	T60.3X3-	T60.3X4-	-	-
noxious, used as food	T62.2X1-	T62.2X2-	T62.2X3-	T62.2X4-	-	-
berries	T62.1X1-	T62.1X2-	T62.1X3-	T62.1X4-	-	-
seeds	T62.2X1-	T62.2X2-	T62.2X3-	T62.2X4-	-	-
specified type NEC	T62.2X1-	T62.2X2-	T62.2X3-	T62.2X4-	-	-
Plasma	T45.8X1-	T45.8X2-	T45.8X3-	T45.8X4-	T45.8X5-	T45.8X6-
expander NEC	T45.8X1-	T45.8X2-	T45.8X3-	T45.8X4-	T45.8X5-	T45.8X6-
protein fraction (human)	T45.8X1-	T45.8X2-	T45.8X3-	T45.8X4-	T45.8X5-	T45.8X6-
Plasmanate	T45.8X1-	T45.8X2-	T45.8X3-	T45.8X4-	T45.8X5-	T45.8X6-
Plasminogen (tissue) **activator**	T45.611-	T45.612-	T45.613-	T45.614-	T45.615-	T45.616-
Plaster dressing	T49.3X1-	T49.3X2-	T49.3X3-	T49.3X4-	T49.3X5-	T49.3X6-
Plastic dressing	T49.3X1-	T49.3X2-	T49.3X3-	T49.3X4-	T49.3X5-	T49.3X6-
Plegicil	T43.3X1-	T43.3X2-	T43.3X3-	T43.3X4-	T43.3X5-	T43.3X6-
Plicamycin	T45.1X1-	T45.1X2-	T45.1X3-	T45.1X4-	T45.1X5-	T45.1X6-
Podophyllotoxin	T49.8X1-	T49.8X2-	T49.8X3-	T49.8X4-	T49.8X5-	T49.8X6-
Podophyllum (resin)	T49.4X1-	T49.4X2-	T49.4X3-	T49.4X4-	T49.4X5-	T49.4X6-
Poison NEC	T65.91X-	T65.92X-	T65.93X-	T65.94X-	-	-
Poisonous berries	T62.1X1-	T62.1X2-	T62.1X3-	T62.1X4-	-	-
Pokeweed (any part)	T62.2X1-	T62.2X2-	T62.2X3-	T62.2X4-	-	-
Poldine metilsulfate	T44.3X1-	T44.3X2-	T44.3X3-	T44.3X4-	T44.3X5-	T44.3X6-
Polidexide (sulfate)	T46.6X1-	T46.6X2-	T46.6X3-	T46.6X4-	T46.6X5-	T46.6X6-
Polidocanol	T46.8X1-	T46.8X2-	T46.8X3-	T46.8X4-	T46.8X5-	T46.8X6-
Poliomyelitis vaccine	T50.B91-	T50.B92-	T50.B93-	T50.B94-	T50.B95-	T50.B96-
Polish (car) (floor) (furni-ture) (metal) (porcelain) (silver)	T65.891-	T65.892-	T65.893-	T65.894-	-	-
abrasive	T65.891-	T65.892-	T65.893-	T65.894-	-	-
porcelain	T65.891-	T65.892-	T65.893-	T65.894-	-	-
Poloxalkol	T47.4X1-	T47.4X2-	T47.4X3-	T47.4X4-	T47.4X5-	T47.4X6-
Poloxamer	T47.4X1-	T47.4X2-	T47.4X3-	T47.4X4-	T47.4X5-	T47.4X6-
Polyaminostyrene resins	T50.3X1-	T50.3X2-	T50.3X3-	T50.3X4-	T50.3X5-	T50.3X6-
Polycarbophil	T47.4X1-	T47.4X2-	T47.4X3-	T47.4X4-	T47.4X5-	T47.4X6-
Polychlorinated biphenyl	T65.891-	T65.892-	T65.893-	T65.894-	-	-
Polycycline	T36.4X1-	T36.4X2-	T36.4X3-	T36.4X4-	T36.4X5-	T36.4X6-

Substance	Poisoning Accidental (unintentional)	Poisoning Intentional self-harm	Poisoning Assault	Poisoning Undetermined	Adverse effect	Underdosing
Polyester fumes	T59.891-	T59.892-	T59.893-	T59.894-	-	-
Polyester resin hardener	T52.91X-	T52.92X-	T52.93X-	T52.94X-	-	-
fumes	T59.891-	T59.892-	T59.893-	T59.894-	-	-
Polyestradiol phosphate	T38.5X1-	T38.5X2-	T38.5X3-	T38.5X4-	T38.5X5-	T38.5X6-
Polyethanolamine alkyl sulfate	T49.2X1-	T49.2X2-	T49.2X3-	T49.2X4-	T49.2X5-	T49.2X6-
Polyethylene adhesive	T49.3X1-	T49.3X2-	T49.3X3-	T49.3X4-	T49.3X5-	T49.3X6-
Polyferose	T45.4X1-	T45.4X2-	T45.4X3-	T45.4X4-	T45.4X5-	T45.4X6-
Polygeline	T45.8X1-	T45.8X2-	T45.8X3-	T45.8X4-	T45.8X5-	T45.8X6-
Polymyxin	T36.8X1-	T36.8X2-	T36.8X3-	T36.8X4-	T36.8X5-	T36.8X6-
B	T36.8X1-	T36.8X2-	T36.8X3-	T36.8X4-	T36.8X5-	T36.8X6-
ENT agent	T49.6X1-	T49.6X2-	T49.6X3-	T49.6X4-	T49.6X5-	T49.6X6-
ophthalmic preparation	T49.5X1-	T49.5X2-	T49.5X3-	T49.5X4-	T49.5X5-	T49.5X6-
topical NEC	T49.0X1-	T49.0X2-	T49.0X3-	T49.0X4-	T49.0X5-	T49.0X6-
E sulfate (eye preparation)	T49.5X1-	T49.5X2-	T49.5X3-	T49.5X4-	T49.5X5-	T49.5X6-
Polynoxylin	T49.0X1-	T49.0X2-	T49.0X3-	T49.0X4-	T49.0X5-	T49.0X6-
Polyoestradiol phosphate	T38.5X1-	T38.5X2-	T38.5X3-	T38.5X4-	T38.5X5-	T38.5X6-
Polyoxymethyleneurea	T49.0X1-	T49.0X2-	T49.0X3-	T49.0X4-	T49.0X5-	T49.0X6-
Polysilane	T47.8X1-	T47.8X2-	T47.8X3-	T47.8X4-	T47.8X5-	T47.8X6-
Polytetrafluoroethylene (inhaled)	T59.891-	T59.892-	T59.893-	T59.894-	-	-
Polythiazide	T50.2X1-	T50.2X2-	T50.2X3-	T50.2X4-	T50.2X5-	T50.2X6-
Polyvidone	T45.8X1-	T45.8X2-	T45.8X3-	T45.8X4-	T45.8X5-	T45.8X6-
Polyvinylpyrrolidone	T45.8X1-	T45.8X2-	T45.8X3-	T45.8X4-	T45.8X5-	T45.8X6-
Pontocaine (hydrochloride) (infiltration) (topical)	T41.3X1-	T41.3X2-	T41.3X3-	T41.3X4-	T41.3X5-	T41.3X6-
nerve block (peripheral) (plexus)	T41.3X1-	T41.3X2-	T41.3X3-	T41.3X4-	T41.3X5-	T41.3X6-
spinal	T41.3X1-	T41.3X2-	T41.3X3-	T41.3X4-	T41.3X5-	T41.3X6-
Porfiromycin	T45.1X1-	T45.1X2-	T45.1X3-	T45.1X4-	T45.1X5-	T45.1X6-
Posterior pituitary hormone NEC	T38.891-	T38.892-	T38.893-	T38.894-	T38.895-	T38.896-
Pot	T40.7X1-	T40.7X2-	T40.7X3-	T40.7X4-	T40.7X5-	T40.7X6-
Potash (caustic)	T54.3X1-	T54.3X2-	T54.3X3-	T54.3X4-	-	-
Potassic saline injection (lactated)	T50.3X1-	T50.3X2-	T50.3X3-	T50.3X4-	T50.3X5-	T50.3X6-
Potassium (salts) **NEC**	T50.3X1-	T50.3X2-	T50.3X3-	T50.3X4-	T50.3X5-	T50.3X6-
aminobenzoate	T45.8X1-	T45.8X2-	T45.8X3-	T45.8X4-	T45.8X5-	T45.8X6-
aminosalicylate	T37.1X1-	T37.1X2-	T37.1X3-	T37.1X4-	T37.1X5-	T37.1X6-
antimony ' tartrate'	T37.8X1-	T37.8X2-	T37.8X3-	T37.8X4-	T37.8X5-	T37.8X6-
arsenite (solution)	T57.0X1-	T57.0X2-	T57.0X3-	T57.0X4-	-	-
bichromate	T56.2X1-	T56.2X2-	T56.2X3-	T56.2X4-	-	-
bisulfate	T47.3X1-	T47.3X2-	T47.3X3-	T47.3X4-	T47.3X5-	T47.3X6-
bromide	T42.6X1-	T42.6X2-	T42.6X3-	T42.6X4-	T42.6X5-	T42.6X6-
canrenoate	T50.0X1-	T50.0X2-	T50.0X3-	T50.0X4-	T50.0X5-	T50.0X6-
carbonate	T54.3X1-	T54.3X2-	T54.3X3-	T54.3X4-	-	-
chlorate NEC	T65.891-	T65.892-	T65.893-	T65.894-	-	-
chloride	T50.3X1-	T50.3X2-	T50.3X3-	T50.3X4-	T50.3X5-	T50.3X6-
citrate	T50.991-	T50.992-	T50.993-	T50.994-	T50.995-	T50.996-
cyanide	T65.0X1-	T65.0X2-	T65.0X3-	T65.0X4-	-	-
ferric hexacyanoferrate (medicinal)	T50.6X1-	T50.6X2-	T50.6X3-	T50.6X4-	T50.6X5-	T50.6X6-
nonmedicinal	T65.891-	T65.892-	T65.893-	T65.894-	-	-
Fluoride	T57.8X1-	T57.8X2-	T57.8X3-	T57.8X4-	-	-
glucaldrate	T47.1X1-	T47.1X2-	T47.1X3-	T47.1X4-	T47.1X5-	T47.1X6-
hydroxide	T54.3X1-	T54.3X2-	T54.3X3-	T54.3X4-	-	-
iodate	T49.0X1-	T49.0X2-	T49.0X3-	T49.0X4-	T49.0X5-	T49.0X6-
iodide	T48.4X1-	T48.4X2-	T48.4X3-	T48.4X4-	T48.4X5-	T48.4X6-
nitrate	T57.8X1-	T57.8X2-	T57.8X3-	T57.8X4-	-	-
oxalate	T65.891-	T65.892-	T65.893-	T65.894-	-	-
perchlorate (nonmedicinal) NEC	T65.891-	T65.892-	T65.893-	T65.894-	-	-
antithyroid	T38.2X1-	T38.2X2-	T38.2X3-	T38.2X4-	T38.2X5-	T38.2X6-
medicinal	T38.2X1-	T38.2X2-	T38.2X3-	T38.2X4-	T38.2X5-	T38.2X6-
Permanganate (nonmedicinal)	T65.891-	T65.892-	T65.893-	T65.894-	-	-
medicinal	T49.0X1-	T49.0X2-	T49.0X3-	T49.0X4-	T49.0X5-	T49.0X6-
sulfate	T47.2X1-	T47.2X2-	T47.2X3-	T47.2X4-	T47.2X5-	T47.2X6-
Potassium-removing resin	T50.3X1-	T50.3X2-	T50.3X3-	T50.3X4-	T50.3X5-	T50.3X6-
Potassium-retaining drug	T50.3X1-	T50.3X2-	T50.3X3-	T50.3X4-	T50.3X5-	T50.3X6-
Povidone	T45.8X1-	T45.8X2-	T45.8X3-	T45.8X4-	T45.8X5-	T45.8X6-
iodine	T49.0X1-	T49.0X2-	T49.0X3-	T49.0X4-	T49.0X5-	T49.0X6-
Practolol	T44.7X1-	T44.7X2-	T44.7X3-	T44.7X4-	T44.7X5-	T44.7X6-
Prajmalium bitartrate	T46.2X1-	T46.2X2-	T46.2X3-	T46.2X4-	T46.2X5-	T46.2X6-
Pralidoxime (iodide)	T50.6X1-	T50.6X2-	T50.6X3-	T50.6X4-	T50.6X5-	T50.6X6-
chloride	T50.6X1-	T50.6X2-	T50.6X3-	T50.6X4-	T50.6X5-	T50.6X6-
Pramiverine	T44.3X1-	T44.3X2-	T44.3X3-	T44.3X4-	T44.3X5-	T44.3X6-
Pramocaine	T49.1X1-	T49.1X2-	T49.1X3-	T49.1X4-	T49.1X5-	T49.1X6-
Pramoxine	T49.1X1-	T49.1X2-	T49.1X3-	T49.1X4-	T49.1X5-	T49.1X6-
Prasterone	T38.7X1-	T38.7X2-	T38.7X3-	T38.7X4-	T38.7X5-	T38.7X6-
Pravastatin	T46.6X1-	T46.6X2-	T46.6X3-	T46.6X4-	T46.6X5-	T46.6X6-

Substance	Poisoning Accidental (unintentional)	Poisoning Intentional self-harm	Poisoning Assault	Poisoning Undetermined	Adverse effect	Underdosing
Prazepam	T42.4X1-	T42.4X2-	T42.4X3-	T42.4X4-	T42.4X5-	T42.4X6-
Praziquantel	T37.4X1-	T37.4X2-	T37.4X3-	T37.4X4-	T37.4X5-	T37.4X6-
Prazitone	T43.291-	T43.292-	T43.293-	T43.294-	T43.295-	T43.296-
Prazosin	T44.6X1-	T44.6X2-	T44.6X3-	T44.6X4-	T44.6X5-	T44.6X6-
Prednicarbate	T49.0X1-	T49.0X2-	T49.0X3-	T49.0X4-	T49.0X5-	T49.0X6-
Prednimustine	T45.1X1-	T45.1X2-	T45.1X3-	T45.1X4-	T45.1X5-	T45.1X6-
Prednisolone	T38.0X1-	T38.0X2-	T38.0X3-	T38.0X4-	T38.0X5-	T38.0X6-
ENT agent	T49.6X1-	T49.6X2-	T49.6X3-	T49.6X4-	T49.6X5-	T49.6X6-
ophthalmic preparation	T49.5X1-	T49.5X2-	T49.5X3-	T49.5X4-	T49.5X5-	T49.5X6-
steaglate	T49.0X1-	T49.0X2-	T49.0X3-	T49.0X4-	T49.0X5-	T49.0X6-
topical NEC	T49.0X1-	T49.0X2-	T49.0X3-	T49.0X4-	T49.0X5-	T49.0X6-
Prednisone	T38.0X1-	T38.0X2-	T38.0X3-	T38.0X4-	T38.0X5-	T38.0X6-
Prednylidene	T38.0X1-	T38.0X2-	T38.0X3-	T38.0X4-	T38.0X5-	T38.0X6-
Pregnandiol	T38.5X1-	T38.5X2-	T38.5X3-	T38.5X4-	T38.5X5-	T38.5X6-
Pregneninolone	T38.5X1-	T38.5X2-	T38.5X3-	T38.5X4-	T38.5X5-	T38.5X6-
Preludin	T43.691-	T43.692-	T43.693-	T43.694-	T43.695-	T43.696-
Premarin	T38.5X1-	T38.5X2-	T38.5X3-	T38.5X4-	T38.5X5-	T38.5X6-
Premedication anesthetic	T41.201-	T41.202-	T41.203-	T41.204-	T41.205-	T41.206-
Prenalterol	T44.5X1-	T44.5X2-	T44.5X3-	T44.5X4-	T44.5X5-	T44.5X6-
Prenoxdiazine	T48.3X1-	T48.3X2-	T48.3X3-	T48.3X4-	T48.3X5-	T48.3X6-
Prenylamine	T46.3X1-	T46.3X2-	T46.3X3-	T46.3X4-	T46.3X5-	T46.3X6-
Preparation H	T49.8X1-	T49.8X2-	T49.8X3-	T49.8X4-	T49.8X5-	T49.8X6-
Preparation, local	T49.4X1-	T49.4X2-	T49.4X3-	T49.4X4-	T49.4X5-	T49.4X6-
Preservative (nonmedicinal)	T65.891-	T65.892-	T65.893-	T65.894-	-	-
medicinal	T50.901-	T50.902-	T50.903-	T50.904-	T50.905-	T50.906-
wood	T60.91X-	T60.92X-	T60.93X-	T60.94X-	-	-
Prethcamide	T50.7X1-	T50.7X2-	T50.7X3-	T50.7X4-	T50.7X5-	T50.7X6-
Pride of China	T62.2X1-	T62.2X2-	T62.2X3-	T62.2X4-	-	-
Pridinol	T44.3X1-	T44.3X2-	T44.3X3-	T44.3X4-	T44.3X5-	T44.3X6-
Prifinium bromide	T44.3X1-	T44.3X2-	T44.3X3-	T44.3X4-	T44.3X5-	T44.3X6-
Prilocaine	T41.3X1-	T41.3X2-	T41.3X3-	T41.3X4-	T41.3X5-	T41.3X6-
infiltration (subcutaneous)	T41.3X1-	T41.3X2-	T41.3X3-	T41.3X4-	T41.3X5-	T41.3X6-
nerve block (peripheral) (plexus)	T41.3X1-	T41.3X2-	T41.3X3-	T41.3X4-	T41.3X5-	T41.3X6-
regional	T41.3X1-	T41.3X2-	T41.3X3-	T41.3X4-	T41.3X5-	T41.3X6-
Primaquine	T37.2X1-	T37.2X2-	T37.2X3-	T37.2X4-	T37.2X5-	T37.2X6-
Primidone	T42.6X1-	T42.6X2-	T42.6X3-	T42.6X4-	T42.6X5-	T42.6X6-
Primula (veris)	T62.2X1-	T62.2X2-	T62.2X3-	T62.2X4-	-	-
Prinadol	T40.2X1-	T40.2X2-	T40.2X3-	T40.2X4-	T40.2X5-	T40.2X6-
Priscol, Priscoline	T44.6X1-	T44.6X2-	T44.6X3-	T44.6X4-	T44.6X5-	T44.6X6-
Pristinamycin	T36.3X1-	T36.3X2-	T36.3X3-	T36.3X4-	T36.3X5-	T36.3X6-
Privet	T62.2X1-	T62.2X2-	T62.2X3-	T62.2X4-	-	-
berries	T62.1X1-	T62.1X2-	T62.1X3-	T62.1X4-	-	-
Privine	T44.4X1-	T44.4X2-	T44.4X3-	T44.4X4-	T44.4X5-	T44.4X6-
Pro-Banthine	T44.3X1-	T44.3X2-	T44.3X3-	T44.3X4-	T44.3X5-	T44.3X6-
Probarbital	T42.3X1-	T42.3X2-	T42.3X3-	T42.3X4-	T42.3X5-	T42.3X6-
Probenecid	T50.4X1-	T50.4X2-	T50.4X3-	T50.4X4-	T50.4X5-	T50.4X6-
Probucol	T46.6X1-	T46.6X2-	T46.6X3-	T46.6X4-	T46.6X5-	T46.6X6-
Procainamide	T46.2X1-	T46.2X2-	T46.2X3-	T46.2X4-	T46.2X5-	T46.2X6-
Procaine	T41.3X1-	T41.3X2-	T41.3X3-	T41.3X4-	T41.3X5-	T41.3X6-
benzylpenicillin	T36.0X1-	T36.0X2-	T36.0X3-	T36.0X4-	T36.0X5-	T36.0X6-
nerve block (periphreal) (plexus)	T41.3X1-	T41.3X2-	T41.3X3-	T41.3X4-	T41.3X5-	T41.3X6-
penicillin G	T36.0X1-	T36.0X2-	T36.0X3-	T36.0X4-	T36.0X5-	T36.0X6-
regional	T41.3X1-	T41.3X2-	T41.3X3-	T41.3X4-	T41.3X5-	T41.3X6-
spinal	T41.3X1-	T41.3X2-	T41.3X3-	T41.3X4-	T41.3X5-	T41.3X6-
Procalmidol	T43.591-	T43.592-	T43.593-	T43.594-	T43.595-	T43.596-
Procarbazine	T45.1X1-	T45.1X2-	T45.1X3-	T45.1X4-	T45.1X5-	T45.1X6-
Procaterol	T44.5X1-	T44.5X2-	T44.5X3-	T44.5X4-	T44.5X5-	T44.5X6-
Prochlorperazine	T43.3X1-	T43.3X2-	T43.3X3-	T43.3X4-	T43.3X5-	T43.3X6-
Procyclidine	T44.3X1-	T44.3X2-	T44.3X3-	T44.3X4-	T44.3X5-	T44.3X6-
Producer gas	T58.8X1-	T58.8X2-	T58.8X3-	T58.8X4-	-	-
Profadol	T40.4X1-	T40.4X2-	T40.4X3-	T40.4X4-	T40.4X5-	T40.4X6-
Profenamine	T44.3X1-	T44.3X2-	T44.3X3-	T44.3X4-	T44.3X5-	T44.3X6-
Profenil	T44.3X1-	T44.3X2-	T44.3X3-	T44.3X4-	T44.3X5-	T44.3X6-
Proflavine	T49.0X1-	T49.0X2-	T49.0X3-	T49.0X4-	T49.0X5-	T49.0X6-
Progabide	T42.6X1-	T42.6X2-	T42.6X3-	T42.6X4-	T42.6X5-	T42.6X6-
Progesterone	T38.5X1-	T38.5X2-	T38.5X3-	T38.5X4-	T38.5X5-	T38.5X6-
Progestin	T38.5X1-	T38.5X2-	T38.5X3-	T38.5X4-	T38.5X5-	T38.5X6-
oral contraceptive	T38.4X1-	T38.4X2-	T38.4X3-	T38.4X4-	T38.4X5-	T38.4X6-
Progestogen NEC	T38.5X1-	T38.5X2-	T38.5X3-	T38.5X4-	T38.5X5-	T38.5X6-
Progestone	T38.5X1-	T38.5X2-	T38.5X3-	T38.5X4-	T38.5X5-	T38.5X6-
Proglumide	T47.1X1-	T47.1X2-	T47.1X3-	T47.1X4-	T47.1X5-	T47.1X6-
Proguanil	T37.2X1-	T37.2X2-	T37.2X3-	T37.2X4-	T37.2X5-	T37.2X6-
Prolactin	T38.811-	T38.812-	T38.813-	T38.814-	T38.815-	T38.816-
Prolintane	T43.691-	T43.692-	T43.693-	T43.694-	T43.695-	T43.696-
Proloid	T38.1X1-	T38.1X2-	T38.1X3-	T38.1X4-	T38.1X5-	T38.1X6-
Proluton	T38.5X1-	T38.5X2-	T38.5X3-	T38.5X4-	T38.5X5-	T38.5X6-

Substance	Poisoning Accidental (unintentional)	Poisoning Intentional self-harm	Poisoning Assault	Poisoning Undetermined	Adverse effect	Underdosing
Promacetin	T37.1X1-	T37.1X2-	T37.1X3-	T37.1X4-	T37.1X5-	T37.1X6-
Promazine	T43.3X1-	T43.3X2-	T43.3X3-	T43.3X4-	T43.3X5-	T43.3X6-
Promedol	T40.2X1-	T40.2X2-	T40.2X3-	T40.2X4-	-	-
Promegestone	T38.5X1-	T38.5X2-	T38.5X3-	T38.5X4-	T38.5X5-	T38.5X6-
Promethazine (teoclate)	T43.3X1-	T43.3X2-	T43.3X3-	T43.3X4-	T43.3X5-	T43.3X6-
Promin	T37.1X1-	T37.1X2-	T37.1X3-	T37.1X4-	T37.1X5-	T37.1X6-
Pronase	T45.3X1-	T45.3X2-	T45.3X3-	T45.3X4-	T45.3X5-	T45.3X6-
Pronestyl (hydrochloride)	T46.2X1-	T46.2X2-	T46.2X3-	T46.2X4-	T46.2X5-	T46.2X6-
Pronetalol	T44.7X1-	T44.7X2-	T44.7X3-	T44.7X4-	T44.7X5-	T44.7X6-
Prontosil	T37.0X1-	T37.0X2-	T37.0X3-	T37.0X4-	T37.0X5-	T37.0X6-
Propachlor	T60.3X1-	T60.3X2-	T60.3X3-	T60.3X4-	-	-
Propafenone	T46.2X1-	T46.2X2-	T46.2X3-	T46.2X4-	T46.2X5-	T46.2X6-
Propallylonal	T42.3X1-	T42.3X2-	T42.3X3-	T42.3X4-	T42.3X5-	T42.3X6-
Propamidine	T49.0X1-	T49.0X2-	T49.0X3-	T49.0X4-	T49.0X5-	T49.0X6-
Propane (distributed in mobile container)	T59.891-	T59.892-	T59.893-	T59.894-	-	-
distributed through pipes	T59.891-	T59.892-	T59.893-	T59.894-	-	-
incomplete combustion	T58.11X-	T58.12X-	T58.13X-	T58.14X-	-	-
Propanidid	T41.291-	T41.292-	T41.293-	T41.294-	T41.295-	T41.296-
Propanil	T60.3X1-	T60.3X2-	T60.3X3-	T60.3X4-	-	-
1-Propanol	T51.3X1-	T51.3X2-	T51.3X3-	T51.3X4-	-	-
2-Propanol	T51.2X1-	T51.2X2-	T51.2X3-	T51.2X4-	-	-
Propantheline	T44.3X1-	T44.3X2-	T44.3X3-	T44.3X4-	T44.3X5-	T44.3X6-
bromide	T44.3X1-	T44.3X2-	T44.3X3-	T44.3X4-	T44.3X5-	T44.3X6-
Proparacaine	T41.3X1-	T41.3X2-	T41.3X3-	T41.3X4-	T41.3X5-	T41.3X6-
Propatylnitrate	T46.3X1-	T46.3X2-	T46.3X3-	T46.3X4-	T46.3X5-	T46.3X6-
Propicillin	T36.0X1-	T36.0X2-	T36.0X3-	T36.0X4-	T36.0X5-	T36.0X6-
Propiolactone	T49.0X1-	T49.0X2-	T49.0X3-	T49.0X4-	T49.0X5-	T49.0X6-
Propiomazine	T45.0X1-	T45.0X2-	T45.0X3-	T45.0X4-	T45.0X5-	T45.0X6-
Propionaldehyde (medicinal)	T42.6X1-	T42.6X2-	T42.6X3-	T42.6X4-	T42.6X5-	T42.6X6-
Propionate (calcium) (sodium)	T49.0X1-	T49.0X2-	T49.0X3-	T49.0X4-	T49.0X5-	T49.0X6-
Propion gel	T49.0X1-	T49.0X2-	T49.0X3-	T49.0X4-	T49.0X5-	T49.0X6-
Propitocaine	T41.3X1-	T41.3X2-	T41.3X3-	T41.3X4-	T41.3X5-	T41.3X6-
infiltration (subcutaneous)	T41.3X1-	T41.3X2-	T41.3X3-	T41.3X4-	T41.3X5-	T41.3X6-
nerve block (peripheral) (plexus)	T41.3X1-	T41.3X2-	T41.3X3-	T41.3X4-	T41.3X5-	T41.3X6-
Propofol	T41.291-	T41.292-	T41.293-	T41.294-	T41.295-	T41.296-
Propoxur	T60.0X1-	T60.0X2-	T60.0X3-	T60.0X4-	-	-
Propoxycaine	T41.3X1-	T41.3X2-	T41.3X3-	T41.3X4-	T41.3X5-	T41.3X6-
infiltration (subcutaneous)	T41.3X1-	T41.3X2-	T41.3X3-	T41.3X4-	T41.3X5-	T41.3X6-
nerve block (peripheral) (plexus)	T41.3X1-	T41.3X2-	T41.3X3-	T41.3X4-	T41.3X5-	T41.3X6-
topical (surface)	T41.3X1-	T41.3X2-	T41.3X3-	T41.3X4-	T41.3X5-	T41.3X6-
Propoxyphene	T40.4X1-	T40.4X2-	T40.4X3-	T40.4X4-	T40.4X5-	T40.4X6-
Propranolol	T44.7X1-	T44.7X2-	T44.7X3-	T44.7X4-	T44.7X5-	T44.7X6-
Propyl						
alcohol	T51.3X1-	T51.3X2-	T51.3X3-	T51.3X4-	-	-
carbinol	T51.3X1-	T51.3X2-	T51.3X3-	T51.3X4-	-	-
hexadrine	T44.4X1-	T44.4X2-	T44.4X3-	T44.4X4-	T44.4X5-	T44.4X6-
iodone	T50.8X1-	T50.8X2-	T50.8X3-	T50.8X4-	T50.8X5-	T50.8X6-
thiouracil	T38.2X1-	T38.2X2-	T38.2X3-	T38.2X4-	T38.2X5-	T38.2X6-
Propylaminopheno-thiazine	T43.3X1-	T43.3X2-	T43.3X3-	T43.3X4-	T43.3X5-	T43.3X6-
Propylene	T59.891-	T59.892-	T59.893-	T59.894-	-	-
Propylhexedrine	T48.5X1-	T48.5X2-	T48.5X3-	T48.5X4-	T48.5X5-	T48.5X6-
Propyliodone	T50.8X1-	T50.8X2-	T50.8X3-	T50.8X4-	T50.8X5-	T50.8X6
Propylparaben (ophthalmic)	T49.5X1-	T49.5X2-	T49.5X3-	T49.5X4-	T49.5X5-	T49.5X6-
Propylthiouracil	T38.2X1-	T38.2X2-	T38.2X3-	T38.2X4-	T38.2X5-	T38.2X6-
Propyphenazone	T39.2X1-	T39.2X2-	T39.2X3-	T39.2X4-	T39.2X5-	T39.2X6-
Proquazone	T39.391-	T39.392-	T39.393-	T39.394-	T39.395-	T39.396-
Proscillaridin	T46.0X1-	T46.0X2-	T46.0X3-	T46.0X4-	T46.0X5-	T46.0X6-
Prostacyclin	T45.521-	T45.522-	T45.523-	T45.524-	T45.525-	T45.526-
Prostaglandin (I2)	T45.521-	T45.522-	T45.523-	T45.524-	T45.525-	T45.526-
E1	T46.7X1-	T46.7X2-	T46.7X3-	T46.7X4-	T46.7X5-	T46.7X6-
E2	T48.0X1-	T48.0X2-	T48.0X3-	T48.0X4-	T48.0X5-	T48.0X6-
F2 alpha	T48.0X1-	T48.0X2-	T48.0X3-	T48.0X4-	T48.0X5-	T48.0X6-
Prostigmin	T44.0X1-	T44.0X2-	T44.0X3-	T44.0X4-	T44.0X5-	T44.0X6-
Prosultiamine	T45.2X1-	T45.2X2-	T45.2X3-	T45.2X4-	T45.2X5-	T45.2X6-
Protamine sulfate	T45.7X1-	T45.7X2-	T45.7X3-	T45.7X4-	T45.7X5-	T45.7X6-
zinc insulin	T38.3X1-	T38.3X2-	T38.3X3-	T38.3X4-	T38.3X5-	T38.3X6-
Protease	T47.5X1-	T47.5X2-	T47.5X3-	T47.5X4-	T47.5X5-	T47.5X6-
Protectant, skin NEC	T49.3X1-	T49.3X2-	T49.3X3-	T49.3X4-	T49.3X5-	T49.3X6-
Protein hydrolysate	T50.991-	T50.992-	T50.993-	T50.994-	T50.995-	T50.996-
Prothiaden — *see* Dothiepin hydrochloride						
Prothionamide	T37.1X1-	T37.1X2-	T37.1X3-	T37.1X4-	T37.1X5-	T37.1X6-
Prothipendyl	T43.591-	T43.592-	T43.593-	T43.594-	T43.595-	T43.596-
Prothoate	T60.0X1-	T60.0X2-	T60.0X3-	T60.0X4-	-	-

Table of Drugs and Chemicals

Prazepam — Prothoate

Substance	Poisoning Accidental (unintentional)	Poisoning Intentional self-harm	Poisoning Assault	Poisoning Undetermined	Adverse effect	Underdosing
Prothrombin						
activator	T45.7X1-	T45.7X2-	T45.7X3-	T45.7X4-	T45.7X5-	T45.7X6-
synthesis inhibitor	T45.511-	T45.512-	T45.513-	T45.514-	T45.515-	T45.516-
Protionamide	T37.1X1-	T37.1X2-	T37.1X3-	T37.1X4-	T37.1X5-	T37.1X6-
Protirelin	T38.891-	T38.892-	T38.893-	T38.894-	T38.895-	T38.896-
Protokylol	T48.6X1-	T48.6X2-	T48.6X3-	T48.6X4-	T48.6X5-	T48.6X6-
Protopam	T50.6X1-	T50.6X2-	T50.6X3-	T50.6X4-	T50.6X5-	T50.6X6-
Protoveratrine (s) (A) (B)	T46.5X1-	T46.5X2-	T46.5X3-	T46.5X4-	T46.5X5-	T46.5X6-
Protriptyline	T43.011-	T43.012-	T43.013-	T43.014-	T43.015-	T43.016-
Provera	T38.5X1-	T38.5X2-	T38.5X3-	T38.5X4-	T38.5X5-	T38.5X6-
Provitamin A	T45.2X1-	T45.2X2-	T45.2X3-	T45.2X4-	T45.2X5-	T45.2X6-
Proxibarbal	T42.3X1-	T42.3X2-	T42.3X3-	T42.3X4-	T42.3X5-	T42.3X6-
Proxymetacaine	T41.3X1-	T41.3X2-	T41.3X3-	T41.3X4-	T41.3X5-	T41.3X6-
Proxyphylline	T48.6X1-	T48.6X2-	T48.6X3-	T48.6X4-	T48.6X5-	T48.6X6-
Prozac — *see* Fluoxetine hydrochloride						
Prunus						
laurocerasus	T62.2X1-	T62.2X2-	T62.2X3-	T62.2X4-	-	-
virginiana	T62.2X1-	T62.2X2-	T62.2X3-	T62.2X4-	-	-
Prussian blue						
commercial	T65.891-	T65.892-	T65.893-	T65.894-	-	-
therapeutic	T50.6X1-	T50.6X2-	T50.6X3-	T50.6X4-	T50.6X5-	T50.6X6-
Prussic acid	T65.0X1-	T65.0X2-	T65.0X3-	T65.0X4-	-	-
vapor	T57.3X1-	T57.3X2-	T57.3X3-	T57.3X4-	-	-
Pseudoephedrine	T44.991-	T44.992-	T44.993-	T44.994-	T44.995-	T44.996-
Psilocin	T40.991-	T40.992-	T40.993-	T40.994-	-	-
Psilocybin	T40.991-	T40.992-	T40.993-	T40.994-	-	-
Psilocybine	T40.991-	T40.992-	T40.993-	T40.994-	-	-
Psoralene (nonmedicinal)	T65.891-	T65.892-	T65.893-	T65.894-	-	-
Psoralens (medicinal)	T50.991-	T50.992-	T50.993-	T50.994-	T50.995-	T50.996-
PSP (phenolsulfonphthalein)	T50.8X1-	T50.8X2-	T50.8X3-	T50.8X4-	T50.8X5-	T50.8X6-
Psychodysleptic drug NEC	T40.901-	T40.902-	T40.903-	T40.904-	T40.905-	T40.906-
Psychostimulant	T43.601-	T43.602-	T43.603-	T43.604-	T43.605-	T43.606-
amphetamine	T43.621-	T43.622-	T43.623-	T43.624-	T43.625-	T43.626-
caffeine	T43.611-	T43.612-	T43.613-	T43.614-	T43.615-	T43.616-
methylphenidate	T43.631-	T43.632-	T43.633-	T43.634-	T43.635-	T43.636-
specified NEC	T43.691-	T43.692-	T43.693-	T43.694-	T43.695-	T43.696-
Psychotherapeutic drug NEC	T43.91X-	T43.92X-	T43.93X-	T43.94X-	T43.95X-	T43.96X-
antidepressants — *see also* Antidepressant	T43.201-	T43.202-	T43.203-	T43.204-	T43.205-	T43.206-
specified NEC	T43.8X1-	T43.8X2-	T43.8X3-	T43.8X4-	T43.8X5-	T43.8X6-
tranquilizers NEC	T43.501-	T43.502-	T43.503-	T43.504-	T43.505-	T43.506-
Psychotomimetic agents	T40.901-	T40.902-	T40.903-	T40.904-	T40.905-	T40.906-
Psychotropic drug NEC	T43.91X-	T43.92X-	T43.93X-	T43.94X-	T43.95X-	T43.96X-
specified NEC	T43.8X1-	T43.8X2-	T43.8X3-	T43.8X4-	T43.8X5-	T43.8X6-
Psyllium hydrophilic mucilloid	T47.4X1-	T47.4X2-	T47.4X3-	T47.4X4-	T47.4X5-	T47.4X6-
Pteroylglutamic acid	T45.8X1-	T45.8X2-	T45.8X3-	T45.8X4-	T45.8X5-	T45.8X6-
Pteroyltriglutamate	T45.1X1-	T45.1X2-	T45.1X3-	T45.1X4-	T45.1X5-	T45.1X6-
PTFE — *see* Polytetrafluoroethylene						
Pulp						
devitalizing paste	T49.7X1-	T49.7X2-	T49.7X3-	T49.7X4-	T49.7X5-	T49.7X6-
dressing	T49.7X1-	T49.7X2-	T49.7X3-	T49.7X4-	T49.7X5-	T49.7X6-
Pulsatilla	T62.2X1-	T62.2X2-	T62.2X3-	T62.2X4-	-	-
Pumpkin seed extract	T37.4X1-	T37.4X2-	T37.4X3-	T37.4X4-	T37.4X5-	T37.4X6-
Purex (bleach)	T54.91X-	T54.92X-	T54.93X-	T54.94X-	-	-
Purgative NEC — *see also* Cathartic	T47.4X1-	T47.4X2-	T47.4X3-	T47.4X4-	T47.4X5-	T47.4X6-
Purine analogue (antineoplastic)	T45.1X1-	T45.1X2-	T45.1X3-	T45.1X4-	T45.1X5-	T45.1X6-
Purine diuretics	T50.2X1-	T50.2X2-	T50.2X3-	T50.2X4-	T50.2X5-	T50.2X6-
Purinethol	T45.1X1-	T45.1X2-	T45.1X3-	T45.1X4-	T45.1X5-	T45.1X6-
PVP	T45.8X1-	T45.8X2-	T45.8X3-	T45.8X4-	T45.8X5-	T45.8X6-
Pyrabital	T39.8X1-	T39.8X2-	T39.8X3-	T39.8X4-	T39.8X5-	T39.8X6-
Pyramidon	T39.2X1-	T39.2X2-	T39.2X3-	T39.2X4-	T39.2X5-	T39.2X6-
Pyrantel	T37.4X1-	T37.4X2-	T37.4X3-	T37.4X4-	T37.4X5-	T37.4X6-
Pyrathiazine	T45.0X1-	T45.0X2-	T45.0X3-	T45.0X4-	T45.0X5-	T45.0X6-
Pyrazinamide	T37.1X1-	T37.1X2-	T37.1X3-	T37.1X4-	T37.1X5-	T37.1X6-
Pyrazinoic acid (amide)	T37.1X1-	T37.1X2-	T37.1X3-	T37.1X4-	T37.1X5-	T37.1X6-
Pyrazole (derivatives)	T39.2X1-	T39.2X2-	T39.2X3-	T39.2X4-	T39.2X5-	T39.2X6-
Pyrazolone analgesic NEC	T39.2X1-	T39.2X2-	T39.2X3-	T39.2X4-	T39.2X5-	T39.2X6-
Pyrethrin, pyrethrum (nonmedicinal)	T60.2X1-	T60.2X2-	T60.2X3-	T60.2X4-	-	-
Pyrethrum extract	T49.0X1-	T49.0X2-	T49.0X3-	T49.0X4-	T49.0X5-	T49.0X6-
Pyribenzamine	T45.0X1-	T45.0X2-	T45.0X3-	T45.0X4-	T45.0X5-	T45.0X6-
Pyridine	T52.8X1-	T52.8X2-	T52.8X3-	T52.8X4-	-	-
aldoxime methiodide	T50.6X1-	T50.6X2-	T50.6X3-	T50.6X4-	T50.6X5-	T50.6X6-
aldoxime methyl chloride	T50.6X1-	T50.6X2-	T50.6X3-	T50.6X4-	T50.6X5-	T50.6X6-
vapor	T59.891-	T59.892-	T59.893-	T59.894-	-	-
Pyridium	T39.8X1-	T39.8X2-	T39.8X3-	T39.8X4-	T39.8X5-	T39.8X6-
Pyridostigmine bromide	T44.0X1-	T44.0X2-	T44.0X3-	T44.0X4-	T44.0X5-	T44.0X6-
Pyridoxal phosphate	T45.2X1-	T45.2X2-	T45.2X3-	T45.2X4-	T45.2X5-	T45.2X6-
Pyridoxine	T45.2X1-	T45.2X2-	T45.2X3-	T45.2X4-	T45.2X5-	T45.2X6-
Pyrilamine	T45.0X1-	T45.0X2-	T45.0X3-	T45.0X4-	T45.0X5-	T45.0X6-
Pyrimethamine	T37.2X1-	T37.2X2-	T37.2X3-	T37.2X4-	T37.2X5-	T37.2X6-
with sulfadoxine	T37.2X1-	T37.2X2-	T37.2X3-	T37.2X4-	T37.2X5-	T37.2X6-
Pyrimidine antagonist	T45.1X1-	T45.1X2-	T45.1X3-	T45.1X4-	T45.1X5-	T45.1X6-
Pyriminil	T60.4X1-	T60.4X2-	T60.4X3-	T60.4X4-	-	-
Pyrithione zinc	T49.4X1-	T49.4X2-	T49.4X3-	T49.4X4-	T49.4X5-	T49.4X6-
Pyrithyldione	T42.6X1-	T42.6X2-	T42.6X3-	T42.6X4-	T42.6X5-	T42.6X6-
Pyrogallic acid	T49.0X1-	T49.0X2-	T49.0X3-	T49.0X4-	T49.0X5-	T49.0X6-
Pyrogallol	T49.0X1-	T49.0X2-	T49.0X3-	T49.0X4-	T49.0X5-	T49.0X6-
Pyroxylin	T49.3X1-	T49.3X2-	T49.3X3-	T49.3X4-	T49.3X5-	T49.3X6-
Pyrrobutamine	T45.0X1-	T45.0X2-	T45.0X3-	T45.0X4-	T45.0X5-	T45.0X6-
Pyrrolizidine alkaloids	T62.8X1-	T62.8X2-	T62.8X3-	T62.8X4-	-	-
Pyrvinium chloride	T37.4X1-	T37.4X2-	T37.4X3-	T37.4X4-	T37.4X5-	T37.4X6-
PZI	T38.3X1-	T38.3X2-	T38.3X3-	T38.3X4-	T38.3X5-	T38.3X6-
Quaalude	T42.6X1-	T42.6X2-	T42.6X3-	T42.6X4-	T42.6X5-	T42.6X6-
Quarternary ammonium						
anti-infective	T49.0X1-	T49.0X2-	T49.0X3-	T49.0X4-	T49.0X5-	T49.0X6-
ganglion blocking	T44.2X1-	T44.2X2-	T44.2X3-	T44.2X4-	T44.2X5-	T44.2X6-
parasympatholytic	T44.3X1-	T44.3X2-	T44.3X3-	T44.3X4-	T44.3X5-	T44.3X6-
Quazepam	T42.4X1-	T42.4X2-	T42.4X3-	T42.4X4-	T42.4X5-	T42.4X6-
Quicklime	T54.3X1-	T54.3X2-	T54.3X3-	T54.3X4-	-	-
Quillaja extract	T48.4X1-	T48.4X2-	T48.4X3-	T48.4X4-	T48.4X5-	T48.4X6-
Quinacrine	T37.2X1-	T37.2X2-	T37.2X3-	T37.2X4-	T37.2X5-	T37.2X6-
Quinaglute	T46.2X1-	T46.2X2-	T46.2X3-	T46.2X4-	T46.2X5-	T46.2X6-
Quinalbarbital	T42.3X1-	T42.3X2-	T42.3X3-	T42.3X4-	T42.3X5-	T42.3X6-
Quinalbarbitone sodium	T42.3X1-	T42.3X2-	T42.3X3-	T42.3X4-	T42.3X5-	T42.3X6-
Quinalphos	T60.0X1-	T60.0X2-	T60.0X3-	T60.0X4-	-	-
Quinapril	T46.4X1-	T46.4X2-	T46.4X3-	T46.4X4-	T46.4X5-	T46.4X6-
Quinestradiol	T38.5X1-	T38.5X2-	T38.5X3-	T38.5X4-	T38.5X5-	T38.5X6-
Quinestradol	T38.5X1-	T38.5X2-	T38.5X3-	T38.5X4-	T38.5X5-	T38.5X6-
Quinestrol	T38.5X1-	T38.5X2-	T38.5X3-	T38.5X4-	T38.5X5-	T38.5X6-
Quinethazone	T50.2X1-	T50.2X2-	T50.2X3-	T50.2X4-	T50.2X5-	T50.2X6-
Quingestanol	T38.4X1-	T38.4X2-	T38.4X3-	T38.4X4-	T38.4X5-	T38.4X6-
Quinidine	T46.2X1-	T46.2X2-	T46.2X3-	T46.2X4-	T46.2X5-	T46.2X6-
Quinine	T37.2X1-	T37.2X2-	T37.2X3-	T37.2X4-	T37.2X5-	T37.2X6-
Quiniobine	T37.8X1-	T37.8X2-	T37.8X3-	T37.8X4-	T37.8X5-	T37.8X6-
Quinisocaine	T49.1X1-	T49.1X2-	T49.1X3-	T49.1X4-	T49.1X5-	T49.1X6-
Quinocide	T37.2X1-	T37.2X2-	T37.2X3-	T37.2X4-	T37.2X5-	T37.2X6-
Quinoline (derivatives) **NEC**	T37.8X1-	T37.8X2-	T37.8X3-	T37.8X4-	T37.8X5-	T37.8X6-
Quinupramine	T43.011-	T43.012-	T43.013-	T43.014-	T43.015-	T43.016-
Quotane	T41.3X1-	T41.3X2-	T41.3X3-	T41.3X4-	T41.3X5-	T41.3X6-
Rabies						
immune globulin (human)	T50.Z11-	T50.Z12-	T50.Z13-	T50.Z14-	T50.Z15-	T50.Z16-
vaccine	T50.B91-	T50.B92-	T50.B93-	T50.B94-	T50.B95-	T50.B96-
Racemoramide	T40.2X1-	T40.2X2-	T40.2X3-	T40.2X4-	-	-
Racemorphan	T40.2X1-	T40.2X2-	T40.2X3-	T40.2X4-	T40.2X5-	T40.2X6-
Racepinefrin	T44.5X1-	T44.5X2-	T44.5X3-	T44.5X4-	T44.5X5-	T44.5X6-
Raclopride	T43.591-	T43.592-	T43.593-	T43.594-	T43.595-	T43.596-
Radiator alcohol	T51.1X1-	T51.1X2-	T51.1X3-	T51.1X4-	-	-
Radioactive drug NEC	T50.8X1-	T50.8X2-	T50.8X3-	T50.8X4-	T50.8X5-	T50.8X6-
Radio-opaque (drugs) (materials)	T50.8X1-	T50.8X2-	T50.8X3-	T50.8X4-	T50.8X5-	T50.8X6-
Ramifenazone	T39.2X1-	T39.2X2-	T39.2X3-	T39.2X4-	T39.2X5-	T39.2X6-
Ramipril	T46.4X1-	T46.4X2-	T46.4X3-	T46.4X4-	T46.4X5-	T46.4X6-
Ranitidine	T47.0X1-	T47.0X2-	T47.0X3-	T47.0X4-	T47.0X5-	T47.0X6-
Ranunculus	T62.2X1-	T62.2X2-	T62.2X3-	T62.2X4-	-	-
Rat poison NEC	T60.4X1-	T60.4X2-	T60.4X3-	T60.4X4-	-	-
Rattlesnake (venom)	T63.011-	T63.012-	T63.013-	T63.014-	-	-
Raubasine	T46.7X1-	T46.7X2-	T46.7X3-	T46.7X4-	T46.7X5-	T46.7X6-
Raudixin	T46.5X1-	T46.5X2-	T46.5X3-	T46.5X4-	T46.5X5-	T46.5X6-
Rautensin	T46.5X1-	T46.5X2-	T46.5X3-	T46.5X4-	T46.5X5-	T46.5X6-
Rautina	T46.5X1-	T46.5X2-	T46.5X3-	T46.5X4-	T46.5X5-	T46.5X6-
Rautotal	T46.5X1-	T46.5X2-	T46.5X3-	T46.5X4-	T46.5X5-	T46.5X6-
Rauwiloid	T46.5X1-	T46.5X2-	T46.5X3-	T46.5X4-	T46.5X5-	T46.5X6-
Rauwoldin	T46.5X1-	T46.5X2-	T46.5X3-	T46.5X4-	T46.5X5-	T46.5X6-
Rauwolfia (alkaloids)	T46.5X1-	T46.5X2-	T46.5X3-	T46.5X4-	T46.5X5-	T46.5X6-
Razoxane	T45.1X1-	T45.1X2-	T45.1X3-	T45.1X4-	T45.1X5-	T45.1X6-
Realgar	T57.0X1-	T57.0X2-	T57.0X3-	T57.0X4-	-	-
Recombinant (R) — *see* specific protein						
Red blood cells, packed	T45.8X1-	T45.8X2-	T45.8X3-	T45.8X4-	T45.8X5-	T45.8X6-
Red squill (scilliroside)	T60.4X1-	T60.4X2-	T60.4X3-	T60.4X4-	-	-
Reducing agent, industrial NEC	T65.891-	T65.892-	T65.893-	T65.894-	-	-

Substance	Poisoning Accidental (unintentional)	Poisoning Intentional self-harm	Poisoning Assault	Poisoning Undetermined	Adverse effect	Underdosing
Refrigerant gas (chlorofluoro-carbon)	T53.5X1-	T53.5X2-	T53.5X3-	T53.5X4-	-	-
not chlorofluoro-carbon	T59.891-	T59.892-	T59.893-	T59.894-	-	-
Regroton	T50.2X1-	T50.2X2-	T50.2X3-	T50.2X4-	T50.2X5-	T50.2X6-
Rehydration salts (oral)	T50.3X1-	T50.3X2-	T50.3X3-	T50.3X4-	T50.3X5-	T50.3X6-
Rela	T42.8X1-	T42.8X2-	T42.8X3-	T42.8X4-	T42.8X5-	T42.8X6-
Relaxant, muscle						
anesthetic	T48.1X1-	T48.1X2-	T48.1X3-	T48.1X4-	T48.1X5-	T48.1X6-
central nervous system	T42.8X1-	T42.8X2-	T42.8X3-	T42.8X4-	T42.8X5-	T42.8X6-
skeletal NEC	T48.1X1-	T48.1X2-	T48.1X3-	T48.1X4-	T48.1X5-	T48.1X6-
smooth NEC	T44.3X1-	T44.3X2-	T44.3X3-	T44.3X4-	T44.3X5-	T44.3X6-
Remoxipride	T43.591-	T43.592-	T43.593-	T43.594-	T43.595-	T43.596-
Renese	T50.2X1-	T50.2X2-	T50.2X3-	T50.2X4-	T50.2X5-	T50.2X6-
Renografin	T50.8X1-	T50.8X2-	T50.8X3-	T50.8X4-	T50.8X5-	T50.8X6-
Replacement solution	T50.3X1-	T50.3X2-	T50.3X3-	T50.3X4-	T50.3X5-	T50.3X6-
Reproterol	T48.6X1-	T48.6X2-	T48.6X3-	T48.6X4-	T48.6X5-	T48.6X6-
Rescinnamine	T46.5X1-	T46.5X2-	T46.5X3-	T46.5X4-	T46.5X5-	T46.5X6-
Reserpin (e)	T46.5X1-	T46.5X2-	T46.5X3-	T46.5X4-	T46.5X5-	T46.5X6-
Resorcin, resorcinol (nonmedicinal)	T65.891-	T65.892-	T65.893-	T65.894-	-	-
medicinal	T49.4X1-	T49.4X2-	T49.4X3-	T49.4X4-	T49.4X5-	T49.4X6-
Respaire	T48.4X1-	T48.4X2-	T48.4X3-	T48.4X4-	T48.4X5-	T48.4X6-
Respiratory drug NEC	T48.901-	T48.902-	T48.903-	T48.904-	T48.905-	T48.906-
antiasthmatic NEC	T48.6X1-	T48.6X2-	T48.6X3-	T48.6X4-	T48.6X5-	T48.6X6-
anti-common-cold NEC	T48.5X1-	T48.5X2-	T48.5X3-	T48.5X4-	T48.5X5-	T48.5X6-
expectorant NEC	T48.4X1-	T48.4X2-	T48.4X3-	T48.4X4-	T48.4X5-	T48.4X6-
stimulant	T48.901-	T48.902-	T48.903-	T48.904-	T48.905-	T48.906-
Retinoic acid	T49.0X1-	T49.0X2-	T49.0X3-	T49.0X4-	T49.0X5-	T49.0X6-
Retinol	T45.2X1-	T45.2X2-	T45.2X3-	T45.2X4-	T45.2X5-	T45.2X6-
Rh (D) **immune globulin** (human)	T50.Z11-	T50.Z12-	T50.Z13-	T50.Z14-	T50.Z15-	T50.Z16-
Rhodine	T39.011-	T39.012-	T39.013-	T39.014-	T39.015-	T39.016-
RhoGAM	T50.Z11-	T50.Z12-	T50.Z13-	T50.Z14-	T50.Z15-	T50.Z16-
Rhubarb						
dry extract	T47.2X1-	T47.2X2-	T47.2X3-	T47.2X4-	T47.2X5-	T47.2X6-
tincture, compound	T47.2X1-	T47.2X2-	T47.2X3-	T47.2X4-	T47.2X5-	T47.2X6-
Ribavirin	T37.5X1-	T37.5X2-	T37.5X3-	T37.5X4-	T37.5X5-	T37.5X6-
Riboflavin	T45.2X1-	T45.2X2-	T45.2X3-	T45.2X4-	T45.2X5-	T45.2X6-
Ribostamycin	T36.5X1-	T36.5X2-	T36.5X3-	T36.5X4-	T36.5X5-	T36.5X6-
Ricin	T62.2X1-	T62.2X2-	T62.2X3-	T62.2X4-	-	-
Ricinus communis	T62.2X1-	T62.2X2-	T62.2X3-	T62.2X4-	-	-
Rickettsial vaccine NEC	T50.A91-	T50.A92-	T50.A93-	T50.A94-	T50.A95-	T50.A96-
Rifabutin	T36.6X1-	T36.6X2-	T36.6X3-	T36.6X4-	T36.6X5-	T36.6X6-
Rifamide	T36.6X1-	T36.6X2-	T36.6X3-	T36.6X4-	T36.6X5-	T36.6X6-
Rifampicin	T36.6X1-	T36.6X2-	T36.6X3-	T36.6X4-	T36.6X5-	T36.6X6-
with isoniazid	T37.1X1-	T37.1X2-	T37.1X3-	T37.1X4-	T37.1X5-	T37.1X6-
Rifampin	T36.6X1-	T36.6X2-	T36.6X3-	T36.6X4-	T36.6X5-	T36.6X6-
Rifamycin	T36.6X1-	T36.6X2-	T36.6X3-	T36.6X4-	T36.6X5-	T36.6X6-
Rifaximin	T36.6X1-	T36.6X2-	T36.6X3-	T36.6X4-	T36.6X5-	T36.6X6-
Rimantadine	T37.5X1-	T37.5X2-	T37.5X3-	T37.5X4-	T37.5X5-	T37.5X6-
Rimazolium metilsulfate	T39.8X1-	T39.8X2-	T39.8X3-	T39.8X4-	T39.8X5-	T39.8X6-
Rimifon	T37.1X1-	T37.1X2-	T37.1X3-	T37.1X4-	T37.1X5-	T37.1X6-
Rimiterol	T48.6X1-	T48.6X2-	T48.6X3-	T48.6X4-	T48.6X5-	T48.6X6-
Ringer (lactate) **solution**	T50.3X1-	T50.3X2-	T50.3X3-	T50.3X4-	T50.3X5-	T50.3X6-
Ristocetin	T36.8X1-	T36.8X2-	T36.8X3-	T36.8X4-	T36.8X5-	T36.8X6-
Ritalin	T43.631-	T43.632-	T43.633-	T43.634-	T43.635-	T43.636-
Ritodrine	T44.5X1-	T44.5X2-	T44.5X3-	T44.5X4-	T44.5X5-	T44.5X6-
Roach killer — *see* Insecticide						
Rociverine	T44.3X1-	T44.3X2-	T44.3X3-	T44.3X4-	T44.3X5-	T44.3X6-
Rocky Mountain spotted fever vaccine	T50.A91-	T50.A92-	T50.A93-	T50.A94-	T50.A95-	T50.A96-
Rodenticide NEC	T60.4X1-	T60.4X2-	T60.4X3-	T60.4X4-	-	-
Rohypnol	T42.4X1-	T42.4X2-	T42.4X3-	T42.4X4-	T42.4X5-	T42.4X6-
Rokitamycin	T36.3X1-	T36.3X2-	T36.3X3-	T36.3X4-	T36.3X5-	T36.3X6-
Rolaids	T47.1X1-	T47.1X2-	T47.1X3-	T47.1X4-	T47.1X5-	T47.1X6-
Rolitetracycline	T36.4X1-	T36.4X2-	T36.4X3-	T36.4X4-	T36.4X5-	T36.4X6-
Romilar	T48.3X1-	T48.3X2-	T48.3X3-	T48.3X4-	T48.3X5-	T48.3X6-
Ronifibrate	T46.6X1-	T46.6X2-	T46.6X3-	T46.6X4-	T46.6X5-	T46.6X6-
Rosaprostol	T47.1X1-	T47.1X2-	T47.1X3-	T47.1X4-	T47.1X5-	T47.1X6-
Rose bengal sodium (131I)	T50.8X1-	T50.8X2-	T50.8X3-	T50.8X4-	T50.8X5-	T50.8X6-
Rose water ointment	T49.3X1-	T49.3X2-	T49.3X3-	T49.3X4-	T49.3X5-	T49.3X6-
Rosoxacin	T37.8X1-	T37.8X2-	T37.8X3-	T37.8X4-	T37.8X5-	T37.8X6-
Rotenone	T60.2X1-	T60.2X2-	T60.2X3-	T60.2X4-	-	-
Rotoxamine	T45.0X1-	T45.0X2-	T45.0X3-	T45.0X4-	T45.0X5-	T45.0X6-
Rough-on-rats	T60.4X1-	T60.4X2-	T60.4X3-	T60.4X4-	-	-
Roxatidine	T47.0X1-	T47.0X2-	T47.0X3-	T47.0X4-	T47.0X5-	T47.0X6-
Roxithromycin	T36.3X1-	T36.3X2-	T36.3X3-	T36.3X4-	T36.3X5-	T36.3X6-
Rt-PA	T45.611-	T45.612-	T45.613-	T45.614-	T45.615-	T45.616-
Rubbing alcohol	T51.2X1-	T51.2X2-	T51.2X3-	T51.2X4-	-	-
Rubefacient	T49.4X1-	T49.4X2-	T49.4X3-	T49.4X4-	T49.4X5-	T49.4X6-
Rubella vaccine	T50.B91-	T50.B92-	T50.B93-	T50.B94-	T50.B95-	T50.B96-
Rubeola vaccine	T50.B91-	T50.B92-	T50.B93-	T50.B94-	T50.B95-	T50.B96-
Rubidium chloride Rb82	T50.8X1-	T50.8X2-	T50.8X3-	T50.8X4-	T50.8X5-	T50.8X6-
Rubidomycin	T45.1X1-	T45.1X2-	T45.1X3-	T45.1X4-	T45.1X5-	T45.1X6-
Rue	T62.2X1-	T62.2X2-	T62.2X3-	T62.2X4-	-	-
Rufocromomycin	T45.1X1-	T45.1X2-	T45.1X3-	T45.1X4-	T45.1X5-	T45.1X6-
Russel's viper venin	T45.7X1-	T45.7X2-	T45.7X3-	T45.7X4-	T45.7X5-	T45.7X6-
Ruta (graveolens)	T62.2X1-	T62.2X2-	T62.2X3-	T62.2X4-	-	-
Rutinum	T46.991-	T46.992-	T46.993-	T46.994-	T46.995-	T46.996-
Rutoside	T46.991-	T46.992-	T46.993-	T46.994-	T46.995-	T46.996-
Sabadilla (plant)	T62.2X1-	T62.2X2-	T62.2X3-	T62.2X4-	-	-
pesticide	T60.2X1-	T60.2X2-	T60.2X3-	T60.2X4-	-	-
Saccharated iron oxide	T45.8X1-	T45.8X2-	T45.8X3-	T45.8X4-	T45.8X5-	T45.8X6-
Saccharin	T50.901-	T50.902-	T50.903-	T50.904-	T50.905-	T50.906-
Saccharomyces boulardii	T47.6X1-	T47.6X2-	T47.6X3-	T47.6X4-	T47.6X5-	T47.6X6-
Safflower oil	T46.6X1-	T46.6X2-	T46.6X3-	T46.6X4-	T46.6X5-	T46.6X6-
Safrazine	T43.1X1-	T43.1X2-	T43.1X3-	T43.1X4-	T43.1X5-	T43.1X6-
Salazosulfapyridine	T37.0X1-	T37.0X2-	T37.0X3-	T37.0X4-	T37.0X5-	T37.0X6-
Salbutamol	T48.6X1-	T48.6X2-	T48.6X3-	T48.6X4-	T48.6X5-	T48.6X6-
Salicylamide	T39.091-	T39.092-	T39.093-	T39.094-	T39.095-	T39.096-
Salicylate NEC	T39.091-	T39.092-	T39.093-	T39.094-	T39.095-	T39.096-
methyl	T49.3X1-	T49.3X2-	T49.3X3-	T49.3X4-	T49.3X5-	T49.3X6-
theobromine calcium	T50.2X1-	T50.2X2-	T50.2X3-	T50.2X4-	T50.2X5-	T50.2X6-
Salicylazosulfapyridine	T37.0X1-	T37.0X2-	T37.0X3-	T37.0X4-	T37.0X5-	T37.0X6-
Salicylhydroxamic acid	T49.0X1-	T49.0X2-	T49.0X3-	T49.0X4-	T49.0X5-	T49.0X6-
Salicylic acid	T49.4X1-	T49.4X2-	T49.4X3-	T49.4X4-	T49.4X5-	T49.4X6-
with benzoic acid	T49.4X1-	T49.4X2-	T49.4X3-	T49.4X4-	T49.4X5-	T49.4X6-
congeners	T39.091-	T39.092-	T39.093-	T39.094-	T39.095-	T39.096-
derivative	T39.091-	T39.092-	T39.093-	T39.094-	T39.095-	T39.096-
salts	T39.091-	T39.092-	T39.093-	T39.094-	T39.095-	T39.096-
Salinazid	T37.1X1-	T37.1X2-	T37.1X3-	T37.1X4-	T37.1X5-	T37.1X6-
Salmeterol	T48.6X1-	T48.6X2-	T48.6X3-	T48.6X4-	T48.6X5-	T48.6X6-
Salol	T49.3X1-	T49.3X2-	T49.3X3-	T49.3X4-	T49.3X5-	T49.3X6-
Salsalate	T39.091-	T39.092-	T39.093-	T39.094-	T39.095-	T39.096-
Salt substitute	T50.901-	T50.902-	T50.903-	T50.904-	T50.905-	T50.906-
Salt-replacing drug	T50.901-	T50.902-	T50.903-	T50.904-	T50.905-	T50.906-
Salt-retaining mineralocorticoid	T50.0X1-	T50.0X2-	T50.0X3-	T50.0X4-	T50.0X5-	T50.0X6-
Saluretic NEC	T50.2X1-	T50.2X2-	T50.2X3-	T50.2X4-	T50.2X5-	T50.2X6-
Saluron	T50.2X1-	T50.2X2-	T50.2X3-	T50.2X4-	T50.2X5-	T50.2X6-
Salvarsan 606 (neosilver) (silver)	T37.8X1-	T37.8X2-	T37.8X3-	T37.8X4-	T37.8X5-	T37.8X6-
Sambucus canadensis	T62.2X1-	T62.2X2-	T62.2X3-	T62.2X4-	-	-
berry	T62.1X1-	T62.1X2-	T62.1X3-	T62.1X4-	-	-
Sandril	T46.5X1-	T46.5X2-	T46.5X3-	T46.5X4-	T46.5X5-	T46.5X6-
Sanguinaria canadensis	T62.2X1-	T62.2X2-	T62.2X3-	T62.2X4-	-	-
Saniflush (cleaner)	T54.2X1-	T54.2X2-	T54.2X3-	T54.2X4-	-	-
Santonin	T37.4X1-	T37.4X2-	T37.4X3-	T37.4X4-	T37.4X5-	T37.4X6-
Santyl	T49.8X1-	T49.8X2-	T49.8X3-	T49.8X4-	T49.8X5-	T49.8X6-
Saralasin	T46.5X1-	T46.5X2-	T46.5X3-	T46.5X4-	T46.5X5-	T46.5X6-
Sarcolysin	T45.1X1-	T45.1X2-	T45.1X3-	T45.1X4-	T45.1X5-	T45.1X6-
Sarkomycin	T45.1X1-	T45.1X2-	T45.1X3-	T45.1X4-	T45.1X5-	T45.1X6-
Saroten	T43.011-	T43.012-	T43.013-	T43.014-	T43.015-	T43.016-
Saturnine — *see* Lead						
Savin (oil)	T49.4X1-	T49.4X2-	T49.4X3-	T49.4X4-	T49.4X5-	T49.4X6-
Scammony	T47.2X1-	T47.2X2-	T47.2X3-	T47.2X4-	T47.2X5-	T47.2X6-
Scarlet red	T49.8X1-	T49.8X2-	T49.8X3-	T49.8X4-	T49.8X5-	T49.8X6-
Scheele's green	T57.0X1-	T57.0X2-	T57.0X3-	T57.0X4-	-	-
insecticide	T57.0X1-	T57.0X2-	T57.0X3-	T57.0X4-	-	-
Schizontozide (blood) (tissue)	T37.2X1-	T37.2X2-	T37.2X3-	T37.2X4-	T37.2X5-	T37.2X6-
Schradan	T60.0X1-	T60.0X2-	T60.0X3-	T60.0X4-	-	-
Schweinfurth green	T57.0X1-	T57.0X2-	T57.0X3-	T57.0X4-	-	-
insecticide	T57.0X1-	T57.0X2-	T57.0X3-	T57.0X4-	-	-
Scilla, rat poison	T60.4X1-	T60.4X2-	T60.4X3-	T60.4X4-	-	-
Scillaren	T60.4X1-	T60.4X2-	T60.4X3-	T60.4X4-	-	-
Sclerosing agent	T46.8X1-	T46.8X2-	T46.8X3-	T46.8X4-	T46.8X5-	T46.8X6-
Scombrotoxin	T61.11X-	T61.12X-	T61.13X-	T61.14X-	-	-
Scopolamine	T44.3X1-	T44.3X2-	T44.3X3-	T44.3X4-	T44.3X5-	T44.3X6-
Scopolia extract	T44.3X1-	T44.3X2-	T44.3X3-	T44.3X4-	T44.3X5-	T44.3X6-
Scouring powder	T65.891-	T65.892-	T65.893-	T65.894-	-	-
Sea						
anemone (sting)	T63.631-	T63.632-	T63.633-	T63.634-	-	-
cucumber (sting)	T63.691-	T63.692-	T63.693-	T63.694-	-	-
snake (bite) (venom)	T63.091-	T63.092-	T63.093-	T63.094-	-	-
urchin spine (puncture)	T63.691-	T63.692-	T63.693-	T63.694-	-	-

Substance	Poisoning Accidental (unintentional)	Poisoning Intentional self-harm	Poisoning Assault	Poisoning Undetermined	Adverse effect	Underdosing
Seafood	T61.91X-	T61.92X-	T61.93X-	T61.94X-	-	-
specified NEC	T61.8X1-	T61.8X2-	T61.8X3-	T61.8X4-	-	-
Secbutabarbital	T42.3X1-	T42.3X2-	T42.3X3-	T42.3X4-	T42.3X5-	T42.3X6-
Secbutabarbitone	T42.3X1-	T42.3X2-	T42.3X3-	T42.3X4-	T42.3X5-	T42.3X6-
Secnidazole	T37.3X1-	T37.3X2-	T37.3X3-	T37.3X4-	T37.3X5-	T37.3X6-
Secobarbital	T42.3X1-	T42.3X2-	T42.3X3-	T42.3X4-	T42.3X5-	T42.3X6-
Seconal	T42.3X1-	T42.3X2-	T42.3X3-	T42.3X4-	T42.3X5-	T42.3X6-
Secretin	T50.8X1-	T50.8X2-	T50.8X3-	T50.8X4-	T50.8X5-	T50.8X6-
Sedative NEC	T42.71X-	T42.72X-	T42.73X-	T42.74X-	T42.75X-	T42.76X-
mixed NEC	T42.6X1-	T42.6X2-	T42.6X3-	T42.6X4-	T42.6X5-	T42.6X6-
Sedormid	T42.6X1-	T42.6X2-	T42.6X3-	T42.6X4-	T42.6X5-	T42.6X6-
Seed disinfectant or dressing	T60.8X1-	T60.8X2-	T60.8X3-	T60.8X4-	-	-
Seeds (poisonous)	T62.2X1-	T62.2X2-	T62.2X3-	T62.2X4-	-	-
Selegiline	T42.8X1-	T42.8X2-	T42.8X3-	T42.8X4-	T42.8X5-	T42.8X6-
Selenium NEC	T56.891-	T56.892-	T56.893-	T56.894-	-	-
disulfide or sulfide	T49.4X1-	T49.4X2-	T49.4X3-	T49.4X4-	T49.4X5-	T49.4X6-
fumes	T59.891-	T59.892-	T59.893-	T59.894-	-	-
sulfide	T49.4X1-	T49.4X2-	T49.4X3-	T49.4X4-	T49.4X5-	T49.4X6-
Selenomethionine (75Se)	T50.8X1-	T50.8X2-	T50.8X3-	T50.8X4-	T50.8X5-	T50.8X6-
Selsun	T49.4X1-	T49.4X2-	T49.4X3-	T49.4X4-	T49.4X5-	T49.4X6-
Semustine	T45.1X1-	T45.1X2-	T45.1X3-	T45.1X4-	T45.1X5-	T45.1X6-
Senega syrup	T48.4X1-	T48.4X2-	T48.4X3-	T48.4X4-	T48.4X5-	T48.4X6-
Senna	T47.2X1-	T47.2X2-	T47.2X3-	T47.2X4-	T47.2X5-	T47.2X6-
Sennoside A+B	T47.2X1-	T47.2X2-	T47.2X3-	T47.2X4-	T47.2X5-	T47.2X6-
Septisol	T49.2X1-	T49.2X2-	T49.2X3-	T49.2X4-	T49.2X5-	T49.2X6-
Seractide	T38.811-	T38.812-	T38.813-	T38.814-	T38.815-	T38.816-
Serax	T42.4X1-	T42.4X2-	T42.4X3-	T42.4X4-	T42.4X5-	T42.4X6-
Serenesil	T42.6X1-	T42.6X2-	T42.6X3-	T42.6X4-	T42.6X5-	T42.6X6-
Serenium (hydrochloride)	T37.91X-	T37.92X-	T37.93X-	T37.94X-	T37.95X-	T37.96X-
Serepax — *see* Oxazepam						
Sermorelin	T38.891-	T38.892-	T38.893-	T38.894-	T38.895-	T38.896-
Sernyl	T41.1X1-	T41.1X2-	T41.1X3-	T41.1X4-	T41.1X5-	T41.1X6-
Serotonin	T50.991-	T50.992-	T50.993-	T50.994-	T50.995-	T50.996-
Serpasil	T46.5X1-	T46.5X2-	T46.5X3-	T46.5X4-	T46.5X5-	T46.5X6-
Serrapeptase	T45.3X1-	T45.3X2-	T45.3X3-	T45.3X4-	T45.3X5-	T45.3X6-
Serum						
antibotulinus	T50.Z11-	T50.Z12-	T50.Z13-	T50.Z14-	T50.Z15-	T50.Z16-
anticytotoxic	T50.Z11-	T50.Z12-	T50.Z13-	T50.Z14-	T50.Z15-	T50.Z16-
antidiphtheria	T50.Z11-	T50.Z12-	T50.Z13-	T50.Z14-	T50.Z15-	T50.Z16-
antimeningococcus	T50.Z11-	T50.Z12-	T50.Z13-	T50.Z14-	T50.Z15-	T50.Z16-
anti-Rh	T50.Z11-	T50.Z12-	T50.Z13-	T50.Z14-	T50.Z15-	T50.Z16-
anti-snake-bite	T50.Z11-	T50.Z12-	T50.Z13-	T50.Z14-	T50.Z15-	T50.Z16-
antitetanic	T50.Z11-	T50.Z12-	T50.Z13-	T50.Z14-	T50.Z15-	T50.Z16-
antitoxic	T50.Z11-	T50.Z12-	T50.Z13-	T50.Z14-	T50.Z15-	T50.Z16-
complement (inhibitor)	T45.8X1-	T45.8X2-	T45.8X3-	T45.8X4-	T45.8X5-	T45.8X6-
convalescent	T50.Z11-	T50.Z12-	T50.Z13-	T50.Z14-	T50.Z15-	T50.Z16-
hemolytic complement	T45.8X1-	T45.8X2-	T45.8X3-	T45.8X4-	T45.8X5-	T45.8X6-
immune (human)	T50.Z11-	T50.Z12-	T50.Z13-	T50.Z14-	T50.Z15-	T50.Z16-
protective NEC	T50.Z11-	T50.Z12-	T50.Z13-	T50.Z14-	T50.Z15-	T50.Z16-
Setastine	T45.0X1-	T45.0X2-	T45.0X3-	T45.0X4-	T45.0X5-	T45.0X6-
Setoperone	T43.591-	T43.592-	T43.593-	T43.594-	T43.595-	T43.596-
Sewer gas	T59.91X-	T59.92X-	T59.93X-	T59.94X-	-	-
Shampoo	T55.0X1-	T55.0X2-	T55.0X3-	T55.0X4-	-	-
Shellfish, noxious, nonbacterial	T61.781-	T61.782-	T61.783-	T61.784-	-	-
Sildenafil	T46.7X1-	T46.7X2-	T46.7X3-	T46.7X4-	T46.7X5-	T46.7X6-
Silibinin	T50.991-	T50.992-	T50.993-	T50.994-	T50.995-	T50.996-
Silicone NEC	T65.891-	T65.892-	T65.893-	T65.894-	-	-
medicinal	T49.3X1-	T49.3X2-	T49.3X3-	T49.3X4-	T49.3X5-	T49.3X6-
Silvadene	T49.0X1-	T49.0X2-	T49.0X3-	T49.0X4-	T49.0X5-	T49.0X6-
Silver	T49.0X1-	T49.0X2-	T49.0X3-	T49.0X4-	T49.0X5-	T49.0X6-
anti-infectives	T49.0X1-	T49.0X2-	T49.0X3-	T49.0X4-	T49.0X5-	T49.0X6-
arsphenamine	T37.8X1-	T37.8X2-	T37.8X3-	T37.8X4-	T37.8X5-	T37.8X6-
colloidal	T49.0X1-	T49.0X2-	T49.0X3-	T49.0X4-	T49.0X5-	T49.0X6-
nitrate	T49.0X1-	T49.0X2-	T49.0X3-	T49.0X4-	T49.0X5-	T49.0X6-
ophthalmic preparation	T49.5X1-	T49.5X2-	T49.5X3-	T49.5X4-	T49.5X5-	T49.5X6-
toughened (keratolytic)	T49.4X1-	T49.4X2-	T49.4X3-	T49.4X4-	T49.4X5-	T49.4X6-
nonmedicinal (dust)	T56.891-	T56.892-	T56.893-	T56.894-	-	-
protein	T49.5X1-	T49.5X2-	T49.5X3-	T49.5X4-	T49.5X5-	T49.5X6-
salvarsan	T37.8X1-	T37.8X2-	T37.8X3-	T37.8X4-	T37.8X5-	T37.8X6-
sulfadiazine	T49.4X1-	T49.4X2-	T49.4X3-	T49.4X4-	T49.4X5-	T49.4X6-
Silymarin	T50.991-	T50.992-	T50.993-	T50.994-	T50.995-	T50.996-
Simaldrate	T47.1X1-	T47.1X2-	T47.1X3-	T47.1X4-	T47.1X5-	T47.1X6-
Simazine	T60.3X1-	T60.3X2-	T60.3X3-	T60.3X4-	-	-
Simethicone	T47.1X1-	T47.1X2-	T47.1X3-	T47.1X4-	T47.1X5-	T47.1X6-
Simfibrate	T46.6X1-	T46.6X2-	T46.6X3-	T46.6X4-	T46.6X5-	T46.6X6-
Simvastatin	T46.6X1-	T46.6X2-	T46.6X3-	T46.6X4-	T46.6X5-	T46.6X6-
Sincalide	T50.8X1-	T50.8X2-	T50.8X3-	T50.8X4-	T50.8X5-	T50.8X6-

Substance	Poisoning Accidental (unintentional)	Poisoning Intentional self-harm	Poisoning Assault	Poisoning Undetermined	Adverse effect	Underdosing
Sinequan	T43.011-	T43.012-	T43.013-	T43.014-	T43.015-	T43.016-
Singoserp	T46.5X1-	T46.5X2-	T46.5X3-	T46.5X4-	T46.5X5-	T46.5X6-
Sintrom	T45.511-	T45.512-	T45.513-	T45.514-	T45.515-	T45.516-
Sisomicin	T36.5X1-	T36.5X2-	T36.5X3-	T36.5X4-	T36.5X5-	T36.5X6-
Sitosterols	T46.6X1-	T46.6X2-	T46.6X3-	T46.6X4-	T46.6X5-	T46.6X6-
Skeletal muscle relaxants	T48.1X1-	T48.1X2-	T48.1X3-	T48.1X4-	T48.1X5-	T48.1X6-
Skin						
agents (external)	T49.91X-	T49.92X-	T49.93X-	T49.94X-	T49.95X-	T49.96X-
specified NEC	T49.8X1-	T49.8X2-	T49.8X3-	T49.8X4-	T49.8X5-	T49.8X6-
test antigen	T50.8X1-	T50.8X2-	T50.8X3-	T50.8X4-	T50.8X5-	T50.8X6-
Sleep-eze	T45.0X1-	T45.0X2-	T45.0X3-	T45.0X4-	T45.0X5-	T45.0X6-
Sleeping draught, pill	T42.71X-	T42.72X-	T42.73X-	T42.74X-	T42.75X-	T42.76X-
Smallpox vaccine	T50.B11-	T50.B12-	T50.B13-	T50.B14-	T50.B15-	T50.B16-
Smelter fumes NEC	T56.91X-	T56.92X-	T56.93X-	T56.94X-	-	-
Smog	T59.1X1-	T59.1X2-	T59.1X3-	T59.1X4-	-	-
Smoke NEC	T59.811-	T59.812-	T59.813-	T59.814-	-	-
Smooth muscle relaxant	T44.3X1-	T44.3X2-	T44.3X3-	T44.3X4-	T44.3X5-	T44.3X6-
Snail killer NEC	T60.8X1-	T60.8X2-	T60.8X3-	T60.8X4-	-	-
Snake venom or bite	T63.001-	T63.002-	T63.003-	T63.004-	-	-
hemocoagulase	T45.7X1-	T45.7X2-	T45.7X3-	T45.7X4-	T45.7X5-	T45.7X6-
Snuff	T65.211-	T65.212-	T65.213-	T65.214-	-	-
Soap (powder) (product)	T55.0X1-	T55.0X2-	T55.0X3-	T55.0X4-	-	-
enema	T47.4X1-	T47.4X2-	T47.4X3-	T47.4X4-	T47.4X5-	T47.4X6-
medicinal, soft	T49.2X1-	T49.2X2-	T49.2X3-	T49.2X4-	T49.2X5-	T49.2X6-
superfatted	T49.2X1-	T49.2X2-	T49.2X3-	T49.2X4-	T49.2X5-	T49.2X6-
Sobrerol	T48.4X1-	T48.4X2-	T48.4X3-	T48.4X4-	T48.4X5-	T48.4X6-
Soda (caustic)	T54.3X1-	T54.3X2-	T54.3X3-	T54.3X4-	-	-
bicarb	T47.1X1-	T47.1X2-	T47.1X3-	T47.1X4-	T47.1X5-	T47.1X6-
chlorinated — *see* Sodium, hypochlorite						
Sodium						
acetosulfone	T37.1X1-	T37.1X2-	T37.1X3-	T37.1X4-	T37.1X5-	T37.1X6-
acetrizoate	T50.8X1-	T50.8X2-	T50.8X3-	T50.8X4-	T50.8X5-	T50.8X6-
acid phosphate	T50.3X1-	T50.3X2-	T50.3X3-	T50.3X4-	T50.3X5-	T50.3X6-
alginate	T47.8X1-	T47.8X2-	T47.8X3-	T47.8X4-	T47.8X5-	T47.8X6-
amidotrizoate	T50.8X1-	T50.8X2-	T50.8X3-	T50.8X4-	T50.8X5-	T50.8X6-
aminopterin	T45.1X1-	T45.1X2-	T45.1X3-	T45.1X4-	T45.1X5-	T45.1X6-
amylosulfate	T47.8X1-	T47.8X2-	T47.8X3-	T47.8X4-	T47.8X5-	T47.8X6-
amytal	T42.3X1-	T42.3X2-	T42.3X3-	T42.3X4-	T42.3X5-	T42.3X6-
antimony gluconate	T37.3X1-	T37.3X2-	T37.3X3-	T37.3X4-	T37.3X5-	T37.3X6-
arsenate	T57.0X1-	T57.0X2-	T57.0X3-	T57.0X4-	-	-
aurothiomalate	T39.4X1-	T39.4X2-	T39.4X3-	T39.4X4-	T39.4X5-	T39.4X6-
aurothiosulfate	T39.4X1-	T39.4X2-	T39.4X3-	T39.4X4-	T39.4X5-	T39.4X6-
barbiturate	T42.3X1-	T42.3X2-	T42.3X3-	T42.3X4-	T42.3X5-	T42.3X6-
basic phosphate	T47.4X1-	T47.4X2-	T47.4X3-	T47.4X4-	T47.4X5-	T47.4X6-
bicarbonate	T47.1X1-	T47.1X2-	T47.1X3-	T47.1X4-	T47.1X5-	T47.1X6-
bichromate	T57.8X1-	T57.8X2-	T57.8X3-	T57.8X4-	-	-
biphosphate	T50.3X1-	T50.3X2-	T50.3X3-	T50.3X4-	T50.3X5-	T50.3X6-
bisulfate	T65.891-	T65.892-	T65.893-	T65.894-	-	-
borate						
cleanser	T57.8X1-	T57.8X2-	T57.8X3-	T57.8X4-	-	-
eye	T49.5X1-	T49.5X2-	T49.5X3-	T49.5X4-	T49.5X5-	T49.5X6-
therapeutic	T49.8X1-	T49.8X2-	T49.8X3-	T49.8X4-	T49.8X5-	T49.8X6-
bromide	T42.6X1-	T42.6X2-	T42.6X3-	T42.6X4-	T42.6X5-	T42.6X6-
cacodylate (nonmedicinal) NEC	T50.8X1-	T50.8X2-	T50.8X3-	T50.8X4-	T50.8X5-	T50.8X6-
anti-infective	T37.8X1-	T37.8X2-	T37.8X3-	T37.8X4-	T37.8X5-	T37.8X6-
herbicide	T60.3X1-	T60.3X2-	T60.3X3-	T60.3X4-	-	-
calcium edetate	T45.8X1-	T45.8X2-	T45.8X3-	T45.8X4-	T45.8X5-	T45.8X6-
carbonate NEC	T54.3X1-	T54.3X2-	T54.3X3-	T54.3X4-	-	-
chlorate NEC	T65.891-	T65.892-	T65.893-	T65.894-	-	-
herbicide	T54.91X-	T54.92X-	T54.93X-	T54.94X-	-	-
chloride	T50.3X1-	T50.3X2-	T50.3X3-	T50.3X4-	T50.3X5-	T50.3X6-
with glucose	T50.3X1-	T50.3X2-	T50.3X3-	T50.3X4-	T50.3X5-	T50.3X6-
chromate	T65.891-	T65.892-	T65.893-	T65.894-	-	-
citrate	T50.991-	T50.992-	T50.993-	T50.994-	T50.995-	T50.996-
cromoglicate	T48.6X1-	T48.6X2-	T48.6X3-	T48.6X4-	T48.6X5-	T48.6X6-
cyanide	T65.0X1-	T65.0X2-	T65.0X3-	T65.0X4-	-	-
cyclamate	T50.3X1-	T50.3X2-	T50.3X3-	T50.3X4-	T50.3X5-	T50.3X6-
dehydrocholate	T45.8X1-	T45.8X2-	T45.8X3-	T45.8X4-	T45.8X5-	T45.8X6-
diatrizoate	T50.8X1-	T50.8X2-	T50.8X3-	T50.8X4-	T50.8X5-	T50.8X6-
dibunate	T48.4X1-	T48.4X2-	T48.4X3-	T48.4X4-	T48.4X5-	T48.4X6-
dioctyl sulfosuccinate	T47.4X1-	T47.4X2-	T47.4X3-	T47.4X4-	T47.4X5-	T47.4X6-
dipantoyl ferrate	T45.8X1-	T45.8X2-	T45.8X3-	T45.8X4-	T45.8X5-	T45.8X6-
edetate	T45.8X1-	T45.8X2-	T45.8X3-	T45.8X4-	T45.8X5-	T45.8X6-
ethacrynate	T50.1X1-	T50.1X2-	T50.1X3-	T50.1X4-	T50.1X5-	T50.1X6-
feredetate	T45.8X1-	T45.8X2-	T45.8X3-	T45.8X4-	T45.8X5-	T45.8X6-
Fluoride — *see* Fluoride						

Substance	Poisoning Accidental (unintentional)	Poisoning Intentional self-harm	Poisoning Assault	Poisoning Undetermined	Adverse effect	Underdosing
Sodium *- continued*						
fluoroacetate (dust) (pesticide)	T60.4X1-	T60.4X2-	T60.4X3-	T60.4X4-	-	-
free salt	T50.3X1-	T50.3X2-	T50.3X3-	T50.3X4-	T50.3X5-	T50.3X6-
fusidate	T36.8X1-	T36.8X2-	T36.8X3-	T36.8X4-	T36.8X5-	T36.8X6-
glucaldrate	T47.1X1-	T47.1X2-	T47.1X3-	T47.1X4-	T47.1X5-	T47.1X6-
glucosulfone	T37.1X1-	T37.1X2-	T37.1X3-	T37.1X4-	T37.1X5-	T37.1X6-
glutamate	T45.8X1-	T45.8X2-	T45.8X3-	T45.8X4-	T45.8X5-	T45.8X6-
hydrogen carbonate	T50.3X1-	T50.3X2-	T50.3X3-	T50.3X4-	T50.3X5-	T50.3X6-
hydroxide	T54.3X1-	T54.3X2-	T54.3X3-	T54.3X4-	-	-
hypochlorite (bleach) NEC	T54.3X1-	T54.3X2-	T54.3X3-	T54.3X4-	-	-
disinfectant	T54.3X1-	T54.3X2-	T54.3X3-	T54.3X4-	-	-
medicinal (anti-infective) (external)	T49.0X1-	T49.0X2-	T49.0X3-	T49.0X4-	T49.0X5-	T49.0X6-
vapor	T54.3X1-	T54.3X2-	T54.3X3-	T54.3X4-	-	-
hyposulfite	T49.0X1-	T49.0X2-	T49.0X3-	T49.0X4-	T49.0X5-	T49.0X6-
indigotin disulfonate	T50.8X1-	T50.8X2-	T50.8X3-	T50.8X4-	T50.8X5-	T50.8X6-
iodide	T50.991-	T50.992-	T50.993-	T50.994-	T50.995-	T50.996-
I-131	T50.8X1-	T50.8X2-	T50.8X3-	T50.8X4-	T50.8X5-	T50.8X6-
therapeutic	T38.2X1-	T38.2X2-	T38.2X3-	T38.2X4-	T38.2X5-	T38.2X6-
iodohippurate (131I)	T50.8X1-	T50.8X2-	T50.8X3-	T50.8X4-	T50.8X5-	T50.8X6-
iopodate	T50.8X1-	T50.8X2-	T50.8X3-	T50.8X4-	T50.8X5-	T50.8X6-
iothalamate	T50.8X1-	T50.8X2-	T50.8X3-	T50.8X4-	T50.8X5-	T50.8X6-
iron edetate	T45.4X1-	T45.4X2-	T45.4X3-	T45.4X4-	T45.4X5-	T45.4X6-
lactate (compound solution)	T45.8X1-	T45.8X2-	T45.8X3-	T45.8X4-	T45.8X5-	T45.8X6-
lauryl (sulfate)	T49.2X1-	T49.2X2-	T49.2X3-	T49.2X4-	T49.2X5-	T49.2X6-
L-triiodothyronine	T38.1X1-	T38.1X2-	T38.1X3-	T38.1X4-	T38.1X5-	T38.1X6-
magnesium citrate	T50.991-	T50.992-	T50.993-	T50.994-	T50.995-	T50.996-
mersalate	T50.2X1-	T50.2X2-	T50.2X3-	T50.2X4-	T50.2X5-	T50.2X6-
metasilicate	T65.891-	T65.892-	T65.893-	T65.894-	-	-
metrizoate	T50.8X1-	T50.8X2-	T50.8X3-	T50.8X4-	T50.8X5-	T50.8X6-
monofluoroacetate (pesticide)	T60.1X1-	T60.1X2-	T60.1X3-	T60.1X4-	-	-
morrhuate	T46.8X1-	T46.8X2-	T46.8X3-	T46.8X4-	T46.8X5-	T46.8X6-
nafcillin	T36.0X1-	T36.0X2-	T36.0X3-	T36.0X4-	T36.0X5-	T36.0X6-
nitrate (oxidizing agent)	T65.891-	T65.892-	T65.893-	T65.894-	-	-
nitrite	T50.6X1-	T50.6X2-	T50.6X3-	T50.6X4-	T50.6X5-	T50.6X6-
nitroferricyanide	T46.5X1-	T46.5X2-	T46.5X3-	T46.5X4-	T46.5X5-	T46.5X6-
nitroprusside	T46.5X1-	T46.5X2-	T46.5X3-	T46.5X4-	T46.5X5-	T46.5X6-
oxalate	T65.891-	T65.892-	T65.893-	T65.894-	-	-
oxide/peroxide	T65.891-	T65.892-	T65.893-	T65.894-	-	-
oxybate	T41.291-	T41.292-	T41.293-	T41.294-	T41.295-	T41.296-
para-aminohippurate	T50.8X1-	T50.8X2-	T50.8X3-	T50.8X4-	T50.8X5-	T50.8X6-
perborate (nonmedicinal) NEC	T65.891-	T65.892-	T65.893-	T65.894-	-	-
medicinal	T49.0X1-	T49.0X2-	T49.0X3-	T49.0X4-	T49.0X5-	T49.0X6-
soap	T55.0X1-	T55.0X2-	T55.0X3-	T55.0X4-	-	-
percarbonate — *see* Sodium, perborate						
pertechnetate Tc99m	T50.8X1-	T50.8X2-	T50.8X3-	T50.8X4-	T50.8X5-	T50.8X6-
phosphate						
cellulose	T45.8X1-	T45.8X2-	T45.8X3-	T45.8X4-	T45.8X5-	T45.8X6-
dibasic	T47.2X1-	T47.2X2-	T47.2X3-	T47.2X4-	T47.2X5-	T47.2X6-
monobasic	T47.2X1-	T47.2X2-	T47.2X3-	T47.2X4-	T47.2X5-	T47.2X6-
phytate	T50.6X1-	T50.6X2-	T50.6X3-	T50.6X4-	T50.6X5-	T50.6X6-
picosulfate	T47.2X1-	T47.2X2-	T47.2X3-	T47.2X4-	T47.2X5-	T47.2X6-
polyhydroxyaluminium monocarbonate	T47.1X1-	T47.1X2-	T47.1X3-	T47.1X4-	T47.1X5-	T47.1X6-
polystyrene sulfonate	T50.3X1-	T50.3X2-	T50.3X3-	T50.3X4-	T50.3X5-	T50.3X6-
propionate	T49.0X1-	T49.0X2-	T49.0X3-	T49.0X4-	T49.0X5-	T49.0X6-
propyl hydroxybenzoate	T50.991-	T50.992-	T50.993-	T50.994-	T50.995-	T50.996-
psylliate	T46.8X1-	T46.8X2-	T46.8X3-	T46.8X4-	T46.8X5-	T46.8X6-
removing resins	T50.3X1-	T50.3X2-	T50.3X3-	T50.3X4-	T50.3X5-	T50.3X6-
salicylate	T39.091-	T39.092-	T39.093-	T39.094-	T39.095-	T39.096-
salt NEC	T50.3X1-	T50.3X2-	T50.3X3-	T50.3X4-	T50.3X5-	T50.3X6-
selenate	T60.2X1-	T60.2X2-	T60.2X3-	T60.2X4-	-	-
stibogluconate	T37.3X1-	T37.3X2-	T37.3X3-	T37.3X4-	T37.3X5-	T37.3X6-
sulfate	T47.4X1-	T47.4X2-	T47.4X3-	T47.4X4-	T47.4X5-	T47.4X6-
sulfoxone	T37.1X1-	T37.1X2-	T37.1X3-	T37.1X4-	T37.1X5-	T37.1X6-
tetradecyl sulfate	T46.8X1-	T46.8X2-	T46.8X3-	T46.8X4-	T46.8X5-	T46.8X6-
thiopental	T41.1X1-	T41.1X2-	T41.1X3-	T41.1X4-	T41.1X5-	T41.1X6-
thiosalicylate	T39.091-	T39.092-	T39.093-	T39.094-	T39.095-	T39.096-
thiosulfate	T50.6X1-	T50.6X2-	T50.6X3-	T50.6X4-	T50.6X5-	T50.6X6-
tolbutamide	T38.3X1-	T38.3X2-	T38.3X3-	T38.3X4-	T38.3X5-	T38.3X6-
(L) -triiodothyronine	T38.1X1-	T38.1X2-	T38.1X3-	T38.1X4-	T38.1X5-	T38.1X6-
tyropanoate	T50.8X1-	T50.8X2-	T50.8X3-	T50.8X4-	T50.8X5-	T50.8X6-
valproate	T42.6X1-	T42.6X2-	T42.6X3-	T42.6X4-	T42.6X5-	T42.6X6-
versenate	T50.6X1-	T50.6X2-	T50.6X3-	T50.6X4-	T50.6X5-	T50.6X6-
Sodium-free salt	T50.901-	T50.902-	T50.903-	T50.904-	T50.905-	T50.906-
Sodium-removing resin	T50.3X1-	T50.3X2-	T50.3X3-	T50.3X4-	T50.3X5-	T50.3X6-
Soft soap	T55.0X1-	T55.0X2-	T55.0X3-	T55.0X4-	-	-

Substance	Poisoning Accidental (unintentional)	Poisoning Intentional self-harm	Poisoning Assault	Poisoning Undetermined	Adverse effect	Underdosing
Solanine	T62.2X1-	T62.2X2-	T62.2X3-	T62.2X4-	-	-
berries	T62.1X1-	T62.1X2-	T62.1X3-	T62.1X4-	-	-
Solanum dulcamara	T62.2X1-	T62.2X2-	T62.2X3-	T62.2X4-	-	-
berries	T62.1X1-	T62.1X2-	T62.1X3-	T62.1X4-	-	-
Solapsone	T37.1X1-	T37.1X2-	T37.1X3-	T37.1X4-	T37.1X5-	T37.1X6-
Solar lotion	T49.3X1-	T49.3X2-	T49.3X3-	T49.3X4-	T49.3X5-	T49.3X6-
Solasulfone	T37.1X1-	T37.1X2-	T37.1X3-	T37.1X4-	T37.1X5-	T37.1X6-
Soldering fluid	T65.891-	T65.892-	T65.893-	T65.894-	-	-
Solid substance	T65.91X-	T65.92X-	T65.93X-	T65.94X-	-	-
specified NEC	T65.891-	T65.892-	T65.893-	T65.894-	-	-
Solvent, industrial NEC	T52.91X-	T52.92X-	T52.93X-	T52.94X-	-	-
naphtha	T52.0X1-	T52.0X2-	T52.0X3-	T52.0X4-	-	-
petroleum	T52.0X1-	T52.0X2-	T52.0X3-	T52.0X4-	-	-
specified NEC	T52.8X1-	T52.8X2-	T52.8X3-	T52.8X4-	-	-
Soma	T42.8X1-	T42.8X2-	T42.8X3-	T42.8X4-	T42.8X5-	T42.8X6-
Somatorelin	T38.891-	T38.892-	T38.893-	T38.894-	T38.895-	T38.896-
Somatostatin	T38.991-	T38.992-	T38.993-	T38.994-	T38.995-	T38.996-
Somatotropin	T38.811-	T38.812-	T38.813-	T38.814-	T38.815-	T38.816-
Somatrem	T38.811-	T38.812-	T38.813-	T38.814-	T38.815-	T38.816-
Somatropin	T38.811-	T38.812-	T38.813-	T38.814-	T38.815-	T38.816-
Sominex	T45.0X1-	T45.0X2-	T45.0X3-	T45.0X4-	T45.0X5-	T45.0X6-
Somnos	T42.6X1-	T42.6X2-	T42.6X3-	T42.6X4-	T42.6X5-	T42.6X6-
Somonal	T42.3X1-	T42.3X2-	T42.3X3-	T42.3X4-	T42.3X5-	T42.3X6-
Soneryl	T42.3X1-	T42.3X2-	T42.3X3-	T42.3X4-	T42.3X5-	T42.3X6-
Soothing syrup	T50.901-	T50.902-	T50.903-	T50.904-	T50.905-	T50.906-
Sopor	T42.6X1-	T42.6X2-	T42.6X3-	T42.6X4-	T42.6X5-	T42.6X6-
Soporific	T42.71X-	T42.72X-	T42.73X-	T42.74X-	T42.75X-	T42.76X-
Soporific drug	T42.71X-	T42.72X-	T42.73X-	T42.74X-	T42.75X-	T42.76X-
specified type NEC	T42.6X1-	T42.6X2-	T42.6X3-	T42.6X4-	T42.6X5-	T42.6X6-
Sorbide nitrate	T46.3X1-	T46.3X2-	T46.3X3-	T46.3X4-	T46.3X5-	T46.3X6-
Sorbitol	T47.4X1-	T47.4X2-	T47.4X3-	T47.4X4-	T47.4X5-	T47.4X6-
Sotalol	T44.7X1-	T44.7X2-	T44.7X3-	T44.7X4-	T44.7X5-	T44.7X6-
Sotradecol	T46.8X1-	T46.8X2-	T46.8X3-	T46.8X4-	T46.8X5-	T46.8X6-
Soysterol	T46.6X1-	T46.6X2-	T46.6X3-	T46.6X4-	T46.6X5-	T46.6X6-
Spacoline	T44.3X1-	T44.3X2-	T44.3X3-	T44.3X4-	T44.3X5-	T44.3X6-
Spanish fly	T49.8X1-	T49.8X2-	T49.8X3-	T49.8X4-	T49.8X5-	T49.8X6-
Sparine	T43.3X1-	T43.3X2-	T43.3X3-	T43.3X4-	T43.3X5-	T43.3X6-
Sparteine	T48.0X1-	T48.0X2-	T48.0X3-	T48.0X4-	T48.0X5-	T48.0X6-
Spasmolytic						
anticholinergics	T44.3X1-	T44.3X2-	T44.3X3-	T44.3X4-	T44.3X5-	T44.3X6-
autonomic	T44.3X1-	T44.3X2-	T44.3X3-	T44.3X4-	T44.3X5-	T44.3X6-
bronchial NEC	T48.6X1-	T48.6X2-	T48.6X3-	T48.6X4-	T48.6X5-	T48.6X6-
quaternary ammonium	T44.3X1-	T44.3X2-	T44.3X3-	T44.3X4-	T44.3X5-	T44.3X6-
skeletal muscle NEC	T48.1X1-	T48.1X2-	T48.1X3-	T48.1X4-	T48.1X5-	T48.1X6-
Spectinomycin	T36.5X1-	T36.5X2-	T36.5X3-	T36.5X4-	T36.5X5-	T36.5X6-
Speed	T43.621-	T43.622-	T43.623-	T43.624-	T43.625-	T43.626-
Spermicide	T49.8X1-	T49.8X2-	T49.8X3-	T49.8X4-	T49.8X5-	T49.8X6-
Spider (bite) (venom)	T63.391-	T63.392-	T63.393-	T63.394-	-	-
antivenin	T50.Z11-	T50.Z12-	T50.Z13-	T50.Z14-	T50.Z15-	T50.Z16-
Spigelia (root)	T37.4X1-	T37.4X2-	T37.4X3-	T37.4X4-	T37.4X5-	T37.4X6-
Spindle inactivator	T50.4X1-	T50.4X2-	T50.4X3-	T50.4X4-	T50.4X5-	T50.4X6-
Spiperone	T43.4X1-	T43.4X2-	T43.4X3-	T43.4X4-	T43.4X5-	T43.4X6-
Spiramycin	T36.3X1-	T36.3X2-	T36.3X3-	T36.3X4-	T36.3X5-	T36.3X6-
Spirapril	T46.4X1-	T46.4X2-	T46.4X3-	T46.4X4-	T46.4X5-	T46.4X6-
Spirilene	T43.591-	T43.592-	T43.593-	T43.594-	T43.595-	T43.596-
Spirit (s) (neutral) **NEC**	T51.0X1-	T51.0X2-	T51.0X3-	T51.0X4-	-	-
beverage	T51.0X1-	T51.0X2-	T51.0X3-	T51.0X4-	-	-
industrial	T51.0X1-	T51.0X2-	T51.0X3-	T51.0X4-	-	-
mineral	T52.0X1-	T52.0X2-	T52.0X3-	T52.0X4-	-	-
of salt — *see* Hydrochloric acid						
surgical	T51.0X1-	T51.0X2-	T51.0X3-	T51.0X4-	-	-
Spironolactone	T50.0X1-	T50.0X2-	T50.0X3-	T50.0X4-	T50.0X5-	T50.0X6-
Spiroperidol	T43.4X1-	T43.4X2-	T43.4X3-	T43.4X4-	T43.4X5-	T43.4X6-
Sponge, absorbable (gelatin)	T45.7X1-	T45.7X2-	T45.7X3-	T45.7X4-	T45.7X5-	T45.7X6-
Sporostacin	T49.0X1-	T49.0X2-	T49.0X3-	T49.0X4-	T49.0X5-	T49.0X6-
Spray (aerosol)	T65.91X-	T65.92X-	T65.93X-	T65.94X-	-	-
cosmetic	T65.891-	T65.892-	T65.893-	T65.894-	-	-
medicinal NEC	T50.901-	T50.902-	T50.903-	T50.904-	T50.905-	T50.906-
pesticides — *see* Pesticides						
specified content — *see* specific substance						
Spurge flax	T62.2X1-	T62.2X2-	T62.2X3-	T62.2X4-	-	-
Spurges	T62.2X1-	T62.2X2-	T62.2X3-	T62.2X4-	-	-
Sputum viscosity-lowering drug	T48.4X1-	T48.4X2-	T48.4X3-	T48.4X4-	T48.4X5-	T48.4X6-
Squill	T46.0X1-	T46.0X2-	T46.0X3-	T46.0X4-	T46.0X5-	T46.0X6-
rat poison	T60.4X1-	T60.4X2-	T60.4X3-	T60.4X4-	-	-
Squirting cucumber (cathartic)	T47.2X1-	T47.2X2-	T47.2X3-	T47.2X4-	T47.2X5-	T47.2X6-

Substance	Poisoning Accidental (unintentional)	Poisoning Intentional self-harm	Poisoning Assault	Poisoning Undetermined	Adverse effect	Underdosing
Stains	T65.6X1-	T65.6X2-	T65.6X3-	T65.6X4-	-	-
Stannous fluoride	T49.7X1-	T49.7X2-	T49.7X3-	T49.7X4-	T49.7X5-	T49.7X6-
Stanolone	T38.7X1-	T38.7X2-	T38.7X3-	T38.7X4-	T38.7X5-	T38.7X6-
Stanozolol	T38.7X1-	T38.7X2-	T38.7X3-	T38.7X4-	T38.7X5-	T38.7X6-
Staphisagria or stavesacre (pediculicide)	T49.0X1-	T49.0X2-	T49.0X3-	T49.0X4-	T49.0X5-	T49.0X6-
Starch	T50.901-	T50.902-	T50.903-	T50.904-	T50.905-	T50.906-
Stelazine	T43.3X1-	T43.3X2-	T43.3X3-	T43.3X4-	T43.3X5-	T43.3X6-
Stemetil	T43.3X1-	T43.3X2-	T43.3X3-	T43.3X4-	T43.3X5-	T43.3X6-
Stepronin	T48.4X1-	T48.4X2-	T48.4X3-	T48.4X4-	T48.4X5-	T48.4X6-
Sterculia	T47.4X1-	T47.4X2-	T47.4X3-	T47.4X4-	T47.4X5-	T47.4X6-
Sternutator gas	T59.891-	T59.892-	T59.893-	T59.894-	-	-
Steroid	T38.0X1-	T38.0X2-	T38.0X3-	T38.0X4-	T38.0X5-	T38.0X6-
anabolic	T38.7X1-	T38.7X2-	T38.7X3-	T38.7X4-	T38.7X5-	T38.7X6-
androgenic	T38.7X1-	T38.7X2-	T38.7X3-	T38.7X4-	T38.7X5-	T38.7X6-
antineoplastic, hormone	T38.7X1-	T38.7X2-	T38.7X3-	T38.7X4-	T38.7X5-	T38.7X6-
estrogen	T38.5X1-	T38.5X2-	T38.5X3-	T38.5X4-	T38.5X5-	T38.5X6-
ENT agent	T49.6X1-	T49.6X2-	T49.6X3-	T49.6X4-	T49.6X5-	T49.6X6-
ophthalmic preparation	T49.5X1-	T49.5X2-	T49.5X3-	T49.5X4-	T49.5X5-	T49.5X6-
topical NEC	T49.0X1-	T49.0X2-	T49.0X3-	T49.0X4-	T49.0X5-	T49.0X6-
Stibine	T56.891-	T56.892-	T56.893-	T56.894-	-	-
Stibogluconate	T37.3X1-	T37.3X2-	T37.3X3-	T37.3X4-	T37.3X5-	T37.3X6-
Stibophen	T37.4X1-	T37.4X2-	T37.4X3-	T37.4X4-	T37.4X5-	T37.4X6-
Stilbamidine (isetionate)	T37.3X1-	T37.3X2-	T37.3X3-	T37.3X4-	T37.3X5-	T37.3X6-
Stilbestrol	T38.5X1-	T38.5X2-	T38.5X3-	T38.5X4-	T38.5X5-	T38.5X6-
Stilboestrol	T38.5X1-	T38.5X2-	T38.5X3-	T38.5X4-	T38.5X5-	T38.5X6-
Stimulant						
central nervous system — *see also* Psychostimulant	T43.601-	T43.602-	T43.603-	T43.604-	T43.605-	T43.606-
analeptics	T50.7X1-	T50.7X2-	T50.7X3-	T50.7X4-	T50.7X5-	T50.7X6-
opiate antagonist	T50.7X1-	T50.7X2-	T50.7X3-	T50.7X4-	T50.7X5-	T50.7X6-
psychotherapeutic NEC — *see also* Psychotherapeutic drug	T43.601-	T43.602-	T43.603-	T43.604-	T43.605-	T43.606-
specified NEC	T43.691-	T43.692-	T43.693-	T43.694-	T43.695-	T43.696-
respiratory	T48.901-	T48.902-	T48.903-	T48.904-	T48.905-	T48.906-
Stone-dissolving drug	T50.901-	T50.902-	T50.903-	T50.904-	T50.905-	T50.906-
Storage battery (cells) (acid)	T54.2X1-	T54.2X2-	T54.2X3-	T54.2X4-	-	-
Stovaine	T41.3X1-	T41.3X2-	T41.3X3-	T41.3X4-	T41.3X5-	T41.3X6-
infiltration (subcutaneous)	T41.3X1-	T41.3X2-	T41.3X3-	T41.3X4-	T41.3X5-	T41.3X6-
nerve block (peripheral) (plexus)	T41.3X1-	T41.3X2-	T41.3X3-	T41.3X4-	T41.3X5-	T41.3X6-
spinal	T41.3X1-	T41.3X2-	T41.3X3-	T41.3X4-	T41.3X5-	T41.3X6-
topical (surface)	T41.3X1-	T41.3X2-	T41.3X3-	T41.3X4-	T41.3X5-	T41.3X6-
Stovarsal	T37.8X1-	T37.8X2-	T37.8X3-	T37.8X4-	T37.8X5-	T37.8X6-
Stove gas — *see* Gas, stove						
Stoxil	T49.5X1-	T49.5X2-	T49.5X3-	T49.5X4-	T49.5X5-	T49.5X6-
Stramonium	T48.6X1-	T48.6X2-	T48.6X3-	T48.6X4-	T48.6X5-	T48.6X6-
natural state	T62.2X1-	T62.2X2-	T62.2X3-	T62.2X4-	-	-
Streptodornase	T45.3X1-	T45.3X2-	T45.3X3-	T45.3X4-	T45.3X5-	T45.3X6-
Streptoduocin	T36.5X1-	T36.5X2-	T36.5X3-	T36.5X4-	T36.5X5-	T36.5X6-
Streptokinase	T45.611-	T45.612-	T45.613-	T45.614-	T45.615-	T45.616-
Streptomycin (derivative)	T36.5X1-	T36.5X2-	T36.5X3-	T36.5X4-	T36.5X5-	T36.5X6-
Streptonivicin	T36.5X1-	T36.5X2-	T36.5X3-	T36.5X4-	T36.5X5-	T36.5X6-
Streptovarycin	T36.5X1-	T36.5X2-	T36.5X3-	T36.5X4-	T36.5X5-	T36.5X6-
Streptozocin	T45.1X1-	T45.1X2-	T45.1X3-	T45.1X4-	T45.1X5-	T45.1X6-
Streptozotocin	T45.1X1-	T45.1X2-	T45.1X3-	T45.1X4-	T45.1X5-	T45.1X6-
Stripper (paint) (solvent)	T52.8X1-	T52.8X2-	T52.8X3-	T52.8X4-	-	-
Strobane	T60.1X1-	T60.1X2-	T60.1X3-	T60.1X4-	-	-
Strofantina	T46.0X1-	T46.0X2-	T46.0X3-	T46.0X4-	T46.0X5-	T46.0X6-
Strophanthin (g) (k)	T46.0X1-	T46.0X2-	T46.0X3-	T46.0X4-	T46.0X5-	T46.0X6-
Strophanthus	T46.0X1-	T46.0X2-	T46.0X3-	T46.0X4-	T46.0X5-	T46.0X6-
Strophantin	T46.0X1-	T46.0X2-	T46.0X3-	T46.0X4-	T46.0X5-	T46.0X6-
Strophantin-g	T46.0X1-	T46.0X2-	T46.0X3-	T46.0X4-	T46.0X5-	T46.0X6-
Strychnine (nonmedicinal) (pesticide) (salts)	T65.1X1-	T65.1X2-	T65.1X3-	T65.1X4-	-	-
medicinal	T48.291-	T48.292-	T48.293-	T48.294-	T48.295-	T48.296-
Strychnos (ignatii) — *see* Strychnine						
Styramate	T42.8X1-	T42.8X2-	T42.8X3-	T42.8X4-	T42.8X5-	T42.8X6-
Styrene	T65.891-	T65.892-	T65.893-	T65.894-	-	-
Succinimide, antiepileptic or anticonvulsant	T42.2X1-	T42.2X2-	T42.2X3-	T42.2X4-	T42.2X5-	T42.2X6-
mercuric — *see* Mercury						
Succinylcholine	T48.1X1-	T48.1X2-	T48.1X3-	T48.1X4-	T48.1X5-	T48.1X6-
Succinylsulfathiazole	T37.0X1-	T37.0X2-	T37.0X3-	T37.0X4-	T37.0X5-	T37.0X6-
Sucralfate	T47.1X1-	T47.1X2-	T47.1X3-	T47.1X4-	T47.1X5-	T47.1X6-
Sucrose	T50.3X1-	T50.3X2-	T50.3X3-	T50.3X4-	T50.3X5-	T50.3X6-
Sufentanil	T40.4X1-	T40.4X2-	T40.4X3-	T40.4X4-	T40.4X5-	T40.4X6-

Substance	Poisoning Accidental (unintentional)	Poisoning Intentional self-harm	Poisoning Assault	Poisoning Undetermined	Adverse effect	Underdosing
Sulbactam	T36.0X1-	T36.0X2-	T36.0X3-	T36.0X4-	T36.0X5-	T36.0X6-
Sulbenicillin	T36.0X1-	T36.0X2-	T36.0X3-	T36.0X4-	T36.0X5-	T36.0X6-
Sulbentine	T49.0X1-	T49.0X2-	T49.0X3-	T49.0X4-	T49.0X5-	T49.0X6-
Sulfacetamide	T49.0X1-	T49.0X2-	T49.0X3-	T49.0X4-	T49.0X5-	T49.0X6-
ophthalmic preparation	T49.5X1-	T49.5X2-	T49.5X3-	T49.5X4-	T49.5X5-	T49.5X6-
Sulfachlorpyridazine	T37.0X1-	T37.0X2-	T37.0X3-	T37.0X4-	T37.0X5-	T37.0X6-
Sulfacitine	T37.0X1-	T37.0X2-	T37.0X3-	T37.0X4-	T37.0X5-	T37.0X6-
Sulfadiasulfone sodium	T37.0X1-	T37.0X2-	T37.0X3-	T37.0X4-	T37.0X5-	T37.0X6-
Sulfadiazine	T37.0X1-	T37.0X2-	T37.0X3-	T37.0X4-	T37.0X5-	T37.0X6-
silver (topical)	T49.0X1-	T49.0X2-	T49.0X3-	T49.0X4-	T49.0X5-	T49.0X6-
Sulfadimethoxine	T37.0X1-	T37.0X2-	T37.0X3-	T37.0X4-	T37.0X5-	T37.0X6-
Sulfadimidine	T37.0X1-	T37.0X2-	T37.0X3-	T37.0X4-	T37.0X5-	T37.0X6-
Sulfadoxine	T37.0X1-	T37.0X2-	T37.0X3-	T37.0X4-	T37.0X5-	T37.0X6-
with pyrimethamine	T37.2X1-	T37.2X2-	T37.2X3-	T37.2X4-	T37.2X5-	T37.2X6-
Sulfaethidole	T37.0X1-	T37.0X2-	T37.0X3-	T37.0X4-	T37.0X5-	T37.0X6-
Sulfafurazole	T37.0X1-	T37.0X2-	T37.0X3-	T37.0X4-	T37.0X5-	T37.0X6-
Sulfaguanidine	T37.0X1-	T37.0X2-	T37.0X3-	T37.0X4-	T37.0X5-	T37.0X6-
Sulfalene	T37.0X1-	T37.0X2-	T37.0X3-	T37.0X4-	T37.0X5-	T37.0X6-
Sulfaloxate	T37.0X1-	T37.0X2-	T37.0X3-	T37.0X4-	T37.0X5-	T37.0X6-
Sulfaloxic acid	T37.0X1-	T37.0X2-	T37.0X3-	T37.0X4-	T37.0X5-	T37.0X6-
Sulfamazone	T39.2X1-	T39.2X2-	T39.2X3-	T39.2X4-	T39.2X5-	T39.2X6-
Sulfamerazine	T37.0X1-	T37.0X2-	T37.0X3-	T37.0X4-	T37.0X5-	T37.0X6-
Sulfameter	T37.0X1-	T37.0X2-	T37.0X3-	T37.0X4-	T37.0X5-	T37.0X6-
Sulfamethazine	T37.0X1-	T37.0X2-	T37.0X3-	T37.0X4-	T37.0X5-	T37.0X6-
Sulfamethizole	T37.0X1-	T37.0X2-	T37.0X3-	T37.0X4-	T37.0X5-	T37.0X6-
Sulfamethoxazole	T37.0X1-	T37.0X2-	T37.0X3-	T37.0X4-	T37.0X5-	T37.0X6-
with trimethoprim	T36.8X1-	T36.8X2-	T36.8X3-	T36.8X4-	T36.8X5-	T36.8X6-
Sulfamethoxydiazine	T37.0X1-	T37.0X2-	T37.0X3-	T37.0X4-	T37.0X5-	T37.0X6-
Sulfamethoxypyridazine	T37.0X1-	T37.0X2-	T37.0X3-	T37.0X4-	T37.0X5-	T37.0X6-
Sulfamethylthiazole	T37.0X1-	T37.0X2-	T37.0X3-	T37.0X4-	T37.0X5-	T37.0X6-
Sulfametoxydiazine	T37.0X1-	T37.0X2-	T37.0X3-	T37.0X4-	T37.0X5-	T37.0X6-
Sulfamidopyrine	T39.2X1-	T39.2X2-	T39.2X3-	T39.2X4-	T39.2X5-	T39.2X6-
Sulfamonomethoxine	T37.0X1-	T37.0X2-	T37.0X3-	T37.0X4-	T37.0X5-	T37.0X6-
Sulfamoxole	T37.0X1-	T37.0X2-	T37.0X3-	T37.0X4-	T37.0X5-	T37.0X6-
Sulfamylon	T49.0X1-	T49.0X2-	T49.0X3-	T49.0X4-	T49.0X5-	T49.0X6-
Sulfan blue (diagnostic dye)	T50.8X1-	T50.8X2-	T50.8X3-	T50.8X4-	T50.8X5-	T50.8X6-
Sulfanilamide	T37.0X1-	T37.0X2-	T37.0X3-	T37.0X4-	T37.0X5-	T37.0X6-
Sulfanilylguanidine	T37.0X1-	T37.0X2-	T37.0X3-	T37.0X4-	T37.0X5-	T37.0X6-
Sulfaperin	T37.0X1-	T37.0X2-	T37.0X3-	T37.0X4-	T37.0X5-	T37.0X6-
Sulfaphenazole	T37.0X1-	T37.0X2-	T37.0X3-	T37.0X4-	T37.0X5-	T37.0X6-
Sulfaphenylthiazole	T37.0X1-	T37.0X2-	T37.0X3-	T37.0X4-	T37.0X5-	T37.0X6-
Sulfaproxyline	T37.0X1-	T37.0X2-	T37.0X3-	T37.0X4-	T37.0X5-	T37.0X6-
Sulfapyridine	T37.0X1-	T37.0X2-	T37.0X3-	T37.0X4-	T37.0X5-	T37.0X6-
Sulfapyrimidine	T37.0X1-	T37.0X2-	T37.0X3-	T37.0X4-	T37.0X5-	T37.0X6-
Sulfarsphenamine	T37.8X1-	T37.8X2-	T37.8X3-	T37.8X4-	T37.8X5-	T37.8X6-
Sulfasalazine	T37.0X1-	T37.0X2-	T37.0X3-	T37.0X4-	T37.0X5-	T37.0X6-
Sulfasuxidine	T37.0X1-	T37.0X2-	T37.0X3-	T37.0X4-	T37.0X5-	T37.0X6-
Sulfasymazine	T37.0X1-	T37.0X2-	T37.0X3-	T37.0X4-	T37.0X5-	T37.0X6-
Sulfated amylopectin	T47.8X1-	T47.8X2-	T47.8X3-	T47.8X4-	T47.8X5-	T47.8X6-
Sulfathiazole	T37.0X1-	T37.0X2-	T37.0X3-	T37.0X4-	T37.0X5-	T37.0X6-
Sulfatostearate	T49.2X1-	T49.2X2-	T49.2X3-	T49.2X4-	T49.2X5-	T49.2X6-
Sulfinpyrazone	T50.4X1-	T50.4X2-	T50.4X3-	T50.4X4-	T50.4X5-	T50.4X6-
Sulfiram	T49.0X1-	T49.0X2-	T49.0X3-	T49.0X4-	T49.0X5-	T49.0X6-
Sulfisomidine	T37.0X1-	T37.0X2-	T37.0X3-	T37.0X4-	T37.0X5-	T37.0X6-
Sulfisoxazole	T37.0X1-	T37.0X2-	T37.0X3-	T37.0X4-	T37.0X5-	T37.0X6-
ophthalmic preparation	T49.5X1-	T49.5X2-	T49.5X3-	T49.5X4-	T49.5X5-	T49.5X6-
Sulfobromophthalein (sodium)	T50.8X1-	T50.8X2-	T50.8X3-	T50.8X4-	T50.8X5-	T50.8X6-
Sulfobromphthalein	T50.8X1-	T50.8X2-	T50.8X3-	T50.8X4-	T50.8X5-	T50.8X6-
Sulfogaiacol	T48.4X1-	T48.4X2-	T48.4X3-	T48.4X4-	T48.4X5-	T48.4X6-
Sulfomyxin	T36.8X1-	T36.8X2-	T36.8X3-	T36.8X4-	T36.8X5-	T36.8X6-
Sulfonal	T42.6X1-	T42.6X2-	T42.6X3-	T42.6X4-	T42.6X5-	T42.6X6-
Sulfonamide NEC	T37.0X1-	T37.0X2-	T37.0X3-	T37.0X4-	T37.0X5-	T37.0X6-
eye	T49.5X1-	T49.5X2-	T49.5X3-	T49.5X4-	T49.5X5-	T49.5X6-
Sulfonazide	T37.1X1-	T37.1X2-	T37.1X3-	T37.1X4-	T37.1X5-	T37.1X6-
Sulfones	T37.1X1-	T37.1X2-	T37.1X3-	T37.1X4-	T37.1X5-	T37.1X6-
Sulfonethylmethane	T42.6X1-	T42.6X2-	T42.6X3-	T42.6X4-	T42.6X5-	T42.6X6-
Sulfonmethane	T42.6X1-	T42.6X2-	T42.6X3-	T42.6X4-	T42.6X5-	T42.6X6-
Sulfonphthal, sulfonphthol	T50.8X1-	T50.8X2-	T50.8X3-	T50.8X4-	T50.8X5-	T50.8X6-
Sulfonylurea derivatives, oral	T38.3X1-	T38.3X2-	T38.3X3-	T38.3X4-	T38.3X5-	T38.3X6-
Sulforidazine	T43.3X1-	T43.3X2-	T43.3X3-	T43.3X4-	T43.3X5-	T43.3X6-
Sulfoxone	T37.1X1-	T37.1X2-	T37.1X3-	T37.1X4-	T37.1X5-	T37.1X6-
Sulfur, sulfurated, sulfuric, sulfurous, sulfuryl (compounds NEC) (medicinal)	T49.4X1-	T49.4X2-	T49.4X3-	T49.4X4-	T49.4X5-	T49.4X6-
acid	T54.2X1-	T54.2X2-	T54.2X3-	T54.2X4-	-	-
dioxide (gas)	T59.1X1-	T59.1X2-	T59.1X3-	T59.1X4-	-	-
ether — *see* Ether(s)						
hydrogen	T59.6X1-	T59.6X2-	T59.6X3-	T59.6X4-	-	-

Substance	Poisoning Accidental (unintentional)	Poisoning Intentional self-harm	Poisoning Assault	Poisoning Undetermined	Adverse effect	Underdosing
Sulfur, sulfurated, sulfuric, sulfurous, sulfuryl - *continued*						
medicinal (keratolytic) (ointment) NEC	T49.4X1-	T49.4X2-	T49.4X3-	T49.4X4-	T49.4X5-	T49.4X6-
ointment	T49.0X1-	T49.0X2-	T49.0X3-	T49.0X4-	T49.0X5-	T49.0X6-
pesticide (vapor)	T60.91X-	T60.92X-	T60.93X-	T60.94X-	-	-
vapor NEC	T59.891-	T59.892-	T59.893-	T59.894-	-	-
Sulfuric acid	T54.2X1-	T54.2X2-	T54.2X3-	T54.2X4-	-	-
Sulglicotide	T47.1X1-	T47.1X2-	T47.1X3-	T47.1X4-	T47.1X5-	T47.1X6-
Sulindac	T39.391-	T39.392-	T39.393-	T39.394-	T39.395-	T39.396-
Sulisatin	T47.2X1-	T47.2X2-	T47.2X3-	T47.2X4-	T47.2X5-	T47.2X6-
Sulisobenzone	T49.3X1-	T49.3X2-	T49.3X3-	T49.3X4-	T49.3X5-	T49.3X6-
Sulkowitch's reagent	T50.8X1-	T50.8X2-	T50.8X3-	T50.8X4-	T50.8X5-	T50.8X6-
Sulmetozine	T44.3X1-	T44.3X2-	T44.3X3-	T44.3X4-	T44.3X5-	T44.3X6-
Suloctidil	T46.7X1-	T46.7X2-	T46.7X3-	T46.7X4-	T46.7X5-	T46.7X6-
Sulph- — *see also* Sulf-						
Sulphadiazine	T37.0X1-	T37.0X2-	T37.0X3-	T37.0X4-	T37.0X5-	T37.0X6-
Sulphadimethoxine	T37.0X1-	T37.0X2-	T37.0X3-	T37.0X4-	T37.0X5-	T37.0X6-
Sulphadimidine	T37.0X1-	T37.0X2-	T37.0X3-	T37.0X4-	T37.0X5-	T37.0X6-
Sulphadione	T37.1X1-	T37.1X2-	T37.1X3-	T37.1X4-	T37.1X5-	T37.1X6-
Sulphafurazole	T37.0X1-	T37.0X2-	T37.0X3-	T37.0X4-	T37.0X5-	T37.0X6-
Sulphamethizole	T37.0X1-	T37.0X2-	T37.0X3-	T37.0X4-	T37.0X5-	T37.0X6-
Sulphamethoxazole	T37.0X1-	T37.0X2-	T37.0X3-	T37.0X4-	T37.0X5-	T37.0X6-
Sulphan blue	T50.8X1-	T50.8X2-	T50.8X3-	T50.8X4-	T50.8X5-	T50.8X6-
Sulphaphenazole	T37.0X1-	T37.0X2-	T37.0X3-	T37.0X4-	T37.0X5-	T37.0X6-
Sulphapyridine	T37.0X1-	T37.0X2-	T37.0X3-	T37.0X4-	T37.0X5-	T37.0X6-
Sulphasalazine	T37.0X1-	T37.0X2-	T37.0X3-	T37.0X4-	T37.0X5-	T37.0X6-
Sulphinpyrazone	T50.4X1-	T50.4X2-	T50.4X3-	T50.4X4-	T50.4X5-	T50.4X6-
Sulpiride	T43.591-	T43.592-	T43.593-	T43.594-	T43.595-	T43.596-
Sulprostone	T48.0X1-	T48.0X2-	T48.0X3-	T48.0X4-	T48.0X5-	T48.0X6-
Sulpyrine	T39.2X1-	T39.2X2-	T39.2X3-	T39.2X4-	T39.2X5-	T39.2X6-
Sultamicillin	T36.0X1-	T36.0X2-	T36.0X3-	T36.0X4-	T36.0X5-	T36.0X6-
Sulthiame	T42.6X1-	T42.6X2-	T42.6X3-	T42.6X4-	T42.6X5-	T42.6X6-
Sultiame	T42.6X1-	T42.6X2-	T42.6X3-	T42.6X4-	T42.6X5-	T42.6X6-
Sultopride	T43.591-	T43.592-	T43.593-	T43.594-	T43.595-	T43.596-
Sumatriptan	T39.8X1-	T39.8X2-	T39.8X3-	T39.8X4-	T39.8X5-	T39.8X6-
Sunflower seed oil	T46.6X1-	T46.6X2-	T46.6X3-	T46.6X4-	T46.6X5-	T46.6X6-
Superinone	T48.4X1-	T48.4X2-	T48.4X3-	T48.4X4-	T48.4X5-	T48.4X6-
Suprofen	T39.311-	T39.312-	T39.313-	T39.314-	T39.315-	T39.316-
Suramin (sodium)	T37.4X1-	T37.4X2-	T37.4X3-	T37.4X4-	T37.4X5-	T37.4X6-
Surfacaine	T41.3X1-	T41.3X2-	T41.3X3-	T41.3X4-	T41.3X5-	T41.3X6-
Surital	T41.1X1-	T41.1X2-	T41.1X3-	T41.1X4-	T41.1X5-	T41.1X6-
Sutilains	T45.3X1-	T45.3X2-	T45.3X3-	T45.3X4-	T45.3X5-	T45.3X6-
Suxamethonium (chloride)	T48.1X1-	T48.1X2-	T48.1X3-	T48.1X4-	T48.1X5-	T48.1X6-
Suxethonium (chloride)	T48.1X1-	T48.1X2-	T48.1X3-	T48.1X4-	T48.1X5-	T48.1X6-
Suxibuzone	T39.2X1-	T39.2X2-	T39.2X3-	T39.2X4-	T39.2X5-	T39.2X6-
Sweet niter spirit	T46.3X1-	T46.3X2-	T46.3X3-	T46.3X4-	T46.3X5-	T46.3X6-
Sweet oil (birch)	T49.3X1-	T49.3X2-	T49.3X3-	T49.3X4-	T49.3X5-	T49.3X6-
Sweetener	T50.901-	T50.902-	T50.903-	T50.904-	T50.905-	T50.906-
Sym-dichloroethyl ether	T53.6X1-	T53.6X2-	T53.6X3-	T53.6X4-	-	-
Sympatholytic NEC	T44.8X1-	T44.8X2-	T44.8X3-	T44.8X4-	T44.8X5-	T44.8X6-
haloalkylamine	T44.8X1-	T44.8X2-	T44.8X3-	T44.8X4-	T44.8X5-	T44.8X6-
Sympathomimetic NEC	T44.901-	T44.902-	T44.903-	T44.904-	T44.905-	T44.906-
anti-common-cold	T48.5X1-	T48.5X2-	T48.5X3-	T48.5X4-	T48.5X5-	T48.5X6-
bronchodilator	T48.6X1-	T48.6X2-	T48.6X3-	T48.6X4-	T48.6X5-	T48.6X6-
specified NEC	T44.991-	T44.992-	T44.993-	T44.994-	T44.995-	T44.996-
Synagis	T50.B91-	T50.B92-	T50.B93-	T50.B94-	T50.B95-	T50.B96-
Synalar	T49.0X1-	T49.0X2-	T49.0X3-	T49.0X4-	T49.0X5-	T49.0X6-
Synthroid	T38.1X1-	T38.1X2-	T38.1X3-	T38.1X4-	T38.1X5-	T38.1X6-
Syntocinon	T48.0X1-	T48.0X2-	T48.0X3-	T48.0X4-	T48.0X5-	T48.0X6-
Syrosingopine	T46.5X1-	T46.5X2-	T46.5X3-	T46.5X4-	T46.5X5-	T46.5X6-
Systemic drug	T45.91X-	T45.92X-	T45.93X-	T45.94X-	T45.95X-	T45.96X-
specified NEC	T45.8X1-	T45.8X2-	T45.8X3-	T45.8X4-	T45.8X5-	T45.8X6-
2,4,5-T	T60.3X1-	T60.3X2-	T60.3X3-	T60.3X4-	-	-
Tablets — *see also* specified substance	T50.901-	T50.902-	T50.903-	T50.904-	T50.905-	T50.906-
Tace	T38.5X1-	T38.5X2-	T38.5X3-	T38.5X4-	T38.5X5-	T38.5X6-
Tacrine	T44.0X1-	T44.0X2-	T44.0X3-	T44.0X4-	T44.0X5-	T44.0X6-
Tadalafil	T46.7X1-	T46.7X2-	T46.7X3-	T46.7X4-	T46.7X5-	T46.7X6-
Talampicillin	T36.0X1-	T36.0X2-	T36.0X3-	T36.0X4-	T36.0X5-	T36.0X6-
Talbutal	T42.3X1-	T42.3X2-	T42.3X3-	T42.3X4-	T42.3X5-	T42.3X6-
Talc powder	T49.3X1-	T49.3X2-	T49.3X3-	T49.3X4-	T49.3X5-	T49.3X6-
Talcum	T49.3X1-	T49.3X2-	T49.3X3-	T49.3X4-	T49.3X5-	T49.3X6-
Taleranol	T38.6X1-	T38.6X2-	T38.6X3-	T38.6X4-	T38.6X5-	T38.6X6-
Tamoxifen	T38.6X1-	T38.6X2-	T38.6X3-	T38.6X4-	T38.6X5-	T38.6X6-
Tamsulosin	T44.6X1-	T44.6X2-	T44.6X3-	T44.6X4-	T44.6X5-	T44.6X6-
Tandearil, tanderil	T39.2X1-	T39.2X2-	T39.2X3-	T39.2X4-	T39.2X5-	T39.2X6-

Substance	Poisoning Accidental (unintentional)	Poisoning Intentional self-harm	Poisoning Assault	Poisoning Undetermined	Adverse effect	Underdosing
Tannic acid	T49.2X1-	T49.2X2-	T49.2X3-	T49.2X4-	T49.2X5-	T49.2X6-
medicinal (astringent)	T49.2X1-	T49.2X2-	T49.2X3-	T49.2X4-	T49.2X5-	T49.2X6-
Tannin — *see* Tannic acid						
Tansy	T62.2X1-	T62.2X2-	T62.2X3-	T62.2X4-	-	-
TAO	T36.3X1-	T36.3X2-	T36.3X3-	T36.3X4-	T36.3X5-	T36.3X6-
Tapazole	T38.2X1-	T38.2X2-	T38.2X3-	T38.2X4-	T38.2X5-	T38.2X6-
Tar NEC	T52.0X1-	T52.0X2-	T52.0X3-	T52.0X4-	-	-
camphor	T60.1X1-	T60.1X2-	T60.1X3-	T60.1X4-	-	-
distillate	T49.1X1-	T49.1X2-	T49.1X3-	T49.1X4-	T49.1X5-	T49.1X6-
fumes	T59.891-	T59.892-	T59.893-	T59.894-	-	-
medicinal	T49.1X1-	T49.1X2-	T49.1X3-	T49.1X4-	T49.1X5-	T49.1X6-
ointment	T49.1X1-	T49.1X2-	T49.1X3-	T49.1X4-	T49.1X5-	T49.1X6-
Taractan	T43.591-	T43.592-	T43.593-	T43.594-	T43.595-	T43.596-
Tarantula (venomous)	T63.321-	T63.322-	T63.323-	T63.324-	-	-
Tartar emetic	T37.8X1-	T37.8X2-	T37.8X3-	T37.8X4-	T37.8X5-	T37.8X6-
Tartaric acid	T65.891-	T65.892-	T65.893-	T65.894-	-	-
Tartrate, laxative	T47.4X1-	T47.4X2-	T47.4X3-	T47.4X4-	T47.4X5-	T47.4X6-
Tartrated antimony (anti-infective)	T37.8X1-	T37.8X2-	T37.8X3-	T37.8X4-	T37.8X5-	T37.8X6-
Tauromustine	T45.1X1-	T45.1X2-	T45.1X3-	T45.1X4-	T45.1X5-	T45.1X6-
TCA — *see* Trichloroacetic acid						
TCDD	T53.7X1-	T53.7X2-	T53.7X3-	T53.7X4-	-	-
TDI (vapor)	T65.0X1-	T65.0X2-	T65.0X3-	T65.0X4-	-	-
Tear						
gas	T59.3X1-	T59.3X2-	T59.3X3-	T59.3X4-	-	-
solution	T49.5X1-	T49.5X2-	T49.5X3-	T49.5X4-	T49.5X5-	T49.5X6-
Teclothiazide	T50.2X1-	T50.2X2-	T50.2X3-	T50.2X4-	T50.2X5-	T50.2X6-
Teclozan	T37.3X1-	T37.3X2-	T37.3X3-	T37.3X4-	T37.3X5-	T37.3X6-
Tegafur	T45.1X1-	T45.1X2-	T45.1X3-	T45.1X4-	T45.1X5-	T45.1X6-
Tegretol	T42.1X1-	T42.1X2-	T42.1X3-	T42.1X4-	T42.1X5-	T42.1X6-
Teicoplanin	T36.8X1-	T36.8X2-	T36.8X3-	T36.8X4-	T36.8X5-	T36.8X6-
Telepaque	T50.8X1-	T50.8X2-	T50.8X3-	T50.8X4-	T50.8X5-	T50.8X6-
Tellurium	T56.891-	T56.892-	T56.893-	T56.894-	-	-
fumes	T56.891-	T56.892-	T56.893-	T56.894-	-	-
TEM	T45.1X1-	T45.1X2-	T45.1X3-	T45.1X4-	T45.1X5-	T45.1X6-
Temazepam	T42.4X1-	T42.4X2-	T42.4X3-	T42.4X4-	T42.4X5-	T42.4X6-
Temocillin	T36.0X1-	T36.0X2-	T36.0X3-	T36.0X4-	T36.0X5-	T36.0X6-
Tenamfetamine	T43.621-	T43.622-	T43.623-	T43.624-	T43.625-	T43.626-
Teniposide	T45.1X1-	T45.1X2-	T45.1X3-	T45.1X4-	T45.1X5-	T45.1X6-
Tenitramine	T46.3X1-	T46.3X2-	T46.3X3-	T46.3X4-	T46.3X5-	T46.3X6-
Tenoglicin	T48.4X1-	T48.4X2-	T48.4X3-	T48.4X4-	T48.4X5-	T48.4X6-
Tenonitrozole	T37.3X1-	T37.3X2-	T37.3X3-	T37.3X4-	T37.3X5-	T37.3X6-
Tenoxicam	T39.391-	T39.392-	T39.393-	T39.394-	T39.395-	T39.396-
TEPA	T45.1X1-	T45.1X2-	T45.1X3-	T45.1X4-	T45.1X5-	T45.1X6-
TEPP	T60.0X1-	T60.0X2-	T60.0X3-	T60.0X4-	-	-
Teprotide	T46.5X1-	T46.5X2-	T46.5X3-	T46.5X4-	T46.5X5-	T46.5X6-
Terazosin	T44.6X1-	T44.6X2-	T44.6X3-	T44.6X4-	T44.6X5-	T44.6X6-
Terbufos	T60.0X1-	T60.0X2-	T60.0X3-	T60.0X4-	-	-
Terbutaline	T48.6X1-	T48.6X2-	T48.6X3-	T48.6X4-	T48.6X5-	T48.6X6-
Terconazole	T49.0X1-	T49.0X2-	T49.0X3-	T49.0X4-	T49.0X5-	T49.0X6-
Terfenadine	T45.0X1-	T45.0X2-	T45.0X3-	T45.0X4-	T45.0X5-	T45.0X6-
Teriparatide (acetate)	T50.991-	T50.992-	T50.993-	T50.994-	T50.995-	T50.996-
Terizidone	T37.1X1-	T37.1X2-	T37.1X3-	T37.1X4-	T37.1X5-	T37.1X6-
Terlipressin	T38.891-	T38.892-	T38.893-	T38.894-	T38.895-	T38.896-
Terodiline	T46.3X1-	T46.3X2-	T46.3X3-	T46.3X4-	T46.3X5-	T46.3X6-
Teroxalene	T37.4X1-	T37.4X2-	T37.4X3-	T37.4X4-	T37.4X5-	T37.4X6-
Terpin (cis) **hydrate**	T48.4X1-	T48.4X2-	T48.4X3-	T48.4X4-	T48.4X5-	T48.4X6-
Terramycin	T36.4X1-	T36.4X2-	T36.4X3-	T36.4X4-	T36.4X5-	T36.4X6-
Tertatolol	T44.7X1-	T44.7X2-	T44.7X3-	T44.7X4-	T44.7X5-	T44.7X6-
Tessalon	T48.3X1-	T48.3X2-	T48.3X3-	T48.3X4-	T48.3X5-	T48.3X6-
Testolactone	T38.7X1-	T38.7X2-	T38.7X3-	T38.7X4-	T38.7X5-	T38.7X6-
Testosterone	T38.7X1-	T38.7X2-	T38.7X3-	T38.7X4-	T38.7X5-	T38.7X6-
Tetanus toxoid or vaccine	T50.A91-	T50.A92-	T50.A93-	T50.A94-	T50.A95-	T50.A96-
antitoxin	T50.Z11-	T50.Z12-	T50.Z13-	T50.Z14-	T50.Z15-	T50.Z16-
immune globulin (human)	T50.Z11-	T50.Z12-	T50.Z13-	T50.Z14-	T50.Z15-	T50.Z16-
toxoid	T50.A91-	T50.A92-	T50.A93-	T50.A94-	T50.A95-	T50.A96-
with diphtheria toxoid	T50.A21-	T50.A22-	T50.A23-	T50.A24-	T50.A25-	T50.A26-
with pertussis	T50.A11-	T50.A12-	T50.A13-	T50.A14-	T50.A15-	T50.A16-
Tetrabenazine	T43.591-	T43.592-	T43.593-	T43.594-	T43.595-	T43.596-
Tetracaine	T41.3X1-	T41.3X2-	T41.3X3-	T41.3X4-	T41.3X5-	T41.3X6-
nerve block (peripheral) (plexus)	T41.3X1-	T41.3X2-	T41.3X3-	T41.3X4-	T41.3X5-	T41.3X6-
regional	T41.3X1-	T41.3X2-	T41.3X3-	T41.3X4-	T41.3X5-	T41.3X6-
spinal	T41.3X1-	T41.3X2-	T41.3X3-	T41.3X4-	T41.3X5-	T41.3X6-
Tetrachlorethylene — *see* Tetrachloroethylene						
Tetrachlormethiazide	T50.2X1-	T50.2X2-	T50.2X3-	T50.2X4-	T50.2X5-	T50.2X6-

Substance	Poisoning Accidental (unintentional)	Poisoning Intentional self-harm	Poisoning Assault	Poisoning Undetermined	Adverse effect	Underdosing
2,3,7,8-Tetrachlorodibenzo-p-dioxin	T53.7X1-	T53.7X2-	T53.7X3-	T53.7X4-	-	-
Tetrachloroethane	T53.6X1-	T53.6X2-	T53.6X3-	T53.6X4-	-	-
vapor	T53.6X1-	T53.6X2-	T53.6X3-	T53.6X4-	-	-
paint or varnish	T53.6X1-	T53.6X2-	T53.6X3-	T53.6X4-	-	-
Tetrachloroethylene (liquid)	T53.3X1-	T53.3X2-	T53.3X3-	T53.3X4-	-	-
medicinal	T37.4X1-	T37.4X2-	T37.4X3-	T37.4X4-	T37.4X5-	T37.4X6-
vapor	T53.3X1-	T53.3X2-	T53.3X3-	T53.3X4-	-	-
Tetrachloromethane — *see* Carbon tetrachloride						
Tetracosactide	T38.811-	T38.812-	T38.813-	T38.814-	T38.815-	T38.816-
Tetracosactrin	T38.811-	T38.812-	T38.813-	T38.814-	T38.815-	T38.816-
Tetracycline	T36.4X1-	T36.4X2-	T36.4X3-	T36.4X4-	T36.4X5-	T36.4X6-
ophthalmic preparation	T49.5X1-	T49.5X2-	T49.5X3-	T49.5X4-	T49.5X5-	T49.5X6-
topical NEC	T49.0X1-	T49.0X2-	T49.0X3-	T49.0X4-	T49.0X5-	T49.0X6-
Tetradifon	T60.8X1-	T60.8X2-	T60.8X3-	T60.8X4-	-	-
Tetradotoxin	T61.771-	T61.772-	T61.773-	T61.774-	-	-
Tetraethyl						
lead	T56.0X1-	T56.0X2-	T56.0X3-	T56.0X4-	-	-
pyrophosphate	T60.0X1-	T60.0X2-	T60.0X3-	T60.0X4-	-	-
Tetraethylammonium chloride	T44.2X1-	T44.2X2-	T44.2X3-	T44.2X4-	T44.2X5-	T44.2X6-
Tetraethylthiuram disulfide	T50.6X1-	T50.6X2-	T50.6X3-	T50.6X4-	T50.6X5-	T50.6X6-
Tetrahydroaminoacridine	T44.0X1-	T44.0X2-	T44.0X3-	T44.0X4-	T44.0X5-	T44.0X6-
Tetrahydrocannabinol	T40.7X1-	T40.7X2-	T40.7X3-	T40.7X4-	T40.7X5-	T40.7X6-
Tetrahydrofuran	T52.8X1-	T52.8X2-	T52.8X3-	T52.8X4-	-	-
Tetrahydronaphthalene	T52.8X1-	T52.8X2-	T52.8X3-	T52.8X4-	-	-
Tetrahydrozoline	T49.5X1-	T49.5X2-	T49.5X3-	T49.5X4-	T49.5X5-	T49.5X6-
Tetralin	T52.8X1-	T52.8X2-	T52.8X3-	T52.8X4-	-	-
Tetramethrin	T60.2X1-	T60.2X2-	T60.2X3-	T60.2X4-	-	-
Tetramethylthiuram (disulfide) **NEC**	T60.3X1-	T60.3X2-	T60.3X3-	T60.3X4-	-	-
medicinal	T49.0X1-	T49.0X2-	T49.0X3-	T49.0X4-	T49.0X5-	T49.0X6-
Tetramisole	T37.4X1-	T37.4X2-	T37.4X3-	T37.4X4-	T37.4X5-	T37.4X6-
Tetranicotinoyl fructose	T46.7X1-	T46.7X2-	T46.7X3-	T46.7X4-	T46.7X5-	T46.7X6-
Tetrazepam	T42.4X1-	T42.4X2-	T42.4X3-	T42.4X4-	T42.4X5-	T42.4X6-
Tetronal	T42.6X1-	T42.6X2-	T42.6X3-	T42.6X4-	T42.6X5-	T42.6X6-
Tetryl	T65.3X1-	T65.3X2-	T65.3X3-	T65.3X4-	-	-
Tetrylammonium chloride	T44.2X1-	T44.2X2-	T44.2X3-	T44.2X4-	T44.2X5-	T44.2X6-
Tetryzoline	T49.5X1-	T49.5X2-	T49.5X3-	T49.5X4-	T49.5X5-	T49.5X6-
Thalidomide	T45.1X1-	T45.1X2-	T45.1X3-	T45.1X4-	T45.1X5-	T45.1X6-
Thallium (compounds) (dust) **NEC**	T56.811-	T56.812-	T56.813-	T56.814-	-	-
pesticide	T60.4X1-	T60.4X2-	T60.4X3-	T60.4X4-	-	-
THC	T40.7X1-	T40.7X2-	T40.7X3-	T40.7X4-	T40.7X5-	T40.7X6-
Thebacon	T48.3X1-	T48.3X2-	T48.3X3-	T48.3X4-	T48.3X5-	T48.3X6-
Thebaine	T40.2X1-	T40.2X2-	T40.2X3-	T40.2X4-	T40.2X5-	T40.2X6-
Thenoic acid	T49.6X1-	T49.6X2-	T49.6X3-	T49.6X4-	T49.6X5-	T49.6X6-
Thenyldiamine	T45.0X1-	T45.0X2-	T45.0X3-	T45.0X4-	T45.0X5-	T45.0X6-
Theobromine (calcium salicylate)	T48.6X1-	T48.6X2-	T48.6X3-	T48.6X4-	T48.6X5-	T48.6X6-
sodium salicylate	T48.6X1-	T48.6X2-	T48.6X3-	T48.6X4-	T48.6X5-	T48.6X6-
Theophyllamine	T48.6X1-	T48.6X2-	T48.6X3-	T48.6X4-	T48.6X5-	T48.6X6-
Theophylline	T48.6X1-	T48.6X2-	T48.6X3-	T48.6X4-	T48.6X5-	T48.6X6-
aminobenzoic acid	T48.6X1-	T48.6X2-	T48.6X3-	T48.6X4-	T48.6X5-	T48.6X6-
ethylenediamine	T48.6X1-	T48.6X2-	T48.6X3-	T48.6X4-	T48.6X5-	T48.6X6-
piperazine p-amino-benzoate	T48.6X1-	T48.6X2-	T48.6X3-	T48.6X4-	T48.6X5-	T48.6X6-
Thiabendazole	T37.4X1-	T37.4X2-	T37.4X3-	T37.4X4-	T37.4X5-	T37.4X6-
Thialbarbital	T41.1X1-	T41.1X2-	T41.1X3-	T41.1X4-	T41.1X5-	T41.1X6-
Thiamazole	T38.2X1-	T38.2X2-	T38.2X3-	T38.2X4-	T38.2X5-	T38.2X6-
Thiambutosine	T37.1X1-	T37.1X2-	T37.1X3-	T37.1X4-	T37.1X5-	T37.1X6-
Thiamine	T45.2X1-	T45.2X2-	T45.2X3-	T45.2X4-	T45.2X5-	T45.2X6-
Thiamphenicol	T36.2X1-	T36.2X2-	T36.2X3-	T36.2X4-	T36.2X5-	T36.2X6-
Thiamylal	T41.1X1-	T41.1X2-	T41.1X3-	T41.1X4-	T41.1X5-	T41.1X6-
sodium	T41.1X1-	T41.1X2-	T41.1X3-	T41.1X4-	T41.1X5-	T41.1X6-
Thiazesim	T43.291-	T43.292-	T43.293-	T43.294-	T43.295-	T43.296-
Thiazides (diuretics)	T50.2X1-	T50.2X2-	T50.2X3-	T50.2X4-	T50.2X5-	T50.2X6-
Thiazinamium metilsulfate	T43.3X1-	T43.3X2-	T43.3X3-	T43.3X4-	T43.3X5-	T43.3X6-
Thiethylperazine	T43.3X1-	T43.3X2-	T43.3X3-	T43.3X4-	T43.3X5-	T43.3X6-
Thimerosal	T49.0X1-	T49.0X2-	T49.0X3-	T49.0X4-	T49.0X5-	T49.0X6-
ophthalmic preparation	T49.5X1-	T49.5X2-	T49.5X3-	T49.5X4-	T49.5X5-	T49.5X6-
Thioacetazone	T37.1X1-	T37.1X2-	T37.1X3-	T37.1X4-	T37.1X5-	T37.1X6-
with isoniazid	T37.1X1-	T37.1X2-	T37.1X3-	T37.1X4-	T37.1X5-	T37.1X6-
Thiobarbital sodium	T41.1X1-	T41.1X2-	T41.1X3-	T41.1X4-	T41.1X5-	T41.1X6-
Thiobarbiturate anesthetic	T41.1X1-	T41.1X2-	T41.1X3-	T41.1X4-	T41.1X5-	T41.1X6-
Thiobismol	T37.8X1-	T37.8X2-	T37.8X3-	T37.8X4-	T37.8X5-	T37.8X6-
Thiobutabarbital sodium	T41.1X1-	T41.1X2-	T41.1X3-	T41.1X4-	T41.1X5-	T41.1X6-
Thiocarbamate (insecticide)	T60.0X1-	T60.0X2-	T60.0X3-	T60.0X4-	-	-
Thiocarbamide	T38.2X1-	T38.2X2-	T38.2X3-	T38.2X4-	T38.2X5-	T38.2X6-
Thiocarbarsone	T37.8X1-	T37.8X2-	T37.8X3-	T37.8X4-	T37.8X5-	T37.8X6-
Thiocarlide	T37.1X1-	T37.1X2-	T37.1X3-	T37.1X4-	T37.1X5-	T37.1X6-
Thioctamide	T50.991-	T50.992-	T50.993-	T50.994-	T50.995-	T50.996-
Thioctic acid	T50.991-	T50.992-	T50.993-	T50.994-	T50.995-	T50.996-
Thiofos	T60.0X1-	T60.0X2-	T60.0X3-	T60.0X4-	-	-
Thioglycolate	T49.4X1-	T49.4X2-	T49.4X3-	T49.4X4-	T49.4X5-	T49.4X6-
Thioglycolic acid	T65.891-	T65.892-	T65.893-	T65.894-	-	-
Thioguanine	T45.1X1-	T45.1X2-	T45.1X3-	T45.1X4-	T45.1X5-	T45.1X6-
Thiomercaptomerin	T50.2X1-	T50.2X2-	T50.2X3-	T50.2X4-	T50.2X5-	T50.2X6-
Thiomerin	T50.2X1-	T50.2X2-	T50.2X3-	T50.2X4-	T50.2X5-	T50.2X6-
Thiomersal	T49.0X1-	T49.0X2-	T49.0X3-	T49.0X4-	T49.0X5-	T49.0X6-
Thionazin	T60.0X1-	T60.0X2-	T60.0X3-	T60.0X4-	-	-
Thiopental (sodium)	T41.1X1-	T41.1X2-	T41.1X3-	T41.1X4-	T41.1X5-	T41.1X6-
Thiopentone (sodium)	T41.1X1-	T41.1X2-	T41.1X3-	T41.1X4-	T41.1X5-	T41.1X6-
Thiopropazate	T43.3X1-	T43.3X2-	T43.3X3-	T43.3X4-	T43.3X5-	T43.3X6-
Thioproperazine	T43.3X1-	T43.3X2-	T43.3X3-	T43.3X4-	T43.3X5-	T43.3X6-
Thioridazine	T43.3X1-	T43.3X2-	T43.3X3-	T43.3X4-	T43.3X5-	T43.3X6-
Thiosinamine	T49.3X1-	T49.3X2-	T49.3X3-	T49.3X4-	T49.3X5-	T49.3X6-
Thiotepa	T45.1X1-	T45.1X2-	T45.1X3-	T45.1X4-	T45.1X5-	T45.1X6-
Thiothixene	T43.4X1-	T43.4X2-	T43.4X3-	T43.4X4-	T43.4X5-	T43.4X6-
Thiouracil (benzyl) (methyl) (propyl)	T38.2X1-	T38.2X2-	T38.2X3-	T38.2X4-	T38.2X5-	T38.2X6-
Thiourea	T38.2X1-	T38.2X2-	T38.2X3-	T38.2X4-	T38.2X5-	T38.2X6-
Thiphenamil	T44.3X1-	T44.3X2-	T44.3X3-	T44.3X4-	T44.3X5-	T44.3X6-
Thiram	T60.3X1-	T60.3X2-	T60.3X3-	T60.3X4-	-	-
medicinal	T49.2X1-	T49.2X2-	T49.2X3-	T49.2X4-	T49.2X5-	T49.2X6-
Thonzylamine (systemic)	T45.0X1-	T45.0X2-	T45.0X3-	T45.0X4-	T45.0X5-	T45.0X6-
mucosal decongestant	T48.5X1-	T48.5X2-	T48.5X3-	T48.5X4-	T48.5X5-	T48.5X6-
Thorazine	T43.3X1-	T43.3X2-	T43.3X3-	T43.3X4-	T43.3X5-	T43.3X6-
Thorium dioxide suspension	T50.8X1-	T50.8X2-	T50.8X3-	T50.8X4-	T50.8X5-	T50.8X6-
Thornapple	T62.2X1-	T62.2X2-	T62.2X3-	T62.2X4-	-	-
Throat drug NEC	T49.6X1-	T49.6X2-	T49.6X3-	T49.6X4-	T49.6X5-	T49.6X6-
Thrombin	T45.7X1-	T45.7X2-	T45.7X3-	T45.7X4-	T45.7X5-	T45.7X6-
Thrombolysin	T45.611-	T45.612-	T45.613-	T45.614-	T45.615-	T45.616-
Thromboplastin	T45.7X1-	T45.7X2-	T45.7X3-	T45.7X4-	T45.7X5-	T45.7X6-
Thurfyl nicotinate	T46.7X1-	T46.7X2-	T46.7X3-	T46.7X4-	T46.7X5-	T46.7X6-
Thymol	T49.0X1-	T49.0X2-	T49.0X3-	T49.0X4-	T49.0X5-	T49.0X6-
Thymopentin	T37.5X1-	T37.5X2-	T37.5X3-	T37.5X4-	T37.5X5-	T37.5X6-
Thymoxamine	T46.7X1-	T46.7X2-	T46.7X3-	T46.7X4-	T46.7X5-	T46.7X6-
Thymus extract	T38.891-	T38.892-	T38.893-	T38.894-	T38.895-	T38.896-
Thyreotrophic hormone	T38.811-	T38.812-	T38.813-	T38.814-	T38.815-	T38.816-
Thyroglobulin	T38.1X1-	T38.1X2-	T38.1X3-	T38.1X4-	T38.1X5-	T38.1X6-
Thyroid (hormone)	T38.1X1-	T38.1X2-	T38.1X3-	T38.1X4-	T38.1X5-	T38.1X6-
Thyrolar	T38.1X1-	T38.1X2-	T38.1X3-	T38.1X4-	T38.1X5-	T38.1X6-
Thyrotrophin	T38.811-	T38.812-	T38.813-	T38.814-	T38.815-	T38.816-
Thyrotropic hormone	T38.811-	T38.812-	T38.813-	T38.814-	T38.815-	T38.816-
Thyroxine	T38.1X1-	T38.1X2-	T38.1X3-	T38.1X4-	T38.1X5-	T38.1X6-
Tiabendazole	T37.4X1-	T37.4X2-	T37.4X3-	T37.4X4-	T37.4X5-	T37.4X6-
Tiamizide	T50.2X1-	T50.2X2-	T50.2X3-	T50.2X4-	T50.2X5-	T50.2X6-
Tianeptine	T43.291-	T43.292-	T43.293-	T43.294-	T43.295-	T43.296-
Tiapamil	T46.1X1-	T46.1X2-	T46.1X3-	T46.1X4-	T46.1X5-	T46.1X6-
Tiapride	T43.591-	T43.592-	T43.593-	T43.594-	T43.595-	T43.596-
Tiaprofenic acid	T39.311-	T39.312-	T39.313-	T39.314-	T39.315-	T39.316-
Tiaramide	T39.8X1-	T39.8X2-	T39.8X3-	T39.8X4-	T39.8X5-	T39.8X6-
Ticarcillin	T36.0X1-	T36.0X2-	T36.0X3-	T36.0X4-	T36.0X5-	T36.0X6-
Ticlatone	T49.0X1-	T49.0X2-	T49.0X3-	T49.0X4-	T49.0X5-	T49.0X6-
Ticlopidine	T45.521-	T45.522-	T45.523-	T45.524-	T45.525-	T45.526-
Ticrynafen	T50.1X1-	T50.1X2-	T50.1X3-	T50.1X4-	T50.1X5-	T50.1X6-
Tidiacic	T50.991-	T50.992-	T50.993-	T50.994-	T50.995-	T50.996-
Tiemonium	T44.3X1-	T44.3X2-	T44.3X3-	T44.3X4-	T44.3X5-	T44.3X6-
iodide	T44.3X1-	T44.3X2-	T44.3X3-	T44.3X4-	T44.3X5-	T44.3X6-
Tienilic acid	T50.1X1-	T50.1X2-	T50.1X3-	T50.1X4-	T50.1X5-	T50.1X6-
Tifenamil	T44.3X1-	T44.3X2-	T44.3X3-	T44.3X4-	T44.3X5-	T44.3X6-
Tigan	T45.0X1-	T45.0X2-	T45.0X3-	T45.0X4-	T45.0X5-	T45.0X6-
Tigloidine	T44.3X1-	T44.3X2-	T44.3X3-	T44.3X4-	T44.3X5-	T44.3X6-
Tilactase	T47.5X1-	T47.5X2-	T47.5X3-	T47.5X4-	T47.5X5-	T47.5X6-
Tiletamine	T41.291-	T41.292-	T41.293-	T41.294-	T41.295-	T41.296-
Tilidine	T40.4X1-	T40.4X2-	T40.4X3-	T40.4X4-	-	-
Timepidium bromide	T44.3X1-	T44.3X2-	T44.3X3-	T44.3X4-	T44.3X5-	T44.3X6-
Timiperone	T43.4X1-	T43.4X2-	T43.4X3-	T43.4X4-	T43.4X5-	T43.4X6-
Timolol	T44.7X1-	T44.7X2-	T44.7X3-	T44.7X4-	T44.7X5-	T44.7X6-
Tin (chloride) (dust) (oxide) **NEC**	T56.6X1-	T56.6X2-	T56.6X3-	T56.6X4-	-	-
anti-infectives	T37.8X1-	T37.8X2-	T37.8X3-	T37.8X4-	T37.8X5-	T37.8X6-
Tincture, iodine — *see* Iodine						
Tindal	T43.3X1-	T43.3X2-	T43.3X3-	T43.3X4-	T43.3X5-	T43.3X6-
Tinidazole	T37.3X1-	T37.3X2-	T37.3X3-	T37.3X4-	T37.3X5-	T37.3X6-
Tinoridine	T39.8X1-	T39.8X2-	T39.8X3-	T39.8X4-	T39.8X5-	T39.8X6-
Tiocarlide	T37.1X1-	T37.1X2-	T37.1X3-	T37.1X4-	T37.1X5-	T37.1X6-

Substance	Poisoning Accidental (unintentional)	Poisoning Intentional self-harm	Poisoning Assault	Poisoning Undetermined	Adverse effect	Underdosing
Tioclomarol	T45.511-	T45.512-	T45.513-	T45.514-	T45.515-	T45.516-
Tioconazole	T49.0X1-	T49.0X2-	T49.0X3-	T49.0X4-	T49.0X5-	T49.0X6-
Tioguanine	T45.1X1-	T45.1X2-	T45.1X3-	T45.1X4-	T45.1X5-	T45.1X6-
Tiopronin	T50.991-	T50.992-	T50.993-	T50.994-	T50.995-	T50.996-
Tiotixene	T43.4X1-	T43.4X2-	T43.4X3-	T43.4X4-	T43.4X5-	T43.4X6-
Tioxolone	T49.4X1-	T49.4X2-	T49.4X3-	T49.4X4-	T49.4X5-	T49.4X6-
Tipepidine	T48.3X1-	T48.3X2-	T48.3X3-	T48.3X4-	T48.3X5-	T48.3X6-
Tiquizium bromide	T44.3X1-	T44.3X2-	T44.3X3-	T44.3X4-	T44.3X5-	T44.3X6-
Tiratricol	T38.1X1-	T38.1X2-	T38.1X3-	T38.1X4-	T38.1X5-	T38.1X6-
Tisopurine	T50.4X1-	T50.4X2-	T50.4X3-	T50.4X4-	T50.4X5-	T50.4X6-
Titanium (compounds) (vapor)	T56.891-	T56.892-	T56.893-	T56.894-	-	-
dioxide	T49.3X1-	T49.3X2-	T49.3X3-	T49.3X4-	T49.3X5-	T49.3X6-
ointment	T49.3X1-	T49.3X2-	T49.3X3-	T49.3X4-	T49.3X5-	T49.3X6-
oxide	T49.3X1-	T49.3X2-	T49.3X3-	T49.3X4-	T49.3X5-	T49.3X6-
tetrachloride	T56.891-	T56.892-	T56.893-	T56.894-	-	-
Titanocene	T56.891-	T56.892-	T56.893-	T56.894-	-	-
Titroid	T38.1X1-	T38.1X2-	T38.1X3-	T38.1X4-	T38.1X5-	T38.1X6-
Tizanidine	T42.8X1-	T42.8X2-	T42.8X3-	T42.8X4-	T42.8X5-	T42.8X6-
TMTD	T60.3X1-	T60.3X2-	T60.3X3-	T60.3X4-	-	-
TNT (fumes)	T65.3X1-	T65.3X2-	T65.3X3-	T65.3X4-	-	-
Toadstool	T62.0X1-	T62.0X2-	T62.0X3-	T62.0X4-	-	-
Tobacco NEC	T65.291-	T65.292-	T65.293-	T65.294-	-	-
cigarettes	T65.221-	T65.222-	T65.223-	T65.224-	-	-
Indian	T62.2X1-	T62.2X2-	T62.2X3-	T62.2X4-	-	-
smoke, second-hand	T65.221-	T65.222-	T65.223-	T65.224-	-	-
Tobramycin	T36.5X1-	T36.5X2-	T36.5X3-	T36.5X4-	T36.5X5-	T36.5X6-
Tocainide	T46.2X1-	T46.2X2-	T46.2X3-	T46.2X4-	T46.2X5-	T46.2X6-
Tocoferol	T45.2X1-	T45.2X2-	T45.2X3-	T45.2X4-	T45.2X5-	T45.2X6-
Tocopherol	T45.2X1-	T45.2X2-	T45.2X3-	T45.2X4-	T45.2X5-	T45.2X6-
acetate	T45.2X1-	T45.2X2-	T45.2X3-	T45.2X4-	T45.2X5-	T45.2X6-
Tocosamine	T48.0X1-	T48.0X2-	T48.0X3-	T48.0X4-	T48.0X5-	T48.0X6-
Todralazine	T46.5X1-	T46.5X2-	T46.5X3-	T46.5X4-	T46.5X5-	T46.5X6-
Tofisopam	T42.4X1-	T42.4X2-	T42.4X3-	T42.4X4-	T42.4X5-	T42.4X6-
Tofranil	T43.011-	T43.012-	T43.013-	T43.014-	T43.015-	T43.016-
Toilet deodorizer	T65.891-	T65.892-	T65.893-	T65.894-	-	-
Tolamolol	T44.7X1-	T44.7X2-	T44.7X3-	T44.7X4-	T44.7X5-	T44.7X6-
Tolazamide	T38.3X1-	T38.3X2-	T38.3X3-	T38.3X4-	T38.3X5-	T38.3X6-
Tolazoline	T46.7X1-	T46.7X2-	T46.7X3-	T46.7X4-	T46.7X5-	T46.7X6-
Tolbutamide (sodium)	T38.3X1-	T38.3X2-	T38.3X3-	T38.3X4-	T38.3X5-	T38.3X6-
Tolciclate	T49.0X1-	T49.0X2-	T49.0X3-	T49.0X4-	T49.0X5-	T49.0X6-
Tolmetin	T39.391-	T39.392-	T39.393-	T39.394-	T39.395-	T39.396-
Tolnaftate	T49.0X1-	T49.0X2-	T49.0X3-	T49.0X4-	T49.0X5-	T49.0X6-
Tolonidine	T46.5X1-	T46.5X2-	T46.5X3-	T46.5X4-	T46.5X5-	T46.5X6-
Toloxatone	T42.6X1-	T42.6X2-	T42.6X3-	T42.6X4-	T42.6X5-	T42.6X6-
Tolperisone	T44.3X1-	T44.3X2-	T44.3X3-	T44.3X4-	T44.3X5-	T44.3X6-
Tolserol	T42.8X1-	T42.8X2-	T42.8X3-	T42.8X4-	T42.8X5-	T42.8X6-
Toluene (liquid)	T52.2X1-	T52.2X2-	T52.2X3-	T52.2X4-	-	-
diisocyanate	T65.0X1-	T65.0X2-	T65.0X3-	T65.0X4-	-	-
Toluidine	T65.891-	T65.892-	T65.893-	T65.894-	-	-
vapor	T59.891-	T59.892-	T59.893-	T59.894-	-	-
Toluol (liquid)	T52.2X1-	T52.2X2-	T52.2X3-	T52.2X4-	-	-
vapor	T52.2X1-	T52.2X2-	T52.2X3-	T52.2X4-	-	-
Toluylenediamine	T65.3X1-	T65.3X2-	T65.3X3-	T65.3X4-	-	-
Tolylene-2,4-diisocyanate	T65.0X1-	T65.0X2-	T65.0X3-	T65.0X4-	-	-
Tonic NEC	T50.901-	T50.902-	T50.903-	T50.904-	T50.905-	T50.906-
Topical action drug NEC	T49.91X-	T49.92X-	T49.93X-	T49.94X-	T49.95X-	T49.96X-
ear, nose or throat	T49.6X1-	T49.6X2-	T49.6X3-	T49.6X4-	T49.6X5-	T49.6X6-
eye	T49.5X1-	T49.5X2-	T49.5X3-	T49.5X4-	T49.5X5-	T49.5X6-
skin	T49.91X-	T49.92X-	T49.93X-	T49.94X-	T49.95X-	T49.96X-
specified NEC	T49.8X1-	T49.8X2-	T49.8X3-	T49.8X4-	T49.8X5-	T49.8X6-
Toquizine	T44.3X1-	T44.3X2-	T44.3X3-	T44.3X4-	T44.3X5-	T44.3X6-
Toremifene	T38.6X1-	T38.6X2-	T38.6X3-	T38.6X4-	T38.6X5-	T38.6X6-
Tosylchloramide sodium	T49.8X1-	T49.8X2-	T49.8X3-	T49.8X4-	T49.8X5-	T49.8X6-
Toxaphene (dust) (spray)	T60.1X1-	T60.1X2-	T60.1X3-	T60.1X4-	-	-
Toxin, diphtheria (Schick Test)	T50.8X1-	T50.8X2-	T50.8X3-	T50.8X4-	T50.8X5-	T50.8X6-
Toxoid						
combined	T50.A21-	T50.A22-	T50.A23-	T50.A24-	T50.A25-	T50.A26-
diphtheria	T50.A91-	T50.A92-	T50.A93-	T50.A94-	T50.A95-	T50.A96-
tetanus	T50.A91-	T50.A92-	T50.A93-	T50.A94-	T50.A95-	T50.A96-
Trace element NEC	T45.8X1-	T45.8X2-	T45.8X3-	T45.8X4-	T45.8X5-	T45.8X6-
Tractor fuel NEC	T52.0X1-	T52.0X2-	T52.0X3-	T52.0X4-	-	-
Tragacanth	T50.991-	T50.992-	T50.993-	T50.994-	T50.995-	T50.996-
Tramadol	T40.4X1-	T40.4X2-	T40.4X3-	T40.4X4-	T40.4X5-	T40.4X6-
Tramazoline	T48.5X1-	T48.5X2-	T48.5X3-	T48.5X4-	T48.5X5-	T48.5X6-
Tranexamic acid	T45.621-	T45.622-	T45.623-	T45.624-	T45.625-	T45.626-
Tranilast	T45.0X1-	T45.0X2-	T45.0X3-	T45.0X4-	T45.0X5-	T45.0X6-
Tranquilizer NEC	T43.501-	T43.502-	T43.503-	T43.504-	T43.505-	T43.506-
with hypnotic or sedative	T42.6X1-	T42.6X2-	T42.6X3-	T42.6X4-	T42.6X5-	T42.6X6-

Substance	Poisoning Accidental (unintentional)	Poisoning Intentional self-harm	Poisoning Assault	Poisoning Undetermined	Adverse effect	Underdosing
Tranquilizer NEC - *continued*						
benzodiazepine NEC	T42.4X1-	T42.4X2-	T42.4X3-	T42.4X4-	T42.4X5-	T42.4X6-
butyrophenone NEC	T43.4X1-	T43.4X2-	T43.4X3-	T43.4X4-	T43.4X5-	T43.4X6-
carbamate	T43.591-	T43.592-	T43.593-	T43.594-	T43.595-	T43.596-
dimethylamine	T43.3X1-	T43.3X2-	T43.3X3-	T43.3X4-	T43.3X5-	T43.3X6-
ethylamine	T43.3X1-	T43.3X2-	T43.3X3-	T43.3X4-	T43.3X5-	T43.3X6-
hydroxyzine	T43.591-	T43.592-	T43.593-	T43.594-	T43.595-	T43.596-
major NEC	T43.501-	T43.502-	T43.503-	T43.504-	T43.505-	T43.506-
penothiazine NEC	T43.3X1-	T43.3X2-	T43.3X3-	T43.3X4-	T43.3X5-	T43.3X6-
phenothiazine-based	T43.3X1-	T43.3X2-	T43.3X3-	T43.3X4-	T43.3X5-	T43.3X6-
piperazine NEC	T43.3X1-	T43.3X2-	T43.3X3-	T43.3X4-	T43.3X5-	T43.3X6-
piperidine	T43.3X1-	T43.3X2-	T43.3X3-	T43.3X4-	T43.3X5-	T43.3X6-
propylamine	T43.3X1-	T43.3X2-	T43.3X3-	T43.3X4-	T43.3X5-	T43.3X6-
specified NEC	T43.591-	T43.592-	T43.593-	T43.594-	T43.595-	T43.596-
thioxanthene NEC	T43.591-	T43.592-	T43.593-	T43.594-	T43.595-	T43.596-
Tranxene	T42.4X1-	T42.4X2-	T42.4X3-	T42.4X4-	T42.4X5-	T42.4X6-
Tranylcypromine	T43.1X1-	T43.1X2-	T43.1X3-	T43.1X4-	T43.1X5-	T43.1X6-
Trapidil	T46.3X1-	T46.3X2-	T46.3X3-	T46.3X4-	T46.3X5-	T46.3X6-
Trasentine	T44.3X1-	T44.3X2-	T44.3X3-	T44.3X4-	T44.3X5-	T44.3X6-
Travert	T50.3X1-	T50.3X2-	T50.3X3-	T50.3X4-	T50.3X5-	T50.3X6-
Trazodone	T43.211-	T43.212-	T43.213-	T43.214-	T43.215-	T43.216-
Trecator	T37.1X1-	T37.1X2-	T37.1X3-	T37.1X4-	T37.1X5-	T37.1X6-
Treosulfan	T45.1X1-	T45.1X2-	T45.1X3-	T45.1X4-	T45.1X5-	T45.1X6-
Tretamine	T45.1X1-	T45.1X2-	T45.1X3-	T45.1X4-	T45.1X5-	T45.1X6-
Tretinoin	T49.0X1-	T49.0X2-	T49.0X3-	T49.0X4-	T49.0X5-	T49.0X6-
Tretoquinol	T48.6X1-	T48.6X2-	T48.6X3-	T48.6X4-	T48.6X5-	T48.6X6-
Triacetin	T49.0X1-	T49.0X2-	T49.0X3-	T49.0X4-	T49.0X5-	T49.0X6-
Triacetoxyanthracene	T49.4X1-	T49.4X2-	T49.4X3-	T49.4X4-	T49.4X5-	T49.4X6-
Triacetyloleandomycin	T36.3X1-	T36.3X2-	T36.3X3-	T36.3X4-	T36.3X5-	T36.3X6-
Triamcinolone	T38.0X1-	T38.0X2-	T38.0X3-	T38.0X4-	T38.0X5-	T38.0X6-
ENT agent	T49.6X1-	T49.6X2-	T49.6X3-	T49.6X4-	T49.6X5-	T49.6X6-
hexacetonide	T49.0X1-	T49.0X2-	T49.0X3-	T49.0X4-	T49.0X5-	T49.0X6-
ophthalmic preparation	T49.5X1-	T49.5X2-	T49.5X3-	T49.5X4-	T49.5X5-	T49.5X6-
topical NEC	T49.0X1-	T49.0X2-	T49.0X3-	T49.0X4-	T49.0X5-	T49.0X6-
Triampyzine	T44.3X1-	T44.3X2-	T44.3X3-	T44.3X4-	T44.3X5-	T44.3X6-
Triamterene	T50.2X1-	T50.2X2-	T50.2X3-	T50.2X4-	T50.2X5-	T50.2X6-
Triazine (herbicide)	T60.3X1-	T60.3X2-	T60.3X3-	T60.3X4-	-	-
Triaziquone	T45.1X1-	T45.1X2-	T45.1X3-	T45.1X4-	T45.1X5-	T45.1X6-
Triazolam	T42.4X1-	T42.4X2-	T42.4X3-	T42.4X4-	T42.4X5-	T42.4X6-
Triazole (herbicide)	T60.3X1-	T60.3X2-	T60.3X3-	T60.3X4-	-	-
Tribenoside	T46.991-	T46.992-	T46.993-	T46.994-	T46.995-	T46.996-
Tribromacetaldehyde	T42.6X1-	T42.6X2-	T42.6X3-	T42.6X4-	T42.6X5-	T42.6X6-
Tribromoethanol, rectal	T41.291-	T41.292-	T41.293-	T41.294-	T41.295-	T41.296-
Tribromomethane	T42.6X1-	T42.6X2-	T42.6X3-	T42.6X4-	T42.6X5-	T42.6X6-
Trichlorethane	T53.2X1-	T53.2X2-	T53.2X3-	T53.2X4-	-	-
Trichlorethylene	T53.2X1-	T53.2X2-	T53.2X3-	T53.2X4-	-	-
Trichlorfon	T60.0X1-	T60.0X2-	T60.0X3-	T60.0X4-	-	-
Trichlormethiazide	T50.2X1-	T50.2X2-	T50.2X3-	T50.2X4-	T50.2X5-	T50.2X6-
Trichlormethine	T45.1X1-	T45.1X2-	T45.1X3-	T45.1X4-	T45.1X5-	T45.1X6-
Trichloroacetic acid, Trichloracetic acid	T54.2X1-	T54.2X2-	T54.2X3-	T54.2X4-	-	-
medicinal	T49.4X1-	T49.4X2-	T49.4X3-	T49.4X4-	T49.4X5-	T49.4X6-
Trichloroethane	T53.2X1-	T53.2X2-	T53.2X3-	T53.2X4-	-	-
Trichloroethanol	T42.6X1-	T42.6X2-	T42.6X3-	T42.6X4-	T42.6X5-	T42.6X6-
Trichloroethyl phosphate	T42.6X1-	T42.6X2-	T42.6X3-	T42.0X4-	T42.6X5-	T42.6X6-
Trichloroethylene (liquid) (vapor)	T53.2X1-	T53.2X2-	T53.2X3-	T53.2X4-	-	-
anesthetic (gas)	T41.0X1-	T41.0X2-	T41.0X3-	T41.0X4-	T41.0X5-	T41.0X6-
vapor NEC	T53.2X1-	T53.2X2-	T53.2X3-	T53.2X4-	-	-
Trichlorofluoromethane NEC	T53.5X1-	T53.5X2-	T53.5X3-	T53.5X4-	-	-
Trichloronate	T60.0X1-	T60.0X2-	T60.0X3-	T60.0X4-	-	-
2,4,5-Trichlorophen-oxyacetic acid	T60.3X1-	T60.3X2-	T60.3X3-	T60.3X4-	-	-
Trichloropropane	T53.6X1-	T53.6X2-	T53.6X3-	T53.6X4-	-	-
Trichlorotriethylamine	T45.1X1-	T45.1X2-	T45.1X3-	T45.1X4-	T45.1X5-	T45.1X6-
Trichomonacides NEC	T37.3X1-	T37.3X2-	T37.3X3-	T37.3X4-	T37.3X5-	T37.3X6-
Trichomycin	T36.7X1-	T36.7X2-	T36.7X3-	T36.7X4-	T36.7X5-	T36.7X6-
Triclobisonium chloride	T49.0X1-	T49.0X2-	T49.0X3-	T49.0X4-	T49.0X5-	T49.0X6-
Triclocarban	T49.0X1-	T49.0X2-	T49.0X3-	T49.0X4-	T49.0X5-	T49.0X6-
Triclofos	T42.6X1-	T42.6X2-	T42.6X3-	T42.6X4-	T42.6X5-	T42.6X6-
Triclosan	T49.0X1-	T49.0X2-	T49.0X3-	T49.0X4-	T49.0X5-	T49.0X6-
Tricresyl phosphate	T65.891-	T65.892-	T65.893-	T65.894-	-	-
solvent	T52.91X-	T52.92X-	T52.93X-	T52.94X-	-	-
Tricyclamol chloride	T44.3X1-	T44.3X2-	T44.3X3-	T44.3X4-	T44.3X5-	T44.3X6-
Tridesilon	T49.0X1-	T49.0X2-	T49.0X3-	T49.0X4-	T49.0X5-	T49.0X6-
Tridihexethyl iodide	T44.3X1-	T44.3X2-	T44.3X3-	T44.3X4-	T44.3X5-	T44.3X6-
Tridione	T42.2X1-	T42.2X2-	T42.2X3-	T42.2X4-	T42.2X5-	T42.2X6-
Trientine	T45.8X1-	T45.8X2-	T45.8X3-	T45.8X4-	T45.8X5-	T45.8X6-

Substance	Poisoning Accidental (unintentional)	Poisoning Intentional self-harm	Poisoning Assault	Poisoning Undetermined	Adverse effect	Underdosing
Triethanolamine NEC	T54.3X1-	T54.3X2-	T54.3X3-	T54.3X4-	-	-
detergent	T54.3X1-	T54.3X2-	T54.3X3-	T54.3X4-	-	-
trinitrate (biphosphate)	T46.3X1-	T46.3X2-	T46.3X3-	T46.3X4-	T46.3X5-	T46.3X6-
Triethanomelamine	T45.1X1-	T45.1X2-	T45.1X3-	T45.1X4-	T45.1X5-	T45.1X6-
Triethylenemelamine	T45.1X1-	T45.1X2-	T45.1X3-	T45.1X4-	T45.1X5-	T45.1X6-
Triethylenephosphoramide	T45.1X1-	T45.1X2-	T45.1X3-	T45.1X4-	T45.1X5-	T45.1X6-
Triethylenethiophosphoramide	T45.1X1-	T45.1X2-	T45.1X3-	T45.1X4-	T45.1X5-	T45.1X6-
Trifluoperazine	T43.3X1-	T43.3X2-	T43.3X3-	T43.3X4-	T43.3X5-	T43.3X6-
Trifluoroethyl vinyl ether	T41.0X1-	T41.0X2-	T41.0X3-	T41.0X4-	T41.0X5-	T41.0X6-
Trifluperidol	T43.4X1-	T43.4X2-	T43.4X3-	T43.4X4-	T43.4X5-	T43.4X6-
Triflupromazine	T43.3X1-	T43.3X2-	T43.3X3-	T43.3X4-	T43.3X5-	T43.3X6-
Trifluridine	T37.5X1-	T37.5X2-	T37.5X3-	T37.5X4-	T37.5X5-	T37.5X6-
Triflusal	T45.521-	T45.522-	T45.523-	T45.524-	T45.525-	T45.526-
Trihexyphenidyl	T44.3X1-	T44.3X2-	T44.3X3-	T44.3X4-	T44.3X5-	T44.3X6-
Triiodothyronine	T38.1X1-	T38.1X2-	T38.1X3-	T38.1X4-	T38.1X5-	T38.1X6-
Trilene	T41.0X1-	T41.0X2-	T41.0X3-	T41.0X4-	T41.0X5-	T41.0X6-
Trilostane	T38.991-	T38.992-	T38.993-	T38.994-	T38.995-	T38.996-
Trimebutine	T44.3X1-	T44.3X2-	T44.3X3-	T44.3X4-	T44.3X5-	T44.3X6-
Trimecaine	T41.3X1-	T41.3X2-	T41.3X3-	T41.3X4-	T41.3X5-	T41.3X6-
Trimeprazine (tartrate)	T44.3X1-	T44.3X2-	T44.3X3-	T44.3X4-	T44.3X5-	T44.3X6-
Trimetaphan camsilate	T44.2X1-	T44.2X2-	T44.2X3-	T44.2X4-	T44.2X5-	T44.2X6-
Trimetazidine	T46.7X1-	T46.7X2-	T46.7X3-	T46.7X4-	T46.7X5-	T46.7X6-
Trimethadione	T42.2X1-	T42.2X2-	T42.2X3-	T42.2X4-	T42.2X5-	T42.2X6-
Trimethaphan	T44.2X1-	T44.2X2-	T44.2X3-	T44.2X4-	T44.2X5-	T44.2X6-
Trimethidinium	T44.2X1-	T44.2X2-	T44.2X3-	T44.2X4-	T44.2X5-	T44.2X6-
Trimethobenzamide	T45.0X1-	T45.0X2-	T45.0X3-	T45.0X4-	T45.0X5-	T45.0X6-
Trimethoprim	T37.8X1-	T37.8X2-	T37.8X3-	T37.8X4-	T37.8X5-	T37.8X6-
with sulfamethoxazole	T36.8X1-	T36.8X2-	T36.8X3-	T36.8X4-	T36.8X5-	T36.8X6-
Trimethylcarbinol	T51.3X1-	T51.3X2-	T51.3X3-	T51.3X4-	-	-
Trimethylpsoralen	T49.3X1-	T49.3X2-	T49.3X3-	T49.3X4-	T49.3X5-	T49.3X6-
Trimeton	T45.0X1-	T45.0X2-	T45.0X3-	T45.0X4-	T45.0X5-	T45.0X6-
Trimetrexate	T45.1X1-	T45.1X2-	T45.1X3-	T45.1X4-	T45.1X5-	T45.1X6-
Trimipramine	T43.011-	T43.012-	T43.013-	T43.014-	T43.015-	T43.016-
Trimustine	T45.1X1-	T45.1X2-	T45.1X3-	T45.1X4-	T45.1X5-	T45.1X6-
Trinitrine	T46.3X1-	T46.3X2-	T46.3X3-	T46.3X4-	T46.3X5-	T46.3X6-
Trinitrobenzol	T65.3X1-	T65.3X2-	T65.3X3-	T65.3X4-	-	-
Trinitrophenol	T65.3X1-	T65.3X2-	T65.3X3-	T65.3X4-	-	-
Trinitrotoluene (fumes)	T65.3X1-	T65.3X2-	T65.3X3-	T65.3X4-	-	-
Trional	T42.6X1-	T42.6X2-	T42.6X3-	T42.6X4-	T42.6X5-	T42.6X6-
Triorthocresyl phosphate	T65.891-	T65.892-	T65.893-	T65.894-	-	-
Trioxide of arsenic	T57.0X1-	T57.0X2-	T57.0X3-	T57.0X4-	-	-
Trioxysalen	T49.4X1-	T49.4X2-	T49.4X3-	T49.4X4-	T49.4X5-	T49.4X6-
Tripamide	T50.2X1-	T50.2X2-	T50.2X3-	T50.2X4-	T50.2X5-	T50.2X6-
Triparanol	T46.6X1-	T46.6X2-	T46.6X3-	T46.6X4-	T46.6X5-	T46.6X6-
Tripelennamine	T45.0X1-	T45.0X2-	T45.0X3-	T45.0X4-	T45.0X5-	T45.0X6-
Triperiden	T44.3X1-	T44.3X2-	T44.3X3-	T44.3X4-	T44.3X5-	T44.3X6-
Triperidol	T43.4X1-	T43.4X2-	T43.4X3-	T43.4X4-	T43.4X5-	T43.4X6-
Triphenylphosphate	T65.891-	T65.892-	T65.893-	T65.894-	-	-
Triple						
bromides	T42.6X1-	T42.6X2-	T42.6X3-	T42.6X4-	T42.6X5-	T42.6X6-
carbonate	T47.1X1-	T47.1X2-	T47.1X3-	T47.1X4-	T47.1X5-	T47.1X6-
vaccine						
DPT	T50.A11-	T50.A12-	T50.A13-	T50.A14-	T50.A15-	T50.A16-
including pertussis	T50.A11-	T50.A12-	T50.A13-	T50.A14-	T50.A15-	T50.A16-
MMR	T50.B91-	T50.B92-	T50.B93-	T50.B94-	T50.B95-	T50.B96-
Triprolidine	T45.0X1-	T45.0X2-	T45.0X3-	T45.0X4-	T45.0X5-	T45.0X6-
Trisodium hydrogen edetate	T50.6X1-	T50.6X2-	T50.6X3-	T50.6X4-	T50.6X5-	T50.6X6-
Trisoralen	T49.3X1-	T49.3X2-	T49.3X3-	T49.3X4-	T49.3X5-	T49.3X6-
Trisulfapyrimidines	T37.0X1-	T37.0X2-	T37.0X3-	T37.0X4-	T37.0X5-	T37.0X6-
Trithiozine	T44.3X1-	T44.3X2-	T44.3X3-	T44.3X4-	T44.3X5-	T44.3X6-
Tritiozine	T44.3X1-	T44.3X2-	T44.3X3-	T44.3X4-	T44.3X5-	T44.3X6-
Tritoqualine	T45.0X1-	T45.0X2-	T45.0X3-	T45.0X4-	T45.0X5-	T45.0X6-
Trofosfamide	T45.1X1-	T45.1X2-	T45.1X3-	T45.1X4-	T45.1X5-	T45.1X6-
Troleandomycin	T36.3X1-	T36.3X2-	T36.3X3-	T36.3X4-	T36.3X5-	T36.3X6-
Trolnitrate (phosphate)	T46.3X1-	T46.3X2-	T46.3X3-	T46.3X4-	T46.3X5-	T46.3X6-
Tromantadine	T37.5X1-	T37.5X2-	T37.5X3-	T37.5X4-	T37.5X5-	T37.5X6-
Trometamol	T50.2X1-	T50.2X2-	T50.2X3-	T50.2X4-	T50.2X5-	T50.2X6-
Tromethamine	T50.2X1-	T50.2X2-	T50.2X3-	T50.2X4-	T50.2X5-	T50.2X6-
Tronothane	T41.3X1-	T41.3X2-	T41.3X3-	T41.3X4-	T41.3X5-	T41.3X6-
Tropacine	T44.3X1-	T44.3X2-	T44.3X3-	T44.3X4-	T44.3X5-	T44.3X6-
Tropatepine	T44.3X1-	T44.3X2-	T44.3X3-	T44.3X4-	T44.3X5-	T44.3X6-
Tropicamide	T44.3X1-	T44.3X2-	T44.3X3-	T44.3X4-	T44.3X5-	T44.3X6-
Trospium chloride	T44.3X1-	T44.3X2-	T44.3X3-	T44.3X4-	T44.3X5-	T44.3X6-
Troxerutin	T46.991-	T46.992-	T46.993-	T46.994-	T46.995-	T46.996-
Troxidone	T42.2X1-	T42.2X2-	T42.2X3-	T42.2X4-	T42.2X5-	T42.2X6-
Tryparsamide	T37.3X1-	T37.3X2-	T37.3X3-	T37.3X4-	T37.3X5-	T37.3X6-
Trypsin	T45.3X1-	T45.3X2-	T45.3X3-	T45.3X4-	T45.3X5-	T45.3X6-
Tryptizol	T43.011-	T43.012-	T43.013-	T43.014-	T43.015-	T43.016-
TSH	T38.811-	T38.812-	T38.813-	T38.814-	T38.815-	T38.816-
Tuaminoheptane	T48.5X1-	T48.5X2-	T48.5X3-	T48.5X4-	T48.5X5-	T48.5X6-
Tuberculin, purified protein derivative (PPD)	T50.8X1-	T50.8X2-	T50.8X3-	T50.8X4-	T50.8X5-	T50.8X6-
Tubocurare	T48.1X1-	T48.1X2-	T48.1X3-	T48.1X4-	T48.1X5-	T48.1X6-
Tubocurarine (chloride)	T48.1X1-	T48.1X2-	T48.1X3-	T48.1X4-	T48.1X5-	T48.1X6-
Tulobuterol	T48.6X1-	T48.6X2-	T48.6X3-	T48.6X4-	T48.6X5-	T48.6X6-
Turpentine (spirits of)	T52.8X1-	T52.8X2-	T52.8X3-	T52.8X4-	-	-
vapor	T52.8X1-	T52.8X2-	T52.8X3-	T52.8X4-	-	-
Tybamate	T43.591-	T43.592-	T43.593-	T43.594-	T43.595-	T43.596-
Tyloxapol	T48.4X1-	T48.4X2-	T48.4X3-	T48.4X4-	T48.4X5-	T48.4X6-
Tymazoline	T48.5X1-	T48.5X2-	T48.5X3-	T48.5X4-	T48.5X5-	T48.5X6-
Typhoid-paratyphoid vaccine	T50.A91-	T50.A92-	T50.A93-	T50.A94-	T50.A95-	T50.A96-
Typhus vaccine	T50.A91-	T50.A92-	T50.A93-	T50.A94-	T50.A95-	T50.A96-
Tyropanoate	T50.8X1-	T50.8X2-	T50.8X3-	T50.8X4-	T50.8X5-	T50.8X6-
Tyrothricin	T49.6X1-	T49.6X2-	T49.6X3-	T49.6X4-	T49.6X5-	T49.6X6-
ENT agent	T49.6X1-	T49.6X2-	T49.6X3-	T49.6X4-	T49.6X5-	T49.6X6-
ophthalmic preparation	T49.5X1-	T49.5X2-	T49.5X3-	T49.5X4-	T49.5X5-	T49.5X6-
Ufenamate	T39.391-	T39.392-	T39.393-	T39.394-	T39.395-	T39.396-
Ultraviolet light protectant	T49.3X1-	T49.3X2-	T49.3X3-	T49.3X4-	T49.3X5-	T49.3X6-
Undecenoic acid	T49.0X1-	T49.0X2-	T49.0X3-	T49.0X4-	T49.0X5-	T49.0X6-
Undecoylium	T49.0X1-	T49.0X2-	T49.0X3-	T49.0X4-	T49.0X5-	T49.0X6-
Undecylenic acid (derivatives)	T49.0X1-	T49.0X2-	T49.0X3-	T49.0X4-	T49.0X5-	T49.0X6-
Unna's boot	T49.3X1-	T49.3X2-	T49.3X3-	T49.3X4-	T49.3X5-	T49.3X6-
Unsaturated fatty acid	T46.6X1-	T46.6X2-	T46.6X3-	T46.6X4-	T46.6X5-	T46.6X6-
Uracil mustard	T45.1X1-	T45.1X2-	T45.1X3-	T45.1X4-	T45.1X5-	T45.1X6-
Uramustine	T45.1X1-	T45.1X2-	T45.1X3-	T45.1X4-	T45.1X5-	T45.1X6-
Urapidil	T46.5X1-	T46.5X2-	T46.5X3-	T46.5X4-	T46.5X5-	T46.5X6-
Urari	T48.1X1-	T48.1X2-	T48.1X3-	T48.1X4-	T48.1X5-	T48.1X6-
Urate oxidase	T50.4X1-	T50.4X2-	T50.4X3-	T50.4X4-	T50.4X5-	T50.4X6-
Urea	T47.3X1-	T47.3X2-	T47.3X3-	T47.3X4-	T47.3X5-	T47.3X6-
peroxide	T49.0X1-	T49.0X2-	T49.0X3-	T49.0X4-	T49.0X5-	T49.0X6-
stibamine	T37.4X1-	T37.4X2-	T37.4X3-	T37.4X4-	T37.4X5-	T37.4X6-
topical	T49.8X1-	T49.8X2-	T49.8X3-	T49.8X4-	T49.8X5-	T49.8X6-
Urethane	T45.1X1-	T45.1X2-	T45.1X3-	T45.1X4-	T45.1X5-	T45.1X6-
Urginea (maritima) (scilla) — *see* Squill						
Uric acid metabolism drug NEC	T50.4X1-	T50.4X2-	T50.4X3-	T50.4X4-	T50.4X5-	T50.4X6-
Uricosuric agent	T50.4X1-	T50.4X2-	T50.4X3-	T50.4X4-	T50.4X5-	T50.4X6-
Urinary anti-infective	T37.8X1-	T37.8X2-	T37.8X3-	T37.8X4-	T37.8X5-	T37.8X6-
Urofollitropin	T38.811-	T38.812-	T38.813-	T38.814-	T38.815-	T38.816-
Urokinase	T45.611-	T45.612-	T45.613-	T45.614-	T45.615-	T45.616-
Urokon	T50.8X1-	T50.8X2-	T50.8X3-	T50.8X4-	T50.8X5-	T50.8X6-
Ursodeoxycholic acid	T50.991-	T50.992-	T50.993-	T50.994-	T50.995-	T50.996-
Ursodiol	T50.991-	T50.992-	T50.993-	T50.994-	T50.995-	T50.996-
Urtica	T62.2X1-	T62.2X2-	T62.2X3-	T62.2X4-	-	-
Utility gas — *see* Gas, utility						
Vaccine NEC	T50.Z91-	T50.Z92-	T50.Z93-	T50.Z94-	T50.Z95-	T50.Z96-
antineoplastic	T50.Z91-	T50.Z92-	T50.Z93-	T50.Z94-	T50.Z95-	T50.Z96-
bacterial NEC	T50.A91-	T50.A92-	T50.A93-	T50.A94-	T50.A95-	T50.A96-
with						
other bacterial component	T50.A21-	T50.A22-	T50.A23-	T50.A24-	T50.A25-	T50.A26-
pertussis component	T50.A11-	T50.A12-	T50.A13-	T50.A14-	T50.A15-	T50.A16-
viral-rickettsial component	T50.A21-	T50.A22-	T50.A23-	T50.A24-	T50.A25-	T50.A26-
mixed NEC	T50.A21-	T50.A22-	T50.A23-	T50.A24-	T50.A25-	T50.A26-
BCG	T50.A91-	T50.A92-	T50.A93-	T50.A94-	T50.A95-	T50.A96-
cholera	T50.A91-	T50.A92-	T50.A93-	T50.A94-	T50.A95-	T50.A96-
diphtheria	T50.A91-	T50.A92-	T50.A93-	T50.A94-	T50.A95-	T50.A96-
with tetanus	T50.A21-	T50.A22-	T50.A23-	T50.A24-	T50.A25-	T50.A26-
and pertussis	T50.A11-	T50.A12-	T50.A13-	T50.A14-	T50.A15-	T50.A16-
influenza	T50.B91-	T50.B92-	T50.B93-	T50.B94-	T50.B95-	T50.B96-
measles	T50.B91-	T50.B92-	T50.B93-	T50.B94-	T50.B95-	T50.B96-
with mumps and rubella	T50.B91-	T50.B92-	T50.B93-	T50.B94-	T50.B95-	T50.B96-
meningococcal	T50.A91-	T50.A92-	T50.A93-	T50.A94-	T50.A95-	T50.A96-
mumps	T50.B91-	T50.B92-	T50.B93-	T50.B94-	T50.B95-	T50.B96-
paratyphoid	T50.A91-	T50.A92-	T50.A93-	T50.A94-	T50.A95-	T50.A96-
pertussis	T50.A11-	T50.A12-	T50.A13-	T50.A14-	T50.A15-	T50.A16-
with diphtheria	T50.A11-	T50.A12-	T50.A13-	T50.A14-	T50.A15-	T50.A16-
and tetanus	T50.A11-	T50.A12-	T50.A13-	T50.A14-	T50.A15-	T50.A16-
with other component	T50.A11-	T50.A12-	T50.A13-	T50.A14-	T50.A15-	T50.A16-
plague	T50.A91-	T50.A92-	T50.A93-	T50.A94-	T50.A95-	T50.A96-
poliomyelitis	T50.B91-	T50.B92-	T50.B93-	T50.B94-	T50.B95-	T50.B96-
poliovirus	T50.B91-	T50.B92-	T50.B93-	T50.B94-	T50.B95-	T50.B96-
rabies	T50.B91-	T50.B92-	T50.B93-	T50.B94-	T50.B95-	T50.B96-
respiratory syncytial virus	T50.B91-	T50.B92-	T50.B93-	T50.B94-	T50.B95-	T50.B96-
rickettsial NEC	T50.A91-	T50.A92-	T50.A93-	T50.A94-	T50.A95-	T50.A96-

Substance	Poisoning Accidental (unintentional)	Poisoning Intentional self-harm	Poisoning Assault	Poisoning Undetermined	Adverse effect	Underdosing
Vaccine NEC - *continued*						
with						
bacterial component	T50.A21-	T50.A22-	T50.A23-	T50.A24-	T50.A25-	T50.A26-
Rocky Mountain spotted fever	T50.A91-	T50.A92-	T50.A93-	T50.A94-	T50.A95-	T50.A96-
rubella	T50.B91-	T50.B92-	T50.B93-	T50.B94-	T50.B95-	T50.B96-
sabin oral	T50.B91-	T50.B92-	T50.B93-	T50.B94-	T50.B95-	T50.B96-
smallpox	T50.B11-	T50.B12-	T50.B13-	T50.B14-	T50.B15-	T50.B16-
TAB	T50.A91-	T50.A92-	T50.A93-	T50.A94-	T50.A95-	T50.A96-
tetanus	T50.A91-	T50.A92-	T50.A93-	T50.A94-	T50.A95-	T50.A96-
typhoid	T50.A91-	T50.A92-	T50.A93-	T50.A94-	T50.A95-	T50.A96-
typhus	T50.A91-	T50.A92-	T50.A93-	T50.A94-	T50.A95-	T50.A96-
viral NEC	T50.B91-	T50.B92-	T50.B93-	T50.B94-	T50.B95-	T50.B96-
yellow fever	T50.B91-	T50.B92-	T50.B93-	T50.B94-	T50.B95-	T50.B96-
Vaccinia immune globulin	T50.Z11-	T50.Z12-	T50.Z13-	T50.Z14-	T50.Z15-	T50.Z16-
Vaginal contraceptives	T49.8X1-	T49.8X2-	T49.8X3-	T49.8X4-	T49.8X5-	T49.8X6-
Valerian						
root	T42.6X1-	T42.6X2-	T42.6X3-	T42.6X4-	T42.6X5-	T42.6X6-
tincture	T42.6X1-	T42.6X2-	T42.6X3-	T42.6X4-	T42.6X5-	T42.6X6-
Valethamate bromide	T44.3X1-	T44.3X2-	T44.3X3-	T44.3X4-	T44.3X5-	T44.3X6-
Valisone	T49.0X1-	T49.0X2-	T49.0X3-	T49.0X4-	T49.0X5-	T49.0X6-
Valium	T42.4X1-	T42.4X2-	T42.4X3-	T42.4X4-	T42.4X5-	T42.4X6-
Valmid	T42.6X1-	T42.6X2-	T42.6X3-	T42.6X4-	T42.6X5-	T42.6X6-
Valnoctamide	T42.6X1-	T42.6X2-	T42.6X3-	T42.6X4-	T42.6X5-	T42.6X6-
Valproate (sodium)	T42.6X1-	T42.6X2-	T42.6X3-	T42.6X4-	T42.6X5-	T42.6X6-
Valproic acid	T42.6X1-	T42.6X2-	T42.6X3-	T42.6X4-	T42.6X5-	T42.6X6-
Valpromide	T42.6X1-	T42.6X2-	T42.6X3-	T42.6X4-	T42.6X5-	T42.6X6-
Vanadium	T56.891-	T56.892-	T56.893-	T56.894-	-	-
Vancomycin	T36.8X1-	T36.8X2-	T36.8X3-	T36.8X4-	T36.8X5-	T36.8X6-
Vapor — *see also* Gas	T59.91X-	T59.92X-	T59.93X-	T59.94X-	-	-
kiln (carbon monoxide)	T58.8X1-	T58.8X2-	T58.8X3-	T58.8X4-	-	-
lead — *see* lead						
specified source NEC	T59.891-	T59.892-	T59.893-	T59.894-	-	-
Vardenafil	T46.7X1-	T46.7X2-	T46.7X3-	T46.7X4-	T46.7X5-	T46.7X6-
Varicose reduction drug	T46.8X1-	T46.8X2-	T46.8X3-	T46.8X4-	T46.8X5-	T46.8X6-
Varnish	T65.4X1-	T65.4X2-	T65.4X3-	T65.4X4-	-	-
cleaner	T52.91X-	T52.92X-	T52.93X-	T52.94X-	-	-
Vaseline	T49.3X1-	T49.3X2-	T49.3X3-	T49.3X4-	T49.3X5-	T49.3X6-
Vasodilan	T46.7X1-	T46.7X2-	T46.7X3-	T46.7X4-	T46.7X5-	T46.7X6-
Vasodilator						
coronary NEC	T46.3X1-	T46.3X2-	T46.3X3-	T46.3X4-	T46.3X5-	T46.3X6-
peripheral NEC	T46.7X1-	T46.7X2-	T46.7X3-	T46.7X4-	T46.7X5-	T46.7X6-
Vasopressin	T38.891-	T38.892-	T38.893-	T38.894-	T38.895-	T38.896-
Vasopressor drugs	T38.891-	T38.892-	T38.893-	T38.894-	T38.895-	T38.896-
Vecuronium bromide	T48.1X1-	T48.1X2-	T48.1X3-	T48.1X4-	T48.1X5-	T48.1X6-
Vegetable extract, astringent	T49.2X1-	T49.2X2-	T49.2X3-	T49.2X4-	T49.2X5-	T49.2X6-
Venlafaxine	T43.211-	T43.212-	T43.213-	T43.214-	T43.215-	T43.216-
Venom, venomous (bite) (sting)	T63.91X-	T63.92X-	T63.93X-	T63.94X-	-	-
amphibian NEC	T63.831-	T63.832-	T63.833-	T63.834-	-	-
animal NEC	T63.891-	T63.892-	T63.893-	T63.894-	-	-
ant	T63.421-	T63.422-	T63.423-	T63.424-	-	-
arthropod NEC	T63.481-	T63.482-	T63.483-	T63.484-	-	-
bee	T63.441-	T63.442-	T63.443-	T63.444-	-	-
centipede	T63.411-	T63.412-	T63.413-	T63.414-	-	-
fish	T63.591-	T63.592-	T63.593-	T63.594-	-	-
frog	T63.811-	T63.812-	T63.813-	T63.814-	-	
hornet	T63.451-	T63.452-	T63.453-	T63.454-	-	-
insect NEC	T63.481-	T63.482-	T63.483-	T63.484-	-	-
lizard	T63.121-	T63.122-	T63.123-	T63.124-	-	-
marine						
animals	T63.691-	T63.692-	T63.693-	T63.694-	-	-
bluebottle	T63.611-	T63.612-	T63.613-	T63.614-	-	-
jellyfish NEC	T63.621-	T63.622-	T63.623-	T63.624-	-	-
Portugese Man-o-war	T63.611-	T63.612-	T63.613-	T63.614-	-	-
sea anemone	T63.631-	T63.632-	T63.633-	T63.634-	-	-
specified NEC	T63.691-	T63.692-	T63.693-	T63.694-	-	-
fish	T63.591-	T63.592-	T63.593-	T63.594-	-	-
plants	T63.711-	T63.712-	T63.713-	T63.714-	-	-
sting ray	T63.511-	T63.512-	T63.513-	T63.514-	-	-
millipede (tropical)	T63.411-	T63.412-	T63.413-	T63.414-	-	-
plant NEC	T63.791-	T63.792-	T63.793-	T63.794-	-	-
marine	T63.711-	T63.712-	T63.713-	T63.714-	-	-
reptile	T63.191-	T63.192-	T63.193-	T63.194-	-	-
gila monster	T63.111-	T63.112-	T63.113-	T63.114-	-	-
lizard NEC	T63.121-	T63.122-	T63.123-	T63.124-	-	-
scorpion	T63.2X1-	T63.2X2-	T63.2X3-	T63.2X4-	-	-
snake	T63.001-	T63.002-	T63.003-	T63.004-	-	-
African NEC	T63.081-	T63.082-	T63.083-	T63.084-	-	-

Substance	Poisoning Accidental (unintentional)	Poisoning Intentional self-harm	Poisoning Assault	Poisoning Undetermined	Adverse effect	Underdosing
Venom, venomous - *continued*						
American (North) (South) NEC	T63.061-	T63.062-	T63.063-	T63.064-	-	-
Asian	T63.081-	T63.082-	T63.083-	T63.084-	-	-
Australian	T63.071-	T63.072-	T63.073-	T63.074-	-	-
cobra	T63.041-	T63.042-	T63.043-	T63.044-	-	-
coral snake	T63.021-	T63.022-	T63.023-	T63.024-	-	-
rattlesnake	T63.011-	T63.012-	T63.013-	T63.014-	-	-
specified NEC	T63.091-	T63.092-	T63.093-	T63.094-	-	-
taipan	T63.031-	T63.032-	T63.033-	T63.034-	-	-
specified NEC	T63.891-	T63.892-	T63.893-	T63.894-	-	-
spider	T63.301-	T63.302-	T63.303-	T63.304-	-	-
black widow	T63.311-	T63.312-	T63.313-	T63.314-	-	-
brown recluse	T63.331-	T63.332-	T63.333-	T63.334-	-	-
specified NEC	T63.391-	T63.392-	T63.393-	T63.394-	-	-
tarantula	T63.321-	T63.322-	T63.323-	T63.324-	-	-
sting ray	T63.511-	T63.512-	T63.513-	T63.514-	-	-
toad	T63.821-	T63.822-	T63.823-	T63.824-	-	-
wasp	T63.461-	T63.462-	T63.463-	T63.464-	-	-
Venous sclerosing drug NEC	T46.8X1-	T46.8X2-	T46.8X3-	T46.8X4-	T46.8X5-	T46.8X6-
Ventolin — *see* Albuterol						
Veramon	T42.3X1-	T42.3X2-	T42.3X3-	T42.3X4-	T42.3X5-	T42.3X6-
Verapamil	T46.1X1-	T46.1X2-	T46.1X3-	T46.1X4-	T46.1X5-	T46.1X6-
Veratrine	T46.5X1-	T46.5X2-	T46.5X3-	T46.5X4-	T46.5X5-	T46.5X6-
Veratrum						
album	T62.2X1-	T62.2X2-	T62.2X3-	T62.2X4-	-	-
alkaloids	T46.5X1-	T46.5X2-	T46.5X3-	T46.5X4-	T46.5X5-	T46.5X6-
viride	T62.2X1-	T62.2X2-	T62.2X3-	T62.2X4-	-	-
Verdigris	T60.3X1-	T60.3X2-	T60.3X3-	T60.3X4-	-	-
Veronal	T42.3X1-	T42.3X2-	T42.3X3-	T42.3X4-	T42.3X5-	T42.3X6-
Veroxil	T37.4X1-	T37.4X2-	T37.4X3-	T37.4X4-	T37.4X5-	T37.4X6-
Versenate	T50.6X1-	T50.6X2-	T50.6X3-	T50.6X4-	T50.6X5-	T50.6X6-
Versidyne	T39.8X1-	T39.8X2-	T39.8X3-	T39.8X4-	T39.8X5-	T39.8X6-
Vetrabutine	T48.0X1-	T48.0X2-	T48.0X3-	T48.0X4-	T48.0X5-	T48.0X6-
Vidarabine	T37.5X1-	T37.5X2-	T37.5X3-	T37.5X4-	T37.5X5-	T37.5X6-
Vienna						
green	T57.0X1-	T57.0X2-	T57.0X3-	T57.0X4-	-	-
insecticide	T60.2X1-	T60.2X2-	T60.2X3-	T60.2X4-	-	-
red	T57.0X1-	T57.0X2-	T57.0X3-	T57.0X4-	-	-
pharmaceutical dye	T50.991-	T50.992-	T50.993-	T50.994-	T50.995-	T50.996-
Vigabatrin	T42.6X1-	T42.6X2-	T42.6X3-	T42.6X4-	T42.6X5-	T42.6X6-
Viloxazine	T43.291-	T43.292-	T43.293-	T43.294-	T43.295-	T43.296-
Viminol	T39.8X1-	T39.8X2-	T39.8X3-	T39.8X4-	T39.8X5-	T39.8X6-
Vinbarbital, vinbarbitone	T42.3X1-	T42.3X2-	T42.3X3-	T42.3X4-	T42.3X5-	T42.3X6-
Vinblastine	T45.1X1-	T45.1X2-	T45.1X3-	T45.1X4-	T45.1X5-	T45.1X6-
Vinburnine	T46.7X1-	T46.7X2-	T46.7X3-	T46.7X4-	T46.7X5-	T46.7X6-
Vincamine	T45.1X1-	T45.1X2-	T45.1X3-	T45.1X4-	T45.1X5-	T45.1X6-
Vincristine	T45.1X1-	T45.1X2-	T45.1X3-	T45.1X4-	T45.1X5-	T45.1X6-
Vindesine	T45.1X1-	T45.1X2-	T45.1X3-	T45.1X4-	T45.1X5-	T45.1X6-
Vinesthene, vinethene	T41.0X1-	T41.0X2-	T41.0X3-	T41.0X4-	T41.0X5-	T41.0X6-
Vinorelbine tartrate	T45.1X1-	T45.1X2-	T45.1X3-	T45.1X4-	T45.1X5-	T45.1X6-
Vinpocetine	T46.7X1-	T46.7X2-	T46.7X3-	T46.7X4-	T46.7X5-	T46.7X6-
Vinyl						
acetate	T65.891-	T65.892-	T65.893-	T65.894-	-	-
bital	T42.3X1-	T42.3X2-	T42.3X3-	T42.3X4-	T42.3X5-	T42.3X6-
bromide	T65.891-	T65.892-	T65.893-	T65.894-	-	-
chloride	T59.891-	T59.892-	T59.893-	T59.894-	-	-
ether	T41.0X1-	T41.0X2-	T41.0X3-	T41.0X4-	T41.0X5-	T41.0X6-
Vinylbital	T42.3X1-	T42.3X2-	T42.3X3-	T42.3X4-	T42.3X5-	T42.3X6-
Vinylidene chloride	T65.891-	T65.892-	T65.893-	T65.894-	-	-
Vioform	T37.8X1-	T37.8X2-	T37.8X3-	T37.8X4-	T37.8X5-	T37.8X6-
topical	T49.0X1-	T49.0X2-	T49.0X3-	T49.0X4-	T49.0X5-	T49.0X6-
Viomycin	T36.8X1-	T36.8X2-	T36.8X3-	T36.8X4-	T36.8X5-	T36.8X6-
Viosterol	T45.2X1-	T45.2X2-	T45.2X3-	T45.2X4-	T45.2X5-	T45.2X6-
Viper (venom)	T63.091-	T63.092-	T63.093-	T63.094-	-	-
Viprynium	T37.4X1-	T37.4X2-	T37.4X3-	T37.4X4-	T37.4X5-	T37.4X6-
Viquidil	T46.7X1-	T46.7X2-	T46.7X3-	T46.7X4-	T46.7X5-	T46.7X6-
Viral vaccine NEC	T50.B91-	T50.B92-	T50.B93-	T50.B94-	T50.B95-	T50.B96-
Virginiamycin	T36.8X1-	T36.8X2-	T36.8X3-	T36.8X4-	T36.8X5-	T36.8X6-
Virugon	T37.5X1-	T37.5X2-	T37.5X3-	T37.5X4-	T37.5X5-	T37.5X6-
Viscous agent	T50.901-	T50.902-	T50.903-	T50.904-	T50.905-	T50.906-
Visine	T49.5X1-	T49.5X2-	T49.5X3-	T49.5X4-	T49.5X5-	T49.5X6-
Visnadine	T46.3X1-	T46.3X2-	T46.3X3-	T46.3X4-	T46.3X5-	T46.3X6-
Vitamin NEC	T45.2X1-	T45.2X2-	T45.2X3-	T45.2X4-	T45.2X5-	T45.2X6-
A	T45.2X1-	T45.2X2-	T45.2X3-	T45.2X4-	T45.2X5-	T45.2X6-
B NEC	T45.2X1-	T45.2X2-	T45.2X3-	T45.2X4-	T45.2X5-	T45.2X6-
nicotinic acid	T46.7X1-	T46.7X2-	T46.7X3-	T46.7X4-	T46.7X5-	T46.7X6-
B1	T45.2X1-	T45.2X2-	T45.2X3-	T45.2X4-	T45.2X5-	T45.2X6-

Substance	Poisoning Accidental (unintentional)	Poisoning Intentional self-harm	Poisoning Assault	Poisoning Undetermined	Adverse effect	Underdosing
Vitamin NEC - *continued*						
B2	T45.2X1-	T45.2X2-	T45.2X3-	T45.2X4-	T45.2X5-	T45.2X6-
B6	T45.2X1-	T45.2X2-	T45.2X3-	T45.2X4-	T45.2X5-	T45.2X6-
B12	T45.2X1-	T45.2X2-	T45.2X3-	T45.2X4-	T45.2X5-	T45.2X6-
B15	T45.2X1-	T45.2X2-	T45.2X3-	T45.2X4-	T45.2X5-	T45.2X6-
C	T45.2X1-	T45.2X2-	T45.2X3-	T45.2X4-	T45.2X5-	T45.2X6-
D	T45.2X1-	T45.2X2-	T45.2X3-	T45.2X4-	T45.2X5-	T45.2X6-
D2	T45.2X1-	T45.2X2-	T45.2X3-	T45.2X4-	T45.2X5-	T45.2X6-
D3	T45.2X1-	T45.2X2-	T45.2X3-	T45.2X4-	T45.2X5-	T45.2X6-
E	T45.2X1-	T45.2X2-	T45.2X3-	T45.2X4-	T45.2X5-	T45.2X6-
E acetate	T45.2X1-	T45.2X2-	T45.2X3-	T45.2X4-	T45.2X5-	T45.2X6-
hematopoietic	T45.8X1-	T45.8X2-	T45.8X3-	T45.8X4-	T45.8X5-	T45.8X6-
K NEC	T45.7X1-	T45.7X2-	T45.7X3-	T45.7X4-	T45.7X5-	T45.7X6-
K1	T45.7X1-	T45.7X2-	T45.7X3-	T45.7X4-	T45.7X5-	T45.7X6-
K2	T45.7X1-	T45.7X2-	T45.7X3-	T45.7X4-	T45.7X5-	T45.7X6-
PP	T45.2X1-	T45.2X2-	T45.2X3-	T45.2X4-	T45.2X5-	T45.2X6-
ulceroprotectant	T47.1X1-	T47.1X2-	T47.1X3-	T47.1X4-	T47.1X5-	T47.1X6-
Vleminckx's solution	T49.4X1-	T49.4X2-	T49.4X3-	T49.4X4-	T49.4X5-	T49.4X6-
Voltaren — *see* Diclofenac sodium						
Warfarin	T45.511-	T45.512-	T45.513-	T45.514-	T45.515-	T45.516-
rodenticide	T60.4X1-	T60.4X2-	T60.4X3-	T60.4X4-	-	-
sodium	T45.511-	T45.512-	T45.513-	T45.514-	T45.515-	T45.516-
Wasp (sting)	T63.461-	T63.462-	T63.463-	T63.464-	-	-
Water						
balance drug	T50.3X1-	T50.3X2-	T50.3X3-	T50.3X4-	T50.3X5-	T50.3X6-
distilled	T50.3X1-	T50.3X2-	T50.3X3-	T50.3X4-	T50.3X5-	T50.3X6-
gas — *see* Gas, water						
incomplete combustion of — *see* Carbon, monoxide, fuel, utility						
hemlock	T62.2X1-	T62.2X2-	T62.2X3-	T62.2X4-	-	-
moccasin (venom)	T63.061-	T63.062-	T63.063-	T63.064-	-	-
purified	T50.3X1-	T50.3X2-	T50.3X3-	T50.3X4-	T50.3X5-	T50.3X6-
Wax (paraffin) (petroleum)	T52.0X1-	T52.0X2-	T52.0X3-	T52.0X4-	-	-
automobile	T65.891-	T65.892-	T65.893-	T65.894-	-	-
floor	T52.0X1-	T52.0X2-	T52.0X3-	T52.0X4-	-	-
Weed killers NEC	T60.3X1-	T60.3X2-	T60.3X3-	T60.3X4-	-	-
Welldorm	T42.6X1-	T42.6X2-	T42.6X3-	T42.6X4-	T42.6X5-	T42.6X6-
White						
arsenic	T57.0X1-	T57.0X2-	T57.0X3-	T57.0X4-	-	-
hellebore	T62.2X1-	T62.2X2-	T62.2X3-	T62.2X4-	-	-
lotion (keratolytic)	T49.4X1-	T49.4X2-	T49.4X3-	T49.4X4-	T49.4X5-	T49.4X6-
spirit	T52.0X1-	T52.0X2-	T52.0X3-	T52.0X4-	-	-
Whitewash	T65.891-	T65.892-	T65.893-	T65.894-	-	-
Whole blood (human)	T45.8X1-	T45.8X2-	T45.8X3-	T45.8X4-	T45.8X5-	T45.8X6-
Wild						
black cherry	T62.2X1-	T62.2X2-	T62.2X3-	T62.2X4-	-	-
poisonous plants NEC	T62.2X1-	T62.2X2-	T62.2X3-	T62.2X4-	-	-
Window cleaning fluid	T65.891-	T65.892-	T65.893-	T65.894-	-	-
Wintergreen (oil)	T49.3X1-	T49.3X2-	T49.3X3-	T49.3X4-	T49.3X5-	T49.3X6-
Wisterine	T62.2X1-	T62.2X2-	T62.2X3-	T62.2X4-	-	-
Witch hazel	T49.2X1-	T49.2X2-	T49.2X3-	T49.2X4-	T49.2X5-	T49.2X6-
Wood alcohol or spirit	T51.1X1-	T51.1X2-	T51.1X3-	T51.1X4-	-	-
Wool fat (hydrous)	T49.3X1-	T49.3X2-	T49.3X3-	T49.3X4-	T49.3X5-	T49.3X6-
Woorali	T48.1X1-	T48.1X2-	T48.1X3-	T48.1X4-	T48.1X5-	T48.1X6-
Wormseed, American	T37.4X1-	T37.4X2-	T37.4X3-	T37.4X4-	T37.4X5-	T37.4X6-
Xamoterol	T44.5X1-	T44.5X2-	T44.5X3-	T44.5X4-	T44.5X5-	T44.5X6-
Xanthine diuretics	T50.2X1-	T50.2X2-	T50.2X3-	T50.2X4-	T50.2X5-	T50.2X6-
Xanthinol nicotinate	T46.7X1-	T46.7X2-	T46.7X3-	T46.7X4-	T46.7X5-	T46.7X6-
Xanthotoxin	T49.3X1-	T49.3X2-	T49.3X3-	T49.3X4-	T49.3X5-	T49.3X6-
Xantinol nicotinate	T46.7X1-	T46.7X2-	T46.7X3-	T46.7X4-	T46.7X5-	T46.7X6-
Xantocillin	T36.0X1-	T36.0X2-	T36.0X3-	T36.0X4-	T36.0X5-	T36.0X6-
Xenon (127Xe) (133Xe)	T50.8X1-	T50.8X2-	T50.8X3-	T50.8X4-	T50.8X5-	T50.8X6-
Xenysalate	T49.4X1-	T49.4X2-	T49.4X3-	T49.4X4-	T49.4X5-	T49.4X6-
Xibornol	T37.8X1-	T37.8X2-	T37.8X3-	T37.8X4-	T37.8X5-	T37.8X6-
Xigris	T45.511-	T45.512-	T45.513-	T45.514-	T45.515-	T45.516-
Xipamide	T50.2X1-	T50.2X2-	T50.2X3-	T50.2X4-	T50.2X5-	T50.2X6-
Xylene (vapor)	T52.2X1-	T52.2X2-	T52.2X3-	T52.2X4-	-	-
Xylocaine (infiltration) (topical)	T41.3X1-	T41.3X2-	T41.3X3-	T41.3X4-	T41.3X5-	T41.3X6-
nerve block (peripheral) (plexus)	T41.3X1-	T41.3X2-	T41.3X3-	T41.3X4-	T41.3X5-	T41.3X6-
spinal	T41.3X1-	T41.3X2-	T41.3X3-	T41.3X4-	T41.3X5-	T41.3X6-
Xylol (vapor)	T52.2X1-	T52.2X2-	T52.2X3-	T52.2X4-	-	-
Xylometazoline	T48.5X1-	T48.5X2-	T48.5X3-	T48.5X4-	T48.5X5-	T48.5X6-
Yeast	T45.2X1-	T45.2X2-	T45.2X3-	T45.2X4-	T45.2X5-	T45.2X6-
dried	T45.2X1-	T45.2X2-	T45.2X3-	T45.2X4-	T45.2X5-	T45.2X6-
Yellow						
fever vaccine	T50.B91-	T50.B92-	T50.B93-	T50.B94-	T50.B95-	T50.B96-
Yellow - *continued*						
jasmine	T62.2X1-	T62.2X2-	T62.2X3-	T62.2X4-	-	-
phenolphthalein	T47.2X1-	T47.2X2-	T47.2X3-	T47.2X4-	T47.2X5-	T47.2X6-
Yew	T62.2X1-	T62.2X2-	T62.2X3-	T62.2X4-	-	-
Yohimbic acid	T40.991-	T40.992-	T40.993-	T40.994-	T40.995-	T40.996-
Zactane	T39.8X1-	T39.8X2-	T39.8X3-	T39.8X4-	T39.8X5-	T39.8X6-
Zalcitabine	T37.5X1-	T37.5X2-	T37.5X3-	T37.5X4-	T37.5X5-	T37.5X6-
Zaroxolyn	T50.2X1-	T50.2X2-	T50.2X3-	T50.2X4-	T50.2X5-	T50.2X6-
Zephiran (topical)	T49.0X1-	T49.0X2-	T49.0X3-	T49.0X4-	T49.0X5-	T49.0X6-
ophthalmic preparation	T49.5X1-	T49.5X2-	T49.5X3-	T49.5X4-	T49.5X5-	T49.5X6-
Zeranol	T38.7X1-	T38.7X2-	T38.7X3-	T38.7X4-	T38.7X5-	T38.7X6-
Zerone	T51.1X1-	T51.1X2-	T51.1X3-	T51.1X4-	-	-
Zidovudine	T37.5X1-	T37.5X2-	T37.5X3-	T37.5X4-	T37.5X5-	T37.5X6-
Zimeldine	T43.221-	T43.222-	T43.223-	T43.224-	T43.225-	T43.226-
Zinc (compounds) (fumes) (vapor) **NEC**	T56.5X1-	T56.5X2-	T56.5X3-	T56.5X4-	-	-
anti-infectives	T49.0X1-	T49.0X2-	T49.0X3-	T49.0X4-	T49.0X5-	T49.0X6-
antivaricose	T46.8X1-	T46.8X2-	T46.8X3-	T46.8X4-	T46.8X5-	T46.8X6-
bacitracin	T49.0X1-	T49.0X2-	T49.0X3-	T49.0X4-	T49.0X5-	T49.0X6-
chloride (mouthwash)	T49.6X1-	T49.6X2-	T49.6X3-	T49.6X4-	T49.6X5-	T49.6X6-
chromate	T56.5X1-	T56.5X2-	T56.5X3-	T56.5X4-	-	-
gelatin	T49.3X1-	T49.3X2-	T49.3X3-	T49.3X4-	T49.3X5-	T49.3X6-
oxide	T49.3X1-	T49.3X2-	T49.3X3-	T49.3X4-	T49.3X5-	T49.3X6-
plaster	T49.3X1-	T49.3X2-	T49.3X3-	T49.3X4-	T49.3X5-	T49.3X6-
peroxide	T49.0X1-	T49.0X2-	T49.0X3-	T49.0X4-	T49.0X5-	T49.0X6-
pesticides	T56.5X1-	T56.5X2-	T56.5X3-	T56.5X4-	-	-
phosphide	T60.4X1-	T60.4X2-	T60.4X3-	T60.4X4-	-	-
pyrithionate	T49.4X1-	T49.4X2-	T49.4X3-	T49.4X4-	T49.4X5-	T49.4X6-
stearate	T49.3X1-	T49.3X2-	T49.3X3-	T49.3X4-	T49.3X5-	T49.3X6-
sulfate	T49.5X1-	T49.5X2-	T49.5X3-	T49.5X4-	T49.5X5-	T49.5X6-
ENT agent	T49.6X1-	T49.6X2-	T49.6X3-	T49.6X4-	T49.6X5-	T49.6X6-
ophthalmic solution	T49.5X1-	T49.5X2-	T49.5X3-	T49.5X4-	T49.5X5-	T49.5X6-
topical NEC	T49.0X1-	T49.0X2-	T49.0X3-	T49.0X4-	T49.0X5-	T49.0X6-
undecylenate	T49.0X1-	T49.0X2-	T49.0X3-	T49.0X4-	T49.0X5-	T49.0X6-
Zineb	T60.0X1-	T60.0X2-	T60.0X3-	T60.0X4-	-	-
Zinostatin	T45.1X1-	T45.1X2-	T45.1X3-	T45.1X4-	T45.1X5-	T45.1X6-
Zipeprol	T48.3X1-	T48.3X2-	T48.3X3-	T48.3X4-	T48.3X5-	T48.3X6-
Zofenopril	T46.4X1-	T46.4X2-	T46.4X3-	T46.4X4-	T46.4X5-	T46.4X6-
Zolpidem	T42.6X1-	T42.6X2-	T42.6X3-	T42.6X4-	T42.6X5-	T42.6X6-
Zomepirac	T39.391-	T39.392-	T39.393-	T39.394-	T39.395-	T39.396-
Zopiclone	T42.6X1-	T42.6X2-	T42.6X3-	T42.6X4-	T42.6X5-	T42.6X6-
Zorubicin	T45.1X1-	T45.1X2-	T45.1X3-	T45.1X4-	T45.1X5-	T45.1X6-
Zotepine	T43.591-	T43.592-	T43.593-	T43.594-	T43.595-	T43.596-
Zovant	T45.511-	T45.512-	T45.513-	T45.514-	T45.515-	T45.516-
Zoxazolamine	T42.8X1-	T42.8X2-	T42.8X3-	T42.8X4-	T42.8X5-	T42.8X6-
Zuclopenthixol	T43.4X1-	T43.4X2-	T43.4X3-	T43.4X4-	T43.4X5-	T43.4X6-
Zygadenus (venenosus)	T62.2X1-	T62.2X2-	T62.2X3-	T62.2X4-	-	-
Zyprexa	T43.591-	T43.592-	T43.593-	T43.594-	T43.595-	T43.596-

A

Abandonment (causing exposure to weather conditions) (with intent to injure or kill) **NEC** X58
Abuse (adult) (child) (mental) (physical) (sexual) X58
Accident (to) X58
 aircraft (in transit) (powered) — *see also* Accident, transport, aircraft
  due to, caused by cataclysm — *see* Forces of nature, by type
 animal-rider — *see* Accident, transport, animal-rider
 animal-drawn vehicle — *see* Accident, transport, animal-drawn vehicle occupant
 automobile — *see* Accident, transport, car occupant
 bare foot water skiier V94.4
 boat, boating — *see also* Accident, watercraft
  striking swimmer
   powered V94.11
   unpowered V94.12
 bus — *see* Accident, transport, bus occupant
 cable car, not on rails V98.0
  on rails — *see* Accident, transport, streetcar occupant
 car — *see* Accident, transport, car occupant
 caused by, due to
  animal NEC W64
  chain hoist W24.0
  cold (excessive) — *see* Exposure, cold
  corrosive liquid, substance — *see* Table of Drugs and Chemicals
  cutting or piercing instrument — *see* Contact, with, by type of instrument
  drive belt W24.0
  electric
   current — *see* Exposure, electric current
   motor — *see also* Contact, with, by type of machine W31.3
    current (of) W86.8
  environmental factor NEC X58
  explosive material — *see* Explosion
  fire, flames — *see* Exposure, fire
  firearm missile — *see* Discharge, firearm by type
  heat (excessive) — *see* Heat
  hot — *see* Contact, with, hot
  ignition — *see* Ignition
  lifting device W24.0
  lightning — *see* subcategory T75.0
   causing fire — *see* Exposure, fire
  machine, machinery — *see* Contact, with, by type of machine
  natural factor NEC X58
  pulley (block) W24.0
  radiation — *see* Radiation
  steam X13.1
   inhalation X13.0
   pipe X16
  thunderbolt — *see* subcategory T75.0
   causing fire — *see* Exposure, fire
  transmission device W24.1
 coach — *see* Accident, transport, bus occupant
 coal car — *see* Accident, transport, industrial vehicle occupant
 diving — *see also* Fall, into, water
  with
   drowning or submersion — *see* Drowning
 forklift — *see* Accident, transport, industrial vehicle occupant
 heavy transport vehicle NOS — *see* Accident, transport, truck occupant
 ice yacht V98.2
 in
  medical, surgical procedure
   as, or due to misadventure — *see* Misadventure
   causing an abnormal reaction or later complication without mention of misadventure — *see also* Complication of or following, by type of procedure Y84.9
 land yacht V98.1
 late effect of — *see* W00-X58 with 7th character S
 logging car — *see* Accident, transport, industrial vehicle occupant
 machine, machinery — *see also* Contact, with, by type of machine
  on board watercraft V93.69
   explosion — *see* Explosion, in, watercraft
   fire — *see* Burn, on board watercraft
   powered craft V93.63
    ferry boat V93.61
    fishing boat V93.62
    jetskis V93.63
    liner V93.61
    merchant ship V93.60
    passenger ship V93.61

Accident (to) - *continued*
 machine, machinery - *continued*
  on board watercraft - *continued*
   powered craft - *continued*
    sailboat V93.64
 mine tram — *see* Accident, transport, industrial vehicle occupant
 mobility scooter (motorized) — *see* Accident, transport, pedestrian, conveyance, specified type NEC
 motor scooter — *see* Accident, transport, motorcyclist
 motor vehicle NOS (traffic) — *see also* Accident, transport V89.2
  nontraffic V89.0
  three-wheeled NOS — *see* Accident, transport, three-wheeled motor vehicle occupant
 motorcycle NOS — *see* Accident, transport, motorcyclist
 nonmotor vehicle NOS (nontraffic) — *see also* Accident, transport V89.1
  traffic NOS V89.3
 nontraffic (victim's mode of transport NOS) V88.9
  collision (between) V88.7
   bus and truck V88.5
   car and:
    bus V88.3
    pickup V88.2
    three-wheeled motor vehicle V88.0
    train V88.6
    truck V88.4
    two-wheeled motor vehicle V88.0
    van V88.2
   specified vehicle NEC and:
    three-wheeled motor vehicle V88.1
    two-wheeled motor vehicle V88.1
  known mode of transport — *see* Accident, transport, by type of vehicle
  noncollision V88.8
 on board watercraft V93.89
  powered craft V93.83
   ferry boat V93.81
   fishing boat V93.82
   jetskis V93.83
   liner V93.81
   merchant ship V93.80
   passenger ship V93.81
  unpowered craft V93.88
   canoe V93.85
   inflatable V93.86
    in tow
     recreational V94.31
     specified NEC V94.32
   kayak V93.85
   sailboat V93.84
   surf-board V93.88
   water skis V93.87
   windsurfer V93.88
 parachutist V97.29
  entangled in object V97.21
  injured on landing V97.22
 pedal cycle — *see* Accident, transport, pedal cyclist
 pedestrian (on foot)
  with
   another pedestrian W51
    with fall W03
     due to ice or snow W00.0
    on pedestrian conveyance NEC V00.09
   roller skater (in-line) V00.01
   skate boarder V00.02
   transport vehicle — *see* Accident, transport
  on pedestrian conveyance — *see* Accident, transport, pedestrian, conveyance
 pick-up truck or van — *see* Accident, transport, pickup truck occupant
 quarry truck — *see* Accident, transport, industrial vehicle occupant
 railway vehicle (any) (in motion) — *see* Accident, transport, railway vehicle occupant
  due to cataclysm — *see* Forces of nature, by type
 scooter (non-motorized) — *see* Accident, transport, pedestrian, conveyance, scooter
 sequelae of — *see* W00-X58 with 7th character S
 skateboard — *see* Accident, transport, pedestrian, conveyance, skateboard
 ski (ing) — *see* Accident, transport, pedestrian, conveyance
  lift V98.3
 specified cause NEC X58
 streetcar — *see* Accident, transport, streetcar occupant
 traffic (victim's mode of transport NOS) V87.9
  collision (between) V87.7

Accident (to) - *continued*
 traffic (victim's mode of transport NOS) - *continued*
  collision (between) - *continued*
   bus and truck V87.5
   car and:
    bus V87.3
    pickup V87.2
    three-wheeled motor vehicle V87.0
    train V87.6
    truck V87.4
    two-wheeled motor vehicle V87.0
    van V87.2
   specified vehicle NEC and:
    three-wheeled motor vehicle V87.1
    two-wheeled motor vehicle V87.1
  known mode of transport — *see* Accident, transport, by type of vehicle
  noncollision V87.8
 transport (involving injury to) V99
  18 wheeler — *see* Accident, transport, truck occupant
  agricultural vehicle occupant (nontraffic) V84.9
   driver V84.5
   hanger-on V84.7
   passenger V84.6
   traffic V84.3
    driver V84.0
    hanger-on V84.2
    passenger V84.1
   while boarding or alighting V84.4
  aircraft NEC V97.89
   military NEC V97.818
    with civlian aircraft V97.810
    civilian injured by V97.811
   occupant injured (in)
    nonpowered craft accident V96.9
     balloon V96.00
      collision V96.03
      crash V96.01
      explosion V96.05
      fire V96.04
      forced landing V96.02
      specified type NEC V96.09
     glider V96.20
      collision V96.23
      crash V96.21
      explosion V96.25
      fire V96.24
      forced landing V96.22
      specified type NEC V96.29
     hang glider V96.10
      collision V96.13
      crash V96.11
      explosion V96.15
      fire V96.14
      forced landing V96.12
      specified type NEC V96.19
     specified craft NEC V96.8
    powered craft accident V95.9
     fixed wing NEC
      commercial V95.30
       collision V95.33
       crash V95.31
       explosion V95.35
       fire V95.34
       forced landing V95.32
       specified type NEC V95.39
      private V95.20
       collision V95.23
       crash V95.21
       explosion V95.25
       fire V95.24
       forced landing V95.22
       specified type NEC V95.29
     glider V95.10
      collision V95.13
      crash V95.11
      explosion V95.15
      fire V95.14
      forced landing V95.12
      specified type NEC V95.19
     helicopter V95.00
      collision V95.03
      crash V95.01
      explosion V95.05
      fire V95.04
      forced landing V95.02
      specified type NEC V95.09
     spacecraft V95.40
      collision V95.43
      crash V95.41
      explosion V95.45
      fire V95.44

- **Accident** (to) - *continued*
  - transport (involving injury to) - *continued*
    - aircraft NEC - *continued*
      - occupant injured (in) - *continued*
        - powered craft accident - *continued*
          - spacecraft - *continued*
            - forced landing V95.42
            - specified type NEC V95.49
          - specified craft NEC V95.8
          - ultralight V95.10
            - collision V95.13
            - crash V95.11
            - explosion V95.15
            - fire V95.14
            - forced landing V95.12
            - specified type NEC V95.19
        - specified accident NEC V97.0
        - while boarding or alighting V97.1
      - person (injured by)
        - falling from, in or on aircraft V97.0
        - machinery on aircraft V97.89
        - on ground with aircraft involvement V97.39
        - rotating propeller V97.32
        - struck by object falling from aircraft V97.31
        - sucked into aircraft jet V97.33
        - while boarding or alighting aircraft V97.1
    - airport (battery-powered) passenger vehicle — *see* Accident, transport, industrial vehicle occupant
    - all-terrain vehicle occupant (nontraffic) V86.95
      - driver V86.55
      - dune buggy — *see* Accident, transport, dune buggy occupant
      - hanger-on V86.75
      - passenger V86.65
      - snowmobile — *see* Accident, transport, snowmobile occupant
      - specified type NEC V86.99
      - traffic V86.35
        - driver V86.05
        - hanger-on V86.25
        - passenger V86.15
      - while boarding or alighting V86.45
    - ambulance occupant (traffic) V86.31
      - driver V86.01
      - hanger-on V86.21
      - nontraffic V86.91
        - driver V86.51
        - hanger-on V86.71
        - passenger V86.61
      - passenger V86.11
      - while boarding or alighting V86.41
    - animal-drawn vehicle occupant (in) V80.929
      - collision (with)
        - animal V80.12
          - being ridden V80.711
        - animal-drawn vehicle V80.721
        - bus V80.42
        - car V80.42
        - fixed or stationary object V80.82
        - military vehicle V80.920
        - nonmotor vehicle V80.791
        - pedal cycle V80.22
        - pedestrian V80.12
        - pickup V80.42
        - railway train or vehicle V80.62
        - specified motor vehicle NEC V80.52
        - streetcar V80.731
        - truck V80.42
        - two- or three-wheeled motor vehicle V80.32
        - van V80.42
      - noncollision V80.02
      - specified circumstance NEC V80.928
    - animal-rider V80.919
      - collision (with)
        - animal V80.11
          - being ridden V80.710
        - animal-drawn vehicle V80.720
        - bus V80.41
        - car V80.41
        - fixed or stationary object V80.81
        - military vehicle V80.910
        - nonmotor vehicle V80.790
        - pedal cycle V80.21
        - pedestrian V80.11
        - pickup V80.41
        - railway train or vehicle V80.61
        - specified motor vehicle NEC V80.51
        - streetcar V80.730
        - truck V80.41
        - two- or three-wheeled motor vehicle V80.31
        - van V80.41
      - noncollision V80.018
        - specified as horse rider V80.010

- **Accident** (to) - *continued*
  - transport (involving injury to) - *continued*
    - animal-rider - *continued*
      - specified circumstance NEC V80.918
    - armored car — *see* Accident, transport, truck occupant
    - battery-powered truck (baggage) (mail) — *see* Accident, transport, industrial vehicle occupant
    - bus occupant V79.9
      - collision (with)
        - animal (traffic) V70.9
          - being ridden (traffic) V76.9
            - nontraffic V76.3
            - while boarding or alighting V76.4
          - nontraffic V70.3
          - while boarding or alighting V70.4
        - animal-drawn vehicle (traffic) V76.9
          - nontraffic V76.3
          - while boarding or alighting V76.4
        - bus (traffic) V74.9
          - nontraffic V74.3
          - while boarding or alighting V74.4
        - car (traffic) V73.9
          - nontraffic V73.3
          - while boarding or alighting V73.4
        - motor vehicle NOS (traffic) V79.60
          - nontraffic V79.20
          - specified type NEC (traffic) V79.69
            - nontraffic V79.29
        - pedal cycle (traffic) V71.9
          - nontraffic V71.3
          - while boarding or alighting V71.4
        - pickup truck (traffic) V73.9
          - nontraffic V73.3
          - while boarding or alighting V73.4
        - railway vehicle (traffic) V75.9
          - nontraffic V75.3
          - while boarding or alighting V75.4
        - specified vehicle NEC (traffic) V76.9
          - nontraffic V76.3
          - while boarding or alighting V76.4
        - stationary object (traffic) V77.9
          - nontraffic V77.3
          - while boarding or alighting V77.4
        - streetcar (traffic) V76.9
          - nontraffic V76.3
          - while boarding or alighting V76.4
        - three wheeled motor vehicle (traffic) V72.9
          - nontraffic V72.3
          - while boarding or alighting V72.4
        - truck (traffic) V74.9
          - nontraffic V74.3
          - while boarding or alighting V74.4
        - two wheeled motor vehicle (traffic) V72.9
          - nontraffic V72.3
          - while boarding or alighting V72.4
        - van (traffic) V73.9
          - nontraffic V73.3
          - while boarding or alighting V73.4
      - driver
        - collision (with)
          - animal (traffic) V70.5
            - being ridden (traffic) V76.5
              - nontraffic V76.0
            - nontraffic V70.0
          - animal-drawn vehicle (traffic) V76.5
            - nontraffic V76.0
          - bus (traffic) V74.5
            - nontraffic V74.0
          - car (traffic) V73.5
            - nontraffic V73.0
          - motor vehicle NOS (traffic) V79.40
            - nontraffic V79.00
            - specified type NEC (traffic) V79.49
              - nontraffic V79.09
          - pedal cycle (traffic) V71.5
            - nontraffic V71.0
          - pickup truck (traffic) V73.5
            - nontraffic V73.0
          - railway vehicle (traffic) V75.5
            - nontraffic V75.0
          - specified vehicle NEC (traffic) V76.5
            - nontraffic V76.0
          - stationary object (traffic) V77.5
            - nontraffic V77.0
          - streetcar (traffic) V76.5
            - nontraffic V76.0
          - three wheeled motor vehicle (traffic) V72.5
            - nontraffic V72.0
          - truck (traffic) V74.5
            - nontraffic V74.0
          - two wheeled motor vehicle (traffic) V72.5
            - nontraffic V72.0

- **Accident** (to) - *continued*
  - transport (involving injury to) - *continued*
    - bus occupant - *continued*
      - driver - *continued*
        - collision (with) - *continued*
          - van (traffic) V73.5
            - nontraffic V73.0
        - noncollision accident (traffic) V78.5
          - nontraffic V78.0
      - noncollision accident (traffic) V78.9
        - nontraffic V78.3
        - while boarding or alighting V78.4
      - nontraffic V79.3
      - hanger-on
        - collision (with)
          - animal (traffic) V70.7
            - being ridden (traffic) V76.7
              - nontraffic V76.2
            - nontraffic V70.2
          - animal-drawn vehicle (traffic) V76.7
            - nontraffic V76.2
          - bus (traffic) V74.7
            - nontraffic V74.2
          - car (traffic) V73.7
            - nontraffic V73.2
          - pedal cycle (traffic) V71.7
            - nontraffic V71.2
          - pickup truck (traffic) V73.7
            - nontraffic V73.2
          - railway vehicle (traffic) V75.7
            - nontraffic V75.2
          - specified vehicle NEC (traffic) V76.7
            - nontraffic V76.2
          - stationary object (traffic) V77.7
            - nontraffic V77.2
          - streetcar (traffic) V76.7
            - nontraffic V76.2
          - three wheeled motor vehicle (traffic) V72.7
            - nontraffic V72.2
          - truck (traffic) V74.7
            - nontraffic V74.2
          - two wheeled motor vehicle (traffic) V72.7
            - nontraffic V72.2
          - van (traffic) V73.7
            - nontraffic V73.2
        - noncollision accident (traffic) V78.7
          - nontraffic V78.2
      - passenger
        - collision (with)
          - animal (traffic) V70.6
            - being ridden (traffic) V76.6
              - nontraffic V76.1
            - nontraffic V70.1
          - animal-drawn vehicle (traffic) V76.6
            - nontraffic V76.1
          - bus (traffic) V74.6
            - nontraffic V74.1
          - car (traffic) V73.6
            - nontraffic V73.1
          - motor vehicle NOS (traffic) V79.50
            - nontraffic V79.10
            - specified type NEC (traffic) V79.59
              - nontraffic V79.19
          - pedal cycle (traffic) V71.6
            - nontraffic V71.1
          - pickup truck (traffic) V73.6
            - nontraffic V73.1
          - railway vehicle (traffic) V75.6
            - nontraffic V75.1
          - specified vehicle NEC (traffic) V76.6
            - nontraffic V76.1
          - stationary object (traffic) V77.6
            - nontraffic V77.1
          - streetcar (traffic) V76.6
            - nontraffic V76.1
          - three wheeled motor vehicle (traffic) V72.6
            - nontraffic V72.1
          - truck (traffic) V74.6
            - nontraffic V74.1
          - two wheeled motor vehicle (traffic) V72.6
            - nontraffic V72.1
          - van (traffic) V73.6
            - nontraffic V73.1
        - noncollision accident (traffic) V78.6
          - nontraffic V78.1
      - specified type NEC V79.88
        - military vehicle V79.81
    - cable car, not on rails V98.0
      - on rails — *see* Accident, transport, streetcar occupant
    - car occupant V49.9
      - ambulance occupant — *see* Accident, transport, ambulance occupant

Accident (to) - *continued*
transport (involving injury to) - *continued*
motorcyclist - *continued*
collision (with) - *continued*
pickup truck (traffic) - *continued*
nontraffic V23.2
while boarding or alighting V23.3
railway vehicle (traffic) V25.9
nontraffic V25.2
while boarding or alighting V25.3
specified vehicle NEC (traffic) V26.9
nontraffic V26.2
while boarding or alighting V26.3
stationary object (traffic) V27.9
nontraffic V27.2
while boarding or alighting V27.3
streetcar (traffic) V26.9
nontraffic V26.2
while boarding or alighting V26.3
three wheeled motor vehicle (traffic) V22.9
nontraffic V22.2
while boarding or alighting V22.3
truck (traffic) V24.9
nontraffic V24.2
while boarding or alighting V24.3
two wheeled motor vehicle (traffic) V22.9
nontraffic V22.2
while boarding or alighting V22.3
van (traffic) V23.9
nontraffic V23.2
while boarding or alighting V23.3
driver
collision (with)
animal (traffic) V20.4
being ridden (traffic) V26.4
nontraffic V26.0
nontraffic V20.0
animal-drawn vehicle (traffic) V26.4
nontraffic V26.0
bus (traffic) V24.4
nontraffic V24.0
car (traffic) V23.4
nontraffic V23.0
motor vehicle NOS (traffic) V29.40
nontraffic V29.00
specified type NEC (traffic) V29.49
nontraffic V29.09
pedal cycle (traffic) V21.4
nontraffic V21.0
pickup truck (traffic) V23.4
nontraffic V23.0
railway vehicle (traffic) V25.4
nontraffic V25.0
specified vehicle NEC (traffic) V26.4
nontraffic V26.0
stationary object (traffic) V27.4
nontraffic V27.0
streetcar (traffic) V26.4
nontraffic V26.0
three wheeled motor vehicle (traffic) V22.4
nontraffic V22.0
truck (traffic) V24.4
nontraffic V24.0
two wheeled motor vehicle (traffic) V22.4
nontraffic V22.0
van (traffic) V23.4
nontraffic V23.0
noncollision accident (traffic) V28.4
nontraffic V28.0
noncollision accident (traffic) V28.9
nontraffic V28.2
while boarding or alighting V28.3
nontraffic V29.3
passenger
collision (with)
animal (traffic) V20.5
being ridden (traffic) V26.5
nontraffic V26.1
nontraffic V20.1
animal-drawn vehicle (traffic) V26.5
nontraffic V26.1
bus (traffic) V24.5
nontraffic V24.1
car (traffic) V23.5
nontraffic V23.1
motor vehicle NOS (traffic) V29.50
nontraffic V29.10
specified type NEC (traffic) V29.59
nontraffic V29.19
pedal cycle (traffic) V21.5
nontraffic V21.1
pickup truck (traffic) V23.5
nontraffic V23.1

Accident (to) - *continued*
transport (involving injury to) - *continued*
motorcyclist - *continued*
passenger - *continued*
collision (with) - *continued*
railway vehicle (traffic) V25.5
nontraffic V25.1
specified vehicle NEC (traffic) V26.5
nontraffic V26.1
stationary object (traffic) V27.5
nontraffic V27.1
streetcar (traffic) V26.5
nontraffic V26.1
three wheeled motor vehicle (traffic) V22.5
nontraffic V22.1
truck (traffic) V24.5
nontraffic V24.1
two wheeled motor vehicle (traffic) V22.5
nontraffic V22.1
van (traffic) V23.5
nontraffic V23.1
noncollision accident (traffic) V28.5
nontraffic V28.1
specified type NEC V29.88
military vehicle V29.81
motor vehicle NEC occupant (traffic) V89.2
occupant (of)
aircraft (powered) V95.9
fixed wing
commercial — *see* Accident, transport, aircraft, occupant, powered, fixed wing, commercial
private — *see* Accident, transport, aircraft, occupant, powered, fixed wing, private
nonpowered V96.9
specified NEC V95.8
airport battery-powered vehicle — *see* Accident, transport, industrial vehicle occupant
all-terrain vehicle (ATV) — *see* Accident, transport, all-terrain vehicle occupant
animal-drawn vehicle — *see* Accident, transport, animal-drawn vehicle occupant
automobile — *see* Accident, transport, car occupant
balloon V96.00
battery-powered vehicle — *see* Accident, transport, industrial vehicle occupant
bicycle — *see* Accident, transport, pedal cyclist
motorized — *see* Accident, transport, motorcycle rider
boat NEC — *see* Accident, watercraft
bulldozer — *see* Accident, transport, construction vehicle occupant
bus — *see* Accident, transport, bus occupant
cable car (on rails) — *see also* Accident, transport, streetcar occupant
not on rails V98.0
car — *see also* Accident, transport, car occupant
cable (on rails) — *see also* Accident, transport, streetcar occupant
not on rails V98.0
coach — *see* Accident, transport, bus occupant
coal-car — *see* Accident, transport, industrial vehicle occupant
digger — *see* Accident, transport, construction vehicle occupant
dump truck — *see* Accident, transport, construction vehicle occupant
earth-leveler — *see* Accident, transport, construction vehicle occupant
farm machinery (self-propelled) — *see* Accident, transport, agricultural vehicle occupant
forklift — *see* Accident, transport, industrial vehicle occupant
glider (unpowered) V96.20
hang V96.10
powered (microlight) (ultralight) — *see* Accident, transport, aircraft, occupant, powered, glider
glider (unpowered) NEC V96.20
hang-glider V96.10
harvester — *see* Accident, transport, agricultural vehicle occupant
heavy (transport) vehicle — *see* Accident, transport, truck occupant
helicopter — *see* Accident, transport, aircraft, occupant, helicopter
ice-yacht V98.2
kite (carrying person) V96.8
land-yacht V98.1
logging car — *see* Accident, transport, industrial vehicle occupant

Accident (to) - *continued*
transport (involving injury to) - *continued*
occupant (of) - *continued*
mechanical shovel — *see* Accident, transport, construction vehicle occupant
microlight — *see* Accident, transport, aircraft, occupant, powered, glider
minibus — *see* Accident, transport, pickup truck occupant
minivan — *see* Accident, transport, pickup truck occupant
moped — *see* Accident, transport, motorcycle
motor scooter — *see* Accident, transport, motorcycle
motorcycle (with sidecar) — *see* Accident, transport, motorcycle
off-road motor-vehicle — *see also* Accident, transport, all-terrain vehicle occupant V86.99
pedal cycle — *see also* Accident, transport, pedal cyclist
pick-up (truck) — *see* Accident, transport, pickup truck occupant
railway (train) (vehicle) (subterranean) (elevated) — *see* Accident, transport, railway vehicle occupant
rickshaw — *see* Accident, transport, pedal cycle
motorized — *see* Accident, transport, three-wheeled motor vehicle
pedal driven — *see* Accident, transport, pedal cyclist
road-roller — *see* Accident, transport, construction vehicle occupant
ship NOS V94.9
ski-lift (chair) (gondola) V98.3
snowmobile — *see* Accident, transport, snowmobile occupant
spacecraft, spaceship — *see* Accident, transport, aircraft, occupant, spacecraft
sport utility vehicle — *see* Accident, transport, pickup truck occupant
streetcar (interurban) (operating on public street or highway) — *see* Accident, transport, streetcar occupant
SUV — *see* Accident, transport, pickup truck occupant
téléférique V98.0
three-wheeled vehicle (motorized) — *see also* Accident, transport, three-wheeled motor vehicle occupant
nonmotorized — *see* Accident, transport, pedal cycle
tractor (farm) (and trailer) — *see* Accident, transport, agricultural vehicle occupant
train — *see* Accident, transport, railway vehicle occupant
tram — *see* Accident, transport, streetcar occupant
in mine or quarry — *see* Accident, transport, industrial vehicle occupant
tricycle — *see* Accident, transport, pedal cycle
motorized — *see* Accident, transport, three-wheeled motor vehicle
trolley — *see* Accident, transport, streetcar occupant
in mine or quarry — *see* Accident, transport, industrial vehicle occupant
tub, in mine or quarry — *see* Accident, transport, industrial vehicle occupant
ultralight — *see* Accident, transport, aircraft, occupant, powered, glider
van — *see* Accident, transport, van occupant
vehicle NEC V89.9
heavy transport — *see* Accident, transport, truck occupant
motor (traffic) NEC V89.2
nontraffic NEC V89.0
watercraft NOS V94.9
causing drowning — *see* Drowning, resulting from accident to boat
off-road motor-vehicle — *see also* Accident, transport, all-terrain vehicle occupant V86.99
parachutist V97.29
after accident to aircraft — *see* Accident, transport, aircraft
entangled in object V97.21
injured on landing V97.22
pedal cyclist V19.9
collision (with)
animal (traffic) V10.9
being ridden (traffic) V16.9
nontraffic V16.2
while boarding or alighting V16.3
nontraffic V10.2

Accident (to) - *continued*
  transport (involving injury to) - *continued*
    pedal cyclist - *continued*
      collision (with) - *continued*
        animal (traffic) - *continued*
          while boarding or alighting V10.3
        animal-drawn vehicle (traffic) V16.9
          nontraffic V16.2
          while boarding or alighting V16.3
        bus (traffic) V14.9
          nontraffic V14.2
          while boarding or alighting V14.3
        car (traffic) V13.9
          nontraffic V13.2
          while boarding or alighting V13.3
        motor vehicle NOS (traffic) V19.60
          nontraffic V19.20
          specified type NEC (traffic) V19.69
            nontraffic V19.29
        pedal cycle (traffic) V11.9
          nontraffic V11.2
          while boarding or alighting V11.3
        pickup truck (traffic) V13.9
          nontraffic V13.2
          while boarding or alighting V13.3
        railway vehicle (traffic) V15.9
          nontraffic V15.2
          while boarding or alighting V15.3
        specified vehicle NEC (traffic) V16.9
          nontraffic V16.2
          while boarding or alighting V16.3
        stationary object (traffic) V17.9
          nontraffic V17.2
          while boarding or alighting V17.3
        streetcar (traffic) V16.9
          nontraffic V16.2
          while boarding or alighting V16.3
        three wheeled motor vehicle (traffic) V12.9
          nontraffic V12.2
          while boarding or alighting V12.3
        truck (traffic) V14.9
          nontraffic V14.2
          while boarding or alighting V14.3
        two wheeled motor vehicle (traffic) V12.9
          nontraffic V12.2
          while boarding or alighting V12.3
        van (traffic) V13.9
          nontraffic V13.2
          while boarding or alighting V13.3
      driver
        collision (with)
          animal (traffic) V10.4
            being ridden (traffic) V16.4
              nontraffic V16.0
            nontraffic V10.0
          animal-drawn vehicle (traffic) V16.4
            nontraffic V16.0
          bus (traffic) V14.4
            nontraffic V14.0
          car (traffic) V13.4
            nontraffic V13.0
          motor vehicle NOS (traffic) V19.40
            nontraffic V19.00
            specified type NEC (traffic) V19.49
              nontraffic V19.09
          pedal cycle (traffic) V11.4
            nontraffic V11.0
          pickup truck (traffic) V13.4
            nontraffic V13.0
          railway vehicle (traffic) V15.4
            nontraffic V15.0
          specified vehicle NEC (traffic) V16.4
            nontraffic V16.0
          stationary object (traffic) V17.4
            nontraffic V17.0
          streetcar (traffic) V16.4
            nontraffic V16.0
          three wheeled motor vehicle (traffic) V12.4
            nontraffic V12.0
          truck (traffic) V14.4
            nontraffic V14.0
          two wheeled motor vehicle (traffic) V12.4
            nontraffic V12.0
          van (traffic) V13.4
            nontraffic V13.0
        noncollision accident (traffic) V18.4
          nontraffic V18.0
      noncollision accident (traffic) V18.9
        nontraffic V18.2
        while boarding or alighting V18.3
      nontraffic V19.3
      passenger
        collision (with)

Accident (to) - *continued*
  transport (involving injury to) - *continued*
    pedal cyclist - *continued*
      passenger - *continued*
        collision (with) - *continued*
          animal (traffic) V10.5
            being ridden (traffic) V16.5
              nontraffic V16.1
            nontraffic V10.1
          animal-drawn vehicle (traffic) V16.5
            nontraffic V16.1
          bus (traffic) V14.5
            nontraffic V14.1
          car (traffic) V13.5
            nontraffic V13.1
          motor vehicle NOS (traffic) V19.50
            nontraffic V19.10
            specified type NEC (traffic) V19.59
              nontraffic V19.19
          pedal cycle (traffic) V11.5
            nontraffic V11.1
          pickup truck (traffic) V13.5
            nontraffic V13.1
          railway vehicle (traffic) V15.5
            nontraffic V15.1
          specified vehicle NEC (traffic) V16.5
            nontraffic V16.1
          stationary object (traffic) V17.5
            nontraffic V17.1
          streetcar (traffic) V16.5
            nontraffic V16.1
          three wheeled motor vehicle (traffic) V12.5
            nontraffic V12.1
          truck (traffic) V14.5
            nontraffic V14.1
          two wheeled motor vehicle (traffic) V12.5
            nontraffic V12.1
          van (traffic) V13.5
            nontraffic V13.1
        noncollision accident (traffic) V18.5
          nontraffic V18.1
      specified type NEC V19.88
        military vehicle V19.81
    pedestrian
      conveyance (occupant) V09.9
        baby stroller V00.828
          collision (with) V09.9
            animal being ridden or animal drawn vehicle V06.99
              nontraffic V06.09
              traffic V06.19
            bus or heavy transport V04.99
              nontraffic V04.09
              traffic V04.19
            car V03.99
              nontraffic V03.09
              traffic V03.19
            pedal cycle V01.99
              nontraffic V01.09
              traffic V01.19
            pick-up truck or van V03.99
              nontraffic V03.09
              traffic V03.19
            railway (train) (vehicle) V05.99
              nontraffic V05.09
              traffic V05.19
            streetcar V06.99
              nontraffic V06.09
              traffic V06.19
            stationary object V00.822
            two- or three-wheeled motor vehicle V02.99
              nontraffic V02.09
              traffic V02.19
            vehicle V09.9
              animal-drawn V06.99
                nontraffic V06.09
                traffic V06.19
              motor
                nontraffic V09.00
                traffic V09.20
          fall V00.821
          nontraffic V09.1
            involving motor vehicle NEC V09.00
          traffic V09.3
            involving motor vehicle NEC V09.20
        flat-bottomed NEC V00.388
          collision (with) V09.9
            animal being ridden or animal drawn vehicle V06.99
              nontraffic V06.09
              traffic V06.19
            bus or heavy transport V04.99
              nontraffic V04.09

Accident (to) - *continued*
  transport (involving injury to) - *continued*
    pedestrian - *continued*
      conveyance (occupant) - *continued*
        flat-bottomed NEC - *continued*
          collision (with) - *continued*
            bus or heavy transport - *continued*
              traffic V04.19
            car V03.99
              nontraffic V03.09
              traffic V03.19
            pedal cycle V01.99
              nontraffic V01.09
              traffic V01.19
            pick-up truck or van V03.99
              nontraffic V03.09
              traffic V03.19
            railway (train) (vehicle) V05.99
              nontraffic V05.09
              traffic V05.19
            stationary object V00.382
            streetcar V06.99
              nontraffic V06.09
              traffic V06.19
            two- or three-wheeled motor vehicle V02.99
              nontraffic V02.09
              traffic V02.19
            vehicle V09.9
              animal-drawn V06.99
                nontraffic V06.09
                traffic V06.19
              motor
                nontraffic V09.00
                traffic V09.20
          fall V00.381
          nontraffic V09.1
            involving motor vehicle NEC V09.00
          snow
            board — *see* Accident, transport, pedestrian, conveyance, snow board
            ski- — *see* Accident, transport, pedestrian, conveyance, skis (snow)
          traffic V09.3
            involving motor vehicle NEC V09.20
        gliding type NEC V00.288
          collision (with) V09.9
            animal being ridden or animal drawn vehicle V06.99
              nontraffic V06.09
              traffic V06.19
            bus or heavy transport V04.99
              nontraffic V04.09
              traffic V04.19
            car V03.99
              nontraffic V03.09
              traffic V03.19
            pedal cycle V01.99
              nontraffic V01.09
              traffic V01.19
            pick-up truck or van V03.99
              nontraffic V03.09
              traffic V03.19
            railway (train) (vehicle) V05.99
              nontraffic V05.09
              traffic V05.19
            stationary object V00.282
            streetcar V06.99
              nontraffic V06.09
              traffic V06.19
            two- or three-wheeled motor vehicle V02.99
              nontraffic V02.09
              traffic V02.19
            vehicle V09.9
              animal-drawn V06.99
                nontraffic V06.09
                traffic V06.19
              motor
                nontraffic V09.00
                traffic V09.20
          fall V00.281
          heelies — *see* Accident, transport, pedestrian, conveyance, heelies
          ice skate — *see* Accident, transport, pedestrian, conveyance, ice skate
          nontraffic V09.1
            involving motor vehicle NEC V09.00
          sled — *see* Accident, transport, pedestrian, conveyance, sled
          traffic V09.3
            involving motor vehicle NEC V09.20
          wheelies — *see* Accident, transport, pedestrian, conveyance, heelies
        heelies V00.158

- **Accident** (to) - *continued*
  - transport (involving injury to) - *continued*
    - pedestrian - *continued*
      - conveyance (occupant) - *continued*
        - heelies - *continued*
          - colliding with stationary object V00.152
          - fall V00.151
        - ice skates V00.218
          - collision (with) V09.9
            - animal being ridden or animal drawn vehicle V06.99
              - nontraffic V06.09
              - traffic V06.19
            - bus or heavy transport V04.99
              - nontraffic V04.09
              - traffic V04.19
            - car V03.99
              - nontraffic V03.09
              - traffic V03.19
            - pedal cycle V01.99
              - nontraffic V01.09
              - traffic V01.19
            - pick-up truck or van V03.99
              - nontraffic V03.09
              - traffic V03.19
            - railway (train) (vehicle) V05.99
              - nontraffic V05.09
              - traffic V05.19
            - streetcar V06.99
              - nontraffic V06.09
              - traffic V06.19
            - stationary object V00.212
            - two- or three-wheeled motor vehicle V02.99
              - nontraffic V02.09
              - traffic V02.19
            - vehicle V09.9
              - animal-drawn V06.99
                - nontraffic V06.09
                - traffic V06.19
              - motor
                - nontraffic V09.00
                - traffic V09.20
          - fall V00.211
          - nontraffic V09.1
            - involving motor vehicle NEC V09.00
          - traffic V09.3
            - involving motor vehicle NEC V09.20
        - motorized mobility scooter V00.838
          - collision with stationary object V00.832
          - fall from V00.831
        - nontraffic V09.1
          - involving motor vehicle V09.00
            - military V09.01
            - specified type NEC V09.09
        - roller skates (non in-line) V00.128
          - collision (with) V09.9
            - animal being ridden or animal drawn vehicle V06.91
              - nontraffic V06.01
              - traffic V06.11
            - bus or heavy transport V04.91
              - nontraffic V04.01
              - traffic V04.11
            - car V03.91
              - nontraffic V03.01
              - traffic V03.11
            - pedal cycle V01.91
              - nontraffic V01.01
              - traffic V01.11
            - pick-up truck or van V03.91
              - nontraffic V03.01
              - traffic V03.11
            - railway (train) (vehicle) V05.91
              - nontraffic V05.01
              - traffic V05.11
            - streetcar V06.91
              - nontraffic V06.01
              - traffic V06.11
            - stationary object V00.122
            - two- or three-wheeled motor vehicle V02.91
              - nontraffic V02.01
              - traffic V02.11
            - vehicle V09.9
              - animal-drawn V06.91
                - nontraffic V06.01
                - traffic V06.11
              - motor
                - nontraffic V09.00
                - traffic V09.20
          - fall V00.121
          - in-line V00.118

- **Accident** (to) - *continued*
  - transport (involving injury to) - *continued*
    - pedestrian - *continued*
      - conveyance (occupant) - *continued*
        - roller skates (non in-line) - *continued*
          - in-line - *continued*
            - collision- — *see* also Accident, transport, pedestrian, conveyance occupant, roller skates, collision
              - with stationary object V00.112
            - fall V00.111
          - nontraffic V09.1
            - involving motor vehicle NEC V09.00
          - traffic V09.3
            - involving motor vehicle NEC V09.20
        - rolling shoes V00.158
          - colliding with stationary object V00.152
          - fall V00.151
        - rolling type NEC V00.188
          - collision (with) V09.9
            - animal being ridden or animal drawn vehicle V06.99
              - nontraffic V06.09
              - traffic V06.19
            - bus or heavy transport V04.99
              - nontraffic V04.09
              - traffic V04.19
            - car V03.99
              - nontraffic V03.09
              - traffic V03.19
            - pedal cycle V01.99
              - nontraffic V01.09
              - traffic V01.19
            - pick-up truck or van V03.99
              - nontraffic V03.09
              - traffic V03.19
            - railway (train) (vehicle) V05.99
              - nontraffic V05.09
              - traffic V05.19
            - stationary object V00.182
            - streetcar V06.99
              - nontraffic V06.09
              - traffic V06.19
            - two- or three-wheeled motor vehicle V02.99
              - nontraffic V02.09
              - traffic V02.19
            - vehicle V09.9
              - animal-drawn V06.99
                - nontraffic V06.09
                - traffic V06.19
              - motor
                - nontraffic V09.00
                - traffic V09.20
          - fall V00.181
          - in-line roller skate — *see* Accident, transport, pedestrian, conveyance, roller skate, in-line
          - nontraffic V09.1
            - involving motor vehicle NEC V09.00
          - roller skate — *see* Accident, transport, pedestrian, conveyance, roller skate
          - scooter (non-motorized) — *see* Accident, transport, pedestrian, conveyance, scooter
          - skateboard — *see* Accident, transport, pedestrian, conveyance, skateboard
          - traffic V09.3
            - involving motor vehicle NEC V09.20
        - scooter (non-motorized) V00.148
          - collision (with) V09.9
            - animal being ridden or animal drawn vehicle V06.99
              - nontraffic V06.09
              - traffic V06.19
            - bus or heavy transport V04.99
              - nontraffic V04.09
              - traffic V04.19
            - car V03.99
              - nontraffic V03.09
              - traffic V03.19
            - pedal cycle V01.99
              - nontraffic V01.09
              - traffic V01.19
            - pick-up truck or van V03.99
              - nontraffic V03.09
              - traffic V03.19
            - railway (train) (vehicle) V05.99
              - nontraffic V05.09
              - traffic V05.19
            - streetcar V06.99
              - nontraffic V06.09
              - traffic V06.19
            - stationary object V00.142
            - two- or three-wheeled motor vehicle V02.99
              - nontraffic V02.09

- **Accident** (to) - *continued*
  - transport (involving injury to) - *continued*
    - pedestrian - *continued*
      - conveyance (occupant) - *continued*
        - scooter (non-motorized) - *continued*
          - collision (with) - *continued*
            - two- or three-wheeled motor vehicle - *continued*
              - traffic V02.19
            - vehicle V09.9
              - animal-drawn V06.99
                - nontraffic V06.09
                - traffic V06.19
              - motor
                - nontraffic V09.00
                - traffic V09.20
          - fall V00.141
          - nontraffic V09.1
            - involving motor vehicle NEC V09.00
          - traffic V09.3
            - involving motor vehicle NEC V09.20
        - skate board V00.138
          - collision (with) V09.9
            - animal being ridden or animal drawn vehicle V06.92
              - nontraffic V06.02
              - traffic V06.12
            - bus or heavy transport V04.92
              - nontraffic V04.02
              - traffic V04.12
            - car V03.92
              - nontraffic V03.02
              - traffic V03.12
            - pedal cycle V01.92
              - nontraffic V01.02
              - traffic V01.12
            - pick-up truck or van V03.92
              - nontraffic V03.02
              - traffic V03.12
            - railway (train) (vehicle) V05.92
              - nontraffic V05.02
              - traffic V05.12
            - streetcar V06.92
              - nontraffic V06.02
              - traffic V06.12
            - stationary object V00.132
            - two- or three-wheeled motor vehicle V02.92
              - nontraffic V02.02
              - traffic V02.12
            - vehicle V09.9
              - animal-drawn V06.92
                - nontraffic V06.02
                - traffic V06.12
              - motor
                - nontraffic V09.00
                - traffic V09.20
          - fall V00.131
          - nontraffic V09.1
            - involving motor vehicle NEC V09.00
          - traffic V09.3
            - involving motor vehicle NEC V09.20
        - sled V00.228
          - collision (with) V09.9
            - animal being ridden or animal drawn vehicle V06.99
              - nontraffic V06.09
              - traffic V06.19
            - bus or heavy transport V04.99
              - nontraffic V04.09
              - traffic V04.19
            - car V03.99
              - nontraffic V03.09
              - traffic V03.19
            - pedal cycle V01.99
              - nontraffic V01.09
              - traffic V01.19
            - pick-up truck or van V03.99
              - nontraffic V03.09
              - traffic V03.19
            - railway (train) (vehicle) V05.99
              - nontraffic V05.09
              - traffic V05.19
            - streetcar V06.99
              - nontraffic V06.09
              - traffic V06.19
            - stationary object V00.222
            - two- or three-wheeled motor vehicle V02.99
              - nontraffic V02.09
              - traffic V02.19
            - vehicle V09.9
              - animal-drawn V06.99
                - nontraffic V06.09
                - traffic V06.19

- **Accident** (to) - *continued*
  - transport (involving injury to) - *continued*
    - pickup truck occupant - *continued*
      - collision (with) - *continued*
        - motor vehicle NOS (traffic) - *continued*
          - specified type NEC (traffic) V59.69
            - nontraffic V59.29
        - pedal cycle (traffic) V51.9
          - nontraffic V51.3
          - while boarding or alighting V51.4
        - pickup truck (traffic) V53.9
          - nontraffic V53.3
          - while boarding or alighting V53.4
        - railway vehicle (traffic) V55.9
          - nontraffic V55.3
          - while boarding or alighting V55.4
        - specified vehicle NEC (traffic) V56.9
          - nontraffic V56.3
          - while boarding or alighting V56.4
        - stationary object (traffic) V57.9
          - nontraffic V57.3
          - while boarding or alighting V57.4
        - streetcar (traffic) V56.9
          - nontraffic V56.3
          - while boarding or alighting V56.4
        - three wheeled motor vehicle (traffic) V52.9
          - nontraffic V52.3
          - while boarding or alighting V52.4
        - truck (traffic) V54.9
          - nontraffic V54.3
          - while boarding or alighting V54.4
        - two wheeled motor vehicle (traffic) V52.9
          - nontraffic V52.3
          - while boarding or alighting V52.4
        - van (traffic) V53.9
          - nontraffic V53.3
          - while boarding or alighting V53.4
      - driver
        - collision (with)
          - animal (traffic) V50.5
            - being ridden (traffic) V56.5
              - nontraffic V56.0
            - nontraffic V50.0
          - animal-drawn vehicle (traffic) V56.5
            - nontraffic V56.0
          - bus (traffic) V54.5
            - nontraffic V54.0
          - car (traffic) V53.5
            - nontraffic V53.0
          - motor vehicle NOS (traffic) V59.40
            - nontraffic V59.00
            - specified type NEC (traffic) V59.49
              - nontraffic V59.09
          - pedal cycle (traffic) V51.5
            - nontraffic V51.0
          - pickup truck (traffic) V53.5
            - nontraffic V53.0
          - railway vehicle (traffic) V55.5
            - nontraffic V55.0
          - specified vehicle NEC (traffic) V56.5
            - nontraffic V56.0
          - stationary object (traffic) V57.5
            - nontraffic V57.0
          - streetcar (traffic) V56.5
            - nontraffic V56.0
          - three wheeled motor vehicle (traffic) V52.5
            - nontraffic V52.0
          - truck (traffic) V54.5
            - nontraffic V54.0
          - two wheeled motor vehicle (traffic) V52.5
            - nontraffic V52.0
          - van (traffic) V53.5
            - nontraffic V53.0
        - noncollision accident (traffic) V58.5
          - nontraffic V58.0
      - noncollision accident (traffic) V58.9
        - nontraffic V58.3
        - while boarding or alighting V58.4
      - nontraffic V59.3
      - hanger-on
        - collision (with)
          - animal (traffic) V50.7
            - being ridden (traffic) V56.7
              - nontraffic V56.2
            - nontraffic V50.2
          - animal-drawn vehicle (traffic) V56.7
            - nontraffic V56.2
          - bus (traffic) V54.7
            - nontraffic V54.2
          - car (traffic) V53.7
            - nontraffic V53.2
          - pedal cycle (traffic) V51.7
            - nontraffic V51.2

- **Accident** (to) - *continued*
  - transport (involving injury to) - *continued*
    - pickup truck occupant - *continued*
      - hanger-on - *continued*
        - collision (with) - *continued*
          - pickup truck (traffic) V53.7
            - nontraffic V53.2
          - railway vehicle (traffic) V55.7
            - nontraffic V55.2
          - specified vehicle NEC (traffic) V56.7
            - nontraffic V56.2
          - stationary object (traffic) V57.7
            - nontraffic V57.2
          - streetcar (traffic) V56.7
            - nontraffic V56.2
          - three wheeled motor vehicle (traffic) V52.7
            - nontraffic V52.2
          - truck (traffic) V54.7
            - nontraffic V54.2
          - two wheeled motor vehicle (traffic) V52.7
            - nontraffic V52.2
          - van (traffic) V53.7
            - nontraffic V53.2
        - noncollision accident (traffic) V58.7
          - nontraffic V58.2
      - passenger
        - collision (with)
          - animal (traffic) V50.6
            - being ridden (traffic) V56.6
              - nontraffic V56.1
            - nontraffic V50.1
          - animal-drawn vehicle (traffic) V56.6
            - nontraffic V56.1
          - bus (traffic) V54.6
            - nontraffic V54.1
          - car (traffic) V53.6
            - nontraffic V53.1
          - motor vehicle NOS (traffic) V59.50
            - nontraffic V59.10
            - specified type NEC (traffic) V59.59
              - nontraffic V59.19
          - pedal cycle (traffic) V51.6
            - nontraffic V51.1
          - pickup truck (traffic) V53.6
            - nontraffic V53.1
          - railway vehicle (traffic) V55.6
            - nontraffic V55.1
          - specified vehicle NEC (traffic) V56.6
            - nontraffic V56.1
          - stationary object (traffic) V57.6
            - nontraffic V57.1
          - streetcar (traffic) V56.6
            - nontraffic V56.1
          - three wheeled motor vehicle (traffic) V52.6
            - nontraffic V52.1
          - truck (traffic) V54.6
            - nontraffic V54.1
          - two wheeled motor vehicle (traffic) V52.6
            - nontraffic V52.1
          - van (traffic) V53.6
            - nontraffic V53.1
        - noncollision accident (traffic) V58.6
          - nontraffic V58.1
      - specified type NEC V59.88
        - military vehicle V59.81
    - quarry truck — *see* Accident, transport, industrial vehicle occupant
    - race car — *see* Accident, transport, motor vehicle NEC occupant
    - railway vehicle occupant V81.9
      - collision (with) V81.3
        - motor vehicle (non-military) (traffic) V81.1
          - military V81.83
          - nontraffic V81.0
        - rolling stock V81.2
        - specified object NEC V81.3
      - during derailment V81.7
        - with antecedent collision — *see* Accident, transport, railway vehicle occupant, collision
      - explosion V81.81
      - fall (in railway vehicle) V81.5
        - during derailment V81.7
          - with antecedent collision — *see* Accident, transport, railway vehicle occupant, collision
        - from railway vehicle V81.6
          - during derailment V81.7
            - with antecedent collision — *see* Accident, transport, railway vehicle occupant, collision
        - while boarding or alighting V81.4
      - fire V81.81
      - object falling onto train V81.82

- **Accident** (to) - *continued*
  - transport (involving injury to) - *continued*
    - railway vehicle occupant - *continued*
      - specified type NEC V81.89
      - while boarding or alighting V81.4
    - ski lift V98.3
    - snowmobile occupant (nontraffic) V86.92
      - driver V86.52
      - hanger-on V86.72
      - passenger V86.62
      - traffic V86.32
        - driver V86.02
        - hanger-on V86.22
        - passenger V86.12
      - while boarding or alighting V86.42
    - specified NEC V98.8
    - sport utility vehicle occupant — *see also* Accident, transport, pickup truck occupant
    - streetcar occupant V82.9
      - collision (with) V82.3
        - motor vehicle (traffic) V82.1
          - nontraffic V82.0
        - rolling stock V82.2
      - during derailment V82.7
        - with antecedent collision — *see* Accident, transport, streetcar occupant, collision
      - fall (in streetcar) V82.5
        - during derailment V82.7
          - with antecedent collision — *see* Accident, transport, streetcar occupant, collision
        - from streetcar V82.6
          - during derailment V82.7
            - with antecedent collision — *see* Accident, transport, streetcar occupant, collision
          - while boarding or alighting V82.4
        - while boarding or alighting V82.4
      - specified type NEC V82.8
      - while boarding or alighting V82.4
    - three-wheeled motor vehicle occupant V39.9
      - collision (with)
        - animal (traffic) V30.9
          - being ridden (traffic) V36.9
            - nontraffic V36.3
            - while boarding or alighting V36.4
          - nontraffic V30.3
          - while boarding or alighting V30.4
        - animal-drawn vehicle (traffic) V36.9
          - nontraffic V36.3
          - while boarding or alighting V36.4
        - bus (traffic) V34.9
          - nontraffic V34.3
          - while boarding or alighting V34.4
        - car (traffic) V33.9
          - nontraffic V33.3
          - while boarding or alighting V33.4
        - motor vehicle NOS (traffic) V39.60
          - nontraffic V39.20
          - specified type NEC (traffic) V39.69
            - nontraffic V39.29
        - pedal cycle (traffic) V31.9
          - nontraffic V31.3
          - while boarding or alighting V31.4
        - pickup truck (traffic) V33.9
          - nontraffic V33.3
          - while boarding or alighting V33.4
        - railway vehicle (traffic) V35.9
          - nontraffic V35.3
          - while boarding or alighting V35.4
        - specified vehicle NEC (traffic) V36.9
          - nontraffic V36.3
          - while boarding or alighting V36.4
        - stationary object (traffic) V37.9
          - nontraffic V37.3
          - while boarding or alighting V37.4
        - streetcar (traffic) V36.9
          - nontraffic V36.3
          - while boarding or alighting V36.4
        - three wheeled motor vehicle (traffic) V32.9
          - nontraffic V32.3
          - while boarding or alighting V32.4
        - truck (traffic) V34.9
          - nontraffic V34.3
          - while boarding or alighting V34.4
        - two wheeled motor vehicle (traffic) V32.9
          - nontraffic V32.3
          - while boarding or alighting V32.4
        - van (traffic) V33.9
          - nontraffic V33.3
          - while boarding or alighting V33.4
      - driver
        - collision (with)
          - animal (traffic) V30.5
            - being ridden (traffic) V36.5

Activity (involving) (of victim at time of event) - *continued*
sleeping (sleep) Y93.84
smoking and grilling food Y93.G2
snorkeling Y93.15
snow NEC Y93.29
boarding Y93.23
shoveling Y93.H1
sledding Y93.23
tubing Y93.23
soccer Y93.66
softball Y93.64
specified NEC Y93.89
spectator at an event Y93.82
sports NEC Y93.79
sports played as a team or group NEC Y93.69
sports played individually NEC Y93.59
springboard diving Y93.12
squash Y93.73
stationary bike Y93.A1
step (stepping) exercise (class) Y93.A3
stepper machine Y93.A1
stove Y93.G3
string instrument playing Y93.J3
surfing Y93.18
wind Y93.18
swimming Y93.11
tackle football Y93.61
tap dancing Y93.41
tennis Y93.73
tobogganing Y93.23
touch football Y93.62
track and field events (non-running) Y93.57
running Y93.02
trampoline Y93.44
treadmill Y93.A1
trimming shrubs Y93.H2
tubing (in calm and turbulent water) Y93.16
snow Y93.23
ultimate frisbee Y93.74
underwater diving Y93.15
unpacking in moving to a new residence Y93.E6
use of stove, oven and microwave oven Y93.G3
vacuuming Y93.E3
volleyball (beach) (court) Y93.68
wake boarding Y93.17
walking an animal Y93.K1
walking (on level or elevated terrain) Y93.01
an animal Y93.K1
wall climbing Y93.31
warm up and cool down exercises Y93.A2
water NEC Y93.19
aerobics Y93.14
craft NEC Y93.19
exercise Y93.14
polo Y93.13
skiing Y93.17
sliding Y93.18
survival training and testing Y93.19
weeding (garden and lawn) Y93.H2
wind instrument playing Y93.J4
windsurfing Y93.18
wrestling Y93.72
yoga Y93.42

Adverse effect of drugs — *see* Table of Drugs and Chemicals
Aerosinusitis - — *see* Air, pressure
After-effect, late — *see* Sequelae
Air
blast in war operations — *see* War operations, air blast
pressure
change, rapid
during
ascent W94.29
while (in) (surfacing from)
aircraft W94.23
deep water diving W94.21
underground W94.22
descent W94.39
in
aircraft W94.31
water W94.32
high, prolonged W94.0
low, prolonged W94.12
due to residence or long visit at high altitude W94.11

Alpine sickness W94.11
Altitude sickness W94.11
Anaphylactic shock, anaphylaxis — *see* Table of Drugs and Chemicals
Andes disease W94.11
Arachnidism, arachnoidism X58
Arson (with intent to injure or kill) X97
Asphyxia, asphyxiation
by
food (bone) (seed) — *see* categories T17 and T18
gas — *see also* Table of Drugs and Chemicals
legal
execution — *see* Legal, intervention, gas
intervention — *see* Legal, intervention, gas
from
fire — *see also* Exposure, fire
in war operations — *see* War operations, fire
ignition — *see* Ignition
vomitus T17.81
in war operations — *see* War operations, restriction of airway

Aspiration
food (any type) (into respiratory tract) (with asphyxia, obstruction respiratory tract, suffocation) — *see* categories T17 and T18
foreign body — *see* Foreign body, aspiration
vomitus (with asphyxia, obstruction respiratory tract, suffocation) T17.81

Assassination (attempt) — *see* Assault
Assault (homicidal) (by) (in) Y09
arson X97
bite (of human being) Y04.1
bodily force Y04.8
bite Y04.1
bumping into Y04.2
sexual — *see* subcategories T74.0, T76.0
unarmed fight Y04.0
bomb X96.9
antipersonnel X96.0
fertilizer X96.3
gasoline X96.1
letter X96.2
petrol X96.1
pipe X96.3
specified NEC X96.8
brawl (hand) (fists) (foot) (unarmed) Y04.0
burning, burns (by fire) NEC X97
acid Y08.89
caustic, corrosive substance Y08.89
chemical from swallowing caustic, corrosive substance — *see* Table of Drugs and Chemicals
cigarette (s) X97
hot object X98.9
fluid NEC X98.2
household appliance X98.3
specified NEC X98.8
steam X98.0
tap water X98.1
vapors X98.0
scalding — *see* Assault, burning
steam X98.0
vitriol Y08.89
caustic, corrosive substance (gas) Y08.89
crashing of
aircraft Y08.81
motor vehicle Y03.8
pushed in front of Y02.0
run over Y03.0
specified NEC Y03.8
cutting or piercing instrument X99.9
dagger X99.2
glass X99.0
knife X99.1
specified NEC X99.8
sword X99.2
dagger X99.2
drowning (in) X92.9
bathtub X92.0
natural water X92.3
specified NEC X92.8
swimming pool X92.1
following fall X92.2
dynamite X96.8
explosive (s) (material) X96.9
fight (hand) (fists) (foot) (unarmed) Y04.0
with weapon — *see* Assault, by type of weapon
fire X97
firearm X95.9
airgun X95.01
handgun X93
hunting rifle X94.1
larger X94.9
specified NEC X94.8
machine gun X94.2
shotgun X94.0
specified NEC X95.8
gunshot (wound) NEC — *see* Assault, firearm, by type
incendiary device X97

Assault (homicidal) (by) (in) - *continued*
injury Y09
to child due to criminal abortion attempt NEC Y08.89
knife X99.1
late effect of — *see* X92-Y08 with 7th character S
placing before moving object NEC Y02.8
motor vehicle Y02.0
poisoning — *see* categories T36-T65 with 7th character S
puncture, any part of body — *see* Assault, cutting or piercing instrument
pushing
before moving object NEC Y02.8
motor vehicle Y02.0
subway train Y02.1
train Y02.1
from high place Y01
rape T74.2-
scalding — *see* Assault, burning
sequelae of — *see* X92-Y08 with 7th character S
sexual (by bodily force) T74.2-
shooting — *see* Assault, firearm
specified means NEC Y08.89
stab, any part of body — *see* Assault, cutting or piercing instrument
steam X98.0
striking against
other person Y04.2
sports equipment Y08.09
baseball bat Y08.02
hockey stick Y08.01
struck by
sports equipment Y08.09
baseball bat Y08.02
hockey stick Y08.01
submersion — *see* Assault, drowning
violence Y09
weapon Y09
blunt Y00
cutting or piercing — *see* Assault, cutting or piercing instrument
firearm — *see* Assault, firearm
wound Y09
cutting — *see* Assault, cutting or piercing instrument
gunshot — *see* Assault, firearm
knife X99.1
piercing — *see* Assault, cutting or piercing instrument
puncture — *see* Assault, cutting or piercing instrument
stab — *see* Assault, cutting or piercing instrument

Attack by mammals NEC W55.89
Avalanche — *see* Landslide
Aviator's disease - — *see* Air, pressure

B

Barotitis, barodontalgia, barosinusitis, barotrauma (otitic) (sinus) - — *see* Air, pressure
Battered (baby) (child) (person) (syndrome) X58
Bayonet wound W26.1
in
legal intervention — *see* Legal, intervention, sharp object, bayonet
war operations — *see* War operations, combat
stated as undetermined whether accidental or intentional Y28.8
suicide (attempt) X78.2

Bean in nose — *see* categories T17 and T18
Bed set on fire NEC — *see* Exposure, fire, uncontrolled, building, bed
Beheading (by guillotine)
homicide X99.9
legal execution — *see* Legal, intervention

Bending, injury in (prolonged) (static) X50.1
Bends - — *see* Air, pressure, change
Bite, bitten by
alligator W58.01
arthropod (nonvenomous) NEC W57
bull W55.21
cat W55.01
cow W55.21
crocodile W58.11
dog W54.0
goat W55.31
hoof stock NEC W55.31
horse W55.11
human being (accidentally) W50.3
with intent to injure or kill Y04.1
as, or caused by, a crowd or human stampede (with fall) W52
assault Y04.1

- **Contact** (accidental) - *continued*
  - with - *continued*
    - machine, machinery - *continued*
      - steam engine W31.3
      - transmission W24.1
      - undercutter W31.0
      - water driven turbine W31.3
      - weaving W31.89
      - woodworking or forming (industrial) W31.2
    - mammal (feces) (urine) W55.89
      - bull — *see* Contact, with, bull
      - cat — *see* Contact, with, cat
      - cow — *see* Contact, with, cow
      - goat — *see* Contact, with, goat
      - hoof stock — *see* Contact, with, hoof stock
      - horse — *see* Contact, with, horse
      - marine W56.39
        - dolphin — *see* Contact, with, dolphin
        - orca — *see* Contact, with, orca
        - sea lion — *see* Contact, with, sea lion
        - specified NEC W56.39
          - bite W56.31
          - strike W56.32
      - pig — *see* Contact, with, pig
      - raccoon — *see* Contact, with, raccoon
      - rodent — *see* Contact, with, rodent
      - sheep — *see* Contact, with, sheep
      - specified NEC W55.89
        - bite W55.81
        - strike W55.82
    - marine
      - animal W56.89
        - bite W56.81
        - dolphin — *see* Contact, with, dolphin
        - fish NEC — *see* Contact, with, fish
        - mammal — *see* Contact, with, mammal, marine
        - orca — *see* Contact, with, orca
        - sea lion — *see* Contact, with, sea lion
        - shark — *see* Contact, with, shark
        - strike W56.82
    - meat
      - grinder (domestic) W29.0
        - industrial W31.82
        - nonpowered W27.4
      - slicer (domestic) W29.0
        - industrial W31.82
    - merry go round W31.81
    - metal, hot (liquid) (molten) NEC X18
    - millipede W57
    - nail W45.0
      - gun W29.4
    - needle (sewing) W27.3
      - hypodermic W46.0
        - contaminated W46.1
    - object (blunt) NEC
      - hot NEC X19
      - legal intervention — *see* Legal, intervention, blunt object
      - sharp NEC W45.8
        - inflicted by other person NEC W45.8
          - stated as
            - intentional homicide (attempt) — *see* Assault, cutting or piercing instrument
        - legal intervention — *see* Legal, intervention, sharp object
        - self-inflicted X78.9
    - orca W56.29
      - bite W56.21
      - strike W56.22
    - overhead plane W31.2
    - paper (as sharp object) W26.2
    - paper-cutter W27.5
    - parrot W61.09
      - bite W61.01
      - strike W61.02
    - pig W55.49
      - bite W55.41
      - strike W55.42
    - pipe, hot X16
    - pitchfork W27.1
    - plane (metal) (wood) W27.0
      - overhead W31.2
    - plant thorns, spines, sharp leaves or other mechanisms W60
    - powered
      - garden cultivator W29.3
      - household appliance, implement, or machine W29.8
      - saw (industrial) W31.2
        - hand W29.8
    - printing machine W31.89
    - psittacine bird W61.29
      - bite W61.21

- **Contact** (accidental) - *continued*
  - with - *continued*
    - psittacine bird - *continued*
      - macaw — *see* Contact, with, macaw
      - parrot — *see* Contact, with, parrot
      - strike W61.22
    - pulley (block) (transmission) W24.0
      - agricultural operations W30.89
    - raccoon W55.59
      - bite W55.51
      - strike W55.52
    - radial-saw (industrial) W31.2
    - radiator (hot) X16
    - rake W27.1
    - rattlesnake X58
    - reaper W30.0
    - reptile W59.89
      - lizard — *see* Contact, with, lizard
      - snake — *see* Contact, with, snake
      - specified NEC W59.89
        - bite W59.81
        - crushing W59.83
        - strike W59.82
      - turtle — *see* Contact, with, turtle
    - rivet gun (powered) W29.4
    - road scraper — *see* Accident, transport, construction vehicle
    - rodent (feces) (urine) W53.89
      - bite W53.81
      - mouse W53.09
        - bite W53.01
      - rat W53.19
        - bite W53.11
      - specified NEC W53.89
        - bite W53.81
      - squirrel W53.29
        - bite W53.21
    - roller coaster W31.81
    - rope NEC W24.0
      - agricultural operations W30.89
    - saliva — *see* Contact, with, by type of animal
    - sander W29.8
      - industrial W31.2
    - saucepan (hot) (glass) (metal) X15.3
    - saw W27.0
      - band (industrial) W31.2
      - bench (industrial) W31.2
      - chain W29.3
      - hand W27.0
    - sawing machine, metal W31.1
    - scissors W27.2
    - scorpion X58
    - screwdriver W27.0
      - powered W29.8
    - sea
      - anemone, cucumber or urchin (spine) X58
      - lion W56.19
        - bite W56.11
        - strike W56.12
    - serpent — *see* Contact, with, snake, by type
    - sewing-machine (electric) (powered) W29.2
      - not powered W27.8
    - shaft (hoist) (lift) (transmission) NEC W24.0
      - agricultural W30.89
    - shark W56.49
      - bite W56.41
      - strike W56.42
    - sharp object (s) W26.9
      - specified NEC W26.8
    - shears (hand) W27.2
      - powered (industrial) W31.1
        - domestic W29.2
    - sheep W55.39
      - bite W55.31
      - strike W55.32
    - shovel W27.8
      - steam — *see* Accident, transport, construction vehicle
    - snake (nonvenomous) W59.19
      - bite W59.11
      - crushing W59.13
      - strike W59.12
    - spade W27.1
    - spider (venomous) X58
    - spin-drier W29.2
    - spinning machine W31.89
    - splinter W45.8
    - sports equipment W21.9
    - staple gun (powered) W29.8
    - steam X13.1
      - engine W31.3
      - inhalation X13.0
      - pipe X16

- **Contact** (accidental) - *continued*
  - with - *continued*
    - steam - *continued*
      - shovel W31.89
    - stove (hot) (kitchen) X15.0
    - substance, hot NEC X19
      - molten (metal) X18
    - sword W26.1
      - assault X99.2
      - stated as undetermined whether accidental or intentional Y28.2
      - suicide (attempt) X78.2
    - tarantula X58
    - thresher W30.0
    - tin can lid W26.8
    - toad W62.1
    - toaster (hot) X15.1
    - tool W27.8
      - hand (not powered) W27.8
        - auger W27.0
        - axe W27.0
        - can opener W27.4
        - chisel W27.0
        - fork W27.4
        - garden W27.1
        - handsaw W27.0
        - hoe W27.1
        - ice-pick W27.4
        - kitchen utensil W27.4
        - manual
          - lawn mower W27.1
          - sewing machine W27.8
        - meat grinder W27.4
        - needle (sewing) W27.3
          - hypodermic W46.0
            - contaminated W46.1
        - paper cutter W27.5
        - pitchfork W27.1
        - rake W27.1
        - scissors W27.2
        - screwdriver W27.0
        - specified NEC W27.8
        - workbench W27.0
      - hot X17
      - powered W29.8
        - blender W29.0
          - commercial W31.82
        - can opener W29.0
          - commercial W31.82
        - chainsaw W29.3
        - clothes dryer W29.2
          - commercial W31.82
        - dishwasher W29.2
          - commercial W31.82
        - edger W29.3
        - electric fan W29.2
          - commercial W31.82
        - electric knife W29.1
        - food processor W29.0
          - commercial W31.82
        - garbage disposal W29.0
          - commercial W31.82
        - garden tool W29.3
        - hedge trimmer W29.3
        - ice maker W29.0
          - commercial W31.82
        - kitchen appliance W29.0
          - commercial W31.82
        - lawn mower W28
        - meat grinder W29.0
          - commercial W31.82
        - mixer W29.0
          - commercial W31.82
        - rototiller W29.3
        - sewing machine W29.2
          - commercial W31.82
        - washing machine W29.2
          - commercial W31.82
    - transmission device (belt, cable, chain, gear, pinion, shaft) W24.1
      - agricultural operations W30.89
    - turbine (gas) (water-driven) W31.3
    - turkey W61.49
      - peck W61.43
      - strike W61.42
    - turtle (nonvenomous) W59.29
      - bite W59.21
      - strike W59.22
      - terrestrial W59.89
        - bite W59.81
        - crushing W59.83
        - strike W59.82
    - under-cutter W31.0

Contact (accidental) - *continued*
with - *continued*
urine — *see* Contact, with, by type of animal
vehicle
agricultural use (transport) — *see* Accident, transport, agricultural vehicle
not on public highway W30.81
industrial use (transport) — *see* Accident, transport, industrial vehicle
not on public highway W31.83
off-road use (transport) — *see* Accident, transport, all-terrain or off-road vehicle
not on public highway W31.83
special construction use (transport) — *see* Accident, transport, construction vehicle
not on public highway W31.83
venomous
animal X58
arthropods X58
lizard X58
marine animal NEC X58
marine plant NEC X58
millipedes (tropical) X58
plant (s) X58
snake X58
spider X58
viper X58
washing-machine (powered) W29.2
wasp X58
weaving-machine W31.89
winch W24.0
agricultural operations W30.89
wire NEC W24.0
agricultural operations W30.89
wood slivers W45.8
yellow jacket X58
zebra — *see* Contact, with, hoof stock NEC
pressure X50.9
stress X50.9
Coup de soleil X32
Crash
aircraft (in transit) (powered) V95.9
balloon V96.01
fixed wing NEC (private) V95.21
commercial V95.31
glider V96.21
hang V96.11
powered V95.11
helicopter V95.01
in war operations — *see* War operations, destruction of aircraft
microlight V95.11
nonpowered V96.9
specified NEC V96.8
powered NEC V95.8
stated as
homicide (attempt) Y08.81
suicide (attempt) X83.0
ultralight V95.11
spacecraft V95.41
transport vehicle NEC — *see also* Accident, transport V89.9
homicide (attempt) Y03.8
motor NEC (traffic) V89.2
homicide (attempt) Y03.8
suicide (attempt) — *see* Suicide, collision
Cruelty (mental) (physical) (sexual) X58
Crushed (accidentally) X58
between objects (moving) (stationary and moving) W23.0
stationary W23.1
by
alligator W58.03
avalanche NEC — *see* Landslide
cave-in W20.0
caused by cataclysmic earth surface movement — *see* Landslide
crocodile W58.13
crowd or human stampede W52
falling
aircraft V97.39
in war operations — *see* War operations, destruction of aircraft
earth, material W20.0
caused by cataclysmic earth surface movement — *see* Landslide
object NEC W20.8
landslide NEC — *see* Landslide
lizard (nonvenomous) W59.09
machinery — *see* Contact, with, by type of machine
reptile NEC W59.89
snake (nonvenomous) W59.13

Crushed (accidentally) - *continued*
in
machinery — *see* Contact, with, by type of machine
Cut, cutting (any part of body) (accidental) — *see also* Contact, with, by object or machine
during medical or surgical treatment as misadventure — *see* Index to Diseases and Injuries, Complications
homicide (attempt) — *see* Assault, cutting or piercing instrument
inflicted by other person — *see* Assault, cutting or piercing instrument
legal
execution — *see* Legal, intervention
intervention — *see* Legal, intervention, sharp object
machine NEC — *see also* Contact, with, by type of machine W31.9
self-inflicted — *see* Suicide, cutting or piercing instrument
suicide (attempt) — *see* Suicide, cutting or piercing instrument
Cyclone (any injury) X37.1

D

Decapitation (accidental circumstances) **NEC** X58
homicide X99.9
legal execution — *see* Legal, intervention
Dehydration from lack of water X58
Deprivation X58
Derailment (accidental)
railway (rolling stock) (train) (vehicle) (without antecedent collision) V81.7
with antecedent collision — *see* Accident, transport, railway vehicle occupant
streetcar (without antecedent collision) V82.7
with antecedent collision — *see* Accident, transport, streetcar occupant
Descent
parachute (voluntary) (without accident to aircraft) V97.29
due to accident to aircraft — *see* Accident, transport, aircraft
Desertion X58
Destitution X58
Disability, late effect or sequela of injury — *see* Sequelae
Discharge (accidental)
airgun W34.010
assault X95.01
homicide (attempt) X95.01
stated as undetermined whether accidental or intentional Y24.0
suicide (attempt) X74.01
BB gun — *see* Discharge, airgun
firearm (accidental) W34.00
assault X95.9
handgun (pistol) (revolver) W32.0
assault X93
homicide (attempt) X93
legal intervention — *see* Legal, intervention, firearm, handgun
stated as undetermined whether accidental or intentional Y22
suicide (attempt) X72
homicide (attempt) X95.9
hunting rifle W33.02
assault X94.1
homicide (attempt) X94.1
legal intervention
injuring
bystander Y35.032
law enforcement personnel Y35.031
suspect Y35.033
stated as undetermined whether accidental or intentional Y23.1
suicide (attempt) X73.1
larger W33.00
assault X94.9
homicide (attempt) X94.9
hunting rifle — *see* Discharge, firearm, hunting rifle
legal intervention — *see* Legal, intervention, firearm by type of firearm
machine gun — *see* Discharge, firearm, machine gun
shotgun — *see* Discharge, firearm, shotgun
specified NEC W33.09
assault X94.8
homicide (attempt) X94.8
legal intervention
injuring

Discharge (accidental) - *continued*
firearm (accidental) - *continued*
larger - *continued*
specified NEC - *continued*
legal intervention - *continued*
injuring - *continued*
bystander Y35.092
law enforcement personnel Y35.091
suspect Y35.093
stated as undetermined whether accidental or intentional Y23.8
suicide (attempt) X73.8
stated as undetermined whether accidental or intentional Y23.9
suicide (attempt) X73.9
legal intervention
injuring
bystander Y35.002
law enforcement personnel Y35.001
suspect Y35.03
using rubber bullet
injuring
bystander Y35.042
law enforcement personnel Y35.041
suspect Y35.043
machine gun W33.03
assault X94.2
homicide (attempt) X94.2
legal intervention — *see* Legal, intervention, firearm, machine gun
stated as undetermined whether accidental or intentional Y23.3
suicide (attempt) X73.2
pellet gun — *see* Discharge, airgun
shotgun W33.01
assault X94.0
homicide (attempt) X94.0
legal intervention — *see* Legal, intervention, firearm, specified NEC
stated as undetermined whether accidental or intentional Y23.0
suicide (attempt) X73.0
specified NEC W34.09
assault X95.8
homicide (attempt) X95.8
legal intervention — *see* Legal, intervention, firearm, specified NEC
stated as undetermined whether accidental or intentional Y24.8
suicide (attempt) X74.8
stated as undetermined whether accidental or intentional Y24.9
suicide (attempt) X74.9
Very pistol W34.09
assault X95.8
homicide (attempt) X95.8
stated as undetermined whether accidental or intentional Y24.8
suicide (attempt) X74.8
firework (s) W39
stated as undetermined whether accidental or intentional Y25
gas-operated gun NEC W34.018
airgun — *see* Discharge, airgun
assault X95.09
homicide (attempt) X95.09
paintball gun — *see* Discharge, paintball gun
stated as undetermined whether accidental or intentional Y24.8
suicide (attempt) X74.09
gun NEC — *see also* Discharge, firearm NEC
air — *see* Discharge, airgun
BB — *see* Discharge, airgun
for single hand use — *see* Discharge, firearm, handgun
hand — *see* Discharge, firearm, handgun
machine — *see* Discharge, firearm, machine gun
other specified — *see* Discharge, firearm NEC
paintball — *see* Discharge, paintball gun
pellet — *see* Discharge, airgun
handgun — *see* Discharge, firearm, handgun
machine gun — *see* Discharge, firearm, machine gun
paintball gun W34.011
assault X95.02
homicide (attempt) X95.02
stated as undetermined whether accidental or intentional Y24.8
suicide (attempt) X74.02
pistol — *see* Discharge, firearm, handgun
flare — *see* Discharge, firearm, Very pistol
pellet — *see* Discharge, airgun
Very — *see* Discharge, firearm, Very pistol

Discharge (accidental) - *continued*
- revolver — *see* Discharge, firearm, handgun
- rifle (hunting) — *see* Discharge, firearm, hunting rifle
- shotgun — *see* Discharge, firearm, shotgun
- spring-operated gun NEC W34.018
  - assault X95.09
  - homicide (attempt) X95.09
  - stated as undetermined whether accidental or intentional Y24.8
  - suicide (attempt) X74.09

Disease
- Andes W94.11
- aviator's - — *see* Air, pressure
- range W94.11

Diver's disease, palsy, paralysis, squeeze - — *see* Air, pressure

Diving (into water) — *see* Accident, diving

Dog bite W54.0

Dragged by transport vehicle NEC — *see also* Accident, transport V09.9

Drinking poison (accidental) — *see* Table of Drugs and Chemicals

Dropped (accidentally) **while being carried or supported by other person** W04

Drowning (accidental) W74
- assault X92.9
- due to
  - accident (to)
    - machinery — *see* Contact, with, by type of machine
    - watercraft V90.89
      - burning V90.29
        - powered V90.23
          - merchant ship V90.20
          - passenger ship V90.21
          - fishing boat V90.22
          - jetskis V90.23
        - unpowered V90.28
          - canoe V90.25
          - inflatable V90.26
          - kayak V90.25
          - sailboat V90.24
          - water skis V90.27
      - crushed V90.39
        - powered V90.33
          - merchant ship V90.30
          - passenger ship V90.31
          - fishing boat V90.32
          - jetskis V90.33
        - unpowered V90.38
          - canoe V90.35
          - inflatable V90.36
          - kayak V90.35
          - sailboat V90.34
          - water skis V90.37
      - overturning V90.09
        - powered V90.03
          - merchant ship V90.00
          - passenger ship V90.01
          - fishing boat V90.02
          - jetskis V90.03
        - unpowered V90.08
          - canoe V90.05
          - inflatable V90.06
          - kayak V90.05
          - sailboat V90.04
      - sinking V90.19
        - powered V90.13
          - merchant ship V90.10
          - passenger ship V90.11
          - fishing boat V90.12
          - jetskis V90.13
        - unpowered V90.18
          - canoe V90.15
          - inflatable V90.16
          - kayak V90.15
          - sailboat V90.14
      - specified type NEC V90.89
        - powered V90.83
          - merchant ship V90.80
          - passenger ship V90.81
          - fishing boat V90.82
          - jetskis V90.83
        - unpowered V90.88
          - canoe V90.85
          - inflatable V90.86
          - kayak V90.85
          - sailboat V90.84
          - water skis V90.87
  - avalanche — *see* Landslide
  - cataclysmic

Drowning (accidental) - *continued*
- due to - *continued*
  - cataclysmic - *continued*
    - earth surface movement NEC — *see* Forces of nature, earth movement
    - storm — *see* Forces of nature, cataclysmic storm
  - cloudburst X37.8
  - cyclone X37.1
  - fall overboard (from) V92.09
    - powered craft V92.03
      - ferry boat V92.01
      - liner V92.01
      - merchant ship V92.00
      - passenger ship V92.01
      - fishing boat V92.02
      - jetskis V92.03
    - unpowered craft V92.08
      - canoe V92.05
      - inflatable V92.06
      - kayak V92.05
      - sailboat V92.04
      - surf-board V92.08
      - water skis V92.07
      - windsurfer V92.08
    - resulting from
      - accident to watercraft — *see* Drowning, due to, accident to, watercraft
      - being washed overboard (from) V92.29
        - powered craft V92.23
          - ferry boat V92.21
          - liner V92.21
          - merchant ship V92.20
          - passenger ship V92.21
          - fishing boat V92.22
          - jetskis V92.23
        - unpowered craft V92.28
          - canoe V92.25
          - inflatable V92.26
          - kayak V92.25
          - sailboat V92.24
          - surf-board V92.28
          - water skis V92.27
          - windsurfer V92.28
      - motion of watercraft V92.19
        - powered craft V92.13
          - ferry boat V92.11
          - liner V92.11
          - merchant ship V92.10
          - passenger ship V92.11
          - fishing boat V92.12
          - jetskis V92.13
        - unpowered craft
          - canoe V92.15
          - inflatable V92.16
          - kayak V92.15
          - sailboat V92.14
  - hurricane X37.0
  - jumping into water from watercraft (involved in accident) — *see also* Drowning, due to, accident to, watercraft
    - without accident to or on watercraft W16.711
  - tidal wave NEC — *see* Forces of nature, tidal wave
  - torrential rain X37.8
- following
  - fall
    - into
      - bathtub W16.211
      - bucket W16.221
      - fountain — *see* Drowning, following, fall, into, water, specified NEC
      - quarry — *see* Drowning, following, fall, into, water, specified NEC
      - reservoir — *see* Drowning, following, fall, into, water, specified NEC
      - swimming-pool W16.011
        - striking
          - bottom W16.021
          - wall W16.031
        - stated as undetermined whether accidental or intentional Y21.3
        - suicide (attempt) X71.2
      - water NOS W16.41
        - natural (lake) (open sea) (river) (stream) (pond) W16.111
          - striking
            - bottom W16.121
            - side W16.131
        - specified NEC W16.311
          - striking
            - bottom W16.321
            - wall W16.331
    - overboard NEC — *see* Drowning, due to, fall overboard

Drowning (accidental) - *continued*
- following - *continued*
  - jump or dive
    - from boat W16.711
      - striking bottom W16.721
    - into
      - fountain — *see* Drowning, following, jump or dive, into, water, specified NEC
      - quarry — *see* Drowning, following, jump or dive, into, water, specified NEC
      - reservoir — *see* Drowning, following, jump or dive, into, water, specified NEC
      - swimming-pool W16.511
        - striking
          - bottom W16.521
          - wall W16.531
        - suicide (attempt) X71.2
      - water NOS W16.91
        - natural (lake) (open sea) (river) (stream) (pond) W16.611
        - specified NEC W16.811
          - striking
            - bottom W16.821
            - wall W16.831
        - striking bottom W16.621
- homicide (attempt) X92.9
- in
  - bathtub (accidental) W65
    - assault X92.0
    - following fall W16.211
      - stated as undetermined whether accidental or intentional Y21.1
    - stated as undetermined whether accidental or intentional Y21.0
    - suicide (attempt) X71.0
  - lake — *see* Drowning, in, natural water
  - natural water (lake) (open sea) (river) (stream) (pond) W69
    - assault X92.3
    - following
      - dive or jump W16.611
        - striking bottom W16.621
      - fall W16.111
        - striking
          - bottom W16.121
          - side W16.131
    - stated as undetermined whether accidental or intentional Y21.4
    - suicide (attempt) X71.3
  - quarry — *see* Drowning, in, specified place NEC
  - quenching tank — *see* Drowning, in, specified place NEC
  - reservoir — *see* Drowning, in, specified place NEC
  - river — *see* Drowning, in, natural water
  - sea — *see* Drowning, in, natural water
  - specified place NEC W73
    - assault X92.8
    - following
      - dive or jump W16.811
        - striking
          - bottom W16.821
          - wall W16.831
      - fall W16.311
        - striking
          - bottom W16.321
          - wall W16.331
    - stated as undetermined whether accidental or intentional Y21.8
    - suicide (attempt) X71.8
  - stream — *see* Drowning, in, natural water
  - swimming-pool W67
    - assault X92.1
      - following fall X92.2
    - following
      - dive or jump W16.511
        - striking
          - bottom W16.521
          - wall W16.531
      - fall W16.011
        - striking
          - bottom W16.021
          - wall W16.031
    - stated as undetermined whether accidental or intentional Y21.2
      - following fall Y21.3
    - suicide (attempt) X71.1
      - following fall X71.2
  - war operations — *see* War operations, restriction of airway
- resulting from accident to watercraftCsee Drowning, due to, accident, watercraft
- self-inflicted X71.9

- **Exposure** (to) - *continued*
  - electric current - *continued*
    - misadventure in medical or surgical procedure in electroshock therapy Y63.4
    - motor (electric) (faulty) W86.8
      - domestic W86.0
    - self-inflicted X83.1
    - specified NEC W86.8
      - domestic W86.0
    - stun gun — *see* Exposure, electric current, taser
    - suicide (attempt) X83.1
    - taser W86.8
      - assault Y08.89
      - legal intervention — *see* category Y35
      - self-harm (intentional) X83.8
      - undetermined intent Y33
    - third rail W86.8
    - transformer (faulty) W86.1
    - transmission lines W85
  - environmental tobacco smoke X58
  - excessive
    - cold — *see* Exposure, cold
    - heat (natural) NEC X30
      - man-made W92
  - factor (s) NOS X58
    - environmental NEC X58
      - man-made NEC W99
      - natural NEC — *see* Forces of nature
    - specified NEC X58
  - fire, flames (accidental) X08.8
    - assault X97
    - campfire — *see* Exposure, fire, controlled, not in building
    - controlled (in)
      - with ignition (of) clothing — *see also* Ignition, clothes X06.2
        - nightwear X05
      - bonfire — *see* Exposure, fire, controlled, not in building
      - brazier (in building or structure) — *see also* Exposure, fire, controlled, building
        - not in building or structure — *see* Exposure, fire, controlled, not in building
      - building or structure X02.0
        - with
          - fall from building X02.3
          - injury due to building collapse X02.2
          - from building X02.5
          - smoke inhalation X02.1
        - hit by object from building X02.4
        - specified mode of injury NEC X02.8
      - fireplace, furnace or stove — *see* Exposure, fire, controlled, building
      - not in building or structure X03.0
        - with
          - fall X03.3
          - smoke inhalation X03.1
        - hit by object X03.4
        - specified mode of injury NEC X03.8
      - trash — *see* Exposure, fire, controlled, not in building
    - fireplace — *see* Exposure, fire, controlled, building
    - fittings or furniture (in building or structure) (uncontrolled) — *see* Exposure, fire, uncontrolled, building
    - forest (uncontrolled) — *see* Exposure, fire, uncontrolled, not in building
    - grass (uncontrolled) — *see* Exposure, fire, uncontrolled, not in building
    - hay (uncontrolled) — *see* Exposure, fire, uncontrolled, not in building
    - homicide (attempt) X97
    - ignition of highly flammable material X04
    - in, of, on, starting in
      - machinery — *see* Contact, with, by type of machine
      - motor vehicle (in motion) — *see also* Accident, transport, occupant by type of vehicle V87.8
        - with collision — *see* Collision
      - railway rolling stock, train, vehicle V81.81
        - with collision — *see* Accident, transport, railway vehicle occupant
      - street car (in motion) V82.8
        - with collision — *see* Accident, transport, streetcar occupant
      - transport vehicle NEC — *see also* Accident, transport
        - with collision — *see* Collision
      - war operations — *see also* War operations, fire
        - from nuclear explosion — *see* War operations, nuclear weapons
      - watercraft (in transit) (not in transit) V91.09

- **Exposure** (to) - *continued*
  - fire, flames (accidental) - *continued*
    - in, of, on, starting in - *continued*
      - watercraft (in transit) (not in transit) - *continued*
        - localized — *see* Burn, on board watercraft, due to, fire on board
        - powered craft V91.03
          - ferry boat V91.01
          - fishing boat V91.02
          - jet skis V91.03
          - liner V91.01
          - merchant ship V91.00
          - passenger ship V91.01
        - unpowered craft V91.08
          - canoe V91.05
          - inflatable V91.06
          - kayak V91.05
          - sailboat V91.04
          - surf-board V91.08
          - waterskis V91.07
          - windsurfer V91.08
    - lumber (uncontrolled) — *see* Exposure, fire, uncontrolled, not in building
    - mine (uncontrolled) — *see* Exposure, fire, uncontrolled, not in building
    - prairie (uncontrolled) — *see* Exposure, fire, uncontrolled, not in building
    - resulting from
      - explosion — *see* Explosion
      - lightning X08.8
    - self-inflicted X76
    - specified NEC X08.8
    - started by other person X97
    - stove — *see* Exposure, fire, controlled, building
    - stated as undetermined whether accidental or intentional Y26
    - suicide (attempt) X76
    - tunnel (uncontrolled) — *see* Exposure, fire, uncontrolled, not in building
    - uncontrolled
      - in building or structure X00.0
        - with
          - fall from building X00.3
          - injury due to building collapse X00.2
          - jump from building X00.5
          - smoke inhalation X00.1
        - bed X08.00
          - due to
            - cigarette X08.01
            - specified material NEC X08.09
        - furniture NEC X08.20
          - due to
            - cigarette X08.21
            - specified material NEC X08.29
        - hit by object from building X00.4
        - sofa X08.10
          - due to
            - cigarette X08.11
            - specified material NEC X08.19
        - specified mode of injury NEC X00.8
      - not in building or structure (any) X01.0
        - with
          - fall X01.3
          - smoke inhalation X01.1
        - hit by object X01.4
        - specified mode of injury NEC X01.8
    - undetermined whether accidental or intentional Y26
  - forces of nature NEC — *see* Forces of nature
  - G-forces (abnormal) W49.9
  - gravitational forces (abnormal) W49.9
  - heat (natural) NEC — *see* Heat
  - high-pressure jet (hydraulic) (pneumatic) W49.9
  - hydraulic jet W49.9
  - inanimate mechanical force W49.9
  - jet, high-pressure (hydraulic) (pneumatic) W49.9
  - lightning — *see* subcategory T75.0
    - causing fire — *see* Exposure, fire
  - mechanical forces NEC W49.9
    - animate NEC W64
    - inanimate NEC W49.9
  - noise W42.9
    - supersonic W42.0
  - noxious substance — *see* Table of Drugs and Chemicals
  - pneumatic jet W49.9
  - prolonged in deep-freeze unit or refrigerator W93.2
  - radiation — *see* Radiation
  - smoke — *see also* Exposure, fire
    - tobacco, second hand Z77.22
  - specified factors NEC X58
  - sunlight X32
    - man-made (sun lamp) W89.8

- **Exposure** (to) - *continued*
  - sunlight - *continued*
    - man-made (sun lamp) - *continued*
      - tanning bed W89.1
  - supersonic waves W42.0
  - transmission line (s) , electric W85
  - vibration W49.9
  - waves
    - infrasound W49.9
    - sound W42.9
    - supersonic W42.0
  - weather NEC — *see* Forces of nature
- **External cause status** Y99.9
  - child assisting in compensated work for family Y99.8
  - civilian activity done for financial or other compensation Y99.0
  - civilian activity done for income or pay Y99.0
  - family member assisting in compensated work for other family member Y99.8
  - hobby not done for income Y99.8
  - leisure activity Y99.8
  - military activity Y99.1
  - off-duty activity of military personnel Y99.8
  - recreation or sport not for income or while a student Y99.8
  - specified NEC Y99.8
  - student activity Y99.8
  - volunteer activity Y99.2

F

- **Factors, supplemental**
  - alcohol
    - blood level
      - less than 20mg/100ml Y90.0
      - presence in blood, level not specified Y90.9
      - 20-39mg/100ml Y90.1
      - 40-59mg/100ml Y90.2
      - 60-79mg/100ml Y90.3
      - 80-99mg/100ml Y90.4
      - 100-119mg/100ml Y90.5
      - 120-199mg/100ml Y90.6
      - 200-239mg/100ml Y90.7
      - 240mg/100ml or more Y90.8
    - presence in blood, but level not specified Y90.9
  - environmental-pollution-related condition- see Z57
  - nosocomial condition Y95
  - work-related condition Y99.0
- **Failure**
  - in suture or ligature during surgical procedure Y65.2
  - mechanical, of instrument or apparatus (any) (during any medical or surgical procedure) Y65.8
  - sterile precautions (during medical and surgical care) — *see* Misadventure, failure, sterile precautions, by type of procedure
  - to
    - introduce tube or instrument Y65.4
      - endotracheal tube during anesthesia Y65.3
    - make curve (transport vehicle) NEC — *see* Accident, transport
    - remove tube or instrument Y65.4
- **Fall, falling** (accidental) W19
  - building W20.1
    - burning (uncontrolled fire) X00.3
  - down
    - embankment W17.81
    - escalator W10.0
    - hill W17.81
    - ladder W11
    - ramp W10.2
    - stairs, steps W10.9
  - due to
    - bumping against
      - object W18.00
        - sharp glass W18.02
        - specified NEC W18.09
        - sports equipment W18.01
      - person W03
        - due to ice or snow W00.0
        - on pedestrian conveyance — *see* Accident, transport, pedestrian, conveyance
    - collision with another person W03
      - due to ice or snow W00.0
      - involving pedestrian conveyance — *see* Accident, transport, pedestrian, conveyance
    - grocery cart tipping over W17.82
    - ice or snow W00.9
      - from one level to another W00.2
        - on stairs or steps W00.1
      - involving pedestrian conveyance — *see* Accident, transport, pedestrian, conveyance
      - on same level W00.0
    - slipping (on moving sidewalk) W01.0

Fall, falling (accidental) - *continued*
  on same level - *continued*
    due to
      specified NEC W18.39
      stepping on an object W18.31
  out of
    bed W06
    building NEC W13.8
    chair W07
    furniture NEC W08
    wheelchair, non-moving W05.0
      powered — *see* Accident, transport, pedestrian, conveyance, specified type NEC
    window W13.4
  over
    animal W01.0
    cliff W15
    embankment W17.81
    small object W01.0
  rock W20.8
  same level W18.30
    from
      being crushed, pushed, or stepped on by a crowd or human stampede W52
      collision, pushing, shoving, by or with other person W03
      slipping, stumbling, tripping W01.0
    involving ice or snow W00.0
      involving skates (ice) (roller) , skateboard, skis — *see* Accident, transport, pedestrian, conveyance
  snowslide (avalanche) — *see* Landslide
  stone W20.8
  structure W20.1
    burning (uncontrolled fire) X00.3
  through
    bridge W13.1
    floor W13.3
    roof W13.2
    wall W13.8
    window W13.4
  timber W20.8
  tree (caused by lightning) W20.8
  while being carried or supported by other person (s) W04
Fallen on by
  animal (not being ridden) NEC W55.89
Felo-de-se — *see* Suicide
Fight (hand) (fists) (foot) — *see* Assault, fight
Fire (accidental) — *see* Exposure, fire
Firearm discharge — *see* Discharge, firearm
Fireball effects from nuclear explosion in war operations — *see* War operations, nuclear weapons
Fireworks (explosion) W39
Flash burns from explosion — *see* Explosion
Flood (any injury) (caused by) X38
  collapse of man-made structure causing earth movement X36.0
  tidal wave — *see* Forces of nature, tidal wave
Food (any type) **in**
  air passages (with asphyxia, obstruction, or suffocation) — *see* categories T17 and T18
  alimentary tract causing asphyxia (due to compression of trachea) — *see* categories T17 and T18
Forces of nature X39.8
  avalanche X36.1
    causing transport accident — *see* Accident, transport, by type of vehicle
  blizzard X37.2
  cataclysmic storm X37.9
    with flood X38
    blizzard X37.2
    cloudburst X37.8
    cyclone X37.1
    dust storm X37.3
    hurricane X37.0
    specified storm NEC X37.8
    storm surge X37.0
    tornado X37.1
    twister X37.1
    typhoon X37.0
  cloudburst X37.8
  cold (natural) X31
  cyclone X37.1
  dam collapse causing earth movement X36.0
  dust storm X37.3
  earth movement X36.1
    earthquake X34
    caused by dam or structure collapse X36.0
  earthquake X34
  flood (caused by) X38

Forces of nature - *continued*
  flood (caused by) - *continued*
    dam collapse X36.0
    tidal wave — *see* Forces of nature, tidal wave
  heat (natural) X30
  hurricane X37.0
  landslide X36.1
    causing transport accident — *see* Accident, transport, by type of vehicle
  lightning — *see* subcategory T75.0
    causing fire — *see* Exposure, fire
  mudslide X36.1
    causing transport accident — *see* Accident, transport, by type of vehicle
  radiation (natural) X39.08
    radon X39.01
  radon X39.01
  specified force NEC X39.8
  storm surge X37.0
  structure collapse causing earth movement X36.0
  sunlight X32
  tidal wave X37.41
    due to
      earthquake X37.41
      landslide X37.43
      storm X37.42
      volcanic eruption X37.41
  tornado X37.1
  tsunami X37.41
  twister X37.1
  typhoon X37.0
  volcanic eruption X35
Foreign body
  aspiration — *see* Index to Diseases and Injuries, Foreign body, respiratory tract
  embedded in skin W45
  entering through skin W45.8
    can lid W26.8
    nail W45.0
    paper W26.2
    specified NEC W45.8
    splinter W45.8
Forest fire (exposure to) — *see* Exposure, fire, uncontrolled, not in building
Found injured X58
  from exposure (to) — *see* Exposure
  on
    highway, road (way) , street V89.9
    railway right of way V81.9
Fracture (circumstances unknown or unspecified) X58
  due to specified cause NEC X58
Freezing — *see* Exposure, cold
Frostbite X31
  due to man-made conditions — *see* Exposure, cold, man-made
Frozen — *see* Exposure, cold

G

Gored by bull W55.22
Gunshot wound W34.00

H

Hailstones, injured by X39.8
Hanged herself or himself — *see* Hanging, self-inflicted
Hanging (accidental) (*see also* category T71)
  legal execution — *see* Legal, intervention, specified means NEC
Heat (effects of) (excessive) X30
  due to
    man-made conditions W92
      on board watercraft V93.29
        fishing boat V93.22
        merchant ship V93.20
        passenger ship V93.21
        sailboat V93.24
        specified powered craft NEC V93.23
    weather (conditions) X30
  from
    electric heating apparatus causing burning X16
    nuclear explosion in war operations — *see* War operations, nuclear weapons
  inappropriate in local application or packing in medical or surgical procedure Y63.5
Hemorrhage
  delayed following medical or surgical treatment without mention of misadventure — *see* Index to Diseases and Injuries, Complication(s)
  during medical or surgical treatment as misadventure — *see* Index to Diseases and Injuries, Complication(s)
High
  altitude (effects) - — *see* Air, pressure, low

High - *continued*
  level of radioactivity, effects — *see* Radiation
  pressure (effects) - — *see* Air, pressure, high
  temperature, effects — *see* Heat
Hit, hitting (accidental) **by** — *see* Struck by
Hitting against — *see* Striking against
Homicide (attempt) (justifiable) — *see* Assault
Hot
  place, effects — *see also* Heat
  weather, effects X30
House fire (uncontrolled) — *see* Exposure, fire, uncontrolled, building
Humidity, causing problem X39.8
Hunger X58
Hurricane (any injury) X37.0
Hypobarism, hypobaropathy - — *see* Air, pressure, low

I

Ictus
  caloris — *see also* Heat
  solaris X30
Ignition (accidental) — *see also* Exposure, fire X08.8
  anesthetic gas in operating room W40.1
  apparel X06.2
    from highly flammable material X04
    nightwear X05
  bed linen (sheets) (spreads) (pillows) (mattress) — *see* Exposure, fire, uncontrolled, building, bed
  benzine X04
  clothes, clothing NEC (from controlled fire) X06.2
    from
      highly flammable material X04
  ether X04
    in operating room W40.1
  explosive material — *see* Explosion
  gasoline X04
  jewelry (plastic) (any) X06.0
  kerosene X04
  material
    explosive — *see* Explosion
    highly flammable with secondary explosion X04
  nightwear X05
  paraffin X04
  petrol X04
Immersion (accidental) — *see also* Drowning
  hand or foot due to cold (excessive) X31
Implantation of quills of porcupine W55.89
Inanition (from) (hunger) X58
  thirst X58
Inappropriate operation performed
  correct operation on wrong side or body part (wrong side) (wrong site) Y65.53
  operation intended for another patient done on wrong patient Y65.52
  wrong operation performed on correct patient Y65.51
Inattention after, at birth (homicidal intent) (infanticidal intent) X58
Incident, adverse
  device
    anesthesiology Y70.8
      accessory Y70.2
      diagnostic Y70.0
      miscellaneous Y70.8
      monitoring Y70.0
      prosthetic Y70.2
      rehabilitative Y70.1
      surgical Y70.3
      therapeutic Y70.1
    cardiovascular Y71.8
      accessory Y71.2
      diagnostic Y71.0
      miscellaneous Y71.8
      monitoring Y71.0
      prosthetic Y71.2
      rehabilitative Y71.1
      surgical Y71.3
      therapeutic Y71.1
    gastroenterology Y73.8
      accessory Y73.2
      diagnostic Y73.0
      miscellaneous Y73.8
      monitoring Y73.0
      prosthetic Y73.2
      rehabilitative Y73.1
      surgical Y73.3
      therapeutic Y73.1
    general
      hospital Y74.8
        accessory Y74.2
        diagnostic Y74.0

Incident, adverse - *continued*
device - *continued*
general - *continued*
hospital - *continued*
miscellaneous Y74.8
monitoring Y74.0
prosthetic Y74.2
rehabilitative Y74.1
surgical Y74.3
therapeutic Y74.1
surgical Y81.8
accessory Y81.2
diagnostic Y81.0
miscellaneous Y81.8
monitoring Y81.0
prosthetic Y81.2
rehabilitative Y81.1
surgical Y81.3
therapeutic Y81.1
gynecological Y76.8
accessory Y76.2
diagnostic Y76.0
miscellaneous Y76.8
monitoring Y76.0
prosthetic Y76.2
rehabilitative Y76.1
surgical Y76.3
therapeutic Y76.1
medical Y82.9
specified type NEC Y82.8
neurological Y75.8
accessory Y75.2
diagnostic Y75.0
miscellaneous Y75.8
monitoring Y75.0
prosthetic Y75.2
rehabilitative Y75.1
surgical Y75.3
therapeutic Y75.1
obstetrical Y76.8
accessory Y76.2
diagnostic Y76.0
miscellaneous Y76.8
monitoring Y76.0
prosthetic Y76.2
rehabilitative Y76.1
surgical Y76.3
therapeutic Y76.1
ophthalmic Y77.8
accessory Y77.2
diagnostic Y77.0
miscellaneous Y77.8
monitoring Y77.0
prosthetic Y77.2
rehabilitative Y77.1
surgical Y77.3
therapeutic Y77.1
orthopedic Y79.8
accessory Y79.2
diagnostic Y79.0
miscellaneous Y79.8
monitoring Y79.0
prosthetic Y79.2
rehabilitative Y79.1
surgical Y79.3
therapeutic Y79.1
otorhinolaryngological Y72.8
accessory Y72.2
diagnostic Y72.0
miscellaneous Y72.8
monitoring Y72.0
prosthetic Y72.2
rehabilitative Y72.1
surgical Y72.3
therapeutic Y72.1
personal use Y74.8
accessory Y74.2
diagnostic Y74.0
miscellaneous Y74.8
monitoring Y74.0
prosthetic Y74.2
rehabilitative Y74.1
surgical Y74.3
therapeutic Y74.1
physical medicine Y80.8
accessory Y80.2
diagnostic Y80.0
miscellaneous Y80.8
monitoring Y80.0
prosthetic Y80.2
rehabilitative Y80.1
surgical Y80.3
therapeutic Y80.1

Incident, adverse - *continued*
device - *continued*
plastic surgical Y81.8
accessory Y81.2
diagnostic Y81.0
miscellaneous Y81.8
monitoring Y81.0
prosthetic Y81.2
rehabilitative Y81.1
surgical Y81.3
therapeutic Y81.1
radiological Y78.8
accessory Y78.2
diagnostic Y78.0
miscellaneous Y78.8
monitoring Y78.0
prosthetic Y78.2
rehabilitative Y78.1
surgical Y78.3
therapeutic Y78.1
urology Y73.8
accessory Y73.2
diagnostic Y73.0
miscellaneous Y73.8
monitoring Y73.0
prosthetic Y73.2
rehabilitative Y73.1
surgical Y73.3
therapeutic Y73.1
Incineration (accidental) — *see* Exposure, fire
Infanticide — *see* Assault
Infrasound waves (causing injury) W49.9
Ingestion
foreign body (causing injury) (with obstruction) — *see* Foreign body, alimentary canal
poisonous
plant (s) X58
substance NEC — *see* Table of Drugs and Chemicals
Inhalation
excessively cold substance, man-made — *see* Exposure, cold, man-made
food (any type) (into respiratory tract) (with asphyxia, obstruction respiratory tract, suffocation) — *see* categories T17 and T18
foreign body — *see* Foreign body, aspiration
gastric contents (with asphyxia, obstruction respiratory passage, suffocation) T17.81-
hot air or gases X14.0
liquid air, hydrogen, nitrogen W93.12
suicide (attempt) X83.2
steam X13.0
assault X98.0
stated as undetermined whether accidental or intentional Y27.0
suicide (attempt) X77.0
toxic gas — *see* Table of Drugs and Chemicals
vomitus (with asphyxia, obstruction respiratory passage, suffocation) T17.81-
Injury, injured (accidental (ly) **) NOS** X58
by, caused by, from
assault — *see* Assault
law-enforcing agent, police, in course of legal intervention — *see* Legal intervention
suicide (attempt) X83.8
due to, in
civil insurrection — *see* War operations
fight — *see also* Assault, fight Y04.0
war operations — *see* War operations
homicide — *see also* Assault Y09
inflicted (by)
in course of arrest (attempted) , suppression of disturbance, maintenance of order, by law-enforcing agents — *see* Legal intervention
other person
stated as
accidental X58
intentional, homicide (attempt) — *see* Assault
undetermined whether accidental or intentional Y33
purposely (inflicted) by other person (s) — *see* Assault
self-inflicted X83.8
stated as accidental X58
specified cause NEC X58
undetermined whether accidental or intentional Y33
Insolation, effects X30
Insufficient nourishment X58
Interruption of respiration (by)
food (lodged in esophagus) — *see* categories T17 and T18
vomitus (lodged in esophagus) T17.81-

Intervention, legal — *see* Legal intervention
Intoxication
drug — *see* Table of Drugs and Chemicals
poison — *see* Table of Drugs and Chemicals

J

Jammed (accidentally)
between objects (moving) (stationary and moving) W23.0
stationary W23.1
Jumped, jumping
before moving object NEC X81.8
motor vehicle X81.0
subway train X81.1
train X81.1
undetermined whether accidental or intentional Y31
from
boat (into water) voluntarily, without accident (to or on boat) W16.712
with
accident to or on boat — *see* Accident, watercraft
drowning or submersion W16.711
suicide (attempt) X71.3
striking bottom W16.722
causing drowning W16.721
building — *see also* Jumped, from, high place W13.9
burning (uncontrolled fire) X00.5
high place NEC W17.89
suicide (attempt) X80
undetermined whether accidental or intentional Y30
structure — *see also* Jumped, from, high place W13.9
burning (uncontrolled fire) X00.5
into water W16.92
causing drowning W16.91
from, off watercraft — *see* Jumped, from, boat
in
natural body W16.612
causing drowning W16.611
striking bottom W16.622
causing drowning W16.621
specified place NEC W16.812
causing drowning W16.811
striking
bottom W16.822
causing drowning W16.821
wall W16.832
causing drowning W16.831
swimming pool W16.512
causing drowning W16.511
striking
bottom W16.522
causing drowning W16.521
wall W16.532
causing drowning W16.531
suicide (attempt) X71.3

K

Kicked by
animal NEC W55.82
person (s) (accidentally) W50.1
with intent to injure or kill Y04.0
as, or caused by, a crowd or human stampede (with fall) W52
assault Y04.0
homicide (attempt) Y04.0
in
fight Y04.0
legal intervention
injuring
bystander Y35.812
law enforcement personnel Y35.811
suspect Y35.813
Kicking
against
object W22.8
sports equipment W21.9
stationary W22.09
sports equipment W21.89
person — *see* Striking against, person
sports equipment W21.9
carpet stretcher with knee X50.3
Killed, killing (accidentally) **NOS** — *see also* Injury X58
in
action — *see* War operations
brawl, fight (hand) (fists) (foot) Y04.0
by weapon — *see also* Assault
cutting, piercing — *see* Assault, cutting or piercing instrument

Killed, killing (accidentally) **NOS** - *continued*
in - *continued*
brawl, fight (hand) (fists) (foot) - *continued*
by weapon - *continued*
firearm — *see* Discharge, firearm, by type, homicide
self
stated as
accident NOS X58
suicide — *see* Suicide
undetermined whether accidental or intentional Y33
Kneeling (prolonged) (static) X50.1
Knocked down (accidentally) (by) **NOS** X58
animal (not being ridden) NEC — *see also* Struck by, by type of animal
crowd or human stampede W52
person W51
in brawl, fight Y04.0
transport vehicle NEC — *see also* Accident, transport V09.9

L

Laceration NEC — *see* Injury
Lack of
care (helpless person) (infant) (newborn) X58
food except as result of abandonment or neglect X58
due to abandonment or neglect X58
water except as result of transport accident X58
due to transport accident — *see* Accident, transport, by type
helpless person, infant, newborn X58
Landslide (falling on transport vehicle) X36.1
caused by collapse of man-made structure X36.0
Late effect — *see* Sequelae
Legal
execution (any method) — *see* Legal, intervention
intervention (by)
baton — *see* Legal, intervention, blunt object, baton
bayonet — *see* Legal, intervention, sharp object, bayonet
blow — *see* Legal, intervention, manhandling
blunt object
baton
injuring
bystander Y35.312
law enforcement personnel Y35.311
suspect Y35.313
injuring
bystander Y35.302
law enforcement personnel Y35.301
suspect Y35.303
specified NEC
injuring
bystander Y35.392
law enforcement personnel Y35.391
suspect Y35.393
stave
injuring
bystander Y35.392
law enforcement personnel Y35.391
suspect Y35.393
bomb — *see* Legal, intervention, explosive
cutting or piercing instrument — *see* Legal, intervention, sharp object
dynamite — *see* Legal, intervention, explosive, dynamite
explosive (s)
dynamite
injuring
bystander Y35.112
law enforcement personnel Y35.111
suspect Y35.113
grenade
injuring
bystander Y35.192
law enforcement personnel Y35.191
suspect Y35.193
injuring
bystander Y35.102
law enforcement personnel Y35.101
suspect Y35.103
mortar bomb
injuring
bystander Y35.192
law enforcement personnel Y35.191
suspect Y35.193
shell
injuring
bystander Y35.122
law enforcement personnel Y35.121
suspect Y35.123

Legal - *continued*
intervention (by) - *continued*
explosive (s) - *continued*
specified NEC
injuring
bystander Y35.192
law enforcement personnel Y35.191
suspect Y35.193
firearm (s) (discharge)
handgun
injuring
bystander Y35.022
law enforcement personnel Y35.021
suspect Y35.023
injuring
bystander Y35.002
law enforcement personnel Y35.001
suspect Y35.003
machine gun
injuring
bystander Y35.012
law enforcement personnel Y35.011
suspect Y35.013
rifle pellet
injuring
bystander Y35.032
law enforcement personnel Y35.031
suspect Y35.033
rubber bullet
injuring
bystander Y35.042
law enforcement personnel Y35.041
suspect Y35.043
shotgun — *see* Legal, intervention, firearm, specified NEC
specified NEC
injuring
bystander Y35.092
law enforcement personnel Y35.091
suspect Y35.093
gas (asphyxiation) (poisoning)
injuring
bystander Y35.202
law enforcement personnel Y35.201
suspect Y35.203
specified NEC
injuring
bystander Y35.292
law enforcement personnel Y35.291
suspect Y35.293
tear gas
injuring
bystander Y35.212
law enforcement personnel Y35.211
suspect Y35.213
grenade — *see* Legal, intervention, explosive, grenade
injuring
bystander Y35.92
law enforcement personnel Y35.91
suspect Y35.93
late effect (of) — *see* with 7th character S Y35
manhandling
injuring
bystander Y35.812
law enforcement personnel Y35.811
suspect Y35.813
sequelae (of) — *see* with 7th character S Y35
sharp objects
bayonet
injuring
bystander Y35.412
law enforcement personnel Y35.411
suspect Y35.413
injuring
bystander Y35.402
law enforcement personnel Y35.401
suspect Y35.403
specified NEC
injuring
bystander Y35.492
law enforcement personnel Y35.491
suspect Y35.493
specified means NEC
injuring
bystander Y35.892
law enforcement personnel Y35.891
suspect Y35.893
stabbing — *see* Legal, intervention, sharp object
stave — *see* Legal, intervention, blunt object, stave
tear gas — *see* Legal, intervention, gas, tear gas
truncheon — *see* Legal, intervention, blunt object, stave

Lifting — *see also* Overexertion
heavy objects X50.0
weights X50.0
Lightning (shock) (stroke) (struck by) — *see* subcategory T75.0
causing fire — *see* Exposure, fire
Loss of control (transport vehicle) **NEC** — *see* Accident, transport
Lost at sea NOS — *see* Drowning, due to, fall overboard
Low
pressure (effects) - — *see* Air, pressure, low
temperature (effects) — *see* Exposure, cold
Lying before train, vehicle or other moving object X81.8
subway train X81.1
train X81.1
undetermined whether accidental or intentional Y31
Lynching — *see* Assault

M

Malfunction (mechanism or component) (of)
firearm W34.10
airgun W34.110
BB gun W34.110
gas, air or spring-operated gun NEC W34.118
handgun W32.1
hunting rifle W33.12
larger firearm W33.10
specified NEC W33.19
machine gun W33.13
paintball gun W34.111
pellet gun W34.110
shotgun W33.11
specified NEC W34.19
Very pistol [flare] W34.19
handgun — *see* Malfunction, firearm, handgun
Maltreatment — *see* Perpetrator
Mangled (accidentally) **NOS** X58
Manhandling (in brawl, fight) Y04.0
legal intervention — *see* Legal, intervention, manhandling
Manslaughter (nonaccidental) — *see* Assault
Mauled by animal NEC W55.89
Medical procedure, complication of (delayed or as an abnormal reaction without mention of misadventure) — *see* Complication of or following, by specified type of procedure
due to or as a result of misadventure — *see* Misadventure
Melting (due to fire) — *see also* Exposure, fire
apparel NEC X06.3
clothes, clothing NEC X06.3
nightwear X05
fittings or furniture (burning building) (uncontrolled fire) X00.8
nightwear X05
plastic jewelry X06.1
Mental cruelty X58
Military operations (injuries to military and civilians occuring during peacetime on military property and during routine military exercises and operations) (by) (from) (involving) Y37.90-
air blast Y37.20-
aircraft
destruction — *see* Military operations, destruction of aircraft
airway restriction — *see* Military operations, restriction of airways
asphyxiation — *see* Military operations, restriction of airways
biological weapons Y37.6X-
blast Y37.20-
blast fragments Y37.20-
blast wave Y37.20-
blast wind Y37.20-
bomb Y37.20-
dirty Y37.50-
gasoline Y37.31-
incendiary Y37.31-
petrol Y37.31-
bullet Y37.43-
incendiary Y37.32-
rubber Y37.41-
chemical weapons Y37.7X-
combat
hand to hand (unarmed) combat Y37.44-
using blunt or piercing object Y37.45-
conflagration — *see* Military operations, fire
conventional warfare NEC Y37.49-
depth-charge Y37.01-
destruction of aircraft Y37.10-
due to

N

O

- **Overturning** (accidental) - *continued*
  - watercraft (causing drowning, submersion) - *continued*
    - causing injury except drowning or submersion — *see* Accident, watercraft, causing, injury NEC

P

- **Parachute descent** (voluntary) (without accident to aircraft) V97.29
  - due to accident to aircraft — *see* Accident, transport, aircraft
- **Pecked by bird** W61.99
- **Perforation during medical or surgical treatment as misadventure** — *see* Index to Diseases and Injuries, Complication(s)
- **Perpetrator, perpetration, of assault, maltreatment and neglect** (by) Y07.9
  - boyfriend Y07.03
  - brother Y07.410
    - stepbrother Y07.435
  - coach Y07.53
  - cousin
    - female Y07.491
    - male Y07.490
  - daycare provider Y07.519
    - at-home
      - adult care Y07.512
      - childcare Y07.510
    - care center
      - adult care Y07.513
      - childcare Y07.511
  - family member NEC Y07.499
  - father Y07.11
    - adoptive Y07.13
    - foster Y07.420
    - stepfather Y07.430
  - foster father Y07.420
  - foster mother Y07.421
  - girl friend Y07.04
  - healthcare provider Y07.529
    - mental health Y07.521
    - specified NEC Y07.528
  - husband Y07.01
  - instructor Y07.53
  - mother Y07.12
    - adoptive Y07.14
    - foster Y07.421
    - stepmother Y07.433
  - multiple perpetrators Y07.6
  - nonfamily member Y07.50
    - specified NEC Y07.59
  - nurse Y07.528
  - occupational therapist Y07.528
  - partner of parent
    - female Y07.434
    - male Y07.432
  - physical therapist Y07.528
  - sister Y07.411
  - speech therapist Y07.528
  - stepbrother Y07.435
  - stepfather Y07.430
  - stepmother Y07.433
  - stepsister Y07.436
  - teacher Y07.53
  - wife Y07.02
- **Piercing** — *see* Contact, with, by type of object or machine
- **Pinched**
  - between objects (moving) (stationary and moving) W23.0
    - stationary W23.1
- **Pinned under machine** (ry) — *see* Contact, with, by type of machine
- **Place of occurrence** Y92.9
  - abandoned house Y92.89
  - airplane Y92.813
  - airport Y92.520
  - ambulatory health services establishment NEC Y92.538
  - ambulatory surgery center Y92.530
  - amusement park Y92.831
  - apartment (co-op) — *see* Place of occurrence, residence, apartment
  - assembly hall Y92.29
  - bank Y92.510
  - barn Y92.71
  - baseball field Y92.320
  - basketball court Y92.310
  - beach Y92.832
  - boarding house — *see* Place of occurrence, residence, boarding house
  - boat Y92.814

- **Place of occurrence** - *continued*
  - bowling alley Y92.39
  - bridge Y92.89
  - building under construction Y92.61
  - bus Y92.811
    - station Y92.521
  - cafe Y92.511
  - campsite Y92.833
  - campus — *see* Place of occurrence, school
  - canal Y92.89
  - car Y92.810
  - casino Y92.59
  - children's home — *see* Place of occurrence, residence, institutional, orphanage
  - church Y92.22
  - cinema Y92.26
  - clubhouse Y92.29
  - coal pit Y92.64
  - college (community) Y92.214
  - condominium — *see* Place of occurrence, residence, apartment
  - construction area — *see* Place of occurrence, industrial and construction area
  - convalescent home — *see* Place of occurrence, residence, institutional, nursing home
  - court-house Y92.240
  - cricket ground Y92.328
  - cultural building Y92.258
    - art gallery Y92.250
    - museum Y92.251
    - music hall Y92.252
    - opera house Y92.253
    - specified NEC Y92.258
    - theater Y92.254
  - dancehall Y92.252
  - day nursery Y92.210
  - dentist office Y92.531
  - derelict house Y92.89
  - desert Y92.820
  - dock NOS Y92.89
  - dockyard Y92.62
  - doctor's office Y92.531
  - dormitory — *see* Place of occurrence, residence, institutional, school dormitory
  - dry dock Y92.62
  - factory (building) (premises) Y92.63
  - farm (land under cultivation) (outbuildings) Y92.79
    - barn Y92.71
    - chicken coop Y92.72
    - field Y92.73
    - hen house Y92.72
    - house — *see* Place of occurrence, residence, house
    - orchard Y92.74
    - specified NEC Y92.79
  - football field Y92.321
  - forest Y92.821
  - freeway Y92.411
  - gallery Y92.250
  - garage (commercial) Y92.59
    - boarding house Y92.044
    - military base Y92.135
    - mobile home Y92.025
    - nursing home Y92.124
    - orphanage Y92.114
    - private house Y92.015
    - reform school Y92.155
  - gas station Y92.524
  - gasworks Y92.69
  - golf course Y92.39
  - gravel pit Y92.64
  - grocery Y92.512
  - gymnasium Y92.39
  - handball court Y92.318
  - harbor Y92.89
  - harness racing course Y92.39
  - healthcare provider office Y92.531
  - highway (interstate) Y92.411
  - hill Y92.828
  - hockey rink Y92.330
  - home — *see* Place of occurrence, residence
  - hospice — *see* Place of occurrence, residence, institutional, nursing home
  - hospital Y92.239
    - cafeteria Y92.233
    - corridor Y92.232
    - operating room Y92.234
    - patient
      - bathroom Y92.231
      - room Y92.230
    - specified NEC Y92.238
  - hotel Y92.59
  - house — *see also* Place of occurrence, residence
    - abandoned Y92.89

- **Place of occurrence** - *continued*
  - house - *continued*
    - under construction Y92.61
  - industrial and construction area (yard) Y92.69
    - building under construction Y92.61
    - dock Y92.62
    - dry dock Y92.62
    - factory Y92.63
    - gasworks Y92.69
    - mine Y92.64
    - oil rig Y92.65
    - pit Y92.64
    - power station Y92.69
    - shipyard Y92.62
    - specified NEC Y92.69
    - tunnel under construction Y92.69
    - workshop Y92.69
  - kindergarten Y92.211
  - lacrosse field Y92.328
  - lake Y92.828
  - library Y92.241
  - mall Y92.59
  - market Y92.512
  - marsh Y92.828
  - military
    - base — *see* Place of occurrence, residence, institutional, military base
    - training ground Y92.84
  - mine Y92.64
  - mosque Y92.22
  - motel Y92.59
  - motorway (interstate) Y92.411
  - mountain Y92.828
  - movie-house Y92.26
  - museum Y92.251
  - music-hall Y92.252
  - not applicable Y92.9
  - nuclear power station Y92.69
  - nursing home — *see* Place of occurrence, residence, institutional, nursing home
  - office building Y92.59
  - offshore installation Y92.65
  - oil rig Y92.65
  - old people's home — *see* Place of occurrence, residence, institutional, specified NEC
  - opera-house Y92.253
  - orphanage — *see* Place of occurrence, residence, institutional, orphanage
  - outpatient surgery center Y92.530
  - park (public) Y92.830
    - amusement Y92.831
  - parking garage Y92.89
    - lot Y92.481
  - pavement Y92.480
  - physician office Y92.531
  - polo field Y92.328
  - pond Y92.828
  - post office Y92.242
  - power station Y92.69
  - prairie Y92.828
  - prison — *see* Place of occurrence, residence, institutional, prison
  - public
    - administration building Y92.248
      - city hall Y92.243
      - courthouse Y92.240
      - library Y92.241
      - post office Y92.242
      - specified NEC Y92.248
    - building NEC Y92.29
    - hall Y92.29
    - place NOS Y92.89
  - race course Y92.39
  - radio station Y92.59
  - railway line (bridge) Y92.85
  - ranch (outbuildings) — *see* Place of occurrence, farm
  - recreation area Y92.838
    - amusement park Y92.831
    - beach Y92.832
    - campsite Y92.833
    - park (public) Y92.830
    - seashore Y92.832
    - specified NEC Y92.838
  - religious institution Y92.22
  - reform school - — *see* Place of occurrence, residence, institutional, reform school
  - residence (non-institutional) (private) Y92.009
    - apartment Y92.039
      - bathroom Y92.031
      - bedroom Y92.032
      - kitchen Y92.030
      - specified NEC Y92.038

- **Place of occurrence** - *continued*
  - residence (non-institutional) (private) - *continued*
    - bathroom Y92.002
    - bedroom Y92.003
    - boarding house Y92.049
      - bathroom Y92.041
      - bedroom Y92.042
      - driveway Y92.043
      - garage Y92.044
      - garden Y92.046
      - kitchen Y92.040
      - specified NEC Y92.048
      - swimming pool Y92.045
      - yard Y92.046
    - dining room Y92.001
    - garden Y92.007
    - home Y92.009
    - house, single family Y92.019
      - bathroom Y92.012
      - bedroom Y92.013
      - dining room Y92.011
      - driveway Y92.014
      - garage Y92.015
      - garden Y92.017
      - kitchen Y92.010
      - specified NEC Y92.018
      - swimming pool Y92.016
      - yard Y92.017
    - institutional Y92.10
      - children's home — *see* Place of occurrence, residence, institutional, orphanage
      - hospice — *see* Place of occurrence, residence, institutional, nursing home
      - military base Y92.139
        - barracks Y92.133
        - garage Y92.135
        - garden Y92.137
        - kitchen Y92.130
        - mess hall Y92.131
        - specified NEC Y92.138
        - swimming pool Y92.136
        - yard Y92.137
      - nursing home Y92.129
        - bathroom Y92.121
        - bedroom Y92.122
        - driveway Y92.123
        - garage Y92.124
        - garden Y92.126
        - kitchen Y92.120
        - specified NEC Y92.128
        - swimming pool Y92.125
        - yard Y92.126
      - orphanage Y92.119
        - bathroom Y92.111
        - bedroom Y92.112
        - driveway Y92.113
        - garage Y92.114
        - garden Y92.116
        - kitchen Y92.110
        - specified NEC Y92.118
        - swimming pool Y92.115
        - yard Y92.116
      - prison Y92.149
        - bathroom Y92.142
        - cell Y92.143
        - courtyard Y92.147
        - dining room Y92.141
        - kitchen Y92.140
        - specified NEC Y92.148
        - swimming pool Y92.146
      - reform school Y92.159
        - bathroom Y92.152
        - bedroom Y92.153
        - dining room Y92.151
        - driveway Y92.154
        - garage Y92.155
        - garden Y92.157
        - kitchen Y92.150
        - specified NEC Y92.158
        - swimming pool Y92.156
        - yard Y92.157
      - school dormitory Y92.169
        - bathroom Y92.162
        - bedroom Y92.163
        - dining room Y92.161
        - kitchen Y92.160
        - specified NEC Y92.168
      - specified NEC Y92.199
        - bathroom Y92.192
        - bedroom Y92.193
        - dining room Y92.191
        - driveway Y92.194
        - garage Y92.195

- **Place of occurrence** - *continued*
  - residence (non-institutional) (private) - *continued*
    - institutional - *continued*
      - specified NEC - *continued*
        - garden Y92.197
        - kitchen Y92.190
        - specified NEC Y92.198
        - swimming pool Y92.196
        - yard Y92.197
    - kitchen Y92.000
    - mobile home Y92.029
      - bathroom Y92.022
      - bedroom Y92.023
      - dining room Y92.021
      - driveway Y92.024
      - garage Y92.025
      - garden Y92.027
      - kitchen Y92.020
      - specified NEC Y92.028
      - swimming pool Y92.026
      - yard Y92.027
    - specified place in residence NEC Y92.008
    - specified residence type NEC Y92.099
      - bathroom Y92.091
      - bedroom Y92.092
      - driveway Y92.093
      - garage Y92.094
      - garden Y92.096
      - kitchen Y92.090
      - specified NEC Y92.098
      - swimming pool Y92.095
      - yard Y92.096
  - restaurant Y92.511
  - riding school Y92.39
  - river Y92.828
  - road Y92.410
  - rodeo ring Y92.39
  - rugby field Y92.328
  - same day surgery center Y92.530
  - sand pit Y92.64
  - school (private) (public) (state) Y92.219
    - college Y92.214
    - daycare center Y92.210
    - elementary school Y92.211
    - high school Y92.213
    - kindergarten Y92.211
    - middle school Y92.212
    - specified NEC Y92.218
    - trace school Y92.215
    - university Y92.214
    - vocational school Y92.215
  - sea (shore) Y92.832
  - senior citizen center Y92.29
  - service area
    - airport Y92.520
    - bus station Y92.521
    - gas station Y92.524
    - highway rest stop Y92.523
    - railway station Y92.522
  - shipyard Y92.62
  - shop (commercial) Y92.513
  - sidewalk Y92.480
  - silo Y92.79
  - skating rink (roller) Y92.331
    - ice Y92.330
  - slaughter house Y92.86
  - soccer field Y92.322
  - specified place NEC Y92.89
  - sports area Y92.39
    - athletic
      - court Y92.318
        - basketball Y92.310
        - specified NEC Y92.318
        - squash Y92.311
        - tennis Y92.312
      - field Y92.328
        - baseball Y92.320
        - cricket ground Y92.328
        - football Y92.321
        - hockey Y92.328
        - soccer Y92.322
        - specified NEC Y92.328
    - golf course Y92.39
    - gymnasium Y92.39
    - riding school Y92.39
    - skating rink (roller) Y92.331
      - ice Y92.330
    - stadium Y92.39
    - swimming pool Y92.34
  - squash court Y92.311
  - stadium Y92.39
  - steeplechasing course Y92.39
  - store Y92.512

- **Place of occurrence** - *continued*
  - stream Y92.828
  - street and highway Y92.410
    - bike path Y92.482
    - freeway Y92.411
    - highway ramp Y92.415
    - interstate highway Y92.411
    - local residential or business street Y92.414
    - motorway Y92.411
    - parkway Y92.412
    - parking lot Y92.481
    - sidewalk Y92.480
    - specified NEC Y92.488
    - state road Y92.413
  - subway car Y92.816
  - supermarket Y92.512
  - swamp Y92.828
  - swimming pool (public) Y92.34
    - private (at) Y92.095
      - boarding house Y92.045
      - military base Y92.136
      - mobile home Y92.026
      - nursing home Y92.125
      - orphanage Y92.115
      - prison Y92.146
      - reform school Y92.156
      - single family residence Y92.016
  - synagogue Y92.22
  - television station Y92.59
  - tennis court Y92.312
  - theater Y92.254
  - trade area Y92.59
    - bank Y92.510
    - cafe Y92.511
    - casino Y92.59
    - garage Y92.59
    - hotel Y92.59
    - market Y92.512
    - office building Y92.59
    - radio station Y92.59
    - restaurant Y92.511
    - shop Y92.513
    - shopping mall Y92.59
    - store Y92.512
    - supermarket Y92.512
    - television station Y92.59
    - warehouse Y92.59
  - trailer park, residential — *see* Place of occurrence, residence, mobile home
  - trailer site NOS Y92.89
  - train Y92.815
    - station Y92.522
  - truck Y92.812
  - tunnel under construction Y92.69
  - urgent (health) care center Y92.532
  - university Y92.214
  - vehicle (transport) Y92.818
    - airplane Y92.813
    - boat Y92.814
    - bus Y92.811
    - car Y92.810
    - specified NEC Y92.818
    - subway car Y92.816
    - train Y92.815
    - truck Y92.812
  - warehouse Y92.59
  - water reservoir Y92.89
  - wilderness area Y92.828
    - desert Y92.820
    - forest Y92.821
    - marsh Y92.828
    - mountain Y92.828
    - prairie Y92.828
    - specified NEC Y92.828
    - swamp Y92.828
  - workshop Y92.69
  - yard, private Y92.096
    - boarding house Y92.046
    - single family house Y92.017
    - mobile home Y92.027
  - youth center Y92.29
  - zoo (zoological garden) Y92.834
- **Plumbism** — *see* Table of Drugs and Chemicals, lead
- **Poisoning** (accidental) (by) — *see also* Table of Drugs and Chemicals
  - by plant, thorns, spines, sharp leaves or other mechanisms NEC X58
  - carbon monoxide
    - generated by
      - motor vehicle — *see* Accident, transport
      - watercraft (in transit) (not in transit) V93.89
        - ferry boat V93.81
        - fishing boat V93.82

Poisoning (accidental) (by) - *continued*
carbon monoxide - *continued*
generated by - *continued*
watercraft (in transit) (not in transit) - *continued*
jet skis V93.83
liner V93.81
merchant ship V93.80
passenger ship V93.81
powered craft NEC V93.83
caused by injection of poisons into skin by plant thorns, spines, sharp leaves X58
marine or sea plants (venomous) X58
exhaust gas
generated by
motor vehicle — *see* Accident, transport
watercraft (in transit) (not in transit) V93.89
ferry boat V93.81
fishing boat V93.82
jet skis V93.83
liner V93.81
merchant ship V93.80
passenger ship V93.81
powered craft NEC V93.83
fumes or smoke due to
explosion — *see also* Explosion W40.9
fire — *see* Exposure, fire
ignition — *see* Ignition
gas
in legal intervention — *see* Legal, intervention, gas
legal execution — *see* Legal, intervention, gas
in war operations — *see* War operations
legal
execution — *see* Legal, intervention, gas
intervention
by gas — *see* Legal, intervention, gas
other specified means — *see* Legal, intervention, specified means NEC
Powder burn (by) (from)
airgun W34.110
BB gun W34.110
firearm NEC W34.19
gas, air or spring-operated gun NEC W34.118
handgun W32.1
hunting rifle W33.12
larger firearm W33.10
specified NEC W33.19
machine gun W33.13
paintball gun W34.111
pellet gun W34.110
shotgun W33.11
Very pistol [flare] W34.19
Premature cessation (of) **surgical and medical care** Y66
Privation (food) (water) X58
Procedure (operation)
correct, on wrong side or body part (wrong side) (wrong site) Y65.53
intended for another patient done on wrong patient Y65.52
performed on patient not scheduled for surgery Y65.52
performed on wrong patient Y65.52
wrong, performed on correct patient Y65.51
Prolonged
sitting in transport vehicle — *see* Travel, by type of vehicle
stay in
high altitude as cause of anoxia, barodontalgia, barotitis or hypoxia W94.11
weightless environment X52
Pulling, excessive — *see also* Overexertion X50.9
Puncture, puncturing — *see also* Contact, with, by type of object or machine
by
plant thorns, spines, sharp leaves or other mechanisms NEC W60
during medical or surgical treatment as misadventure — *see* Index to Diseases and Injuries, Complication(s)
Pushed, pushing (accidental) (injury in)
by other person (s) (accidental) W51
with fall W03
due to ice or snow W00.0
as, or caused by, a crowd or human stampede (with fall) W52
before moving object NEC Y02.8
motor vehicle Y02.0
subway train Y02.1
train Y02.1
from
high place NEC
in accidental circumstances W17.89
stated as

Pushed, pushing (accidental) (injury in) - *continued*
by other person (s) (accidental) - *continued*
from - *continued*
high place NEC - *continued*
stated as - *continued*
intentional, homicide (attempt) Y01
undetermined whether accidental or intentional Y30
transport vehicle NEC — *see also* Accident, transport V89.9
stated as
intentional, homicide (attempt) Y08.89
overexertion X50.9

R

Radiation (exposure to)
arc lamps W89.0
atomic power plant (malfunction) NEC W88.1
complication of or abnormal reaction to medical radiotherapy Y84.2
electromagnetic, ionizing W88.0
gamma rays W88.1
in
war operations (from or following nuclear explosion) — *see* War operations
inadvertent exposure of patient (receiving test or therapy) Y63.3
infrared (heaters and lamps) W90.1
excessive heat from W92
ionized, ionizing (particles, artificially accelerated)
radioisotopes W88.1
specified NEC W88.8
x-rays W88.0
isotopes, radioactive — *see* Radiation, radioactive isotopes
laser (s) W90.2
in war operations — *see* War operations
misadventure in medical care Y63.2
light sources (man-made visible and ultraviolet) W89.9
natural X32
specified NEC W89.8
tanning bed W89.1
welding light W89.0
man-made visible light W89.9
specified NEC W89.8
tanning bed W89.1
welding light W89.0
microwave W90.8
misadventure in medical or surgical procedure Y63.2
natural NEC X39.08
radon X39.01
overdose (in medical or surgical procedure) Y63.2
radar W90.0
radioactive isotopes (any) W88.1
atomic power plant malfunction W88.1
misadventure in medical or surgical treatment Y63.2
radiofrequency W90.0
radium NEC W88.1
sun X32
ultraviolet (light) (man-made) W89.9
natural X32
specified NEC W89.8
tanning bed W89.1
welding light W89.0
welding arc, torch, or light W89.0
excessive heat from W92
x-rays (hard) (soft) W88.0
Range disease W94.11
Rape (attempted) T74.2-
Rat bite W53.11
Reaching (prolonged) (static) X50.1
Reaction, abnormal to medical procedure — *see also* Complication of or following, by type of procedure Y84.9
with misadventure — *see* Misadventure
biologicals — *see* Table of Drugs and Chemicals
drugs — *see* Table of Drugs and Chemicals
vaccine — *see* Table of Drugs and Chemicals
Recoil
airgun W34.110
BB gun W34.110
firearm NEC W34.19
gas, air or spring-operated gun NEC W34.118
handgun W32.1
hunting rifle W33.12
larger firearm W33.10
specified NEC W33.19
machine gun W33.13
paintball gun W34.111
pellet W34.110
shotgun W33.11

Recoil - *continued*
Very pistol [flare] W34.19
Reduction in
atmospheric pressure - — *see* Air, pressure, change
Rock falling on or hitting (accidentally) (person) W20.8
in cave-in W20.0
Run over (accidentally) (by)
animal (not being ridden) NEC W55.89
machinery — *see* Contact, with, by specified type of machine
transport vehicle NEC — *see also* Accident, transport V09.9
intentional homicide (attempt) Y03.0
motor NEC V09.20
intentional homicide (attempt) Y03.0
Running
before moving object X81.8
motor vehicle X81.0
Running off, away
animal (being ridden) — *see also* Accident, transport V80.918
not being ridden W55.89
animal-drawn vehicle NEC — *see also* Accident, transport V80.928
highway, road (way) , street
transport vehicle NEC — *see also* Accident, transport V89.9
Rupture pressurized devices — *see* Explosion, by type of device

S

Saturnism — *see* Table of Drugs and Chemicals, lead
Scald, scalding (accidental) (by) (from) (in) X19
air (hot) X14.1
gases (hot) X14.1
homicide (attempt) — *see* Assault, burning, hot object
inflicted by other person
stated as intentional, homicide (attempt) — *see* Assault, burning, hot object
liquid (boiling) (hot) NEC X12
stated as undetermined whether accidental or intentional Y27.2
suicide (attempt) X77.2
local application of externally applied substance in medical or surgical care Y63.5
metal (molten) (liquid) (hot) NEC X18
self-inflicted X77.9
stated as undetermined whether accidental or intentional Y27.8
steam X13.1
assault X98.0
stated as undetermined whether accidental or intentional Y27.0
suicide (attempt) X77.0
suicide (attempt) X77.9
vapor (hot) X13.1
assault X98.0
stated as undetermined whether accidental or intentional Y27.0
suicide (attempt) X77.0
Scratched by
cat W55.03
person (s) (accidentally) W50.4
with intent to injure or kill Y04.0
as, or caused by, a crowd or human stampede (with fall) W52
assault Y04.0
homicide (attempt) Y04.0
in
fight Y04.0
legal intervention
injuring
bystander Y35.892
law enforcement personnel Y35.891
suspect Y35.893
Seasickness T75.3
Self-harm NEC — *see also* External cause by type, undetermined whether accidental or intentional
intentional — *see* Suicide
poisoning NEC — *see* Table of drugs and biologicals, accident
Self-inflicted (injury) **NEC** — *see also* External cause by type, undetermined whether accidental or intentional
intentional — *see* Suicide
poisoning NEC — *see* Table of drugs and biologicals, accident
Sequelae (of)
accident NEC — *see* W00-X58 with 7th character S
assault (homicidal) (any means) — *see* X92-Y08 with 7th character S

Sequelae (of) - *continued*
- homicide, attempt (any means) — *see* X92-Y08 with 7th character S
- injury undetermined whether accidentally or purposely inflicted — *see* Y21-Y33 with 7th character S
- intentional self-harm (classifiable to X71-X83) — *see* X71-X83 with 7th character S
- legal intervention — *see* with 7th character S Y35
- motor vehicle accident — *see* V00-V99 with 7th character S
- suicide, attempt (any means) — *see* X71-X83 with 7th character S
- transport accident — *see* V00-V99 with 7th character S
- war operations — *see* War operations

Shock
- electric — *see* Exposure, electric current
- from electric appliance (any) (faulty) W86.8
  - domestic W86.0
  - suicide (attempt) X83.1

Shooting, shot (accidental (ly) **)** — *see also* Discharge, firearm, by type
- herself or himself — *see* Discharge, firearm by type, self-inflicted
- homicide (attempt) — *see* Discharge, firearm by type, homicide
- in war operations — *see* War operations
- inflicted by other person — *see* Discharge, firearm by type, homicide
  - accidental — *see* Discharge, firearm, by type of firearm
- legal
  - execution — *see* Legal, intervention, firearm
  - intervention — *see* Legal, intervention, firearm
- self-inflicted — *see* Discharge, firearm by type, suicide
  - accidental — *see* Discharge, firearm, by type of firearm
- suicide (attempt) — *see* Discharge, firearm by type, suicide

Shoving (accidentally) **by other person** — *see* Pushed, by other person

Sickness
- alpine W94.11
- motion — *see* Motion
- mountain W94.11

Sinking (accidental)
- watercraft (causing drowning, submersion) — *see also* Drowning, due to, accident to, watercraft, sinking
  - causing injury except drowning or submersion — *see* Accident, watercraft, causing, injury NEC

Siriasis X32

Sitting (prolonged) (static) X50.1

Slashed wrists — *see* Cut, self-inflicted

Slipping (accidental) (on same level) (with fall) W01.0
- on
  - ice W00.0
    - with skates — *see* Accident, transport, pedestrian, conveyance
  - mud W01.0
  - oil W01.0
  - snow W00.0
    - with skis — *see* Accident, transport, pedestrian, conveyance
  - surface (slippery) (wet) NEC W01.0
- without fall W18.40
  - due to
    - specified NEC W18.49
    - stepping from one level to another W18.43
    - stepping into hole or opening W18.42
    - stepping on object W18.41

Sliver, wood, contact with W45.8

Smoldering (due to fire) — *see* Exposure, fire

Sodomy (attempted) **by force** T74.2-

Sound waves (causing injury) W42.9
- supersonic W42.0

Splinter, contact with W45.8

Stab, stabbing — *see* Cut

Standing (prolonged) (static) X50.1

Starvation X58

Status of external cause Y99.9
- child assisting in compensated work for family Y99.8
- civilian activity done for financial or other compensation Y99.0
- civilian activity done for income or pay Y99.0
- family member assisting in compensated work for other family member Y99.8
- hobby not done for income Y99.8

Status of external cause - *continued*
- leisure activity Y99.8
- military activity Y99.1
- off-duty activity of military personnel Y99.8
- recreation or sport not for income or while a student Y99.8
- specified NEC Y99.8
- student activity Y99.8
- volunteer activity Y99.2

Stepped on
- by
  - animal (not being ridden) NEC W55.89
  - crowd or human stampede W52
  - person W50.0

Stepping on
- object W22.8
  - with fall W18.31
  - sports equipment W21.9
  - stationary W22.09
    - sports equipment W21.89
- person W51
  - by crowd or human stampede W52
- sports equipment W21.9

Sting
- arthropod, nonvenomous W57
- insect, nonvenomous W57

Storm (cataclysmic) — *see* Forces of nature, cataclysmic storm

Straining, excessive — *see also* Overexertion X50.9

Strangling — *see* Strangulation

Strangulation (accidental) — *see* category T71

Strenuous movements — *see also* Overexertion X50.9

Striking against
- airbag (automobile) W22.10
  - driver side W22.11
  - front passenger side W22.12
  - specified NEC W22.19
- bottom when
  - diving or jumping into water (in) W16.822
    - causing drowning W16.821
    - from boat W16.722
      - causing drowning W16.721
    - natural body W16.622
      - causing drowning W16.821
    - swimming pool W16.522
      - causing drowning W16.521
  - falling into water (in) W16.322
    - causing drowning W16.321
    - fountain — *see* Striking against, bottom when, falling into water, specified NEC
    - natural body W16.122
      - causing drowning W16.121
    - reservoir — *see* Striking against, bottom when, falling into water, specified NEC
    - specified NEC W16.322
      - causing drowning W16.321
    - swimming pool W16.022
      - causing drowning W16.021
- diving board (swimming-pool) W21.4
- object W22.8
  - with
    - drowning or submersion — *see* Drowning
    - fall — *see* Fall, due to, bumping against, object
  - caused by crowd or human stampede (with fall) W52
  - furniture W22.03
  - lamppost W22.02
  - sports equipment W21.9
  - stationary W22.09
    - sports equipment W21.89
  - wall W22.01
- person (s) W51
  - with fall W03
    - due to ice or snow W00.0
  - as, or caused by, a crowd or human stampede (with fall) W52
  - assault Y04.2
  - homicide (attempt) Y04.2
- sports equipment W21.9
- wall (when) W22.01
  - diving or jumping into water (in) W16.832
    - causing drowning W16.831
    - swimming pool W16.532
      - causing drowning W16.531
  - falling into water (in) W16.332
    - causing drowning W16.331
    - fountain — *see* Striking against, wall when, falling into water, specified NEC
    - natural body W16.132
      - causing drowning W16.131
    - reservoir — *see* Striking against, wall when, falling into water, specified NEC

Striking against - *continued*
- wall (when) - *continued*
  - falling into water (in) - *continued*
    - specified NEC W16.332
      - causing drowning W16.331
    - swimming pool W16.032
      - causing drowning W16.031
  - swimming pool (when) W22.042
    - causing drowning W22.041
    - diving or jumping into water W16.532
      - causing drowning W16.531
    - falling into water W16.032
      - causing drowning W16.031

Struck (accidentally) **by**
- airbag (automobile) W22.10
  - driver side W22.11
  - front passenger side W22.12
  - specified NEC W22.19
- alligator W58.02
- animal (not being ridden) NEC W55.89
- avalanche — *see* Landslide
- ball (hit) (thrown) W21.00
  - assault Y08.09
  - baseball W21.03
  - basketball W21.05
  - golf ball W21.04
  - football W21.01
  - soccer W21.02
  - softball W21.07
  - specified NEC W21.09
  - volleyball W21.06
- bat or racquet
  - baseball bat W21.11
    - assault Y08.02
  - golf club W21.13
    - assault Y08.09
  - specified NEC W21.19
    - assault Y08.09
  - tennis racquet W21.12
    - assault Y08.09
- bullet — *see also* Discharge, firearm by type
  - in war operations — *see* War operations
- crocodile W58.12
- dog W54.1
- flare, Very pistol — *see* Discharge, firearm NEC
- hailstones X39.8
- hockey (ice)
  - field
    - puck W21.221
    - stick W21.211
  - puck W21.220
  - stick W21.210
    - assault Y08.01
- landslide — *see* Landslide
- law-enforcement agent (on duty) — *see* Legal, intervention, manhandling
  - with blunt object — *see* Legal, intervention, blunt object
- lightning — *see* subcategory T75.0
  - causing fire — *see* Exposure, fire
- machine — *see* Contact, with, by type of machine
- mammal NEC W55.89
  - marine W56.32
- marine animal W56.82
- missile
  - firearm — *see* Discharge, firearm by type
  - in war operations — *see* War operations, missile
- object W22.8
  - blunt W22.8
    - assault Y00
    - suicide (attempt) X79
    - undetermined whether accidental or intentional Y29
  - falling W20.8
    - from, in, on
      - building W20.1
        - burning (uncontrolled fire) X00.4
      - cataclysmic
        - earth surface movement NEC — *see* Landslide
        - storm — *see* Forces of nature, cataclysmic storm
      - cave-in W20.0
      - earthquake X34
      - machine (in operation) — *see* Contact, with, by type of machine
      - structure W20.1
        - burning X00.4
      - transport vehicle (in motion) — *see* Accident, transport, by type of vehicle
      - watercraft V93.49
        - due to
          - accident to craft V91.39
            - powered craft V91.33

CHAPTER 1: CERTAIN INFECTIOUS AND PARASITIC DISEASES (A00-B99)

INCLUDES diseases generally recognized as communicable or transmissible

Use additional code to identify resistance to antimicrobial drugs (Z16.-)

EXCLUDES 1 *certain localized infections - see body system-related chapters*

EXCLUDES 2 *carrier or suspected carrier of infectious disease (Z22.-)*
infectious and parasitic diseases complicating pregnancy, childbirth and the puerperium (O98.-)
infectious and parasitic diseases specific to the perinatal period (P35-P39)
influenza and other acute respiratory infections (J00-J22)

This chapter contains the following blocks:

A00-A09	Intestinal infectious diseases
A15-A19	Tuberculosis
A20-A28	Certain zoonotic bacterial diseases
A30-A49	Other bacterial diseases
A50-A64	Infections with a predominantly sexual mode of transmission
A65-A69	Other spirochetal diseases
A70-A74	Other diseases caused by chlamydiae
A75-A79	Rickettsioses
A80-A89	Viral and prion infections of the central nervous system
A90-A99	Arthropod-borne viral fevers and viral hemorrhagic fevers
B00-B09	Viral infections characterized by skin and mucous membrane lesions
B10	Other human herpesviruses
B15-B19	Viral hepatitis
B20	Human immunodeficiency virus [HIV] disease
B25-B34	Other viral diseases
B35-B49	Mycoses
B50-B64	Protozoal diseases
B65-B83	Helminthiases
B85-B89	Pediculosis, acariasis and other infestations
B90-B94	Sequelae of infectious and parasitic diseases
B95-B97	Bacterial and viral infectious agents
B99	Other infectious diseases

Intestinal infectious diseases (A00-A09)

4 **A00 Cholera**
- **A00.0 Cholera due to Vibrio cholerae 01, biovar cholerae**
  Classical cholera
- **A00.1 Cholera due to Vibrio cholerae 01, biovar eltor**
  Cholera eltor
- **A00.9 Cholera, unspecified**

4 **A01 Typhoid and paratyphoid fevers**
- 5 **A01.0 Typhoid fever**
  Infection due to Salmonella typhi
  - **A01.00 Typhoid fever, unspecified**
  - **A01.01 Typhoid meningitis**
  - **A01.02 Typhoid fever with heart involvement**
    Typhoid endocarditis
    Typhoid myocarditis
  - **A01.03 Typhoid pneumonia** HCC
  - **A01.04 Typhoid arthritis** HCC
  - **A01.05 Typhoid osteomyelitis** HCC
  - **A01.09 Typhoid fever with other complications**
- **A01.1 Paratyphoid fever A**
- **A01.2 Paratyphoid fever B**
- **A01.3 Paratyphoid fever C**
- **A01.4 Paratyphoid fever, unspecified**
  Infection due to Salmonella paratyphi NOS

4 **A02 Other salmonella infections**

INCLUDES infection or foodborne intoxication due to any Salmonella species other than S. typhi and S. paratyphi

- **A02.0 Salmonella enteritis**
  Salmonellosis
- **A02.1 Salmonella sepsis** HCC HIV
- 5 **A02.2 Localized salmonella infections**
  - **A02.20 Localized salmonella infection, unspecified** HIV
  - **A02.21 Salmonella meningitis** HIV
  - **A02.22 Salmonella pneumonia** HCC HIV
  - **A02.23 Salmonella arthritis** HCC HIV

    CODING TIP✓ Salmonella arthritis is a reactive arthritis. Code A02.23 indicates the arthritis and its cause. Do not assign an additional code for arthritis.
  - **A02.24 Salmonella osteomyelitis** HCC HIV
  - **A02.25 Salmonella pyelonephritis** HIV
    Salmonella tubulo-interstitial nephropathy
  - **A02.29 Salmonella with other localized infection** HIV
- **A02.8 Other specified salmonella infections** HIV
- **A02.9 Salmonella infection, unspecified** HIV

4 **A03 Shigellosis**
- **A03.0 Shigellosis due to Shigella dysenteriae**
  Group A shigellosis [Shiga-Kruse dysentery]
- **A03.1 Shigellosis due to Shigella flexneri**
  Group B shigellosis
- **A03.2 Shigellosis due to Shigella boydii**
  Group C shigellosis
- **A03.3 Shigellosis due to Shigella sonnei**
  Group D shigellosis
- **A03.8 Other shigellosis**
- **A03.9 Shigellosis, unspecified**
  Bacillary dysentery NOS

4 **A04 Other bacterial intestinal infections**

EXCLUDES 1 *bacterial foodborne intoxications, NEC (A05.-)*
tuberculous enteritis (A18.32)

- **A04.0 Enteropathogenic Escherichia coli infection**
- **A04.1 Enterotoxigenic Escherichia coli infection**
- **A04.2 Enteroinvasive Escherichia coli infection**
- **A04.3 Enterohemorrhagic Escherichia coli infection**
- **A04.4 Other intestinal Escherichia coli infections**
  Escherichia coli enteritis NOS
- **A04.5 Campylobacter enteritis**
- **A04.6 Enteritis due to Yersinia enterocolitica**

  EXCLUDES 1 *extraintestinal yersiniosis (A28.2)*

  CODING TIP✓ Arthropathy associated with Yersinia requires an additional code from M02.-.
- 5 **A04.7 Enterocolitis due to Clostridium difficile**
  Foodborne intoxication by Clostridium difficile
  Pseudomembraneous colitis
  - **A04.71 Enterocolitis due to Clostridium difficile, recurrent**

    CODING TIP✓ Recurrence is defined by complete abatement of CDI symptoms while on appropriate therapy, followed by subsequent reappearance of diarrhea and other symptoms after treatment has been stopped. Recurrence typically occurs within one week after treatment cessation, however recurrence may occur up to 8 weeks later.
    AHA: 4Q 2017, 4
  - **A04.72 Enterocolitis due to Clostridium difficile, not specified as recurrent**

    CODING TIP✓ A04.72 is the default code for C. difficile enteritis. Use this code when there is no documentation of recurrence.
    AHA. 4Q 2017, 4
- **A04.8 Other specified bacterial intestinal infections**
- **A04.9 Bacterial intestinal infection, unspecified**
  Bacterial enteritis NOS

4 **A05 Other bacterial foodborne intoxications, not elsewhere classified**

EXCLUDES 1 *Clostridium difficile foodborne intoxication and infection (A04.7-)*
Escherichia coli infection (A04.0-A04.4)
listeriosis (A32.-)
salmonella foodborne intoxication and infection (A02.-)
toxic effect of noxious foodstuffs (T61-T62)

- **A05.0 Foodborne staphylococcal intoxication**

A05.1 **Botulism food poisoning**
Botulism NOS
Classical foodborne intoxication due to Clostridium botulinum
EXCLUDES 1 *infant botulism (A48.51)*
wound botulism (A48.52)

DEFINITION Muscle-paralyzing disease caused by ingesting the neurotoxins produced by the bacteria Clostridium botulinum.

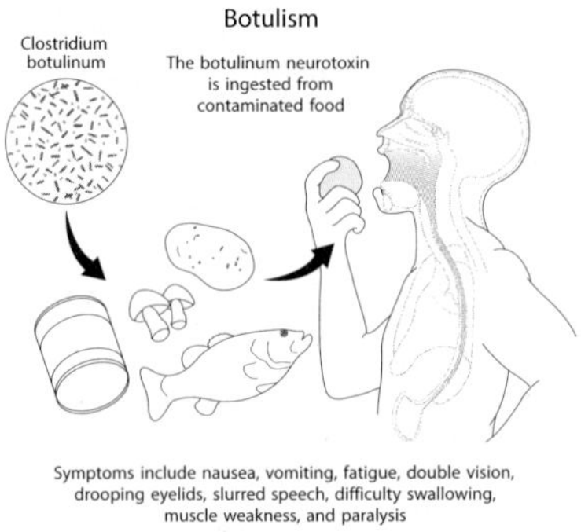
Botulism
Clostridium botulinum
The botulinum neurotoxin is ingested from contaminated food
Symptoms include nausea, vomiting, fatigue, double vision, drooping eyelids, slurred speech, difficulty swallowing, muscle weakness, and paralysis

A05.2 **Foodborne Clostridium perfringens [Clostridium welchii] intoxication**
Enteritis necroticans
Pig-bel
A05.3 **Foodborne Vibrio parahaemolyticus intoxication**
A05.4 **Foodborne Bacillus cereus intoxication**
A05.5 **Foodborne Vibrio vulnificus intoxication**
A05.8 **Other specified bacterial foodborne intoxications**
A05.9 **Bacterial foodborne intoxication, unspecified**

4 **A06** **Amebiasis**
INCLUDES infection due to Entamoeba histolytica
EXCLUDES 1 *other protozoal intestinal diseases (A07.-)*
EXCLUDES 2 *acanthamebiasis (B60.1-)*
Naegleriasis (B60.2)

A06.0 **Acute amebic dysentery**
Acute amebiasis
Intestinal amebiasis NOS
A06.1 **Chronic intestinal amebiasis**
A06.2 **Amebic nondysenteric colitis**
A06.3 **Ameboma of intestine**
Ameboma NOS
A06.4 **Amebic liver abscess**
Hepatic amebiasis
A06.5 **Amebic lung abscess** HCC
Amebic abscess of lung (and liver)
A06.6 **Amebic brain abscess**
Amebic abscess of brain (and liver) (and lung)
A06.7 **Cutaneous amebiasis**
5 **A06.8** **Amebic infection of other sites**
A06.81 **Amebic cystitis**
A06.82 **Other amebic genitourinary infections**
Amebic balanitis
Amebic vesiculitis
Amebic vulvovaginitis
A06.89 **Other amebic infections**
Amebic appendicitis
Amebic splenic abscess
A06.9 **Amebiasis, unspecified**

4 **A07** **Other protozoal intestinal diseases**
A07.0 **Balantidiasis**
Balantidial dysentery
A07.1 **Giardiasis [lambliasis]**

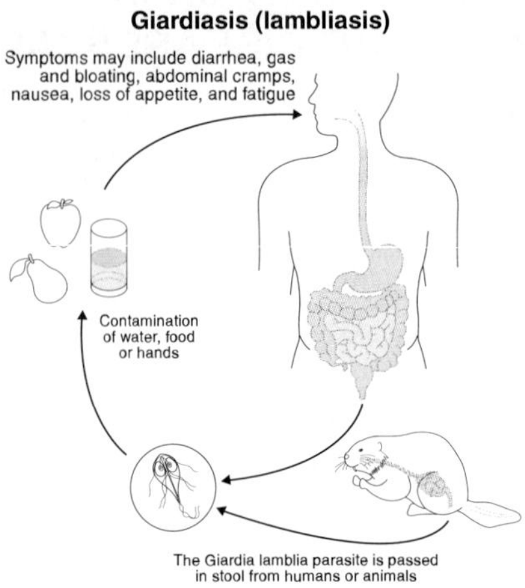
Giardiasis (lambliasis)
Symptoms may include diarrhea, gas and bloating, abdominal cramps, nausea, loss of appetite, and fatigue
Contamination of water, food or hands
The Giardia lamblia parasite is passed in stool from humans or animals

A07.2 **Cryptosporidiosis** HCC
A07.3 **Isosporiasis** HIV
Infection due to Isospora belli and Isospora hominis
Intestinal coccidiosis
Isosporosis
A07.4 **Cyclosporiasis**
A07.8 **Other specified protozoal intestinal diseases**
Intestinal microsporidiosis
Intestinal trichomoniasis
Sarcocystosis
Sarcosporidiosis
A07.9 **Protozoal intestinal disease, unspecified**
Flagellate diarrhea
Protozoal colitis
Protozoal diarrhea
Protozoal dysentery

4 **A08** **Viral and other specified intestinal infections**
EXCLUDES 1 *influenza with involvement of gastrointestinal tract (J09.X3, J10.2, J11.2)*

A08.0 **Rotaviral enteritis**
5 **A08.1** **Acute gastroenteropathy due to Norwalk agent and other small round viruses**
A08.11 **Acute gastroenteropathy due to Norwalk agent**
Acute gastroenteropathy due to Norovirus
Acute gastroenteropathy due to Norwalk-like agent
A08.19 **Acute gastroenteropathy due to other small round viruses**
Acute gastroenteropathy due to small round virus [SRV] NOS
A08.2 **Adenoviral enteritis**
5 **A08.3** **Other viral enteritis**
A08.31 **Calicivirus enteritis**
A08.32 **Astrovirus enteritis**
A08.39 **Other viral enteritis**
Coxsackie virus enteritis
Echovirus enteritis
Enterovirus enteritis NEC
Torovirus enteritis
A08.4 **Viral intestinal infection, unspecified**
Viral enteritis NOS
Viral gastroenteritis NOS
Viral gastroenteropathy NOS
AHA: 3Q 2016, 8
AHA: 3Q 2016, 12
A08.8 **Other specified intestinal infections**

A09 **Infectious gastroenteritis and colitis, unspecified**
Infectious colitis NOS
Infectious enteritis NOS
Infectious gastroenteritis NOS
EXCLUDES 1 *colitis NOS (K52.9)*
diarrhea NOS (R19.7)
enteritis NOS (K52.9)
gastroenteritis NOS (K52.9)
noninfective gastroenteritis and colitis, unspecified (K52.9)

Tuberculosis (A15-A19)

INCLUDES infections due to Mycobacterium tuberculosis and Mycobacterium bovis

EXCLUDES 1 *congenital tuberculosis (P37.0)*
nonspecific reaction to test for tuberculosis without active tuberculosis (R76.1-)
pneumoconiosis associated with tuberculosis, any type in A15 (J65)
positive PPD (R76.11)
positive tuberculin skin test without active tuberculosis (R76.11)
sequelae of tuberculosis (B90.-)
silicotuberculosis (J65)

CODING TIP ✓ Codes from A15-A19 should not be assigned to report a positive PPD (Mantoux) test. A positive PPD (Mantoux) skin test without active tuberculosis should be coded to R76.11.

4 A15 Respiratory tuberculosis

A15.0 Tuberculosis of lung HIV
Tuberculous bronchiectasis
Tuberculous fibrosis of lung
Tuberculous pneumonia
Tuberculous pneumothorax

A15.4 Tuberculosis of intrathoracic lymph nodes HIV
Tuberculosis of hilar lymph nodes
Tuberculosis of mediastinal lymph nodes
Tuberculosis of tracheobronchial lymph nodes
EXCLUDES 1 *tuberculosis specified as primary (A15.7)*

A15.5 Tuberculosis of larynx, trachea and bronchus HIV
Tuberculosis of bronchus
Tuberculosis of glottis
Tuberculosis of larynx
Tuberculosis of trachea

A15.6 Tuberculous pleurisy HIV
Tuberculosis of pleura Tuberculous empyema
EXCLUDES 1 *primary respiratory tuberculosis (A15.7)*

A15.7 Primary respiratory tuberculosis HIV

A15.8 Other respiratory tuberculosis HIV
Mediastinal tuberculosis
Nasopharyngeal tuberculosis
Tuberculosis of nose
Tuberculosis of sinus [any nasal]

A15.9 Respiratory tuberculosis unspecified HIV

4 A17 Tuberculosis of nervous system

A17.0 Tuberculous meningitis HIV
Tuberculosis of meninges (cerebral)(spinal)
Tuberculous leptomeningitis
EXCLUDES 1 *tuberculous meningoencephalitis (A17.82)*

A17.1 Meningeal tuberculoma HIV
Tuberculoma of meninges (cerebral) (spinal)
EXCLUDES 2 *tuberculoma of brain and spinal cord (A17.81)*

5 A17.8 Other tuberculosis of nervous system

A17.81 Tuberculoma of brain and spinal cord HIV
Tuberculous abscess of brain and spinal cord

A17.82 Tuberculous meningoencephalitis HIV
Tuberculous myelitis

A17.83 Tuberculous neuritis HIV
Tuberculous mononeuropathy

A17.89 Other tuberculosis of nervous system HIV
Tuberculous polyneuropathy

A17.9 Tuberculosis of nervous system, unspecified HIV

4 A18 Tuberculosis of other organs

5 A18.0 Tuberculosis of bones and joints

A18.01 Tuberculosis of spine HIV
Pott's disease or curvature of spine
Tuberculous arthritis
Tuberculous osteomyelitis of spine
Tuberculous spondylitis

A18.02 Tuberculous arthritis of other joints HIV
Tuberculosis of hip (joint)
Tuberculosis of knee (joint)

A18.03 Tuberculosis of other bones HIV
Tuberculous mastoiditis
Tuberculous osteomyelitis

A18.09 Other musculoskeletal tuberculosis HIV
Tuberculous myositis
Tuberculous synovitis
Tuberculous tenosynovitis

5 A18.1 Tuberculosis of genitourinary system

A18.10 Tuberculosis of genitourinary system, unspecified HIV

A18.11 Tuberculosis of kidney and ureter HIV

A18.12 Tuberculosis of bladder HIV

A18.13 Tuberculosis of other urinary organs HIV
Tuberculous urethritis

A18.14 Tuberculosis of prostate ♂ A HIV

A18.15 Tuberculosis of other male genital organs ♂ HIV

A18.16 Tuberculosis of cervix ♀ HIV

A18.17 Tuberculous female pelvic inflammatory disease ♀ HIV
Tuberculous endometritis
Tuberculous oophoritis and salpingitis

A18.18 Tuberculosis of other female genital organs ♀ HIV
Tuberculous ulceration of vulva

A18.2 Tuberculous peripheral lymphadenopathy HIV
Tuberculous adenitis
EXCLUDES 2 *tuberculosis of bronchial and mediastinal lymph nodes (A15.4)*
tuberculosis of mesenteric and retroperitoneal lymph nodes (A18.39)
tuberculous tracheobronchial adenopathy (A15.4)

5 A18.3 Tuberculosis of intestines, peritoneum and mesenteric glands

A18.31 Tuberculous peritonitis HIV
Tuberculous ascites

A18.32 Tuberculous enteritis HIV
Tuberculosis of anus and rectum
Tuberculosis of intestine (large) (small)

A18.39 Retroperitoneal tuberculosis HIV
Tuberculosis of mesenteric glands
Tuberculosis of retroperitoneal (lymph glands)

A18.4 Tuberculosis of skin and subcutaneous tissue HIV
Erythema induratum, tuberculous
Lupus excedens
Lupus vulgaris NOS
Lupus vulgaris of eyelid
Scrofuloderma
Tuberculosis of external ear
EXCLUDES 2 *lupus erythematosus (L93.-)*
lupus NOS (M32.9)
systemic (M32.-)

5 A18.5 Tuberculosis of eye
EXCLUDES 2 *lupus vulgaris of eyelid (A18.4)*

A18.50 Tuberculosis of eye, unspecified HIV

A18.51 Tuberculous episcleritis HIV

A18.52 Tuberculous keratitis HIV
Tuberculous interstitial keratitis
Tuberculous keratoconjunctivitis (interstitial) (phlyctenular)

A18.53 Tuberculous chorioretinitis HIV

A18.54 Tuberculous iridocyclitis HIV

A18.59 Other tuberculosis of eye HIV
Tuberculous conjunctivitis

A18.6 Tuberculosis of (inner) (middle) ear HIV
Tuberculous otitis media
EXCLUDES 2 *tuberculosis of external ear (A18.4)*
tuberculous mastoiditis (A18.03)

A18.7 Tuberculosis of adrenal glands HIV
Tuberculous Addison's disease

5 A18.8 Tuberculosis of other specified organs

A18.81 Tuberculosis of thyroid gland HIV

A18.82 Tuberculosis of other endocrine glands HIV
Tuberculosis of pituitary gland
Tuberculosis of thymus gland

A18.83 Tuberculosis of digestive tract organs, not elsewhere classified HIV
EXCLUDES 1 *tuberculosis of intestine (A18.32)*

A18.84 **Tuberculosis of heart** HIV
Tuberculous cardiomyopathy
Tuberculous endocarditis
Tuberculous myocarditis
Tuberculous pericarditis
A18.85 **Tuberculosis of spleen** HIV
A18.89 **Tuberculosis of other sites** HIV
Tuberculosis of muscle
Tuberculous cerebral arteritis

A19 Miliary tuberculosis
INCLUDES disseminated tuberculosis
generalized tuberculosis
tuberculous polyserositis
A19.0 **Acute miliary tuberculosis of a single specified site** HIV
A19.1 **Acute miliary tuberculosis of multiple sites** HIV
A19.2 **Acute miliary tuberculosis, unspecified** HIV
A19.8 **Other miliary tuberculosis** HIV
A19.9 **Miliary tuberculosis, unspecified** HIV

Certain zoonotic bacterial diseases (A20-A28)

A20 Plague
INCLUDES infection due to Yersinia pestis
A20.0 **Bubonic plague**
DEFINITION Infection with the Yersinia pestis bacillus, transmitted via flea, tick, and lice bites and by contact with infected persons or materials, causing severe inflammation and death of skin cells.
A20.1 **Cellulocutaneous plague**
A20.2 **Pneumonic plague** HCC
DEFINITION Rapidly progressive, often fatal plague pneumonia caused by direct inhalation of bacteria with severe cough producing frothy, bloody, mucoid sputum.
A20.3 **Plague meningitis**
A20.7 **Septicemic plague** HCC
DEFINITION High-density bloodstream infection in acute bubonic plague; may cause death before the appearance of buboes or pulmonary manifestations.
A20.8 **Other forms of plague**
Abortive plague
Asymptomatic plague
Pestis minor
A20.9 **Plague, unspecified**

A21 Tularemia
INCLUDES deer-fly fever
infection due to Francisella tularensis
rabbit fever
A21.0 **Ulceroglandular tularemia**
A21.1 **Oculoglandular tularemia**
Ophthalmic tularemia
A21.2 **Pulmonary tularemia** HCC
A21.3 **Gastrointestinal tularemia**
Abdominal tularemia
A21.7 **Generalized tularemia**
A21.8 **Other forms of tularemia**
A21.9 **Tularemia, unspecified**

A22 Anthrax
INCLUDES infection due to Bacillus anthracis
A22.0 **Cutaneous anthrax**
Malignant carbuncle
Malignant pustule
A22.1 **Pulmonary anthrax** HCC
Inhalation anthrax
Ragpicker's disease
Woolsorter's disease
A22.2 **Gastrointestinal anthrax**
A22.7 **Anthrax sepsis** HCC
A22.8 **Other forms of anthrax**
Anthrax meningitis
A22.9 **Anthrax, unspecified**

A23 Brucellosis
INCLUDES Malta fever
Mediterranean fever
undulant fever
A23.0 **Brucellosis due to Brucella melitensis**
A23.1 **Brucellosis due to Brucella abortus**
A23.2 **Brucellosis due to Brucella suis**
A23.3 **Brucellosis due to Brucella canis**
A23.8 **Other brucellosis**
A23.9 **Brucellosis, unspecified**

A24 Glanders and melioidosis
A24.0 **Glanders**
Infection due to Pseudomonas mallei
Malleus
A24.1 **Acute and fulminating melioidosis**
Melioidosis pneumonia
Melioidosis sepsis
A24.2 **Subacute and chronic melioidosis**
A24.3 **Other melioidosis**
A24.9 **Melioidosis, unspecified**
Infection due to Pseudomonas pseudomallei NOS
Whitmore's disease

A25 Rat-bite fevers
A25.0 **Spirillosis**
Sodoku
A25.1 **Streptobacillosis**
Epidemic arthritic erythema
Haverhill fever
Streptobacillary rat-bite fever
A25.9 **Rat-bite fever, unspecified**

A26 Erysipeloid
A26.0 **Cutaneous erysipeloid**
Erythema migrans
A26.7 **Erysipelothrix sepsis** HCC
A26.8 **Other forms of erysipeloid**
A26.9 **Erysipeloid, unspecified**

A27 Leptospirosis
A27.0 **Leptospirosis icterohemorrhagica**
Leptospiral or spirochetal jaundice (hemorrhagic)
Weil's disease
A27.8 **Other forms of leptospirosis**
A27.81 **Aseptic meningitis in leptospirosis**
A27.89 **Other forms of leptospirosis**
A27.9 **Leptospirosis, unspecified**

A28 Other zoonotic bacterial diseases, not elsewhere classified
A28.0 **Pasteurellosis**
A28.1 **Cat-scratch disease**
Cat-scratch fever
A28.2 **Extraintestinal yersiniosis**
EXCLUDES 1 *enteritis due to Yersinia enterocolitica (A04.6)*
plague (A20.-)
A28.8 **Other specified zoonotic bacterial diseases, not elsewhere classified**
A28.9 **Zoonotic bacterial disease, unspecified**

Other bacterial diseases (A30-A49)

A30 Leprosy [Hansen's disease]
INCLUDES infection due to Mycobacterium leprae
EXCLUDES 1 *sequelae of leprosy (B92)*
CODING TIP ✓ Arthropathy associated with leprosy requires an additional code from M01.-.
A30.0 **Indeterminate leprosy**
I leprosy
A30.1 **Tuberculoid leprosy**
TT leprosy
A30.2 **Borderline tuberculoid leprosy**
BT leprosy
A30.3 **Borderline leprosy**
BB leprosy
A30.4 **Borderline lepromatous leprosy**
BL leprosy
A30.5 **Lepromatous leprosy**
LL leprosy
A30.8 **Other forms of leprosy**
A30.9 **Leprosy, unspecified**

A31 Infection due to other mycobacteria

EXCLUDES 2 *leprosy (A30.-)*
tuberculosis (A15-A19)

A31.0 Pulmonary mycobacterial infection HCC
Infection due to Mycobacterium avium
Infection due to Mycobacterium intracellulare [Battey bacillus]
Infection due to Mycobacterium kansasii

A31.1 Cutaneous mycobacterial infection
Buruli ulcer
Infection due to Mycobacterium marinum
Infection due to Mycobacterium ulcerans

A31.2 Disseminated mycobacterium avium-intracellulare complex (DMAC) HCC HIV
MAC sepsis

A31.8 Other mycobacterial infections HIV

A31.9 Mycobacterial infection, unspecified HIV
Atypical mycobacterial infection NOS
Mycobacteriosis NOS

A32 Listeriosis

INCLUDES listerial foodborne infection

EXCLUDES 1 *neonatal (disseminated) listeriosis (P37.2)*

A32.0 Cutaneous listeriosis

A32.1 Listerial meningitis and meningoencephalitis

A32.11 Listerial meningitis

A32.12 Listerial meningoencephalitis

A32.7 Listerial sepsis HCC

A32.8 Other forms of listeriosis

A32.81 Oculoglandular listeriosis

A32.82 Listerial endocarditis

A32.89 Other forms of listeriosis
Listerial cerebral arteritis

A32.9 Listeriosis, unspecified

A33 Tetanus neonatorum N

A34 Obstetrical tetanus ♀ M

A35 Other tetanus
Tetanus NOS

EXCLUDES 1 *obstetrical tetanus (A34)*
tetanus neonatorum (A33)

DEFINITION Potentially fatal disease due to the neurotoxin of Clostridium tetani, entering the body through contaminated wound, burn, or ulcer; causes muscular contractions, hyperreflexia, lockjaw, respiratory spasm, seizures, and paralysis.

A36 Diphtheria

A36.0 Pharyngeal diphtheria
Diphtheritic membranous angina
Tonsillar diphtheria

DEFINITION An acute infectious disease usually confined to the upper respiratory tract, caused by toxigenic strains of Corynebacterium diphtheriae, and acquired by contact with an infected person or carrier of the disease.

A36.1 Nasopharyngeal diphtheria

A36.2 Laryngeal diphtheria
Diphtheritic laryngotracheitis

A36.3 Cutaneous diphtheria

EXCLUDES 2 *erythrasma (L08.1)*

A36.8 Other diphtheria

A36.81 Diphtheritic cardiomyopathy HCC
Diphtheritic myocarditis

A36.82 Diphtheritic radiculomyelitis

A36.83 Diphtheritic polyneuritis

A36.84 Diphtheritic tubulo-interstitial nephropathy

A36.85 Diphtheritic cystitis

A36.86 Diphtheritic conjunctivitis

A36.89 Other diphtheritic complications
Diphtheritic peritonitis

A36.9 Diphtheria, unspecified

A37 Whooping cough

A37.0 Whooping cough due to Bordetella pertussis

DEFINITION Infectious disease caused by Bordetella pertussis, marked by inflammation of mucous membranes and cough, ending in a prolonged crowing or whooping respiration.

A37.00 Whooping cough due to Bordetella pertussis without pneumonia

A37.01 Whooping cough due to Bordetella pertussis with pneumonia

A37.1 Whooping cough due to Bordetella parapertussis

A37.10 Whooping cough due to Bordetella parapertussis without pneumonia

A37.11 Whooping cough due to Bordetella parapertussis with pneumonia

A37.8 Whooping cough due to other Bordetella species

A37.80 Whooping cough due to other Bordetella species without pneumonia

A37.81 Whooping cough due to other Bordetella species with pneumonia

A37.9 Whooping cough, unspecified species

A37.90 Whooping cough, unspecified species without pneumonia

A37.91 Whooping cough, unspecified species with pneumonia

A38 Scarlet fever

INCLUDES scarlatina

EXCLUDES 2 *streptococcal sore throat (J02.0)*

A38.0 Scarlet fever with otitis media

DEFINITION Infection with group A beta-hemolytic streptococcal bacteria causing sore throat, fever, and rough, bright red "sandpaper" rash over most of the body.

A38.1 Scarlet fever with myocarditis

A38.8 Scarlet fever with other complications

A38.9 Scarlet fever, uncomplicated
Scarlet fever, NOS

A39 Meningococcal infection

A39.0 Meningococcal meningitis

DEFINITION Inflammation of the membranes (meninges) around the brain or spinal cord causing fever, headache, stiff neck, muscle aches, and skin rashes.

A39.1 Waterhouse-Friderichsen syndrome HCC
Meningococcal hemorrhagic adrenalitis
Meningococcic adrenal syndrome

DEFINITION Syndrome associated with meningococcal meningitis, marked by sudden fever, purple skin discoloration, and hemorrhage into the adrenal glands with cardiovascular collapse.

A39.2 Acute meningococcemia HCC

A39.3 Chronic meningococcemia HCC

A39.4 Meningococcemia, unspecified HCC

A39.5 Meningococcal heart disease

A39.50 Meningococcal carditis, unspecified

A39.51 Meningococcal endocarditis

A39.52 Meningococcal myocarditis

A39.53 Meningococcal pericarditis

A39.8 Other meningococcal infections

A39.81 Meningococcal encephalitis

A39.82 Meningococcal retrobulbar neuritis

A39.83 Meningococcal arthritis HCC

A39.84 Postmeningococcal arthritis HCC

A39.89 Other meningococcal infections
Meningococcal conjunctivitis

A39.9 Meningococcal infection, unspecified
Meningococcal disease NOS

A40 Streptococcal sepsis

Code first:
postprocedural streptococcal sepsis (T81.4-)
streptococcal sepsis during labor (O75.3)
streptococcal sepsis following abortion or ectopic or molar pregnancy (O03-O07, O08.0)
streptococcal sepsis following immunization (T88.0)
streptococcal sepsis following infusion, transfusion or therapeutic injection (T80.2-)

EXCLUDES 1 *neonatal (P36.0-P36.1)*
puerperal sepsis (O85)
sepsis due to Streptococcus, group D (A41.81)

GUIDELINES **Section I.C.1.d.1)(a)(i-iii)**
Negative or inconclusive blood cultures do not preclude a diagnosis of sepsis in patients with clinical evidence of the condition, however, the provider should be queried.

The term urosepsis is a nonspecific term. It is not to be considered synonymous with sepsis. It has no default code in the Alphabetic Index. Should a provider use this term, he/she must be queried for clarification.

If a patient has sepsis and associated acute organ dysfunction or multiple organ dysfunction (MOD), follow the instructions for coding severe sepsis.

GUIDELINES **Section I.C.1.d.1)(a)(iv)**
If a patient has sepsis and an acute organ dysfunction, but the medical record documentation indicates that the acute organ dysfunction is related to a medical condition other than the sepsis, do not assign a code from subcategory R65.2, Severe sepsis. An acute organ dysfunction must be associated with the sepsis in order to assign the severe sepsis code. If the documentation is not clear as to whether an acute organ dysfunction is related to the sepsis or another medical condition, query the provider.

GUIDELINES **Section I.C.15.k**
Code O85, Puerperal sepsis, should be assigned with a secondary code to identify the causal organism (e.g., for a bacterial infection, assign a code from category B95-B96, Bacterial infections in conditions classified elsewhere). A code from category A40, Streptococcal sepsis, or A41, Other sepsis, should not be used for puerperal sepsis. If applicable, use additional codes to identify severe sepsis (R65.2-) and any associated acute organ dysfunction.

CODING TIP✓ When sepsis is present with a localized infection, such as UTI or pneumonia, sequence the sepsis and then the localized infection. The causative organism may be identified in the sepsis code, and therefore doesn't need to be repeated with the localized infection, except in the case of combination codes that identify the organism. Use the combination code for the pneumonia, if the localized infection is pneumonia.

CODING TIP✓ Do not assign a code from A40-A41 to indicate a bacterial infection in conditions classified elsewhere, e.g., a localized infection. Codes classified in A40-A41 are used to indicate systemic infection.

A40.0 **Sepsis due to streptococcus, group A** HCC

A40.1 **Sepsis due to streptococcus, group B** HCC

A40.3 **Sepsis due to Streptococcus pneumoniae** HCC
Pneumococcal sepsis

A40.8 **Other streptococcal sepsis** HCC

A40.9 **Streptococcal sepsis, unspecified** HCC HIV

4 **A41** **Other sepsis**
Code first:
- postprocedural sepsis (T81.4-)
- sepsis during labor (O75.3)
- sepsis following abortion, ectopic or molar pregnancy (O03-O07, O08.0)
- sepsis following immunization (T88.0)
- sepsis following infusion, transfusion or therapeutic injection (T80.2-)

EXCLUDES 1
bacteremia NOS (R78.81)
neonatal (P36.-)
puerperal sepsis (O85)
streptococcal sepsis (A40.-)

EXCLUDES 2
sepsis (due to) (in) actinomycotic (A42.7)
sepsis (due to) (in) anthrax (A22.7)
sepsis (due to) (in) candidal (B37.7)
sepsis (due to) (in) Erysipelothrix (A26.7)
sepsis (due to) (in) extraintestinal yersiniosis (A28.2)
sepsis (due to) (in) gonococcal (A54.86)
sepsis (due to) (in) herpesviral (B00.7)
sepsis (due to) (in) listerial (A32.7)
sepsis (due to) (in) melioidosis (A24.1)
sepsis (due to) (in) meningococcal (A39.2-A39.4)
sepsis (due to) (in) plague (A20.7)
sepsis (due to) (in) tularemia (A21.7)
toxic shock syndrome (A48.3)

GUIDELINES **Section I.C.1.d.1)(a)**
For a diagnosis of sepsis, assign the appropriate code for the underlying systemic infection. If the type of infection or causal organism is not further specified, assign code A41.9, Sepsis, unspecified organism. A code from subcategory R65.2, Severe sepsis, should not be assigned unless severe sepsis or an associated acute organ dysfunction is documented.

GUIDELINES **Section I.C.1.d.1)(b)**
The coding of severe sepsis requires a minimum of two codes: first a code for the underlying systemic infection, followed by a code from subcategory R65.2, Severe sepsis. If the causal organism is not documented, assign code A41.9, Sepsis, unspecified organism, for the infection. Additional code(s) for the associated acute organ dysfunction are also required. Due to the complex nature of severe sepsis, some cases may require querying the provider prior to assignment of the codes.

GUIDELINES **Section I.C.15.k**
Code O85, Puerperal sepsis, should be assigned with a secondary code to identify the causal organism (e.g., for a bacterial infection, assign a code from category B95-B96, Bacterial infections in conditions classified elsewhere). A code from category A40, Streptococcal sepsis, or A41, Other sepsis, should not be used for puerperal sepsis. If applicable, use additional codes to identify severe sepsis (R65.2-) and any associated acute organ dysfunction.

CODING TIP✓ When sepsis is present with a localized infection, such as UTI or pneumonia, sequence the sepsis and then the localized infection. The causative organism may be identified in the sepsis code, and therefore doesn't need to be repeated with the localized infection, except in the case of combination codes that identify the organism. Use the combination code for the pneumonia, if the localized infection is pneumonia.

CODING TIP✓ Do not assign a code from A40-A41 to indicate a bacterial infection in conditions classified elsewhere, e.g., a localized infection. Codes classified in A40-A41 are used to indicate systemic infection.

5 **A41.0** **Sepsis due to Staphylococcus aureus**

A41.01 **Sepsis due to Methicillin susceptible Staphylococcus aureus** HCC HIV
MSSA sepsis
Staphylococcus aureus sepsis NOS

A41.02 **Sepsis due to Methicillin resistant Staphylococcus aureus** HCC HIV

GUIDELINES **Section I.C.1.e.1)(a).**
When a patient is diagnosed with an infection that is due to methicillin resistant Staphylococcus aureus (MRSA), and that infection has a combination code that includes the causal organism (e.g., sepsis, pneumonia) assign the appropriate combination code for the condition (e.g., code A41.02 ...). Do not assign code B95.62, Methicillin resistant Staphylococcus aureus infection as the cause of diseases classified elsewhere, as an additional code because the combination code includes the type of infection and the MRSA organism.

A41.1 **Sepsis due to other specified staphylococcus** HCC HIV
Coagulase negative staphylococcus sepsis

A41.2 **Sepsis due to unspecified staphylococcus** HCC HIV

A41.3 **Sepsis due to Hemophilus influenzae** HCC HIV

A41.4 **Sepsis due to anaerobes** HCC HIV
EXCLUDES 1 *gas gangrene (A48.0)*

5 **A41.5** **Sepsis due to other Gram-negative organisms**

A41.50 **Gram-negative sepsis, unspecified** HCC HIV
Gram-negative sepsis NOS

A41.51 **Sepsis due to Escherichia coli [E. coli]** HCC HIV
AHA: 1Q 2018, 13

A41.52 **Sepsis due to Pseudomonas** HCC HIV
Pseudomonas aeroginosa

A41.53 **Sepsis due to Serratia** HCC HIV

A41.59 **Other Gram-negative sepsis** HCC HIV

5 **A41.8** **Other specified sepsis**

A41.81 **Sepsis due to Enterococcus** HCC HIV

A41.89 **Other specified sepsis** HCC HIV
AHA: 3Q 2016, 8-14

A41.9 **Sepsis, unspecified organism** HCC HIV
Septicemia NOS

4 A42 **Actinomycosis**
EXCLUDES 1 *actinomycetoma (B47.1)*

A42.0 **Pulmonary actinomycosis** HCC HIV
A42.1 **Abdominal actinomycosis** HIV
A42.2 **Cervicofacial actinomycosis** HIV
A42.7 **Actinomycotic sepsis** HCC HIV
5 A42.8 **Other forms of actinomycosis**
A42.81 **Actinomycotic meningitis** HIV
A42.82 **Actinomycotic encephalitis** HIV
A42.89 **Other forms of actinomycosis** HIV
A42.9 **Actinomycosis, unspecified** HIV

4 A43 **Nocardiosis**
A43.0 **Pulmonary nocardiosis** HCC HIV
A43.1 **Cutaneous nocardiosis** HIV
A43.8 **Other forms of nocardiosis** HIV
A43.9 **Nocardiosis, unspecified** HIV

4 A44 **Bartonellosis**
A44.0 **Systemic bartonellosis**
Oroya fever
A44.1 **Cutaneous and mucocutaneous bartonellosis**
Verruga peruana
A44.8 **Other forms of bartonellosis**
A44.9 **Bartonellosis, unspecified**

A46 **Erysipelas**
EXCLUDES 1 *postpartum or puerperal erysipelas (O86.89)*

DEFINITION Superficial cellulitis with dermal lymphatic involvement, commonly caused by group A beta-hemolytic streptococci; presents with shiny, raised, indurated, tender lesions with distinct margins, commonly on the legs and face.

4 A48 **Other bacterial diseases, not elsewhere classified**
EXCLUDES 1 *actinomycetoma (B47.1)*

A48.0 **Gas gangrene** HCC
Clostridial cellulitis
Clostridial myonecrosis

CODING TIP ✓ Gas gangrene is a medical emergency caused by the bacterial organism clostridium. This code should not be used when the documentation simply states gangrene.
AHA: 4Q 2017, 80

A48.1 **Legionnaires' disease** HCC HIV
A48.2 **Nonpneumonic Legionnaires' disease [Pontiac fever]**
A48.3 **Toxic shock syndrome** HCC
Use additional code to identify the organism (B95, B96)
EXCLUDES 1 *endotoxic shock NOS (R57.8)*
sepsis NOS (A41.9)
A48.4 **Brazilian purpuric fever**
Systemic Hemophilus aegyptius infection
5 A48.5 **Other specified botulism**
Non-foodborne intoxication due to toxins of Clostridium botulinum [C. botulinum]
EXCLUDES 1 *food poisoning due to toxins of Clostridium botulinum (A05.1)*
A48.51 **Infant botulism** P
A48.52 **Wound botulism**
Non-foodborne botulism NOS
Use additional code for associated wound

DEFINITION Wound infection with Clostridium botulinum producing neurological effects of severe hypotonia and paralysis without gastrointestinal symptoms of food poisoning.

A48.8 **Other specified bacterial diseases**

4 A49 **Bacterial infection of unspecified site**
EXCLUDES 1 *bacterial agents as the cause of diseases classified elsewhere (B95-B96)*
chlamydial infection NOS (A74.9)
meningococcal infection NOS (A39.9)
rickettsial infection NOS (A79.9)
spirochetal infection NOS (A69.9)

5 A49.0 **Staphylococcal infection, unspecified site**
A49.01 **Methicillin susceptible Staphylococcus aureus infection, unspecified site**
Methicillin susceptible Staphylococcus aureus (MSSA) infection
Staphylococcus aureus infection NOS
A49.02 **Methicillin resistant Staphylococcus aureus infection, unspecified site**
Methicillin resistant Staphylococcus aureus (MRSA) infection
A49.1 **Streptococcal infection, unspecified site**
A49.2 **Hemophilus influenzae infection, unspecified site**
A49.3 **Mycoplasma infection, unspecified site**
A49.8 **Other bacterial infections of unspecified site**
A49.9 **Bacterial infection, unspecified**
EXCLUDES 1 *bacteremia NOS (R78.81)*

Infections with a predominantly sexual mode of transmission (A50-A64)

EXCLUDES 1 *human immunodeficiency virus [HIV] disease (B20)*
nonspecific and nongonococcal urethritis (N34.1)
Reiter's disease (M02.3-)

4 A50 **Congenital syphilis**
5 A50.0 **Early congenital syphilis, symptomatic**
Any congenital syphilitic condition specified as early or manifest less than two years after birth.
A50.01 **Early congenital syphilitic oculopathy**
A50.02 **Early congenital syphilitic osteochondropathy**
A50.03 **Early congenital syphilitic pharyngitis**
Early congenital syphilitic laryngitis
A50.04 **Early congenital syphilitic pneumonia**
A50.05 **Early congenital syphilitic rhinitis**
A50.06 **Early cutaneous congenital syphilis**
A50.07 **Early mucocutaneous congenital syphilis**
A50.08 **Early visceral congenital syphilis**
A50.09 **Other early congenital syphilis, symptomatic**
A50.1 **Early congenital syphilis, latent**
Congenital syphilis without clinical manifestations, with positive serological reaction and negative spinal fluid test, less than two years after birth.
A50.2 **Early congenital syphilis, unspecified**
Congenital syphilis NOS less than two years after birth.
5 A50.3 **Late congenital syphilitic oculopathy**
EXCLUDES 1 *Hutchinson's triad (A50.53)*
A50.30 **Late congenital syphilitic oculopathy, unspecified**
A50.31 **Late congenital syphilitic interstitial keratitis**
A50.32 **Late congenital syphilitic chorioretinitis**
A50.39 **Other late congenital syphilitic oculopathy**
5 A50.4 **Late congenital neurosyphilis [juvenile neurosyphilis]**
Use additional code to identify any associated mental disorder
EXCLUDES 1 *Hutchinson's triad (A50.53)*
A50.40 **Late congenital neurosyphilis, unspecified**
Juvenile neurosyphilis NOS
A50.41 **Late congenital syphilitic meningitis**
A50.42 **Late congenital syphilitic encephalitis**
A50.43 **Late congenital syphilitic polyneuropathy**
A50.44 **Late congenital syphilitic optic nerve atrophy**
A50.45 **Juvenile general paresis**
Dementia paralytica juvenilis
Juvenile tabetoparetic neurosyphilis
A50.49 **Other late congenital neurosyphilis**
Juvenile tabes dorsalis
5 A50.5 **Other late congenital syphilis, symptomatic**
Any congenital syphilitic condition specified as late or manifest two years or more after birth.
A50.51 **Clutton's joints**
A50.52 **Hutchinson's teeth**
A50.53 **Hutchinson's triad**
A50.54 **Late congenital cardiovascular syphilis**
A50.55 **Late congenital syphilitic arthropathy** HCC

A50.56 **Late congenital syphilitic osteochondropathy**
A50.57 **Syphilitic saddle nose**
A50.59 **Other late congenital syphilis, symptomatic**
A50.6 **Late congenital syphilis, latent**
Congenital syphilis without clinical manifestations, with positive serological reaction and negative spinal fluid test, two years or more after birth.
A50.7 **Late congenital syphilis, unspecified**
Congenital syphilis NOS two years or more after birth.
A50.9 **Congenital syphilis, unspecified**

A51 Early syphilis
A51.0 **Primary genital syphilis**
Syphilitic chancre NOS
A51.1 **Primary anal syphilis**
A51.2 **Primary syphilis of other sites**
A51.3 **Secondary syphilis of skin and mucous membranes**
A51.31 **Condyloma latum**
A51.32 **Syphilitic alopecia**
A51.39 **Other secondary syphilis of skin**
Syphilitic leukoderma
Syphilitic mucous patch
EXCLUDES 1 *late syphilitic leukoderma (A52.79)*
A51.4 **Other secondary syphilis**
A51.41 **Secondary syphilitic meningitis**
A51.42 **Secondary syphilitic female pelvic disease** ♀
A51.43 **Secondary syphilitic oculopathy**
Secondary syphilitic chorioretinitis
Secondary syphilitic iridocyclitis, iritis
Secondary syphilitic uveitis
A51.44 **Secondary syphilitic nephritis**
A51.45 **Secondary syphilitic hepatitis**
A51.46 **Secondary syphilitic osteopathy**
A51.49 **Other secondary syphilitic conditions**
Secondary syphilitic lymphadenopathy
Secondary syphilitic myositis
A51.5 **Early syphilis, latent**
Syphilis (acquired) without clinical manifestations, with positive serological reaction and negative spinal fluid test, less than two years after infection.
A51.9 **Early syphilis, unspecified**

A52 Late syphilis
A52.0 **Cardiovascular and cerebrovascular syphilis**
A52.00 **Cardiovascular syphilis, unspecified**
A52.01 **Syphilitic aneurysm of aorta**
A52.02 **Syphilitic aortitis**
A52.03 **Syphilitic endocarditis**
Syphilitic aortic valve incompetence or stenosis
Syphilitic mitral valve stenosis
Syphilitic pulmonary valve regurgitation
A52.04 **Syphilitic cerebral arteritis**
A52.05 **Other cerebrovascular syphilis**
Syphilitic cerebral aneurysm (ruptured) (non-ruptured)
Syphilitic cerebral thrombosis
A52.06 **Other syphilitic heart involvement**
Syphilitic coronary artery disease
Syphilitic myocarditis
Syphilitic pericarditis
A52.09 **Other cardiovascular syphilis**
A52.1 **Symptomatic neurosyphilis**
A52.10 **Symptomatic neurosyphilis, unspecified**
A52.11 **Tabes dorsalis**
Locomotor ataxia (progressive)
Tabetic neurosyphilis
A52.12 **Other cerebrospinal syphilis**
A52.13 **Late syphilitic meningitis**
A52.14 **Late syphilitic encephalitis**
A52.15 **Late syphilitic neuropathy**
Late syphilitic acoustic neuritis
Late syphilitic optic (nerve) atrophy
Late syphilitic polyneuropathy
Late syphilitic retrobulbar neuritis
A52.16 **Charcôt's arthropathy (tabetic)**
A52.17 **General paresis**
Dementia paralytica
A52.19 **Other symptomatic neurosyphilis**
Syphilitic parkinsonism
A52.2 **Asymptomatic neurosyphilis**
A52.3 **Neurosyphilis, unspecified**
Gumma (syphilitic)
Syphilis (late)
Syphiloma
A52.7 **Other symptomatic late syphilis**
A52.71 **Late syphilitic oculopathy**
Late syphilitic chorioretinitis
Late syphilitic episcleritis
A52.72 **Syphilis of lung and bronchus**
A52.73 **Symptomatic late syphilis of other respiratory organs**
A52.74 **Syphilis of liver and other viscera**
Late syphilitic peritonitis
A52.75 **Syphilis of kidney and ureter**
Syphilitic glomerular disease
A52.76 **Other genitourinary symptomatic late syphilis**
Late syphilitic female pelvic inflammatory disease
A52.77 **Syphilis of bone and joint**
A52.78 **Syphilis of other musculoskeletal tissue**
Late syphilitic bursitis
Syphilis [stage unspecified] of bursa
Syphilis [stage unspecified] of muscle
Syphilis [stage unspecified] of synovium
Syphilis [stage unspecified] of tendon
A52.79 **Other symptomatic late syphilis**
Late syphilitic leukoderma
Syphilis of adrenal gland
Syphilis of pituitary gland
Syphilis of thyroid gland
Syphilitic splenomegaly
EXCLUDES 1 *syphilitic leukoderma (secondary) (A51.39)*
A52.8 **Late syphilis, latent**
Syphilis (acquired) without clinical manifestations, with positive serological reaction and negative spinal fluid test, two years or more after infection
A52.9 **Late syphilis, unspecified**

A53 Other and unspecified syphilis
A53.0 **Latent syphilis, unspecified as early or late**
Latent syphilis NOS
Positive serological reaction for syphilis
A53.9 **Syphilis, unspecified**
Infection due to Treponema pallidum NOS
Syphilis (acquired) NOS
EXCLUDES 1 *syphilis NOS under two years of age (A50.2)*

A54 Gonococcal infection
A54.0 **Gonococcal infection of lower genitourinary tract without periurethral or accessory gland abscess**
EXCLUDES 1 *gonococcal infection with genitourinary gland abscess (A54.1)*
gonococcal infection with periurethral abscess (A54.1)
A54.00 **Gonococcal infection of lower genitourinary tract, unspecified**
A54.01 **Gonococcal cystitis and urethritis, unspecified**
A54.02 **Gonococcal vulvovaginitis, unspecified** ♀
A54.03 **Gonococcal cervicitis, unspecified** ♀
A54.09 **Other gonococcal infection of lower genitourinary tract**
A54.1 **Gonococcal infection of lower genitourinary tract with periurethral and accessory gland abscess**
Gonococcal Bartholin's gland abscess
A54.2 **Gonococcal pelviperitonitis and other gonococcal genitourinary infection**
A54.21 **Gonococcal infection of kidney and ureter**
A54.22 **Gonococcal prostatitis** ♂
A54.23 **Gonococcal infection of other male genital organs** ♂
Gonococcal epididymitis
Gonococcal orchitis
A54.24 **Gonococcal female pelvic inflammatory disease** ♀
Gonococcal pelviperitonitis
EXCLUDES 1 *gonococcal peritonitis (A54.85)*
A54.29 **Other gonococcal genitourinary infections**
A54.3 **Gonococcal infection of eye**

A54.30 **Gonococcal infection of eye, unspecified**
A54.31 **Gonococcal conjunctivitis**
Ophthalmia neonatorum due to gonococcus
A54.32 **Gonococcal iridocyclitis**
A54.33 **Gonococcal keratitis**
A54.39 **Other gonococcal eye infection**
Gonococcal endophthalmia

A54.4 **Gonococcal infection of musculoskeletal system**
A54.40 **Gonococcal infection of musculoskeletal system, unspecified** HCC
A54.41 **Gonococcal spondylopathy** HCC
A54.42 **Gonococcal arthritis** HCC
EXCLUDES 2 *gonococcal infection of spine (A54.41)*
A54.43 **Gonococcal osteomyelitis** HCC
EXCLUDES 2 *gonococcal infection of spine (A54.41)*
A54.49 **Gonococcal infection of other musculoskeletal tissue** HCC
Gonococcal bursitis
Gonococcal myositis
Gonococcal synovitis
Gonococcal tenosynovitis

A54.5 **Gonococcal pharyngitis**
A54.6 **Gonococcal infection of anus and rectum**
A54.8 **Other gonococcal infections**
A54.81 **Gonococcal meningitis**
A54.82 **Gonococcal brain abscess**
A54.83 **Gonococcal heart infection**
Gonococcal endocarditis
Gonococcal myocarditis
Gonococcal pericarditis
A54.84 **Gonococcal pneumonia** HCC
A54.85 **Gonococcal peritonitis** HCC
EXCLUDES 1 *gonococcal pelviperitonitis (A54.24)*
A54.86 **Gonococcal sepsis** HCC
A54.89 **Other gonococcal infections**
Gonococcal keratoderma
Gonococcal lymphadenitis
A54.9 **Gonococcal infection, unspecified**

A55 **Chlamydial lymphogranuloma (venereum)**
Climatic or tropical bubo
Durand-Nicolas-Favre disease
Esthiomene
Lymphogranuloma inguinale

DEFINITION Sexually transmitted infection by Chlamydia trachomatis, seen in warm climates; presents with primary cutaneous or mucosal lesion at infection site and acute unilateral or bilateral lymphadenopathy.

A56 **Other sexually transmitted chlamydial diseases**
INCLUDES sexually transmitted diseases due to Chlamydia trachomatis
EXCLUDES 1 *neonatal chlamydial conjunctivitis (P39.1)*
neonatal chlamydial pneumonia (P23.1)
EXCLUDES 2 *chlamydial lymphogranuloma (A55)*
conditions classified to A74.-

A56.0 **Chlamydial infection of lower genitourinary tract**
A56.00 **Chlamydial infection of lower genitourinary tract, unspecified**
A56.01 **Chlamydial cystitis and urethritis**
A56.02 **Chlamydial vulvovaginitis** ♀
A56.09 **Other chlamydial infection of lower genitourinary tract**
Chlamydial cervicitis

A56.1 **Chlamydial infection of pelviperitoneum and other genitourinary organs**
A56.11 **Chlamydial female pelvic inflammatory disease** ♀
A56.19 **Other chlamydial genitourinary infection**
Chlamydial epididymitis
Chlamydial orchitis

A56.2 **Chlamydial infection of genitourinary tract, unspecified**
A56.3 **Chlamydial infection of anus and rectum**
A56.4 **Chlamydial infection of pharynx**
A56.8 **Sexually transmitted chlamydial infection of other sites**

A57 **Chancroid**
Ulcus molle

DEFINITION Sexually transmitted disease, characterized by a painful, primary ulcer, usually on the external genitalia.

A58 **Granuloma inguinale**
Donovanosis

A59 **Trichomoniasis**
EXCLUDES 2 *intestinal trichomoniasis (A07.8)*

A59.0 **Urogenital trichomoniasis**
A59.00 **Urogenital trichomoniasis, unspecified**
Fluor (vaginalis) due to Trichomonas
Leukorrhea (vaginalis) due to Trichomonas
A59.01 **Trichomonal vulvovaginitis** ♀

DEFINITION Sexually transmitted disease caused by the protozoan Trichomonas vaginalis infecting the vagina and external female genitalia.

A59.02 **Trichomonal prostatitis** ♂
A59.03 **Trichomonal cystitis and urethritis**

Trichomonal cystitis and urethritis

A sexually transmitted disease caused by the protozoan Trichomonas vaginalis infecting the urethra

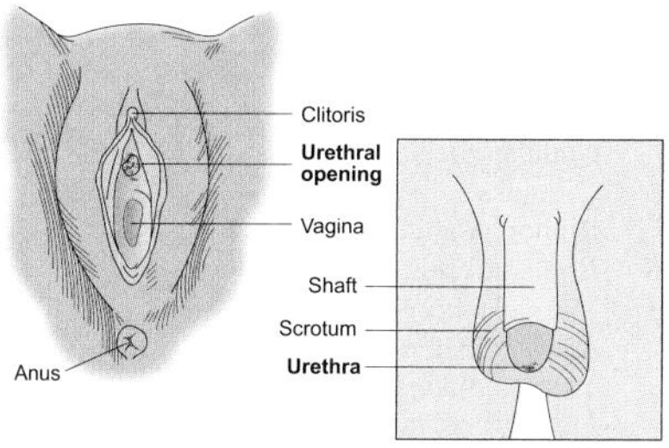

A59.09 **Other urogenital trichomoniasis**
Trichomonas cervicitis
A59.8 **Trichomoniasis of other sites**
A59.9 **Trichomoniasis, unspecified**

A60 **Anogenital herpesviral [herpes simplex] infections**

A60.0 **Herpesviral infection of genitalia and urogenital tract**
A60.00 **Herpesviral infection of urogenital system, unspecified** HIV
A60.01 **Herpesviral infection of penis** ♂ HIV
A60.02 **Herpesviral infection of other male genital organs** ♂
A60.03 **Herpesviral cervicitis** ♀
A60.04 **Herpesviral vulvovaginitis** ♀ HIV
Herpesviral [herpes simplex] ulceration
Herpesviral [herpes simplex] vaginitis
Herpesviral [herpes simplex] vulvitis
A60.09 **Herpesviral infection of other urogenital tract** HIV
A60.1 **Herpesviral infection of perianal skin and rectum** HIV
A60.9 **Anogenital herpesviral infection, unspecified** HIV

A63 **Other predominantly sexually transmitted diseases, not elsewhere classified**
EXCLUDES 2 *molluscum contagiosum (B08.1)*
papilloma of cervix (D26.0)
A63.0 **Anogenital (venereal) warts**
Anogenital warts due to (human) papillomavirus [HPV]
Condyloma acuminatum

DEFINITION A wartlike growth on the skin or mucous membrane, in the area of the anus or external genitalia.

A63.8 **Other specified predominantly sexually transmitted diseases**

A64 **Unspecified sexually transmitted disease**

Other spirochetal diseases (A65-A69)

EXCLUDES 2 *leptospirosis (A27.-)*
syphilis (A50-A53)

A65 **Nonvenereal syphilis**
Bejel
Endemic syphilis
Njovera

4 A66 Yaws
INCLUDES bouba
frambesia (tropica)
pian

A66.0 Initial lesions of yaws
Chancre of yaws
Frambesia, initial or primary
Initial frambesial ulcer
Mother yaw

A66.1 Multiple papillomata and wet crab yaws
Frambesioma
Pianoma
Plantar or palmar papilloma of yaws

A66.2 Other early skin lesions of yaws
Cutaneous yaws, less than five years after infection
Early yaws (cutaneous)(macular)(maculopapular)(micropapular)(papular)
Frambeside of early yaws

A66.3 Hyperkeratosis of yaws
Ghoul hand
Hyperkeratosis, palmar or plantar (early) (late) due to yaws
Worm-eaten soles

A66.4 Gummata and ulcers of yaws
Gummatous frambeside
Nodular late yaws (ulcerated)

A66.5 Gangosa
Rhinopharyngitis mutilans

A66.6 Bone and joint lesions of yaws HCC
Yaws ganglion
Yaws goundou
Yaws gumma, bone
Yaws gummatous osteitis or periostitis
Yaws hydrarthrosis
Yaws osteitis
Yaws periostitis (hypertrophic)

A66.7 Other manifestations of yaws
Juxta-articular nodules of yaws
Mucosal yaws

A66.8 Latent yaws
Yaws without clinical manifestations, with positive serology

A66.9 Yaws, unspecified

4 A67 Pinta [carate]

A67.0 Primary lesions of pinta
Chancre (primary) of pinta
Papule (primary) of pinta

A67.1 Intermediate lesions of pinta
Erythematous plaques of pinta
Hyperchromic lesions of pinta
Hyperkeratosis of pinta
Pintids

A67.2 Late lesions of pinta
Achromic skin lesions of pinta
Cicatricial skin lesions of pinta
Dyschromic skin lesions of pinta

A67.3 Mixed lesions of pinta
Achromic with hyperchromic skin lesions of pinta [carate]

A67.9 Pinta, unspecified

4 A68 Relapsing fevers
INCLUDES recurrent fever
EXCLUDES 2 *Lyme disease (A69.2-)*

A68.0 Louse-borne relapsing fever
Relapsing fever due to Borrelia recurrentis

A68.1 Tick-borne relapsing fever
Relapsing fever due to any Borrelia species other than Borrelia recurrentis

A68.9 Relapsing fever, unspecified

4 A69 Other spirochetal infections

A69.0 Necrotizing ulcerative stomatitis
Cancrum oris
Fusospirochetal gangrene
Noma
Stomatitis gangrenosa

A69.1 Other Vincent's infections
Fusospirochetal pharyngitis
Necrotizing ulcerative (acute) gingivitis
Necrotizing ulcerative (acute) gingivostomatitis
Spirochetal stomatitis
Trench mouth
Vincent's angina
Vincent's gingivitis

5 A69.2 Lyme disease
Erythema chronicum migrans due to Borrelia burgdorferi

DEFINITION Tick-transmitted infection caused by Borrelia burgdorferi, manifesting with erythema chronicum migrans, myalgia, arthritis of the large joints, and nervous and cardiovascular system involvement.

A69.20 Lyme disease, unspecified

Lyme disease

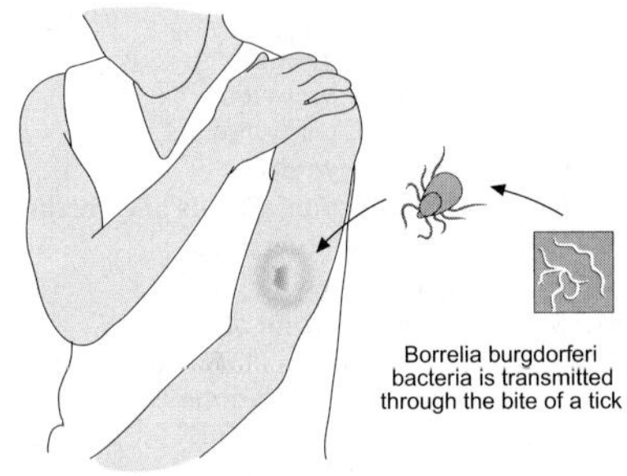
Borrelia burgdorferi bacteria is transmitted through the bite of a tick

A69.21 Meningitis due to Lyme disease

A69.22 Other neurologic disorders in Lyme disease
Cranial neuritis
Meningoencephalitis
Polyneuropathy

A69.23 Arthritis due to Lyme disease HCC

A69.29 Other conditions associated with Lyme disease
Myopericarditis due to Lyme disease
AHA: 3Q 2016, 8
AHA: 3Q 2016, 12

A69.8 Other specified spirochetal infections

A69.9 Spirochetal infection, unspecified

Other diseases caused by chlamydiae (A70-A74)

EXCLUDES 1 *sexually transmitted chlamydial diseases (A55-A56)*

A70 Chlamydia psittaci infections
Ornithosis
Parrot fever
Psittacosis

4 A71 Trachoma
EXCLUDES 1 *sequelae of trachoma (B94.0)*

A71.0 Initial stage of trachoma
Trachoma dubium

A71.1 Active stage of trachoma
Granular conjunctivitis (trachomatous)
Trachomatous follicular conjunctivitis
Trachomatous pannus

A71.9 Trachoma, unspecified

4 A74 Other diseases caused by chlamydiae
EXCLUDES 1 *neonatal chlamydial conjunctivitis (P39.1)*
neonatal chlamydial pneumonia (P23.1)
Reiter's disease (M02.3-)
sexually transmitted chlamydial diseases (A55-A56)
EXCLUDES 2 *chlamydial pneumonia (J16.0)*

A74.0 Chlamydial conjunctivitis
Paratrachoma

5 A74.8 Other chlamydial diseases

A74.81 Chlamydial peritonitis

A74.89 Other chlamydial diseases

A74.9 **Chlamydial infection, unspecified**
Chlamydiosis NOS

Rickettsioses (A75-A79)

A75 **Typhus fever**
EXCLUDES 1 *rickettsiosis due to Ehrlichia sennetsu (A79.81)*

A75.0 **Epidemic louse-borne typhus fever due to Rickettsia prowazekii**
Classical typhus (fever)
Epidemic (louse-borne) typhus

A75.1 **Recrudescent typhus [Brill's disease]**
Brill-Zinsser disease

A75.2 **Typhus fever due to Rickettsia typhi**
Murine (flea-borne) typhus

A75.3 **Typhus fever due to Rickettsia tsutsugamushi**
Scrub (mite-borne) typhus
Tsutsugamushi fever

A75.9 **Typhus fever, unspecified**
Typhus (fever) NOS

A77 **Spotted fever [tick-borne rickettsioses]**

A77.0 **Spotted fever due to Rickettsia rickettsii**
Rocky Mountain spotted fever
Sao Paulo fever

A77.1 **Spotted fever due to Rickettsia conorii**
African tick typhus
Boutonneuse fever
India tick typhus
Kenya tick typhus
Marseilles fever
Mediterranean tick fever

A77.2 **Spotted fever due to Rickettsia siberica**
North Asian tick fever
Siberian tick typhus

A77.3 **Spotted fever due to Rickettsia australis**
Queensland tick typhus

A77.4 **Ehrlichiosis**
EXCLUDES 1 *Rickettsiosis due to Ehrlichia sennetsu (A79.81)*

A77.40 **Ehrlichiosis, unspecified**

A77.41 **Ehrlichiosis chafeensis [E. chafeensis]**

A77.49 **Other ehrlichiosis**

A77.8 **Other spotted fevers**

A77.9 **Spotted fever, unspecified**
Tick-borne typhus NOS

A78 **Q fever**
Infection due to Coxiella burnetii
Nine Mile fever
Quadrilateral fever

A79 **Other rickettsioses**

A79.0 **Trench fever**
Quintan fever
Wolhynian fever

A79.1 **Rickettsialpox due to Rickettsia akari**
Kew Garden fever
Vesicular rickettsiosis

A79.8 **Other specified rickettsioses**

A79.81 **Rickettsiosis due to Ehrlichia sennetsu**

A79.89 **Other specified rickettsioses**

A79.9 **Rickettsiosis, unspecified**
Rickettsial infection NOS

Viral and prion infections of the central nervous system (A80-A89)

EXCLUDES 1 *postpolio syndrome (G14)*
sequelae of poliomyelitis (B91)
sequelae of viral encephalitis (B94.1)

A80 **Acute poliomyelitis**

CODING TIP ✓ Assign a code from category A80 to indicate acute poliomyelitis, not a sequela of polio, or post polio syndrome. A80- codes are used to report acute, active poliomyelitis only. Use B91 for sequelae of polio, or G14 for post polio syndrome, which must be documented by the physician.

A80.0 **Acute paralytic poliomyelitis, vaccine-associated**

A80.1 **Acute paralytic poliomyelitis, wild virus, imported**

A80.2 **Acute paralytic poliomyelitis, wild virus, indigenous**

A80.3 **Acute paralytic poliomyelitis, other and unspecified**

A80.30 **Acute paralytic poliomyelitis, unspecified**

A80.39 **Other acute paralytic poliomyelitis**

A80.4 **Acute nonparalytic poliomyelitis**

A80.9 **Acute poliomyelitis, unspecified**

A81 **Atypical virus infections of central nervous system**
INCLUDES diseases of the central nervous system caused by prions
Use additional code to identify:
dementia with behavioral disturbance (F02.81)
dementia without behavioral disturbance (F02.80)

A81.0 **Creutzfeldt-Jakob disease**

DEFINITION Degenerative neural disease caused by a prion (an infectious protein); presents with loss of muscular control, balance, and memory, twitching movements, nervousness and agitation, changes in personality, and dementia.

A81.00 **Creutzfeldt-Jakob disease, unspecified**
Jakob-Creutzfeldt disease, unspecified

A81.01 **Variant Creutzfeldt-Jakob disease**
vCJD

DEFINITION Rare, transmissible form of fatal Jakob-Creutzfeldt disease, affecting younger people with a longer duration, causing spongiform degeneration of the brain with unusual psychiatric and sensory symptoms.

A81.09 **Other Creutzfeldt-Jakob disease**
CJD
Familial Creutzfeldt-Jakob disease
Iatrogenic Creutzfeldt-Jakob disease
Sporadic Creutzfeldt-Jakob disease
Subacute spongiform encephalopathy (with dementia)

A81.1 **Subacute sclerosing panencephalitis**
Dawson's inclusion body encephalitis
Van Bogaert's sclerosing leukoencephalopathy

A81.2 **Progressive multifocal leukoencephalopathy** HIV
Multifocal leukoencephalopathy NOS

A81.8 **Other atypical virus infections of central nervous system**

A81.81 **Kuru**

A81.82 **Gerstmann-Sträussler-Scheinker syndrome** HIV
GSS syndrome

DEFINITION Extremely rare, inherited, fatal disease of the brain that progresses slowly, causing lack of muscle coordination, unsteady gait, dementia, slurred speech, spasticity, and coma before death.

A81.83 **Fatal familial insomnia** HIV
FFI

DEFINITION Very rare, inherited brain disease caused by prion protein mutation from soluble to insoluble, resulting in plaques forming in the thalamus, causing insomnia that progresses to dementia, unresponsiveness, and death.

A81.89 **Other atypical virus infections of central nervous system** HIV

A81.9 **Atypical virus infection of central nervous system, unspecified** HIV
Prion diseases of the central nervous system NOS

A82 **Rabies**

A82.0 **Sylvatic rabies**

A82.1 **Urban rabies**

A82.9 **Rabies, unspecified**

A83 **Mosquito-borne viral encephalitis**
INCLUDES mosquito-borne viral meningoencephalitis
EXCLUDES 2 *Venezuelan equine encephalitis (A92.2)*
West Nile fever (A92.3-)
West Nile virus (A92.3-)

A83.0 **Japanese encephalitis**

A83.1 **Western equine encephalitis**

A83.2 **Eastern equine encephalitis**

A83.3 **St Louis encephalitis**

A83.4 **Australian encephalitis**
Kunjin virus disease

A83.5 **California encephalitis**
California meningoencephalitis
La Crosse encephalitis
A83.6 **Rocio virus disease**
A83.8 **Other mosquito-borne viral encephalitis**
A83.9 **Mosquito-borne viral encephalitis, unspecified**

4 **A84 Tick-borne viral encephalitis**
INCLUDES tick-borne viral meningoencephalitis
A84.0 **Far Eastern tick-borne encephalitis [Russian spring-summer encephalitis]**
A84.1 **Central European tick-borne encephalitis**
A84.8 **Other tick-borne viral encephalitis**
Louping ill
Powassan virus disease
A84.9 **Tick-borne viral encephalitis, unspecified**

4 **A85 Other viral encephalitis, not elsewhere classified**
INCLUDES specified viral encephalomyelitis NEC
specified viral meningoencephalitis NEC
EXCLUDES 1 *benign myalgic encephalomyelitis (G93.3)*
encephalitis due to cytomegalovirus (B25.8)
encephalitis due to herpesvirus NEC (B10.0-)
encephalitis due to herpesvirus [herpes simplex] (B00.4)
encephalitis due to measles virus (B05.0)
encephalitis due to mumps virus (B26.2)
encephalitis due to poliomyelitis virus (A80.-)
encephalitis due to zoster (B02.0)
lymphocytic choriomeningitis (A87.2)
A85.0 **Enteroviral encephalitis** HIV
Enteroviral encephalomyelitis
A85.1 **Adenoviral encephalitis** HIV
Adenoviral meningoencephalitis
A85.2 **Arthropod-borne viral encephalitis, unspecified**
EXCLUDES 1 *West nile virus with encephalitis (A92.31)*
A85.8 **Other specified viral encephalitis** HIV
Encephalitis lethargica
Von Economo-Cruchet disease

A86 Unspecified viral encephalitis HIV
Viral encephalomyelitis NOS
Viral meningoencephalitis NOS

4 **A87 Viral meningitis**
EXCLUDES 1 *meningitis due to herpesvirus [herpes simplex] (B00.3)*
meningitis due to herpesvirus [herpes simplex] (B00.3)
meningitis due to measles virus (B05.1)
meningitis due to mumps virus (B26.1)
meningitis due to poliomyelitis virus (A80.-)
meningitis due to zoster (B02.1)
A87.0 **Enteroviral meningitis**
Coxsackievirus meningitis
Echovirus meningitis
A87.1 **Adenoviral meningitis**
A87.2 **Lymphocytic choriomeningitis**
Lymphocytic meningoencephalitis
A87.8 **Other viral meningitis**
A87.9 **Viral meningitis, unspecified**

4 **A88 Other viral infections of central nervous system, not elsewhere classified**
EXCLUDES 1 *viral encephalitis NOS (A86)*
viral meningitis NOS (A87.9)
A88.0 **Enteroviral exanthematous fever [Boston exanthem]**
A88.1 **Epidemic vertigo**
A88.8 **Other specified viral infections of central nervous system** HIV

A89 Unspecified viral infection of central nervous system HIV

Arthropod-borne viral fevers and viral hemorrhagic fevers (A90-A99)

A90 Dengue fever [classical dengue]
EXCLUDES 1 *dengue hemorrhagic fever (A91)*
AHA: 3Q 2016, 8
AHA: 3Q 2016, 13

A91 Dengue hemorrhagic fever

4 **A92 Other mosquito-borne viral fevers**
EXCLUDES 1 *Ross River disease (B33.1)*
A92.0 **Chikungunya virus disease**
Chikungunya (hemorrhagic) fever
A92.1 **O'nyong-nyong fever**
A92.2 **Venezuelan equine fever**
Venezuelan equine encephalitis
Venezuelan equine encephalomyelitis virus disease
5 A92.3 **West Nile virus infection**
West Nile fever

West Nile virus infection

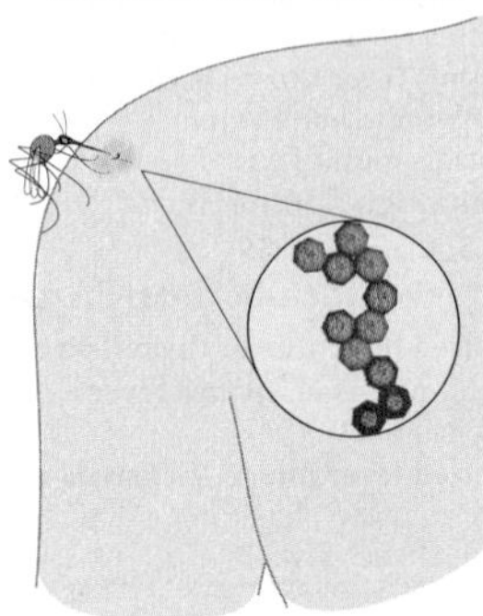

A92.30 **West Nile virus infection, unspecified**
West Nile fever NOS
West Nile fever without complications
West Nile virus NOS
A92.31 **West Nile virus infection with encephalitis**
West Nile encephalitis
West Nile encephalomyelitis
AHA: 3Q 2016, 8
AHA: 3Q 2016, 13
A92.32 **West Nile virus infection with other neurologic manifestation**
Use additional code to specify the neurologic manifestation
A92.39 **West Nile virus infection with other complications**
Use additional code to specify the other conditions
A92.4 **Rift Valley fever**
▲ A92.5 **Zika virus disease**
Zika virus fever
Zika virus infection
Zika NOS
EXCLUDES 1 *congenital Zika virus disease (P35.4)*

CODING TIP ✓ Zika virus must be documented by the physician. Suspected or probable Zika should not be coded as Zika. In that case, code the symptoms/signs experienced by the patient.

DEFINITION Disease caused by infection with the Zika virus most commonly presents with fever, rash, joint pain, reddening of the eyes, muscle pain, and headache. Zika viral infection is primarily spread by the bite of infected mosquitoes.
AHA: 4Q 2016, 4

A92.8 **Other specified mosquito-borne viral fevers**
A92.9 **Mosquito-borne viral fever, unspecified**

4 **A93 Other arthropod-borne viral fevers, not elsewhere classified**
A93.0 **Oropouche virus disease**
Oropouche fever
A93.1 **Sandfly fever**
Pappataci fever
Phlebotomus fever
A93.2 **Colorado tick fever**
A93.8 **Other specified arthropod-borne viral fevers**
Piry virus disease
Vesicular stomatitis virus disease [Indiana fever]

A94 Unspecified arthropod-borne viral fever
Arboviral fever NOS
Arbovirus infection NOS

4 A95 Yellow fever
- A95.0 **Sylvatic yellow fever**
  Jungle yellow fever
- A95.1 **Urban yellow fever**
- A95.9 **Yellow fever, unspecified**

4 A96 Arenaviral hemorrhagic fever
- A96.0 **Junin hemorrhagic fever**
  Argentinian hemorrhagic fever
- A96.1 **Machupo hemorrhagic fever**
  Bolivian hemorrhagic fever
- A96.2 **Lassa fever**
- A96.8 **Other arenaviral hemorrhagic fevers**
- A96.9 **Arenaviral hemorrhagic fever, unspecified**

4 A98 Other viral hemorrhagic fevers, not elsewhere classified
EXCLUDES 1 *chikungunya hemorrhagic fever (A92.0)*
dengue hemorrhagic fever (A91)
- A98.0 **Crimean-Congo hemorrhagic fever**
  Central Asian hemorrhagic fever
- A98.1 **Omsk hemorrhagic fever**
- A98.2 **Kyasanur Forest disease**
- A98.3 **Marburg virus disease**
- A98.4 **Ebola virus disease**
- A98.5 **Hemorrhagic fever with renal syndrome**
  Epidemic hemorrhagic fever
  Korean hemorrhagic fever
  Russian hemorrhagic fever
  Hantaan virus disease
  Hantavirus disease with renal manifestations
  Nephropathia epidemica
  Songo fever
  EXCLUDES 1 *hantavirus (cardio) -pulmonary syndrome (B33.4)*
- A98.8 **Other specified viral hemorrhagic fevers**

A99 Unspecified viral hemorrhagic fever

Viral infections characterized by skin and mucous membrane lesions (B00-B09)

4 B00 Herpesviral [herpes simplex] infections
EXCLUDES 1 *congenital herpesviral infections (P35.2)*
EXCLUDES 2 *anogenital herpesviral infection (A60.-)*
gammaherpesviral mononucleosis (B27.0-)
herpangina (B08.5)

CODING TIP✓ Conditions classified to B00 are due to herpes simplex virus, not those due to herpes zoster virus (such as shingles). Category B02- includes infections due to herpes zoster virus.

- B00.0 **Eczema herpeticum** HIV
  Kaposi's varicelliform eruption
  DEFINITION Potentially fatal infection with the herpes simplex virus at the site of an existing skin condition, often atopic dermatitis, causing severe rash, fever, and fatigue.
- B00.1 **Herpesviral vesicular dermatitis** HIV
  Herpes simplex facialis
  Herpes simplex labialis
  Herpes simplex otitis externa
  Vesicular dermatitis of ear
  Vesicular dermatitis of lip
- B00.2 **Herpesviral gingivostomatitis and pharyngotonsillitis** HIV
  Herpesviral pharyngitis
- B00.3 **Herpesviral meningitis** HIV
- B00.4 **Herpesviral encephalitis** HIV
  Herpesviral meningoencephalitis
  Simian B disease
  EXCLUDES 1 *herpesviral encephalitis due to herpesvirus 6 and 7 (B10.01, B10.09)*
  non-simplex herpesviral encephalitis (B10.0-)
- 5 B00.5 **Herpesviral ocular disease**
  - B00.50 **Herpesviral ocular disease, unspecified** HIV
  - B00.51 **Herpesviral iridocyclitis** HIV
    Herpesviral iritis
    Herpesviral uveitis, anterior
  - B00.52 **Herpesviral keratitis** HIV
    Herpesviral keratoconjunctivitis
  - B00.53 **Herpesviral conjunctivitis** HIV
  - B00.59 **Other herpesviral disease of eye** HIV
    Herpesviral dermatitis of eyelid
- B00.7 **Disseminated herpesviral disease** HCC HIV
  Herpesviral sepsis
- 5 B00.8 **Other forms of herpesviral infections**
  - B00.81 **Herpesviral hepatitis** HIV
  - B00.82 **Herpes simplex myelitis** HCC
  - B00.89 **Other herpesviral infection** HIV
    Herpesviral whitlow
    DEFINITION Viral infection that results in a painful, blistery eruption on one of the digits.
- B00.9 **Herpesviral infection, unspecified** HIV
  Herpes simplex infection NOS

4 B01 Varicella [chickenpox]
- B01.0 **Varicella meningitis**
- 5 B01.1 **Varicella encephalitis, myelitis and encephalomyelitis**
  Postchickenpox encephalitis, myelitis and encephalomyelitis
  - B01.11 **Varicella encephalitis and encephalomyelitis**
    Postchickenpox encephalitis and encephalomyelitis
  - B01.12 **Varicella myelitis** HCC
    Postchickenpox myelitis
- B01.2 **Varicella pneumonia**
- 5 B01.8 **Varicella with other complications**
  - B01.81 **Varicella keratitis**
  - B01.89 **Other varicella complications**
- B01.9 **Varicella without complication**
  Varicella NOS

4 B02 Zoster [herpes zoster]
INCLUDES shingles
zona

Zoster (herpes zoster)

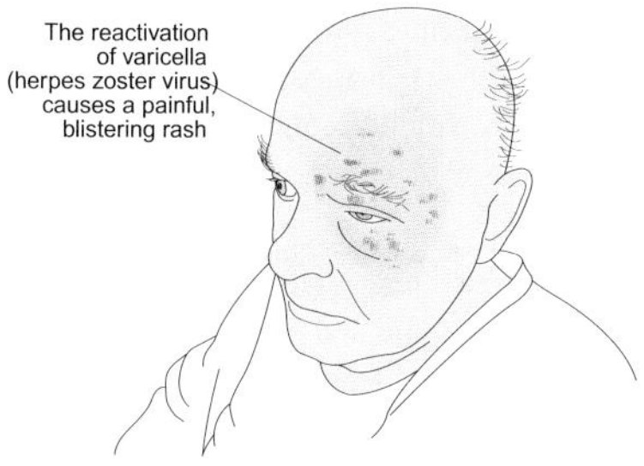
The reactivation of varicella (herpes zoster virus) causes a painful, blistering rash

- B02.0 **Zoster encephalitis** HIV
  Zoster meningoencephalitis
- B02.1 **Zoster meningitis** HIV
- 5 B02.2 **Zoster with other nervous system involvement**
  - B02.21 **Postherpetic geniculate ganglionitis** HIV
  - B02.22 **Postherpetic trigeminal neuralgia** HIV
  - B02.23 **Postherpetic polyneuropathy** HIV
  - B02.24 **Postherpetic myelitis** HCC
    Herpes zoster myelitis
  - B02.29 **Other postherpetic nervous system involvement** HIV
    Postherpetic radiculopathy
- 5 B02.3 **Zoster ocular disease**
  - B02.30 **Zoster ocular disease, unspecified** HIV
  - B02.31 **Zoster conjunctivitis** HIV
  - B02.32 **Zoster iridocyclitis** HIV
  - B02.33 **Zoster keratitis** HIV
    Herpes zoster keratoconjunctivitis
  - B02.34 **Zoster scleritis** HIV

B02.39 Other herpes zoster eye disease HIV
Zoster blepharitis

B02.7 Disseminated zoster HIV

B02.8 Zoster with other complications HIV
Herpes zoster otitis externa

B02.9 Zoster without complications HIV
Zoster NOS

B03 Smallpox
Note: In 1980 the 33rd World Health Assembly declared that smallpox had been eradicated.
The classification is maintained for surveillance purposes.

B04 Monkeypox

4 **B05 Measles**
INCLUDES morbilli
EXCLUDES 1 *subacute sclerosing panencephalitis (A81.1)*

B05.0 Measles complicated by encephalitis
Postmeasles encephalitis

B05.1 Measles complicated by meningitis
Postmeasles meningitis

B05.2 Measles complicated by pneumonia
Postmeasles pneumonia

B05.3 Measles complicated by otitis media
Postmeasles otitis media

B05.4 Measles with intestinal complications

5 **B05.8** Measles with other complications

B05.81 Measles keratitis and keratoconjunctivitis

B05.89 Other measles complications

B05.9 Measles without complication
Measles NOS

4 **B06 Rubella [German measles]**
EXCLUDES 1 *congenital rubella (P35.0)*

5 **B06.0** Rubella with neurological complications

B06.00 Rubella with neurological complication, unspecified

B06.01 Rubella encephalitis
Rubella meningoencephalitis

B06.02 Rubella meningitis

B06.09 Other neurological complications of rubella

5 **B06.8** Rubella with other complications

B06.81 Rubella pneumonia

B06.82 Rubella arthritis HCC

B06.89 Other rubella complications

B06.9 Rubella without complication
Rubella NOS

4 **B07 Viral warts**
INCLUDES verruca simplex
verruca vulgaris
viral warts due to human papillomavirus
EXCLUDES 2 *anogenital (venereal) warts (A63.0)*
papilloma of bladder (D41.4)
papilloma of cervix (D26.0)
papilloma larynx (D14.1)

B07.0 Plantar wart
Verruca plantaris
DEFINITION Noncancerous skin growths on the soles of the feet, often under pressure points, caused by the human papilloma virus that enters through tiny cuts or cracks in the skin.

B07.8 Other viral warts
Common wart
Flat wart
Verruca plana

B07.9 Viral wart, unspecified

4 **B08 Other viral infections characterized by skin and mucous membrane lesions, not elsewhere classified**
EXCLUDES 1 *vesicular stomatitis virus disease (A93.8)*

5 **B08.0** Other orthopoxvirus infections
EXCLUDES 2 *monkeypox (B04)*

6 **B08.01** Cowpox and vaccinia not from vaccine

B08.010 Cowpox

B08.011 Vaccinia not from vaccine
EXCLUDES 1 *vaccinia (from vaccination) (generalized) (T88.1)*

B08.02 Orf virus disease
Contagious pustular dermatitis
Ecthyma contagiosum
DEFINITION Skin disease closely related to smallpox, manifesting with localized, small, red, fluid-filled pustules that scab and heal, providing immunity to smallpox.

B08.03 Pseudocowpox [milker's node]

B08.04 Paravaccinia, unspecified

B08.09 Other orthopoxvirus infections
Orthopoxvirus infection NOS

B08.1 Molluscum contagiosum

5 **B08.2** Exanthema subitum [sixth disease]
Roseola infantum

B08.20 Exanthema subitum [sixth disease], unspecified P
Roseola infantum, unspecified
DEFINITION Common childhood herpes viral illness of mild upper respiratory symptoms, swollen glands, high fever lasting 3-7 days ending abruptly, followed by a rash.

B08.21 Exanthema subitum [sixth disease] due to human herpesvirus 6 P
Roseola infantum due to human herpesvirus 6

B08.22 Exanthema subitum [sixth disease] due to human herpesvirus 7 P
Roseola infantum due to human herpesvirus 7

B08.3 Erythema infectiosum [fifth disease]
DEFINITION A mild infectious disease occurring mainly in early childhood, marked by a rosy-red rash on the cheeks, often spreading to the trunk and limbs. Fever and arthritis may also be present.

B08.4 Enteroviral vesicular stomatitis with exanthem
Hand, foot and mouth disease

B08.5 Enteroviral vesicular pharyngitis
Herpangina

5 **B08.6** Parapoxvirus infections

B08.60 Parapoxvirus infection, unspecified

B08.61 Bovine stomatitis

B08.62 Sealpox

B08.69 Other parapoxvirus infections

5 **B08.7** Yatapoxvirus infections

B08.70 Yatapoxvirus infection, unspecified

B08.71 Tanapox virus disease

B08.72 Yaba pox virus disease
Yaba monkey tumor disease

B08.79 Other yatapoxvirus infections

B08.8 Other specified viral infections characterized by skin and mucous membrane lesions
Enteroviral lymphonodular pharyngitis
Foot-and-mouth disease
Poxvirus NEC

B09 Unspecified viral infection characterized by skin and mucous membrane lesions
Viral enanthema NOS
Viral exanthema NOS

Other human herpesviruses (B10)

4 **B10 Other human herpesviruses**
EXCLUDES 2 *cytomegalovirus (B25.9)*
Epstein-Barr virus (B27.0-)
herpes NOS (B00.9)
herpes simplex (B00.-)
herpes zoster (B02.-)
human herpesvirus NOS (B00.-)
human herpesvirus 1 and 2 (B00.-)
human herpesvirus 3 (B01.-, B02.-)
human herpesvirus 4 (B27.0-)
human herpesvirus 5 (B25.-)
varicella (B01.-)
zoster (B02.-)

5 **B10.0 Other human herpesvirus encephalitis**
EXCLUDES 2 *herpes encephalitis NOS (B00.4)*
herpes simplex encephalitis (B00.4)
human herpesvirus encephalitis (B00.4)
simian B herpes virus encephalitis (B00.4)
B10.01 Human herpesvirus 6 encephalitis HIV
B10.09 Other human herpesvirus encephalitis HIV
Human herpesvirus 7 encephalitis
5 **B10.8 Other human herpesvirus infection**
B10.81 Human herpesvirus 6 infection
B10.82 Human herpesvirus 7 infection
B10.89 Other human herpesvirus infection
Human herpesvirus 8 infection
Kaposi's sarcoma-associated herpesvirus infection

Viral hepatitis (B15-B19)

EXCLUDES 1 *sequelae of viral hepatitis (B94.2)*
EXCLUDES 2 *cytomegaloviral hepatitis (B25.1)*
herpesviral [herpes simplex] hepatitis (B00.81)

CODING TIP✓ When viral hepatitis is also documented as a confirmed diagnosis in a patient with any diagnosis classifiable to K74.-, the appropriate code from B15-B19 should also be assigned. The sequencing of the K74.- and the viral hepatitis code is according to focus of care.

4 **B15 Acute hepatitis A**
B15.0 Hepatitis A with hepatic coma
B15.9 Hepatitis A without hepatic coma
Hepatitis A (acute)(viral) NOS
4 **B16 Acute hepatitis B**
B16.0 Acute hepatitis B with delta-agent with hepatic coma
B16.1 Acute hepatitis B with delta-agent without hepatic coma
B16.2 Acute hepatitis B without delta-agent with hepatic coma
B16.9 Acute hepatitis B without delta-agent and without hepatic coma
Hepatitis B (acute) (viral) NOS
AHA: 3Q 2016, 13
4 **B17 Other acute viral hepatitis**
B17.0 Acute delta-(super) infection of hepatitis B carrier
5 **B17.1 Acute hepatitis C**
B17.10 Acute hepatitis C without hepatic coma
Acute hepatitis C NOS
B17.11 Acute hepatitis C with hepatic coma
B17.2 Acute hepatitis E
B17.8 Other specified acute viral hepatitis
Hepatitis non-A non-B (acute) (viral) NEC
B17.9 Acute viral hepatitis, unspecified
Acute hepatitis NOS
Acute infectious hepatitis NOS
4 **B18 Chronic viral hepatitis**
INCLUDES Carrier of viral hepatitis
B18.0 Chronic viral hepatitis B with delta-agent HCC
B18.1 Chronic viral hepatitis B without delta-agent HCC
Carrier of viral hepatitis B
Chronic (viral) hepatitis B
B18.2 Chronic viral hepatitis C HCC
Carrier of viral hepatitis C
AHA: 1Q 2017, 41
B18.8 Other chronic viral hepatitis HCC
Carrier of other viral hepatitis
B18.9 Chronic viral hepatitis, unspecified HCC
Carrier of unspecified viral hepatitis
4 **B19 Unspecified viral hepatitis**
B19.0 Unspecified viral hepatitis with hepatic coma
5 **B19.1 Unspecified viral hepatitis B**
B19.10 Unspecified viral hepatitis B without hepatic coma
Unspecified viral hepatitis B NOS
B19.11 Unspecified viral hepatitis B with hepatic coma
5 **B19.2 Unspecified viral hepatitis C**
B19.20 Unspecified viral hepatitis C without hepatic coma
Viral hepatitis C NOS
B19.21 Unspecified viral hepatitis C with hepatic coma
B19.9 Unspecified viral hepatitis without hepatic coma
Viral hepatitis NOS

Human immunodeficiency virus [HIV] disease (B20)

B20 Human immunodeficiency virus [HIV] disease HCC HIV
INCLUDES acquired immune deficiency syndrome [AIDS]
AIDS-related complex [ARC]
HIV infection, symptomatic
Code first:
Human immunodeficiency virus [HIV] disease complicating pregnancy, childbirth and the puerperium, if applicable (O98.7-)
Use additional code(s) to identify all manifestations of HIV infection
EXCLUDES 1 *asymptomatic human immunodeficiency virus [HIV] infection status (Z21)*
exposure to HIV virus (Z20.6)
inconclusive serologic evidence of HIV (R75)

GUIDELINES **Section I.C.1.a.1)**
Code only confirmed cases of HIV infection/illness: This [guideline] is an exception to the hospital inpatient guideline Section II, H. In this context, "confirmation" does not require documentation of positive serology or culture for HIV; the provider's diagnostic statement that the patient is HIV positive, or has an HIV-related illness is sufficient. B20, Human immunideficiency virus (HIV) disease should be assigned.

GUIDELINES **Section I.C.1.a.2)(a)**
If a patient is admitted for an HIV-related condition, the principal diagnosis should be B20, Human immunodeficiency virus [HIV] disease followed by additional diagnosis codes for all reported HIV-related conditions.

GUIDELINES **Section I.C.1.a.2)(b)**
If a patient with HIV disease is admitted for an unrelated condition (such as a traumatic injury), the code for the unrelated condition (e.g., the nature of injury code) should be the principal diagnosis. Other diagnoses would be B20 followed by additional diagnosis codes for all reported HIV-related conditions.

GUIDELINES **Section I.C.1.a.2)(c)**
Whether the patient is newly diagnosed or has had previous admissions/encounters for HIV conditions is irrelevant to the sequencing decision.

GUIDELINES **Section I.C.1.a.2)(e)**
Patients with inconclusive HIV serology, but no definitive diagnosis or manifestations of the illness, may be assigned code R75, Inconclusive laboratory evidence of human immunodeficiency virus [HIV].

GUIDELINES **Section I.C.1.a.2)(f)**
Patients previously diagnosed with any HIV illness (B20) should never be assigned to R75 or Z21, Asymptomatic human immunodeficiency virus [HIV] infection status.

Other viral diseases (B25-B34)

4 **B25 Cytomegaloviral disease**
EXCLUDES 1 *congenital cytomegalovirus infection (P35.1)*
cytomegaloviral mononucleosis (B27.1-)
B25.0 Cytomegaloviral pneumonitis HCC
B25.1 Cytomegaloviral hepatitis HCC
B25.2 Cytomegaloviral pancreatitis HCC
B25.8 Other cytomegaloviral diseases HCC HIV
Cytomegaloviral encephalitis
B25.9 Cytomegaloviral disease, unspecified HCC HIV
4 **B26 Mumps**
INCLUDES epidemic parotitis
infectious parotitis
B26.0 Mumps orchitis ♂
B26.1 Mumps meningitis
B26.2 Mumps encephalitis
B26.3 Mumps pancreatitis
5 **B26.8 Mumps with other complications**
B26.81 Mumps hepatitis
B26.82 Mumps myocarditis
B26.83 Mumps nephritis
B26.84 Mumps polyneuropathy

B26.85 Mumps arthritis HCC

B26.89 Other mumps complications

B26.9 Mumps without complication
Mumps NOS
Mumps parotitis NOS

B27 Infectious mononucleosis
INCLUDES glandular fever
monocytic angina
Pfeiffer's disease

B27.0 Gammaherpesviral mononucleosis
Mononucleosis due to Epstein-Barr virus

B27.00 Gammaherpesviral mononucleosis without complication

B27.01 Gammaherpesviral mononucleosis with polyneuropathy

B27.02 Gammaherpesviral mononucleosis with meningitis

B27.09 Gammaherpesviral mononucleosis with other complications
Hepatomegaly in gammaherpesviral mononucleosis

B27.1 Cytomegaloviral mononucleosis

B27.10 Cytomegaloviral mononucleosis without complications

B27.11 Cytomegaloviral mononucleosis with polyneuropathy

B27.12 Cytomegaloviral mononucleosis with meningitis

B27.19 Cytomegaloviral mononucleosis with other complication
Hepatomegaly in cytomegaloviral mononucleosis

B27.8 Other infectious mononucleosis

B27.80 Other infectious mononucleosis without complication

B27.81 Other infectious mononucleosis with polyneuropathy

B27.82 Other infectious mononucleosis with meningitis

B27.89 Other infectious mononucleosis with other complication
Hepatomegaly in other infectious mononucleosis

B27.9 Infectious mononucleosis, unspecified

B27.90 Infectious mononucleosis, unspecified without complication

B27.91 Infectious mononucleosis, unspecified with polyneuropathy

B27.92 Infectious mononucleosis, unspecified with meningitis

B27.99 Infectious mononucleosis, unspecified with other complication
Hepatomegaly in unspecified infectious mononucleosis

B30 Viral conjunctivitis
EXCLUDES 1 *herpesviral [herpes simplex] ocular disease (B00.5)*
ocular zoster (B02.3)

B30.0 Keratoconjunctivitis due to adenovirus
Epidemic keratoconjunctivitis
Shipyard eye

B30.1 Conjunctivitis due to adenovirus
Acute adenoviral follicular conjunctivitis
Swimming-pool conjunctivitis

B30.2 Viral pharyngoconjunctivitis

B30.3 Acute epidemic hemorrhagic conjunctivitis (enteroviral)
Conjunctivitis due to coxsackievirus 24
Conjunctivitis due to enterovirus 70
Hemorrhagic conjunctivitis (acute)(epidemic)

B30.8 Other viral conjunctivitis
Newcastle conjunctivitis

B30.9 Viral conjunctivitis, unspecified

B33 Other viral diseases, not elsewhere classified

B33.0 Epidemic myalgia
Bornholm disease

B33.1 Ross River disease
Epidemic polyarthritis and exanthema
Ross River fever

B33.2 Viral carditis
Coxsackie (virus) carditis

B33.20 Viral carditis, unspecified

B33.21 Viral endocarditis

B33.22 Viral myocarditis

B33.23 Viral pericarditis

B33.24 Viral cardiomyopathy HCC

B33.3 Retrovirus infections, not elsewhere classified
Retrovirus infection NOS

B33.4 Hantavirus (cardio)-pulmonary syndrome [HPS] [HCPS]
Hantavirus disease with pulmonary manifestations
Sin nombre virus disease
Use additional code to identify any associated acute kidney failure (N17.9)
EXCLUDES 1 *hantavirus disease with renal manifestations (A98.5)*
hemorrhagic fever with renal manifestations (A98.5)

B33.8 Other specified viral diseases
EXCLUDES 1 *anogenital human papillomavirus infection (A63.0)*
viral warts due to human papillomavirus infection (B07)

B34 Viral infection of unspecified site
EXCLUDES 1 *anogenital human papillomavirus infection (A63.0)*
cytomegaloviral disease NOS (B25.9)
herpesvirus [herpes simplex] infection NOS (B00.9)
retrovirus infection NOS (B33.3)
viral agents as the cause of diseases classified elsewhere (B97.-)
viral warts due to human papillomavirus infection (B07)

CODING TIP ✓ Avoid using these codes for viral-caused infections. Most viral infections have combination codes.

B34.0 Adenovirus infection, unspecified

B34.1 Enterovirus infection, unspecified
Coxsackievirus infection NOS
Echovirus infection NOS

B34.2 Coronavirus infection, unspecified
EXCLUDES 1 *pneumonia due to SARS-associated coronavirus (J12.81)*

B34.3 Parvovirus infection, unspecified

B34.4 Papovavirus infection, unspecified

B34.8 Other viral infections of unspecified site

B34.9 Viral infection, unspecified
Viremia NOS
AHA: 3Q 2016, 10

Mycoses (B35-B49)

EXCLUDES 2 *hypersensitivity pneumonitis due to organic dust (J67.-)*
mycosis fungoides (C84.0-)

B35 Dermatophytosis
INCLUDES favus
infections due to species of Epidermophyton, Micro-sporum and Trichophyton
tinea, any type except those in B36.-

B35.0 Tinea barbae and tinea capitis
Beard ringworm
Kerion
Scalp ringworm
Sycosis, mycotic

DEFINITION Superficial fungal infections of the skin of bearded parts of the face and neck, and the scalp.

B35.1 Tinea unguium
Dermatophytic onychia
Dermatophytosis of nail
Onychomycosis
Ringworm of nails

DEFINITION Fungal infection of the nails, first the surface, lateral and distal edges, and later, the part beneath the nail plate.

B35.2 Tinea manuum
Dermatophytosis of hand
Hand ringworm

B35.3 Tinea pedis
Athlete's foot
Dermatophytosis of foot
Foot ringworm

B35.4 Tinea corporis
Ringworm of the body

B35.5 Tinea imbricata
Tokelau

DEFINITION A fungal infection which affects skin with few or no hair follicles, typically seen in humid climates. The early lesion is annular with a circle of scales at the outside boundary.

B35.6 Tinea cruris
Dhobi itch
Groin ringworm
Jock itch

DEFINITION Fungal infection of the groin commonly known as jock itch.

B35.8 Other dermatophytoses
Disseminated dermatophytosis
Granulomatous dermatophytosis

B35.9 Dermatophytosis, unspecified
Ringworm NOS

4 B36 Other superficial mycoses

B36.0 Pityriasis versicolor
Tinea flava
Tinea versicolor

B36.1 Tinea nigra
Keratomycosis nigricans palmaris
Microsporosis nigra
Pityriasis nigra

DEFINITION A minor fungal infection having dark lesions with the appearance of spattered silver nitrate on the skin.

B36.2 White piedra
Tinea blanca

DEFINITION A fungal disease of hair covered skin, marked by pale patches and bald spot where the infection occurred.

B36.3 Black piedra
B36.8 Other specified superficial mycoses
B36.9 Superficial mycosis, unspecified

4 B37 Candidiasis

INCLUDES candidosis
moniliasis

EXCLUDES 1 *neonatal candidiasis (P37.5)*

B37.0 Candidal stomatitis HIV
Oral thrush

DEFINITION Fungal infection located in the mouth.

Candidal stomatitis
Candidiasis of the mouth (thrush)

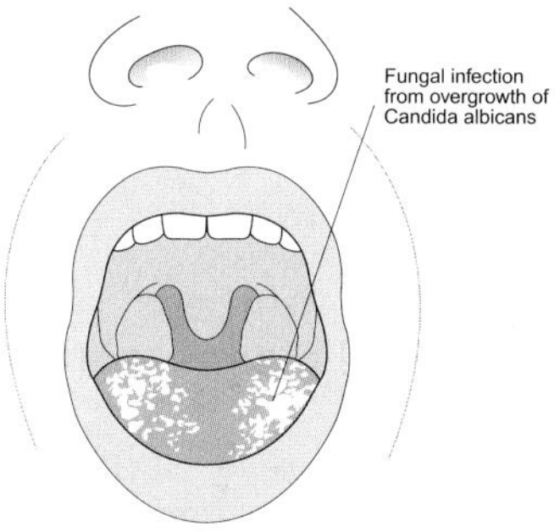

B37.1 Pulmonary candidiasis HCC HIV
Candidal bronchitis
Candidal pneumonia

B37.2 Candidiasis of skin and nail HIV
Candidal onychia
Candidal paronychia

EXCLUDES 2 *diaper dermatitis (L22)*

B37.3 Candidiasis of vulva and vagina ♀
Candidal vulvovaginitis
Monilial vulvovaginitis
Vaginal thrush

5 B37.4 Candidiasis of other urogenital sites

B37.41 Candidal cystitis and urethritis

CODING TIP ✓ B37.41 is a combination code that includes both the infection of the urinary tract and candida as the infectious cause. No additional codes should be assigned for urinary infection.

B37.42 Candidal balanitis ♂

B37.49 Other urogenital candidiasis
Candidal pyelonephritis

B37.5 Candidal meningitis HIV
B37.6 Candidal endocarditis HIV
B37.7 Candidal sepsis HCC
Disseminated candidiasis
Systemic candidiasis
AHA: 4Q 2014, 46

5 B37.8 Candidiasis of other sites

B37.81 Candidal esophagitis HCC HIV

DEFINITION Fungal infection of the esophagus, usually occurring in patients with immunocompromised states.

B37.82 Candidal enteritis HIV
Candidal proctitis
B37.83 Candidal cheilitis HIV
B37.84 Candidal otitis externa HIV
B37.89 Other sites of candidiasis HIV
Candidal osteomyelitis

B37.9 Candidiasis, unspecified HIV
Thrush NOS

4 B38 Coccidioidomycosis

Primary coccidioidomycosis (pulmonary)
A respiratory disease caused by inhaling the fungal spores of Coccidioides immitis or Coccidioides posadasii

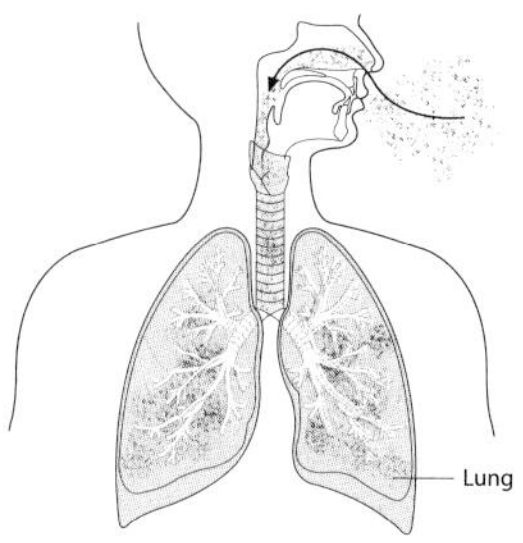

B38.0 Acute pulmonary coccidioidomycosis HCC HIV
B38.1 Chronic pulmonary coccidioidomycosis HCC HIV
B38.2 Pulmonary coccidioidomycosis, unspecified HCC HIV
B38.3 Cutaneous coccidioidomycosis HIV
B38.4 Coccidioidomycosis meningitis HIV
B38.7 Disseminated coccidioidomycosis HIV
Generalized coccidioidomycosis

5 B38.8 Other forms of coccidioidomycosis

B38.81 Prostatic coccidioidomycosis ♂ HIV
B38.89 Other forms of coccidioidomycosis HIV

B38.9 Coccidioidomycosis, unspecified HIV

▲ 4 B39 Histoplasmosis

Code first:
associated AIDS (B20)
Use additional code for any associated manifestations, such as:
endocarditis (I39)
meningitis (G02)
pericarditis (I32)
retinitis (H32)

CODING TIP ✓ Histoplasmosis (B39) is usually associated with HIV/AIDS. If so, then B20 is coded prior to using the B39 category code, unless other restrictions apply. (*See coding tip at category B20*).

B39.0 Acute pulmonary histoplasmosis capsulati HCC HIV
B39.1 Chronic pulmonary histoplasmosis capsulati HCC HIV
B39.2 Pulmonary histoplasmosis capsulati, unspecified HCC HIV
B39.3 Disseminated histoplasmosis capsulati HIV
Generalized histoplasmosis capsulati

B39.4 **Histoplasmosis capsulati, unspecified** HIV
American histoplasmosis
B39.5 **Histoplasmosis duboisii** HIV
African histoplasmosis
B39.9 **Histoplasmosis, unspecified** HIV

4 B40 Blastomycosis
EXCLUDES 1 *Brazilian blastomycosis (B41.-)*
keloidal blastomycosis (B48.0)
B40.0 **Acute pulmonary blastomycosis** HCC
B40.1 **Chronic pulmonary blastomycosis** HCC
B40.2 **Pulmonary blastomycosis, unspecified** HCC
B40.3 **Cutaneous blastomycosis**
B40.7 **Disseminated blastomycosis**
Generalized blastomycosis
5 B40.8 **Other forms of blastomycosis**
B40.81 **Blastomycotic meningoencephalitis**
Meningomyelitis due to blastomycosis
B40.89 **Other forms of blastomycosis**
B40.9 **Blastomycosis, unspecified**

4 B41 Paracoccidioidomycosis
INCLUDES Brazilian blastomycosis
Lutz' disease
B41.0 **Pulmonary paracoccidioidomycosis** HCC
B41.7 **Disseminated paracoccidioidomycosis**
Generalized paracoccidioidomycosis
B41.8 **Other forms of paracoccidioidomycosis**
B41.9 **Paracoccidioidomycosis, unspecified**

4 B42 Sporotrichosis
B42.0 **Pulmonary sporotrichosis**
B42.1 **Lymphocutaneous sporotrichosis**
B42.7 **Disseminated sporotrichosis**
Generalized sporotrichosis
5 B42.8 **Other forms of sporotrichosis**
B42.81 **Cerebral sporotrichosis**
Meningitis due to sporotrichosis
B42.82 **Sporotrichosis arthritis** HCC
B42.89 **Other forms of sporotrichosis**
B42.9 **Sporotrichosis, unspecified**

4 B43 Chromomycosis and pheomycotic abscess
B43.0 **Cutaneous chromomycosis**
Dermatitis verrucosa
B43.1 **Pheomycotic brain abscess**
Cerebral chromomycosis
B43.2 **Subcutaneous pheomycotic abscess and cyst**
B43.8 **Other forms of chromomycosis**
B43.9 **Chromomycosis, unspecified**

4 B44 Aspergillosis
INCLUDES aspergilloma
B44.0 **Invasive pulmonary aspergillosis** HCC
B44.1 **Other pulmonary aspergillosis** HCC
B44.2 **Tonsillar aspergillosis** HCC
B44.7 **Disseminated aspergillosis** HCC
Generalized aspergillosis
5 B44.8 **Other forms of aspergillosis**
B44.81 **Allergic bronchopulmonary aspergillosis** HCC
B44.89 **Other forms of aspergillosis** HCC
B44.9 **Aspergillosis, unspecified** HCC

4 B45 Cryptococcosis
B45.0 **Pulmonary cryptococcosis** HCC HIV
DEFINITION Yeastlike fungus infection, by cryptococcus neoformans, commonly occurring in the soil, which infects via the lungs and may spread to the brain and meninges.
B45.1 **Cerebral cryptococcosis** HCC
Cryptococcal meningitis
Cryptococcosis meningocerebralis
DEFINITION Infection of the brain and/or its surrounding tissues causing hydrocephalus and intracerebral cysts due to infection with cryptococcus fungus.
B45.2 **Cutaneous cryptococcosis** HCC HIV
B45.3 **Osseous cryptococcosis** HCC HIV
B45.7 **Disseminated cryptococcosis** HCC HIV
Generalized cryptococcosis
B45.8 **Other forms of cryptococcosis** HCC HIV
B45.9 **Cryptococcosis, unspecified** HCC HIV

4 B46 Zygomycosis
B46.0 **Pulmonary mucormycosis** HCC
B46.1 **Rhinocerebral mucormycosis** HCC
B46.2 **Gastrointestinal mucormycosis** HCC
B46.3 **Cutaneous mucormycosis** HCC
Subcutaneous mucormycosis
B46.4 **Disseminated mucormycosis** HCC
Generalized mucormycosis
B46.5 **Mucormycosis, unspecified** HCC
B46.8 **Other zygomycoses** HCC
Entomophthoromycosis
B46.9 **Zygomycosis, unspecified** HCC
Phycomycosis NOS

4 B47 Mycetoma
B47.0 **Eumycetoma**
Madura foot, mycotic
Maduromycosis
B47.1 **Actinomycetoma** HIV
B47.9 **Mycetoma, unspecified** HIV
Madura foot NOS
DEFINITION Chronic infection involving the feet, characterized by formation of localized lesions, with swelling and multiple draining sinuses.

4 B48 Other mycoses, not elsewhere classified
B48.0 **Lobomycosis**
Keloidal blastomycosis
Lobo's disease
DEFINITION A fungal infection of the skin caused by Lobo loboi and characterized by keloidal nodular lesions occurring on the face, ears, and extremities.
B48.1 **Rhinosporidiosis**
B48.2 **Allescheriasis**
Infection due to Pseudallescheria boydii
EXCLUDES 1 *eumycetoma (B47.0)*
B48.3 **Geotrichosis**
Geotrichum stomatitis
B48.4 **Penicillosis** HCC
B48.8 **Other specified mycoses** HCC HIV
Adiaspiromycosis
Infection of tissue and organs by Alternaria
Infection of tissue and organs by Drechslera
Infection of tissue and organs by Fusarium
Infection of tissue and organs by saprophytic fungi NEC
AHA: 2Q 2014, 13
AHA: 4Q 2014, 46

B49 Unspecified mycosis
Fungemia NOS

Protozoal diseases (B50-B64)

EXCLUDES 1 *amebiasis (A06.-)*
other protozoal intestinal diseases (A07.-)

4 B50 Plasmodium falciparum malaria
INCLUDES mixed infections of Plasmodium falciparum with any other Plasmodium species
B50.0 **Plasmodium falciparum malaria with cerebral complications**
Cerebral malaria NOS
B50.8 **Other severe and complicated Plasmodium falciparum malaria**
Severe or complicated Plasmodium falciparum malaria NOS
B50.9 **Plasmodium falciparum malaria, unspecified**

▲ 4 B51 Plasmodium vivax malaria
INCLUDES mixed infections of Plasmodium vivax with other Plasmodium species, except Plasmodium falciparum
EXCLUDES 1 *plasmodium vivax with Plasmodium falciparum (B50.-)*
B51.0 **Plasmodium vivax malaria with rupture of spleen**
B51.8 **Plasmodium vivax malaria with other complications**

B51.9 **Plasmodium vivax malaria without complication**
Plasmodium vivax malaria NOS

4 **B52 Plasmodium malariae malaria**
INCLUDES mixed infections of Plasmodium malariae with other Plasmodium species, except Plasmodium falciparum and Plasmodium vivax
EXCLUDES 1 *Plasmodium falciparum (B50.-)*
Plasmodium vivax (B51.-)

B52.0 **Plasmodium malariae malaria with nephropathy**
B52.8 **Plasmodium malariae malaria with other complications**
B52.9 **Plasmodium malariae malaria without complication**
Plasmodium malariae malaria NOS

4 **B53 Other specified malaria**
B53.0 **Plasmodium ovale malaria**
EXCLUDES 1 *Plasmodium ovale with Plasmodium falciparum (B50.-)*
Plasmodium ovale with Plasmodium malariae (B52.-)
Plasmodium ovale with Plasmodium vivax (B51.-)

B53.1 **Malaria due to simian plasmodia**
EXCLUDES 1 *Malaria due to simian plasmodia with Plasmodium falciparum (B50.-)*
Malaria due to simian plasmodia with Plasmodium malariae (B52.-)
Malaria due to simian plasmodia with Plasmodium ovale (B53.0)
Malaria due to simian plasmodia with Plasmodium vivax (B51.-)

B53.8 **Other malaria, not elsewhere classified**

B54 Unspecified malaria

Malaria Life Cycle

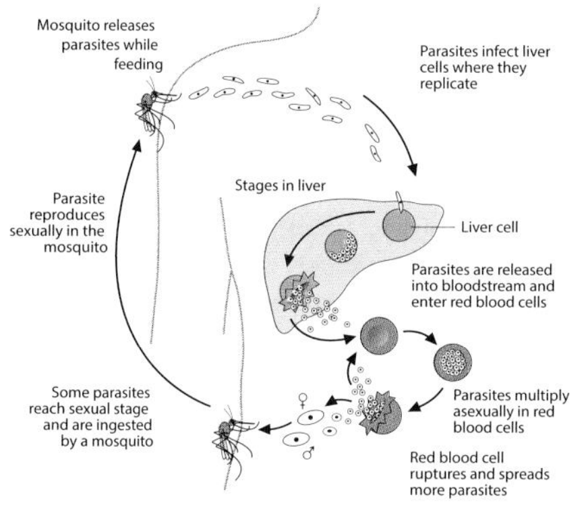

4 **B55 Leishmaniasis**
B55.0 **Visceral leishmaniasis**
Kala-azar
Post-kala-azar dermal leishmaniasis
B55.1 **Cutaneous leishmaniasis**
B55.2 **Mucocutaneous leishmaniasis**
B55.9 **Leishmaniasis, unspecified**

4 **B56 African trypanosomiasis**
B56.0 **Gambiense trypanosomiasis**
Infection due to Trypanosoma brucei gambiense
West African sleeping sickness
B56.1 **Rhodesiense trypanosomiasis**
East African sleeping sickness
Infection due to Trypanosoma brucei rhodesiense
B56.9 **African trypanosomiasis, unspecified**
Sleeping sickness NOS

4 **B57 Chagas' disease**
INCLUDES American trypanosomiasis
infection due to Trypanosoma cruzi

B57.0 **Acute Chagas' disease with heart involvement**
Acute Chagas' disease with myocarditis
B57.1 **Acute Chagas' disease without heart involvement**
Acute Chagas' disease NOS
B57.2 **Chagas' disease (chronic) with heart involvement**
American trypanosomiasis NOS
Chagas' disease (chronic) NOS
Chagas' disease (chronic) with myocarditis
Trypanosomiasis NOS
5 B57.3 **Chagas' disease (chronic) with digestive system involvement**
B57.30 **Chagas' disease with digestive system involvement, unspecified**
B57.31 **Megaesophagus in Chagas' disease**
B57.32 **Megacolon in Chagas' disease**
B57.39 **Other digestive system involvement in Chagas' disease**
5 B57.4 **Chagas' disease (chronic) with nervous system involvement**
B57.40 **Chagas' disease with nervous system involvement, unspecified**
B57.41 **Meningitis in Chagas' disease**
B57.42 **Meningoencephalitis in Chagas' disease**
B57.49 **Other nervous system involvement in Chagas' disease**
B57.5 **Chagas' disease (chronic) with other organ involvement**

4 **B58 Toxoplasmosis**
INCLUDES infection due to Toxoplasma gondii
EXCLUDES 1 *congenital toxoplasmosis (P37.1)*

5 B58.0 **Toxoplasma oculopathy**
B58.00 **Toxoplasma oculopathy, unspecified** HIV
B58.01 **Toxoplasma chorioretinitis** HIV
B58.09 **Other toxoplasma oculopathy** HIV
Toxoplasma uveitis
B58.1 **Toxoplasma hepatitis** HIV
B58.2 **Toxoplasma meningoencephalitis** HCC HIV
B58.3 **Pulmonary toxoplasmosis** HCC HIV
5 B58.8 **Toxoplasmosis with other organ involvement**
B58.81 **Toxoplasma myocarditis** HIV
B58.82 **Toxoplasma myositis** HIV
B58.83 **Toxoplasma tubulo-interstitial nephropathy** HIV
Toxoplasma pyelonephritis
B58.89 **Toxoplasmosis with other organ involvement** HIV
B58.9 **Toxoplasmosis, unspecified** HIV

B59 Pneumocystosis HCC HIV
Pneumonia due to Pneumocystis carinii
Pneumonia due to Pneumocystis jiroveci

CODING TIP ✓ Pneumocystosis is usually associated with HIV/AIDS. If so, then B20 is coded prior to using the B59 category code, unless other restrictions apply. (*See coding tip at category B20.*)

4 **B60 Other protozoal diseases, not elsewhere classified**
EXCLUDES 1 *cryptosporidiosis (A07.2)*
intestinal microsporidiosis (A07.8)
isosporiasis (A07.3)

B60.0 **Babesiosis**
Piroplasmosis
5 B60.1 **Acanthamebiasis**
B60.10 **Acanthamebiasis, unspecified**
B60.11 **Meningoencephalitis due to Acanthamoeba (culbertsoni)**
B60.12 **Conjunctivitis due to Acanthamoeba**
B60.13 **Keratoconjunctivitis due to Acanthamoeba**
B60.19 **Other acanthamebic disease**
B60.2 **Naegleriasis**
Primary amebic meningoencephalitis
B60.8 **Other specified protozoal diseases** HIV
Microsporidiosis

B64 Unspecified protozoal disease

Helminthiases (B65-B83)

4 **B65 Schistosomiasis [bilharziasis]**
INCLUDES snail fever

B65.0 **Schistosomiasis due to Schistosoma haematobium [urinary schistosomiasis]**
B65.1 **Schistosomiasis due to Schistosoma mansoni [intestinal schistosomiasis]**

B65.2 **Schistosomiasis due to Schistosoma japonicum**
Asiatic schistosomiasis
B65.3 **Cercarial dermatitis**
Swimmer's itch
DEFINITION An itching inflammation of the skin due to penetration of larval forms of schistosomes (parasitic worms), occurring in bathers of infested waters.
B65.8 **Other schistosomiasis**
Infection due to Schistosoma intercalatum
Infection due to Schistosoma mattheei
Infection due to Schistosoma mekongi
B65.9 **Schistosomiasis, unspecified**

B66 Other fluke infections
B66.0 **Opisthorchiasis**
Infection due to cat liver fluke
Infection due to Opisthorchis (felineus)(viverrini)
B66.1 **Clonorchiasis**
Chinese liver fluke disease
Infection due to Clonorchis sinensis
Oriental liver fluke disease
B66.2 **Dicroceliasis**
Infection due to Dicrocoelium dendriticum
Lancet fluke infection
B66.3 **Fascioliasis**
Infection due to Fasciola gigantica
Infection due to Fasciola hepatica
Infection due to Fasciola indica
Sheep liver fluke disease
B66.4 **Paragonimiasis** HCC
Infection due to Paragonimus species
Lung fluke disease
Pulmonary distomiasis
B66.5 **Fasciolopsiasis**
Infection due to Fasciolopsis buski
Intestinal distomiasis
B66.8 **Other specified fluke infections**
Echinostomiasis
Heterophyiasis
Metagonimiasis
Nanophyetiasis
Watsoniasis
B66.9 **Fluke infection, unspecified**

B67 Echinococcosis
INCLUDES hydatidosis
B67.0 **Echinococcus granulosus infection of liver**
DEFINITION A genus of parasitic tapeworm passed from dogs. The larvae form large cysts in the liver, causing serious and sometimes fatal disease.
B67.1 **Echinococcus granulosus infection of lung** HCC
B67.2 **Echinococcus granulosus infection of bone**
B67.3 **Echinococcus granulosus infection, other and multiple sites**
B67.31 **Echinococcus granulosus infection, thyroid gland**
B67.32 **Echinococcus granulosus infection, multiple sites**
B67.39 **Echinococcus granulosus infection, other sites**
B67.4 **Echinococcus granulosus infection, unspecified**
Dog tapeworm (infection)
B67.5 **Echinococcus multilocularis infection of liver**
B67.6 **Echinococcus multilocularis infection, other and multiple sites**
B67.61 **Echinococcus multilocularis infection, multiple sites**
B67.69 **Echinococcus multilocularis infection, other sites**
B67.7 **Echinococcus multilocularis infection, unspecified**
B67.8 **Echinococcosis, unspecified, of liver**
B67.9 **Echinococcosis, other and unspecified**
B67.90 **Echinococcosis, unspecified**
Echinococcosis NOS
B67.99 **Other echinococcosis**

B68 Taeniasis
EXCLUDES 1 *cysticercosis (B69.-)*
B68.0 **Taenia solium taeniasis**
Pork tapeworm (infection)
B68.1 **Taenia saginata taeniasis**
Beef tapeworm (infection)
Infection due to adult tapeworm Taenia saginata
B68.9 **Taeniasis, unspecified**

B69 Cysticercosis
INCLUDES cysticerciasis infection due to larval form of Taenia solium
B69.0 **Cysticercosis of central nervous system**
B69.1 **Cysticercosis of eye**
B69.8 **Cysticercosis of other sites**
B69.81 **Myositis in cysticercosis**
B69.89 **Cysticercosis of other sites**
B69.9 **Cysticercosis, unspecified**
DEFINITION Infection caused by the pork tapeworm when its larvae enter the body and form cysts.

B70 Diphyllobothriasis and sparganosis
B70.0 **Diphyllobothriasis**
Diphyllobothrium (adult) (latum) (pacificum) infection
Fish tapeworm (infection)
EXCLUDES 2 *larval diphyllobothriasis (B70.1)*
B70.1 **Sparganosis**
Infection due to Sparganum (mansoni) (proliferum)
Infection due to Spirometra larva
Larval diphyllobothriasis
Spirometrosis

B71 Other cestode infections
B71.0 **Hymenolepiasis**
Dwarf tapeworm infection
Rat tapeworm (infection)
B71.1 **Dipylidiasis**
B71.8 **Other specified cestode infections**
Coenurosis
B71.9 **Cestode infection, unspecified**
Tapeworm (infection) NOS

B72 Dracunculiasis
INCLUDES guinea worm infection
infection due to Dracunculus medinensis

B73 Onchocerciasis
INCLUDES onchocerca volvulus infection
onchocercosis
river blindness
B73.0 **Onchocerciasis with eye disease**
B73.00 **Onchocerciasis with eye involvement, unspecified**
B73.01 **Onchocerciasis with endophthalmitis**
B73.02 **Onchocerciasis with glaucoma**
B73.09 **Onchocerciasis with other eye involvement**
Infestation of eyelid due to onchocerciasis
B73.1 **Onchocerciasis without eye disease**

B74 Filariasis
EXCLUDES 2 *onchocerciasis (B73)*
tropical (pulmonary) eosinophilia NOS (J82)
B74.0 **Filariasis due to Wuchereria bancrofti**
Bancroftian elephantiasis
Bancroftian filariasis
B74.1 **Filariasis due to Brugia malayi**
B74.2 **Filariasis due to Brugia timori**
B74.3 **Loiasis**
Calabar swelling
Eyeworm disease of Africa
Loa loa infection
B74.4 **Mansonelliasis**
Infection due to Mansonella ozzardi
Infection due to Mansonella perstans
Infection due to Mansonella streptocerca
B74.8 **Other filariases**
Dirofilariasis
B74.9 **Filariasis, unspecified**

B75 Trichinellosis
INCLUDES infection due to Trichinella species
trichiniasis

B76 Hookworm diseases
INCLUDES uncinariasis
B76.0 **Ancylostomiasis**
Infection due to Ancylostoma species
B76.1 **Necatoriasis**
Infection due to Necator americanus
B76.8 **Other hookworm diseases**
B76.9 **Hookworm disease, unspecified**
Cutaneous larva migrans NOS

B77 Ascariasis
INCLUDES ascaridiasis
roundworm infection
B77.0 Ascariasis with intestinal complications
B77.8 Ascariasis with other complications
B77.81 Ascariasis pneumonia
B77.89 Ascariasis with other complications
B77.9 Ascariasis, unspecified

B78 Strongyloidiasis
EXCLUDES 1 *trichostrongyliasis (B81.2)*
B78.0 Intestinal strongyloidiasis HIV
B78.1 Cutaneous strongyloidiasis
B78.7 Disseminated strongyloidiasis HIV
B78.9 Strongyloidiasis, unspecified HIV

B79 Trichuriasis
INCLUDES trichocephaliasis
whipworm (disease) (infection)

B80 Enterobiasis
INCLUDES oxyuriasis
pinworm infection
threadworm infection

B81 Other intestinal helminthiases, not elsewhere classified
EXCLUDES 1 *angiostrongyliasis due to:*
Angiostrongylus cantonensis (B83.2)
Parastrongylus cantonensis (B83.2)
B81.0 Anisakiasis
Infection due to Anisakis larva
B81.1 Intestinal capillariasis
Capillariasis NOS
Infection due to Capillaria philippinensis
EXCLUDES 2 *hepatic capillariasis (B83.8)*
B81.2 Trichostrongyliasis
B81.3 Intestinal angiostrongyliasis
Angiostrongyliasis due to:
Angiostrongylus costaricensis
Parastrongylus costaricensis
B81.4 Mixed intestinal helminthiases
Infection due to intestinal helminths classified to more than one of the categories B65.0-B81.3 and B81.8
Mixed helminthiasis NOS
B81.8 Other specified intestinal helminthiases
Infection due to Oesophagostomum species [esophagostomiasis]
Infection due to Ternidens diminutus [ternidensiasis]

B82 Unspecified intestinal parasitism
B82.0 Intestinal helminthiasis, unspecified
B82.9 Intestinal parasitism, unspecified

B83 Other helminthiases
EXCLUDES 1 *capillariasis NOS (B81.1)*
EXCLUDES 2 *intestinal capillariasis (B81.1)*
B83.0 Visceral larva migrans
Toxocariasis
B83.1 Gnathostomiasis
Wandering swelling
B83.2 Angiostrongyliasis due to Parastrongylus cantonensis
Eosinophilic meningoencephalitis due to Parastrongylus cantonensis
EXCLUDES 2 *intestinal angiostrongyliasis (B81.3)*
B83.3 Syngamiasis
Syngamosis
B83.4 Internal hirudiniasis
EXCLUDES 2 *external hirudiniasis (B88.3)*
B83.8 Other specified helminthiases
Acanthocephaliasis
Gongylonemiasis
Hepatic capillariasis
Metastrongyliasis
Thelaziasis
B83.9 Helminthiasis, unspecified
Worms NOS
EXCLUDES 1 *intestinal helminthiasis NOS (B82.0)*

Pediculosis, acariasis and other infestations (B85-B89)

B85 Pediculosis and phthiriasis
B85.0 Pediculosis due to Pediculus humanus capitis
Head-louse infestation
B85.1 Pediculosis due to Pediculus humanus corporis
Body-louse infestation
B85.2 Pediculosis, unspecified
B85.3 Phthiriasis
Infestation by crab-louse
Infestation by Phthirus pubis
B85.4 Mixed pediculosis and phthiriasis
Infestation classifiable to more than one of the categories B85.0-B85.3

B86 Scabies
Sarcoptic itch

B87 Myiasis
INCLUDES infestation by larva of flies
B87.0 Cutaneous myiasis
Creeping myiasis
DEFINITION Infestation by the fly larvae of the genus Oestrus causing inflamed furuncles where the larvae are maturing beneath the skin.
B87.1 Wound myiasis
Traumatic myiasis
B87.2 Ocular myiasis
B87.3 Nasopharyngeal myiasis
Laryngeal myiasis
B87.4 Aural myiasis
B87.8 Myiasis of other sites
B87.81 Genitourinary myiasis
B87.82 Intestinal myiasis
B87.89 Myiasis of other sites
B87.9 Myiasis, unspecified

B88 Other infestations
B88.0 Other acariasis
Acarine dermatitis
Dermatitis due to Demodex species
Dermatitis due to Dermanyssus gallinae
Dermatitis due to Liponyssoides sanguineus
Trombiculosis
EXCLUDES 2 *scabies (B86)*
B88.1 Tungiasis [sandflea infestation]
B88.2 Other arthropod infestations
Scarabiasis
B88.3 External hirudiniasis
Leech infestation NOS
EXCLUDES 2 *internal hirudiniasis (B83.4)*
B88.8 Other specified infestations
Ichthyoparasitism due to Vandellia cirrhosa
Linguatulosis
Porocephaliasis
B88.9 Infestation, unspecified
Infestation (skin) NOS
Infestation by mites NOS
Skin parasites NOS

B89 Unspecified parasitic disease

Sequelae of infectious and parasitic diseases (B90-B94)

Note: Categories B90-B94 are to be used to indicate conditions in categories A00-B89 as the cause of sequelae, which are themselves classified elsewhere. The 'sequelae' include conditions specified as such; they also include residuals of diseases classifiable to the above categories if there is evidence that the disease itself is no longer present. Codes from these categories are not to be used for chronic infections. Code chronic current infections to active infectious disease as appropriate.
Code first:
condition resulting from (sequela) the infectious or parasitic disease

B90 Sequelae of tuberculosis

CODING TIP ✓ Conditions classified here are specifically reportable as sequelae or late effects of tuberculosis. The active disease is no longer present. Acute tuberculosis should be coded to A15-A19.

B90.0 **Sequelae of central nervous system tuberculosis**

B90.1 **Sequelae of genitourinary tuberculosis**

B90.2 **Sequelae of tuberculosis of bones and joints**

B90.8 **Sequelae of tuberculosis of other organs**

EXCLUDES 2 *sequelae of respiratory tuberculosis (B90.9)*

B90.9 **Sequelae of respiratory and unspecified tuberculosis**

Sequelae of tuberculosis NOS

B91 **Sequelae of poliomyelitis**

EXCLUDES 1 *postpolio syndrome (G14)*

CODING TIP ✓ Conditions classified here are specifically reportable as sequelae of poliomyelitis. Acute poliomyelitis should be coded to A80. When postpolio syndrome is specified, report code G14 rather than B91.

B92 **Sequelae of leprosy**

4 **B94** **Sequelae of other and unspecified infectious and parasitic diseases**

B94.0 **Sequelae of trachoma**

B94.1 **Sequelae of viral encephalitis**

B94.2 **Sequelae of viral hepatitis**

B94.8 **Sequelae of other specified infectious and parasitic diseases**

AHA: 4Q 2017, 85

B94.9 **Sequelae of unspecified infectious and parasitic disease**

Bacterial and viral infectious agents (B95-B97)

Note: These categories are provided for use as supplementary or additional codes to identify the infectious agent(s) in diseases classified elsewhere.

GUIDELINES **Section I.C.1.b**

Certain infections are classified in chapters other than Chapter 1 and no organism is identified as part of the infection code. In these instances, it is necessary to use an additional code from Chapter 1 to identify the organism. A code from category B95, Streptococcus, Staphylococcus, and Enterococcus as the cause of diseases classified to other chapters, B96, Other bacterial agents as the cause of diseases classified to other chapters, or B97, Viral agents as the cause of diseases classified to other chapters, is to be used as an additional code to identify the organism. An instructional note will be found at the infection code advising that an additional organism code is required.

Section I.C.1.c

Many bacterial infections are resistant to current antibiotics. It is necessary to identify all infections documented as antibiotic resistant. Assign a code from category Z16, Resistance to antimicrobial drugs, following the infection code only if the infection code does not identify drug resistance.

CODING TIP ✓ Conditions classified here are specifically reportable as additional codes to identify infectious agents in diseases classified elsewhere. Do not assign codes from B95-B97 without a code for the underlying disease process first.

4 **B95** **Streptococcus, Staphylococcus, and Enterococcus as the cause of diseases classified elsewhere**

B95.0 **Streptococcus, group A, as the cause of diseases classified elsewhere**

B95.1 **Streptococcus, group B, as the cause of diseases classified elsewhere**

B95.2 **Enterococcus as the cause of diseases classified elsewhere**

B95.3 **Streptococcus pneumoniae as the cause of diseases classified elsewhere**

B95.4 **Other streptococcus as the cause of diseases classified elsewhere**

B95.5 **Unspecified streptococcus as the cause of diseases classified elsewhere**

5 **B95.6** **Staphylococcus aureus as the cause of diseases classified elsewhere**

B95.61 **Methicillin susceptible Staphylococcus aureus infection as the cause of diseases classified elsewhere**

Methicillin susceptible Staphylococcus aureus (MSSA) infection as the cause of diseases classified elsewhere

Staphylococcus aureus infection NOS as the cause of diseases classified elsewhere

B95.62 **Methicillin resistant Staphylococcus aureus infection as the cause of diseases classified elsewhere**

Methicillin resistant staphylococcus aureus (MRSA) infection as the cause of diseases classified elsewhere

GUIDELINES **Section I.C.1.e.1)**

Selection and sequencing of MRSA codes:

(a) Combination codes for MRSA infection. When a patient is diagnosed with an infection that is due to MRSA, and that infection has a combination code that includes the causal organism (e.g., sepsis, pneumonia) assign the appropriate combination code for the condition (e.g., code A41.02, Sepsis due to Methicillin resistant Staphylococcus aureus or code J15.212, Pneumonia due to Methicillin resistant Staphylococcus aureus). Do not assign code B95.62, Methicillin resistant Staphylococcus aureus infection as the cause of diseases classified elsewhere, as an additional code because the combination code includes the type of infection and the MRSA organism. Do not assign a code from subcategory Z16.11, Resistance to penicillins, as an additional diagnosis.

(b) Other codes for MRSA infection. When there is documentation of a current infection (e.g., wound infection, stitch abscess, urinary tract infection) due to MRSA, and that infection does not have a combination code that includes the causal organism, assign the appropriate code to identify the condition along with code B95.62, Methicillin resistant Staphylococcus aureus infection as the cause of diseases classified elsewhere for the MRSA infection. Do not assign a code from subcategory Z16.11, Resistance to penicillins.

AHA: 1Q 2016, 12-13

B95.7 **Other staphylococcus as the cause of diseases classified elsewhere**

CODING TIP ✓ Use this code when another staph is identified, such as Staphyloccus epidermidis.

B95.8 **Unspecified staphylococcus as the cause of diseases classified elsewhere**

4 **B96** **Other bacterial agents as the cause of diseases classified elsewhere**

B96.0 **Mycoplasma pneumoniae [M. pneumoniae] as the cause of diseases classified elsewhere**

Pleuro-pneumonia-like-organism [PPLO]

B96.1 **Klebsiella pneumoniae [K. pneumoniae] as the cause of diseases classified elsewhere**

5 **B96.2** **Escherichia coli [E. coli] as the cause of diseases classified elsewhere**

B96.20 **Unspecified Escherichia coli [E. coli] as the cause of diseases classified elsewhere**

Escherichia coli [E. coli] NOS

B96.21 **Shiga toxin-producing Escherichia coli [E. coli] (STEC) O157 as the cause of diseases classified elsewhere**

E. coli O157:H- (nonmotile) with confirmation of Shiga toxin

E. coli O157 with confirmation of Shiga toxin when H antigen is unknown, or is not H7

O157:H7 Escherichia coli [E.coli] with or without confirmation of Shiga toxin-production

Shiga toxin-producing Escherichia coli [E.coli] O157:H7 with or without confirmation of Shiga toxin-production

STEC O157:H7 with or without confirmation of Shiga toxin-production

B96.22 **Other specified Shiga toxin-producing Escherichia coli [E. coli] (STEC) as the cause of diseases classified elsewhere**

Non-O157 Shiga toxin-producing Escherichia coli [E.coli]

Non-O157 Shiga toxin-producing Escherichia coli [E.coli] with known O group

B96.23 Unspecified Shiga toxin-producing Escherichia coli [E. coli] (STEC) as the cause of diseases classified elsewhere
Shiga toxin-producing Escherichia coli [E. coli] with unspecified O group
STEC NOS

B96.29 Other Escherichia coli [E. coli] as the cause of diseases classified elsewhere
Non-Shiga toxin-producing E. coli

B96.3 Hemophilus influenzae [H. influenzae] as the cause of diseases classified elsewhere

B96.4 Proteus (mirabilis) (morganii) as the cause of diseases classified elsewhere

B96.5 Pseudomonas (aeruginosa) (mallei) (pseudomallei) as the cause of diseases classified elsewhere
AHA: 1Q 2015, 18

B96.6 Bacteroides fragilis [B. fragilis] as the cause of diseases classified elsewhere

B96.7 Clostridium perfringens [C. perfringens] as the cause of diseases classified elsewhere
CODING TIP✓ Clostridium difficile is coded to A04.7-.

5 B96.8 Other specified bacterial agents as the cause of diseases classified elsewhere

B96.81 Helicobacter pylori [H. pylori] as the cause of diseases classified elsewhere
DEFINITION Common gastric pathogen causing dyspepsia, gastritis, peptic ulcer disease, gastric adenocarcinoma, and gastric lymphoma.

B96.82 Vibrio vulnificus as the cause of diseases classified elsewhere

B96.89 Other specified bacterial agents as the cause of diseases classified elsewhere
CODING TIP✓ Do not use to indicate an unknown bacteria causing a localized infection. If the bacteria is unknown, there is no need to add a code for the bacteria.

4 B97 Viral agents as the cause of diseases classified elsewhere
CODING TIP✓ Most viral conditions use combination codes. Search the index for the specific condition before choosing B97 codes.

B97.0 Adenovirus as the cause of diseases classified elsewhere

5 B97.1 Enterovirus as the cause of diseases classified elsewhere

B97.10 Unspecified enterovirus as the cause of diseases classified elsewhere

B97.11 Coxsackievirus as the cause of diseases classified elsewhere

B97.12 Echovirus as the cause of diseases classified elsewhere
DEFINITION A group of DNA-containing viruses that affect the tissue linings of the respiratory tract, eyes, intestines, and urinary tract. There are approximately 50 serotypes.

B97.19 Other enterovirus as the cause of diseases classified elsewhere

5 B97.2 Coronavirus as the cause of diseases classified elsewhere

B97.21 SARS-associated coronavirus as the cause of diseases classified elsewhere
EXCLUDES 1 *pneumonia due to SARS-associated coronavirus (J12.81)*

B97.29 Other coronavirus as the cause of diseases classified elsewhere

5 B97.3 Retrovirus as the cause of diseases classified elsewhere
EXCLUDES 1 *Human immunodeficiency virus [HIV] disease (B20)*

B97.30 Unspecified retrovirus as the cause of diseases classified elsewhere

B97.31 Lentivirus as the cause of diseases classified elsewhere

B97.32 Oncovirus as the cause of diseases classified elsewhere

B97.33 Human T-cell lymphotrophic virus, type I [HTLV-I] as the cause of diseases classified elsewhere

B97.34 Human T-cell lymphotrophic virus, type II [HTLV-II] as the cause of diseases classified elsewhere

B97.35 Human immunodeficiency virus, type 2 [HIV 2] as the cause of diseases classified elsewhere HCC

B97.39 Other retrovirus as the cause of diseases classified elsewhere

B97.4 Respiratory syncytial virus as the cause of diseases classified elsewhere

B97.5 Reovirus as the cause of diseases classified elsewhere

B97.6 Parvovirus as the cause of diseases classified elsewhere

B97.7 Papillomavirus as the cause of diseases classified elsewhere

5 B97.8 Other viral agents as the cause of diseases classified elsewhere

B97.81 Human metapneumovirus as the cause of diseases classified elsewhere

B97.89 Other viral agents as the cause of diseases classified elsewhere
AHA: 3Q 2016, 8-9
AHA: 3Q 2016, 14

Other infectious diseases (B99)

4 B99 Other and unspecified infectious diseases
CODING TIP✓ Do not use to indicate an unknown bacteria causing a localized infection. If the bacteria is unknown, there is no need to add a code for the bacteria.

B99.8 Other infectious disease HIV

B99.9 Unspecified infectious disease

CHAPTER 2: NEOPLASMS (C00-D49)

Note: Functional activity

All neoplasms are classified in this chapter, whether they are functionally active or not. An additional code from Chapter 4 may be used, to identify functional activity associated with any neoplasm.

Morphology [Histology]

Chapter 2 classifies neoplasms primarily by site (topography), with broad groupings for behavior, malignant, in situ, benign, etc. The Table of Neoplasms should be used to identify the correct topography code. In a few cases, such as for malignant melanoma and certain neuroendocrine tumors, the morphology (histologic type) is included in the category and codes.

Primary malignant neoplasms overlapping site boundaries

A primary malignant neoplasm that overlaps two or more contiguous (next to each other) sites should be classified to the subcategory/code .8 ('overlapping lesion'), unless the combination is specifically indexed elsewhere. For multiple neoplasms of the same site that are not contiguous, such as tumors in different quadrants of the same breast, codes for each site should be assigned.

Malignant neoplasm of ectopic tissue

Malignant neoplasms of ectopic tissue are to be coded to the site mentioned, e.g., ectopic pancreatic malignant neoplasms are coded to pancreas, unspecified (C25.9).

GUIDELINES **Section I.C.2**

Chapter 2 of the ICD-10-CM contains the codes for most benign and all malignant neoplasms. Certain benign neoplasms, such as prostatic adenomas, may be found in the specific body system chapters. To properly code a neoplasm it is necessary to determine from the record if the neoplasm is benign, in-situ, malignant, or of uncertain histologic behavior. If malignant, any secondary (metastatic) sites should also be determined.

GUIDELINES **Section I.C.2**

The neoplasm table in the Alphabetic Index should be referenced first. However, if the histological term is documented, that term should be referenced first, rather than going immediately to the Neoplasm Table, in order to determine which column in the Neoplasm Table is appropriate. For example, if the documentation indicates "adenoma," refer to the term in the Alphabetic Index to review the entries under this term and the instructional note to "see also neoplasm, by site, benign." The table provides the proper code based on the type of neoplasm and the site.

This chapter contains the following blocks:

C00-C14	Malignant neoplasms of lip, oral cavity and pharynx
C15-C26	Malignant neoplasms of digestive organs
C30-C39	Malignant neoplasms of respiratory and intrathoracic organs
C40-C41	Malignant neoplasms of bone and articular cartilage
C43-C44	Melanoma and other malignant neoplasms of skin
C45-C49	Malignant neoplasms of mesothelial and soft tissue
C50	Malignant neoplasms of breast
C51-C58	Malignant neoplasms of female genital organs
C60-C63	Malignant neoplasms of male genital organs
C64-C68	Malignant neoplasms of urinary tract
C69-C72	Malignant neoplasms of eye, brain and other parts of central nervous system
C73-C75	Malignant neoplasms of thyroid and other endocrine glands
C7A	Malignant neuroendocrine tumors
C7B	Secondary neuroendocrine tumors
C76-C80	Malignant neoplasms of ill-defined, other secondary and unspecified sites
C81-C96	Malignant neoplasms of lymphoid, hematopoietic and related tissue
D00-D09	In situ neoplasms
D10-D36	Benign neoplasms, except benign neuroendocrine tumors
D3A	Benign neuroendocrine tumors
D37-D48	Neoplasms of uncertain behavior, polycythemia vera and myelodysplastic syndromes
D49	Neoplasms of unspecified behavior

Malignant neoplasms (C00-C96)

Malignant neoplasms, stated or presumed to be primary (of specified sites), and certain specified histologies, except neuroendocrine, and of lymphoid, hematopoietic and related tissue (C00-C75)

Malignant neoplasms of lip, oral cavity and pharynx (C00-C14)

CODING TIP✓ Codes classifiable to C00-C14 include active cancer. History of cancer to the lip, pharynx, or oral cavity should be coded to Z85.81-.

4 C00 Malignant neoplasm of lip

Use additional code to identify:
alcohol abuse and dependence (F10.-)
history of tobacco dependence (Z87.891)
tobacco dependence (F17.-)
tobacco use (Z72.0)

EXCLUDES 1 *malignant melanoma of lip (C43.0)*
Merkel cell carcinoma of lip (C4A.0)
other and unspecified malignant neoplasm of skin of lip (C44.0-)

C00.0 Malignant neoplasm of external upper lip
Malignant neoplasm of lipstick area of upper lip
Malignant neoplasm of upper lip NOS
Malignant neoplasm of vermilion border of upper lip

C00.1 Malignant neoplasm of external lower lip
Malignant neoplasm of lower lip NOS
Malignant neoplasm of lipstick area of lower lip
Malignant neoplasm of vermilion border of lower lip

C00.2 Malignant neoplasm of external lip, unspecified
Malignant neoplasm of vermilion border of lip NOS

C00.3 Malignant neoplasm of upper lip, inner aspect
Malignant neoplasm of buccal aspect of upper lip
Malignant neoplasm of frenulum of upper lip
Malignant neoplasm of mucosa of upper lip
Malignant neoplasm of oral aspect of upper lip

C00.4 Malignant neoplasm of lower lip, inner aspect
Malignant neoplasm of buccal aspect of lower lip
Malignant neoplasm of frenulum of lower lip
Malignant neoplasm of mucosa of lower lip
Malignant neoplasm of oral aspect of lower lip

C00.5 Malignant neoplasm of lip, unspecified, inner aspect
Malignant neoplasm of buccal aspect of lip, unspecified
Malignant neoplasm of frenulum of lip, unspecified
Malignant neoplasm of mucosa of lip, unspecified
Malignant neoplasm of oral aspect of lip, unspecified

C00.6 Malignant neoplasm of commissure of lip, unspecified

C00.8 Malignant neoplasm of overlapping sites of lip

C00.9 Malignant neoplasm of lip, unspecified

C01 Malignant neoplasm of base of tongue HCC
Malignant neoplasm of dorsal surface of base of tongue
Malignant neoplasm of fixed part of tongue NOS
Malignant neoplasm of posterior third of tongue
Use additional code to identify:
alcohol abuse and dependence (F10.-)
history of tobacco dependence (Z87.891)
tobacco dependence (F17.-)
tobacco use (Z72.0)

4 C02 Malignant neoplasm of other and unspecified parts of tongue
Use additional code to identify:
alcohol abuse and dependence (F10.-)
history of tobacco dependence (Z87.891)
tobacco dependence (F17.-)
tobacco use (Z72.0)

C02.0 Malignant neoplasm of dorsal surface of tongue HCC
Malignant neoplasm of anterior two-thirds of tongue, dorsal surface

EXCLUDES 2 *malignant neoplasm of dorsal surface of base of tongue (C01)*

C02.1 **Malignant neoplasm of border of tongue** HCC
Malignant neoplasm of tip of tongue

C02.2 **Malignant neoplasm of ventral surface of tongue** HCC
Malignant neoplasm of anterior two-thirds of tongue, ventral surface
Malignant neoplasm of frenulum linguae

C02.3 **Malignant neoplasm of anterior two-thirds of tongue, part unspecified** HCC
Malignant neoplasm of middle third of tongue NOS
Malignant neoplasm of mobile part of tongue NOS

C02.4 **Malignant neoplasm of lingual tonsil** HCC
EXCLUDES 2 *malignant neoplasm of tonsil NOS (C09.9)*

C02.8 **Malignant neoplasm of overlapping sites of tongue** HCC
Malignant neoplasm of two or more contiguous sites of tongue

C02.9 **Malignant neoplasm of tongue, unspecified** HCC

4 C03 Malignant neoplasm of gum

INCLUDES malignant neoplasm of alveolar (ridge) mucosa
malignant neoplasm of gingiva

Use additional code to identify:
alcohol abuse and dependence (F10.-)
history of tobacco dependence (Z87.891)
tobacco dependence (F17.-)
tobacco use (Z72.0)

EXCLUDES 2 *malignant odontogenic neoplasms (C41.0-C41.1)*

C03.0 **Malignant neoplasm of upper gum** HCC

C03.1 **Malignant neoplasm of lower gum** HCC

C03.9 **Malignant neoplasm of gum, unspecified** HCC

4 C04 Malignant neoplasm of floor of mouth

Use additional code to identify:
alcohol abuse and dependence (F10.-)
history of tobacco dependence (Z87.891)
tobacco dependence (F17.-)
tobacco use (Z72.0)

C04.0 **Malignant neoplasm of anterior floor of mouth** HCC
Malignant neoplasm of anterior to the premolar-canine junction

C04.1 **Malignant neoplasm of lateral floor of mouth** HCC

C04.8 **Malignant neoplasm of overlapping sites of floor of mouth** HCC

C04.9 **Malignant neoplasm of floor of mouth, unspecified** HCC

4 C05 Malignant neoplasm of palate

Use additional code to identify:
alcohol abuse and dependence (F10.-)
history of tobacco dependence (Z87.891)
tobacco dependence (F17.-)
tobacco use (Z72.0)

EXCLUDES 1 *Kaposi's sarcoma of palate (C46.2)*

C05.0 **Malignant neoplasm of hard palate** HCC

C05.1 **Malignant neoplasm of soft palate** HCC
EXCLUDES 2 *malignant neoplasm of nasopharyngeal surface of soft palate (C11.3)*

C05.2 **Malignant neoplasm of uvula** HCC

C05.8 **Malignant neoplasm of overlapping sites of palate** HCC

C05.9 **Malignant neoplasm of palate, unspecified** HCC
Malignant neoplasm of roof of mouth

4 C06 Malignant neoplasm of other and unspecified parts of mouth

Use additional code to identify:
alcohol abuse and dependence (F10.-)
history of tobacco dependence (Z87.891)
tobacco dependence (F17.-)
tobacco use (Z72.0)

C06.0 **Malignant neoplasm of cheek mucosa** HCC
Malignant neoplasm of buccal mucosa NOS
Malignant neoplasm of internal cheek

C06.1 **Malignant neoplasm of vestibule of mouth** HCC
Malignant neoplasm of buccal sulcus (upper) (lower)
Malignant neoplasm of labial sulcus (upper) (lower)

C06.2 **Malignant neoplasm of retromolar area** HCC

5 **C06.8** **Malignant neoplasm of overlapping sites of other and unspecified parts of mouth**

C06.80 **Malignant neoplasm of overlapping sites of unspecified parts of mouth** HCC

C06.89 **Malignant neoplasm of overlapping sites of other parts of mouth** HCC
'book leaf' neoplasm [ventral surface of tongue and floor of mouth]

C06.9 **Malignant neoplasm of mouth, unspecified** HCC
Malignant neoplasm of minor salivary gland, unspecified site
Malignant neoplasm of oral cavity NOS

C07 Malignant neoplasm of parotid gland HCC

Use additional code to identify:
alcohol abuse and dependence (F10.-)
exposure to environmental tobacco smoke (Z77.22)
exposure to tobacco smoke in the perinatal period (P96.81)
history of tobacco dependence (Z87.891)
occupational exposure to environmental tobacco smoke (Z57.31)
tobacco dependence (F17.-)
tobacco use (Z72.0)

4 C08 Malignant neoplasm of other and unspecified major salivary glands

INCLUDES malignant neoplasm of salivary ducts

Use additional code to identify:
alcohol abuse and dependence (F10.-)
exposure to environmental tobacco smoke (Z77.22)
exposure to tobacco smoke in the perinatal period (P96.81)
history of tobacco dependence (Z87.891)
occupational exposure to environmental tobacco smoke (Z57.31)
tobacco dependence (F17.-)
tobacco use (Z72.0)

EXCLUDES 1 *malignant neoplasms of specified minor salivary glands which are classified according to their anatomical location*

EXCLUDES 2 *malignant neoplasms of minor salivary glands NOS (C06.9)*
malignant neoplasm of parotid gland (C07)

C08.0 **Malignant neoplasm of submandibular gland** HCC
Malignant neoplasm of submaxillary gland

C08.1 **Malignant neoplasm of sublingual gland** HCC

C08.9 **Malignant neoplasm of major salivary gland, unspecified** HCC
Malignant neoplasm of salivary gland (major) NOS

4 C09 Malignant neoplasm of tonsil

Use additional code to identify:
alcohol abuse and dependence (F10.-)
exposure to environmental tobacco smoke (Z77.22)
exposure to tobacco smoke in the perinatal period (P96.81)
history of tobacco dependence (Z87.891)
occupational exposure to environmental tobacco smoke (Z57.31)
tobacco dependence (F17.-)
tobacco use (Z72.0)

EXCLUDES 2 *malignant neoplasm of lingual tonsil (C02.4)*
malignant neoplasm of pharyngeal tonsil (C11.1)

C09.0 **Malignant neoplasm of tonsillar fossa** HCC

C09.1 **Malignant neoplasm of tonsil lar pillar (anterior) (posterior)** HCC

C09.8 **Malignant neoplasm of overlapping sites of tonsil** HCC

C09.9 **Malignant neoplasm of tonsil, unspecified** HCC
Malignant neoplasm of tonsil NOS
Malignant neoplasm of faucial tonsils
Malignant neoplasm of palatine tonsils

4 C10 Malignant neoplasm of oropharynx

Use additional code to identify:
alcohol abuse and dependence (F10.-)
exposure to environmental tobacco smoke (Z77.22)
exposure to tobacco smoke in the perinatal period (P96.81)
history of tobacco dependence (Z87.891)
occupational exposure to environmental tobacco smoke (Z57.31)
tobacco dependence (F17.-)
tobacco use (Z72.0)

EXCLUDES 2 *malignant neoplasm of tonsil (C09.-)*

C10.0 **Malignant neoplasm of vallecula** HCC

C10.1 **Malignant neoplasm of anterior surface of epiglottis** HCC
Malignant neoplasm of epiglottis, free border [margin]
Malignant neoplasm of glossoepiglottic fold(s)
EXCLUDES 2 *malignant neoplasm of epiglottis (suprahyoid portion) NOS (C32.1)*

C10.2 Malignant neoplasm of lateral wall of oropharynx HCC

C10.3 Malignant neoplasm of posterior wall of oropharynx HCC

C10.4 Malignant neoplasm of branchial cleft HCC
Malignant neoplasm of branchial cyst [site of neoplasm]

C10.8 Malignant neoplasm of overlapping sites of oropharynx HCC
Malignant neoplasm of junctional region of oropharynx

C10.9 Malignant neoplasm of oropharynx, unspecified HCC

C11 Malignant neoplasm of nasopharynx
Use additional code to identify:
exposure to environmental tobacco smoke (Z77.22)
exposure to tobacco smoke in the perinatal period (P96.81)
history of tobacco dependence (Z87.891)
occupational exposure to environmental tobacco smoke (Z57.31)
tobacco dependence (F17.-)
tobacco use (Z72.0)

C11.0 Malignant neoplasm of superior wall of nasopharynx HCC
Malignant neoplasm of roof of nasopharynx

C11.1 Malignant neoplasm of posterior wall of nasopharynx HCC
Malignant neoplasm of adenoid
Malignant neoplasm of pharyngeal tonsil

C11.2 Malignant neoplasm of lateral wall of nasopharynx HCC
Malignant neoplasm of fossa of Rosenmüller
Malignant neoplasm of opening of auditory tube
Malignant neoplasm of pharyngeal recess

C11.3 Malignant neoplasm of anterior wall of nasopharynx HCC
Malignant neoplasm of floor of nasopharynx
Malignant neoplasm of nasopharyngeal (anterior) (posterior) surface of soft palate
Malignant neoplasm of posterior margin of nasal choana
Malignant neoplasm of posterior margin of nasal septum

C11.8 Malignant neoplasm of overlapping sites of nasopharynx HCC

C11.9 Malignant neoplasm of nasopharynx, unspecified HCC
Malignant neoplasm of nasopharyngeal wall NOS

C12 Malignant neoplasm of pyriform sinus HCC
Malignant neoplasm of pyriform fossa
Use additional code to identify:
exposure to environmental tobacco smoke (Z77.22)
exposure to tobacco smoke in the perinatal period (P96.81)
history of tobacco dependence (Z87.891)
occupational exposure to environmental tobacco smoke (Z57.31)
tobacco dependence (F17.-)
tobacco use (Z72.0)

C13 Malignant neoplasm of hypopharynx
Use additional code to identify:
exposure to environmental tobacco smoke (Z77.22)
exposure to tobacco smoke in the perinatal period (P96.81)
history of tobacco dependence (Z87.891)
occupational exposure to environmental tobacco smoke (Z57.31)
tobacco dependence (F17.-)
tobacco use (Z72.0)
EXCLUDES 2 *malignant neoplasm of pyriform sinus (C12)*

C13.0 Malignant neoplasm of postcricoid region HCC

C13.1 Malignant neoplasm of aryepiglottic fold, hypopharyngeal aspect HCC
Malignant neoplasm of aryepiglottic fold, marginal zone
Malignant neoplasm of aryepiglottic fold NOS
Malignant neoplasm of interarytenoid fold, marginal zone
Malignant neoplasm of interarytenoid fold NOS
EXCLUDES 2 *malignant neoplasm of aryepiglottic fold or interarytenoid fold, laryngeal aspect (C32.1)*

C13.2 Malignant neoplasm of posterior wall of hypopharynx HCC

C13.8 Malignant neoplasm of overlapping sites of hypopharynx HCC

C13.9 Malignant neoplasm of hypopharynx, unspecified HCC
Malignant neoplasm of hypopharyngeal wall NOS

C14 Malignant neoplasm of other and ill-defined sites in the lip, oral cavity and pharynx
Use additional code to identify:
alcohol abuse and dependence (F10.-)
exposure to environmental tobacco smoke (Z77.22)
exposure to tobacco smoke in the perinatal period (P96.81)
history of tobacco dependence (Z87.891)
occupational exposure to environmental tobacco smoke (Z57.31)
tobacco dependence (F17.-)
tobacco use (Z72.0)
EXCLUDES 1 *malignant neoplasm of oral cavity NOS (C06.9)*

C14.0 Malignant neoplasm of pharynx, unspecified HCC

C14.2 Malignant neoplasm of Waldeyer's ring HCC

C14.8 Malignant neoplasm of overlapping sites of lip, oral cavity and pharynx HCC
Primary malignant neoplasm of two or more contiguous sites of lip, oral cavity and pharynx
EXCLUDES 1 *'book leaf' neoplasm [ventral surface of tongue and floor of mouth] (C06.89)*

Malignant neoplasms of digestive organs (C15-C26)

EXCLUDES 1 *Kaposi's sarcoma of gastrointestinal sites (C46.4)*
EXCLUDES 2 *gastrointestinal stromal tumors (C49.A-)*

CODING TIP✓ Codes classifiable to C15-C26 include active cancer. History of cancer to digestive organs should be coded to Z85.0-.

C15 Malignant neoplasm of esophagus
Use additional code to identify:
alcohol abuse and dependence (F10.-)

C15.3 Malignant neoplasm of upper third of esophagus HCC

C15.4 Malignant neoplasm of middle third of esophagus HCC

C15.5 Malignant neoplasm of lower third of esophagus HCC
EXCLUDES 1 *malignant neoplasm of cardio-esophageal junction (C16.0)*

C15.8 Malignant neoplasm of overlapping sites of esophagus HCC

C15.9 Malignant neoplasm of esophagus, unspecified HCC

C16 Malignant neoplasm of stomach
Use additional code to identify:
alcohol abuse and dependence (F10.-)
EXCLUDES 2 *malignant carcinoid tumor of the stomach (C7A.092)*

C16.0 Malignant neoplasm of cardia HCC
Malignant neoplasm of cardiac orifice
Malignant neoplasm of cardio-esophageal junction
Malignant neoplasm of esophagus and stomach
Malignant neoplasm of gastro-esophageal junction

C16.1 Malignant neoplasm of fundus of stomach HCC

C16.2 Malignant neoplasm of body of stomach HCC

C16.3 Malignant neoplasm of pyloric antrum HCC
Malignant neoplasm of gastric antrum

C16.4 Malignant neoplasm of pylorus HCC
Malignant neoplasm of prepylorus
Malignant neoplasm of pyloric canal

C16.5 Malignant neoplasm of lesser curvature of stomach, unspecified HCC
Malignant neoplasm of lesser curvature of stomach, not classifiable to C16.1-C16.4

C16.6 Malignant neoplasm of greater curvature of stomach, unspecified HCC
Malignant neoplasm of greater curvature of stomach, not classifiable to C16.0-C16.4

C16.8 Malignant neoplasm of overlapping sites of stomach HCC

C16.9 Malignant neoplasm of stomach, unspecified HCC
Gastric cancer NOS

C17 Malignant neoplasm of small intestine
EXCLUDES 1 *malignant carcinoid tumors of the small intestine (C7A.01)*

C17.0 Malignant neoplasm of duodenum HCC

C17.1 Malignant neoplasm of jejunum HCC

C17.2 Malignant neoplasm of ileum HCC
EXCLUDES 1 *malignant neoplasm of ileocecal valve (C18.0)*

C17.3 **Meckel's diverticulum, malignant** HCC
EXCLUDES 1 *Meckel's diverticulum, congenital (Q43.0)*

C17.8 **Malignant neoplasm of overlapping sites of small intestine** HCC

C17.9 **Malignant neoplasm of small intestine, unspecified** HCC

C18 Malignant neoplasm of colon
EXCLUDES 1 *malignant carcinoid tumors of the colon (C7A.02-)*

C18.0 **Malignant neoplasm of cecum** HCC
Malignant neoplasm of ileocecal valve

C18.1 **Malignant neoplasm of appendix** HCC

C18.2 **Malignant neoplasm of ascending colon** HCC

C18.3 **Malignant neoplasm of hepatic flexure** HCC

C18.4 **Malignant neoplasm of transverse colon** HCC

C18.5 **Malignant neoplasm of splenic flexure** HCC

C18.6 **Malignant neoplasm of descending colon** HCC

C18.7 **Malignant neoplasm of sigmoid colon** HCC
Malignant neoplasm of sigmoid (flexure)
EXCLUDES 1 *malignant neoplasm of rectosigmoid junction (C19)*

C18.8 **Malignant neoplasm of overlapping sites of colon** HCC

C18.9 **Malignant neoplasm of colon, unspecified** HCC
Malignant neoplasm of large intestine NOS

C19 Malignant neoplasm of rectosigmoid junction HCC
Malignant neoplasm of colon with rectum
Malignant neoplasm of rectosigmoid (colon)
EXCLUDES 1 *malignant carcinoid tumors of the colon (C7A.02-)*

C20 Malignant neoplasm of rectum HCC
Malignant neoplasm of rectal ampulla
EXCLUDES 1 *malignant carcinoid tumor of the rectum (C7A.026)*

C21 Malignant neoplasm of anus and anal canal
EXCLUDES 2 *malignant carcinoid tumors of the colon (C7A.02-)*
malignant melanoma of anal margin (C43.51)
malignant melanoma of anal skin (C43.51)
malignant melanoma of perianal skin (C43.51)
other and unspecified malignant neoplasm of anal margin (C44.500, C44.510, C44.520, C44.590)
other and unspecified malignant neoplasm of anal skin (C44.500, C44.510, C44.520, C44.590)
other and unspecified malignant neoplasm of perianal skin (C44.500, C44.510, C44.520, C44.590)

C21.0 **Malignant neoplasm of anus, unspecified** HCC

C21.1 **Malignant neoplasm of anal canal** HCC
Malignant neoplasm of anal sphincter

C21.2 **Malignant neoplasm of cloacogenic zone** HCC

C21.8 **Malignant neoplasm of overlapping sites of rectum, anus and anal canal** HCC
Malignant neoplasm of anorectal junction
Malignant neoplasm of anorectum
Primary malignant neoplasm of two or more contiguous sites of rectum, anus and anal canal

C22 Malignant neoplasm of liver and intrahepatic bile ducts
Use additional code to identify:
alcohol abuse and dependence (F10.-)
hepatitis B (B16.-, B18.0-B18.1)
hepatitis C (B17.1-, B18.2)
EXCLUDES 1 *malignant neoplasm of biliary tract NOS (C24.9)*
secondary malignant neoplasm of liver and intrahepatic bile duct (C78.7)

C22.0 **Liver cell carcinoma** HCC
Hepatocellular carcinoma
Hepatoma
AHA: 1Q 2016, 18-19

C22.1 **Intrahepatic bile duct carcinoma** HCC
Cholangiocarcinoma
EXCLUDES 1 *malignant neoplasm of hepatic duct (C24.0)*

C22.2 **Hepatoblastoma** HCC

C22.3 **Angiosarcoma of liver** HCC
Kupffer cell sarcoma

C22.4 **Other sarcomas of liver** HCC

C22.7 **Other specified carcinomas of liver** HCC

C22.8 **Malignant neoplasm of liver, primary, unspecified as to type** HCC

C22.9 **Malignant neoplasm of liver, not specified as primary or secondary** HCC

C23 Malignant neoplasm of gallbladder HCC

C24 Malignant neoplasm of other and unspecified parts of biliary tract
EXCLUDES 1 *malignant neoplasm of intrahepatic bile duct (C22.1)*

C24.0 **Malignant neoplasm of extrahepatic bile duct** HCC
Malignant neoplasm of biliary duct or passage NOS
Malignant neoplasm of common bile duct
Malignant neoplasm of cystic duct
Malignant neoplasm of hepatic duct

C24.1 **Malignant neoplasm of ampulla of Vater** HCC

C24.8 **Malignant neoplasm of overlapping sites of biliary tract** HCC
Malignant neoplasm involving both intrahepatic and extrahepatic bile ducts
Primary malignant neoplasm of two or more contiguous sites of biliary tract

C24.9 **Malignant neoplasm of biliary tract, unspecified** HCC

C25 Malignant neoplasm of pancreas
Code also:
exocrine pancreatic insufficiency (K86.81)
Use additional code to identify:
alcohol abuse and dependence (F10.-)

C25.0 **Malignant neoplasm of head of pancreas** HCC

C25.1 **Malignant neoplasm of body of pancreas** HCC

C25.2 **Malignant neoplasm of tail of pancreas** HCC

C25.3 **Malignant neoplasm of pancreatic duct** HCC

C25.4 **Malignant neoplasm of endocrine pancreas** HCC
Malignant neoplasm of islets of Langerhans
Use additional code to identify any functional activity.

C25.7 **Malignant neoplasm of other parts of pancreas** HCC
Malignant neoplasm of neck of pancreas

C25.8 **Malignant neoplasm of overlapping sites of pancreas** HCC

C25.9 **Malignant neoplasm of pancreas, unspecified** HCC

C26 Malignant neoplasm of other and ill-defined digestive organs
EXCLUDES 1 *malignant neoplasm of peritoneum and retroperitoneum (C48.-)*

C26.0 **Malignant neoplasm of intestinal tract, part unspecified** HCC
Malignant neoplasm of intestine NOS

C26.1 **Malignant neoplasm of spleen** HCC
EXCLUDES 1 *Hodgkin lymphoma (C81.-)*
non-Hodgkin lymphoma (C82-C85)

C26.9 **Malignant neoplasm of ill-defined sites within the digestive system** HCC
Malignant neoplasm of alimentary canal or tract NOS
Malignant neoplasm of gastrointestinal tract NOS
EXCLUDES 1 *malignant neoplasm of abdominal NOS (C76.2)*
malignant neoplasm of intra-abdominal NOS (C76.2)

Malignant neoplasms of respiratory and intrathoracic organs (C30-C39)

INCLUDES malignant neoplasm of middle ear

EXCLUDES 1 *mesothelioma (C45.-)*

CODING TIP ✓ Codes classifiable to C30-C39 include active cancer. History of cancer to respiratory system and other intrathoracic organs should be coded using codes from Z85.1- and Z85.2-.

C30 Malignant neoplasm of nasal cavity and middle ear

C30.0 Malignant neoplasm of nasal cavity HCC
Malignant neoplasm of cartilage of nose
Malignant neoplasm of nasal concha
Malignant neoplasm of internal nose
Malignant neoplasm of septum of nose
Malignant neoplasm of vestibule of nose
EXCLUDES 1 *malignant neoplasm of nasal bone (C41.0)*
malignant neoplasm of nose NOS (C76.0)
malignant neoplasm of olfactory bulb (C72.2-)
malignant neoplasm of posterior margin of nasal septum and choana (C11.3)
malignant melanoma of skin of nose (C43.31)
malignant neoplasm of turbinates (C41.0)
other and unspecified malignant neoplasm of skin of nose C44.301, C44.311, C44.321, C44.391)

C30.1 Malignant neoplasm of middle ear HCC
Malignant neoplasm of antrum tympanicum
Malignant neoplasm of auditory tube
Malignant neoplasm of eustachian tube
Malignant neoplasm of inner ear
Malignant neoplasm of mastoid air cells
Malignant neoplasm of tympanic cavity
EXCLUDES 1 *malignant neoplasm of auricular canal (external) (C43.2-,C44.2-)*
malignant neoplasm of bone of ear (meatus) (C41.0)
malignant neoplasm of cartilage of ear (C49.0)
malignant melanoma of skin of (external) ear (C43.2-)
other and unspecified malignant neoplasm of skin of (external) ear (C44.2-)

4 C31 Malignant neoplasm of accessory sinuses

C31.0 Malignant neoplasm of maxillary sinus HCC
Malignant neoplasm of antrum (Highmore) (maxillary)

C31.1 Malignant neoplasm of ethmoidal sinus HCC

C31.2 Malignant neoplasm of frontal sinus HCC

C31.3 Malignant neoplasm of sphenoid sinus HCC

C31.8 Malignant neoplasm of overlapping sites of accessory sinuses HCC

C31.9 Malignant neoplasm of accessory sinus, unspecified HCC

4 C32 Malignant neoplasm of larynx

Use additional code to identify:
alcohol abuse and dependence (F10.-)
exposure to environmental tobacco smoke (Z77.22)
exposure to tobacco smoke in the perinatal period (P96.81)
history of tobacco dependence (Z87.891)
occupational exposure to environmental tobacco smoke (Z57.31)
tobacco dependence (F17.-)
tobacco use (Z72.0)

C32.0 Malignant neoplasm of glottis HCC
Malignant neoplasm of intrinsic larynx
Malignant neoplasm of laryngeal commissure (anterior)(posterior)
Malignant neoplasm of vocal cord (true) NOS

C32.1 Malignant neoplasm of supraglottis HCC
Malignant neoplasm of aryepiglottic fold or interarytenoid fold, laryngeal aspect
Malignant neoplasm of epiglottis (suprahyoid portion) NOS
Malignant neoplasm of extrinsic larynx
Malignant neoplasm of false vocal cord
Malignant neoplasm of posterior (laryngeal) surface of epiglottis
Malignant neoplasm of ventricular bands
EXCLUDES 2 *malignant neoplasm of anterior surface of epiglottis (C10.1)*
malignant neoplasm of aryepiglottic fold or interarytenoid fold, hypopharyngeal aspect (C13.1)
malignant neoplasm of aryepiglottic fold or interarytenoid fold, marginal zone (C13.1)
malignant neoplasm of aryepiglottic fold or interarytenoid fold NOS (C13.1)

C32.2 Malignant neoplasm of subglottis HCC

C32.3 Malignant neoplasm of laryngeal cartilage HCC

C32.8 Malignant neoplasm of overlapping sites of larynx HCC

C32.9 Malignant neoplasm of larynx, unspecified HCC

C33 Malignant neoplasm of trachea HCC

Use additional code to identify:
exposure to environmental tobacco smoke (Z77.22)
exposure to tobacco smoke in the perinatal period (P96.81)
history of tobacco dependence (Z87.891)
occupational exposure to environmental tobacco smoke (Z57.31)
tobacco dependence (F17.-)
tobacco use (Z72.0)

4 C34 Malignant neoplasm of bronchus and lung

Use additional code to identify:
exposure to environmental tobacco smoke (Z77.22)
exposure to tobacco smoke in the perinatal period (P96.81)
history of tobacco dependence (Z87.891)
occupational exposure to environmental tobacco smoke (Z57.31)
tobacco dependence (F17.-)
tobacco use (Z72.0)
EXCLUDES 1 *Kaposi's sarcoma of lung (C46.5-)*
malignant carcinoid tumor of the bronchus and lung (C7A.090)

5 C34.0 Malignant neoplasm of main bronchus
Malignant neoplasm of carina
Malignant neoplasm of hilus (of lung)

C34.00 Malignant neoplasm of unspecified main bronchus HCC

C34.01 Malignant neoplasm of right main bronchus HCC

C34.02 Malignant neoplasm of left main bronchus HCC

5 C34.1 Malignant neoplasm of upper lobe, bronchus or lung

C34.10 Malignant neoplasm of upper lobe, unspecified bronchus or lung HCC

C34.11 Malignant neoplasm of upper lobe, right bronchus or lung HCC

C34.12 Malignant neoplasm of upper lobe, left bronchus or lung HCC

C34.2 Malignant neoplasm of middle lobe, bronchus or lung HCC

5 C34.3 Malignant neoplasm of lower lobe, bronchus or lung

C34.30 Malignant neoplasm of lower lobe, unspecified bronchus or lung HCC

C34.31 Malignant neoplasm of lower lobe, right bronchus or lung HCC

C34.32 Malignant neoplasm of lower lobe, left bronchus or lung HCC

5 C34.8 Malignant neoplasm of overlapping sites of bronchus and lung

C34.80 Malignant neoplasm of overlapping sites of unspecified bronchus and lung HCC

C34.81 Malignant neoplasm of overlapping sites of right bronchus and lung HCC

C34.82 Malignant neoplasm of overlapping sites of left bronchus and lung HCC

5 C34.9 Malignant neoplasm of unspecified part of bronchus or lung

C34.90 Malignant neoplasm of unspecified part of unspecified bronchus or lung HCC
Lung cancer NOS
AHA: 2Q 2014, 10

C34.91 Malignant neoplasm of unspecified part of right bronchus or lung HCC

C34.92 Malignant neoplasm of unspecified part of left bronchus or lung HCC

C37 Malignant neoplasm of thymus HCC

EXCLUDES 1 *malignant carcinoid tumor of the thymus (C7A.091)*

4 C38 Malignant neoplasm of heart, mediastinum and pleura

EXCLUDES 1 *mesothelioma (C45.-)*

C38.0 Malignant neoplasm of heart HCC
Malignant neoplasm of pericardium
EXCLUDES 1 *malignant neoplasm of great vessels (C49.3)*

C38.1 Malignant neoplasm of anterior mediastinum HCC

C38.2 Malignant neoplasm of posterior mediastinum HCC

C38.3 Malignant neoplasm of mediastinum, part unspecified HCC

C38.4 Malignant neoplasm of pleura HCC
C38.8 Malignant neoplasm of overlapping sites of heart, mediastinum and pleura HCC

4 C39 Malignant neoplasm of other and ill-defined sites in the respiratory system and intrathoracic organs

Use additional code to identify:
exposure to environmental tobacco smoke (Z77.22)
exposure to tobacco smoke in the perinatal period (P96.81)
history of tobacco dependence (Z87.891)
occupational exposure to environmental tobacco smoke (Z57.31)
tobacco dependence (F17.-)
tobacco use (Z72.0)

EXCLUDES 1 *intrathoracic malignant neoplasm NOS (C76.1)*
thoracic malignant neoplasm NOS (C76.1)

C39.0 Malignant neoplasm of upper respiratory tract, part unspecified HCC
C39.9 Malignant neoplasm of lower respiratory tract, part unspecified HCC
Malignant neoplasm of respiratory tract NOS

Malignant neoplasms of bone and articular cartilage (C40-C41)

INCLUDES malignant neoplasm of cartilage (articular) (joint)
malignant neoplasm of periosteum

EXCLUDES 1 *malignant neoplasm of bone marrow NOS (C96.9)*
malignant neoplasm of synovia (C49.-)

CODING TIP ✓ Codes classifiable to C40-C41 include active cancer. History of cancer to bone or soft tissue should be coded to Z85.83-.

4 C40 Malignant neoplasm of bone and articular cartilage of limbs

Use additional code to identify major osseous defect, if applicable (M89.7-)

5 C40.0 Malignant neoplasm of scapula and long bones of upper limb
⊟ C40.00 Malignant neoplasm of scapula and long bones of unspecified upper limb HCC
⊟ C40.01 Malignant neoplasm of scapula and long bones of right upper limb HCC
⊟ C40.02 Malignant neoplasm of scapula and long bones of left upper limb HCC

5 C40.1 Malignant neoplasm of short bones of upper limb
⊟ C40.10 Malignant neoplasm of short bones of unspecified upper limb HCC
⊟ C40.11 Malignant neoplasm of short bones of right upper limb HCC
⊟ C40.12 Malignant neoplasm of short bones of left upper limb HCC

5 C40.2 Malignant neoplasm of long bones of lower limb
⊟ C40.20 Malignant neoplasm of long bones of unspecified lower limb HCC
⊟ C40.21 Malignant neoplasm of long bones of right lower limb HCC
⊟ C40.22 Malignant neoplasm of long bones of left lower limb HCC

5 C40.3 Malignant neoplasm of short bones of lower limb
⊟ C40.30 Malignant neoplasm of short bones of unspecified lower limb HCC
⊟ C40.31 Malignant neoplasm of short bones of right lower limb HCC
⊟ C40.32 Malignant neoplasm of short bones of left lower limb HCC

5 C40.8 Malignant neoplasm of overlapping sites of bone and articular cartilage of limb
⊟ C40.80 Malignant neoplasm of overlapping sites of bone and articular cartilage of unspecified limb HCC
⊟ C40.81 Malignant neoplasm of overlapping sites of bone and articular cartilage of right limb HCC
⊟ C40.82 Malignant neoplasm of overlapping sites of bone and articular cartilage of left limb HCC

5 C40.9 Malignant neoplasm of unspecified bones and articular cartilage of limb
⊟ C40.90 Malignant neoplasm of unspecified bones and articular cartilage of unspecified limb HCC
⊟ C40.91 Malignant neoplasm of unspecified bones and articular cartilage of right limb HCC
⊟ C40.92 Malignant neoplasm of unspecified bones and articular cartilage of left limb HCC

4 C41 Malignant neoplasm of bone and articular cartilage of other and unspecified sites

EXCLUDES 1 *malignant neoplasm of bones of limbs (C40.-)*
malignant neoplasm of cartilage of ear (C49.0)
malignant neoplasm of cartilage of eyelid (C49.0)
malignant neoplasm of cartilage of larynx (C32.3)
malignant neoplasm of cartilage of limbs (C40.-)
malignant neoplasm of cartilage of nose (C30.0)

C41.0 Malignant neoplasm of bones of skull and face HCC
Malignant neoplasm of maxilla (superior)
Malignant neoplasm of orbital bone
EXCLUDES 2 *carcinoma, any type except intraosseous or odontogenic of:*
maxillary sinus (C31.0)
upper jaw (C03.0)
malignant neoplasm of jaw bone (lower) (C41.1)

C41.1 Malignant neoplasm of mandible HCC
Malignant neoplasm of inferior maxilla
Malignant neoplasm of lower jaw bone
EXCLUDES 2 *carcinoma, any type except intraosseous or odontogenic of:*
jaw NOS (C03.9)
lower (C03.1)
malignant neoplasm of upper jaw bone (C41.0)

C41.2 Malignant neoplasm of vertebral column HCC
EXCLUDES 1 *malignant neoplasm of sacrum and coccyx (C41.4)*

C41.3 Malignant neoplasm of ribs, sternum and clavicle HCC
C41.4 Malignant neoplasm of pelvic bones, sacrum and coccyx HCC
C41.9 Malignant neoplasm of bone and articular cartilage, unspecified HCC

Melanoma and other malignant neoplasms of skin (C43-C44)

CODING TIP ✓ Codes classifiable to C43-C44 include active cancer. History of cancer to skin should be coded to Z85.82-.

4 C43 Malignant melanoma of skin

EXCLUDES 1 *melanoma in situ (D03.-)*

EXCLUDES 2 *malignant melanoma of skin of genital organs (C51-C52, C60.-, C63.-)*
Merkel cell carcinoma (C4A.-)
sites other than skin-code to malignant neoplasm of the site

C43.0 Malignant melanoma of lip HCC
EXCLUDES 1 *malignant neoplasm of vermilion border of lip (C00.0-C00.2)*

5 C43.1 Malignant melanoma of eyelid, including canthus
⊟ C43.10 Malignant melanoma of unspecified eyelid, including canthus HCC
▲ 6 C43.11 Malignant melanoma of right eyelid, including canthus HCC
● ⊟ C43.111 Malignant melanoma of right upper eyelid, including canthus
● ⊟ C43.112 Malignant melanoma of right lower eyelid, including canthus
▲ 6 C43.12 Malignant melanoma of left eyelid, including canthus HCC
● ⊟ C43.121 Malignant melanoma of left upper eyelid, including canthus
● ⊟ C43.122 Malignant melanoma of left lower eyelid, including canthus

5 C43.2 Malignant melanoma of ear and external auricular canal
⊟ C43.20 Malignant melanoma of unspecified ear and external auricular canal HCC
⊟ C43.21 Malignant melanoma of right ear and external auricular canal HCC
⊟ C43.22 Malignant melanoma of left ear and external auricular canal HCC

5 C43.3 Malignant melanoma of other and unspecified parts of face

C43.30 Malignant melanoma of unspecified part of face HCC

C43.31 Malignant melanoma of nose HCC

C43.39 Malignant melanoma of other parts of face HCC

Malignant melanoma of cheek

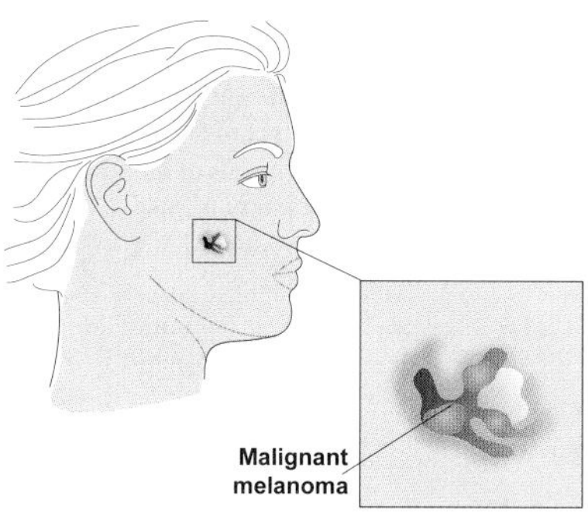

C43.4 Malignant melanoma of scalp and neck HCC

5 C43.5 Malignant melanoma of trunk

EXCLUDES 2 *malignant neoplasm of anus NOS (C21.0)*
malignant neoplasm of scrotum (C63.2)

C43.51 Malignant melanoma of anal skin HCC
Malignant melanoma of anal margin
Malignant melanoma of perianal skin

C43.52 Malignant melanoma of skin of breast HCC

C43.59 Malignant melanoma of other part of trunk HCC

5 C43.6 Malignant melanoma of upper limb, including shoulder

C43.60 Malignant melanoma of unspecified upper limb, including shoulder HCC

C43.61 Malignant melanoma of right upper limb, including shoulder HCC

C43.62 Malignant melanoma of left upper limb, including shoulder HCC

5 C43.7 Malignant melanoma of lower limb, including hip

C43.70 Malignant melanoma of unspecified lower limb, including hip HCC

C43.71 Malignant melanoma of right lower limb, including hip HCC

C43.72 Malignant melanoma of left lower limb, including hip HCC

C43.8 Malignant melanoma of overlapping sites of skin HCC

C43.9 Malignant melanoma of skin, unspecified HCC
Malignant melanoma of unspecified site of skin
Melanoma (malignant) NOS

4 C4A Merkel cell carcinoma

C4A.0 Merkel cell carcinoma of lip HCC

EXCLUDES 1 *malignant neoplasm of vermilion border of lip (C00.0-C00.2)*

5 C4A.1 Merkel cell carcinoma of eyelid, including canthus

C4A.10 Merkel cell carcinoma of unspecified eyelid, including canthus HCC

▲ 6 C4A.11 Merkel cell carcinoma of right eyelid, including canthus HCC

● C4A.111 Merkel cell carcinoma of right upper eyelid, including canthus

● C4A.112 Merkel cell carcinoma of right lower eyelid, including canthus

▲ 6 C4A.12 Merkel cell carcinoma of left eyelid, including canthus HCC

● C4A.121 Merkel cell carcinoma of left upper eyelid, including canthus

● C4A.122 Merkel cell carcinoma of left lower eyelid, including canthus

5 C4A.2 Merkel cell carcinoma of ear and external auricular canal

C4A.20 Merkel cell carcinoma of unspecified ear and external auricular canal HCC

C4A.21 Merkel cell carcinoma of right ear and external auricular canal HCC

C4A.22 Merkel cell carcinoma of left ear and external auricular canal HCC

5 C4A.3 Merkel cell carcinoma of other and unspecified parts of face

C4A.30 Merkel cell carcinoma of unspecified part of face HCC

C4A.31 Merkel cell carcinoma of nose HCC

C4A.39 Merkel cell carcinoma of other parts of face HCC

C4A.4 Merkel cell carcinoma of scalp and neck HCC

5 C4A.5 Merkel cell carcinoma of trunk

EXCLUDES 2 *malignant neoplasm of anus NOS (C21.0)*
malignant neoplasm of scrotum (C63.2)

C4A.51 Merkel cell carcinoma of anal skin HCC
Merkel cell carcinoma of anal margin
Merkel cell carcinoma of perianal skin

C4A.52 Merkel cell carcinoma of skin of breast HCC

C4A.59 Merkel cell carcinoma of other part of trunk HCC

5 C4A.6 Merkel cell carcinoma of upper limb, including shoulder

C4A.60 Merkel cell carcinoma of unspecified upper limb, including shoulder HCC

C4A.61 Merkel cell carcinoma of right upper limb, including shoulder HCC

C4A.62 Merkel cell carcinoma of left upper limb, including shoulder HCC

5 C4A.7 Merkel cell carcinoma of lower limb, including hip

C4A.70 Merkel cell carcinoma of unspecified lower limb, including hip HCC

C4A.71 Merkel cell carcinoma of right lower limb, including hip HCC

C4A.72 Merkel cell carcinoma of left lower limb, including hip HCC

C4A.8 Merkel cell carcinoma of overlapping sites HCC

C4A.9 Merkel cell carcinoma, unspecified HCC
Merkel cell carcinoma of unspecified site
Merkel cell carcinoma NOS

4 C44 Other and unspecified malignant neoplasm of skin

INCLUDES malignant neoplasm of sebaceous glands
malignant neoplasm of sweat glands

EXCLUDES 1 *Kaposi's sarcoma of skin (C46.0)*
malignant melanoma of skin (C43.-)
malignant neoplasm of skin of genital organs (C51-C52, C60.-, C63.2)
Merkel cell carcinoma (C4A.-)

5 C44.0 Other and unspecified malignant neoplasm of skin of lip

EXCLUDES 1 *malignant neoplasm of lip (C00.-)*

C44.00 Unspecified malignant neoplasm of skin of lip

C44.01 Basal cell carcinoma of skin of lip

C44.02 Squamous cell carcinoma of skin of lip

C44.09 Other specified malignant neoplasm of skin of lip

5 C44.1 Other and unspecified malignant neoplasm of skin of eyelid, including canthus

EXCLUDES 1 *connective tissue of eyelid (C49.0)*

6 C44.10 Unspecified malignant neoplasm of skin of eyelid, including canthus

C44.101 Unspecified malignant neoplasm of skin of unspecified eyelid, including canthus

▲ 7 C44.102 Unspecified malignant neoplasm of skin of right eyelid, including canthus

CODING TIP ✓ There was no 7th character table published with codes C44.102- and C44.109-. A 7th character of 1 denotes "upper" and a 7th character of 2 denotes "lower".

▲ 7 C44.109 Unspecified malignant neoplasm of skin of left eyelid, including canthus

6 C44.11 Basal cell carcinoma of skin of eyelid, including canthus

C44.111 Basal cell carcinoma of skin of unspecified eyelid, including canthus

▲ 7 C44.112 Basal cell carcinoma of skin of right eyelid, including canthus

CODING TIP ✓ There was no 7th character table published with codes C44.112- and C44.119-. A 7th character of 1 denotes "upper" and a 7th character of 2 denotes "lower".

▲ 7 ⊟ **C44.119** **Basal cell carcinoma of skin of left eyelid, including canthus**

6 **C44.12** **Squamous cell carcinoma of skin of eyelid, including canthus**

⊟ **C44.121** **Squamous cell carcinoma of skin of unspecified eyelid, including canthus**

▲ 7 ⊟ **C44.122** **Squamous cell carcinoma of skin of right eyelid, including canthus**

CODING TIP ✓ There was no 7th character table published with codes C44.122- and C44.129-. A 7th character of 1 denotes "upper" and a 7th character of 2 denotes "lower".

▲ 7 ⊟ **C44.129** **Squamous cell carcinoma of skin of left eyelid, including canthus**

● 6 **C44.13** **Sebaceous cell carcinoma of skin of eyelid, including canthus**

● ⊟ **C44.131** **Sebaceous cell carcinoma of skin of unspecified eyelid, including canthus**

● 7 ⊟ **C44.132** **Sebaceous cell carcinoma of skin of right eyelid, including canthus**

CODING TIP ✓ There was no 7th character table published with codes C44.132- and C44.139-. A 7th character of 1 denotes "upper" and a 7th character of 2 denotes "lower".

● 7 ⊟ **C44.139** **Sebaceous cell carcinoma of skin of left eyelid, including canthus**

6 **C44.19** **Other specified malignant neoplasm of skin of eyelid, including canthus**

⊟ **C44.191** **Other specified malignant neoplasm of skin of unspecified eyelid, including canthus**

▲ 7 ⊟ **C44.192** **Other specified malignant neoplasm of skin of right eyelid, including canthus**

CODING TIP ✓ There was no 7th character table published with codes C44.192- and C44.199-. A 7th character of 1 denotes "upper" and a 7th character of 2 denotes "lower".

▲ 7 ⊟ **C44.199** **Other specified malignant neoplasm of skin of left eyelid, including canthus**

5 **C44.2** **Other and unspecified malignant neoplasm of skin of ear and external auricular canal**

EXCLUDES 1 *connective tissue of ear (C49.0)*

6 **C44.20** **Unspecified malignant neoplasm of skin of ear and external auricular canal**

⊟ **C44.201** **Unspecified malignant neoplasm of skin of unspecified ear and external auricular canal**

⊟ **C44.202** **Unspecified malignant neoplasm of skin of right ear and external auricular canal**

⊟ **C44.209** **Unspecified malignant neoplasm of skin of left ear and external auricular canal**

6 **C44.21** **Basal cell carcinoma of skin of ear and external auricular canal**

⊟ **C44.211** **Basal cell carcinoma of skin of unspecified ear and external auricular canal**

⊟ **C44.212** **Basal cell carcinoma of skin of right ear and external auricular canal**

⊟ **C44.219** **Basal cell carcinoma of skin of left ear and external auricular canal**

6 **C44.22** **Squamous cell carcinoma of skin of ear and external auricular canal**

⊟ **C44.221** **Squamous cell carcinoma of skin of unspecified ear and external auricular canal**

⊟ **C44.222** **Squamous cell carcinoma of skin of right ear and external auricular canal**

⊟ **C44.229** **Squamous cell carcinoma of skin of left ear and external auricular canal**

6 **C44.29** **Other specified malignant neoplasm of skin of ear and external auricular canal**

⊟ **C44.291** **Other specified malignant neoplasm of skin of unspecified ear and external auricular canal**

⊟ **C44.292** **Other specified malignant neoplasm of skin of right ear and external auricular canal**

⊟ **C44.299** **Other specified malignant neoplasm of skin of left ear and external auricular canal**

5 **C44.3** **Other and unspecified malignant neoplasm of skin of other and unspecified parts of face**

6 **C44.30** **Unspecified malignant neoplasm of skin of other and unspecified parts of face**

C44.300 **Unspecified malignant neoplasm of skin of unspecified part of face**

C44.301 **Unspecified malignant neoplasm of skin of nose**

C44.309 **Unspecified malignant neoplasm of skin of other parts of face**

6 **C44.31** **Basal cell carcinoma of skin of other and unspecified parts of face**

C44.310 **Basal cell carcinoma of skin of unspecified parts of face**

C44.311 **Basal cell carcinoma of skin of nose**

C44.319 **Basal cell carcinoma of skin of other parts of face**

6 **C44.32** **Squamous cell carcinoma of skin of other and unspecified parts of face**

C44.320 **Squamous cell carcinoma of skin of unspecified parts of face**

C44.321 **Squamous cell carcinoma of skin of nose**

C44.329 **Squamous cell carcinoma of skin of other parts of face**

6 **C44.39** **Other specified malignant neoplasm of skin of other and unspecified parts of face**

C44.390 **Other specified malignant neoplasm of skin of unspecified parts of face**

C44.391 **Other specified malignant neoplasm of skin of nose**

C44.399 **Other specified malignant neoplasm of skin of other parts of face**

5 **C44.4** **Other and unspecified malignant neoplasm of skin of scalp and neck**

C44.40 **Unspecified malignant neoplasm of skin of scalp and neck**

C44.41 **Basal cell carcinoma of skin of scalp and neck**

C44.42 **Squamous cell carcinoma of skin of scalp and neck**

C44.49 **Other specified malignant neoplasm of skin of scalp and neck**

5 **C44.5** **Other and unspecified malignant neoplasm of skin of trunk**

EXCLUDES 1 *anus NOS (C21.0)*
scrotum (C63.2)

6 **C44.50** **Unspecified malignant neoplasm of skin of trunk**

C44.500 **Unspecified malignant neoplasm of anal skin**
Unspecified malignant neoplasm of anal margin
Unspecified malignant neoplasm of perianal skin

C44.501 **Unspecified malignant neoplasm of skin of breast**

C44.509 **Unspecified malignant neoplasm of skin of other part of trunk**

6 **C44.51** **Basal cell carcinoma of skin of trunk**

C44.510 **Basal cell carcinoma of anal skin**
Basal cell carcinoma of anal margin
Basal cell carcinoma of perianal skin

C44.511 **Basal cell carcinoma of skin of breast**

C44.519 **Basal cell carcinoma of skin of other part of trunk**

6 **C44.52** **Squamous cell carcinoma of skin of trunk**

C44.520 **Squamous cell carcinoma of anal skin**
Squamous cell carcinoma of anal margin
Squamous cell carcinoma of perianal skin

C44.521 **Squamous cell carcinoma of skin of breast**

C44.529 **Squamous cell carcinoma of skin of other part of trunk**

6 **C44.59** **Other specified malignant neoplasm of skin of trunk**

C44.590 **Other specified malignant neoplasm of anal skin**
Other specified malignant neoplasm of anal margin
Other specified malignant neoplasm of perianal skin

C44.591 **Other specified malignant neoplasm of skin of breast**

C44.599 **Other specified malignant neoplasm of skin of other part of trunk**

5 C44.6 **Other and unspecified malignant neoplasm of skin of upper limb, including shoulder**

6 C44.60 **Unspecified malignant neoplasm of skin of upper limb, including shoulder**

C44.601 **Unspecified malignant neoplasm of skin of unspecified upper limb, including shoulder**

C44.602 **Unspecified malignant neoplasm of skin of right upper limb, including shoulder**

C44.609 **Unspecified malignant neoplasm of skin of left upper limb, including shoulder**

6 C44.61 **Basal cell carcinoma of skin of upper limb, including shoulder**

C44.611 **Basal cell carcinoma of skin of unspecified upper limb, including shoulder**

C44.612 **Basal cell carcinoma of skin of right upper limb, including shoulder**

C44.619 **Basal cell carcinoma of skin of left upper limb, including shoulder**

6 C44.62 **Squamous cell carcinoma of skin of upper limb, including shoulder**

C44.621 **Squamous cell carcinoma of skin of unspecified upper limb, including shoulder**

C44.622 **Squamous cell carcinoma of skin of right upper limb, including shoulder**

C44.629 **Squamous cell carcinoma of skin of left upper limb, including shoulder**

6 C44.69 **Other specified malignant neoplasm of skin of upper limb, including shoulder**

C44.691 **Other specified malignant neoplasm of skin of unspecified upper limb, including shoulder**

C44.692 **Other specified malignant neoplasm of skin of right upper limb, including shoulder**

C44.699 **Other specified malignant neoplasm of skin of left upper limb, including shoulder**

5 C44.7 **Other and unspecified malignant neoplasm of skin of lower limb, including hip**

6 C44.70 **Unspecified malignant neoplasm of skin of lower limb, including hip**

C44.701 **Unspecified malignant neoplasm of skin of unspecified lower limb, including hip**

C44.702 **Unspecified malignant neoplasm of skin of right lower limb, including hip**

C44.709 **Unspecified malignant neoplasm of skin of left lower limb, including hip**

6 C44.71 **Basal cell carcinoma of skin of lower limb, including hip**

C44.711 **Basal cell carcinoma of skin of unspecified lower limb, including hip**

C44.712 **Basal cell carcinoma of skin of right lower limb, including hip**

C44.719 **Basal cell carcinoma of skin of left lower limb, including hip**

6 C44.72 **Squamous cell carcinoma of skin of lower limb, including hip**

C44.721 **Squamous cell carcinoma of skin of unspecified lower limb, including hip**

C44.722 **Squamous cell carcinoma of skin of right lower limb, including hip**

C44.729 **Squamous cell carcinoma of skin of left lower limb, including hip**

6 C44.79 **Other specified malignant neoplasm of skin of lower limb, including hip**

C44.791 **Other specified malignant neoplasm of skin of unspecified lower limb, including hip**

C44.792 **Other specified malignant neoplasm of skin of right lower limb, including hip**

C44.799 **Other specified malignant neoplasm of skin of left lower limb, including hip**

5 C44.8 **Other and unspecified malignant neoplasm of overlapping sites of skin**

C44.80 **Unspecified malignant neoplasm of overlapping sites of skin**

C44.81 **Basal cell carcinoma of overlapping sites of skin**

C44.82 **Squamous cell carcinoma of overlapping sites of skin**

C44.89 **Other specified malignant neoplasm of overlapping sites of skin**

5 C44.9 **Other and unspecified malignant neoplasm of skin, unspecified**

C44.90 **Unspecified malignant neoplasm of skin, unspecified**
Malignant neoplasm of unspecified site of skin

C44.91 **Basal cell carcinoma of skin, unspecified**

C44.92 **Squamous cell carcinoma of skin, unspecified**

C44.99 **Other specified malignant neoplasm of skin, unspecified**

Malignant neoplasms of mesothelial and soft tissue (C45-C49)

CODING TIP ✓ Codes classifiable to C45-C49 include active cancer. History of cancer to soft tissue should be coded to Z85.83-.

4 C45 **Mesothelioma**

C45.0 **Mesothelioma of pleura** HCC
EXCLUDES 1 *other malignant neoplasm of pleura (C38.4)*
AHA: 2Q 2017, 11

C45.1 **Mesothelioma of peritoneum** HCC
Mesothelioma of cul-de-sac
Mesothelioma of mesentery
Mesothelioma of mesocolon
Mesothelioma of omentum
Mesothelioma of peritoneum (parietal) (pelvic)
EXCLUDES 1 *other malignant neoplasm of soft tissue of peritoneum (C48.-)*

C45.2 **Mesothelioma of pericardium** HCC
EXCLUDES 1 *other malignant neoplasm of pericardium (C38.0)*

C45.7 **Mesothelioma of other sites** HCC

C45.9 **Mesothelioma, unspecified** HCC

4 C46 **Kaposi's sarcoma**
Code first:
any human immunodeficiency virus [HIV] disease (B20)

C46.0 **Kaposi's sarcoma of skin** HCC HIV

C46.1 **Kaposi's sarcoma of soft tissue** HCC HIV
Kaposi's sarcoma of blood vessel
Kaposi's sarcoma of connective tissue
Kaposi's sarcoma of fascia
Kaposi's sarcoma of ligament
Kaposi's sarcoma of lymphatic(s) NEC
Kaposi's sarcoma of muscle
EXCLUDES 2 *Kaposi's sarcoma of lymph glands and nodes (C46.3)*

C46.2 **Kaposi's sarcoma of palate** HCC HIV

C46.3 **Kaposi's sarcoma of lymph nodes** HCC HIV

C46.4 **Kaposi's sarcoma of gastrointestinal sites** HCC HIV

5 C46.5 **Kaposi's sarcoma of lung**

C46.50 **Kaposi's sarcoma of unspecified lung** HCC HIV

C46.51 **Kaposi's sarcoma of right lung** HCC HIV

C46.52 **Kaposi's sarcoma of left lung** HCC HIV

C46.7 **Kaposi's sarcoma of other sites** HCC HIV

C46.9 **Kaposi's sarcoma, unspecified** HCC HIV
Kaposi's sarcoma of unspecified site

4 C47 **Malignant neoplasm of peripheral nerves and autonomic nervous system**
INCLUDES malignant neoplasm of sympathetic and parasympathetic nerves and ganglia
EXCLUDES 1 *Kaposi's sarcoma of soft tissue (C46.1)*

C47.0 **Malignant neoplasm of peripheral nerves of head, face and neck** HCC
EXCLUDES 1 *malignant neoplasm of peripheral nerves of orbit (C69.6-)*

5 C47.1 **Malignant neoplasm of peripheral nerves of upper limb, including shoulder**

C47.10 **Malignant neoplasm of peripheral nerves of unspecified upper limb, including shoulder** HCC

C47.11 **Malignant neoplasm of peripheral nerves of right upper limb, including shoulder** HCC

C47.12 **Malignant neoplasm of peripheral nerves of left upper limb, including shoulder** HCC

5 C47.2 **Malignant neoplasm of peripheral nerves of lower limb, including hip**

C47.20 **Malignant neoplasm of peripheral nerves of unspecified lower limb, including hip** HCC

⊟ C47.21 **Malignant neoplasm of peripheral nerves of right lower limb, including hip** HCC

⊟ C47.22 **Malignant neoplasm of peripheral nerves of left lower limb, including hip** HCC

C47.3 **Malignant neoplasm of peripheral nerves of thorax** HCC

C47.4 **Malignant neoplasm of peripheral nerves of abdomen** HCC

C47.5 **Malignant neoplasm of peripheral nerves of pelvis** HCC

C47.6 **Malignant neoplasm of peripheral nerves of trunk, unspecified** HCC

Malignant neoplasm of peripheral nerves of unspecified part of trunk

C47.8 **Malignant neoplasm of overlapping sites of peripheral nerves and autonomic nervous system** HCC

C47.9 **Malignant neoplasm of peripheral nerves and autonomic nervous system, unspecified** HCC

Malignant neoplasm of unspecified site of peripheral nerves and autonomic nervous system

④ C48 **Malignant neoplasm of retroperitoneum and peritoneum**

EXCLUDES 1 *Kaposi's sarcoma of connective tissue (C46.1)*
mesothelioma (C45.-)

C48.0 **Malignant neoplasm of retroperitoneum** HCC

C48.1 **Malignant neoplasm of specified parts of peritoneum** HCC

Malignant neoplasm of cul-de-sac
Malignant neoplasm of mesentery
Malignant neoplasm of mesocolon
Malignant neoplasm of omentum
Malignant neoplasm of parietal peritoneum
Malignant neoplasm of pelvic peritoneum

C48.2 **Malignant neoplasm of peritoneum, unspecified** HCC

C48.8 **Malignant neoplasm of overlapping sites of retroperitoneum and peritoneum** HCC

④ C49 **Malignant neoplasm of other connective and soft tissue**

INCLUDES malignant neoplasm of blood vessel
malignant neoplasm of bursa
malignant neoplasm of cartilage
malignant neoplasm of fascia
malignant neoplasm of fat
malignant neoplasm of ligament, except uterine
malignant neoplasm of lymphatic vessel
malignant neoplasm of muscle
malignant neoplasm of synovia
malignant neoplasm of tendon (sheath)

EXCLUDES 1 *malignant neoplasm of cartilage (of) :*
articular (C40-C41)
larynx (C32.3)
nose (C30.0)
malignant neoplasm of connective tissue of breast (C50.-)

EXCLUDES 2 *Kaposi's sarcoma of soft tissue (C46.1)*
malignant neoplasm of heart (C38.0)
malignant neoplasm of peripheral nerves and autonomic nervous system (C47.-)
malignant neoplasm of peritoneum (C48.2)
malignant neoplasm of retroperitoneum (C48.0)
malignant neoplasm of uterine ligament (C57.3)
mesothelioma (C45.-)

C49.0 **Malignant neoplasm of connective and soft tissue of head, face and neck** HCC

Malignant neoplasm of connective tissue of ear
Malignant neoplasm of connective tissue of eyelid

EXCLUDES 1 *connective tissue of orbit (C69.6-)*

⑤ C49.1 **Malignant neoplasm of connective and soft tissue of upper limb, including shoulder**

⊟ C49.10 **Malignant neoplasm of connective and soft tissue of unspecified upper limb, including shoulder** HCC

⊟ C49.11 **Malignant neoplasm of connective and soft tissue of right upper limb, including shoulder** HCC

⊟ C49.12 **Malignant neoplasm of connective and soft tissue of left upper limb, including shoulder** HCC

⑤ C49.2 **Malignant neoplasm of connective and soft tissue of lower limb, including hip**

⊟ C49.20 **Malignant neoplasm of connective and soft tissue of unspecified lower limb, including hip** HCC

⊟ C49.21 **Malignant neoplasm of connective and soft tissue of right lower limb, including hip** HCC

⊟ C49.22 **Malignant neoplasm of connective and soft tissue of left lower limb, including hip** HCC

C49.3 **Malignant neoplasm of connective and soft tissue of thorax** HCC

Malignant neoplasm of axilla
Malignant neoplasm of diaphragm
Malignant neoplasm of great vessels

EXCLUDES 1 *malignant neoplasm of breast (C50.-)*
malignant neoplasm of heart (C38.0)
malignant neoplasm of mediastinum (C38.1-C38.3)
malignant neoplasm of thymus (C37)

AHA: 3Q 2015, 19

C49.4 **Malignant neoplasm of connective and soft tissue of abdomen** HCC

Malignant neoplasm of abdominal wall
Malignant neoplasm of hypochondrium

C49.5 **Malignant neoplasm of connective and soft tissue of pelvis** HCC

Malignant neoplasm of buttock
Malignant neoplasm of groin
Malignant neoplasm of perineum

C49.6 **Malignant neoplasm of connective and soft tissue of trunk, unspecified** HCC

Malignant neoplasm of back NOS

C49.8 **Malignant neoplasm of overlapping sites of connective and soft tissue** HCC

Primary malignant neoplasm of two or more contiguous sites of connective and soft tissue

C49.9 **Malignant neoplasm of connective and soft tissue, unspecified** HCC

⑤ C49.A **Gastrointestinal stromal tumor**

AHA: 4Q 2016, 8

C49.A0 **Gastrointestinal stromal tumor, unspecified site** HCC

C49.A1 **Gastrointestinal stromal tumor of esophagus** HCC

C49.A2 **Gastrointestinal stromal tumor of stomach** HCC

C49.A3 **Gastrointestinal stromal tumor of small intestine** HCC

C49.A4 **Gastrointestinal stromal tumor of large intestine** HCC

C49.A5 **Gastrointestinal stromal tumor of rectum** HCC

C49.A9 **Gastrointestinal stromal tumor of other sites** HCC

Malignant neoplasms of breast (C50)

CODING TIP✓ Code C50 indicates active cancer. History of cancer to the breast should be coded to Z85.3. Add a Z79.81- code for treatment agents affecting estrogen receptors and estrogen levels.

④ C50 **Malignant neoplasm of breast**

INCLUDES connective tissue of breast
Paget's disease of breast
Paget's disease of nipple

Use additional code to identify estrogen receptor status (Z17.0, Z17.1)

EXCLUDES 1 *skin of breast (C44.501, C44.511, C44.521, C44.591)*

⑤ C50.0 **Malignant neoplasm of nipple and areola**

⑥ C50.01 **Malignant neoplasm of nipple and areola, female**

⊟ C50.011 **Malignant neoplasm of nipple and areola, right female breast** ♀HCC

⊟ C50.012 **Malignant neoplasm of nipple and areola, left female breast** ♀HCC

⊟ C50.019 **Malignant neoplasm of nipple and areola, unspecified female breast** ♀HCC

⑥ C50.02 **Malignant neoplasm of nipple and areola, male**

⊟ C50.021 **Malignant neoplasm of nipple and areola, right male breast** ♂HCC

⊟ C50.022 **Malignant neoplasm of nipple and areola, left male breast** ♂HCC

⊟ C50.029 **Malignant neoplasm of nipple and areola, unspecified male breast** ♂HCC

⑤ C50.1 **Malignant neoplasm of central portion of breast**

⑥ C50.11 **Malignant neoplasm of central portion of breast, female**

⊟ C50.111 **Malignant neoplasm of central portion of right female breast** ♀HCC

C50.112 Malignant neoplasm of central portion of left female breast ♀ HCC
C50.119 Malignant neoplasm of central portion of unspecified female breast ♀ HCC
C50.12 Malignant neoplasm of central portion of breast, male
C50.121 Malignant neoplasm of central portion of right male breast ♂ HCC
C50.122 Malignant neoplasm of central portion of left male breast ♂ HCC
C50.129 Malignant neoplasm of central portion of unspecified male breast ♂ HCC
C50.2 Malignant neoplasm of upper-inner quadrant of breast
C50.21 Malignant neoplasm of upper-inner quadrant of breast, female
C50.211 Malignant neoplasm of upper-inner quadrant of right female breast ♀ HCC
C50.212 Malignant neoplasm of upper-inner quadrant of left female breast ♀ HCC
C50.219 Malignant neoplasm of upper-inner quadrant of unspecified female breast ♀ HCC
C50.22 Malignant neoplasm of upper-inner quadrant of breast, male
C50.221 Malignant neoplasm of upper-inner quadrant of right male breast ♂ HCC
C50.222 Malignant neoplasm of upper-inner quadrant of left male breast ♂ HCC
C50.229 Malignant neoplasm of upper-inner quadrant of unspecified male breast ♂ HCC
C50.3 Malignant neoplasm of lower-inner quadrant of breast
C50.31 Malignant neoplasm of lower-inner quadrant of breast, female
C50.311 Malignant neoplasm of lower-inner quadrant of right female breast ♀ HCC
C50.312 Malignant neoplasm of lower-inner quadrant of left female breast ♀ HCC
C50.319 Malignant neoplasm of lower-inner quadrant of unspecified female breast ♀ HCC
C50.32 Malignant neoplasm of lower-inner quadrant of breast, male
C50.321 Malignant neoplasm of lower-inner quadrant of right male breast ♂ HCC
C50.322 Malignant neoplasm of lower-inner quadrant of left male breast ♂ HCC
C50.329 Malignant neoplasm of lower-inner quadrant of unspecified male breast ♂ HCC
C50.4 Malignant neoplasm of upper-outer quadrant of breast
C50.41 Malignant neoplasm of upper-outer quadrant of breast, female
C50.411 Malignant neoplasm of upper-outer quadrant of right female breast ♀ HCC
C50.412 Malignant neoplasm of upper-outer quadrant of left female breast ♀ HCC
C50.419 Malignant neoplasm of upper-outer quadrant of unspecified female breast ♀ HCC
C50.42 Malignant neoplasm of upper-outer quadrant of breast, male
C50.421 Malignant neoplasm of upper-outer quadrant of right male breast ♂ HCC
C50.422 Malignant neoplasm of upper-outer quadrant of left male breast ♂ HCC
C50.429 Malignant neoplasm of upper-outer quadrant of unspecified male breast ♂ HCC
C50.5 Malignant neoplasm of lower-outer quadrant of breast
C50.51 Malignant neoplasm of lower-outer quadrant of breast, female
C50.511 Malignant neoplasm of lower-outer quadrant of right female breast ♀ HCC
C50.512 Malignant neoplasm of lower-outer quadrant of left female breast ♀ HCC
C50.519 Malignant neoplasm of lower-outer quadrant of unspecified female breast ♀ HCC
C50.52 Malignant neoplasm of lower-outer quadrant of breast, male
C50.521 Malignant neoplasm of lower-outer quadrant of right male breast ♂ HCC
C50.522 Malignant neoplasm of lower-outer quadrant of left male breast ♂ HCC
C50.529 Malignant neoplasm of lower-outer quadrant of unspecified male breast ♂ HCC
C50.6 Malignant neoplasm of axillary tail of breast
C50.61 Malignant neoplasm of axillary tail of breast, female
C50.611 Malignant neoplasm of axillary tail of right female breast ♀ HCC
C50.612 Malignant neoplasm of axillary tail of left female breast ♀ HCC
C50.619 Malignant neoplasm of axillary tail of unspecified female breast ♀ HCC
C50.62 Malignant neoplasm of axillary tail of breast, male
C50.621 Malignant neoplasm of axillary tail of right male breast ♂ HCC
C50.622 Malignant neoplasm of axillary tail of left male breast ♂ HCC
C50.629 Malignant neoplasm of axillary tail of unspecified male breast ♂ HCC
C50.8 Malignant neoplasm of overlapping sites of breast
C50.81 Malignant neoplasm of overlapping sites of breast, female
C50.811 Malignant neoplasm of overlapping sites of right female breast ♀ HCC
C50.812 Malignant neoplasm of overlapping sites of left female breast ♀ HCC
C50.819 Malignant neoplasm of overlapping sites of unspecified female breast ♀ HCC
C50.82 Malignant neoplasm of overlapping sites of breast, male
C50.821 Malignant neoplasm of overlapping sites of right male breast ♂ HCC
C50.822 Malignant neoplasm of overlapping sites of left male breast ♂ HCC
C50.829 Malignant neoplasm of overlapping sites of unspecified male breast ♂ HCC
C50.9 Malignant neoplasm of breast of unspecified site
C50.91 Malignant neoplasm of breast of unspecified site, female
C50.911 Malignant neoplasm of unspecified site of right female breast ♀ HCC
C50.912 Malignant neoplasm of unspecified site of left female breast ♀ HCC
C50.919 Malignant neoplasm of unspecified site of unspecified female breast ♀ HCC
C50.92 Malignant neoplasm of breast of unspecified site, male
C50.921 Malignant neoplasm of unspecified site of right male breast ♂ HCC
C50.922 Malignant neoplasm of unspecified site of left male breast ♂ HCC
C50.929 Malignant neoplasm of unspecified site of unspecified male breast ♂ HCC

Malignant neoplasms of female genital organs (C51-C58)

INCLUDES malignant neoplasm of skin of female genital organs

CODING TIP ✓ Categories C51-C58 indicate active cancer. See Z85.40-Z85.44 for personal history of primary malignancy of female genital organs and Z85.45-Z85.49 for personal history of primary malignancy of male genital organs.

C51 Malignant neoplasm of vulva
EXCLUDES 1 *carcinoma in situ of vulva (D07.1)*
C51.0 Malignant neoplasm of labium majus ♀ HCC
Malignant neoplasm of Bartholin's [greater vestibular] gland
C51.1 Malignant neoplasm of labium minus ♀ HCC
C51.2 Malignant neoplasm of clitoris ♀ HCC
C51.8 Malignant neoplasm of overlapping sites of vulva ♀ HCC
C51.9 Malignant neoplasm of vulva, unspecified ♀ HCC
Malignant neoplasm of external female genitalia NOS
Malignant neoplasm of pudendum

C52 Malignant neoplasm of vagina ♀ HCC
EXCLUDES 1 *carcinoma in situ of vagina (D07.2)*

4 **C53 Malignant neoplasm of cervix uteri**
EXCLUDES 1 *carcinoma in situ of cervix uteri (D06.-)*

C53.0 Malignant neoplasm of endocervix ♀ HCC
C53.1 Malignant neoplasm of exocervix ♀ HCC
C53.8 Malignant neoplasm of overlapping sites of cervix uteri ♀ HCC
C53.9 Malignant neoplasm of cervix uteri, unspecified ♀ HCC
AHA: 4Q 2017, 81

4 **C54 Malignant neoplasm of corpus uteri**
C54.0 Malignant neoplasm of isthmus uteri ♀ HCC
Malignant neoplasm of lower uterine segment
C54.1 Malignant neoplasm of endometrium ♀ HCC
C54.2 Malignant neoplasm of myometrium ♀ HCC
C54.3 Malignant neoplasm of fundus uteri ♀ HCC
C54.8 Malignant neoplasm of overlapping sites of corpus uteri ♀ HCC
C54.9 Malignant neoplasm of corpus uteri, unspecified ♀ HCC

C55 Malignant neoplasm of uterus, part unspecified ♀ HCC

4 **C56 Malignant neoplasm of ovary**
Use additional code to identify any functional activity
C56.1 Malignant neoplasm of right ovary ♀ HCC
C56.2 Malignant neoplasm of left ovary ♀ HCC
C56.9 Malignant neoplasm of unspecified ovary ♀ HCC

4 **C57 Malignant neoplasm of other and unspecified female genital organs**
5 **C57.0 Malignant neoplasm of fallopian tube**
Malignant neoplasm of oviduct
Malignant neoplasm of uterine tube
C57.00 Malignant neoplasm of unspecified fallopian tube ♀ HCC
C57.01 Malignant neoplasm of right fallopian tube ♀ HCC
C57.02 Malignant neoplasm of left fallopian tube ♀ HCC
5 **C57.1 Malignant neoplasm of broad ligament**
C57.10 Malignant neoplasm of unspecified broad ligament ♀ HCC
C57.11 Malignant neoplasm of right broad ligament ♀ HCC
C57.12 Malignant neoplasm of left broad ligament ♀ HCC
5 **C57.2 Malignant neoplasm of round ligament**
C57.20 Malignant neoplasm of unspecified round ligament ♀ HCC
C57.21 Malignant neoplasm of right round ligament ♀ HCC
C57.22 Malignant neoplasm of left round ligament ♀ HCC
C57.3 Malignant neoplasm of parametrium ♀ HCC
Malignant neoplasm of uterine ligament NOS
C57.4 Malignant neoplasm of uterine adnexa, unspecified ♀ HCC
C57.7 Malignant neoplasm of other specified female genital organs ♀ HCC
Malignant neoplasm of wolffian body or duct
C57.8 Malignant neoplasm of overlapping sites of female genital organs ♀ HCC
Primary malignant neoplasm of two or more contiguous sites of the female genital organs whose point of origin cannot be determined
Primary tubo-ovarian malignant neoplasm whose point of origin cannot be determined
Primary utero-ovarian malignant neoplasm whose point of origin cannot be determined
C57.9 Malignant neoplasm of female genital organ, unspecified ♀ HCC
Malignant neoplasm of female genitourinary tract NOS

C58 Malignant neoplasm of placenta ♀ M HCC
INCLUDES choriocarcinoma NOS
chorionepithelioma NOS
EXCLUDES 1 *chorioadenoma (destruens) (D39.2)*
hydatidiform mole NOS (O01.9)
invasive hydatidiform mole (D39.2)
male choriocarcinoma NOS (C62.9-)
malignant hydatidiform mole (D39.2)

Malignant neoplasms of male genital organs (C60-C63)

INCLUDES malignant neoplasm of skin of male genital organs

CODING TIP ✓ Codes classifiable to C60-C63 include active cancer. History of cancer to the male genital organs should be coded to Z85.4-.

4 **C60 Malignant neoplasm of penis**
C60.0 Malignant neoplasm of prepuce ♂ HCC
Malignant neoplasm of foreskin
C60.1 Malignant neoplasm of glans penis ♂ HCC
C60.2 Malignant neoplasm of body of penis ♂ HCC
Malignant neoplasm of corpus cavernosum
C60.8 Malignant neoplasm of overlapping sites of penis ♂ HCC
C60.9 Malignant neoplasm of penis, unspecified ♂ HCC
Malignant neoplasm of skin of penis NOS

C61 Malignant neoplasm of prostate ♂ HCC
Use additional code to identify:
hormone sensitivity status (Z19.1-Z19.2)
rising PSA following treatment for malignant neoplasm of prostate (R97.21)
EXCLUDES 1 *malignant neoplasm of seminal vesicle (C63.7)*

4 **C62 Malignant neoplasm of testis**
Use additional code to identify any functional activity
5 **C62.0 Malignant neoplasm of undescended testis**
Malignant neoplasm of ectopic testis
Malignant neoplasm of retained testis
C62.00 Malignant neoplasm of unspecified undescended testis ♂ HCC
C62.01 Malignant neoplasm of undescended right testis ♂ HCC
C62.02 Malignant neoplasm of undescended left testis ♂ HCC
5 **C62.1 Malignant neoplasm of descended testis**
Malignant neoplasm of scrotal testis
C62.10 Malignant neoplasm of unspecified descended testis ♂ HCC
C62.11 Malignant neoplasm of descended right testis ♂ HCC
C62.12 Malignant neoplasm of descended left testis ♂ HCC
5 **C62.9 Malignant neoplasm of testis, unspecified whether descended or undescended**
C62.90 Malignant neoplasm of unspecified testis, unspecified whether descended or undescended ♂ HCC
Malignant neoplasm of testis NOS
C62.91 Malignant neoplasm of right testis, unspecified whether descended or undescended ♂ HCC
C62.92 Malignant neoplasm of left testis, unspecified whether descended or undescended ♂ HCC

4 **C63 Malignant neoplasm of other and unspecified male genital organs**
5 **C63.0 Malignant neoplasm of epididymis**
C63.00 Malignant neoplasm of unspecified epididymis ♂ HCC
C63.01 Malignant neoplasm of right epididymis ♂ HCC
C63.02 Malignant neoplasm of left epididymis ♂ HCC
5 **C63.1 Malignant neoplasm of spermatic cord**
C63.10 Malignant neoplasm of unspecified spermatic cord ♂ HCC
C63.11 Malignant neoplasm of right spermatic cord ♂ HCC
C63.12 Malignant neoplasm of left spermatic cord ♂ HCC
C63.2 Malignant neoplasm of scrotum ♂ HCC
Malignant neoplasm of skin of scrotum
C63.7 Malignant neoplasm of other specified male genital organs ♂ HCC
Malignant neoplasm of seminal vesicle
Malignant neoplasm of tunica vaginalis
C63.8 Malignant neoplasm of overlapping sites of male genital organs ♂ HCC
Primary malignant neoplasm of two or more contiguous sites of male genital organs whose point of origin cannot be determined

C63.9 **Malignant neoplasm of male genital organ, unspecified** ♂ HCC
Malignant neoplasm of male genitourinary tract NOS

Malignant neoplasms of urinary tract (C64-C68)

CODING TIP ✓ Codes classifiable to C64-C68 include active cancer. History of cancer to the urinary tract should be coded to Z85.5-.

C64 Malignant neoplasm of kidney, except renal pelvis
EXCLUDES 1 *malignant carcinoid tumor of the kidney (C7A.093)*
malignant neoplasm of renal calyces (C65.-)
malignant neoplasm of renal pelvis (C65.-)
C64.1 **Malignant neoplasm of right kidney, except renal pelvis** HCC
C64.2 **Malignant neoplasm of left kidney, except renal pelvis** HCC
C64.9 **Malignant neoplasm of unspecified kidney, except renal pelvis** HCC

C65 Malignant neoplasm of renal pelvis
INCLUDES malignant neoplasm of pelviureteric junction
malignant neoplasm of renal calyces
C65.1 **Malignant neoplasm of right renal pelvis** HCC
C65.2 **Malignant neoplasm of left renal pelvis** HCC
C65.9 **Malignant neoplasm of unspecified renal pelvis** HCC

C66 Malignant neoplasm of ureter
EXCLUDES 1 *malignant neoplasm of ureteric orifice of bladder (C67.6)*
C66.1 **Malignant neoplasm of right ureter** HCC
C66.2 **Malignant neoplasm of left ureter** HCC
C66.9 **Malignant neoplasm of unspecified ureter** HCC

C67 Malignant neoplasm of bladder
C67.0 **Malignant neoplasm of trigone of bladder** HCC
C67.1 **Malignant neoplasm of dome of bladder** HCC
C67.2 **Malignant neoplasm of lateral wall of bladder** HCC
C67.3 **Malignant neoplasm of anterior wall of bladder** HCC
C67.4 **Malignant neoplasm of posterior wall of bladder** HCC
C67.5 **Malignant neoplasm of bladder neck** HCC
Malignant neoplasm of internal urethral orifice
C67.6 **Malignant neoplasm of ureteric orifice** HCC
C67.7 **Malignant neoplasm of urachus** HCC
C67.8 **Malignant neoplasm of overlapping sites of bladder** HCC
C67.9 **Malignant neoplasm of bladder, unspecified** HCC
AHA: 1Q 2016, 19

C68 Malignant neoplasm of other and unspecified urinary organs
EXCLUDES 1 *malignant neoplasm of female genitourinary tract NOS (C57.9)*
malignant neoplasm of male genitourinary tract NOS (C63.9)
C68.0 **Malignant neoplasm of urethra** HCC
EXCLUDES 1 *malignant neoplasm of urethral orifice of bladder (C67.5)*
C68.1 **Malignant neoplasm of paraurethral glands** HCC
C68.8 **Malignant neoplasm of overlapping sites of urinary organs** HCC
Primary malignant neoplasm of two or more contiguous sites of urinary organs whose point of origin cannot be determined
C68.9 **Malignant neoplasm of urinary organ, unspecified** HCC
Malignant neoplasm of urinary system NOS

Malignant neoplasms of eye, brain and other parts of central nervous system (C69-C72)

CODING TIP ✓ Codes classifiable to C69-C72 include active cancer. History of cancer to eye, brain, or other area of nervous system should be coded to Z85.84-.

C69 Malignant neoplasm of eye and adnexa
EXCLUDES 1 *malignant neoplasm of connective tissue of eyelid (C49.0)*
malignant neoplasm of eyelid (skin) (C43.1-, C44.1-)
malignant neoplasm of optic nerve (C72.3-)

C69.0 **Malignant neoplasm of conjunctiva**
C69.00 **Malignant neoplasm of unspecified conjunctiva** HCC
C69.01 **Malignant neoplasm of right conjunctiva** HCC
C69.02 **Malignant neoplasm of left conjunctiva** HCC
C69.1 **Malignant neoplasm of cornea**
C69.10 **Malignant neoplasm of unspecified cornea** HCC
C69.11 **Malignant neoplasm of right cornea** HCC
C69.12 **Malignant neoplasm of left cornea** HCC
C69.2 **Malignant neoplasm of retina**
EXCLUDES 1 *dark area on retina (D49.81)*
neoplasm of unspecified behavior of retina and choroid (D49.81)
retinal freckle (D49.81)
C69.20 **Malignant neoplasm of unspecified retina** HCC
C69.21 **Malignant neoplasm of right retina** HCC
C69.22 **Malignant neoplasm of left retina** HCC
C69.3 **Malignant neoplasm of choroid**
C69.30 **Malignant neoplasm of unspecified choroid** HCC
C69.31 **Malignant neoplasm of right choroid** HCC
C69.32 **Malignant neoplasm of left choroid** HCC
C69.4 **Malignant neoplasm of ciliary body**
C69.40 **Malignant neoplasm of unspecified ciliary body** HCC
C69.41 **Malignant neoplasm of right ciliary body** HCC
C69.42 **Malignant neoplasm of left ciliary body** HCC
C69.5 **Malignant neoplasm of lacrimal gland and duct**
Malignant neoplasm of lacrimal sac
Malignant neoplasm of nasolacrimal duct
C69.50 **Malignant neoplasm of unspecified lacrimal gland and duct** HCC
C69.51 **Malignant neoplasm of right lacrimal gland and duct** HCC
C69.52 **Malignant neoplasm of left lacrimal gland and duct** HCC
C69.6 **Malignant neoplasm of orbit**
Malignant neoplasm of connective tissue of orbit
Malignant neoplasm of extraocular muscle
Malignant neoplasm of peripheral nerves of orbit
Malignant neoplasm of retrobulbar tissue
Malignant neoplasm of retro-ocular tissue
EXCLUDES 1 *malignant neoplasm of orbital bone (C41.0)*
C69.60 **Malignant neoplasm of unspecified orbit** HCC
C69.61 **Malignant neoplasm of right orbit** HCC
C69.62 **Malignant neoplasm of left orbit** HCC
C69.8 **Malignant neoplasm of overlapping sites of eye and adnexa**
C69.80 **Malignant neoplasm of overlapping sites of unspecified eye and adnexa** HCC
C69.81 **Malignant neoplasm of overlapping sites of right eye and adnexa** HCC
C69.82 **Malignant neoplasm of overlapping sites of left eye and adnexa** HCC
C69.9 **Malignant neoplasm of unspecified site of eye**
Malignant neoplasm of eyeball
C69.90 **Malignant neoplasm of unspecified site of unspecified eye** HCC
C69.91 **Malignant neoplasm of unspecified site of right eye** HCC
C69.92 **Malignant neoplasm of unspecified site of left eye** HCC

C70 Malignant neoplasm of meninges
C70.0 **Malignant neoplasm of cerebral meninges** HCC
C70.1 **Malignant neoplasm of spinal meninges** HCC
C70.9 **Malignant neoplasm of meninges, unspecified** HCC

C71 Malignant neoplasm of brain
EXCLUDES 1 *malignant neoplasm of cranial nerves (C72.2-C72.5)*
retrobulbar malignant neoplasm (C69.6-)
C71.0 **Malignant neoplasm of cerebrum, except lobes and ventricles** HCC
Malignant neoplasm of supratentorial NOS
C71.1 **Malignant neoplasm of frontal lobe** HCC
C71.2 **Malignant neoplasm of temporal lobe** HCC
C71.3 **Malignant neoplasm of parietal lobe** HCC
C71.4 **Malignant neoplasm of occipital lobe** HCC

C71.5 **Malignant neoplasm of cerebral ventricle** HCC
EXCLUDES 1 *malignant neoplasm of fourth cerebral ventricle (C71.7)*
C71.6 **Malignant neoplasm of cerebellum** HCC
C71.7 **Malignant neoplasm of brain stem** HCC
Malignant neoplasm of fourth cerebral ventricle
Infratentorial malignant neoplasm NOS
C71.8 **Malignant neoplasm of overlapping sites of brain** HCC
C71.9 **Malignant neoplasm of brain, unspecified** HCC
AHA: 3Q 2014, 4

4 C72 **Malignant neoplasm of spinal cord, cranial nerves and other parts of central nervous system**
EXCLUDES 1 *malignant neoplasm of meninges (C70.-)*
malignant neoplasm of peripheral nerves and autonomic nervous system (C47.-)
C72.0 **Malignant neoplasm of spinal cord** HCC
C72.1 **Malignant neoplasm of cauda equina** HCC
5 C72.2 **Malignant neoplasm of olfactory nerve**
Malignant neoplasm of olfactory bulb
C72.20 **Malignant neoplasm of unspecified olfactory nerve** HCC
C72.21 **Malignant neoplasm of right olfactory nerve** HCC
C72.22 **Malignant neoplasm of left olfactory nerve** HCC
5 C72.3 **Malignant neoplasm of optic nerve**
C72.30 **Malignant neoplasm of unspecified optic nerve** HCC
C72.31 **Malignant neoplasm of right optic nerve** HCC
C72.32 **Malignant neoplasm of left optic nerve** HCC
5 C72.4 **Malignant neoplasm of acoustic nerve**
C72.40 **Malignant neoplasm of unspecified acoustic nerve** HCC
C72.41 **Malignant neoplasm of right acoustic nerve** HCC
C72.42 **Malignant neoplasm of left acoustic nerve** HCC
5 C72.5 **Malignant neoplasm of other and unspecified cranial nerves**
C72.50 **Malignant neoplasm of unspecified cranial nerve** HCC
Malignant neoplasm of cranial nerve NOS
C72.59 **Malignant neoplasm of other cranial nerves** HCC
C72.9 **Malignant neoplasm of central nervous system, unspecified** HCC
Malignant neoplasm of unspecified site of central nervous system
Malignant neoplasm of nervous system NOS

Malignant neoplasms of thyroid and other endocrine glands (C73-C75)

CODING TIP ✓ Codes classifiable to C73-C75 include active cancer. History of cancer to endocrine glands should be coded to Z85.85-.

C73 **Malignant neoplasm of thyroid gland** HCC
Use additional code to identify any functional activity

4 C74 **Malignant neoplasm of adrenal gland**
5 C74.0 **Malignant neoplasm of cortex of adrenal gland**
C74.00 **Malignant neoplasm of cortex of unspecified adrenal gland** HCC
C74.01 **Malignant neoplasm of cortex of right adrenal gland** HCC
C74.02 **Malignant neoplasm of cortex of left adrenal gland** HCC
5 C74.1 **Malignant neoplasm of medulla of adrenal gland**
C74.10 **Malignant neoplasm of medulla of unspecified adrenal gland** HCC
C74.11 **Malignant neoplasm of medulla of right adrenal gland** HCC
C74.12 **Malignant neoplasm of medulla of left adrenal gland** HCC
5 C74.9 **Malignant neoplasm of unspecified part of adrenal gland**
C74.90 **Malignant neoplasm of unspecified part of unspecified adrenal gland** HCC
C74.91 **Malignant neoplasm of unspecified part of right adrenal gland** HCC
C74.92 **Malignant neoplasm of unspecified part of left adrenal gland** HCC

4 C75 **Malignant neoplasm of other endocrine glands and related structures**
EXCLUDES 1 *malignant carcinoid tumors (C7A.0-)*
malignant neoplasm of adrenal gland (C74.-)
malignant neoplasm of endocrine pancreas (C25.4)
malignant neoplasm of islets of Langerhans (C25.4)
malignant neoplasm of ovary (C56.-)
malignant neoplasm of testis (C62.-)
malignant neoplasm of thymus (C37)
malignant neoplasm of thyroid gland (C73)
malignant neuroendocrine tumors (C7A.-)
C75.0 **Malignant neoplasm of parathyroid gland** HCC
C75.1 **Malignant neoplasm of pituitary gland** HCC
C75.2 **Malignant neoplasm of craniopharyngeal duct** HCC
C75.3 **Malignant neoplasm of pineal gland** HCC
C75.4 **Malignant neoplasm of carotid body** HCC
C75.5 **Malignant neoplasm of aortic body and other paraganglia** HCC
C75.8 **Malignant neoplasm with pluriglandular involvement, unspecified** HCC
C75.9 **Malignant neoplasm of endocrine gland, unspecified** HCC

Malignant neuroendocrine tumors (C7A)

4 C7A **Malignant neuroendocrine tumors**
Code also:
any associated multiple endocrine neoplasia [MEN] syndromes (E31.2-)
Use additional code to identify any associated endocrine syndrome, such as:
carcinoid syndrome (E34.0)
EXCLUDES 2 *malignant pancreatic islet cell tumors (C25.4)*
Merkel cell carcinoma (C4A.-)

CODING TIP ✓ Codes classifiable to C7A- include primary neuroendocrine tumors, which are considered active malignant carcinoid tumors. Neoplasms that have been previously excised or eradicated and have no further treatment directed at that site should have a code from category Z85- for the anatomical location and not a code from C7A-.

5 C7A.0 **Malignant carcinoid tumors**
C7A.00 **Malignant carcinoid tumor of unspecified site** HCC
6 C7A.01 **Malignant carcinoid tumors of the small intestine**
C7A.010 **Malignant carcinoid tumor of the duodenum** HCC
C7A.011 **Malignant carcinoid tumor of the jejunum** HCC
C7A.012 **Malignant carcinoid tumor of the ileum** HCC
C7A.019 **Malignant carcinoid tumor of the small intestine, unspecified portion** HCC
6 C7A.02 **Malignant carcinoid tumors of the appendix, large intestine, and rectum**
C7A.020 **Malignant carcinoid tumor of the appendix** HCC
C7A.021 **Malignant carcinoid tumor of the cecum** HCC
C7A.022 **Malignant carcinoid tumor of the ascending colon** HCC
C7A.023 **Malignant carcinoid tumor of the transverse colon** HCC
C7A.024 **Malignant carcinoid tumor of the descending colon** HCC
C7A.025 **Malignant carcinoid tumor of the sigmoid colon** HCC
C7A.026 **Malignant carcinoid tumor of the rectum** HCC
C7A.029 **Malignant carcinoid tumor of the large intestine, unspecified portion** HCC
Malignant carcinoid tumor of the colon NOS
6 C7A.09 **Malignant carcinoid tumors of other sites**
C7A.090 **Malignant carcinoid tumor of the bronchus and lung** HCC
C7A.091 **Malignant carcinoid tumor of the thymus** HCC
C7A.092 **Malignant carcinoid tumor of the stomach** HCC
C7A.093 **Malignant carcinoid tumor of the kidney** HCC
C7A.094 **Malignant carcinoid tumor of the foregut, unspecified** HCC

C7A.095 **Malignant carcinoid tumor of the midgut, unspecified** HCC

C7A.096 **Malignant carcinoid tumor of the hindgut, unspecified** HCC

C7A.098 **Malignant carcinoid tumors of other sites** HCC

C7A.1 **Malignant poorly differentiated neuroendocrine tumors** HCC
Malignant poorly differentiated neuroendocrine tumor NOS
Malignant poorly differentiated neuroendocrine carcinoma, any site
High grade neuroendocrine carcinoma, any site

C7A.8 **Other malignant neuroendocrine tumors** HCC

Secondary neuroendocrine tumors (C7B)

4 C7B **Secondary neuroendocrine tumors**
Use additional code to identify any functional activity

CODING TIP✓ Codes classifiable to C7B- include secondary (metastasic) neuroendocrine tumors, which are considered active malignant carcinoid tumors. Neoplasms that have been previously excised or eradicated and have no further treatment directed at that site should have a code from category Z85- for the anatomical location and not a code from C7B-.

5 C7B.0 **Secondary carcinoid tumors**

C7B.00 **Secondary carcinoid tumors, unspecified site** HCC

C7B.01 **Secondary carcinoid tumors of distant lymph nodes** HCC

C7B.02 **Secondary carcinoid tumors of liver** HCC

C7B.03 **Secondary carcinoid tumors of bone** HCC

C7B.04 **Secondary carcinoid tumors of peritoneum** HCC
Mesentary metastasis of carcinoid tumor

C7B.09 **Secondary carcinoid tumors of other sites** HCC

C7B.1 **Secondary Merkel cell carcinoma** HCC
Merkel cell carcinoma nodal presentation
Merkel cell carcinoma visceral metastatic presentation

C7B.8 **Other secondary neuroendocrine tumors** HCC

Malignant neoplasms of ill-defined, other secondary and unspecified sites (C76-C80)

4 C76 **Malignant neoplasm of other and ill-defined sites**

EXCLUDES 1 *malignant neoplasm of female genitourinary tract NOS (C57.9)*
malignant neoplasm of male genitourinary tract NOS (C63.9)
malignant neoplasm of lymphoid, hematopoietic and related tissue (C81-C96)
malignant neoplasm of skin (C44.-)
malignant neoplasm of unspecified site NOS (C80.1)

C76.0 **Malignant neoplasm of head, face and neck** HCC
Malignant neoplasm of cheek NOS
Malignant neoplasm of nose NOS

C76.1 **Malignant neoplasm of thorax** HCC
Intrathoracic malignant neoplasm NOS
Malignant neoplasm of axilla NOS
Thoracic malignant neoplasm NOS

C76.2 **Malignant neoplasm of abdomen** HCC

C76.3 **Malignant neoplasm of pelvis** HCC
Malignant neoplasm of groin NOS
Malignant neoplasm of sites overlapping systems within the pelvis
Rectovaginal (septum) malignant neoplasm
Rectovesical (septum) malignant neoplasm

5 C76.4 **Malignant neoplasm of upper limb**

C76.40 **Malignant neoplasm of unspecified upper limb** HCC

C76.41 **Malignant neoplasm of right upper limb** HCC

C76.42 **Malignant neoplasm of left upper limb** HCC

5 C76.5 **Malignant neoplasm of lower limb**

C76.50 **Malignant neoplasm of unspecified lower limb** HCC

C76.51 **Malignant neoplasm of right lower limb** HCC

C76.52 **Malignant neoplasm of left lower limb** HCC

C76.8 **Malignant neoplasm of other specified ill-defined sites** HCC
Malignant neoplasm of overlapping ill-defined sites

4 C77 **Secondary and unspecified malignant neoplasm of lymph nodes**

EXCLUDES 1 *malignant neoplasm of lymph nodes, specified as primary (C81-C86, C88, C96.-)*
mesentary metastasis of carcinoid tumor (C7B.04)
secondary carcinoid tumors of distant lymph nodes (C7B.01)

CODING TIP✓ Codes classifiable to C77- include neoplasms specified as secondary active neoplasms of lymph nodes. Primary neoplasms of lymphatic tissue should not be coded using codes from C77-. Neoplasms that have been previously excised or eradicated and have no further treatment directed at that site should have a code from category Z85- and not a code from C77-.

C77.0 **Secondary and unspecified malignant neoplasm of lymph nodes of head, face and neck** HCC
Secondary and unspecified malignant neoplasm of supraclavicular lymph nodes

C77.1 **Secondary and unspecified malignant neoplasm of intrathoracic lymph nodes** HCC

C77.2 **Secondary and unspecified malignant neoplasm of intra-abdominal lymph nodes** HCC

C77.3 **Secondary and unspecified malignant neoplasm of axilla and upper limb lymph nodes** HCC
Secondary and unspecified malignant neoplasm of pectoral lymph nodes

C77.4 **Secondary and unspecified malignant neoplasm of inguinal and lower limb lymph nodes** HCC

C77.5 **Secondary and unspecified malignant neoplasm of intrapelvic lymph nodes** HCC

C77.8 **Secondary and unspecified malignant neoplasm of lymph nodes of multiple regions** HCC

C77.9 **Secondary and unspecified malignant neoplasm of lymph node, unspecified** HCC

4 C78 **Secondary malignant neoplasm of respiratory and digestive organs**

EXCLUDES 1 *secondary carcinoid tumors of liver (C7B.02)*
secondary carcinoid tumors of peritoneum (C7B.04)

EXCLUDES 2 *lymph node metastases (C77.0)*

CODING TIP✓ Codes classifiable to C78 and C79 include neoplasms specified as secondary active neoplasms. Primary neoplasms should not be coded to category C78 or C79. Neoplasms that have been previously excised or eradicated and have no further treatment directed at that site should have a code from category Z85 assigned for the anatomical location and not a code from C78 or C79.

5 C78.0 **Secondary malignant neoplasm of lung**

C78.00 **Secondary malignant neoplasm of unspecified lung** HCC

C78.01 **Secondary malignant neoplasm of right lung** HCC

C78.02 **Secondary malignant neoplasm of left lung** HCC

C78.1 **Secondary malignant neoplasm of mediastinum** HCC

C78.2 **Secondary malignant neoplasm of pleura** HCC

5 C78.3 **Secondary malignant neoplasm of other and unspecified respiratory organs**

C78.30 **Secondary malignant neoplasm of unspecified respiratory organ** HCC

C78.39 **Secondary malignant neoplasm of other respiratory organs** HCC

C78.4 **Secondary malignant neoplasm of small intestine** HCC

C78.5 **Secondary malignant neoplasm of large intestine and rectum** HCC

C78.6 **Secondary malignant neoplasm of retroperitoneum and peritoneum** HCC
AHA: 2Q 2017, 12

C78.7 **Secondary malignant neoplasm of liver and intrahepatic bile duct** HCC

5 C78.8 **Secondary malignant neoplasm of other and unspecified digestive organs**

C78.80 **Secondary malignant neoplasm of unspecified digestive organ** HCC

C78.89 **Secondary malignant neoplasm of other digestive organs** HCC
Code also:
exocrine pancreatic insufficiency (K86.81)

C79 Secondary malignant neoplasm of other and unspecified sites

EXCLUDES 1 *secondary carcinoid tumors (C7B.-)*
secondary neuroendocrine tumors (C7B.-)

CODING TIP ✓ Codes classifiable to C78 and C79 include neoplasms specified as secondary active neoplasms. Primary neoplasms should not be coded to category C78 or C79. Neoplasms that have been previously excised or eradicated and have no further treatment directed at that site should have a code from category Z85 assigned for the anatomical location and not a code from C78 or C79.

C79.0 **Secondary malignant neoplasm of kidney and renal pelvis**
- C79.00 **Secondary malignant neoplasm of unspecified kidney and renal pelvis** HCC
- C79.01 **Secondary malignant neoplasm of right kidney and renal pelvis** HCC
- C79.02 **Secondary malignant neoplasm of left kidney and renal pelvis** HCC

C79.1 **Secondary malignant neoplasm of bladder and other and unspecified urinary organs**
- C79.10 **Secondary malignant neoplasm of unspecified urinary organs** HCC
- C79.11 **Secondary malignant neoplasm of bladder** HCC
  EXCLUDES 2 *lymph node metastases (C77.0)*
- C79.19 **Secondary malignant neoplasm of other urinary organs** HCC

C79.2 **Secondary malignant neoplasm of skin** HCC
EXCLUDES 1 *secondary Merkel cell carcinoma (C7B.1)*

C79.3 **Secondary malignant neoplasm of brain and cerebral meninges**
- C79.31 **Secondary malignant neoplasm of brain** HCC
- C79.32 **Secondary malignant neoplasm of cerebral meninges** HCC

C79.4 **Secondary malignant neoplasm of other and unspecified parts of nervous system**
- C79.40 **Secondary malignant neoplasm of unspecified part of nervous system** HCC
- C79.49 **Secondary malignant neoplasm of other parts of nervous system** HCC

C79.5 **Secondary malignant neoplasm of bone and bone marrow**
EXCLUDES 1 *secondary carcinoid tumors of bone (C7B.03)*
- C79.51 **Secondary malignant neoplasm of bone** HCC
- C79.52 **Secondary malignant neoplasm of bone marrow** HCC

C79.6 **Secondary malignant neoplasm of ovary**
- C79.60 **Secondary malignant neoplasm of unspecified ovary** ♀ HCC
- C79.61 **Secondary malignant neoplasm of right ovary** ♀ HCC
- C79.62 **Secondary malignant neoplasm of left ovary** ♀ HCC

C79.7 **Secondary malignant neoplasm of adrenal gland**
- C79.70 **Secondary malignant neoplasm of unspecified adrenal gland** HCC
- C79.71 **Secondary malignant neoplasm of right adrenal gland** HCC
- C79.72 **Secondary malignant neoplasm of left adrenal gland** HCC

C79.8 **Secondary malignant neoplasm of other specified sites**
- C79.81 **Secondary malignant neoplasm of breast** HCC
- C79.82 **Secondary malignant neoplasm of genital organs** HCC
- C79.89 **Secondary malignant neoplasm of other specified sites** HCC
  AHA: 2Q 2017, 11

C79.9 **Secondary malignant neoplasm of unspecified site** HCC
Metastatic cancer NOS
Metastatic disease NOS
EXCLUDES 1 *carcinomatosis NOS (C80.0)*
generalized cancer NOS (C80.0)
malignant (primary) neoplasm of unspecified site (C80.1)

C80 Malignant neoplasm without specification of site

EXCLUDES 1 *malignant carcinoid tumor of unspecified site (C7A.00)*
malignant neoplasm of specified multiple sites- code to each site

C80.0 **Disseminated malignant neoplasm, unspecified** HCC
Carcinomatosis NOS
Generalized cancer, unspecified site (primary) (secondary)
Generalized malignancy, unspecified site (primary) (secondary)

GUIDELINES **Section I.C.2.j**
Code C80.0 is for use only in those cases where the patient has advanced metastatic disease and no known primary or secondary sites are specified. It should not be used in place of assigning codes for the primary site and all known secondary sites.

C80.1 **Malignant (primary) neoplasm, unspecified** HCC
Cancer NOS
Cancer unspecified site (primary)
Carcinoma unspecified site (primary)
Malignancy unspecified site (primary)
EXCLUDES 1 *secondary malignant neoplasm of unspecified site (C79.9)*

GUIDELINES **Section I.C.2.k**
Code C80.1 equates to Cancer, unspecified. This code should only be used when no determination can be made as to the primary site of a malignancy. This code should rarely be used in the inpatient setting.

CODING TIP ✓ When coding a secondary site of the cancer and the primary site is unknown, C80.1 should be added for unknown primary site. A biopsy-proven malignancy for which a primary site cannot be found constitutes 0.5% to 7% of all cancer patients.

C80.2 **Malignant neoplasm associated with transplanted organ** HCC
Code first:
complication of transplanted organ (T86.-)
Use additional code to identify the specific malignancy

GUIDELINES **Section I.C.2.r**
A malignant neoplasm of a transplanted organ should be coded as a transplant complication. Assign first the appropriate code from category T86.-, Complications of transplanted organs and tissue, followed by code C80.2. Use an additional code for the specific malignancy.

Malignant neoplasms of lymphoid, hematopoietic and related tissue (C81-C96)

EXCLUDES 2 *Kaposi's sarcoma of lymph nodes (C46.3)*
secondary and unspecified neoplasm of lymph nodes (C77.-)
secondary neoplasm of bone marrow (C79.52)
secondary neoplasm of spleen (C78.89)

CODING TIP ✓ Codes classifiable to C81-C96 include active malignancy of lymphoid, hematopeotic and related tissues. Secondary neoplastic disease of lymph tissue should not be coded using codes from C81-C96.

C81 Hodgkin lymphoma

EXCLUDES 1 *personal history of Hodgkin lymphoma (Z85.71)*

C81.0 **Nodular lymphocyte predominant Hodgkin lymphoma**
- C81.00 **Nodular lymphocyte predominant Hodgkin lymphoma, unspecified site** HCC
- C81.01 **Nodular lymphocyte predominant Hodgkin lymphoma, lymph nodes of head, face, and neck** HCC
- C81.02 **Nodular lymphocyte predominant Hodgkin lymphoma, intrathoracic lymph nodes** HCC
- C81.03 **Nodular lymphocyte predominant Hodgkin lymphoma, intra-abdominal lymph nodes** HCC
- C81.04 **Nodular lymphocyte predominant Hodgkin lymphoma, lymph nodes of axilla and upper limb** HCC
- C81.05 **Nodular lymphocyte predominant Hodgkin lymphoma, lymph nodes of inguinal region and lower limb** HCC
- C81.06 **Nodular lymphocyte predominant Hodgkin lymphoma, intrapelvic lymph nodes** HCC

C81.07 Nodular lymphocyte predominant Hodgkin lymphoma, spleen HCC
C81.08 Nodular lymphocyte predominant Hodgkin lymphoma, lymph nodes of multiple sites HCC
C81.09 Nodular lymphocyte predominant Hodgkin lymphoma, extranodal and solid organ sites HCC

5 C81.1 Nodular sclerosis Hodgkin lymphoma
Nodular sclerosis classical Hodgkin lymphoma
C81.10 Nodular sclerosis Hodgkin lymphoma, unspecified site HCC
C81.11 Nodular sclerosis Hodgkin lymphoma, lymph nodes of head, face, and neck HCC
C81.12 Nodular sclerosis Hodgkin lymphoma, intrathoracic lymph nodes HCC
C81.13 Nodular sclerosis Hodgkin lymphoma, intra-abdominal lymph nodes HCC
C81.14 Nodular sclerosis Hodgkin lymphoma, lymph nodes of axilla and upper limb HCC
C81.15 Nodular sclerosis Hodgkin lymphoma, lymph nodes of inguinal region and lower limb HCC
C81.16 Nodular sclerosis Hodgkin lymphoma, intrapelvic lymph nodes HCC
C81.17 Nodular sclerosis Hodgkin lymphoma, spleen HCC
C81.18 Nodular sclerosis Hodgkin lymphoma, lymph nodes of multiple sites HCC
C81.19 Nodular sclerosis Hodgkin lymphoma, extranodal and solid organ sites HCC

5 C81.2 Mixed cellularity Hodgkin lymphoma
Mixed cellularity classical Hodgkin lymphoma
C81.20 Mixed cellularity Hodgkin lymphoma, unspecified site HCC
C81.21 Mixed cellularity Hodgkin lymphoma, lymph nodes of head, face, and neck HCC
C81.22 Mixed cellularity Hodgkin lymphoma, intrathoracic lymph nodes HCC
C81.23 Mixed cellularity Hodgkin lymphoma, intra-abdominal lymph nodes HCC
C81.24 Mixed cellularity Hodgkin lymphoma, lymph nodes of axilla and upper limb HCC
C81.25 Mixed cellularity Hodgkin lymphoma, lymph nodes of inguinal region and lower limb HCC
C81.26 Mixed cellularity Hodgkin lymphoma, intrapelvic lymph nodes HCC
C81.27 Mixed cellularity Hodgkin lymphoma, spleen HCC
C81.28 Mixed cellularity Hodgkin lymphoma, lymph nodes of multiple sites HCC
C81.29 Mixed cellularity Hodgkin lymphoma, extranodal and solid organ sites HCC

5 C81.3 Lymphocyte depleted Hodgkin lymphoma
Lymphocyte depleted classical Hodgkin lymphoma
C81.30 Lymphocyte depleted Hodgkin lymphoma, unspecified site HCC
C81.31 Lymphocyte depleted Hodgkin lymphoma, lymph nodes of head, face, and neck HCC
C81.32 Lymphocyte depleted Hodgkin lymphoma, intrathoracic lymph nodes HCC
C81.33 Lymphocyte depleted Hodgkin lymphoma, intra-abdominal lymph nodes HCC
C81.34 Lymphocyte depleted Hodgkin lymphoma, lymph nodes of axilla and upper limb HCC
C81.35 Lymphocyte depleted Hodgkin lymphoma, lymph nodes of inguinal region and lower limb HCC
C81.36 Lymphocyte depleted Hodgkin lymphoma, intrapelvic lymph nodes HCC
C81.37 Lymphocyte depleted Hodgkin lymphoma, spleen HCC
C81.38 Lymphocyte depleted Hodgkin lymphoma, lymph nodes of multiple sites HCC
C81.39 Lymphocyte depleted Hodgkin lymphoma, extranodal and solid organ sites HCC

5 C81.4 Lymphocyte-rich Hodgkin lymphoma
Lymphocyte-rich classical Hodgkin lymphoma
EXCLUDES 1 *nodular lymphocyte predominant Hodgkin lymphoma (C81.0-)*
C81.40 Lymphocyte-rich Hodgkin lymphoma, unspecified site HCC
C81.41 Lymphocyte-rich Hodgkin lymphoma, lymph nodes of head, face, and neck HCC
C81.42 Lymphocyte-rich Hodgkin lymphoma, intrathoracic lymph nodes HCC
C81.43 Lymphocyte-rich Hodgkin lymphoma, intra-abdominal lymph nodes HCC
C81.44 Lymphocyte-rich Hodgkin lymphoma, lymph nodes of axilla and upper limb HCC
C81.45 Lymphocyte-rich Hodgkin lymphoma, lymph nodes of inguinal region and lower limb HCC
C81.46 Lymphocyte-rich Hodgkin lymphoma, intrapelvic lymph nodes HCC
C81.47 Lymphocyte-rich Hodgkin lymphoma, spleen HCC
C81.48 Lymphocyte-rich Hodgkin lymphoma, lymph nodes of multiple sites HCC
C81.49 Lymphocyte-rich Hodgkin lymphoma, extranodal and solid organ sites HCC

5 C81.7 Other Hodgkin lymphoma
Classical Hodgkin lymphoma NOS
Other classical Hodgkin lymphoma
C81.70 Other Hodgkin lymphoma, unspecified site HCC
C81.71 Other Hodgkin lymphoma, lymph nodes of head, face, and neck HCC
C81.72 Other Hodgkin lymphoma, intrathoracic lymph nodes HCC
C81.73 Other Hodgkin lymphoma, intra-abdominal lymph nodes HCC
C81.74 Other Hodgkin lymphoma, lymph nodes of axilla and upper limb HCC
C81.75 Other Hodgkin lymphoma, lymph nodes of inguinal region and lower limb HCC
C81.76 Other Hodgkin lymphoma, intrapelvic lymph nodes HCC
C81.77 Other Hodgkin lymphoma, spleen HCC
C81.78 Other Hodgkin lymphoma, lymph nodes of multiple sites HCC
C81.79 Other Hodgkin lymphoma, extranodal and solid organ sites HCC

5 C81.9 Hodgkin lymphoma, unspecified
C81.90 Hodgkin lymphoma, unspecified, unspecified site HCC
C81.91 Hodgkin lymphoma, unspecified, lymph nodes of head, face, and neck HCC
C81.92 Hodgkin lymphoma, unspecified, intrathoracic lymph nodes HCC
C81.93 Hodgkin lymphoma, unspecified, intra-abdominal lymph nodes HCC
C81.94 Hodgkin lymphoma, unspecified, lymph nodes of axilla and upper limb HCC
C81.95 Hodgkin lymphoma, unspecified, lymph nodes of inguinal region and lower limb HCC
C81.96 Hodgkin lymphoma, unspecified, intrapelvic lymph nodes HCC
C81.97 Hodgkin lymphoma, unspecified, spleen HCC
C81.98 Hodgkin lymphoma, unspecified, lymph nodes of multiple sites HCC
C81.99 Hodgkin lymphoma, unspecified, extranodal and solid organ sites HCC

4 C82 Follicular lymphoma
INCLUDES follicular lymphoma with or without diffuse areas
EXCLUDES 1 *mature T/NK-cell lymphomas (C84.-)*
personal history of non-Hodgkin lymphoma (Z85.72)

5 C82.0 Follicular lymphoma grade I
C82.00 Follicular lymphoma grade I, unspecified site HCC
C82.01 Follicular lymphoma grade I, lymph nodes of head, face, and neck HCC
C82.02 Follicular lymphoma grade I, intrathoracic lymph nodes HCC
C82.03 Follicular lymphoma grade I, intra-abdominal lymph nodes HCC
C82.04 Follicular lymphoma grade I, lymph nodes of axilla and upper limb HCC

C82.05 Follicular lymphoma grade I, lymph nodes of inguinal region and lower limb HCC
C82.06 Follicular lymphoma grade I, intrapelvic lymph nodes HCC
C82.07 Follicular lymphoma grade I, spleen HCC
C82.08 Follicular lymphoma grade I, lymph nodes of multiple sites HCC
C82.09 Follicular lymphoma grade I, extranodal and solid organ sites HCC

5 C82.1 Follicular lymphoma grade II
C82.10 Follicular lymphoma grade II, unspecified site HCC
C82.11 Follicular lymphoma grade II, lymph nodes of head, face, and neck HCC
C82.12 Follicular lymphoma grade II, intrathoracic lymph nodes HCC
C82.13 Follicular lymphoma grade II, intra-abdominal lymph nodes HCC
C82.14 Follicular lymphoma grade II, lymph nodes of axilla and upper limb HCC
C82.15 Follicular lymphoma grade II, lymph nodes of inguinal region and lower limb HCC
C82.16 Follicular lymphoma grade II, intrapelvic lymph nodes HCC
C82.17 Follicular lymphoma grade II, spleen HCC
C82.18 Follicular lymphoma grade II, lymph nodes of multiple sites HCC
C82.19 Follicular lymphoma grade II, extranodal and solid organ sites HCC

5 C82.2 Follicular lymphoma grade III, unspecified
C82.20 Follicular lymphoma grade III, unspecified, unspecified site HCC
C82.21 Follicular lymphoma grade III, unspecified, lymph nodes of head, face, and neck HCC
C82.22 Follicular lymphoma grade III, unspecified, intrathoracic lymph nodes HCC
C82.23 Follicular lymphoma grade III, unspecified, intra-abdominal lymph nodes HCC
C82.24 Follicular lymphoma grade III, unspecified, lymph nodes of axilla and upper limb HCC
C82.25 Follicular lymphoma grade III, unspecified, lymph nodes of inguinal region and lower limb HCC
C82.26 Follicular lymphoma grade III, unspecified, intrapelvic lymph nodes HCC
C82.27 Follicular lymphoma grade III, unspecified, spleen HCC
C82.28 Follicular lymphoma grade III, unspecified, lymph nodes of multiple sites HCC
C82.29 Follicular lymphoma grade III, unspecified, extranodal and solid organ sites HCC

5 C82.3 Follicular lymphoma grade IIIa
C82.30 Follicular lymphoma grade IIIa, unspecified site HCC
C82.31 Follicular lymphoma grade IIIa, lymph nodes of head, face, and neck HCC
C82.32 Follicular lymphoma grade IIIa, intrathoracic lymph nodes HCC
C82.33 Follicular lymphoma grade IIIa, intra-abdominal lymph nodes HCC
C82.34 Follicular lymphoma grade IIIa, lymph nodes of axilla and upper limb HCC
C82.35 Follicular lymphoma grade IIIa, lymph nodes of inguinal region and lower limb HCC
C82.36 Follicular lymphoma grade IIIa, intrapelvic lymph nodes HCC
C82.37 Follicular lymphoma grade IIIa, spleen HCC
C82.38 Follicular lymphoma grade IIIa, lymph nodes of multiple sites HCC
C82.39 Follicular lymphoma grade IIIa, extranodal and solid organ sites HCC

5 C82.4 Follicular lymphoma grade IIIb
C82.40 Follicular lymphoma grade IIIb, unspecified site HCC
C82.41 Follicular lymphoma grade IIIb, lymph nodes of head, face, and neck HCC
C82.42 Follicular lymphoma grade IIIb, intrathoracic lymph nodes HCC
C82.43 Follicular lymphoma grade IIIb, intra-abdominal lymph nodes HCC
C82.44 Follicular lymphoma grade IIIb, lymph nodes of axilla and upper limb HCC
C82.45 Follicular lymphoma grade IIIb, lymph nodes of inguinal region and lower limb HCC
C82.46 Follicular lymphoma grade IIIb, intrapelvic lymph nodes HCC
C82.47 Follicular lymphoma grade IIIb, spleen HCC
C82.48 Follicular lymphoma grade IIIb, lymph nodes of multiple sites HCC
C82.49 Follicular lymphoma grade IIIb, extranodal and solid organ sites HCC

5 C82.5 Diffuse follicle center lymphoma
C82.50 Diffuse follicle center lymphoma, unspecified site HCC HIV
C82.51 Diffuse follicle center lymphoma, lymph nodes of head, face, and neck HCC HIV
C82.52 Diffuse follicle center lymphoma, intrathoracic lymph nodes HCC HIV
C82.53 Diffuse follicle center lymphoma, intra-abdominal lymph nodes HCC HIV
C82.54 Diffuse follicle center lymphoma, lymph nodes of axilla and upper limb HCC HIV
C82.55 Diffuse follicle center lymphoma, lymph nodes of inguinal region and lower limb HCC HIV
C82.56 Diffuse follicle center lymphoma, intrapelvic lymph nodes HCC HIV
C82.57 Diffuse follicle center lymphoma, spleen HCC HIV
C82.58 Diffuse follicle center lymphoma, lymph nodes of multiple sites HCC HIV
C82.59 Diffuse follicle center lymphoma, extranodal and solid organ sites HCC HIV

5 C82.6 Cutaneous follicle center lymphoma
C82.60 Cutaneous follicle center lymphoma, unspecified site HCC
C82.61 Cutaneous follicle center lymphoma, lymph nodes of head, face, and neck HCC
C82.62 Cutaneous follicle center lymphoma, intrathoracic lymph nodes HCC
C82.63 Cutaneous follicle center lymphoma, intra-abdominal lymph nodes HCC
C82.64 Cutaneous follicle center lymphoma, lymph nodes of axilla and upper limb HCC
C82.65 Cutaneous follicle center lymphoma, lymph nodes of inguinal region and lower limb HCC
C82.66 Cutaneous follicle center lymphoma, intrapelvic lymph nodes HCC
C82.67 Cutaneous follicle center lymphoma, spleen HCC
C82.68 Cutaneous follicle center lymphoma, lymph nodes of multiple sites HCC
C82.69 Cutaneous follicle center lymphoma, extranodal and solid organ sites HCC

5 C82.8 Other types of follicular lymphoma
C82.80 Other types of follicular lymphoma, unspecified site HCC
C82.81 Other types of follicular lymphoma, lymph nodes of head, face, and neck HCC
C82.82 Other types of follicular lymphoma, intrathoracic lymph nodes HCC
C82.83 Other types of follicular lymphoma, intra-abdominal lymph nodes HCC
C82.84 Other types of follicular lymphoma, lymph nodes of axilla and upper limb HCC
C82.85 Other types of follicular lymphoma, lymph nodes of inguinal region and lower limb HCC
C82.86 Other types of follicular lymphoma, intrapelvic lymph nodes HCC
C82.87 Other types of follicular lymphoma, spleen HCC
C82.88 Other types of follicular lymphoma, lymph nodes of multiple sites HCC
C82.89 Other types of follicular lymphoma, extranodal and solid organ sites HCC

5 C82.9 Follicular lymphoma, unspecified

C82.90 **Follicular lymphoma, unspecified, unspecified site** HCC

C82.91 **Follicular lymphoma, unspecified, lymph nodes of head, face, and neck** HCC

C82.92 **Follicular lymphoma, unspecified, intrathoracic lymph nodes** HCC

C82.93 **Follicular lymphoma, unspecified, intra-abdominal lymph nodes** HCC

C82.94 **Follicular lymphoma, unspecified, lymph nodes of axilla and upper limb** HCC

C82.95 **Follicular lymphoma, unspecified, lymph nodes of inguinal region and lower limb** HCC

C82.96 **Follicular lymphoma, unspecified, intrapelvic lymph nodes** HCC

C82.97 **Follicular lymphoma, unspecified, spleen** HCC

C82.98 **Follicular lymphoma, unspecified, lymph nodes of multiple sites** HCC

C82.99 **Follicular lymphoma, unspecified, extranodal and solid organ sites** HCC

4 C83 Non-follicular **lymphoma**

EXCLUDES 1 *personal history of non-Hodgkin lymphoma (Z85.72)*

5 C83.0 Small cell B- **lymphoma**

Lymphoplasmacytic lymphoma
Nodal marginal zone lymphoma
Non-leukemic variant of B-CLL
Splenic marginal zone lymphoma

EXCLUDES 1 *chronic lymphocytic leukemia (C91.1)*
mature T/NK-cell lymphomas (C84.-)
Waldenström macroglobulinemia (C88.0)

DEFINITION Uncommon, low-grade, slow-growing B-cell non-Hodgkin's lymphoma involving the marginal, patchy area of the lymph node outside the mantle zone; not very responsive to traditional therapy.

C83.00 **Small cell B-cell lymphoma, unspecified site** HCC HIV

C83.01 **Small cell B-cell lymphoma, lymph nodes of head, face, and neck** HCC HIV

C83.02 **Small cell B-cell lymphoma, intrathoracic lymph nodes** HCC HIV

C83.03 **Small cell B-cell lymphoma, intra-abdominal lymph nodes** HCC HIV

C83.04 **Small cell B-cell lymphoma, lymph nodes of axilla and upper limb** HCC HIV

C83.05 **Small cell B-cell lymphoma, lymph nodes of inguinal region and lower limb** HCC HIV

C83.06 **Small cell B-cell lymphoma, intrapelvic lymph nodes** HCC HIV

C83.07 **Small cell B-cell lymphoma, spleen** HCC HIV

C83.08 **Small cell B-cell lymphoma, lymph nodes of multiple sites** HCC HIV

C83.09 **Small cell B-cell lymphoma, extranodal and solid organ sites** HCC HIV

5 C83.1 Mantle cell **lymphoma**

Centrocytic lymphoma
Malignant lymphomatous polyposis

C83.10 **Mantle cell lymphoma, unspecified site** HCC HIV

C83.11 **Mantle cell lymphoma, lymph nodes of head, face, and neck** HCC HIV

C83.12 **Mantle cell lymphoma, intrathoracic lymph nodes** HCC HIV

C83.13 **Mantle cell lymphoma, intra-abdominal lymph nodes** HCC HIV

C83.14 **Mantle cell lymphoma, lymph nodes of axilla and upper limb** HCC HIV

C83.15 **Mantle cell lymphoma, lymph nodes of inguinal region and lower limb** HCC HIV

C83.16 **Mantle cell lymphoma, intrapelvic lymph nodes** HCC HIV

C83.17 **Mantle cell lymphoma, spleen** HCC HIV

C83.18 **Mantle cell lymphoma, lymph nodes of multiple sites** HCC HIV

C83.19 **Mantle cell lymphoma, extranodal and solid organ sites** HCC HIV

5 C83.3 Diffuse large B-cell **lymphoma**

Anaplastic diffuse large B-cell lymphoma
CD30-positive diffuse large B-cell lymphoma
Centroblastic diffuse large B-cell lymphoma
Diffuse large B-cell lymphoma, subtype not specified
Immunoblastic diffuse large B-cell lymphoma
Plasmablastic diffuse large B-cell lymphoma
Diffuse large B-cell lymphoma, subtype not specified
T-cell rich diffuse large B-cell lymphoma

EXCLUDES 1 *mediastinal (thymic) large B-cell lymphoma (C85.2-)*
mature T/NK-cell lymphomas (C84.-)

C83.30 **Diffuse large B-cell lymphoma, unspecified site** HCC HIV

C83.31 **Diffuse large B-cell lymphoma, lymph nodes of head, face, and neck** HCC HIV

C83.32 **Diffuse large B-cell lymphoma, intrathoracic lymph nodes** HCC HIV

C83.33 **Diffuse large B-cell lymphoma, intra-abdominal lymph nodes** HCC HIV

C83.34 **Diffuse large B-cell lymphoma, lymph nodes of axilla and upper limb** HCC HIV

C83.35 **Diffuse large B-cell lymphoma, lymph nodes of inguinal region and lower limb** HCC HIV

C83.36 **Diffuse large B-cell lymphoma, intrapelvic lymph nodes** HCC HIV

C83.37 **Diffuse large B-cell lymphoma, spleen** HCC HIV

C83.38 **Diffuse large B-cell lymphoma, lymph nodes of multiple sites** HCC HIV

C83.39 **Diffuse large B-cell lymphoma, extranodal and solid organ sites** HCC HIV

5 C83.5 **Lymphoblastic** (diffuse) **lymphoma**

B-precursor lymphoma
Lymphoblastic B-cell lymphoma
Lymphoblastic lymphoma NOS
Lymphoblastic T-cell lymphoma
T-precursor lymphoma

C83.50 **Lymphoblastic (diffuse) lymphoma, unspecified site** HCC

C83.51 **Lymphoblastic (diffuse) lymphoma, lymph nodes of head, face, and neck** HCC

C83.52 **Lymphoblastic (diffuse) lymphoma, intrathoracic lymph nodes** HCC

C83.53 **Lymphoblastic (diffuse) lymphoma, intra-abdominal lymph nodes** HCC

C83.54 **Lymphoblastic (diffuse) lymphoma, lymph nodes of axilla and upper limb** HCC

C83.55 **Lymphoblastic (diffuse) lymphoma, lymph nodes of inguinal region and lower limb** HCC

C83.56 **Lymphoblastic (diffuse) lymphoma, intrapelvic lymph nodes** HCC

C83.57 **Lymphoblastic (diffuse) lymphoma, spleen** HCC

C83.58 **Lymphoblastic (diffuse) lymphoma, lymph nodes of multiple sites** HCC

C83.59 **Lymphoblastic (diffuse) lymphoma, extranodal and solid organ sites** HCC

5 C83.7 Burkitt **lymphoma**

Atypical Burkitt lymphoma
Burkitt-like lymphoma

EXCLUDES 1 *mature B-cell leukemia Burkitt type (C91.A-)*

C83.70 **Burkitt lymphoma, unspecified site** HCC HIV

C83.71 **Burkitt lymphoma, lymph nodes of head, face, and neck** HCC HIV

C83.72 **Burkitt lymphoma, intrathoracic lymph nodes** HCC HIV

C83.73 **Burkitt lymphoma, intra-abdominal lymph nodes** HCC HIV

C83.74 **Burkitt lymphoma, lymph nodes of axilla and upper limb** HCC HIV

C83.75 **Burkitt lymphoma, lymph nodes of inguinal region and lower limb** HCC HIV

C83.76 **Burkitt lymphoma, intrapelvic lymph nodes** HCC HIV

C83.77 **Burkitt lymphoma, spleen** HCC HIV

C83.78 **Burkitt lymphoma, lymph nodes of multiple sites** HCC HIV

C83.79 **Burkitt lymphoma, extranodal and solid organ sites** HCC HIV

5 C83.8 **Other non-follicular lymphoma**
Intravascular large B-cell lymphoma
Lymphoid granulomatosis
Primary effusion B-cell lymphoma
EXCLUDES 1 *mediastinal (thymic) large B-cell lymphoma (C85.2-)*
T-cell rich B-cell lymphoma (C83.3-)

C83.80 **Other non-follicular lymphoma, unspecified site** HCC HIV
C83.81 **Other non-follicular lymphoma, lymph nodes of head, face, and neck** HCC HIV
C83.82 **Other non-follicular lymphoma, intrathoracic lymph nodes** HCC HIV
C83.83 **Other non-follicular lymphoma, intra-abdominal lymph nodes** HCC HIV
C83.84 **Other non-follicular lymphoma, lymph nodes of axilla and upper limb** HCC HIV
C83.85 **Other non-follicular lymphoma, lymph nodes of inguinal region and lower limb** HCC HIV
C83.86 **Other non-follicular lymphoma, intrapelvic lymph nodes** HCC HIV
C83.87 **Other non-follicular lymphoma, spleen** HCC HIV
C83.88 **Other non-follicular lymphoma, lymph nodes of multiple sites** HCC HIV
C83.89 **Other non-follicular lymphoma, extranodal and solid organ sites** HCC HIV

5 C83.9 **Non-follicular (diffuse) lymphoma, unspecified**

C83.90 **Non-follicular (diffuse) lymphoma, unspecified, unspecified site** HCC HIV
C83.91 **Non-follicular (diffuse) lymphoma, unspecified, lymph nodes of head, face, and neck** HCC HIV
C83.92 **Non-follicular (diffuse) lymphoma, unspecified, intrathoracic lymph nodes** HCC HIV
C83.93 **Non-follicular (diffuse) lymphoma, unspecified, intra-abdominal lymph nodes** HCC HIV
C83.94 **Non-follicular (diffuse) lymphoma, unspecified, lymph nodes of axilla and upper limb** HCC HIV
C83.95 **Non-follicular (diffuse) lymphoma, unspecified, lymph nodes of inguinal region and lower limb** HCC HIV
C83.96 **Non-follicular (diffuse) lymphoma, unspecified, intrapelvic lymph nodes** HCC HIV
C83.97 **Non-follicular (diffuse) lymphoma, unspecified, spleen** HCC HIV
C83.98 **Non-follicular (diffuse) lymphoma, unspecified, lymph nodes of multiple sites** HCC HIV
C83.99 **Non-follicular (diffuse) lymphoma, unspecified, extranodal and solid organ sites** HCC HIV

4 C84 **Mature T/NK-cell lymphomas**
EXCLUDES 1 *personal history of non-Hodgkin lymphoma (Z85.72)*

5 C84.0 **Mycosis fungoides**
EXCLUDES 1 *peripheral T-cell lymphoma, not classified (C84.4-)*
DEFINITION A rare, progressive form of slow-growing cutaneous T-cell lymphoma associated with a chromosome abnormality that evolves into a generalized, high grade, aggressive systemic form of lymphoma.

C84.00 **Mycosis fungoides, unspecified site** HCC
C84.01 **Mycosis fungoides, lymph nodes of head, face, and neck** HCC
C84.02 **Mycosis fungoides, intrathoracic lymph nodes** HCC
C84.03 **Mycosis fungoides, intra-abdominal lymph nodes** HCC
C84.04 **Mycosis fungoides, lymph nodes of axilla and upper limb** HCC
C84.05 **Mycosis fungoides, lymph nodes of inguinal region and lower limb** HCC
C84.06 **Mycosis fungoides, intrapelvic lymph nodes** HCC
C84.07 **Mycosis fungoides, spleen** HCC
C84.08 **Mycosis fungoides, lymph nodes of multiple sites** HCC
C84.09 **Mycosis fungoides, extranodal and solid organ sites** HCC

5 C84.1 **Sézary disease**

C84.10 **Sézary disease, unspecified site** HCC
C84.11 **Sézary disease, lymph nodes of head, face, and neck** HCC
C84.12 **Sézary disease, intrathoracic lymph nodes** HCC
C84.13 **Sézary disease, intra-abdominal lymph nodes** HCC
C84.14 **Sézary disease, lymph nodes of axilla and upper limb** HCC
C84.15 **Sézary disease, lymph nodes of inguinal region and lower limb** HCC
C84.16 **Sézary disease, intrapelvic lymph nodes** HCC
C84.17 **Sézary disease, spleen** HCC
C84.18 **Sézary disease, lymph nodes of multiple sites** HCC
C84.19 **Sézary disease, extranodal and solid organ sites** HCC

5 C84.4 **Peripheral T-cell lymphoma, not classified**
Lennert's lymphoma
Lymphoepithelioid lymphoma
Mature T-cell lymphoma, not elsewhere classified
DEFINITION Aggressive, non-Hodgkin's lymphoma derived from mature neoplastic T-cell lymphocytes that have moved to other tissue, causing site-related symptoms and generalized lymphadenopathy.

C84.40 **Peripheral T-cell lymphoma, not classified, unspecified site** HCC HIV
C84.41 **Peripheral T-cell lymphoma, not classified, lymph nodes of head, face, and neck** HCC HIV
C84.42 **Peripheral T-cell lymphoma, not classified, intrathoracic lymph nodes** HCC HIV
C84.43 **Peripheral T-cell lymphoma, not classified, intra-abdominal lymph nodes** HCC HIV
C84.44 **Peripheral T-cell lymphoma, not classified, lymph nodes of axilla and upper limb** HCC HIV
C84.45 **Peripheral T-cell lymphoma, not classified, lymph nodes of inguinal region and lower limb** HCC HIV
C84.46 **Peripheral T-cell lymphoma, not classified, intrapelvic lymph nodes** HCC HIV
C84.47 **Peripheral T-cell lymphoma, not classified, spleen** HCC HIV
C84.48 **Peripheral T-cell lymphoma, not classified, lymph nodes of multiple sites** HCC HIV
C84.49 **Peripheral T-cell lymphoma, not classified, extranodal and solid organ sites** HCC HIV

5 C84.6 **Anaplastic large cell lymphoma, ALK-positive**
Anaplastic large cell lymphoma, CD30-positive

C84.60 **Anaplastic large cell lymphoma, ALK-positive, unspecified site** HCC HIV
C84.61 **Anaplastic large cell lymphoma, ALK-positive, lymph nodes of head, face, and neck** HCC HIV
C84.62 **Anaplastic large cell lymphoma, ALK-positive, intrathoracic lymph nodes** HCC HIV
C84.63 **Anaplastic large cell lymphoma, ALK-positive, intra-abdominal lymph nodes** HCC HIV
C84.64 **Anaplastic large cell lymphoma, ALK-positive, lymph nodes of axilla and upper limb** HCC HIV
C84.65 **Anaplastic large cell lymphoma, ALK-positive, lymph nodes of inguinal region and lower limb** HCC HIV
C84.66 **Anaplastic large cell lymphoma, ALK-positive, intrapelvic lymph nodes** HCC HIV
C84.67 **Anaplastic large cell lymphoma, ALK-positive, spleen** HCC HIV

C84.68 Anaplastic large cell lymphoma, ALK-positive, lymph nodes of multiple sites HCC HIV

C84.69 Anaplastic large cell lymphoma, ALK-positive, extranodal and solid organ sites HCC HIV

5 C84.7 Anaplastic large cell lymphoma, ALK-negative

EXCLUDES 1 *primary cutaneous CD30-positive T-cell proliferations (C86.6-)*

C84.70 Anaplastic large cell lymphoma, ALK-negative, unspecified site HCC HIV

C84.71 Anaplastic large cell lymphoma, ALK-negative, lymph nodes of head, face, and neck HCC HIV

C84.72 Anaplastic large cell lymphoma, ALK-negative, intrathoracic lymph nodes HCC HIV

C84.73 Anaplastic large cell lymphoma, ALK-negative, intra-abdominal lymph nodes HCC HIV

C84.74 Anaplastic large cell lymphoma, ALK-negative, lymph nodes of axilla and upper limb HCC HIV

C84.75 Anaplastic large cell lymphoma, ALK-negative, lymph nodes of inguinal region and lower limb HCC HIV

C84.76 Anaplastic large cell lymphoma, ALK-negative, intrapelvic lymph nodes HCC HIV

C84.77 Anaplastic large cell lymphoma, ALK-negative, spleen HCC HIV

C84.78 Anaplastic large cell lymphoma, ALK-negative, lymph nodes of multiple sites HCC HIV

C84.79 Anaplastic large cell lymphoma, ALK-negative, extranodal and solid organ sites HCC HIV

5 C84.A Cutaneous T-cell lymphoma, unspecified

C84.A0 Cutaneous T-cell lymphoma, unspecified, unspecified site HCC HIV

C84.A1 Cutaneous T-cell lymphoma, unspecified lymph nodes of head, face, and neck HCC HIV

C84.A2 Cutaneous T-cell lymphoma, unspecified, intrathoracic lymph nodes HCC HIV

C84.A3 Cutaneous T-cell lymphoma, unspecified, intra-abdominal lymph nodes HCC HIV

C84.A4 Cutaneous T-cell lymphoma, unspecified, lymph nodes of axilla and upper limb HCC HIV

C84.A5 Cutaneous T-cell lymphoma, unspecified, lymph nodes of inguinal region and lower limb HCC HIV

C84.A6 Cutaneous T-cell lymphoma, unspecified, intrapelvic lymph nodes HCC HIV

C84.A7 Cutaneous T-cell lymphoma, unspecified, spleen HCC HIV

C84.A8 Cutaneous T-cell lymphoma, unspecified, lymph nodes of multiple sites HCC HIV

C84.A9 Cutaneous T-cell lymphoma, unspecified, extranodal and solid organ sites HCC HIV

5 C84.Z Other mature T/NK-cell lymphomas

Note: If T-cell lineage or involvement is mentioned in conjunction with a specific lymphoma, code to the more specific description.

EXCLUDES 1 *angioimmunoblastic T-cell lymphoma (C86.5)*
blastic NK-cell lymphoma (C86.4)
enteropathy-type T-cell lymphoma (C86.2)
extranodal NK-cell lymphoma, nasal type (C86.0)
hepatosplenic T-cell lymphoma (C86.1)
primary cutaneous CD30-positive T-cell proliferations (C86.6)
subcutaneous panniculitis-like T-cell lymphoma (C86.3)
T-cell leukemia (C91.1-)

C84.Z0 Other mature T/NK-cell lymphomas, unspecified site HCC HIV

C84.Z1 Other mature T/NK-cell lymphomas, lymph nodes of head, face, and neck HCC HIV

C84.Z2 Other mature T/NK-cell lymphomas, intrathoracic lymph nodes HCC HIV

C84.Z3 Other mature T/NK-cell lymphomas, intra-abdominal lymph nodes HCC HIV

C84.Z4 Other mature T/NK-cell lymphomas, lymph nodes of axilla and upper limb HCC HIV

C84.Z5 Other mature T/NK-cell lymphomas, lymph nodes of inguinal region and lower limb HCC HIV

C84.Z6 Other mature T/NK-cell lymphomas, intrapelvic lymph nodes HCC HIV

C84.Z7 Other mature T/NK-cell lymphomas, spleen HCC HIV

C84.Z8 Other mature T/NK-cell lymphomas, lymph nodes of multiple sites HCC HIV

C84.Z9 Other mature T/NK-cell lymphomas, extranodal and solid organ sites HCC HIV

5 C84.9 Mature T/NK-cell lymphomas, unspecified

NK/T cell lymphoma NOS

EXCLUDES 1 *mature T-cell lymphoma, not elsewhere classified (C84.4-)*

C84.90 Mature T/NK-cell lymphomas, unspecified, unspecified site HCC HIV

C84.91 Mature T/NK-cell lymphomas, unspecified, lymph nodes of head, face, and neck HCC HIV

C84.92 Mature T/NK-cell lymphomas, unspecified, intrathoracic lymph nodes HCC HIV

C84.93 Mature T/NK-cell lymphomas, unspecified, intra-abdominal lymph nodes HCC HIV

C84.94 Mature T/NK-cell lymphomas, unspecified, lymph nodes of axilla and upper limb HCC HIV

C84.95 Mature T/NK-cell lymphomas, unspecified, lymph nodes of inguinal region and lower limb HCC HIV

C84.96 Mature T/NK-cell lymphomas, unspecified, intrapelvic lymph nodes HCC HIV

C84.97 Mature T/NK-cell lymphomas, unspecified, spleen HCC HIV

C84.98 Mature T/NK-cell lymphomas, unspecified, lymph nodes of multiple sites HCC HIV

C84.99 Mature T/NK-cell lymphomas, unspecified, extranodal and solid organ sites HCC HIV

4 C85 Other specified and unspecified types of non-Hodgkin lymphoma

EXCLUDES 1 *other specified types of T/NK-cell lymphoma (C86.-)*
personal history of non-Hodgkin lymphoma (Z85.72)

5 C85.1 Unspecified B-cell lymphoma

Note: If B-cell lineage or involvement is mentioned in conjunction with a specific lymphoma, code to the more specific description.

C85.10 Unspecified B-cell lymphoma, unspecified site HCC HIV

C85.11 Unspecified B-cell lymphoma, lymph nodes of head, face, and neck HCC HIV

C85.12 Unspecified B-cell lymphoma, intrathoracic lymph nodes HCC HIV

C85.13 Unspecified B-cell lymphoma, intra-abdominal lymph nodes HCC HIV

C85.14 Unspecified B-cell lymphoma, lymph nodes of axilla and upper limb HCC HIV

C85.15 Unspecified B-cell lymphoma, lymph nodes of inguinal region and lower limb HCC HIV

C85.16 Unspecified B-cell lymphoma, intrapelvic lymph nodes HCC HIV

C85.17 Unspecified B-cell lymphoma, spleen HCC HIV

C85.18 Unspecified B-cell lymphoma, lymph nodes of multiple sites HCC HIV

C85.19 Unspecified B-cell lymphoma, extranodal and solid organ sites HCC HIV

5 C85.2 Mediastinal (thymic) large B-cell lymphoma

C85.20 Mediastinal (thymic) large B-cell lymphoma, unspecified site HCC HIV

C85.21 **Mediastinal (thymic) large B-cell lymphoma, lymph nodes of head, face, and neck** HCC HIV

C85.22 **Mediastinal (thymic) large B-cell lymphoma, intrathoracic lymph nodes** HCC HIV

C85.23 **Mediastinal (thymic) large B-cell lymphoma, intra-abdominal lymph nodes** HCC HIV

C85.24 **Mediastinal (thymic) large B-cell lymphoma, lymph nodes of axilla and upper limb** HCC HIV

C85.25 **Mediastinal (thymic) large B-cell lymphoma, lymph nodes of inguinal region and lower limb** HCC HIV

C85.26 **Mediastinal (thymic) large B-cell lymphoma, intrapelvic lymph nodes** HCC HIV

C85.27 **Mediastinal (thymic) large B-cell lymphoma, spleen** HCC HIV

C85.28 **Mediastinal (thymic) large B-cell lymphoma, lymph nodes of multiple sites** HCC HIV

C85.29 **Mediastinal (thymic) large B-cell lymphoma, extranodal and solid organ sites** HCC HIV

5 C85.8 **Other specified types of non-Hodgkin lymphoma**

C85.80 **Other specified types of non-Hodgkin lymphoma, unspecified site** HCC HIV

C85.81 **Other specified types of non-Hodgkin lymphoma, lymph nodes of head, face, and neck** HCC HIV

C85.82 **Other specified types of non-Hodgkin lymphoma, intrathoracic lymph nodes** HCC HIV

C85.83 **Other specified types of non-Hodgkin lymphoma, intra-abdominal lymph nodes** HCC HIV

C85.84 **Other specified types of non-Hodgkin lymphoma, lymph nodes of axilla and upper limb** HCC HIV

C85.85 **Other specified types of non-Hodgkin lymphoma, lymph nodes of inguinal region and lower limb** HCC HIV

C85.86 **Other specified types of non-Hodgkin lymphoma, intrapelvic lymph nodes** HCC HIV

C85.87 **Other specified types of non-Hodgkin lymphoma, spleen** HCC HIV

C85.88 **Other specified types of non-Hodgkin lymphoma, lymph nodes of multiple sites** HCC HIV

C85.89 **Other specified types of non-Hodgkin lymphoma, extranodal and solid organ sites** HCC HIV

5 C85.9 **Non-Hodgkin lymphoma, unspecified**

Lymphoma NOS
Malignant lymphoma NOS
Non-Hodgkin lymphoma NOS

C85.90 **Non-Hodgkin lymphoma, unspecified, unspecified site** HCC HIV

C85.91 **Non-Hodgkin lymphoma, unspecified, lymph nodes of head, face, and neck** HCC HIV

C85.92 **Non-Hodgkin lymphoma, unspecified, intrathoracic lymph nodes** HCC HIV

C85.93 **Non-Hodgkin lymphoma, unspecified, intra-abdominal lymph nodes** HCC HIV

C85.94 **Non-Hodgkin lymphoma, unspecified, lymph nodes of axilla and upper limb** HCC HIV

C85.95 **Non-Hodgkin lymphoma, unspecified, lymph nodes of inguinal region and lower limb** HCC HIV

C85.96 **Non-Hodgkin lymphoma, unspecified, intrapelvic lymph nodes** HCC HIV

C85.97 **Non-Hodgkin lymphoma, unspecified, spleen** HCC HIV

C85.98 **Non-Hodgkin lymphoma, unspecified, lymph nodes of multiple sites** HCC HIV

C85.99 **Non-Hodgkin lymphoma, unspecified, extranodal and solid organ sites** HCC HIV

4 C86 Other specified types of T/NK-cell lymphoma

EXCLUDES 1 *anaplastic large cell lymphoma, ALK negative (C84.7-)*
anaplastic large cell lymphoma, ALK positive (C84.6-)
mature T/NK-cell lymphomas (C84.-)
other specified types of non-Hodgkin lymphoma (C85.8-)

C86.0 **Extranodal NK/T-cell lymphoma, nasal type** HCC HIV

C86.1 **Hepatosplenic T-cell lymphoma** HCC HIV
Alpha-beta and gamma delta types

C86.2 **Enteropathy-type (intestinal) T-cell lymphoma** HCC HIV
Enteropathy associated T-cell lymphoma

C86.3 **Subcutaneous panniculitis-like T-cell lymphoma** HCC HIV

C86.4 **Blastic NK-cell lymphoma** HCC HIV
Blastic plasmacytoid dendritic cell neoplasm (BPDCN)

C86.5 **Angioimmunoblastic T-cell lymphoma** HCC HIV
Angioimmunoblastic lymphadenopathy with dysproteinemia (AILD)

C86.6 **Primary cutaneous CD30-positive T-cell proliferations** HCC HIV
Lymphomatoid papulosis
Primary cutaneous anaplastic large cell lymphoma
Primary cutaneous CD30-positive large T-cell lymphoma

4 C88 Malignant immunoproliferative diseases and certain other B-cell lymphomas

EXCLUDES 1 *B-cell lymphoma, unspecified (C85.1-)*
personal history of other malignant neoplasms of lymphoid, hematopoietic and related tissues (Z85.79)

C88.0 **Waldenström macroglobulinemia** HCC
Lymphoplasmacytic lymphoma with IgM-production
Macroglobulinemia (idiopathic) (primary)
EXCLUDES 1 *small cell B-cell lymphoma (C83.0)*

C88.2 **Heavy chain disease** HCC
Franklin disease
Gamma heavy chain disease
Mu heavy chain disease

C88.3 **Immunoproliferative small intestinal disease** HCC
Alpha heavy chain disease
Mediterranean lymphoma

C88.4 **Extranodal marginal zone B-cell lymphoma of mucosa-associated lymphoid tissue [MALT-lymphoma]** HCC HIV
Lymphoma of skin-associated lymphoid tissue [SALT-lymphoma]
Lymphoma of bronchial-associated lymphoid tissue [BALT-lymphoma]
EXCLUDES 1 *high malignant (diffuse large B-cell) lymphoma (C83.3-)*

C88.8 **Other malignant immunoproliferative diseases** HCC

C88.9 **Malignant immunoproliferative disease, unspecified** HCC
Immunoproliferative disease NOS

4 C90 Multiple myeloma and malignant plasma cell neoplasms

EXCLUDES 1 *personal history of other malignant neoplasms of lymphoid, hematopoietic and related tissues (Z85.79)*

GUIDELINES **Section I.C.2.n**
The categories for leukemia [C91 - C95], and category C90, Multiple myeloma and malignant plasma cell neoplasms, have codes indicating whether or not the leukemia has achieved remission. There are also codes Z85.6, Personal history of leukemia, and Z85.79, Personal history of other malignant neoplasms of lymphoid, hematopoietic and related tissues. If the documentation is unclear, as to whether the leukemia has achieved remission, the provider should be queried.

CODING TIP ✓ Terms such as "in remission" and "in relapse" must be specified by the physician in order to indicate assignment of a code specifying these terms. If the physician has not specified one of these terms, select the code for "not having achieved remission."

5 C90.0 Multiple myeloma
Kahler's disease
Medullary plasmacytoma
Myelomatosis
Plasma cell myeloma
EXCLUDES 1 *solitary myeloma (C90.3-)*
solitary plasmactyoma (C90.3-)

Multiple myeloma

A type of cancer characterized by excessive numbers of malignant plasma cells in the bone marrow

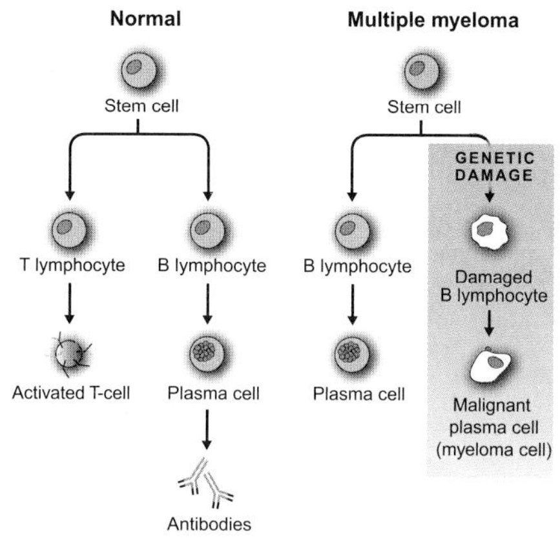

C90.00 Multiple myeloma not having achieved remission HCC
Multiple myeloma with failed remission
Multiple myeloma NOS

C90.01 Multiple myeloma in remission HCC

C90.02 Multiple myeloma in relapse HCC

5 C90.1 Plasma cell leukemia
Plasmacytic leukemia

C90.10 Plasma cell leukemia not having achieved remission HCC
Plasma cell leukemia with failed remission
Plasma cell leukemia NOS

C90.11 Plasma cell leukemia in remission HCC

C90.12 Plasma cell leukemia in relapse HCC

5 C90.2 Extramedullary plasmacytoma

C90.20 Extramedullary plasmacytoma not having achieved remission HCC
Extramedullary plasmacytoma with failed remission
Extramedullary plasmacytoma NOS

C90.21 Extramedullary plasmacytoma in remission HCC

C90.22 Extramedullary plasmacytoma in relapse HCC

5 C90.3 Solitary plasmacytoma
Localized malignant plasma cell tumor NOS
Plasmacytoma NOS
Solitary myeloma

C90.30 Solitary plasmacytoma not having achieved remission HCC
Solitary plasmacytoma with failed remission
Solitary plasmacytoma NOS

C90.31 Solitary plasmacytoma in remission HCC

C90.32 Solitary plasmacytoma in relapse HCC

4 C91 Lymphoid leukemia
EXCLUDES 1 *personal history of leukemia (Z85.6)*

CODING TIP✓ Terms such as "in remission" and "in relapse" must be specified by the physician in order to indicate assignment of a code specifying these terms. If the physician has not specified one of these terms, select the code for "not having achieved remission."

5 C91.0 Acute lymphoblastic leukemia [ALL]
Note: Code C91.0 should only be used for T-cell and B-cell precursor leukemia

C91.00 Acute lymphoblastic leukemia not having achieved remission HCC
Acute lymphoblastic leukemia with failed remission
Acute lymphoblastic leukemia NOS

C91.01 Acute lymphoblastic leukemia, in remission HCC

C91.02 Acute lymphoblastic leukemia, in relapse HCC

5 C91.1 Chronic lymphocytic leukemia of B-cell type
Lymphoplasmacytic leukemia
Richter syndrome
EXCLUDES 1 *lymphoplasmacytic lymphoma (C83.0-)*

C91.10 Chronic lymphocytic leukemia of B-cell type not having achieved remission HCC
Chronic lymphocytic leukemia of B-cell type with failed remission
Chronic lymphocytic leukemia of B-cell type NOS

C91.11 Chronic lymphocytic leukemia of B-cell type in remission HCC

C91.12 Chronic lymphocytic leukemia of B-cell type in relapse HCC

5 C91.3 Prolymphocytic leukemia of B-cell type

C91.30 Prolymphocytic leukemia of B-cell type not having achieved remission HCC
Prolymphocytic leukemia of B-cell type with failed remission
Prolymphocytic leukemia of B-cell type NOS

C91.31 Prolymphocytic leukemia of B-cell type, in remission HCC

C91.32 Prolymphocytic leukemia of B-cell type, in relapse HCC

5 C91.4 Hairy cell leukemia
Leukemic reticuloendotheliosis

C91.40 Hairy cell leukemia not having achieved remission HCC
Hairy cell leukemia with failed remission
Hairy cell leukemia NOS

C91.41 Hairy cell leukemia, in remission HCC

C91.42 Hairy cell leukemia, in relapse HCC

5 C91.5 Adult T-cell lymphoma/leukemia (HTLV-1-associated)
Acute variant of adult T-cell lymphoma/leukemia (HTLV-1-associated)
Chronic variant of adult T-cell lymphoma/leukemia (HTLV-1-associated)
Lymphomatoid variant of adult T-cell lymphoma/leukemia (HTLV-1-associated)
Smouldering variant of adult T-cell lymphoma/leukemia (HTLV-1-associated)

C91.50 Adult T-cell lymphoma/leukemia (HTLV-1-associated) not having achieved remission A HCC
Adult T-cell lymphoma/leukemia (HTLV-1-associated) with failed remission
Adult T-cell lymphoma/leukemia (HTLV-1-associated) NOS

C91.51 Adult T-cell lymphoma/leukemia (HTLV-1-associated), in remission A HCC

C91.52 Adult T-cell lymphoma/leukemia (HTLV-1-associated), in relapse A HCC

5 C91.6 Prolymphocytic leukemia of T-cell type

C91.60 Prolymphocytic leukemia of T-cell type not having achieved remission HCC
Prolymphocytic leukemia of T-cell type with failed remission
Prolymphocytic leukemia of T-cell type NOS

C91.61 Prolymphocytic leukemia of T-cell type, in remission HCC

C91.62 Prolymphocytic leukemia of T-cell type, in relapse HCC

5 C91.A Mature B-cell leukemia Burkitt-type
EXCLUDES 1 *Burkitt lymphoma (C83.7-)*

C91.A0 Mature B-cell leukemia Burkitt-type not having achieved remission HCC
Mature B-cell leukemia Burkitt-type with failed remission
Mature B-cell leukemia Burkitt-type NOS

C91.A1 Mature B-cell leukemia Burkitt-type, in remission HCC

C91.A2 Mature B-cell leukemia Burkitt-type, in relapse HCC

5 C91.Z Other lymphoid leukemia
T-cell large granular lymphocytic leukemia (associated with rheumatoid arthritis)

C91.Z0 Other lymphoid leukemia not having achieved remission HCC
Other lymphoid leukemia with failed remission
Other lymphoid leukemia NOS

C91.Z1 Other lymphoid leukemia, in remission HCC

C91.Z2 **Other lymphoid leukemia, in relapse** HCC

C91.9 **Lymphoid leukemia, unspecified**

C91.90 **Lymphoid leukemia, unspecified not having achieved remission** HCC
Lymphoid leukemia with failed remission
Lymphoid leukemia NOS

C91.91 **Lymphoid leukemia, unspecified, in remission** HCC

C91.92 **Lymphoid leukemia, unspecified, in relapse** HCC

C92 Myeloid leukemia

INCLUDES granulocytic leukemia
myelogenous leukemia

EXCLUDES 1 *personal history of leukemia (Z85.6)*

CODING TIP ✓ Terms such as "in remission" and "in relapse" must be specified by the physician to indicate assignment of a code specifying these terms. If the physician has not specified one of these terms, select the code for "not having achieved remission."

C92.0 **Acute myeloblastic leukemia**
Acute myeloblastic leukemia, minimal differentiation
Acute myeloblastic leukemia (with maturation)
Acute myeloblastic leukemia 1/ETO
Acute myeloblastic leukemia M0
Acute myeloblastic leukemia M1
Acute myeloblastic leukemia M2
Acute myeloblastic leukemia with t(8;21)
Acute myeloblastic leukemia (without a FAB classification) NOS
Refractory anemia with excess blasts in transformation [RAEB T]

EXCLUDES 1 *acute exacerbation of chronic myeloid leukemia (C92.10)*
refractory anemia with excess of blasts not in transformation (D46.2-)

C92.00 **Acute myeloblastic leukemia, not having achieved remission** HCC
Acute myeloblastic leukemia with failed remission
Acute myeloblastic leukemia NOS

C92.01 **Acute myeloblastic leukemia, in remission** HCC

C92.02 **Acute myeloblastic leukemia, in relapse** HCC

C92.1 **Chronic myeloid leukemia, BCR/ABL-positive**
Chronic myelogenous leukemia, Philadelphia chromosome (Ph1) positive
Chronic myelogenous leukemia, t(9;22) (q34;q11)
Chronic myelogenous leukemia with crisis of blast cells

EXCLUDES 1 *atypical chronic myeloid leukemia BCR/ABL-negative (C92.2-)*
chronic myelomonocytic leukemia (C93.1-)
chronic myeloproliferative disease (D47.1)

C92.10 **Chronic myeloid leukemia, BCR/ABL-positive, not having achieved remission** HCC
Chronic myeloid leukemia, BCR/ABL-positive with failed remission
Chronic myeloid leukemia, BCR/ABL-positive NOS

C92.11 **Chronic myeloid leukemia, BCR/ABL-positive, in remission** HCC

C92.12 **Chronic myeloid leukemia, BCR/ABL-positive, in relapse** HCC

C92.2 **Atypical chronic myeloid leukemia, BCR/ABL-negative**

C92.20 **Atypical chronic myeloid leukemia, BCR/ABL-negative, not having achieved remission** HCC
Atypical chronic myeloid leukemia, BCR/ABL-negative with failed remission
Atypical chronic myeloid leukemia, BCR/ABL-negative NOS

C92.21 **Atypical chronic myeloid leukemia, BCR/ABL-negative, in remission** HCC

C92.22 **Atypical chronic myeloid leukemia, BCR/ABL-negative, in relapse** HCC

C92.3 **Myeloid sarcoma**
A malignant tumor of immature myeloid cells
Chloroma
Granulocytic sarcoma

C92.30 **Myeloid sarcoma, not having achieved remission** HCC
Myeloid sarcoma with failed remission
Myeloid sarcoma NOS

C92.31 **Myeloid sarcoma, in remission** HCC

C92.32 **Myeloid sarcoma, in relapse** HCC

C92.4 **Acute promyelocytic leukemia**
AML M3
AML Me with t(15;17) and variants

C92.40 **Acute promyelocytic leukemia, not having achieved remission** HCC
Acute promyelocytic leukemia with failed remission
Acute promyelocytic leukemia NOS

C92.41 **Acute promyelocytic leukemia, in remission** HCC

C92.42 **Acute promyelocytic leukemia, in relapse** HCC

C92.5 **Acute myelomonocytic leukemia**
AML M4
AML M4 Eo with inv(16) or t(16;16)

C92.50 **Acute myelomonocytic leukemia, not having achieved remission** HCC
Acute myelomonocytic leukemia with failed remission
Acute myelomonocytic leukemia NOS

C92.51 **Acute myelomonocytic leukemia, in remission** HCC

C92.52 **Acute myelomonocytic leukemia, in relapse** HCC

C92.6 **Acute myeloid leukemia with 11q23-abnormality**
Acute myeloid leukemia with variation of MLL-gene

C92.60 **Acute myeloid leukemia with 11q23-abnormality not having achieved remission** HCC
Acute myeloid leukemia with 11q23-abnormality with failed remission
Acute myeloid leukemia with 11q23-abnormality NOS

C92.61 **Acute myeloid leukemia with 11q23-abnormality in remission** HCC

C92.62 **Acute myeloid leukemia with 11q23-abnormality in relapse** HCC

C92.A **Acute myeloid leukemia with multilineage dysplasia**
Acute myeloid leukemia with dysplasia of remaining hematopoesis and/or myelodysplastic disease in its history

C92.A0 **Acute myeloid leukemia with multilineage dysplasia, not having achieved remission** HCC
Acute myeloid leukemia with multilineage dysplasia with failed remission
Acute myeloid leukemia with multilineage dysplasia NOS

C92.A1 **Acute myeloid leukemia with multilineage dysplasia, in remission** HCC

C92.A2 **Acute myeloid leukemia with multilineage dysplasia, in relapse** HCC

C92.Z **Other myeloid leukemia**

C92.Z0 **Other myeloid leukemia not having achieved remission** HCC
Myeloid leukemia NEC with failed remission
Myeloid leukemia NEC

C92.Z1 **Other myeloid leukemia, in remission** HCC

C92.Z2 **Other myeloid leukemia, in relapse** HCC

C92.9 **Myeloid leukemia, unspecified**

C92.90 **Myeloid leukemia, unspecified, not having achieved remission** HCC
Myeloid leukemia, unspecified with failed remission
Myeloid leukemia, unspecified NOS

C92.91 **Myeloid leukemia, unspecified in remission** HCC

C92.92 **Myeloid leukemia, unspecified in relapse** HCC

C93 Monocytic leukemia

INCLUDES monocytoid leukemia

EXCLUDES 1 *personal history of leukemia (Z85.6)*

CODING TIP ✓ Terms such as "in remission" and "in relapse" must be specified by the physician to indicate assignment of a code specifying these terms. If the physician has not specified one of these terms, select the code for "not having achieved remission."

C93.0 **Acute monoblastic/monocytic leukemia**
AML M5
AML M5a
AML M5b

C93.00 **Acute monoblastic/monocytic leukemia, not having achieved remission** HCC
Acute monoblastic/monocytic leukemia with failed remission
Acute monoblastic/monocytic leukemia NOS

C93.01 **Acute monoblastic/monocytic leukemia, in remission** HCC

C93.02 **Acute monoblastic/monocytic leukemia, in relapse** HCC

5 **C93.1 Chronic myelomonocytic leukemia**
Chronic monocytic leukemia
CMML-1
CMML-2
CMML with eosinophilia

C93.10 Chronic myelomonocytic leukemia not having achieved remission HCC
Chronic myelomonocytic leukemia with failed remission
Chronic myelomonocytic leukemia NOS

C93.11 Chronic myelomonocytic leukemia, in remission HCC

C93.12 Chronic myelomonocytic leukemia, in relapse HCC

5 **C93.3 Juvenile myelomonocytic leukemia**

C93.30 Juvenile myelomonocytic leukemia, not having achieved remission P HCC
Juvenile myelomonocytic leukemia with failed remission
Juvenile myelomonocytic leukemia NOS

C93.31 Juvenile myelomonocytic leukemia, in remission P HCC

C93.32 Juvenile myelomonocytic leukemia, in relapse P HCC

5 **C93.Z Other monocytic leukemia**

C93.Z0 Other monocytic leukemia, not having achieved remission HCC
Other monocytic leukemia NOS

C93.Z1 Other monocytic leukemia, in remission HCC

C93.Z2 Other monocytic leukemia, in relapse HCC

5 **C93.9 Monocytic leukemia, unspecified**

C93.90 Monocytic leukemia, unspecified, not having achieved remission HCC
Monocytic leukemia, unspecified with failed remission
Monocytic leukemia, unspecified NOS

C93.91 Monocytic leukemia, unspecified in remission HCC

C93.92 Monocytic leukemia, unspecified in relapse HCC

4 **C94 Other leukemias of specified cell type**

EXCLUDES 1 *leukemic reticuloendotheliosis (C91.4-)*
myelodysplastic syndromes (D46.-)
personal history of leukemia (Z85.6)
plasma cell leukemia (C90.1-)

CODING TIP✓ Terms such as "in remission" and "in relapse" must be specified by the physician to indicate assignment of a code specifying these terms. If the physician has not specified one of these terms, select the code for "not having achieved remission."

5 **C94.0 Acute erythroid leukemia**
Acute myeloid leukemia M6(a)(b)
Erythroleukemia

C94.00 Acute erythroid leukemia, not having achieved remission HCC
Acute erythroid leukemia with failed remission
Acute erythroid leukemia NOS

C94.01 Acute erythroid leukemia, in remission HCC

C94.02 Acute erythroid leukemia, in relapse HCC

5 **C94.2 Acute megakaryoblastic leukemia**
Acute myeloid leukemia M7
Acute megakaryocytic leukemia

C94.20 Acute megakaryoblastic leukemia not having achieved remission HCC
Acute megakaryoblastic leukemia with failed remission
Acute megakaryoblastic leukemia NOS

C94.21 Acute megakaryoblastic leukemia, in remission HCC

C94.22 Acute megakaryoblastic leukemia, in relapse HCC

5 **C94.3 Mast cell leukemia**

C94.30 Mast cell leukemia not having achieved remission HCC
Mast cell leukemia with failed remission
Mast cell leukemia NOS

C94.31 Mast cell leukemia, in remission HCC

C94.32 Mast cell leukemia, in relapse HCC

5 **C94.4 Acute panmyelosis with myelofibrosis**
Acute myelofibrosis

EXCLUDES 1 *myelofibrosis NOS (D75.81)*
secondary myelofibrosis NOS (D75.81)

C94.40 Acute panmyelosis with myelofibrosis not having achieved remission HCC
Acute myelofibrosis NOS
Acute panmyelosis with myelofibrosis with failed remission
Acute panmyelosis NOS

C94.41 Acute panmyelosis with myelofibrosis, in remission HCC

C94.42 Acute panmyelosis with myelofibrosis, in relapse HCC

C94.6 Myelodysplastic disease, not classified HCC
Myeloproliferative disease, not classified

5 **C94.8 Other specified leukemias**
Aggressive NK-cell leukemia
Acute basophilic leukemia

C94.80 Other specified leukemias not having achieved remission HCC
Other specified leukemia with failed remission
Other specified leukemias NOS

C94.81 Other specified leukemias, in remission HCC

C94.82 Other specified leukemias, in relapse HCC

4 **C95 Leukemia of unspecified cell type**

EXCLUDES 1 *personal history of leukemia (Z85.6)*

CODING TIP✓ Terms such as "in remission" and "in relapse" must be specified by the physician to indicate assignment of a code specifying these terms. If the physician has not specified one of these terms, select the code for "not having achieved remission."

Leukemia of unspecified cell type

Leukemia begins in a cell in the bone marrow. The cell undergoes a leukemic change and it multiplies into many cells. The leukemia cells grow and survive better than normal cells and eventually crowd out the normal cells.

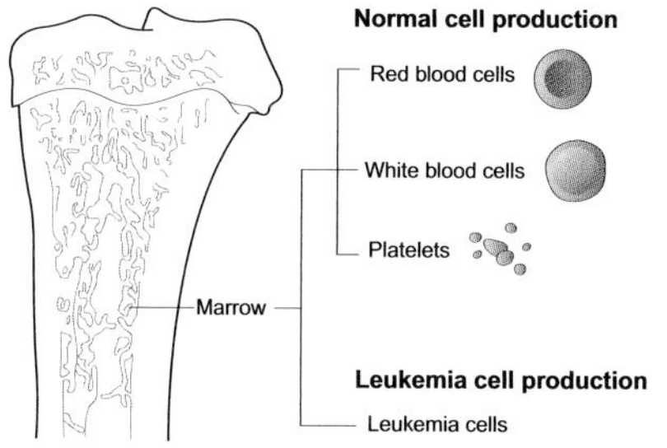

5 **C95.0 Acute leukemia of unspecified cell type**
Acute bilineal leukemia
Acute mixed lineage leukemia
Biphenotypic acute leukemia
Stem cell leukemia of unclear lineage

EXCLUDES 1 *acute exacerbation of unspecified chronic leukemia (C95.10)*

C95.00 Acute leukemia of unspecified cell type not having achieved remission HCC
Acute leukemia of unspecified cell type with failed remission
Acute leukemia NOS

C95.01 Acute leukemia of unspecified cell type, in remission HCC

C95.02 Acute leukemia of unspecified cell type, in relapse HCC

5 **C95.1 Chronic leukemia of unspecified cell type**

C95.10 Chronic leukemia of unspecified cell type not having achieved remission HCC
Chronic leukemia of unspecified cell type with failed remission
Chronic leukemia NOS

C95.11 Chronic leukemia of unspecified cell type, in remission HCC

C95.12 Chronic leukemia of unspecified cell type, in relapse HCC

5 **C95.9 Leukemia, unspecified**

C95.90 Leukemia, unspecified not having achieved remission HCC
Leukemia, unspecified with failed remission
Leukemia NOS

C95.91 **Leukemia, unspecified, in remission** HCC

C95.92 **Leukemia, unspecified, in relapse** HCC

4 C96 Other and unspecified malignant neoplasms of lymphoid, hematopoietic and related tissue

EXCLUDES 1 *personal history of other malignant neoplasms of lymphoid, hematopoietic and related tissues (Z85.79)*

C96.0 **Multifocal and multisystemic (disseminated) Langerhans-cell histiocytosis** HCC
Histiocytosis X, multisystemic
Letterer-Siwe disease
EXCLUDES 1 *adult pulmonary Langerhans cell histiocytosis (J84.82)*
multifocal and unisystemic Langerhans-cell histiocytosis (C96.5)
unifocal Langerhans-cell histiocytosis (C96.6)

5 C96.2 **Malignant mast cell neoplasm** HCC
EXCLUDES 1 *indolent mastocytosis (D47.02)*
mast cell leukemia (C94.30)
mastocytosis (congenital) (cutaneous) (Q82.2)

C96.20 **Malignant mast cell neoplasm, unspecified** HCC
AHA: 4Q 2017, 4

C96.21 **Aggressive systemic mastocytosis** HCC
AHA: 4Q 2017, 4

C96.22 **Mast cell sarcoma** HCC
AHA: 4Q 2017, 4

C96.29 **Other malignant mast cell neoplasm** HCC
AHA: 4Q 2017, 4

C96.4 **Sarcoma of dendritic cells (accessory cells)** HCC
Follicular dendritic cell sarcoma
Interdigitating dendritic cell sarcoma
Langerhans cell sarcoma

C96.5 **Multifocal and unisystemic Langerhans-cell histiocytosis** HCC
Hand-Schüller-Christian disease
Histiocytosis X, multifocal
EXCLUDES 1 *multifocal and multisystemic (disseminated) Langerhans-cell histiocytosis (C96.0)*
unifocal Langerhans-cell histiocytosis (C96.6)

C96.6 **Unifocal Langerhans-cell histiocytosis** HCC
Eosinophilic granuloma
Histiocytosis X, unifocal
Histiocytosis X NOS
Langerhans-cell histiocytosis NOS
EXCLUDES 1 *multifocal and multisysemic (disseminated) Langerhans-cell histiocytosis (C96.0)*
multifocal and unisystemic Langerhans-cell histiocytosis (C96.5)

C96.A **Histiocytic sarcoma** HCC
Malignant histiocytosis

C96.Z **Other specified malignant neoplasms of lymphoid, hematopoietic and related tissue** HCC

C96.9 **Malignant neoplasm of lymphoid, hematopoietic and related tissue, unspecified** HCC

In situ neoplasms (D00-D09)

INCLUDES Bowen's disease
erythroplasia
grade III intraepithelial neoplasia
Queyrat's erythroplasia

CODING TIP ✓ Carcinomas in situ are defined as cancer that has stayed in place in the specific location of origin and not spread or invaded any neighboring tissue. The physician must state "in situ" or pre-cancerous/pre-malignant lesion in order to indicate the correct assignment of any D00-D09 codes.

4 D00 Carcinoma in situ of oral cavity, esophagus and stomach

EXCLUDES 1 *melanoma in situ (D03.-)*

5 D00.0 **Carcinoma in situ of lip, oral cavity and pharynx**
Use additional code to identify:
exposure to environmental tobacco smoke (Z77.22)
exposure to tobacco smoke in the perinatal period (P96.81)
history of tobacco dependence (Z87.891)
occupational exposure to environmental tobacco smoke (Z57.31)
tobacco dependence (F17.-)
tobacco use (Z72.0)
EXCLUDES 1 *carcinoma in situ of aryepiglottic fold or interarytenoid fold, laryngeal aspect (D02.0)*
carcinoma in situ of epiglottis NOS (D02.0)
carcinoma in situ of epiglottis suprahyoid portion (D02.0)
carcinoma in situ of skin of lip (D03.0, D04.0)

D00.00 **Carcinoma in situ of oral cavity, unspecified site**

D00.01 **Carcinoma in situ of labial mucosa and vermilion border**

D00.02 **Carcinoma in situ of buccal mucosa**

D00.03 **Carcinoma in situ of gingiva and edentulous alveolar ridge**

D00.04 **Carcinoma in situ of soft palate**

D00.05 **Carcinoma in situ of hard palate**

D00.06 **Carcinoma in situ of floor of mouth**

D00.07 **Carcinoma in situ of tongue**

D00.08 **Carcinoma in situ of pharynx**
Carcinoma in situ of aryepiglottic fold NOS
Carcinoma in situ of hypopharyngeal aspect of aryepiglottic fold
Carcinoma in situ of marginal zone of aryepiglottic fold

D00.1 **Carcinoma in situ of esophagus**

D00.2 **Carcinoma in situ of stomach**

4 D01 Carcinoma in situ of other and unspecified digestive organs

EXCLUDES 1 *melanoma in situ (D03.-)*

D01.0 **Carcinoma in situ of colon**
EXCLUDES 1 *carcinoma in situ of rectosigmoid junction (D01.1)*

D01.1 **Carcinoma in situ of rectosigmoid junction**

D01.2 **Carcinoma in situ of rectum**

D01.3 **Carcinoma in situ of anus and anal canal**
Anal intraepithelial neoplasia III [AIN III]
Severe dysplasia of anus
EXCLUDES 1 *anal intraepithelial neoplasia I and II [AIN I and AIN II] (K62.82)*
carcinoma in situ of anal margin (D04.5)
carcinoma in situ of anal skin (D04.5)
carcinoma in situ of perianal skin (D04.5)

5 D01.4 **Carcinoma in situ of other and unspecified parts of intestine**
EXCLUDES 1 *carcinoma in situ of ampulla of Vater (D01.5)*

D01.40 **Carcinoma in situ of unspecified part of intestine**

D01.49 **Carcinoma in situ of other parts of intestine**

D01.5 **Carcinoma in situ of liver, gallbladder and bile ducts**
Carcinoma in situ of ampulla of Vater

D01.7 **Carcinoma in situ of other specified digestive organs**
Carcinoma in situ of pancreas

D01.9 **Carcinoma in situ of digestive organ, unspecified**

4 D02 Carcinoma in situ of middle ear and respiratory system

Use additional code to identify:
exposure to environmental tobacco smoke (Z77.22)
exposure to tobacco smoke in the perinatal period (P96.81)
history of tobacco dependence (Z87.891)
occupational exposure to environmental tobacco smoke (Z57.31)
tobacco dependence (F17.-)
tobacco use (Z72.0)

EXCLUDES 1 *melanoma in situ (D03.-)*

D02.0 **Carcinoma in situ of larynx**
Carcinoma in situ of aryepiglottic fold or interarytenoid fold, laryngeal aspect
Carcinoma in situ of epiglottis (suprahyoid portion)
EXCLUDES 1 *carcinoma in situ of aryepiglottic fold or interarytenoid fold NOS (D00.08)*
carcinoma in situ of hypopharyngeal aspect (D00.08)
carcinoma in situ of marginal zone (D00.08)

D02.1 **Carcinoma in situ of trachea**

5 **D02.2** **Carcinoma in situ of bronchus and lung**
- **D02.20** **Carcinoma in situ of unspecified bronchus and lung**
- **D02.21** **Carcinoma in situ of right bronchus and lung**
- **D02.22** **Carcinoma in situ of left bronchus and lung**

D02.3 **Carcinoma in situ of other parts of respiratory system**
Carcinoma in situ of accessory sinuses
Carcinoma in situ of middle ear
Carcinoma in situ of nasal cavities
EXCLUDES 1 *carcinoma in situ of ear (external) (skin) (D04.2-)*
carcinoma in situ of nose NOS D09.8
carcinoma in situ of skin of nose (D04.3)

D02.4 **Carcinoma in situ of respiratory system, unspecified**

4 **D03** **Melanoma in situ**

D03.0 **Melanoma in situ of lip** HCC

5 **D03.1** **Melanoma in situ of eyelid, including canthus**
- **D03.10** **Melanoma in situ of unspecified eyelid, including canthus** HCC
- ▲6 **D03.11** **Melanoma in situ of right eyelid, including canthus** HCC
  - ● **D03.111** **Melanoma in situ of right upper eyelid, including canthus**
  - ● **D03.112** **Melanoma in situ of right lower eyelid, including canthus**
- ▲6 **D03.12** **Melanoma in situ of left eyelid, including canthus** HCC
  - ● **D03.121** **Melanoma in situ of left upper eyelid, including canthus**
  - ● **D03.122** **Melanoma in situ of left lower eyelid, including canthus**

5 **D03.2** **Melanoma in situ of ear and external auricular canal**
- **D03.20** **Melanoma in situ of unspecified ear and external auricular canal** HCC
- **D03.21** **Melanoma in situ of right ear and external auricular canal** HCC
- **D03.22** **Melanoma in situ of left ear and external auricular canal** HCC

5 **D03.3** **Melanoma in situ of other and unspecified parts of face**
- **D03.30** **Melanoma in situ of unspecified part of face** HCC
- **D03.39** **Melanoma in situ of other parts of face** HCC

D03.4 **Melanoma in situ of scalp and neck** HCC

5 **D03.5** **Melanoma in situ of trunk**
- **D03.51** **Melanoma in situ of anal skin** HCC
  Melanoma in situ of anal margin
  Melanoma in situ of perianal skin
- **D03.52** **Melanoma in situ of breast (skin) (soft tissue)** HCC
- **D03.59** **Melanoma in situ of other part of trunk** HCC

5 **D03.6** **Melanoma in situ of upper limb, including shoulder**
- **D03.60** **Melanoma in situ of unspecified upper limb, including shoulder** HCC
- **D03.61** **Melanoma in situ of right upper limb, including shoulder** HCC
- **D03.62** **Melanoma in situ of left upper limb, including shoulder** HCC

5 **D03.7** **Melanoma in situ of lower limb, including hip**
- **D03.70** **Melanoma in situ of unspecified lower limb, including hip** HCC
- **D03.71** **Melanoma in situ of right lower limb, including hip** HCC
- **D03.72** **Melanoma in situ of left lower limb, including hip** HCC

D03.8 **Melanoma in situ of other sites** HCC
Melanoma in situ of scrotum
EXCLUDES 1 *carcinoma in situ of scrotum (D07.61)*

D03.9 **Melanoma in situ, unspecified** HCC

4 **D04** **Carcinoma in situ of skin**
EXCLUDES 1 *erythroplasia of Queyrat (penis) NOS (D07.4)*
melanoma in situ (D03.-)

D04.0 **Carcinoma in situ of skin of lip**
EXCLUDES 1 *carcinoma in situ of vermilion border of lip (D00.01)*

5 **D04.1** **Carcinoma in situ of skin of eyelid, including canthus**
- **D04.10** **Carcinoma in situ of skin of unspecified eyelid, including canthus**

Carcinoma in situ of skin; eyelid

Skin cancer confined to the epidermis that has not spread into nearby normal tissue

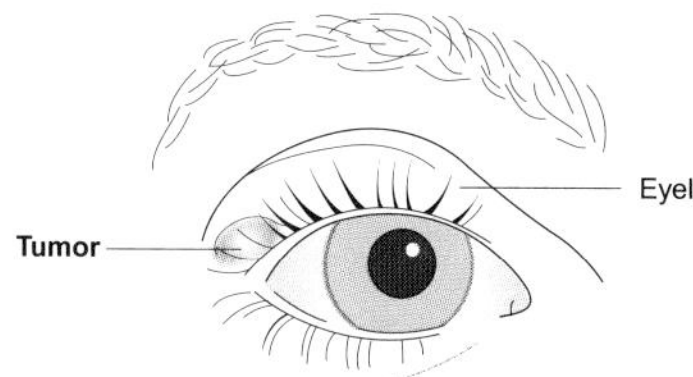

- ▲6 **D04.11** **Carcinoma in situ of skin of right eyelid, including canthus**
  - ● **D04.111** **Carcinoma in situ of skin of right upper eyelid, including canthus**
  - ● **D04.112** **Carcinoma in situ of skin of right lower eyelid, including canthus**
- ▲6 **D04.12** **Carcinoma in situ of skin of left eyelid, including canthus**
  - ● **D04.121** **Carcinoma in situ of skin of left upper eyelid, including canthus**
  - ● **D04.122** **Carcinoma in situ of skin of left lower eyelid, including canthus**

5 **D04.2** **Carcinoma in situ of skin of ear and external auricular canal**
- **D04.20** **Carcinoma in situ of skin of unspecified ear and external auricular canal**
- **D04.21** **Carcinoma in situ of skin of right ear and external auricular canal**
- **D04.22** **Carcinoma in situ of skin of left ear and external auricular canal**

5 **D04.3** **Carcinoma in situ of skin of other and unspecified parts of face**
- **D04.30** **Carcinoma in situ of skin of unspecified part of face**
- **D04.39** **Carcinoma in situ of skin of other parts of face**

D04.4 **Carcinoma in situ of skin of scalp and neck**

D04.5 **Carcinoma in situ of skin of trunk**
Carcinoma in situ of anal margin
Carcinoma in situ of anal skin
Carcinoma in situ of perianal skin
Carcinoma in situ of skin of breast
EXCLUDES 1 *carcinoma in situ of anus NOS (D01.3)*
carcinoma in situ of scrotum (D07.61)
carcinoma in situ of skin of genital organs (D07.-)

5 **D04.6** **Carcinoma in situ of skin of upper limb, including shoulder**
- **D04.60** **Carcinoma in situ of skin of unspecified upper limb, including shoulder**
- **D04.61** **Carcinoma in situ of skin of right upper limb, including shoulder**
- **D04.62** **Carcinoma in situ of skin of left upper limb, including shoulder**

5 **D04.7** **Carcinoma in situ of skin of lower limb, including hip**
- **D04.70** **Carcinoma in situ of skin of unspecified lower limb, including hip**
- **D04.71** **Carcinoma in situ of skin of right lower limb, including hip**
- **D04.72** **Carcinoma in situ of skin of left lower limb, including hip**

D04.8 **Carcinoma in situ of skin of other sites**

D04.9 **Carcinoma in situ of skin, unspecified**

4 D05 Carcinoma in situ of breast

EXCLUDES 1 *carcinoma in situ of skin of breast (D04.5)*
melanoma in situ of breast (skin) (D03.5)
Paget's disease of breast or nipple (C50.-)

5 D05.0 Lobular carcinoma in situ of breast

D05.00 Lobular carcinoma in situ of unspecified breast

D05.01 Lobular carcinoma in situ of right breast

D05.02 Lobular carcinoma in situ of left breast

5 D05.1 Intraductal carcinoma in situ of breast

D05.10 Intraductal carcinoma in situ of unspecified breast

D05.11 Intraductal carcinoma in situ of right breast

D05.12 Intraductal carcinoma in situ of left breast

5 D05.8 Other specified type of carcinoma in situ of breast

D05.80 Other specified type of carcinoma in situ of unspecified breast

D05.81 Other specified type of carcinoma in situ of right breast

D05.82 Other specified type of carcinoma in situ of left breast

5 D05.9 Unspecified type of carcinoma in situ of breast

D05.90 Unspecified type of carcinoma in situ of unspecified breast

D05.91 Unspecified type of carcinoma in situ of right breast

D05.92 Unspecified type of carcinoma in situ of left breast

4 D06 Carcinoma in situ of cervix uteri

INCLUDES cervical adenocarcinoma in situ
cervical intraepithelial glandular neoplasia
cervical intraepithelial neoplasia III [CIN III]
severe dysplasia of cervix uteri

EXCLUDES 1 *cervical intraepithelial neoplasia II [CIN II] (N87.1)*
cytologic evidence of malignancy of cervix without histologic confirmation (R87.614)
high grade squamous intraepithelial lesion (HGSIL) of cervix (R87.613)
melanoma in situ of cervix (D03.5)
moderate cervical dysplasia (N87.1)

D06.0 Carcinoma in situ of endocervix ♀

D06.1 Carcinoma in situ of exocervix ♀

D06.7 Carcinoma in situ of other parts of cervix ♀

D06.9 Carcinoma in situ of cervix, unspecified ♀

4 D07 Carcinoma in situ of other and unspecified genital organs

EXCLUDES 1 *melanoma in situ of trunk (D03.5)*

D07.0 Carcinoma in situ of endometrium ♀

D07.1 Carcinoma in situ of vulva ♀
Severe dysplasia of vulva
Vulvar intraepithelial neoplasia III [VIN III]

EXCLUDES 1 *moderate dysplasia of vulva (N90.1)*
vulvar intraepithelial neoplasia II [VIN II] (N90.1)

D07.2 Carcinoma in situ of vagina ♀
Severe dysplasia of vagina
Vaginal intraepithelial neoplasia III [VAIN III]

EXCLUDES 1 *moderate dysplasia of vagina (N89.1)*
vaginal intraepithelial neoplasia II [VIN II] (N89.1)

5 D07.3 Carcinoma in situ of other and unspecified female genital organs

D07.30 Carcinoma in situ of unspecified female genital organs ♀

D07.39 Carcinoma in situ of other female genital organs ♀

D07.4 Carcinoma in situ of penis ♂
Erythroplasia of Queyrat NOS

D07.5 Carcinoma in situ of prostate ♂
Prostatic intraepithelial neoplasia III (PIN III)
Severe dysplasia of prostate

EXCLUDES 1 *dysplasia (mild) (moderate) of prostate (N42.3-)*
prostatic intraepithelial neoplasia II [PIN II] (N42.3-)

5 D07.6 Carcinoma in situ of other and unspecified male genital organs

D07.60 Carcinoma in situ of unspecified male genital organs ♂

D07.61 Carcinoma in situ of scrotum ♂

D07.69 Carcinoma in situ of other male genital organs ♂

4 D09 Carcinoma in situ of other and unspecified sites

EXCLUDES 1 *melanoma in situ (D03.-)*

D09.0 Carcinoma in situ of bladder

5 D09.1 Carcinoma in situ of other and unspecified urinary organs

D09.10 Carcinoma in situ of unspecified urinary organ

D09.19 Carcinoma in situ of other urinary organs

5 D09.2 Carcinoma in situ of eye

EXCLUDES 1 *carcinoma in situ of skin of eyelid (D04.1-)*

D09.20 Carcinoma in situ of unspecified eye

D09.21 Carcinoma in situ of right eye

D09.22 Carcinoma in situ of left eye

D09.3 Carcinoma in situ of thyroid and other endocrine glands

EXCLUDES 1 *carcinoma in situ of endocrine pancreas (D01.7)*
carcinoma in situ of ovary (D07.39)
carcinoma in situ of testis (D07.69)

D09.8 Carcinoma in situ of other specified sites

D09.9 Carcinoma in situ, unspecified

Benign neoplasms, except benign neuroendocrine tumors (D10-D36)

4 D10 Benign neoplasm of mouth and pharynx

D10.0 Benign neoplasm of lip
Benign neoplasm of lip (frenulum) (inner aspect) (mucosa) (vermilion border)

EXCLUDES 1 *benign neoplasm of skin of lip (D22.0, D23.0)*

D10.1 Benign neoplasm of tongue
Benign neoplasm of lingual tonsil

D10.2 Benign neoplasm of floor of mouth

5 D10.3 Benign neoplasm of other and unspecified parts of mouth

D10.30 Benign neoplasm of unspecified part of mouth

D10.39 Benign neoplasm of other parts of mouth
Benign neoplasm of minor salivary gland NOS

EXCLUDES 1 *benign odontogenic neoplasms (D16.4-D16.5)*
benign neoplasm of mucosa of lip (D10.0)
benign neoplasm of nasopharyngeal surface of soft palate (D10.6)

D10.4 Benign neoplasm of tonsil
Benign neoplasm of tonsil (faucial) (palatine)

EXCLUDES 1 *benign neoplasm of lingual tonsil (D10.1)*
benign neoplasm of pharyngeal tonsil (D10.6)
benign neoplasm of tonsillar fossa (D10.5)
benign neoplasm of tonsillar pillars (D10.5)

D10.5 Benign neoplasm of other parts of oropharynx
Benign neoplasm of epiglottis, anterior aspect
Benign neoplasm of tonsillar fossa
Benign neoplasm of tonsillar pillars
Benign neoplasm of vallecula

EXCLUDES 1 *benign neoplasm of epiglottis NOS (D14.1)*
benign neoplasm of epiglottis, suprahyoid portion (D14.1)

D10.6 Benign neoplasm of nasopharynx
Benign neoplasm of pharyngeal tonsil
Benign neoplasm of posterior margin of septum and choanae

D10.7 Benign neoplasm of hypopharynx

D10.9 Benign neoplasm of pharynx, unspecified

4 D11 Benign neoplasm of major salivary glands

EXCLUDES 1 *benign neoplasms of specified minor salivary glands which are classified according to their anatomical location*
benign neoplasms of minor salivary glands NOS (D10.39)

D11.0 Benign neoplasm of parotid gland

D11.7 **Benign neoplasm of other major salivary glands**
Benign neoplasm of sublingual salivary gland
Benign neoplasm of submandibular salivary gland
D11.9 **Benign neoplasm of major salivary gland, unspecified**

4 D12 **Benign neoplasm of colon, rectum, anus and anal canal**
EXCLUDES 1 *benign carcinoid tumors of the large intestine, and rectum (D3A.02-)*
CODING TIP ✓ Adenomatous polyps are coded to D12. Hyperplastic polyps are coded to K63.5.

D12.0 **Benign neoplasm of cecum**
Benign neoplasm of ileocecal valve
D12.1 **Benign neoplasm of appendix**
EXCLUDES 1 *benign carcinoid tumor of the appendix (D3A.020)*
D12.2 **Benign neoplasm of ascending colon**
AHA: 2Q 2018, 11
D12.3 **Benign neoplasm of transverse colon**
Benign neoplasm of hepatic flexure
Benign neoplasm of splenic flexure
D12.4 **Benign neoplasm of descending colon**
AHA: 2Q 2015, 14
D12.5 **Benign neoplasm of sigmoid colon**
D12.6 **Benign neoplasm of colon, unspecified**
Adenomatosis of colon
Benign neoplasm of large intestine NOS
Polyposis (hereditary) of colon
EXCLUDES 1 *inflammatory polyp of colon (K51.4-)*
polyp of colon NOS (K63.5)
AHA: 1Q 2017, 8
D12.7 **Benign neoplasm of rectosigmoid junction**
D12.8 **Benign neoplasm of rectum**
EXCLUDES 1 *benign carcinoid tumor of the rectum (D3A.026)*
D12.9 **Benign neoplasm of anus and anal canal**
Benign neoplasm of anus NOS
EXCLUDES 1 *benign neoplasm of anal margin (D22.5, D23.5)*
benign neoplasm of anal skin (D22.5, D23.5)
benign neoplasm of perianal skin (D22.5, D23.5)

4 D13 **Benign neoplasm of other and ill-defined parts of digestive system**
EXCLUDES 1 *benign stromal tumors of digestive system (D21.4)*

D13.0 **Benign neoplasm of esophagus**
D13.1 **Benign neoplasm of stomach**
EXCLUDES 1 *benign carcinoid tumor of the stomach (D3A.092)*
D13.2 **Benign neoplasm of duodenum**
EXCLUDES 1 *benign carcinoid tumor of the duodenum (D3A.010)*
5 D13.3 **Benign neoplasm of other and unspecified parts of small intestine**
EXCLUDES 1 *benign carcinoid tumors of the small intestine (D3A.01-)*
benign neoplasm of ileocecal valve (D12.0)
D13.30 **Benign neoplasm of unspecified part of small intestine**
D13.39 **Benign neoplasm of other parts of small intestine**
D13.4 **Benign neoplasm of liver**
Benign neoplasm of intrahepatic bile ducts
D13.5 **Benign neoplasm of extrahepatic bile ducts**
D13.6 **Benign neoplasm of pancreas**
EXCLUDES 1 *benign neoplasm of endocrine pancreas (D13.7)*
D13.7 **Benign neoplasm of endocrine pancreas**
Islet cell tumor
Benign neoplasm of islets of Langerhans
Use additional code to identify any functional activity.
D13.9 **Benign neoplasm of ill-defined sites within the digestive system**
Benign neoplasm of digestive system NOS
Benign neoplasm of intestine NOS
Benign neoplasm of spleen

4 D14 **Benign neoplasm of middle ear and respiratory system**

D14.0 **Benign neoplasm of middle ear, nasal cavity and accessory sinuses**
Benign neoplasm of cartilage of nose
EXCLUDES 1 *benign neoplasm of auricular canal (external) (D22.2-, D23.2-)*
benign neoplasm of bone of ear (D16.4)
benign neoplasm of bone of nose (D16.4)
benign neoplasm of cartilage of ear (D21.0)
benign neoplasm of ear (external) (skin) (D22.2-, D23.2-)
benign neoplasm of nose NOS (D36.7)
benign neoplasm of skin of nose (D22.39, D23.39)
benign neoplasm of olfactory bulb (D33.3)
benign neoplasm of posterior margin of septum and choanae (D10.6)
polyp of accessory sinus (J33.8)
polyp of ear (middle) (H74.4)
polyp of nasal (cavity) (J33.-)
D14.1 **Benign neoplasm of larynx**
Adenomatous polyp of larynx
Benign neoplasm of epiglottis (suprahyoid portion)
EXCLUDES 1 *benign neoplasm of epiglottis, anterior aspect (D10.5)*
polyp (nonadenomatous) of vocal cord or larynx (J38.1)
D14.2 **Benign neoplasm of trachea**
5 D14.3 **Benign neoplasm of bronchus and lung**
EXCLUDES 1 *benign carcinoid tumor of the bronchus and lung (D3A.090)*
D14.30 **Benign neoplasm of unspecified bronchus and lung**
D14.31 **Benign neoplasm of right bronchus and lung**
D14.32 **Benign neoplasm of left bronchus and lung**
D14.4 **Benign neoplasm of respiratory system, unspecified**

4 D15 **Benign neoplasm of other and unspecified intrathoracic organs**
EXCLUDES 1 *benign neoplasm of mesothelial tissue (D19.-)*

D15.0 **Benign neoplasm of thymus**
EXCLUDES 1 *benign carcinoid tumor of the thymus (D3A.091)*
D15.1 **Benign neoplasm of heart**
EXCLUDES 1 *benign neoplasm of great vessels (D21.3)*
D15.2 **Benign neoplasm of mediastinum**
D15.7 **Benign neoplasm of other specified intrathoracic organs**
D15.9 **Benign neoplasm of intrathoracic organ, unspecified**

4 D16 **Benign neoplasm of bone and articular cartilage**
EXCLUDES 1 *benign neoplasm of connective tissue of ear (D21.0)*
benign neoplasm of connective tissue of eyelid (D21.0)
benign neoplasm of connective tissue of larynx (D14.1)
benign neoplasm of connective tissue of nose (D14.0)
benign neoplasm of synovia (D21.-)

5 D16.0 **Benign neoplasm of scapula and long bones of upper limb**
D16.00 **Benign neoplasm of scapula and long bones of unspecified upper limb**
D16.01 **Benign neoplasm of scapula and long bones of right upper limb**
D16.02 **Benign neoplasm of scapula and long bones of left upper limb**
5 D16.1 **Benign neoplasm of short bones of upper limb**
D16.10 **Benign neoplasm of short bones of unspecified upper limb**
D16.11 **Benign neoplasm of short bones of right upper limb**
D16.12 **Benign neoplasm of short bones of left upper limb**
5 D16.2 **Benign neoplasm of long bones of lower limb**
D16.20 **Benign neoplasm of long bones of unspecified lower limb**
D16.21 **Benign neoplasm of long bones of right lower limb**
D16.22 **Benign neoplasm of long bones of left lower limb**
5 D16.3 **Benign neoplasm of short bones of lower limb**
D16.30 **Benign neoplasm of short bones of unspecified lower limb**
D16.31 **Benign neoplasm of short bones of right lower limb**
D16.32 **Benign neoplasm of short bones of left lower limb**

D16.4 Benign neoplasm of bones of skull and face
Benign neoplasm of maxilla (superior)
Benign neoplasm of orbital bone
Keratocyst of maxilla
Keratocystic odontogenic tumor of maxilla
EXCLUDES 2 *benign neoplasm of lower jaw bone (D16.5)*

D16.5 Benign neoplasm of lower jaw bone
Keratocyst of mandible
Keratocystic odontogenic tumor of mandible

D16.6 Benign neoplasm of vertebral column
EXCLUDES 1 *benign neoplasm of sacrum and coccyx (D16.8)*

D16.7 Benign neoplasm of ribs, sternum and clavicle

D16.8 Benign neoplasm of pelvic bones, sacrum and coccyx

D16.9 Benign neoplasm of bone and articular cartilage, unspecified

4 D17 Benign lipomatous neoplasm

D17.0 Benign lipomatous neoplasm of skin and subcutaneous tissue of head, face and neck

Benign lipomatous neoplasm

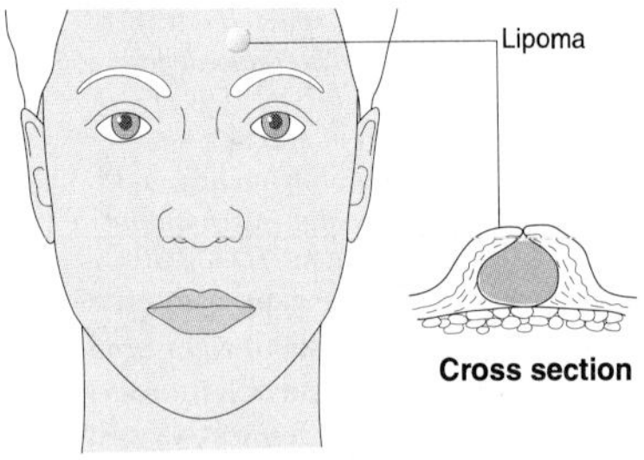

D17.1 Benign lipomatous neoplasm of skin and subcutaneous tissue of trunk

5 D17.2 Benign lipomatous neoplasm of skin and subcutaneous tissue of limb

Laterality D17.20 Benign lipomatous neoplasm of skin and subcutaneous tissue of unspecified limb

Laterality D17.21 Benign lipomatous neoplasm of skin and subcutaneous tissue of right arm

Laterality D17.22 Benign lipomatous neoplasm of skin and subcutaneous tissue of left arm

Laterality D17.23 Benign lipomatous neoplasm of skin and subcutaneous tissue of right leg

Laterality D17.24 Benign lipomatous neoplasm of skin and subcutaneous tissue of left leg

5 D17.3 Benign lipomatous neoplasm of skin and subcutaneous tissue of other and unspecified sites

D17.30 Benign lipomatous neoplasm of skin and subcutaneous tissue of unspecified sites

D17.39 Benign lipomatous neoplasm of skin and subcutaneous tissue of other sites

D17.4 Benign lipomatous neoplasm of intrathoracic organs

D17.5 Benign lipomatous neoplasm of intra-abdominal organs
EXCLUDES 1 *benign lipomatous neoplasm of peritoneum and retroperitoneum (D17.79)*

D17.6 Benign lipomatous neoplasm of spermatic cord ♂

5 D17.7 Benign lipomatous neoplasm of other sites

D17.71 Benign lipomatous neoplasm of kidney

D17.72 Benign lipomatous neoplasm of other genitourinary organ

D17.79 Benign lipomatous neoplasm of other sites
Benign lipomatous neoplasm of peritoneum
Benign lipomatous neoplasm of retroperitoneum

D17.9 Benign lipomatous neoplasm, unspecified
Lipoma NOS

4 D18 Hemangioma and lymphangioma, any site

EXCLUDES 1 *benign neoplasm of glomus jugulare (D35.6)*
blue or pigmented nevus (D22.-)
nevus NOS (D22.-)
vascular nevus (Q82.5)

5 D18.0 Hemangioma
Angioma NOS
Cavernous nevus

D18.00 Hemangioma unspecified site

D18.01 Hemangioma of skin and subcutaneous tissue

D18.02 Hemangioma of intracranial structures HCC

D18.03 Hemangioma of intra-abdominal structures

D18.09 Hemangioma of other sites

D18.1 Lymphangioma, any site

4 D19 Benign neoplasm of mesothelial tissue

D19.0 Benign neoplasm of mesothelial tissue of pleura

D19.1 Benign neoplasm of mesothelial tissue of peritoneum

D19.7 Benign neoplasm of mesothelial tissue of other sites

D19.9 Benign neoplasm of mesothelial tissue, unspecified
Benign mesothelioma NOS

4 D20 Benign neoplasm of soft tissue of retroperitoneum and peritoneum

EXCLUDES 1 *benign lipomatous neoplasm of peritoneum and retroperitoneum (D17.79)*
benign neoplasm of mesothelial tissue (D19.-)

D20.0 Benign neoplasm of soft tissue of retroperitoneum

D20.1 Benign neoplasm of soft tissue of peritoneum

4 D21 Other benign neoplasms of connective and Other soft tissue

INCLUDES benign neoplasm of blood vessel
benign neoplasm of bursa
benign neoplasm of cartilage
benign neoplasm of fascia
benign neoplasm of fat
benign neoplasm of ligament, except uterine
benign neoplasm of lymphatic channel
benign neoplasm of muscle
benign neoplasm of synovia
benign neoplasm of tendon (sheath)
benign stromal tumors

EXCLUDES 1 *benign neoplasm of articular cartilage (D16.-)*
benign neoplasm of cartilage of larynx (D14.1)
benign neoplasm of cartilage of nose (D14.0)
benign neoplasm of connective tissue of breast (D24.-)
benign neoplasm of peripheral nerves and autonomic nervous system (D36.1-)
benign neoplasm of peritoneum (D20.1)
benign neoplasm of retroperitoneum (D20.0)
benign neoplasm of uterine ligament, any (D28.2)
benign neoplasm of vascular tissue (D18.-)
hemangioma (D18.0-)
lipomatous neoplasm (D17.-)
lymphangioma (D18.1)
uterine leiomyoma (D25.-)

D21.0 Benign neoplasm of connective and other soft tissue of head, face and neck
Benign neoplasm of connective tissue of ear
Benign neoplasm of connective tissue of eyelid
EXCLUDES 1 *benign neoplasm of connective tissue of orbit (D31.6-)*

5 D21.1 Benign neoplasm of connective and other soft tissue of upper limb, including shoulder

Laterality D21.10 Benign neoplasm of connective and other soft tissue of unspecified upper limb, including shoulder

Laterality D21.11 Benign neoplasm of connective and other soft tissue of right upper limb, including shoulder

Laterality D21.12 Benign neoplasm of connective and other soft tissue of left upper limb, including shoulder

5 D21.2 Benign neoplasm of connective and other soft tissue of lower limb, including hip

Laterality D21.20 Benign neoplasm of connective and other soft tissue of unspecified lower limb, including hip

Laterality D21.21 Benign neoplasm of connective and other soft tissue of right lower limb, including hip

Laterality D21.22 Benign neoplasm of connective and other soft tissue of left lower limb, including hip

D21.3 Benign neoplasm of connective and other soft tissue of thorax
Benign neoplasm of axilla
Benign neoplasm of diaphragm
Benign neoplasm of great vessels
EXCLUDES 1 *benign neoplasm of heart (D15.1)*
benign neoplasm of mediastinum (D15.2)
benign neoplasm of thymus (D15.0)

D21.4 **Benign neoplasm of connective and other soft tissue of abdomen**
Benign stromal tumors of abdomen

D21.5 **Benign neoplasm of connective and other soft tissue of pelvis**
EXCLUDES 1 *benign neoplasm of any uterine ligament (D28.2)*
uterine leiomyoma (D25.-)

D21.6 **Benign neoplasm of connective and other soft tissue of trunk, unspecified**
Benign neoplasm of back NOS

D21.9 **Benign neoplasm of connective and other soft tissue, unspecified**

D22 Melanocytic nevi
INCLUDES atypical nevus
blue hairy pigmented nevus
nevus NOS

D22.0 **Melanocytic nevi of lip**
D22.1 **Melanocytic nevi of eyelid, including canthus**
D22.10 **Melanocytic nevi of unspecified eyelid, including canthus**
▲ D22.11 **Melanocytic nevi of right eyelid, including canthus**
● D22.111 **Melanocytic nevi of right upper eyelid, including canthus**
● D22.112 **Melanocytic nevi of right lower eyelid, including canthus**
▲ D22.12 **Melanocytic nevi of left eyelid, including canthus**
● D22.121 **Melanocytic nevi of left upper eyelid, including canthus**
● D22.122 **Melanocytic nevi of left lower eyelid, including canthus**
D22.2 **Melanocytic nevi of ear and external auricular canal**
D22.20 **Melanocytic nevi of unspecified ear and external auricular canal**
D22.21 **Melanocytic nevi of right ear and external auricular canal**
D22.22 **Melanocytic nevi of left ear and external auricular canal**
D22.3 **Melanocytic nevi of other and unspecified parts of face**
D22.30 **Melanocytic nevi of unspecified part of face**
D22.39 **Melanocytic nevi of other parts of face**
D22.4 **Melanocytic nevi of scalp and neck**
D22.5 **Melanocytic nevi of trunk**
Melanocytic nevi of anal margin
Melanocytic nevi of anal skin
Melanocytic nevi of perianal skin
Melanocytic nevi of skin of breast
D22.6 **Melanocytic nevi of upper limb, including shoulder**
D22.60 **Melanocytic nevi of unspecified upper limb, including shoulder**
D22.61 **Melanocytic nevi of right upper limb, including shoulder**
D22.62 **Melanocytic nevi of left upper limb, including shoulder**
D22.7 **Melanocytic nevi of lower limb, including hip**
D22.70 **Melanocytic nevi of unspecified lower limb, including hip**
D22.71 **Melanocytic nevi of right lower limb, including hip**
D22.72 **Melanocytic nevi of left lower limb, including hip**
D22.9 **Melanocytic nevi, unspecified**

D23 Other benign neoplasms of skin
INCLUDES benign neoplasm of hair follicles
benign neoplasm of sebaceous glands
benign neoplasm of sweat glands
EXCLUDES 1 *benign lipomatous neoplasms of skin (D17.0-D17.3)*
melanocytic nevi (D22.-)

D23.0 **Other benign neoplasm of skin of lip**
EXCLUDES 1 *benign neoplasm of vermilion border of lip (D10.0)*
D23.1 **Other benign neoplasm of skin of eyelid, including canthus**
D23.10 **Other benign neoplasm of skin of unspecified eyelid, including canthus**
▲ D23.11 **Other benign neoplasm of skin of right eyelid, including canthus**
● D23.111 **Other benign neoplasm of skin of right upper eyelid, including canthus**
● D23.112 **Other benign neoplasm of skin of right lower eyelid, including canthus**
▲ D23.12 **Other benign neoplasm of skin of left eyelid, including canthus**
● D23.121 **Other benign neoplasm of skin of left upper eyelid, including canthus**
● D23.122 **Other benign neoplasm of skin of left lower eyelid, including canthus**
D23.2 **Other benign neoplasm of skin of ear and external auricular canal**
D23.20 **Other benign neoplasm of skin of unspecified ear and external auricular canal**
D23.21 **Other benign neoplasm of skin of right ear and external auricular canal**
D23.22 **Other benign neoplasm of skin of left ear and external auricular canal**
D23.3 **Other benign neoplasm of skin of other and unspecified parts of face**
D23.30 **Other benign neoplasm of skin of unspecified part of face**
D23.39 **Other benign neoplasm of skin of other parts of face**
D23.4 **Other benign neoplasm of skin of scalp and neck**
D23.5 **Other benign neoplasm of skin of trunk**
Other benign neoplasm of anal margin
Other benign neoplasm of anal skin
Other benign neoplasm of perianal skin
Other benign neoplasm of skin of breast
EXCLUDES 1 *benign neoplasm of anus NOS (D12.9)*
D23.6 **Other benign neoplasm of skin of upper limb, including shoulder**
D23.60 **Other benign neoplasm of skin of unspecified upper limb, including shoulder**
D23.61 **Other benign neoplasm of skin of right upper limb, including shoulder**
D23.62 **Other benign neoplasm of skin of left upper limb, including shoulder**
D23.7 **Other benign neoplasm of skin of lower limb, including hip**
D23.70 **Other benign neoplasm of skin of unspecified lower limb, including hip**
D23.71 **Other benign neoplasm of skin of right lower limb, including hip**
D23.72 **Other benign neoplasm of skin of left lower limb, including hip**
D23.9 **Other benign neoplasm of skin, unspecified**

D24 Benign neoplasm of breast
INCLUDES benign neoplasm of connective tissue of breast
benign neoplasm of soft parts of breast
fibroadenoma of breast
EXCLUDES 2 *adenofibrosis of breast (N60.2)*
benign cyst of breast (N60.-)
benign mammary dysplasia (N60.-)
benign neoplasm of skin of breast (D22.5, D23.5)
fibrocystic disease of breast (N60.-)

D24.1 **Benign neoplasm of right breast**
D24.2 **Benign neoplasm of left breast**
D24.9 **Benign neoplasm of unspecified breast**

D25 Leiomyoma of uterus
INCLUDES uterine fibroid
uterine fibromyoma
uterine myoma

D25.0 **Submucous leiomyoma of uterus** ♀
D25.1 **Intramural leiomyoma of uterus** ♀
Interstitial leiomyoma of uterus
D25.2 **Subserosal leiomyoma of uterus** ♀
Subperitoneal leiomyoma of uterus
D25.9 **Leiomyoma of uterus, unspecified** ♀

D26 Other benign neoplasms of uterus
D26.0 **Other benign neoplasm of cervix uteri** ♀
D26.1 **Other benign neoplasm of corpus uteri** ♀
D26.7 **Other benign neoplasm of other parts of uterus** ♀
D26.9 **Other benign neoplasm of uterus, unspecified** ♀

● New | Manifestation | 4-7 Digit Indicators | Laterality | A Adult | M Maternity | N Newborn | P Pediatric | ♂ Male
▲ Revised | Unspecified | AHA Coding Clinic | HCC Hierarchical Condition Categories | HIV HIV Related Conditions | ♀ Female

D27 Benign neoplasm of ovary
Use additional code to identify any functional activity.
EXCLUDES 2 *corpus albicans cyst (N83.2-)*
corpus luteum cyst (N83.1-)
endometrial cyst (N80.1)
follicular (atretic) cyst (N83.0-)
graafian follicle cyst (N83.0-)
ovarian cyst NEC (N83.2-)
ovarian retention cyst (N83.2-)

D27.0 Benign neoplasm of right ovary ♀
D27.1 Benign neoplasm of left ovary ♀
D27.9 Benign neoplasm of unspecified ovary ♀

D28 Benign neoplasm of other and unspecified female genital organs
INCLUDES adenomatous polyp
benign neoplasm of skin of female genital organs
benign teratoma
EXCLUDES 1 *epoophoron cyst (Q50.5)*
fimbrial cyst (Q50.4)
Gartner's duct cyst (Q52.4)
parovarian cyst (Q50.5)

D28.0 Benign neoplasm of vulva ♀
D28.1 Benign neoplasm of vagina ♀
D28.2 Benign neoplasm of uterine tubes and ligaments ♀
Benign neoplasm of fallopian tube
Benign neoplasm of uterine ligament (broad) (round)
D28.7 Benign neoplasm of other specified female genital organs ♀
D28.9 Benign neoplasm of female genital organ, unspecified ♀

D29 Benign neoplasm of male genital organs
INCLUDES benign neoplasm of skin of male genital organs

D29.0 Benign neoplasm of penis ♂
D29.1 Benign neoplasm of prostate ♂
EXCLUDES 1 *enlarged prostate (N40.-)*
D29.2 Benign neoplasm of testis
Use additional code to identify any functional activity.
D29.20 Benign neoplasm of unspecified testis ♂
D29.21 Benign neoplasm of right testis ♂
D29.22 Benign neoplasm of left testis ♂
D29.3 Benign neoplasm of epididymis
D29.30 Benign neoplasm of unspecified epididymis ♂
D29.31 Benign neoplasm of right epididymis ♂
D29.32 Benign neoplasm of left epididymis ♂
D29.4 Benign neoplasm of scrotum ♂
Benign neoplasm of skin of scrotum
D29.8 Benign neoplasm of other specified male genital organs ♂
Benign neoplasm of seminal vesicle
Benign neoplasm of spermatic cord
Benign neoplasm of tunica vaginalis
D29.9 Benign neoplasm of male genital organ, unspecified ♂

D30 Benign neoplasm of urinary organs
D30.0 Benign neoplasm of kidney
EXCLUDES 1 *benign carcinoid tumor of the kidney (D3A.093)*
benign neoplasm of renal calyces (D30.1-)
benign neoplasm of renal pelvis (D30.1-)
D30.00 Benign neoplasm of unspecified kidney
D30.01 Benign neoplasm of right kidney
D30.02 Benign neoplasm of left kidney
D30.1 Benign neoplasm of renal pelvis
D30.10 Benign neoplasm of unspecified renal pelvis
D30.11 Benign neoplasm of right renal pelvis
D30.12 Benign neoplasm of left renal pelvis
D30.2 Benign neoplasm of ureter
EXCLUDES 1 *benign neoplasm of ureteric orifice of bladder (D30.3)*
D30.20 Benign neoplasm of unspecified ureter
D30.21 Benign neoplasm of right ureter
D30.22 Benign neoplasm of left ureter
D30.3 Benign neoplasm of bladder
Benign neoplasm of ureteric orifice of bladder
Benign neoplasm of urethral orifice of bladder
D30.4 Benign neoplasm of urethra
EXCLUDES 1 *benign neoplasm of urethral orifice of bladder (D30.3)*
D30.8 Benign neoplasm of other specified urinary organs
Benign neoplasm of paraurethral glands
D30.9 Benign neoplasm of urinary organ, unspecified
Benign neoplasm of urinary system NOS

D31 Benign neoplasm of eye and adnexa
EXCLUDES 1 *benign neoplasm of connective tissue of eyelid (D21.0)*
benign neoplasm of optic nerve (D33.3)
benign neoplasm of skin of eyelid (D22.1-, D23.1-)

D31.0 Benign neoplasm of conjunctiva
D31.00 Benign neoplasm of unspecified conjunctiva
D31.01 Benign neoplasm of right conjunctiva
D31.02 Benign neoplasm of left conjunctiva
D31.1 Benign neoplasm of cornea
D31.10 Benign neoplasm of unspecified cornea
D31.11 Benign neoplasm of right cornea
D31.12 Benign neoplasm of left cornea
D31.2 Benign neoplasm of retina
EXCLUDES 1 *dark area on retina (D49.81)*
hemangioma of retina (D49.81)
neoplasm of unspecified behavior of retina and choroid (D49.81)
retinal freckle (D49.81)
D31.20 Benign neoplasm of unspecified retina
D31.21 Benign neoplasm of right retina
D31.22 Benign neoplasm of left retina
D31.3 Benign neoplasm of choroid
D31.30 Benign neoplasm of unspecified choroid
D31.31 Benign neoplasm of right choroid
D31.32 Benign neoplasm of left choroid
D31.4 Benign neoplasm of ciliary body
D31.40 Benign neoplasm of unspecified ciliary body
D31.41 Benign neoplasm of right ciliary body
D31.42 Benign neoplasm of left ciliary body
D31.5 Benign neoplasm of lacrimal gland and duct
Benign neoplasm of lacrimal sac
Benign neoplasm of nasolacrimal duct
D31.50 Benign neoplasm of unspecified lacrimal gland and duct
D31.51 Benign neoplasm of right lacrimal gland and duct
D31.52 Benign neoplasm of left lacrimal gland and duct
D31.6 Benign neoplasm of unspecified site of orbit
Benign neoplasm of connective tissue of orbit
Benign neoplasm of extraocular muscle
Benign neoplasm of peripheral nerves of orbit
Benign neoplasm of retrobulbar tissue
Benign neoplasm of retro-ocular tissue
EXCLUDES 1 *benign neoplasm of orbital bone (D16.4)*
D31.60 Benign neoplasm of unspecified site of unspecified orbit
D31.61 Benign neoplasm of unspecified site of right orbit
D31.62 Benign neoplasm of unspecified site of left orbit
D31.9 Benign neoplasm of unspecified part of eye
Benign neoplasm of eyeball
D31.90 Benign neoplasm of unspecified part of unspecified eye
D31.91 Benign neoplasm of unspecified part of right eye
D31.92 Benign neoplasm of unspecified part of left eye

D32 Benign neoplasm of meninges
D32.0 Benign neoplasm of cerebral meninges HCC
D32.1 Benign neoplasm of spinal meninges HCC
D32.9 Benign neoplasm of meninges, unspecified HCC
Meningioma NOS

4 D33 Benign neoplasm of brain and other parts of central nervous system

EXCLUDES 1 *angioma (D18.0-)*
benign neoplasm of meninges (D32.-)
benign neoplasm of peripheral nerves and autonomic nervous system (D36.1-)
hemangioma (D18.0-)
neurofibromatosis (Q85.0-)
retro-ocular benign neoplasm (D31.6-)

D33.0 Benign neoplasm of brain, supratentorial HCC
Benign neoplasm of cerebral ventricle
Benign neoplasm of cerebrum
Benign neoplasm of frontal lobe
Benign neoplasm of occipital lobe
Benign neoplasm of parietal lobe
Benign neoplasm of temporal lobe
EXCLUDES 1 *benign neoplasm of fourth ventricle (D33.1)*

D33.1 Benign neoplasm of brain, infratentorial HCC
Benign neoplasm of brain stem
Benign neoplasm of cerebellum
Benign neoplasm of fourth ventricle

D33.2 Benign neoplasm of brain, unspecified HCC

D33.3 Benign neoplasm of cranial nerves HCC
Benign neoplasm of olfactory bulb

D33.4 Benign neoplasm of spinal cord HCC

D33.7 Benign neoplasm of other specified parts of central nervous system HCC

D33.9 Benign neoplasm of central nervous system, unspecified HCC
Benign neoplasm of nervous system (central) NOS

D34 Benign neoplasm of thyroid gland
Use additional code to identify any functional activity

4 D35 Benign neoplasm of other and unspecified endocrine glands
Use additional code to identify any functional activity
EXCLUDES 1 *benign neoplasm of endocrine pancreas (D13.7)*
benign neoplasm of ovary (D27.-)
benign neoplasm of testis (D29.2.-)
benign neoplasm of thymus (D15.0)

5 D35.0 Benign neoplasm of adrenal gland
D35.00 Benign neoplasm of unspecified adrenal gland
D35.01 Benign neoplasm of right adrenal gland
D35.02 Benign neoplasm of left adrenal gland

D35.1 Benign neoplasm of parathyroid gland

D35.2 Benign neoplasm of pituitary gland HCC
AHA: 3Q 2014, 22

D35.3 Benign neoplasm of craniopharyngeal duct HCC

D35.4 Benign neoplasm of pineal gland HCC

D35.5 Benign neoplasm of carotid body

D35.6 Benign neoplasm of aortic body and other paraganglia
Benign tumor of glomus jugulare

D35.7 Benign neoplasm of other specified endocrine glands

D35.9 Benign neoplasm of endocrine gland, unspecified
Benign neoplasm of unspecified endocrine gland

4 D36 Benign neoplasm of other and unspecified sites

D36.0 Benign neoplasm of lymph nodes
EXCLUDES 1 *lymphangioma (D18.1)*

5 D36.1 Benign neoplasm of peripheral nerves and autonomic nervous system
EXCLUDES 1 *benign neoplasm of peripheral nerves of orbit (D31.6-)*
neurofibromatosis (Q85.0-)

D36.10 Benign neoplasm of peripheral nerves and autonomic nervous system, unspecified
D36.11 Benign neoplasm of peripheral nerves and autonomic nervous system of face, head, and neck
D36.12 Benign neoplasm of peripheral nerves and autonomic nervous system, upper limb, including shoulder
D36.13 Benign neoplasm of peripheral nerves and autonomic nervous system of lower limb, including hip
D36.14 Benign neoplasm of peripheral nerves and autonomic nervous system of thorax
D36.15 Benign neoplasm of peripheral nerves and autonomic nervous system of abdomen
D36.16 Benign neoplasm of peripheral nerves and autonomic nervous system of pelvis
D36.17 Benign neoplasm of peripheral nerves and autonomic nervous system of trunk, unspecified

D36.7 Benign neoplasm of other specified sites
Benign neoplasm of nose NOS

D36.9 Benign neoplasm, unspecified site

Benign neuroendocrine tumors (D3A)

4 D3A Benign neuroendocrine tumors
Code also:
any associated multiple endocrine neoplasia [MEN] syndromes (E31.2-)
Use additional code to identify any associated endocrine syndrome, such as:
carcinoid syndrome (E34.0)
EXCLUDES 2 *benign pancreatic islet cell tumors (D13.7)*

5 D3A.0 Benign carcinoid tumors

D3A.00 Benign carcinoid tumor of unspecified site
Carcinoid tumor NOS

6 D3A.01 Benign carcinoid tumors of the small intestine
D3A.010 Benign carcinoid tumor of the duodenum
D3A.011 Benign carcinoid tumor of the jejunum
D3A.012 Benign carcinoid tumor of the ileum
D3A.019 Benign carcinoid tumor of the small intestine, unspecified portion

6 D3A.02 Benign carcinoid tumors of the appendix, large intestine, and rectum
D3A.020 Benign carcinoid tumor of the appendix
D3A.021 Benign carcinoid tumor of the cecum
D3A.022 Benign carcinoid tumor of the ascending colon
D3A.023 Benign carcinoid tumor of the transverse colon
D3A.024 Benign carcinoid tumor of the descending colon
D3A.025 Benign carcinoid tumor of the sigmoid colon
D3A.026 Benign carcinoid tumor of the rectum
D3A.029 Benign carcinoid tumor of the large intestine, unspecified portion
Benign carcinoid tumor of the colon NOS

6 D3A.09 Benign carcinoid tumors of other sites
D3A.090 Benign carcinoid tumor of the bronchus and lung
D3A.091 Benign carcinoid tumor of the thymus
D3A.092 Benign carcinoid tumor of the stomach
D3A.093 Benign carcinoid tumor of the kidney
D3A.094 Benign carcinoid tumor of the foregut, unspecified
D3A.095 Benign carcinoid tumor of the midgut, unspecified
D3A.096 Benign carcinoid tumor of the hindgut, unspecified
D3A.098 Benign carcinoid tumors of other sites

D3A.8 Other benign neuroendocrine tumors
Neuroendocrine tumor NOS

Neoplasms of uncertain behavior, polycythemia vera and myelodysplastic syndromes (D37-D48)

Note: Categories D37-D44, and D48 classify by site neoplasms of uncertain behavior, i.e., histologic confirmation whether the neoplasm is malignant or benign cannot be made.

EXCLUDES 1 *neoplasms of unspecified behavior (D49.-)*

CODING TIP ✓ Codes classifiable to D37-D48 include tumors specifically reported as those of "uncertain behavior." This term is a specific diagnostic statement that must be reported by the physician in order to support assignment of any code from D37-D48, as these tumors include lesions whose behavior cannot be predicted. The status is currently benign, but the tumor could undergo a malignant transformation. These codes are not to be used when a biopsy has not been performed or results are not confirmed.

D37 Neoplasm of uncertain behavior of oral cavity and digestive organs

EXCLUDES 1 *stromal tumors of uncertain behavior of digestive system (D48.1)*

D37.0 Neoplasm of uncertain behavior of lip, oral cavity and pharynx

EXCLUDES 1 *neoplasm of uncertain behavior of aryepiglottic fold or interarytenoid fold, laryngeal aspect (D38.0)*
neoplasm of uncertain behavior of epiglottis NOS (D38.0)
neoplasm of uncertain behavior of skin of lip (D48.5)
neoplasm of uncertain behavior of suprahyoid portion of epiglottis (D38.0)

D37.01 Neoplasm of uncertain behavior of lip
Neoplasm of uncertain behavior of vermilion border of lip

D37.02 Neoplasm of uncertain behavior of tongue

D37.03 Neoplasm of uncertain behavior of the major salivary glands

D37.030 Neoplasm of uncertain behavior of the parotid salivary glands

D37.031 Neoplasm of uncertain behavior of the sublingual salivary glands

D37.032 Neoplasm of uncertain behavior of the submandibular salivary glands

D37.039 Neoplasm of uncertain behavior of the major salivary glands, unspecified

D37.04 Neoplasm of uncertain behavior of the minor salivary glands
Neoplasm of uncertain behavior of submucosal salivary glands of lip
Neoplasm of uncertain behavior of submucosal salivary glands of cheek
Neoplasm of uncertain behavior of submucosal salivary glands of hard palate
Neoplasm of uncertain behavior of submucosal salivary glands of soft palate

D37.05 Neoplasm of uncertain behavior of pharynx
Neoplasm of uncertain behavior of aryepiglottic fold of pharynx NOS
Neoplasm of uncertain behavior of hypopharyngeal aspect of aryepiglottic fold of pharynx
Neoplasm of uncertain behavior of marginal zone of aryepiglottic fold of pharynx

D37.09 Neoplasm of uncertain behavior of other specified sites of the oral cavity

D37.1 Neoplasm of uncertain behavior of stomach

D37.2 Neoplasm of uncertain behavior of small intestine

D37.3 Neoplasm of uncertain behavior of appendix

D37.4 Neoplasm of uncertain behavior of colon

D37.5 Neoplasm of uncertain behavior of rectum
Neoplasm of uncertain behavior of rectosigmoid junction

D37.6 Neoplasm of uncertain behavior of liver, gallbladder and bile ducts
Neoplasm of uncertain behavior of ampulla of Vater

D37.8 Neoplasm of uncertain behavior of other specified digestive organs
Neoplasm of uncertain behavior of anal canal
Neoplasm of uncertain behavior of anal sphincter
Neoplasm of uncertain behavior of anus NOS
Neoplasm of uncertain behavior of esophagus
Neoplasm of uncertain behavior of intestine NOS
Neoplasm of uncertain behavior of pancreas

EXCLUDES 1 *neoplasm of uncertain behavior of anal margin (D48.5)*
neoplasm of uncertain behavior of anal skin (D48.5)
neoplasm of uncertain behavior of perianal skin (D48.5)

D37.9 Neoplasm of uncertain behavior of digestive organ, unspecified

D38 Neoplasm of uncertain behavior of middle ear and respiratory and intrathoracic organs

EXCLUDES 1 *neoplasm of uncertain behavior of heart (D48.7)*

D38.0 Neoplasm of uncertain behavior of larynx
Neoplasm of uncertain behavior of aryepiglottic fold or interarytenoid fold, laryngeal aspect
Neoplasm of uncertain behavior of epiglottis (suprahyoid portion)

EXCLUDES 1 *neoplasm of uncertain behavior of aryepiglottic fold or interarytenoid fold NOS (D37.05)*
neoplasm of uncertain behavior of hypopharyngeal aspect of aryepiglottic fold (D37.05)
neoplasm of uncertain behavior of marginal zone of aryepiglottic fold (D37.05)

D38.1 Neoplasm of uncertain behavior of trachea, bronchus and lung

D38.2 Neoplasm of uncertain behavior of pleura

D38.3 Neoplasm of uncertain behavior of mediastinum

D38.4 Neoplasm of uncertain behavior of thymus

D38.5 Neoplasm of uncertain behavior of other respiratory organs
Neoplasm of uncertain behavior of accessory sinuses
Neoplasm of uncertain behavior of cartilage of nose
Neoplasm of uncertain behavior of middle ear
Neoplasm of uncertain behavior of nasal cavities

EXCLUDES 1 *neoplasm of uncertain behavior of ear (external) (skin) (D48.5)*
neoplasm of uncertain behavior of nose NOS (D48.7)
neoplasm of uncertain behavior of skin of nose (D48.5)

D38.6 Neoplasm of uncertain behavior of respiratory organ, unspecified

D39 Neoplasm of uncertain behavior of female genital organs

D39.0 Neoplasm of uncertain behavior of uterus ♀

D39.1 Neoplasm of uncertain behavior of ovary
Use additional code to identify any functional activity.

D39.10 Neoplasm of uncertain behavior of unspecified ovary ♀

D39.11 Neoplasm of uncertain behavior of right ovary ♀

D39.12 Neoplasm of uncertain behavior of left ovary ♀

D39.2 Neoplasm of uncertain behavior of placenta ♀ M
Chorioadenoma destruens
Invasive hydatidiform mole
Malignant hydatidiform mole

EXCLUDES 1 *hydatidiform mole NOS (O01.9)*

D39.8 Neoplasm of uncertain behavior of other specified female genital organs ♀
Neoplasm of uncertain behavior of skin of female genital organs

D39.9 Neoplasm of uncertain behavior of female genital organ, unspecified ♀

D40 Neoplasm of uncertain behavior of male genital organs

D40.0 Neoplasm of uncertain behavior of prostate ♂

D40.1 Neoplasm of uncertain behavior of testis

D40.10 Neoplasm of uncertain behavior of unspecified testis ♂

D40.11 Neoplasm of uncertain behavior of right testis ♂

D40.12 Neoplasm of uncertain behavior of left testis ♂

D40.8 Neoplasm of uncertain behavior of other specified male genital organs ♂
Neoplasm of uncertain behavior of skin of male genital organs

D40.9 Neoplasm of uncertain behavior of male genital organ, unspecified ♂

D41 Neoplasm of uncertain behavior of urinary organs

D41.0 Neoplasm of uncertain behavior of kidney

EXCLUDES 1 *neoplasm of uncertain behavior of renal pelvis (D41.1-)*

D41.00 Neoplasm of uncertain behavior of unspecified kidney

D41.01 Neoplasm of uncertain behavior of right kidney

D41.02 Neoplasm of uncertain behavior of left kidney

D41.1 Neoplasm of uncertain behavior of renal pelvis

D41.10 Neoplasm of uncertain behavior of unspecified renal pelvis

D41.11 **Neoplasm of uncertain behavior of right renal pelvis**
D41.12 **Neoplasm of uncertain behavior of left renal pelvis**
D41.2 **Neoplasm of uncertain behavior of ureter**
D41.20 **Neoplasm of uncertain behavior of unspecified ureter**
D41.21 **Neoplasm of uncertain behavior of right ureter**
D41.22 **Neoplasm of uncertain behavior of left ureter**
D41.3 **Neoplasm of uncertain behavior of urethra**
D41.4 **Neoplasm of uncertain behavior of bladder**
D41.8 **Neoplasm of uncertain behavior of other specified urinary organs**
D41.9 **Neoplasm of uncertain behavior of unspecified urinary organ**

D42 **Neoplasm of uncertain behavior of meninges**
D42.0 **Neoplasm of uncertain behavior of cerebral meninges** HCC
D42.1 **Neoplasm of uncertain behavior of spinal meninges** HCC
D42.9 **Neoplasm of uncertain behavior of meninges, unspecified** HCC

D43 **Neoplasm of uncertain behavior of brain and central nervous system**
EXCLUDES 1 *neoplasm of uncertain behavior of peripheral nerves and autonomic nervous system (D48.2)*
D43.0 **Neoplasm of uncertain behavior of brain, supratentorial** HCC
Neoplasm of uncertain behavior of cerebral ventricle
Neoplasm of uncertain behavior of cerebrum
Neoplasm of uncertain behavior of frontal lobe
Neoplasm of uncertain behavior of occipital lobe
Neoplasm of uncertain behavior of parietal lobe
Neoplasm of uncertain behavior of temporal lobe
EXCLUDES 1 *neoplasm of uncertain behavior of fourth ventricle (D43.1)*
D43.1 **Neoplasm of uncertain behavior of brain, infratentorial** HCC
Neoplasm of uncertain behavior of brain stem
Neoplasm of uncertain behavior of cerebellum
Neoplasm of uncertain behavior of fourth ventricle
D43.2 **Neoplasm of uncertain behavior of brain, unspecified** HCC
D43.3 **Neoplasm of uncertain behavior of cranial nerves** HCC
D43.4 **Neoplasm of uncertain behavior of spinal cord** HCC
D43.8 **Neoplasm of uncertain behavior of other specified parts of central nervous system** HCC
D43.9 **Neoplasm of uncertain behavior of central nervous system, unspecified** HCC
Neoplasm of uncertain behavior of nervous system (central) NOS

D44 **Neoplasm of uncertain behavior of endocrine glands**
EXCLUDES 1 *multiple endocrine adenomatosis (E31.2-)*
multiple endocrine neoplasia (E31.2-)
neoplasm of uncertain behavior of endocrine pancreas (D37.8)
neoplasm of uncertain behavior of ovary (D39.1-)
neoplasm of uncertain behavior of testis (D40.1-)
neoplasm of uncertain behavior of thymus (D38.4)
D44.0 **Neoplasm of uncertain behavior of thyroid gland**
D44.1 **Neoplasm of uncertain behavior of adrenal gland**
Use additional code to identify any functional activity.
D44.10 **Neoplasm of uncertain behavior of unspecified adrenal gland**
D44.11 **Neoplasm of uncertain behavior of right adrenal gland**
D44.12 **Neoplasm of uncertain behavior of left adrenal gland**
D44.2 **Neoplasm of uncertain behavior of parathyroid gland**
D44.3 **Neoplasm of uncertain behavior of pituitary gland** HCC
Use additional code to identify any functional activity.
D44.4 **Neoplasm of uncertain behavior of craniopharyngeal duct** HCC
D44.5 **Neoplasm of uncertain behavior of pineal gland** HCC
D44.6 **Neoplasm of uncertain behavior of carotid body** HCC
D44.7 **Neoplasm of uncertain behavior of aortic body and other paraganglia** HCC
D44.9 **Neoplasm of uncertain behavior of unspecified endocrine gland**

D45 **Polycythemia vera** HCC
EXCLUDES 1 *familial polycythemia (D75.0)*
secondary polycythemia (D75.1)

D46 **Myelodysplastic syndromes**
Use additional code for adverse effect, if applicable, to identify drug (T36-T50 with fifth or sixth character 5)
EXCLUDES 2 *drug-induced aplastic anemia (D61.1)*
D46.0 **Refractory anemia without ring sideroblasts, so stated** HCC
Refractory anemia without sideroblasts, without excess of blasts
D46.1 **Refractory anemia with ring sideroblasts** HCC
RARS
D46.2 **Refractory anemia with excess of blasts [RAEB]**
D46.20 **Refractory anemia with excess of blasts, unspecified** HCC
RAEB NOS
D46.21 **Refractory anemia with excess of blasts 1** HCC
RAEB 1
D46.22 **Refractory anemia with excess of blasts 2** HCC
RAEB 2
D46.A **Refractory cytopenia with multilineage dysplasia** HCC
D46.B **Refractory cytopenia with multilineage dysplasia and ring sideroblasts** HCC
RCMD RS
D46.C **Myelodysplastic syndrome with isolated del(5q) chromosomal abnormality** HCC
Myelodysplastic syndrome with 5q deletion
5q minus syndrome NOS
D46.4 **Refractory anemia, unspecified** HCC
D46.Z **Other myelodysplastic syndromes** HCC
EXCLUDES 1 *chronic myelomonocytic leukemia (C93.1-)*
D46.9 **Myelodysplastic syndrome, unspecified** HCC
Myelodysplasia NOS

D47 **Other neoplasms of uncertain behavior of lymphoid, hematopoietic and related tissue**
▲ D47.0 **Mast cell neoplasms of uncertain behavior**
EXCLUDES 1 *congenital cutaneous mastocytosis (Q82.2)*
histiocytic neoplasms of uncertain behavior (D47.Z9)
malignant mast cell neoplasm (C96.2-)
D47.01 **Cutaneous mastocytosis**
Diffuse cutaneous mastocytosis
Maculopapular cutaneous mastocytosis
Solitary mastocytoma
Telangiectasia macularis eruptiva perstans
Urticaria pigmentosa
EXCLUDES 1 *congenital (diffuse) (maculopapular) cutaneous mastocytosis (Q82.2)*
congenital urticaria pigmentosa (Q82.2)
extracutaneous mastocytoma (D47.09)
AHA: 4Q 2017, 4
D47.02 **Systemic mastocytosis**
Indolent systemic mastocytosis
Isolated bone marrow mastocytosis
Smoldering systemic mastocytosis
Systemic mastocytosis, with an associated hematological non-mast cell lineage disease (SM-AHNMD)
Code also, if applicable, any associated hematological non-mast cell lineage disease, such as:
acute myeloid leukemia (C92.6-, C92.A-)
chronic myelomonocytic leukemia (C93.1-)
essential thrombocytosis (D47.3)
hypereosinophilic syndrome (D72.1)
myelodysplastic syndrome (D46.9)
myeloproliferative syndrome (D47.1)
non-Hodgkin lymphoma (C82-C85)
plasma cell myeloma (C90.0-)
polycythemia vera (D45)
EXCLUDES 1 *aggressive systemic mastocytosis (C96.21)*
mast cell leukemia (C94.3-)
AHA: 4Q 2017, 4

D47.09 Other **mast cell neoplasms of uncertain behavior**
Extracutaneous mastocytoma
Mast cell tumor NOS
Mastocytoma NOS
Mastocytosis NOS
AHA: 4Q 2017, 4

D47.1 **Chronic myeloproliferative disease** HCC
Chronic neutrophilic leukemia
Myeloproliferative disease, unspecified
EXCLUDES 1 *atypical chronic myeloid leukemia BCR/ABL-negative (C92.2-)*
chronic myeloid leukemia BCR/ABL-positive (C92.1-)
myelofibrosis NOS (D75.81)
myelophthisic anemia (D61.82)
myelophthisis (D61.82)
secondary myelofibrosis NOS (D75.81)

D47.2 **Monoclonal gammopathy**
Monoclonal gammopathy of undetermined significance [MGUS]

D47.3 **Essential (hemorrhagic) thrombocythemia** HCC
Essential thrombocytosis
Idiopathic hemorrhagic thrombocythemia
DEFINITION Rare myeloproliferative disorder characterized by uncontrolled over-production of blood platelet precursor cells, leading to splenomegaly, hemorrhaging from the intestines, gums, or nose, and blood vessel thrombosis.

D47.4 **Osteomyelofibrosis** HCC
Chronic idiopathic myelofibrosis
Myelofibrosis (idiopathic) (with myeloid metaplasia)
Myelosclerosis (megakaryocytic) with myeloid metaplasia
Secondary myelofibrosis in myeloproliferative disease
EXCLUDES 1 *acute myelofibrosis (C94.4-)*

5 **D47.Z** **Other specified neoplasms of uncertain behavior of lymphoid, hematopoietic and related tissue**
AHA: 4Q 2016, 8

D47.Z1 **Post-transplant lymphoproliferative disorder (PTLD)** HCC
Code first:
complications of transplanted organs and tissue (T86.-)

D47.Z2 **Castleman disease** HCC
Code also:
if applicable human herpesvirus 8 infection (B10.89)
EXCLUDES 2 *Kaposi's sarcoma (C46-)*

D47.Z9 **Other specified neoplasms of uncertain behavior of lymphoid, hematopoietic and related tissue** HCC
Histiocytic tumors of uncertain behavior

D47.9 **Neoplasm of uncertain behavior of lymphoid, hematopoietic and related tissue, unspecified** HCC
Lymphoproliferative disease NOS

4 **D48** **Neoplasm of uncertain behavior of other and unspecified sites**
EXCLUDES 1 *neurofibromatosis (nonmalignant) (Q85.0-)*

D48.0 **Neoplasm of uncertain behavior of bone and articular cartilage**
EXCLUDES 1 *neoplasm of uncertain behavior of cartilage of ear (D48.1)*
neoplasm of uncertain behavior of cartilage of larynx (D38.0)
neoplasm of uncertain behavior of cartilage of nose (D38.5)
neoplasm of uncertain behavior of connective tissue of eyelid (D48.1)
neoplasm of uncertain behavior of synovia (D48.1)

D48.1 **Neoplasm of uncertain behavior of connective and other soft tissue**
Neoplasm of uncertain behavior of connective tissue of ear
Neoplasm of uncertain behavior of connective tissue of eyelid
Stromal tumors of uncertain behavior of digestive system
EXCLUDES 1 *neoplasm of uncertain behavior of articular cartilage (D48.0)*
neoplasm of uncertain behavior of cartilage of larynx (D38.0)
neoplasm of uncertain behavior of cartilage of nose (D38.5)
neoplasm of uncertain behavior of connective tissue of breast (D48.6-)

D48.2 **Neoplasm of uncertain behavior of peripheral nerves and autonomic nervous system**
EXCLUDES 1 *neoplasm of uncertain behavior of peripheral nerves of orbit (D48.7)*

D48.3 **Neoplasm of uncertain behavior of retroperitoneum**

D48.4 **Neoplasm of uncertain behavior of peritoneum**

D48.5 **Neoplasm of uncertain behavior of skin**
Neoplasm of uncertain behavior of anal margin
Neoplasm of uncertain behavior of anal skin
Neoplasm of uncertain behavior of perianal skin
Neoplasm of uncertain behavior of skin of breast
EXCLUDES 1 *neoplasm of uncertain behavior of anus NOS (D37.8)*
neoplasm of uncertain behavior of skin of genital organs (D39.8, D40.8)
neoplasm of uncertain behavior of vermilion border of lip (D37.0)

5 **D48.6** **Neoplasm of uncertain behavior of breast**
Neoplasm of uncertain behavior of connective tissue of breast
Cystosarcoma phyllodes
EXCLUDES 1 *neoplasm of uncertain behavior of skin of breast (D48.5)*

D48.60 **Neoplasm of uncertain behavior of unspecified breast**

D48.61 **Neoplasm of uncertain behavior of right breast**

D48.62 **Neoplasm of uncertain behavior of left breast**

D48.7 **Neoplasm of uncertain behavior of other specified sites**
Neoplasm of uncertain behavior of eye
Neoplasm of uncertain behavior of heart
Neoplasm of uncertain behavior of peripheral nerves of orbit
EXCLUDES 1 *neoplasm of uncertain behavior of connective tissue (D48.1)*
neoplasm of uncertain behavior of skin of eyelid (D48.5)

D48.9 **Neoplasm of uncertain behavior, unspecified**

Neoplasms of unspecified behavior (D49)

4 **D49** **Neoplasms of unspecified behavior**
Note: Category D49 classifies by site neoplasms of unspecified morphology and behavior. The term 'mass', unless otherwise stated, is not to be regarded as a neoplastic growth.
INCLUDES 'growth' NOS
neoplasm NOS
new growth NOS
tumor NOS
EXCLUDES 1 *neoplasms of uncertain behavior (D37-D44, D48)*
CODING TIP ✓ Codes classifiable to D49 include tumors that have not been defined as malignant or benign. Unspecified behavior is a specific diagnostic criterion that must be indicated in the documentation. It is not equivalent to NEC/NOS.

D49.0 **Neoplasm of unspecified behavior of digestive system**
EXCLUDES 1 *neoplasm of unspecified behavior of margin of anus (D49.2)*
neoplasm of unspecified behavior of perianal skin (D49.2)
neoplasm of unspecified behavior of skin of anus (D49.2)

D49.1 **Neoplasm of unspecified behavior of respiratory system**

D49.2 **Neoplasm of unspecified behavior of bone, soft tissue, and skin**

EXCLUDES 1 *neoplasm of unspecified behavior of anal canal (D49.0)*
neoplasm of unspecified behavior of anus NOS (D49.0)
neoplasm of unspecified behavior of bone marrow (D49.89)
neoplasm of unspecified behavior of cartilage of larynx (D49.1)
neoplasm of unspecified behavior of cartilage of nose (D49.1)
neoplasm of unspecified behavior of connective tissue of breast (D49.3)
neoplasm of unspecified behavior of skin of genital organs (D49.59)
neoplasm of unspecified behavior of vermilion border of lip (D49.0)

D49.3 **Neoplasm of unspecified behavior of breast**

EXCLUDES 1 *neoplasm of unspecified behavior of skin of breast (D49.2)*

D49.4 **Neoplasm of unspecified behavior of bladder**

5 **D49.5** **Neoplasm of unspecified behavior of other genitourinary organs**

6 **D49.51** **Neoplasm of unspecified behavior of kidney**

AHA: 4Q 2016, 9

D49.511 **Neoplasm of unspecified behavior of right kidney**

D49.512 **Neoplasm of unspecified behavior of left kidney**

D49.519 **Neoplasm of unspecified behavior of unspecified kidney**

D49.59 **Neoplasm of unspecified behavior of other genitourinary organ**

AHA: 4Q 2016, 9

D49.6 **Neoplasm of unspecified behavior of brain** HCC

EXCLUDES 1 *neoplasm of unspecified behavior of cerebral meninges (D49.7)*
neoplasm of unspecified behavior of cranial nerves (D49.7)

D49.7 **Neoplasm of unspecified behavior of endocrine glands and other parts of nervous system**

EXCLUDES 1 *neoplasm of unspecified behavior of peripheral, sympathetic, and parasympathetic nerves and ganglia (D49.2)*

5 **D49.8** **Neoplasm of unspecified behavior of other specified sites**

EXCLUDES 1 *neoplasm of unspecified behavior of eyelid (skin) (D49.2)*
neoplasm of unspecified behavior of eyelid cartilage (D49.2)
neoplasm of unspecified behavior of great vessels (D49.2)
neoplasm of unspecified behavior of optic nerve (D49.7)

D49.81 **Neoplasm of unspecified behavior of retina and choroid**

Dark area on retina
Retinal freckle

D49.89 **Neoplasm of unspecified behavior of other specified sites**

D49.9 **Neoplasm of unspecified behavior of unspecified site**

CHAPTER 3: DISEASES OF THE BLOOD AND BLOOD-FORMING ORGANS AND CERTAIN DISORDERS INVOLVING THE IMMUNE MECHANISM (D50-D89)

EXCLUDES 2 *autoimmune disease (systemic) NOS (M35.9)*
certain conditions originating in the perinatal period (P00-P96)
complications of pregnancy, childbirth and the puerperium (O00-O9A)
congenital malformations, deformations and chromosomal abnormalities (Q00-Q99)
endocrine, nutritional and metabolic diseases (E00-E88)
human immunodeficiency virus [HIV] disease (B20)
injury, poisoning and certain other consequences of external causes (S00-T88)
neoplasms (C00-D49)
symptoms, signs and abnormal clinical and laboratory findings, not elsewhere classified (R00-R94)

This chapter contains the following blocks:

D50-D53	Nutritional anemias
D55-D59	Hemolytic anemias
D60-D64	Aplastic and other anemias and other bone marrow failure syndromes
D65-D69	Coagulation defects, purpura and other hemorrhagic conditions
D70-D77	Other disorders of blood and blood-forming organs
D78	Intraoperative and postprocedural complications of the spleen
D80-D89	Certain disorders involving the immune mechanism

Nutritional anemias (D50-D53)

4 D50 Iron deficiency anemia

INCLUDES asiderotic anemia
hypochromic anemia

CODING TIP✓ Do not assign codes from category D50 when the record only reports "iron deficiency" but does not specifically state "iron deficiency anemia" or "anemia due to iron deficiency." Iron deficiency (without anemia) should be coded to E61.1.

D50.0 Iron deficiency anemia secondary to blood loss (chronic)
Posthemorrhagic anemia (chronic)
EXCLUDES 1 *acute posthemorrhagic anemia (D62)*
congenital anemia from fetal blood loss (P61.3)

CODING TIP✓ The term "chronic" is a non-essential modifier in the code title for iron deficiency anemia secondary to blood loss (chronic). When the record specifies posthemorrhagic anemia (not specified as acute), D50.0 should be assigned. No time period is specifically required for the condition.

DEFINITION Iron depletion from sustained RBC loss in long-term bleeding, often from an ulcerous lesion, causing decreased hemoglobin and insufficient tissue oxygenation.

D50.1 Sideropenic dysphagia
Kelly-Paterson syndrome
Plummer-Vinson syndrome

D50.8 Other iron deficiency anemias
Iron deficiency anemia due to inadequate dietary iron intake

CODING TIP✓ Code D50.8 should be used to report anemia due to dietary iron deficiency.

D50.9 Iron deficiency anemia, unspecified

CODING TIP✓ When the record specifies only "hypochromic anemia" with no cause provided, report code D50.9.

DEFINITION Insufficient stores of iron in the body causing decreased hemoglobin and a reduction in red blood cell oxygen carrying capacity.

4 D51 Vitamin B12 deficiency anemia
EXCLUDES 1 *vitamin B12 deficiency (E53.8)*

CODING TIP✓ Do not assign codes from category D51 when the record only reports "vitamin B12 deficiency" but does not specifically state "vitamin B12 deficiency anemia" or "anemia due to vitamin B12 deficiency." A deficiency (without anemia) should be coded to E53.8.

D51.0 Vitamin B12 deficiency anemia due to intrinsic factor deficiency
Addison anemia
Biermer anemia
Pernicious (congenital) anemia
Congenital intrinsic factor deficiency

DEFINITION Anemia due to underlying Vitamin B12 malabsorption caused by inadequate production of intrinsic factor in the gastric mucosa.

D51.1 Vitamin B12 deficiency anemia due to selective vitamin B12 malabsorption with proteinuria
Imerslund (Gräsbeck) syndrome
Megaloblastic hereditary anemia

D51.2 Transcobalamin II deficiency

D51.3 Other dietary vitamin B12 deficiency anemia
Vegan anemia

Dietary vitamin B_{12} deficiency anemia

Symptoms include fatigue, weakness, tingling and numbness in extremities, balance and memory problems, even irreversible nerve damage

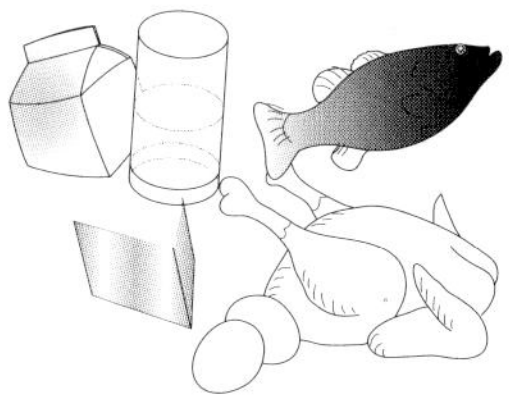

Beef, poultry, fish, dairy products, and eggs are the best sources of Vitamin B_{12}

D51.8 Other vitamin B12 deficiency anemias

D51.9 Vitamin B12 deficiency anemia, unspecified

4 D52 Folate deficiency anemia
EXCLUDES 1 *folate deficiency without anemia (E53.8)*

DEFINITION Lack of folic acid causing large, immature, misshapen red blood cells, called megaloblasts, to form in the bone marrow.

D52.0 Dietary folate deficiency anemia
Nutritional megaloblastic anemia

D52.1 Drug-induced folate deficiency anemia
Use additional code for adverse effect, if applicable, to identify drug (T36-T50 with fifth or sixth character 5)

D52.8 Other folate deficiency anemias

D52.9 Folate deficiency anemia, unspecified
Folic acid deficiency anemia NOS

4 D53 Other nutritional anemias

INCLUDES megaloblastic anemia unresponsive to vitamin B12 or folate therapy

D53.0 Protein deficiency anemia
Amino-acid deficiency anemia
Orotaciduric anemia
EXCLUDES 1 *Lesch-Nyhan syndrome (E79.1)*

D53.1 Other megaloblastic anemias, not elsewhere classified
Megaloblastic anemia NOS
EXCLUDES 1 *Di Guglielmo's disease (C94.0)*

D53.2 Scorbutic anemia
EXCLUDES 1 *scurvy (E54)*

D53.8 Other specified nutritional anemias
Anemia associated with deficiency of copper
Anemia associated with deficiency of molybdenum
Anemia associated with deficiency of zinc
EXCLUDES 1 *nutritional deficiencies without anemia, such as:*
copper deficiency NOS (E61.0)
molybdenum deficiency NOS (E61.5)
zinc deficiency NOS (E60)

D53.9 Nutritional anemia, unspecified
Simple chronic anemia
EXCLUDES 1 *anemia NOS (D64.9)*

Hemolytic anemias (D55-D59)

4 D55 Anemia due to enzyme disorders

EXCLUDES 1 *drug-induced enzyme deficiency anemia (D59.2)*

D55.0 Anemia due to glucose-6-phosphate dehydrogenase [G6PD] deficiency HCC
Favism
G6PD deficiency anemia

D55.1 Anemia due to other disorders of glutathione metabolism HCC
Anemia (due to) enzyme deficiencies, except G6PD, related to the hexose monophosphate [HMP] shunt pathway
Anemia (due to) hemolytic nonspherocytic (hereditary), type I

DEFINITION Anemia resulting from damage or destruction of RBCs in high numbers due to insufficient glutathione, a tripeptide used by RBCs to protect against oxidative damage.

D55.2 Anemia due to disorders of glycolytic enzymes HCC
Hemolytic nonspherocytic (hereditary) anemia, type II
Hexokinase deficiency anemia
Pyruvate kinase [PK] deficiency anemia
Triose-phosphate isomerase deficiency anemia

EXCLUDES 1 *disorders of glycolysis not associated with anemia (E74.8)*

D55.3 Anemia due to disorders of nucleotide metabolism HCC

D55.8 Other anemias due to enzyme disorders HCC

D55.9 Anemia due to enzyme disorder, unspecified HCC

4 D56 Thalassemia

EXCLUDES 1 *sickle-cell thalassemia (D57.4-)*

D56.0 Alpha thalassemia HCC
Alpha thalassemia major
Hemoglobin H Constant Spring
Hemoglobin H disease
Hydrops fetalis due to alpha thalassemia
Severe alpha thalassemia
Triple gene defect alpha thalassemia
Use additional code, if applicable, for hydrops fetalis due to alpha thalassemia (P56.99)

EXCLUDES 1 *alpha thalassemia trait or minor (D56.3)*
asymptomatic alpha thalassemia (D56.3)
hydrops fetalis due to isoimmunization (P56.0)
hydrops fetalis not due to immune hemolysis (P83.2)

DEFINITION Hemoglobinopathy caused by genetic decrease in alpha globin chain formation needed for normal hemoglobin A (2 alpha and 2 beta chains), forming unstable hemoglobin and leading to RBC breakage.

D56.1 Beta thalassemia HCC
Beta thalassemia major
Cooley's anemia
Homozygous beta thalassemia
Severe beta thalassemia
Thalassemia intermedia
Thalassemia major

EXCLUDES 1 *beta thalassemia minor (D56.3)*
beta thalassemia trait (D56.3)
delta-beta thalassemia (D56.2)
hemoglobin E-beta thalassemia (D56.5)
sickle-cell beta thalassemia (D57.4-)

DEFINITION Hemoglobinopathy caused by genetic decrease in beta globin chain formation needed for normal hemoglobin A (2 alpha and 2 beta chains), leaving insoluble alpha chain aggregates that interfere with RBC production, maturation, and membrane function.

D56.2 Delta-beta thalassemia HCC
Homozygous delta-beta thalassemia

EXCLUDES 1 *delta-beta thalassemia minor (D56.3)*
delta-beta thalassemia trait (D56.3)

D56.3 Thalassemia minor
Alpha thalassemia minor
Alpha thalassemia silent carrier
Alpha thalassemia trait
Beta thalassemia minor
Beta thalassemia trait
Delta-beta thalassemia minor
Delta-beta thalassemia trait
Thalassemia trait NOS

EXCLUDES 1 *alpha thalassemia (D56.0)*
beta thalassemia (D56.1)
delta-beta thalassemia (D56.2)
hemoglobin E-beta thalassemia (D56.5)
sickle-cell trait (D57.3)

DEFINITION Alpha, beta, and delta-beta hemoglobinopathies caused by small gene mutations resulting in mild signs and symptoms of anemia, or asymptomatic trait or silent carrier forms.

D56.4 Hereditary persistence of fetal hemoglobin [HPFH] HCC

D56.5 Hemoglobin E-beta thalassemia HCC

EXCLUDES 1 *beta thalassemia (D56.1)*
beta thalassemia minor (D56.3)
beta thalassemia trait (D56.3)
delta-beta thalassemia (D56.2)
delta-beta thalassemia trait (D56.3)
hemoglobin E disease (D58.2)
other hemoglobinopathies (D58.2)
sickle-cell beta thalassemia (D57.4-)

DEFINITION Hemoglobinopathy caused by variations in beta globin chain formation, producing unstable hemoglobin E and causing microcytic anemia, poor growth, splenomegaly, and heart failure.

D56.8 Other thalassemias HCC
Dominant thalassemia
Hemoglobin C thalassemia
Mixed thalassemia
Thalassemia with other hemoglobinopathy

EXCLUDES 1 *hemoglobin C disease (D58.2)*
hemoglobin E disease (D58.2)
other hemoglobinopathies (D58.2)
sickle-cell anemia (D57.-)
sickle-cell thalassemia (D57.4)

D56.9 Thalassemia, unspecified
Mediterranean anemia (with other hemoglobinopathy)

DEFINITION Inherited blood disease causing disruption in the normal production of hemoglobin and a high rate of red blood cell destruction.

4 D57 Sickle-cell disorders

Use additional code for any associated fever (R50.81)

EXCLUDES 1 *other hemoglobinopathies (D58.-)*

5 D57.0 Hb-SS disease with crisis
Sickle-cell disease NOS with crisis
Hb-SS disease with vasoocclusive pain

D57.00 Hb-SS disease with crisis, unspecified HCC

DEFINITION Hereditary disease in which RBCs contain abnormal hemoglobin S, making them elongated and crescent-shaped. The fragile, sickled cells become blocked in tiny blood vessels and break apart, causing vaso-occlusive pain.

D57.01 Hb-SS disease with acute chest syndrome HCC

DEFINITION Life-threatening complication of sickle-cell disease in which blood clots form in the tiny blood vessels of the lungs with repeated episodes of bleeding from the alveoli and hemosiderin buildup.

D57.02 Hb-SS disease with splenic sequestration HCC

CODING TIP ✓ Sickle cell with splenic sequestration crisis occurs when the sickle red blood cells block the blood vessels inside the spleen, preventing blood from leaving the spleen and causing splenomegaly and anemia. In Hb-SS disease, a sickle cell gene "S" is inherited from each parent. Commonly called sickle cell anemia, this is the most severe form.

DEFINITION Life-threatening complication of sickle-cell disease in which sickled cells become trapped in the spleen, causing acute swelling, high fever, intense abdominal pain, jaundice, leukocytosis, and tissue infarction.

D57.1 Sickle-cell disease without crisis HCC
Hb-SS disease without crisis
Sickle-cell anemia NOS
Sickle-cell disease NOS
Sickle-cell disorder NOS

DEFINITION Chronic, hereditary disease in which red blood cells contain abnormal hemoglobin S and are stiff and misshapen like a crescent, inhibiting blood flow through small blood vessels.

Sickle-cell disease without crisis

Normal red blood cells
Cells are compact and flexible, enabling them to squeeze through small capillaries

Sickled red blood cells
Cells are stiff and angular, causing them to become stuck in small capillaries

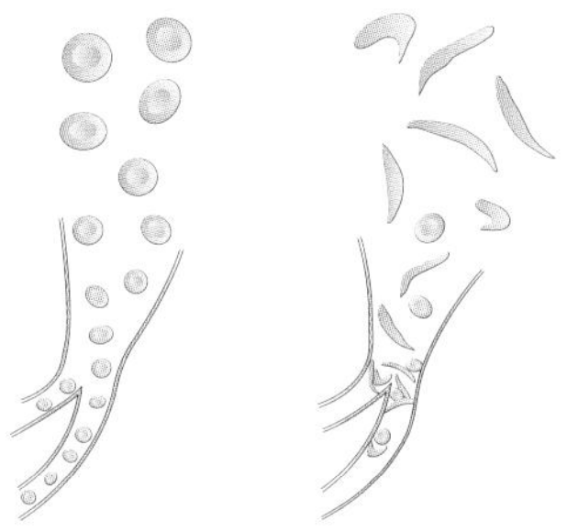

5 **D57.2 Sickle-cell/Hb-C disease**
Hb-SC disease
Hb-S/Hb-C disease

D57.20 Sickle-cell/Hb-C disease without crisis HCC

6 **D57.21 Sickle-cell/Hb-C disease with crisis**

D57.211 Sickle-cell/Hb-C disease with acute chest syndrome HCC

D57.212 Sickle-cell/Hb-C disease with splenic sequestration HCC

CODING TIP ✓ Sickle cell with splenic sequestration crisis occurs when the sickle red blood cells block the blood vessels inside the spleen, preventing blood from leaving the spleen and causing splenomegaly and anemia. In Hb-C disease, a sickle cell "S" gene is inherited from one parent and a gene for abnormal hemoglobin "C" is inherited from the other parent. This is usually a milder form of SCD.

D57.219 Sickle-cell/Hb-C disease with crisis, unspecified HCC
Sickle-cell/Hb-C disease with crisis NOS

D57.3 Sickle-cell trait HCC
Hb-S trait
Heterozygous hemoglobin S

CODING TIP ✓ When a patient is reported only to have sickle cell "trait" but no sickle cell disease is stated, report only D57.3. A person who carries the sickle cell trait rarely exhibits any disease symptoms, but can pass the gene on.

DEFINITION Condition in which a person carries one gene for normal hemoglobin and one for abnormal hemoglobin S that sickles red blood cells, producing only mild anemia or remaining asymptomatic.

5 **D57.4 Sickle-cell thalassemia**
Sickle-cell beta thalassemia
Thalassemia Hb-S disease

CODING TIP ✓ Sickle cell thalassemia is a form of sickle cell disease that affects the production of hemoglobin in red blood cells, resulting in a reduction or absence of normal hemoglobin.

D57.40 Sickle-cell thalassemia without crisis HCC
Microdrepanocytosis
Sickle-cell thalassemia NOS

DEFINITION Inherited form of anemia, occurring mainly among people of Mediterranean descent, caused by faulty synthesis of part of the hemoglobin molecule.

6 **D57.41 Sickle-cell thalassemia with crisis**
Sickle-cell thalassemia with vasoocclusive pain

D57.411 Sickle-cell thalassemia with acute chest syndrome HCC

D57.412 Sickle-cell thalassemia with splenic sequestration HCC

D57.419 Sickle-cell thalassemia with crisis, unspecified HCC
Sickle-cell thalassemia with crisis NOS

5 **D57.8 Other sickle-cell disorders**
Hb-SD disease
Hb-SE disease

D57.80 Other sickle-cell disorders without crisis HCC

6 **D57.81 Other sickle-cell disorders with crisis**

D57.811 Other sickle-cell disorders with acute chest syndrome HCC

D57.812 Other sickle-cell disorders with splenic sequestration HCC

D57.819 Other sickle-cell disorders with crisis, unspecified HCC
Other sickle-cell disorders with crisis NOS

4 D58 Other hereditary hemolytic anemias

EXCLUDES 1 *hemolytic anemia of the newborn (P55.-)*

D58.0 Hereditary spherocytosis HCC
Acholuric (familial) jaundice
Congenital (spherocytic) hemolytic icterus
Minkowski-Chauffard syndrome

DEFINITION Congenital form of spherocytosis with hemolytic anemia, abnormal fragility of erythrocytes, jaundice, and splenomegaly.

D58.1 Hereditary elliptocytosis HCC
Elliptocytosis (congenital)
Ovalocytosis (congenital) (hereditary)

D58.2 Other hemoglobinopathies HCC
Abnormal hemoglobin NOS
Congenital Heinz body anemia
Hb-C disease
Hb-D disease
Hb-E disease
Hemoglobinopathy NOS
Unstable hemoglobin hemolytic disease

EXCLUDES 1 *familial polycythemia (D75.0)*
Hb-M disease (D74.0)
hemoglobin E-beta thalassemia (D56.5)
hereditary persistence of fetal hemoglobin [HPFH] (D56.4)
high-altitude polycythemia (D75.1)
methemoglobinemia (D74.-)
other hemoglobinopathies with thalassemia (D56.8)

D58.8 Other specified hereditary hemolytic anemias HCC
Stomatocytosis

D58.9 Hereditary hemolytic anemia, unspecified HCC

4 D59 Acquired hemolytic anemia

D59.0 Drug-induced autoimmune hemolytic anemia HCC
Use additional code for adverse effect, if applicable, to identify drug (T36-T50 with fifth or sixth character 5)

D59.1 Other autoimmune hemolytic anemias HCC
Autoimmune hemolytic disease (cold type) (warm type)
Chronic cold hemagglutinin disease
Cold agglutinin disease
Cold agglutinin hemoglobinuria
Cold type (secondary) (symptomatic) hemolytic anemia
Warm type (secondary) (symptomatic) hemolytic anemia

EXCLUDES 1 *Evans syndrome (D69.41)*
hemolytic disease of newborn (P55.-)
paroxysmal cold hemoglobinuria (D59.6)

D59.2 Drug-induced nonautoimmune hemolytic anemia HCC
Drug-induced enzyme deficiency anemia
Use additional code for adverse effect, if applicable, to identify drug (T36-T50 with fifth or sixth character 5)

● New | Manifestation | 4-7 Digit Indicators | Laterality | A Adult | M Maternity | N Newborn | P Pediatric | ♂ Male
▲ Revised | Unspecified | AHA Coding Clinic | HCC Hierarchical Condition Categories | HIV HIV Related Conditions | ♀ Female

D59.3 Hemolytic-uremic syndrome HCC
Use additional code to identify associated:
E. coli infection (B96.2-)
Pneumococcal pneumonia (J13)
Shigella dysenteriae (A03.9)

DEFINITION Condition in which platelets become clogged in narrow renal blood vessels, leading to the destruction of red blood cells and kidney failure. Symptoms include severe abdominal pain, diarrhea, nausea, and vomiting.

D59.4 Other nonautoimmune hemolytic anemias HCC
Mechanical hemolytic anemia
Microangiopathic hemolytic anemia
Toxic hemolytic anemia

D59.5 Paroxysmal nocturnal hemoglobinuria [Marchiafava-Micheli] HCC
EXCLUDES 1 *hemoglobinuria NOS (R82.3)*

D59.6 Hemoglobinuria due to hemolysis from other external causes HCC
Hemoglobinuria from exertion
March hemoglobinuria
Paroxysmal cold hemoglobinuria
Use additional code (Chapter 20) to identify external cause
EXCLUDES 1 *hemoglobinuria NOS (R82.3)*

CODING TIP✓ Hemoglobinuria is a condition where excess hemoglobin is found in high concentrations in the urine. Code D59.6 only when the hemoglobinuria is stated as due to hemolysis related to a specific other cause (the hemolysis of red blood cells due to another specific cause or condition is resulting in the hemoglobinuria). An external cause code (from Chapter 20) should be assigned to identify the external cause.

D59.8 Other acquired hemolytic anemias HCC

D59.9 Acquired hemolytic anemia, unspecified HCC
Idiopathic hemolytic anemia, chronic

Aplastic and other anemias and other bone marrow failure syndromes (D60-D64)

4 D60 Acquired pure red cell aplasia [erythroblastopenia]
INCLUDES red cell aplasia (acquired) (adult) (with thymoma)
EXCLUDES 1 *congenital red cell aplasia (D61.01)*

D60.0 Chronic acquired pure red cell aplasia HCC

DEFINITION Decline of RBC precursor cells in the bone marrow until nearly absent while WBC precursors are present at normal levels; causes normochromic, normoblastic anemia.

D60.1 Transient acquired pure red cell aplasia HCC

D60.8 Other acquired pure red cell aplasias HCC

D60.9 Acquired pure red cell aplasia, unspecified HCC

4 D61 Other aplastic anemias and other bone marrow failure syndromes
EXCLUDES 1 *neutropenia (D70.-)*

5 D61.0 Constitutional aplastic anemia

D61.01 Constitutional (pure) red blood cell aplasia HCC
Blackfan-Diamond syndrome
Congenital (pure) red cell aplasia
Familial hypoplastic anemia
Primary (pure) red cell aplasia
Red cell (pure) aplasia of infants
EXCLUDES 1 *acquired red cell aplasia (D60.9)*

D61.09 Other constitutional aplastic anemia HCC
Fanconi's anemia
Pancytopenia with malformations

D61.1 Drug-induced aplastic anemia HCC
Use additional code for adverse effect, if applicable, to identify drug (T36-T50 with fifth or sixth character 5)

CODING TIP✓ When the record specifies only "anemia due to antineoplastic chemotherapy" but does not specify it as aplastic anemia due to the antineoplastic chemotherapy, report code D64.81.

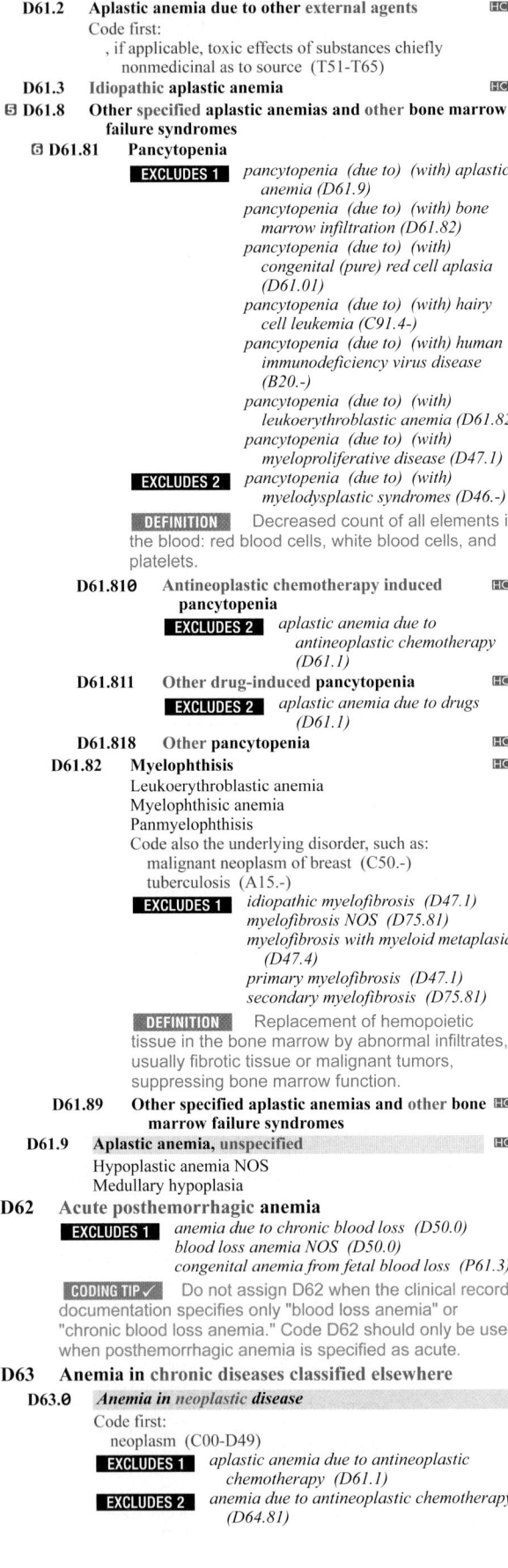

D61.2 Aplastic anemia due to other external agents HCC
Code first:
, if applicable, toxic effects of substances chiefly nonmedicinal as to source (T51-T65)

D61.3 Idiopathic aplastic anemia HCC

5 D61.8 Other specified aplastic anemias and other bone marrow failure syndromes

6 D61.81 Pancytopenia
EXCLUDES 1 *pancytopenia (due to) (with) aplastic anemia (D61.9)*
pancytopenia (due to) (with) bone marrow infiltration (D61.82)
pancytopenia (due to) (with) congenital (pure) red cell aplasia (D61.01)
pancytopenia (due to) (with) hairy cell leukemia (C91.4-)
pancytopenia (due to) (with) human immunodeficiency virus disease (B20.-)
pancytopenia (due to) (with) leukoerythroblastic anemia (D61.82)
pancytopenia (due to) (with) myeloproliferative disease (D47.1)
EXCLUDES 2 *pancytopenia (due to) (with) myelodysplastic syndromes (D46.-)*

DEFINITION Decreased count of all elements in the blood: red blood cells, white blood cells, and platelets.

D61.810 Antineoplastic chemotherapy induced pancytopenia HCC
EXCLUDES 2 *aplastic anemia due to antineoplastic chemotherapy (D61.1)*

D61.811 Other drug-induced pancytopenia HCC
EXCLUDES 2 *aplastic anemia due to drugs (D61.1)*

D61.818 Other pancytopenia HCC

D61.82 Myelophthisis HCC
Leukoerythroblastic anemia
Myelophthisic anemia
Panmyelophthisis
Code also the underlying disorder, such as:
malignant neoplasm of breast (C50.-)
tuberculosis (A15.-)
EXCLUDES 1 *idiopathic myelofibrosis (D47.1)*
myelofibrosis NOS (D75.81)
myelofibrosis with myeloid metaplasia (D47.4)
primary myelofibrosis (D47.1)
secondary myelofibrosis (D75.81)

DEFINITION Replacement of hemopoietic tissue in the bone marrow by abnormal infiltrates, usually fibrotic tissue or malignant tumors, suppressing bone marrow function.

D61.89 Other specified aplastic anemias and other bone marrow failure syndromes HCC

D61.9 Aplastic anemia, unspecified HCC
Hypoplastic anemia NOS
Medullary hypoplasia

D62 Acute posthemorrhagic anemia
EXCLUDES 1 *anemia due to chronic blood loss (D50.0)*
blood loss anemia NOS (D50.0)
congenital anemia from fetal blood loss (P61.3)

CODING TIP✓ Do not assign D62 when the clinical record documentation specifies only "blood loss anemia" or "chronic blood loss anemia." Code D62 should only be used when posthemorrhagic anemia is specified as acute.

4 D63 Anemia in chronic diseases classified elsewhere

D63.0 *Anemia in neoplastic disease*
Code first:
neoplasm (C00-D49)
EXCLUDES 1 *aplastic anemia due to antineoplastic chemotherapy (D61.1)*
EXCLUDES 2 *anemia due to antineoplastic chemotherapy (D64.81)*

GUIDELINES **Section 1.C.2.c.1** When admission/encounter is for management of an anemia associated with the malignancy, and the treatment is only for anemia, the appropriate code for the malignancy is sequenced as the principal or first-listed diagnosis followed by the appropriate code for the anemia (such as code D63.0, Anemia in neoplastic disease).

CODING TIP✓ When a patient is admitted for anemia due to neoplastic disease (D63.0), a code for the appropriate neoplasm must be first assigned, regardless of whether the focus of care is the neoplastic disease or the anemia. Anemia is assumed related to the neoplastic disease.

D63.1 ***Anemia in chronic kidney disease***
Erythropoietin resistant anemia (EPO resistant anemia)
Code first:
underlying chronic kidney disease (CKD) (N18.-)

D63.8 ***Anemia in other chronic diseases classified elsewhere***
Code first underlying disease, such as:
diphyllobothriasis (B70.0)
hookworm disease (B76.0-B76.9)
hypothyroidism (E00.0-E03.9)
malaria (B50.0-B54)
symptomatic late syphilis (A52.79)
tuberculosis (A18.89)

4 D64 Other anemias
EXCLUDES 1 *refractory anemia (D46.-)*
refractory anemia with excess blasts in transformation [RAEB T] (C92.0-)

D64.0 **Hereditary sideroblastic anemia** HCC
Sex-linked hypochromic sideroblastic anemia

DEFINITION Group of blood disorders in which the bone marrow's ability to produce normal red blood cells is impaired and sideroblasts, or deformed red blood cells, are present in the bloodstream.

D64.1 ***Secondary sideroblastic anemia due to disease*** HCC
Code first:
underlying disease

D64.2 **Secondary sideroblastic anemia due to drugs and toxins** HCC
Code first:
poisoning due to drug or toxin, if applicable (T36-T65 with fifth or sixth character 1-4 or 6)
Use additional code for adverse effect, if applicable, to identify drug (T36-T50 with fifth or sixth character 5)

D64.3 **Other sideroblastic anemias** HCC
Sideroblastic anemia NOS
Pyridoxine-responsive sideroblastic anemia NEC

D64.4 **Congenital dyserythropoietic anemia**
Dyshematopoietic anemia (congenital)
EXCLUDES 1 *Blackfan-Diamond syndrome (D61.01)*
Di Guglielmo's disease (C94.0)

CODING TIP✓ Congenital dyserythropoietic anemia is defined as a congenital condition resulting in immature red blood cells that are unusually shaped and cannot develop into functional mature cells, leading to a shortage of healthy red blood cells. These patients also frequently have thrombocytopenia, which should be additionally coded if present.

5 D64.8 **Other specified anemias**

D64.81 **Anemia due to antineoplastic chemotherapy**
Antineoplastic chemotherapy induced anemia
EXCLUDES 1 *aplastic anemia due to antineoplastic chemotherapy (D61.1)*
EXCLUDES 2 *anemia in neoplastic disease (D63.0)*

GUIDELINES **Section I.C.2.c.2)** When the admission/encounter is for management of an anemia associated with an adverse effect of the administration of chemotherapy or immunotherapy and the only treatment is for the anemia, the anemia code is sequenced first followed by the appropriate codes for the neoplasm and the adverse effect (T45.1X5, Adverse effect of antineoplastic and immunosuppressive drugs).

When the admission/encounter is for management of an anemia associated with an adverse effect of radiotherapy, the anemia code should be sequenced first, followed by the appropriate neoplasm code and code Y84.2, radiological procedure and radiotherapy as the cause of abnormal reaction of the patient, or of later complication, without mention of misadventure at the time of the procedure.

CODING TIP✓ Do not assign D64.81 to indicate aplastic anemia due to antineoplastic chemotherapy. If the diagnostic statements specifically report aplastic anemia due to antineoplastic chemotherapy, assign D61.1.

CODING TIP✓ Do not assign D64.81 to indicate anemia due to neoplastic disease. Anemia due to neoplastic disease should be coded to D63.0. D64.81 is for the management of anemia due to chemotherapy. Reference the guidelines for sequencing information since anemia secondary to chemotherapy is different than anemia due to neoplasm.
AHA: 4Q 2014, 22

D64.89 **Other specified anemias**
Infantile pseudoleukemia

D64.9 **Anemia, unspecified**

Coagulation defects, purpura and other hemorrhagic conditions (D65-D69)

CODING TIP✓ The codes in D65-D69 are used for different kinds of hemophilias. If bleeds are related to anticoagulant drugs, see D68.32.

D65 **Disseminated intravascular coagulation [defibrination syndrome]** HCC
Afibrinogenemia, acquired
Consumption coagulopathy
Diffuse or disseminated intravascular coagulation [DIC]
Fibrinolytic hemorrhage, acquired
Fibrinolytic purpura
Purpura fulminans
EXCLUDES 1 *disseminated intravascular coagulation (complicating) :*
abortion or ectopic or molar pregnancy (O00-O07, O08.1)
in newborn (P60)
pregnancy, childbirth and the puerperium (O45.0, O46.0, O67.0, O72.3)

DEFINITION Bleeding disorder characterized by an abnormal reduction in the elements involved in blood clotting; marked by profuse hemorrhaging in the late stages.

D66 **Hereditary factor VIII deficiency** HCC
Classical hemophilia
Deficiency factor VIII (with functional defect)
Hemophilia NOS
Hemophilia A
EXCLUDES 1 *factor VIII deficiency with vascular defect (D68.0)*

DEFINITION Most common form of hemophilia, referred to as classic hemophilia or hemophilia A; characterized by profuse bleeding from injuries, as well as bleeding from the joints, muscles, digestive tract, and brain.

Congenital factor VIII disorder
(Also known as hemophilia A or classic hemophilia)

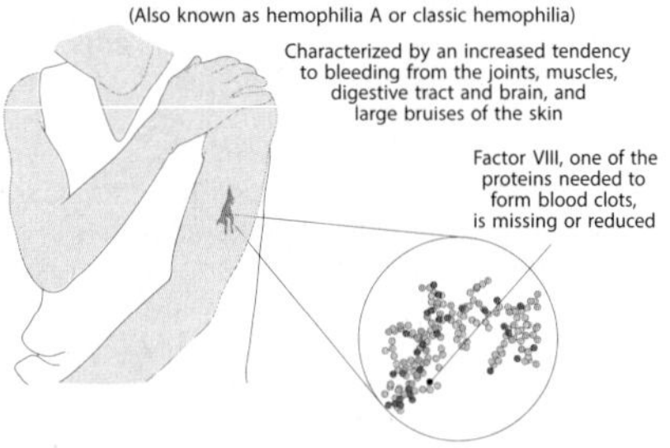
Characterized by an increased tendency to bleeding from the joints, muscles, digestive tract and brain, and large bruises of the skin
Factor VIII, one of the proteins needed to form blood clots, is missing or reduced

D67 Hereditary factor IX deficiency HCC
Christmas disease
Factor IX deficiency (with functional defect)
Hemophilia B
Plasma thromboplastin component [PTC] deficiency

DEFINITION A clotting disorder of blood, caused by hereditary deficiency of factor IX.

4 D68 Other coagulation defects

EXCLUDES 1 *abnormal coagulation profile (R79.1)*
coagulation defects complicating abortion or ectopic or molar pregnancy (O00-O07, O08.1)
coagulation defects complicating pregnancy, childbirth and the puerperium (O45.0, O46.0, O67.0, O72.3)

D68.0 Von Willebrand's disease HCC
Angiohemophilia
Factor VIII deficiency with vascular defect
Vascular hemophilia

EXCLUDES 1 *capillary fragility (hereditary) (D69.8)*
factor VIII deficiency NOS (D66)
factor VIII deficiency with functional defect (D66)

D68.1 Hereditary factor XI deficiency HCC
Hemophilia C
Plasma thromboplastin antecedent [PTA] deficiency
Rosenthal's disease

D68.2 Hereditary deficiency of other clotting factors HCC
AC globulin deficiency
Congenital afibrinogenemia
Deficiency of factor I [fibrinogen]
Deficiency of factor II [prothrombin]
Deficiency of factor V [labile]
Deficiency of factor VII [stable]
Deficiency of factor X [Stuart-Prower]
Deficiency of factor XII [Hageman]
Deficiency of factor XIII [fibrin stabilizing]
Dysfibrinogenemia (congenital)
Hypoproconvertinemia
Owren's disease
Proaccelerin deficiency

5 D68.3 Hemorrhagic disorder due to circulating anticoagulants

6 D68.31 Hemorrhagic disorder due to intrinsic circulating anticoagulants, antibodies, or inhibitors

D68.311 Acquired hemophilia HCC
Autoimmune hemophilia
Autoimmune inhibitors to clotting factors
Secondary hemophilia

D68.312 Antiphospholipid antibody with hemorrhagic disorder HCC
Lupus anticoagulant (LAC) with hemorrhagic disorder
Systemic lupus erythematosus [SLE] inhibitor with hemorrhagic disorder

EXCLUDES 1 *antiphospholipid antibody, finding without diagnosis (R76.0)*
antiphospholipid antibody syndrome (D68.61)
antiphospholipid antibody with hypercoagulable state (D68.61)
lupus anticoagulant (LAC) finding without diagnosis (R76.0)
lupus anticoagulant (LAC) with hypercoagulable state (D68.62)
systemic lupus erythematosus [SLE] inhibitor finding without diagnosis (R76.0)
systemic lupus erythematosus [SLE] inhibitor with hypercoagulable state (D68.62)

D68.318 Other hemorrhagic disorder due to intrinsic circulating anticoagulants, antibodies, or inhibitors HCC
Antithromboplastinemia
Antithromboplastinogenemia
Hemorrhagic disorder due to intrinsic increase in antithrombin
Hemorrhagic disorder due to intrinsic increase in anti-VIIIa
Hemorrhagic disorder due to intrinsic increase in anti-IXa
Hemorrhagic disorder due to intrinsic increase in anti-XIa

D68.32 Hemorrhagic disorder due to extrinsic circulating anticoagulants HCC
Drug-induced hemorrhagic disorder
Hemorrhagic disorder due to increase in anti-IIa
Hemorrhagic disorder due to increase in anti-Xa
Hyperheparinemia
Use additional code for adverse effect, if applicable, to identify drug (T45.515, T45.525)
AHA: 1Q 2016, 14

D68.4 Acquired coagulation factor deficiency HCC
Deficiency of coagulation factor due to liver disease
Deficiency of coagulation factor due to vitamin K deficiency

EXCLUDES 1 *vitamin K deficiency of newborn (P53)*

5 D68.5 Primary thrombophilia
Primary hypercoagulable states

EXCLUDES 1 *antiphospholipid syndrome (D68.61)*
lupus anticoagulant (D68.62)
secondary activated protein C resistance (D68.69)
secondary antiphospholipid antibody syndrome (D68.69)
secondary lupus anticoagulant with hypercoagulable state (D68.69)
secondary systemic lupus erythematosus [SLE] inhibitor with hypercoagulable state (D68.69)
systemic lupus erythematosus [SLE] inhibitor finding without diagnosis (R76.0)
systemic lupus erythematosus [SLE] inhibitor with hemorrhagic disorder (D68.312)
thrombotic thrombocytopenic purpura (M31.1)

DEFINITION Abnormal development of blood clots in arteries or veins.

D68.51 Activated protein C resistance HCC
Factor V Leiden mutation

D68.52 Prothrombin gene mutation HCC

D68.59 Other **primary thrombophilia** HCC
Antithrombin III deficiency
Hypercoagulable state NOS
Primary hypercoagulable state NEC
Primary thrombophilia NEC
Protein C deficiency
Protein S deficiency
Thrombophilia NOS

5 **D68.6** **Other** thrombophilia
Other hypercoagulable states
EXCLUDES 1 *diffuse or disseminated intravascular coagulation [DIC] (D65)*
heparin induced thrombocytopenia (HIT) (D75.82)
hyperhomocysteinemia (E72.11)

D68.61 **Antiphospholipid syndrome** HCC
Anticardiolipin syndrome
Antiphospholipid antibody syndrome
EXCLUDES 1 *anti-phospholipid antibody, finding without diagnosis (R76.0)*
anti-phospholipid antibody with hemorrhagic disorder (D68.312)
lupus anticoagulant syndrome (D68.62)

D68.62 **Lupus anticoagulant syndrome** HCC
Lupus anticoagulant
Presence of systemic lupus erythematosus [SLE] inhibitor
EXCLUDES 1 *anticardiolipin syndrome (D68.61)*
antiphospholipid syndrome (D68.61)
lupus anticoagulant (LAC) finding without diagnosis (R76.0)
lupus anticoagulant (LAC) with hemorrhagic disorder (D68.312)

D68.69 **Other thrombophilia** HCC
Hypercoagulable states NEC
Secondary hypercoagulable state NOS

D68.8 **Other** specified **coagulation defects** HCC
EXCLUDES 1 *hemorrhagic disease of newborn (P53)*

D68.9 **Coagulation defect,** unspecified HCC

4 **D69** **Purpura and other hemorrhagic conditions**
EXCLUDES 1 *benign hypergammaglobulinemic purpura (D89.0)*
cryoglobulinemic purpura (D89.1)
essential (hemorrhagic) thrombocythemia (D47.3)
hemorrhagic thrombocythemia (D47.3)
purpura fulminans (D65)
thrombotic thrombocytopenic purpura (M31.1)
Waldenström hypergammaglobulinemic purpura (D89.0)

D69.0 Allergic **purpura** HCC
Allergic vasculitis
Nonthrombocytopenic hemorrhagic purpura
Nonthrombocytopenic idiopathic purpura
Purpura anaphylactoid
Purpura Henoch(-Schönlein)
Purpura rheumatica
Vascular purpura
EXCLUDES 1 *thrombocytopenic hemorrhagic purpura (D69.3)*
DEFINITION Allergic reaction causing hemorrhaging of the skin and mucous membranes; produces purple discolorations on the skin surface.

Allergic purpura

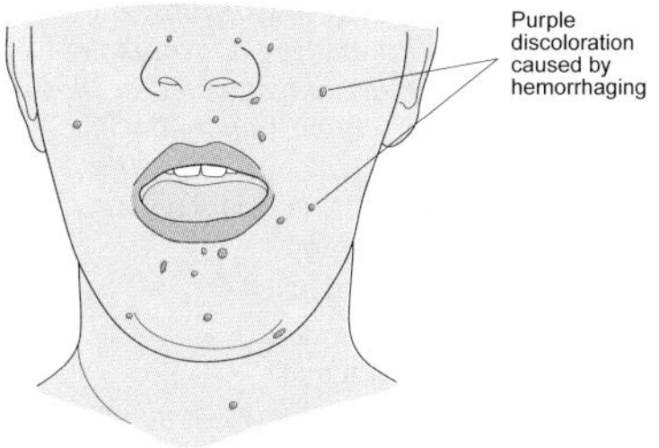

D69.1 **Qualitative platelet defects** HCC
Bernard-Soulier [giant platelet] syndrome
Glanzmann's disease
Grey platelet syndrome
Thromboasthenia (hemorrhagic) (hereditary)
Thrombocytopathy
EXCLUDES 1 *von Willebrand's disease (D68.0)*

D69.2 **Other** nonthrombocytopenic **purpura** HCC
Purpura NOS
Purpura simplex
Senile purpura

D69.3 Immune thrombocytopenic **purpura** HCC
Hemorrhagic (thrombocytopenic) purpura
Idiopathic thrombocytopenic purpura
Tidal platelet dysgenesis

5 **D69.4** **Other** primary thrombocytopenia
EXCLUDES 1 *transient neonatal thrombocytopenia (P61.0)*
Wiskott-Aldrich syndrome (D82.0)

D69.41 **Evans syndrome** HCC

D69.42 Congenital and hereditary **thrombocytopenia purpura** HCC
Congenital thrombocytopenia
Hereditary thrombocytopenia
Code first congential or hereditary disorder, such as:
thrombocytopenia with absent radius (TAR syndrome) (Q87.2)

D69.49 **Other primary thrombocytopenia** HCC
Megakaryocytic hypoplasia
Primary thrombocytopenia NOS

5 **D69.5** **Secondary thrombocytopenia**
EXCLUDES 1 *heparin induced thrombocytopenia (HIT) (D75.82)*
transient thrombocytopenia of newborn (P61.0)
DEFINITION Uncommon but life-threatening adverse reaction in which arterial or venous thrombotic complications develop that can lead to pulmonary embolism, amputation, stroke, or acute myocardial infarction.

D69.51 **Posttransfusion purpura**
Posttransfusion purpura from whole blood (fresh) or blood products
PTP

D69.59 Other **secondary thrombocytopenia**
AHA: 4Q 2014, 22

D69.6 **Thrombocytopenia, unspecified** HCC

D69.8 **Other** specified **hemorrhagic conditions** HCC
Capillary fragility (hereditary)
Vascular pseudohemophilia

D69.9 **Hemorrhagic condition,** unspecified HCC

Other disorders of blood and blood-forming organs (D70-D77)

4 **D70** **Neutropenia**
INCLUDES agranulocytosis
decreased absolute neurophile count (ANC)
Use additional code for any associated:
fever (R50.81)
mucositis (J34.81, K12.3-, K92.81, N76.81)
EXCLUDES 1 *neutropenic splenomegaly (D73.81)*
transient neonatal neutropenia (P61.5)

D70.0 **Congenital agranulocytosis** HCC
Congenital neutropenia
Infantile genetic agranulocytosis
Kostmann's disease

D70.1 **Agranulocytosis secondary to cancer chemotherapy** HCC
Code also:
underlying neoplasm
Use additional code for adverse effect, if applicable, to identify drug (T45.1X5)
AHA: 4Q 2014, 22

D70.2 **Other drug-induced agranulocytosis** HCC
Use additional code for adverse effect, if applicable, to identify drug (T36-T50 with fifth or sixth character 5)

D70.3 **Neutropenia** due to infection HCC

D70.4 **Cyclic neutropenia** HCC
Cyclic hematopoiesis
Periodic neutropenia

D70.8 **Other neutropenia** HCC

D70.9 **Neutropenia, unspecified** HCC

D71 **Functional disorders of polymorphonuclear neutrophils** HCC
Cell membrane receptor complex [CR3] defect
Chronic (childhood) granulomatous disease
Congenital dysphagocytosis
Progressive septic granulomatosis

D72 **Other disorders of white blood cells**
EXCLUDES 1 *basophilia (D72.824)*
immunity disorders (D80-D89)
neutropenia (D70)
preleukemia (syndrome) (D46.9)

D72.0 **Genetic anomalies of leukocytes** HCC
Alder (granulation) (granulocyte) anomaly
Alder syndrome
Hereditary leukocytic hypersegmentation
Hereditary leukocytic hyposegmentation
Hereditary leukomelanopathy
May-Hegglin (granulation) (granulocyte) anomaly
May-Hegglin syndrome
Pelger-Huët (granulation) (granulocyte) anomaly
Pelger-Huët syndrome
EXCLUDES 1 *Chédiak (-Steinbrinck) -Higashi syndrome (E70.330)*

D72.1 **Eosinophilia**
Allergic eosinophilia
Hereditary eosinophilia
EXCLUDES 1 *Löffler's syndrome (J82)*
pulmonary eosinophilia (J82)

D72.8 **Other specified disorders of white blood cells**
EXCLUDES 1 *leukemia (C91-C95)*

D72.81 **Decreased white blood cell count**
EXCLUDES 1 *neutropenia (D70.-)*

D72.810 **Lymphocytopenia**
Decreased lymphocytes

D72.818 **Other decreased white blood cell count**
Basophilic leukopenia
Eosinophilic leukopenia
Monocytopenia
Other decreased leukocytes
Plasmacytopenia

D72.819 **Decreased white blood cell count, unspecified**
Decreased leukocytes, unspecified
Leukocytopenia, unspecified
Leukopenia
EXCLUDES 1 *malignant leukopenia (D70.9)*

D72.82 **Elevated white blood cell count**
EXCLUDES 1 *eosinophilia (D72.1)*

D72.820 **Lymphocytosis (symptomatic)**
Elevated lymphocytes

D72.821 **Monocytosis (symptomatic)**
EXCLUDES 1 *infectious mononucleosis (B27.-)*

D72.822 **Plasmacytosis**

D72.823 **Leukemoid reaction**
Basophilic leukemoid reaction
Leukemoid reaction NOS
Lymphocytic leukemoid reaction
Monocytic leukemoid reaction
Myelocytic leukemoid reaction
Neutrophilic leukemoid reaction

DEFINITION A state of circulating blood presenting a clinical picture resembling or indistinguishable from leukemia due to a condition such as infection, bone marrow compromise, liver failure, and inflammatory disorders.

D72.824 **Basophilia**

DEFINITION Abnormally increased number of basophils in the blood, which release histamine and serotonin upon stimulation.

D72.825 **Bandemia**
Bandemia without diagnosis of specific infection
EXCLUDES 1 *confirmed infection - code to infection*
leukemia (C91.-, C92.-, C93.-, C94.-, C95.-)

DEFINITION Nonspecific elevated count of immature white blood cells when other white blood cell counts are normal.

D72.828 **Other elevated white blood cell count**

D72.829 **Elevated white blood cell count, unspecified**
Elevated leukocytes, unspecified
Leukocytosis, unspecified

D72.89 **Other specified disorders of white blood cells**
Abnormality of white blood cells NEC

D72.9 **Disorder of white blood cells, unspecified**
Abnormal leukocyte differential NOS

D73 **Diseases of spleen**

D73.0 **Hyposplenism**
Atrophy of spleen
EXCLUDES 1 *asplenia (congenital) (Q89.01)*
postsurgical absence of spleen (Z90.81)

D73.1 **Hypersplenism**
EXCLUDES 1 *neutropenic splenomegaly (D73.81)*
primary splenic neutropenia (D73.81)
splenitis, splenomegaly in late syphilis (A52.79)
splenitis, splenomegaly in tuberculosis (A18.85)
splenomegaly NOS (R16.1)
splenomegaly congenital (Q89.0)

D73.2 **Chronic congestive splenomegaly**

D73.3 **Abscess of spleen**

D73.4 **Cyst of spleen**

D73.5 **Infarction of spleen**
Splenic rupture, nontraumatic
Torsion of spleen
EXCLUDES 1 *rupture of spleen due to Plasmodium vivax malaria (B51.0)*
traumatic rupture of spleen (S36.03-)

D73.8 **Other diseases of spleen**

D73.81 **Neutropenic splenomegaly**
Werner-Schultz disease

D73.89 **Other diseases of spleen**
Fibrosis of spleen NOS
Perisplenitis
Splenitis NOS

D73.9 **Disease of spleen, unspecified**

D74 **Methemoglobinemia**

D74.0 **Congenital methemoglobinemia**
Congenital NADH-methemoglobin reductase deficiency
Hemoglobin-M [Hb-M] disease
Methemoglobinemia, hereditary

D74.8 **Other methemoglobinemias**
Acquired methemoglobinemia (with sulfhemoglobinemia)
Toxic methemoglobinemia

D74.9 **Methemoglobinemia, unspecified**

DEFINITION Presence of a higher than normal level of methemoglobin, a form of hemoglobin that does not bind oxygen, in the blood. When its concentration is elevated in red blood cells, anemia and hypoxia may occur.

D75 **Other and unspecified diseases of blood and blood-forming organs**
EXCLUDES 2 *acute lymphadenitis (L04.-)*
chronic lymphadenitis (I88.1)
enlarged lymph nodes (R59.-)
hypergammaglobulinemia NOS (D89.2)
lymphadenitis NOS (I88.9)
mesenteric lymphadenitis (acute) (chronic) (I88.0)

D75.0 **Familial erythrocytosis**
Benign polycythemia
Familial polycythemia
EXCLUDES 1 *hereditary ovalocytosis (D58.1)*

D75.1 Secondary polycythemia
Acquired polycythemia
Emotional polycythemia
Erythrocytosis NOS
Hypoxemic polycythemia
Nephrogenous polycythemia
Polycythemia due to erythropoietin
Polycythemia due to fall in plasma volume
Polycythemia due to high altitude
Polycythemia due to stress
Polycythemia NOS
Relative polycythemia
EXCLUDES 1 *polycythemia neonatorum (P61.1)*
polycythemia vera (D45)

5 D75.8 Other specified diseases of blood and blood-forming organs

D75.81 *Myelofibrosis* HCC
Myelofibrosis NOS
Secondary myelofibrosis NOS
Code first the underlying disorder, such as:
malignant neoplasm of breast (C50.-)
Use additional code, if applicable, for associated therapy-related myelodysplastic syndrome (D46.-)
Use additional code for adverse effect, if applicable, to identify drug (T45.1X5)
EXCLUDES 1 *acute myelofibrosis (C94.4-)*
idiopathic myelofibrosis (D47.1)
leukoerythroblastic anemia (D61.82)
myelofibrosis with myeloid metaplasia (D47.4)
myelophthisic anemia (D61.82)
myelophthisis (D61.82)
primary myelofibrosis (D47.1)

D75.82 Heparin induced thrombocytopenia (HIT) HCC

D75.89 Other specified diseases of blood and blood-forming organs

D75.9 Disease of blood and blood-forming organs, unspecified

4 D76 Other specified diseases with participation of lymphoreticular and reticulohistiocytic tissue
EXCLUDES 1 *(Abt-) Letterer-Siwe disease (C96.0)*
eosinophilic granuloma (C96.6)
Hand-Schüller-Christian disease (C96.5)
histiocytic medullary reticulosis (C96.9)
histiocytic sarcoma (C96.A)
histiocytosis X, multifocal (C96.5)
histiocytosis X, unifocal (C96.6)
Langerhans-cell histiocytosis, multifocal (C96.5)
Langerhans-cell histiocytosis NOS (C96.6)
Langerhans-cell histiocytosis, unifocal (C96.6)
leukemic reticuloendotheliosis (C91.4-)
lipomelanotic reticulosis (I89.8)
malignant histiocytosis (C96.A)
malignant reticulosis (C86.0)
nonlipid reticuloendotheliosis (C96.0)

D76.1 Hemophagocytic lymphohistiocytosis HCC
Familial hemophagocytic reticulosis
Histiocytoses of mononuclear phagocytes

D76.2 Hemophagocytic syndrome, infection-associated HCC
Use additional code to identify infectious agent or disease.

D76.3 Other histiocytosis syndromes HCC
Reticulohistiocytoma (giant-cell)
Sinus histiocytosis with massive lymphadenopathy
Xanthogranuloma

D77 *Other disorders of blood and blood-forming organs in diseases classified elsewhere*
Code first underlying disease, such as:
amyloidosis (E85.-)
congenital early syphilis (A50.0)
echinococcosis (B67.0-B67.9)
malaria (B50.0-B54)
schistosomiasis [bilharziasis] (B65.0-B65.9)
vitamin C deficiency (E54)
EXCLUDES 1 *rupture of spleen due to Plasmodium vivax malaria (B51.0)*
splenitis, splenomegaly in late syphilis (A52.79)
splenitis, splenomegaly in tuberculosis (A18.85)

Intraoperative and postprocedural complications of the spleen (D78)

CODING TIP ✓ Conditions classifiable to D78- are classifiable as intraoperative and postprocedural complications. These conditions should only be assigned when diagnostic statements clearly indicate that the condition is a complication of a procedure.

4 D78 Intraoperative and postprocedural complications of the spleen

5 D78.0 Intraoperative hemorrhage and hematoma of the spleen complicating a procedure
EXCLUDES 1 *intraoperative hemorrhage and hematoma of the spleen due to accidental puncture or laceration during a procedure (D78.1-)*

D78.01 Intraoperative hemorrhage and hematoma of the spleen complicating a procedure on the spleen

D78.02 Intraoperative hemorrhage and hematoma of the spleen complicating other procedure

5 D78.1 Accidental puncture and laceration of the spleen during a procedure

D78.11 Accidental puncture and laceration of the spleen during a procedure on the spleen

D78.12 Accidental puncture and laceration of the spleen during other procedure

5 D78.2 Postprocedural hemorrhage of the spleen following a procedure

D78.21 Postprocedural hemorrhage of the spleen following a procedure on the spleen

D78.22 Postprocedural hemorrhage of the spleen following other procedure

5 D78.3 Postprocedural hematoma and seroma of the spleen following a procedure

D78.31 Postprocedural hematoma of the spleen following a procedure on the spleen

D78.32 Postprocedural hematoma of the spleen following other procedure

D78.33 Postprocedural seroma of the spleen following a procedure on the spleen

D78.34 Postprocedural seroma of the spleen following other procedure

5 D78.8 Other intraoperative and postprocedural complications of the spleen
Use additional code, if applicable, to further specify disorder

D78.81 Other intraoperative complications of the spleen

D78.89 Other postprocedural complications of the spleen

Certain disorders involving the immune mechanism (D80-D89)

INCLUDES defects in the complement system
immunodeficiency disorders, except human immunodeficiency virus [HIV] disease
sarcoidosis

EXCLUDES 1 *autoimmune disease (systemic) NOS (M35.9)*
functional disorders of polymorphonuclear neutrophils (D71)
human immunodeficiency virus [HIV] disease (B20)

4 D80 Immunodeficiency with predominantly antibody defects

D80.0 Hereditary hypogammaglobulinemia HCC
Autosomal recessive agammaglobulinemia (Swiss type)
X-linked agammaglobulinemia [Bruton] (with growth hormone deficiency)

D80.1 Nonfamilial hypogammaglobulinemia HCC
Agammaglobulinemia with immunoglobulin-bearing B-lymphocytes
Common variable agammaglobulinemia [CVAgamma]
Hypogammaglobulinemia NOS
DEFINITION Loss of the body's ability to respond to infection because of a lack of immunoglobulins (antibodies) in the blood.

D80.2 Selective deficiency of immunoglobulin A [IgA] HCC

D80.3 Selective deficiency of immunoglobulin G [IgG] subclasses HCC

D80.4 Selective deficiency of immunoglobulin M [IgM] HCC

D80.5 Immunodeficiency with increased immunoglobulin M [IgM] HCC

D80.6 **Antibody deficiency with near-normal immunoglobulins or with hyperimmunoglobulinemia** HCC

D80.7 **Transient hypogammaglobulinemia of infancy** HCC

D80.8 **Other immunodeficiencies with predominantly antibody defects** HCC
Kappa light chain deficiency

D80.9 **Immunodeficiency with predominantly antibody defects, unspecified** HCC

4 D81 Combined immunodeficiencies

EXCLUDES 1 *autosomal recessive agammaglobulinemia (Swiss type) (D80.0)*

D81.0 **Severe combined immunodeficiency [SCID] with reticular dysgenesis** HCC

D81.1 **Severe combined immunodeficiency [SCID] with low T- and B-cell numbers** HCC

D81.2 **Severe combined immunodeficiency [SCID] with low or normal B-cell numbers** HCC

D81.3 **Adenosine deaminase [ADA] deficiency** HCC

D81.4 **Nezelof's syndrome** HCC

D81.5 **Purine nucleoside phosphorylase [PNP] deficiency** HCC

D81.6 **Major histocompatibility complex class I deficiency** HCC
Bare lymphocyte syndrome

D81.7 **Major histocompatibility complex class II deficiency** HCC

5 **D81.8** **Other combined immunodeficiencies**

6 **D81.81** **Biotin-dependent carboxylase deficiency**
Multiple carboxylase deficiency
EXCLUDES 1 *biotin-dependent carboxylase deficiency due to dietary deficiency of biotin (E53.8)*

D81.810 **Biotinidase deficiency**

D81.818 **Other biotin-dependent carboxylase deficiency**
Holocarboxylase synthetase deficiency
Other multiple carboxylase deficiency

D81.819 **Biotin-dependent carboxylase deficiency, unspecified**
Multiple carboxylase deficiency, unspecified

D81.89 **Other combined immunodeficiencies** HCC

D81.9 **Combined immunodeficiency, unspecified** HCC
Severe combined immunodeficiency disorder [SCID] NOS

4 D82 Immunodeficiency associated with other major defects

EXCLUDES 1 *ataxia telangiectasia [Louis-Bar] (G11.3)*

D82.0 **Wiskott-Aldrich syndrome** HCC
Immunodeficiency with thrombocytopenia and eczema

DEFINITION X-linked immunodeficiency syndrome presenting with eczema, thrombocytopenia, and recurrent pyogenic infection.

D82.1 **Di George's syndrome** HCC
Pharyngeal pouch syndrome
Thymic alymphoplasia
Thymic aplasia or hypoplasia with immunodeficiency

DEFINITION Congenital disorder with hypoplasia or aplasia of the thymus and parathyroid glands; associated with congenital heart defects, great vessel anomalies, esophageal atresia, and abnormal facial structure.

D82.2 **Immunodeficiency with short-limbed stature** HCC

D82.3 **Immunodeficiency following hereditary defective response to Epstein-Barr virus** HCC
X-linked lymphoproliferative disease

D82.4 **Hyperimmunoglobulin E [IgE] syndrome** HCC

CODING TIP✓ Patients with hyperimmunoglobulin E [IgE] syndrome have a lifelong condition characterized by elevated IgE levels, which may also be referred to as "Job syndrome." These patients are highly prone to problematic skin conditions such as eczema, skin lesions and infections (abscesses), sinus infections, and other respiratory infections, which should be additionally coded when present.

D82.8 **Immunodeficiency associated with other specified major defects** HCC

D82.9 **Immunodeficiency associated with major defect, unspecified** HCC

4 D83 Common variable immunodeficiency

D83.0 **Common variable immunodeficiency with predominant abnormalities of B-cell numbers and function** HCC

D83.1 **Common variable immunodeficiency with predominant immunoregulatory T-cell disorders** HCC

D83.2 **Common variable immunodeficiency with autoantibodies to B- or T-cells** HCC

D83.8 **Other common variable immunodeficiencies** HCC

D83.9 **Common variable immunodeficiency, unspecified** HCC

4 D84 Other immunodeficiencies

D84.0 **Lymphocyte function antigen-1 [LFA-1] defect** HCC

D84.1 **Defects in the complement system** HCC
C1 esterase inhibitor [C1-INH] deficiency

D84.8 **Other specified immunodeficiencies** HCC

D84.9 **Immunodeficiency, unspecified** HCC

4 D86 Sarcoidosis

D86.0 **Sarcoidosis of lung** HCC

D86.1 **Sarcoidosis of lymph nodes**

D86.2 **Sarcoidosis of lung with sarcoidosis of lymph nodes** HCC

D86.3 **Sarcoidosis of skin**

5 **D86.8** **Sarcoidosis of other sites**

D86.81 **Sarcoid meningitis**

D86.82 **Multiple cranial nerve palsies in sarcoidosis** HCC

D86.83 **Sarcoid iridocyclitis**

D86.84 **Sarcoid pyelonephritis**
Tubulo-interstitial nephropathy in sarcoidosis

D86.85 **Sarcoid myocarditis**

D86.86 **Sarcoid arthropathy**
Polyarthritis in sarcoidosis

D86.87 **Sarcoid myositis**

D86.89 **Sarcoidosis of other sites**
Hepatic granuloma
Uveoparotid fever [Heerfordt]

D86.9 **Sarcoidosis, unspecified**

4 D89 Other disorders involving the immune mechanism, not elsewhere classified

EXCLUDES 1 *hyperglobulinemia NOS (R77.1)*
monoclonal gammopathy (of undetermined significance) (D47.2)

EXCLUDES 2 *transplant failure and rejection (T86.-)*

D89.0 **Polyclonal hypergammaglobulinemia**
Benign hypergammaglobulinemic purpura
Polyclonal gammopathy NOS

D89.1 **Cryoglobulinemia** HCC
Cryoglobulinemic purpura
Cryoglobulinemic vasculitis
Essential cryoglobulinemia
Idiopathic cryoglobulinemia
Mixed cryoglobulinemia
Primary cryoglobulinemia
Secondary cryoglobulinemia

D89.2 **Hypergammaglobulinemia, unspecified**

D89.3 **Immune reconstitution syndrome** HCC
Immune reconstitution inflammatory syndrome [IRIS]
Use additional code for adverse effect, if applicable, to identify drug (T36-T50 with fifth or sixth character 5)

5 **D89.4** **Mast cell activation syndrome and related disorders**

EXCLUDES 1 *aggressive systemic mastocytosis (C96.21)*
congenital cutaneous mastocytosis (Q82.2)
(non-congenital) cutaneous mastocytosis (D47.01)
(indolent) systemic mastocytosis (D47.02)
malignant mast cell neoplasm (C96.2-)
malignant mastocytoma (C96.29)
mast cell leukemia (C94.3-)
mast cell sarcoma (C96.22)
mastocytoma NOS (D47.09)
other mast cell neoplasms of uncertain behavior (D47.09)
systemic mastocytosis associated with a clonal hematologic non-mast cell lineage disease (SM-AHNMD) (D47.02)

D89.40 **Mast cell activation, unspecified** HCC
Mast cell activation disorder, unspecified
Mast cell activation syndrome, NOS

D89.41 **Monoclonal mast cell activation syndrome** HCC

D89.42 **Idiopathic mast cell activation syndrome** HCC

D89.43 **Secondary mast cell activation** HCC

Secondary mast cell activation syndrome

Code also:

underlying etiology, if known

D89.49 **Other mast cell activation disorder** HCC

Other mast cell activation syndrome

5 **D89.8** **Other specified disorders involving the immune mechanism, not elsewhere classified**

6 **D89.81** **Graft-versus-host disease**

Code first underlying cause, such as:

complications of transplanted organs and tissue (T86.-)

complications of blood transfusion (T80.89)

Use additional code to identify associated manifestations, such as:

desquamative dermatitis (L30.8)

diarrhea (R19.7)

elevated bilirubin (R17)

hair loss (L65.9)

CODING TIP✓ Code D89.81 may only be assigned when the provider specifically indicates this condition. Development of complicating disease, such as ESRD or neoplasm in a transplanted organ, should not be assumed to indicate graft versus host disease.

D89.810 **Acute graft-versus-host disease** HCC

D89.811 **Chronic graft-versus-host disease** HCC

D89.812 **Acute on chronic graft-versus-host disease** HCC

D89.813 **Graft-versus-host disease, unspecified** HCC

D89.82 **Autoimmune lymphoproliferative syndrome [ALPS]** HCC

D89.89 **Other specified disorders involving the immune mechanism, not elsewhere classified** HCC

EXCLUDES 1 *human immunodeficiency virus disease (B20)*

AHA: 4Q 2017, 85

D89.9 **Disorder involving the immune mechanism, unspecified** HCC

Immune disease NOS

AHA: 3Q 2015, 22

CHAPTER 4: ENDOCRINE, NUTRITIONAL AND METABOLIC DISEASES (E00-E89)

Note: All neoplasms, whether functionally active or not, are classified in Chapter 2. Appropriate codes in this chapter (i.e. E05.8, E07.0, E16-E31, E34.-) may be used as additional codes to indicate either functional activity by neoplasms and ectopic endocrine tissue or hyperfunction and hypofunction of endocrine glands associated with neoplasms and other conditions classified elsewhere.

EXCLUDES 1 *transitory endocrine and metabolic disorders specific to newborn (P70-P74)*

This chapter contains the following blocks:

E00-E07	Disorders of thyroid gland
E08-E13	Diabetes mellitus
E15-E16	Other disorders of glucose regulation and pancreatic internal secretion
E20-E35	Disorders of other endocrine glands
E36	Intraoperative complications of endocrine system
E40-E46	Malnutrition
E50-E64	Other nutritional deficiencies
E65-E68	Overweight, obesity and other hyperalimentation
E70-E88	Metabolic disorders
E89	Postprocedural endocrine and metabolic complications and disorders, not elsewhere classified

Disorders of thyroid gland (E00-E07)

E00 Congenital iodine-deficiency syndrome

Use additional code (F70-F79) to identify associated intellectual disabilities.

EXCLUDES 1 *subclinical iodine-deficiency hypothyroidism (E02)*

CODING TIP ✓ Do not assign a code from E00 to identify any condition that is not reported as "congenital" (present from birth).

DEFINITION Congenital iodine-deficiency syndrome is a congenital disorder often referred to as "cretinism." Congenital iodine-deficiency syndrome results from a thyroid hormone deficiency during fetal development and marked in childhood by dwarfed stature, mental retardation, dystrophy of the bones, and a low basal metabolism.

E00.0 Congenital iodine-deficiency syndrome, neurological type

Endemic cretinism, neurological type

DEFINITION Underactive thyroid gland present at birth with inadequate hormone production and slowed metabolic processes. Untreated, it can cause brain damage, mental retardation, and developmental delays.

E00.1 Congenital iodine-deficiency syndrome, myxedematous type

Endemic hypothyroid cretinism

Endemic cretinism, myxedematous type

E00.2 Congenital iodine-deficiency syndrome, mixed type

Endemic cretinism, mixed type

E00.9 Congenital iodine-deficiency syndrome, unspecified

Congenital iodine-deficiency hypothyroidism NOS

Endemic cretinism NOS

E01 Iodine-deficiency related thyroid disorders and allied conditions

EXCLUDES 1 *congenital iodine-deficiency syndrome (E00.-)*
subclinical iodine-deficiency hypothyroidism (E02)

E01.0 Iodine-deficiency related diffuse (endemic) goiter

E01.1 Iodine-deficiency related multinodular (endemic) goiter

Iodine-deficiency related nodular goiter

E01.2 Iodine-deficiency related (endemic) goiter, unspecified

Endemic goiter NOS

E01.8 Other iodine-deficiency related thyroid disorders and allied conditions

Acquired iodine-deficiency hypothyroidism NOS

E02 Subclinical iodine-deficiency hypothyroidism

DEFINITION Early stage of hypothyroidism marked by increased TSH levels and normal free thyroxin T4 levels; occurs when the body requires additional TSH in order to produce enough thyroxin, and developing into overt hypothyroidism in a few years.

E03 Other hypothyroidism

EXCLUDES 1 *iodine-deficiency related hypothyroidism (E00-E02)*
postprocedural hypothyroidism (E89.0)

E03.0 Congenital hypothyroidism with diffuse goiter

Congenital parenchymatous goiter (nontoxic)

Congenital goiter (nontoxic) NOS

EXCLUDES 1 *transitory congenital goiter with normal function (P72.0)*

DEFINITION Abnormal hormone production or blocked TSH receptors in the fetus causing underactive thyroid with diffuse enlargement at birth, tracheal compression, difficulty breathing, and dysphagia.

E03.1 Congenital hypothyroidism without goiter

Aplasia of thyroid (with myxedema)

Congenital atrophy of thyroid

Congenital hypothyroidism NOS

E03.2 Hypothyroidism due to medicaments and other exogenous substances

Code first:
poisoning due to drug or toxin, if applicable (T36-T65 with fifth or sixth character 1-4 or 6)

Use additional code for adverse effect, if applicable, to identify drug (T36-T50 with fifth or sixth character 5)

E03.3 Postinfectious hypothyroidism

DEFINITION Damage to normal thyroid function from a previous infection, resulting in tiredness, weight gain, constipation, cold intolerance, dry skin, slowed mental function, and depression.

E03.4 Atrophy of thyroid (acquired)

EXCLUDES 1 *congenital atrophy of thyroid (E03.1)*

DEFINITION Abnormally small thyroid due to tissue degeneration and wasting; the gland becomes nonviable or severely reduced in function.

E03.5 Myxedema coma HCC

DEFINITION Fully symptomatic hypothyroid disease manifesting with coma in a seriously decompensated state, mostly in the elderly, accompanied by hypothermia, hypoventilation with hypoxia, hypercapnia, hyponatremia, and bradycardia.

E03.8 Other specified hypothyroidism

E03.9 Hypothyroidism, unspecified

Myxedema NOS

DEFINITION Failure of the thyroid gland to produce enough hormone to maintain the body's metabolism, causing fatigue, weight gain, muscle aches and cramps, cold intolerance, memory loss, and depression.

E04 Other nontoxic goiter

EXCLUDES 1 *congenital goiter (NOS) (diffuse) (parenchymatous) (E03.0)*
iodine-deficiency related goiter (E00-E02)

E04.0 Nontoxic diffuse goiter

Diffuse (colloid) nontoxic goiter

Simple nontoxic goiter

DEFINITION Generalized, simple, painless thyroid enlargement without impairment of glandular function due to an overload of thyroid-stimulating hormone (TSH) from the pituitary gland.

E04.1 Nontoxic single thyroid nodule

Colloid nodule (cystic) (thyroid)

Nontoxic uninodular goiter

Thyroid (cystic) nodule NOS

DEFINITION A simple, painless, cyst-like node or singular goiter on the thyroid that is not impairing the normal glandular function.

E04.2 Nontoxic multinodular goiter

Cystic goiter NOS

Multinodular (cystic) goiter NOS

DEFINITION Multiple hard knobs, or cysts, in the thyroid detected by palpation but not impairing function or causing disease.

E04.8 Other specified nontoxic goiter

E04.9 Nontoxic goiter, unspecified

Goiter NOS

Nodular goiter (nontoxic) NOS

4 E05 Thyrotoxicosis [hyperthyroidism]

EXCLUDES 1 *chronic thyroiditis with transient thyrotoxicosis (E06.2)*
neonatal thyrotoxicosis (P72.1)

CODING TIP✓ Thyrotoxicosis is another term for hyperthyroidism, and these terms may frequently be used interchangeably in clinical records. Unspecified hyperthyroidism should be coded to E05.9-.

CODING TIP✓ Codes from category E05 are combination codes that indicate the presence or absence of thyrotoxic crisis or storm. A thyrotoxic crisis (also called "thyroid storm") is a condition that may occur among individuals with hyperthyroidism and is marked by tachycardia, fever, and hypertension, which may or may not result in congestive heart failure and/or shock. Thyrotoxic crisis should only be coded when specified by the physician and cannot be assumed based upon other symptoms alone.

5 E05.0 Thyrotoxicosis with diffuse goiter
Exophthalmic or toxic goiter NOS
Graves' disease
Toxic diffuse goiter

DEFINITION Thyrotropin receptor antibody production that mimics the pituitary's normal regulatory hormone, overriding it and increasing thyroid hormone production, marked by enlarged thyroid and bulging eyes.

E05.00 Thyrotoxicosis with diffuse goiter without thyrotoxic crisis or storm

DEFINITION Hyperthyroid conditions with excessive hormone production and speeding up of body functions; increased heart rate and blood pressure, excessive sweating, hand tremors, nervousness and anxiety, insomnia, and weight loss with increased appetite.

E05.01 Thyrotoxicosis with diffuse goiter with thyrotoxic crisis or storm

DEFINITION Severe, sudden worsening of hyperthyroid conditions from injury, stress, or gland removal that can lead to coma and death, manifesting with tachycardia, arrhythmia, vomiting, high fever, diarrhea, and dehydration.

5 E05.1 Thyrotoxicosis with toxic single thyroid nodule
Thyrotoxicosis with toxic uninodular goiter

E05.10 Thyrotoxicosis with toxic single thyroid nodule without thyrotoxic crisis or storm

E05.11 Thyrotoxicosis with toxic single thyroid nodule with thyrotoxic crisis or storm

5 E05.2 Thyrotoxicosis with toxic multinodular goiter
Toxic nodular goiter NOS

E05.20 Thyrotoxicosis with toxic multinodular goiter without thyrotoxic crisis or storm

E05.21 Thyrotoxicosis with toxic multinodular goiter with thyrotoxic crisis or storm

5 E05.3 Thyrotoxicosis from ectopic thyroid tissue

E05.30 Thyrotoxicosis from ectopic thyroid tissue without thyrotoxic crisis or storm

E05.31 Thyrotoxicosis from ectopic thyroid tissue with thyrotoxic crisis or storm

5 E05.4 Thyrotoxicosis factitia

DEFINITION Thyrotoxicosis factitia is a condition of higher than normal thyroid hormones (T3 and T4) resulting from excess ingestion of thyroid hormone (medication). The condition may be iatrogenic (adverse effect resulting from taking prescription correctly) or due to intentional ingestion of excess medication (poisoning). The cause of the condition should be identified and the coder should follow guidelines for coding of adverse effects and poisoning when assigning a code from E05.4-.

E05.40 Thyrotoxicosis factitia without thyrotoxic crisis or storm

E05.41 Thyrotoxicosis factitia with thyrotoxic crisis or storm

5 E05.8 Other thyrotoxicosis
Overproduction of thyroid-stimulating hormone

E05.80 Other thyrotoxicosis without thyrotoxic crisis or storm

E05.81 Other thyrotoxicosis with thyrotoxic crisis or storm

5 E05.9 Thyrotoxicosis, unspecified
Hyperthyroidism NOS

E05.90 Thyrotoxicosis, unspecified without thyrotoxic crisis or storm

E05.91 Thyrotoxicosis, unspecified with thyrotoxic crisis or storm

4 E06 Thyroiditis

EXCLUDES 1 *postpartum thyroiditis (O90.5)*

CODING TIP✓ Thyroiditis is a condition marked by inflammation of the thyroid (may or may not be infectious in nature), and should not be confused with hyperthyroidism. Various forms of thyroiditis may result in either hyper- or hypothyroidism.

E06.0 Acute thyroiditis
Abscess of thyroid
Pyogenic thyroiditis
Suppurative thyroiditis
Use additional code (B95-B97) to identify infectious agent.

DEFINITION Painful infection of the thyroid gland, often with abscess and pus formation.

Acute thyroiditis

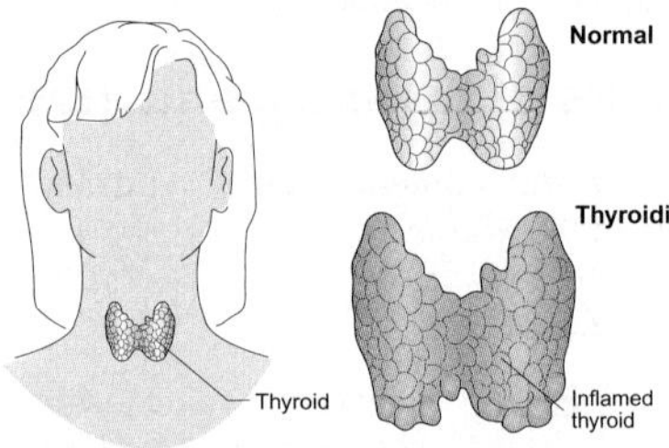

E06.1 Subacute thyroiditis
de Quervain thyroiditis
Giant-cell thyroiditis
Granulomatous thyroiditis
Nonsuppurative thyroiditis
Viral thyroiditis

EXCLUDES 1 *autoimmune thyroiditis (E06.3)*

DEFINITION Thyroid inflammation often resulting from another disease, such as mumps or flu, presenting with fever, radiating neck pain, and hyperthyroidism symptoms than can last months.

E06.2 Chronic thyroiditis with transient thyrotoxicosis

EXCLUDES 1 *autoimmune thyroiditis (E06.3)*

E06.3 Autoimmune thyroiditis
Hashimoto's thyroiditis
Hashitoxicosis (transient)
Lymphadenoid goiter
Lymphocytic thyroiditis
Struma lymphomatosa

DEFINITION Autoimmune inflammation of the thyroid with lymphocyte infiltration that presents with painless thyroid enlargement and hypothyroid symptoms.

E06.4 Drug-induced thyroiditis
Use additional code for adverse effect, if applicable, to identify drug (T36-T50 with fifth or sixth character 5)

CODING TIP✓ Drug-induced thyroiditis should only be coded when clinical record documentation clearly indicates thyroiditis (inflammation of the thyroid), resulting from the administration of a specific drug or chemical. The causative drug or chemical should be identified and the coder should follow guidelines for coding of adverse effects and poisoning when assigning a code from E06.4. If the physician uses the term "hypothyroidism, due to drugs or toxins," see E03.2.

DEFINITION Iatrogenic inflammation of the thyroid due to taking certain medications, such as lithium, or an overdose of iodine.

E06.5 Other chronic **thyroiditis**
Chronic fibrous thyroiditis
Chronic thyroiditis NOS
Ligneous thyroiditis
Riedel thyroiditis

E06.9 **Thyroiditis,** unspecified

DEFINITION Inflammation of the thyroid with noticeable swelling, often on one side, possibly inducing symptoms of hyper- or hypothyroidism, from unspecified causation or acuity.

4 E07 Other **disorders of thyroid**

E07.0 **Hypersecretion of calcitonin**
C-cell hyperplasia of thyroid
Hypersecretion of thyrocalcitonin

E07.1 **Dyshormogenetic goiter**
Familial dyshormogenetic goiter
Pendred's syndrome
EXCLUDES 1 *transitory congenital goiter with normal function (P72.0)*

5 E07.8 **Other** specified **disorders of thyroid**

E07.81 **Sick-euthyroid syndrome**
Euthyroid sick-syndrome
DEFINITION Condition in which thyroid hormone levels are off due to a non-thyroid related problem.

E07.89 **Other specified disorders of thyroid**
Abnormality of thyroid-binding globulin
Hemorrhage of thyroid
Infarction of thyroid

E07.9 **Disorder of thyroid,** unspecified

Diabetes mellitus (E08-E13)

GUIDELINES **Section I.C.4.a.1)-3)**
The diabetes mellitus codes are combination codes that include the type of diabetes mellitus, the body system affected, and the complications affecting that body system. As many codes within a particular category as are necessary to describe all of the complications of the disease may be used. They should be sequenced based on the reason for a particular encounter. Assign as many codes from categories E08 – E13 as needed to identify all of the associated conditions that the patient has.

The age of a patient is not the sole determining factor, though most type 1 diabetics develop the condition before reaching puberty. For this reason type 1 diabetes mellitus is also referred to as juvenile diabetes.

If the type of diabetes mellitus is not documented in the medical record the default is E11.-, Type 2 diabetes mellitus.

If the documentation in a medical record does not indicate the type of diabetes but does indicate that the patient uses insulin, code E11, Type 2 diabetes mellitus, should be assigned. An additional code should be assigned from category Z79 to identify the long-term (current) use of insulin or oral hypoglycemic drugs. If the patient is treated with both oral medications and insulin, only the code for long-term (current) use of insulin should be assigned. Code Z79.4 should not be assigned if insulin is given temporarily to bring a type 2 patient's blood sugar under control during an encounter.

GUIDELINES **Section I.C.4.a.6)**
Codes under categories E08, Diabetes mellitus due to underlying condition, E09, Drug or chemical induced diabetes mellitus, and E13, Other specified diabetes mellitus, identify complications/manifestations associated with secondary diabetes mellitus. Secondary diabetes is always caused by another condition or event (e.g., cystic fibrosis, malignant neoplasm of pancreas, pancreatectomy, adverse effect of drug, or poisoning).

CODING TIP✓ Codes E08-E13 are combination codes that generally do not require a second code to describe the manifestation unless specified by the code specific convention. Specifically, when coding diabetes with an ulcer, diabetic chronic kidney disease, or speciified manifestations that do not belong in a specific subcategory, a second code is required. A second code to identify gastroparesis (K31.84) may be assigned, optionally, when coding diabetic gastroparesis.

CODING TIP✓ Reference the alphabetical index to review conditions that the classification assumes are related to diabetes. All manifestations/complications listed under the word 'with' in the index are presumed related unless the physician specified a different cause in documentation. The 'with' convention does not apply to "not elsewhere classified (NEC)" index entries that cover broad categories of conditions. Coding professionals should not assume a causal relationship when the diabetic complication is "NEC."

CODING TIP✓ When hyperglycemia, poorly controlled, inadequately controlled, or out of control, is documented, diabetes with hyperglycemia should be coded. The clinical record should support the hyperglycemia.

4 E08 **Diabetes mellitus** due to underlying condition
Code first the underlying condition, such as:
congenital rubella (P35.0)
Cushing's syndrome (E24.-)
cystic fibrosis (E84.-)
malignant neoplasm (C00-C96)
malnutrition (E40-E46)
pancreatitis and other diseases of the pancreas (K85-K86.-)
Use additional code to identify control using:
insulin (Z79.4)
oral antidiabetic drugs (Z79.84)
oral hypoglycemic drugs (Z79.84)
EXCLUDES 1 *drug or chemical induced diabetes mellitus (E09.-)*
gestational diabetes (O24.4-)
neonatal diabetes mellitus (P70.2)
postpancreatectomy diabetes mellitus (E13.-)
postprocedural diabetes mellitus (E13.-)
secondary diabetes mellitus NEC (E13.-)
type 1 diabetes mellitus (E10.-)
type 2 diabetes mellitus (E11.-)

GUIDELINES **Section 1.C.4.a.3**
An additional code should be assigned from category Z79 to identify the long-term (current) use of insulin or oral hypoglycemic drugs. If the patient is treated with both oral medications and insulin, only the code for long-term (current) use of insulin should be assigned. Code Z79.4 should not be assigned if insulin is given temporarily to bring a type 2 patient's blood sugar under control during an encounter.

GUIDELINES **Section I.C.4.a.6)(a)**
Secondary diabetes mellitus and the use of insulin or oral hypoglycemic drugs. For patients with secondary diabetes mellitus who routinely use insulin or oral hypoglycemic drugs, an additional code from category Z79 should be assigned to identify the long-term (current) use of insulin or oral hypoglycemic drugs. If the patient is treated with both oral medications and insulin, only the code for long-term (current) use of insulin should be assigned. Code Z79.4 should not be assigned if insulin is given temporarily to bring a type 2 patient's blood sugar under control during an encounter.

GUIDELINES **Section I.C.4.a.6)**
Codes under categories E08, Diabetes mellitus due to underlying condition, E09, Drug or chemical induced diabetes mellitus, and E13, Other specified diabetes mellitus, identify complications/manifestations associated with secondary diabetes mellitus. Secondary diabetes is always caused by another condition or event (e.g., cystic fibrosis, malignant neoplasm of pancreas, pancreatectomy, adverse effect of drug, or poisoning).

CODING TIP✓ If the patient uses an insulin pump, use Z96.41 as an additional code. If there is a complication involving the insulin pump, use a code from T85.6- or T85.7- instead of the Z code.

CODING TIP✓ When coding diabetes mellitus due to an underlying condition, the underlying condition and relationship to diabetes should be specified by the provider. This category does not include unspecified secondary diabetes, postprocedural/postpancreatectomy diabetes, or diabetes due to the effects of drugs or chemicals.

5 E08.0 **Diabetes mellitus due to underlying condition with hyperosmolarity**

E08.00 ***Diabetes mellitus due to underlying condition with hyperosmolarity*** HCC
without nonketotic hyperglycemic-hyperosmolar coma (NKHHC)

E08.01 *Diabetes mellitus due to underlying condition with hyperosmolarity with coma* HCC

E08.1 **Diabetes mellitus due to underlying condition with ketoacidosis**

E08.10 *Diabetes mellitus due to underlying condition with ketoacidosis without coma* HCC

E08.11 *Diabetes mellitus due to underlying condition with ketoacidosis with coma* HCC

E08.2 **Diabetes mellitus due to underlying condition with kidney complications**

CODING TIP✓ Diabetic triopathy refers to the three most common types of manifestations of diabetes--nephropathy, retinopathy and neuropathy.

E08.21 *Diabetes mellitus due to underlying condition with diabetic nephropathy* HCC

Diabetes mellitus due to underlying condition with intercapillary glomerulosclerosis

Diabetes mellitus due to underlying condition with intracapillary glomerulonephrosis

Diabetes mellitus due to underlying condition with Kimmelstiel-Wilson disease

E08.22 *Diabetes mellitus due to underlying condition with diabetic chronic kidney disease* HCC

Use additional code to identify stage of chronic kidney disease (N18.1-N18.6)

CODING TIP✓ When diabetes, CKD and hypertension are documented, sequence the appropriate category of diabetes with CKD (E--.22) and the appropriate hypertension code (I12 or I13) prior to N18. The hypertension or the diabetes may be sequenced first depending on the focus of care. Use N18.1-N18.6 or N18.9 to indicate the CKD. The only time that the conditions should be coded differently is if the physician specifically documents that the conditions are not related.

CODING TIP✓ Assign an additional code from N18- to indicate the stage of CKD. When diabetic nephropathy and CKD are documented, code diabetic CKD, not nephropathy, because CKD is more specific.

E08.29 *Diabetes mellitus due to underlying condition with other diabetic kidney complication* HCC

Renal tubular degeneration in diabetes mellitus due to underlying condition

E08.3 **Diabetes mellitus due to underlying condition with ophthalmic complications**

CODING TIP✓ When coding diabetes with ophthalmic manifestations, review the clinical record and plan of care to ensure that the functional impact of visual impairments is reported.

CODING TIP✓ Diabetic triopathy refers to the three most common types of manifestations of diabetes--nephropathy, retinopathy and neuropathy.

AHA: 4Q 2016, 11

E08.31 **Diabetes mellitus due to underlying condition with unspecified diabetic retinopathy**

E08.311 *Diabetes mellitus due to underlying condition with unspecified diabetic retinopathy with macular edema* HCC

E08.319 *Diabetes mellitus due to underlying condition with unspecified diabetic retinopathy without macular edema* HCC

E08.32 **Diabetes mellitus due to underlying condition with mild nonproliferative diabetic retinopathy**

Diabetes mellitus due to underlying condition with nonproliferative diabetic retinopathy NOS

One of the following 7th characters is to be assigned to codes in subcategory E08.32 to designate laterality of the disease:

1	right eye
2	left eye
3	bilateral
9	unspecified eye

E08.321- **Diabetes mellitus due to underlying condition with mild nonproliferative diabetic retinopathy with macular edema** HCC

E08.329- **Diabetes mellitus due to underlying condition with mild nonproliferative diabetic retinopathy without macular edema** HCC

E08.33 **Diabetes mellitus due to underlying condition with moderate nonproliferative diabetic retinopathy**

One of the following 7th characters is to be assigned to codes in subcategory E08.33 to designate laterality of the disease:

1	right eye
2	left eye
3	bilateral
9	unspecified eye

E08.331- **Diabetes mellitus due to underlying condition with moderate nonproliferative diabetic retinopathy with macular edema** HCC

E08.339- **Diabetes mellitus due to underlying condition with moderate nonproliferative diabetic retinopathy without macular edema** HCC

E08.34 **Diabetes mellitus due to underlying condition with severe nonproliferative diabetic retinopathy**

One of the following 7th characters is to be assigned to codes in subcategory E08.34 to designate laterality of the disease:

1	right eye
2	left eye
3	bilateral
9	unspecified eye

E08.341- **Diabetes mellitus due to underlying condition with severe nonproliferative diabetic retinopathy with macular edema** HCC

E08.349- **Diabetes mellitus due to underlying condition with severe nonproliferative diabetic retinopathy without macular edema** HCC

E08.35 **Diabetes mellitus due to underlying condition with proliferative diabetic retinopathy**

One of the following 7th characters is to be assigned to codes in subcategory E08.35 to designate laterality of the disease:

1	right eye
2	left eye
3	bilateral
9	unspecified eye

E08.351- **Diabetes mellitus due to underlying condition with proliferative diabetic retinopathy with macular edema** HCC

E08.352- **Diabetes mellitus due to underlying condition with proliferative diabetic retinopathy with traction retinal detachment involving the macula** HCC

E08.353- **Diabetes mellitus due to underlying condition with proliferative diabetic retinopathy with traction retinal detachment not involving the macula** HCC

E08.354- **Diabetes mellitus due to underlying condition with proliferative diabetic retinopathy with combined traction retinal detachment and rhegmatogenous retinal detachment** HCC

E08.355- **Diabetes mellitus due to underlying condition with stable proliferative diabetic retinopathy** HCC

E08.359- **Diabetes mellitus due to underlying condition with proliferative diabetic retinopathy without macular edema** HCC

E08.36 ***Diabetes mellitus due to underlying condition with diabetic cataract*** HCC

CODING TIP✓ Cataracts are more common in diabetic patients. The classification assumes a relationship between cataracts and diabetes, when the patient has diabetes, unless the physician specified a different cause.

7 E08.37X- **Diabetes mellitus due to underlying condition with diabetic macular edema, resolved following treatment** HCC

One of the following 7th characters is to be assigned to code E08.37 to designate laterality of the disease:

1	right eye
2	left eye
3	bilateral
9	unspecified eye

CODING TIP✓ The macular edema may be resolved, but the retinopathy remains. This code is like a history code for the macular edema.

E08.39 ***Diabetes mellitus due to underlying condition with other diabetic ophthalmic complication*** HCC

Use additional code to identify manifestation, such as: diabetic glaucoma (H40-H42)

CODING TIP✓ When a diagnosis of diabetes mellitus due to an underlying condition with diabetic glaucoma is reported, assign E08.39. The most common type of diabetic glaucoma is open angle glaucoma coded with H40.1-.

5 E08.4 **Diabetes mellitus due to underlying condition with neurological complications**

CODING TIP✓ When coding diabetes with neurological conditions, whether a causal relationship can be assumed depends on the type of neurological condition. For diagnoses of neuropathy and neuralgia with diabetes, assume a causal relationship (unless the provider states another cause) because they are listed specifically under "with" in the ICD-10-CM index. However, a causal relationship cannot be assumed for NEC diagnoses such as "other stated neurological complication" and a linkage to diabetes must be documented.

E08.40 ***Diabetes mellitus due to underlying condition with diabetic neuropathy, unspecified*** HCC

E08.41 ***Diabetes mellitus due to underlying condition with diabetic mononeuropathy*** HCC

E08.42 ***Diabetes mellitus due to underlying condition with diabetic polyneuropathy*** HCC

Diabetes mellitus due to underlying condition with diabetic neuralgia

E08.43 ***Diabetes mellitus due to underlying condition with diabetic autonomic (poly)neuropathy*** HCC

Diabetes mellitus due to underlying condition with diabetic gastroparesis

AHA: 4Q 2013, 115

E08.44 ***Diabetes mellitus due to underlying condition with diabetic amyotrophy*** HCC

E08.49 ***Diabetes mellitus due to underlying condition with other diabetic neurological complication*** HCC

5 E08.5 **Diabetes mellitus due to underlying condition with circulatory complications**

CODING TIP✓ Peripheral arteriosclerosis, peripheral vascular disease and peripheral arterial disease in a diabetic patient should be linked and coded as "diabetic peripheral angiopathy."

E08.51 ***Diabetes mellitus due to underlying condition with diabetic peripheral angiopathy without gangrene*** HCC

E08.52 ***Diabetes mellitus due to underlying condition with diabetic peripheral angiopathy with gangrene*** HCC

Diabetes mellitus due to underlying condition with diabetic gangrene

E08.59 ***Diabetes mellitus due to underlying condition with other circulatory complications*** HCC

5 E08.6 **Diabetes mellitus due to underlying condition with other specified complications**

6 E08.61 **Diabetes mellitus due to underlying condition with diabetic arthropathy**

E08.610 ***Diabetes mellitus due to underlying condition with diabetic neuropathic arthropathy*** HCC

Diabetes mellitus due to underlying condition with Charcôt's joints

E08.618 ***Diabetes mellitus due to underlying condition with other diabetic arthropathy*** HCC

CODING TIP✓ The "with" causality guideline does not apply to "not elsewhere classified (NEC)" codes such as "other diabetic arthropathy" that cover broad categories of conditions. Instead, the provider must document that a condition such as arthritis is a diabetic complication.

6 E08.62 **Diabetes mellitus due to underlying condition with skin complications**

E08.620 ***Diabetes mellitus due to underlying condition with diabetic dermatitis*** HCC

Diabetes mellitus due to underlying condition with diabetic necrobiosis lipoidica

E08.621 ***Diabetes mellitus due to underlying condition with foot ulcer*** HCC

Use additional code to identify site of ulcer (L97.4-, L97.5-)

E08.622 ***Diabetes mellitus due to underlying condition with other skin ulcer*** HCC

Use additional code to identify site of ulcer (L97.1-L97.9, L98.41-L98.49)

CODING TIP✓ Diabetes codes with 4th, 5th and 6th characters .622 are used when an ulcer is located on the lower extremity, beginning at the ankle, and not including the foot.

E08.628 ***Diabetes mellitus due to underlying condition with other skin complications*** HCC

6 E08.63 **Diabetes mellitus due to underlying condition with oral complications**

E08.630 ***Diabetes mellitus due to underlying condition with periodontal disease*** HCC

E08.638 ***Diabetes mellitus due to underlying condition with other oral complications*** HCC

6 E08.64 **Diabetes mellitus due to underlying condition with hypoglycemia**

E08.641 ***Diabetes mellitus due to underlying condition with hypoglycemia with coma*** HCC

E08.649 ***Diabetes mellitus due to underlying condition with hypoglycemia without coma*** HCC

CODING TIP✓ The physician should be queried when the term "uncontrolled" is used to determine whether the patient has hyperglycemia, hypoglycemia or both.

CODING TIP✓ If encephalopathy is due to hypoglycemia, use G93.41 as an additional code.

CODING TIP✓ When hyperglycemia, poorly controlled, inadequately controlled, or out of control, is documented, diabetes with hyperglycemia should be coded. The clinical record should support the hyperglycemia.

E08.65 ***Diabetes mellitus due to underlying condition with hyperglycemia*** HCC

E08.69 ***Diabetes mellitus due to underlying condition with other specified complication*** HCC

Use additional code to identify complication

CODING TIP ✓ When osteomyelitis is specified as due to diabetes mellitus due to an underlying condition, code first the underlying condition, and assign code E08.69, followed by the appropriate code to specify the type and location of the osteomyelitis. This classification presumes a cause and effect relationship between osteomyelitis and diabetes when no other cause is documented. Use the appropriate code for the osteomyelitis after coding diabetes with other specified manifestations.

E08.8 ***Diabetes mellitus due to underlying condition with unspecified complications*** HCC

E08.9 ***Diabetes mellitus due to underlying condition without complications*** HCC

4 E09 Drug or chemical induced diabetes mellitus

Code first:
poisoning due to drug or toxin, if applicable (T36-T65 with fifth or sixth character 1-4 or 6)
Use additional code for adverse effect, if applicable, to identify drug (T36-T50 with fifth or sixth character 5)
Use additional code to identify control using:
insulin (Z79.4)
oral antidiabetic drugs (Z79.84)
oral hypoglycemic drugs (Z79.84)

EXCLUDES 1 *diabetes mellitus due to underlying condition (E08.-)*
gestational diabetes (O24.4-)
neonatal diabetes mellitus (P70.2)
postpancreatectomy diabetes mellitus (E13.-)
postprocedural diabetes mellitus (E13.-)
secondary diabetes mellitus NEC (E13.-)
type 1 diabetes mellitus (E10.-)
type 2 diabetes mellitus (E11.-)

GUIDELINES **Section 1.C.4.a.3**
An additional code should be assigned from category Z79 to identify the long-term (current) use of insulin or oral hypoglycemic drugs. If the patient is treated with both oral medications and insulin, only the code for long-term (current) use of insulin should be assigned. Code Z79.4 should not be assigned if insulin is given temporarily to bring a type 2 patient's blood sugar under control during an encounter.

GUIDELINES **Section I.C.4.a.6(a)**
Codes under categories E08, Diabetes mellitus due to underlying condition, E09, Drug or chemical induced diabetes mellitus, and E13, Other specified diabetes mellitus, identify complications/manifestations associated with secondary diabetes mellitus. Secondary diabetes is always caused by another condition or event (e.g., cystic fibrosis, malignant neoplasm of pancreas, pancreatectomy, adverse effect of drug, or poisoning).
For patients with secondary diabetes mellitus who routinely use insulin or oral hypoglycemic drugs, an additional code from category Z79 should be assigned to identify the long-term (current) use of insulin or oral hypoglycemic drugs. If the patient is treated with both oral medications and insulin, only the code for long-term (current) use of insulin should be assigned. Code Z79.4 should not be assigned if insulin is given temporarily to bring a secondary diabetic patient's blood sugar under control during an encounter.

GUIDELINES **Section I.C.4.a**
The diabetes mellitus codes are combination codes that include the type of diabetes mellitus, the body system affected, and the complications affecting that body system. As many codes within a particular category as are necessary to describe all of the complications of the disease may be used. They should be sequenced based on the reason for a particular encounter. Assign as many codes from categories E08 – E13 as needed to identify all of the associated conditions that the patient has.

CODING TIP ✓ If the patient uses an insulin pump, use Z96.41 as an additional code. If there is a complication involving the insulin pump, use a code from T85.6- or T85.7- instead of the Z code.

5 E09.0 Drug or chemical induced diabetes mellitus with hyperosmolarity

E09.00 **Drug or chemical induced diabetes mellitus with hyperosmolarity without nonketotic hyperglycemic-hyperosmolar coma (NKHHC)** HCC

E09.01 **Drug or chemical induced diabetes mellitus with hyperosmolarity with coma** HCC

5 E09.1 Drug or chemical induced diabetes mellitus with ketoacidosis

E09.10 **Drug or chemical induced diabetes mellitus with ketoacidosis without coma** HCC

E09.11 **Drug or chemical induced diabetes mellitus with ketoacidosis with coma** HCC

5 E09.2 Drug or chemical induced diabetes mellitus with kidney complications

CODING TIP ✓ Diabetic triopathy refers to the three most common types of manifestations of diabetes--nephropathy, retinopathy and neuropathy.

E09.21 **Drug or chemical induced diabetes mellitus with diabetic nephropathy** HCC
Drug or chemical induced diabetes mellitus with intercapillary glomerulosclerosis
Drug or chemical induced diabetes mellitus with intracapillary glomerulonephrosis
Drug or chemical induced diabetes mellitus with Kimmelstiel-Wilson disease

E09.22 **Drug or chemical induced diabetes mellitus with diabetic chronic kidney disease** HCC
Use additional code to identify stage of chronic kidney disease (N18.1-N18.6)

CODING TIP ✓ When diabetes, CKD and hypertension are documented, sequence the appropriate category of diabetes with CKD (E--.22) and the appropriate hypertension code (I12 or I13) prior to N18. The hypertension or the diabetes may be sequenced first depending on the focus of care. Use N18.1-N18.6 or N18.9 to indicate the CKD. The only time that the conditions should be coded differently is if the physician specifically documents that the conditions are not related.

CODING TIP ✓ Assign an additional code from N18- to indicate the stage of CKD. When diabetic nephropathy and CKD are documented, code diabetic CKD, not nephropathy, because CKD is more specific.

E09.29 **Drug or chemical induced diabetes mellitus with other diabetic kidney complication** HCC
Drug or chemical induced diabetes mellitus with renal tubular degeneration

5 E09.3 Drug or chemical induced diabetes mellitus with ophthalmic complications

CODING TIP ✓ Diabetic triopathy refers to the three most common types of manifestations of diabetes--nephropathy, retinopathy and neuropathy.

CODING TIP ✓ When coding diabetes with ophthalmic manifestations, review the clinical record and plan of care to ensure that the functional impact of visual impairments is reported.
AHA: 4Q 2016, 11

6 E09.31 **Drug or chemical induced diabetes mellitus with unspecified diabetic retinopathy**

E09.311 **Drug or chemical induced diabetes mellitus with unspecified diabetic retinopathy with macular edema** HCC

E09.319 **Drug or chemical induced diabetes mellitus with unspecified diabetic retinopathy without macular edema** HCC

6 E09.32 **Drug or chemical induced diabetes mellitus with mild nonproliferative diabetic retinopathy**
Drug or chemical induced diabetes mellitus with nonproliferative diabetic retinopathy NOS

One of the following 7th characters is to be assigned to codes in subcategory E09.32 to designate laterality of the disease:

1	right eye
2	left eye
3	bilateral
9	unspecified eye

7 ⊟ **E09.321- Drug or chemical induced diabetes mellitus with mild nonproliferative diabetic retinopathy with macular edema** HCC

7 ⊟ **E09.329- Drug or chemical induced diabetes mellitus with mild nonproliferative diabetic retinopathy without macular edema** HCC

6 **E09.33 Drug or chemical induced diabetes mellitus with moderate nonproliferative diabetic retinopathy**

One of the following 7th characters is to be assigned to codes in subcategory E09.33 to designate laterality of the disease:
1 right eye
2 left eye
3 bilateral
9 unspecified eye

7 ⊟ **E09.331- Drug or chemical induced diabetes mellitus with moderate nonproliferative diabetic retinopathy with macular edema** HCC

7 ⊟ **E09.339- Drug or chemical induced diabetes mellitus with moderate nonproliferative diabetic retinopathy without macular edema** HCC

6 **E09.34 Drug or chemical induced diabetes mellitus with severe nonproliferative diabetic retinopathy**

One of the following 7th characters is to be assigned to codes in subcategory E09.34 to designate laterality of the disease:
1 right eye
2 left eye
3 bilateral
9 unspecified eye

7 ⊟ **E09.341- Drug or chemical induced diabetes mellitus with severe nonproliferative diabetic retinopathy with macular edema** HCC

7 ⊟ **E09.349- Drug or chemical induced diabetes mellitus with severe nonproliferative diabetic retinopathy without macular edema** HCC

6 **E09.35 Drug or chemical induced diabetes mellitus with proliferative diabetic retinopathy**

One of the following 7th characters is to be assigned to codes in subcategory E09.35 to designate laterality of the disease:
1 right eye
2 left eye
3 bilateral
9 unspecified eye

7 ⊟ **E09.351- Drug or chemical induced diabetes mellitus with proliferative diabetic retinopathy with macular edema** HCC

7 ⊟ **E09.352- Drug or chemical induced diabetes mellitus with proliferative diabetic retinopathy with traction retinal detachment involving the macula** HCC

7 ⊟ **E09.353- Drug or chemical induced diabetes mellitus with proliferative diabetic retinopathy with traction retinal detachment not involving the macula** HCC

7 ⊟ **E09.354- Drug or chemical induced diabetes mellitus with proliferative diabetic retinopathy with combined traction retinal detachment and rhegmatogenous retinal detachment** HCC

7 ⊟ **E09.355- Drug or chemical induced diabetes mellitus with stable proliferative diabetic retinopathy** HCC

7 ⊟ **E09.359- Drug or chemical induced diabetes mellitus with proliferative diabetic retinopathy without macular edema** HCC

E09.36 Drug or chemical induced diabetes mellitus with diabetic cataract HCC

CODING TIP ✓ Cataracts are more common in diabetic patients. The classification assumes a relationship between cataracts and diabetes, when the patient has diabetes, unless the physician specified a different cause.

7 ⊟ **E09.37X- Drug or chemical induced diabetes mellitus with diabetic macular edema, resolved following treatment** HCC

One of the following 7th characters is to be assigned to code E09.37 to designate laterality of the disease:
1 right eye
2 left eye
3 bilateral
9 unspecified eye

CODING TIP ✓ The macular edema may be resolved, but the retinopathy remains. This code is like a history code for the macular edema.

E09.39 Drug or chemical induced diabetes mellitus with other diabetic ophthalmic complication HCC

Use additional code to identify manifestation, such as: diabetic glaucoma (H40-H42)

CODING TIP ✓ When a diagnosis of drug or chemical induced diabetes mellitus with diabetic glaucoma is reported, assign E09.39. The most common type of diabetic glaucoma is open angle glaucoma coded with H40.1-.

5 **E09.4 Drug or chemical induced diabetes mellitus with neurological complications**

CODING TIP ✓ When coding diabetes with neurological conditions, whether a causal relationship can be assumed depends on the type of neurological condition. For diagnoses of neuropathy and neuralgia with diabetes, assume a causal relationship (unless the provider states another cause) because they are listed specifically under "with" in the ICD-10-CM index. However, a causal relationship cannot be assumed for NEC diagnoses such as "other stated neurological complication" and a linkage to diabetes must be documented.

E09.40 Drug or chemical induced diabetes mellitus with neurological complications with diabetic neuropathy, unspecified HCC

E09.41 Drug or chemical induced diabetes mellitus with neurological complications with diabetic mononeuropathy HCC

E09.42 Drug or chemical induced diabetes mellitus with neurological complications with diabetic polyneuropathy HCC

Drug or chemical induced diabetes mellitus with diabetic neuralgia

E09.43 Drug or chemical induced diabetes mellitus with neurological complications with diabetic autonomic (poly)neuropathy HCC

Drug or chemical induced diabetes mellitus with diabetic gastroparesis

AHA: 4Q 2013, 115

E09.44 Drug or chemical induced diabetes mellitus with neurological complications with diabetic amyotrophy HCC

E09.49 Drug or chemical induced diabetes mellitus with neurological complications with other diabetic neurological complication HCC

5 **E09.5 Drug or chemical induced diabetes mellitus with circulatory complications**

CODING TIP ✓ Peripheral arteriosclerosis, peripheral vascular disease and peripheral arterial disease in a diabetic patient should be linked and coded as "diabetic peripheral angiopathy."

E09.51 Drug or chemical induced diabetes mellitus with diabetic peripheral angiopathy without gangrene HCC

E09.52 Drug or chemical induced diabetes mellitus with diabetic peripheral angiopathy with gangrene HCC

Drug or chemical induced diabetes mellitus with diabetic gangrene

E09.59 **Drug or chemical induced diabetes mellitus with other circulatory complications** HCC

5 **E09.6** **Drug or chemical induced diabetes mellitus with other specified complications**

6 **E09.61** **Drug or chemical induced diabetes mellitus with diabetic arthropathy**

E09.610 **Drug or chemical induced diabetes mellitus with diabetic neuropathic arthropathy** HCC
Drug or chemical induced diabetes mellitus with Charcôt's joints

E09.618 **Drug or chemical induced diabetes mellitus with other diabetic arthropathy** HCC

CODING TIP ✓ The "with" causality guideline does not apply to "not elsewhere classified (NEC)" codes such as "other diabetic arthropathy" that cover broad categories of conditions. Instead, the provider must document that a condition such as arthritis is a diabetic complication.

6 **E09.62** **Drug or chemical induced diabetes mellitus with skin complications**

E09.620 **Drug or chemical induced diabetes mellitus with diabetic dermatitis** HCC
Drug or chemical induced diabetes mellitus with diabetic necrobiosis lipoidica

E09.621 **Drug or chemical induced diabetes mellitus with foot ulcer** HCC
Use additional code to identify site of ulcer (L97.4-, L97.5-)

E09.622 **Drug or chemical induced diabetes mellitus with other skin ulcer** HCC
Use additional code to identify site of ulcer (L97.1-L97.9, L98.41-L98.49)

CODING TIP ✓ Diabetes codes with 4th, 5th and 6th characters .622 are used when an ulcer is located on the lower extremity, beginning at the ankle, and not including the foot.

E09.628 **Drug or chemical induced diabetes mellitus with other skin complications** HCC

6 **E09.63** **Drug or chemical induced diabetes mellitus with oral complications**

E09.630 **Drug or chemical induced diabetes mellitus with periodontal disease** HCC

E09.638 **Drug or chemical induced diabetes mellitus with other oral complications** HCC

6 **E09.64** **Drug or chemical induced diabetes mellitus with hypoglycemia**

E09.641 **Drug or chemical induced diabetes mellitus with hypoglycemia with coma** HCC

E09.649 **Drug or chemical induced diabetes mellitus with hypoglycemia without coma** HCC

CODING TIP ✓ The physician should be queried when the term "uncontrolled" is used to determine whether the patient has hyperglycemia, hypoglycemia or both.

CODING TIP ✓ If encephalopathy is due to hypoglycemia, use G93.41 as an additional code.

CODING TIP ✓ When hyperglycemia, poorly controlled, inadequately controlled, or out of control, is documented, diabetes with hyperglycemia should be coded. The clinical record should support the hyperglycemia.

E09.65 **Drug or chemical induced diabetes mellitus with hyperglycemia** HCC

E09.69 **Drug or chemical induced diabetes mellitus with other specified complication** HCC
Use additional code to identify complication

CODING TIP ✓ When osteomyelitis is specified as due to drug or chemical-induced diabetes mellitus, code first any applicable poisoning by the toxin and assign code E09.69, or assign code E09.69 followed by the appropriate code to identify an adverse effect by the drug, and then assign the appropriate code to specify the type and location of the osteomyelitis. This classification presumes a cause and effect relationship between osteomyelitis and diabetes, when no other cause is documented. Use the appropriate code for the osteomyelitis after coding diabetes with other specified manifestations.

E09.8 **Drug or chemical induced diabetes mellitus with unspecified complications** HCC

E09.9 **Drug or chemical induced diabetes mellitus without complications** HCC

4 **E10** **Type 1 diabetes mellitus**

INCLUDES brittle diabetes (mellitus)
diabetes (mellitus) due to autoimmune process
diabetes (mellitus) due to immune mediated pancreatic islet beta-cell destruction
idiopathic diabetes (mellitus)
juvenile onset diabetes (mellitus)
ketosis-prone diabetes (mellitus)

EXCLUDES 1 *diabetes mellitus due to underlying condition (E08.-)*
drug or chemical induced diabetes mellitus (E09.-)
gestational diabetes (O24.4-)
hyperglycemia NOS (R73.9)
neonatal diabetes mellitus (P70.2)
postpancreatectomy diabetes mellitus (E13.-)
postprocedural diabetes mellitus (E13.-)
secondary diabetes mellitus NEC (E13.-)
type 2 diabetes mellitus (E11.-)

GUIDELINES **Section I.C.4.a.1)**
The age of a patient is not the sole determining factor, though most type 1 diabetics develop the condition before reaching puberty. For this reason type 1 diabetes mellitus is also referred to as juvenile diabetes.

CODING TIP ✓ If the patient uses an insulin pump, use Z96.41 as an additional code. If there is a complication involving the insulin pump, use a code from T85.6- or T85.7- instead of the Z code.

5 **E10.1** **Type 1 diabetes mellitus with ketoacidosis**

DEFINITION Diabetic complication characterized by hyperglycemia, hyperketonemia, and metabolic acidosis; often presents with nausea, vomiting, and abdominal pain; may progress to cerebral edema or lead to coma and/or death.

E10.10 **Type 1 diabetes mellitus with ketoacidosis without coma** HCC
AHA: 3Q 2013, 20

E10.11 **Type 1 diabetes mellitus with ketoacidosis with coma** HCC

5 **E10.2** **Type 1 diabetes mellitus with kidney complications**

E10.21 **Type 1 diabetes mellitus with diabetic nephropathy** HCC
Type 1 diabetes mellitus with intercapillary glomerulosclerosis
Type 1 diabetes mellitus with intracapillary glomerulonephrosis
Type 1 diabetes mellitus with Kimmelstiel-Wilson disease

E10.22 **Type 1 diabetes mellitus with diabetic chronic kidney disease** HCC
Use additional code to identify stage of chronic kidney disease (N18.1-N18.6)

CODING TIP When diabetes, CKD and hypertension are documented, sequence the appropriate category of diabetes with CKD (E--.22) and the appropriate hypertension code (I12 or I13) prior to N18. The hypertension or the diabetes may be sequenced first depending on the focus of care. Use N18.1-N18.6 or N18.9 to indicate the CKD. The only time that the conditions should be coded differently is if the physician specifically documents that the conditions are not related.

CODING TIP Assign an additional code from N18- to indicate the stage of CKD. When diabetic nephropathy and CKD are documented, code diabetic CKD, not nephropathy, because CKD is more specific.

E10.29 **Type 1 diabetes mellitus with other diabetic kidney complication** HCC
Type 1 diabetes mellitus with renal tubular degeneration
AHA: 1Q 2016, 13

5 **E10.3** **Type 1 diabetes mellitus with ophthalmic complications**

CODING TIP When coding diabetes with ophthalmic manifestations, review the clinical record and plan of care to ensure that the functional impact of visual impairments is reported.

CODING TIP Diabetic triopathy refers to the most common types of manifestations of diabetes--nephropathy, retinopathy and neuropathy.
AHA: 4Q 2016, 11

6 **E10.31** **Type 1 diabetes mellitus with unspecified diabetic retinopathy**

E10.311 **Type 1 diabetes mellitus with unspecified diabetic retinopathy with macular edema** HCC

E10.319 **Type 1 diabetes mellitus with unspecified diabetic retinopathy without macular edema** HCC

6 **E10.32** **Type 1 diabetes mellitus with mild nonproliferative diabetic retinopathy**
Type 1 diabetes mellitus with nonproliferative diabetic retinopathy NOS

One of the following 7th characters is to be assigned to codes in subcategory E10.32 to designate laterality of the disease:
1 right eye
2 left eye
3 bilateral
9 unspecified eye

7 ⊟ **E10.321-** **Type 1 diabetes mellitus with mild nonproliferative diabetic retinopathy with macular edema** HCC

7 ⊟ **E10.329-** **Type 1 diabetes mellitus with mild nonproliferative diabetic retinopathy without macular edema** HCC

6 **E10.33** **Type 1 diabetes mellitus with moderate nonproliferative diabetic retinopathy**

One of the following 7th characters is to be assigned to codes in subcategory E10.33 to designate laterality of the disease:
1 right eye
2 left eye
3 bilateral
9 unspecified eye

7 ⊟ **E10.331-** **Type 1 diabetes mellitus with moderate nonproliferative diabetic retinopathy with macular edema** HCC

7 ⊟ **E10.339-** **Type 1 diabetes mellitus with moderate nonproliferative diabetic retinopathy without macular edema** HCC

6 **E10.34** **Type 1 diabetes mellitus with severe nonproliferativediabetic retinopathy**

One of the following 7th characters is to be assigned to codes in subcategory E10.34 to designate laterality of the disease:
1 right eye
2 left eye
3 bilateral
9 unspecified eye

7 ⊟ **E10.341-** **Type 1 diabetes mellitus with severe nonproliferative diabetic retinopathy with macular edema** HCC

7 ⊟ **E10.349-** **Type 1 diabetes mellitus with severe nonproliferative diabetic retinopathy without macular edema** HCC

6 **E10.35** **Type 1 diabetes mellitus with proliferative diabetic retinopathy**

One of the following 7th characters is to be assigned to codes in subcategory E10.35 to designate laterality of the disease:
1 right eye
2 left eye
3 bilateral
9 unspecified eye

7 ⊟ **E10.351-** **Type 1 diabetes mellitus with proliferative diabetic retinopathy with macular edema** HCC

7 ⊟ **E10.352-** **Type 1 diabetes mellitus with proliferative diabetic retinopathy with traction retinal detachment involving the macula** HCC

7 ⊟ **E10.353-** **Type 1 diabetes mellitus with proliferative diabetic retinopathy with traction retinal detachment not involving the macula** HCC

7 ⊟ **E10.354-** **Type 1 diabetes mellitus with proliferative diabetic retinopathy with combined traction retinal detachment and rhegmatogenous retinal detachment** HCC

7 ⊟ **E10.355-** **Type 1 diabetes mellitus with stable proliferative diabetic retinopathy** HCC

7 ⊟ **E10.359-** **Type 1 diabetes mellitus with proliferative diabetic retinopathy without macular edema** HCC

E10.36 **Type 1 diabetes mellitus with diabetic cataract** HCC

CODING TIP Cataracts are more common in diabetic patients. The classification assumes a relationship between cataracts and diabetes, when the patient has diabetes, unless the physician specified a different cause.

7 ⊟ **E10.37X-** **Type 1 diabetes mellitus with diabetic macular edema, resolved following treatment** HCC

One of the following 7th characters is to be assigned to code E10.37 to designate laterality of the disease:
1 right eye
2 left eye
3 bilateral
9 unspecified eye

CODING TIP The macular edema may be resolved, but the retinopathy remains. This code is like a history code for the macular edema.

E10.39 **Type 1 diabetes mellitus with other diabetic ophthalmic complication** HCC
Use additional code to identify manifestation, such as: diabetic glaucoma (H40-H42)

CODING TIP When a diagnosis of Type 1 diabetes mellitus with diabetic glaucoma is reported, assign E10.39. The most common type is open angle glaucoma coded with H40.1-.

5 **E10.4** **Type 1 diabetes mellitus with neurological complications**

CODING TIP✓ When coding diabetes with neurological conditions, whether a causal relationship can be assumed depends on the type of neurological condition. For diagnoses of neuropathy and neuralgia with diabetes, assume a causal relationship (unless the provider states another cause) because they are listed specifically under "with" in the ICD-10-CM index. However, a causal relationship cannot be assumed for NEC diagnoses such as "other stated neurological complication" and a linkage to diabetes must be documented.

CODING TIP✓ Use E10.4- or E11.4- for diabetic neurological complications. Amyotrophy is a neurogenic muscle weakness that begins in the sacrum and hips. Polyneuropathy is known as stocking-glove numbness to describe numbness/tingling in hands, feet and ankles. Peripheral autonomic neuropathy is neuropathy of the peripheral autonomic nervous system and affects everyday body functions such as blood pressure, heart rate, bowel and bladder emptying, digestion and other involuntary responses. It may be responsible for the orthostatic hypotension in the diabetic. Neurogenic arthropathy is also known as Charcot arthropathy or rocker foot.

E10.40 **Type 1 diabetes mellitus with diabetic neuropathy, unspecified** HCC

E10.41 **Type 1 diabetes mellitus with diabetic mononeuropathy** HCC

E10.42 **Type 1 diabetes mellitus with diabetic polyneuropathy** HCC
Type 1 diabetes mellitus with diabetic neuralgia

E10.43 **Type 1 diabetes mellitus with diabetic autonomic (poly)neuropathy** HCC
Type 1 diabetes mellitus with diabetic gastroparesis
AHA: 4Q 2013, 115

E10.44 **Type 1 diabetes mellitus with diabetic amyotrophy** HCC

E10.49 **Type 1 diabetes mellitus with other diabetic neurological complication** HCC

5 **E10.5** **Type 1 diabetes mellitus with circulatory complications**

CODING TIP✓ Peripheral arteriosclerosis, peripheral vascular disease and peripheral arterial disease in a diabetic patient should be linked and coded as "diabetic peripheral angiopathy."

E10.51 **Type 1 diabetes mellitus with diabetic peripheral angiopathy without gangrene** HCC

E10.52 **Type 1 diabetes mellitus with diabetic peripheral angiopathy with gangrene** HCC
Type 1 diabetes mellitus with diabetic gangrene

E10.59 **Type 1 diabetes mellitus with other circulatory complications** HCC

5 **E10.6** **Type 1 diabetes mellitus with other specified complications**

6 **E10.61** **Type 1 diabetes mellitus with diabetic arthropathy**

E10.610 **Type 1 diabetes mellitus with diabetic neuropathic arthropathy** HCC
Type 1 diabetes mellitus with Charcôt's joints

E10.618 **Type 1 diabetes mellitus with other diabetic arthropathy** HCC

CODING TIP✓ The "with" causality guideline does not apply to "not elsewhere classified (NEC)" codes such as "other diabetic arthropathy" that cover broad categories of conditions. Instead, the provider must document that a condition such as arthritis is a diabetic complication.

6 **E10.62** **Type 1 diabetes mellitus with skin complications**

E10.620 **Type 1 diabetes mellitus with diabetic dermatitis** HCC
Type 1 diabetes mellitus with diabetic necrobiosis lipoidica

E10.621 **Type 1 diabetes mellitus with foot ulcer** HCC
Use additional code to identify site of ulcer (L97.4-, L97.5-)

E10.622 **Type 1 diabetes mellitus with other skin ulcer** HCC
Use additional code to identify site of ulcer (L97.1-L97.9, L98.41-L98.49)

CODING TIP✓ Diabetes codes with 4th, 5th and 6th characters .622 are used when an ulcer is located on the lower extremity, beginning at the ankle, and not including the foot.

E10.628 **Type 1 diabetes mellitus with other skin complications** HCC

6 **E10.63** **Type 1 diabetes mellitus with oral complications**

E10.630 **Type 1 diabetes mellitus with periodontal disease** HCC

E10.638 **Type 1 diabetes mellitus with other oral complications** HCC

6 **E10.64** **Type 1 diabetes mellitus with hypoglycemia**

E10.641 **Type 1 diabetes mellitus with hypoglycemia with coma** HCC

E10.649 **Type 1 diabetes mellitus with hypoglycemia without coma** HCC

CODING TIP✓ The physician should be queried when the term "uncontrolled" is used to determine whether the patient has hyperglycemia, hypoglycemia or both.

CODING TIP✓ If encephalopathy is due to hypoglycemia, use G93.41 as an additional code.
AHA: 1Q 2016, 13

E10.65 **Type 1 diabetes mellitus with hyperglycemia** HCC

CODING TIP✓ When hyperglycemia, poorly controlled, inadequately controlled, or out of control, is documented, diabetes with hyperglycemia should be coded. The clinical record should support the hyperglycemia.

E10.69 **Type 1 diabetes mellitus with other specified complication** HCC
Use additional code to identify complication

CODING TIP✓ When osteomyelitis is specified as due to type 1 diabetes mellitus, assign code E10.69, followed by the appropriate code to specify the type and location of the osteomyelitis. This classification presumes a cause and effect relationship between osteomyelitis and diabetes, when no other cause is documented. Use the appropriate code for the osteomyelitis after coding diabetes with other specified manifestations.

E10.8 **Type 1 diabetes mellitus with unspecified complications** HCC

E10.9 **Type 1 diabetes mellitus without complications** HCC

CODING TIP✓ Report code E10.9 when documentation does not mention a complication or when manifestations cannot be confirmed with the physician. Do not use this code with any other codes from category E10 or with a manifestation. At times when a manifestation is suspected but cannot be confirmed, E10.9 may be coded to indicate no causal relationship between diabetes and the possible manifestation.

4 **E11** **Type 2 diabetes mellitus**

INCLUDES diabetes (mellitus) due to insulin secretory defect
diabetes NOS
insulin resistant diabetes (mellitus)

Use additional code to identify control using:
insulin (Z79.4)
oral antidiabetic drugs (Z79.84)
oral hypoglycemic drugs (Z79.84)

EXCLUDES 1 *diabetes mellitus due to underlying condition (E08.-)*
drug or chemical induced diabetes mellitus (E09.-)
gestational diabetes (O24.4-)
neonatal diabetes mellitus (P70.2)
postpancreatectomy diabetes mellitus (E13.-)
postprocedural diabetes mellitus (E13.-)
secondary diabetes mellitus NEC (E13.-)
type 1 diabetes mellitus (E10.-)

GUIDELINES **Section 1.C.4.a.3**
An additional code should be assigned from category Z79 to identify the long-term (current) use of insulin or oral hypoglycemic drugs. If the patient is treated with both oral medications and insulin, only the code for long-term (current) use of insulin should be assigned. Code Z79.4 should not be assigned if insulin is given temporarily to bring a type 2 patient's blood sugar under control during an encounter.

GUIDELINES **Section I.C.4.a.2)-3)**
If the type of diabetes mellitus is not documented in the medical record the default is E11.-, Type 2 diabetes mellitus. If the documentation in a medical record does not indicate the type of diabetes but does indicate that the patient uses insulin, code E11, Type 2 diabetes mellitus, should be assigned.
An additional code should be assigned from category Z79 to identify the long-term (current) use of insulin or oral hypoglycemic drugs. If the patient is treated with both oral medications and insulin, only the code for long-term (current) use of insulin should be assigned. Code Z79.4 should not be assigned if insulin is given temporarily to bring a type 2 patient's blood sugar under control during an encounter.

CODING TIP✓ If the patient uses an insulin pump, use Z96.41 as an additional code. If there is a complication involving the insulin pump, use a code from T85.6- or T85.7- instead of the Z code.

5 **E11.0 Type 2 diabetes mellitus with hyperosmolarity**

DEFINITION Metabolic diabetic emergency presenting with altered consciousness varying from confusion or disorientation to coma, with extreme dehydration, and high blood concentrations of sugar and sodium.

E11.00 Type 2 diabetes mellitus with hyperosmolarity without nonketotic hyperglycemic-hyperosmolar coma (NKHHC) HCC

E11.01 Type 2 diabetes mellitus with hyperosmolarity with coma HCC

5 **E11.1 Type 2 diabetes mellitus with ketoacidosis**

E11.10 Type 2 diabetes mellitus with ketoacidosis without coma HCC
AHA: 4Q 2017, 5

E11.11 Type 2 diabetes mellitus with ketoacidosis with coma HCC
AHA: 4Q 2017, 5

5 **E11.2 Type 2 diabetes mellitus with kidney complications**

CODING TIP✓ Diabetic triopathy refers to the most common types of manifestations of diabetes--nephropathy, retinopathy and neuropathy.

E11.21 Type 2 diabetes mellitus with diabetic nephropathy HCC
Type 2 diabetes mellitus with intercapillary glomerulosclerosis
Type 2 diabetes mellitus with intracapillary glomerulonephrosis
Type 2 diabetes mellitus with Kimmelstiel-Wilson disease

E11.22 Type 2 diabetes mellitus with diabetic chronic kidney disease HCC
Use additional code to identify stage of chronic kidney disease (N18.1-N18.6)

CODING TIP✓ When diabetes, CKD and hypertension are documented, sequence the appropriate category of diabetes with CKD (E--.22) and the appropriate hypertension code (I12 or I13) prior to N18. The hypertension or the diabetes may be sequenced first depending on the focus of care. Use N18.1-N18.6 or N18.9 to indicate the CKD. The only time that the conditions should be coded differently is if the physician specifically documents that the conditions are not related.

CODING TIP✓ Assign an additional code from N18- to indicate the stage of CKD. When diabetic nephropathy and CKD are documented, code diabetic CKD, not nephropathy, because CKD is more specific.
AHA: 1Q 2016, 12-13
AHA: 2Q 2016, 36

E11.29 Type 2 diabetes mellitus with other diabetic kidney complication HCC
Type 2 diabetes mellitus with renal tubular degeneration

5 **E11.3 Type 2 diabetes mellitus with ophthalmic complications**

CODING TIP✓ When coding diabetes with ophthalmic manifestations, review the clinical record and plan of care to ensure that the functional impact of visual impairments is reported.

CODING TIP✓ Diabetic triopathy refers to the most common types of manifestations of diabetes--nephropathy, retinopathy and neuropathy.
AHA: 4Q 2016, 11

6 **E11.31 Type 2 diabetes mellitus with unspecified diabetic retinopathy**

E11.311 Type 2 diabetes mellitus with unspecified diabetic retinopathy with macular edema HCC

E11.319 Type 2 diabetes mellitus with unspecified diabetic retinopathy without macular edema HCC
AHA: 3Q 2013, 20

6 **E11.32 Type 2 diabetes mellitus with mild nonproliferative diabetic retinopathy**
Type 2 diabetes mellitus with nonproliferative diabetic retinopathy NOS

One of the following 7th characters is to be assigned to codes in subcategory E11.32 to designate laterality of the disease:

1	right eye
2	left eye
3	bilateral
9	unspecified eye

7 ⊟ **E11.321- Type 2 diabetes mellitus with mild nonproliferative diabetic retinopathy with macular edema** HCC

7 ⊟ **E11.329- Type 2 diabetes mellitus with mild nonproliferative diabetic retinopathy without macular edema** HCC

6 **E11.33 Type 2 diabetes mellitus with moderate nonproliferative diabetic retinopathy**

One of the following 7th characters is to be assigned to codes in subcategory E11.33 to designate laterality of the disease:

1	right eye
2	left eye
3	bilateral
9	unspecified eye

7 ⊟ **E11.331- Type 2 diabetes mellitus with moderate nonproliferative diabetic retinopathy with macular edema** HCC

7 ⊟ **E11.339- Type 2 diabetes mellitus with moderate nonproliferative diabetic retinopathy without macular edema** HCC

6 **E11.34 Type 2 diabetes mellitus with severe nonproliferative diabetic retinopathy**

One of the following 7th characters is to be assigned to codes in subcategory E11.34 to designate laterality of the disease:

1	right eye
2	left eye
3	bilateral
9	unspecified eye

7 ⊟ **E11.341- Type 2 diabetes mellitus with severe nonproliferative diabetic retinopathy with macular edema** HCC

7 ⊟ **E11.349- Type 2 diabetes mellitus with severe nonproliferative diabetic retinopathy without macular edema** HCC

6 **E11.35** **Type 2 diabetes mellitus with proliferative diabetic retinopathy**

One of the following 7th characters is to be assigned to codes in subcategory E11.35 to designate laterality of the disease:
1 right eye
2 left eye
3 bilateral
9 unspecified eye

7 **E11.351-** **Type 2 diabetes mellitus with proliferative diabetic retinopathy with macular edema** HCC

7 **E11.352-** **Type 2 diabetes mellitus with proliferative diabetic retinopathy with traction retinal detachment involving the macula** HCC

7 **E11.353-** **Type 2 diabetes mellitus with proliferative diabetic retinopathy with traction retinal detachment not involving the macula** HCC

7 **E11.354-** **Type 2 diabetes mellitus with proliferative diabetic retinopathy with combined traction retinal detachment and rhegmatogenous retinal detachment** HCC

7 **E11.355-** **Type 2 diabetes mellitus with stable proliferative diabetic retinopathy** HCC

7 **E11.359-** **Type 2 diabetes mellitus with proliferative diabetic retinopathy without macular edema** HCC

E11.36 **Type 2 diabetes mellitus with diabetic cataract** HCC

CODING TIP✓ Cataracts are more common in diabetic patients. The classification assumes a relationship between cataracts and diabetes, when the patient has diabetes, unless the physician specified a different cause.

AHA: 2Q 2016, 36

7 **E11.37X-** **Type 2 diabetes mellitus with diabetic macular edema, resolved following treatment** HCC

One of the following 7th characters is to be assigned to code E11.37 to designate laterality of the disease:
1 right eye
2 left eye
3 bilateral
9 unspecified eye

CODING TIP✓ The macular edema may be resolved, but the retinopathy remains. This code is like a history code for the macular edema.

E11.39 **Type 2 diabetes mellitus with other diabetic ophthalmic complication** HCC

Use additional code to identify manifestation, such as: diabetic glaucoma (H40-H42)

CODING TIP✓ When a diagnosis of Type 2 or unspecified diabetes mellitus with diabetic glaucoma is reported, assign E11.39. The most common type of diabetic glaucoma is open angle glaucoma coded with H40.1-.

5 **E11.4** **Type 2 diabetes mellitus with neurological complications**

CODING TIP✓ When coding diabetes with neurological conditions, whether a causal relationship can be assumed depends on the type of neurological condition. For diagnoses of neuropathy and neuralgia with diabetes, assume a causal relationship (unless the provider states another cause) because they are listed specifically under "with" in the ICD-10-CM index. However, a causal relationship cannot be assumed for NEC diagnoses such as "other stated neurological complication" and a linkage to diabetes must be documented.

CODING TIP✓ Use E10.4- or E11.4- for diabetic neurological complications. Amyotrophy is a neurogenic muscle weakness that begins in the sacrum and hips. Polyneuropathy is known as stocking-glove numbness to describe numbness/tingling in hands, feet and ankles. Peripheral autonomic neuropathy is neuropathy of the peripheral autonomic nervous system and affects everyday body functions such as blood pressure, heart rate, bowel and bladder emptying, digestion and other involuntary responses. It may be responsible for the orthostatic hypotension in the diabetic. Neurogenic arthropathy is also known as Charcot arthropathy or rocker foot.

E11.40 **Type 2 diabetes mellitus with diabetic neuropathy, unspecified** HCC

AHA: 4Q 2013, 129

E11.41 **Type 2 diabetes mellitus with diabetic mononeuropathy** HCC

E11.42 **Type 2 diabetes mellitus with diabetic polyneuropathy** HCC

Type 2 diabetes mellitus with diabetic neuralgia

AHA: 1Q 2016, 12-13

E11.43 **Type 2 diabetes mellitus with diabetic autonomic (poly)neuropathy** HCC

Type 2 diabetes mellitus with diabetic gastroparesis

AHA: 4Q 2013, 115

AHA: 2Q 2016, 36

E11.44 **Type 2 diabetes mellitus with diabetic amyotrophy** HCC

AHA: 2Q 2016, 36

E11.49 **Type 2 diabetes mellitus with other diabetic neurological complication** HCC

5 **E11.5** **Type 2 diabetes mellitus with circulatory complications**

CODING TIP✓ Peripheral arteriosclerosis, peripheral vascular disease and peripheral arterial disease in a diabetic patient should be linked and coded as "diabetic peripheral angiopathy."

E11.51 **Type 2 diabetes mellitus with diabetic peripheral angiopathy without gangrene** HCC

E11.52 **Type 2 diabetes mellitus with diabetic peripheral angiopathy with gangrene** HCC

Type 2 diabetes mellitus with diabetic gangrene

AHA: 4Q 2017, 80

E11.59 **Type 2 diabetes mellitus with other circulatory complications** HCC

5 **E11.6** **Type 2 diabetes mellitus with other specified complications**

6 **E11.61** **Type 2 diabetes mellitus with diabetic arthropathy**

E11.610 **Type 2 diabetes mellitus with diabetic neuropathic arthropathy** HCC

Type 2 diabetes mellitus with Charcôt's joints

AHA: 2Q 2016, 36

E11.618 **Type 2 diabetes mellitus with other diabetic arthropathy** HCC

CODING TIP✓ The "with" causality guideline does not apply to "not elsewhere classified (NEC)" codes such as "other diabetic arthropathy" that cover broad categories of conditions. Instead, the provider must document that a condition such as arthritis is a diabetic complication.

AHA: 2Q 2016, 36

6 **E11.62** **Type 2 diabetes mellitus with skin complications**

E11.620 **Type 2 diabetes mellitus with diabetic dermatitis** HCC

Type 2 diabetes mellitus with diabetic necrobiosis lipoidica

E11.621 **Type 2 diabetes mellitus with foot ulcer** HCC

Use additional code to identify site of ulcer (L97.4-, L97.5-)

AHA: 1Q 2016, 12-13

E11.622 **Type 2 diabetes mellitus with other skin ulcer** HCC

Use additional code to identify site of ulcer (L97.1-L97.9, L98.41-L98.49)

CODING TIP✓ Diabetes codes with 4th, 5th and 6th characters .622 are used when an ulcer is located on the lower extremity, beginning at the ankle, and not including the foot.

AHA: 4Q 2017, 13

E11.628 **Type 2 diabetes mellitus with other skin complications** HCC

Ⓖ **E11.63** **Type 2 diabetes mellitus with oral complications**

E11.630 **Type 2 diabetes mellitus with periodontal disease** HCC

E11.638 **Type 2 diabetes mellitus with other oral complications** HCC

Ⓖ **E11.64** **Type 2 diabetes mellitus with hypoglycemia**

E11.641 **Type 2 diabetes mellitus with hypoglycemia with coma** HCC

E11.649 **Type 2 diabetes mellitus with hypoglycemia without coma** HCC

CODING TIP✓ The physician should be queried when the term "uncontrolled" is used to determine whether the patient has hyperglycemia, hypoglycemia or both.

CODING TIP✓ If encephalopathy is due to hypoglycemia, use G93.41 as an additional code.

AHA: 3Q 2015, 21
AHA: 3Q 2016, 42
AHA: 2Q 2017, 8

E11.65 **Type 2 diabetes mellitus with hyperglycemia** HCC

CODING TIP✓ When hyperglycemia, poorly controlled, inadequately controlled, or out of control, is documented, diabetes with hyperglycemia should be coded. The clinical record should support the hyperglycemia.

AHA: 3Q 2013, 20

E11.69 **Type 2 diabetes mellitus with other specified complication** HCC

Use additional code to identify complication

CODING TIP✓ When osteomyelitis is specified as due to type 2 or uspecified diabetes mellitus, assign code E11.69, followed by the appropriate code to specify the type and location of the osteomyelitis. This classification presumes a cause and effect relationship between osteomyelitis and diabetes, when no other cause is documented. Use the appropriate code for the osteomyelitis after coding diabetes with other specified manifestations.

AHA: 4Q 2016, 141

E11.8 **Type 2 diabetes mellitus with unspecified complications** HCC

E11.9 **Type 2 diabetes mellitus without complications** HCC

CODING TIP✓ Report code E11.9 when documentation does not mention a complication or manifestations cannot be confirmed with the physician. Do not use this code with any other codes from category E11 or with a manifestation. At times when a manifestation is suspected, but cannot be confirmed, E11.9 may be coded to indicate no causal relationship between diabetes and the possible manifestation.

DEFINITION Underproduction or underutilization of insulin; presents with abnormally high blood sugar (glucose) levels, resulting in impaired carbohydrate and fat metabolism.

AHA: 4Q 2013, 128
AHA: 2Q 2016, 36

Type 2 diabetes mellitus

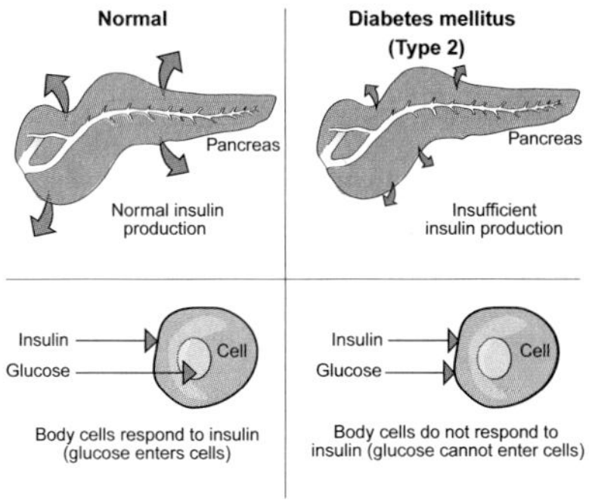

④ **E13** **Other specified diabetes mellitus**

INCLUDES diabetes mellitus due to genetic defects of beta-cell function
diabetes mellitus due to genetic defects in insulin action
postpancreatectomy diabetes mellitus
postprocedural diabetes mellitus
secondary diabetes mellitus NEC

Use additional code to identify control using:
insulin (Z79.4)
oral antidiabetic drugs (Z79.84)
oral hypoglycemic drugs (Z79.84)

EXCLUDES 1 *diabetes (mellitus) due to autoimmune process (E10.-)*
diabetes (mellitus) due to immune mediated pancreatic islet beta-cell destruction (E10.-)
diabetes mellitus due to underlying condition (E08.-)
drug or chemical induced diabetes mellitus (E09.-)
gestational diabetes (O24.4-)
neonatal diabetes mellitus (P70.2)
type 1 diabetes mellitus (E10.-)

GUIDELINES **Section 1.C.4.a.3**

An additional code should be assigned from category Z79 to identify the long-term (current) use of insulin or oral hypoglycemic drugs. If the patient is treated with both oral medications and insulin, only the code for long-term (current) use of insulin should be assigned. Code Z79.4 should not be assigned if insulin is given temporarily to bring a type 2 patient's blood sugar under control during an encounter.

GUIDELINES **Section I.C.4.a.6(a)**

Codes under categories E08, Diabetes mellitus due to underlying condition, E09, Drug or chemical induced diabetes mellitus, and E13, Other specified diabetes mellitus, identify complications/manifestations associated with secondary diabetes mellitus. Secondary diabetes is always caused by another condition or event (e.g., cystic fibrosis, malignant neoplasm of pancreas, pancreatectomy, adverse effect of drug, or poisoning).

For patients with secondary diabetes mellitus who routinely use insulin or oral hypoglycemic drugs, an additional code from category Z79 should be assigned to identify the long-term (current) use of insulin or oral hypoglycemic drugs. If the patient is treated with both oral medications and insulin, only the code for long-term (current) use of insulin should be assigned. Code Z79.4 should not be assigned if insulin is given temporarily to bring a secondary diabetic patient's blood sugar under control during an encounter.

GUIDELINES **Section I.C.4.a.6)(b)(i)**

For postpancreatectomy diabetes mellitus (lack of insulin due to the surgical removal of all or part of the pancreas), assign code E89.1, Postprocedural hypoinsulinemia. Assign a code from category E13 and a code from subcategory Z90.41-, Acquired absence of pancreas, as additional codes.

CODING TIP✓ If the patient uses an insulin pump, use Z96.41 as an additional code. If there is a complication involving the insulin pump, use a code from T85.6- or T85.7- instead of the Z code.

CODING TIP✓ When diabetes is specified as due to surgical removal of the pancreas (causing a lack of insulin), proper sequencing requires the coder to assign first code E89.1 Postprocedural hypoinsulinemia, followed by the appropriate code from category E13, as well as a code for acquired absence of pancreas (Z90.41-), and insulin use (Z79.4).

5 **E13.0 Other specified diabetes mellitus with hyperosmolarity**

E13.00 Other specified diabetes mellitus with hyperosmolarity without nonketotic hyperglycemic-hyperosmolar coma (NKHHC) HCC

EXCLUDES 2 *type 2 diabetes mellitus (E11.-)*

E13.01 Other specified diabetes mellitus with hyperosmolarity with coma HCC

5 **E13.1 Other specified diabetes mellitus with ketoacidosis**

E13.10 Other specified diabetes mellitus with ketoacidosis without coma HCC

AHA: 1Q 2013, 26

AHA: 2Q 2016, 10

E13.11 Other specified diabetes mellitus with ketoacidosis with coma HCC

5 **E13.2 Other specified diabetes mellitus with kidney complications**

CODING TIP✓ Diabetic triopathy refers to the most common types of manifestations of diabetes--nephropathy, retinopathy and neuropathy.

E13.21 Other specified diabetes mellitus with diabetic nephropathy HCC

Other specified diabetes mellitus with intercapillary glomerulosclerosis

Other specified diabetes mellitus with intracapillary glomerulonephrosis

Other specified diabetes mellitus with Kimmelstiel-Wilson disease

E13.22 Other specified diabetes mellitus with diabetic chronic kidney disease HCC

Use additional code to identify stage of chronic kidney disease (N18.1-N18.6)

CODING TIP✓ When diabetes, CKD and hypertension are documented, sequence the appropriate category of diabetes with CKD (E--.22) and the appropriate hypertension code (I12 or I13) prior to N18. The hypertension or the diabetes may be sequenced first depending on the focus of care. Use N18.1-N18.6 or N18.9 to indicate the CKD. The only time that the conditions should be coded differently is if the physician specifically documents that the conditions are not related.

CODING TIP✓ Assign an additional code from N18- to indicate the stage of CKD. When diabetic nephropathy and CKD are documented, code diabetic CKD, not nephropathy, because CKD is more specific.

E13.29 Other specified diabetes mellitus with other diabetic kidney complication HCC

Other specified diabetes mellitus with renal tubular degeneration

5 **E13.3 Other specified diabetes mellitus with ophthalmic complications**

CODING TIP✓ Diabetic triopathy refers to the most common types of manifestations of diabetes--nephropathy, retinopathy and neuropathy.

AHA: 4Q 2016, 11

6 **E13.31 Other specified diabetes mellitus with unspecified diabetic retinopathy**

E13.311 Other specified diabetes mellitus with unspecified diabetic retinopathy with macular edema HCC

E13.319 Other specified diabetes mellitus with unspecified diabetic retinopathy without macular edema HCC

6 **E13.32 Other specified diabetes mellitus with mild nonproliferative diabetic retinopathy**

Other specified diabetes mellitus with nonproliferative diabetic retinopathy NOS

One of the following 7th characters is to be assigned to codes in subcategory E13.32 to designate laterality of the disease:

1 right eye
2 left eye
3 bilateral
9 unspecified eye

7 ⊟ **E13.321- Other specified diabetes mellitus with mild nonproliferative diabetic retinopathy with macular edema** HCC

7 ⊟ **E13.329- Other specified diabetes mellitus with mild nonproliferative diabetic retinopathy without macular edema** HCC

6 **E13.33 Other specified diabetes mellitus with moderate nonproliferative diabetic retinopathy**

One of the following 7th characters is to be assigned to codes in subcategory E13.33 to designate laterality of the disease:

1 right eye
2 left eye
3 bilateral
9 unspecified eye

7 ⊟ **E13.331- Other specified diabetes mellitus with moderate nonproliferative diabetic retinopathy with macular edema** HCC

7 ⊟ **E13.339- Other specified diabetes mellitus with moderate nonproliferative diabetic retinopathy without macular edema** HCC

6 **E13.34 Other specified diabetes mellitus with severe nonproliferative diabetic retinopathy**

One of the following 7th characters is to be assigned to codes in subcategory E13.34 to designate laterality of the disease:

1 right eye
2 left eye
3 bilateral
9 unspecified eye

7 ⊟ **E13.341- Other specified diabetes mellitus with severe nonproliferative diabetic retinopathy with macular edema** HCC

7 ⊟ **E13.349- Other specified diabetes mellitus with severe nonproliferative diabetic retinopathy without macular edema** HCC

6 **E13.35 Other specified diabetes mellitus with proliferative diabetic retinopathy**

One of the following 7th characters is to be assigned to codes in subcategory E13.35 to designate laterality of the disease:

1 right eye
2 left eye
3 bilateral
9 unspecified eye

7 ⊟ **E13.351- Other specified diabetes mellitus with proliferative diabetic retinopathy with macular edema** HCC

7 ⊟ **E13.352- Other specified diabetes mellitus with proliferative diabetic retinopathy with traction retinal detachment involving the macula** HCC

7 ⊟ **E13.353- Other specified diabetes mellitus with proliferative diabetic retinopathy with traction retinal detachment not involving the macula** HCC

7 ⊟ **E13.354- Other specified diabetes mellitus with proliferative diabetic retinopathy with combined traction retinal detachment and rhegmatogenous retinal detachment** HCC

7 ⊟ **E13.355- Other specified diabetes mellitus with stable proliferative diabetic retinopathy** HCC

7 ⊟ E13.359- **Other specified diabetes mellitus with proliferative diabetic retinopathy without macular edema** HCC

E13.36 **Other specified diabetes mellitus with diabetic cataract** HCC

CODING TIP ✓ Cataracts are more common in diabetic patients. The classification assumes a relationship between cataracts and diabetes, when the patient has diabetes, unless the physician specified a different cause.

7 ⊟ E13.37X- **Other specified diabetes mellitus with diabetic macular edema, resolved following treatment** HCC

One of the following 7th characters is to be assigned to code E13.37 to designate laterality of the disease:

1 right eye
2 left eye
3 bilateral
9 unspecified eye

CODING TIP ✓ The macular edema may be resolved, but the retinopathy remains. This code is like a history code for the macular edema.

E13.39 **Other specified diabetes mellitus with other diabetic ophthalmic complication** HCC

Use additional code to identify manifestation, such as: diabetic glaucoma (H40-H42)

CODING TIP ✓ When a diagnosis of other specified diabetes mellitus with diabetic glaucoma is reported, assign code E13.39. The most common type of diabetic glaucoma is open angle glaucoma coded with H40.1-.

5 E13.4 **Other specified diabetes mellitus with neurological complications**

CODING TIP ✓ When coding diabetes with neurological conditions, whether a causal relationship can be assumed depends on the type of neurological condition. For diagnoses of neuropathy and neuralgia with diabetes, assume a causal relationship (unless the provider states another cause) because they are listed specifically under "with" in the ICD-10-CM index. However, a causal relationship cannot be assumed for NEC diagnoses such as "other stated neurological complication" and a linkage to diabetes must be documented.

E13.40 **Other specified diabetes mellitus with diabetic neuropathy, unspecified** HCC

E13.41 **Other specified diabetes mellitus with diabetic mononeuropathy** HCC

E13.42 **Other specified diabetes mellitus with diabetic polyneuropathy** HCC

Other specified diabetes mellitus with diabetic neuralgia

E13.43 **Other specified diabetes mellitus with diabetic autonomic (poly)neuropathy** HCC

Other specified diabetes mellitus with diabetic gastroparesis

AHA: 4Q 2013, 115

E13.44 **Other specified diabetes mellitus with diabetic amyotrophy** HCC

E13.49 **Other specified diabetes mellitus with other diabetic neurological complication** HCC

5 E13.5 **Other specified diabetes mellitus with circulatory complications**

CODING TIP ✓ Peripheral arteriosclerosis, peripheral vascular disease and peripheral arterial disease in a diabetic patient should be linked and coded as "diabetic peripheral angiopathy."

E13.51 **Other specified diabetes mellitus with diabetic peripheral angiopathy without gangrene** HCC

E13.52 **Other specified diabetes mellitus with diabetic peripheral angiopathy with gangrene** HCC

Other specified diabetes mellitus with diabetic gangrene

E13.59 **Other specified diabetes mellitus with other circulatory complications** HCC

5 E13.6 **Other specified diabetes mellitus with other specified complications**

6 E13.61 **Other specified diabetes mellitus with diabetic arthropathy**

E13.610 **Other specified diabetes mellitus with diabetic neuropathic arthropathy** HCC

Other specified diabetes mellitus with Charcôt's joints

E13.618 **Other specified diabetes mellitus with other diabetic arthropathy** HCC

CODING TIP ✓ The "with" causality guideline does not apply to "not elsewhere classified (NEC)" codes such as "other diabetic arthropathy" that cover broad categories of conditions. Instead, the provider must document that a condition such as arthritis is a diabetic complication.

6 E13.62 **Other specified diabetes mellitus with skin complications**

E13.620 **Other specified diabetes mellitus with diabetic dermatitis** HCC

Other specified diabetes mellitus with diabetic necrobiosis lipoidica

E13.621 **Other specified diabetes mellitus with foot ulcer** HCC

Use additional code to identify site of ulcer (L97.4-, L97.5-)

E13.622 **Other specified diabetes mellitus with other skin ulcer** HCC

Use additional code to identify site of ulcer (L97.1-L97.9, L98.41-L98.49)

CODING TIP ✓ Diabetes codes with 4th, 5th and 6th characters .622 are used when an ulcer is located on the lower extremity, beginning at the ankle, and not including the foot.

E13.628 **Other specified diabetes mellitus with other skin complications** HCC

6 E13.63 **Other specified diabetes mellitus with oral complications**

E13.630 **Other specified diabetes mellitus with periodontal disease** HCC

E13.638 **Other specified diabetes mellitus with other oral complications** HCC

6 E13.64 **Other specified diabetes mellitus with hypoglycemia**

E13.641 **Other specified diabetes mellitus with hypoglycemia with coma** HCC

E13.649 **Other specified diabetes mellitus with hypoglycemia without coma** HCC

CODING TIP ✓ The physician should be queried when the term "uncontrolled" is used to determine whether the patient has hyperglycemia, hypoglycemia or both.

CODING TIP ✓ If encephalopathy is due to hypoglycemia, use G93.41 as an additional code.

E13.65 **Other specified diabetes mellitus with hyperglycemia** HCC

CODING TIP ✓ When hyperglycemia, poorly controlled, inadequately controlled, or out of control, is documented, diabetes with hyperglycemia should be coded. The clinical record should support the hyperglycemia.

E13.69 **Other specified diabetes mellitus with other specified complication** HCC

Use additional code to identify complication

CODING TIP ✓ When osteomyelitis is specified as due to other specified diabetes mellitus, assign code E13.69, followed by the appropriate code to specify the type and location of the osteomyelitis. This classification presumes a cause and effect relationship between osteomyelitis and diabetes, when no other cause is documented. Use the appropriate code for the osteomyelitis after coding diabetes with other specified manifestations.

E13.8 **Other specified diabetes mellitus with unspecified complications** HCC

E13.9 **Other specified diabetes mellitus without complications** HCC

Other disorders of glucose regulation and pancreatic internal secretion (E15-E16)

E15 Nondiabetic hypoglycemic coma HCC

INCLUDES drug-induced insulin coma in nondiabetic
hyperinsulinism with hypoglycemic coma
hypoglycemic coma NOS

CODING TIP ✓ Do not assign code category E15 for patients with diabetes mellitus.

CODING TIP ✓ Do not use E15 for Type 1, Type 2 or secondary diabetes patients.

4 E16 Other disorders of pancreatic internal secretion

E16.0 Drug-induced hypoglycemia without coma
Use additional code for adverse effect, if applicable, to identify drug (T36-T50 with fifth or sixth character 5)

EXCLUDES 1 *diabetes with hypoglycemia without coma (E09.649)*

CODING TIP ✓ Do not use E16.0, E16.1, E16.3, E16.4, E16.8, E16.9 for Type 1, Type 2 or secondary diabetes patients.

E16.1 Other hypoglycemia
Functional hyperinsulinism
Functional nonhyperinsulinemic hypoglycemia
Hyperinsulinism NOS
Hyperplasia of pancreatic islet beta cells NOS

EXCLUDES 1 *diabetes with hypoglycemia (E08.649, E10.649, E11.649, E13.649)*
hypoglycemia in infant of diabetic mother (P70.1)
neonatal hypoglycemia (P70.4)

CODING TIP ✓ Do not assign E16.1 to report hypoglycemia in a patient with a known diagnosis of diabetes, including post-procedural hypoinsulinemia.

CODING TIP ✓ Do not use E16.0, E16.1, E16.3, E16.4, E16.8, E16.9 for Type 1, Type 2 or secondary diabetes patients.

E16.2 Hypoglycemia, unspecified

EXCLUDES 1 *diabetes with hypoglycemia (E08.649, E10.649, E11.649, E13.649)*

CODING TIP ✓ Do not use E16.2 for Type 1, Type 2 or secondary diabetes patients.

DEFINITION Condition in which blood sugar levels are too low for normal functioning, manifesting as weakness, trembling, hunger, headache, irritability, racing heartbeat, confusion, even convulsions or coma.

AHA: 2Q 2017, 8

E16.3 Increased secretion of glucagon
Hyperplasia of pancreatic endocrine cells with glucagon excess

CODING TIP ✓ Do not use E16.0, E16.1, E16.3, E16.4, E16.8, E16.9 for Type 1, Type 2 or secondary diabetes patients.

E16.4 Increased secretion of gastrin
Hypergastrinemia
Hyperplasia of pancreatic endocrine cells with gastrin excess
Zollinger-Ellison syndrome

CODING TIP ✓ Do not use E16.0, E16.1, E16.3, E16.4, E16.8, E16.9 for Type 1, Type 2 or secondary diabetes patients.

E16.8 Other specified disorders of pancreatic internal secretion
Increased secretion from endocrine pancreas of growth hormone-releasing hormone
Increased secretion from endocrine pancreas of pancreatic polypeptide
Increased secretion from endocrine pancreas of somatostatin
Increased secretion from endocrine pancreas of vasoactive-intestinal polypeptide

CODING TIP ✓ Do not use E16.0, E16.1, E16.3, E16.4, E16.8, E16.9 for Type 1, Type 2 or secondary diabetes patients.

CODING TIP ✓ Do not use E16.8 for steroid induced diabetes. Use category E09 instead.

E16.9 Disorder of pancreatic internal secretion, unspecified
Islet-cell hyperplasia NOS
Pancreatic endocrine cell hyperplasia NOS

CODING TIP ✓ Do not use E16.0, E16.1, E16.3, E16.4, E16.8, E16.9 for Type 1, Type 2 or secondary diabetes patients.

Disorders of other endocrine glands (E20-E35)

EXCLUDES 1 *galactorrhea (N64.3)*
gynecomastia (N62)

4 E20 Hypoparathyroidism

EXCLUDES 1 *Di George's syndrome (D82.1)*
postprocedural hypoparathyroidism (E89.2)
tetany NOS (R29.0)
transitory neonatal hypoparathyroidism (P71.4)

DEFINITION Reduced production of parathyroid hormone causing tingling of the hands, fingers, and mouth, muscle cramps, and possibly convulsions.

E20.0 Idiopathic hypoparathyroidism HCC

E20.1 Pseudohypoparathyroidism

CODING TIP ✓ Patients with pseudohypoparathyroidism produce adequate levels of PTH, but are resistant to its effects due to a genetic abnormality. These patients typically exhibit low blood calcium and elevated phosphorus, which are characteristic of hypoparathyroidism and should not be separately coded.

DEFINITION Condition of hypoparathyroidism symptoms manifesting due to an inadequate response to the parathyroid hormone, rather than an insufficient amount of the hormone.

E20.8 Other hypoparathyroidism HCC

E20.9 Hypoparathyroidism, unspecified HCC
Parathyroid tetany

4 E21 Hyperparathyroidism and other disorders of parathyroid gland

EXCLUDES 1 *adult osteomalacia (M83.-)*
ectopic hyperparathyroidism (E34.2)
familial hypocalciuric hypercalcemia (E83.52)
hungry bone syndrome (E83.81)
infantile and juvenile osteomalacia (E55.0)

E21.0 Primary hyperparathyroidism HCC
Hyperplasia of parathyroid
Osteitis fibrosa cystica generalisata [von Recklinghausen's disease of bone]

DEFINITION Excessive production of parathyroid hormone, usually caused by hyperplasia of the gland itself, causing decreased calcium levels in bones.

E21.1 Secondary hyperparathyroidism, not elsewhere classified HCC

EXCLUDES 1 *secondary hyperparathyroidism of renal origin (N25.81)*

CODING TIP ✓ Do not assign E21.1 if the causative mechanism of the diagnosed secondary hyperparathyroid disease is of renal (kidney) origin.

E21.2 Other hyperparathyroidism HCC
Tertiary hyperparathyroidism

EXCLUDES 1 *familial hypocalciuric hypercalcemia (E83.52)*

E21.3 Hyperparathyroidism, unspecified HCC

E21.4 Other specified disorders of parathyroid gland HCC

E21.5 Disorder of parathyroid gland, unspecified HCC

4 E22 Hyperfunction of pituitary gland

EXCLUDES 1 *Cushing's syndrome (E24.-)*
Nelson's syndrome (E24.1)
overproduction of ACTH not associated with Cushing's disease (E27.0)
overproduction of pituitary ACTH (E24.0)
overproduction of thyroid-stimulating hormone (E05.8-)

E22.0 Acromegaly and pituitary gigantism HCC
Overproduction of growth hormone

EXCLUDES 1 *constitutional gigantism (E34.4)*
constitutional tall stature (E34.4)
increased secretion from endocrine pancreas of growth hormone-releasing hormone (E16.8)

DEFINITION Acromegaly: Abnormally large growth of the hands, feet and facial features due to the production of too much growth hormone in adults by the pituitary gland.

E22.1 **Hyperprolactinemia** HCC
Use additional code for adverse effect, if applicable, to identify drug (T36-T50 with fifth or sixth character 5)

E22.2 **Syndrome of inappropriate secretion of antidiuretic hormone** HCC

E22.8 **Other hyperfunction of pituitary gland** HCC
Central precocious puberty

E22.9 **Hyperfunction of pituitary gland, unspecified** HCC

E23 Hypofunction and other disorders of the pituitary gland

INCLUDES the listed conditions whether the disorder is in the pituitary or the hypothalamus

EXCLUDES 1 *postprocedural hypopituitarism (E89.3)*

E23.0 **Hypopituitarism** HCC
Fertile eunuch syndrome
Hypogonadotropic hypogonadism
Idiopathic growth hormone deficiency
Isolated deficiency of gonadotropin
Isolated deficiency of growth hormone
Isolated deficiency of pituitary hormone
Kallmann's syndrome
Lorain-Levi short stature
Necrosis of pituitary gland (postpartum)
Panhypopituitarism
Pituitary cachexia
Pituitary insufficiency NOS
Pituitary short stature
Sheehan's syndrome
Simmonds' disease

DEFINITION A type of dwarfism with retention of infantile characteristics, due to undersecretion of growth hormone and gonadotropin deficiency.

E23.1 **Drug-induced hypopituitarism** HCC
Use additional code for adverse effect, if applicable, to identify drug (T36-T50 with fifth or sixth character 5)

E23.2 **Diabetes insipidus** HCC
EXCLUDES 1 *nephrogenic diabetes insipidus (N25.1)*

DEFINITION Insufficient vasopressin production/secretion of antidiuretic hormone (ADH) resulting in intense thirst and excretion of large amounts of urine.

E23.3 **Hypothalamic dysfunction, not elsewhere classified** HCC
EXCLUDES 1 *Prader-Willi syndrome (Q87.1)*
Russell-Silver syndrome (Q87.1)

E23.6 **Other disorders of pituitary gland** HCC
Abscess of pituitary
Adiposogenital dystrophy

E23.7 **Disorder of pituitary gland, unspecified** HCC

E24 Cushing's syndrome

EXCLUDES 1 *congenital adrenal hyperplasia (E25.0)*

CODING TIP✓ When Cushing's syndrome is stated as the cause of diabetes mellitus in the patient, assign the appropriate code for Cushing's syndrome, followed by the appropriate code from category E08 for diabetes mellitus due to an underlying condition.

E24.0 **Pituitary-dependent Cushing's disease** HCC
Overproduction of pituitary ACTH
Pituitary-dependent hypercorticalism

E24.1 **Nelson's syndrome** HCC

E24.2 **Drug-induced Cushing's syndrome** HCC
Use additional code for adverse effect, if applicable, to identify drug (T36-T50 with fifth or sixth character 5)

CODING TIP✓ Code E24.2 should only be assigned when documentation clearly indicates a relationship between Cushing's syndrome and a drug or chemical as the underlying cause.

E24.3 **Ectopic ACTH syndrome** HCC

E24.4 **Alcohol-induced pseudo-Cushing's syndrome** HCC

E24.8 **Other Cushing's syndrome** HCC

E24.9 **Cushing's syndrome, unspecified** HCC

DEFINITION Disorder caused by prolonged exposure of body tissues to high levels of cortisol, presenting with upper body obesity, thinning arms and legs, brittle bones, severe fatigue, weakness, high blood pressure, and high blood sugar.

E25 Adrenogenital disorders

INCLUDES adrenogenital syndromes, virilizing or feminizing, whether acquired or due to adrenal hyperplasia consequent on inborn enzyme defects in hormone synthesis
Female adrenal pseudohermaphroditism
Female heterosexual precocious pseudopuberty
Male isosexual precocious pseudopuberty
Male macrogenitosomia praecox
Male sexual precocity with adrenal hyperplasia
Male virilization (female)

EXCLUDES 1 *indeterminate sex and pseudohermaphroditism (Q56)*
chromosomal abnormalities (Q90-Q99)

E25.0 **Congenital adrenogenital disorders associated with enzyme deficiency** HCC
Congenital adrenal hyperplasia
21-Hydroxylase deficiency
Salt-losing congenital adrenal hyperplasia

E25.8 **Other adrenogenital disorders** HCC
Idiopathic adrenogenital disorder
Use additional code for adverse effect, if applicable, to identify drug (T36-T50 with fifth or sixth character 5)

E25.9 **Adrenogenital disorder, unspecified** HCC
Adrenogenital syndrome NOS

E26 Hyperaldosteronism

E26.0 **Primary hyperaldosteronism**

DEFINITION Excessive aldosterone production; typically presents with loss of potassium, muscular weakness, and elevated blood pressure.

E26.01 **Conn's syndrome** HCC
Code also:
adrenal adenoma (D35.0-)

DEFINITION Excess secretion of aldosterone due to an adrenocortical adenoma, causing hypokalemia, alkalosis, muscular weakness, polyuria, polydipsia, and hypertension.

E26.02 **Glucocorticoid-remediable aldosteronism** HCC
Familial aldosteronism type I

E26.09 **Other primary hyperaldosteronism** HCC
Primary aldosteronism due to adrenal hyperplasia (bilateral)

E26.1 **Secondary hyperaldosteronism** HCC

E26.8 **Other hyperaldosteronism**

E26.81 **Bartter's syndrome** HCC

DEFINITION Group of symptoms caused by the kidneys' inability to reabsorb potassium, also known as urinary potassium wasting; causes renal cell enlargement, alkalosis, hyperaldosteronism, cramping, constipation, urinary frequency, and weakness.

E26.89 **Other hyperaldosteronism** HCC

E26.9 **Hyperaldosteronism, unspecified** HCC
Aldosteronism NOS
Hyperaldosteronism NOS

E27 Other disorders of adrenal gland

E27.0 **Other adrenocortical overactivity** HCC
Overproduction of ACTH, not associated with Cushing's disease
Premature adrenarche
EXCLUDES 1 *Cushing's syndrome (E24.-)*

E27.1 **Primary adrenocortical insufficiency** HCC
Addison's disease
Autoimmune adrenalitis
EXCLUDES 1 *Addison only phenotype adrenoleukodystrophy (E71.528)*
amyloidosis (E85.-)
tuberculous Addison's disease (A18.7)
Waterhouse-Friderichsen syndrome (A39.1)

E27.2 **Addisonian crisis** HCC
Adrenal crisis
Adrenocortical crisis

CODING TIP✓ Do not assign E27.2 to indicate Addison's disease. Code E27.2 indicates Addisonian crisis, a severe and life-threatening condition that may occur in individuals with Addison's disease or other conditions resulting in severely elevated cortisol levels. Addison's disease in the absence of crisis should be coded to E27.1.

DEFINITION Low levels of the glucocorticoid hormone, cortisol, secreted by the adrenal glands and responsible for regulating blood pressure, cardiovascular function, inflammatory response, insulin effects, and metabolism.

E27.3 Drug-induced adrenocortical insufficiency HCC
Use additional code for adverse effect, if applicable, to identify drug (T36-T50 with fifth or sixth character 5)

CODING TIP✓ Code E27.3 should only be assigned when documentation clearly indicates a relationship between adrenocortical insufficiency and a drug or chemical as the underlying cause. Assign a code from T36-T50 following E27.3 to indicate the drug and adverse effect.

5 **E27.4 Other and unspecified adrenocortical insufficiency**
EXCLUDES 1 *adrenoleukodystrophy [Addison-Schilder] (E71.528)*
Waterhouse-Friderichsen syndrome (A39.1)

E27.40 Unspecified adrenocortical insufficiency HCC
Adrenocortical insufficiency NOS
Hypoaldosteronism

E27.49 Other adrenocortical insufficiency HCC
Adrenal hemorrhage
Adrenal infarction

E27.5 Adrenomedullary hyperfunction HCC
Adrenomedullary hyperplasia
Catecholamine hypersecretion

DEFINITION Overproduction of adrenaline hormones by the adrenal medulla, causing heart disease, high blood pressure, and related problems.

E27.8 Other specified disorders of adrenal gland HCC
Abnormality of cortisol-binding globulin

E27.9 Disorder of adrenal gland, unspecified HCC

4 **E28 Ovarian dysfunction**
EXCLUDES 1 *isolated gonadotropin deficiency (E23.0)*
postprocedural ovarian failure (E89.4-)

E28.0 Estrogen excess ♀
Use additional code for adverse effect, if applicable, to identify drug (T36-T50 with fifth or sixth character 5)

E28.1 Androgen excess ♀
Hypersecretion of ovarian androgens
Use additional code for adverse effect, if applicable, to identify drug (T36-T50 with fifth or sixth character 5)

E28.2 Polycystic ovarian syndrome ♀
Sclerocystic ovary syndrome
Stein-Leventhal syndrome

CODING TIP✓ Polycystic ovarian syndrome (PCOS) is associated with increased risk for a number of other endocrine disorders, including insulin resistance, hypothyroidism and obesity. When present, these other diagnoses should also be reported.

DEFINITION Syndrome in which the ovaries produce too many androgens, causing ovarian cysts and interfering with the menstrual cycle; results in missed, heavy, or irregular periods, infertility, abdominal discomfort, acne, weight gain, and uterine bleeding.

5 **E28.3 Primary ovarian failure**
EXCLUDES 1 *pure gonadal dysgenesis (Q99.1)*
Turner's syndrome (Q96.-)

6 **E28.31 Premature menopause**

E28.310 Symptomatic premature menopause ♀ A
Symptoms such as flushing, sleeplessness, headache, lack of concentration, associated with premature menopause

E28.319 Asymptomatic premature menopause ♀ A
Premature menopause NOS

E28.39 Other primary ovarian failure ♀
Decreased estrogen
Resistant ovary syndrome

E28.8 Other ovarian dysfunction ♀
Ovarian hyperfunction NOS
EXCLUDES 1 *postprocedural ovarian failure (E89.4-)*

E28.9 Ovarian dysfunction, unspecified ♀

4 **E29 Testicular dysfunction**
EXCLUDES 1 *androgen insensitivity syndrome (E34.5-)*
azoospermia or oligospermia NOS (N46.0-N46.1)
isolated gonadotropin deficiency (E23.0)
Klinefelter's syndrome (Q98.0-Q98.1, Q98.4)

E29.0 Testicular hyperfunction ♂
Hypersecretion of testicular hormones

DEFINITION Excessive testosterone production, often due to an active tumor on the testicle. Commonly presents with increased muscle and bone growth in children and increased secondary sex characteristics.

Testicular hyperfunction

The secretion of too much testosterone into the body

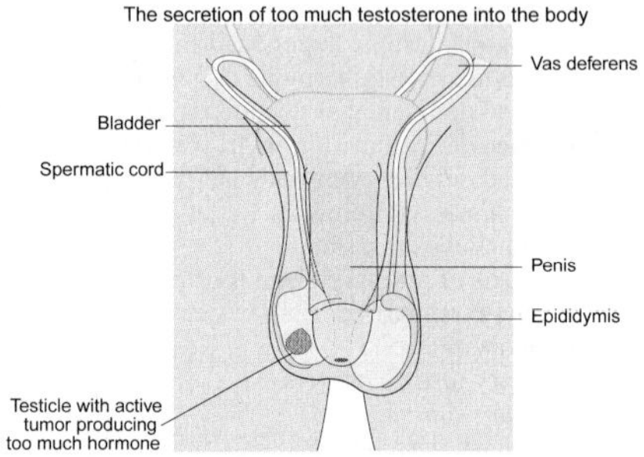

E29.1 Testicular hypofunction ♂
Defective biosynthesis of testicular androgen NOS
5-delta-Reductase deficiency (with male pseudohermaphroditism)
Testicular hypogonadism NOS
Use additional code for adverse effect, if applicable, to identify drug (T36-T50 with fifth or sixth character 5)
EXCLUDES 1 *postprocedural testicular hypofunction (E89.5)*

DEFINITION Underdevelopment of all the genital tissues with decreased functional activities of the gonads.

E29.8 Other testicular dysfunction ♂

E29.9 Testicular dysfunction, unspecified ♂

4 **E30 Disorders of puberty, not elsewhere classified**

E30.0 Delayed puberty
Constitutional delay of puberty
Delayed sexual development

E30.1 Precocious puberty P
Precocious menstruation
EXCLUDES 1 *Albright (-McCune) (-Sternberg) syndrome (Q78.1)*
central precocious puberty (E22.8)
congenital adrenal hyperplasia (E25.0)
female heterosexual precocious pseudopuberty (E25.-)
male isosexual precocious pseudopuberty (E25.-)

E30.8 Other disorders of puberty P
Premature thelarche

E30.9 Disorder of puberty, unspecified

4 **E31 Polyglandular dysfunction**
EXCLUDES 1 *ataxia telangiectasia [Louis-Bar] (G11.3)*
dystrophia myotonica [Steinert] (G71.11)
pseudohypoparathyroidism (E20.1)

E31.0 Autoimmune polyglandular failure HCC
Schmidt's syndrome

DEFINITION Schmidt's syndrome: hypofunction of more than one endocrine gland in different combinations, including the thyroid, adrenals, gonads, parathyroid, and pancreas; occurs primarily in adult females.

E31.1 **Polyglandular hyperfunction** HCC
EXCLUDES 1 *multiple endocrine adenomatosis (E31.2-)*
multiple endocrine neoplasia (E31.2-)

5 E31.2 **Multiple endocrine neoplasia [MEN] syndromes**
Multiple endocrine adenomatosis
Code also:
any associated malignancies and other conditions associated with the syndromes

CODING TIP ✓ MEN syndromes are distinct, inherited autosomal disorders, which may present in conjunction with endocrine tumors.

E31.20 **Multiple endocrine neoplasia [MEN] syndrome, unspecified** HCC
Multiple endocrine adenomatosis NOS
Multiple endocrine neoplasia [MEN] syndrome NOS

E31.21 **Multiple endocrine neoplasia [MEN] type I** HCC
Wermer's syndrome

DEFINITION Hyperplasia or tumors of the parathyroid, pancreatic islet cells, and pituitary gland; causes oversecretion of hormones, kidney stones, infertility, and severe peptic ulcers.

E31.22 **Multiple endocrine neoplasia [MEN] type IIA** HCC
Sipple's syndrome

DEFINITION Triad of thyroid medullary carcinoma, adrenal gland tumor, and parathyroid hyperplasia.

E31.23 **Multiple endocrine neoplasia [MEN] type IIB** HCC

E31.8 **Other polyglandular dysfunction** HCC

E31.9 **Polyglandular dysfunction, unspecified** HCC

4 E32 **Diseases of thymus**
EXCLUDES 1 *aplasia or hypoplasia of thymus with immunodeficiency (D82.1)*
myasthenia gravis (G70.0)

E32.0 **Persistent hyperplasia of thymus** HCC
Hypertrophy of thymus

Persistent hyperplasia of thymus
Continued abnormal growth of the thymus gland

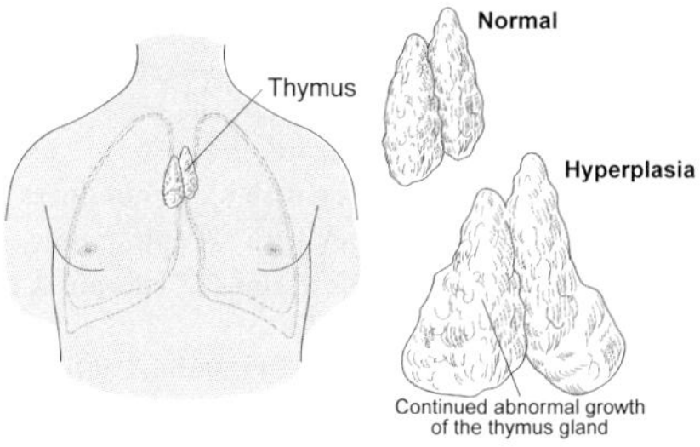

E32.1 **Abscess of thymus** HCC

E32.8 **Other diseases of thymus** HCC
EXCLUDES 1 *aplasia or hypoplasia with immunodeficiency (D82.1)*
thymoma (D15.0)

E32.9 **Disease of thymus, unspecified** HCC

4 E34 **Other endocrine disorders**
EXCLUDES 1 *pseudohypoparathyroidism (E20.1)*

E34.0 **Carcinoid syndrome** HCC
Note: May be used as an additional code to identify functional activity associated with a carcinoid tumor.

CODING TIP ✓ Carcinoid syndrome is a specific syndrome causing a variety of symptoms in patients with advanced stage malignant carcinoid tumors. When coding carcinoid syndrome, the specific type and location of the carcinoid tumor should be identified and additionally coded by assigning the appropriate code(s) from category C7A and/or C7B.

DEFINITION Condition in which cancerous cells secrete hormones into the bloodstream causing chemical imbalances in the body with symptoms of periodic flushing, diarrhea, abdominal pain, and high blood pressure.

E34.1 **Other hypersecretion of intestinal hormones**

E34.2 **Ectopic hormone secretion, not elsewhere classified**
EXCLUDES 1 *ectopic ACTH syndrome (E24.3)*

DEFINITION Condition that occurs when a glandular tumor metastasizes, moving from its original location to another area of the body, and continues to secrete hormones.

E34.3 **Short stature due to endocrine disorder**
Constitutional short stature
Laron-type short stature
EXCLUDES 1 *achondroplastic short stature (Q77.4)*
hypochondroplastic short stature (Q77.4)
nutritional short stature (E45)
pituitary short stature (E23.0)
progeria (E34.8)
renal short stature (N25.0)
Russell-Silver syndrome (Q87.1)
short-limbed stature with immunodeficiency (D82.2)
short stature in specific dysmorphic syndromes - code to syndrome - see Alphabetical Index
short stature NOS (R62.52)

E34.4 **Constitutional tall stature** HCC
Constitutional gigantism

5 E34.5 **Androgen insensitivity syndrome**

DEFINITION Defects in androgen action causing feminization of external genitalia, abnormal sexual development, infertility, and pseudohermaphroditism in males.

E34.50 **Androgen insensitivity syndrome, unspecified**
Androgen insensitivity NOS

E34.51 **Complete androgen insensitivity syndrome**
Complete androgen insensitivity
de Quervain syndrome
Goldberg-Maxwell syndrome

E34.52 **Partial androgen insensitivity syndrome**
Partial androgen insensitivity
Reifenstein syndrome

E34.8 **Other specified endocrine disorders**
Pineal gland dysfunction
Progeria
EXCLUDES 2 *pseudohypoparathyroidism (E20.1)*

E34.9 **Endocrine disorder, unspecified**
Endocrine disturbance NOS
Hormone disturbance NOS

E35 ***Disorders of endocrine glands in diseases classified elsewhere***
Code first underlying disease, such as:
late congenital syphilis of thymus gland [Dubois disease] (A50.5)
Use additional code, if applicable, to identify:
sequelae of tuberculosis of other organs (B90.8)
EXCLUDES 1 *Echinococcus granulosus infection of thyroid gland (B67.3)*
meningococcal hemorrhagic adrenalitis (A39.1)
syphilis of endocrine gland (A52.79)
tuberculosis of adrenal gland, except calcification (A18.7)
tuberculosis of endocrine gland NEC (A18.82)
tuberculosis of thyroid gland (A18.81)
Waterhouse-Friderichsen syndrome (A39.1)

Intraoperative complications of endocrine system (E36)

CODING TIP ✓ Codes classifiable to E36 are complication codes (intraoperative complications) and should only be coded when the physician specifically indicates a relationship between the operative procedure and the specific complication. If no relationship between the condition suspected to be a complication and the operative procedure is stated, the provider may be queried to clarify if the condition is classifiable as a complication.

4 E36 **Intraoperative complications of endocrine system**
EXCLUDES 2 *postprocedural endocrine and metabolic complications and disorders, not elsewhere classified (E89.-)*

5 E36.0 Intraoperative hemorrhage and hematoma of an endocrine system organ or structure complicating a procedure

EXCLUDES 1 *intraoperative hemorrhage and hematoma of an endocrine system organ or structure due to accidental puncture or laceration during a procedure (E36.1-)*

E36.01 Intraoperative hemorrhage and hematoma of an endocrine system organ or structure complicating an endocrine system procedure

E36.02 Intraoperative hemorrhage and hematoma of an endocrine system organ or structure complicating other procedure

5 E36.1 Accidental puncture and laceration of an endocrine system organ or structure during a procedure

E36.11 Accidental puncture and laceration of an endocrine system organ or structure during an endocrine system procedure

E36.12 Accidental puncture and laceration of an endocrine system organ or structure during other procedure

E36.8 Other intraoperative complications of endocrine system
Use additional code, if applicable, to further specify disorder

Malnutrition (E40-E46)

EXCLUDES 1 *intestinal malabsorption (K90.-)*
sequelae of protein-calorie malnutrition (E64.0)

EXCLUDES 2 *nutritional anemias (D50-D53)*
starvation (T73.0)

CODING TIP✓ Malnutrition is defined as insufficient, excessive or imbalanced nutrient consumption. Not all patients experiencing malnutrition will present with inadequate intake or low body weight/BMI. The specific type of malnutrition (such as severe, moderate, Kwashiorkor, etc.) must be indicated by the patient's provider and cannot be assumed. When documentation only states "malnutrition," assign E46.

E40 Kwashiorkor HCC
Severe malnutrition with nutritional edema with dyspigmentation of skin and hair
EXCLUDES 1 *marasmic kwashiorkor (E42)*

E41 Nutritional marasmus HCC
Severe malnutrition with marasmus
EXCLUDES 1 *marasmic kwashiorkor (E42)*

CODING TIP✓ The description of "emaciated" or "emaciation" without being documented with the term malnutrition should be assigned code R64, Cachexia.

DEFINITION Chronic wasting of body tissues, especially in young children, commonly due to prolonged dietary deficiency of protein and calories.

E42 Marasmic kwashiorkor HCC
Intermediate form severe protein-calorie malnutrition
Severe protein-calorie malnutrition with signs of both kwashiorkor and marasmus

E43 Unspecified severe protein-calorie malnutrition HCC
Starvation edema
AHA: 4Q 2017, 85

4 E44 Protein-calorie malnutrition of moderate and mild degree

E44.0 Moderate protein-calorie malnutrition HCC

E44.1 Mild protein-calorie malnutrition HCC

E45 Retarded development following protein-calorie malnutrition HCC
Nutritional short stature
Nutritional stunting
Physical retardation due to malnutrition

E46 Unspecified protein-calorie malnutrition HCC
Malnutrition NOS
Protein-calorie imbalance NOS
EXCLUDES 1 *nutritional deficiency NOS (E63.9)*
AHA: 3Q 2017, 25

Unspecified protein calorie malnutrition

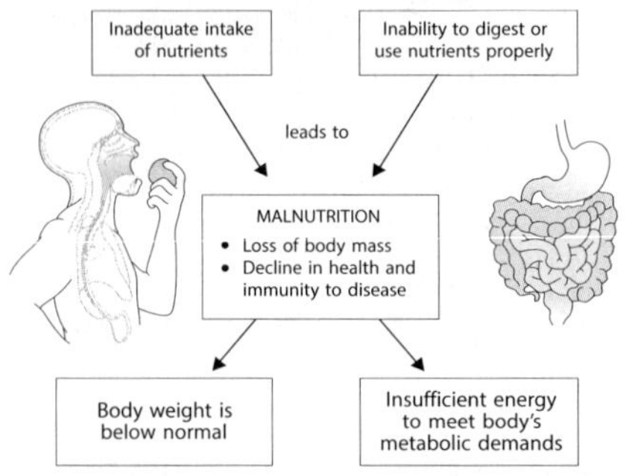
Inadequate intake of nutrients
Inability to digest or use nutrients properly
leads to
MALNUTRITION
• Loss of body mass
• Decline in health and immunity to disease
Body weight is below normal
Insufficient energy to meet body's metabolic demands

Other nutritional deficiencies (E50-E64)

EXCLUDES 2 *nutritional anemias (D50-D53)*

CODING TIP✓ E50-E64 include nutritional deficiencies of vitamins and minerals. Anemia relating to nutritional deficiencies are in Chapter 3.

4 E50 Vitamin A deficiency
EXCLUDES 1 *sequelae of vitamin A deficiency (E64.1)*

E50.0 Vitamin A deficiency with conjunctival xerosis

DEFINITION Vitamin A deficiency with dryness of the membrane that lines eyelids and covers the exposed surface of the sclera.

E50.1 Vitamin A deficiency with Bitot's spot and conjunctival xerosis
Bitot's spot in the young child

DEFINITION Vitamin A deficiency with superficial spots of keratinized epithelium on the conjunctiva, accompanied by dryness.

E50.2 Vitamin A deficiency with corneal xerosis

E50.3 Vitamin A deficiency with corneal ulceration and xerosis

E50.4 Vitamin A deficiency with keratomalacia

DEFINITION Vitamin A deficiency with softening of the corneas that may lead to corneal infection or rupture.

E50.5 Vitamin A deficiency with night blindness

E50.6 Vitamin A deficiency with xerophthalmic scars of cornea

E50.7 Other ocular manifestations of vitamin A deficiency
Xerophthalmia NOS

E50.8 Other manifestations of vitamin A deficiency
Follicular keratosis
Xeroderma

E50.9 Vitamin A deficiency, unspecified
Hypovitaminosis A NOS

Vitamin A deficiency

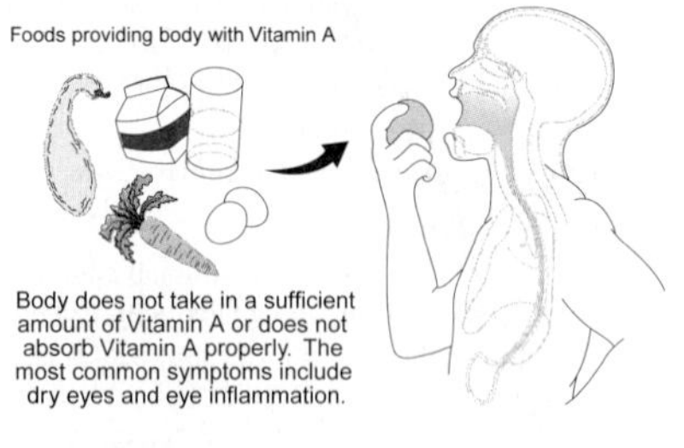
Foods providing body with Vitamin A
Body does not take in a sufficient amount of Vitamin A or does not absorb Vitamin A properly. The most common symptoms include dry eyes and eye inflammation.

4 E51 Thiamine deficiency
EXCLUDES 1 *sequelae of thiamine deficiency (E64.8)*

5 E51.1 Beriberi

DEFINITION Severe Vitamin B1 (thiamine) deficiency causing nerve, heart, and/or brain abnormalities.

E51.11 Dry beriberi
Beriberi NOS
Beriberi with polyneuropathy

E51.12 **Wet beriberi**
Beriberi with cardiovascular manifestations
Cardiovascular beriberi
Shoshin disease

E51.2 **Wernicke's encephalopathy**

E51.8 **Other manifestations of thiamine deficiency**

E51.9 **Thiamine deficiency, unspecified**

E52 **Niacin deficiency [pellagra]**
Niacin (-tryptophan) deficiency
Nicotinamide deficiency
Pellagra (alcoholic)
EXCLUDES 1 *sequelae of niacin deficiency (E64.8)*

DEFINITION Niacin and amino acid tryptophan deficiency affecting the skin, digestive tract, and brain.

4 E53 **Deficiency of other B group vitamins**
EXCLUDES 1 *sequelae of vitamin B deficiency (E64.8)*

E53.0 **Riboflavin deficiency**
Ariboflavinosis
Vitamin B2 deficiency

DEFINITION Riboflavin deficiency causing dry throat and nasal passages, mouth sores, magenta-colored tongue, and overproduction of oil on the skin.

E53.1 **Pyridoxine deficiency**
Vitamin B6 deficiency
EXCLUDES 1 *pyridoxine-responsive sideroblastic anemia (D64.3)*

E53.8 **Deficiency of other specified B group vitamins**
Biotin deficiency
Cyanocobalamin deficiency
Folate deficiency
Folic acid deficiency
Pantothenic acid deficiency
Vitamin B12 deficiency
EXCLUDES 1 *folate deficiency anemia (D52.-)*
vitamin B12 deficiency anemia (D51.-)

E53.9 **Vitamin B deficiency, unspecified**

E54 **Ascorbic acid deficiency**
Deficiency of vitamin C
Scurvy
EXCLUDES 1 *scorbutic anemia (D53.2)*
sequelae of vitamin C deficiency (E64.2)

DEFINITION Condition known as scurvy caused by deficiency of ascorbic acid (vitamin C) and marked by weakness, anemia, spongy gums, and mucocutaneous hemorrhages.

4 E55 **Vitamin D deficiency**
EXCLUDES 1 *adult osteomalacia (M83.-)*
osteoporosis (M80.-)
sequelae of rickets (E64.3)

E55.0 **Rickets, active**
Infantile osteomalacia
Juvenile osteomalacia
EXCLUDES 1 *celiac rickets (K90.0)*
Crohn's rickets (K50.-)
hereditary vitamin D-dependent rickets (E83.32)
inactive rickets (E64.3)
renal rickets (N25.0)
sequelae of rickets (E64.3)
vitamin D-resistant rickets (E83.31)

DEFINITION Childhood disease caused by a lack of vitamin D, resulting in soft, spongy bones and bone pain as well as skeletal deformities (e.g., bowlegs, scoliosis), distortion of the rib cage, and oddly-shaped skull.

E55.9 **Vitamin D deficiency, unspecified**
Avitaminosis D

4 E56 **Other vitamin deficiencies**
EXCLUDES 1 *sequelae of other vitamin deficiencies (E64.8)*

E56.0 **Deficiency of vitamin E**

E56.1 **Deficiency of vitamin K**
EXCLUDES 1 *deficiency of coagulation factor due to vitamin K deficiency (D68.4)*
vitamin K deficiency of newborn (P53)

E56.8 **Deficiency of other vitamins**

E56.9 **Vitamin deficiency, unspecified**

E58 **Dietary calcium deficiency**
EXCLUDES 1 *disorders of calcium metabolism (E83.5-)*
sequelae of calcium deficiency (E64.8)

E59 **Dietary selenium deficiency**
Keshan disease
EXCLUDES 1 *sequelae of selenium deficiency (E64.8)*

E60 **Dietary zinc deficiency**

4 E61 **Deficiency of other nutrient elements**
Use additional code for adverse effect, if applicable, to identify drug (T36-T50 with fifth or sixth character 5)
EXCLUDES 1 *disorders of mineral metabolism (E83.-)*
iodine deficiency related thyroid disorders (E00-E02)
sequelae of malnutrition and other nutritional deficiencies (E64.-)

E61.0 **Copper deficiency**

E61.1 **Iron deficiency**
EXCLUDES 1 *iron deficiency anemia (D50.-)*

E61.2 **Magnesium deficiency**

E61.3 **Manganese deficiency**

E61.4 **Chromium deficiency**

E61.5 **Molybdenum deficiency**

E61.6 **Vanadium deficiency**

E61.7 **Deficiency of multiple nutrient elements**

E61.8 **Deficiency of other specified nutrient elements**

E61.9 **Deficiency of nutrient element, unspecified**

4 E63 **Other nutritional deficiencies**
EXCLUDES 1 *dehydration (E86.0)*
failure to thrive, adult (R62.7)
failure to thrive, child (R62.51)
feeding problems in newborn (P92.-)
sequelae of malnutrition and other nutritional deficiencies (E64.-)

E63.0 **Essential fatty acid [EFA] deficiency**

E63.1 **Imbalance of constituents of food intake**

E63.8 **Other specified nutritional deficiencies**

E63.9 **Nutritional deficiency, unspecified**

4 E64 **Sequelae of malnutrition and other nutritional deficiencies**
Note: This category is to be used to indicate conditions in categories E43, E44, E46, E50-E63 as the cause of sequelae, which are themselves classified elsewhere. The 'sequelae' include conditions specified as such; they also include the late effects of diseases classifiable to the above categories if the disease itself is no longer present
Code first:
condition resulting from (sequela) of malnutrition and other nutritional deficiencies

E64.0 **Sequelae of protein-calorie malnutrition** HCC
EXCLUDES 2 *retarded development following protein-calorie malnutrition (E45)*

E64.1 **Sequelae of vitamin A deficiency**

E64.2 **Sequelae of vitamin C deficiency**

E64.3 **Sequelae of rickets**

E64.8 **Sequelae of other nutritional deficiencies**

E64.9 **Sequelae of unspecified nutritional deficiency**

Overweight, obesity and other hyperalimentation (E65-E68)

E65 **Localized adiposity**
Fat pad

4 E66 **Overweight and obesity**
Code first:
obesity complicating pregnancy, childbirth and the puerperium, if applicable (O99.21-)
Use additional code to identify body mass index (BMI), if known (Z68.-)
EXCLUDES 1 *adiposogenital dystrophy (E23.6)*
lipomatosis NOS (E88.2)
lipomatosis dolorosa [Dercum] (E88.2)
Prader-Willi syndrome (Q87.1)

GUIDELINES **Section I.B.14**
For the Body Mass Index (BMI), depth of non-pressure chronic ulcers, pressure ulcer stage, coma scale, and NIH stroke scale (NIHSS) codes, code assignment may be based on medical record documentation from clinicians who are not the patient's provider (i.e., physician or other qualified healthcare practitioner legally accountable for establishing the patient's diagnosis), since this information is typically documented by other clinicians involved in the care of the patient (e.g., a dietitian often documents the BMI, a nurse often documents the pressure ulcer stages, and an emergency medical technician often documents the coma scale). However, the associated diagnosis (such as overweight, obesity, acute stroke, or pressure ulcer) must be documented by the patient's provider.

CODING TIP✓ The provider must provide documentation of a clinical condition, such as obesity, to justify reporting a code for the body mass index.

5 **E66.0 Obesity due to excess calories**

DEFINITION Increased body weight with excessive accumulation of fat caused by overeating and/or a sedentary lifestyle.

E66.01 Morbid (severe) obesity due to excess calories HCC

EXCLUDES 1 *morbid (severe) obesity with alveolar hypoventilation (E66.2)*

CODING TIP✓ Note that the alphabetical index refers to this code for morbid obesity as well as severe obesity.

E66.09 Other obesity due to excess calories

E66.1 Drug-induced obesity

Use additional code for adverse effect, if applicable, to identify drug (T36-T50 with fifth or sixth character 5)

CODING TIP✓ This code should only be assigned when documentation clearly indicates a relationship between obesity and a drug or chemical as the underlying cause. Assign a code from T36-T50 following E66.1 to indicate the drug and adverse effect.

E66.2 Morbid (severe) obesity with alveolar hypoventilation HCC

Obesity hypoventilation syndrome (OHS)
Pickwickian syndrome

E66.3 Overweight

E66.8 Other obesity

E66.9 Obesity, unspecified

Obesity NOS
AHA: 4Q 2013, 129

4 **E67 Other hyperalimentation**

EXCLUDES 1 *hyperalimentation NOS (R63.2)*
sequelae of hyperalimentation (E68)

E67.0 Hypervitaminosis A

▲ **E67.1 Hypercarotenemia**

DEFINITION Elevated beta-carotene levels in the blood that presents with yellowing of the skin, caused by excessive ingestion of carotene-rich foods, or the inability to convert carotenoids to vitamin A.

E67.2 Megavitamin-B6 syndrome

E67.3 Hypervitaminosis D

E67.8 Other specified hyperalimentation

E68 Sequelae of hyperalimentation

Code first:
condition resulting from (sequela) of hyperalimentation

Metabolic disorders (E70-E88)

EXCLUDES 1 *androgen insensitivity syndrome (E34.5-)*
congenital adrenal hyperplasia (E25.0)
Ehlers-Danlos syndrome (Q79.6)
hemolytic anemias attributable to enzyme disorders (D55.-)
Marfan's syndrome (Q87.4)
5-alpha-reductase deficiency (E29.1)

4 **E70 Disorders of aromatic amino-acid metabolism**

E70.0 Classical phenylketonuria HCC

DEFINITION Inherited metabolic disorder caused by an enzyme deficiency resulting in accumulation of phenylalanine and its metabolites in the blood with excess excretion in the urine; causes mental retardation, seizures, eczema, and abnormal body odor.

E70.1 Other hyperphenylalaninemias HCC

5 **E70.2 Disorders of tyrosine metabolism**

EXCLUDES 1 *transitory tyrosinemia of newborn (P74.5)*

E70.20 Disorder of tyrosine metabolism, unspecified HCC

E70.21 Tyrosinemia HCC

Hypertyrosinemia

E70.29 Other disorders of tyrosine metabolism HCC

Alkaptonuria
Ochronosis

5 **E70.3 Albinism**

E70.30 Albinism, unspecified HCC

6 **E70.31 Ocular albinism**

E70.310 X-linked ocular albinism HCC

E70.311 Autosomal recessive ocular albinism HCC

E70.318 Other ocular albinism HCC

E70.319 Ocular albinism, unspecified HCC

6 **E70.32 Oculocutaneous albinism**

EXCLUDES 1 *Chediak-Higashi syndrome (E70.330)*
Hermansky-Pudlak syndrome (E70.331)

E70.320 Tyrosinase negative oculocutaneous albinism HCC

Albinism I
Oculocutaneous albinism ty-neg

E70.321 Tyrosinase positive oculocutaneous albinism HCC

Albinism II
Oculocutaneous albinism ty-pos

E70.328 Other oculocutaneous albinism HCC

Cross syndrome

E70.329 Oculocutaneous albinism, unspecified HCC

6 **E70.33 Albinism with hematologic abnormality**

E70.330 Chediak-Higashi syndrome HCC

E70.331 Hermansky-Pudlak syndrome HCC

E70.338 Other albinism with hematologic abnormality HCC

E70.339 Albinism with hematologic abnormality, unspecified HCC

E70.39 Other specified albinism HCC

Piebaldism

5 **E70.4 Disorders of histidine metabolism**

E70.40 Disorders of histidine metabolism, unspecified HCC

E70.41 Histidinemia HCC

E70.49 Other disorders of histidine metabolism HCC

E70.5 Disorders of tryptophan metabolism HCC

E70.8 Other disorders of aromatic amino-acid metabolism HCC

E70.9 Disorder of aromatic amino-acid metabolism, unspecified HCC

4 **E71 Disorders of branched-chain amino-acid metabolism and fatty-acid metabolism**

E71.0 Maple-syrup-urine disease HCC

5 **E71.1 Other disorders of branched-chain amino-acid metabolism**

6 **E71.11 Branched-chain organic acidurias**

E71.110 Isovaleric acidemia HCC

E71.111 3-methylglutaconic aciduria HCC

E71.118 Other branched-chain organic acidurias HCC

6 **E71.12 Disorders of propionate metabolism**

E71.120 Methylmalonic acidemia HCC

E71.121 Propionic acidemia HCC

E71.128 Other disorders of propionate metabolism HCC

E71.19 Other disorders of branched-chain amino-acid metabolism HCC

Hyperleucine-isoleucinemia
Hypervalinemia

E71.2 Disorder of branched-chain amino-acid metabolism, unspecified HCC

5 E71.3 Disorders of fatty-acid metabolism
EXCLUDES 1 *peroxisomal disorders (E71.5)*
Refsum's disease (G60.1)
Schilder's disease (G37.0)
EXCLUDES 2 *carnitine deficiency due to inborn error of metabolism (E71.42)*

E71.30 Disorder of fatty-acid metabolism, unspecified

6 E71.31 Disorders of fatty-acid oxidation

E71.310 Long chain/very long chain acyl CoA dehydrogenase deficiency HCC
LCAD
VLCAD

E71.311 Medium chain acyl CoA dehydrogenase deficiency HCC
MCAD

E71.312 Short chain acyl CoA dehydrogenase deficiency HCC
SCAD

E71.313 Glutaric aciduria type II HCC
Glutaric aciduria type II A
Glutaric aciduria type II B
Glutaric aciduria type II C
EXCLUDES 1 *glutaric aciduria (type 1) NOS (E72.3)*

E71.314 Muscle carnitine palmitoyltransferase deficiency HCC

E71.318 Other disorders of fatty-acid oxidation HCC

E71.32 Disorders of ketone metabolism HCC

E71.39 Other disorders of fatty-acid metabolism HCC

5 E71.4 Disorders of carnitine metabolism
EXCLUDES 1 *Muscle carnitine palmitoyltransferase deficiency (E71.314)*

E71.40 Disorder of carnitine metabolism, unspecified HCC

E71.41 Primary carnitine deficiency HCC

E71.42 Carnitine deficiency due to inborn errors of metabolism HCC
Code also:
associated inborn error or metabolism

E71.43 Iatrogenic carnitine deficiency HCC
Carnitine deficiency due to hemodialysis
Carnitine deficiency due to Valproic acid therapy

6 E71.44 Other secondary carnitine deficiency

E71.440 Ruvalcaba-Myhre-Smith syndrome HCC

E71.448 Other secondary carnitine deficiency HCC

5 E71.5 Peroxisomal disorders
EXCLUDES 1 *Schilder's disease (G37.0)*

E71.50 Peroxisomal disorder, unspecified HCC

6 E71.51 Disorders of peroxisome biogenesis
Group 1 peroxisomal disorders
EXCLUDES 1 *Refsum's disease (G60.1)*

E71.510 Zellweger syndrome HCC

E71.511 Neonatal adrenoleukodystrophy HCC
EXCLUDES 1 *X-linked adrenoleukodystrophy (E71.42-)*

E71.518 Other disorders of peroxisome biogenesis HCC

6 E71.52 X-linked adrenoleukodystrophy

E71.520 Childhood cerebral X-linked adrenoleukodystrophy HCC

E71.521 Adolescent X-linked adrenoleukodystrophy HCC

E71.522 Adrenomyeloneuropathy HCC

E71.528 Other X-linked adrenoleukodystrophy HCC
Addison only phenotype adrenoleukodystrophy
Addison-Schilder adrenoleukodystrophy

E71.529 X-linked adrenoleukodystrophy, unspecified type HCC

E71.53 Other group 2 peroxisomal disorders HCC

6 E71.54 Other peroxisomal disorders

E71.540 Rhizomelic chondrodysplasia punctata HCC
EXCLUDES 1 *chondrodysplasia punctata NOS (Q77.3)*

E71.541 Zellweger-like syndrome HCC

E71.542 Other group 3 peroxisomal disorders HCC

E71.548 Other peroxisomal disorders HCC

4 E72 Other disorders of amino-acid metabolism
EXCLUDES 1 *disorders of:*
aromatic amino-acid metabolism (E70.-)
branched-chain amino-acid metabolism (E71.0-E71.2)
fatty-acid metabolism (E71.3)
purine and pyrimidine metabolism (E79.-)
gout (M1A.-, M10.-)

5 E72.0 Disorders of amino-acid transport
EXCLUDES 1 *disorders of tryptophan metabolism (E70.5)*

E72.00 Disorders of amino-acid transport, unspecified HCC

E72.01 Cystinuria HCC

E72.02 Hartnup's disease HCC

E72.03 Lowe's syndrome HCC
Use additional code for associated glaucoma (H42)

E72.04 Cystinosis HCC
Fanconi (-de Toni) (-Debré) syndrome with cystinosis
EXCLUDES 1 *Fanconi (-de Toni) (-Debré) syndrome without cystinosis (E72.09)*

E72.09 Other disorders of amino-acid transport HCC
Fanconi (-de Toni) (-Debré) syndrome, unspecified

5 E72.1 Disorders of sulfur-bearing amino-acid metabolism
EXCLUDES 1 *cystinosis (E72.04)*
cystinuria (E72.01)
transcobalamin II deficiency (D51.2)

E72.10 Disorders of sulfur-bearing amino-acid metabolism, unspecified HCC

E72.11 Homocystinuria HCC
Cystathionine synthase deficiency

E72.12 Methylenetetrahydrofolate reductase deficiency HCC

E72.19 Other disorders of sulfur-bearing amino-acid metabolism HCC
Cystathioninuria
Methioninemia
Sulfite oxidase deficiency

5 E72.2 Disorders of urea cycle metabolism
EXCLUDES 1 *disorders of ornithine metabolism (E72.4)*

E72.20 Disorder of urea cycle metabolism, unspecified HCC
Hyperammonemia
EXCLUDES 1 *hyperammonemia- hyperornithinemia- homocitrullinemia syndrome E72.4*
transient hyperammonemia of newborn (P74.6)

E72.21 Argininemia HCC

E72.22 Arginosuccinic aciduria HCC

E72.23 Citrullinemia HCC

E72.29 Other disorders of urea cycle metabolism HCC

E72.3 Disorders of lysine and hydroxylysine metabolism HCC
Glutaric aciduria NOS
Glutaric aciduria (type I)
Hydroxylysinemia
Hyperlysinemia
EXCLUDES 1 *glutaric aciduria type II (E71.313)*
Refsum's disease (G60.1)
Zellweger syndrome (E71.510)

E72.4 Disorders of ornithine metabolism HCC
Hyperammonemia-Hyperornithinemia-Homocitrullinemia syndrome
Ornithinemia (types I, II)
Ornithine transcarbamylase deficiency
EXCLUDES 1 *hereditary choroidal dystrophy (H31.2-)*

5 E72.5 Disorders of glycine metabolism

E72.50 Disorder of glycine metabolism, unspecified HCC

E72.51 Non-ketotic hyperglycinemia HCC

E72.52 Trimethylaminuria HCC

▲ E72.53 Primary hyperoxaluria HCC
Oxalosis
Oxaluria

E72.59 Other disorders of glycine metabolism HCC
D-glycericacidemia
Hyperhydroxyprolinemia
Hyperprolinemia (types I, II)
Sarcosinemia

▲ 5 E72.8 Other specified disorders of amino-acid metabolism HCC

● **E72.81 Disorders of gamma aminobutyric acid metabolism**
4-hydroxybutyric aciduria
Disorders of GABA metabolism
GABA metabolic defect
GABA transaminase deficiency
GABA-T deficiency
Gamma-hydroxybutyric aciduria
SSADHD
Succinic semialdehyde dehydrogenase deficiency

● **E72.89 Other specified disorders of amino-acid metabolism**
Disorders of beta-amino-acid metabolism
Disorders of gamma-glutamyl cycle

E72.9 Disorder of amino-acid metabolism, unspecified HCC

4 E73 Lactose intolerance

E73.0 Congenital lactase deficiency
E73.1 Secondary lactase deficiency
E73.8 Other lactose intolerance
E73.9 Lactose intolerance, unspecified

4 E74 Other disorders of carbohydrate metabolism

EXCLUDES 1 *diabetes mellitus (E08-E13)*
hypoglycemia NOS (E16.2)
increased secretion of glucagon (E16.3)
mucopolysaccharidosis (E76.0-E76.3)

5 E74.0 Glycogen storage disease

E74.00 Glycogen storage disease, unspecified HCC

E74.01 von Gierke disease HCC
Type I glycogen storage disease

E74.02 Pompe disease HCC
Cardiac glycogenosis
Type II glycogen storage disease

DEFINITION Pompe disease is also called type II glycogen storage disease and is a congenital disease caused by a metabolic error in which the body deposits an abnormally high amount of glycogen in the kidneys and liver. The disease produces symptoms such as hypoglycemia (low blood sugar) and hyperlipemia (an excess of lipid molecules in the blood, which can lead to problems such as clogged arteries and heart attacks).

E74.03 Cori disease HCC
Forbes disease
Type III glycogen storage disease

E74.04 McArdle disease HCC
Type V glycogen storage disease

E74.09 Other glycogen storage disease HCC
Andersen disease
Hers disease
Tauri disease
Glycogen storage disease, types 0, IV, VI-XI
Liver phosphorylase deficiency
Muscle phosphofructokinase deficiency

5 E74.1 Disorders of fructose metabolism

EXCLUDES 1 *muscle phosphofructokinase deficiency (E74.09)*

E74.10 Disorder of fructose metabolism, unspecified

E74.11 Essential fructosuria
Fructokinase deficiency

E74.12 Hereditary fructose intolerance
Fructosemia

E74.19 Other disorders of fructose metabolism
Fructose-1, 6-diphosphatase deficiency

5 E74.2 Disorders of galactose metabolism

E74.20 Disorders of galactose metabolism, unspecified HCC
E74.21 Galactosemia HCC
E74.29 Other disorders of galactose metabolism HCC
Galactokinase deficiency

5 E74.3 Other disorders of intestinal carbohydrate absorption

EXCLUDES 2 *lactose intolerance (E73.-)*

E74.31 Sucrase-isomaltase deficiency

E74.39 Other disorders of intestinal carbohydrate absorption
Disorder of intestinal carbohydrate absorption NOS
Glucose-galactose malabsorption
Sucrase deficiency

E74.4 Disorders of pyruvate metabolism and gluconeogenesis HCC
Deficiency of phosphoenolpyruvate carboxykinase
Deficiency of pyruvate carboxylase
Deficiency of pyruvate dehydrogenase

EXCLUDES 1 *disorders of pyruvate metabolism and gluconeogenesis with anemia (D55.-)*
Leigh's syndrome (G31.82)

E74.8 Other specified disorders of carbohydrate metabolism HCC
Essential pentosuria
Renal glycosuria

DEFINITION Excess glucose in the urine with normal levels in the blood, due to renal tubules' inability to reabsorb glucose completely.

E74.9 Disorder of carbohydrate metabolism, unspecified HCC

4 E75 Disorders of sphingolipid metabolism and other lipid storage disorders

EXCLUDES 1 *mucolipidosis, types I-III (E77.0-E77.1)*
Refsum's disease (G60.1)

5 E75.0 GM2 gangliosidosis

E75.00 GM2 gangliosidosis, unspecified
E75.01 Sandhoff disease
E75.02 Tay-Sachs disease
E75.09 Other GM2 gangliosidosis
Adult GM2 gangliosidosis
Juvenile GM2 gangliosidosis

5 E75.1 Other and unspecified gangliosidosis

E75.10 Unspecified gangliosidosis
Gangliosidosis NOS

E75.11 Mucolipidosis IV

E75.19 Other gangliosidosis
GM1 gangliosidosis
GM3 gangliosidosis

5 E75.2 Other sphingolipidosis

EXCLUDES 1 *adrenoleukodystrophy [Addison-Schilder] (E71.528)*

E75.21 Fabry (-Anderson) disease HCC
E75.22 Gaucher disease HCC
E75.23 Krabbe disease

6 E75.24 Niemann-Pick disease

E75.240 Niemann-Pick disease type A HCC
E75.241 Niemann-Pick disease type B HCC
E75.242 Niemann-Pick disease type C HCC
E75.243 Niemann-Pick disease type D HCC
E75.248 Other Niemann-Pick disease HCC
E75.249 Niemann-Pick disease, unspecified HCC

E75.25 Metachromatic leukodystrophy

● **E75.26 Sulfatase deficiency**
Multiple sulfatase deficiency (MSD)

▲ **E75.29 Other sphingolipidosis**
Farber's syndrome
Sulfatide lipidosis

E75.3 Sphingolipidosis, unspecified HCC

E75.4 Neuronal ceroid lipofuscinosis
Batten disease
Bielschowsky-Jansky disease
Kufs disease
Spielmeyer-Vogt disease

E75.5 Other lipid storage disorders
Cerebrotendinous cholesterosis [van Bogaert-Scherer-Epstein]
Wolman's disease

E75.6 Lipid storage disorder, unspecified

4 E76 Disorders of glycosaminoglycan metabolism

5 E76.0 Mucopolysaccharidosis, type I

E76.01 Hurler's syndrome HCC
E76.02 Hurler-Scheie syndrome HCC
E76.03 Scheie's syndrome HCC

E76.1 Mucopolysaccharidosis, type II HCC
Hunter's syndrome

5 E76.2 Other mucopolysaccharidoses

6 E76.21 Morquio mucopolysaccharidoses

E76.210 **Morquio A mucopolysaccharidoses** HCC
Classic Morquio syndrome
Morquio syndrome A
Mucopolysaccharidosis, type IVA

E76.211 **Morquio B mucopolysaccharidoses** HCC
Morquio-like mucopolysaccharidoses
Morquio-like syndrome
Morquio syndrome B
Mucopolysaccharidosis, type IVB

E76.219 **Morquio mucopolysaccharidoses, unspecified** HCC
Morquio syndrome
Mucopolysaccharidosis, type IV

E76.22 **Sanfilippo mucopolysaccharidoses** HCC
Mucopolysaccharidosis, type III (A) (B) (C) (D)
Sanfilippo A syndrome
Sanfilippo B syndrome
Sanfilippo C syndrome
Sanfilippo D syndrome

E76.29 **Other mucopolysaccharidoses** HCC
beta-Glucuronidase deficiency
Maroteaux-Lamy (mild) (severe) syndrome
Mucopolysaccharidosis, types VI, VII

E76.3 **Mucopolysaccharidosis, unspecified** HCC

E76.8 **Other disorders of glucosaminoglycan metabolism** HCC

E76.9 **Glucosaminoglycan metabolism disorder, unspecified** HCC

4 E77 Disorders of glycoprotein metabolism

E77.0 **Defects in post-translational modification of lysosomal enzymes** HCC
Mucolipidosis II [I-cell disease]
Mucolipidosis III [pseudo-Hurler polydystrophy]

E77.1 **Defects in glycoprotein degradation** HCC
Aspartylglucosaminuria
Fucosidosis
Mannosidosis
Sialidosis [mucolipidosis I]

E77.8 **Other disorders of glycoprotein metabolism** HCC

E77.9 **Disorder of glycoprotein metabolism, unspecified** HCC

4 E78 Disorders of lipoprotein metabolism and other lipidemias

EXCLUDES 1 *sphingolipidosis (E75.0-E75.3)*

5 E78.0 **Pure hypercholesterolemia**
AHA: 4Q 2016, 13

E78.00 **Pure hypercholesterolemia, unspecified**
Fredrickson's hyperlipoproteinemia, type IIa
Hyperbetalipoproteinemia
Low-density-lipoprotein-type [LDL] hyperlipoproteinemia
(Pure) hypercholesterolemia NOS

E78.01 **Familial hypercholesterolemia**

E78.1 **Pure hyperglyceridemia**
Elevated fasting triglycerides
Endogenous hyperglyceridemia
Fredrickson's hyperlipoproteinemia, type IV
Hyperlipidemia, group B
Hyperprebetalipoproteinemia
Very-low-density-lipoprotein-type [VLDL] hyperlipoproteinemia

▲ E78.2 **Mixed hyperlipidemia**
Broad- or floating-betalipoproteinemia
Combined hyperlipidemia NOS
Elevated cholesterol with elevated triglycerides NEC
Fredrickson's hyperlipoproteinemia, type IIb or III
Hyperbetalipoproteinemia with prebetalipoproteinemia
Hypercholesteremia with endogenous hyperglyceridemia
Hyperlipidemia, group C
Tubo-eruptive xanthoma
Xanthoma tuberosum

EXCLUDES 1 *cerebrotendinous cholesterosis [van Bogaert-Scherer- Epstein] (E75.5)*
familial combined hyperlipidemia (E78.49)

E78.3 **Hyperchylomicronemia**
Chylomicron retention disease
Fredrickson's hyperlipoproteinemia, type I or V
Hyperlipidemia, group D
Mixed hyperglyceridemia

▲ 5 E78.4 **Other hyperlipidemia**

● E78.41 **Elevated Lipoprotein(a)**
Elevated Lp(a)

● E78.49 **Other hyperlipidemia**
Familial combined hyperlipidemia

E78.5 **Hyperlipidemia, unspecified**

DEFINITION An excess of lipids or fats in the blood.

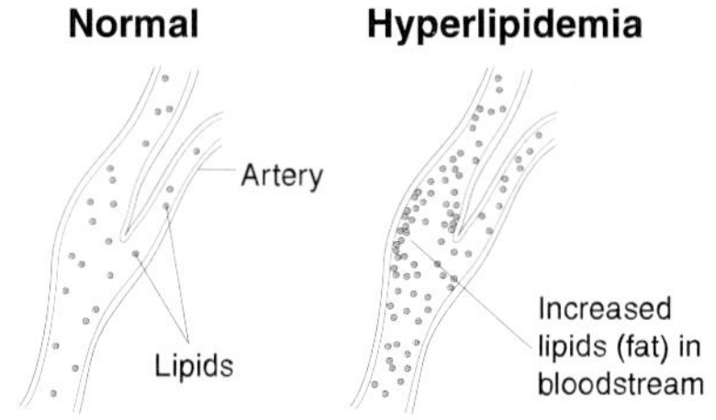

E78.6 **Lipoprotein deficiency**
Abetalipoproteinemia
Depressed HDL cholesterol
High-density lipoprotein deficiency
Hypoalphalipoproteinemia
Hypobetalipoproteinemia (familial)
Lecithin cholesterol acyltransferase deficiency
Tangier disease

5 E78.7 **Disorders of bile acid and cholesterol metabolism**

EXCLUDES 1 *Niemann-Pick disease type C (E75.242)*

E78.70 **Disorder of bile acid and cholesterol metabolism, unspecified**

E78.71 **Barth syndrome**

E78.72 **Smith-Lemli-Opitz syndrome**

E78.79 **Other disorders of bile acid and cholesterol metabolism**

5 E78.8 **Other disorders of lipoprotein metabolism**

E78.81 **Lipoid dermatoarthritis**

E78.89 **Other lipoprotein metabolism disorders**

E78.9 **Disorder of lipoprotein metabolism, unspecified**

4 E79 Disorders of purine and pyrimidine metabolism

EXCLUDES 1 *Ataxia-telangiectasia (Q87.1)*
Bloom's syndrome (Q82.8)
Cockayne's syndrome (Q87.1)
calculus of kidney (N20.0)
combined immunodeficiency disorders (D81.-)
Fanconi's anemia (D61.09)
gout (M1A.-, M10.-)
orotaciduric anemia (D53.0)
progeria (E34.8)
Werner's syndrome (E34.8)
xeroderma pigmentosum (Q82.1)

E79.0 **Hyperuricemia without signs of inflammatory arthritis and tophaceous disease**
Asymptomatic hyperuricemia

E79.1 **Lesch-Nyhan syndrome** HCC
HGPRT deficiency

E79.2 **Myoadenylate deaminase deficiency** HCC

E79.8 **Other disorders of purine and pyrimidine metabolism** HCC
Hereditary xanthinuria

E79.9 **Disorder of purine and pyrimidine metabolism, unspecified** HCC

4 E80 Disorders of porphyrin and bilirubin metabolism

INCLUDES defects of catalase and peroxidase

E80.0 **Hereditary erythropoietic porphyria** HCC
Congenital erythropoietic porphyria
Erythropoietic protoporphyria

E80.1 **Porphyria cutanea tarda** HCC

5 E80.2 **Other and unspecified porphyria**

E80.20 **Unspecified porphyria** HCC
Porphyria NOS

E80.21 **Acute intermittent (hepatic) porphyria** HCC

E80.29 **Other porphyria** HCC
Hereditary coproporphyria

E80.3 **Defects of catalase and peroxidase** HCC
Acatalasia [Takahara]

E80.4 **Gilbert syndrome**

DEFINITION A harmless inborn error of bilirubin metabolism from an abnormal liver enzyme causing a benign elevation of unconjugated bilirubin with no liver damage or hematologic abnormalities.

E80.5 Crigler-Najjar syndrome

E80.6 Other disorders of bilirubin metabolism
Dubin-Johnson syndrome
Rotor's syndrome

E80.7 Disorder of bilirubin metabolism, unspecified

4 E83 Disorders of mineral metabolism

EXCLUDES 1 *dietary mineral deficiency (E58-E61)*
parathyroid disorders (E20-E21)
vitamin D deficiency (E55.-)

5 E83.0 Disorders of copper metabolism

E83.00 Disorder of copper metabolism, unspecified

E83.01 Wilson's disease
Code also:
associated Kayser Fleischer ring (H18.04-)

E83.09 Other disorders of copper metabolism
Menkes' (kinky hair) (steely hair) disease

5 E83.1 Disorders of iron metabolism

EXCLUDES 1 *iron deficiency anemia (D50.-)*
sideroblastic anemia (D64.0-D64.3)

E83.10 Disorder of iron metabolism, unspecified

6 E83.11 Hemochromatosis

EXCLUDES 1 *GALD (P78.84)*
Gestational alloimmune liver disease (P78.84)
Neonatal hemochromatosis (P78.84)

E83.110 Hereditary hemochromatosis HCC
Bronzed diabetes
Pigmentary cirrhosis (of liver)
Primary (hereditary) hemochromatosis

DEFINITION A genetic problem causing the body to store too much iron, resulting in liver swelling, skin bronzing, and development of diabetes, arthritis, and organ failure.

E83.111 Hemochromatosis due to repeated red blood cell transfusions
Iron overload due to repeated red blood cell transfusions
Transfusion (red blood cell) associated hemochromatosis

E83.118 Other hemochromatosis

E83.119 Hemochromatosis, unspecified

E83.19 Other disorders of iron metabolism
Use additional code, if applicable, for idiopathic pulmonary hemosiderosis (J84.03)

E83.2 Disorders of zinc metabolism
Acrodermatitis enteropathica

5 E83.3 Disorders of phosphorus metabolism and phosphatases

EXCLUDES 1 *adult osteomalacia (M83.-)*
osteoporosis (M80.-)

E83.30 Disorder of phosphorus metabolism, unspecified

E83.31 Familial hypophosphatemia
Vitamin D-resistant osteomalacia
Vitamin D-resistant rickets

EXCLUDES 1 *vitamin D-deficiency rickets (E55.0)*

E83.32 Hereditary vitamin D-dependent rickets (type 1) (type 2)
25-hydroxyvitamin D 1-alpha-hydroxylase deficiency
Pseudovitamin D deficiency
Vitamin D receptor defect

E83.39 Other disorders of phosphorus metabolism
Acid phosphatase deficiency
Hypophosphatasia

5 E83.4 Disorders of magnesium metabolism

E83.40 Disorders of magnesium metabolism, unspecified

E83.41 Hypermagnesemia

E83.42 Hypomagnesemia

E83.49 Other disorders of magnesium metabolism

5 E83.5 Disorders of calcium metabolism

EXCLUDES 1 *chondrocalcinosis (M11.1-M11.2)*
hungry bone syndrome (E83.81)
hyperparathyroidism (E21.0-E21.3)

E83.50 Unspecified disorder of calcium metabolism

E83.51 Hypocalcemia

DEFINITION Reduced calcium levels in the blood causing hyperactive deep tendon reflexes, Chvostek's sign, muscle and abdominal cramps, and carpopedal spasm.

E83.52 Hypercalcemia
Familial hypocalciuric hypercalcemia

DEFINITION Excess calcium levels in the blood causing fatigue, muscle weakness, depression, anorexia, nausea, and constipation.

▲ **E83.59 Other disorders of calcium metabolism**

5 E83.8 Other disorders of mineral metabolism

E83.81 Hungry bone syndrome

DEFINITION Low levels of calcium due to elevated parathyroid hormone levels or thyrotoxicosis that later return to normal or lower levels after treatment, causing bones to hoard calcium, resulting in increased bone density.

E83.89 Other disorders of mineral metabolism

E83.9 Disorder of mineral metabolism, unspecified

4 E84 Cystic fibrosis

INCLUDES mucoviscidosis

Code also:
exocrine pancreatic insufficiency (K86.81)

CODING TIP✓ When reporting a E84 code, do not use an additional code for other disease of the lung. Chronic lung disease with bronchiectasis is an integral part of cystic fibrosis and is not reported separately. However, an infection, such as pneumonia, should be coded separately. A patient with both pulmonary manifestations and gastrointestinal manifestations is coded with E84.0 and E84.1. Other manifestations (E84.8) include diabetes (E08) and right ventricular hypertrophy (I51.7).

E84.0 Cystic fibrosis with pulmonary manifestations HCC
Use additional code to identify any infectious organism present, such as:
Pseudomonas (B96.5)

5 E84.1 Cystic fibrosis with intestinal manifestations

E84.11 Meconium ileus in cystic fibrosis N HCC

EXCLUDES 1 *meconium ileus not due to cystic fibrosis (P76.0)*

E84.19 Cystic fibrosis with other intestinal manifestations HCC
Distal intestinal obstruction syndrome

E84.8 Cystic fibrosis with other manifestations HCC

E84.9 Cystic fibrosis, unspecified HCC

DEFINITION Defective gene causing overproduction of mucous that builds up in lung passages, resulting in life-threatening respiratory problems.

Cystic fibrosis, unspecified

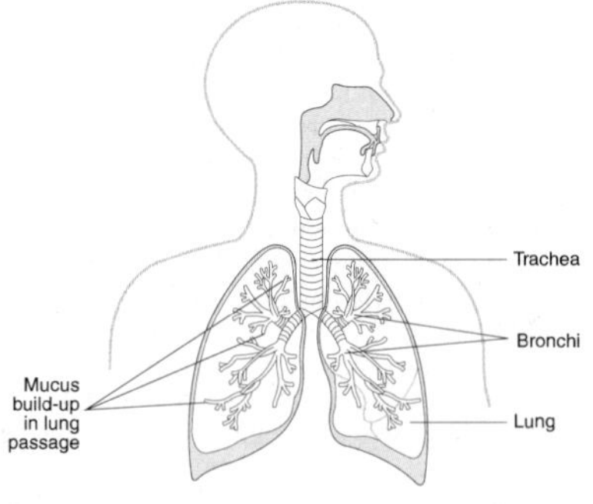

4 E85 Amyloidosis

EXCLUDES 2 *Alzheimer's disease (G30.0-)*

E85.0 Non-neuropathic heredofamilial amyloidosis HCC
Hereditary amyloid nephropathy
Code also associated disorders, such as:
autoinflammatory syndromes (M04.-)

EXCLUDES 2 *Transthyretin-related (ATTR) familial amyloid cardiomyopathy (E85.4)*

E85.1 **Neuropathic heredofamilial amyloidosis** HCC
Amyloid polyneuropathy (Portuguese)
Transthyretin-related (ATTR) familial amyloid polyneuropathy
AHA: 4Q 2012, 99-100

E85.2 **Heredofamilial amyloidosis, unspecified** HCC

E85.3 **Secondary systemic amyloidosis** HCC
Hemodialysis-associated amyloidosis
DEFINITION Secondary amyloidosis is also known as reactive systemic amyloidosis, in which the deposited protein fibrils are of the AA type caused by a reaction to a chronic infection or other condition, such as osteomyelitis, rheumatoid arthritis, or a noninfectious disease process such as kidney failure with long term hemodialysis.

E85.4 **Organ-limited amyloidosis** HCC
Localized amyloidosis
Transthyretin-related (ATTR) familial amyloid cardiomyopathy

5 E85.8 **Other amyloidosis** HCC

E85.81 **Light chain (AL) amyloidosis** HCC
AHA: 4Q 2017, 6

E85.82 **Wild-type transthyretin-related (ATTR) amyloidosis** HCC
Senile systemic amyloidosis (SSA)
AHA: 4Q 2017, 6

E85.89 **Other amyloidosis** HCC
AHA: 4Q 2017, 6

E85.9 **Amyloidosis, unspecified** HCC
DEFINITION Abnormal accumulation of amyloid-like proteins in tissues.

4 E86 Volume depletion

Use additional code(s) for any associated disorders of electrolyte and acid-base balance (E87.-)

EXCLUDES 1 *dehydration of newborn (P74.1)*
hypovolemic shock NOS (R57.1)
postprocedural hypovolemic shock (T81.19)
traumatic hypovolemic shock (T79.4)

E86.0 **Dehydration**
GUIDELINES **Section I.C.2.c.3)**
When the admission/encounter is for management of dehydration due to the malignancy and only the dehydration is being treated (intravenous rehydration), the dehydration is sequenced first, followed by the code(s) for the malignancy.
AHA: 1Q 2014, 7

E86.1 **Hypovolemia**
Depletion of volume of plasma
DEFINITION Abnormal decrease in the total volume of circulating blood with a corresponding loss of sodium electrolytes.

E86.9 **Volume depletion, unspecified**

4 E87 Other disorders of fluid, electrolyte and acid-base balance

EXCLUDES 1 *diabetes insipidus (E23.2)*
electrolyte imbalance associated with hyperemesis gravidarum (O21.1)
electrolyte imbalance following ectopic or molar pregnancy (O08.5)
familial periodic paralysis (G72.3)

E87.0 **Hyperosmolality and hypernatremia**
Sodium [Na] excess
Sodium [Na] overload
AHA: 1Q 2014, 7

E87.1 **Hypo-osmolality and hyponatremia**
Sodium [Na] deficiency
EXCLUDES 1 *syndrome of inappropriate secretion of antidiuretic hormone (E22.2)*
AHA: 1Q 2014, 7

E87.2 **Acidosis**
Acidosis NOS
Lactic acidosis
Metabolic acidosis
Respiratory acidosis
EXCLUDES 1 *diabetic acidosis - see categories E08-E10, E13 with ketoacidosis*
DEFINITION An abnormal increase in the acidity of body fluids, caused either by accumulation of acids or by depletion of bicarbonates.

E87.3 **Alkalosis**
Alkalosis NOS
Metabolic alkalosis
Respiratory alkalosis

E87.4 **Mixed disorder of acid-base balance**

E87.5 **Hyperkalemia**
Potassium [K] excess
Potassium [K] overload
DEFINITION An abnormally high concentration of potassium ions in the blood.

E87.6 **Hypokalemia**
Potassium [K] deficiency
DEFINITION Low potassium level in the blood causing neuromuscular disorders ranging from weakness to paralysis, electrocardiographic abnormalities, renal disease, and gastrointestinal disorders.

5 E87.7 **Fluid overload**
EXCLUDES 1 *edema NOS (R60.9)*
fluid retention (R60.9)
DEFINITION High infusion rates or transfusion volumes not processed effectively by the recipient, causing circulatory system overload marked by acute respiratory distress.

E87.70 **Fluid overload, unspecified**

E87.71 **Transfusion associated circulatory overload**
Fluid overload due to transfusion (blood) (blood components)
TACO

E87.79 **Other fluid overload**

E87.8 **Other disorders of electrolyte and fluid balance, not elsewhere classified**
Electrolyte imbalance NOS
Hyperchloremia
Hypochloremia

4 E88 Other and unspecified metabolic disorders

Use additional codes for associated conditions

EXCLUDES 1 *histiocytosis X (chronic) (C96.6)*

5 E88.0 **Disorders of plasma-protein metabolism, not elsewhere classified**
EXCLUDES 1 *disorder of lipoprotein metabolism (E78.-)*
monoclonal gammopathy (of undetermined significance) (D47.2)
polyclonal hypergammaglobulinemia (D89.0)
Waldenström macroglobulinemia (C88.0)

E88.01 **Alpha-1-antitrypsin deficiency** HCC
AAT deficiency

● E88.02 **Plasminogen deficiency**
Dysplasminogenemia
Hypoplasminogenemia
Type 1 plasminogen deficiency
Type 2 plasminogen deficiency
Code also:
, if applicable, ligneous conjunctivitis (H10.51)
Use additional code for associated findings, such as:
hydrocephalus (G91.4)
ligneous conjunctivitis (H10.51)
otitis media (H67.-)
respiratory disorder related to plasminogen deficiency (J99)

E88.09 **Other disorders of plasma-protein metabolism, not elsewhere classified**
Bisalbuminemia

E88.1 **Lipodystrophy, not elsewhere classified**
Lipodystrophy NOS
EXCLUDES 1 *Whipple's disease (K90.81)*
DEFINITION Defective fat metabolism resulting in abnormal or degenerative subcutaneous fat deposits that appear as lumps or dents under the skin.

E88.2 **Lipomatosis, not elsewhere classified**
Lipomatosis NOS
Lipomatosis (Check) dolorosa [Dercum]

E88.3 Tumor lysis syndrome
Tumor lysis syndrome (spontaneous)
Tumor lysis syndrome following antineoplastic drug chemotherapy
Use additional code for adverse effect, if applicable, to identify drug (T45.1X5)

E88.4 Mitochondrial metabolism disorders
EXCLUDES 1 *disorders of pyruvate metabolism (E74.4)*
Kearns-Sayre syndrome (H49.81)
Leber's disease (H47.22)
Leigh's encephalopathy (G31.82)
Mitochondrial myopathy, NEC (G71.3)
Reye's syndrome (G93.7)

E88.40 Mitochondrial metabolism disorder, unspecified HCC

E88.41 MELAS syndrome HCC
Mitochondrial myopathy, encephalopathy, lactic acidosis and stroke-like episodes

E88.42 MERRF syndrome HCC
Myoclonic epilepsy associated with ragged-red fibers
Code also:
progressive myoclonic epilepsy (G40.3-)

E88.49 Other mitochondrial metabolism disorders HCC

E88.8 Other specified metabolic disorders

E88.81 Metabolic syndrome
Dysmetabolic syndrome X
Use additional codes for associated manifestations, such as:
obesity (E66.-)

CODING TIP ✓ Metabolic syndrome (also called dysmetabolic syndrome X) involves a cluster of symptoms placing individuals at risk for development of a number of disease processes. Manifestations of metabolic syndrome confirmed by the physician, such as obesity (and BMI as calculated by the clinical record documentation), should additionally be coded following E88.81.

E88.89 Other specified metabolic disorders HCC
Launois-Bensaude adenolipomatosis
EXCLUDES 1 *adult pulmonary Langerhans cell histiocytosis (J84.82)*

E88.9 Metabolic disorder, unspecified

Postprocedural endocrine and metabolic complications and disorders, not elsewhere classified (E89)

CODING TIP ✓ Conditions classifiable to E89 are classifiable as postprocedural complications. These conditions should only be assigned when diagnostic statements clearly indicate that the condition is a complication of a procedure.

E89 Postprocedural endocrine and metabolic complications and disorders, not elsewhere classified
EXCLUDES 2 *intraoperative complications of endocrine system organ or structure (E36.0-, E36.1-, E36.8)*

E89.0 Postprocedural hypothyroidism
Postirradiation hypothyroidism
Postsurgical hypothyroidism

DEFINITION Underactive thyroid gland due to surgery or radiation, causing an inadequate production of thyroid hormone and a slowing of metabolic processes.

E89.1 Postprocedural hypoinsulinemia
Postpancreatectomy hyperglycemia
Postsurgical hypoinsulinemia
Use additional code, if applicable, to identify:
acquired absence of pancreas (Z90.41-)
diabetes mellitus (postpancreatectomy) (postprocedural) (E13.-)
insulin use (Z79.4)
EXCLUDES 1 *transient postprocedural hyperglycemia (R73.9)*
transient postprocedural hypoglycemia (E16.2)

GUIDELINES **Section I.C.4.a.6)(b)(i)**
For postpancreatectomy diabetes mellitus (lack of insulin due to the surgical removal of all or part of the pancreas), assign code E89.1, Postprocedural hypoinsulinemia. Assign a code from category E13 and a code from subcategory Z90.41-, Acquired absence of pancreas, as additional codes.

CODING TIP ✓ Because the pancreas is the organ that produces insulin, the removal of even a portion of the pancreas can produce diabetic-like symptoms. If manifestations are produced because of the hyperglycemia and lack of insulin, the provider must document support for adding the codes for manifestations after E89.1 with the appropriate E13 code(s). Also add the acquired absence of pancreas (Z90.41-) and use of insulin (Z79.4).

E89.2 Postprocedural hypoparathyroidism HCC
Parathyroprival tetany

E89.3 Postprocedural hypopituitarism HCC
Postirradiation hypopituitarism

E89.4 Postprocedural ovarian failure

E89.40 Asymptomatic postprocedural ovarian failure ♀
Postprocedural ovarian failure NOS

E89.41 Symptomatic postprocedural ovarian failure ♀
Symptoms such as flushing, sleeplessness, headache, lack of concentration, associated with postprocedural menopause

E89.5 Postprocedural testicular hypofunction ♂

E89.6 Postprocedural adrenocortical (-medullary) hypofunction HCC

E89.8 Other postprocedural endocrine and metabolic complications and disorders

E89.81 Postprocedural hemorrhage of an endocrine system organ or structure following a procedure

E89.810 Postprocedural hemorrhage of an endocrine system organ or structure following an endocrine system procedure

E89.811 Postprocedural hemorrhage of an endocrine system organ or structure following other procedure

E89.82 Postprocedural hematoma and seroma of an endocrine system organ or structure

E89.820 Postprocedural hematoma of an endocrine system organ or structure following an endocrine system procedure

E89.821 Postprocedural hematoma of an endocrine system organ or structure following other procedure

E89.822 Postprocedural seroma of an endocrine system organ or structure following an endocrine system procedure

E89.823 Postprocedural seroma of an endocrine system organ or structure following other procedure

E89.89 Other postprocedural endocrine and metabolic complications and disorders
Use additional code, if applicable, to further specify disorder

CHAPTER 5: MENTAL, BEHAVIORAL AND NEURODEVELOPMENTAL DISORDERS (F01-F99)

INCLUDES disorders of psychological development

EXCLUDES 2 *symptoms, signs and abnormal clinical laboratory findings, not elsewhere classified (R00-R99)*

This chapter contains the following blocks:

F01-F09	Mental disorders due to known physiological conditions
F10-F19	Mental and behavioral disorders due to psychoactive substance use
F20-F29	Schizophrenia, schizotypal, delusional, and other non-mood psychotic disorders
F30-F39	Mood [affective] disorders
F40-F48	Anxiety, dissociative, stress-related, somatoform and other nonpsychotic mental disorders
F50-F59	Behavioral syndromes associated with physiological disturbances and physical factors
F60-F69	Disorders of adult personality and behavior
F70-F79	Intellectual disabilities
F80-F89	Pervasive and specific developmental disorders
F90-F98	Behavioral and emotional disorders with onset usually occurring in childhood and adolescence
F99	Unspecified mental disorder

Mental disorders due to known physiological conditions (F01-F09)

Note: This block comprises a range of mental disorders grouped together on the basis of their having in common a demonstrable etiology in cerebral disease, brain injury, or other insult leading to cerebral dysfunction. The dysfunction may be primary, as in diseases, injuries, and insults that affect the brain directly and selectively; or secondary, as in systemic diseases and disorders that attack the brain only as one of the multiple organs or systems of the body that are involved.

CODING TIP✓ Conditions classifiable here are specifically reportable as due to an underlying cause or condition.

4 F01 Vascular dementia

Vascular dementia as a result of infarction of the brain due to vascular disease, including hypertensive cerebrovascular disease.

INCLUDES arteriosclerotic dementia

Code first:
the underlying physiological condition or sequelae of cerebrovascular disease.

5 F01.5 Vascular dementia

CODING TIP✓ Vascular dementia must be specified by the physician and may also be reported as "multi-infarct dementia." In this case it should be coded as a sequela of cerebrovascular accident (stroke). This type of dementia also may be related to other cerebral vascular disorders including vascular hypertension and cerebral atherosclerosis. Major neurocognitive disorder is coded as vascular dementia if the physician does not specify another cause.

F01.50 Vascular dementia without behavioral disturbance A

Major neurocognitive disorder without behavioral disturbance

F01.51 Vascular dementia with behavioral disturbance A

Major neurocognitive disorder due to vascular disease, with behavioral disturbance
Major neurocognitive disorder with aggressive behavior
Major neurocognitive disorder with combative behavior
Major neurocognitive disorder with violent behavior
Vascular dementia with aggressive behavior
Vascular dementia with combative behavior
Vascular dementia with violent behavior
Use additional code, if applicable, to identify wandering in vascular dementia (Z91.83)

CODING TIP✓ Anxiety is not considered a behavior indicated by a 5th character of 1. Anxiety, when documented by the physician, in addition to dementia, should be coded separately.

4 F02 Dementia in other diseases classified elsewhere

INCLUDES Major neurocognitive disorder in other diseases classified elsewhere

Code first the underlying physiological condition, such as:
Alzheimer's (G30.-)
cerebral lipidosis (E75.4)
Creutzfeldt-Jakob disease (A81.0-)
dementia with Lewy bodies (G31.83)
dementia with Parkinsonism (G31.83)
epilepsy and recurrent seizures (G40.-)
frontotemporal dementia (G31.09)
hepatolenticular degeneration (E83.0)
human immunodeficiency virus [HIV] disease (B20)
Huntington's disease (G10)
hypercalcemia (E83.52)
hypothyroidism, acquired (E00-E03.-)
intoxications (T36-T65)
Jakob-Creutzfeldt disease (A81.0-)
multiple sclerosis (G35)
neurosyphilis (A52.17)
niacin deficiency [pellagra] (E52)
Parkinson's disease (G20)
Pick's disease (G31.01)
polyarteritis nodosa (M30.0)
prion disease (A81.9)
systemic lupus erythematosus (M32.-)
traumatic brain injury (S06.-)
trypanosomiasis (B56.-, B57.-)
vitamin B deficiency (E53.8)

EXCLUDES 2 *dementia in alcohol and psychoactive substance disorders (F10-F19, with .17, .27, .97)*
vascular dementia (F01.5-)

5 F02.8 Dementia in other diseases classified elsewhere

CODING TIP✓ Codes F02.80 and F02.81 are manifestation-only codes and should be used only to report dementia in an etiology/manifestation pairing. An F02.8- code should never be used alone and inappropriate use of these codes may result in claims edits. Always code the etiology first, followed by the appropriate F02.8- code to specify dementia with or without behavioral disturbance. The physician must document a diagnosis of dementia and the presence of behavioral disturbances.

F02.80 *Dementia in other diseases classified elsewhere without behavioral disturbance*

Dementia in other diseases classified elsewhere NOS
Major neurocognitive disorder in other diseases classified elsewhere
AHA: 2Q 2016, 6
AHA: 4Q 2016, 141
AHA: 1Q 2017, 43

F02.81 *Dementia in other diseases classified elsewhere with behavioral disturbance*

Dementia in other diseases classified elsewhere with aggressive behavior
Dementia in other diseases classified elsewhere with combative behavior
Dementia in other diseases classified elsewhere with violent behavior
Major neurocognitive disorder in other diseases classified elsewhere with aggressive behavior
Major neurocognitive disorder in other diseases classified elsewhere with combative behavior
Major neurocognitive disorder in other diseases classified elsewhere with violent behavior
Use additional code, if applicable, to identify wandering in dementia in conditions classified elsewhere (Z91.83)

CODING TIP✓ Anxiety is not considered a behavior indicated by a 5th character of 1. Anxiety, when documented by the physician, in addition to dementia, should be coded separately.
AHA: 2Q 2017, 7

F03 Unspecified dementia
Presenile dementia NOS
Presenile psychosis NOS
Primary degenerative dementia NOS
Senile dementia NOS
Senile dementia depressed or paranoid type
Senile psychosis NOS
EXCLUDES 1 *senility NOS (R41.81)*
EXCLUDES 2 *mild memory disturbance due to known physiological condition (F06.8)*
senile dementia with delirium or acute confusional state (F05)
DEFINITION Loss of cognitive and intellectual functions, such as impaired memory, judgment, and intellect, without impaired perception or consciousness.

F03.9 Unspecified dementia
CODING TIP✓ Codes F03.90 and F03.91 are to be used for dementia that is not specified as due to another condition, and is reported as unspecified, senile psychosis, senile dementia (may also state depressed or paranoid type), primary degenerative dementia, or presenile dementia/psychosis. Do not confuse these conditions with organic brain disease or senility NOS. Senility NOS should not be coded with an F03.9- code (see excludes 1 notes) as this is less specific. When senile dementia is specified, the appropriate F03.9- code should be used. If the physician documentation states major neurocognitive disorder, do not code as unspecified dementia.

F03.90 Unspecified dementia without behavioral disturbance A HIV
Dementia NOS
AHA: 4Q 2012, 92

F03.91 Unspecified dementia with behavioral disturbance A
Unspecified dementia with aggressive behavior
Unspecified dementia with combative behavior
Unspecified dementia with violent behavior
Use additional code, if applicable, to identify wandering in unspecified dementia (Z91.83)
CODING TIP✓ Anxiety is not considered a behavior indicated by a 5th character of 1. Anxiety, when documented by the physician, in addition to dementia, should be coded separately.

F04 Amnestic disorder due to known physiological condition
Korsakov's psychosis or syndrome, nonalcoholic
Code first:
the underlying physiological condition
EXCLUDES 1 *amnesia NOS (R41.3)*
anterograde amnesia (R41.1)
dissociative amnesia (F44.0)
retrograde amnesia (R41.2)
EXCLUDES 2 *alcohol-induced or unspecified Korsakov's syndrome (F10.26, F10.96)*
Korsakov's syndrome induced by other psychoactive substances (F13.26, F13.96, F19.16, F19.26, F19.96)

F05 Delirium due to known physiological condition
Acute or subacute brain syndrome
Acute or subacute confusional state (nonalcoholic)
Acute or subacute infective psychosis
Acute or subacute organic reaction
Acute or subacute psycho-organic syndrome
Delirium of mixed etiology
Delirium superimposed on dementia
Sundowning
Code first:
the underlying physiological condition
EXCLUDES 1 *delirium NOS (R41.0)*
EXCLUDES 2 *delirium tremens alcohol-induced or unspecified (F10.231, F10.921)*
CODING TIP✓ Patients with dementia may also have delirium or sundowning. When appropriate, add F05 when dementia is coded.

F06 Other mental disorders due to known physiological condition
INCLUDES mental disorders due to endocrine disorder
mental disorders due to exogenous hormone
mental disorders due to exogenous toxic substance
mental disorders due to primary cerebral disease
mental disorders due to somatic illness
mental disorders due to systemic disease affecting the brain
Code first:
the underlying physiological condition
EXCLUDES 1 *unspecified dementia (F03)*
EXCLUDES 2 *delirium due to known physiological condition (F05)*
dementia as classified in F01-F02
other mental disorders associated with alcohol and other psychoactive substances (F10-F19)

F06.0 Psychotic disorder with hallucinations due to known physiological condition
Organic hallucinatory state (nonalcoholic)
EXCLUDES 2 *hallucinations and perceptual disturbance induced by alcohol and other psychoactive substances (F10-F19 with .151, .251, .951)*
schizophrenia (F20.-)

F06.1 Catatonic disorder due to known physiological condition
Catatonia associated with another mental disorder
Catatonia NOS
EXCLUDES 1 *catatonic stupor (R40.1)*
stupor NOS (R40.1)
EXCLUDES 2 *catatonic schizophrenia (F20.2)*
dissociative stupor (F44.2)

F06.2 Psychotic disorder with delusions due to known physiological condition
Paranoid and paranoid-hallucinatory organic states
Schizophrenia-like psychosis in epilepsy
EXCLUDES 2 *alcohol and drug-induced psychotic disorder (F10-F19 with .150, .250, .950)*
brief psychotic disorder (F23)
delusional disorder (F22)
schizophrenia (F20.-)

F06.3 Mood disorder due to known physiological condition
EXCLUDES 2 *mood disorders due to alcohol and other psychoactive substances (F10-F19 with .14, .24, .94)*
mood disorders, not due to known physiological condition or unspecified (F30-F39)

F06.30 Mood disorder due to known physiological condition, unspecified

F06.31 Mood disorder due to known physiological condition with depressive features
Depressive disorder due to known physiological condition, with depressive features

F06.32 Mood disorder due to known physiological condition with major depressive-like episode
Depressive disorder due to known physiological condition, with major depressive-like episode

F06.33 Mood disorder due to known physiological condition with manic features
Bipolar and related disorder due to a known physiological condition, with manic features
Bipolar and related disorder due to known physiological condition, with manic- or hypomanic-like episodes

F06.34 Mood disorder due to known physiological condition with mixed features
Bipolar and related disorder due to known physiological condition, with mixed features
Depressive disorder due to known physiological condition, with mixed features

F06.4 Anxiety disorder due to known physiological condition
EXCLUDES 2 *anxiety disorders due to alcohol and other psychoactive substances (F10-F19 with .180, .280, .980)*
anxiety disorders, not due to known physiological condition or unspecified (F40.-, F41.-)

F06.8 Other specified mental disorders due to known physiological condition HIV
Epileptic psychosis NOS
Obsessive-compulsive and related disorder due to a known physiological condition
Organic dissociative disorder
Organic emotionally labile [asthenic] disorder

4 F07 Personality and behavioral disorders due to known physiological condition
Code first:
the underlying physiological condition

F07.0 Personality change due to known physiological condition
Frontal lobe syndrome
Limbic epilepsy personality syndrome
Lobotomy syndrome
Organic personality disorder
Organic pseudopsychopathic personality
Organic pseudoretarded personality
Postleucotomy syndrome
Code first:
underlying physiological condition

EXCLUDES 1 *mild cognitive impairment (G31.84)*
postconcussional syndrome (F07.81)
postencephalitic syndrome (F07.89)
signs and symptoms involving emotional state (R45.-)

EXCLUDES 2 *specific personality disorder (F60.-)*

DEFINITION Frontal lobe syndrome: Damage to the frontal lobe of the brain, typically manifesting as apathy, a lack of planning, emotional bluntness, the absence of abstract thought and attention, and judgment changes.

5 F07.8 Other personality and behavioral disorders due to known physiological condition

F07.81 Postconcussional syndrome
Postcontusional syndrome (encephalopathy)
Post-traumatic brain syndrome, nonpsychotic
Use additional code to identify associated post-traumatic headache, if applicable (G44.3-)

EXCLUDES 1 *current concussion (brain) (S06.0-)*
postencephalitic syndrome (F07.89)

CODING TIP ✓ Code F07.81 should not be used for the patient who has a current concussion (see the Excludes 1 notes). Postconcussional syndrome is a complex disorder resulting from traumatic brain injury and is not associated with the severity of the initial injury. No documented loss of consciousness with the initial injury is necessary for a diagnosis of postconcussional syndrome, but the physician must specify this disorder.

DEFINITION Symptoms such as headache, amnesia, and lack of concentration due to a severe blow to the skull.

F07.89 Other personality and behavioral disorders due to known physiological condition
Postencephalitic syndrome
Right hemispheric organic affective disorder

F07.9 Unspecified personality and behavioral disorder due to known physiological condition HIV
Organic psychosyndrome

F09 Unspecified mental disorder due to known physiological condition HIV
Mental disorder NOS due to known physiological condition
Organic brain syndrome NOS
Organic mental disorder NOS
Organic psychosis NOS
Symptomatic psychosis NOS
Code first:
the underlying physiological condition

EXCLUDES 1 *psychosis NOS (F29)*

Mental and behavioral disorders due to psychoactive substance use (F10-F19)

GUIDELINES **Section I.C.5.b.1)-3)**
Selection of codes for "in remission" for categories F10-F19, Mental and behavioral disorders due to psychoactive substance use (categories F10-F19 with -.21), requires the provider's clinical judgment. The appropriate codes for "in remission" are assigned only on the basis of provider documentation (as defined in the Official Guidelines for Coding and Reporting) unless otherwise instructed by the classification.

Mild substance use disorders in early or sustained remission are classified to the appropriate codes for substance abuse in remission, and moderate or severe substance use disorders in early or sustained remission are classified to the appropriate codes for substance dependence in remission.

When the provider documentation refers to use, abuse and dependence of the same substance (e.g. alcohol, opioid, cannabis, etc.), only one code should be assigned to identify the pattern of use based on the following hierarchy:

- If both use and abuse are documented, assign only the code for abuse
- If both abuse and dependence are documented, assign only the code for dependence
- If use, abuse and dependence are all documented, assign only the code for dependence
- If both use and dependence are documented, assign only the code for dependence.

As with all other unspecified diagnoses, the codes for unspecified psychoactive substance use disorders (F10.9-, F11.9-, F12.9-, F13.9-, F14.9-, F15.9-, F16.9-, F18.9-, F19.9-) should only be assigned based on provider documentation and when they meet the definition of a reportable diagnosis (see Section III, Reporting Additional Diagnoses). The codes are to be used only when the psychoactive substance use is associated with a physical, mental or behavioral disorder, and such a relationship is documented by the provider.

CODING TIP ✓ When coding disorders due to psychoactive use, abuse and dependence, refer to provider documentation to determine the appropriate code selection for either use, abuse, or dependence. Only one code should be used to specify use or abuse of or dependence on a substance, even when documentation uses multiple terms to refer to use, abuse and/or dependence. Coders should refer to the appropriate hierarchy to determine code selection. When coding tobacco use NOS, do not use a code from F10-F19. Instead report code Z72.0 (Tobacco use).

4 F10 Alcohol related disorders
Use additional code for blood alcohol level, if applicable (Y90.-)

5 F10.1 Alcohol abuse

EXCLUDES 1 *alcohol dependence (F10.2-)*
alcohol use, unspecified (F10.9-)

F10.10 Alcohol abuse, uncomplicated
Alcohol use disorder, mild

F10.11 Alcohol abuse, in remission
Alcohol use disorder, mild, in early remission
Alcohol use disorder, mild, in sustained remission
AHA: 4Q 2017, 6

6 F10.12 Alcohol abuse with intoxication

F10.120 Alcohol abuse with intoxication, uncomplicated HCC

F10.121 Alcohol abuse with intoxication delirium HCC

F10.129 Alcohol abuse with intoxication, unspecified HCC

F10.14 Alcohol abuse with alcohol-induced mood disorder HCC
Alcohol use disorder, mild, with alcohol-induced bipolar or related disorder
Alcohol use disorder, mild, with alcohol-induced depressive disorder

6 F10.15 Alcohol abuse with alcohol-induced psychotic disorder

F10.150 Alcohol abuse with alcohol-induced psychotic disorder with delusions HCC

F10.151 Alcohol abuse with alcohol-induced psychotic disorder with hallucinations HCC

F10.159 Alcohol abuse with alcohol-induced psychotic disorder, unspecified HCC

6 F10.18 Alcohol abuse with other alcohol-induced disorders

F10.180 **Alcohol abuse with alcohol-induced anxiety disorder** HCC

F10.181 **Alcohol abuse with alcohol-induced sexual dysfunction** HCC

F10.182 **Alcohol abuse with alcohol-induced sleep disorder** HCC

F10.188 **Alcohol abuse with other alcohol-induced disorder** HCC

F10.19 **Alcohol abuse with unspecified alcohol-induced disorder** HCC

5 **F10.2** **Alcohol dependence**

EXCLUDES 1 *alcohol abuse (F10.1-)*
alcohol use, unspecified (F10.9-)

EXCLUDES 2 *toxic effect of alcohol (T51.0-)*

F10.20 **Alcohol dependence, uncomplicated** HCC
Alcohol use disorder, moderate
Alcohol use disorder, severe

F10.21 **Alcohol dependence, in remission** HCC
Alcohol use disorder, moderate, in early remission
Alcohol use disorder, moderate, in sustained remission
Alcohol use disorder, severe, in early remission
Alcohol use disorder, severe, in sustained remission

6 **F10.22** **Alcohol dependence with intoxication**
Acute drunkenness (in alcoholism)

EXCLUDES 2 *alcohol dependence with withdrawal (F10.23-)*

F10.220 **Alcohol dependence with intoxication, uncomplicated** HCC

F10.221 **Alcohol dependence with intoxication delirium** HCC

F10.229 **Alcohol dependence with intoxication, unspecified** HCC

6 **F10.23** **Alcohol dependence with withdrawal**

EXCLUDES 2 *Alcohol dependence with intoxication (F10.22-)*

F10.230 **Alcohol dependence with withdrawal, uncomplicated** HCC

F10.231 **Alcohol dependence with withdrawal delirium** HCC

DEFINITION Delirium occurring when an alcoholic is denied alcohol for a significant period of time.

F10.232 **Alcohol dependence with withdrawal with perceptual disturbance** HCC

F10.239 **Alcohol dependence with withdrawal, unspecified** HCC
AHA: 2Q 2015, 15

F10.24 **Alcohol dependence with alcohol-induced mood disorder** HCC
Alcohol use disorder, moderate, with alcohol-induced bipolar or related disorder
Alcohol use disorder, moderate, with alcohol-induced depressive disorder
Alcohol use disorder, severe, with alcohol-induced bipolar or related disorder
Alcohol use disorder, severe, with alcohol-induced depressive disorder

6 **F10.25** **Alcohol dependence with alcohol-induced psychotic disorder**

F10.250 **Alcohol dependence with alcohol-induced psychotic disorder with delusions** HCC

F10.251 **Alcohol dependence with alcohol-induced psychotic disorder with hallucinations** HCC

F10.259 **Alcohol dependence with alcohol-induced psychotic disorder, unspecified** HCC

F10.26 **Alcohol dependence with alcohol-induced persisting amnestic disorder** HCC
Alcohol use disorder, moderate, with alcohol-induced major neurocognitive disorder, amnestic-confabulatory type
Alcohol use disorder, severe, with alcohol-induced major neurocognitive disorder, amnestic-confabulatory type

F10.27 **Alcohol dependence with alcohol-induced persisting dementia** HCC
Alcohol use disorder, moderate, with alcohol-induced major neurocognitive disorder, nonamnestic-confabulatory type
Alcohol use disorder, severe, with alcohol-induced major neurocognitive disorder, nonamnestic-confabulatory type

DEFINITION Lasting state of dementia due to chronic alcoholism.

6 **F10.28** **Alcohol dependence with other alcohol-induced disorders**

F10.280 **Alcohol dependence with alcohol-induced anxiety disorder** HCC

F10.281 **Alcohol dependence with alcohol-induced sexual dysfunction** HCC

F10.282 **Alcohol dependence with alcohol-induced sleep disorder** HCC

F10.288 **Alcohol dependence with other alcohol-induced disorder** HCC
Alcohol use disorder, moderate, with alcohol-induced mild neurocognitive disorder
Alcohol use disorder, severe, with alcohol-induced mild neurocognitive disorder

F10.29 **Alcohol dependence with unspecified alcohol-induced disorder** HCC

5 **F10.9** **Alcohol use, unspecified**

EXCLUDES 1 *alcohol abuse (F10.1-)*
alcohol dependence (F10.2-)

6 **F10.92** **Alcohol use, unspecified with intoxication**

F10.920 **Alcohol use, unspecified with intoxication, uncomplicated** HCC

F10.921 **Alcohol use, unspecified with intoxication delirium** HCC

F10.929 **Alcohol use, unspecified with intoxication, unspecified** HCC

F10.94 **Alcohol use, unspecified with alcohol-induced mood disorder** HCC
Alcohol induced bipolar or related disorder, without use disorder
Alcohol induced depressive disorder, without use disorder

6 **F10.95** **Alcohol use, unspecified with alcohol-induced psychotic disorder**

F10.950 **Alcohol use, unspecified with alcohol-induced psychotic disorder with delusions** HCC

F10.951 **Alcohol use, unspecified with alcohol-induced psychotic disorder with hallucinations** HCC

F10.959 **Alcohol use, unspecified with alcohol-induced psychotic disorder, unspecified** HCC
Alcohol-induced psychotic disorder without use disorder

F10.96 **Alcohol use, unspecified with alcohol-induced persisting amnestic disorder** HCC
Alcohol-induced major neurocognitive disorder, amnestic-confabulatory type, without use disorder

F10.97 **Alcohol use, unspecified with alcohol-induced persisting dementia** HCC
Alcohol-induced major neurocognitive disorder, nonamnestic-confabulatory type, without use disorder

6 **F10.98** **Alcohol use, unspecified with other alcohol-induced disorders**

F10.980 **Alcohol use, unspecified with alcohol-induced anxiety disorder** HCC
Alcohol induced anxiety disorder, without use disorder

F10.981 **Alcohol use, unspecified with alcohol-induced sexual dysfunction** HCC
Alcohol induced sexual dysfunction, without use disorder

F10.982 **Alcohol use, unspecified with alcohol-induced sleep disorder** HCC
Alcohol induced sleep disorder, without use disorder

DEFINITION Disruption of normal sleep patterns due to the consumption of alcohol.

F10.988 **Alcohol use, unspecified with other alcohol-induced disorder** HCC
Alcohol induced mild neurocognitive disorder, without use disorder

F10.99 **Alcohol use, unspecified with unspecified alcohol-induced disorder** HCC

4 F11 Opioid related disorders

CODING TIP✓ Do not assign a code from F11 for prescribed opioid use alone. Without provider documentation of an associated physical, mental or behavioral disorder, "opioid use" is not coded.

5 F11.1 Opioid abuse
EXCLUDES 1 *opioid dependence (F11.2-)*
opioid use, unspecified (F11.9-)

F11.10 **Opioid abuse, uncomplicated** HCC
Opioid use disorder, mild

F11.11 **Opioid abuse, in remission** HCC
Opioid use disorder, mild, in early remission
Opioid use disorder, mild, in sustained remission
AHA: 4Q 2017, 6

6 F11.12 Opioid abuse with intoxication

F11.120 **Opioid abuse with intoxication, uncomplicated** HCC
F11.121 **Opioid abuse with intoxication delirium** HCC
F11.122 **Opioid abuse with intoxication with perceptual disturbance** HCC
F11.129 **Opioid abuse with intoxication, unspecified** HCC

F11.14 **Opioid abuse with opioid-induced mood disorder** HCC
Opioid use disorder, mild, with opioid-induced depressive disorder

6 F11.15 Opioid abuse with opioid-induced psychotic disorder

F11.150 **Opioid abuse with opioid-induced psychotic disorder with delusions** HCC
F11.151 **Opioid abuse with opioid-induced psychotic disorder with hallucinations** HCC
F11.159 **Opioid abuse with opioid-induced psychotic disorder, unspecified** HCC

6 F11.18 Opioid abuse with other opioid-induced disorder

F11.181 **Opioid abuse with opioid-induced sexual dysfunction** HCC
F11.182 **Opioid abuse with opioid-induced sleep disorder** HCC
F11.188 **Opioid abuse with other opioid-induced disorder** HCC

F11.19 **Opioid abuse with unspecified opioid-induced disorder** HCC

5 F11.2 Opioid dependence
EXCLUDES 1 *opioid abuse (F11.1-)*
opioid use, unspecified (F11.9-)
EXCLUDES 2 *opioid poisoning (T40.0-T40.2-)*

F11.20 **Opioid dependence, uncomplicated** HCC
Opioid use disorder, moderate
Opioid use disorder, severe

F11.21 **Opioid dependence, in remission** HCC
Opioid use disorder, moderate, in early remission
Opioid use disorder, moderate, in sustained remission
Opioid use disorder, severe, in early remission
Opioid use disorder, severe, in sustained remission

6 F11.22 Opioid dependence with intoxication
EXCLUDES 1 *opioid dependence with withdrawal (F11.23)*

F11.220 **Opioid dependence with intoxication, uncomplicated** HCC
F11.221 **Opioid dependence with intoxication delirium** HCC
F11.222 **Opioid dependence with intoxication with perceptual disturbance** HCC
F11.229 **Opioid dependence with intoxication, unspecified** HCC

F11.23 **Opioid dependence with withdrawal** HCC
EXCLUDES 1 *opioid dependence with intoxication (F11.22-)*

F11.24 **Opioid dependence with opioid-induced mood disorder** HCC
Opioid use disorder, moderate, with opioid induced depressive disorder

6 F11.25 Opioid dependence with opioid-induced psychotic disorder

F11.250 **Opioid dependence with opioid-induced psychotic disorder with delusions** HCC
F11.251 **Opioid dependence with opioid-induced psychotic disorder with hallucinations** HCC
F11.259 **Opioid dependence with opioid-induced psychotic disorder, unspecified** HCC

6 F11.28 Opioid dependence with other opioid-induced disorder

F11.281 **Opioid dependence with opioid-induced sexual dysfunction** HCC
F11.282 **Opioid dependence with opioid-induced sleep disorder** HCC
F11.288 **Opioid dependence with other opioid-induced disorder** HCC

F11.29 **Opioid dependence with unspecified opioid-induced disorder** HCC

5 F11.9 Opioid use, unspecified
EXCLUDES 1 *opioid abuse (F11.1-)*
opioid dependence (F11.2-)

CODING TIP✓ Use disorder is coded to abuse or dependence depending on the severity. Mild is coded to abuse, and moderate and severe are coded to dependence.

F11.90 **Opioid use, unspecified, uncomplicated**

6 F11.92 Opioid use, unspecified with intoxication
EXCLUDES 1 *opioid use, unspecified with withdrawal (F11.93)*

F11.920 **Opioid use, unspecified with intoxication, uncomplicated** HCC
F11.921 **Opioid use, unspecified with intoxication delirium** HCC
Opioid-induced delirium
F11.922 **Opioid use, unspecified with intoxication with perceptual disturbance** HCC
F11.929 **Opioid use, unspecified with intoxication, unspecified** HCC

F11.93 **Opioid use, unspecified with withdrawal** HCC
EXCLUDES 1 *opioid use, unspecified with intoxication (F11.92-)*

F11.94 **Opioid use, unspecified with opioid-induced mood disorder** HCC
Opioid induced depressive disorder, without use disorder

6 F11.95 Opioid use, unspecified with opioid-induced psychotic disorder

F11.950 **Opioid use, unspecified with opioid-induced psychotic disorder with delusions** HCC
F11.951 **Opioid use, unspecified with opioid-induced psychotic disorder with hallucinations** HCC
F11.959 **Opioid use, unspecified with opioid-induced psychotic disorder, unspecified** HCC

6 F11.98 Opioid use, unspecified with other specified opioid-induced disorder

F11.981 **Opioid use, unspecified with opioid-induced sexual dysfunction** HCC
Opioid induced sexual dysfunction, without use disorder
F11.982 **Opioid use, unspecified with opioid-induced sleep disorder** HCC
Opioid induced sleep disorder, without use disorder
F11.988 **Opioid use, unspecified with other opioid-induced disorder** HCC
Opioid induced anxiety disorder, without use disorder

F11.99 **Opioid use, unspecified with unspecified opioid-induced disorder** HCC

4 F12 Cannabis related disorders

INCLUDES marijuana

CODING TIP✓ Recreational marijuana use or medical use of marijuana should not ordinarily be coded. Do not assign a code for marijuana use, without an associated physical, mental or behavioral disorder documented by the provider.

5 F12.1 **Cannabis abuse**

EXCLUDES 1 *cannabis dependence (F12.2-)*
cannabis use, unspecified (F12.9-)

F12.10 **Cannabis abuse, uncomplicated**
Cannabis use disorder, mild

F12.11 **Cannabis abuse, in remission**
Cannabis use disorder, mild, in early remission
Cannabis use disorder, mild, in sustained remission
AHA: 4Q 2017, 6

6 F12.12 **Cannabis abuse with intoxication**

F12.120 **Cannabis abuse with intoxication, uncomplicated** HCC

F12.121 **Cannabis abuse with intoxication delirium** HCC

F12.122 **Cannabis abuse with intoxication with perceptual disturbance** HCC

F12.129 **Cannabis abuse with intoxication, unspecified** HCC

6 F12.15 **Cannabis abuse with psychotic disorder**

F12.150 **Cannabis abuse with psychotic disorder with delusions** HCC

F12.151 **Cannabis abuse with psychotic disorder with hallucinations** HCC

F12.159 **Cannabis abuse with psychotic disorder, unspecified** HCC

6 F12.18 **Cannabis abuse with other cannabis-induced disorder**

F12.180 **Cannabis abuse with cannabis-induced anxiety disorder** HCC

F12.188 **Cannabis abuse with other cannabis-induced disorder** HCC
Cannabis use disorder, mild, with cannabis-induced sleep disorder

F12.19 **Cannabis abuse with unspecified cannabis-induced disorder** HCC

5 F12.2 **Cannabis dependence**

EXCLUDES 1 *cannabis abuse (F12.1-)*
cannabis use, unspecified (F12.9-)

EXCLUDES 2 *cannabis poisoning (T40.7-)*

F12.20 **Cannabis dependence, uncomplicated** HCC
Cannabis use disorder, moderate
Cannabis use disorder, severe

F12.21 **Cannabis dependence, in remission** HCC
Cannabis use disorder, moderate, in early remission
Cannabis use disorder, moderate, in sustained remission
Cannabis use disorder, severe, in early remission
Cannabis use disorder, severe, in sustained remission

6 F12.22 **Cannabis dependence with intoxication**

F12.220 **Cannabis dependence with intoxication, uncomplicated** HCC

F12.221 **Cannabis dependence with intoxication delirium** HCC

F12.222 **Cannabis dependence with intoxication with perceptual disturbance** HCC

F12.229 **Cannabis dependence with intoxication, unspecified** HCC

● F12.23 **Cannabis dependence with withdrawal**

6 F12.25 **Cannabis dependence with psychotic disorder**

F12.250 **Cannabis dependence with psychotic disorder with delusions** HCC

F12.251 **Cannabis dependence with psychotic disorder with hallucinations** HCC

F12.259 **Cannabis dependence with psychotic disorder, unspecified** HCC

6 F12.28 **Cannabis dependence with other cannabis-induced disorder**

F12.280 **Cannabis dependence with cannabis-induced anxiety disorder** HCC

▲ F12.288 **Cannabis dependence with other cannabis-induced disorder** HCC
Cannabis use disorder, moderate, with cannabis-induced sleep disorder
Cannabis use disorder, severe, with cannabis-induced sleep disorder

F12.29 **Cannabis dependence with unspecified cannabis-induced disorder** HCC

5 F12.9 **Cannabis use, unspecified**

EXCLUDES 1 *cannabis abuse (F12.1-)*
cannabis dependence (F12.2-)

CODING TIP✓ Use disorder is coded to abuse or dependence depending on the severity. Mild is coded to abuse, and moderate and severe are coded to dependence.

F12.90 **Cannabis use, unspecified, uncomplicated**

6 F12.92 **Cannabis use, unspecified with intoxication**

F12.920 **Cannabis use, unspecified with intoxication, uncomplicated** HCC

F12.921 **Cannabis use, unspecified with intoxication delirium** HCC

F12.922 **Cannabis use, unspecified with intoxication with perceptual disturbance** HCC

F12.929 **Cannabis use, unspecified with intoxication, unspecified** HCC

● F12.93 **Cannabis use, unspecified with withdrawal**

6 F12.95 **Cannabis use, unspecified with psychotic disorder**

F12.950 **Cannabis use, unspecified with psychotic disorder with delusions** HCC

F12.951 **Cannabis use, unspecified with psychotic disorder with hallucinations** HCC

F12.959 **Cannabis use, unspecified with psychotic disorder, unspecified** HCC
Cannabis induced psychotic disorder, without use disorder

6 F12.98 **Cannabis use, unspecified with other cannabis-induced disorder**

F12.980 **Cannabis use, unspecified with anxiety disorder** HCC
Cannabis induced anxiety disorder, without use disorder

F12.988 **Cannabis use, unspecified with other cannabis-induced disorder** HCC
Cannabis induced sleep disorder, without use disorder

F12.99 **Cannabis use, unspecified with unspecified cannabis-induced disorder** HCC

4 F13 Sedative, hypnotic, or anxiolytic related disorders

5 F13.1 **Sedative, hypnotic or anxiolytic-related abuse**

EXCLUDES 1 *sedative, hypnotic or anxiolytic-related dependence (F13.2-)*
sedative, hypnotic, or anxiolytic use, unspecified (F13.9-)

F13.10 **Sedative, hypnotic or anxiolytic abuse, uncomplicated** HCC
Sedative, hypnotic, or anxiolytic use disorder, mild

F13.11 **Sedative, hypnotic or anxiolytic abuse, in remission** HCC
Sedative, hypnotic or anxiolytic use disorder, mild, in early remission
Sedative, hypnotic or anxiolytic use disorder, mild, in sustained remission
AHA: 4Q 2017, 6

6 F13.12 **Sedative, hypnotic or anxiolytic abuse with intoxication**

F13.120 **Sedative, hypnotic or anxiolytic abuse with intoxication, uncomplicated** HCC

F13.121 **Sedative, hypnotic or anxiolytic abuse with intoxication delirium** HCC

F13.129 **Sedative, hypnotic or anxiolytic abuse with intoxication, unspecified** HCC

F13.14 **Sedative, hypnotic or anxiolytic abuse with sedative, hypnotic or anxiolytic-induced mood disorder** HCC
Sedative, hypnotic, or anxiolytic use disorder, mild, with sedative, hypnotic, or anxiolytic-induced bipolar or related disorder
Sedative, hypnotic, or anxiolytic use disorder, mild, with sedative, hypnotic, or anxiolytic-induced depressive disorder

6 F13.15 **Sedative, hypnotic or anxiolytic abuse with sedative, hypnotic or anxiolytic-induced psychotic disorder**

● New | Manifestation | 4-7 Digit Indicators | Laterality | A Adult | M Maternity | N Newborn | P Pediatric | ♂ Male
▲ Revised | Unspecified | AHA Coding Clinic | HCC Hierarchical Condition Categories | HIV HIV Related Conditions | ♀ Female

F13.150 Sedative, hypnotic or anxiolytic abuse with sedative, hypnotic or anxiolytic-induced psychotic disorder with delusions HCC

F13.151 Sedative, hypnotic or anxiolytic abuse with sedative, hypnotic or anxiolytic-induced psychotic disorder with hallucinations HCC

F13.159 Sedative, hypnotic or anxiolytic abuse with sedative, hypnotic or anxiolytic-induced psychotic disorder, unspecified HCC

6 F13.18 Sedative, hypnotic or anxiolytic abuse with other sedative, hypnotic or anxiolytic-induced disorders

F13.180 Sedative, hypnotic or anxiolytic abuse with sedative, hypnotic or anxiolytic-induced anxiety disorder HCC

F13.181 Sedative, hypnotic or anxiolytic abuse with sedative, hypnotic or anxiolytic-induced sexual dysfunction HCC

F13.182 Sedative, hypnotic or anxiolytic abuse with sedative, hypnotic or anxiolytic-induced sleep disorder HCC

F13.188 Sedative, hypnotic or anxiolytic abuse with other sedative, hypnotic or anxiolytic-induced disorder HCC

F13.19 Sedative, hypnotic or anxiolytic abuse with unspecified sedative, hypnotic or anxiolytic-induced disorder HCC

5 F13.2 Sedative, hypnotic or anxiolytic-related dependence

EXCLUDES 1 *sedative, hypnotic or anxiolytic-related abuse (F13.1-)*
sedative, hypnotic, or anxiolytic use, unspecified (F13.9-)

EXCLUDES 2 *sedative, hypnotic, or anxiolytic poisoning (T42.-)*

F13.20 Sedative, hypnotic or anxiolytic dependence, uncomplicated HCC

F13.21 Sedative, hypnotic or anxiolytic dependence, in remission HCC
Sedative, hypnotic or anxiolytic use disorder, moderate, in early remission
Sedative, hypnotic or anxiolytic use disorder, moderate, in sustained remission
Sedative, hypnotic or anxiolytic use disorder, severe, in early remission
Sedative, hypnotic or anxiolytic use disorder, severe, in sustained remission

6 F13.22 Sedative, hypnotic or anxiolytic dependence with intoxication

EXCLUDES 1 *sedative, hypnotic or anxiolytic dependence with withdrawal (F13.23-)*

F13.220 Sedative, hypnotic or anxiolytic dependence with intoxication, uncomplicated HCC

F13.221 Sedative, hypnotic or anxiolytic dependence with intoxication delirium HCC

F13.229 Sedative, hypnotic or anxiolytic dependence with intoxication, unspecified HCC

6 F13.23 Sedative, hypnotic or anxiolytic dependence with withdrawal
Sedative, hypnotic, or anxiolytic use disorder, moderate
Sedative, hypnotic, or anxiolytic use disorder, severe

EXCLUDES 1 *sedative, hypnotic or anxiolytic dependence with intoxication (F13.22-)*

DEFINITION Curtailed drug use, resulting in physical or psychological symptoms lasting hours to weeks, commonly featuring headache, anxiety, depression, chills, sweats, and tremors.

F13.230 Sedative, hypnotic or anxiolytic dependence with withdrawal, uncomplicated HCC

F13.231 Sedative, hypnotic or anxiolytic dependence with withdrawal delirium HCC

F13.232 Sedative, hypnotic or anxiolytic dependence with withdrawal with perceptual disturbance HCC
Sedative, hypnotic, or anxiolytic withdrawal with perceptual disturbances

F13.239 Sedative, hypnotic or anxiolytic dependence with withdrawal, unspecified HCC
Sedative, hypnotic, or anxiolytic withdrawal without perceptual disturbances

F13.24 Sedative, hypnotic or anxiolytic dependence with sedative, hypnotic or anxiolytic-induced mood disorder HCC
Sedative, hypnotic, or anxiolytic use disorder, moderate, with sedative, hypnotic, or anxiolytic-induced bipolar or related disorder
Sedative, hypnotic, or anxiolytic use disorder, moderate, with sedative, hypnotic, or anxiolytic-induced depressive disorder
Sedative, hypnotic, or anxiolytic use disorder, severe, with sedative, hypnotic, or anxiolytic-induced bipolar or related disorder
Sedative, hypnotic, or anxiolytic use disorder, severe, with sedative, hypnotic, or anxiolytic-induced depressive disorder

6 F13.25 Sedative, hypnotic or anxiolytic dependence with sedative, hypnotic or anxiolytic-induced psychotic disorder

F13.250 Sedative, hypnotic or anxiolytic dependence with sedative, hypnotic or anxiolytic-induced psychotic disorder with delusions HCC

F13.251 Sedative, hypnotic or anxiolytic dependence with sedative, hypnotic or anxiolytic-induced psychotic disorder with hallucinations HCC

F13.259 Sedative, hypnotic or anxiolytic dependence with sedative, hypnotic or anxiolytic-induced psychotic disorder, unspecified HCC

F13.26 Sedative, hypnotic or anxiolytic dependence with sedative, hypnotic or anxiolytic-induced persisting amnestic disorder HCC

F13.27 Sedative, hypnotic or anxiolytic dependence with sedative, hypnotic or anxiolytic-induced persisting dementia HCC
Sedative, hypnotic, or anxiolytic use disorder, moderate, with sedative, hypnotic, or anxiolytic-induced major neurocognitive disorder
Sedative, hypnotic, or anxiolytic use disorder, severe, with sedative, hypnotic, or anxiolytic-induced major neurocognitive disorder

6 F13.28 Sedative, hypnotic or anxiolytic dependence with other sedative, hypnotic or anxiolytic-induced disorders

F13.280 Sedative, hypnotic or anxiolytic dependence with sedative, hypnotic or anxiolytic-induced anxiety disorder HCC

F13.281 Sedative, hypnotic or anxiolytic dependence with sedative, hypnotic or anxiolytic-induced sexual dysfunction HCC

F13.282 Sedative, hypnotic or anxiolytic dependence with sedative, hypnotic or anxiolytic-induced sleep disorder HCC

F13.288 Sedative, hypnotic or anxiolytic dependence with other sedative, hypnotic or anxiolytic-induced disorder HCC
Sedative, hypnotic, or anxiolytic use disorder, moderate, with sedative, hypnotic, or anxiolytic-induced mild neurocognitive disorder
Sedative, hypnotic, or anxiolytic use disorder, severe, with sedative, hypnotic, or anxiolytic-induced mild neurocognitive disorder

F13.29 Sedative, hypnotic or anxiolytic dependence with unspecified sedative, hypnotic or anxiolytic-induced disorder HCC

5 F13.9 Sedative, hypnotic or anxiolytic-related use, unspecified

EXCLUDES 1 *sedative, hypnotic or anxiolytic-related abuse (F13.1-)*
sedative, hypnotic or anxiolytic-related dependence (F13.2-)

CODING TIP ✓ Use disorder is coded to abuse or dependence depending on the severity. Mild is coded to abuse, and moderate and severe are coded to dependence.

F13.90 **Sedative, hypnotic, or anxiolytic use, unspecified, uncomplicated**

6 **F13.92** **Sedative, hypnotic or anxiolytic use, unspecified with intoxication**

EXCLUDES 1 *sedative, hypnotic or anxiolytic use, unspecified with withdrawal (F13.93-)*

F13.920 **Sedative, hypnotic or anxiolytic use, unspecified with intoxication, uncomplicated** HCC

F13.921 **Sedative, hypnotic or anxiolytic use, unspecified with intoxication delirium** HCC

Sedative, hypnotic, or anxiolytic-induced delirium

F13.929 **Sedative, hypnotic or anxiolytic use, unspecified with intoxication, unspecified** HCC

6 **F13.93** **Sedative, hypnotic or anxiolytic use, unspecified with withdrawal**

EXCLUDES 1 *sedative, hypnotic or anxiolytic use, unspecified with intoxication (F13.92-)*

F13.930 **Sedative, hypnotic or anxiolytic use, unspecified with withdrawal, uncomplicated** HCC

F13.931 **Sedative, hypnotic or anxiolytic use, unspecified with withdrawal delirium** HCC

F13.932 **Sedative, hypnotic or anxiolytic use, unspecified with withdrawal with perceptual disturbances** HCC

F13.939 **Sedative, hypnotic or anxiolytic use, unspecified with withdrawal, unspecified** HCC

F13.94 **Sedative, hypnotic or anxiolytic use, unspecified with sedative, hypnotic or anxiolytic-induced mood disorder** HCC

Sedative, hypnotic, or anxiolytic-induced bipolar or related disorder, without use disorder

Sedative, hypnotic, or anxiolytic-induced depressive disorder, without use disorder

6 **F13.95** **Sedative, hypnotic or anxiolytic use, unspecified with sedative, hypnotic or anxiolytic-induced psychotic disorder**

F13.950 **Sedative, hypnotic or anxiolytic use, unspecified with sedative, hypnotic or anxiolytic-induced psychotic disorder with delusions** HCC

F13.951 **Sedative, hypnotic or anxiolytic use, unspecified with sedative, hypnotic or anxiolytic-induced psychotic disorder with hallucinations** HCC

F13.959 **Sedative, hypnotic or anxiolytic use, unspecified with sedative, hypnotic or anxiolytic-induced psychotic disorder, unspecified** HCC

Sedative, hypnotic, or anxiolytic-induced psychotic disorder, without use disorder

F13.96 **Sedative, hypnotic or anxiolytic use, unspecified with sedative, hypnotic or anxiolytic-induced persisting amnestic disorder** HCC

F13.97 **Sedative, hypnotic or anxiolytic use, unspecified with sedative, hypnotic or anxiolytic-induced persisting dementia** HCC

Sedative, hypnotic, or anxiolytic-induced major neurocognitive disorder, without use disorder

6 **F13.98** **Sedative, hypnotic or anxiolytic use, unspecified with other sedative, hypnotic or anxiolytic-induced disorders**

F13.980 **Sedative, hypnotic or anxiolytic use, unspecified with sedative, hypnotic or anxiolytic-induced anxiety disorder** HCC

Sedative, hypnotic, or anxiolytic-induced anxiety disorder, without use disorder

F13.981 **Sedative, hypnotic or anxiolytic use, unspecified with sedative, hypnotic or anxiolytic-induced sexual dysfunction** HCC

Sedative, hypnotic, or anxiolytic-induced sexual dysfunction disorder, without use disorder

F13.982 **Sedative, hypnotic or anxiolytic use, unspecified with sedative, hypnotic or anxiolytic-induced sleep disorder** HCC

Sedative, hypnotic, or anxiolytic-induced sleep disorder, without use disorder

F13.988 **Sedative, hypnotic or anxiolytic use, unspecified with other sedative, hypnotic or anxiolytic-induced disorder** HCC

Sedative, hypnotic, or anxiolytic-induced mild neurocognitive disorder

F13.99 **Sedative, hypnotic or anxiolytic use, unspecified with unspecified sedative, hypnotic or anxiolytic-induced disorder** HCC

4 **F14** **Cocaine related disorders**

EXCLUDES 2 *other stimulant-related disorders (F15.-)*

5 **F14.1** **Cocaine abuse**

EXCLUDES 1 *cocaine dependence (F14.2-)*
cocaine use, unspecified (F14.9-)

F14.10 **Cocaine abuse, uncomplicated** HCC

Cocaine use disorder, mild

F14.11 **Cocaine abuse, in remission** HCC

Cocaine use disorder, mild, in early remission

Cocaine use disorder, mild, in sustained remission

AHA: 4Q 2017, 6

6 **F14.12** **Cocaine abuse with intoxication**

F14.120 **Cocaine abuse with intoxication, uncomplicated** HCC

F14.121 **Cocaine abuse with intoxication with delirium** HCC

F14.122 **Cocaine abuse with intoxication with perceptual disturbance** HCC

F14.129 **Cocaine abuse with intoxication, unspecified** HCC

F14.14 **Cocaine abuse with cocaine-induced mood disorder** HCC

Cocaine use disorder, mild, with cocaine-induced bipolar or related disorder

Cocaine use disorder, mild, with cocaine-induced depressive disorder

6 **F14.15** **Cocaine abuse with cocaine-induced psychotic disorder**

F14.150 **Cocaine abuse with cocaine-induced psychotic disorder with delusions** HCC

F14.151 **Cocaine abuse with cocaine-induced psychotic disorder with hallucinations** HCC

F14.159 **Cocaine abuse with cocaine-induced psychotic disorder, unspecified** HCC

6 **F14.18** **Cocaine abuse with other cocaine-induced disorder**

F14.180 **Cocaine abuse with cocaine-induced anxiety disorder** HCC

F14.181 **Cocaine abuse with cocaine-induced sexual dysfunction** HCC

F14.182 **Cocaine abuse with cocaine-induced sleep disorder** HCC

F14.188 **Cocaine abuse with other cocaine-induced disorder** HCC

Cocaine use disorder, mild, with cocaine-induced obsessive compulsive or related disorder

F14.19 **Cocaine abuse with unspecified cocaine-induced disorder** HCC

5 **F14.2** **Cocaine dependence**

EXCLUDES 1 *cocaine abuse (F14.1-)*
cocaine use, unspecified (F14.9-)

EXCLUDES 2 *cocaine poisoning (T40.5-)*

F14.20 **Cocaine dependence, uncomplicated** HCC

Cocaine use disorder, moderate

Cocaine use disorder, severe

F14.21 **Cocaine dependence, in remission** HCC

Cocaine use disorder, moderate, in early remission

Cocaine use disorder, moderate, in sustained remission

Cocaine use disorder, severe, in early remission

Cocaine use disorder, severe, in sustained remission

6 **F14.22** **Cocaine dependence with intoxication**

EXCLUDES 1 *cocaine dependence with withdrawal (F14.23)*

F14.220 **Cocaine dependence with intoxication, uncomplicated** HCC

F14.221 **Cocaine dependence with intoxication delirium** HCC

F14.222 **Cocaine dependence with intoxication with perceptual disturbance** HCC

F14.229 **Cocaine dependence with intoxication, unspecified** HCC

F14.23 **Cocaine dependence with withdrawal** HCC

EXCLUDES 1 *cocaine dependence with intoxication (F14.22-)*

F14.24 **Cocaine dependence with cocaine-induced mood disorder** HCC

Cocaine use disorder, moderate, with cocaine-induced bipolar or related disorder

Cocaine use disorder, moderate, with cocaine-induced depressive disorder

Cocaine use disorder, severe, with cocaine-induced bipolar or related disorder

Cocaine use disorder, severe, with cocaine-induced depressive disorder

6 **F14.25** **Cocaine dependence with cocaine-induced psychotic disorder**

F14.250 **Cocaine dependence with cocaine-induced psychotic disorder with delusions** HCC

F14.251 **Cocaine dependence with cocaine-induced psychotic disorder with hallucinations** HCC

F14.259 **Cocaine dependence with cocaine-induced psychotic disorder, unspecified** HCC

6 **F14.28** **Cocaine dependence with other cocaine-induced disorder**

F14.280 **Cocaine dependence with cocaine-induced anxiety disorder** HCC

F14.281 **Cocaine dependence with cocaine-induced sexual dysfunction** HCC

F14.282 **Cocaine dependence with cocaine-induced sleep disorder** HCC

F14.288 **Cocaine dependence with other cocaine-induced disorder** HCC

Cocaine use disorder, moderate, with cocaine-induced obsessive compulsive or related disorder

Cocaine use disorder, severe, with cocaine-induced obsessive compulsive or related disorder

F14.29 **Cocaine dependence with unspecified cocaine-induced disorder** HCC

5 **F14.9** **Cocaine use, unspecified**

EXCLUDES 1 *cocaine abuse (F14.1-)*
cocaine dependence (F14.2-)

CODING TIP✓ Use disorder is coded to abuse or dependence depending on the severity. Mild is coded to abuse, and moderate and severe are coded to dependence.

F14.90 **Cocaine use, unspecified, uncomplicated**

AHA: 2Q 2018, 8

6 **F14.92** **Cocaine use, unspecified with intoxication**

F14.920 **Cocaine use, unspecified with intoxication, uncomplicated** HCC

F14.921 **Cocaine use, unspecified with intoxication delirium** HCC

F14.922 **Cocaine use, unspecified with intoxication with perceptual disturbance** HCC

F14.929 **Cocaine use, unspecified with intoxication, unspecified** HCC

F14.94 **Cocaine use, unspecified with cocaine-induced mood disorder** HCC

Cocaine induced bipolar or related disorder, without use disorder

Cocaine induced depressive disorder, without use disorder

6 **F14.95** **Cocaine use, unspecified with cocaine-induced psychotic disorder**

F14.950 **Cocaine use, unspecified with cocaine-induced psychotic disorder with delusions** HCC

F14.951 **Cocaine use, unspecified with cocaine-induced psychotic disorder with hallucinations** HCC

F14.959 **Cocaine use, unspecified with cocaine-induced psychotic disorder, unspecified** HCC

Cocaine induced psychotic disorder, without use disorder

6 **F14.98** **Cocaine use, unspecified with other specified cocaine-induced disorder**

F14.980 **Cocaine use, unspecified with cocaine-induced anxiety disorder** HCC

Cocaine induced anxiety disorder, without use disorder

F14.981 **Cocaine use, unspecified with cocaine-induced sexual dysfunction** HCC

Cocaine induced sexual dysfunction, without use disorder

F14.982 **Cocaine use, unspecified with cocaine-induced sleep disorder** HCC

Cocaine induced sleep disorder, without use disorder

F14.988 **Cocaine use, unspecified with other cocaine-induced disorder** HCC

Cocaine induced obsessive compulsive or related disorder

F14.99 **Cocaine use, unspecified with unspecified cocaine-induced disorder** HCC

4 **F15** **Other stimulant related disorders**

INCLUDES amphetamine-related disorders
caffeine

EXCLUDES 2 *cocaine-related disorders (F14.-)*

CODING TIP✓ Use this category of codes for methamphetamines and "bath salts" abuse and dependence.

5 **F15.1** **Other stimulant abuse**

EXCLUDES 1 *other stimulant dependence (F15.2-)*
other stimulant use, unspecified (F15.9-)

F15.10 **Other stimulant abuse, uncomplicated** HCC

Amphetamine type substance use disorder, mild

Other or unspecified stimulant use disorder, mild

F15.11 **Other stimulant abuse, in remission** HCC

Amphetamine type substance use disorder, mild, in early remission

Amphetamine type substance use disorder, mild, in sustained remission

Other or unspecified stimulant use disorder, mild, in early remission

Other or unspecified stimulant use disorder, mild, in sustained remission

AHA: 4Q 2017, 6

6 **F15.12** **Other stimulant abuse with intoxication**

F15.120 **Other stimulant abuse with intoxication, uncomplicated** HCC

F15.121 **Other stimulant abuse with intoxication delirium** HCC

F15.122 **Other stimulant abuse with intoxication with perceptual disturbance** HCC

Amphetamine or other stimulant use disorder, mild, with amphetamine or other stimulant intoxication, with perceptual disturbances

F15.129 **Other stimulant abuse with intoxication, unspecified** HCC

Amphetamine or other stimulant use disorder, mild, with amphetamine or other stimulant intoxication, without perceptual disturbances

F15.14 **Other stimulant abuse with stimulant-induced mood disorder** HCC

Amphetamine or other stimulant use disorder, mild, with amphetamine or other stimulant induced bipolar or related disorder

Amphetamine or other stimulant use disorder, mild, with amphetamine or other stimulant induced depressive disorder

6 **F15.15** **Other stimulant abuse with stimulant-induced psychotic disorder**

F15.150 **Other stimulant abuse with stimulant-induced psychotic disorder with delusions** HCC

F15.151 **Other stimulant abuse with stimulant-induced psychotic disorder with hallucinations** HCC

F15.159 **Other stimulant abuse with stimulant-induced psychotic disorder, unspecified** HCC

6 F15.18 **Other stimulant abuse with other stimulant-induced disorder**

F15.180 **Other stimulant abuse with stimulant-induced anxiety disorder** HCC

F15.181 **Other stimulant abuse with stimulant-induced sexual dysfunction** HCC

F15.182 **Other stimulant abuse with stimulant-induced sleep disorder** HCC

F15.188 **Other stimulant abuse with other stimulant-induced disorder** HCC

Amphetamine or other stimulant use disorder, mild, with amphetamine or other stimulant induced obsessive-compulsive or related disorder

F15.19 **Other stimulant abuse with unspecified stimulant-induced disorder** HCC

5 F15.2 **Other stimulant dependence**

EXCLUDES 1 *other stimulant abuse (F15.1-)*
other stimulant use, unspecified (F15.9-)

F15.20 **Other stimulant dependence, uncomplicated** HCC

Amphetamine type substance use disorder, moderate
Amphetamine type substance use disorder, severe
Other or unspecified stimulant use disorder, moderate
Other or unspecified stimulant use disorder, severe

F15.21 **Other stimulant dependence, in remission** HCC

Amphetamine type substance use disorder, moderate, in early remission
Amphetamine type substance use disorder, moderate, in sustained remission
Amphetamine type substance use disorder, severe, in early remission
Amphetamine type substance use disorder, severe, in sustained remission
Other or unspecified stimulant use disorder, moderate, in early remission
Other or unspecified stimulant use disorder, moderate, in sustained remission
Other or unspecified stimulant use disorder, severe, in early remission
Other or unspecified stimulant use disorder, severe, in sustained remission

6 F15.22 **Other stimulant dependence with intoxication**

EXCLUDES 1 *other stimulant dependence with withdrawal (F15.23)*

F15.220 **Other stimulant dependence with intoxication, uncomplicated** HCC

F15.221 **Other stimulant dependence with intoxication delirium** HCC

F15.222 **Other stimulant dependence with intoxication with perceptual disturbance** HCC

Amphetamine or other stimulant use disorder, moderate, with amphetamine or other stimulant intoxication, with perceptual disturbances
Amphetamine or other stimulant use disorder, severe, with amphetamine or other stimulant intoxication, with perceptual disturbances

F15.229 **Other stimulant dependence with intoxication, unspecified** HCC

Amphetamine or other stimulant use disorder, moderate, with amphetamine or other stimulant intoxication, without perceptual disturbances
Amphetamine or other stimulant use disorder, severe, with amphetamine or other stimulant intoxication, without perceptual disturbances

F15.23 **Other stimulant dependence with withdrawal** HCC

Amphetamine or other stimulant withdrawal

EXCLUDES 1 *other stimulant dependence with intoxication (F15.22-)*

F15.24 **Other stimulant dependence with stimulant-induced mood disorder** HCC

Amphetamine or other stimulant use disorder, moderate, with amphetamine or other stimulant-induced bipolar or related disorder
Amphetamine or other stimulant use disorder, moderate, with amphetamine or other stimulant induced depressive disorder
Amphetamine or other stimulant use disorder, severe, with amphetamine or other stimulant-induced bipolar or related disorder
Amphetamine or other stimulant use disorder, severe, with amphetamine or other stimulant-induced depressive disorder

6 F15.25 **Other stimulant dependence with stimulant-induced psychotic disorder**

F15.250 **Other stimulant dependence with stimulant-induced psychotic disorder with delusions** HCC

F15.251 **Other stimulant dependence with stimulant-induced psychotic disorder with hallucinations** HCC

F15.259 **Other stimulant dependence with stimulant-induced psychotic disorder, unspecified** HCC

6 F15.28 **Other stimulant dependence with other stimulant-induced disorder**

F15.280 **Other stimulant dependence with stimulant-induced anxiety disorder** HCC

F15.281 **Other stimulant dependence with stimulant-induced sexual dysfunction** HCC

F15.282 **Other stimulant dependence with stimulant-induced sleep disorder** HCC

F15.288 **Other stimulant dependence with other stimulant-induced disorder** HCC

Amphetamine or other stimulant use disorder, moderate, with amphetamine or other stimulant induced obsessive compulsive or related disorder
Amphetamine or other stimulant use disorder, severe, with amphetamine or other stimulant induced obsessive compulsive or related disorder

F15.29 **Other stimulant dependence with unspecified stimulant-induced disorder** HCC

5 F15.9 **Other stimulant use, unspecified**

EXCLUDES 1 *other stimulant abuse (F15.1-)*
other stimulant dependence (F15.2-)

CODING TIP ✓ Use disorder is coded to abuse or dependence depending on the severity. Mild is coded to abuse, and moderate and severe are coded to dependence.

F15.90 **Other stimulant use, unspecified, uncomplicated**

6 F15.92 **Other stimulant use, unspecified with intoxication**

EXCLUDES 1 *other stimulant use, unspecified with withdrawal (F15.93)*

F15.920 **Other stimulant use, unspecified with intoxication, uncomplicated** HCC

F15.921 **Other stimulant use, unspecified with intoxication delirium** HCC

Amphetamine or other stimulant-induced delirium

F15.922 **Other stimulant use, unspecified with intoxication with perceptual disturbance** HCC

F15.929 **Other stimulant use, unspecified with intoxication, unspecified** HCC

Caffeine intoxication

F15.93 **Other stimulant use, unspecified with withdrawal** HCC

Caffeine withdrawal

EXCLUDES 1 *other stimulant use, unspecified with intoxication (F15.92-)*

F15.94 **Other stimulant use, unspecified with stimulant-induced mood disorder** HCC

Amphetamine or other stimulant-induced bipolar or related disorder, without use disorder
Amphetamine or other stimulant-induced depressive disorder, without use disorder

6 F15.95 **Other stimulant use, unspecified with stimulant-induced psychotic disorder**

F15.950 **Other stimulant use, unspecified with stimulant-induced psychotic disorder with delusions** HCC

F15.951 **Other stimulant use, unspecified with stimulant-induced psychotic disorder with hallucinations** HCC

F15.959 **Other stimulant use, unspecified with stimulant-induced psychotic disorder, unspecified** HCC

Amphetamine or other stimulant-induced psychotic disorder, without use disorder

6 **F15.98** **Other stimulant use, unspecified with other stimulant-induced disorder**

F15.980 **Other stimulant use, unspecified with stimulant-induced anxiety disorder** HCC

Amphetamine or other stimulant-induced anxiety disorder, without use disorder

Caffeine induced anxiety disorder, without use disorder

F15.981 **Other stimulant use, unspecified with stimulant-induced sexual dysfunction** HCC

Amphetamine or other stimulant-induced sexual dysfunction, without use disorder

F15.982 **Other stimulant use, unspecified with stimulant-induced sleep disorder** HCC

Amphetamine or other stimulant-induced sleep disorder, without use disorder

Caffeine induced sleep disorder, without use disorder

F15.988 **Other stimulant use, unspecified with other stimulant-induced disorder** HCC

Amphetamine or other stimulant-induced obsessive compulsive or related disorder, without use disorder

F15.99 **Other stimulant use, unspecified with unspecified stimulant-induced disorder** HCC

4 F16 Hallucinogen related disorders

INCLUDES ecstasy
PCP
phencyclidine

5 **F16.1** **Hallucinogen abuse**

EXCLUDES 1 *hallucinogen dependence (F16.2-)*
hallucinogen use, unspecified (F16.9-)

F16.10 **Hallucinogen abuse, uncomplicated** HCC

Other hallucinogen use disorder, mild
Phencyclidine use disorder, mild

F16.11 **Hallucinogen abuse, in remission** HCC

Other hallucinogen use disorder, mild, in early remission
Other hallucinogen use disorder, mild, in sustained remission
Phencyclidine use disorder, mild, in early remission
Phencyclidine use disorder, mild, in sustained remission
AHA: 4Q 2017, 6

6 **F16.12** **Hallucinogen abuse with intoxication**

F16.120 **Hallucinogen abuse with intoxication, uncomplicated** HCC

F16.121 **Hallucinogen abuse with intoxication with delirium** HCC

F16.122 **Hallucinogen abuse with intoxication with perceptual disturbance** HCC

F16.129 **Hallucinogen abuse with intoxication, unspecified** HCC

F16.14 **Hallucinogen abuse with hallucinogen-induced mood disorder** HCC

Other hallucinogen use disorder, mild, with other hallucinogen induced bipolar or related disorder
Other hallucinogen use disorder, mild, with other hallucinogen induced depressive disorder
Phencyclidine use disorder, mild, with phencyclidine induced bipolar or related disorder
Phencyclidine use disorder, mild, with phencyclidine induced depressive disorder

6 **F16.15** **Hallucinogen abuse with hallucinogen-induced psychotic disorder**

F16.150 **Hallucinogen abuse with hallucinogen-induced psychotic disorder with delusions** HCC

F16.151 **Hallucinogen abuse with hallucinogen-induced psychotic disorder with hallucinations** HCC

F16.159 **Hallucinogen abuse with hallucinogen-induced psychotic disorder, unspecified** HCC

6 **F16.18** **Hallucinogen abuse with other hallucinogen-induced disorder**

F16.180 **Hallucinogen abuse with hallucinogen-induced anxiety disorder** HCC

F16.183 **Hallucinogen abuse with hallucinogen persisting perception disorder (flashbacks)** HCC

F16.188 **Hallucinogen abuse with other hallucinogen-induced disorder** HCC

F16.19 **Hallucinogen abuse with unspecified hallucinogen-induced disorder** HCC

5 **F16.2** **Hallucinogen dependence**

EXCLUDES 1 *hallucinogen abuse (F16.1-)*
hallucinogen use, unspecified (F16.9-)

F16.20 **Hallucinogen dependence, uncomplicated** HCC

Other hallucinogen use disorder, moderate
Other hallucinogen use disorder, severe
Phencyclidine use disorder, moderate
Phencyclidine use disorder, severe

F16.21 **Hallucinogen dependence, in remission** HCC

Other hallucinogen use disorder, moderate, in early remission
Other hallucinogen use disorder, moderate, in sustained remission
Other hallucinogen use disorder, severe, in early remission
Other hallucinogen use disorder, severe, in sustained remission
Phencyclidine use disorder, moderate, in early remission
Phencyclidine use disorder, moderate, in sustained remission
Phencyclidine use disorder, severe, in early remission
Phencyclidine use disorder, severe, in sustained remission

6 **F16.22** **Hallucinogen dependence with intoxication**

F16.220 **Hallucinogen dependence with intoxication, uncomplicated** HCC

F16.221 **Hallucinogen dependence with intoxication with delirium** HCC

F16.229 **Hallucinogen dependence with intoxication, unspecified** HCC

F16.24 **Hallucinogen dependence with hallucinogen-induced mood disorder** HCC

Other hallucinogen use disorder, moderate, with other hallucinogen induced bipolar or related disorder
Other hallucinogen use disorder, moderate, with other hallucinogen induced depressive disorder
Other hallucinogen use disorder, severe, with other hallucinogen-induced bipolar or related disorder
Other hallucinogen use disorder, severe, with other hallucinogen-induced depressive disorder
Phencyclidine use disorder, moderate, with phencyclidine induced bipolar or related disorder
Phencyclidine use disorder, moderate, with phencyclidine induced depressive disorder
Phencyclidine use disorder, severe, with phencyclidine induced bipolar or related disorder
Phencyclidine use disorder, severe, with phencyclidine-induced depressive disorder

6 **F16.25** **Hallucinogen dependence with hallucinogen-induced psychotic disorder**

F16.250 **Hallucinogen dependence with hallucinogen-induced psychotic disorder with delusions** HCC

F16.251 **Hallucinogen dependence with hallucinogen-induced psychotic disorder with hallucinations** HCC

F16.259 **Hallucinogen dependence with hallucinogen-induced psychotic disorder, unspecified** HCC

6 **F16.28** **Hallucinogen dependence with other hallucinogen-induced disorder**

F16.280 **Hallucinogen dependence with hallucinogen-induced anxiety disorder** HCC

F16.283 **Hallucinogen dependence with hallucinogen persisting perception disorder (flashbacks)** HCC

F16.288 **Hallucinogen dependence with other hallucinogen-induced disorder** HCC

F16.29 **Hallucinogen dependence with unspecified hallucinogen-induced disorder** HCC

5 F16.9 **Hallucinogen use, unspecified**

EXCLUDES 1 *hallucinogen abuse (F16.1-)*
hallucinogen dependence (F16.2-)

CODING TIP ✓ Use disorder is coded to abuse or dependence depending on the severity. Mild is coded to abuse, and moderate and severe are coded to dependence.

F16.90 **Hallucinogen use, unspecified, uncomplicated**

6 F16.92 **Hallucinogen use, unspecified with intoxication**

F16.920 **Hallucinogen use, unspecified with intoxication, uncomplicated** HCC

F16.921 **Hallucinogen use, unspecified with intoxication with delirium** HCC

Other hallucinogen intoxication delirium

F16.929 **Hallucinogen use, unspecified with intoxication, unspecified** HCC

F16.94 **Hallucinogen use, unspecified with hallucinogen-induced mood disorder** HCC

Other hallucinogen induced bipolar or related disorder, without use disorder
Other hallucinogen induced depressive disorder, without use disorder
Phencyclidine induced bipolar or related disorder, without use disorder
Phencyclidine induced depressive disorder, without use disorder

6 F16.95 **Hallucinogen use, unspecified with hallucinogen-induced psychotic disorder**

F16.950 **Hallucinogen use, unspecified with hallucinogen-induced psychotic disorder with delusions** HCC

F16.951 **Hallucinogen use, unspecified with hallucinogen-induced psychotic disorder with hallucinations** HCC

F16.959 **Hallucinogen use, unspecified with hallucinogen-induced psychotic disorder, unspecified** HCC

Other hallucinogen induced psychotic disorder, without use disorder
Phencyclidine induced psychotic disorder, without use disorder

6 F16.98 **Hallucinogen use, unspecified with other specified hallucinogen-induced disorder**

F16.980 **Hallucinogen use, unspecified with hallucinogen-induced anxiety disorder** HCC

Other hallucinogen-induced anxiety disorder, without use disorder
Phencyclidine induced anxiety disorder, without use disorder

F16.983 **Hallucinogen use, unspecified with hallucinogen persisting perception disorder (flashbacks)** HCC

F16.988 **Hallucinogen use, unspecified with other hallucinogen-induced disorder** HCC

F16.99 **Hallucinogen use, unspecified with unspecified hallucinogen-induced disorder** HCC

4 F17 **Nicotine dependence**

EXCLUDES 1 *history of tobacco dependence (Z87.891)*
tobacco use NOS (Z72.0)

EXCLUDES 2 *tobacco use (smoking) during pregnancy, childbirth and the puerperium (O99.33-)*
toxic effect of nicotine (T65.2-)

CODING TIP ✓ Use disorder, regardless of the severity (mild, moderate or severe), is coded to dependence. There is no separate code to indicate abuse.

5 F17.2 **Nicotine dependence**

CODING TIP ✓ Use the appropriate code to specify nicotine product when known. ICD-10 codes provide for greater specificity, allowing the coder to specify dependence on a specific nicotine product.

6 F17.20 **Nicotine dependence, unspecified**

F17.200 **Nicotine dependence, unspecified, uncomplicated**

Tobacco use disorder, mild
Tobacco use disorder, moderate
Tobacco use disorder, severe

CODING TIP ✓ Use code F17.200 if the physician documents "smoker" or tobacco/nicotine dependence.

AHA: 4Q 2013, 108
AHA: 1Q 2016, 36-37

F17.201 **Nicotine dependence, unspecified, in remission**

Tobacco use disorder, mild, in early remission
Tobacco use disorder, mild, in sustained remission
Tobacco use disorder, moderate, in early remission
Tobacco use disorder, moderate, in sustained remission
Tobacco use disorder, severe, in early remission
Tobacco use disorder, severe, in sustained remission

F17.203 **Nicotine dependence unspecified, with withdrawal**

Tobacco withdrawal

F17.208 **Nicotine dependence, unspecified, with other nicotine-induced disorders**

F17.209 **Nicotine dependence, unspecified, with unspecified nicotine-induced disorders**

6 F17.21 **Nicotine dependence, cigarettes**

F17.210 **Nicotine dependence, cigarettes, uncomplicated**

CODING TIP ✓ Assign codes F17.210 and F17.290 for a patient who both smokes cigarettes and uses an electronic cigarette. Only assign F17.290 if a person is only using an e-cigarette or "vaping" when nicotine is used.

CODING TIP ✓ Do not use code F17.210 to report tobacco use. The provider/physician must specify tobacco dependence.

AHA: 4Q 2013, 109
AHA: 2Q 2017, 28

F17.211 **Nicotine dependence, cigarettes, in remission**

Tobacco use disorder, cigarettes, mild, in early remission
Tobacco use disorder, cigarettes, mild, in sustained remission
Tobacco use disorder, cigarettes, moderate, in early remission
Tobacco use disorder, cigarettes, moderate, in sustained remission
Tobacco use disorder, cigarettes, severe, in early remission
Tobacco use disorder, cigarettes, severe, in sustained remission

CODING TIP ✓ Do not use code F17.211 to report a history of tobacco use in a patient who has discontinued the use of cigarettes/quit smoking. History of smoking should be coded to Z87.891.

F17.213 **Nicotine dependence, cigarettes, with withdrawal**

F17.218 **Nicotine dependence, cigarettes, with other nicotine-induced disorders**

AHA: 4Q 2013, 109

F17.219 **Nicotine dependence, cigarettes, with unspecified nicotine-induced disorders**

6 F17.22 **Nicotine dependence, chewing tobacco**

F17.220 **Nicotine dependence, chewing tobacco, uncomplicated**

F17.221 Nicotine dependence, chewing tobacco, in remission HCC
Tobacco use disorder, chewing tobacco, mild, in early remission
Tobacco use disorder, chewing tobacco, mild, in sustained remission
Tobacco use disorder, chewing tobacco, moderate, in early remission
Tobacco use disorder, chewing tobacco, moderate, in sustained remission
Tobacco use disorder, chewing tobacco, severe, in early remission
Tobacco use disorder, chewing tobacco, severe, in sustained remission

F17.223 Nicotine dependence, chewing tobacco, with withdrawal

F17.228 Nicotine dependence, chewing tobacco, with other nicotine-induced disorders

F17.229 Nicotine dependence, chewing tobacco, with unspecified nicotine-induced disorders

6 **F17.29 Nicotine dependence, other tobacco product**

F17.290 Nicotine dependence, other tobacco product, uncomplicated

CODING TIP ✓ Assign codes F17.210 and F17.290 for a patient who both smokes cigarettes and uses an electronic cigarette. Only assign F17.290 if a person is only using an e-cigarette or "vaping" when nicotine is used.
AHA: 2Q 2017, 28

F17.291 Nicotine dependence, other tobacco product, in remission
Tobacco use disorder, other tobacco product, mild, in early remission
Tobacco use disorder, other tobacco product, mild, in sustained remission
Tobacco use disorder, other tobacco product, moderate, in early remission
Tobacco use disorder, other tobacco product, moderate, in sustained remission
Tobacco use disorder, other tobacco product, severe, in early remission
Tobacco use disorder, other tobacco product, severe, in sustained remission

F17.293 Nicotine dependence, other tobacco product, with withdrawal

F17.298 Nicotine dependence, other tobacco product, with other nicotine-induced disorders

F17.299 Nicotine dependence, other tobacco product, with unspecified nicotine-induced disorders

4 F18 Inhalant related disorders

INCLUDES volatile solvents

5 **F18.1 Inhalant abuse**

EXCLUDES 1 *inhalant dependence (F18.2-)*
inhalant use, unspecified (F18.9-)

F18.10 Inhalant abuse, uncomplicated HCC
Inhalant use disorder, mild

F18.11 Inhalant abuse, in remission HCC
Inhalant use disorder, mild, in early remission
Inhalant use disorder, mild, in sustained remission
AHA: 4Q 2017, 6

6 **F18.12 Inhalant abuse with intoxication**

F18.120 Inhalant abuse with intoxication, uncomplicated HCC

F18.121 Inhalant abuse with intoxication delirium HCC

F18.129 Inhalant abuse with intoxication, unspecified HCC

F18.14 Inhalant abuse with inhalant-induced mood disorder HCC
Inhalant use disorder, mild, with inhalant induced depressive disorder

6 **F18.15 Inhalant abuse with inhalant-induced psychotic disorder**

F18.150 Inhalant abuse with inhalant-induced psychotic disorder with delusions HCC

F18.151 Inhalant abuse with inhalant-induced psychotic disorder with hallucinations HCC

F18.159 Inhalant abuse with inhalant-induced psychotic disorder, unspecified HCC

F18.17 Inhalant abuse with inhalant-induced dementia HCC
Inhalant use disorder, mild, with inhalant induced major neurocognitive disorder

6 **F18.18 Inhalant abuse with other inhalant-induced disorders**

F18.180 Inhalant abuse with inhalant-induced anxiety disorder HCC

F18.188 Inhalant abuse with other inhalant-induced disorder HCC
Inhalant use disorder, mild, with inhalant induced mild neurocognitive disorder

F18.19 Inhalant abuse with unspecified inhalant-induced disorder HCC

5 **F18.2 Inhalant dependence**

EXCLUDES 1 *inhalant abuse (F18.1-)*
inhalant use, unspecified (F18.9-)

F18.20 Inhalant dependence, uncomplicated HCC
Inhalant use disorder, moderate
Inhalant use disorder, severe

F18.21 Inhalant dependence, in remission HCC
Inhalant use disorder, moderate, in early remission
Inhalant use disorder, moderate, in sustained remission
Inhalant use disorder, severe, in early remission
Inhalant use disorder, severe, in sustained remission

6 **F18.22 Inhalant dependence with intoxication**

F18.220 Inhalant dependence with intoxication, uncomplicated HCC

F18.221 Inhalant dependence with intoxication delirium HCC

F18.229 Inhalant dependence with intoxication, unspecified HCC

F18.24 Inhalant dependence with inhalant-induced mood disorder HCC
Inhalant use disorder, moderate, with inhalant induced depressive disorder
Inhalant use disorder, severe, with inhalant induced depressive disorder

6 **F18.25 Inhalant dependence with inhalant-induced psychotic disorder**

F18.250 Inhalant dependence with inhalant-induced psychotic disorder with delusions HCC

F18.251 Inhalant dependence with inhalant-induced psychotic disorder with hallucinations HCC

F18.259 Inhalant dependence with inhalant-induced psychotic disorder, unspecified HCC

F18.27 Inhalant dependence with inhalant-induced dementia HCC
Inhalant use disorder, moderate, with inhalant induced major neurocognitive disorder
Inhalant use disorder, severe, with inhalant induced major neurocognitive disorder

6 **F18.28 Inhalant dependence with other inhalant-induced disorders**

F18.280 Inhalant dependence with inhalant-induced anxiety disorder HCC

F18.288 Inhalant dependence with other inhalant-induced disorder HCC
Inhalant use disorder, moderate, with inhalant-induced mild neurocognitive disorder
Inhalant use disorder, severe, with inhalant-induced mild neurocognitive disorder

F18.29 Inhalant dependence with unspecified inhalant-induced disorder HCC

5 **F18.9 Inhalant use, unspecified**

EXCLUDES 1 *inhalant abuse (F18.1-)*
inhalant dependence (F18.2-)

CODING TIP ✓ Use disorder is coded to abuse or dependence depending on the severity. Mild is coded to abuse, and moderate and severe are coded to dependence.

F18.90 Inhalant use, unspecified, uncomplicated

6 **F18.92 Inhalant use, unspecified with intoxication**

F18.920 Inhalant use, unspecified with intoxication, uncomplicated HCC

F18.921 Inhalant use, unspecified with intoxication with delirium HCC

F18.929 Inhalant use, unspecified with intoxication, unspecified HCC

F18.94 **Inhalant use, unspecified with inhalant-induced mood disorder** HCC
Inhalant induced depressive disorder

F18.95 **Inhalant use, unspecified with inhalant-induced psychotic disorder**

F18.950 **Inhalant use, unspecified with inhalant-induced psychotic disorder with delusions** HCC

F18.951 **Inhalant use, unspecified with inhalant-induced psychotic disorder with hallucinations** HCC

F18.959 **Inhalant use, unspecified with inhalant-induced psychotic disorder, unspecified** HCC

F18.97 **Inhalant use, unspecified with inhalant-induced persisting dementia** HCC
Inhalant-induced major neurocognitive disorder

F18.98 **Inhalant use, unspecified with other inhalant-induced disorders**

F18.980 **Inhalant use, unspecified with inhalant-induced anxiety disorder** HCC

F18.988 **Inhalant use, unspecified with other inhalant-induced disorder** HCC
Inhalant-induced mild neurocognitive disorder

F18.99 **Inhalant use, unspecified with unspecified inhalant-induced disorder** HCC

F19 Other psychoactive substance related disorders

INCLUDES polysubstance drug use (indiscriminate drug use)

F19.1 **Other psychoactive substance abuse**

EXCLUDES 1 *other psychoactive substance dependence (F19.2-)*
other psychoactive substance use, unspecified (F19.9-)

F19.10 **Other psychoactive substance abuse, uncomplicated** HCC
Other (or unknown) substance use disorder, mild

F19.11 **Other psychoactive substance abuse, in remission** HCC
Other (or unknown) substance use disorder, mild, in early remission
Other (or unknown) substance use disorder, mild, in sustained remission
AHA: 4Q 2017, 6

F19.12 **Other psychoactive substance abuse with intoxication**

F19.120 **Other psychoactive substance abuse with intoxication, uncomplicated** HCC

F19.121 **Other psychoactive substance abuse with intoxication delirium** HCC

F19.122 **Other psychoactive substance abuse with intoxication with perceptual disturbances** HCC

F19.129 **Other psychoactive substance abuse with intoxication, unspecified** HCC

F19.14 **Other psychoactive substance abuse with psychoactive substance-induced mood disorder** HCC
Other (or unknown) substance use disorder, mild, with other (or unknown) substance-induced bipolar or related disorder
Other (or unknown) substance use disorder, mild, with other (or unknown) substance-induced depressive disorder

F19.15 **Other psychoactive substance abuse with psychoactive substance-induced psychotic disorder**

F19.150 **Other psychoactive substance abuse with psychoactive substance-induced psychotic disorder with delusions** HCC

F19.151 **Other psychoactive substance abuse with psychoactive substance-induced psychotic disorder with hallucinations** HCC

F19.159 **Other psychoactive substance abuse with psychoactive substance-induced psychotic disorder, unspecified** HCC

F19.16 **Other psychoactive substance abuse with psychoactive substance-induced persisting amnestic disorder** HCC

F19.17 **Other psychoactive substance abuse with psychoactive substance-induced persisting dementia** HCC
Other (or unknown) substance use disorder, mild, with other (or unknown) substance-induced major neurocognitive disorder

F19.18 **Other psychoactive substance abuse with other psychoactive substance-induced disorders**

F19.180 **Other psychoactive substance abuse with psychoactive substance-induced anxiety disorder** HCC

F19.181 **Other psychoactive substance abuse with psychoactive substance-induced sexual dysfunction** HCC

F19.182 **Other psychoactive substance abuse with psychoactive substance-induced sleep disorder** HCC

F19.188 **Other psychoactive substance abuse with other psychoactive substance-induced disorder** HCC
Other (or unknown) substance use disorder, mild, with other (or unknown) substance induced mild neurocognitive disorder
Other (or unknown) substance use disorder, mild, with other (or unknown) substance induced obsessive-compulsive or related disorder

F19.19 **Other psychoactive substance abuse with unspecified psychoactive substance-induced disorder** HCC

F19.2 **Other psychoactive substance dependence**

EXCLUDES 1 *other psychoactive substance abuse (F19.1-)*
other psychoactive substance use, unspecified (F19.9-)

F19.20 **Other psychoactive substance dependence, uncomplicated** HCC
Other (or unknown) substance use disorder, moderate
Other (or unknown) substance use disorder, severe

▲ F19.21 **Other psychoactive substance dependence, in remission** HCC
Other (or unknown) substance use disorder, moderate, in early remission
Other (or unknown) substance use disorder, moderate, in sustained remission
Other (or unknown) substance use disorder, severe, in early remission
Other (or unknown) substance use disorder, severe, in sustained remission

F19.22 **Other psychoactive substance dependence with intoxication**

EXCLUDES 1 *other psychoactive substance dependence with withdrawal (F19.23-)*

F19.220 **Other psychoactive substance dependence with intoxication, uncomplicated** HCC

F19.221 **Other psychoactive substance dependence with intoxication delirium** HCC

F19.222 **Other psychoactive substance dependence with intoxication with perceptual disturbance** HCC

F19.229 **Other psychoactive substance dependence with intoxication, unspecified** HCC

F19.23 **Other psychoactive substance dependence with withdrawal**

EXCLUDES 1 *other psychoactive substance dependence with intoxication (F19.22-)*

F19.230 **Other psychoactive substance dependence with withdrawal, uncomplicated** HCC

F19.231 **Other psychoactive substance dependence with withdrawal delirium** HCC

F19.232 **Other psychoactive substance dependence with withdrawal with perceptual disturbance** HCC

F19.239 **Other psychoactive substance dependence with withdrawal, unspecified** HCC

F19.24 **Other psychoactive substance dependence with psychoactive substance-induced mood disorder** HCC
Other (or unknown) substance use disorder, moderate, with other (or unknown) substance induced bipolar or related disorder
Other (or unknown) substance use disorder, moderate, with other (or unknown) substance induced depressive disorder
Other (or unknown) substance use disorder, severe, with other (or unknown) substance induced bipolar or related disorder
Other (or unknown) substance use disorder, severe, with other (or unknown) substance induced depressive disorder

6 F19.25 **Other psychoactive substance dependence with psychoactive substance-induced psychotic disorder**

F19.250 **Other psychoactive substance dependence with psychoactive substance-induced psychotic disorder with delusions** HCC

F19.251 **Other psychoactive substance dependence with psychoactive substance-induced psychotic disorder with hallucinations** HCC

F19.259 **Other psychoactive substance dependence with psychoactive substance-induced psychotic disorder, unspecified** HCC

F19.26 **Other psychoactive substance dependence with psychoactive substance-induced persisting amnestic disorder** HCC

F19.27 **Other psychoactive substance dependence with psychoactive substance-induced persisting dementia** HCC
Other (or unknown) substance use disorder, moderate, with other (or unknown) substance induced major neurocognitive disorder
Other (or unknown) substance use disorder, severe, with other (or unknown) substance induced major neurocognitive disorder

6 F19.28 **Other psychoactive substance dependence with other psychoactive substance-induced disorders**

F19.280 **Other psychoactive substance dependence with psychoactive substance-induced anxiety disorder** HCC

F19.281 **Other psychoactive substance dependence with psychoactive substance-induced sexual dysfunction** HCC

F19.282 **Other psychoactive substance dependence with psychoactive substance-induced sleep disorder** HCC

F19.288 **Other psychoactive substance dependence with other psychoactive substance-induced disorder** HCC
Other (or unknown) substance use disorder, moderate, with other (or unknown) substance induced mild neurocognitive disorder
Other (or unknown) substance use disorder, severe, with other (or unknown) substance induced mild neurocognitive disorder
Other (or unknown) substance use disorder, moderate, with other (or unknown) substance induced obsessive compulsive or related disorder
Other (or unknown) substance use disorder, severe, with other (or unknown) substance induced obsessive-compulsive or related disorder

F19.29 **Other psychoactive substance dependence with unspecified psychoactive substance-induced disorder** HCC

5 F19.9 **Other psychoactive substance use, unspecified**

EXCLUDES 1 *other psychoactive substance abuse (F19.1-)*
other psychoactive substance dependence (F19.2-)

CODING TIP ✓ Use disorder is coded to abuse or dependence depending on the severity. Mild is coded to abuse, and moderate and severe are coded to dependence.

F19.90 **Other psychoactive substance use, unspecified, uncomplicated**

6 F19.92 **Other psychoactive substance use, unspecified with intoxication**

EXCLUDES 1 *other psychoactive substance use, unspecified with withdrawal (F19.93)*

F19.920 **Other psychoactive substance use, unspecified with intoxication, uncomplicated** HCC

F19.921 **Other psychoactive substance use, unspecified with intoxication with delirium** HCC
Other (or unknown) substance-induced delirium

F19.922 **Other psychoactive substance use, unspecified with intoxication with perceptual disturbance** HCC

F19.929 **Other psychoactive substance use, unspecified with intoxication, unspecified** HCC

6 F19.93 **Other psychoactive substance use, unspecified with withdrawal**

EXCLUDES 1 *other psychoactive substance use, unspecified with intoxication (F19.92-)*

F19.930 **Other psychoactive substance use, unspecified with withdrawal, uncomplicated** HCC

F19.931 **Other psychoactive substance use, unspecified with withdrawal delirium** HCC

F19.932 **Other psychoactive substance use, unspecified with withdrawal with perceptual disturbance** HCC

F19.939 **Other psychoactive substance use, unspecified with withdrawal, unspecified** HCC

F19.94 **Other psychoactive substance use, unspecified with psychoactive substance-induced mood disorder** HCC
Other (or unknown) substance-induced bipolar or related disorder, without use disorder
Other (or unknown) substance-induced depressive disorder, without use disorder

6 F19.95 **Other psychoactive substance use, unspecified with psychoactive substance-induced psychotic disorder**

F19.950 **Other psychoactive substance use, unspecified with psychoactive substance-induced psychotic disorder with delusions** HCC

F19.951 **Other psychoactive substance use, unspecified with psychoactive substance-induced psychotic disorder with hallucinations** HCC

F19.959 **Other psychoactive substance use, unspecified with psychoactive substance-induced psychotic disorder, unspecified** HCC
Other or unknown substance-induced psychotic disorder, without use disorder

F19.96 **Other psychoactive substance use, unspecified with psychoactive substance-induced persisting amnestic disorder** HCC

F19.97 **Other psychoactive substance use, unspecified with psychoactive substance-induced persisting dementia** HCC
Other (or unknown) substance-induced major neurocognitive disorder, without use disorder

6 F19.98 **Other psychoactive substance use, unspecified with other psychoactive substance-induced disorders**

F19.980 **Other psychoactive substance use, unspecified with psychoactive substance-induced anxiety disorder** HCC
Other (or unknown) substance-induced anxiety disorder, without use disorder

F19.981 **Other psychoactive substance use, unspecified with psychoactive substance-induced sexual dysfunction** HCC
Other (or unknown) substance-induced sexual dysfunction, without use disorder

F19.982 **Other psychoactive substance use, unspecified with psychoactive substance-induced sleep disorder** HCC
Other (or unknown) substance-induced sleep disorder, without use disorder

F19.988 **Other psychoactive substance use, unspecified with other psychoactive substance-induced disorder** HCC
Other (or unknown) substance-induced mild neurocognitive disorder, without use disorder
Other (or unknown) substance-induced obsessive-compulsive or related disorder, without use disorder

F19.99 **Other psychoactive substance use, unspecified with unspecified psychoactive substance-induced disorder** HCC

Schizophrenia, schizotypal, delusional, and other non-mood psychotic disorders (F20-F29)

4 **F20 Schizophrenia**
EXCLUDES 1 *brief psychotic disorder (F23)*
cyclic schizophrenia (F25.0)
mood [affective] disorders with psychotic symptoms (F30.2, F31.2, F31.5, F31.64, F32.3, F33.3)
schizoaffective disorder (F25.-)
schizophrenic reaction NOS (F23)
EXCLUDES 2 *schizophrenic reaction in:*
alcoholism (F10.15-, F10.25-, F10.95-)
brain disease (F06.2)
epilepsy (F06.2)
psychoactive drug use (F11-F19 with .15. .25, .95)
schizotypal disorder (F21)

F20.0 **Paranoid schizophrenia** HCC
Paraphrenic schizophrenia
EXCLUDES 1 *involutional paranoid state (F22)*
paranoia (F22)
DEFINITION Schizophrenia marked by displays of megalomania, delusions of persecution and/or grandeur, hallucinations, and aggressive behavior.

F20.1 **Disorganized schizophrenia** HCC
Hebephrenic schizophrenia
Hebephrenia

F20.2 **Catatonic schizophrenia** HCC
Schizophrenic catalepsy
Schizophrenic catatonia
Schizophrenic flexibilitas cerea
EXCLUDES 1 *catatonic stupor (R40.1)*

F20.3 **Undifferentiated schizophrenia** HCC
Atypical schizophrenia
EXCLUDES 1 *acute schizophrenia-like psychotic disorder (F23)*
EXCLUDES 2 *post-schizophrenic depression (F32.89)*

F20.5 **Residual schizophrenia** HCC
Restzustand (schizophrenic)
Schizophrenic residual state

5 F20.8 **Other schizophrenia**

F20.81 **Schizophreniform disorder** HCC
Schizophreniform psychosis NOS

F20.89 **Other schizophrenia** HCC
Cenesthopathic schizophrenia
Simple schizophrenia

F20.9 **Schizophrenia, unspecified** HCC

F21 Schizotypal disorder HCC
Borderline schizophrenia
Latent schizophrenia
Latent schizophrenic reaction
Prepsychotic schizophrenia
Prodromal schizophrenia
Pseudoneurotic schizophrenia
Pseudopsychopathic schizophrenia
Schizotypal personality disorder
EXCLUDES 2 *Asperger's syndrome (F84.5)*
schizoid personality disorder (F60.1)

CODING TIP ✓ Do not use code F21 when schizophrenia or schizoaffective disorder is specified by the physician. Schizotypal disorder is a personality disorder characterized by behaviors that impact interpersonal relationships, affect appearance and often exacerbate depressive and/or anxious symptoms.

F22 Delusional disorders HCC
Delusional dysmorphophobia
Involutional paranoid state
Paranoia
Paranoia querulans
Paranoid psychosis
Paranoid state
Paraphrenia (late)
Sensitiver Beziehungswahn
EXCLUDES 1 *mood [affective] disorders with psychotic symptoms (F30.2, F31.2, F31.5, F31.64, F32.3, F33.3)*
paranoid schizophrenia (F20.0)
EXCLUDES 2 *paranoid personality disorder (F60.0)*
paranoid psychosis, psychogenic (F23)
paranoid reaction (F23)
DEFINITION Paranoia: Extreme, irrational distrust of others.

F23 Brief psychotic disorder HCC
Paranoid reaction
Psychogenic paranoid psychosis
EXCLUDES 2 *mood [affective] disorders with psychotic symptoms (F30.2, F31.2, F31.5, F31.64, F32.3, F33.3)*

F24 Shared psychotic disorder HCC
Folie à deux
Induced paranoid disorder
Induced psychotic disorder

4 **F25 Schizoaffective disorders**
EXCLUDES 1 *mood [affective] disorders with psychotic symptoms (F30.2, F31.2, F31.5, F31.64, F32.3, F33.3)*
schizophrenia (F20.-)
CODING TIP ✓ Do not use F25.- codes when schizophrenia is specified by the physician. Schizoaffective disorder is diagnosed in patients who do not meet the criteria for either schizophrenia or bipolar disorder but often demonstrate characteristics of both disorders.

F25.0 **Schizoaffective disorder, bipolar type** HCC
Cyclic schizophrenia
Schizoaffective disorder, manic type
Schizoaffective disorder, mixed type
Schizoaffective psychosis, bipolar type

F25.1 **Schizoaffective disorder, depressive type** HCC
Schizoaffective psychosis, depressive type

F25.8 **Other schizoaffective disorders** HCC

F25.9 **Schizoaffective disorder, unspecified** HCC
Schizoaffective psychosis NOS

F28 Other psychotic disorder not due to a substance or known physiological condition HCC HIV
Chronic hallucinatory psychosis
Other specified schizophrenia spectrum and other psychotic disorder

F29 Unspecified psychosis not due to a substance or known physiological condition HCC HIV
Psychosis NOS
Unspecified schizophrenia spectrum and other psychotic disorder
EXCLUDES 1 *mental disorder NOS (F99)*
unspecified mental disorder due to known physiological condition (F09)

Mood [affective] disorders (F30-F39)

4 **F30 Manic episode**
INCLUDES bipolar disorder, single manic episode
mixed affective episode
EXCLUDES 1 *bipolar disorder (F31.-)*
major depressive disorder, single episode (F32.-)
major depressive disorder, recurrent (F33.-)

5 F30.1 **Manic episode without psychotic symptoms**

F30.10 **Manic episode without psychotic symptoms, unspecified** HCC

F30.11 **Manic episode without psychotic symptoms, mild** HCC

F30.12 **Manic episode without psychotic symptoms, moderate** HCC

F30.13 **Manic episode, severe, without psychotic symptoms** HCC

F30.2 **Manic episode, severe with psychotic symptoms** HCC
Manic stupor
Mania with mood-congruent psychotic symptoms
Mania with mood-incongruent psychotic symptoms

F30.3 **Manic episode in partial remission** HCC

F30.4 **Manic episode in full remission** HCC

F30.8 **Other manic episodes** HCC
Hypomania

F30.9 **Manic episode, unspecified** HCC
Mania NOS

4 F31 Bipolar disorder

INCLUDES bipolar I disorder
bipolar type I disorder
manic-depressive illness
manic-depressive psychosis
manic-depressive reaction

EXCLUDES 1 *bipolar disorder, single manic episode (F30.-)*
major depressive disorder, single episode (F32.-)
major depressive disorder, recurrent (F33.-)

EXCLUDES 2 *cyclothymia (F34.0)*

CODING TIP✓ When assigning a code for bipolar disorder, no additional code for depression or depressive disorder should be assigned if the patient is also reported to have depression and/or depressive symptoms. Individuals with bipolar disorder may have alternating periods of emotional highs and lows reported as cyclothymic features. When cyclothymic features are additionally reported by the physician, cyclothymia (F34.0) should be additionally coded.

F31.0 **Bipolar disorder, current episode hypomanic** HCC

5 **F31.1** **Bipolar disorder, current episode manic without psychotic features**

F31.10 **Bipolar disorder, current episode manic without psychotic features, unspecified** HCC

F31.11 **Bipolar disorder, current episode manic without psychotic features, mild** HCC

F31.12 **Bipolar disorder, current episode manic without psychotic features, moderate** HCC

F31.13 **Bipolar disorder, current episode manic without psychotic features, severe** HCC

F31.2 **Bipolar disorder, current episode manic severe with psychotic features** HCC
Bipolar disorder, current episode manic with mood-congruent psychotic symptoms
Bipolar disorder, current episode manic with mood-incongruent psychotic symptoms
Bipolar I disorder, current or most recent episode manic with psychotic features

5 **F31.3** **Bipolar disorder, current episode depressed, mild or moderate severity**

F31.30 **Bipolar disorder, current episode depressed, mild or moderate severity, unspecified** HCC

F31.31 **Bipolar disorder, current episode depressed, mild** HCC

F31.32 **Bipolar disorder, current episode depressed, moderate** HCC

F31.4 **Bipolar disorder, current episode depressed, severe, without psychotic features** HCC

CODING TIP✓ Depression documented as with anxiety is not coded to dysthymic disorder. When physician documentation reports depression with anxiety, use F41.8, Other specified anxiety disorders.

F31.5 **Bipolar disorder, current episode depressed, severe, with psychotic features** HCC
Bipolar disorder, current episode depressed with mood-incongruent psychotic symptoms
Bipolar disorder, current episode depressed with mood-congruent psychotic symptoms
Bipolar I disorder, current or most recent episode depressed, with psychotic features

5 **F31.6** **Bipolar disorder, current episode mixed**

F31.60 **Bipolar disorder, current episode mixed, unspecified** HCC

F31.61 **Bipolar disorder, current episode mixed, mild** HCC

F31.62 **Bipolar disorder, current episode mixed, moderate** HCC

F31.63 **Bipolar disorder, current episode mixed, severe, without psychotic features** HCC

F31.64 **Bipolar disorder, current episode mixed, severe, with psychotic features** HCC
Bipolar disorder, current episode mixed with mood-congruent psychotic symptoms
Bipolar disorder, current episode mixed with mood-incongruent psychotic symptoms

5 **F31.7** **Bipolar disorder, currently in remission**

F31.70 **Bipolar disorder, currently in remission, most recent episode unspecified** HCC

F31.71 **Bipolar disorder, in partial remission, most recent episode hypomanic** HCC

F31.72 **Bipolar disorder, in full remission, most recent episode hypomanic** HCC

F31.73 **Bipolar disorder, in partial remission, most recent episode manic** HCC

F31.74 **Bipolar disorder, in full remission, most recent episode manic** HCC

F31.75 **Bipolar disorder, in partial remission, most recent episode depressed** HCC

F31.76 **Bipolar disorder, in full remission, most recent episode depressed** HCC

F31.77 **Bipolar disorder, in partial remission, most recent episode mixed** HCC

F31.78 **Bipolar disorder, in full remission, most recent episode mixed** HCC

5 **F31.8** **Other bipolar disorders**

F31.81 **Bipolar II disorder** HCC
Bipolar disorder, type 2

F31.89 **Other bipolar disorder** HCC
Recurrent manic episodes NOS

F31.9 **Bipolar disorder, unspecified** HCC
Manic depression

4 F32 Major depressive disorder, single episode

INCLUDES single episode of agitated depression
single episode of depressive reaction
single episode of major depression
single episode of psychogenic depression
single episode of reactive depression
single episode of vital depression

EXCLUDES 1 *bipolar disorder (F31.-)*
manic episode (F30.-)
recurrent depressive disorder (F33.-)

EXCLUDES 2 *adjustment disorder (F43.2)*

F32.0 **Major depressive disorder, single episode, mild** HCC

F32.1 **Major depressive disorder, single episode, moderate** HCC

F32.2 **Major depressive disorder, single episode, severe without psychotic features** HCC

F32.3 **Major depressive disorder, single episode, severe with psychotic features** HCC
Single episode of major depression with mood-congruent psychotic symptoms
Single episode of major depression with mood-incongruent psychotic symptoms
Single episode of major depression with psychotic symptoms
Single episode of psychogenic depressive psychosis
Single episode of psychotic depression
Single episode of reactive depressive psychosis

F32.4 **Major depressive disorder, single episode, in partial remission** HCC

F32.5 **Major depressive disorder, single episode, in full remission** HCC

5 **F32.8** **Other depressive episodes**

F32.81 **Premenstrual dysphoric disorder** ♀

EXCLUDES 1 *premenstrual tension syndrome (N94.3)*

DEFINITION Premenstrual dysphoric disorder (PMDD) is a severe form of premenstrual syndrome (PMS). PMDD is characterized by depression, anxiety, tension and irritability that typically begins after release of the ovum.
AHA: 4Q 2016, 14

F32.89 **Other specified depressive episodes**
Atypical depression
Post-schizophrenic depression
Single episode of 'masked' depression NOS
AHA: 4Q 2016, 14

F32.9 **Major depressive disorder, single episode, unspecified**
Depression NOS
Depressive disorder NOS
Major depression NOS
CODING TIP✓ Documentation: Unspecified and chronic depression should be coded to F32.9. A physician must provide confirmation of the diagnosis of depression to assign this code, and it should not be assigned based upon the presence of symptoms alone.
AHA: 4Q 2013, 107, 108

4 F33 **Major depressive disorder, recurrent**
INCLUDES recurrent episodes of depressive reaction
recurrent episodes of endogenous depression
recurrent episodes of major depression
recurrent episodes of psychogenic depression
recurrent episodes of reactive depression
recurrent episodes of seasonal depressive disorder
recurrent episodes of vital depression
EXCLUDES 1 *bipolar disorder (F31.-)*
manic episode (F30.-)

F33.0 **Major depressive disorder, recurrent, mild** HCC
F33.1 **Major depressive disorder, recurrent, moderate** HCC
F33.2 **Major depressive disorder, recurrent severe without psychotic features** HCC
F33.3 **Major depressive disorder, recurrent, severe with psychotic symptoms** HCC
Endogenous depression with psychotic symptoms
Major depressive disorder, recurrent, with psychotic features
Recurrent severe episodes of major depression with mood-congruent psychotic symptoms
Recurrent severe episodes of major depression with mood-incongruent psychotic symptoms
Recurrent severe episodes of major depression with psychotic symptoms
Recurrent severe episodes of psychogenic depressive psychosis
Recurrent severe episodes of psychotic depression
Recurrent severe episodes of reactive depressive psychosis

5 F33.4 **Major depressive disorder, recurrent, in remission**
F33.40 **Major depressive disorder, recurrent, in remission, unspecified** HCC
F33.41 **Major depressive disorder, recurrent, in partial remission** HCC
F33.42 **Major depressive disorder, recurrent, in full remission** HCC

F33.8 **Other recurrent depressive disorders** HCC
Recurrent brief depressive episodes
F33.9 **Major depressive disorder, recurrent, unspecified** HCC
Monopolar depression NOS

4 F34 **Persistent mood [affective] disorders**
F34.0 **Cyclothymic disorder**
Affective personality disorder
Cycloid personality
Cyclothymia
Cyclothymic personality
DEFINITION Mild mood swings between elevated mood and mild depression.

F34.1 **Dysthymic disorder**
Depressive neurosis
Depressive personality disorder
Dysthymia
Neurotic depression
Persistent anxiety depression
Persistent depressive disorder
EXCLUDES 2 *anxiety depression (mild or not persistent) (F41.8)*

5 F34.8 **Other persistent mood [affective] disorders**
F34.81 **Disruptive mood dysregulation disorder** HCC
AHA: 4Q 2016, 14
F34.89 **Other specified persistent mood disorders** HCC
AHA: 4Q 2016, 14
F34.9 **Persistent mood [affective] disorder, unspecified** HCC

F39 **Unspecified mood [affective] disorder** HCC
Affective psychosis NOS

Anxiety, dissociative, stress-related, somatoform and other nonpsychotic mental disorders (F40-F48)

4 F40 **Phobic anxiety disorders**
5 F40.0 **Agoraphobia**
F40.00 **Agoraphobia, unspecified**
F40.01 **Agoraphobia with panic disorder**
Panic disorder with agoraphobia
EXCLUDES 1 *panic disorder without agoraphobia (F41.0)*
DEFINITION Fear of open spaces or crowds, traveling, or leaving a safe place, accompanied by panic attacks.
F40.02 **Agoraphobia without panic disorder**

5 F40.1 **Social phobias**
Anthropophobia
Social anxiety disorder
Social anxiety disorder of childhood
Social neurosis
DEFINITION Intense fear of appearing in public, especially in situations where one is the center of attention.
F40.10 **Social phobia, unspecified**
F40.11 **Social phobia, generalized**

5 F40.2 **Specific (isolated) phobias**
EXCLUDES 2 *dysmorphophobia (nondelusional) (F45.22)*
nosophobia (F45.22)
6 F40.21 **Animal type phobia**
F40.210 **Arachnophobia**
Fear of spiders
F40.218 **Other animal type phobia**
6 F40.22 **Natural environment type phobia**
F40.220 **Fear of thunderstorms**
F40.228 **Other natural environment type phobia**
6 F40.23 **Blood, injection, injury type phobia**
F40.230 **Fear of blood**
F40.231 **Fear of injections and transfusions**
F40.232 **Fear of other medical care**
F40.233 **Fear of injury**
6 F40.24 **Situational type phobia**
F40.240 **Claustrophobia**
F40.241 **Acrophobia**
F40.242 **Fear of bridges**
F40.243 **Fear of flying**
F40.248 **Other situational type phobia**
6 F40.29 **Other specified phobia**
F40.290 **Androphobia**
Fear of men
F40.291 **Gynephobia**
Fear of women
F40.298 **Other specified phobia**

F40.8 **Other phobic anxiety disorders**
Phobic anxiety disorder of childhood
F40.9 **Phobic anxiety disorder, unspecified**
Phobia NOS
Phobic state NOS

4 F41 **Other anxiety disorders**
EXCLUDES 2 *anxiety in:*
acute stress reaction (F43.0)
transient adjustment reaction (F43.2)
neurasthenia (F48.8)
psychophysiologic disorders (F45.-)
separation anxiety (F93.0)
F41.0 **Panic disorder [episodic paroxysmal anxiety]**
Panic attack
Panic state
EXCLUDES 1 *panic disorder with agoraphobia (F40.01)*

DEFINITION Unexplained bouts of intense fear or anxiety, accompanied by physiological symptoms of elevated heart rate, sweating, trembling, dizziness, and dyspnea.

F41.1 Generalized anxiety disorder
Anxiety neurosis
Anxiety reaction
Anxiety state
Overanxious disorder
EXCLUDES 2 *neurasthenia (F48.8)*

DEFINITION Persistent, uncontrollable worry about aspects of a person's life; diagnosed when symptoms last longer than six months, with anxiety present on the majority of days in that time.

F41.3 Other mixed anxiety disorders

F41.8 Other specified anxiety disorders
Anxiety depression (mild or not persistent)
Anxiety hysteria
Mixed anxiety and depressive disorder

CODING TIP ✓ **Documentation:** When physician documentation specifies depression with anxiety, F41.8 should be assigned. The term "with" is considered a relational term and is interpreted to mean "associated with" or "due to."

F41.9 Anxiety disorder, unspecified
Anxiety NOS

F42 Obsessive-compulsive disorder
EXCLUDES 2 *obsessive-compulsive personality (disorder) (F60.5)*
obsessive-compulsive symptoms occurring in depression (F32-F33)
obsessive-compulsive symptoms occurring in schizophrenia (F20.-)

DEFINITION Recurrent obsessions of thought or action that are time-consuming or disruptive to daily life and can produce anxiety or distress.

F42.2 Mixed obsessional thoughts and acts

F42.3 Hoarding disorder
AHA: 4Q 2016, 14

F42.4 Excoriation (skin-picking) disorder
EXCLUDES 1 *factitial dermatitis (L98.1)*
other specified behavioral and emotional disorders with onset usually occurring in early childhood and adolescence (F98.8)
AHA: 4Q 2016, 14

F42.8 Other obsessive-compulsive disorder
Anancastic neurosis
Obsessive-compulsive neurosis

F42.9 Obsessive-compulsive disorder, unspecified

F43 Reaction to severe stress, and adjustment disorders

F43.0 Acute stress reaction
Acute crisis reaction
Acute reaction to stress
Combat and operational stress reaction
Combat fatigue
Crisis state
Psychic shock

F43.1 Post-traumatic stress disorder (PTSD)
Traumatic neurosis

DEFINITION Chronic stressful response to traumatic events such as combat, rape, physical assault, and natural disasters with sudden, powerful memories (flashbacks) of the event, anxiety, and panic.

F43.10 Post-traumatic stress disorder, unspecified

F43.11 Post-traumatic stress disorder, acute

F43.12 Post-traumatic stress disorder, chronic

F43.2 Adjustment disorders
Culture shock
Grief reaction
Hospitalism in children
EXCLUDES 2 *separation anxiety disorder of childhood (F93.0)*

F43.20 Adjustment disorder, unspecified

F43.21 Adjustment disorder with depressed mood

CODING TIP ✓ Complicated bereavement of any nature is coded to F43.21. Bereavement (uncomplicated) due to loss of a family member only is coded Z63.4.

DEFINITION Prolonged depressive state as a reaction to an event or change in the patient's life.
AHA: 1Q 2014, 25

F43.22 Adjustment disorder with anxiety

F43.23 Adjustment disorder with mixed anxiety and depressed mood

F43.24 Adjustment disorder with disturbance of conduct

F43.25 Adjustment disorder with mixed disturbance of emotions and conduct

F43.29 Adjustment disorder with other symptoms

F43.8 Other reactions to severe stress
Other specified trauma and stressor-related disorder

F43.9 Reaction to severe stress, unspecified
Trauma and stressor-related disorder, NOS

F44 Dissociative and conversion disorders
INCLUDES conversion hysteria
conversion reaction
hysteria
hysterical psychosis
EXCLUDES 2 *malingering [conscious simulation] (Z76.5)*

F44.0 Dissociative amnesia
EXCLUDES 1 *amnesia NOS (R41.3)*
anterograde amnesia (R41.1)
dissociative amnesia with dissociative fugue (F44.1)
retrograde amnesia (R41.2)
EXCLUDES 2 *alcohol-or other psychoactive substance-induced amnestic disorder (F10, F13, F19 with .26, .96)*
amnestic disorder due to known physiological condition (F04)
postictal amnesia in epilepsy (G40.-)

DEFINITION Psychological trauma causing temporary forgetting of personal information and inability to perform complex tasks, like driving or cooking.

F44.1 Dissociative fugue
Dissociative amnesia with dissociative fugue
EXCLUDES 2 *postictal fugue in epilepsy (G40.-)*

DEFINITION Disorder occurring in response to a severe, recent stressor, in which the patient invents a new personality and becomes unable to remember his/her previous identity, lasting days or months.

F44.2 Dissociative stupor
EXCLUDES 1 *catatonic stupor (R40.1)*
stupor NOS (R40.1)
EXCLUDES 2 *catatonic disorder due to known physiological condition (F06.1)*
depressive stupor (F32, F33)
manic stupor (F30, F31)

F44.4 Conversion disorder with motor symptom or deficit
Conversion disorder with abnormal movement
Conversion disorder with speech symptoms
Conversion disorder with swallowing symptoms
Conversion disorder with weakness/paralysis
Dissociative motor disorders
Psychogenic aphonia
Psychogenic dysphonia

F44.5 Conversion disorder with seizures or convulsions
Conversion disorder with attacks or seizures
Dissociative convulsions

F44.6 Conversion disorder with sensory symptom or deficit
Conversion disorder with anesthesia or sensory loss
Conversion disorder with special sensory symptoms
Dissociative anesthesia and sensory loss
Psychogenic deafness

F44.7 Conversion disorder with mixed symptom presentation

F44.8 Other dissociative and conversion disorders

F44.81 Dissociative identity disorder
Multiple personality disorder

F44.89 Other dissociative and conversion disorders
Ganser's syndrome
Psychogenic confusion
Psychogenic twilight state
Trance and possession disorders

F44.9 Dissociative and conversion disorder, unspecified
Dissociative disorder NOS

▲ 4 **F45 Somatoform disorders**
EXCLUDES 2 *dissociative and conversion disorders (F44.-)*
factitious disorders (F68.1-, F68.A)
hair-plucking (F63.3)
lalling (F80.0)
lisping (F80.0)
malingering [conscious simulation] (Z76.5)
nail-biting (F98.8)
psychological or behavioral factors associated with disorders or diseases classified elsewhere (F54)
sexual dysfunction, not due to a substance or known physiological condition (F52.-)
thumb-sucking (F98.8)
tic disorders (in childhood and adolescence) (F95.-)
Tourette's syndrome (F95.2)
trichotillomania (F63.3)

F45.0 Somatization disorder
Briquet's disorder
Multiple psychosomatic disorder

F45.1 Undifferentiated somatoform disorder
Somatic symptom disorder
Undifferentiated psychosomatic disorder

5 **F45.2 Hypochondriacal disorders**
EXCLUDES 2 *delusional dysmorphophobia (F22)*
fixed delusions about bodily functions or shape (F22)

DEFINITION Chronic worry about nonexistent illnesses that one believes one may have.

F45.20 Hypochondriacal disorder, unspecified

F45.21 Hypochondriasis
Hypochondriacal neurosis
Illness anxiety disorder

F45.22 Body dysmorphic disorder
Dysmorphophobia (nondelusional)
Nosophobia

F45.29 Other hypochondriacal disorders

5 **F45.4 Pain disorders related to psychological factors**
EXCLUDES 1 *pain NOS (R52)*

F45.41 Pain disorder exclusively related to psychological factors
Somatoform pain disorder (persistent)

GUIDELINES Section I.C.5.a
Assign code F45.41 for pain that is exclusively related to psychological disorders. As indicated by the Excludes 1 note under category G89, a code from category G89 should not be assigned with code F45.41.

CODING TIP✓ Do not use F45.41 to report somatoform disorder not related to pain, chronic pain syndrome, or psychological factors related to chronic pain disorders (G89.-, F45.42).

F45.42 Pain disorder with related psychological factors
Code also:
associated acute or chronic pain (G89.-)

GUIDELINES Section I.C.5.a
Code F45.42 should be used with a code from category G89, Pain, not elsewhere classified, if there is documentation of a psychological component for a patient with acute or chronic pain.

CODING TIP✓ When the clinical record specifies that the patient has a pain disorder with related psychological factors, this code should be assigned with an additional code from G89.-.

F45.8 Other somatoform disorders
Psychogenic dysmenorrhea
Psychogenic dysphagia, including 'globus hystericus'
Psychogenic pruritus
Psychogenic torticollis
Somatoform autonomic dysfunction
Teeth grinding
EXCLUDES 1 *sleep related teeth grinding (G47.63)*

F45.9 Somatoform disorder, unspecified
Psychosomatic disorder NOS

4 **F48 Other nonpsychotic mental disorders**

F48.1 Depersonalization-derealization syndrome

F48.2 Pseudobulbar affect
Involuntary emotional expression disorder
Code first underlying cause, if known, such as:
amyotrophic lateral sclerosis (G12.21)
multiple sclerosis (G35)
sequelae of cerebrovascular disease (I69.-)
sequelae of traumatic intracranial injury (S06.-)

F48.8 Other specified nonpsychotic mental disorders
Dhat syndrome
Neurasthenia
Occupational neurosis, including writer's cramp
Psychasthenia
Psychasthenic neurosis
Psychogenic syncope

F48.9 Nonpsychotic mental disorder, unspecified
Neurosis NOS

Behavioral syndromes associated with physiological disturbances and physical factors (F50-F59)

4 **F50 Eating disorders**
EXCLUDES 1 *anorexia NOS (R63.0)*
feeding difficulties (R63.3)
feeding problems of newborn (P92.-)
polyphagia (R63.2)
EXCLUDES 2 *feeding disorder in infancy or childhood (F98.2-)*

5 **F50.0 Anorexia nervosa**
EXCLUDES 1 *loss of appetite (R63.0)*
psychogenic loss of appetite (F50.89)

CODING TIP✓ This code can be assigned only if specified as "anorexia nervosa," which is differentiated from simple anorexia (loss of appetite) due to psychological features, including intense fear of weight gain, body image distortions, and a refusal to maintain normal body weight.

F50.00 Anorexia nervosa, unspecified

F50.01 Anorexia nervosa, restricting type

F50.02 Anorexia nervosa, binge eating/purging type
EXCLUDES 1 *bulimia nervosa (F50.2)*

F50.2 Bulimia nervosa
Bulimia NOS
Hyperorexia nervosa
EXCLUDES 1 *anorexia nervosa, binge eating/purging type (F50.02)*

DEFINITION Repetitive episodes of binge eating followed by excessive measures to avoid gaining weight, such as self-induced vomiting and extreme exercising.

5 **F50.8 Other eating disorders**
EXCLUDES 2 *pica of infancy and childhood (F98.3)*

F50.81 Binge eating disorder
AHA: 4Q 2016, 14

F50.82 Avoidant/restrictive food intake disorder
AHA: 4Q 2017, 7

F50.89 Other specified eating disorder
Pica in adults
Psychogenic loss of appetite

DEFINITION This code includes pica in adults. Pica is the urge to eat nonfood substances, such as dirt, paper, paint, and rocks. It also includes the psychogenic loss of appetite characterized by an aversion to food or eating with no pathologic or physiologic explanation.

F50.9 **Eating disorder, unspecified**
Atypical anorexia nervosa
Atypical bulimia nervosa
Feeding or eating disorder, unspecified
Other specified feeding disorder

4 F51 **Sleep disorders not due to a substance or known physiological condition**
EXCLUDES 2 *organic sleep disorders (G47.-)*

5 F51.0 **Insomnia not due to a substance or known physiological condition**
EXCLUDES 2 *alcohol related insomnia (F10.182, F10.282, F10.982)*
drug-related insomnia (F11.182, F11.282, F11.982, F13.182, F13.282, F13.982, F14.182, F14.282, F14.982, F15.182, F15.282, F15.982, F19.182, F19.282, F19.982)
insomnia NOS (G47.0-)
insomnia due to known physiological condition (G47.0-)
organic insomnia (G47.0-)
sleep deprivation (Z72.820)

F51.01 **Primary insomnia**
Idiopathic insomnia

F51.02 **Adjustment insomnia**

F51.03 **Paradoxical insomnia**

F51.04 **Psychophysiologic insomnia**

F51.05 **Insomnia due to other mental disorder**
Code also:
associated mental disorder

F51.09 **Other insomnia not due to a substance or known physiological condition**

5 F51.1 **Hypersomnia not due to a substance or known physiological condition**
EXCLUDES 2 *alcohol related hypersomnia (F10.182, F10.282, F10.982)*
drug-related hypersomnia (F11.182, F11.282, F11.982, F13.182, F13.282, F13.982, F14.182, F14.282, F14.982, F15.182, F15.282, F15.982, F19.182, F19.282, F19.982)
hypersomnia NOS (G47.10)
hypersomnia due to known physiological condition (G47.10)
idiopathic hypersomnia (G47.11, G47.12)
narcolepsy (G47.4-)

F51.11 **Primary hypersomnia**

F51.12 **Insufficient sleep syndrome**
EXCLUDES 1 *sleep deprivation (Z72.820)*

F51.13 **Hypersomnia due to other mental disorder**
Code also:
associated mental disorder

F51.19 **Other hypersomnia not due to a substance or known physiological condition**

F51.3 **Sleepwalking [somnambulism]**
Non-rapid eye movement sleep arousal disorders, sleepwalking type

F51.4 **Sleep terrors [night terrors]**
Non-rapid eye movement sleep arousal disorders, sleep terror type

F51.5 **Nightmare disorder**
Dream anxiety disorder

F51.8 **Other sleep disorders not due to a substance or known physiological condition**

F51.9 **Sleep disorder not due to a substance or known physiological condition, unspecified**
Emotional sleep disorder NOS

4 F52 **Sexual dysfunction not due to a substance or known physiological condition**
EXCLUDES 2 *Dhat syndrome (F48.8)*

F52.0 **Hypoactive sexual desire disorder**
Lack or loss of sexual desire
Male hypoactive sexual desire disorder
Sexual anhedonia
EXCLUDES 1 *decreased libido (R68.82)*

DEFINITION Markedly decreased sexual desire.

F52.1 **Sexual aversion disorder**
Sexual aversion and lack of sexual enjoyment

5 F52.2 **Sexual arousal disorders**
Failure of genital response

F52.21 **Male erectile disorder** ♂
Erectile disorder
Psychogenic impotence
EXCLUDES 1 *impotence of organic origin (N52.-)*
impotence NOS (N52.-)

F52.22 **Female sexual arousal disorder** ♀
Female sexual interest/arousal disorder

5 F52.3 **Orgasmic disorder**
Inhibited orgasm
Psychogenic anorgasmy

F52.31 **Female orgasmic disorder** ♀

F52.32 **Male orgasmic disorder** ♂
Delayed ejaculation

F52.4 **Premature ejaculation** ♂

F52.5 **Vaginismus not due to a substance or known physiological condition** ♀
Psychogenic vaginismus
EXCLUDES 2 *vaginismus (due to a known physiological condition) (N94.2)*

F52.6 **Dyspareunia not due to a substance or known physiological condition**
Genito-pelvic pain penetration disorder
Psychogenic dyspareunia
EXCLUDES 2 *dyspareunia (due to a known physiological condition) (N94.1-)*

F52.8 **Other sexual dysfunction not due to a substance or known physiological condition**
Excessive sexual drive
Nymphomania
Satyriasis

F52.9 **Unspecified sexual dysfunction not due to a substance or known physiological condition**
Sexual dysfunction NOS

▲ 4 F53 **Mental and behavioral disorders associated with the puerperium, not elsewhere classified**
EXCLUDES 1 *mood disorders with psychotic features (F30.2, F31.2, F31.5, F31.64, F32.3, F33.3)*
postpartum dysphoria (O90.6)
psychosis in schizophrenia, schizotypal, delusional, and other psychotic disorders (F20-F29)

● F53.0 **Postpartum depression** ♀ M
Postnatal depression, NOS
Postpartum depression, NOS

● F53.1 **Puerperal psychosis** ♀ M
Postpartum psychosis
Puerperal psychosis, NOS

F54 ***Psychological and behavioral factors associated with disorders or diseases classified elsewhere***
Psychological factors affecting physical conditions
Code first the associated physical disorder, such as:
asthma (J45.-)
dermatitis (L23-L25)
gastric ulcer (K25.-)
mucous colitis (K58.-)
ulcerative colitis (K51.-)
urticaria (L50.-)
EXCLUDES 2 *tension-type headache (G44.2)*

CODING TIP ✓ Assign code F54 when a psychological condition causes exacerbation of a specific physical condition, such as asthma or ulcers. This code may not be used alone, and documentation should specify that the psychological condition has caused exacerbation of the physical state. Code the physical condition first, followed by F54.

F55 Abuse of non-psychoactive substances

EXCLUDES 2 *abuse of psychoactive substances (F10-F19)*

F55.0 Abuse of antacids
F55.1 Abuse of herbal or folk remedies
F55.2 Abuse of laxatives
F55.3 Abuse of steroids or hormones
F55.4 Abuse of vitamins
F55.8 Abuse of other non-psychoactive substances

F59 Unspecified behavioral syndromes associated with physiological disturbances and physical factors

Psychogenic physiological dysfunction NOS

CODING TIP ✓ Do not use F59 to report psychosomatic disorder. Psychosomatic disorder has a specific code and should be coded to F45.9.

Disorders of adult personality and behavior (F60-F69)

F60 Specific personality disorders

F60.0 Paranoid personality disorder HCC
Expansive paranoid personality (disorder)
Fanatic personality (disorder)
Querulant personality (disorder)
Paranoid personality (disorder)
Sensitive paranoid personality (disorder)

EXCLUDES 2 *paranoia (F22)*
paranoia querulans (F22)
paranoid psychosis (F22)
paranoid schizophrenia (F20.0)
paranoid state (F22)

F60.1 Schizoid personality disorder HCC

EXCLUDES 2 *Asperger's syndrome (F84.5)*
delusional disorder (F22)
schizoid disorder of childhood (F84.5)
schizophrenia (F20.-)
schizotypal disorder (F21)

F60.2 Antisocial personality disorder HCC
Amoral personality (disorder)
Asocial personality (disorder)
Dissocial personality disorder
Psychopathic personality (disorder)
Sociopathic personality (disorder)

EXCLUDES 1 *conduct disorders (F91.-)*

EXCLUDES 2 *borderline personality disorder (F60.3)*

F60.3 Borderline personality disorder
Aggressive personality (disorder)
Emotionally unstable personality disorder
Explosive personality (disorder)

EXCLUDES 2 *antisocial personality disorder (F60.2)*

DEFINITION Disorder in which a person is quick to anger, aggressive, abnormally emotional, and argumentative.

F60.4 Histrionic personality disorder HCC
Hysterical personality (disorder)
Psychoinfantile personality (disorder)

F60.5 Obsessive-compulsive personality disorder
Anankastic personality (disorder)
Compulsive personality (disorder)
Obsessional personality (disorder)

EXCLUDES 2 *obsessive-compulsive disorder (F42-)*

F60.6 Avoidant personality disorder HCC
Anxious personality disorder

F60.7 Dependent personality disorder HCC
Asthenic personality (disorder)
Inadequate personality (disorder)
Passive personality (disorder)

F60.8 Other specific personality disorders

F60.81 Narcissistic personality disorder HCC

F60.89 Other specific personality disorders HCC
Eccentric personality disorder
'Haltlose' type personality disorder
Immature personality disorder
Passive-aggressive personality disorder
Psychoneurotic personality disorder
Self-defeating personality disorder

F60.9 Personality disorder, unspecified HCC
Character disorder NOS
Character neurosis NOS
Pathological personality NOS

F63 Impulse disorders

EXCLUDES 2 *habitual excessive use of alcohol or psychoactive substances (F10-F19)*
impulse disorders involving sexual behavior (F65.-)

F63.0 Pathological gambling
Compulsive gambling
Gambling disorder

EXCLUDES 1 *gambling and betting NOS (Z72.6)*

EXCLUDES 2 *excessive gambling by manic patients (F30, F31)*
gambling in antisocial personality disorder (F60.2)

F63.1 Pyromania
Pathological fire-setting

EXCLUDES 2 *fire-setting (by) (in):*
adult with antisocial personality disorder (F60.2)
alcohol or psychoactive substance intoxication (F10-F19)
conduct disorders (F91.-)
mental disorders due to known physiological condition (F01-F09)
schizophrenia (F20.-)

DEFINITION Uncontrollable impulse to set fires.

F63.2 Kleptomania
Pathological stealing

EXCLUDES 1 *shoplifting as the reason for observation for suspected mental disorder (Z03.8)*

EXCLUDES 2 *depressive disorder with stealing (F31-F33)*
stealing due to underlying mental condition-code to mental condition
stealing in mental disorders due to known physiological condition (F01-F09)

DEFINITION Irresistible impulse to steal.

F63.3 Trichotillomania
Hair plucking

EXCLUDES 2 *other stereotyped movement disorder (F98.4)*

F63.8 Other impulse disorders

F63.81 Intermittent explosive disorder

F63.89 Other impulse disorders

F63.9 Impulse disorder, unspecified
Impulse control disorder NOS

F64 Gender identity disorders

F64.0 Transsexualism
Gender identity disorder in adolescence and adulthood
Gender dysphoria in adolescents and adults
AHA: 4Q 2016, 14

F64.1 Dual role transvestism
Use additional code to identify sex reassignment status (Z87.890)

EXCLUDES 1 *gender identity disorder in childhood (F64.2)*

EXCLUDES 2 *fetishistic transvestism (F65.1)*

F64.2 Gender identity disorder of childhood P
Gender dysphoria in children

EXCLUDES 1 *gender identity disorder in adolescence and adulthood (F64.0)*

EXCLUDES 2 *sexual maturation disorder (F66)*

F64.8 Other gender identity disorders
Other specified gender dysphoria

F64.9 Gender identity disorder, unspecified
Gender dysphoria, unspecified
Gender-role disorder NOS

F65 Paraphilias

F65.0 Fetishism
Fetishistic disorder
F65.1 Transvestic fetishism
Fetishistic transvestism
Transvestic disorder
F65.2 Exhibitionism
Exhibitionistic disorder
DEFINITION Compulsion to expose genitals in public.
F65.3 Voyeurism
Voyeuristic disorder
DEFINITION Uncontrollable compulsion to covertly observe others who are nude or engaged in sexual activity.
F65.4 Pedophilia
Pedophilic disorder
5 F65.5 Sadomasochism
F65.50 Sadomasochism, unspecified
F65.51 Sexual masochism
Sexual masochism disorder
DEFINITION Psychosexual disorder marked by the need to be humiliated or hurt to achieve sexual gratification.
F65.52 Sexual sadism
Sexual sadism disorder
DEFINITION Psychosexual disorder marked by the need to humiliate or injure others to achieve sexual gratification.
5 F65.8 Other paraphilias
F65.81 Frotteurism
Frotteuristic disorder
F65.89 Other paraphilias
Necrophilia
Other specified paraphilic disorder
DEFINITION Sexual attraction to corpses.
F65.9 Paraphilia, unspecified
Paraphilic disorder, unspecified
Sexual deviation NOS
F66 Other sexual disorders
Sexual maturation disorder
Sexual relationship disorder
4 F68 Other disorders of adult personality and behavior
▲ 5 F68.1 Factitious disorder imposed on self
Compensation neurosis
Elaboration of physical symptoms for psychological reasons
Hospital hopper syndrome
Münchausen's syndrome
Peregrinating patient
EXCLUDES 2 *factitial dermatitis (L98.1)*
person feigning illness (with obvious motivation) (Z76.5)
▲ F68.10 Factitious disorder imposed on self, unspecified
▲ F68.11 Factitious disorder imposed on self, with predominantly psychological signs and symptoms
▲ F68.12 Factitious disorder imposed on self, with predominantly physical signs and symptoms
▲ F68.13 Factitious disorder imposed on self, with combined psychological and physical signs and symptoms
● F68.A Factitious disorder imposed on another
Factitious disorder by proxy
Münchausen's by proxy
F68.8 Other specified disorders of adult personality and behavior
F69 Unspecified disorder of adult personality and behavior A

Intellectual Disabilities (F70-F79)

Code first:
any associated physical or developmental disorders
EXCLUDES 1 *borderline intellectual functioning, IQ above 70 to 84 (R41.83)*

CODING TIP✓ When IQ is specified, use the appropriate code from F70-F79 to specify level of intellectual disability based upon reported IQ. When developmental delays or disorders are additionally noted in a patient with Intellectual disability, these should be coded first.

F70 Mild intellectual disabilities
IQ level 50-55 to approximately 70
Mild mental subnormality
F71 Moderate intellectual disabilities
IQ level 35-40 to 50-55
Moderate mental subnormality
F72 Severe intellectual disabilities
IQ 20-25 to 35-40
Severe mental subnormality
F73 Profound intellectual disabilities
IQ level below 20-25
Profound mental subnormality
F78 Other intellectual disabilities
F79 Unspecified intellectual disabilities
Mental deficiency NOS
Mental subnormality NOS

Pervasive and specific developmental disorders (F80-F89)

CODING TIP✓ Disorders coded to categories F80-F89 should be specified as related to a developmental origin.

4 F80 Specific developmental disorders of speech and language
F80.0 Phonological disorder
Dyslalia
Functional speech articulation disorder
Lalling
Lisping
Phonological developmental disorder
Speech articulation developmental disorder
Speech-sound disorder
EXCLUDES 1 *speech articulation impairment due to aphasia NOS (R47.01)*
speech articulation impairment due to apraxia (R48.2)
EXCLUDES 2 *speech articulation impairment due to hearing loss (F80.4)*
speech articulation impairment due to intellectual disabilities (F70-F79)
speech articulation impairment with expressive language developmental disorder (F80.1)
speech articulation impairment with mixed receptive expressive language developmental disorder (F80.2)
CODING TIP✓ Code any additional speech articulation disorders in addition, when applicable.
F80.1 Expressive language disorder
Developmental dysphasia or aphasia, expressive type
EXCLUDES 1 *mixed receptive-expressive language disorder (F80.2)*
dysphasia and aphasia NOS (R47.-)
EXCLUDES 2 *acquired aphasia with epilepsy [Landau-Kleffner] (G40.80-)*
selective mutism (F94.0)
intellectual disabilities (F70-F79)
pervasive developmental disorders (F84.-)
CODING TIP✓ Language disorders should not be coded here unless specified as related to a developmental cause.

F80.2 Mixed receptive-expressive language disorder
Developmental dysphasia or aphasia, receptive type
Developmental Wernicke's aphasia
EXCLUDES 1 *central auditory processing disorder (H93.25)*
dysphasia or aphasia NOS (R47.-)
expressive language disorder (F80.1)
expressive type dysphasia or aphasia (F80.1)
word deafness (H93.25)
EXCLUDES 2 *acquired aphasia with epilepsy [Landau-Kleffner] (G40.80-)*
pervasive developmental disorders (F84.-)
selective mutism (F94.0)
intellectual disabilities (F70-F79)

DEFINITION Problems comprehending as well as expressing verbal language.

F80.4 Speech and language development delay due to hearing loss
Code also:
type of hearing loss (H90.-, H91.-)

5 **F80.8 Other developmental disorders of speech and language**

F80.81 Childhood onset fluency disorder
Cluttering NOS
Stuttering NOS
EXCLUDES 1 *adult onset fluency disorder (F98.5)*
fluency disorder in conditions classified elsewhere (R47.82)
fluency disorder (stuttering) following cerebrovascular disease (I69. with final characters -23)

F80.82 Social pragmatic communication disorder
EXCLUDES 1 *Asperger's syndrome (F84.5)*
autistic disorder (F84.0)

F80.89 Other developmental disorders of speech and language
AHA: 1Q 2017, 27

F80.9 Developmental disorder of speech and language, unspecified
Communication disorder NOS
Language disorder NOS

4 **F81 Specific developmental disorders of scholastic skills**

F81.0 Specific reading disorder
'Backward reading'
Developmental dyslexia
Specific learning disorder, with impairment in reading
Specific reading retardation
EXCLUDES 1 *alexia NOS (R48.0)*
dyslexia NOS (R48.0)

F81.2 Mathematics disorder
Developmental acalculia
Developmental arithmetical disorder
Developmental Gerstmann's syndrome
Specific learning disorder, with impairment in mathematics
EXCLUDES 1 *acalculia NOS (R48.8)*
EXCLUDES 2 *arithmetical difficulties associated with a reading disorder (F81.0)*
arithmetical difficulties associated with a spelling disorder (F81.81)
arithmetical difficulties due to inadequate teaching (Z55.8)

5 **F81.8 Other developmental disorders of scholastic skills**

F81.81 Disorder of written expression
Specific learning disorder, with impairment in written expression
Specific spelling disorder

F81.89 Other developmental disorders of scholastic skills

F81.9 Developmental disorder of scholastic skills, unspecified
Knowledge acquisition disability NOS
Learning disability NOS
Learning disorder NOS

F82 Specific developmental disorder of motor function
Clumsy child syndrome
Developmental coordination disorder
Developmental dyspraxia
EXCLUDES 1 *abnormalities of gait and mobility (R26.-)*
lack of coordination (R27.-)
EXCLUDES 2 *lack of coordination secondary to intellectual disabilities (F70-F79)*

4 **F84 Pervasive developmental disorders**
Use additional code to identify any associated medical condition and intellectual disabilities.

F84.0 Autistic disorder
Autism spectrum disorder
Infantile autism
Infantile psychosis
Kanner's syndrome
EXCLUDES 1 *Asperger's syndrome (F84.5)*

DEFINITION Neurological disorder appearing at a young age that impairs social development and communication skills, and resulting in abnormal behavior that varies in degree of severity and ability to function.

F84.2 Rett's syndrome
EXCLUDES 1 *Asperger's syndrome (F84.5)*
Autistic disorder (F84.0)
Other childhood disintegrative disorder (F84.3)

F84.3 Other childhood disintegrative disorder P
Dementia infantilis
Disintegrative psychosis
Heller's syndrome
Symbiotic psychosis
Use additional code to identify any associated neurological condition.
EXCLUDES 1 *Asperger's syndrome (F84.5)*
Autistic disorder (F84.0)
Rett's syndrome (F84.2)

F84.5 Asperger's syndrome
Asperger's disorder
Autistic psychopathy
Schizoid disorder of childhood

F84.8 Other pervasive developmental disorders
Overactive disorder associated with intellectual disabilities and stereotyped movements

F84.9 Pervasive developmental disorder, unspecified
Atypical autism

F88 Other disorders of psychological development
Developmental agnosia
Global developmental delay
Other specified neurodevelopmental disorder

F89 Unspecified disorder of psychological development
Developmental disorder NOS
Neurodevelopmental disorder NOS

Behavioral and emotional disorders with onset usually occurring in childhood and adolescence (F90-F98)

Note: Codes within categories F90-F98 may be used regardless of the age of a patient. These disorders generally have onset within the childhood or adolescent years, but may continue throughout life or not be diagnosed until adulthood

CODING TIP ✓ Disorders classified to categories F90-F98 are frequently diagnosed in childhood and adolescence. However, a diagnosis may be made at any time during an individual's lifetime and may still be reported here when the diagnosis criteria are applicable.

4 **F90 Attention-deficit hyperactivity disorders**
INCLUDES attention deficit disorder with hyperactivity
attention deficit syndrome with hyperactivity
EXCLUDES 2 *anxiety disorders (F40.-, F41.-)*
mood [affective] disorders (F30-F39)
pervasive developmental disorders (F84.-)
schizophrenia (F20.-)

F90.0 Attention-deficit hyperactivity disorder, predominantly inattentive type
Attention-deficit/hyperactivity disorder, predominantly inattentive presentation

F90.1 Attention-deficit hyperactivity disorder, predominantly hyperactive type
Attention-deficit/hyperactivity disorder, predominantly hyperactive impulsive presentation

F90.2 Attention-deficit hyperactivity disorder, combined type
Attention-deficit/hyperactivity disorder, combined presentation

F90.8 Attention-deficit hyperactivity disorder, other type

F90.9 Attention-deficit hyperactivity disorder, unspecified type
Attention-deficit hyperactivity disorder of childhood or adolescence NOS
Attention-deficit hyperactivity disorder NOS

4 F91 Conduct disorders
EXCLUDES 1 *antisocial behavior (Z72.81-)*
antisocial personality disorder (F60.2)
EXCLUDES 2 *conduct problems associated with attention-deficit hyperactivity disorder (F90.-)*
mood [affective] disorders (F30-F39)
pervasive developmental disorders (F84.-)
schizophrenia (F20.-)

F91.0 Conduct disorder confined to family context

F91.1 Conduct disorder, childhood-onset type
Unsocialized conduct disorder
Conduct disorder, solitary aggressive type
Unsocialized aggressive disorder

F91.2 Conduct disorder, adolescent-onset type
Socialized conduct disorder
Conduct disorder, group type

F91.3 Oppositional defiant disorder

F91.8 Other conduct disorders
Other specified conduct disorder
Other specified disruptive disorder

F91.9 Conduct disorder, unspecified
Behavioral disorder NOS
Conduct disorder NOS
Disruptive behavior disorder NOS
Disruptive disorder NOS

4 F93 Emotional disorders with onset specific to childhood

F93.0 Separation anxiety disorder of childhood
EXCLUDES 2 *mood [affective] disorders (F30-F39)*
nonpsychotic mental disorders (F40-F48)
phobic anxiety disorder of childhood (F40.8)
social phobia (F40.1)

DEFINITION Abnormal anxiety when separated from a parent, guardian, or usual environment.

F93.8 Other childhood emotional disorders
Identity disorder
EXCLUDES 2 *gender identity disorder of childhood (F64.2)*

F93.9 Childhood emotional disorder, unspecified

4 F94 Disorders of social functioning with onset specific to childhood and adolescence

F94.0 Selective mutism
Elective mutism
EXCLUDES 2 *pervasive developmental disorders (F84.-)*
schizophrenia (F20.-)
specific developmental disorders of speech and language (F80.-)
transient mutism as part of separation anxiety in young children (F93.0)

F94.1 Reactive attachment disorder of childhood
Use additional code to identify any associated failure to thrive or growth retardation
EXCLUDES 1 *disinhibited attachment disorder of childhood (F94.2)*
normal variation in pattern of selective attachment
EXCLUDES 2 *Asperger's syndrome (F84.5)*
maltreatment syndromes (T74.-)
sexual or physical abuse in childhood, resulting in psychosocial problems (Z62.81-)

F94.2 Disinhibited attachment disorder of childhood
Affectionless psychopathy
Institutional syndrome
EXCLUDES 1 *reactive attachment disorder of childhood (F94.1)*
EXCLUDES 2 *Asperger's syndrome (F84.5)*
attention-deficit hyperactivity disorders (F90.-)
hospitalism in children (F43.2-)

F94.8 Other childhood disorders of social functioning

F94.9 Childhood disorder of social functioning, unspecified

4 F95 Tic disorder

F95.0 Transient tic disorder
Provisional tic disorder

F95.1 Chronic motor or vocal tic disorder

F95.2 Tourette's disorder
Combined vocal and multiple motor tic disorder [de la Tourette]
Tourette's syndrome

F95.8 Other tic disorders

F95.9 Tic disorder, unspecified
Tic NOS

4 F98 Other behavioral and emotional disorders with onset usually occurring in childhood and adolescence
EXCLUDES 2 *breath-holding spells (R06.89)*
gender identity disorder of childhood (F64.2)
Kleine-Levin syndrome (G47.13)
obsessive-compulsive disorder (F42-)
sleep disorders not due to a substance or known physiological condition (F51.-)

F98.0 Enuresis not due to a substance or known physiological condition
Enuresis (primary) (secondary) of nonorganic origin
Functional enuresis
Psychogenic enuresis
Urinary incontinence of nonorganic origin
EXCLUDES 1 *enuresis NOS (R32)*

F98.1 Encopresis not due to a substance or known physiological condition
Functional encopresis
Incontinence of feces of nonorganic origin
Psychogenic encopresis
Use additional code to identify the cause of any coexisting constipation.
EXCLUDES 1 *encopresis NOS (R15.-)*

5 F98.2 Other feeding disorders of infancy and childhood
EXCLUDES 1 *feeding difficulties (R63.3)*
EXCLUDES 2 *anorexia nervosa and other eating disorders (F50.-)*
feeding problems of newborn (P92.-)
pica of infancy or childhood (F98.3)

F98.21 Rumination disorder of infancy

F98.29 Other feeding disorders of infancy and early childhood

F98.3 Pica of infancy and childhood
DEFINITION Compulsion to eat inedible substances, such as dirt or rocks.

F98.4 Stereotyped movement disorders
Stereotype/habit disorder
EXCLUDES 1 *abnormal involuntary movements (R25.-)*
EXCLUDES 2 *compulsions in obsessive-compulsive disorder (F42-)*
hair plucking (F63.3)
movement disorders of organic origin (G20-G25)
nail-biting (F98.8)
nose-picking (F98.8)
stereotypies that are part of a broader psychiatric condition (F01-F95)
thumb-sucking (F98.8)
tic disorders (F95.-)
trichotillomania (F63.3)

F98.5 Adult onset fluency disorder
EXCLUDES 1 *childhood onset fluency disorder (F80.81)*
dysphasia (R47.02)
fluency disorder in conditions classified elsewhere (R47.82)
fluency disorder (stuttering) following cerebrovascular disease (I69. with final characters -23)
tic disorders (F95.-)

CODING TIP ✓ This code is used for post-childhood onset of stuttering symptoms secondary to emotional stress or trauma. Do not assign F98.5 to report fluency disorder as a sequela of cerebral vascular disease or another cause or to identify dysphasia.

DEFINITION Normal flow of speech disrupted by repeated sounds or pauses.

F98.8 **Other specified behavioral and emotional disorders with onset usually occurring in childhood and adolescence**
Excessive masturbation
Nail-biting
Nose-picking
Thumb-sucking

F98.9 **Unspecified behavioral and emotional disorders with onset usually occurring in childhood and adolescence**

Unspecified mental disorder (F99)

F99 **Mental disorder, not otherwise specified**
Mental illness NOS
EXCLUDES 1 *unspecified mental disorder due to known physiological condition (F09)*

CODING TIP ✓ Use F99 only when the clinical documentation from the provider reports mental illness but does not specify anything further.

CHAPTER 6: DISEASES OF THE NERVOUS SYSTEM (G00-G99)

EXCLUDES 2 *certain conditions originating in the perinatal period (P04-P96)*
certain infectious and parasitic diseases (A00-B99)
complications of pregnancy, childbirth and the puerperium (O00-O9A)
congenital malformations, deformations, and chromosomal abnormalities (Q00-Q99)
endocrine, nutritional and metabolic diseases (E00-E88)
injury, poisoning and certain other consequences of external causes (S00-T88)
neoplasms (C00-D49)
symptoms, signs and abnormal clinical and laboratory findings, not elsewhere classified (R00-R94)

This chapter contains the following blocks:

G00-G09	Inflammatory diseases of the central nervous system
G10-G14	Systemic atrophies primarily affecting the central nervous system
G20-G26	Extrapyramidal and movement disorders
G30-G32	Other degenerative diseases of the nervous system
G35-G37	Demyelinating diseases of the central nervous system
G40-G47	Episodic and paroxysmal disorders
G50-G59	Nerve, nerve root and plexus disorders
G60-G65	Polyneuropathies and other disorders of the peripheral nervous system
G70-G73	Diseases of myoneural junction and muscle
G80-G83	Cerebral palsy and other paralytic syndromes
G89-G99	Other disorders of the nervous system

Inflammatory diseases of the central nervous system (G00-G09)

CODING TIP✓ If the central nervous system infection (CNS) is resolved but has a potential for reoccurence, use Z86.61, personal history of CNS infections. If the CNS infection is resolved, but the patient suffers neurological deficits, code the residual deficit followed by the sequela code G09.

4 G00 Bacterial meningitis, not elsewhere classified

INCLUDES bacterial arachnoiditis
bacterial leptomeningitis
bacterial meningitis
bacterial pachymeningitis

EXCLUDES 1 *bacterial meningoencephalitis (G04.2)*
bacterial meningomyelitis (G04.2)

G00.0 Hemophilus meningitis
Meningitis due to Hemophilus influenzae

DEFINITION Bacterial infection of the tissues (meninges) surrounding the brain and spinal cord, causing fever, headache, vomiting, malaise, and stiff neck and may progress to confusion, stupor, convulsions, coma, and death.

G00.1 Pneumococcal meningitis
Meningtitis due to Streptococcal pneumoniae

G00.2 Streptococcal meningitis
Use additional code to further identify organism (B95.0-B95.5)

G00.3 Staphylococcal meningitis
Use additional code to further identify organism (B95.61-B95.8)

Staphylococcal meningitis

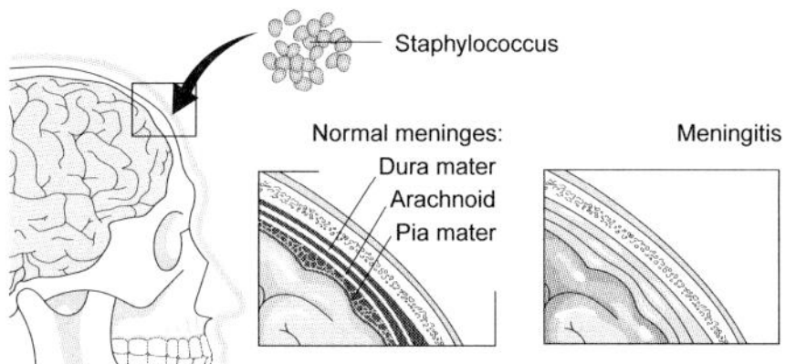

Meningitis, an infection of the lining of the brain and spinal cord, caused by the bacteria staphylococcus

G00.8 Other bacterial meningitis
Meningitis due to Escherichia coli
Meningitis due to Friedländer's bacillus
Meningitis due to Klebsiella
Use additional code to further identify organism (B96.-)

G00.9 Bacterial meningitis, unspecified
Meningitis due to gram-negative bacteria, unspecified
Purulent meningitis NOS
Pyogenic meningitis NOS
Suppurative meningitis NOS

G01 *Meningitis in bacterial diseases classified elsewhere*
Code first:
underlying disease

EXCLUDES 1 *meningitis (in) :*
gonococcal (A54.81)
leptospirosis (A27.81)
listeriosis (A32.11)
Lyme disease (A69.21)
meningococcal (A39.0)
neurosyphilis (A52.13)
tuberculosis (A17.0)
meningoencephalitis and meningomyelitis in bacterial diseases classified elsewhere (G05)

G02 *Meningitis in other infectious and parasitic diseases classified elsewhere*
Code first underlying disease, such as:
African trypanosomiasis (B56.-)
poliovirus infection (A80.-)

EXCLUDES 1 *candidal meningitis (B37.5)*
coccidioidomycosis meningitis (B38.4)
cryptococcal meningitis (B45.1)
herpesviral [herpes simplex] meningitis (B00.3)
infectious mononucleosis complicated by meningitis (B27.- with fourth character 2)
measles complicated by meningitis (B05.1)
meningoencephalitis and meningomyelitis in other infectious and parasitic diseases classified elsewhere (G05)
mumps meningitis (B26.1)
rubella meningitis (B06.02)
varicella [chickenpox] meningitis (B01.0)
zoster meningitis (B02.1)

4 G03 Meningitis due to other and unspecified causes

INCLUDES arachnoiditis NOS
leptomeningitis NOS
meningitis NOS
pachymeningitis NOS

EXCLUDES 1 *meningoencephalitis (G04.-)*
meningomyelitis (G04.-)

G03.0 Nonpyogenic meningitis
Aseptic meningitis
Nonbacterial meningitis

G03.1 Chronic meningitis

G03.2 Benign recurrent meningitis [Mollaret]

CODING TIP✓ Do not confuse chronic meningitis with benign recurrent Mollaret's meningitis. Mollaret's meningitis is a rare disorder characterized by a recurrent, mild, and aseptic inflammation of the meninges due to an unknown cause.

G03.8 Meningitis due to other specified causes

G03.9 Meningitis, unspecified
Arachnoiditis (spinal) NOS

CODING TIP✓ Meningitis that is not specified as acute, chronic, or due to a specified cause should be coded to G03.9.

4 G04 Encephalitis, myelitis and encephalomyelitis

INCLUDES acute ascending myelitis
meningoencephalitis
meningomyelitis

EXCLUDES 1 *encephalopathy NOS (G93.40)*

EXCLUDES 2 *acute transverse myelitis (G37.3-)*
alcoholic encephalopathy (G31.2)
benign myalgic encephalomyelitis (G93.3)
multiple sclerosis (G35)
subacute necrotizing myelitis (G37.4)
toxic encephalitis (G92)
toxic encephalopathy (G92)

5 G04.0 Acute disseminated encephalitis and encephalomyelitis (ADEM)

EXCLUDES 1 *acute necrotizing hemorrhagic encephalopathy (G04.3-)*
other noninfectious acute disseminated encephalomyelitis (noninfectious ADEM) (G04.81)

G04.00 Acute disseminated encephalitis and encephalomyelitis, unspecified

G04.01 Postinfectious acute disseminated encephalitis and encephalomyelitis (Postinfectious ADEM)

EXCLUDES 1 *post chickenpox encephalitis (B01.1)*
post measles encephalitis (B05.0)
post measles myelitis (B05.1)

G04.02 Postimmunization acute disseminated encephalitis, myelitis and encephalomyelitis

Encephalitis, post immunization
Encephalomyelitis, post immunization
Use additional code to identify the vaccine (T50.A-, T50.B-, T50.Z-)

CODING TIP ✓ G04.02 should be assigned for encephalitis, myelitis, and encephalomyelitis that is reported to be caused by the administration of vaccines. Use an additional code from T36-T50 to identify the adverse effect from the vaccine.

G04.1 Tropical spastic paraplegia HCC

G04.2 Bacterial meningoencephalitis and meningomyelitis, not elsewhere classified

5 G04.3 Acute necrotizing hemorrhagic encephalopathy

EXCLUDES 1 *acute disseminated encephalitis and encephalomyelitis (G04.0-)*

G04.30 Acute necrotizing hemorrhagic encephalopathy, unspecified

G04.31 Postinfectious acute necrotizing hemorrhagic encephalopathy

G04.32 Postimmunization acute necrotizing hemorrhagic encephalopathy

Use additional code to identify the vaccine (T50.A-, T50.B-, T50.Z-)

G04.39 Other acute necrotizing hemorrhagic encephalopathy

Code also:
underlying etiology, if applicable

5 G04.8 Other encephalitis, myelitis and encephalomyelitis

Code also:
any associated seizure (G40.-, R56.9)

G04.81 Other encephalitis and encephalomyelitis HIV

Noninfectious acute disseminated encephalomyelitis (noninfectious ADEM)

G04.89 Other myelitis HCC HIV

5 G04.9 Encephalitis, myelitis and encephalomyelitis, unspecified

G04.90 Encephalitis and encephalomyelitis, unspecified HIV

Ventriculitis (cerebral) NOS

G04.91 Myelitis, unspecified HCC HIV

4 G05 Encephalitis, myelitis and encephalomyelitis in diseases classified elsewhere

Code first underlying disease, such as:
human immunodeficiency virus [HIV] disease (B20)
poliovirus (A80.-)
suppurative otitis media (H66.01-H66.4)
trichinellosis (B75)

EXCLUDES 1 *adenoviral encephalitis, myelitis and encephalomyelitis (A85.1)*
congenital toxoplasmosis encephalitis, myelitis and encephalomyelitis (P37.1)
cytomegaloviral encephalitis, myelitis and encephalomyelitis (B25.8)
encephalitis, myelitis and encephalomyelitis (in) measles (B05.0)
encephalitis, myelitis and encephalomyelitis (in) systemic lupus erythematosus (M32.19)
enteroviral encephalitis, myelitis and encephalomyelitis (A85.0)
eosinophilic meningoencephalitis (B83.2)
herpesviral [herpes simplex] encephalitis, myelitis and encephalomyelitis (B00.4)
listerial encephalitis, myelitis and encephalomyelitis (A32.12)
meningococcal encephalitis, myelitis and encephalomyelitis (A39.81)
mumps encephalitis, myelitis and encephalomyelitis (B26.2)
postchickenpox encephalitis, myelitis and encephalomyelitis (B01.1-)
rubella encephalitis, myelitis and encephalomyelitis (B06.01)
toxoplasmosis encephalitis, myelitis and encephalomyelitis (B58.2)
zoster encephalitis, myelitis and encephalomyelitis (B02.0)

G05.3 ***Encephalitis and encephalomyelitis in diseases classified elsewhere***

Meningoencephalitis in diseases classified elsewhere

G05.4 ***Myelitis in diseases classified elsewhere*** HCC

Meningomyelitis in diseases classified elsewhere

4 G06 Intracranial and intraspinal abscess and granuloma

Use additional code (B95-B97) to identify infectious agent.

G06.0 Intracranial abscess and granuloma

Brain [any part] abscess (embolic)
Cerebellar abscess (embolic)
Cerebral abscess (embolic)
Intracranial epidural abscess or granuloma
Intracranial extradural abscess or granuloma
Intracranial subdural abscess or granuloma
Otogenic abscess (embolic)

EXCLUDES 1 *tuberculous intracranial abscess and granuloma (A17.81)*

Intracranial abscess and granuloma

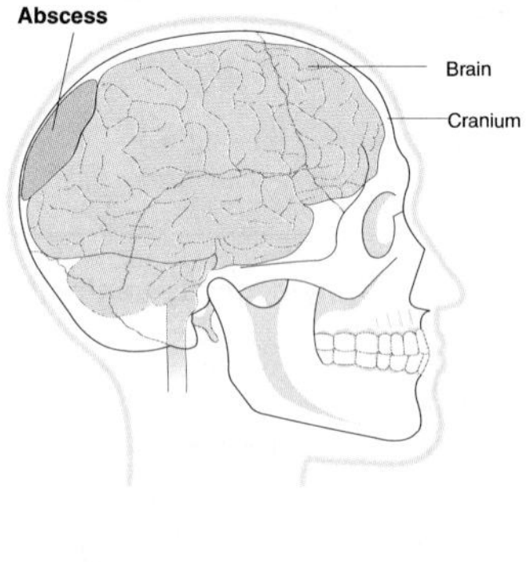

G06.1 Intraspinal abscess and granuloma

Abscess (embolic) of spinal cord [any part]
Intraspinal epidural abscess or granuloma
Intraspinal extradural abscess or granuloma
Intraspinal subdural abscess or granuloma

EXCLUDES 1 *tuberculous intraspinal abscess and granuloma (A17.81)*

G06.2 Extradural and subdural **abscess,** unspecified

G07 ***Intracranial and intraspinal abscess and granuloma in diseases** classified elsewhere*

Code first underlying disease, such as:
schistosomiasis granuloma of brain (B65.-)

EXCLUDES 1 *abscess of brain:*
amebic (A06.6)
chromomycotic (B43.1)
gonococcal (A54.82)
tuberculous (A17.81)
tuberculoma of meninges (A17.1)

G08 Intracranial and intraspinal phlebitis and thrombophlebitis

Septic embolism of intracranial or intraspinal venous sinuses and veins
Septic endophlebitis of intracranial or intraspinal venous sinuses and veins
Septic phlebitis of intracranial or intraspinal venous sinuses and veins
Septic thrombophlebitis of intracranial or intraspinal venous sinuses and veins
Septic thrombosis of intracranial or intraspinal venous sinuses and veins

EXCLUDES 1 *intracranial phlebitis and thrombophlebitis complicating:*
abortion, ectopic or molar pregnancy (O00-O07, O08.7)
pregnancy, childbirth and the puerperium (O22.5, O87.3)
nonpyogenic intracranial phlebitis and thrombophlebitis (I67.6)

EXCLUDES 2 *intracranial phlebitis and thrombophlebitis complicating nonpyogenic intraspinal phlebitis and thrombophlebitis (G95.1)*

DEFINITION Inflammation and/or blood clot formation in a large vein or channel for venous blood circulation in the brain or spine.

G09 Sequelae **of inflammatory diseases of central nervous system**

Note: Category G09 is to be used to indicate conditions whose primary classification is to G00-G08 as the cause of sequelae, themselves classifiable elsewhere. The 'sequelae' include conditions specified as residuals.
Code first:
condition resulting from (sequela) of inflammatory diseases of central nervous system

Systemic atrophies primarily affecting the central nervous system (G10-G14)

G10 Huntington's disease HCC

Huntington's chorea
Huntington's dementia
Code also:
dementia in other diseases classified elsewhere without behavioral disturbance (F02.80)

CODING TIP✓ Huntington's disease is a progressive neurological disorder that includes dementia and mental deterioration as part of its progressive course. An additional code (F02-) should be assigned to identify dementia with or without behavioral disturbance.

DEFINITION A genetic, degenerative disorder of the neurons of the brain, characterized by progressive difficulty with physical and mental tasks until death occurs.

4 **G11 Hereditary ataxia**

EXCLUDES 2 *cerebral palsy (G80.-)*
hereditary and idiopathic neuropathy (G60.-)
metabolic disorders (E70-E88)

CODING TIP✓ **Documentation:** When assigning a code from category G11.-, the coder should review the record in full and assign the most specific code. Coders should not, however, assign codes for early vs. late onset or a hereditary vs. congenital condition unless specifically reported as confirmed by the patient's physician in the record.

G11.0 Congenital nonprogressive **ataxia** HCC

G11.1 Early-onset cerebellar **ataxia** HCC

Early-onset cerebellar ataxia with essential tremor
Early-onset cerebellar ataxia with myoclonus [Hunt's ataxia]
Early-onset cerebellar ataxia with retained tendon reflexes
Friedreich's ataxia (autosomal recessive)
X-linked recessive spinocerebellar ataxia

G11.2 Late-onset cerebellar **ataxia** A HCC

G11.3 Cerebellar **ataxia with** defective DNA repair HCC

Ataxia telangiectasia [Louis-Bar]

EXCLUDES 2 *Cockayne's syndrome (Q87.1)*
other disorders of purine and pyrimidine metabolism (E79.-)
xeroderma pigmentosum (Q82.1)

G11.4 Hereditary spastic paraplegia HCC

DEFINITION Hereditary disorder characterized by lower-limb spasticity and near total loss of joint flexibility while the upper limbs remain unaffected.

G11.8 Other **hereditary ataxias** HCC

G11.9 Hereditary ataxia, unspecified HCC

Hereditary cerebellar ataxia NOS
Hereditary cerebellar degeneration
Hereditary cerebellar disease
Hereditary cerebellar syndrome

4 **G12** Spinal muscular **atrophy and** related syndromes

G12.0 Infantile **spinal muscular atrophy,** type I [Werdnig-Hoffman] HCC

G12.1 Other inherited **spinal muscular atrophy** HCC

Adult form spinal muscular atrophy
Childhood form, type II spinal muscular atrophy
Distal spinal muscular atrophy
Juvenile form, type III spinal muscular atrophy [Kugelberg-Welander]
Progressive bulbar palsy of childhood [Fazio-Londe]
Scapuloperoneal form spinal muscular atrophy

5 **G12.2 Motor neuron disease**

G12.20 Motor neuron disease, unspecified HCC

G12.21 Amyotrophic lateral sclerosis A HCC

Amyotrophic lateral sclerosis (ALS)

Also known as Lou Gehrig's disease, ALS is caused by the degeneration and death of motor neurons in the spinal cord and brain

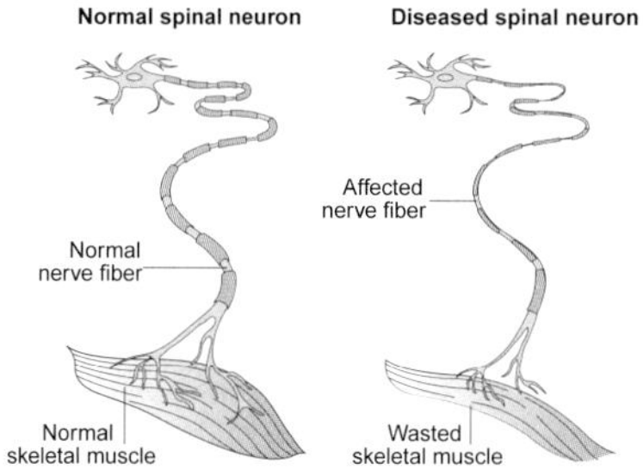

G12.22 Progressive bulbar palsy HCC

G12.23 Primary lateral sclerosis HCC
AHA: 4Q 2017, 8

G12.24 Familial **motor neuron disease** HCC
AHA: 4Q 2017, 8

G12.25 Progressive spinal muscle atrophy HCC
AHA: 4Q 2017, 8

G12.29 Other **motor neuron disease** HCC

G12.8 Other **spinal muscular atrophies and related syndromes** HCC

G12.9 Spinal muscular atrophy, unspecified HCC

4 **G13 Systemic atrophies primarily affecting central nervous system in** diseases classified elsewhere

G13.0 *Paraneoplastic neuromyopathy and neuropathy* HCC

Carcinomatous neuromyopathy
Sensorial paraneoplastic neuropathy [Denny Brown]
Code first:
underlying neoplasm (C00-D49)

G13.1 ***Other systemic atrophy primarily affecting central nervous system in** neoplastic **disease*** HCC

Paraneoplastic limbic encephalopathy
Code first:
underlying neoplasm (C00-D49)

G13.2 ***Systemic atrophy primarily affecting the central nervous system in myxedema***
Code first underlying disease, such as:
hypothyroidism (E03.-)
myxedematous congenital iodine deficiency (E00.1)

G13.8 ***Systemic atrophy primarily affecting central nervous system in other diseases classified elsewhere***
Code first:
underlying disease

G14 Postpolio syndrome
INCLUDES postpolio myelitic syndrome
EXCLUDES 1 *sequelae of poliomyelitis (B91)*

CODING TIP✓ Post polio syndrome is differentiated from sequelae of poliomyelitis or residual deficits related to resolved poliomyelitis. When the record only specifies residual deficits related to resolved poliomyelitis, but does not specify post polio syndrome, coders should assign B91, Sequelae of poliomyelitis.

Extrapyramidal and movement disorders (G20-G26)

G20 Parkinson's disease HCC
Hemiparkinsonism
Idiopathic Parkinsonism or Parkinson's disease
Paralysis agitans
Parkinsonism or Parkinson's disease NOS
Primary Parkinsonism or Parkinson's disease
EXCLUDES 1 *dementia with Parkinsonism (G31.83)*

CODING TIP✓ Parkinsonism disorders are representative of multiple primary and secondary disorders that result in Parkinsonian traits, but not all patients with Parkinsonism disorders have Parkinson's disease. Only when the physician specifies Parkinson's disease should G20 be coded. Do not assign code G20 for a patient with a Parkinsonism disorder.

CODING TIP✓ When a patient is reported to have Parkinson's disease with related dementia, assign G20 followed by a code from category F02.8-, Dementia in diseases classified elsewhere. The physician must report the dementia as related to the Parkinson's disease in order to code the dementia as a manifestation.
AHA: 2Q 2016, 7
AHA: 2Q 2017, 7

4 **G21 Secondary parkinsonism**
EXCLUDES 1 *dementia with Parkinsonism (G31.83)*
Huntington's disease (G10)
Shy-Drager syndrome (G90.3)
syphilitic Parkinsonism (A52.19)

G21.0 **Malignant neuroleptic syndrome**
Use additional code for adverse effect, if applicable, to identify drug (T43.3X5, T43.4X5, T43.505, T43.595)
EXCLUDES 1 *neuroleptic induced parkinsonism (G21.11)*

5 G21.1 **Other drug-induced secondary parkinsonism**
CODING TIP✓ Drug-induced Parkinsonism is considered an adverse effect of a drug. The causative relationship must be stated by the physician. Assign an additional code to identify the drug.

G21.11 **Neuroleptic induced parkinsonism** HCC
Use additional code for adverse effect, if applicable, to identify drug (T43.3X5, T43.4X5, T43.505, T43.595)
EXCLUDES 1 *malignant neuroleptic syndrome (G21.0)*

G21.19 **Other drug induced secondary parkinsonism** HCC
Other medication-induced parkinsonism
Use additional code for adverse effect, if applicable, to identify drug (T36-T50 with fifth or sixth character 5)

G21.2 **Secondary parkinsonism due to other external agents** HCC
Code first:
(T51-T65) to identify external agent

G21.3 **Postencephalitic parkinsonism** HCC
G21.4 **Vascular parkinsonism** HCC
G21.8 **Other secondary parkinsonism** HCC
G21.9 **Secondary parkinsonism, unspecified** HCC

4 **G23 Other degenerative diseases of basal ganglia**
EXCLUDES 2 *multi-system degeneration of the autonomic nervous system (G90.3)*

G23.0 **Hallervorden-Spatz disease** HCC
Pigmentary pallidal degeneration
G23.1 **Progressive supranuclear ophthalmoplegia [Steele-Richardson-Olszewski]** HCC
Progressive supranuclear palsy
G23.2 **Striatonigral degeneration** HCC
G23.8 **Other specified degenerative diseases of basal ganglia** HCC
Calcification of basal ganglia
G23.9 **Degenerative disease of basal ganglia, unspecified** HCC

4 **G24 Dystonia**
INCLUDES dyskinesia
EXCLUDES 2 *athetoid cerebral palsy (G80.3)*

CODING TIP✓ Dystonias may be specified to congenital or acquired, primary or secondary, and may be anatomically specific. When coding dystonias, the coder should attempt to obtain specific information regarding the origin of the dystonia and the specific type of movement disorder so that the most specific code may be assigned.

▲ 5 G24.0 **Drug induced dystonia**
Use additional code for adverse effect, if applicable, to identify drug (T36-T50 with fifth or sixth character 5)

G24.01 **Drug induced subacute dyskinesia**
Drug induced blepharospasm
Drug induced orofacial dyskinesia
Neuroleptic induced tardive dyskinesia
Tardive dyskinesia
CODING TIP✓ Tardive dyskinesia due to use of medications, also referred to as lingual-facial-buccal dyskinesia, which presents as uncontrollable movements of the mouth, tongue, jaw, and cheeks, should be coded using G24.01 followed by the appropriate code to identify the drug causing the dyskinesia. This effect is commonly found following the use of neuroleptic medications.
DEFINITION Involuntary repetitive movements of facial, buccal, oral, and cervical muscles, induced by long-term use of antipsychotic agent, sometimes persisting after withdrawal of the agent.

G24.02 **Drug induced acute dystonia**
Acute dystonic reaction to drugs
Neuroleptic induced acute dystonia
G24.09 **Other drug induced dystonia**

G24.1 **Genetic torsion dystonia**
Dystonia deformans progressiva
Dystonia musculorum deformans
Familial torsion dystonia
Idiopathic familial dystonia
Idiopathic (torsion) dystonia NOS
(Schwalbe-) Ziehen-Oppenheim disease
G24.2 **Idiopathic nonfamilial dystonia**
G24.3 **Spasmodic torticollis**
EXCLUDES 1 *congenital torticollis (Q68.0)*
hysterical torticollis (F44.4)
ocular torticollis (R29.891)
psychogenic torticollis (F45.8)
torticollis NOS (M43.6)
traumatic recurrent torticollis (S13.4)
DEFINITION Contractions of the neck muscles causing contortion, pain, and abnormal head posture.
G24.4 **Idiopathic orofacial dystonia**
Orofacial dyskinesia
EXCLUDES 1 *drug induced orofacial dyskinesia (G24.01)*
G24.5 **Blepharospasm**
EXCLUDES 1 *drug induced blepharospasm (G24.01)*
DEFINITION Spasm of the orbicularis oculi muscle, causing uncontrolled winking or blinking.
G24.8 **Other dystonia**
Acquired torsion dystonia NOS
G24.9 **Dystonia, unspecified**
Dyskinesia NOS

4 G25 Other extrapyramidal and movement disorders
EXCLUDES 2 *sleep related movement disorders (G47.6-)*

G25.0 **Essential tremor**
Familial tremor
EXCLUDES 1 *tremor NOS (R25.1)*

CODING TIP ✓ Do not assign G25.0 to report unspecified tremors or tremors in a patient with a confirmed diagnosis of Parkinson's disease.

G25.1 **Drug-induced tremor**
Use additional code for adverse effect, if applicable, to identify drug (T36-T50 with fifth or sixth character 5)

G25.2 **Other specified forms of tremor**
Intention tremor

G25.3 **Myoclonus**
Drug-induced myoclonus
Palatal myoclonus
Use additional code for adverse effect, if applicable, to identify drug (T36-T50 with fifth or sixth character 5)
EXCLUDES 1 *facial myokymia (G51.4)*
myoclonic epilepsy (G40.-)

CODING TIP ✓ Myoclonus is also reported as muscle twitching and is often a symptom of a more specific disease process. When the specific disease process is known, code the underlying disease. If myoclonus is related to the adverse effect of a medication, use an additional code to identify the drug. This code should not be assigned for myoclonic epilepsy or seizures.

DEFINITION Spontaneous contractions of a muscle or group of muscles as a part of a disease process, drug side effect, or abnormal physiological response.

G25.4 **Drug-induced chorea**
Use additional code for adverse effect, if applicable, to identify drug (T36-T50 with fifth or sixth character 5)

G25.5 **Other chorea**
Chorea NOS
EXCLUDES 1 *chorea NOS with heart involvement (I02.0)*
Huntington's chorea (G10)
rheumatic chorea (I02.-)
Sydenham's chorea (I02.-)

5 G25.6 **Drug induced tics and other tics of organic origin**

G25.61 **Drug induced tics**
Use additional code for adverse effect, if applicable, to identify drug (T36-T50 with fifth or sixth character 5)

G25.69 **Other tics of organic origin**
EXCLUDES 1 *habit spasm (F95.9)*
tic NOS (F95.9)
Tourette's syndrome (F95.2)

5 G25.7 **Other and unspecified drug induced movement disorders**
Use additional code for adverse effect, if applicable, to identify drug (T36-T50 with fifth or sixth character 5)

G25.70 **Drug induced movement disorder, unspecified**

G25.71 **Drug induced akathisia**
Drug induced acathisia
Neuroleptic induced acute akathisia
Tardive akathisia

CODING TIP ✓ Akathisia is a syndrome characterized by a restless inability to maintain stillness or to "sit still" and is frequently induced by the use of various medications, including antipsychotics. When caused by the effect of a drug, an additional code should be assigned to identify the drug.

G25.79 **Other drug induced movement disorders**

5 G25.8 **Other specified extrapyramidal and movement disorders**

G25.81 **Restless legs syndrome**

DEFINITION Irresistible urge to move legs, particularly when sitting or lying down, with leg sensations such as creeping, crawling, itching, tugging, tightening, or pulling alleviated upon movement.

G25.82 **Stiff-man syndrome**

DEFINITION Progressive fluctuating rigidity of axial and limb muscles in the absence of any signs of cerebral and/or spinal cord disease.

G25.83 **Benign shuddering attacks**

G25.89 **Other specified extrapyramidal and movement disorders**

G25.9 **Extrapyramidal and movement disorder, unspecified**

G26 ***Extrapyramidal and movement disorders in diseases classified elsewhere***
Code first:
underlying disease

Other degenerative diseases of the nervous system (G30-G32)

4 G30 **Alzheimer's disease**
INCLUDES Alzheimer's dementia senile and presenile forms
Use additional code to identify:
delirium, if applicable (F05)
dementia with behavioral disturbance (F02.81)
dementia without behavioral disturbance (F02.80)
EXCLUDES 1 *senile degeneration of brain NEC (G31.1)*
senile dementia NOS (F03)
senility NOS (R41.81)

CODING TIP ✓ **Documentation:** Alzheimer's disease is a particular neurological condition and must be specifically confirmed by a physician. Early onset Alzheimer's is defined as diagnosis prior to the age of 65; however, the designation of early and late onset must be documented by, or confirmed with, the patient's physician and may not be assumed. Query the physician if the information is not readily available and, if unable to make a determination, assign code G30.9 for Alzheimer's disease, unspecified. Dementia is part of the disease, so the physician does not have to specifically mention dementia with Alzheimer's. The Alzheimers is paired with the F02.8- code as a manifestation of Alzheimer's.

DEFINITION Progressive degenerative disease of the brain of unknown cause with diffuse atrophy throughout the cerebral cortex; it initially presents with slight memory disturbance or personality changes that progressively deteriorate to profound memory loss and dementia.

G30.0 **Alzheimer's disease with early onset**

CODING TIP ✓ Early onset Alzheimer's is very uncommon and is diagnosed prior to the age of 65. Coders may not assume a diagnosis of early onset Alzheimer's disease, but must have confirmed evidence of this from the patient's physician in order to assign the diagnosis appropriately.

G30.1 **Alzheimer's disease with late onset** A

CODING TIP ✓ Late onset Alzheimer's is the most common type and presents with symptoms after the age of 65. Coders may not assume a diagnosis of late onset Alzheimer's disease but must have confirmed evidence of this from the patient's physician to assign the diagnosis appropriately.

G30.8 **Other Alzheimer's disease**

G30.9 **Alzheimer's disease, unspecified**
AHA: 4Q 2012, 95
AHA: 2Q 2016, 6
AHA: 1Q 2017, 43

4 G31 **Other degenerative diseases of nervous system, not elsewhere classified**
Use additional code to identify:
dementia with behavioral disturbance (F02.81)
dementia without behavioral disturbance (F02.80)
EXCLUDES 2 *Reye's syndrome (G93.7)*

5 G31.0 **Frontotemporal dementia**

G31.01 **Pick's disease**
Primary progressive aphasia
Progressive isolated aphasia

DEFINITION Rare, progressive, degenerative disease of the brain, similar to Alzheimer's disease but with cortical atrophy confined to the frontal and temporal lobes.

G31.09 **Other frontotemporal dementia**
Frontal dementia

G31.1 **Senile degeneration of brain, not elsewhere classified**
EXCLUDES 1 *Alzheimer's disease (G30.-)*
senility NOS (R41.81)

G31.2 Degeneration of nervous system due to alcohol
Alcoholic cerebellar ataxia
Alcoholic cerebellar degeneration
Alcoholic cerebral degeneration
Alcoholic encephalopathy
Dysfunction of the autonomic nervous system due to alcohol
Code also:
associated alcoholism (F10.-)

CODING TIP ✓ Cerebellar ataxia, encephalopathy, cerebellar degeneration, and autonomic dysfunction/degeneration, when specified as due to alcohol, should be coded to G31.2. Also assign the appropriate F10.- code to identify alcohol dependence/alcoholism, and, when applicable, a code to specify dementia (with or without behavior disturbance) as a manifestation (F02.8-). The dementia in alcohol dependence with alcohol-induced dementia code can be coded with F02.8-.

5 **G31.8 Other specified degenerative diseases of nervous system**

G31.81 Alpers disease
Grey-matter degeneration

G31.82 Leigh's disease
Subacute necrotizing encephalopathy

G31.83 Dementia with Lewy bodies
Dementia with Parkinsonism
Lewy body dementia
Lewy body disease
AHA: 4Q 2016, 141

G31.84 Mild cognitive impairment, so stated
Mild neurocognitive disorder
EXCLUDES 1 *age related cognitive decline (R41.81)*
altered mental status (R41.82)
cerebral degeneration (G31.9)
change in mental status (R41.82)
cognitive deficits following (sequelae of) cerebral hemorrhage or infarction (I69.01-, I69.11-, I69.21-, I69.31-, I69.81-, I69.91-)
cognitive impairment due to intracranial or head injury (S06.-)
dementia (F01.-, F02.-, F03)
mild memory disturbance (F06.8)
neurologic neglect syndrome (R41.4)
personality change, nonpsychotic (F68.8)

DEFINITION Impairment in memory or other specific cognitive function, beyond what is normally seen at a given age, but with function remaining relatively intact in the other cognitive domains.

G31.85 Corticobasal degeneration

G31.89 Other specified degenerative diseases of nervous system

G31.9 Degenerative disease of nervous system, unspecified

4 **G32 Other degenerative disorders of nervous system in diseases classified elsewhere**

G32.0 *Subacute combined degeneration of spinal cord in diseases classified elsewhere* HCC
Dana-Putnam syndrome
Sclerosis of spinal cord (combined) (dorsolateral) (posterolateral)
Code first underlying disease, such as:
anemia (D51.9)
dietary (D51.3)
pernicious (D51.0)
vitamin B12 deficiency (E53.8)
EXCLUDES 1 *syphilitic combined degeneration of spinal cord (A52.11)*

5 **G32.8 Other specified degenerative disorders of nervous system in diseases classified elsewhere**
Code first underlying disease, such as:
amyloidosis cerebral degeneration (E85.-)
cerebral degeneration (due to) hypothyroidism (E00.0-E03.9)
cerebral degeneration (due to) neoplasm (C00-D49)
cerebral degeneration (due to) vitamin B deficiency, except thiamine (E52-E53.-)
EXCLUDES 1 *superior hemorrhagic polioencephalitis [Wernicke's encephalopathy] (E51.2)*

G32.81 *Cerebellar ataxia in diseases classified elsewhere* HCC
Code first underlying disease, such as:
celiac disease (with gluten ataxia) (K90.0)
cerebellar ataxia (in) neoplastic disease (paraneoplastic cerebellar degeneration) (C00-D49)
non-celiac gluten ataxia (M35.9)
EXCLUDES 1 *systemic atrophy primarily affecting the central nervous system in alcoholic cerebellar ataxia (G31.2)*
systemic atrophy primarily affecting the central nervous system in myxedema (G13.2)

G32.89 *Other specified degenerative disorders of nervous system in diseases classified elsewhere*
Degenerative encephalopathy in diseases classified elsewhere

Demyelinating diseases of the central nervous system (G35-G37)

G35 Multiple sclerosis HCC
Disseminated multiple sclerosis
Generalized multiple sclerosis
Multiple sclerosis NOS
Multiple sclerosis of brain stem
Multiple sclerosis of cord

Multiple sclerosis (MS)

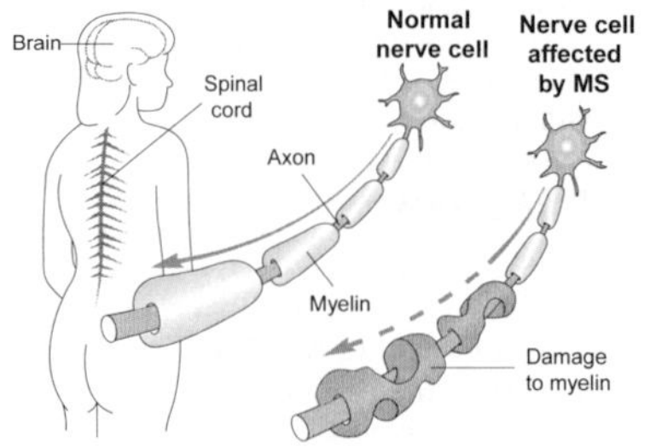

4 **G36 Other acute disseminated demyelination**
EXCLUDES 1 *postinfectious encephalitis and encephalomyelitis NOS (G04.01)*

G36.0 Neuromyelitis optica [Devic] HCC
Demyelination in optic neuritis
EXCLUDES 1 *optic neuritis NOS (H46)*

G36.1 Acute and subacute hemorrhagic leukoencephalitis [Hurst] HCC

G36.8 Other specified acute disseminated demyelination HCC

G36.9 Acute disseminated demyelination, unspecified HCC HIV

4 **G37 Other demyelinating diseases of central nervous system**

G37.0 Diffuse sclerosis of central nervous system HCC
Periaxial encephalitis
Schilder's disease
EXCLUDES 1 *X linked adrenoleukodystrophy (E71.52-)*

G37.1 Central demyelination of corpus callosum HCC

G37.2 Central pontine myelinolysis HCC

G37.3 Acute transverse myelitis in demyelinating disease of central nervous system HCC
Acute transverse myelitis NOS
Acute transverse myelopathy
EXCLUDES 1 *multiple sclerosis (G35)*
neuromyelitis optica [Devic] (G36.0)

DEFINITION Spinal cord disorder with inflammatory lesions across the entire width of one level; numbness, back pain, weakness, sensory loss, motor and sphincter deficits, loss of bladder and bowel control appear quickly and progress to paraplegia.

G37.4 Subacute necrotizing myelitis of central nervous system HCC HIV

G37.5 Concentric sclerosis [Balo] of central nervous system HCC

G37.8 **Other specified demyelinating diseases of central nervous system** HCC

G37.9 **Demyelinating disease of central nervous system, unspecified** HCC HIV

Episodic and paroxysmal disorders (G40-G47)

4 G40 **Epilepsy and recurrent seizures**

Note: the following terms are to be considered equivalent to intractable: pharmacoresistant (pharmacologically resistant), treatment resistant, refractory (medically) and poorly controlled

EXCLUDES 1 *conversion disorder with seizures (F44.5)*
convulsions NOS (R56.9)
post traumatic seizures (R56.1)
seizure (convulsive) NOS (R56.9)
seizure of newborn (P90)

EXCLUDES 2 *hippocampal sclerosis (G93.81)*
mesial temporal sclerosis (G93.81)
temporal sclerosis (G93.81)
Todd's paralysis (G83.84)

CODING TIP✓ When coding epileptic syndromes, coders should note that seizure(s)/epileptic disorders noted by the physician as treatment- or medication-resistant, refractory, or poorly controlled should be coded to intractable. Coders should not assign R56.9, Unspecified convulsions, for patients experiencing seizure disorders or recurrent seizures. Recurrent seizures and unspecified seizure disorders, when not reported as intractable, should be coded to G40.909.

5 G40.0 **Localization-related (focal) (partial) idiopathic epilepsy and epileptic syndromes with seizures of localized onset**

Benign childhood epilepsy with centrotemporal EEG spikes
Childhood epilepsy with occipital EEG paroxysms

EXCLUDES 1 *adult onset localization-related epilepsy (G40.1-, G40.2-)*

6 G40.00 **Localization-related (focal) (partial) idiopathic epilepsy and epileptic syndromes with seizures of localized onset, not intractable**

Localization-related (focal) (partial) idiopathic epilepsy and epileptic syndromes with seizures of localized onset without intractability

G40.001 **Localization-related (focal) (partial) idiopathic epilepsy and epileptic syndromes with seizures of localized onset, not intractable, with status epilepticus** HCC

G40.009 **Localization-related (focal) (partial) idiopathic epilepsy and epileptic syndromes with seizures of localized onset, not intractable, without status epilepticus** HCC

Localization-related (focal) (partial) idiopathic epilepsy and epileptic syndromes with seizures of localized onset NOS

6 G40.01 **Localization-related (focal) (partial) idiopathic epilepsy and epileptic syndromes with seizures of localized onset, intractable**

G40.011 **Localization-related (focal) (partial) idiopathic epilepsy and epileptic syndromes with seizures of localized onset, intractable, with status epilepticus** HCC

G40.019 **Localization-related (focal) (partial) idiopathic epilepsy and epileptic syndromes with seizures of localized onset, intractable, without status epilepticus** HCC

5 G40.1 **Localization-related (focal) (partial) symptomatic epilepsy and epileptic syndromes with simple partial seizures**

Attacks without alteration of consciousness
Epilepsia partialis continua [Kozhevnikof]
Simple partial seizures developing into secondarily generalized seizures

6 G40.10 **Localization-related (focal) (partial) symptomatic epilepsy and epileptic syndromes with simple partial seizures, not intractable**

Localization-related (focal) (partial) symptomatic epilepsy and epileptic syndromes with simple partial seizures without intractability

G40.101 **Localization-related (focal) (partial) symptomatic epilepsy and epileptic syndromes with simple partial seizures, not intractable, with status epilepticus** HCC

G40.109 **Localization-related (focal) (partial) symptomatic epilepsy and epileptic syndromes with simple partial seizures, not intractable, without status epilepticus** HCC

Localization-related (focal) (partial) symptomatic epilepsy and epileptic syndromes with simple partial seizures NOS

6 G40.11 **Localization-related (focal) (partial) symptomatic epilepsy and epileptic syndromes with simple partial seizures, intractable**

G40.111 **Localization-related (focal) (partial) symptomatic epilepsy and epileptic syndromes with simple partial seizures, intractable, with status epilepticus** HCC

G40.119 **Localization-related (focal) (partial) symptomatic epilepsy and epileptic syndromes with simple partial seizures, intractable, without status epilepticus** HCC

5 G40.2 **Localization-related (focal) (partial) symptomatic epilepsy and epileptic syndromes with complex partial seizures**

Attacks with alteration of consciousness, often with automatisms
Complex partial seizures developing into secondarily generalized seizures

6 G40.20 **Localization-related (focal) (partial) symptomatic epilepsy and epileptic syndromes with complex partial seizures, not intractable**

Localization-related (focal) (partial) symptomatic epilepsy and epileptic syndromes with complex partial seizures without intractability

G40.201 **Localization-related (focal) (partial) symptomatic epilepsy and epileptic syndromes with complex partial seizures, not intractable, with status epilepticus** HCC

G40.209 **Localization-related (focal) (partial) symptomatic epilepsy and epileptic syndromes with complex partial seizures, not intractable, without status epilepticus** HCC

Localization-related (focal) (partial) symptomatic epilepsy and epileptic syndromes with complex partial seizures NOS

6 G40.21 **Localization-related (focal) (partial) symptomatic epilepsy and epileptic syndromes with complex partial seizures, intractable**

G40.211 **Localization-related (focal) (partial) symptomatic epilepsy and epileptic syndromes with complex partial seizures, intractable, with status epilepticus** HCC

G40.219 **Localization-related (focal) (partial) symptomatic epilepsy and epileptic syndromes with complex partial seizures, intractable, without status epilepticus** HCC

5 G40.3 **Generalized idiopathic epilepsy and epileptic syndromes**

Code also:
MERRF syndrome, if applicable (E88.42)

6 G40.30 **Generalized idiopathic epilepsy and epileptic syndromes, not intractable**

Generalized idiopathic epilepsy and epileptic syndromes without intractability

G40.301 **Generalized idiopathic epilepsy and epileptic syndromes, not intractable, with status epilepticus** HCC

G40.309 **Generalized idiopathic epilepsy and epileptic syndromes, not intractable, without status epilepticus** HCC

Generalized idiopathic epilepsy and epileptic syndromes NOS

6 G40.31 **Generalized idiopathic epilepsy and epileptic syndromes, intractable**

G40.311 **Generalized idiopathic epilepsy and epileptic syndromes, intractable, with status epilepticus** HCC

G40.319 **Generalized idiopathic epilepsy and epileptic syndromes, intractable, without status epilepticus** HCC

5 G40.A Absence epileptic syndrome
Childhood absence epilepsy [pyknolepsy]
Juvenile absence epilepsy
Absence epileptic syndrome, NOS

6 G40.A0 Absence epileptic syndrome, not intractable

G40.A01 Absence epileptic syndrome, not intractable, with status epilepticus HCC

G40.A09 Absence epileptic syndrome, not intractable, without status epilepticus HCC

6 G40.A1 Absence epileptic syndrome, intractable

G40.A11 Absence epileptic syndrome, intractable, with status epilepticus HCC

G40.A19 Absence epileptic syndrome, intractable, without status epilepticus HCC

5 G40.B Juvenile myoclonic epilepsy [impulsive petit mal]

6 G40.B0 Juvenile myoclonic epilepsy, not intractable

G40.B01 Juvenile myoclonic epilepsy, not intractable, with status epilepticus HCC

G40.B09 Juvenile myoclonic epilepsy, not intractable, without status epilepticus HCC

6 G40.B1 Juvenile myoclonic epilepsy, intractable

G40.B11 Juvenile myoclonic epilepsy, intractable, with status epilepticus HCC

G40.B19 Juvenile myoclonic epilepsy, intractable, without status epilepticus HCC

5 G40.4 Other generalized epilepsy and epileptic syndromes
Epilepsy with grand mal seizures on awakening
Epilepsy with myoclonic absences
Epilepsy with myoclonic-astatic seizures
Grand mal seizure NOS
Nonspecific atonic epileptic seizures
Nonspecific clonic epileptic seizures
Nonspecific myoclonic epileptic seizures
Nonspecific tonic epileptic seizures
Nonspecific tonic-clonic epileptic seizures
Symptomatic early myoclonic encephalopathy

6 G40.40 Other generalized epilepsy and epileptic syndromes, not intractable
Other generalized epilepsy and epileptic syndromes without intractability
Other generalized epilepsy and epileptic syndromes NOS

G40.401 Other generalized epilepsy and epileptic syndromes, not intractable, with status epilepticus HCC

G40.409 Other generalized epilepsy and epileptic syndromes, not intractable, without status epilepticus HCC

6 G40.41 Other generalized epilepsy and epileptic syndromes, intractable

G40.411 Other generalized epilepsy and epileptic syndromes, intractable, with status epilepticus HCC

G40.419 Other generalized epilepsy and epileptic syndromes, intractable, without status epilepticus HCC

5 G40.5 Epileptic seizures related to external causes
Epileptic seizures related to alcohol
Epileptic seizures related to drugs
Epileptic seizures related to hormonal changes
Epileptic seizures related to sleep deprivation
Epileptic seizures related to stress
Code also:
, if applicable, associated epilepsy and recurrent seizures (G40.-)
Use additional code for adverse effect, if applicable, to identify drug (T36-T50 with fifth or sixth character 5)

6 G40.50 Epileptic seizures related to external causes, not intractable

G40.501 Epileptic seizures related to external causes, not intractable, with status epilepticus HCC

G40.509 Epileptic seizures related to external causes, not intractable, without status epilepticus HCC
Epileptic seizures related to external causes, NOS

5 G40.8 Other epilepsy and recurrent seizures
Epilepsies and epileptic syndromes undetermined as to whether they are focal or generalized
Landau-Kleffner syndrome

6 G40.80 Other epilepsy

G40.801 Other epilepsy, not intractable, with status epilepticus HCC
Other epilepsy without intractability with status epilepticus

G40.802 Other epilepsy, not intractable, without status epilepticus HCC
Other epilepsy NOS
Other epilepsy without intractability without status epilepticus

G40.803 Other epilepsy, intractable, with status epilepticus HCC

G40.804 Other epilepsy, intractable, without status epilepticus HCC

6 G40.81 Lennox-Gastaut syndrome

G40.811 Lennox-Gastaut syndrome, not intractable, with status epilepticus HCC

G40.812 Lennox-Gastaut syndrome, not intractable, without status epilepticus HCC

G40.813 Lennox-Gastaut syndrome, intractable, with status epilepticus HCC

G40.814 Lennox-Gastaut syndrome, intractable, without status epilepticus HCC

6 G40.82 Epileptic spasms
Infantile spasms
Salaam attacks
West's syndrome

G40.821 Epileptic spasms, not intractable, with status epilepticus HCC

G40.822 Epileptic spasms, not intractable, without status epilepticus HCC

G40.823 Epileptic spasms, intractable, with status epilepticus HCC

G40.824 Epileptic spasms, intractable, without status epilepticus HCC

G40.89 Other seizures HCC

EXCLUDES 1 *post traumatic seizures (R56.1)*
recurrent seizures NOS (G40.909)
seizure NOS (R56.9)

5 G40.9 Epilepsy, unspecified

6 G40.90 Epilepsy, unspecified, not intractable
Epilepsy, unspecified, without intractability

G40.901 Epilepsy, unspecified, not intractable, with status epilepticus HCC

G40.909 Epilepsy, unspecified, not intractable, without status epilepticus HCC
Epilepsy NOS
Epileptic convulsions NOS
Epileptic fits NOS
Epileptic seizures NOS
Recurrent seizures NOS
Seizure disorder NOS

CODING TIP✓ Recurrent seizures and unspecified seizure disorders, when not identified as intractable, should be reported using this code. Do not assign R56.9, Unspecified convulsions, to report a diagnosis of recurrent seizures or seizure disorder.

6 G40.91 Epilepsy, unspecified, intractable
Intractable seizure disorder NOS

G40.911 Epilepsy, unspecified, intractable, with status epilepticus HCC

G40.919 Epilepsy, unspecified, intractable, without status epilepticus HCC

4 G43 Migraine
Note: the following terms are to be considered equivalent to intractable: pharmacoresistant (pharmacologically resistant), treatment resistant, refractory (medically) and poorly controlled
Use additional code for adverse effect, if applicable, to identify drug (T36-T50 with fifth or sixth character 5)

EXCLUDES 1 *headache NOS (R51)*
lower half migraine (G44.00)

EXCLUDES 2 *headache syndromes (G44.-)*

5 **G43.0 Migraine without aura**
Common migraine
EXCLUDES 1 *chronic migraine without aura (G43.7-)*

6 **G43.00 Migraine without aura, not intractable**
Migraine without aura without mention of refractory migraine

G43.001 Migraine without aura, not intractable, with status migrainosus

G43.009 Migraine without aura, not intractable, without status migrainosus
Migraine without aura NOS

6 **G43.01 Migraine without aura, intractable**
Migraine without aura with refractory migraine

G43.011 Migraine without aura, intractable, with status migrainosus

G43.019 Migraine without aura, intractable, without status migrainosus

5 **G43.1 Migraine with aura**
Basilar migraine
Classical migraine
Migraine equivalents
Migraine preceded or accompanied by transient focal neurological phenomena
Migraine triggered seizures
Migraine with acute-onset aura
Migraine with aura without headache (migraine equivalents)
Migraine with prolonged aura
Migraine with typical aura
Retinal migraine
Code also:
any associated seizure (G40.-, R56.9)
EXCLUDES 1 *persistent migraine aura (G43.5-, G43.6-)*

6 **G43.10 Migraine with aura, not intractable**
Migraine with aura without mention of refractory migraine

G43.101 Migraine with aura, not intractable, with status migrainosus

G43.109 Migraine with aura, not intractable, without status migrainosus
Migraine with aura NOS

6 **G43.11 Migraine with aura, intractable**
Migraine with aura with refractory migraine

G43.111 Migraine with aura, intractable, with status migrainosus

G43.119 Migraine with aura, intractable, without status migrainosus

5 **G43.4 Hemiplegic migraine**
Familial migraine
Sporadic migraine

6 **G43.40 Hemiplegic migraine, not intractable**
Hemiplegic migraine without refractory migraine

G43.401 Hemiplegic migraine, not intractable, with status migrainosus

G43.409 Hemiplegic migraine, not intractable, without status migrainosus
Hemiplegic migraine NOS

6 **G43.41 Hemiplegic migraine, intractable**
Hemiplegic migraine with refractory migraine

G43.411 Hemiplegic migraine, intractable, with status migrainosus

G43.419 Hemiplegic migraine, intractable, without status migrainosus

5 **G43.5 Persistent migraine aura without cerebral infarction**

6 **G43.50 Persistent migraine aura without cerebral infarction, not intractable**
Persistent migraine aura without cerebral infarction, without refractory migraine

G43.501 Persistent migraine aura without cerebral infarction, not intractable, with status migrainosus

G43.509 Persistent migraine aura without cerebral infarction, not intractable, without status migrainosus
Persistent migraine aura NOS

6 **G43.51 Persistent migraine aura without cerebral infarction, intractable**
Persistent migraine aura without cerebral infarction, with refractory migraine

G43.511 Persistent migraine aura without cerebral infarction, intractable, with status migrainosus

G43.519 Persistent migraine aura without cerebral infarction, intractable, without status migrainosus

5 **G43.6 Persistent migraine aura with cerebral infarction**
Code also:
the type of cerebral infarction (I63.-)

6 **G43.60 Persistent migraine aura with cerebral infarction, not intractable**
Persistent migraine aura with cerebral infarction, without refractory migraine

G43.601 Persistent migraine aura with cerebral infarction, not intractable, with status migrainosus

G43.609 Persistent migraine aura with cerebral infarction, not intractable, without status migrainosus

6 **G43.61 Persistent migraine aura with cerebral infarction, intractable**
Persistent migraine aura with cerebral infarction, with refractory migraine

G43.611 Persistent migraine aura with cerebral infarction, intractable, with status migrainosus

G43.619 Persistent migraine aura with cerebral infarction, intractable, without status migrainosus

5 **G43.7 Chronic migraine without aura**
Transformed migraine
EXCLUDES 1 *migraine without aura (G43.0-)*

6 **G43.70 Chronic migraine without aura, not intractable**
Chronic migraine without aura, without refractory migraine

G43.701 Chronic migraine without aura, not intractable, with status migrainosus

G43.709 Chronic migraine without aura, not intractable, without status migrainosus
Chronic migraine without aura NOS

6 **G43.71 Chronic migraine without aura, intractable**
Chronic migraine without aura, with refractory migraine

G43.711 Chronic migraine without aura, intractable, with status migrainosus

G43.719 Chronic migraine without aura, intractable, without status migrainosus

5 **G43.A Cyclical vomiting**

G43.A0 Cyclical vomiting, not intractable
Cyclical vomiting, without refractory migraine

G43.A1 Cyclical vomiting, intractable
Cyclical vomiting, with refractory migraine

5 **G43.B Ophthalmoplegic migraine**

G43.B0 Ophthalmoplegic migraine, not intractable
Ophthalmoplegic migraine, without refractory migraine

G43.B1 Ophthalmoplegic migraine, intractable
Ophthalmoplegic migraine, with refractory migraine

5 **G43.C Periodic headache syndromes in child or adult**

G43.C0 Periodic headache syndromes in child or adult, not intractable
Periodic headache syndromes in child or adult, without refractory migraine

G43.C1 Periodic headache syndromes in child or adult, intractable
Periodic headache syndromes in child or adult, with refractory migraine

5 **G43.D Abdominal migraine**

G43.D0 Abdominal migraine, not intractable
Abdominal migraine, without refractory migraine

G43.D1 Abdominal migraine, intractable
Abdominal migraine, with refractory migraine

5 **G43.8 Other migraine**

6 **G43.80 Other migraine, not intractable**
Other migraine, without refractory migraine

G43.801 Other migraine, not intractable, with status migrainosus

G43.809 Other migraine, not intractable, without status migrainosus

6 G43.81 Other migraine, intractable
Other migraine, with refractory migraine

G43.811 Other migraine, intractable, with status migrainosus

G43.819 Other migraine, intractable, without status migrainosus

6 G43.82 Menstrual migraine, not intractable
Menstrual headache, not intractable
Menstrual migraine, without refractory migraine
Menstrually related migraine, not intractable
Pre-menstrual headache, not intractable
Pre-menstrual migraine, not intractable
Pure menstrual migraine, not intractable
Code also:
associated premenstrual tension syndrome (N94.3)

G43.821 Menstrual migraine, not intractable, with status migrainosus ♀

G43.829 Menstrual migraine, not intractable, without status migrainosus ♀
Menstrual migraine NOS

6 G43.83 Menstrual migraine, intractable
Menstrual headache, intractable
Menstrual migraine, with refractory migraine
Menstrually related migraine, intractable
Pre-menstrual headache, intractable
Pre-menstrual migraine, intractable
Pure menstrual migraine, intractable
Code also:
associated premenstrual tension syndrome (N94.3)

G43.831 Menstrual migraine, intractable, with status migrainosus ♀

G43.839 Menstrual migraine, intractable, without status migrainosus ♀

5 G43.9 Migraine, unspecified

6 G43.90 Migraine, unspecified, not intractable
Migraine, unspecified, without refractory migraine

G43.901 Migraine, unspecified, not intractable, with status migrainosus
Status migrainosus NOS

G43.909 Migraine, unspecified, not intractable, without status migrainosus
Migraine NOS

6 G43.91 Migraine, unspecified, intractable
Migraine, unspecified, with refractory migraine

G43.911 Migraine, unspecified, intractable, with status migrainosus

G43.919 Migraine, unspecified, intractable, without status migrainosus

4 G44 Other headache syndromes

EXCLUDES 1 *headache NOS (R51)*

EXCLUDES 2 *atypical facial pain (G50.1)*
headache due to lumbar puncture (G97.1)
migraines (G43.-)
trigeminal neuralgia (G50.0)

5 G44.0 Cluster headaches and other trigeminal autonomic cephalgias (TAC)

6 G44.00 Cluster headache syndrome, unspecified
Ciliary neuralgia
Cluster headache NOS
Histamine cephalgia
Lower half migraine
Migrainous neuralgia

G44.001 Cluster headache syndrome, unspecified, intractable

G44.009 Cluster headache syndrome, unspecified, not intractable
Cluster headache syndrome NOS

6 G44.01 Episodic cluster headache

DEFINITION Distinctive headache marked by excruciating, searing pain that develops quickly without warning on one side and occurs in frequent attacks lasting from 15 minutes to 3 hours, in cyclical patterns of up to 12 weeks, followed by remission periods.

G44.011 Episodic cluster headache, intractable

G44.019 Episodic cluster headache, not intractable
Episodic cluster headache NOS

6 G44.02 Chronic cluster headache

G44.021 Chronic cluster headache, intractable

G44.029 Chronic cluster headache, not intractable
Chronic cluster headache NOS

6 G44.03 Episodic paroxysmal hemicrania
Paroxysmal hemicrania NOS

DEFINITION Rare headache with severe throbbing or boring pain in the eye or temple on one side and accompanying autonomic responses; occurring in frequent, daily attacks with relatively long headache-free periods.

G44.031 Episodic paroxysmal hemicrania, intractable

G44.039 Episodic paroxysmal hemicrania, not intractable
Episodic paroxysmal hemicrania NOS

6 G44.04 Chronic paroxysmal hemicrania

G44.041 Chronic paroxysmal hemicrania, intractable

G44.049 Chronic paroxysmal hemicrania, not intractable
Chronic paroxysmal hemicrania NOS

6 G44.05 Short lasting unilateral neuralgiform headache with conjunctival injection and tearing (SUNCT)

G44.051 Short lasting unilateral neuralgiform headache with conjunctival injection and tearing (SUNCT), intractable

G44.059 Short lasting unilateral neuralgiform headache with conjunctival injection and tearing (SUNCT), not intractable
Short lasting unilateral neuralgiform headache with conjunctival injection and tearing (SUNCT) NOS

6 G44.09 Other trigeminal autonomic cephalgias (TAC)

G44.091 Other trigeminal autonomic cephalgias (TAC), intractable

G44.099 Other trigeminal autonomic cephalgias (TAC), not intractable

G44.1 Vascular headache, not elsewhere classified

EXCLUDES 2 *cluster headache (G44.0)*
complicated headache syndromes (G44.5-)
drug-induced headache (G44.4-)
migraine (G43.-)
other specified headache syndromes (G44.8-)
post-traumatic headache (G44.3-)
tension-type headache (G44.2-)

5 G44.2 Tension-type headache

6 G44.20 Tension-type headache, unspecified

DEFINITION Common, muscular contraction headaches, that produce a mild to moderate, dull, achy tightening pain over the forehead and sides like a band encircling the head or pain at the back of the neck or base of the skull.

G44.201 Tension-type headache, unspecified, intractable

G44.209 Tension-type headache, unspecified, not intractable
Tension headache NOS

6 G44.21 Episodic tension-type headache

G44.211 Episodic tension-type headache, intractable

G44.219 Episodic tension-type headache, not intractable
Episodic tension-type headache NOS

6 G44.22 Chronic tension-type headache

G44.221 Chronic tension-type headache, intractable

G44.229 Chronic tension-type headache, not intractable
Chronic tension-type headache NOS

5 G44.3 Post-traumatic headache

6 G44.30 Post-traumatic headache, unspecified

DEFINITION Headache as a result of head trauma or injury, with frequency and severity diminishing over time; symptoms such as insomnia, concentration problems, personality changes, and dizziness often accompany the headache.

G44.301 Post-traumatic headache, unspecified, intractable

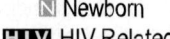

G44.309 Post-traumatic headache, unspecified, not intractable
Post-traumatic headache NOS

6 G44.31 Acute post-traumatic headache
G44.311 Acute post-traumatic headache, intractable
G44.319 Acute post-traumatic headache, not intractable
Acute post-traumatic headache NOS
6 G44.32 Chronic post-traumatic headache
G44.321 Chronic post-traumatic headache, intractable
G44.329 Chronic post-traumatic headache, not intractable
Chronic post-traumatic headache NOS
5 G44.4 Drug-induced headache, not elsewhere classified
Medication overuse headache
Use additional code for adverse effect, if applicable, to identify drug (T36-T50 with fifth or sixth character 5)

DEFINITION Most common type of chronic daily headache caused by overuse of migraine-abortive ergot alkaloids and analgesic drugs.

G44.40 Drug-induced headache, not elsewhere classified, not intractable
G44.41 Drug-induced headache, not elsewhere classified, intractable
5 G44.5 Complicated headache syndromes
G44.51 Hemicrania continua
G44.52 New daily persistent headache (NDPH)
G44.53 Primary thunderclap headache

DEFINITION Dramatic, sudden, severe headache coming without warning, peaking within 60 seconds, then fading over several hours; sometimes signaling a potentially life-threatening condition, such as a ruptured cerebral aneurysm or subarachnoid hemorrhage.

G44.59 Other complicated headache syndrome
5 G44.8 Other specified headache syndromes
G44.81 Hypnic headache

DEFINITION Relatively rare headache connected to REM sleep, marked by being awakened with intense throbbing or dull type pain through the head, accompanied by nausea, and lasting about an hour.

G44.82 Headache associated with sexual activity
Orgasmic headache
Preorgasmic headache
G44.83 Primary cough headache

DEFINITION Headache triggered by bouts of coughing or physically straining movements, such as laughing or sneezing, often described as sharp, stabbing, or splitting on both sides of the head and back of the skull.

G44.84 Primary exertional headache
G44.85 Primary stabbing headache
G44.89 Other headache syndrome

4 G45 Transient cerebral ischemic attacks and related syndromes
EXCLUDES 1 *neonatal cerebral ischemia (P91.0)*
transient retinal artery occlusion (H34.0-)
G45.0 Vertebro-basilar artery syndrome

DEFINITION Obstruction of the vertebral or basilar artery temporarily blocking blood flow to the brain, causing vertigo, diplopia, nystagmus, and muscle weakness.

G45.1 Carotid artery syndrome (hemispheric)
G45.2 Multiple and bilateral precerebral artery syndromes
G45.3 Amaurosis fugax

CODING TIP✓ Amaurosis fugax is a sudden loss of vision in one eye related to impaired carotid blood flow and impaired retinal blood supply and is generally temporary. The condition may signal pending stroke and should not be confused with blindness. Coders should not code blindness in a patient with this condition.

G45.4 Transient global amnesia
EXCLUDES 1 *amnesia NOS (R41.3)*
G45.8 Other transient cerebral ischemic attacks and related syndromes
G45.9 Transient cerebral ischemic attack, unspecified
Spasm of cerebral artery
TIA
Transient cerebral ischemia NOS

CODING TIP✓ There is no code to report sequelae of a TIA, as these are considered to be "transient" and should not cause residual effects. If residual effects are noted, the coder should query the physician to determine if the patient experienced a CVA. A history of TIA (or CVA) with no residual neurological deficits may be coded to Z86.73, Personal history of transient ischemic attack, and cerebral infarction, without residual deficits.

4 G46 Vascular syndromes of brain in cerebrovascular diseases
Code first:
underlying cerebrovascular disease (I60-I69)

CODING TIP✓ Conditions classified to G46.- include syndromes occurring as a result of specific types of cerebral vascular disease and cerebral vascular accidents (CVA). When a syndrome classifiable to G46.- occurs as a residual of a non-traumatic CVA, assign the appropriate I69 code to indicate sequelae of cerebrovascular disease. These syndromes may be coded as "other sequelae" of CVAs and should then be coded following the appropriate I69 code with the 6th character "8."

G46.0 Middle cerebral artery syndrome
G46.1 Anterior cerebral artery syndrome
G46.2 Posterior cerebral artery syndrome
G46.3 Brain stem stroke syndrome
Benedikt syndrome
Claude syndrome
Foville syndrome
Millard-Gubler syndrome
Wallenberg syndrome
Weber syndrome
G46.4 Cerebellar stroke syndrome
G46.5 Pure motor lacunar syndrome
G46.6 Pure sensory lacunar syndrome
G46.7 Other lacunar syndromes
G46.8 Other vascular syndromes of brain in cerebrovascular diseases

4 G47 Sleep disorders
EXCLUDES 2 *nightmares (F51.5)*
nonorganic sleep disorders (F51.-)
sleep terrors (F51.4)
sleepwalking (F51.3)
5 G47.0 Insomnia
EXCLUDES 2 *alcohol related insomnia (F10.182, F10.282, F10.982)*
drug-related insomnia (F11.182, F11.282, F11.982, F13.182, F13.282, F13.982, F14.182, F14.282, F14.982, F15.182, F15.282, F15.982, F19.182, F19.282, F19.982)
idiopathic insomnia (F51.01)
insomnia due to a mental disorder (F51.05)
insomnia not due to a substance or known physiological condition (F51.0-)
nonorganic insomnia (F51.0-)
primary insomnia (F51.01)
sleep apnea (G47.3-)
G47.00 Insomnia, unspecified
Insomnia NOS
G47.01 Insomnia due to medical condition
Code also:
associated medical condition
G47.09 Other insomnia
5 G47.1 Hypersomnia
EXCLUDES 2 *alcohol-related hypersomnia (F10.182, F10.282, F10.982)*
drug-related hypersomnia (F11.182, F11.282, F11.982, F13.182, F13.282, F13.982, F14.182, F14.282, F14.982, F15.182, F15.282, F15.982, F19.182, F19.282, F19.982)
hypersomnia due to a mental disorder (F51.13)
hypersomnia not due to a substance or known physiological condition (F51.1-)
primary hypersomnia (F51.11)
sleep apnea (G47.3-)

G47.10 **Hypersomnia, unspecified**
Hypersomnia NOS
G47.11 **Idiopathic hypersomnia with long sleep time**
Idiopathic hypersomnia NOS
G47.12 **Idiopathic hypersomnia without long sleep time**
G47.13 **Recurrent hypersomnia**
Kleine-Levin syndrome
Menstrual related hypersomnia
G47.14 **Hypersomnia due to medical condition**
Code also:
associated medical condition
G47.19 **Other hypersomnia**
5 G47.2 **Circadian rhythm sleep disorders**
Disorders of the sleep wake schedule
Inversion of nyctohemeral rhythm
Inversion of sleep rhythm
G47.20 **Circadian rhythm sleep disorder, unspecified type**
Sleep wake schedule disorder NOS
G47.21 **Circadian rhythm sleep disorder, delayed sleep phase type**
Delayed sleep phase syndrome
G47.22 **Circadian rhythm sleep disorder, advanced sleep phase type**
G47.23 **Circadian rhythm sleep disorder, irregular sleep wake type**
Irregular sleep-wake pattern
G47.24 **Circadian rhythm sleep disorder, free running type**
Circadian rhythm sleep disorder, non-24-hour sleep-wake type
G47.25 **Circadian rhythm sleep disorder, jet lag type**
G47.26 **Circadian rhythm sleep disorder, shift work type**
G47.27 ***Circadian rhythm sleep disorder in conditions classified elsewhere***
Code first:
underlying condition
G47.29 **Other circadian rhythm sleep disorder**
5 G47.3 **Sleep apnea**
Code also:
any associated underlying condition
EXCLUDES 1 *apnea NOS (R06.81)*
Cheyne-Stokes breathing (R06.3)
pickwickian syndrome (E66.2)
sleep apnea of newborn (P28.3)
G47.30 **Sleep apnea, unspecified**
Sleep apnea NOS
G47.31 **Primary central sleep apnea**
Idiopathic central sleep apnea
G47.32 **High altitude periodic breathing**
G47.33 **Obstructive sleep apnea (adult) (pediatric)**
Obstructive sleep apnea hypopnea
EXCLUDES 1 *obstructive sleep apnea of newborn (P28.3)*
G47.34 **Idiopathic sleep related nonobstructive alveolar hypoventilation**
Sleep related hypoxia
G47.35 **Congenital central alveolar hypoventilation syndrome**
G47.36 ***Sleep related hypoventilation in conditions classified elsewhere***
Sleep related hypoxemia in conditions classified elsewhere
Code first:
underlying condition
G47.37 ***Central sleep apnea in conditions classified elsewhere***
Code first:
underlying condition
G47.39 **Other sleep apnea**
5 G47.4 **Narcolepsy and cataplexy**
6 G47.41 **Narcolepsy**
G47.411 **Narcolepsy with cataplexy**
G47.419 **Narcolepsy without cataplexy**
Narcolepsy NOS
6 G47.42 **Narcolepsy in conditions classified elsewhere**
Code first:
underlying condition
G47.421 ***Narcolepsy in conditions classified elsewhere with cataplexy***
G47.429 ***Narcolepsy in conditions classified elsewhere without cataplexy***

5 G47.5 **Parasomnia**
EXCLUDES 1 *alcohol induced parasomnia (F10.182, F10.282, F10.982)*
drug induced parasomnia (F11.182, F11.282, F11.982, F13.182, F13.282, F13.982, F14.182, F14.282, F14.982, F15.182, F15.282, F15.982, F19.182, F19.282, F19.982)
parasomnia not due to a substance or known physiological condition (F51.8)
G47.50 **Parasomnia, unspecified**
Parasomnia NOS
G47.51 **Confusional arousals**
G47.52 **REM sleep behavior disorder**
G47.53 **Recurrent isolated sleep paralysis**
G47.54 ***Parasomnia in conditions classified elsewhere***
Code first:
underlying condition
G47.59 **Other parasomnia**
5 G47.6 **Sleep related movement disorders**
EXCLUDES 2 *restless legs syndrome (G25.81)*
G47.61 **Periodic limb movement disorder**
DEFINITION Involuntary limb movement or jerking during or just before sleep.
G47.62 **Sleep related leg cramps**
G47.63 **Sleep related bruxism**
EXCLUDES 1 *psychogenic bruxism (F45.8)*
DEFINITION Grinding the teeth during sleep.
G47.69 **Other sleep related movement disorders**
G47.8 **Other sleep disorders**
Other specified sleep-wake disorder
G47.9 **Sleep disorder, unspecified**
Sleep disorder NOS
Unspecified sleep-wake disorder

Nerve, nerve root and plexus disorders (G50-G59)

EXCLUDES 1 *current traumatic nerve, nerve root and plexus disorders - see Injury, nerve by body region*
neuralgia NOS (M79.2)
neuritis NOS (M79.2)
peripheral neuritis in pregnancy (O26.82-)
radiculitis NOS (M54.1-)

CODING TIP ✓ When coding neuralgias and neuropathy, coders should understand the definitions of the terms neuralgia, neuritis, and neuropathy. Neuritis is an inflammation of the nerve and should not be coded unless specifically noted in the "includes" notes for the code selected. Neuralgia indicates nerve pain, which may or may not be the result of neuritis or other disease or damage to the nerve, such as phantom limb pain/syndrome with pain (G54.6). Neuropathy indicates pain related to damaged and diseased nerve pathways.

4 G50 **Disorders of trigeminal nerve**
INCLUDES disorders of 5th cranial nerve
G50.0 **Trigeminal neuralgia**
Syndrome of paroxysmal facial pain
Tic douloureux
G50.1 **Atypical facial pain**
G50.8 **Other disorders of trigeminal nerve**
G50.9 **Disorder of trigeminal nerve, unspecified**
4 G51 **Facial nerve disorders**
INCLUDES disorders of 7th cranial nerve
G51.0 **Bell's palsy**
Facial palsy
DEFINITION Temporary, unilateral facial muscle weakness or paralysis resulting from damage or trauma to one of the paired facial nerves.
G51.1 **Geniculate ganglionitis**
EXCLUDES 1 *postherpetic geniculate ganglionitis (B02.21)*
DEFINITION Inflammation of the facial nerve ganglion.
G51.2 **Melkersson's syndrome**
Melkersson-Rosenthal syndrome

▲ G51.3 **Clonic hemifacial spasm**
- ● G51.31 **Clonic hemifacial spasm, right**
- ● G51.32 **Clonic hemifacial spasm, left**
- ● G51.33 **Clonic hemifacial spasm, bilateral**
- ● G51.39 **Clonic hemifacial spasm, unspecified**

G51.4 **Facial myokymia**
G51.8 **Other disorders of facial nerve**
G51.9 **Disorder of facial nerve, unspecified**

G52 Disorders of other cranial nerves

EXCLUDES 2 *disorders of acoustic [8th] nerve (H93.3)*
disorders of optic [2nd] nerve (H46, H47.0)
paralytic strabismus due to nerve palsy (H49.0-H49.2)

G52.0 **Disorders of olfactory nerve**
Disorders of 1st cranial nerve

G52.1 **Disorders of glossopharyngeal nerve**
Disorder of 9th cranial nerve
Glossopharyngeal neuralgia

G52.2 **Disorders of vagus nerve**
Disorders of pneumogastric [10th] nerve

G52.3 **Disorders of hypoglossal nerve**
Disorders of 12th cranial nerve

G52.7 **Disorders of multiple cranial nerves**
Polyneuritis cranialis

G52.8 **Disorders of other specified cranial nerves**
G52.9 **Cranial nerve disorder, unspecified**

G53 *Cranial nerve disorders in diseases classified elsewhere*

Code first underlying disease, such as:
neoplasm (C00-D49)

EXCLUDES 1 *multiple cranial nerve palsy in sarcoidosis (D86.82)*
multiple cranial nerve palsy in syphilis (A52.15)
postherpetic geniculate ganglionitis (B02.21)
postherpetic trigeminal neuralgia (B02.22)

G54 Nerve root and plexus disorders

EXCLUDES 1 *current traumatic nerve root and plexus disorders - see nerve injury by body region*
intervertebral disc disorders (M50-M51)
neuralgia or neuritis NOS (M79.2)
neuritis or radiculitis brachial NOS (M54.13)
neuritis or radiculitis lumbar NOS (M54.16)
neuritis or radiculitis lumbosacral NOS (M54.17)
neuritis or radiculitis thoracic NOS (M54.14)
radiculitis NOS (M54.10)
radiculopathy NOS (M54.10)
spondylosis (M47.-)

G54.0 **Brachial plexus disorders**
Thoracic outlet syndrome

G54.1 **Lumbosacral plexus disorders**
G54.2 **Cervical root disorders, not elsewhere classified**
G54.3 **Thoracic root disorders, not elsewhere classified**
G54.4 **Lumbosacral root disorders, not elsewhere classified**
G54.5 **Neuralgic amyotrophy**
Parsonage-Aldren-Turner syndrome
Shoulder-girdle neuritis

EXCLUDES 1 *neuralgic amyotrophy in diabetes mellitus (E08-E13 with .44)*

CODING TIP ✓ Do not assign code G54.5 for diabetic amyotrophy. Diabetes with amyotrophy should be coded with the appropriate combination code to specify the type of diabetes and the neuralgic amyotrophy manifestation (E08-E13 with 4th and 5th character .44).

G54.6 **Phantom limb syndrome with pain** HCC
G54.7 **Phantom limb syndrome without pain** HCC
Phantom limb syndrome NOS

G54.8 **Other nerve root and plexus disorders**
G54.9 **Nerve root and plexus disorder, unspecified**

G55 *Nerve root and plexus compressions in diseases classified elsewhere*

Code first underlying disease, such as:
neoplasm (C00-D49)

EXCLUDES 1 *nerve root compression (due to) (in) ankylosing spondylitis (M45.-)*
nerve root compression (due to) (in) dorsopathies (M53.-, M54.-)
nerve root compression (due to) (in) intervertebral disc disorders (M50.1.-, M51.1.-)
nerve root compression (due to) (in) spondylopathies (M46.-, M48.-)
nerve root compression (due to) (in) spondylosis (M47.0-M47.2.-)

G56 Mononeuropathies of upper limb

EXCLUDES 1 *current traumatic nerve disorder - see nerve injury by body region*

CODING TIP ✓ Complex regional pain syndromes (CRPS Type I or II or unspecified) are no longer classified and coded to causalgias and mononeuropathies. When CRPS Type I, Type II or unspecified is reported, it should be coded to the appropriate G90.5- code.

G56.0 **Carpal tunnel syndrome**

DEFINITION Pain, burning, tingling and/or numbness in the fingers and hand, often extending to the elbow, due to compression of the median nerve within the carpal tunnel.

- G56.00 **Carpal tunnel syndrome, unspecified upper limb**
- G56.01 **Carpal tunnel syndrome, right upper limb**
- G56.02 **Carpal tunnel syndrome, left upper limb**
- G56.03 **Carpal tunnel syndrome, bilateral upper limbs**
  AHA: 4Q 2016, 17

G56.1 **Other lesions of median nerve**
- G56.10 **Other lesions of median nerve, unspecified upper limb**
- G56.11 **Other lesions of median nerve, right upper limb**
- G56.12 **Other lesions of median nerve, left upper limb**
- G56.13 **Other lesions of median nerve, bilateral upper limbs**
  AHA: 4Q 2016, 17

G56.2 **Lesion of ulnar nerve**
Tardy ulnar nerve palsy
- G56.20 **Lesion of ulnar nerve, unspecified upper limb**
- G56.21 **Lesion of ulnar nerve, right upper limb**
- G56.22 **Lesion of ulnar nerve, left upper limb**
- G56.23 **Lesion of ulnar nerve, bilateral upper limbs**
  AHA: 4Q 2016, 17

G56.3 **Lesion of radial nerve**
- G56.30 **Lesion of radial nerve, unspecified upper limb**
- G56.31 **Lesion of radial nerve, right upper limb**
- G56.32 **Lesion of radial nerve, left upper limb**
- G56.33 **Lesion of radial nerve, bilateral upper limbs**
  AHA: 4Q 2016, 17

G56.4 **Causalgia of upper limb**
Complex regional pain syndrome II of upper limb

EXCLUDES 1 *complex regional pain syndrome I of lower limb (G90.52-)*
complex regional pain syndrome I of upper limb (G90.51-)
complex regional pain syndrome II of lower limb (G57.7-)
reflex sympathetic dystrophy of lower limb (G90.52-)
reflex sympathetic dystrophy of upper limb (G90.51-)

DEFINITION A burning pain in the arm along the course of a peripheral nerve usually associated with skin changes.

- G56.40 **Causalgia of unspecified upper limb**
- G56.41 **Causalgia of right upper limb**
- G56.42 **Causalgia of left upper limb**
- G56.43 **Causalgia of bilateral upper limbs**
  AHA: 4Q 2016, 17

G56.8 **Other specified mononeuropathies of upper limb**
Interdigital neuroma of upper limb

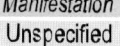

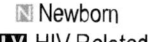

Diseases of the Nervous System

- G56.80 **Other specified mononeuropathies of unspecified upper limb**
- G56.81 **Other specified mononeuropathies of right upper limb**
- G56.82 **Other specified mononeuropathies of left upper limb**
- G56.83 **Other specified mononeuropathies of bilateral upper limbs**
  AHA: 4Q 2016, 17

G56.9 **Unspecified mononeuropathy of upper limb**

- G56.90 **Unspecified mononeuropathy of unspecified upper limb**
- G56.91 **Unspecified mononeuropathy of right upper limb**
- G56.92 **Unspecified mononeuropathy of left upper limb**
- G56.93 **Unspecified mononeuropathy of bilateral upper limbs**
  AHA: 4Q 2016, 17

G57 Mononeuropathies of lower limb

EXCLUDES 1 *current traumatic nerve disorder - see nerve injury by body region*

G57.0 **Lesion of sciatic nerve**

EXCLUDES 1 *sciatica NOS (M54.3-)*

EXCLUDES 2 *sciatica attributed to intervertebral disc disorder (M51.1.-)*

- G57.00 **Lesion of sciatic nerve, unspecified lower limb**
- G57.01 **Lesion of sciatic nerve, right lower limb**
- G57.02 **Lesion of sciatic nerve, left lower limb**
- G57.03 **Lesion of sciatic nerve, bilateral lower limbs**
  AHA: 4Q 2016, 17

G57.1 **Meralgia paresthetica**
Lateral cutaneous nerve of thigh syndrome

- G57.10 **Meralgia paresthetica, unspecified lower limb**
- G57.11 **Meralgia paresthetica, right lower limb**
- G57.12 **Meralgia paresthetica, left lower limb**
- G57.13 **Meralgia paresthetica, bilateral lower limbs**
  AHA: 4Q 2016, 17

G57.2 **Lesion of femoral nerve**

- G57.20 **Lesion of femoral nerve, unspecified lower limb**
- G57.21 **Lesion of femoral nerve, right lower limb**
- G57.22 **Lesion of femoral nerve, left lower limb**
- G57.23 **Lesion of femoral nerve, bilateral lower limbs**
  AHA: 4Q 2016, 17

G57.3 **Lesion of lateral popliteal nerve**
Peroneal nerve palsy

- G57.30 **Lesion of lateral popliteal nerve, unspecified lower limb**
- G57.31 **Lesion of lateral popliteal nerve, right lower limb**
- G57.32 **Lesion of lateral popliteal nerve, left lower limb**
- G57.33 **Lesion of lateral popliteal nerve, bilateral lower limbs**
  AHA: 4Q 2016, 17

G57.4 **Lesion of medial popliteal nerve**

- G57.40 **Lesion of medial popliteal nerve, unspecified lower limb**
- G57.41 **Lesion of medial popliteal nerve, right lower limb**
- G57.42 **Lesion of medial popliteal nerve, left lower limb**
- G57.43 **Lesion of medial popliteal nerve, bilateral lower limbs**
  AHA: 4Q 2016, 17

G57.5 **Tarsal tunnel syndrome**

DEFINITION Pain, burning, tingling, and/or numbness of the sole of the foot, often extending to the ankle, due to compression of the posterior tibial nerve or plantar nerves within the tarsal tunnel.

- G57.50 **Tarsal tunnel syndrome, unspecified lower limb**
- G57.51 **Tarsal tunnel syndrome, right lower limb**
- G57.52 **Tarsal tunnel syndrome, left lower limb**
- G57.53 **Tarsal tunnel syndrome, bilateral lower limbs**
  AHA: 4Q 2016, 17

G57.6 **Lesion of plantar nerve**
Morton's metatarsalgia

DEFINITION Thickening of tissue that surrounds the digital nerve leading to the toes. Most frequently develops between the third and fourth toes, usually in response to irritation, trauma or excessive pressure.

- G57.60 **Lesion of plantar nerve, unspecified lower limb**
- G57.61 **Lesion of plantar nerve, right lower limb**
- G57.62 **Lesion of plantar nerve, left lower limb**
- G57.63 **Lesion of plantar nerve, bilateral lower limbs**
  AHA: 4Q 2016, 17

G57.7 **Causalgia of lower limb**
Complex regional pain syndrome II of lower limb

EXCLUDES 1 *complex regional pain syndrome I of lower limb (G90.52-)*
complex regional pain syndrome I of upper limb (G90.51-)
complex regional pain syndrome II of upper limb (G56.4-)
reflex sympathetic dystrophy of lower limb (G90.52-)
reflex sympathetic dystrophy of upper limb (G90.51-)

- G57.70 **Causalgia of unspecified lower limb**
- G57.71 **Causalgia of right lower limb**
- G57.72 **Causalgia of left lower limb**
- G57.73 **Causalgia of bilateral lower limbs**
  AHA: 4Q 2016, 17

G57.8 **Other specified mononeuropathies of lower limb**
Interdigital neuroma of lower limb

- G57.80 **Other specified mononeuropathies of unspecified lower limb**
- G57.81 **Other specified mononeuropathies of right lower limb**
- G57.82 **Other specified mononeuropathies of left lower limb**
- G57.83 **Other specified mononeuropathies of bilateral lower limbs**
  AHA: 4Q 2016, 17

G57.9 **Unspecified mononeuropathy of lower limb**

- G57.90 **Unspecified mononeuropathy of unspecified lower limb**
- G57.91 **Unspecified mononeuropathy of right lower limb**
- G57.92 **Unspecified mononeuropathy of left lower limb**
- G57.93 **Unspecified mononeuropathy of bilateral lower limbs**
  AHA: 4Q 2016, 17

G58 Other mononeuropathies

- G58.0 **Intercostal neuropathy**
- G58.7 **Mononeuritis multiplex**
- G58.8 **Other specified mononeuropathies**
- G58.9 **Mononeuropathy, unspecified**

G59 *Mononeuropathy in diseases classified elsewhere*

Code first:
underlying disease

EXCLUDES 1 *diabetic mononeuropathy (E08-E13 with .41)*
syphilitic nerve paralysis (A52.19)
syphilitic neuritis (A52.15)
tuberculous mononeuropathy (A17.83)

Polyneuropathies and other disorders of the peripheral nervous system (G60-G65)

EXCLUDES 1 *neuralgia NOS (M79.2)*
neuritis NOS (M79.2)
peripheral neuritis in pregnancy (O26.82-)
radiculitis NOS (M54.10)

G60 Hereditary and idiopathic neuropathy

G60.0 **Hereditary motor and sensory neuropathy**
Charcot-Marie-Tooth disease
Déjérine-Sottas disease
Hereditary motor and sensory neuropathy, types I-IV
Hypertrophic neuropathy of infancy
Peroneal muscular atrophy (axonal type) (hypertrophic type)
Roussy-Levy syndrome

G60.1 **Refsum's disease**
Infantile Refsum disease

G60.2 **Neuropathy in association with hereditary ataxia**

G60.3 **Idiopathic progressive neuropathy**

G60.8 **Other hereditary and idiopathic neuropathies**
Dominantly inherited sensory neuropathy
Morvan's disease
Nelaton's syndrome
Recessively inherited sensory neuropathy

G60.9 **Hereditary and idiopathic neuropathy, unspecified**

CODING TIP ✓ The physician should document hereditary and/or idiopathic neuropathy to assign G60.9. If polyneuropathy is documented without a type or cause, assign G62.9.

4 G61 Inflammatory polyneuropathy

CODING TIP ✓ When an inflammatory neuropathy is reported as unresolved, assign the appropriate code from G61.-. If inflammatory neuropathy is documented as resolved but residual neurologic deficits remain as sequelae, assign the appropriate code from category G65.-, Sequelae of inflammatory and toxic polyneuropathies.

G61.0 **Guillain-Barre syndrome** HCC
Acute (post-)infective polyneuritis
Miller Fisher Syndrome

CODING TIP ✓ When Guillain-Barre syndrome is reported as unresolved, assign code G61.0. If a Guillain-Barre syndrome is documented as resolved but residual neurologic deficits remain as sequelae, assign code G65.0, Sequelae of Guillain-Barre syndrome (code first the residual defects when coding G65.0). Acute inflammatory demyelinating polyneuropathy is included in this code.

DEFINITION Disorder that causes the body's immune system to attack the nerves; paralysis begins at the feet and progresses upwards through the legs and torso to the arms and face.
AHA: 2Q 2014, 4

Guillain-Barre Syndrome (GBS)

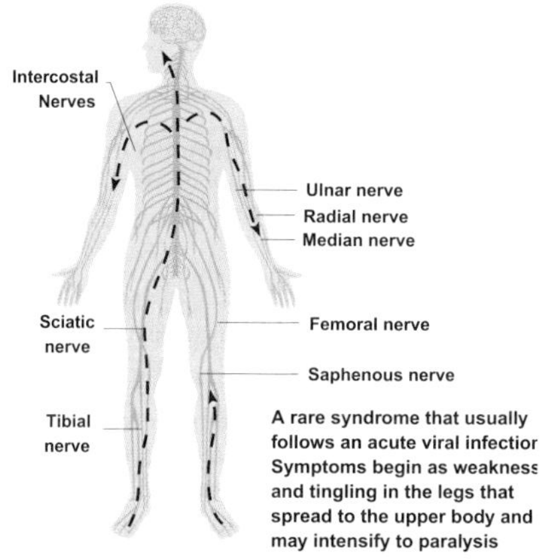
Intercostal
Nerves
Ulnar nerve
Radial nerve
Median nerve
Sciatic
nerve
Femoral nerve
Saphenous nerve
Tibial
nerve
A rare syndrome that usually follows an acute viral infectior Symptoms begin as weakness and tingling in the legs that spread to the upper body and may intensify to paralysis

G61.1 **Serum neuropathy** HCC
Use additional code for adverse effect, if applicable, to identify serum (T50.-)

5 **G61.8** **Other inflammatory polyneuropathies**

G61.81 **Chronic inflammatory demyelinating polyneuritis** HCC

G61.82 **Multifocal motor neuropathy** HCC
MMN
AHA: 4Q 2016, 18

G61.89 **Other inflammatory polyneuropathies** HCC

G61.9 **Inflammatory polyneuropathy, unspecified** HCC

4 G62 Other and unspecified polyneuropathies

G62.0 **Drug-induced polyneuropathy** HCC
Use additional code for adverse effect, if applicable, to identify drug (T36-T50 with fifth or sixth character 5)

CODING TIP ✓ Assign G62.0 when the polyneuropathy is specifically reported by the physician as related to the use of a drug. An additional code should be assigned to identify the drug.

G62.1 **Alcoholic polyneuropathy** HCC

CODING TIP ✓ Assign G62.1 when the physician specifically reports that the polyneuropathy results from alcohol use. The coder should also code any history of, or current use, of alcohol.

DEFINITION Loss of nerve function due to damage from prolonged, excessive alcohol consumption; commonly presents with numbness, weakness, and burning in the feet.

G62.2 **Polyneuropathy due to other toxic agents** HCC
Code first:
(T51-T65) to identify toxic agent

5 **G62.8** **Other specified polyneuropathies**

G62.81 **Critical illness polyneuropathy** HCC
Acute motor neuropathy

G62.82 **Radiation-induced polyneuropathy** HCC
Use additional external cause code (W88-W90, X39.0-) to identify cause

G62.89 **Other specified polyneuropathies**
AHA: 2Q 2016, 11

G62.9 **Polyneuropathy, unspecified**
Neuropathy NOS

CODING TIP ✓ The physician should document hereditary and/or idiopathic neuropathy to assign G60.9. If polyneuropathy is documented without a type or cause, assign G62.9.

G63 *Polyneuropathy in diseases classified elsewhere* HCC

Code first underlying disease, such as:
amyloidosis (E85.-)
endocrine disease, except diabetes (E00-E07, E15-E16, E20-E34)
metabolic diseases (E70-E88)
neoplasm (C00-D49)
nutritional deficiency (E40-E64)

EXCLUDES 1 *polyneuropathy (in) :*
diabetes mellitus (E08-E13 with .42)
diphtheria (A36.83)
infectious mononucleosis (B27.0-B27.9 with 1)
Lyme disease (A69.22)
mumps (B26.84)
postherpetic (B02.23)
rheumatoid arthritis (M05.33)
scleroderma (M34.83)
systemic lupus erythematosus (M32.19)

CODING TIP ✓ Do not assign code G63 for diabetic polyneuropathy. Diabetes with polyneuropathy should be coded with the appropriate combination code to specify the type of diabetes and the polyneuropathy manifestation.

CODING TIP ✓ Code G63 is a manifestation code and must be sequenced following the code for the underlying disease process identified as the etiological cause for the polyneuropathy.
AHA: 4Q 2012, 99-100

G64 Other disorders of peripheral nervous system

Disorder of peripheral nervous system NOS

4 G65 Sequelae of inflammatory and toxic polyneuropathies

Code first:
condition resulting from (sequela) of inflammatory and toxic polyneuropathies

G65.0 **Sequelae of Guillain-Barré syndrome** HCC

G65.1 **Sequelae of other inflammatory polyneuropathy** HCC

G65.2 **Sequelae of toxic polyneuropathy** HCC

Diseases of myoneural junction and muscle (G70-G73)

4 G70 Myasthenia gravis and other myoneural disorders

EXCLUDES 1 *botulism (A05.1, A48.51-A48.52)*
transient neonatal myasthenia gravis (P94.0)

5 **G70.0** **Myasthenia gravis**

CODING TIP ✓ When myasthenia gravis is not documented as with or without exacerbation (no exacerbation is specified), assign code G70.00, without (acute) exacerbation.

G70.00 **Myasthenia gravis without (acute) exacerbation** HCC
Myasthenia gravis NOS

G70.01 **Myasthenia gravis with (acute) exacerbation** HCC
Myasthenia gravis in crisis

G70.1 **Toxic myoneural disorders** HCC
Code first:
(T51-T65) to identify toxic agent

G70.2 **Congenital and developmental myasthenia** HCC

5 G70.8 **Other specified myoneural disorders**

G70.80 **Lambert-Eaton syndrome, unspecified** HCC
Lambert-Eaton syndrome NOS

G70.81 ***Lambert-Eaton syndrome in disease classified elsewhere*** HCC
Code first:
underlying disease
EXCLUDES 1 *Lambert-Eaton syndrome in neoplastic disease (G73.1)*

G70.89 **Other specified myoneural disorders** HCC

G70.9 **Myoneural disorder, unspecified** HCC

4 G71 Primary disorders of muscles

EXCLUDES 2 *arthrogryposis multiplex congenita (Q74.3)*
metabolic disorders (E70-E88)
myositis (M60.-)

▲ 5 G71.0 **Muscular dystrophy** HCC

● G71.00 **Muscular dystrophy, unspecified**

● G71.01 **Duchenne or Becker muscular dystrophy**
Autosomal recessive, childhood type, muscular dystrophy resembling Duchenne or Becker muscular dystrophy
Benign [Becker] muscular dystrophy
Severe [Duchenne] muscular dystrophy

● G71.02 **Facioscapulohumeral muscular dystrophy**
Scapulohumeral muscular dystrophy

● G71.09 **Other specified muscular dystrophies**
Benign scapuloperoneal muscular dystrophy with early contractures [Emery-Dreifuss]
Congenital muscular dystrophy NOS
Congenital muscular dystrophy with specific morphological abnormalities of the muscle fiber
Distal muscular dystrophy
Limb-girdle muscular dystrophy
Ocular muscular dystrophy
Oculopharyngeal muscular dystrophy
Scapuloperoneal muscular dystrophy

5 G71.1 **Myotonic disorders**

G71.11 **Myotonic muscular dystrophy** HCC
Dystrophia myotonica [Steinert]
Myotonia atrophica
Myotonic dystrophy
Proximal myotonic myopathy (PROMM)
Steinert disease

G71.12 **Myotonia congenita**
Acetazolamide responsive myotonia congenita
Dominant myotonia congenita [Thomsen disease]
Myotonia levior
Recessive myotonia congenita [Becker disease]

G71.13 **Myotonic chondrodystrophy**
Chondrodystrophic myotonia
Congenital myotonic chondrodystrophy
Schwartz-Jampel disease

DEFINITION Muscle disorder of late infancy with distinctive signs: mask-like face with small features, short stature or dwarfism, limited joint mobility, hip dysplasia, and generalized myotonia with hypertrophied diaphragmatic muscles. Death usually occurs due to respiratory compromise.

G71.14 **Drug induced myotonia**
Use additional code for adverse effect, if applicable, to identify drug (T36-T50 with fifth or sixth character 5)

G71.19 **Other specified myotonic disorders**
Myotonia fluctuans
Myotonia permanens
Neuromyotonia [Isaacs]
Paramyotonia congenita (of von Eulenburg)
Pseudomyotonia
Symptomatic myotonia

G71.2 **Congenital myopathies** HCC
Central core disease
Fiber-type disproportion
Minicore disease
Multicore disease
Myotubular (centronuclear) myopathy
Nemaline myopathy
EXCLUDES 1 *arthrogryposis multiplex congenita (Q74.3)*

G71.3 **Mitochondrial myopathy, not elsewhere classified**
EXCLUDES 1 *Kearns-Sayre syndrome (H49.81)*
Leber's disease (H47.21)
Leigh's encephalopathy (G31.82)
mitochondrial metabolism disorders (E88.4.-)
Reye's syndrome (G93.7)

G71.8 **Other primary disorders of muscles**

G71.9 **Primary disorder of muscle, unspecified**
Hereditary myopathy NOS

4 G72 Other and unspecified myopathies

EXCLUDES 1 *arthrogryposis multiplex congenita (Q74.3)*
dermatopolymyositis (M33.-)
ischemic infarction of muscle (M62.2-)
myositis (M60.-)
polymyositis (M33.2.-)

G72.0 **Drug-induced myopathy**
Use additional code for adverse effect, if applicable, to identify drug (T36-T50 with fifth or sixth character 5)

G72.1 **Alcoholic myopathy**
Use additional code to identify alcoholism (F10.-)

G72.2 **Myopathy due to other toxic agents**
Code first:
(T51-T65) to identify toxic agent

G72.3 **Periodic paralysis**
Familial periodic paralysis
Hyperkalemic periodic paralysis (familial)
Hypokalemic periodic paralysis (familial)
Myotonic periodic paralysis (familial)
Normokalemic paralysis (familial)
Potassium sensitive periodic paralysis
EXCLUDES 1 *paramyotonia congenita (of von Eulenburg) (G71.19)*

5 G72.4 **Inflammatory and immune myopathies, not elsewhere classified**

G72.41 **Inclusion body myositis [IBM]**

G72.49 **Other inflammatory and immune myopathies, not elsewhere classified**
Inflammatory myopathy NOS

5 G72.8 **Other specified myopathies**

G72.81 **Critical illness myopathy**
Acute necrotizing myopathy
Acute quadriplegic myopathy
Intensive care (ICU) myopathy
Myopathy of critical illness

G72.89 **Other specified myopathies**

G72.9 **Myopathy, unspecified**

4 G73 Disorders of myoneural junction and muscle in diseases classified elsewhere

G73.1 ***Lambert-Eaton syndrome in neoplastic disease*** HCC
Code first:
underlying neoplasm (C00-D49)
EXCLUDES 1 *Lambert-Eaton syndrome not associated with neoplasm (G70.80-G70.81)*

G73.3 ***Myasthenic syndromes in other diseases classified elsewhere*** HCC
Code first underlying disease, such as:
neoplasm (C00-D49)
thyrotoxicosis (E05.-)

G73.7 ***Myopathy in diseases classified elsewhere***
Code first underlying disease, such as:
hyperparathyroidism (E21.0, E21.3)
hypoparathyroidism (E20.-)
glycogen storage disease (E74.0)
lipid storage disorders (E75.-)
EXCLUDES 1 *myopathy in:*
rheumatoid arthritis (M05.32)
sarcoidosis (D86.87)
scleroderma (M34.82)
sicca syndrome [Sjögren] (M35.03)
systemic lupus erythematosus (M32.19)

Cerebral palsy and other paralytic syndromes (G80-G83)

GUIDELINES Section I.C.6.a
Codes from category G81, Hemiplegia and hemiparesis, and subcategories, G83.1, Monoplegia of lower limb, G83.2, Monoplegia of upper limb, and G83.3, Monoplegia, unspecified, identify whether the dominant or nondominant side is affected. Should the affected side be documented, but not specified as dominant or nondominant, and the classification system does not indicate a default, code selection is as follows:
- For ambidextrous patients, the default should be dominant.
- If the left side is affected, the default is non-dominant.
- If the right side is affected, the default is dominant.

4 G80 Cerebral palsy
EXCLUDES 1 *hereditary spastic paraplegia (G11.4)*

G80.0 Spastic quadriplegic cerebral palsy HCC
Congenital spastic paralysis (cerebral)
DEFINITION Palsy presenting with spastic paralysis of all four limbs from early brain damage.

G80.1 Spastic diplegic cerebral palsy HCC
Spastic cerebral palsy NOS

G80.2 Spastic hemiplegic cerebral palsy HCC
DEFINITION Palsy affecting the limbs on either the left or the right side (e.g., the right arm and right leg).

G80.3 Athetoid cerebral palsy HCC
Double athetosis (syndrome)
Dyskinetic cerebral palsy
Dystonic cerebral palsy
Vogt disease
DEFINITION Permanent, nonprogressive, motor disorder caused by brain damage usually occurring shortly before, during, or after birth and characterized by uncontrolled, writhing movements of the hands, feet, arms, or legs.

G80.4 Ataxic cerebral palsy HCC

G80.8 Other cerebral palsy HCC
Mixed cerebral palsy syndromes

G80.9 Cerebral palsy, unspecified HCC
Cerebral palsy NOS

4 G81 Hemiplegia and hemiparesis
Note: This category is to be used only when hemiplegia (complete)(incomplete) is reported without further specification, or is stated to be old or longstanding but of unspecified cause. The category is also for use in multiple coding to identify these types of hemiplegia resulting from any cause.
EXCLUDES 1 *congenital cerebral palsy (G80.-)*
hemiplegia and hemiparesis due to sequela of cerebrovascular disease (I69.05-, I69.15-, I69.25-, I69.35-, I69.85-, I69.95-)

CODING TIP✓ When coding hemiplegia and monoplegia, the dominance rule stated in the guidelines applies. Coders should note that there is no option to code unspecified side since the classification assumes dominant side.

CODING TIP✓ When paraplegia, hemiplegia, hemiparesis or another paralytic state results from a brain or spinal cord injury, code the paralysis/paresis followed by the code for the brain or spinal injury with the 7th character "S" to report a sequela of the injury.
AHA: 4Q 2012, 106

5 G81.0 Flaccid hemiplegia

G81.00 Flaccid hemiplegia affecting unspecified side HCC

G81.01 Flaccid hemiplegia affecting right dominant side HCC

G81.02 Flaccid hemiplegia affecting left dominant side HCC

G81.03 Flaccid hemiplegia affecting right nondominant side HCC

G81.04 Flaccid hemiplegia affecting left nondominant side HCC

5 G81.1 Spastic hemiplegia

G81.10 Spastic hemiplegia affecting unspecified side HCC

G81.11 Spastic hemiplegia affecting right dominant side HCC

G81.12 Spastic hemiplegia affecting left dominant side HCC

G81.13 Spastic hemiplegia affecting right nondominant side HCC

G81.14 Spastic hemiplegia affecting left nondominant side HCC

5 G81.9 Hemiplegia, unspecified

G81.90 Hemiplegia, unspecified affecting unspecified side HCC

G81.91 Hemiplegia, unspecified affecting right dominant side HCC

G81.92 Hemiplegia, unspecified affecting left dominant side HCC

G81.93 Hemiplegia, unspecified affecting right nondominant side HCC

G81.94 Hemiplegia, unspecified affecting left nondominant side HCC
AHA: 1Q 2015, 26

4 G82 Paraplegia (paraparesis) and quadriplegia (quadriparesis)
Note: This category is to be used only when the listed conditions are reported without further specification, or are stated to be old or longstanding but of unspecified cause. The category is also for use in multiple coding to identify these conditions resulting from any cause
EXCLUDES 1 *congenital cerebral palsy (G80.-)*
functional quadriplegia (R53.2)
hysterical paralysis (F44.4)

CODING TIP✓ When paraplegia, hemiplegia, hemiparesis or another paralytic state results from a brain or spinal cord injury, code the paralysis/paresis followed by the code for the brain or spinal injury with the 7th character "S" to report a sequela of the injury.

5 G82.2 Paraplegia
Paralysis of both lower limbs NOS
Paraparesis (lower) NOS
Paraplegia (lower) NOS

G82.20 Paraplegia, unspecified HCC
AHA: 3Q 2017, 3

G82.21 Paraplegia, complete HCC

G82.22 Paraplegia, incomplete HCC

5 G82.5 Quadriplegia

G82.50 Quadriplegia, unspecified HCC

G82.51 Quadriplegia, C1-C4 complete HCC

G82.52 Quadriplegia, C1-C4 incomplete HCC

G82.53 Quadriplegia, C5-C7 complete HCC

G82.54 Quadriplegia, C5-C7 incomplete HCC

4 G83 Other paralytic syndromes
Note: This category is to be used only when the listed conditions are reported without further specification, or are stated to be old or longstanding but of unspecified cause. The category is also for use in multiple coding to identify these conditions resulting from any cause.
INCLUDES paralysis (complete) (incomplete), except as in G80-G82

CODING TIP✓ When coding hemiplegia and monoplegia, the dominance rule stated in the guidelines applies. Coders should note that there is no option to code unspecified side since the classification assumes dominant side.

CODING TIP✓ When paraplegia, hemiplegia, hemiparesis or another paralytic state results from a brain or spinal cord injury, code the paralysis/paresis followed by the code for the brain or spinal injury with the 7th character "S" to report a sequela of the injury.

G83.0 Diplegia of upper limbs HCC
Diplegia (upper)
Paralysis of both upper limbs

5 G83.1 Monoplegia of lower limb
Paralysis of lower limb
EXCLUDES 1 *monoplegia of lower limbs due to sequela of cerebrovascular disease (I69.04-, I69.14-, I69.24-, I69.34-, I69.84-, I69.94-)*
AHA: 4Q 2012, 106

G83.10 Monoplegia of lower limb affecting unspecified side HCC

⊟ **G83.11 Monoplegia of lower limb affecting right dominant side** HCC
⊟ **G83.12 Monoplegia of lower limb affecting left dominant side** HCC
⊟ **G83.13 Monoplegia of lower limb affecting right nondominant side** HCC
⊟ **G83.14 Monoplegia of lower limb affecting left nondominant side** HCC

5 **G83.2 Monoplegia of upper limb**
Paralysis of upper limb
EXCLUDES 1 *monoplegia of upper limbs due to sequela of cerebrovascular disease (I69.03-, I69.13-, I69.23-, I69.33-, I69.83-, I69.93-)*
AHA: 4Q 2012, 106

⊟ **G83.20 Monoplegia of upper limb affecting unspecified side** HCC
⊟ **G83.21 Monoplegia of upper limb affecting right dominant side** HCC
⊟ **G83.22 Monoplegia of upper limb affecting left dominant side** HCC
⊟ **G83.23 Monoplegia of upper limb affecting right nondominant side** HCC
⊟ **G83.24 Monoplegia of upper limb affecting left nondominant side** HCC

5 **G83.3 Monoplegia, unspecified**
AHA: 4Q 2012, 106

⊟ **G83.30 Monoplegia, unspecified affecting unspecified side** HCC
⊟ **G83.31 Monoplegia, unspecified affecting right dominant side** HCC
⊟ **G83.32 Monoplegia, unspecified affecting left dominant side** HCC
⊟ **G83.33 Monoplegia, unspecified affecting right nondominant side** HCC
⊟ **G83.34 Monoplegia, unspecified affecting left nondominant side** HCC

G83.4 Cauda equina syndrome HCC
Neurogenic bladder due to cauda equina syndrome
EXCLUDES 1 *cord bladder NOS (G95.89)*
neurogenic bladder NOS (N31.9)

CODING TIP ✓ Assign G83.4 only when the physician specifically reports cauda equina syndrome. This code includes neurogenic bladder, and no additional code for neurogenic bladder should be assigned when present.

DEFINITION Emergent condition due to compression of spinal nerve roots causing dull aching pain in the perineum, bladder, and sacrum with associated paresthesia, bladder dysfunction, and/or paralysis.

G83.5 Locked-in state HCC

5 **G83.8 Other specified paralytic syndromes**
EXCLUDES 1 *paralytic syndromes due to current spinal cord injury-code to spinal cord injury (S14, S24, S34)*

G83.81 Brown-Séquard syndrome HCC
G83.82 Anterior cord syndrome HCC
G83.83 Posterior cord syndrome HCC
G83.84 Todd's paralysis (postepileptic) HCC
G83.89 Other specified paralytic syndromes HCC

G83.9 Paralytic syndrome, unspecified HCC

Other disorders of the nervous system (G89-G99)

▲ 4 **G89 Pain, not elsewhere classified**
Code also:
related psychological factors associated with pain (F45.42)
EXCLUDES 1 *generalized pain NOS (R52)*
pain disorders exclusively related to psychological factors (F45.41)
pain NOS (R52)
EXCLUDES 2 *atypical face pain (G50.1)*
headache syndromes (G44.-)
localized pain, unspecified type - code to pain by site, such as:
abdomen pain (R10.-)
back pain (M54.9)
breast pain (N64.4)
chest pain (R07.1-R07.9)
ear pain (H92.0-)
eye pain (H57.1)
headache (R51)
joint pain (M25.5-)
limb pain (M79.6-)
lumbar region pain (M54.5)
painful urination (R30.9)
pelvic and perineal pain (R10.2)
shoulder pain (M25.51-)
spine pain (M54.-)
throat pain (R07.0)
tongue pain (K14.6)
tooth pain (K08.8)
renal colic (N23)
migraines (G43.-)
myalgia (M79.1-)
pain from prosthetic devices, implants, and grafts (T82.84, T83.84, T84.84, T85.84-)
phantom limb syndrome with pain (G54.6)
vulvar vestibulitis (N94.810)
vulvodynia (N94.81-)

GUIDELINES **Section I.C.5.a**
Assign code F45.41 for pain that is exclusively related to psychological disorders. As indicated by the Excludes 1 note under category G89, a code from category G89 should not be assigned with code F45.41. Code F45.42, Pain disorders with related psychological factors, should be used with a code from category G89 if there is documentation of a psychological component for a patient with acute or chronic pain.

GUIDELINES **Section I.C.6.b.1)**
Codes in category G89 may be used in conjunction with codes from other categories and chapters to provide more detail about acute or chronic pain and neoplasm-related pain, unless otherwise indicated below. If the pain is not specified as acute or chronic, postthoracotomy, postprocedural, or neoplasm-related, do not assign codes from category G89. A code from category G89 should not be assigned if the underlying (definitive) diagnosis is known, unless the reason for the encounter is pain control/management and not management of the underlying condition.

When an admission or encounter is for a procedure aimed at treating the underlying condition (e.g., spinal fusion, kyphoplasty), a code for the underlying condition (e.g., vertebral fracture, spinal stenosis) should be assigned as the principal diagnosis. No code from category G89 should be assigned.

CODING TIP ✓ **Documentation:** Pain disorders should be coded only when specified by the physician and when the plan of care specifically addresses pain with interventions and goals to address the pain as a focus of care.

G89.0 Central pain syndrome
Déjérine-Roussy syndrome
Myelopathic pain syndrome
Thalamic pain syndrome (hyperesthetic)

GUIDELINES **Section I.C.6.b.6)**
Central pain syndrome (G89.0) and chronic pain syndrome (G89.4) are different than the term "chronic pain," and therefore codes should only be used when the provider has specifically documented this condition.

CODING TIP✓ Do not code G89.0 unless the physician specifies central pain syndrome. Use G89.0 if: 1) Traumatic or brain-related damage to the central nervous system (e.g., damage from stroke, MS, tumors, epilepsy, Parkinson's); 2) The character and extent of the pain is partly related to a variety of causes; 3) Treatment includes pain medications. It also might be appropriate for patients on antidepressants and anticonvulsants.

5 **G89.1 Acute pain, not elsewhere classified**

CODING TIP✓ When the clinical record specifies that the patient has a pain disorder with related psychological factors, F45.42 should be additionally assigned.

G89.11 Acute pain due to trauma

G89.12 Acute post-thoracotomy pain
Post-thoracotomy pain NOS

GUIDELINES **Section I.C.6.b.3)(a)-(b)**
The provider's documentation should be used to guide the coding of postoperative pain. The default for post-thoracotomy and other postoperative pain not specified as acute or chronic is the code for the acute form. Routine or expected postoperative pain immediately after surgery should not be coded.

(a) Postoperative pain not associated with a specific postoperative complication is assigned to the appropriate postoperative pain code in category G89.

(b) Postoperative pain associated with specific postoperative complication (such as painful wire sutures) is assigned to the appropriate code(s) found in Chapter 19, Injury, poisoning, and certain other consequences of external causes. If appropriate, use additional code(s) from category G89 to identify acute or chronic pain (G89.18 or G89.28).

G89.18 Other acute postprocedural pain
Postoperative pain NOS
Postprocedural pain NOS

CODING TIP✓ G89.18 is the default code for post-operative/post-procedural pain when not specified as acute or chronic. G89.18 should not be coded in all patients who experience pain following a procedure. It is expected that some pain would be experienced following a procedure, and these codes are used for unusual pain.

5 **G89.2 Chronic pain, not elsewhere classified**

EXCLUDES 1
causalgia, lower limb (G57.7-)
causalgia, upper limb (G56.4-)
central pain syndrome (G89.0)
chronic pain syndrome (G89.4)
complex regional pain syndrome II, lower limb (G57.7-)
complex regional pain syndrome II, upper limb (G56.4-)
neoplasm related chronic pain (G89.3)
reflex sympathetic dystrophy (G90.5-)

GUIDELINES **Section I.C.6.b.4)**
Chronic pain is classified to subcategory G89.2. There is no time frame defining when pain becomes chronic pain. The provider's documentation should be used to guide use of these codes.

CODING TIP✓ When the clinical record specifies that the patient has a pain disorder with related psychological factors, F45.42 should be additionally assigned.

CODING TIP✓ No specific time frame is required in order to code chronic pain

G89.21 Chronic pain due to trauma

G89.22 Chronic post-thoracotomy pain

G89.28 Other chronic postprocedural pain
Other chronic postoperative pain

CODING TIP✓ Post-procedural pain that is not specified as acute or chronic should not be coded to G89.28, or to G89.18, Other acute postprocedural pain. Post operative pain should not be coded in all patients who experience pain following a procedure. It is expected that some pain would be experienced following a procedure.

G89.29 Other chronic pain

G89.3 Neoplasm related pain (acute) (chronic)
Cancer associated pain
Pain due to malignancy (primary) (secondary)
Tumor associated pain

GUIDELINES **Section I.C.6.b.5)**
Code G89.3 is assigned to pain documented as being related, associated or due to cancer, primary or secondary malignancy, or tumor. This code is assigned regardless of whether the pain is acute or chronic. This code may be assigned as the principal or first listed code when the stated reason for the admission/encounter is documented as pain control/pain management. The underlying neoplasm should be reported as an additional diagnosis.

When the reason for the admission/encounter is management of the neoplasm and the pain associated with the neoplasm is also documented, code G89.3 may be assigned as an additional diagnosis. It is not necessary to assign an additional code for the site of the pain.

CODING TIP✓ When pain is known to be associated with a known neoplasm and the plan of care will include interventions to address the pain, first code the neoplasm, then follow with code G89.3.

G89.4 Chronic pain syndrome
Chronic pain associated with significant psychosocial dysfunction

GUIDELINES **Section I.C.6.b.6)**
Central pain syndrome (G89.0) and chronic pain syndrome (G89.4) are different than the term "chronic pain," and therefore codes should only be used when the provider has specifically documented this condition.

CODING TIP✓ Do not confuse chronic pain syndrome with chronic pain (unspecified). Chronic pain syndrome is a specifically diagnosed condition that must be reported by the patient's physician and includes a cycle of psychological and physical components.

4 **G90 Disorders of autonomic nervous system**

EXCLUDES 1 *dysfunction of the autonomic nervous system due to alcohol (G31.2)*

5 **G90.0 Idiopathic peripheral autonomic neuropathy**

G90.01 Carotid sinus syncope
Carotid sinus syndrome

DEFINITION Exaggerated response to carotid sinus baroreceptor stimulation causing bradycardia, hypotension, and dizziness.

G90.09 Other idiopathic peripheral autonomic neuropathy
Idiopathic peripheral autonomic neuropathy NOS

CODING TIP✓ Do not assign G90.09 for polyneuropathy or unspecified peripheral neuropathy. G90.09 is assigned to specify peripheral autonomic neuropathy, a condition that impairs nervous system function between the autonomic nervous system and the brain, resulting in autonomic dysregulation.

G90.1 Familial dysautonomia [Riley-Day] HCC

G90.2 Horner's syndrome
Bernard(-Horner) syndrome
Cervical sympathetic dystrophy or paralysis

G90.3 Multi-system degeneration of the autonomic nervous system HCC
Neurogenic orthostatic hypotension [Shy-Drager]

EXCLUDES 1 *orthostatic hypotension NOS (I95.1)*

G90.4 **Autonomic dysreflexia**
Use additional code to identify the cause, such as:
fecal impaction (K56.41)
pressure ulcer (pressure area) (L89.-)
urinary tract infection (N39.0)

[5] **G90.5** **Complex regional pain syndrome I (CRPS I)**
Reflex sympathetic dystrophy
EXCLUDES 1 *causalgia of lower limb (G57.7-)*
causalgia of upper limb (G56.4-)
complex regional pain syndrome II of lower limb (G57.7-)
complex regional pain syndrome II of upper limb (G56.4-)

G90.50 **Complex regional pain syndrome I, unspecified**
[6] **G90.51** **Complex regional pain syndrome I of upper limb**
[Laterality] **G90.511** **Complex regional pain syndrome I of right upper limb**
[Laterality] **G90.512** **Complex regional pain syndrome I of left upper limb**
[Laterality] **G90.513** **Complex regional pain syndrome I of upper limb, bilateral**
[Laterality] **G90.519** **Complex regional pain syndrome I of unspecified upper limb**
[6] **G90.52** **Complex regional pain syndrome I of lower limb**
[Laterality] **G90.521** **Complex regional pain syndrome I of right lower limb**
[Laterality] **G90.522** **Complex regional pain syndrome I of left lower limb**
[Laterality] **G90.523** **Complex regional pain syndrome I of lower limb, bilateral**
[Laterality] **G90.529** **Complex regional pain syndrome I of unspecified lower limb**
G90.59 **Complex regional pain syndrome I of other specified site**

G90.8 **Other disorders of autonomic nervous system**
G90.9 **Disorder of the autonomic nervous system, unspecified**

[4] **G91** **Hydrocephalus**
INCLUDES acquired hydrocephalus
EXCLUDES 1 *Arnold-Chiari syndrome with hydrocephalus (Q07.-)*
congenital hydrocephalus (Q03.-)
spina bifida with hydrocephalus (Q05.-)

G91.0 **Communicating hydrocephalus**
Secondary normal pressure hydrocephalus
G91.1 **Obstructive hydrocephalus**
G91.2 **(Idiopathic) normal pressure hydrocephalus**
Normal pressure hydrocephalus NOS
DEFINITION Disruption of normal cerebrospinal fluid circulation and gradual ventricular enlargement without known cause resulting in abnormal gait, cognitive impairment, and urinary incontinence.
G91.3 **Post-traumatic hydrocephalus, unspecified**
▲ **G91.4** ***Hydrocephalus in diseases classified elsewhere***
Code first underlying condition, such as:
congenital syphilis (A50.4-)
neoplasm (C00-D49)
plasminogen deficiency (E88.02)
EXCLUDES 1 *hydrocephalus due to congenital toxoplasmosis (P37.1)*
AHA: 3Q 2014, 4
G91.8 **Other hydrocephalus**
G91.9 **Hydrocephalus, unspecified**

G92 **Toxic encephalopathy**
Toxic encephalitis
Toxic metabolic encephalopathy
Code first:
, if applicable, drug induced (T36-T50)
(T51-T65) to identify toxic agent
AHA: 1Q 2017, 39
AHA: 1Q 2017, 40

Toxic encephalopathy

Deterioration of neurological function due to toxic substance

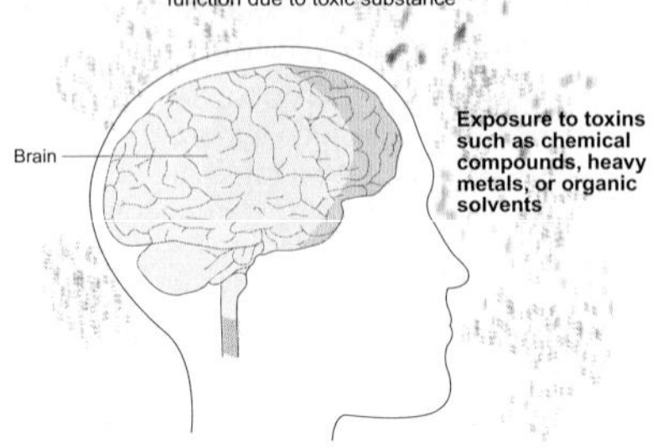

[4] **G93** **Other disorders of brain**

G93.0 **Cerebral cysts**
Arachnoid cyst
Porencephalic cyst, acquired
EXCLUDES 1 *acquired periventricular cysts of newborn (P91.1)*
congenital cerebral cysts (Q04.6)

G93.1 **Anoxic brain damage, not elsewhere classified** HCC
EXCLUDES 1 *cerebral anoxia due to anesthesia during labor and delivery (O74.3)*
cerebral anoxia due to anesthesia during the puerperium (O89.2)
neonatal anoxia (P84)
CODING TIP ✓ When the anoxic brain damage is noted as a sequelae of an injury, a code from Chapter 19, Injury, Poisoning and Certain Other Consequences of External Causes should be additionally assigned (with a 7th character "S").

G93.2 **Benign intracranial hypertension**
EXCLUDES 1 *hypertensive encephalopathy (I67.4)*

G93.3 **Postviral fatigue syndrome**
Benign myalgic encephalomyelitis
EXCLUDES 1 *chronic fatigue syndrome NOS (R53.82)*

[5] **G93.4** **Other and unspecified encephalopathy**
EXCLUDES 1 *alcoholic encephalopathy (G31.2)*
encephalopathy in diseases classified elsewhere (G94)
hypertensive encephalopathy (I67.4)
toxic (metabolic) encephalopathy (G92)

G93.40 **Encephalopathy, unspecified** HIV

Encephalopathy

Any disease or disorder of the brain that alters brain function or structure

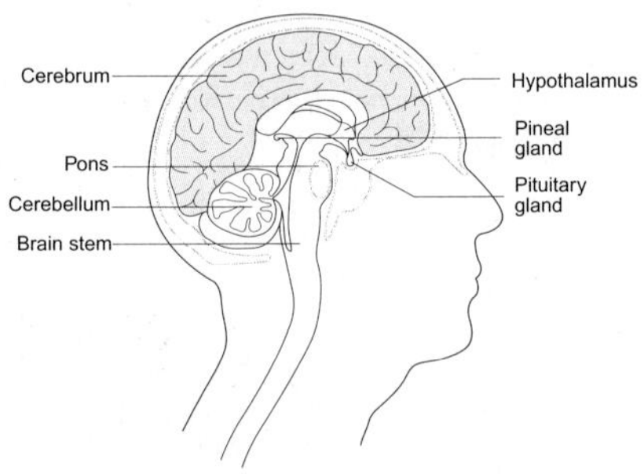

G93.41 **Metabolic encephalopathy** HIV
Septic encephalopathy
CODING TIP ✓ Assign G93.41 when encephalopathy is documented related to sepsis.
DEFINITION Neuropsychiatric disturbances due to metabolic brain disease, commonly caused by hypoxia, ischemia, hypoglycemia, or diseases of other organs.
AHA: 3Q 2015, 21
AHA: 3Q 2016, 42
AHA: 2Q 2017, 8

G93.49 Other encephalopathy HIV
Encephalopathy NEC
CODING TIP ✓ Assign G93.49 when encephalopathy is documented related to a CVA or stroke.
AHA: 2Q 2017, 9
AHA: 2Q 2018, 17
AHA: 2Q 2018, 19

G93.5 Compression of brain HCC
Arnold-Chiari type 1 compression of brain
Compression of brain (stem)
Herniation of brain (stem)
EXCLUDES 1 *diffuse traumatic compression of brain (S06.2-)*
focal traumatic compression of brain (S06.3-)

G93.6 Cerebral edema HCC
EXCLUDES 1 *cerebral edema due to birth injury (P11.0)*
traumatic cerebral edema (S06.1-)

G93.7 Reye's syndrome P
Code first:
poisoning due to salicylates, if applicable (T39.0-, with sixth character 1-4)
Use additional code for adverse effect due to salicylates, if applicable (T39.0-, with sixth character 5)
DEFINITION Rare, acute, sometimes fatal childhood disease with recurrent vomiting, elevated serum transaminase levels and liver changes, then acute brain swelling, consciousness disturbances and seizures.

5 **G93.8 Other specified disorders of brain**
G93.81 Temporal sclerosis
Hippocampal sclerosis
Mesial temporal sclerosis
G93.82 Brain death
G93.89 Other specified disorders of brain
Postradiation encephalopathy

G93.9 Disorder of brain, unspecified HIV

G94 *Other disorders of brain in diseases classified elsewhere*
Code first:
underlying disease
EXCLUDES 1 *encephalopathy in congenital syphilis (A50.49)*
encephalopathy in influenza (J09.X9, J10.81, J11.81)
encephalopathy in syphilis (A52.19)
hydrocephalus in diseases classified elsewhere (G91.4)

4 **G95 Other and unspecified diseases of spinal cord**
EXCLUDES 2 *myelitis (G04.-)*

G95.0 Syringomyelia and syringobulbia HCC
DEFINITION Cyst formation within the spinal cord resulting from trauma, hemorrhage, meningitis, tumor, or Chiari 1 malformation. The growing cyst destroys the cord's center, causing neurologic deficits that progress to greater degrees when not treated surgically.

5 **G95.1 Vascular myelopathies**
EXCLUDES 2 *intraspinal phlebitis and thrombophlebitis, except non-pyogenic (G08)*
G95.11 Acute infarction of spinal cord (embolic) (nonembolic) HCC
Anoxia of spinal cord
Arterial thrombosis of spinal cord
G95.19 Other vascular myelopathies HCC
Edema of spinal cord
Hematomyelia
Nonpyogenic intraspinal phlebitis and thrombophlebitis
Subacute necrotic myelopathy

5 **G95.2 Other and unspecified cord compression**
G95.20 Unspecified cord compression HCC HIV
G95.29 Other cord compression HCC HIV

5 **G95.8 Other specified diseases of spinal cord**
EXCLUDES 1 *neurogenic bladder NOS (N31.9)*
neurogenic bladder due to cauda equina syndrome (G83.4)
neuromuscular dysfunction of bladder without spinal cord lesion (N31.-)
G95.81 Conus medullaris syndrome HCC
G95.89 Other specified diseases of spinal cord HCC
Cord bladder NOS
Drug-induced myelopathy
Radiation-induced myelopathy
EXCLUDES 1 *myelopathy NOS (G95.9)*

G95.9 Disease of spinal cord, unspecified HCC HIV
Myelopathy NOS

4 **G96 Other disorders of central nervous system**

G96.0 Cerebrospinal fluid leak
EXCLUDES 1 *cerebrospinal fluid leak from spinal puncture (G97.0)*
AHA: 2Q 2018, 10
AHA: 2Q 2018, 10

5 **G96.1 Disorders of meninges, not elsewhere classified**
G96.11 Dural tear
EXCLUDES 1 *accidental puncture or laceration of dura during a procedure (G97.41)*
AHA: 4Q 2014, 24
G96.12 Meningeal adhesions (cerebral) (spinal)
G96.19 Other disorders of meninges, not elsewhere classified

G96.8 Other specified disorders of central nervous system
G96.9 Disorder of central nervous system, unspecified HIV

4 **G97 Intraoperative and postprocedural complications and disorders of nervous system, not elsewhere classified**
EXCLUDES 2 *intraoperative and postprocedural cerebrovascular infarction (I97.81-, I97.82-)*
CODING TIP ✓ **Documentation:** Do not assign any code for intraoperative and postprocedural complications and disorders of the nervous system without specific documentation from the patient's physician providing a specific relationship between the complication and the procedure.

G97.0 Cerebrospinal fluid leak from spinal puncture
G97.1 Other reaction to spinal and lumbar puncture
Headache due to lumbar puncture
G97.2 Intracranial hypotension following ventricular shunting

5 **G97.3 Intraoperative hemorrhage and hematoma of a nervous system organ or structure complicating a procedure**
EXCLUDES 1 *intraoperative hemorrhage and hematoma of a nervous system organ or structure due to accidental puncture and laceration during a procedure (G97.4-)*
G97.31 Intraoperative hemorrhage and hematoma of a nervous system organ or structure complicating a nervous system procedure
G97.32 Intraoperative hemorrhage and hematoma of a nervous system organ or structure complicating other procedure

5 **G97.4 Accidental puncture and laceration of a nervous system organ or structure during a procedure**
G97.41 Accidental puncture or laceration of dura during a procedure
Incidental (inadvertent) durotomy
AHA: 4Q 2014, 24
G97.48 Accidental puncture and laceration of other nervous system organ or structure during a nervous system procedure
G97.49 Accidental puncture and laceration of other nervous system organ or structure during other procedure

5 **G97.5 Postprocedural hemorrhage of a nervous system organ or structure following a procedure**
G97.51 Postprocedural hemorrhage of a nervous system organ or structure following a nervous system procedure
G97.52 Postprocedural hemorrhage of a nervous system organ or structure following other procedure

5 **G97.6 Postprocedural hematoma and seroma of a nervous system organ or structure following a procedure**
G97.61 Postprocedural hematoma of a nervous system organ or structure following a nervous system procedure
G97.62 Postprocedural hematoma of a nervous system organ or structure following other procedure
G97.63 Postprocedural seroma of a nervous system organ or structure following a nervous system procedure
G97.64 Postprocedural seroma of a nervous system organ or structure following other procedure

5 G97.8 Other intraoperative and postprocedural complications and disorders of nervous system

Use additional code to further specify disorder

G97.81 Other intraoperative complications of nervous system

G97.82 Other postprocedural complications and disorders of nervous system

4 G98 Other disorders of nervous system not elsewhere classified

INCLUDES nervous system disorder NOS

G98.0 Neurogenic arthritis, not elsewhere classified

Nonsyphilitic neurogenic arthropathy NEC

Nonsyphilitic neurogenic spondylopathy NEC

EXCLUDES 1 *spondylopathy (in) :*
syringomyelia and syringobulbia (G95.0)
tabes dorsalis (A52.11)

G98.8 Other disorders of nervous system HIV

Nervous system disorder NOS

4 G99 Other disorders of nervous system in diseases classified elsewhere

G99.0 Autonomic neuropathy in diseases classified elsewhere

Code first underlying disease, such as:
amyloidosis (E85.-)
gout (M1A.-, M10.-)
hyperthyroidism (E05.-)

EXCLUDES 1 *diabetic autonomic neuropathy (E08-E13 with .43)*

G99.2 Myelopathy in diseases classified elsewhere HCC

Code first underlying disease, such as:
neoplasm (C00-D49)

EXCLUDES 1 *myelopathy in:*
intervertebral disease (M50.0-, M51.0-)
spondylosis (M47.0-, M47.1-)

G99.8 Other specified disorders of nervous system in diseases classified elsewhere

Code first underlying disorder, such as:
amyloidosis (E85.-)
avitaminosis (E56.9)

EXCLUDES 1 *nervous system involvement in:*
cysticercosis (B69.0)
rubella (B06.0-)
syphilis (A52.1-)

CHAPTER 7: DISEASES OF THE EYE AND ADNEXA (H00-H59)

Note: Use an external cause code following the code for the eye condition, if applicable, to identify the cause of the eye condition

EXCLUDES 2 *certain conditions originating in the perinatal period (P04-P96)*
certain infectious and parasitic diseases (A00-B99)
complications of pregnancy, childbirth and the puerperium (O00-O9A)
congenital malformations, deformations, and chromosomal abnormalities (Q00-Q99)
diabetes mellitus related eye conditions (E09.3-, E10.3-, E11.3-, E13.3-)
endocrine, nutritional and metabolic diseases (E00-E88)
injury (trauma) of eye and orbit (S05.-)
injury, poisoning and certain other consequences of external causes (S00-T88)
neoplasms (C00-D49)
symptoms, signs and abnormal clinical and laboratory findings, not elsewhere classified (R00-R94)
syphilis related eye disorders (A50.01, A50.3-, A51.43, A52.71)

This chapter contains the following blocks:

H00-H05	Disorders of eyelid, lacrimal system and orbit
H10-H11	Disorders of conjunctiva
H15-H22	Disorders of sclera, cornea, iris and ciliary body
H25-H28	Disorders of lens
H30-H36	Disorders of choroid and retina
H40-H42	Glaucoma
H43-H44	Disorders of vitreous body and globe
H46-H47	Disorders of optic nerve and visual pathways
H49-H52	Disorders of ocular muscles, binocular movement, accommodation and refraction
H53-H54	Visual disturbances and blindness
H55-H57	Other disorders of eye and adnexa
H59	Intraoperative and postprocedural complications and disorders of eye and adnexa, not elsewhere classified

Disorders of eyelid, lacrimal system and orbit (H00-H05)

EXCLUDES 2 *open wound of eyelid (S01.1-)*
superficial injury of eyelid (S00.1-, S00.2-)

4 **H00 Hordeolum and chalazion**

5 **H00.0 Hordeolum (externum) (internum) of eyelid**

6 **H00.01 Hordeolum externum**
Hordeolum NOS
Stye
DEFINITION Staph infection of an oil gland in an eyelash follicle.

- ⊟ **H00.011 Hordeolum externum right upper eyelid**
- ⊟ **H00.012 Hordeolum externum right lower eyelid**
- ⊟ **H00.013 Hordeolum externum right eye, unspecified eyelid**
- ⊟ **H00.014 Hordeolum externum left upper eyelid**
- ⊟ **H00.015 Hordeolum externum left lower eyelid**
- ⊟ **H00.016 Hordeolum externum left eye, unspecified eyelid**
- ⊟ **H00.019 Hordeolum externum unspecified eye, unspecified eyelid**

6 **H00.02 Hordeolum internum**
Infection of meibomian gland

- ⊟ **H00.021 Hordeolum internum right upper eyelid**
- ⊟ **H00.022 Hordeolum internum right lower eyelid**
- ⊟ **H00.023 Hordeolum internum right eye, unspecified eyelid**
- ⊟ **H00.024 Hordeolum internum left upper eyelid**
- ⊟ **H00.025 Hordeolum internum left lower eyelid**
- ⊟ **H00.026 Hordeolum internum left eye, unspecified eyelid**
- ⊟ **H00.029 Hordeolum internum unspecified eye, unspecified eyelid**

6 **H00.03 Abscess of eyelid**
Furuncle of eyelid

- ⊟ **H00.031 Abscess of right upper eyelid**
- ⊟ **H00.032 Abscess of right lower eyelid**
- ⊟ **H00.033 Abscess of eyelid right eye, unspecified eyelid**
- ⊟ **H00.034 Abscess of left upper eyelid**
- ⊟ **H00.035 Abscess of left lower eyelid**
- ⊟ **H00.036 Abscess of eyelid left eye, unspecified eyelid**
- ⊟ **H00.039 Abscess of eyelid unspecified eye, unspecified eyelid**

5 **H00.1 Chalazion**
Meibomian (gland) cyst
EXCLUDES 2 *infected meibomian gland (H00.02-)*
DEFINITION Cyst of the tarsal (eyelid) gland.

- ⊟ **H00.11 Chalazion right upper eyelid**
- ⊟ **H00.12 Chalazion right lower eyelid**
- ⊟ **H00.13 Chalazion right eye, unspecified eyelid**
- ⊟ **H00.14 Chalazion left upper eyelid**
- ⊟ **H00.15 Chalazion left lower eyelid**
- ⊟ **H00.16 Chalazion left eye, unspecified eyelid**
- ⊟ **H00.19 Chalazion unspecified eye, unspecified eyelid**

4 **H01 Other inflammation of eyelid**

5 **H01.0 Blepharitis**
EXCLUDES 1 *blepharoconjunctivitis (H10.5-)*

6 **H01.00 Unspecified blepharitis**
DEFINITION An inflammation of the eyelids or lid margins.

- ⊟ **H01.001 Unspecified blepharitis right upper eyelid**
- ⊟ **H01.002 Unspecified blepharitis right lower eyelid**
- ⊟ **H01.003 Unspecified blepharitis right eye, unspecified eyelid**
- ⊟ **H01.004 Unspecified blepharitis left upper eyelid**
- ⊟ **H01.005 Unspecified blepharitis left lower eyelid**
- ⊟ **H01.006 Unspecified blepharitis left eye, unspecified eyelid**
- ⊟ **H01.009 Unspecified blepharitis unspecified eye, unspecified eyelid**
- ● ⊟ **H01.00A Unspecified blepharitis right eye, upper and lower eyelids**
- ● ⊟ **H01.00B Unspecified blepharitis left eye, upper and lower eyelids**

6 **H01.01 Ulcerative blepharitis**

- ⊟ **H01.011 Ulcerative blepharitis right upper eyelid**
- ⊟ **H01.012 Ulcerative blepharitis right lower eyelid**
- ⊟ **H01.013 Ulcerative blepharitis right eye, unspecified eyelid**
- ⊟ **H01.014 Ulcerative blepharitis left upper eyelid**
- ⊟ **H01.015 Ulcerative blepharitis left lower eyelid**
- ⊟ **H01.016 Ulcerative blepharitis left eye, unspecified eyelid**
- ⊟ **H01.019 Ulcerative blepharitis unspecified eye, unspecified eyelid**
- ● ⊟ **H01.01A Ulcerative blepharitis right eye, upper and lower eyelids**
- ● ⊟ **H01.01B Ulcerative blepharitis left eye, upper and lower eyelids**

6 **H01.02 Squamous blepharitis**

- ⊟ **H01.021 Squamous blepharitis right upper eyelid**
- ⊟ **H01.022 Squamous blepharitis right lower eyelid**
- ⊟ **H01.023 Squamous blepharitis right eye, unspecified eyelid**
- ⊟ **H01.024 Squamous blepharitis left upper eyelid**
- ⊟ **H01.025 Squamous blepharitis left lower eyelid**
- ⊟ **H01.026 Squamous blepharitis left eye, unspecified eyelid**
- ⊟ **H01.029 Squamous blepharitis unspecified eye, unspecified eyelid**
- ● ⊟ **H01.02A Squamous blepharitis right eye, upper and lower eyelids**
- ● ⊟ **H01.02B Squamous blepharitis left eye, upper and lower eyelids**

5 **H01.1 Noninfectious dermatoses of eyelid**

6 **H01.11** Allergic dermatitis of eyelid
Contact dermatitis of eyelid
- **H01.111** Allergic dermatitis of right upper eyelid
- **H01.112** Allergic dermatitis of right lower eyelid
- **H01.113** Allergic dermatitis of right eye, unspecified eyelid
- **H01.114** Allergic dermatitis of left upper eyelid
- **H01.115** Allergic dermatitis of left lower eyelid
- **H01.116** Allergic dermatitis of left eye, unspecified eyelid
- **H01.119** Allergic dermatitis of unspecified eye, unspecified eyelid

6 **H01.12** Discoid lupus erythematosus of eyelid
- **H01.121** Discoid lupus erythematosus of right upper eyelid
- **H01.122** Discoid lupus erythematosus of right lower eyelid
- **H01.123** Discoid lupus erythematosus of right eye, unspecified eyelid
- **H01.124** Discoid lupus erythematosus of left upper eyelid
- **H01.125** Discoid lupus erythematosus of left lower eyelid
- **H01.126** Discoid lupus erythematosus of left eye, unspecified eyelid
- **H01.129** Discoid lupus erythematosus of unspecified eye, unspecified eyelid

6 **H01.13** Eczematous dermatitis of eyelid
- **H01.131** Eczematous dermatitis of right upper eyelid
- **H01.132** Eczematous dermatitis of right lower eyelid
- **H01.133** Eczematous dermatitis of right eye, unspecified eyelid
- **H01.134** Eczematous dermatitis of left upper eyelid
- **H01.135** Eczematous dermatitis of left lower eyelid
- **H01.136** Eczematous dermatitis of left eye, unspecified eyelid
- **H01.139** Eczematous dermatitis of unspecified eye, unspecified eyelid

6 **H01.14** Xeroderma of eyelid
- **H01.141** Xeroderma of right upper eyelid
- **H01.142** Xeroderma of right lower eyelid
- **H01.143** Xeroderma of right eye, unspecified eyelid
- **H01.144** Xeroderma of left upper eyelid
- **H01.145** Xeroderma of left lower eyelid
- **H01.146** Xeroderma of left eye, unspecified eyelid
- **H01.149** Xeroderma of unspecified eye, unspecified eyelid

H01.8 Other specified inflammations of eyelid

H01.9 Unspecified inflammation of eyelid
Inflammation of eyelid NOS

4 H02 Other disorders of eyelid

EXCLUDES 1 *congenital malformations of eyelid (Q10.0-Q10.3)*

5 **H02.0** Entropion and trichiasis of eyelid

6 **H02.00** Unspecified entropion of eyelid

DEFINITION Inward curling of the eyelid margin, usually the bottom, so the lashes irritate the surface of the eyeball.

- **H02.001** Unspecified entropion of right upper eyelid
- **H02.002** Unspecified entropion of right lower eyelid
- **H02.003** Unspecified entropion of right eye, unspecified eyelid
- **H02.004** Unspecified entropion of left upper eyelid
- **H02.005** Unspecified entropion of left lower eyelid
- **H02.006** Unspecified entropion of left eye, unspecified eyelid
- **H02.009** Unspecified entropion of unspecified eye, unspecified eyelid

6 **H02.01** Cicatricial entropion of eyelid
- **H02.011** Cicatricial entropion of right upper eyelid
- **H02.012** Cicatricial entropion of right lower eyelid
- **H02.013** Cicatricial entropion of right eye, unspecified eyelid
- **H02.014** Cicatricial entropion of left upper eyelid
- **H02.015** Cicatricial entropion of left lower eyelid
- **H02.016** Cicatricial entropion of left eye, unspecified eyelid
- **H02.019** Cicatricial entropion of unspecified eye, unspecified eyelid

6 **H02.02** Mechanical entropion of eyelid
- **H02.021** Mechanical entropion of right upper eyelid
- **H02.022** Mechanical entropion of right lower eyelid
- **H02.023** Mechanical entropion of right eye, unspecified eyelid
- **H02.024** Mechanical entropion of left upper eyelid
- **H02.025** Mechanical entropion of left lower eyelid
- **H02.026** Mechanical entropion of left eye, unspecified eyelid
- **H02.029** Mechanical entropion of unspecified eye, unspecified eyelid

6 **H02.03** Senile entropion of eyelid
- **H02.031** Senile entropion of right upper eyelid A
- **H02.032** Senile entropion of right lower eyelid A
- **H02.033** Senile entropion of right eye, unspecified eyelid A
- **H02.034** Senile entropion of left upper eyelid A
- **H02.035** Senile entropion of left lower eyelid A
- **H02.036** Senile entropion of left eye, unspecified eyelid A
- **H02.039** Senile entropion of unspecified eye, unspecified eyelid A

6 **H02.04** Spastic entropion of eyelid
- **H02.041** Spastic entropion of right upper eyelid
- **H02.042** Spastic entropion of right lower eyelid
- **H02.043** Spastic entropion of right eye, unspecified eyelid
- **H02.044** Spastic entropion of left upper eyelid
- **H02.045** Spastic entropion of left lower eyelid
- **H02.046** Spastic entropion of left eye, unspecified eyelid
- **H02.049** Spastic entropion of unspecified eye, unspecified eyelid

6 **H02.05** Trichiasis without entropion
- **H02.051** Trichiasis without entropion right upper eyelid
- **H02.052** Trichiasis without entropion right lower eyelid
- **H02.053** Trichiasis without entropion right eye, unspecified eyelid
- **H02.054** Trichiasis without entropion left upper eyelid
- **H02.055** Trichiasis without entropion left lower eyelid
- **H02.056** Trichiasis without entropion left eye, unspecified eyelid
- **H02.059** Trichiasis without entropion unspecified eye, unspecified eyelid

5 **H02.1** Ectropion of eyelid

6 **H02.10** Unspecified ectropion of eyelid

DEFINITION Outward curling of the eyelid away from the eye, usually the lower, exposing the inner surface and causing irritation, dryness, pain and possible conjunctivitis and keratitis.

- **H02.101** Unspecified ectropion of right upper eyelid
- **H02.102** Unspecified ectropion of right lower eyelid
- **H02.103** Unspecified ectropion of right eye, unspecified eyelid
- **H02.104** Unspecified ectropion of left upper eyelid
- **H02.105** Unspecified ectropion of left lower eyelid
- **H02.106** Unspecified ectropion of left eye, unspecified eyelid
- **H02.109** Unspecified ectropion of unspecified eye, unspecified eyelid

6 **H02.11** Cicatricial ectropion of eyelid
- **H02.111** Cicatricial ectropion of right upper eyelid
- **H02.112** Cicatricial ectropion of right lower eyelid

- H02.113 Cicatricial ectropion of right eye, unspecified eyelid
- H02.114 Cicatricial ectropion of left upper eyelid
- H02.115 Cicatricial ectropion of left lower eyelid
- H02.116 Cicatricial ectropion of left eye, unspecified eyelid
- H02.119 Cicatricial ectropion of unspecified eye, unspecified eyelid

H02.12 Mechanical ectropion of eyelid

- H02.121 Mechanical ectropion of right upper eyelid
- H02.122 Mechanical ectropion of right lower eyelid
- H02.123 Mechanical ectropion of right eye, unspecified eyelid
- H02.124 Mechanical ectropion of left upper eyelid
- H02.125 Mechanical ectropion of left lower eyelid
- H02.126 Mechanical ectropion of left eye, unspecified eyelid
- H02.129 Mechanical ectropion of unspecified eye, unspecified eyelid

H02.13 Senile ectropion of eyelid

- H02.131 Senile ectropion of right upper eyelid A
- H02.132 Senile ectropion of right lower eyelid A
- H02.133 Senile ectropion of right eye, unspecified eyelid A
- H02.134 Senile ectropion of left upper eyelid A
- H02.135 Senile ectropion of left lower eyelid A
- H02.136 Senile ectropion of left eye, unspecified eyelid A
- H02.139 Senile ectropion of unspecified eye, unspecified eyelid A

H02.14 Spastic ectropion of eyelid

- H02.141 Spastic ectropion of right upper eyelid
- H02.142 Spastic ectropion of right lower eyelid
- H02.143 Spastic ectropion of right eye, unspecified eyelid
- H02.144 Spastic ectropion of left upper eyelid
- H02.145 Spastic ectropion of left lower eyelid
- H02.146 Spastic ectropion of left eye, unspecified eyelid
- H02.149 Spastic ectropion of unspecified eye, unspecified eyelid

● H02.15 Paralytic ectropion of eyelid

- ● H02.151 Paralytic ectropion of right upper eyelid
- ● H02.152 Paralytic ectropion of right lower eyelid
- ● H02.153 Paralytic ectropion of right eye, unspecified eyelid
- ● H02.154 Paralytic ectropion of left upper eyelid
- ● H02.155 Paralytic ectropion of left lower eyelid
- ● H02.156 Paralytic ectropion of left eye, unspecified eyelid
- ● H02.159 Paralytic ectropion of unspecified eye, unspecified eyelid

H02.2 Lagophthalmos

H02.20 Unspecified lagophthalmos

- H02.201 Unspecified lagophthalmos right upper eyelid
- H02.202 Unspecified lagophthalmos right lower eyelid
- H02.203 Unspecified lagophthalmos right eye, unspecified eyelid
- H02.204 Unspecified lagophthalmos left upper eyelid
- H02.205 Unspecified lagophthalmos left lower eyelid
- H02.206 Unspecified lagophthalmos left eye, unspecified eyelid
- H02.209 Unspecified lagophthalmos unspecified eye, unspecified eyelid
- ● H02.20A Unspecified lagophthalmos right eye, upper and lower eyelids
- ● H02.20B Unspecified lagophthalmos left eye, upper and lower eyelids
- ● H02.20C Unspecified lagophthalmos, bilateral, upper and lower eyelids

H02.21 Cicatricial lagophthalmos

DEFINITION Inability to completely close the eye due to the presence of scar tissue.

- H02.211 Cicatricial lagophthalmos right upper eyelid
- H02.212 Cicatricial lagophthalmos right lower eyelid
- H02.213 Cicatricial lagophthalmos right eye, unspecified eyelid
- H02.214 Cicatricial lagophthalmos left upper eyelid
- H02.215 Cicatricial lagophthalmos left lower eyelid
- H02.216 Cicatricial lagophthalmos left eye, unspecified eyelid
- H02.219 Cicatricial lagophthalmos unspecified eye, unspecified eyelid
- ● H02.21A Cicatricial lagophthalmos right eye, upper and lower eyelids
- ● H02.21B Cicatricial lagophthalmos left eye, upper and lower eyelids
- ● H02.21C Cicatricial lagophthalmos, bilateral, upper and lower eyelids

H02.22 Mechanical lagophthalmos

- H02.221 Mechanical lagophthalmos right upper eyelid
- H02.222 Mechanical lagophthalmos right lower eyelid
- H02.223 Mechanical lagophthalmos right eye, unspecified eyelid
- H02.224 Mechanical lagophthalmos left upper eyelid
- H02.225 Mechanical lagophthalmos left lower eyelid
- H02.226 Mechanical lagophthalmos left eye, unspecified eyelid
- H02.229 Mechanical lagophthalmos unspecified eye, unspecified eyelid
- ● H02.22A Mechanical lagophthalmos right eye, upper and lower eyelids
- ● H02.22B Mechanical lagophthalmos left eye, upper and lower eyelids
- ● H02.22C Mechanical lagophthalmos, bilateral, upper and lower eyelids

H02.23 Paralytic lagophthalmos

- H02.231 Paralytic lagophthalmos right upper eyelid
- H02.232 Paralytic lagophthalmos right lower eyelid
- H02.233 Paralytic lagophthalmos right eye, unspecified eyelid
- H02.234 Paralytic lagophthalmos left upper eyelid
- H02.235 Paralytic lagophthalmos left lower eyelid
- H02.236 Paralytic lagophthalmos left eye, unspecified eyelid
- H02.239 Paralytic lagophthalmos unspecified eye, unspecified eyelid
- ● H02.23A Paralytic lagophthalmos right eye, upper and lower eyelids
- ● H02.23B Paralytic lagophthalmos left eye, upper and lower eyelids
- ● H02.23C Paralytic lagophthalmos, bilateral, upper and lower eyelids

H02.3 Blepharochalasis

Pseudoptosis

DEFINITION Sagging of the skin of the eyelid. In the upper eyelid, the skin sags over the eye obstructing vision; usually due to changes in elastin and collagen, affecting the skin's elasticity.

- H02.30 Blepharochalasis unspecified eye, unspecified eyelid
- H02.31 Blepharochalasis right upper eyelid
- H02.32 Blepharochalasis right lower eyelid
- H02.33 Blepharochalasis right eye, unspecified eyelid
- H02.34 Blepharochalasis left upper eyelid
- H02.35 Blepharochalasis left lower eyelid
- H02.36 Blepharochalasis left eye, unspecified eyelid

H02.4 Ptosis of eyelid

H02.40 Unspecified ptosis of eyelid

- H02.401 Unspecified ptosis of right eyelid
- H02.402 Unspecified ptosis of left eyelid
- H02.403 Unspecified ptosis of bilateral eyelids
- H02.409 Unspecified ptosis of unspecified eyelid

6 **H02.41 Mechanical ptosis of eyelid**
- **H02.411 Mechanical ptosis of right eyelid**
- **H02.412 Mechanical ptosis of left eyelid**
- **H02.413 Mechanical ptosis of bilateral eyelids**
- **H02.419 Mechanical ptosis of unspecified eyelid**

6 **H02.42 Myogenic ptosis of eyelid**
- **H02.421 Myogenic ptosis of right eyelid**
- **H02.422 Myogenic ptosis of left eyelid**
- **H02.423 Myogenic ptosis of bilateral eyelids**
- **H02.429 Myogenic ptosis of unspecified eyelid**

6 **H02.43 Paralytic ptosis of eyelid**
Neurogenic ptosis of eyelid
- **H02.431 Paralytic ptosis of right eyelid**
- **H02.432 Paralytic ptosis of left eyelid**
- **H02.433 Paralytic ptosis of bilateral eyelids**
- **H02.439 Paralytic ptosis unspecified eyelid**

5 **H02.5 Other disorders affecting eyelid function**
EXCLUDES 2 *blepharospasm (G24.5)*
organic tic (G25.69)
psychogenic tic (F95.-)

6 **H02.51 Abnormal innervation syndrome**
- **H02.511 Abnormal innervation syndrome right upper eyelid**
- **H02.512 Abnormal innervation syndrome right lower eyelid**
- **H02.513 Abnormal innervation syndrome right eye, unspecified eyelid**
- **H02.514 Abnormal innervation syndrome left upper eyelid**
- **H02.515 Abnormal innervation syndrome left lower eyelid**
- **H02.516 Abnormal innervation syndrome left eye, unspecified eyelid**
- **H02.519 Abnormal innervation syndrome unspecified eye, unspecified eyelid**

6 **H02.52 Blepharophimosis**
Ankyloblepharon
DEFINITION Hereditary disorder in which the palpebral fissures (space between the eyelids) is narrowed, giving the appearance of continually squinting.
- **H02.521 Blepharophimosis right upper eyelid**
- **H02.522 Blepharophimosis right lower eyelid**
- **H02.523 Blepharophimosis right eye, unspecified eyelid**
- **H02.524 Blepharophimosis left upper eyelid**
- **H02.525 Blepharophimosis left lower eyelid**
- **H02.526 Blepharophimosis left eye, unspecified eyelid**
- **H02.529 Blepharophimosis unspecified eye, unspecified lid**

6 **H02.53 Eyelid retraction**
Eyelid lag
- **H02.531 Eyelid retraction right upper eyelid**
- **H02.532 Eyelid retraction right lower eyelid**
- **H02.533 Eyelid retraction right eye, unspecified eyelid**
- **H02.534 Eyelid retraction left upper eyelid**
- **H02.535 Eyelid retraction left lower eyelid**
- **H02.536 Eyelid retraction left eye, unspecified eyelid**
- **H02.539 Eyelid retraction unspecified eye, unspecified lid**

H02.59 Other disorders affecting eyelid function
Deficient blink reflex
Sensory disorders

5 **H02.6 Xanthelasma of eyelid**
- **H02.60 Xanthelasma of unspecified eye, unspecified eyelid**
- **H02.61 Xanthelasma of right upper eyelid**
- **H02.62 Xanthelasma of right lower eyelid**
- **H02.63 Xanthelasma of right eye, unspecified eyelid**
- **H02.64 Xanthelasma of left upper eyelid**
- **H02.65 Xanthelasma of left lower eyelid**
- **H02.66 Xanthelasma of left eye, unspecified eyelid**

5 **H02.7 Other and unspecified degenerative disorders of eyelid and periocular area**

H02.70 Unspecified degenerative disorders of eyelid and periocular area

6 **H02.71 Chloasma of eyelid and periocular area**
Dyspigmentation of eyelid
Hyperpigmentation of eyelid
- **H02.711 Chloasma of right upper eyelid and periocular area**
- **H02.712 Chloasma of right lower eyelid and periocular area**
- **H02.713 Chloasma of right eye, unspecified eyelid and periocular area**
- **H02.714 Chloasma of left upper eyelid and periocular area**
- **H02.715 Chloasma of left lower eyelid and periocular area**
- **H02.716 Chloasma of left eye, unspecified eyelid and periocular area**
- **H02.719 Chloasma of unspecified eye, unspecified eyelid and periocular area**

6 **H02.72 Madarosis of eyelid and periocular area**
Hypotrichosis of eyelid
- **H02.721 Madarosis of right upper eyelid and periocular area**
- **H02.722 Madarosis of right lower eyelid and periocular area**
- **H02.723 Madarosis of right eye, unspecified eyelid and periocular area**
- **H02.724 Madarosis of left upper eyelid and periocular area**
- **H02.725 Madarosis of left lower eyelid and periocular area**
- **H02.726 Madarosis of left eye, unspecified eyelid and periocular area**
- **H02.729 Madarosis of unspecified eye, unspecified eyelid and periocular area**

6 **H02.73 Vitiligo of eyelid and periocular area**
Hypopigmentation of eyelid
- **H02.731 Vitiligo of right upper eyelid and periocular area**
- **H02.732 Vitiligo of right lower eyelid and periocular area**
- **H02.733 Vitiligo of right eye, unspecified eyelid and periocular area**
- **H02.734 Vitiligo of left upper eyelid and periocular area**
- **H02.735 Vitiligo of left lower eyelid and periocular area**
- **H02.736 Vitiligo of left eye, unspecified eyelid and periocular area**
- **H02.739 Vitiligo of unspecified eye, unspecified eyelid and periocular area**

H02.79 Other degenerative disorders of eyelid and periocular area

5 **H02.8 Other specified disorders of eyelid**

6 **H02.81 Retained foreign body in eyelid**
Use additional code to identify the type of retained foreign body (Z18.-)
EXCLUDES 1 *laceration of eyelid with foreign body (S01.12-)*
retained intraocular foreign body (H44.6-, H44.7-)
superficial foreign body of eyelid and periocular area (S00.25-)
- **H02.811 Retained foreign body in right upper eyelid**
- **H02.812 Retained foreign body in right lower eyelid**
- **H02.813 Retained foreign body in right eye, unspecified eyelid**
- **H02.814 Retained foreign body in left upper eyelid**
- **H02.815 Retained foreign body in left lower eyelid**
- **H02.816 Retained foreign body in left eye, unspecified eyelid**
- **H02.819 Retained foreign body in unspecified eye, unspecified eyelid**

6 **H02.82 Cysts of eyelid**
Sebaceous cyst of eyelid

- H02.821 Cysts of right upper eyelid
- H02.822 Cysts of right lower eyelid
- H02.823 Cysts of right eye, unspecified eyelid
- H02.824 Cysts of left upper eyelid
- H02.825 Cysts of left lower eyelid
- H02.826 Cysts of left eye, unspecified eyelid
- H02.829 Cysts of unspecified eye, unspecified eyelid

H02.83 Dermatochalasis of eyelid
- H02.831 Dermatochalasis of right upper eyelid
- H02.832 Dermatochalasis of right lower eyelid
- H02.833 Dermatochalasis of right eye, unspecified eyelid
- H02.834 Dermatochalasis of left upper eyelid
- H02.835 Dermatochalasis of left lower eyelid
- H02.836 Dermatochalasis of left eye, unspecified eyelid
- H02.839 Dermatochalasis of unspecified eye, unspecified eyelid

H02.84 Edema of eyelid
Hyperemia of eyelid
- H02.841 Edema of right upper eyelid
- H02.842 Edema of right lower eyelid
- H02.843 Edema of right eye, unspecified eyelid
- H02.844 Edema of left upper eyelid
- H02.845 Edema of left lower eyelid
- H02.846 Edema of left eye, unspecified eyelid
- H02.849 Edema of unspecified eye, unspecified eyelid

H02.85 Elephantiasis of eyelid
- H02.851 Elephantiasis of right upper eyelid
- H02.852 Elephantiasis of right lower eyelid
- H02.853 Elephantiasis of right eye, unspecified eyelid
- H02.854 Elephantiasis of left upper eyelid
- H02.855 Elephantiasis of left lower eyelid
- H02.856 Elephantiasis of left eye, unspecified eyelid
- H02.859 Elephantiasis of unspecified eye, unspecified eyelid

H02.86 Hypertrichosis of eyelid
- H02.861 Hypertrichosis of right upper eyelid
- H02.862 Hypertrichosis of right lower eyelid
- H02.863 Hypertrichosis of right eye, unspecified eyelid
- H02.864 Hypertrichosis of left upper eyelid
- H02.865 Hypertrichosis of left lower eyelid
- H02.866 Hypertrichosis of left eye, unspecified eyelid
- H02.869 Hypertrichosis of unspecified eye, unspecified eyelid

H02.87 Vascular anomalies of eyelid
- H02.871 Vascular anomalies of right upper eyelid
- H02.872 Vascular anomalies of right lower eyelid
- H02.873 Vascular anomalies of right eye, unspecified eyelid
- H02.874 Vascular anomalies of left upper eyelid
- H02.875 Vascular anomalies of left lower eyelid
- H02.876 Vascular anomalies of left eye, unspecified eyelid
- H02.879 Vascular anomalies of unspecified eye, unspecified eyelid

● **H02.88 Meibomian gland dysfunction of eyelid**
- ● H02.881 Meibomian gland dysfunction right upper eyelid
- ● H02.882 Meibomian gland dysfunction right lower eyelid
- ● H02.883 Meibomian gland dysfunction of right eye, unspecified eyelid
- ● H02.884 Meibomian gland dysfunction left upper eyelid
- ● H02.885 Meibomian gland dysfunction left lower eyelid
- ● H02.886 Meibomian gland dysfunction of left eye, unspecified eyelid
- ● H02.889 Meibomian gland dysfunction of unspecified eye, unspecified eyelid
- ● H02.88A Meibomian gland dysfunction right eye, upper and lower eyelids
- ● H02.88B Meibomian gland dysfunction left eye, upper and lower eyelids

H02.89 Other specified disorders of eyelid
Hemorrhage of eyelid

H02.9 Unspecified disorder of eyelid
Disorder of eyelid NOS

H04 Disorders of lacrimal system

EXCLUDES 1 *congenital malformations of lacrimal system (Q10.4-Q10.6)*

H04.0 Dacryoadenitis

H04.00 Unspecified dacryoadenitis

DEFINITION Inflammation of the lacrimal gland.

- H04.001 Unspecified dacryoadenitis, right lacrimal gland
- H04.002 Unspecified dacryoadenitis, left lacrimal gland
- H04.003 Unspecified dacryoadenitis, bilateral lacrimal glands
- H04.009 Unspecified dacryoadenitis, unspecified lacrimal gland

H04.01 Acute dacryoadenitis
- H04.011 Acute dacryoadenitis, right lacrimal gland
- H04.012 Acute dacryoadenitis, left lacrimal gland
- H04.013 Acute dacryoadenitis, bilateral lacrimal glands
- H04.019 Acute dacryoadenitis, unspecified lacrimal gland

H04.02 Chronic dacryoadenitis
- H04.021 Chronic dacryoadenitis, right lacrimal gland
- H04.022 Chronic dacryoadenitis, left lacrimal gland
- H04.023 Chronic dacryoadenitis, bilateral lacrimal gland
- H04.029 Chronic dacryoadenitis, unspecified lacrimal gland

H04.03 Chronic enlargement of lacrimal gland
- H04.031 Chronic enlargement of right lacrimal gland
- H04.032 Chronic enlargement of left lacrimal gland
- H04.033 Chronic enlargement of bilateral lacrimal glands
- H04.039 Chronic enlargement of unspecified lacrimal gland

H04.1 Other disorders of lacrimal gland

H04.11 Dacryops
- H04.111 Dacryops of right lacrimal gland
- H04.112 Dacryops of left lacrimal gland
- H04.113 Dacryops of bilateral lacrimal glands
- H04.119 Dacryops of unspecified lacrimal gland

H04.12 Dry eye syndrome
Tear film insufficiency, NOS
- H04.121 Dry eye syndrome of right lacrimal gland
- H04.122 Dry eye syndrome of left lacrimal gland
- H04.123 Dry eye syndrome of bilateral lacrimal glands
- H04.129 Dry eye syndrome of unspecified lacrimal gland

H04.13 Lacrimal cyst
Lacrimal cystic degeneration
- H04.131 Lacrimal cyst, right lacrimal gland
- H04.132 Lacrimal cyst, left lacrimal gland
- H04.133 Lacrimal cyst, bilateral lacrimal glands
- H04.139 Lacrimal cyst, unspecified lacrimal gland

H04.14 Primary lacrimal gland atrophy

DEFINITION Wasting of the lacrimal glands causing severe dryness with decreased tear production.

- H04.141 Primary lacrimal gland atrophy, right lacrimal gland
- H04.142 Primary lacrimal gland atrophy, left lacrimal gland
- H04.143 Primary lacrimal gland atrophy, bilateral lacrimal glands
- H04.149 Primary lacrimal gland atrophy, unspecified lacrimal gland

H04.15 Secondary lacrimal gland atrophy

H04.151 Secondary lacrimal gland atrophy, right lacrimal gland
H04.152 Secondary lacrimal gland atrophy, left lacrimal gland
H04.153 Secondary lacrimal gland atrophy, bilateral lacrimal glands
H04.159 Secondary lacrimal gland atrophy, unspecified lacrimal gland

H04.16 Lacrimal gland dislocation

DEFINITION Lacrimal gland separated from the tear ducts, preventing tears from passing normally to the eye.

H04.161 Lacrimal gland dislocation, right lacrimal gland
H04.162 Lacrimal gland dislocation, left lacrimal gland
H04.163 Lacrimal gland dislocation, bilateral lacrimal glands
H04.169 Lacrimal gland dislocation, unspecified lacrimal gland

H04.19 Other specified disorders of lacrimal gland

H04.2 Epiphora

H04.20 Unspecified epiphora
▲ H04.201 Unspecified epiphora, right side
▲ H04.202 Unspecified epiphora, left side
▲ H04.203 Unspecified epiphora, bilateral
▲ H04.209 Unspecified epiphora, unspecified side

H04.21 Epiphora due to excess lacrimation
H04.211 Epiphora due to excess lacrimation, right lacrimal gland
H04.212 Epiphora due to excess lacrimation, left lacrimal gland
H04.213 Epiphora due to excess lacrimation, bilateral lacrimal glands
H04.219 Epiphora due to excess lacrimation, unspecified lacrimal gland

H04.22 Epiphora due to insufficient drainage
▲ H04.221 Epiphora due to insufficient drainage, right side
▲ H04.222 Epiphora due to insufficient drainage, left side
▲ H04.223 Epiphora due to insufficient drainage, bilateral
▲ H04.229 Epiphora due to insufficient drainage, unspecified side

H04.3 Acute and unspecified inflammation of lacrimal passages

EXCLUDES 1 *neonatal dacryocystitis (P39.1)*

H04.30 Unspecified dacryocystitis

DEFINITION Inflammation of the lacrimal sac in the eye causing obstruction of the tube draining tears into the nose.

H04.301 Unspecified dacryocystitis of right lacrimal passage
H04.302 Unspecified dacryocystitis of left lacrimal passage
H04.303 Unspecified dacryocystitis of bilateral lacrimal passages
H04.309 Unspecified dacryocystitis of unspecified lacrimal passage

H04.31 Phlegmonous dacryocystitis
H04.311 Phlegmonous dacryocystitis of right lacrimal passage
H04.312 Phlegmonous dacryocystitis of left lacrimal passage
H04.313 Phlegmonous dacryocystitis of bilateral lacrimal passages
H04.319 Phlegmonous dacryocystitis of unspecified lacrimal passage

H04.32 Acute dacryocystitis
Acute dacryopericystitis

DEFINITION Sudden, severe inflammation of the tear sac, usually due to blockage of the tear ducts.

H04.321 Acute dacryocystitis of right lacrimal passage
H04.322 Acute dacryocystitis of left lacrimal passage
H04.323 Acute dacryocystitis of bilateral lacrimal passages
H04.329 Acute dacryocystitis of unspecified lacrimal passage

H04.33 Acute lacrimal canaliculitis

DEFINITION Sudden, severe inflammation of the lacrimal passages or tear ducts.

H04.331 Acute lacrimal canaliculitis of right lacrimal passage
H04.332 Acute lacrimal canaliculitis of left lacrimal passage
H04.333 Acute lacrimal canaliculitis of bilateral lacrimal passages
H04.339 Acute lacrimal canaliculitis of unspecified lacrimal passage

H04.4 Chronic inflammation of lacrimal passages

H04.41 Chronic dacryocystitis
H04.411 Chronic dacryocystitis of right lacrimal passage
H04.412 Chronic dacryocystitis of left lacrimal passage
H04.413 Chronic dacryocystitis of bilateral lacrimal passages
H04.419 Chronic dacryocystitis of unspecified lacrimal passage

H04.42 Chronic lacrimal canaliculitis
H04.421 Chronic lacrimal canaliculitis of right lacrimal passage
H04.422 Chronic lacrimal canaliculitis of left lacrimal passage
H04.423 Chronic lacrimal canaliculitis of bilateral lacrimal passages
H04.429 Chronic lacrimal canaliculitis of unspecified lacrimal passage

H04.43 Chronic lacrimal mucocele

DEFINITION Inflammation of the lacrimal system in which the tear ducts, and then the eyes, become filled with mucous.

H04.431 Chronic lacrimal mucocele of right lacrimal passage
H04.432 Chronic lacrimal mucocele of left lacrimal passage
H04.433 Chronic lacrimal mucocele of bilateral lacrimal passages
H04.439 Chronic lacrimal mucocele of unspecified lacrimal passage

H04.5 Stenosis and insufficiency of lacrimal passages

H04.51 Dacryolith
H04.511 Dacryolith of right lacrimal passage
H04.512 Dacryolith of left lacrimal passage
H04.513 Dacryolith of bilateral lacrimal passages
H04.519 Dacryolith of unspecified lacrimal passage

H04.52 Eversion of lacrimal punctum

DEFINITION Tear duct exit turned away from the eye, causing tears to flow directly onto the face instead of moistening the eyeball.

H04.521 Eversion of right lacrimal punctum
H04.522 Eversion of left lacrimal punctum
H04.523 Eversion of bilateral lacrimal punctum
H04.529 Eversion of unspecified lacrimal punctum

H04.53 Neonatal obstruction of nasolacrimal duct

EXCLUDES 1 *congenital stenosis and stricture of lacrimal duct (Q10.5)*

H04.531 Neonatal obstruction of right nasolacrimal duct N
H04.532 Neonatal obstruction of left nasolacrimal duct N
H04.533 Neonatal obstruction of bilateral nasolacrimal duct N
H04.539 Neonatal obstruction of unspecified nasolacrimal duct N

H04.54 Stenosis of lacrimal canaliculi
H04.541 Stenosis of right lacrimal canaliculi
H04.542 Stenosis of left lacrimal canaliculi
H04.543 Stenosis of bilateral lacrimal canaliculi
H04.549 Stenosis of unspecified lacrimal canaliculi

- 6 H04.55 Acquired stenosis of nasolacrimal duct
  - 7 H04.551 Acquired stenosis of right nasolacrimal duct
  - 7 H04.552 Acquired stenosis of left nasolacrimal duct
  - 7 H04.553 Acquired stenosis of bilateral nasolacrimal duct
  - 7 H04.559 Acquired stenosis of unspecified nasolacrimal duct
- 6 H04.56 Stenosis of lacrimal punctum
  - 7 H04.561 Stenosis of right lacrimal punctum
  - 7 H04.562 Stenosis of left lacrimal punctum
  - 7 H04.563 Stenosis of bilateral lacrimal punctum
  - 7 H04.569 Stenosis of unspecified lacrimal punctum
- 6 H04.57 Stenosis of lacrimal sac
  - 7 H04.571 Stenosis of right lacrimal sac
  - 7 H04.572 Stenosis of left lacrimal sac
  - 7 H04.573 Stenosis of bilateral lacrimal sac
  - 7 H04.579 Stenosis of unspecified lacrimal sac
- 5 H04.6 Other changes of lacrimal passages
  - 6 H04.61 Lacrimal fistula
    - 7 H04.611 Lacrimal fistula right lacrimal passage
    - 7 H04.612 Lacrimal fistula left lacrimal passage
    - 7 H04.613 Lacrimal fistula bilateral lacrimal passages
    - 7 H04.619 Lacrimal fistula unspecified lacrimal passage
  - H04.69 Other changes of lacrimal passages
- 5 H04.8 Other disorders of lacrimal system
  - 6 H04.81 Granuloma of lacrimal passages
    - 7 H04.811 Granuloma of right lacrimal passage
    - 7 H04.812 Granuloma of left lacrimal passage
    - 7 H04.813 Granuloma of bilateral lacrimal passages
    - 7 H04.819 Granuloma of unspecified lacrimal passage
  - H04.89 Other disorders of lacrimal system
- H04.9 Disorder of lacrimal system, unspecified

4 H05 Disorders of orbit

EXCLUDES 1 *congenital malformation of orbit (Q10.7)*

- 5 H05.0 Acute inflammation of orbit
  - H05.00 Unspecified acute inflammation of orbit
  - 6 H05.01 Cellulitis of orbit
    Abscess of orbit
    - 7 H05.011 Cellulitis of right orbit
    - 7 H05.012 Cellulitis of left orbit
    - 7 H05.013 Cellulitis of bilateral orbits
    - 7 H05.019 Cellulitis of unspecified orbit
  - 6 H05.02 Osteomyelitis of orbit
    - 7 H05.021 Osteomyelitis of right orbit
    - 7 H05.022 Osteomyelitis of left orbit
    - 7 H05.023 Osteomyelitis of bilateral orbits
    - 7 H05.029 Osteomyelitis of unspecified orbit
  - 6 H05.03 Periostitis of orbit
    - 7 H05.031 Periostitis of right orbit
    - 7 H05.032 Periostitis of left orbit
    - 7 H05.033 Periostitis of bilateral orbits
    - 7 H05.039 Periostitis of unspecified orbit
  - 6 H05.04 Tenonitis of orbit
    - 7 H05.041 Tenonitis of right orbit
    - 7 H05.042 Tenonitis of left orbit
    - 7 H05.043 Tenonitis of bilateral orbits
    - 7 H05.049 Tenonitis of unspecified orbit
- 5 H05.1 Chronic inflammatory disorders of orbit
  - H05.10 Unspecified chronic inflammatory disorders of orbit
  - 6 H05.11 Granuloma of orbit
    Pseudotumor (inflammatory) of orbit
    - 7 H05.111 Granuloma of right orbit
    - 7 H05.112 Granuloma of left orbit
    - 7 H05.113 Granuloma of bilateral orbits
    - 7 H05.119 Granuloma of unspecified orbit
  - 6 H05.12 Orbital myositis
    DEFINITION Inflammation of one of the muscles that moves the eyeball.
    - 7 H05.121 Orbital myositis, right orbit
    - 7 H05.122 Orbital myositis, left orbit
    - 7 H05.123 Orbital myositis, bilateral
    - 7 H05.129 Orbital myositis, unspecified orbit
- 5 H05.2 Exophthalmic conditions
  - H05.20 Unspecified exophthalmos
  - 6 H05.21 Displacement (lateral) of globe
    DEFINITION Condition in which the eyeball is situated towards the side of the head, away from the nose.
    - 7 H05.211 Displacement (lateral) of globe, right eye
    - 7 H05.212 Displacement (lateral) of globe, left eye
    - 7 H05.213 Displacement (lateral) of globe, bilateral
    - 7 H05.219 Displacement (lateral) of globe, unspecified eye
  - 6 H05.22 Edema of orbit
    Orbital congestion
    - 7 H05.221 Edema of right orbit
    - 7 H05.222 Edema of left orbit
    - 7 H05.223 Edema of bilateral orbit
    - 7 H05.229 Edema of unspecified orbit
  - 6 H05.23 Hemorrhage of orbit
    - 7 H05.231 Hemorrhage of right orbit
    - 7 H05.232 Hemorrhage of left orbit
    - 7 H05.233 Hemorrhage of bilateral orbit
    - 7 H05.239 Hemorrhage of unspecified orbit
  - 6 H05.24 Constant exophthalmos
    - 7 H05.241 Constant exophthalmos, right eye
    - 7 H05.242 Constant exophthalmos, left eye
    - 7 H05.243 Constant exophthalmos, bilateral
    - 7 H05.249 Constant exophthalmos, unspecified eye
  - 6 H05.25 Intermittent exophthalmos
    - 7 H05.251 Intermittent exophthalmos, right eye
    - 7 H05.252 Intermittent exophthalmos, left eye
    - 7 H05.253 Intermittent exophthalmos, bilateral
    - 7 H05.259 Intermittent exophthalmos, unspecified eye
  - 6 H05.26 Pulsating exophthalmos
    - 7 H05.261 Pulsating exophthalmos, right eye
    - 7 H05.262 Pulsating exophthalmos, left eye
    - 7 H05.263 Pulsating exophthalmos, bilateral
    - 7 H05.269 Pulsating exophthalmos, unspecified eye
- 5 H05.3 Deformity of orbit
  EXCLUDES 1 *congenital deformity of orbit (Q10.7)*
  hypertelorism (Q75.2)
  - H05.30 Unspecified deformity of orbit
  - 6 H05.31 Atrophy of orbit
    - 7 H05.311 Atrophy of right orbit
    - 7 H05.312 Atrophy of left orbit
    - 7 H05.313 Atrophy of bilateral orbit
    - 7 H05.319 Atrophy of unspecified orbit
  - 6 H05.32 Deformity of orbit due to bone disease
    Code also:
    associated bone disease
    - 7 H05.321 Deformity of right orbit due to bone disease
    - 7 H05.322 Deformity of left orbit due to bone disease
    - 7 H05.323 Deformity of bilateral orbits due to bone disease
    - 7 H05.329 Deformity of unspecified orbit due to bone disease
  - 6 H05.33 Deformity of orbit due to trauma or surgery
    - 7 H05.331 Deformity of right orbit due to trauma or surgery
    - 7 H05.332 Deformity of left orbit due to trauma or surgery
    - 7 H05.333 Deformity of bilateral orbits due to trauma or surgery
    - 7 H05.339 Deformity of unspecified orbit due to trauma or surgery

6 H05.34 Enlargement of orbit
- H05.341 Enlargement of right orbit
- H05.342 Enlargement of left orbit
- H05.343 Enlargement of bilateral orbits
- H05.349 Enlargement of unspecified orbit

6 H05.35 Exostosis of orbit

DEFINITION Abnormal bone growth of the eye socket; can impair vision and prevent the eye from moving properly.

- H05.351 Exostosis of right orbit
- H05.352 Exostosis of left orbit
- H05.353 Exostosis of bilateral orbits
- H05.359 Exostosis of unspecified orbit

5 H05.4 Enophthalmos

6 H05.40 Unspecified enophthalmos

DEFINITION Condition in which the eye is recessed abnormally deep within the eye socket.

- H05.401 Unspecified enophthalmos, right eye
- H05.402 Unspecified enophthalmos, left eye
- H05.403 Unspecified enophthalmos, bilateral
- H05.409 Unspecified enophthalmos, unspecified eye

6 H05.41 Enophthalmos due to atrophy of orbital tissue
- H05.411 Enophthalmos due to atrophy of orbital tissue, right eye
- H05.412 Enophthalmos due to atrophy of orbital tissue, left eye
- H05.413 Enophthalmos due to atrophy of orbital tissue, bilateral
- H05.419 Enophthalmos due to atrophy of orbital tissue, unspecified eye

6 H05.42 Enophthalmos due to trauma or surgery
- H05.421 Enophthalmos due to trauma or surgery, right eye
- H05.422 Enophthalmos due to trauma or surgery, left eye
- H05.423 Enophthalmos due to trauma or surgery, bilateral
- H05.429 Enophthalmos due to trauma or surgery, unspecified eye

5 H05.5 Retained (old) foreign body following penetrating wound of orbit

Retrobulbar foreign body

Use additional code to identify the type of retained foreign body (Z18.-)

EXCLUDES 1 *current penetrating wound of orbit (S05.4-)*

EXCLUDES 2 *retained foreign body of eyelid (H02.81-)*
retained intraocular foreign body (H44.6-, H44.7-)

- H05.50 Retained (old) foreign body following penetrating wound of unspecified orbit
- H05.51 Retained (old) foreign body following penetrating wound of right orbit
- H05.52 Retained (old) foreign body following penetrating wound of left orbit
- H05.53 Retained (old) foreign body following penetrating wound of bilateral orbits

5 H05.8 Other disorders of orbit

6 H05.81 Cyst of orbit

Encephalocele of orbit
- H05.811 Cyst of right orbit
- H05.812 Cyst of left orbit
- H05.813 Cyst of bilateral orbits
- H05.819 Cyst of unspecified orbit

6 H05.82 Myopathy of extraocular muscles
- H05.821 Myopathy of extraocular muscles, right orbit
- H05.822 Myopathy of extraocular muscles, left orbit
- H05.823 Myopathy of extraocular muscles, bilateral
- H05.829 Myopathy of extraocular muscles, unspecified orbit

H05.89 Other disorders of orbit

H05.9 Unspecified disorder of orbit

Disorders of conjunctiva (H10-H11)

4 H10 Conjunctivitis

EXCLUDES 1 *keratoconjunctivitis (H16.2-)*

CODING TIP ✓ Consider codes from H10 when an infectious organism is not identified and the documentation only supports a clinical picture of conjunctivitis. If a certain bacterial or viral cause is known, a code from the Infectious and parasitic disease chapter may be more appropriate.

5 H10.0 Mucopurulent conjunctivitis

6 H10.01 Acute follicular conjunctivitis
- H10.011 Acute follicular conjunctivitis, right eye
- H10.012 Acute follicular conjunctivitis, left eye
- H10.013 Acute follicular conjunctivitis, bilateral
- H10.019 Acute follicular conjunctivitis, unspecified eye

6 H10.02 Other mucopurulent conjunctivitis

CODING TIP ✓ Subcategory H10.02 is commonly referred to as pink eye.

DEFINITION Inflammation of the conjunctiva with the production of mucous and pus.

- H10.021 Other mucopurulent conjunctivitis, right eye
- H10.022 Other mucopurulent conjunctivitis, left eye
- H10.023 Other mucopurulent conjunctivitis, bilateral
- H10.029 Other mucopurulent conjunctivitis, unspecified eye

5 H10.1 Acute atopic conjunctivitis

Acute papillary conjunctivitis

DEFINITION Sudden, severe case of conjunctivitis caused by allergies.

- H10.10 Acute atopic conjunctivitis, unspecified eye
- H10.11 Acute atopic conjunctivitis, right eye
- H10.12 Acute atopic conjunctivitis, left eye
- H10.13 Acute atopic conjunctivitis, bilateral

5 H10.2 Other acute conjunctivitis

CODING TIP ✓ Consider subcategory H10.2 when light or noxious chemicals cause conjunctivitis.

6 H10.21 Acute toxic conjunctivitis

Acute chemical conjunctivitis

Code first:

(T51-T65) to identify chemical and intent

EXCLUDES 1 *burn and corrosion of eye and adnexa (T26.-)*

- H10.211 Acute toxic conjunctivitis, right eye
- H10.212 Acute toxic conjunctivitis, left eye
- H10.213 Acute toxic conjunctivitis, bilateral
- H10.219 Acute toxic conjunctivitis, unspecified eye

6 H10.22 Pseudomembranous conjunctivitis
- H10.221 Pseudomembranous conjunctivitis, right eye
- H10.222 Pseudomembranous conjunctivitis, left eye
- H10.223 Pseudomembranous conjunctivitis, bilateral
- H10.229 Pseudomembranous conjunctivitis, unspecified eye

6 H10.23 Serous conjunctivitis, except viral

EXCLUDES 1 *viral conjunctivitis (B30.-)*

- H10.231 Serous conjunctivitis, except viral, right eye
- H10.232 Serous conjunctivitis, except viral, left eye
- H10.233 Serous conjunctivitis, except viral, bilateral
- H10.239 Serous conjunctivitis, except viral, unspecified eye

5 H10.3 Unspecified acute conjunctivitis

EXCLUDES 1 *ophthalmia neonatorum NOS (P39.1)*

- H10.30 Unspecified acute conjunctivitis, unspecified eye
- H10.31 Unspecified acute conjunctivitis, right eye
- H10.32 Unspecified acute conjunctivitis, left eye
- H10.33 Unspecified acute conjunctivitis, bilateral

5 H10.4 Chronic conjunctivitis

6 H10.40 Unspecified chronic conjunctivitis

H10.401 Unspecified chronic conjunctivitis, right eye
H10.402 Unspecified chronic conjunctivitis, left eye
H10.403 Unspecified chronic conjunctivitis, bilateral
H10.409 Unspecified chronic conjunctivitis, unspecified eye
H10.41 Chronic giant papillary conjunctivitis
H10.411 Chronic giant papillary conjunctivitis, right eye
H10.412 Chronic giant papillary conjunctivitis, left eye
H10.413 Chronic giant papillary conjunctivitis, bilateral
H10.419 Chronic giant papillary conjunctivitis, unspecified eye
H10.42 Simple chronic conjunctivitis
H10.421 Simple chronic conjunctivitis, right eye
H10.422 Simple chronic conjunctivitis, left eye
H10.423 Simple chronic conjunctivitis, bilateral
H10.429 Simple chronic conjunctivitis, unspecified eye
H10.43 Chronic follicular conjunctivitis
H10.431 Chronic follicular conjunctivitis, right eye
H10.432 Chronic follicular conjunctivitis, left eye
H10.433 Chronic follicular conjunctivitis, bilateral
H10.439 Chronic follicular conjunctivitis, unspecified eye
H10.44 Vernal conjunctivitis
EXCLUDES 1 *vernal keratoconjunctivitis with limbar and corneal involvement (H16.26-)*
DEFINITION Seasonal inflammation of the conjunctiva due to an allergic reaction to pollen, mold, or another seasonal factor.
H10.45 Other chronic allergic conjunctivitis
H10.5 Blepharoconjunctivitis
H10.50 Unspecified blepharoconjunctivitis
H10.501 Unspecified blepharoconjunctivitis, right eye
H10.502 Unspecified blepharoconjunctivitis, left eye
H10.503 Unspecified blepharoconjunctivitis, bilateral
H10.509 Unspecified blepharoconjunctivitis, unspecified eye
▲ H10.51 Ligneous conjunctivitis
Code also underlying condition if known, such as: plasminogen deficiency (E88.02)
H10.511 Ligneous conjunctivitis, right eye
H10.512 Ligneous conjunctivitis, left eye
H10.513 Ligneous conjunctivitis, bilateral
H10.519 Ligneous conjunctivitis, unspecified eye
H10.52 Angular blepharoconjunctivitis
H10.521 Angular blepharoconjunctivitis, right eye
H10.522 Angular blepharoconjunctivitis, left eye
H10.523 Angular blepharoconjunctivitis, bilateral
H10.529 Angular blepharoconjunctivitis, unspecified eye
H10.53 Contact blepharoconjunctivitis
H10.531 Contact blepharoconjunctivitis, right eye
H10.532 Contact blepharoconjunctivitis, left eye
H10.533 Contact blepharoconjunctivitis, bilateral
H10.539 Contact blepharoconjunctivitis, unspecified eye
H10.8 Other conjunctivitis
H10.81 Pingueculitis
EXCLUDES 1 *pinguecula (H11.15-)*
DEFINITION Yellowish, raised areas of limbal conjunctival tissue, usually seen with chronic sun exposure, that become acutely vascularized, irritated, and inflamed.
H10.811 Pingueculitis, right eye
H10.812 Pingueculitis, left eye
H10.813 Pingueculitis, bilateral
H10.819 Pingueculitis, unspecified eye
● H10.82 Rosacea conjunctivitis
Code first:
underlying rosacea dermatitis (L71.-)
● H10.821 Rosacea conjunctivitis, right eye
● H10.822 Rosacea conjunctivitis, left eye
● H10.823 Rosacea conjunctivitis, bilateral
● H10.829 Rosacea conjunctivitis, unspecified eye
H10.89 Other conjunctivitis
H10.9 Unspecified conjunctivitis

H11 Other disorders of conjunctiva

EXCLUDES 1 *keratoconjunctivitis (H16.2-)*

H11.0 Pterygium of eye
EXCLUDES 1 *pseudopterygium (H11.81-)*
H11.00 Unspecified pterygium of eye
DEFINITION Raised, wedge-shaped overgrowth of the conjunctiva onto the cornea of the eye.
H11.001 Unspecified pterygium of right eye
H11.002 Unspecified pterygium of left eye
H11.003 Unspecified pterygium of eye, bilateral
H11.009 Unspecified pterygium of unspecified eye
H11.01 Amyloid pterygium
H11.011 Amyloid pterygium of right eye
H11.012 Amyloid pterygium of left eye
H11.013 Amyloid pterygium of eye, bilateral
H11.019 Amyloid pterygium of unspecified eye
H11.02 Central pterygium of eye
H11.021 Central pterygium of right eye
H11.022 Central pterygium of left eye
H11.023 Central pterygium of eye, bilateral
H11.029 Central pterygium of unspecified eye
H11.03 Double pterygium of eye
H11.031 Double pterygium of right eye
H11.032 Double pterygium of left eye
H11.033 Double pterygium of eye, bilateral
H11.039 Double pterygium of unspecified eye
H11.04 Peripheral pterygium of eye, stationary
H11.041 Peripheral pterygium, stationary, right eye
H11.042 Peripheral pterygium, stationary, left eye
H11.043 Peripheral pterygium, stationary, bilateral
H11.049 Peripheral pterygium, stationary, unspecified eye
H11.05 Peripheral pterygium of eye, progressive
H11.051 Peripheral pterygium, progressive, right eye
H11.052 Peripheral pterygium, progressive, left eye
H11.053 Peripheral pterygium, progressive, bilateral
H11.059 Peripheral pterygium, progressive, unspecified eye
H11.06 Recurrent pterygium of eye
H11.061 Recurrent pterygium of right eye
H11.062 Recurrent pterygium of left eye
H11.063 Recurrent pterygium of eye, bilateral
H11.069 Recurrent pterygium of unspecified eye
H11.1 Conjunctival degenerations and deposits
EXCLUDES 2 *pseudopterygium (H11.81)*
H11.10 Unspecified conjunctival degenerations
H11.11 Conjunctival deposits
H11.111 Conjunctival deposits, right eye
H11.112 Conjunctival deposits, left eye
H11.113 Conjunctival deposits, bilateral
H11.119 Conjunctival deposits, unspecified eye
H11.12 Conjunctival concretions
DEFINITION Yellow-white granules or cysts which form just beneath the conjunctiva, wearing it away and causing the sensation of a foreign body in the eye.
H11.121 Conjunctival concretions, right eye
H11.122 Conjunctival concretions, left eye
H11.123 Conjunctival concretions, bilateral
H11.129 Conjunctival concretions, unspecified eye
H11.13 Conjunctival pigmentations
Conjunctival argyrosis [argyria]

- H11.131 Conjunctival pigmentations, right eye
- H11.132 Conjunctival pigmentations, left eye
- H11.133 Conjunctival pigmentations, bilateral
- H11.139 Conjunctival pigmentations, unspecified eye

H11.14 Conjunctival xerosis, unspecified

EXCLUDES 1 *xerosis of conjunctiva due to vitamin A deficiency (E50.0, E50.1)*

- H11.141 Conjunctival xerosis, unspecified, right eye
- H11.142 Conjunctival xerosis, unspecified, left eye
- H11.143 Conjunctival xerosis, unspecified, bilateral
- H11.149 Conjunctival xerosis, unspecified, unspecified eye

H11.15 Pinguecula

EXCLUDES 1 *pingueculitis (H10.81-)*

DEFINITION Small, nonmalignant, yellowish growth on the conjunctiva often asymptomatic and requiring no treatment but may cause irritation.

- H11.151 Pinguecula, right eye
- H11.152 Pinguecula, left eye
- H11.153 Pinguecula, bilateral
- H11.159 Pinguecula, unspecified eye

H11.2 Conjunctival scars

H11.21 Conjunctival adhesions and strands (localized)

- H11.211 Conjunctival adhesions and strands (localized), right eye
- H11.212 Conjunctival adhesions and strands (localized), left eye
- H11.213 Conjunctival adhesions and strands (localized), bilateral
- H11.219 Conjunctival adhesions and strands (localized), unspecified eye

H11.22 Conjunctival granuloma

- H11.221 Conjunctival granuloma, right eye
- H11.222 Conjunctival granuloma, left eye
- H11.223 Conjunctival granuloma, bilateral
- H11.229 Conjunctival granuloma, unspecified

H11.23 Symblepharon

DEFINITION Conjunctiva of the eyelid that has adhered to the eye, sometimes over the cornea, requiring surgical removal.

- H11.231 Symblepharon, right eye
- H11.232 Symblepharon, left eye
- H11.233 Symblepharon, bilateral
- H11.239 Symblepharon, unspecified eye

H11.24 Scarring of conjunctiva

- H11.241 Scarring of conjunctiva, right eye
- H11.242 Scarring of conjunctiva, left eye
- H11.243 Scarring of conjunctiva, bilateral
- H11.249 Scarring of conjunctiva, unspecified eye

H11.3 Conjunctival hemorrhage

Subconjunctival hemorrhage

- H11.30 Conjunctival hemorrhage, unspecified eye
- H11.31 Conjunctival hemorrhage, right eye
- H11.32 Conjunctival hemorrhage, left eye
- H11.33 Conjunctival hemorrhage, bilateral

H11.4 Other conjunctival vascular disorders and cysts

H11.41 Vascular abnormalities of conjunctiva

Conjunctival aneurysm

- H11.411 Vascular abnormalities of conjunctiva, right eye
- H11.412 Vascular abnormalities of conjunctiva, left eye
- H11.413 Vascular abnormalities of conjunctiva, bilateral
- H11.419 Vascular abnormalities of conjunctiva, unspecified eye

H11.42 Conjunctival edema

- H11.421 Conjunctival edema, right eye
- H11.422 Conjunctival edema, left eye
- H11.423 Conjunctival edema, bilateral
- H11.429 Conjunctival edema, unspecified eye

H11.43 Conjunctival hyperemia

- H11.431 Conjunctival hyperemia, right eye
- H11.432 Conjunctival hyperemia, left eye
- H11.433 Conjunctival hyperemia, bilateral
- H11.439 Conjunctival hyperemia, unspecified eye

H11.44 Conjunctival cysts

- H11.441 Conjunctival cysts, right eye
- H11.442 Conjunctival cysts, left eye
- H11.443 Conjunctival cysts, bilateral
- H11.449 Conjunctival cysts, unspecified eye

H11.8 Other specified disorders of conjunctiva

H11.81 Pseudopterygium of conjunctiva

- H11.811 Pseudopterygium of conjunctiva, right eye
- H11.812 Pseudopterygium of conjunctiva, left eye
- H11.813 Pseudopterygium of conjunctiva, bilateral
- H11.819 Pseudopterygium of conjunctiva, unspecified eye

H11.82 Conjunctivochalasis

DEFINITION Loosening of the conjunctiva's attachment to the eye, causing wrinkling, dryness, and a tendency to trap particles in the folds, causing chronic inflammation.

- H11.821 Conjunctivochalasis, right eye
- H11.822 Conjunctivochalasis, left eye
- H11.823 Conjunctivochalasis, bilateral
- H11.829 Conjunctivochalasis, unspecified eye

H11.89 Other specified disorders of conjunctiva

H11.9 Unspecified disorder of conjunctiva

Disorders of sclera, cornea, iris and ciliary body (H15-H22)

H15 Disorders of sclera

H15.0 Scleritis

H15.00 Unspecified scleritis

- H15.001 Unspecified scleritis, right eye
- H15.002 Unspecified scleritis, left eye
- H15.003 Unspecified scleritis, bilateral
- H15.009 Unspecified scleritis, unspecified eye

H15.01 Anterior scleritis

- H15.011 Anterior scleritis, right eye
- H15.012 Anterior scleritis, left eye
- H15.013 Anterior scleritis, bilateral
- H15.019 Anterior scleritis, unspecified eye

H15.02 Brawny scleritis

DEFINITION Severe inflammation of the sclera affecting the border between the sclera and the cornea.

- H15.021 Brawny scleritis, right eye
- H15.022 Brawny scleritis, left eye
- H15.023 Brawny scleritis, bilateral
- H15.029 Brawny scleritis, unspecified eye

H15.03 Posterior scleritis

Sclerotenonitis

- H15.031 Posterior scleritis, right eye
- H15.032 Posterior scleritis, left eye
- H15.033 Posterior scleritis, bilateral
- H15.039 Posterior scleritis, unspecified eye

H15.04 Scleritis with corneal involvement

- H15.041 Scleritis with corneal involvement, right eye
- H15.042 Scleritis with corneal involvement, left eye
- H15.043 Scleritis with corneal involvement, bilateral
- H15.049 Scleritis with corneal involvement, unspecified eye

H15.05 Scleromalacia perforans

- H15.051 Scleromalacia perforans, right eye
- H15.052 Scleromalacia perforans, left eye
- H15.053 Scleromalacia perforans, bilateral
- H15.059 Scleromalacia perforans, unspecified eye

H15.09 Other scleritis

Scleral abscess

- H15.091 Other scleritis, right eye

- H15.092 Other scleritis, left eye
- H15.093 Other scleritis, bilateral
- H15.099 Other scleritis, unspecified eye

H15.1 Episcleritis

H15.10 Unspecified episcleritis
- H15.101 Unspecified episcleritis, right eye
- H15.102 Unspecified episcleritis, left eye
- H15.103 Unspecified episcleritis, bilateral
- H15.109 Unspecified episcleritis, unspecified eye

H15.11 Episcleritis periodica fugax

DEFINITION Periodic attacks of inflammation of the sclera; typically of rapid onset and short duration.

- H15.111 Episcleritis periodica fugax, right eye
- H15.112 Episcleritis periodica fugax, left eye
- H15.113 Episcleritis periodica fugax, bilateral
- H15.119 Episcleritis periodica fugax, unspecified eye

H15.12 Nodular episcleritis
- H15.121 Nodular episcleritis, right eye
- H15.122 Nodular episcleritis, left eye
- H15.123 Nodular episcleritis, bilateral
- H15.129 Nodular episcleritis, unspecified eye

H15.8 Other disorders of sclera

EXCLUDES 2 *blue sclera (Q13.5)*
degenerative myopia (H44.2-)

H15.81 Equatorial staphyloma
- H15.811 Equatorial staphyloma, right eye
- H15.812 Equatorial staphyloma, left eye
- H15.813 Equatorial staphyloma, bilateral
- H15.819 Equatorial staphyloma, unspecified eye

H15.82 Localized anterior staphyloma
- H15.821 Localized anterior staphyloma, right eye
- H15.822 Localized anterior staphyloma, left eye
- H15.823 Localized anterior staphyloma, bilateral
- H15.829 Localized anterior staphyloma, unspecified eye

H15.83 Staphyloma posticum
- H15.831 Staphyloma posticum, right eye
- H15.832 Staphyloma posticum, left eye
- H15.833 Staphyloma posticum, bilateral
- H15.839 Staphyloma posticum, unspecified eye

H15.84 Scleral ectasia

DEFINITION Contents of the eyeball protrude through an abnormally thin section of the sclera.

- H15.841 Scleral ectasia, right eye
- H15.842 Scleral ectasia, left eye
- H15.843 Scleral ectasia, bilateral
- H15.849 Scleral ectasia, unspecified eye

H15.85 Ring staphyloma
- H15.851 Ring staphyloma, right eye
- H15.852 Ring staphyloma, left eye
- H15.853 Ring staphyloma, bilateral
- H15.859 Ring staphyloma, unspecified eye

H15.89 Other disorders of sclera

H15.9 Unspecified disorder of sclera

H16 Keratitis

H16.0 Corneal ulcer

H16.00 Unspecified corneal ulcer
- H16.001 Unspecified corneal ulcer, right eye
- H16.002 Unspecified corneal ulcer, left eye
- H16.003 Unspecified corneal ulcer, bilateral
- H16.009 Unspecified corneal ulcer, unspecified eye

H16.01 Central corneal ulcer
- H16.011 Central corneal ulcer, right eye
- H16.012 Central corneal ulcer, left eye
- H16.013 Central corneal ulcer, bilateral
- H16.019 Central corneal ulcer, unspecified eye

H16.02 Ring corneal ulcer

DEFINITION Ring of ulceration encircling the entire edge of the cornea.

- H16.021 Ring corneal ulcer, right eye
- H16.022 Ring corneal ulcer, left eye
- H16.023 Ring corneal ulcer, bilateral
- H16.029 Ring corneal ulcer, unspecified eye

H16.03 Corneal ulcer with hypopyon
- H16.031 Corneal ulcer with hypopyon, right eye
- H16.032 Corneal ulcer with hypopyon, left eye
- H16.033 Corneal ulcer with hypopyon, bilateral
- H16.039 Corneal ulcer with hypopyon, unspecified eye

H16.04 Marginal corneal ulcer
- H16.041 Marginal corneal ulcer, right eye
- H16.042 Marginal corneal ulcer, left eye
- H16.043 Marginal corneal ulcer, bilateral
- H16.049 Marginal corneal ulcer, unspecified eye

H16.05 Mooren's corneal ulcer
- H16.051 Mooren's corneal ulcer, right eye
- H16.052 Mooren's corneal ulcer, left eye
- H16.053 Mooren's corneal ulcer, bilateral
- H16.059 Mooren's corneal ulcer, unspecified eye

H16.06 Mycotic corneal ulcer

DEFINITION Corneal ulcer caused by a fungal infection.

- H16.061 Mycotic corneal ulcer, right eye
- H16.062 Mycotic corneal ulcer, left eye
- H16.063 Mycotic corneal ulcer, bilateral
- H16.069 Mycotic corneal ulcer, unspecified eye

H16.07 Perforated corneal ulcer

Perforated corneal ulcer

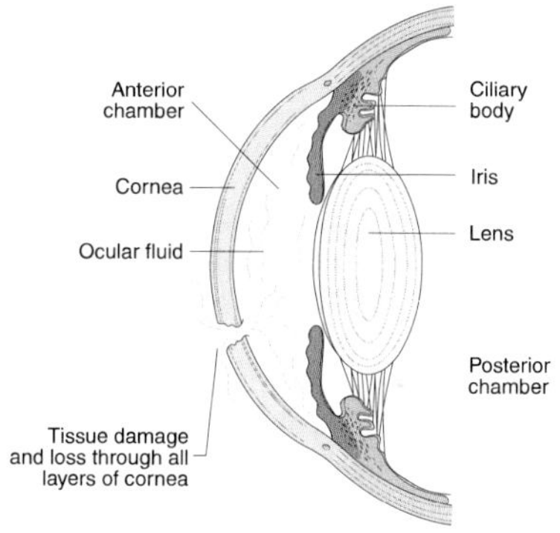

- H16.071 Perforated corneal ulcer, right eye
- H16.072 Perforated corneal ulcer, left eye
- H16.073 Perforated corneal ulcer, bilateral
- H16.079 Perforated corneal ulcer, unspecified eye

H16.1 Other and unspecified superficial keratitis without conjunctivitis

H16.10 Unspecified superficial keratitis
- H16.101 Unspecified superficial keratitis, right eye
- H16.102 Unspecified superficial keratitis, left eye
- H16.103 Unspecified superficial keratitis, bilateral
- H16.109 Unspecified superficial keratitis, unspecified eye

H16.11 Macular keratitis
Areolar keratitis
Nummular keratitis
Stellate keratitis
Striate keratitis
- H16.111 Macular keratitis, right eye
- H16.112 Macular keratitis, left eye
- H16.113 Macular keratitis, bilateral
- H16.119 Macular keratitis, unspecified eye

H16.12 Filamentary keratitis

DEFINITION Keratitis with twisted filaments of mucoid material on the surface of the cornea.

- H16.121 Filamentary keratitis, right eye
- H16.122 Filamentary keratitis, left eye
- H16.123 Filamentary keratitis, bilateral
- H16.129 Filamentary keratitis, unspecified eye

H16.13 Photokeratitis
Snow blindness
Welders keratitis

DEFINITION Painful, inflamed cornea that develops due to over-exposure to ultraviolet light.

- H16.131 Photokeratitis, right eye
- H16.132 Photokeratitis, left eye
- H16.133 Photokeratitis, bilateral
- H16.139 Photokeratitis, unspecified eye

H16.14 Punctate keratitis
- H16.141 Punctate keratitis, right eye
- H16.142 Punctate keratitis, left eye
- H16.143 Punctate keratitis, bilateral
- H16.149 Punctate keratitis, unspecified eye

H16.2 Keratoconjunctivitis

DEFINITION Inflammation of both the cornea and the conjunctiva; presents with burning, bloodshot, watery eyes sensitive to bright light, blurred vision, and a sensation of something in the eye.

H16.20 Unspecified keratoconjunctivitis
Superficial keratitis with conjunctivitis NOS
- H16.201 Unspecified keratoconjunctivitis, right eye
- H16.202 Unspecified keratoconjunctivitis, left eye
- H16.203 Unspecified keratoconjunctivitis, bilateral
- H16.209 Unspecified keratoconjunctivitis, unspecified eye

H16.21 Exposure keratoconjunctivitis

DEFINITION Dryness and inflammation of the cornea and conjunctiva caused by the failure of the eyelid to completely close during sleep and/or blinking.

- H16.211 Exposure keratoconjunctivitis, right eye
- H16.212 Exposure keratoconjunctivitis, left eye
- H16.213 Exposure keratoconjunctivitis, bilateral
- H16.219 Exposure keratoconjunctivitis, unspecified eye

H16.22 Keratoconjunctivitis sicca, not specified as Sjögren's
EXCLUDES 1 *Sjögren's syndrome (M35.01)*
- H16.221 Keratoconjunctivitis sicca, not specified as Sjögren's, right eye
- H16.222 Keratoconjunctivitis sicca, not specified as Sjögren's, left eye
- H16.223 Keratoconjunctivitis sicca, not specified as Sjögren's, bilateral
- H16.229 Keratoconjunctivitis sicca, not specified as Sjögren's, unspecified eye

H16.23 Neurotrophic keratoconjunctivitis
- H16.231 Neurotrophic keratoconjunctivitis, right eye
- H16.232 Neurotrophic keratoconjunctivitis, left eye
- H16.233 Neurotrophic keratoconjunctivitis, bilateral
- H16.239 Neurotrophic keratoconjunctivitis, unspecified eye

H16.24 Ophthalmia nodosa
- H16.241 Ophthalmia nodosa, right eye
- H16.242 Ophthalmia nodosa, left eye
- H16.243 Ophthalmia nodosa, bilateral
- H16.249 Ophthalmia nodosa, unspecified eye

H16.25 Phlyctenular keratoconjunctivitis
- H16.251 Phlyctenular keratoconjunctivitis, right eye
- H16.252 Phlyctenular keratoconjunctivitis, left eye
- H16.253 Phlyctenular keratoconjunctivitis, bilateral
- H16.259 Phlyctenular keratoconjunctivitis, unspecified eye

H16.26 Vernal keratoconjunctivitis, with limbar and corneal involvement
EXCLUDES 1 *vernal conjunctivitis without limbar and corneal involvement (H10.44)*
- H16.261 Vernal keratoconjunctivitis, with limbar and corneal involvement, right eye
- H16.262 Vernal keratoconjunctivitis, with limbar and corneal involvement, left eye
- H16.263 Vernal keratoconjunctivitis, with limbar and corneal involvement, bilateral
- H16.269 Vernal keratoconjunctivitis, with limbar and corneal involvement, unspecified eye

H16.29 Other keratoconjunctivitis
- H16.291 Other keratoconjunctivitis, right eye
- H16.292 Other keratoconjunctivitis, left eye
- H16.293 Other keratoconjunctivitis, bilateral
- H16.299 Other keratoconjunctivitis, unspecified eye

H16.3 Interstitial and deep keratitis

H16.30 Unspecified interstitial keratitis
- H16.301 Unspecified interstitial keratitis, right eye
- H16.302 Unspecified interstitial keratitis, left eye
- H16.303 Unspecified interstitial keratitis, bilateral
- H16.309 Unspecified interstitial keratitis, unspecified eye

H16.31 Corneal abscess
- H16.311 Corneal abscess, right eye
- H16.312 Corneal abscess, left eye
- H16.313 Corneal abscess, bilateral
- H16.319 Corneal abscess, unspecified eye

H16.32 Diffuse interstitial keratitis
Cogan's syndrome

DEFINITION Rare disorder characterized by recurrent inflammation of the cornea with episodes of dizziness and hearing loss that can lead to blindness and deafness if left untreated.

- H16.321 Diffuse interstitial keratitis, right eye
- H16.322 Diffuse interstitial keratitis, left eye
- H16.323 Diffuse interstitial keratitis, bilateral
- H16.329 Diffuse interstitial keratitis, unspecified eye

H16.33 Sclerosing keratitis
- H16.331 Sclerosing keratitis, right eye
- H16.332 Sclerosing keratitis, left eye
- H16.333 Sclerosing keratitis, bilateral
- H16.339 Sclerosing keratitis, unspecified eye

H16.39 Other interstitial and deep keratitis
- H16.391 Other interstitial and deep keratitis, right eye
- H16.392 Other interstitial and deep keratitis, left eye
- H16.393 Other interstitial and deep keratitis, bilateral
- H16.399 Other interstitial and deep keratitis, unspecified eye

H16.4 Corneal neovascularization

H16.40 Unspecified corneal neovascularization
- H16.401 Unspecified corneal neovascularization, right eye
- H16.402 Unspecified corneal neovascularization, left eye
- H16.403 Unspecified corneal neovascularization, bilateral
- H16.409 Unspecified corneal neovascularization, unspecified eye

H16.41 Ghost vessels (corneal)
- H16.411 Ghost vessels (corneal), right eye
- H16.412 Ghost vessels (corneal), left eye
- H16.413 Ghost vessels (corneal), bilateral
- H16.419 Ghost vessels (corneal), unspecified eye

H16.42 Pannus (corneal)
- H16.421 Pannus (corneal), right eye
- H16.422 Pannus (corneal), left eye
- H16.423 Pannus (corneal), bilateral
- H16.429 Pannus (corneal), unspecified eye

H16.43 Localized vascularization of cornea
- H16.431 Localized vascularization of cornea, right eye
- H16.432 Localized vascularization of cornea, left eye
- H16.433 Localized vascularization of cornea, bilateral
- H16.439 Localized vascularization of cornea, unspecified eye

H16.44 Deep vascularization of cornea
- H16.441 Deep vascularization of cornea, right eye

H16.442 Deep vascularization of cornea, left eye
H16.443 Deep vascularization of cornea, bilateral
H16.449 Deep vascularization of cornea, unspecified eye
H16.8 Other keratitis
H16.9 Unspecified keratitis

H17 Corneal scars and opacities
H17.0 Adherent leukoma
H17.00 Adherent leukoma, unspecified eye
H17.01 Adherent leukoma, right eye
H17.02 Adherent leukoma, left eye
H17.03 Adherent leukoma, bilateral
H17.1 Central corneal opacity
H17.10 Central corneal opacity, unspecified eye
H17.11 Central corneal opacity, right eye
H17.12 Central corneal opacity, left eye
H17.13 Central corneal opacity, bilateral
H17.8 Other corneal scars and opacities
H17.81 Minor opacity of cornea
Corneal nebula
H17.811 Minor opacity of cornea, right eye
H17.812 Minor opacity of cornea, left eye
H17.813 Minor opacity of cornea, bilateral
H17.819 Minor opacity of cornea, unspecified eye
H17.82 Peripheral opacity of cornea
H17.821 Peripheral opacity of cornea, right eye
H17.822 Peripheral opacity of cornea, left eye
H17.823 Peripheral opacity of cornea, bilateral
H17.829 Peripheral opacity of cornea, unspecified eye
H17.89 Other corneal scars and opacities
H17.9 Unspecified corneal scar and opacity

H18 Other disorders of cornea
H18.0 Corneal pigmentations and deposits
H18.00 Unspecified corneal deposit
H18.001 Unspecified corneal deposit, right eye
H18.002 Unspecified corneal deposit, left eye
H18.003 Unspecified corneal deposit, bilateral
H18.009 Unspecified corneal deposit, unspecified eye
H18.01 Anterior corneal pigmentations
Staehli's line
H18.011 Anterior corneal pigmentations, right eye
H18.012 Anterior corneal pigmentations, left eye
H18.013 Anterior corneal pigmentations, bilateral
H18.019 Anterior corneal pigmentations, unspecified eye
H18.02 Argentous corneal deposits
H18.021 Argentous corneal deposits, right eye
H18.022 Argentous corneal deposits, left eye
H18.023 Argentous corneal deposits, bilateral
H18.029 Argentous corneal deposits, unspecified eye
H18.03 Corneal deposits in metabolic disorders
Code also:
associated metabolic disorder
H18.031 Corneal deposits in metabolic disorders, right eye
H18.032 Corneal deposits in metabolic disorders, left eye
H18.033 Corneal deposits in metabolic disorders, bilateral
H18.039 Corneal deposits in metabolic disorders, unspecified eye
H18.04 Kayser-Fleischer ring
Code also:
associated Wilson's disease (E83.01)
DEFINITION Gray-green or brownish ring of copper deposits on the exterior of the cornea that grow slowly inward; often seen with liver disorders.
H18.041 Kayser-Fleischer ring, right eye
H18.042 Kayser-Fleischer ring, left eye
H18.043 Kayser-Fleischer ring, bilateral
H18.049 Kayser-Fleischer ring, unspecified eye
H18.05 Posterior corneal pigmentations
Krukenberg's spindle
H18.051 Posterior corneal pigmentations, right eye
H18.052 Posterior corneal pigmentations, left eye
H18.053 Posterior corneal pigmentations, bilateral
H18.059 Posterior corneal pigmentations, unspecified eye
H18.06 Stromal corneal pigmentations
Hematocornea
H18.061 Stromal corneal pigmentations, right eye
H18.062 Stromal corneal pigmentations, left eye
H18.063 Stromal corneal pigmentations, bilateral
H18.069 Stromal corneal pigmentations, unspecified eye
H18.1 Bullous keratopathy
H18.10 Bullous keratopathy, unspecified eye
H18.11 Bullous keratopathy, right eye
H18.12 Bullous keratopathy, left eye
H18.13 Bullous keratopathy, bilateral
H18.2 Other and unspecified corneal edema
H18.20 Unspecified corneal edema
H18.21 Corneal edema secondary to contact lens
EXCLUDES 2 *other corneal disorders due to contact lens (H18.82-)*
H18.211 Corneal edema secondary to contact lens, right eye
H18.212 Corneal edema secondary to contact lens, left eye
H18.213 Corneal edema secondary to contact lens, bilateral
H18.219 Corneal edema secondary to contact lens, unspecified eye
H18.22 Idiopathic corneal edema
H18.221 Idiopathic corneal edema, right eye
H18.222 Idiopathic corneal edema, left eye
H18.223 Idiopathic corneal edema, bilateral
H18.229 Idiopathic corneal edema, unspecified eye
H18.23 Secondary corneal edema
H18.231 Secondary corneal edema, right eye
H18.232 Secondary corneal edema, left eye
H18.233 Secondary corneal edema, bilateral
H18.239 Secondary corneal edema, unspecified eye
H18.3 Changes of corneal membranes
H18.30 Unspecified corneal membrane change
H18.31 Folds and rupture in Bowman's membrane
H18.311 Folds and rupture in Bowman's membrane, right eye
H18.312 Folds and rupture in Bowman's membrane, left eye
H18.313 Folds and rupture in Bowman's membrane, bilateral
H18.319 Folds and rupture in Bowman's membrane, unspecified eye
H18.32 Folds in Descemet's membrane
DEFINITION Fold in the membrane between the innermost layer of the cornea and the stroma (strong, supportive layer), affecting vision and preventing the flow of nutrients out of the cornea.
H18.321 Folds in Descemet's membrane, right eye
H18.322 Folds in Descemet's membrane, left eye
H18.323 Folds in Descemet's membrane, bilateral
H18.329 Folds in Descemet's membrane, unspecified eye
H18.33 Rupture in Descemet's membrane
H18.331 Rupture in Descemet's membrane, right eye
H18.332 Rupture in Descemet's membrane, left eye
H18.333 Rupture in Descemet's membrane, bilateral
H18.339 Rupture in Descemet's membrane, unspecified eye
H18.4 Corneal degeneration
EXCLUDES 1 *Mooren's ulcer (H16.0-)*
recurrent erosion of cornea (H18.83-)
H18.40 Unspecified corneal degeneration
H18.41 Arcus senilis
Senile corneal changes
H18.411 Arcus senilis, right eye
H18.412 Arcus senilis, left eye

H18.413 Arcus senilis, bilateral
H18.419 Arcus senilis, unspecified eye
H18.42 Band keratopathy

DEFINITION Degeneration of the cornea in which calcium deposits are laid in horizontal band-like layers, obscuring the patient's vision.

H18.421 Band keratopathy, right eye
H18.422 Band keratopathy, left eye
H18.423 Band keratopathy, bilateral
H18.429 Band keratopathy, unspecified eye
H18.43 Other calcerous corneal degeneration
H18.44 Keratomalacia

EXCLUDES 1 *keratomalacia due to vitamin A deficiency (E50.4)*

H18.441 Keratomalacia, right eye
H18.442 Keratomalacia, left eye
H18.443 Keratomalacia, bilateral
H18.449 Keratomalacia, unspecified eye
H18.45 Nodular corneal degeneration
H18.451 Nodular corneal degeneration, right eye
H18.452 Nodular corneal degeneration, left eye
H18.453 Nodular corneal degeneration, bilateral
H18.459 Nodular corneal degeneration, unspecified eye
H18.46 Peripheral corneal degeneration
H18.461 Peripheral corneal degeneration, right eye
H18.462 Peripheral corneal degeneration, left eye
H18.463 Peripheral corneal degeneration, bilateral
H18.469 Peripheral corneal degeneration, unspecified eye
H18.49 Other corneal degeneration
H18.5 Hereditary corneal dystrophies
H18.50 Unspecified hereditary corneal dystrophies
H18.51 Endothelial corneal dystrophy
Fuchs' dystrophy
H18.52 Epithelial (juvenile) corneal dystrophy

DEFINITION Multiple lesions on the outermost layer of the cornea occurring in the early years, which gradually grow together and obscure vision.

H18.53 Granular corneal dystrophy
H18.54 Lattice corneal dystrophy
H18.55 Macular corneal dystrophy
H18.59 Other hereditary corneal dystrophies
H18.6 Keratoconus
H18.60 Keratoconus, unspecified
H18.601 Keratoconus, unspecified, right eye
H18.602 Keratoconus, unspecified, left eye
H18.603 Keratoconus, unspecified, bilateral
H18.609 Keratoconus, unspecified, unspecified eye
H18.61 Keratoconus, stable
H18.611 Keratoconus, stable, right eye
H18.612 Keratoconus, stable, left eye
H18.613 Keratoconus, stable, bilateral
H18.619 Keratoconus, stable, unspecified eye
H18.62 Keratoconus, unstable
Acute hydrops
H18.621 Keratoconus, unstable, right eye
H18.622 Keratoconus, unstable, left eye
H18.623 Keratoconus, unstable, bilateral
H18.629 Keratoconus, unstable, unspecified eye
H18.7 Other and unspecified corneal deformities

EXCLUDES 1 *congenital malformations of cornea (Q13.3-Q13.4)*

H18.70 Unspecified corneal deformity
H18.71 Corneal ectasia
H18.711 Corneal ectasia, right eye
H18.712 Corneal ectasia, left eye
H18.713 Corneal ectasia, bilateral
H18.719 Corneal ectasia, unspecified eye
H18.72 Corneal staphyloma
H18.721 Corneal staphyloma, right eye
H18.722 Corneal staphyloma, left eye
H18.723 Corneal staphyloma, bilateral
H18.729 Corneal staphyloma, unspecified eye
H18.73 Descemetocele
H18.731 Descemetocele, right eye
H18.732 Descemetocele, left eye
H18.733 Descemetocele, bilateral
H18.739 Descemetocele, unspecified eye
H18.79 Other corneal deformities
H18.791 Other corneal deformities, right eye
H18.792 Other corneal deformities, left eye
H18.793 Other corneal deformities, bilateral
H18.799 Other corneal deformities, unspecified eye
H18.8 Other specified disorders of cornea
H18.81 Anesthesia and hypoesthesia of cornea

DEFINITION Decreased or complete loss of corneal sensitivity to pain and irritation.

H18.811 Anesthesia and hypoesthesia of cornea, right eye
H18.812 Anesthesia and hypoesthesia of cornea, left eye
H18.813 Anesthesia and hypoesthesia of cornea, bilateral
H18.819 Anesthesia and hypoesthesia of cornea, unspecified eye
H18.82 Corneal disorder due to contact lens

EXCLUDES 2 *corneal edema due to contact lens (H18.21-)*

H18.821 Corneal disorder due to contact lens, right eye
H18.822 Corneal disorder due to contact lens, left eye
H18.823 Corneal disorder due to contact lens, bilateral
H18.829 Corneal disorder due to contact lens, unspecified eye
H18.83 Recurrent erosion of cornea
H18.831 Recurrent erosion of cornea, right eye
H18.832 Recurrent erosion of cornea, left eye
H18.833 Recurrent erosion of cornea, bilateral
H18.839 Recurrent erosion of cornea, unspecified eye
H18.89 Other specified disorders of cornea
H18.891 Other specified disorders of cornea, right eye
H18.892 Other specified disorders of cornea, left eye
H18.893 Other specified disorders of cornea, bilateral
H18.899 Other specified disorders of cornea, unspecified eye
H18.9 Unspecified disorder of cornea

H20 Iridocyclitis

H20.0 Acute and subacute iridocyclitis
Acute anterior uveitis
Acute cyclitis
Acute iritis
Subacute anterior uveitis
Subacute cyclitis
Subacute iritis

EXCLUDES 1 *iridocyclitis, iritis, uveitis (due to) (in) diabetes mellitus (E08-E13 with .39)*
iridocyclitis, iritis, uveitis (due to) (in) diphtheria (A36.89)
iridocyclitis, iritis, uveitis (due to) (in) gonococcal (A54.32)
iridocyclitis, iritis, uveitis (due to) (in) herpes (simplex) (B00.51)
iridocyclitis, iritis, uveitis (due to) (in) herpes zoster (B02.32)
iridocyclitis, iritis, uveitis (due to) (in) late congenital syphilis (A50.39)
iridocyclitis, iritis, uveitis (due to) (in) late syphilis (A52.71)
iridocyclitis, iritis, uveitis (due to) (in) sarcoidosis (D86.83)
iridocyclitis, iritis, uveitis (due to) (in) syphilis (A51.43)
iridocyclitis, iritis, uveitis (due to) (in) toxoplasmosis (B58.09)
iridocyclitis, iritis, uveitis (due to) (in) tuberculosis (A18.54)

H20.00 Unspecified acute and subacute iridocyclitis
H20.01 Primary iridocyclitis
H20.011 Primary iridocyclitis, right eye
H20.012 Primary iridocyclitis, left eye
H20.013 Primary iridocyclitis, bilateral

H20.019 Primary iridocyclitis, unspecified eye
H20.02 Recurrent acute iridocyclitis
H20.021 Recurrent acute iridocyclitis, right eye
H20.022 Recurrent acute iridocyclitis, left eye
H20.023 Recurrent acute iridocyclitis, bilateral
H20.029 Recurrent acute iridocyclitis, unspecified eye
H20.03 Secondary infectious iridocyclitis
H20.031 Secondary infectious iridocyclitis, right eye
H20.032 Secondary infectious iridocyclitis, left eye
H20.033 Secondary infectious iridocyclitis, bilateral
H20.039 Secondary infectious iridocyclitis, unspecified eye
H20.04 Secondary noninfectious iridocyclitis
H20.041 Secondary noninfectious iridocyclitis, right eye
H20.042 Secondary noninfectious iridocyclitis, left eye
H20.043 Secondary noninfectious iridocyclitis, bilateral
H20.049 Secondary noninfectious iridocyclitis, unspecified eye
H20.05 Hypopyon
DEFINITION Accumulation of pus in the anterior chamber of the eye between the cornea and the iris and lens.
H20.051 Hypopyon, right eye
H20.052 Hypopyon, left eye
H20.053 Hypopyon, bilateral
H20.059 Hypopyon, unspecified eye
H20.1 Chronic iridocyclitis
Use additional code for any associated cataract (H26.21-)
EXCLUDES 2 *posterior cyclitis (H30.2-)*
H20.10 Chronic iridocyclitis, unspecified eye
H20.11 Chronic iridocyclitis, right eye
H20.12 Chronic iridocyclitis, left eye
H20.13 Chronic iridocyclitis, bilateral
H20.2 Lens-induced iridocyclitis
H20.20 Lens-induced iridocyclitis, unspecified eye
H20.21 Lens-induced iridocyclitis, right eye
H20.22 Lens-induced iridocyclitis, left eye
H20.23 Lens-induced iridocyclitis, bilateral
H20.8 Other iridocyclitis
EXCLUDES 2 *glaucomatocyclitis crises (H40.4-)*
posterior cyclitis (H30.2-)
sympathetic uveitis (H44.13-)
H20.81 Fuchs' heterochromic cyclitis
H20.811 Fuchs' heterochromic cyclitis, right eye
H20.812 Fuchs' heterochromic cyclitis, left eye
H20.813 Fuchs' heterochromic cyclitis, bilateral
H20.819 Fuchs' heterochromic cyclitis, unspecified eye
H20.82 Vogt-Koyanagi syndrome
H20.821 Vogt-Koyanagi syndrome, right eye
H20.822 Vogt-Koyanagi syndrome, left eye
H20.823 Vogt-Koyanagi syndrome, bilateral
H20.829 Vogt-Koyanagi syndrome, unspecified eye
H20.9 Unspecified iridocyclitis
Uveitis NOS
H21 Other disorders of iris and ciliary body
EXCLUDES 2 *sympathetic uveitis (H44.1-)*
H21.0 Hyphema
EXCLUDES 1 *traumatic hyphema (S05.1-)*
DEFINITION Bleeding in the iris that pools in the bottom of the cornea causing vision to be extremely blurred.
H21.00 Hyphema, unspecified eye
H21.01 Hyphema, right eye
H21.02 Hyphema, left eye
H21.03 Hyphema, bilateral
H21.1 Other vascular disorders of iris and ciliary body
Neovascularization of iris or ciliary body
Rubeosis iridis
Rubeosis of iris
H21.1X Other vascular disorders of iris and ciliary body
H21.1X1 Other vascular disorders of iris and ciliary body, right eye
H21.1X2 Other vascular disorders of iris and ciliary body, left eye
H21.1X3 Other vascular disorders of iris and ciliary body, bilateral
H21.1X9 Other vascular disorders of iris and ciliary body, unspecified eye
H21.2 Degeneration of iris and ciliary body
H21.21 Degeneration of chamber angle
H21.211 Degeneration of chamber angle, right eye
H21.212 Degeneration of chamber angle, left eye
H21.213 Degeneration of chamber angle, bilateral
H21.219 Degeneration of chamber angle, unspecified eye
H21.22 Degeneration of ciliary body
H21.221 Degeneration of ciliary body, right eye
H21.222 Degeneration of ciliary body, left eye
H21.223 Degeneration of ciliary body, bilateral
H21.229 Degeneration of ciliary body, unspecified eye
H21.23 Degeneration of iris (pigmentary)
Translucency of iris
DEFINITION Fading of the pigmentation (color) of the iris, allowing light to seep in rather than being blocked; presents with light-sensitivity and blurred vision.
H21.231 Degeneration of iris (pigmentary), right eye
H21.232 Degeneration of iris (pigmentary), left eye
H21.233 Degeneration of iris (pigmentary), bilateral
H21.239 Degeneration of iris (pigmentary), unspecified eye
H21.24 Degeneration of pupillary margin
H21.241 Degeneration of pupillary margin, right eye
H21.242 Degeneration of pupillary margin, left eye
H21.243 Degeneration of pupillary margin, bilateral
H21.249 Degeneration of pupillary margin, unspecified eye
H21.25 Iridoschisis
H21.251 Iridoschisis, right eye
H21.252 Iridoschisis, left eye
H21.253 Iridoschisis, bilateral
H21.259 Iridoschisis, unspecified eye
H21.26 Iris atrophy (essential) (progressive)
H21.261 Iris atrophy (essential) (progressive), right eye
H21.262 Iris atrophy (essential) (progressive), left eye
H21.263 Iris atrophy (essential) (progressive), bilateral
H21.269 Iris atrophy (essential) (progressive), unspecified eye
H21.27 Miotic pupillary cyst
DEFINITION Fluid-filled pockets in the iris at the pupil's edge, causing the iris to contract and interfering with vision when light is less than optimal.
H21.271 Miotic pupillary cyst, right eye
H21.272 Miotic pupillary cyst, left eye
H21.273 Miotic pupillary cyst, bilateral
H21.279 Miotic pupillary cyst, unspecified eye
H21.29 Other iris atrophy
H21.3 Cyst of iris, ciliary body and anterior chamber
EXCLUDES 2 *miotic pupillary cyst (H21.27-)*
H21.30 Idiopathic cysts of iris, ciliary body or anterior chamber
Cyst of iris, ciliary body or anterior chamber NOS
H21.301 Idiopathic cysts of iris, ciliary body or anterior chamber, right eye
H21.302 Idiopathic cysts of iris, ciliary body or anterior chamber, left eye
H21.303 Idiopathic cysts of iris, ciliary body or anterior chamber, bilateral

H21.309 Idiopathic cysts of iris, ciliary body or anterior chamber, unspecified eye

H21.31 Exudative cysts of iris or anterior chamber
- H21.311 Exudative cysts of iris or anterior chamber, right eye
- H21.312 Exudative cysts of iris or anterior chamber, left eye
- H21.313 Exudative cysts of iris or anterior chamber, bilateral
- H21.319 Exudative cysts of iris or anterior chamber, unspecified eye

H21.32 Implantation cysts of iris, ciliary body or anterior chamber
- H21.321 Implantation cysts of iris, ciliary body or anterior chamber, right eye
- H21.322 Implantation cysts of iris, ciliary body or anterior chamber, left eye
- H21.323 Implantation cysts of iris, ciliary body or anterior chamber, bilateral
- H21.329 Implantation cysts of iris, ciliary body or anterior chamber, unspecified eye

H21.33 Parasitic cyst of iris, ciliary body or anterior chamber
- H21.331 Parasitic cyst of iris, ciliary body or anterior chamber, right eye
- H21.332 Parasitic cyst of iris, ciliary body or anterior chamber, left eye
- H21.333 Parasitic cyst of iris, ciliary body or anterior chamber, bilateral
- H21.339 Parasitic cyst of iris, ciliary body or anterior chamber, unspecified eye

H21.34 Primary cyst of pars plana
- H21.341 Primary cyst of pars plana, right eye
- H21.342 Primary cyst of pars plana, left eye
- H21.343 Primary cyst of pars plana, bilateral
- H21.349 Primary cyst of pars plana, unspecified eye

H21.35 Exudative cyst of pars plana
- H21.351 Exudative cyst of pars plana, right eye
- H21.352 Exudative cyst of pars plana, left eye
- H21.353 Exudative cyst of pars plana, bilateral
- H21.359 Exudative cyst of pars plana, unspecified eye

H21.4 Pupillary membranes

Iris bombé
Pupillary occlusion
Pupillary seclusion

EXCLUDES 1 *congenital pupillary membranes (Q13.8)*

- H21.40 Pupillary membranes, unspecified eye
- H21.41 Pupillary membranes, right eye
- H21.42 Pupillary membranes, left eye
- H21.43 Pupillary membranes, bilateral

H21.5 Other and unspecified adhesions and disruptions of iris and ciliary body

EXCLUDES 1 *corectopia (Q13.2)*

H21.50 Unspecified adhesions of iris

Synechia (iris) NOS
- H21.501 Unspecified adhesions of iris, right eye
- H21.502 Unspecified adhesions of iris, left eye
- H21.503 Unspecified adhesions of iris, bilateral
- H21.509 Unspecified adhesions of iris and ciliary body, unspecified eye

H21.51 Anterior synechiae (iris)
- H21.511 Anterior synechiae (iris), right eye
- H21.512 Anterior synechiae (iris), left eye
- H21.513 Anterior synechiae (iris), bilateral
- H21.519 Anterior synechiae (iris), unspecified eye

H21.52 Goniosynechiae

DEFINITION Adhesion of the iris to the posterior surface of the cornea, in the angle of the anterior chamber of the eye.
- H21.521 Goniosynechiae, right eye
- H21.522 Goniosynechiae, left eye
- H21.523 Goniosynechiae, bilateral
- H21.529 Goniosynechiae, unspecified eye

H21.53 Iridodialysis

DEFINITION Separation or loosening of the iris from its root at the ciliary body, usually from trauma or surgical accident.
- H21.531 Iridodialysis, right eye
- H21.532 Iridodialysis, left eye
- H21.533 Iridodialysis, bilateral
- H21.539 Iridodialysis, unspecified eye

H21.54 Posterior synechiae (iris)

DEFINITION Adhesion where the lens and the iris grow together, preventing the iris from dilating and contracting properly.
- H21.541 Posterior synechiae (iris), right eye
- H21.542 Posterior synechiae (iris), left eye
- H21.543 Posterior synechiae (iris), bilateral
- H21.549 Posterior synechiae (iris), unspecified eye

H21.55 Recession of chamber angle
- H21.551 Recession of chamber angle, right eye
- H21.552 Recession of chamber angle, left eye
- H21.553 Recession of chamber angle, bilateral
- H21.559 Recession of chamber angle, unspecified eye

H21.56 Pupillary abnormalities

Deformed pupil
Ectopic pupil
Rupture of sphincter, pupil

EXCLUDES 1 *congenital deformity of pupil (Q13.2-)*
- H21.561 Pupillary abnormality, right eye
- H21.562 Pupillary abnormality, left eye
- H21.563 Pupillary abnormality, bilateral
- H21.569 Pupillary abnormality, unspecified eye

H21.8 Other specified disorders of iris and ciliary body

H21.81 Floppy iris syndrome

Intraoperative floppy iris syndrome (IFIS)

Use additional code for adverse effect, if applicable, to identify drug (T36-T50 with fifth or sixth character 5)

DEFINITION Syndrome occurring in one who has taken alpha-blockers; a dilated iris does not stay dilated, causing potentially injurious surgical complications.

H21.82 Plateau iris syndrome (post-iridectomy) (postprocedural)

H21.89 Other specified disorders of iris and ciliary body

H21.9 Unspecified disorder of iris and ciliary body

H22 ***Disorders of iris and ciliary body in diseases classified elsewhere***

Code first underlying disease, such as:
gout (M1A.-, M10.-)
leprosy (A30.-)
parasitic disease (B89)

Disorders of lens (H25-H28)

H25 Age-related cataract

Senile cataract

EXCLUDES 2 *capsular glaucoma with pseudoexfoliation of lens (H40.1-)*

H25.0 Age-related incipient cataract

H25.01 Cortical age-related cataract
- H25.011 Cortical age-related cataract, right eye A
- H25.012 Cortical age-related cataract, left eye A
- H25.013 Cortical age-related cataract, bilateral A
- H25.019 Cortical age-related cataract, unspecified eye A

H25.03 Anterior subcapsular polar age-related cataract
- H25.031 Anterior subcapsular polar age-related cataract, right eye A
- H25.032 Anterior subcapsular polar age-related cataract, left eye A
- H25.033 Anterior subcapsular polar age-related cataract, bilateral A
- H25.039 Anterior subcapsular polar age-related cataract, unspecified eye A

H25.04 Posterior subcapsular polar age-related cataract
- H25.041 Posterior subcapsular polar age-related cataract, right eye A

H25.042 Posterior subcapsular polar age-related cataract, left eye A
H25.043 Posterior subcapsular polar age-related cataract, bilateral A
H25.049 Posterior subcapsular polar age-related cataract, unspecified eye A

H25.09 Other age-related incipient cataract
Coronary age-related cataract
Punctate age-related cataract
Water clefts

H25.091 Other age-related incipient cataract, right eye A
H25.092 Other age-related incipient cataract, left eye A
H25.093 Other age-related incipient cataract, bilateral A
H25.099 Other age-related incipient cataract, unspecified eye A

H25.1 Age-related nuclear cataract
Cataracta brunescens
Nuclear sclerosis cataract

H25.10 Age-related nuclear cataract, unspecified eye A
H25.11 Age-related nuclear cataract, right eye A
H25.12 Age-related nuclear cataract, left eye A
AHA: 1Q 2016, 32-33
H25.13 Age-related nuclear cataract, bilateral A
AHA: 1Q 2016, 32-33

H25.2 Age-related cataract, morgagnian type
Age-related hypermature cataract

H25.20 Age-related cataract, morgagnian type, unspecified eye A
H25.21 Age-related cataract, morgagnian type, right eye A
H25.22 Age-related cataract, morgagnian type, left eye A
H25.23 Age-related cataract, morgagnian type, bilateral A

H25.8 Other age-related cataract

H25.81 Combined forms of age-related cataract

H25.811 Combined forms of age-related cataract, right eye A
H25.812 Combined forms of age-related cataract, left eye A
H25.813 Combined forms of age-related cataract, bilateral A
H25.819 Combined forms of age-related cataract, unspecified eye A

H25.89 Other age-related cataract A

H25.9 Unspecified age-related cataract A

H26 Other cataract

EXCLUDES 1 *congenital cataract (Q12.0)*

DEFINITION Partial or complete clouding on or in the lens or lens capsule of the eye, obscuring vision.

H26.0 Infantile and juvenile cataract

H26.00 Unspecified infantile and juvenile cataract

H26.001 Unspecified infantile and juvenile cataract, right eye P
H26.002 Unspecified infantile and juvenile cataract, left eye P
H26.003 Unspecified infantile and juvenile cataract, bilateral P
H26.009 Unspecified infantile and juvenile cataract, unspecified eye P

H26.01 Infantile and juvenile cortical, lamellar, or zonular cataract

H26.011 Infantile and juvenile cortical, lamellar, or zonular cataract, right eye P
H26.012 Infantile and juvenile cortical, lamellar, or zonular cataract, left eye P
H26.013 Infantile and juvenile cortical, lamellar, or zonular cataract, bilateral P
H26.019 Infantile and juvenile cortical, lamellar, or zonular cataract, unspecified eye P

H26.03 Infantile and juvenile nuclear cataract

H26.031 Infantile and juvenile nuclear cataract, right eye P
H26.032 Infantile and juvenile nuclear cataract, left eye P
H26.033 Infantile and juvenile nuclear cataract, bilateral P
H26.039 Infantile and juvenile nuclear cataract, unspecified eye P

H26.04 Anterior subcapsular polar infantile and juvenile cataract

H26.041 Anterior subcapsular polar infantile and juvenile cataract, right eye P
H26.042 Anterior subcapsular polar infantile and juvenile cataract, left eye P
H26.043 Anterior subcapsular polar infantile and juvenile cataract, bilateral P
H26.049 Anterior subcapsular polar infantile and juvenile cataract, unspecified eye P

H26.05 Posterior subcapsular polar infantile and juvenile cataract

H26.051 Posterior subcapsular polar infantile and juvenile cataract, right eye P
H26.052 Posterior subcapsular polar infantile and juvenile cataract, left eye P
H26.053 Posterior subcapsular polar infantile and juvenile cataract, bilateral P
H26.059 Posterior subcapsular polar infantile and juvenile cataract, unspecified eye P

H26.06 Combined forms of infantile and juvenile cataract

H26.061 Combined forms of infantile and juvenile cataract, right eye P
H26.062 Combined forms of infantile and juvenile cataract, left eye P
H26.063 Combined forms of infantile and juvenile cataract, bilateral P
H26.069 Combined forms of infantile and juvenile cataract, unspecified eye P

H26.09 Other infantile and juvenile cataract P

H26.1 Traumatic cataract
Use additional code (Chapter 20) to identify external cause

H26.10 Unspecified traumatic cataract

H26.101 Unspecified traumatic cataract, right eye
H26.102 Unspecified traumatic cataract, left eye
H26.103 Unspecified traumatic cataract, bilateral
H26.109 Unspecified traumatic cataract, unspecified eye

H26.11 Localized traumatic opacities

H26.111 Localized traumatic opacities, right eye
H26.112 Localized traumatic opacities, left eye
H26.113 Localized traumatic opacities, bilateral
H26.119 Localized traumatic opacities, unspecified eye

H26.12 Partially resolved traumatic cataract

H26.121 Partially resolved traumatic cataract, right eye
H26.122 Partially resolved traumatic cataract, left eye
H26.123 Partially resolved traumatic cataract, bilateral
H26.129 Partially resolved traumatic cataract, unspecified eye

H26.13 Total traumatic cataract

H26.131 Total traumatic cataract, right eye
H26.132 Total traumatic cataract, left eye
H26.133 Total traumatic cataract, bilateral
H26.139 Total traumatic cataract, unspecified eye

H26.2 Complicated cataract

H26.20 Unspecified complicated cataract
Cataracta complicata NOS

H26.21 Cataract with neovascularization
Code also associated condition, such as:
chronic iridocyclitis (H20.1-)

H26.211 Cataract with neovascularization, right eye
H26.212 Cataract with neovascularization, left eye
H26.213 Cataract with neovascularization, bilateral
H26.219 Cataract with neovascularization, unspecified eye

H26.22 Cataract secondary to ocular disorders (degenerative) (inflammatory)
Code also:
associated ocular disorder

H26.221 Cataract secondary to ocular disorders (degenerative) (inflammatory), right eye
H26.222 Cataract secondary to ocular disorders (degenerative) (inflammatory), left eye

☐ **H26.223** **Cataract secondary to ocular disorders (degenerative) (inflammatory), bilateral**

☐ **H26.229** **Cataract secondary to ocular disorders (degenerative) (inflammatory), unspecified eye**

⑤ **H26.23** **Glaucomatous flecks (subcapsular)**
Code first:
  underlying glaucoma (H40-H42)

☐ **H26.231** **Glaucomatous flecks (subcapsular), right eye**

☐ **H26.232** **Glaucomatous flecks (subcapsular), left eye**

☐ **H26.233** **Glaucomatous flecks (subcapsular), bilateral**

☐ **H26.239** **Glaucomatous flecks (subcapsular), unspecified eye**

⑤ **H26.3** **Drug-induced cataract**
Toxic cataract
Use additional code for adverse effect, if applicable, to identify drug (T36-T50 with fifth or sixth character 5)
DEFINITION Cataract caused by exposure to a drug or other toxic substance, such as a miotic, antimiotic, corticosteroid, metal, nitro compound, or substituted hydrocarbon.

☐ **H26.30** **Drug-induced cataract, unspecified eye**

☐ **H26.31** **Drug-induced cataract, right eye**

☐ **H26.32** **Drug-induced cataract, left eye**

☐ **H26.33** **Drug-induced cataract, bilateral**

⑤ **H26.4** **Secondary cataract**

H26.40 **Unspecified secondary cataract**

⑤ **H26.41** **Soemmering's ring**
DEFINITION Doughnut-shaped remnant of lens behind the pupil, occurring after cataract surgery or secondary to trauma.

☐ **H26.411** **Soemmering's ring, right eye**

☐ **H26.412** **Soemmering's ring, left eye**

☐ **H26.413** **Soemmering's ring, bilateral**

☐ **H26.419** **Soemmering's ring, unspecified eye**

⑤ **H26.49** **Other secondary cataract**

☐ **H26.491** **Other secondary cataract, right eye**

☐ **H26.492** **Other secondary cataract, left eye**
AHA: 2Q 2018, 11

☐ **H26.493** **Other secondary cataract, bilateral**

☐ **H26.499** **Other secondary cataract, unspecified eye**

H26.8 **Other specified cataract**

H26.9 **Unspecified cataract**

④ **H27** **Other disorders of lens**
EXCLUDES 1 *congenital lens malformations (Q12.-)*
mechanical complications of intraocular lens implant (T85.2)
pseudophakia (Z96.1)

⑤ **H27.0** **Aphakia**
Acquired absence of lens
Acquired aphakia
Aphakia due to trauma
EXCLUDES 1 *cataract extraction status (Z98.4-)*
congenital absence of lens (Q12.3)
congenital aphakia (Q12.3)
DEFINITION Absence of the crystalline lens of the eye.

☐ **H27.00** **Aphakia, unspecified eye**

☐ **H27.01** **Aphakia, right eye**

☐ **H27.02** **Aphakia, left eye**

☐ **H27.03** **Aphakia, bilateral**

⑤ **H27.1** **Dislocation of lens**

H27.10 **Unspecified dislocation of lens**

⑥ **H27.11** **Subluxation of lens**

☐ **H27.111** **Subluxation of lens, right eye**

☐ **H27.112** **Subluxation of lens, left eye**

☐ **H27.113** **Subluxation of lens, bilateral**

☐ **H27.119** **Subluxation of lens, unspecified eye**

⑥ **H27.12** **Anterior dislocation of lens**

☐ **H27.121** **Anterior dislocation of lens, right eye**

☐ **H27.122** **Anterior dislocation of lens, left eye**

☐ **H27.123** **Anterior dislocation of lens, bilateral**

☐ **H27.129** **Anterior dislocation of lens, unspecified eye**

⑥ **H27.13** **Posterior dislocation of lens**

☐ **H27.131** **Posterior dislocation of lens, right eye**

☐ **H27.132** **Posterior dislocation of lens, left eye**

☐ **H27.133** **Posterior dislocation of lens, bilateral**

☐ **H27.139** **Posterior dislocation of lens, unspecified eye**

H27.8 **Other specified disorders of lens**

H27.9 **Unspecified disorder of lens**

H28 *Cataract in diseases classified elsewhere*
Code first underlying disease, such as:
  hypoparathyroidism (E20.-)
  myotonia (G71.1-)
  myxedema (E03.-)
  protein-calorie malnutrition (E40-E46)
EXCLUDES 1 *cataract in diabetes mellitus*
(E08.36, E09.36, E10.36, E11.36, E13.36)

Disorders of choroid and retina (H30-H36)

④ **H30** **Chorioretinal inflammation**

⑤ **H30.0** **Focal chorioretinal inflammation**
Focal chorioretinitis
Focal choroiditis
Focal retinitis
Focal retinochoroiditis

⑥ **H30.00** **Unspecified focal chorioretinal inflammation**
Focal chorioretinitis NOS
Focal choroiditis NOS
Focal retinitis NOS
Focal retinochoroiditis NOS

☐ **H30.001** **Unspecified focal chorioretinal inflammation, right eye**

☐ **H30.002** **Unspecified focal chorioretinal inflammation, left eye**

☐ **H30.003** **Unspecified focal chorioretinal inflammation, bilateral**

☐ **H30.009** **Unspecified focal chorioretinal inflammation, unspecified eye**

⑥ **H30.01** **Focal chorioretinal inflammation, juxtapapillary**

☐ **H30.011** **Focal chorioretinal inflammation, juxtapapillary, right eye**

☐ **H30.012** **Focal chorioretinal inflammation, juxtapapillary, left eye**

☐ **H30.013** **Focal chorioretinal inflammation, juxtapapillary, bilateral**

☐ **H30.019** **Focal chorioretinal inflammation, juxtapapillary, unspecified eye**

⑥ **H30.02** **Focal chorioretinal inflammation of posterior pole**

☐ **H30.021** **Focal chorioretinal inflammation of posterior pole, right eye**

☐ **H30.022** **Focal chorioretinal inflammation of posterior pole, left eye**

☐ **H30.023** **Focal chorioretinal inflammation of posterior pole, bilateral**

☐ **H30.029** **Focal chorioretinal inflammation of posterior pole, unspecified eye**

⑥ **H30.03** **Focal chorioretinal inflammation, peripheral**

☐ **H30.031** **Focal chorioretinal inflammation, peripheral, right eye**

☐ **H30.032** **Focal chorioretinal inflammation, peripheral, left eye**

☐ **H30.033** **Focal chorioretinal inflammation, peripheral, bilateral**

☐ **H30.039** **Focal chorioretinal inflammation, peripheral, unspecified eye**

⑥ **H30.04** **Focal chorioretinal inflammation, macular or paramacular**

☐ **H30.041** **Focal chorioretinal inflammation, macular or paramacular, right eye**

☐ **H30.042** **Focal chorioretinal inflammation, macular or paramacular, left eye**

☐ **H30.043** **Focal chorioretinal inflammation, macular or paramacular, bilateral**

☐ **H30.049** **Focal chorioretinal inflammation, macular or paramacular, unspecified eye**

● New	*Manifestation*	④-⑦ Digit Indicators	☐ Laterality	Ⓐ Adult	Ⓜ Maternity	Ⓝ Newborn	Ⓟ Pediatric	♂ Male
▲ Revised	Unspecified	AHA Coding Clinic	HCC Hierarchical Condition Categories			HIV HIV Related Conditions		♀ Female

H30.1 Disseminated chorioretinal inflammation
Disseminated chorioretinitis
Disseminated choroiditis
Disseminated retinitis
Disseminated retinochoroiditis
EXCLUDES 2 *exudative retinopathy (H35.02-)*

H30.10 Unspecified disseminated chorioretinal inflammation
Disseminated chorioretinitis NOS
Disseminated choroiditis NOS
Disseminated retinitis NOS
Disseminated retinochoroiditis NOS

H30.101 Unspecified disseminated chorioretinal inflammation, right eye
H30.102 Unspecified disseminated chorioretinal inflammation, left eye
H30.103 Unspecified disseminated chorioretinal inflammation, bilateral
H30.109 Unspecified disseminated chorioretinal inflammation, unspecified eye

H30.11 Disseminated chorioretinal inflammation of posterior pole
H30.111 Disseminated chorioretinal inflammation of posterior pole, right eye
H30.112 Disseminated chorioretinal inflammation of posterior pole, left eye
H30.113 Disseminated chorioretinal inflammation of posterior pole, bilateral
H30.119 Disseminated chorioretinal inflammation of posterior pole, unspecified eye

H30.12 Disseminated chorioretinal inflammation, peripheral
H30.121 Disseminated chorioretinal inflammation, peripheral right eye
H30.122 Disseminated chorioretinal inflammation, peripheral, left eye
H30.123 Disseminated chorioretinal inflammation, peripheral, bilateral
H30.129 Disseminated chorioretinal inflammation, peripheral, unspecified eye

H30.13 Disseminated chorioretinal inflammation, generalized
H30.131 Disseminated chorioretinal inflammation, generalized, right eye
H30.132 Disseminated chorioretinal inflammation, generalized, left eye
H30.133 Disseminated chorioretinal inflammation, generalized, bilateral
H30.139 Disseminated chorioretinal inflammation, generalized, unspecified eye

H30.14 Acute posterior multifocal placoid pigment epitheliopathy
H30.141 Acute posterior multifocal placoid pigment epitheliopathy, right eye
H30.142 Acute posterior multifocal placoid pigment epitheliopathy, left eye
H30.143 Acute posterior multifocal placoid pigment epitheliopathy, bilateral
H30.149 Acute posterior multifocal placoid pigment epitheliopathy, unspecified eye

H30.2 Posterior cyclitis
Pars planitis
DEFINITION Inflammation of the peripheral retina and the ciliary body, the hair-like structures that hold the lens of the eye in place.

H30.20 Posterior cyclitis, unspecified eye
H30.21 Posterior cyclitis, right eye
H30.22 Posterior cyclitis, left eye
H30.23 Posterior cyclitis, bilateral

H30.8 Other chorioretinal inflammations
H30.81 Harada's disease
H30.811 Harada's disease, right eye
H30.812 Harada's disease, left eye
H30.813 Harada's disease, bilateral
H30.819 Harada's disease, unspecified eye

H30.89 Other chorioretinal inflammations
H30.891 Other chorioretinal inflammations, right eye
H30.892 Other chorioretinal inflammations, left eye
H30.893 Other chorioretinal inflammations, bilateral
H30.899 Other chorioretinal inflammations, unspecified eye

H30.9 Unspecified chorioretinal inflammation
Chorioretinitis NOS
Choroiditis NOS
Neuroretinitis NOS
Retinitis NOS
Retinochoroiditis NOS

H30.90 Unspecified chorioretinal inflammation, unspecified eye
H30.91 Unspecified chorioretinal inflammation, right eye
H30.92 Unspecified chorioretinal inflammation, left eye
H30.93 Unspecified chorioretinal inflammation, bilateral

H31 Other disorders of choroid

H31.0 Chorioretinal scars
EXCLUDES 2 *postsurgical chorioretinal scars (H59.81-)*

H31.00 Unspecified chorioretinal scars
H31.001 Unspecified chorioretinal scars, right eye
H31.002 Unspecified chorioretinal scars, left eye
H31.003 Unspecified chorioretinal scars, bilateral
H31.009 Unspecified chorioretinal scars, unspecified eye

H31.01 Macula scars of posterior pole (postinflammatory) (post-traumatic)
EXCLUDES 1 *postprocedural chorioretentinal scar (H59.81-)*

H31.011 Macula scars of posterior pole (postinflammatory) (post-traumatic), right eye
H31.012 Macula scars of posterior pole (postinflammatory) (post-traumatic), left eye
H31.013 Macula scars of posterior pole (postinflammatory) (post-traumatic), bilateral
H31.019 Macula scars of posterior pole (postinflammatory) (post-traumatic), unspecified eye

H31.02 Solar retinopathy
DEFINITION Scar on the retina resulting from solar radiation.

H31.021 Solar retinopathy, right eye
H31.022 Solar retinopathy, left eye
H31.023 Solar retinopathy, bilateral
H31.029 Solar retinopathy, unspecified eye

H31.09 Other chorioretinal scars
H31.091 Other chorioretinal scars, right eye
H31.092 Other chorioretinal scars, left eye
H31.093 Other chorioretinal scars, bilateral
H31.099 Other chorioretinal scars, unspecified eye

H31.1 Choroidal degeneration
EXCLUDES 2 *angioid streaks of macula (H35.33)*

H31.10 Unspecified choroidal degeneration
Choroidal sclerosis NOS

H31.101 Choroidal degeneration, unspecified, right eye
H31.102 Choroidal degeneration, unspecified, left eye
H31.103 Choroidal degeneration, unspecified, bilateral
H31.109 Choroidal degeneration, unspecified, unspecified eye

H31.11 Age-related choroidal atrophy
H31.111 Age-related choroidal atrophy, right eye A
H31.112 Age-related choroidal atrophy, left eye A
H31.113 Age-related choroidal atrophy, bilateral A
H31.119 Age-related choroidal atrophy, unspecified eye A

H31.12 Diffuse secondary atrophy of choroid
H31.121 Diffuse secondary atrophy of choroid, right eye
H31.122 Diffuse secondary atrophy of choroid, left eye
H31.123 Diffuse secondary atrophy of choroid, bilateral

H31.129 Diffuse secondary atrophy of choroid, unspecified eye

H31.2 Hereditary choroidal dystrophy

EXCLUDES 2 *hyperornithinemia (E72.4)*
ornithinemia (E72.4)

H31.20 Hereditary choroidal dystrophy, unspecified

H31.21 Choroideremia

H31.22 Choroidal dystrophy (central areolar) (generalized) (peripapillary)

H31.23 Gyrate atrophy, choroid

H31.29 Other hereditary choroidal dystrophy

H31.3 Choroidal hemorrhage and rupture

H31.30 Unspecified choroidal hemorrhage

H31.301 Unspecified choroidal hemorrhage, right eye

H31.302 Unspecified choroidal hemorrhage, left eye

H31.303 Unspecified choroidal hemorrhage, bilateral

H31.309 Unspecified choroidal hemorrhage, unspecified eye

H31.31 Expulsive choroidal hemorrhage

H31.311 Expulsive choroidal hemorrhage, right eye

H31.312 Expulsive choroidal hemorrhage, left eye

H31.313 Expulsive choroidal hemorrhage, bilateral

H31.319 Expulsive choroidal hemorrhage, unspecified eye

H31.32 Choroidal rupture

H31.321 Choroidal rupture, right eye

H31.322 Choroidal rupture, left eye

H31.323 Choroidal rupture, bilateral

H31.329 Choroidal rupture, unspecified eye

H31.4 Choroidal detachment

H31.40 Unspecified choroidal detachment

H31.401 Unspecified choroidal detachment, right eye

H31.402 Unspecified choroidal detachment, left eye

H31.403 Unspecified choroidal detachment, bilateral

H31.409 Unspecified choroidal detachment, unspecified eye

H31.41 Hemorrhagic choroidal detachment

H31.411 Hemorrhagic choroidal detachment, right eye

H31.412 Hemorrhagic choroidal detachment, left eye

H31.413 Hemorrhagic choroidal detachment, bilateral

H31.419 Hemorrhagic choroidal detachment, unspecified eye

H31.42 Serous choroidal detachment

H31.421 Serous choroidal detachment, right eye

H31.422 Serous choroidal detachment, left eye

H31.423 Serous choroidal detachment, bilateral

H31.429 Serous choroidal detachment, unspecified eye

H31.8 Other specified disorders of choroid

H31.9 Unspecified disorder of choroid

H32 ***Chorioretinal disorders in diseases classified elsewhere***

Code first underlying disease, such as:
congenital toxoplasmosis (P37.1)
histoplasmosis (B39.-)
leprosy (A30.-)

EXCLUDES 1 *chorioretinitis (in) :*
toxoplasmosis (acquired) (B58.01)
tuberculosis (A18.53)

H33 **Retinal detachments and breaks**

EXCLUDES 1 *detachment of retinal pigment epithelium (H35.72-, H35.73-)*

DEFINITION Condition in which the retina separates from its underlying layer of cells in the back of the eye, resulting in a decrease in the visual field or blindness.

H33.0 Retinal detachment with retinal break

Rhegmatogenous retinal detachment

EXCLUDES 1 *serous retinal detachment (without retinal break) (H33.2-)*

H33.00 Unspecified retinal detachment with retinal break

H33.001 Unspecified retinal detachment with retinal break, right eye

H33.002 Unspecified retinal detachment with retinal break, left eye

H33.003 Unspecified retinal detachment with retinal break, bilateral

H33.009 Unspecified retinal detachment with retinal break, unspecified eye

H33.01 Retinal detachment with single break

H33.011 Retinal detachment with single break, right eye

H33.012 Retinal detachment with single break, left eye

H33.013 Retinal detachment with single break, bilateral

H33.019 Retinal detachment with single break, unspecified eye

H33.02 Retinal detachment with multiple breaks

H33.021 Retinal detachment with multiple breaks, right eye

H33.022 Retinal detachment with multiple breaks, left eye

H33.023 Retinal detachment with multiple breaks, bilateral

H33.029 Retinal detachment with multiple breaks, unspecified eye

H33.03 Retinal detachment with giant retinal tear

H33.031 Retinal detachment with giant retinal tear, right eye

H33.032 Retinal detachment with giant retinal tear, left eye

H33.033 Retinal detachment with giant retinal tear, bilateral

H33.039 Retinal detachment with giant retinal tear, unspecified eye

H33.04 Retinal detachment with retinal dialysis

H33.041 Retinal detachment with retinal dialysis, right eye

H33.042 Retinal detachment with retinal dialysis, left eye

H33.043 Retinal detachment with retinal dialysis, bilateral

H33.049 Retinal detachment with retinal dialysis, unspecified eye

H33.05 Total retinal detachment

H33.051 Total retinal detachment, right eye

H33.052 Total retinal detachment, left eye

H33.053 Total retinal detachment, bilateral

H33.059 Total retinal detachment, unspecified eye

H33.1 Retinoschisis and retinal cysts

EXCLUDES 1 *congenital retinoschisis (Q14.1)*
microcystoid degeneration of retina (H35.42-)

H33.10 Unspecified retinoschisis

H33.101 Unspecified retinoschisis, right eye

H33.102 Unspecified retinoschisis, left eye

H33.103 Unspecified retinoschisis, bilateral

H33.109 Unspecified retinoschisis, unspecified eye

H33.11 Cyst of ora serrata

H33.111 Cyst of ora serrata, right eye

H33.112 Cyst of ora serrata, left eye

H33.113 Cyst of ora serrata, bilateral

H33.119 Cyst of ora serrata, unspecified eye

H33.12 Parasitic cyst of retina

H33.121 Parasitic cyst of retina, right eye

H33.122 Parasitic cyst of retina, left eye

H33.123 Parasitic cyst of retina, bilateral

H33.129 Parasitic cyst of retina, unspecified eye

H33.19 Other retinoschisis and retinal cysts

Pseudocyst of retina

H33.191 Other retinoschisis and retinal cysts, right eye

H33.192 Other retinoschisis and retinal cysts, left eye

H33.193 Other retinoschisis and retinal cysts, bilateral

H33.199 Other retinoschisis and retinal cysts, unspecified eye

H33.2 Serous retinal detachment

Retinal detachment NOS
Retinal detachment without retinal break

EXCLUDES 1 *central serous chorioretinopathy (H35.71-)*

H33.20 Serous retinal detachment, unspecified eye

H33.21 Serous retinal detachment, right eye
H33.22 Serous retinal detachment, left eye
H33.23 Serous retinal detachment, bilateral

H33.3 Retinal breaks without detachment
EXCLUDES 1 *chorioretinal scars after surgery for detachment (H59.81-)*
peripheral retinal degeneration without break (H35.4-)

H33.30 Unspecified retinal break
H33.301 Unspecified retinal break, right eye
H33.302 Unspecified retinal break, left eye
H33.303 Unspecified retinal break, bilateral
H33.309 Unspecified retinal break, unspecified eye

H33.31 Horseshoe tear of retina without detachment
Operculum of retina without detachment
H33.311 Horseshoe tear of retina without detachment, right eye
H33.312 Horseshoe tear of retina without detachment, left eye
H33.313 Horseshoe tear of retina without detachment, bilateral
H33.319 Horseshoe tear of retina without detachment, unspecified eye

H33.32 Round hole of retina without detachment
H33.321 Round hole, right eye
H33.322 Round hole, left eye
H33.323 Round hole, bilateral
H33.329 Round hole, unspecified eye

H33.33 Multiple defects of retina without detachment
H33.331 Multiple defects of retina without detachment, right eye
H33.332 Multiple defects of retina without detachment, left eye
H33.333 Multiple defects of retina without detachment, bilateral
H33.339 Multiple defects of retina without detachment, unspecified eye

H33.4 Traction detachment of retina
Proliferative vitreo-retinopathy with retinal detachment
H33.40 Traction detachment of retina, unspecified eye
H33.41 Traction detachment of retina, right eye
H33.42 Traction detachment of retina, left eye
H33.43 Traction detachment of retina, bilateral

H33.8 Other retinal detachments

H34 Retinal vascular occlusions
EXCLUDES 1 *amaurosis fugax (G45.3)*

H34.0 Transient retinal artery occlusion
H34.00 Transient retinal artery occlusion, unspecified eye
H34.01 Transient retinal artery occlusion, right eye
H34.02 Transient retinal artery occlusion, left eye
H34.03 Transient retinal artery occlusion, bilateral

H34.1 Central retinal artery occlusion
H34.10 Central retinal artery occlusion, unspecified eye
H34.11 Central retinal artery occlusion, right eye
H34.12 Central retinal artery occlusion, left eye
H34.13 Central retinal artery occlusion, bilateral

H34.2 Other retinal artery occlusions
H34.21 Partial retinal artery occlusion
Hollenhorst's plaque
Retinal microembolism
H34.211 Partial retinal artery occlusion, right eye
H34.212 Partial retinal artery occlusion, left eye
H34.213 Partial retinal artery occlusion, bilateral
H34.219 Partial retinal artery occlusion, unspecified eye

H34.23 Retinal artery branch occlusion
H34.231 Retinal artery branch occlusion, right eye
H34.232 Retinal artery branch occlusion, left eye
H34.233 Retinal artery branch occlusion, bilateral
H34.239 Retinal artery branch occlusion, unspecified eye

H34.8 Other retinal vascular occlusions
AHA: 4Q 2016, 19

H34.81 Central retinal vein occlusion
One of the following 7th characters is to be assigned to codes in subcategory H34.81 to designate the severity of the occlusion:
0 with macular edema
1 with retinal neovascularization
2 stable

H34.811- Central retinal vein occlusion, right eye
H34.812- Central retinal vein occlusion, left eye
H34.813- Central retinal vein occlusion, bilateral
H34.819- Central retinal vein occlusion, unspecified eye

H34.82 Venous engorgement
Incipient retinal vein occlusion
Partial retinal vein occlusion
H34.821 Venous engorgement, right eye
H34.822 Venous engorgement, left eye
H34.823 Venous engorgement, bilateral
H34.829 Venous engorgement, unspecified eye

H34.83 Tributary (branch) retinal vein occlusion
One of the following 7th characters is to be assigned to codes in subcategory H34.83 to designate the severity of the occlusion:
0 with macular edema
1 with retinal neovascularization
2 stable

H34.831- Tributary (branch) retinal vein occlusion, right eye
H34.832- Tributary (branch) retinal vein occlusion, left eye
H34.833- Tributary (branch) retinal vein occlusion, bilateral
H34.839- Tributary (branch) retinal vein occlusion, unspecified eye

H34.9 Unspecified retinal vascular occlusion

H35 Other retinal disorders
EXCLUDES 2 *diabetic retinal disorders (E08.311-E08.359, E09.311-E09.359, E10.311-E10.359, E11.311-E11.359, E13.311-E13.359)*

H35.0 Background retinopathy and retinal vascular changes
Code also:
any associated hypertension (I10.-)

GUIDELINES **Section I.C.9.a.5)**
Subcategory H35.0, Background retinopathy and retinal vascular changes, should be used with a code from category I10-I15, Hypertensive disease to include the systemic hypertension. The sequencing is based on the reason for the encounter.

H35.00 Unspecified background retinopathy

H35.01 Changes in retinal vascular appearance
Retinal vascular sheathing
H35.011 Changes in retinal vascular appearance, right eye
H35.012 Changes in retinal vascular appearance, left eye
H35.013 Changes in retinal vascular appearance, bilateral
H35.019 Changes in retinal vascular appearance, unspecified eye

H35.02 Exudative retinopathy
Coats retinopathy
H35.021 Exudative retinopathy, right eye
H35.022 Exudative retinopathy, left eye
H35.023 Exudative retinopathy, bilateral
H35.029 Exudative retinopathy, unspecified eye

H35.03 Hypertensive retinopathy
H35.031 Hypertensive retinopathy, right eye
H35.032 Hypertensive retinopathy, left eye
H35.033 Hypertensive retinopathy, bilateral
H35.039 Hypertensive retinopathy, unspecified eye

H35.04 Retinal micro-aneurysms, unspecified
H35.041 Retinal micro-aneurysms, unspecified, right eye
H35.042 Retinal micro-aneurysms, unspecified, left eye
H35.043 Retinal micro-aneurysms, unspecified, bilateral

H35.049 **Retinal micro-aneurysms, unspecified, unspecified eye**

H35.05 **Retinal neovascularization, unspecified**

H35.051 **Retinal neovascularization, unspecified, right eye**

H35.052 **Retinal neovascularization, unspecified, left eye**

H35.053 **Retinal neovascularization, unspecified, bilateral**

H35.059 **Retinal neovascularization, unspecified, unspecified eye**

H35.06 **Retinal vasculitis**

Eales disease
Retinal perivasculitis

H35.061 **Retinal vasculitis, right eye**

H35.062 **Retinal vasculitis, left eye**

H35.063 **Retinal vasculitis, bilateral**

H35.069 **Retinal vasculitis, unspecified eye**

H35.07 **Retinal telangiectasis**

H35.071 **Retinal telangiectasis, right eye**

H35.072 **Retinal telangiectasis, left eye**

H35.073 **Retinal telangiectasis, bilateral**

H35.079 **Retinal telangiectasis, unspecified eye**

H35.09 **Other intraretinal microvascular abnormalities**

Retinal varices

H35.1 **Retinopathy of prematurity**

H35.10 **Retinopathy of prematurity, unspecified**

Retinopathy of prematurity NOS

H35.101 **Retinopathy of prematurity, unspecified, right eye**

H35.102 **Retinopathy of prematurity, unspecified, left eye**

H35.103 **Retinopathy of prematurity, unspecified, bilateral**

H35.109 **Retinopathy of prematurity, unspecified, unspecified eye**

H35.11 **Retinopathy of prematurity, stage 0**

H35.111 **Retinopathy of prematurity, stage 0, right eye**

H35.112 **Retinopathy of prematurity, stage 0, left eye**

H35.113 **Retinopathy of prematurity, stage 0, bilateral**

H35.119 **Retinopathy of prematurity, stage 0, unspecified eye**

H35.12 **Retinopathy of prematurity, stage 1**

H35.121 **Retinopathy of prematurity, stage 1, right eye**

H35.122 **Retinopathy of prematurity, stage 1, left eye**

H35.123 **Retinopathy of prematurity, stage 1, bilateral**

H35.129 **Retinopathy of prematurity, stage 1, unspecified eye**

H35.13 **Retinopathy of prematurity, stage 2**

H35.131 **Retinopathy of prematurity, stage 2, right eye**

H35.132 **Retinopathy of prematurity, stage 2, left eye**

H35.133 **Retinopathy of prematurity, stage 2, bilateral**

H35.139 **Retinopathy of prematurity, stage 2, unspecified eye**

H35.14 **Retinopathy of prematurity, stage 3**

H35.141 **Retinopathy of prematurity, stage 3, right eye**

H35.142 **Retinopathy of prematurity, stage 3, left eye**

H35.143 **Retinopathy of prematurity, stage 3, bilateral**

H35.149 **Retinopathy of prematurity, stage 3, unspecified eye**

H35.15 **Retinopathy of prematurity, stage 4**

H35.151 **Retinopathy of prematurity, stage 4, right eye**

H35.152 **Retinopathy of prematurity, stage 4, left eye**

H35.153 **Retinopathy of prematurity, stage 4, bilateral**

H35.159 **Retinopathy of prematurity, stage 4, unspecified eye**

H35.16 **Retinopathy of prematurity, stage 5**

H35.161 **Retinopathy of prematurity, stage 5, right eye**

H35.162 **Retinopathy of prematurity, stage 5, left eye**

H35.163 **Retinopathy of prematurity, stage 5, bilateral**

H35.169 **Retinopathy of prematurity, stage 5, unspecified eye**

H35.17 **Retrolental fibroplasia**

H35.171 **Retrolental fibroplasia, right eye**

H35.172 **Retrolental fibroplasia, left eye**

H35.173 **Retrolental fibroplasia, bilateral**

H35.179 **Retrolental fibroplasia, unspecified eye**

H35.2 **Other non-diabetic proliferative retinopathy**

Proliferative vitreo-retinopathy

EXCLUDES 1 *proliferative vitreo-retinopathy with retinal detachment (H33.4-)*

H35.20 **Other non-diabetic proliferative retinopathy, unspecified eye**

H35.21 **Other non-diabetic proliferative retinopathy, right eye**

H35.22 **Other non-diabetic proliferative retinopathy, left eye**

H35.23 **Other non-diabetic proliferative retinopathy, bilateral**

H35.3 **Degeneration of macula and posterior pole**

H35.30 **Unspecified macular degeneration** A

Age-related macular degeneration

H35.31 **Nonexudative age-related macular degeneration**

Atrophic age-related macular degeneration
Dry age-related macular degeneration

One of the following 7th characters is to be assigned to codes in subcategory H35.31 to designate the stage of the disease:

0	stage unspecified
1	early dry stage
2	intermediate dry stage
3	advanced atrophic without subfoveal involvement
4	advanced atrophic with subfoveal involvement

AHA: 4Q 2016, 20

H35.311- **Nonexudative age-related macular degeneration, right eye** A

H35.312- **Nonexudative age-related macular degeneration, left eye** A

H35.313- **Nonexudative age-related macular degeneration, bilateral** A

H35.319- **Nonexudative age-related macular degeneration, unspecified eye** A

H35.32 **Exudative age-related macular degeneration**

Wet age-related macular degeneration

One of the following 7th characters is to be assigned to codes in subcategory H35.32 to designate the stage of the disease:

0	stage unspecified
1	with active choroidal neovascularization
2	with inactive choroidal neovascularization
3	with inactive scar

AHA: 4Q 2016, 20

H35.321- **Exudative age-related macular degeneration, right eye** A HCC

H35.322- **Exudative age-related macular degeneration, left eye** A HCC

H35.323- **Exudative age-related macular degeneration, bilateral** A HCC

H35.329- **Exudative age-related macular degeneration, unspecified eye** A HCC

H35.33 **Angioid streaks of macula**

H35.34 **Macular cyst, hole, or pseudohole**

H35.341 **Macular cyst, hole, or pseudohole, right eye**

H35.342 **Macular cyst, hole, or pseudohole, left eye**

H35.343 **Macular cyst, hole, or pseudohole, bilateral**

H35.349 **Macular cyst, hole, or pseudohole, unspecified eye**

H35.35 **Cystoid macular degeneration**

EXCLUDES 1 *cystoid macular edema following cataract surgery (H59.03-)*

H35.351 **Cystoid macular degeneration, right eye**

H35.352 **Cystoid macular degeneration, left eye**

H35.353 **Cystoid macular degeneration, bilateral**

H35.359 **Cystoid macular degeneration, unspecified eye**

H35.36 **Drusen (degenerative) of macula**

DEFINITION Small, bright deposits or accumulations of material seen in the retina and/or optic disc that are associated with a variety of eye diseases including macular degeneration, hereditary retinal degeneration, and loss of peripheral vision.

- H35.361 **Drusen (degenerative) of macula, right eye**
- H35.362 **Drusen (degenerative) of macula, left eye**
- H35.363 **Drusen (degenerative) of macula, bilateral**
  AHA: 1Q 2017, 51
- H35.369 **Drusen (degenerative) of macula, unspecified eye**

6 H35.37 **Puckering of macula**
- H35.371 **Puckering of macula, right eye**
- H35.372 **Puckering of macula, left eye**
- H35.373 **Puckering of macula, bilateral**
- H35.379 **Puckering of macula, unspecified eye**

6 H35.38 **Toxic maculopathy**
Code first:
poisoning due to drug or toxin, if applicable (T36-T65 with fifth or sixth character 1-4 or 6)
Use additional code for adverse effect, if applicable, to identify drug (T36-T50 with fifth or sixth character 5)
- H35.381 **Toxic maculopathy, right eye**
- H35.382 **Toxic maculopathy, left eye**
- H35.383 **Toxic maculopathy, bilateral**
- H35.389 **Toxic maculopathy, unspecified eye**

5 H35.4 **Peripheral retinal degeneration**
EXCLUDES 1 *hereditary retinal degeneration (dystrophy) (H35.5-)*
peripheral retinal degeneration with retinal break (H33.3-)

H35.40 **Unspecified peripheral retinal degeneration**

6 H35.41 **Lattice degeneration of retina**
Palisade degeneration of retina
- H35.411 **Lattice degeneration of retina, right eye**
- H35.412 **Lattice degeneration of retina, left eye**
- H35.413 **Lattice degeneration of retina, bilateral**
- H35.419 **Lattice degeneration of retina, unspecified eye**

6 H35.42 **Microcystoid degeneration of retina**
- H35.421 **Microcystoid degeneration of retina, right eye**
- H35.422 **Microcystoid degeneration of retina, left eye**
- H35.423 **Microcystoid degeneration of retina, bilateral**
- H35.429 **Microcystoid degeneration of retina, unspecified eye**

6 H35.43 **Paving stone degeneration of retina**
- H35.431 **Paving stone degeneration of retina, right eye**
- H35.432 **Paving stone degeneration of retina, left eye**
- H35.433 **Paving stone degeneration of retina, bilateral**
- H35.439 **Paving stone degeneration of retina, unspecified eye**

6 H35.44 **Age-related reticular degeneration of retina**
- H35.441 **Age-related reticular degeneration of retina, right eye** A
- H35.442 **Age-related reticular degeneration of retina, left eye** A
- H35.443 **Age-related reticular degeneration of retina, bilateral** A
- H35.449 **Age-related reticular degeneration of retina, unspecified eye** A

6 H35.45 **Secondary pigmentary degeneration**
- H35.451 **Secondary pigmentary degeneration, right eye**
- H35.452 **Secondary pigmentary degeneration, left eye**
- H35.453 **Secondary pigmentary degeneration, bilateral**
- H35.459 **Secondary pigmentary degeneration, unspecified eye**

6 H35.46 **Secondary vitreoretinal degeneration**
- H35.461 **Secondary vitreoretinal degeneration, right eye**
- H35.462 **Secondary vitreoretinal degeneration, left eye**
- H35.463 **Secondary vitreoretinal degeneration, bilateral**
- H35.469 **Secondary vitreoretinal degeneration, unspecified eye**

5 H35.5 **Hereditary retinal dystrophy**
EXCLUDES 1 *dystrophies primarily involving Bruch's membrane (H31.1-)*

H35.50 **Unspecified hereditary retinal dystrophy**
H35.51 **Vitreoretinal dystrophy**
H35.52 **Pigmentary retinal dystrophy**
Albipunctate retinal dystrophy
Retinitis pigmentosa
Tapetoretinal dystrophy
H35.53 **Other dystrophies primarily involving the sensory retina**
Stargardt's disease

DEFINITION Stargardt's disease: genetic condition causing degeneration of the macula, occurring by age 20, with rapid loss of visual acuity and abnormal pigmentation of the macula.

H35.54 **Dystrophies primarily involving the retinal pigment epithelium**
Vitelliform retinal dystrophy

5 H35.6 **Retinal hemorrhage**
- H35.60 **Retinal hemorrhage, unspecified eye**
- H35.61 **Retinal hemorrhage, right eye**
- H35.62 **Retinal hemorrhage, left eye**
- H35.63 **Retinal hemorrhage, bilateral**

5 H35.7 **Separation of retinal layers**
EXCLUDES 1 *retinal detachment (serous) (H33.2-)*
rhegmatogenous retinal detachment (H33.0-)

H35.70 **Unspecified separation of retinal layers**

6 H35.71 **Central serous chorioretinopathy**

DEFINITION Fluid seepage from the choroid into the retina, causing the retinal layers to fill and separate from each other.

- H35.711 **Central serous chorioretinopathy, right eye**
- H35.712 **Central serous chorioretinopathy, left eye**
- H35.713 **Central serous chorioretinopathy, bilateral**
- H35.719 **Central serous chorioretinopathy, unspecified eye**

6 H35.72 **Serous detachment of retinal pigment epithelium**
- H35.721 **Serous detachment of retinal pigment epithelium, right eye**
- H35.722 **Serous detachment of retinal pigment epithelium, left eye**
- H35.723 **Serous detachment of retinal pigment epithelium, bilateral**
- H35.729 **Serous detachment of retinal pigment epithelium, unspecified eye**

6 H35.73 **Hemorrhagic detachment of retinal pigment epithelium**
- H35.731 **Hemorrhagic detachment of retinal pigment epithelium, right eye**
- H35.732 **Hemorrhagic detachment of retinal pigment epithelium, left eye**
- H35.733 **Hemorrhagic detachment of retinal pigment epithelium, bilateral**
- H35.739 **Hemorrhagic detachment of retinal pigment epithelium, unspecified eye**

5 H35.8 **Other specified retinal disorders**
EXCLUDES 2 *retinal hemorrhage (H35.6-)*

H35.81 **Retinal edema**
Retinal cotton wool spots
H35.82 **Retinal ischemia**
H35.89 **Other specified retinal disorders**

H35.9 **Unspecified retinal disorder**

H36 ***Retinal disorders in diseases classified elsewhere***
Code first underlying disease, such as:
lipid storage disorders (E75.-)
sickle-cell disorders (D57.-)
EXCLUDES 1 *arteriosclerotic retinopathy (H35.0-)*
diabetic retinopathy (E08.3-, E09.3-, E10.3-, E11.3-, E13.3-)

Glaucoma (H40-H42)

4 H40 **Glaucoma**
EXCLUDES 1 *absolute glaucoma (H44.51-)*
congenital glaucoma (Q15.0)
traumatic glaucoma due to birth injury (P15.3)

Diseases of the Eye and Adnexa

H35.36 — H40

GUIDELINES **Section I.C.7.a.1)**
Assign as many codes from category H40, Glaucoma, as needed to identify the type of glaucoma, the affected eye, and the glaucoma stage.

GUIDELINES **Section I.C.7.a.2)-3)**
When a patient has bilateral glaucoma and both eyes are documented as being the same type and stage, and there is a code for bilateral glaucoma, report only the code for the type of glaucoma, bilateral, with the seventh character for the stage.

When a patient has bilateral glaucoma and each eye is documented as having a different type or stage, and the classification distinguishes laterality, assign the appropriate code for each eye rather than the code for bilateral glaucoma.

5 **H40.0** **Glaucoma** suspect

DEFINITION Increase in intraocular pressure causing pathologic changes in the optic disk and defects in the field of vision.

6 **H40.00** **Preglaucoma, unspecified**
- **H40.001** **Preglaucoma, unspecified,** right eye
- **H40.002** **Preglaucoma, unspecified,** left eye
- **H40.003** **Preglaucoma, unspecified,** bilateral
- **H40.009** **Preglaucoma, unspecified,** unspecified eye

6 **H40.01** **Open angle with borderline findings, low risk**
Open angle, low risk
- **H40.011** **Open angle with borderline findings, low risk, right eye**
- **H40.012** **Open angle with borderline findings, low risk, left eye**
- **H40.013** **Open angle with borderline findings, low risk, bilateral**
- **H40.019** **Open angle with borderline findings, low risk, unspecified eye**

6 **H40.02** **Open angle with borderline findings, high risk**
Open angle, high risk
- **H40.021** **Open angle with borderline findings, high risk, right eye**
- **H40.022** **Open angle with borderline findings, high risk, left eye**
- **H40.023** **Open angle with borderline findings, high risk, bilateral**
- **H40.029** **Open angle with borderline findings, high risk, unspecified eye**

6 **H40.03** **Anatomical narrow angle**
Primary angle closure suspect
- **H40.031** **Anatomical narrow angle,** right eye
- **H40.032** **Anatomical narrow angle,** left eye
- **H40.033** **Anatomical narrow angle,** bilateral
- **H40.039** **Anatomical narrow angle,** unspecified eye

6 **H40.04** **Steroid responder**
- **H40.041** **Steroid responder,** right eye
- **H40.042** **Steroid responder,** left eye
- **H40.043** **Steroid responder,** bilateral
- **H40.049** **Steroid responder,** unspecified eye

6 **H40.05** **Ocular hypertension**
- **H40.051** **Ocular hypertension,** right eye
- **H40.052** **Ocular hypertension,** left eye
- **H40.053** **Ocular hypertension,** bilateral
- **H40.059** **Ocular hypertension,** unspecified eye

6 **H40.06** Primary angle closure without **glaucoma** damage
- **H40.061** **Primary angle closure without glaucoma damage,** right eye
- **H40.062** **Primary angle closure without glaucoma damage,** left eye
- **H40.063** **Primary angle closure without glaucoma damage,** bilateral
- **H40.069** **Primary angle closure without glaucoma damage,** unspecified eye

5 **H40.1** Open-angle **glaucoma**

Open-angle glaucoma

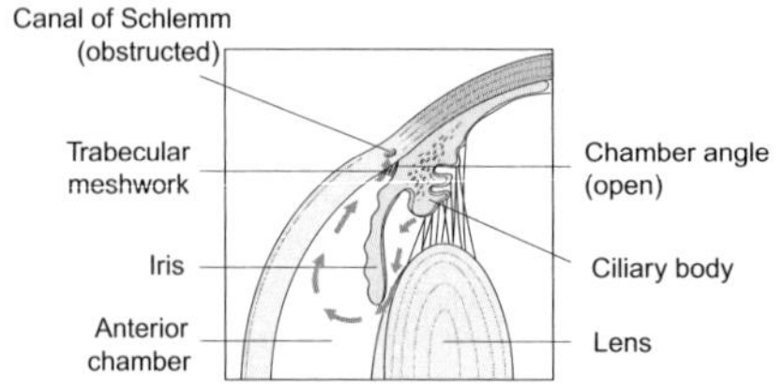

7 **H40.10X-** Unspecified **open-angle glaucoma**

One of the following 7th characters is to be assigned to code H40.10 to designate the stage of glaucoma
- 0 stage unspecified
- 1 mild stage
- 2 moderate stage
- 3 severe stage
- 4 indeterminate stage

GUIDELINES **Section I.C.7.a.2)-3)** When a patient has bilateral glaucoma and both eyes are documented as being the same type and stage, and the classification does not provide a code for bilateral glaucoma, report only one code for the type of glaucoma with the appropriate seventh character for the stage. When a patient has bilateral glaucoma and each eye is documented as having a different type, and the classification does not distinguish laterality, assign one code for each type of glaucoma with the appropriate seventh character for the stage. When a patient has bilateral glaucoma and each eye is documented as having the same type, but different stage, and the classification does not distinguish laterality, assign a code for the type of glaucoma for each eye with the seventh character for the specific glaucoma stage documented for each eye.

6 **H40.11** Primary **open-angle glaucoma**
Chronic simple glaucoma

One of the following 7th characters is to be assigned to each code in subcategory H40.11 to designate the stage of glaucoma
- 0 stage unspecified
- 1 mild stage
- 2 moderate stage
- 3 severe stage
- 4 indeterminate stage

AHA: 4Q 2016, 22

- 7 **H40.111-** **Primary open-angle glaucoma,** right eye
- 7 **H40.112-** **Primary open-angle glaucoma,** left eye
- 7 **H40.113-** **Primary open-angle glaucoma,** bilateral
- 7 **H40.119-** **Primary open-angle glaucoma,** unspecified eye

6 **H40.12** Low-tension **glaucoma**

One of the following 7th characters is to be assigned to each code in subcategory H40.12 to designate the stage of glaucoma
- 0 stage unspecified
- 1 mild stage
- 2 moderate stage
- 3 severe stage
- 4 indeterminate stage

- 7 **H40.121-** **Low-tension glaucoma,** right eye
- 7 **H40.122-** **Low-tension glaucoma,** left eye
- 7 **H40.123-** **Low-tension glaucoma,** bilateral
- 7 **H40.129-** **Low-tension glaucoma,** unspecified eye

6 **H40.13** Pigmentary **glaucoma**

One of the following 7th characters is to be assigned to each code in subcategory H40.13 to designate the stage of glaucoma
0 stage unspecified
1 mild stage
2 moderate stage
3 severe stage
4 indeterminate stage

DEFINITION Granules of pigment coloring the eye break off and block drainage canals, increasing intraocular pressure.

7 **H40.131-** **Pigmentary glaucoma,** right eye
7 **H40.132-** **Pigmentary glaucoma,** left eye
7 **H40.133-** **Pigmentary glaucoma,** bilateral
7 **H40.139-** **Pigmentary glaucoma,** unspecified eye

6 **H40.14** Capsular **glaucoma with** pseudoexfoliation **of lens**

One of the following 7th characters is to be assigned to each code in subcategory H40.14 to designate the stage of glaucoma
0 stage unspecified
1 mild stage
2 moderate stage
3 severe stage
4 indeterminate stage

7 **H40.141-** **Capsular glaucoma with pseudoexfoliation of lens,** right eye
7 **H40.142-** **Capsular glaucoma with pseudoexfoliation of lens,** left eye
7 **H40.143-** **Capsular glaucoma with pseudoexfoliation of lens,** bilateral
7 **H40.149-** **Capsular glaucoma with pseudoexfoliation of lens,** unspecified eye

6 **H40.15** Residual stage of **open-angle glaucoma**
H40.151 **Residual stage of open-angle glaucoma,** right eye
H40.152 **Residual stage of open-angle glaucoma,** left eye
H40.153 **Residual stage of open-angle glaucoma,** bilateral
H40.159 **Residual stage of open-angle glaucoma,** unspecified eye

5 **H40.2** Primary angle-closure **glaucoma**
EXCLUDES 1 *aqueous misdirection (H40.83-)*
malignant glaucoma (H40.83-)

7 **H40.20X-** Unspecified **primary angle-closure glaucoma**

One of the following 7th characters is to be assigned to code H40.20 to designate the stage of glaucoma
0 stage unspecified
1 mild stage
2 moderate stage
3 severe stage
4 indeterminate stage

GUIDELINES **Section I.C.7.a.2)-3)** When a patient has bilateral glaucoma and both eyes are documented as being the same type and stage, and the classification does not provide a code for bilateral glaucoma, report only one code for the type of glaucoma with the appropriate seventh character for the stage. When a patient has bilateral glaucoma and each eye is documented as having a different type, and the classification does not distinguish laterality, assign one code for each type of glaucoma with the appropriate seventh character for the stage. When a patient has bilateral glaucoma and each eye is documented as having the same type, but different stage, and the classification does not distinguish laterality, assign a code for the type of glaucoma for each eye with the seventh character for the specific glaucoma stage documented for each eye.

6 **H40.21** Acute **angle-closure glaucoma**
Acute angle-closure glaucoma attack
Acute angle-closure glaucoma crisis

DEFINITION Severe, sudden increase in intraocular pressure due to a blockage of the chamber angle at the junction of the iris and cornea, preventing normal aqueous fluid drainage and causing rapid loss of vision.

H40.211 **Acute angle-closure glaucoma,** right eye
H40.212 **Acute angle-closure glaucoma,** left eye
H40.213 **Acute angle-closure glaucoma,** bilateral
H40.219 **Acute angle-closure glaucoma,** unspecified eye

6 **H40.22** Chronic **angle-closure glaucoma**
Chronic primary angle closure glaucoma

One of the following 7th characters is to be assigned to each code in subcategory H40.22 to designate the stage of glaucoma
0 stage unspecified
1 mild stage
2 moderate stage
3 severe stage
4 indeterminate stage

7 **H40.221-** **Chronic angle-closure glaucoma,** right eye
7 **H40.222-** **Chronic angle-closure glaucoma,** left eye
7 **H40.223-** **Chronic angle-closure glaucoma,** bilateral
7 **H40.229-** **Chronic angle-closure glaucoma,** unspecified eye

6 **H40.23** Intermittent **angle-closure glaucoma**
H40.231 **Intermittent angle-closure glaucoma,** right eye
H40.232 **Intermittent angle-closure glaucoma,** left eye
H40.233 **Intermittent angle-closure glaucoma,** bilateral
H40.239 **Intermittent angle-closure glaucoma,** unspecified eye

6 **H40.24** Residual stage **of angle-closure glaucoma**
H40.241 **Residual stage of angle-closure glaucoma,** right eye
H40.242 **Residual stage of angle-closure glaucoma,** left eye
H40.243 **Residual stage of angle-closure glaucoma,** bilateral
H40.249 **Residual stage of angle-closure glaucoma,** unspecified eye

5 **H40.3** **Glaucoma** secondary to eye trauma
Code also:
underlying condition

One of the following 7th characters is to be assigned to each code in subcategory H40.3 to designate the stage of glaucoma
0 stage unspecified
1 mild stage
2 moderate stage
3 severe stage
4 indeterminate stage

7 **H40.30X-** **Glaucoma secondary to eye trauma,** unspecified eye
7 **H40.31X-** **Glaucoma secondary to eye trauma,** right eye
7 **H40.32X-** **Glaucoma secondary to eye trauma,** left eye
7 **H40.33X-** **Glaucoma secondary to eye trauma,** bilateral

5 **H40.4** **Glaucoma** secondary to eye inflammation
Code also:
underlying condition

One of the following 7th characters is to be assigned to each code in subcategory H40.4 to designate the stage of glaucoma
0 stage unspecified
1 mild stage
2 moderate stage
3 severe stage
4 indeterminate stage

7 **H40.40X-** **Glaucoma secondary to eye inflammation,** unspecified eye
7 **H40.41X-** **Glaucoma secondary to eye inflammation,** right eye

H40.42X- Glaucoma secondary to eye inflammation, left eye

H40.43X- Glaucoma secondary to eye inflammation, bilateral

H40.5 Glaucoma secondary to other eye disorders

Code also:
underlying eye disorder

One of the following 7th characters is to be assigned to each code in subcategory H40.5 to designate the stage of glaucoma
0 stage unspecified
1 mild stage
2 moderate stage
3 severe stage
4 indeterminate stage

H40.50X- Glaucoma secondary to other eye disorders, unspecified eye

H40.51X- Glaucoma secondary to other eye disorders, right eye

H40.52X- Glaucoma secondary to other eye disorders, left eye

H40.53X- Glaucoma secondary to other eye disorders, bilateral

H40.6 Glaucoma secondary to drugs

Use additional code for adverse effect, if applicable, to identify drug (T36-T50 with fifth or sixth character 5)

One of the following 7th characters is to be assigned to each code in subcategory H40.6 to designate the stage of glaucoma
0 stage unspecified
1 mild stage
2 moderate stage
3 severe stage
4 indeterminate stage

H40.60X- Glaucoma secondary to drugs, unspecified eye

H40.61X- Glaucoma secondary to drugs, right eye

H40.62X- Glaucoma secondary to drugs, left eye

H40.63X- Glaucoma secondary to drugs, bilateral

H40.8 Other glaucoma

H40.81 Glaucoma with increased episcleral venous pressure

DEFINITION Blood pressure of the veins in the white of the eye increases as the pressure of intraocular fluid increases.

H40.811 Glaucoma with increased episcleral venous pressure, right eye

H40.812 Glaucoma with increased episcleral venous pressure, left eye

H40.813 Glaucoma with increased episcleral venous pressure, bilateral

H40.819 Glaucoma with increased episcleral venous pressure, unspecified eye

H40.82 Hypersecretion glaucoma

DEFINITION Overproduction of ocular fluid rather than insufficient drainage that causes increased intraocular pressure.

H40.821 Hypersecretion glaucoma, right eye

H40.822 Hypersecretion glaucoma, left eye

H40.823 Hypersecretion glaucoma, bilateral

H40.829 Hypersecretion glaucoma, unspecified eye

H40.83 Aqueous misdirection

Malignant glaucoma

H40.831 Aqueous misdirection, right eye

H40.832 Aqueous misdirection, left eye

H40.833 Aqueous misdirection, bilateral

H40.839 Aqueous misdirection, unspecified eye

H40.89 Other specified glaucoma

H40.9 Unspecified glaucoma

H42 *Glaucoma in diseases classified elsewhere*

Code first underlying condition, such as:
amyloidosis (E85.-)
aniridia (Q13.1)
glaucoma (in) diabetes mellitus (E08.39, E09.39, E10.39, E11.39, E13.39)
Lowe's syndrome (E72.03)
Reiger's anomaly (Q13.81)
specified metabolic disorder (E70-E88)

EXCLUDES 1 *glaucoma (in) onchocerciasis (B73.02)*
glaucoma (in) syphilis (A52.71)
glaucoma (in) tuberculous (A18.59)

Disorders of vitreous body and globe (H43-H44)

H43 Disorders of vitreous body

H43.0 Vitreous prolapse

EXCLUDES 1 *vitreous syndrome following cataract surgery (H59.0-)*
traumatic vitreous prolapse (S05.2-)

H43.00 Vitreous prolapse, unspecified eye

H43.01 Vitreous prolapse, right eye

H43.02 Vitreous prolapse, left eye

H43.03 Vitreous prolapse, bilateral

H43.1 Vitreous hemorrhage

H43.10 Vitreous hemorrhage, unspecified eye HCC

H43.11 Vitreous hemorrhage, right eye HCC

H43.12 Vitreous hemorrhage, left eye HCC

H43.13 Vitreous hemorrhage, bilateral HCC

H43.2 Crystalline deposits in vitreous body

H43.20 Crystalline deposits in vitreous body, unspecified eye

H43.21 Crystalline deposits in vitreous body, right eye

H43.22 Crystalline deposits in vitreous body, left eye

H43.23 Crystalline deposits in vitreous body, bilateral

H43.3 Other vitreous opacities

H43.31 Vitreous membranes and strands

H43.311 Vitreous membranes and strands, right eye

H43.312 Vitreous membranes and strands, left eye

H43.313 Vitreous membranes and strands, bilateral

H43.319 Vitreous membranes and strands, unspecified eye

H43.39 Other vitreous opacities

Vitreous floaters

H43.391 Other vitreous opacities, right eye

H43.392 Other vitreous opacities, left eye

H43.393 Other vitreous opacities, bilateral

H43.399 Other vitreous opacities, unspecified eye

H43.8 Other disorders of vitreous body

EXCLUDES 1 *proliferative vitreo-retinopathy with retinal detachment (H33.4-)*

EXCLUDES 2 *vitreous abscess (H44.02-)*

H43.81 Vitreous degeneration

Vitreous detachment

H43.811 Vitreous degeneration, right eye

H43.812 Vitreous degeneration, left eye

H43.813 Vitreous degeneration, bilateral

H43.819 Vitreous degeneration, unspecified eye

H43.82 Vitreomacular adhesion

Vitreomacular traction

H43.821 Vitreomacular adhesion, right eye A

H43.822 Vitreomacular adhesion, left eye A

H43.823 Vitreomacular adhesion, bilateral A

H43.829 Vitreomacular adhesion, unspecified eye A

H43.89 Other disorders of vitreous body

H43.9 Unspecified disorder of vitreous body

H44 Disorders of globe

INCLUDES disorders affecting multiple structures of eye

H44.0 Purulent endophthalmitis

Use additional code to identify organism

EXCLUDES 1 *bleb associated endophthalmitis (H59.4-)*

6 H44.00 Unspecified purulent endophthalmitis

Purulent endophthalmitis

An inflammation of the tissues of the eye resulting in pus formation

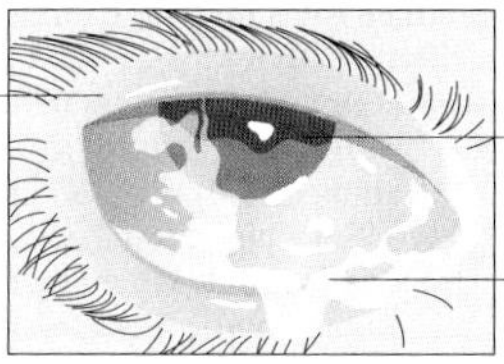

7 H44.001 **Unspecified purulent endophthalmitis, right eye**
7 H44.002 **Unspecified purulent endophthalmitis, left eye**
7 H44.003 **Unspecified purulent endophthalmitis, bilateral**
7 H44.009 **Unspecified purulent endophthalmitis, unspecified eye**

6 H44.01 **Panophthalmitis (acute)**

DEFINITION Inflammation affecting all the structures or tissues of the eye.

7 H44.011 **Panophthalmitis (acute), right eye**
7 H44.012 **Panophthalmitis (acute), left eye**
7 H44.013 **Panophthalmitis (acute), bilateral**
7 H44.019 **Panophthalmitis (acute), unspecified eye**

6 H44.02 **Vitreous abscess (chronic)**
7 H44.021 **Vitreous abscess (chronic), right eye**
7 H44.022 **Vitreous abscess (chronic), left eye**
7 H44.023 **Vitreous abscess (chronic), bilateral**
7 H44.029 **Vitreous abscess (chronic), unspecified eye**

5 H44.1 **Other endophthalmitis**

EXCLUDES 1 *bleb associated endophthalmitis (H59.4-)*

EXCLUDES 2 *ophthalmia nodosa (H16.2-)*

6 H44.11 **Panuveitis**

DEFINITION Inflammation of the entire pigmented layer of the eye (uveal tract).

7 H44.111 **Panuveitis, right eye**
7 H44.112 **Panuveitis, left eye**
7 H44.113 **Panuveitis, bilateral**
7 H44.119 **Panuveitis, unspecified eye**

6 H44.12 **Parasitic endophthalmitis, unspecified**
7 H44.121 **Parasitic endophthalmitis, unspecified, right eye**
7 H44.122 **Parasitic endophthalmitis, unspecified, left eye**
7 H44.123 **Parasitic endophthalmitis, unspecified, bilateral**
7 H44.129 **Parasitic endophthalmitis, unspecified, unspecified eye**

6 H44.13 **Sympathetic uveitis**
7 H44.131 **Sympathetic uveitis, right eye**
7 H44.132 **Sympathetic uveitis, left eye**
7 H44.133 **Sympathetic uveitis, bilateral**
7 H44.139 **Sympathetic uveitis, unspecified eye**

H44.19 **Other endophthalmitis**

5 H44.2 **Degenerative myopia**
Malignant myopia

6 H44.20 **Degenerative myopia, unspecified eye**
6 H44.21 **Degenerative myopia, right eye**
6 H44.22 **Degenerative myopia, left eye**
6 H44.23 **Degenerative myopia, bilateral**

6 H44.2A **Degenerative myopia with choroidal neovascularization**
Use additional code for any associated choroid disorders (H31.-)
AHA: 4Q 2017, 8

7 H44.2A1 **Degenerative myopia with choroidal neovascularization, right eye**
AHA: 4Q 2017, 8
7 H44.2A2 **Degenerative myopia with choroidal neovascularization, left eye**
AHA: 4Q 2017, 8
7 H44.2A3 **Degenerative myopia with choroidal neovascularization, bilateral eye**
AHA: 4Q 2017, 8
7 H44.2A9 **Degenerative myopia with choroidal neovascularization, unspecified eye**
AHA: 4Q 2017, 8

6 H44.2B **Degenerative myopia with macular hole**
AHA: 4Q 2017, 8
7 H44.2B1 **Degenerative myopia with macular hole, right eye**
AHA: 4Q 2017, 8
7 H44.2B2 **Degenerative myopia with macular hole, left eye**
AHA: 4Q 2017, 8
7 H44.2B3 **Degenerative myopia with macular hole, bilateral eye**
AHA: 4Q 2017, 8
7 H44.2B9 **Degenerative myopia with macular hole, unspecified eye**
AHA: 4Q 2017, 8

6 H44.2C **Degenerative myopia with retinal detachment**
Use additional code to identify the retinal detachment (H33.-)
AHA: 4Q 2017, 8
7 H44.2C1 **Degenerative myopia with retinal detachment, right eye**
AHA: 4Q 2017, 8
7 H44.2C2 **Degenerative myopia with retinal detachment, left eye**
AHA: 4Q 2017, 8
7 H44.2C3 **Degenerative myopia with retinal detachment, bilateral eye**
AHA: 4Q 2017, 8
7 H44.2C9 **Degenerative myopia with retinal detachment, unspecified eye**
AHA: 4Q 2017, 8

6 H44.2D **Degenerative myopia with foveoschisis**
AHA: 4Q 2017, 8
7 H44.2D1 **Degenerative myopia with foveoschisis, right eye**
AHA: 4Q 2017, 8
7 H44.2D2 **Degenerative myopia with foveoschisis, left eye**
AHA: 4Q 2017, 8
7 H44.2D3 **Degenerative myopia with foveoschisis, bilateral eye**
AHA: 4Q 2017, 8
7 H44.2D9 **Degenerative myopia with foveoschisis, unspecified eye**
AHA: 4Q 2017, 8

6 H44.2E **Degenerative myopia with other maculopathy**
AHA: 4Q 2017, 8
7 H44.2E1 **Degenerative myopia with other maculopathy, right eye**
7 H44.2E2 **Degenerative myopia with other maculopathy, left eye**
7 H44.2E3 **Degenerative myopia with other maculopathy, bilateral eye**
7 H44.2E9 **Degenerative myopia with other maculopathy, unspecified eye**

5 H44.3 **Other and unspecified degenerative disorders of globe**
H44.30 **Unspecified degenerative disorder of globe**
6 H44.31 **Chalcosis**
7 H44.311 **Chalcosis, right eye**
7 H44.312 **Chalcosis, left eye**
7 H44.313 **Chalcosis, bilateral**
7 H44.319 **Chalcosis, unspecified eye**
6 H44.32 **Siderosis of eye**
7 H44.321 **Siderosis of eye, right eye**
7 H44.322 **Siderosis of eye, left eye**
7 H44.323 **Siderosis of eye, bilateral**
7 H44.329 **Siderosis of eye, unspecified eye**

● New *Manifestation* 4-7 Digit Indicators Laterality A Adult M Maternity N Newborn P Pediatric ♂ Male
▲ Revised Unspecified AHA Coding Clinic HCC Hierarchical Condition Categories HIV HIV Related Conditions ♀ Female

- H44.39 Other degenerative disorders of globe
  - H44.391 Other degenerative disorders of globe, right eye
  - H44.392 Other degenerative disorders of globe, left eye
  - H44.393 Other degenerative disorders of globe, bilateral
  - H44.399 Other degenerative disorders of globe, unspecified eye
- H44.4 Hypotony of eye
  - H44.40 Unspecified hypotony of eye
  - H44.41 Flat anterior chamber hypotony of eye
    - H44.411 Flat anterior chamber hypotony of right eye
    - H44.412 Flat anterior chamber hypotony of left eye
    - H44.413 Flat anterior chamber hypotony of eye, bilateral
    - H44.419 Flat anterior chamber hypotony of unspecified eye
  - H44.42 Hypotony of eye due to ocular fistula
    - H44.421 Hypotony of right eye due to ocular fistula
    - H44.422 Hypotony of left eye due to ocular fistula
    - H44.423 Hypotony of eye due to ocular fistula, bilateral
    - H44.429 Hypotony of unspecified eye due to ocular fistula
  - H44.43 Hypotony of eye due to other ocular disorders
    - H44.431 Hypotony of eye due to other ocular disorders, right eye
    - H44.432 Hypotony of eye due to other ocular disorders, left eye
    - H44.433 Hypotony of eye due to other ocular disorders, bilateral
    - H44.439 Hypotony of eye due to other ocular disorders, unspecified eye
  - H44.44 Primary hypotony of eye
    - H44.441 Primary hypotony of right eye
    - H44.442 Primary hypotony of left eye
    - H44.443 Primary hypotony of eye, bilateral
    - H44.449 Primary hypotony of unspecified eye
- H44.5 Degenerated conditions of globe
  - H44.50 Unspecified degenerated conditions of globe
  - H44.51 Absolute glaucoma
    - H44.511 Absolute glaucoma, right eye
    - H44.512 Absolute glaucoma, left eye
    - H44.513 Absolute glaucoma, bilateral
    - H44.519 Absolute glaucoma, unspecified eye
  - H44.52 Atrophy of globe
    Phthisis bulbi
    - H44.521 Atrophy of globe, right eye
    - H44.522 Atrophy of globe, left eye
    - H44.523 Atrophy of globe, bilateral
    - H44.529 Atrophy of globe, unspecified eye
  - H44.53 Leucocoria
    - H44.531 Leucocoria, right eye
    - H44.532 Leucocoria, left eye
    - H44.533 Leucocoria, bilateral
    - H44.539 Leucocoria, unspecified eye
- H44.6 Retained (old) intraocular foreign body, magnetic
  Use additional code to identify magnetic foreign body (Z18.11)
  EXCLUDES 1 *current intraocular foreign body (S05.-)*
  EXCLUDES 2 *retained foreign body in eyelid (H02.81-)*
  retained (old) foreign body following penetrating wound of orbit (H05.5-)
  retained (old) intraocular foreign body, nonmagnetic (H44.7-)
  - H44.60 Unspecified retained (old) intraocular foreign body, magnetic
    - H44.601 Unspecified retained (old) intraocular foreign body, magnetic, right eye
    - H44.602 Unspecified retained (old) intraocular foreign body, magnetic, left eye
    - H44.603 Unspecified retained (old) intraocular foreign body, magnetic, bilateral
    - H44.609 Unspecified retained (old) intraocular foreign body, magnetic, unspecified eye
  - H44.61 Retained (old) magnetic foreign body in anterior chamber
    - H44.611 Retained (old) magnetic foreign body in anterior chamber, right eye
    - H44.612 Retained (old) magnetic foreign body in anterior chamber, left eye
    - H44.613 Retained (old) magnetic foreign body in anterior chamber, bilateral
    - H44.619 Retained (old) magnetic foreign body in anterior chamber, unspecified eye
  - H44.62 Retained (old) magnetic foreign body in iris or ciliary body
    - H44.621 Retained (old) magnetic foreign body in iris or ciliary body, right eye
    - H44.622 Retained (old) magnetic foreign body in iris or ciliary body, left eye
    - H44.623 Retained (old) magnetic foreign body in iris or ciliary body, bilateral
    - H44.629 Retained (old) magnetic foreign body in iris or ciliary body, unspecified eye
  - H44.63 Retained (old) magnetic foreign body in lens
    - H44.631 Retained (old) magnetic foreign body in lens, right eye
    - H44.632 Retained (old) magnetic foreign body in lens, left eye
    - H44.633 Retained (old) magnetic foreign body in lens, bilateral
    - H44.639 Retained (old) magnetic foreign body in lens, unspecified eye
  - H44.64 Retained (old) magnetic foreign body in posterior wall of globe
    - H44.641 Retained (old) magnetic foreign body in posterior wall of globe, right eye
    - H44.642 Retained (old) magnetic foreign body in posterior wall of globe, left eye
    - H44.643 Retained (old) magnetic foreign body in posterior wall of globe, bilateral
    - H44.649 Retained (old) magnetic foreign body in posterior wall of globe, unspecified eye
  - H44.65 Retained (old) magnetic foreign body in vitreous body
    - H44.651 Retained (old) magnetic foreign body in vitreous body, right eye
    - H44.652 Retained (old) magnetic foreign body in vitreous body, left eye
    - H44.653 Retained (old) magnetic foreign body in vitreous body, bilateral
    - H44.659 Retained (old) magnetic foreign body in vitreous body, unspecified eye
  - H44.69 Retained (old) intraocular foreign body, magnetic, in other or multiple sites
    - H44.691 Retained (old) intraocular foreign body, magnetic, in other or multiple sites, right eye
    - H44.692 Retained (old) intraocular foreign body, magnetic, in other or multiple sites, left eye
    - H44.693 Retained (old) intraocular foreign body, magnetic, in other or multiple sites, bilateral
    - H44.699 Retained (old) intraocular foreign body, magnetic, in other or multiple sites, unspecified eye
- H44.7 Retained (old) intraocular foreign body, nonmagnetic
  Use additional code to identify nonmagnetic foreign body (Z18.01-Z18.10, Z18.12, Z18.2-Z18.9)
  EXCLUDES 1 *current intraocular foreign body (S05.-)*
  EXCLUDES 2 *retained foreign body in eyelid (H02.81-)*
  retained (old) foreign body following penetrating wound of orbit (H05.5-)
  retained (old) intraocular foreign body, magnetic (H44.6-)
  - H44.70 Unspecified retained (old) intraocular foreign body, nonmagnetic
    - H44.701 Unspecified retained (old) intraocular foreign body, nonmagnetic, right eye
    - H44.702 Unspecified retained (old) intraocular foreign body, nonmagnetic, left eye
    - H44.703 Unspecified retained (old) intraocular foreign body, nonmagnetic, bilateral
    - H44.709 Unspecified retained (old) intraocular foreign body, nonmagnetic, unspecified eye
      Retained (old) intraocular foreign body NOS

6 H44.71 Retained (nonmagnetic) (old) foreign body in anterior chamber
- H44.711 Retained (nonmagnetic) (old) foreign body in anterior chamber, right eye
- H44.712 Retained (nonmagnetic) (old) foreign body in anterior chamber, left eye
- H44.713 Retained (nonmagnetic) (old) foreign body in anterior chamber, bilateral
- H44.719 Retained (nonmagnetic) (old) foreign body in anterior chamber, unspecified eye

6 H44.72 Retained (nonmagnetic) (old) foreign body in iris or ciliary body
- H44.721 Retained (nonmagnetic) (old) foreign body in iris or ciliary body, right eye
- H44.722 Retained (nonmagnetic) (old) foreign body in iris or ciliary body, left eye
- H44.723 Retained (nonmagnetic) (old) foreign body in iris or ciliary body, bilateral
- H44.729 Retained (nonmagnetic) (old) foreign body in iris or ciliary body, unspecified eye

6 H44.73 Retained (nonmagnetic) (old) foreign body in lens
- H44.731 Retained (nonmagnetic) (old) foreign body in lens, right eye
- H44.732 Retained (nonmagnetic) (old) foreign body in lens, left eye
- H44.733 Retained (nonmagnetic) (old) foreign body in lens, bilateral
- H44.739 Retained (nonmagnetic) (old) foreign body in lens, unspecified eye

6 H44.74 Retained (nonmagnetic) (old) foreign body in posterior wall of globe
- H44.741 Retained (nonmagnetic) (old) foreign body in posterior wall of globe, right eye
- H44.742 Retained (nonmagnetic) (old) foreign body in posterior wall of globe, left eye
- H44.743 Retained (nonmagnetic) (old) foreign body in posterior wall of globe, bilateral
- H44.749 Retained (nonmagnetic) (old) foreign body in posterior wall of globe, unspecified eye

6 H44.75 Retained (nonmagnetic) (old) foreign body in vitreous body
- H44.751 Retained (nonmagnetic) (old) foreign body in vitreous body, right eye
- H44.752 Retained (nonmagnetic) (old) foreign body in vitreous body, left eye
- H44.753 Retained (nonmagnetic) (old) foreign body in vitreous body, bilateral
- H44.759 Retained (nonmagnetic) (old) foreign body in vitreous body, unspecified eye

6 H44.79 Retained (old) intraocular foreign body, nonmagnetic, in other or multiple sites
- H44.791 Retained (old) intraocular foreign body, nonmagnetic, in other or multiple sites, right eye
- H44.792 Retained (old) intraocular foreign body, nonmagnetic, in other or multiple sites, left eye
- H44.793 Retained (old) intraocular foreign body, nonmagnetic, in other or multiple sites, bilateral
- H44.799 Retained (old) intraocular foreign body, nonmagnetic, in other or multiple sites, unspecified eye

5 H44.8 Other disorders of globe

6 H44.81 Hemophthalmos

DEFINITION Accumulation of blood within the eyeball that is not due to a current injury.

- H44.811 Hemophthalmos, right eye
- H44.812 Hemophthalmos, left eye
- H44.813 Hemophthalmos, bilateral
- H44.819 Hemophthalmos, unspecified eye

6 H44.82 Luxation of globe
- H44.821 Luxation of globe, right eye
- H44.822 Luxation of globe, left eye
- H44.823 Luxation of globe, bilateral
- H44.829 Luxation of globe, unspecified eye

H44.89 Other disorders of globe

H44.9 Unspecified disorder of globe

Disorders of optic nerve and visual pathways (H46-H47)

4 H46 Optic neuritis

EXCLUDES 2 *ischemic optic neuropathy (H47.01-)*
neuromyelitis optica [Devic] (G36.0)

5 H46.0 Optic papillitis

DEFINITION Swelling of the optic disc where the optic nerve connects to the retina.

- H46.00 Optic papillitis, unspecified eye
- H46.01 Optic papillitis, right eye
- H46.02 Optic papillitis, left eye
- H46.03 Optic papillitis, bilateral

5 H46.1 Retrobulbar neuritis

Retrobulbar neuritis NOS

EXCLUDES 1 *syphilitic retrobulbar neuritis (A52.15)*

DEFINITION Inflammation of the optic nerve directly behind the eye.

- H46.10 Retrobulbar neuritis, unspecified eye
- H46.11 Retrobulbar neuritis, right eye
- H46.12 Retrobulbar neuritis, left eye
- H46.13 Retrobulbar neuritis, bilateral

H46.2 Nutritional optic neuropathy

H46.3 Toxic optic neuropathy

Code first:
(T51-T65) to identify cause

H46.8 Other optic neuritis

H46.9 Unspecified optic neuritis

4 H47 Other disorders of optic [2nd] nerve and visual pathways

5 H47.0 Disorders of optic nerve, not elsewhere classified

6 H47.01 Ischemic optic neuropathy
- H47.011 Ischemic optic neuropathy, right eye
- H47.012 Ischemic optic neuropathy, left eye
- H47.013 Ischemic optic neuropathy, bilateral
- H47.019 Ischemic optic neuropathy, unspecified eye

6 H47.02 Hemorrhage in optic nerve sheath
- H47.021 Hemorrhage in optic nerve sheath, right eye
- H47.022 Hemorrhage in optic nerve sheath, left eye
- H47.023 Hemorrhage in optic nerve sheath, bilateral
- H47.029 Hemorrhage in optic nerve sheath, unspecified eye

6 H47.03 Optic nerve hypoplasia
- H47.031 Optic nerve hypoplasia, right eye
- H47.032 Optic nerve hypoplasia, left eye
- H47.033 Optic nerve hypoplasia, bilateral
- H47.039 Optic nerve hypoplasia, unspecified eye

6 H47.09 Other disorders of optic nerve, not elsewhere classified

Compression of optic nerve
- H47.091 Other disorders of optic nerve, not elsewhere classified, right eye
- H47.092 Other disorders of optic nerve, not elsewhere classified, left eye
- H47.093 Other disorders of optic nerve, not elsewhere classified, bilateral
- H47.099 Other disorders of optic nerve, not elsewhere classified, unspecified eye

5 H47.1 Papilledema

H47.10 Unspecified papilledema

H47.11 Papilledema associated with increased intracranial pressure

DEFINITION Swelling of the optic disk (the part of the retina that connects to the optic nerve) caused by increased intracranial pressure.

H47.12 Papilledema associated with decreased ocular pressure

H47.13 Papilledema associated with retinal disorder

6 H47.14 Foster-Kennedy syndrome

● New | Manifestation | 4-7 Digit Indicators | Laterality | A Adult | M Maternity | N Newborn | P Pediatric | ♂ Male
▲ Revised | Unspecified | AHA Coding Clinic | HCC Hierarchical Condition Categories | HIV HIV Related Conditions | ♀ Female

DEFINITION Disease that presents with papilledema in one eye and atrophy of the optic nerve of the other; caused by increased intracranial pressure from a tumor.

- H47.141 **Foster-Kennedy syndrome, right eye**
- H47.142 **Foster-Kennedy syndrome, left eye**
- H47.143 **Foster-Kennedy syndrome, bilateral**
- H47.149 **Foster-Kennedy syndrome, unspecified eye**

H47.2 **Optic atrophy**

- H47.20 **Unspecified optic atrophy**
- H47.21 **Primary optic atrophy**
  - H47.211 **Primary optic atrophy, right eye**
  - H47.212 **Primary optic atrophy, left eye**
  - H47.213 **Primary optic atrophy, bilateral**
  - H47.219 **Primary optic atrophy, unspecified eye**
- H47.22 **Hereditary optic atrophy**
  Leber's optic atrophy
- H47.23 **Glaucomatous optic atrophy**
  - H47.231 **Glaucomatous optic atrophy, right eye**
  - H47.232 **Glaucomatous optic atrophy, left eye**
  - H47.233 **Glaucomatous optic atrophy, bilateral**
  - H47.239 **Glaucomatous optic atrophy, unspecified eye**
- H47.29 **Other optic atrophy**
  Temporal pallor of optic disc
  - H47.291 **Other optic atrophy, right eye**
  - H47.292 **Other optic atrophy, left eye**
  - H47.293 **Other optic atrophy, bilateral**
  - H47.299 **Other optic atrophy, unspecified eye**

H47.3 **Other disorders of optic disc**

- H47.31 **Coloboma of optic disc**

  DEFINITION Congenital defect of the iris in which there is a gap, hole, or cleft that failed to close; may cause ghost images, blurred or decreased visual activity.

  - H47.311 **Coloboma of optic disc, right eye**
  - H47.312 **Coloboma of optic disc, left eye**
  - H47.313 **Coloboma of optic disc, bilateral**
  - H47.319 **Coloboma of optic disc, unspecified eye**
- H47.32 **Drusen of optic disc**
  - H47.321 **Drusen of optic disc, right eye**
  - H47.322 **Drusen of optic disc, left eye**
  - H47.323 **Drusen of optic disc, bilateral**
  - H47.329 **Drusen of optic disc, unspecified eye**
- H47.33 **Pseudopapilledema of optic disc**
  - H47.331 **Pseudopapilledema of optic disc, right eye**
  - H47.332 **Pseudopapilledema of optic disc, left eye**
  - H47.333 **Pseudopapilledema of optic disc, bilateral**
  - H47.339 **Pseudopapilledema of optic disc, unspecified eye**
- H47.39 **Other disorders of optic disc**
  - H47.391 **Other disorders of optic disc, right eye**
  - H47.392 **Other disorders of optic disc, left eye**
  - H47.393 **Other disorders of optic disc, bilateral**
  - H47.399 **Other disorders of optic disc, unspecified eye**

H47.4 **Disorders of optic chiasm**

Code also:
underlying condition

- H47.41 **Disorders of optic chiasm in (due to) inflammatory disorders**
- H47.42 **Disorders of optic chiasm in (due to) neoplasm**
- H47.43 **Disorders of optic chiasm in (due to) vascular disorders**
- H47.49 **Disorders of optic chiasm in (due to) other disorders**

H47.5 **Disorders of other visual pathways**

Disorders of optic tracts, geniculate nuclei and optic radiations
Code also:
underlying condition

- H47.51 **Disorders of visual pathways in (due to) inflammatory disorders**
  - H47.511 **Disorders of visual pathways in (due to) inflammatory disorders, right side**
  - H47.512 **Disorders of visual pathways in (due to) inflammatory disorders, left side**
  - H47.519 **Disorders of visual pathways in (due to) inflammatory disorders, unspecified side**
- H47.52 **Disorders of visual pathways in (due to) neoplasm**
  - H47.521 **Disorders of visual pathways in (due to) neoplasm, right side**
  - H47.522 **Disorders of visual pathways in (due to) neoplasm, left side**
  - H47.529 **Disorders of visual pathways in (due to) neoplasm, unspecified side**
- H47.53 **Disorders of visual pathways in (due to) vascular disorders**
  - H47.531 **Disorders of visual pathways in (due to) vascular disorders, right side**
  - H47.532 **Disorders of visual pathways in (due to) vascular disorders, left side**
  - H47.539 **Disorders of visual pathways in (due to) vascular disorders, unspecified side**

H47.6 **Disorders of visual cortex**

Code also:
underlying condition

EXCLUDES 1 *injury to visual cortex S04.04*

- H47.61 **Cortical blindness**

  DEFINITION Blindness caused by a defect of the brain and not the eyes.

  - H47.611 **Cortical blindness, right side of brain**
  - H47.612 **Cortical blindness, left side of brain**
  - H47.619 **Cortical blindness, unspecified side of brain**
- H47.62 **Disorders of visual cortex in (due to) inflammatory disorders**
  - H47.621 **Disorders of visual cortex in (due to) inflammatory disorders, right side of brain**
  - H47.622 **Disorders of visual cortex in (due to) inflammatory disorders, left side of brain**
  - H47.629 **Disorders of visual cortex in (due to) inflammatory disorders, unspecified side of brain**
- H47.63 **Disorders of visual cortex in (due to) neoplasm**
  - H47.631 **Disorders of visual cortex in (due to) neoplasm, right side of brain**
  - H47.632 **Disorders of visual cortex in (due to) neoplasm, left side of brain**
  - H47.639 **Disorders of visual cortex in (due to) neoplasm, unspecified side of brain**
- H47.64 **Disorders of visual cortex in (due to) vascular disorders**
  - H47.641 **Disorders of visual cortex in (due to) vascular disorders, right side of brain**
  - H47.642 **Disorders of visual cortex in (due to) vascular disorders, left side of brain**
  - H47.649 **Disorders of visual cortex in (due to) vascular disorders, unspecified side of brain**

H47.9 **Unspecified disorder of visual pathways**

Disorders of ocular muscles, binocular movement, accommodation and refraction (H49-H52)

EXCLUDES 2 *nystagmus and other irregular eye movements (H55)*

H49 Paralytic strabismus

EXCLUDES 2 *internal ophthalmoplegia (H52.51-)*
internuclear ophthalmoplegia (H51.2-)
progressive supranuclear ophthalmoplegia (G23.1)

H49.0 **Third [oculomotor] nerve palsy**

- H49.00 **Third [oculomotor] nerve palsy, unspecified eye**
- H49.01 **Third [oculomotor] nerve palsy, right eye**
- H49.02 **Third [oculomotor] nerve palsy, left eye**
- H49.03 **Third [oculomotor] nerve palsy, bilateral**

H49.1 **Fourth [trochlear] nerve palsy**

- H49.10 **Fourth [trochlear] nerve palsy, unspecified eye**
- H49.11 **Fourth [trochlear] nerve palsy, right eye**
- H49.12 **Fourth [trochlear] nerve palsy, left eye**
- H49.13 **Fourth [trochlear] nerve palsy, bilateral**

H49.2 **Sixth [abducent] nerve palsy**

H49.20 **Sixth [abducent] nerve palsy, unspecified eye**
H49.21 **Sixth [abducent] nerve palsy, right eye**
H49.22 **Sixth [abducent] nerve palsy, left eye**
H49.23 **Sixth [abducent] nerve palsy, bilateral**

H49.3 **Total (external) ophthalmoplegia**

DEFINITION Paralysis of all of the muscles that move the eye as well as the muscles controlling the diameter of the pupil and shape of the lens.

H49.30 **Total (external) ophthalmoplegia, unspecified eye**
H49.31 **Total (external) ophthalmoplegia, right eye**
H49.32 **Total (external) ophthalmoplegia, left eye**
H49.33 **Total (external) ophthalmoplegia, bilateral**

H49.4 **Progressive external ophthalmoplegia**

EXCLUDES 1 *Kearns-Sayre syndrome (H49.81-)*

H49.40 **Progressive external ophthalmoplegia, unspecified eye**
H49.41 **Progressive external ophthalmoplegia, right eye**
H49.42 **Progressive external ophthalmoplegia, left eye**
H49.43 **Progressive external ophthalmoplegia, bilateral**

H49.8 **Other paralytic strabismus**

H49.81 **Kearns-Sayre syndrome**
Progressive external ophthalmoplegia with pigmentary retinopathy
Use additional code for other manifestation, such as: heart block (I45.9)

H49.811 **Kearns-Sayre syndrome, right eye** HCC
H49.812 **Kearns-Sayre syndrome, left eye** HCC
H49.813 **Kearns-Sayre syndrome, bilateral** HCC
H49.819 **Kearns-Sayre syndrome, unspecified eye** HCC

H49.88 **Other paralytic strabismus**
External ophthalmoplegia NOS

H49.881 **Other paralytic strabismus, right eye**
H49.882 **Other paralytic strabismus, left eye**
H49.883 **Other paralytic strabismus, bilateral**
H49.889 **Other paralytic strabismus, unspecified eye**

H49.9 **Unspecified paralytic strabismus**

H50 Other strabismus

H50.0 **Esotropia**
Convergent concomitant strabismus

EXCLUDES 1 *intermittent esotropia (H50.31-, H50.32)*

DEFINITION Deviation of the visual axis of one or both eyes inward toward that of the other eye.

H50.00 **Unspecified esotropia**

H50.01 **Monocular esotropia**
H50.011 **Monocular esotropia, right eye**
H50.012 **Monocular esotropia, left eye**

H50.02 **Monocular esotropia with A pattern**
H50.021 **Monocular esotropia with A pattern, right eye**
H50.022 **Monocular esotropia with A pattern, left eye**

H50.03 **Monocular esotropia with V pattern**
H50.031 **Monocular esotropia with V pattern, right eye**
H50.032 **Monocular esotropia with V pattern, left eye**

H50.04 **Monocular esotropia with other noncomitancies**
H50.041 **Monocular esotropia with other noncomitancies, right eye**
H50.042 **Monocular esotropia with other noncomitancies, left eye**

H50.05 **Alternating esotropia**
H50.06 **Alternating esotropia with A pattern**
H50.07 **Alternating esotropia with V pattern**
H50.08 **Alternating esotropia with other noncomitancies**

H50.1 **Exotropia**
Divergent concomitant strabismus

EXCLUDES 1 *intermittent exotropia (H50.33-, H50.34)*

DEFINITION An abnormal alignment of one or both eyes in which one or both eyes deviate outward.

H50.10 **Unspecified exotropia**

Exotropia

A type of strabismus in which one or both eyes turn outwards

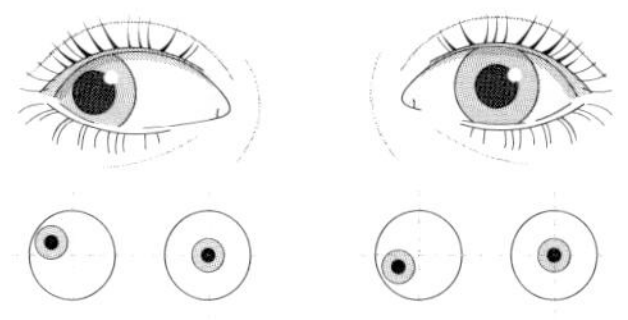
Exotropia with V pattern: outward deviation is greater in upgaze
Exotropia with A pattern: outward deviatiion is greater in downgaze

H50.11 **Monocular exotropia**
H50.111 **Monocular exotropia, right eye**
H50.112 **Monocular exotropia, left eye**

H50.12 **Monocular exotropia with A pattern**
H50.121 **Monocular exotropia with A pattern, right eye**
H50.122 **Monocular exotropia with A pattern, left eye**

H50.13 **Monocular exotropia with V pattern**
H50.131 **Monocular exotropia with V pattern, right eye**
H50.132 **Monocular exotropia with V pattern, left eye**

H50.14 **Monocular exotropia with other noncomitancies**
H50.141 **Monocular exotropia with other noncomitancies, right eye**
H50.142 **Monocular exotropia with other noncomitancies, left eye**

H50.15 **Alternating exotropia**
H50.16 **Alternating exotropia with A pattern**
H50.17 **Alternating exotropia with V pattern**
H50.18 **Alternating exotropia with other noncomitancies**

H50.2 **Vertical strabismus**
Hypertropia

H50.21 **Vertical strabismus, right eye**
H50.22 **Vertical strabismus, left eye**

H50.3 **Intermittent heterotropia**

H50.30 **Unspecified intermittent heterotropia**

H50.31 **Intermittent monocular esotropia**
H50.311 **Intermittent monocular esotropia, right eye**
H50.312 **Intermittent monocular esotropia, left eye**

H50.32 **Intermittent alternating esotropia**

H50.33 **Intermittent monocular exotropia**
H50.331 **Intermittent monocular exotropia, right eye**
H50.332 **Intermittent monocular exotropia, left eye**

H50.34 **Intermittent alternating exotropia**

H50.4 **Other and unspecified heterotropia**

H50.40 **Unspecified heterotropia**

H50.41 **Cyclotropia**
H50.411 **Cyclotropia, right eye**
H50.412 **Cyclotropia, left eye**

H50.42 **Monofixation syndrome**
H50.43 **Accommodative component in esotropia**

H50.5 **Heterophoria**

H50.50 **Unspecified heterophoria**
H50.51 **Esophoria**
H50.52 **Exophoria**
H50.53 **Vertical heterophoria**
H50.54 **Cyclophoria**
H50.55 **Alternating heterophoria**

H50.6 **Mechanical strabismus**

H50.60 **Mechanical strabismus, unspecified**
H50.61 **Brown's sheath syndrome**

● New ▲ Revised *Manifestation* *Unspecified* 4-7 Digit Indicators AHA Coding Clinic Laterality HCC Hierarchical Condition Categories A Adult M Maternity N Newborn HIV HIV Related Conditions P Pediatric ♂ Male ♀ Female

DEFINITION Condition in which the muscle that moves the eye upward and inward is too short, impairing eye movement.

H50.611 Brown's sheath syndrome, right eye
H50.612 Brown's sheath syndrome, left eye
H50.69 Other mechanical strabismus
Strabismus due to adhesions
Traumatic limitation of duction of eye muscle
H50.8 Other specified strabismus
H50.81 Duane's syndrome
DEFINITION Congenital eye muscle disorder due to cranial nerve dysfunction that inhibits normal rotation of one or both eyes inward and outward, also causing abnormal inward turning with distant viewing and eye retraction when viewing up close.
H50.811 Duane's syndrome, right eye
H50.812 Duane's syndrome, left eye
H50.89 Other specified strabismus
H50.9 Unspecified strabismus

H51 Other disorders of binocular movement
H51.0 Palsy (spasm) of conjugate gaze
H51.1 Convergence insufficiency and excess
H51.11 Convergence insufficiency
H51.12 Convergence excess
DEFINITION Eyes fail to move in a coordinated fashion when viewing objects up close.
H51.2 Internuclear ophthalmoplegia
H51.20 Internuclear ophthalmoplegia, unspecified eye
H51.21 Internuclear ophthalmoplegia, right eye
H51.22 Internuclear ophthalmoplegia, left eye
H51.23 Internuclear ophthalmoplegia, bilateral
H51.8 Other specified disorders of binocular movement
H51.9 Unspecified disorder of binocular movement

H52 Disorders of refraction and accommodation
H52.0 Hypermetropia
H52.00 Hypermetropia, unspecified eye
H52.01 Hypermetropia, right eye
H52.02 Hypermetropia, left eye
H52.03 Hypermetropia, bilateral
H52.1 Myopia
EXCLUDES 1 *degenerative myopia (H44.2-)*
H52.10 Myopia, unspecified eye
H52.11 Myopia, right eye
H52.12 Myopia, left eye
H52.13 Myopia, bilateral
H52.2 Astigmatism
DEFINITION Condition in which the cornea is not shaped perfectly round, causing light to focus on more than one point of the retina and resulting in blurred vision.
H52.20 Unspecified astigmatism
H52.201 Unspecified astigmatism, right eye
H52.202 Unspecified astigmatism, left eye
H52.203 Unspecified astigmatism, bilateral
H52.209 Unspecified astigmatism, unspecified eye
H52.21 Irregular astigmatism
H52.211 Irregular astigmatism, right eye
H52.212 Irregular astigmatism, left eye
H52.213 Irregular astigmatism, bilateral
H52.219 Irregular astigmatism, unspecified eye
H52.22 Regular astigmatism
H52.221 Regular astigmatism, right eye
H52.222 Regular astigmatism, left eye
H52.223 Regular astigmatism, bilateral
H52.229 Regular astigmatism, unspecified eye
H52.3 Anisometropia and aniseikonia
H52.31 Anisometropia
DEFINITION Each eye has a different refractive power.
H52.32 Aniseikonia
DEFINITION One eye sees an object differently in size and shape than the way the other eye sees it.
H52.4 Presbyopia
DEFINITION Lens of the eye loses its elasticity due to age, making it more difficult to focus on near points.
H52.5 Disorders of accommodation
H52.51 Internal ophthalmoplegia (complete) (total)
H52.511 Internal ophthalmoplegia (complete) (total), right eye
H52.512 Internal ophthalmoplegia (complete) (total), left eye
H52.513 Internal ophthalmoplegia (complete) (total), bilateral
H52.519 Internal ophthalmoplegia (complete) (total), unspecified eye
H52.52 Paresis of accommodation
DEFINITION Paralysis of the ciliary muscles of the eye that results in the loss of visual accommodation.
H52.521 Paresis of accommodation, right eye
H52.522 Paresis of accommodation, left eye
H52.523 Paresis of accommodation, bilateral
H52.529 Paresis of accommodation, unspecified eye
H52.53 Spasm of accommodation
DEFINITION Abnormal, uncontrolled contraction of the ciliary muscle, usually initially presenting as near-sightedness.
H52.531 Spasm of accommodation, right eye
H52.532 Spasm of accommodation, left eye
H52.533 Spasm of accommodation, bilateral
H52.539 Spasm of accommodation, unspecified eye
H52.6 Other disorders of refraction
H52.7 Unspecified disorder of refraction

Visual disturbances and blindness (H53-H54)

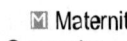

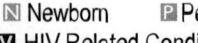

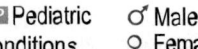

H53 Visual disturbances
H53.0 Amblyopia ex anopsia
EXCLUDES 1 *amblyopia due to vitamin A deficiency (E50.5)*
H53.00 Unspecified amblyopia
H53.001 Unspecified amblyopia, right eye
H53.002 Unspecified amblyopia, left eye
H53.003 Unspecified amblyopia, bilateral
H53.009 Unspecified amblyopia, unspecified eye
H53.01 Deprivation amblyopia
H53.011 Deprivation amblyopia, right eye
H53.012 Deprivation amblyopia, left eye
H53.013 Deprivation amblyopia, bilateral
H53.019 Deprivation amblyopia, unspecified eye
H53.02 Refractive amblyopia
H53.021 Refractive amblyopia, right eye
H53.022 Refractive amblyopia, left eye
H53.023 Refractive amblyopia, bilateral
H53.029 Refractive amblyopia, unspecified eye
H53.03 Strabismic amblyopia
EXCLUDES 1 *strabismus (H50.-)*
H53.031 Strabismic amblyopia, right eye
H53.032 Strabismic amblyopia, left eye
H53.033 Strabismic amblyopia, bilateral
H53.039 Strabismic amblyopia, unspecified eye
H53.04 Amblyopia suspect
AHA: 4Q 2016, 22
H53.041 Amblyopia suspect, right eye
H53.042 Amblyopia suspect, left eye
H53.043 Amblyopia suspect, bilateral
H53.049 Amblyopia suspect, unspecified eye

5 H53.1 Subjective visual disturbances
EXCLUDES 1 *subjective visual disturbances due to vitamin A deficiency (E50.5)*
visual hallucinations (R44.1)
H53.10 Unspecified subjective visual disturbances
H53.11 Day blindness
Hemeralopia
6 H53.12 Transient visual loss
Scintillating scotoma
EXCLUDES 1 *amaurosis fugax (G45.3-)*
transient retinal artery occlusion (H34.0-)
H53.121 Transient visual loss, right eye
H53.122 Transient visual loss, left eye
H53.123 Transient visual loss, bilateral
H53.129 Transient visual loss, unspecified eye
6 H53.13 Sudden visual loss
H53.131 Sudden visual loss, right eye
H53.132 Sudden visual loss, left eye
H53.133 Sudden visual loss, bilateral
H53.139 Sudden visual loss, unspecified eye
6 H53.14 Visual discomfort
Asthenopia
Photophobia
H53.141 Visual discomfort, right eye
H53.142 Visual discomfort, left eye
H53.143 Visual discomfort, bilateral
H53.149 Visual discomfort, unspecified
H53.15 Visual distortions of shape and size
Metamorphopsia
H53.16 Psychophysical visual disturbances
H53.19 Other subjective visual disturbances
Visual halos
DEFINITION Photopsia: sparks or flashes in the field of vision, due to retinal irritation.
H53.2 Diplopia
Double vision
5 H53.3 Other and unspecified disorders of binocular vision
H53.30 Unspecified disorder of binocular vision
H53.31 Abnormal retinal correspondence
H53.32 Fusion with defective stereopsis
H53.33 Simultaneous visual perception without fusion
DEFINITION Imaging from both eyes reaches the brain and are both processed, but without being merged into a single image; the patient sees two side-by-side images instead of one.
H53.34 Suppression of binocular vision
5 H53.4 Visual field defects
H53.40 Unspecified visual field defects
6 H53.41 Scotoma involving central area
Central scotoma
H53.411 Scotoma involving central area, right eye
H53.412 Scotoma involving central area, left eye
H53.413 Scotoma involving central area, bilateral
H53.419 Scotoma involving central area, unspecified eye
6 H53.42 Scotoma of blind spot area
Enlarged blind spot
DEFINITION Blind spot (scotoma) in the central five degrees of the patient's vision.
H53.421 Scotoma of blind spot area, right eye
H53.422 Scotoma of blind spot area, left eye
H53.423 Scotoma of blind spot area, bilateral
H53.429 Scotoma of blind spot area, unspecified eye
6 H53.43 Sector or arcuate defects
Arcuate scotoma
Bjerrum scotoma
H53.431 Sector or arcuate defects, right eye
H53.432 Sector or arcuate defects, left eye
H53.433 Sector or arcuate defects, bilateral
H53.439 Sector or arcuate defects, unspecified eye
6 H53.45 Other localized visual field defect
Peripheral visual field defect
Ring scotoma NOS
Scotoma NOS
H53.451 Other localized visual field defect, right eye
H53.452 Other localized visual field defect, left eye
H53.453 Other localized visual field defect, bilateral
H53.459 Other localized visual field defect, unspecified eye
6 H53.46 Homonymous bilateral field defects
Homonymous hemianopia
Homonymous hemianopsia
Quadrant anopia
Quadrant anopsia
H53.461 Homonymous bilateral field defects, right side
H53.462 Homonymous bilateral field defects, left side
H53.469 Homonymous bilateral field defects, unspecified side
Homonymous bilateral field defects NOS
H53.47 Heteronymous bilateral field defects
Heteronymous hemianop(s)ia
6 H53.48 Generalized contraction of visual field
H53.481 Generalized contraction of visual field, right eye
H53.482 Generalized contraction of visual field, left eye
H53.483 Generalized contraction of visual field, bilateral
H53.489 Generalized contraction of visual field, unspecified eye
5 H53.5 Color vision deficiencies
Color blindness
EXCLUDES 2 *day blindness (H53.11)*
H53.50 Unspecified color vision deficiencies
Color blindness NOS
H53.51 Achromatopsia
DEFINITION Nonprogressive, hereditary visual disorder and retinal abnormality causing decreased vision, light sensitivity, nystagmus, and complete color blindness.
H53.52 Acquired color vision deficiency
H53.53 Deuteranomaly
Deuteranopia
DEFINITION A deficiency in color perception primarily affecting red-green hues due to deficient pigment sensitive to green wavelengths, a common form of color blindness.
H53.54 Protanomaly
Protanopia
H53.55 Tritanomaly
Tritanopia
DEFINITION A deficiency in color perception characterized by an inability to discern blue and yellow due to an absence of blue-sensitive pigment in the retina.
H53.59 Other color vision deficiencies
5 H53.6 Night blindness
EXCLUDES 1 *night blindness due to vitamin A deficiency (E50.5)*
H53.60 Unspecified night blindness
H53.61 Abnormal dark adaptation curve
H53.62 Acquired night blindness
H53.63 Congenital night blindness
H53.69 Other night blindness
5 H53.7 Vision sensitivity deficiencies
H53.71 Glare sensitivity
H53.72 Impaired contrast sensitivity
H53.8 Other visual disturbances
H53.9 Unspecified visual disturbance

4 H54 Blindness and low vision
Note: For definition of visual impairment categories see table below
Code first:
any associated underlying cause of the blindness
EXCLUDES 1 *amaurosis fugax (G45.3)*

GUIDELINES **Section I.C.7.b**
If "blindness" or "low vision" of both eyes is documented but the visual impairment category is not documented, assign code H54.3, Unqualified visual loss, both eyes. If "blindness" or "low vision" in one eye is documented but the visual impairment category is not documented, assign a code from H54.6-, Unqualified visual loss, one eye. If "blindness" or "visual loss" is documented without any information about whether one or both eyes are affected, assign code H54.7, Unspecified visual loss.

CODING TIP✓ Do not use H54 codes for patients with common refractive errors, e.g. farsightedness, nearsightedness, astigmatism, etc. These codes are to indicate the level of vision for those with other eye conditions such as cataracts, retinopathy, glaucoma, hemianopsia, etc.

5 **H54.0 Blindness, both eyes**
Visual impairment categories 3, 4, 5 in both eyes.
CODING TIP✓ Do not use H54.0 to indicate blindness in the USA. See H54.3 or H54.8, depending on the physician's documentation.
AHA: 4Q 2017, 9

6 **H54.0X Blindness, both eyes, different category levels**
CODING TIP✓ The sixth character represents the category of vision in the right eye, and a seventh character represents the category of vision in the left eye.

7 **H54.0X3 Blindness right eye, category 3**
7 **H54.0X4 Blindness right eye, category 4**
7 **H54.0X5 Blindness right eye, category 5**

5 **H54.1 Blindness, one eye, low vision other eye**
Visual impairment categories 3, 4, 5 in one eye, with categories 1 or 2 in the other eye.

H54.10 Blindness, one eye, low vision other eye, unspecified eyes

6 **H54.11 Blindness, right eye, low vision left eye**
CODING TIP✓ The sixth character represents the category of vision in the right eye, and a seventh character represents the category of vision in the left eye.
AHA: 4Q 2017, 9

7 **H54.113 Blindness right eye category 3, low vision left eye**
7 **H54.114 Blindness right eye category 4, low vision left eye**
7 **H54.115 Blindness right eye category 5, low vision left eye**

6 **H54.12 Blindness, left eye, low vision right eye**
CODING TIP✓ The sixth character represents the category of vision in the right eye, and a seventh character represents the category of vision in the left eye.
AHA: 4Q 2017, 9

7 **H54.121 Low vision right eye category 1, blindness left eye**
7 **H54.122 Low vision right eye category 2, blindness left eye**

5 **H54.2 Low vision, both eyes**
Visual impairment categories 1 or 2 in both eyes.
AHA: 4Q 2017, 9

6 **H54.2X Low vision, both eyes, different category levels**
CODING TIP✓ The sixth character represents the category of vision in the right eye, and a seventh character represents the category of vision in the left eye.

7 **H54.2X1 Low vision, right eye, category 1**
7 **H54.2X2 Low vision, right eye, category 2**

H54.3 Unqualified visual loss, both eyes
Visual impairment category 9 in both eyes.

5 **H54.4 Blindness, one eye**
Visual impairment categories 3, 4, 5 in one eye [normal vision in other eye]

H54.40 Blindness, one eye, unspecified eye

6 **H54.41 Blindness, right eye, normal vision left eye**
CODING TIP✓ The sixth character represents the category of vision in the right eye, and a seventh character represents the category of vision in the left eye.
AHA: 4Q 2017, 9

7 **H54.413 Blindness, right eye, category 3**
7 **H54.414 Blindness, right eye, category 4**
7 **H54.415 Blindness, right eye, category 5**

6 **H54.42 Blindness, left eye, normal vision right eye**
AHA: 4Q 2017, 9

7 **H54.42A Blindness, left eye, category 3-5**
CODING TIP✓ The sixth character represents the category of vision in the right eye, and a seventh character represents the category of vision in the left eye.

5 **H54.5 Low vision, one eye**
Visual impairment categories 1 or 2 in one eye [normal vision in other eye].

H54.50 Low vision, one eye, unspecified eye

6 **H54.51 Low vision, right eye, normal vision left eye**
CODING TIP✓ The sixth character represents the category of vision in the right eye, and a seventh character represents the category of vision in the left eye.
AHA: 4Q 2017, 9

7 **H54.511 Low vision, right eye, category 1-2**

6 **H54.52 Low vision, left eye, normal vision right eye**
AHA: 4Q 2017, 9

7 **H54.52A Low vision, left eye, category 1-2**
CODING TIP✓ The sixth character represents the category of vision in the right eye, and a seventh character represents the category of vision in the left eye.

5 **H54.6 Unqualified visual loss, one eye**
Visual impairment category 9 in one eye [normal vision in other eye].

H54.60 Unqualified visual loss, one eye, unspecified
H54.61 Unqualified visual loss, right eye, normal vision left eye
H54.62 Unqualified visual loss, left eye, normal vision right eye

H54.7 Unspecified visual loss
Visual impairment category 9 NOS

H54.8 Legal blindness, as defined in USA
Blindness NOS according to USA definition
Note: The table below gives a classification of severity of visual impairment recommended by a WHO Study Group on the Prevention of Blindness, Geneva, 6-10 November 1972.
The term 'low vision' in category H54 comprises categories 1 and 2 of the table, the term 'blindness' categories 3, 4 and 5, and the term 'unqualified visual loss' category 9.
If the extent of the visual field is taken into account, patients with a field no greater than 10 but greater than 5 around central fixation should be placed in category 3 and patients with a field no greater than 5 around central fixation should be placed in category 4, even if the central acuity is not impaired.

EXCLUDES 1 *legal blindness with specification of impairment level (H54.0-H54.7)*

Category of visual impairment	Visual acuity with best possible correction	
	Maximum less than:	Minimum equal to or better than:
1	6/18 3/10(0.3) 20/70	6/60 1/10(0.1) 20/200
2	6/60 1/10(0.1) 20/200	3/60 1/20(0.05) 20/400
3	3/60 1/20(0.05) 20/400	1/60(finger counting at one meter) 1/50(0.02) 5/300(20/1200)
4	1/60(finger counting at one meter) 1/50(0.02) 5/300	Light perception
5	No light perception	
9	Undetermined or unspecified	

CODING TIP✓ Use this code when the physician documents blindness without an indication of eyes involved. If "blindness" or "low vision" of both eyes is documented but the visual impairment category is not documented, assign code H54.3, Unqualified visual loss, both eyes.

CODING TIP✓ Use this code to indicate blindness in both eyes.

Other disorders of eye and adnexa (H55-H57)

H55 Nystagmus and other irregular eye movements

H55.0 Nystagmus

- **H55.00** Unspecified nystagmus
- **H55.01** Congenital nystagmus
- **H55.02** Latent nystagmus

DEFINITION Involuntary rapid movement of the eyeball occurring only when one eye is covered.

- **H55.03** Visual deprivation nystagmus
- **H55.04** Dissociated nystagmus

DEFINITION Involuntary rhythmic movements in both eyes that are dissimilar in direction, extent, and frequency of movement.

- **H55.09** Other forms of nystagmus

H55.8 Other irregular eye movements

- **H55.81** Saccadic eye movements

DEFINITION Rapid and involuntary eye movement while changing focus on stationary objects.

- **H55.89** Other irregular eye movements

H57 Other disorders of eye and adnexa

H57.0 Anomalies of pupillary function

- **H57.00** Unspecified anomaly of pupillary function
- **H57.01** Argyll Robertson pupil, atypical

EXCLUDES 1 *syphilitic Argyll Robertson pupil (A52.19)*

- **H57.02** Anisocoria

DEFINITION Pupils of unequal size.

- **H57.03** Miosis

DEFINITION Constriction of the pupil.

- **H57.04** Mydriasis

H57.05 Tonic pupil

- **H57.051** Tonic pupil, right eye
- **H57.052** Tonic pupil, left eye
- **H57.053** Tonic pupil, bilateral
- **H57.059** Tonic pupil, unspecified eye

- **H57.09** Other anomalies of pupillary function

H57.1 Ocular pain

- **H57.10** Ocular pain, unspecified eye
- **H57.11** Ocular pain, right eye
- **H57.12** Ocular pain, left eye
- **H57.13** Ocular pain, bilateral

▲ **H57.8 Other specified disorders of eye and adnexa**

● **H57.81 Brow ptosis**

- ● **H57.811** Brow ptosis, right
- ● **H57.812** Brow ptosis, left
- ● **H57.813** Brow ptosis, bilateral
- ● **H57.819** Brow ptosis, unspecified

● **H57.89** Other specified disorders of eye and adnexa

H57.9 Unspecified disorder of eye and adnexa

Intraoperative and postprocedural complications and disorders of eye and adnexa, not elsewhere classified (H59)

H59 Intraoperative and postprocedural complications and disorders of eye and adnexa, not elsewhere classified

EXCLUDES 1 *mechanical complication of intraocular lens (T85.2)*
mechanical complication of other ocular prosthetic devices, implants and grafts (T85.3)
pseudophakia (Z96.1)
secondary cataracts (H26.4-)

H59.0 Disorders of the eye following cataract surgery

H59.01 Keratopathy (bullous aphakic) following cataract surgery

Vitreal corneal syndrome
Vitreous (touch) syndrome

- **H59.011** Keratopathy (bullous aphakic) following cataract surgery, right eye
- **H59.012** Keratopathy (bullous aphakic) following cataract surgery, left eye
- **H59.013** Keratopathy (bullous aphakic) following cataract surgery, bilateral
- **H59.019** Keratopathy (bullous aphakic) following cataract surgery, unspecified eye

H59.02 Cataract (lens) fragments in eye following cataract surgery

- **H59.021** Cataract (lens) fragments in eye following cataract surgery, right eye
- **H59.022** Cataract (lens) fragments in eye following cataract surgery, left eye
- **H59.023** Cataract (lens) fragments in eye following cataract surgery, bilateral
- **H59.029** Cataract (lens) fragments in eye following cataract surgery, unspecified eye

H59.03 Cystoid macular edema following cataract surgery

- **H59.031** Cystoid macular edema following cataract surgery, right eye
- **H59.032** Cystoid macular edema following cataract surgery, left eye
- **H59.033** Cystoid macular edema following cataract surgery, bilateral
- **H59.039** Cystoid macular edema following cataract surgery, unspecified eye

H59.09 Other disorders of the eye following cataract surgery

- **H59.091** Other disorders of the right eye following cataract surgery
- **H59.092** Other disorders of the left eye following cataract surgery
- **H59.093** Other disorders of the eye following cataract surgery, bilateral
- **H59.099** Other disorders of unspecified eye following cataract surgery

H59.1 Intraoperative hemorrhage and hematoma of eye and adnexa complicating a procedure

EXCLUDES 1 *intraoperative hemorrhage and hematoma of eye and adnexa due to accidental puncture or laceration during a procedure (H59.2-)*

6 **H59.11** Intraoperative hemorrhage and hematoma of eye and adnexa complicating an ophthalmic procedure
- **H59.111** Intraoperative hemorrhage and hematoma of right eye and adnexa complicating an ophthalmic procedure
- **H59.112** Intraoperative hemorrhage and hematoma of left eye and adnexa complicating an ophthalmic procedure
- **H59.113** Intraoperative hemorrhage and hematoma of eye and adnexa complicating an ophthalmic procedure, bilateral
- **H59.119** Intraoperative hemorrhage and hematoma of unspecified eye and adnexa complicating an ophthalmic procedure

6 **H59.12** Intraoperative hemorrhage and hematoma of eye and adnexa complicating other procedure
- **H59.121** Intraoperative hemorrhage and hematoma of right eye and adnexa complicating other procedure
- **H59.122** Intraoperative hemorrhage and hematoma of left eye and adnexa complicating other procedure
- **H59.123** Intraoperative hemorrhage and hematoma of eye and adnexa complicating other procedure, bilateral
- **H59.129** Intraoperative hemorrhage and hematoma of unspecified eye and adnexa complicating other procedure

5 **H59.2** Accidental puncture and laceration of eye and adnexa during a procedure

6 **H59.21** Accidental puncture and laceration of eye and adnexa during an ophthalmic procedure
- **H59.211** Accidental puncture and laceration of right eye and adnexa during an ophthalmic procedure
- **H59.212** Accidental puncture and laceration of left eye and adnexa during an ophthalmic procedure
- **H59.213** Accidental puncture and laceration of eye and adnexa during an ophthalmic procedure, bilateral
- **H59.219** Accidental puncture and laceration of unspecified eye and adnexa during an ophthalmic procedure

6 **H59.22** Accidental puncture and laceration of eye and adnexa during other procedure
- **H59.221** Accidental puncture and laceration of right eye and adnexa during other procedure
- **H59.222** Accidental puncture and laceration of left eye and adnexa during other procedure
- **H59.223** Accidental puncture and laceration of eye and adnexa during other procedure, bilateral
- **H59.229** Accidental puncture and laceration of unspecified eye and adnexa during other procedure

5 **H59.3** Postprocedural hemorrhage, hematoma, and seroma of eye and adnexa following a procedure

6 **H59.31** Postprocedural hemorrhage of eye and adnexa following an ophthalmic procedure
- **H59.311** Postprocedural hemorrhage of right eye and adnexa following an ophthalmic procedure
- **H59.312** Postprocedural hemorrhage of left eye and adnexa following an ophthalmic procedure
- **H59.313** Postprocedural hemorrhage of eye and adnexa following an ophthalmic procedure, bilateral
- **H59.319** Postprocedural hemorrhage of unspecified eye and adnexa following an ophthalmic procedure

6 **H59.32** Postprocedural hemorrhage of eye and adnexa following other procedure
- **H59.321** Postprocedural hemorrhage of right eye and adnexa following other procedure
- **H59.322** Postprocedural hemorrhage of left eye and adnexa following other procedure
- **H59.323** Postprocedural hemorrhage of eye and adnexa following other procedure, bilateral
- **H59.329** Postprocedural hemorrhage of unspecified eye and adnexa following other procedure

6 **H59.33** Postprocedural hematoma of eye and adnexa following an ophthalmic procedure
- **H59.331** Postprocedural hematoma of right eye and adnexa following an ophthalmic procedure
- **H59.332** Postprocedural hematoma of left eye and adnexa following an ophthalmic procedure
- **H59.333** Postprocedural hematoma of eye and adnexa following an ophthalmic procedure, bilateral
- **H59.339** Postprocedural hematoma of unspecified eye and adnexa following an ophthalmic procedure

6 **H59.34** Postprocedural hematoma of eye and adnexa following other procedure
- **H59.341** Postprocedural hematoma of right eye and adnexa following other procedure
- **H59.342** Postprocedural hematoma of left eye and adnexa following other procedure
- **H59.343** Postprocedural hematoma of eye and adnexa following other procedure, bilateral
- **H59.349** Postprocedural hematoma of unspecified eye and adnexa following other procedure

6 **H59.35** Postprocedural seroma of eye and adnexa following an ophthalmic procedure
- **H59.351** Postprocedural seroma of right eye and adnexa following an ophthalmic procedure
- **H59.352** Postprocedural seroma of left eye and adnexa following an ophthalmic procedure
- **H59.353** Postprocedural seroma of eye and adnexa following an ophthalmic procedure, bilateral
- **H59.359** Postprocedural seroma of unspecified eye and adnexa following an ophthalmic procedure

6 **H59.36** Postprocedural seroma of eye and adnexa following other procedure
- **H59.361** Postprocedural seroma of right eye and adnexa following other procedure
- **H59.362** Postprocedural seroma of left eye and adnexa following other procedure
- **H59.363** Postprocedural seroma of eye and adnexa following other procedure, bilateral
- **H59.369** Postprocedural seroma of unspecified eye and adnexa following other procedure

5 **H59.4** Inflammation (infection) of postprocedural bleb

Postprocedural blebitis

EXCLUDES 1 *filtering (vitreous) bleb after glaucoma surgery status (Z98.83)*

- **H59.40** Inflammation (infection) of postprocedural bleb, unspecified
- **H59.41** Inflammation (infection) of postprocedural bleb, stage 1
- **H59.42** Inflammation (infection) of postprocedural bleb, stage 2
- **H59.43** Inflammation (infection) of postprocedural bleb, stage 3

  Bleb endophthalmitis

5 **H59.8** Other intraoperative and postprocedural complications and disorders of eye and adnexa, not elsewhere classified

6 **H59.81** Chorioretinal scars after surgery for detachment
- **H59.811** Chorioretinal scars after surgery for detachment, right eye
- **H59.812** Chorioretinal scars after surgery for detachment, left eye
- **H59.813** Chorioretinal scars after surgery for detachment, bilateral
- **H59.819** Chorioretinal scars after surgery for detachment, unspecified eye

- **H59.88** Other intraoperative complications of eye and adnexa, not elsewhere classified
- **H59.89** Other postprocedural complications and disorders of eye and adnexa, not elsewhere classified

CHAPTER 8: DISEASES OF THE EAR AND MASTOID PROCESS (H60-H95)

Note: Use an external cause code following the code for the ear condition, if applicable, to identify the cause of the ear condition

EXCLUDES 2 *certain conditions originating in the perinatal period (P04-P96)*
certain infectious and parasitic diseases (A00-B99)
complications of pregnancy, childbirth and the puerperium (O00-O9A)
congenital malformations, deformations and chromosomal abnormalities (Q00-Q99)
endocrine, nutritional and metabolic diseases (E00-E88)
injury, poisoning and certain other consequences of external causes (S00-T88)
neoplasms (C00-D49)
symptoms, signs and abnormal clinical and laboratory findings, not elsewhere classified (R00-R94)

This chapter contains the following blocks:

H60-H62	Diseases of external ear
H65-H75	Diseases of middle ear and mastoid
H80-H83	Diseases of inner ear
H90-H94	Other disorders of ear
H95	Intraoperative and postprocedural complications and disorders of ear and mastoid process, not elsewhere classified

Diseases of external ear (H60-H62)

④ **H60 Otitis externa**

Ear anatomy

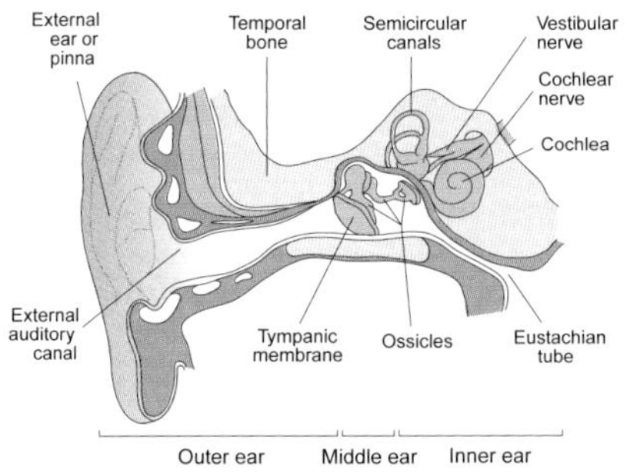

⑤ **H60.0 Abscess of external ear**
Boil of external ear
Carbuncle of auricle or external auditory canal
Furuncle of external ear
⊟ **H60.00 Abscess of external ear, unspecified ear**
⊟ **H60.01 Abscess of right external ear**
⊟ **H60.02 Abscess of left external ear**
⊟ **H60.03 Abscess of external ear, bilateral**

⑤ **H60.1 Cellulitis of external ear**
Cellulitis of auricle
Cellulitis of external auditory canal
⊟ **H60.10 Cellulitis of external ear, unspecified ear**
⊟ **H60.11 Cellulitis of right external ear**
⊟ **H60.12 Cellulitis of left external ear**
⊟ **H60.13 Cellulitis of external ear, bilateral**

⑤ **H60.2 Malignant otitis externa**
⊟ **H60.20 Malignant otitis externa, unspecified ear**
⊟ **H60.21 Malignant otitis externa, right ear**
⊟ **H60.22 Malignant otitis externa, left ear**
⊟ **H60.23 Malignant otitis externa, bilateral**

⑤ **H60.3 Other infective otitis externa**
⑥ **H60.31 Diffuse otitis externa**
⊟ **H60.311 Diffuse otitis externa, right ear**
⊟ **H60.312 Diffuse otitis externa, left ear**
⊟ **H60.313 Diffuse otitis externa, bilateral**
⊟ **H60.319 Diffuse otitis externa, unspecified ear**
⑥ **H60.32 Hemorrhagic otitis externa**
⊟ **H60.321 Hemorrhagic otitis externa, right ear**
⊟ **H60.322 Hemorrhagic otitis externa, left ear**
⊟ **H60.323 Hemorrhagic otitis externa, bilateral**
⊟ **H60.329 Hemorrhagic otitis externa, unspecified ear**
⑥ **H60.33 Swimmer's ear**
⊟ **H60.331 Swimmer's ear, right ear**
⊟ **H60.332 Swimmer's ear, left ear**
⊟ **H60.333 Swimmer's ear, bilateral**
⊟ **H60.339 Swimmer's ear, unspecified ear**
⑥ **H60.39 Other infective otitis externa**
⊟ **H60.391 Other infective otitis externa, right ear**
⊟ **H60.392 Other infective otitis externa, left ear**
⊟ **H60.393 Other infective otitis externa, bilateral**
⊟ **H60.399 Other infective otitis externa, unspecified ear**

⑤ **H60.4 Cholesteatoma of external ear**
Keratosis obturans of external ear (canal)
EXCLUDES 2 *cholesteatoma of middle ear (H71.-)*
recurrent cholesteatoma of postmastoidectomy cavity (H95.0-)
⊟ **H60.40 Cholesteatoma of external ear, unspecified ear**
⊟ **H60.41 Cholesteatoma of right external ear**
⊟ **H60.42 Cholesteatoma of left external ear**
⊟ **H60.43 Cholesteatoma of external ear, bilateral**

⑤ **H60.5 Acute noninfective otitis externa**
⑥ **H60.50 Unspecified acute noninfective otitis externa**
Acute otitis externa NOS
⊟ **H60.501 Unspecified acute noninfective otitis externa, right ear**
⊟ **H60.502 Unspecified acute noninfective otitis externa, left ear**
⊟ **H60.503 Unspecified acute noninfective otitis externa, bilateral**
⊟ **H60.509 Unspecified acute noninfective otitis externa, unspecified ear**
⑥ **H60.51 Acute actinic otitis externa**
⊟ **H60.511 Acute actinic otitis externa, right ear**
⊟ **H60.512 Acute actinic otitis externa, left ear**
⊟ **H60.513 Acute actinic otitis externa, bilateral**
⊟ **H60.519 Acute actinic otitis externa, unspecified ear**
⑥ **H60.52 Acute chemical otitis externa**
⊟ **H60.521 Acute chemical otitis externa, right ear**
⊟ **H60.522 Acute chemical otitis externa, left ear**
⊟ **H60.523 Acute chemical otitis externa, bilateral**
⊟ **H60.529 Acute chemical otitis externa, unspecified ear**
⑥ **H60.53 Acute contact otitis externa**
⊟ **H60.531 Acute contact otitis externa, right ear**
⊟ **H60.532 Acute contact otitis externa, left ear**
⊟ **H60.533 Acute contact otitis externa, bilateral**
⊟ **H60.539 Acute contact otitis externa, unspecified ear**
⑥ **H60.54 Acute eczematoid otitis externa**
⊟ **H60.541 Acute eczematoid otitis externa, right ear**
⊟ **H60.542 Acute eczematoid otitis externa, left ear**
⊟ **H60.543 Acute eczematoid otitis externa, bilateral**
⊟ **H60.549 Acute eczematoid otitis externa, unspecified ear**
⑥ **H60.55 Acute reactive otitis externa**
⊟ **H60.551 Acute reactive otitis externa, right ear**
⊟ **H60.552 Acute reactive otitis externa, left ear**
⊟ **H60.553 Acute reactive otitis externa, bilateral**
⊟ **H60.559 Acute reactive otitis externa, unspecified ear**
⑥ **H60.59 Other noninfective acute otitis externa**
⊟ **H60.591 Other noninfective acute otitis externa, right ear**
⊟ **H60.592 Other noninfective acute otitis externa, left ear**
⊟ **H60.593 Other noninfective acute otitis externa, bilateral**
⊟ **H60.599 Other noninfective acute otitis externa, unspecified ear**

⑤ **H60.6 Unspecified chronic otitis externa**
⊟ **H60.60 Unspecified chronic otitis externa, unspecified ear**

H60.61 Unspecified chronic otitis externa, right ear
H60.62 Unspecified chronic otitis externa, left ear
H60.63 Unspecified chronic otitis externa, bilateral
H60.8 Other otitis externa
H60.8X Other otitis externa
H60.8X1 Other otitis externa, right ear
H60.8X2 Other otitis externa, left ear
H60.8X3 Other otitis externa, bilateral
H60.8X9 Other otitis externa, unspecified ear
H60.9 Unspecified otitis externa
H60.90 Unspecified otitis externa, unspecified ear
H60.91 Unspecified otitis externa, right ear
H60.92 Unspecified otitis externa, left ear
H60.93 Unspecified otitis externa, bilateral

H61 Other disorders of external ear

H61.0 Chondritis and perichondritis of external ear
Chondrodermatitis nodularis chronica helicis
Perichondritis of auricle
Perichondritis of pinna
DEFINITION Inflammation of the cartilage of the outer, visible part of the ear.
H61.00 Unspecified perichondritis of external ear
H61.001 Unspecified perichondritis of right external ear
H61.002 Unspecified perichondritis of left external ear
H61.003 Unspecified perichondritis of external ear, bilateral
H61.009 Unspecified perichondritis of external ear, unspecified ear
H61.01 Acute perichondritis of external ear
H61.011 Acute perichondritis of right external ear
H61.012 Acute perichondritis of left external ear
H61.013 Acute perichondritis of external ear, bilateral
H61.019 Acute perichondritis of external ear, unspecified ear
H61.02 Chronic perichondritis of external ear
H61.021 Chronic perichondritis of right external ear
H61.022 Chronic perichondritis of left external ear
H61.023 Chronic perichondritis of external ear, bilateral
H61.029 Chronic perichondritis of external ear, unspecified ear
H61.03 Chondritis of external ear
Chondritis of auricle
Chondritis of pinna
H61.031 Chondritis of right external ear
H61.032 Chondritis of left external ear
AHA: 1Q 2015, 18
H61.033 Chondritis of external ear, bilateral
H61.039 Chondritis of external ear, unspecified ear
H61.1 Noninfective disorders of pinna
EXCLUDES 2 *cauliflower ear (M95.1-)*
gouty tophi of ear (M1A.-)
H61.10 Unspecified noninfective disorders of pinna
Disorder of pinna NOS
H61.101 Unspecified noninfective disorders of pinna, right ear
H61.102 Unspecified noninfective disorders of pinna, left ear
H61.103 Unspecified noninfective disorders of pinna, bilateral
H61.109 Unspecified noninfective disorders of pinna, unspecified ear
H61.11 Acquired deformity of pinna
Acquired deformity of auricle
EXCLUDES 2 *cauliflower ear (M95.1-)*
H61.111 Acquired deformity of pinna, right ear
H61.112 Acquired deformity of pinna, left ear
H61.113 Acquired deformity of pinna, bilateral
H61.119 Acquired deformity of pinna, unspecified ear
H61.12 Hematoma of pinna
Hematoma of auricle
DEFINITION Swelling filled with blood on the outer ear.
H61.121 Hematoma of pinna, right ear
H61.122 Hematoma of pinna, left ear
H61.123 Hematoma of pinna, bilateral
H61.129 Hematoma of pinna, unspecified ear
H61.19 Other noninfective disorders of pinna
H61.191 Noninfective disorders of pinna, right ear
H61.192 Noninfective disorders of pinna, left ear
H61.193 Noninfective disorders of pinna, bilateral
H61.199 Noninfective disorders of pinna, unspecified ear
H61.2 Impacted cerumen
Wax in ear
DEFINITION Ear wax blocking the external ear canal.
H61.20 Impacted cerumen, unspecified ear
H61.21 Impacted cerumen, right ear
H61.22 Impacted cerumen, left ear
H61.23 Impacted cerumen, bilateral
H61.3 Acquired stenosis of external ear canal
Collapse of external ear canal
EXCLUDES 1 *postprocedural stenosis of external ear canal (H95.81-)*
H61.30 Acquired stenosis of external ear canal, unspecified
H61.301 Acquired stenosis of right external ear canal, unspecified
H61.302 Acquired stenosis of left external ear canal, unspecified
H61.303 Acquired stenosis of external ear canal, unspecified, bilateral
H61.309 Acquired stenosis of external ear canal, unspecified, unspecified ear
H61.31 Acquired stenosis of external ear canal secondary to trauma
H61.311 Acquired stenosis of right external ear canal secondary to trauma
H61.312 Acquired stenosis of left external ear canal secondary to trauma
H61.313 Acquired stenosis of external ear canal secondary to trauma, bilateral
H61.319 Acquired stenosis of external ear canal secondary to trauma, unspecified ear
H61.32 Acquired stenosis of external ear canal secondary to inflammation and infection
H61.321 Acquired stenosis of right external ear canal secondary to inflammation and infection
H61.322 Acquired stenosis of left external ear canal secondary to inflammation and infection
H61.323 Acquired stenosis of external ear canal secondary to inflammation and infection, bilateral
H61.329 Acquired stenosis of external ear canal secondary to inflammation and infection, unspecified ear
H61.39 Other acquired stenosis of external ear canal
H61.391 Other acquired stenosis of right external ear canal
H61.392 Other acquired stenosis of left external ear canal
H61.393 Other acquired stenosis of external ear canal, bilateral
H61.399 Other acquired stenosis of external ear canal, unspecified ear
H61.8 Other specified disorders of external ear
H61.81 Exostosis of external canal
DEFINITION A bony growth covered with cartilage on the outer ear.
H61.811 Exostosis of right external canal
H61.812 Exostosis of left external canal
H61.813 Exostosis of external canal, bilateral
H61.819 Exostosis of external canal, unspecified ear
H61.89 Other specified disorders of external ear
H61.891 Other specified disorders of right external ear
H61.892 Other specified disorders of left external ear

H61.893 Other specified disorders of external ear, bilateral
H61.899 Other specified disorders of external ear, unspecified ear
H61.9 Disorder of external ear, unspecified
H61.90 Disorder of external ear, unspecified, unspecified ear
H61.91 Disorder of right external ear, unspecified
H61.92 Disorder of left external ear, unspecified
H61.93 Disorder of external ear, unspecified, bilateral
H62 Disorders of external ear in diseases classified elsewhere
H62.4 Otitis externa in other diseases classified elsewhere
Code first underlying disease, such as:
erysipelas (A46)
impetigo (L01.0)
EXCLUDES 1 *otitis externa (in) :*
candidiasis (B37.84)
herpes viral [herpes simplex] (B00.1)
herpes zoster (B02.8)
H62.40 *Otitis externa in other diseases classified elsewhere, unspecified ear*
H62.41 *Otitis externa in other diseases classified elsewhere, right ear*
H62.42 *Otitis externa in other diseases classified elsewhere, left ear*
H62.43 *Otitis externa in other diseases classified elsewhere, bilateral*
H62.8 Other disorders of external ear in diseases classified elsewhere
Code first underlying disease, such as:
gout (M1A.-, M10.-)
H62.8X Other disorders of external ear in diseases classified elsewhere
H62.8X1 *Other disorders of right external ear in diseases classified elsewhere*
H62.8X2 *Other disorders of left external ear in diseases classified elsewhere*
H62.8X3 *Other disorders of external ear in diseases classified elsewhere, bilateral*
H62.8X9 *Other disorders of external ear in diseases classified elsewhere, unspecified ear*

Diseases of middle ear and mastoid (H65-H75)

H65 Nonsuppurative otitis media
INCLUDES nonsuppurative otitis media with myringitis
Use additional code for any associated perforated tympanic membrane (H72.-)
Use additional code to identify:
exposure to environmental tobacco smoke (Z77.22)
exposure to tobacco smoke in the perinatal period (P96.81)
history of tobacco dependence (Z87.891)
occupational exposure to environmental tobacco smoke (Z57.31)
tobacco dependence (F17.-)
tobacco use (Z72.0)
H65.0 Acute serous otitis media
Acute and subacute secretory otitis
H65.00 Acute serous otitis media, unspecified ear
H65.01 Acute serous otitis media, right ear
H65.02 Acute serous otitis media, left ear
H65.03 Acute serous otitis media, bilateral
H65.04 Acute serous otitis media, recurrent, right ear
H65.05 Acute serous otitis media, recurrent, left ear
H65.06 Acute serous otitis media, recurrent, bilateral
H65.07 Acute serous otitis media, recurrent, unspecified ear
H65.1 Other acute nonsuppurative otitis media
EXCLUDES 1 *otitic barotrauma (T70.0)*
otitis media (acute) NOS (H66.9)
H65.11 Acute and subacute allergic otitis media (mucoid) (sanguinous) (serous)
H65.111 Acute and subacute allergic otitis media (mucoid) (sanguinous) (serous), right ear
H65.112 Acute and subacute allergic otitis media (mucoid) (sanguinous) (serous), left ear
H65.113 Acute and subacute allergic otitis media (mucoid) (sanguinous) (serous), bilateral
H65.114 Acute and subacute allergic otitis media (mucoid) (sanguinous) (serous), recurrent, right ear
H65.115 Acute and subacute allergic otitis media (mucoid) (sanguinous) (serous), recurrent, left ear
H65.116 Acute and subacute allergic otitis media (mucoid) (sanguinous) (serous), recurrent, bilateral
H65.117 Acute and subacute allergic otitis media (mucoid) (sanguinous) (serous), recurrent, unspecified ear
H65.119 Acute and subacute allergic otitis media (mucoid) (sanguinous) (serous), unspecified ear
H65.19 Other acute nonsuppurative otitis media
Acute and subacute mucoid otitis media
Acute and subacute nonsuppurative otitis media NOS
Acute and subacute sanguinous otitis media
Acute and subacute seromucinous otitis media
H65.191 Other acute nonsuppurative otitis media, right ear
H65.192 Other acute nonsuppurative otitis media, left ear
H65.193 Other acute nonsuppurative otitis media, bilateral
H65.194 Other acute nonsuppurative otitis media, recurrent, right ear
H65.195 Other acute nonsuppurative otitis media, recurrent, left ear
H65.196 Other acute nonsuppurative otitis media, recurrent, bilateral
H65.197 Other acute nonsuppurative otitis media recurrent, unspecified ear
H65.199 Other acute nonsuppurative otitis media, unspecified ear
H65.2 Chronic serous otitis media
Chronic tubotympanal catarrh
H65.20 Chronic serous otitis media, unspecified ear
H65.21 Chronic serous otitis media, right ear
H65.22 Chronic serous otitis media, left ear
H65.23 Chronic serous otitis media, bilateral
H65.3 Chronic mucoid otitis media
Chronic mucinous otitis media
Chronic secretory otitis media
Chronic transudative otitis media
Glue ear
EXCLUDES 1 *adhesive middle ear disease (H74.1)*
DEFINITION Long-term middle ear infection causing mucous to become trapped in the middle ear.
H65.30 Chronic mucoid otitis media, unspecified ear
H65.31 Chronic mucoid otitis media, right ear
H65.32 Chronic mucoid otitis media, left ear
H65.33 Chronic mucoid otitis media, bilateral
H65.4 Other chronic nonsuppurative otitis media
H65.41 Chronic allergic otitis media
H65.411 Chronic allergic otitis media, right ear
H65.412 Chronic allergic otitis media, left ear
H65.413 Chronic allergic otitis media, bilateral
H65.419 Chronic allergic otitis media, unspecified ear
H65.49 Other chronic nonsuppurative otitis media
Chronic exudative otitis media
Chronic nonsuppurative otitis media NOS
Chronic otitis media with effusion (nonpurulent)
Chronic seromucinous otitis media
H65.491 Other chronic nonsuppurative otitis media, right ear
H65.492 Other chronic nonsuppurative otitis media, left ear
H65.493 Other chronic nonsuppurative otitis media, bilateral
H65.499 Other chronic nonsuppurative otitis media, unspecified ear

H65.9 Unspecified nonsuppurative otitis media
Allergic otitis media NOS
Catarrhal otitis media NOS
Exudative otitis media NOS
Mucoid otitis media NOS
Otitis media with effusion (nonpurulent) NOS
Secretory otitis media NOS
Seromucinous otitis media NOS
Serous otitis media NOS
Transudative otitis media NOS

H65.90 Unspecified nonsuppurative otitis media, unspecified ear
H65.91 Unspecified nonsuppurative otitis media, right ear
H65.92 Unspecified nonsuppurative otitis media, left ear
H65.93 Unspecified nonsuppurative otitis media, bilateral

H66 Suppurative and unspecified otitis media

INCLUDES suppurative and unspecified otitis media with myringitis

Use additional code to identify:
exposure to environmental tobacco smoke (Z77.22)
exposure to tobacco smoke in the perinatal period (P96.81)
history of tobacco dependence (Z87.891)
occupational exposure to environmental tobacco smoke (Z57.31)
tobacco dependence (F17.-)
tobacco use (Z72.0)

H66.0 Acute suppurative otitis media

H66.00 Acute suppurative otitis media without spontaneous rupture of ear drum
H66.001 Acute suppurative otitis media without spontaneous rupture of ear drum, right ear
AHA: 1Q 2016, 34
H66.002 Acute suppurative otitis media without spontaneous rupture of ear drum, left ear
H66.003 Acute suppurative otitis media without spontaneous rupture of ear drum, bilateral
H66.004 Acute suppurative otitis media without spontaneous rupture of ear drum, recurrent, right ear
H66.005 Acute suppurative otitis media without spontaneous rupture of ear drum, recurrent, left ear
H66.006 Acute suppurative otitis media without spontaneous rupture of ear drum, recurrent, bilateral
H66.007 Acute suppurative otitis media without spontaneous rupture of ear drum, recurrent, unspecified ear
H66.009 Acute suppurative otitis media without spontaneous rupture of ear drum, unspecified ear

H66.01 Acute suppurative otitis media with spontaneous rupture of ear drum
H66.011 Acute suppurative otitis media with spontaneous rupture of ear drum, right ear
H66.012 Acute suppurative otitis media with spontaneous rupture of ear drum, left ear
H66.013 Acute suppurative otitis media with spontaneous rupture of ear drum, bilateral
H66.014 Acute suppurative otitis media with spontaneous rupture of ear drum, recurrent, right ear
H66.015 Acute suppurative otitis media with spontaneous rupture of ear drum, recurrent, left ear
H66.016 Acute suppurative otitis media with spontaneous rupture of ear drum, recurrent, bilateral
H66.017 Acute suppurative otitis media with spontaneous rupture of ear drum, recurrent, unspecified ear
H66.019 Acute suppurative otitis media with spontaneous rupture of ear drum, unspecified ear

H66.1 Chronic tubotympanic suppurative otitis media
Benign chronic suppurative otitis media
Chronic tubotympanic disease
Use additional code for any associated perforated tympanic membrane (H72.-)

H66.10 Chronic tubotympanic suppurative otitis media, unspecified
H66.11 Chronic tubotympanic suppurative otitis media, right ear
H66.12 Chronic tubotympanic suppurative otitis media, left ear
H66.13 Chronic tubotympanic suppurative otitis media, bilateral

H66.2 Chronic atticoantral suppurative otitis media
Chronic atticoantral disease
Use additional code for any associated perforated tympanic membrane (H72.-)

H66.20 Chronic atticoantral suppurative otitis media, unspecified ear
H66.21 Chronic atticoantral suppurative otitis media, right ear
H66.22 Chronic atticoantral suppurative otitis media, left ear
H66.23 Chronic atticoantral suppurative otitis media, bilateral

H66.3 Other chronic suppurative otitis media
Chronic suppurative otitis media NOS
Use additional code for any associated perforated tympanic membrane (H72.-)
EXCLUDES 1 *tuberculous otitis media (A18.6)*

H66.3X Other chronic suppurative otitis media
H66.3X1 Other chronic suppurative otitis media, right ear
H66.3X2 Other chronic suppurative otitis media, left ear
H66.3X3 Other chronic suppurative otitis media, bilateral
H66.3X9 Other chronic suppurative otitis media, unspecified ear

H66.4 Suppurative otitis media, unspecified
Purulent otitis media NOS
Use additional code for any associated perforated tympanic membrane (H72.-)

H66.40 Suppurative otitis media, unspecified, unspecified ear
H66.41 Suppurative otitis media, unspecified, right ear
H66.42 Suppurative otitis media, unspecified, left ear
H66.43 Suppurative otitis media, unspecified, bilateral

H66.9 Otitis media, unspecified
Otitis media NOS
Acute otitis media NOS
Chronic otitis media NOS
Use additional code for any associated perforated tympanic membrane (H72.-)

H66.90 Otitis media, unspecified, unspecified ear
H66.91 Otitis media, unspecified, right ear
H66.92 Otitis media, unspecified, left ear
H66.93 Otitis media, unspecified, bilateral

▲ H67 Otitis media in diseases classified elsewhere

Code first underlying disease, such as:
plasminogen deficiency (E88.02)
viral disease NEC (B00-B34)
Use additional code for any associated perforated tympanic membrane (H72.-)
EXCLUDES 1 *otitis media in:*
influenza (J09.X9, J10.83, J11.83)
measles (B05.3)
scarlet fever (A38.0)
tuberculosis (A18.6)

H67.1 Otitis media in diseases classified elsewhere, right ear
H67.2 Otitis media in diseases classified elsewhere, left ear
H67.3 Otitis media in diseases classified elsewhere, bilateral
H67.9 Otitis media in diseases classified elsewhere, unspecified ear

H68 Eustachian salpingitis and obstruction

H68.0 Eustachian salpingitis

H68.00 Unspecified Eustachian salpingitis
H68.001 Unspecified Eustachian salpingitis, right ear
H68.002 Unspecified Eustachian salpingitis, left ear
H68.003 Unspecified Eustachian salpingitis, bilateral

H68.009 Unspecified Eustachian salpingitis, unspecified ear
H68.01 Acute Eustachian salpingitis
H68.011 Acute Eustachian salpingitis, right ear
H68.012 Acute Eustachian salpingitis, left ear
H68.013 Acute Eustachian salpingitis, bilateral
H68.019 Acute Eustachian salpingitis, unspecified ear
H68.02 Chronic Eustachian salpingitis
H68.021 Chronic Eustachian salpingitis, right ear
H68.022 Chronic Eustachian salpingitis, left ear
H68.023 Chronic Eustachian salpingitis, bilateral
H68.029 Chronic Eustachian salpingitis, unspecified ear
H68.1 Obstruction of Eustachian tube
Stenosis of Eustachian tube
Stricture of Eustachian tube
H68.10 Unspecified obstruction of Eustachian tube
H68.101 Unspecified obstruction of Eustachian tube, right ear
H68.102 Unspecified obstruction of Eustachian tube, left ear
H68.103 Unspecified obstruction of Eustachian tube, bilateral
H68.109 Unspecified obstruction of Eustachian tube, unspecified ear
H68.11 Osseous obstruction of Eustachian tube
H68.111 Osseous obstruction of Eustachian tube, right ear
H68.112 Osseous obstruction of Eustachian tube, left ear
H68.113 Osseous obstruction of Eustachian tube, bilateral
H68.119 Osseous obstruction of Eustachian tube, unspecified ear
H68.12 Intrinsic cartilagenous obstruction of Eustachian tube
H68.121 Intrinsic cartilagenous obstruction of Eustachian tube, right ear
H68.122 Intrinsic cartilagenous obstruction of Eustachian tube, left ear
H68.123 Intrinsic cartilagenous obstruction of Eustachian tube, bilateral
H68.129 Intrinsic cartilagenous obstruction of Eustachian tube, unspecified ear
H68.13 Extrinsic cartilagenous obstruction of Eustachian tube
Compression of Eustachian tube
H68.131 Extrinsic cartilagenous obstruction of Eustachian tube, right ear
H68.132 Extrinsic cartilagenous obstruction of Eustachian tube, left ear
H68.133 Extrinsic cartilagenous obstruction of Eustachian tube, bilateral
H68.139 Extrinsic cartilagenous obstruction of Eustachian tube, unspecified ear

H69 Other and unspecified disorders of Eustachian tube

H69.0 Patulous Eustachian tube
H69.00 Patulous Eustachian tube, unspecified ear
H69.01 Patulous Eustachian tube, right ear
H69.02 Patulous Eustachian tube, left ear
H69.03 Patulous Eustachian tube, bilateral
H69.8 Other specified disorders of Eustachian tube
H69.80 Other specified disorders of Eustachian tube, unspecified ear
H69.81 Other specified disorders of Eustachian tube, right ear
H69.82 Other specified disorders of Eustachian tube, left ear
H69.83 Other specified disorders of Eustachian tube, bilateral
H69.9 Unspecified Eustachian tube disorder
H69.90 Unspecified Eustachian tube disorder, unspecified ear
H69.91 Unspecified Eustachian tube disorder, right ear
H69.92 Unspecified Eustachian tube disorder, left ear
H69.93 Unspecified Eustachian tube disorder, bilateral

H70 Mastoiditis and related conditions

H70.0 Acute mastoiditis
Abscess of mastoid
Empyema of mastoid
H70.00 Acute mastoiditis without complications
H70.001 Acute mastoiditis without complications, right ear
H70.002 Acute mastoiditis without complications, left ear
H70.003 Acute mastoiditis without complications, bilateral
H70.009 Acute mastoiditis without complications, unspecified ear
H70.01 Subperiosteal abscess of mastoid
H70.011 Subperiosteal abscess of mastoid, right ear
H70.012 Subperiosteal abscess of mastoid, left ear
H70.013 Subperiosteal abscess of mastoid, bilateral
H70.019 Subperiosteal abscess of mastoid, unspecified ear
H70.09 Acute mastoiditis with other complications
H70.091 Acute mastoiditis with other complications, right ear
H70.092 Acute mastoiditis with other complications, left ear
H70.093 Acute mastoiditis with other complications, bilateral
H70.099 Acute mastoiditis with other complications, unspecified ear
H70.1 Chronic mastoiditis
Caries of mastoid
Fistula of mastoid
EXCLUDES 1 *tuberculous mastoiditis (A18.03)*
H70.10 Chronic mastoiditis, unspecified ear
H70.11 Chronic mastoiditis, right ear
H70.12 Chronic mastoiditis, left ear
H70.13 Chronic mastoiditis, bilateral
H70.2 Petrositis
Inflammation of petrous bone
H70.20 Unspecified petrositis
DEFINITION Inflammation of the dense, hard bone behind the temple protecting the inner ear.
H70.201 Unspecified petrositis, right ear
H70.202 Unspecified petrositis, left ear
H70.203 Unspecified petrositis, bilateral
H70.209 Unspecified petrositis, unspecified ear
H70.21 Acute petrositis
H70.211 Acute petrositis, right ear
H70.212 Acute petrositis, left ear
H70.213 Acute petrositis, bilateral
H70.219 Acute petrositis, unspecified ear
H70.22 Chronic petrositis
H70.221 Chronic petrositis, right ear
H70.222 Chronic petrositis, left ear
H70.223 Chronic petrositis, bilateral
H70.229 Chronic petrositis, unspecified ear
H70.8 Other mastoiditis and related conditions
EXCLUDES 1 *preauricular sinus and cyst (Q18.1)*
sinus, fistula, and cyst of branchial cleft (Q18.0)
H70.81 Postauricular fistula
H70.811 Postauricular fistula, right ear
H70.812 Postauricular fistula, left ear
H70.813 Postauricular fistula, bilateral
H70.819 Postauricular fistula, unspecified ear
H70.89 Other mastoiditis and related conditions
H70.891 Other mastoiditis and related conditions, right ear
H70.892 Other mastoiditis and related conditions, left ear
H70.893 Other mastoiditis and related conditions, bilateral

H70.899 **Other mastoiditis and related conditions, unspecified ear**

H70.9 Unspecified **mastoiditis**

H70.90 **Unspecified mastoiditis,** unspecified ear

H70.91 **Unspecified mastoiditis,** right ear

H70.92 **Unspecified mastoiditis,** left ear

H70.93 **Unspecified mastoiditis,** bilateral

H71 Cholesteatoma of middle ear

EXCLUDES 2 *cholesteatoma of external ear (H60.4-)*
recurrent cholesteatoma of postmastoidectomy cavity (H95.0-)

DEFINITION Cyst-like mass filled with cell debris and cholesterol crystals in the middle ear and/or mastoid process that can damage the ossicles, causing deafness, vertigo, and nerve deterioration.

H71.0 **Cholesteatoma of** attic

H71.00 **Cholesteatoma of attic,** unspecified ear

H71.01 **Cholesteatoma of attic,** right ear

H71.02 **Cholesteatoma of attic,** left ear

H71.03 **Cholesteatoma of attic,** bilateral

H71.1 **Cholesteatoma of** tympanum

H71.10 **Cholesteatoma of tympanum,** unspecified ear

H71.11 **Cholesteatoma of tympanum,** right ear

H71.12 **Cholesteatoma of tympanum,** left ear

H71.13 **Cholesteatoma of tympanum,** bilateral

H71.2 **Cholesteatoma of** mastoid

H71.20 **Cholesteatoma of mastoid,** unspecified ear

H71.21 **Cholesteatoma of mastoid,** right ear

H71.22 **Cholesteatoma of mastoid,** left ear

H71.23 **Cholesteatoma of mastoid,** bilateral

H71.3 Diffuse **cholesteatosis**

H71.30 **Diffuse cholesteatosis,** unspecified ear

H71.31 **Diffuse cholesteatosis,** right ear

H71.32 **Diffuse cholesteatosis,** left ear

H71.33 **Diffuse cholesteatosis,** bilateral

H71.9 Unspecified **cholesteatoma**

H71.90 **Unspecified cholesteatoma,** unspecified ear

H71.91 **Unspecified cholesteatoma,** right ear

H71.92 **Unspecified cholesteatoma,** left ear

H71.93 **Unspecified cholesteatoma,** bilateral

H72 Perforation of tympanic membrane

INCLUDES persistent post-traumatic perforation of ear drum
postinflammatory perforation of ear drum

Code first:
any associated otitis media (H65.-, H66.1-, H66.2-, H66.3-, H66.4-, H66.9-, H67.-)

EXCLUDES 1 *acute suppurative otitis media with rupture of the tympanic membrane (H66.01-)*
traumatic rupture of ear drum (S09.2-)

Perforation of tympanic membrane

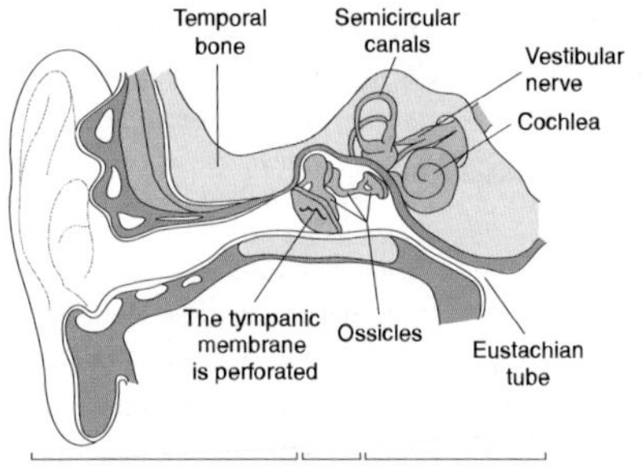

H72.0 Central **perforation of tympanic membrane**

H72.00 **Central perforation of tympanic membrane,** unspecified ear

H72.01 **Central perforation of tympanic membrane,** right ear

H72.02 **Central perforation of tympanic membrane,** left ear

H72.03 **Central perforation of tympanic membrane,** bilateral

H72.1 Attic **perforation of tympanic membrane**
Perforation of pars flaccida

H72.10 **Attic perforation of tympanic membrane,** unspecified ear

H72.11 **Attic perforation of tympanic membrane,** right ear

H72.12 **Attic perforation of tympanic membrane,** left ear

H72.13 **Attic perforation of tympanic membrane,** bilateral

H72.2 Other marginal **perforations of tympanic membrane**

H72.2X **Other marginal perforations of tympanic membrane**

H72.2X1 **Other marginal perforations of tympanic membrane,** right ear

H72.2X2 **Other marginal perforations of tympanic membrane,** left ear

H72.2X3 **Other marginal perforations of tympanic membrane,** bilateral

H72.2X9 **Other marginal perforations of tympanic membrane,** unspecified ear

H72.8 Other **perforations of tympanic membrane**

H72.81 Multiple **perforations of tympanic membrane**

H72.811 **Multiple perforations of tympanic membrane,** right ear

H72.812 **Multiple perforations of tympanic membrane,** left ear

H72.813 **Multiple perforations of tympanic membrane,** bilateral

H72.819 **Multiple perforations of tympanic membrane,** unspecified ear

H72.82 Total **perforations of tympanic membrane**

H72.821 **Total perforations of tympanic membrane,** right ear

H72.822 **Total perforations of tympanic membrane,** left ear

H72.823 **Total perforations of tympanic membrane,** bilateral

H72.829 **Total perforations of tympanic membrane,** unspecified ear

H72.9 Unspecified **perforation of tympanic membrane**

H72.90 **Unspecified perforation of tympanic membrane,** unspecified ear

H72.91 **Unspecified perforation of tympanic membrane,** right ear

H72.92 **Unspecified perforation of tympanic membrane,** left ear

H72.93 **Unspecified perforation of tympanic membrane,** bilateral

H73 Other disorders of tympanic membrane

H73.0 **Acute myringitis**

EXCLUDES 1 *acute myringitis with otitis media (H65, H66)*

H73.00 Unspecified **acute myringitis**
Acute tympanitis NOS

H73.001 **Acute myringitis,** right ear

H73.002 **Acute myringitis,** left ear

H73.003 **Acute myringitis,** bilateral

H73.009 **Acute myringitis,** unspecified ear

H73.01 Bullous **myringitis**

DEFINITION Inflammation of the eardrum caused by a virus and characterized by blood-filled blisters.

H73.011 **Bullous myringitis,** right ear

H73.012 **Bullous myringitis,** left ear

H73.013 **Bullous myringitis,** bilateral

H73.019 **Bullous myringitis,** unspecified ear

H73.09 Other **acute myringitis**

H73.091 **Other acute myringitis,** right ear

H73.092 **Other acute myringitis,** left ear

H73.093 **Other acute myringitis,** bilateral

H73.099 **Other acute myringitis,** unspecified ear

H73.1 Chronic myringitis
Chronic tympanitis
EXCLUDES 1 *chronic myringitis with otitis media (H65, H66)*
- H73.10 Chronic myringitis, unspecified ear
- H73.11 Chronic myringitis, right ear
- H73.12 Chronic myringitis, left ear
- H73.13 Chronic myringitis, bilateral

H73.2 Unspecified myringitis
- H73.20 Unspecified myringitis, unspecified ear
- H73.21 Unspecified myringitis, right ear
- H73.22 Unspecified myringitis, left ear
- H73.23 Unspecified myringitis, bilateral

H73.8 Other specified disorders of tympanic membrane
H73.81 Atrophic flaccid tympanic membrane
DEFINITION Eardrum that has wasted away and lost its tension, resulting in severe hearing loss.
- H73.811 Atrophic flaccid tympanic membrane, right ear
- H73.812 Atrophic flaccid tympanic membrane, left ear
- H73.813 Atrophic flaccid tympanic membrane, bilateral
- H73.819 Atrophic flaccid tympanic membrane, unspecified ear

H73.82 Atrophic nonflaccid tympanic membrane
- H73.821 Atrophic nonflaccid tympanic membrane, right ear
- H73.822 Atrophic nonflaccid tympanic membrane, left ear
- H73.823 Atrophic nonflaccid tympanic membrane, bilateral
- H73.829 Atrophic nonflaccid tympanic membrane, unspecified ear

H73.89 Other specified disorders of tympanic membrane
- H73.891 Other specified disorders of tympanic membrane, right ear
- H73.892 Other specified disorders of tympanic membrane, left ear
- H73.893 Other specified disorders of tympanic membrane, bilateral
- H73.899 Other specified disorders of tympanic membrane, unspecified ear

H73.9 Unspecified disorder of tympanic membrane
- H73.90 Unspecified disorder of tympanic membrane, unspecified ear
- H73.91 Unspecified disorder of tympanic membrane, right ear
- H73.92 Unspecified disorder of tympanic membrane, left ear
- H73.93 Unspecified disorder of tympanic membrane, bilateral

H74 Other disorders of middle ear mastoid
EXCLUDES 2 *mastoiditis (H70.-)*

H74.0 Tympanosclerosis
DEFINITION Thickening and hardening of the eardrum, reducing its ability to vibrate and transmit sound.
- H74.01 Tympanosclerosis, right ear
- H74.02 Tympanosclerosis, left ear
- H74.03 Tympanosclerosis, bilateral
- H74.09 Tympanosclerosis, unspecified ear

H74.1 Adhesive middle ear disease
Adhesive otitis
EXCLUDES 1 *glue ear (H65.3-)*
- H74.11 Adhesive right middle ear disease
- H74.12 Adhesive left middle ear disease
- H74.13 Adhesive middle ear disease, bilateral
- H74.19 Adhesive middle ear disease, unspecified ear

H74.2 Discontinuity and dislocation of ear ossicles
- H74.20 Discontinuity and dislocation of ear ossicles, unspecified ear
- H74.21 Discontinuity and dislocation of right ear ossicles
- H74.22 Discontinuity and dislocation of left ear ossicles
- H74.23 Discontinuity and dislocation of ear ossicles, bilateral

H74.3 Other acquired abnormalities of ear ossicles
H74.31 Ankylosis of ear ossicles
- H74.311 Ankylosis of ear ossicles, right ear
- H74.312 Ankylosis of ear ossicles, left ear
- H74.313 Ankylosis of ear ossicles, bilateral
- H74.319 Ankylosis of ear ossicles, unspecified ear

H74.32 Partial loss of ear ossicles
- H74.321 Partial loss of ear ossicles, right ear
- H74.322 Partial loss of ear ossicles, left ear
- H74.323 Partial loss of ear ossicles, bilateral
- H74.329 Partial loss of ear ossicles, unspecified ear

H74.39 Other acquired abnormalities of ear ossicles
- H74.391 Other acquired abnormalities of right ear ossicles
- H74.392 Other acquired abnormalities of left ear ossicles
- H74.393 Other acquired abnormalities of ear ossicles, bilateral
- H74.399 Other acquired abnormalities of ear ossicles, unspecified ear

H74.4 Polyp of middle ear
- H74.40 Polyp of middle ear, unspecified ear
- H74.41 Polyp of right middle ear
- H74.42 Polyp of left middle ear
- H74.43 Polyp of middle ear, bilateral

H74.8 Other specified disorders of middle ear and mastoid
H74.8X Other specified disorders of middle ear and mastoid
- H74.8X1 Other specified disorders of right middle ear and mastoid
- H74.8X2 Other specified disorders of left middle ear and mastoid
- H74.8X3 Other specified disorders of middle ear and mastoid, bilateral
- H74.8X9 Other specified disorders of middle ear and mastoid, unspecified ear

H74.9 Unspecified disorder of middle ear and mastoid
- H74.90 Unspecified disorder of middle ear and mastoid, unspecified ear
- H74.91 Unspecified disorder of right middle ear and mastoid
- H74.92 Unspecified disorder of left middle ear and mastoid
- H74.93 Unspecified disorder of middle ear and mastoid, bilateral

H75 Other disorders of middle ear and mastoid in diseases classified elsewhere
Code first:
underlying disease

H75.0 Mastoiditis in infectious and parasitic diseases classified elsewhere
EXCLUDES 1 *mastoiditis (in) :*
syphilis (A52.77)
tuberculosis (A18.03)
- H75.00 *Mastoiditis in infectious and parasitic diseases classified elsewhere, unspecified ear*
- H75.01 *Mastoiditis in infectious and parasitic diseases classified elsewhere, right ear*
- H75.02 *Mastoiditis in infectious and parasitic diseases classified elsewhere, left ear*
- H75.03 *Mastoiditis in infectious and parasitic diseases classified elsewhere, bilateral*

H75.8 Other specified disorders of middle ear and mastoid in diseases classified elsewhere
- H75.80 *Other specified disorders of middle ear and mastoid in diseases classified elsewhere, unspecified ear*
- H75.81 *Other specified disorders of right middle ear and mastoid in diseases classified elsewhere*
- H75.82 *Other specified disorders of left middle ear and mastoid in diseases classified elsewhere*
- H75.83 *Other specified disorders of middle ear and mastoid in diseases classified elsewhere, bilateral*

Diseases of inner ear (H80-H83)

H80 Otosclerosis

INCLUDES Otospongiosis

H80.0 Otosclerosis involving oval window, nonobliterative
- **H80.00 Otosclerosis involving oval window, nonobliterative, unspecified ear**
- **H80.01 Otosclerosis involving oval window, nonobliterative, right ear**
- **H80.02 Otosclerosis involving oval window, nonobliterative, left ear**
- **H80.03 Otosclerosis involving oval window, nonobliterative, bilateral**

H80.1 Otosclerosis involving oval window, obliterative
- **H80.10 Otosclerosis involving oval window, obliterative, unspecified ear**
- **H80.11 Otosclerosis involving oval window, obliterative, right ear**
- **H80.12 Otosclerosis involving oval window, obliterative, left ear**
- **H80.13 Otosclerosis involving oval window, obliterative, bilateral**

H80.2 Cochlear otosclerosis

Otosclerosis involving otic capsule
Otosclerosis involving round window

DEFINITION Formation of bony tissue in the cochlea, causing hearing loss.

- **H80.20 Cochlear otosclerosis, unspecified ear**
- **H80.21 Cochlear otosclerosis, right ear**
- **H80.22 Cochlear otosclerosis, left ear**
- **H80.23 Cochlear otosclerosis, bilateral**

H80.8 Other otosclerosis
- **H80.80 Other otosclerosis, unspecified ear**
- **H80.81 Other otosclerosis, right ear**
- **H80.82 Other otosclerosis, left ear**
- **H80.83 Other otosclerosis, bilateral**

H80.9 Unspecified otosclerosis
- **H80.90 Unspecified otosclerosis, unspecified ear**
- **H80.91 Unspecified otosclerosis, right ear**
- **H80.92 Unspecified otosclerosis, left ear**
- **H80.93 Unspecified otosclerosis, bilateral**

H81 Disorders of vestibular function

EXCLUDES 1 *epidemic vertigo (A88.1)*
vertigo NOS (R42)

H81.0 Ménière's disease

Labyrinthine hydrops
Ménière's syndrome or vertigo

DEFINITION Disorder of the inner ear causing attacks of vertigo, tinnitus, and progressive hearing loss involving all tones.

- **H81.01 Ménière's disease, right ear**
- **H81.02 Ménière's disease, left ear**
- **H81.03 Ménière's disease, bilateral**
- **H81.09 Ménière's disease, unspecified ear**

H81.1 Benign paroxysmal vertigo
- **H81.10 Benign paroxysmal vertigo, unspecified ear**
- **H81.11 Benign paroxysmal vertigo, right ear**
- **H81.12 Benign paroxysmal vertigo, left ear**
- **H81.13 Benign paroxysmal vertigo, bilateral**

H81.2 Vestibular neuronitis
- **H81.20 Vestibular neuronitis, unspecified ear**
- **H81.21 Vestibular neuronitis, right ear**
- **H81.22 Vestibular neuronitis, left ear**
- **H81.23 Vestibular neuronitis, bilateral**

H81.3 Other peripheral vertigo

H81.31 Aural vertigo
- **H81.311 Aural vertigo, right ear**
- **H81.312 Aural vertigo, left ear**
- **H81.313 Aural vertigo, bilateral**
- **H81.319 Aural vertigo, unspecified ear**

H81.39 Other peripheral vertigo

Lermoyez' syndrome
Otogenic vertigo
Peripheral vertigo NOS

- **H81.391 Other peripheral vertigo, right ear**
- **H81.392 Other peripheral vertigo, left ear**
- **H81.393 Other peripheral vertigo, bilateral**
- **H81.399 Other peripheral vertigo, unspecified ear**

H81.4 Vertigo of central origin

Central positional nystagmus

- **H81.41 Vertigo of central origin, right ear**
- **H81.42 Vertigo of central origin, left ear**
- **H81.43 Vertigo of central origin, bilateral**
- **H81.49 Vertigo of central origin, unspecified ear**

H81.8 Other disorders of vestibular function

H81.8X Other disorders of vestibular function
- **H81.8X1 Other disorders of vestibular function, right ear**
- **H81.8X2 Other disorders of vestibular function, left ear**
- **H81.8X3 Other disorders of vestibular function, bilateral**
- **H81.8X9 Other disorders of vestibular function, unspecified ear**

H81.9 Unspecified disorder of vestibular function

Vertiginous syndrome NOS

- **H81.90 Unspecified disorder of vestibular function, unspecified ear**
- **H81.91 Unspecified disorder of vestibular function, right ear**
- **H81.92 Unspecified disorder of vestibular function, left ear**
- **H81.93 Unspecified disorder of vestibular function, bilateral**

H82 Vertiginous syndromes in diseases classified elsewhere

Code first:
underlying disease

EXCLUDES 1 *epidemic vertigo (A88.1)*

- H82.1 ***Vertiginous syndromes in diseases classified elsewhere, right ear***
- H82.2 ***Vertiginous syndromes in diseases classified elsewhere, left ear***
- H82.3 ***Vertiginous syndromes in diseases classified elsewhere, bilateral***
- H82.9 ***Vertiginous syndromes in diseases classified elsewhere, unspecified ear***

H83 Other diseases of inner ear

H83.0 Labyrinthitis
- **H83.01 Labyrinthitis, right ear**
- **H83.02 Labyrinthitis, left ear**
- **H83.03 Labyrinthitis, bilateral**
- **H83.09 Labyrinthitis, unspecified ear**

H83.1 Labyrinthine fistula
- **H83.11 Labyrinthine fistula, right ear**
- **H83.12 Labyrinthine fistula, left ear**
- **H83.13 Labyrinthine fistula, bilateral**
- **H83.19 Labyrinthine fistula, unspecified ear**

H83.2 Labyrinthine dysfunction

Labyrinthine hypersensitivity
Labyrinthine hypofunction
Labyrinthine loss of function

H83.2X Labyrinthine dysfunction
- **H83.2X1 Labyrinthine dysfunction, right ear**
- **H83.2X2 Labyrinthine dysfunction, left ear**
- **H83.2X3 Labyrinthine dysfunction, bilateral**
- **H83.2X9 Labyrinthine dysfunction, unspecified ear**

H83.3 Noise effects on inner ear

Acoustic trauma of inner ear
Noise-induced hearing loss of inner ear

H83.3X Noise effects on inner ear
- **H83.3X1 Noise effects on right inner ear**
- **H83.3X2 Noise effects on left inner ear**
- **H83.3X3 Noise effects on inner ear, bilateral**
- **H83.3X9 Noise effects on inner ear, unspecified ear**

H83.8 Other specified diseases of inner ear

H83.8X Other specified diseases of inner ear
- **H83.8X1 Other specified diseases of right inner ear**

H83.8X2 Other specified diseases of left inner ear
H83.8X3 Other specified diseases of inner ear, bilateral
H83.8X9 Other specified diseases of inner ear, unspecified ear
H83.9 Unspecified disease of inner ear
H83.90 Unspecified disease of inner ear, unspecified ear
H83.91 Unspecified disease of right inner ear
H83.92 Unspecified disease of left inner ear
H83.93 Unspecified disease of inner ear, bilateral

Other disorders of ear (H90-H94)

H90 Conductive and sensorineural hearing loss

EXCLUDES 1 *deaf nonspeaking NEC (H91.3)*
deafness NOS (H91.9-)
hearing loss NOS (H91.9-)
noise-induced hearing loss (H83.3-)
ototoxic hearing loss (H91.0-)
sudden (idiopathic) hearing loss (H91.2-)

H90.0 Conductive hearing loss, bilateral
H90.1 Conductive hearing loss, unilateral with unrestricted hearing on the contralateral side
H90.11 Conductive hearing loss, unilateral, right ear, with unrestricted hearing on the contralateral side
H90.12 Conductive hearing loss, unilateral, left ear, with unrestricted hearing on the contralateral side
H90.2 Conductive hearing loss, unspecified
Conductive deafness NOS
DEFINITION Loss of audio acuity caused by transmission interference of sound waves before they can reach the inner ear and the auditory nerve.
H90.3 Sensorineural hearing loss, bilateral
H90.4 Sensorineural hearing loss, unilateral with unrestricted hearing on the contralateral side
H90.41 Sensorineural hearing loss, unilateral, right ear, with unrestricted hearing on the contralateral side
H90.42 Sensorineural hearing loss, unilateral, left ear, with unrestricted hearing on the contralateral side
H90.5 Unspecified sensorineural hearing loss
Central hearing loss NOS
Congenital deafness NOS
Neural hearing loss NOS
Perceptive hearing loss NOS
Sensorineural deafness NOS
Sensory hearing loss NOS
EXCLUDES 1 *abnormal auditory perception (H93.2-)*
psychogenic deafness (F44.6)
DEFINITION Sensory-nerve based hearing loss caused by a disorder affecting the VIII cranial nerve, the inner ear sensory perception, or the central processing area of the brain.
H90.6 Mixed conductive and sensorineural hearing loss, bilateral
AHA: 2Q 2015, 7
H90.7 Mixed conductive and sensorineural hearing loss, unilateral with unrestricted hearing on the contralateral side
H90.71 Mixed conductive and sensorineural hearing loss, unilateral, right ear, with unrestricted hearing on the contralateral side
H90.72 Mixed conductive and sensorineural hearing loss, unilateral, left ear, with unrestricted hearing on the contralateral side
H90.8 Mixed conductive and sensorineural hearing loss, unspecified
H90.A Conductive and sensorineural hearing loss with restricted hearing on the contralateral side
H90.A1 Conductive hearing loss, unilateral, with restricted hearing on the contralateral side
AHA: 4Q 2016, 23
H90.A11 Conductive hearing loss, unilateral, right ear with restricted hearing on the contralateral side
H90.A12 Conductive hearing loss, unilateral, left ear with restricted hearing on the contralateral side
H90.A2 Sensorineural hearing loss, unilateral, with restricted hearing on the contralateral side
H90.A21 Sensorineural hearing loss, unilateral, right ear, with restricted hearing on the contralateral side
H90.A22 Sensorineural hearing loss, unilateral, left ear, with restricted hearing on the contralateral side
H90.A3 Mixed conductive and sensorineural hearing loss, unilateral with restricted hearing on the contralateral side
H90.A31 Mixed conductive and sensorineural hearing loss, unilateral, right ear with restricted hearing on the contralateral side
H90.A32 Mixed conductive and sensorineural hearing loss, unilateral, left ear with restricted hearing on the contralateral side

H91 Other and unspecified hearing loss

EXCLUDES 1 *abnormal auditory perception (H93.2-)*
hearing loss as classified in H90.-
impacted cerumen (H61.2-)
noise-induced hearing loss (H83.3-)
psychogenic deafness (F44.6)
transient ischemic deafness (H93.01-)

H91.0 Ototoxic hearing loss
Code first:
poisoning due to drug or toxin, if applicable (T36-T65 with fifth or sixth character 1-4 or 6)
Use additional code for adverse effect, if applicable, to identify drug (T36-T50 with fifth or sixth character 5)
H91.01 Ototoxic hearing loss, right ear
H91.02 Ototoxic hearing loss, left ear
H91.03 Ototoxic hearing loss, bilateral
H91.09 Ototoxic hearing loss, unspecified ear
H91.1 Presbycusis
Presbyacusia
DEFINITION Gradual hearing loss that normally occurs with age.
H91.10 Presbycusis, unspecified ear
H91.11 Presbycusis, right ear
H91.12 Presbycusis, left ear
H91.13 Presbycusis, bilateral
H91.2 Sudden idiopathic hearing loss
Sudden hearing loss NOS
H91.20 Sudden idiopathic hearing loss, unspecified ear
H91.21 Sudden idiopathic hearing loss, right ear
H91.22 Sudden idiopathic hearing loss, left ear
H91.23 Sudden idiopathic hearing loss, bilateral
H91.3 Deaf nonspeaking, not elsewhere classified
H91.8 Other specified hearing loss
H91.8X Other specified hearing loss
H91.8X1 Other specified hearing loss, right ear
H91.8X2 Other specified hearing loss, left ear
H91.8X3 Other specified hearing loss, bilateral
H91.8X9 Other specified hearing loss, unspecified ear
H91.9 Unspecified hearing loss
Deafness NOS
High frequency deafness
Low frequency deafness
H91.90 Unspecified hearing loss, unspecified ear
H91.91 Unspecified hearing loss, right ear
H91.92 Unspecified hearing loss, left ear
H91.93 Unspecified hearing loss, bilateral

H92 Otalgia and effusion of ear

H92.0 Otalgia
H92.01 Otalgia, right ear
H92.02 Otalgia, left ear
H92.03 Otalgia, bilateral
H92.09 Otalgia, unspecified ear
H92.1 Otorrhea
EXCLUDES 1 *leakage of cerebrospinal fluid through ear (G96.0)*
DEFINITION Fluid leaking from the ear.
H92.10 Otorrhea, unspecified ear

H92.11 **Otorrhea, right ear**
H92.12 **Otorrhea, left ear**
H92.13 **Otorrhea, bilateral**

H92.2 **Otorrhagia**
EXCLUDES 1 *traumatic otorrhagia - code to injury*
H92.20 **Otorrhagia, unspecified ear**
H92.21 **Otorrhagia, right ear**
H92.22 **Otorrhagia, left ear**
H92.23 **Otorrhagia, bilateral**

H93 Other disorders of ear, not elsewhere classified

H93.0 **Degenerative and vascular disorders of ear**
EXCLUDES 1 *presbycusis (H91.1)*

H93.01 **Transient ischemic deafness**
DEFINITION A passing hearing loss that occurs when blood flow to the auditory organs is decreased due to injury or disease.
H93.011 **Transient ischemic deafness, right ear**
H93.012 **Transient ischemic deafness, left ear**
H93.013 **Transient ischemic deafness, bilateral**
H93.019 **Transient ischemic deafness, unspecified ear**

H93.09 **Unspecified degenerative and vascular disorders of ear**
H93.091 **Unspecified degenerative and vascular disorders of right ear**
H93.092 **Unspecified degenerative and vascular disorders of left ear**
H93.093 **Unspecified degenerative and vascular disorders of ear, bilateral**
H93.099 **Unspecified degenerative and vascular disorders of unspecified ear**

H93.1 **Tinnitus**
DEFINITION Ringing, hissing, roaring or other sound in the ear in the absence of any apparent stimulus.
H93.11 **Tinnitus, right ear**
H93.12 **Tinnitus, left ear**
H93.13 **Tinnitus, bilateral**
H93.19 **Tinnitus, unspecified ear**

H93.A **Pulsatile tinnitus**
AHA: 4Q 2016, 25
H93.A1 **Pulsatile tinnitus, right ear**
H93.A2 **Pulsatile tinnitus, left ear**
H93.A3 **Pulsatile tinnitus, bilateral**
H93.A9 **Pulsatile tinnitus, unspecified ear**

H93.2 **Other abnormal auditory perceptions**
EXCLUDES 2 *auditory hallucinations (R44.0)*

H93.21 **Auditory recruitment**
H93.211 **Auditory recruitment, right ear**
H93.212 **Auditory recruitment, left ear**
H93.213 **Auditory recruitment, bilateral**
H93.219 **Auditory recruitment, unspecified ear**

H93.22 **Diplacusis**
DEFINITION One sound is heard as two separate sounds at different tones or pitches.
H93.221 **Diplacusis, right ear**
H93.222 **Diplacusis, left ear**
H93.223 **Diplacusis, bilateral**
H93.229 **Diplacusis, unspecified ear**

H93.23 **Hyperacusis**
DEFINITION Hearing is abnormally heightened; normal sounds seem amplified, even cause ear pain.
H93.231 **Hyperacusis, right ear**
H93.232 **Hyperacusis, left ear**
H93.233 **Hyperacusis, bilateral**
H93.239 **Hyperacusis, unspecified ear**

H93.24 **Temporary auditory threshold shift**
H93.241 **Temporary auditory threshold shift, right ear**
H93.242 **Temporary auditory threshold shift, left ear**
H93.243 **Temporary auditory threshold shift, bilateral**
H93.249 **Temporary auditory threshold shift, unspecified ear**

H93.25 **Central auditory processing disorder**
Congenital auditory imperception
Word deafness
EXCLUDES 1 *mixed receptive-expressive language disorder (F80.2)*

H93.29 **Other abnormal auditory perceptions**
H93.291 **Other abnormal auditory perceptions, right ear**
H93.292 **Other abnormal auditory perceptions, left ear**
H93.293 **Other abnormal auditory perceptions, bilateral**
H93.299 **Other abnormal auditory perceptions, unspecified ear**

H93.3 **Disorders of acoustic nerve**
Disorder of 8th cranial nerve
EXCLUDES 1 *acoustic neuroma (D33.3)*
syphilitic acoustic neuritis (A52.15)

H93.3X **Disorders of acoustic nerve**
H93.3X1 **Disorders of right acoustic nerve**
H93.3X2 **Disorders of left acoustic nerve**
H93.3X3 **Disorders of bilateral acoustic nerves**
H93.3X9 **Disorders of unspecified acoustic nerve**

H93.8 **Other specified disorders of ear**
H93.8X **Other specified disorders of ear**
H93.8X1 **Other specified disorders of right ear**
H93.8X2 **Other specified disorders of left ear**
H93.8X3 **Other specified disorders of ear, bilateral**
H93.8X9 **Other specified disorders of ear, unspecified ear**

H93.9 **Unspecified disorder of ear**
H93.90 **Unspecified disorder of ear, unspecified ear**
H93.91 **Unspecified disorder of right ear**
H93.92 **Unspecified disorder of left ear**
H93.93 **Unspecified disorder of ear, bilateral**

H94 Other disorders of ear in diseases classified elsewhere

H94.0 **Acoustic neuritis in infectious and parasitic diseases classified elsewhere**
Code first underlying disease, such as:
parasitic disease (B65-B89)
EXCLUDES 1 *acoustic neuritis (in) :*
herpes zoster (B02.29)
syphilis (A52.15)
H94.00 ***Acoustic neuritis in infectious and parasitic diseases classified elsewhere, unspecified ear***
H94.01 ***Acoustic neuritis in infectious and parasitic diseases classified elsewhere, right ear***
H94.02 ***Acoustic neuritis in infectious and parasitic diseases classified elsewhere, left ear***
H94.03 ***Acoustic neuritis in infectious and parasitic diseases classified elsewhere, bilateral***

H94.8 **Other specified disorders of ear in diseases classified elsewhere**
Code first underlying disease, such as:
congenital syphilis (A50.0)
EXCLUDES 1 *aural myiasis (B87.4)*
syphilitic labyrinthitis (A52.79)
H94.80 ***Other specified disorders of ear in diseases classified elsewhere, unspecified ear***
H94.81 ***Other specified disorders of right ear in diseases classified elsewhere***
H94.82 ***Other specified disorders of left ear in diseases classified elsewhere***
H94.83 ***Other specified disorders of ear in diseases classified elsewhere, bilateral***

Intraoperative and postprocedural complications and disorders of ear and mastoid process, not elsewhere classified (H95)

H95 Intraoperative and postprocedural complications and disorders of ear and mastoid process, not elsewhere classified

H95.0 **Recurrent cholesteatoma of postmastoidectomy cavity**

H95.00 Recurrent cholesteatoma of postmastoidectomy cavity, unspecified ear

H95.01 Recurrent cholesteatoma of postmastoidectomy cavity, right ear

H95.02 Recurrent cholesteatoma of postmastoidectomy cavity, left ear

H95.03 Recurrent cholesteatoma of postmastoidectomy cavity, bilateral ears

H95.1 Other disorders of ear and mastoid process following mastoidectomy

H95.11 Chronic inflammation of postmastoidectomy cavity

H95.111 Chronic inflammation of postmastoidectomy cavity, right ear

H95.112 Chronic inflammation of postmastoidectomy cavity, left ear

H95.113 Chronic inflammation of postmastoidectomy cavity, bilateral ears

H95.119 Chronic inflammation of postmastoidectomy cavity, unspecified ear

H95.12 Granulation of postmastoidectomy cavity

H95.121 Granulation of postmastoidectomy cavity, right ear

H95.122 Granulation of postmastoidectomy cavity, left ear

H95.123 Granulation of postmastoidectomy cavity, bilateral ears

H95.129 Granulation of postmastoidectomy cavity, unspecified ear

H95.13 Mucosal cyst of postmastoidectomy cavity

H95.131 Mucosal cyst of postmastoidectomy cavity, right ear

H95.132 Mucosal cyst of postmastoidectomy cavity, left ear

H95.133 Mucosal cyst of postmastoidectomy cavity, bilateral ears

H95.139 Mucosal cyst of postmastoidectomy cavity, unspecified ear

H95.19 Other disorders following mastoidectomy

H95.191 Other disorders following mastoidectomy, right ear

H95.192 Other disorders following mastoidectomy, left ear

H95.193 Other disorders following mastoidectomy, bilateral ears

H95.199 Other disorders following mastoidectomy, unspecified ear

H95.2 Intraoperative hemorrhage and hematoma of ear and mastoid process complicating a procedure

EXCLUDES 1 *intraoperative hemorrhage and hematoma of ear and mastoid process due to accidental puncture or laceration during a procedure (H95.3-)*

H95.21 Intraoperative hemorrhage and hematoma of ear and mastoid process complicating a procedure on the ear and mastoid process

H95.22 Intraoperative hemorrhage and hematoma of ear and mastoid process complicating other procedure

H95.3 Accidental puncture and laceration of ear and mastoid process during a procedure

H95.31 Accidental puncture and laceration of the ear and mastoid process during a procedure on the ear and mastoid process

H95.32 Accidental puncture and laceration of the ear and mastoid process during other procedure

H95.4 Postprocedural hemorrhage of ear and mastoid process following a procedure

H95.41 Postprocedural hemorrhage of ear and mastoid process following a procedure on the ear and mastoid process

H95.42 Postprocedural hemorrhage of ear and mastoid process following other procedure

H95.5 Postprocedural hematoma and seroma of ear and mastoid process following a procedure

H95.51 Postprocedural hematoma of ear and mastoid process following a procedure on the ear and mastoid process

H95.52 Postprocedural hematoma of ear and mastoid process following other procedure

H95.53 Postprocedural seroma of ear and mastoid process following a procedure on the ear and mastoid process

H95.54 Postprocedural seroma of ear and mastoid process following other procedure

H95.8 Other intraoperative and postprocedural complications and disorders of the ear and mastoid process, not elsewhere classified

EXCLUDES 2 *postprocedural complications and disorders following mastoidectomy (H95.0-, H95.1-)*

H95.81 Postprocedural stenosis of external ear canal

H95.811 Postprocedural stenosis of right external ear canal

H95.812 Postprocedural stenosis of left external ear canal

H95.813 Postprocedural stenosis of external ear canal, bilateral

H95.819 Postprocedural stenosis of unspecified external ear canal

H95.88 Other intraoperative complications and disorders of the ear and mastoid process, not elsewhere classified

Use additional code, if applicable, to further specify disorder

H95.89 Other postprocedural complications and disorders of the ear and mastoid process, not elsewhere classified

Use additional code, if applicable, to further specify disorder

CHAPTER 9: DISEASES OF THE CIRCULATORY SYSTEM (I00-I99)

EXCLUDES 2 *certain conditions originating in the perinatal period (P04-P96)*
certain infectious and parasitic diseases (A00-B99)
complications of pregnancy, childbirth and the puerperium (O00-O9A)
congenital malformations, deformations, and chromosomal abnormalities (Q00-Q99)
endocrine, nutritional and metabolic diseases (E00-E88)
injury, poisoning and certain other consequences of external causes (S00-T88)
neoplasms (C00-D49)
symptoms, signs and abnormal clinical and laboratory findings, not elsewhere classified (R00-R94)
systemic connective tissue disorders (M30-M36)
transient cerebral ischemic attacks and related syndromes (G45.-)

This chapter contains the following blocks:

I00-I02	Acute rheumatic fever
I05-I09	Chronic rheumatic heart diseases
I10-I16	Hypertensive diseases
I20-I25	Ischemic heart diseases
I26-I28	Pulmonary heart disease and diseases of pulmonary circulation
I30-I52	Other forms of heart disease
I60-I69	Cerebrovascular diseases
I70-I79	Diseases of arteries, arterioles and capillaries
I80-I89	Diseases of veins, lymphatic vessels and lymph nodes, not elsewhere classified
I95-I99	Other and unspecified disorders of the circulatory system

Acute rheumatic fever (I00-I02)

CODING TIP✓ Pericarditis, endocarditis, and myocarditis are only coded here when specified as "rheumatic." Do not assign a code for acute, chronic, infective, or other non-rheumatic pericarditis, endocarditis, or myocarditis using a code from I00-I02.

I00 **Rheumatic fever without heart involvement**

INCLUDES arthritis, rheumatic, acute or subacute

EXCLUDES 1 *rheumatic fever with heart involvement (I01.0 -I01.9)*

DEFINITION Delayed, febrile, inflammatory disease resulting about 20 days after streptococcal infection; presents with joint pain, migratory arthritis, skin rash on the trunk and proximal extremities, and nosebleeds; can cause cardiac damage.

I01 **Rheumatic fever with heart involvement**

EXCLUDES 1 *chronic diseases of rheumatic origin (I05-I09) unless rheumatic fever is also present or there is evidence of reactivation or activity of the rheumatic process.*

CODING TIP✓ Pericarditis, endocarditis, and myocarditis are coded with I01-I02 when specified as rheumatic, or associated with rheumatic fever.

I01.0 **Acute rheumatic pericarditis**
Any condition in I00 with pericarditis
Rheumatic pericarditis (acute)
EXCLUDES 1 *acute pericarditis not specified as rheumatic (I30.-)*

I01.1 **Acute rheumatic endocarditis**
Any condition in I00 with endocarditis or valvulitis
Acute rheumatic valvulitis

I01.2 **Acute rheumatic myocarditis**
Any condition in I00 with myocarditis

I01.8 **Other acute rheumatic heart disease**
Any condition in I00 with other or multiple types of heart involvement
Acute rheumatic pancarditis

I01.9 **Acute rheumatic heart disease, unspecified**
Any condition in I00 with unspecified type of heart involvement
Rheumatic carditis, acute
Rheumatic heart disease, active or acute

I02 **Rheumatic chorea**

INCLUDES Sydenham's chorea

EXCLUDES 1 *chorea NOS (G25.5)*
Huntington's chorea (G10)

CODING TIP✓ Pericarditis, endocarditis, and myocarditis are coded with I01-I02 when specified as rheumatic, or associated with rheumatic fever.

CODING TIP✓ Rheumatic chorea may also be referred to as "St. Vitus dance" and is more frequently diagnosed in children and adolescents.

I02.0 **Rheumatic chorea with heart involvement**
Chorea NOS with heart involvement
Rheumatic chorea with heart involvement of any type classifiable under I01.-

I02.9 **Rheumatic chorea without heart involvement**
Rheumatic chorea NOS

Chronic rheumatic heart diseases (I05-I09)

CODING TIP✓ When coding both mitral valve disease and tricuspid valve disease, the provider should specify whether the condition is rheumatic in nature. If the origin of the disease is unspecified, the default code for both valves is rheumatic.

CODING TIP✓ Categories I05-I09 include disease of the heart valve(s) specified as rheumatic.

I05 **Rheumatic mitral valve diseases**

INCLUDES conditions classifiable to both I05.0 and I05.2-I05.9, whether specified as rheumatic or not

EXCLUDES 1 *mitral valve disease specified as nonrheumatic (I34.-)*
mitral valve disease with aortic and/or tricuspid valve involvement (I08.-)

I05.0 **Rheumatic mitral stenosis**
Mitral (valve) obstruction (rheumatic)

I05.1 **Rheumatic mitral insufficiency**
Rheumatic mitral incompetence
Rheumatic mitral regurgitation
EXCLUDES 1 *mitral insufficiency not specified as rheumatic (I34.0)*

I05.2 **Rheumatic mitral stenosis with insufficiency**
Rheumatic mitral stenosis with incompetence or regurgitation

I05.8 **Other rheumatic mitral valve diseases**
Rheumatic mitral (valve) failure

I05.9 **Rheumatic mitral valve disease, unspecified**
Rheumatic mitral (valve) disorder (chronic) NOS

I06 **Rheumatic aortic valve diseases**

EXCLUDES 1 *aortic valve disease not specified as rheumatic (I35.-)*
aortic valve disease with mitral and/or tricuspid valve involvement (I08.-)

I06.0 **Rheumatic aortic stenosis**
Rheumatic aortic (valve) obstruction

I06.1 **Rheumatic aortic insufficiency**
Rheumatic aortic incompetence
Rheumatic aortic regurgitation

I06.2 **Rheumatic aortic stenosis with insufficiency**
Rheumatic aortic stenosis with incompetence or regurgitation

I06.8 **Other rheumatic aortic valve diseases**

I06.9 **Rheumatic aortic valve disease, unspecified**
Rheumatic aortic (valve) disease NOS

I07 **Rheumatic tricuspid valve diseases**

INCLUDES rheumatic tricuspid valve diseases specified as rheumatic or unspecified

EXCLUDES 1 *tricuspid valve disease specified as nonrheumatic (I36.-)*
tricuspid valve disease with aortic and/or mitral valve involvement (I08.-)

I07.0 **Rheumatic tricuspid stenosis**
Tricuspid (valve) stenosis (rheumatic)

I07.1 **Rheumatic tricuspid insufficiency**
Tricuspid (valve) insufficiency (rheumatic)

I07.2 **Rheumatic tricuspid stenosis and insufficiency**

I07.8 **Other rheumatic tricuspid valve diseases**

I07.9 **Rheumatic tricuspid valve disease, unspecified**
Rheumatic tricuspid valve disorder NOS

4 I08 Multiple valve diseases

INCLUDES multiple valve diseases specified as rheumatic or unspecified

EXCLUDES 1 *endocarditis, valve unspecified (I38)*
multiple valve disease specified a nonrheumatic (I34.-, I35.-, I36.-, I37.-, I38.-, Q22.-, Q23.-, Q24.8-)
rheumatic valve disease NOS (I09.1)

I08.0 Rheumatic disorders of both mitral and aortic valves
Involvement of both mitral and aortic valves specified as rheumatic or unspecified

I08.1 Rheumatic disorders of both mitral and tricuspid valves

I08.2 Rheumatic disorders of both aortic and tricuspid valves

I08.3 Combined rheumatic disorders of mitral, aortic and tricuspid valves

I08.8 Other rheumatic multiple valve diseases

I08.9 Rheumatic multiple valve disease, unspecified

CODING TIP ✓ When the clinical record reports rheumatic disease of multiple valves, but the affected valves are not specified, assign code I08.9.

4 I09 Other rheumatic heart diseases

I09.0 Rheumatic myocarditis

EXCLUDES 1 *myocarditis not specified as rheumatic (I51.4)*

DEFINITION Chronic inflammation and degeneration of heart muscle due to rheumatic heart disease.

I09.1 Rheumatic diseases of endocardium, valve unspecified
Rheumatic endocarditis (chronic)
Rheumatic valvulitis (chronic)

EXCLUDES 1 *endocarditis, valve unspecified (I38)*

I09.2 Chronic rheumatic pericarditis
Adherent pericardium, rheumatic
Chronic rheumatic mediastinopericarditis
Chronic rheumatic myopericarditis

EXCLUDES 1 *chronic pericarditis not specified as rheumatic (I31.-)*

5 I09.8 Other specified rheumatic heart diseases

I09.81 Rheumatic heart failure HCC
Use additional code to identify type of heart failure (I50.-)

DEFINITION Severe rheumatic damage to heart valves causing heart failure.

I09.89 Other specified rheumatic heart diseases
Rheumatic disease of pulmonary valve

I09.9 Rheumatic heart disease, unspecified
Rheumatic carditis

EXCLUDES 1 *rheumatoid carditis (M05.31)*

Hypertensive diseases (I10-I16)

Use additional code to identify:
exposure to environmental tobacco smoke (Z77.22)
history of tobacco dependence (Z87.891)
occupational exposure to environmental tobacco smoke (Z57.31)
tobacco dependence (F17.-)
tobacco use (Z72.0)

EXCLUDES 1 *neonatal hypertension (P29.2)*
primary pulmonary hypertension (I27.0)

EXCLUDES 2 *hypertensive disease complicating pregnancy, childbirth and the puerperium (O10-O11, O13-O16)*

GUIDELINES **Section I.C.9.a.**
The classification presumes a causal relationship between hypertension and heart involvement and between hypertension and kidney involvement, as the two conditions are linked by the term "with" in the Alphabetic Index. These conditions should be coded as related even in the absence of provider documentation explicitly linking them, unless the documentation clearly states the conditions are unrelated.
For hypertension and conditions not specifically linked by relational terms such as "with," "associated with" or "due to" in the classification, provider documentation must link the conditions in order to code them as related.

I10 Essential (primary) hypertension

INCLUDES high blood pressure
hypertension (arterial) (benign) (essential) (malignant) (primary) (systemic)

EXCLUDES 1 *hypertensive disease complicating pregnancy, childbirth and the puerperium (O10-O11, O13-O16)*

EXCLUDES 2 *essential (primary) hypertension involving vessels of brain (I60-I69)*
essential (primary) hypertension involving vessels of eye (H35.0-)

AHA: 4Q 2013, 128
AHA: 2Q 2018, 7

4 I11 Hypertensive heart disease

INCLUDES any condition in I50.-, I51.4-I51.9 due to hypertension

GUIDELINES **Section I.C.9.a.1)**
Hypertension with heart conditions classified to I50.- or I51.4-I51.7, I51.89, I51.9, are assigned to a code from category I11, Hypertensive heart disease. Use additional code(s) from category I50, Heart failure, to identify the type(s) of heart failure in those patients with heart failure.

The same heart conditions (I50.-, I51.4-I51.7, I51.89, I51.9) with hypertension are coded separately if the provider has documented they are unrelated to the hypertension. Sequence according to the circumstances of the admission/encounter.

GUIDELINES **Section I.C.9.a.**
The classification presumes a causal relationship between hypertension and heart involvement and between hypertension and kidney involvement, as the two conditions are linked by the term "with" in the Alphabetic Index. These conditions should be coded as related even in the absence of provider documentation explicitly linking them, unless the documentation clearly states the conditions are unrelated.

I11.0 Hypertensive heart disease with heart failure HCC
Hypertensive heart failure
Use additional code to identify type of heart failure (I50.-)
AHA: 1Q 2017, 47

I11.9 Hypertensive heart disease without heart failure
Hypertensive heart disease NOS

4 I12 Hypertensive chronic kidney disease

INCLUDES any condition in N18 and N26 - due to hypertension
arteriosclerosis of kidney
arteriosclerotic nephritis (chronic) (interstitial)
hypertensive nephropathy
nephrosclerosis

EXCLUDES 1 *hypertension due to kidney disease (I15.0, I15.1)*
renovascular hypertension (I15.0)
secondary hypertension (I15.-)

EXCLUDES 2 *acute kidney failure (N17.-)*

GUIDELINES **Section I.C.9.a.2)**
Assign codes from category I12, Hypertensive chronic kidney disease, when both hypertension and a condition classifiable to category N18, Chronic kidney disease (CKD), are present. CKD should not be coded as hypertensive if the provider indicates the CKD is not related to the hypertension.
The appropriate code from category N18 should be used as a secondary code with a code from category I12 to identify the stage of chronic kidney disease.
See Section I.C.14. Chronic kidney disease.
If a patient has hypertensive chronic kidney disease and acute renal failure, an additional code for the acute renal failure is required.

CODING TIP ✓ A relationship may be assumed between hypertension and any condition classifiable to N18.- or N26.-. This is due to the pathology of hypertension, which impacts renal function, often resulting in kidney dysfunction. The exception to this assumption is when clinical record documentation reports that hypertension has been caused secondary to the kidney dysfunction (renovascular hypertension). When this is the case, the hypertension is secondary to the renal dysfunction and is coded using a code from I15.-.

I12.0 Hypertensive chronic kidney disease with stage 5 chronic kidney disease or end stage renal disease HCC

Use additional code to identify the stage of chronic kidney disease (N18.5, N18.6)

AHA: 3Q 2016, 22

AHA: 3Q 2016, 23

I12.9 Hypertensive chronic kidney disease with stage 1 through stage 4 chronic kidney disease, or unspecified chronic kidney disease

Hypertensive chronic kidney disease NOS

Hypertensive renal disease NOS

Use additional code to identify the stage of chronic kidney disease (N18.1-N18.4, N18.9)

4 I13 Hypertensive heart and chronic kidney disease

INCLUDES any condition in I11.- with any condition in I12.-

cardiorenal disease

cardiovascular renal disease

GUIDELINES **Section I.C.9.a.3)**

Assign codes from combination category I13, Hypertensive heart and chronic kidney disease, when there is hypertension with both heart and kidney involvement. If heart failure is present, assign an additional code from category I50 to identify the type of heart failure.

The appropriate code from category N18, Chronic kidney disease, should be used as a secondary code with a code from category I13 to identify the stage of chronic kidney disease.

The codes in category I13 are combination codes that include hypertension, heart disease and chronic kidney disease. The Includes note at I13 specifies that the conditions included at I11 and I12 are included together in I13. If a patient has hypertension, heart disease and chronic kidney disease, then a code from I13 should be used, not individual codes for hypertension, heart disease and chronic kidney disease, or codes from I11 or I12.

CODING TIP✓ I13 is a combination code that includes hypertensive heart disease and hypertensive chronic kidney disease. Additional codes should be assigned for the type of heart failure (I50.-) and the stage of chronic kidney disease (N18.-). The heart conditions in codes I51.4-I51.9 are inclusive in the I13.1- category.

I13.0 Hypertensive heart and chronic kidney disease with heart failure and stage 1 through stage 4 chronic kidney disease, or unspecified chronic kidney disease HCC

Use additional code to identify type of heart failure (I50.-)

Use additional code to identify stage of chronic kidney disease (N18.1-N18.4, N18.9)

5 I13.1 Hypertensive heart and chronic kidney disease without heart failure

I13.10 Hypertensive heart and chronic kidney disease without heart failure, with stage 1 through stage 4 chronic kidney disease, or unspecified chronic kidney disease

Hypertensive heart disease and hypertensive chronic kidney disease NOS

Use additional code to identify the stage of chronic kidney disease (N18.1-N18.4, N18.9)

I13.11 Hypertensive heart and chronic kidney disease without heart failure, with stage 5 chronic kidney disease, or end stage renal disease HCC

Use additional code to identify the stage of chronic kidney disease (N18.5, N18.6)

I13.2 Hypertensive heart and chronic kidney disease with heart failure and with stage 5 chronic kidney disease, or end stage renal disease HCC

Use additional code to identify type of heart failure (I50.-)

Use additional code to identify the stage of chronic kidney disease (N18.5, N18.6)

4 I15 Secondary hypertension

Code also:

underlying condition

EXCLUDES 1 *postprocedural hypertension (I97.3)*

EXCLUDES 2 *secondary hypertension involving vessels of brain (I60-I69)*

secondary hypertension involving vessels of eye (H35.0-)

GUIDELINES **Section I.C.9.a.6)**

Secondary hypertension is due to an underlying condition. Two codes are required: one to identify the underlying etiology and one from category I15 to identify the hypertension. Sequencing of codes is determined by the reason for admission/encounter.

CODING TIP✓ It is more common for hypertension to cause the renal dysfunction, however when hypertension is confirmed caused by the kidney (renal) dysfunction, assign a code from I15.-.

I15.0 Renovascular hypertension

CODING TIP✓ Do not confuse hypertensive chronic kidney disease with renovascular hypertension, a condition in which the kidney dysfunction causes the hypertension. When this is the case, the hypertension is secondary to the renal dysfunction and is coded using I15.0. The two conditions may be coded in either order. An additional code for the underlying condition should also be assigned.

I15.1 Hypertension secondary to other renal disorders

AHA: 3Q 2016, 22

AHA: 3Q 2016, 23

I15.2 Hypertension secondary to endocrine disorders

CODING TIP✓ Assign I15.2 when hypertension is specified as due to Cushing's syndrome, primary aldosteronism, acromegaly, hypo/hyperthyroidism, or another specified endocrine disorder. Do not assign a code from I10-I13.0 when hypertension is specified as secondary to one of these causes.

I15.8 Other secondary hypertension

I15.9 Secondary hypertension, unspecified

4 I16 Hypertensive crisis

Code also:

any identified hypertensive disease (I10-I15)

AHA: 4Q 2016, 26

I16.0 Hypertensive urgency

I16.1 Hypertensive emergency

I16.9 Hypertensive crisis, unspecified

Ischemic heart diseases (I20-I25)

Use additional code to identify presence of hypertension (I10-I16)

4 I20 Angina pectoris

Use additional code to identify:

exposure to environmental tobacco smoke (Z77.22)

history of tobacco dependence (Z87.891)

occupational exposure to environmental tobacco smoke (Z57.31)

tobacco dependence (F17.-)

tobacco use (Z72.0)

EXCLUDES 1 *angina pectoris with atherosclerotic heart disease of native coronary arteries (I25.1-)*

atherosclerosis of coronary artery bypass graft (s) and coronary artery of transplanted heart with angina pectoris (I25.7-)

postinfarction angina (I23.7)

GUIDELINES **Section I.C.9.b.** ICD-10-CM has combination codes for atherosclerotic heart disease with angina pectoris. The subcategories for these codes are I25.11, Atherosclerotic heart disease of native coronary artery with angina pectoris and I25.7, Atherosclerosis of coronary artery bypass graft(s) and coronary artery of transplanted heart with angina pectoris.
When using one of these combination codes it is not necessary to use an additional code for angina pectoris. A causal relationship can be assumed in a patient with both atherosclerosis and angina pectoris, unless the documentation indicates the angina is due to something other than the atherosclerosis. If a patient with coronary artery disease is admitted due to an acute myocardial infarction (AMI), the AMI should be sequenced before the coronary artery disease.

CODING TIP✓ Do not assign a code from I20.- for a patient who also has coronary artery disease (CAD)/atherosclerotic heart disease (ASHD). Angina in a patient with CAD/ASHD should be coded to the appropriate I25.11- code.

I20.0 Unstable angina HCC
Accelerated angina
Crescendo angina
De novo effort angina
Intermediate coronary syndrome
Preinfarction syndrome
Worsening effort angina

I20.1 Angina pectoris with documented spasm HCC
Angiospastic angina
Prinzmetal angina
Spasm-induced angina
Variant angina

I20.8 Other forms of angina pectoris HCC
Angina equivalent
Angina of effort
Coronary slow flow syndrome
Stenocardia
Stable angina
Use additional code(s) for symptoms associated with angina equivalent

I20.9 Angina pectoris, unspecified HCC
Angina NOS
Anginal syndrome
Cardiac angina
Ischemic chest pain

4 I21 Acute myocardial infarction

INCLUDES cardiac infarction
coronary (artery) embolism
coronary (artery) occlusion
coronary (artery) rupture
coronary (artery) thrombosis
infarction of heart, myocardium, or ventricle
myocardial infarction specified as acute or with a stated duration of 4 weeks (28 days) or less from onset

Use additional code, if applicable, to identify:
exposure to environmental tobacco smoke (Z77.22)
history of tobacco dependence (Z87.891)
occupational exposure to environmental tobacco smoke (Z57.31)
status post administration of tPA (rtPA) in a different facility within the last 24 hours prior to admission to current facility (Z92.82)
tobacco dependence (F17.-)
tobacco use (Z72.0)

EXCLUDES 2 *old myocardial infarction (I25.2)*
postmyocardial infarction syndrome (I24.1)
subsequent type 1 myocardial infarction (I22.-)

GUIDELINES **Section I.C.9.e.1)**
The ICD-10-CM codes for type 1 acute myocardial infarction (AMI) identify the site, such as anterolateral wall or true posterior wall. Subcategories I21.0-I21.2 and code I21.3 are used for type 1 ST elevation myocardial infarction (STEMI). Code I21.4, Non-ST elevation (NSTEMI) myocardial infarction, is used for type 1 non ST elevation myocardial infarction (NSTEMI) and nontransmural MIs.

If a type 1 NSTEMI evolves to a STEMI, assign the STEMI code. If a type 1 STEMI converts to NSTEMI due to thrombolytic therapy, it is still coded as a STEMI.

For encounters occurring while the myocardial infarction is equal to, or less than, four weeks old, including transfers to another acute setting or a postacute setting, and the myocardial infarction meets the definition for "other diagnoses" (see Section III, Reporting Additional Diagnoses), codes from category I21 may continue to be reported. For encounters after the 4 week time frame and the patient is still receiving care related to the myocardial infarction, the appropriate aftercare code should be assigned, rather than a code from category I21. For old or healed myocardial infarctions not requiring further care, code I25.2, Old myocardial infarction, may be assigned.

GUIDELINES **Section I.C.9.b**
If a patient with coronary artery disease is admitted due to an acute myocardial infarction (AMI), the AMI should be sequenced before the coronary artery disease.

CODING TIP✓ When assigning any code from I21.- to report STEMI or NSTEMI, note that ICD-10 coding guidelines only allow assignment of these codes for 4 weeks following the occurrence of the MI.

AHA: 4Q 2012, 97, 103-104
AHA: 1Q 2013, 25-26

5 I21.0 ST elevation (STEMI) myocardial infarction of anterior wall
Type 1 ST elevation myocardial infarction of anterior wall

I21.01 ST elevation (STEMI) myocardial infarction involving left main coronary artery HCC

I21.02 ST elevation (STEMI) myocardial infarction involving left anterior descending coronary artery HCC
ST elevation (STEMI) myocardial infarction involving diagonal coronary artery
AHA: 1Q 2013, 26

I21.09 ST elevation (STEMI) myocardial infarction involving other coronary artery of anterior wall HCC
Acute transmural myocardial infarction of anterior wall
Anteroapical transmural (Q wave) infarction (acute)
Anterolateral transmural (Q wave) infarction (acute)
Anteroseptal transmural (Q wave) infarction (acute)
Transmural (Q wave) infarction (acute) (of) anterior (wall) NOS
AHA: 4Q 2012, 102

5 I21.1 ST elevation (STEMI) myocardial infarction of inferior wall
Type 1 ST elevation myocardial infarction of inferior wall

I21.11 ST elevation (STEMI) myocardial infarction involving right coronary artery HCC
Inferoposterior transmural (Q wave) infarction (acute)

I21.19 ST elevation (STEMI) myocardial infarction involving other coronary artery of inferior wall HCC
Acute transmural myocardial infarction of inferior wall
Inferolateral transmural (Q wave) infarction (acute)
Transmural (Q wave) infarction (acute) (of) diaphragmatic wall
Transmural (Q wave) infarction (acute) (of) inferior (wall) NOS

EXCLUDES 2 *ST elevation (STEMI) myocardial infarction involving left circumflex coronary artery (I21.21)*

AHA: 4Q 2012, 97

5 I21.2 ST elevation (STEMI) myocardial infarction of other sites
Type 1 ST elevation myocardial infarction of other sites

I21.21 ST elevation (STEMI) myocardial infarction involving left circumflex coronary artery HCC
ST elevation (STEMI) myocardial infarction involving oblique marginal coronary artery

I21.29 ST elevation (STEMI) myocardial infarction involving other sites HCC
Acute transmural myocardial infarction of other sites
Apical-lateral transmural (Q wave) infarction (acute)
Basal-lateral transmural (Q wave) infarction (acute)
High lateral transmural (Q wave) infarction (acute)
Lateral (wall) NOS transmural (Q wave) infarction (acute)
Posterior (true) transmural (Q wave) infarction (acute)
Posterobasal transmural (Q wave) infarction (acute)
Posterolateral transmural (Q wave) infarction (acute)
Posteroseptal transmural (Q wave) infarction (acute)
Septal transmural (Q wave) infarction (acute) NOS

I21.3 ST elevation (STEMI) myocardial infarction of unspecified site HCC
Acute transmural myocardial infarction of unspecified site
Transmural (Q wave) myocardial infarction NOS
Type 1 ST elevation myocardial infarction of unspecified site

GUIDELINES **Section I.C.9.e.2)**
Code I21.9, Acute myocardial infarction, unspecified, is the default for the unspecified term acute myocardial infarction or unspecified type. If only type 1 STEMI or transmural MI without the site is documented, query the provider as to the site, or assign code I21.3, ST elevation (STEMI) myocardial infarction of unspecified site.

I21.4 Non-ST elevation (NSTEMI) myocardial infarction HCC
Acute subendocardial myocardial infarction
Non-Q wave myocardial infarction NOS
Nontransmural myocardial infarction NOS
Type 1 non-ST elevation myocardial infarction

GUIDELINES **Section I.C.9.e.1)**
Code I21.4, Non-ST elevation (NSTEMI) myocardial infarction, is used for type 1 non ST elevation myocardial infarction (NSTEMI) and nontransmural MIs.

GUIDELINES **Section I.C.9.e.3)**
If an AMI is documented as nontransmural or subendocardial, but the site is provided, it is still coded as a subendocardial AMI.
AHA: 2Q 2015, 16
AHA: 1Q 2017, 44

I21.9 Acute myocardial infarction, unspecified HCC
Myocardial infarction (acute) NOS

GUIDELINES **Section I.C.9.e.2)**
Code I21.9, Acute myocardial infarction, unspecified, is the default for the unspecified term acute myocardial infarction or unspecified type. If only type 1 STEMI or transmural MI without the site is documented, query the provider as to the site, or assign code I21.3, ST elevation (STEMI) myocardial infarction of unspecified site.

5 I21.A Other type of myocardial infarction

I21.A1 Myocardial infarction type 2 HCC
Myocardial infarction due to demand ischemia
Myocardial infarction secondary to ischemic imbalance
Code also the underlying cause, if known and applicable, such as:
- anemia (D50.0-D64.9)
- chronic obstructive pulmonary disease (J44.-)
- heart failure (I50.-)
- paroxysmal tachycardia (I47.0-I47.9)
- renal failure (N17.0-N19)
- shock (R57.0-R57.9)

GUIDELINES **Section I.C.9.e.5)**
The ICD-10-CM provides codes for different types of myocardial infarction. Type 1 myocardial infarctions are assigned to codes I21.0-I21.4, and I21.9.
Type 2 myocardial infarction, and myocardial infarction due to demand ischemia or secondary to ischemic balance, is assigned to code I21.A1, Myocardial infarction type 2 with a code for the underlying cause. Do not assign code I24.8, Other forms of acute ischemic heart disease for the demand ischemia. Sequencing of type 2 AMI or the underlying cause is dependent on the circumstances of admission. When a type 2 AMI code is described as NSTEMI or STEMI, only assign code I21.A1. Codes I21.01-I21.4 should only be assigned for type 1 AMIs.
Acute myocardial infarctions type 3, 4a, 4b, 4c and 5 are assigned to code I21.A9, Other myocardial infarction type.
The "Code also" and "Code first" notes should be followed related to complications, and for coding of postprocedural myocardial infarctions during or following cardiac surgery.
AHA: 4Q 2017, 10

I21.A9 Other myocardial infarction type HCC
Myocardial infarction associated with revascularization procedure
Myocardial infarction type 3
Myocardial infarction type 4a
Myocardial infarction type 4b
Myocardial infarction type 4c
Myocardial infarction type 5
Code first:
- , if applicable, postprocedural myocardial infarction following cardiac surgery (I97.190) , or postprocedural myocardial infarction during cardiac surgery (I97.790)

Code also complication, if known and applicable, such as:
- (acute) stent occlusion (T82.897-)
- (acute) stent stenosis (T82.857-)
- (acute) stent thrombosis (T82.867-)
- cardiac arrest due to underlying cardiac condition (I46.2)
- complication of percutaneous coronary intervention (PCI) (I97.89)
- occlusion of coronary artery bypass graft (T82.218-)

AHA: 4Q 2017, 10

4 I22 Subsequent ST elevation (STEMI) and non-ST elevation (NSTEMI) myocardial infarction

INCLUDES acute myocardial infarction occurring within four weeks (28 days) of a previous acute myocardial infarction, regardless of site
cardiac infarction
coronary (artery) embolism
coronary (artery) occlusion
coronary (artery) rupture
coronary (artery) thrombosis
infarction of heart, myocardium, or ventricle
recurrent myocardial infarction
reinfarction of myocardium
rupture of heart, myocardium, or ventricle
subsequent type 1 myocardial infarction

Use additional code, if applicable, to identify:
- *exposure to environmental tobacco smoke (Z77.22)*
- *history of tobacco dependence (Z87.891)*
- *occupational exposure to environmental tobacco smoke (Z57.31)*
- *status post administration of tPA (rtPA) in a different facility within the last 24 hours prior to admission to current facility (Z92.82)*
- *tobacco dependence (F17.-)*
- *tobacco use (Z72.0)*

EXCLUDES 1 *subsequent myocardial infarction, type 2 (I21.A1)*
subsequent myocardial infarction of other type (type 3) (type 4) (type 5) (I21.A9)

GUIDELINES Section I.C.9.e.4)
Do not assign code I22 for subsequent myocardial infarctions other than type 1 or unspecified. For subsequent type 2 AMI assign only code I21.A1. For subsequent type 4 or type 5 AMI, assign only code I21.A9.

GUIDELINES **Section I.C.9.e.4)**
A code from category I22, Subsequent ST elevation (STEMI) and non-ST elevation (NSTEMI) myocardial infarction, is to be used when a patient who has suffered a type 1 or unspecified AMI has a new AMI within the 4 week time frame of the initial AMI. A code from category I22 must be used in conjunction with a code from category I21. The sequencing of the I22 and I21 codes depends on the circumstances of the encounter.
Do not assign code I22 for subsequent myocardial infarctions other than type 1 or unspecified. For subsequent type 2 AMI assign only code I21.A1. For subsequent type 4 or type 5 AMI, assign only code I21.A9.

CODING TIP ✓ A code from category I22 must be used in conjunction with a code from category I21. The sequencing of the codes will depend on the circumstances of the encounter.

CODING TIP ✓ A code from category I22 should not be used for subsequent MIs other than type I or unspecified. For subsequent type 2 AMIs, assign only code I21.A1. For subsequent type 4 or 5 AMIs, assign only code I21.A9.
AHA: 4Q 2012, 97, 103-104
AHA: 1Q 2013, 25

I22.0 Subsequent ST elevation (STEMI) myocardial infarction of anterior wall HCC
Subsequent acute transmural myocardial infarction of anterior wall
Subsequent transmural (Q wave) infarction (acute)(of) anterior (wall) NOS
Subsequent anteroapical transmural (Q wave) infarction (acute)
Subsequent anterolateral transmural (Q wave) infarction (acute)
Subsequent anteroseptal transmural (Q wave) infarction (acute)

I22.1 Subsequent ST elevation (STEMI) myocardial infarction of inferior wall HCC
Subsequent acute transmural myocardial infarction of inferior wall
Subsequent transmural (Q wave) infarction (acute)(of) diaphragmatic wall
Subsequent transmural (Q wave) infarction (acute)(of) inferior (wall) NOS
Subsequent inferolateral transmural (Q wave) infarction (acute)
Subsequent inferoposterior transmural (Q wave) infarction (acute)
AHA: 4Q 2012, 97, 102, 103-104

I22.2 Subsequent non-ST elevation (NSTEMI) myocardial infarction HCC
Subsequent acute subendocardial myocardial infarction
Subsequent non-Q wave myocardial infarction NOS
Subsequent nontransmural myocardial infarction NOS

I22.8 Subsequent ST elevation (STEMI) myocardial infarction of other sites HCC
Subsequent acute transmural myocardial infarction of other sites
Subsequent apical-lateral transmural (Q wave) myocardial infarction (acute)
Subsequent basal-lateral transmural (Q wave) myocardial infarction (acute)
Subsequent high lateral transmural (Q wave) myocardial infarction (acute)
Subsequent transmural (Q wave) myocardial infarction (acute)(of) lateral (wall) NOS
Subsequent posterior (true) transmural (Q wave) myocardial infarction (acute)
Subsequent posterobasal transmural (Q wave) myocardial infarction (acute)
Subsequent posterolateral transmural (Q wave) myocardial infarction (acute)
Subsequent posteroseptal transmural (Q wave) myocardial infarction (acute)
Subsequent septal NOS transmural (Q wave) myocardial infarction (acute)

I22.9 Subsequent ST elevation (STEMI) myocardial infarction of unspecified site HCC
Subsequent acute myocardial infarction of unspecified site
Subsequent myocardial infarction (acute) NOS

4 I23 Certain current complications following ST elevation (STEMI) and non-ST elevation (NSTEMI) myocardial infarction (within the 28 day period)

CODING TIP ✓ When assigning a code from category I23.-, also assign a code from category I21.-, and I22.-, as appropriate, if the encounter is within 4 weeks of the AMI. Use of codes from category I23.- may be appropriate after the 4 week period has lapsed. "Within the 28 day period" is a non-essential modifier in the category title.

I23.0 Hemopericardium as current complication following acute myocardial infarction A HCC
EXCLUDES 1 *hemopericardium not specified as current complication following acute myocardial infarction (I31.2)*

CODING TIP ✓ **Documentation**: Hemopericardium is frequently documented with cardiac wall rupture, including ventricular rupture, following MI, and results in pooling of blood in the pericardial space, leading to tamponade. This life-threatening condition may occur during or shortly after an MI.

I23.1 Atrial septal defect as current complication following acute myocardial infarction A HCC
EXCLUDES 1 *acquired atrial septal defect not specified as current complication following acute myocardial infarction (I51.0)*

I23.2 Ventricular septal defect as current complication following acute myocardial infarction A HCC
EXCLUDES 1 *acquired ventricular septal defect not specified as current complication following acute myocardial infarction (I51.0)*

I23.3 Rupture of cardiac wall without hemopericardium as current complication following acute myocardial infarction A HCC
AHA: 2Q 2017, 11

I23.4 Rupture of chordae tendineae as current complication following acute myocardial infarction HCC
EXCLUDES 1 *rupture of chordae tendineae not specified as current complication following acute myocardial infarction (I51.1)*

DEFINITION Tear in the fibrous, cord-like tissue connecting the papillary muscles to the valves, holding the valve flaps in place to prevent their eversion.

I23.5 Rupture of papillary muscle as current complication following acute myocardial infarction HCC
EXCLUDES 1 *rupture of papillary muscle not specified as current complication following acute myocardial infarction (I51.2)*

I23.6 Thrombosis of atrium, auricular appendage, and ventricle as current complications following acute myocardial infarction A HCC
EXCLUDES 1 *thrombosis of atrium, auricular appendage, and ventricle not specified as current complication following acute myocardial infarction (I51.3)*

I23.7 Postinfarction angina A HCC

CODING TIP ✓ Post-infarction angina includes a syndrome of ischemic chest pain occurring either at rest or during minimal activity 24 hours or more following an acute MI. It is more common after NSTEMI. Post infarction angina is considered a complication (not simply angina after an MI) and must be documented by the physician.
AHA: 2Q 2015, 16-17

I23.8 Other current complications following acute myocardial infarction A HCC

4 I24 Other acute ischemic heart diseases

EXCLUDES 1 *angina pectoris (I20.-)*
transient myocardial ischemia in newborn (P29.4)

I24.0 **Acute coronary thrombosis not resulting in myocardial infarction** HCC
Acute coronary (artery) (vein) embolism not resulting in myocardial infarction
Acute coronary (artery) (vein) occlusion not resulting in myocardial infarction
Acute coronary (artery) (vein) thromboembolism not resulting in myocardial infarction
EXCLUDES 1 *atherosclerotic heart disease (I25.1-)*
AHA: 1Q 2013, 24

I24.1 **Dressler's syndrome** HCC
Postmyocardial infarction syndrome
EXCLUDES 1 *postinfarction angina (I23.7)*

DEFINITION Fever, chest pain, pleuritis, and pericarditis weeks or months after heart injury caused by surgery or myocardial infarction.

I24.8 **Other forms of acute ischemic heart disease** HCC
EXCLUDES 1 *myocardial infarction due to demand ischemia (I21.A1)*

I24.9 **Acute ischemic heart disease, unspecified** HCC
EXCLUDES 1 *ischemic heart disease (chronic) NOS (I25.9)*

4 I25 **Chronic ischemic heart disease**
Use additional code to identify:
chronic total occlusion of coronary artery (I25.82)
exposure to environmental tobacco smoke (Z77.22)
history of tobacco dependence (Z87.891)
occupational exposure to environmental tobacco smoke (Z57.31)
tobacco dependence (F17.-)
tobacco use (Z72.0)

GUIDELINES **Section I.C.9.b**
ICD-10-CM has combination codes for atherosclerotic heart disease with angina pectoris. The subcategories for these codes are I25.11, Atherosclerotic heart disease of native coronary artery with angina pectoris, and I25.7, Atherosclerosis of coronary artery bypass graft(s) and coronary artery of transplanted heart with angina pectoris.

When using one of these combination codes it is not necessary to use an additional code for angina pectoris. A causal relationship can be assumed in a patient with both atherosclerosis and angina pectoris, unless the documentation indicates the angina is due to something other than the atherosclerosis.

If a patient with coronary artery disease is admitted due to an acute myocardial infarction (AMI), the AMI should be sequenced before the coronary artery disease.

5 I25.1 **Atherosclerotic heart disease of native coronary artery**
Atherosclerotic cardiovascular disease
Coronary (artery) atheroma
Coronary (artery) atherosclerosis
Coronary (artery) disease
Coronary (artery) sclerosis
Use additional code, if applicable, to identify:
coronary atherosclerosis due to calcified coronary lesion (I25.84)
coronary atherosclerosis due to lipid rich plaque (I25.83)
EXCLUDES 2 *atheroembolism (I75.-)*
atherosclerosis of coronary artery bypass graft (s) and transplanted heart (I25.7-)

I25.10 **Atherosclerotic heart disease of native coronary artery without angina pectoris** A
Atherosclerotic heart disease NOS

DEFINITION Clogging of coronary arteries with fatty plaque build-up, restricting blood flow and hardening the arteries.
AHA: 4Q 2012, 92
AHA: 4Q 2013, 128
AHA: 2Q 2015, 17

Coronary atherosclerosis

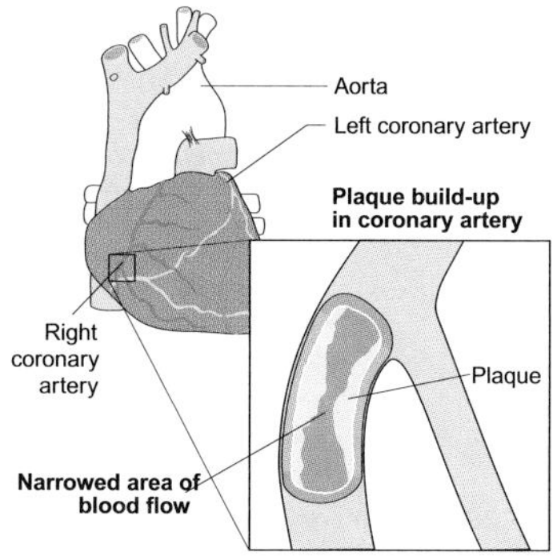

6 I25.11 **Atherosclerotic heart disease of native coronary artery with angina pectoris**
CODING TIP ✓ When a patient presents with both coronary artery disease (CAD) / atherosclerotic heart disease and angina, a code from I25.11- should be assigned. If the specific type of angina is not specified in the clinical record, assign code I25.119.

I25.110 **Atherosclerotic heart disease of native coronary artery with unstable angina pectoris** A HCC
EXCLUDES 1 *unstable angina without atherosclerotic heart disease (I20.0)*

I25.111 **Atherosclerotic heart disease of native coronary artery with angina pectoris with documented spasm** A HCC
EXCLUDES 1 *angina pectoris with documented spasm without atherosclerotic heart disease (I20.1)*

I25.118 **Atherosclerotic heart disease of native coronary artery with other forms of angina pectoris** A HCC
EXCLUDES 1 *other forms of angina pectoris without atherosclerotic heart disease (I20.8)*
AHA: 2Q 2015, 16-17

I25.119 **Atherosclerotic heart disease of native coronary artery with unspecified angina pectoris** A HCC
Atherosclerotic heart disease with angina NOS
Atherosclerotic heart disease with ischemic chest pain
EXCLUDES 1 *unspecified angina pectoris without atherosclerotic heart disease (I20.9)*

I25.2 **Old myocardial infarction**
Healed myocardial infarction
Past myocardial infarction diagnosed by ECG or other investigation, but currently presenting no symptoms
GUIDELINES **Section I.C.9.e.1)**
For old or healed myocardial infarctions not requiring further care, code I25.2 may be assigned.

I25.3 **Aneurysm of heart**
Mural aneurysm
Ventricular aneurysm

5 I25.4 **Coronary artery aneurysm and dissection**

I25.41 **Coronary artery aneurysm**
Coronary arteriovenous fistula, acquired
EXCLUDES 1 *congenital coronary (artery) aneurysm (Q24.5)*

I25.42 **Coronary artery dissection**

I25.5 **Ischemic cardiomyopathy**
EXCLUDES 2 *coronary atherosclerosis (I25.1-, I25.7-)*

I25.6 **Silent myocardial ischemia**

I25.7 Atherosclerosis of coronary artery bypass graft(s) and coronary artery of transplanted heart with angina pectoris

Use additional code, if applicable, to identify:
coronary atherosclerosis due to calcified coronary lesion (I25.84)
coronary atherosclerosis due to lipid rich plaque (I25.83)

EXCLUDES 1 *atherosclerosis of bypass graft (s) of transplanted heart without angina pectoris (I25.812)*
atherosclerosis of coronary artery bypass graft (s) without angina pectoris (I25.810)
atherosclerosis of native coronary artery of transplanted heart without angina pectoris (I25.811)

I25.70 Atherosclerosis of coronary artery bypass graft(s), unspecified, with angina pectoris

I25.700 Atherosclerosis of coronary artery bypass graft(s), unspecified, with unstable angina pectoris A HCC

EXCLUDES 1 *unstable angina pectoris without atherosclerosis of coronary artery bypass graft (I20.0)*

I25.701 Atherosclerosis of coronary artery bypass graft(s), unspecified, with angina pectoris with documented spasm A HCC

EXCLUDES 1 *angina pectoris with documented spasm without atherosclerosis of coronary artery bypass graft (I20.1)*

I25.708 Atherosclerosis of coronary artery bypass graft(s), unspecified, with other forms of angina pectoris A HCC

EXCLUDES 1 *other forms of angina pectoris without atherosclerosis of coronary artery bypass graft (I20.8)*

I25.709 Atherosclerosis of coronary artery bypass graft(s), unspecified, with unspecified angina pectoris A HCC

EXCLUDES 1 *unspecified angina pectoris without atherosclerosis of coronary artery bypass graft (I20.9)*

I25.71 Atherosclerosis of autologous vein coronary artery bypass graft(s) with angina pectoris

I25.710 Atherosclerosis of autologous vein coronary artery bypass graft(s) with unstable angina pectoris A HCC

EXCLUDES 1 *unstable angina without atherosclerosis of autologous vein coronary artery bypass graft (s) (I20.0)*

EXCLUDES 2 *embolism or thrombus of coronary artery bypass graft (s) (T82.8-)*

I25.711 Atherosclerosis of autologous vein coronary artery bypass graft(s) with angina pectoris with documented spasm A HCC

EXCLUDES 1 *angina pectoris with documented spasm without atherosclerosis of autologous vein coronary artery bypass graft (s) (I20.1)*

I25.718 Atherosclerosis of autologous vein coronary artery bypass graft(s) with other forms of angina pectoris A HCC

EXCLUDES 1 *other forms of angina pectoris without atherosclerosis of autologous vein coronary artery bypass graft (s) (I20.8)*

I25.719 Atherosclerosis of autologous vein coronary artery bypass graft(s) with unspecified angina pectoris A HCC

EXCLUDES 1 *unspecified angina pectoris without atherosclerosis of autologous vein coronary artery bypass graft (s) (I20.9)*

I25.72 Atherosclerosis of autologous artery coronary artery bypass graft(s) with angina pectoris

Atherosclerosis of internal mammary artery graft with angina pectoris

I25.720 Atherosclerosis of autologous artery coronary artery bypass graft(s) with unstable angina pectoris A HCC

EXCLUDES 1 *unstable angina without atherosclerosis of autologous artery coronary artery bypass graft (s) (I20.0)*

I25.721 Atherosclerosis of autologous artery coronary artery bypass graft(s) with angina pectoris with documented spasm A HCC

EXCLUDES 1 *angina pectoris with documented spasm without atherosclerosis of autologous artery coronary artery bypass graft (s) (I20.1)*

I25.728 Atherosclerosis of autologous artery coronary artery bypass graft(s) with other forms of angina pectoris A HCC

EXCLUDES 1 *other forms of angina pectoris without atherosclerosis of autologous artery coronary artery bypass graft (s) (I20.8)*

I25.729 Atherosclerosis of autologous artery coronary artery bypass graft(s) with unspecified angina pectoris A HCC

EXCLUDES 1 *unspecified angina pectoris without atherosclerosis of autologous artery coronary artery bypass graft (s) (I20.9)*

I25.73 Atherosclerosis of nonautologous biological coronary artery bypass graft(s) with angina pectoris

I25.730 Atherosclerosis of nonautologous biological coronary artery bypass graft(s) with unstable angina pectoris A HCC

EXCLUDES 1 *unstable angina without atherosclerosis of nonautologous biological coronary artery bypass graft (s) (I20.0)*

I25.731 Atherosclerosis of nonautologous biological coronary artery bypass graft(s) with angina pectoris with documented spasm A HCC

EXCLUDES 1 *angina pectoris with documented spasm without atherosclerosis of nonautologous biological coronary artery bypass graft (s) (I20.1)*

I25.738 Atherosclerosis of nonautologous biological coronary artery bypass graft(s) with other forms of angina pectoris A HCC

EXCLUDES 1 *other forms of angina pectoris without atherosclerosis of nonautologous biological coronary artery bypass graft (s) (I20.8)*

I25.739 Atherosclerosis of nonautologous biological coronary artery bypass graft(s) with unspecified angina pectoris A HCC

EXCLUDES 1 *unspecified angina pectoris without atherosclerosis of nonautologous biological coronary artery bypass graft (s) (I20.9)*

I25.75 Atherosclerosis of native coronary artery of transplanted heart with angina pectoris

EXCLUDES 1 *atherosclerosis of native coronary artery of transplanted heart without angina pectoris (I25.811)*

I25.750 Atherosclerosis of native coronary artery of transplanted heart with unstable angina HCC

I25.751 Atherosclerosis of native coronary artery of transplanted heart with angina pectoris with documented spasm HCC

I25.758 Atherosclerosis of native coronary artery of transplanted heart with other forms of angina pectoris HCC

I25.759 Atherosclerosis of native coronary artery of transplanted heart with unspecified angina pectoris HCC

6 **I25.76 Atherosclerosis of bypass graft of coronary artery of transplanted heart with angina pectoris**

EXCLUDES 1 *atherosclerosis of bypass graft of coronary artery of transplanted heart without angina pectoris (I25.812)*

I25.760 Atherosclerosis of bypass graft of coronary artery of transplanted heart with unstable angina A HCC

I25.761 Atherosclerosis of bypass graft of coronary artery of transplanted heart with angina pectoris with documented spasm A HCC

I25.768 Atherosclerosis of bypass graft of coronary artery of transplanted heart with other forms of angina pectoris A HCC

I25.769 Atherosclerosis of bypass graft of coronary artery of transplanted heart with unspecified angina pectoris A HCC

6 **I25.79 Atherosclerosis of other coronary artery bypass graft(s) with angina pectoris**

I25.790 Atherosclerosis of other coronary artery bypass graft(s) with unstable angina pectoris A HCC

EXCLUDES 1 *unstable angina without atherosclerosis of other coronary artery bypass graft (s) (I20.0)*

I25.791 Atherosclerosis of other coronary artery bypass graft(s) with angina pectoris with documented spasm A HCC

EXCLUDES 1 *angina pectoris with documented spasm without atherosclerosis of other coronary artery bypass graft (s) (I20.1)*

I25.798 Atherosclerosis of other coronary artery bypass graft(s) with other forms of angina pectoris A HCC

EXCLUDES 1 *other forms of angina pectoris without atherosclerosis of other coronary artery bypass graft (s) (I20.8)*

I25.799 Atherosclerosis of other coronary artery bypass graft(s) with unspecified angina pectoris A HCC

EXCLUDES 1 *unspecified angina pectoris without atherosclerosis of other coronary artery bypass graft (s) (I20.9)*

5 **I25.8 Other forms of chronic ischemic heart disease**

6 **I25.81 Atherosclerosis of other coronary vessels without angina pectoris**

Use additional code, if applicable, to identify:
coronary atherosclerosis due to calcified coronary lesion (I25.84)
coronary atherosclerosis due to lipid rich plaque (I25.83)

EXCLUDES 1 *atherosclerotic heart disease of native coronary artery without angina pectoris (I25.10)*

I25.810 Atherosclerosis of coronary artery bypass graft(s) without angina pectoris A

Atherosclerosis of coronary artery bypass graft NOS

EXCLUDES 1 *atherosclerosis of coronary bypass graft (s) with angina pectoris (I25.70-I25.73-, I25.79-)*

I25.811 Atherosclerosis of native coronary artery of transplanted heart without angina pectoris

Atherosclerosis of native coronary artery of transplanted heart NOS

EXCLUDES 1 *atherosclerosis of native coronary artery of transplanted heart with angina pectoris (I25.75-)*

I25.812 Atherosclerosis of bypass graft of coronary artery of transplanted heart without angina pectoris A

Atherosclerosis of bypass graft of transplanted heart NOS

EXCLUDES 1 *atherosclerosis of bypass graft of transplanted heart with angina pectoris (I25.76)*

I25.82 Chronic total occlusion of coronary artery

Complete occlusion of coronary artery
Total occlusion of coronary artery
Code first:
coronary atherosclerosis (I25.1-, I25.7-, I25.81-)

EXCLUDES 1 *acute coronary occlusion with myocardial infarction (I21.0-I21.9, I22.-)*
acute coronary occlusion without myocardial infarction (I24.0)

I25.83 Coronary atherosclerosis due to lipid rich plaque A

Code first:
coronary atherosclerosis (I25.1-, I25.7-, I25.81-)

I25.84 Coronary atherosclerosis due to calcified coronary lesion

Coronary atherosclerosis due to severely calcified coronary lesion
Code first:
coronary atherosclerosis (I25.1-, I25.7-, I25.81-)

I25.89 Other forms of chronic ischemic heart disease

I25.9 Chronic ischemic heart disease, unspecified

Ischemic heart disease (chronic) NOS

Pulmonary heart disease and diseases of pulmonary circulation (I26-I28)

4 **I26 Pulmonary embolism**

INCLUDES pulmonary (acute) (artery)(vein) infarction
pulmonary (acute) (artery)(vein) thromboembolism
pulmonary (acute) (artery)(vein) thrombosis

EXCLUDES 2 *chronic pulmonary embolism (I27.82)*
personal history of pulmonary embolism (Z86.711)
pulmonary embolism complicating abortion, ectopic or molar pregnancy (O00-O07, O08.2)
pulmonary embolism complicating pregnancy, childbirth and the puerperium (O88.-)
pulmonary embolism due to trauma (T79.0, T79.1)
pulmonary embolism due to complications of surgical and medical care (T80.0, T81.7-, T82.8-)
septic (non-pulmonary) arterial embolism (I76)

5 **I26.0 Pulmonary embolism with acute cor pulmonale**

CODING TIP ✓ Category I26.0- codes should be assigned only when cor pulmonale is reported as occurring and associated with a pulmonary embolus. Cor pulmonale is a right ventricular dysfunction and failure.

I26.01 Septic pulmonary embolism with acute cor pulmonale HCC

Code first:
underlying infection

CODING TIP ✓ The term septic pulmonary embolism indicates a pulmonary embolus resulting from embolization of infectious particles which enter the lungs in the pulmonary arterial system. This can occur as a result of infectious DVT, periodontal disease, infected venous catheters, endocarditis, or other systemic infections. This code should only be assigned when the embolus is stated as septic and related to an infectious cause. A second code for the underlying/causative infection must be assigned.

I26.02 Saddle embolus of pulmonary artery with acute cor pulmonale HCC

I26.09 Other pulmonary embolism with acute cor pulmonale HCC

Acute cor pulmonale NOS
AHA: 4Q 2014, 22

5 **I26.9 Pulmonary embolism without acute cor pulmonale**

I26.90 Septic pulmonary embolism without acute cor pulmonale HCC
Code first:
underlying infection

I26.92 Saddle embolus of pulmonary artery without acute cor pulmonale HCC

I26.99 Other pulmonary embolism without acute cor pulmonale HCC
Acute pulmonary embolism NOS
Pulmonary embolism NOS

CODING TIP ✓ Documentation indicating pulmonary embolism, without further information, is assigned I26.99.

4 **I27 Other pulmonary heart diseases**

GUIDELINES **Section I.C.9.a.11)**
Pulmonary hypertension is classified to category I27, Other pulmonary heart diseases. For secondary pulmonary hypertension (I27.1, I27.2-), code also any associated conditions or adverse effects of drugs or toxins. The sequencing is based on the reason for the encounter, except for adverse effects of drugs (See Section I.C.19.e.).

I27.0 Primary pulmonary hypertension HCC
Heritable pulmonary arterial hypertension
Idiopathic pulmonary arterial hypertension
Primary group 1 pulmonary hypertension
Primary pulmonary arterial hypertension
EXCLUDES 1 *persistent pulmonary hypertension of newborn (P29.30)*
pulmonary hypertension NOS (I27.20)
secondary pulmonary arterial hypertension (I27.21)
secondary pulmonary hypertension (I27.29)
AHA: 4Q 2017, 11

I27.1 Kyphoscoliotic heart disease HCC
AHA: 4Q 2017, 11

5 **I27.2 Other secondary pulmonary hypertension** HCC
Code also:
associated underlying condition
EXCLUDES 1 *Eisenmenger's syndrome (I27.83)*
AHA: 4Q 2014, 21, 22
AHA: 2Q 2016, 8
AHA: 4Q 2017, 11

I27.20 Pulmonary hypertension, unspecified HCC
Pulmonary hypertension NOS
AHA: 4Q 2017, 11

I27.21 Secondary pulmonary arterial hypertension HCC
(Associated) (drug-induced) (toxin-induced) pulmonary arterial hypertension NOS
(Associated) (drug-induced) (toxin-induced) (secondary) group 1 pulmonary hypertension
Code also associated conditions if applicable, or adverse effects of drugs or toxins, such as:
adverse effect of appetite depressants (T50.5X5)
congenital heart disease (Q20-Q28)
human immunodeficiency virus [HIV] disease (B20)
polymyositis (M33.2-)
portal hypertension (K76.6)
rheumatoid arthritis (M05.-)
schistosomiasis (B65.-)
Sjögren syndrome (M35.0-)
systemic sclerosis (M34.-)
AHA: 4Q 2017, 11

I27.22 Pulmonary hypertension due to left heart disease HCC
Group 2 pulmonary hypertension
Code also associated left heart disease, if known, such as:
multiple valve disease (I08.-)
rheumatic mitral valve diseases (I05.-)
rheumatic aortic valve diseases (I06.-)
AHA: 4Q 2017, 11

I27.23 Pulmonary hypertension due to lung diseasesand hypoxia HCC
Group 3 pulmonary hypertension
Code also associated lung disease, if known, such as:
bronchiectasis (J47.-)
cystic fibrosis with pulmonary manifestations (E84.0)
interstitial lung disease (J84.-)
pleural effusion (J90)
sleep apnea (G47.3-)
AHA: 4Q 2017, 11

I27.24 Chronic thromboembolic pulmonary hypertension HCC
Group 4 pulmonary hypertension
Code also:
associated pulmonary embolism, if applicable (I26.-, I27.82)
AHA: 4Q 2017, 11

▲ **I27.29 Other secondary pulmonary hypertension** HCC
Group 5 pulmonary hypertension
Pulmonary hypertension with unclear multifactorial mechanisms
Pulmonary hypertension due to hematologic disorders
Pulmonary hypertension due to metabolic disorders
Pulmonary hypertension due to other systemic disorders
Code also other associated disorders, if known, such as:
chronic myeloid leukemia (C92.10- C92.22)
essential thrombocythemia (D47.3)
Gaucher disease (E75.22)
hypertensive chronic kidney disease with end stage renal disease (I12.0, I13.11, I13.2)
hyperthyroidism (E05.-)
hypothyroidism (E00-E03)
polycythemia vera (D45)
sarcoidosis (D86.-)
AHA: 4Q 2017, 11

5 **I27.8 Other specified pulmonary heart diseases**
AHA: 4Q 2017, 11

I27.81 Cor pulmonale (chronic) HCC
Cor pulmonale NOS
EXCLUDES 1 *acute cor pulmonale (I26.0-)*
AHA: 4Q 2014, 21
AHA: 4Q 2017, 11

I27.82 Chronic pulmonary embolism HCC
Use additional code, if applicable, for associated long-term (current) use of anticoagulants (Z79.01)
EXCLUDES 1 *personal history of pulmonary embolism (Z86.711)*
AHA: 4Q 2017, 11

I27.83 Eisenmenger's syndrome HCC
Eisenmenger's complex
(Irreversible) Eisenmenger's disease
Pulmonary hypertension with right to left shunt related to congenital heart disease
Code also underlying heart defect, if known, such as:
atrial septal defect (Q21.1)
Eisenmenger's defect (Q21.8)
patent ductus arteriosus (Q25.0)
ventricular septal defect (Q21.0)
AHA: 4Q 2017, 11

I27.89 Other specified pulmonary heart diseases HCC
AHA: 4Q 2017, 11

I27.9 Pulmonary heart disease, unspecified HCC
Chronic cardiopulmonary disease
AHA: 4Q 2017, 11

4 **I28 Other diseases of pulmonary vessels**

I28.0 Arteriovenous fistula of pulmonary vessels HCC
EXCLUDES 1 *congenital arteriovenous fistula (Q25.72)*

DEFINITION Abnormal passage between the pulmonary arterial and venous systems, which causes unoxygenated blood to enter systemic circulation.

I28.1 Aneurysm of pulmonary artery HCC
EXCLUDES 1 *congenital aneurysm (Q25.79)*
congenital arteriovenous aneurysm (Q25.72)

DEFINITION Bulging in one portion of the arterial wall that brings blood to the lungs, forming a pouch or sac with the potential for rupture.

I28.8 **Other diseases of pulmonary vessels** HCC
Pulmonary arteritis
Pulmonary endarteritis
Rupture of pulmonary vessels
Stenosis of pulmonary vessels
Stricture of pulmonary vessels

I28.9 **Disease of pulmonary vessels, unspecified** HCC

Other forms of heart disease (I30-I52)

4 I30 Acute pericarditis

INCLUDES acute mediastinopericarditis
acute myopericarditis
acute pericardial effusion
acute pleuropericarditis
acute pneumopericarditis

EXCLUDES 1 *Dressler's syndrome (I24.1)*
rheumatic pericarditis (acute) (I01.0)
viral pericarditis due to Coxsakie virus (B33.23)

I30.0 **Acute nonspecific idiopathic pericarditis**

I30.1 **Infective pericarditis**
Pneumococcal pericarditis
Pneumopyopericardium
Purulent pericarditis
Pyopericarditis
Pyopericardium
Pyopneumopericardium
Staphylococcal pericarditis
Streptococcal pericarditis
Suppurative pericarditis
Viral pericarditis
Use additional code (B95-B97) to identify infectious agent

I30.8 **Other forms of acute pericarditis**

I30.9 **Acute pericarditis, unspecified**

4 I31 Other diseases of pericardium

EXCLUDES 1 *diseases of pericardium specified as rheumatic (I09.2)*
postcardiotomy syndrome (I97.0)
traumatic injury to pericardium (S26.-)

I31.0 **Chronic adhesive pericarditis**
Accretio cordis
Adherent pericardium
Adhesive mediastinopericarditis

DEFINITION Pericardial inflammation with adhesion between the two pericardial layers or between the pericardium and the heart or neighboring structures.

I31.1 **Chronic constrictive pericarditis**
Concretio cordis
Pericardial calcification

I31.2 **Hemopericardium, not elsewhere classified**

EXCLUDES 1 *hemopericardium as current complication following acute myocardial infarction (I23.0)*

DEFINITION Bleeding causing the sac around the heart to fill with blood.

I31.3 **Pericardial effusion (noninflammatory)**
Chylopericardium

EXCLUDES 1 *acute pericardial effusion (I30.9)*

I31.4 **Cardiac tamponade**
Code first:
underlying cause

DEFINITION Increased pressure on the heart due to fluid in the pericardial sac, impairing ventricular filling action and causing decreased cardiac output.

I31.8 **Other specified diseases of pericardium**
Epicardial plaques
Focal pericardial adhesions

I31.9 **Disease of pericardium, unspecified**
Pericarditis (chronic) NOS

I32 ***Pericarditis in diseases classified elsewhere***
Code first:
underlying disease

EXCLUDES 1 *pericarditis (in) :*
coxsackie (virus) (B33.23)
gonococcal (A54.83)
meningococcal (A39.53)
rheumatoid (arthritis) (M05.31)
syphilitic (A52.06)
systemic lupus erythematosus (M32.12)
tuberculosis (A18.84)

DEFINITION Inflammation of the membranous sac around the heart occurring with another underlying disease process, causing chest pain, coughing, fatigue, and fever.

4 I33 Acute and subacute endocarditis

EXCLUDES 1 *acute rheumatic endocarditis (I01.1)*
endocarditis NOS (I38)

I33.0 **Acute and subacute infective endocarditis** HIV
Bacterial endocarditis (acute) (subacute)
Infective endocarditis (acute) (subacute) NOS
Endocarditis lenta (acute) (subacute)
Malignant endocarditis (acute) (subacute)
Purulent endocarditis (acute) (subacute)
Septic endocarditis (acute) (subacute)
Ulcerative endocarditis (acute) (subacute)
Vegetative endocarditis (acute) (subacute)
Use additional code (B95-B97) to identify infectious agent

I33.9 **Acute and subacute endocarditis, unspecified** HIV
Acute endocarditis NOS
Acute myoendocarditis NOS
Acute periendocarditis NOS
Subacute endocarditis NOS
Subacute myoendocarditis NOS
Subacute periendocarditis NOS

4 I34 Nonrheumatic mitral valve disorders

EXCLUDES 1 *mitral valve disease (I05.9)*
mitral valve failure (I05.8)
mitral valve stenosis (I05.0)
mitral valve disorder of unspecified cause with diseases of aortic and/or tricuspid valve (s) (I08.-)
mitral valve disorder of unspecified cause with mitral stenosis or obstruction (I05.0)
mitral valve disorder specified as congenital (Q23.2, Q23.9)
mitral valve disorder specified as rheumatic (I05.-)

I34.0 **Nonrheumatic mitral (valve) insufficiency**
Nonrheumatic mitral (valve) incompetence NOS
Nonrheumatic mitral (valve) regurgitation NOS

I34.1 **Nonrheumatic mitral (valve) prolapse**
Floppy nonrheumatic mitral valve syndrome

EXCLUDES 1 *Marfan's syndrome (Q87.4-)*

I34.2 **Nonrheumatic mitral (valve) stenosis**

I34.8 **Other nonrheumatic mitral valve disorders**

I34.9 **Nonrheumatic mitral valve disorder, unspecified**

4 I35 Nonrheumatic aortic valve disorders

EXCLUDES 1 *aortic valve disorder of unspecified cause but with diseases of mitral and/or tricuspid valve (s) (I08.-)*
aortic valve disorder specified as congenital (Q23.0, Q23.1)
aortic valve disorder specified as rheumatic (I06.-)
hypertrophic subaortic stenosis (I42.1)

I35.0 **Nonrheumatic aortic (valve) stenosis**

Nonrheumatic aortic (valve) stenosis

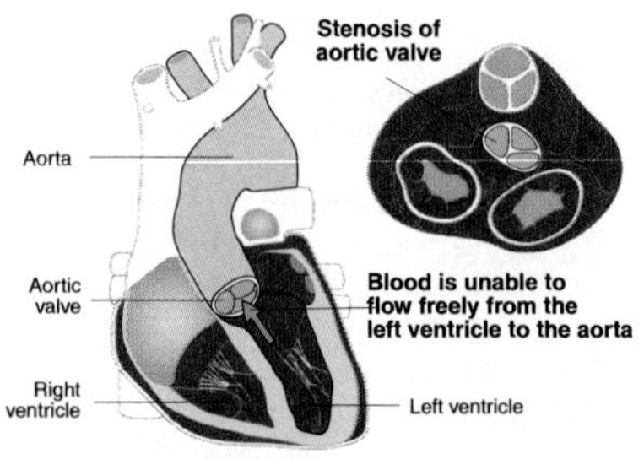

I35.1 **Nonrheumatic aortic (valve) insufficiency**
Nonrheumatic aortic (valve) incompetence NOS
Nonrheumatic aortic (valve) regurgitation NOS

I35.2 **Nonrheumatic aortic (valve) stenosis with insufficiency**

I35.8 **Other nonrheumatic aortic valve disorders**

I35.9 **Nonrheumatic aortic valve disorder, unspecified**

I36 Nonrheumatic tricuspid valve disorders

EXCLUDES 1 *tricuspid valve disorders of unspecified cause (I07.-)*
tricuspid valve disorders specified as congenital (Q22.4, Q22.8, Q22.9)
tricuspid valve disorders specified as rheumatic (I07.-)
tricuspid valve disorders with aortic and/or mitral valve involvement (I08.-)

I36.0 **Nonrheumatic tricuspid (valve) stenosis**

I36.1 **Nonrheumatic tricuspid (valve) insufficiency**
Nonrheumatic tricuspid (valve) incompetence
Nonrheumatic tricuspid (valve) regurgitation

I36.2 **Nonrheumatic tricuspid (valve) stenosis with insufficiency**

I36.8 **Other nonrheumatic tricuspid valve disorders**

I36.9 **Nonrheumatic tricuspid valve disorder, unspecified**

I37 Nonrheumatic pulmonary valve disorders

EXCLUDES 1 *pulmonary valve disorder specified as congenital (Q22.1, Q22.2, Q22.3)*
pulmonary valve disorder specified as rheumatic (I09.89)

I37.0 **Nonrheumatic pulmonary valve stenosis**

I37.1 **Nonrheumatic pulmonary valve insufficiency**
Nonrheumatic pulmonary valve incompetence
Nonrheumatic pulmonary valve regurgitation

I37.2 **Nonrheumatic pulmonary valve stenosis with insufficiency**

I37.8 **Other nonrheumatic pulmonary valve disorders**

I37.9 **Nonrheumatic pulmonary valve disorder, unspecified**

I38 Endocarditis, valve unspecified

INCLUDES endocarditis (chronic) NOS
valvular incompetence NOS
valvular insufficiency NOS
valvular regurgitation NOS
valvular stenosis NOS
valvulitis (chronic) NOS

EXCLUDES 1 *congenital insufficiency of cardiac valve NOS (Q24.8)*
congenital stenosis of cardiac valve NOS (Q24.8)
endocardial fibroelastosis (I42.4)
endocarditis specified as rheumatic (I09.1)

I39 *Endocarditis and heart valve disorders in diseases classified elsewhere*

Code first underlying disease, such as:
Q fever (A78)

EXCLUDES 1 *endocardial involvement in:*
candidiasis (B37.6)
gonococcal infection (A54.83)
Libman-Sacks disease (M32.11)
listerosis (A32.82)
meningococcal infection (A39.51)
rheumatoid arthritis (M05.31)
syphilis (A52.03)
tuberculosis (A18.84)
typhoid fever (A01.02)

CODING TIP ✓ I39 is a manifestation code. A code for the causative underlying disease process must be sequenced first.

CODING TIP ✓ **Documentation:** Assign this code only when the clinical record supports a cause and effect relationship between the underlying disease process and the endocarditis/valve disorder.

I40 Acute myocarditis

INCLUDES subacute myocarditis

EXCLUDES 1 *acute rheumatic myocarditis (I01.2)*

DEFINITION Severe inflammation of heart muscle tissue.

I40.0 **Infective myocarditis** HIV
Septic myocarditis
Use additional code (B95-B97) to identify infectious agent

I40.1 **Isolated myocarditis** HIV
Fiedler's myocarditis
Giant cell myocarditis
Idiopathic myocarditis

I40.8 **Other acute myocarditis** HIV

I40.9 **Acute myocarditis, unspecified** HIV

I41 *Myocarditis in diseases classified elsewhere*

Code first underlying disease, such as:
typhus (A75.0-A75.9)

EXCLUDES 1 *myocarditis (in):*
Chagas' disease (chronic) (B57.2)
acute (B57.0)
coxsackie (virus) infection (B33.22)
diphtheritic (A36.81)
gonococcal (A54.83)
influenzal (J09.X9, J10.82, J11.82)
meningococcal (A39.52)
mumps (B26.82)
rheumatoid arthritis (M05.31)
sarcoid (D86.85)
syphilis (A52.06)
toxoplasmosis (B58.81)
tuberculous (A18.84)

CODING TIP ✓ I41 is a manifestation code. A code for the causative underlying disease process must be sequenced first.

CODING TIP ✓ **Documentation:** Assign this code only when the clinical record supports a cause and effect relationship between the underlying disease process and myocarditis.

I42 Cardiomyopathy

INCLUDES myocardiopathy

Code first:
pre-existing cardiomyopathy complicating pregnancy and puerperium (O99.4)

EXCLUDES 2 *ischemic cardiomyopathy (I25.5)*
peripartum cardiomyopathy (O90.3)
ventricular hypertrophy (I51.7)

I42.0 **Dilated cardiomyopathy** HCC
Congestive cardiomyopathy

I42.1 **Obstructive hypertrophic cardiomyopathy** HCC
Hypertrophic subaortic stenosis (idiopathic)

I42.2 **Other hypertrophic cardiomyopathy** HCC
Nonobstructive hypertrophic cardiomyopathy

I42.3 **Endomyocardial (eosinophilic) disease** HCC
Endomyocardial (tropical) fibrosis
Löffler's endocarditis

I42.4 **Endocardial fibroelastosis** HCC
Congenital cardiomyopathy
Elastomyofibrosis

I42.5 **Other restrictive cardiomyopathy** HCC
Constrictive cardiomyopathy NOS

I42.6 **Alcoholic cardiomyopathy** HCC
Code also:
presence of alcoholism (F10.-)

DEFINITION Dilated disease of the heart muscle due to alcohol abuse.

I42.7 Cardiomyopathy due to drug and external agent HCC
Code first:
poisoning due to drug or toxin, if applicable (T36-T65 with fifth or sixth character 1-4 or 6)
Use additional code for adverse effect, if applicable, to identify drug (T36-T50 with fifth or sixth character 5)

I42.8 Other cardiomyopathies HCC

I42.9 Cardiomyopathy, unspecified HCC
Cardiomyopathy (primary) (secondary) NOS

I43 *Cardiomyopathy in diseases classified elsewhere* HCC
Code first underlying disease, such as:
amyloidosis (E85.-)
glycogen storage disease (E74.0)
gout (M10.0-)
thyrotoxicosis (E05.0-E05.9-)

EXCLUDES 1 *cardiomyopathy (in) :*
coxsackie (virus) (B33.24)
diphtheria (A36.81)
sarcoidosis (D86.85)
tuberculosis (A18.84)

CODING TIP✓ I43 is a manifestation code. A code for the causative underlying disease process must be sequenced first.

CODING TIP✓ **Documentation:** Assign this code only when the clinical record supports a cause and effect relationship between the underlying disease process and cardiomyopathy.

4 I44 Atrioventricular and left bundle-branch block
CODING TIP✓ When reviewing documentation for heart block, it is important to differentiate heart block degree from heart block type.

I44.0 Atrioventricular block, first degree

▲ **I44.1 Atrioventricular block, second degree**
Atrioventricular block, type I and II
Möbitz block, type I and II
Second degree block, type I and II
Wenckebach's block

I44.2 Atrioventricular block, complete HCC
Complete heart block NOS
Third degree block

DEFINITION No conduction of electrical impulses occurs between the atria and ventricles, requiring a pacemaker to maintain rhythm.

5 **I44.3 Other and unspecified atrioventricular block**
Atrioventricular block NOS

I44.30 Unspecified atrioventricular block

I44.39 Other atrioventricular block

I44.4 Left anterior fascicular block

I44.5 Left posterior fascicular block

5 **I44.6 Other and unspecified fascicular block**

I44.60 Unspecified fascicular block
Left bundle-branch hemiblock NOS

I44.69 Other fascicular block

I44.7 Left bundle-branch block, unspecified

4 I45 Other conduction disorders
CODING TIP✓ When reviewing documentation for heart block, it is important to differentiate heart block degree from heart block type.

I45.0 Right fascicular block

5 **I45.1 Other and unspecified right bundle-branch block**

I45.10 Unspecified right bundle-branch block
Right bundle-branch block NOS

I45.19 Other right bundle-branch block

I45.2 Bifascicular block

I45.3 Trifascicular block

I45.4 Nonspecific intraventricular block
Bundle-branch block NOS

DEFINITION A condition in which portions of the heart's conduction system are defective and either slow or block the electrical impulses traveling through specialized conduction tissue on the way to the ventricles.

I45.5 Other specified heart block
Sinoatrial block
Sinoauricular block

EXCLUDES 1 *heart block NOS (I45.9)*

I45.6 Pre-excitation syndrome
Accelerated atrioventricular conduction
Accessory atrioventricular conduction
Anomalous atrioventricular excitation
Lown-Ganong-Levine syndrome
Pre-excitation atrioventricular conduction
Wolff-Parkinson-White syndrome

5 **I45.8 Other specified conduction disorders**

I45.81 Long QT syndrome

DEFINITION Hereditary defect of the heart's electrical conduction system with an abnormally long gap in the time it takes for the ventricles to contract.

I45.89 Other specified conduction disorders
Atrioventricular [AV] dissociation
Interference dissociation
Isorhythmic dissociation
Nonparoxysmal AV nodal tachycardia
AHA: 2Q 2013, 31-32

I45.9 Conduction disorder, unspecified
Heart block NOS
Stokes-Adams syndrome

4 I46 Cardiac arrest
EXCLUDES 1 *cardiogenic shock (R57.0)*

I46.2 Cardiac arrest due to underlying cardiac condition HCC
Code first:
underlying cardiac condition

I46.8 Cardiac arrest due to other underlying condition HCC
Code first:
underlying condition

I46.9 Cardiac arrest, cause unspecified HCC

4 I47 Paroxysmal tachycardia
Code first tachycardia complicating:
abortion or ectopic or molar pregnancy (O00-O07, O08.8)
obstetric surgery and procedures (O75.4)

EXCLUDES 1 *tachycardia NOS (R00.0)*
sinoauricular tachycardia NOS (R00.0)
sinus [sinusal] tachycardia NOS (R00.0)

CODING TIP✓ Do not assign a code from I47.- when only tachycardia is reported in the record and is not specified, or is reported in the record as sinus tachycardia or sinoauricular. When tachycardia is reported as sinus tachycardia or is not specified, report code R00.0 rather than a code from I47.-.

I47.0 Re-entry ventricular arrhythmia HCC

I47.1 Supraventricular tachycardia HCC
Atrial (paroxysmal) tachycardia
Atrioventricular [AV] (paroxysmal) tachycardia
Atrioventricular re-entrant (nodal) tachycardia [AVNRT] [AVRT]
Junctional (paroxysmal) tachycardia
Nodal (paroxysmal) tachycardia

DEFINITION Abnormally rapid atrial rhythm occurring from time to time, most often in the young.

I47.2 Ventricular tachycardia HCC

DEFINITION Potentially lethal rapid heart beat initiating in the ventricles marked by three of more consecutive premature beats.
AHA: 3Q 2013, 23

I47.9 Paroxysmal tachycardia, unspecified HCC
Bouveret (-Hoffman) syndrome

4 I48 Atrial fibrillation and flutter
CODING TIP✓ When assigning a code for atrial fibrillation or flutter, assign the most specific code according to the diagnostic statements given by the patient's physician.

DEFINITION Abnormal heart rhythm that occurs in the atria of the heart.

I48.0 Paroxysmal atrial fibrillation HCC

I48.1 Persistent atrial fibrillation HCC

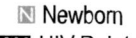

CODING TIP✓ Do not assume a diagnosis of persistent atrial fibrillation in a patient who has a longstanding history of atrial fibrillation. This code may be assigned only when documented by the physician.

I48.2 Chronic atrial fibrillation HCC
Permanent atrial fibrillation

CODING TIP✓ **Documentation:** Do not assume a diagnosis of chronic atrial fibrillation in a patient who has a longstanding history of atrial fibrillation or has simply had atrial fibrillation for a long period of time. This code may only be assigned with a supportive confirmation diagnosis by the physician. Without such a diagnostic statement, an unspecified code (I48.91) must be assigned.
AHA: 4Q 2013, 128

I48.3 Typical atrial flutter HCC
Type I atrial flutter

I48.4 Atypical atrial flutter HCC
Type II atrial flutter

5 **I48.9 Unspecified atrial fibrillation and atrial flutter**

I48.91 Unspecified atrial fibrillation HCC

I48.92 Unspecified atrial flutter HCC

4 **I49 Other cardiac arrhythmias**
Code first cardiac arrhythmia complicating:
abortion or ectopic or molar pregnancy (O00-O07, O08.8)
obstetric surgery and procedures (O75.4)
EXCLUDES 1 *neonatal dysrhythmia (P29.1-)*
sinoatrial bradycardia (R00.1)
sinus bradycardia (R00.1)
vagal bradycardia (R00.1)
EXCLUDES 2 *bradycardia NOS (R00.1)*

5 **I49.0 Ventricular fibrillation and flutter**

I49.01 Ventricular fibrillation HCC

I49.02 Ventricular flutter HCC

I49.1 Atrial premature depolarization
Atrial premature beats

I49.2 Junctional premature depolarization HCC

I49.3 Ventricular premature depolarization

5 **I49.4 Other and unspecified premature depolarization**

I49.40 Unspecified premature depolarization
Premature beats NOS

I49.49 Other premature depolarization
Ectopic beats
Extrasystoles
Extrasystolic arrhythmias
Premature contractions

I49.5 Sick sinus syndrome HCC
Tachycardia-bradycardia syndrome

I49.8 Other specified cardiac arrhythmias
Brugada syndrome
Coronary sinus rhythm disorder
Ectopic rhythm disorder
Nodal rhythm disorder

I49.9 Cardiac arrhythmia, unspecified
Arrhythmia (cardiac) NOS

4 **I50 Heart failure**
Code first:
heart failure complicating abortion or ectopic or molar pregnancy (O00-O07, O08.8)
heart failure due to hypertension (I11.0)
heart failure due to hypertension with chronic kidney disease (I13.-)
heart failure following surgery (I97.13-)
obstetric surgery and procedures (O75.4)
rheumatic heart failure (I09.81)
EXCLUDES 1 *neonatal cardiac failure (P29.0)*
EXCLUDES 2 *cardiac arrest (I46.-)*

GUIDELINES **Section I.C.9.a.1)**
Hypertension with heart conditions classified to I50.- or I51.4-I51.7, I51.89, I51.9, are assigned to a code from category I11, Hypertensive heart disease. Use additional code(s) from category I50, Heart failure, to identify the type(s) of heart failure in those patients with heart failure.

The same heart conditions (I50.-, I51.4-I51.7, I51.89, I51.9) with hypertension are coded separately if the provider has documented they are unrelated to the hypertension. Sequence according to the circumstances of the admission/encounter.

CODING TIP✓ Stage A of the ABCD Heart Failure Classification of the American College of Cardiology (ACC)/American Heart Association (AHA) is the presence of heart failure risk factors but no heart disease and no symptoms. This should not be coded to the regular heart failure codes, but rather to code Z91.89, Other specified personal risk factors, not elsewhere classified.

CODING TIP✓ The term "congestive" is a non-essential modifier for heart failure codes. When coding heart failure, note the non-essential modifier (congestive) and that no additional code should be used if a patient has both CHF and a more specific form of heart failure, such as diastolic heart failure.

I50.1 Left ventricular failure, unspecified HCC
Cardiac asthma
Edema of lung with heart disease NOS
Edema of lung with heart failure
Left heart failure
Pulmonary edema with heart disease NOS
Pulmonary edema with heart failure
EXCLUDES 1 *edema of lung without heart disease or heart failure (J81.-)*
pulmonary edema without heart disease or failure (J81.-)

5 **I50.2 Systolic (congestive) heart failure**
Heart failure with reduced ejection fraction [HFrEF]
Systolic left ventricular heart failure
Code also:
end stage heart failure, if applicable (I50.84)
EXCLUDES 1 *combined systolic (congestive) and diastolic (congestive) heart failure (I50.4-)*

DEFINITION Heart muscle fails to contract with adequate force and not enough oxygen-rich blood is pumped to the body.

I50.20 Unspecified systolic (congestive) heart failure HCC

I50.21 Acute systolic (congestive) heart failure HCC

I50.22 Chronic systolic (congestive) heart failure HCC

I50.23 Acute on chronic systolic (congestive) heart failure HCC
AHA: 2Q 2013, 33

5 **I50.3 Diastolic (congestive) heart failure**
Diastolic left ventricular heart failure
Heart failure with normal ejection fraction
Heart failure with preserved ejection fraction [HFpEF]
Code also:
end stage heart failure, if applicable (I50.84)
EXCLUDES 1 *combined systolic (congestive) and diastolic (congestive) heart failure (I50.4-)*

DEFINITION Heart muscle contracts normally but ventricles fail to relax properly after contraction, resulting in less blood entering the heart.

I50.30 Unspecified diastolic (congestive) heart failure HCC

I50.31 Acute diastolic (congestive) heart failure HCC
AHA: 1Q 2017, 46

I50.32 Chronic diastolic (congestive) heart failure HCC

I50.33 Acute on chronic diastolic (congestive) heart failure HCC

5 **I50.4 Combined systolic (congestive) and diastolic (congestive) heart failure**
Combined systolic and diastolic left ventricular heart failure
Heart failure with reduced ejection fraction and diastolic dysfunction
Code also:
end stage heart failure, if applicable (I50.84)

DEFINITION Heart fails both to contract and relax properly, resulting in an insufficient amount of blood moving through the circulatory system.

I50.40 **Unspecified combined systolic (congestive) and diastolic (congestive) heart failure** HCC

I50.41 **Acute combined systolic (congestive) and diastolic (congestive) heart failure** HCC

I50.42 **Chronic combined systolic (congestive) and diastolic (congestive) heart failure** HCC

I50.43 **Acute on chronic combined systolic (congestive) and diastolic (congestive) heart failure** HCC

5 I50.8 **Other heart failure**

6 I50.81 **Right heart failure**
Right ventricular failure

I50.810 **Right heart failure, unspecified** HCC
Right heart failure without mention of left heart failure
Right ventricular failure NOS
AHA: 4Q 2017, 12

I50.811 **Acute right heart failure** HCC
Acute isolated right heart failure
Acute (isolated) right ventricular failure
AHA: 4Q 2017, 12

I50.812 **Chronic right heart failure** HCC
Chronic isolated right heart failure
Chronic (isolated) right ventricular failure
AHA: 4Q 2017, 12

I50.813 **Acute on chronic right heart failure** HCC
Acute on chronic isolated right heart failure
Acute on chronic (isolated) right ventricular failure
Acute decompensation of chronic (isolated) right ventricular failure
Acute exacerbation of chronic (isolated) right ventricular failure
AHA: 4Q 2017, 12

I50.814 **Right heart failure due to left heart failure** HCC
Right ventricular failure secondary to left ventricular failure
Code also:
the type of left ventricular failure, if known (I50.2-I50.43)
EXCLUDES 1 *Right heart failure with but not due to left heart failure (I50.82)*
AHA: 4Q 2017, 12

I50.82 **Biventricular heart failure** HCC
Code also:
the type of left ventricular failure as systolic, diastolic, or combined, if known (I50.2-I50.43)
AHA: 4Q 2017, 12

I50.83 **High output heart failure** HCC
AHA: 4Q 2017, 12

I50.84 **End stage heart failure** HCC
Stage D heart failure
Code also:
the type of heart failure as systolic, diastolic, or combined, if known (I50.2-I50.43)
AHA: 4Q 2017, 12

I50.89 **Other heart failure** HCC

I50.9 **Heart failure, unspecified** HCC
Cardiac, heart or myocardial failure NOS
Congestive heart disease
Congestive heart failure NOS
EXCLUDES 2 *fluid overload (E87.70)*
AHA: 4Q 2012, 92
AHA: 4Q 2014, 21
AHA: 2Q 2015, 15
AHA: 1Q 2017, 46

4 I51 **Complications and ill-defined descriptions of heart disease**
EXCLUDES 1 *any condition in I51.4-I51.9 due to hypertension (I11.-)*
any condition in I51.4-I51.9 due to hypertension and chronic kidney disease (I13.-)
heart disease specified as rheumatic (I00-I09)

I51.0 **Cardiac septal defect, acquired** A
Acquired septal atrial defect (old)
Acquired septal auricular defect (old)
Acquired septal ventricular defect (old)
EXCLUDES 1 *cardiac septal defect as current complication following acute myocardial infarction (I23.1, I23.2)*

I51.1 **Rupture of chordae tendineae, not elsewhere classified** HCC
EXCLUDES 1 *rupture of chordae tendineae as current complication following acute myocardial infarction (I23.4)*
DEFINITION Tear in the fibrous, cord-like tissue connecting the papillary muscles to the valves, holding the valve flaps in place to prevent their eversion.

I51.2 **Rupture of papillary muscle, not elsewhere classified** HCC
EXCLUDES 1 *rupture of papillary muscle as current complication following acute myocardial infarction (I23.5)*

I51.3 **Intracardiac thrombosis, not elsewhere classified**
Apical thrombosis (old)
Atrial thrombosis (old)
Auricular thrombosis (old)
Mural thrombosis (old)
Ventricular thrombosis (old)
EXCLUDES 1 *intracardiac thrombosis as current complication following acute myocardial infarction (I23.6)*
AHA: 1Q 2013, 24

I51.4 **Myocarditis, unspecified** HCC
Chronic (interstitial) myocarditis
Myocardial fibrosis
Myocarditis NOS
EXCLUDES 1 *acute or subacute myocarditis (I40.-)*

I51.5 **Myocardial degeneration** HCC
Fatty degeneration of heart or myocardium
Myocardial disease
Senile degeneration of heart or myocardium
DEFINITION Wasting away of the heart muscle.

I51.7 **Cardiomegaly**
Cardiac dilatation
Cardiac hypertrophy
Ventricular dilatation

5 I51.8 **Other ill-defined heart diseases**

I51.81 **Takotsubo syndrome**
Reversible left ventricular dysfunction following sudden emotional stress
Stress induced cardiomyopathy
Takotsubo cardiomyopathy
Transient left ventricular apical ballooning syndrome
AHA: 2Q 2018, 7

I51.89 **Other ill-defined heart diseases**
Carditis (acute)(chronic)
Pancarditis (acute)(chronic)
CODING TIP ✓ Diastolic dysfunction or systolic dysfunction is coded to I51.89 if not related to heart failure. If related to heart failure, then diastolic heart failure or systolic heart failure should be coded.

I51.9 **Heart disease, unspecified**
CODING TIP ✓ This code is assigned for end stage heart disease, but the physician should always be queried for additional information regarding the type of heart disease.

I52 ***Other heart disorders in diseases classified elsewhere***
Code first underlying disease, such as:
congenital syphilis (A50.5)
mucopolysaccharidosis (E76.3)
schistosomiasis (B65.0-B65.9)
EXCLUDES 1 *heart disease (in) :*
gonococcal infection (A54.83)
meningococcal infection (A39.50)
rheumatoid arthritis (M05.31)
syphilis (A52.06)

Cerebrovascular diseases (I60-I69)

Use additional code to identify presence of:
alcohol abuse and dependence (F10.-)
exposure to environmental tobacco smoke (Z77.22)
history of tobacco dependence (Z87.891)
hypertension (I10-I16)
occupational exposure to environmental tobacco smoke (Z57.31)
tobacco dependence (F17.-)
tobacco use (Z72.0)

EXCLUDES 1 *traumatic intracranial hemorrhage (S06.-)*

GUIDELINES C. 9.a.4
For hypertensive cerebrovascular disease, first assign the appropriate code from categories I60-I69, followed by the appropriate hypertension code.

4 I60 Nontraumatic subarachnoid hemorrhage
EXCLUDES 1 *syphilitic ruptured cerebral aneurysm (A52.05)*
EXCLUDES 2 *sequelae of subarachnoid hemorrhage (I69.0-)*
AHA: 4Q 2012, 92

5 I60.0 Nontraumatic subarachnoid hemorrhage from carotid siphon and bifurcation
- **6 I60.00 Nontraumatic subarachnoid hemorrhage from unspecified carotid siphon and bifurcation** HCC
- **6 I60.01 Nontraumatic subarachnoid hemorrhage from right carotid siphon and bifurcation** HCC
- **6 I60.02 Nontraumatic subarachnoid hemorrhage from left carotid siphon and bifurcation** HCC

5 I60.1 Nontraumatic subarachnoid hemorrhage from middle cerebral artery
- **6 I60.10 Nontraumatic subarachnoid hemorrhage from unspecified middle cerebral artery** HCC
- **6 I60.11 Nontraumatic subarachnoid hemorrhage from right middle cerebral artery** HCC
- **6 I60.12 Nontraumatic subarachnoid hemorrhage from left middle cerebral artery** HCC

I60.2 Nontraumatic subarachnoid hemorrhage from anterior communicating artery HCC

5 I60.3 Nontraumatic subarachnoid hemorrhage from posterior communicating artery
- **6 I60.30 Nontraumatic subarachnoid hemorrhage from unspecified posterior communicating artery** HCC
- **6 I60.31 Nontraumatic subarachnoid hemorrhage from right posterior communicating artery** HCC
- **6 I60.32 Nontraumatic subarachnoid hemorrhage from left posterior communicating artery** HCC

I60.4 Nontraumatic subarachnoid hemorrhage from basilar artery HCC

5 I60.5 Nontraumatic subarachnoid hemorrhage from vertebral artery
- **6 I60.50 Nontraumatic subarachnoid hemorrhage from unspecified vertebral artery** HCC
- **6 I60.51 Nontraumatic subarachnoid hemorrhage from right vertebral artery** HCC
- **6 I60.52 Nontraumatic subarachnoid hemorrhage from left vertebral artery** HCC

I60.6 Nontraumatic subarachnoid hemorrhage from other intracranial arteries HCC

I60.7 Nontraumatic subarachnoid hemorrhage from unspecified intracranial artery HCC
Ruptured (congenital) berry aneurysm
Ruptured (congenital) cerebral aneurysm
Subarachnoid hemorrhage (nontraumatic) from cerebral artery NOS
Subarachnoid hemorrhage (nontraumatic) from communicating artery NOS
EXCLUDES 1 *berry aneurysm, nonruptured (I67.1)*

I60.8 Other nontraumatic subarachnoid hemorrhage HCC
Meningeal hemorrhage
Rupture of cerebral arteriovenous malformation

I60.9 Nontraumatic subarachnoid hemorrhage, unspecified HCC

4 I61 Nontraumatic intracerebral hemorrhage
EXCLUDES 2 *sequelae of intracerebral hemorrhage (I69.1-)*
AHA: 2Q 2017, 9
AHA: 2Q 2017, 10

I61.0 Nontraumatic intracerebral hemorrhage in hemisphere, subcortical HCC
Deep intracerebral hemorrhage (nontraumatic)

I61.1 Nontraumatic intracerebral hemorrhage in hemisphere, cortical HCC
Cerebral lobe hemorrhage (nontraumatic)
Superficial intracerebral hemorrhage (nontraumatic)

I61.2 Nontraumatic intracerebral hemorrhage in hemisphere, unspecified HCC

I61.3 Nontraumatic intracerebral hemorrhage in brain stem HCC

I61.4 Nontraumatic intracerebral hemorrhage in cerebellum HCC

I61.5 Nontraumatic intracerebral hemorrhage, intraventricular HCC

I61.6 Nontraumatic intracerebral hemorrhage, multiple localized HCC

I61.8 Other nontraumatic intracerebral hemorrhage HCC

I61.9 Nontraumatic intracerebral hemorrhage, unspecified HCC
AHA: 4Q 2012, 92

4 I62 Other and unspecified nontraumatic intracranial hemorrhage
EXCLUDES 2 *sequelae of intracranial hemorrhage (I69.2)*

5 I62.0 Nontraumatic subdural hemorrhage
- **I62.00 Nontraumatic subdural hemorrhage, unspecified** HCC
- **I62.01 Nontraumatic acute subdural hemorrhage** HCC
- **I62.02 Nontraumatic subacute subdural hemorrhage** HCC
- **I62.03 Nontraumatic chronic subdural hemorrhage** HCC

I62.1 Nontraumatic extradural hemorrhage HCC
Nontraumatic epidural hemorrhage

I62.9 Nontraumatic intracranial hemorrhage, unspecified HCC
AHA: 4Q 2012, 92

4 I63 Cerebral infarction
INCLUDES occlusion and stenosis of cerebral and precerebral arteries, resulting in cerebral infarction
Use additional code, if applicable, to identify status post administration of tPA (rtPA) in a different facility within the last 24 hours prior to admission to current facility (Z92.82)
Use additional code, if known, to indicate National Institutes of Health Stroke Scale (NIHSS) score (R29.7-)
EXCLUDES 2 *sequelae of cerebral infarction (I69.3-)*
AHA: 4Q 2012, 92
AHA: 4Q 2016, 28

5 I63.0 Cerebral infarction due to thrombosis of precerebral arteries
- **I63.00 Cerebral infarction due to thrombosis of unspecified precerebral artery** HCC
- **6 I63.01 Cerebral infarction due to thrombosis of vertebral artery**
  - **7 I63.011 Cerebral infarction due to thrombosis of right vertebral artery** HCC
  - **7 I63.012 Cerebral infarction due to thrombosis of left vertebral artery** HCC
  - **7 I63.013 Cerebral infarction due to thrombosis of bilateral vertebral arteries** HCC
  - **7 I63.019 Cerebral infarction due to thrombosis of unspecified vertebral artery** HCC
- **I63.02 Cerebral infarction due to thrombosis of basilar artery** HCC
- **6 I63.03 Cerebral infarction due to thrombosis of carotid artery**
  - **7 I63.031 Cerebral infarction due to thrombosis of right carotid artery** HCC
  - **7 I63.032 Cerebral infarction due to thrombosis of left carotid artery** HCC
  - **7 I63.033 Cerebral infarction due to thrombosis of bilateral carotid arteries** HCC
  - **7 I63.039 Cerebral infarction due to thrombosis of unspecified carotid artery** HCC
- **I63.09 Cerebral infarction due to thrombosis of other precerebral artery** HCC

5 I63.1 Cerebral infarction due to embolism of precerebral arteries
I63.10 Cerebral infarction due to embolism of unspecified precerebral artery HCC
6 I63.11 Cerebral infarction due to embolism of vertebral artery
I63.111 Cerebral infarction due to embolism of right vertebral artery HCC
I63.112 Cerebral infarction due to embolism of left vertebral artery HCC
I63.113 Cerebral infarction due to embolism of bilateral vertebral arteries HCC
I63.119 Cerebral infarction due to embolism of unspecified vertebral artery HCC
I63.12 Cerebral infarction due to embolism of basilar artery HCC
6 I63.13 Cerebral infarction due to embolism of carotid artery
I63.131 Cerebral infarction due to embolism of right carotid artery HCC
I63.132 Cerebral infarction due to embolism of left carotid artery HCC
I63.133 Cerebral infarction due to embolism of bilateral carotid arteries HCC
I63.139 Cerebral infarction due to embolism of unspecified carotid artery HCC
I63.19 Cerebral infarction due to embolism of other precerebral artery HCC
5 I63.2 Cerebral infarction due to unspecified occlusion or stenosis of precerebral arteries
I63.20 Cerebral infarction due to unspecified occlusion or stenosis of unspecified precerebral arteries HCC
6 I63.21 Cerebral infarction due to unspecified occlusion or stenosis of vertebral arteries
I63.211 Cerebral infarction due to unspecified occlusion or stenosis of right vertebral artery HCC
I63.212 Cerebral infarction due to unspecified occlusion or stenosis of left vertebral artery HCC
I63.213 Cerebral infarction due to unspecified occlusion or stenosis of bilateral vertebral arteries HCC
▲ I63.219 Cerebral infarction due to unspecified occlusion or stenosis of unspecified vertebral artery HCC
I63.22 Cerebral infarction due to unspecified occlusion or stenosis of basilar artery HCC
6 I63.23 Cerebral infarction due to unspecified occlusion or stenosis of carotid arteries
I63.231 Cerebral infarction due to unspecified occlusion or stenosis of right carotid arteries HCC
I63.232 Cerebral infarction due to unspecified occlusion or stenosis of left carotid arteries HCC
I63.233 Cerebral infarction due to unspecified occlusion or stenosis of bilateral carotid arteries HCC
▲ I63.239 Cerebral infarction due to unspecified occlusion or stenosis of unspecified carotid artery HCC
I63.29 Cerebral infarction due to unspecified occlusion or stenosis of other precerebral arteries HCC
5 I63.3 Cerebral infarction due to thrombosis of cerebral arteries
I63.30 Cerebral infarction due to thrombosis of unspecified cerebral artery HCC
6 I63.31 Cerebral infarction due to thrombosis of middle cerebral artery
I63.311 Cerebral infarction due to thrombosis of right middle cerebral artery HCC
I63.312 Cerebral infarction due to thrombosis of left middle cerebral artery HCC
I63.313 Cerebral infarction due to thrombosis of bilateral middle cerebral arteries HCC
I63.319 Cerebral infarction due to thrombosis of unspecified middle cerebral artery HCC
6 I63.32 Cerebral infarction due to thrombosis of anterior cerebral artery
I63.321 Cerebral infarction due to thrombosis of right anterior cerebral artery HCC
I63.322 Cerebral infarction due to thrombosis of left anterior cerebral artery HCC
I63.323 Cerebral infarction due to thrombosis of bilateral anterior cerebral arteries HCC
I63.329 Cerebral infarction due to thrombosis of unspecified anterior cerebral artery HCC
6 I63.33 Cerebral infarction due to thrombosis of posterior cerebral artery
I63.331 Cerebral infarction due to thrombosis of right posterior cerebral artery HCC
I63.332 Cerebral infarction due to thrombosis of left posterior cerebral artery HCC
▲ I63.333 Cerebral infarction due to thrombosis of bilateral posterior cerebral arteries HCC
I63.339 Cerebral infarction due to thrombosis of unspecified posterior cerebral artery HCC
6 I63.34 Cerebral infarction due to thrombosis of cerebellar artery
I63.341 Cerebral infarction due to thrombosis of right cerebellar artery HCC
I63.342 Cerebral infarction due to thrombosis of left cerebellar artery HCC
▲ I63.343 Cerebral infarction due to thrombosis of bilateral cerebellar arteries HCC
I63.349 Cerebral infarction due to thrombosis of unspecified cerebellar artery HCC
I63.39 Cerebral infarction due to thrombosis of other cerebral artery HCC
5 I63.4 Cerebral infarction due to embolism of cerebral arteries
I63.40 Cerebral infarction due to embolism of unspecified cerebral artery HCC
6 I63.41 Cerebral infarction due to embolism of middle cerebral artery
I63.411 Cerebral infarction due to embolism of right middle cerebral artery HCC
I63.412 Cerebral infarction due to embolism of left middle cerebral artery HCC
I63.413 Cerebral infarction due to embolism of bilateral middle cerebral arteries HCC
I63.419 Cerebral infarction due to embolism of unspecified middle cerebral artery HCC
6 I63.42 Cerebral infarction due to embolism of anterior cerebral artery
I63.421 Cerebral infarction due to embolism of right anterior cerebral artery HCC
I63.422 Cerebral infarction due to embolism of left anterior cerebral artery HCC
I63.423 Cerebral infarction due to embolism of bilateral anterior cerebral arteries HCC
I63.429 Cerebral infarction due to embolism of unspecified anterior cerebral artery HCC
6 I63.43 Cerebral infarction due to embolism of posterior cerebral artery
I63.431 Cerebral infarction due to embolism of right posterior cerebral artery HCC
I63.432 Cerebral infarction due to embolism of left posterior cerebral artery HCC
I63.433 Cerebral infarction due to embolism of bilateral posterior cerebral arteries HCC
I63.439 Cerebral infarction due to embolism of unspecified posterior cerebral artery HCC
6 I63.44 Cerebral infarction due to embolism of cerebellar artery
I63.441 Cerebral infarction due to embolism of right cerebellar artery HCC
I63.442 Cerebral infarction due to embolism of left cerebellar artery HCC
I63.443 Cerebral infarction due to embolism of bilateral cerebellar arteries HCC
I63.449 Cerebral infarction due to embolism of unspecified cerebellar artery HCC
I63.49 Cerebral infarction due to embolism of other cerebral artery HCC

5 I63.5 Cerebral infarction due to unspecified occlusion or stenosis of cerebral arteries

I63.50 Cerebral infarction due to unspecified occlusion or stenosis of unspecified cerebral artery HCC

6 I63.51 Cerebral infarction due to unspecified occlusion or stenosis of middle cerebral artery

I63.511 Cerebral infarction due to unspecified occlusion or stenosis of right middle cerebral artery HCC

I63.512 Cerebral infarction due to unspecified occlusion or stenosis of left middle cerebral artery HCC

I63.513 Cerebral infarction due to unspecified occlusion or stenosis of bilateral middle cerebral arteries HCC

I63.519 Cerebral infarction due to unspecified occlusion or stenosis of unspecified middle cerebral artery HCC

6 I63.52 Cerebral infarction due to unspecified occlusion or stenosis of anterior cerebral artery

I63.521 Cerebral infarction due to unspecified occlusion or stenosis of right anterior cerebral artery HCC

I63.522 Cerebral infarction due to unspecified occlusion or stenosis of left anterior cerebral artery HCC

I63.523 Cerebral infarction due to unspecified occlusion or stenosis of bilateral anterior cerebral arteries HCC

I63.529 Cerebral infarction due to unspecified occlusion or stenosis of unspecified anterior cerebral artery HCC

6 I63.53 Cerebral infarction due to unspecified occlusion or stenosis of posterior cerebral artery

I63.531 Cerebral infarction due to unspecified occlusion or stenosis of right posterior cerebral artery HCC

I63.532 Cerebral infarction due to unspecified occlusion or stenosis of left posterior cerebral artery HCC

AHA: 2Q 2017, 10

I63.533 Cerebral infarction due to unspecified occlusion or stenosis of bilateral posterior cerebral arteries HCC

I63.539 Cerebral infarction due to unspecified occlusion or stenosis of unspecified posterior cerebral artery HCC

6 I63.54 Cerebral infarction due to unspecified occlusion or stenosis of cerebellar artery

I63.541 Cerebral infarction due to unspecified occlusion or stenosis of right cerebellar artery HCC

I63.542 Cerebral infarction due to unspecified occlusion or stenosis of left cerebellar artery HCC

I63.543 Cerebral infarction due to unspecified occlusion or stenosis of bilateral cerebellar arteries HCC

I63.549 Cerebral infarction due to unspecified occlusion or stenosis of unspecified cerebellar artery HCC

I63.59 Cerebral infarction due to unspecified occlusion or stenosis of other cerebral artery HCC

I63.6 Cerebral infarction due to cerebral venous thrombosis, nonpyogenic HCC

▲ **5 I63.8 Other cerebral infarction** HCC

AHA: 2Q 2017, 9

● **I63.81 Other cerebral infarction due to occlusion or stenosis of small artery**

Lacunar infarction

● **I63.89 Other cerebral infarction**

I63.9 Cerebral infarction, unspecified HCC

Stroke NOS

EXCLUDES 2 *transient cerebral ischemic attacks and related syndromes (G45.-)*

AHA: 1Q 2015, 26

4 I65 Occlusion and stenosis of precerebral arteries, not resulting in cerebral infarction

INCLUDES embolism of precerebral artery
narrowing of precerebral artery
obstruction (complete) (partial) of precerebral artery
thrombosis of precerebral artery

EXCLUDES 1 *insufficiency, NOS, of precerebral artery (G45.-)*
insufficiency of precerebral arteries causing cerebral infarction (I63.0-I63.2)

CODING TIP✓ Codes from categories I65.- and I66.- are used to indicate stenosis and occlusion that do not result in infarction. Assign the most specific code as appropriate according to diagnostic statements provided by the physician. If the affected artery is not specified, do not assume a code for an affected location, but rather use an unspecified code. If more than one arterial location is affected and a specific code is available for separate locations, separate codes should be assigned.

AHA: 4Q 2012, 92

5 I65.0 Occlusion and stenosis of vertebral artery

I65.01 Occlusion and stenosis of right vertebral artery

I65.02 Occlusion and stenosis of left vertebral artery

I65.03 Occlusion and stenosis of bilateral vertebral arteries

I65.09 Occlusion and stenosis of unspecified vertebral artery

I65.1 Occlusion and stenosis of basilar artery

5 I65.2 Occlusion and stenosis of carotid artery

I65.21 Occlusion and stenosis of right carotid artery

I65.22 Occlusion and stenosis of left carotid artery

I65.23 Occlusion and stenosis of bilateral carotid arteries

AHA: 2Q 2018, 7

I65.29 Occlusion and stenosis of unspecified carotid artery

I65.8 Occlusion and stenosis of other precerebral arteries

I65.9 Occlusion and stenosis of unspecified precerebral artery

Occlusion and stenosis of precerebral artery NOS

4 I66 Occlusion and stenosis of cerebral arteries, not resulting in cerebral infarction

INCLUDES embolism of cerebral artery
narrowing of cerebral artery
obstruction (complete) (partial) of cerebral artery
thrombosis of cerebral artery

EXCLUDES 1 *Occlusion and stenosis of cerebral artery causing cerebral infarction (I63.3-I63.5)*

CODING TIP✓ Codes from categories I65.- and I66.- are used to indicate stenosis and occlusion that do not result in infarction. Assign the most specific code as appropriate according to diagnostic statements provided by the physician. If the affected artery is not specified, do not assume a code for an affected location, but rather use an unspecified code. If more than one arterial location is affected and a specific code is available for separate locations, separate codes should be assigned.

AHA: 4Q 2012, 92

5 I66.0 Occlusion and stenosis of middle cerebral artery

I66.01 Occlusion and stenosis of right middle cerebral artery

I66.02 Occlusion and stenosis of left middle cerebral artery

I66.03 Occlusion and stenosis of bilateral middle cerebral arteries

I66.09 Occlusion and stenosis of unspecified middle cerebral artery

5 I66.1 Occlusion and stenosis of anterior cerebral artery

I66.11 Occlusion and stenosis of right anterior cerebral artery

I66.12 Occlusion and stenosis of left anterior cerebral artery

I66.13 Occlusion and stenosis of bilateral anterior cerebral arteries

I66.19 Occlusion and stenosis of unspecified anterior cerebral artery

5 I66.2 Occlusion and stenosis of posterior cerebral artery

I66.21 Occlusion and stenosis of right posterior cerebral artery

I66.22 **Occlusion and stenosis of left posterior cerebral artery**

I66.23 **Occlusion and stenosis of bilateral posterior cerebral arteries**

I66.29 **Occlusion and stenosis of unspecified posterior cerebral artery**

I66.3 **Occlusion and stenosis of cerebellar arteries**

I66.8 **Occlusion and stenosis of other cerebral arteries**
Occlusion and stenosis of perforating arteries

I66.9 **Occlusion and stenosis of unspecified cerebral artery**

I67 Other cerebrovascular diseases

EXCLUDES 2 *sequelae of the listed conditions (I69.8)*

AHA: 4Q 2012, 92

I67.0 **Dissection of cerebral arteries, nonruptured** HCC
EXCLUDES 1 *ruptured cerebral arteries (I60.7)*

I67.1 **Cerebral aneurysm, nonruptured**
Cerebral aneurysm NOS
Cerebral arteriovenous fistula, acquired
Internal carotid artery aneurysm, intracranial portion
Internal carotid artery aneurysm, NOS
EXCLUDES 1 *congenital cerebral aneurysm, nonruptured (Q28.-)*
ruptured cerebral aneurysm (I60.7)

I67.2 **Cerebral atherosclerosis** A
Atheroma of cerebral and precerebral arteries

I67.3 **Progressive vascular leukoencephalopathy** HIV
Binswanger's disease

I67.4 **Hypertensive encephalopathy**
EXCLUDES 2 *insufficiency, NOS, of precerebral arteries (G45.2)*

I67.5 **Moyamoya disease**

I67.6 **Nonpyogenic thrombosis of intracranial venous system**
Nonpyogenic thrombosis of cerebral vein
Nonpyogenic thrombosis of intracranial venous sinus
EXCLUDES 1 *nonpyogenic thrombosis of intracranial venous system causing infarction (I63.6)*

I67.7 **Cerebral arteritis, not elsewhere classified**
Granulomatous angiitis of the nervous system
EXCLUDES 1 *allergic granulomatous angiitis (M30.1)*

DEFINITION Inflammation of an artery in the head.

I67.8 **Other specified cerebrovascular diseases**

I67.81 **Acute cerebrovascular insufficiency**
Acute cerebrovascular insufficiency unspecified as to location or reversibility

I67.82 **Cerebral ischemia**
Chronic cerebral ischemia

I67.83 **Posterior reversible encephalopathy syndrome** HIV
PRES

I67.84 **Cerebral vasospasm and vasoconstriction**

I67.841 **Reversible cerebrovascular vasoconstriction syndrome**
Call-Fleming syndrome
Code first:
underlying condition, if applicable, such as eclampsia (O15.00-O15.9)

I67.848 **Other cerebrovascular vasospasm and vasoconstriction**

● I67.85 **Hereditary cerebrovascular diseases**

● I67.850 **Cerebral autosomal dominant arteriopathy with subcortical infarcts and leukoencephalopathy**
CADASIL
Code also any associated diagnoses, such as:
epilepsy (G40.-)
stroke (I63.-)
vascular dementia (F01.-)

● I67.858 **Other hereditary cerebrovascular disease**

I67.89 **Other cerebrovascular disease**

I67.9 **Cerebrovascular disease, unspecified**

CODING TIP ✓ Do not assign I67.9 for sequelae of cerebral vascular accident. Do not assign I67.9 for cerebral atherosclerosis or any other known type of cerebral vascular disorder. If the type of cerebral vascular disease is not specified in the record, query the physician to attempt to obtain a more specific diagnosis.

I68 Cerebrovascular disorders in diseases classified elsewhere

I68.0 ***Cerebral amyloid angiopathy***
Code first:
underlying amyloidosis (E85.-)

I68.2 ***Cerebral arteritis in other diseases classified elsewhere***
Code first:
underlying disease
EXCLUDES 1 *cerebral arteritis (in) :*
listerosis (A32.89)
systemic lupus erythematosus (M32.19)
syphilis (A52.04)
tuberculosis (A18.89)

I68.8 ***Other cerebrovascular disorders in diseases classified elsewhere***
Code first:
underlying disease
EXCLUDES 1 *syphilitic cerebral aneurysm (A52.05)*

I69 Sequelae of cerebrovascular disease

Note: Category I69 is to be used to indicate conditions in I60-I67 as the cause of sequelae. The 'sequelae' include conditions specified as such or as residuals which may occur at any time after the onset of the causal condition

EXCLUDES 1 *personal history of cerebral infarction without residual deficit (Z86.73)*
personal history of prolonged reversible ischemic neurologic deficit (PRIND) (Z86.73)
personal history of reversible ischemic neurologcial deficit (RIND) (Z86.73)
sequelae of traumatic intracranial injury (S06.-)

GUIDELINES **Section I.C.9.d.1)**
Category I69 is used to indicate conditions classifiable to categories I60-I67 as the causes of sequela (neurologic deficits), themselves classified elsewhere. These "late effects" include neurologic deficits that persist after initial onset of conditions classifiable to categories I60-I67. The neurologic deficits caused by cerebrovascular disease may be present from the onset or may arise at any time after the onset or may arise at any time after the onset of the condition classifiable to categories I60-I67.

Codes from category I69, Sequelae of cerebrovascular disease, that specify hemiplegia, hemiparesis and monoplegia identify whether the dominant or nondominant side is affected. Should the affected side be documented, but not specified as dominant or nondominant, and the classification system does not indicate a default, code selection is as follows:
- For ambidextrous patients, the default should be dominant.
- If the left side is affected, the default is non-dominant.
- If the right side is affected, the default is dominant.

GUIDELINES **Section I.C.9.d.3)**
Codes from category I69 should not be assigned if the patient does not have neurologic deficits.
AHA: 4Q 2012, 92, 107
AHA: 4Q 2016, 28

I69.0 **Sequelae of nontraumatic subarachnoid hemorrhage**

CODING TIP ✓ Use subcategory I69.0, I69.1 or I69.2 for patients who have had a cerebrovascular accident (CVA) involving a bleed when residual neurological deficits are apparent. If there are no neurological deficits, use Z86.73 instead. The neurologic deficits caused by cerebrovascular disease may be present from the onset or may arise at any time after the onset of the condition. Some I69.- codes are combination codes that include the residual deficit within the code, e.g., I69.351. Others are combination codes that require additional information in the form of a secondary code to further specify the deficit, e.g., I69.391, which has an instructional note to use an additional code to identify the type of dysphagia, if known (R13.1-).

I69.00 **Unspecified sequelae of nontraumatic subarachnoid hemorrhage**

I69.01 **Cognitive deficits following nontraumatic subarachnoid hemorrhage**

I69.010 **Attention and concentration deficit following nontraumatic subarachnoid hemorrhage**

I69.011 **Memory deficit following nontraumatic subarachnoid hemorrhage**

I69.012 Visuospatial deficit and spatial neglect following nontraumatic subarachnoid hemorrhage

I69.013 Psychomotor deficit following nontraumatic subarachnoid hemorrhage

I69.014 Frontal lobe and executive function deficit following nontraumatic subarachnoid hemorrhage

I69.015 Cognitive social or emotional deficit following nontraumatic subarachnoid hemorrhage

I69.018 Other symptoms and signs involving cognitive functions following nontraumatic subarachnoid hemorrhage

I69.019 Unspecified symptoms and signs involving cognitive functions following nontraumatic subarachnoid hemorrhage

6 I69.02 Speech and language deficits following nontraumatic subarachnoid hemorrhage

I69.020 Aphasia following nontraumatic subarachnoid hemorrhage

I69.021 Dysphasia following nontraumatic subarachnoid hemorrhage

I69.022 Dysarthria following nontraumatic subarachnoid hemorrhage

I69.023 Fluency disorder following nontraumatic subarachnoid hemorrhage
Stuttering following nontraumatic subarachnoid hemorrhage

I69.028 Other speech and language deficits following nontraumatic subarachnoid hemorrhage

6 I69.03 Monoplegia of upper limb following nontraumatic subarachnoid hemorrhage
AHA: 4Q 2012, 105-106

Laterality I69.031 Monoplegia of upper limb following nontraumatic subarachnoid hemorrhage affecting right dominant side HCC

Laterality I69.032 Monoplegia of upper limb following nontraumatic subarachnoid hemorrhage affecting left dominant side HCC

Laterality I69.033 Monoplegia of upper limb following nontraumatic subarachnoid hemorrhage affecting right non-dominant side HCC

Laterality I69.034 Monoplegia of upper limb following nontraumatic subarachnoid hemorrhage affecting left non-dominant side HCC

Laterality I69.039 Monoplegia of upper limb following nontraumatic subarachnoid hemorrhage affecting unspecified side HCC

6 I69.04 Monoplegia of lower limb following nontraumatic subarachnoid hemorrhage
AHA: 4Q 2012, 105-106

Laterality I69.041 Monoplegia of lower limb following nontraumatic subarachnoid hemorrhage affecting right dominant side HCC

Laterality I69.042 Monoplegia of lower limb following nontraumatic subarachnoid hemorrhage affecting left dominant side HCC

Laterality I69.043 Monoplegia of lower limb following nontraumatic subarachnoid hemorrhage affecting right non-dominant side HCC

Laterality I69.044 Monoplegia of lower limb following nontraumatic subarachnoid hemorrhage affecting left non-dominant side HCC

Laterality I69.049 Monoplegia of lower limb following nontraumatic subarachnoid hemorrhage affecting unspecified side HCC

6 I69.05 Hemiplegia and hemiparesis following nontraumatic subarachnoid hemorrhage

Laterality I69.051 Hemiplegia and hemiparesis following nontraumatic subarachnoid hemorrhage affecting right dominant side HCC

Laterality I69.052 Hemiplegia and hemiparesis following nontraumatic subarachnoid hemorrhage affecting left dominant side HCC

Laterality I69.053 Hemiplegia and hemiparesis following nontraumatic subarachnoid hemorrhage affecting right non-dominant side HCC

Laterality I69.054 Hemiplegia and hemiparesis following nontraumatic subarachnoid hemorrhage affecting left non-dominant side HCC

Laterality I69.059 Hemiplegia and hemiparesis following nontraumatic subarachnoid hemorrhage affecting unspecified side HCC

6 I69.06 Other paralytic syndrome following nontraumatic subarachnoid hemorrhage
Use additional code to identify type of paralytic syndrome, such as:
locked-in state (G83.5)
quadriplegia (G82.5-)

EXCLUDES 1 *hemiplegia/hemiparesis following nontraumatic subarachnoid hemorrhage (I69.05-)*
monoplegia of lower limb following nontraumatic subarachnoid hemorrhage (I69.04-)
monoplegia of upper limb following nontraumatic subarachnoid hemorrhage (I69.03-)

Laterality I69.061 Other paralytic syndrome following nontraumatic subarachnoid hemorrhage affecting right dominant side HCC

Laterality I69.062 Other paralytic syndrome following nontraumatic subarachnoid hemorrhage affecting left dominant side HCC

Laterality I69.063 Other paralytic syndrome following nontraumatic subarachnoid hemorrhage affecting right non-dominant side HCC

Laterality I69.064 Other paralytic syndrome following nontraumatic subarachnoid hemorrhage affecting left non-dominant side HCC

Laterality I69.065 Other paralytic syndrome following nontraumatic subarachnoid hemorrhage, bilateral HCC

Laterality I69.069 Other paralytic syndrome following nontraumatic subarachnoid hemorrhage affecting unspecified side HCC

6 I69.09 Other sequelae of nontraumatic subarachnoid hemorrhage

I69.090 Apraxia following nontraumatic subarachnoid hemorrhage

I69.091 Dysphagia following nontraumatic subarachnoid hemorrhage
Use additional code to identify the type of dysphagia, if known (R13.1-)

I69.092 Facial weakness following nontraumatic subarachnoid hemorrhage
Facial droop following nontraumatic subarachnoid hemorrhage

I69.093 Ataxia following nontraumatic subarachnoid hemorrhage

I69.098 Other sequelae following nontraumatic subarachnoid hemorrhage
Alterations of sensation following nontraumatic subarachnoid hemorrhage
Disturbance of vision following nontraumatic subarachnoid hemorrhage
Use additional code to identify the sequelae

5 I69.1 Sequelae of nontraumatic intracerebral hemorrhage

CODING TIP ✓ Use subcategory I69.0, I69.1 or I69.2 for patients who have had a cerebrovascular accident (CVA) involving a bleed when residual neurological deficits are apparent. If there are no neurological deficits, use Z86.73 instead. The neurologic deficits caused by cerebrovascular disease may be present from the onset or may arise at any time after the onset of the condition. Some I69.- codes are combination codes that include the residual deficit within the code, e.g., I69.351. Others are combination codes that require additional information in the form of a secondary code to further specify the deficit, e.g., I69.391, which has an instructional note to use an additional code to identify the type of dysphagia, if known (R13.1-).

I69.10 Unspecified sequelae of nontraumatic intracerebral hemorrhage

6 I69.11 Cognitive deficits following nontraumatic intracerebral hemorrhage

I69.110 Attention and concentration deficit following nontraumatic intracerebral hemorrhage

I69.111 Memory deficit following nontraumatic intracerebral hemorrhage

I69.112 Visuospatial deficit and spatial neglect following nontraumatic intracerebral hemorrhage

I69.113 Psychomotor deficit following nontraumatic intracerebral hemorrhage

I69.114 Frontal lobe and executive function deficit following nontraumatic intracerebral hemorrhage

I69.115 Cognitive social or emotional deficit following nontraumatic intracerebral hemorrhage

I69.118 Other symptoms and signs involving cognitive functions following nontraumatic intracerebral hemorrhage

I69.119 Unspecified symptoms and signs involving cognitive functions following nontraumatic intracerebral hemorrhage

6 I69.12 Speech and language deficits following nontraumatic intracerebral hemorrhage

I69.120 Aphasia following nontraumatic intracerebral hemorrhage

I69.121 Dysphasia following nontraumatic intracerebral hemorrhage

I69.122 Dysarthria following nontraumatic intracerebral hemorrhage

I69.123 Fluency disorder following nontraumatic intracerebral hemorrhage
Stuttering following nontraumatic intracerebral hemorrhage

I69.128 Other speech and language deficits following nontraumatic intracerebral hemorrhage

6 I69.13 Monoplegia of upper limb following nontraumatic intracerebral hemorrhage
AHA: 4Q 2012, 105-106

I69.131 Monoplegia of upper limb following nontraumatic intracerebral hemorrhage affecting right dominant side HCC

I69.132 Monoplegia of upper limb following nontraumatic intracerebral hemorrhage affecting left dominant side HCC

I69.133 Monoplegia of upper limb following nontraumatic intracerebral hemorrhage affecting right non-dominant side HCC

I69.134 Monoplegia of upper limb following nontraumatic intracerebral hemorrhage affecting left non-dominant side HCC

I69.139 Monoplegia of upper limb following nontraumatic intracerebral hemorrhage affecting unspecified side HCC

6 I69.14 Monoplegia of lower limb following nontraumatic intracerebral hemorrhage
AHA: 4Q 2012, 105-106

I69.141 Monoplegia of lower limb following nontraumatic intracerebral hemorrhage affecting right dominant side HCC

I69.142 Monoplegia of lower limb following nontraumatic intracerebral hemorrhage affecting left dominant side HCC

I69.143 Monoplegia of lower limb following nontraumatic intracerebral hemorrhage affecting right non-dominant side HCC

I69.144 Monoplegia of lower limb following nontraumatic intracerebral hemorrhage affecting left non-dominant side HCC

I69.149 Monoplegia of lower limb following nontraumatic intracerebral hemorrhage affecting unspecified side HCC

6 I69.15 Hemiplegia and hemiparesis following nontraumatic intracerebral hemorrhage

I69.151 Hemiplegia and hemiparesis following nontraumatic intracerebral hemorrhage affecting right dominant side HCC

I69.152 Hemiplegia and hemiparesis following nontraumatic intracerebral hemorrhage affecting left dominant side HCC

I69.153 Hemiplegia and hemiparesis following nontraumatic intracerebral hemorrhage affecting right non-dominant side HCC

I69.154 Hemiplegia and hemiparesis following nontraumatic intracerebral hemorrhage affecting left non-dominant side HCC

I69.159 Hemiplegia and hemiparesis following nontraumatic intracerebral hemorrhage affecting unspecified side HCC

6 I69.16 Other paralytic syndrome following nontraumatic intracerebral hemorrhage
Use additional code to identify type of paralytic syndrome, such as:
locked-in state (G83.5)
quadriplegia (G82.5-)

EXCLUDES 1 *hemiplegia/hemiparesis following nontraumatic intracerebral hemorrhage (I69.15-)*
monoplegia of lower limb following nontraumatic intracerebral hemorrhage (I69.14-)
monoplegia of upper limb following nontraumatic intracerebral hemorrhage (I69.13-)

I69.161 Other paralytic syndrome following nontraumatic intracerebral hemorrhage affecting right dominant side HCC

I69.162 Other paralytic syndrome following nontraumatic intracerebral hemorrhage affecting left dominant side HCC

I69.163 Other paralytic syndrome following nontraumatic intracerebral hemorrhage affecting right non-dominant side HCC

I69.164 Other paralytic syndrome following nontraumatic intracerebral hemorrhage affecting left non-dominant side HCC

I69.165 Other paralytic syndrome following nontraumatic intracerebral hemorrhage, bilateral HCC

I69.169 Other paralytic syndrome following nontraumatic intracerebral hemorrhage affecting unspecified side HCC

6 I69.19 Other sequelae of nontraumatic intracerebral hemorrhage

I69.190 Apraxia following nontraumatic intracerebral hemorrhage

I69.191 Dysphagia following nontraumatic intracerebral hemorrhage
Use additional code to identify the type of dysphagia, if known (R13.1-)

I69.192 Facial weakness following nontraumatic intracerebral hemorrhage
Facial droop following nontraumatic intracerebral hemorrhage

I69.193 Ataxia following nontraumatic intracerebral hemorrhage

I69.198 Other sequelae of nontraumatic intracerebral hemorrhage
Alteration of sensations following nontraumatic intracerebral hemorrhage
Disturbance of vision following nontraumatic intracerebral hemorrhage
Use additional code to identify the sequelae

5 I69.2 Sequelae of other nontraumatic intracranial hemorrhage

CODING TIP ✓ Use subcategory I69.0, I69.1 or I69.2 for patients who have had a cerebrovascular accident (CVA) involving a bleed when residual neurological deficits are apparent. If there are no neurological deficits, use Z86.73 instead. The neurologic deficits caused by cerebrovascular disease may be present from the onset or may arise at any time after the onset of the condition. Some I69.- codes are combination codes that include the residual deficit within the code, e.g., I69.351. Others are combination codes that require additional information in the form of a secondary code to further specify the deficit, e.g., I69.391, which has an instructional note to use an additional code to identify the type of dysphagia, if known (R13.1-).

I69.20 Unspecified sequelae of other nontraumatic intracranial hemorrhage

6 I69.21 Cognitive deficits following other nontraumatic intracranial hemorrhage

I69.210 Attention and concentration deficit following other nontraumatic intracranial hemorrhage

I69.211 Memory deficit following other nontraumatic intracranial hemorrhage

I69.212 **Visuospatial deficit and spatial neglect following other nontraumatic intracranial hemorrhage**

I69.213 **Psychomotor deficit following other nontraumatic intracranial hemorrhage**

I69.214 **Frontal lobe and executive function deficit following other nontraumatic intracranial hemorrhage**

I69.215 **Cognitive social or emotional deficit following other nontraumatic intracranial hemorrhage**

I69.218 **Other symptoms and signs involving cognitive functions following other nontraumatic intracranial hemorrhage**

I69.219 **Unspecified symptoms and signs involving cognitive functions following other nontraumatic intracranial hemorrhage**

6 I69.22 **Speech and language deficits following other nontraumatic intracranial hemorrhage**

I69.220 **Aphasia following other nontraumatic intracranial hemorrhage**

I69.221 **Dysphasia following other nontraumatic intracranial hemorrhage**

I69.222 **Dysarthria following other nontraumatic intracranial hemorrhage**

I69.223 **Fluency disorder following other nontraumatic intracranial hemorrhage**
Stuttering following other nontraumatic intracranial hemorrhage

I69.228 **Other speech and language deficits following Other nontraumatic intracranial hemorrhage**

6 I69.23 **Monoplegia of upper limb following other nontraumatic intracranial hemorrhage**

I69.231 **Monoplegia of upper limb following other nontraumatic intracranial hemorrhage affecting right dominant side** HCC

I69.232 **Monoplegia of upper limb following other nontraumatic intracranial hemorrhage affecting left dominant side** HCC

I69.233 **Monoplegia of upper limb following other nontraumatic intracranial hemorrhage affecting right non-dominant side** HCC

I69.234 **Monoplegia of upper limb following other nontraumatic intracranial hemorrhage affecting left non-dominant side** HCC

I69.239 **Monoplegia of upper limb following other nontraumatic intracranial hemorrhage affecting unspecified side** HCC

6 I69.24 **Monoplegia of lower limb following other nontraumatic intracranial hemorrhage**

I69.241 **Monoplegia of lower limb following other nontraumatic intracranial hemorrhage affecting right dominant side** HCC

I69.242 **Monoplegia of lower limb following other nontraumatic intracranial hemorrhage affecting left dominant side** HCC

I69.243 **Monoplegia of lower limb following other nontraumatic intracranial hemorrhage affecting right non-dominant side** HCC

I69.244 **Monoplegia of lower limb following other nontraumatic intracranial hemorrhage affecting left non-dominant side** HCC

I69.249 **Monoplegia of lower limb following other nontraumatic intracranial hemorrhage affecting unspecified side** HCC

6 I69.25 **Hemiplegia and hemiparesis following other nontraumatic intracranial hemorrhage**

I69.251 **Hemiplegia and hemiparesis following other nontraumatic intracranial hemorrhage affecting right dominant side** HCC

I69.252 **Hemiplegia and hemiparesis following other nontraumatic intracranial hemorrhage affecting left dominant side** HCC

I69.253 **Hemiplegia and hemiparesis following other nontraumatic intracranial hemorrhage affecting right non-dominant side** HCC

I69.254 **Hemiplegia and hemiparesis following other nontraumatic intracranial hemorrhage affecting left non-dominant side** HCC

I69.259 **Hemiplegia and hemiparesis following other nontraumatic intracranial hemorrhage affecting unspecified side** HCC

6 I69.26 **Other paralytic syndrome following other nontraumatic intracranial hemorrhage**
Use additional code to identify type of paralytic syndrome, such as:
locked-in state (G83.5)
quadriplegia (G82.5-)

EXCLUDES 1 *hemiplegia/hemiparesis following other nontraumatic intracranial hemorrhage (I69.25-)*
monoplegia of lower limb following other nontraumatic intracranial hemorrhage (I69.24-)
monoplegia of upper limb following other nontraumatic intracranial hemorrhage (I69.23-)

I69.261 **Other paralytic syndrome following other nontraumatic intracranial hemorrhage affecting right dominant side** HCC

I69.262 **Other paralytic syndrome following other nontraumatic intracranial hemorrhage affecting left dominant side** HCC

I69.263 **Other paralytic syndrome following other nontraumatic intracranial hemorrhage affecting right non-dominant side** HCC

I69.264 **Other paralytic syndrome following other nontraumatic intracranial hemorrhage affecting left non-dominant side** HCC

I69.265 **Other paralytic syndrome following other nontraumatic intracranial hemorrhage, bilateral** HCC

I69.269 **Other paralytic syndrome following other nontraumatic intracranial hemorrhage affecting unspecified side** HCC

6 I69.29 **Other sequelae of Other nontraumatic intracranial hemorrhage**

I69.290 **Apraxia following other nontraumatic intracranial hemorrhage**

I69.291 **Dysphagia following other nontraumatic intracranial hemorrhage**
Use additional code to identify the type of dysphagia, if known (R13.1-)

I69.292 **Facial weakness following other nontraumatic intracranial hemorrhage**
Facial droop following other nontraumatic intracranial hemorrhage

I69.293 **Ataxia following other nontraumatic intracranial hemorrhage**

I69.298 **Other sequelae of other nontraumatic intracranial hemorrhage**
Alteration of sensation following other nontraumatic intracranial hemorrhage
Disturbance of vision following other nontraumatic intracranial hemorrhage
Use additional code to identify the sequelae

5 I69.3 **Sequelae of cerebral infarction**
Sequelae of stroke NOS
AHA: 4Q 2012, 92, 95
AHA: 4Q 2013, 127

I69.30 **Unspecified sequelae of cerebral infarction**

6 I69.31 **Cognitive deficits following cerebral infarction**

I69.310 **Attention and concentration deficit following cerebral infarction**

I69.311 **Memory deficit following cerebral infarction**

I69.312 **Visuospatial deficit and spatial neglect following cerebral infarction**

I69.313 **Psychomotor deficit following cerebral infarction**

I69.314 **Frontal lobe and executive function deficit following cerebral infarction**

I69.315 **Cognitive social or emotional deficit following cerebral infarction**

I69.318 **Other symptoms and signs involving cognitive functions following cerebral infarction**

I69.319 **Unspecified symptoms and signs involving cognitive functions following cerebral infarction**

6 I69.32 **Speech and language deficits following cerebral infarction**

I69.320 Aphasia following cerebral infarction
AHA: 4Q 2013, 128
I69.321 Dysphasia following cerebral infarction
AHA: 4Q 2012, 91-92, 95
I69.322 Dysarthria following cerebral infarction
EXCLUDES 2 *transient ischemic attack (TIA) (G45.9)*
I69.323 Fluency disorder following cerebral infarction
Stuttering following cerebral infarction
I69.328 Other speech and language deficits following cerebral infarction

6 I69.33 Monoplegia of upper limb following cerebral infarction
AHA: 1Q 2017, 47
I69.331 Monoplegia of upper limb following cerebral infarction affecting right dominant side HCC
I69.332 Monoplegia of upper limb following cerebral infarction affecting left dominant side HCC
I69.333 Monoplegia of upper limb following cerebral infarction affecting right non-dominant side HCC
I69.334 Monoplegia of upper limb following cerebral infarction affecting left non-dominant side HCC
I69.339 Monoplegia of upper limb following cerebral infarction affecting unspecified side HCC

6 I69.34 Monoplegia of lower limb following cerebral infarction
AHA: 1Q 2017, 47
I69.341 Monoplegia of lower limb following cerebral infarction affecting right dominant side HCC
I69.342 Monoplegia of lower limb following cerebral infarction affecting left dominant side HCC
I69.343 Monoplegia of lower limb following cerebral infarction affecting right non-dominant side HCC
I69.344 Monoplegia of lower limb following cerebral infarction affecting left non-dominant side HCC
I69.349 Monoplegia of lower limb following cerebral infarction affecting unspecified side HCC

6 I69.35 Hemiplegia and hemiparesis following cerebral infarction
I69.351 Hemiplegia and hemiparesis following cerebral infarction affecting right dominant side HCC
EXCLUDES 2 *transient ischemic attack (TIA) (G45.9)*
AHA: 4Q 2013, 128
AHA: 1Q 2015, 25
I69.352 Hemiplegia and hemiparesis following cerebral infarction affecting left dominant side HCC
I69.353 Hemiplegia and hemiparesis following cerebral infarction affecting right non-dominant side HCC
I69.354 Hemiplegia and hemiparesis following cerebral infarction affecting left non-dominant side HCC
AHA: 4Q 2012, 91-92, 95
I69.359 Hemiplegia and hemiparesis following cerebral infarction affecting unspecified side HCC

6 I69.36 Other paralytic syndrome following cerebral infarction
Use additional code to identify type of paralytic syndrome, such as:
locked-in state (G83.5)
quadriplegia (G82.5-)
EXCLUDES 1 *hemiplegia/hemiparesis following cerebral infarction (I69.35-)*
monoplegia of lower limb following cerebral infarction (I69.34-)
monoplegia of upper limb following cerebral infarction (I69.33-)
I69.361 Other paralytic syndrome following cerebral infarction affecting right dominant side HCC
I69.362 Other paralytic syndrome following cerebral infarction affecting left dominant side HCC
I69.363 Other paralytic syndrome following cerebral infarction affecting right non-dominant side HCC
I69.364 Other paralytic syndrome following cerebral infarction affecting left non-dominant side HCC
I69.365 Other paralytic syndrome following cerebral infarction, bilateral HCC
I69.369 Other paralytic syndrome following cerebral infarction affecting unspecified side HCC

6 I69.39 Other sequelae of cerebral infarction
I69.390 Apraxia following cerebral infarction
I69.391 Dysphagia following cerebral infarction
Use additional code to identify the type of dysphagia, if known (R13.1-)
I69.392 Facial weakness following cerebral infarction
Facial droop following cerebral infarction
I69.393 Ataxia following cerebral infarction
I69.398 Other sequelae of cerebral infarction
Alteration of sensation following cerebral infarction
Disturbance of vision following cerebral infarction
Use additional code to identify the sequelae

5 I69.8 Sequelae of other cerebrovascular diseases
EXCLUDES 1 *sequelae of traumatic intracranial injury (S06.-)*
I69.80 Unspecified sequelae of other cerebrovascular disease

6 I69.81 Cognitive deficits following other cerebrovascular disease
I69.810 Attention and concentration deficit following other cerebrovascular disease
I69.811 Memory deficit following other cerebrovascular disease
I69.812 Visuospatial deficit and spatial neglect following other cerebrovascular disease
I69.813 Psychomotor deficit following other cerebrovascular disease
I69.814 Frontal lobe and executive function deficit following other cerebrovascular disease
I69.815 Cognitive social or emotional deficit following other cerebrovascular disease
I69.818 Other symptoms and signs involving cognitive functions following other cerebrovascular disease
I69.819 Unspecified symptoms and signs involving cognitive functions following other cerebrovascular disease

6 I69.82 Speech and language deficits following other cerebrovascular disease
I69.820 Aphasia following other cerebrovascular disease
I69.821 Dysphasia following other cerebrovascular disease
I69.822 Dysarthria following other cerebrovascular disease
I69.823 Fluency disorder following other cerebrovascular disease
Stuttering following other cerebrovascular disease
I69.828 Other speech and language deficits following Other cerebrovascular disease

6 I69.83 Monoplegia of upper limb following other cerebrovascular disease
I69.831 Monoplegia of upper limb following other cerebrovascular disease affecting right dominant side HCC
I69.832 Monoplegia of upper limb following other cerebrovascular disease affecting left dominant side HCC
I69.833 Monoplegia of upper limb following other cerebrovascular disease affecting right non-dominant side HCC

I69.834 Monoplegia of upper limb following other cerebrovascular disease affecting left non-dominant side HCC

I69.839 Monoplegia of upper limb following other cerebrovascular disease affecting unspecified side HCC

I69.84 Monoplegia of lower limb following other cerebrovascular disease

I69.841 Monoplegia of lower limb following other cerebrovascular disease affecting right dominant side HCC

I69.842 Monoplegia of lower limb following other cerebrovascular disease affecting left dominant side HCC

I69.843 Monoplegia of lower limb following other cerebrovascular disease affecting right non-dominant side HCC

I69.844 Monoplegia of lower limb following other cerebrovascular disease affecting left non-dominant side HCC

I69.849 Monoplegia of lower limb following other cerebrovascular disease affecting unspecified side HCC

I69.85 Hemiplegia and hemiparesis following other cerebrovascular disease

I69.851 Hemiplegia and hemiparesis following other cerebrovascular disease affecting right dominant side HCC

I69.852 Hemiplegia and hemiparesis following other cerebrovascular disease affecting left dominant side HCC

I69.853 Hemiplegia and hemiparesis following other cerebrovascular disease affecting right non-dominant side HCC

I69.854 Hemiplegia and hemiparesis following other cerebrovascular disease affecting left non-dominant side HCC

I69.859 Hemiplegia and hemiparesis following other cerebrovascular disease affecting unspecified side HCC

I69.86 Other paralytic syndrome following other cerebrovascular disease

Use additional code to identify type of paralytic syndrome, such as:
locked-in state (G83.5)
quadriplegia (G82.5-)

EXCLUDES 1 *hemiplegia/hemiparesis following other cerebrovascular disease (I69.85-)*
monoplegia of lower limb following other cerebrovascular disease (I69.84-)
monoplegia of upper limb following other cerebrovascular disease (I69.83-)

I69.861 Other paralytic syndrome following other cerebrovascular disease affecting right dominant side HCC

I69.862 Other paralytic syndrome following other cerebrovascular disease affecting left dominant side HCC

I69.863 Other paralytic syndrome following other cerebrovascular disease affecting right non-dominant side HCC

I69.864 Other paralytic syndrome following other cerebrovascular disease affecting left non-dominant side HCC

I69.865 Other paralytic syndrome following other cerebrovascular disease, bilateral HCC

I69.869 Other paralytic syndrome following other cerebrovascular disease affecting unspecified side HCC

I69.89 Other sequelae of other cerebrovascular disease

I69.890 Apraxia following other cerebrovascular disease

I69.891 Dysphagia following other cerebrovascular disease

Use additional code to identify the type of dysphagia, if known (R13.1-)

I69.892 Facial weakness following other cerebrovascular disease

Facial droop following other cerebrovascular disease

I69.893 Ataxia following other cerebrovascular disease

I69.898 Other sequelae of other cerebrovascular disease

Alteration of sensation following other cerebrovascular disease
Disturbance of vision following other cerebrovascular disease
Use additional code to identify the sequelae

I69.9 Sequelae of unspecified cerebrovascular diseases

EXCLUDES 1 *sequelae of stroke (I69.3)*
sequelae of traumatic intracranial injury (S06.-)

I69.90 Unspecified sequelae of unspecified cerebrovascular disease

I69.91 Cognitive deficits following unspecified cerebrovascular disease

I69.910 Attention and concentration deficit following unspecified cerebrovascular disease

I69.911 Memory deficit following unspecified cerebrovascular disease

I69.912 Visuospatial deficit and spatial neglect following unspecified cerebrovascular disease

I69.913 Psychomotor deficit following unspecified cerebrovascular disease

I69.914 Frontal lobe and executive function deficit following unspecified cerebrovascular disease

I69.915 Cognitive social or emotional deficit following unspecified cerebrovascular disease

I69.918 Other symptoms and signs involving cognitive functions following unspecified cerebrovascular disease

I69.919 Unspecified symptoms and signs involving cognitive functions following unspecified cerebrovascular disease

I69.92 Speech and language deficits following unspecified cerebrovascular disease

I69.920 Aphasia following unspecified cerebrovascular disease

DEFINITION Impaired or complete loss of the ability to communicate with language or symbols resulting from brain damage.

I69.921 Dysphasia following unspecified cerebrovascular disease

DEFINITION Impairment in the ability to speak or understand words resulting from brain damage.

I69.922 Dysarthria following unspecified cerebrovascular disease

I69.923 Fluency disorder following unspecified cerebrovascular disease

Stuttering following unspecified cerebrovascular disease

I69.928 Other speech and language deficits following unspecified cerebrovascular disease

I69.93 Monoplegia of upper limb following unspecified cerebrovascular disease

I69.931 Monoplegia of upper limb following unspecified cerebrovascular disease affecting right dominant side HCC

I69.932 Monoplegia of upper limb following unspecified cerebrovascular disease affecting left dominant side HCC

I69.933 Monoplegia of upper limb following unspecified cerebrovascular disease affecting right non-dominant side HCC

I69.934 Monoplegia of upper limb following unspecified cerebrovascular disease affecting left non-dominant side HCC

I69.939 Monoplegia of upper limb following unspecified cerebrovascular disease affecting unspecified side HCC

I69.94 Monoplegia of lower limb following unspecified cerebrovascular disease

⊟ **I69.941** **Monoplegia of lower limb following unspecified cerebrovascular disease affecting right dominant side** HCC

⊟ **I69.942** **Monoplegia of lower limb following unspecified cerebrovascular disease affecting left dominant side** HCC

⊟ **I69.943** **Monoplegia of lower limb following unspecified cerebrovascular disease affecting right non-dominant side** HCC

⊟ **I69.944** **Monoplegia of lower limb following unspecified cerebrovascular disease affecting left non-dominant side** HCC

⊟ **I69.949** **Monoplegia of lower limb following unspecified cerebrovascular disease affecting unspecified side** HCC

6 **I69.95** **Hemiplegia and hemiparesis following unspecified cerebrovascular disease**

DEFINITION Paralysis affecting one side of the body.

⊟ **I69.951** **Hemiplegia and hemiparesis following unspecified cerebrovascular disease affecting right dominant side** HCC

⊟ **I69.952** **Hemiplegia and hemiparesis following unspecified cerebrovascular disease affecting left dominant side** HCC

⊟ **I69.953** **Hemiplegia and hemiparesis following unspecified cerebrovascular disease affecting right non-dominant side** HCC

⊟ **I69.954** **Hemiplegia and hemiparesis following unspecified cerebrovascular disease affecting left non-dominant side** HCC

⊟ **I69.959** **Hemiplegia and hemiparesis following unspecified cerebrovascular disease affecting unspecified side** HCC

6 **I69.96** **Other paralytic syndrome following unspecified cerebrovascular disease**

Use additional code to identify type of paralytic syndrome, such as:
locked-in state (G83.5)
quadriplegia (G82.5-)

EXCLUDES 1 *hemiplegia/hemiparesis following unspecified cerebrovascular disease (I69.95-)*
monoplegia of lower limb following unspecified cerebrovascular disease (I69.94-)
monoplegia of upper limb following unspecified cerebrovascular disease (I69.93-)

⊟ **I69.961** **Other paralytic syndrome following unspecified cerebrovascular disease affecting right dominant side** HCC

⊟ **I69.962** **Other paralytic syndrome following unspecified cerebrovascular disease affecting left dominant side** HCC

⊟ **I69.963** **Other paralytic syndrome following unspecified cerebrovascular disease affecting right non-dominant side** HCC

⊟ **I69.964** **Other paralytic syndrome following unspecified cerebrovascular disease affecting left non-dominant side** HCC

⊟ **I69.965** **Other paralytic syndrome following unspecified cerebrovascular disease, bilateral** HCC

⊟ **I69.969** **Other paralytic syndrome following unspecified cerebrovascular disease affecting unspecified side** HCC

6 **I69.99** **Other sequelae of unspecified cerebrovascular disease**

I69.990 **Apraxia following unspecified cerebrovascular disease**

I69.991 **Dysphagia following unspecified cerebrovascular disease**

Use additional code to identify the type of dysphagia, if known (R13.1-)

I69.992 **Facial weakness following unspecified cerebrovascular disease**

Facial droop following unspecified cerebrovascular disease

I69.993 **Ataxia following unspecified cerebrovascular disease**

DEFINITION Inability to coordinate muscle movement.

I69.998 **Other sequelae following unspecified cerebrovascular disease**

Alteration in sensation following unspecified cerebrovascular disease
Disturbance of vision following unspecified cerebrovascular disease
Use additional code to identify the sequelae

Diseases of arteries, arterioles and capillaries (I70-I79)

4 **I70** **Atherosclerosis**

INCLUDES arteriolosclerosis
arterial degeneration
arteriosclerosis
arteriosclerotic vascular disease
arteriovascular degeneration
atheroma
endarteritis deformans or obliterans
senile arteritis
senile endarteritis
vascular degeneration

Use additional code to identify:
exposure to environmental tobacco smoke (Z77.22)
history of tobacco dependence (Z87.891)
occupational exposure to environmental tobacco smoke (Z57.31)
tobacco dependence (F17.-)
tobacco use (Z72.0)

EXCLUDES 2 *arteriosclerotic cardiovascular disease (I25.1-)*
arteriosclerotic heart disease (I25.1-)
atheroembolism (I75.-)
cerebral atherosclerosis (I67.2)
coronary atherosclerosis (I25.1-)
mesenteric atherosclerosis (K55.1)
precerebral atherosclerosis (I67.2)
primary pulmonary atherosclerosis (I27.0)

I70.0 **Atherosclerosis of aorta** A HCC

DEFINITION Fatty plaque deposits in the aorta that reduce its diameter and elasticity.

I70.1 **Atherosclerosis of renal artery** A HCC

Goldblatt's kidney

EXCLUDES 2 *atherosclerosis of renal arterioles (I12.-)*

CODING TIP ✓ Atherosclerosis of renal artery may also be reported as renal artery stenosis. When renal artery stenosis is reported as causative of hypertension, an additional code of I15.0, Renovascular hypertension, should be reported.

5 **I70.2** **Atherosclerosis of native arteries of the extremities**

Mönckeberg's (medial) sclerosis
Use additional code, if applicable, to identify chronic total occlusion of artery of extremity (I70.92)

EXCLUDES 2 *atherosclerosis of bypass graft of extremities (I70.30-I70.79)*

6 **I70.20** **Unspecified atherosclerosis of native arteries of extremities**

⊟ **I70.201** **Unspecified atherosclerosis of native arteries of extremities, right leg** A HCC

⊟ **I70.202** **Unspecified atherosclerosis of native arteries of extremities, left leg** A HCC

⊟ **I70.203** **Unspecified atherosclerosis of native arteries of extremities, bilateral legs** A HCC

⊟ **I70.208** **Unspecified atherosclerosis of native arteries of extremities, other extremity** A HCC

⊟ **I70.209** **Unspecified atherosclerosis of native arteries of extremities, unspecified extremity** A HCC

6 **I70.21** **Atherosclerosis of native arteries of extremities with intermittent claudication**

- I70.211 Atherosclerosis of native arteries of extremities with intermittent claudication, right leg A HCC
- I70.212 Atherosclerosis of native arteries of extremities with intermittent claudication, left leg A HCC
- I70.213 Atherosclerosis of native arteries of extremities with intermittent claudication, bilateral legs A HCC
- I70.218 Atherosclerosis of native arteries of extremities with intermittent claudication, other extremity A HCC
- I70.219 Atherosclerosis of native arteries of extremities with intermittent claudication, unspecified extremity A HCC

6 I70.22 Atherosclerosis of native arteries of extremities with rest pain

INCLUDES any condition classifiable to I70.21-

- I70.221 Atherosclerosis of native arteries of extremities with rest pain, right leg A HCC
- I70.222 Atherosclerosis of native arteries of extremities with rest pain, left leg A HCC
- I70.223 Atherosclerosis of native arteries of extremities with rest pain, bilateral legs A HCC
- I70.228 Atherosclerosis of native arteries of extremities with rest pain, other extremity A HCC
- I70.229 Atherosclerosis of native arteries of extremities with rest pain, unspecified extremity A HCC

6 I70.23 Atherosclerosis of native arteries of right leg with ulceration

INCLUDES any condition classifiable to I70.211 and I70.221

Use additional code to identify severity of ulcer (L97.-)

CODING TIP✓ When bilateral ulcers are present or ulcers of multiple specified areas classifiable in a patient with atherosclerosis of the extremities, assign a code for each specific site, taking laterality into account. A second code from category L97.- or L98.49- to specify the severity of the ulcer must be used following each reported site of atherosclerosis to the extremity with ulceration.

- I70.231 Atherosclerosis of native arteries of right leg with ulceration of thigh A HCC
- I70.232 Atherosclerosis of native arteries of right leg with ulceration of calf A HCC
- I70.233 Atherosclerosis of native arteries of right leg with ulceration of ankle A HCC
- I70.234 Atherosclerosis of native arteries of right leg with ulceration of heel and midfoot A HCC
  Atherosclerosis of native arteries of right leg with ulceration of plantar surface of midfoot
- I70.235 Atherosclerosis of native arteries of right leg with ulceration of other part of foot A HCC
  Atherosclerosis of native arteries of right leg extremities with ulceration of toe
- I70.238 Atherosclerosis of native arteries of right leg with ulceration of other part of lower right leg A HCC
- I70.239 Atherosclerosis of native arteries of right leg with ulceration of unspecified site A HCC

6 I70.24 Atherosclerosis of native arteries of left leg with ulceration

INCLUDES any condition classifiable to I70.212 and I70.222

Use additional code to identify severity of ulcer (L97.-)

CODING TIP✓ When bilateral ulcers are present or ulcers of multiple specified areas classifiable in a patient with atherosclerosis of the extremities, assign a code for each specific site, taking laterality into account. A second code from category L97.- or L98.49- to specify the severity of the ulcer must be used following each reported site of atherosclerosis to the extremity with ulceration.

- I70.241 Atherosclerosis of native arteries of left leg with ulceration of thigh A HCC
- I70.242 Atherosclerosis of native arteries of left leg with ulceration of calf A HCC
- I70.243 Atherosclerosis of native arteries of left leg with ulceration of ankle A HCC
- I70.244 Atherosclerosis of native arteries of left leg with ulceration of heel and midfoot A HCC
  Atherosclerosis of native arteries of left leg with ulceration of plantar surface of midfoot
- I70.245 Atherosclerosis of native arteries of left leg with ulceration of other part of foot A HCC
  Atherosclerosis of native arteries of left leg extremities with ulceration of toe
- I70.248 Atherosclerosis of native arteries of left leg with ulceration of other part of lower left leg A HCC
- I70.249 Atherosclerosis of native arteries of left leg with ulceration of unspecified site A HCC

I70.25 Atherosclerosis of native arteries of other extremities with ulceration A HCC

INCLUDES any condition classifiable to I70.218 and I70.228

Use additional code to identify the severity of the ulcer (L98.49-)

CODING TIP✓ When bilateral ulcers are present or ulcers of multiple specified areas classifiable in a patient with atherosclerosis of the extremities, assign a code for each specific site, taking laterality into account. A second code from category L97.- or L98.49- to specify the severity of the ulcer must be used following each reported site of atherosclerosis to the extremity with ulceration.

6 I70.26 Atherosclerosis of native arteries of extremities with gangrene

INCLUDES any condition classifiable to I70.21-, I70.22-, I70.23-, I70.24-, and I70.25-

Use additional code to identify the severity of any ulcer (L97.-, L98.49-), if applicable

CODING TIP✓ When the clinical record reports atherosclerosis of the lower extremities with ulceration and gangrene, assign a code from I70.26-. Do not code the gangrene separately. An additional code from category L97.- should be assigned to report the severity of any ulceration.

- I70.261 Atherosclerosis of native arteries of extremities with gangrene, right leg A HCC
- I70.262 Atherosclerosis of native arteries of extremities with gangrene, left leg A HCC
- I70.263 Atherosclerosis of native arteries of extremities with gangrene, bilateral legs A HCC
- I70.268 Atherosclerosis of native arteries of extremities with gangrene, other extremity A HCC
- I70.269 Atherosclerosis of native arteries of extremities with gangrene, unspecified extremity A HCC

6 I70.29 Other atherosclerosis of native arteries of extremities

- I70.291 Other atherosclerosis of native arteries of extremities, right leg A HCC
- I70.292 Other atherosclerosis of native arteries of extremities, left leg A HCC
- I70.293 Other atherosclerosis of native arteries of extremities, bilateral legs A HCC
- I70.298 Other atherosclerosis of native arteries of extremities, other extremity A HCC
- I70.299 Other atherosclerosis of native arteries of extremities, unspecified extremity A HCC

5 I70.3 Atherosclerosis of unspecified type of bypass graft(s) of the extremities

Use additional code, if applicable, to identify chronic total occlusion of artery of extremity (I70.92)

EXCLUDES 1 *embolism or thrombus of bypass graft (s) of extremities (T82.8-)*

6 I70.30 Unspecified atherosclerosis of Unspecified type of bypass graft(s) of the extremities

I70.301 Unspecified atherosclerosis of unspecified type of bypass graft(s) of the extremities, right leg A HCC

I70.302 Unspecified atherosclerosis of unspecified type of bypass graft(s) of the extremities, left leg A HCC

I70.303 Unspecified atherosclerosis of unspecified type of bypass graft(s) of the extremities, bilateral legs A HCC

I70.308 Unspecified atherosclerosis of unspecified type of bypass graft(s) of the extremities, other extremity A HCC

I70.309 Unspecified atherosclerosis of unspecified type of bypass graft(s) of the extremities, unspecified extremity A HCC

I70.31 Atherosclerosis of unspecified type of bypass graft(s) of the extremities with intermittent claudication

I70.311 Atherosclerosis of unspecified type of bypass graft(s) of the extremities with intermittent claudication, right leg A HCC

I70.312 Atherosclerosis of unspecified type of bypass graft(s) of the extremities with intermittent claudication, left leg A HCC

I70.313 Atherosclerosis of unspecified type of bypass graft(s) of the extremities with intermittent claudication, bilateral legs A HCC

I70.318 Atherosclerosis of unspecified type of bypass graft(s) of the extremities with intermittent claudication, other extremity A HCC

I70.319 Atherosclerosis of unspecified type of bypass graft(s) of the extremities with intermittent claudication, unspecified extremity A HCC

I70.32 Atherosclerosis of unspecified type of bypass graft(s) of the extremities with rest pain

INCLUDES any condition classifiable to I70.31-

I70.321 Atherosclerosis of unspecified type of bypass graft(s) of the extremities with rest pain, right leg A HCC

I70.322 Atherosclerosis of unspecified type of bypass graft(s) of the extremities with rest pain, left leg A HCC

I70.323 Atherosclerosis of unspecified type of bypass graft(s) of the extremities with rest pain, bilateral legs A HCC

I70.328 Atherosclerosis of unspecified type of bypass graft(s) of the extremities with rest pain, other extremity A HCC

I70.329 Atherosclerosis of unspecified type of bypass graft(s) of the extremities with rest pain, unspecified extremity A HCC

I70.33 Atherosclerosis of unspecified type of bypass graft(s) of the right leg with ulceration

INCLUDES any condition classifiable to I70.311 and I70.321

Use additional code to identify severity of ulcer (L97.-)

I70.331 Atherosclerosis of unspecified type of bypass graft(s) of the right leg with ulceration of thigh A HCC

I70.332 Atherosclerosis of unspecified type of bypass graft(s) of the right leg with ulceration of calf A HCC

I70.333 Atherosclerosis of unspecified type of bypass graft(s) of the right leg with ulceration of ankle A HCC

I70.334 Atherosclerosis of unspecified type of bypass graft(s) of the right leg with ulceration of heel and midfoot A HCC

Atherosclerosis of unspecified type of bypass graft(s) of right leg with ulceration of plantar surface of midfoot

I70.335 Atherosclerosis of unspecified type of bypass graft(s) of the right leg with ulceration of other part of foot A HCC

Atherosclerosis of unspecified type of bypass graft(s) of the right leg with ulceration of toe

I70.338 Atherosclerosis of unspecified type of bypass graft(s) of the right leg with ulceration of other part of lower leg A HCC

I70.339 Atherosclerosis of unspecified type of bypass graft(s) of the right leg with ulceration of unspecified site A HCC

I70.34 Atherosclerosis of unspecified type of bypass graft(s) of the left leg with ulceration

INCLUDES any condition classifiable to I70.312 and I70.322

Use additional code to identify severity of ulcer (L97.-)

I70.341 Atherosclerosis of unspecified type of bypass graft(s) of the left leg with ulceration of thigh A HCC

I70.342 Atherosclerosis of unspecified type of bypass graft(s) of the left leg with ulceration of calf A HCC

I70.343 Atherosclerosis of unspecified type of bypass graft(s) of the left leg with ulceration of ankle A HCC

I70.344 Atherosclerosis of unspecified type of bypass graft(s) of the left leg with ulceration of heel and midfoot A HCC

Atherosclerosis of unspecified type of bypass graft(s) of left leg with ulceration of plantar surface of midfoot

I70.345 Atherosclerosis of unspecified type of bypass graft(s) of the left leg with ulceration of other part of foot A HCC

Atherosclerosis of unspecified type of bypass graft(s) of the left leg with ulceration of toe

I70.348 Atherosclerosis of unspecified type of bypass graft(s) of the left leg with ulceration of other part of lower leg A HCC

I70.349 Atherosclerosis of unspecified type of bypass graft(s) of the left leg with ulceration of unspecified site A HCC

I70.35 Atherosclerosis of unspecified type of bypass graft(s) of other extremity with ulceration A HCC

INCLUDES any condition classifiable to I70.318 and I70.328

Use additional code to identify severity of ulcer (L98.49-)

I70.36 Atherosclerosis of unspecified type of bypass graft(s) of the extremities with gangrene

INCLUDES any condition classifiable to I70.31-, I70.32-, I70.33-, I70.34-, I70.35

Use additional code to identify the severity of any ulcer (L97.-, L98.49-), if applicable

I70.361 Atherosclerosis of unspecified type of bypass graft(s) of the extremities with gangrene, right leg A HCC

I70.362 Atherosclerosis of unspecified type of bypass graft(s) of the extremities with gangrene, left leg A HCC

I70.363 Atherosclerosis of unspecified type of bypass graft(s) of the extremities with gangrene, bilateral legs A HCC

I70.368 Atherosclerosis of unspecified type of bypass graft(s) of the extremities with gangrene, other extremity A HCC

I70.369 Atherosclerosis of unspecified type of bypass graft(s) of the extremities with gangrene, unspecified extremity A HCC

I70.39 Other atherosclerosis of unspecified type of bypass graft(s) of the extremities

I70.391 Other atherosclerosis of unspecified type of bypass graft(s) of the extremities, right leg A HCC

I70.392 Other atherosclerosis of unspecified type of bypass graft(s) of the extremities, left leg A HCC

I70.393 Other atherosclerosis of unspecified type of bypass graft(s) of the extremities, bilateral legs A HCC

I70.398 Other atherosclerosis of unspecified type of bypass graft(s) of the extremities, other extremity A HCC

I70.399 Other atherosclerosis of unspecified type of bypass graft(s) of the extremities, unspecified extremity A HCC

I70.4 Atherosclerosis of autologous vein bypass graft(s) of the extremities

Use additional code, if applicable, to identify chronic total occlusion of artery of extremity (I70.92)

I70.40 Unspecified atherosclerosis of autologous vein bypass graft(s) of the extremities

I70.401 Unspecified atherosclerosis of autologous vein bypass graft(s) of the extremities, right leg A HCC

I70.402 Unspecified atherosclerosis of autologous vein bypass graft(s) of the extremities, left leg A HCC

I70.403 Unspecified atherosclerosis of autologous vein bypass graft(s) of the extremities, bilateral legs A HCC

I70.408 Unspecified atherosclerosis of autologous vein bypass graft(s) of the extremities, other extremity A HCC

I70.409 Unspecified atherosclerosis of autologous vein bypass graft(s) of the extremities, unspecified extremity A HCC

I70.41 Atherosclerosis of autologous vein bypass graft(s) of the extremities with intermittent claudication

I70.411 Atherosclerosis of autologous vein bypass graft(s) of the extremities with intermittent claudication, right leg A HCC

I70.412 Atherosclerosis of autologous vein bypass graft(s) of the extremities with intermittent claudication, left leg A HCC

I70.413 Atherosclerosis of autologous vein bypass graft(s) of the extremities with intermittent claudication, bilateral legs A HCC

I70.418 Atherosclerosis of autologous vein bypass graft(s) of the extremities with intermittent claudication, other extremity A HCC

I70.419 Atherosclerosis of autologous vein bypass graft(s) of the extremities with intermittent claudication, unspecified extremity A HCC

I70.42 Atherosclerosis of autologous vein bypass graft(s) of the extremities with rest pain

INCLUDES any condition classifiable to I70.41-

I70.421 Atherosclerosis of autologous vein bypass graft(s) of the extremities with rest pain, right leg A HCC

I70.422 Atherosclerosis of autologous vein bypass graft(s) of the extremities with rest pain, left leg A HCC

I70.423 Atherosclerosis of autologous vein bypass graft(s) of the extremities with rest pain, bilateral legs A HCC

I70.428 Atherosclerosis of autologous vein bypass graft(s) of the extremities with rest pain, other extremity A HCC

I70.429 Atherosclerosis of autologous vein bypass graft(s) of the extremities with rest pain, unspecified extremity A HCC

I70.43 Atherosclerosis of autologous vein bypass graft(s) of the right leg with ulceration

INCLUDES any condition classifiable to I70.411 and I70.421

Use additional code to identify severity of ulcer (L97.-)

I70.431 Atherosclerosis of autologous vein bypass graft(s) of the right leg with ulceration of thigh A HCC

I70.432 Atherosclerosis of autologous vein bypass graft(s) of the right leg with ulceration of calf A HCC

I70.433 Atherosclerosis of autologous vein bypass graft(s) of the right leg with ulceration of ankle A HCC

I70.434 Atherosclerosis of autologous vein bypass graft(s) of the right leg with ulceration of heel and midfoot A HCC

Atherosclerosis of autologous vein bypass graft(s) of right leg with ulceration of plantar surface of midfoot

I70.435 Atherosclerosis of autologous vein bypass graft(s) of the right leg with ulceration of other part of foot A HCC

Atherosclerosis of autologous vein bypass graft(s) of right leg with ulceration of toe

I70.438 Atherosclerosis of autologous vein bypass graft(s) of the right leg with ulceration of other part of lower leg A HCC

I70.439 Atherosclerosis of autologous vein bypass graft(s) of the right leg with ulceration of unspecified site A HCC

I70.44 Atherosclerosis of autologous vein bypass graft(s) of the left leg with ulceration

INCLUDES any condition classifiable to I70.412 and I70.422

Use additional code to identify severity of ulcer (L97.-)

I70.441 Atherosclerosis of autologous vein bypass graft(s) of the left leg with ulceration of thigh A HCC

I70.442 Atherosclerosis of autologous vein bypass graft(s) of the left leg with ulceration of calf A HCC

I70.443 Atherosclerosis of autologous vein bypass graft(s) of the left leg with ulceration of ankle A HCC

I70.444 Atherosclerosis of autologous vein bypass graft(s) of the left leg with ulceration of heel and midfoot A HCC

Atherosclerosis of autologous vein bypass graft(s) of left leg with ulceration of plantar surface of midfoot

I70.445 Atherosclerosis of autologous vein bypass graft(s) of the left leg with ulceration of other part of foot A HCC

Atherosclerosis of autologous vein bypass graft(s) of left leg with ulceration of toe

I70.448 Atherosclerosis of autologous vein bypass graft(s) of the left leg with ulceration of other part of lower leg A HCC

I70.449 Atherosclerosis of autologous vein bypass graft(s) of the left leg with ulceration of unspecified site A HCC

I70.45 Atherosclerosis of autologous vein bypass graft(s) of other extremity with ulceration A HCC

INCLUDES any condition classifiable to I70.418, I70.428, and I70.438

Use additional code to identify severity of ulcer (L98.49)

I70.46 Atherosclerosis of autologous vein bypass graft(s) of the extremities with gangrene

INCLUDES any condition classifiable to I70.41-, I70.42-, and I70.43-, I70.44-, I70.45

Use additional code to identify the severity of any ulcer (L97.-, L98.49-), if applicable

I70.461 Atherosclerosis of autologous vein bypass graft(s) of the extremities with gangrene, right leg A HCC

I70.462 Atherosclerosis of autologous vein bypass graft(s) of the extremities with gangrene, left leg A HCC

I70.463 Atherosclerosis of autologous vein bypass graft(s) of the extremities with gangrene, bilateral legs A HCC

I70.468 Atherosclerosis of autologous vein bypass graft(s) of the extremities with gangrene, other extremity A HCC

I70.469 Atherosclerosis of autologous vein bypass graft(s) of the extremities with gangrene, unspecified extremity A HCC

I70.49 Other atherosclerosis of autologous vein bypass graft(s) of the extremities

I70.491 Other atherosclerosis of autologous vein bypass graft(s) of the extremities, right leg A HCC

I70.492 Other atherosclerosis of autologous vein bypass graft(s) of the extremities, left leg A HCC

I70.493 Other atherosclerosis of autologous vein bypass graft(s) of the extremities, bilateral legs A HCC

I70.498 Other atherosclerosis of autologous vein bypass graft(s) of the extremities, other extremity A HCC

I70.499 Other atherosclerosis of autologous vein bypass graft(s) of the extremities, unspecified extremity A HCC

I70.5 Atherosclerosis of nonautologous biological bypass graft(s) of the extremities

Use additional code, if applicable, to identify chronic total occlusion of artery of extremity (I70.92)

I70.50 Unspecified atherosclerosis of nonautologous biological bypass graft(s) of the extremities

I70.501 Unspecified atherosclerosis of nonautologous biological bypass graft(s) of the extremities, right leg A HCC

I70.502 Unspecified atherosclerosis of nonautologous biological bypass graft(s) of the extremities, left leg A HCC

I70.503 Unspecified atherosclerosis of nonautologous biological bypass graft(s) of the extremities, bilateral legs A HCC

I70.508 Unspecified atherosclerosis of nonautologous biological bypass graft(s) of the extremities, other extremity A HCC

I70.509 Unspecified atherosclerosis of nonautologous biological bypass graft(s) of the extremities, unspecified extremity A HCC

I70.51 Atherosclerosis of nonautologous biological bypass graft(s) of the extremities intermittent claudication

I70.511 Atherosclerosis of nonautologous biological bypass graft(s) of the extremities with intermittent claudication, right leg A HCC

I70.512 Atherosclerosis of nonautologous biological bypass graft(s) of the extremities with intermittent claudication, left leg A HCC

I70.513 Atherosclerosis of nonautologous biological bypass graft(s) of the extremities with intermittent claudication, bilateral legs A HCC

I70.518 Atherosclerosis of nonautologous biological bypass graft(s) of the extremities with intermittent claudication, other extremity A HCC

I70.519 Atherosclerosis of nonautologous biological bypass graft(s) of the extremities with intermittent claudication, unspecified extremity A HCC

I70.52 Atherosclerosis of nonautologous biological bypass graft(s) of the extremities with rest pain

INCLUDES any condition classifiable to I70.51-

I70.521 Atherosclerosis of nonautologous biological bypass graft(s) of the extremities with rest pain, right leg A HCC

I70.522 Atherosclerosis of nonautologous biological bypass graft(s) of the extremities with rest pain, left leg A HCC

I70.523 Atherosclerosis of nonautologous biological bypass graft(s) of the extremities with rest pain, bilateral legs A HCC

I70.528 Atherosclerosis of nonautologous biological bypass graft(s) of the extremities with rest pain, other extremity A HCC

I70.529 Atherosclerosis of nonautologous biological bypass graft(s) of the extremities with rest pain, unspecified extremity A HCC

I70.53 Atherosclerosis of nonautologous biological bypass graft(s) of the right leg with ulceration

INCLUDES any condition classifiable to I70.511 and I70.521

Use additional code to identify severity of ulcer (L97.-)

I70.531 Atherosclerosis of nonautologous biological bypass graft(s) of the right leg with ulceration of thigh A HCC

I70.532 Atherosclerosis of nonautologous biological bypass graft(s) of the right leg with ulceration of calf A HCC

I70.533 Atherosclerosis of nonautologous biological bypass graft(s) of the right leg with ulceration of ankle A HCC

I70.534 Atherosclerosis of nonautologous biological bypass graft(s) of the right leg with ulceration of heel and midfoot A HCC

Atherosclerosis of nonautologous biological bypass graft(s) of right leg with ulceration of plantar surface of midfoot

I70.535 Atherosclerosis of nonautologous biological bypass graft(s) of the right leg with ulceration of other part of foot A HCC

Atherosclerosis of nonautologous biological bypass graft(s) of the right leg with ulceration of toe

I70.538 Atherosclerosis of nonautologous biological bypass graft(s) of the right leg with ulceration of other part of lower leg A HCC

I70.539 Atherosclerosis of nonautologous biological bypass graft(s) of the right leg with ulceration of unspecified site A HCC

I70.54 Atherosclerosis of nonautologous biological bypass graft(s) of the left leg with ulceration

INCLUDES any condition classifiable to I70.512 and I70.522

Use additional code to identify severity of ulcer (L97.-)

I70.541 Atherosclerosis of nonautologous biological bypass graft(s) of the left leg with ulceration of thigh A HCC

I70.542 Atherosclerosis of nonautologous biological bypass graft(s) of the left leg with ulceration of calf A HCC

I70.543 Atherosclerosis of nonautologous biological bypass graft(s) of the left leg with ulceration of ankle A HCC

I70.544 Atherosclerosis of nonautologous biological bypass graft(s) of the left leg with ulceration of heel and midfoot A HCC

Atherosclerosis of nonautologous biological bypass graft(s) of left leg with ulceration of plantar surface of midfoot

I70.545 Atherosclerosis of nonautologous biological bypass graft(s) of the left leg with ulceration of other part of foot A HCC

Atherosclerosis of nonautologous biological bypass graft(s) of the left leg with ulceration of toe

I70.548 Atherosclerosis of nonautologous biological bypass graft(s) of the left leg with ulceration of other part of lower leg A HCC

I70.549 Atherosclerosis of nonautologous biological bypass graft(s) of the left leg with ulceration of unspecified site A HCC

I70.55 Atherosclerosis of nonautologous biological bypass graft(s) of other extremity with ulceration A HCC

INCLUDES any condition classifiable to I70.518, I70.528, and I70.538

Use additional code to identify severity of ulcer (L98.49)

6 I70.56 **Atherosclerosis of nonautologous biological bypass graft(s) of the extremities with gangrene**
INCLUDES any condition classifiable to I70.51-, I70.52-, and I70.53-, I70.54-, I70.55
Use additional code to identify the severity of any ulcer (L97.-, L98.49-), if applicable

- **I70.561** **Atherosclerosis of nonautologous biological bypass graft(s) of the extremities with gangrene, right leg** A HCC
- **I70.562** **Atherosclerosis of nonautologous biological bypass graft(s) of the extremities with gangrene, left leg** A HCC
- **I70.563** **Atherosclerosis of nonautologous biological bypass graft(s) of the extremities with gangrene, bilateral legs** A HCC
- **I70.568** **Atherosclerosis of nonautologous biological bypass graft(s) of the extremities with gangrene, other extremity** A HCC
- **I70.569** **Atherosclerosis of nonautologous biological bypass graft(s) of the extremities with gangrene, unspecified extremity** A HCC

6 I70.59 **Other atherosclerosis of nonautologous biological bypass graft(s) of the extremities**

- **I70.591** **Other atherosclerosis of nonautologous biological bypass graft(s) of the extremities, right leg** A HCC
- **I70.592** **Other atherosclerosis of nonautologous biological bypass graft(s) of the extremities, left leg** A HCC
- **I70.593** **Other atherosclerosis of nonautologous biological bypass graft(s) of the extremities, bilateral legs** A HCC
- **I70.598** **Other atherosclerosis of nonautologous biological bypass graft(s) of the extremities, other extremity** A HCC
- **I70.599** **Other atherosclerosis of nonautologous biological bypass graft(s) of the extremities, unspecified extremity** A HCC

5 I70.6 **Atherosclerosis of nonbiological bypass graft(s) of the extremities**
Use additional code, if applicable, to identify chronic total occlusion of artery of extremity (I70.92)

6 I70.60 **Unspecified atherosclerosis of nonbiological bypass graft(s) of the extremities**

- **I70.601** **Unspecified atherosclerosis of nonbiological bypass graft(s) of the extremities, right leg** A HCC
- **I70.602** **Unspecified atherosclerosis of nonbiological bypass graft(s) of the extremities, left leg** A HCC
- **I70.603** **Unspecified atherosclerosis of nonbiological bypass graft(s) of the extremities, bilateral legs** A HCC
- **I70.608** **Unspecified atherosclerosis of nonbiological bypass graft(s) of the extremities, other extremity** A HCC
- **I70.609** **Unspecified atherosclerosis of nonbiological bypass graft(s) of the extremities, unspecified extremity** A HCC

6 I70.61 **Atherosclerosis of nonbiological bypass graft(s) of the extremities with intermittent claudication**

- **I70.611** **Atherosclerosis of nonbiological bypass graft(s) of the extremities with intermittent claudication, right leg** A HCC
- **I70.612** **Atherosclerosis of nonbiological bypass graft(s) of the extremities with intermittent claudication, left leg** A HCC
- **I70.613** **Atherosclerosis of nonbiological bypass graft(s) of the extremities with intermittent claudication, bilateral legs** A HCC
- **I70.618** **Atherosclerosis of nonbiological bypass graft(s) of the extremities with intermittent claudication, other extremity** A HCC
- **I70.619** **Atherosclerosis of nonbiological bypass graft(s) of the extremities with intermittent claudication, unspecified extremity** A HCC

6 I70.62 **Atherosclerosis of nonbiological bypass graft(s) of the extremities with rest pain**
INCLUDES any condition classifiable to I70.61-

- **I70.621** **Atherosclerosis of nonbiological bypass graft(s) of the extremities with rest pain, right leg** A HCC
- **I70.622** **Atherosclerosis of nonbiological bypass graft(s) of the extremities with rest pain, left leg** A HCC
- **I70.623** **Atherosclerosis of nonbiological bypass graft(s) of the extremities with rest pain, bilateral legs** A HCC
- **I70.628** **Atherosclerosis of nonbiological bypass graft(s) of the extremities with rest pain, other extremity** A HCC
- **I70.629** **Atherosclerosis of nonbiological bypass graft(s) of the extremities with rest pain, unspecified extremity** A HCC

6 I70.63 **Atherosclerosis of nonbiological bypass graft(s) of the right leg with ulceration**
INCLUDES any condition classifiable to I70.611 and I70.621
Use additional code to identify severity of ulcer (L97.-)

- **I70.631** **Atherosclerosis of nonbiological bypass graft(s) of the right leg with ulceration of thigh** A HCC
- **I70.632** **Atherosclerosis of nonbiological bypass graft(s) of the right leg with ulceration of calf** A HCC
- **I70.633** **Atherosclerosis of nonbiological bypass graft(s) of the right leg with ulceration of ankle** A HCC
- **I70.634** **Atherosclerosis of nonbiological bypass graft(s) of the right leg with ulceration of heel and midfoot** A HCC
  Atherosclerosis of nonbiological bypass graft(s) of right leg with ulceration of plantar surface of midfoot
- **I70.635** **Atherosclerosis of nonbiological bypass graft(s) of the right leg with ulceration of other part of foot** A HCC
  Atherosclerosis of nonbiological bypass graft(s) of the right leg with ulceration of toe
- **I70.638** **Atherosclerosis of nonbiological bypass graft(s) of the right leg with ulceration of other part of lower leg** A HCC
- **I70.639** **Atherosclerosis of nonbiological bypass graft(s) of the right leg with ulceration of unspecified site** A HCC

6 I70.64 **Atherosclerosis of nonbiological bypass graft(s) of the left leg with ulceration**
INCLUDES any condition classifiable to I70.612 and I70.622
Use additional code to identify severity of ulcer (L97.-)

- **I70.641** **Atherosclerosis of nonbiological bypass graft(s) of the left leg with ulceration of thigh** A HCC
- **I70.642** **Atherosclerosis of nonbiological bypass graft(s) of the left leg with ulceration of calf** A HCC
- **I70.643** **Atherosclerosis of nonbiological bypass graft(s) of the left leg with ulceration of ankle** A HCC
- **I70.644** **Atherosclerosis of nonbiological bypass graft(s) of the left leg with ulceration of heel and midfoot** A HCC
  Atherosclerosis of nonbiological bypass graft(s) of left leg with ulceration of plantar surface of midfoot
- **I70.645** **Atherosclerosis of nonbiological bypass graft(s) of the left leg with ulceration of other part of foot** A HCC
  Atherosclerosis of nonbiological bypass graft(s) of the left leg with ulceration of toe

I70.648 Atherosclerosis of nonbiological bypass graft(s) of the left leg with ulceration of other part of lower leg A HCC

I70.649 Atherosclerosis of nonbiological bypass graft(s) of the left leg with ulceration of unspecified site A HCC

I70.65 Atherosclerosis of nonbiological bypass graft(s) of other extremity with ulceration A HCC
INCLUDES any condition classifiable to I70.618 and I70.628
Use additional code to identify severity of ulcer (L98.49)

I70.66 Atherosclerosis of nonbiological bypass graft(s) of the extremities with gangrene
INCLUDES any condition classifiable to I70.61-, I70.62-, I70.63-, I70.64-, I70.65
Use additional code to identify the severity of any ulcer (L97.-, L98.49-), if applicable

I70.661 Atherosclerosis of nonbiological bypass graft(s) of the extremities with gangrene, right leg A HCC

I70.662 Atherosclerosis of nonbiological bypass graft(s) of the extremities with gangrene, left leg A HCC

I70.663 Atherosclerosis of nonbiological bypass graft(s) of the extremities with gangrene, bilateral legs A HCC

I70.668 Atherosclerosis of nonbiological bypass graft(s) of the extremities with gangrene, other extremity A HCC

I70.669 Atherosclerosis of nonbiological bypass graft(s) of the extremities with gangrene, unspecified extremity A HCC

I70.69 Other atherosclerosis of nonbiological bypass graft(s) of the extremities

I70.691 Other atherosclerosis of nonbiological bypass graft(s) of the extremities, right leg A HCC

I70.692 Other atherosclerosis of nonbiological bypass graft(s) of the extremities, left leg A HCC

I70.693 Other atherosclerosis of nonbiological bypass graft(s) of the extremities, bilateral legs A HCC

I70.698 Other atherosclerosis of nonbiological bypass graft(s) of the extremities, other extremity A HCC

I70.699 Other atherosclerosis of nonbiological bypass graft(s) of the extremities, unspecified extremity A HCC

I70.7 Atherosclerosis of other type of bypass graft(s) of the extremities
Use additional code, if applicable, to identify chronic total occlusion of artery of extremity (I70.92)

I70.70 Unspecified atherosclerosis of other type of bypass graft(s) of the extremities

I70.701 Unspecified atherosclerosis of other type of bypass graft(s) of the extremities, right leg A HCC

I70.702 Unspecified atherosclerosis of other type of bypass graft(s) of the extremities, left leg A HCC

I70.703 Unspecified atherosclerosis of other type of bypass graft(s) of the extremities, bilateral legs A HCC

I70.708 Unspecified atherosclerosis of other type of bypass graft(s) of the extremities, other extremity A HCC

I70.709 Unspecified atherosclerosis of other type of bypass graft(s) of the extremities, unspecified extremity A HCC

I70.71 Atherosclerosis of other type of bypass graft(s) of the extremities with intermittent claudication

I70.711 Atherosclerosis of other type of bypass graft(s) of the extremities with intermittent claudication, right leg A HCC

I70.712 Atherosclerosis of other type of bypass graft(s) of the extremities with intermittent claudication, left leg A HCC

I70.713 Atherosclerosis of other type of bypass graft(s) of the extremities with intermittent claudication, bilateral legs A HCC

I70.718 Atherosclerosis of other type of bypass graft(s) of the extremities with intermittent claudication, other extremity A HCC

I70.719 Atherosclerosis of other type of bypass graft(s) of the extremities with intermittent claudication, unspecified extremity A HCC

I70.72 Atherosclerosis of other type of bypass graft(s) of the extremities with rest pain
INCLUDES any condition classifiable to I70.71-

I70.721 Atherosclerosis of other type of bypass graft(s) of the extremities with rest pain, right leg A HCC

I70.722 Atherosclerosis of other type of bypass graft(s) of the extremities with rest pain, left leg A HCC

I70.723 Atherosclerosis of other type of bypass graft(s) of the extremities with rest pain, bilateral legs A HCC

I70.728 Atherosclerosis of other type of bypass graft(s) of the extremities with rest pain, other extremity A HCC

I70.729 Atherosclerosis of other type of bypass graft(s) of the extremities with rest pain, unspecified extremity A HCC

I70.73 Atherosclerosis of other type of bypass graft(s) of the right leg with ulceration
INCLUDES any condition classifiable to I70.711 and I70.721
Use additional code to identify severity of ulcer (L97.-)

I70.731 Atherosclerosis of other type of bypass graft(s) of the right leg with ulceration of thigh A HCC

I70.732 Atherosclerosis of other type of bypass graft(s) of the right leg with ulceration of calf A HCC

I70.733 Atherosclerosis of other type of bypass graft(s) of the right leg with ulceration of ankle A HCC

I70.734 Atherosclerosis of other type of bypass graft(s) of the right leg with ulceration of heel and midfoot A HCC
Atherosclerosis of other type of bypass graft(s) of right leg with ulceration of plantar surface of midfoot

I70.735 Atherosclerosis of other type of bypass graft(s) of the right leg with ulceration of other part of foot A HCC
Atherosclerosis of other type of bypass graft(s) of right leg with ulceration of toe

I70.738 Atherosclerosis of other type of bypass graft(s) of the right leg with ulceration of other part of lower leg A HCC

I70.739 Atherosclerosis of other type of bypass graft(s) of the right leg with ulceration of unspecified site A HCC

I70.74 Atherosclerosis of other type of bypass graft(s) of the left leg with ulceration
INCLUDES any condition classifiable to I70.712 and I70.722
Use additional code to identify severity of ulcer (L97.-)

I70.741 Atherosclerosis of other type of bypass graft(s) of the left leg with ulceration of thigh A HCC

I70.742 Atherosclerosis of other type of bypass graft(s) of the left leg with ulceration of calf A HCC

I70.743 Atherosclerosis of other type of bypass graft(s) of the left leg with ulceration of ankle A HCC

I70.744 Atherosclerosis of other type of bypass graft(s) of the left leg with ulceration of heel and midfoot A HCC
Atherosclerosis of other type of bypass graft(s) of left leg with ulceration of plantar surface of midfoot

I70.745 **Atherosclerosis of other type of bypass graft(s) of the left leg with ulceration of other part of foot** A HCC
Atherosclerosis of other type of bypass graft(s) of left leg with ulceration of toe

I70.748 **Atherosclerosis of other type of bypass graft(s) of the left leg with ulceration of other part of lower leg** A HCC

I70.749 **Atherosclerosis of other type of bypass graft(s) of the left leg with ulceration of unspecified site** A HCC

I70.75 **Atherosclerosis of other type of bypass graft(s) of other extremity with ulceration** A HCC
INCLUDES any condition classifiable to I70.718 and I70.728
Use additional code to identify severity of ulcer (L98.49)

6 I70.76 **Atherosclerosis of other type of bypass graft(s) of the extremities with gangrene**
INCLUDES any condition classifiable to I70.71-, I70.72-, I70.73-, I70.74-, I70.75
Use additional code to identify the severity of any ulcer (L97.-, L98.49-), if applicable

I70.761 **Atherosclerosis of other type of bypass graft(s) of the extremities with gangrene, right leg** A HCC

I70.762 **Atherosclerosis of other type of bypass graft(s) of the extremities with gangrene, left leg** A HCC

I70.763 **Atherosclerosis of other type of bypass graft(s) of the extremities with gangrene, bilateral legs** A HCC

I70.768 **Atherosclerosis of other type of bypass graft(s) of the extremities with gangrene, other extremity** A HCC

I70.769 **Atherosclerosis of other type of bypass graft(s) of the extremities with gangrene, unspecified extremity** A HCC

6 I70.79 **Other atherosclerosis of Other type of bypass graft(s) of the extremities**

I70.791 **Other atherosclerosis of other type of bypass graft(s) of the extremities, right leg** A HCC

I70.792 **Other atherosclerosis of other type of bypass graft(s) of the extremities, left leg** A HCC

I70.793 **Other atherosclerosis of other type of bypass graft(s) of the extremities, bilateral legs** A HCC

I70.798 **Other atherosclerosis of other type of bypass graft(s) of the extremities, other extremity** A HCC

I70.799 **Other atherosclerosis of other type of bypass graft(s) of the extremities, unspecified extremity** A HCC

I70.8 **Atherosclerosis of other arteries** A

5 I70.9 **Other and unspecified atherosclerosis**

I70.90 **Unspecified atherosclerosis** A

I70.91 **Generalized atherosclerosis** A

I70.92 **Chronic total occlusion of artery of the extremities** A HCC
Complete occlusion of artery of the extremities
Total occlusion of artery of the extremities
Code first:
atherosclerosis of arteries of the extremities (I70.2-, I70.3-, I70.4-, I70.5-, I70.6-, I70.7-)

4 I71 Aortic aneurysm and dissection

EXCLUDES 1 *aortic ectasia (I77.81-)*
syphilitic aortic aneurysm (A52.01)
traumatic aortic aneurysm (S25.09, S35.09)

5 I71.0 **Dissection of aorta**

I71.00 **Dissection of unspecified site of aorta** HCC

I71.01 **Dissection of thoracic aorta** HCC

I71.02 **Dissection of abdominal aorta** HCC

I71.03 **Dissection of thoracoabdominal aorta** HCC

I71.1 **Thoracic aortic aneurysm, ruptured** HCC

I71.2 **Thoracic aortic aneurysm, without rupture** HCC

I71.3 **Abdominal aortic aneurysm, ruptured** HCC

I71.4 **Abdominal aortic aneurysm, without rupture** HCC

Abdominal aortic aneurysm, without rupture

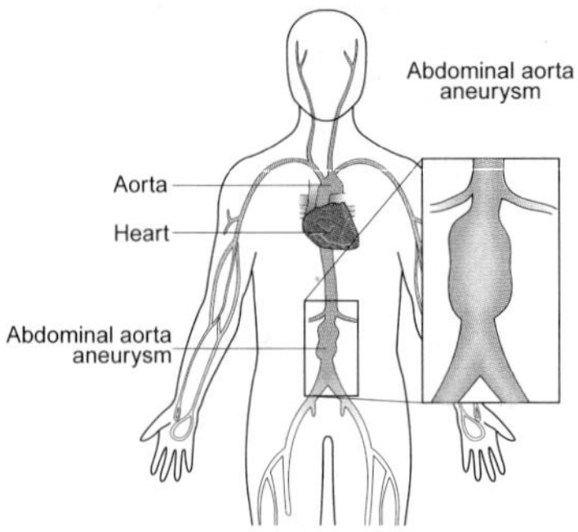

I71.5 **Thoracoabdominal aortic aneurysm, ruptured** HCC

I71.6 **Thoracoabdominal aortic aneurysm, without rupture** HCC

I71.8 **Aortic aneurysm of unspecified site, ruptured** HCC
Rupture of aorta NOS

I71.9 **Aortic aneurysm of unspecified site, without rupture** HCC
Aneurysm of aorta
Dilatation of aorta
Hyaline necrosis of aorta

4 I72 Other aneurysm

INCLUDES aneurysm (cirsoid) (false) (ruptured)

EXCLUDES 2 *acquired aneurysm (I77.0)*
aneurysm (of) aorta (I71.-)
aneurysm (of) arteriovenous NOS (Q27.3-)
carotid artery dissection (I77.71)
cerebral (nonruptured) aneurysm (I67.1)
coronary aneurysm (I25.4)
coronary artery dissection (I25.42)
dissection of artery NEC (I77.79)
dissection of precerebral artery, congenital (nonruptured) (Q28.1)
heart aneurysm (I25.3)
iliac artery dissection (I77.72)
precerebral artery, congenital (nonruptured) (Q28.1)
pulmonary artery aneurysm (I28.1)
renal artery dissection (I77.73)
retinal aneurysm (H35.0)
ruptured cerebral aneurysm (I60.7)
varicose aneurysm (I77.0)
vertebral artery dissection (I77.74)

AHA: 4Q 2016, 28

I72.0 **Aneurysm of carotid artery** HCC
Aneurysm of common carotid artery
Aneurysm of external carotid artery
Aneurysm of internal carotid artery, extracranial portion
EXCLUDES 1 *aneurysm of internal carotid artery, intracranial portion (I67.1)*
aneurysm of internal carotid artery NOS (I67.1)

I72.1 **Aneurysm of artery of upper extremity** HCC

I72.2 **Aneurysm of renal artery** HCC

I72.3 **Aneurysm of iliac artery** HCC

I72.4 **Aneurysm of artery of lower extremity** HCC

I72.5 **Aneurysm of other precerebral arteries** HCC
Aneurysm of basilar artery (trunk)
EXCLUDES 2 *aneurysm of carotid artery (I72.0)*
aneurysm of vertebral artery (I72.6)
dissection of carotid artery (I77.71)
dissection of other precerebral arteries (I77.75)
dissection of vertebral artery (I77.74)

I72.6 **Aneurysm of vertebral artery** HCC
EXCLUDES 2 *dissection of vertebral artery (I77.74)*

I72.8 **Aneurysm of other specified arteries** HCC

I72.9 **Aneurysm of unspecified site** HCC

I73 Other peripheral vascular diseases

EXCLUDES 2 *chilblains (T69.1)*
frostbite (T33-T34)
immersion hand or foot (T69.0-)
spasm of cerebral artery (G45.9)

I73.0 Raynaud's syndrome
Raynaud's disease
Raynaud's phenomenon (secondary)

I73.00 Raynaud's syndrome without gangrene

I73.01 Raynaud's syndrome with gangrene HCC

DEFINITION Medium-sized blood vessels of the hands and feet become inflamed and blocked by blood clots, causing gangrene of the extremities.

I73.1 Thromboangiitis obliterans [Buerger's disease] HCC

I73.8 Other specified peripheral vascular diseases

EXCLUDES 1 *diabetic (peripheral) angiopathy (E08-E13 with .51-.52)*

I73.81 Erythromelalgia HCC

DEFINITION Abnormal dilation of extremity blood vessels, especially in the feet, causing a painful, burning sensation, and redness.

I73.89 Other specified peripheral vascular diseases HCC
Acrocyanosis
Erythrocyanosis
Simple acroparesthesia [Schultze's type]
Vasomotor acroparesthesia [Nothnagel's type]

I73.9 Peripheral vascular disease, unspecified HCC
Intermittent claudication
Peripheral angiopathy NOS
Spasm of artery

EXCLUDES 1 *atherosclerosis of the extremities (I70.2--I70.7-)*

CODING TIP✓ Do not assign I73.9 when peripheral atherosclerosis is reported in the clinical record. Note, atherosclerosis of the extremities is a more specific diagnosis and should be coded using a code from I70.2- through I70.7-.

Peripheral vascular disease, unspecified

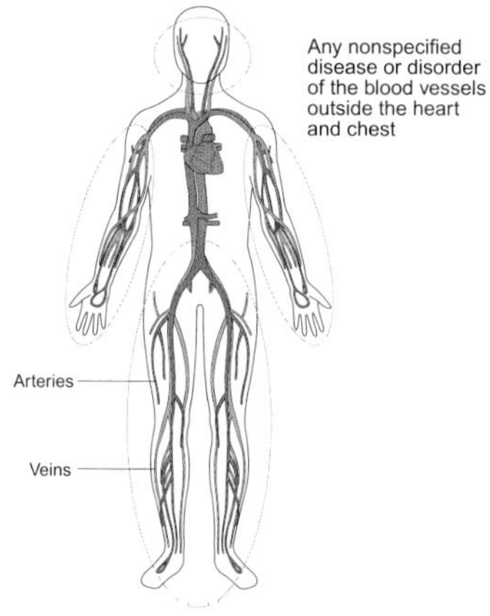
Any nonspecified disease or disorder of the blood vessels outside the heart and chest
Arteries
Veins

I74 Arterial embolism and thrombosis

INCLUDES embolic infarction
embolic occlusion
thrombotic infarction
thrombotic occlusion

Code first:
embolism and thrombosis complicating abortion or ectopic or molar pregnancy (O00-O07, O08.2)
embolism and thrombosis complicating pregnancy, childbirth and the puerperium (O88.-)

EXCLUDES 2 *atheroembolism (I75.-)*
basilar embolism and thrombosis (I63.0-I63.2, I65.1)
carotid embolism and thrombosis (I63.0-I63.2, I65.2)
cerebral embolism and thrombosis (I63.3-I63.5, I66.-)
coronary embolism and thrombosis (I21-I25)
mesenteric embolism and thrombosis (K55.0-)
ophthalmic embolism and thrombosis (H34.-)
precerebral embolism and thrombosis NOS (I63.0-I63.2, I65.9)
pulmonary embolism and thrombosis (I26.-)
renal embolism and thrombosis (N28.0)
retinal embolism and thrombosis (H34.-)
septic embolism and thrombosis (I76)
vertebral embolism and thrombosis (I63.0-I63.2, I65.0)

I74.0 Embolism and thrombosis of abdominal aorta

I74.01 Saddle embolus of abdominal aorta HCC

I74.09 Other arterial embolism and thrombosis of abdominal aorta HCC
Aortic bifurcation syndrome
Aortoiliac obstruction
Leriche's syndrome

I74.1 Embolism and thrombosis of other and unspecified parts of aorta

I74.10 Embolism and thrombosis of unspecified parts of aorta HCC

I74.11 Embolism and thrombosis of thoracic aorta HCC

I74.19 Embolism and thrombosis of other parts of aorta HCC

I74.2 Embolism and thrombosis of arteries of the upper extremities HCC

I74.3 Embolism and thrombosis of arteries of the lower extremities HCC

I74.4 Embolism and thrombosis of arteries of extremities, unspecified HCC
Peripheral arterial embolism NOS

I74.5 Embolism and thrombosis of iliac artery HCC

I74.8 Embolism and thrombosis of other arteries HCC

I74.9 Embolism and thrombosis of unspecified artery HCC

I75 Atheroembolism

INCLUDES atherothrombotic microembolism
cholesterol embolism

I75.0 Atheroembolism of extremities

I75.01 Atheroembolism of upper extremity

I75.011 Atheroembolism of right upper extremity HCC

I75.012 Atheroembolism of left upper extremity HCC

I75.013 Atheroembolism of bilateral upper extremities HCC

I75.019 Atheroembolism of unspecified upper extremity HCC

I75.02 Atheroembolism of lower extremity

I75.021 Atheroembolism of right lower extremity HCC

I75.022 Atheroembolism of left lower extremity HCC

I75.023 Atheroembolism of bilateral lower extremities HCC

I75.029 Atheroembolism of unspecified lower extremity HCC

I75.8 Atheroembolism of other sites

I75.81 Atheroembolism of kidney HCC
Use additional code for any associated acute kidney failure and chronic kidney disease (N17.-, N18.-)

I75.89 Atheroembolism of other site HCC

I76 Septic arterial embolism HCC
Code first underlying infection, such as:
infective endocarditis (I33.0)
lung abscess (J85.-)
Use additional code to identify the site of the embolism (I74.-)
EXCLUDES 2 *septic pulmonary embolism (I26.01, I26.90)*

DEFINITION Dislodged material from a centralized infection lodged in a small arteriole, causing tissue death due to bacteria and lack of blood supply.

4 I77 Other disorders of arteries and arterioles
EXCLUDES 2 *collagen (vascular) diseases (M30-M36)*
hypersensitivity angiitis (M31.0)
pulmonary artery (I28.-)

I77.0 Arteriovenous fistula, acquired HCC
Aneurysmal varix
Arteriovenous aneurysm, acquired
EXCLUDES 1 *arteriovenous aneurysm NOS (Q27.3-)*
presence of arteriovenous shunt (fistula) for dialysis (Z99.2)
traumatic - see injury of blood vessel by body region
EXCLUDES 2 *cerebral (I67.1)*
coronary (I25.4)

I77.1 Stricture of artery HCC
Narrowing of artery

I77.2 Rupture of artery HCC
Erosion of artery
Fistula of artery
Ulcer of artery
EXCLUDES 1 *traumatic rupture of artery - see injury of blood vessel by body region*

CODING TIP ✓ Do not assign code I77.2 for a traumatic rupture of the artery. A fistula, ulcer, or arterial erosion would be coded to I77.2.

I77.3 Arterial fibromuscular dysplasia HCC
Fibromuscular hyperplasia (of) carotid artery
Fibromuscular hyperplasia (of) renal artery

I77.4 Celiac artery compression syndrome HCC

I77.5 Necrosis of artery HCC

▲ **I77.6 Arteritis, unspecified** HCC
Aortitis NOS
Endarteritis NOS
EXCLUDES 1 *arteritis or endarteritis:*
aortic arch (M31.4)
cerebral NEC (I67.7)
coronary (I25.89)
deformans (I70.-)
giant cell (M31.5, M31.6)
obliterans (I70.-)
senile (I70.-)

5 I77.7 Other arterial dissection
EXCLUDES 2 *dissection of aorta (I71.0-)*
dissection of coronary artery (I25.42)
AHA: 4Q 2016, 28

I77.70 Dissection of unspecified artery HCC

I77.71 Dissection of carotid artery HCC

I77.72 Dissection of iliac artery HCC

I77.73 Dissection of renal artery HCC

I77.74 Dissection of vertebral artery HCC
EXCLUDES 2 *aneurysm of vertebral artery (I72.6)*

I77.75 Dissection of other precerebral arteries HCC
Dissection of basilar artery (trunk)
EXCLUDES 2 *aneurysm of carotid artery (I72.0)*
aneurysm of other precerebral arteries (I72.5)
aneurysm of vertebral artery (I72.6)
dissection of carotid artery (I77.71)
dissection of vertebral artery (I77.74)

I77.76 Dissection of artery of upper extremity HCC

I77.77 Dissection of artery of lower extremity HCC

I77.79 Dissection of other specified artery HCC

5 I77.8 Other specified disorders of arteries and arterioles

6 I77.81 Aortic ectasia
Ectasis aorta
EXCLUDES 1 *aortic aneurysm and dissection (I71.0-)*

I77.810 Thoracic aortic ectasia HCC

I77.811 Abdominal aortic ectasia HCC

I77.812 Thoracoabdominal aortic ectasia HCC

I77.819 Aortic ectasia, unspecified site HCC

I77.89 Other specified disorders of arteries and arterioles HCC

I77.9 Disorder of arteries and arterioles, unspecified HCC

4 I78 Diseases of capillaries

I78.0 Hereditary hemorrhagic telangiectasia HCC
Rendu-Osler-Weber disease

I78.1 Nevus, non-neoplastic
Araneus nevus
Senile nevus
Spider nevus
Stellar nevus
EXCLUDES 1 *nevus NOS (D22.-)*
vascular NOS (Q82.5)
EXCLUDES 2 *blue nevus (D22.-)*
flammeus nevus (Q82.5)
hairy nevus (D22.-)
melanocytic nevus (D22.-)
pigmented nevus (D22.-)
portwine nevus (Q82.5)
sanguineous nevus (Q82.5)
strawberry nevus (Q82.5)
verrucous nevus (Q82.5)

I78.8 Other diseases of capillaries

I78.9 Disease of capillaries, unspecified

4 I79 Disorders of arteries, arterioles and capillaries in diseases classified elsewhere

CODING TIP ✓ Codes from category I79.- should be coded only when the arterial disease/dysfunction is specified as due to another primary disease process. The causative disease process should be coded first.

I79.0 ***Aneurysm of aorta in diseases classified elsewhere*** HCC
Code first:
underlying disease
EXCLUDES 1 *syphilitic aneurysm (A52.01)*

CODING TIP ✓ I79.0 should be coded only when an aortic aneurysm is specified as due to another primary disease process. The causative disease process should be coded first.

I79.1 ***Aortitis in diseases classified elsewhere*** HCC
Code first:
underlying disease
EXCLUDES 1 *syphilitic aortitis (A52.02)*

I79.8 ***Other disorders of arteries, arterioles and capillaries in diseases classified elsewhere*** HCC
Code first underlying disease, such as:
amyloidosis (E85.-)
EXCLUDES 1 *diabetic (peripheral) angiopathy (E08-E13 with .51-.52)*
syphilitic endarteritis (A52.09)
tuberculous endarteritis (A18.89)

Diseases of veins, lymphatic vessels and lymph nodes, not elsewhere classified (I80-I89)

4 I80 Phlebitis and thrombophlebitis
INCLUDES endophlebitis
inflammation, vein
periphlebitis
suppurative phlebitis
Code first:
phlebitis and thrombophlebitis complicating abortion, ectopic or molar pregnancy (O00-O07, O08.7)
phlebitis and thrombophlebitis complicating pregnancy, childbirth and the puerperium (O22.-, O87.-)
EXCLUDES 1 *venous embolism and thrombosis of lower extremities (I82.4-, I82.5-, I82.81-)*

5 I80.0 Phlebitis and thrombophlebitis of superficial vessels of lower extremities
Phlebitis and thrombophlebitis of femoropopliteal vein

⊟ I80.00 Phlebitis and thrombophlebitis of superficial vessels of unspecified lower extremity

I80.01 Phlebitis and thrombophlebitis of superficial vessels of right lower extremity
I80.02 Phlebitis and thrombophlebitis of superficial vessels of left lower extremity
I80.03 Phlebitis and thrombophlebitis of superficial vessels of lower extremities, bilateral

I80.1 Phlebitis and thrombophlebitis of femoral vein
I80.10 Phlebitis and thrombophlebitis of unspecified femoral vein HCC
I80.11 Phlebitis and thrombophlebitis of right femoral vein HCC
I80.12 Phlebitis and thrombophlebitis of left femoral vein HCC
I80.13 Phlebitis and thrombophlebitis of femoral vein, bilateral HCC

I80.2 Phlebitis and thrombophlebitis of other and unspecified deep vessels of lower extremities
I80.20 Phlebitis and thrombophlebitis of unspecified deep vessels of lower extremities
I80.201 Phlebitis and thrombophlebitis of unspecified deep vessels of right lower extremity HCC
I80.202 Phlebitis and thrombophlebitis of unspecified deep vessels of left lower extremity HCC
I80.203 Phlebitis and thrombophlebitis of unspecified deep vessels of lower extremities, bilateral HCC
I80.209 Phlebitis and thrombophlebitis of unspecified deep vessels of unspecified lower extremity HCC

I80.21 Phlebitis and thrombophlebitis of iliac vein
I80.211 Phlebitis and thrombophlebitis of right iliac vein HCC
I80.212 Phlebitis and thrombophlebitis of left iliac vein HCC
I80.213 Phlebitis and thrombophlebitis of iliac vein, bilateral HCC
I80.219 Phlebitis and thrombophlebitis of unspecified iliac vein HCC

I80.22 Phlebitis and thrombophlebitis of popliteal vein
I80.221 Phlebitis and thrombophlebitis of right popliteal vein HCC
I80.222 Phlebitis and thrombophlebitis of left popliteal vein HCC
I80.223 Phlebitis and thrombophlebitis of popliteal vein, bilateral HCC
I80.229 Phlebitis and thrombophlebitis of unspecified popliteal vein HCC

I80.23 Phlebitis and thrombophlebitis of tibial vein
I80.231 Phlebitis and thrombophlebitis of right tibial vein HCC
I80.232 Phlebitis and thrombophlebitis of left tibial vein HCC
I80.233 Phlebitis and thrombophlebitis of tibial vein, bilateral HCC
I80.239 Phlebitis and thrombophlebitis of unspecified tibial vein HCC

I80.29 Phlebitis and thrombophlebitis of other deep vessels of lower extremities
I80.291 Phlebitis and thrombophlebitis of other deep vessels of right lower extremity HCC
I80.292 Phlebitis and thrombophlebitis of other deep vessels of left lower extremity HCC
I80.293 Phlebitis and thrombophlebitis of other deep vessels of lower extremity, bilateral HCC
I80.299 Phlebitis and thrombophlebitis of other deep vessels of unspecified lower extremity HCC

I80.3 Phlebitis and thrombophlebitis of lower extremities, unspecified
I80.8 Phlebitis and thrombophlebitis of other sites
I80.9 Phlebitis and thrombophlebitis of unspecified site

I81 Portal vein thrombosis

Portal (vein) obstruction

EXCLUDES 2 *hepatic vein thrombosis (I82.0)*
phlebitis of portal vein (K75.1)

CODING TIP ✓ Portal vein thrombosis is a specific clinical condition caused by the occlusion/obstruction of the portal vein but does not include occlusion of the hepatic vein, and is relatively common in cirrhosis patients. It often leads to portal hypertension. When this condition occurs, any comorbid hepatic vein thrombosis and/or portal hypertension should also be coded.

I82 Other venous embolism and thrombosis

Code first venous embolism and thrombosis complicating:
abortion, ectopic or molar pregnancy (O00-O07, O08.7)
pregnancy, childbirth and the puerperium (O22.-, O87.-)

EXCLUDES 2 *venous embolism and thrombosis (of) :*
cerebral (I63.6, I67.6)
coronary (I21-I25)
intracranial and intraspinal, septic or NOS (G08)
intracranial, nonpyogenic (I67.6)
intraspinal, nonpyogenic (G95.1)
mesenteric (K55.0-)
portal (I81)
pulmonary (I26.-)

I82.0 Budd-Chiari syndrome HCC
Hepatic vein thrombosis

DEFINITION Obstruction or occlusion of the hepatic veins, causing an enlarged liver, abdominal pain/tenderness, intractable ascites, mild jaundice, portal hypertension, and liver failure.

I82.1 Thrombophlebitis migrans

I82.2 Embolism and thrombosis of vena cava and other thoracic veins
I82.21 Embolism and thrombosis of superior vena cava
I82.210 Acute embolism and thrombosis of superior vena cava HCC
Embolism and thrombosis of superior vena cava NOS
I82.211 Chronic embolism and thrombosis of superior vena cava HCC
I82.22 Embolism and thrombosis of inferior vena cava
I82.220 Acute embolism and thrombosis of inferior vena cava HCC
Embolism and thrombosis of inferior vena cava NOS
I82.221 Chronic embolism and thrombosis of inferior vena cava HCC
I82.29 Embolism and thrombosis of other thoracic veins
Embolism and thrombosis of brachiocephalic (innominate) vein
I82.290 Acute embolism and thrombosis of other thoracic veins HCC
I82.291 Chronic embolism and thrombosis of other thoracic veins HCC

I82.3 Embolism and thrombosis of renal vein HCC

I82.4 Acute embolism and thrombosis of deep veins of lower extremity
I82.40 Acute embolism and thrombosis of unspecified deep veins of lower extremity
Deep vein thrombosis NOS
DVT NOS

EXCLUDES 1 *acute embolism and thrombosis of unspecified deep veins of distal lower extremity (I82.4Z-)*
acute embolism and thrombosis of unspecified deep veins of proximal lower extremity (I82.4Y-)

I82.401 Acute embolism and thrombosis of unspecified deep veins of right lower extremity HCC
I82.402 Acute embolism and thrombosis of unspecified deep veins of left lower extremity HCC
I82.403 Acute embolism and thrombosis of unspecified deep veins of lower extremity, bilateral HCC

Diseases of the Circulatory System
I80.01 — I82.403

● New | Manifestation | 4-7 Digit Indicators | Laterality | A Adult | M Maternity | N Newborn | P Pediatric | ♂ Male
▲ Revised | Unspecified | AHA Coding Clinic | HCC Hierarchical Condition Categories | HIV HIV Related Conditions | ♀ Female

I82.409 Acute embolism and thrombosis of unspecified deep veins of unspecified lower extremity HCC

I82.41 Acute embolism and thrombosis of femoral vein
- I82.411 Acute embolism and thrombosis of right femoral vein HCC
- I82.412 Acute embolism and thrombosis of left femoral vein HCC
- I82.413 Acute embolism and thrombosis of femoral vein, bilateral HCC
- I82.419 Acute embolism and thrombosis of unspecified femoral vein HCC

I82.42 Acute embolism and thrombosis of iliac vein
- I82.421 Acute embolism and thrombosis of right iliac vein HCC
- I82.422 Acute embolism and thrombosis of left iliac vein HCC
- I82.423 Acute embolism and thrombosis of iliac vein, bilateral HCC
- I82.429 Acute embolism and thrombosis of unspecified iliac vein HCC

I82.43 Acute embolism and thrombosis of popliteal vein
- I82.431 Acute embolism and thrombosis of right popliteal vein HCC
- I82.432 Acute embolism and thrombosis of left popliteal vein HCC
- I82.433 Acute embolism and thrombosis of popliteal vein, bilateral HCC
- I82.439 Acute embolism and thrombosis of unspecified popliteal vein HCC

I82.44 Acute embolism and thrombosis of tibial vein
- I82.441 Acute embolism and thrombosis of right tibial vein HCC
- I82.442 Acute embolism and thrombosis of left tibial vein HCC
- I82.443 Acute embolism and thrombosis of tibial vein, bilateral HCC
- I82.449 Acute embolism and thrombosis of unspecified tibial vein HCC

I82.49 Acute embolism and thrombosis of other specified deep vein of lower extremity
- I82.491 Acute embolism and thrombosis of other specified deep vein of right lower extremity HCC
- I82.492 Acute embolism and thrombosis of other specified deep vein of left lower extremity HCC
- I82.493 Acute embolism and thrombosis of other specified deep vein of lower extremity, bilateral HCC
- I82.499 Acute embolism and thrombosis of other specified deep vein of unspecified lower extremity HCC

I82.4Y Acute embolism and thrombosis of unspecified deep veins of proximal lower extremity

Acute embolism and thrombosis of deep vein of thigh NOS

Acute embolism and thrombosis of deep vein of upper leg NOS

- I82.4Y1 Acute embolism and thrombosis of unspecified deep veins of right proximal lower extremity HCC
- I82.4Y2 Acute embolism and thrombosis of unspecified deep veins of left proximal lower extremity HCC
- I82.4Y3 Acute embolism and thrombosis of unspecified deep veins of proximal lower extremity, bilateral HCC
- I82.4Y9 Acute embolism and thrombosis of unspecified deep veins of unspecified proximal lower extremity HCC

I82.4Z Acute embolism and thrombosis of unspecified deep veins of distal lower extremity

Acute embolism and thrombosis of deep vein of calf NOS

Acute embolism and thrombosis of deep vein of lower leg NOS

- I82.4Z1 Acute embolism and thrombosis of unspecified deep veins of right distal lower extremity HCC
- I82.4Z2 Acute embolism and thrombosis of unspecified deep veins of left distal lower extremity HCC
- I82.4Z3 Acute embolism and thrombosis of unspecified deep veins of distal lower extremity, bilateral HCC
- I82.4Z9 Acute embolism and thrombosis of unspecified deep veins of unspecified distal lower extremity HCC

I82.5 Chronic embolism and thrombosis of deep veins of lower extremity

Use additional code, if applicable, for associated long-term (current) use of anticoagulants (Z79.01)

EXCLUDES 1 *personal history of venous embolism and thrombosis (Z86.718)*

I82.50 Chronic embolism and thrombosis of unspecified deep veins of lower extremity

EXCLUDES 1 *chronic embolism and thrombosis of unspecified deep veins of distal lower extremity (I82.5Z-)*
chronic embolism and thrombosis of unspecified deep veins of proximal lower extremity (I82.5Y-)

- I82.501 Chronic embolism and thrombosis of unspecified deep veins of right lower extremity HCC
- I82.502 Chronic embolism and thrombosis of unspecified deep veins of left lower extremity HCC
- I82.503 Chronic embolism and thrombosis of unspecified deep veins of lower extremity, bilateral HCC
- I82.509 Chronic embolism and thrombosis of unspecified deep veins of unspecified lower extremity HCC

I82.51 Chronic embolism and thrombosis of femoral vein
- I82.511 Chronic embolism and thrombosis of right femoral vein HCC
- I82.512 Chronic embolism and thrombosis of left femoral vein HCC
- I82.513 Chronic embolism and thrombosis of femoral vein, bilateral HCC
- I82.519 Chronic embolism and thrombosis of unspecified femoral vein HCC

I82.52 Chronic embolism and thrombosis of iliac vein
- I82.521 Chronic embolism and thrombosis of right iliac vein HCC
- I82.522 Chronic embolism and thrombosis of left iliac vein HCC
- I82.523 Chronic embolism and thrombosis of iliac vein, bilateral HCC
- I82.529 Chronic embolism and thrombosis of unspecified iliac vein HCC

I82.53 Chronic embolism and thrombosis of popliteal vein
- I82.531 Chronic embolism and thrombosis of right popliteal vein HCC
- I82.532 Chronic embolism and thrombosis of left popliteal vein HCC
- I82.533 Chronic embolism and thrombosis of popliteal vein, bilateral HCC
- I82.539 Chronic embolism and thrombosis of unspecified popliteal vein HCC

I82.54 Chronic embolism and thrombosis of tibial vein
- I82.541 Chronic embolism and thrombosis of right tibial vein HCC
- I82.542 Chronic embolism and thrombosis of left tibial vein HCC
- I82.543 Chronic embolism and thrombosis of tibial vein, bilateral HCC
- I82.549 Chronic embolism and thrombosis of unspecified tibial vein HCC

I82.59 Chronic embolism and thrombosis of other specified deep vein of lower extremity
- I82.591 Chronic embolism and thrombosis of other specified deep vein of right lower extremity HCC
- I82.592 Chronic embolism and thrombosis of other specified deep vein of left lower extremity HCC

I82.593 **Chronic embolism and thrombosis of other specified deep vein of lower extremity, bilateral** HCC

I82.599 **Chronic embolism and thrombosis of other specified deep vein of unspecified lower extremity** HCC

I82.5Y **Chronic embolism and thrombosis of unspecified deep veins of proximal lower extremity**
Chronic embolism and thrombosis of deep veins of thigh NOS
Chronic embolism and thrombosis of deep veins of upper leg NOS

I82.5Y1 **Chronic embolism and thrombosis of unspecified deep veins of right proximal lower extremity** HCC

I82.5Y2 **Chronic embolism and thrombosis of unspecified deep veins of left proximal lower extremity** HCC

I82.5Y3 **Chronic embolism and thrombosis of unspecified deep veins of proximal lower extremity, bilateral** HCC

I82.5Y9 **Chronic embolism and thrombosis of unspecified deep veins of unspecified proximal lower extremity** HCC

I82.5Z **Chronic embolism and thrombosis of unspecified deep veins of distal lower extremity**
Chronic embolism and thrombosis of deep veins of calf NOS
Chronic embolism and thrombosis of deep veins of lower leg NOS

I82.5Z1 **Chronic embolism and thrombosis of unspecified deep veins of right distal lower extremity** HCC

I82.5Z2 **Chronic embolism and thrombosis of unspecified deep veins of left distal lower extremity** HCC

I82.5Z3 **Chronic embolism and thrombosis of unspecified deep veins of distal lower extremity, bilateral** HCC

I82.5Z9 **Chronic embolism and thrombosis of unspecified deep veins of unspecified distal lower extremity** HCC

I82.6 **Acute embolism and thrombosis of veins of upper extremity**

I82.60 **Acute embolism and thrombosis of unspecified veins of upper extremity**

I82.601 **Acute embolism and thrombosis of unspecified veins of right upper extremity**

I82.602 **Acute embolism and thrombosis of unspecified veins of left upper extremity**

I82.603 **Acute embolism and thrombosis of unspecified veins of upper extremity, bilateral**

I82.609 **Acute embolism and thrombosis of unspecified veins of unspecified upper extremity**

I82.61 **Acute embolism and thrombosis of superficial veins of upper extremity**
Acute embolism and thrombosis of antecubital vein
Acute embolism and thrombosis of basilic vein
Acute embolism and thrombosis of cephalic vein

I82.611 **Acute embolism and thrombosis of superficial veins of right upper extremity**

I82.612 **Acute embolism and thrombosis of superficial veins of left upper extremity**

I82.613 **Acute embolism and thrombosis of superficial veins of upper extremity, bilateral**

I82.619 **Acute embolism and thrombosis of superficial veins of unspecified upper extremity**

I82.62 **Acute embolism and thrombosis of deep veins of upper extremity**
Acute embolism and thrombosis of brachial vein
Acute embolism and thrombosis of radial vein
Acute embolism and thrombosis of ulnar vein

I82.621 **Acute embolism and thrombosis of deep veins of right upper extremity** HCC

I82.622 **Acute embolism and thrombosis of deep veins of left upper extremity** HCC

I82.623 **Acute embolism and thrombosis of deep veins of upper extremity, bilateral** HCC

I82.629 **Acute embolism and thrombosis of deep veins of unspecified upper extremity** HCC

I82.7 **Chronic embolism and thrombosis of veins of upper extremity**
Use additional code, if applicable, for associated long-term (current) use of anticoagulants (Z79.01)
EXCLUDES 1 *personal history of venous embolism and thrombosis (Z86.718)*

I82.70 **Chronic embolism and thrombosis of unspecified veins of upper extremity**

I82.701 **Chronic embolism and thrombosis of unspecified veins of right upper extremity**

I82.702 **Chronic embolism and thrombosis of unspecified veins of left upper extremity**

I82.703 **Chronic embolism and thrombosis of unspecified veins of upper extremity, bilateral**

I82.709 **Chronic embolism and thrombosis of unspecified veins of unspecified upper extremity**

I82.71 **Chronic embolism and thrombosis of superficial veins of upper extremity**
Chronic embolism and thrombosis of antecubital vein
Chronic embolism and thrombosis of basilic vein
Chronic embolism and thrombosis of cephalic vein

I82.711 **Chronic embolism and thrombosis of superficial veins of right upper extremity**

I82.712 **Chronic embolism and thrombosis of superficial veins of left upper extremity**

I82.713 **Chronic embolism and thrombosis of superficial veins of upper extremity, bilateral**

I82.719 **Chronic embolism and thrombosis of superficial veins of unspecified upper extremity**

I82.72 **Chronic embolism and thrombosis of deep veins of upper extremity**
Chronic embolism and thrombosis of brachial vein
Chronic embolism and thrombosis of radial vein
Chronic embolism and thrombosis of ulnar vein

I82.721 **Chronic embolism and thrombosis of deep veins of right upper extremity** HCC

I82.722 **Chronic embolism and thrombosis of deep veins of left upper extremity** HCC

I82.723 **Chronic embolism and thrombosis of deep veins of upper extremity, bilateral** HCC

I82.729 **Chronic embolism and thrombosis of deep veins of unspecified upper extremity** HCC

I82.A **Embolism and thrombosis of axillary vein**

I82.A1 **Acute embolism and thrombosis of axillary vein**

I82.A11 **Acute embolism and thrombosis of right axillary vein** HCC

I82.A12 **Acute embolism and thrombosis of left axillary vein** HCC

I82.A13 **Acute embolism and thrombosis of axillary vein, bilateral** HCC

I82.A19 **Acute embolism and thrombosis of unspecified axillary vein** HCC

I82.A2 **Chronic embolism and thrombosis of axillary vein**

I82.A21 **Chronic embolism and thrombosis of right axillary vein** HCC

I82.A22 **Chronic embolism and thrombosis of left axillary vein** HCC

I82.A23 **Chronic embolism and thrombosis of axillary vein, bilateral** HCC

I82.A29 **Chronic embolism and thrombosis of unspecified axillary vein** HCC

I82.B **Embolism and thrombosis of subclavian vein**

I82.B1 **Acute embolism and thrombosis of subclavian vein**

I82.B11 **Acute embolism and thrombosis of right subclavian vein** HCC

I82.B12 **Acute embolism and thrombosis of left subclavian vein** HCC

I82.B13 **Acute embolism and thrombosis of subclavian vein, bilateral** HCC

I82.B19 **Acute embolism and thrombosis of unspecified subclavian vein** HCC

I82.B2 **Chronic embolism and thrombosis of subclavian vein**

I82.B21 Chronic embolism and thrombosis of right subclavian vein HCC
I82.B22 Chronic embolism and thrombosis of left subclavian vein HCC
I82.B23 Chronic embolism and thrombosis of subclavian vein, bilateral HCC
I82.B29 Chronic embolism and thrombosis of unspecified subclavian vein HCC

I82.C Embolism and thrombosis of internal jugular vein

I82.C1 Acute embolism and thrombosis of internal jugular vein
I82.C11 Acute embolism and thrombosis of right internal jugular vein HCC
I82.C12 Acute embolism and thrombosis of left internal jugular vein HCC
I82.C13 Acute embolism and thrombosis of internal jugular vein, bilateral HCC
I82.C19 Acute embolism and thrombosis of unspecified internal jugular vein HCC

I82.C2 Chronic embolism and thrombosis of internal jugular vein
I82.C21 Chronic embolism and thrombosis of right internal jugular vein HCC
I82.C22 Chronic embolism and thrombosis of left internal jugular vein HCC
I82.C23 Chronic embolism and thrombosis of internal jugular vein, bilateral HCC
I82.C29 Chronic embolism and thrombosis of unspecified internal jugular vein HCC

I82.8 Embolism and thrombosis of other specified veins
Use additional code, if applicable, for associated long-term (current) use of anticoagulants (Z79.01)

I82.81 Embolism and thrombosis of superficial veins of lower extremities
Embolism and thrombosis of saphenous vein (greater) (lesser)
I82.811 Embolism and thrombosis of superficial veins of right lower extremity
I82.812 Embolism and thrombosis of superficial veins of left lower extremity
I82.813 Embolism and thrombosis of superficial veins of lower extremities, bilateral
I82.819 Embolism and thrombosis of superficial veins of unspecified lower extremity

I82.89 Embolism and thrombosis of other specified veins
I82.890 Acute embolism and thrombosis of other specified veins
I82.891 Chronic embolism and thrombosis of other specified veins

I82.9 Embolism and thrombosis of unspecified vein
I82.90 Acute embolism and thrombosis of unspecified vein
Embolism of vein NOS
Thrombosis (vein) NOS
I82.91 Chronic embolism and thrombosis of unspecified vein

I83 Varicose veins of lower extremities

EXCLUDES 1 *varicose veins complicating pregnancy (O22.0-)*
varicose veins complicating the puerperium (O87.4)

CODING TIP✓ **Documentation:** When assigning a code from I83.-, coders should assign the most specific code applicable, but cannot assume a specific code. A relationship between a lower extremity wound and varicosity must be stated in the clinical record as a cause and effect relationship by the patient's physician in order to assign a code from I83.2- or I83.0-. Inflammation should not be assumed to be related to varicosities but should be verified by a physician as related before assigning a code from category I83.1-. An additional code from category L97.- should be assigned to report the severity of the ulceration.

I83.0 Varicose veins of lower extremities with ulcer
Use additional code to identify severity of ulcer (L97.-)

I83.00 Varicose veins of unspecified lower extremity with ulcer
I83.001 Varicose veins of unspecified lower extremity with ulcer of thigh A HCC
I83.002 Varicose veins of unspecified lower extremity with ulcer of calf A HCC
I83.003 Varicose veins of unspecified lower extremity with ulcer of ankle A HCC
I83.004 Varicose veins of unspecified lower extremity with ulcer of heel and midfoot A HCC
Varicose veins of unspecified lower extremity with ulcer of plantar surface of midfoot
I83.005 Varicose veins of unspecified lower extremity with ulcer other part of foot A HCC
Varicose veins of unspecified lower extremity with ulcer of toe
I83.008 Varicose veins of unspecified lower extremity with ulcer other part of lower leg A HCC
I83.009 Varicose veins of unspecified lower extremity with ulcer of unspecified site A HCC

I83.01 Varicose veins of right lower extremity with ulcer
I83.011 Varicose veins of right lower extremity with ulcer of thigh A HCC
I83.012 Varicose veins of right lower extremity with ulcer of calf A HCC
I83.013 Varicose veins of right lower extremity with ulcer of ankle A HCC
I83.014 Varicose veins of right lower extremity with ulcer of heel and midfoot A HCC
Varicose veins of right lower extremity with ulcer of plantar surface of midfoot
I83.015 Varicose veins of right lower extremity with ulcer other part of foot A HCC
Varicose veins of right lower extremity with ulcer of toe
I83.018 Varicose veins of right lower extremity with ulcer other part of lower leg A HCC
I83.019 Varicose veins of right lower extremity with ulcer of unspecified site A HCC

I83.02 Varicose veins of left lower extremity with ulcer
I83.021 Varicose veins of left lower extremity with ulcer of thigh A HCC
I83.022 Varicose veins of left lower extremity with ulcer of calf A HCC
I83.023 Varicose veins of left lower extremity with ulcer of ankle A HCC
I83.024 Varicose veins of left lower extremity with ulcer of heel and midfoot A HCC
Varicose veins of left lower extremity with ulcer of plantar surface of midfoot
I83.025 Varicose veins of left lower extremity with ulcer other part of foot A HCC
Varicose veins of left lower extremity with ulcer of toe
I83.028 Varicose veins of left lower extremity with ulcer other part of lower leg A HCC
I83.029 Varicose veins of left lower extremity with ulcer of unspecified site A HCC

I83.1 Varicose veins of lower extremities with inflammation

CODING TIP✓ **Documentation:** Do not assume inflammation of the lower extremities to be related to varicosities when present. A cause and effect relationship should be confirmed in order to assign a code from category I83.1-.

I83.10 Varicose veins of unspecified lower extremity with inflammation A
I83.11 Varicose veins of right lower extremity with inflammation A
I83.12 Varicose veins of left lower extremity with inflammation A

I83.2 Varicose veins of lower extremities with both ulcer and inflammation
Use additional code to identify severity of ulcer (L97.-)

CODING TIP✓ If the clinical record reports a confirmed diagnosis of ulcers due to varicosity (condition classifiable to I83.0), as well as inflammation due to varicosity (condition classifiable to I83.1-), then a code from category I83.2- should be reported instead. An additional code is required to indicate the severity of the ulcer.

6 I83.20 **Varicose veins of unspecified lower extremity with both ulcer and inflammation**

I83.201 **Varicose veins of unspecified lower extremity with both ulcer of thigh and inflammation** A HCC

I83.202 **Varicose veins of unspecified lower extremity with both ulcer of calf and inflammation** A HCC

I83.203 **Varicose veins of unspecified lower extremity with both ulcer of ankle and inflammation** A HCC

I83.204 **Varicose veins of unspecified lower extremity with both ulcer of heel and midfoot and inflammation** A HCC
Varicose veins of unspecified lower extremity with both ulcer of plantar surface of midfoot and inflammation

I83.205 **Varicose veins of unspecified lower extremity with both ulcer other part of foot and inflammation** A HCC
Varicose veins of unspecified lower extremity with both ulcer of toe and inflammation

I83.208 **Varicose veins of unspecified lower extremity with both ulcer of other part of lower extremity and inflammation** A HCC

I83.209 **Varicose veins of unspecified lower extremity with both ulcer of unspecified site and inflammation** A HCC

6 I83.21 **Varicose veins of right lower extremity with both ulcer and inflammation**

I83.211 **Varicose veins of right lower extremity with both ulcer of thigh and inflammation** A HCC

I83.212 **Varicose veins of right lower extremity with both ulcer of calf and inflammation** A HCC

I83.213 **Varicose veins of right lower extremity with both ulcer of ankle and inflammation** A HCC

I83.214 **Varicose veins of right lower extremity with both ulcer of heel and midfoot and inflammation** A HCC
Varicose veins of right lower extremity with both ulcer of plantar surface of midfoot and inflammation

I83.215 **Varicose veins of right lower extremity with both ulcer other part of foot and inflammation** A HCC
Varicose veins of right lower extremity with both ulcer of toe and inflammation

I83.218 **Varicose veins of right lower extremity with both ulcer of other part of lower extremity and inflammation** A HCC

I83.219 **Varicose veins of right lower extremity with both ulcer of unspecified site and inflammation** A HCC

6 I83.22 **Varicose veins of left lower extremity with both ulcer and inflammation**

I83.221 **Varicose veins of left lower extremity with both ulcer of thigh and inflammation** A HCC

I83.222 **Varicose veins of left lower extremity with both ulcer of calf and inflammation** A HCC

I83.223 **Varicose veins of left lower extremity with both ulcer of ankle and inflammation** A HCC

I83.224 **Varicose veins of left lower extremity with both ulcer of heel and midfoot and inflammation** A HCC
Varicose veins of left lower extremity with both ulcer of plantar surface of midfoot and inflammation

I83.225 **Varicose veins of left lower extremity with both ulcer other part of foot and inflammation** A HCC
Varicose veins of left lower extremity with both ulcer of toe and inflammation

I83.228 **Varicose veins of left lower extremity with both ulcer of other part of lower extremity and inflammation** A HCC

I83.229 **Varicose veins of left lower extremity with both ulcer of unspecified site and inflammation** A HCC

5 I83.8 **Varicose veins of lower extremities with other complications**

6 I83.81 **Varicose veins of lower extremities with pain**

I83.811 **Varicose veins of right lower extremity with pain** A

I83.812 **Varicose veins of left lower extremity with pain** A

I83.813 **Varicose veins of bilateral lower extremities with pain** A

I83.819 **Varicose veins of unspecified lower extremity with pain** A

6 I83.89 **Varicose veins of lower extremities with other complications**
Varicose veins of lower extremities with edema
Varicose veins of lower extremities with swelling

I83.891 **Varicose veins of right lower extremity with other complications** A

I83.892 **Varicose veins of left lower extremity with other complications** A

I83.893 **Varicose veins of bilateral lower extremities with other complications** A

I83.899 **Varicose veins of unspecified lower extremity with other complications** A

5 I83.9 **Asymptomatic varicose veins of lower extremities**
Phlebectasia of lower extremities
Varicose veins of lower extremities
Varix of lower extremities

Varicose veins

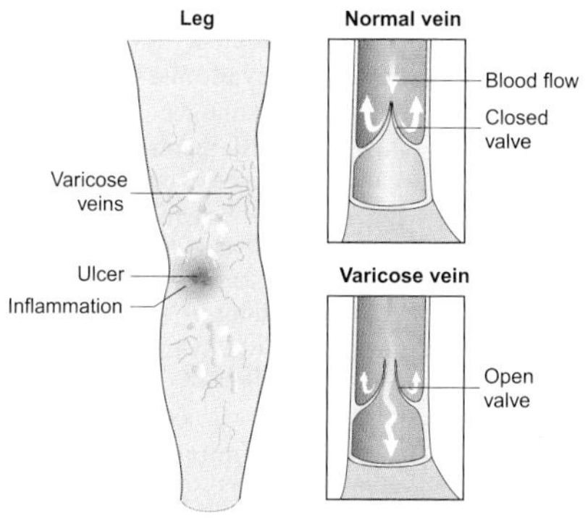

I83.90 **Asymptomatic varicose veins of unspecified lower extremity** A
Varicose veins NOS

I83.91 **Asymptomatic varicose veins of right lower extremity** A

I83.92 **Asymptomatic varicose veins of left lower extremity** A

I83.93 **Asymptomatic varicose veins of bilateral lower extremities** A

4 I85 **Esophageal varices**
Use additional code to identify:
alcohol abuse and dependence (F10.-)

CODING TIP ✓ Esophageal varices are coded to vascular disorders, rather than gastrointestinal disorders, due to the nature of their pathophysiology. Bleeding varices can be life-threatening and cause additional complex cardiovascular complications.

5 I85.0 **Esophageal varices**
Idiopathic esophageal varices
Primary esophageal varices

I85.00 **Esophageal varices without bleeding** HCC
Esophageal varices NOS

CODING TIP ✓ When the clinical record does not specify bleeding or absence of bleeding in a patient with esophageal varices, assign code I85.00, when the varices are not specified as related to any other cause.

I85.01 **Esophageal varices with bleeding** HCC

I85.1 **Secondary esophageal varices**
Esophageal varices secondary to alcoholic liver disease
Esophageal varices secondary to cirrhosis of liver
Esophageal varices secondary to schistosomiasis
Esophageal varices secondary to toxic liver disease
Code first:
underlying disease

I85.10 **Secondary esophageal varices without bleeding** HCC

I85.11 **Secondary esophageal varices with bleeding** HCC

I86 Varicose veins of other sites

EXCLUDES 1 *varicose veins of unspecified site (I83.9-)*

EXCLUDES 2 *retinal varices (H35.0-)*

I86.0 **Sublingual varices**

I86.1 **Scrotal varices** ♂
Varicocele

I86.2 **Pelvic varices**

I86.3 **Vulval varices** ♀
EXCLUDES 1 *vulval varices complicating childbirth and the puerperium (O87.8)*
vulval varices complicating pregnancy (O22.1-)

I86.4 **Gastric varices**

I86.8 **Varicose veins of other specified sites** A
Varicose ulcer of nasal septum

I87 Other disorders of veins

I87.0 **Postthrombotic syndrome**
Chronic venous hypertension due to deep vein thrombosis
Postphlebitic syndrome
EXCLUDES 1 *chronic venous hypertension without deep vein thrombosis (I87.3-)*

I87.00 **Postthrombotic syndrome without complications**
Asymptomatic Postthrombotic syndrome

I87.001 **Postthrombotic syndrome without complications of right lower extremity**

I87.002 **Postthrombotic syndrome without complications of left lower extremity**

I87.003 **Postthrombotic syndrome without complications of bilateral lower extremity**

I87.009 **Postthrombotic syndrome without complications of unspecified extremity**
Postthrombotic syndrome NOS

I87.01 **Postthrombotic syndrome with ulcer**
Use additional code to specify site and severity of ulcer (L97.-)

I87.011 **Postthrombotic syndrome with ulcer of right lower extremity** HCC

I87.012 **Postthrombotic syndrome with ulcer of left lower extremity** HCC

I87.013 **Postthrombotic syndrome with ulcer of bilateral lower extremity** HCC

I87.019 **Postthrombotic syndrome with ulcer of unspecified lower extremity** HCC

I87.02 **Postthrombotic syndrome with inflammation**

I87.021 **Postthrombotic syndrome with inflammation of right lower extremity**

I87.022 **Postthrombotic syndrome with inflammation of left lower extremity**

I87.023 **Postthrombotic syndrome with inflammation of bilateral lower extremity**

I87.029 **Postthrombotic syndrome with inflammation of unspecified lower extremity**

I87.03 **Postthrombotic syndrome with ulcer and inflammation**
Use additional code to specify site and severity of ulcer (L97.-)

I87.031 **Postthrombotic syndrome with ulcer and inflammation of right lower extremity** HCC

I87.032 **Postthrombotic syndrome with ulcer and inflammation of left lower extremity** HCC

I87.033 **Postthrombotic syndrome with ulcer and inflammation of bilateral lower extremity** HCC

I87.039 **Postthrombotic syndrome with ulcer and inflammation of unspecified lower extremity** HCC

I87.09 **Postthrombotic syndrome with other complications**

I87.091 **Postthrombotic syndrome with other complications of right lower extremity**

I87.092 **Postthrombotic syndrome with other complications of left lower extremity**

I87.093 **Postthrombotic syndrome with other complications of bilateral lower extremity**

I87.099 **Postthrombotic syndrome with other complications of unspecified lower extremity**

I87.1 **Compression of vein**
Stricture of vein
Vena cava syndrome (inferior) (superior)
EXCLUDES 2 *compression of pulmonary vein (I28.8)*

I87.2 **Venous insufficiency (chronic) (peripheral)**
Stasis dermatitis
EXCLUDES 1 *stasis dermatitis with varicose veins of lower extremities (I83.1-, I83.2-)*

I87.3 **Chronic venous hypertension (idiopathic)**
Stasis edema
EXCLUDES 1 *chronic venous hypertension due to deep vein thrombosis (I87.0-)*
varicose veins of lower extremities (I83.-)

I87.30 **Chronic venous hypertension (idiopathic) without complications**
Asymptomatic chronic venous hypertension (idiopathic)

I87.301 **Chronic venous hypertension (idiopathic) without complications of right lower extremity**

I87.302 **Chronic venous hypertension (idiopathic) without complications of left lower extremity**

I87.303 **Chronic venous hypertension (idiopathic) without complications of bilateral lower extremity**

I87.309 **Chronic venous hypertension (idiopathic) without complications of unspecified lower extremity**
Chronic venous hypertension NOS

I87.31 **Chronic venous hypertension (idiopathic) with ulcer**
Use additional code to specify site and severity of ulcer (L97.-)

I87.311 **Chronic venous hypertension (idiopathic) with ulcer of right lower extremity** HCC

I87.312 **Chronic venous hypertension (idiopathic) with ulcer of left lower extremity** HCC

I87.313 **Chronic venous hypertension (idiopathic) with ulcer of bilateral lower extremity** HCC

I87.319 **Chronic venous hypertension (idiopathic) with ulcer of unspecified lower extremity** HCC

I87.32 **Chronic venous hypertension (idiopathic) with inflammation**

I87.321 **Chronic venous hypertension (idiopathic) with inflammation of right lower extremity**

I87.322 **Chronic venous hypertension (idiopathic) with inflammation of left lower extremity**

I87.323 **Chronic venous hypertension (idiopathic) with inflammation of bilateral lower extremity**

I87.329 **Chronic venous hypertension (idiopathic) with inflammation of unspecified lower extremity**

I87.33 **Chronic venous hypertension (idiopathic) with ulcer and inflammation**
Use additional code to specify site and severity of ulcer (L97.-)

I87.331 **Chronic venous hypertension (idiopathic) with ulcer and inflammation of right lower extremity** HCC

I87.332 **Chronic venous hypertension (idiopathic) with ulcer and inflammation of left lower extremity** HCC

I87.333 **Chronic venous hypertension (idiopathic) with ulcer and inflammation of bilateral lower extremity** HCC

I87.339 **Chronic venous hypertension (idiopathic) with ulcer and inflammation of unspecified lower extremity** HCC

I87.39 Chronic venous hypertension (idiopathic) with other complications

I87.391 Chronic venous hypertension (idiopathic) with other complications of right lower extremity

I87.392 Chronic venous hypertension (idiopathic) with other complications of left lower extremity

I87.393 Chronic venous hypertension (idiopathic) with other complications of bilateral lower extremity

I87.399 Chronic venous hypertension (idiopathic) with other complications of unspecified lower extremity

I87.8 Other specified disorders of veins
Phlebosclerosis
Venofibrosis

I87.9 Disorder of vein, unspecified

I88 Nonspecific lymphadenitis

EXCLUDES 1 *acute lymphadenitis, except mesenteric (L04.-)*
enlarged lymph nodes NOS (R59.-)
human immunodeficiency virus [HIV] disease resulting in generalized lymphadenopathy (B20)

I88.0 Nonspecific mesenteric lymphadenitis
Mesenteric lymphadenitis (acute)(chronic)

I88.1 Chronic lymphadenitis, except mesenteric
Adenitis
Lymphadenitis

DEFINITION Chronic enlargement of the lymphatic glands.

I88.8 Other nonspecific lymphadenitis

I88.9 Nonspecific lymphadenitis, unspecified
Lymphadenitis NOS

Nonspecific lymphadenitis, unspecified

Inflammation of one or more lymph nodes

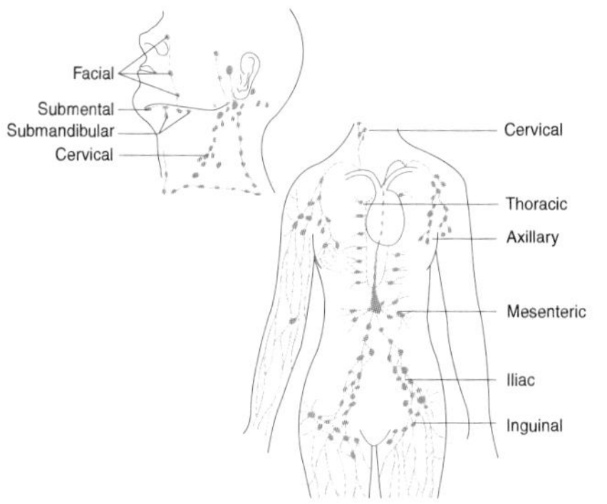

I89 Other noninfective disorders of lymphatic vessels and lymph nodes

EXCLUDES 1 *chylocele, tunica vaginalis (nonfilarial) NOS (N50.89)*
enlarged lymph nodes NOS (R59.-)
filarial chylocele (B74.-)
hereditary lymphedema (Q82.0)

I89.0 Lymphedema, not elsewhere classified
Elephantiasis (nonfilarial) NOS
Lymphangiectasis
Obliteration, lymphatic vessel
Praecox lymphedema
Secondary lymphedema

EXCLUDES 1 *postmastectomy lymphedema (I97.2)*

I89.1 Lymphangitis
Chronic lymphangitis
Lymphangitis NOS
Subacute lymphangitis

EXCLUDES 1 *acute lymphangitis (L03.-)*

I89.8 Other specified noninfective disorders of lymphatic vessels and lymph nodes
Chylocele (nonfilarial)
Chylous ascites
Chylous cyst
Lipomelanotic reticulosis
Lymph node or vessel fistula
Lymph node or vessel infarction
Lymph node or vessel rupture

I89.9 Noninfective disorder of lymphatic vessels and lymph nodes, unspecified
Disease of lymphatic vessels NOS

Other and unspecified disorders of the circulatory system (I95-I99)

I95 Hypotension

EXCLUDES 1 *cardiovascular collapse (R57.9)*
maternal hypotension syndrome (O26.5-)
nonspecific low blood pressure reading NOS (R03.1)

CODING TIP ✓ A low blood pressure reading in the absence of a diagnosis of hypotension should not be coded to I95.-. A singular low blood pressure reading with no diagnosis of hypotension should be coded to R03.1.

I95.0 Idiopathic hypotension

CODING TIP ✓ **Documentation:** Idiopathic hypotension requires a confirmed diagnosis by the patient's physician and may not be assumed. Do not assign I95.0 for a patient with hypotension of uncertain cause, with no physician report of idiopathic etiology, and do not assign for a singular low blood pressure reading.

I95.1 Orthostatic hypotension
Hypotension, postural

EXCLUDES 1 *neurogenic orthostatic hypotension [Shy-Drager] (G90.3)*
orthostatic hypotension due to drugs (I95.2)

CODING TIP ✓ Do not assign code I95.1 for orthostasis resulting from medication effects. Hypotension secondary to medication/drug effects is coded to I95.2 and is coded as an adverse effect.

DEFINITION Abnormally low blood pressure that occurs when the patient moves to a standing or upright position.

I95.2 Hypotension due to drugs
Orthostatic hypotension due to drugs
Use additional code for adverse effect, if applicable, to identify drug (T36-T50 with fifth or sixth character 5)

CODING TIP ✓ When hypotension or orthostasis is confirmed and reported in the medical record as resulting from the effects of medications or other drugs, code I95.2 should be assigned. An additional code from category T36-T50 should be assigned to identify the drug.

I95.3 Hypotension of hemodialysis
Intra-dialytic hypotension

I95.8 Other hypotension

I95.81 Postprocedural hypotension

I95.89 Other hypotension
Chronic hypotension

I95.9 Hypotension, unspecified

I96 Gangrene, not elsewhere classified HCC
Gangrenous cellulitis

EXCLUDES 1 *gangrene in atherosclerosis of native arteries of the extremities (I70.26)*
gangrene in hernia (K40.1, K40.4, K41.1, K41.4, K42.1, K43.1-, K44.1, K45.1, K46.1)
gangrene in other peripheral vascular diseases (I73.-)
gangrene of certain specified sites - see Alphabetical Index
gas gangrene (A48.0)
pyoderma gangrenosum (L88)

EXCLUDES 2 *gangrene in diabetes mellitus (E08-E13 with .52)*

CODING TIP✓ Code I96 should be assigned to indicate gangrenous cellulitis, such as in the case of gangrene in a pressure ulcer. The L89.- codes for pressure ulcers indicate that coders should "code first" any associated gangrene. In this case, I96 should be assigned. Do not use I96 to indicate gangrene in diabetes, atherosclerosis or other vascular disease, pyoderma gangrenosum, gas gangrene, or gangrene in a hernia.

DEFINITION Complication of cell death (necrosis), characterized by tissue decay, which becomes black and malodorous, caused by infection or ischemia, resulting from insufficient blood supply.

AHA: 2Q 2013, 34-35
AHA: 3Q 2017, 6

4 I97 Intraoperative and postprocedural complications and disorders of circulatory system, not elsewhere classified

EXCLUDES 2 *postprocedural shock (T81.1-)*

CODING TIP✓ **Documentation:** Codes in category I97.- are complication codes and require physician documentation and confirmation of a cause and effect relationship between the procedure and the complicated condition.

I97.0 Postcardiotomy syndrome

5 I97.1 Other postprocedural cardiac functional disturbances

EXCLUDES 2 *acute pulmonary insufficiency following thoracic surgery (J95.1)*
intraoperative cardiac functional disturbances (I97.7-)

6 I97.11 Postprocedural cardiac insufficiency

I97.110 Postprocedural cardiac insufficiency following cardiac surgery

I97.111 Postprocedural cardiac insufficiency following other surgery

6 I97.12 Postprocedural cardiac arrest

I97.120 Postprocedural cardiac arrest following cardiac surgery

I97.121 Postprocedural cardiac arrest following other surgery

6 I97.13 Postprocedural heart failure

Use additional code to identify the heart failure (I50.-)

I97.130 Postprocedural heart failure following cardiac surgery

I97.131 Postprocedural heart failure following other surgery

6 I97.19 Other postprocedural cardiac functional disturbances

Use additional code, if applicable, to further specify disorder

I97.190 Other postprocedural cardiac functional disturbances following cardiac surgery

Use additional code, if applicable, for type 4 or type 5 myocardial infarction, to further specify disorder

I97.191 Other postprocedural cardiac functional disturbances following other surgery

I97.2 Postmastectomy lymphedema syndrome A

Elephantiasis due to mastectomy
Obliteration of lymphatic vessels

CODING TIP✓ Assign code I97.2 only when lymphedema is specifically reported as related to the effects of a mastectomy.

DEFINITION Localized edema in the arm following breast and lymph node removal due to lack of lymph circulation through the chest area.

I97.3 Postprocedural hypertension

5 I97.4 Intraoperative hemorrhage and hematoma of a circulatory system organ or structure complicating a procedure

EXCLUDES 1 *intraoperative hemorrhage and hematoma of a circulatory system organ or structure due to accidental puncture and laceration during a procedure (I97.5-)*

EXCLUDES 2 *intraoperative cerebrovascular hemorrhage complicating a procedure (G97.3-)*

6 I97.41 Intraoperative hemorrhage and hematoma of a circulatory system organ or structure complicating a circulatory system procedure

I97.410 Intraoperative hemorrhage and hematoma of a circulatory system organ or structure complicating a cardiac catheterization

I97.411 Intraoperative hemorrhage and hematoma of a circulatory system organ or structure complicating a cardiac bypass

I97.418 Intraoperative hemorrhage and hematoma of a circulatory system organ or structure complicating other circulatory system procedure

I97.42 Intraoperative hemorrhage and hematoma of a circulatory system organ or structure complicating other procedure

5 I97.5 Accidental puncture and laceration of a circulatory system organ or structure during a procedure

EXCLUDES 2 *accidental puncture and laceration of brain during a procedure (G97.4-)*

I97.51 Accidental puncture and laceration of a circulatory system organ or structure during a circulatory system procedure

I97.52 Accidental puncture and laceration of a circulatory system organ or structure during other procedure

5 I97.6 Postprocedural hemorrhage, hematoma and seroma of a circulatory system organ or structure following a procedure

EXCLUDES 2 *postprocedural cerebrovascular hemorrhage complicating a procedure (G97.5-)*

AHA: 1Q 2014, 7

6 I97.61 Postprocedural hemorrhage of a circulatory system organ or structure following a circulatory system procedure

I97.610 Postprocedural hemorrhage of a circulatory system organ or structure following a cardiac catheterization

I97.611 Postprocedural hemorrhage of a circulatory system organ or structure following cardiac bypass

I97.618 Postprocedural hemorrhage of a circulatory system organ or structure following other circulatory system procedure

6 I97.62 Postprocedural hemorrhage, hematoma and seroma of a circulatory system organ or structure following other procedure

I97.620 Postprocedural hemorrhage of a circulatory system organ or structure following other procedure

I97.621 Postprocedural hematoma of a circulatory system organ or structure following other procedure

I97.622 Postprocedural seroma of a circulatory system organ or structure following other procedure

6 I97.63 Postprocedural hematoma of a circulatory system organ or structure following a circulatory system procedure

I97.630 Postprocedural hematoma of a circulatory system organ or structure following a cardiac catheterization

I97.631 Postprocedural hematoma of a circulatory system organ or structure following cardiac bypass

I97.638 Postprocedural hematoma of a circulatory system organ or structure following other circulatory system procedure

6 I97.64 Postprocedural seroma of a circulatory system organ or structure following a circulatory system procedure

I97.640 Postprocedural seroma of a circulatory system organ or structure following a cardiac catheterization

I97.641 Postprocedural seroma of a circulatory system organ or structure following cardiac bypass

I97.648 Postprocedural seroma of a circulatory system organ or structure following other circulatory system procedure

5 I97.7 Intraoperative cardiac functional disturbances

EXCLUDES 2 *acute pulmonary insufficiency following thoracic surgery (J95.1)*
postprocedural cardiac functional disturbances (I97.1-)

6 I97.71 Intraoperative cardiac arrest

I97.710 Intraoperative cardiac arrest during cardiac surgery

I97.711 Intraoperative cardiac arrest during other surgery

6 I97.79 Other intraoperative cardiac functional disturbances

Use additional code, if applicable, to further specify disorder

I97.790 Other intraoperative cardiac functional disturbances during cardiac surgery

I97.791 Other intraoperative cardiac functional disturbances during other surgery

5 I97.8 Other intraoperative and postprocedural complications and disorders of the circulatory system, not elsewhere classified

Use additional code, if applicable, to further specify disorder

6 I97.81 Intraoperative cerebrovascular infarction

I97.810 Intraoperative cerebrovascular infarction during cardiac surgery HCC

I97.811 Intraoperative cerebrovascular infarction during other surgery HCC

6 I97.82 Postprocedural cerebrovascular infarction

I97.820 Postprocedural cerebrovascular infarction following cardiac surgery HCC

I97.821 Postprocedural cerebrovascular infarction following other surgery HCC

I97.88 Other intraoperative complications of the circulatory system, not elsewhere classified

I97.89 Other postprocedural complications and disorders of the circulatory system, not elsewhere classified

4 I99 **Other and unspecified disorders of circulatory system**

I99.8 Other disorder of circulatory system

I99.9 Unspecified disorder of circulatory system

CHAPTER 10: DISEASES OF THE RESPIRATORY SYSTEM (J00-J99)

Note: When a respiratory condition is described as occurring in more than one site and is not specifically indexed, it should be classified to the lower anatomic site (e.g. tracheobronchitis to bronchitis in J40).

Use additional code, where applicable, to identify:
exposure to environmental tobacco smoke (Z77.22)
exposure to tobacco smoke in the perinatal period (P96.81)
history of tobacco dependence (Z87.891)
occupational exposure to environmental tobacco smoke (Z57.31)
tobacco dependence (F17.-)
tobacco use (Z72.0)

EXCLUDES 2 *certain conditions originating in the perinatal period (P04-P96)*
certain infectious and parasitic diseases (A00-B99)
complications of pregnancy, childbirth and the puerperium (O00-O9A)
congenital malformations, deformations and chromosomal abnormalities (Q00-Q99)
endocrine, nutritional and metabolic diseases (E00-E88)
injury, poisoning and certain other consequences of external causes (S00-T88)
neoplasms (C00-D49)
smoke inhalation (T59.81-)
symptoms, signs and abnormal clinical and laboratory findings, not elsewhere classified (R00-R94)

This chapter contains the following blocks:

J00-J06	Acute upper respiratory infections
J09-J18	Influenza and pneumonia
J20-J22	Other acute lower respiratory infections
J30-J39	Other diseases of upper respiratory tract
J40-J47	Chronic lower respiratory diseases
J60-J70	Lung diseases due to external agents
J80-J84	Other respiratory diseases principally affecting the interstitium
J85-J86	Suppurative and necrotic conditions of the lower respiratory tract
J90-J94	Other diseases of the pleura
J95	Intraoperative and postprocedural complications and disorders of respiratory system, not elsewhere classified
J96-J99	Other diseases of the respiratory system

Acute upper respiratory infections (J00-J06)

EXCLUDES 1 *chronic obstructive pulmonary disease with acute lower respiratory infection (J44.0)*
influenza virus with other respiratory manifestations (J09.X2, J10.1, J11.1)

J00 Acute nasopharyngitis [common cold]
Acute rhinitis
Coryza (acute)
Infective nasopharyngitis NOS
Infective rhinitis
Nasal catarrh, acute
Nasopharyngitis NOS

EXCLUDES 1 *acute pharyngitis (J02.-)*
acute sore throat NOS (J02.9)
pharyngitis NOS (J02.9)
rhinitis NOS (J31.0)
sore throat NOS (J02.9)

EXCLUDES 2 *allergic rhinitis (J30.1-J30.9)*
chronic pharyngitis (J31.2)
chronic rhinitis (J31.0)
chronic sore throat (J31.2)
nasopharyngitis, chronic (J31.1)
vasomotor rhinitis (J30.0)

Upper respiratory system

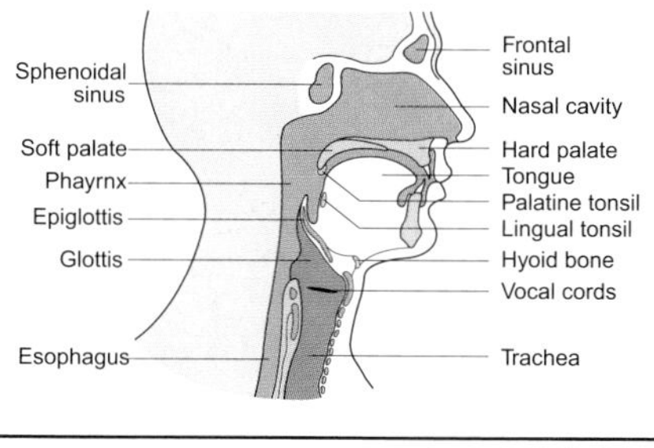

4 **J01 Acute sinusitis**

INCLUDES acute abscess of sinus
acute empyema of sinus
acute infection of sinus
acute inflammation of sinus
acute suppuration of sinus

Use additional code (B95-B97) to identify infectious agent.

EXCLUDES 1 *sinusitis NOS (J32.9)*

EXCLUDES 2 *chronic sinusitis (J32.0-J32.8)*

5 **J01.0 Acute maxillary sinusitis**
Acute antritis

Acute maxillary sinusitis

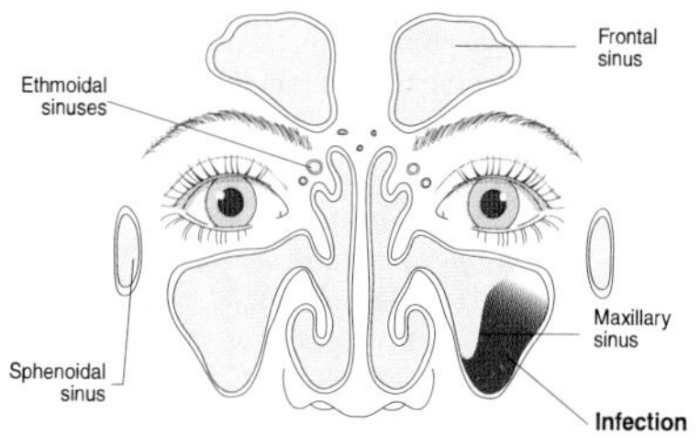

J01.00 Acute maxillary sinusitis, unspecified
J01.01 Acute recurrent maxillary sinusitis

5 **J01.1 Acute frontal sinusitis**
J01.10 Acute frontal sinusitis, unspecified
J01.11 Acute recurrent frontal sinusitis

5 **J01.2 Acute ethmoidal sinusitis**
J01.20 Acute ethmoidal sinusitis, unspecified
J01.21 Acute recurrent ethmoidal sinusitis

5 **J01.3 Acute sphenoidal sinusitis**
J01.30 Acute sphenoidal sinusitis, unspecified
J01.31 Acute recurrent sphenoidal sinusitis

5 **J01.4 Acute pansinusitis**
J01.40 Acute pansinusitis, unspecified
J01.41 Acute recurrent pansinusitis

5 **J01.8 Other acute sinusitis**
J01.80 Other acute sinusitis
Acute sinusitis involving more than one sinus but not pansinusitis
J01.81 Other acute recurrent sinusitis
Acute recurrent sinusitis involving more than one sinus but not pansinusitis

5 **J01.9 Acute sinusitis, unspecified**
J01.90 Acute sinusitis, unspecified
J01.91 Acute recurrent sinusitis, unspecified

4 **J02 Acute pharyngitis**

INCLUDES acute sore throat

EXCLUDES 1 *acute laryngopharyngitis (J06.0)*
peritonsillar abscess (J36)
pharyngeal abscess (J39.1)
retropharyngeal abscess (J39.0)

EXCLUDES 2 *chronic pharyngitis (J31.2)*

CODING TIP✓ Note the anatomical differences between pharyngitis and laryngitis. Pharyngitis involves inflammation of the pharynx, the area of the back of the throat between the tonsils and the larynx. Laryngitis involves inflammation of the vocal cords. These are inflammatory conditions, which may involve infection but indicate inflammation in different anatomical areas. Do not assume that because the patient has pharyngitis, the larynx is also inflamed.

J02.0 Streptococcal pharyngitis
Septic pharyngitis
Streptococcal sore throat

EXCLUDES 2 *scarlet fever (A38.-)*

J02.8 **Acute pharyngitis due to other specified organisms**
Use additional code (B95-B97) to identify infectious agent
EXCLUDES 1 *acute pharyngitis due to coxsackie virus (B08.5)*
acute pharyngitis due to gonococcus (A54.5)
acute pharyngitis due to herpes [simplex] virus (B00.2)
acute pharyngitis due to infectious mononucleosis (B27.-)
enteroviral vesicular pharyngitis (B08.5)

J02.9 **Acute pharyngitis, unspecified**
Gangrenous pharyngitis (acute)
Infective pharyngitis (acute) NOS
Pharyngitis (acute) NOS
Sore throat (acute) NOS
Suppurative pharyngitis (acute)
Ulcerative pharyngitis (acute)

4 J03 **Acute tonsillitis**
EXCLUDES 1 *acute sore throat (J02.-)*
hypertrophy of tonsils (J35.1)
peritonsillar abscess (J36)
sore throat NOS (J02.9)
streptococcal sore throat (J02.0)
EXCLUDES 2 *chronic tonsillitis (J35.0)*

5 J03.0 **Streptococcal tonsillitis**
J03.00 **Acute streptococcal tonsillitis, unspecified**
J03.01 **Acute recurrent streptococcal tonsillitis**

5 J03.8 **Acute tonsillitis due to other specified organisms**
Use additional code (B95-B97) to identify infectious agent.
EXCLUDES 1 *diphtheritic tonsillitis (A36.0)*
herpesviral pharyngotonsillitis (B00.2)
streptococcal tonsillitis (J03.0)
tuberculous tonsillitis (A15.8)
Vincent's tonsillitis (A69.1)
J03.80 **Acute tonsillitis due to other specified organisms**
J03.81 **Acute recurrent tonsillitis due to other specified organisms**

5 J03.9 **Acute tonsillitis, unspecified**
Follicular tonsillitis (acute)
Gangrenous tonsillitis (acute)
Infective tonsillitis (acute)
Tonsillitis (acute) NOS
Ulcerative tonsillitis (acute)
J03.90 **Acute tonsillitis, unspecified**
J03.91 **Acute recurrent tonsillitis, unspecified**

4 J04 **Acute laryngitis and tracheitis**
Use additional code (B95-B97) to identify infectious agent.
EXCLUDES 1 *acute obstructive laryngitis [croup] and epiglottitis (J05.-)*
EXCLUDES 2 *laryngismus (stridulus) (J38.5)*

J04.0 **Acute laryngitis**
Edematous laryngitis (acute)
Laryngitis (acute) NOS
Subglottic laryngitis (acute)
Suppurative laryngitis (acute)
Ulcerative laryngitis (acute)
EXCLUDES 1 *acute obstructive laryngitis (J05.0)*
EXCLUDES 2 *chronic laryngitis (J37.0)*

5 J04.1 **Acute tracheitis**
Acute viral tracheitis
Catarrhal tracheitis (acute)
Tracheitis (acute) NOS
EXCLUDES 2 *chronic tracheitis (J42)*
J04.10 **Acute tracheitis without obstruction**
J04.11 **Acute tracheitis with obstruction**

J04.2 **Acute laryngotracheitis**
Laryngotracheitis NOS
Tracheitis (acute) with laryngitis (acute)
EXCLUDES 1 *acute obstructive laryngotracheitis (J05.0)*
EXCLUDES 2 *chronic laryngotracheitis (J37.1)*

CODING TIP✓ J04.2 is a specific code and should be assigned when the patient is reported as specifically having laryngotracheitis by the physician. This involves inflammation of both the larynx and trachea.

5 J04.3 **Supraglottitis, unspecified**

CODING TIP✓ Supraglottitis is a potentially life-threatening inflammation of the supraglottic area of the airway. If airway obstruction is documented, assign J04.31.

J04.30 **Supraglottitis, unspecified, without obstruction**
J04.31 **Supraglottitis, unspecified, with obstruction**

4 J05 **Acute obstructive laryngitis [croup] and epiglottitis**
Use additional code (B95-B97) to identify infectious agent.

J05.0 **Acute obstructive laryngitis [croup]**
Obstructive laryngitis (acute) NOS
Obstructive laryngotracheitis NOS

5 J05.1 **Acute epiglottitis**
EXCLUDES 2 *epiglottitis, chronic (J37.0)*
J05.10 **Acute epiglottitis without obstruction**
Epiglottitis NOS
J05.11 **Acute epiglottitis with obstruction**

4 J06 **Acute upper respiratory infections of multiple and unspecified sites**
EXCLUDES 1 *acute respiratory infection NOS (J22)*
streptococcal pharyngitis (J02.0)

J06.0 **Acute laryngopharyngitis**
J06.9 **Acute upper respiratory infection, unspecified**
Upper respiratory disease, acute
Upper respiratory infection NOS

CODING TIP✓ Assign J06.9 for upper respiratory infection NOS only when a more specific diagnosis to identify the type of infection cannot be identified.

Influenza and pneumonia (J09-J18)

EXCLUDES 2 *allergic or eosinophilic pneumonia (J82)*
aspiration pneumonia NOS (J69.0)
meconium pneumonia (P24.01)
neonatal aspiration pneumonia (P24.-)
pneumonia due to solids and liquids (J69.-)
congenital pneumonia (P23.9)
lipid pneumonia (J69.1)
rheumatic pneumonia (I00)
ventilator associated pneumonia (J95.851)

CODING TIP✓ Influenza is not considered a lower respiratory infection for the purposes of coding COPD with J44.0. If influenza results in pneumonia, code the COPD as J44.0, and the influenza. Sequence according to the focus of care.

CODING TIP✓ Pneumonia should be coded to the specific causative organism using a combination code when a specific code is available. Evaluate all available clinical documentation and assign the most specific code for pneumonia. When the causative organism of bacterial pneumonia is known but no combination code exists, assign J15.8.

CODING TIP✓ When pneumonia is diagnosed in a patient who also has COPD, the coder should assign J44.0 (Chronic obstructive pulmonary disease with lower respiratory tract infection) and the specific code to indicate the type of pneumonia. Sequence according to the focus of care.

4 J09 **Influenza due to certain identified influenza viruses**
EXCLUDES 1 *influenza A/H1N1 (J10.-)*
influenza due to other identified influenza virus (J10.-)
influenza due to unidentified influenza virus (J11.-)
seasonal influenza due to other identified influenza virus (J10.-)
seasonal influenza due to unidentified influenza virus (J11.-)

GUIDELINES Section I.C.10.c
Code only confirmed cases of influenza due to certain identified influenza viruses (category J09), and due to other identified influenza virus (category J10) ... coding should be based on the provider's diagnostic statement that the patient has avian influenza, or other novel influenza A, for category J09, or has another particular identified strain of influenza, such as H1N1 or H3N2, but not identified as novel or variant, for category J10.

If the provider records "suspected" or "possible" or "probable" avian influenza, or novel influenza, or other identified influenza, then the appropriate influenza code from category J11, Influenza due to unidentified influenza virus, should be assigned.

CODING TIP ✓ J09 is not used for influenza type A. Influenza due to **novel** influenza A is coded to J09 along with manifestations of other respiratory, gastrointestinal and other manifestations. Use additional codes to identify the manifestations.

5 **J09.X Influenza due to identified novel influenza A virus**
Avian influenza
Bird influenza
Influenza A/H5N1
Influenza of other animal origin, not bird or swine
Swine influenza virus (viruses that normally cause infections in pigs)

J09.X1 Influenza due to identified novel influenza A virus with pneumonia HIV
Code also, if applicable, associated:
lung abscess (J85.1)
other specified type of pneumonia

J09.X2 Influenza due to identified novel influenza A virus with other respiratory manifestations
Influenza due to identified novel influenza A virus NOS
Influenza due to identified novel influenza A virus with laryngitis
Influenza due to identified novel influenza A virus with pharyngitis
Influenza due to identified novel influenza A virus with upper respiratory symptoms
Use additional code, if applicable, for associated:
pleural effusion (J91.8)
sinusitis (J01.-)

J09.X3 Influenza due to identified novel influenza A virus with gastrointestinal manifestations
Influenza due to identified novel influenza A virus gastroenteritis
EXCLUDES 1 *'intestinal flu' [viral gastroenteritis] (A08.-)*

J09.X9 Influenza due to identified novel influenza A virus with other manifestations
Influenza due to identified novel influenza A virus with encephalopathy
Influenza due to identified novel influenza A virus with myocarditis
Influenza due to identified novel influenza A virus with otitis media
Use additional code to identify manifestation

4 **J10 Influenza due to other identified influenza virus**
EXCLUDES 1 *influenza due to avian influenza virus (J09.X-)*
influenza due to swine flu (J09.X-)
influenza due to unidentifed influenza virus (J11.-)

GUIDELINES Section I.C.10.c
Code only confirmed cases of influenza due to certain identified influenza viruses (category J09), and due to other identified influenza virus (category J10) ... coding should be based on the provider's diagnostic statement that the patient has avian influenza, or other novel influenza A, for category J09, or has another particular identified strain of influenza, such as H1N1 or H3N2, but not identified as novel or variant, for category J10.

If the provider records "suspected" or "possible" or "probable" avian influenza, or novel influenza, or other identified influenza, then the appropriate influenza code from category J11, Influenza due to unidentified influenza virus, should be assigned.

5 **J10.0 Influenza due to other identified influenza virus with pneumonia**
Code also:
associated lung abscess, if applicable (J85.1)

J10.00 Influenza due to other identified influenza virus with unspecified type of pneumonia

J10.01 Influenza due to other identified influenza virus with the same other identified influenza virus pneumonia

J10.08 Influenza due to other identified influenza virus with other specified pneumonia HIV
Code also:
other specified type of pneumonia
AHA: 4Q 2017, 75

J10.1 Influenza due to other identified influenza virus with other respiratory manifestations
Influenza due to other identified influenza virus NOS
Influenza due to other identified influenza virus with laryngitis
Influenza due to other identified influenza virus with pharyngitis
Influenza due to other identified influenza virus with upper respiratory symptoms
Use additional code for associated pleural effusion, if applicable (J91.8)
Use additional code for associated sinusitis, if applicable (J01.-)
AHA: 3Q 2016, 11

J10.2 Influenza due to other identified influenza virus with gastrointestinal manifestations
Influenza due to other identified influenza virus gastroenteritis
EXCLUDES 1 *'intestinal flu' [viral gastroenteritis] (A08.-)*

5 **J10.8 Influenza due to other identified influenza virus with other manifestations**

J10.81 Influenza due to other identified influenza virus with encephalopathy

J10.82 Influenza due to other identified influenza virus with myocarditis

J10.83 Influenza due to other identified influenza virus with otitis media
Use additional code for any associated perforated tympanic membrane (H72.-)

J10.89 Influenza due to other identified influenza virus with other manifestations
Use additional codes to identify the manifestations

4 **J11 Influenza due to unidentified influenza virus**

5 **J11.0 Influenza due to unidentified influenza virus with pneumonia**
Code also:
associated lung abscess, if applicable (J85.1)

J11.00 Influenza due to unidentified influenza virus with unspecified type of pneumonia
Influenza with pneumonia NOS
AHA: 3Q 2016, 12

J11.08 Influenza due to unidentified influenza virus with specified pneumonia
Code also:
other specified type of pneumonia

J11.1 Influenza due to unidentified influenza virus with other respiratory manifestations
Influenza NOS
Influenzal laryngitis NOS
Influenzal pharyngitis NOS
Influenza with upper respiratory symptoms NOS
Use additional code for associated pleural effusion, if applicable (J91.8)
Use additional code for associated sinusitis, if applicable (J01.-)

J11.2 Influenza due to unidentified influenza virus with gastrointestinal manifestations
Influenza gastroenteritis NOS
EXCLUDES 1 *'intestinal flu' [viral gastroenteritis] (A08.-)*

5 **J11.8 Influenza due to unidentified influenza virus with other manifestations**

J11.81 Influenza due to unidentified influenza virus with encephalopathy
Influenzal encephalopathy NOS

J11.82 **Influenza due to unidentified influenza virus with myocarditis**
Influenzal myocarditis NOS

J11.83 **Influenza due to unidentified influenza virus with otitis media**
Influenzal otitis media NOS
Use additional code for any associated perforated tympanic membrane (H72.-)

J11.89 **Influenza due to unidentified influenza virus with other manifestations**
Use additional codes to identify the manifestations

4 J12 **Viral pneumonia, not elsewhere classified**
INCLUDES bronchopneumonia due to viruses other than influenza viruses
Code first:
associated influenza, if applicable (J09.X1, J10.0-, J11.0-)
Code also:
associated abscess, if applicable (J85.1)
EXCLUDES 1 *aspiration pneumonia due to anesthesia during labor and delivery (O74.0)*
aspiration pneumonia due to anesthesia during pregnancy (O29)
aspiration pneumonia due to anesthesia during puerperium (O89.0)
aspiration pneumonia due to solids and liquids (J69.-)
aspiration pneumonia NOS (J69.0)
congenital pneumonia (P23.0)
congenital rubella pneumonitis (P35.0)
interstitial pneumonia NOS (J84.9)
lipid pneumonia (J69.1)
neonatal aspiration pneumonia (P24.-)

J12.0 **Adenoviral pneumonia**
J12.1 **Respiratory syncytial virus pneumonia**
J12.2 **Parainfluenza virus pneumonia**
J12.3 **Human metapneumovirus pneumonia** HIV
5 J12.8 **Other viral pneumonia**
J12.81 **Pneumonia due to SARS-associated coronavirus** HIV
Severe acute respiratory syndrome NOS
J12.89 **Other viral pneumonia** HIV
J12.9 **Viral pneumonia, unspecified** HIV

J13 **Pneumonia due to Streptococcus pneumoniae** HCC HIV
Bronchopneumonia due to S. pneumoniae
Code first:
associated influenza, if applicable (J09.X1, J10.0-, J11.0-)
Code also:
associated abscess, if applicable (J85.1)
EXCLUDES 1 *congenital pneumonia due to S. pneumoniae (P23.6)*
lobar pneumonia, unspecified organism (J18.1)
pneumonia due to other streptococci (J15.3-J15.4)

Pneumonia due to *S. pneumoniae*

A culture has determined the pneumonia is caused by ***Streptococcus pneumoniae***

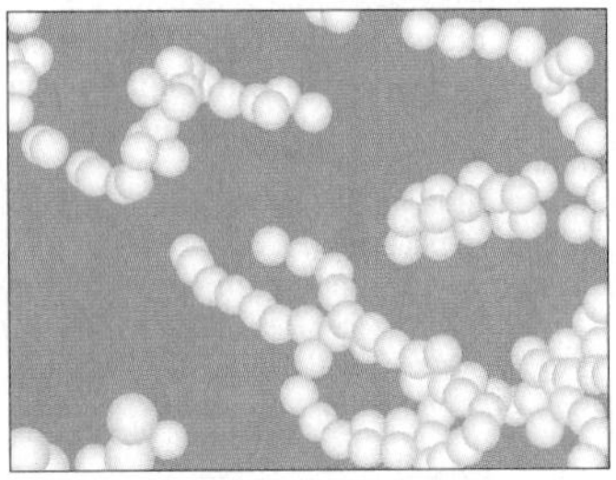

Streptococcus bacteria

J14 **Pneumonia due to Hemophilus influenzae** HCC HIV
Bronchopneumonia due to H. influenzae
Code first:
associated influenza, if applicable (J09.X1, J10.0-, J11.0-)
Code also:
associated abscess, if applicable (J85.1)
EXCLUDES 1 *congenital pneumonia due to H. influenzae (P23.6)*

4 J15 **Bacterial pneumonia, not elsewhere classified**
INCLUDES bronchopneumonia due to bacteria other than S. pneumoniae and H. influenzae
Code first:
associated influenza, if applicable (J09.X1, J10.0-, J11.0-)
Code also:
associated abscess, if applicable (J85.1)
EXCLUDES 1 *chlamydial pneumonia (J16.0)*
congenital pneumonia (P23.-)
Legionnaires' disease (A48.1)
spirochetal pneumonia (A69.8)

J15.0 **Pneumonia due to Klebsiella pneumoniae** HCC HIV
J15.1 **Pneumonia due to Pseudomonas** HCC HIV
5 J15.2 **Pneumonia due to staphylococcus**
J15.20 **Pneumonia due to staphylococcus, unspecified** HCC HIV
6 J15.21 **Pneumonia due to staphylococcus aureus**
J15.211 **Pneumonia due to Methicillin susceptible Staphylococcus aureus** HCC HIV
MSSA pneumonia
Pneumonia due to Staphylococcus aureus NOS
J15.212 **Pneumonia due to Methicillin resistant Staphylococcus aureus** HCC HIV

GUIDELINES **Section I.C.1.e.1)**
When a patient is diagnosed with an infection that is due to methicillin resistant Staphylococcus aureus (MRSA), and that infection has a combination code that includes the causal organism (e.g., sepsis, pneumonia) assign the appropriate combination code for the condition (e.g., code A41.02, Sepsis due to Methicillin resistant Staphylococcus aureus or code J15.212, Pneumonia due to Methicillin resistant Staphylococcus aureus). Do not assign code B95.62, Methicillin resistant Staphylococcus aureus infection as the cause of diseases classified elsewhere, as an additional code because the combination code includes the type of infection and the MRSA organism. Do not assign a code from subcategory Z16.11, Resistance to penicillins, as an additional diagnosis.

J15.29 **Pneumonia due to other staphylococcus** HCC HIV
J15.3 **Pneumonia due to streptococcus, group B** HCC HIV
J15.4 **Pneumonia due to other streptococci** HCC HIV
EXCLUDES 1 *pneumonia due to streptococcus, group B (J15.3)*
pneumonia due to Streptococcus pneumoniae (J13)
J15.5 **Pneumonia due to Escherichia coli** HCC HIV
J15.6 **Pneumonia due to other Gram-negative bacteria** HCC HIV
Pneumonia due to other aerobic Gram-negative bacteria
Pneumonia due to Serratia marcescens
J15.7 **Pneumonia due to Mycoplasma pneumoniae**
J15.8 **Pneumonia due to other specified bacteria** HCC HIV

CODING TIP ✓ Do not assign code J15.8 for unspecified pneumonia. J15.8 indicates pneumonia with a specified organism for which no combination code exists.

J15.9 **Unspecified bacterial pneumonia** HIV
Pneumonia due to gram-positive bacteria
AHA: 4Q 2017, 75

J16 Pneumonia due to other infectious organisms, not elsewhere classified

Code first:
associated influenza, if applicable (J09.X1, J10.0-, J11.0-)
Code also:
associated abscess, if applicable (J85.1)

EXCLUDES 1 *congenital pneumonia (P23.-)*
ornithosis (A70)
pneumocystosis (B59)
pneumonia NOS (J18.9)

J16.0 Chlamydial pneumonia

J16.8 Pneumonia due to other specified infectious organisms

J17 *Pneumonia in diseases classified elsewhere*

Code first underlying disease, such as:
Q fever (A78)
rheumatic fever (I00)
schistosomiasis (B65.0-B65.9)

EXCLUDES 1 *candidial pneumonia (B37.1)*
chlamydial pneumonia (J16.0)
gonorrheal pneumonia (A54.84)
histoplasmosis pneumonia (B39.0-B39.2)
measles pneumonia (B05.2)
nocardiosis pneumonia (A43.0)
pneumocystosis (B59)
pneumonia due to Pneumocystis carinii (B59)
pneumonia due to Pneumocystis jiroveci (B59)
pneumonia in actinomycosis (A42.0)
pneumonia in anthrax (A22.1)
pneumonia in ascariasis (B77.81)
pneumonia in aspergillosis (B44.0-B44.1)
pneumonia in coccidioidomycosis (B38.0-B38.2)
pneumonia in cytomegalovirus disease (B25.0)
pneumonia in toxoplasmosis (B58.3)
rubella pneumonia (B06.81)
salmonella pneumonia (A02.22)
spirochetal infection NEC with pneumonia (A69.8)
tularemia pneumonia (A21.2)
typhoid fever with pneumonia (A01.03)
varicella pneumonia (B01.2)
whooping cough with pneumonia (A37 with fifth-character 1)

J18 Pneumonia, unspecified organism

Code first:
associated influenza, if applicable (J09.X1, J10.0-, J11.0-)

EXCLUDES 1 *abscess of lung with pneumonia (J85.1)*
aspiration pneumonia due to anesthesia during labor and delivery (O74.0)
aspiration pneumonia due to anesthesia during pregnancy (O29)
aspiration pneumonia due to anesthesia during puerperium (O89.0)
aspiration pneumonia due to solids and liquids (J69.-)
aspiration pneumonia NOS (J69.0)
congenital pneumonia (P23.0)
drug-induced interstitial lung disorder (J70.2-J70.4)
interstitial pneumonia NOS (J84.9)
lipid pneumonia (J69.1)
neonatal aspiration pneumonia (P24.-)
pneumonitis due to external agents (J67-J70)
pneumonitis due to fumes and vapors (J68.0)
usual interstitial pneumonia (J84.17)

J18.0 Bronchopneumonia, unspecified organism

EXCLUDES 1 *hypostatic bronchopneumonia (J18.2)*
lipid pneumonia (J69.1)

EXCLUDES 2 *acute bronchiolitis (J21.-)*
chronic bronchiolitis (J44.9)

J18.1 Lobar pneumonia, unspecified organism HCC HIV

AHA: 3Q 2016, 15-16
AHA: 1Q 2017, 26

J18.2 Hypostatic pneumonia, unspecified organism

Hypostatic bronchopneumonia
Passive pneumonia

J18.8 Other pneumonia, unspecified organism HIV

J18.9 Pneumonia, unspecified organism HIV

CODING TIP ✓ Do not assign J18.9 when the causative organism or underlying cause of pneumonia is reported in the clinical record. If the organism or cause of pneumonia is known, a combination code should be assigned. When pneumonia is diagnosed in a patient who also has COPD, the coder should assign J44.0 (COPD with lower respiratory tract infection) and the type of pneumonia, and sequence according to the focus of care.

AHA: 4Q 2012, 94
AHA: 3Q 2014, 4
AHA: 3Q 2016, 15-16
AHA: 1Q 2017, 26

Other acute lower respiratory infections (J20-J22)

EXCLUDES 2 *chronic obstructive pulmonary disease with acute lower respiratory infection (J44.0)*

CODING TIP ✓ The presence of conditions in J20-J22 along with COPD, require the COPD be coded with J44.0 with the lower respiratory infection code. Sequence according to the focus of care.

CODING TIP ✓ **Documentation:** Be cautious to differentiate the diagnostic differences between bronchitis and bronchiolitis. These are not interchangeable and are not the same disease process. Bronchitis is inflammation of the mucous membranes of the bronchi, while bronchiolitis involves inflammation of the smaller bronchioles which lead directly to the lungs. Bronchiolitis is more commonly diagnosed in children.

J20 Acute bronchitis

INCLUDES acute and subacute bronchitis (with) bronchospasm
acute and subacute bronchitis (with) tracheitis
acute and subacute bronchitis (with) tracheobronchitis, acute
acute and subacute fibrinous bronchitis
acute and subacute membranous bronchitis
acute and subacute purulent bronchitis
acute and subacute septic bronchitis

EXCLUDES 1 *bronchitis NOS (J40)*
tracheobronchitis NOS (J40)

EXCLUDES 2 *acute bronchitis with bronchiectasis (J47.0)*
acute bronchitis with chronic obstructive asthma (J44.0)
acute bronchitis with chronic obstructive pulmonary disease (J44.0)
allergic bronchitis NOS (J45.909-)
bronchitis due to chemicals, fumes and vapors (J68.0)
chronic bronchitis NOS (J42)
chronic mucopurulent bronchitis (J41.1)
chronic obstructive bronchitis (J44.-)
chronic obstructive tracheobronchitis (J44.-)
chronic simple bronchitis (J41.0)
chronic tracheobronchitis (J42)

J20.0 Acute bronchitis due to Mycoplasma pneumoniae

J20.1 Acute bronchitis due to Hemophilus influenzae

J20.2 Acute bronchitis due to streptococcus

J20.3 Acute bronchitis due to coxsackievirus

J20.4 Acute bronchitis due to parainfluenza virus

J20.5 Acute bronchitis due to respiratory syncytial virus

J20.6 Acute bronchitis due to rhinovirus

AHA: 3Q 2016, 10

J20.7 Acute bronchitis due to echovirus

J20.8 Acute bronchitis due to other specified organisms

AHA: 3Q 2016, 11

J20.9 Acute bronchitis, unspecified

AHA: 3Q 2016, 15-16
AHA: 1Q 2017, 26

J21 Acute bronchiolitis

INCLUDES acute bronchiolitis with bronchospasm

EXCLUDES 2 *respiratory bronchiolitis interstitial lung disease (J84.115)*

J21.0 Acute bronchiolitis due to respiratory syncytial virus

J21.1 Acute bronchiolitis due to human metapneumovirus

J21.8 Acute bronchiolitis due to other specified organisms

J21.9 Acute bronchiolitis, unspecified
Bronchiolitis (acute)
EXCLUDES 1 *chronic bronchiolitis (J44.-)*

J22 Unspecified acute lower respiratory infection
Acute (lower) respiratory (tract) infection NOS
EXCLUDES 1 *upper respiratory infection (acute) (J06.9)*

Other diseases of upper respiratory tract (J30-J39)

4 J30 Vasomotor and allergic rhinitis
INCLUDES spasmodic rhinorrhea
EXCLUDES 1 *allergic rhinitis with asthma (bronchial) (J45.909)*
rhinitis NOS (J31.0)

J30.0 Vasomotor rhinitis

J30.1 Allergic rhinitis due to pollen
Allergy NOS due to pollen
Hay fever
Pollinosis

J30.2 Other seasonal allergic rhinitis

J30.5 Allergic rhinitis due to food

5 J30.8 Other allergic rhinitis

J30.81 Allergic rhinitis due to animal (cat) (dog) hair and dander

J30.89 Other allergic rhinitis
Perennial allergic rhinitis

J30.9 Allergic rhinitis, unspecified

4 J31 Chronic rhinitis, nasopharyngitis and pharyngitis
Use additional code to identify:
exposure to environmental tobacco smoke (Z77.22)
exposure to tobacco smoke in the perinatal period (P96.81)
history of tobacco dependence (Z87.891)
occupational exposure to environmental tobacco smoke (Z57.31)
tobacco dependence (F17.-)
tobacco use (Z72.0)

J31.0 Chronic rhinitis
Atrophic rhinitis (chronic)
Granulomatous rhinitis (chronic)
Hypertrophic rhinitis (chronic)
Obstructive rhinitis (chronic)
Ozena
Purulent rhinitis (chronic)
Rhinitis (chronic) NOS
Ulcerative rhinitis (chronic)
EXCLUDES 1 *allergic rhinitis (J30.1-J30.9)*
vasomotor rhinitis (J30.0)

DEFINITION Long-term inflammation of the nasal mucous membrane, with wasting of the mucous membrane and glands.

J31.1 Chronic nasopharyngitis
EXCLUDES 2 *acute nasopharyngitis (J00)*

DEFINITION Long-term inflammation of the nasal and pharyngeal (throat) mucous membranes.

J31.2 Chronic pharyngitis
Chronic sore throat
Atrophic pharyngitis (chronic)
Granular pharyngitis (chronic)
Hypertrophic pharyngitis (chronic)
EXCLUDES 2 *acute pharyngitis (J02.9)*

4 J32 Chronic sinusitis
INCLUDES sinus abscess
sinus empyema
sinus infection
sinus suppuration
Use additional code to identify:
exposure to environmental tobacco smoke (Z77.22)
exposure to tobacco smoke in the perinatal period (P96.81)
history of tobacco dependence (Z87.891)
infectious agent (B95-B97)
occupational exposure to environmental tobacco smoke (Z57.31)
tobacco dependence (F17.-)
tobacco use (Z72.0)
EXCLUDES 2 *acute sinusitis (J01.-)*

CODING TIP ✓ Do not assign a code from J32.- when sinusitis is reported as acute or infectious, unless the patient is reported to have both the chronic and acute form of sinusitis. If both forms are reported as confirmed in the medical record, assign separate and specific codes for each.

J32.0 Chronic maxillary sinusitis
Antritis (chronic)
Maxillary sinusitis NOS

J32.1 Chronic frontal sinusitis
Frontal sinusitis NOS

J32.2 Chronic ethmoidal sinusitis
Ethmoidal sinusitis NOS
EXCLUDES 1 *Woakes' ethmoiditis (J33.1)*

J32.3 Chronic sphenoidal sinusitis
Sphenoidal sinusitis NOS

J32.4 Chronic pansinusitis
Pansinusitis NOS

J32.8 Other chronic sinusitis
Sinusitis (chronic) involving more than one sinus but not pansinusitis

J32.9 Chronic sinusitis, unspecified
Sinusitis (chronic) NOS

4 J33 Nasal polyp
Use additional code to identify:
exposure to environmental tobacco smoke (Z77.22)
exposure to tobacco smoke in the perinatal period (P96.81)
history of tobacco dependence (Z87.891)
occupational exposure to environmental tobacco smoke (Z57.31)
tobacco dependence (F17.-)
tobacco use (Z72.0)
EXCLUDES 1 *adenomatous polyps (D14.0)*

J33.0 Polyp of nasal cavity
Choanal polyp
Nasopharyngeal polyp

J33.1 Polypoid sinus degeneration
Woakes' syndrome or ethmoiditis

J33.8 Other polyp of sinus
Accessory polyp of sinus
Ethmoidal polyp of sinus
Maxillary polyp of sinus
Sphenoidal polyp of sinus

J33.9 Nasal polyp, unspecified

4 J34 Other and unspecified disorders of nose and nasal sinuses
EXCLUDES 2 *varicose ulcer of nasal septum (I86.8)*

J34.0 Abscess, furuncle and carbuncle of nose
Cellulitis of nose
Necrosis of nose
Ulceration of nose

J34.1 Cyst and mucocele of nose and nasal sinus

J34.2 Deviated nasal septum
Deflection or deviation of septum (nasal) (acquired)
EXCLUDES 1 *congenital deviated nasal septum (Q67.4)*

DEFINITION Cartilage separating the nostrils is shifted out of position, usually due to an old traumatic injury.

J34.3 Hypertrophy of nasal turbinates

5 J34.8 Other specified disorders of nose and nasal sinuses

J34.81 Nasal mucositis (ulcerative)
Code also type of associated therapy, such as:
antineoplastic and immunosuppressive drugs (T45.1X-)
radiological procedure and radiotherapy (Y84.2)
EXCLUDES 2 *gastrointestinal mucositis (ulcerative) (K92.81)*
mucositis (ulcerative) of vagina and vulva (N76.81)
oral mucositis (ulcerative) (K12.3-)

J34.89 Other specified disorders of nose and nasal sinuses
Perforation of nasal septum NOS
Rhinolith

J34.9 Unspecified disorder of nose and nasal sinuses

J35 Chronic diseases of tonsils and adenoids
Use additional code to identify:
exposure to environmental tobacco smoke (Z77.22)
exposure to tobacco smoke in the perinatal period (P96.81)
history of tobacco dependence (Z87.891)
occupational exposure to environmental tobacco smoke (Z57.31)
tobacco dependence (F17.-)
tobacco use (Z72.0)

J35.0 Chronic tonsillitis and adenoiditis
EXCLUDES 2 *acute tonsillitis (J03.-)*

J35.01 Chronic tonsillitis

Chronic tonsillitis

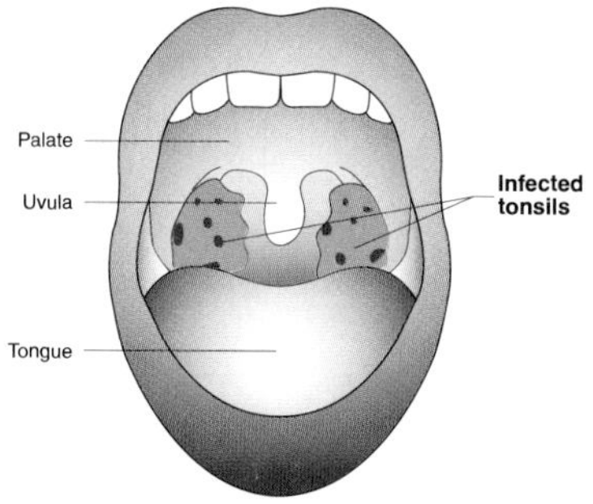

J35.02 Chronic adenoiditis

J35.03 Chronic tonsillitis and adenoiditis

J35.1 Hypertrophy of tonsils
Enlargement of tonsils
EXCLUDES 1 *hypertrophy of tonsils with tonsillitis (J35.0-)*

J35.2 Hypertrophy of adenoids
Enlargement of adenoids
EXCLUDES 1 *hypertrophy of adenoids with adenoiditis (J35.0-)*

J35.3 Hypertrophy of tonsils with Hypertrophy of adenoids
EXCLUDES 1 *hypertrophy of tonsils and adenoids with tonsillitis and adenoiditis (J35.03)*

J35.8 Other chronic diseases of tonsils and adenoids
Adenoid vegetations
Amygdalolith
Calculus, tonsil
Cicatrix of tonsil (and adenoid)
Tonsillar tag
Ulcer of tonsil

J35.9 Chronic disease of tonsils and adenoids, unspecified
Disease (chronic) of tonsils and adenoids NOS

J36 Peritonsillar abscess
INCLUDES abscess of tonsil
peritonsillar cellulitis
quinsy
Use additional code (B95-B97) to identify infectious agent.
EXCLUDES 1 *acute tonsillitis (J03.-)*
chronic tonsillitis (J35.0)
retropharyngeal abscess (J39.0)
tonsillitis NOS (J03.9-)

J37 Chronic laryngitis and laryngotracheitis
Use additional code to identify:
exposure to environmental tobacco smoke (Z77.22)
exposure to tobacco smoke in the perinatal period (P96.81)
history of tobacco dependence (Z87.891)
infectious agent (B95-B97)
occupational exposure to environmental tobacco smoke (Z57.31)
tobacco dependence (F17.-)
tobacco use (Z72.0)

CODING TIP ✓ Assign a code from J37.- only when the physician specifies laryngitis or laryngotracheitis as "chronic."

J37.0 Chronic laryngitis
Catarrhal laryngitis
Hypertrophic laryngitis
Sicca laryngitis
EXCLUDES 2 *acute laryngitis (J04.0)*
obstructive (acute) laryngitis (J05.0)

J37.1 Chronic laryngotracheitis
Laryngitis, chronic, with tracheitis (chronic)
Tracheitis, chronic, with laryngitis
EXCLUDES 1 *chronic tracheitis (J42)*
EXCLUDES 2 *acute laryngotracheitis (J04.2)*
acute tracheitis (J04.1)
DEFINITION Long-term inflammation extending past the vocal cords and into the trachea.

J38 Diseases of vocal cords and larynx, not elsewhere classified
Use additional code to identify:
exposure to environmental tobacco smoke (Z77.22)
exposure to tobacco smoke in the perinatal period (P96.81)
history of tobacco dependence (Z87.891)
occupational exposure to environmental tobacco smoke (Z57.31)
tobacco dependence (F17.-)
tobacco use (Z72.0)
EXCLUDES 1 *congenital laryngeal stridor (P28.89)*
obstructive laryngitis (acute) (J05.0)
postprocedural subglottic stenosis (J95.5)
stridor (R06.1)
ulcerative laryngitis (J04.0)

J38.0 Paralysis of vocal cords and larynx
Laryngoplegia
Paralysis of glottis

J38.00 Paralysis of vocal cords and larynx, unspecified

J38.01 Paralysis of vocal cords and larynx, unilateral

J38.02 Paralysis of vocal cords and larynx, bilateral

J38.1 Polyp of vocal cord and larynx
EXCLUDES 1 *adenomatous polyps (D14.1)*

J38.2 Nodules of vocal cords
Chorditis (fibrinous)(nodosa)(tuberosa)
Singer's nodes
Teacher's nodes

J38.3 Other diseases of vocal cords
Abscess of vocal cords
Cellulitis of vocal cords
Granuloma of vocal cords
Leukokeratosis of vocal cords
Leukoplakia of vocal cords

J38.4 Edema of larynx
Edema (of) glottis
Subglottic edema
Supraglottic edema
EXCLUDES 1 *acute obstructive laryngitis [croup] (J05.0)*
edematous laryngitis (J04.0)

J38.5 Laryngeal spasm
Laryngismus (stridulus)

J38.6 **Stenosis of larynx**

Stenosis of larynx

Abnormal narrowing or constriction of larynx

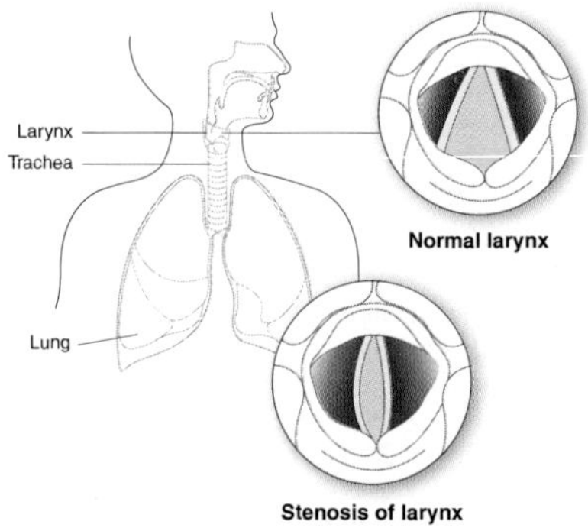

J38.7 **Other diseases of larynx**
Abscess of larynx
Cellulitis of larynx
Disease of larynx NOS
Necrosis of larynx
Pachyderma of larynx
Perichondritis of larynx
Ulcer of larynx

4 J39 **Other diseases of upper respiratory tract**

EXCLUDES 1 *acute respiratory infection NOS (J22)*
acute upper respiratory infection (J06.9)
upper respiratory inflammation due to chemicals, gases, fumes or vapors (J68.2)

J39.0 **Retropharyngeal and parapharyngeal abscess**
Peripharyngeal abscess

EXCLUDES 1 *peritonsillar abscess (J36)*

DEFINITION Pus-filled sore at the back of the throat.

J39.1 **Other abscess of pharynx**
Cellulitis of pharynx
Nasopharyngeal abscess

CODING TIP ✓ Do not assign J39.1 for a diagnosis of pharyngitis. Acute pharyngitis should be coded to J02.-

J39.2 **Other diseases of pharynx**
Cyst of pharynx
Edema of pharynx

EXCLUDES 2 *chronic pharyngitis (J31.2)*
ulcerative pharyngitis (J02.9)

J39.3 **Upper respiratory tract hypersensitivity reaction, site unspecified**

EXCLUDES 1 *hypersensitivity reaction of upper respiratory tract, such as:*
extrinsic allergic alveolitis (J67.9)
pneumoconiosis (J60-J67.9)

J39.8 **Other specified diseases of upper respiratory tract**
J39.9 **Disease of upper respiratory tract, unspecified**

Chronic lower respiratory diseases (J40-J47)

EXCLUDES 1 *bronchitis due to chemicals, gases, fumes and vapors (J68.0)*
EXCLUDES 2 *cystic fibrosis (E84.-)*

J40 **Bronchitis, not specified as acute or chronic**
Bronchitis NOS
Bronchitis with tracheitis NOS
Catarrhal bronchitis
Tracheobronchitis NOS
Use additional code to identify:
exposure to environmental tobacco smoke (Z77.22)
exposure to tobacco smoke in the perinatal period (P96.81)
history of tobacco dependence (Z87.891)
occupational exposure to environmental tobacco smoke (Z57.31)
tobacco dependence (F17.-)
tobacco use (Z72.0)

EXCLUDES 1 *acute bronchitis (J20.-)*
allergic bronchitis NOS (J45.909-)
asthmatic bronchitis NOS (J45.9-)
bronchitis due to chemicals, gases, fumes and vapors (J68.0)

CODING TIP ✓ Do not assign code J40 for chronic, chronic obstructive, or acute bronchitis. J40 should be assigned only when no diagnostic information is available to differentiate the type of bronchitis.

Bronchitis, not specified as acute or chronic

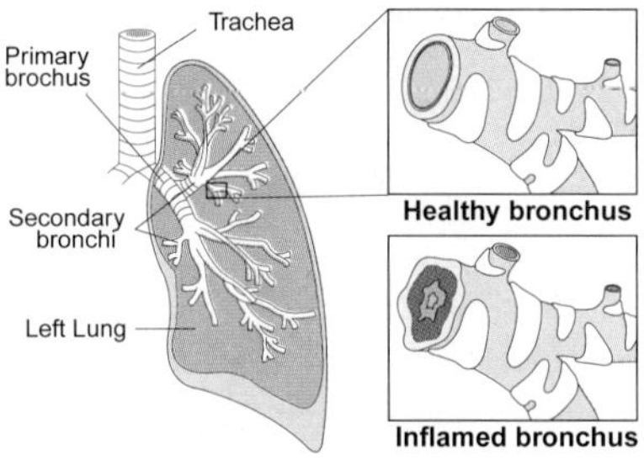

4 J41 **Simple and mucopurulent chronic bronchitis**
Use additional code to identify:
exposure to environmental tobacco smoke (Z77.22)
exposure to tobacco smoke in the perinatal period (P96.81)
history of tobacco dependence (Z87.891)
occupational exposure to environmental tobacco smoke (Z57.31)
tobacco dependence (F17.-)
tobacco use (Z72.0)

EXCLUDES 1 *chronic bronchitis NOS (J42)*
chronic obstructive bronchitis (J44.-)

CODING TIP ✓ Chronic bronchitis not specified as "obstructive" should be coded to J41.0-J42. Chronic bronchitis that is specified as obstructive is coded to category J44.-. Chronic indicates cough with mucus most days of the month for at least 3 months out of the year.

J41.0 **Simple chronic bronchitis** HCC
J41.1 **Mucopurulent chronic bronchitis** HCC
J41.8 **Mixed simple and mucopurulent chronic bronchitis** HCC

J42 **Unspecified chronic bronchitis** HCC
Chronic bronchitis NOS
Chronic tracheitis
Chronic tracheobronchitis
Use additional code to identify:
exposure to environmental tobacco smoke (Z77.22)
exposure to tobacco smoke in the perinatal period (P96.81)
history of tobacco dependence (Z87.891)
occupational exposure to environmental tobacco smoke (Z57.31)
tobacco dependence (F17.-)
tobacco use (Z72.0)

EXCLUDES 1 *chronic asthmatic bronchitis (J44.-)*
chronic bronchitis with airways obstruction (J44.-)
chronic emphysematous bronchitis (J44.-)
chronic obstructive pulmonary disease NOS (J44.9)
simple and mucopurulent chronic bronchitis (J41.-)

CODING TIP ✓ Chronic bronchitis not specified as "obstructive" should be coded to J41.0-J42. Chronic bronchitis that is specified as obstructive is coded to category J44.-. Chronic indicates cough with mucus most days of the month for at least 3 months out of the year.

J43 Emphysema

Use additional code to identify:
exposure to environmental tobacco smoke (Z77.22)
history of tobacco dependence (Z87.891)
occupational exposure to environmental tobacco smoke (Z57.31)
tobacco dependence (F17.-)
tobacco use (Z72.0)

EXCLUDES 1
compensatory emphysema (J98.3)
emphysema due to inhalation of chemicals, gases, fumes or vapors (J68.4)
emphysema with chronic (obstructive) bronchitis (J44.-)
emphysematous (obstructive) bronchitis (J44.-)
interstitial emphysema (J98.2)
mediastinal emphysema (J98.2)
neonatal interstitial emphysema (P25.0)
surgical (subcutaneous) emphysema (T81.82)
traumatic subcutaneous emphysema (T79.7)

CODING TIP ✓ Emphysema and COPD is coded to J43. Emphysema is a type of COPD.

CODING TIP ✓ Do not assign a code from J43.- when the physician documentation reports emphysema with COPD, chronic obstructive bronchitis or emphysematous bronchitis. Emphysema with COPD, bronchitis and emphysematous bronchitis should be coded to J44.- and cannot be coded on the same claim as J43.-.

CODING TIP ✓ When a diagnosis supports coding a more specific code for emphysema, such as interstitial emphysema (J98.2), compensatory emphysema (J98.3), or subcutaneous emphysema due to trauma (T79.7), then do not assign J43.-, but assign the more specific code.

J43.0 Unilateral pulmonary emphysema [MacLeod's syndrome] HCC
Swyer-James syndrome
Unilateral emphysema
Unilateral hyperlucent lung
Unilateral pulmonary artery functional hypoplasia
Unilateral transparency of lung

J43.1 Panlobular emphysema HCC
Panacinar emphysema

J43.2 Centrilobular emphysema HCC

J43.8 Other emphysema HCC

J43.9 Emphysema, unspecified HCC
Bullous emphysema (lung)(pulmonary)
Emphysema (lung)(pulmonary) NOS
Emphysematous bleb
Vesicular emphysema (lung)(pulmonary)

DEFINITION Abnormal enlargement of the air sacs in the lungs, which lose their elasticity, making breathing increasingly difficult.
AHA: 4Q 2017, 76
AHA: 4Q 2017, 77

Emphysema, unspecified

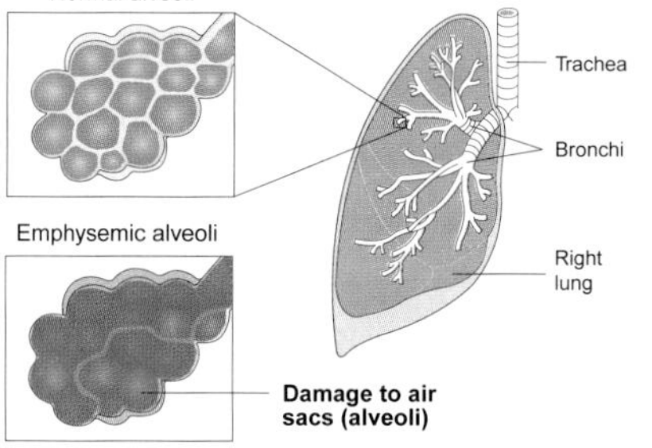

J44 Other chronic obstructive pulmonary disease

INCLUDES
asthma with chronic obstructive pulmonary disease
chronic asthmatic (obstructive) bronchitis
chronic bronchitis with airways obstruction
chronic bronchitis with emphysema
chronic emphysematous bronchitis
chronic obstructive asthma
chronic obstructive bronchitis
chronic obstructive tracheobronchitis

Code also:
type of asthma, if applicable (J45.-)

Use additional code to identify:
exposure to environmental tobacco smoke (Z77.22)
history of tobacco dependence (Z87.891)
occupational exposure to environmental tobacco smoke (Z57.31)
tobacco dependence (F17.-)
tobacco use (Z72.0)

EXCLUDES 1
bronchiectasis (J47.-)
chronic bronchitis NOS (J42)
chronic simple and mucopurulent bronchitis (J41.-)
chronic tracheitis (J42)
chronic tracheobronchitis (J42)
emphysema without chronic bronchitis (J43.-)

GUIDELINES **Section I.C.10.a**
The codes in categories J44 and J45 distinguish between uncomplicated cases and those in acute exacerbation. An acute exacerbation is a worsening or a decompensation of a chronic condition. An acute exacerbation is not equivalent to an infection superimposed on a chronic condition, though an exacerbation may be triggered by an infection.

CODING TIP ✓ When the physician reports chronic obstructive asthma or chronic asthmatic bronchitis, and the type of asthma is specified, an additional code from category J45.- should be reported.
AHA: 1Q 2017, 25
AHA: 2Q 2017, 30

Chronic obstructive pulmonary disease

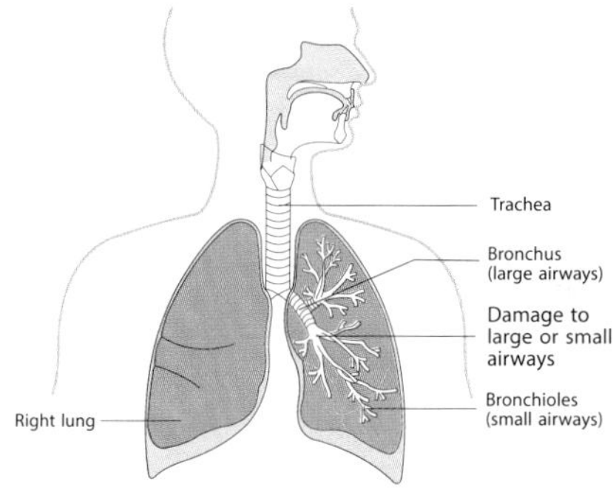

J44.0 Chronic obstructive pulmonary disease with acute lower respiratory infection HCC
Code also:
to identify the infection

CODING TIP ✓ Assign a code from J44.0 when a patient has both chronic obstructive pulmonary disease (COPD) and a diagnosis of a lower respiratory tract infection. An additional code should be assigned to report the infection. If the physician confirms both a diagnosis of a lower respiratory tract infection and exacerbation of the COPD, both J44.1, Chronic obstructive pulmonary disease with acute exacerbation, and J44.0, Chronic obstructive pulmonary disease with acute lower respiratory infection, should be assigned, followed by a code for the specific lower respiratory infection. Lower respiratory infections include pneumonia, bronchitis and bronchiolitis.
AHA: 3Q 2016, 15-16
AHA: 1Q 2017, 26
AHA: 2Q 2017, 30
AHA: 4Q 2017, 75

J44.1 Chronic obstructive pulmonary disease with (acute) exacerbation HCC
Decompensated COPD
Decompensated COPD with (acute) exacerbation
EXCLUDES 2 *chronic obstructive pulmonary disease [COPD] with acute bronchitis (J44.0)*
lung diseases due to external agents (J60-J70)

CODING TIP ✓ **Documentation:** Do not assign J44.1 unless the physician has confirmed that the condition is exacerbated. An exacerbation may not be assumed without physician confirmation, and changes in treatment and medication regimen do not presume an exacerbation.

AHA: 1Q 2016, 36
AHA: 3Q 2016, 15-16
AHA: 1Q 2017, 26
AHA: 4Q 2017, 75

J44.9 Chronic obstructive pulmonary disease, unspecified HCC
Chronic obstructive airway disease NOS
Chronic obstructive lung disease NOS
EXCLUDES 2 *lung diseases due to external agents (J60-J70)*

AHA: 4Q 2013, 109, 129
AHA: 4Q 2014, 21
AHA: 1Q 2016, 36-37
AHA: 1Q 2017, 24
AHA: 1Q 2017, 25
AHA: 4Q 2017, 76
AHA: 4Q 2017, 76

4 J45 Asthma

INCLUDES allergic (predominantly) asthma
allergic bronchitis NOS
allergic rhinitis with asthma
atopic asthma
extrinsic allergic asthma
hay fever with asthma
idiosyncratic asthma
intrinsic nonallergic asthma
nonallergic asthma

Use additional code to identify:
exposure to environmental tobacco smoke (Z77.22)
exposure to tobacco smoke in the perinatal period (P96.81)
history of tobacco dependence (Z87.891)
occupational exposure to environmental tobacco smoke (Z57.31)
tobacco dependence (F17.-)
tobacco use (Z72.0)

EXCLUDES 1 *detergent asthma (J69.8)*
eosinophilic asthma (J82)
miner's asthma (J60)
wheezing NOS (R06.2)
wood asthma (J67.8)

EXCLUDES 2 *asthma with chronic obstructive pulmonary disease (J44.9)*
chronic asthmatic (obstructive) bronchitis (J44.9)
chronic obstructive asthma (J44.9)

GUIDELINES **Section I.C.10.a**
The codes in categories J44 and J45 distinguish between uncomplicated cases and those in acute exacerbation. An acute exacerbation is a worsening or a decompensation of a chronic condition. An acute exacerbation is not equivalent to an infection superimposed on a chronic condition, though an exacerbation may be triggered by an infection.

CODING TIP ✓ **Documentation:** When reporting a code from category J45.-, do not report the condition as exacerbated without physician confirmation of the diagnosis. An exacerbation may not be assumed without physician confirmation, and changes in treatment and medication regimen do not presume an exacerbation.

DEFINITION Asthma is also known as reactive airway disease. It is an inflammatory process of the lining of the airways of the lungs and is considered reversible. Patients with asthma typically develop wheezing, shortness of breath and cough. Because the inflammation of the lining of the airways is considered reversible, asthma symptoms are intermittent and cover a spectrum from mild-to-severe disease. Several symptoms overlap in patients with COPD and asthma. A history of wheezing strongly suggests a diagnosis of asthma, whereas chronic cough productive of sputum is more indicative of COPD.

Asthma

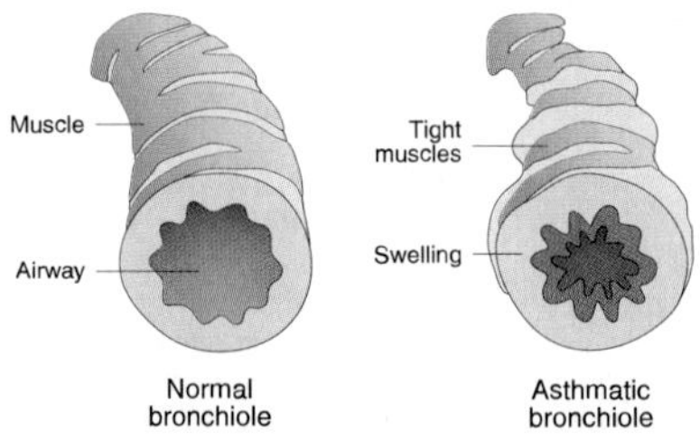

5 J45.2 Mild intermittent asthma
J45.20 Mild intermittent asthma, uncomplicated
Mild intermittent asthma NOS
J45.21 Mild intermittent asthma with (acute) exacerbation
J45.22 Mild intermittent asthma with status asthmaticus

5 J45.3 Mild persistent asthma
J45.30 Mild persistent asthma, uncomplicated
Mild persistent asthma NOS
J45.31 Mild persistent asthma with (acute) exacerbation
AHA: 1Q 2016, 35
J45.32 Mild persistent asthma with status asthmaticus

5 J45.4 Moderate persistent asthma
J45.40 Moderate persistent asthma, uncomplicated
Moderate persistent asthma NOS
J45.41 Moderate persistent asthma with (acute) exacerbation
AHA: 1Q 2017, 26
J45.42 Moderate persistent asthma with status asthmaticus

5 J45.5 Severe persistent asthma
J45.50 Severe persistent asthma, uncomplicated
Severe persistent asthma NOS
J45.51 Severe persistent asthma with (acute) exacerbation
J45.52 Severe persistent asthma with status asthmaticus

5 J45.9 Other and unspecified asthma
6 J45.90 Unspecified asthma
Asthmatic bronchitis NOS
Childhood asthma NOS
Late onset asthma
J45.901 Unspecified asthma with (acute) exacerbation
AHA: 4Q 2017, 76
J45.902 Unspecified asthma with status asthmaticus
J45.909 Unspecified asthma, uncomplicated
Asthma NOS
EXCLUDES 2 *lung diseases due to external agents (J60-J70)*
6 J45.99 Other asthma
J45.990 Exercise induced bronchospasm
J45.991 Cough variant asthma
J45.998 Other asthma

J47 Bronchiectasis
INCLUDES bronchiolectasis
Use additional code to identify:
exposure to environmental tobacco smoke (Z77.22)
exposure to tobacco smoke in the perinatal period (P96.81)
history of tobacco dependence (Z87.891)
occupational exposure to environmental tobacco smoke (Z57.31)
tobacco dependence (F17.-)
tobacco use (Z72.0)
EXCLUDES 1 *congenital bronchiectasis (Q33.4)*
tuberculous bronchiectasis (current disease) (A15.0)

J47.0 Bronchiectasis with acute lower respiratory infection HCC
Bronchiectasis with acute bronchitis
Use additional code to identify the infection

J47.1 Bronchiectasis with (acute) exacerbation HCC

J47.9 Bronchiectasis, uncomplicated HCC
Bronchiectasis NOS
DEFINITION Destruction and widening of the large airways, often due to recurrent, severe infection or inflammation, or following foreign body obstruction.

Lung diseases due to external agents (J60-J70)

EXCLUDES 2 *asthma (J45.-)*
malignant neoplasm of bronchus and lung (C34.-)

J60 Coalworker's pneumoconiosis A HCC
Anthracosilicosis
Anthracosis
Black lung disease
Coalworker's lung
EXCLUDES 1 *coalworker pneumoconiosis with tuberculosis, any type in A15 (J65)*
DEFINITION Silicotic nodules and scar-tissue formation in the lungs due to prolonged inhalation and collection of coal dust particles in the bronchioles.

J61 Pneumoconiosis due to asbestos and other mineral fibers A HCC
Asbestosis
EXCLUDES 1 *pleural plaque with asbestosis (J92.0)*
pneumoconiosis with tuberculosis, any type in A15 (J65)
DEFINITION Chronic lung disease caused by inhaling asbestos particles over a prolonged period.

J62 Pneumoconiosis due to dust containing silica
INCLUDES silicotic fibrosis (massive) of lung
EXCLUDES 1 *pneumoconiosis with tuberculosis, any type in A15 (J65)*

J62.0 Pneumoconiosis due to talc dust HCC

J62.8 Pneumoconiosis due to other dust containing silica HCC
Silicosis NOS

J63 Pneumoconiosis due to other inorganic dusts
EXCLUDES 1 *pneumoconiosis with tuberculosis, any type in A15 (J65)*

J63.0 Aluminosis (of lung) HCC

J63.1 Bauxite fibrosis (of lung) HCC

J63.2 Berylliosis HCC

J63.3 Graphite fibrosis (of lung) HCC

J63.4 Siderosis HCC

J63.5 Stannosis HCC

J63.6 Pneumoconiosis due to other specified inorganic dusts HCC

J64 Unspecified pneumoconiosis HCC
EXCLUDES 1 *pneumonoconiosis with tuberculosis, any type in A15 (J65)*

J65 Pneumoconiosis associated with tuberculosis HCC
Any condition in J60-J64 with tuberculosis, any type in A15
Silicotuberculosis

J66 Airway disease due to specific organic dust
EXCLUDES 2 *allergic alveolitis (J67.-)*
asbestosis (J61)
bagassosis (J67.1)
farmer's lung (J67.0)
hypersensitivity pneumonitis due to organic dust (J67.-)
reactive airways dysfunction syndrome (J68.3)

J66.0 Byssinosis HCC
Airway disease due to cotton dust

J66.1 Flax-dressers' disease HCC

J66.2 Cannabinosis HCC

J66.8 Airway disease due to other specific organic dusts HCC

J67 Hypersensitivity pneumonitis due to organic dust
INCLUDES allergic alveolitis and pneumonitis due to inhaled organic dust and particles of fungal, actinomycetic or other origin
EXCLUDES 1 *pneumonitis due to inhalation of chemicals, gases, fumes or vapors (J68.0)*

J67.0 Farmer's lung HCC
Harvester's lung
Haymaker's lung
Moldy hay disease
DEFINITION Inflammation of the small, inner air sacs in the lungs, due to an allergic reaction triggered by inhaled organic substances or microorganisms.

J67.1 Bagassosis HCC
Bagasse disease
Bagasse pneumonitis

J67.2 Bird fancier's lung HCC
Budgerigar fancier's disease or lung
Pigeon fancier's disease or lung

J67.3 Suberosis HCC
Corkhandler's disease or lung
Corkworker's disease or lung

J67.4 Maltworker's lung HCC
Alveolitis due to Aspergillus clavatus

J67.5 Mushroom-worker's lung HCC

J67.6 Maple-bark-stripper's lung HCC
Alveolitis due to Cryptostroma corticale
Cryptostromosis

J67.7 Air conditioner and humidifier lung HCC
Allergic alveolitis due to fungal, thermophilic actinomycetes and other organisms growing in ventilation [air conditioning] systems

J67.8 Hypersensitivity pneumonitis due to other organic dusts HCC
Cheese-washer's lung
Coffee-worker's lung
Fish-meal worker's lung
Furrier's lung
Sequoiosis

J67.9 Hypersensitivity pneumonitis due to unspecified organic dust HCC
Allergic alveolitis (extrinsic) NOS
Hypersensitivity pneumonitis NOS

J68 Respiratory conditions due to inhalation of chemicals, gases, fumes and vapors
Code first:
(T51-T65) to identify cause
Use additional code to identify associated respiratory conditions, such as:
acute respiratory failure (J96.0-)

J68.0 Bronchitis and pneumonitis due to chemicals, gases, fumes and vapors HCC
Chemical bronchitis (acute)

J68.1 Pulmonary edema due to chemicals, gases, fumes and vapors HCC
Chemical pulmonary edema (acute) (chronic)
EXCLUDES 1 *pulmonary edema (acute) (chronic) NOS (J81.-)*

J68.2 Upper respiratory inflammation due to chemicals, gases, fumes and vapors, not elsewhere classified HCC

J68.3 Other acute and subacute respiratory conditions due to chemicals, gases, fumes and vapors HCC
Reactive airways dysfunction syndrome

J68.4 **Chronic respiratory conditions due to chemicals, gases, fumes and vapors** HCC
Emphysema (diffuse) (chronic) due to inhalation of chemicals, gases, fumes and vapors
Obliterative bronchiolitis (chronic) (subacute) due to inhalation of chemicals, gases, fumes and vapors
Pulmonary fibrosis (chronic) due to inhalation of chemicals, gases, fumes and vapors
EXCLUDES 1 *chronic pulmonary edema due to chemicals, gases, fumes and vapors (J68.1)*

J68.8 **Other respiratory conditions due to chemicals, gases, fumes and vapors** HCC

J68.9 **Unspecified respiratory condition due to chemicals, gases, fumes and vapors** HCC

4 J69 **Pneumonitis due to solids and liquids**
EXCLUDES 1 *neonatal aspiration syndromes (P24.-)*
postprocedural pneumonitis (J95.4)

J69.0 **Pneumonitis due to inhalation of food and vomit** HCC
Aspiration pneumonia NOS
Aspiration pneumonia (due to) food (regurgitated)
Aspiration pneumonia (due to) gastric secretions
Aspiration pneumonia (due to) milk
Aspiration pneumonia (due to) vomit
Code also:
any associated foreign body in respiratory tract (T17.-)
EXCLUDES 1 *chemical pneumonitis due to anesthesia (J95.4)*
obstetric aspiration pneumonitis (O74.0)
AHA: 1Q 2017, 24

J69.1 **Pneumonitis due to inhalation of oils and essences** HCC
Exogenous lipoid pneumonia
Lipid pneumonia NOS
Code first:
(T51-T65) to identify substance
EXCLUDES 1 *endogenous lipoid pneumonia (J84.89)*

J69.8 **Pneumonitis due to inhalation of other solids and liquids** HCC
Pneumonitis due to aspiration of blood
Pneumonitis due to aspiration of detergent
Code first:
(T51-T65) to identify substance

4 J70 **Respiratory conditions due to other external agents**

J70.0 **Acute pulmonary manifestations due to radiation** HCC
Radiation pneumonitis
Use additional code (W88-W90, X39.0-) to identify the external cause

J70.1 **Chronic and other pulmonary manifestations due to radiation** HCC
Fibrosis of lung following radiation
Use additional code (W88-W90, X39.0-) to identify the external cause

J70.2 **Acute drug-induced interstitial lung disorders** HCC
Use additional code for adverse effect, if applicable, to identify drug (T36-T50 with fifth or sixth character 5)
EXCLUDES 1 *interstitial pneumonia NOS (J84.9)*
lymphoid interstitial pneumonia (J84.2)

J70.3 **Chronic drug-induced interstitial lung disorders** HCC
Use additional code for adverse effect, if applicable, to identify drug (T36-T50 with fifth or sixth character 5)
EXCLUDES 1 *interstitial pneumonia NOS (J84.9)*
lymphoid interstitial pneumonia (J84.2)

J70.4 **Drug-induced interstitial lung disorders, unspecified** HCC
Use additional code for adverse effect, if applicable, to identify drug (T36-T50 with fifth or sixth character 5)
EXCLUDES 1 *interstitial pneumonia NOS (J84.9)*
lymphoid interstitial pneumonia (J84.2)

J70.5 **Respiratory conditions due to smoke inhalation** HCC
Smoke inhalation NOS
EXCLUDES 1 *smoke inhalation due to chemicals, gases, fumes and vapors (J68.9)*
AHA: 4Q 2013, 121

J70.8 **Respiratory conditions due to other specified external agents** HCC
Code first:
(T51-T65) to identify the external agent

J70.9 **Respiratory conditions due to unspecified external agent** HCC
Code first:
(T51-T65) to identify the external agent

Other respiratory diseases principally affecting the interstitium (J80-J84)

J80 **Acute respiratory distress syndrome** HCC
Acute respiratory distress syndrome in adult or child
Adult hyaline membrane disease
EXCLUDES 1 *respiratory distress syndrome in newborn (perinatal) (P22.0)*

CODING TIP ✓ ARDS is a rapidly progressive, life-threatening condition that has symptoms of dyspnea, tachypnea, and hypoxemia. Fluid builds up in the alveoli and decreases the amount of oxygen that is circulated through the bloodstream. Low levels of oxygen in the blood impairs organ function. ARDS differs from acute respiratory distress (R06.03).

4 J81 **Pulmonary edema**
Use additional code to identify:
exposure to environmental tobacco smoke (Z77.22)
history of tobacco dependence (Z87.891)
occupational exposure to environmental tobacco smoke (Z57.31)
tobacco dependence (F17.-)
tobacco use (Z72.0)
EXCLUDES 1 *chemical (acute) pulmonary edema (J68.1)*
hypostatic pneumonia (J18.2)
passive pneumonia (J18.2)
pulmonary edema due to external agents (J60-J70)
pulmonary edema with heart disease NOS (I50.1)
pulmonary edema with heart failure (I50.1)

J81.0 **Acute pulmonary edema** HCC
Acute edema of lung
DEFINITION Sudden, severe accumulation of fluid in the lungs.

J81.1 **Chronic pulmonary edema**
Pulmonary congestion (chronic) (passive)
Pulmonary edema NOS

J82 **Pulmonary eosinophilia, not elsewhere classified** HCC
Allergic pneumonia
Eosinophilic asthma
Eosinophilic pneumonia
Löffler's pneumonia
Tropical (pulmonary) eosinophilia NOS
EXCLUDES 1 *pulmonary eosinophilia due to aspergillosis (B44.-)*
pulmonary eosinophilia due to drugs (J70.2-J70.4)
pulmonary eosinophilia due to specified parasitic infection (B50-B83)
pulmonary eosinophilia due to systemic connective tissue disorders (M30-M36)
pulmonary infiltrate NOS (R91.8)

4 J84 **Other interstitial pulmonary diseases**
EXCLUDES 1 *drug-induced interstitial lung disorders (J70.2-J70.4)*
interstitial emphysema (J98.2)
EXCLUDES 2 *lung diseases due to external agents (J60-J70)*

5 J84.0 **Alveolar and parieto-alveolar conditions**

J84.01 **Alveolar proteinosis** HCC

J84.02 **Pulmonary alveolar microlithiasis** HCC

J84.03 ***Idiopathic pulmonary hemosiderosis*** HCC
Essential brown induration of lung
Code first underlying disease, such as:
disorders of iron metabolism (E83.1-)
EXCLUDES 1 *acute idiopathic pulmonary hemorrhage in infants [AIPHI] (R04.81)*

J84.09 **Other alveolar and parieto-alveolar conditions** HCC

5 J84.1 **Other interstitial pulmonary diseases with fibrosis**
EXCLUDES 1 *pulmonary fibrosis (chronic) due to inhalation of chemicals, gases, fumes or vapors (J68.4)*
pulmonary fibrosis (chronic) following radiation (J70.1)

DEFINITION Formation of fibrous tissue and scarring in the lungs after the lungs have been inflamed for a significant period of time.

J84.10 Pulmonary fibrosis, unspecified HCC
Capillary fibrosis of lung
Cirrhosis of lung (chronic) NOS
Fibrosis of lung (atrophic) (chronic) (confluent) (massive) (perialveolar) (peribronchial) NOS
Induration of lung (chronic) NOS
Postinflammatory pulmonary fibrosis

6 **J84.11 Idiopathic interstitial pneumonia**
EXCLUDES 1 *lymphoid interstitial pneumonia (J84.2)*
pneumocystis pneumonia (B59)

J84.111 Idiopathic interstitial pneumonia, not otherwise specified HCC

J84.112 Idiopathic pulmonary fibrosis HCC
Cryptogenic fibrosing alveolitis
Idiopathic fibrosing alveolitis

J84.113 Idiopathic non-specific interstitial pneumonitis HCC
EXCLUDES 1 *non-specific interstitial pneumonia NOS, or due to known underlying cause (J84.89)*

J84.114 Acute interstitial pneumonitis HCC
Hamman-Rich syndrome
EXCLUDES 1 *pneumocystis pneumonia (B59)*

J84.115 Respiratory bronchiolitis interstitial lung disease HCC

J84.116 Cryptogenic organizing pneumonia HCC
EXCLUDES 1 *organizing pneumonia NOS, or due to known underlying cause (J84.89)*

J84.117 Desquamative interstitial pneumonia HCC

J84.17 *Other interstitial pulmonary diseases with fibrosis in diseases classified elsewhere* HCC
Interstitial pneumonia (nonspecific) (usual) due to collagen vascular disease
Interstitial pneumonia (nonspecific) (usual) in diseases classified elsewhere
Organizing pneumonia due to collagen vascular disease
Organizing pneumonia in diseases classified elsewhere
Code first underlying disease, such as:
progressive systemic sclerosis (M34.0)
rheumatoid arthritis (M05.00-M06.9)
systemic lupus erythematosis (M32.0-M32.9)

J84.2 Lymphoid interstitial pneumonia HCC
Lymphoid interstitial pneumonitis

5 **J84.8 Other specified interstitial pulmonary diseases**
EXCLUDES 1 *exogenous lipoid pneumonia (J69.1)*
unspecified lipoid pneumonia (J69.1)

J84.81 Lymphangioleiomyomatosis HCC
Lymphangiomyomatosis

J84.82 Adult pulmonary Langerhans cell histiocytosis A HCC
Adult PLCH

J84.83 Surfactant mutations of the lung HCC

6 **J84.84 Other interstitial lung diseases of childhood**

J84.841 Neuroendocrine cell hyperplasia of infancy HCC

J84.842 Pulmonary interstitial glycogenosis HCC

J84.843 Alveolar capillary dysplasia with vein misalignment HCC

J84.848 Other interstitial lung diseases of childhood HCC

J84.89 Other specified interstitial pulmonary diseases HCC
Endogenous lipoid pneumonia
Interstitial pneumonitis
Non-specific interstitial pneumonitis NOS
Organizing pneumonia NOS
Code first, if applicable:
poisoning due to drug or toxin (T51-T65 with fifth or sixth character to indicate intent) , for toxic pneumonopathy
underlying cause of pneumonopathy, if known
Use additional code, for adverse effect, to identify drug (T36-T50 with fifth or sixth character 5), if drug-induced
EXCLUDES 1 *cryptogenic organizing pneumonia (J84.116)*
idiopathic non-specific interstitial pneumonitis (J84.113)
lipoid pneumonia, exogenous or unspecified (J69.1)
lymphoid interstitial pneumonia (J84.2)

J84.9 Interstitial pulmonary disease, unspecified HCC
Interstitial pneumonia NOS

Suppurative and necrotic conditions of the lower respiratory tract (J85-J86)

CODING TIP ✓ When the record specifies the causative organism, use an additional code to report the organism specified, following the instructions to "use an additional code."

4 **J85 Abscess of lung and mediastinum**
Use additional code (B95-B97) to identify infectious agent.

J85.0 Gangrene and necrosis of lung HCC

J85.1 Abscess of lung with pneumonia HCC
Code also:
the type of pneumonia

J85.2 Abscess of lung without pneumonia HCC
Abscess of lung NOS

J85.3 Abscess of mediastinum HCC

4 **J86 Pyothorax**
Use additional code (B95-B97) to identify infectious agent.
EXCLUDES 1 *abscess of lung (J85.-)*
pyothorax due to tuberculosis (A15.6)

J86.0 Pyothorax with fistula HCC
Bronchocutaneous fistula
Bronchopleural fistula
Hepatopleural fistula
Mediastinal fistula
Pleural fistula
Thoracic fistula
Any condition classifiable to J86.9 with fistula

J86.9 Pyothorax without fistula HCC
Abscess of pleura
Abscess of thorax
Empyema (chest) (lung) (pleura)
Fibrinopurulent pleurisy
Purulent pleurisy
Pyopneumothorax
Septic pleurisy
Seropurulent pleurisy
Suppurative pleurisy

Other diseases of the pleura (J90-J94)

J90 Pleural effusion, not elsewhere classified
Encysted pleurisy
Pleural effusion NOS
Pleurisy with effusion (exudative) (serous)
EXCLUDES 1 *chylous (pleural) effusion (J94.0)*
malignant pleural effusion (J91.0))
pleurisy NOS (R09.1)
tuberculous pleural effusion (A15.6)

CODING TIP ✓ Pleural effusion indicates excess pleural fluid built up and accumulated in the pleural lining causing respiratory distress.

J91 Pleural effusion in conditions classified elsewhere

EXCLUDES 2 *pleural effusion in heart failure (I50.-)*
pleural effusion in systemic lupus erythematosus (M32.13)

CODING TIP ✓ Pleural effusion in systemic lupus erythematosus and in heart failure are to be coded as J91.8. Code first the causative condition. However, if the pleural effusion requires separate treatment, i.e. chest tube for drainage, then add the code for pleural effusion.

J91.0 *Malignant pleural effusion*
Code first:
underlying neoplasm

DEFINITION Dangerous fluid accumulation between the layers of the membrane lining the chest cavity and lungs, most often caused by cancers of the breast, lung, or lymph nodes.

J91.8 *Pleural effusion in other conditions classified elsewhere*
Code first underlying disease, such as:
filariasis (B74.0-B74.9)
influenza (J09.X2, J10.1, J11.1)
AHA: 2Q 2015, 16

J92 Pleural plaque

INCLUDES pleural thickening

J92.0 Pleural plaque with presence of asbestos
J92.9 Pleural plaque without asbestos
Pleural plaque NOS

J93 Pneumothorax and air leak

EXCLUDES 1 *congenital or perinatal pneumothorax (P25.1)*
postprocedural air leak (J95.812)
postprocedural pneumothorax (J95.811)
traumatic pneumothorax (S27.0)
tuberculous (current disease) pneumothorax (A15.-)
pyopneumothorax (J86.-)

J93.0 Spontaneous tension pneumothorax
J93.1 Other spontaneous pneumothorax
J93.11 Primary spontaneous pneumothorax

Primary spontaneous pneumothorax
A lung collapses due to an accumulation of air between lungs and the chest cavity

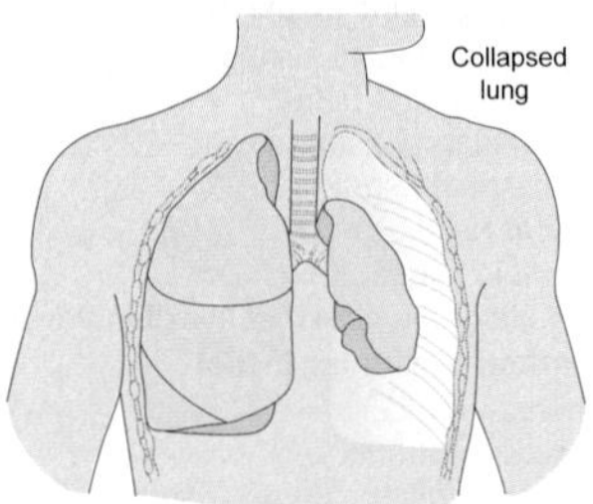

J93.12 Secondary spontaneous pneumothorax
Code first underlying condition, such as:
catamenial pneumothorax due to endometriosis (N80.8)
cystic fibrosis (E84.-)
eosinophilic pneumonia (J82)
lymphangioleiomyomatosis (J84.81)
malignant neoplasm of bronchus and lung (C34.-)
Marfan's syndrome (Q87.4)
pneumonia due to Pneumocystis carinii (B59)
secondary malignant neoplasm of lung (C78.0-)
spontaneous rupture of the esophagus (K22.3)

J93.8 Other pneumothorax and air leak
J93.81 Chronic pneumothorax
J93.82 Other air leak
Persistent air leak
J93.83 Other pneumothorax
Acute pneumothorax
Spontaneous pneumothorax NOS
J93.9 Pneumothorax, unspecified
Pneumothorax NOS

J94 Other pleural conditions

EXCLUDES 1 *pleurisy NOS (R09.1)*
traumatic hemopneumothorax (S27.2)
traumatic hemothorax (S27.1)
tuberculous pleural conditions (current disease) (A15.-)

J94.0 Chylous effusion
Chyliform effusion
J94.1 Fibrothorax
J94.2 Hemothorax
Hemopneumothorax
J94.8 Other specified pleural conditions
Hydropneumothorax
Hydrothorax
J94.9 Pleural condition, unspecified

Intraoperative and postprocedural complications and disorders of respiratory system, not elsewhere classified (J95)

J95 Intraoperative and postprocedural complications and disorders of respiratory system, not elsewhere classified

EXCLUDES 2 *aspiration pneumonia (J69.-)*
emphysema (subcutaneous) resulting from a procedure (T81.82)
hypostatic pneumonia (J18.2)
pulmonary manifestations due to radiation (J70.0-J70.1)

CODING TIP ✓ Codes in category J95.- are complication codes and require physician documentation and confirmation of a cause and effect relationship between the procedure and the complicated condition.

J95.0 Tracheostomy complications
J95.00 Unspecified tracheostomy complication HCC
J95.01 Hemorrhage from tracheostomy stoma HCC
J95.02 Infection of tracheostomy stoma HCC
Use additional code to identify type of infection, such as:
cellulitis of neck (L03.221)
sepsis (A40, A41.-)

CODING TIP ✓ When coding J95.02, use an additional code to indicate the infection, such as cellulitis, sepsis, or the infectious organism, when the specific information is available.

J95.03 Malfunction of tracheostomy stoma HCC
Mechanical complication of tracheostomy stoma
Obstruction of tracheostomy airway
Tracheal stenosis due to tracheostomy
J95.04 Tracheo-esophageal fistula following tracheostomy HCC
J95.09 Other tracheostomy complication HCC
J95.1 Acute pulmonary insufficiency following thoracic surgery HCC

EXCLUDES 2 *Functional disturbances following cardiac surgery (I97.0, I97.1-)*

J95.2 Acute pulmonary insufficiency following nonthoracic surgery HCC

EXCLUDES 2 *Functional disturbances following cardiac surgery (I97.0, I97.1-)*

J95.3 Chronic pulmonary insufficiency following surgery HCC

EXCLUDES 2 *Functional disturbances following cardiac surgery (I97.0, I97.1-)*

J95.4 Chemical pneumonitis due to anesthesia
Mendelson's syndrome
Postprocedural aspiration pneumonia
Use additional code for adverse effect, if applicable, to identify drug (T41.- with fifth or sixth character 5)

EXCLUDES 1 *aspiration pneumonitis due to anesthesia complicating labor and delivery (O74.0)*
aspiration pneumonitis due to anesthesia complicating pregnancy (O29)
aspiration pneumonitis due to anesthesia complicating the puerperium (O89.01)

J95.5 Postprocedural subglottic stenosis

5 **J95.6 Intraoperative hemorrhage and hematoma of a respiratory system organ or structure complicating a procedure**
EXCLUDES 1 *intraoperative hemorrhage and hematoma of a respiratory system organ or structure due to accidental puncture and laceration during procedure (J95.7-)*

J95.61 Intraoperative hemorrhage and hematoma of a respiratory system organ or structure complicating a respiratory system procedure

J95.62 Intraoperative hemorrhage and hematoma of a respiratory system organ or structure complicating other procedure

5 **J95.7 Accidental puncture and laceration of a respiratory system organ or structure during a procedure**
EXCLUDES 2 *postprocedural pneumothorax (J95.811)*

J95.71 Accidental puncture and laceration of a respiratory system organ or structure during a respiratory system procedure

J95.72 Accidental puncture and laceration of a respiratory system organ or structure during other procedure

5 **J95.8 Other intraoperative and postprocedural complications and disorders of respiratory system, not elsewhere classified**

6 **J95.81 Postprocedural pneumothorax and air leak**

J95.811 Postprocedural pneumothorax

J95.812 Postprocedural air leak

6 **J95.82 Postprocedural respiratory failure**
EXCLUDES 1 *Respiratory failure in other conditions (J96.-)*

J95.821 Acute postprocedural respiratory failure HCC
Postprocedural respiratory failure NOS

J95.822 Acute and chronic postprocedural respiratory failure HCC

6 **J95.83 Postprocedural hemorrhage of a respiratory system organ or structure following a procedure**

J95.830 Postprocedural hemorrhage of a respiratory system organ or structure following a respiratory system procedure

J95.831 Postprocedural hemorrhage of a respiratory system organ or structure following other procedure

J95.84 Transfusion-related acute lung injury (TRALI)

6 **J95.85 Complication of respirator [ventilator]**

J95.850 Mechanical complication of respirator HCC
EXCLUDES 1 *encounter for respirator [ventilator] dependence during power failure (Z99.12)*

J95.851 Ventilator associated pneumonia HCC
Ventilator associated pneumonitis
Use additional code to identify the organism, if known (B95.-, B96.-, B97.-)
EXCLUDES 1 *ventilator lung in newborn (P27.8)*
AHA: 1Q 2017, 25

J95.859 Other complication of respirator [ventilator] HCC

6 **J95.86 Postprocedural hematoma and seroma of a respiratory system organ or structure following a procedure**

J95.860 Postprocedural hematoma of a respiratory system organ or structure following a respiratory system procedure

J95.861 Postprocedural hematoma of a respiratory system organ or structure following other procedure

J95.862 Postprocedural seroma of a respiratory system organ or structure following a respiratory system procedure

J95.863 Postprocedural seroma of a respiratory system organ or structure following other procedure

J95.88 Other intraoperative complications of respiratory system, not elsewhere classified

J95.89 Other postprocedural complications and disorders of respiratory system, not elsewhere classified
Use additional code to identify disorder, such as:
aspiration pneumonia (J69.-)
bacterial or viral pneumonia (J12-J18)
EXCLUDES 2 *acute pulmonary insufficiency following thoracic surgery (J95.1)*
postprocedural subglottic stenosis (J95.5)

Other diseases of the respiratory system (J96-J99)

4 **J96 Respiratory failure, not elsewhere classified**
EXCLUDES 1 *acute respiratory distress syndrome (J80)*
cardiorespiratory failure (R09.2)
newborn respiratory distress syndrome (P22.0)
postprocedural respiratory failure (J95.82-)
respiratory arrest (R09.2)
respiratory arrest of newborn (P28.81)
respiratory failure of newborn (P28.5)

5 **J96.0 Acute respiratory failure**

J96.00 Acute respiratory failure, unspecified whether with hypoxia or hypercapnia HCC
AHA: 4Q 2013, 121
AHA: 3Q 2016, 14

J96.01 Acute respiratory failure with hypoxia HCC

J96.02 Acute respiratory failure with hypercapnia HCC

5 **J96.1 Chronic respiratory failure**

J96.10 Chronic respiratory failure, unspecified whether with hypoxia or hypercapnia HCC
AHA: 1Q 2015, 21
AHA: 1Q 2016, 38

J96.11 Chronic respiratory failure with hypoxia HCC
AHA: 4Q 2013, 129

J96.12 Chronic respiratory failure with hypercapnia HCC

5 **J96.2 Acute and chronic respiratory failure**
Acute on chronic respiratory failure

J96.20 Acute and chronic respiratory failure, unspecified whether with hypoxia or hypercapnia HCC

J96.21 Acute and chronic respiratory failure with hypoxia HCC

J96.22 Acute and chronic respiratory failure with hypercapnia HCC

5 **J96.9 Respiratory failure, unspecified**

J96.90 Respiratory failure, unspecified, unspecified whether with hypoxia or hypercapnia HCC

J96.91 Respiratory failure, unspecified with hypoxia HCC

J96.92 Respiratory failure, unspecified with hypercapnia HCC

4 **J98 Other respiratory disorders**
Use additional code to identify:
exposure to environmental tobacco smoke (Z77.22)
exposure to tobacco smoke in the perinatal period (P96.81)
history of tobacco dependence (Z87.891)
occupational exposure to environmental tobacco smoke (Z57.31)
tobacco dependence (F17.-)
tobacco use (Z72.0)
EXCLUDES 1 *newborn apnea (P28.4)*
newborn sleep apnea (P28.3)
EXCLUDES 2 *apnea NOS (R06.81)*
sleep apnea (G47.3-)

5 **J98.0 Diseases of bronchus, not elsewhere classified**

J98.01 Acute bronchospasm
EXCLUDES 1 *acute bronchiolitis with bronchospasm (J21.-)*
acute bronchitis with bronchospasm (J20.-)
asthma (J45.-)
exercise induced bronchospasm (J45.990)

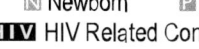

DEFINITION Constriction or contraction of the smooth muscle in the large air passages, severely limiting airflow.

J98.09 Other diseases of bronchus, not elsewhere classified
Broncholithiasis
Calcification of bronchus
Stenosis of bronchus
Tracheobronchial collapse
Tracheobronchial dyskinesia
Ulcer of bronchus

5 **J98.1 Pulmonary collapse**
EXCLUDES 1 *therapeutic collapse of lung status (Z98.3)*

J98.11 Atelectasis
EXCLUDES 1 *newborn atelectasis*
tuberculous atelectasis (current disease) (A15)

J98.19 Other pulmonary collapse

J98.2 Interstitial emphysema HCC
Mediastinal emphysema
EXCLUDES 1 *emphysema NOS (J43.9)*
emphysema in newborn (P25.0)
surgical emphysema (subcutaneous) (T81.82)
traumatic subcutaneous emphysema (T79.7)

J98.3 Compensatory emphysema HCC

J98.4 Other disorders of lung
Calcification of lung
Cystic lung disease (acquired)
Lung disease NOS
Pulmolithiasis
EXCLUDES 1 *acute interstitial pneumonitis (J84.114)*
pulmonary insufficiency following surgery (J95.1-J95.2)

5 **J98.5 Diseases of mediastinum, not elsewhere classified**
EXCLUDES 2 *abscess of mediastinum (J85.3)*
AHA: 4Q 2016, 29

J98.51 Mediastinitis
Code first:
underlying condition, if applicable, such as postoperative mediastinitis (T81.-)

J98.59 Other diseases of mediastinum, not elsewhere classified
Fibrosis of mediastinum
Hernia of mediastinum
Retraction of mediastinum

J98.6 Disorders of diaphragm
Diaphragmatitis
Paralysis of diaphragm
Relaxation of diaphragm
EXCLUDES 1 *congenital malformation of diaphragm NEC (Q79.1)*
congenital diaphragmatic hernia (Q79.0)
EXCLUDES 2 *diaphragmatic hernia (K44.-)*

J98.8 Other specified respiratory disorders

J98.9 Respiratory disorder, unspecified
Respiratory disease (chronic) NOS

▲ **J99 *Respiratory disorders in diseases classified elsewhere*** HCC
Code first underlying disease, such as:
amyloidosis (E85.-)
ankylosing spondylitis (M45)
congenital syphilis (A50.5)
cryoglobulinemia (D89.1)
early congenital syphilis (A50.0)
plasminogen deficiency (E88.02)
schistosomiasis (B65.0-B65.9)
EXCLUDES 1 *respiratory disorders in:*
amebiasis (A06.5)
blastomycosis (B40.0-B40.2)
candidiasis (B37.1)
coccidioidomycosis (B38.0-B38.2)
cystic fibrosis with pulmonary manifestations (E84.0)
dermatomyositis (M33.01, M33.11)
histoplasmosis (B39.0-B39.2)
late syphilis (A52.72, A52.73)
polymyositis (M33.21)
sicca syndrome (M35.02)
systemic lupus erythematosus (M32.13)
systemic sclerosis (M34.81)
Wegener's granulomatosis (M31.30-M31.31)

CHAPTER 11: DISEASES OF THE DIGESTIVE SYSTEM (K00-K95)

EXCLUDES 2 *certain conditions originating in the perinatal period (P04-P96)*
certain infectious and parasitic diseases (A00-B99)
complications of pregnancy, childbirth and the puerperium (O00-O9A)
congenital malformations, deformations and chromosomal abnormalities (Q00-Q99)
endocrine, nutritional and metabolic diseases (E00-E88)
injury, poisoning and certain other consequences of external causes (S00-T88)
neoplasms (C00-D49)
symptoms, signs and abnormal clinical and laboratory findings, not elsewhere classified (R00-R94)

This chapter contains the following blocks:

K00-K14	Diseases of oral cavity and salivary glands
K20-K31	Diseases of esophagus, stomach and duodenum
K35-K38	Diseases of appendix
K40-K46	Hernia
K50-K52	Noninfective enteritis and colitis
K55-K64	Other diseases of intestines
K65-K68	Diseases of peritoneum and retroperitoneum
K70-K77	Diseases of liver
K80-K87	Disorders of gallbladder, biliary tract and pancreas
K90-K95	Other diseases of the digestive system

Diseases of oral cavity and salivary glands (K00-K14)

4 **K00 Disorders of tooth development and eruption**
EXCLUDES 2 *embedded and impacted teeth (K01.-)*

Oral cavity anatomy

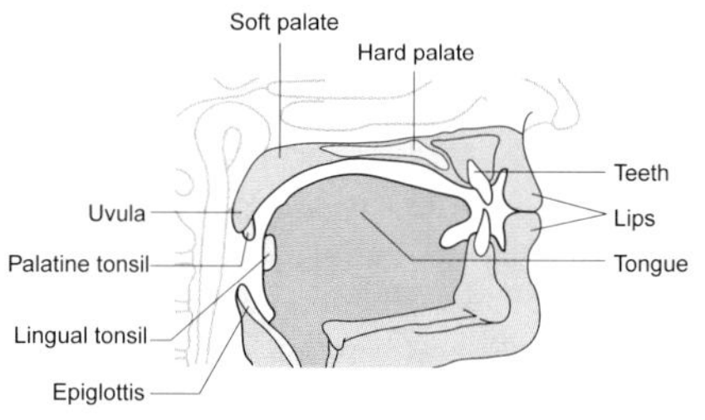

K00.0 Anodontia
Hypodontia
Oligodontia
EXCLUDES 1 *acquired absence of teeth (K08.1-)*

DEFINITION Defect in which many or all of the teeth do not develop and are absent from the mouth.

K00.1 Supernumerary teeth
Distomolar
Fourth molar
Mesiodens
Paramolar
Supplementary teeth
EXCLUDES 2 *supernumerary roots (K00.2)*

K00.2 Abnormalities of size and form of teeth
Concrescence of teeth
Fusion of teeth
Gemination of teeth
Dens evaginatus
Dens in dente
Dens invaginatus
Enamel pearls
Macrodontia
Microdontia
Peg-shaped [conical] teeth
Supernumerary roots
Taurodontism
Tuberculum paramolare
EXCLUDES 1 *abnormalities of teeth due to congenital syphilis (A50.5)*
tuberculum Carabelli, which is regarded as a normal variation and should not be coded

K00.3 Mottled teeth
Dental fluorosis
Mottling of enamel
Nonfluoride enamel opacities
EXCLUDES 2 *deposits [accretions] on teeth (K03.6)*

K00.4 Disturbances in tooth formation
Aplasia and hypoplasia of cementum
Dilaceration of tooth
Enamel hypoplasia (neonatal) (postnatal) (prenatal)
Regional odontodysplasia
Turner's tooth
EXCLUDES 1 *Hutchinson's teeth and mulberry molars in congenital syphilis (A50.5)*
EXCLUDES 2 *mottled teeth (K00.3)*

K00.5 Hereditary disturbances in tooth structure, not elsewhere classified
Amelogenesis imperfecta
Dentinogenesis imperfecta
Odontogenesis imperfecta
Dentinal dysplasia
Shell teeth

K00.6 Disturbances in tooth eruption
Dentia praecox
Natal tooth
Neonatal tooth
Premature eruption of tooth
Premature shedding of primary [deciduous] tooth
Prenatal teeth
Retained [persistent] primary tooth
EXCLUDES 2 *embedded and impacted teeth (K01.-)*

K00.7 Teething syndrome

K00.8 Other disorders of tooth development
Color changes during tooth formation
Intrinsic staining of teeth NOS
EXCLUDES 2 *posteruptive color changes (K03.7)*

K00.9 Disorder of tooth development, unspecified
Disorder of odontogenesis NOS

4 **K01 Embedded and impacted teeth**
EXCLUDES 1 *abnormal position of fully erupted teeth (M26.3-)*

K01.0 Embedded teeth

K01.1 Impacted teeth

4 **K02 Dental caries**
INCLUDES caries of dentine
dental cavities
early childhood caries
pre-eruptive caries
recurrent caries (dentino enamel junction) (enamel) (to the pulp)
tooth decay

K02.3 Arrested dental caries
Arrested coronal and root caries

5 **K02.5 Dental caries on pit and fissure surface**
Dental caries on chewing surface of tooth

K02.51 Dental caries on pit and fissure surface limited to enamel
White spot lesions [initial caries] on pit and fissure surface of tooth

K02.52 **Dental caries on pit and fissure surface penetrating into dentin**
Primary dental caries, cervical origin

K02.53 **Dental caries on pit and fissure surface penetrating into pulp**

K02.6 **Dental caries on smooth surface**

K02.61 **Dental caries on smooth surface limited to enamel**
White spot lesions [initial caries] on smooth surface of tooth

K02.62 **Dental caries on smooth surface penetrating into dentin**

K02.63 **Dental caries on smooth surface penetrating into pulp**

K02.7 **Dental root caries**

K02.9 **Dental caries, unspecified**

K03 Other diseases of hard tissues of teeth

EXCLUDES 2 *bruxism (F45.8)*
dental caries (K02.-)
teeth-grinding NOS (F45.8)

K03.0 **Excessive attrition of teeth**
Approximal wear of teeth
Occlusal wear of teeth

DEFINITION Teeth exhibit excessive wear and tear as a result of tooth-to-tooth contact, often due to grinding the teeth.

K03.1 **Abrasion of teeth**
Dentifrice abrasion of teeth
Habitual abrasion of teeth
Occupational abrasion of teeth
Ritual abrasion of teeth
Traditional abrasion of teeth
Wedge defect NOS

DEFINITION Teeth exhibit specific wear and tear as a result of tooth contact with another object.

K03.2 **Erosion of teeth**
Erosion of teeth due to diet
Erosion of teeth due to drugs and medicaments
Erosion of teeth due to persistent vomiting
Erosion of teeth NOS
Idiopathic erosion of teeth
Occupational erosion of teeth

K03.3 **Pathological resorption of teeth**
Internal granuloma of pulp
Resorption of teeth (external)

K03.4 **Hypercementosis**
Cementation hyperplasia

K03.5 **Ankylosis of teeth**

DEFINITION Roots of the teeth grow into and merge with the bone of the jaw; most often occurring during development of baby teeth.

K03.6 **Deposits [accretions] on teeth**
Betel deposits [accretions] on teeth
Black deposits [accretions] on teeth
Extrinsic staining of teeth NOS
Green deposits [accretions] on teeth
Materia alba deposits [accretions] on teeth
Orange deposits [accretions] on teeth
Staining of teeth NOS
Subgingival dental calculus
Supragingival dental calculus
Tobacco deposits [accretions] on teeth

DEFINITION Calculous deposits or tartar build-up that resists removal by normal brushing and requires professional cleaning.

K03.7 **Posteruptive color changes of dental hard tissues**

EXCLUDES 2 *deposits [accretions] on teeth (K03.6)*

K03.8 **Other specified diseases of hard tissues of teeth**

K03.81 **Cracked tooth**

EXCLUDES 1 *asymptomatic craze lines in enamel - omit code*
broken or fractured tooth due to trauma (S02.5)

K03.89 **Other specified diseases of hard tissues of teeth**

K03.9 **Disease of hard tissues of teeth, unspecified**

K04 Diseases of pulp and periapical tissues

AHA: 4Q 2016, 29

K04.0 **Pulpitis**
Acute pulpitis
Chronic (hyperplastic) (ulcerative) pulpitis

DEFINITION Painful inflammation of the soft living tissue containing nerves within the center of the tooth.

K04.01 **Reversible pulpitis**

K04.02 **Irreversible pulpitis**

K04.1 **Necrosis of pulp**
Pulpal gangrene

K04.2 **Pulp degeneration**
Denticles
Pulpal calcifications
Pulpal stones

K04.3 **Abnormal hard tissue formation in pulp**
Secondary or irregular dentine

K04.4 **Acute apical periodontitis of pulpal origin**
Acute apical periodontitis NOS

EXCLUDES 1 *acute periodontitis (K05.2-)*

DEFINITION Severe inflammation of the periodontal ligament connecting the tooth to the jawbone due to infection or necrosis of the soft, living tissue in the center of the tooth.

K04.5 **Chronic apical periodontitis**
Apical or periapical granuloma
Apical periodontitis NOS

EXCLUDES 1 *chronic periodontitis (K05.3-)*

K04.6 **Periapical abscess with sinus**
Dental abscess with sinus
Dentoalveolar abscess with sinus

K04.7 **Periapical abscess without sinus**
Dental abscess without sinus
Dentoalveolar abscess without sinus

K04.8 **Radicular cyst**
Apical (periodontal) cyst
Periapical cyst
Residual radicular cyst

EXCLUDES 2 *lateral periodontal cyst (K09.0)*

K04.9 **Other and unspecified diseases of pulp and periapical tissues**

K04.90 **Unspecified diseases of pulp and periapical tissues**

K04.99 **Other diseases of pulp and periapical tissues**

K05 Gingivitis and periodontal diseases

Use additional code to identify:
alcohol abuse and dependence (F10.-)
exposure to environmental tobacco smoke (Z77.22)
exposure to tobacco smoke in the perinatal period (P96.81)
history of tobacco dependence (Z87.891)
occupational exposure to environmental tobacco smoke (Z57.31)
tobacco dependence (F17.-)
tobacco use (Z72.0)

AHA: 4Q 2016, 29

K05.0 **Acute gingivitis**

EXCLUDES 1 *acute necrotizing ulcerative gingivitis (A69.1)*
herpesviral [herpes simplex] gingivostomatitis (B00.2)

K05.00 **Acute gingivitis, plaque induced**
Acute gingivitis NOS
Plaque induced gingival disease

Plaque-induced acute gingivitis
An inflammation of the gums caused by bacterial biofilm of plaque

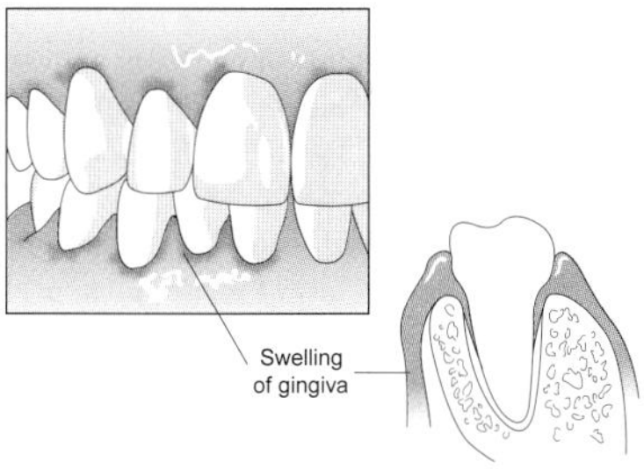

K05.01 **Acute gingivitis, non-plaque induced**

5 **K05.1** **Chronic gingivitis**
Desquamative gingivitis (chronic)
Gingivitis (chronic) NOS
Hyperplastic gingivitis (chronic)
Pregnancy associated gingivitis
Simple marginal gingivitis (chronic)
Ulcerative gingivitis (chronic)
Code first:
, if applicable, diseases of the digestive system complicating pregnancy (O99.61-)

K05.10 **Chronic gingivitis, plaque induced**
Chronic gingivitis NOS
Gingivitis NOS

K05.11 **Chronic gingivitis, non-plaque induced**

5 **K05.2** **Aggressive periodontitis**
Acute pericoronitis
EXCLUDES 1 *acute apical periodontitis (K04.4)*
periapical abscess (K04.7)
periapical abscess with sinus (K04.6)

K05.20 **Aggressive periodontitis, unspecified**
DEFINITION Serious and destructive inflammation and infection of the ligaments and bones supporting the teeth, leading to tooth loss.

6 **K05.21** **Aggressive periodontitis, localized**
Periodontal abscess

K05.211 **Aggressive periodontitis, localized, slight**
K05.212 **Aggressive periodontitis, localized, moderate**
K05.213 **Aggressive periodontitis, localized, severe**
K05.219 **Aggressive periodontitis, localized, unspecified severity**

6 **K05.22** **Aggressive periodontitis, generalized**

K05.221 **Aggressive periodontitis, generalized, slight**
K05.222 **Aggressive periodontitis, generalized, moderate**
K05.223 **Aggressive periodontitis, generalized, severe**
K05.229 **Aggressive periodontitis, generalized, unspecified severity**

5 **K05.3** **Chronic periodontitis**
Chronic pericoronitis
Complex periodontitis
Periodontitis NOS
Simplex periodontitis
EXCLUDES 1 *chronic apical periodontitis (K04.5)*

K05.30 **Chronic periodontitis, unspecified**

6 **K05.31** **Chronic periodontitis, localized**

K05.311 **Chronic periodontitis, localized, slight**
K05.312 **Chronic periodontitis, localized, moderate**
K05.313 **Chronic periodontitis, localized, severe**
K05.319 **Chronic periodontitis, localized, unspecified severity**

6 **K05.32** **Chronic periodontitis, generalized**

K05.321 **Chronic periodontitis, generalized, slight**
K05.322 **Chronic periodontitis, generalized, moderate**
K05.323 **Chronic periodontitis, generalized, severe**
K05.329 **Chronic periodontitis, generalized, unspecified severity**

K05.4 **Periodontosis**
Juvenile periodontosis

K05.5 **Other periodontal diseases**
Combined periodontic-endodontic lesion
Narrow gingival width (of periodontal soft tissue)
EXCLUDES 2 *leukoplakia of gingiva (K13.21)*

K05.6 **Periodontal disease, unspecified**

4 **K06** **Other disorders of gingiva and edentulous alveolar ridge**
EXCLUDES 2 *acute gingivitis (K05.0)*
atrophy of edentulous alveolar ridge (K08.2)
chronic gingivitis (K05.1)
gingivitis NOS (K05.1)
AHA: 4Q 2016, 29

5 **K06.0** **Gingival recession**
Gingival recession (postinfective) (postprocedural)
DEFINITION Gums that have receded, exposing more tooth.

6 **K06.01** **Gingival recession, localized**
AHA: 4Q 2017, 13

K06.010 **Localized gingival recession, unspecified**
Localized gingival recession, NOS
K06.011 **Localized gingival recession, minimal**
K06.012 **Localized gingival recession, moderate**
K06.013 **Localized gingival recession, severe**

6 **K06.02** **Gingival recession, generalized**
AHA: 4Q 2017, 13

K06.020 **Generalized gingival recession, unspecified**
Generalized gingival recession, NOS
K06.021 **Generalized gingival recession, minimal**
K06.022 **Generalized gingival recession, moderate**
K06.023 **Generalized gingival recession, severe**

K06.1 **Gingival enlargement**
Gingival fibromatosis

K06.2 **Gingival and edentulous alveolar ridge lesions associated with trauma**
Irritative hyperplasia of edentulous ridge [denture hyperplasia]
Use additional code (Chapter 20) to identify external cause or denture status (Z97.2)

K06.3 **Horizontal alveolar bone loss**

K06.8 **Other specified disorders of gingiva and edentulous alveolar ridge**
Fibrous epulis
Flabby alveolar ridge
Giant cell epulis
Peripheral giant cell granuloma of gingiva
Pyogenic granuloma of gingiva
Vertical ridge deficiency
EXCLUDES 2 *gingival cyst (K09.0)*

K06.9 **Disorder of gingiva and edentulous alveolar ridge, unspecified**

4 **K08** **Other disorders of teeth and supporting structures**
EXCLUDES 2 *dentofacial anomalies [including malocclusion] (M26.-)*
disorders of jaw (M27.-)
AHA: 4Q 2016, 29

K08.0 **Exfoliation of teeth due to systemic causes**
Code also:
underlying systemic condition

5 **K08.1** **Complete loss of teeth**
Acquired loss of teeth, complete
EXCLUDES 1 *congenital absence of teeth (K00.0)*
exfoliation of teeth due to systemic causes (K08.0)
partial loss of teeth (K08.4-)

6 **K08.10** **Complete loss of teeth, unspecified cause**

K08.101 **Complete loss of teeth, unspecified cause, class I**
K08.102 **Complete loss of teeth, unspecified cause, class II**

K08.103 Complete loss of teeth, unspecified cause, class III
K08.104 Complete loss of teeth, unspecified cause, class IV
K08.109 Complete loss of teeth, unspecified cause, unspecified class
Edentulism NOS

6 K08.11 Complete loss of teeth due to trauma
K08.111 Complete loss of teeth due to trauma, class I
K08.112 Complete loss of teeth due to trauma, class II
K08.113 Complete loss of teeth due to trauma, class III
K08.114 Complete loss of teeth due to trauma, class IV
K08.119 Complete loss of teeth due to trauma, unspecified class

6 K08.12 Complete loss of teeth due to periodontal diseases
K08.121 Complete loss of teeth due to periodontal diseases, class I
K08.122 Complete loss of teeth due to periodontal diseases, class II
K08.123 Complete loss of teeth due to periodontal diseases, class III
K08.124 Complete loss of teeth due to periodontal diseases, class IV
K08.129 Complete loss of teeth due to periodontal diseases, unspecified class

6 K08.13 Complete loss of teeth due to caries
K08.131 Complete loss of teeth due to caries, class I
K08.132 Complete loss of teeth due to caries, class II
K08.133 Complete loss of teeth due to caries, class III
K08.134 Complete loss of teeth due to caries, class IV
K08.139 Complete loss of teeth due to caries, unspecified class

6 K08.19 Complete loss of teeth due to other specified cause
K08.191 Complete loss of teeth due to other specified cause, class I
K08.192 Complete loss of teeth due to other specified cause, class II
K08.193 Complete loss of teeth due to other specified cause, class III
K08.194 Complete loss of teeth due to other specified cause, class IV
K08.199 Complete loss of teeth due to other specified cause, unspecified class

5 K08.2 Atrophy of edentulous alveolar ridge
K08.20 Unspecified atrophy of edentulous alveolar ridge
Atrophy of the mandible NOS
Atrophy of the maxilla NOS
K08.21 Minimal atrophy of the mandible
Minimal atrophy of the edentulous mandible
K08.22 Moderate atrophy of the mandible
Moderate atrophy of the edentulous mandible
K08.23 Severe atrophy of the mandible
Severe atrophy of the edentulous mandible
K08.24 Minimal atrophy of maxilla
Minimal atrophy of the edentulous maxilla
K08.25 Moderate atrophy of the maxilla
Moderate atrophy of the edentulous maxilla
K08.26 Severe atrophy of the maxilla
Severe atrophy of the edentulous maxilla

K08.3 Retained dental root
DEFINITION Part or all of the root structure of a tooth remains in the jaw after the tooth is extracted or otherwise lost.

5 K08.4 Partial loss of teeth
Acquired loss of teeth, partial
EXCLUDES 1 *complete loss of teeth (K08.1-)*
congenital absence of teeth (K00.0)
EXCLUDES 2 *exfoliation of teeth due to systemic causes (K08.0)*

6 K08.40 Partial loss of teeth, unspecified cause
K08.401 Partial loss of teeth, unspecified cause, class I
K08.402 Partial loss of teeth, unspecified cause, class II
K08.403 Partial loss of teeth, unspecified cause, class III
K08.404 Partial loss of teeth, unspecified cause, class IV
K08.409 Partial loss of teeth, unspecified cause, unspecified class
Tooth extraction status NOS

6 K08.41 Partial loss of teeth due to trauma
K08.411 Partial loss of teeth due to trauma, class I
K08.412 Partial loss of teeth due to trauma, class II
K08.413 Partial loss of teeth due to trauma, class III
K08.414 Partial loss of teeth due to trauma, class IV
K08.419 Partial loss of teeth due to trauma, unspecified class

6 K08.42 Partial loss of teeth due to periodontal diseases
K08.421 Partial loss of teeth due to periodontal diseases, class I
K08.422 Partial loss of teeth due to periodontal diseases, class II
K08.423 Partial loss of teeth due to periodontal diseases, class III
K08.424 Partial loss of teeth due to periodontal diseases, class IV
K08.429 Partial loss of teeth due to periodontal diseases, unspecified class

6 K08.43 Partial loss of teeth due to caries
K08.431 Partial loss of teeth due to caries, class I
K08.432 Partial loss of teeth due to caries, class II
K08.433 Partial loss of teeth due to caries, class III
K08.434 Partial loss of teeth due to caries, class IV
K08.439 Partial loss of teeth due to caries, unspecified class

6 K08.49 Partial loss of teeth due to other specified cause
K08.491 Partial loss of teeth due to other specified cause, class I
K08.492 Partial loss of teeth due to other specified cause, class II
K08.493 Partial loss of teeth due to other specified cause, class III
K08.494 Partial loss of teeth due to other specified cause, class IV
K08.499 Partial loss of teeth due to other specified cause, unspecified class

5 K08.5 Unsatisfactory restoration of tooth
Defective bridge, crown, filling
Defective dental restoration
EXCLUDES 1 *dental restoration status (Z98.811)*
EXCLUDES 2 *endosseous dental implant failure (M27.6-)*
unsatisfactory endodontic treatment (M27.5-)

K08.50 Unsatisfactory restoration of tooth, unspecified
Defective dental restoration NOS
K08.51 Open restoration margins of tooth
Dental restoration failure of marginal integrity
Open margin on tooth restoration
Poor gingival margin to tooth restoration
K08.52 Unrepairable overhanging of dental restorative materials
Overhanging of tooth restoration

6 K08.53 Fractured dental restorative material
EXCLUDES 1 *cracked tooth (K03.81)*
traumatic fracture of tooth (S02.5)
K08.530 Fractured dental restorative material without loss of material
K08.531 Fractured dental restorative material with loss of material
K08.539 Fractured dental restorative material, unspecified

K08.54 Contour of existing restoration of tooth biologically incompatible with oral health
Dental restoration failure of periodontal anatomical integrity
Unacceptable contours of existing restoration of tooth
Unacceptable morphology of existing restoration of tooth
K08.55 Allergy to existing dental restorative material
Use additional code to identify the specific type of allergy

K08.56 **Poor aesthetic of existing restoration of tooth**
Dental restoration aesthetically inadequate or displeasing

K08.59 **Other unsatisfactory restoration of tooth**
Other defective dental restoration

5 **K08.8** **Other specified disorders of teeth and supporting structures**

K08.81 **Primary occlusal trauma**

K08.82 **Secondary occlusal trauma**

K08.89 **Other specified disorders of teeth and supporting structures**
Enlargement of alveolar ridge NOS
Insufficient anatomic crown height
Insufficient clinical crown length
Irregular alveolar process
Toothache NOS

K08.9 **Disorder of teeth and supporting structures, unspecified**

4 **K09** **Cysts of oral region, not elsewhere classified**

INCLUDES lesions showing histological features both of aneurysmal cyst and of another fibro-osseous lesion

EXCLUDES 2 *cysts of jaw (M27.0-, M27.4-)*
radicular cyst (K04.8)

K09.0 **Developmental odontogenic cysts**
Dentigerous cyst
Eruption cyst
Follicular cyst
Gingival cyst
Lateral periodontal cyst
Primordial cyst

EXCLUDES 2 *keratocysts (D16.4, D16.5)*
odontogenic keratocystic tumors (D16.4, D16.5)

K09.1 **Developmental (nonodontogenic) cysts of oral region**
Cyst (of) incisive canal
Cyst (of) palatine of papilla
Globulomaxillary cyst
Median palatal cyst
Nasoalveolar cyst
Nasolabial cyst
Nasopalatine duct cyst

K09.8 **Other cysts of oral region, not elsewhere classified**
Dermoid cyst
Epidermoid cyst
Lymphoepithelial cyst
Epstein's pearl

K09.9 **Cyst of oral region, unspecified**

4 **K11** **Diseases of salivary glands**

Use additional code to identify:
alcohol abuse and dependence (F10.-)
exposure to environmental tobacco smoke (Z77.22)
exposure to tobacco smoke in the perinatal period (P96.81)
history of tobacco dependence (Z87.891)
occupational exposure to environmental tobacco smoke (Z57.31)
tobacco dependence (F17.-)
tobacco use (Z72.0)

K11.0 **Atrophy of salivary gland**

DEFINITION Wasting of the saliva glands, resulting in insufficient saliva production.

K11.1 **Hypertrophy of salivary gland**

5 **K11.2** **Sialoadenitis**
Parotitis

EXCLUDES 1 *epidemic parotitis (B26.-)*
mumps (B26.-)
uveoparotid fever [Heerfordt] (D86.89)

K11.20 **Sialoadenitis, unspecified**

K11.21 **Acute sialoadenitis**

EXCLUDES 1 *acute recurrent sialoadenitis (K11.22)*

K11.22 **Acute recurrent sialoadenitis**

K11.23 **Chronic sialoadenitis**

K11.3 **Abscess of salivary gland**

K11.4 **Fistula of salivary gland**

EXCLUDES 1 *congenital fistula of salivary gland (Q38.4)*

K11.5 **Sialolithiasis**
Calculus of salivary gland or duct
Stone of salivary gland or duct

K11.6 **Mucocele of salivary gland**
Mucous extravasation cyst of salivary gland
Mucous retention cyst of salivary gland
Ranula

Mucocele of salivary gland

A mucus-filled cyst often on the lower lip caused by a plugged salivary gland

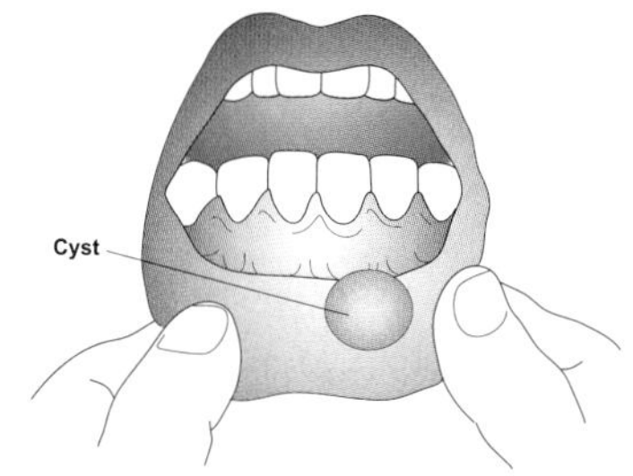

K11.7 **Disturbances of salivary secretion**
Hypoptyalism
Ptyalism
Xerostomia

EXCLUDES 2 *dry mouth NOS (R68.2)*

K11.8 **Other diseases of salivary glands**
Benign lymphoepithelial lesion of salivary gland
Mikulicz' disease
Necrotizing sialometaplasia
Sialectasia
Stenosis of salivary duct
Stricture of salivary duct

EXCLUDES 1 *sicca syndrome [Sjögren] (M35.0-)*

K11.9 **Disease of salivary gland, unspecified**
Sialoadenopathy NOS

4 **K12** **Stomatitis and related lesions**

Use additional code to identify:
alcohol abuse and dependence (F10.-)
exposure to environmental tobacco smoke (Z77.22)
exposure to tobacco smoke in the perinatal period (P96.81)
history of tobacco dependence (Z87.891)
occupational exposure to environmental tobacco smoke (Z57.31)
tobacco dependence (F17.-)
tobacco use (Z72.0)

EXCLUDES 1 *cancrum oris (A69.0)*
cheilitis (K13.0)
gangrenous stomatitis (A69.0)
herpesviral [herpes simplex] gingivostomatitis (B00.2)
noma (A69.0)

K12.0 **Recurrent oral aphthae**
Aphthous stomatitis (major) (minor)
Bednar's aphthae
Periadenitis mucosa necrotica recurrens
Recurrent aphthous ulcer
Stomatitis herpetiformis

K12.1 **Other forms of stomatitis**
Stomatitis NOS
Denture stomatitis
Ulcerative stomatitis
Vesicular stomatitis

EXCLUDES 1 *acute necrotizing ulcerative stomatitis (A69.1)*
Vincent's stomatitis (A69.1)

DEFINITION Painful inflammation of the mucosal soft tissues of the mouth, usually from a viral infection that can lead to ulcers or vesicular lesions.

K12.2 **Cellulitis and abscess of mouth**
Cellulitis of mouth (floor)
Submandibular abscess

EXCLUDES 2 *abscess of salivary gland (K11.3)*
abscess of tongue (K14.0)
periapical abscess (K04.6-K04.7)
periodontal abscess (K05.21)
peritonsillar abscess (J36)

K12.3 Oral mucositis (ulcerative)
Mucositis (oral) (oropharyneal)
EXCLUDES 2 *gastrointestinal mucositis (ulcerative) (K92.81)*
mucositis (ulcerative) of vagina and vulva (N76.81)
nasal mucositis (ulcerative) (J34.81)

K12.30 Oral mucositis (ulcerative), unspecified

K12.31 Oral mucositis (ulcerative) due to antineoplastic therapy
Use additional code for adverse effect, if applicable, to identify antineoplastic and immunosuppressive drugs (T45.1X5)
Use additional code for other antineoplastic therapy, such as:
radiological procedure and radiotherapy (Y84.2)

K12.32 Oral mucositis (ulcerative) due to other drugs
Use additional code for adverse effect, if applicable, to identify drug (T36-T50 with fifth or sixth character 5)

K12.33 Oral mucositis (ulcerative) due to radiation
Use additional external cause code (W88-W90, X39.0-) to identify cause

K12.39 Other oral mucositis (ulcerative)
Viral oral mucositis (ulcerative)

K13 Other diseases of lip and oral mucosa

INCLUDES epithelial disturbances of tongue

Use additional code to identify:
alcohol abuse and dependence (F10.-)
exposure to environmental tobacco smoke (Z77.22)
exposure to tobacco smoke in the perinatal period (P96.81)
history of tobacco dependence (Z87.891)
occupational exposure to environmental tobacco smoke (Z57.31)
tobacco dependence (F17.-)
tobacco use (Z72.0)

EXCLUDES 2 *certain disorders of gingiva and edentulous alveolar ridge (K05-K06)*
cysts of oral region (K09.-)
diseases of tongue (K14.-)
stomatitis and related lesions (K12.-)

K13.0 Diseases of lips
Abscess of lips
Angular cheilitis
Cellulitis of lips
Cheilitis NOS
Cheilodynia
Cheilosis
Exfoliative cheilitis
Fistula of lips
Glandular cheilitis
Hypertrophy of lips
Perlèche NEC
EXCLUDES 1 *ariboflavinosis (E53.0)*
cheilitis due to radiation-related disorders (L55-L59)
congenital fistula of lips (Q38.0)
congenital hypertrophy of lips (Q18.6)
Perlèche due to candidiasis (B37.83)
Perlèche due to riboflavin deficiency (E53.0)

K13.1 Cheek and lip biting

K13.2 Leukoplakia and other disturbances of oral epithelium, including tongue
EXCLUDES 1 *carcinoma in situ of oral epithelium (D00.0-)*
hairy leukoplakia (K13.3)

K13.21 Leukoplakia of oral mucosa, including tongue
Leukokeratosis of oral mucosa
Leukoplakia of gingiva, lips, tongue
EXCLUDES 1 *hairy leukoplakia (K13.3)*
leukokeratosis nicotina palati (K13.24)

Leukoplakia of oral mucosa, including tongue

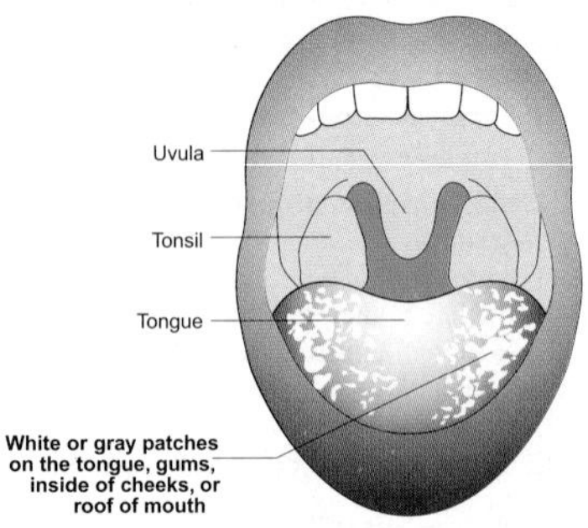

K13.22 Minimal keratinized residual ridge mucosa
Minimal keratinization of alveolar ridge mucosa

K13.23 Excessive keratinized residual ridge mucosa
Excessive keratinization of alveolar ridge mucosa

K13.24 Leukokeratosis nicotina palati
Smoker's palate

K13.29 Other disturbances of oral epithelium, including tongue
Erythroplakia of mouth or tongue
Focal epithelial hyperplasia of mouth or tongue
Leukoedema of mouth or tongue
Other oral epithelium disturbances

K13.3 Hairy leukoplakia

K13.4 Granuloma and granuloma-like lesions of oral mucosa
Eosinophilic granuloma
Granuloma pyogenicum
Verrucous xanthoma

K13.5 Oral submucous fibrosis
Submucous fibrosis of tongue

DEFINITION Build-up of fibrous (scar-like) tissue within the soft tissues of the mouth, causing rigidity and inability to open the mouth.

K13.6 Irritative hyperplasia of oral mucosa
EXCLUDES 2 *irritative hyperplasia of edentulous ridge [denture hyperplasia] (K06.2)*

K13.7 Other and unspecified lesions of oral mucosa

K13.70 Unspecified lesions of oral mucosa

K13.79 Other lesions of oral mucosa
Focal oral mucinosis

K14 Diseases of tongue

Use additional code to identify:
alcohol abuse and dependence (F10.-)
exposure to environmental tobacco smoke (Z77.22)
history of tobacco dependence (Z87.891)
occupational exposure to environmental tobacco smoke (Z57.31)
tobacco dependence (F17.-)
tobacco use (Z72.0)

EXCLUDES 2 *erythroplakia (K13.29)*
focal epithelial hyperplasia (K13.29)
leukedema of tongue (K13.29)
leukoplakia of tongue (K13.21)
hairy leukoplakia (K13.3)
macroglossia (congenital) (Q38.2)
submucous fibrosis of tongue (K13.5)

K14.0 Glossitis
Abscess of tongue
Ulceration (traumatic) of tongue
EXCLUDES 1 *atrophic glossitis (K14.4)*

DEFINITION Changes in the appearance of the tongue due to inflammation.

K14.1 Geographic tongue
Benign migratory glossitis
Glossitis areata exfoliativa

K14.2 Median rhomboid glossitis

K14.3 Hypertrophy of tongue papillae
Black hairy tongue
Coated tongue
Hypertrophy of foliate papillae
Lingua villosa nigra

K14.4 Atrophy of tongue papillae
Atrophic glossitis

K14.5 Plicated tongue
Fissured tongue
Furrowed tongue
Scrotal tongue
EXCLUDES 1 *fissured tongue, congenital (Q38.3)*

K14.6 Glossodynia
Glossopyrosis
Painful tongue
DEFINITION Pain and/or a burning sensation in the tongue.

K14.8 Other diseases of tongue
Atrophy of tongue
Crenated tongue
Enlargement of tongue
Glossocele
Glossoptosis
Hypertrophy of tongue

K14.9 Disease of tongue, unspecified
Glossopathy NOS

Diseases of esophagus, stomach and duodenum (K20-K31)

EXCLUDES 2 *hiatus hernia (K44.-)*

4 K20 Esophagitis
Use additional code to identify:
alcohol abuse and dependence (F10.-)
EXCLUDES 1 *erosion of esophagus (K22.1-)*
esophagitis with gastro-esophageal reflux disease (K21.0)
reflux esophagitis (K21.0)
ulcerative esophagitis (K22.1-)
EXCLUDES 2 *eosinophilic gastritis or gastroenteritis (K52.81)*

CODING TIP✓ Do not assign a code from K20.- if gastroesophageal reflux is also diagnosed. When a patient has confirmed diagnoses of both gastroesophageal reflux and esophagitis, code K21.0 should be assigned.

K20.0 Eosinophilic esophagitis

K20.8 Other esophagitis
Abscess of esophagus

K20.9 Esophagitis, unspecified
Esophagitis NOS

4 K21 Gastro-esophageal reflux disease
EXCLUDES 1 *newborn esophageal reflux (P78.83)*

K21.0 Gastro-esophageal reflux disease with esophagitis
Reflux esophagitis
DEFINITION Esophageal inflammation due to reflux of gastric acid from the stomach back up into the esophagus.

K21.9 Gastro-esophageal reflux disease without esophagitis
Esophageal reflux NOS
DEFINITION A burning sensation, usually centered in the middle of the chest near the breast bone, caused by the reflux of acidic stomach fluids that enter the lower end of the esophagus.
AHA: 1Q 2016, 18

4 K22 Other diseases of esophagus
EXCLUDES 2 *esophageal varices (I85.-)*

Esophageal anatomy

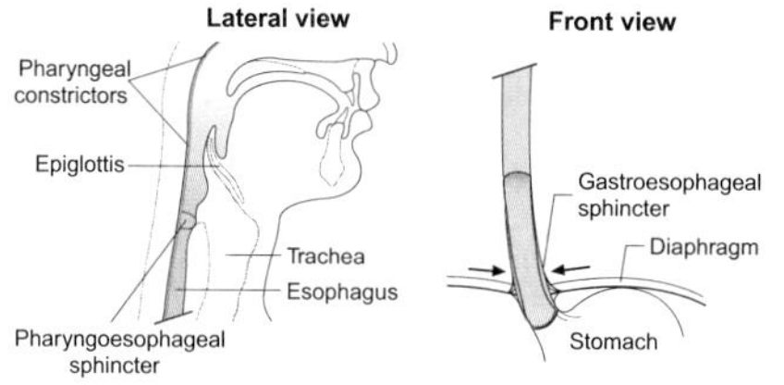

K22.0 Achalasia of cardia
Achalasia NOS
Cardiospasm
EXCLUDES 1 *congenital cardiospasm (Q39.5)*

5 K22.1 Ulcer of esophagus
Barrett's ulcer
Erosion of esophagus
Fungal ulcer of esophagus
Peptic ulcer of esophagus
Ulcer of esophagus due to ingestion of chemicals
Ulcer of esophagus due to ingestion of drugs and medicaments
Ulcerative esophagitis
Code first:
poisoning due to drug or toxin, if applicable (T36-T65 with fifth or sixth character 1-4 or 6)
Use additional code for adverse effect, if applicable, to identify drug (T36-T50 with fifth or sixth character 5)
EXCLUDES 1 *Barrett's esophagus (K22.7-)*

K22.10 Ulcer of esophagus without bleeding
Ulcer of esophagus NOS

K22.11 Ulcer of esophagus with bleeding
EXCLUDES 2 *bleeding esophageal varices (I85.01, I85.11)*

Ulcer of esophagus with bleeding
A lesion that develops on the interior wall of the esophagus

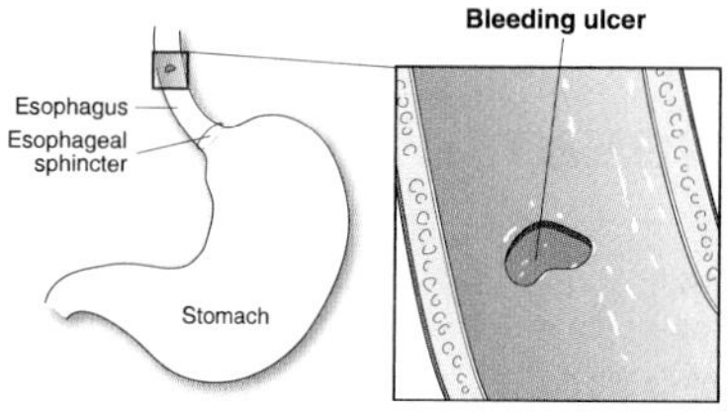

K22.2 Esophageal obstruction
Compression of esophagus
Constriction of esophagus
Stenosis of esophagus
Stricture of esophagus
EXCLUDES 1 *congenital stenosis or stricture of esophagus (Q39.3)*

K22.3 Perforation of esophagus
Rupture of esophagus
EXCLUDES 1 *traumatic perforation of (thoracic) esophagus (S27.8-)*

K22.4 Dyskinesia of esophagus
Corkscrew esophagus
Diffuse esophageal spasm
Spasm of esophagus
EXCLUDES 1 *cardiospasm (K22.0)*
DEFINITION Weakened, paralyzed, or uncoordinated movement of esophageal muscles, causing difficulty swallowing.

K22.5 Diverticulum of esophagus, acquired
Esophageal pouch, acquired
EXCLUDES 1 *diverticulum of esophagus (congenital) (Q39.6)*

K22.6 Gastro-esophageal laceration-hemorrhage syndrome
Mallory-Weiss syndrome

CODING TIP ✓ Code K22.6 should be assigned only for patients diagnosed with Mallory-Weiss syndrome or esophageal laceration and bleeding due to Mallory-Weiss tears. When esophageal bleeding is documented as due to esophageal varices, assign a code from I85.-.

DEFINITION Esophagus becomes torn and bleeds near its connection to the stomach due to prolonged vomiting, hiccupping, or other spasmodic activity.

5 **K22.7 Barrett's esophagus**
Barrett's disease
Barrett's syndrome
EXCLUDES 1 *Barrett's ulcer (K22.1)*
malignant neoplasm of esophagus (C15.-)

K22.70 Barrett's esophagus without dysplasia
Barrett's esophagus NOS

6 **K22.71 Barrett's esophagus with dysplasia**

K22.710 Barrett's esophagus with low grade dysplasia

K22.711 Barrett's esophagus with high grade dysplasia

K22.719 Barrett's esophagus with dysplasia, unspecified

K22.8 Other specified diseases of esophagus
Hemorrhage of esophagus NOS
EXCLUDES 2 *esophageal varices (I85.-)*
Paterson-Kelly syndrome (D50.1)

CODING TIP ✓ Do not assign K22.8 when esophageal hemorrhage is documented as due to Mallory-Weiss syndrome. When Mallory-Weiss syndrome causes laceration and esophageal hemorrhage, assign code K22.6. Also do not assign for esophageal bleeding due to varices. When esophageal bleeding is documented as due to esophageal varices, assign a code from I85.-.

K22.9 Disease of esophagus, unspecified

K23 *Disorders of esophagus in diseases classified elsewhere*
Code first underlying disease, such as:
congenital syphilis (A50.5)
EXCLUDES 1 *late syphilis (A52.79)*
megaesophagus due to Chagas' disease (B57.31)
tuberculosis (A18.83)

4 **K25 Gastric ulcer**
INCLUDES erosion (acute) of stomach
pylorus ulcer (peptic)
stomach ulcer (peptic)
Use additional code to identify:
alcohol abuse and dependence (F10.-)
EXCLUDES 1 *acute gastritis (K29.0-)*
peptic ulcer NOS (K27.-)

CODING TIP ✓ Gastric ulcers are often documented as stomach ulcers. Carefully read all documentation in order to code ulcers to the proper anatomic location.

CODING TIP ✓ When documentation specifies that any gastric, duodenal or peptic ulcer is related to alcohol abuse or dependence, coders should assign an additional code to specify the abuse/dependence as specified.

Gastric ulcer

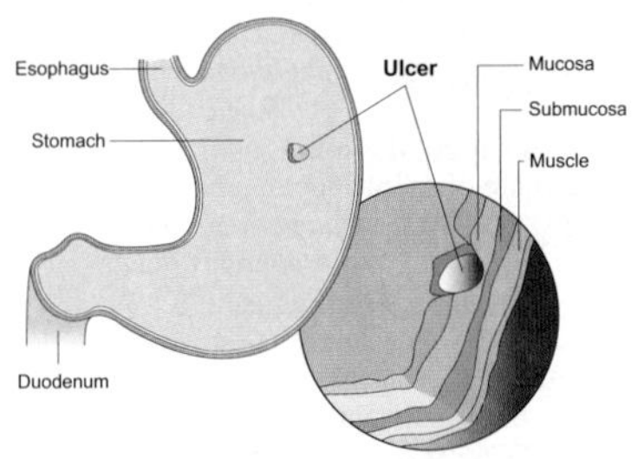

K25.0 Acute gastric ulcer with hemorrhage

K25.1 Acute gastric ulcer with perforation HCC

K25.2 Acute gastric ulcer with both hemorrhage and perforation HCC

K25.3 Acute gastric ulcer without hemorrhage or perforation

K25.4 Chronic or unspecified gastric ulcer with hemorrhage
AHA: 3Q 2017, 27

K25.5 Chronic or unspecified gastric ulcer with perforation HCC

K25.6 Chronic or unspecified gastric ulcer with both hemorrhage and perforation HCC

K25.7 Chronic gastric ulcer without hemorrhage or perforation

K25.9 Gastric ulcer, unspecified as acute or chronic, without hemorrhage or perforation

4 **K26 Duodenal ulcer**
INCLUDES erosion (acute) of duodenum
duodenum ulcer (peptic)
postpyloric ulcer (peptic)
Use additional code to identify:
alcohol abuse and dependence (F10.-)
EXCLUDES 1 *peptic ulcer NOS (K27.-)*

CODING TIP ✓ A peptic ulcer should be coded to K26.- only when specified as duodenal or postpyloric. When documentation reports an ulcer as peptic and does not specify to one of these locations, assign a code from K27.-

CODING TIP ✓ When documentation specifies that any gastric, duodenal or peptic ulcer is related to alcohol abuse or dependence, coders should assign an additional code to specify the abuse/dependence as specified.

K26.0 Acute duodenal ulcer with hemorrhage

K26.1 Acute duodenal ulcer with perforation HCC

K26.2 Acute duodenal ulcer with both hemorrhage and perforation HCC

K26.3 Acute duodenal ulcer without hemorrhage or perforation

K26.4 Chronic or unspecified duodenal ulcer with hemorrhage
AHA: 1Q 2016, 14

K26.5 Chronic or unspecified duodenal ulcer with perforation HCC

K26.6 Chronic or unspecified duodenal ulcer with both hemorrhage and perforation HCC

K26.7 Chronic duodenal ulcer without hemorrhage or perforation

K26.9 Duodenal ulcer, unspecified as acute or chronic, without hemorrhage or perforation

4 **K27 Peptic ulcer, site unspecified**
INCLUDES gastroduodenal ulcer NOS
peptic ulcer NOS
Use additional code to identify:
alcohol abuse and dependence (F10.-)
EXCLUDES 1 *peptic ulcer of newborn (P78.82)*

CODING TIP ✓ When documentation specifies that any gastric, duodenal or peptic ulcer is related to alcohol abuse or dependence, coders should assign an additional code to specify the abuse/dependence as specified.

K27.0 Acute peptic ulcer, site unspecified, with hemorrhage

K27.1 Acute peptic ulcer, site unspecified, with perforation HCC

K27.2 Acute peptic ulcer, site unspecified, with both hemorrhage and perforation HCC

K27.3 Acute peptic ulcer, site unspecified, without hemorrhage or perforation

K27.4 Chronic or unspecified peptic ulcer, site unspecified, with hemorrhage

K27.5 Chronic or unspecified peptic ulcer, site unspecified, with perforation HCC

K27.6 Chronic or unspecified peptic ulcer, site unspecified, with both hemorrhage and perforation HCC

K27.7 Chronic peptic ulcer, site unspecified, without hemorrhage or perforation

K27.9 Peptic ulcer, site unspecified, unspecified as acute or chronic, without hemorrhage or perforation

4 **K28 Gastrojejunal ulcer**
INCLUDES anastomotic ulcer (peptic) or erosion
gastrocolic ulcer (peptic) or erosion
gastrointestinal ulcer (peptic) or erosion
gastrojejunal ulcer (peptic) or erosion
jejunal ulcer (peptic) or erosion
marginal ulcer (peptic) or erosion
stomal ulcer (peptic) or erosion
Use additional code to identify:
alcohol abuse and dependence (F10.-)
EXCLUDES 1 *primary ulcer of small intestine (K63.3)*

K28.0 Acute gastrojejunal ulcer with hemorrhage
K28.1 Acute gastrojejunal ulcer with perforation HCC
K28.2 Acute gastrojejunal ulcer with both hemorrhage and perforation HCC
K28.3 Acute gastrojejunal ulcer without hemorrhage or perforation
K28.4 Chronic or unspecified gastrojejunal ulcer with hemorrhage
K28.5 Chronic or unspecified gastrojejunal ulcer with perforation HCC
K28.6 Chronic or unspecified gastrojejunal ulcer with both hemorrhage and perforation HCC
K28.7 Chronic gastrojejunal ulcer without hemorrhage or perforation
K28.9 Gastrojejunal ulcer, unspecified as acute or chronic, without hemorrhage or perforation

4 **K29 Gastritis and duodenitis**
EXCLUDES 1 *eosinophilic gastritis or gastroenteritis (K52.81)*
Zollinger-Ellison syndrome (E16.4)

5 K29.0 Acute gastritis
Use additional code to identify:
alcohol abuse and dependence (F10.-)
EXCLUDES 1 *erosion (acute) of stomach (K25.-)*
K29.00 Acute gastritis without bleeding
K29.01 Acute gastritis with bleeding

5 K29.2 Alcoholic gastritis
Use additional code to identify:
alcohol abuse and dependence (F10.-)
K29.20 Alcoholic gastritis without bleeding
K29.21 Alcoholic gastritis with bleeding

5 K29.3 Chronic superficial gastritis
K29.30 Chronic superficial gastritis without bleeding
K29.31 Chronic superficial gastritis with bleeding

5 K29.4 Chronic atrophic gastritis
Gastric atrophy
K29.40 Chronic atrophic gastritis without bleeding
K29.41 Chronic atrophic gastritis with bleeding

5 K29.5 Unspecified chronic gastritis
Chronic antral gastritis
Chronic fundal gastritis
K29.50 Unspecified chronic gastritis without bleeding
K29.51 Unspecified chronic gastritis with bleeding

5 K29.6 Other gastritis
Giant hypertrophic gastritis
Granulomatous gastritis
Ménétrier's disease
K29.60 Other gastritis without bleeding
K29.61 Other gastritis with bleeding

5 K29.7 Gastritis, unspecified
K29.70 Gastritis, unspecified, without bleeding
K29.71 Gastritis, unspecified, with bleeding

5 K29.8 Duodenitis
K29.80 Duodenitis without bleeding
K29.81 Duodenitis with bleeding

5 K29.9 Gastroduodenitis, unspecified
K29.90 Gastroduodenitis, unspecified, without bleeding
K29.91 Gastroduodenitis, unspecified, with bleeding

K30 Functional dyspepsia
Indigestion
EXCLUDES 1 *dyspepsia NOS (R10.13)*
heartburn (R12)
nervous dyspepsia (F45.8)
neurotic dyspepsia (F45.8)
psychogenic dyspepsia (F45.8)

4 **K31 Other diseases of stomach and duodenum**
INCLUDES functional disorders of stomach
EXCLUDES 2 *diabetic gastroparesis*
(E08.43, E09.43, E10.43, E11.43, E13.43)
diverticulum of duodenum (K57.00-K57.13)

K31.0 Acute dilatation of stomach
Acute distention of stomach
DEFINITION Distention of the stomach due to excessive gas build-up or bowel obstruction, preventing passage of food.

K31.1 Adult hypertrophic pyloric stenosis A
Pyloric stenosis NOS
EXCLUDES 1 *congenital or infantile pyloric stenosis (Q40.0)*

K31.2 Hourglass stricture and stenosis of stomach
EXCLUDES 1 *congenital hourglass stomach (Q40.2)*
hourglass contraction of stomach (K31.89)

K31.3 Pylorospasm, not elsewhere classified
EXCLUDES 1 *congenital or infantile pylorospasm (Q40.0)*
neurotic pylorospasm (F45.8)
psychogenic pylorospasm (F45.8)

K31.4 Gastric diverticulum
EXCLUDES 1 *congenital diverticulum of stomach (Q40.2)*

K31.5 Obstruction of duodenum
Constriction of duodenum
Duodenal ileus (chronic)
Stenosis of duodenum
Stricture of duodenum
Volvulus of duodenum
EXCLUDES 1 *congenital stenosis of duodenum (Q41.0)*

K31.6 Fistula of stomach and duodenum
Gastrocolic fistula
Gastrojejunocolic fistula

K31.7 Polyp of stomach and duodenum
EXCLUDES 1 *adenomatous polyp of stomach (D13.1)*

5 K31.8 Other specified diseases of stomach and duodenum
6 K31.81 Angiodysplasia of stomach and duodenum
K31.811 Angiodysplasia of stomach and duodenum with bleeding
K31.819 Angiodysplasia of stomach and duodenum without bleeding
Angiodysplasia of stomach and duodenum NOS
K31.82 Dieulafoy lesion (hemorrhagic) of stomach and duodenum
EXCLUDES 2 *Dieulafoy lesion of intestine (K63.81)*
DEFINITION Abnormality of arteriole within the digestive tract protruding through a tiny mucosal defect, usually near the gastroesophageal junction, that can cause massive gastrointestinal bleeding.
K31.83 Achlorhydria
DEFINITION Absence of hydrochloric acid in the stomach's gastric secretions, most often from antibodies against cells producing gastric acid, or a symptom of H. pylori infection, atrophic gastritis, or cancer.
K31.84 Gastroparesis
Gastroparalysis
Code first underlying disease, if known, such as:
anorexia nervosa (F50.0-)
diabetes mellitus
(E08.43, E09.43, E10.43, E11.43, E13.43)
scleroderma (M34.-)
AHA: 4Q 2013, 115
K31.89 Other diseases of stomach and duodenum
AHA: 1Q 2017, 28
K31.9 Disease of stomach and duodenum, unspecified

Diseases of appendix (K35-K38)

4 **K35 Acute appendicitis**
CODING TIP ✓ With acute appendicitis, the single most important distinction is between perforation (bacterial contamination of the peritoneal space) and no perforation (no bacterial contamination), rather than the presence or absence of sterile inflammation of the peritoneum. The term peritonitis is used by different surgeons to mean different things.

▲ 5 K35.2 Acute appendicitis with generalized peritonitis
Appendicitis (acute) with generalized (diffuse) peritonitis following rupture or perforation of appendix
● K35.20 Acute appendicitis with generalized peritonitis, without abscess
(Acute) appendicitis with generalized peritonitis NOS

● K35.21 **Acute appendicitis with generalized peritonitis, with abscess**

▲ K35.3 **Acute appendicitis with localized peritonitis**

Appendicitis

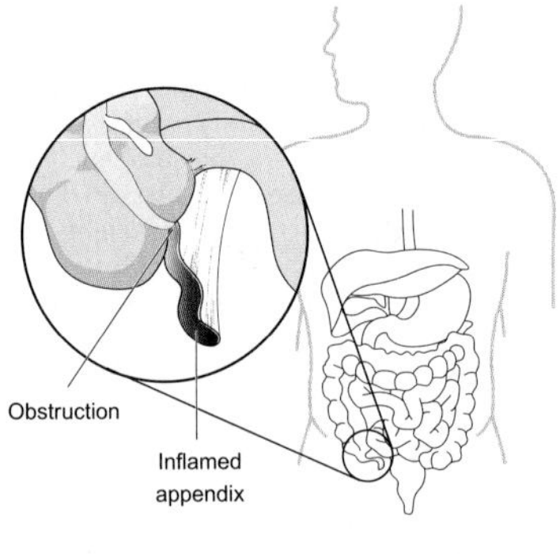

● K35.30 **Acute appendicitis with localized peritonitis, without perforation or gangrene**
Acute appendicitis with localized peritonitis NOS

● K35.31 **Acute appendicitis with localized peritonitis and gangrene, without perforation**

● K35.32 **Acute appendicitis with perforation and localized peritonitis, without abscess**
(Acute) appendicitis with perforation NOS
Perforated appendix NOS
Ruptured appendix (with localized peritonitis) NOS

● K35.33 **Acute appendicitis with perforation and localized peritonitis, with abscess**
(Acute) appendicitis with (peritoneal) abscess NOS
Ruptured appendix with localized peritonitis and abscess

K35.8 **Other and unspecified acute appendicitis**

K35.80 **Unspecified acute appendicitis**
Acute appendicitis NOS
Acute appendicitis without (localized) (generalized) peritonitis

▲ K35.89 **Other acute appendicitis**

● K35.890 **Other acute appendicitis without perforation or gangrene**

● K35.891 **Other acute appendicitis without perforation, with gangrene**
(Acute) appendicitis with gangrene NOS

K36 **Other appendicitis**
Chronic appendicitis
Recurrent appendicitis

▲ K37 **Unspecified appendicitis**
EXCLUDES 1 *-unspecified appendicitis with peritonitis (K35.2-, K35.3-)*

K38 **Other diseases of appendix**

K38.0 **Hyperplasia of appendix**

K38.1 **Appendicular concretions**
Fecalith of appendix
Stercolith of appendix

K38.2 **Diverticulum of appendix**

K38.3 **Fistula of appendix**

K38.8 **Other specified diseases of appendix**
Intussusception of appendix

K38.9 **Disease of appendix, unspecified**

Hernia (K40-K46)

Note: Hernia with both gangrene and obstruction is classified to hernia with gangrene.

INCLUDES acquired hernia
congenital [except diaphragmatic or hiatus] hernia
recurrent hernia

K40 **Inguinal hernia**

INCLUDES bubonocele
direct inguinal hernia
double inguinal hernia
indirect inguinal hernia
inguinal hernia NOS
oblique inguinal hernia
scrotal hernia

DEFINITION Weakness in the muscles in the groin area between the abdomen and thigh, allowing part of the intestine to bulge through the muscle wall.

Inguinal hernia

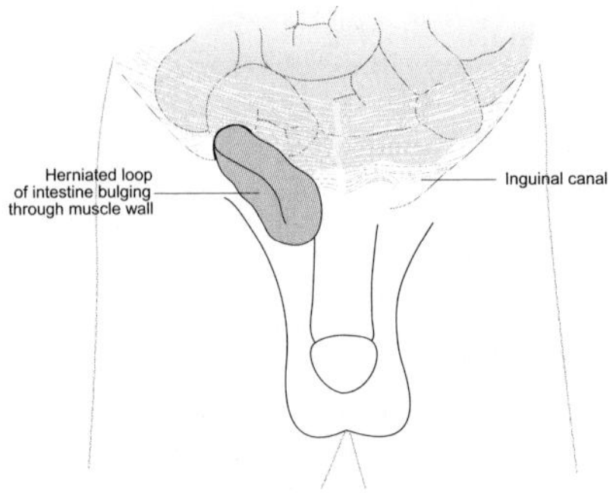

K40.0 **Bilateral inguinal hernia, with obstruction, without gangrene**
Inguinal hernia (bilateral) causing obstruction without gangrene
Incarcerated inguinal hernia (bilateral) without gangrene
Irreducible inguinal hernia (bilateral) without gangrene
Strangulated inguinal hernia (bilateral) without gangrene

K40.00 **Bilateral inguinal hernia, with obstruction, without gangrene, not specified as recurrent**
Bilateral inguinal hernia, with obstruction, without gangrene NOS

K40.01 **Bilateral inguinal hernia, with obstruction, without gangrene, recurrent**

K40.1 **Bilateral inguinal hernia, with gangrene**

K40.10 **Bilateral inguinal hernia, with gangrene, not specified as recurrent**
Bilateral inguinal hernia, with gangrene NOS

K40.11 **Bilateral inguinal hernia, with gangrene, recurrent**

K40.2 **Bilateral inguinal hernia, without obstruction or gangrene**

K40.20 **Bilateral inguinal hernia, without obstruction or gangrene, not specified as recurrent**
Bilateral inguinal hernia NOS

K40.21 **Bilateral inguinal hernia, without obstruction or gangrene, recurrent**

K40.3 **Unilateral inguinal hernia, with obstruction, without gangrene**
Inguinal hernia (unilateral) causing obstruction without gangrene
Incarcerated inguinal hernia (unilateral) without gangrene
Irreducible inguinal hernia (unilateral) without gangrene
Strangulated inguinal hernia (unilateral) without gangrene

K40.30 **Unilateral inguinal hernia, with obstruction, without gangrene, not specified as recurrent**
Inguinal hernia, with obstruction NOS
Unilateral inguinal hernia, with obstruction, without gangrene NOS

K40.31 **Unilateral inguinal hernia, with obstruction, without gangrene, recurrent**

K40.4 **Unilateral inguinal hernia, with gangrene**

K40.40 **Unilateral inguinal hernia, with gangrene, not specified as recurrent**
Inguinal hernia with gangrene NOS
Unilateral inguinal hernia with gangrene NOS

K40.41 **Unilateral inguinal hernia, with gangrene, recurrent**

K40.9 **Unilateral inguinal hernia, without obstruction or gangrene**

K40.90 Unilateral inguinal hernia, without obstruction or gangrene, not specified as recurrent
Inguinal hernia NOS
Unilateral inguinal hernia NOS

K40.91 Unilateral inguinal hernia, without obstruction or gangrene, recurrent

K41 Femoral hernia

K41.0 Bilateral femoral hernia, with obstruction, without gangrene
Femoral hernia (bilateral) causing obstruction, without gangrene
Incarcerated femoral hernia (bilateral), without gangrene
Irreducible femoral hernia (bilateral), without gangrene
Strangulated femoral hernia (bilateral), without gangrene

K41.00 Bilateral femoral hernia, with obstruction, without gangrene, not specified as recurrent
Bilateral femoral hernia, with obstruction, without gangrene NOS

K41.01 Bilateral femoral hernia, with obstruction, without gangrene, recurrent

K41.1 Bilateral femoral hernia, with gangrene

K41.10 Bilateral femoral hernia, with gangrene, not specified as recurrent
Bilateral femoral hernia, with gangrene NOS

K41.11 Bilateral femoral hernia, with gangrene, recurrent

K41.2 Bilateral femoral hernia, without obstruction or gangrene

K41.20 Bilateral femoral hernia, without obstruction or gangrene, not specified as recurrent
Bilateral femoral hernia NOS

K41.21 Bilateral femoral hernia, without obstruction or gangrene, recurrent

K41.3 Unilateral femoral hernia, with obstruction, without gangrene
Femoral hernia (unilateral) causing obstruction, without gangrene
Incarcerated femoral hernia (unilateral), without gangrene
Irreducible femoral hernia (unilateral), without gangrene
Strangulated femoral hernia (unilateral), without gangrene

K41.30 Unilateral femoral hernia, with obstruction, without gangrene, not specified as recurrent
Femoral hernia, with obstruction NOS
Unilateral femoral hernia, with obstruction NOS

K41.31 Unilateral femoral hernia, with obstruction, without gangrene, recurrent

K41.4 Unilateral femoral hernia, with gangrene

K41.40 Unilateral femoral hernia, with gangrene, not specified as recurrent
Femoral hernia, with gangrene NOS
Unilateral femoral hernia, with gangrene NOS

K41.41 Unilateral femoral hernia, with gangrene, recurrent

K41.9 Unilateral femoral hernia, without obstruction or gangrene

K41.90 Unilateral femoral hernia, without obstruction or gangrene, not specified as recurrent
Femoral hernia NOS
Unilateral femoral hernia NOS

K41.91 Unilateral femoral hernia, without obstruction or gangrene, recurrent

K42 Umbilical hernia

INCLUDES paraumbilical hernia

EXCLUDES 1 *omphalocele (Q79.2)*

K42.0 Umbilical hernia with obstruction, without gangrene
Umbilical hernia causing obstruction, without gangrene
Incarcerated umbilical hernia, without gangrene
Irreducible umbilical hernia, without gangrene
Strangulated umbilical hernia, without gangrene

K42.1 Umbilical hernia with gangrene
Gangrenous umbilical hernia

K42.9 Umbilical hernia without obstruction or gangrene
Umbilical hernia NOS

K43 Ventral hernia

Ventral hernia

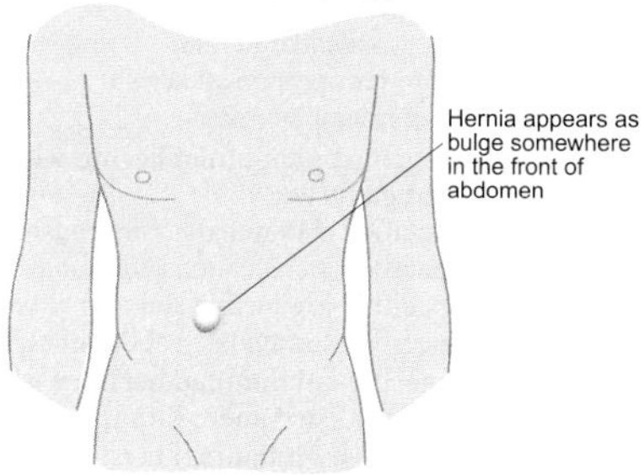
Hernia appears as bulge somewhere in the front of abdomen

K43.0 Incisional hernia with obstruction, without gangrene
Incisional hernia causing obstruction, without gangrene
Incarcerated incisional hernia, without gangrene
Irreducible incisional hernia, without gangrene
Strangulated incisional hernia, without gangrene

K43.1 Incisional hernia with gangrene
Gangrenous incisional hernia

K43.2 Incisional hernia without obstruction or gangrene
Incisional hernia NOS

K43.3 Parastomal hernia with obstruction, without gangrene
Incarcerated parastomal hernia, without gangrene
Irreducible parastomal hernia, without gangrene
Parastomal hernia causing obstruction, without gangrene
Strangulated parastomal hernia, without gangrene

K43.4 Parastomal hernia with gangrene
Gangrenous parastomal hernia

K43.5 Parastomal hernia without obstruction or gangrene
Parastomal hernia NOS

K43.6 Other and unspecified ventral hernia with obstruction, without gangrene
Epigastric hernia causing obstruction, without gangrene
Hypogastric hernia causing obstruction, without gangrene
Incarcerated epigastric hernia without gangrene
Incarcerated hypogastric hernia without gangrene
Incarcerated midline hernia without gangrene
Incarcerated spigelian hernia without gangrene
Incarcerated subxiphoid hernia without gangrene
Irreducible epigastric hernia without gangrene
Irreducible hypogastric hernia without gangrene
Irreducible midline hernia without gangrene
Irreducible spigelian hernia without gangrene
Irreducible subxiphoid hernia without gangrene
Midline hernia causing obstruction, without gangrene
Spigelian hernia causing obstruction, without gangrene
Strangulated epigastric hernia without gangrene
Strangulated hypogastric hernia without gangrene
Strangulated midline hernia without gangrene
Strangulated spigelian hernia without gangrene
Strangulated subxiphoid hernia without gangrene
Subxiphoid hernia causing obstruction, without gangrene

K43.7 Other and unspecified ventral hernia with gangrene
Any condition listed under K43.6 specified as gangrenous

K43.9 Ventral hernia without obstruction or gangrene
Epigastric hernia
Ventral hernia NOS

K44 Diaphragmatic hernia

INCLUDES hiatus hernia (esophageal) (sliding)
paraesophageal hernia

EXCLUDES 1 *congenital diaphragmatic hernia (Q79.0)*
congenital hiatus hernia (Q40.1)

K44.0 Diaphragmatic hernia with obstruction, without gangrene
Diaphragmatic hernia causing obstruction
Incarcerated diaphragmatic hernia
Irreducible diaphragmatic hernia
Strangulated diaphragmatic hernia

K44.1 Diaphragmatic hernia with gangrene
Gangrenous diaphragmatic hernia

K44.9 Diaphragmatic hernia without obstruction or gangrene
Diaphragmatic hernia NOS

4 K45 Other abdominal hernia

INCLUDES abdominal hernia, specified site NEC
lumbar hernia
obturator hernia
pudendal hernia
retroperitoneal hernia
sciatic hernia

K45.0 Other specified abdominal hernia with obstruction, without gangrene
Other specified abdominal hernia causing obstruction
Other specified incarcerated abdominal hernia
Other specified irreducible abdominal hernia
Other specified strangulated abdominal hernia

K45.1 Other specified abdominal hernia with gangrene
Any condition listed under K45 specified as gangrenous

K45.8 Other specified abdominal hernia without obstruction or gangrene

4 K46 Unspecified abdominal hernia

INCLUDES enterocele
epiplocele
hernia NOS
interstitial hernia
intestinal hernia
intra-abdominal hernia

EXCLUDES 1 *vaginal enterocele (N81.5)*

K46.0 Unspecified abdominal hernia with obstruction, without gangrene
Unspecified abdominal hernia causing obstruction
Unspecified incarcerated abdominal hernia
Unspecified irreducible abdominal hernia
Unspecified strangulated abdominal hernia

K46.1 Unspecified abdominal hernia with gangrene
Any condition listed under K46 specified as gangrenous

K46.9 Unspecified abdominal hernia without obstruction or gangrene
Abdominal hernia NOS

Noninfective enteritis and colitis (K50-K52)

INCLUDES noninfective inflammatory bowel disease

EXCLUDES 1 *irritable bowel syndrome (K58.-)*
megacolon (K59.3-)

CODING TIP ✓ Do not assign a code from K50-K52 when enteritis/colitis is specified as infectious. Infectious colitis requires assignment of a code from Chapter 1, Certain Infectious and Parasitic Diseases.

4 K50 Crohn's disease [regional enteritis]

INCLUDES granulomatous enteritis

Use additional code to identify manifestations, such as: pyoderma gangrenosum (L88)

EXCLUDES 1 *ulcerative colitis (K51.-)*

5 K50.0 Crohn's disease of small intestine
Crohn's disease [regional enteritis] of duodenum
Crohn's disease [regional enteritis] of ileum
Crohn's disease [regional enteritis] of jejunum
Regional ileitis
Terminal ileitis

EXCLUDES 1 *Crohn's disease of both small and large intestine (K50.8-)*

Crohn's disease of small intestine

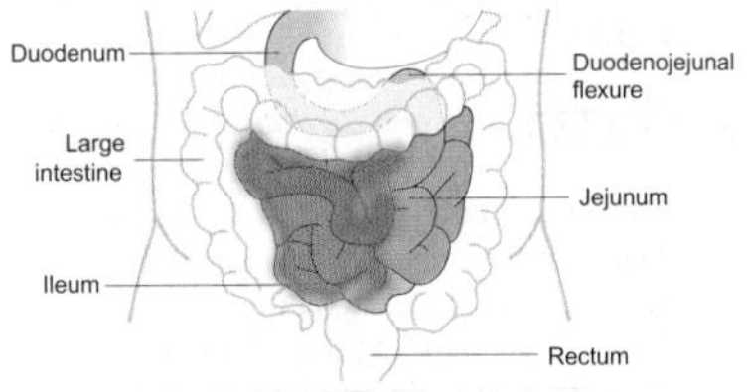

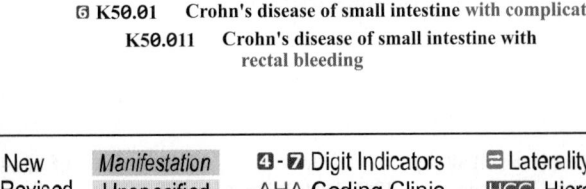

K50.00 Crohn's disease of small intestine without complications HCC

6 K50.01 Crohn's disease of small intestine with complications

K50.011 Crohn's disease of small intestine with rectal bleeding HCC

K50.012 Crohn's disease of small intestine with intestinal obstruction HCC

K50.013 Crohn's disease of small intestine with fistula HCC

K50.014 Crohn's disease of small intestine with abscess HCC
AHA: 4Q 2012, 104

K50.018 Crohn's disease of small intestine with other complication HCC

K50.019 Crohn's disease of small intestine with unspecified complications HCC

5 K50.1 Crohn's disease of large intestine
Crohn's disease [regional enteritis] of colon
Crohn's disease [regional enteritis] of large bowel
Crohn's disease [regional enteritis] of rectum
Granulomatous colitis
Regional colitis

EXCLUDES 1 *Crohn's disease of both small and large intestine (K50.8)*

Crohn's disease of large intestine

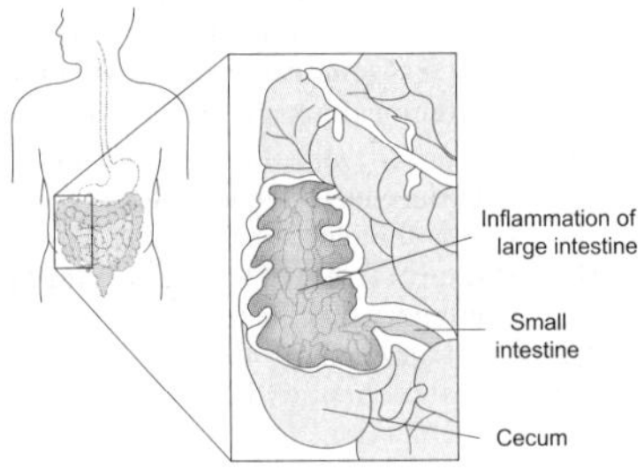

K50.10 Crohn's disease of large intestine without complications HCC

6 K50.11 Crohn's disease of large intestine with complications

K50.111 Crohn's disease of large intestine with rectal bleeding HCC

K50.112 Crohn's disease of large intestine with intestinal obstruction HCC

K50.113 Crohn's disease of large intestine with fistula HCC

K50.114 Crohn's disease of large intestine with abscess HCC
AHA: 4Q 2012, 104

K50.118 Crohn's disease of large intestine with other complication HCC

K50.119 Crohn's disease of large intestine with unspecified complications HCC

5 K50.8 Crohn's disease of both small and large intestine

K50.80 Crohn's disease of both small and large intestine without complications HCC

6 K50.81 Crohn's disease of both small and large intestine with complications

K50.811 Crohn's disease of both small and large intestine with rectal bleeding HCC

K50.812 Crohn's disease of both small and large intestine with intestinal obstruction HCC

K50.813 Crohn's disease of both small and large intestine with fistula HCC

K50.814 Crohn's disease of both small and large intestine with abscess HCC
AHA: 4Q 2012, 104

K50.818 Crohn's disease of both small and large intestine with other complication HCC

K50.819 Crohn's disease of both small and large intestine with unspecified complications HCC

5 K50.9 Crohn's disease, unspecified

K50.90 Crohn's disease, unspecified, without complications HCC
Crohn's disease NOS
Regional enteritis NOS

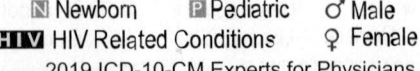

6 K50.91 Crohn's disease, unspecified, with complications

K50.911 Crohn's disease, unspecified, with rectal bleeding HCC

K50.912 Crohn's disease, unspecified, with intestinal obstruction HCC

K50.913 Crohn's disease, unspecified, with fistula HCC

K50.914 Crohn's disease, unspecified, with abscess HCC

AHA: 4Q 2012, 104

K50.918 Crohn's disease, unspecified, with other complication HCC

K50.919 Crohn's disease, unspecified, with unspecified complications HCC

K51 Ulcerative colitis

Use additional code to identify manifestations, such as: pyoderma gangrenosum (L88)

EXCLUDES 1 *Crohn's disease [regional enteritis] (K50.-)*

K51.0 Ulcerative (chronic) pancolitis

Backwash ileitis

K51.00 Ulcerative (chronic) pancolitis without complications HCC

Ulcerative (chronic) pancolitis NOS

K51.01 Ulcerative (chronic) pancolitis with complications

K51.011 Ulcerative (chronic) pancolitis with rectal bleeding HCC

K51.012 Ulcerative (chronic) pancolitis with intestinal obstruction HCC

K51.013 Ulcerative (chronic) pancolitis with fistula HCC

K51.014 Ulcerative (chronic) pancolitis with abscess HCC

K51.018 Ulcerative (chronic) pancolitis with other complication HCC

K51.019 Ulcerative (chronic) pancolitis with unspecified complications HCC

K51.2 Ulcerative (chronic) proctitis

K51.20 Ulcerative (chronic) proctitis without complications HCC

Ulcerative (chronic) proctitis NOS

K51.21 Ulcerative (chronic) proctitis with complications

K51.211 Ulcerative (chronic) proctitis with rectal bleeding HCC

K51.212 Ulcerative (chronic) proctitis with intestinal obstruction HCC

K51.213 Ulcerative (chronic) proctitis with fistula HCC

K51.214 Ulcerative (chronic) proctitis with abscess HCC

K51.218 Ulcerative (chronic) proctitis with other complication HCC

K51.219 Ulcerative (chronic) proctitis with unspecified complications HCC

K51.3 Ulcerative (chronic) rectosigmoiditis

K51.30 Ulcerative (chronic) rectosigmoiditis without complications HCC

Ulcerative (chronic) rectosigmoiditis NOS

K51.31 Ulcerative (chronic) rectosigmoiditis with complications

K51.311 Ulcerative (chronic) rectosigmoiditis with rectal bleeding HCC

K51.312 Ulcerative (chronic) rectosigmoiditis with intestinal obstruction HCC

K51.313 Ulcerative (chronic) rectosigmoiditis with fistula HCC

K51.314 Ulcerative (chronic) rectosigmoiditis with abscess HCC

K51.318 Ulcerative (chronic) rectosigmoiditis with other complication HCC

K51.319 Ulcerative (chronic) rectosigmoiditis with unspecified complications HCC

K51.4 Inflammatory polyps of colon

EXCLUDES 1 *adenomatous polyp of colon (D12.6)*
polyposis of colon (D12.6)
polyps of colon NOS (K63.5)

K51.40 Inflammatory polyps of colon without complications HCC

Inflammatory polyps of colon NOS

K51.41 Inflammatory polyps of colon with complications

K51.411 Inflammatory polyps of colon with rectal bleeding HCC

K51.412 Inflammatory polyps of colon with intestinal obstruction HCC

K51.413 Inflammatory polyps of colon with fistula HCC

K51.414 Inflammatory polyps of colon with abscess HCC

K51.418 Inflammatory polyps of colon with other complication HCC

K51.419 Inflammatory polyps of colon with unspecified complications HCC

K51.5 Left sided colitis

Left hemicolitis

K51.50 Left sided colitis without complications HCC

Left sided colitis NOS

K51.51 Left sided colitis with complications

K51.511 Left sided colitis with rectal bleeding HCC

K51.512 Left sided colitis with intestinal obstruction HCC

K51.513 Left sided colitis with fistula HCC

K51.514 Left sided colitis with abscess HCC

K51.518 Left sided colitis with other complication HCC

K51.519 Left sided colitis with unspecified complications HCC

K51.8 Other ulcerative colitis

K51.80 Other ulcerative colitis without complications HCC

DEFINITION Inflammation of the intestinal lining with ulcer formation, causing diarrhea as the colon empties frequently.

K51.81 Other ulcerative colitis with complications

K51.811 Other ulcerative colitis with rectal bleeding HCC

K51.812 Other ulcerative colitis with intestinal obstruction HCC

K51.813 Other ulcerative colitis with fistula HCC

K51.814 Other ulcerative colitis with abscess HCC

K51.818 Other ulcerative colitis with other complication HCC

K51.819 Other ulcerative colitis with unspecified complications HCC

K51.9 Ulcerative colitis, unspecified

K51.90 Ulcerative colitis, unspecified, without complications HCC

K51.91 Ulcerative colitis, unspecified, with complications

K51.911 Ulcerative colitis, unspecified with rectal bleeding HCC

K51.912 Ulcerative colitis, unspecified with intestinal obstruction HCC

K51.913 Ulcerative colitis, unspecified with fistula HCC

K51.914 Ulcerative colitis, unspecified with abscess HCC

K51.918 Ulcerative colitis, unspecified with other complication HCC

K51.919 Ulcerative colitis, unspecified with unspecified complications HCC

K52 Other and unspecified noninfective gastroenteritis and colitis

K52.0 Gastroenteritis and colitis due to radiation

K52.1 Toxic gastroenteritis and colitis

Drug-induced gastroenteritis and colitis

Code first:
(T51-T65) to identify toxic agent

Use additional code for adverse effect, if applicable, to identify drug (T36-T50 with fifth or sixth character 5)

K52.2 Allergic and dietetic gastroenteritis and colitis

Food hypersensitivity gastroenteritis or colitis

Use additional code to identify type of food allergy (Z91.01-, Z91.02-)

EXCLUDES 2 *allergic eosinophilic colitis (K52.82)*
allergic eosinophilic esophagitis (K20.0)
allergic eosinophilic gastritis (K52.81)
allergic eosinophilic gastroenteritis (K52.81)
food protein-induced proctocolitis (K52.82)

▲ K52.21 Food protein-induced enterocolitis syndrome

FPIES

Use additional code for hypovolemic shock, if present (R57.1)

DEFINITION A nontypical, non-IgE, food allergy affecting infants and young children with serious gastrointestinal effects that result in profound vomiting, severe diarrhea involving both the large and small intestine, and dehydration as well as severe lethargy and dangerous changes in body temperature and blood pressure. Symptoms may not be immediate or show up on standard allergy tests, but will appear after ingesting a food trigger.
AHA: 4Q 2016, 30

K52.22 Food protein-induced enteropathy
DEFINITION A type of food protein intolerance with gastrointestinal manifestations, typically occurring in the pediatric population in the first 6 months of life and most often as intolerance to cow's milk or soy milk protein.
AHA: 4Q 2016, 30

K52.29 Other allergic and dietetic gastroenteritis and colitis
Food hypersensitivity gastroenteritis or colitis
Immediate gastrointestinal hypersensitivity
AHA: 4Q 2016, 30

K52.3 Indeterminate colitis
Colonic inflammatory bowel disease unclassified (IBDU)
EXCLUDES 1 *unspecified colitis (K52.9)*
AHA: 4Q 2016, 30

5 K52.8 Other specified noninfective gastroenteritis and colitis

K52.81 Eosinophilic gastritis or gastroenteritis
Eosinophilic enteritis
EXCLUDES 2 *eosinophilic esophagitis (K20.0)*

K52.82 Eosinophilic colitis
Allergic proctocolitis
Food-induced eosinophilic proctocolitis
Food protein-induced proctocolitis
Milk protein-induced proctocolitis

6 K52.83 Microscopic colitis
AHA: 4Q 2016, 30

K52.831 Collagenous colitis
K52.832 Lymphocytic colitis
K52.838 Other microscopic colitis
K52.839 Microscopic colitis, unspecified

K52.89 Other specified noninfective gastroenteritis and colitis

K52.9 Noninfective gastroenteritis and colitis, unspecified
Colitis NOS
Enteritis NOS
Gastroenteritis NOS
Ileitis NOS
Jejunitis NOS
Sigmoiditis NOS
EXCLUDES 1 *diarrhea NOS (R19.7)*
functional diarrhea (K59.1)
infectious gastroenteritis and colitis NOS (A09)
neonatal diarrhea (noninfective) (P78.3)
psychogenic diarrhea (F45.8)

Other diseases of intestines (K55-K64)

4 K55 Vascular disorders of intestine
EXCLUDES 1 *necrotizing enterocolitis of newborn (P77.-)*

5 K55.0 Acute vascular disorders of intestine
Infarction of appendices epiploicae
Mesenteric (artery) (vein) embolism
Mesenteric (artery) (vein) infarction
Mesenteric (artery) (vein) thrombosis

6 K55.01 Acute (reversible) ischemia of small intestine

K55.011 Focal (segmental) acute (reversible) ischemia of small intestine HCC
K55.012 Diffuse acute (reversible) ischemia of small intestine HCC
K55.019 Acute (reversible) ischemia of small intestine, extent unspecified HCC

6 K55.02 Acute infarction of small intestine
Gangrene of small intestine
Necrosis of small intestine

K55.021 Focal (segmental) acute infarction of small intestine HCC
K55.022 Diffuse acute infarction of small intestine HCC
K55.029 Acute infarction of small intestine, extent unspecified HCC

6 K55.03 Acute (reversible) ischemia of large intestine
Acute fulminant ischemic colitis
Subacute ischemic colitis

K55.031 Focal (segmental) acute (reversible) ischemia of large intestine HCC
K55.032 Diffuse acute (reversible) ischemia of large intestine HCC
K55.039 Acute (reversible) ischemia of large intestine, extent unspecified HCC

6 K55.04 Acute infarction of large intestine
Gangrene of large intestine
Necrosis of large intestine

K55.041 Focal (segmental) acute infarction of large intestine HCC
K55.042 Diffuse acute infarction of large intestine HCC
K55.049 Acute infarction of large intestine, extent unspecified HCC

6 K55.05 Acute (reversible) ischemia of intestine, part unspecified

K55.051 Focal (segmental) acute (reversible) ischemia of intestine, part unspecified HCC
K55.052 Diffuse acute (reversible) ischemia of intestine, part unspecified HCC
K55.059 Acute (reversible) ischemia of intestine, part and extent unspecified HCC

6 K55.06 Acute infarction of intestine, part unspecified
Acute intestinal infarction
Gangrene of intestine
Necrosis of intestine

K55.061 Focal (segmental) acute infarction of intestine, part unspecified HCC
K55.062 Diffuse acute infarction of intestine, part unspecified HCC
K55.069 Acute infarction of intestine, part and extent unspecified HCC

K55.1 Chronic vascular disorders of intestine HCC
Chronic ischemic colitis
Chronic ischemic enteritis
Chronic ischemic enterocolitis
Ischemic stricture of intestine
Mesenteric atherosclerosis
Mesenteric vascular insufficiency

5 K55.2 Angiodysplasia of colon

K55.20 Angiodysplasia of colon without hemorrhage
K55.21 Angiodysplasia of colon with hemorrhage
DEFINITION Dilated intestinal blood vessels with corresponding thinning and weakening of vessel walls and bleeding into the intestinal tract.

5 K55.3 Necrotizing enterocolitis
EXCLUDES 1 *necrotizing enterocolitis of newborn (P77.-)*
EXCLUDES 2 *necrotizing enterocolitis due to Clostridium difficile (A04.7-)*
AHA: 4Q 2016, 32

K55.30 Necrotizing enterocolitis, unspecified HCC
Necrotizing enterocolitis, NOS

K55.31 Stage 1 necrotizing enterocolitis HCC
Necrotizing enterocolitis without pneumatosis, without perforation

K55.32 Stage 2 necrotizing enterocolitis HCC
Necrotizing enterocolitis with pneumatosis, without perforation

K55.33 Stage 3 necrotizing enterocolitis HCC
Necrotizing enterocolitis with perforation
Necrotizing enterocolitis with pneumatosis and perforation

K55.8 Other vascular disorders of intestine HCC

K55.9 Vascular disorder of intestine, unspecified HCC
Ischemic colitis
Ischemic enteritis
Ischemic enterocolitis

K56 Paralytic ileus and intestinal obstruction without hernia

EXCLUDES 1 *congenital stricture or stenosis of intestine (Q41-Q42)*
cystic fibrosis with meconium ileus (E84.11)
ischemic stricture of intestine (K55.1)
meconium ileus NOS (P76.0)
neonatal intestinal obstructions classifiable to P76.-
obstruction of duodenum (K31.5)
postprocedural intestinal obstruction (K91.3-)
stenosis of anus or rectum (K62.4)

K56.0 Paralytic ileus HCC
Paralysis of bowel
Paralysis of colon
Paralysis of intestine
EXCLUDES 1 *gallstone ileus (K56.3)*
ileus NOS (K56.7)
obstructive ileus NOS (K56.69-)

DEFINITION Blockage in the small or large intestine due to nonfunctioning muscle wall; may occur due to fluid imbalance, nerve damage, decreased blood supply, or toxins.

K56.1 Intussusception HCC
Intussusception or invagination of bowel
Intussusception or invagination of colon
Intussusception or invagination of intestine
Intussusception or invagination of rectum
EXCLUDES 2 *intussusception of appendix (K38.8)*

Intussusception

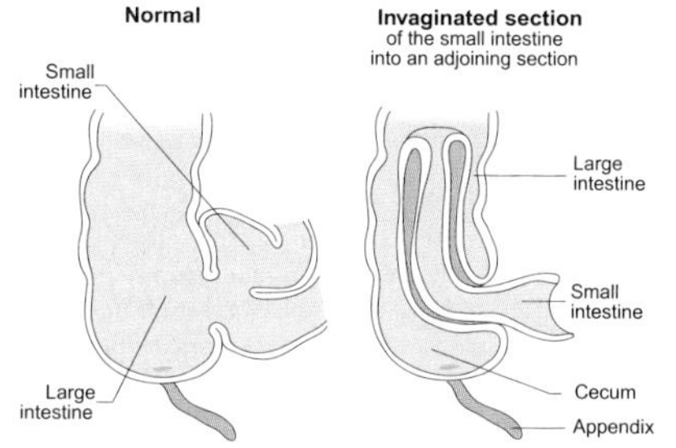

K56.2 Volvulus HCC
Strangulation of colon or intestine
Torsion of colon or intestine
Twist of colon or intestine
EXCLUDES 2 *volvulus of duodenum (K31.5)*

DEFINITION Twisting of the intestine, constricting the passageway and cutting off blood supply to the area; presents with sudden, severe abdominal pain, vomiting, and abdominal distention.

K56.3 Gallstone ileus HCC
Obstruction of intestine by gallstone

K56.4 Other impaction of intestine

K56.41 Fecal impaction HCC
EXCLUDES 1 *constipation (K59.0-)*
incomplete defecation (R15.0)

K56.49 Other impaction of intestine HCC

K56.5 Intestinal adhesions [bands] with obstruction (postinfection) HCC
Abdominal hernia due to adhesions with obstruction
Peritoneal adhesions [bands] with intestinal obstruction (postinfection)

CODING TIP✓ Intestinal obstruction varies in severity, from partial or intermittent obstruction that usually resolves without intervention to complete obstruction that requires surgery and may lead to intestinal gangrene and perforation. Physicians frequently describe intestinal obstruction as partial versus complete. In addition to partial and complete, these codes define the obstruction as due to adhesions which generally are a result of surgery or infection.

K56.50 Intestinal adhesions [bands], unspecified as to partial versus complete obstruction HCC
Intestinal adhesions with obstruction NOS
AHA: 4Q 2017, 13

K56.51 Intestinal adhesions [bands], with partial obstruction HCC
Intestinal adhesions with incomplete obstruction
AHA: 4Q 2017, 13

K56.52 Intestinal adhesions [bands] with complete obstruction HCC
AHA: 4Q 2017, 13

K56.6 Other and unspecified intestinal obstruction

CODING TIP✓ Intestinal obstruction varies in severity, from partial or intermittent obstruction that usually resolves without intervention to complete obstruction that requires surgery and may lead to intestinal gangrene and perforation. Physicians frequently describe intestinal obstruction as partial versus complete. In addition to partial and complete, these codes are used when the cause of the obstruction is not documented or the type of obstruction is not due to adhesions.

K56.60 Unspecified intestinal obstruction HCC
EXCLUDES 1 *intestinal obstruction due to specified condition-code to condition*

K56.600 Partial intestinal obstruction, unspecified as to cause HCC
Incomplete intestinal obstruction, NOS
AHA: 4Q 2017, 13

K56.601 Complete intestinal obstruction, unspecified as to cause HCC
AHA: 4Q 2017, 13

K56.609 Unspecified intestinal obstruction, unspecified as to partial versus complete obstruction HCC
Intestinal obstruction NOS
AHA: 4Q 2017, 13

K56.69 Other intestinal obstruction HCC
Enterostenosis NOS
Obstructive ileus NOS
Occlusion of colon or intestine NOS
Stenosis of colon or intestine NOS
Stricture of colon or intestine NOS
EXCLUDES 1 *intestinal obstruction due to specified condition-code to condition*

K56.690 Other partial intestinal obstruction HCC
Other incomplete intestinal obstruction
AHA: 4Q 2017, 13

K56.691 Other complete intestinal obstruction HCC
AHA: 4Q 2017, 13

K56.699 Other intestinal obstruction unspecified as to partial versus complete obstruction HCC
Other intestinal obstruction, NEC
AHA: 4Q 2017, 13

K56.7 Ileus, unspecified HCC
EXCLUDES 1 *obstructive ileus (K56.69-)*
EXCLUDES 2 *intestinal obstruction with hernia (K40-K46)*
AHA: 1Q 2017, 40

▲ **K57 Diverticular disease of intestine**
Code also:
if applicable peritonitis K65.-
EXCLUDES 1 *congenital diverticulum of intestine (Q43.8)*
Meckel's diverticulum (Q43.0)
EXCLUDES 2 *diverticulum of appendix (K38.2)*

CODING TIP✓ Do not assign a code from K57.- for diverticular conditions reported as congenital. Congenital diverticulum should be coded to the appropriate Q43.- code.

K57.0 Diverticulitis of small intestine with perforation and abscess
Diverticulitis of small intestine with peritonitis
EXCLUDES 1 *diverticulitis of both small and large intestine with perforation and abscess (K57.4-)*

K57.00 **Diverticulitis of small intestine with perforation and abscess without bleeding**

K57.01 **Diverticulitis of small intestine with perforation and abscess with bleeding**

5 **K57.1** **Diverticular disease of small intestine without perforation or abscess**

EXCLUDES 1 *diverticular disease of both small and large intestine without perforation or abscess (K57.5-)*

K57.10 **Diverticulosis of small intestine without perforation or abscess without bleeding**
Diverticular disease of small intestine NOS

K57.11 **Diverticulosis of small intestine without perforation or abscess with bleeding**

K57.12 **Diverticulitis of small intestine without perforation or abscess without bleeding**

Diverticulitis of small intestine without perforation or abscess, without bleeding

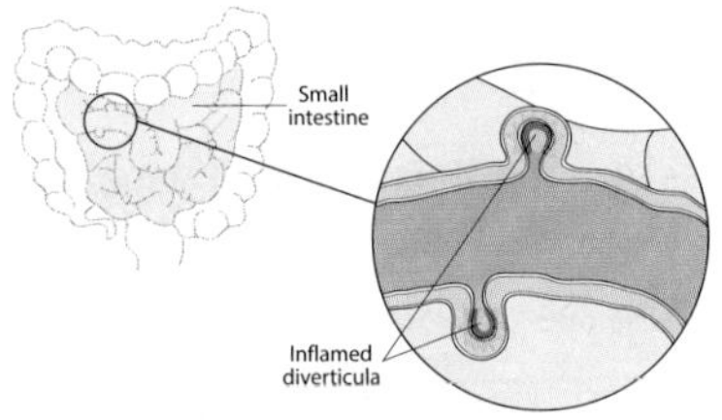

K57.13 **Diverticulitis of small intestine without perforation or abscess with bleeding**

5 **K57.2** **Diverticulitis of large intestine with perforation and abscess**
Diverticulitis of colon with peritonitis

EXCLUDES 1 *diverticulitis of both small and large intestine with perforation and abscess (K57.4-)*

K57.20 **Diverticulitis of large intestine with perforation and abscess without bleeding**

K57.21 **Diverticulitis of large intestine with perforation and abscess with bleeding**

5 **K57.3** **Diverticular disease of large intestine without perforation or abscess**

EXCLUDES 1 *diverticular disease of both small and large intestine without perforation or abscess (K57.5-)*

K57.30 **Diverticulosis of large intestine without perforation or abscess without bleeding**
Diverticular disease of colon NOS

K57.31 **Diverticulosis of large intestine without perforation or abscess with bleeding**

K57.32 **Diverticulitis of large intestine without perforation or abscess without bleeding**

K57.33 **Diverticulitis of large intestine without perforation or abscess with bleeding**

5 **K57.4** **Diverticulitis of both small and large intestine with perforation and abscess**
Diverticulitis of both small and large intestine with peritonitis

K57.40 **Diverticulitis of both small and large intestine with perforation and abscess without bleeding**

K57.41 **Diverticulitis of both small and large intestine with perforation and abscess with bleeding**

5 **K57.5** **Diverticular disease of both small and large intestine without perforation or abscess**

K57.50 **Diverticulosis of both small and large intestine without perforation or abscess without bleeding**
Diverticular disease of both small and large intestine NOS

K57.51 **Diverticulosis of both small and large intestine without perforation or abscess with bleeding**

K57.52 **Diverticulitis of both small and large intestine without perforation or abscess without bleeding**

K57.53 **Diverticulitis of both small and large intestine without perforation or abscess with bleeding**

5 **K57.8** **Diverticulitis of intestine, part unspecified, with perforation and abscess**
Diverticulitis of intestine NOS with peritonitis

K57.80 **Diverticulitis of intestine, part unspecified, with perforation and abscess without bleeding**

K57.81 **Diverticulitis of intestine, part unspecified, with perforation and abscess with bleeding**

5 **K57.9** **Diverticular disease of intestine, part unspecified, without perforation or abscess**

K57.90 **Diverticulosis of intestine, part unspecified, without perforation or abscess without bleeding**
Diverticular disease of intestine NOS

K57.91 **Diverticulosis of intestine, part unspecified, without perforation or abscess with bleeding**

K57.92 **Diverticulitis of intestine, part unspecified, without perforation or abscess without bleeding**

K57.93 **Diverticulitis of intestine, part unspecified, without perforation or abscess with bleeding**

4 **K58** **Irritable bowel syndrome**

INCLUDES irritable colon
spastic colon

DEFINITION Functional disorder of hypersensitive nerves and muscles in the colon, causing cramping, pain, diarrhea, and/or constipation.

AHA: 4Q 2016, 32

K58.0 **Irritable bowel syndrome with diarrhea**

CODING TIP ✓ Do not assign an additional code for the diarrhea. K58.0 is a combination code and does not require additional coding of the included symptom.

K58.1 **Irritable bowel syndrome with constipation**

K58.2 **Mixed irritable bowel syndrome**

K58.8 **Other irritable bowel syndrome**

K58.9 **Irritable bowel syndrome without diarrhea**
Irritable bowel syndrome NOS

4 **K59** **Other functional intestinal disorders**

EXCLUDES 1 *change in bowel habit NOS (R19.4)*
intestinal malabsorption (K90.-)
psychogenic intestinal disorders (F45.8)

EXCLUDES 2 *functional disorders of stomach (K31.-)*

5 **K59.0** **Constipation**
Use additional code for adverse effect, if applicable, to identify drug (T36-T50 with fifth or sixth character 5)

EXCLUDES 1 *fecal impaction (K56.41)*
incomplete defecation (R15.0)

AHA: 4Q 2016, 33

K59.00 **Constipation, unspecified**

K59.01 **Slow transit constipation**

DEFINITION Dysfunction of intestinal smooth muscles that move fecal matter, causing slow stool movement.

K59.02 **Outlet dysfunction constipation**

K59.03 **Drug induced constipation**
Use additional code for adverse effect, if applicable, to identify drug (T36-T50 with fifth or sixth character 5

K59.04 **Chronic idiopathic constipation**
Functional constipation

DEFINITION Chronic idiopathic constipation, also known as functional constipation, is a long-lasting or recurring reduction in stool frequency, usually less than 3 times per week, difficulty passing stools, or both without any underlying illness, medication, or physiological cause, such as hormonal imbalance.

K59.09 **Other constipation**
Chronic constipation

K59.1 **Functional diarrhea**

EXCLUDES 1 *diarrhea NOS (R19.7)*
irritable bowel syndrome with diarrhea (K58.0)

K59.2 **Neurogenic bowel, not elsewhere classified**

DEFINITION Intestinal dysfunction due to spinal cord damage.

5 **K59.3 Megacolon, not elsewhere classified**
Dilatation of colon
Code first:
, if applicable (T51-T65) to identify toxic agent
EXCLUDES 1 *congenital megacolon (aganglionic) (Q43.1)*
megacolon (due to) (in) Chagas' disease (B57.32)
megacolon (due to) (in) Clostridium difficile (A04.7-)
megacolon (due to) (in) Hirschsprung's disease (Q43.1)

CODING TIP✓ Megacolon is an abnormal dilation of the colon, generally accompanied by reduced peristalsis. Do not assign a code from K59.3- if the cause is known to be due to another condition such as *Clostridium difficile* (A04.7), Hirschsprung's disease (Q43.1), or other congenital or known cause. When the cause is known, code the cause of the megacolon.

DEFINITION Enlargement or dilation of the sigmoid colon.

AHA: 4Q 2016, 33

K59.31 Toxic megacolon HCC
K59.39 Other megacolon
Megacolon NOS
DEFINITION A condition in which the large intestine becomes extremely distended and stretched so that it is much larger than usual. This may be an acute, sudden and severe condition due to infection, or a chronic condition due to abnormal growth. Note: Congenital megacolon and that due to exposure to toxins is classified by other codes.

K59.4 Anal spasm
Proctalgia fugax
K59.8 Other specified functional intestinal disorders
Atony of colon
Pseudo-obstruction (acute) (chronic) of intestine
K59.9 Functional intestinal disorder, unspecified

4 **K60 Fissure and fistula of anal and rectal regions**
EXCLUDES 1 *fissure and fistula of anal and rectal regions with abscess or cellulitis (K61.-)*
EXCLUDES 2 *anal sphincter tear (healed) (nontraumatic) (old) (K62.81)*

K60.0 Acute anal fissure
K60.1 Chronic anal fissure
K60.2 Anal fissure, unspecified
K60.3 Anal fistula
DEFINITION An abnormal passage from the anus to the skin.
K60.4 Rectal fistula
Fistula of rectum to skin
EXCLUDES 1 *rectovaginal fistula (N82.3)*
vesicorectal fistual (N32.1)
K60.5 Anorectal fistula

4 **K61 Abscess of anal and rectal regions**
INCLUDES abscess of anal and rectal regions
cellulitis of anal and rectal regions

▲ **K61.0 Anal abscess**
Perianal abscess
EXCLUDES 2 *intrasphincteric abscess (K61.4)*
▲ **K61.1 Rectal abscess**
Perirectal abscess
EXCLUDES 1 *ischiorectal abscess (K61.39)*
AHA: 4Q 2012, 104
K61.2 Anorectal abscess
▲ 5 **K61.3 Ischiorectal abscess**
● **K61.31 Horseshoe abscess**
● **K61.39 Other ischiorectal abscess**
Abscess of ischiorectal fossa
Ischiorectal abscess, NOS
▲ **K61.4 Intrasphincteric abscess**
Intersphincteric abscess
● **K61.5 Supralevator abscess**

4 **K62 Other diseases of anus and rectum**
INCLUDES anal canal
EXCLUDES 2 *colostomy and enterostomy malfunction (K94.0-, K94.1-)*
fecal incontinence (R15.-)
hemorrhoids (K64.-)

K62.0 Anal polyp
K62.1 Rectal polyp
EXCLUDES 1 *adenomatous polyp (D12.8)*
K62.2 Anal prolapse
Prolapse of anal canal
K62.3 Rectal prolapse
Prolapse of rectal mucosa
DEFINITION Rectal tissue falls from its usual position, turning itself inside out and protruding from the body in late stages.

Rectal prolapse

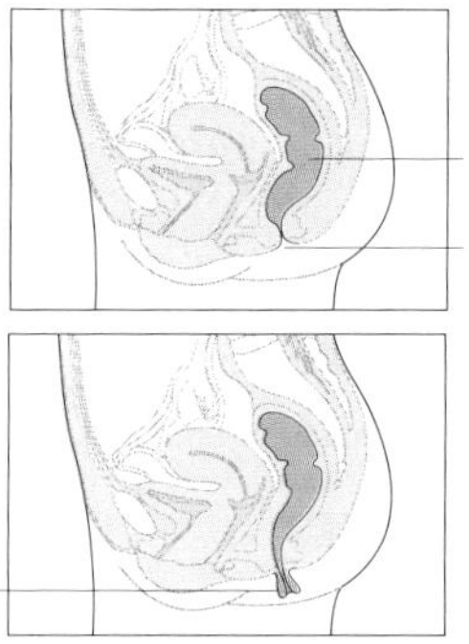

K62.4 Stenosis of anus and rectum
Stricture of anus (sphincter)
K62.5 Hemorrhage of anus and rectum
EXCLUDES 1 *gastrointestinal bleeding NOS (K92.2)*
melena (K92.1)
neonatal rectal hemorrhage (P54.2)
K62.6 Ulcer of anus and rectum
Solitary ulcer of anus and rectum
Stercoral ulcer of anus and rectum
EXCLUDES 1 *fissure and fistula of anus and rectum (K60.-)*
ulcerative colitis (K51.-)
DEFINITION Open sore in the rectum and/or anus causing pain that worsens during defecation and blood or mucous in the stool.
K62.7 Radiation proctitis
Use additional code to identify the type of radiation (W90.-)
CODING TIP✓ Radiation proctitis includes ulceration of the rectal lining due to the adverse effects of radiation. Assign an additional code from W90.- to identify radiation exposure.
5 **K62.8 Other specified diseases of anus and rectum**
EXCLUDES 2 *ulcerative proctitis (K51.2)*
K62.81 Anal sphincter tear (healed) (nontraumatic) (old)
Tear of anus, nontraumatic
Use additional code for any associated fecal incontinence (R15.-)
EXCLUDES 2 *anal fissure (K60.-)*
anal sphincter tear (healed) (old) complicating delivery (O34.7-)
traumatic tear of anal sphincter (S31.831)

K62.82 **Dysplasia of anus**
Anal intraepithelial neoplasia I and II (AIN I and II) (histologically confirmed)
Dysplasia of anus NOS
Mild and moderate dysplasia of anus (histologically confirmed)
EXCLUDES 1 *abnormal results from anal cytologic examination without histologic confirmation (R85.61-)*
anal intraepithelial neoplasia III (D01.3)
carcinoma in situ of anus (D01.3)
HGSIL of anus (R85.613)
severe dysplasia of anus (D01.3)

K62.89 **Other specified diseases of anus and rectum**
Proctitis NOS
Use additional code for any associated fecal incontinence (R15.-)

K62.9 **Disease of anus and rectum, unspecified**

4 K63 Other diseases of intestine

▲ K63.0 **Abscess of intestine**
EXCLUDES 1 *abscess of intestine with Crohn's disease (K50.014, K50.114, K50.814, K50.914,)*
abscess of intestine with diverticular disease (K57.0, K57.2, K57.4, K57.8)
abscess of intestine with ulcerative colitis (K51.014, K51.214, K51.314, K51.414, K51.514, K51.814, K51.914)
EXCLUDES 2 *abscess of anal and rectal regions (K61.-)*
abscess of appendix (K35.3-)

▲ K63.1 **Perforation of intestine (nontraumatic)** HCC
Perforation (nontraumatic) of rectum
EXCLUDES 1 *perforation (nontraumatic) of duodenum (K26.-)*
perforation (nontraumatic) of intestine with diverticular disease (K57.0, K57.2, K57.4, K57.8)
EXCLUDES 2 *perforation (nontraumatic) of appendix (K35.2-, K35.3-)*
DEFINITION Hole in the intestinal wall allowing food and/or fecal matter to leak into the abdominal cavity.

Perforation of intestine

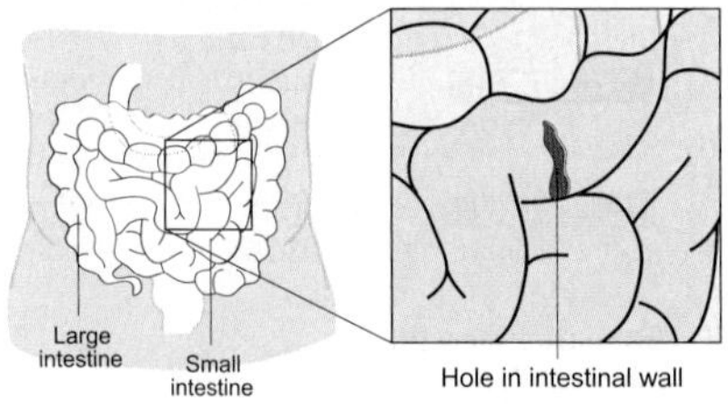

K63.2 **Fistula of intestine**
EXCLUDES 1 *fistula of duodenum (K31.6)*
fistula of intestine with Crohn's disease (K50.013, K50.113, K50.813, K50.913,)
fistula of intestine with ulcerative colitis (K51.013, K51.213, K51.313, K51.413, K51.513, K51.813, K51.913)
EXCLUDES 2 *fistula of anal and rectal regions (K60.-)*
fistula of appendix (K38.3)
intestinal-genital fistula, female (N82.2-N82.4)
vesicointestinal fistula (N32.1)
DEFINITION Abnormal passageway between loops of the intestine or the intestine and another organ or the abdominal wall.

Fistula of intestine

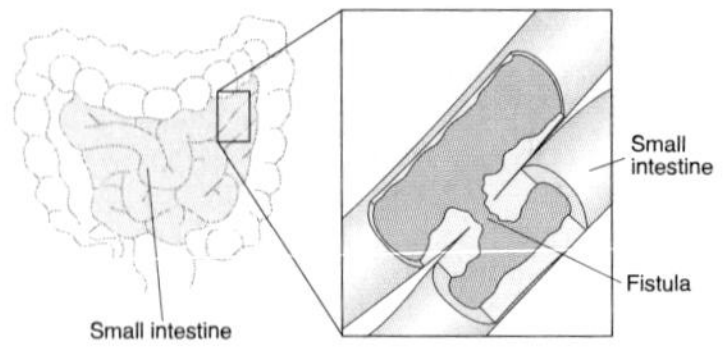

K63.3 **Ulcer of intestine**
Primary ulcer of small intestine
EXCLUDES 1 *duodenal ulcer (K26.-)*
gastrointestinal ulcer (K28.-)
gastrojejunal ulcer (K28.-)
jejunal ulcer (K28.-)
peptic ulcer, site unspecified (K27.-)
ulcer of intestine with perforation (K63.1)
ulcer of anus or rectum (K62.6)
ulcerative colitis (K51.-)

K63.4 **Enteroptosis**

K63.5 **Polyp of colon**
EXCLUDES 1 *adenomatous polyp of colon (D12.6)*
inflammatory polyp of colon (K51.4-)
polyposis of colon (D12.6)
AHA: 2Q 2015, 14
AHA: 1Q 2017, 15

5 K63.8 **Other specified diseases of intestine**

K63.81 **Dieulafoy lesion of intestine**
EXCLUDES 2 *Dieulafoy lesion of stomach and duodenum (K31.82)*

K63.89 **Other specified diseases of intestine**
AHA: 2Q 2013, 31

K63.9 **Disease of intestine, unspecified**

4 K64 Hemorrhoids and perianal venous thrombosis
INCLUDES piles
EXCLUDES 1 *hemorrhoids complicating childbirth and the puerperium (O87.2)*
hemorrhoids complicating pregnancy (O22.4)

K64.0 **First degree hemorrhoids**
Grade/stage I hemorrhoids
Hemorrhoids (bleeding) without prolapse outside of anal canal

K64.1 **Second degree hemorrhoids**
Grade/stage II hemorrhoids
Hemorrhoids (bleeding) that prolapse with straining, but retract spontaneously

K64.2 **Third degree hemorrhoids**
Grade/stage III hemorrhoids
Hemorrhoids (bleeding) that prolapse with straining and require manual replacement back inside anal canal

K64.3 **Fourth degree hemorrhoids**
Grade/stage IV hemorrhoids
Hemorrhoids (bleeding) with prolapsed tissue that cannot be manually replaced

K64.4 **Residual hemorrhoidal skin tags**
External hemorrhoids, NOS
Skin tags of anus

K64.5 **Perianal venous thrombosis**
External hemorrhoids with thrombosis
Perianal hematoma
Thrombosed hemorrhoids NOS

K64.8 **Other hemorrhoids**
Internal hemorrhoids, without mention of degree
Prolapsed hemorrhoids, degree not specified

K64.9 **Unspecified hemorrhoids**
Hemorrhoids (bleeding) NOS
Hemorrhoids (bleeding) without mention of degree

Diseases of peritoneum and retroperitoneum (K65-K68)

▲ 4 **K65 Peritonitis**
Code also:
if applicable diverticular disease of intestine (K57.-)
Use additional code (B95-B97), to identify infectious agent, if known
EXCLUDES 1 *acute appendicitis with generalized peritonitis (K35.2-)*
aseptic peritonitis (T81.6)
benign paroxysmal peritonitis (E85.0)
chemical peritonitis (T81.6)
gonococcal peritonitis (A54.85)
neonatal peritonitis (P78.0-P78.1)
pelvic peritonitis, female (N73.3-N73.5)
periodic familial peritonitis (E85.0)
peritonitis due to talc or other foreign substance (T81.6)
peritonitis in chlamydia (A74.81)
peritonitis in diphtheria (A36.89)
peritonitis in syphilis (late) (A52.74)
peritonitis in tuberculosis (A18.31)
peritonitis with or following abortion or ectopic or molar pregnancy (O00-O07, O08.0)
peritonitis with or following appendicitis (K35.-)
puerperal peritonitis (O85)
retroperitoneal infections (K68.-)

CODING TIP ✓ When the causative infectious organism is known, always assign an additional code from B95-B97 to identify the infectious agent.

K65.0 Generalized (acute) peritonitis HCC
Pelvic peritonitis (acute), male
Subphrenic peritonitis (acute)
Suppurative peritonitis (acute)

K65.1 Peritoneal abscess HCC
Abdominopelvic abscess
Abscess (of) omentum
Abscess (of) peritoneum
Mesenteric abscess
Retrocecal abscess
Subdiaphragmatic abscess
Subhepatic abscess
Subphrenic abscess

K65.2 Spontaneous bacterial peritonitis HCC
EXCLUDES 1 *bacterial peritonitis NOS (K65.9)*

CODING TIP ✓ Do not assign K65.2 unless the physician has specifically provided a diagnosis of "spontaneous" bacterial peritonitis. Bacterial peritonitis not specified as spontaneous is classified to K65.9 (Peritonitis NOS).

K65.3 Choleperitonitis HCC
Peritonitis due to bile

K65.4 Sclerosing mesenteritis HCC
Fat necrosis of peritoneum
(Idiopathic) sclerosing mesenteric fibrosis
Mesenteric lipodystrophy
Mesenteric panniculitis
Retractile mesenteritis

DEFINITION Rare, idiopathic lesions of fat necrosis, fibrosis, and chronic inflammation causing single or multiple lesions, with diffuse thickening of the mesentery.

K65.8 Other peritonitis HCC
Chronic proliferative peritonitis
Peritonitis due to urine

K65.9 Peritonitis, unspecified HCC
Bacterial peritonitis NOS
AHA: 2Q 2013, 31

4 **K66 Other disorders of peritoneum**
EXCLUDES 2 *ascites (R18.-)*
peritoneal effusion (chronic) (R18.8)

K66.0 Peritoneal adhesions (postprocedural) (postinfection)
Adhesions (of) abdominal (wall)
Adhesions (of) diaphragm
Adhesions (of) intestine
Adhesions (of) male pelvis
Adhesions (of) omentum
Adhesions (of) stomach
Adhesive bands
Mesenteric adhesions
EXCLUDES 1 *female pelvic adhesions [bands] (N73.6)*
peritoneal adhesions with intestinal obstruction (K56.5-)

Peritoneal adhesions (postprocedural) (postinfection)

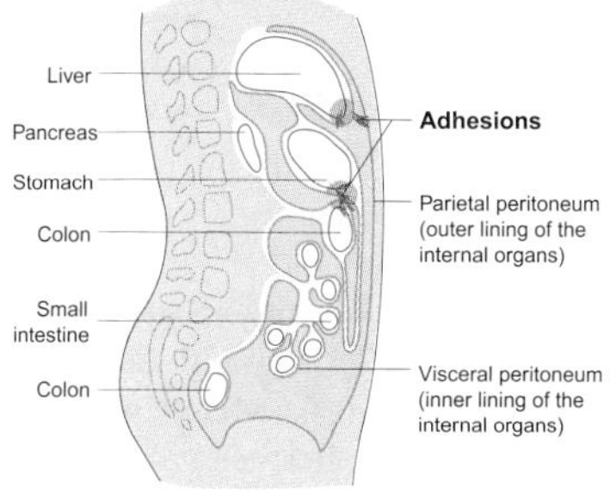

K66.1 Hemoperitoneum
EXCLUDES 1 *traumatic hemoperitoneum (S36.8-)*

K66.8 Other specified disorders of peritoneum

K66.9 Disorder of peritoneum, unspecified

K67 *Disorders of peritoneum in infectious diseases classified elsewhere* HCC
Code first underlying disease, such as:
congenital syphilis (A50.0)
helminthiasis (B65.0 -B83.9)
EXCLUDES 1 *peritonitis in chlamydia (A74.81)*
peritonitis in diphtheria (A36.89)
peritonitis in gonococcal (A54.85)
peritonitis in syphilis (late) (A52.74)
peritonitis in tuberculosis (A18.31)

4 **K68 Disorders of retroperitoneum**

5 **K68.1 Retroperitoneal abscess**

▲ **K68.11 Postprocedural retroperitoneal abscess**
EXCLUDES 2 *infection following procedure (T81.4-)*

K68.12 Psoas muscle abscess HCC

K68.19 Other retroperitoneal abscess HCC

K68.9 Other disorders of retroperitoneum

Diseases of liver (K70-K77)

EXCLUDES 1 *jaundice NOS (R17)*
EXCLUDES 2 *hemochromatosis (E83.11-)*
Reye's syndrome (G93.7)
viral hepatitis (B15-B19)
Wilson's disease (E83.0)

4 **K70 Alcoholic liver disease**
Use additional code to identify:
alcohol abuse and dependence (F10.-)

CODING TIP ✓ Codes from category K70.- indicate liver disease resulting from alcohol use. An additional code should be assigned to identify alcohol abuse or dependence.

Liver anatomy

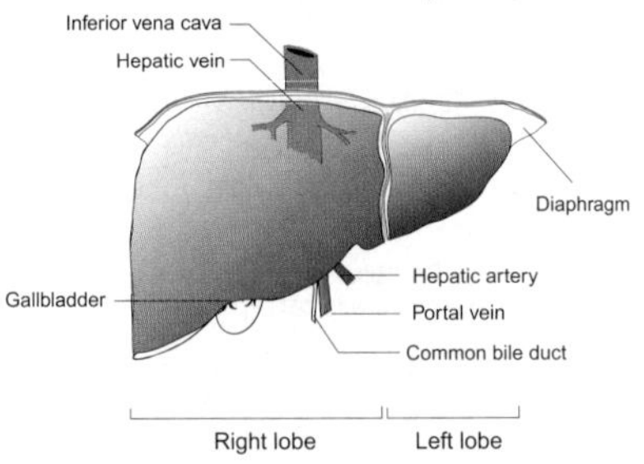

K70.0 **Alcoholic fatty liver** A

5 **K70.1** **Alcoholic hepatitis**

- **K70.10** **Alcoholic hepatitis without ascites** A
- **K70.11** **Alcoholic hepatitis with ascites** A

K70.2 **Alcoholic fibrosis and sclerosis of liver** A

DEFINITION Intermediate stage liver disease in which normal, healthy tissue of the liver is replaced by scar tissue due to long-term, excessive alcohol consumption.

5 **K70.3** **Alcoholic cirrhosis of liver**
Alcoholic cirrhosis NOS

DEFINITION Late stage liver disease characterized by inflammation, debilitating scar tissue, and damaged membranes due to long-term, excessive alcohol consumption.

- **K70.30** **Alcoholic cirrhosis of liver without ascites** A HCC

Alcoholic cirrhosis of liver without ascites

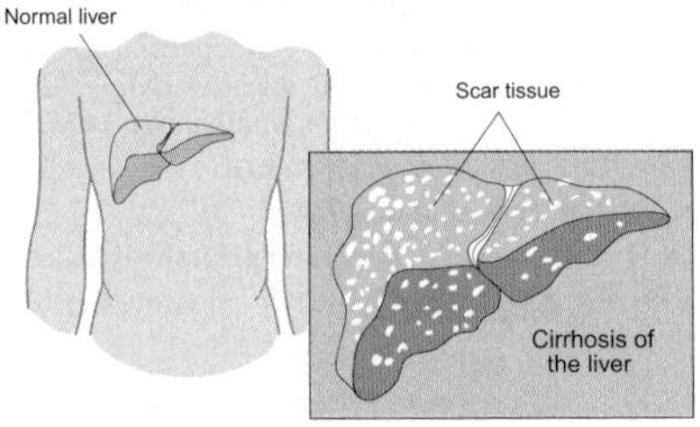

- **K70.31** **Alcoholic cirrhosis of liver with ascites** A HCC

5 **K70.4** **Alcoholic hepatic failure**
Acute alcoholic hepatic failure
Alcoholic hepatic failure NOS
Chronic alcoholic hepatic failure
Subacute alcoholic hepatic failure

- **K70.40** **Alcoholic hepatic failure without coma** A HCC
- **K70.41** **Alcoholic hepatic failure with coma** A HCC

K70.9 **Alcoholic liver disease, unspecified** A HCC

4 **K71** **Toxic liver disease**

INCLUDES drug-induced idiosyncratic (unpredictable) liver disease
drug-induced toxic (predictable) liver disease

Code first:
poisoning due to drug or toxin, if applicable (T36-T65 with fifth or sixth character 1-4 or 6)

Use additional code for adverse effect, if applicable, to identify drug (T36-T50 with fifth or sixth character 5)

EXCLUDES 2 *alcoholic liver disease (K70.-)*
Budd-Chiari syndrome (I82.0)

CODING TIP ✓ Codes from category K71.- indicate liver disease resulting from toxicity or toxic damage to the liver due to chemical exposure, including drugs. When a condition from K71.- is caused by poisoning, code first the appropriate T36-T65 code to indicate poisoning. When the condition is diagnosed as an adverse effect, code the appropriate K71.- code followed by the appropriate code from categories T36-T50 to indicate adverse effect.

K71.0 **Toxic liver disease with cholestasis**
Cholestasis with hepatocyte injury
'Pure' cholestasis

5 **K71.1** **Toxic liver disease with hepatic necrosis**
Hepatic failure (acute) (chronic) due to drugs

- **K71.10** **Toxic liver disease with hepatic necrosis, without coma**
- **K71.11** **Toxic liver disease with hepatic necrosis, with coma** HCC

K71.2 **Toxic liver disease with acute hepatitis**

K71.3 **Toxic liver disease with chronic persistent hepatitis**

K71.4 **Toxic liver disease with chronic lobular hepatitis**

5 **K71.5** **Toxic liver disease with chronic active hepatitis**
Toxic liver disease with lupoid hepatitis

- **K71.50** **Toxic liver disease with chronic active hepatitis without ascites**
- **K71.51** **Toxic liver disease with chronic active hepatitis with ascites**

K71.6 **Toxic liver disease with hepatitis, not elsewhere classified**

K71.7 **Toxic liver disease with fibrosis and cirrhosis of liver**

K71.8 **Toxic liver disease with other disorders of liver**
Toxic liver disease with focal nodular hyperplasia
Toxic liver disease with hepatic granulomas
Toxic liver disease with peliosis hepatis
Toxic liver disease with veno-occlusive disease of liver

K71.9 **Toxic liver disease, unspecified**

4 **K72** **Hepatic failure, not elsewhere classified**

INCLUDES fulminant hepatitis NEC, with hepatic failure
hepatic encephalopathy NOS
liver (cell) necrosis with hepatic failure
malignant hepatitis NEC, with hepatic failure
yellow liver atrophy or dystrophy

EXCLUDES 1 *alcoholic hepatic failure (K70.4)*
hepatic failure with toxic liver disease (K71.1-)
icterus of newborn (P55-P59)
postprocedural hepatic failure (K91.82)

EXCLUDES 2 *hepatic failure complicating abortion or ectopic or molar pregnancy (O00-O07, O08.8)*
hepatic failure complicating pregnancy, childbirth and the puerperium (O26.6-)
viral hepatitis with hepatic coma (B15-B19)

5 **K72.0** **Acute and subacute hepatic failure**
Acute non-viral hepatitis NOS
AHA: 2Q 2014, 13

- **K72.00** **Acute and subacute hepatic failure without coma**
  AHA: 2Q 2015, 17
- **K72.01** **Acute and subacute hepatic failure with coma** HCC

5 **K72.1** **Chronic hepatic failure**

- **K72.10** **Chronic hepatic failure without coma** HCC
  AHA: 1Q 2017, 41
- **K72.11** **Chronic hepatic failure with coma** HCC

5 **K72.9** **Hepatic failure, unspecified**

- **K72.90** **Hepatic failure, unspecified without coma** HCC
  AHA: 2Q 2016, 35
- **K72.91** **Hepatic failure, unspecified with coma** HCC
  Hepatic coma NOS

4 **K73** **Chronic hepatitis, not elsewhere classified**

EXCLUDES 1 *alcoholic hepatitis (chronic) (K70.1-)*
drug-induced hepatitis (chronic) (K71.-)
granulomatous hepatitis (chronic) NEC (K75.3)
reactive, nonspecific hepatitis (chronic) (K75.2)
viral hepatitis (chronic) (B15-B19)

CODING TIP ✓ Do not assign a code from category K73.- when hepatitis is specified as viral or due to a specific cause, such as alcohol use or toxicity.

K73.0 **Chronic persistent hepatitis, not elsewhere classified** HCC

K73.1 **Chronic lobular hepatitis, not elsewhere classified** HCC

K73.2 **Chronic active hepatitis, not elsewhere classified** HCC

K73.8 **Other chronic hepatitis, not elsewhere classified** HCC

K73.9 **Chronic hepatitis, unspecified** HCC

K74 Fibrosis and cirrhosis of liver

Code also:

, if applicable, viral hepatitis (acute) (chronic) (B15-B19)

EXCLUDES 1 *alcoholic cirrhosis (of liver) (K70.3)*
alcoholic fibrosis of liver (K70.2)
cardiac sclerosis of liver (K76.1)
cirrhosis (of liver) with toxic liver disease (K71.7)
congenital cirrhosis (of liver) (P78.81)
pigmentary cirrhosis (of liver) (E83.110)

CODING TIP ✓ When viral hepatitis is also documented as a confirmed diagnosis in a patient with any diagnosis classifiable to K74.-, the appropriate code from B15-B19 should also be assigned. The sequencing of the K74.- and the viral hepatitis code is according to focus of care.

K74.0 **Hepatic fibrosis**

K74.1 **Hepatic sclerosis**

K74.2 **Hepatic fibrosis with Hepatic sclerosis**

▲ K74.3 **Primary biliary cirrhosis** HCC
Chronic nonsuppurative destructive cholangitis
Primary biliary cholangitis

EXCLUDES 2 *primary schlerosing cholangitis (K83.01)*

DEFINITION Scar tissue formation of the ducts carrying bile from the liver to the small intestine, resulting in bile build-up and liver damage leading to cirrhosis.

K74.4 **Secondary biliary cirrhosis** HCC

K74.5 **Biliary cirrhosis, unspecified** HCC

K74.6 **Other and unspecified cirrhosis of liver**

K74.60 **Unspecified cirrhosis of liver** HCC
Cirrhosis (of liver) NOS

K74.69 **Other cirrhosis of liver** HCC
Cryptogenic cirrhosis (of liver)
Macronodular cirrhosis (of liver)
Micronodular cirrhosis (of liver)
Mixed type cirrhosis (of liver)
Portal cirrhosis (of liver)
Postnecrotic cirrhosis (of liver)

K75 Other inflammatory liver diseases

EXCLUDES 2 *toxic liver disease (K71.-)*

▲ K75.0 **Abscess of liver**
Cholangitic hepatic abscess
Hematogenic hepatic abscess
Hepatic abscess NOS
Lymphogenic hepatic abscess
Pylephlebitic hepatic abscess

EXCLUDES 1 *amebic liver abscess (A06.4)*
cholangitis without liver abscess (K83.09)
pylephlebitis without liver abscess (K75.1)

EXCLUDES 2 *acute or subacute hepatitis NOS (B17.9)*
acute or subacute non-viral hepatitis (K72.0)
chronic hepatitis NEC (K73.8)

K75.1 **Phlebitis of portal vein**
Pylephlebitis

EXCLUDES 1 *pylephlebitic liver abscess (K75.0)*

K75.2 **Nonspecific reactive hepatitis**

EXCLUDES 1 *acute or subacute hepatitis (K72.0-)*
chronic hepatitis NEC (K73.-)
viral hepatitis (B15-B19)

K75.3 **Granulomatous hepatitis, not elsewhere classified**

EXCLUDES 1 *acute or subacute hepatitis (K72.0-)*
chronic hepatitis NEC (K73.-)
viral hepatitis (B15-B19)

K75.4 **Autoimmune hepatitis** HCC
Lupoid hepatitis NEC

DEFINITION Continuous inflammation and necrosis of liver cells that progresses to cirrhosis, in association with autoimmune diseases and not infection, alcohol consumption, or toxic exposure.

K75.8 **Other specified inflammatory liver diseases**

K75.81 **Nonalcoholic steatohepatitis (NASH)**

K75.89 **Other specified inflammatory liver diseases**

K75.9 **Inflammatory liver disease, unspecified**
Hepatitis NOS

EXCLUDES 1 *acute or subacute hepatitis (K72.0-)*
chronic hepatitis NEC (K73.-)
viral hepatitis (B15-B19)

CODING TIP ✓ **Documentation:** When documentation confirms only that a patient has hepatitis but does not provide any further detail, assign K75.9 to indicate hepatitis NOS. Do not assign this code if specific cause/type of hepatitis is specified in diagnostic information.

AHA: 2Q 2015, 17

K76 Other diseases of liver

EXCLUDES 2 *alcoholic liver disease (K70.-)*
amyloid degeneration of liver (E85.-)
cystic disease of liver (congenital) (Q44.6)
hepatic vein thrombosis (I82.0)
hepatomegaly NOS (R16.0)
pigmentary cirrhosis (of liver) (E83.110)
portal vein thrombosis (I81)
toxic liver disease (K71.-)

K76.0 **Fatty (change of) liver, not elsewhere classified**
Nonalcoholic fatty liver disease (NAFLD)

EXCLUDES 1 *nonalcoholic steatohepatitis (NASH) (K75.81)*

K76.1 **Chronic passive congestion of liver**
Cardiac cirrhosis
Cardiac sclerosis

K76.2 **Central hemorrhagic necrosis of liver**

EXCLUDES 1 *liver necrosis with hepatic failure (K72.-)*

K76.3 **Infarction of liver**

K76.4 **Peliosis hepatis**
Hepatic angiomatosis

K76.5 **Hepatic veno-occlusive disease**

EXCLUDES 1 *Budd-Chiari syndrome (I82.0)*

K76.6 **Portal hypertension** HCC

Use additional code for any associated complications, such as:
portal hypertensive gastropathy (K31.89)

DEFINITION Increase in the pressure within the portal vein which carries blood from the digestive organs to the liver, caused by a blockage of blood flow through the liver.

K76.7 **Hepatorenal syndrome** HCC

EXCLUDES 1 *hepatorenal syndrome following labor and delivery (O90.4)*
postprocedural hepatorenal syndrome (K91.83)

K76.8 **Other specified diseases of liver**

K76.81 **Hepatopulmonary syndrome** HCC
Code first underlying liver disease, such as:
alcoholic cirrhosis of liver (K70.3-)
cirrhosis of liver without mention of alcohol (K74.6-)

K76.89 **Other specified diseases of liver**
Cyst (simple) of liver
Focal nodular hyperplasia of liver
Hepatoptosis

K76.9 **Liver disease, unspecified**

K77 ***Liver disorders in diseases classified elsewhere***

Code first underlying disease, such as:
amyloidosis (E85.-)
congenital syphilis (A50.0, A50.5)
congenital toxoplasmosis (P37.1)
schistosomiasis (B65.0-B65.9)

EXCLUDES 1 *alcoholic hepatitis (K70.1-)*
alcoholic liver disease (K70.-)
cytomegaloviral hepatitis (B25.1)
herpesviral [herpes simplex] hepatitis (B00.81)
infectious mononucleosis with liver disease (B27.0-B27.9 with .9)
mumps hepatitis (B26.81)
sarcoidosis with liver disease (D86.89)
secondary syphilis with liver disease (A51.45)
syphilis (late) with liver disease (A52.74)
toxoplasmosis (acquired) hepatitis (B58.1)
tuberculosis with liver disease (A18.83)

Disorders of gallbladder, biliary tract and pancreas (K80-K87)

4 K80 Cholelithiasis

EXCLUDES 1 *retained cholelithiasis following cholecystectomy (K91.86)*

▲ 5 **K80.0** **Calculus of gallbladder with acute cholecystitis**
Any condition listed in K80.2 with acute cholecystitis
Use additional code if applicable for associated gangrene of gallbladder (K82.A1), or perforation of gallbladder (K82.A2)

K80.00 **Calculus of gallbladder with acute cholecystitis without obstruction**

K80.01 **Calculus of gallbladder with acute cholecystitis with obstruction**

▲ 5 **K80.1** **Calculus of gallbladder with other cholecystitis**
Use additional code if applicable for associated gangrene of gallbladder (K82.A1), or perforation of gallbladder (K82.A2)

K80.10 **Calculus of gallbladder with chronic cholecystitis without obstruction**
Cholelithiasis with cholecystitis NOS

K80.11 **Calculus of gallbladder with chronic cholecystitis with obstruction**

K80.12 **Calculus of gallbladder with acute and chronic cholecystitis without obstruction**

K80.13 **Calculus of gallbladder with acute and chronic cholecystitis with obstruction**

K80.18 **Calculus of gallbladder with other cholecystitis without obstruction**

K80.19 **Calculus of gallbladder with other cholecystitis with obstruction**

5 **K80.2** **Calculus of gallbladder without cholecystitis**
Cholecystolithiasis without cholecystitis
Cholelithiasis (without cholecystitis)
Colic (recurrent) of gallbladder (without cholecystitis)
Gallstone (impacted) of cystic duct (without cholecystitis)
Gallstone (impacted) of gallbladder (without cholecystitis)

K80.20 **Calculus of gallbladder without cholecystitis without obstruction**

K80.21 **Calculus of gallbladder without cholecystitis with obstruction**

Calculus of gallbladder without cholecystitis with obstruction

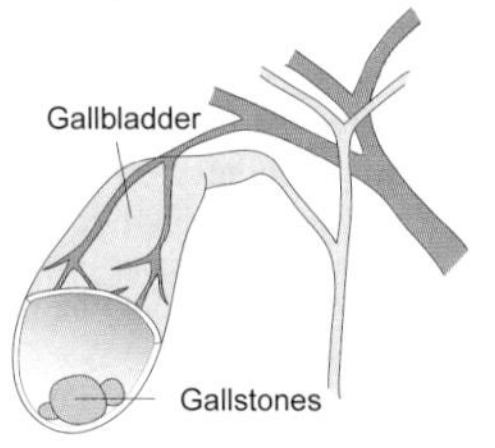

5 **K80.3** **Calculus of bile duct with cholangitis**
Any condition listed in K80.5 with cholangitis

K80.30 **Calculus of bile duct with cholangitis, unspecified, without obstruction**

K80.31 **Calculus of bile duct with cholangitis, unspecified, with obstruction**

K80.32 **Calculus of bile duct with acute cholangitis without obstruction**

K80.33 **Calculus of bile duct with acute cholangitis with obstruction**

K80.34 **Calculus of bile duct with chronic cholangitis without obstruction**

K80.35 **Calculus of bile duct with chronic cholangitis with obstruction**

K80.36 **Calculus of bile duct with acute and chronic cholangitis without obstruction**

K80.37 **Calculus of bile duct with acute and chronic cholangitis with obstruction**

▲ 5 **K80.4** **Calculus of bile duct with cholecystitis**
Any condition listed in K80.5 with cholecystitis (with cholangitis)
Use additional code if applicable for associated gangrene of gallbladder (K82.A1), or perforation of gallbladder (K82.A2)

K80.40 **Calculus of bile duct with cholecystitis, unspecified, without obstruction**

K80.41 **Calculus of bile duct with cholecystitis, unspecified, with obstruction**

K80.42 **Calculus of bile duct with acute cholecystitis without obstruction**

K80.43 **Calculus of bile duct with acute cholecystitis with obstruction**

K80.44 **Calculus of bile duct with chronic cholecystitis without obstruction**

K80.45 **Calculus of bile duct with chronic cholecystitis with obstruction**

K80.46 **Calculus of bile duct with acute and chronic cholecystitis without obstruction**

K80.47 **Calculus of bile duct with acute and chronic cholecystitis with obstruction**

5 **K80.5** **Calculus of bile duct without cholangitis or cholecystitis**
Choledocholithiasis (without cholangitis or cholecystitis)
Gallstone (impacted) of bile duct NOS (without cholangitis or cholecystitis)
Gallstone (impacted) of common duct (without cholangitis or cholecystitis)
Gallstone (impacted) of hepatic duct (without cholangitis or cholecystitis)
Hepatic cholelithiasis (without cholangitis or cholecystitis)
Hepatic colic (recurrent) (without cholangitis or cholecystitis)

K80.50 **Calculus of bile duct without cholangitis or cholecystitis without obstruction**

K80.51 **Calculus of bile duct without cholangitis or cholecystitis with obstruction**

▲ 5 **K80.6** **Calculus of gallbladder and bile duct with cholecystitis**
Use additional code if applicable for associated gangrene of gallbladder (K82.A1), or perforation of gallbladder (K82.A2)

K80.60 **Calculus of gallbladder and bile duct with cholecystitis, unspecified, without obstruction**

K80.61 **Calculus of gallbladder and bile duct with cholecystitis, unspecified, with obstruction**

K80.62 **Calculus of gallbladder and bile duct with acute cholecystitis without obstruction**

K80.63 **Calculus of gallbladder and bile duct with acute cholecystitis with obstruction**

K80.64 **Calculus of gallbladder and bile duct with chronic cholecystitis without obstruction**

K80.65 **Calculus of gallbladder and bile duct with chronic cholecystitis with obstruction**

K80.66 **Calculus of gallbladder and bile duct with acute and chronic cholecystitis without obstruction**

K80.67 **Calculus of gallbladder and bile duct with acute and chronic cholecystitis with obstruction**

5 **K80.7** **Calculus of gallbladder and bile duct without cholecystitis**

K80.70 **Calculus of gallbladder and bile duct without cholecystitis without obstruction**

K80.71 **Calculus of gallbladder and bile duct without cholecystitis with obstruction**

5 **K80.8** **Other cholelithiasis**

K80.80 **Other cholelithiasis without obstruction**

K80.81 **Other cholelithiasis with obstruction**

▲ 4 **K81** **Cholecystitis**
Use additional code if applicable for associated gangrene of gallbladder (K82.A1), or perforation of gallbladder (K82.A2)

EXCLUDES 1 *cholecystitis with cholelithiasis (K80.-)*

K81.0 **Acute cholecystitis**
Abscess of gallbladder
Angiocholecystitis
Emphysematous (acute) cholecystitis
Empyema of gallbladder
Gangrene of gallbladder
Gangrenous cholecystitis
Suppurative cholecystitis

K81.1 **Chronic cholecystitis**

K81.2 Acute cholecystitis with chronic cholecystitis
K81.9 Cholecystitis, unspecified

K82 Other diseases of gallbladder

EXCLUDES 1 *nonvisualization of gallbladder (R93.2)*
postcholecystectomy syndrome (K91.5)

K82.0 Obstruction of gallbladder
Occlusion of cystic duct or gallbladder without cholelithiasis
Stenosis of cystic duct or gallbladder without cholelithiasis
Stricture of cystic duct or gallbladder without cholelithiasis
EXCLUDES 1 *obstruction of gallbladder with cholelithiasis (K80.-)*

Obstruction of gallbladder

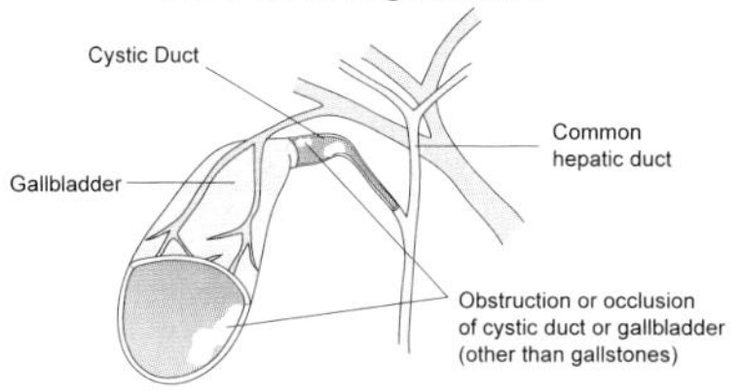

K82.1 Hydrops of gallbladder
Mucocele of gallbladder
DEFINITION Overly full, distended gallbladder due to accumulation of mucous and watery material rather than stone formation.

▲ **K82.2 Perforation of gallbladder**
Rupture of cystic duct or gallbladder
EXCLUDES 1 *Perforation of gallbladder in cholecystitis (K82.A2)*

K82.3 Fistula of gallbladder
Cholecystocolic fistula
Cholecystoduodenal fistula

K82.4 Cholesterolosis of gallbladder
Strawberry gallbladder
EXCLUDES 1 *cholesterolosis of gallbladder with cholecystitis (K81.-)*
cholesterolosis of gallbladder with cholelithiasis (K80.-)
DEFINITION Build-up of cholesterol deposits on the surface of the gallbladder, giving it a 'strawberry' appearance.

K82.8 Other specified diseases of gallbladder
Adhesions of cystic duct or gallbladder
Atrophy of cystic duct or gallbladder
Cyst of cystic duct or gallbladder
Dyskinesia of cystic duct or gallbladder
Hypertrophy of cystic duct or gallbladder
Nonfunctioning of cystic duct or gallbladder
Ulcer of cystic duct or gallbladder

K82.9 Disease of gallbladder, unspecified

● **K82.A Disorders of gallbladder in diseases classified elsewhere**
Code first:
the type of cholecystitis (K81.-) , or cholelithiasis with cholecystitis (K80.00-K80.19, K80.40-K80.47, K80.60-K80.67)

● K82.A1 *Gangrene of gallbladder in cholecystitis*
● K82.A2 *Perforation of gallbladder in cholecystitis*

K83 Other diseases of biliary tract

EXCLUDES 1 *postcholecystectomy syndrome (K91.5)*
EXCLUDES 2 *conditions involving the gallbladder (K81-K82)*
conditions involving the cystic duct (K81-K82)

▲ **K83.0 Cholangitis**
EXCLUDES 1 *cholangitic liver abscess (K75.0)*
cholangitis with choledocholithiasis (K80.3-, K80.4-)
EXCLUDES 2 *chronic nonsuppurative destructive cholangitis (K74.3)*
primary biliary cholangitis (K74.3)
primary biliary cirrhosis (K74.3)
DEFINITION Infection of the biliary tract; presents with pain in the upper-right abdomen which may grow worse after a fatty meal, fever, nausea, vomiting, flatulence, pale-colored stool, and yellowing of the eyes and skin.

● **K83.01 Primary sclerosing cholangitis**
● **K83.09 Other cholangitis**
Ascending cholangitis
Cholangitis NOS
Primary cholangitis
Recurrent cholangitis
Sclerosing cholangitis
Secondary cholangitis
Stenosing cholangitis
Suppurative cholangitis

K83.1 Obstruction of bile duct
Occlusion of bile duct without cholelithiasis
Stenosis of bile duct without cholelithiasis
Stricture of bile duct without cholelithiasis
EXCLUDES 1 *congenital obstruction of bile duct (Q44.3)*
obstruction of bile duct with cholelithiasis (K80.-)
AHA: 1Q 2016, 18-19

Obstruction of bile duct

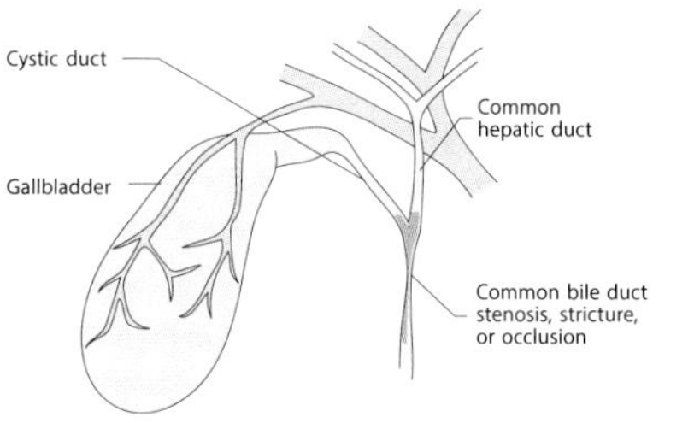

K83.2 Perforation of bile duct
Rupture of bile duct

K83.3 Fistula of bile duct
Choledochoduodenal fistula

K83.4 Spasm of sphincter of Oddi

K83.5 Biliary cyst

K83.8 Other specified diseases of biliary tract
Adhesions of biliary tract
Atrophy of biliary tract
Hypertrophy of biliary tract
Ulcer of biliary tract

K83.9 Disease of biliary tract, unspecified

K85 Acute pancreatitis

INCLUDES acute (recurrent) pancreatitis
subacute pancreatitis
AHA: 4Q 2016, 34

K85.0 Idiopathic acute pancreatitis
K85.00 Idiopathic acute pancreatitis without necrosis or infection
K85.01 Idiopathic acute pancreatitis with uninfected necrosis
K85.02 Idiopathic acute pancreatitis with infected necrosis

K85.1 Biliary acute pancreatitis
Gallstone pancreatitis
K85.10 Biliary acute pancreatitis without necrosis or infection
K85.11 Biliary acute pancreatitis with uninfected necrosis
K85.12 Biliary acute pancreatitis with infected necrosis

K85.2 Alcohol induced acute pancreatitis
EXCLUDES 2 *alcohol induced chronic pancreatitis (K86.0)*
CODING TIP ✓ Assign a code from K85.2- only when physician documentation clearly confirms chronic pancreatitis due to alcohol use. The appropriate F10 code with 5th and 6th digits .88 (F10.188, F10.288, F10.988) should also be added.
K85.20 Alcohol induced acute pancreatitis without necrosis or infection
K85.21 Alcohol induced acute pancreatitis with uninfected necrosis
K85.22 Alcohol induced acute pancreatitis with infected necrosis

5 K85.3 **Drug induced acute pancreatitis**
Use additional code for adverse effect, if applicable, to identify drug (T36-T50 with fifth or sixth character 5)
Use additional code to identify drug abuse and dependence (F11.-F17.-)
K85.30 **Drug induced acute pancreatitis without necrosis or infection**
K85.31 **Drug induced acute pancreatitis with uninfected necrosis**
K85.32 **Drug induced acute pancreatitis with infected necrosis**
5 K85.8 **Other acute pancreatitis**
K85.80 **Other acute pancreatitis without necrosis or infection**
K85.81 **Other acute pancreatitis with uninfected necrosis**
K85.82 **Other acute pancreatitis with infected necrosis**
5 K85.9 **Acute pancreatitis, unspecified**
Pancreatitis NOS
K85.90 **Acute pancreatitis without necrosis or infection, unspecified**
K85.91 **Acute pancreatitis with uninfected necrosis, unspecified**
K85.92 **Acute pancreatitis with infected necrosis, unspecified**

4 **K86 Other diseases of pancreas**
EXCLUDES 2 *fibrocystic disease of pancreas (E84.-)*
islet cell tumor (of pancreas) (D13.7)
pancreatic steatorrhea (K90.3)

K86.0 **Alcohol-induced chronic pancreatitis** HCC
Code also:
exocrine pancreatic insufficiency (K86.81)
Use additional code to identify:
alcohol abuse and dependence (F10.-)
EXCLUDES 2 *alcohol induced acute pancreatitis (K85.2-)*

CODING TIP ✓ Assign a code from K86.0- only when physician documentation clearly confirms acute pancreatitis due to alcohol use. The appropriate F10 code with 5th and 6th digits .88 (F10.188, F10.288, F10.988) should also be added.

K86.1 **Other chronic pancreatitis** HCC
Chronic pancreatitis NOS
Infectious chronic pancreatitis
Recurrent chronic pancreatitis
Relapsing chronic pancreatitis
Code also:
exocrine pancreatic insufficiency (K86.81)
K86.2 **Cyst of pancreas**

Cyst of pancreas

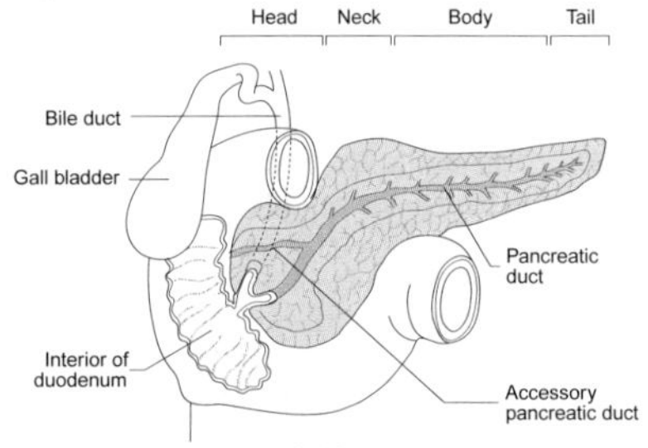

Cysts are a collection of fluid in the head, body, or tail of the pancreas

K86.3 **Pseudocyst of pancreas**
5 K86.8 **Other specified diseases of pancreas**
AHA: 4Q 2016, 34
K86.81 **Exocrine pancreatic insufficiency**
CODING TIP ✓ Exocrine pancreatic insufficiency results in an inability to digest food properly due to insufficient production of enzymes. It is common in patients with cystic fibrosis and chronic pancreatitis.

DEFINITION Insufficient pancreatic secretory functioning causes malfunctioning digestion and the malabsorption of fats in particular, which leads to malnutrition, and associated diseases of nutritional deficiencies. It is common in cystic fibrosis patients. Symptoms include chronic diarrhea or passing foul-smelling, voluminous stools, bloating, abdominal pain and cramping, weight loss, and steatorrhea.

K86.89 **Other specified diseases of pancreas**
Aseptic pancreatic necrosis, unrelated to acute pancreatitis
Atrophy of pancreas
Calculus of pancreas
Cirrhosis of pancreas
Fibrosis of pancreas
Pancreatic fat necrosis, unrelated to acute pancreatitis
Pancreatic infantilism
Pancreatic necrosis NOS, unrelated to acute pancreatitis
K86.9 **Disease of pancreas, unspecified**

K87 *Disorders of gallbladder, biliary tract and pancreas in diseases classified elsewhere*
Code first:
underlying disease
EXCLUDES 1 *cytomegaloviral pancreatitis (B25.2)*
mumps pancreatitis (B26.3)
syphilitic gallbladder (A52.74)
syphilitic pancreas (A52.74)
tuberculosis of gallbladder (A18.83)
tuberculosis of pancreas (A18.83)

Other diseases of the digestive system (K90-K95)

4 **K90 Intestinal malabsorption**
EXCLUDES 1 *intestinal malabsorption following gastrointestinal surgery (K91.2)*

CODING TIP ✓ Do not assign a code from K90.- when malabsorption is reported as post-surgical or post-procedural. Post-procedural / post-surgical complications affecting the gastrointestinal system are coded to category K91.-

K90.0 **Celiac disease**
Celiac disease with steatorrhea
Celiac gluten-sensitive enteropathy
Nontropical sprue
Code also:
exocrine pancreatic insufficiency (K86.81)
Use additional code for associated disorders including:
dermatitis herpetiformis (L13.0)
gluten ataxia (G32.81)

DEFINITION Malabsorption syndrome precipitated by ingestion of gluten with loss of villous projections of the intestinal mucosa; manifests with bulky, frothy diarrhea, abdominal distention, flatulence, weight loss, and vitamin and electrolyte depletion.

K90.1 **Tropical sprue**
Sprue NOS
Tropical steatorrhea

DEFINITION A malabsorption syndrome occurring in the tropics and subtropics, marked by inflammation of the mucous tissue of the mouth, diarrhea, and anemia.

K90.2 **Blind loop syndrome, not elsewhere classified**
Blind loop syndrome NOS
EXCLUDES 1 *congenital blind loop syndrome (Q43.8)*
postsurgical blind loop syndrome (K91.2)
K90.3 **Pancreatic steatorrhea**

DEFINITION Insufficient pancreatic enzyme excretions causing severe malabsorption and nutrient deficiencies with loose stools containing unabsorbed fat.

5 K90.4 **Other malabsorption due to intolerance**
EXCLUDES 2 *celiac gluten-sensitive enteropathy (K90.0)*
lactose intolerance (E73.-)
K90.41 **Non-celiac gluten sensitivity**
Gluten sensitivity NOS
Non-celiac gluten sensitive enteropathy

AHA: 4Q 2016, 35

K90.49 Malabsorption due to intolerance, not elsewhere classified
Malabsorption due to intolerance to carbohydrate
Malabsorption due to intolerance to fat
Malabsorption due to intolerance to protein
Malabsorption due to intolerance to starch

5 **K90.8 Other intestinal malabsorption**

K90.81 Whipple's disease

K90.89 Other intestinal malabsorption

K90.9 Intestinal malabsorption, unspecified
AHA: 4Q 2017, 85

4 **K91 Intraoperative and postprocedural complications and disorders of digestive system, not elsewhere classified**

EXCLUDES 2 *complications of artificial opening of digestive system (K94.-)*
complications of bariatric procedures (K95.-)
gastrojejunal ulcer (K28.-)
postprocedural (radiation) retroperitoneal abscess (K68.11)
radiation colitis (K52.0)
radiation gastroenteritis (K52.0)
radiation proctitis (K62.7)

CODING TIP ✓ Documentation: Codes in category K91.- are complication codes and require physician documentation and confirmation of a cause and effect relationship between the procedure and the complicated condition. Documentation must also support this relationship.

K91.0 Vomiting following gastrointestinal surgery

K91.1 Postgastric surgery syndromes
Dumping syndrome
Postgastrectomy syndrome
Postvagotomy syndrome

K91.2 Postsurgical malabsorption, not elsewhere classified
Postsurgical blind loop syndrome
EXCLUDES 1 *malabsorption osteomalacia in adults (M83.2)*
malabsorption osteoporosis, postsurgical (M80.8-, M81.8)

5 **K91.3 Postprocedural intestinal obstruction**

CODING TIP ✓ Intestinal obstruction varies in severity, from partial or intermittent obstruction that usually resolves without intervention to complete obstruction that requires surgery and may lead to intestinal gangrene and perforation. Assign a code from subcategory K91.3- when the documentation indicates the obstruction is a complication following a procedure, based on whether the obstruction is partial, complete or unspecified.
AHA: 1Q 2017, 40

K91.30 Postprocedural intestinal obstruction, unspecified as to partial versus complete
Postprocedural intestinal obstruction NOS
AHA: 4Q 2017, 13

K91.31 Postprocedural partial intestinal obstruction
Postprocedural incomplete intestinal obstruction
AHA: 4Q 2017, 13

K91.32 Postprocedural complete intestinal obstruction
AHA: 4Q 2017, 13

K91.5 Postcholecystectomy syndrome

5 **K91.6 Intraoperative hemorrhage and hematoma of a digestive system organ or structure complicating a procedure**
EXCLUDES 1 *intraoperative hemorrhage and hematoma of a digestive system organ or structure due to accidental puncture and laceration during a procedure (K91.7-)*

K91.61 Intraoperative hemorrhage and hematoma of a digestive system organ or structure complicating a digestive system procedure

K91.62 Intraoperative hemorrhage and hematoma of a digestive system organ or structure complicating other procedure

5 **K91.7 Accidental puncture and laceration of a digestive system organ or structure during a procedure**

K91.71 Accidental puncture and laceration of a digestive system organ or structure during a digestive system procedure

K91.72 Accidental puncture and laceration of a digestive system organ or structure during other procedure

5 **K91.8 Other intraoperative and postprocedural complications and disorders of digestive system**

K91.81 Other intraoperative complications of digestive system

K91.82 Postprocedural hepatic failure

K91.83 Postprocedural hepatorenal syndrome

6 **K91.84 Postprocedural hemorrhage of a digestive system organ or structure following a procedure**

K91.840 Postprocedural hemorrhage of a digestive system organ or structure following a digestive system procedure
AHA: 1Q 2016, 15

K91.841 Postprocedural hemorrhage of a digestive system organ or structure following other procedure

6 **K91.85 Complications of intestinal pouch**

K91.850 Pouchitis HCC
Inflammation of internal ileoanal pouch

K91.858 Other complications of intestinal pouch HCC

K91.86 Retained cholelithiasis following cholecystectomy

6 **K91.87 Postprocedural hematoma and seroma of a digestive system organ or structure following a procedure**

K91.870 Postprocedural hematoma of a digestive system organ or structure following a digestive system procedure

K91.871 Postprocedural hematoma of a digestive system organ or structure following other procedure

K91.872 Postprocedural seroma of a digestive system organ or structure following a digestive system procedure

K91.873 Postprocedural seroma of a digestive system organ or structure following other procedure

K91.89 Other postprocedural complications and disorders of digestive system
Use additional code, if applicable, to further specify disorder
EXCLUDES 2 *postprocedural retroperitoneal abscess (K68.11)*
AHA: 1Q 2017, 40

4 **K92 Other diseases of digestive system**
EXCLUDES 1 *neonatal gastrointestinal hemorrhage (P54.0-P54.3)*

K92.0 Hematemesis

K92.1 Melena
EXCLUDES 1 *occult blood in feces (R19.5)*

K92.2 Gastrointestinal hemorrhage, unspecified
Gastric hemorrhage NOS
Intestinal hemorrhage NOS
EXCLUDES 1 *acute hemorrhagic gastritis (K29.01)*
hemorrhage of anus and rectum (K62.5)
angiodysplasia of stomach with hemorrhage (K31.811)
diverticular disease with hemorrhage (K57.-)
gastritis and duodenitis with hemorrhage (K29.-)
peptic ulcer with hemorrhage (K25-K28)

5 **K92.8 Other specified diseases of the digestive system**

K92.81 Gastrointestinal mucositis (ulcerative)
Code also type of associated therapy, such as:
antineoplastic and immunosuppressive drugs (T45.1X-)
radiological procedure and radiotherapy (Y84.2)
EXCLUDES 2 *mucositis (ulcerative) of vagina and vulva (N76.81)*
nasal mucositis (ulcerative) (J34.81)
oral mucositis (ulcerative) (K12.3-)

K92.89 Other specified diseases of the digestive system

K92.9 Disease of digestive system, unspecified

4 **K94 Complications of artificial openings of the digestive system**

CODING TIP✓ All colostomy, gastrostomy, enterostomy, and esophagostomy complications are coded to category K94.- . This includes excoriation and denuding of the skin surrounding the ostomy, infection of the ostomy site, hemorrhage of the ostomy site, and other complications. No additional code should be used when coding skin complications unless an infection is present, in which case an additional code should be used to specify the infection. When an ostomy complication is present, do not assign a Z code for the ostomy. Z codes indicate routine ostomy care and are not appropriate in the case of a complicated ostomy.

5 K94.0 Colostomy complications

K94.00 Colostomy complication, unspecified HCC

K94.01 Colostomy hemorrhage HCC

K94.02 Colostomy infection HCC

Use additional code to specify type of infection, such as:
cellulitis of abdominal wall (L03.311)
sepsis (A40.-, A41.-)

K94.03 Colostomy malfunction HCC

Mechanical complication of colostomy

K94.09 Other complications of colostomy HCC

5 K94.1 Enterostomy complications

K94.10 Enterostomy complication, unspecified HCC

K94.11 Enterostomy hemorrhage HCC

K94.12 Enterostomy infection HCC

Use additional code to specify type of infection, such as:
cellulitis of abdominal wall (L03.311)
sepsis (A40.-, A41.-)

K94.13 Enterostomy malfunction HCC

Mechanical complication of enterostomy

K94.19 Other complications of enterostomy HCC

5 K94.2 Gastrostomy complications

K94.20 Gastrostomy complication, unspecified HCC

K94.21 Gastrostomy hemorrhage HCC

K94.22 Gastrostomy infection HCC

Use additional code to specify type of infection, such as:
cellulitis of abdominal wall (L03.311)
sepsis (A40.-, A41.-)

K94.23 Gastrostomy malfunction HCC

Mechanical complication of gastrostomy

K94.29 Other complications of gastrostomy HCC

5 K94.3 Esophagostomy complications

K94.30 Esophagostomy complications, unspecified HCC

K94.31 Esophagostomy hemorrhage HCC

K94.32 Esophagostomy infection HCC

Use additional code to identify the infection

K94.33 Esophagostomy malfunction HCC

Mechanical complication of esophagostomy

K94.39 Other complications of esophagostomy HCC

4 K95 Complications of bariatric procedures

CODING TIP✓ Infection due to gastric band or other bariatric procedure with a POA indicator of "N" or "U" will be flagged as a hospital-acquired condition (HAC) under the Medicare program when identified during inpatient admission for bariatric surgery performed for morbid obesity (E66.01).

CODING TIP✓ **Documentation:** Codes in category K95.- are complication codes and require physician documentation and confirmation of a cause and effect relationship between the procedure and the complicated condition. Documentation must also support this relationship. Codes from K95 should be used instead of Z98.84, bariatric surgery status, if a complication exists as a direct result of the surgery.

5 K95.0 Complications of gastric band procedure

K95.01 Infection due to gastric band procedure

Use additional code to specify type of infection or organism, such as:
bacterial and viral infectious agents (B95.-, B96.-)
cellulitis of abdominal wall (L03.311)
sepsis (A40.-, A41.-)

K95.09 Other complications of gastric band procedure

Use additional code, if applicable, to further specify complication

5 K95.8 Complications of other bariatric procedure

EXCLUDES 1 *complications of gastric band surgery (K95.0-)*

K95.81 Infection due to other bariatric procedure

Use additional code to specify type of infection or organism, such as:
bacterial and viral infectious agents (B95.-, B96.-)
cellulitis of abdominal wall (L03.311)
sepsis (A40.-, A41.-)

K95.89 Other complications of Other bariatric procedure

Use additional code, if applicable, to further specify complication

CHAPTER 12: DISEASES OF THE SKIN AND SUBCUTANEOUS TISSUE (L00 -L99)

EXCLUDES 2 *certain conditions originating in the perinatal period (P04-P96)*
certain infectious and parasitic diseases (A00-B99)
complications of pregnancy, childbirth and the puerperium (O00-O9A)
congenital malformations, deformations, and chromosomal abnormalities (Q00-Q99)
endocrine, nutritional and metabolic diseases (E00-E88)
lipomelanotic reticulosis (I89.8)
neoplasms (C00-D49)
symptoms, signs and abnormal clinical and laboratory findings, not elsewhere classified (R00-R94)
systemic connective tissue disorders (M30-M36)
viral warts (B07.-)

This chapter contains the following blocks:

L00-L08	Infections of the skin and subcutaneous tissue
L10-L14	Bullous disorders
L20-L30	Dermatitis and eczema
L40-L45	Papulosquamous disorders
L49-L54	Urticaria and erythema
L55-L59	Radiation-related disorders of the skin and subcutaneous tissue
L60-L75	Disorders of skin appendages
L76	Intraoperative and postprocedural complications of skin and subcutaneous tissue
L80-L99	Other disorders of the skin and subcutaneous tissue

Infections of the skin and subcutaneous tissue (L00-L08)

Use additional code (B95-B97) to identify infectious agent.

EXCLUDES 2 *hordeolum (H00.0)*
infective dermatitis (L30.3)
local infections of skin classified in Chapter 1
lupus panniculitis (L93.2)
panniculitis NOS (M79.3)
panniculitis of neck and back (M54.0-)
Perlèche NOS (K13.0)
Perlèche due to candidiasis (B37.0)
Perlèche due to riboflavin deficiency (E53.0)
pyogenic granuloma (L98.0)
relapsing panniculitis [Weber-Christian] (M35.6)
viral warts (B07.-)
zoster (B02.-)

L00 Staphylococcal scalded skin syndrome
Ritter's disease
Use additional code to identify percentage of skin exfoliation (L49.-)

EXCLUDES 1 *bullous impetigo (L01.03)*
pemphigus neonatorum (L01.03)
toxic epidermal necrolysis [Lyell] (L51.2)

DEFINITION The breakdown of dermal layer cellular structure by staph bacteria causing large sections of skin to slough off and peel away, leaving raw, exposed areas.

4 **L01 Impetigo**

EXCLUDES 1 *impetigo herpetiformis (L40.1)*

5 **L01.0 Impetigo**
Impetigo contagiosa
Impetigo vulgaris

DEFINITION Bacterial skin infection in children; small pustules form over a reddish rash and burst, leaving an itchy, yellow crust over the affected area.

L01.00 Impetigo, unspecified
Impetigo NOS

L01.01 Non-bullous impetigo

DEFINITION Most common type of impetigo due to staph or strep bacteria, in which tiny blisters form (particularly on the face), burst quickly, and leave a small, wet, weeping spot that crusts over and disappears, leaving a red mark that later heals.

L01.02 Bockhart's impetigo
Impetigo follicularis
Perifolliculitis NOS
Superficial pustular perifolliculitis

DEFINITION Superficial, pustular folliculitis caused by *S. aureus*; characterized by small, painful, tense, yellowish-white domed pustules in crops around follicular orifices that heal in a few days.

L01.03 Bullous impetigo
Impetigo neonatorum
Pemphigus neonatorum

DEFINITION Impetigo of longer duration (generally due to *S. aureus*), in which large, clear, fluid-filled blisters form on red sores, become cloudy, then burst and ooze, leaving a large, yellowish, crusty scab.

L01.09 Other impetigo
Ulcerative impetigo

DEFINITION Ulcerative impetigo: A deeper dermis form of impetigo with small, shallow, purulent ulcers that form under a thick, brownish-black crusted surface infection, surrounded by erythema.

L01.1 Impetiginization of other dermatoses

DEFINITION Impetigo occurring in an area already experiencing a dermatosis; the infected blisters burst, leaving a weeping wet patch that crusts over, worsening the existing condition.

4 **L02 Cutaneous abscess, furuncle and carbuncle**
Use additional code to identify organism (B95-B96)

EXCLUDES 2 *abscess of anus and rectal regions (K61.-)*
abscess of female genital organs (external) (N76.4)
abscess of male genital organs (external) (N48.2, N49.-)

CODING TIP ✓ Abscesses, carbuncles and furuncles are coded separately from cellulitis (L03). Furuncles are commonly known as boils. Use an additional code to identify the causative organism.

DEFINITION Abscess: A pocket of pus that collects within an infected area of skin and is generally red and sore.

DEFINITION Carbuncle: A group of several infected hair follicles, or furuncles, that join together with more than one opening to drain pus, often extending into deeper tissue.

DEFINITION Furuncle: A bacterial infection of a hair follicle characterized by a painful, red, swollen bump filled with fluid, pus, and cellular debris; also called a boil.

5 **L02.0 Cutaneous abscess, furuncle and carbuncle of face**

EXCLUDES 2 *abscess of ear, external (H60.0)*
abscess of eyelid (H00.0)
abscess of head [any part, except face] (L02.8)
abscess of lacrimal gland (H04.0)
abscess of lacrimal passages (H04.3)
abscess of mouth (K12.2)
abscess of nose (J34.0)
abscess of orbit (H05.0)
submandibular abscess (K12.2)

L02.01 Cutaneous abscess of face

L02.02 Furuncle of face
Boil of face
Folliculitis of face

L02.03 Carbuncle of face

5 **L02.1 Cutaneous abscess, furuncle and carbuncle of neck**

L02.11 Cutaneous abscess of neck

L02.12 Furuncle of neck
Boil of neck
Folliculitis of neck

L02.13 Carbuncle of neck

5 **L02.2 Cutaneous abscess, furuncle and carbuncle of trunk**
EXCLUDES 1 *non-newborn omphalitis (L08.82)*
omphalitis of newborn (P38.-)
EXCLUDES 2 *abscess of breast (N61.1)*
abscess of buttocks (L02.3)
abscess of female external genital organs (N76.4)
abscess of male external genital organs (N48.2, N49.-)
abscess of hip (L02.4)

6 **L02.21 Cutaneous abscess of trunk**
L02.211 Cutaneous abscess of abdominal wall
L02.212 Cutaneous abscess of back [any part, except buttock]
L02.213 Cutaneous abscess of chest wall
L02.214 Cutaneous abscess of groin
L02.215 Cutaneous abscess of perineum
L02.216 Cutaneous abscess of umbilicus
L02.219 Cutaneous abscess of trunk, unspecified

6 **L02.22 Furuncle of trunk**
Boil of trunk
Folliculitis of trunk
L02.221 Furuncle of abdominal wall
L02.222 Furuncle of back [any part, except buttock]
L02.223 Furuncle of chest wall
L02.224 Furuncle of groin
L02.225 Furuncle of perineum
L02.226 Furuncle of umbilicus
L02.229 Furuncle of trunk, unspecified

6 **L02.23 Carbuncle of trunk**
L02.231 Carbuncle of abdominal wall
L02.232 Carbuncle of back [any part, except buttock]
L02.233 Carbuncle of chest wall
L02.234 Carbuncle of groin
L02.235 Carbuncle of perineum
L02.236 Carbuncle of umbilicus
L02.239 Carbuncle of trunk, unspecified

5 **L02.3 Cutaneous abscess, furuncle and carbuncle of buttock**
EXCLUDES 1 *pilonidal cyst with abscess (L05.01)*

L02.31 Cutaneous abscess of buttock
Cutaneous abscess of gluteal region
L02.32 Furuncle of buttock
Boil of buttock
Folliculitis of buttock
Furuncle of gluteal region
L02.33 Carbuncle of buttock
Carbuncle of gluteal region

5 **L02.4 Cutaneous abscess, furuncle and carbuncle of limb**
EXCLUDES 2 *Cutaneous abscess, furuncle and carbuncle of groin (L02.214, L02.224, L02.234)*
Cutaneous abscess, furuncle and carbuncle of hand (L02.5-)
Cutaneous abscess, furuncle and carbuncle of foot (L02.6-)

6 **L02.41 Cutaneous abscess of limb**
⊟ **L02.411 Cutaneous abscess of right axilla**
⊟ **L02.412 Cutaneous abscess of left axilla**
⊟ **L02.413 Cutaneous abscess of right upper limb**
⊟ **L02.414 Cutaneous abscess of left upper limb**
⊟ **L02.415 Cutaneous abscess of right lower limb**
⊟ **L02.416 Cutaneous abscess of left lower limb**
⊟ **L02.419 Cutaneous abscess of limb, unspecified**

6 **L02.42 Furuncle of limb**
Boil of limb
Folliculitis of limb
⊟ **L02.421 Furuncle of right axilla**
⊟ **L02.422 Furuncle of left axilla**
⊟ **L02.423 Furuncle of right upper limb**
⊟ **L02.424 Furuncle of left upper limb**
⊟ **L02.425 Furuncle of right lower limb**
⊟ **L02.426 Furuncle of left lower limb**
⊟ **L02.429 Furuncle of limb, unspecified**

6 **L02.43 Carbuncle of limb**
⊟ **L02.431 Carbuncle of right axilla**
⊟ **L02.432 Carbuncle of left axilla**
⊟ **L02.433 Carbuncle of right upper limb**
⊟ **L02.434 Carbuncle of left upper limb**
⊟ **L02.435 Carbuncle of right lower limb**
⊟ **L02.436 Carbuncle of left lower limb**
⊟ **L02.439 Carbuncle of limb, unspecified**

5 **L02.5 Cutaneous abscess, furuncle and carbuncle of hand**
6 **L02.51 Cutaneous abscess of hand**
⊟ **L02.511 Cutaneous abscess of right hand**
⊟ **L02.512 Cutaneous abscess of left hand**
⊟ **L02.519 Cutaneous abscess of unspecified hand**

6 **L02.52 Furuncle hand**
Boil of hand
Folliculitis of hand
⊟ **L02.521 Furuncle right hand**
⊟ **L02.522 Furuncle left hand**
⊟ **L02.529 Furuncle unspecified hand**

6 **L02.53 Carbuncle of hand**
⊟ **L02.531 Carbuncle of right hand**
⊟ **L02.532 Carbuncle of left hand**
⊟ **L02.539 Carbuncle of unspecified hand**

5 **L02.6 Cutaneous abscess, furuncle and carbuncle of foot**
6 **L02.61 Cutaneous abscess of foot**
⊟ **L02.611 Cutaneous abscess of right foot**
⊟ **L02.612 Cutaneous abscess of left foot**
⊟ **L02.619 Cutaneous abscess of unspecified foot**

6 **L02.62 Furuncle of foot**
Boil of foot
Folliculitis of foot
⊟ **L02.621 Furuncle of right foot**
⊟ **L02.622 Furuncle of left foot**
⊟ **L02.629 Furuncle of unspecified foot**

6 **L02.63 Carbuncle of foot**
⊟ **L02.631 Carbuncle of right foot**
⊟ **L02.632 Carbuncle of left foot**
⊟ **L02.639 Carbuncle of unspecified foot**

5 **L02.8 Cutaneous abscess, furuncle and carbuncle of other sites**
6 **L02.81 Cutaneous abscess of other sites**
L02.811 Cutaneous abscess of head [any part, except face]
L02.818 Cutaneous abscess of other sites

6 **L02.82 Furuncle of other sites**
Boil of other sites
Folliculitis of other sites
L02.821 Furuncle of head [any part, except face]
L02.828 Furuncle of other sites

6 **L02.83 Carbuncle of other sites**
L02.831 Carbuncle of head [any part, except face]
L02.838 Carbuncle of other sites

5 **L02.9 Cutaneous abscess, furuncle and carbuncle, unspecified**
L02.91 Cutaneous abscess, unspecified
L02.92 Furuncle, unspecified
Boil NOS
Furunculosis NOS
L02.93 Carbuncle, unspecified

L03 Cellulitis and acute lymphangitis

EXCLUDES 2 *cellulitis of anal and rectal region (K61.-)*
cellulitis of external auditory canal (H60.1)
cellulitis of eyelid (H00.0)
cellulitis of female external genital organs (N76.4)
cellulitis of lacrimal apparatus (H04.3)
cellulitis of male external genital organs (N48.2, N49.-)
cellulitis of mouth (K12.2)
cellulitis of nose (J34.0)
eosinophilic cellulitis [Wells] (L98.3)
febrile neutrophilic dermatosis [Sweet] (L98.2)
lymphangitis (chronic) (subacute) (I89.1)

CODING TIP ✓ L03 includes codes for cellulitis. When diagnostic statements indicate abscess, a code from L02 should be coded.

CODING TIP ✓ Cellulitis usually presents as an abrupt onset of redness, swelling, pain, or heat in the affected area. Unless a diagnosis of cellulitis is documented by the physician, a code from category L03 should not be assigned. If cellulitis is associated with a wound or ostomy, code the wound or complicated ostomy first, followed by the appropriate L03 code for cellulitis.

DEFINITION Acute lymphangitis: A quickly spreading bacterial infection of the lymph vessels appearing as painful, red streaks visible through the skin surface.

DEFINITION Cellulitis: A spreading bacterial infection of connective soft tissue extending into deep dermal and subcutaneous layers; produces circumscribed swelling, fever, and swollen lymph nodes.

L03.0 Cellulitis and acute lymphangitis of finger and toe
Infection of nail
Onychia
Paronychia
Perionychia

L03.01 Cellulitis of finger
Felon
Whitlow
EXCLUDES 1 *herpetic whitlow (B00.89)*

L03.011 Cellulitis of right finger
L03.012 Cellulitis of left finger
L03.019 Cellulitis of unspecified finger

L03.02 Acute lymphangitis of finger
Hangnail with lymphangitis of finger

L03.021 Acute lymphangitis of right finger
L03.022 Acute lymphangitis of left finger
L03.029 Acute lymphangitis of unspecified finger

L03.03 Cellulitis of toe

L03.031 Cellulitis of right toe
L03.032 Cellulitis of left toe
L03.039 Cellulitis of unspecified toe

L03.04 Acute lymphangitis of toe
Hangnail with lymphangitis of toe

L03.041 Acute lymphangitis of right toe
L03.042 Acute lymphangitis of left toe
L03.049 Acute lymphangitis of unspecified toe

L03.1 Cellulitis and acute lymphangitis of other parts of limb

L03.11 Cellulitis of other parts of limb
EXCLUDES 2 *cellulitis of fingers (L03.01-)*
cellulitis of toes (L03.03-)
groin (L03.314)

L03.111 Cellulitis of right axilla
L03.112 Cellulitis of left axilla
L03.113 Cellulitis of right upper limb
L03.114 Cellulitis of left upper limb
L03.115 Cellulitis of right lower limb
L03.116 Cellulitis of left lower limb
L03.119 Cellulitis of unspecified part of limb

L03.12 Acute lymphangitis of other parts of limb
EXCLUDES 2 *acute lymphangitis of fingers (L03.2-)*
acute lymphangitis of toes (L03.04-)
acute lymphangitis of groin (L03.324)

L03.121 Acute lymphangitis of right axilla
L03.122 Acute lymphangitis of left axilla
L03.123 Acute lymphangitis of right upper limb
L03.124 Acute lymphangitis of left upper limb
L03.125 Acute lymphangitis of right lower limb
L03.126 Acute lymphangitis of left lower limb
L03.129 Acute lymphangitis of unspecified part of limb

L03.2 Cellulitis and acute lymphangitis of face and neck

L03.21 Cellulitis and acute lymphangitis of face

L03.211 Cellulitis of face
EXCLUDES 2 *abscess of orbit (H05.01-)*
cellulitis of ear (H60.1-)
cellulitis of eyelid (H00.0-)
cellulitis of head (L03.81)
cellulitis of lacrimal apparatus (H04.3)
cellulitis of lip (K13.0)
cellulitis of mouth (K12.2)
cellulitis of nose (internal) (J34.0)
cellulitis of orbit (H05.01-)
cellulitis of scalp (L03.81)

L03.212 Acute lymphangitis of face
L03.213 Periorbital cellulitis
Preseptal cellulitis
AHA: 4Q 2016, 36

L03.22 Cellulitis and acute lymphangitis of neck

L03.221 Cellulitis of neck
L03.222 Acute lymphangitis of neck

L03.3 Cellulitis and acute lymphangitis of trunk

L03.31 Cellulitis of trunk
EXCLUDES 2 *cellulitis of anal and rectal regions (K61.-)*
cellulitis of breast NOS (N61.0)
cellulitis of female external genital organs (N76.4)
cellulitis of male external genital organs (N48.2, N49.-)
omphalitis of newborn (P38.-)
puerperal cellulitis of breast (O91.2)

L03.311 Cellulitis of abdominal wall
EXCLUDES 2 *cellulitis of umbilicus (L03.316)*
cellulitis of groin (L03.314)

L03.312 Cellulitis of back [any part except buttock]
L03.313 Cellulitis of chest wall
L03.314 Cellulitis of groin
L03.315 Cellulitis of perineum
L03.316 Cellulitis of umbilicus
L03.317 Cellulitis of buttock
L03.319 Cellulitis of trunk, unspecified

L03.32 Acute lymphangitis of trunk

L03.321 Acute lymphangitis of abdominal wall
L03.322 Acute lymphangitis of back [any part except buttock]
L03.323 Acute lymphangitis of chest wall
L03.324 Acute lymphangitis of groin
L03.325 Acute lymphangitis of perineum
L03.326 Acute lymphangitis of umbilicus
L03.327 Acute lymphangitis of buttock
L03.329 Acute lymphangitis of trunk, unspecified

L03.8 Cellulitis and acute lymphangitis of other sites

L03.81 Cellulitis of other sites

L03.811 Cellulitis of head [any part, except face]
Cellulitis of scalp
EXCLUDES 2 *cellulitis of face (L03.211)*

L03.818 Cellulitis of other sites

L03.89 Acute lymphangitis of other sites

L03.891 Acute lymphangitis of head [any part, except face]
L03.898 Acute lymphangitis of other sites

L03.9 Cellulitis and acute lymphangitis, unspecified

L03.90 Cellulitis, unspecified

L03.91 **Acute lymphangitis, unspecified**
EXCLUDES 1 *lymphangitis NOS (I89.1)*

L04 **Acute lymphadenitis**
INCLUDES abscess (acute) of lymph nodes, except mesenteric
acute lymphadenitis, except mesenteric
EXCLUDES 1 *chronic or subacute lymphadenitis, except mesenteric (I88.1)*
enlarged lymph nodes (R59.-)
human immunodeficiency virus [HIV] disease resulting in generalized lymphadenopathy (B20)
lymphadenitis NOS (I88.9)
nonspecific mesenteric lymphadenitis (I88.0)

L04.0 **Acute lymphadenitis of face, head and neck**
L04.1 **Acute lymphadenitis of trunk**

Acute lymphadenitis of trunk

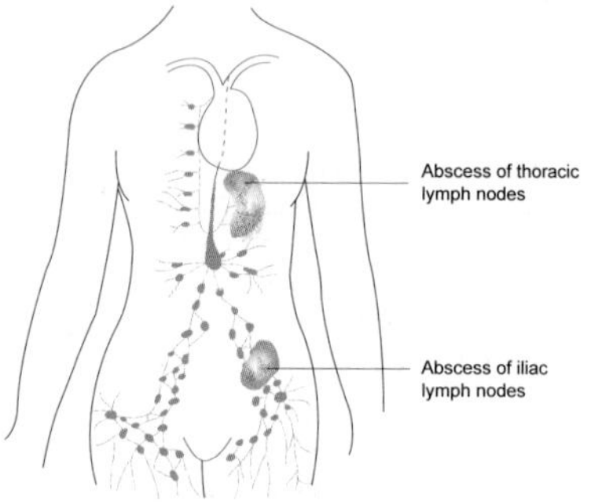

L04.2 **Acute lymphadenitis of upper limb**
Acute lymphadenitis of axilla
Acute lymphadenitis of shoulder
L04.3 **Acute lymphadenitis of lower limb**
Acute lymphadenitis of hip
EXCLUDES 2 *acute lymphadenitis of groin (L04.1)*
L04.8 **Acute lymphadenitis of other sites**
L04.9 **Acute lymphadenitis, unspecified**

L05 **Pilonidal cyst and sinus**
L05.0 **Pilonidal cyst and sinus with abscess**
DEFINITION An abscessed sinus tract draining to the surface and located in the tailbone area, often associated with ingrown hairs.
L05.01 **Pilonidal cyst with abscess**
Pilonidal abscess
Pilonidal dimple with abscess
Postanal dimple with abscess
EXCLUDES 2 *congenital sacral dimple (Q82.6)*
parasacral dimple (Q82.6)
L05.02 **Pilonidal sinus with abscess**
Coccygeal fistula with abscess
Coccygeal sinus with abscess
Pilonidal fistula with abscess
L05.9 **Pilonidal cyst and sinus without abscess**
L05.91 **Pilonidal cyst without abscess**
Pilonidal dimple
Postanal dimple
Pilonidal cyst NOS
EXCLUDES 2 *congenital sacral dimple (Q82.6)*
parasacral dimple (Q82.6)
L05.92 **Pilonidal sinus without abscess**
Coccygeal fistula
Coccygeal sinus without abscess
Pilonidal fistula

L08 **Other local infections of skin and subcutaneous tissue**
L08.0 **Pyoderma**
Dermatitis gangrenosa
Purulent dermatitis
Septic dermatitis
Suppurative dermatitis
EXCLUDES 1 *pyoderma gangrenosum (L88)*
pyoderma vegetans (L08.81)
DEFINITION A skin condition producing pus.
L08.1 **Erythrasma** HIV
DEFINITION Skin infection caused by Corynebacterium minutissimum in which pink-red patches with fine scales and wrinkling appear in perpetually moist skin folds (intergluteal fold, inframammary fold, armpits, groin) and later turn brown and scaly.
L08.8 **Other specified local infections of the skin and subcutaneous tissue**
L08.81 **Pyoderma vegetans**
EXCLUDES 1 *pyoderma gangrenosum (L88)*
pyoderma NOS (L08.0)
L08.82 **Omphalitis not of newborn**
EXCLUDES 1 *omphalitis of newborn (P38.-)*
L08.89 **Other specified local infections of the skin and subcutaneous tissue**
L08.9 **Local infection of the skin and subcutaneous tissue, unspecified**

Bullous disorders (L10-L14)

EXCLUDES 1 *benign familial pemphigus [Hailey-Hailey] (Q82.8)*
staphylococcal scalded skin syndrome (L00)
toxic epidermal necrolysis [Lyell] (L51.2)

L10 **Pemphigus**
EXCLUDES 1 *pemphigus neonatorum (L01.03)*
L10.0 **Pemphigus vulgaris**
L10.1 **Pemphigus vegetans**
L10.2 **Pemphigus foliaceous**
L10.3 **Brazilian pemphigus [fogo selvagem]**
L10.4 **Pemphigus erythematosus**
Senear-Usher syndrome
L10.5 **Drug-induced pemphigus**
Use additional code for adverse effect, if applicable, to identify drug (T36-T50 with fifth or sixth character 5)
CODING TIP✓ Code L10.5 should only be assigned when documentation clearly indicates a relationship between pemphigus and a drug or chemical as the underlying cause. Assign a code from T36-T50 following L10.5 to indicate the drug and adverse effect.
L10.8 **Other pemphigus**
L10.81 **Paraneoplastic pemphigus**
L10.89 **Other pemphigus**
L10.9 **Pemphigus, unspecified**

L11 **Other acantholytic disorders**
L11.0 **Acquired keratosis follicularis**
EXCLUDES 1 *keratosis follicularis (congenital) [Darier-White] (Q82.8)*
L11.1 **Transient acantholytic dermatosis [Grover]**
L11.8 **Other specified acantholytic disorders**
L11.9 **Acantholytic disorder, unspecified**

L12 **Pemphigoid**
EXCLUDES 1 *herpes gestationis (O26.4-)*
impetigo herpetiformis (L40.1)
L12.0 **Bullous pemphigoid**
L12.1 **Cicatricial pemphigoid**
Benign mucous membrane pemphigoid
L12.2 **Chronic bullous disease of childhood** P
Juvenile dermatitis herpetiformis
L12.3 **Acquired epidermolysis bullosa**
EXCLUDES 1 *epidermolysis bullosa (congenital) (Q81.-)*
L12.30 **Acquired epidermolysis bullosa, unspecified** HCC
L12.31 **Epidermolysis bullosa due to drug** HCC
Use additional code for adverse effect, if applicable, to identify drug (T36-T50 with fifth or sixth character 5)
L12.35 **Other acquired epidermolysis bullosa** HCC
L12.8 **Other pemphigoid**
L12.9 **Pemphigoid, unspecified**

L13 **Other bullous disorders**

L13.0 Dermatitis herpetiformis
Duhring's disease
Hydroa herpetiformis
EXCLUDES 1 *juvenile dermatitis herpetiformis (L12.2)*
senile dermatitis herpetiformis (L12.0)
DEFINITION Chronic skin disease that can persist indefinitely, characterized by intensely itchy, symmetrical excoriations on the elbows, knees, lower back, buttocks, and shoulders, often accompanied by burning and stinging hours before an eruption.

L13.1 Subcorneal pustular dermatitis
Sneddon-Wilkinson disease

L13.8 Other specified bullous disorders

L13.9 Bullous disorder, unspecified

L14 *Bullous disorders in diseases classified elsewhere*
Code first:
underlying disease

Dermatitis and eczema (L20-L30)

Note: In this block the terms dermatitis and eczema are used synonymously and interchangeably.
EXCLUDES 2 *chronic (childhood) granulomatous disease (D71)*
dermatitis gangrenosa (L08.0)
dermatitis herpetiformis (L13.0)
dry skin dermatitis (L85.3)
factitial dermatitis (L98.1)
perioral dermatitis (L71.0)
radiation-related disorders of the skin and subcutaneous tissue (L55-L59)
stasis dermatitis (I87.2)

4 **L20 Atopic dermatitis**

L20.0 Besnier's prurigo

5 **L20.8 Other atopic dermatitis**
EXCLUDES 2 *circumscribed neurodermatitis (L28.0)*

L20.81 Atopic neurodermatitis
Diffuse neurodermatitis

L20.82 Flexural eczema

L20.83 Infantile (acute) (chronic) eczema P

L20.84 Intrinsic (allergic) eczema

L20.89 Other atopic dermatitis

L20.9 Atopic dermatitis, unspecified

4 **L21 Seborrheic dermatitis**
EXCLUDES 2 *infective dermatitis (L30.3)*
seborrheic keratosis (L82.-)

L21.0 Seborrhea capitis
Cradle cap
DEFINITION Inflammatory skin rash on the scalp of infants, characterized by flaky or scaly skin with redness.
AHA: 1Q 2018, 5

L21.1 Seborrheic infantile dermatitis P

L21.8 Other seborrheic dermatitis

L21.9 Seborrheic dermatitis, unspecified
Seborrhea NOS
DEFINITION Overactivity of the sebaceous (fat) glands, resulting in an inflammatory skin rash.

L22 Diaper dermatitis
Diaper erythema
Diaper rash
Psoriasiform diaper rash

4 **L23 Allergic contact dermatitis**
EXCLUDES 1 *allergy NOS (T78.40)*
contact dermatitis NOS (L25.9)
dermatitis NOS (L30.9)
EXCLUDES 2 *dermatitis due to substances taken internally (L27.-)*
dermatitis of eyelid (H01.1-)
diaper dermatitis (L22)
eczema of external ear (H60.5-)
irritant contact dermatitis (L24.-)
perioral dermatitis (L71.0)
radiation-related disorders of the skin and subcutaneous tissue (L55-L59)

CODING TIP✓ Do not assign a code from L23 to report a skin reaction or allergy due to drugs or other medications that are ingested (internally). A code from category L27 should be assigned to indicate a skin reaction or allergy due to drugs or other medications ingested internally (with an additional code from T36-T50 assigned to indicate the adverse effect and specific drug).

CODING TIP✓ Contact dermatitis indicates that the inflammation of the skin is related to contact with a substance. The specific causative substance that resulted in the condition should be documented and the plan of care should include appropriate interventions for skin care and instruction on prevention of contact with irritants. If the patient had contact with substances and had a non-allergic type reaction, see L24.

DEFINITION Inflammation of the skin upon contact with an allergen, due to hypersensitization.

L23.0 Allergic contact dermatitis due to metals
Allergic contact dermatitis due to chromium
Allergic contact dermatitis due to nickel

L23.1 Allergic contact dermatitis due to adhesives

L23.2 Allergic contact dermatitis due to cosmetics

L23.3 Allergic contact dermatitis due to drugs in contact with skin
Use additional code for adverse effect, if applicable, to identify drug (T36-T50 with fifth or sixth character 5)
EXCLUDES 2 *dermatitis due to ingested drugs and medicaments (L27.0-L27.1)*

L23.4 Allergic contact dermatitis due to dyes

L23.5 Allergic contact dermatitis due to other chemical products
Allergic contact dermatitis due to cement
Allergic contact dermatitis due to insecticide
Allergic contact dermatitis due to plastic
Allergic contact dermatitis due to rubber

L23.6 Allergic contact dermatitis due to food in contact with the skin
EXCLUDES 2 *dermatitis due to ingested food (L27.2)*

L23.7 Allergic contact dermatitis due to plants, except food
EXCLUDES 2 *allergy NOS due to pollen (J30.1)*

5 **L23.8 Allergic contact dermatitis due to other agents**

L23.81 Allergic contact dermatitis due to animal (cat) (dog) dander
Allergic contact dermatitis due to animal (cat) (dog) hair

L23.89 Allergic contact dermatitis due to other agents

L23.9 Allergic contact dermatitis, unspecified cause
Allergic contact eczema NOS

4 **L24 Irritant contact dermatitis**
EXCLUDES 1 *allergy NOS (T78.40)*
contact dermatitis NOS (L25.9)
dermatitis NOS (L30.9)
EXCLUDES 2 *allergic contact dermatitis (L23.-)*
dermatitis due to substances taken internally (L27.-)
dermatitis of eyelid (H01.1-)
diaper dermatitis (L22)
eczema of external ear (H60.5-)
perioral dermatitis (L71.0)
radiation-related disorders of the skin and subcutaneous tissue (L55-L59)

CODING TIP✓ Contact dermatitis indicates that the inflammation of the skin is related to contact with a substance. The specific causative substance that resulted in the condition should be documented, and the plan of care should include appropriate interventions for skin care and instruction on prevention of contact with irritants.

L24.0 Irritant contact dermatitis due to detergents

L24.1 Irritant contact dermatitis due to oils and greases

L24.2 Irritant contact dermatitis due to solvents
Irritant contact dermatitis due to chlorocompound
Irritant contact dermatitis due to cyclohexane
Irritant contact dermatitis due to ester
Irritant contact dermatitis due to glycol
Irritant contact dermatitis due to hydrocarbon
Irritant contact dermatitis due to ketone

L24.3 Irritant contact dermatitis due to cosmetics

L24.4 **Irritant contact dermatitis due to drugs in contact with skin**
Use additional code for adverse effect, if applicable, to identify drug (T36-T50 with fifth or sixth character 5)

L24.5 **Irritant contact dermatitis due to other chemical products**
Irritant contact dermatitis due to cement
Irritant contact dermatitis due to insecticide
Irritant contact dermatitis due to plastic
Irritant contact dermatitis due to rubber

L24.6 **Irritant contact dermatitis due to food in contact with skin**
EXCLUDES 2 *dermatitis due to ingested food (L27.2)*

L24.7 **Irritant contact dermatitis due to plants, except food**
EXCLUDES 2 *allergy NOS to pollen (J30.1)*

5 L24.8 **Irritant contact dermatitis due to other agents**

L24.81 **Irritant contact dermatitis due to metals**
Irritant contact dermatitis due to chromium
Irritant contact dermatitis due to nickel

L24.89 **Irritant contact dermatitis due to other agents**
Irritant contact dermatitis due to dyes

L24.9 **Irritant contact dermatitis, unspecified cause**
Irritant contact eczema NOS

4 L25 **Unspecified contact dermatitis**
EXCLUDES 1 *allergic contact dermatitis (L23.-)*
allergy NOS (T78.40)
dermatitis NOS (L30.9)
irritant contact dermatitis (L24.-)
EXCLUDES 2 *dermatitis due to ingested substances (L27.-)*
dermatitis of eyelid (H01.1-)
eczema of external ear (H60.5-)
perioral dermatitis (L71.0)
radiation-related disorders of the skin and subcutaneous tissue (L55-L59)

CODING TIP ✓ Contact dermatitis indicates that the inflammation of the skin is related to contact with a substance. The specific causative substance that resulted in the condition should be documented, and the plan of care should include appropriate interventions for skin care and instruction on prevention of contact with irritants.

L25.0 **Unspecified contact dermatitis due to cosmetics**

L25.1 **Unspecified contact dermatitis due to drugs in contact with skin**
Use additional code for adverse effect, if applicable, to identify drug (T36-T50 with fifth or sixth character 5)
EXCLUDES 2 *dermatitis due to ingested drugs and medicaments (L27.0-L27.1)*

L25.2 **Unspecified contact dermatitis due to dyes**

L25.3 **Unspecified contact dermatitis due to other chemical products**
Unspecified contact dermatitis due to cement
Unspecified contact dermatitis due to insecticide

L25.4 **Unspecified contact dermatitis due to food in contact with skin**
EXCLUDES 2 *dermatitis due to ingested food (L27.2)*

L25.5 **Unspecified contact dermatitis due to plants, except food**
EXCLUDES 1 *nettle rash (L50.9)*
EXCLUDES 2 *allergy NOS due to pollen (J30.1)*

L25.8 **Unspecified contact dermatitis due to other agents**

L25.9 **Unspecified contact dermatitis, unspecified cause**
Contact dermatitis (occupational) NOS
Contact eczema (occupational) NOS

L26 **Exfoliative dermatitis**
Hebra's pityriasis
EXCLUDES 1 *Ritter's disease (L00)*

4 L27 **Dermatitis due to substances taken internally**
EXCLUDES 1 *allergy NOS (T78.40)*
EXCLUDES 2 *adverse food reaction, except dermatitis (T78.0-T78.1)*
contact dermatitis (L23-L25)
drug photoallergic response (L56.1)
drug phototoxic response (L56.0)
urticaria (L50.-)

L27.0 **Generalized skin eruption due to drugs and medicaments taken internally**
Use additional code for adverse effect, if applicable, to identify drug (T36-T50 with fifth or sixth character 5)

L27.1 **Localized skin eruption due to drugs and medicaments taken internally**
Use additional code for adverse effect, if applicable, to identify drug (T36-T50 with fifth or sixth character 5)

L27.2 **Dermatitis due to ingested food**
EXCLUDES 2 *dermatitis due to food in contact with skin (L23.6, L24.6, L25.4)*

L27.8 **Dermatitis due to other substances taken internally**

L27.9 **Dermatitis due to unspecified substance taken internally**

4 L28 **Lichen simplex chronicus and prurigo**

L28.0 **Lichen simplex chronicus**
Circumscribed neurodermatitis
Lichen NOS

L28.1 **Prurigo nodularis**

L28.2 **Other prurigo**
Prurigo NOS
Prurigo Hebra
Prurigo mitis
Urticaria papulosa

DEFINITION Chronic inflammatory skin disease featuring blistering papules and severe itching.

4 L29 **Pruritus**
EXCLUDES 1 *neurotic excoriation (L98.1)*
psychogenic pruritus (F45.8)

CODING TIP ✓ Do not confuse pruritis with urticaria. Pruritis refers to "itch" or "itching" while urticaria refers to hives. Urticaria should be coded to L50.

L29.0 **Pruritus ani**

DEFINITION Severe itching of the perianal region.

L29.1 **Pruritus scroti** ♂

L29.2 **Pruritus vulvae** ♀

L29.3 **Anogenital pruritus, unspecified**

L29.8 **Other pruritus**

L29.9 **Pruritus, unspecified**
Itch NOS

4 L30 **Other and unspecified dermatitis**
EXCLUDES 2 *contact dermatitis (L23-L25)*
dry skin dermatitis (L85.3)
small plaque parapsoriasis (L41.3)
stasis dermatitis (I87.2)

L30.0 **Nummular dermatitis**

L30.1 **Dyshidrosis [pompholyx]**

L30.2 **Cutaneous autosensitization**
Candidid [levurid]
Dermatophytid
Eczematid

L30.3 **Infective dermatitis**
Infectious eczematoid dermatitis

L30.4 **Erythema intertrigo**

L30.5 **Pityriasis alba**

L30.8 **Other specified dermatitis**

L30.9 **Dermatitis, unspecified**
Eczema NOS

Papulosquamous disorders (L40-L45)

4 L40 **Psoriasis**

L40.0 **Psoriasis vulgaris**
Nummular psoriasis
Plaque psoriasis

L40.1 **Generalized pustular psoriasis**
Impetigo herpetiformis
Von Zumbusch's disease

L40.2 **Acrodermatitis continua**

L40.3 **Pustulosis palmaris et plantaris**

L40.4 **Guttate psoriasis**

5 L40.5 **Arthropathic psoriasis**

L40.50 **Arthropathic psoriasis, unspecified** HCC

L40.51 **Distal interphalangeal psoriatic arthropathy** HCC

L40.52 **Psoriatic arthritis mutilans** HCC

L40.53 **Psoriatic spondylitis** HCC

L40.54 **Psoriatic juvenile arthropathy** HCC

L40.59 **Other psoriatic arthropathy** HCC

L40.8 Other psoriasis
Flexural psoriasis
L40.9 Psoriasis, unspecified

L41 Parapsoriasis
EXCLUDES 1 *poikiloderma vasculare atrophicans (L94.5)*
L41.0 Pityriasis lichenoides et varioliformis acuta
Mucha-Habermann disease
L41.1 Pityriasis lichenoides chronica
L41.3 Small plaque parapsoriasis
L41.4 Large plaque parapsoriasis
L41.5 Retiform parapsoriasis
L41.8 Other parapsoriasis
L41.9 Parapsoriasis, unspecified

L42 Pityriasis rosea
DEFINITION Skin that is marked with scaling, pink, oval macules, arranged with the long axes parallel to the cleavage lines of the skin.

L43 Lichen planus
EXCLUDES 1 *lichen planopilaris (L66.1)*
L43.0 Hypertrophic lichen planus
L43.1 Bullous lichen planus
L43.2 Lichenoid drug reaction
Use additional code for adverse effect, if applicable, to identify drug (T36-T50 with fifth or sixth character 5)
L43.3 Subacute (active) lichen planus
Lichen planus tropicus
L43.8 Other lichen planus
L43.9 Lichen planus, unspecified

L44 Other papulosquamous disorders
L44.0 Pityriasis rubra pilaris
DEFINITION Rare skin condition of red-orange, scaly patches spreading over the body, thickened palms and soles, and rough, dry plugs within the rash.
L44.1 Lichen nitidus
L44.2 Lichen striatus
L44.3 Lichen ruber moniliformis
L44.4 Infantile papular acrodermatitis [Gianotti-Crosti] P
L44.8 Other specified papulosquamous disorders
L44.9 Papulosquamous disorder, unspecified

L45 *Papulosquamous disorders in diseases classified elsewhere*
Code first:
underlying disease.

Urticaria and erythema (L49-L54)

EXCLUDES 1 *Lyme disease (A69.2-)*
rosacea (L71.-)

L49 Exfoliation due to erythematous conditions according to extent of body surface involved
Code first erythematous condition causing exfoliation, such as:
Ritter's disease (L00)
(Staphylococcal) scalded skin syndrom (L00)
Stevens-Johnson syndrome (L51.1)
Stevens-Johnson syndrome-toxic epidermal necrolysis overlap syndrome (L51.3)
Toxic epidermal necrolysis (L51.2)
L49.0 Exfoliation due to erythematous condition involving less than 10 percent of body surface
Exfoliation due to erythematous condition NOS
L49.1 Exfoliation due to erythematous condition involving 10-19 percent of body surface
L49.2 Exfoliation due to erythematous condition involving 20-29 percent of body surface
L49.3 Exfoliation due to erythematous condition involving 30-39 percent of body surface
L49.4 Exfoliation due to erythematous condition involving 40-49 percent of body surface
L49.5 Exfoliation due to erythematous condition involving 50-59 percent of body surface
L49.6 Exfoliation due to erythematous condition involving 60-69 percent of body surface
L49.7 Exfoliation due to erythematous condition involving 70-79 percent of body surface
L49.8 Exfoliation due to erythematous condition involving 80-89 percent of body surface
L49.9 Exfoliation due to erythematous condition involving 90 or more percent of body surface

L50 Urticaria
EXCLUDES 1 *allergic contact dermatitis (L23.-)*
angioneurotic edema (T78.3)
giant urticaria (T78.3)
hereditary angio-edema (D84.1)
Quincke's edema (T78.3)
serum urticaria (T80.6-)
solar urticaria (L56.3)
urticaria neonatorum (P83.8)
urticaria papulosa (L28.2)
urticaria pigmentosa (Q82.2)
CODING TIP✓ Do not confuse urticaria with pruritis. Pruritis refers to "itch" or "itching" while urticaria refers to hives. Pruritis should be coded to L29.
L50.0 Allergic urticaria
DEFINITION The most common form of hives in which smooth, raised, pink or white, itchy welts appear on or beneath the skin as a hypersensitivity response of the immune system to an allergic trigger.

Allergic urticaria

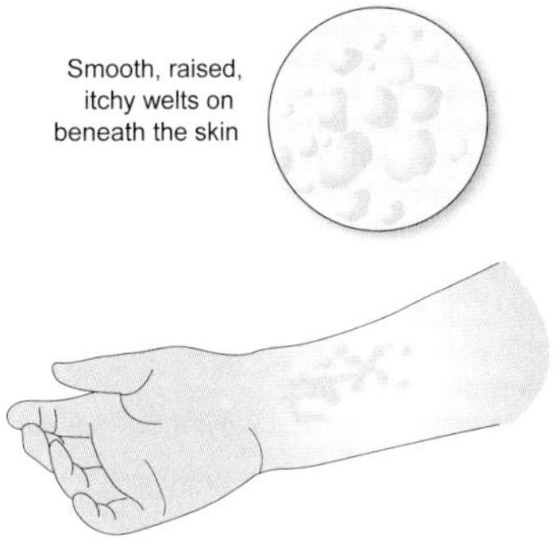

L50.1 Idiopathic urticaria
DEFINITION The appearance of hives with no known, apparent cause.
L50.2 Urticaria due to cold and heat
EXCLUDES 2 *familial cold urticaria (M04.2)*
DEFINITION The appearance of hives in response to external heat or cold that typically fade after moving to a comfortable temperature.
L50.3 Dermatographic urticaria
DEFINITION The appearance of hives in only one particular area of the body.
L50.4 Vibratory urticaria
DEFINITION Hives brought on by intense, prolonged vibration, such as that which occurs with the use of heavy mechanical equipment.
L50.5 Cholinergic urticaria
DEFINITION Hives that occur in response to a rise in body temperature, such as from exercise, stress, or overheating.
L50.6 Contact urticaria
L50.8 Other urticaria
Chronic urticaria
Recurrent periodic urticaria
L50.9 Urticaria, unspecified

Diseases of the Skin and Subcutaneous Tissue

▲ 4 **L51 Erythema multiforme**
Use additional code for adverse effect, if applicable, to identify drug (T36-T50 with fifth or sixth character 5)
Use additional code to identify associated manifestations, such as:
arthropathy associated with dermatological disorders (M14.8-)
conjunctival edema (H11.42)
conjunctivitis (H10.22-)
corneal scars and opacities (H17.-)
corneal ulcer (H16.0-)
edema of eyelid (H02.84-)
inflammation of eyelid (H01.8)
keratoconjunctivitis sicca (H16.22-)
mechanical lagophthalmos (H02.22-)
stomatitis (K12.-)
symblepharon (H11.23-)
Use additional code to identify percentage of skin exfoliation (L49.-)
EXCLUDES 1 *staphylococcal scalded skin syndrome (L00)*
Ritter's disease (L00)

L51.0 Nonbullous erythema multiforme
L51.1 Stevens-Johnson syndrome HCC
L51.2 Toxic epidermal necrolysis [Lyell] HCC
L51.3 Stevens-Johnson syndrome-toxic epidermal necrolysis overlap syndrome HCC
SJS-TEN overlap syndrome
L51.8 Other erythema multiforme
L51.9 Erythema multiforme, unspecified
Erythema iris
Erythema multiforme major NOS
Erythema multiforme minor NOS
Herpes iris
DEFINITION Erythema multiforme minor NOS: Acute, localized, self-limiting eruption marked by distinctive, classical target lesions of pink-red blotches with a ring around a pale center.

L52 Erythema nodosum
EXCLUDES 1 *tuberculous erythema nodosum (A18.4)*
DEFINITION An inflammatory skin disorder marked by flat, firm, warm, red, tender, or painful nodules about an inch across under the skin that turn purple and fade to brown after several weeks, commonly found on anterior lower legs.

4 **L53 Other erythematous conditions**
EXCLUDES 1 *erythema ab igne (L59.0)*
erythema due to external agents in contact with skin (L23-L25)
erythema intertrigo (L30.4)

L53.0 Toxic erythema
Code first:
poisoning due to drug or toxin, if applicable (T36-T65 with fifth or sixth character 1-4 or 6)
Use additional code for adverse effect, if applicable, to identify drug (T36-T50 with fifth or sixth character 5)
EXCLUDES 1 *neonatal erythema toxicum (P83.1)*
L53.1 Erythema annulare centrifugum
L53.2 Erythema marginatum
L53.3 Other chronic figurate erythema
L53.8 Other specified erythematous conditions
L53.9 Erythematous condition, unspecified
Erythema NOS
Erythroderma NOS

L54 *Erythema in diseases classified elsewhere*
Code first:
underlying disease.

Radiation-related disorders of the skin and subcutaneous tissue (L55-L59)

4 **L55 Sunburn**
L55.0 Sunburn of first degree
L55.1 Sunburn of second degree
L55.2 Sunburn of third degree
L55.9 Sunburn, unspecified

4 **L56 Other acute skin changes due to ultraviolet radiation**
Use additional code to identify the source of the ultraviolet radiation (W89, X32)

L56.0 Drug phototoxic response
Use additional code for adverse effect, if applicable, to identify drug (T36-T50 with fifth or sixth character 5)
L56.1 Drug photoallergic response
Use additional code for adverse effect, if applicable, to identify drug (T36-T50 with fifth or sixth character 5)
L56.2 Photocontact dermatitis [berloque dermatitis]
L56.3 Solar urticaria
L56.4 Polymorphous light eruption
L56.5 Disseminated superficial actinic porokeratosis (DSAP)
L56.8 Other specified acute skin changes due to ultraviolet radiation
L56.9 Acute skin change due to ultraviolet radiation, unspecified

4 **L57 Skin changes due to chronic exposure to nonionizing radiation**
Use additional code to identify the source of the ultraviolet radiation (W89)
L57.0 Actinic keratosis
Keratosis NOS
Senile keratosis
Solar keratosis

Actinic keratosis
A rough growth on the skin due to chronic exposure to nonionizing radiation

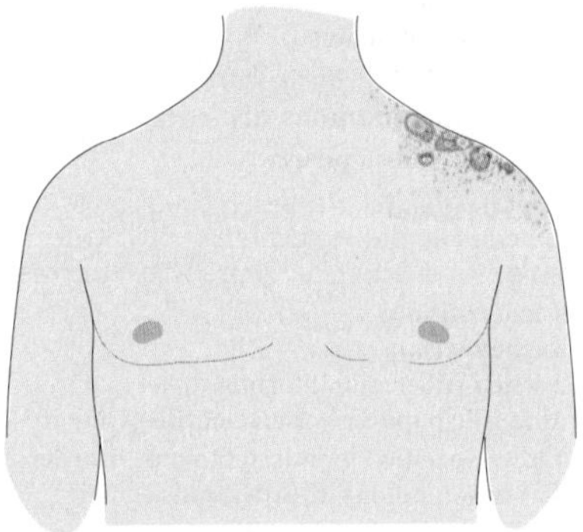

L57.1 Actinic reticuloid
L57.2 Cutis rhomboidalis nuchae
L57.3 Poikiloderma of Civatte
L57.4 Cutis laxa senilis
Elastosis senilis
L57.5 Actinic granuloma
L57.8 Other skin changes due to chronic exposure to nonionizing radiation
Farmer's skin
Sailor's skin
Solar dermatitis
DEFINITION Solar dermatitis: Premature aging of the skin and degeneration of the elastic tissue of the dermis due to prolonged exposure to sunlight.
L57.9 Skin changes due to chronic exposure to nonionizing radiation, unspecified

4 **L58 Radiodermatitis**
Use additional code to identify the source of the radiation (W88, W90)
L58.0 Acute radiodermatitis
L58.1 Chronic radiodermatitis
L58.9 Radiodermatitis, unspecified

4 **L59 Other disorders of skin and subcutaneous tissue related to radiation**
L59.0 Erythema ab igne [dermatitis ab igne]
L59.8 Other specified disorders of the skin and subcutaneous tissue related to radiation
AHA: 1Q 2017, 33
L59.9 Disorder of the skin and subcutaneous tissue related to radiation, unspecified

Disorders of skin appendages (L60-L75)

EXCLUDES 1 *congenital malformations of integument (Q84.-)*

L60 Nail disorders

EXCLUDES 2 *clubbing of nails (R68.3)*
onychia and paronychia (L03.0-)

L60.0 **Ingrowing nail**

Ingrowing nail

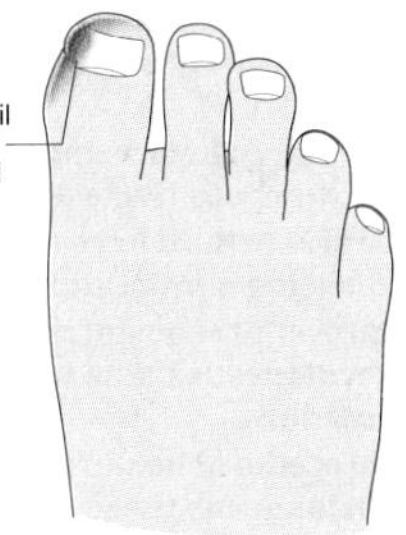

L60.1 **Onycholysis**
L60.2 **Onychogryphosis**
L60.3 **Nail dystrophy**
L60.4 **Beau's lines**
L60.5 **Yellow nail syndrome**
L60.8 **Other nail disorders**
L60.9 **Nail disorder, unspecified**

L62 *Nail disorders in diseases classified elsewhere*
Code first underlying disease, such as:
pachydermoperiostosis (M89.4-)

L63 Alopecia areata

DEFINITION Patchy loss of hair on the head or body.

L63.0 **Alopecia (capitis) totalis**
L63.1 **Alopecia universalis**
L63.2 **Ophiasis**
L63.8 **Other alopecia areata**
L63.9 **Alopecia areata, unspecified**

L64 Androgenic alopecia

INCLUDES male-pattern baldness

L64.0 **Drug-induced androgenic alopecia**
Use additional code for adverse effect, if applicable, to identify drug (T36-T50 with fifth or sixth character 5)
L64.8 **Other androgenic alopecia**
L64.9 **Androgenic alopecia, unspecified**

L65 Other nonscarring hair loss
Use additional code for adverse effect, if applicable, to identify drug (T36-T50 with fifth or sixth character 5)

EXCLUDES 1 *trichotillomania (F63.3)*

L65.0 **Telogen effluvium**
L65.1 **Anagen effluvium**
L65.2 **Alopecia mucinosa**
L65.8 **Other specified nonscarring hair loss**
L65.9 **Nonscarring hair loss, unspecified**
Alopecia NOS

L66 Cicatricial alopecia [scarring hair loss]

L66.0 **Pseudopelade**
L66.1 **Lichen planopilaris**
Follicular lichen planus
L66.2 **Folliculitis decalvans**
L66.3 **Perifolliculitis capitis abscedens**
L66.4 **Folliculitis ulerythematosa reticulata**
L66.8 **Other cicatricial alopecia**
AHA: 1Q 2015, 19
L66.9 **Cicatricial alopecia, unspecified**

L67 Hair color and hair shaft abnormalities

EXCLUDES 1 *monilethrix (Q84.1)*
pili annulati (Q84.1)
telogen effluvium (L65.0)

L67.0 **Trichorrhexis nodosa**
L67.1 **Variations in hair color**
Canities
Greyness, hair (premature)
Heterochromia of hair
Poliosis circumscripta, acquired
Poliosis NOS
L67.8 **Other hair color and hair shaft abnormalities**
Fragilitas crinium
L67.9 **Hair color and hair shaft abnormality, unspecified**

L68 Hypertrichosis

INCLUDES excess hair

EXCLUDES 1 *congenital hypertrichosis (Q84.2)*
persistent lanugo (Q84.2)

L68.0 **Hirsutism**
L68.1 **Acquired hypertrichosis lanuginosa**
L68.2 **Localized hypertrichosis**
L68.3 **Polytrichia**
L68.8 **Other hypertrichosis**
L68.9 **Hypertrichosis, unspecified**

L70 Acne

EXCLUDES 2 *acne keloid (L73.0)*

L70.0 **Acne vulgaris**
L70.1 **Acne conglobata**
L70.2 **Acne varioliformis**
Acne necrotica miliaris
L70.3 **Acne tropica**
L70.4 **Infantile acne** P
L70.5 **Acné excoriée**
Acné excoriée des jeunes filles
Picker's acne
L70.8 **Other acne**
L70.9 **Acne, unspecified**

L71 Rosacea
Use additional code for adverse effect, if applicable, to identify drug (T36-T50 with fifth or sixth character 5)

L71.0 **Perioral dermatitis**
L71.1 **Rhinophyma**
L71.8 **Other rosacea**

Rosacea

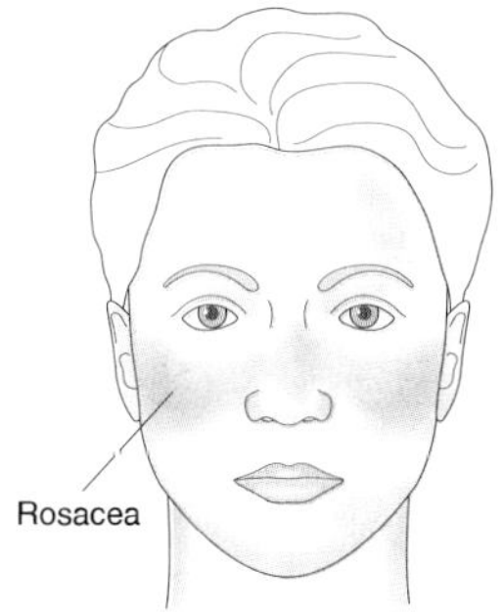

L71.9 **Rosacea, unspecified**

L72 Follicular cysts of skin and subcutaneous tissue

L72.0 **Epidermal cyst**
L72.1 **Pilar and trichodermal cyst**
L72.11 **Pilar cyst**
L72.12 **Trichodermal cyst**
Trichilemmal (proliferating) cyst
L72.2 **Steatocystoma multiplex**

L72.3 Sebaceous cyst
EXCLUDES 2 *pilar cyst (L72.11)*
trichilemmal (proliferating) cyst (L72.12)

Sebaceous cyst

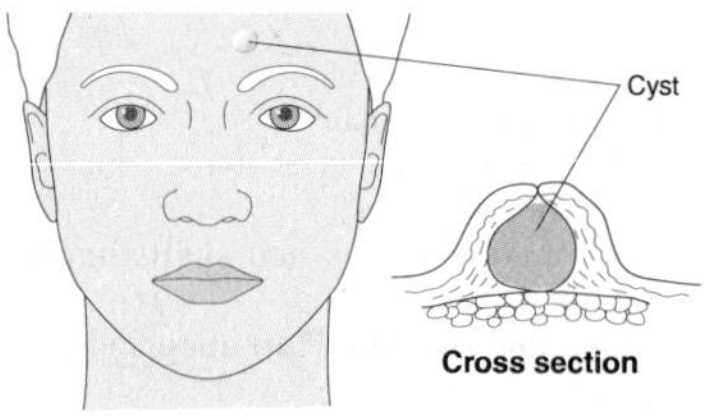

L72.8 **Other follicular cysts of the skin and subcutaneous tissue**
L72.9 **Follicular cyst of the skin and subcutaneous tissue, unspecified**

L73 **Other follicular disorders**
L73.0 **Acne keloid**
L73.1 **Pseudofolliculitis barbae**
L73.2 **Hidradenitis suppurativa**
L73.8 **Other specified follicular disorders**
Sycosis barbae
L73.9 **Follicular disorder, unspecified**

L74 **Eccrine sweat disorders**
EXCLUDES 2 *generalized hyperhidrosis (R61)*
L74.0 **Miliaria rubra**
DEFINITION Inflammatory heat rash caused by obstruction of the sweat glands with resultant skin rash of small clusters of red pimples on the skin.
L74.1 **Miliaria crystallina**
L74.2 **Miliaria profunda**
Miliaria tropicalis
L74.3 **Miliaria, unspecified**
L74.4 **Anhidrosis**
Hypohidrosis
L74.5 **Focal hyperhidrosis**
L74.51 **Primary focal hyperhidrosis**
L74.510 **Primary focal hyperhidrosis, axilla**
L74.511 **Primary focal hyperhidrosis, face**
L74.512 **Primary focal hyperhidrosis, palms**
L74.513 **Primary focal hyperhidrosis, soles**
L74.519 **Primary focal hyperhidrosis, unspecified**
L74.52 **Secondary focal hyperhidrosis**
Frey's syndrome
L74.8 **Other eccrine sweat disorders**
L74.9 **Eccrine sweat disorder, unspecified**
Sweat gland disorder NOS

L75 **Apocrine sweat disorders**
EXCLUDES 1 *dyshidrosis (L30.1)*
hidradenitis suppurativa (L73.2)
L75.0 **Bromhidrosis**
L75.1 **Chromhidrosis**
L75.2 **Apocrine miliaria**
Fox-Fordyce disease
L75.8 **Other apocrine sweat disorders**
L75.9 **Apocrine sweat disorder, unspecified**

Intraoperative and postprocedural complications of skin and subcutaneous tissue (L76)

L76 **Intraoperative and postprocedural complications of skin and subcutaneous tissue**
CODING TIP ✓ Conditions classifiable to L76 are classifiable as intraoperative and postprocedural complications. These conditions should only be assigned when diagnostic statements clearly indicate that the condition is a complication of a procedure.

L76.0 **Intraoperative hemorrhage and hematoma of skin and subcutaneous tissue complicating a procedure**
EXCLUDES 1 *intraoperative hemorrhage and hematoma of skin and subcutaneous tissue due to accidental puncture and laceration during a procedure (L76.1-)*
L76.01 **Intraoperative hemorrhage and hematoma of skin and subcutaneous tissue complicating a dermatologic procedure**
L76.02 **Intraoperative hemorrhage and hematoma of skin and subcutaneous tissue complicating other procedure**
L76.1 **Accidental puncture and laceration of skin and subcutaneous tissue during a procedure**
L76.11 **Accidental puncture and laceration of skin and subcutaneous tissue during a dermatologic procedure**
L76.12 **Accidental puncture and laceration of skin and subcutaneous tissue during other procedure**
L76.2 **Postprocedural hemorrhage of skin and subcutaneous tissue following a procedure**
L76.21 **Postprocedural hemorrhage of skin and subcutaneous tissue following a dermatologic procedure**
L76.22 **Postprocedural hemorrhage of skin and subcutaneous tissue following other procedure**
L76.3 **Postprocedural hematoma and seroma of skin and subcutaneous tissue following a procedure**
L76.31 **Postprocedural hematoma of skin and subcutaneous tissue following a dermatologic procedure**
L76.32 **Postprocedural hematoma of skin and subcutaneous tissue following other procedure**
L76.33 **Postprocedural seroma of skin and subcutaneous tissue following a dermatologic procedure**
L76.34 **Postprocedural seroma of skin and subcutaneous tissue following other procedure**
L76.8 **Other intraoperative and postprocedural complications of skin and subcutaneous tissue**
Use additional code, if applicable, to further specify disorder
L76.81 **Other intraoperative complications of skin and subcutaneous tissue**
L76.82 **Other postprocedural complications of skin and subcutaneous tissue**
AHA: 3Q 2017, 6

Other disorders of the skin and subcutaneous tissue (L80-L99)

L80 **Vitiligo**
EXCLUDES 2 *vitiligo of eyelids (H02.73-)*
vitiligo of vulva (N90.89)
DEFINITION White patches devoid of pigmentation appearing on otherwise normal skin.

L81 **Other disorders of pigmentation**
EXCLUDES 1 *birthmark NOS (Q82.5)*
Peutz-Jeghers syndrome (Q85.8)
EXCLUDES 2 *nevus - see Alphabetical Index*
L81.0 **Postinflammatory hyperpigmentation**
L81.1 **Chloasma**
L81.2 **Freckles**
L81.3 **Café au lait spots**
L81.4 **Other melanin hyperpigmentation**
Lentigo
L81.5 **Leukoderma, not elsewhere classified**
L81.6 **Other disorders of diminished melanin formation**
L81.7 **Pigmented purpuric dermatosis**
Angioma serpiginosum
L81.8 **Other specified disorders of pigmentation**
Iron pigmentation
Tattoo pigmentation
L81.9 **Disorder of pigmentation, unspecified**

L82 **Seborrheic keratosis**
INCLUDES basal cell papilloma
dermatosis papulosa nigra
Leser-Trélat disease
EXCLUDES 2 *seborrheic dermatitis (L21.-)*
L82.0 **Inflamed seborrheic keratosis**

DEFINITION Noncancerous, barnacle-like skin lesions appearing in areas of long-term sun exposure in the elderly. Growths are irritated, itchy, inflamed, and may even bleed.

L82.1 Other seborrheic keratosis
Seborrheic keratosis NOS

DEFINITION Noncancerous skin lesion associated with aging and long periods of sun exposure. Growths appear round or oval, slightly elevated, black, brown, or pale in appearance with a crusty or scaly surface.

Seborrheic keratosis

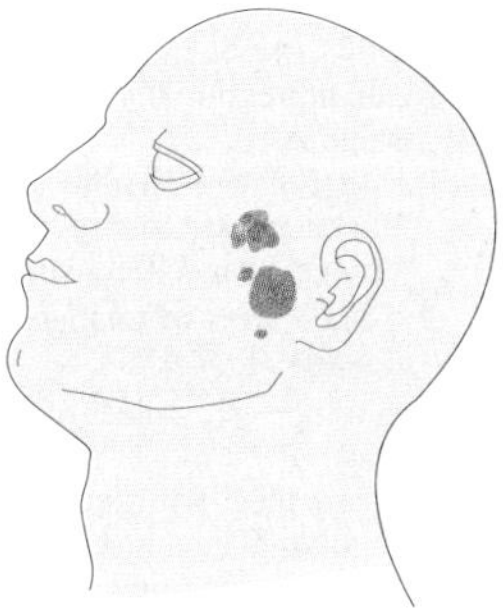

L83 Acanthosis nigricans
Confluent and reticulated papillomatosis

L84 Corns and callosities
Callus
Clavus

4 L85 Other epidermal thickening
EXCLUDES 2 *hypertrophic disorders of the skin (L91.-)*

L85.0 Acquired ichthyosis
EXCLUDES 1 *congenital ichthyosis (Q80.-)*

L85.1 Acquired keratosis [keratoderma] palmaris et plantaris
EXCLUDES 1 *inherited keratosis palmaris et plantaris (Q82.8)*

L85.2 Keratosis punctata (palmaris et plantaris)

L85.3 Xerosis cutis
Dry skin dermatitis

L85.8 Other specified epidermal thickening
Cutaneous horn

L85.9 Epidermal thickening, unspecified

L86 *Keratoderma in diseases classified elsewhere*
Code first underlying disease, such as:
Reiter's disease (M02.3-)
EXCLUDES 1 *gonococcal keratoderma (A54.89)*
gonococcal keratosis (A54.89)
keratoderma due to vitamin A deficiency (E50.8)
keratosis due to vitamin A deficiency (E50.8)
xeroderma due to vitamin A deficiency (E50.8)

4 L87 Transepidermal elimination disorders
EXCLUDES 1 *granuloma annulare (perforating) (L92.0)*

L87.0 Keratosis follicularis et parafollicularis in cutem penetrans
Kyrle disease
Hyperkeratosis follicularis penetrans

L87.1 Reactive perforating collagenosis

L87.2 Elastosis perforans serpiginosa

L87.8 Other transepidermal elimination disorders

L87.9 Transepidermal elimination disorder, unspecified

L88 Pyoderma gangrenosum
Phagedenic pyoderma
EXCLUDES 1 *dermatitis gangrenosa (L08.0)*

4 L89 Pressure ulcer
INCLUDES bed sore
decubitus ulcer
plaster ulcer
pressure area
pressure sore

Code first:
any associated gangrene (I96)

EXCLUDES 2 *decubitus (trophic) ulcer of cervix (uteri) (N86)*
diabetic ulcers (E08.621, E08.622, E09.621, E09.622, E10.621, E10.622, E11.621, E11.622, E13.621, E13.622)
non-pressure chronic ulcer of skin (L97.-)
skin infections (L00-L08)
varicose ulcer (I83.0, I83.2)

GUIDELINES **Section I.B.14**
For the Body Mass Index (BMI), depth of non-pressure chronic ulcers, pressure ulcer stage, coma scale, and NIH stroke scale (NIHSS) codes, code assignment may be based on medical record documentation from clinicians who are not the patient's provider (i.e., physician or other qualified healthcare practitioner legally accountable for establishing the patient's diagnosis), since this information is typically documented by other clinicians involved in the care of the patient (e.g., a dietitian often documents the BMI, a nurse often documents the pressure ulcer stages, and an emergency medical technician often documents the coma scale). However, the associated diagnosis (such as overweight, obesity, acute stroke, or pressure ulcer) must be documented by the patient's provider.

GUIDELINES **Section I.C.12.a.1)**
Codes from category L89 are combination codes that identify the site of the pressure ulcer as well as the stage of the ulcer. ... Assign as many codes from category L89 as needed to identify all the pressure ulcers the patient has, if applicable.

GUIDELINES **Section I.C.12.a.2)**
Assignment of the code for unstageable pressure ulcer (L89.-- 0) should be based on the clinical documentation. These codes are used for pressure ulcers whose stage cannot be clinically determined (e.g., the ulcer is covered by eschar or has been treated with a skin or muscle graft) and pressure ulcers that are documented as deep tissue injury but not documented as due to trauma. This code should not be confused with the codes for unspecified stage (L89.--9). When there is no documentation regarding the stage of the pressure ulcer, assign the appropriate code for unspecified stage (L89.--9).

GUIDELINES **Section I.C.12.a.4)**
No code is assigned if the documentation states that the pressure ulcer is completely healed.

CODING TIP✓ Unstageable means that the pressure ulcer cannot be staged as the underlying tissue is not visible due to the presence of eschar or slough, nonremovable wound coverings or casts and ulcers treated with skin or muscle grafts.

CODING TIP✓ Pressure injury is equivalent to pressure ulcer and should be coded based upon the site and stage of the pressure injury. Deep tissue injury is coded as unstageable pressure ulcer based upon site.

CODING TIP✓ When assigning a code for any overweight, obesity, or morbid obesity, physician documentation indicating obesity as a diagnosis is required. If suspected, but not present, the coder may query the provider to obtain confirmation of the condition, but may not code obesity without confirmation from the provider. BMI Z68.- may be calculated and coded based upon documentation from other clinicians and calculated BMI may be coded alone without a diagnosis of obesity. BMI may only be reported as secondary code.

DEFINITION A pressure-induced ulceration or sore of the skin usually occurring when a patient is confined to bed for long periods of time, due to lack of circulation and oxygenation to the affected tissue.
AHA: 2Q 2018, 16

5 L89.0 Pressure ulcer of elbow

6 L89.00 **Pressure ulcer of unspecified elbow**

L89.000 **Pressure ulcer of unspecified elbow, unstageable** HCC

L89.001 **Pressure ulcer of unspecified elbow, stage 1**
Healing pressure ulcer of unspecified elbow, stage 1
Pressure pre-ulcer skin changes limited to persistent focal edema, unspecified elbow

L89.002 **Pressure ulcer of unspecified elbow, stage 2**
Healing pressure ulcer of unspecified elbow, stage 2
Pressure ulcer with abrasion, blister, partial thickness skin loss involving epidermis and/or dermis, unspecified elbow

L89.003 **Pressure ulcer of unspecified elbow, stage 3** HCC
Healing pressure ulcer of unspecified elbow, stage 3
Pressure ulcer with full thickness skin loss involving damage or necrosis of subcutaneous tissue, unspecified elbow

L89.004 **Pressure ulcer of unspecified elbow, stage 4** HCC
Healing pressure ulcer of unspecified elbow, stage 4
Pressure ulcer with necrosis of soft tissues through to underlying muscle, tendon, or bone, unspecified elbow

L89.009 **Pressure ulcer of unspecified elbow, unspecified stage**
Healing pressure ulcer of elbow NOS
Healing pressure ulcer of unspecified elbow, unspecified stage

6 L89.01 **Pressure ulcer of right elbow**

L89.010 **Pressure ulcer of right elbow, unstageable** HCC

L89.011 **Pressure ulcer of right elbow, stage 1**
Healing pressure ulcer of right elbow, stage 1
Pressure pre-ulcer skin changes limited to persistent focal edema, right elbow

L89.012 **Pressure ulcer of right elbow, stage 2**
Healing pressure ulcer of right elbow, stage 2
Pressure ulcer with abrasion, blister, partial thickness skin loss involving epidermis and/or dermis, right elbow

L89.013 **Pressure ulcer of right elbow, stage 3** HCC
Healing pressure ulcer of right elbow, stage 3
Pressure ulcer with full thickness skin loss involving damage or necrosis of subcutaneous tissue, right elbow

L89.014 **Pressure ulcer of right elbow, stage 4** HCC
Healing pressure ulcer of right elbow, stage 4
Pressure ulcer with necrosis of soft tissues through to underlying muscle, tendon, or bone, right elbow

L89.019 **Pressure ulcer of right elbow, unspecified stage**
Healing pressure right of elbow NOS
Healing pressure ulcer of right elbow, unspecified stage

6 L89.02 **Pressure ulcer of left elbow**

L89.020 **Pressure ulcer of left elbow, unstageable** HCC

L89.021 **Pressure ulcer of left elbow, stage 1**
Healing pressure ulcer of left elbow, stage 1
Pressure pre-ulcer skin changes limited to persistent focal edema, left elbow

L89.022 **Pressure ulcer of left elbow, stage 2**
Healing pressure ulcer of left elbow, stage 2
Pressure ulcer with abrasion, blister, partial thickness skin loss involving epidermis and/or dermis, left elbow

L89.023 **Pressure ulcer of left elbow, stage 3** HCC
Healing pressure ulcer of left elbow, stage 3
Pressure ulcer with full thickness skin loss involving damage or necrosis of subcutaneous tissue, left elbow

L89.024 **Pressure ulcer of left elbow, stage 4** HCC
Healing pressure ulcer of left elbow, stage 4
Pressure ulcer with necrosis of soft tissues through to underlying muscle, tendon, or bone, left elbow

L89.029 **Pressure ulcer of left elbow, unspecified stage**
Healing pressure ulcer of left of elbow NOS
Healing pressure ulcer of left elbow, unspecified stage

5 L89.1 **Pressure ulcer of back**

6 L89.10 **Pressure ulcer of unspecified part of back**

L89.100 **Pressure ulcer of unspecified part of back, unstageable** HCC

L89.101 **Pressure ulcer of unspecified part of back, stage 1**
Healing pressure ulcer of unspecified part of back, stage 1
Pressure pre-ulcer skin changes limited to persistent focal edema, unspecified part of back

L89.102 **Pressure ulcer of unspecified part of back, stage 2**
Healing pressure ulcer of unspecified part of back, stage 2
Pressure ulcer with abrasion, blister, partial thickness skin loss involving epidermis and/or dermis, unspecified part of back

L89.103 **Pressure ulcer of unspecified part of back, stage 3** HCC
Healing pressure ulcer of unspecified part of back, stage 3
Pressure ulcer with full thickness skin loss involving damage or necrosis of subcutaneous tissue, unspecified part of back

L89.104 **Pressure ulcer of unspecified part of back, stage 4** HCC
Healing pressure ulcer of unspecified part of back, stage 4
Pressure ulcer with necrosis of soft tissues through to underlying muscle, tendon, or bone, unspecified part of back

L89.109 **Pressure ulcer of unspecified part of back, unspecified stage**
Healing pressure ulcer of unspecified part of back NOS
Healing pressure ulcer of unspecified part of back, unspecified stage

6 L89.11 **Pressure ulcer of right upper back**
Pressure ulcer of right shoulder blade

L89.110 **Pressure ulcer of right upper back, unstageable** HCC

L89.111 **Pressure ulcer of right upper back, stage 1**
Healing pressure ulcer of right upper back, stage 1
Pressure pre-ulcer skin changes limited to persistent focal edema, right upper back

L89.112 **Pressure ulcer of right upper back, stage 2**
Healing pressure ulcer of right upper back, stage 2
Pressure ulcer with abrasion, blister, partial thickness skin loss involving epidermis and/or dermis, right upper back

L89.113 **Pressure ulcer of right upper back, stage 3** HCC
Healing pressure ulcer of right upper back, stage 3
Pressure ulcer with full thickness skin loss involving damage or necrosis of subcutaneous tissue, right upper back

L89.114 **Pressure ulcer of right upper back, stage 4** HCC
Healing pressure ulcer of right upper back, stage 4
Pressure ulcer with necrosis of soft tissues through to underlying muscle, tendon, or bone, right upper back

L89.119 **Pressure ulcer of right upper back, unspecified stage**
Healing pressure ulcer of right upper back NOS
Healing pressure ulcer of right upper back, unspecified stage

6 L89.12 **Pressure ulcer of left upper back**
Pressure ulcer of left shoulder blade

L89.120 **Pressure ulcer of left upper back, unstageable** HCC

L89.121 **Pressure ulcer of left upper back, stage 1**
Healing pressure ulcer of left upper back, stage 1
Pressure pre-ulcer skin changes limited to persistent focal edema, left upper back

L89.122 **Pressure ulcer of left upper back, stage 2**
Healing pressure ulcer of left upper back, stage 2
Pressure ulcer with abrasion, blister, partial thickness skin loss involving epidermis and/or dermis, left upper back

L89.123 **Pressure ulcer of left upper back, stage 3** HCC
Healing pressure ulcer of left upper back, stage 3
Pressure ulcer with full thickness skin loss involving damage or necrosis of subcutaneous tissue, left upper back

L89.124 **Pressure ulcer of left upper back, stage 4** HCC
Healing pressure ulcer of left upper back, stage 4
Pressure ulcer with necrosis of soft tissues through to underlying muscle, tendon, or bone, left upper back

L89.129 **Pressure ulcer of left upper back, unspecified stage**
Healing pressure ulcer of left upper back NOS
Healing pressure ulcer of left upper back, unspecified stage

L89.13 **Pressure ulcer of right lower back**

L89.130 **Pressure ulcer of right lower back, unstageable** HCC

L89.131 **Pressure ulcer of right lower back, stage 1**
Healing pressure ulcer of right lower back, stage 1
Pressure pre-ulcer skin changes limited to persistent focal edema, right lower back

L89.132 **Pressure ulcer of right lower back, stage 2**
Healing pressure ulcer of right lower back, stage 2
Pressure ulcer with abrasion, blister, partial thickness skin loss involving epidermis and/or dermis, right lower back

L89.133 **Pressure ulcer of right lower back, stage 3** HCC
Healing pressure ulcer of right lower back, stage 3
Pressure ulcer with full thickness skin loss involving damage or necrosis of subcutaneous tissue, right lower back

L89.134 **Pressure ulcer of right lower back, stage 4** HCC
Healing pressure ulcer of right lower back, stage 4
Pressure ulcer with necrosis of soft tissues through to underlying muscle, tendon, or bone, right lower back

L89.139 **Pressure ulcer of right lower back, unspecified stage**
Healing pressure ulcer of right lower back NOS
Healing pressure ulcer of right lower back, unspecified stage

L89.14 **Pressure ulcer of left lower back**

L89.140 **Pressure ulcer of left lower back, unstageable** HCC

L89.141 **Pressure ulcer of left lower back, stage 1**
Healing pressure ulcer of left lower back, stage 1
Pressure pre-ulcer skin changes limited to persistent focal edema, left lower back

L89.142 **Pressure ulcer of left lower back, stage 2**
Healing pressure ulcer of left lower back, stage 2
Pressure ulcer with abrasion, blister, partial thickness skin loss involving epidermis and/or dermis, left lower back

L89.143 **Pressure ulcer of left lower back, stage 3** HCC
Healing pressure ulcer of left lower back, stage 3
Pressure ulcer with full thickness skin loss involving damage or necrosis of subcutaneous tissue, left lower back

L89.144 **Pressure ulcer of left lower back, stage 4** HCC
Healing pressure ulcer of left lower back, stage 4
Pressure ulcer with necrosis of soft tissues through to underlying muscle, tendon, or bone, left lower back

L89.149 **Pressure ulcer of left lower back, unspecified stage**
Healing pressure ulcer of left lower back NOS
Healing pressure ulcer of left lower back, unspecified stage

L89.15 **Pressure ulcer of sacral region**
Pressure ulcer of coccyx
Pressure ulcer of tailbone

L89.150 **Pressure ulcer of sacral region, unstageable** HCC

L89.151 **Pressure ulcer of sacral region, stage 1**
Healing pressure ulcer of sacral region, stage 1
Pressure pre-ulcer skin changes limited to persistent focal edema, sacral region

L89.152 **Pressure ulcer of sacral region, stage 2**
Healing pressure ulcer of sacral region, stage 2
Pressure ulcer with abrasion, blister, partial thickness skin loss involving epidermis and/or dermis, sacral region

L89.153 **Pressure ulcer of sacral region, stage 3** HCC
Healing pressure ulcer of sacral region, stage 3
Pressure ulcer with full thickness skin loss involving damage or necrosis of subcutaneous tissue, sacral region

L89.154 **Pressure ulcer of sacral region, stage 4** HCC
Healing pressure ulcer of sacral region, stage 4
Pressure ulcer with necrosis of soft tissues through to underlying muscle, tendon, or bone, sacral region

L89.159 **Pressure ulcer of sacral region, unspecified stage**
Healing pressure ulcer of sacral region NOS
Healing pressure ulcer of sacral region, unspecified stage

L89.2 **Pressure ulcer of hip**

L89.20 **Pressure ulcer of unspecified hip**

L89.200 **Pressure ulcer of unspecified hip, unstageable** HCC

L89.201 **Pressure ulcer of unspecified hip, stage 1**
Healing pressure ulcer of unspecified hip back, stage 1
Pressure pre-ulcer skin changes limited to persistent focal edema, unspecified hip

L89.202 **Pressure ulcer of unspecified hip, stage 2**
Healing pressure ulcer of unspecified hip, stage 2
Pressure ulcer with abrasion, blister, partial thickness skin loss involving epidermis and/or dermis, unspecified hip

L89.203 **Pressure ulcer of unspecified hip, stage 3** HCC
Healing pressure ulcer of unspecified hip, stage 3
Pressure ulcer with full thickness skin loss involving damage or necrosis of subcutaneous tissue, unspecified hip

L89.204 **Pressure ulcer of unspecified hip, stage 4** HCC
Healing pressure ulcer of unspecified hip, stage 4
Pressure ulcer with necrosis of soft tissues through to underlying muscle, tendon, or bone, unspecified hip

L89.209 **Pressure ulcer of unspecified hip, unspecified stage**
Healing pressure ulcer of unspecified hip NOS
Healing pressure ulcer of unspecified hip, unspecified stage

L89.21 **Pressure ulcer of right hip**

L89.210 **Pressure ulcer of right hip, unstageable** HCC

L89.211 **Pressure ulcer of right hip, stage 1**
Healing pressure ulcer of right hip back, stage 1
Pressure pre-ulcer skin changes limited to persistent focal edema, right hip

L89.212 **Pressure ulcer of right hip, stage 2**
Healing pressure ulcer of right hip, stage 2
Pressure ulcer with abrasion, blister, partial thickness skin loss involving epidermis and/or dermis, right hip

L89.213 **Pressure ulcer of right hip, stage 3** HCC
Healing pressure ulcer of right hip, stage 3
Pressure ulcer with full thickness skin loss involving damage or necrosis of subcutaneous tissue, right hip

L89.214 **Pressure ulcer of right hip, stage 4** HCC
Healing pressure ulcer of right hip, stage 4
Pressure ulcer with necrosis of soft tissues through to underlying muscle, tendon, or bone, right hip

L89.219 **Pressure ulcer of right hip, unspecified stage**
Healing pressure ulcer of right hip NOS
Healing pressure ulcer of right hip, unspecified stage

L89.22 **Pressure ulcer of left hip**

L89.220 **Pressure ulcer of left hip, unstageable** HCC

L89.221 **Pressure ulcer of left hip, stage 1**
Healing pressure ulcer of left hip back, stage 1
Pressure pre-ulcer skin changes limited to persistent focal edema, left hip

L89.222 **Pressure ulcer of left hip, stage 2**
Healing pressure ulcer of left hip, stage 2
Pressure ulcer with abrasion, blister, partial thickness skin loss involving epidermis and/or dermis, left hip

L89.223 **Pressure ulcer of left hip, stage 3** HCC
Healing pressure ulcer of left hip, stage 3
Pressure ulcer with full thickness skin loss involving damage or necrosis of subcutaneous tissue, left hip

L89.224 **Pressure ulcer of left hip, stage 4** HCC
Healing pressure ulcer of left hip, stage 4
Pressure ulcer with necrosis of soft tissues through to underlying muscle, tendon, or bone, left hip

L89.229 **Pressure ulcer of left hip, unspecified stage**
Healing pressure ulcer of left hip NOS
Healing pressure ulcer of left hip, unspecified stage

L89.3 **Pressure ulcer of buttock**

L89.30 **Pressure ulcer of unspecified buttock**

L89.300 **Pressure ulcer of unspecified buttock, unstageable** HCC

L89.301 **Pressure ulcer of unspecified buttock, stage 1**
Healing pressure ulcer of unspecified buttock, stage 1
Pressure pre-ulcer skin changes limited to persistent focal edema, unspecified buttock

L89.302 **Pressure ulcer of unspecified buttock, stage 2**
Healing pressure ulcer of unspecified buttock, stage 2
Pressure ulcer with abrasion, blister, partial thickness skin loss involving epidermis and/or dermis, unspecified buttock

L89.303 **Pressure ulcer of unspecified buttock, stage 3** HCC
Healing pressure ulcer of unspecified buttock, stage 3
Pressure ulcer with full thickness skin loss involving damage or necrosis of subcutaneous tissue, unspecified buttock

L89.304 **Pressure ulcer of unspecified buttock, stage 4** HCC
Healing pressure ulcer of unspecified buttock, stage 4
Pressure ulcer with necrosis of soft tissues through to underlying muscle, tendon, or bone, unspecified buttock

L89.309 **Pressure ulcer of unspecified buttock, unspecified stage**
Healing pressure ulcer of unspecified buttock NOS
Healing pressure ulcer of unspecified buttock, unspecified stage

L89.31 **Pressure ulcer of right buttock**

L89.310 **Pressure ulcer of right buttock, unstageable** HCC

L89.311 **Pressure ulcer of right buttock, stage 1**
Healing pressure ulcer of right buttock, stage 1
Pressure pre-ulcer skin changes limited to persistent focal edema, right buttock

L89.312 **Pressure ulcer of right buttock, stage 2**
Healing pressure ulcer of right buttock, stage 2
Pressure ulcer with abrasion, blister, partial thickness skin loss involving epidermis and/or dermis, right buttock

L89.313 **Pressure ulcer of right buttock, stage 3** HCC
Healing pressure ulcer of right buttock, stage 3
Pressure ulcer with full thickness skin loss involving damage or necrosis of subcutaneous tissue, right buttock

L89.314 **Pressure ulcer of right buttock, stage 4** HCC
Healing pressure ulcer of right buttock, stage 4
Pressure ulcer with necrosis of soft tissues through to underlying muscle, tendon, or bone, right buttock

L89.319 **Pressure ulcer of right buttock, unspecified stage**
Healing pressure ulcer of right buttock NOS
Healing pressure ulcer of right buttock, unspecified stage

L89.32 **Pressure ulcer of left buttock**

L89.320 **Pressure ulcer of left buttock, unstageable** HCC

L89.321 **Pressure ulcer of left buttock, stage 1**
Healing pressure ulcer of left buttock, stage 1
Pressure pre-ulcer skin changes limited to persistent focal edema, left buttock

L89.322 **Pressure ulcer of left buttock, stage 2**
Healing pressure ulcer of left buttock, stage 2
Pressure ulcer with abrasion, blister, partial thickness skin loss involving epidermis and/or dermis, left buttock

L89.323 **Pressure ulcer of left buttock, stage 3** HCC
Healing pressure ulcer of left buttock, stage 3
Pressure ulcer with full thickness skin loss involving damage or necrosis of subcutaneous tissue, left buttock

L89.324 **Pressure ulcer of left buttock, stage 4** HCC
Healing pressure ulcer of left buttock, stage 4
Pressure ulcer with necrosis of soft tissues through to underlying muscle, tendon, or bone, left buttock

L89.329 **Pressure ulcer of left buttock, unspecified stage**
Healing pressure ulcer of left buttock NOS
Healing pressure ulcer of left buttock, unspecified stage

L89.4 **Pressure ulcer of contiguous site of back, buttock and hip**

CODING TIP ✓ When a patient presents with a pressure ulcer that is contiguous to the surface area of the back, buttock, and/or hip, a code from L89.4- should be assigned. The stage of the ulcer should be assigned as the worst stage identifiable (the area of the ulcer which has deteriorated to its worst stage).

L89.40 **Pressure ulcer of contiguous site of back, buttock and hip, unspecified stage**
Healing pressure ulcer of contiguous site of back, buttock and hip NOS
Healing pressure ulcer of contiguous site of back, buttock and hip, unspecified stage

L89.41 **Pressure ulcer of contiguous site of back, buttock and hip, stage 1**
Healing pressure ulcer of contiguous site of back, buttock and hip, stage 1
Pressure pre-ulcer skin changes limited to persistent focal edema, contiguous site of back, buttock and hip

L89.42 **Pressure ulcer of contiguous site of back, buttock and hip, stage 2**
Healing pressure ulcer of contiguous site of back, buttock and hip, stage 2
Pressure ulcer with abrasion, blister, partial thickness skin loss involving epidermis and/or dermis, contiguous site of back, buttock and hip

L89.43 **Pressure ulcer of contiguous site of back, buttock and hip, stage 3** HCC
Healing pressure ulcer of contiguous site of back, buttock and hip, stage 3
Pressure ulcer with full thickness skin loss involving damage or necrosis of subcutaneous tissue, contiguous site of back, buttock and hip

L89.44 **Pressure ulcer of contiguous site of back, buttock and hip, stage 4** HCC
Healing pressure ulcer of contiguous site of back, buttock and hip, stage 4
Pressure ulcer with necrosis of soft tissues through to underlying muscle, tendon, or bone, contiguous site of back, buttock and hip

L89.45 **Pressure ulcer of contiguous site of back, buttock and hip, unstageable** HCC

L89.5 **Pressure ulcer of ankle**

L89.50 **Pressure ulcer of unspecified ankle**

L89.500 **Pressure ulcer of unspecified ankle, unstageable** HCC

L89.501 **Pressure ulcer of unspecified ankle, stage 1**
Healing pressure ulcer of unspecified ankle, stage 1
Pressure pre-ulcer skin changes limited to persistent focal edema, unspecified ankle

L89.502 **Pressure ulcer of unspecified ankle, stage 2**
Healing pressure ulcer of unspecified ankle, stage 2
Pressure ulcer with abrasion, blister, partial thickness skin loss involving epidermis and/or dermis, unspecified ankle

L89.503 **Pressure ulcer of unspecified ankle, stage 3** HCC
Healing pressure ulcer of unspecified ankle, stage 3
Pressure ulcer with full thickness skin loss involving damage or necrosis of subcutaneous tissue, unspecified ankle

L89.504 **Pressure ulcer of unspecified ankle, stage 4** HCC
Healing pressure ulcer of unspecified ankle, stage 4
Pressure ulcer with necrosis of soft tissues through to underlying muscle, tendon, or bone, unspecified ankle

L89.509 **Pressure ulcer of unspecified ankle, unspecified stage**
Healing pressure ulcer of unspecified ankle NOS
Healing pressure ulcer of unspecified ankle, unspecified stage

6 L89.51 **Pressure ulcer of right ankle**

L89.510 **Pressure ulcer of right ankle, unstageable** HCC

L89.511 **Pressure ulcer of right ankle, stage 1**
Healing pressure ulcer of right ankle, stage 1
Pressure pre-ulcer skin changes limited to persistent focal edema, right ankle

L89.512 **Pressure ulcer of right ankle, stage 2**
Healing pressure ulcer of right ankle, stage 2
Pressure ulcer with abrasion, blister, partial thickness skin loss involving epidermis and/or dermis, right ankle

L89.513 **Pressure ulcer of right ankle, stage 3** HCC
Healing pressure ulcer of right ankle, stage 3
Pressure ulcer with full thickness skin loss involving damage or necrosis of subcutaneous tissue, right ankle

L89.514 **Pressure ulcer of right ankle, stage 4** HCC
Healing pressure ulcer of right ankle, stage 4
Pressure ulcer with necrosis of soft tissues through to underlying muscle, tendon, or bone, right ankle

L89.519 **Pressure ulcer of right ankle, unspecified stage**
Healing pressure ulcer of right ankle NOS
Healing pressure ulcer of right ankle, unspecified stage

6 L89.52 **Pressure ulcer of left ankle**

L89.520 **Pressure ulcer of left ankle, unstageable** HCC

L89.521 **Pressure ulcer of left ankle, stage 1**
Healing pressure ulcer of left ankle, stage 1
Pressure pre-ulcer skin changes limited to persistent focal edema, left ankle

L89.522 **Pressure ulcer of left ankle, stage 2**
Healing pressure ulcer of left ankle, stage 2
Pressure ulcer with abrasion, blister, partial thickness skin loss involving epidermis and/or dermis, left ankle

L89.523 **Pressure ulcer of left ankle, stage 3** HCC
Healing pressure ulcer of left ankle, stage 3
Pressure ulcer with full thickness skin loss involving damage or necrosis of subcutaneous tissue, left ankle

L89.524 **Pressure ulcer of left ankle, stage 4** HCC
Healing pressure ulcer of left ankle, stage 4
Pressure ulcer with necrosis of soft tissues through to underlying muscle, tendon, or bone, left ankle

L89.529 **Pressure ulcer of left ankle, unspecified stage**
Healing pressure ulcer of left ankle NOS
Healing pressure ulcer of left ankle, unspecified stage

5 L89.6 **Pressure ulcer of heel**

6 L89.60 **Pressure ulcer of unspecified heel**

L89.600 **Pressure ulcer of unspecified heel, unstageable** HCC

L89.601 **Pressure ulcer of unspecified heel, stage 1**
Healing pressure ulcer of unspecified heel, stage 1
Pressure pre-ulcer skin changes limited to persistent focal edema, unspecified heel

L89.602 **Pressure ulcer of unspecified heel, stage 2**
Healing pressure ulcer of unspecified heel, stage 2
Pressure ulcer with abrasion, blister, partial thickness skin loss involving epidermis and/or dermis, unspecified heel

L89.603 **Pressure ulcer of unspecified heel, stage 3** HCC
Healing pressure ulcer of unspecified heel, stage 3
Pressure ulcer with full thickness skin loss involving damage or necrosis of subcutaneous tissue, unspecified heel

L89.604 **Pressure ulcer of unspecified heel, stage 4** HCC
Healing pressure ulcer of unspecified heel, stage 4
Pressure ulcer with necrosis of soft tissues through to underlying muscle, tendon, or bone, unspecified heel

L89.609 **Pressure ulcer of unspecified heel, unspecified stage**
Healing pressure ulcer of unspecified heel NOS
Healing pressure ulcer of unspecified heel, unspecified stage

6 L89.61 **Pressure ulcer of right heel**

L89.610 **Pressure ulcer of right heel, unstageable** HCC

L89.611 **Pressure ulcer of right heel, stage 1**
Healing pressure ulcer of right heel, stage 1
Pressure pre-ulcer skin changes limited to persistent focal edema, right heel

L89.612 **Pressure ulcer of right heel, stage 2**
Healing pressure ulcer of right heel, stage 2
Pressure ulcer with abrasion, blister, partial thickness skin loss involving epidermis and/or dermis, right heel

L89.613 **Pressure ulcer of right heel, stage 3** HCC
Healing pressure ulcer of right heel, stage 3
Pressure ulcer with full thickness skin loss involving damage or necrosis of subcutaneous tissue, right heel

L89.614 **Pressure ulcer of right heel, stage 4** HCC
Healing pressure ulcer of right heel, stage 4
Pressure ulcer with necrosis of soft tissues through to underlying muscle, tendon, or bone, right heel

L89.619 **Pressure ulcer of right heel, unspecified stage**
Healing pressure ulcer of right heel NOS
Healing pressure ulcer of right heel, unspecified stage

6 L89.62 **Pressure ulcer of left heel**

L89.620 **Pressure ulcer of left heel, unstageable** HCC

L89.621 **Pressure ulcer of left heel, stage 1**
Healing pressure ulcer of left heel, stage 1
Pressure pre-ulcer skin changes limited to persistent focal edema, left heel

L89.622 **Pressure ulcer of left heel, stage 2**
Healing pressure ulcer of left heel, stage 2
Pressure ulcer with abrasion, blister, partial thickness skin loss involving epidermis and/or dermis, left heel
AHA: 4Q 2016, 143

L89.623 **Pressure ulcer of left heel, stage 3** HCC
Healing pressure ulcer of left heel, stage 3
Pressure ulcer with full thickness skin loss involving damage or necrosis of subcutaneous tissue, left heel
AHA: 4Q 2016, 143

L89.624 **Pressure ulcer of left heel, stage 4** HCC
Healing pressure ulcer of left heel, stage 4
Pressure ulcer with necrosis of soft tissues through to underlying muscle, tendon, or bone, left heel

L89.629 **Pressure ulcer of left heel, unspecified stage**
Healing pressure ulcer of left heel NOS
Healing pressure ulcer of left heel, unspecified stage

5 L89.8 **Pressure ulcer of other site**

6 L89.81 **Pressure ulcer of head**
Pressure ulcer of face

L89.810 **Pressure ulcer of head, unstageable** HCC

L89.811 **Pressure ulcer of head, stage 1**
Healing pressure ulcer of head, stage 1
Pressure pre-ulcer skin changes limited to persistent focal edema, head

L89.812 **Pressure ulcer of head, stage 2**
Healing pressure ulcer of head, stage 2
Pressure ulcer with abrasion, blister, partial thickness skin loss involving epidermis and/or dermis, head

L89.813 **Pressure ulcer of head, stage 3** HCC
Healing pressure ulcer of head, stage 3
Pressure ulcer with full thickness skin loss involving damage or necrosis of subcutaneous tissue, head

L89.814 **Pressure ulcer of head, stage 4** HCC
Healing pressure ulcer of head, stage 4
Pressure ulcer with necrosis of soft tissues through to underlying muscle, tendon, or bone, head

L89.819 **Pressure ulcer of head, unspecified stage**
Healing pressure ulcer of head NOS
Healing pressure ulcer of head, unspecified stage

6 L89.89 **Pressure ulcer of other site**

L89.890 **Pressure ulcer of other site, unstageable** HCC

L89.891 **Pressure ulcer of other site, stage 1**
Healing pressure ulcer of other site, stage 1
Pressure pre-ulcer skin changes limited to persistent focal edema, other site

L89.892 **Pressure ulcer of other site, stage 2**
Healing pressure ulcer of other site, stage 2
Pressure ulcer with abrasion, blister, partial thickness skin loss involving epidermis and/or dermis, other site

L89.893 **Pressure ulcer of other site, stage 3** HCC
Healing pressure ulcer of other site, stage 3
Pressure ulcer with full thickness skin loss involving damage or necrosis of subcutaneous tissue, other site

L89.894 **Pressure ulcer of other site, stage 4** HCC
Healing pressure ulcer of other site, stage 4
Pressure ulcer with necrosis of soft tissues through to underlying muscle, tendon, or bone, other site

L89.899 **Pressure ulcer of other site, unspecified stage**
Healing pressure ulcer of other site NOS
Healing pressure ulcer of other site, unspecified stage

5 L89.9 **Pressure ulcer of unspecified site**

L89.90 **Pressure ulcer of unspecified site, unspecified stage**
Healing pressure ulcer of unspecified site NOS
Healing pressure ulcer of unspecified site, unspecified stage

L89.91 **Pressure ulcer of unspecified site, stage 1**
Healing pressure ulcer of unspecified site, stage 1
Pressure pre-ulcer skin changes limited to persistent focal edema, unspecified site

L89.92 **Pressure ulcer of unspecified site, stage 2**
Healing pressure ulcer of unspecified site, stage 2
Pressure ulcer with abrasion, blister, partial thickness skin loss involving epidermis and/or dermis, unspecified site

L89.93 **Pressure ulcer of unspecified site, stage 3** HCC
Healing pressure ulcer of unspecified site, stage 3
Pressure ulcer with full thickness skin loss involving damage or necrosis of subcutaneous tissue, unspecified site

L89.94 **Pressure ulcer of unspecified site, stage 4** HCC
Healing pressure ulcer of unspecified site, stage 4
Pressure ulcer with necrosis of soft tissues through to underlying muscle, tendon, or bone, unspecified site

L89.95 **Pressure ulcer of unspecified site, unstageable** HCC

4 L90 **Atrophic disorders of skin**

L90.0 **Lichen sclerosus et atrophicus**
EXCLUDES 2 *lichen sclerosus of external female genital organs (N90.4)*
lichen sclerosus of external male genital organs (N48.0)

L90.1 **Anetoderma of Schweninger-Buzzi**

L90.2 **Anetoderma of Jadassohn-Pellizzari**

L90.3 **Atrophoderma of Pasini and Pierini**

L90.4 **Acrodermatitis chronica atrophicans**

L90.5 **Scar conditions and fibrosis of skin**
Adherent scar (skin)
Cicatrix
Disfigurement of skin due to scar
Fibrosis of skin NOS
Scar NOS
EXCLUDES 2 *hypertrophic scar (L91.0)*
keloid scar (L91.0)
AHA: 1Q 2015, 19
AHA: 2Q 2016, 5

L90.6 **Striae atrophicae**

L90.8 **Other atrophic disorders of skin**

L90.9 **Atrophic disorder of skin, unspecified**

4 L91 **Hypertrophic disorders of skin**

L91.0 **Hypertrophic scar**
Keloid
Keloid scar
EXCLUDES 2 *acne keloid (L73.0)*
scar NOS (L90.5)

L91.8 **Other hypertrophic disorders of the skin**

L91.9 **Hypertrophic disorder of the skin, unspecified**

4 L92 **Granulomatous disorders of skin and subcutaneous tissue**
EXCLUDES 2 *actinic granuloma (L57.5)*

L92.0 **Granuloma annulare**
Perforating granuloma annulare

L92.1 **Necrobiosis lipoidica, not elsewhere classified**
EXCLUDES 1 *necrobiosis lipoidica associated with diabetes mellitus (E08-E13 with .620)*

L92.2 **Granuloma faciale [eosinophilic granuloma of skin]**

L92.3 **Foreign body granuloma of the skin and subcutaneous tissue**
Use additional code to identify the type of retained foreign body (Z18.-)

L92.8 **Other granulomatous disorders of the skin and subcutaneous tissue**

L92.9 **Granulomatous disorder of the skin and subcutaneous tissue, unspecified**
EXCLUDES 2 *umbilical granuloma (P83.81)*

4 L93 **Lupus erythematosus**
Use additional code for adverse effect, if applicable, to identify drug (T36-T50 with fifth or sixth character 5)
EXCLUDES 1 *lupus exedens (A18.4)*
lupus vulgaris (A18.4)
scleroderma (M34.-)
systemic lupus erythematosus (M32.-)

L93.0 **Discoid lupus erythematosus**
Lupus erythematosus NOS

L93.1 **Subacute cutaneous lupus erythematosus**

L93.2 **Other local lupus erythematosus**
Lupus erythematosus profundus
Lupus panniculitis

4 L94 **Other localized connective tissue disorders**
EXCLUDES 1 *systemic connective tissue disorders (M30-M36)*

L94.0 **Localized scleroderma [morphea]**
Circumscribed scleroderma

L94.1 **Linear scleroderma**
En coup de sabre lesion

L94.2 **Calcinosis cutis**

L94.3 **Sclerodactyly**

L94.4 **Gottron's papules**

L94.5 **Poikiloderma vasculare atrophicans**

L94.6 **Ainhum**

L94.8 **Other specified localized connective tissue disorders**

L94.9 **Localized connective tissue disorder, unspecified**

L95 Vasculitis limited to skin, not elsewhere classified

EXCLUDES 1 *angioma serpiginosum (L81.7)*
Henoch (-Schönlein) purpura (D69.0)
hypersensitivity angiitis (M31.0)
lupus panniculitis (L93.2)
panniculitis NOS (M79.3)
panniculitis of neck and back (M54.0-)
polyarteritis nodosa (M30.0)
relapsing panniculitis (M35.6)
rheumatoid vasculitis (M05.2)
serum sickness (T80.6-)
urticaria (L50.-)
Wegener's granulomatosis (M31.3-)

L95.0 Livedoid vasculitis
Atrophie blanche (en plaque)
L95.1 Erythema elevatum diutinum
L95.8 Other vasculitis limited to the skin
L95.9 Vasculitis limited to the skin, unspecified

L97 Non-pressure chronic ulcer of lower limb, not elsewhere classified

INCLUDES chronic ulcer of skin of lower limb NOS
non-healing ulcer of skin
non-infected sinus of skin
trophic ulcer NOS
tropical ulcer NOS
ulcer of skin of lower limb NOS

Code first any associated underlying condition, such as:
any associated gangrene (I96)
atherosclerosis of the lower extremities
(I70.23-, I70.24-, I70.33-, I70.34-, I70.43-, I70.44-, I70.53-, I70.54-, I70.63-, I70.64-, I70.73-, I70.74-)
chronic venous hypertension (I87.31-, I87.33-)
diabetic ulcers
(E08.621, E08.622, E09.621, E09.622, E10.621, E10.622, E11.621, E11.622, E13.621, E13.622)
postphlebitic syndrome (I87.01-, I87.03-)
postthrombotic syndrome (I87.01-, I87.03-)
varicose ulcer (I83.0-, I83.2-)

EXCLUDES 2 *pressure ulcer (pressure area) (L89.-)*
skin infections (L00-L08)
specific infections classified to A00-B99

GUIDELINES **Section I.B.14**
For the Body Mass Index (BMI), depth of non-pressure chronic ulcers, pressure ulcer stage, coma scale, and NIH stroke scale (NIHSS) codes, code assignment may be based on medical record documentation from clinicians who are not the patient's provider (i.e., physician or other qualified healthcare practitioner legally accountable for establishing the patient's diagnosis), since this information is typically documented by other clinicians involved in the care of the patient (e.g., a dietitian often documents the BMI, a nurse often documents the pressure ulcer stages, and an emergency medical technician often documents the coma scale). However, the associated diagnosis (such as overweight, obesity, acute stroke, or pressure ulcer) must be documented by the patient's provider.

CODING TIP✓ A causal relationship is assumed between diabetes and non-pressure ulcers unless otherwise specified by the provider. Code first the combination code for the type of diabetes and ulcer E08.6-E13.6 with the fifth and sixth character defining foot (E13.621) or other skin (E13.622) followed by the location and severity of the ulcer (L97). Code also any other coexisting pathology such as polyneuropathy or gangrene.

CODING TIP✓ When coding any non-pressure chronic ulcer classifiable to L97, first code the underlying cause of the ulcer, if known, followed by the appropriate L97 code to identify the ulcer location, site and severity. Any gangrene associated with the ulcer should also be coded first (prior to sequencing of the L97 code). Skin ulceration in a diabetic is assumed related to the diabetes, unless otherwise specified by the physician.

CODING TIP✓ L97 codes are specific for site, laterality, and severity (e.g., skin, fat layer exposed, necrosis of muscle, necrosis of bone). The severity of the ulcer may be coded based upon documentation from other clinicians (Official Coding Guidlines I.B.15), but confirmation of necrosis of bone should be obtained by diagnostic testing such as MRI (cannot determine through visualization alone). These codes are for non-pressure chronic ulcers and not for nonhealing surgical wounds.

L97.1 Non-pressure chronic ulcer of thigh

L97.10 Non-pressure chronic ulcer of unspecified thigh

L97.101 Non-pressure chronic ulcer of unspecified thigh limited to breakdown of skin HCC
L97.102 Non-pressure chronic ulcer of unspecified thigh with fat layer exposed HCC
L97.103 Non-pressure chronic ulcer of unspecified thigh with necrosis of muscle HCC
L97.104 Non-pressure chronic ulcer of unspecified thigh with necrosis of bone HCC
L97.105 Non-pressure chronic ulcer of unspecified thigh with muscle involvement without evidence of necrosis HCC
L97.106 Non-pressure chronic ulcer of unspecified thigh with bone involvement without evidence of necrosis HCC
L97.108 Non-pressure chronic ulcer of unspecified thigh with other specified severity HCC
L97.109 Non-pressure chronic ulcer of unspecified thigh with unspecified severity HCC

L97.11 Non-pressure chronic ulcer of right thigh

L97.111 Non-pressure chronic ulcer of right thigh limited to breakdown of skin HCC
L97.112 Non-pressure chronic ulcer of right thigh with fat layer exposed HCC
L97.113 Non-pressure chronic ulcer of right thigh with necrosis of muscle HCC
L97.114 Non-pressure chronic ulcer of right thigh with necrosis of bone HCC
L97.115 Non-pressure chronic ulcer of right thigh with muscle involvement without evidence of necrosis HCC
L97.116 Non-pressure chronic ulcer of right thigh with bone involvement without evidence of necrosis HCC
L97.118 Non-pressure chronic ulcer of right thigh with other specified severity HCC
L97.119 Non-pressure chronic ulcer of right thigh with unspecified severity HCC

L97.12 Non-pressure chronic ulcer of left thigh

L97.121 Non-pressure chronic ulcer of left thigh limited to breakdown of skin HCC
L97.122 Non-pressure chronic ulcer of left thigh with fat layer exposed HCC
L97.123 Non-pressure chronic ulcer of left thigh with necrosis of muscle HCC
L97.124 Non-pressure chronic ulcer of left thigh with necrosis of bone HCC
L97.125 Non-pressure chronic ulcer of left thigh with muscle involvement without evidence of necrosis HCC
L97.126 Non-pressure chronic ulcer of left thigh with bone involvement without evidence of necrosis HCC
L97.128 Non-pressure chronic ulcer of left thigh with other specified severity HCC
L97.129 Non-pressure chronic ulcer of left thigh with unspecified severity HCC

L97.2 Non-pressure chronic ulcer of calf

L97.20 Non-pressure chronic ulcer of unspecified calf

L97.201 Non-pressure chronic ulcer of unspecified calf limited to breakdown of skin HCC
L97.202 Non-pressure chronic ulcer of unspecified calf with fat layer exposed HCC
L97.203 Non-pressure chronic ulcer of unspecified calf with necrosis of muscle HCC

L97.204 Non-pressure chronic ulcer of unspecified calf with necrosis of bone HCC
L97.205 Non-pressure chronic ulcer of unspecified calf with muscle involvement without evidence of necrosis HCC
L97.206 Non-pressure chronic ulcer of unspecified calf with bone involvement without evidence of necrosis HCC
L97.208 Non-pressure chronic ulcer of unspecified calf with other specified severity HCC
L97.209 Non-pressure chronic ulcer of unspecified calf with unspecified severity HCC

6 L97.21 Non-pressure chronic ulcer of right calf
L97.211 Non-pressure chronic ulcer of right calf limited to breakdown of skin HCC
L97.212 Non-pressure chronic ulcer of right calf with fat layer exposed HCC
L97.213 Non-pressure chronic ulcer of right calf with necrosis of muscle HCC
L97.214 Non-pressure chronic ulcer of right calf with necrosis of bone HCC
L97.215 Non-pressure chronic ulcer of right calf with muscle involvement without evidence of necrosis HCC
L97.216 Non-pressure chronic ulcer of right calf with bone involvement without evidence of necrosis HCC
L97.218 Non-pressure chronic ulcer of right calf with other specified severity HCC
L97.219 Non-pressure chronic ulcer of right calf with unspecified severity HCC

6 L97.22 Non-pressure chronic ulcer of left calf
L97.221 Non-pressure chronic ulcer of left calf limited to breakdown of skin HCC
L97.222 Non-pressure chronic ulcer of left calf with fat layer exposed HCC
L97.223 Non-pressure chronic ulcer of left calf with necrosis of muscle HCC
L97.224 Non-pressure chronic ulcer of left calf with necrosis of bone HCC
L97.225 Non-pressure chronic ulcer of left calf with muscle involvement without evidence of necrosis HCC
L97.226 Non-pressure chronic ulcer of left calf with bone involvement without evidence of necrosis HCC
L97.228 Non-pressure chronic ulcer of left calf with other specified severity HCC
L97.229 Non-pressure chronic ulcer of left calf with unspecified severity HCC

5 L97.3 Non-pressure chronic ulcer of ankle

6 L97.30 Non-pressure chronic ulcer of unspecified ankle
L97.301 Non-pressure chronic ulcer of unspecified ankle limited to breakdown of skin HCC
L97.302 Non-pressure chronic ulcer of unspecified ankle with fat layer exposed HCC
L97.303 Non-pressure chronic ulcer of unspecified ankle with necrosis of muscle HCC
L97.304 Non-pressure chronic ulcer of unspecified ankle with necrosis of bone HCC
L97.305 Non-pressure chronic ulcer of unspecified ankle with muscle involvement without evidence of necrosis HCC
L97.306 Non-pressure chronic ulcer of unspecified ankle with bone involvement without evidence of necrosis HCC
L97.308 Non-pressure chronic ulcer of unspecified ankle with other specified severity HCC
L97.309 Non-pressure chronic ulcer of unspecified ankle with unspecified severity HCC

6 L97.31 Non-pressure chronic ulcer of right ankle
L97.311 Non-pressure chronic ulcer of right ankle limited to breakdown of skin HCC
L97.312 Non-pressure chronic ulcer of right ankle with fat layer exposed HCC
L97.313 Non-pressure chronic ulcer of right ankle with necrosis of muscle HCC
L97.314 Non-pressure chronic ulcer of right ankle with necrosis of bone HCC
L97.315 Non-pressure chronic ulcer of right ankle with muscle involvement without evidence of necrosis HCC
AHA: 4Q 2017, 13
L97.316 Non-pressure chronic ulcer of right ankle with bone involvement without evidence of necrosis HCC
L97.318 Non-pressure chronic ulcer of right ankle with other specified severity HCC
L97.319 Non-pressure chronic ulcer of right ankle with unspecified severity HCC

6 L97.32 Non-pressure chronic ulcer of left ankle
L97.321 Non-pressure chronic ulcer of left ankle limited to breakdown of skin HCC
L97.322 Non-pressure chronic ulcer of left ankle with fat layer exposed HCC
L97.323 Non-pressure chronic ulcer of left ankle with necrosis of muscle HCC
L97.324 Non-pressure chronic ulcer of left ankle with necrosis of bone HCC
L97.325 Non-pressure chronic ulcer of left ankle with muscle involvement without evidence of necrosis HCC
L97.326 Non-pressure chronic ulcer of left ankle with bone involvement without evidence of necrosis HCC
L97.328 Non-pressure chronic ulcer of left ankle with other specified severity HCC
L97.329 Non-pressure chronic ulcer of left ankle with unspecified severity HCC

5 L97.4 Non-pressure chronic ulcer of heel and midfoot
Non-pressure chronic ulcer of plantar surface of midfoot

6 L97.40 Non-pressure chronic ulcer of unspecified heel and midfoot
L97.401 Non-pressure chronic ulcer of unspecified heel and midfoot limited to breakdown of skin HCC
L97.402 Non-pressure chronic ulcer of unspecified heel and midfoot with fat layer exposed HCC
L97.403 Non-pressure chronic ulcer of unspecified heel and midfoot with necrosis of muscle HCC
L97.404 Non-pressure chronic ulcer of unspecified heel and midfoot with necrosis of bone HCC
L97.405 Non-pressure chronic ulcer of unspecified heel and midfoot with muscle involvement without evidence of necrosis HCC
L97.406 Non-pressure chronic ulcer of unspecified heel and midfoot with bone involvement without evidence of necrosis HCC
L97.408 Non-pressure chronic ulcer of unspecified heel and midfoot with other specified severity HCC
L97.409 Non-pressure chronic ulcer of unspecified heel and midfoot with unspecified severity HCC

6 L97.41 Non-pressure chronic ulcer of right heel and midfoot
L97.411 Non-pressure chronic ulcer of right heel and midfoot limited to breakdown of skin HCC
L97.412 Non-pressure chronic ulcer of right heel and midfoot with fat layer exposed HCC
L97.413 Non-pressure chronic ulcer of right heel and midfoot with necrosis of muscle HCC
L97.414 Non-pressure chronic ulcer of right heel and midfoot with necrosis of bone HCC
L97.415 Non-pressure chronic ulcer of right heel and midfoot with muscle involvement without evidence of necrosis HCC

L97.416 Non-pressure chronic ulcer of right heel and midfoot with bone involvement without evidence of necrosis HCC
L97.418 Non-pressure chronic ulcer of right heel and midfoot with other specified severity HCC
L97.419 Non-pressure chronic ulcer of right heel and midfoot with unspecified severity HCC
L97.42 Non-pressure chronic ulcer of left heel and midfoot
L97.421 Non-pressure chronic ulcer of left heel and midfoot limited to breakdown of skin HCC
AHA: 1Q 2016, 12-13
L97.422 Non-pressure chronic ulcer of left heel and midfoot with fat layer exposed HCC
L97.423 Non-pressure chronic ulcer of left heel and midfoot with necrosis of muscle HCC
L97.424 Non-pressure chronic ulcer of left heel and midfoot with necrosis of bone HCC
L97.425 Non-pressure chronic ulcer of left heel and midfoot with muscle involvement without evidence of necrosis HCC
L97.426 Non-pressure chronic ulcer of left heel and midfoot with bone involvement without evidence of necrosis HCC
L97.428 Non-pressure chronic ulcer of left heel and midfoot with other specified severity HCC
L97.429 Non-pressure chronic ulcer of left heel and midfoot with unspecified severity HCC
L97.5 Non-pressure chronic ulcer of other part of foot
Non-pressure chronic ulcer of toe
L97.50 Non-pressure chronic ulcer of other part of unspecified foot
L97.501 Non-pressure chronic ulcer of other part of unspecified foot limited to breakdown of skin HCC
L97.502 Non-pressure chronic ulcer of other part of unspecified foot with fat layer exposed HCC
L97.503 Non-pressure chronic ulcer of other part of unspecified foot with necrosis of muscle HCC
L97.504 Non-pressure chronic ulcer of other part of unspecified foot with necrosis of bone HCC
L97.505 Non-pressure chronic ulcer of other part of unspecified foot with muscle involvement without evidence of necrosis HCC
L97.506 Non-pressure chronic ulcer of other part of unspecified foot with bone involvement without evidence of necrosis HCC
L97.508 Non-pressure chronic ulcer of other part of unspecified foot with other specified severity HCC
L97.509 Non-pressure chronic ulcer of other part of unspecified foot with unspecified severity HCC
L97.51 Non-pressure chronic ulcer of other part of right foot
L97.511 Non-pressure chronic ulcer of other part of right foot limited to breakdown of skin HCC
L97.512 Non-pressure chronic ulcer of other part of right foot with fat layer exposed HCC
L97.513 Non-pressure chronic ulcer of other part of right foot with necrosis of muscle HCC
L97.514 Non-pressure chronic ulcer of other part of right foot with necrosis of bone HCC
L97.515 Non-pressure chronic ulcer of other part of right foot with muscle involvement without evidence of necrosis HCC
L97.516 Non-pressure chronic ulcer of other part of right foot with bone involvement without evidence of necrosis HCC
L97.518 Non-pressure chronic ulcer of other part of right foot with other specified severity HCC
L97.519 Non-pressure chronic ulcer of other part of right foot with unspecified severity HCC
L97.52 Non-pressure chronic ulcer of other part of left foot
L97.521 Non-pressure chronic ulcer of other part of left foot limited to breakdown of skin HCC
L97.522 Non-pressure chronic ulcer of other part of left foot with fat layer exposed HCC
L97.523 Non-pressure chronic ulcer of other part of left foot with necrosis of muscle HCC
L97.524 Non-pressure chronic ulcer of other part of left foot with necrosis of bone HCC
L97.525 Non-pressure chronic ulcer of other part of left foot with muscle involvement without evidence of necrosis HCC
L97.526 Non-pressure chronic ulcer of other part of left foot with bone involvement without evidence of necrosis HCC
L97.528 Non-pressure chronic ulcer of other part of left foot with other specified severity HCC
L97.529 Non-pressure chronic ulcer of other part of left foot with unspecified severity HCC
L97.8 Non-pressure chronic ulcer of other part of lower leg
L97.80 Non-pressure chronic ulcer of other part of unspecified lower leg
L97.801 Non-pressure chronic ulcer of other part of unspecified lower leg limited to breakdown of skin HCC
L97.802 Non-pressure chronic ulcer of other part of unspecified lower leg with fat layer exposed HCC
L97.803 Non-pressure chronic ulcer of other part of unspecified lower leg with necrosis of muscle HCC
L97.804 Non-pressure chronic ulcer of other part of unspecified lower leg with necrosis of bone HCC
L97.805 Non-pressure chronic ulcer of other part of unspecified lower leg with muscle involvement without evidence of necrosis HCC
L97.806 Non-pressure chronic ulcer of other part of unspecified lower leg with bone involvement without evidence of necrosis HCC
L97.808 Non-pressure chronic ulcer of other part of unspecified lower leg with other specified severity HCC
L97.809 Non-pressure chronic ulcer of other part of unspecified lower leg with unspecified severity HCC
L97.81 Non-pressure chronic ulcer of other part of right lower leg
L97.811 Non-pressure chronic ulcer of other part of right lower leg limited to breakdown of skin HCC
L97.812 Non-pressure chronic ulcer of other part of right lower leg with fat layer exposed HCC
L97.813 Non-pressure chronic ulcer of other part of right lower leg with necrosis of muscle HCC
L97.814 Non-pressure chronic ulcer of other part of right lower leg with necrosis of bone HCC
L97.815 Non-pressure chronic ulcer of other part of right lower leg with muscle involvement without evidence of necrosis HCC
L97.816 Non-pressure chronic ulcer of other part of right lower leg with bone involvement without evidence of necrosis HCC
L97.818 Non-pressure chronic ulcer of other part of right lower leg with other specified severity HCC
L97.819 Non-pressure chronic ulcer of other part of right lower leg with unspecified severity HCC
L97.82 Non-pressure chronic ulcer of other part of left lower leg
L97.821 Non-pressure chronic ulcer of other part of left lower leg limited to breakdown of skin HCC

L97.822 Non-pressure chronic ulcer of other part of left lower leg with fat layer exposed HCC
L97.823 Non-pressure chronic ulcer of other part of left lower leg with necrosis of muscle HCC
L97.824 Non-pressure chronic ulcer of other part of left lower leg with necrosis of bone HCC
L97.825 Non-pressure chronic ulcer of other part of left lower leg with muscle involvement without evidence of necrosis HCC
L97.826 Non-pressure chronic ulcer of other part of left lower leg with bone involvement without evidence of necrosis HCC
L97.828 Non-pressure chronic ulcer of other part of left lower leg with other specified severity HCC
L97.829 Non-pressure chronic ulcer of other part of left lower leg with unspecified severity HCC

L97.9 Non-pressure chronic ulcer of unspecified part of lower leg

L97.90 Non-pressure chronic ulcer of unspecified part of unspecified lower leg

L97.901 Non-pressure chronic ulcer of unspecified part of unspecified lower leg limited to breakdown of skin HCC
L97.902 Non-pressure chronic ulcer of unspecified part of unspecified lower leg with fat layer exposed HCC
L97.903 Non-pressure chronic ulcer of unspecified part of unspecified lower leg with necrosis of muscle HCC
L97.904 Non-pressure chronic ulcer of unspecified part of unspecified lower leg with necrosis of bone HCC
L97.905 Non-pressure chronic ulcer of unspecified part of unspecified lower leg with muscle involvement without evidence of necrosis HCC
L97.906 Non-pressure chronic ulcer of unspecified part of unspecified lower leg with bone involvement without evidence of necrosis HCC
L97.908 Non-pressure chronic ulcer of unspecified part of unspecified lower leg with other specified severity HCC
L97.909 Non-pressure chronic ulcer of unspecified part of unspecified lower leg with unspecified severity HCC

L97.91 Non-pressure chronic ulcer of unspecified part of right lower leg

L97.911 Non-pressure chronic ulcer of unspecified part of right lower leg limited to breakdown of skin HCC
L97.912 Non-pressure chronic ulcer of unspecified part of right lower leg with fat layer exposed HCC
L97.913 Non-pressure chronic ulcer of unspecified part of right lower leg with necrosis of muscle HCC
L97.914 Non-pressure chronic ulcer of unspecified part of right lower leg with necrosis of bone HCC
L97.915 Non-pressure chronic ulcer of unspecified part of right lower leg with muscle involvement without evidence of necrosis HCC
L97.916 Non-pressure chronic ulcer of unspecified part of right lower leg with bone involvement without evidence of necrosis HCC
L97.918 Non-pressure chronic ulcer of unspecified part of right lower leg with other specified severity HCC
L97.919 Non-pressure chronic ulcer of unspecified part of right lower leg with unspecified severity HCC

L97.92 Non-pressure chronic ulcer of unspecified part of left lower leg

L97.921 Non-pressure chronic ulcer of unspecified part of left lower leg limited to breakdown of skin HCC
L97.922 Non-pressure chronic ulcer of unspecified part of left lower leg with fat layer exposed HCC
L97.923 Non-pressure chronic ulcer of unspecified part of left lower leg with necrosis of muscle HCC
L97.924 Non-pressure chronic ulcer of unspecified part of left lower leg with necrosis of bone HCC
L97.925 Non-pressure chronic ulcer of unspecified part of left lower leg with muscle involvement without evidence of necrosis HCC
L97.926 Non-pressure chronic ulcer of unspecified part of left lower leg with bone involvement without evidence of necrosis HCC
L97.928 Non-pressure chronic ulcer of unspecified part of left lower leg with other specified severity HCC
L97.929 Non-pressure chronic ulcer of unspecified part of left lower leg with unspecified severity HCC

L98 Other disorders of skin and subcutaneous tissue, not elsewhere classified

L98.0 Pyogenic granuloma

EXCLUDES 2 *pyogenic granuloma of gingiva (K06.8)*
pyogenic granuloma of maxillary alveolar ridge (K04.5)
pyogenic granuloma of oral mucosa (K13.4)

L98.1 Factitial dermatitis

Neurotic excoriation

EXCLUDES 1 *Excoriation (skin-picking) disorder (F42.4)*

CODING TIP ✓ Factitial dermatitis, L98.1, may also be referred to as neurotic excoriation or dermatitis artefacta and is characterized by deliberate, self-inflicted skin lesions produced as a result of underlying psychological conditions. When specified, any underlying or additional psychological conditions should also be coded. An example of a psychological condition is obsessive-compulsive disorder (F42).

L98.2 Febrile neutrophilic dermatosis [Sweet]

L98.3 Eosinophilic cellulitis [Wells]

L98.4 Non-pressure chronic ulcer of skin, not elsewhere classified

Chronic ulcer of skin NOS
Tropical ulcer NOS
Ulcer of skin NOS

EXCLUDES 2 *pressure ulcer (pressure area) (L89.-)*
gangrene (I96)
skin infections (L00-L08)
specific infections classified to A00-B99
ulcer of lower limb NEC (L97.-)
varicose ulcer (I83.0-I82.2)

L98.41 Non-pressure chronic ulcer of buttock

L98.411 Non-pressure chronic ulcer of buttock limited to breakdown of skin HCC
L98.412 Non-pressure chronic ulcer of buttock with fat layer exposed HCC
L98.413 Non-pressure chronic ulcer of buttock with necrosis of muscle HCC
L98.414 Non-pressure chronic ulcer of buttock with necrosis of bone HCC
L98.415 Non-pressure chronic ulcer of buttock with muscle involvement without evidence of necrosis HCC
L98.416 Non-pressure chronic ulcer of buttock with bone involvement without evidence of necrosis HCC
L98.418 Non-pressure chronic ulcer of buttock with other specified severity HCC
L98.419 Non-pressure chronic ulcer of buttock with unspecified severity HCC

L98.42 Non-pressure chronic ulcer of back

L98.421 Non-pressure chronic ulcer of back limited to breakdown of skin HCC

● New | Manifestation | 4-7 Digit Indicators | Laterality | A Adult | M Maternity | N Newborn | P Pediatric | ♂ Male
▲ Revised | Unspecified | AHA Coding Clinic | HCC Hierarchical Condition Categories | HIV HIV Related Conditions | ♀ Female

L98.422 Non-pressure chronic ulcer of back with fat layer exposed HCC

L98.423 Non-pressure chronic ulcer of back with necrosis of muscle HCC

L98.424 Non-pressure chronic ulcer of back with necrosis of bone HCC

L98.425 Non-pressure chronic ulcer of back with muscle involvement without evidence of necrosis HCC

L98.426 Non-pressure chronic ulcer of back with bone involvement without evidence of necrosis HCC

L98.428 Non-pressure chronic ulcer of back with other specified severity HCC

L98.429 Non-pressure chronic ulcer of back with unspecified severity HCC

6 **L98.49 Non-pressure chronic ulcer of skin of other sites**

Non-pressure chronic ulcer of skin NOS

L98.491 Non-pressure chronic ulcer of skin of other sites limited to breakdown of skin HCC

L98.492 Non-pressure chronic ulcer of skin of other sites with fat layer exposed HCC

L98.493 Non-pressure chronic ulcer of skin of other sites with necrosis of muscle HCC

L98.494 Non-pressure chronic ulcer of skin of other sites with necrosis of bone HCC

▲ L98.495 Non-pressure chronic ulcer of skin of other sites with muscle involvement without evidence of necrosis HCC

▲ L98.496 Non-pressure chronic ulcer of skin of other sites with bone involvement without evidence of necrosis HCC

▲ L98.498 Non-pressure chronic ulcer of skin of other sites with other specified severity HCC

L98.499 Non-pressure chronic ulcer of skin of other sites with unspecified severity HCC

L98.5 Mucinosis of the skin

Focal mucinosis

Lichen myxedematosus

Reticular erythematous mucinosis

EXCLUDES 1 *focal oral mucinosis (K13.79)*
myxedema (E03.9)

L98.6 Other infiltrative disorders of the skin and subcutaneous tissue

EXCLUDES 1 *hyalinosis cutis et mucosae (E78.89)*

L98.7 Excessive and redundant skin and subcutaneous tissue

Loose or sagging skin following bariatric surgery weight loss

Loose or sagging skin following dietary weight loss

Loose or sagging skin, NOS

EXCLUDES 2 *acquired excess or redundant skin of eyelid (H02.3-)*
congenital excess or redundant skin of eyelid (Q10.3)
skin changes due to chronic exposure to nonionizing radiation (L57.-)

AHA: 4Q 2016, 36

L98.8 Other specified disorders of the skin and subcutaneous tissue

AHA: 2Q 2013, 31-32

L98.9 Disorder of the skin and subcutaneous tissue, unspecified

L99 *Other disorders of skin and subcutaneous tissue in diseases classified elsewhere*

Code first underlying disease, such as:
amyloidosis (E85.-)

EXCLUDES 1 *skin disorders in diabetes (E08-E13 with .62)*
skin disorders in gonorrhea (A54.89)
skin disorders in syphilis (A51.31, A52.79)

CHAPTER 13: DISEASES OF THE MUSCULOSKELETAL SYSTEM AND CONNECTIVE TISSUE (M00-M99)

Note: Use an external cause code following the code for the musculoskeletal condition, if applicable, to identify the cause of the musculoskeletal condition

EXCLUDES 2 *arthropathic psoriasis (L40.5-)*
certain conditions originating in the perinatal period (P04-P96)
certain infectious and parasitic diseases (A00-B99)
compartment syndrome (traumatic) (T79.A-)
complications of pregnancy, childbirth and the puerperium (O00-O9A)
congenital malformations, deformations, and chromosomal abnormalities (Q00-Q99)
endocrine, nutritional and metabolic diseases (E00-E88)
injury, poisoning and certain other consequences of external causes (S00-T88)
neoplasms (C00-D49)
symptoms, signs and abnormal clinical and laboratory findings, not elsewhere classified (R00-R94)

GUIDELINES **Section I.C.13.a**
Most of the codes within Chapter 13 have site and laterality designations. The site represents the bone, joint or the muscle involved. For some conditions where more than one bone, joint or muscle is usually involved, such as osteoarthritis, there is a "multiple sites" code available. For categories where no multiple site code is provided and more than one bone, joint or muscle is involved, multiple codes should be used to indicate the different sites involved.

GUIDELINES **Section I.C.13.a.1)**
For certain conditions, the bone may be affected at the upper or lower end, (e.g., avascular necrosis of bone, M87, Osteoporosis, M80, M81). Though the portion of the bone affected may be at the joint, the site designation will be the bone, not the joint.

GUIDELINES **Section I.C.13.b**
Many musculoskeletal conditions are a result of previous injury or trauma to a site, or are recurrent conditions. Bone, joint or muscle conditions that are the result of a healed injury are usually found in chapter 13. Recurrent bone, joint or muscle conditions are also usually found in chapter 13. Any current, acute injury should be coded to the appropriate injury code from chapter 19. Chronic or recurrent conditions should generally be coded with a code from chapter 13. If it is difficult to determine from the documentation in the record which code is best to describe a condition, query the provider.

This chapter contains the following blocks:

M00-M02	Infectious arthropathies
M04	Autoinflammatory syndromes
M05-M14	Inflammatory polyarthropathies
M15-M19	Osteoarthritis
M20-M25	Other joint disorders
M26-M27	Dentofacial anomalies [including malocclusion] and other disorders of jaw
M30-M36	Systemic connective tissue disorders
M40-M43	Deforming dorsopathies
M45-M49	Spondylopathies
M50-M54	Other dorsopathies
M60-M63	Disorders of muscles
M65-M67	Disorders of synovium and tendon
M70-M79	Other soft tissue disorders
M80-M85	Disorders of bone density and structure
M86-M90	Other osteopathies
M91-M94	Chondropathies
M95	Other disorders of the musculoskeletal system and connective tissue
M96	Intraoperative and postprocedural complications and disorders of musculoskeletal system, not elsewhere classified
M97	Periprosthetic fracture around internal prosthetic joint
M99	Biomechanical lesions, not elsewhere classified

Arthropathies (M00-M25)

INCLUDES Disorders affecting predominantly peripheral (limb) joints

Infectious arthropathies (M00-M02)

Note: This block comprises arthropathies due to microbiological agents.
Distinction is made between the following types of etiological relationship:
a) direct infection of joint, where organisms invade synovial tissue and microbial antigen is present in the joint;
b) indirect infection, which may be of two types: a reactive arthropathy, where microbial infection of the body is established but neither organisms nor antigens can be identified in the joint, and a postinfective arthropathy, where microbial antigen is present but recovery of an organism is inconstant and evidence of local multiplication is lacking.

4 **M00 Pyogenic arthritis**

5 **M00.0 Staphylococcal arthritis and polyarthritis**
Use additional code (B95.61-B95.8) to identify bacterial agent
EXCLUDES 2 *infection and inflammatory reaction due to internal joint prosthesis (T84.5-)*

M00.00 Staphylococcal arthritis, unspecified joint HCC
6 **M00.01 Staphylococcal arthritis, shoulder**
- **M00.011 Staphylococcal arthritis, right shoulder** HCC
- **M00.012 Staphylococcal arthritis, left shoulder** HCC
- **M00.019 Staphylococcal arthritis, unspecified shoulder** HCC

6 **M00.02 Staphylococcal arthritis, elbow**
- **M00.021 Staphylococcal arthritis, right elbow** HCC
- **M00.022 Staphylococcal arthritis, left elbow** HCC
- **M00.029 Staphylococcal arthritis, unspecified elbow** HCC

6 **M00.03 Staphylococcal arthritis, wrist**
Staphylococcal arthritis of carpal bones
- **M00.031 Staphylococcal arthritis, right wrist** HCC
- **M00.032 Staphylococcal arthritis, left wrist** HCC
- **M00.039 Staphylococcal arthritis, unspecified wrist** HCC

6 **M00.04 Staphylococcal arthritis, hand**
Staphylococcal arthritis of metacarpus and phalanges
- **M00.041 Staphylococcal arthritis, right hand** HCC
- **M00.042 Staphylococcal arthritis, left hand** HCC
- **M00.049 Staphylococcal arthritis, unspecified hand** HCC

6 **M00.05 Staphylococcal arthritis, hip**
- **M00.051 Staphylococcal arthritis, right hip** HCC
- **M00.052 Staphylococcal arthritis, left hip** HCC
- **M00.059 Staphylococcal arthritis, unspecified hip** HCC

6 **M00.06 Staphylococcal arthritis, knee**
- **M00.061 Staphylococcal arthritis, right knee** HCC
- **M00.062 Staphylococcal arthritis, left knee** HCC
- **M00.069 Staphylococcal arthritis, unspecified knee** HCC

6 **M00.07 Staphylococcal arthritis, ankle and foot**
Staphylococcal arthritis, tarsus, metatarsus and phalanges
- **M00.071 Staphylococcal arthritis, right ankle and foot** HCC
- **M00.072 Staphylococcal arthritis, left ankle and foot** HCC
- **M00.079 Staphylococcal arthritis, unspecified ankle and foot** HCC

M00.08 Staphylococcal arthritis, vertebrae HCC
M00.09 Staphylococcal polyarthritis HCC

5 **M00.1 Pneumococcal arthritis and polyarthritis**

M00.10 Pneumococcal arthritis, unspecified joint HCC
6 **M00.11 Pneumococcal arthritis, shoulder**
- **M00.111 Pneumococcal arthritis, right shoulder** HCC
- **M00.112 Pneumococcal arthritis, left shoulder** HCC
- **M00.119 Pneumococcal arthritis, unspecified shoulder** HCC

6 **M00.12 Pneumococcal arthritis, elbow**
- **M00.121 Pneumococcal arthritis, right elbow** HCC
- **M00.122 Pneumococcal arthritis, left elbow** HCC
- **M00.129 Pneumococcal arthritis, unspecified elbow** HCC

6 **M00.13 Pneumococcal arthritis, wrist**
Pneumococcal arthritis of carpal bones
- **M00.131 Pneumococcal arthritis, right wrist** HCC
- **M00.132 Pneumococcal arthritis, left wrist** HCC

M00.139 Pneumococcal arthritis, unspecified wrist HCC

M00.14 Pneumococcal arthritis, hand
Pneumococcal arthritis of metacarpus and phalanges

M00.141 Pneumococcal arthritis, right hand HCC

M00.142 Pneumococcal arthritis, left hand HCC

M00.149 Pneumococcal arthritis, unspecified hand HCC

M00.15 Pneumococcal arthritis, hip

M00.151 Pneumococcal arthritis, right hip HCC

M00.152 Pneumococcal arthritis, left hip HCC

M00.159 Pneumococcal arthritis, unspecified hip HCC

M00.16 Pneumococcal arthritis, knee

M00.161 Pneumococcal arthritis, right knee HCC

M00.162 Pneumococcal arthritis, left knee HCC

M00.169 Pneumococcal arthritis, unspecified knee HCC

M00.17 Pneumococcal arthritis, ankle and foot
Pneumococcal arthritis, tarsus, metatarsus and phalanges

M00.171 Pneumococcal arthritis, right ankle and foot HCC

M00.172 Pneumococcal arthritis, left ankle and foot HCC

M00.179 Pneumococcal arthritis, unspecified ankle and foot HCC

M00.18 Pneumococcal arthritis, vertebrae HCC

M00.19 Pneumococcal polyarthritis HCC

M00.2 Other streptococcal arthritis and polyarthritis
Use additional code (B95.0-B95.2, B95.4-B95.5) to identify bacterial agent

M00.20 Other streptococcal arthritis, unspecified joint HCC

M00.21 Other streptococcal arthritis, shoulder

M00.211 Other streptococcal arthritis, right shoulder HCC

M00.212 Other streptococcal arthritis, left shoulder HCC

M00.219 Other streptococcal arthritis, unspecified shoulder HCC

M00.22 Other streptococcal arthritis, elbow

M00.221 Other streptococcal arthritis, right elbow HCC

M00.222 Other streptococcal arthritis, left elbow HCC

M00.229 Other streptococcal arthritis, unspecified elbow HCC

M00.23 Other streptococcal arthritis, wrist
Other streptococcal arthritis of carpal bones

M00.231 Other streptococcal arthritis, right wrist HCC

M00.232 Other streptococcal arthritis, left wrist HCC

M00.239 Other streptococcal arthritis, unspecified wrist HCC

M00.24 Other streptococcal arthritis, hand
Other streptococcal arthritis metacarpus and phalanges

M00.241 Other streptococcal arthritis, right hand HCC

M00.242 Other streptococcal arthritis, left hand HCC

M00.249 Other streptococcal arthritis, unspecified hand HCC

M00.25 Other streptococcal arthritis, hip

M00.251 Other streptococcal arthritis, right hip HCC

M00.252 Other streptococcal arthritis, left hip HCC

M00.259 Other streptococcal arthritis, unspecified hip HCC

M00.26 Other streptococcal arthritis, knee

M00.261 Other streptococcal arthritis, right knee HCC

M00.262 Other streptococcal arthritis, left knee HCC

M00.269 Other streptococcal arthritis, unspecified knee HCC

M00.27 Other streptococcal arthritis, ankle and foot
Other streptococcal arthritis, tarsus, metatarsus and phalanges

M00.271 Other streptococcal arthritis, right ankle and foot HCC

M00.272 Other streptococcal arthritis, left ankle and foot HCC

M00.279 Other streptococcal arthritis, unspecified ankle and foot HCC

M00.28 Other streptococcal arthritis, vertebrae HCC

M00.29 Other streptococcal polyarthritis HCC

M00.8 Arthritis and polyarthritis due to other bacteria
Use additional code (B96) to identify bacteria

M00.80 Arthritis due to other bacteria, unspecified joint HCC

M00.81 Arthritis due to other bacteria, shoulder

M00.811 Arthritis due to other bacteria, right shoulder HCC

M00.812 Arthritis due to other bacteria, left shoulder HCC

M00.819 Arthritis due to other bacteria, unspecified shoulder HCC

M00.82 Arthritis due to other bacteria, elbow

M00.821 Arthritis due to other bacteria, right elbow HCC

M00.822 Arthritis due to other bacteria, left elbow HCC

M00.829 Arthritis due to other bacteria, unspecified elbow HCC

M00.83 Arthritis due to other bacteria, wrist
Arthritis due to other bacteria, carpal bones

M00.831 Arthritis due to other bacteria, right wrist HCC

M00.832 Arthritis due to other bacteria, left wrist HCC

M00.839 Arthritis due to other bacteria, unspecified wrist HCC

M00.84 Arthritis due to other bacteria, hand
Arthritis due to other bacteria, metacarpus and phalanges

M00.841 Arthritis due to other bacteria, right hand HCC

M00.842 Arthritis due to other bacteria, left hand HCC

M00.849 Arthritis due to other bacteria, unspecified hand HCC

M00.85 Arthritis due to other bacteria, hip

M00.851 Arthritis due to other bacteria, right hip HCC

M00.852 Arthritis due to other bacteria, left hip HCC

M00.859 Arthritis due to other bacteria, unspecified hip HCC

M00.86 Arthritis due to other bacteria, knee

M00.861 Arthritis due to other bacteria, right knee HCC

M00.862 Arthritis due to other bacteria, left knee HCC

M00.869 Arthritis due to other bacteria, unspecified knee HCC

M00.87 Arthritis due to other bacteria, ankle and foot
Arthritis due to other bacteria, tarsus, metatarsus, and phalanges

M00.871 Arthritis due to other bacteria, right ankle and foot HCC

M00.872 Arthritis due to other bacteria, left ankle and foot HCC

M00.879 Arthritis due to other bacteria, unspecified ankle and foot HCC

M00.88 Arthritis due to other bacteria, vertebrae HCC

M00.89 Polyarthritis due to other bacteria HCC

M00.9 Pyogenic arthritis, unspecified HCC
Infective arthritis NOS

M01 Direct infections of joint in infectious and parasitic diseases classified elsewhere

Code first underlying disease, such as:
leprosy [Hansen's disease] (A30.-)
mycoses (B35-B49)
O'nyong-nyong fever (A92.1)
paratyphoid fever (A01.1-A01.4)

EXCLUDES 1
arthropathy in Lyme disease (A69.23)
gonococcal arthritis (A54.42)
meningococcal arthritis (A39.83)
mumps arthritis (B26.85)
postinfective arthropathy (M02.-)
postmeningococcal arthritis (A39.84)
reactive arthritis (M02.3)
rubella arthritis (B06.82)
sarcoidosis arthritis (D86.86)
typhoid fever arthritis (A01.04)
tuberculosis arthritis (A18.01-A18.02)

M01.X Direct infection of joint in infectious and parasitic diseases classified elsewhere

● New ▲ Revised *Manifestation* Unspecified 4-7 Digit Indicators AHA Coding Clinic Laterality HCC Hierarchical Condition Categories A Adult M Maternity N Newborn HIV HIV Related Conditions P Pediatric ♂ Male ♀ Female

M01.X0 *Direct infection of unspecified joint in infectious and parasitic diseases classified elsewhere* HCC

M01.X1 Direct infection of shoulder joint in infectious and parasitic diseases classified elsewhere

- **M01.X11** *Direct infection of right shoulder in infectious and parasitic diseases classified elsewhere* HCC
- **M01.X12** *Direct infection of left shoulder in infectious and parasitic diseases classified elsewhere* HCC
- **M01.X19** *Direct infection of unspecified shoulder in infectious and parasitic diseases classified elsewhere* HCC

M01.X2 Direct infection of elbow in infectious and parasitic diseases classified elsewhere

- **M01.X21** *Direct infection of right elbow in infectious and parasitic diseases classified elsewhere* HCC
- **M01.X22** *Direct infection of left elbow in infectious and parasitic diseases classified elsewhere* HCC
- **M01.X29** *Direct infection of unspecified elbow in infectious and parasitic diseases classified elsewhere* HCC

M01.X3 Direct infection of wrist in infectious and parasitic diseases classified elsewhere

Direct infection of carpal bones in infectious and parasitic diseases classified elsewhere

- **M01.X31** *Direct infection of right wrist in infectious and parasitic diseases classified elsewhere* HCC
- **M01.X32** *Direct infection of left wrist in infectious and parasitic diseases classified elsewhere* HCC
- **M01.X39** *Direct infection of unspecified wrist in infectious and parasitic diseases classified elsewhere* HCC

M01.X4 Direct infection of hand in infectious and parasitic diseases classified elsewhere

Direct infection of metacarpus and phalanges in infectious and parasitic diseases classified elsewhere

- **M01.X41** *Direct infection of right hand in infectious and parasitic diseases classified elsewhere* HCC
- **M01.X42** *Direct infection of left hand in infectious and parasitic diseases classified elsewhere* HCC
- **M01.X49** *Direct infection of unspecified hand in infectious and parasitic diseases classified elsewhere* HCC

M01.X5 Direct infection of hip in infectious and parasitic diseases classified elsewhere

- **M01.X51** *Direct infection of right hip in infectious and parasitic diseases classified elsewhere* HCC
- **M01.X52** *Direct infection of left hip in infectious and parasitic diseases classified elsewhere* HCC
- **M01.X59** *Direct infection of unspecified hip in infectious and parasitic diseases classified elsewhere* HCC

M01.X6 Direct infection of knee in infectious and parasitic diseases classified elsewhere

- **M01.X61** *Direct infection of right knee in infectious and parasitic diseases classified elsewhere* HCC
- **M01.X62** *Direct infection of left knee in infectious and parasitic diseases classified elsewhere* HCC
- **M01.X69** *Direct infection of unspecified knee in infectious and parasitic diseases classified elsewhere* HCC

M01.X7 Direct infection of ankle and foot in infectious and parasitic diseases classified elsewhere

Direct infection of tarsus, metatarsus and phalanges in infectious and parasitic diseases classified elsewhere

- **M01.X71** *Direct infection of right ankle and foot in infectious and parasitic diseases classified elsewhere* HCC
- **M01.X72** *Direct infection of left ankle and foot in infectious and parasitic diseases classified elsewhere* HCC
- **M01.X79** *Direct infection of unspecified ankle and foot in infectious and parasitic diseases classified elsewhere* HCC

M01.X8 *Direct infection of vertebrae in infectious and parasitic diseases classified elsewhere* HCC

M01.X9 *Direct infection of multiple joints in infectious and parasitic diseases classified elsewhere* HCC

M02 Postinfective and reactive arthropathies

Code first underlying disease, such as:
- congenital syphilis [Clutton's joints] (A50.5)
- enteritis due to Yersinia enterocolitica (A04.6)
- infective endocarditis (I33.0)
- viral hepatitis (B15-B19)

EXCLUDES 1 *Behçet's disease (M35.2)*
direct infections of joint in infectious and parasitic diseases classified elsewhere (M01.-)
postmeningococcal arthritis (A39.84)
mumps arthritis (B26.85)
rubella arthritis (B06.82)
syphilis arthritis (late) (A52.77)
rheumatic fever (I00)
tabetic arthropathy [Charcôt's] (A52.16)

CODING TIP ✓ M02.- codes indicate arthropathy due to another cause. The identified underlying cause should be coded first.

M02.0 Arthropathy following intestinal bypass

M02.00 Arthropathy following intestinal bypass, unspecified site

M02.01 Arthropathy following intestinal bypass, shoulder

- **M02.011 Arthropathy following intestinal bypass, right shoulder**
- **M02.012 Arthropathy following intestinal bypass, left shoulder**
- **M02.019 Arthropathy following intestinal bypass, unspecified shoulder**

M02.02 Arthropathy following intestinal bypass, elbow

- **M02.021 Arthropathy following intestinal bypass, right elbow**
- **M02.022 Arthropathy following intestinal bypass, left elbow**
- **M02.029 Arthropathy following intestinal bypass, unspecified elbow**

M02.03 Arthropathy following intestinal bypass, wrist

Arthropathy following intestinal bypass, carpal bones

- **M02.031 Arthropathy following intestinal bypass, right wrist**
- **M02.032 Arthropathy following intestinal bypass, left wrist**
- **M02.039 Arthropathy following intestinal bypass, unspecified wrist**

M02.04 Arthropathy following intestinal bypass, hand

Arthropathy following intestinal bypass, metacarpals and phalanges

- **M02.041 Arthropathy following intestinal bypass, right hand**
- **M02.042 Arthropathy following intestinal bypass, left hand**
- **M02.049 Arthropathy following intestinal bypass, unspecified hand**

M02.05 Arthropathy following intestinal bypass, hip

- **M02.051 Arthropathy following intestinal bypass, right hip**
- **M02.052 Arthropathy following intestinal bypass, left hip**
- **M02.059 Arthropathy following intestinal bypass, unspecified hip**

M02.06 Arthropathy following intestinal bypass, knee

- **M02.061 Arthropathy following intestinal bypass, right knee**
- **M02.062 Arthropathy following intestinal bypass, left knee**
- **M02.069 Arthropathy following intestinal bypass, unspecified knee**

M02.07 Arthropathy following intestinal bypass, ankle and foot

Arthropathy following intestinal bypass, tarsus, metatarsus and phalanges

- **M02.071 Arthropathy following intestinal bypass, right ankle and foot**

Diseases of the Musculoskeletal System and Connective Tissue

M01.X0 — M02.071

M02.072 Arthropathy following intestinal bypass, left ankle and foot
M02.079 Arthropathy following intestinal bypass, unspecified ankle and foot
M02.08 Arthropathy following intestinal bypass, vertebrae
M02.09 Arthropathy following intestinal bypass, multiple sites
M02.1 Postdysenteric arthropathy
M02.10 Postdysenteric arthropathy, unspecified site HCC
M02.11 Postdysenteric arthropathy, shoulder
M02.111 Postdysenteric arthropathy, right shoulder HCC
M02.112 Postdysenteric arthropathy, left shoulder HCC
M02.119 Postdysenteric arthropathy, unspecified shoulder HCC
M02.12 Postdysenteric arthropathy, elbow
M02.121 Postdysenteric arthropathy, right elbow HCC
M02.122 Postdysenteric arthropathy, left elbow HCC
M02.129 Postdysenteric arthropathy, unspecified elbow HCC
M02.13 Postdysenteric arthropathy, wrist
Postdysenteric arthropathy, carpal bones
M02.131 Postdysenteric arthropathy, right wrist HCC
M02.132 Postdysenteric arthropathy, left wrist HCC
M02.139 Postdysenteric arthropathy, unspecified wrist HCC
M02.14 Postdysenteric arthropathy, hand
Postdysenteric arthropathy, metacarpus and phalanges
M02.141 Postdysenteric arthropathy, right hand HCC
M02.142 Postdysenteric arthropathy, left hand HCC
M02.149 Postdysenteric arthropathy, unspecified hand HCC
M02.15 Postdysenteric arthropathy, hip
M02.151 Postdysenteric arthropathy, right hip HCC
M02.152 Postdysenteric arthropathy, left hip HCC
M02.159 Postdysenteric arthropathy, unspecified hip HCC
M02.16 Postdysenteric arthropathy, knee
M02.161 Postdysenteric arthropathy, right knee HCC
M02.162 Postdysenteric arthropathy, left knee HCC
M02.169 Postdysenteric arthropathy, unspecified knee HCC
M02.17 Postdysenteric arthropathy, ankle and foot
Postdysenteric arthropathy, tarsus, metatarsus and phalanges
M02.171 Postdysenteric arthropathy, right ankle and foot HCC
M02.172 Postdysenteric arthropathy, left ankle and foot HCC
M02.179 Postdysenteric arthropathy, unspecified ankle and foot HCC
M02.18 Postdysenteric arthropathy, vertebrae HCC
M02.19 Postdysenteric arthropathy, multiple sites HCC
M02.2 Postimmunization arthropathy
M02.20 Postimmunization arthropathy, unspecified site
M02.21 Postimmunization arthropathy, shoulder
M02.211 Postimmunization arthropathy, right shoulder
M02.212 Postimmunization arthropathy, left shoulder
M02.219 Postimmunization arthropathy, unspecified shoulder
M02.22 Postimmunization arthropathy, elbow
M02.221 Postimmunization arthropathy, right elbow
M02.222 Postimmunization arthropathy, left elbow
M02.229 Postimmunization arthropathy, unspecified elbow
M02.23 Postimmunization arthropathy, wrist
Postimmunization arthropathy, carpal bones
M02.231 Postimmunization arthropathy, right wrist
M02.232 Postimmunization arthropathy, left wrist
M02.239 Postimmunization arthropathy, unspecified wrist
M02.24 Postimmunization arthropathy, hand
Postimmunization arthropathy, metacarpus and phalanges
M02.241 Postimmunization arthropathy, right hand
M02.242 Postimmunization arthropathy, left hand
M02.249 Postimmunization arthropathy, unspecified hand
M02.25 Postimmunization arthropathy, hip
M02.251 Postimmunization arthropathy, right hip
M02.252 Postimmunization arthropathy, left hip
M02.259 Postimmunization arthropathy, unspecified hip
M02.26 Postimmunization arthropathy, knee
M02.261 Postimmunization arthropathy, right knee
M02.262 Postimmunization arthropathy, left knee
M02.269 Postimmunization arthropathy, unspecified knee
M02.27 Postimmunization arthropathy, ankle and foot
Postimmunization arthropathy, tarsus, metatarsus and phalanges
M02.271 Postimmunization arthropathy, right ankle and foot
M02.272 Postimmunization arthropathy, left ankle and foot
M02.279 Postimmunization arthropathy, unspecified ankle and foot
M02.28 Postimmunization arthropathy, vertebrae
M02.29 Postimmunization arthropathy, multiple sites
M02.3 Reiter's disease
Reactive arthritis
M02.30 Reiter's disease, unspecified site HCC
M02.31 Reiter's disease, shoulder
M02.311 Reiter's disease, right shoulder HCC
M02.312 Reiter's disease, left shoulder HCC
M02.319 Reiter's disease, unspecified shoulder HCC
M02.32 Reiter's disease, elbow
M02.321 Reiter's disease, right elbow HCC
M02.322 Reiter's disease, left elbow HCC
M02.329 Reiter's disease, unspecified elbow HCC
M02.33 Reiter's disease, wrist
Reiter's disease, carpal bones
M02.331 Reiter's disease, right wrist HCC
M02.332 Reiter's disease, left wrist HCC
M02.339 Reiter's disease, unspecified wrist HCC
M02.34 Reiter's disease, hand
Reiter's disease, metacarpus and phalanges
M02.341 Reiter's disease, right hand HCC
M02.342 Reiter's disease, left hand HCC
M02.349 Reiter's disease, unspecified hand HCC
M02.35 Reiter's disease, hip
M02.351 Reiter's disease, right hip HCC
M02.352 Reiter's disease, left hip HCC
M02.359 Reiter's disease, unspecified hip HCC
M02.36 Reiter's disease, knee
M02.361 Reiter's disease, right knee HCC
M02.362 Reiter's disease, left knee HCC
M02.369 Reiter's disease, unspecified knee HCC
M02.37 Reiter's disease, ankle and foot
Reiter's disease, tarsus, metatarsus and phalanges
M02.371 Reiter's disease, right ankle and foot HCC
M02.372 Reiter's disease, left ankle and foot HCC
M02.379 Reiter's disease, unspecified ankle and foot HCC
M02.38 Reiter's disease, vertebrae HCC
M02.39 Reiter's disease, multiple sites HCC
M02.8 Other reactive arthropathies
M02.80 *Other reactive arthropathies, unspecified site* HCC
M02.81 Other reactive arthropathies, shoulder
M02.811 *Other reactive arthropathies, right shoulder* HCC
M02.812 *Other reactive arthropathies, left shoulder* HCC

M02.819 *Other reactive arthropathies, unspecified shoulder* HCC

M02.82 **Other reactive arthropathies, elbow**

M02.821 *Other reactive arthropathies, right elbow* HCC

M02.822 *Other reactive arthropathies, left elbow* HCC

M02.829 *Other reactive arthropathies, unspecified elbow* HCC

M02.83 **Other reactive arthropathies, wrist**

Other reactive arthropathies, carpal bones

M02.831 *Other reactive arthropathies, right wrist* HCC

M02.832 *Other reactive arthropathies, left wrist* HCC

M02.839 *Other reactive arthropathies, unspecified wrist* HCC

M02.84 **Other reactive arthropathies, hand**

Other reactive arthropathies, metacarpus and phalanges

M02.841 *Other reactive arthropathies, right hand* HCC

M02.842 *Other reactive arthropathies, left hand* HCC

M02.849 *Other reactive arthropathies, unspecified hand* HCC

M02.85 **Other reactive arthropathies, hip**

M02.851 *Other reactive arthropathies, right hip* HCC

M02.852 *Other reactive arthropathies, left hip* HCC

M02.859 *Other reactive arthropathies, unspecified hip* HCC

M02.86 **Other reactive arthropathies, knee**

M02.861 *Other reactive arthropathies, right knee* HCC

M02.862 *Other reactive arthropathies, left knee* HCC

M02.869 *Other reactive arthropathies, unspecified knee* HCC

M02.87 **Other reactive arthropathies, ankle and foot**

Other reactive arthropathies, tarsus, metatarsus and phalanges

M02.871 *Other reactive arthropathies, right ankle and foot* HCC

M02.872 *Other reactive arthropathies, left ankle and foot* HCC

M02.879 *Other reactive arthropathies, unspecified ankle and foot* HCC

M02.88 *Other reactive arthropathies, vertebrae* HCC

M02.89 *Other reactive arthropathies, multiple sites* HCC

M02.9 *Reactive arthropathy, unspecified* HCC

Autoinflammatory syndromes (M04)

M04 **Autoinflammatory syndromes**

EXCLUDES 2 *Crohn's disease (K50.-)*

AHA: 4Q 2016, 37

M04.1 **Periodic fever syndromes** HCC

Familial Mediterranean fever
Hyperimmunoglobin D syndrome
Mevalonate kinase deficiency
Tumor necrosis factor receptor associated periodic syndrome [TRAPS]

DEFINITION The disease is characterized by recurrent attacks of fever; intense inflammatory response pain in the abdomen, joints, and chest; and red, swollen skin lesions; it often leads to kidney failure.

M04.2 **Cryopyrin-associated periodic syndromes** HCC

Chronic infantile neurological, cutaneous and articular syndrome [CINCA]
Familial cold autoinflammatory syndrome
Familial cold urticaria
Muckle-Wells syndrome
Neonatal onset multisystemic inflammatory disorder [NOMID]

M04.8 **Other autoinflammatory syndromes** HCC

Blau syndrome
Deficiency of interleukin 1 receptor antagonist [DIRA]
Majeed syndrome
Periodic fever, aphthous stomatitis, pharyngitis, and adenopathy syndrome [PFAPA]
Pyogenic arthritis, pyoderma gangrenosum, and acne syndrome [PAPA]

M04.9 **Autoinflammatory syndrome, unspecified** HCC

Inflammatory polyarthropathies (M05-M14)

M05 **Rheumatoid arthritis with rheumatoid factor**

EXCLUDES 1 *rheumatic fever (I00)*
juvenile rheumatoid arthritis (M08.-)
rheumatoid arthritis of spine (M45.-)

CODING TIP ✓ Rheumatoid arthritis classified here includes rheumatoid arthritis and associated conditions (see combination codes) that have an identified rheumatoid factor present. Do not assume the presence of rheumatoid factor when a diagnosis of rheumatoid arthritis is noted in the clinical record. Rheumatoid arthritis that is not specified with rheumatoid factor is coded to M06.-. There are many associated conditions that the classification assumes are related to rheumatoid arthritis. Consult the alphabetic index "arthritis, rheumatoid, with."

M05.0 **Felty's syndrome**

Rheumatoid arthritis with splenoadenomegaly and leukopenia

DEFINITION Atypical form of rheumatoid arthritis presenting with fever, enlarged spleen, recurring infections, and decreased white cell count.

M05.00 **Felty's syndrome, unspecified site** HCC

M05.01 **Felty's syndrome, shoulder**

M05.011 **Felty's syndrome, right shoulder** HCC

M05.012 **Felty's syndrome, left shoulder** HCC

M05.019 **Felty's syndrome, unspecified shoulder** HCC

M05.02 **Felty's syndrome, elbow**

M05.021 **Felty's syndrome, right elbow** HCC

M05.022 **Felty's syndrome, left elbow** HCC

M05.029 **Felty's syndrome, unspecified elbow** HCC

M05.03 **Felty's syndrome, wrist**

Felty's syndrome, carpal bones

M05.031 **Felty's syndrome, right wrist** HCC

M05.032 **Felty's syndrome, left wrist** HCC

M05.039 **Felty's syndrome, unspecified wrist** HCC

M05.04 **Felty's syndrome, hand**

Felty's syndrome, metacarpus and phalanges

M05.041 **Felty's syndrome, right hand** HCC

M05.042 **Felty's syndrome, left hand** HCC

M05.049 **Felty's syndrome, unspecified hand** HCC

M05.05 **Felty's syndrome, hip**

M05.051 **Felty's syndrome, right hip** HCC

M05.052 **Felty's syndrome, left hip** HCC

M05.059 **Felty's syndrome, unspecified hip** HCC

M05.06 **Felty's syndrome, knee**

M05.061 **Felty's syndrome, right knee** HCC

M05.062 **Felty's syndrome, left knee** HCC

M05.069 **Felty's syndrome, unspecified knee** HCC

M05.07 **Felty's syndrome, ankle and foot**

Felty's syndrome, tarsus, metatarsus and phalanges

M05.071 **Felty's syndrome, right ankle and foot** HCC

M05.072 **Felty's syndrome, left ankle and foot** HCC

M05.079 **Felty's syndrome, unspecified ankle and foot** HCC

M05.09 **Felty's syndrome, multiple sites** HCC

M05.1 **Rheumatoid lung disease with rheumatoid arthritis**

M05.10 **Rheumatoid lung disease with rheumatoid arthritis of unspecified site** HCC

M05.11 **Rheumatoid lung disease with rheumatoid arthritis of shoulder**

M05.111 Rheumatoid lung disease with rheumatoid arthritis of right shoulder HCC
M05.112 Rheumatoid lung disease with rheumatoid arthritis of left shoulder HCC
M05.119 Rheumatoid lung disease with rheumatoid arthritis of unspecified shoulder HCC
M05.12 Rheumatoid lung disease with rheumatoid arthritis of elbow
M05.121 Rheumatoid lung disease with rheumatoid arthritis of right elbow HCC
M05.122 Rheumatoid lung disease with rheumatoid arthritis of left elbow HCC
M05.129 Rheumatoid lung disease with rheumatoid arthritis of unspecified elbow HCC
M05.13 Rheumatoid lung disease with rheumatoid arthritis of wrist
Rheumatoid lung disease with rheumatoid arthritis, carpal bones
M05.131 Rheumatoid lung disease with rheumatoid arthritis of right wrist HCC
M05.132 Rheumatoid lung disease with rheumatoid arthritis of left wrist HCC
M05.139 Rheumatoid lung disease with rheumatoid arthritis of unspecified wrist HCC
M05.14 Rheumatoid lung disease with rheumatoid arthritis of hand
Rheumatoid lung disease with rheumatoid arthritis, metacarpus and phalanges
M05.141 Rheumatoid lung disease with rheumatoid arthritis of right hand HCC
M05.142 Rheumatoid lung disease with rheumatoid arthritis of left hand HCC
M05.149 Rheumatoid lung disease with rheumatoid arthritis of unspecified hand HCC
M05.15 Rheumatoid lung disease with rheumatoid arthritis of hip
M05.151 Rheumatoid lung disease with rheumatoid arthritis of right hip HCC
M05.152 Rheumatoid lung disease with rheumatoid arthritis of left hip HCC
M05.159 Rheumatoid lung disease with rheumatoid arthritis of unspecified hip HCC
M05.16 Rheumatoid lung disease with rheumatoid arthritis of knee
M05.161 Rheumatoid lung disease with rheumatoid arthritis of right knee HCC
M05.162 Rheumatoid lung disease with rheumatoid arthritis of left knee HCC
M05.169 Rheumatoid lung disease with rheumatoid arthritis of unspecified knee HCC
M05.17 Rheumatoid lung disease with rheumatoid arthritis of ankle and foot
Rheumatoid lung disease with rheumatoid arthritis, tarsus, metatarsus and phalanges
M05.171 Rheumatoid lung disease with rheumatoid arthritis of right ankle and foot HCC
M05.172 Rheumatoid lung disease with rheumatoid arthritis of left ankle and foot HCC
M05.179 Rheumatoid lung disease with rheumatoid arthritis of unspecified ankle and foot HCC
M05.19 Rheumatoid lung disease with rheumatoid arthritis of multiple sites HCC
M05.2 Rheumatoid vasculitis with rheumatoid arthritis
M05.20 Rheumatoid vasculitis with rheumatoid arthritis of unspecified site HCC
M05.21 Rheumatoid vasculitis with rheumatoid arthritis of shoulder
M05.211 Rheumatoid vasculitis with rheumatoid arthritis of right shoulder HCC
M05.212 Rheumatoid vasculitis with rheumatoid arthritis of left shoulder HCC
M05.219 Rheumatoid vasculitis with rheumatoid arthritis of unspecified shoulder HCC
M05.22 Rheumatoid vasculitis with rheumatoid arthritis of elbow
M05.221 Rheumatoid vasculitis with rheumatoid arthritis of right elbow HCC
M05.222 Rheumatoid vasculitis with rheumatoid arthritis of left elbow HCC
M05.229 Rheumatoid vasculitis with rheumatoid arthritis of unspecified elbow HCC
M05.23 Rheumatoid vasculitis with rheumatoid arthritis of wrist
Rheumatoid vasculitis with rheumatoid arthritis, carpal bones
M05.231 Rheumatoid vasculitis with rheumatoid arthritis of right wrist HCC
M05.232 Rheumatoid vasculitis with rheumatoid arthritis of left wrist HCC
M05.239 Rheumatoid vasculitis with rheumatoid arthritis of unspecified wrist HCC
M05.24 Rheumatoid vasculitis with rheumatoid arthritis of hand
Rheumatoid vasculitis with rheumatoid arthritis, metacarpus and phalanges
M05.241 Rheumatoid vasculitis with rheumatoid arthritis of right hand HCC
M05.242 Rheumatoid vasculitis with rheumatoid arthritis of left hand HCC
M05.249 Rheumatoid vasculitis with rheumatoid arthritis of unspecified hand HCC
M05.25 Rheumatoid vasculitis with rheumatoid arthritis of hip
M05.251 Rheumatoid vasculitis with rheumatoid arthritis of right hip HCC
M05.252 Rheumatoid vasculitis with rheumatoid arthritis of left hip HCC
M05.259 Rheumatoid vasculitis with rheumatoid arthritis of unspecified hip HCC
M05.26 Rheumatoid vasculitis with rheumatoid arthritis of knee
M05.261 Rheumatoid vasculitis with rheumatoid arthritis of right knee HCC
M05.262 Rheumatoid vasculitis with rheumatoid arthritis of left knee HCC
M05.269 Rheumatoid vasculitis with rheumatoid arthritis of unspecified knee HCC
M05.27 Rheumatoid vasculitis with rheumatoid arthritis of ankle and foot
Rheumatoid vasculitis with rheumatoid arthritis, tarsus, metatarsus and phalanges
M05.271 Rheumatoid vasculitis with rheumatoid arthritis of right ankle and foot HCC
M05.272 Rheumatoid vasculitis with rheumatoid arthritis of left ankle and foot HCC
M05.279 Rheumatoid vasculitis with rheumatoid arthritis of unspecified ankle and foot HCC
M05.29 Rheumatoid vasculitis with rheumatoid arthritis of multiple sites HCC
M05.3 Rheumatoid heart disease with rheumatoid arthritis
Rheumatoid carditis
Rheumatoid endocarditis
Rheumatoid myocarditis
Rheumatoid pericarditis
M05.30 Rheumatoid heart disease with rheumatoid arthritis of unspecified site HCC
M05.31 Rheumatoid heart disease with rheumatoid arthritis of shoulder
M05.311 Rheumatoid heart disease with rheumatoid arthritis of right shoulder HCC
M05.312 Rheumatoid heart disease with rheumatoid arthritis of left shoulder HCC
M05.319 Rheumatoid heart disease with rheumatoid arthritis of unspecified shoulder HCC
M05.32 Rheumatoid heart disease with rheumatoid arthritis of elbow
M05.321 Rheumatoid heart disease with rheumatoid arthritis of right elbow HCC
M05.322 Rheumatoid heart disease with rheumatoid arthritis of left elbow HCC
M05.329 Rheumatoid heart disease with rheumatoid arthritis of unspecified elbow HCC

6 M05.33 Rheumatoid heart disease with rheumatoid arthritis of wrist
Rheumatoid heart disease with rheumatoid arthritis, carpal bones
- **M05.331 Rheumatoid heart disease with rheumatoid arthritis of right wrist** HCC
- **M05.332 Rheumatoid heart disease with rheumatoid arthritis of left wrist** HCC
- **M05.339 Rheumatoid heart disease with rheumatoid arthritis of unspecified wrist** HCC

6 M05.34 Rheumatoid heart disease with rheumatoid arthritis of hand
Rheumatoid heart disease with rheumatoid arthritis, metacarpus and phalanges
- **M05.341 Rheumatoid heart disease with rheumatoid arthritis of right hand** HCC
- **M05.342 Rheumatoid heart disease with rheumatoid arthritis of left hand** HCC
- **M05.349 Rheumatoid heart disease with rheumatoid arthritis of unspecified hand** HCC

6 M05.35 Rheumatoid heart disease with rheumatoid arthritis of hip
- **M05.351 Rheumatoid heart disease with rheumatoid arthritis of right hip** HCC
- **M05.352 Rheumatoid heart disease with rheumatoid arthritis of left hip** HCC
- **M05.359 Rheumatoid heart disease with rheumatoid arthritis of unspecified hip** HCC

6 M05.36 Rheumatoid heart disease with rheumatoid arthritis of knee
- **M05.361 Rheumatoid heart disease with rheumatoid arthritis of right knee** HCC
- **M05.362 Rheumatoid heart disease with rheumatoid arthritis of left knee** HCC
- **M05.369 Rheumatoid heart disease with rheumatoid arthritis of unspecified knee** HCC

6 M05.37 Rheumatoid heart disease with rheumatoid arthritis of ankle and foot
Rheumatoid heart disease with rheumatoid arthritis, tarsus, metatarsus and phalanges
- **M05.371 Rheumatoid heart disease with rheumatoid arthritis of right ankle and foot** HCC
- **M05.372 Rheumatoid heart disease with rheumatoid arthritis of left ankle and foot** HCC
- **M05.379 Rheumatoid heart disease with rheumatoid arthritis of unspecified ankle and foot** HCC

M05.39 Rheumatoid heart disease with rheumatoid arthritis of multiple sites HCC

5 M05.4 Rheumatoid myopathy with rheumatoid arthritis

M05.40 Rheumatoid myopathy with rheumatoid arthritis of unspecified site HCC

6 M05.41 Rheumatoid myopathy with rheumatoid arthritis of shoulder
- **M05.411 Rheumatoid myopathy with rheumatoid arthritis of right shoulder** HCC
- **M05.412 Rheumatoid myopathy with rheumatoid arthritis of left shoulder** HCC
- **M05.419 Rheumatoid myopathy with rheumatoid arthritis of unspecified shoulder** HCC

6 M05.42 Rheumatoid myopathy with rheumatoid arthritis of elbow
- **M05.421 Rheumatoid myopathy with rheumatoid arthritis of right elbow** HCC
- **M05.422 Rheumatoid myopathy with rheumatoid arthritis of left elbow** HCC
- **M05.429 Rheumatoid myopathy with rheumatoid arthritis of unspecified elbow** HCC

6 M05.43 Rheumatoid myopathy with rheumatoid arthritis of wrist
Rheumatoid myopathy with rheumatoid arthritis, carpal bones
- **M05.431 Rheumatoid myopathy with rheumatoid arthritis of right wrist** HCC
- **M05.432 Rheumatoid myopathy with rheumatoid arthritis of left wrist** HCC
- **M05.439 Rheumatoid myopathy with rheumatoid arthritis of unspecified wrist** HCC

6 M05.44 Rheumatoid myopathy with rheumatoid arthritis of hand
Rheumatoid myopathy with rheumatoid arthritis, metacarpus and phalanges
- **M05.441 Rheumatoid myopathy with rheumatoid arthritis of right hand** HCC
- **M05.442 Rheumatoid myopathy with rheumatoid arthritis of left hand** HCC
- **M05.449 Rheumatoid myopathy with rheumatoid arthritis of unspecified hand** HCC

6 M05.45 Rheumatoid myopathy with rheumatoid arthritis of hip
- **M05.451 Rheumatoid myopathy with rheumatoid arthritis of right hip** HCC
- **M05.452 Rheumatoid myopathy with rheumatoid arthritis of left hip** HCC
- **M05.459 Rheumatoid myopathy with rheumatoid arthritis of unspecified hip** HCC

6 M05.46 Rheumatoid myopathy with rheumatoid arthritis of knee
- **M05.461 Rheumatoid myopathy with rheumatoid arthritis of right knee** HCC
- **M05.462 Rheumatoid myopathy with rheumatoid arthritis of left knee** HCC
- **M05.469 Rheumatoid myopathy with rheumatoid arthritis of unspecified knee** HCC

6 M05.47 Rheumatoid myopathy with rheumatoid arthritis of ankle and foot
Rheumatoid myopathy with rheumatoid arthritis, tarsus, metatarsus and phalanges
- **M05.471 Rheumatoid myopathy with rheumatoid arthritis of right ankle and foot** HCC
- **M05.472 Rheumatoid myopathy with rheumatoid arthritis of left ankle and foot** HCC
- **M05.479 Rheumatoid myopathy with rheumatoid arthritis of unspecified ankle and foot** HCC

M05.49 Rheumatoid myopathy with rheumatoid arthritis of multiple sites HCC

5 M05.5 Rheumatoid polyneuropathy with rheumatoid arthritis

M05.50 Rheumatoid polyneuropathy with rheumatoid arthritis of unspecified site HCC

6 M05.51 Rheumatoid polyneuropathy with rheumatoid arthritis of shoulder
- **M05.511 Rheumatoid polyneuropathy with rheumatoid arthritis of right shoulder** HCC
- **M05.512 Rheumatoid polyneuropathy with rheumatoid arthritis of left shoulder** HCC
- **M05.519 Rheumatoid polyneuropathy with rheumatoid arthritis of unspecified shoulder** HCC

6 M05.52 Rheumatoid polyneuropathy with rheumatoid arthritis of elbow
- **M05.521 Rheumatoid polyneuropathy with rheumatoid arthritis of right elbow** HCC
- **M05.522 Rheumatoid polyneuropathy with rheumatoid arthritis of left elbow** HCC
- **M05.529 Rheumatoid polyneuropathy with rheumatoid arthritis of unspecified elbow** HCC

6 M05.53 Rheumatoid polyneuropathy with rheumatoid arthritis of wrist
Rheumatoid polyneuropathy with rheumatoid arthritis, carpal bones
- **M05.531 Rheumatoid polyneuropathy with rheumatoid arthritis of right wrist** HCC
- **M05.532 Rheumatoid polyneuropathy with rheumatoid arthritis of left wrist** HCC
- **M05.539 Rheumatoid polyneuropathy with rheumatoid arthritis of unspecified wrist** HCC

6 M05.54 Rheumatoid polyneuropathy with rheumatoid arthritis of hand
Rheumatoid polyneuropathy with rheumatoid arthritis, metacarpus and phalanges
- **M05.541 Rheumatoid polyneuropathy with rheumatoid arthritis of right hand** HCC
- **M05.542 Rheumatoid polyneuropathy with rheumatoid arthritis of left hand** HCC

M05.549 Rheumatoid polyneuropathy with rheumatoid arthritis of unspecified hand HCC

M05.55 Rheumatoid polyneuropathy with rheumatoid arthritis of hip

M05.551 Rheumatoid polyneuropathy with rheumatoid arthritis of right hip HCC

M05.552 Rheumatoid polyneuropathy with rheumatoid arthritis of left hip HCC

M05.559 Rheumatoid polyneuropathy with rheumatoid arthritis of unspecified hip HCC

M05.56 Rheumatoid polyneuropathy with rheumatoid arthritis of knee

M05.561 Rheumatoid polyneuropathy with rheumatoid arthritis of right knee HCC

M05.562 Rheumatoid polyneuropathy with rheumatoid arthritis of left knee HCC

M05.569 Rheumatoid polyneuropathy with rheumatoid arthritis of unspecified knee HCC

M05.57 Rheumatoid polyneuropathy with rheumatoid arthritis of ankle and foot
Rheumatoid polyneuropathy with rheumatoid arthritis, tarsus, metatarsus and phalanges

M05.571 Rheumatoid polyneuropathy with rheumatoid arthritis of right ankle and foot HCC

M05.572 Rheumatoid polyneuropathy with rheumatoid arthritis of left ankle and foot HCC

M05.579 Rheumatoid polyneuropathy with rheumatoid arthritis of unspecified ankle and foot HCC

M05.59 Rheumatoid polyneuropathy with rheumatoid arthritis of multiple sites HCC

M05.6 Rheumatoid arthritis with involvement of other organs and systems

M05.60 Rheumatoid arthritis of unspecified site with involvement of other organs and systems HCC

M05.61 Rheumatoid arthritis of shoulder with involvement of other organs and systems

M05.611 Rheumatoid arthritis of right shoulder with involvement of other organs and systems HCC

M05.612 Rheumatoid arthritis of left shoulder with involvement of other organs and systems HCC

M05.619 Rheumatoid arthritis of unspecified shoulder with involvement of other organs and systems HCC

M05.62 Rheumatoid arthritis of elbow with involvement of other organs and systems

M05.621 Rheumatoid arthritis of right elbow with involvement of other organs and systems HCC

M05.622 Rheumatoid arthritis of left elbow with involvement of other organs and systems HCC

M05.629 Rheumatoid arthritis of unspecified elbow with involvement of other organs and systems HCC

M05.63 Rheumatoid arthritis of wrist with involvement of other organs and systems
Rheumatoid arthritis of carpal bones with involvement of other organs and systems

M05.631 Rheumatoid arthritis of right wrist with involvement of other organs and systems HCC

M05.632 Rheumatoid arthritis of left wrist with involvement of other organs and systems HCC

M05.639 Rheumatoid arthritis of unspecified wrist with involvement of other organs and systems HCC

M05.64 Rheumatoid arthritis of hand with involvement of other organs and systems
Rheumatoid arthritis of metacarpus and phalanges with involvement of other organs and systems

M05.641 Rheumatoid arthritis of right hand with involvement of other organs and systems HCC

M05.642 Rheumatoid arthritis of left hand with involvement of other organs and systems HCC

M05.649 Rheumatoid arthritis of unspecified hand with involvement of other organs and systems HCC

M05.65 Rheumatoid arthritis of hip with involvement of other organs and systems

M05.651 Rheumatoid arthritis of right hip with involvement of other organs and systems HCC

M05.652 Rheumatoid arthritis of left hip with involvement of other organs and systems HCC

M05.659 Rheumatoid arthritis of unspecified hip with involvement of other organs and systems HCC

M05.66 Rheumatoid arthritis of knee with involvement of other organs and systems

M05.661 Rheumatoid arthritis of right knee with involvement of other organs and systems HCC

M05.662 Rheumatoid arthritis of left knee with involvement of other organs and systems HCC

M05.669 Rheumatoid arthritis of unspecified knee with involvement of other organs and systems HCC

M05.67 Rheumatoid arthritis of ankle and foot with involvement of other organs and systems
Rheumatoid arthritis of tarsus, metatarsus and phalanges with involvement of other organs and systems

M05.671 Rheumatoid arthritis of right ankle and foot with involvement of other organs and systems HCC

M05.672 Rheumatoid arthritis of left ankle and foot with involvement of other organs and systems HCC

M05.679 Rheumatoid arthritis of unspecified ankle and foot with involvement of other organs and systems HCC

M05.69 Rheumatoid arthritis of multiple sites with involvement of other organs and systems HCC

M05.7 Rheumatoid arthritis with rheumatoid factor without organ or systems involvement

M05.70 Rheumatoid arthritis with rheumatoid factor of unspecified site without organ or systems involvement HCC

M05.71 Rheumatoid arthritis with rheumatoid factor of shoulder without organ or systems involvement

M05.711 Rheumatoid arthritis with rheumatoid factor of right shoulder without organ or systems involvement HCC

M05.712 Rheumatoid arthritis with rheumatoid factor of left shoulder without organ or systems involvement HCC

M05.719 Rheumatoid arthritis with rheumatoid factor of unspecified shoulder without organ or systems involvement HCC

M05.72 Rheumatoid arthritis with rheumatoid factor of elbow without organ or systems involvement

M05.721 Rheumatoid arthritis with rheumatoid factor of right elbow without organ or systems involvement HCC

M05.722 Rheumatoid arthritis with rheumatoid factor of left elbow without organ or systems involvement HCC

M05.729 Rheumatoid arthritis with rheumatoid factor of unspecified elbow without organ or systems involvement HCC

M05.73 Rheumatoid arthritis with rheumatoid factor of wrist without organ or systems involvement

M05.731 Rheumatoid arthritis with rheumatoid factor of right wrist without organ or systems involvement HCC

M05.732 Rheumatoid arthritis with rheumatoid factor of left wrist without organ or systems involvement HCC

M05.739 Rheumatoid arthritis with rheumatoid factor of unspecified wrist without organ or systems involvement HCC

M05.74 Rheumatoid arthritis with rheumatoid factor of hand without organ or systems involvement

M05.741 Rheumatoid arthritis with rheumatoid factor of right hand without organ or systems involvement HCC

M05.742 Rheumatoid arthritis with rheumatoid factor of left hand without organ or systems involvement HCC
M05.749 Rheumatoid arthritis with rheumatoid factor of unspecified hand without organ or systems involvement HCC
M05.75 Rheumatoid arthritis with rheumatoid factor of hip without organ or systems involvement
M05.751 Rheumatoid arthritis with rheumatoid factor of right hip without organ or systems involvement HCC
M05.752 Rheumatoid arthritis with rheumatoid factor of left hip without organ or systems involvement HCC
M05.759 Rheumatoid arthritis with rheumatoid factor of unspecified hip without organ or systems involvement HCC
M05.76 Rheumatoid arthritis with rheumatoid factor of knee without organ or systems involvement
M05.761 Rheumatoid arthritis with rheumatoid factor of right knee without organ or systems involvement HCC
M05.762 Rheumatoid arthritis with rheumatoid factor of left knee without organ or systems involvement HCC
M05.769 Rheumatoid arthritis with rheumatoid factor of unspecified knee without organ or systems involvement HCC
M05.77 Rheumatoid arthritis with rheumatoid factor of ankle and foot without organ or systems involvement
M05.771 Rheumatoid arthritis with rheumatoid factor of right ankle and foot without organ or systems involvement HCC
M05.772 Rheumatoid arthritis with rheumatoid factor of left ankle and foot without organ or systems involvement HCC
M05.779 Rheumatoid arthritis with rheumatoid factor of unspecified ankle and foot without organ or systems involvement HCC
M05.79 Rheumatoid arthritis with rheumatoid factor of multiple sites without organ or systems involvement HCC
M05.8 Other rheumatoid arthritis with rheumatoid factor
M05.80 Other rheumatoid arthritis with rheumatoid factor of unspecified site HCC
M05.81 Other rheumatoid arthritis with rheumatoid factor of shoulder
M05.811 Other rheumatoid arthritis with rheumatoid factor of right shoulder HCC
M05.812 Other rheumatoid arthritis with rheumatoid factor of left shoulder HCC
M05.819 Other rheumatoid arthritis with rheumatoid factor of unspecified shoulder HCC
M05.82 Other rheumatoid arthritis with rheumatoid factor of elbow
M05.821 Other rheumatoid arthritis with rheumatoid factor of right elbow HCC
M05.822 Other rheumatoid arthritis with rheumatoid factor of left elbow HCC
M05.829 Other rheumatoid arthritis with rheumatoid factor of unspecified elbow HCC
M05.83 Other rheumatoid arthritis with rheumatoid factor of wrist
M05.831 Other rheumatoid arthritis with rheumatoid factor of right wrist HCC
M05.832 Other rheumatoid arthritis with rheumatoid factor of left wrist HCC
M05.839 Other rheumatoid arthritis with rheumatoid factor of unspecified wrist HCC
M05.84 Other rheumatoid arthritis with rheumatoid factor of hand
M05.841 Other rheumatoid arthritis with rheumatoid factor of right hand HCC
M05.842 Other rheumatoid arthritis with rheumatoid factor of left hand HCC
M05.849 Other rheumatoid arthritis with rheumatoid factor of unspecified hand HCC
M05.85 Other rheumatoid arthritis with rheumatoid factor of hip
M05.851 Other rheumatoid arthritis with rheumatoid factor of right hip HCC
M05.852 Other rheumatoid arthritis with rheumatoid factor of left hip HCC
M05.859 Other rheumatoid arthritis with rheumatoid factor of unspecified hip HCC
M05.86 Other rheumatoid arthritis with rheumatoid factor of knee
M05.861 Other rheumatoid arthritis with rheumatoid factor of right knee HCC
M05.862 Other rheumatoid arthritis with rheumatoid factor of left knee HCC
M05.869 Other rheumatoid arthritis with rheumatoid factor of unspecified knee HCC
M05.87 Other rheumatoid arthritis with rheumatoid factor of ankle and foot
M05.871 Other rheumatoid arthritis with rheumatoid factor of right ankle and foot HCC
M05.872 Other rheumatoid arthritis with rheumatoid factor of left ankle and foot HCC
M05.879 Other rheumatoid arthritis with rheumatoid factor of unspecified ankle and foot HCC
M05.89 Other rheumatoid arthritis with rheumatoid factor of multiple sites HCC
M05.9 Rheumatoid arthritis with rheumatoid factor, unspecified HCC

M06 Other rheumatoid arthritis

CODING TIP ✓ M06 includes the rheumatoid arthritis codes without rheumatoid factor, with site and comorbidity.

M06.0 Rheumatoid arthritis without rheumatoid factor
M06.00 Rheumatoid arthritis without rheumatoid factor, unspecified site HCC
M06.01 Rheumatoid arthritis without rheumatoid factor, shoulder
M06.011 Rheumatoid arthritis without rheumatoid factor, right shoulder HCC
M06.012 Rheumatoid arthritis without rheumatoid factor, left shoulder HCC
M06.019 Rheumatoid arthritis without rheumatoid factor, unspecified shoulder HCC
M06.02 Rheumatoid arthritis without rheumatoid factor, elbow
M06.021 Rheumatoid arthritis without rheumatoid factor, right elbow HCC
M06.022 Rheumatoid arthritis without rheumatoid factor, left elbow HCC
M06.029 Rheumatoid arthritis without rheumatoid factor, unspecified elbow HCC
M06.03 Rheumatoid arthritis without rheumatoid factor, wrist
M06.031 Rheumatoid arthritis without rheumatoid factor, right wrist HCC
M06.032 Rheumatoid arthritis without rheumatoid factor, left wrist HCC
M06.039 Rheumatoid arthritis without rheumatoid factor, unspecified wrist HCC
M06.04 Rheumatoid arthritis without rheumatoid factor, hand
M06.041 Rheumatoid arthritis without rheumatoid factor, right hand HCC
M06.042 Rheumatoid arthritis without rheumatoid factor, left hand HCC
M06.049 Rheumatoid arthritis without rheumatoid factor, unspecified hand HCC
M06.05 Rheumatoid arthritis without rheumatoid factor, hip
M06.051 Rheumatoid arthritis without rheumatoid factor, right hip HCC
M06.052 Rheumatoid arthritis without rheumatoid factor, left hip HCC
M06.059 Rheumatoid arthritis without rheumatoid factor, unspecified hip HCC

6 **M06.06** **Rheumatoid arthritis without rheumatoid factor, knee**
- **M06.061** **Rheumatoid arthritis without rheumatoid factor, right knee** HCC
- **M06.062** **Rheumatoid arthritis without rheumatoid factor, left knee** HCC
- **M06.069** **Rheumatoid arthritis without rheumatoid factor, unspecified knee** HCC

6 **M06.07** **Rheumatoid arthritis without rheumatoid factor, ankle and foot**
- **M06.071** **Rheumatoid arthritis without rheumatoid factor, right ankle and foot** HCC
- **M06.072** **Rheumatoid arthritis without rheumatoid factor, left ankle and foot** HCC
- **M06.079** **Rheumatoid arthritis without rheumatoid factor, unspecified ankle and foot** HCC

M06.08 **Rheumatoid arthritis without rheumatoid factor, vertebrae** HCC

M06.09 **Rheumatoid arthritis without rheumatoid factor, multiple sites** HCC

M06.1 **Adult-onset Still's disease** A HCC

EXCLUDES 1 *Still's disease NOS (M08.2-)*

5 **M06.2** **Rheumatoid bursitis**

M06.20 **Rheumatoid bursitis, unspecified site** HCC

6 **M06.21** **Rheumatoid bursitis, shoulder**
- **M06.211** **Rheumatoid bursitis, right shoulder** HCC
- **M06.212** **Rheumatoid bursitis, left shoulder** HCC
- **M06.219** **Rheumatoid bursitis, unspecified shoulder** HCC

6 **M06.22** **Rheumatoid bursitis, elbow**
- **M06.221** **Rheumatoid bursitis, right elbow** HCC
- **M06.222** **Rheumatoid bursitis, left elbow** HCC
- **M06.229** **Rheumatoid bursitis, unspecified elbow** HCC

6 **M06.23** **Rheumatoid bursitis, wrist**
- **M06.231** **Rheumatoid bursitis, right wrist** HCC
- **M06.232** **Rheumatoid bursitis, left wrist** HCC
- **M06.239** **Rheumatoid bursitis, unspecified wrist** HCC

6 **M06.24** **Rheumatoid bursitis, hand**
- **M06.241** **Rheumatoid bursitis, right hand** HCC
- **M06.242** **Rheumatoid bursitis, left hand** HCC
- **M06.249** **Rheumatoid bursitis, unspecified hand** HCC

6 **M06.25** **Rheumatoid bursitis, hip**
- **M06.251** **Rheumatoid bursitis, right hip** HCC
- **M06.252** **Rheumatoid bursitis, left hip** HCC
- **M06.259** **Rheumatoid bursitis, unspecified hip** HCC

6 **M06.26** **Rheumatoid bursitis, knee**
- **M06.261** **Rheumatoid bursitis, right knee** HCC
- **M06.262** **Rheumatoid bursitis, left knee** HCC
- **M06.269** **Rheumatoid bursitis, unspecified knee** HCC

6 **M06.27** **Rheumatoid bursitis, ankle and foot**
- **M06.271** **Rheumatoid bursitis, right ankle and foot** HCC
- **M06.272** **Rheumatoid bursitis, left ankle and foot** HCC
- **M06.279** **Rheumatoid bursitis, unspecified ankle and foot** HCC

M06.28 **Rheumatoid bursitis, vertebrae** HCC

M06.29 **Rheumatoid bursitis, multiple sites** HCC

5 **M06.3** **Rheumatoid nodule**

M06.30 **Rheumatoid nodule, unspecified site** HCC

6 **M06.31** **Rheumatoid nodule, shoulder**
- **M06.311** **Rheumatoid nodule, right shoulder** HCC
- **M06.312** **Rheumatoid nodule, left shoulder** HCC
- **M06.319** **Rheumatoid nodule, unspecified shoulder** HCC

6 **M06.32** **Rheumatoid nodule, elbow**
- **M06.321** **Rheumatoid nodule, right elbow** HCC
- **M06.322** **Rheumatoid nodule, left elbow** HCC
- **M06.329** **Rheumatoid nodule, unspecified elbow** HCC

6 **M06.33** **Rheumatoid nodule, wrist**
- **M06.331** **Rheumatoid nodule, right wrist** HCC
- **M06.332** **Rheumatoid nodule, left wrist** HCC
- **M06.339** **Rheumatoid nodule, unspecified wrist** HCC

6 **M06.34** **Rheumatoid nodule, hand**
- **M06.341** **Rheumatoid nodule, right hand** HCC
- **M06.342** **Rheumatoid nodule, left hand** HCC
- **M06.349** **Rheumatoid nodule, unspecified hand** HCC

6 **M06.35** **Rheumatoid nodule, hip**
- **M06.351** **Rheumatoid nodule, right hip** HCC
- **M06.352** **Rheumatoid nodule, left hip** HCC
- **M06.359** **Rheumatoid nodule, unspecified hip** HCC

6 **M06.36** **Rheumatoid nodule, knee**
- **M06.361** **Rheumatoid nodule, right knee** HCC
- **M06.362** **Rheumatoid nodule, left knee** HCC
- **M06.369** **Rheumatoid nodule, unspecified knee** HCC

6 **M06.37** **Rheumatoid nodule, ankle and foot**
- **M06.371** **Rheumatoid nodule, right ankle and foot** HCC
- **M06.372** **Rheumatoid nodule, left ankle and foot** HCC
- **M06.379** **Rheumatoid nodule, unspecified ankle and foot** HCC

M06.38 **Rheumatoid nodule, vertebrae** HCC

M06.39 **Rheumatoid nodule, multiple sites** HCC

M06.4 **Inflammatory polyarthropathy** HCC

EXCLUDES 1 *polyarthritis NOS (M13.0)*

5 **M06.8** **Other specified rheumatoid arthritis**

M06.80 **Other specified rheumatoid arthritis, unspecified site** HCC

6 **M06.81** **Other specified rheumatoid arthritis, shoulder**
- **M06.811** **Other specified rheumatoid arthritis, right shoulder** HCC
- **M06.812** **Other specified rheumatoid arthritis, left shoulder** HCC
- **M06.819** **Other specified rheumatoid arthritis, unspecified shoulder** HCC

6 **M06.82** **Other specified rheumatoid arthritis, elbow**
- **M06.821** **Other specified rheumatoid arthritis, right elbow** HCC
- **M06.822** **Other specified rheumatoid arthritis, left elbow** HCC
- **M06.829** **Other specified rheumatoid arthritis, unspecified elbow** HCC

6 **M06.83** **Other specified rheumatoid arthritis, wrist**
- **M06.831** **Other specified rheumatoid arthritis, right wrist** HCC
- **M06.832** **Other specified rheumatoid arthritis, left wrist** HCC
- **M06.839** **Other specified rheumatoid arthritis, unspecified wrist** HCC

6 **M06.84** **Other specified rheumatoid arthritis, hand**
- **M06.841** **Other specified rheumatoid arthritis, right hand** HCC
- **M06.842** **Other specified rheumatoid arthritis, left hand** HCC
- **M06.849** **Other specified rheumatoid arthritis, unspecified hand** HCC

6 **M06.85** **Other specified rheumatoid arthritis, hip**
- **M06.851** **Other specified rheumatoid arthritis, right hip** HCC
- **M06.852** **Other specified rheumatoid arthritis, left hip** HCC
- **M06.859** **Other specified rheumatoid arthritis, unspecified hip** HCC

6 **M06.86** **Other specified rheumatoid arthritis, knee**
- **M06.861** **Other specified rheumatoid arthritis, right knee** HCC
- **M06.862** **Other specified rheumatoid arthritis, left knee** HCC
- **M06.869** **Other specified rheumatoid arthritis, unspecified knee** HCC

6 **M06.87** **Other specified rheumatoid arthritis, ankle and foot**
- **M06.871** **Other specified rheumatoid arthritis, right ankle and foot** HCC

⊟ M06.872 Other specified rheumatoid arthritis, left ankle and foot HCC
⊟ M06.879 Other specified rheumatoid arthritis, unspecified ankle and foot HCC
M06.88 Other specified rheumatoid arthritis, vertebrae HCC
M06.89 Other specified rheumatoid arthritis, multiple sites HCC
M06.9 Rheumatoid arthritis, unspecified HCC

4 **M07 Enteropathic arthropathies**
Code also associated enteropathy, such as:
regional enteritis [Crohn's disease] (K50.-)
ulcerative colitis (K51.-)
EXCLUDES 1 *psoriatic arthropathies (L40.5-)*

5 **M07.6 Enteropathic arthropathies**
M07.60 Enteropathic arthropathies, unspecified site
6 M07.61 Enteropathic arthropathies, shoulder
⊟ M07.611 Enteropathic arthropathies, right shoulder
⊟ M07.612 Enteropathic arthropathies, left shoulder
⊟ M07.619 Enteropathic arthropathies, unspecified shoulder
6 M07.62 Enteropathic arthropathies, elbow
⊟ M07.621 Enteropathic arthropathies, right elbow
⊟ M07.622 Enteropathic arthropathies, left elbow
⊟ M07.629 Enteropathic arthropathies, unspecified elbow
6 M07.63 Enteropathic arthropathies, wrist
⊟ M07.631 Enteropathic arthropathies, right wrist
⊟ M07.632 Enteropathic arthropathies, left wrist
⊟ M07.639 Enteropathic arthropathies, unspecified wrist
6 M07.64 Enteropathic arthropathies, hand
⊟ M07.641 Enteropathic arthropathies, right hand
⊟ M07.642 Enteropathic arthropathies, left hand
⊟ M07.649 Enteropathic arthropathies, unspecified hand
6 M07.65 Enteropathic arthropathies, hip
⊟ M07.651 Enteropathic arthropathies, right hip
⊟ M07.652 Enteropathic arthropathies, left hip
⊟ M07.659 Enteropathic arthropathies, unspecified hip
6 M07.66 Enteropathic arthropathies, knee
⊟ M07.661 Enteropathic arthropathies, right knee
⊟ M07.662 Enteropathic arthropathies, left knee
⊟ M07.669 Enteropathic arthropathies, unspecified knee
6 M07.67 Enteropathic arthropathies, ankle and foot
⊟ M07.671 Enteropathic arthropathies, right ankle and foot
⊟ M07.672 Enteropathic arthropathies, left ankle and foot
⊟ M07.679 Enteropathic arthropathies, unspecified ankle and foot
M07.68 Enteropathic arthropathies, vertebrae
M07.69 Enteropathic arthropathies, multiple sites

4 **M08 Juvenile arthritis**
Code also any associated underlying condition, such as:
regional enteritis [Crohn's disease] (K50.-)
ulcerative colitis (K51.-)
EXCLUDES 1 *arthropathy in Whipple's disease (M14.8)*
Felty's syndrome (M05.0)
juvenile dermatomyositis (M33.0-)
psoriatic juvenile arthropathy (L40.54)

CODING TIP ✓ Juvenile arthritis generally indicates arthritic conditions that have developed in individuals under 16 years of age. Autoimmune disorders are often the cause of these conditions, and all available records should be carefully reviewed to assign the most specific diagnosis and identify any underlying conditions.

5 **M08.0 Unspecified juvenile rheumatoid arthritis**
Juvenile rheumatoid arthritis with or without rheumatoid factor
M08.00 Unspecified juvenile rheumatoid arthritis of unspecified site HCC
6 M08.01 Unspecified juvenile rheumatoid arthritis, shoulder
⊟ M08.011 Unspecified juvenile rheumatoid arthritis, right shoulder HCC
⊟ M08.012 Unspecified juvenile rheumatoid arthritis, left shoulder HCC
⊟ M08.019 Unspecified juvenile rheumatoid arthritis, unspecified shoulder HCC
6 M08.02 Unspecified juvenile rheumatoid arthritis of elbow
⊟ M08.021 Unspecified juvenile rheumatoid arthritis, right elbow HCC
⊟ M08.022 Unspecified juvenile rheumatoid arthritis, left elbow HCC
⊟ M08.029 Unspecified juvenile rheumatoid arthritis, unspecified elbow HCC
6 M08.03 Unspecified juvenile rheumatoid arthritis, wrist
⊟ M08.031 Unspecified juvenile rheumatoid arthritis, right wrist HCC
⊟ M08.032 Unspecified juvenile rheumatoid arthritis, left wrist HCC
⊟ M08.039 Unspecified juvenile rheumatoid arthritis, unspecified wrist HCC
6 M08.04 Unspecified juvenile rheumatoid arthritis, hand
⊟ M08.041 Unspecified juvenile rheumatoid arthritis, right hand HCC
⊟ M08.042 Unspecified juvenile rheumatoid arthritis, left hand HCC
⊟ M08.049 Unspecified juvenile rheumatoid arthritis, unspecified hand HCC
6 M08.05 Unspecified juvenile rheumatoid arthritis, hip
⊟ M08.051 Unspecified juvenile rheumatoid arthritis, right hip HCC
⊟ M08.052 Unspecified juvenile rheumatoid arthritis, left hip HCC
⊟ M08.059 Unspecified juvenile rheumatoid arthritis, unspecified hip HCC
6 M08.06 Unspecified juvenile rheumatoid arthritis, knee
⊟ M08.061 Unspecified juvenile rheumatoid arthritis, right knee HCC
⊟ M08.062 Unspecified juvenile rheumatoid arthritis, left knee HCC
⊟ M08.069 Unspecified juvenile rheumatoid arthritis, unspecified knee HCC
6 M08.07 Unspecified juvenile rheumatoid arthritis, ankle and foot
⊟ M08.071 Unspecified juvenile rheumatoid arthritis, right ankle and foot HCC
⊟ M08.072 Unspecified juvenile rheumatoid arthritis, left ankle and foot HCC
⊟ M08.079 Unspecified juvenile rheumatoid arthritis, unspecified ankle and foot HCC
M08.08 Unspecified juvenile rheumatoid arthritis, vertebrae HCC
M08.09 Unspecified juvenile rheumatoid arthritis, multiple sites HCC

M08.1 Juvenile ankylosing spondylitis HCC
EXCLUDES 1 *ankylosing spondylitis in adults (M45.0-)*

5 **M08.2 Juvenile rheumatoid arthritis with systemic onset**
Still's disease NOS
EXCLUDES 1 *adult-onset Still's disease (M06.1-)*
M08.20 Juvenile rheumatoid arthritis with systemic onset, unspecified site HCC
6 M08.21 Juvenile rheumatoid arthritis with systemic onset, shoulder
⊟ M08.211 Juvenile rheumatoid arthritis with systemic onset, right shoulder HCC
⊟ M08.212 Juvenile rheumatoid arthritis with systemic onset, left shoulder HCC
⊟ M08.219 Juvenile rheumatoid arthritis with systemic onset, unspecified shoulder HCC
6 M08.22 Juvenile rheumatoid arthritis with systemic onset, elbow
⊟ M08.221 Juvenile rheumatoid arthritis with systemic onset, right elbow HCC
⊟ M08.222 Juvenile rheumatoid arthritis with systemic onset, left elbow HCC

Diseases of the Musculoskeletal System and Connective Tissue

M08.229 Juvenile rheumatoid arthritis with systemic onset, unspecified elbow HCC

M08.23 Juvenile rheumatoid arthritis with systemic onset, wrist

M08.231 Juvenile rheumatoid arthritis with systemic onset, right wrist HCC

M08.232 Juvenile rheumatoid arthritis with systemic onset, left wrist HCC

M08.239 Juvenile rheumatoid arthritis with systemic onset, unspecified wrist HCC

M08.24 Juvenile rheumatoid arthritis with systemic onset, hand

M08.241 Juvenile rheumatoid arthritis with systemic onset, right hand HCC

M08.242 Juvenile rheumatoid arthritis with systemic onset, left hand HCC

M08.249 Juvenile rheumatoid arthritis with systemic onset, unspecified hand HCC

M08.25 Juvenile rheumatoid arthritis with systemic onset, hip

M08.251 Juvenile rheumatoid arthritis with systemic onset, right hip HCC

M08.252 Juvenile rheumatoid arthritis with systemic onset, left hip HCC

M08.259 Juvenile rheumatoid arthritis with systemic onset, unspecified hip HCC

M08.26 Juvenile rheumatoid arthritis with systemic onset, knee

M08.261 Juvenile rheumatoid arthritis with systemic onset, right knee HCC

M08.262 Juvenile rheumatoid arthritis with systemic onset, left knee HCC

M08.269 Juvenile rheumatoid arthritis with systemic onset, unspecified knee HCC

M08.27 Juvenile rheumatoid arthritis with systemic onset, ankle and foot

M08.271 Juvenile rheumatoid arthritis with systemic onset, right ankle and foot HCC

M08.272 Juvenile rheumatoid arthritis with systemic onset, left ankle and foot HCC

M08.279 Juvenile rheumatoid arthritis with systemic onset, unspecified ankle and foot HCC

M08.28 Juvenile rheumatoid arthritis with systemic onset, vertebrae HCC

M08.29 Juvenile rheumatoid arthritis with systemic onset, multiple sites HCC

M08.3 Juvenile rheumatoid polyarthritis (seronegative) HCC

M08.4 Pauciarticular juvenile rheumatoid arthritis

CODING TIP ✓ Pauciarticular juvenile rheumatoid arthritis, also called oligoarticular juvenile idiopathic arthritis, affects five or fewer joints and is asymmetric. These codes require site and laterality.

M08.40 Pauciarticular juvenile rheumatoid arthritis, unspecified site HCC

M08.41 Pauciarticular juvenile rheumatoid arthritis, shoulder

M08.411 Pauciarticular juvenile rheumatoid arthritis, right shoulder HCC

M08.412 Pauciarticular juvenile rheumatoid arthritis, left shoulder HCC

M08.419 Pauciarticular juvenile rheumatoid arthritis, unspecified shoulder HCC

M08.42 Pauciarticular juvenile rheumatoid arthritis, elbow

M08.421 Pauciarticular juvenile rheumatoid arthritis, right elbow HCC

M08.422 Pauciarticular juvenile rheumatoid arthritis, left elbow HCC

M08.429 Pauciarticular juvenile rheumatoid arthritis, unspecified elbow HCC

M08.43 Pauciarticular juvenile rheumatoid arthritis, wrist

M08.431 Pauciarticular juvenile rheumatoid arthritis, right wrist HCC

M08.432 Pauciarticular juvenile rheumatoid arthritis, left wrist HCC

M08.439 Pauciarticular juvenile rheumatoid arthritis, unspecified wrist HCC

M08.44 Pauciarticular juvenile rheumatoid arthritis, hand

M08.441 Pauciarticular juvenile rheumatoid arthritis, right hand HCC

M08.442 Pauciarticular juvenile rheumatoid arthritis, left hand HCC

M08.449 Pauciarticular juvenile rheumatoid arthritis, unspecified hand HCC

M08.45 Pauciarticular juvenile rheumatoid arthritis, hip

M08.451 Pauciarticular juvenile rheumatoid arthritis, right hip HCC

M08.452 Pauciarticular juvenile rheumatoid arthritis, left hip HCC

M08.459 Pauciarticular juvenile rheumatoid arthritis, unspecified hip HCC

M08.46 Pauciarticular juvenile rheumatoid arthritis, knee

M08.461 Pauciarticular juvenile rheumatoid arthritis, right knee HCC

M08.462 Pauciarticular juvenile rheumatoid arthritis, left knee HCC

M08.469 Pauciarticular juvenile rheumatoid arthritis, unspecified knee HCC

M08.47 Pauciarticular juvenile rheumatoid arthritis, ankle and foot

M08.471 Pauciarticular juvenile rheumatoid arthritis, right ankle and foot HCC

M08.472 Pauciarticular juvenile rheumatoid arthritis, left ankle and foot HCC

M08.479 Pauciarticular juvenile rheumatoid arthritis, unspecified ankle and foot HCC

M08.48 Pauciarticular juvenile rheumatoid arthritis, vertebrae HCC

M08.8 Other juvenile arthritis

M08.80 Other juvenile arthritis, unspecified site HCC

M08.81 Other juvenile arthritis, shoulder

M08.811 Other juvenile arthritis, right shoulder HCC

M08.812 Other juvenile arthritis, left shoulder HCC

M08.819 Other juvenile arthritis, unspecified shoulder HCC

M08.82 Other juvenile arthritis, elbow

M08.821 Other juvenile arthritis, right elbow HCC

M08.822 Other juvenile arthritis, left elbow HCC

M08.829 Other juvenile arthritis, unspecified elbow HCC

M08.83 Other juvenile arthritis, wrist

M08.831 Other juvenile arthritis, right wrist HCC

M08.832 Other juvenile arthritis, left wrist HCC

M08.839 Other juvenile arthritis, unspecified wrist HCC

M08.84 Other juvenile arthritis, hand

M08.841 Other juvenile arthritis, right hand HCC

M08.842 Other juvenile arthritis, left hand HCC

M08.849 Other juvenile arthritis, unspecified hand HCC

M08.85 Other juvenile arthritis, hip

M08.851 Other juvenile arthritis, right hip HCC

M08.852 Other juvenile arthritis, left hip HCC

M08.859 Other juvenile arthritis, unspecified hip HCC

M08.86 Other juvenile arthritis, knee

M08.861 Other juvenile arthritis, right knee HCC

M08.862 Other juvenile arthritis, left knee HCC

M08.869 Other juvenile arthritis, unspecified knee HCC

M08.87 Other juvenile arthritis, ankle and foot

M08.871 Other juvenile arthritis, right ankle and foot HCC

M08.872 Other juvenile arthritis, left ankle and foot HCC

M08.879 Other juvenile arthritis, unspecified ankle and foot HCC

M08.88 Other juvenile arthritis, other specified site HCC

Other juvenile arthritis, vertebrae

M08.89 Other juvenile arthritis, multiple sites HCC

M08.9 **Juvenile arthritis, unspecified**

EXCLUDES 1 *juvenile rheumatoid arthritis, unspecified (M08.0-)*

M08.90 **Juvenile arthritis, unspecified, unspecified site** HCC

M08.91 **Juvenile arthritis, unspecified, shoulder**

M08.911 **Juvenile arthritis, unspecified, right shoulder** HCC

M08.912 **Juvenile arthritis, unspecified, left shoulder** HCC

M08.919 **Juvenile arthritis, unspecified, unspecified shoulder** HCC

M08.92 **Juvenile arthritis, unspecified, elbow**

M08.921 **Juvenile arthritis, unspecified, right elbow** HCC

M08.922 **Juvenile arthritis, unspecified, left elbow** HCC

M08.929 **Juvenile arthritis, unspecified, unspecified elbow** HCC

M08.93 **Juvenile arthritis, unspecified, wrist**

M08.931 **Juvenile arthritis, unspecified, right wrist** HCC

M08.932 **Juvenile arthritis, unspecified, left wrist** HCC

M08.939 **Juvenile arthritis, unspecified, unspecified wrist** HCC

M08.94 **Juvenile arthritis, unspecified, hand**

M08.941 **Juvenile arthritis, unspecified, right hand** HCC

M08.942 **Juvenile arthritis, unspecified, left hand** HCC

M08.949 **Juvenile arthritis, unspecified, unspecified hand** HCC

M08.95 **Juvenile arthritis, unspecified, hip**

M08.951 **Juvenile arthritis, unspecified, right hip** HCC

M08.952 **Juvenile arthritis, unspecified, left hip** HCC

M08.959 **Juvenile arthritis, unspecified, unspecified hip** HCC

M08.96 **Juvenile arthritis, unspecified, knee**

M08.961 **Juvenile arthritis, unspecified, right knee** HCC

M08.962 **Juvenile arthritis, unspecified, left knee** HCC

M08.969 **Juvenile arthritis, unspecified, unspecified knee** HCC

M08.97 **Juvenile arthritis, unspecified, ankle and foot**

M08.971 **Juvenile arthritis, unspecified, right ankle and foot** HCC

M08.972 **Juvenile arthritis, unspecified, left ankle and foot** HCC

M08.979 **Juvenile arthritis, unspecified, unspecified ankle and foot** HCC

M08.98 **Juvenile arthritis, unspecified, vertebrae** HCC

M08.99 **Juvenile arthritis, unspecified, multiple sites** HCC

M1A Chronic gout

Use additional code to identify:
Autonomic neuropathy in diseases classified elsewhere (G99.0)
Calculus of urinary tract in diseases classified elsewhere (N22)
Cardiomyopathy in diseases classified elsewhere (I43)
Disorders of external ear in diseases classified elsewhere (H61.1-, H62.8-)
Disorders of iris and ciliary body in diseases classified elsewhere (H22)
Glomerular disorders in diseases classified elsewhere (N08)

EXCLUDES 1 *gout NOS (M10.-)*

EXCLUDES 2 *acute gout (M10.-)*

The appropriate 7th character is to be added to each code from category M1A
0 without tophus (tophi)
1 with tophus (tophi)

CODING TIP ✓ Do not assign a code from category M1A.- unless the physician has specifically provided a diagnosis of "chronic" gout or there is documentation of the presence of tophi.

M1A.0 **Idiopathic chronic gout**
Chronic gouty bursitis
Primary chronic gout

M1A.00X- **Idiopathic chronic gout, unspecified site**

M1A.01 **Idiopathic chronic gout, shoulder**

M1A.011- **Idiopathic chronic gout, right shoulder**

M1A.012- **Idiopathic chronic gout, left shoulder**

M1A.019- **Idiopathic chronic gout, unspecified shoulder**

M1A.02 **Idiopathic chronic gout, elbow**

M1A.021- **Idiopathic chronic gout, right elbow**

M1A.022- **Idiopathic chronic gout, left elbow**

M1A.029- **Idiopathic chronic gout, unspecified elbow**

M1A.03 **Idiopathic chronic gout, wrist**

M1A.031- **Idiopathic chronic gout, right wrist**

M1A.032- **Idiopathic chronic gout, left wrist**

M1A.039- **Idiopathic chronic gout, unspecified wrist**

M1A.04 **Idiopathic chronic gout, hand**

M1A.041- **Idiopathic chronic gout, right hand**

M1A.042- **Idiopathic chronic gout, left hand**

M1A.049- **Idiopathic chronic gout, unspecified hand**

M1A.05 **Idiopathic chronic gout, hip**

M1A.051- **Idiopathic chronic gout, right hip**

M1A.052- **Idiopathic chronic gout, left hip**

M1A.059- **Idiopathic chronic gout, unspecified hip**

M1A.06 **Idiopathic chronic gout, knee**

M1A.061- **Idiopathic chronic gout, right knee**

M1A.062- **Idiopathic chronic gout, left knee**

M1A.069- **Idiopathic chronic gout, unspecified knee**

M1A.07 **Idiopathic chronic gout, ankle and foot**

Idiopathic chronic gout

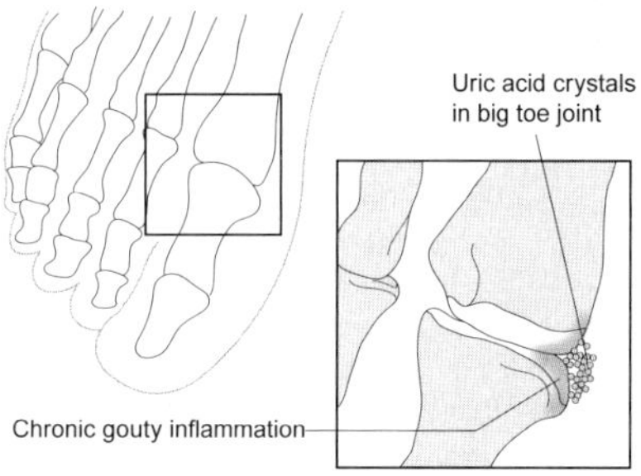

M1A.071- **Idiopathic chronic gout, right ankle and foot**

M1A.072- **Idiopathic chronic gout, left ankle and foot**

M1A.079- **Idiopathic chronic gout, unspecified ankle and foot**

M1A.08X- **Idiopathic chronic gout, vertebrae**

M1A.09X- **Idiopathic chronic gout, multiple sites**

M1A.1 **Lead-induced chronic gout**
Code first:
toxic effects of lead and its compounds (T56.0-)

M1A.10X- **Lead-induced chronic gout, unspecified site**

M1A.11 **Lead-induced chronic gout, shoulder**

M1A.111- **Lead-induced chronic gout, right shoulder**

M1A.112- **Lead-induced chronic gout, left shoulder**

M1A.119- **Lead-induced chronic gout, unspecified shoulder**

M1A.12 **Lead-induced chronic gout, elbow**

M1A.121- **Lead-induced chronic gout, right elbow**

M1A.122- **Lead-induced chronic gout, left elbow**

M1A.129- **Lead-induced chronic gout, unspecified elbow**

M1A.13 **Lead-induced chronic gout, wrist**

M1A.131- **Lead-induced chronic gout, right wrist**

M1A.132- **Lead-induced chronic gout, left wrist**

M1A.139- **Lead-induced chronic gout, unspecified wrist**

M1A.14 **Lead-induced chronic gout, hand**

M1A.141- **Lead-induced chronic gout, right hand**

M1A.142- **Lead-induced chronic gout, left hand**

M1A.149- **Lead-induced chronic gout, unspecified hand**

M1A.15 **Lead-induced chronic gout, hip**

7 ⊟ M1A.151- Lead-induced chronic gout, right hip
7 ⊟ M1A.152- Lead-induced chronic gout, left hip
7 ⊟ M1A.159- Lead-induced chronic gout, unspecified hip
6 M1A.16 Lead-induced chronic gout, knee
7 ⊟ M1A.161- Lead-induced chronic gout, right knee
7 ⊟ M1A.162- Lead-induced chronic gout, left knee
7 ⊟ M1A.169- Lead-induced chronic gout, unspecified knee
6 M1A.17 Lead-induced chronic gout, ankle and foot
7 ⊟ M1A.171- Lead-induced chronic gout, right ankle and foot
7 ⊟ M1A.172- Lead-induced chronic gout, left ankle and foot
7 ⊟ M1A.179- Lead-induced chronic gout, unspecified ankle and foot
7 M1A.18X- Lead-induced chronic gout, vertebrae
7 M1A.19X- Lead-induced chronic gout, multiple sites
5 M1A.2 Drug-induced chronic gout
Use additional code for adverse effect, if applicable, to identify drug (T36-T50 with fifth or sixth character 5)
7 M1A.20X- Drug-induced chronic gout, unspecified site
6 M1A.21 Drug-induced chronic gout, shoulder
7 ⊟ M1A.211- Drug-induced chronic gout, right shoulder
7 ⊟ M1A.212- Drug-induced chronic gout, left shoulder
7 ⊟ M1A.219- Drug-induced chronic gout, unspecified shoulder
6 M1A.22 Drug-induced chronic gout, elbow
7 ⊟ M1A.221- Drug-induced chronic gout, right elbow
7 ⊟ M1A.222- Drug-induced chronic gout, left elbow
7 ⊟ M1A.229- Drug-induced chronic gout, unspecified elbow
6 M1A.23 Drug-induced chronic gout, wrist
7 ⊟ M1A.231- Drug-induced chronic gout, right wrist
7 ⊟ M1A.232- Drug-induced chronic gout, left wrist
7 ⊟ M1A.239- Drug-induced chronic gout, unspecified wrist
6 M1A.24 Drug-induced chronic gout, hand
7 ⊟ M1A.241- Drug-induced chronic gout, right hand
7 ⊟ M1A.242- Drug-induced chronic gout, left hand
7 ⊟ M1A.249- Drug-induced chronic gout, unspecified hand
6 M1A.25 Drug-induced chronic gout, hip
7 ⊟ M1A.251- Drug-induced chronic gout, right hip
7 ⊟ M1A.252- Drug-induced chronic gout, left hip
7 ⊟ M1A.259- Drug-induced chronic gout, unspecified hip
6 M1A.26 Drug-induced chronic gout, knee
7 ⊟ M1A.261- Drug-induced chronic gout, right knee
7 ⊟ M1A.262- Drug-induced chronic gout, left knee
7 ⊟ M1A.269- Drug-induced chronic gout, unspecified knee
6 M1A.27 Drug-induced chronic gout, ankle and foot
7 ⊟ M1A.271- Drug-induced chronic gout, right ankle and foot
7 ⊟ M1A.272- Drug-induced chronic gout, left ankle and foot
7 ⊟ M1A.279- Drug-induced chronic gout, unspecified ankle and foot
7 M1A.28X- Drug-induced chronic gout, vertebrae
7 M1A.29X- Drug-induced chronic gout, multiple sites
5 M1A.3 Chronic gout due to renal impairment
Code first:
associated renal disease
7 M1A.30X- Chronic gout due to renal impairment, unspecified site
6 M1A.31 Chronic gout due to renal impairment, shoulder
7 ⊟ M1A.311- Chronic gout due to renal impairment, right shoulder
7 ⊟ M1A.312- Chronic gout due to renal impairment, left shoulder
7 ⊟ M1A.319- Chronic gout due to renal impairment, unspecified shoulder
6 M1A.32 Chronic gout due to renal impairment, elbow
7 ⊟ M1A.321- Chronic gout due to renal impairment, right elbow
7 ⊟ M1A.322- Chronic gout due to renal impairment, left elbow
7 ⊟ M1A.329- Chronic gout due to renal impairment, unspecified elbow
6 M1A.33 Chronic gout due to renal impairment, wrist
7 ⊟ M1A.331- Chronic gout due to renal impairment, right wrist
7 ⊟ M1A.332- Chronic gout due to renal impairment, left wrist
7 ⊟ M1A.339- Chronic gout due to renal impairment, unspecified wrist
6 M1A.34 Chronic gout due to renal impairment, hand
7 ⊟ M1A.341- Chronic gout due to renal impairment, right hand
7 ⊟ M1A.342- Chronic gout due to renal impairment, left hand
7 ⊟ M1A.349- Chronic gout due to renal impairment, unspecified hand
6 M1A.35 Chronic gout due to renal impairment, hip
7 ⊟ M1A.351- Chronic gout due to renal impairment, right hip
7 ⊟ M1A.352- Chronic gout due to renal impairment, left hip
7 ⊟ M1A.359- Chronic gout due to renal impairment, unspecified hip
6 M1A.36 Chronic gout due to renal impairment, knee
7 ⊟ M1A.361- Chronic gout due to renal impairment, right knee
7 ⊟ M1A.362- Chronic gout due to renal impairment, left knee
7 ⊟ M1A.369- Chronic gout due to renal impairment, unspecified knee
6 M1A.37 Chronic gout due to renal impairment, ankle and foot
7 ⊟ M1A.371- Chronic gout due to renal impairment, right ankle and foot
7 ⊟ M1A.372- Chronic gout due to renal impairment, left ankle and foot
7 ⊟ M1A.379- Chronic gout due to renal impairment, unspecified ankle and foot
7 M1A.38X- Chronic gout due to renal impairment, vertebrae
7 M1A.39X- Chronic gout due to renal impairment, multiple sites
5 M1A.4 Other secondary chronic gout
Code first:
associated condition
7 M1A.40X- Other secondary chronic gout, unspecified site
6 M1A.41 Other secondary chronic gout, shoulder
7 ⊟ M1A.411- Other secondary chronic gout, right shoulder
7 ⊟ M1A.412- Other secondary chronic gout, left shoulder
7 ⊟ M1A.419- Other secondary chronic gout, unspecified shoulder
6 M1A.42 Other secondary chronic gout, elbow
7 ⊟ M1A.421- Other secondary chronic gout, right elbow
7 ⊟ M1A.422- Other secondary chronic gout, left elbow
7 ⊟ M1A.429- Other secondary chronic gout, unspecified elbow
6 M1A.43 Other secondary chronic gout, wrist
7 ⊟ M1A.431- Other secondary chronic gout, right wrist
7 ⊟ M1A.432- Other secondary chronic gout, left wrist
7 ⊟ M1A.439- Other secondary chronic gout, unspecified wrist
6 M1A.44 Other secondary chronic gout, hand
7 ⊟ M1A.441- Other secondary chronic gout, right hand
7 ⊟ M1A.442- Other secondary chronic gout, left hand
7 ⊟ M1A.449- Other secondary chronic gout, unspecified hand
6 M1A.45 Other secondary chronic gout, hip
7 ⊟ M1A.451- Other secondary chronic gout, right hip
7 ⊟ M1A.452- Other secondary chronic gout, left hip
7 ⊟ M1A.459- Other secondary chronic gout, unspecified hip
6 M1A.46 Other secondary chronic gout, knee
7 ⊟ M1A.461- Other secondary chronic gout, right knee
7 ⊟ M1A.462- Other secondary chronic gout, left knee
7 ⊟ M1A.469- Other secondary chronic gout, unspecified knee
6 M1A.47 Other secondary chronic gout, ankle and foot
7 ⊟ M1A.471- Other secondary chronic gout, right ankle and foot
7 ⊟ M1A.472- Other secondary chronic gout, left ankle and foot
7 ⊟ M1A.479- Other secondary chronic gout, unspecified ankle and foot
7 M1A.48X- Other secondary chronic gout, vertebrae

7 M1A.49X- Other secondary chronic gout, multiple sites
7 M1A.9XX- Chronic gout, unspecified

4 **M10 Gout**
Acute gout
Gout attack
Gout flare
Podagra
Use additional code to identify:
Autonomic neuropathy in diseases classified elsewhere (G99.0)
Calculus of urinary tract in diseases classified elsewhere (N22)
Cardiomyopathy in diseases classified elsewhere (I43)
Disorders of external ear in diseases classified elsewhere (H61.1-, H62.8-)
Disorders of iris and ciliary body in diseases classified elsewhere (H22)
Glomerular disorders in diseases classified elsewhere (N08)
EXCLUDES 2 *chronic gout (M1A.-)*

Acute Gout

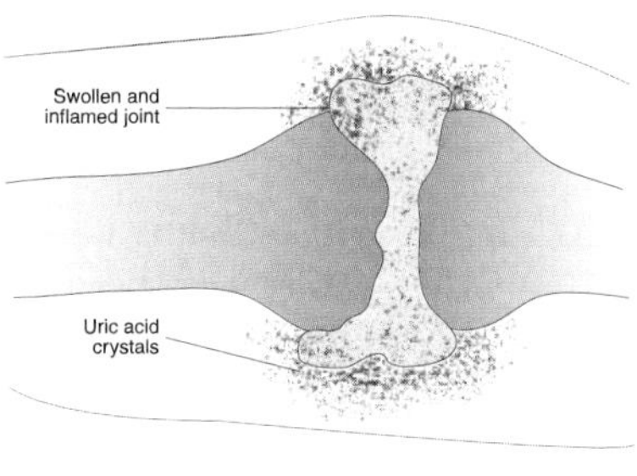

5 M10.0 Idiopathic gout
Gouty bursitis
Primary gout
M10.00 Idiopathic gout, unspecified site
6 M10.01 Idiopathic gout, shoulder
M10.011 Idiopathic gout, right shoulder
M10.012 Idiopathic gout, left shoulder
M10.019 Idiopathic gout, unspecified shoulder
6 M10.02 Idiopathic gout, elbow
M10.021 Idiopathic gout, right elbow
M10.022 Idiopathic gout, left elbow
M10.029 Idiopathic gout, unspecified elbow
6 M10.03 Idiopathic gout, wrist
M10.031 Idiopathic gout, right wrist
M10.032 Idiopathic gout, left wrist
M10.039 Idiopathic gout, unspecified wrist
6 M10.04 Idiopathic gout, hand
M10.041 Idiopathic gout, right hand
M10.042 Idiopathic gout, left hand
M10.049 Idiopathic gout, unspecified hand
6 M10.05 Idiopathic gout, hip
M10.051 Idiopathic gout, right hip
M10.052 Idiopathic gout, left hip
M10.059 Idiopathic gout, unspecified hip
6 M10.06 Idiopathic gout, knee
M10.061 Idiopathic gout, right knee
M10.062 Idiopathic gout, left knee
M10.069 Idiopathic gout, unspecified knee
6 M10.07 Idiopathic gout, ankle and foot
M10.071 Idiopathic gout, right ankle and foot
M10.072 Idiopathic gout, left ankle and foot
M10.079 Idiopathic gout, unspecified ankle and foot
M10.08 Idiopathic gout, vertebrae
M10.09 Idiopathic gout, multiple sites
5 M10.1 Lead-induced gout
Code first:
toxic effects of lead and its compounds (T56.0-)
M10.10 Lead-induced gout, unspecified site
6 M10.11 Lead-induced gout, shoulder
M10.111 Lead-induced gout, right shoulder
M10.112 Lead-induced gout, left shoulder
M10.119 Lead-induced gout, unspecified shoulder
6 M10.12 Lead-induced gout, elbow
M10.121 Lead-induced gout, right elbow
M10.122 Lead-induced gout, left elbow
M10.129 Lead-induced gout, unspecified elbow
6 M10.13 Lead-induced gout, wrist
M10.131 Lead-induced gout, right wrist
M10.132 Lead-induced gout, left wrist
M10.139 Lead-induced gout, unspecified wrist
6 M10.14 Lead-induced gout, hand
M10.141 Lead-induced gout, right hand
M10.142 Lead-induced gout, left hand
M10.149 Lead-induced gout, unspecified hand
6 M10.15 Lead-induced gout, hip
M10.151 Lead-induced gout, right hip
M10.152 Lead-induced gout, left hip
M10.159 Lead-induced gout, unspecified hip
6 M10.16 Lead-induced gout, knee
M10.161 Lead-induced gout, right knee
M10.162 Lead-induced gout, left knee
M10.169 Lead-induced gout, unspecified knee
6 M10.17 Lead-induced gout, ankle and foot
M10.171 Lead-induced gout, right ankle and foot
M10.172 Lead-induced gout, left ankle and foot
M10.179 Lead-induced gout, unspecified ankle and foot
M10.18 Lead-induced gout, vertebrae
M10.19 Lead-induced gout, multiple sites
5 M10.2 Drug-induced gout
Use additional code for adverse effect, if applicable, to identify drug (T36-T50 with fifth or sixth character 5)
M10.20 Drug-induced gout, unspecified site
6 M10.21 Drug-induced gout, shoulder
M10.211 Drug-induced gout, right shoulder
M10.212 Drug-induced gout, left shoulder
M10.219 Drug-induced gout, unspecified shoulder
6 M10.22 Drug-induced gout, elbow
M10.221 Drug-induced gout, right elbow
M10.222 Drug-induced gout, left elbow
M10.229 Drug-induced gout, unspecified elbow
6 M10.23 Drug-induced gout, wrist
M10.231 Drug-induced gout, right wrist
M10.232 Drug-induced gout, left wrist
M10.239 Drug-induced gout, unspecified wrist
6 M10.24 Drug-induced gout, hand
M10.241 Drug-induced gout, right hand
M10.242 Drug-induced gout, left hand
M10.249 Drug-induced gout, unspecified hand
6 M10.25 Drug-induced gout, hip
M10.251 Drug-induced gout, right hip
M10.252 Drug-induced gout, left hip
M10.259 Drug-induced gout, unspecified hip
6 M10.26 Drug-induced gout, knee
M10.261 Drug-induced gout, right knee
M10.262 Drug-induced gout, left knee
M10.269 Drug-induced gout, unspecified knee
6 M10.27 Drug-induced gout, ankle and foot
M10.271 Drug-induced gout, right ankle and foot
M10.272 Drug-induced gout, left ankle and foot
M10.279 Drug-induced gout, unspecified ankle and foot
M10.28 Drug-induced gout, vertebrae
M10.29 Drug-induced gout, multiple sites
5 M10.3 Gout due to renal impairment
Code first:
associated renal disease

M10.30 Gout due to renal impairment, unspecified site
6 M10.31 Gout due to renal impairment, shoulder
M10.311 Gout due to renal impairment, right shoulder
M10.312 Gout due to renal impairment, left shoulder
M10.319 Gout due to renal impairment, unspecified shoulder
6 M10.32 Gout due to renal impairment, elbow
M10.321 Gout due to renal impairment, right elbow
M10.322 Gout due to renal impairment, left elbow
M10.329 Gout due to renal impairment, unspecified elbow
6 M10.33 Gout due to renal impairment, wrist
M10.331 Gout due to renal impairment, right wrist
M10.332 Gout due to renal impairment, left wrist
M10.339 Gout due to renal impairment, unspecified wrist
6 M10.34 Gout due to renal impairment, hand
M10.341 Gout due to renal impairment, right hand
M10.342 Gout due to renal impairment, left hand
M10.349 Gout due to renal impairment, unspecified hand
6 M10.35 Gout due to renal impairment, hip
M10.351 Gout due to renal impairment, right hip
M10.352 Gout due to renal impairment, left hip
M10.359 Gout due to renal impairment, unspecified hip
6 M10.36 Gout due to renal impairment, knee
M10.361 Gout due to renal impairment, right knee
M10.362 Gout due to renal impairment, left knee
M10.369 Gout due to renal impairment, unspecified knee
6 M10.37 Gout due to renal impairment, ankle and foot
M10.371 Gout due to renal impairment, right ankle and foot
M10.372 Gout due to renal impairment, left ankle and foot
M10.379 Gout due to renal impairment, unspecified ankle and foot
M10.38 Gout due to renal impairment, vertebrae
M10.39 Gout due to renal impairment, multiple sites
5 M10.4 Other secondary gout
Code first:
associated condition
M10.40 Other secondary gout, unspecified site
6 M10.41 Other secondary gout, shoulder
M10.411 Other secondary gout, right shoulder
M10.412 Other secondary gout, left shoulder
M10.419 Other secondary gout, unspecified shoulder
6 M10.42 Other secondary gout, elbow
M10.421 Other secondary gout, right elbow
M10.422 Other secondary gout, left elbow
M10.429 Other secondary gout, unspecified elbow
6 M10.43 Other secondary gout, wrist
M10.431 Other secondary gout, right wrist
M10.432 Other secondary gout, left wrist
M10.439 Other secondary gout, unspecified wrist
6 M10.44 Other secondary gout, hand
M10.441 Other secondary gout, right hand
M10.442 Other secondary gout, left hand
M10.449 Other secondary gout, unspecified hand
6 M10.45 Other secondary gout, hip
M10.451 Other secondary gout, right hip
M10.452 Other secondary gout, left hip
M10.459 Other secondary gout, unspecified hip
6 M10.46 Other secondary gout, knee
M10.461 Other secondary gout, right knee
M10.462 Other secondary gout, left knee
M10.469 Other secondary gout, unspecified knee
6 M10.47 Other secondary gout, ankle and foot
M10.471 Other secondary gout, right ankle and foot
M10.472 Other secondary gout, left ankle and foot
M10.479 Other secondary gout, unspecified ankle and foot
M10.48 Other secondary gout, vertebrae
M10.49 Other secondary gout, multiple sites
M10.9 Gout, unspecified
Gout NOS

4 M11 Other crystal arthropathies
5 M11.0 Hydroxyapatite deposition disease
M11.00 Hydroxyapatite deposition disease, unspecified site
6 M11.01 Hydroxyapatite deposition disease, shoulder
M11.011 Hydroxyapatite deposition disease, right shoulder
M11.012 Hydroxyapatite deposition disease, left shoulder
M11.019 Hydroxyapatite deposition disease, unspecified shoulder
6 M11.02 Hydroxyapatite deposition disease, elbow
M11.021 Hydroxyapatite deposition disease, right elbow
M11.022 Hydroxyapatite deposition disease, left elbow
M11.029 Hydroxyapatite deposition disease, unspecified elbow
6 M11.03 Hydroxyapatite deposition disease, wrist
M11.031 Hydroxyapatite deposition disease, right wrist
M11.032 Hydroxyapatite deposition disease, left wrist
M11.039 Hydroxyapatite deposition disease, unspecified wrist
6 M11.04 Hydroxyapatite deposition disease, hand
M11.041 Hydroxyapatite deposition disease, right hand
M11.042 Hydroxyapatite deposition disease, left hand
M11.049 Hydroxyapatite deposition disease, unspecified hand
6 M11.05 Hydroxyapatite deposition disease, hip
M11.051 Hydroxyapatite deposition disease, right hip
M11.052 Hydroxyapatite deposition disease, left hip
M11.059 Hydroxyapatite deposition disease, unspecified hip
6 M11.06 Hydroxyapatite deposition disease, knee
M11.061 Hydroxyapatite deposition disease, right knee
M11.062 Hydroxyapatite deposition disease, left knee
M11.069 Hydroxyapatite deposition disease, unspecified knee
6 M11.07 Hydroxyapatite deposition disease, ankle and foot
M11.071 Hydroxyapatite deposition disease, right ankle and foot
M11.072 Hydroxyapatite deposition disease, left ankle and foot
M11.079 Hydroxyapatite deposition disease, unspecified ankle and foot
M11.08 Hydroxyapatite deposition disease, vertebrae
M11.09 Hydroxyapatite deposition disease, multiple sites
5 M11.1 Familial chondrocalcinosis
M11.10 Familial chondrocalcinosis, unspecified site
6 M11.11 Familial chondrocalcinosis, shoulder
M11.111 Familial chondrocalcinosis, right shoulder
M11.112 Familial chondrocalcinosis, left shoulder
M11.119 Familial chondrocalcinosis, unspecified shoulder
6 M11.12 Familial chondrocalcinosis, elbow
M11.121 Familial chondrocalcinosis, right elbow
M11.122 Familial chondrocalcinosis, left elbow
M11.129 Familial chondrocalcinosis, unspecified elbow
6 M11.13 Familial chondrocalcinosis, wrist
M11.131 Familial chondrocalcinosis, right wrist
M11.132 Familial chondrocalcinosis, left wrist
M11.139 Familial chondrocalcinosis, unspecified wrist
6 M11.14 Familial chondrocalcinosis, hand
M11.141 Familial chondrocalcinosis, right hand
M11.142 Familial chondrocalcinosis, left hand
M11.149 Familial chondrocalcinosis, unspecified hand

● New | Manifestation | 4-7 Digit Indicators | Laterality | A Adult | M Maternity | N Newborn | P Pediatric | ♂ Male
▲ Revised | Unspecified | AHA Coding Clinic | HCC Hierarchical Condition Categories | HIV HIV Related Conditions | ♀ Female

- M11.15 Familial chondrocalcinosis, hip
  - M11.151 Familial chondrocalcinosis, right hip
  - M11.152 Familial chondrocalcinosis, left hip
  - M11.159 Familial chondrocalcinosis, unspecified hip
- M11.16 Familial chondrocalcinosis, knee
  - M11.161 Familial chondrocalcinosis, right knee
  - M11.162 Familial chondrocalcinosis, left knee
  - M11.169 Familial chondrocalcinosis, unspecified knee
- M11.17 Familial chondrocalcinosis, ankle and foot
  - M11.171 Familial chondrocalcinosis, right ankle and foot
  - M11.172 Familial chondrocalcinosis, left ankle and foot
  - M11.179 Familial chondrocalcinosis, unspecified ankle and foot
- M11.18 Familial chondrocalcinosis, vertebrae
- M11.19 Familial chondrocalcinosis, multiple sites

M11.2 Other chondrocalcinosis
Chondrocalcinosis NOS

- M11.20 Other chondrocalcinosis, unspecified site
- M11.21 Other chondrocalcinosis, shoulder
  - M11.211 Other chondrocalcinosis, right shoulder
  - M11.212 Other chondrocalcinosis, left shoulder
  - M11.219 Other chondrocalcinosis, unspecified shoulder
- M11.22 Other chondrocalcinosis, elbow
  - M11.221 Other chondrocalcinosis, right elbow
  - M11.222 Other chondrocalcinosis, left elbow
  - M11.229 Other chondrocalcinosis, unspecified elbow
- M11.23 Other chondrocalcinosis, wrist
  - M11.231 Other chondrocalcinosis, right wrist
  - M11.232 Other chondrocalcinosis, left wrist
  - M11.239 Other chondrocalcinosis, unspecified wrist
- M11.24 Other chondrocalcinosis, hand
  - M11.241 Other chondrocalcinosis, right hand
  - M11.242 Other chondrocalcinosis, left hand
  - M11.249 Other chondrocalcinosis, unspecified hand
- M11.25 Other chondrocalcinosis, hip
  - M11.251 Other chondrocalcinosis, right hip
  - M11.252 Other chondrocalcinosis, left hip
  - M11.259 Other chondrocalcinosis, unspecified hip
- M11.26 Other chondrocalcinosis, knee
  - M11.261 Other chondrocalcinosis, right knee
  - M11.262 Other chondrocalcinosis, left knee
  - M11.269 Other chondrocalcinosis, unspecified knee
- M11.27 Other chondrocalcinosis, ankle and foot
  - M11.271 Other chondrocalcinosis, right ankle and foot
  - M11.272 Other chondrocalcinosis, left ankle and foot
  - M11.279 Other chondrocalcinosis, unspecified ankle and foot
- M11.28 Other chondrocalcinosis, vertebrae
- M11.29 Other chondrocalcinosis, multiple sites

M11.8 Other specified crystal arthropathies

- M11.80 Other specified crystal arthropathies, unspecified site
- M11.81 Other specified crystal arthropathies, shoulder
  - M11.811 Other specified crystal arthropathies, right shoulder
  - M11.812 Other specified crystal arthropathies, left shoulder
  - M11.819 Other specified crystal arthropathies, unspecified shoulder
- M11.82 Other specified crystal arthropathies, elbow
  - M11.821 Other specified crystal arthropathies, right elbow
  - M11.822 Other specified crystal arthropathies, left elbow
  - M11.829 Other specified crystal arthropathies, unspecified elbow
- M11.83 Other specified crystal arthropathies, wrist
  - M11.831 Other specified crystal arthropathies, right wrist
  - M11.832 Other specified crystal arthropathies, left wrist
  - M11.839 Other specified crystal arthropathies, unspecified wrist
- M11.84 Other specified crystal arthropathies, hand
  - M11.841 Other specified crystal arthropathies, right hand
  - M11.842 Other specified crystal arthropathies, left hand
  - M11.849 Other specified crystal arthropathies, unspecified hand
- M11.85 Other specified crystal arthropathies, hip
  - M11.851 Other specified crystal arthropathies, right hip
  - M11.852 Other specified crystal arthropathies, left hip
  - M11.859 Other specified crystal arthropathies, unspecified hip
- M11.86 Other specified crystal arthropathies, knee
  - M11.861 Other specified crystal arthropathies, right knee
  - M11.862 Other specified crystal arthropathies, left knee
  - M11.869 Other specified crystal arthropathies, unspecified knee
- M11.87 Other specified crystal arthropathies, ankle and foot
  - M11.871 Other specified crystal arthropathies, right ankle and foot
  - M11.872 Other specified crystal arthropathies, left ankle and foot
  - M11.879 Other specified crystal arthropathies, unspecified ankle and foot
- M11.88 Other specified crystal arthropathies, vertebrae
- M11.89 Other specified crystal arthropathies, multiple sites

M11.9 Crystal arthropathy, unspecified

M12 Other and unspecified arthropathy

EXCLUDES 1 *arthrosis (M15-M19)*
cricoarytenoid arthropathy (J38.7)

M12.0 Chronic postrheumatic arthropathy [Jaccoud]

- M12.00 Chronic postrheumatic arthropathy [Jaccoud], unspecified site HCC
- M12.01 Chronic postrheumatic arthropathy [Jaccoud], shoulder
  - M12.011 Chronic postrheumatic arthropathy [Jaccoud], right shoulder HCC
  - M12.012 Chronic postrheumatic arthropathy [Jaccoud], left shoulder HCC
  - M12.019 Chronic postrheumatic arthropathy [Jaccoud], unspecified shoulder HCC
- M12.02 Chronic postrheumatic arthropathy [Jaccoud], elbow
  - M12.021 Chronic postrheumatic arthropathy [Jaccoud], right elbow HCC
  - M12.022 Chronic postrheumatic arthropathy [Jaccoud], left elbow HCC
  - M12.029 Chronic postrheumatic arthropathy [Jaccoud], unspecified elbow HCC
- M12.03 Chronic postrheumatic arthropathy [Jaccoud], wrist
  - M12.031 Chronic postrheumatic arthropathy [Jaccoud], right wrist HCC
  - M12.032 Chronic postrheumatic arthropathy [Jaccoud], left wrist HCC
  - M12.039 Chronic postrheumatic arthropathy [Jaccoud], unspecified wrist HCC
- M12.04 Chronic postrheumatic arthropathy [Jaccoud], hand
  - M12.041 Chronic postrheumatic arthropathy [Jaccoud], right hand HCC
  - M12.042 Chronic postrheumatic arthropathy [Jaccoud], left hand HCC
  - M12.049 Chronic postrheumatic arthropathy [Jaccoud], unspecified hand HCC
- M12.05 Chronic postrheumatic arthropathy [Jaccoud], hip
  - M12.051 Chronic postrheumatic arthropathy [Jaccoud], right hip HCC
  - M12.052 Chronic postrheumatic arthropathy [Jaccoud], left hip HCC
  - M12.059 Chronic postrheumatic arthropathy [Jaccoud], unspecified hip HCC
- M12.06 Chronic postrheumatic arthropathy [Jaccoud], knee
  - M12.061 Chronic postrheumatic arthropathy [Jaccoud], right knee HCC
  - M12.062 Chronic postrheumatic arthropathy [Jaccoud], left knee HCC
  - M12.069 Chronic postrheumatic arthropathy [Jaccoud], unspecified knee HCC

Diseases of the Musculoskeletal System and Connective Tissue

M12.07 Chronic postrheumatic arthropathy [Jaccoud], ankle and foot
M12.071 Chronic postrheumatic arthropathy [Jaccoud], right ankle and foot HCC
M12.072 Chronic postrheumatic arthropathy [Jaccoud], left ankle and foot HCC
M12.079 Chronic postrheumatic arthropathy [Jaccoud], unspecified ankle and foot HCC
M12.08 Chronic postrheumatic arthropathy [Jaccoud], other specified site HCC
Chronic postrheumatic arthropathy [Jaccoud], vertebrae
M12.09 Chronic postrheumatic arthropathy [Jaccoud], multiple sites HCC
M12.1 Kaschin-Beck disease
Osteochondroarthrosis deformans endemica
M12.10 Kaschin-Beck disease, unspecified site
M12.11 Kaschin-Beck disease, shoulder
M12.111 Kaschin-Beck disease, right shoulder
M12.112 Kaschin-Beck disease, left shoulder
M12.119 Kaschin-Beck disease, unspecified shoulder
M12.12 Kaschin-Beck disease, elbow
M12.121 Kaschin-Beck disease, right elbow
M12.122 Kaschin-Beck disease, left elbow
M12.129 Kaschin-Beck disease, unspecified elbow
M12.13 Kaschin-Beck disease, wrist
M12.131 Kaschin-Beck disease, right wrist
M12.132 Kaschin-Beck disease, left wrist
M12.139 Kaschin-Beck disease, unspecified wrist
M12.14 Kaschin-Beck disease, hand
M12.141 Kaschin-Beck disease, right hand
M12.142 Kaschin-Beck disease, left hand
M12.149 Kaschin-Beck disease, unspecified hand
M12.15 Kaschin-Beck disease, hip
M12.151 Kaschin-Beck disease, right hip
M12.152 Kaschin-Beck disease, left hip
M12.159 Kaschin-Beck disease, unspecified hip
M12.16 Kaschin-Beck disease, knee
M12.161 Kaschin-Beck disease, right knee
M12.162 Kaschin-Beck disease, left knee
M12.169 Kaschin-Beck disease, unspecified knee
M12.17 Kaschin-Beck disease, ankle and foot
M12.171 Kaschin-Beck disease, right ankle and foot
M12.172 Kaschin-Beck disease, left ankle and foot
M12.179 Kaschin-Beck disease, unspecified ankle and foot
M12.18 Kaschin-Beck disease, vertebrae
M12.19 Kaschin-Beck disease, multiple sites
M12.2 Villonodular synovitis (pigmented)
M12.20 Villonodular synovitis (pigmented), unspecified site
M12.21 Villonodular synovitis (pigmented), shoulder
M12.211 Villonodular synovitis (pigmented), right shoulder
M12.212 Villonodular synovitis (pigmented), left shoulder
M12.219 Villonodular synovitis (pigmented), unspecified shoulder
M12.22 Villonodular synovitis (pigmented), elbow
M12.221 Villonodular synovitis (pigmented), right elbow
M12.222 Villonodular synovitis (pigmented), left elbow
M12.229 Villonodular synovitis (pigmented), unspecified elbow
M12.23 Villonodular synovitis (pigmented), wrist
M12.231 Villonodular synovitis (pigmented), right wrist
M12.232 Villonodular synovitis (pigmented), left wrist
M12.239 Villonodular synovitis (pigmented), unspecified wrist
M12.24 Villonodular synovitis (pigmented), hand
M12.241 Villonodular synovitis (pigmented), right hand
M12.242 Villonodular synovitis (pigmented), left hand
M12.249 Villonodular synovitis (pigmented), unspecified hand
M12.25 Villonodular synovitis (pigmented), hip
M12.251 Villonodular synovitis (pigmented), right hip
M12.252 Villonodular synovitis (pigmented), left hip
M12.259 Villonodular synovitis (pigmented), unspecified hip
M12.26 Villonodular synovitis (pigmented), knee
M12.261 Villonodular synovitis (pigmented), right knee
M12.262 Villonodular synovitis (pigmented), left knee
M12.269 Villonodular synovitis (pigmented), unspecified knee
M12.27 Villonodular synovitis (pigmented), ankle and foot
M12.271 Villonodular synovitis (pigmented), right ankle and foot
M12.272 Villonodular synovitis (pigmented), left ankle and foot
M12.279 Villonodular synovitis (pigmented), unspecified ankle and foot
M12.28 Villonodular synovitis (pigmented), other specified site
Villonodular synovitis (pigmented), vertebrae
M12.29 Villonodular synovitis (pigmented), multiple sites
M12.3 Palindromic rheumatism
M12.30 Palindromic rheumatism, unspecified site
M12.31 Palindromic rheumatism, shoulder
M12.311 Palindromic rheumatism, right shoulder
M12.312 Palindromic rheumatism, left shoulder
M12.319 Palindromic rheumatism, unspecified shoulder
M12.32 Palindromic rheumatism, elbow
M12.321 Palindromic rheumatism, right elbow
M12.322 Palindromic rheumatism, left elbow
M12.329 Palindromic rheumatism, unspecified elbow
M12.33 Palindromic rheumatism, wrist
M12.331 Palindromic rheumatism, right wrist
M12.332 Palindromic rheumatism, left wrist
M12.339 Palindromic rheumatism, unspecified wrist
M12.34 Palindromic rheumatism, hand
M12.341 Palindromic rheumatism, right hand
M12.342 Palindromic rheumatism, left hand
M12.349 Palindromic rheumatism, unspecified hand
M12.35 Palindromic rheumatism, hip
M12.351 Palindromic rheumatism, right hip
M12.352 Palindromic rheumatism, left hip
M12.359 Palindromic rheumatism, unspecified hip
M12.36 Palindromic rheumatism, knee
M12.361 Palindromic rheumatism, right knee
M12.362 Palindromic rheumatism, left knee
M12.369 Palindromic rheumatism, unspecified knee
M12.37 Palindromic rheumatism, ankle and foot
M12.371 Palindromic rheumatism, right ankle and foot
M12.372 Palindromic rheumatism, left ankle and foot
M12.379 Palindromic rheumatism, unspecified ankle and foot
M12.38 Palindromic rheumatism, other specified site
Palindromic rheumatism, vertebrae
M12.39 Palindromic rheumatism, multiple sites
M12.4 Intermittent hydrarthrosis
M12.40 Intermittent hydrarthrosis, unspecified site
M12.41 Intermittent hydrarthrosis, shoulder
M12.411 Intermittent hydrarthrosis, right shoulder
M12.412 Intermittent hydrarthrosis, left shoulder
M12.419 Intermittent hydrarthrosis, unspecified shoulder
M12.42 Intermittent hydrarthrosis, elbow
M12.421 Intermittent hydrarthrosis, right elbow
M12.422 Intermittent hydrarthrosis, left elbow
M12.429 Intermittent hydrarthrosis, unspecified elbow
M12.43 Intermittent hydrarthrosis, wrist
M12.431 Intermittent hydrarthrosis, right wrist
M12.432 Intermittent hydrarthrosis, left wrist
M12.439 Intermittent hydrarthrosis, unspecified wrist
M12.44 Intermittent hydrarthrosis, hand
M12.441 Intermittent hydrarthrosis, right hand
M12.442 Intermittent hydrarthrosis, left hand
M12.449 Intermittent hydrarthrosis, unspecified hand
M12.45 Intermittent hydrarthrosis, hip
M12.451 Intermittent hydrarthrosis, right hip

M12.452 Intermittent hydrarthrosis, left hip
M12.459 Intermittent hydrarthrosis, unspecified hip
M12.46 Intermittent hydrarthrosis, knee
M12.461 Intermittent hydrarthrosis, right knee
M12.462 Intermittent hydrarthrosis, left knee
M12.469 Intermittent hydrarthrosis, unspecified knee
M12.47 Intermittent hydrarthrosis, ankle and foot
M12.471 Intermittent hydrarthrosis, right ankle and foot
M12.472 Intermittent hydrarthrosis, left ankle and foot
M12.479 Intermittent hydrarthrosis, unspecified ankle and foot
M12.48 Intermittent hydrarthrosis, other site
M12.49 Intermittent hydrarthrosis, multiple sites
M12.5 Traumatic arthropathy
EXCLUDES 1 *current injury-see Alphabetic Index*
post-traumatic osteoarthritis of first carpometacarpal joint (M18.2-M18.3)
post-traumatic osteoarthritis of hip (M16.4-M16.5)
post-traumatic osteoarthritis of knee (M17.2-M17.3)
post-traumatic osteoarthritis NOS (M19.1-)
post-traumatic osteoarthritis of other single joints (M19.1-)
M12.50 Traumatic arthropathy, unspecified site
M12.51 Traumatic arthropathy, shoulder
M12.511 Traumatic arthropathy, right shoulder
M12.512 Traumatic arthropathy, left shoulder
M12.519 Traumatic arthropathy, unspecified shoulder
M12.52 Traumatic arthropathy, elbow
M12.521 Traumatic arthropathy, right elbow
M12.522 Traumatic arthropathy, left elbow
M12.529 Traumatic arthropathy, unspecified elbow
M12.53 Traumatic arthropathy, wrist
M12.531 Traumatic arthropathy, right wrist
M12.532 Traumatic arthropathy, left wrist
M12.539 Traumatic arthropathy, unspecified wrist
M12.54 Traumatic arthropathy, hand
M12.541 Traumatic arthropathy, right hand
M12.542 Traumatic arthropathy, left hand
M12.549 Traumatic arthropathy, unspecified hand
M12.55 Traumatic arthropathy, hip
M12.551 Traumatic arthropathy, right hip
M12.552 Traumatic arthropathy, left hip
AHA: 1Q 2015, 17
M12.559 Traumatic arthropathy, unspecified hip
M12.56 Traumatic arthropathy, knee
M12.561 Traumatic arthropathy, right knee
M12.562 Traumatic arthropathy, left knee
M12.569 Traumatic arthropathy, unspecified knee
M12.57 Traumatic arthropathy, ankle and foot
M12.571 Traumatic arthropathy, right ankle and foot
M12.572 Traumatic arthropathy, left ankle and foot
M12.579 Traumatic arthropathy, unspecified ankle and foot
M12.58 Traumatic arthropathy, other specified site
Traumatic arthropathy, vertebrae
M12.59 Traumatic arthropathy, multiple sites
M12.8 Other specific arthropathies, not elsewhere classified
Transient arthropathy
M12.80 Other specific arthropathies, not elsewhere classified, unspecified site
M12.81 Other specific arthropathies, not elsewhere classified, shoulder
M12.811 Other specific arthropathies, not elsewhere classified, right shoulder
M12.812 Other specific arthropathies, not elsewhere classified, left shoulder
M12.819 Other specific arthropathies, not elsewhere classified, unspecified shoulder
M12.82 Other specific arthropathies, not elsewhere classified, elbow
M12.821 Other specific arthropathies, not elsewhere classified, right elbow
M12.822 Other specific arthropathies, not elsewhere classified, left elbow
M12.829 Other specific arthropathies, not elsewhere classified, unspecified elbow
M12.83 Other specific arthropathies, not elsewhere classified, wrist
M12.831 Other specific arthropathies, not elsewhere classified, right wrist
M12.832 Other specific arthropathies, not elsewhere classified, left wrist
M12.839 Other specific arthropathies, not elsewhere classified, unspecified wrist
M12.84 Other specific arthropathies, not elsewhere classified, hand
M12.841 Other specific arthropathies, not elsewhere classified, right hand
M12.842 Other specific arthropathies, not elsewhere classified, left hand
M12.849 Other specific arthropathies, not elsewhere classified, unspecified hand
M12.85 Other specific arthropathies, not elsewhere classified, hip
M12.851 Other specific arthropathies, not elsewhere classified, right hip
M12.852 Other specific arthropathies, not elsewhere classified, left hip
M12.859 Other specific arthropathies, not elsewhere classified, unspecified hip
M12.86 Other specific arthropathies, not elsewhere classified, knee
M12.861 Other specific arthropathies, not elsewhere classified, right knee
M12.862 Other specific arthropathies, not elsewhere classified, left knee
M12.869 Other specific arthropathies, not elsewhere classified, unspecified knee
M12.87 Other specific arthropathies, not elsewhere classified, ankle and foot
M12.871 Other specific arthropathies, not elsewhere classified, right ankle and foot
M12.872 Other specific arthropathies, not elsewhere classified, left ankle and foot
M12.879 Other specific arthropathies, not elsewhere classified, unspecified ankle and foot
M12.88 Other specific arthropathies, not elsewhere classified, other specified site
Other specific arthropathies, not elsewhere classified, vertebrae
M12.89 Other specific arthropathies, not elsewhere classified, multiple sites
M12.9 Arthropathy, unspecified

M13 Other arthritis

EXCLUDES 1 *arthrosis (M15-M19)*
osteoarthritis (M15-M19)
M13.0 Polyarthritis, unspecified
M13.1 Monoarthritis, not elsewhere classified
M13.10 Monoarthritis, not elsewhere classified, unspecified site
M13.11 Monoarthritis, not elsewhere classified, shoulder
M13.111 Monoarthritis, not elsewhere classified, right shoulder
M13.112 Monoarthritis, not elsewhere classified, left shoulder
M13.119 Monoarthritis, not elsewhere classified, unspecified shoulder
M13.12 Monoarthritis, not elsewhere classified, elbow
M13.121 Monoarthritis, not elsewhere classified, right elbow
M13.122 Monoarthritis, not elsewhere classified, left elbow
M13.129 Monoarthritis, not elsewhere classified, unspecified elbow
M13.13 Monoarthritis, not elsewhere classified, wrist
M13.131 Monoarthritis, not elsewhere classified, right wrist
M13.132 Monoarthritis, not elsewhere classified, left wrist

M13.139 Monoarthritis, not elsewhere classified, unspecified wrist

M13.14 Monoarthritis, not elsewhere classified, hand

M13.141 Monoarthritis, not elsewhere classified, right hand

M13.142 Monoarthritis, not elsewhere classified, left hand

M13.149 Monoarthritis, not elsewhere classified, unspecified hand

M13.15 Monoarthritis, not elsewhere classified, hip

M13.151 Monoarthritis, not elsewhere classified, right hip

M13.152 Monoarthritis, not elsewhere classified, left hip

M13.159 Monoarthritis, not elsewhere classified, unspecified hip

M13.16 Monoarthritis, not elsewhere classified, knee

M13.161 Monoarthritis, not elsewhere classified, right knee

M13.162 Monoarthritis, not elsewhere classified, left knee

M13.169 Monoarthritis, not elsewhere classified, unspecified knee

M13.17 Monoarthritis, not elsewhere classified, ankle and foot

M13.171 Monoarthritis, not elsewhere classified, right ankle and foot

M13.172 Monoarthritis, not elsewhere classified, left ankle and foot

M13.179 Monoarthritis, not elsewhere classified, unspecified ankle and foot

M13.8 Other specified arthritis

Allergic arthritis

EXCLUDES 1 *osteoarthritis (M15-M19)*

M13.80 Other specified arthritis, unspecified site

M13.81 Other specified arthritis, shoulder

M13.811 Other specified arthritis, right shoulder

M13.812 Other specified arthritis, left shoulder

M13.819 Other specified arthritis, unspecified shoulder

M13.82 Other specified arthritis, elbow

M13.821 Other specified arthritis, right elbow

M13.822 Other specified arthritis, left elbow

M13.829 Other specified arthritis, unspecified elbow

M13.83 Other specified arthritis, wrist

M13.831 Other specified arthritis, right wrist

M13.832 Other specified arthritis, left wrist

M13.839 Other specified arthritis, unspecified wrist

M13.84 Other specified arthritis, hand

M13.841 Other specified arthritis, right hand

M13.842 Other specified arthritis, left hand

M13.849 Other specified arthritis, unspecified hand

M13.85 Other specified arthritis, hip

M13.851 Other specified arthritis, right hip

M13.852 Other specified arthritis, left hip

M13.859 Other specified arthritis, unspecified hip

M13.86 Other specified arthritis, knee

M13.861 Other specified arthritis, right knee

M13.862 Other specified arthritis, left knee

M13.869 Other specified arthritis, unspecified knee

M13.87 Other specified arthritis, ankle and foot

M13.871 Other specified arthritis, right ankle and foot

M13.872 Other specified arthritis, left ankle and foot

M13.879 Other specified arthritis, unspecified ankle and foot

M13.88 Other specified arthritis, other site

M13.89 Other specified arthritis, multiple sites

M14 Arthropathies in other diseases classified elsewhere

EXCLUDES 1 *arthropathy in:*
diabetes mellitus (E08-E13 with .61-)
hematological disorders (M36.2-M36.3)
hypersensitivity reactions (M36.4)
neoplastic disease (M36.1)
neurosyphillis (A52.16)
sarcoidosis (D86.86)
enteropathic arthropathies (M07.-)
juvenile psoriatic arthropathy (L40.54)
lipoid dermatoarthritis (E78.81)

M14.6 Charcôt's joint

Neuropathic arthropathy

EXCLUDES 1 *Charcôt's joint in diabetes mellitus (E08-E13 with .610)*
Charcôt's joint in tabes dorsalis (A52.16)

CODING TIP ✓ Do not assign a code from M14.6- to report Charcot arthropathy in diabetes or syphilis. Charcot's joint in diabetes mellitus should be coded to the appropriate combination code from E08-E13 indicating the manifestation.

M14.60 Charcôt's joint, unspecified site

M14.61 Charcôt's joint, shoulder

M14.611 Charcôt's joint, right shoulder

M14.612 Charcôt's joint, left shoulder

M14.619 Charcôt's joint, unspecified shoulder

M14.62 Charcôt's joint, elbow

M14.621 Charcôt's joint, right elbow

M14.622 Charcôt's joint, left elbow

M14.629 Charcôt's joint, unspecified elbow

M14.63 Charcôt's joint, wrist

M14.631 Charcôt's joint, right wrist

M14.632 Charcôt's joint, left wrist

M14.639 Charcôt's joint, unspecified wrist

M14.64 Charcôt's joint, hand

M14.641 Charcôt's joint, right hand

M14.642 Charcôt's joint, left hand

M14.649 Charcôt's joint, unspecified hand

M14.65 Charcôt's joint, hip

M14.651 Charcôt's joint, right hip

M14.652 Charcôt's joint, left hip

M14.659 Charcôt's joint, unspecified hip

M14.66 Charcôt's joint, knee

M14.661 Charcôt's joint, right knee

M14.662 Charcôt's joint, left knee

M14.669 Charcôt's joint, unspecified knee

M14.67 Charcôt's joint, ankle and foot

M14.671 Charcôt's joint, right ankle and foot

M14.672 Charcôt's joint, left ankle and foot

M14.679 Charcôt's joint, unspecified ankle and foot

M14.68 Charcôt's joint, vertebrae

M14.69 Charcôt's joint, multiple sites

M14.8 Arthropathies in other specified diseases classified elsewhere

Code first underlying disease, such as:
amyloidosis (E85.-)
erythema multiforme (L51.-)
erythema nodosum (L52)
hemochromatosis (E83.11-)
hyperparathyroidism (E21.-)
hypothyroidism (E00-E03)
sickle-cell disorders (D57.-)
thyrotoxicosis [hyperthyroidism] (E05.-)
Whipple's disease (K90.81)

M14.80 *Arthropathies in other specified diseases classified elsewhere, unspecified site*

M14.81 Arthropathies in other specified diseases classified elsewhere, shoulder

M14.811 *Arthropathies in other specified diseases classified elsewhere, right shoulder*

M14.812 *Arthropathies in other specified diseases classified elsewhere, left shoulder*

M14.819 *Arthropathies in other specified diseases classified elsewhere, unspecified shoulder*

M14.82 Arthropathies in other specified diseases classified elsewhere, elbow

M14.821 *Arthropathies in other specified diseases classified elsewhere, right elbow*

M14.822 *Arthropathies in other specified diseases classified elsewhere, left elbow*

M14.829 *Arthropathies in other specified diseases classified elsewhere, unspecified elbow*

M14.83 Arthropathies in other specified diseases classified elsewhere, wrist

M14.831 *Arthropathies in other specified diseases classified elsewhere, right wrist*

M14.832 *Arthropathies in other specified diseases classified elsewhere, left wrist*

M14.839 *Arthropathies in other specified diseases classified elsewhere, unspecified wrist*

M14.84 **Arthropathies in other specified diseases classified elsewhere, hand**

M14.841 *Arthropathies in other specified diseases classified elsewhere, right hand*

M14.842 *Arthropathies in other specified diseases classified elsewhere, left hand*

M14.849 *Arthropathies in other specified diseases classified elsewhere, unspecified hand*

M14.85 **Arthropathies in other specified diseases classified elsewhere, hip**

M14.851 *Arthropathies in other specified diseases classified elsewhere, right hip*

M14.852 *Arthropathies in other specified diseases classified elsewhere, left hip*

M14.859 *Arthropathies in other specified diseases classified elsewhere, unspecified hip*

M14.86 **Arthropathies in other specified diseases classified elsewhere, knee**

M14.861 *Arthropathies in other specified diseases classified elsewhere, right knee*

M14.862 *Arthropathies in other specified diseases classified elsewhere, left knee*

M14.869 *Arthropathies in other specified diseases classified elsewhere, unspecified knee*

M14.87 **Arthropathies in other specified diseases classified elsewhere, ankle and foot**

M14.871 *Arthropathies in other specified diseases classified elsewhere, right ankle and foot*

M14.872 *Arthropathies in other specified diseases classified elsewhere, left ankle and foot*

M14.879 *Arthropathies in other specified diseases classified elsewhere, unspecified ankle and foot*

M14.88 *Arthropathies in other specified diseases classified elsewhere, vertebrae*

M14.89 *Arthropathies in other specified diseases classified elsewhere, multiple sites*

Osteoarthritis (M15-M19)

EXCLUDES 2 *osteoarthritis of spine (M47.-)*

CODING TIP ✓ Osteoarthritis/degenerative joint disease (Categories M15-M19) is the most common type of arthritis in the elderly. If the arthritis is in the spine, refer to Category M47. When coding osteoarthrosis, review the medical records to determine whether the OA is localized or generalized; primary or secondary. Bilateral osteoarthrosis of the same site is considered localized. Generalized OA affects multiple joints (M15). Code joints affected separately and avoid the M15 for multiple joints, if multiple joint sites have been identified. Primary osteoarthritis is caused by aging. Secondary OA is caused by other conditions such as obesity.

M15 **Polyosteoarthritis**

INCLUDES arthritis of multiple sites

EXCLUDES 1 *bilateral involvement of single joint (M16-M19)*

CODING TIP ✓ Osteoarthritis/degenerative joint disease (Categories M15-M19) is the most common type of arthritis in the elderly. If the arthritis is in the spine, refer to Category M47. When coding osteoarthrosis, review the medical records to determine whether the OA is localized or generalized; primary or secondary. Bilateral osteoarthrosis of the same site is considered localized. Generalized OA affects multiple joints. Code joints affected separately. Primary osteoarthritis is caused by aging. Secondary OA is caused by other conditions such as avascular necrosis.

M15.0 **Primary generalized (osteo)arthritis**

M15.1 **Heberden's nodes (with arthropathy)**
Interphalangeal distal osteoarthritis

M15.2 **Bouchard's nodes (with arthropathy)**
Juxtaphalangeal distal osteoarthritis

M15.3 **Secondary multiple arthritis**
Post-traumatic polyosteoarthritis

M15.4 **Erosive (osteo)arthritis**

M15.8 **Other polyosteoarthritis**

M15.9 **Polyosteoarthritis, unspecified**
Generalized osteoarthritis NOS

M16 **Osteoarthritis of hip**

CODING TIP ✓ Assign a code for primary osteoarthritis when the diagnostic statement states arthritis of a specified joint but does not define the type of arthritis. The default code for osteoarthritis without specified type is primary.

M16.0 **Bilateral primary osteoarthritis of hip**
AHA: 4Q 2016, 146
AHA: 2Q 2018, 12

M16.1 **Unilateral primary osteoarthritis of hip**
Primary osteoarthritis of hip NOS

M16.10 **Unilateral primary osteoarthritis, unspecified hip**

M16.11 **Unilateral primary osteoarthritis, right hip**

M16.12 **Unilateral primary osteoarthritis, left hip**

M16.2 **Bilateral osteoarthritis resulting from hip dysplasia**

M16.3 **Unilateral osteoarthritis resulting from hip dysplasia**
Dysplastic osteoarthritis of hip NOS

M16.30 **Unilateral osteoarthritis resulting from hip dysplasia, unspecified hip**

M16.31 **Unilateral osteoarthritis resulting from hip dysplasia, right hip**

M16.32 **Unilateral osteoarthritis resulting from hip dysplasia, left hip**

M16.4 **Bilateral post-traumatic osteoarthritis of hip**

M16.5 **Unilateral post-traumatic osteoarthritis of hip**
Post-traumatic osteoarthritis of hip NOS

M16.50 **Unilateral post-traumatic osteoarthritis, unspecified hip**

M16.51 **Unilateral post-traumatic osteoarthritis, right hip**

M16.52 **Unilateral post-traumatic osteoarthritis, left hip**

M16.6 **Other bilateral secondary osteoarthritis of hip**

M16.7 **Other unilateral secondary osteoarthritis of hip**
Secondary osteoarthritis of hip NOS

M16.9 **Osteoarthritis of hip, unspecified**

M17 **Osteoarthritis of knee**

CODING TIP ✓ Assign a code for primary osteoarthritis when the diagnostic statement states arthritis of a specified joint but does not define the type of arthritis. The default code for osteoarthritis without specified type is primary.

M17.0 **Bilateral primary osteoarthritis of knee**

M17.1 **Unilateral primary osteoarthritis of knee**
Primary osteoarthritis of knee NOS

M17.10 **Unilateral primary osteoarthritis, unspecified knee**
AHA: 4Q 2016, 147

M17.11 **Unilateral primary osteoarthritis, right knee**

M17.12 **Unilateral primary osteoarthritis, left knee**
AHA: 4Q 2016, 146

M17.2 **Bilateral post-traumatic osteoarthritis of knee**

M17.3 **Unilateral post-traumatic osteoarthritis of knee**
Post-traumatic osteoarthritis of knee NOS

M17.30 **Unilateral post-traumatic osteoarthritis, unspecified knee**

M17.31 **Unilateral post-traumatic osteoarthritis, right knee**

M17.32 **Unilateral post-traumatic osteoarthritis, left knee**

M17.4 **Other bilateral secondary osteoarthritis of knee**

M17.5 **Other unilateral secondary osteoarthritis of knee**
Secondary osteoarthritis of knee NOS

M17.9 **Osteoarthritis of knee, unspecified**

M18 **Osteoarthritis of first carpometacarpal joint**

CODING TIP ✓ Assign a code for primary osteoarthritis when the diagnostic statement states arthritis of a specified joint but does not define the type of arthritis. The default code for osteoarthritis without specified type is primary.

M18.0 **Bilateral primary osteoarthritis of first carpometacarpal joints**

M18.1 **Unilateral primary osteoarthritis of first carpometacarpal joint**
Primary osteoarthritis of first carpometacarpal joint NOS

M18.10 **Unilateral primary osteoarthritis of first carpometacarpal joint, unspecified hand**

M18.11 **Unilateral primary osteoarthritis of first carpometacarpal joint, right hand**

M18.12 **Unilateral primary osteoarthritis of first carpometacarpal joint, left hand**

M18.2 Bilateral post-traumatic osteoarthritis of first carpometacarpal joints
5 M18.3 Unilateral post-traumatic osteoarthritis of first carpometacarpal joint
Post-traumatic osteoarthritis of first carpometacarpal joint NOS
M18.30 Unilateral post-traumatic osteoarthritis of first carpometacarpal joint, unspecified hand
M18.31 Unilateral post-traumatic osteoarthritis of first carpometacarpal joint, right hand
M18.32 Unilateral post-traumatic osteoarthritis of first carpometacarpal joint, left hand
M18.4 Other bilateral secondary osteoarthritis of first carpometacarpal joints
5 M18.5 Other unilateral secondary osteoarthritis of first carpometacarpal joint
Secondary osteoarthritis of first carpometacarpal joint NOS
M18.50 Other unilateral secondary osteoarthritis of first carpometacarpal joint, unspecified hand
M18.51 Other unilateral secondary osteoarthritis of first carpometacarpal joint, right hand
M18.52 Other unilateral secondary osteoarthritis of first carpometacarpal joint, left hand
M18.9 Osteoarthritis of first carpometacarpal joint, unspecified

4 **M19 Other and unspecified osteoarthritis**

EXCLUDES 1 *polyarthritis (M15.-)*

EXCLUDES 2 *arthrosis of spine (M47.-)*
hallux rigidus (M20.2)
osteoarthritis of spine (M47.-)

CODING TIP✓ Assign a code for primary osteoarthritis when the diagnostic statement states arthritis of a specified joint but does not define the type of arthritis. The default code for osteoarthritis without specified type is primary.

5 M19.0 Primary osteoarthritis of other joints
6 M19.01 Primary osteoarthritis, shoulder
M19.011 Primary osteoarthritis, right shoulder
AHA: 4Q 2016, 145
M19.012 Primary osteoarthritis, left shoulder
M19.019 Primary osteoarthritis, unspecified shoulder
6 M19.02 Primary osteoarthritis, elbow
M19.021 Primary osteoarthritis, right elbow
M19.022 Primary osteoarthritis, left elbow
M19.029 Primary osteoarthritis, unspecified elbow
6 M19.03 Primary osteoarthritis, wrist
M19.031 Primary osteoarthritis, right wrist
M19.032 Primary osteoarthritis, left wrist
M19.039 Primary osteoarthritis, unspecified wrist
6 M19.04 Primary osteoarthritis, hand
EXCLUDES 2 *primary osteoarthritis of first carpometacarpal joint (M18.0-, M18.1-)*
M19.041 Primary osteoarthritis, right hand
M19.042 Primary osteoarthritis, left hand
M19.049 Primary osteoarthritis, unspecified hand
6 M19.07 Primary osteoarthritis ankle and foot
M19.071 Primary osteoarthritis, right ankle and foot
M19.072 Primary osteoarthritis, left ankle and foot
M19.079 Primary osteoarthritis, unspecified ankle and foot
5 M19.1 Post-traumatic osteoarthritis of other joints
6 M19.11 Post-traumatic osteoarthritis, shoulder
M19.111 Post-traumatic osteoarthritis, right shoulder
M19.112 Post-traumatic osteoarthritis, left shoulder
M19.119 Post-traumatic osteoarthritis, unspecified shoulder
6 M19.12 Post-traumatic osteoarthritis, elbow
M19.121 Post-traumatic osteoarthritis, right elbow
M19.122 Post-traumatic osteoarthritis, left elbow
M19.129 Post-traumatic osteoarthritis, unspecified elbow
6 M19.13 Post-traumatic osteoarthritis, wrist
M19.131 Post-traumatic osteoarthritis, right wrist
M19.132 Post-traumatic osteoarthritis, left wrist
M19.139 Post-traumatic osteoarthritis, unspecified wrist
6 M19.14 Post-traumatic osteoarthritis, hand
EXCLUDES 2 *post-traumatic osteoarthritis of first carpometacarpal joint (M18.2-, M18.3-)*
M19.141 Post-traumatic osteoarthritis, right hand
M19.142 Post-traumatic osteoarthritis, left hand
M19.149 Post-traumatic osteoarthritis, unspecified hand
6 M19.17 Post-traumatic osteoarthritis, ankle and foot
M19.171 Post-traumatic osteoarthritis, right ankle and foot
M19.172 Post-traumatic osteoarthritis, left ankle and foot
M19.179 Post-traumatic osteoarthritis, unspecified ankle and foot
5 M19.2 Secondary osteoarthritis of other joints
6 M19.21 Secondary osteoarthritis, shoulder
M19.211 Secondary osteoarthritis, right shoulder
M19.212 Secondary osteoarthritis, left shoulder
M19.219 Secondary osteoarthritis, unspecified shoulder
6 M19.22 Secondary osteoarthritis, elbow
M19.221 Secondary osteoarthritis, right elbow
M19.222 Secondary osteoarthritis, left elbow
M19.229 Secondary osteoarthritis, unspecified elbow
6 M19.23 Secondary osteoarthritis, wrist
M19.231 Secondary osteoarthritis, right wrist
M19.232 Secondary osteoarthritis, left wrist
M19.239 Secondary osteoarthritis, unspecified wrist
6 M19.24 Secondary osteoarthritis, hand
M19.241 Secondary osteoarthritis, right hand
M19.242 Secondary osteoarthritis, left hand
M19.249 Secondary osteoarthritis, unspecified hand
6 M19.27 Secondary osteoarthritis, ankle and foot
M19.271 Secondary osteoarthritis, right ankle and foot
M19.272 Secondary osteoarthritis, left ankle and foot
M19.279 Secondary osteoarthritis, unspecified ankle and foot
5 M19.9 Osteoarthritis, unspecified site

CODING TIP✓ If the site is known, do not use M19.9- codes. The default is primary coded to the site.

M19.90 Unspecified osteoarthritis, Unspecified site
Arthrosis NOS
Arthritis NOS
Osteoarthritis NOS
AHA: 4Q 2016, 147
M19.91 Primary osteoarthritis, unspecified site
Primary osteoarthritis NOS
M19.92 Post-traumatic osteoarthritis, unspecified site
Post-traumatic osteoarthritis NOS
M19.93 Secondary osteoarthritis, unspecified site
Secondary osteoarthritis NOS

Other joint disorders (M20-M25)

EXCLUDES 2 *joints of the spine (M40-M54)*

4 **M20 Acquired deformities of fingers and toes**

EXCLUDES 1 *acquired absence of fingers and toes (Z89.-)*
congenital absence of fingers and toes (Q71.3-, Q72.3-)
congenital deformities and malformations of fingers and toes (Q66.-, Q68-Q70, Q74.-)

5 M20.0 Deformity of finger(s)
EXCLUDES 1 *clubbing of fingers (R68.3)*
palmar fascial fibromatosis [Dupuytren] (M72.0)
trigger finger (M65.3)
6 M20.00 Unspecified deformity of finger(s)
M20.001 Unspecified deformity of right finger(s)
M20.002 Unspecified deformity of left finger(s)
M20.009 Unspecified deformity of unspecified finger(s)
6 M20.01 Mallet finger
M20.011 Mallet finger of right finger(s)
M20.012 Mallet finger of left finger(s)

M20.019 **Mallet finger of unspecified finger(s)**

M20.02 Boutonnière deformity

M20.021 Boutonnière deformity of right finger(s)

M20.022 Boutonnière deformity of left finger(s)

M20.029 **Boutonnière deformity of unspecified finger(s)**

M20.03 Swan-neck deformity

M20.031 Swan-neck deformity of right finger(s)

M20.032 Swan-neck deformity of left finger(s)

M20.039 **Swan-neck deformity of unspecified finger(s)**

M20.09 Other deformity of finger(s)

M20.091 Other deformity of right finger(s)

M20.092 Other deformity of left finger(s)

M20.099 **Other deformity of finger(s), unspecified finger(s)**

M20.1 Hallux valgus (acquired)

EXCLUDES 2 *bunion (M21.6-)*

M20.10 **Hallux valgus (acquired), unspecified foot**

Hallux valgus

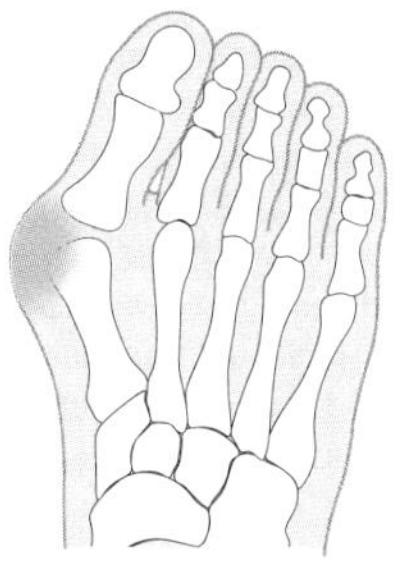

M20.11 Hallux valgus (acquired), right foot

M20.12 Hallux valgus (acquired), left foot

M20.2 Hallux rigidus

DEFINITION Inflexible, stiff great toe, with limited motion at the metatarsophalangeal joint.

M20.20 **Hallux rigidus, unspecified foot**

M20.21 Hallux rigidus, right foot

M20.22 Hallux rigidus, left foot

M20.3 Hallux varus (acquired)

DEFINITION Displaced joint of the big toe which is pointed away from the rest of the toes.

M20.30 **Hallux varus (acquired), unspecified foot**

M20.31 Hallux varus (acquired), right foot

M20.32 Hallux varus (acquired), left foot

M20.4 Other hammer toe(s) (acquired)

M20.40 **Other hammer toe(s) (acquired), unspecified foot**

M20.41 Other hammer toe(s) (acquired), right foot

M20.42 Other hammer toe(s) (acquired), left foot

M20.5 Other deformities of toe(s) (acquired)

M20.5X Other deformities of toe(s) (acquired)

M20.5X1 Other deformities of toe(s) (acquired), right foot

M20.5X2 Other deformities of toe(s) (acquired), left foot

M20.5X9 **Other deformities of toe(s) (acquired), unspecified foot**

M20.6 **Acquired deformities of toe(s), unspecified**

M20.60 **Acquired deformities of toe(s), unspecified, unspecified foot**

M20.61 **Acquired deformities of toe(s), unspecified, right foot**

M20.62 **Acquired deformities of toe(s), unspecified, left foot**

M21 Other acquired deformities of limbs

EXCLUDES 1 *acquired absence of limb (Z89.-)*
congenital absence of limbs (Q71-Q73)
congenital deformities and malformations of limbs (Q65-Q66, Q68-Q74)

EXCLUDES 2 *acquired deformities of fingers or toes (M20.-)*
coxa plana (M91.2)

M21.0 Valgus deformity, not elsewhere classified

EXCLUDES 1 *metatarsus valgus (Q66.6)*
talipes calcaneovalgus (Q66.4)

M21.00 **Valgus deformity, not elsewhere classified, unspecified site**

M21.02 Valgus deformity, not elsewhere classified, elbow
Cubitus valgus

M21.021 Valgus deformity, not elsewhere classified, right elbow

M21.022 Valgus deformity, not elsewhere classified, left elbow

M21.029 **Valgus deformity, not elsewhere classified, unspecified elbow**

M21.05 Valgus deformity, not elsewhere classified, hip

M21.051 Valgus deformity, not elsewhere classified, right hip

M21.052 Valgus deformity, not elsewhere classified, left hip

M21.059 **Valgus deformity, not elsewhere classified, unspecified hip**

M21.06 Valgus deformity, not elsewhere classified, knee
Genu valgum
Knock knee

DEFINITION Deformity in which the knees are angled abnormally close together with the ankles apart when standing erect with the legs straightened.

M21.061 Valgus deformity, not elsewhere classified, right knee

M21.062 Valgus deformity, not elsewhere classified, left knee

M21.069 **Valgus deformity, not elsewhere classified, unspecified knee**

M21.07 Valgus deformity, not elsewhere classified, ankle

M21.071 Valgus deformity, not elsewhere classified, right ankle

M21.072 Valgus deformity, not elsewhere classified, left ankle

M21.079 **Valgus deformity, not elsewhere classified, unspecified ankle**

M21.1 Varus deformity, not elsewhere classified

EXCLUDES 1 *metatarsus varus (Q66.22)*
tibia vara (M92.5)

M21.10 **Varus deformity, not elsewhere classified, unspecified site**

M21.12 Varus deformity, not elsewhere classified, elbow
Cubitus varus, elbow

M21.121 Varus deformity, not elsewhere classified, right elbow

M21.122 Varus deformity, not elsewhere classified, left elbow

M21.129 **Varus deformity, not elsewhere classified, unspecified elbow**

M21.15 Varus deformity, not elsewhere classified, hip

M21.151 Varus deformity, not elsewhere classified, right hip

M21.152 Varus deformity, not elsewhere classified, left hip

M21.159 **Varus deformity, not elsewhere classified, unspecified**

M21.16 Varus deformity, not elsewhere classified, knee
Bow leg
Genu varum

M21.161 Varus deformity, not elsewhere classified, right knee

M21.162 Varus deformity, not elsewhere classified, left knee

M21.169 **Varus deformity, not elsewhere classified, unspecified knee**

M21.17 Varus deformity, not elsewhere classified, ankle

DEFINITION Inward angulation of the tibia and fibula on the talus generally due to trauma or overpull by the tibialis posterior and anterior tendons.

M21.171 Varus deformity, not elsewhere classified, right ankle
M21.172 Varus deformity, not elsewhere classified, left ankle
M21.179 Varus deformity, not elsewhere classified, unspecified ankle

M21.2 Flexion deformity
M21.20 Flexion deformity, unspecified site
M21.21 Flexion deformity, shoulder
M21.211 Flexion deformity, right shoulder
M21.212 Flexion deformity, left shoulder
M21.219 Flexion deformity, unspecified shoulder
M21.22 Flexion deformity, elbow
M21.221 Flexion deformity, right elbow
M21.222 Flexion deformity, left elbow
M21.229 Flexion deformity, unspecified elbow
M21.23 Flexion deformity, wrist
M21.231 Flexion deformity, right wrist
M21.232 Flexion deformity, left wrist
M21.239 Flexion deformity, unspecified wrist
M21.24 Flexion deformity, finger joints
M21.241 Flexion deformity, right finger joints
M21.242 Flexion deformity, left finger joints
M21.249 Flexion deformity, unspecified finger joints
M21.25 Flexion deformity, hip
M21.251 Flexion deformity, right hip
M21.252 Flexion deformity, left hip
M21.259 Flexion deformity, unspecified hip
M21.26 Flexion deformity, knee
M21.261 Flexion deformity, right knee
M21.262 Flexion deformity, left knee
M21.269 Flexion deformity, unspecified knee
M21.27 Flexion deformity, ankle and toes
M21.271 Flexion deformity, right ankle and toes
M21.272 Flexion deformity, left ankle and toes
M21.279 Flexion deformity, unspecified ankle and toes

M21.3 Wrist or foot drop (acquired)
M21.33 Wrist drop (acquired)
M21.331 Wrist drop, right wrist
M21.332 Wrist drop, left wrist
M21.339 Wrist drop, unspecified wrist
M21.37 Foot drop (acquired)
M21.371 Foot drop, right foot
M21.372 Foot drop, left foot
M21.379 Foot drop, unspecified foot

M21.4 Flat foot [pes planus] (acquired)
EXCLUDES 1 *congenital pes planus (Q66.5-)*
M21.40 Flat foot [pes planus] (acquired), unspecified foot
M21.41 Flat foot [pes planus] (acquired), right foot
M21.42 Flat foot [pes planus] (acquired), left foot

M21.5 Acquired clawhand, clubhand, clawfoot and clubfoot
EXCLUDES 1 *clubfoot, not specified as acquired (Q66.89)*
M21.51 Acquired clawhand
M21.511 Acquired clawhand, right hand
M21.512 Acquired clawhand, left hand
M21.519 Acquired clawhand, unspecified hand
M21.52 Acquired clubhand
M21.521 Acquired clubhand, right hand
M21.522 Acquired clubhand, left hand
M21.529 Acquired clubhand, unspecified hand
M21.53 Acquired clawfoot
M21.531 Acquired clawfoot, right foot
M21.532 Acquired clawfoot, left foot
M21.539 Acquired clawfoot, unspecified foot
M21.54 Acquired clubfoot
M21.541 Acquired clubfoot, right foot
M21.542 Acquired clubfoot, left foot
M21.549 Acquired clubfoot, unspecified foot

M21.6 Other acquired deformities of foot
EXCLUDES 2 *deformities of toe (acquired) (M20.1-M20.6-)*
M21.61 Bunion
AHA: 4Q 2016, 38
M21.611 Bunion of right foot
M21.612 Bunion of left foot
M21.619 Bunion of unspecified foot
M21.62 Bunionette
AHA: 4Q 2016, 38
M21.621 Bunionette of right foot
M21.622 Bunionette of left foot
M21.629 Bunionette of unspecified foot
M21.6X Other acquired deformities of foot
M21.6X1 Other acquired deformities of right foot
M21.6X2 Other acquired deformities of left foot
M21.6X9 Other acquired deformities of unspecified foot

M21.7 Unequal limb length (acquired)
Note: The site used should correspond to the shorter limb
CODING TIP ✓ Acquired unequal limb length is usually due to an injury. When causation is documented, consider adding the injury with 7th character S.
M21.70 Unequal limb length (acquired), unspecified site
M21.72 Unequal limb length (acquired), humerus
M21.721 Unequal limb length (acquired), right humerus
M21.722 Unequal limb length (acquired), left humerus
M21.729 Unequal limb length (acquired), unspecified humerus
M21.73 Unequal limb length (acquired), ulna and radius
M21.731 Unequal limb length (acquired), right ulna
M21.732 Unequal limb length (acquired), left ulna
M21.733 Unequal limb length (acquired), right radius
M21.734 Unequal limb length (acquired), left radius
M21.739 Unequal limb length (acquired), unspecified ulna and radius
M21.75 Unequal limb length (acquired), femur
M21.751 Unequal limb length (acquired), right femur
M21.752 Unequal limb length (acquired), left femur
M21.759 Unequal limb length (acquired), unspecified femur
M21.76 Unequal limb length (acquired), tibia and fibula
M21.761 Unequal limb length (acquired), right tibia
M21.762 Unequal limb length (acquired), left tibia
M21.763 Unequal limb length (acquired), right fibula
M21.764 Unequal limb length (acquired), left fibula
M21.769 Unequal limb length (acquired), unspecified tibia and fibula

M21.8 Other specified acquired deformities of limbs
EXCLUDES 2 *coxa plana (M91.2)*
M21.80 Other specified acquired deformities of unspecified limb
M21.82 Other specified acquired deformities of upper arm
M21.821 Other specified acquired deformities of right upper arm
M21.822 Other specified acquired deformities of left upper arm
M21.829 Other specified acquired deformities of unspecified upper arm
M21.83 Other specified acquired deformities of forearm
M21.831 Other specified acquired deformities of right forearm
M21.832 Other specified acquired deformities of left forearm
M21.839 Other specified acquired deformities of unspecified forearm
M21.85 Other specified acquired deformities of thigh
M21.851 Other specified acquired deformities of right thigh
M21.852 Other specified acquired deformities of left thigh
M21.859 Other specified acquired deformities of unspecified thigh
M21.86 Other specified acquired deformities of lower leg

● New | Manifestation | 4-7 Digit Indicators | Laterality | A Adult | M Maternity | N Newborn | P Pediatric | ♂ Male
▲ Revised | Unspecified | AHA Coding Clinic | HCC Hierarchical Condition Categories | HIV HIV Related Conditions | ♀ Female

M21.861 Other specified acquired deformities of right lower leg
M21.862 Other specified acquired deformities of left lower leg
M21.869 Other specified acquired deformities of unspecified lower leg
M21.9 Unspecified acquired deformity of limb and hand
M21.90 Unspecified acquired deformity of unspecified limb
M21.92 Unspecified acquired deformity of upper arm
M21.921 Unspecified acquired deformity of right upper arm
M21.922 Unspecified acquired deformity of left upper arm
M21.929 Unspecified acquired deformity of unspecified upper arm
M21.93 Unspecified acquired deformity of forearm
M21.931 Unspecified acquired deformity of right forearm
M21.932 Unspecified acquired deformity of left forearm
M21.939 Unspecified acquired deformity of unspecified forearm
M21.94 Unspecified acquired deformity of hand
M21.941 Unspecified acquired deformity of hand, right hand
M21.942 Unspecified acquired deformity of hand, left hand
M21.949 Unspecified acquired deformity of hand, unspecified hand
M21.95 Unspecified acquired deformity of thigh
M21.951 Unspecified acquired deformity of right thigh
M21.952 Unspecified acquired deformity of left thigh
M21.959 Unspecified acquired deformity of unspecified thigh
M21.96 Unspecified acquired deformity of lower leg
M21.961 Unspecified acquired deformity of right lower leg
M21.962 Unspecified acquired deformity of left lower leg
M21.969 Unspecified acquired deformity of unspecified lower leg

M22 Disorder of patella

EXCLUDES 1 *traumatic dislocation of patella (S83.0-)*

M22.0 Recurrent dislocation of patella
M22.00 Recurrent dislocation of patella, unspecified knee
M22.01 Recurrent dislocation of patella, right knee
M22.02 Recurrent dislocation of patella, left knee
M22.1 Recurrent subluxation of patella
Incomplete dislocation of patella
M22.10 Recurrent subluxation of patella, unspecified knee
M22.11 Recurrent subluxation of patella, right knee
M22.12 Recurrent subluxation of patella, left knee
M22.2 Patellofemoral disorders
M22.2X Patellofemoral disorders
M22.2X1 Patellofemoral disorders, right knee
M22.2X2 Patellofemoral disorders, left knee
M22.2X9 Patellofemoral disorders, unspecified knee
M22.3 Other derangements of patella
M22.3X Other derangements of patella
M22.3X1 Other derangements of patella, right knee
M22.3X2 Other derangements of patella, left knee
M22.3X9 Other derangements of patella, unspecified knee
M22.4 Chondromalacia patellae
M22.40 Chondromalacia patellae, unspecified knee
M22.41 Chondromalacia patellae, right knee
M22.42 Chondromalacia patellae, left knee
M22.8 Other disorders of patella
M22.8X Other disorders of patella
M22.8X1 Other disorders of patella, right knee
M22.8X2 Other disorders of patella, left knee
M22.8X9 Other disorders of patella, unspecified knee
M22.9 Unspecified disorder of patella
M22.90 Unspecified disorder of patella, unspecified knee
M22.91 Unspecified disorder of patella, right knee
M22.92 Unspecified disorder of patella, left knee

M23 Internal derangement of knee

EXCLUDES 1 *ankylosis (M24.66)*
current injury - see injury of knee and lower leg (S80-S89)
deformity of knee (M21.-)
osteochondritis dissecans (M93.2)
recurrent dislocation or subluxation of joints (M24.4)
recurrent dislocation or subluxation of patella (M22.0-M22.1)

M23.0 Cystic meniscus
M23.00 Cystic meniscus, unspecified meniscus
Cystic meniscus, unspecified lateral meniscus
Cystic meniscus, unspecified medial meniscus
M23.000 Cystic meniscus, unspecified lateral meniscus, right knee
M23.001 Cystic meniscus, unspecified lateral meniscus, left knee
M23.002 Cystic meniscus, unspecified lateral meniscus, unspecified knee
M23.003 Cystic meniscus, unspecified medial meniscus, right knee
M23.004 Cystic meniscus, unspecified medial meniscus, left knee
M23.005 Cystic meniscus, unspecified medial meniscus, unspecified knee
M23.006 Cystic meniscus, unspecified meniscus, right knee
M23.007 Cystic meniscus, unspecified meniscus, left knee
M23.009 Cystic meniscus, unspecified meniscus, unspecified knee
M23.01 Cystic meniscus, anterior horn of medial meniscus
M23.011 Cystic meniscus, anterior horn of medial meniscus, right knee
M23.012 Cystic meniscus, anterior horn of medial meniscus, left knee
M23.019 Cystic meniscus, anterior horn of medial meniscus, unspecified knee
M23.02 Cystic meniscus, posterior horn of medial meniscus
M23.021 Cystic meniscus, posterior horn of medial meniscus, right knee
M23.022 Cystic meniscus, posterior horn of medial meniscus, left knee
M23.029 Cystic meniscus, posterior horn of medial meniscus, unspecified knee
M23.03 Cystic meniscus, other medial meniscus
M23.031 Cystic meniscus, other medial meniscus, right knee
M23.032 Cystic meniscus, other medial meniscus, left knee
M23.039 Cystic meniscus, other medial meniscus, unspecified knee
M23.04 Cystic meniscus, anterior horn of lateral meniscus
M23.041 Cystic meniscus, anterior horn of lateral meniscus, right knee
M23.042 Cystic meniscus, anterior horn of lateral meniscus, left knee
M23.049 Cystic meniscus, anterior horn of lateral meniscus, unspecified knee
M23.05 Cystic meniscus, posterior horn of lateral meniscus
M23.051 Cystic meniscus, posterior horn of lateral meniscus, right knee
M23.052 Cystic meniscus, posterior horn of lateral meniscus, left knee
M23.059 Cystic meniscus, posterior horn of lateral meniscus, unspecified knee
M23.06 Cystic meniscus, other lateral meniscus
M23.061 Cystic meniscus, other lateral meniscus, right knee
M23.062 Cystic meniscus, other lateral meniscus, left knee

M23.069 Cystic meniscus, other lateral meniscus, unspecified knee

M23.2 Derangement of meniscus due to old tear or injury
Old bucket-handle tear

CODING TIP ✓ When a meniscus tear is unspecified as to acute or chronic, query the provider. Otherwise, report the default code from S83.2-.

M23.20 Derangement of unspecified meniscus due to old tear or injury
Derangement of unspecified lateral meniscus due to old tear or injury
Derangement of unspecified medial meniscus due to old tear or injury

M23.200 Derangement of unspecified lateral meniscus due to old tear or injury, right knee
M23.201 Derangement of unspecified lateral meniscus due to old tear or injury, left knee
M23.202 Derangement of unspecified lateral meniscus due to old tear or injury, unspecified knee
M23.203 Derangement of unspecified medial meniscus due to old tear or injury, right knee
M23.204 Derangement of unspecified medial meniscus due to old tear or injury, left knee
M23.205 Derangement of unspecified medial meniscus due to old tear or injury, unspecified knee
M23.206 Derangement of unspecified meniscus due to old tear or injury, right knee
M23.207 Derangement of unspecified meniscus due to old tear or injury, left knee
M23.209 Derangement of unspecified meniscus due to old tear or injury, unspecified knee

M23.21 Derangement of anterior horn of medial meniscus due to old tear or injury
M23.211 Derangement of anterior horn of medial meniscus due to old tear or injury, right knee
M23.212 Derangement of anterior horn of medial meniscus due to old tear or injury, left knee
M23.219 Derangement of anterior horn of medial meniscus due to old tear or injury, unspecified knee

M23.22 Derangement of posterior horn of medial meniscus due to old tear or injury
M23.221 Derangement of posterior horn of medial meniscus due to old tear or injury, right knee
M23.222 Derangement of posterior horn of medial meniscus due to old tear or injury, left knee
M23.229 Derangement of posterior horn of medial meniscus due to old tear or injury, unspecified knee

M23.23 Derangement of other medial meniscus due to old tear or injury
M23.231 Derangement of other medial meniscus due to old tear or injury, right knee
M23.232 Derangement of other medial meniscus due to old tear or injury, left knee
M23.239 Derangement of other medial meniscus due to old tear or injury, unspecified knee

M23.24 Derangement of anterior horn of lateral meniscus due to old tear or injury
M23.241 Derangement of anterior horn of lateral meniscus due to old tear or injury, right knee
M23.242 Derangement of anterior horn of lateral meniscus due to old tear or injury, left knee
M23.249 Derangement of anterior horn of lateral meniscus due to old tear or injury, unspecified knee

M23.25 Derangement of posterior horn of lateral meniscus due to old tear or injury
M23.251 Derangement of posterior horn of lateral meniscus due to old tear or injury, right knee
M23.252 Derangement of posterior horn of lateral meniscus due to old tear or injury, left knee
M23.259 Derangement of posterior horn of lateral meniscus due to old tear or injury, unspecified knee

M23.26 Derangement of other lateral meniscus due to old tear or injury
M23.261 Derangement of other lateral meniscus due to old tear or injury, right knee
M23.262 Derangement of other lateral meniscus due to old tear or injury, left knee
M23.269 Derangement of other lateral meniscus due to old tear or injury, unspecified knee

M23.3 Other meniscus derangements
Degenerate meniscus
Detached meniscus
Retained meniscus

M23.30 Other meniscus derangements, unspecified meniscus
Other meniscus derangements, unspecified lateral meniscus
Other meniscus derangements, unspecified medial meniscus

M23.300 Other meniscus derangements, unspecified lateral meniscus, right knee
M23.301 Other meniscus derangements, unspecified lateral meniscus, left knee
M23.302 Other meniscus derangements, unspecified lateral meniscus, unspecified knee
M23.303 Other meniscus derangements, unspecified medial meniscus, right knee
M23.304 Other meniscus derangements, unspecified medial meniscus, left knee
M23.305 Other meniscus derangements, unspecified medial meniscus, unspecified knee
M23.306 Other meniscus derangements, unspecified meniscus, right knee
M23.307 Other meniscus derangements, unspecified meniscus, left knee
M23.309 Other meniscus derangements, unspecified meniscus, unspecified knee

M23.31 Other meniscus derangements, anterior horn of medial meniscus
M23.311 Other meniscus derangements, anterior horn of medial meniscus, right knee
M23.312 Other meniscus derangements, anterior horn of medial meniscus, left knee
M23.319 Other meniscus derangements, anterior horn of medial meniscus, unspecified knee

M23.32 Other meniscus derangements, posterior horn of medial meniscus
M23.321 Other meniscus derangements, posterior horn of medial meniscus, right knee
M23.322 Other meniscus derangements, posterior horn of medial meniscus, left knee
M23.329 Other meniscus derangements, posterior horn of medial meniscus, unspecified knee

M23.33 Other meniscus derangements, other medial meniscus
M23.331 Other meniscus derangements, other medial meniscus, right knee
M23.332 Other meniscus derangements, other medial meniscus, left knee
M23.339 Other meniscus derangements, other medial meniscus, unspecified knee

M23.34 Other meniscus derangements, anterior horn of lateral meniscus
M23.341 Other meniscus derangements, anterior horn of lateral meniscus, right knee
M23.342 Other meniscus derangements, anterior horn of lateral meniscus, left knee
M23.349 Other meniscus derangements, anterior horn of lateral meniscus, unspecified knee

M23.35 Other meniscus derangements, posterior horn of lateral meniscus
M23.351 Other meniscus derangements, posterior horn of lateral meniscus, right knee
M23.352 Other meniscus derangements, posterior horn of lateral meniscus, left knee
M23.359 Other meniscus derangements, posterior horn of lateral meniscus, unspecified knee

M23.36 Other meniscus derangements, other lateral meniscus
M23.361 Other meniscus derangements, other lateral meniscus, right knee

M23.362 Other meniscus derangements, other lateral meniscus, left knee
M23.369 Other meniscus derangements, other lateral meniscus, unspecified knee
M23.4 Loose body in knee
M23.40 Loose body in knee, unspecified knee
M23.41 Loose body in knee, right knee
M23.42 Loose body in knee, left knee
M23.5 Chronic instability of knee
M23.50 Chronic instability of knee, unspecified knee
M23.51 Chronic instability of knee, right knee
M23.52 Chronic instability of knee, left knee
M23.6 Other spontaneous disruption of ligament(s) of knee
M23.60 Other spontaneous disruption of unspecified ligament of knee
M23.601 Other spontaneous disruption of unspecified ligament of right knee
M23.602 Other spontaneous disruption of unspecified ligament of left knee
M23.609 Other spontaneous disruption of unspecified ligament of unspecified knee
M23.61 Other spontaneous disruption of anterior cruciate ligament of knee
M23.611 Other spontaneous disruption of anterior cruciate ligament of right knee
M23.612 Other spontaneous disruption of anterior cruciate ligament of left knee
M23.619 Other spontaneous disruption of anterior cruciate ligament of unspecified knee
M23.62 Other spontaneous disruption of posterior cruciate ligament of knee
M23.621 Other spontaneous disruption of posterior cruciate ligament of right knee
M23.622 Other spontaneous disruption of posterior cruciate ligament of left knee
M23.629 Other spontaneous disruption of posterior cruciate ligament of unspecified knee
M23.63 Other spontaneous disruption of medial collateral ligament of knee
M23.631 Other spontaneous disruption of medial collateral ligament of right knee
M23.632 Other spontaneous disruption of medial collateral ligament of left knee
M23.639 Other spontaneous disruption of medial collateral ligament of unspecified knee
M23.64 Other spontaneous disruption of lateral collateral ligament of knee
M23.641 Other spontaneous disruption of lateral collateral ligament of right knee
M23.642 Other spontaneous disruption of lateral collateral ligament of left knee
M23.649 Other spontaneous disruption of lateral collateral ligament of unspecified knee
M23.67 Other spontaneous disruption of capsular ligament of knee
M23.671 Other spontaneous disruption of capsular ligament of right knee
M23.672 Other spontaneous disruption of capsular ligament of left knee
M23.679 Other spontaneous disruption of capsular ligament of unspecified knee
M23.8 Other internal derangements of knee
Laxity of ligament of knee
Snapping knee
M23.8X Other internal derangements of knee
M23.8X1 Other internal derangements of right knee
M23.8X2 Other internal derangements of left knee
M23.8X9 Other internal derangements of unspecified knee
M23.9 Unspecified internal derangement of knee
M23.90 Unspecified internal derangement of unspecified knee
M23.91 Unspecified internal derangement of right knee
M23.92 Unspecified internal derangement of left knee

M24 Other specific joint derangements
EXCLUDES 1 *current injury - see injury of joint by body region*
EXCLUDES 2 *ganglion (M67.4)*
snapping knee (M23.8-)
temporomandibular joint disorders (M26.6-)

M24.0 Loose body in joint
EXCLUDES 2 *loose body in knee (M23.4)*
M24.00 Loose body in unspecified joint
M24.01 Loose body in shoulder
M24.011 Loose body in right shoulder
M24.012 Loose body in left shoulder
M24.019 Loose body in unspecified shoulder
M24.02 Loose body in elbow
M24.021 Loose body in right elbow
M24.022 Loose body in left elbow
M24.029 Loose body in unspecified elbow
M24.03 Loose body in wrist
M24.031 Loose body in right wrist
M24.032 Loose body in left wrist
M24.039 Loose body in unspecified wrist
M24.04 Loose body in finger joints
M24.041 Loose body in right finger joint(s)
M24.042 Loose body in left finger joint(s)
M24.049 Loose body in unspecified finger joint(s)
M24.05 Loose body in hip
M24.051 Loose body in right hip
M24.052 Loose body in left hip
M24.059 Loose body in unspecified hip
M24.07 Loose body in ankle and toe joints
M24.071 Loose body in right ankle
M24.072 Loose body in left ankle
M24.073 Loose body in unspecified ankle
M24.074 Loose body in right toe joint(s)
M24.075 Loose body in left toe joint(s)
M24.076 Loose body in unspecified toe joints
M24.08 Loose body, other site
M24.1 Other articular cartilage disorders
EXCLUDES 2 *chondrocalcinosis (M11.1, M11.2-)*
internal derangement of knee (M23.-)
metastatic calcification (E83.5)
ochronosis (E70.2)
M24.10 Other articular cartilage disorders, unspecified site
M24.11 Other articular cartilage disorders, shoulder
M24.111 Other articular cartilage disorders, right shoulder
M24.112 Other articular cartilage disorders, left shoulder
M24.119 Other articular cartilage disorders, unspecified shoulder
M24.12 Other articular cartilage disorders, elbow
M24.121 Other articular cartilage disorders, right elbow
M24.122 Other articular cartilage disorders, left elbow
M24.129 Other articular cartilage disorders, unspecified elbow
M24.13 Other articular cartilage disorders, wrist
M24.131 Other articular cartilage disorders, right wrist
M24.132 Other articular cartilage disorders, left wrist
M24.139 Other articular cartilage disorders, unspecified wrist
M24.14 Other articular cartilage disorders, hand
M24.141 Other articular cartilage disorders, right hand
M24.142 Other articular cartilage disorders, left hand
M24.149 Other articular cartilage disorders, unspecified hand
M24.15 Other articular cartilage disorders, hip
M24.151 Other articular cartilage disorders, right hip
M24.152 Other articular cartilage disorders, left hip
M24.159 Other articular cartilage disorders, unspecified hip
M24.17 Other articular cartilage disorders, ankle and foot
M24.171 Other articular cartilage disorders, right ankle

M24.172 Other articular cartilage disorders, left ankle
M24.173 Other articular cartilage disorders, unspecified ankle
M24.174 Other articular cartilage disorders, right foot
M24.175 Other articular cartilage disorders, left foot
M24.176 Other articular cartilage disorders, unspecified foot

M24.2 Disorder of ligament
Instability secondary to old ligament injury
Ligamentous laxity NOS
EXCLUDES 1 *familial ligamentous laxity (M35.7)*
EXCLUDES 2 *internal derangement of knee (M23.5-M23.89)*

M24.20 Disorder of ligament, unspecified site
M24.21 Disorder of ligament, shoulder
M24.211 Disorder of ligament, right shoulder
M24.212 Disorder of ligament, left shoulder
M24.219 Disorder of ligament, unspecified shoulder
M24.22 Disorder of ligament, elbow
M24.221 Disorder of ligament, right elbow
M24.222 Disorder of ligament, left elbow
M24.229 Disorder of ligament, unspecified elbow
M24.23 Disorder of ligament, wrist
M24.231 Disorder of ligament, right wrist
M24.232 Disorder of ligament, left wrist
M24.239 Disorder of ligament, unspecified wrist
M24.24 Disorder of ligament, hand
M24.241 Disorder of ligament, right hand
M24.242 Disorder of ligament, left hand
M24.249 Disorder of ligament, unspecified hand
M24.25 Disorder of ligament, hip
M24.251 Disorder of ligament, right hip
M24.252 Disorder of ligament, left hip
M24.259 Disorder of ligament, unspecified hip
M24.27 Disorder of ligament, ankle and foot
M24.271 Disorder of ligament, right ankle
M24.272 Disorder of ligament, left ankle
M24.273 Disorder of ligament, unspecified ankle
M24.274 Disorder of ligament, right foot
M24.275 Disorder of ligament, left foot
M24.276 Disorder of ligament, unspecified foot
M24.28 Disorder of ligament, vertebrae

M24.3 Pathological dislocation of joint, not elsewhere classified
EXCLUDES 1 *congenital dislocation or displacement of joint- see congenital malformations and deformations of the musculoskeletal system (Q65-Q79)*
current injury - see injury of joints and ligaments by body region
recurrent dislocation of joint (M24.4-)

M24.30 Pathological dislocation of unspecified joint, not elsewhere classified
M24.31 Pathological dislocation of shoulder, not elsewhere classified
M24.311 Pathological dislocation of right shoulder, not elsewhere classified
M24.312 Pathological dislocation of left shoulder, not elsewhere classified
M24.319 Pathological dislocation of unspecified shoulder, not elsewhere classified
M24.32 Pathological dislocation of elbow, not elsewhere classified
M24.321 Pathological dislocation of right elbow, not elsewhere classified
M24.322 Pathological dislocation of left elbow, not elsewhere classified
M24.329 Pathological dislocation of unspecified elbow, not elsewhere classified
M24.33 Pathological dislocation of wrist, not elsewhere classified
M24.331 Pathological dislocation of right wrist, not elsewhere classified
M24.332 Pathological dislocation of left wrist, not elsewhere classified
M24.339 Pathological dislocation of unspecified wrist, not elsewhere classified
M24.34 Pathological dislocation of hand, not elsewhere classified
M24.341 Pathological dislocation of right hand, not elsewhere classified
M24.342 Pathological dislocation of left hand, not elsewhere classified
M24.349 Pathological dislocation of unspecified hand, not elsewhere classified
M24.35 Pathological dislocation of hip, not elsewhere classified
M24.351 Pathological dislocation of right hip, not elsewhere classified
M24.352 Pathological dislocation of left hip, not elsewhere classified
M24.359 Pathological dislocation of unspecified hip, not elsewhere classified
M24.36 Pathological dislocation of knee, not elsewhere classified
M24.361 Pathological dislocation of right knee, not elsewhere classified
M24.362 Pathological dislocation of left knee, not elsewhere classified
M24.369 Pathological dislocation of unspecified knee, not elsewhere classified
M24.37 Pathological dislocation of ankle and foot, not elsewhere classified
M24.371 Pathological dislocation of right ankle, not elsewhere classified
M24.372 Pathological dislocation of left ankle, not elsewhere classified
M24.373 Pathological dislocation of unspecified ankle, not elsewhere classified
M24.374 Pathological dislocation of right foot, not elsewhere classified
M24.375 Pathological dislocation of left foot, not elsewhere classified
M24.376 Pathological dislocation of unspecified foot, not elsewhere classified

M24.4 Recurrent dislocation of joint
Recurrent subluxation of joint
EXCLUDES 2 *recurrent dislocation of patella (M22.0-M22.1)*
recurrent vertebral dislocation (M43.3-, M43.4, M43.5-)

M24.40 Recurrent dislocation, unspecified joint
M24.41 Recurrent dislocation, shoulder
M24.411 Recurrent dislocation, right shoulder
M24.412 Recurrent dislocation, left shoulder
M24.419 Recurrent dislocation, unspecified shoulder
M24.42 Recurrent dislocation, elbow
M24.421 Recurrent dislocation, right elbow
M24.422 Recurrent dislocation, left elbow
M24.429 Recurrent dislocation, unspecified elbow
M24.43 Recurrent dislocation, wrist
M24.431 Recurrent dislocation, right wrist
M24.432 Recurrent dislocation, left wrist
M24.439 Recurrent dislocation, unspecified wrist
M24.44 Recurrent dislocation, hand and finger(s)
M24.441 Recurrent dislocation, right hand
M24.442 Recurrent dislocation, left hand
M24.443 Recurrent dislocation, unspecified hand
M24.444 Recurrent dislocation, right finger
M24.445 Recurrent dislocation, left finger
M24.446 Recurrent dislocation, unspecified finger
M24.45 Recurrent dislocation, hip
M24.451 Recurrent dislocation, right hip
M24.452 Recurrent dislocation, left hip
M24.459 Recurrent dislocation, unspecified hip
M24.46 Recurrent dislocation, knee
M24.461 Recurrent dislocation, right knee
M24.462 Recurrent dislocation, left knee
M24.469 Recurrent dislocation, unspecified knee
M24.47 Recurrent dislocation, ankle, foot and toes
M24.471 Recurrent dislocation, right ankle

M24.472 Recurrent dislocation, left ankle
M24.473 Recurrent dislocation, unspecified ankle
M24.474 Recurrent dislocation, right foot
M24.475 Recurrent dislocation, left foot
M24.476 Recurrent dislocation, unspecified foot
M24.477 Recurrent dislocation, right toe(s)
M24.478 Recurrent dislocation, left toe(s)
M24.479 Recurrent dislocation, unspecified toe(s)

M24.5 Contracture of joint

EXCLUDES 1 *contracture of muscle without contracture of joint (M62.4-)*
contracture of tendon (sheath) without contracture of joint (M62.4-)
Dupuytren's contracture (M72.0)

EXCLUDES 2 *acquired deformities of limbs (M20-M21)*

CODING TIP ✓ Contracture of joint is a joint dysfunction that results from prolonged immobility or improper positioning, leading to joint stiffness and decreased range of movement. It may be caused by injury or disease, nerve injury (peripheral nerve damage and spinal cord injury), muscle tendon injury or ligament disease.

M24.50 Contracture, unspecified joint
M24.51 Contracture, shoulder
M24.511 Contracture, right shoulder
M24.512 Contracture, left shoulder
M24.519 Contracture, unspecified shoulder
M24.52 Contracture, elbow
M24.521 Contracture, right elbow
M24.522 Contracture, left elbow
M24.529 Contracture, unspecified elbow
M24.53 Contracture, wrist
M24.531 Contracture, right wrist
M24.532 Contracture, left wrist
M24.539 Contracture, unspecified wrist
M24.54 Contracture, hand
M24.541 Contracture, right hand
M24.542 Contracture, left hand
M24.549 Contracture, unspecified hand
M24.55 Contracture, hip
M24.551 Contracture, right hip
AHA: 2Q 2016, 6
M24.552 Contracture, left hip
AHA: 2Q 2016, 6
M24.559 Contracture, unspecified hip
M24.56 Contracture, knee
M24.561 Contracture, right knee
AHA: 2Q 2016, 6
M24.562 Contracture, left knee
AHA: 2Q 2016, 6
M24.569 Contracture, unspecified knee
M24.57 Contracture, ankle and foot
M24.571 Contracture, right ankle
M24.572 Contracture, left ankle
M24.573 Contracture, unspecified ankle
M24.574 Contracture, right foot
M24.575 Contracture, left foot
M24.576 Contracture, unspecified foot

M24.6 Ankylosis of joint

EXCLUDES 1 *stiffness of joint without ankylosis (M25.6-)*

EXCLUDES 2 *spine (M43.2-)*

M24.60 Ankylosis, unspecified joint
M24.61 Ankylosis, shoulder
M24.611 Ankylosis, right shoulder
M24.612 Ankylosis, left shoulder
M24.619 Ankylosis, unspecified shoulder
M24.62 Ankylosis, elbow
M24.621 Ankylosis, right elbow
M24.622 Ankylosis, left elbow
M24.629 Ankylosis, unspecified elbow
M24.63 Ankylosis, wrist
M24.631 Ankylosis, right wrist
M24.632 Ankylosis, left wrist
M24.639 Ankylosis, unspecified wrist
M24.64 Ankylosis, hand
M24.641 Ankylosis, right hand
M24.642 Ankylosis, left hand
M24.649 Ankylosis, unspecified hand
M24.65 Ankylosis, hip
M24.651 Ankylosis, right hip
M24.652 Ankylosis, left hip
M24.659 Ankylosis, unspecified hip
M24.66 Ankylosis, knee
M24.661 Ankylosis, right knee
M24.662 Ankylosis, left knee
M24.669 Ankylosis, unspecified knee
M24.67 Ankylosis, ankle and foot
M24.671 Ankylosis, right ankle
M24.672 Ankylosis, left ankle
M24.673 Ankylosis, unspecified ankle
M24.674 Ankylosis, right foot
M24.675 Ankylosis, left foot
M24.676 Ankylosis, unspecified foot

M24.7 Protrusio acetabuli

M24.8 Other specific joint derangements, not elsewhere classified

EXCLUDES 2 *iliotibial band syndrome (M76.3)*

M24.80 Other specific joint derangements of unspecified joint, not elsewhere classified
M24.81 Other specific joint derangements of shoulder, not elsewhere classified
M24.811 Other specific joint derangements of right shoulder, not elsewhere classified
M24.812 Other specific joint derangements of left shoulder, not elsewhere classified
M24.819 Other specific joint derangements of unspecified shoulder, not elsewhere classified
M24.82 Other specific joint derangements of elbow, not elsewhere classified
M24.821 Other specific joint derangements of right elbow, not elsewhere classified
M24.822 Other specific joint derangements of left elbow, not elsewhere classified
M24.829 Other specific joint derangements of unspecified elbow, not elsewhere classified
M24.83 Other specific joint derangements of wrist, not elsewhere classified
M24.831 Other specific joint derangements of right wrist, not elsewhere classified
M24.832 Other specific joint derangements of left wrist, not elsewhere classified
M24.839 Other specific joint derangements of unspecified wrist, not elsewhere classified
M24.84 Other specific joint derangements of hand, not elsewhere classified
M24.841 Other specific joint derangements of right hand, not elsewhere classified
M24.842 Other specific joint derangements of left hand, not elsewhere classified
M24.849 Other specific joint derangements of unspecified hand, not elsewhere classified
M24.85 Other specific joint derangements of hip, not elsewhere classified
Irritable hip
M24.851 Other specific joint derangements of right hip, not elsewhere classified
M24.852 Other specific joint derangements of left hip, not elsewhere classified
M24.859 Other specific joint derangements of unspecified hip, not elsewhere classified
M24.87 Other specific joint derangements of ankle and foot, not elsewhere classified
M24.871 Other specific joint derangements of right ankle, not elsewhere classified
M24.872 Other specific joint derangements of left ankle, not elsewhere classified

M24.873 Other specific joint derangements of unspecified ankle, not elsewhere classified
M24.874 Other specific joint derangements of right foot, not elsewhere classified
M24.875 Other specific joint derangements left foot, not elsewhere classified
M24.876 Other specific joint derangements of unspecified foot, not elsewhere classified
M24.9 Joint derangement, unspecified

M25 Other joint disorder, not elsewhere classified

EXCLUDES 2 *abnormality of gait and mobility (R26.-)*
acquired deformities of limb (M20-M21)
calcification of bursa (M71.4-)
calcification of shoulder (joint) (M75.3)
calcification of tendon (M65.2-)
difficulty in walking (R26.2)
temporomandibular joint disorder (M26.6-)

M25.0 Hemarthrosis
EXCLUDES 1 *current injury - see injury of joint by body region*
hemophilic arthropathy (M36.2)
M25.00 Hemarthrosis, unspecified joint
M25.01 Hemarthrosis, shoulder
M25.011 Hemarthrosis, right shoulder
M25.012 Hemarthrosis, left shoulder
M25.019 Hemarthrosis, unspecified shoulder
M25.02 Hemarthrosis, elbow
M25.021 Hemarthrosis, right elbow
M25.022 Hemarthrosis, left elbow
M25.029 Hemarthrosis, unspecified elbow
M25.03 Hemarthrosis, wrist
M25.031 Hemarthrosis, right wrist
M25.032 Hemarthrosis, left wrist
M25.039 Hemarthrosis, unspecified wrist
M25.04 Hemarthrosis, hand
M25.041 Hemarthrosis, right hand
M25.042 Hemarthrosis, left hand
M25.049 Hemarthrosis, unspecified hand
M25.05 Hemarthrosis, hip
M25.051 Hemarthrosis, right hip
M25.052 Hemarthrosis, left hip
M25.059 Hemarthrosis, unspecified hip
M25.06 Hemarthrosis, knee
M25.061 Hemarthrosis, right knee
M25.062 Hemarthrosis, left knee
M25.069 Hemarthrosis, unspecified knee
M25.07 Hemarthrosis, ankle and foot
M25.071 Hemarthrosis, right ankle
M25.072 Hemarthrosis, left ankle
M25.073 Hemarthrosis, unspecified ankle
M25.074 Hemarthrosis, right foot
M25.075 Hemarthrosis, left foot
M25.076 Hemarthrosis, unspecified foot
M25.08 Hemarthrosis, other specified site
Hemarthrosis, vertebrae

M25.1 Fistula of joint
M25.10 Fistula, unspecified joint
M25.11 Fistula, shoulder
M25.111 Fistula, right shoulder
M25.112 Fistula, left shoulder
M25.119 Fistula, unspecified shoulder
M25.12 Fistula, elbow
M25.121 Fistula, right elbow
M25.122 Fistula, left elbow
M25.129 Fistula, unspecified elbow
M25.13 Fistula, wrist
M25.131 Fistula, right wrist
M25.132 Fistula, left wrist
M25.139 Fistula, unspecified wrist
M25.14 Fistula, hand
M25.141 Fistula, right hand
M25.142 Fistula, left hand
M25.149 Fistula, unspecified hand
M25.15 Fistula, hip
M25.151 Fistula, right hip
M25.152 Fistula, left hip
M25.159 Fistula, unspecified hip
M25.16 Fistula, knee
M25.161 Fistula, right knee
M25.162 Fistula, left knee
M25.169 Fistula, unspecified knee
M25.17 Fistula, ankle and foot
M25.171 Fistula, right ankle
M25.172 Fistula, left ankle
M25.173 Fistula, unspecified ankle
M25.174 Fistula, right foot
M25.175 Fistula, left foot
M25.176 Fistula, unspecified foot
M25.18 Fistula, other specified site
Fistula, vertebrae

M25.2 Flail joint
M25.20 Flail joint, unspecified joint
M25.21 Flail joint, shoulder
M25.211 Flail joint, right shoulder
M25.212 Flail joint, left shoulder
M25.219 Flail joint, unspecified shoulder
M25.22 Flail joint, elbow
M25.221 Flail joint, right elbow
M25.222 Flail joint, left elbow
M25.229 Flail joint, unspecified elbow
M25.23 Flail joint, wrist
M25.231 Flail joint, right wrist
M25.232 Flail joint, left wrist
M25.239 Flail joint, unspecified wrist
M25.24 Flail joint, hand
M25.241 Flail joint, right hand
M25.242 Flail joint, left hand
M25.249 Flail joint, unspecified hand
M25.25 Flail joint, hip
M25.251 Flail joint, right hip
M25.252 Flail joint, left hip
M25.259 Flail joint, unspecified hip
M25.26 Flail joint, knee
M25.261 Flail joint, right knee
M25.262 Flail joint, left knee
M25.269 Flail joint, unspecified knee
M25.27 Flail joint, ankle and foot
M25.271 Flail joint, right ankle and foot
M25.272 Flail joint, left ankle and foot
M25.279 Flail joint, unspecified ankle and foot
M25.28 Flail joint, other site

M25.3 Other instability of joint
EXCLUDES 1 *instability of joint secondary to old ligament injury (M24.2-)*
instability of joint secondary to removal of joint prosthesis (M96.8-)
EXCLUDES 2 *spinal instabilities (M53.2-)*
M25.30 Other instability, unspecified joint
M25.31 Other instability, shoulder
M25.311 Other instability, right shoulder
M25.312 Other instability, left shoulder
M25.319 Other instability, unspecified shoulder
M25.32 Other instability, elbow
M25.321 Other instability, right elbow
M25.322 Other instability, left elbow
M25.329 Other instability, unspecified elbow
M25.33 Other instability, wrist
M25.331 Other instability, right wrist
M25.332 Other instability, left wrist
M25.339 Other instability, unspecified wrist
M25.34 Other instability, hand

M25.341 Other instability, right hand
M25.342 Other instability, left hand
M25.349 Other instability, unspecified hand
M25.35 Other instability, hip
M25.351 Other instability, right hip
M25.352 Other instability, left hip
M25.359 Other instability, unspecified hip
M25.36 Other instability, knee
M25.361 Other instability, right knee
M25.362 Other instability, left knee
M25.369 Other instability, unspecified knee
M25.37 Other instability, ankle and foot
M25.371 Other instability, right ankle
M25.372 Other instability, left ankle
M25.373 Other instability, unspecified ankle
M25.374 Other instability, right foot
M25.375 Other instability, left foot
M25.376 Other instability, unspecified foot
M25.4 Effusion of joint
EXCLUDES 1 *hydrarthrosis in yaws (A66.6)*
intermittent hydrarthrosis (M12.4-)
other infective (teno) synovitis (M65.1-)
M25.40 Effusion, unspecified joint
M25.41 Effusion, shoulder
M25.411 Effusion, right shoulder
M25.412 Effusion, left shoulder
M25.419 Effusion, unspecified shoulder
M25.42 Effusion, elbow
M25.421 Effusion, right elbow
M25.422 Effusion, left elbow
M25.429 Effusion, unspecified elbow
M25.43 Effusion, wrist
M25.431 Effusion, right wrist
M25.432 Effusion, left wrist
M25.439 Effusion, unspecified wrist
M25.44 Effusion, hand
M25.441 Effusion, right hand
M25.442 Effusion, left hand
M25.449 Effusion, unspecified hand
M25.45 Effusion, hip
M25.451 Effusion, right hip
M25.452 Effusion, left hip
M25.459 Effusion, unspecified hip
M25.46 Effusion, knee
M25.461 Effusion, right knee
M25.462 Effusion, left knee
M25.469 Effusion, unspecified knee
M25.47 Effusion, ankle and foot
M25.471 Effusion, right ankle
M25.472 Effusion, left ankle
M25.473 Effusion, unspecified ankle
M25.474 Effusion, right foot
M25.475 Effusion, left foot
M25.476 Effusion, unspecified foot
M25.48 Effusion, other site
M25.5 Pain in joint
EXCLUDES 2 *pain in hand (M79.64-)*
pain in fingers (M79.64-)
pain in foot (M79.67-)
pain in limb (M79.6-)
pain in toes (M79.67-)
CODING TIP ✓ These codes should be used when 1) the cause of the pain is unknown; 2) the pain is a sequela of an injury; or 3) in conjunction with a G89 code. Do not use these codes with conditions that result in the pain such as arthritis or injuries.
M25.50 Pain in unspecified joint
M25.51 Pain in shoulder
M25.511 Pain in right shoulder
M25.512 Pain in left shoulder
M25.519 Pain in unspecified shoulder
M25.52 Pain in elbow
M25.521 Pain in right elbow
M25.522 Pain in left elbow
M25.529 Pain in unspecified elbow
M25.53 Pain in wrist
M25.531 Pain in right wrist
M25.532 Pain in left wrist
M25.539 Pain in unspecified wrist
M25.54 Pain in joints of hand
AHA: 4Q 2016, 38
M25.541 Pain in joints of right hand
M25.542 Pain in joints of left hand
M25.549 Pain in joints of unspecified hand
Pain in joints of hand NOS
M25.55 Pain in hip
M25.551 Pain in right hip
M25.552 Pain in left hip
M25.559 Pain in unspecified hip
M25.56 Pain in knee
M25.561 Pain in right knee
M25.562 Pain in left knee
M25.569 Pain in unspecified knee
M25.57 Pain in ankle and joints of foot
M25.571 Pain in right ankle and joints of right foot
M25.572 Pain in left ankle and joints of left foot
M25.579 Pain in unspecified ankle and joints of unspecified foot
M25.6 Stiffness of joint, not elsewhere classified
EXCLUDES 1 *ankylosis of joint (M24.6-)*
contracture of joint (M24.5-)
CODING TIP ✓ These codes should be used when 1) the cause of the stiffness is unknown; 2) the stiffness is a sequela of an injury. Do not use these codes with conditions like arthritis.
M25.60 Stiffness of unspecified joint, not elsewhere classified
M25.61 Stiffness of shoulder, not elsewhere classified
M25.611 Stiffness of right shoulder, not elsewhere classified
M25.612 Stiffness of left shoulder, not elsewhere classified
M25.619 Stiffness of unspecified shoulder, not elsewhere classified
M25.62 Stiffness of elbow, not elsewhere classified
M25.621 Stiffness of right elbow, not elsewhere classified
M25.622 Stiffness of left elbow, not elsewhere classified
M25.629 Stiffness of unspecified elbow, not elsewhere classified
M25.63 Stiffness of wrist, not elsewhere classified
M25.631 Stiffness of right wrist, not elsewhere classified
M25.632 Stiffness of left wrist, not elsewhere classified
M25.639 Stiffness of unspecified wrist, not elsewhere classified
M25.64 Stiffness of hand, not elsewhere classified
M25.641 Stiffness of right hand, not elsewhere classified
M25.642 Stiffness of left hand, not elsewhere classified
M25.649 Stiffness of unspecified hand, not elsewhere classified
M25.65 Stiffness of hip, not elsewhere classified
M25.651 Stiffness of right hip, not elsewhere classified
M25.652 Stiffness of left hip, not elsewhere classified
M25.659 Stiffness of unspecified hip, not elsewhere classified
M25.66 Stiffness of knee, not elsewhere classified
M25.661 Stiffness of right knee, not elsewhere classified
M25.662 Stiffness of left knee, not elsewhere classified
M25.669 Stiffness of unspecified knee, not elsewhere classified
M25.67 Stiffness of ankle and foot, not elsewhere classified
M25.671 Stiffness of right ankle, not elsewhere classified
M25.672 Stiffness of left ankle, not elsewhere classified
M25.673 Stiffness of unspecified ankle, not elsewhere classified
M25.674 Stiffness of right foot, not elsewhere classified
M25.675 Stiffness of left foot, not elsewhere classified

M25.676 Stiffness of unspecified foot, not elsewhere classified

M25.7 Osteophyte

M25.70 Osteophyte, unspecified joint

M25.71 Osteophyte, shoulder

M25.711 Osteophyte, right shoulder

M25.712 Osteophyte, left shoulder

M25.719 Osteophyte, unspecified shoulder

M25.72 Osteophyte, elbow

M25.721 Osteophyte, right elbow

M25.722 Osteophyte, left elbow

M25.729 Osteophyte, unspecified elbow

M25.73 Osteophyte, wrist

M25.731 Osteophyte, right wrist

M25.732 Osteophyte, left wrist

M25.739 Osteophyte, unspecified wrist

M25.74 Osteophyte, hand

M25.741 Osteophyte, right hand

M25.742 Osteophyte, left hand

M25.749 Osteophyte, unspecified hand

M25.75 Osteophyte, hip

M25.751 Osteophyte, right hip

M25.752 Osteophyte, left hip

M25.759 Osteophyte, unspecified hip

M25.76 Osteophyte, knee

M25.761 Osteophyte, right knee

M25.762 Osteophyte, left knee

M25.769 Osteophyte, unspecified knee

M25.77 Osteophyte, ankle and foot

M25.771 Osteophyte, right ankle

M25.772 Osteophyte, left ankle

M25.773 Osteophyte, unspecified ankle

M25.774 Osteophyte, right foot

M25.775 Osteophyte, left foot

M25.776 Osteophyte, unspecified foot

M25.78 Osteophyte, vertebrae

M25.8 Other specified joint disorders

M25.80 Other specified joint disorders, unspecified joint

M25.81 Other specified joint disorders, shoulder

M25.811 Other specified joint disorders, right shoulder

M25.812 Other specified joint disorders, left shoulder

M25.819 Other specified joint disorders, unspecified shoulder

M25.82 Other specified joint disorders, elbow

M25.821 Other specified joint disorders, right elbow

M25.822 Other specified joint disorders, left elbow

M25.829 Other specified joint disorders, unspecified elbow

M25.83 Other specified joint disorders, wrist

M25.831 Other specified joint disorders, right wrist

M25.832 Other specified joint disorders, left wrist

M25.839 Other specified joint disorders, unspecified wrist

M25.84 Other specified joint disorders, hand

M25.841 Other specified joint disorders, right hand

M25.842 Other specified joint disorders, left hand

M25.849 Other specified joint disorders, unspecified hand

M25.85 Other specified joint disorders, hip

M25.851 Other specified joint disorders, right hip

M25.852 Other specified joint disorders, left hip
AHA: 4Q 2014, 25

M25.859 Other specified joint disorders, unspecified hip

M25.86 Other specified joint disorders, knee

M25.861 Other specified joint disorders, right knee

M25.862 Other specified joint disorders, left knee

M25.869 Other specified joint disorders, unspecified knee

M25.87 Other specified joint disorders, ankle and foot

M25.871 Other specified joint disorders, right ankle and foot

M25.872 Other specified joint disorders, left ankle and foot

M25.879 Other specified joint disorders, unspecified ankle and foot

M25.9 Joint disorder, unspecified

Dentofacial anomalies [including malocclusion] and other disorders of jaw (M26-M27)

EXCLUDES 1 *hemifacial atrophy or hypertrophy (Q67.4)*
unilateral condylar hyperplasia or hypoplasia (M27.8)

M26 Dentofacial anomalies [including malocclusion]

M26.0 Major anomalies of jaw size

EXCLUDES 1 *acromegaly (E22.0)*
Robin's syndrome (Q87.0)

M26.00 Unspecified anomaly of jaw size

M26.01 Maxillary hyperplasia

M26.02 Maxillary hypoplasia
AHA: 3Q 2014, 23

M26.03 Mandibular hyperplasia

Mandibular hyperplasia

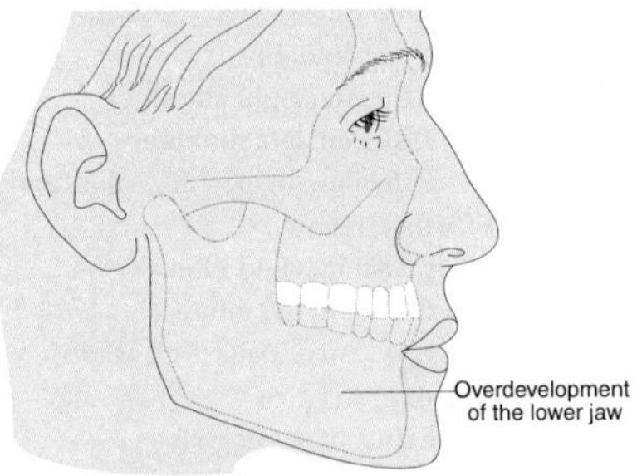

M26.04 Mandibular hypoplasia

M26.05 Macrogenia

DEFINITION Abnormally large chin.

M26.06 Microgenia

M26.07 Excessive tuberosity of jaw
Entire maxillary tuberosity

M26.09 Other specified anomalies of jaw size

M26.1 Anomalies of jaw-cranial base relationship

M26.10 Unspecified anomaly of jaw-cranial base relationship

M26.11 Maxillary asymmetry

M26.12 Other jaw asymmetry

M26.19 Other specified anomalies of jaw-cranial base relationship

M26.2 Anomalies of dental arch relationship

M26.20 Unspecified anomaly of dental arch relationship

M26.21 Malocclusion, Angle's class

M26.211 Malocclusion, Angle's class I
Neutro-occlusion

Malocclusion, Angle's Class 1

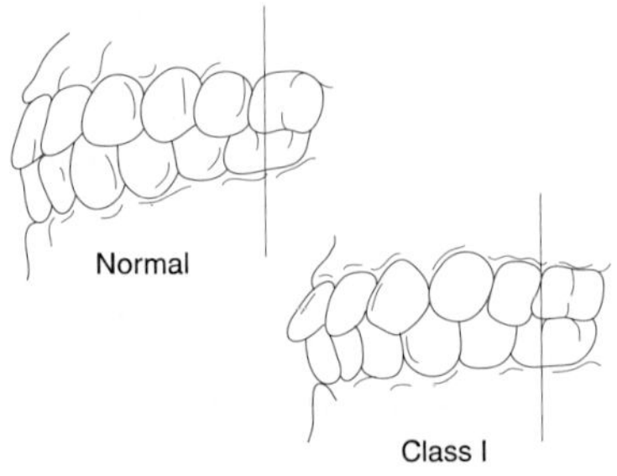

M26.212 Malocclusion, Angle's class II
Disto-occlusion Division I
Disto-occlusion Division II

M26.213 **Malocclusion, Angle's class III**
Mesio-occlusion
M26.219 **Malocclusion, Angle's class, unspecified**
6 M26.22 **Open occlusal relationship**
▲ M26.220 **Open anterior occlusal relationship**
Anterior open bite
▲ M26.221 **Open posterior occlusal relationship**
Posterior open bite
M26.23 **Excessive horizontal overlap**
Excessive horizontal overjet
M26.24 **Reverse articulation**
Crossbite (anterior) (posterior)
M26.25 **Anomalies of interarch distance**
M26.29 **Other anomalies of dental arch relationship**
Midline deviation of dental arch
Overbite (excessive) deep
Overbite (excessive) horizontal
Overbite (excessive) vertical
Posterior lingual occlusion of mandibular teeth
5 M26.3 **Anomalies of tooth position of fully erupted tooth or teeth**
EXCLUDES 2 *embedded and impacted teeth (K01.-)*
M26.30 **Unspecified anomaly of tooth position of fully erupted tooth or teeth**
Abnormal spacing of fully erupted tooth or teeth NOS
Displacement of fully erupted tooth or teeth NOS
Transposition of fully erupted tooth or teeth NOS
M26.31 **Crowding of fully erupted teeth**
M26.32 **Excessive spacing of fully erupted teeth**
Diastema of fully erupted tooth or teeth NOS
M26.33 **Horizontal displacement of fully erupted tooth or teeth**
Tipped tooth or teeth
Tipping of fully erupted tooth
M26.34 **Vertical displacement of fully erupted tooth or teeth**
Extruded tooth
Infraeruption of tooth or teeth
Supraeruption of tooth or teeth
M26.35 **Rotation of fully erupted tooth or teeth**
M26.36 **Insufficient interocclusal distance of fully erupted teeth (ridge)**
Lack of adequate intermaxillary vertical dimension of fully erupted teeth
M26.37 **Excessive interocclusal distance of fully erupted teeth**
Excessive intermaxillary vertical dimension of fully erupted teeth
Loss of occlusal vertical dimension of fully erupted teeth
M26.39 **Other anomalies of tooth position of fully erupted tooth or teeth**
M26.4 **Malocclusion, unspecified**
5 M26.5 **Dentofacial functional abnormalities**
EXCLUDES 1 *bruxism (F45.8)*
teeth-grinding NOS (F45.8)
M26.50 **Dentofacial functional abnormalities, unspecified**
M26.51 **Abnormal jaw closure**
M26.52 **Limited mandibular range of motion**
M26.53 **Deviation in opening and closing of the mandible**
M26.54 **Insufficient anterior guidance**
Insufficient anterior occlusal guidance
M26.55 **Centric occlusion maximum intercuspation discrepancy**
EXCLUDES 1 *centric occlusion NOS (M26.59)*
M26.56 **Non-working side interference**
Balancing side interference
M26.57 **Lack of posterior occlusal support**
M26.59 **Other dentofacial functional abnormalities**
Centric occlusion (of teeth) NOS
Malocclusion due to abnormal swallowing
Malocclusion due to mouth breathing
Malocclusion due to tongue, lip or finger habits
5 M26.6 **Temporomandibular joint disorders**
EXCLUDES 2 *current temporomandibular joint dislocation (S03.0)*
current temporomandibular joint sprain (S03.4)
AHA: 4Q 2016, 38
6 M26.60 **Temporomandibular joint disorder, unspecified**
⊟ M26.601 **Right temporomandibular joint disorder, unspecified**
⊟ M26.602 **Left temporomandibular joint disorder, unspecified**
⊟ M26.603 **Bilateral temporomandibular joint disorder, unspecified**
⊟ M26.609 **Unspecified temporomandibular joint disorder, Unspecified side**
Temporomandibular joint disorder NOS
6 M26.61 **Adhesions and ankylosis of temporomandibular joint**
⊟ M26.611 **Adhesions and ankylosis of right temporomandibular joint**
⊟ M26.612 **Adhesions and ankylosis of left temporomandibular joint**
⊟ M26.613 **Adhesions and ankylosis of bilateral temporomandibular joint**
⊟ M26.619 **Adhesions and ankylosis of temporomandibular joint, unspecified side**
6 M26.62 **Arthralgia of temporomandibular joint**

Arthralgia of temporomandibular joint

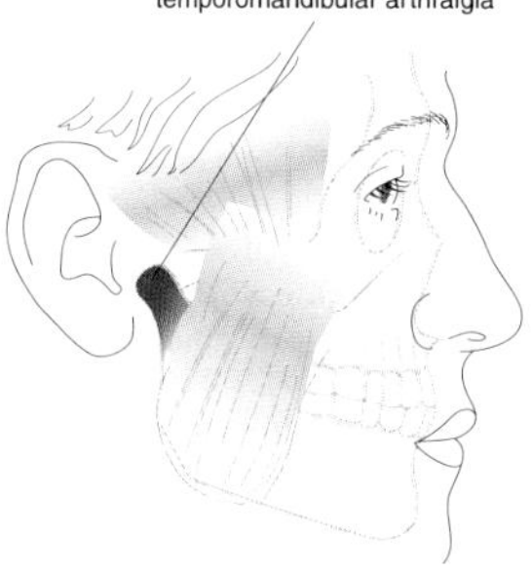
Pain, redness, swelling, and/or stiffness of the joint may accompany temporomandibular arthralgia

⊟ M26.621 **Arthralgia of right temporomandibular joint**
⊟ M26.622 **Arthralgia of left temporomandibular joint**
⊟ M26.623 **Arthralgia of bilateral temporomandibular joint**
⊟ M26.629 **Arthralgia of temporomandibular joint, unspecified side**
6 M26.63 **Articular disc disorder of temporomandibular joint**
⊟ M26.631 **Articular disc disorder of right temporomandibular joint**
⊟ M26.632 **Articular disc disorder of left temporomandibular joint**
⊟ M26.633 **Articular disc disorder of bilateral temporomandibular joint**
⊟ M26.639 **Articular disc disorder of temporomandibular joint, unspecified side**
M26.69 **Other specified disorders of temporomandibular joint**
5 M26.7 **Dental alveolar anomalies**
M26.70 **Unspecified alveolar anomaly**
M26.71 **Alveolar maxillary hyperplasia**
M26.72 **Alveolar mandibular hyperplasia**
M26.73 **Alveolar maxillary hypoplasia**
M26.74 **Alveolar mandibular hypoplasia**
M26.79 **Other specified alveolar anomalies**
5 M26.8 **Other dentofacial anomalies**
M26.81 **Anterior soft tissue impingement**
Anterior soft tissue impingement on teeth
M26.82 **Posterior soft tissue impingement**
Posterior soft tissue impingement on teeth
M26.89 **Other dentofacial anomalies**
M26.9 **Dentofacial anomaly, unspecified**

4 M27 Other diseases of jaws

M27.0 **Developmental disorders of jaws**
Latent bone cyst of jaw
Stafne's cyst
Torus mandibularis
Torus palatinus

M27.1 Giant cell granuloma, central
Giant cell granuloma NOS
EXCLUDES 1 *peripheral giant cell granuloma (K06.8)*

M27.2 Inflammatory conditions of jaws
Osteitis of jaw(s)
Osteomyelitis (neonatal) jaw(s)
Osteoradionecrosis jaw(s)
Periostitis jaw(s)
Sequestrum of jaw bone
Use additional code (W88-W90, X39.0) to identify radiation, if radiation-induced
EXCLUDES 2 *osteonecrosis of jaw due to drug (M87.180)*

M27.3 Alveolitis of jaws
Alveolar osteitis
Dry socket
DEFINITION Inflammation of the tooth sockets.

5 **M27.4 Other and unspecified cysts of jaw**
EXCLUDES 1 *cysts of oral region (K09.-)*
latent bone cyst of jaw (M27.0)
Stafne's cyst (M27.0)

M27.40 Unspecified cyst of jaw
Cyst of jaw NOS

M27.49 Other cysts of jaw
Aneurysmal cyst of jaw
Hemorrhagic cyst of jaw
Traumatic cyst of jaw

5 **M27.5 Periradicular pathology associated with previous endodontic treatment**

M27.51 Perforation of root canal space due to endodontic treatment

M27.52 Endodontic overfill

M27.53 Endodontic underfill

M27.59 Other periradicular pathology associated with previous endodontic treatment

5 **M27.6 Endosseous dental implant failure**

M27.61 Osseointegration failure of dental implant
Hemorrhagic complications of dental implant placement
Iatrogenic osseointegration failure of dental implant
Osseointegration failure of dental implant due to complications of systemic disease
Osseointegration failure of dental implant due to poor bone quality
Pre-integration failure of dental implant NOS
Pre-osseointegration failure of dental implant

M27.62 Post-osseointegration biological failure of dental implant
Failure of dental implant due to lack of attached gingiva
Failure of dental implant due to occlusal trauma (caused by poor prosthetic design)
Failure of dental implant due to parafunctional habits
Failure of dental implant due to periodontal infection (peri-implantitis)
Failure of dental implant due to poor oral hygiene
Iatrogenic post-osseointegration failure of dental implant
Post-osseointegration failure of dental implant due to complications of systemic disease

M27.63 Post-osseointegration mechanical failure of dental implant
Failure of dental prosthesis causing loss of dental implant
Fracture of dental implant
EXCLUDES 2 *cracked tooth (K03.81)*
fractured dental restorative material with loss of material (K08.531)
fractured dental restorative material without loss of material (K08.530)
fractured tooth (S02.5)

M27.69 Other endosseous dental implant failure
Dental implant failure NOS

M27.8 Other specified diseases of jaws
Cherubism
Exostosis
Fibrous dysplasia
Unilateral condylar hyperplasia
Unilateral condylar hypoplasia
EXCLUDES 1 *jaw pain (R68.84)*

M27.9 Disease of jaws, unspecified

Systemic connective tissue disorders (M30-M36)

INCLUDES autoimmune disease NOS
collagen (vascular) disease NOS
systemic autoimmune disease
systemic collagen (vascular) disease
EXCLUDES 1 *autoimmune disease, single organ or single cell-type -code to relevant condition category*

4 **M30 Polyarteritis nodosa and related conditions**
EXCLUDES 1 *microscopic polyarteritis (M31.7)*

M30.0 Polyarteritis nodosa HCC
DEFINITION The body's immune system mistakenly attacks small and medium-sized blood vessels, resulting in tissue death.

M30.1 Polyarteritis with lung involvement [Churg-Strauss] HCC
Allergic granulomatous angiitis

M30.2 Juvenile polyarteritis HCC

M30.3 Mucocutaneous lymph node syndrome [Kawasaki] HCC

M30.8 Other conditions related to polyarteritis nodosa HCC
Polyangiitis overlap syndrome

4 **M31 Other necrotizing vasculopathies**

M31.0 Hypersensitivity angiitis HCC
Goodpasture's syndrome

M31.1 Thrombotic microangiopathy HCC
Thrombotic thrombocytopenic purpura

M31.2 Lethal midline granuloma HCC
DEFINITION Tumor associated with infection that appears in the nose or sinuses that may be fatal if not diagnosed and treated in time.

5 **M31.3 Wegener's granulomatosis**
Necrotizing respiratory granulomatosis

M31.30 Wegener's granulomatosis without renal involvement HCC
Wegener's granulomatosis NOS

M31.31 Wegener's granulomatosis with renal involvement HCC

M31.4 Aortic arch syndrome [Takayasu] HCC

M31.5 Giant cell arteritis with polymyalgia rheumatica HCC

M31.6 Other giant cell arteritis HCC

M31.7 Microscopic polyangiitis HCC
Microscopic polyarteritis
EXCLUDES 1 *polyarteritis nodosa (M30.0)*

M31.8 Other specified necrotizing vasculopathies HCC
Hypocomplementemic vasculitis
Septic vasculitis

M31.9 Necrotizing vasculopathy, unspecified HCC

4 **M32 Systemic lupus erythematosus (SLE)**
EXCLUDES 1 *lupus erythematosus (discoid) (NOS) (L93.0)*
CODING TIP✓ Do not assign a code from category M32.- unless lupus is specified as systemic.

M32.0 Drug-induced systemic lupus erythematosus HCC
Use additional code for adverse effect, if applicable, to identify drug (T36-T50 with fifth or sixth character 5)
CODING TIP✓ Assign code M32.0 only when documentation clearly confirms that the systemic lupus diagnosis is secondary to the effects of a drug. An additional code from categories T36-T50 should be used to identify the drug.

5 **M32.1 Systemic lupus erythematosus with organ or system involvement**

M32.10 Systemic lupus erythematosus, organ or system involvement unspecified HCC

M32.11 Endocarditis in systemic lupus erythematosus HCC
Libman-Sacks disease

M32.12 Pericarditis in systemic lupus erythematosus HCC
Lupus pericarditis

M32.13 Lung involvement in systemic lupus erythematosus HCC
Pleural effusion due to systemic lupus erythematosus

M32.14 Glomerular disease in systemic lupus erythematosus HCC
Lupus renal disease NOS
AHA: 4Q 2013, 125

M32.15 **Tubulo-interstitial nephropathy in systemic lupus erythematosus** HCC
M32.19 **Other organ or system involvement in systemic lupus erythematosus** HCC
M32.8 **Other forms of systemic lupus erythematosus** HCC
M32.9 **Systemic lupus erythematosus, unspecified** HCC
SLE NOS
Systemic lupus erythematosus NOS
Systemic lupus erythematosus without organ involvement

4 M33 Dermatopolymyositis

5 M33.0 **Juvenile dermatomyositis**

M33.00 **Juvenile dermatomyositis, organ involvement unspecified** HCC
M33.01 **Juvenile dermatomyositis with respiratory involvement** HCC
M33.02 **Juvenile dermatomyositis with myopathy** HCC
M33.03 **Juvenile dermatomyositis without myopathy** HCC
AHA: 4Q 2017, 14
M33.09 **Juvenile dermatomyositis with other organ involvement** HCC

5 M33.1 **Other dermatomyositis**
Adult dermatomyositis

M33.10 **Other dermatomyositis, organ involvement unspecified** HCC
M33.11 **Other dermatomyositis with respiratory involvement** HCC
M33.12 **Other dermatomyositis with myopathy** HCC
M33.13 **Other dermatomyositis without myopathy** HCC
Dermatomyositis NOS
AHA: 4Q 2017, 14
M33.19 **Other dermatomyositis with other organ involvement** HCC

5 M33.2 **Polymyositis**

M33.20 **Polymyositis, organ involvement unspecified** HCC
M33.21 **Polymyositis with respiratory involvement** HCC
M33.22 **Polymyositis with myopathy** HCC
M33.29 **Polymyositis with other organ involvement** HCC

5 M33.9 **Dermatopolymyositis, unspecified**

M33.90 **Dermatopolymyositis, unspecified, organ involvement unspecified** HCC
M33.91 **Dermatopolymyositis, unspecified with respiratory involvement** HCC
M33.92 **Dermatopolymyositis, unspecified with myopathy** HCC
M33.93 **Dermatopolymyositis, unspecified without myopathy** HCC
AHA: 4Q 2017, 14
M33.99 **Dermatopolymyositis, unspecified with other organ involvement** HCC

4 M34 Systemic sclerosis [scleroderma]

EXCLUDES 1 *circumscribed scleroderma (L94.0)*
neonatal scleroderma (P83.8)

M34.0 **Progressive systemic sclerosis** HCC
M34.1 **CR(E)ST syndrome** HCC
Combination of calcinosis, Raynaud's phenomenon, esophageal dysfunction, sclerodactyly, telangiectasia
M34.2 **Systemic sclerosis induced by drug and chemical** HCC
Code first:
poisoning due to drug or toxin, if applicable (T36-T65 with fifth or sixth character 1-4 or 6)
Use additional code for adverse effect, if applicable, to identify drug (T36-T50 with fifth or sixth character 5)

5 M34.8 **Other forms of systemic sclerosis**

M34.81 **Systemic sclerosis with lung involvement** HCC
M34.82 **Systemic sclerosis with myopathy** HCC
M34.83 **Systemic sclerosis with polyneuropathy** HCC
M34.89 **Other systemic sclerosis** HCC

M34.9 **Systemic sclerosis, unspecified** HCC

4 M35 Other systemic involvement of connective tissue

EXCLUDES 1 *reactive perforating collagenosis (L87.1)*

5 M35.0 **Sicca syndrome [Sjögren]**

M35.00 **Sicca syndrome, unspecified** HCC
M35.01 **Sicca syndrome with keratoconjunctivitis** HCC
M35.02 **Sicca syndrome with lung involvement** HCC
M35.03 **Sicca syndrome with myopathy** HCC
M35.04 **Sicca syndrome with tubulo-interstitial nephropathy** HCC
Renal tubular acidosis in sicca syndrome
M35.09 **Sicca syndrome with other organ involvement** HCC

M35.1 **Other overlap syndromes** HCC
Mixed connective tissue disease
EXCLUDES 1 *polyangiitis overlap syndrome (M30.8)*
M35.2 **Behçet's disease** HCC
DEFINITION Relapsing inflammatory disorder with recurring painful sores of the mouth, skin, and genitals, swollen joints, severe uveitis, retinal vasculitis, optic atrophy, and digestive system involvement.
M35.3 **Polymyalgia rheumatica** HCC
EXCLUDES 1 *polymyalgia rheumatica with giant cell arteritis (M31.5)*
CODING TIP ✓ Polymyalgia rheumatica is a disorder that almost always occurs in people older than 50. The cause is unknown. Although symptoms are located predominantly in the muscles and there are no outward signs of arthritis, in some cases, there is evidence of inflammatory arthritis.
M35.4 **Diffuse (eosinophilic) fasciitis**
M35.5 **Multifocal fibrosclerosis** HCC
M35.6 **Relapsing panniculitis [Weber-Christian]**
EXCLUDES 1 *lupus panniculitis (L93.2)*
panniculitis NOS (M79.3-)
M35.7 **Hypermobility syndrome**
Familial ligamentous laxity
EXCLUDES 1 *Ehlers-Danlos syndrome (Q79.6)*
ligamentous laxity, NOS (M24.2-)
M35.8 **Other specified systemic involvement of connective tissue** HCC
M35.9 **Systemic involvement of connective tissue, unspecified** HCC
Autoimmune disease (systemic) NOS
Collagen (vascular) disease NOS

4 M36 Systemic disorders of connective tissue in diseases classified elsewhere

EXCLUDES 2 *arthropathies in diseases classified elsewhere (M14.-)*

M36.0 ***Dermato(poly)myositis in neoplastic disease*** HCC
Code first:
underlying neoplasm (C00-D49)
M36.1 ***Arthropathy in neoplastic disease***
Code first underlying neoplasm, such as:
leukemia (C91-C95)
malignant histiocytosis (C96.A)
multiple myeloma (C90.0)
M36.2 ***Hemophilic arthropathy***
Hemarthrosis in hemophilic arthropathy
Code first underlying disease, such as:
factor VIII deficiency (D66)
with vascular defect (D68.0)
factor IX deficiency (D67)
hemophilia (classical) (D66)
hemophilia B (D67)
hemophilia C (D68.1)
M36.3 ***Arthropathy in other blood disorders***
M36.4 ***Arthropathy in hypersensitivity reactions classified elsewhere***
Code first underlying disease, such as:
Henoch (-Schönlein) purpura (D69.0)
serum sickness (T80.6-)
M36.8 ***Systemic disorders of connective tissue in other diseases classified elsewhere*** HCC
Code first underlying disease, such as:
alkaptonuria (E70.2)
hypogammaglobulinemia (D80.-)
ochronosis (E70.2)

Dorsopathies (M40-M54)

Deforming dorsopathies (M40-M43)

4 **M40 Kyphosis and lordosis**

EXCLUDES 1 *congenital kyphosis and lordosis (Q76.4)*
kyphoscoliosis (M41.-)
postprocedural kyphosis and lordosis (M96.-)

5 **M40.0 Postural kyphosis**

EXCLUDES 1 *osteochondrosis of spine (M42.-)*

- **M40.00 Postural kyphosis, site unspecified**
- **M40.03 Postural kyphosis, cervicothoracic region**
- **M40.04 Postural kyphosis, thoracic region**
- **M40.05 Postural kyphosis, thoracolumbar region**

5 **M40.1 Other secondary kyphosis**

CODING TIP✓ Secondary kyphosis (spinal curvature) develops as a result of another condition, such as osteoporosis, endocrine disease or muscular dystrophy. The term "hyperkyphosis" may also be used to describe extreme spinal rounding.

- **M40.10 Other secondary kyphosis, site unspecified**
- **M40.12 Other secondary kyphosis, cervical region**
- **M40.13 Other secondary kyphosis, cervicothoracic region**
- **M40.14 Other secondary kyphosis, thoracic region**
- **M40.15 Other secondary kyphosis, thoracolumbar region**

5 **M40.2 Other and unspecified kyphosis**

6 **M40.20 Unspecified kyphosis**

- **M40.202 Unspecified kyphosis, cervical region**
- **M40.203 Unspecified kyphosis, cervicothoracic region**
- **M40.204 Unspecified kyphosis, thoracic region**
- **M40.205 Unspecified kyphosis, thoracolumbar region**
- **M40.209 Unspecified kyphosis, site unspecified**

6 **M40.29 Other kyphosis**

- **M40.292 Other kyphosis, cervical region**
- **M40.293 Other kyphosis, cervicothoracic region**
- **M40.294 Other kyphosis, thoracic region**
- **M40.295 Other kyphosis, thoracolumbar region**
- **M40.299 Other kyphosis, site unspecified**

5 **M40.3 Flatback syndrome**

- **M40.30 Flatback syndrome, site unspecified**
- **M40.35 Flatback syndrome, thoracolumbar region**
- **M40.36 Flatback syndrome, lumbar region**
- **M40.37 Flatback syndrome, lumbosacral region**

5 **M40.4 Postural lordosis**

Acquired lordosis

- **M40.40 Postural lordosis, site unspecified**
- **M40.45 Postural lordosis, thoracolumbar region**
- **M40.46 Postural lordosis, lumbar region**
- **M40.47 Postural lordosis, lumbosacral region**

5 **M40.5 Lordosis, unspecified**

- **M40.50 Lordosis, unspecified, site unspecified**
- **M40.55 Lordosis, unspecified, thoracolumbar region**
- **M40.56 Lordosis, unspecified, lumbar region**
- **M40.57 Lordosis, unspecified, lumbosacral region**

4 **M41 Scoliosis**

INCLUDES kyphoscoliosis

EXCLUDES 1 *congenital scoliosis NOS (Q67.5)*
congenital scoliosis due to bony malformation (Q76.3)
postural congenital scoliosis (Q67.5)
kyphoscoliotic heart disease (I27.1)
postprocedural scoliosis (M96.-)

CODING TIP✓ Do not use these codes following scoliosis surgery. The correct aftercare code to use following surgery to treat scoliosis is Z47.82.

5 **M41.0 Infantile idiopathic scoliosis**

- **M41.00 Infantile idiopathic scoliosis, site unspecified**
- **M41.02 Infantile idiopathic scoliosis, cervical region**
- **M41.03 Infantile idiopathic scoliosis, cervicothoracic region**
- **M41.04 Infantile idiopathic scoliosis, thoracic region**
  AHA: 4Q 2014, 27
- **M41.05 Infantile idiopathic scoliosis, thoracolumbar region**
- **M41.06 Infantile idiopathic scoliosis, lumbar region**
- **M41.07 Infantile idiopathic scoliosis, lumbosacral region**
- **M41.08 Infantile idiopathic scoliosis, sacral and sacrococcygeal region**

5 **M41.1 Juvenile and adolescent idiopathic scoliosis**

6 **M41.11 Juvenile idiopathic scoliosis**

- **M41.112 Juvenile idiopathic scoliosis, cervical region**
- **M41.113 Juvenile idiopathic scoliosis, cervicothoracic region**
- **M41.114 Juvenile idiopathic scoliosis, thoracic region**
- **M41.115 Juvenile idiopathic scoliosis, thoracolumbar region**
- **M41.116 Juvenile idiopathic scoliosis, lumbar region**
- **M41.117 Juvenile idiopathic scoliosis, lumbosacral region**
- **M41.119 Juvenile idiopathic scoliosis, site unspecified**
  AHA: 4Q 2014, 29

6 **M41.12 Adolescent scoliosis**

- **M41.122 Adolescent idiopathic scoliosis, cervical region**
- **M41.123 Adolescent idiopathic scoliosis, cervicothoracic region**
- **M41.124 Adolescent idiopathic scoliosis, thoracic region**
- **M41.125 Adolescent idiopathic scoliosis, thoracolumbar region**
- **M41.126 Adolescent idiopathic scoliosis, lumbar region**
- **M41.127 Adolescent idiopathic scoliosis, lumbosacral region**
- **M41.129 Adolescent idiopathic scoliosis, site unspecified**

5 **M41.2 Other idiopathic scoliosis**

- **M41.20 Other idiopathic scoliosis, site unspecified**
- **M41.22 Other idiopathic scoliosis, cervical region**
- **M41.23 Other idiopathic scoliosis, cervicothoracic region**
- **M41.24 Other idiopathic scoliosis, thoracic region**

Scoliosis, thoracic region

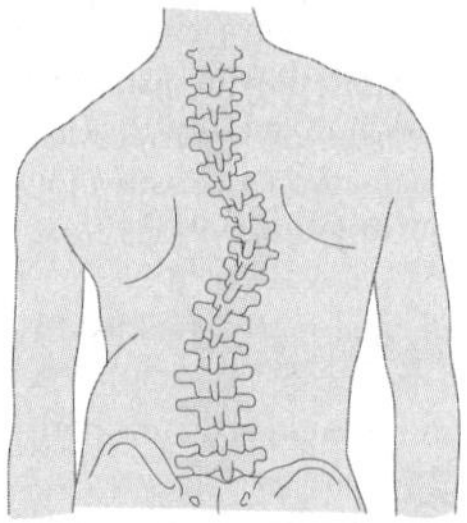

- **M41.25 Other idiopathic scoliosis, thoracolumbar region**
- **M41.26 Other idiopathic scoliosis, lumbar region**
- **M41.27 Other idiopathic scoliosis, lumbosacral region**

5 **M41.3 Thoracogenic scoliosis**

- **M41.30 Thoracogenic scoliosis, site unspecified**
- **M41.34 Thoracogenic scoliosis, thoracic region**
- **M41.35 Thoracogenic scoliosis, thoracolumbar region**

5 **M41.4 Neuromuscular scoliosis**

Scoliosis secondary to cerebral palsy, Friedreich's ataxia, poliomyelitis and other neuromuscular disorders
Code also:
underlying condition

- **M41.40 Neuromuscular scoliosis, site unspecified**
- **M41.41 Neuromuscular scoliosis, occipito-atlanto-axial region**
- **M41.42 Neuromuscular scoliosis, cervical region**
- **M41.43 Neuromuscular scoliosis, cervicothoracic region**
- **M41.44 Neuromuscular scoliosis, thoracic region**
- **M41.45 Neuromuscular scoliosis, thoracolumbar region**
  AHA: 4Q 2014, 28
- **M41.46 Neuromuscular scoliosis, lumbar region**

M41.47 Neuromuscular scoliosis, lumbosacral region

5 M41.5 Other secondary scoliosis

M41.50 Other secondary scoliosis, site unspecified

M41.52 Other secondary scoliosis, cervical region

M41.53 Other secondary scoliosis, cervicothoracic region

M41.54 Other secondary scoliosis, thoracic region

M41.55 Other secondary scoliosis, thoracolumbar region

M41.56 Other secondary scoliosis, lumbar region

M41.57 Other secondary scoliosis, lumbosacral region

5 M41.8 Other forms of scoliosis

M41.80 Other forms of scoliosis, site unspecified

M41.82 Other forms of scoliosis, cervical region

M41.83 Other forms of scoliosis, cervicothoracic region

M41.84 Other forms of scoliosis, thoracic region

M41.85 Other forms of scoliosis, thoracolumbar region

M41.86 Other forms of scoliosis, lumbar region

M41.87 Other forms of scoliosis, lumbosacral region

M41.9 Scoliosis, unspecified

4 M42 Spinal osteochondrosis

5 M42.0 Juvenile osteochondrosis of spine

Calvé's disease

Scheuermann's disease

EXCLUDES 1 *postural kyphosis (M40.0)*

M42.00 Juvenile osteochondrosis of spine, site unspecified

M42.01 Juvenile osteochondrosis of spine, occipito-atlanto-axial region

M42.02 Juvenile osteochondrosis of spine, cervical region

M42.03 Juvenile osteochondrosis of spine, cervicothoracic region

M42.04 Juvenile osteochondrosis of spine, thoracic region

M42.05 Juvenile osteochondrosis of spine, thoracolumbar region

M42.06 Juvenile osteochondrosis of spine, lumbar region

M42.07 Juvenile osteochondrosis of spine, lumbosacral region

M42.08 Juvenile osteochondrosis of spine, sacral and sacrococcygeal region

M42.09 Juvenile osteochondrosis of spine, multiple sites in spine

5 M42.1 Adult osteochondrosis of spine

M42.10 Adult osteochondrosis of spine, site unspecified A

M42.11 Adult osteochondrosis of spine, occipito-atlanto-axial region A

M42.12 Adult osteochondrosis of spine, cervical region A

M42.13 Adult osteochondrosis of spine, cervicothoracic region A

M42.14 Adult osteochondrosis of spine, thoracic region A

M42.15 Adult osteochondrosis of spine, thoracolumbar region A

M42.16 Adult osteochondrosis of spine, lumbar region A

M42.17 Adult osteochondrosis of spine, lumbosacral region A

M42.18 Adult osteochondrosis of spine, sacral and sacrococcygeal region A

M42.19 Adult osteochondrosis of spine, multiple sites in spine A

M42.9 Spinal osteochondrosis, unspecified

4 M43 Other deforming dorsopathies

EXCLUDES 1 *congenital spondylolysis and spondylolisthesis (Q76.2)*
hemivertebra (Q76.3-Q76.4)
Klippel-Feil syndrome (Q76.1)
lumbarization and sacralization (Q76.4)
platyspondylisis (Q76.4)
spina bifida occulta (Q76.0)
spinal curvature in osteoporosis (M80.-)
spinal curvature in Paget's disease of bone [osteitis deformans] (M88.-)

5 M43.0 Spondylolysis

EXCLUDES 1 *congenital spondylolysis (Q76.2)*
spondylolisthesis (M43.1)

DEFINITION A defect of the pars interarticularis segment of vertebral bone that connects the facet joints, causing stress fracture and predisposing to slippage; occurs most commonly in the lumbar region (specifically L5) during adolescence.

M43.00 Spondylolysis, site unspecified

M43.01 Spondylolysis, occipito-atlanto-axial region

M43.02 Spondylolysis, cervical region

M43.03 Spondylolysis, cervicothoracic region

M43.04 Spondylolysis, thoracic region

M43.05 Spondylolysis, thoracolumbar region

M43.06 Spondylolysis, lumbar region

M43.07 Spondylolysis, lumbosacral region

M43.08 Spondylolysis, sacral and sacrococcygeal region

M43.09 Spondylolysis, multiple sites in spine

5 M43.1 Spondylolisthesis

EXCLUDES 1 *acute traumatic of lumbosacral region (S33.1)*
acute traumatic of sites other than lumbosacral- code to Fracture, vertebra, by region
congenital spondylolisthesis (Q76.2)

DEFINITION An acquired condition in which one vertebra slips forward over the one below it, often from degenerative aging or a small fracture in the piece of bone (pars interarticularis) connecting the facet joint above to the one below.

M43.10 Spondylolisthesis, site unspecified

M43.11 Spondylolisthesis, occipito-atlanto-axial region

M43.12 Spondylolisthesis, cervical region

M43.13 Spondylolisthesis, cervicothoracic region

M43.14 Spondylolisthesis, thoracic region

M43.15 Spondylolisthesis, thoracolumbar region

M43.16 Spondylolisthesis, lumbar region

M43.17 Spondylolisthesis, lumbosacral region

M43.18 Spondylolisthesis, sacral and sacrococcygeal region

M43.19 Spondylolisthesis, multiple sites in spine

5 M43.2 Fusion of spine

Ankylosis of spinal joint

EXCLUDES 1 *ankylosing spondylitis (M45.0-)*
congenital fusion of spine (Q76.4)

EXCLUDES 2 *arthrodesis status (Z98.1)*
pseudoarthrosis after fusion or arthrodesis (M96.0)

CODING TIP✓ Ankylosis of the joint is caused by arthritis, traumatic injury or infection. The joint will assume the least painful position and become permanently fixed. This code should not be used for a surgical fusion which is coded as Z98.1.

M43.20 Fusion of spine, site unspecified

M43.21 Fusion of spine, occipito-atlanto-axial region

M43.22 Fusion of spine, cervical region

M43.23 Fusion of spine, cervicothoracic region

M43.24 Fusion of spine, thoracic region

M43.25 Fusion of spine, thoracolumbar region

M43.26 Fusion of spine, lumbar region

M43.27 Fusion of spine, lumbosacral region

M43.28 Fusion of spine, sacral and sacrococcygeal region

M43.3 Recurrent atlantoaxial dislocation with myelopathy

M43.4 Other recurrent atlantoaxial dislocation

5 M43.5 Other recurrent vertebral dislocation

EXCLUDES 1 *biomechanical lesions NEC (M99.-)*

6 M43.5X Other recurrent vertebral dislocation

M43.5X2 Other recurrent vertebral dislocation, cervical region

M43.5X3 Other recurrent vertebral dislocation, cervicothoracic region

M43.5X4 Other recurrent vertebral dislocation, thoracic region

M43.5X5 Other recurrent vertebral dislocation, thoracolumbar region

M43.5X6 Other recurrent vertebral dislocation, lumbar region

M43.5X7 Other recurrent vertebral dislocation, lumbosacral region

M43.5X8 Other recurrent vertebral dislocation, sacral and sacrococcygeal region

M43.5X9 Other recurrent vertebral dislocation, site unspecified

M43.6 Torticollis

EXCLUDES 1 *congenital (sternomastoid) torticollis (Q68.0)*
current injury - see Injury, of spine, by body region
ocular torticollis (R29.891)
psychogenic torticollis (F45.8)
spasmodic torticollis (G24.3)
torticollis due to birth injury (P15.2)

DEFINITION Contraction of the neck muscles causing limited neck motion and head positioned to one side.

5 **M43.8 Other specified deforming dorsopathies**

EXCLUDES 2 *kyphosis and lordosis (M40.-)*
scoliosis (M41.-)

6 **M43.8X Other specified deforming dorsopathies**

M43.8X1 Other specified deforming dorsopathies, occipito-atlanto-axial region
M43.8X2 Other specified deforming dorsopathies, cervical region
M43.8X3 Other specified deforming dorsopathies, cervicothoracic region
M43.8X4 Other specified deforming dorsopathies, thoracic region
M43.8X5 Other specified deforming dorsopathies, thoracolumbar region
M43.8X6 Other specified deforming dorsopathies, lumbar region
M43.8X7 Other specified deforming dorsopathies, lumbosacral region
M43.8X8 Other specified deforming dorsopathies, sacral and sacrococcygeal region
M43.8X9 Other specified deforming dorsopathies, site unspecified

M43.9 Deforming dorsopathy, unspecified
Curvature of spine NOS

Spondylopathies (M45-M49)

4 **M45 Ankylosing spondylitis**
Rheumatoid arthritis of spine

EXCLUDES 1 *arthropathy in Reiter's disease (M02.3-)*
juvenile (ankylosing) spondylitis (M08.1)

EXCLUDES 2 *Behçet's disease (M35.2)*

CODING TIP ✓ Ankylosing spondylosis is a specific inflammatory disease that causes fusion of the vertebrae and reduced mobility/flexion. It may impact more than one area of the vertebrae.

DEFINITION Autoimmune arthritis causing chronic inflammation of the spine and sacroiliac joints, eventually leading to spinal fusion from calcification of ligaments and discs that progresses up the spine, possibly affecting other organs.

M45.0 Ankylosing spondylitis of multiple sites in spine HCC
M45.1 Ankylosing spondylitis of occipito-atlanto-axial region HCC
M45.2 Ankylosing spondylitis of cervical region HCC
M45.3 Ankylosing spondylitis of cervicothoracic region HCC
M45.4 Ankylosing spondylitis of thoracic region HCC
M45.5 Ankylosing spondylitis of thoracolumbar region HCC
M45.6 Ankylosing spondylitis lumbar region HCC
M45.7 Ankylosing spondylitis of lumbosacral region HCC
M45.8 Ankylosing spondylitis sacral and sacrococcygeal region HCC
M45.9 Ankylosing spondylitis of unspecified sites in spine HCC

4 **M46 Other inflammatory spondylopathies**

5 **M46.0 Spinal enthesopathy**
Disorder of ligamentous or muscular attachments of spine

M46.00 Spinal enthesopathy, site unspecified HCC
M46.01 Spinal enthesopathy, occipito-atlanto-axial region HCC
M46.02 Spinal enthesopathy, cervical region HCC
M46.03 Spinal enthesopathy, cervicothoracic region HCC
M46.04 Spinal enthesopathy, thoracic region HCC
M46.05 Spinal enthesopathy, thoracolumbar region HCC
M46.06 Spinal enthesopathy, lumbar region HCC
M46.07 Spinal enthesopathy, lumbosacral region HCC
M46.08 Spinal enthesopathy, sacral and sacrococcygeal region HCC
M46.09 Spinal enthesopathy, multiple sites in spine HCC

M46.1 Sacroiliitis, not elsewhere classified HCC

5 **M46.2 Osteomyelitis of vertebra**

M46.20 Osteomyelitis of vertebra, site unspecified HCC
M46.21 Osteomyelitis of vertebra, occipito-atlanto-axial region HCC
M46.22 Osteomyelitis of vertebra, cervical region HCC
M46.23 Osteomyelitis of vertebra, cervicothoracic region HCC
M46.24 Osteomyelitis of vertebra, thoracic region HCC
M46.25 Osteomyelitis of vertebra, thoracolumbar region HCC
M46.26 Osteomyelitis of vertebra, lumbar region HCC
M46.27 Osteomyelitis of vertebra, lumbosacral region HCC
M46.28 Osteomyelitis of vertebra, sacral and sacrococcygeal region HCC

5 **M46.3 Infection of intervertebral disc (pyogenic)**
Use additional code (B95-B97) to identify infectious agent.

M46.30 Infection of intervertebral disc (pyogenic), site unspecified HCC
M46.31 Infection of intervertebral disc (pyogenic), occipito-atlanto-axial region HCC
M46.32 Infection of intervertebral disc (pyogenic), cervical region HCC
M46.33 Infection of intervertebral disc (pyogenic), cervicothoracic region HCC
M46.34 Infection of intervertebral disc (pyogenic), thoracic region HCC
M46.35 Infection of intervertebral disc (pyogenic), thoracolumbar region HCC
M46.36 Infection of intervertebral disc (pyogenic), lumbar region HCC
M46.37 Infection of intervertebral disc (pyogenic), lumbosacral region HCC
M46.38 Infection of intervertebral disc (pyogenic), sacral and sacrococcygeal region HCC
M46.39 Infection of intervertebral disc (pyogenic), multiple sites in spine HCC

5 **M46.4 Discitis, unspecified**

M46.40 Discitis, unspecified, site unspecified
M46.41 Discitis, unspecified, occipito-atlanto-axial region
M46.42 Discitis, unspecified, cervical region
M46.43 Discitis, unspecified, cervicothoracic region
M46.44 Discitis, unspecified, thoracic region
M46.45 Discitis, unspecified, thoracolumbar region
M46.46 Discitis, unspecified, lumbar region
M46.47 Discitis, unspecified, lumbosacral region
M46.48 Discitis, unspecified, sacral and sacrococcygeal region
M46.49 Discitis, unspecified, multiple sites in spine

5 **M46.5 Other infective spondylopathies**

M46.50 Other infective spondylopathies, site unspecified HCC
M46.51 Other infective spondylopathies, occipito-atlanto-axial region HCC
M46.52 Other infective spondylopathies, cervical region HCC
M46.53 Other infective spondylopathies, cervicothoracic region HCC
M46.54 Other infective spondylopathies, thoracic region HCC
M46.55 Other infective spondylopathies, thoracolumbar region HCC
M46.56 Other infective spondylopathies, lumbar region HCC
M46.57 Other infective spondylopathies, lumbosacral region HCC
M46.58 Other infective spondylopathies, sacral and sacrococcygeal region HCC
M46.59 Other infective spondylopathies, multiple sites in spine HCC

5 **M46.8 Other specified inflammatory spondylopathies**

M46.80 Other specified inflammatory spondylopathies, site unspecified HCC
M46.81 Other specified inflammatory spondylopathies, occipito-atlanto-axial region HCC

M46.82 Other specified inflammatory spondylopathies, cervical region HCC
M46.83 Other specified inflammatory spondylopathies, cervicothoracic region HCC
M46.84 Other specified inflammatory spondylopathies, thoracic region HCC
M46.85 Other specified inflammatory spondylopathies, thoracolumbar region HCC
M46.86 Other specified inflammatory spondylopathies, lumbar region HCC
M46.87 Other specified inflammatory spondylopathies, lumbosacral region HCC
M46.88 Other specified inflammatory spondylopathies, sacral and sacrococcygeal region HCC
M46.89 Other specified inflammatory spondylopathies, multiple sites in spine HCC

5 M46.9 Unspecified inflammatory spondylopathy
M46.90 Unspecified inflammatory spondylopathy, site unspecified HCC
M46.91 Unspecified inflammatory spondylopathy, occipito-atlanto-axial region HCC
M46.92 Unspecified inflammatory spondylopathy, cervical region HCC
M46.93 Unspecified inflammatory spondylopathy, cervicothoracic region HCC
M46.94 Unspecified inflammatory spondylopathy, thoracic region HCC
M46.95 Unspecified inflammatory spondylopathy, thoracolumbar region HCC
M46.96 Unspecified inflammatory spondylopathy, lumbar region HCC
M46.97 Unspecified inflammatory spondylopathy, lumbosacral region HCC
M46.98 Unspecified inflammatory spondylopathy, sacral and sacrococcygeal region HCC
M46.99 Unspecified inflammatory spondylopathy, multiple sites in spine HCC

4 M47 Spondylosis

INCLUDES arthrosis or osteoarthritis of spine
degeneration of facet joints

CODING TIP ✓ OA of spine is coded M47.-. OA of the spine causing weakness, spasticity, clumsiness, altered tonus, but generally no pain, should be coded M47.1-. OA of the spine causing pain, numbness and weakness is coded as M47.2. Query the physician for more specificity when clinical documentation includes those symptoms.

5 M47.0 Anterior spinal and vertebral artery compression syndromes
6 M47.01 Anterior spinal artery compression syndromes
M47.011 Anterior spinal artery compression syndromes, occipito-atlanto-axial region
M47.012 Anterior spinal artery compression syndromes, cervical region
M47.013 Anterior spinal artery compression syndromes, cervicothoracic region
M47.014 Anterior spinal artery compression syndromes, thoracic region
M47.015 Anterior spinal artery compression syndromes, thoracolumbar region
M47.016 Anterior spinal artery compression syndromes, lumbar region
M47.019 Anterior spinal artery compression syndromes, site unspecified
6 M47.02 Vertebral artery compression syndromes
M47.021 Vertebral artery compression syndromes, occipito-atlanto-axial region
M47.022 Vertebral artery compression syndromes, cervical region
M47.029 Vertebral artery compression syndromes, site unspecified

5 M47.1 Other spondylosis with myelopathy
Spondylogenic compression of spinal cord
EXCLUDES 1 *vertebral subluxation (M43.3-M43.59)*

CODING TIP ✓ Myelopathy refers to weakness, spasticity, clumsiness, altered tonus, hyperreflexia and pathological reflexes, but generally no pain.

M47.10 Other spondylosis with myelopathy, site unspecified
M47.11 Other spondylosis with myelopathy, occipito-atlanto-axial region
M47.12 Other spondylosis with myelopathy, cervical region
M47.13 Other spondylosis with myelopathy, cervicothoracic region
M47.14 Other spondylosis with myelopathy, thoracic region
M47.15 Other spondylosis with myelopathy, thoracolumbar region
M47.16 Other spondylosis with myelopathy, lumbar region

5 M47.2 Other spondylosis with radiculopathy

CODING TIP ✓ Radiculopathy refers to symptoms of pain, numbness and weakness in a pattern consistent with the distribution of a particular nerve root.

M47.20 Other spondylosis with radiculopathy, site unspecified
M47.21 Other spondylosis with radiculopathy, occipito-atlanto-axial region
M47.22 Other spondylosis with radiculopathy, cervical region
M47.23 Other spondylosis with radiculopathy, cervicothoracic region
M47.24 Other spondylosis with radiculopathy, thoracic region
M47.25 Other spondylosis with radiculopathy, thoracolumbar region
M47.26 Other spondylosis with radiculopathy, lumbar region
M47.27 Other spondylosis with radiculopathy, lumbosacral region
M47.28 Other spondylosis with radiculopathy, sacral and sacrococcygeal region

5 M47.8 Other spondylosis
6 M47.81 Spondylosis without myelopathy or radiculopathy
M47.811 Spondylosis without myelopathy or radiculopathy, occipito-atlanto-axial region
M47.812 Spondylosis without myelopathy or radiculopathy, cervical region
AHA: 2Q 2018, 11
M47.813 Spondylosis without myelopathy or radiculopathy, cervicothoracic region
M47.814 Spondylosis without myelopathy or radiculopathy, thoracic region
M47.815 Spondylosis without myelopathy or radiculopathy, thoracolumbar region
M47.816 Spondylosis without myelopathy or radiculopathy, lumbar region
M47.817 Spondylosis without myelopathy or radiculopathy, lumbosacral region
M47.818 Spondylosis without myelopathy or radiculopathy, sacral and sacrococcygeal region
M47.819 Spondylosis without myelopathy or radiculopathy, site unspecified
6 M47.89 Other spondylosis
M47.891 Other spondylosis, occipito-atlanto-axial region
M47.892 Other spondylosis, cervical region
M47.893 Other spondylosis, cervicothoracic region
M47.894 Other spondylosis, thoracic region
M47.895 Other spondylosis, thoracolumbar region
M47.896 Other spondylosis, lumbar region
M47.897 Other spondylosis, lumbosacral region
M47.898 Other spondylosis, sacral and sacrococcygeal region
M47.899 Other spondylosis, site unspecified
M47.9 Spondylosis, unspecified

4 M48 Other spondylopathies

5 M48.0 Spinal stenosis
Caudal stenosis
M48.00 Spinal stenosis, site unspecified
M48.01 Spinal stenosis, occipito-atlanto-axial region
M48.02 Spinal stenosis, cervical region
M48.03 Spinal stenosis, cervicothoracic region
M48.04 Spinal stenosis, thoracic region
M48.05 Spinal stenosis, thoracolumbar region
6 M48.06 Spinal stenosis, lumbar region

CODING TIP ✓ Neurogenic claudication is a commonly used term for a syndrome associated with significant lumbar spinal stenosis leading to compression of the cauda equina (lumbar nerves). Symptoms experienced are buttock and lower extremity cramping, pain, and fatigue. There is no separate code for neurogenic claudication.
AHA: 3Q 2017, 24

M48.061 **Spinal stenosis, lumbar region without neurogenic claudication**
Spinal stenosis, lumbar region NOS
AHA: 4Q 2017, 14

M48.062 **Spinal stenosis, lumbar region with neurogenic claudication**
AHA: 4Q 2017, 14

M48.07 **Spinal stenosis, lumbosacral region**

M48.08 **Spinal stenosis, sacral and sacrococcygeal region**

5 **M48.1** **Ankylosing hyperostosis [Forestier]**
Diffuse idiopathic skeletal hyperostosis [DISH]

M48.10 **Ankylosing hyperostosis [Forestier], site unspecified**
M48.11 **Ankylosing hyperostosis [Forestier], occipito-atlanto-axial region**
M48.12 **Ankylosing hyperostosis [Forestier], cervical region**
M48.13 **Ankylosing hyperostosis [Forestier], cervicothoracic region**
M48.14 **Ankylosing hyperostosis [Forestier], thoracic region**
M48.15 **Ankylosing hyperostosis [Forestier], thoracolumbar region**
M48.16 **Ankylosing hyperostosis [Forestier], lumbar region**
M48.17 **Ankylosing hyperostosis [Forestier], lumbosacral region**
M48.18 **Ankylosing hyperostosis [Forestier], sacral and sacrococcygeal region**
M48.19 **Ankylosing hyperostosis [Forestier], multiple sites in spine**

5 **M48.2** **Kissing spine**

M48.20 **Kissing spine, site unspecified**
M48.21 **Kissing spine, occipito-atlanto-axial region**
M48.22 **Kissing spine, cervical region**
M48.23 **Kissing spine, cervicothoracic region**
M48.24 **Kissing spine, thoracic region**
M48.25 **Kissing spine, thoracolumbar region**
M48.26 **Kissing spine, lumbar region**
M48.27 **Kissing spine, lumbosacral region**

5 **M48.3** Traumatic spondylopathy

M48.30 **Traumatic spondylopathy, site unspecified**
M48.31 **Traumatic spondylopathy, occipito-atlanto-axial region**
M48.32 **Traumatic spondylopathy, cervical region**
M48.33 **Traumatic spondylopathy, cervicothoracic region**
M48.34 **Traumatic spondylopathy, thoracic region**
M48.35 **Traumatic spondylopathy, thoracolumbar region**
M48.36 **Traumatic spondylopathy, lumbar region**
M48.37 **Traumatic spondylopathy, lumbosacral region**
M48.38 **Traumatic spondylopathy, sacral and sacrococcygeal region**

5 **M48.4** **Fatigue fracture of vertebra**
Stress fracture of vertebra

EXCLUDES 1 *pathological fracture NOS (M84.4-)*
pathological fracture of vertebra due to neoplasm (M84.58)
pathological fracture of vertebra due to other diagnosis (M84.68)
pathological fracture of vertebra due to osteoporosis (M80.-)
traumatic fracture of vertebrae (S12.0-S12.3-, S22.0-, S32.0-)

The appropriate 7th character is to be added to each code from subcategory M48.4:

A	initial encounter for fracture
D	subsequent encounter for fracture with routine healing
G	subsequent encounter for fracture with delayed healing
S	sequela of fracture

7 **M48.40X-** **Fatigue fracture of vertebra, site unspecified**
7 **M48.41X-** **Fatigue fracture of vertebra, occipito-atlanto-axial region**
7 **M48.42X-** **Fatigue fracture of vertebra, cervical region**
7 **M48.43X-** **Fatigue fracture of vertebra, cervicothoracic region**
7 **M48.44X-** **Fatigue fracture of vertebra, thoracic region**
7 **M48.45X-** **Fatigue fracture of vertebra, thoracolumbar region**
7 **M48.46X-** **Fatigue fracture of vertebra, lumbar region**
7 **M48.47X-** **Fatigue fracture of vertebra, lumbosacral region**
7 **M48.48X-** **Fatigue fracture of vertebra, sacral and sacrococcygeal region**

5 **M48.5** **Collapsed vertebra, not elsewhere classified**
Collapsed vertebra NOS
Compression fracture of vertebra NOS
Wedging of vertebra NOS

EXCLUDES 1 *current injury - see Injury of spine, by body region*
fatigue fracture of vertebra (M48.4)
pathological fracture of vertebra due to neoplasm (M84.58)
pathological fracture of vertebra due to other diagnosis (M84.68)
pathological fracture of vertebra due to osteoporosis (M80.-)
pathological fracture NOS (M84.4-)
stress fracture of vertebra (M48.4-)
traumatic fracture of vertebra (S12.-, S22.-, S32.-)

The appropriate 7th character is to be added to each code from subcategory M48.5:

A	initial encounter for fracture
D	subsequent encounter for fracture with routine healing
G	subsequent encounter for fracture with delayed healing
S	sequela of fracture

7 **M48.50X-** **Collapsed vertebra, not elsewhere classified, site unspecified** HCC
7 **M48.51X-** **Collapsed vertebra, not elsewhere classified, occipito-atlanto-axial region** HCC
7 **M48.52X-** **Collapsed vertebra, not elsewhere classified, cervical region** HCC
7 **M48.53X-** **Collapsed vertebra, not elsewhere classified, cervicothoracic region** HCC
7 **M48.54X-** **Collapsed vertebra, not elsewhere classified, thoracic region** HCC
7 **M48.55X-** **Collapsed vertebra, not elsewhere classified, thoracolumbar region** HCC
7 **M48.56X-** **Collapsed vertebra, not elsewhere classified, lumbar region** HCC
7 **M48.57X-** **Collapsed vertebra, not elsewhere classified, lumbosacral region** HCC
7 **M48.58X-** **Collapsed vertebra, not elsewhere classified, sacral and sacrococcygeal region** HCC

5 **M48.8** **Other specified spondylopathies**
Ossification of posterior longitudinal ligament

6 **M48.8X** **Other specified spondylopathies**

M48.8X1 **Other specified spondylopathies, occipito-atlanto-axial region** HCC
M48.8X2 **Other specified spondylopathies, cervical region** HCC
M48.8X3 **Other specified spondylopathies, cervicothoracic region** HCC
M48.8X4 **Other specified spondylopathies, thoracic region** HCC
M48.8X5 **Other specified spondylopathies, thoracolumbar region** HCC
M48.8X6 **Other specified spondylopathies, lumbar region** HCC
M48.8X7 **Other specified spondylopathies, lumbosacral region** HCC
M48.8X8 **Other specified spondylopathies, sacral and sacrococcygeal region** HCC
M48.8X9 **Other specified spondylopathies, site unspecified** HCC

M48.9 **Spondylopathy, unspecified**

M49 Spondylopathies in diseases classified elsewhere

INCLUDES curvature of spine in diseases classified elsewhere
deformity of spine in diseases classified elsewhere
kyphosis in diseases classified elsewhere
scoliosis in diseases classified elsewhere
spondylopathy in diseases classified elsewhere

Code first underlying disease, such as:
brucellosis (A23.-)
Charcot-Marie-Tooth disease (G60.0)
enterobacterial infections (A01-A04)
osteitis fibrosa cystica (E21.0)

EXCLUDES 1 *curvature of spine in tuberculosis [Pott's] (A18.01)*
enteropathic arthropathies (M07.-)
gonococcal spondylitis (A54.41)
neuropathic [tabes dorsalis] spondylitis (A52.11)
neuropathic spondylopathy in syringomyelia (G95.0)
neuropathic spondylopathy in tabes dorsalis (A52.11)
nonsyphilitic neuropathic spondylopathy NEC (G98.0)
spondylitis in syphilis (acquired) (A52.77)
tuberculous spondylitis (A18.01)
typhoid fever spondylitis (A01.05)

M49.8 Spondylopathy in diseases classified elsewhere

CODING TIP ✓ M49.8- codes indicate spondylopathy due to an underlying condition. The underlying condition should be identified and coded first.

M49.80 ***Spondylopathy in diseases classified elsewhere, site unspecified*** HCC

M49.81 ***Spondylopathy in diseases classified elsewhere, occipito-atlanto-axial region*** HCC

M49.82 ***Spondylopathy in diseases classified elsewhere, cervical region*** HCC

M49.83 ***Spondylopathy in diseases classified elsewhere, cervicothoracic region*** HCC

M49.84 ***Spondylopathy in diseases classified elsewhere, thoracic region*** HCC

M49.85 ***Spondylopathy in diseases classified elsewhere, thoracolumbar region*** HCC

M49.86 ***Spondylopathy in diseases classified elsewhere, lumbar region*** HCC

M49.87 ***Spondylopathy in diseases classified elsewhere, lumbosacral region*** HCC

M49.88 ***Spondylopathy in diseases classified elsewhere, sacral and sacrococcygeal region*** HCC

M49.89 ***Spondylopathy in diseases classified elsewhere, multiple sites in spine*** HCC

Other dorsopathies (M50-M54)

EXCLUDES 1 *current injury - see injury of spine by body region*
discitis NOS (M46.4-)

M50 Cervical disc disorders

Note: code to the most superior level of disorder

INCLUDES cervicothoracic disc disorders with cervicalgia
cervicothoracic disc disorders

CODING TIP ✓ If the patient has a disc disorder at more than one region, code to the highest level of each region. Note the excludes 2 note at M51.

M50.0 Cervical disc disorder with myelopathy

CODING TIP ✓ Myelopathy refers to weakness, spasticity, clumsiness, altered tonus, hyperreflexia and pathological reflexes, but generally no pain.
AHA: 1Q 2016, 17

M50.00 Cervical disc disorder with myelopathy, unspecified cervical region

M50.01 Cervical disc disorder with myelopathy, high cervical region
C2-C3 disc disorder with myelopathy
C3-C4 disc disorder with myelopathy

M50.02 Cervical disc disorder with myelopathy, mid-cervical region
AHA: 4Q 2016, 39

M50.020 Cervical disc disorder with myelopathy, mid-cervical region, unspecified level

M50.021 Cervical disc disorder at C4-C5 level with myelopathy
C4-C5 disc disorder with myelopathy

M50.022 Cervical disc disorder at C5-C6 level with myelopathy
C5-C6 disc disorder with myelopathy

M50.023 Cervical disc disorder at C6-C7 level with myelopathy
C6-C7 disc disorder with myelopathy

M50.03 Cervical disc disorder with myelopathy, cervicothoracic region
C7-T1 disc disorder with myelopathy

M50.1 Cervical disc disorder with radiculopathy

EXCLUDES 2 *brachial radiculitis NOS (M54.13)*

CODING TIP ✓ Radiculopathy refers to symptoms of pain, numbness and weakness in a pattern consistent with the distribution of a particular nerve root.
AHA: 1Q 2016, 17

M50.10 Cervical disc disorder with radiculopathy, unspecified cervical region

M50.11 Cervical disc disorder with radiculopathy, high cervical region
C2-C3 disc disorder with radiculopathy
C3 radiculopathy due to disc disorder
C3-C4 disc disorder with radiculopathy
C4 radiculopathy due to disc disorder

M50.12 Cervical disc disorder with radiculopathy, mid-cervical region
AHA: 4Q 2016, 39

M50.120 Mid-cervical disc disorder, unspecified

M50.121 Cervical disc disorder at C4-C5 level with radiculopathy
C4-C5 disc disorder with radiculopathy
C5 radiculopathy due to disc disorder

M50.122 Cervical disc disorder at C5-C6 level with radiculopathy
C5-C6 disc disorder with radiculopathy
C6 radiculopathy due to disc disorder

M50.123 Cervical disc disorder at C6-C7 level with radiculopathy
C6-C7 disc disorder with radiculopathy
C7 radiculopathy due to disc disorder

M50.13 Cervical disc disorder with radiculopathy, cervicothoracic region
C7-T1 disc disorder with radiculopathy
C8 radiculopathy due to disc disorder

M50.2 Other cervical disc displacement

M50.20 Other cervical disc displacement, unspecified cervical region

M50.21 Other cervical disc displacement, high cervical region
Other C2-C3 cervical disc displacement
Other C3-C4 cervical disc displacement

M50.22 Other cervical disc displacement, mid-cervical region

M50.220 Other cervical disc displacement, mid-cervical region, unspecified level

M50.221 Other cervical disc displacement at C4-C5 level
Other C4-C5 cervical disc displacement

M50.222 Other cervical disc displacement at C5-C6 level
Other C5-C6 cervical disc displacement

M50.223 Other cervical disc displacement at C6-C7 level
Other C6-C7 cervical disc displacement

M50.23 Other cervical disc displacement, cervicothoracic region
Other C7-T1 cervical disc displacement

M50.3 Other cervical disc degeneration

M50.30 Other cervical disc degeneration, unspecified cervical region

M50.31 Other cervical disc degeneration, high cervical region
Other C2-C3 cervical disc degeneration
Other C3-C4 cervical disc degeneration

M50.32 Other cervical disc degeneration, mid-cervical region

M50.320 **Other cervical disc degeneration, mid-cervical region, unspecified level**
M50.321 **Other cervical disc degeneration at C4-C5 level**
Other C4-C5 cervical disc degeneration
M50.322 **Other cervical disc degeneration at C5-C6 level**
Other C5-C6 cervical disc degeneration
M50.323 **Other cervical disc degeneration at C6-C7 level**
Other C6-C7 cervical disc degeneration
M50.33 **Other cervical disc degeneration, cervicothoracic region**
Other C7-T1 cervical disc degeneration

5 **M50.8** **Other cervical disc disorders**
M50.80 **Other cervical disc disorders, unspecified cervical region**
M50.81 **Other cervical disc disorders, high cervical region**
Other C2-C3 cervical disc disorders
Other C3-C4 cervical disc disorders
6 **M50.82** **Other cervical disc disorders, mid-cervical region**
M50.820 **Other cervical disc disorders, mid-cervical region, unspecified level**
M50.821 **Other cervical disc disorders at C4-C5 level**
Other C4-C5 cervical disc disorders
M50.822 **Other cervical disc disorders at C5-C6 level**
Other C5-C6 cervical disc disorders
M50.823 **Other cervical disc disorders at C6-C7 level**
Other C6-C7 cervical disc disorders
M50.83 **Other cervical disc disorders, cervicothoracic region**
Other C7-T1 cervical disc disorders

5 **M50.9** **Cervical disc disorder, unspecified**
M50.90 **Cervical disc disorder, unspecified, unspecified cervical region**
M50.91 **Cervical disc disorder, unspecified, high cervical region**
C2-C3 cervical disc disorder, unspecified
C3-C4 cervical disc disorder, unspecified
6 **M50.92** **Cervical disc disorder, unspecified, mid-cervical region**
M50.920 **Unspecified cervical disc disorder, mid-cervical region, unspecified level**
M50.921 **Unspecified cervical disc disorder at C4-C5 level**
Unspecified C4-C5 cervical disc disorder
M50.922 **Unspecified cervical disc disorder at C5-C6 level**
Unspecified C5-C6 cervical disc disorder
M50.923 **Unspecified cervical disc disorder at C6-C7 level**
Unspecified C6-C7 cervical disc disorder
M50.93 **Cervical disc disorder, unspecified, cervicothoracic region**
C7-T1 cervical disc disorder, unspecified

4 M51 Thoracic, thoracolumbar, and lumbosacral intervertebral disc disorders

EXCLUDES 2 *cervical and cervicothoracic disc disorders (M50.-)*
sacral and sacrococcygeal disorders (M53.3)

CODING TIP ✓ If the patient has a disc disorder at more than one region, code to the highest level of each region. Note the excludes 2 note at M51.

5 **M51.0** **Thoracic, thoracolumbar and lumbosacral intervertebral disc disorders with myelopathy**

CODING TIP ✓ Myelopathy refers to weakness, spasticity, clumsiness, altered tonus, hyperreflexia and pathological reflexes, but generally no pain.

M51.04 **Intervertebral disc disorders with myelopathy, thoracic region**
M51.05 **Intervertebral disc disorders with myelopathy, thoracolumbar region**
M51.06 **Intervertebral disc disorders with myelopathy, lumbar region**

5 **M51.1** **Thoracic, thoracolumbar and lumbosacral intervertebral disc disorders with radiculopathy**
Sciatica due to intervertebral disc disorder

EXCLUDES 1 *lumbar radiculitis NOS (M54.16)*
sciatica NOS (M54.3)

CODING TIP ✓ Radiculopathy refers to symptoms of pain, numbness and weakness in a pattern consistent with the distribution of a particular nerve root.

M51.14 **Intervertebral disc disorders with radiculopathy, thoracic region**
M51.15 **Intervertebral disc disorders with radiculopathy, thoracolumbar region**
M51.16 **Intervertebral disc disorders with radiculopathy, lumbar region**
M51.17 **Intervertebral disc disorders with radiculopathy, lumbosacral region**

5 **M51.2** **Other thoracic, thoracolumbar and lumbosacral intervertebral disc displacement**
Lumbago due to displacement of intervertebral disc
M51.24 **Other intervertebral disc displacement, thoracic region**
M51.25 **Other intervertebral disc displacement, thoracolumbar region**
M51.26 **Other intervertebral disc displacement, lumbar region**
M51.27 **Other intervertebral disc displacement, lumbosacral region**

5 **M51.3** **Other thoracic, thoracolumbar and lumbosacral intervertebral disc degeneration**
M51.34 **Other intervertebral disc degeneration, thoracic region**
M51.35 **Other intervertebral disc degeneration, thoracolumbar region**
M51.36 **Other intervertebral disc degeneration, lumbar region**
AHA: 2Q 2018, 12
M51.37 **Other intervertebral disc degeneration, lumbosacral region**

5 **M51.4** **Schmorl's nodes**
M51.44 **Schmorl's nodes, thoracic region**
M51.45 **Schmorl's nodes, thoracolumbar region**
M51.46 **Schmorl's nodes, lumbar region**
M51.47 **Schmorl's nodes, lumbosacral region**

5 **M51.8** **Other thoracic, thoracolumbar and lumbosacral intervertebral disc disorders**
M51.84 **Other intervertebral disc disorders, thoracic region**
M51.85 **Other intervertebral disc disorders, thoracolumbar region**
M51.86 **Other intervertebral disc disorders, lumbar region**
M51.87 **Other intervertebral disc disorders, lumbosacral region**

M51.9 **Unspecified thoracic, thoracolumbar and lumbosacral intervertebral disc disorder**

4 M53 Other and unspecified dorsopathies, not elsewhere classified

M53.0 **Cervicocranial syndrome**
Posterior cervical sympathetic syndrome
M53.1 **Cervicobrachial syndrome**

EXCLUDES 2 *cervical disc disorder (M50.-)*
thoracic outlet syndrome (G54.0)

5 **M53.2** **Spinal instabilities**
6 **M53.2X** **Spinal instabilities**
M53.2X1 **Spinal instabilities, occipito-atlanto-axial region**
M53.2X2 **Spinal instabilities, cervical region**
M53.2X3 **Spinal instabilities, cervicothoracic region**
M53.2X4 **Spinal instabilities, thoracic region**
M53.2X5 **Spinal instabilities, thoracolumbar region**
M53.2X6 **Spinal instabilities, lumbar region**
M53.2X7 **Spinal instabilities, lumbosacral region**
M53.2X8 **Spinal instabilities, sacral and sacrococcygeal region**
M53.2X9 **Spinal instabilities, site unspecified**

M53.3 **Sacrococcygeal disorders, not elsewhere classified**
Coccygodynia

5 **M53.8** **Other specified dorsopathies**
M53.80 **Other specified dorsopathies, site unspecified**
M53.81 **Other specified dorsopathies, occipito-atlanto-axial region**
M53.82 **Other specified dorsopathies, cervical region**
M53.83 **Other specified dorsopathies, cervicothoracic region**
M53.84 **Other specified dorsopathies, thoracic region**
M53.85 **Other specified dorsopathies, thoracolumbar region**
M53.86 **Other specified dorsopathies, lumbar region**

M53.87 **Other specified dorsopathies, lumbosacral region**

M53.88 **Other specified dorsopathies, sacral and sacrococcygeal region**

M53.9 **Dorsopathy, unspecified**

4 **M54** **Dorsalgia**

EXCLUDES 1 *psychogenic dorsalgia (F45.41)*

5 **M54.0** **Panniculitis affecting regions of neck and back**

EXCLUDES 1 *lupus panniculitis (L93.2)*
panniculitis NOS (M79.3)
relapsing [Weber-Christian] panniculitis (M35.6)

M54.00 **Panniculitis affecting regions of neck and back, site unspecified**

M54.01 **Panniculitis affecting regions of neck and back, occipito-atlanto-axial region**

M54.02 **Panniculitis affecting regions of neck and back, cervical region**

M54.03 **Panniculitis affecting regions of neck and back, cervicothoracic region**

M54.04 **Panniculitis affecting regions of neck and back, thoracic region**

M54.05 **Panniculitis affecting regions of neck and back, thoracolumbar region**

M54.06 **Panniculitis affecting regions of neck and back, lumbar region**

M54.07 **Panniculitis affecting regions of neck and back, lumbosacral region**

M54.08 **Panniculitis affecting regions of neck and back, sacral and sacrococcygeal region**

M54.09 **Panniculitis affecting regions, neck and back, multiple sites in spine**

5 **M54.1** **Radiculopathy**

Brachial neuritis or radiculitis NOS
Lumbar neuritis or radiculitis NOS
Lumbosacral neuritis or radiculitis NOS
Thoracic neuritis or radiculitis NOS
Radiculitis NOS

EXCLUDES 1 *neuralgia and neuritis NOS (M79.2)*
radiculopathy with cervical disc disorder (M50.1)
radiculopathy with lumbar and other intervertebral disc disorder (M51.1-)
radiculopathy with spondylosis (M47.2-)

CODING TIP ✓ Radiculopathy associated with a disc disorder should not be coded to M54.1. Note the excludes 1 note.

M54.10 **Radiculopathy, site unspecified**

M54.11 **Radiculopathy, occipito-atlanto-axial region**

M54.12 **Radiculopathy, cervical region**

M54.13 **Radiculopathy, cervicothoracic region**

M54.14 **Radiculopathy, thoracic region**

M54.15 **Radiculopathy, thoracolumbar region**

M54.16 **Radiculopathy, lumbar region**

M54.17 **Radiculopathy, lumbosacral region**

M54.18 **Radiculopathy, sacral and sacrococcygeal region**

M54.2 **Cervicalgia**

EXCLUDES 1 *cervicalgia due to intervertebral cervical disc disorder (M50.-)*

CODING TIP ✓ Cervicalgia associated with a disc disorder should not be coded to M54.2. Note the excludes 1 note.

5 **M54.3** **Sciatica**

EXCLUDES 1 *lesion of sciatic nerve (G57.0)*
sciatica due to intervertebral disc disorder (M51.1-)
sciatica with lumbago (M54.4-)

CODING TIP ✓ Sciatica associated with a disc disorder should not be coded to M54.3. Note the excludes 1 note.

DEFINITION Severe pain in the sciatic nerve running down the lower back through the leg; usually resulting from nerve compression or pinching.

⊟ **M54.30** **Sciatica, unspecified side**

⊟ **M54.31** **Sciatica, right side**

⊟ **M54.32** **Sciatica, left side**

5 **M54.4** **Lumbago with sciatica**

EXCLUDES 1 *lumbago with sciatica due to intervertebral disc disorder (M51.1-)*

CODING TIP ✓ Lumbago associated with a disc disorder should not be coded with this code. Note the excludes 1 note.

⊟ **M54.40** **Lumbago with sciatica, unspecified side**

⊟ **M54.41** **Lumbago with sciatica, right side**

⊟ **M54.42** **Lumbago with sciatica, left side**

AHA: 2Q 2016, 7

M54.5 **Low back pain**

Loin pain
Lumbago NOS

EXCLUDES 1 *low back strain (S39.012)*
lumbago due to intervertebral disc displacement (M51.2-)
lumbago with sciatica (M54.4-)

CODING TIP ✓ Lumbago associated with a disc disorder should not be coded with this code. Note the excludes 1 note.

M54.6 **Pain in thoracic spine**

EXCLUDES 1 *pain in thoracic spine due to intervertebral disc disorder (M51.-)*

5 **M54.8** **Other dorsalgia**

EXCLUDES 1 *dorsalgia in thoracic region (M54.6)*
low back pain (M54.5)

M54.81 **Occipital neuralgia**

M54.89 **Other dorsalgia**

M54.9 **Dorsalgia, unspecified**

Backache NOS
Back pain NOS

Soft tissue disorders (M60-M79)

Disorders of muscles (M60-M63)

EXCLUDES 1 *dermatopolymyositis (M33.-)*
muscular dystrophies and myopathies (G71-G72)
myopathy in amyloidosis (E85.-)
myopathy in polyarteritis nodosa (M30.0)
myopathy in rheumatoid arthritis (M05.32)
myopathy in scleroderma (M34.-)
myopathy in Sjögren's syndrome (M35.03)
myopathy in systemic lupus erythematosus (M32.-)

4 **M60** **Myositis**

EXCLUDES 2 *inclusion body myositis [IBM] (G72.41)*

CODING TIP ✓ **Documentation:** Myositis indicates inflammation of the muscles. This may be caused by inflammatory disorders/autoimmune conditions, infection, or injury. Review all clinical documentation carefully to identify any cause and assign the most specific code for the condition.

5 **M60.0** **Infective myositis**

Tropical pyomyositis
Use additional code (B95-B97) to identify infectious agent

6 **M60.00** **Infective myositis, unspecified site**

⊟ **M60.000** **Infective myositis, unspecified right arm**

Infective myositis, right upper limb NOS

⊟ **M60.001** **Infective myositis, unspecified left arm**

Infective myositis, left upper limb NOS

⊟ **M60.002** **Infective myositis, unspecified arm**

Infective myositis, upper limb NOS

⊟ **M60.003** **Infective myositis, unspecified right leg**

Infective myositis, right lower limb NOS

⊟ **M60.004** **Infective myositis, unspecified left leg**

Infective myositis, left lower limb NOS

⊟ **M60.005** **Infective myositis, unspecified leg**

Infective myositis, lower limb NOS

⊟ **M60.009** **Infective myositis, unspecified site**

6 **M60.01** **Infective myositis, shoulder**

⊟ **M60.011** **Infective myositis, right shoulder**

⊟ **M60.012** **Infective myositis, left shoulder**

⊟ **M60.019** **Infective myositis, unspecified shoulder**

M60.02 Infective myositis, upper arm
M60.021 Infective myositis, right upper arm
M60.022 Infective myositis, left upper arm
M60.029 Infective myositis, unspecified upper arm
M60.03 Infective myositis, forearm
M60.031 Infective myositis, right forearm
M60.032 Infective myositis, left forearm
M60.039 Infective myositis, unspecified forearm
M60.04 Infective myositis, hand and fingers
M60.041 Infective myositis, right hand
M60.042 Infective myositis, left hand
M60.043 Infective myositis, unspecified hand
M60.044 Infective myositis, right finger(s)
M60.045 Infective myositis, left finger(s)
M60.046 Infective myositis, unspecified finger(s)
M60.05 Infective myositis, thigh
M60.051 Infective myositis, right thigh
M60.052 Infective myositis, left thigh
M60.059 Infective myositis, unspecified thigh
M60.06 Infective myositis, lower leg
M60.061 Infective myositis, right lower leg
M60.062 Infective myositis, left lower leg
M60.069 Infective myositis, unspecified lower leg
M60.07 Infective myositis, ankle, foot and toes
M60.070 Infective myositis, right ankle
M60.071 Infective myositis, left ankle
M60.072 Infective myositis, unspecified ankle
M60.073 Infective myositis, right foot
M60.074 Infective myositis, left foot
M60.075 Infective myositis, unspecified foot
M60.076 Infective myositis, right toe(s)
M60.077 Infective myositis, left toe(s)
M60.078 Infective myositis, unspecified toe(s)
M60.08 Infective myositis, other site
M60.09 Infective myositis, multiple sites
M60.1 Interstitial myositis
M60.10 Interstitial myositis of unspecified site
M60.11 Interstitial myositis, shoulder
M60.111 Interstitial myositis, right shoulder
M60.112 Interstitial myositis, left shoulder
M60.119 Interstitial myositis, unspecified shoulder
M60.12 Interstitial myositis, upper arm
M60.121 Interstitial myositis, right upper arm
M60.122 Interstitial myositis, left upper arm
M60.129 Interstitial myositis, unspecified upper arm
M60.13 Interstitial myositis, forearm
M60.131 Interstitial myositis, right forearm
M60.132 Interstitial myositis, left forearm
M60.139 Interstitial myositis, unspecified forearm
M60.14 Interstitial myositis, hand
M60.141 Interstitial myositis, right hand
M60.142 Interstitial myositis, left hand
M60.149 Interstitial myositis, unspecified hand
M60.15 Interstitial myositis, thigh
M60.151 Interstitial myositis, right thigh
M60.152 Interstitial myositis, left thigh
M60.159 Interstitial myositis, unspecified thigh
M60.16 Interstitial myositis, lower leg
M60.161 Interstitial myositis, right lower leg
M60.162 Interstitial myositis, left lower leg
M60.169 Interstitial myositis, unspecified lower leg
M60.17 Interstitial myositis, ankle and foot
M60.171 Interstitial myositis, right ankle and foot
M60.172 Interstitial myositis, left ankle and foot
M60.179 Interstitial myositis, unspecified ankle and foot
M60.18 Interstitial myositis, other site
M60.19 Interstitial myositis, multiple sites
M60.2 Foreign body granuloma of soft tissue, not elsewhere classified
Use additional code to identify the type of retained foreign body (Z18.-)
EXCLUDES 1 *foreign body granuloma of skin and subcutaneous tissue (L92.3)*
M60.20 Foreign body granuloma of soft tissue, not elsewhere classified, unspecified site
M60.21 Foreign body granuloma of soft tissue, not elsewhere classified, shoulder
M60.211 Foreign body granuloma of soft tissue, not elsewhere classified, right shoulder
M60.212 Foreign body granuloma of soft tissue, not elsewhere classified, left shoulder
M60.219 Foreign body granuloma of soft tissue, not elsewhere classified, unspecified shoulder
M60.22 Foreign body granuloma of soft tissue, not elsewhere classified, upper arm
M60.221 Foreign body granuloma of soft tissue, not elsewhere classified, right upper arm
M60.222 Foreign body granuloma of soft tissue, not elsewhere classified, left upper arm
M60.229 Foreign body granuloma of soft tissue, not elsewhere classified, unspecified upper arm
M60.23 Foreign body granuloma of soft tissue, not elsewhere classified, forearm
M60.231 Foreign body granuloma of soft tissue, not elsewhere classified, right forearm
M60.232 Foreign body granuloma of soft tissue, not elsewhere classified, left forearm
M60.239 Foreign body granuloma of soft tissue, not elsewhere classified, unspecified forearm
M60.24 Foreign body granuloma of soft tissue, not elsewhere classified, hand
M60.241 Foreign body granuloma of soft tissue, not elsewhere classified, right hand
M60.242 Foreign body granuloma of soft tissue, not elsewhere classified, left hand
M60.249 Foreign body granuloma of soft tissue, not elsewhere classified, unspecified hand
M60.25 Foreign body granuloma of soft tissue, not elsewhere classified, thigh
M60.251 Foreign body granuloma of soft tissue, not elsewhere classified, right thigh
M60.252 Foreign body granuloma of soft tissue, not elsewhere classified, left thigh
M60.259 Foreign body granuloma of soft tissue, not elsewhere classified, unspecified thigh
M60.26 Foreign body granuloma of soft tissue, not elsewhere classified, lower leg
M60.261 Foreign body granuloma of soft tissue, not elsewhere classified, right lower leg
M60.262 Foreign body granuloma of soft tissue, not elsewhere classified, left lower leg
M60.269 Foreign body granuloma of soft tissue, not elsewhere classified, unspecified lower leg
M60.27 Foreign body granuloma of soft tissue, not elsewhere classified, ankle and foot
M60.271 Foreign body granuloma of soft tissue, not elsewhere classified, right ankle and foot
M60.272 Foreign body granuloma of soft tissue, not elsewhere classified, left ankle and foot
M60.279 Foreign body granuloma of soft tissue, not elsewhere classified, unspecified ankle and foot
M60.28 Foreign body granuloma of soft tissue, not elsewhere classified, other site
M60.8 Other myositis
M60.80 Other myositis, unspecified site
M60.81 Other myositis shoulder
M60.811 Other myositis, right shoulder
M60.812 Other myositis, left shoulder
M60.819 Other myositis, unspecified shoulder
M60.82 Other myositis, upper arm

M60.821 Other myositis, right upper arm
M60.822 Other myositis, left upper arm
M60.829 Other myositis, unspecified upper arm
M60.83 Other myositis, forearm
M60.831 Other myositis, right forearm
M60.832 Other myositis, left forearm
M60.839 Other myositis, unspecified forearm
M60.84 Other myositis, hand
M60.841 Other myositis, right hand
M60.842 Other myositis, left hand
M60.849 Other myositis, unspecified hand
M60.85 Other myositis, thigh
M60.851 Other myositis, right thigh
M60.852 Other myositis, left thigh
M60.859 Other myositis, unspecified thigh
M60.86 Other myositis, lower leg
M60.861 Other myositis, right lower leg
M60.862 Other myositis, left lower leg
M60.869 Other myositis, unspecified lower leg
M60.87 Other myositis, ankle and foot
M60.871 Other myositis, right ankle and foot
M60.872 Other myositis, left ankle and foot
M60.879 Other myositis, unspecified ankle and foot
M60.88 Other myositis, other site
M60.89 Other myositis, multiple sites
M60.9 Myositis, unspecified

M61 Calcification and ossification of muscle

M61.0 Myositis ossificans traumatica
M61.00 Myositis ossificans traumatica, unspecified site
M61.01 Myositis ossificans traumatica, shoulder
M61.011 Myositis ossificans traumatica, right shoulder
M61.012 Myositis ossificans traumatica, left shoulder
M61.019 Myositis ossificans traumatica, unspecified shoulder
M61.02 Myositis ossificans traumatica, upper arm
M61.021 Myositis ossificans traumatica, right upper arm
M61.022 Myositis ossificans traumatica, left upper arm
M61.029 Myositis ossificans traumatica, unspecified upper arm
M61.03 Myositis ossificans traumatica, forearm
M61.031 Myositis ossificans traumatica, right forearm
M61.032 Myositis ossificans traumatica, left forearm
M61.039 Myositis ossificans traumatica, unspecified forearm
M61.04 Myositis ossificans traumatica, hand
M61.041 Myositis ossificans traumatica, right hand
M61.042 Myositis ossificans traumatica, left hand
M61.049 Myositis ossificans traumatica, unspecified hand
M61.05 Myositis ossificans traumatica, thigh
M61.051 Myositis ossificans traumatica, right thigh
M61.052 Myositis ossificans traumatica, left thigh
M61.059 Myositis ossificans traumatica, unspecified thigh
M61.06 Myositis ossificans traumatica, lower leg
M61.061 Myositis ossificans traumatica, right lower leg
M61.062 Myositis ossificans traumatica, left lower leg
M61.069 Myositis ossificans traumatica, unspecified lower leg
M61.07 Myositis ossificans traumatica, ankle and foot
M61.071 Myositis ossificans traumatica, right ankle and foot
M61.072 Myositis ossificans traumatica, left ankle and foot
M61.079 Myositis ossificans traumatica, unspecified ankle and foot
M61.08 Myositis ossificans traumatica, other site
M61.09 Myositis ossificans traumatica, multiple sites
M61.1 Myositis ossificans progressiva
Fibrodysplasia ossificans progressiva
M61.10 Myositis ossificans progressiva, unspecified site
M61.11 Myositis ossificans progressiva, shoulder
M61.111 Myositis ossificans progressiva, right shoulder
M61.112 Myositis ossificans progressiva, left shoulder
M61.119 Myositis ossificans progressiva, unspecified shoulder
M61.12 Myositis ossificans progressiva, upper arm
M61.121 Myositis ossificans progressiva, right upper arm
M61.122 Myositis ossificans progressiva, left upper arm
M61.129 Myositis ossificans progressiva, unspecified arm
M61.13 Myositis ossificans progressiva, forearm
M61.131 Myositis ossificans progressiva, right forearm
M61.132 Myositis ossificans progressiva, left forearm
M61.139 Myositis ossificans progressiva, unspecified forearm
M61.14 Myositis ossificans progressiva, hand and finger(s)
M61.141 Myositis ossificans progressiva, right hand
M61.142 Myositis ossificans progressiva, left hand
M61.143 Myositis ossificans progressiva, unspecified hand
M61.144 Myositis ossificans progressiva, right finger(s)
M61.145 Myositis ossificans progressiva, left finger(s)
M61.146 Myositis ossificans progressiva, unspecified finger(s)
M61.15 Myositis ossificans progressiva, thigh
M61.151 Myositis ossificans progressiva, right thigh
M61.152 Myositis ossificans progressiva, left thigh
M61.159 Myositis ossificans progressiva, unspecified thigh
M61.16 Myositis ossificans progressiva, lower leg
M61.161 Myositis ossificans progressiva, right lower leg
M61.162 Myositis ossificans progressiva, left lower leg
M61.169 Myositis ossificans progressiva, unspecified lower leg
M61.17 Myositis ossificans progressiva, ankle, foot and toe(s)
M61.171 Myositis ossificans progressiva, right ankle
M61.172 Myositis ossificans progressiva, left ankle
M61.173 Myositis ossificans progressiva, unspecified ankle
M61.174 Myositis ossificans progressiva, right foot
M61.175 Myositis ossificans progressiva, left foot
M61.176 Myositis ossificans progressiva, unspecified foot
M61.177 Myositis ossificans progressiva, right toe(s)
M61.178 Myositis ossificans progressiva, left toe(s)
M61.179 Myositis ossificans progressiva, unspecified toe(s)
M61.18 Myositis ossificans progressiva, other site
M61.19 Myositis ossificans progressiva, multiple sites
M61.2 Paralytic calcification and ossification of muscle
Myositis ossificans associated with quadriplegia or paraplegia
M61.20 Paralytic calcification and ossification of muscle, unspecified site
M61.21 Paralytic calcification and ossification of muscle, shoulder
M61.211 Paralytic calcification and ossification of muscle, right shoulder
M61.212 Paralytic calcification and ossification of muscle, left shoulder
M61.219 Paralytic calcification and ossification of muscle, unspecified shoulder
M61.22 Paralytic calcification and ossification of muscle, upper arm
M61.221 Paralytic calcification and ossification of muscle, right upper arm
M61.222 Paralytic calcification and ossification of muscle, left upper arm
M61.229 Paralytic calcification and ossification of muscle, unspecified upper arm
M61.23 Paralytic calcification and ossification of muscle, forearm
M61.231 Paralytic calcification and ossification of muscle, right forearm

M61.232 Paralytic calcification and ossification of muscle, left forearm
M61.239 Paralytic calcification and ossification of muscle, unspecified forearm
M61.24 Paralytic calcification and ossification of muscle, hand
M61.241 Paralytic calcification and ossification of muscle, right hand
M61.242 Paralytic calcification and ossification of muscle, left hand
M61.249 Paralytic calcification and ossification of muscle, unspecified hand
M61.25 Paralytic calcification and ossification of muscle, thigh
M61.251 Paralytic calcification and ossification of muscle, right thigh
M61.252 Paralytic calcification and ossification of muscle, left thigh
M61.259 Paralytic calcification and ossification of muscle, unspecified thigh
M61.26 Paralytic calcification and ossification of muscle, lower leg
M61.261 Paralytic calcification and ossification of muscle, right lower leg
M61.262 Paralytic calcification and ossification of muscle, left lower leg
M61.269 Paralytic calcification and ossification of muscle, unspecified lower leg
M61.27 Paralytic calcification and ossification of muscle, ankle and foot
M61.271 Paralytic calcification and ossification of muscle, right ankle and foot
M61.272 Paralytic calcification and ossification of muscle, left ankle and foot
M61.279 Paralytic calcification and ossification of muscle, unspecified ankle and foot
M61.28 Paralytic calcification and ossification of muscle, other site
M61.29 Paralytic calcification and ossification of muscle, multiple sites
M61.3 Calcification and ossification of muscles associated with burns
Myositis ossificans associated with burns
M61.30 Calcification and ossification of muscles associated with burns, unspecified site
M61.31 Calcification and ossification of muscles associated with burns, shoulder
M61.311 Calcification and ossification of muscles associated with burns, right shoulder
M61.312 Calcification and ossification of muscles associated with burns, left shoulder
M61.319 Calcification and ossification of muscles associated with burns, unspecified shoulder
M61.32 Calcification and ossification of muscles associated with burns, upper arm
M61.321 Calcification and ossification of muscles associated with burns, right upper arm
M61.322 Calcification and ossification of muscles associated with burns, left upper arm
M61.329 Calcification and ossification of muscles associated with burns, unspecified upper arm
M61.33 Calcification and ossification of muscles associated with burns, forearm
M61.331 Calcification and ossification of muscles associated with burns, right forearm
M61.332 Calcification and ossification of muscles associated with burns, left forearm
M61.339 Calcification and ossification of muscles associated with burns, unspecified forearm
M61.34 Calcification and ossification of muscles associated with burns, hand
M61.341 Calcification and ossification of muscles associated with burns, right hand
M61.342 Calcification and ossification of muscles associated with burns, left hand
M61.349 Calcification and ossification of muscles associated with burns, unspecified hand
M61.35 Calcification and ossification of muscles associated with burns, thigh
M61.351 Calcification and ossification of muscles associated with burns, right thigh
M61.352 Calcification and ossification of muscles associated with burns, left thigh
M61.359 Calcification and ossification of muscles associated with burns, unspecified thigh
M61.36 Calcification and ossification of muscles associated with burns, lower leg
M61.361 Calcification and ossification of muscles associated with burns, right lower leg
M61.362 Calcification and ossification of muscles associated with burns, left lower leg
M61.369 Calcification and ossification of muscles associated with burns, unspecified lower leg
M61.37 Calcification and ossification of muscles associated with burns, ankle and foot
M61.371 Calcification and ossification of muscles associated with burns, right ankle and foot
M61.372 Calcification and ossification of muscles associated with burns, left ankle and foot
M61.379 Calcification and ossification of muscles associated with burns, unspecified ankle and foot
M61.38 Calcification and ossification of muscles associated with burns, other site
M61.39 Calcification and ossification of muscles associated with burns, multiple sites
M61.4 Other calcification of muscle
EXCLUDES 1 *calcific tendinitis NOS (M65.2-)*
calcific tendinitis of shoulder (M75.3)
M61.40 Other calcification of muscle, unspecified site
M61.41 Other calcification of muscle, shoulder
M61.411 Other calcification of muscle, right shoulder
M61.412 Other calcification of muscle, left shoulder
M61.419 Other calcification of muscle, unspecified shoulder
M61.42 Other calcification of muscle, upper arm
M61.421 Other calcification of muscle, right upper arm
M61.422 Other calcification of muscle, left upper arm
M61.429 Other calcification of muscle, unspecified upper arm
M61.43 Other calcification of muscle, forearm
M61.431 Other calcification of muscle, right forearm
M61.432 Other calcification of muscle, left forearm
M61.439 Other calcification of muscle, unspecified forearm
M61.44 Other calcification of muscle, hand
M61.441 Other calcification of muscle, right hand
M61.442 Other calcification of muscle, left hand
M61.449 Other calcification of muscle, unspecified hand
M61.45 Other calcification of muscle, thigh
M61.451 Other calcification of muscle, right thigh
M61.452 Other calcification of muscle, left thigh
M61.459 Other calcification of muscle, unspecified thigh
M61.46 Other calcification of muscle, lower leg
M61.461 Other calcification of muscle, right lower leg
M61.462 Other calcification of muscle, left lower leg
M61.469 Other calcification of muscle, unspecified lower leg
M61.47 Other calcification of muscle, ankle and foot
M61.471 Other calcification of muscle, right ankle and foot
M61.472 Other calcification of muscle, left ankle and foot
M61.479 Other calcification of muscle, unspecified ankle and foot
M61.48 Other calcification of muscle, other site
M61.49 Other calcification of muscle, multiple sites
M61.5 Other ossification of muscle
M61.50 Other ossification of muscle, unspecified site
M61.51 Other ossification of muscle, shoulder
M61.511 Other ossification of muscle, right shoulder
M61.512 Other ossification of muscle, left shoulder
M61.519 Other ossification of muscle, unspecified shoulder
M61.52 Other ossification of muscle, upper arm

M61.521 Other ossification of muscle, right upper arm
M61.522 Other ossification of muscle, left upper arm
M61.529 Other ossification of muscle, unspecified upper arm
M61.53 Other ossification of muscle, forearm
M61.531 Other ossification of muscle, right forearm
M61.532 Other ossification of muscle, left forearm
M61.539 Other ossification of muscle, unspecified forearm
M61.54 Other ossification of muscle, hand
M61.541 Other ossification of muscle, right hand
M61.542 Other ossification of muscle, left hand
M61.549 Other ossification of muscle, unspecified hand
M61.55 Other ossification of muscle, thigh
M61.551 Other ossification of muscle, right thigh
M61.552 Other ossification of muscle, left thigh
M61.559 Other ossification of muscle, unspecified thigh
M61.56 Other ossification of muscle, lower leg
M61.561 Other ossification of muscle, right lower leg
M61.562 Other ossification of muscle, left lower leg
M61.569 Other ossification of muscle, unspecified lower leg
M61.57 Other ossification of muscle, ankle and foot
M61.571 Other ossification of muscle, right ankle and foot
M61.572 Other ossification of muscle, left ankle and foot
M61.579 Other ossification of muscle, unspecified ankle and foot
M61.58 Other ossification of muscle, other site
M61.59 Other ossification of muscle, multiple sites
M61.9 Calcification and ossification of muscle, unspecified

▲ M62 Other disorders of muscle

EXCLUDES 1 *alcoholic myopathy (G72.1)*
cramp and spasm (R25.2)
drug-induced myopathy (G72.0)
myalgia (M79.1-)
stiff-man syndrome (G25.82)
EXCLUDES 2 *nontraumatic hematoma of muscle (M79.81)*

M62.0 Separation of muscle (nontraumatic)
Diastasis of muscle
EXCLUDES 1 *diastasis recti complicating pregnancy, labor and delivery (O71.8)*
traumatic separation of muscle- see strain of muscle by body region

CODING TIP✓ Codes classified in M62.0- through M62.28 indicate muscle separation, rupture and ischemia of a non-traumatic origin. When a traumatic muscle injury is reported, do not assign a code from M62.0- through M62.28, but instead assign a code from Chapter 19, Injury, Poisoning and Certain Other Consequences of External Causes.

M62.00 Separation of muscle (nontraumatic), unspecified site
M62.01 Separation of muscle (nontraumatic), shoulder
M62.011 Separation of muscle (nontraumatic), right shoulder
M62.012 Separation of muscle (nontraumatic), left shoulder
M62.019 Separation of muscle (nontraumatic), unspecified shoulder
M62.02 Separation of muscle (nontraumatic), upper arm
M62.021 Separation of muscle (nontraumatic), right upper arm
M62.022 Separation of muscle (nontraumatic), left upper arm
M62.029 Separation of muscle (nontraumatic), unspecified upper arm
M62.03 Separation of muscle (nontraumatic), forearm
M62.031 Separation of muscle (nontraumatic), right forearm
M62.032 Separation of muscle (nontraumatic), left forearm
M62.039 Separation of muscle (nontraumatic), unspecified forearm
M62.04 Separation of muscle (nontraumatic), hand
M62.041 Separation of muscle (nontraumatic), right hand
M62.042 Separation of muscle (nontraumatic), left hand
M62.049 Separation of muscle (nontraumatic), unspecified hand
M62.05 Separation of muscle (nontraumatic), thigh
M62.051 Separation of muscle (nontraumatic), right thigh
M62.052 Separation of muscle (nontraumatic), left thigh
M62.059 Separation of muscle (nontraumatic), unspecified thigh
M62.06 Separation of muscle (nontraumatic), lower leg
M62.061 Separation of muscle (nontraumatic), right lower leg
M62.062 Separation of muscle (nontraumatic), left lower leg
M62.069 Separation of muscle (nontraumatic), unspecified lower leg
M62.07 Separation of muscle (nontraumatic), ankle and foot
M62.071 Separation of muscle (nontraumatic), right ankle and foot
M62.072 Separation of muscle (nontraumatic), left ankle and foot
M62.079 Separation of muscle (nontraumatic), unspecified ankle and foot
M62.08 Separation of muscle (nontraumatic), other site

M62.1 Other rupture of muscle (nontraumatic)
EXCLUDES 1 *traumatic rupture of muscle - see strain of muscle by body region*
EXCLUDES 2 *rupture of tendon (M66.-)*

CODING TIP✓ Codes classified in M62.0- through M62.28 indicate muscle separation, rupture and ischemia of a non-traumatic origin. When a traumatic muscle injury is reported, do not assign a code from M62.0- through M62.28, but instead assign a code from Chapter 19, Injury, Poisoning and Certain Other Consequences of External Causes.

M62.10 Other rupture of muscle (nontraumatic), unspecified site
M62.11 Other rupture of muscle (nontraumatic), shoulder
M62.111 Other rupture of muscle (nontraumatic), right shoulder
M62.112 Other rupture of muscle (nontraumatic), left shoulder
M62.119 Other rupture of muscle (nontraumatic), unspecified shoulder
M62.12 Other rupture of muscle (nontraumatic), upper arm
M62.121 Other rupture of muscle (nontraumatic), right upper arm
M62.122 Other rupture of muscle (nontraumatic), left upper arm
M62.129 Other rupture of muscle (nontraumatic), unspecified upper arm
M62.13 Other rupture of muscle (nontraumatic), forearm
M62.131 Other rupture of muscle (nontraumatic), right forearm
M62.132 Other rupture of muscle (nontraumatic), left forearm
M62.139 Other rupture of muscle (nontraumatic), unspecified forearm
M62.14 Other rupture of muscle (nontraumatic), hand
M62.141 Other rupture of muscle (nontraumatic), right hand
M62.142 Other rupture of muscle (nontraumatic), left hand
M62.149 Other rupture of muscle (nontraumatic), unspecified hand
M62.15 Other rupture of muscle (nontraumatic), thigh
M62.151 Other rupture of muscle (nontraumatic), right thigh
M62.152 Other rupture of muscle (nontraumatic), left thigh
M62.159 Other rupture of muscle (nontraumatic), unspecified thigh
M62.16 Other rupture of muscle (nontraumatic), lower leg

M62.161 Other rupture of muscle (nontraumatic), right lower leg
M62.162 Other rupture of muscle (nontraumatic), left lower leg
M62.169 Other rupture of muscle (nontraumatic), unspecified lower leg
M62.17 Other rupture of muscle (nontraumatic), ankle and foot
M62.171 Other rupture of muscle (nontraumatic), right ankle and foot
M62.172 Other rupture of muscle (nontraumatic), left ankle and foot
M62.179 Other rupture of muscle (nontraumatic), unspecified ankle and foot
M62.18 Other rupture of muscle (nontraumatic), other site
M62.2 Nontraumatic ischemic infarction of muscle

EXCLUDES 1 *compartment syndrome (traumatic) (T79.A-)*
nontraumatic compartment syndrome (M79.A-)
traumatic ischemia of muscle (T79.6)
rhabdomyolysis (M62.82)
Volkmann's ischemic contracture (T79.6)

CODING TIP ✓ Codes classified in M62.0- through M62.28 indicate muscle separation, rupture and ischemia of a non-traumatic origin. When a traumatic muscle injury is reported, do not assign a code from M62.0- through M62.28, but instead assign a code from Chapter 19, Injury, Poisoning and Certain Other Consequences of External Causes.

M62.20 Nontraumatic ischemic infarction of muscle, unspecified site
M62.21 Nontraumatic ischemic infarction of muscle, shoulder
M62.211 Nontraumatic ischemic infarction of muscle, right shoulder
M62.212 Nontraumatic ischemic infarction of muscle, left shoulder
M62.219 Nontraumatic ischemic infarction of muscle, unspecified shoulder
M62.22 Nontraumatic ischemic infarction of muscle, upper arm
M62.221 Nontraumatic ischemic infarction of muscle, right upper arm
M62.222 Nontraumatic ischemic infarction of muscle, left upper arm
M62.229 Nontraumatic ischemic infarction of muscle, unspecified upper arm
M62.23 Nontraumatic ischemic infarction of muscle, forearm
M62.231 Nontraumatic ischemic infarction of muscle, right forearm
M62.232 Nontraumatic ischemic infarction of muscle, left forearm
M62.239 Nontraumatic ischemic infarction of muscle, unspecified forearm
M62.24 Nontraumatic ischemic infarction of muscle, hand
M62.241 Nontraumatic ischemic infarction of muscle, right hand
M62.242 Nontraumatic ischemic infarction of muscle, left hand
M62.249 Nontraumatic ischemic infarction of muscle, unspecified hand
M62.25 Nontraumatic ischemic infarction of muscle, thigh
M62.251 Nontraumatic ischemic infarction of muscle, right thigh
M62.252 Nontraumatic ischemic infarction of muscle, left thigh
M62.259 Nontraumatic ischemic infarction of muscle, unspecified thigh
M62.26 Nontraumatic ischemic infarction of muscle, lower leg
M62.261 Nontraumatic ischemic infarction of muscle, right lower leg
M62.262 Nontraumatic ischemic infarction of muscle, left lower leg
M62.269 Nontraumatic ischemic infarction of muscle, unspecified lower leg
M62.27 Nontraumatic ischemic infarction of muscle, ankle and foot
M62.271 Nontraumatic ischemic infarction of muscle, right ankle and foot
M62.272 Nontraumatic ischemic infarction of muscle, left ankle and foot
M62.279 Nontraumatic ischemic infarction of muscle, unspecified ankle and foot
M62.28 Nontraumatic ischemic infarction of muscle, other site
M62.3 Immobility syndrome (paraplegic)

CODING TIP ✓ Do not assign M62.3 for paraplegia that is due to a neurologic condition or injury. M62.3 indicates paraplegia of a non-neurologic origin due to immobility.

M62.4 Contracture of muscle
Contracture of tendon (sheath)

EXCLUDES 1 *contracture of joint (M24.5-)*

M62.40 Contracture of muscle, unspecified site
M62.41 Contracture of muscle, shoulder
M62.411 Contracture of muscle, right shoulder
M62.412 Contracture of muscle, left shoulder
M62.419 Contracture of muscle, unspecified shoulder
M62.42 Contracture of muscle, upper arm
M62.421 Contracture of muscle, right upper arm
M62.422 Contracture of muscle, left upper arm
M62.429 Contracture of muscle, unspecified upper arm
M62.43 Contracture of muscle, forearm
M62.431 Contracture of muscle, right forearm
M62.432 Contracture of muscle, left forearm
M62.439 Contracture of muscle, unspecified forearm
M62.44 Contracture of muscle, hand
M62.441 Contracture of muscle, right hand
M62.442 Contracture of muscle, left hand
M62.449 Contracture of muscle, unspecified hand
M62.45 Contracture of muscle, thigh
M62.451 Contracture of muscle, right thigh
M62.452 Contracture of muscle, left thigh
M62.459 Contracture of muscle, unspecified thigh
M62.46 Contracture of muscle, lower leg
M62.461 Contracture of muscle, right lower leg
M62.462 Contracture of muscle, left lower leg
M62.469 Contracture of muscle, unspecified lower leg
M62.47 Contracture of muscle, ankle and foot
M62.471 Contracture of muscle, right ankle and foot
M62.472 Contracture of muscle, left ankle and foot
M62.479 Contracture of muscle, unspecified ankle and foot
M62.48 Contracture of muscle, other site
M62.49 Contracture of muscle, multiple sites
M62.5 Muscle wasting and atrophy, not elsewhere classified
Disuse atrophy NEC

EXCLUDES 1 *neuralgic amyotrophy (G54.5)*
progressive muscular atrophy (G12.21)
sarcopenia (M62.84)

EXCLUDES 2 *pelvic muscle wasting (N81.84)*

M62.50 Muscle wasting and atrophy, not elsewhere classified, unspecified site
M62.51 Muscle wasting and atrophy, not elsewhere classified, shoulder
M62.511 Muscle wasting and atrophy, not elsewhere classified, right shoulder
M62.512 Muscle wasting and atrophy, not elsewhere classified, left shoulder
M62.519 Muscle wasting and atrophy, not elsewhere classified, unspecified shoulder
M62.52 Muscle wasting and atrophy, not elsewhere classified, upper arm
M62.521 Muscle wasting and atrophy, not elsewhere classified, right upper arm
M62.522 Muscle wasting and atrophy, not elsewhere classified, left upper arm
M62.529 Muscle wasting and atrophy, not elsewhere classified, unspecified upper arm

6 M62.53 Muscle wasting and atrophy, not elsewhere classified, forearm
- **M62.531** Muscle wasting and atrophy, not elsewhere classified, right forearm
- **M62.532** Muscle wasting and atrophy, not elsewhere classified, left forearm
- **M62.539** Muscle wasting and atrophy, not elsewhere classified, unspecified forearm

6 M62.54 Muscle wasting and atrophy, not elsewhere classified, hand
- **M62.541** Muscle wasting and atrophy, not elsewhere classified, right hand
- **M62.542** Muscle wasting and atrophy, not elsewhere classified, left hand
- **M62.549** Muscle wasting and atrophy, not elsewhere classified, unspecified hand

6 M62.55 Muscle wasting and atrophy, not elsewhere classified, thigh
- **M62.551** Muscle wasting and atrophy, not elsewhere classified, right thigh
- **M62.552** Muscle wasting and atrophy, not elsewhere classified, left thigh
- **M62.559** Muscle wasting and atrophy, not elsewhere classified, unspecified thigh

6 M62.56 Muscle wasting and atrophy, not elsewhere classified, lower leg
- **M62.561** Muscle wasting and atrophy, not elsewhere classified, right lower leg
- **M62.562** Muscle wasting and atrophy, not elsewhere classified, left lower leg
- **M62.569** Muscle wasting and atrophy, not elsewhere classified, unspecified lower leg

6 M62.57 Muscle wasting and atrophy, not elsewhere classified, ankle and foot
- **M62.571** Muscle wasting and atrophy, not elsewhere classified, right ankle and foot
- **M62.572** Muscle wasting and atrophy, not elsewhere classified, left ankle and foot
- **M62.579** Muscle wasting and atrophy, not elsewhere classified, unspecified ankle and foot

M62.58 Muscle wasting and atrophy, not elsewhere classified, other site

M62.59 Muscle wasting and atrophy, not elsewhere classified, multiple sites

5 M62.8 Other specified disorders of muscle

EXCLUDES 2 *nontraumatic hematoma of muscle (M79.81)*

M62.81 Muscle weakness (generalized)

EXCLUDES 1 *muscle weakness in sarcopenia (M62.84)*

CODING TIP ✓ Use M62.81 for true muscle weakness as a result of musculoskeletal disorders, neuromuscular disease or degenerative disease otherwise unidentified. Unilateral weakness associated with stroke, brain disorders or injury is coded to hemiplegia/hemiparesis, not M62.81. Muscle group measurements are not required, but measurable muscle weakness must be documented.

M62.82 Rhabdomyolysis

EXCLUDES 1 *traumatic rhabdomyolysis (T79.6)*

6 M62.83 Muscle spasm
- **M62.830** Muscle spasm of back
- **M62.831** Muscle spasm of calf
  - Charley-horse
- **M62.838** Other muscle spasm

M62.84 Sarcopenia

Age-related sarcopenia

Code first underlying disease, if applicable, such as:
- disorders of myoneural junction and muscle disease in diseases classified elsewhere (G73.-)
- other and unspecified myopathies (G72.-)
- primary disorders of muscles (G71.-)

AHA: 4Q 2016, 41

M62.89 Other specified disorders of muscle

Muscle (sheath) hernia

M62.9 Disorder of muscle, unspecified

4 M63 Disorders of muscle in diseases classified elsewhere

Code first underlying disease, such as:
- leprosy (A30.-)
- neoplasm (C49.-, C79.89, D21.-, D48.1)
- schistosomiasis (B65.-)
- trichinellosis (B75)

EXCLUDES 1
- *myopathy in cysticercosis (B69.81)*
- *myopathy in endocrine diseases (G73.7)*
- *myopathy in metabolic diseases (G73.7)*
- *myopathy in sarcoidosis (D86.87)*
- *myopathy in secondary syphilis (A51.49)*
- *myopathy in syphilis (late) (A52.78)*
- *myopathy in toxoplasmosis (B58.82)*
- *myopathy in tuberculosis (A18.09)*

5 M63.8 Disorders of muscle in diseases classified elsewhere

M63.80 *Disorders of muscle in diseases classified elsewhere, unspecified site*

6 M63.81 Disorders of muscle in diseases classified elsewhere, shoulder
- **M63.811** *Disorders of muscle in diseases classified elsewhere, right shoulder*
- **M63.812** *Disorders of muscle in diseases classified elsewhere, left shoulder*
- **M63.819** *Disorders of muscle in diseases classified elsewhere, unspecified shoulder*

6 M63.82 Disorders of muscle in diseases classified elsewhere, upper arm
- **M63.821** *Disorders of muscle in diseases classified elsewhere, right upper arm*
- **M63.822** *Disorders of muscle in diseases classified elsewhere, left upper arm*
- **M63.829** *Disorders of muscle in diseases classified elsewhere, unspecified upper arm*

6 M63.83 Disorders of muscle in diseases classified elsewhere, forearm
- **M63.831** *Disorders of muscle in diseases classified elsewhere, right forearm*
- **M63.832** *Disorders of muscle in diseases classified elsewhere, left forearm*
- **M63.839** *Disorders of muscle in diseases classified elsewhere, unspecified forearm*

6 M63.84 Disorders of muscle in diseases classified elsewhere, hand
- **M63.841** *Disorders of muscle in diseases classified elsewhere, right hand*
- **M63.842** *Disorders of muscle in diseases classified elsewhere, left hand*
- **M63.849** *Disorders of muscle in diseases classified elsewhere, unspecified hand*

6 M63.85 Disorders of muscle in diseases classified elsewhere, thigh
- **M63.851** *Disorders of muscle in diseases classified elsewhere, right thigh*
- **M63.852** *Disorders of muscle in diseases classified elsewhere, left thigh*
- **M63.859** *Disorders of muscle in diseases classified elsewhere, unspecified thigh*

6 M63.86 Disorders of muscle in diseases classified elsewhere, lower leg
- **M63.861** *Disorders of muscle in diseases classified elsewhere, right lower leg*
- **M63.862** *Disorders of muscle in diseases classified elsewhere, left lower leg*
- **M63.869** *Disorders of muscle in diseases classified elsewhere, unspecified lower leg*

6 M63.87 Disorders of muscle in diseases classified elsewhere, ankle and foot
- **M63.871** *Disorders of muscle in diseases classified elsewhere, right ankle and foot*
- **M63.872** *Disorders of muscle in diseases classified elsewhere, left ankle and foot*
- **M63.879** *Disorders of muscle in diseases classified elsewhere, unspecified ankle and foot*

M63.88 *Disorders of muscle in diseases classified elsewhere, other site*

M63.89 *Disorders of muscle in diseases classified elsewhere, multiple sites*

Disorders of synovium and tendon (M65-M67)

M65 Synovitis and tenosynovitis

EXCLUDES 1 *chronic crepitant synovitis of hand and wrist (M70.0-)*
current injury - see injury of ligament or tendon by body region
soft tissue disorders related to use, overuse and pressure (M70.-)

M65.0 Abscess of tendon sheath
Use additional code (B95-B96) to identify bacterial agent.
- M65.00 Abscess of tendon sheath, unspecified site
- M65.01 Abscess of tendon sheath, shoulder
  - M65.011 Abscess of tendon sheath, right shoulder
  - M65.012 Abscess of tendon sheath, left shoulder
  - M65.019 Abscess of tendon sheath, unspecified shoulder
- M65.02 Abscess of tendon sheath, upper arm
  - M65.021 Abscess of tendon sheath, right upper arm
  - M65.022 Abscess of tendon sheath, left upper arm
  - M65.029 Abscess of tendon sheath, unspecified upper arm
- M65.03 Abscess of tendon sheath, forearm
  - M65.031 Abscess of tendon sheath, right forearm
  - M65.032 Abscess of tendon sheath, left forearm
  - M65.039 Abscess of tendon sheath, unspecified forearm
- M65.04 Abscess of tendon sheath, hand
  - M65.041 Abscess of tendon sheath, right hand
  - M65.042 Abscess of tendon sheath, left hand
  - M65.049 Abscess of tendon sheath, unspecified hand
- M65.05 Abscess of tendon sheath, thigh
  - M65.051 Abscess of tendon sheath, right thigh
  - M65.052 Abscess of tendon sheath, left thigh
  - M65.059 Abscess of tendon sheath, unspecified thigh
- M65.06 Abscess of tendon sheath, lower leg
  - M65.061 Abscess of tendon sheath, right lower leg
  - M65.062 Abscess of tendon sheath, left lower leg
  - M65.069 Abscess of tendon sheath, unspecified lower leg
- M65.07 Abscess of tendon sheath, ankle and foot
  - M65.071 Abscess of tendon sheath, right ankle and foot
  - M65.072 Abscess of tendon sheath, left ankle and foot
  - M65.079 Abscess of tendon sheath, unspecified ankle and foot
- M65.08 Abscess of tendon sheath, other site

M65.1 Other infective (teno)synovitis
- M65.10 Other infective (teno)synovitis, unspecified site
- M65.11 Other infective (teno)synovitis, shoulder
  - M65.111 Other infective (teno)synovitis, right shoulder
  - M65.112 Other infective (teno)synovitis, left shoulder
  - M65.119 Other infective (teno)synovitis, unspecified shoulder
- M65.12 Other infective (teno)synovitis, elbow
  - M65.121 Other infective (teno)synovitis, right elbow
  - M65.122 Other infective (teno)synovitis, left elbow
  - M65.129 Other infective (teno)synovitis, unspecified elbow
- M65.13 Other infective (teno)synovitis, wrist
  - M65.131 Other infective (teno)synovitis, right wrist
  - M65.132 Other infective (teno)synovitis, left wrist
  - M65.139 Other infective (teno)synovitis, unspecified wrist
- M65.14 Other infective (teno)synovitis, hand
  - M65.141 Other infective (teno)synovitis, right hand
  - M65.142 Other infective (teno)synovitis, left hand
  - M65.149 Other infective (teno)synovitis, unspecified hand
- M65.15 Other infective (teno)synovitis, hip
  - M65.151 Other infective (teno)synovitis, right hip
  - M65.152 Other infective (teno)synovitis, left hip
  - M65.159 Other infective (teno)synovitis, unspecified hip
- M65.16 Other infective (teno)synovitis, knee
  - M65.161 Other infective (teno)synovitis, right knee
  - M65.162 Other infective (teno)synovitis, left knee
  - M65.169 Other infective (teno)synovitis, unspecified knee
- M65.17 Other infective (teno)synovitis, ankle and foot
  - M65.171 Other infective (teno)synovitis, right ankle and foot
  - M65.172 Other infective (teno)synovitis, left ankle and foot
  - M65.179 Other infective (teno)synovitis, unspecified ankle and foot
- M65.18 Other infective (teno)synovitis, other site
- M65.19 Other infective (teno)synovitis, multiple sites

M65.2 Calcific tendinitis

EXCLUDES 1 *tendinitis as classified in M75-M77*
calcified tendinitis of shoulder (M75.3)
- M65.20 Calcific tendinitis, unspecified site
- M65.22 Calcific tendinitis, upper arm
  - M65.221 Calcific tendinitis, right upper arm
  - M65.222 Calcific tendinitis, left upper arm
  - M65.229 Calcific tendinitis, unspecified upper arm
- M65.23 Calcific tendinitis, forearm
  - M65.231 Calcific tendinitis, right forearm
  - M65.232 Calcific tendinitis, left forearm
  - M65.239 Calcific tendinitis, unspecified forearm
- M65.24 Calcific tendinitis, hand
  - M65.241 Calcific tendinitis, right hand
  - M65.242 Calcific tendinitis, left hand
  - M65.249 Calcific tendinitis, unspecified hand
- M65.25 Calcific tendinitis, thigh
  - M65.251 Calcific tendinitis, right thigh
  - M65.252 Calcific tendinitis, left thigh
  - M65.259 Calcific tendinitis, unspecified thigh
- M65.26 Calcific tendinitis, lower leg
  - M65.261 Calcific tendinitis, right lower leg
  - M65.262 Calcific tendinitis, left lower leg
  - M65.269 Calcific tendinitis, unspecified lower leg
- M65.27 Calcific tendinitis, ankle and foot
  - M65.271 Calcific tendinitis, right ankle and foot
  - M65.272 Calcific tendinitis, left ankle and foot
  - M65.279 Calcific tendinitis, unspecified ankle and foot
- M65.28 Calcific tendinitis, other site
- M65.29 Calcific tendinitis, multiple sites

M65.3 Trigger finger
Nodular tendinous disease
- M65.30 Trigger finger, unspecified finger
- M65.31 Trigger thumb
  - M65.311 Trigger thumb, right thumb
  - M65.312 Trigger thumb, left thumb
  - M65.319 Trigger thumb, unspecified thumb
- M65.32 Trigger finger, index finger
  - M65.321 Trigger finger, right index finger
  - M65.322 Trigger finger, left index finger
  - M65.329 Trigger finger, unspecified index finger
- M65.33 Trigger finger, middle finger
  - M65.331 Trigger finger, right middle finger
  - M65.332 Trigger finger, left middle finger
  - M65.339 Trigger finger, unspecified middle finger
- M65.34 Trigger finger, ring finger
  - M65.341 Trigger finger, right ring finger
  - M65.342 Trigger finger, left ring finger
  - M65.349 Trigger finger, unspecified ring finger
- M65.35 Trigger finger, little finger
  - M65.351 Trigger finger, right little finger
  - M65.352 Trigger finger, left little finger
  - M65.359 Trigger finger, unspecified little finger

M65.4 Radial styloid tenosynovitis [de Quervain]

M65.8 Other synovitis and tenosynovitis
- M65.80 Other synovitis and tenosynovitis, unspecified site
- M65.81 Other synovitis and tenosynovitis, shoulder
  - M65.811 Other synovitis and tenosynovitis, right shoulder
  - M65.812 Other synovitis and tenosynovitis, left shoulder

M65.819 Other synovitis and tenosynovitis, unspecified shoulder
M65.82 Other synovitis and tenosynovitis, upper arm
M65.821 Other synovitis and tenosynovitis, right upper arm
M65.822 Other synovitis and tenosynovitis, left upper arm
M65.829 Other synovitis and tenosynovitis, unspecified upper arm
M65.83 Other synovitis and tenosynovitis, forearm
M65.831 Other synovitis and tenosynovitis, right forearm
M65.832 Other synovitis and tenosynovitis, left forearm
M65.839 Other synovitis and tenosynovitis, unspecified forearm
M65.84 Other synovitis and tenosynovitis, hand
M65.841 Other synovitis and tenosynovitis, right hand
M65.842 Other synovitis and tenosynovitis, left hand
M65.849 Other synovitis and tenosynovitis, unspecified hand
M65.85 Other synovitis and tenosynovitis, thigh
M65.851 Other synovitis and tenosynovitis, right thigh
M65.852 Other synovitis and tenosynovitis, left thigh
M65.859 Other synovitis and tenosynovitis, unspecified thigh
M65.86 Other synovitis and tenosynovitis, lower leg
M65.861 Other synovitis and tenosynovitis, right lower leg
M65.862 Other synovitis and tenosynovitis, left lower leg
M65.869 Other synovitis and tenosynovitis, unspecified lower leg
M65.87 Other synovitis and tenosynovitis, ankle and foot
M65.871 Other synovitis and tenosynovitis, right ankle and foot
M65.872 Other synovitis and tenosynovitis, left ankle and foot
M65.879 Other synovitis and tenosynovitis, unspecified ankle and foot
M65.88 Other synovitis and tenosynovitis, other site
M65.89 Other synovitis and tenosynovitis, multiple sites
M65.9 Synovitis and tenosynovitis, unspecified

M66 Spontaneous rupture of synovium and tendon

INCLUDES rupture that occurs when a normal force is applied to tissues that are inferred to have less than normal strength

EXCLUDES 2 *rotator cuff syndrome (M75.1-)*
rupture where an abnormal force is applied to normal tissue - see injury of tendon by body region

M66.0 Rupture of popliteal cyst
M66.1 Rupture of synovium
Rupture of synovial cyst
EXCLUDES 2 *rupture of popliteal cyst (M66.0)*
M66.10 Rupture of synovium, unspecified joint
M66.11 Rupture of synovium, shoulder
M66.111 Rupture of synovium, right shoulder
M66.112 Rupture of synovium, left shoulder
M66.119 Rupture of synovium, unspecified shoulder
M66.12 Rupture of synovium, elbow
M66.121 Rupture of synovium, right elbow
M66.122 Rupture of synovium, left elbow
M66.129 Rupture of synovium, unspecified elbow
M66.13 Rupture of synovium, wrist
M66.131 Rupture of synovium, right wrist
M66.132 Rupture of synovium, left wrist
M66.139 Rupture of synovium, unspecified wrist
M66.14 Rupture of synovium, hand and fingers
M66.141 Rupture of synovium, right hand
M66.142 Rupture of synovium, left hand
M66.143 Rupture of synovium, unspecified hand
M66.144 Rupture of synovium, right finger(s)
M66.145 Rupture of synovium, left finger(s)
M66.146 Rupture of synovium, unspecified finger(s)
M66.15 Rupture of synovium, hip
M66.151 Rupture of synovium, right hip
M66.152 Rupture of synovium, left hip
M66.159 Rupture of synovium, unspecified hip
M66.17 Rupture of synovium, ankle, foot and toes
M66.171 Rupture of synovium, right ankle
M66.172 Rupture of synovium, left ankle
M66.173 Rupture of synovium, unspecified ankle
M66.174 Rupture of synovium, right foot
M66.175 Rupture of synovium, left foot
M66.176 Rupture of synovium, unspecified foot
M66.177 Rupture of synovium, right toe(s)
M66.178 Rupture of synovium, left toe(s)
M66.179 Rupture of synovium, unspecified toe(s)
M66.18 Rupture of synovium, other site
M66.2 Spontaneous rupture of extensor tendons
M66.20 Spontaneous rupture of extensor tendons, unspecified site
M66.21 Spontaneous rupture of extensor tendons, shoulder
M66.211 Spontaneous rupture of extensor tendons, right shoulder
M66.212 Spontaneous rupture of extensor tendons, left shoulder
M66.219 Spontaneous rupture of extensor tendons, unspecified shoulder
M66.22 Spontaneous rupture of extensor tendons, upper arm
M66.221 Spontaneous rupture of extensor tendons, right upper arm
M66.222 Spontaneous rupture of extensor tendons, left upper arm
M66.229 Spontaneous rupture of extensor tendons, unspecified upper arm
M66.23 Spontaneous rupture of extensor tendons, forearm
M66.231 Spontaneous rupture of extensor tendons, right forearm
M66.232 Spontaneous rupture of extensor tendons, left forearm
M66.239 Spontaneous rupture of extensor tendons, unspecified forearm
M66.24 Spontaneous rupture of extensor tendons, hand
M66.241 Spontaneous rupture of extensor tendons, right hand
M66.242 Spontaneous rupture of extensor tendons, left hand
M66.249 Spontaneous rupture of extensor tendons, unspecified hand
M66.25 Spontaneous rupture of extensor tendons, thigh
M66.251 Spontaneous rupture of extensor tendons, right thigh
M66.252 Spontaneous rupture of extensor tendons, left thigh
M66.259 Spontaneous rupture of extensor tendons, unspecified thigh
M66.26 Spontaneous rupture of extensor tendons, lower leg
M66.261 Spontaneous rupture of extensor tendons, right lower leg
M66.262 Spontaneous rupture of extensor tendons, left lower leg
M66.269 Spontaneous rupture of extensor tendons, unspecified lower leg
M66.27 Spontaneous rupture of extensor tendons, ankle and foot
M66.271 Spontaneous rupture of extensor tendons, right ankle and foot
M66.272 Spontaneous rupture of extensor tendons, left ankle and foot
M66.279 Spontaneous rupture of extensor tendons, unspecified ankle and foot
M66.28 Spontaneous rupture of extensor tendons, other site
M66.29 Spontaneous rupture of extensor tendons, multiple sites
M66.3 Spontaneous rupture of flexor tendons
M66.30 Spontaneous rupture of flexor tendons, unspecified site
M66.31 Spontaneous rupture of flexor tendons, shoulder
M66.311 Spontaneous rupture of flexor tendons, right shoulder

M66.312 Spontaneous rupture of flexor tendons, left shoulder
M66.319 Spontaneous rupture of flexor tendons, unspecified shoulder
M66.32 Spontaneous rupture of flexor tendons, upper arm
M66.321 Spontaneous rupture of flexor tendons, right upper arm
M66.322 Spontaneous rupture of flexor tendons, left upper arm
M66.329 Spontaneous rupture of flexor tendons, unspecified upper arm
M66.33 Spontaneous rupture of flexor tendons, forearm
M66.331 Spontaneous rupture of flexor tendons, right forearm
M66.332 Spontaneous rupture of flexor tendons, left forearm
M66.339 Spontaneous rupture of flexor tendons, unspecified forearm
M66.34 Spontaneous rupture of flexor tendons, hand
M66.341 Spontaneous rupture of flexor tendons, right hand
M66.342 Spontaneous rupture of flexor tendons, left hand
M66.349 Spontaneous rupture of flexor tendons, unspecified hand
M66.35 Spontaneous rupture of flexor tendons, thigh
M66.351 Spontaneous rupture of flexor tendons, right thigh
M66.352 Spontaneous rupture of flexor tendons, left thigh
M66.359 Spontaneous rupture of flexor tendons, unspecified thigh
M66.36 Spontaneous rupture of flexor tendons, lower leg
M66.361 Spontaneous rupture of flexor tendons, right lower leg
M66.362 Spontaneous rupture of flexor tendons, left lower leg
M66.369 Spontaneous rupture of flexor tendons, unspecified lower leg
M66.37 Spontaneous rupture of flexor tendons, ankle and foot
M66.371 Spontaneous rupture of flexor tendons, right ankle and foot
M66.372 Spontaneous rupture of flexor tendons, left ankle and foot
M66.379 Spontaneous rupture of flexor tendons, unspecified ankle and foot
M66.38 Spontaneous rupture of flexor tendons, other site
M66.39 Spontaneous rupture of flexor tendons, multiple sites
M66.8 Spontaneous rupture of other tendons
M66.80 Spontaneous rupture of other tendons, unspecified site
M66.81 Spontaneous rupture of other tendons, shoulder
M66.811 Spontaneous rupture of other tendons, right shoulder
M66.812 Spontaneous rupture of other tendons, left shoulder
M66.819 Spontaneous rupture of other tendons, unspecified shoulder
M66.82 Spontaneous rupture of other tendons, upper arm
M66.821 Spontaneous rupture of other tendons, right upper arm
M66.822 Spontaneous rupture of other tendons, left upper arm
M66.829 Spontaneous rupture of other tendons, unspecified upper arm
M66.83 Spontaneous rupture of other tendons, forearm
M66.831 Spontaneous rupture of other tendons, right forearm
M66.832 Spontaneous rupture of other tendons, left forearm
M66.839 Spontaneous rupture of other tendons, unspecified forearm
M66.84 Spontaneous rupture of other tendons, hand
M66.841 Spontaneous rupture of other tendons, right hand
M66.842 Spontaneous rupture of other tendons, left hand
M66.849 Spontaneous rupture of other tendons, unspecified hand
M66.85 Spontaneous rupture of other tendons, thigh
M66.851 Spontaneous rupture of other tendons, right thigh
M66.852 Spontaneous rupture of other tendons, left thigh
M66.859 Spontaneous rupture of other tendons, unspecified thigh
M66.86 Spontaneous rupture of other tendons, lower leg
M66.861 Spontaneous rupture of other tendons, right lower leg
M66.862 Spontaneous rupture of other tendons, left lower leg
M66.869 Spontaneous rupture of other tendons, unspecified lower leg
M66.87 Spontaneous rupture of other tendons, ankle and foot
M66.871 Spontaneous rupture of other tendons, right ankle and foot
M66.872 Spontaneous rupture of other tendons, left ankle and foot
M66.879 Spontaneous rupture of other tendons, unspecified ankle and foot
M66.88 Spontaneous rupture of other tendons, other
M66.89 Spontaneous rupture of other tendons, multiple sites
M66.9 Spontaneous rupture of unspecified tendon
Rupture at musculotendinous junction, nontraumatic

M67 Other disorders of synovium and tendon

EXCLUDES 1 *palmar fascial fibromatosis [Dupuytren] (M72.0)*
tendinitis NOS (M77.9-)
xanthomatosis localized to tendons (E78.2)

M67.0 Short Achilles tendon (acquired)
M67.00 Short Achilles tendon (acquired), unspecified ankle
M67.01 Short Achilles tendon (acquired), right ankle
M67.02 Short Achilles tendon (acquired), left ankle
M67.2 Synovial hypertrophy, not elsewhere classified
EXCLUDES 1 *villonodular synovitis (pigmented) (M12.2-)*
M67.20 Synovial hypertrophy, not elsewhere classified, unspecified site
M67.21 Synovial hypertrophy, not elsewhere classified, shoulder
M67.211 Synovial hypertrophy, not elsewhere classified, right shoulder
M67.212 Synovial hypertrophy, not elsewhere classified, left shoulder
M67.219 Synovial hypertrophy, not elsewhere classified, unspecified shoulder
M67.22 Synovial hypertrophy, not elsewhere classified, upper arm
M67.221 Synovial hypertrophy, not elsewhere classified, right upper arm
M67.222 Synovial hypertrophy, not elsewhere classified, left upper arm
M67.229 Synovial hypertrophy, not elsewhere classified, unspecified upper arm
M67.23 Synovial hypertrophy, not elsewhere classified, forearm
M67.231 Synovial hypertrophy, not elsewhere classified, right forearm
M67.232 Synovial hypertrophy, not elsewhere classified, left forearm
M67.239 Synovial hypertrophy, not elsewhere classified, unspecified forearm
M67.24 Synovial hypertrophy, not elsewhere classified, hand
M67.241 Synovial hypertrophy, not elsewhere classified, right hand
M67.242 Synovial hypertrophy, not elsewhere classified, left hand
M67.249 Synovial hypertrophy, not elsewhere classified, unspecified hand
M67.25 Synovial hypertrophy, not elsewhere classified, thigh
M67.251 Synovial hypertrophy, not elsewhere classified, right thigh
M67.252 Synovial hypertrophy, not elsewhere classified, left thigh
M67.259 Synovial hypertrophy, not elsewhere classified, unspecified thigh

6 M67.26 Synovial hypertrophy, not elsewhere classified, lower leg
- 7 M67.261 Synovial hypertrophy, not elsewhere classified, right lower leg
- 7 M67.262 Synovial hypertrophy, not elsewhere classified, left lower leg
- 7 M67.269 Synovial hypertrophy, not elsewhere classified, unspecified lower leg

6 M67.27 Synovial hypertrophy, not elsewhere classified, ankle and foot
- 7 M67.271 Synovial hypertrophy, not elsewhere classified, right ankle and foot
- 7 M67.272 Synovial hypertrophy, not elsewhere classified, left ankle and foot
- 7 M67.279 Synovial hypertrophy, not elsewhere classified, unspecified ankle and foot

M67.28 Synovial hypertrophy, not elsewhere classified, other site

M67.29 Synovial hypertrophy, not elsewhere classified, multiple sites

5 M67.3 Transient synovitis

Toxic synovitis

EXCLUDES 1 *palindromic rheumatism (M12.3-)*

M67.30 Transient synovitis, unspecified site

6 M67.31 Transient synovitis, shoulder
- 7 M67.311 Transient synovitis, right shoulder
- 7 M67.312 Transient synovitis, left shoulder
- 7 M67.319 Transient synovitis, unspecified shoulder

6 M67.32 Transient synovitis, elbow
- 7 M67.321 Transient synovitis, right elbow
- 7 M67.322 Transient synovitis, left elbow
- 7 M67.329 Transient synovitis, unspecified elbow

6 M67.33 Transient synovitis, wrist
- 7 M67.331 Transient synovitis, right wrist
- 7 M67.332 Transient synovitis, left wrist
- 7 M67.339 Transient synovitis, unspecified wrist

6 M67.34 Transient synovitis, hand
- 7 M67.341 Transient synovitis, right hand
- 7 M67.342 Transient synovitis, left hand
- 7 M67.349 Transient synovitis, unspecified hand

6 M67.35 Transient synovitis, hip
- 7 M67.351 Transient synovitis, right hip
- 7 M67.352 Transient synovitis, left hip
- 7 M67.359 Transient synovitis, unspecified hip

6 M67.36 Transient synovitis, knee
- 7 M67.361 Transient synovitis, right knee
- 7 M67.362 Transient synovitis, left knee
- 7 M67.369 Transient synovitis, unspecified knee

6 M67.37 Transient synovitis, ankle and foot
- 7 M67.371 Transient synovitis, right ankle and foot
- 7 M67.372 Transient synovitis, left ankle and foot
- 7 M67.379 Transient synovitis, unspecified ankle and foot

M67.38 Transient synovitis, other site

M67.39 Transient synovitis, multiple sites

5 M67.4 Ganglion

Ganglion of joint or tendon (sheath)

EXCLUDES 1 *ganglion in yaws (A66.6)*

EXCLUDES 2 *cyst of bursa (M71.2-M71.3)*
cyst of synovium (M71.2-M71.3)

M67.40 Ganglion, unspecified site

6 M67.41 Ganglion, shoulder
- 7 M67.411 Ganglion, right shoulder
- 7 M67.412 Ganglion, left shoulder
- 7 M67.419 Ganglion, unspecified shoulder

6 M67.42 Ganglion, elbow
- 7 M67.421 Ganglion, right elbow
- 7 M67.422 Ganglion, left elbow
- 7 M67.429 Ganglion, unspecified elbow

6 M67.43 Ganglion, wrist

Ganglion, wrist

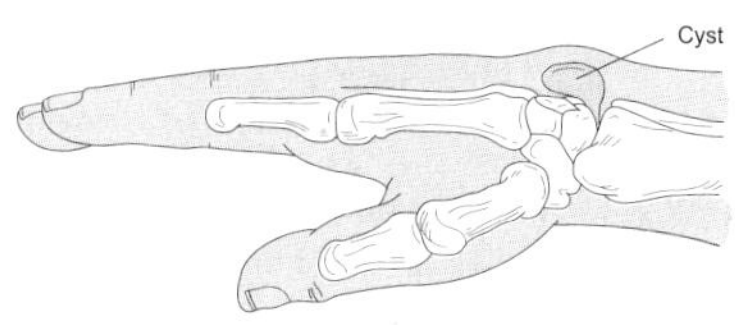

- 7 M67.431 Ganglion, right wrist
- 7 M67.432 Ganglion, left wrist
- 7 M67.439 Ganglion, unspecified wrist

6 M67.44 Ganglion, hand
- 7 M67.441 Ganglion, right hand
- 7 M67.442 Ganglion, left hand
- 7 M67.449 Ganglion, unspecified hand

6 M67.45 Ganglion, hip
- 7 M67.451 Ganglion, right hip
- 7 M67.452 Ganglion, left hip
- 7 M67.459 Ganglion, unspecified hip

6 M67.46 Ganglion, knee
- 7 M67.461 Ganglion, right knee
- 7 M67.462 Ganglion, left knee
- 7 M67.469 Ganglion, unspecified knee

6 M67.47 Ganglion, ankle and foot
- 7 M67.471 Ganglion, right ankle and foot
- 7 M67.472 Ganglion, left ankle and foot
- 7 M67.479 Ganglion, unspecified ankle and foot

M67.48 Ganglion, other site

M67.49 Ganglion, multiple sites

5 M67.5 Plica syndrome

Plica knee
- 7 M67.50 Plica syndrome, unspecified knee
- 7 M67.51 Plica syndrome, right knee
- 7 M67.52 Plica syndrome, left knee

5 M67.8 Other specified disorders of synovium and tendon

M67.80 Other specified disorders of synovium and tendon, unspecified site

6 M67.81 Other specified disorders of synovium and tendon, shoulder
- 7 M67.811 Other specified disorders of synovium, right shoulder
- 7 M67.812 Other specified disorders of synovium, left shoulder
- 7 M67.813 Other specified disorders of tendon, right shoulder
- 7 M67.814 Other specified disorders of tendon, left shoulder
- 7 M67.819 Other specified disorders of synovium and tendon, unspecified shoulder

6 M67.82 Other specified disorders of synovium and tendon, elbow
- 7 M67.821 Other specified disorders of synovium, right elbow
- 7 M67.822 Other specified disorders of synovium, left elbow
- 7 M67.823 Other specified disorders of tendon, right elbow
- 7 M67.824 Other specified disorders of tendon, left elbow
- 7 M67.829 Other specified disorders of synovium and tendon, unspecified elbow

6 M67.83 Other specified disorders of synovium and tendon, wrist
- 7 M67.831 Other specified disorders of synovium, right wrist
- 7 M67.832 Other specified disorders of synovium, left wrist
- 7 M67.833 Other specified disorders of tendon, right wrist
- 7 M67.834 Other specified disorders of tendon, left wrist
- 7 M67.839 Other specified disorders of synovium and tendon, unspecified forearm

6 M67.84 Other specified disorders of synovium and tendon, hand
- 7 M67.841 Other specified disorders of synovium, right hand

M67.842 Other specified disorders of synovium, left hand
M67.843 Other specified disorders of tendon, right hand
M67.844 Other specified disorders of tendon, left hand
M67.849 Other specified disorders of synovium and tendon, unspecified hand
M67.85 Other specified disorders of synovium and tendon, hip
M67.851 Other specified disorders of synovium, right hip
M67.852 Other specified disorders of synovium, left hip
M67.853 Other specified disorders of tendon, right hip
M67.854 Other specified disorders of tendon, left hip
M67.859 Other specified disorders of synovium and tendon, unspecified hip
M67.86 Other specified disorders of synovium and tendon, knee
M67.861 Other specified disorders of synovium, right knee
M67.862 Other specified disorders of synovium, left knee
M67.863 Other specified disorders of tendon, right knee
M67.864 Other specified disorders of tendon, left knee
M67.869 Other specified disorders of synovium and tendon, unspecified knee
M67.87 Other specified disorders of synovium and tendon, ankle and foot
M67.871 Other specified disorders of synovium, right ankle and foot
M67.872 Other specified disorders of synovium, left ankle and foot
M67.873 Other specified disorders of tendon, right ankle and foot
M67.874 Other specified disorders of tendon, left ankle and foot
M67.879 Other specified disorders of synovium and tendon, unspecified ankle and foot
M67.88 Other specified disorders of synovium and tendon, other site
M67.89 Other specified disorders of synovium and tendon, multiple sites
M67.9 Unspecified disorder of synovium and tendon
M67.90 Unspecified disorder of synovium and tendon, unspecified site
M67.91 Unspecified disorder of synovium and tendon, shoulder
M67.911 Unspecified disorder of synovium and tendon, right shoulder
M67.912 Unspecified disorder of synovium and tendon, left shoulder
M67.919 Unspecified disorder of synovium and tendon, unspecified shoulder
M67.92 Unspecified disorder of synovium and tendon, upper arm
M67.921 Unspecified disorder of synovium and tendon, right upper arm
M67.922 Unspecified disorder of synovium and tendon, left upper arm
M67.929 Unspecified disorder of synovium and tendon, unspecified upper arm
M67.93 Unspecified disorder of synovium and tendon, forearm
M67.931 Unspecified disorder of synovium and tendon, right forearm
M67.932 Unspecified disorder of synovium and tendon, left forearm
M67.939 Unspecified disorder of synovium and tendon, unspecified forearm
M67.94 Unspecified disorder of synovium and tendon, hand
M67.941 Unspecified disorder of synovium and tendon, right hand
M67.942 Unspecified disorder of synovium and tendon, left hand
M67.949 Unspecified disorder of synovium and tendon, unspecified hand
M67.95 Unspecified disorder of synovium and tendon, thigh
M67.951 Unspecified disorder of synovium and tendon, right thigh
M67.952 Unspecified disorder of synovium and tendon, left thigh
M67.959 Unspecified disorder of synovium and tendon, unspecified thigh
M67.96 Unspecified disorder of synovium and tendon, lower leg
M67.961 Unspecified disorder of synovium and tendon, right lower leg
M67.962 Unspecified disorder of synovium and tendon, left lower leg
M67.969 Unspecified disorder of synovium and tendon, unspecified lower leg
M67.97 Unspecified disorder of synovium and tendon, ankle and foot
M67.971 Unspecified disorder of synovium and tendon, right ankle and foot
M67.972 Unspecified disorder of synovium and tendon, left ankle and foot
M67.979 Unspecified disorder of synovium and tendon, unspecified ankle and foot
M67.98 Unspecified disorder of synovium and tendon, other site
M67.99 Unspecified disorder of synovium and tendon, multiple sites

Other soft tissue disorders (M70-M79)

M70 Soft tissue disorders related to use, overuse and pressure

INCLUDES soft tissue disorders of occupational origin

Use additional external cause code to identify activity causing disorder (Y93.-)

EXCLUDES 1 *bursitis NOS (M71.9-)*

EXCLUDES 2 *bursitis of shoulder (M75.5)*
enthesopathies (M76-M77)
pressure ulcer (pressure area) (L89.-)

M70.0 Crepitant synovitis (acute) (chronic) of hand and wrist
M70.03 Crepitant synovitis (acute) (chronic), wrist
M70.031 Crepitant synovitis (acute) (chronic), right wrist
M70.032 Crepitant synovitis (acute) (chronic), left wrist
M70.039 Crepitant synovitis (acute) (chronic), unspecified wrist
M70.04 Crepitant synovitis (acute) (chronic), hand
M70.041 Crepitant synovitis (acute) (chronic), right hand
M70.042 Crepitant synovitis (acute) (chronic), left hand
M70.049 Crepitant synovitis (acute) (chronic), unspecified hand
M70.1 Bursitis of hand
M70.10 Bursitis, unspecified hand
M70.11 Bursitis, right hand
M70.12 Bursitis, left hand
M70.2 Olecranon bursitis
M70.20 Olecranon bursitis, unspecified elbow
M70.21 Olecranon bursitis, right elbow
M70.22 Olecranon bursitis, left elbow
M70.3 Other bursitis of elbow
M70.30 Other bursitis of elbow, unspecified elbow
M70.31 Other bursitis of elbow, right elbow
M70.32 Other bursitis of elbow, left elbow
M70.4 Prepatellar bursitis
M70.40 Prepatellar bursitis, unspecified knee
M70.41 Prepatellar bursitis, right knee
M70.42 Prepatellar bursitis, left knee
M70.5 Other bursitis of knee
M70.50 Other bursitis of knee, unspecified knee
M70.51 Other bursitis of knee, right knee
M70.52 Other bursitis of knee, left knee
M70.6 Trochanteric bursitis
Trochanteric tendinitis
M70.60 Trochanteric bursitis, unspecified hip

M70.61 Trochanteric bursitis, right hip
M70.62 Trochanteric bursitis, left hip
M70.7 Other bursitis of hip
Ischial bursitis
M70.70 Other bursitis of hip, unspecified hip
M70.71 Other bursitis of hip, right hip
M70.72 Other bursitis of hip, left hip
M70.8 Other soft tissue disorders related to use, overuse and pressure
M70.80 Other soft tissue disorders related to use, overuse and pressure of unspecified site
M70.81 Other soft tissue disorders related to use, overuse and pressure of shoulder
M70.811 Other soft tissue disorders related to use, overuse and pressure, right shoulder
M70.812 Other soft tissue disorders related to use, overuse and pressure, left shoulder
M70.819 Other soft tissue disorders related to use, overuse and pressure, unspecified shoulder
M70.82 Other soft tissue disorders related to use, overuse and pressure of upper arm
M70.821 Other soft tissue disorders related to use, overuse and pressure, right upper arm
M70.822 Other soft tissue disorders related to use, overuse and pressure, left upper arm
M70.829 Other soft tissue disorders related to use, overuse and pressure, unspecified upper arms
M70.83 Other soft tissue disorders related to use, overuse and pressure of forearm
M70.831 Other soft tissue disorders related to use, overuse and pressure, right forearm
M70.832 Other soft tissue disorders related to use, overuse and pressure, left forearm
M70.839 Other soft tissue disorders related to use, overuse and pressure, unspecified forearm
M70.84 Other soft tissue disorders related to use, overuse and pressure of hand
M70.841 Other soft tissue disorders related to use, overuse and pressure, right hand
M70.842 Other soft tissue disorders related to use, overuse and pressure, left hand
M70.849 Other soft tissue disorders related to use, overuse and pressure, unspecified hand
M70.85 Other soft tissue disorders related to use, overuse and pressure of thigh
M70.851 Other soft tissue disorders related to use, overuse and pressure, right thigh
M70.852 Other soft tissue disorders related to use, overuse and pressure, left thigh
M70.859 Other soft tissue disorders related to use, overuse and pressure, unspecified thigh
M70.86 Other soft tissue disorders related to use, overuse and pressure lower leg
M70.861 Other soft tissue disorders related to use, overuse and pressure, right lower leg
M70.862 Other soft tissue disorders related to use, overuse and pressure, left lower leg
M70.869 Other soft tissue disorders related to use, overuse and pressure, unspecified leg
M70.87 Other soft tissue disorders related to use, overuse and pressure of ankle and foot
M70.871 Other soft tissue disorders related to use, overuse and pressure, right ankle and foot
M70.872 Other soft tissue disorders related to use, overuse and pressure, left ankle and foot
M70.879 Other soft tissue disorders related to use, overuse and pressure, unspecified ankle and foot
M70.88 Other soft tissue disorders related to use, overuse and pressure other site
M70.89 Other soft tissue disorders related to use, overuse and pressure multiple sites
M70.9 Unspecified soft tissue disorder related to use, overuse and pressure
M70.90 Unspecified soft tissue disorder related to use, overuse and pressure of unspecified site
M70.91 Unspecified soft tissue disorder related to use, overuse and pressure of shoulder
M70.911 Unspecified soft tissue disorder related to use, overuse and pressure, right shoulder
M70.912 Unspecified soft tissue disorder related to use, overuse and pressure, left shoulder
M70.919 Unspecified soft tissue disorder related to use, overuse and pressure, unspecified shoulder
M70.92 Unspecified soft tissue disorder related to use, overuse and pressure of upper arm
M70.921 Unspecified soft tissue disorder related to use, overuse and pressure, right upper arm
M70.922 Unspecified soft tissue disorder related to use, overuse and pressure, left upper arm
M70.929 Unspecified soft tissue disorder related to use, overuse and pressure, unspecified upper arm
M70.93 Unspecified soft tissue disorder related to use, overuse and pressure of forearm
M70.931 Unspecified soft tissue disorder related to use, overuse and pressure, right forearm
M70.932 Unspecified soft tissue disorder related to use, overuse and pressure, left forearm
M70.939 Unspecified soft tissue disorder related to use, overuse and pressure, unspecified forearm
M70.94 Unspecified soft tissue disorder related to use, overuse and pressure of hand
M70.941 Unspecified soft tissue disorder related to use, overuse and pressure, right hand
M70.942 Unspecified soft tissue disorder related to use, overuse and pressure, left hand
M70.949 Unspecified soft tissue disorder related to use, overuse and pressure, unspecified hand
M70.95 Unspecified soft tissue disorder related to use, overuse and pressure of thigh
M70.951 Unspecified soft tissue disorder related to use, overuse and pressure, right thigh
M70.952 Unspecified soft tissue disorder related to use, overuse and pressure, left thigh
M70.959 Unspecified soft tissue disorder related to use, overuse and pressure, unspecified thigh
M70.96 Unspecified soft tissue disorder related to use, overuse and pressure lower leg
M70.961 Unspecified soft tissue disorder related to use, overuse and pressure, right lower leg
M70.962 Unspecified soft tissue disorder related to use, overuse and pressure, left lower leg
M70.969 Unspecified soft tissue disorder related to use, overuse and pressure, unspecified lower leg
M70.97 Unspecified soft tissue disorder related to use, overuse and pressure of ankle and foot
M70.971 Unspecified soft tissue disorder related to use, overuse and pressure, right ankle and foot
M70.972 Unspecified soft tissue disorder related to use, overuse and pressure, left ankle and foot
M70.979 Unspecified soft tissue disorder related to use, overuse and pressure, unspecified ankle and foot
M70.98 Unspecified soft tissue disorder related to use, overuse and pressure other
M70.99 Unspecified soft tissue disorder related to use, overuse and pressure multiple sites

M71 Other bursopathies

EXCLUDES 1 *bunion (M20.1)*
bursitis related to use, overuse or pressure (M70.-)
enthesopathies (M76-M77)

M71.0 Abscess of bursa
Use additional code (B95.-, B96.-) to identify causative organism
M71.00 Abscess of bursa, unspecified site
M71.01 Abscess of bursa, shoulder

- M71.011 Abscess of bursa, right shoulder
- M71.012 Abscess of bursa, left shoulder
- M71.019 Abscess of bursa, unspecified shoulder
- M71.02 Abscess of bursa, elbow
  - M71.021 Abscess of bursa, right elbow
  - M71.022 Abscess of bursa, left elbow
  - M71.029 Abscess of bursa, unspecified elbow
- M71.03 Abscess of bursa, wrist
  - M71.031 Abscess of bursa, right wrist
  - M71.032 Abscess of bursa, left wrist
  - M71.039 Abscess of bursa, unspecified wrist
- M71.04 Abscess of bursa, hand
  - M71.041 Abscess of bursa, right hand
  - M71.042 Abscess of bursa, left hand
  - M71.049 Abscess of bursa, unspecified hand
- M71.05 Abscess of bursa, hip
  - M71.051 Abscess of bursa, right hip
  - M71.052 Abscess of bursa, left hip
  - M71.059 Abscess of bursa, unspecified hip
- M71.06 Abscess of bursa, knee
  - M71.061 Abscess of bursa, right knee
  - M71.062 Abscess of bursa, left knee
  - M71.069 Abscess of bursa, unspecified knee
- M71.07 Abscess of bursa, ankle and foot
  - M71.071 Abscess of bursa, right ankle and foot
  - M71.072 Abscess of bursa, left ankle and foot
  - M71.079 Abscess of bursa, unspecified ankle and foot
- M71.08 Abscess of bursa, other site
- M71.09 Abscess of bursa, multiple sites

M71.1 Other infective bursitis

Use additional code (B95.-, B96.-) to identify causative organism

- M71.10 Other infective bursitis, unspecified site
- M71.11 Other infective bursitis, shoulder
  - M71.111 Other infective bursitis, right shoulder
  - M71.112 Other infective bursitis, left shoulder
  - M71.119 Other infective bursitis, unspecified shoulder
- M71.12 Other infective bursitis, elbow
  - M71.121 Other infective bursitis, right elbow
  - M71.122 Other infective bursitis, left elbow
  - M71.129 Other infective bursitis, unspecified elbow
- M71.13 Other infective bursitis, wrist
  - M71.131 Other infective bursitis, right wrist
  - M71.132 Other infective bursitis, left wrist
  - M71.139 Other infective bursitis, unspecified wrist
- M71.14 Other infective bursitis, hand
  - M71.141 Other infective bursitis, right hand
  - M71.142 Other infective bursitis, left hand
  - M71.149 Other infective bursitis, unspecified hand
- M71.15 Other infective bursitis, hip
  - M71.151 Other infective bursitis, right hip
  - M71.152 Other infective bursitis, left hip
  - M71.159 Other infective bursitis, unspecified hip
- M71.16 Other infective bursitis, knee
  - M71.161 Other infective bursitis, right knee
  - M71.162 Other infective bursitis, left knee
  - M71.169 Other infective bursitis, unspecified knee
- M71.17 Other infective bursitis, ankle and foot
  - M71.171 Other infective bursitis, right ankle and foot
  - M71.172 Other infective bursitis, left ankle and foot
  - M71.179 Other infective bursitis, unspecified ankle and foot
- M71.18 Other infective bursitis, other site
- M71.19 Other infective bursitis, multiple sites

M71.2 Synovial cyst of popliteal space [Baker]

EXCLUDES 1 *synovial cyst of popliteal space with rupture (M66.0)*

DEFINITION Collection of synovial fluid that has escaped from the knee joint or bursa and has formed a synovial-lined sac behind the knee.

- M71.20 Synovial cyst of popliteal space [Baker], unspecified knee
- M71.21 Synovial cyst of popliteal space [Baker], right knee
- M71.22 Synovial cyst of popliteal space [Baker], left knee

M71.3 Other bursal cyst

Synovial cyst NOS

EXCLUDES 1 *synovial cyst with rupture (M66.1-)*

- M71.30 Other bursal cyst, unspecified site
- M71.31 Other bursal cyst, shoulder
  - M71.311 Other bursal cyst, right shoulder
  - M71.312 Other bursal cyst, left shoulder
  - M71.319 Other bursal cyst, unspecified shoulder
- M71.32 Other bursal cyst, elbow
  - M71.321 Other bursal cyst, right elbow
  - M71.322 Other bursal cyst, left elbow
  - M71.329 Other bursal cyst, unspecified elbow
- M71.33 Other bursal cyst, wrist
  - M71.331 Other bursal cyst, right wrist
  - M71.332 Other bursal cyst, left wrist
  - M71.339 Other bursal cyst, unspecified wrist
- M71.34 Other bursal cyst, hand
  - M71.341 Other bursal cyst, right hand
  - M71.342 Other bursal cyst, left hand
  - M71.349 Other bursal cyst, unspecified hand
- M71.35 Other bursal cyst, hip
  - M71.351 Other bursal cyst, right hip
  - M71.352 Other bursal cyst, left hip
  - M71.359 Other bursal cyst, unspecified hip
- M71.37 Other bursal cyst, ankle and foot
  - M71.371 Other bursal cyst, right ankle and foot
  - M71.372 Other bursal cyst, left ankle and foot
  - M71.379 Other bursal cyst, unspecified ankle and foot
- M71.38 Other bursal cyst, other site
- M71.39 Other bursal cyst, multiple sites

M71.4 Calcium deposit in bursa

EXCLUDES 2 *calcium deposit in bursa of shoulder (M75.3)*

- M71.40 Calcium deposit in bursa, unspecified site
- M71.42 Calcium deposit in bursa, elbow
  - M71.421 Calcium deposit in bursa, right elbow
  - M71.422 Calcium deposit in bursa, left elbow
  - M71.429 Calcium deposit in bursa, unspecified elbow
- M71.43 Calcium deposit in bursa, wrist
  - M71.431 Calcium deposit in bursa, right wrist
  - M71.432 Calcium deposit in bursa, left wrist
  - M71.439 Calcium deposit in bursa, unspecified wrist
- M71.44 Calcium deposit in bursa, hand
  - M71.441 Calcium deposit in bursa, right hand
  - M71.442 Calcium deposit in bursa, left hand
  - M71.449 Calcium deposit in bursa, unspecified hand
- M71.45 Calcium deposit in bursa, hip
  - M71.451 Calcium deposit in bursa, right hip
  - M71.452 Calcium deposit in bursa, left hip
  - M71.459 Calcium deposit in bursa, unspecified hip
- M71.46 Calcium deposit in bursa, knee
  - M71.461 Calcium deposit in bursa, right knee
  - M71.462 Calcium deposit in bursa, left knee
  - M71.469 Calcium deposit in bursa, unspecified knee
- M71.47 Calcium deposit in bursa, ankle and foot
  - M71.471 Calcium deposit in bursa, right ankle and foot
  - M71.472 Calcium deposit in bursa, left ankle and foot
  - M71.479 Calcium deposit in bursa, unspecified ankle and foot
- M71.48 Calcium deposit in bursa, other site
- M71.49 Calcium deposit in bursa, multiple sites

5 **M71.5** Other bursitis, not elsewhere classified
EXCLUDES 1 *bursitis NOS (M71.9-)*
EXCLUDES 2 *bursitis of shoulder (M75.5)*
bursitis of tibial collateral [Pellegrini-Stieda] (M76.4-)
M71.50 **Other bursitis, not elsewhere classified, unspecified site**
6 **M71.52** Other bursitis, not elsewhere classified, elbow
- **M71.521** Other bursitis, not elsewhere classified, right elbow
- **M71.522** Other bursitis, not elsewhere classified, left elbow
- **M71.529** **Other bursitis, not elsewhere classified, unspecified elbow**

6 **M71.53** Other bursitis, not elsewhere classified, wrist
- **M71.531** Other bursitis, not elsewhere classified, right wrist
- **M71.532** Other bursitis, not elsewhere classified, left wrist
- **M71.539** **Other bursitis, not elsewhere classified, unspecified wrist**

6 **M71.54** Other bursitis, not elsewhere classified, hand
- **M71.541** Other bursitis, not elsewhere classified, right hand
- **M71.542** Other bursitis, not elsewhere classified, left hand
- **M71.549** **Other bursitis, not elsewhere classified, unspecified hand**

6 **M71.55** Other bursitis, not elsewhere classified, hip
- **M71.551** Other bursitis, not elsewhere classified, right hip
- **M71.552** Other bursitis, not elsewhere classified, left hip
- **M71.559** **Other bursitis, not elsewhere classified, unspecified hip**

6 **M71.56** Other bursitis, not elsewhere classified, knee
- **M71.561** Other bursitis, not elsewhere classified, right knee
- **M71.562** Other bursitis, not elsewhere classified, left knee
- **M71.569** **Other bursitis, not elsewhere classified, unspecified knee**

6 **M71.57** Other bursitis, not elsewhere classified, ankle and foot
- **M71.571** Other bursitis, not elsewhere classified, right ankle and foot
- **M71.572** Other bursitis, not elsewhere classified, left ankle and foot
- **M71.579** **Other bursitis, not elsewhere classified, unspecified ankle and foot**

M71.58 Other bursitis, not elsewhere classified, other site

5 **M71.8** Other specified bursopathies
M71.80 **Other specified bursopathies, unspecified site**
6 **M71.81** Other specified bursopathies, shoulder
- **M71.811** Other specified bursopathies, right shoulder
- **M71.812** Other specified bursopathies, left shoulder
- **M71.819** **Other specified bursopathies, unspecified shoulder**

6 **M71.82** Other specified bursopathies, elbow
- **M71.821** Other specified bursopathies, right elbow
- **M71.822** Other specified bursopathies, left elbow
- **M71.829** **Other specified bursopathies, unspecified elbow**

6 **M71.83** Other specified bursopathies, wrist
- **M71.831** Other specified bursopathies, right wrist
- **M71.832** Other specified bursopathies, left wrist
- **M71.839** **Other specified bursopathies, unspecified wrist**

6 **M71.84** Other specified bursopathies, hand
- **M71.841** Other specified bursopathies, right hand
- **M71.842** Other specified bursopathies, left hand
- **M71.849** **Other specified bursopathies, unspecified hand**

6 **M71.85** Other specified bursopathies, hip
- **M71.851** Other specified bursopathies, right hip
- **M71.852** Other specified bursopathies, left hip
- **M71.859** **Other specified bursopathies, unspecified hip**

6 **M71.86** Other specified bursopathies, knee
- **M71.861** Other specified bursopathies, right knee
- **M71.862** Other specified bursopathies, left knee
- **M71.869** **Other specified bursopathies, unspecified knee**

6 **M71.87** Other specified bursopathies, ankle and foot
- **M71.871** Other specified bursopathies, right ankle and foot
- **M71.872** Other specified bursopathies, left ankle and foot
- **M71.879** **Other specified bursopathies, unspecified ankle and foot**

M71.88 Other specified bursopathies, other site
M71.89 Other specified bursopathies, multiple sites
M71.9 **Bursopathy, unspecified**
Bursitis NOS

4 **M72** **Fibroblastic disorders**
EXCLUDES 2 *retroperitoneal fibromatosis (D48.3)*
M72.0 **Palmar fascial fibromatosis [Dupuytren]** A
M72.1 **Knuckle pads**
M72.2 **Plantar fascial fibromatosis**
Plantar fasciitis

Plantar fascial fibromatosis

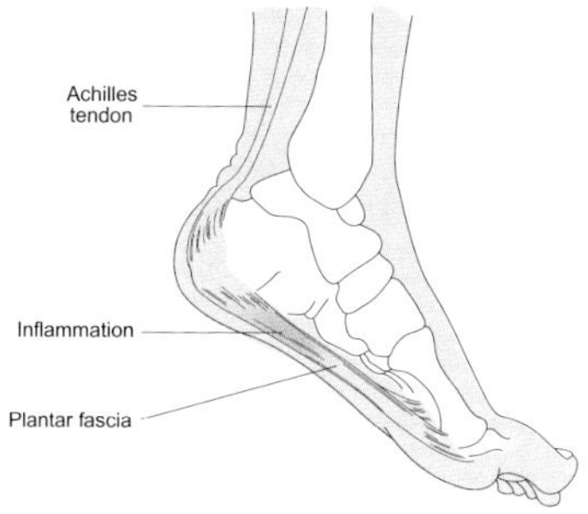

M72.4 **Pseudosarcomatous fibromatosis**
Nodular fasciitis
M72.6 **Necrotizing fasciitis** HCC
Use additional code (B95.-, B96.-) to identify causative organism
M72.8 **Other fibroblastic disorders**
Abscess of fascia
Fasciitis NEC
Other infective fasciitis
Use additional code to (B95.-, B96.-) identify causative organism
EXCLUDES 1 *diffuse (eosinophilic) fasciitis (M35.4)*
necrotizing fasciitis (M72.6)
nodular fasciitis (M72.4)
perirenal fasciitis NOS (N13.5)
perirenal fasciitis with infection (N13.6)
plantar fasciitis (M72.2)
M72.9 **Fibroblastic disorder, unspecified**
Fasciitis NOS
Fibromatosis NOS

4 **M75** **Shoulder lesions**
EXCLUDES 2 *shoulder-hand syndrome (M89.0-)*
5 **M75.0** **Adhesive capsulitis of shoulder**
Frozen shoulder
Periarthritis of shoulder
- **M75.00** **Adhesive capsulitis of unspecified shoulder**
- **M75.01** **Adhesive capsulitis of right shoulder**
- **M75.02** **Adhesive capsulitis of left shoulder**
  AHA: 2Q 2015, 23

5 **M75.1 Rotator cuff tear or rupture, not specified as traumatic**
Rotator cuff syndrome
Supraspinatus tear or rupture, not specified as traumatic
Supraspinatus syndrome
EXCLUDES 1 *tear of rotator cuff, traumatic (S46.01-)*

Rotator cuff tear or rupture
not specified as traumatic

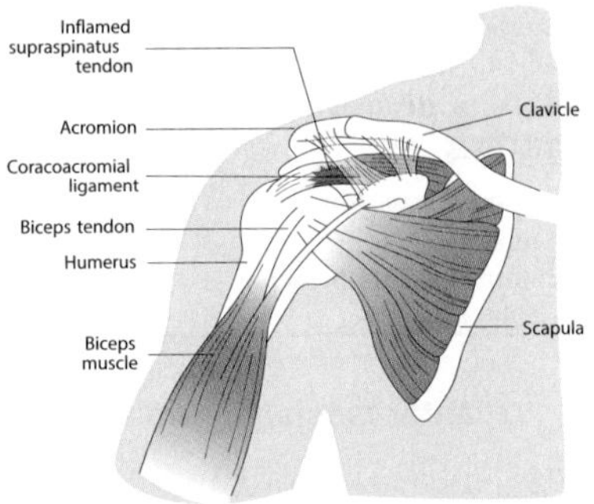

6 **M75.10 Unspecified rotator cuff tear or rupture, not specified as traumatic**
- **M75.100 Unspecified rotator cuff tear or rupture of unspecified shoulder, not specified as traumatic**
- **M75.101 Unspecified rotator cuff tear or rupture of right shoulder, not specified as traumatic**
- **M75.102 Unspecified rotator cuff tear or rupture of left shoulder, not specified as traumatic**

6 **M75.11 Incomplete rotator cuff tear or rupture not specified as traumatic**
- **M75.110 Incomplete rotator cuff tear or rupture of unspecified shoulder, not specified as traumatic**
- **M75.111 Incomplete rotator cuff tear or rupture of right shoulder, not specified as traumatic**
- **M75.112 Incomplete rotator cuff tear or rupture of left shoulder, not specified as traumatic**

6 **M75.12 Complete rotator cuff tear or rupture not specified as traumatic**
CODING TIP✓ A complete tear of the rotator cuff is a complete tear of one or more of the four tendons. For rotator cuff tears due to trauma, use S46.01-.

Complete rotator cuff tear or rupture

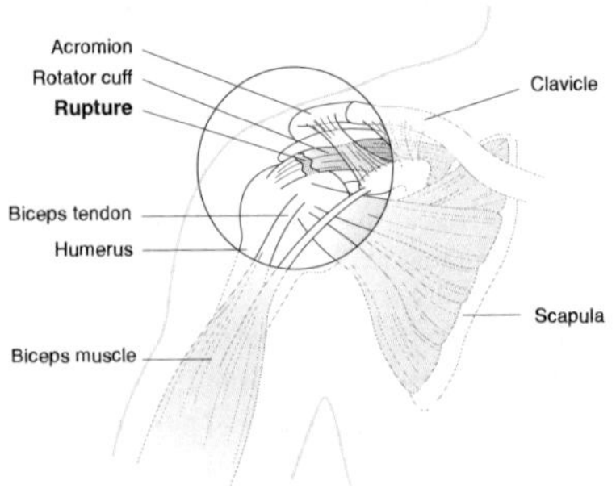

- **M75.120 Complete rotator cuff tear or rupture of unspecified shoulder, not specified as traumatic**
- **M75.121 Complete rotator cuff tear or rupture of right shoulder, not specified as traumatic**
- **M75.122 Complete rotator cuff tear or rupture of left shoulder, not specified as traumatic**

5 **M75.2 Bicipital tendinitis**
- **M75.20 Bicipital tendinitis, unspecified shoulder**
- **M75.21 Bicipital tendinitis, right shoulder**
- **M75.22 Bicipital tendinitis, left shoulder**

5 **M75.3 Calcific tendinitis of shoulder**
Calcified bursa of shoulder
- **M75.30 Calcific tendinitis of unspecified shoulder**
- **M75.31 Calcific tendinitis of right shoulder**
- **M75.32 Calcific tendinitis of left shoulder**

5 **M75.4 Impingement syndrome of shoulder**
- **M75.40 Impingement syndrome of unspecified shoulder**
- **M75.41 Impingement syndrome of right shoulder**
- **M75.42 Impingement syndrome of left shoulder**

5 **M75.5 Bursitis of shoulder**
- **M75.50 Bursitis of unspecified shoulder**
- **M75.51 Bursitis of right shoulder**
- **M75.52 Bursitis of left shoulder**

5 **M75.8 Other shoulder lesions**
- **M75.80 Other shoulder lesions, unspecified shoulder**
- **M75.81 Other shoulder lesions, right shoulder**
- **M75.82 Other shoulder lesions, left shoulder**

5 **M75.9 Shoulder lesion, unspecified**
- **M75.90 Shoulder lesion, unspecified, unspecified shoulder**
- **M75.91 Shoulder lesion, unspecified, right shoulder**
- **M75.92 Shoulder lesion, unspecified, left shoulder**

4 M76 Enthesopathies, lower limb, excluding foot
EXCLUDES 2 *bursitis due to use, overuse and pressure (M70.-)*
enthesopathies of ankle and foot (M77.5-)

5 **M76.0 Gluteal tendinitis**
- **M76.00 Gluteal tendinitis, unspecified hip**
- **M76.01 Gluteal tendinitis, right hip**
- **M76.02 Gluteal tendinitis, left hip**

5 **M76.1 Psoas tendinitis**
- **M76.10 Psoas tendinitis, unspecified hip**
- **M76.11 Psoas tendinitis, right hip**
- **M76.12 Psoas tendinitis, left hip**

5 **M76.2 Iliac crest spur**
- **M76.20 Iliac crest spur, unspecified hip**
- **M76.21 Iliac crest spur, right hip**
- **M76.22 Iliac crest spur, left hip**

5 **M76.3 Iliotibial band syndrome**
- **M76.30 Iliotibial band syndrome, unspecified leg**
- **M76.31 Iliotibial band syndrome, right leg**
- **M76.32 Iliotibial band syndrome, left leg**

5 **M76.4 Tibial collateral bursitis [Pellegrini-Stieda]**
- **M76.40 Tibial collateral bursitis [Pellegrini-Stieda], unspecified leg**
- **M76.41 Tibial collateral bursitis [Pellegrini-Stieda], right leg**
- **M76.42 Tibial collateral bursitis [Pellegrini-Stieda], left leg**

5 **M76.5 Patellar tendinitis**
- **M76.50 Patellar tendinitis, unspecified knee**
- **M76.51 Patellar tendinitis, right knee**
- **M76.52 Patellar tendinitis, left knee**

5 **M76.6 Achilles tendinitis**
Achilles bursitis
- **M76.60 Achilles tendinitis, unspecified leg**
- **M76.61 Achilles tendinitis, right leg**
- **M76.62 Achilles tendinitis, left leg**

5 **M76.7 Peroneal tendinitis**
- **M76.70 Peroneal tendinitis, unspecified leg**
- **M76.71 Peroneal tendinitis, right leg**
- **M76.72 Peroneal tendinitis, left leg**

5 **M76.8 Other specified enthesopathies of lower limb, excluding foot**

6 **M76.81 Anterior tibial syndrome**
- **M76.811 Anterior tibial syndrome, right leg**
- **M76.812 Anterior tibial syndrome, left leg**
- **M76.819 Anterior tibial syndrome, unspecified leg**

6 **M76.82 Posterior tibial tendinitis**
- **M76.821 Posterior tibial tendinitis, right leg**
- **M76.822 Posterior tibial tendinitis, left leg**
- **M76.829 Posterior tibial tendinitis, unspecified leg**

6 **M76.89 Other specified enthesopathies of lower limb, excluding foot**

M76.891 Other specified enthesopathies of right lower limb, excluding foot
M76.892 Other specified enthesopathies of left lower limb, excluding foot
M76.899 Other specified enthesopathies of unspecified lower limb, excluding foot
M76.9 Unspecified enthesopathy, lower limb, excluding foot

M77 Other enthesopathies

EXCLUDES 1 *bursitis NOS (M71.9-)*

EXCLUDES 2 *bursitis due to use, overuse and pressure (M70.-)*
osteophyte (M25.7)
spinal enthesopathy (M46.0-)

M77.0 Medial epicondylitis
M77.00 Medial epicondylitis, unspecified elbow
M77.01 Medial epicondylitis, right elbow
M77.02 Medial epicondylitis, left elbow
M77.1 Lateral epicondylitis
Tennis elbow

DEFINITION A painful inflammation of the tendons that anchor the extensor carpi radialis brevis muscle to the outer aspect of the humerus at the elbow.

M77.10 Lateral epicondylitis, unspecified elbow
M77.11 Lateral epicondylitis, right elbow
M77.12 Lateral epicondylitis, left elbow
M77.2 Periarthritis of wrist
M77.20 Periarthritis, unspecified wrist
M77.21 Periarthritis, right wrist
M77.22 Periarthritis, left wrist
M77.3 Calcaneal spur

Calcaneal spur

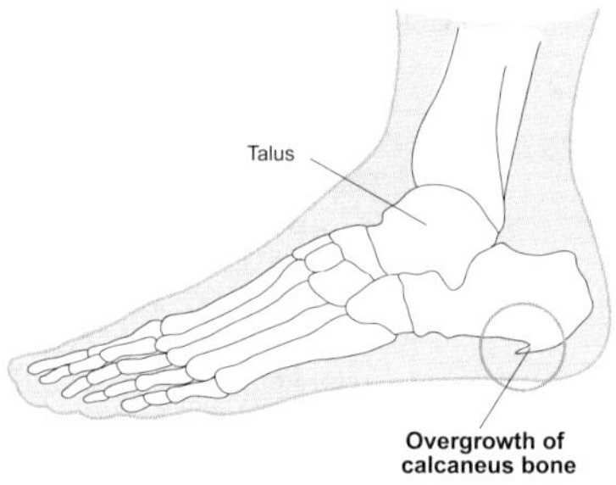

M77.30 Calcaneal spur, unspecified foot
M77.31 Calcaneal spur, right foot
M77.32 Calcaneal spur, left foot
M77.4 Metatarsalgia

EXCLUDES 1 *Morton's metatarsalgia (G57.6)*

M77.40 Metatarsalgia, unspecified foot
M77.41 Metatarsalgia, right foot
M77.42 Metatarsalgia, left foot
M77.5 Other enthesopathy of foot
M77.50 Other enthesopathy of unspecified foot
M77.51 Other enthesopathy of right foot
M77.52 Other enthesopathy of left foot
M77.8 Other enthesopathies, not elsewhere classified
M77.9 Enthesopathy, unspecified
Bone spur NOS
Capsulitis NOS
Periarthritis NOS
Tendinitis NOS

M79 Other and unspecified soft tissue disorders, not elsewhere classified

EXCLUDES 1 *psychogenic rheumatism (F45.8)*
soft tissue pain, psychogenic (F45.41)

M79.0 Rheumatism, unspecified

EXCLUDES 1 *fibromyalgia (M79.7)*
palindromic rheumatism (M12.3-)

▲ M79.1 Myalgia
Myofascial pain syndrome

EXCLUDES 1 *fibromyalgia (M79.7)*
myositis (M60.-)

● M79.10 Myalgia, unspecified site
● M79.11 Myalgia of mastication muscle
● M79.12 Myalgia of auxiliary muscles, head and neck
● M79.18 Myalgia, other site
M79.2 Neuralgia and neuritis, unspecified

EXCLUDES 1 *brachial radiculitis NOS (M54.1)*
lumbosacral radiculitis NOS (M54.1)
mononeuropathies (G56-G58)
radiculitis NOS (M54.1)
sciatica (M54.3-M54.4)

M79.3 Panniculitis, unspecified

EXCLUDES 1 *lupus panniculitis (L93.2)*
neck and back panniculitis (M54.0-)
relapsing [Weber-Christian] panniculitis (M35.6)

M79.4 Hypertrophy of (infrapatellar) fat pad
M79.5 Residual foreign body in soft tissue

EXCLUDES 1 *foreign body granuloma of skin and subcutaneous tissue (L92.3)*
foreign body granuloma of soft tissue (M60.2-)

CODING TIP ✓ Foreign body refers to something that is not meant to be part of the soft tissue.

M79.6 Pain in limb, hand, foot, fingers and toes

EXCLUDES 2 *pain in joint (M25.5-)*

CODING TIP ✓ These codes should be used when 1) the cause of the pain is unknown; 2) the pain is a sequela of an injury; or 3) in conjunction with a G89 code. Do not use these codes with conditions where pain is integral.

M79.60 Pain in limb, unspecified
M79.601 Pain in right arm
Pain in right upper limb NOS
M79.602 Pain in left arm
Pain in left upper limb NOS
M79.603 Pain in arm, unspecified
Pain in upper limb NOS
M79.604 Pain in right leg
Pain in right lower limb NOS
M79.605 Pain in left leg
Pain in left lower limb NOS
M79.606 Pain in leg, unspecified
Pain in lower limb NOS
M79.609 Pain in unspecified limb
Pain in limb NOS
M79.62 Pain in upper arm
Pain in axillary region
M79.621 Pain in right upper arm
M79.622 Pain in left upper arm
M79.629 Pain in unspecified upper arm
M79.63 Pain in forearm
M79.631 Pain in right forearm
M79.632 Pain in left forearm
M79.639 Pain in unspecified forearm
M79.64 Pain in hand and fingers
M79.641 Pain in right hand
M79.642 Pain in left hand
M79.643 Pain in unspecified hand
M79.644 Pain in right finger(s)
M79.645 Pain in left finger(s)
M79.646 Pain in unspecified finger(s)
M79.65 Pain in thigh
M79.651 Pain in right thigh
M79.652 Pain in left thigh
M79.659 Pain in unspecified thigh
M79.66 Pain in lower leg
M79.661 Pain in right lower leg
M79.662 Pain in left lower leg
M79.669 Pain in unspecified lower leg
M79.67 Pain in foot and toes

M79.671 Pain in right foot
M79.672 Pain in left foot
M79.673 Pain in unspecified foot
M79.674 Pain in right toe(s)
M79.675 Pain in left toe(s)
M79.676 Pain in unspecified toe(s)

M79.7 Fibromyalgia
Fibromyositis
Fibrositis
Myofibrositis

M79.A Nontraumatic compartment syndrome
Code first:
, if applicable, associated postprocedural complication
EXCLUDES 1 *compartment syndrome NOS (T79.A-)*
fibromyalgia (M79.7)
nontraumatic ischemic infarction of muscle (M62.2-)
traumatic compartment syndrome (T79.A-)

M79.A1 Nontraumatic compartment syndrome of upper extremity
Nontraumatic compartment syndrome of shoulder, arm, forearm, wrist, hand, and fingers
M79.A11 Nontraumatic compartment syndrome of right upper extremity
M79.A12 Nontraumatic compartment syndrome of left upper extremity
M79.A19 Nontraumatic compartment syndrome of unspecified upper extremity

M79.A2 Nontraumatic compartment syndrome of lower extremity
Nontraumatic compartment syndrome of hip, buttock, thigh, leg, foot, and toes
M79.A21 Nontraumatic compartment syndrome of right lower extremity
M79.A22 Nontraumatic compartment syndrome of left lower extremity
M79.A29 Nontraumatic compartment syndrome of unspecified lower extremity

M79.A3 Nontraumatic compartment syndrome of abdomen
M79.A9 Nontraumatic compartment syndrome of other sites

M79.8 Other specified soft tissue disorders
M79.81 Nontraumatic hematoma of soft tissue
Nontraumatic hematoma of muscle
Nontraumatic seroma of muscle and soft tissue
DEFINITION A spontaneous, nontraumatic localized collection of partially clotted blood within a soft tissue such as muscle.
M79.89 Other specified soft tissue disorders
Polyalgia

M79.9 Soft tissue disorder, unspecified

Osteopathies and chondropathies (M80-M94)

Disorders of bone density and structure (M80-M85)

M80 Osteoporosis with current pathological fracture
INCLUDES osteoporosis with current fragility fracture
Use additional code to identify major osseous defect, if applicable (M89.7-)
EXCLUDES 1 *collapsed vertebra NOS (M48.5)*
pathological fracture NOS (M84.4)
wedging of vertebra NOS (M48.5)
EXCLUDES 2 *personal history of (healed) osteoporosis fracture (Z87.310)*

The appropriate 7th character is to be added to each code from category M80:

A	initial encounter for fracture
D	subsequent encounter for fracture with routine healing
G	subsequent encounter for fracture with delayed healing
K	subsequent encounter for fracture with nonunion
P	subsequent encounter for fracture with malunion
S	sequela

GUIDELINES **Section I.C.13.c**
Coding of Pathologic Fractures: 7th character D is to be used for encounters after the patient has completed active treatment for the fracture and is receiving routine care for the fracture during the healing or recovery phase. The other 7th characters, listed under each subcategory in the Tabular List, are to be used for subsequent encounters for treatment of problems associated with the healing, such as malunions, nonunions, and sequelae.
Care for complications of surgical treatment for fracture repairs during the healing or recovery phase should be coded with the appropriate complication codes.

GUIDELINES **Section I.C.13.d.2)**
Category M80, Osteoporosis with current pathological fracture, is for patients who have a current pathologic fracture at the time of an encounter. The codes under M80 identify the site of the fracture. A code from category M80, not a traumatic fracture code, should be used for any patient with known osteoporosis who suffers a fracture, even if the patient had a minor fall or trauma, if that fall or trauma would not usually break a normal, healthy bone.

CODING TIP When a patient with osteoporosis is noted to have an active fracture, use the osteoporosis fracture codes, even if the patient had a minor fall or trauma (fall from standing height or less), unless the physician has identified the fracture as a traumatic fracture. Age-related osteoporosis includes post-menopausal and senile osteoporosis, as well as unspecified. Age-related osteoporosis is the default if the type of osteoporosis is not identified. Code Z87.310 is assigned only for an osteoporosis fracture that has healed.

M80.0 Age-related osteoporosis with current pathological fracture
Involutional osteoporosis with current pathological fracture
Osteoporosis NOS with current pathological fracture
Postmenopausal osteoporosis with current pathological fracture
Senile osteoporosis with current pathological fracture

M80.00X- Age-related osteoporosis with current pathological fracture, unspecified site

M80.01 Age-related osteoporosis with current pathological fracture, shoulder
M80.011- Age-related osteoporosis with current pathological fracture, right shoulder
M80.012- Age-related osteoporosis with current pathological fracture, left shoulder
M80.019- Age-related osteoporosis with current pathological fracture, unspecified shoulder

M80.02 Age-related osteoporosis with current pathological fracture, humerus
M80.021- Age-related osteoporosis with current pathological fracture, right humerus
M80.022- Age-related osteoporosis with current pathological fracture, left humerus
M80.029- Age-related osteoporosis with current pathological fracture, unspecified humerus

M80.03 Age-related osteoporosis with current pathological fracture, forearm
Age-related osteoporosis with current pathological fracture of wrist
M80.031- Age-related osteoporosis with current pathological fracture, right forearm
M80.032- Age-related osteoporosis with current pathological fracture, left forearm
M80.039- Age-related osteoporosis with current pathological fracture, unspecified forearm

M80.04 Age-related osteoporosis with current pathological fracture, hand
M80.041- Age-related osteoporosis with current pathological fracture, right hand
M80.042- Age-related osteoporosis with current pathological fracture, left hand
M80.049- Age-related osteoporosis with current pathological fracture, unspecified hand

6 **M80.05 Age-related osteoporosis with current pathological fracture, femur**
Age-related osteoporosis with current pathological fracture of hip

7 ⊟ **M80.051- Age-related osteoporosis with current pathological fracture, right femur** A HCC

7 ⊟ **M80.052- Age-related osteoporosis with current pathological fracture, left femur** A HCC

7 ⊟ **M80.059- Age-related osteoporosis with current pathological fracture, unspecified femur** A HCC

6 **M80.06 Age-related osteoporosis with current pathological fracture, lower leg**

7 ⊟ **M80.061- Age-related osteoporosis with current pathological fracture, right lower leg** A

7 ⊟ **M80.062- Age-related osteoporosis with current pathological fracture, left lower leg** A

7 ⊟ **M80.069- Age-related osteoporosis with current pathological fracture, unspecified lower leg** A

6 **M80.07 Age-related osteoporosis with current pathological fracture, ankle and foot**

7 ⊟ **M80.071- Age-related osteoporosis with current pathological fracture, right ankle and foot** A

7 ⊟ **M80.072- Age-related osteoporosis with current pathological fracture, left ankle and foot** A

7 ⊟ **M80.079- Age-related osteoporosis with current pathological fracture, unspecified ankle and foot** A

7 **M80.08X- Age-related osteoporosis with current pathological fracture, vertebra(e)** A HCC

Age-related osteoporosis with current pathological fracture, vertebra(e)

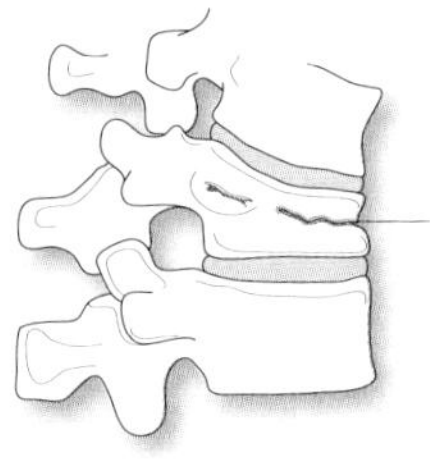

5 **M80.8 Other osteoporosis with current pathological fracture**
Drug-induced osteoporosis with current pathological fracture
Idiopathic osteoporosis with current pathological fracture
Osteoporosis of disuse with current pathological fracture
Postoophorectomy osteoporosis with current pathological fracture
Postsurgical malabsorption osteoporosis with current pathological fracture
Post-traumatic osteoporosis with current pathological fracture
Use additional code for adverse effect, if applicable, to identify drug (T36-T50 with fifth or sixth character 5)

7 **M80.80X- Other osteoporosis with current pathological fracture, unspecified site**

6 **M80.81 Other osteoporosis with pathological fracture, shoulder**

7 ⊟ **M80.811- Other osteoporosis with current pathological fracture, right shoulder**

7 ⊟ **M80.812- Other osteoporosis with current pathological fracture, left shoulder**

7 ⊟ **M80.819- Other osteoporosis with current pathological fracture, unspecified shoulder**

6 **M80.82 Other osteoporosis with current pathological fracture, humerus**

7 ⊟ **M80.821- Other osteoporosis with current pathological fracture, right humerus**

7 ⊟ **M80.822- Other osteoporosis with current pathological fracture, left humerus**

7 ⊟ **M80.829- Other osteoporosis with current pathological fracture, unspecified humerus**

6 **M80.83 Other osteoporosis with current pathological fracture, forearm**
Other osteoporosis with current pathological fracture of wrist

7 ⊟ **M80.831- Other osteoporosis with current pathological fracture, right forearm**

7 ⊟ **M80.832- Other osteoporosis with current pathological fracture, left forearm**

7 ⊟ **M80.839- Other osteoporosis with current pathological fracture, unspecified forearm**

6 **M80.84 Other osteoporosis with current pathological fracture, hand**

7 ⊟ **M80.841- Other osteoporosis with current pathological fracture, right hand**

7 ⊟ **M80.842- Other osteoporosis with current pathological fracture, left hand**

7 ⊟ **M80.849- Other osteoporosis with current pathological fracture, unspecified hand**

6 **M80.85 Other osteoporosis with current pathological fracture, femur**
Other osteoporosis with current pathological fracture of hip

7 ⊟ **M80.851- Other osteoporosis with current pathological fracture, right femur** HCC

7 ⊟ **M80.852- Other osteoporosis with current pathological fracture, left femur** HCC

7 ⊟ **M80.859- Other osteoporosis with current pathological fracture, unspecified femur** HCC

6 **M80.86 Other osteoporosis with current pathological fracture, lower leg**

7 ⊟ **M80.861- Other osteoporosis with current pathological fracture, right lower leg**

7 ⊟ **M80.862- Other osteoporosis with current pathological fracture, left lower leg**

7 ⊟ **M80.869- Other osteoporosis with current pathological fracture, unspecified lower leg**

6 **M80.87 Other osteoporosis with current pathological fracture, ankle and foot**

7 ⊟ **M80.871- Other osteoporosis with current pathological fracture, right ankle and foot**

7 ⊟ **M80.872- Other osteoporosis with current pathological fracture, left ankle and foot**

7 ⊟ **M80.879- Other osteoporosis with current pathological fracture, unspecified ankle and foot**

7 **M80.88X- Other osteoporosis with current pathological fracture, vertebra(e)** HCC

4 **M81 Osteoporosis without current pathological fracture**
Use additional code to identify:
major osseous defect, if applicable (M89.7-)
personal history of (healed) osteoporosis fracture, if applicable (Z87.310)

EXCLUDES 1 *osteoporosis with current pathological fracture (M80.-)*
Sudeck's atrophy (M89.0)

GUIDELINES **Section I.C.13.d.1)**
Category M81, Osteoporosis without current pathological fracture, is for use for patients with osteoporosis who do not currently have a pathologic fracture due to the osteoporosis, even if they have had a fracture in the past. For patients with a history of osteoporosis fractures, status code Z87.310, Personal history of (healed) osteoporosis fracture, should follow the code from M81.

CODING TIP ✓ M81 is coded for patients with osteoporosis with no current fracture. Osteoporosis is not site-specific since it's considered a systemic condition.

Osteoporosis without current pathological fracture

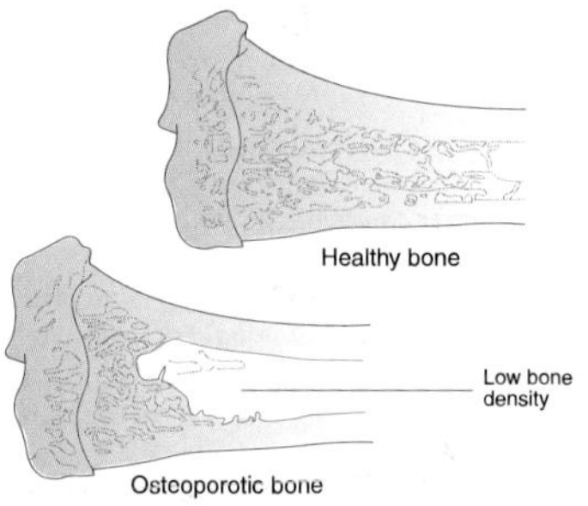

M81.0 **Age-related osteoporosis without current pathological fracture** [A]
Involutional osteoporosis without current pathological fracture
Osteoporosis NOS
Postmenopausal osteoporosis without current pathological fracture
Senile osteoporosis without current pathological fracture

M81.6 **Localized osteoporosis [Lequesne]**
EXCLUDES 1 *Sudeck's atrophy (M89.0)*

M81.8 **Other osteoporosis without current pathological fracture**
Drug-induced osteoporosis without current pathological fracture
Idiopathic osteoporosis without current pathological fracture
Osteoporosis of disuse without current pathological fracture
Postoophorectomy osteoporosis without current pathological fracture
Postsurgical malabsorption osteoporosis without current pathological fracture
Post-traumatic osteoporosis without current pathological fracture
Use additional code for adverse effect, if applicable, to identify drug (T36-T50 with fifth or sixth character 5)

[4] **M83** **Adult osteomalacia**
EXCLUDES 1 *infantile and juvenile osteomalacia (E55.0)*
renal osteodystrophy (N25.0)
rickets (active) (E55.0)
rickets (active) sequelae (E64.3)
vitamin D-resistant osteomalacia (E83.3)
vitamin D-resistant rickets (active) (E83.3)

CODING TIP ✓ Osteomalacia differs from osteoporosis in that osteomalacia implies softening of the bone due to demineralization. Osteoporosis indicates a clear reduction in bone density/mass with porousness of the bones.

DEFINITION Deficient levels of calcium in the bone, resulting in bone softening.

M83.0 **Puerperal osteomalacia** ♀ [M]
M83.1 **Senile osteomalacia** [A]
M83.2 **Adult osteomalacia due to malabsorption** [A]
Postsurgical malabsorption osteomalacia in adults
M83.3 **Adult osteomalacia due to malnutrition** [A]
M83.4 **Aluminum bone disease**
M83.5 **Other drug-induced osteomalacia in adults** [A]
Use additional code for adverse effect, if applicable, to identify drug (T36-T50 with fifth or sixth character 5)
M83.8 **Other adult osteomalacia** [A]
M83.9 **Adult osteomalacia, unspecified** [A]

[4] **M84** **Disorder of continuity of bone**
EXCLUDES 2 *traumatic fracture of bone-see fracture, by site*

GUIDELINES **Section I.C.13.c**
Coding of Pathologic Fractures: 7th character D is to be used for encounters after the patient has completed active treatment for the fracture and is receiving routine care for the fracture during the healing or recovery phase. The other 7th characters, listed under each subcategory in the Tabular List, are to be used for subsequent encounters for treatment of problems associated with the healing, such as malunions, nonunions, and sequelae.
Care for complications of surgical treatment for fracture repairs during the healing or recovery phase should be coded with the appropriate complication codes.

[5] **M84.3** **Stress fracture**
Fatigue fracture
March fracture
Stress fracture NOS
Stress reaction
Use additional external cause code(s) to identify the cause of the stress fracture
EXCLUDES 1 *pathological fracture NOS (M84.4.-)*
pathological fracture due to osteoporosis (M80.-)
traumatic fracture (S12.-, S22.-, S32.-, S42.-, S52.-, S62.-, S72.-, S82.-, S92.-)
EXCLUDES 2 *personal history of (healed) stress (fatigue) fracture (Z87.312)*
stress fracture of vertebra (M48.4-)

The appropriate 7th character is to be added to each code from subcategory M84.3:

A	initial encounter for fracture
D	subsequent encounter for fracture with routine healing
G	subsequent encounter for fracture with delayed healing
K	subsequent encounter for fracture with nonunion
P	subsequent encounter for fracture with malunion
S	sequela

DEFINITION Small, hairline crack(s) in the surface of a bone due to overuse or activity that applies a repetitive force to a particular area, most commonly occurring in the lower legs and feet.

[7] **M84.30X-** **Stress fracture, unspecified site**
[6] **M84.31** **Stress fracture, shoulder**
[7] [L] **M84.311-** **Stress fracture, right shoulder**
[7] [L] **M84.312-** **Stress fracture, left shoulder**
[7] [L] **M84.319-** **Stress fracture, unspecified shoulder**
[6] **M84.32** **Stress fracture, humerus**
[7] [L] **M84.321-** **Stress fracture, right humerus**
[7] [L] **M84.322-** **Stress fracture, left humerus**
[7] [L] **M84.329-** **Stress fracture, unspecified humerus**
[6] **M84.33** **Stress fracture, ulna and radius**
[7] [L] **M84.331-** **Stress fracture, right ulna**
[7] [L] **M84.332-** **Stress fracture, left ulna**
[7] [L] **M84.333-** **Stress fracture, right radius**
[7] [L] **M84.334-** **Stress fracture, left radius**
[7] [L] **M84.339-** **Stress fracture, unspecified ulna and radius**
[6] **M84.34** **Stress fracture, hand and fingers**
[7] [L] **M84.341-** **Stress fracture, right hand**
[7] [L] **M84.342-** **Stress fracture, left hand**
[7] [L] **M84.343-** **Stress fracture, unspecified hand**
[7] [L] **M84.344-** **Stress fracture, right finger(s)**
[7] [L] **M84.345-** **Stress fracture, left finger(s)**
[7] [L] **M84.346-** **Stress fracture, unspecified finger(s)**
[6] **M84.35** **Stress fracture, pelvis and femur**
Stress fracture, hip
[7] [L] **M84.350-** **Stress fracture, pelvis**
[7] [L] **M84.351-** **Stress fracture, right femur**
[7] [L] **M84.352-** **Stress fracture, left femur**
[7] [L] **M84.353-** **Stress fracture, unspecified femur**
[7] [L] **M84.359-** **Stress fracture, hip, unspecified**
[6] **M84.36** **Stress fracture, tibia and fibula**

- M84.361- Stress fracture, right tibia
- M84.362- Stress fracture, left tibia
- M84.363- Stress fracture, right fibula
- M84.364- Stress fracture, left fibula
- M84.369- Stress fracture, unspecified tibia and fibula

M84.37 Stress fracture, ankle, foot and toes
- M84.371- Stress fracture, right ankle
- M84.372- Stress fracture, left ankle
- M84.373- Stress fracture, unspecified ankle
- M84.374- Stress fracture, right foot
- M84.375- Stress fracture, left foot
- M84.376- Stress fracture, unspecified foot
- M84.377- Stress fracture, right toe(s)
- M84.378- Stress fracture, left toe(s)
- M84.379- Stress fracture, unspecified toe(s)

M84.38X- Stress fracture, other site

EXCLUDES 2 *stress fracture of vertebra (M48.4-)*

M84.4 Pathological fracture, not elsewhere classified

Chronic fracture
Pathological fracture NOS

EXCLUDES 1 *collapsed vertebra NEC (M48.5)*
pathological fracture in neoplastic disease (M84.5-)
pathological fracture in osteoporosis (M80.-)
pathological fracture in other disease (M84.6-)
stress fracture (M84.3-)
traumatic fracture (S12.-, S22.-, S32.-, S42.-, S52.-, S62.-, S72.-, S82.-, S92.-)

EXCLUDES 2 *personal history of (healed) pathological fracture (Z87.311)*

The appropriate 7th character is to be added to each code from subcategory M84.4:

A	initial encounter for fracture
D	subsequent encounter for fracture with routine healing
G	subsequent encounter for fracture with delayed healing
K	subsequent encounter for fracture with nonunion
P	subsequent encounter for fracture with malunion
S	sequela

CODING TIP ✓ Spontaneous fractures are always considered pathologic fractures. Compression fractures may be considered pathologic fractures. If the patient falls and has a compression fracture or unusual fracture, ask the physician whether it is considered traumatic or pathologic.

DEFINITION A break resulting from widespread lesions or disease process that destroys normal bone mass, causing the weakened bone to break spontaneously without obvious external force.

M84.40X- Pathological fracture, unspecified site

M84.41 Pathological fracture, shoulder
- M84.411- Pathological fracture, right shoulder
- M84.412- Pathological fracture, left shoulder
- M84.419- Pathological fracture, unspecified shoulder

M84.42 Pathological fracture, humerus
- M84.421- Pathological fracture, right humerus
- M84.422- Pathological fracture, left humerus
- M84.429- Pathological fracture, unspecified humerus

M84.43 Pathological fracture, ulna and radius
- M84.431- Pathological fracture, right ulna
- M84.432- Pathological fracture, left ulna
- M84.433- Pathological fracture, right radius
- M84.434- Pathological fracture, left radius
- M84.439- Pathological fracture, unspecified ulna and radius

M84.44 Pathological fracture, hand and fingers
- M84.441- Pathological fracture, right hand
- M84.442- Pathological fracture, left hand
- M84.443- Pathological fracture, unspecified hand
- M84.444- Pathological fracture, right finger(s)
- M84.445- Pathological fracture, left finger(s)
- M84.446- Pathological fracture, unspecified finger(s)

M84.45 Pathological fracture, femur and pelvis
- M84.451- Pathological fracture, right femur HCC
- M84.452- Pathological fracture, left femur HCC
- M84.453- Pathological fracture, unspecified femur HCC
- M84.454- Pathological fracture, pelvis
  AHA: 4Q 2016, 42
- M84.459- Pathological fracture, hip, unspecified HCC

M84.46 Pathological fracture, tibia and fibula
- M84.461- Pathological fracture, right tibia
- M84.462- Pathological fracture, left tibia
- M84.463- Pathological fracture, right fibula
- M84.464- Pathological fracture, left fibula
- M84.469- Pathological fracture, unspecified tibia and fibula

M84.47 Pathological fracture, ankle, foot and toes
- M84.471- Pathological fracture, right ankle
- M84.472- Pathological fracture, left ankle
- M84.473- Pathological fracture, unspecified ankle
- M84.474- Pathological fracture, right foot
- M84.475- Pathological fracture, left foot
- M84.476- Pathological fracture, unspecified foot
- M84.477- Pathological fracture, right toe(s)
- M84.478- Pathological fracture, left toe(s)
- M84.479- Pathological fracture, unspecified toe(s)

M84.48X- Pathological fracture, other site

M84.5 Pathological fracture in neoplastic disease

Code also:
underlying neoplasm

The appropriate 7th character is to be added to each code from subcategory M84.5:

A	initial encounter for fracture
D	subsequent encounter for fracture with routine healing
G	subsequent encounter for fracture with delayed healing
K	subsequent encounter for fracture with nonunion
P	subsequent encounter for fracture with malunion
S	sequela

GUIDELINES **Section I.C.2.l.6)**

When an encounter is for a pathological fracture due to a neoplasm, and the focus of treatment is the fracture, a code from subcategory M84.5, Pathological fracture in neoplastic disease, should be sequenced first, followed by the code for the neoplasm. If the focus of treatment is the neoplasm with an associated pathological fracture, the neoplasm code should be sequenced first, followed by a code from M84.5 for the pathological fracture.

DEFINITION A break resulting from metastatic invasion or tumor growth that destroys normal bone mass, resulting in fracture without obvious trauma to the bone.

M84.50X- Pathological fracture in neoplastic disease, unspecified site

M84.51 Pathological fracture in neoplastic disease, shoulder
- M84.511- Pathological fracture in neoplastic disease, right shoulder
- M84.512- Pathological fracture in neoplastic disease, left shoulder
- M84.519- Pathological fracture in neoplastic disease, unspecified shoulder

M84.52 Pathological fracture in neoplastic disease, humerus
- M84.521- Pathological fracture in neoplastic disease, right humerus
- M84.522- Pathological fracture in neoplastic disease, left humerus
- M84.529- Pathological fracture in neoplastic disease, unspecified humerus

M84.53 Pathological fracture in neoplastic disease, ulna and radius
- M84.531- Pathological fracture in neoplastic disease, right ulna

7 ⊟ M84.532- Pathological fracture in neoplastic disease, left ulna
7 ⊟ M84.533- Pathological fracture in neoplastic disease, right radius
7 ⊟ M84.534- Pathological fracture in neoplastic disease, left radius
7 ⊟ M84.539- Pathological fracture in neoplastic disease, unspecified ulna and radius

6 M84.54 Pathological fracture in neoplastic disease, hand
7 ⊟ M84.541- Pathological fracture in neoplastic disease, right hand
7 ⊟ M84.542- Pathological fracture in neoplastic disease, left hand
7 ⊟ M84.549- Pathological fracture in neoplastic disease, unspecified hand

6 M84.55 Pathological fracture in neoplastic disease, pelvis and femur
7 ⊟ M84.550- Pathological fracture in neoplastic disease, pelvis
7 ⊟ M84.551- Pathological fracture in neoplastic disease, right femur HCC
7 ⊟ M84.552- Pathological fracture in neoplastic disease, left femur HCC
7 ⊟ M84.553- Pathological fracture in neoplastic disease, unspecified femur HCC
7 ⊟ M84.559- Pathological fracture in neoplastic disease, hip, unspecified HCC

6 M84.56 Pathological fracture in neoplastic disease, tibia and fibula
7 ⊟ M84.561- Pathological fracture in neoplastic disease, right tibia
7 ⊟ M84.562- Pathological fracture in neoplastic disease, left tibia
7 ⊟ M84.563- Pathological fracture in neoplastic disease, right fibula
7 ⊟ M84.564- Pathological fracture in neoplastic disease, left fibula
7 ⊟ M84.569- Pathological fracture in neoplastic disease, unspecified tibia and fibula

6 M84.57 Pathological fracture in neoplastic disease, ankle and foot
7 ⊟ M84.571- Pathological fracture in neoplastic disease, right ankle
7 ⊟ M84.572- Pathological fracture in neoplastic disease, left ankle
7 ⊟ M84.573- Pathological fracture in neoplastic disease, unspecified ankle
7 ⊟ M84.574- Pathological fracture in neoplastic disease, right foot
7 ⊟ M84.575- Pathological fracture in neoplastic disease, left foot
7 ⊟ M84.576- Pathological fracture in neoplastic disease, unspecified foot

7 M84.58X- Pathological fracture in neoplastic disease, other specified site
Pathological fracture in neoplastic disease, vertebrae

5 M84.6 Pathological fracture in other disease
Code also:
underlying condition
EXCLUDES 1 *pathological fracture in osteoporosis (M80.-)*

The appropriate 7th character is to be added to each code from subcategory M84.6:

A	initial encounter for fracture
D	subsequent encounter for fracture with routine healing
G	subsequent encounter for fracture with delayed healing
K	subsequent encounter for fracture with nonunion
P	subsequent encounter for fracture with malunion
S	sequela

7 M84.60X- Pathological fracture in other disease, unspecified site

6 M84.61 Pathological fracture in other disease, shoulder
7 ⊟ M84.611- Pathological fracture in other disease, right shoulder
7 ⊟ M84.612- Pathological fracture in other disease, left shoulder
7 ⊟ M84.619- Pathological fracture in other disease, unspecified shoulder

6 M84.62 Pathological fracture in other disease, humerus
7 ⊟ M84.621- Pathological fracture in other disease, right humerus
7 ⊟ M84.622- Pathological fracture in other disease, left humerus
7 ⊟ M84.629- Pathological fracture in other disease, unspecified humerus

6 M84.63 Pathological fracture in other disease, ulna and radius
7 ⊟ M84.631- Pathological fracture in other disease, right ulna
7 ⊟ M84.632- Pathological fracture in other disease, left ulna
7 ⊟ M84.633- Pathological fracture in other disease, right radius
7 ⊟ M84.634- Pathological fracture in other disease, left radius
7 ⊟ M84.639- Pathological fracture in other disease, unspecified ulna and radius

6 M84.64 Pathological fracture in other disease, hand
7 ⊟ M84.641- Pathological fracture in other disease, right hand
7 ⊟ M84.642- Pathological fracture in other disease, left hand
7 ⊟ M84.649- Pathological fracture in other disease, unspecified hand

6 M84.65 Pathological fracture in other disease, pelvis and femur
7 ⊟ M84.650- Pathological fracture in other disease, pelvis
7 ⊟ M84.651- Pathological fracture in other disease, right femur HCC
7 ⊟ M84.652- Pathological fracture in other disease, left femur HCC
7 ⊟ M84.653- Pathological fracture in other disease, unspecified femur HCC
7 ⊟ M84.659- Pathological fracture in other disease, hip, unspecified HCC

6 M84.66 Pathological fracture in other disease, tibia and fibula
7 ⊟ M84.661- Pathological fracture in other disease, right tibia
7 ⊟ M84.662- Pathological fracture in other disease, left tibia
7 ⊟ M84.663- Pathological fracture in other disease, right fibula
7 ⊟ M84.664- Pathological fracture in other disease, left fibula
7 ⊟ M84.669- Pathological fracture in other disease, unspecified tibia and fibula

6 M84.67 Pathological fracture in other disease, ankle and foot
7 ⊟ M84.671- Pathological fracture in other disease, right ankle
7 ⊟ M84.672- Pathological fracture in other disease, left ankle
7 ⊟ M84.673- Pathological fracture in other disease, unspecified ankle
7 ⊟ M84.674- Pathological fracture in other disease, right foot
7 ⊟ M84.675- Pathological fracture in other disease, left foot
7 ⊟ M84.676- Pathological fracture in other disease, unspecified foot

7 M84.68X- Pathological fracture in other disease, other site

5 M84.7 Nontraumatic fracture, not elsewhere classified
6 M84.75 Atypical femoral fracture

The appropriate 7th character is to be added to each code from M84.75:

A	initial encounter for fracture
D	subsequent encounter for fracture with routine healing
G	subsequent encounter for fracture with delayed healing
K	subsequent encounter for fracture with nonunion
P	subsequent encounter for fracture with malunion
S	sequela

AHA: 4Q 2016, 41

7 M84.750- Atypical femoral fracture, unspecified
7 M84.751- Incomplete atypical femoral fracture, right leg
7 M84.752- Incomplete atypical femoral fracture, left leg
7 M84.753- Incomplete atypical femoral fracture, unspecified leg
7 M84.754- Complete transverse atypical femoral fracture, right leg HCC
7 M84.755- Complete transverse atypical femoral fracture, left leg HCC
7 M84.756- Complete transverse atypical femoral fracture, unspecified leg HCC
7 M84.757- Complete oblique atypical femoral fracture, right leg HCC
7 M84.758- Complete oblique atypical femoral fracture, left leg HCC
7 M84.759- Complete oblique atypical femoral fracture, unspecified leg HCC

5 M84.8 Other disorders of continuity of bone
M84.80 Other disorders of continuity of bone, unspecified site
6 M84.81 Other disorders of continuity of bone, shoulder
M84.811 Other disorders of continuity of bone, right shoulder
M84.812 Other disorders of continuity of bone, left shoulder
M84.819 Other disorders of continuity of bone, unspecified shoulder
6 M84.82 Other disorders of continuity of bone, humerus
M84.821 Other disorders of continuity of bone, right humerus
M84.822 Other disorders of continuity of bone, left humerus
M84.829 Other disorders of continuity of bone, unspecified humerus
6 M84.83 Other disorders of continuity of bone, ulna and radius
M84.831 Other disorders of continuity of bone, right ulna
M84.832 Other disorders of continuity of bone, left ulna
M84.833 Other disorders of continuity of bone, right radius
M84.834 Other disorders of continuity of bone, left radius
M84.839 Other disorders of continuity of bone, unspecified ulna and radius
6 M84.84 Other disorders of continuity of bone, hand
M84.841 Other disorders of continuity of bone, right hand
M84.842 Other disorders of continuity of bone, left hand
M84.849 Other disorders of continuity of bone, unspecified hand
6 M84.85 Other disorders of continuity of bone, pelvic region and thigh
M84.851 Other disorders of continuity of bone, right pelvic region and thigh
M84.852 Other disorders of continuity of bone, left pelvic region and thigh
M84.859 Other disorders of continuity of bone, unspecified pelvic region and thigh
6 M84.86 Other disorders of continuity of bone, tibia and fibula
M84.861 Other disorders of continuity of bone, right tibia
M84.862 Other disorders of continuity of bone, left tibia
M84.863 Other disorders of continuity of bone, right fibula
M84.864 Other disorders of continuity of bone, left fibula
M84.869 Other disorders of continuity of bone, unspecified tibia and fibula
6 M84.87 Other disorders of continuity of bone, ankle and foot
M84.871 Other disorders of continuity of bone, right ankle and foot
M84.872 Other disorders of continuity of bone, left ankle and foot
M84.879 Other disorders of continuity of bone, unspecified ankle and foot
M84.88 Other disorders of continuity of bone, other site
M84.9 Disorder of continuity of bone, unspecified

4 M85 Other disorders of bone density and structure
EXCLUDES 1 *osteogenesis imperfecta (Q78.0)*
osteopetrosis (Q78.2)
osteopoikilosis (Q78.8)
polyostotic fibrous dysplasia (Q78.1)

5 M85.0 Fibrous dysplasia (monostotic)
EXCLUDES 2 *fibrous dysplasia of jaw (M27.8)*
M85.00 Fibrous dysplasia (monostotic), unspecified site
6 M85.01 Fibrous dysplasia (monostotic), shoulder
M85.011 Fibrous dysplasia (monostotic), right shoulder
M85.012 Fibrous dysplasia (monostotic), left shoulder
M85.019 Fibrous dysplasia (monostotic), unspecified shoulder
6 M85.02 Fibrous dysplasia (monostotic), upper arm
M85.021 Fibrous dysplasia (monostotic), right upper arm
M85.022 Fibrous dysplasia (monostotic), left upper arm
M85.029 Fibrous dysplasia (monostotic), unspecified upper arm
6 M85.03 Fibrous dysplasia (monostotic), forearm
M85.031 Fibrous dysplasia (monostotic), right forearm
M85.032 Fibrous dysplasia (monostotic), left forearm
M85.039 Fibrous dysplasia (monostotic), unspecified forearm
6 M85.04 Fibrous dysplasia (monostotic), hand
M85.041 Fibrous dysplasia (monostotic), right hand
M85.042 Fibrous dysplasia (monostotic), left hand
M85.049 Fibrous dysplasia (monostotic), unspecified hand
6 M85.05 Fibrous dysplasia (monostotic), thigh
M85.051 Fibrous dysplasia (monostotic), right thigh
M85.052 Fibrous dysplasia (monostotic), left thigh
M85.059 Fibrous dysplasia (monostotic), unspecified thigh
6 M85.06 Fibrous dysplasia (monostotic), lower leg
M85.061 Fibrous dysplasia (monostotic), right lower leg
M85.062 Fibrous dysplasia (monostotic), left lower leg
M85.069 Fibrous dysplasia (monostotic), unspecified lower leg
6 M85.07 Fibrous dysplasia (monostotic), ankle and foot
M85.071 Fibrous dysplasia (monostotic), right ankle and foot
M85.072 Fibrous dysplasia (monostotic), left ankle and foot
M85.079 Fibrous dysplasia (monostotic), unspecified ankle and foot
M85.08 Fibrous dysplasia (monostotic), other site
M85.09 Fibrous dysplasia (monostotic), multiple sites

5 M85.1 Skeletal fluorosis
M85.10 Skeletal fluorosis, unspecified site
6 M85.11 Skeletal fluorosis, shoulder
M85.111 Skeletal fluorosis, right shoulder
M85.112 Skeletal fluorosis, left shoulder
M85.119 Skeletal fluorosis, unspecified shoulder
6 M85.12 Skeletal fluorosis, upper arm
M85.121 Skeletal fluorosis, right upper arm
M85.122 Skeletal fluorosis, left upper arm
M85.129 Skeletal fluorosis, unspecified upper arm
6 M85.13 Skeletal fluorosis, forearm
M85.131 Skeletal fluorosis, right forearm
M85.132 Skeletal fluorosis, left forearm
M85.139 Skeletal fluorosis, unspecified forearm
6 M85.14 Skeletal fluorosis, hand
M85.141 Skeletal fluorosis, right hand
M85.142 Skeletal fluorosis, left hand
M85.149 Skeletal fluorosis, unspecified hand
6 M85.15 Skeletal fluorosis, thigh
M85.151 Skeletal fluorosis, right thigh
M85.152 Skeletal fluorosis, left thigh
M85.159 Skeletal fluorosis, unspecified thigh
6 M85.16 Skeletal fluorosis, lower leg

M85.161 Skeletal fluorosis, right lower leg
M85.162 Skeletal fluorosis, left lower leg
M85.169 Skeletal fluorosis, unspecified lower leg
M85.17 Skeletal fluorosis, ankle and foot
M85.171 Skeletal fluorosis, right ankle and foot
M85.172 Skeletal fluorosis, left ankle and foot
M85.179 Skeletal fluorosis, unspecified ankle and foot
M85.18 Skeletal fluorosis, other site
M85.19 Skeletal fluorosis, multiple sites
M85.2 Hyperostosis of skull
M85.3 Osteitis condensans
M85.30 Osteitis condensans, unspecified site
M85.31 Osteitis condensans, shoulder
M85.311 Osteitis condensans, right shoulder
M85.312 Osteitis condensans, left shoulder
M85.319 Osteitis condensans, unspecified shoulder
M85.32 Osteitis condensans, upper arm
M85.321 Osteitis condensans, right upper arm
M85.322 Osteitis condensans, left upper arm
M85.329 Osteitis condensans, unspecified upper arm
M85.33 Osteitis condensans, forearm
M85.331 Osteitis condensans, right forearm
M85.332 Osteitis condensans, left forearm
M85.339 Osteitis condensans, unspecified forearm
M85.34 Osteitis condensans, hand
M85.341 Osteitis condensans, right hand
M85.342 Osteitis condensans, left hand
M85.349 Osteitis condensans, unspecified hand
M85.35 Osteitis condensans, thigh
M85.351 Osteitis condensans, right thigh
M85.352 Osteitis condensans, left thigh
M85.359 Osteitis condensans, unspecified thigh
M85.36 Osteitis condensans, lower leg
M85.361 Osteitis condensans, right lower leg
M85.362 Osteitis condensans, left lower leg
M85.369 Osteitis condensans, unspecified lower leg
M85.37 Osteitis condensans, ankle and foot
M85.371 Osteitis condensans, right ankle and foot
M85.372 Osteitis condensans, left ankle and foot
M85.379 Osteitis condensans, unspecified ankle and foot
M85.38 Osteitis condensans, other site
M85.39 Osteitis condensans, multiple sites
M85.4 Solitary bone cyst
EXCLUDES 2 *solitary cyst of jaw (M27.4)*
M85.40 Solitary bone cyst, unspecified site
M85.41 Solitary bone cyst, shoulder
M85.411 Solitary bone cyst, right shoulder
M85.412 Solitary bone cyst, left shoulder
M85.419 Solitary bone cyst, unspecified shoulder
M85.42 Solitary bone cyst, humerus
M85.421 Solitary bone cyst, right humerus
M85.422 Solitary bone cyst, left humerus
M85.429 Solitary bone cyst, unspecified humerus
M85.43 Solitary bone cyst, ulna and radius
M85.431 Solitary bone cyst, right ulna and radius
M85.432 Solitary bone cyst, left ulna and radius
M85.439 Solitary bone cyst, unspecified ulna and radius
M85.44 Solitary bone cyst, hand
M85.441 Solitary bone cyst, right hand
M85.442 Solitary bone cyst, left hand
M85.449 Solitary bone cyst, unspecified hand
M85.45 Solitary bone cyst, pelvis
M85.451 Solitary bone cyst, right pelvis
M85.452 Solitary bone cyst, left pelvis
M85.459 Solitary bone cyst, unspecified pelvis
M85.46 Solitary bone cyst, tibia and fibula
M85.461 Solitary bone cyst, right tibia and fibula
M85.462 Solitary bone cyst, left tibia and fibula
M85.469 Solitary bone cyst, unspecified tibia and fibula
M85.47 Solitary bone cyst, ankle and foot
M85.471 Solitary bone cyst, right ankle and foot
M85.472 Solitary bone cyst, left ankle and foot
M85.479 Solitary bone cyst, unspecified ankle and foot
M85.48 Solitary bone cyst, other site
M85.5 Aneurysmal bone cyst
EXCLUDES 2 *aneurysmal cyst of jaw (M27.4)*
M85.50 Aneurysmal bone cyst, unspecified site
M85.51 Aneurysmal bone cyst, shoulder
M85.511 Aneurysmal bone cyst, right shoulder
M85.512 Aneurysmal bone cyst, left shoulder
M85.519 Aneurysmal bone cyst, unspecified shoulder
M85.52 Aneurysmal bone cyst, upper arm
M85.521 Aneurysmal bone cyst, right upper arm
M85.522 Aneurysmal bone cyst, left upper arm
M85.529 Aneurysmal bone cyst, unspecified upper arm
M85.53 Aneurysmal bone cyst, forearm
M85.531 Aneurysmal bone cyst, right forearm
M85.532 Aneurysmal bone cyst, left forearm
M85.539 Aneurysmal bone cyst, unspecified forearm
M85.54 Aneurysmal bone cyst, hand
M85.541 Aneurysmal bone cyst, right hand
M85.542 Aneurysmal bone cyst, left hand
M85.549 Aneurysmal bone cyst, unspecified hand
M85.55 Aneurysmal bone cyst, thigh
M85.551 Aneurysmal bone cyst, right thigh
M85.552 Aneurysmal bone cyst, left thigh
M85.559 Aneurysmal bone cyst, unspecified thigh
M85.56 Aneurysmal bone cyst, lower leg
M85.561 Aneurysmal bone cyst, right lower leg
M85.562 Aneurysmal bone cyst, left lower leg
M85.569 Aneurysmal bone cyst, unspecified lower leg
M85.57 Aneurysmal bone cyst, ankle and foot
M85.571 Aneurysmal bone cyst, right ankle and foot
M85.572 Aneurysmal bone cyst, left ankle and foot
M85.579 Aneurysmal bone cyst, unspecified ankle and foot
M85.58 Aneurysmal bone cyst, other site
M85.59 Aneurysmal bone cyst, multiple sites
M85.6 Other cyst of bone
EXCLUDES 1 *cyst of jaw NEC (M27.4)*
osteitis fibrosa cystica generalisata [von Recklinghausen's disease of bone] (E21.0)
M85.60 Other cyst of bone, unspecified site
M85.61 Other cyst of bone, shoulder
M85.611 Other cyst of bone, right shoulder
M85.612 Other cyst of bone, left shoulder
M85.619 Other cyst of bone, unspecified shoulder
M85.62 Other cyst of bone, upper arm
M85.621 Other cyst of bone, right upper arm
M85.622 Other cyst of bone, left upper arm
M85.629 Other cyst of bone, unspecified upper arm
M85.63 Other cyst of bone, forearm
M85.631 Other cyst of bone, right forearm
M85.632 Other cyst of bone, left forearm
M85.639 Other cyst of bone, unspecified forearm
M85.64 Other cyst of bone, hand
M85.641 Other cyst of bone, right hand
M85.642 Other cyst of bone, left hand
M85.649 Other cyst of bone, unspecified hand
M85.65 Other cyst of bone, thigh
M85.651 Other cyst of bone, right thigh
M85.652 Other cyst of bone, left thigh
M85.659 Other cyst of bone, unspecified thigh
M85.66 Other cyst of bone, lower leg
M85.661 Other cyst of bone, right lower leg
M85.662 Other cyst of bone, left lower leg
M85.669 Other cyst of bone, unspecified lower leg
M85.67 Other cyst of bone, ankle and foot
M85.671 Other cyst of bone, right ankle and foot
M85.672 Other cyst of bone, left ankle and foot
M85.679 Other cyst of bone, unspecified ankle and foot

M85.68 **Other cyst of bone, other site**
M85.69 **Other cyst of bone, multiple sites**
M85.8 **Other specified disorders of bone density and structure**
Hyperostosis of bones, except skull
Osteosclerosis, acquired
EXCLUDES 1 *diffuse idiopathic skeletal hyperostosis [DISH] (M48.1)*
osteosclerosis congenita (Q77.4)
osteosclerosis fragilitas (generalista) (Q78.2)
osteosclerosis myelofibrosis (D75.81)
M85.80 **Other specified disorders of bone density and structure, unspecified site**
M85.81 **Other specified disorders of bone density and structure, shoulder**
M85.811 **Other specified disorders of bone density and structure, right shoulder**
M85.812 **Other specified disorders of bone density and structure, left shoulder**
M85.819 **Other specified disorders of bone density and structure, unspecified shoulder**
M85.82 **Other specified disorders of bone density and structure, upper arm**
M85.821 **Other specified disorders of bone density and structure, right upper arm**
M85.822 **Other specified disorders of bone density and structure, left upper arm**
M85.829 **Other specified disorders of bone density and structure, unspecified upper arm**
M85.83 **Other specified disorders of bone density and structure, forearm**
M85.831 **Other specified disorders of bone density and structure, right forearm**
M85.832 **Other specified disorders of bone density and structure, left forearm**
M85.839 **Other specified disorders of bone density and structure, unspecified forearm**
M85.84 **Other specified disorders of bone density and structure, hand**
M85.841 **Other specified disorders of bone density and structure, right hand**
M85.842 **Other specified disorders of bone density and structure, left hand**
M85.849 **Other specified disorders of bone density and structure, unspecified hand**
M85.85 **Other specified disorders of bone density and structure, thigh**
M85.851 **Other specified disorders of bone density and structure, right thigh**
M85.852 **Other specified disorders of bone density and structure, left thigh**
M85.859 **Other specified disorders of bone density and structure, unspecified thigh**
M85.86 **Other specified disorders of bone density and structure, lower leg**
M85.861 **Other specified disorders of bone density and structure, right lower leg**
M85.862 **Other specified disorders of bone density and structure, left lower leg**
M85.869 **Other specified disorders of bone density and structure, unspecified lower leg**
M85.87 **Other specified disorders of bone density and structure, ankle and foot**
M85.871 **Other specified disorders of bone density and structure, right ankle and foot**
M85.872 **Other specified disorders of bone density and structure, left ankle and foot**
M85.879 **Other specified disorders of bone density and structure, unspecified ankle and foot**
M85.88 **Other specified disorders of bone density and structure, other site**
M85.89 **Other specified disorders of bone density and structure, multiple sites**
M85.9 **Disorder of bone density and structure, unspecified**

Other osteopathies (M86-M90)

EXCLUDES 1 *postprocedural osteopathies (M96.-)*

M86 **Osteomyelitis**
Use additional code (B95-B97) to identify infectious agent
Use additional code to identify major osseous defect, if applicable (M89.7-)
EXCLUDES 1 *osteomyelitis due to:*
echinococcus (B67.2)
gonococcus (A54.43)
salmonella (A02.24)
EXCLUDES 2 *ostemyelitis of:*
orbit (H05.0-)
petrous bone (H70.2-)
vertebra (M46.2-)

CODING TIP ✓ ICD-10-CM assumes a relationship between diabetes mellitus and osteomyelitis when both conditions are present, unless the physician states otherwise. However, no manifestation combination code pairing for diabetic osteomyelitis exists. When osteomyelitis occurs in a diabetic patient, the appropriate code from E08-E13 should be assigned with 4th & 5th characters -.69 followed by the appropriate code for osteomyelitis, unless the provider specifies that the two conditions are separate. Documentation must include the type (acute or chronic) and site.

CODING TIP ✓ If not documented, query the physician on the timing of the osteomyelitis (acute, subacute, chronic).

CODING TIP ✓ Osteomyelitis commonly occurs in diabetic patients. However, no manifestation combination code pairing for diabetic osteomyelitis exists. When osteomyelitis occurs in a diabetic patient and is confirmed as due to diabetes, the appropriate code from E08-E13 should be assigned with 4th & 5th characters -.69 followed by the appropriate code for osteomyelitis. Documentation must include the type (acute or chronic) and site.

CODING TIP ✓ Codes classified to M86.- do not include osteomyelitis of the orbit, petrous bone, or vertebrae. Look for other causes of the osteomyelitis in the record, besides diabetes.

M86.0 **Acute hematogenous osteomyelitis**
M86.00 **Acute hematogenous osteomyelitis, unspecified site** HCC
M86.01 **Acute hematogenous osteomyelitis, shoulder**
M86.011 **Acute hematogenous osteomyelitis, right shoulder** HCC
M86.012 **Acute hematogenous osteomyelitis, left shoulder** HCC
M86.019 **Acute hematogenous osteomyelitis, unspecified shoulder** HCC
M86.02 **Acute hematogenous osteomyelitis, humerus**
M86.021 **Acute hematogenous osteomyelitis, right humerus** HCC
M86.022 **Acute hematogenous osteomyelitis, left humerus** HCC
M86.029 **Acute hematogenous osteomyelitis, unspecified humerus** HCC
M86.03 **Acute hematogenous osteomyelitis, radius and ulna**
M86.031 **Acute hematogenous osteomyelitis, right radius and ulna** HCC
M86.032 **Acute hematogenous osteomyelitis, left radius and ulna** HCC
M86.039 **Acute hematogenous osteomyelitis, unspecified radius and ulna** HCC
M86.04 **Acute hematogenous osteomyelitis, hand**
M86.041 **Acute hematogenous osteomyelitis, right hand** HCC
M86.042 **Acute hematogenous osteomyelitis, left hand** HCC
M86.049 **Acute hematogenous osteomyelitis, unspecified hand** HCC
M86.05 **Acute hematogenous osteomyelitis, femur**
M86.051 **Acute hematogenous osteomyelitis, right femur** HCC
M86.052 **Acute hematogenous osteomyelitis, left femur** HCC
M86.059 **Acute hematogenous osteomyelitis, unspecified femur** HCC
M86.06 **Acute hematogenous osteomyelitis, tibia and fibula**

M86.061 Acute hematogenous osteomyelitis, right tibia and fibula HCC
M86.062 Acute hematogenous osteomyelitis, left tibia and fibula HCC
M86.069 Acute hematogenous osteomyelitis, unspecified tibia and fibula HCC
M86.07 Acute hematogenous osteomyelitis, ankle and foot
M86.071 Acute hematogenous osteomyelitis, right ankle and foot HCC
M86.072 Acute hematogenous osteomyelitis, left ankle and foot HCC
M86.079 Acute hematogenous osteomyelitis, unspecified ankle and foot HCC
M86.08 Acute hematogenous osteomyelitis, other sites HCC
M86.09 Acute hematogenous osteomyelitis, multiple sites HCC
M86.1 Other acute osteomyelitis
M86.10 Other acute osteomyelitis, unspecified site HCC
M86.11 Other acute osteomyelitis, shoulder
M86.111 Other acute osteomyelitis, right shoulder HCC
M86.112 Other acute osteomyelitis, left shoulder HCC
M86.119 Other acute osteomyelitis, unspecified shoulder HCC
M86.12 Other acute osteomyelitis, humerus
M86.121 Other acute osteomyelitis, right humerus HCC
M86.122 Other acute osteomyelitis, left humerus HCC
M86.129 Other acute osteomyelitis, unspecified humerus HCC
M86.13 Other acute osteomyelitis, radius and ulna
M86.131 Other acute osteomyelitis, right radius and ulna HCC
M86.132 Other acute osteomyelitis, left radius and ulna HCC
M86.139 Other acute osteomyelitis, unspecified radius and ulna HCC
M86.14 Other acute osteomyelitis, hand
M86.141 Other acute osteomyelitis, right hand HCC
M86.142 Other acute osteomyelitis, left hand HCC
M86.149 Other acute osteomyelitis, unspecified hand HCC
M86.15 Other acute osteomyelitis, femur
M86.151 Other acute osteomyelitis, right femur HCC
M86.152 Other acute osteomyelitis, left femur HCC
M86.159 Other acute osteomyelitis, unspecified femur HCC
M86.16 Other acute osteomyelitis, tibia and fibula
M86.161 Other acute osteomyelitis, right tibia and fibula HCC
M86.162 Other acute osteomyelitis, left tibia and fibula HCC
M86.169 Other acute osteomyelitis, unspecified tibia and fibula HCC
M86.17 Other acute osteomyelitis, ankle and foot
M86.171 Other acute osteomyelitis, right ankle and foot HCC
M86.172 Other acute osteomyelitis, left ankle and foot HCC
M86.179 Other acute osteomyelitis, unspecified ankle and foot HCC
M86.18 Other acute osteomyelitis, other site HCC
M86.19 Other acute osteomyelitis, multiple sites HCC
M86.2 Subacute osteomyelitis
M86.20 Subacute osteomyelitis, unspecified site HCC
M86.21 Subacute osteomyelitis, shoulder
M86.211 Subacute osteomyelitis, right shoulder HCC
M86.212 Subacute osteomyelitis, left shoulder HCC
M86.219 Subacute osteomyelitis, unspecified shoulder HCC
M86.22 Subacute osteomyelitis, humerus
M86.221 Subacute osteomyelitis, right humerus HCC
M86.222 Subacute osteomyelitis, left humerus HCC
M86.229 Subacute osteomyelitis, unspecified humerus HCC
M86.23 Subacute osteomyelitis, radius and ulna
M86.231 Subacute osteomyelitis, right radius and ulna HCC
M86.232 Subacute osteomyelitis, left radius and ulna HCC
M86.239 Subacute osteomyelitis, unspecified radius and ulna HCC
M86.24 Subacute osteomyelitis, hand
M86.241 Subacute osteomyelitis, right hand HCC
M86.242 Subacute osteomyelitis, left hand HCC
M86.249 Subacute osteomyelitis, unspecified hand HCC
M86.25 Subacute osteomyelitis, femur
M86.251 Subacute osteomyelitis, right femur HCC
M86.252 Subacute osteomyelitis, left femur HCC
M86.259 Subacute osteomyelitis, unspecified femur HCC
M86.26 Subacute osteomyelitis, tibia and fibula
M86.261 Subacute osteomyelitis, right tibia and fibula HCC
M86.262 Subacute osteomyelitis, left tibia and fibula HCC
M86.269 Subacute osteomyelitis, unspecified tibia and fibula HCC
M86.27 Subacute osteomyelitis, ankle and foot
M86.271 Subacute osteomyelitis, right ankle and foot HCC
M86.272 Subacute osteomyelitis, left ankle and foot HCC
M86.279 Subacute osteomyelitis, unspecified ankle and foot HCC
M86.28 Subacute osteomyelitis, other site HCC
M86.29 Subacute osteomyelitis, multiple sites HCC
M86.3 Chronic multifocal osteomyelitis
M86.30 Chronic multifocal osteomyelitis, unspecified site HCC
M86.31 Chronic multifocal osteomyelitis, shoulder
M86.311 Chronic multifocal osteomyelitis, right shoulder HCC
M86.312 Chronic multifocal osteomyelitis, left shoulder HCC
M86.319 Chronic multifocal osteomyelitis, unspecified shoulder HCC
M86.32 Chronic multifocal osteomyelitis, humerus
M86.321 Chronic multifocal osteomyelitis, right humerus HCC
M86.322 Chronic multifocal osteomyelitis, left humerus HCC
M86.329 Chronic multifocal osteomyelitis, unspecified humerus HCC
M86.33 Chronic multifocal osteomyelitis, radius and ulna
M86.331 Chronic multifocal osteomyelitis, right radius and ulna HCC
M86.332 Chronic multifocal osteomyelitis, left radius and ulna HCC
M86.339 Chronic multifocal osteomyelitis, unspecified radius and ulna HCC
M86.34 Chronic multifocal osteomyelitis, hand
M86.341 Chronic multifocal osteomyelitis, right hand HCC
M86.342 Chronic multifocal osteomyelitis, left hand HCC
M86.349 Chronic multifocal osteomyelitis, unspecified hand HCC
M86.35 Chronic multifocal osteomyelitis, femur
M86.351 Chronic multifocal osteomyelitis, right femur HCC
M86.352 Chronic multifocal osteomyelitis, left femur HCC
M86.359 Chronic multifocal osteomyelitis, unspecified femur HCC
M86.36 Chronic multifocal osteomyelitis, tibia and fibula
M86.361 Chronic multifocal osteomyelitis, right tibia and fibula HCC
M86.362 Chronic multifocal osteomyelitis, left tibia and fibula HCC
M86.369 Chronic multifocal osteomyelitis, unspecified tibia and fibula HCC
M86.37 Chronic multifocal osteomyelitis, ankle and foot
M86.371 Chronic multifocal osteomyelitis, right ankle and foot HCC
M86.372 Chronic multifocal osteomyelitis, left ankle and foot HCC
M86.379 Chronic multifocal osteomyelitis, unspecified ankle and foot HCC

M86.38 Chronic multifocal osteomyelitis, other site HCC
M86.39 Chronic multifocal osteomyelitis, multiple sites HCC
5 M86.4 Chronic osteomyelitis with draining sinus
M86.40 Chronic osteomyelitis with draining sinus, unspecified site HCC
6 M86.41 Chronic osteomyelitis with draining sinus, shoulder
M86.411 Chronic osteomyelitis with draining sinus, right shoulder HCC
M86.412 Chronic osteomyelitis with draining sinus, left shoulder HCC
M86.419 Chronic osteomyelitis with draining sinus, unspecified shoulder HCC
6 M86.42 Chronic osteomyelitis with draining sinus, humerus
M86.421 Chronic osteomyelitis with draining sinus, right humerus HCC
M86.422 Chronic osteomyelitis with draining sinus, left humerus HCC
M86.429 Chronic osteomyelitis with draining sinus, unspecified humerus HCC
6 M86.43 Chronic osteomyelitis with draining sinus, radius and ulna
M86.431 Chronic osteomyelitis with draining sinus, right radius and ulna HCC
M86.432 Chronic osteomyelitis with draining sinus, left radius and ulna HCC
M86.439 Chronic osteomyelitis with draining sinus, unspecified radius and ulna HCC
6 M86.44 Chronic osteomyelitis with draining sinus, hand
M86.441 Chronic osteomyelitis with draining sinus, right hand HCC
M86.442 Chronic osteomyelitis with draining sinus, left hand HCC
M86.449 Chronic osteomyelitis with draining sinus, unspecified hand HCC
6 M86.45 Chronic osteomyelitis with draining sinus, femur
M86.451 Chronic osteomyelitis with draining sinus, right femur HCC
M86.452 Chronic osteomyelitis with draining sinus, left femur HCC
M86.459 Chronic osteomyelitis with draining sinus, unspecified femur HCC
6 M86.46 Chronic osteomyelitis with draining sinus, tibia and fibula
M86.461 Chronic osteomyelitis with draining sinus, right tibia and fibula HCC
M86.462 Chronic osteomyelitis with draining sinus, left tibia and fibula HCC
M86.469 Chronic osteomyelitis with draining sinus, unspecified tibia and fibula HCC
6 M86.47 Chronic osteomyelitis with draining sinus, ankle and foot
M86.471 Chronic osteomyelitis with draining sinus, right ankle and foot HCC
M86.472 Chronic osteomyelitis with draining sinus, left ankle and foot HCC
M86.479 Chronic osteomyelitis with draining sinus, unspecified ankle and foot HCC
M86.48 Chronic osteomyelitis with draining sinus, other site HCC
M86.49 Chronic osteomyelitis with draining sinus, multiple sites HCC
5 M86.5 Other chronic hematogenous osteomyelitis
M86.50 Other chronic hematogenous osteomyelitis, unspecified site HCC
6 M86.51 Other chronic hematogenous osteomyelitis, shoulder
M86.511 Other chronic hematogenous osteomyelitis, right shoulder HCC
M86.512 Other chronic hematogenous osteomyelitis, left shoulder HCC
M86.519 Other chronic hematogenous osteomyelitis, unspecified shoulder HCC
6 M86.52 Other chronic hematogenous osteomyelitis, humerus
M86.521 Other chronic hematogenous osteomyelitis, right humerus HCC
M86.522 Other chronic hematogenous osteomyelitis, left humerus HCC
M86.529 Other chronic hematogenous osteomyelitis, unspecified humerus HCC
6 M86.53 Other chronic hematogenous osteomyelitis, radius and ulna
M86.531 Other chronic hematogenous osteomyelitis, right radius and ulna HCC
M86.532 Other chronic hematogenous osteomyelitis, left radius and ulna HCC
M86.539 Other chronic hematogenous osteomyelitis, unspecified radius and ulna HCC
6 M86.54 Other chronic hematogenous osteomyelitis, hand
M86.541 Other chronic hematogenous osteomyelitis, right hand HCC
M86.542 Other chronic hematogenous osteomyelitis, left hand HCC
M86.549 Other chronic hematogenous osteomyelitis, unspecified hand HCC
6 M86.55 Other chronic hematogenous osteomyelitis, femur
M86.551 Other chronic hematogenous osteomyelitis, right femur HCC
M86.552 Other chronic hematogenous osteomyelitis, left femur HCC
M86.559 Other chronic hematogenous osteomyelitis, unspecified femur HCC
6 M86.56 Other chronic hematogenous osteomyelitis, tibia and fibula
M86.561 Other chronic hematogenous osteomyelitis, right tibia and fibula HCC
M86.562 Other chronic hematogenous osteomyelitis, left tibia and fibula HCC
M86.569 Other chronic hematogenous osteomyelitis, unspecified tibia and fibula HCC
6 M86.57 Other chronic hematogenous osteomyelitis, ankle and foot
M86.571 Other chronic hematogenous osteomyelitis, right ankle and foot HCC
M86.572 Other chronic hematogenous osteomyelitis, left ankle and foot HCC
M86.579 Other chronic hematogenous osteomyelitis, unspecified ankle and foot HCC
M86.58 Other chronic hematogenous osteomyelitis, other site HCC
M86.59 Other chronic hematogenous osteomyelitis, multiple sites HCC
5 M86.6 Other chronic osteomyelitis
M86.60 Other chronic osteomyelitis, unspecified site HCC
6 M86.61 Other chronic osteomyelitis, shoulder
M86.611 Other chronic osteomyelitis, right shoulder HCC
M86.612 Other chronic osteomyelitis, left shoulder HCC
M86.619 Other chronic osteomyelitis, unspecified shoulder HCC
6 M86.62 Other chronic osteomyelitis, humerus
M86.621 Other chronic osteomyelitis, right humerus HCC
M86.622 Other chronic osteomyelitis, left humerus HCC
M86.629 Other chronic osteomyelitis, unspecified humerus HCC
6 M86.63 Other chronic osteomyelitis, radius and ulna
M86.631 Other chronic osteomyelitis, right radius and ulna HCC
M86.632 Other chronic osteomyelitis, left radius and ulna HCC
M86.639 Other chronic osteomyelitis, unspecified radius and ulna HCC
6 M86.64 Other chronic osteomyelitis, hand
M86.641 Other chronic osteomyelitis, right hand HCC
M86.642 Other chronic osteomyelitis, left hand HCC
M86.649 Other chronic osteomyelitis, unspecified hand HCC
6 M86.65 Other chronic osteomyelitis, thigh
M86.651 Other chronic osteomyelitis, right thigh HCC
M86.652 Other chronic osteomyelitis, left thigh HCC
M86.659 Other chronic osteomyelitis, unspecified thigh HCC
6 M86.66 Other chronic osteomyelitis, tibia and fibula
M86.661 Other chronic osteomyelitis, right tibia and fibula HCC
M86.662 Other chronic osteomyelitis, left tibia and fibula HCC

M86.669 Other chronic osteomyelitis, unspecified tibia and fibula HCC

M86.67 Other chronic osteomyelitis, ankle and foot

M86.671 Other chronic osteomyelitis, right ankle and foot HCC
AHA: 1Q 2016, 13

M86.672 Other chronic osteomyelitis, left ankle and foot HCC

M86.679 Other chronic osteomyelitis, unspecified ankle and foot HCC

M86.68 Other chronic osteomyelitis, other site HCC

M86.69 Other chronic osteomyelitis, multiple sites HCC

M86.8 Other osteomyelitis
Brodie's abscess

M86.8X Other osteomyelitis

M86.8X0 Other osteomyelitis, multiple sites HCC

M86.8X1 Other osteomyelitis, shoulder HCC

M86.8X2 Other osteomyelitis, upper arm HCC

M86.8X3 Other osteomyelitis, forearm HCC

M86.8X4 Other osteomyelitis, hand HCC

M86.8X5 Other osteomyelitis, thigh HCC

M86.8X6 Other osteomyelitis, lower leg HCC

M86.8X7 Other osteomyelitis, ankle and foot HCC

M86.8X8 Other osteomyelitis, other site HCC

M86.8X9 Other osteomyelitis, unspecified sites HCC

M86.9 Osteomyelitis, unspecified HCC
Infection of bone NOS
Periostitis without osteomyelitis

M87 Osteonecrosis

INCLUDES avascular necrosis of bone

Use additional code to identify major osseous defect, if applicable (M89.7-)

EXCLUDES 1 *juvenile osteonecrosis (M91-M92)*
osteochondropathies (M90-M93)

GUIDELINES **Section I.C.13.a.1)**
For certain conditions, the bone may be affected at the upper or lower end, (e.g., avascular necrosis of bone, M87, Osteoporosis, M80, M81). Though the portion of the bone affected may be at the joint, the site designation will be the bone, not the joint.

CODING TIP ✓ **Documentation:** Osteonecrosis also may be termed avascular necrosis or aseptic necrosis of the bone. The condition indicates a necrosis of bone due to impaired blood supply and may be related to trauma, use of drugs or another cause. Review documentation carefully to determine if a causative condition is known.

DEFINITION The death of bone tissue from an interruption of its blood supply.

M87.0 Idiopathic aseptic necrosis of bone

DEFINITION The death of bone tissue from ischemia of unknown cause.

M87.00 Idiopathic aseptic necrosis of unspecified bone HCC

M87.01 Idiopathic aseptic necrosis of shoulder
Idiopathic aseptic necrosis of clavicle and scapula

M87.011 Idiopathic aseptic necrosis of right shoulder HCC

M87.012 Idiopathic aseptic necrosis of left shoulder HCC

M87.019 Idiopathic aseptic necrosis of unspecified shoulder HCC

M87.02 Idiopathic aseptic necrosis of humerus

M87.021 Idiopathic aseptic necrosis of right humerus HCC

M87.022 Idiopathic aseptic necrosis of left humerus HCC

M87.029 Idiopathic aseptic necrosis of unspecified humerus HCC

M87.03 Idiopathic aseptic necrosis of radius, ulna and carpus

M87.031 Idiopathic aseptic necrosis of right radius HCC

M87.032 Idiopathic aseptic necrosis of left radius HCC

M87.033 Idiopathic aseptic necrosis of unspecified radius HCC

M87.034 Idiopathic aseptic necrosis of right ulna HCC

M87.035 Idiopathic aseptic necrosis of left ulna HCC

M87.036 Idiopathic aseptic necrosis of unspecified ulna HCC

M87.037 Idiopathic aseptic necrosis of right carpus HCC

M87.038 Idiopathic aseptic necrosis of left carpus HCC

M87.039 Idiopathic aseptic necrosis of unspecified carpus HCC

M87.04 Idiopathic aseptic necrosis of hand and fingers
Idiopathic aseptic necrosis of metacarpals and phalanges of hands

M87.041 Idiopathic aseptic necrosis of right hand HCC

M87.042 Idiopathic aseptic necrosis of left hand HCC

M87.043 Idiopathic aseptic necrosis of unspecified hand HCC

M87.044 Idiopathic aseptic necrosis of right finger(s) HCC

M87.045 Idiopathic aseptic necrosis of left finger(s) HCC

M87.046 Idiopathic aseptic necrosis of unspecified finger(s) HCC

M87.05 Idiopathic aseptic necrosis of pelvis and femur

M87.050 Idiopathic aseptic necrosis of pelvis HCC

M87.051 Idiopathic aseptic necrosis of right femur HCC

M87.052 Idiopathic aseptic necrosis of left femur HCC

M87.059 Idiopathic aseptic necrosis of unspecified femur HCC
Idiopathic aseptic necrosis of hip NOS

M87.06 Idiopathic aseptic necrosis of tibia and fibula

M87.061 Idiopathic aseptic necrosis of right tibia HCC

M87.062 Idiopathic aseptic necrosis of left tibia HCC

M87.063 Idiopathic aseptic necrosis of unspecified tibia HCC

M87.064 Idiopathic aseptic necrosis of right fibula HCC

M87.065 Idiopathic aseptic necrosis of left fibula HCC

M87.066 Idiopathic aseptic necrosis of unspecified fibula HCC

M87.07 Idiopathic aseptic necrosis of ankle, foot and toes
Idiopathic aseptic necrosis of metatarsus, tarsus, and phalanges of toes

M87.071 Idiopathic aseptic necrosis of right ankle HCC

M87.072 Idiopathic aseptic necrosis of left ankle HCC

M87.073 Idiopathic aseptic necrosis of unspecified ankle HCC

M87.074 Idiopathic aseptic necrosis of right foot HCC

M87.075 Idiopathic aseptic necrosis of left foot HCC

M87.076 Idiopathic aseptic necrosis of unspecified foot HCC

M87.077 Idiopathic aseptic necrosis of right toe(s) HCC

M87.078 Idiopathic aseptic necrosis of left toe(s) HCC

M87.079 Idiopathic aseptic necrosis of unspecified toe(s) HCC

M87.08 Idiopathic aseptic necrosis of bone, other site HCC

M87.09 Idiopathic aseptic necrosis of bone, multiple sites HCC

M87.1 Osteonecrosis due to drugs
Use additional code for adverse effect, if applicable, to identify drug (T36-T50 with fifth or sixth character 5)

M87.10 Osteonecrosis due to drugs, unspecified bone HCC

M87.11 Osteonecrosis due to drugs, shoulder

M87.111 Osteonecrosis due to drugs, right shoulder HCC

M87.112 Osteonecrosis due to drugs, left shoulder HCC

M87.119 Osteonecrosis due to drugs, unspecified shoulder HCC

M87.12 Osteonecrosis due to drugs, humerus

M87.121 Osteonecrosis due to drugs, right humerus HCC

M87.122 Osteonecrosis due to drugs, left humerus HCC

M87.129 Osteonecrosis due to drugs, unspecified humerus HCC

M87.13 Osteonecrosis due to drugs of radius, ulna and carpus

M87.131 Osteonecrosis due to drugs of right radius HCC

M87.132 Osteonecrosis due to drugs of left radius HCC

M87.133 Osteonecrosis due to drugs of unspecified radius HCC

M87.134 Osteonecrosis due to drugs of right ulna HCC
M87.135 Osteonecrosis due to drugs of left ulna HCC
M87.136 Osteonecrosis due to drugs of unspecified ulna HCC
M87.137 Osteonecrosis due to drugs of right carpus HCC
M87.138 Osteonecrosis due to drugs of left carpus HCC
M87.139 Osteonecrosis due to drugs of unspecified carpus HCC
M87.14 Osteonecrosis due to drugs, hand and fingers
M87.141 Osteonecrosis due to drugs, right hand HCC
M87.142 Osteonecrosis due to drugs, left hand HCC
M87.143 Osteonecrosis due to drugs, unspecified hand HCC
M87.144 Osteonecrosis due to drugs, right finger(s) HCC
M87.145 Osteonecrosis due to drugs, left finger(s) HCC
M87.146 Osteonecrosis due to drugs, unspecified finger(s) HCC
M87.15 Osteonecrosis due to drugs, pelvis and femur
M87.150 Osteonecrosis due to drugs, pelvis HCC
M87.151 Osteonecrosis due to drugs, right femur HCC
M87.152 Osteonecrosis due to drugs, left femur HCC
M87.159 Osteonecrosis due to drugs, unspecified femur HCC
M87.16 Osteonecrosis due to drugs, tibia and fibula
M87.161 Osteonecrosis due to drugs, right tibia HCC
M87.162 Osteonecrosis due to drugs, left tibia HCC
M87.163 Osteonecrosis due to drugs, unspecified tibia HCC
M87.164 Osteonecrosis due to drugs, right fibula HCC
M87.165 Osteonecrosis due to drugs, left fibula HCC
M87.166 Osteonecrosis due to drugs, unspecified fibula HCC
M87.17 Osteonecrosis due to drugs, ankle, foot and toes
M87.171 Osteonecrosis due to drugs, right ankle HCC
M87.172 Osteonecrosis due to drugs, left ankle HCC
M87.173 Osteonecrosis due to drugs, unspecified ankle HCC
M87.174 Osteonecrosis due to drugs, right foot HCC
M87.175 Osteonecrosis due to drugs, left foot HCC
M87.176 Osteonecrosis due to drugs, unspecified foot HCC
M87.177 Osteonecrosis due to drugs, right toe(s) HCC
M87.178 Osteonecrosis due to drugs, left toe(s) HCC
M87.179 Osteonecrosis due to drugs, unspecified toe(s) HCC
M87.18 Osteonecrosis due to drugs, other site
M87.180 Osteonecrosis due to drugs, jaw HCC
M87.188 Osteonecrosis due to drugs, other site HCC
M87.19 Osteonecrosis due to drugs, multiple sites HCC
M87.2 Osteonecrosis due to previous trauma
M87.20 Osteonecrosis due to previous trauma, unspecified bone HCC
M87.21 Osteonecrosis due to previous trauma, shoulder
M87.211 Osteonecrosis due to previous trauma, right shoulder HCC
M87.212 Osteonecrosis due to previous trauma, left shoulder HCC
M87.219 Osteonecrosis due to previous trauma, unspecified shoulder HCC
M87.22 Osteonecrosis due to previous trauma, humerus
M87.221 Osteonecrosis due to previous trauma, right humerus HCC
M87.222 Osteonecrosis due to previous trauma, left humerus HCC
M87.229 Osteonecrosis due to previous trauma, unspecified humerus HCC
M87.23 Osteonecrosis due to previous trauma of radius, ulna and carpus
M87.231 Osteonecrosis due to previous trauma of right radius HCC
M87.232 Osteonecrosis due to previous trauma of left radius HCC
M87.233 Osteonecrosis due to previous trauma of unspecified radius HCC
M87.234 Osteonecrosis due to previous trauma of right ulna HCC
M87.235 Osteonecrosis due to previous trauma of left ulna HCC
M87.236 Osteonecrosis due to previous trauma of unspecified ulna HCC
M87.237 Osteonecrosis due to previous trauma of right carpus HCC
M87.238 Osteonecrosis due to previous trauma of left carpus HCC
M87.239 Osteonecrosis due to previous trauma of unspecified carpus HCC
M87.24 Osteonecrosis due to previous trauma, hand and fingers
M87.241 Osteonecrosis due to previous trauma, right hand HCC
M87.242 Osteonecrosis due to previous trauma, left hand HCC
M87.243 Osteonecrosis due to previous trauma, unspecified hand HCC
M87.244 Osteonecrosis due to previous trauma, right finger(s) HCC
M87.245 Osteonecrosis due to previous trauma, left finger(s) HCC
M87.246 Osteonecrosis due to previous trauma, unspecified finger(s) HCC
M87.25 Osteonecrosis due to previous trauma, pelvis and femur
M87.250 Osteonecrosis due to previous trauma, pelvis HCC
M87.251 Osteonecrosis due to previous trauma, right femur HCC
M87.252 Osteonecrosis due to previous trauma, left femur HCC
M87.256 Osteonecrosis due to previous trauma, unspecified femur HCC
M87.26 Osteonecrosis due to previous trauma, tibia and fibula
M87.261 Osteonecrosis due to previous trauma, right tibia HCC
M87.262 Osteonecrosis due to previous trauma, left tibia HCC
M87.263 Osteonecrosis due to previous trauma, unspecified tibia HCC
M87.264 Osteonecrosis due to previous trauma, right fibula HCC
M87.265 Osteonecrosis due to previous trauma, left fibula HCC
M87.266 Osteonecrosis due to previous trauma, unspecified fibula HCC
M87.27 Osteonecrosis due to previous trauma, ankle, foot and toes
M87.271 Osteonecrosis due to previous trauma, right ankle HCC
M87.272 Osteonecrosis due to previous trauma, left ankle HCC
M87.273 Osteonecrosis due to previous trauma, unspecified ankle HCC
M87.274 Osteonecrosis due to previous trauma, right foot HCC
M87.275 Osteonecrosis due to previous trauma, left foot HCC
M87.276 Osteonecrosis due to previous trauma, unspecified foot HCC
M87.277 Osteonecrosis due to previous trauma, right toe(s) HCC
M87.278 Osteonecrosis due to previous trauma, left toe(s) HCC
M87.279 Osteonecrosis due to previous trauma, unspecified toe(s) HCC
M87.28 Osteonecrosis due to previous trauma, other site HCC
M87.29 Osteonecrosis due to previous trauma, multiple sites HCC
M87.3 Other secondary osteonecrosis
M87.30 Other secondary osteonecrosis, unspecified bone HCC
M87.31 Other secondary osteonecrosis, shoulder
M87.311 Other secondary osteonecrosis, right shoulder HCC

M87.312 Other secondary osteonecrosis, left shoulder HCC
M87.319 Other secondary osteonecrosis, unspecified shoulder HCC
M87.32 Other secondary osteonecrosis, humerus
M87.321 Other secondary osteonecrosis, right humerus HCC
M87.322 Other secondary osteonecrosis, left humerus HCC
M87.329 Other secondary osteonecrosis, unspecified humerus HCC
M87.33 Other secondary osteonecrosis of radius, ulna and carpus
M87.331 Other secondary osteonecrosis of right radius HCC
M87.332 Other secondary osteonecrosis of left radius HCC
M87.333 Other secondary osteonecrosis of unspecified radius HCC
M87.334 Other secondary osteonecrosis of right ulna HCC
M87.335 Other secondary osteonecrosis of left ulna HCC
M87.336 Other secondary osteonecrosis of unspecified ulna HCC
M87.337 Other secondary osteonecrosis of right carpus HCC
M87.338 Other secondary osteonecrosis of left carpus HCC
M87.339 Other secondary osteonecrosis of unspecified carpus HCC
M87.34 Other secondary osteonecrosis, hand and fingers
M87.341 Other secondary osteonecrosis, right hand HCC
M87.342 Other secondary osteonecrosis, left hand HCC
M87.343 Other secondary osteonecrosis, unspecified hand HCC
M87.344 Other secondary osteonecrosis, right finger(s) HCC
M87.345 Other secondary osteonecrosis, left finger(s) HCC
M87.346 Other secondary osteonecrosis, unspecified finger(s) HCC
M87.35 Other secondary osteonecrosis, pelvis and femur
M87.350 Other secondary osteonecrosis, pelvis HCC
M87.351 Other secondary osteonecrosis, right femur HCC
M87.352 Other secondary osteonecrosis, left femur HCC
M87.353 Other secondary osteonecrosis, unspecified femur HCC
M87.36 Other secondary osteonecrosis, tibia and fibula
M87.361 Other secondary osteonecrosis, right tibia HCC
M87.362 Other secondary osteonecrosis, left tibia HCC
M87.363 Other secondary osteonecrosis, unspecified tibia HCC
M87.364 Other secondary osteonecrosis, right fibula HCC
M87.365 Other secondary osteonecrosis, left fibula HCC
M87.366 Other secondary osteonecrosis, unspecified fibula HCC
M87.37 Other secondary osteonecrosis, ankle and foot
M87.371 Other secondary osteonecrosis, right ankle HCC
M87.372 Other secondary osteonecrosis, left ankle HCC
M87.373 Other secondary osteonecrosis, unspecified ankle HCC
M87.374 Other secondary osteonecrosis, right foot HCC
M87.375 Other secondary osteonecrosis, left foot HCC
M87.376 Other secondary osteonecrosis, unspecified foot HCC
M87.377 Other secondary osteonecrosis, right toe(s) HCC
M87.378 Other secondary osteonecrosis, left toe(s) HCC
M87.379 Other secondary osteonecrosis, unspecified toe(s) HCC
M87.38 Other secondary osteonecrosis, other site HCC
M87.39 Other secondary osteonecrosis, multiple sites HCC
M87.8 Other osteonecrosis
M87.80 Other osteonecrosis, unspecified bone HCC
M87.81 Other osteonecrosis, shoulder
M87.811 Other osteonecrosis, right shoulder HCC
M87.812 Other osteonecrosis, left shoulder HCC
M87.819 Other osteonecrosis, unspecified shoulder HCC
M87.82 Other osteonecrosis, humerus
M87.821 Other osteonecrosis, right humerus HCC
M87.822 Other osteonecrosis, left humerus HCC
M87.829 Other osteonecrosis, unspecified humerus HCC
M87.83 Other osteonecrosis of radius, ulna and carpus
M87.831 Other osteonecrosis of right radius HCC
M87.832 Other osteonecrosis of left radius HCC
M87.833 Other osteonecrosis of unspecified radius HCC
M87.834 Other osteonecrosis of right ulna HCC
M87.835 Other osteonecrosis of left ulna HCC
M87.836 Other osteonecrosis of unspecified ulna HCC
M87.837 Other osteonecrosis of right carpus HCC
M87.838 Other osteonecrosis of left carpus HCC
M87.839 Other osteonecrosis of unspecified carpus HCC
M87.84 Other osteonecrosis, hand and fingers
M87.841 Other osteonecrosis, right hand HCC
M87.842 Other osteonecrosis, left hand HCC
M87.843 Other osteonecrosis, unspecified hand HCC
M87.844 Other osteonecrosis, right finger(s) HCC
M87.845 Other osteonecrosis, left finger(s) HCC
M87.849 Other osteonecrosis, unspecified finger(s) HCC
M87.85 Other osteonecrosis, pelvis and femur
M87.850 Other osteonecrosis, pelvis HCC
M87.851 Other osteonecrosis, right femur HCC
M87.852 Other osteonecrosis, left femur HCC
M87.859 Other osteonecrosis, unspecified femur HCC
M87.86 Other osteonecrosis, tibia and fibula
M87.861 Other osteonecrosis, right tibia HCC
M87.862 Other osteonecrosis, left tibia HCC
M87.863 Other osteonecrosis, unspecified tibia HCC
M87.864 Other osteonecrosis, right fibula HCC
M87.865 Other osteonecrosis, left fibula HCC
M87.869 Other osteonecrosis, unspecified fibula HCC
M87.87 Other osteonecrosis, ankle, foot and toes
M87.871 Other osteonecrosis, right ankle HCC
M87.872 Other osteonecrosis, left ankle HCC
M87.873 Other osteonecrosis, unspecified ankle HCC
M87.874 Other osteonecrosis, right foot HCC
M87.875 Other osteonecrosis, left foot HCC
M87.876 Other osteonecrosis, unspecified foot HCC
M87.877 Other osteonecrosis, right toe(s) HCC
M87.878 Other osteonecrosis, left toe(s) HCC
M87.879 Other osteonecrosis, unspecified toe(s) HCC
M87.88 Other osteonecrosis, other site HCC
M87.89 Other osteonecrosis, multiple sites HCC
M87.9 Osteonecrosis, unspecified HCC
Necrosis of bone NOS

M88 Osteitis deformans [Paget's disease of bone]

EXCLUDES 1 *osteitis deformans in neoplastic disease (M90.6)*

DEFINITION A bone disorder characterized by cycles of bone loss followed by excessive attempts at repair; results in painful, deformed, enlarged bones of porous tissue prone to fractures and arthritic affected joints.

M88.0 Osteitis deformans of skull

DEFINITION Excessive breakdown and rebuilding of bone tissue in the skull, resulting in an enlarged head with abnormally remodeled skull bones that may press on nerves causing headache, vertigo, tinnitus, or hearing loss.

M88.1 Osteitis deformans of vertebrae

DEFINITION Excessive breakdown and rebuilding of the vertebrae with bone material that is less dense, resulting in an abnormally remodeled, thickened spine prone to fracture that may compress nerve roots causing pain, numbness, and tingling in arms or legs.

M88.8 Osteitis deformans of other bones
M88.81 Osteitis deformans of shoulder
M88.811 Osteitis deformans of right shoulder
M88.812 Osteitis deformans of left shoulder
M88.819 Osteitis deformans of unspecified shoulder
M88.82 Osteitis deformans of upper arm

M88.821 Osteitis deformans of right upper arm
M88.822 Osteitis deformans of left upper arm
M88.829 Osteitis deformans of unspecified upper arm
M88.83 Osteitis deformans of forearm
M88.831 Osteitis deformans of right forearm
M88.832 Osteitis deformans of left forearm
M88.839 Osteitis deformans of unspecified forearm
M88.84 Osteitis deformans of hand
M88.841 Osteitis deformans of right hand
M88.842 Osteitis deformans of left hand
M88.849 Osteitis deformans of unspecified hand
M88.85 Osteitis deformans of thigh
M88.851 Osteitis deformans of right thigh
M88.852 Osteitis deformans of left thigh
M88.859 Osteitis deformans of unspecified thigh
M88.86 Osteitis deformans of lower leg
M88.861 Osteitis deformans of right lower leg
M88.862 Osteitis deformans of left lower leg
M88.869 Osteitis deformans of unspecified lower leg
M88.87 Osteitis deformans of ankle and foot
M88.871 Osteitis deformans of right ankle and foot
M88.872 Osteitis deformans of left ankle and foot
M88.879 Osteitis deformans of unspecified ankle and foot
M88.88 Osteitis deformans of other bones
EXCLUDES 2 *osteitis deformans of skull (M88.0)*
osteitis deformans of vertebrae (M88.1)
M88.89 Osteitis deformans of multiple sites
M88.9 Osteitis deformans of unspecified bone

M89 Other disorders of bone

M89.0 Algoneurodystrophy
Shoulder-hand syndrome
Sudeck's atrophy
EXCLUDES 1 *causalgia, lower limb (G57.7-)*
causalgia, upper limb (G56.4-)
complex regional pain syndrome II, lower limb (G57.7-)
complex regional pain syndrome II, upper limb (G56.4-)
reflex sympathetic dystrophy (G90.5-)
DEFINITION Acute wasting away of bone(s) following relatively minor injury; presents with severe burning pain in the affected extremity, trophic changes in bone, and vasomotor disturbances without specific nerve injury.
M89.00 Algoneurodystrophy, unspecified site
M89.01 Algoneurodystrophy, shoulder
M89.011 Algoneurodystrophy, right shoulder
M89.012 Algoneurodystrophy, left shoulder
M89.019 Algoneurodystrophy, unspecified shoulder
M89.02 Algoneurodystrophy, upper arm
M89.021 Algoneurodystrophy, right upper arm
M89.022 Algoneurodystrophy, left upper arm
M89.029 Algoneurodystrophy, unspecified upper arm
M89.03 Algoneurodystrophy, forearm
M89.031 Algoneurodystrophy, right forearm
M89.032 Algoneurodystrophy, left forearm
M89.039 Algoneurodystrophy, unspecified forearm
M89.04 Algoneurodystrophy, hand
M89.041 Algoneurodystrophy, right hand
M89.042 Algoneurodystrophy, left hand
M89.049 Algoneurodystrophy, unspecified hand
M89.05 Algoneurodystrophy, thigh
M89.051 Algoneurodystrophy, right thigh
M89.052 Algoneurodystrophy, left thigh
M89.059 Algoneurodystrophy, unspecified thigh
M89.06 Algoneurodystrophy, lower leg
M89.061 Algoneurodystrophy, right lower leg
M89.062 Algoneurodystrophy, left lower leg
M89.069 Algoneurodystrophy, unspecified lower leg
M89.07 Algoneurodystrophy, ankle and foot
M89.071 Algoneurodystrophy, right ankle and foot
M89.072 Algoneurodystrophy, left ankle and foot
M89.079 Algoneurodystrophy, unspecified ankle and foot
M89.08 Algoneurodystrophy, other site
M89.09 Algoneurodystrophy, multiple sites
M89.1 Physeal arrest
Arrest of growth plate
Epiphyseal arrest
Growth plate arrest
M89.12 Physeal arrest, humerus
M89.121 Complete physeal arrest, right proximal humerus
M89.122 Complete physeal arrest, left proximal humerus
M89.123 Partial physeal arrest, right proximal humerus
M89.124 Partial physeal arrest, left proximal humerus
M89.125 Complete physeal arrest, right distal humerus
M89.126 Complete physeal arrest, left distal humerus
M89.127 Partial physeal arrest, right distal humerus
M89.128 Partial physeal arrest, left distal humerus
M89.129 Physeal arrest, humerus, unspecified
M89.13 Physeal arrest, forearm
M89.131 Complete physeal arrest, right distal radius
M89.132 Complete physeal arrest, left distal radius
M89.133 Partial physeal arrest, right distal radius
M89.134 Partial physeal arrest, left distal radius
M89.138 Other physeal arrest of forearm
M89.139 Physeal arrest, forearm, unspecified
M89.15 Physeal arrest, femur
M89.151 Complete physeal arrest, right proximal femur
M89.152 Complete physeal arrest, left proximal femur
M89.153 Partial physeal arrest, right proximal femur
M89.154 Partial physeal arrest, left proximal femur
M89.155 Complete physeal arrest, right distal femur
M89.156 Complete physeal arrest, left distal femur
M89.157 Partial physeal arrest, right distal femur
M89.158 Partial physeal arrest, left distal femur
M89.159 Physeal arrest, femur, unspecified
M89.16 Physeal arrest, lower leg
M89.160 Complete physeal arrest, right proximal tibia
M89.161 Complete physeal arrest, left proximal tibia
M89.162 Partial physeal arrest, right proximal tibia
M89.163 Partial physeal arrest, left proximal tibia
M89.164 Complete physeal arrest, right distal tibia
M89.165 Complete physeal arrest, left distal tibia
M89.166 Partial physeal arrest, right distal tibia
M89.167 Partial physeal arrest, left distal tibia
M89.168 Other physeal arrest of lower leg
M89.169 Physeal arrest, lower leg, unspecified
M89.18 Physeal arrest, other site
M89.2 Other disorders of bone development and growth
M89.20 Other disorders of bone development and growth, unspecified site
M89.21 Other disorders of bone development and growth, shoulder
M89.211 Other disorders of bone development and growth, right shoulder
M89.212 Other disorders of bone development and growth, left shoulder
M89.219 Other disorders of bone development and growth, unspecified shoulder
M89.22 Other disorders of bone development and growth, humerus
M89.221 Other disorders of bone development and growth, right humerus
M89.222 Other disorders of bone development and growth, left humerus
M89.229 Other disorders of bone development and growth, unspecified humerus
M89.23 Other disorders of bone development and growth, ulna and radius
M89.231 Other disorders of bone development and growth, right ulna

M89.232 Other disorders of bone development and growth, left ulna
M89.233 Other disorders of bone development and growth, right radius
M89.234 Other disorders of bone development and growth, left radius
M89.239 Other disorders of bone development and growth, unspecified ulna and radius
M89.24 Other disorders of bone development and growth, hand
M89.241 Other disorders of bone development and growth, right hand
M89.242 Other disorders of bone development and growth, left hand
M89.249 Other disorders of bone development and growth, unspecified hand
M89.25 Other disorders of bone development and growth, femur
M89.251 Other disorders of bone development and growth, right femur
M89.252 Other disorders of bone development and growth, left femur
M89.259 Other disorders of bone development and growth, unspecified femur
M89.26 Other disorders of bone development and growth, tibia and fibula
M89.261 Other disorders of bone development and growth, right tibia
M89.262 Other disorders of bone development and growth, left tibia
M89.263 Other disorders of bone development and growth, right fibula
M89.264 Other disorders of bone development and growth, left fibula
M89.269 Other disorders of bone development and growth, unspecified lower leg
M89.27 Other disorders of bone development and growth, ankle and foot
M89.271 Other disorders of bone development and growth, right ankle and foot
M89.272 Other disorders of bone development and growth, left ankle and foot
M89.279 Other disorders of bone development and growth, unspecified ankle and foot
M89.28 Other disorders of bone development and growth, other site
M89.29 Other disorders of bone development and growth, multiple sites
M89.3 Hypertrophy of bone
M89.30 Hypertrophy of bone, unspecified site
M89.31 Hypertrophy of bone, shoulder
M89.311 Hypertrophy of bone, right shoulder
M89.312 Hypertrophy of bone, left shoulder
M89.319 Hypertrophy of bone, unspecified shoulder
M89.32 Hypertrophy of bone, humerus
M89.321 Hypertrophy of bone, right humerus
M89.322 Hypertrophy of bone, left humerus
M89.329 Hypertrophy of bone, unspecified humerus
M89.33 Hypertrophy of bone, ulna and radius
M89.331 Hypertrophy of bone, right ulna
M89.332 Hypertrophy of bone, left ulna
M89.333 Hypertrophy of bone, right radius
M89.334 Hypertrophy of bone, left radius
M89.339 Hypertrophy of bone, unspecified ulna and radius
M89.34 Hypertrophy of bone, hand
M89.341 Hypertrophy of bone, right hand
M89.342 Hypertrophy of bone, left hand
M89.349 Hypertrophy of bone, unspecified hand
M89.35 Hypertrophy of bone, femur
M89.351 Hypertrophy of bone, right femur
M89.352 Hypertrophy of bone, left femur
M89.359 Hypertrophy of bone, unspecified femur
M89.36 Hypertrophy of bone, tibia and fibula
M89.361 Hypertrophy of bone, right tibia
M89.362 Hypertrophy of bone, left tibia
M89.363 Hypertrophy of bone, right fibula
M89.364 Hypertrophy of bone, left fibula
M89.369 Hypertrophy of bone, unspecified tibia and fibula
M89.37 Hypertrophy of bone, ankle and foot
M89.371 Hypertrophy of bone, right ankle and foot
M89.372 Hypertrophy of bone, left ankle and foot
M89.379 Hypertrophy of bone, unspecified ankle and foot
M89.38 Hypertrophy of bone, other site
M89.39 Hypertrophy of bone, multiple sites
M89.4 Other hypertrophic osteoarthropathy
Marie-Bamberger disease
Pachydermoperiostosis
M89.40 Other hypertrophic osteoarthropathy, unspecified site
M89.41 Other hypertrophic osteoarthropathy, shoulder
M89.411 Other hypertrophic osteoarthropathy, right shoulder
M89.412 Other hypertrophic osteoarthropathy, left shoulder
M89.419 Other hypertrophic osteoarthropathy, unspecified shoulder
M89.42 Other hypertrophic osteoarthropathy, upper arm
M89.421 Other hypertrophic osteoarthropathy, right upper arm
M89.422 Other hypertrophic osteoarthropathy, left upper arm
M89.429 Other hypertrophic osteoarthropathy, unspecified upper arm
M89.43 Other hypertrophic osteoarthropathy, forearm
M89.431 Other hypertrophic osteoarthropathy, right forearm
M89.432 Other hypertrophic osteoarthropathy, left forearm
M89.439 Other hypertrophic osteoarthropathy, unspecified forearm
M89.44 Other hypertrophic osteoarthropathy, hand
M89.441 Other hypertrophic osteoarthropathy, right hand
M89.442 Other hypertrophic osteoarthropathy, left hand
M89.449 Other hypertrophic osteoarthropathy, unspecified hand
M89.45 Other hypertrophic osteoarthropathy, thigh
M89.451 Other hypertrophic osteoarthropathy, right thigh
M89.452 Other hypertrophic osteoarthropathy, left thigh
M89.459 Other hypertrophic osteoarthropathy, unspecified thigh
M89.46 Other hypertrophic osteoarthropathy, lower leg
M89.461 Other hypertrophic osteoarthropathy, right lower leg
M89.462 Other hypertrophic osteoarthropathy, left lower leg
M89.469 Other hypertrophic osteoarthropathy, unspecified lower leg
M89.47 Other hypertrophic osteoarthropathy, ankle and foot
M89.471 Other hypertrophic osteoarthropathy, right ankle and foot
M89.472 Other hypertrophic osteoarthropathy, left ankle and foot
M89.479 Other hypertrophic osteoarthropathy, unspecified ankle and foot
M89.48 Other hypertrophic osteoarthropathy, other site
M89.49 Other hypertrophic osteoarthropathy, multiple sites
M89.5 Osteolysis
Use additional code to identify major osseous defect, if applicable (M89.7-)
EXCLUDES 2 *periprosthetic osteolysis of internal prosthetic joint (T84.05-)*
M89.50 Osteolysis, unspecified site
M89.51 Osteolysis, shoulder
M89.511 Osteolysis, right shoulder
M89.512 Osteolysis, left shoulder
M89.519 Osteolysis, unspecified shoulder
M89.52 Osteolysis, upper arm

M89.521 Osteolysis, right upper arm
M89.522 Osteolysis, left upper arm
M89.529 Osteolysis, unspecified upper arm
M89.53 Osteolysis, forearm
M89.531 Osteolysis, right forearm
M89.532 Osteolysis, left forearm
M89.539 Osteolysis, unspecified forearm
M89.54 Osteolysis, hand
M89.541 Osteolysis, right hand
M89.542 Osteolysis, left hand
M89.549 Osteolysis, unspecified hand
M89.55 Osteolysis, thigh
M89.551 Osteolysis, right thigh
M89.552 Osteolysis, left thigh
M89.559 Osteolysis, unspecified thigh
M89.56 Osteolysis, lower leg
M89.561 Osteolysis, right lower leg
M89.562 Osteolysis, left lower leg
M89.569 Osteolysis, unspecified lower leg
M89.57 Osteolysis, ankle and foot
M89.571 Osteolysis, right ankle and foot
M89.572 Osteolysis, left ankle and foot
M89.579 Osteolysis, unspecified ankle and foot
M89.58 Osteolysis, other site
M89.59 Osteolysis, multiple sites
M89.6 Osteopathy after poliomyelitis
Use additional code (B91) to identify previous poliomyelitis
EXCLUDES 1 *postpolio syndrome (G14)*
M89.60 Osteopathy after poliomyelitis, unspecified site HCC
M89.61 Osteopathy after poliomyelitis, shoulder
M89.611 Osteopathy after poliomyelitis, right shoulder HCC
M89.612 Osteopathy after poliomyelitis, left shoulder HCC
M89.619 Osteopathy after poliomyelitis, unspecified shoulder HCC
M89.62 Osteopathy after poliomyelitis, upper arm
M89.621 Osteopathy after poliomyelitis, right upper arm HCC
M89.622 Osteopathy after poliomyelitis, left upper arm HCC
M89.629 Osteopathy after poliomyelitis, unspecified upper arm HCC
M89.63 Osteopathy after poliomyelitis, forearm
M89.631 Osteopathy after poliomyelitis, right forearm HCC
M89.632 Osteopathy after poliomyelitis, left forearm HCC
M89.639 Osteopathy after poliomyelitis, unspecified forearm HCC
M89.64 Osteopathy after poliomyelitis, hand
M89.641 Osteopathy after poliomyelitis, right hand HCC
M89.642 Osteopathy after poliomyelitis, left hand HCC
M89.649 Osteopathy after poliomyelitis, unspecified hand HCC
M89.65 Osteopathy after poliomyelitis, thigh
M89.651 Osteopathy after poliomyelitis, right thigh HCC
M89.652 Osteopathy after poliomyelitis, left thigh HCC
M89.659 Osteopathy after poliomyelitis, unspecified thigh HCC
M89.66 Osteopathy after poliomyelitis, lower leg
M89.661 Osteopathy after poliomyelitis, right lower leg HCC
M89.662 Osteopathy after poliomyelitis, left lower leg HCC
M89.669 Osteopathy after poliomyelitis, unspecified lower leg HCC
M89.67 Osteopathy after poliomyelitis, ankle and foot
M89.671 Osteopathy after poliomyelitis, right ankle and foot HCC
M89.672 Osteopathy after poliomyelitis, left ankle and foot HCC
M89.679 Osteopathy after poliomyelitis, unspecified ankle and foot HCC
M89.68 Osteopathy after poliomyelitis, other site HCC
M89.69 Osteopathy after poliomyelitis, multiple sites HCC
M89.7 Major osseous defect
Code first underlying disease, if known, such as:
aseptic necrosis of bone (M87.-)
malignant neoplasm of bone (C40.-)
osteolysis (M89.5)
osteomyelitis (M86.-)
osteonecrosis (M87.-)
osteoporosis (M80.-, M81.-)
periprosthetic osteolysis (T84.05-)
M89.70 Major osseous defect, unspecified site
M89.71 Major osseous defect, shoulder region
Major osseous defect clavicle or scapula
M89.711 Major osseous defect, right shoulder region
M89.712 Major osseous defect, left shoulder region
M89.719 Major osseous defect, unspecified shoulder region
M89.72 Major osseous defect, humerus
M89.721 Major osseous defect, right humerus
M89.722 Major osseous defect, left humerus
M89.729 Major osseous defect, unspecified humerus
M89.73 Major osseous defect, forearm
Major osseous defect of radius and ulna
M89.731 Major osseous defect, right forearm
M89.732 Major osseous defect, left forearm
M89.739 Major osseous defect, unspecified forearm
M89.74 Major osseous defect, hand
Major osseous defect of carpus, fingers, metacarpus
M89.741 Major osseous defect, right hand
M89.742 Major osseous defect, left hand
M89.749 Major osseous defect, unspecified hand
M89.75 Major osseous defect, pelvic region and thigh
Major osseous defect of femur and pelvis
M89.751 Major osseous defect, right pelvic region and thigh
M89.752 Major osseous defect, left pelvic region and thigh
M89.759 Major osseous defect, unspecified pelvic region and thigh
M89.76 Major osseous defect, lower leg
Major osseous defect of fibula and tibia
M89.761 Major osseous defect, right lower leg
M89.762 Major osseous defect, left lower leg
M89.769 Major osseous defect, unspecified lower leg
M89.77 Major osseous defect, ankle and foot
Major osseous defect of metatarsus, tarsus, toes
M89.771 Major osseous defect, right ankle and foot
M89.772 Major osseous defect, left ankle and foot
M89.779 Major osseous defect, unspecified ankle and foot
M89.78 Major osseous defect, other site
M89.79 Major osseous defect, multiple sites
M89.8 Other specified disorders of bone
Infantile cortical hyperostoses
Post-traumatic subperiosteal ossification
M89.8X Other specified disorders of bone
M89.8X0 Other specified disorders of bone, multiple sites
M89.8X1 Other specified disorders of bone, shoulder
M89.8X2 Other specified disorders of bone, upper arm
M89.8X3 Other specified disorders of bone, forearm
M89.8X4 Other specified disorders of bone, hand
M89.8X5 Other specified disorders of bone, thigh
M89.8X6 Other specified disorders of bone, lower leg
M89.8X7 Other specified disorders of bone, ankle and foot
M89.8X8 Other specified disorders of bone, other site
M89.8X9 Other specified disorders of bone, unspecified site
M89.9 Disorder of bone, unspecified

4 M90 Osteopathies in diseases classified elsewhere

EXCLUDES 1 *osteochondritis, osteomyelitis, and osteopathy (in) :*
cryptococcosis (B45.3)
diabetes mellitus (E08-E13 with .69-)
gonococcal (A54.43)
neurogenic syphilis (A52.11)
renal osteodystrophy (N25.0)
salmonellosis (A02.24)
secondary syphilis (A51.46)
syphilis (late) (A52.77)

5 M90.5 Osteonecrosis in diseases classified elsewhere
Code first underlying disease, such as:
caisson disease (T70.3)
hemoglobinopathy (D50-D64)

M90.50 *Osteonecrosis in diseases classified elsewhere, unspecified site* HCC

6 M90.51 Osteonecrosis in diseases classified elsewhere, shoulder
- **M90.511** *Osteonecrosis in diseases classified elsewhere, right shoulder* HCC
- **M90.512** *Osteonecrosis in diseases classified elsewhere, left shoulder* HCC
- **M90.519** *Osteonecrosis in diseases classified elsewhere, unspecified shoulder* HCC

6 M90.52 Osteonecrosis in diseases classified elsewhere, upper arm
- **M90.521** *Osteonecrosis in diseases classified elsewhere, right upper arm* HCC
- **M90.522** *Osteonecrosis in diseases classified elsewhere, left upper arm* HCC
- **M90.529** *Osteonecrosis in diseases classified elsewhere, unspecified upper arm* HCC

6 M90.53 Osteonecrosis in diseases classified elsewhere, forearm
- **M90.531** *Osteonecrosis in diseases classified elsewhere, right forearm* HCC
- **M90.532** *Osteonecrosis in diseases classified elsewhere, left forearm* HCC
- **M90.539** *Osteonecrosis in diseases classified elsewhere, unspecified forearm* HCC

6 M90.54 Osteonecrosis in diseases classified elsewhere, hand
- **M90.541** *Osteonecrosis in diseases classified elsewhere, right hand* HCC
- **M90.542** *Osteonecrosis in diseases classified elsewhere, left hand* HCC
- **M90.549** *Osteonecrosis in diseases classified elsewhere, unspecified hand* HCC

6 M90.55 Osteonecrosis in diseases classified elsewhere, thigh
- **M90.551** *Osteonecrosis in diseases classified elsewhere, right thigh* HCC
- **M90.552** *Osteonecrosis in diseases classified elsewhere, left thigh* HCC
- **M90.559** *Osteonecrosis in diseases classified elsewhere, unspecified thigh* HCC

6 M90.56 Osteonecrosis in diseases classified elsewhere, lower leg
- **M90.561** *Osteonecrosis in diseases classified elsewhere, right lower leg* HCC
- **M90.562** *Osteonecrosis in diseases classified elsewhere, left lower leg* HCC
- **M90.569** *Osteonecrosis in diseases classified elsewhere, unspecified lower leg* HCC

6 M90.57 Osteonecrosis in diseases classified elsewhere, ankle and foot
- **M90.571** *Osteonecrosis in diseases classified elsewhere, right ankle and foot* HCC
- **M90.572** *Osteonecrosis in diseases classified elsewhere, left ankle and foot* HCC
- **M90.579** *Osteonecrosis in diseases classified elsewhere, unspecified ankle and foot* HCC

M90.58 *Osteonecrosis in diseases classified elsewhere, other site* HCC

M90.59 *Osteonecrosis in diseases classified elsewhere, multiple sites* HCC

5 M90.6 Osteitis deformans in neoplastic diseases
Osteitis deformans in malignant neoplasm of bone
Code first:
the neoplasm (C40.-, C41.-)

EXCLUDES 1 *osteitis deformans [Paget's disease of bone] (M88.-)*

DEFINITION Excessive breakdown with abnormal reformation of bone tissue in the presence of a malignant neoplasm of the bone; results in painful, deformed bones prone to pathological fractures.

M90.60 *Osteitis deformans in neoplastic diseases, unspecified site*

6 M90.61 Osteitis deformans in neoplastic diseases, shoulder
- **M90.611** *Osteitis deformans in neoplastic diseases, right shoulder*
- **M90.612** *Osteitis deformans in neoplastic diseases, left shoulder*
- **M90.619** *Osteitis deformans in neoplastic diseases, unspecified shoulder*

6 M90.62 Osteitis deformans in neoplastic diseases, upper arm
- **M90.621** *Osteitis deformans in neoplastic diseases, right upper arm*
- **M90.622** *Osteitis deformans in neoplastic diseases, left upper arm*
- **M90.629** *Osteitis deformans in neoplastic diseases, unspecified upper arm*

6 M90.63 Osteitis deformans in neoplastic diseases, forearm
- **M90.631** *Osteitis deformans in neoplastic diseases, right forearm*
- **M90.632** *Osteitis deformans in neoplastic diseases, left forearm*
- **M90.639** *Osteitis deformans in neoplastic diseases, unspecified forearm*

6 M90.64 Osteitis deformans in neoplastic diseases, hand
- **M90.641** *Osteitis deformans in neoplastic diseases, right hand*
- **M90.642** *Osteitis deformans in neoplastic diseases, left hand*
- **M90.649** *Osteitis deformans in neoplastic diseases, unspecified hand*

6 M90.65 Osteitis deformans in neoplastic diseases, thigh
- **M90.651** *Osteitis deformans in neoplastic diseases, right thigh*
- **M90.652** *Osteitis deformans in neoplastic diseases, left thigh*
- **M90.659** *Osteitis deformans in neoplastic diseases, unspecified thigh*

6 M90.66 Osteitis deformans in neoplastic diseases, lower leg
- **M90.661** *Osteitis deformans in neoplastic diseases, right lower leg*
- **M90.662** *Osteitis deformans in neoplastic diseases, left lower leg*
- **M90.669** *Osteitis deformans in neoplastic diseases, unspecified lower leg*

6 M90.67 Osteitis deformans in neoplastic diseases, ankle and foot
- **M90.671** *Osteitis deformans in neoplastic diseases, right ankle and foot*
- **M90.672** *Osteitis deformans in neoplastic diseases, left ankle and foot*
- **M90.679** *Osteitis deformans in neoplastic diseases, unspecified ankle and foot*

M90.68 *Osteitis deformans in neoplastic diseases, other site*

M90.69 *Osteitis deformans in neoplastic diseases, multiple sites*

5 M90.8 Osteopathy in diseases classified elsewhere
Code first underlying disease, such as:
rickets (E55.0)
vitamin-D-resistant rickets (E83.3)

M90.80 *Osteopathy in diseases classified elsewhere, unspecified site*

6 M90.81 Osteopathy in diseases classified elsewhere, shoulder

M90.811 *Osteopathy in diseases classified elsewhere, right shoulder*

M90.812 *Osteopathy in diseases classified elsewhere, left shoulder*

M90.819 *Osteopathy in diseases classified elsewhere, unspecified shoulder*

M90.82 Osteopathy in diseases classified elsewhere, upper arm

M90.821 *Osteopathy in diseases classified elsewhere, right upper arm*

M90.822 *Osteopathy in diseases classified elsewhere, left upper arm*

M90.829 *Osteopathy in diseases classified elsewhere, unspecified upper arm*

M90.83 Osteopathy in diseases classified elsewhere, forearm

M90.831 *Osteopathy in diseases classified elsewhere, right forearm*

M90.832 *Osteopathy in diseases classified elsewhere, left forearm*

M90.839 *Osteopathy in diseases classified elsewhere, unspecified forearm*

M90.84 Osteopathy in diseases classified elsewhere, hand

M90.841 *Osteopathy in diseases classified elsewhere, right hand*

M90.842 *Osteopathy in diseases classified elsewhere, left hand*

M90.849 *Osteopathy in diseases classified elsewhere, unspecified hand*

M90.85 Osteopathy in diseases classified elsewhere, thigh

M90.851 *Osteopathy in diseases classified elsewhere, right thigh*

M90.852 *Osteopathy in diseases classified elsewhere, left thigh*

M90.859 *Osteopathy in diseases classified elsewhere, unspecified thigh*

M90.86 Osteopathy in diseases classified elsewhere, lower leg

M90.861 *Osteopathy in diseases classified elsewhere, right lower leg*

M90.862 *Osteopathy in diseases classified elsewhere, left lower leg*

M90.869 *Osteopathy in diseases classified elsewhere, unspecified lower leg*

M90.87 Osteopathy in diseases classified elsewhere, ankle and foot

M90.871 *Osteopathy in diseases classified elsewhere, right ankle and foot*

M90.872 *Osteopathy in diseases classified elsewhere, left ankle and foot*

M90.879 *Osteopathy in diseases classified elsewhere, unspecified ankle and foot*

M90.88 *Osteopathy in diseases classified elsewhere, other site*

M90.89 *Osteopathy in diseases classified elsewhere, multiple sites*

Chondropathies (M91-M94)

EXCLUDES 1 *postprocedural chondropathies (M96.-)*

M91 Juvenile osteochondrosis of hip and pelvis

EXCLUDES 1 *slipped upper femoral epiphysis (nontraumatic) (M93.0)*

M91.0 Juvenile osteochondrosis of pelvis

Osteochondrosis (juvenile) of acetabulum
Osteochondrosis (juvenile) of iliac crest [Buchanan]
Osteochondrosis (juvenile) of ischiopubic synchondrosis [van Neck]
Osteochondrosis (juvenile) of symphysis pubis [Pierson]

M91.1 Juvenile osteochondrosis of head of femur [Legg-Calvé-Perthes]

DEFINITION Disruption of blood supply to the femoral head epiphysis in children, resulting in death of bone; occurs most commonly in boys age 4-8.

M91.10 **Juvenile osteochondrosis of head of femur [Legg-Calvé-Perthes], unspecified leg**

M91.11 **Juvenile osteochondrosis of head of femur [Legg-Calvé-Perthes], right leg**

M91.12 **Juvenile osteochondrosis of head of femur [Legg-Calvé-Perthes], left leg**

M91.2 Coxa plana

Hip deformity due to previous juvenile osteochondrosis

DEFINITION Residual effect of Legg-Calve-Perthes in which the necrotic bone of the normally rounded femoral head is flattened due to gradual bone replacement; secondary deformity of the acetabulum occurs with growth.

M91.20 **Coxa plana, unspecified hip**

M91.21 **Coxa plana, right hip**

M91.22 **Coxa plana, left hip**

M91.3 Pseudocoxalgia

M91.30 **Pseudocoxalgia, unspecified hip**

M91.31 **Pseudocoxalgia, right hip**

M91.32 **Pseudocoxalgia, left hip**

M91.4 Coxa magna

DEFINITION Residual effect of Legg-Calve-Perthes in which the femoral head is enlarged, becoming broad and overgrown due to the gradual bone replacement process.

M91.40 **Coxa magna, unspecified hip**

M91.41 **Coxa magna, right hip**

M91.42 **Coxa magna, left hip**

M91.8 Other juvenile osteochondrosis of hip and pelvis

Juvenile osteochondrosis after reduction of congenital dislocation of hip

M91.80 **Other juvenile osteochondrosis of hip and pelvis, unspecified leg**

M91.81 **Other juvenile osteochondrosis of hip and pelvis, right leg**

M91.82 **Other juvenile osteochondrosis of hip and pelvis, left leg**

M91.9 Juvenile osteochondrosis of hip and pelvis, unspecified

M91.90 **Juvenile osteochondrosis of hip and pelvis, unspecified, unspecified leg**

M91.91 **Juvenile osteochondrosis of hip and pelvis, unspecified, right leg**

M91.92 **Juvenile osteochondrosis of hip and pelvis, unspecified, left leg**

M92 Other juvenile osteochondrosis

DEFINITION Condition of unknown etiology affecting the developing growth plate and ossification centers in children where increased stress occurs; genetics, repeated trauma, mechanical factors, hormone imbalances, and vascular abnormalities may be a factor.

M92.0 Juvenile osteochondrosis of humerus

Osteochondrosis (juvenile) of capitulum of humerus [Panner]
Osteochondrosis (juvenile) of head of humerus [Haas]

M92.00 **Juvenile osteochondrosis of humerus, unspecified arm**

M92.01 **Juvenile osteochondrosis of humerus, right arm**

M92.02 **Juvenile osteochondrosis of humerus, left arm**

M92.1 Juvenile osteochondrosis of radius and ulna

Osteochondrosis (juvenile) of lower ulna [Burns]
Osteochondrosis (juvenile) of radial head [Brailsford]

M92.10 **Juvenile osteochondrosis of radius and ulna, unspecified arm**

M92.11 **Juvenile osteochondrosis of radius and ulna, right arm**

M92.12 **Juvenile osteochondrosis of radius and ulna, left arm**

M92.2 Juvenile osteochondrosis, hand

M92.20 **Unspecified juvenile osteochondrosis, hand**

M92.201 **Unspecified juvenile osteochondrosis, right hand**

M92.202 **Unspecified juvenile osteochondrosis, left hand**

M92.209 **Unspecified juvenile osteochondrosis, unspecified hand**

M92.21 **Osteochondrosis (juvenile) of carpal lunate [Kienböck]**

M92.211 **Osteochondrosis (juvenile) of carpal lunate [Kienböck], right hand**

M92.212 Osteochondrosis (juvenile) of carpal lunate [Kienböck], left hand
M92.219 Osteochondrosis (juvenile) of carpal lunate [Kienböck], unspecified hand
M92.22 Osteochondrosis (juvenile) of metacarpal heads [Mauclaire]
M92.221 Osteochondrosis (juvenile) of metacarpal heads [Mauclaire], right hand
M92.222 Osteochondrosis (juvenile) of metacarpal heads [Mauclaire], left hand
M92.229 Osteochondrosis (juvenile) of metacarpal heads [Mauclaire], unspecified hand
M92.29 Other juvenile osteochondrosis, hand
M92.291 Other juvenile osteochondrosis, right hand
M92.292 Other juvenile osteochondrosis, left hand
M92.299 Other juvenile osteochondrosis, unspecified hand
M92.3 Other juvenile osteochondrosis, upper limb
M92.30 Other juvenile osteochondrosis, unspecified upper limb
M92.31 Other juvenile osteochondrosis, right upper limb
M92.32 Other juvenile osteochondrosis, left upper limb
M92.4 Juvenile osteochondrosis of patella
Osteochondrosis (juvenile) of primary patellar center [Köhler]
Osteochondrosis (juvenile) of secondary patellar centre [Sinding Larsen]
M92.40 Juvenile osteochondrosis of patella, unspecified knee
M92.41 Juvenile osteochondrosis of patella, right knee
M92.42 Juvenile osteochondrosis of patella, left knee
M92.5 Juvenile osteochondrosis of tibia and fibula
Osteochondrosis (juvenile) of proximal tibia [Blount]
Osteochondrosis (juvenile) of tibial tubercle [Osgood-Schlatter]
Tibia vara
M92.50 Juvenile osteochondrosis of tibia and fibula, unspecified leg
M92.51 Juvenile osteochondrosis of tibia and fibula, right leg
M92.52 Juvenile osteochondrosis of tibia and fibula, left leg
M92.6 Juvenile osteochondrosis of tarsus
Osteochondrosis (juvenile) of calcaneum [Sever]
Osteochondrosis (juvenile) of os tibiale externum [Haglund]
Osteochondrosis (juvenile) of talus [Diaz]
Osteochondrosis (juvenile) of tarsal navicular [Köhler]
M92.60 Juvenile osteochondrosis of tarsus, unspecified ankle
M92.61 Juvenile osteochondrosis of tarsus, right ankle
M92.62 Juvenile osteochondrosis of tarsus, left ankle
M92.7 Juvenile osteochondrosis of metatarsus
Osteochondrosis (juvenile) of fifth metatarsus [Iselin]
Osteochondrosis (juvenile) of second metatarsus [Freiberg]
M92.70 Juvenile osteochondrosis of metatarsus, unspecified foot
M92.71 Juvenile osteochondrosis of metatarsus, right foot
M92.72 Juvenile osteochondrosis of metatarsus, left foot
M92.8 Other specified juvenile osteochondrosis
Calcaneal apophysitis
M92.9 Juvenile osteochondrosis, unspecified
Juvenile apophysitis NOS
Juvenile epiphysitis NOS
Juvenile osteochondritis NOS
Juvenile osteochondrosis NOS

M93 Other osteochondropathies

EXCLUDES 2 *osteochondrosis of spine (M42.-)*

M93.0 Slipped upper femoral epiphysis (nontraumatic)
Use additional code for associated chondrolysis (M94.3)
DEFINITION Nontraumatic slippage of the femoral head of the epiphysis occurring in adolescence.
M93.00 Unspecified slipped upper femoral epiphysis (nontraumatic)
M93.001 Unspecified slipped upper femoral epiphysis (nontraumatic), right hip
M93.002 Unspecified slipped upper femoral epiphysis (nontraumatic), left hip
M93.003 Unspecified slipped upper femoral epiphysis (nontraumatic), unspecified hip
M93.01 Acute slipped upper femoral epiphysis (nontraumatic)
M93.011 Acute slipped upper femoral epiphysis (nontraumatic), right hip
M93.012 Acute slipped upper femoral epiphysis (nontraumatic), left hip
M93.013 Acute slipped upper femoral epiphysis (nontraumatic), unspecified hip
M93.02 Chronic slipped upper femoral epiphysis (nontraumatic)
M93.021 Chronic slipped upper femoral epiphysis (nontraumatic), right hip
M93.022 Chronic slipped upper femoral epiphysis (nontraumatic), left hip
M93.023 Chronic slipped upper femoral epiphysis (nontraumatic), unspecified hip
M93.03 Acute on chronic slipped upper femoral epiphysis (nontraumatic)
M93.031 Acute on chronic slipped upper femoral epiphysis (nontraumatic), right hip
M93.032 Acute on chronic slipped upper femoral epiphysis (nontraumatic), left hip
M93.033 Acute on chronic slipped upper femoral epiphysis (nontraumatic), unspecified hip
M93.1 Kienböck's disease of adults A
Adult osteochondrosis of carpal lunates
DEFINITION Idiopathic disruption of blood supply to the carpal lunate bone in adults, resulting in death of the bone tissue.
M93.2 Osteochondritis dissecans
DEFINITION Joint condition in which a piece of cartilage and thin, underlying bone detaches from the bone's end; occurs most often in boys age 10-20 after a joint injury, and commonly affecting the knee.
M93.20 Osteochondritis dissecans of unspecified site
M93.21 Osteochondritis dissecans of shoulder
M93.211 Osteochondritis dissecans, right shoulder
M93.212 Osteochondritis dissecans, left shoulder
M93.219 Osteochondritis dissecans, unspecified shoulder
M93.22 Osteochondritis dissecans of elbow
M93.221 Osteochondritis dissecans, right elbow
M93.222 Osteochondritis dissecans, left elbow
M93.229 Osteochondritis dissecans, unspecified elbow
M93.23 Osteochondritis dissecans of wrist
M93.231 Osteochondritis dissecans, right wrist
M93.232 Osteochondritis dissecans, left wrist
M93.239 Osteochondritis dissecans, unspecified wrist
M93.24 Osteochondritis dissecans of joints of hand
M93.241 Osteochondritis dissecans, joints of right hand
M93.242 Osteochondritis dissecans, joints of left hand
M93.249 Osteochondritis dissecans, joints of unspecified hand
M93.25 Osteochondritis dissecans of hip
M93.251 Osteochondritis dissecans, right hip
M93.252 Osteochondritis dissecans, left hip
M93.259 Osteochondritis dissecans, unspecified hip
M93.26 Osteochondritis dissecans knee
M93.261 Osteochondritis dissecans, right knee
M93.262 Osteochondritis dissecans, left knee
M93.269 Osteochondritis dissecans, unspecified knee
M93.27 Osteochondritis dissecans of ankle and joints of foot
M93.271 Osteochondritis dissecans, right ankle and joints of right foot
M93.272 Osteochondritis dissecans, left ankle and joints of left foot
M93.279 Osteochondritis dissecans, unspecified ankle and joints of foot
M93.28 Osteochondritis dissecans other site
M93.29 Osteochondritis dissecans multiple sites
M93.8 Other specified osteochondropathies

DEFINITION Other conditions affecting bone and cartilage at any age, noted by abnormal endochondral ossification.

M93.80 Other specified osteochondropathies of unspecified site
M93.81 Other specified osteochondropathies of shoulder
M93.811 Other specified osteochondropathies, right shoulder
M93.812 Other specified osteochondropathies, left shoulder
M93.819 Other specified osteochondropathies, unspecified shoulder
M93.82 Other specified osteochondropathies of upper arm
M93.821 Other specified osteochondropathies, right upper arm
M93.822 Other specified osteochondropathies, left upper arm
M93.829 Other specified osteochondropathies, unspecified upper arm
M93.83 Other specified osteochondropathies of forearm
M93.831 Other specified osteochondropathies, right forearm
M93.832 Other specified osteochondropathies, left forearm
M93.839 Other specified osteochondropathies, unspecified forearm
M93.84 Other specified osteochondropathies of hand
M93.841 Other specified osteochondropathies, right hand
M93.842 Other specified osteochondropathies, left hand
M93.849 Other specified osteochondropathies, unspecified hand
M93.85 Other specified osteochondropathies of thigh
M93.851 Other specified osteochondropathies, right thigh
M93.852 Other specified osteochondropathies, left thigh
M93.859 Other specified osteochondropathies, unspecified thigh
M93.86 Other specified osteochondropathies lower leg
M93.861 Other specified osteochondropathies, right lower leg
M93.862 Other specified osteochondropathies, left lower leg
M93.869 Other specified osteochondropathies, unspecified lower leg
M93.87 Other specified osteochondropathies of ankle and foot
M93.871 Other specified osteochondropathies, right ankle and foot
M93.872 Other specified osteochondropathies, left ankle and foot
M93.879 Other specified osteochondropathies, unspecified ankle and foot
M93.88 other specified osteochondropathies other
M93.89 Other specified osteochondropathies multiple sites

M93.9 Osteochondropathy, unspecified
Apophysitis NOS
Epiphysitis NOS
Osteochondritis NOS
Osteochondrosis NOS

M93.90 Osteochondropathy, unspecified of unspecified site
M93.91 Osteochondropathy, unspecified of shoulder
M93.911 Osteochondropathy, unspecified, right shoulder
M93.912 Osteochondropathy, unspecified, left shoulder
M93.919 Osteochondropathy, unspecified, unspecified shoulder
M93.92 Osteochondropathy, unspecified of upper arm
M93.921 Osteochondropathy, unspecified, right upper arm
M93.922 Osteochondropathy, unspecified, left upper arm
M93.929 Osteochondropathy, unspecified, unspecified upper arm
M93.93 Osteochondropathy, unspecified of forearm
M93.931 Osteochondropathy, unspecified, right forearm
M93.932 Osteochondropathy, unspecified, left forearm
M93.939 Osteochondropathy, unspecified, unspecified forearm
M93.94 Osteochondropathy, unspecified of hand
M93.941 Osteochondropathy, unspecified, right hand
M93.942 Osteochondropathy, unspecified, left hand
M93.949 Osteochondropathy, unspecified, unspecified hand
M93.95 Osteochondropathy, unspecified of thigh
M93.951 Osteochondropathy, unspecified, right thigh
M93.952 Osteochondropathy, unspecified, left thigh
M93.959 Osteochondropathy, unspecified, unspecified thigh
M93.96 Osteochondropathy, unspecified lower leg
M93.961 Osteochondropathy, unspecified, right lower leg
M93.962 Osteochondropathy, unspecified, left lower leg
M93.969 Osteochondropathy, unspecified, unspecified lower leg
M93.97 Osteochondropathy, unspecified of ankle and foot
M93.971 Osteochondropathy, unspecified, right ankle and foot
M93.972 Osteochondropathy, unspecified, left ankle and foot
M93.979 Osteochondropathy, unspecified, unspecified ankle and foot
M93.98 Osteochondropathy, unspecified other
M93.99 Osteochondropathy, unspecified multiple sites

M94 Other disorders of cartilage

M94.0 Chondrocostal junction syndrome [Tietze]
Costochondritis
M94.1 Relapsing polychondritis
M94.2 Chondromalacia

EXCLUDES 1 *chondromalacia patellae (M22.4)*

DEFINITION Joint cartilage softens and degenerates, causing tenderness, pain, and a grinding sensation.

M94.20 Chondromalacia, unspecified site
M94.21 Chondromalacia, shoulder
M94.211 Chondromalacia, right shoulder
M94.212 Chondromalacia, left shoulder
M94.219 Chondromalacia, unspecified shoulder
M94.22 Chondromalacia, elbow
M94.221 Chondromalacia, right elbow
M94.222 Chondromalacia, left elbow
M94.229 Chondromalacia, unspecified elbow
M94.23 Chondromalacia, wrist
M94.231 Chondromalacia, right wrist
M94.232 Chondromalacia, left wrist
M94.239 Chondromalacia, unspecified wrist
M94.24 Chondromalacia, joints of hand
M94.241 Chondromalacia, joints of right hand
M94.242 Chondromalacia, joints of left hand
M94.249 Chondromalacia, joints of unspecified hand
M94.25 Chondromalacia, hip
M94.251 Chondromalacia, right hip
M94.252 Chondromalacia, left hip
M94.259 Chondromalacia, unspecified hip
M94.26 Chondromalacia, knee

CODING TIP ✓ Do not assign M94.26- for chondromalacia patellae (also called "runner's knee" or CMP). Chondromalacia patellae is an inflammation of the underside of the patella and is coded to M22.4.

M94.261 Chondromalacia, right knee
M94.262 Chondromalacia, left knee
M94.269 Chondromalacia, unspecified knee
M94.27 Chondromalacia, ankle and joints of foot
M94.271 Chondromalacia, right ankle and joints of right foot
M94.272 Chondromalacia, left ankle and joints of left foot
M94.279 Chondromalacia, unspecified ankle and joints of foot
M94.28 Chondromalacia, other site
M94.29 Chondromalacia, multiple sites

M94.3 Chondrolysis
Code first:
any associated slipped upper femoral epiphysis (nontraumatic) (M93.0-)

DEFINITION Sudden, severe damage to joint cartilage causing rapid death of normal cartilage cells and abrupt loss of the joint's cartilage layer.

M94.35 Chondrolysis, hip
M94.351 Chondrolysis, right hip
M94.352 Chondrolysis, left hip
M94.359 Chondrolysis, unspecified hip
M94.8 Other specified disorders of cartilage
M94.8X Other specified disorders of cartilage
M94.8X0 Other specified disorders of cartilage, multiple sites
M94.8X1 Other specified disorders of cartilage, shoulder
M94.8X2 Other specified disorders of cartilage, upper arm
M94.8X3 Other specified disorders of cartilage, forearm
M94.8X4 Other specified disorders of cartilage, hand
M94.8X5 Other specified disorders of cartilage, thigh
M94.8X6 Other specified disorders of cartilage, lower leg
M94.8X7 Other specified disorders of cartilage, ankle and foot
M94.8X8 Other specified disorders of cartilage, other site
M94.8X9 Other specified disorders of cartilage, unspecified sites
M94.9 Disorder of cartilage, unspecified

Other disorders of the musculoskeletal system and connective tissue (M95)

M95 Other acquired deformities of musculoskeletal system and connective tissue

EXCLUDES 2
acquired absence of limbs and organs (Z89-Z90)
acquired deformities of limbs (M20-M21)
congenital malformations and deformations of the musculoskeletal system (Q65-Q79)
deforming dorsopathies (M40-M43)
dentofacial anomalies [including malocclusion] (M26.-)
postprocedural musculoskeletal disorders (M96.-)

M95.0 Acquired deformity of nose
EXCLUDES 2 *deviated nasal septum (J34.2)*

M95.1 Cauliflower ear
EXCLUDES 2 *other acquired deformities of ear (H61.1)*

Cauliflower ear

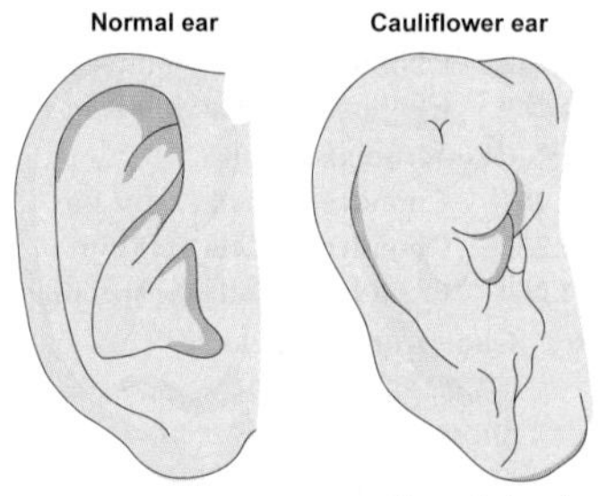

Abnormal external ear as a result of injury

M95.10 Cauliflower ear, unspecified ear
M95.11 Cauliflower ear, right ear
M95.12 Cauliflower ear, left ear
M95.2 Other acquired deformity of head
M95.3 Acquired deformity of neck
M95.4 Acquired deformity of chest and rib
AHA: 4Q 2014, 26, 27
M95.5 Acquired deformity of pelvis
EXCLUDES 1 *maternal care for known or suspected disproportion (O33.-)*

M95.8 Other specified acquired deformities of musculoskeletal system
M95.9 Acquired deformity of musculoskeletal system, unspecified

Intraoperative and postprocedural complications and disorders of musculoskeletal system, not elsewhere classified (M96)

M96 Intraoperative and postprocedural complications and disorders of musculoskeletal system, not elsewhere classified

EXCLUDES 2
arthropathy following intestinal bypass (M02.0-)
complications of internal orthopedic prosthetic devices, implants and grafts (T84.-)
disorders associated with osteoporosis (M80)
periprosthetic fracture around internal prosthetic joint (M97.-)
presence of functional implants and other devices (Z96-Z97)

CODING TIP ✓ **Documentation:** Codes in category M96.- are complication codes and require physician documentation and confirmation of a cause and effect relationship between the procedure and the complicated condition.

M96.0 Pseudarthrosis after fusion or arthrodesis
M96.1 Postlaminectomy syndrome, not elsewhere classified
M96.2 Postradiation kyphosis
M96.3 Postlaminectomy kyphosis
M96.4 Postsurgical lordosis
M96.5 Postradiation scoliosis
M96.6 Fracture of bone following insertion of orthopedic implant, joint prosthesis, or bone plate
Intraoperative fracture of bone during insertion of orthopedic implant, joint prosthesis, or bone plate
EXCLUDES 2 *complication of internal orthopedic devices, implants or grafts (T84.-)*

M96.62 Fracture of humerus following insertion of orthopedic implant, joint prosthesis, or bone plate
M96.621 Fracture of humerus following insertion of orthopedic implant, joint prosthesis, or bone plate, right arm HCC
M96.622 Fracture of humerus following insertion of orthopedic implant, joint prosthesis, or bone plate, left arm HCC
M96.629 Fracture of humerus following insertion of orthopedic implant, joint prosthesis, or bone plate, unspecified arm HCC
M96.63 Fracture of radius or ulna following insertion of orthopedic implant, joint prosthesis, or bone plate
M96.631 Fracture of radius or ulna following insertion of orthopedic implant, joint prosthesis, or bone plate, right arm HCC
M96.632 Fracture of radius or ulna following insertion of orthopedic implant, joint prosthesis, or bone plate, left arm HCC
M96.639 Fracture of radius or ulna following insertion of orthopedic implant, joint prosthesis, or bone plate, unspecified arm HCC
M96.65 Fracture of pelvis following insertion of orthopedic implant, joint prosthesis, or bone plate HCC
M96.66 Fracture of femur following insertion of orthopedic implant, joint prosthesis, or bone plate
M96.661 Fracture of femur following insertion of orthopedic implant, joint prosthesis, or bone plate, right leg HCC
M96.662 Fracture of femur following insertion of orthopedic implant, joint prosthesis, or bone plate, left leg HCC
M96.669 Fracture of femur following insertion of orthopedic implant, joint prosthesis, or bone plate, unspecified leg HCC
M96.67 Fracture of tibia or fibula following insertion of orthopedic implant, joint prosthesis, or bone plate

M96.671 Fracture of tibia or fibula following insertion of orthopedic implant, joint prosthesis, or bone plate, right leg HCC

M96.672 Fracture of tibia or fibula following insertion of orthopedic implant, joint prosthesis, or bone plate, left leg HCC

M96.679 Fracture of tibia or fibula following insertion of orthopedic implant, joint prosthesis, or bone plate, unspecified leg HCC

M96.69 Fracture of other bone following insertion of orthopedic implant, joint prosthesis, or bone plate HCC

M96.8 Other intraoperative and postprocedural complications and disorders of musculoskeletal system, not elsewhere classified

M96.81 Intraoperative hemorrhage and hematoma of a musculoskeletal structure complicating a procedure

EXCLUDES 1 *intraoperative hemorrhage and hematoma of a musculoskeletal structure due to accidental puncture and laceration during a procedure (M96.82-)*

M96.810 Intraoperative hemorrhage and hematoma of a musculoskeletal structure complicating a musculoskeletal system procedure

M96.811 Intraoperative hemorrhage and hematoma of a musculoskeletal structure complicating other procedure

M96.82 Accidental puncture and laceration of a musculoskeletal structure during a procedure

CODING TIP ✓ Use additional code for the organ injured.

M96.820 Accidental puncture and laceration of a musculoskeletal structure during a musculoskeletal system procedure

M96.821 Accidental puncture and laceration of a musculoskeletal structure during other procedure

M96.83 Postprocedural hemorrhage of a musculoskeletal structure following a procedure

M96.830 Postprocedural hemorrhage of a musculoskeletal structure following a musculoskeletal system procedure

M96.831 Postprocedural hemorrhage of a musculoskeletal structure following other procedure

M96.84 Postprocedural hematoma and seroma of a musculoskeletal structure following a procedure

M96.840 Postprocedural hematoma of a musculoskeletal structure following a musculoskeletal system procedure

M96.841 Postprocedural hematoma of a musculoskeletal structure following other procedure

M96.842 Postprocedural seroma of a musculoskeletal structure following a musculoskeletal system procedure

M96.843 Postprocedural seroma of a musculoskeletal structure following other procedure

M96.89 Other intraoperative and postprocedural complications and disorders of the musculoskeletal system

Instability of joint secondary to removal of joint prosthesis

Use additional code, if applicable, to further specify disorder

Periprosthetic fracture around internal prosthetic joint (M97)

M97 Periprosthetic fracture around internal prosthetic joint

EXCLUDES 2 *fracture of bone following insertion of orthopedic implant, joint prosthesis or bone plate (M96.6-)*

breakage (fracture) of prosthetic joint (T84.01-)

The appropriate 7th character is to be added to each code from category M97

A	initial encounter
D	subsequent encounter
S	sequela

CODING TIP ✓ For more specific reporting of a periprosthetic fracture, in addition to a code from M97, code also the appropriate traumatic fracture code from Chapter 19 or a code from category M84 if the fracture is pathological in origin.

AHA: 4Q 2016, 42

M97.0 Periprosthetic fracture around internal prosthetic hip joint

M97.01X- Periprosthetic fracture around internal prosthetic right hip joint HCC

M97.02X- Periprosthetic fracture around internal prosthetic left hip joint HCC

M97.1 Periprosthetic fracture around internal prosthetic knee joint

M97.11X- Periprosthetic fracture around internal prosthetic right knee joint

M97.12X- Periprosthetic fracture around internal prosthetic left knee joint

M97.2 Periprosthetic fracture around internal prosthetic ankle joint

M97.21X- Periprosthetic fracture around internal prosthetic right ankle joint

M97.22X- Periprosthetic fracture around internal prosthetic left ankle joint

M97.3 Periprosthetic fracture around internal prosthetic shoulder joint

M97.31X- Periprosthetic fracture around internal prosthetic right shoulder joint

M97.32X- Periprosthetic fracture around internal prosthetic left shoulder joint

M97.4 Periprosthetic fracture around internal prosthetic elbow joint

M97.41X- Periprosthetic fracture around internal prosthetic right elbow joint

M97.42X- Periprosthetic fracture around internal prosthetic left elbow joint

M97.8XX- Periprosthetic fracture around other internal prosthetic joint

Periprosthetic fracture around internal prosthetic finger joint

Periprosthetic fracture around internal prosthetic spinal joint

Periprosthetic fracture around internal prosthetic toe joint

Periprosthetic fracture around internal prosthetic wrist joint

Use additional code to identify the joint (Z96.6-)

M97.9XX- Periprosthetic fracture around unspecified internal prosthetic joint

Biomechanical lesions, not elsewhere classified (M99)

M99 Biomechanical lesions, not elsewhere classified

Note: This category should not be used if the condition can be classified elsewhere.

M99.0 Segmental and somatic dysfunction

M99.00 Segmental and somatic dysfunction of head region

M99.01 Segmental and somatic dysfunction of cervical region

M99.02 Segmental and somatic dysfunction of thoracic region

M99.03 Segmental and somatic dysfunction of lumbar region

M99.04 Segmental and somatic dysfunction of sacral region

M99.05 Segmental and somatic dysfunction of pelvic region

M99.06 Segmental and somatic dysfunction of lower extremity

M99.07 Segmental and somatic dysfunction of upper extremity

M99.08 Segmental and somatic dysfunction of rib cage

M99.09 Segmental and somatic dysfunction of abdomen and other regions

M99.1 Subluxation complex (vertebral)

M99.10 Subluxation complex (vertebral) of head region

M99.11 Subluxation complex (vertebral) of cervical region

M99.12 Subluxation complex (vertebral) of thoracic region

M99.13 Subluxation complex (vertebral) of lumbar region

M99.14 Subluxation complex (vertebral) of sacral region

M99.15 Subluxation complex (vertebral) of pelvic region
M99.16 Subluxation complex (vertebral) of lower extremity
M99.17 Subluxation complex (vertebral) of upper extremity
M99.18 Subluxation complex (vertebral) of rib cage
M99.19 Subluxation complex (vertebral) of abdomen and other regions

M99.2 Subluxation stenosis of neural canal
M99.20 Subluxation stenosis of neural canal of head region
M99.21 Subluxation stenosis of neural canal of cervical region
M99.22 Subluxation stenosis of neural canal of thoracic region
M99.23 Subluxation stenosis of neural canal of lumbar region
M99.24 Subluxation stenosis of neural canal of sacral region
M99.25 Subluxation stenosis of neural canal of pelvic region
M99.26 Subluxation stenosis of neural canal of lower extremity
M99.27 Subluxation stenosis of neural canal of upper extremity
M99.28 Subluxation stenosis of neural canal of rib cage
M99.29 Subluxation stenosis of neural canal of abdomen and other regions

M99.3 Osseous stenosis of neural canal
M99.30 Osseous stenosis of neural canal of head region
M99.31 Osseous stenosis of neural canal of cervical region
M99.32 Osseous stenosis of neural canal of thoracic region
M99.33 Osseous stenosis of neural canal of lumbar region
M99.34 Osseous stenosis of neural canal of sacral region
M99.35 Osseous stenosis of neural canal of pelvic region
M99.36 Osseous stenosis of neural canal of lower extremity
M99.37 Osseous stenosis of neural canal of upper extremity
M99.38 Osseous stenosis of neural canal of rib cage
M99.39 Osseous stenosis of neural canal of abdomen and other regions

M99.4 Connective tissue stenosis of neural canal
M99.40 Connective tissue stenosis of neural canal of head region
M99.41 Connective tissue stenosis of neural canal of cervical region
M99.42 Connective tissue stenosis of neural canal of thoracic region
M99.43 Connective tissue stenosis of neural canal of lumbar region
M99.44 Connective tissue stenosis of neural canal of sacral region
M99.45 Connective tissue stenosis of neural canal of pelvic region
M99.46 Connective tissue stenosis of neural canal of lower extremity
M99.47 Connective tissue stenosis of neural canal of upper extremity
M99.48 Connective tissue stenosis of neural canal of rib cage
M99.49 Connective tissue stenosis of neural canal of abdomen and other regions

M99.5 Intervertebral disc stenosis of neural canal
M99.50 Intervertebral disc stenosis of neural canal of head region
M99.51 Intervertebral disc stenosis of neural canal of cervical region
M99.52 Intervertebral disc stenosis of neural canal of thoracic region
M99.53 Intervertebral disc stenosis of neural canal of lumbar region
M99.54 Intervertebral disc stenosis of neural canal of sacral region
M99.55 Intervertebral disc stenosis of neural canal of pelvic region
M99.56 Intervertebral disc stenosis of neural canal of lower extremity
M99.57 Intervertebral disc stenosis of neural canal of upper extremity
M99.58 Intervertebral disc stenosis of neural canal of rib cage
M99.59 Intervertebral disc stenosis of neural canal of abdomen and other regions

M99.6 Osseous and subluxation stenosis of intervertebral foramina
M99.60 Osseous and subluxation stenosis of intervertebral foramina of head region
M99.61 Osseous and subluxation stenosis of intervertebral foramina of cervical region
M99.62 Osseous and subluxation stenosis of intervertebral foramina of thoracic region
M99.63 Osseous and subluxation stenosis of intervertebral foramina of lumbar region
M99.64 Osseous and subluxation stenosis of intervertebral foramina of sacral region
M99.65 Osseous and subluxation stenosis of intervertebral foramina of pelvic region
M99.66 Osseous and subluxation stenosis of intervertebral foramina of lower extremity
M99.67 Osseous and subluxation stenosis of intervertebral foramina of upper extremity
M99.68 Osseous and subluxation stenosis of intervertebral foramina of rib cage
M99.69 Osseous and subluxation stenosis of intervertebral foramina of abdomen and other regions

M99.7 Connective tissue and disc stenosis of intervertebral foramina
M99.70 Connective tissue and disc stenosis of intervertebral foramina of head region
M99.71 Connective tissue and disc stenosis of intervertebral foramina of cervical region
M99.72 Connective tissue and disc stenosis of intervertebral foramina of thoracic region
M99.73 Connective tissue and disc stenosis of intervertebral foramina of lumbar region
M99.74 Connective tissue and disc stenosis of intervertebral foramina of sacral region
M99.75 Connective tissue and disc stenosis of intervertebral foramina of pelvic region
M99.76 Connective tissue and disc stenosis of intervertebral foramina of lower extremity
M99.77 Connective tissue and disc stenosis of intervertebral foramina of upper extremity
M99.78 Connective tissue and disc stenosis of intervertebral foramina of rib cage
M99.79 Connective tissue and disc stenosis of intervertebral foramina of abdomen and other regions

M99.8 Other biomechanical lesions
M99.80 Other biomechanical lesions of head region
M99.81 Other biomechanical lesions of cervical region
M99.82 Other biomechanical lesions of thoracic region
M99.83 Other biomechanical lesions of lumbar region
M99.84 Other biomechanical lesions of sacral region
M99.85 Other biomechanical lesions of pelvic region
M99.86 Other biomechanical lesions of lower extremity
M99.87 Other biomechanical lesions of upper extremity
M99.88 Other biomechanical lesions of rib cage
M99.89 Other biomechanical lesions of abdomen and other regions

M99.9 Biomechanical lesion, unspecified

CHAPTER 14: DISEASES OF THE GENITOURINARY SYSTEM (N00-N99)

EXCLUDES 2 *certain conditions originating in the perinatal period (P04-P96)*
certain infectious and parasitic diseases (A00-B99)
complications of pregnancy, childbirth and the puerperium (O00-O9A)
congenital malformations, deformations and chromosomal abnormalities (Q00-Q99)
endocrine, nutritional and metabolic diseases (E00-E88)
injury, poisoning and certain other consequences of external causes (S00-T88)
neoplasms (C00-D49)
symptoms, signs and abnormal clinical and laboratory findings, not elsewhere classified (R00-R94)

This chapter contains the following blocks:

N00-N08	Glomerular diseases
N10-N16	Renal tubulo-interstitial diseases
N17-N19	Acute kidney failure and chronic kidney disease
N20-N23	Urolithiasis
N25-N29	Other disorders of kidney and ureter
N30-N39	Other diseases of the urinary system
N40-N53	Diseases of male genital organs
N60-N65	Disorders of breast
N70-N77	Inflammatory diseases of female pelvic organs
N80-N98	Noninflammatory disorders of female genital tract
N99	Intraoperative and postprocedural complications and disorders of genitourinary system, not elsewhere classified

Glomerular diseases (N00-N08)

Code also:
any associated kidney failure (N17-N19) .

EXCLUDES 1 *hypertensive chronic kidney disease (I12.-)*

4 N00 Acute nephritic syndrome

INCLUDES acute glomerular disease
acute glomerulonephritis
acute nephritis

EXCLUDES 1 *acute tubulo-interstitial nephritis (N10)*
nephritic syndrome NOS (N05.-)

N00.0 Acute nephritic syndrome with minor glomerular abnormality
Acute nephritic syndrome with minimal change lesion

N00.1 Acute nephritic syndrome with focal and segmental glomerular lesions
Acute nephritic syndrome with focal and segmental hyalinosis
Acute nephritic syndrome with focal and segmental sclerosis
Acute nephritic syndrome with focal glomerulonephritis

N00.2 Acute nephritic syndrome with diffuse membranous glomerulonephritis

N00.3 Acute nephritic syndrome with diffuse mesangial proliferative glomerulonephritis

N00.4 Acute nephritic syndrome with diffuse endocapillary proliferative glomerulonephritis

N00.5 Acute nephritic syndrome with diffuse mesangiocapillary glomerulonephritis
Acute nephritic syndrome with membranoproliferative glomerulonephritis, types 1 and 3, or NOS

N00.6 Acute nephritic syndrome with dense deposit disease
Acute nephritic syndrome with membranoproliferative glomerulonephritis, type 2

N00.7 Acute nephritic syndrome with diffuse crescentic glomerulonephritis
Acute nephritic syndrome with extracapillary glomerulonephritis

N00.8 Acute nephritic syndrome with other morphologic changes
Acute nephritic syndrome with proliferative glomerulonephritis NOS

N00.9 Acute nephritic syndrome with unspecified morphologic changes

4 N01 Rapidly progressive nephritic syndrome

INCLUDES rapidly progressive glomerular disease
rapidly progressive glomerulonephritis
rapidly progressive nephritis

EXCLUDES 1 *nephritic syndrome NOS (N05.-)*

N01.0 Rapidly progressive nephritic syndrome with minor glomerular abnormality
Rapidly progressive nephritic syndrome with minimal change lesion

N01.1 Rapidly progressive nephritic syndrome with focal and segmental glomerular lesions
Rapidly progressive nephritic syndrome with focal and segmental hyalinosis
Rapidly progressive nephritic syndrome with focal and segmental sclerosis
Rapidly progressive nephritic syndrome with focal glomerulonephritis

N01.2 Rapidly progressive nephritic syndrome with diffuse membranous glomerulonephritis

N01.3 Rapidly progressive nephritic syndrome with diffuse mesangial proliferative glomerulonephritis

N01.4 Rapidly progressive nephritic syndrome with diffuse endocapillary proliferative glomerulonephritis

N01.5 Rapidly progressive nephritic syndrome with diffuse mesangiocapillary glomerulonephritis
Rapidly progressive nephritic syndrome with membranoproliferative glomerulonephritis, types 1 and 3, or NOS

N01.6 Rapidly progressive nephritic syndrome with dense deposit disease
Rapidly progressive nephritic syndrome with membranoproliferative glomerulonephritis, type 2

N01.7 Rapidly progressive nephritic syndrome with diffuse crescentic glomerulonephritis
Rapidly progressive nephritic syndrome with extracapillary glomerulonephritis

N01.8 Rapidly progressive nephritic syndrome with other morphologic changes
Rapidly progressive nephritic syndrome with proliferative glomerulonephritis NOS

N01.9 Rapidly progressive nephritic syndrome with unspecified morphologic changes

4 N02 Recurrent and persistent hematuria

EXCLUDES 1 *acute cystitis with hematuria (N30.01)*
hematuria NOS (R31.9)
hematuria not associated with specified morphologic lesions (R31.-)

N02.0 Recurrent and persistent hematuria with minor glomerular abnormality
Recurrent and persistent hematuria with minimal change lesion

N02.1 Recurrent and persistent hematuria with focal and segmental glomerular lesions
Recurrent and persistent hematuria with focal and segmental hyalinosis
Recurrent and persistent hematuria with focal and segmental sclerosis
Recurrent and persistent hematuria with focal glomerulonephritis

N02.2 Recurrent and persistent hematuria with diffuse membranous glomerulonephritis

N02.3 Recurrent and persistent hematuria with diffuse mesangial proliferative glomerulonephritis

N02.4 Recurrent and persistent hematuria with diffuse endocapillary proliferative glomerulonephritis

N02.5 Recurrent and persistent hematuria with diffuse mesangiocapillary glomerulonephritis
Recurrent and persistent hematuria with membranoproliferative glomerulonephritis, types 1 and 3, or NOS

N02.6 Recurrent and persistent hematuria with dense deposit disease
Recurrent and persistent hematuria with membranoproliferative glomerulonephritis, type 2

N02.7 Recurrent and persistent hematuria with diffuse crescentic glomerulonephritis
Recurrent and persistent hematuria with extracapillary glomerulonephritis

N02.8 **Recurrent and persistent hematuria with other morphologic changes**
Recurrent and persistent hematuria with proliferative glomerulonephritis NOS

N02.9 **Recurrent and persistent hematuria with unspecified morphologic changes**
AHA: 2Q 2017, 5

N03 **Chronic nephritic syndrome**

INCLUDES chronic glomerular disease
chronic glomerulonephritis
chronic nephritis

EXCLUDES 1 *chronic tubulo-interstitial nephritis (N11.-)*
diffuse sclerosing glomerulonephritis (N05.8-)
nephritic syndrome NOS (N05.-)

N03.0 **Chronic nephritic syndrome with minor glomerular abnormality**
Chronic nephritic syndrome with minimal change lesion

N03.1 **Chronic nephritic syndrome with focal and segmental glomerular lesions**
Chronic nephritic syndrome with focal and segmental hyalinosis
Chronic nephritic syndrome with focal and segmental sclerosis
Chronic nephritic syndrome with focal glomerulonephritis

N03.2 **Chronic nephritic syndrome with diffuse membranous glomerulonephritis**

N03.3 **Chronic nephritic syndrome with diffuse mesangial proliferative glomerulonephritis**

N03.4 **Chronic nephritic syndrome with diffuse endocapillary proliferative glomerulonephritis**

N03.5 **Chronic nephritic syndrome with diffuse mesangiocapillary glomerulonephritis**
Chronic nephritic syndrome with membranoproliferative glomerulonephritis, types 1 and 3, or NOS

N03.6 **Chronic nephritic syndrome with dense deposit disease**
Chronic nephritic syndrome with membranoproliferative glomerulonephritis, type 2

N03.7 **Chronic nephritic syndrome with diffuse crescentic glomerulonephritis**
Chronic nephritic syndrome with extracapillary glomerulonephritis

N03.8 **Chronic nephritic syndrome with other morphologic changes**
Chronic nephritic syndrome with proliferative glomerulonephritis NOS

N03.9 **Chronic nephritic syndrome with unspecified morphologic changes**

N04 **Nephrotic syndrome**

INCLUDES congenital nephrotic syndrome
lipoid nephrosis

N04.0 **Nephrotic syndrome with minor glomerular abnormality**
Nephrotic syndrome with minimal change lesion

N04.1 **Nephrotic syndrome with focal and segmental glomerular lesions**
Nephrotic syndrome with focal and segmental hyalinosis
Nephrotic syndrome with focal and segmental sclerosis
Nephrotic syndrome with focal glomerulonephritis

N04.2 **Nephrotic syndrome with diffuse membranous glomerulonephritis**

N04.3 **Nephrotic syndrome with diffuse mesangial proliferative glomerulonephritis**

N04.4 **Nephrotic syndrome with diffuse endocapillary proliferative glomerulonephritis**

N04.5 **Nephrotic syndrome with diffuse mesangiocapillary glomerulonephritis**
Nephrotic syndrome with membranoproliferative glomerulonephritis, types 1 and 3, or NOS

N04.6 **Nephrotic syndrome with dense deposit disease**
Nephrotic syndrome with membranoproliferative glomerulonephritis, type 2

N04.7 **Nephrotic syndrome with diffuse crescentic glomerulonephritis**
Nephrotic syndrome with extracapillary glomerulonephritis

N04.8 **Nephrotic syndrome with other morphologic changes**
Nephrotic syndrome with proliferative glomerulonephritis NOS

N04.9 **Nephrotic syndrome with unspecified morphologic changes**

Nephrotic syndrome with unspecified morphologic changes

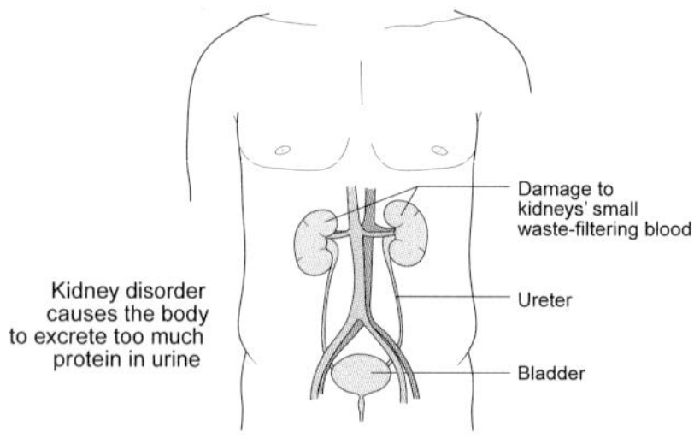
Damage to kidneys' small waste-filtering blood
Kidney disorder causes the body to excrete too much protein in urine
Ureter
Bladder

N05 **Unspecified nephritic syndrome**

INCLUDES glomerular disease NOS
glomerulonephritis NOS
nephritis NOS
nephropathy NOS and renal disease NOS with morphological lesion specified in .0-.8

EXCLUDES 1 *nephropathy NOS with no stated morphological lesion (N28.9)*
renal disease NOS with no stated morphological lesion (N28.9)
tubulo-interstitial nephritis NOS (N12)

N05.0 **Unspecified nephritic syndrome with minor glomerular abnormality**
Unspecified nephritic syndrome with minimal change lesion

N05.1 **Unspecified nephritic syndrome with focal and segmental glomerular lesions**
Unspecified nephritic syndrome with focal and segmental hyalinosis
Unspecified nephritic syndrome with focal and segmental sclerosis
Unspecified nephritic syndrome with focal glomerulonephritis

N05.2 **Unspecified nephritic syndrome with diffuse membranous glomerulonephritis**

N05.3 **Unspecified nephritic syndrome with diffuse mesangial proliferative glomerulonephritis**

N05.4 **Unspecified nephritic syndrome with diffuse endocapillary proliferative glomerulonephritis**

N05.5 **Unspecified nephritic syndrome with diffuse mesangiocapillary glomerulonephritis**
Unspecified nephritic syndrome with membranoproliferative glomerulonephritis, types 1 and 3, or NOS

N05.6 **Unspecified nephritic syndrome with dense deposit disease**
Unspecified nephritic syndrome with membranoproliferative glomerulonephritis, type 2

N05.7 **Unspecified nephritic syndrome with diffuse crescentic glomerulonephritis**
Unspecified nephritic syndrome with extracapillary glomerulonephritis

N05.8 **Unspecified nephritic syndrome with other morphologic changes**
Unspecified nephritic syndrome with proliferative glomerulonephritis NOS

N05.9 **Unspecified nephritic syndrome with unspecified morphologic changes**

N06 **Isolated proteinuria with specified morphological lesion**

EXCLUDES 1 *Proteinuria not associated with specific morphologic lesions (R80.0)*

N06.0 **Isolated proteinuria with minor glomerular abnormality**
Isolated proteinuria with minimal change lesion

N06.1 **Isolated proteinuria with focal and segmental glomerular lesions**
Isolated proteinuria with focal and segmental hyalinosis
Isolated proteinuria with focal and segmental sclerosis
Isolated proteinuria with focal glomerulonephritis

N06.2 **Isolated proteinuria with diffuse membranous glomerulonephritis**

N06.3 Isolated proteinuria with diffuse mesangial proliferative glomerulonephritis

N06.4 Isolated proteinuria with diffuse endocapillary proliferative glomerulonephritis

N06.5 Isolated proteinuria with diffuse mesangiocapillary glomerulonephritis
Isolated proteinuria with membranoproliferative glomerulonephritis, types 1 and 3, or NOS

N06.6 Isolated proteinuria with dense deposit disease
Isolated proteinuria with membranoproliferative glomerulonephritis, type 2

N06.7 Isolated proteinuria with diffuse crescentic glomerulonephritis
Isolated proteinuria with extracapillary glomerulonephritis

N06.8 Isolated proteinuria with other morphologic lesion
Isolated proteinuria with proliferative glomerulonephritis NOS

N06.9 Isolated proteinuria with unspecified morphologic lesion

4 N07 Hereditary nephropathy, not elsewhere classified

EXCLUDES 2 *Alport's syndrome (Q87.81-)*
hereditary amyloid nephropathy (E85.-)
nail patella syndrome (Q87.2)
non-neuropathic heredofamilial amyloidosis (E85.-)

N07.0 Hereditary nephropathy, not elsewhere classified with minor glomerular abnormality
Hereditary nephropathy, not elsewhere classified with minimal change lesion

N07.1 Hereditary nephropathy, not elsewhere classified with focal and segmental glomerular lesions
Hereditary nephropathy, not elsewhere classified with focal and segmental hyalinosis
Hereditary nephropathy, not elsewhere classified with focal and segmental sclerosis
Hereditary nephropathy, not elsewhere classified with focal glomerulonephritis

N07.2 Hereditary nephropathy, not elsewhere classified with diffuse membranous glomerulonephritis

N07.3 Hereditary nephropathy, not elsewhere classified with diffuse mesangial proliferative glomerulonephritis

N07.4 Hereditary nephropathy, not elsewhere classified with diffuse endocapillary proliferative glomerulonephritis

N07.5 Hereditary nephropathy, not elsewhere classified with diffuse mesangiocapillary glomerulonephritis
Hereditary nephropathy, not elsewhere classified with membranoproliferative glomerulonephritis, types 1 and 3, or NOS

N07.6 Hereditary nephropathy, not elsewhere classified with dense deposit disease
Hereditary nephropathy, not elsewhere classified with membranoproliferative glomerulonephritis, type 2

N07.7 Hereditary nephropathy, not elsewhere classified with diffuse crescentic glomerulonephritis
Hereditary nephropathy, not elsewhere classified with extracapillary glomerulonephritis

N07.8 Hereditary nephropathy, not elsewhere classified with other morphologic lesions
Hereditary nephropathy, not elsewhere classified with proliferative glomerulonephritis NOS

N07.9 Hereditary nephropathy, not elsewhere classified with unspecified morphologic lesions

N08 *Glomerular disorders in diseases classified elsewhere*

Glomerulonephritis
Nephritis
Nephropathy
Code first underlying disease, such as:
amyloidosis (E85.-)
congenital syphilis (A50.5)
cryoglobulinemia (D89.1)
disseminated intravascular coagulation (D65)
gout (M1A.-, M10.-)
microscopic polyangiitis (M31.7)
multiple myeloma (C90.0-)
sepsis (A40.0-A41.9)
sickle-cell disease (D57.0-D57.8)

EXCLUDES 1 *glomerulonephritis, nephritis and nephropathy (in) :*
antiglomerular basement membrane disease (M31.0)
diabetes (E08-E13 with .21)
gonococcal (A54.21)
Goodpasture's syndrome (M31.0)
hemolytic-uremic syndrome (D59.3)
lupus (M32.14)
mumps (B26.83)
syphilis (A52.75)
systemic lupus erythematosus (M32.14)
Wegener's granulomatosis (M31.31)
pyelonephritis in diseases classified elsewhere (N16)
renal tubulo-interstitial disorders classified elsewhere (N16)

CODING TIP✓ Do not assign code N08 for a patient diagnosed with diabetic nephropathy. For a patient diagnosed with diabetic nephropathy, choose and assign the appropriate combination code to specify the manifestation from categories E08-E13 with 4th and 5th characters .21.

Renal tubulo-interstitial diseases (N10-N16)

INCLUDES pyelonephritis

EXCLUDES 1 *pyeloureteritis cystica (N28.85)*

CODING TIP✓ If the urinary tract infection is resolved, or if the patient has recurrent infections, consider the use of Z87.440

N10 Acute pyelonephritis

Acute infectious interstitial nephritis
Acute pyelitis
Acute tubulo-interstitial nephritis
Hemoglobin nephrosis
Myoglobin nephrosis
Use additional code (B95-B97), to identify infectious agent.

4 N11 Chronic tubulo-interstitial nephritis

INCLUDES chronic infectious interstitial nephritis
chronic pyelitis
chronic pyelonephritis

Use additional code (B95-B97), to identify infectious agent.

N11.0 Nonobstructive reflux-associated chronic pyelonephritis
Pyelonephritis (chronic) associated with (vesicoureteral) reflux
EXCLUDES 1 *vesicoureteral reflux NOS (N13.70)*

N11.1 Chronic obstructive pyelonephritis
Pyelonephritis (chronic) associated with anomaly of pelviureteric junction
Pyelonephritis (chronic) associated with anomaly of pyeloureteric junction
Pyelonephritis (chronic) associated with crossing of vessel
Pyelonephritis (chronic) associated with kinking of ureter
Pyelonephritis (chronic) associated with obstruction of ureter
Pyelonephritis (chronic) associated with stricture of pelviureteric junction
Pyelonephritis (chronic) associated with stricture of ureter
EXCLUDES 1 *calculous pyelonephritis (N20.9)*
obstructive uropathy (N13.-)

N11.8 Other chronic tubulo-interstitial nephritis
Nonobstructive chronic pyelonephritis NOS

N11.9 Chronic tubulo-interstitial nephritis, unspecified
Chronic interstitial nephritis NOS
Chronic pyelitis NOS
Chronic pyelonephritis NOS

N12 Tubulo-interstitial nephritis, not specified as acute or chronic
Interstitial nephritis NOS
Pyelitis NOS
Pyelonephritis NOS
EXCLUDES 1 *calculous pyelonephritis (N20.9)*

[4] **N13 Obstructive and reflux uropathy**
EXCLUDES 2 *calculus of kidney and ureter without hydronephrosis (N20.-)*
congenital obstructive defects of renal pelvis and ureter (Q62.0-Q62.3)
hydronephrosis with ureteropelvic junction obstruction (Q62.11)
obstructive pyelonephritis (N11.1)

N13.0 Hydronephrosis with ureteropelvic junction obstruction
Hydronephrosis due to acquired occlusion of ureteropelvic junction
EXCLUDES 2 *Hydronephrosis with ureteropelvic junction obstruction due to calculus (N13.2)*
AHA: 4Q 2016, 43

N13.1 Hydronephrosis with ureteral stricture, not elsewhere classified
EXCLUDES 1 *Hydronephrosis with ureteral stricture with infection (N13.6)*

N13.2 Hydronephrosis with renal and ureteral calculous obstruction
EXCLUDES 1 *Hydronephrosis with renal and ureteral calculous obstruction with infection (N13.6)*

[5] **N13.3 Other and unspecified hydronephrosis**
EXCLUDES 1 *hydronephrosis with infection (N13.6)*

N13.30 Unspecified hydronephrosis

N13.39 Other hydronephrosis

N13.4 Hydroureter
EXCLUDES 1 *congenital hydroureter (Q62.3-)*
hydroureter with infection (N13.6)
vesicoureteral-reflux with hydroureter (N13.73-)

N13.5 Crossing vessel and stricture of ureter without hydronephrosis
Kinking and stricture of ureter without hydronephrosis
EXCLUDES 1 *Crossing vessel and stricture of ureter without hydronephrosis with infection (N13.6)*

Crossing vessel and stricture of ureter without hydronephrosis

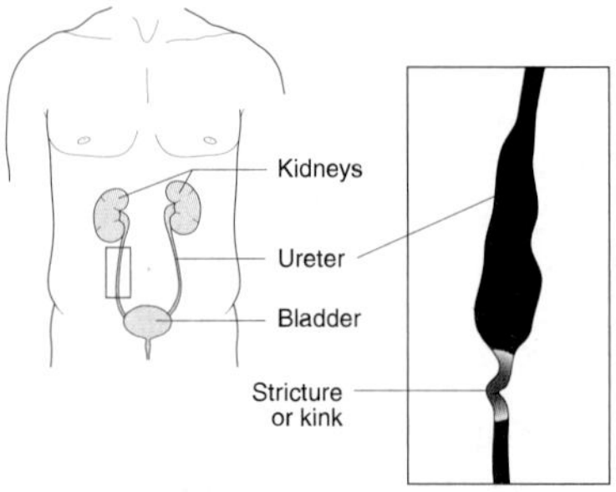

N13.6 Pyonephrosis
Conditions in N13.0-N13.5 with infection
Obstructive uropathy with infection
Use additional code (B95-B97), to identify infectious agent.
AHA: 2Q 2018, 16

[5] **N13.7 Vesicoureteral-reflux**
EXCLUDES 1 *reflux-associated pyelonephritis (N11.0)*

N13.70 Vesicoureteral-reflux, unspecified
Vesicoureteral-reflux NOS
DEFINITION Abnormal retrograde flow of urine from bladder back into the ureter and kidney; may cause progressive, long-term damage.

N13.71 Vesicoureteral-reflux without reflux nephropathy

[6] **N13.72 Vesicoureteral-reflux with reflux nephropathy without hydroureter**

N13.721 Vesicoureteral-reflux with reflux nephropathy without hydroureter, unilateral

N13.722 Vesicoureteral-reflux with reflux nephropathy without hydroureter, bilateral

N13.729 Vesicoureteral-reflux with reflux nephropathy without hydroureter, unspecified

[6] **N13.73 Vesicoureteral-reflux with reflux nephropathy with hydroureter**

N13.731 Vesicoureteral-reflux with reflux nephropathy with hydroureter, unilateral

N13.732 Vesicoureteral-reflux with reflux nephropathy with hydroureter, bilateral

N13.739 Vesicoureteral-reflux with reflux nephropathy with hydroureter, unspecified

N13.8 Other obstructive and reflux uropathy
Urinary tract obstruction due to specified cause
Code first, if applicable, any causal condition, such as:
enlarged prostate (N40.1)

N13.9 Obstructive and reflux uropathy, unspecified
Urinary tract obstruction NOS

Obstructive and reflux uropathy, unspecified

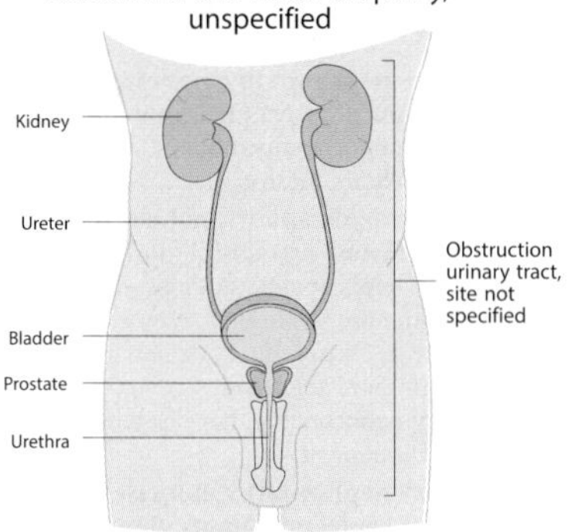

[4] **N14 Drug- and heavy-metal-induced tubulo-interstitial and tubular conditions**
Code first:
poisoning due to drug or toxin, if applicable (T36-T65 with fifth or sixth character 1-4 or 6)
Use additional code for adverse effect, if applicable, to identify drug (T36-T50 with fifth or sixth character 5)

CODING TIP ✓ Conditions classified to N14.- indicate nephropathy due to drugs, metals, or other toxic exposure. When one of these conditions has been specifically reported, first assign the appropriate code from T36-T65 when the condition is due to a poisoning. Or, to indicate adverse effect, assign a second code from T36-T50 following the appropriate N14.- code.

N14.0 Analgesic nephropathy

N14.1 Nephropathy induced by other drugs, medicaments and biological substances

N14.2 Nephropathy induced by unspecified drug, medicament or biological substance

N14.3 Nephropathy induced by heavy metals

N14.4 Toxic nephropathy, not elsewhere classified

[4] **N15 Other renal tubulo-interstitial diseases**

N15.0 Balkan nephropathy
Balkan endemic nephropathy

N15.1 Renal and perinephric abscess

N15.8 Other specified renal tubulo-interstitial diseases

N15.9 Renal tubulo-interstitial disease, unspecified
Infection of kidney NOS
EXCLUDES 1 *urinary tract infection NOS (N39.0)*

N16 ***Renal tubulo-interstitial disorders in diseases classified elsewhere***
Pyelonephritis
Tubulo-interstitial nephritis
Code first underlying disease, such as:
brucellosis (A23.0-A23.9)
cryoglobulinemia (D89.1)
glycogen storage disease (E74.0)
leukemia (C91-C95)
lymphoma (C81.0-C85.9, C96.0-C96.9)
multiple myeloma (C90.0-)
sepsis (A40.0-A41.9)
Wilson's disease (E83.0)

EXCLUDES 1 *diphtheritic pyelonephritis and tubulo-interstitial nephritis (A36.84)*
pyelonephritis and tubulo-interstitial nephritis in candidiasis (B37.49)
pyelonephritis and tubulo-interstitial nephritis in cystinosis (E72.04)
pyelonephritis and tubulo-interstitial nephritis in salmonella infection (A02.25)
pyelonephritis and tubulo-interstitial nephritis in sarcoidosis (D86.84)
pyelonephritis and tubulo-interstitial nephritis in sicca syndrome [Sjogren's] (M35.04)
pyelonephritis and tubulo-interstitial nephritis in systemic lupus erythematosus (M32.15)
pyelonephritis and tubulo-interstitial nephritis in toxoplasmosis (B58.83)
renal tubular degeneration in diabetes (E08-E13 with .29)
syphilitic pyelonephritis and tubulo-interstitial nephritis (A52.75)

Acute kidney failure and chronic kidney disease (N17-N19)

EXCLUDES 2 *congenital renal failure (P96.0)*
drug- and heavy-metal-induced tubulo-interstitial and tubular conditions (N14.-)
extrarenal uremia (R39.2)
hemolytic-uremic syndrome (D59.3)
hepatorenal syndrome (K76.7)
postpartum hepatorenal syndrome (O90.4)
posttraumatic renal failure (T79.5)
prerenal uremia (R39.2)
renal failure complicating abortion or ectopic or molar pregnancy (O00-O07, O08.4)
renal failure following labor and delivery (O90.4)
renal failure postprocedural (N99.0)

4 N17 **Acute kidney failure**
Code also:
associated underlying condition

EXCLUDES 1 *posttraumatic renal failure (T79.5)*

GUIDELINES **Section I.C.9.a.2)**
If a patient has hypertensive chronic kidney disease and acute renal failure, an additional code for the acute renal failure [category N17] is required.

CODING TIP ✓ When both acute kidney failure and chronic kidney disease (CKD) are present, both conditions should be coded.

N17.0 **Acute kidney failure with tubular necrosis** HCC
Acute tubular necrosis
Renal tubular necrosis
Tubular necrosis NOS

Acute kidney failure with tubular necrosis

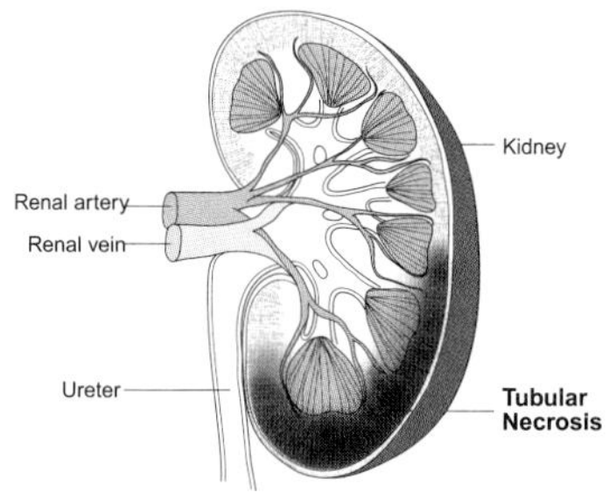

N17.1 **Acute kidney failure with acute cortical necrosis** HCC
Acute cortical necrosis
Cortical necrosis NOS
Renal cortical necrosis

N17.2 **Acute kidney failure with medullary necrosis** HCC
Medullary [papillary] necrosis NOS
Acute medullary [papillary] necrosis
Renal medullary [papillary] necrosis

N17.8 **Other acute kidney failure** HCC

N17.9 **Acute kidney failure, unspecified** HCC
Acute kidney injury (nontraumatic)

EXCLUDES 2 *traumatic kidney injury (S37.0-)*

4 N18 **Chronic kidney disease (CKD)**
Code first any associated:
diabetic chronic kidney disease (E08.22, E09.22, E10.22, E11.22, E13.22)
hypertensive chronic kidney disease (I12.-, I13.-)
Use additional code to identify kidney transplant status, if applicable, (Z94.0)

GUIDELINES **Section I.C.14.a.1)**
The ICD-10-CM classifies CKD based on severity. The severity of CKD is designated by stages 1-5. Stage 2, code N18.2, equates to mild CKD; stage 3, code N18.3, equates to moderate CKD; and stage 4, code N18.4, equates to severe CKD. Code N18.6, End stage renal disease (ESRD), is assigned when the provider has documented end-stage-renal disease (ESRD). If both a stage of CKD and ESRD are documented, assign code N18.6 only.

GUIDELINES **Section I.C.14.a.2)**
Patients who have undergone kidney transplant may still have some form of chronic kidney disease (CKD) because the kidney transplant may not fully restore kidney function. Therefore, the presence of CKD alone does not constitute a transplant complication. Assign the appropriate N18 code for the patient's stage of CKD and code Z94.0, Kidney transplant status. If a transplant complication such as failure or rejection or other transplant complication is documented, see section I.C.19.g for information on coding complications of a kidney transplant. If the documentation is unclear as to whether the patient has a complication of the transplant, query the provider.

GUIDELINES **Section I.C.14.a.3)**
Patients with CKD may also suffer from other serious conditions, most commonly diabetes mellitus and hypertension. The sequencing of the CKD code in relationship to codes for other contributing conditions is based on the conventions in the Tabular List.

CODING TIP ✓ Note that when assigning a code from N18.- as a confirmed manifestation of diabetes mellitus, the code N18.9 is not an allowed pairing. Only N18.1-N18.6 may be assigned as additional diagnoses to identify the stage of chronic kidney disease when this is a confirmed manifestation of diabetes mellitus.

N18.1 **Chronic kidney disease, stage 1**
N18.2 **Chronic kidney disease, stage 2 (mild)**
N18.3 **Chronic kidney disease, stage 3 (moderate)**
N18.4 **Chronic kidney disease, stage 4 (severe)** HCC
AHA: 1Q 2013, 24

N18.5 **Chronic kidney disease, stage 5** HCC
EXCLUDES 1 *chronic kidney disease, stage 5 requiring chronic dialysis (N18.6)*

N18.6 **End stage renal disease** HCC
Chronic kidney disease requiring chronic dialysis
Use additional code to identify dialysis status (Z99.2)
AHA: 4Q 2013, 124, 125
AHA: 1Q 2016, 12-13
AHA: 3Q 2016, 22
AHA: 3Q 2016, 23

N18.9 **Chronic kidney disease, unspecified**
Chronic renal disease
Chronic renal failure NOS
Chronic renal insufficiency
Chronic uremia NOS
Diffuse sclerosing glomerulonephritis NOS

N19 **Unspecified kidney failure**
Uremia NOS
EXCLUDES 1 *acute kidney failure (N17.-)*
chronic kidney disease (N18.-)
chronic uremia (N18.9)
extrarenal uremia (R39.2)
prerenal uremia (R39.2)
renal insufficiency (acute) (N28.9)
uremia of newborn (P96.0)

Urolithiasis (N20-N23)

4 N20 **Calculus of kidney and ureter**
Calculous pyelonephritis
EXCLUDES 1 *nephrocalcinosis (E83.5)*
that with hydronephrosis (N13.2)

CODING TIP ✓ If the renal calculi is resolved, or if the patient has a history of recurrent kidney stones, consider the use of Z87.442.

N20.0 **Calculus of kidney**
Nephrolithiasis NOS
Renal calculus
Renal stone
Staghorn calculus
Stone in kidney

N20.1 **Calculus of ureter**
Ureteric stone
AHA: 3Q 2016, 23
AHA: 3Q 2016, 24

Calculus of ureter

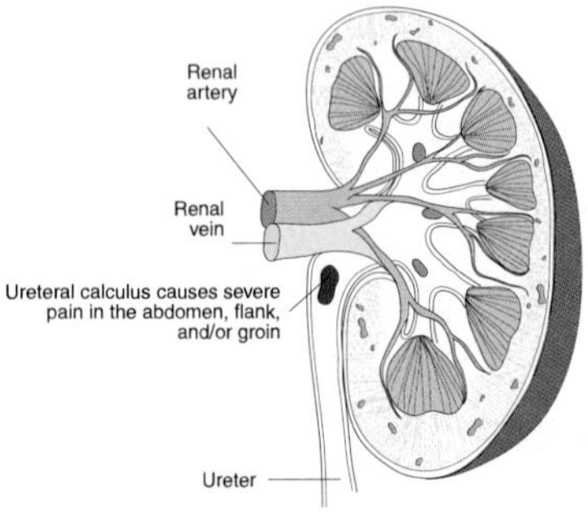

N20.2 **Calculus of kidney with calculus of ureter**
N20.9 **Urinary calculus, unspecified**

4 N21 **Calculus of lower urinary tract**
INCLUDES calculus of lower urinary tract with cystitis and urethritis

N21.0 **Calculus in bladder**
Calculus in diverticulum of bladder
Urinary bladder stone
EXCLUDES 2 *staghorn calculus (N20.0)*

DEFINITION An abnormal concretion of mineral salts, occurring in the bladder.

N21.1 **Calculus in urethra**
EXCLUDES 2 *calculus of prostate (N42.0)*

Calculus in urethra

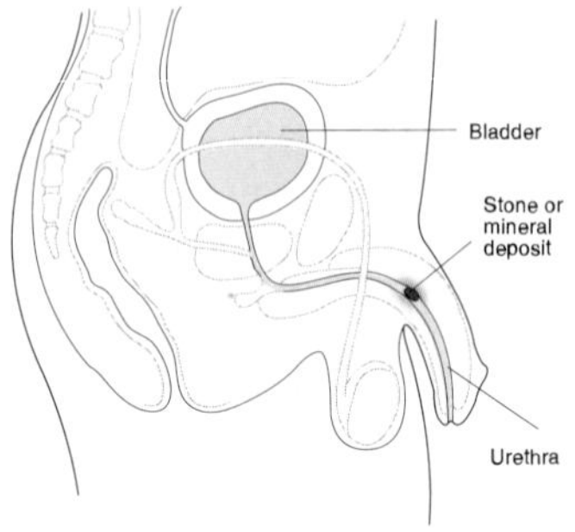

N21.8 **Other lower urinary tract calculus**
N21.9 **Calculus of lower urinary tract, unspecified**
EXCLUDES 1 *calculus of urinary tract NOS (N20.9)*

N22 ***Calculus of urinary tract in diseases classified elsewhere***
Code first underlying disease, such as:
gout (M1A.-, M10.-)
schistosomiasis (B65.0-B65.9)

N23 **Unspecified renal colic**

Other disorders of kidney and ureter (N25-N29)

EXCLUDES 2 *disorders of kidney and ureter with urolithiasis (N20-N23)*

4 N25 **Disorders resulting from impaired renal tubular function**

N25.0 **Renal osteodystrophy**
Azotemic osteodystrophy
Phosphate-losing tubular disorders
Renal rickets
Renal short stature
EXCLUDES 2 *metabolic disorders classifiable to E70-E88*

N25.1 **Nephrogenic diabetes insipidus** HCC
EXCLUDES 1 *diabetes insipidus NOS (E23.2)*

5 N25.8 **Other disorders resulting from impaired renal tubular function**

N25.81 **Secondary hyperparathyroidism of renal origin** HCC
EXCLUDES 1 *secondary hyperparathyroidism, non-renal (E21.1)*
EXCLUDES 2 *metabolic disorders classifiable to E70-E88*

N25.89 **Other disorders resulting from impaired renal tubular function**
Hypokalemic nephropathy
Lightwood-Albright syndrome
Renal tubular acidosis NOS

N25.9 **Disorder resulting from impaired renal tubular function, unspecified**

4 N26 **Unspecified contracted kidney**
EXCLUDES 1 *contracted kidney due to hypertension (I12.-)*
diffuse sclerosing glomerulonephritis (N05.8.-)
hypertensive nephrosclerosis (arteriolar) (arteriosclerotic) (I12.-)
small kidney of unknown cause (N27.-)

CODING TIP ✓ When a condition classifiable to N26.- is present in combination with a diagnosis of hypertension, I12.9 should be assigned followed by the appropriate N26.- code.

N26.1 **Atrophy of kidney (terminal)**
N26.2 **Page kidney**

N26.9 Renal sclerosis, unspecified

Renal sclerosis

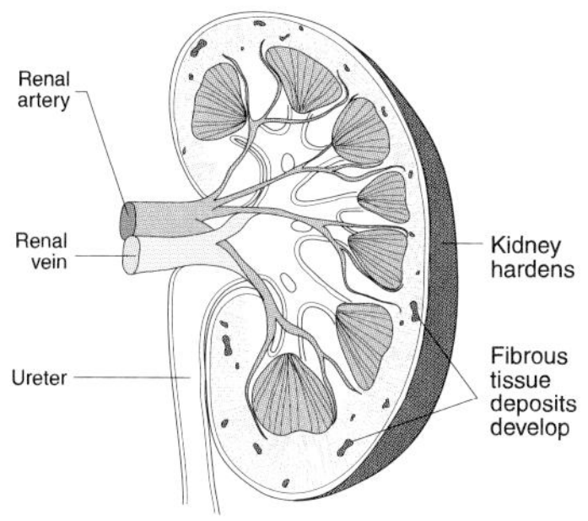

N27 Small kidney of unknown cause

INCLUDES oligonephronia

N27.0 Small kidney, unilateral
N27.1 Small kidney, bilateral
N27.9 Small kidney, unspecified

N28 Other disorders of kidney and ureter, not elsewhere classified

N28.0 Ischemia and infarction of kidney HCC

Renal artery embolism
Renal artery obstruction
Renal artery occlusion
Renal artery thrombosis
Renal infarct

EXCLUDES 1 *atherosclerosis of renal artery (extrarenal part) (I70.1)*
congenital stenosis of renal artery (Q27.1)
Goldblatt's kidney (I70.1)

N28.1 Cyst of kidney, acquired

Cyst (multiple) (solitary) of kidney (acquired)

EXCLUDES 1 *cystic kidney disease (congenital) (Q61.-)*

CODING TIP✓ N28.1 is coded only for acquired renal cysts. Note that cysts documented as single or solitary are considered congenital while those documented as simple are considered acquired. If the medical record is not clear as to whether the cyst is acquired or congenital, the provider should be queried. Carefully review documentation provided to ensure the cyst is in the kidney. Cysts noted to be present in the ureters are not classified here.

N28.8 Other specified disorders of kidney and ureter

EXCLUDES 1 *hydroureter (N13.4)*
ureteric stricture with hydronephrosis (N13.1)
ureteric stricture without hydronephrosis (N13.5)

N28.81 Hypertrophy of kidney
N28.82 Megaloureter
N28.83 Nephroptosis
N28.84 Pyelitis cystica
N28.85 Pyeloureteritis cystica

DEFINITION Infection of the renal pelvis and ureter with development of small cysts in the kidney and ureter.

N28.86 Ureteritis cystica
N28.89 Other specified disorders of kidney and ureter

N28.9 Disorder of kidney and ureter, unspecified

Nephropathy NOS
Renal disease (acute) NOS
Renal insufficiency (acute)

EXCLUDES 1 *chronic renal insufficiency (N18.9)*
unspecified nephritic syndrome (N05.-)

AHA: 1Q 2016, 13

N29 *Other disorders of kidney and ureter in diseases classified elsewhere*

Code first underlying disease, such as:
amyloidosis (E85.-)
nephrocalcinosis (E83.5)
schistosomiasis (B65.0-B65.9)

EXCLUDES 1 *disorders of kidney and ureter in:*
cystinosis (E72.0)
gonorrhea (A54.21)
syphilis (A52.75)
tuberculosis (A18.11)

Other diseases of the urinary system (N30-N39)

EXCLUDES 1 *urinary infection (complicating) :*
abortion or ectopic or molar pregnancy (O00-O07, O08.8)
pregnancy, childbirth and the puerperium (O23.-, O75.3, O86.2-)

N30 Cystitis

Use additional code to identify infectious agent (B95-B97)

EXCLUDES 1 *prostatocystitis (N41.3)*

CODING TIP✓ Cystitis indicates inflammation and/or infection localized to the bladder. When a urinary tract infection is specified as cystitis, assign the appropriate N30.- code. Also assign a code for the causative organism, when known. An unspecified urinary tract infection should be coded to N39.0.

N30.0 Acute cystitis

EXCLUDES 1 *irradiation cystitis (N30.4-)*
trigonitis (N30.3-)

N30.00 Acute cystitis without hematuria
N30.01 Acute cystitis with hematuria

N30.1 Interstitial cystitis (chronic)

N30.10 Interstitial cystitis (chronic) without hematuria
N30.11 Interstitial cystitis (chronic) with hematuria

N30.2 Other chronic cystitis

N30.20 Other chronic cystitis without hematuria
N30.21 Other chronic cystitis with hematuria

N30.3 Trigonitis

Urethrotrigonitis

DEFINITION Inflammation of the mouth of the bladder where it drains into the urethra.

N30.30 Trigonitis without hematuria
N30.31 Trigonitis with hematuria

N30.4 Irradiation cystitis

N30.40 Irradiation cystitis without hematuria
N30.41 Irradiation cystitis with hematuria

N30.8 Other cystitis

Abscess of bladder

N30.80 Other cystitis without hematuria
N30.81 Other cystitis with hematuria

DEFINITION Bullous (cystic) cystitis: Inflammation of the bladder with formation of cysts on the interior bladder wall.

N30.9 Cystitis, unspecified

N30.90 Cystitis, unspecified without hematuria
N30.91 Cystitis, unspecified with hematuria

N31 Neuromuscular dysfunction of bladder, not elsewhere classified

Use additional code to identify any associated urinary incontinence (N39.3-N39.4-)

EXCLUDES 1 *cord bladder NOS (G95.89)*
neurogenic bladder due to cauda equina syndrome (G83.4)
neuromuscular dysfunction due to spinal cord lesion (G95.89)

N31.0 Uninhibited neuropathic bladder, not elsewhere classified
N31.1 Reflex neuropathic bladder, not elsewhere classified

N31.2 Flaccid neuropathic bladder, not elsewhere classified
Atonic (motor) (sensory) neuropathic bladder
Autonomous neuropathic bladder
Nonreflex neuropathic bladder

Flaccid neuropathic bladder, not elsewhere classified

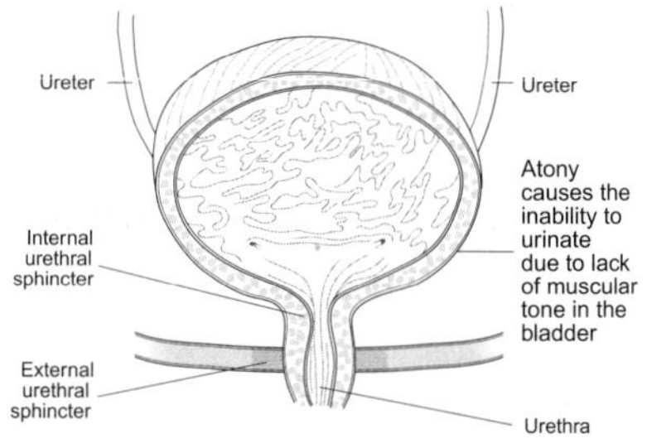

N31.8 Other neuromuscular dysfunction of bladder

N31.9 Neuromuscular dysfunction of bladder, unspecified
Neurogenic bladder dysfunction NOS

4 N32 Other disorders of bladder

EXCLUDES 2 *calculus of bladder (N21.0)*
cystocele (N81.1-)
hernia or prolapse of bladder, female (N81.1-)

N32.0 Bladder-neck obstruction
Bladder-neck stenosis (acquired)
EXCLUDES 1 *congenital bladder-neck obstruction (Q64.3-)*
DEFINITION Blockage in the opening between the bladder and the urethra, causing bladder distention and decreased urine output.

N32.1 Vesicointestinal fistula
Vesicorectal fistula
DEFINITION Abnormal passage between the bladder and the intestines.

N32.2 Vesical fistula, not elsewhere classified
EXCLUDES 1 *fistula between bladder and female genital tract (N82.0-N82.1)*

N32.3 Diverticulum of bladder
EXCLUDES 1 *congenital diverticulum of bladder (Q64.6)*
diverticulitis of bladder (N30.8-)

5 N32.8 Other specified disorders of bladder

N32.81 Overactive bladder
Detrusor muscle hyperactivity
EXCLUDES 1 *frequent urination due to specified bladder condition- code to condition*

N32.89 Other specified disorders of bladder
Bladder hemorrhage
Bladder hypertrophy
Calcified bladder
Contracted bladder

N32.9 Bladder disorder, unspecified

N33 *Bladder disorders in diseases classified elsewhere*

Code first underlying disease, such as:
schistosomiasis (B65.0-B65.9)
EXCLUDES 1 *bladder disorder in syphilis (A52.76)*
bladder disorder in tuberculosis (A18.12)
candidal cystitis (B37.41)
chlamydial cystitis (A56.01)
cystitis in gonorrhea (A54.01)
cystitis in neurogenic bladder (N31.-)
diphtheritic cystitis (A36.85)
syphilitic cystitis (A52.76)
trichomonal cystitis (A59.03)

4 N34 Urethritis and urethral syndrome

Use additional code (B95-B97), to identify infectious agent.
EXCLUDES 2 *Reiter's disease (M02.3-)*
urethritis in diseases with a predominantly sexual mode of transmission (A50-A64)
urethrotrigonitis (N30.3-)

N34.0 Urethral abscess
Abscess (of) Cowper's gland
Abscess (of) Littré's gland
Abscess (of) urethral (gland)
Periurethral abscess
EXCLUDES 1 *urethral caruncle (N36.2)*

Urethral abscess

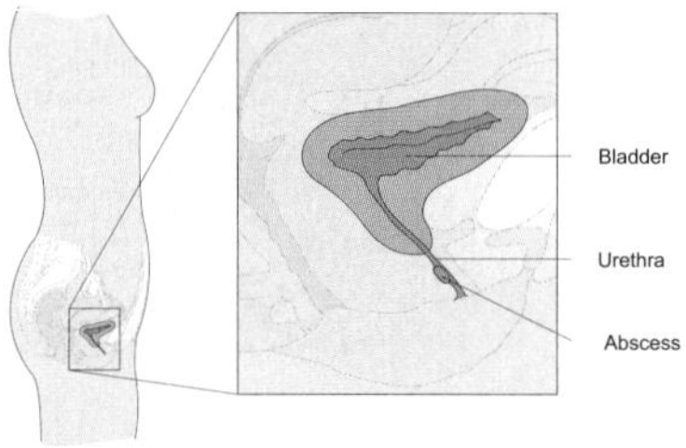

N34.1 Nonspecific urethritis
Nongonococcal urethritis
Nonvenereal urethritis

N34.2 Other urethritis
Meatitis, urethral
Postmenopausal urethritis
Ulcer of urethra (meatus)
Urethritis NOS

N34.3 Urethral syndrome, unspecified

4 N35 Urethral stricture

EXCLUDES 1 *congenital urethral stricture (Q64.3-)*
postprocedural urethral stricture (N99.1-)

5 N35.0 Post-traumatic urethral stricture
Urethral stricture due to injury
EXCLUDES 1 *postprocedural urethral stricture (N99.1-)*

6 N35.01 Post-traumatic urethral stricture, male

N35.010 Post-traumatic urethral stricture, male, meatal ♂

N35.011 Post-traumatic bulbous urethral stricture ♂

N35.012 Post-traumatic membranous urethral stricture ♂

N35.013 Post-traumatic anterior urethral stricture ♂

N35.014 Post-traumatic urethral stricture, male, unspecified ♂

● **N35.016 Post-traumatic urethral stricture, male, overlapping sites** ♂

6 N35.02 Post-traumatic urethral stricture, female

N35.021 Urethral stricture due to childbirth ♀

N35.028 Other post-traumatic urethral stricture, female ♀

5 N35.1 Postinfective urethral stricture, not elsewhere classified
EXCLUDES 1 *urethral stricture associated with schistosomiasis (B65.-, N29)*
gonococcal urethral stricture (A54.01)
syphilitic urethral stricture (A52.76)

6 N35.11 Postinfective urethral stricture, not elsewhere classified, male

N35.111 Postinfective urethral stricture, not elsewhere classified, male, meatal ♂

N35.112 Postinfective bulbous urethral stricture, not elsewhere classified, male ♂

N35.113 Postinfective membranous urethral stricture, not elsewhere classified, male ♂

N35.114 Postinfective anterior urethral stricture, not elsewhere classified, male ♂

● **N35.116 Postinfective urethral stricture, not elsewhere classified, male, overlapping sites** ♂

N35.119 Postinfective urethral stricture, not elsewhere classified, male, unspecified ♂

N35.12 Postinfective urethral stricture, not elsewhere classified, female ♀

▲ **5 N35.8 Other urethral stricture**
EXCLUDES 1 *postprocedural urethral stricture (N99.1-)*

● **6 N35.81 Other urethral stricture, male**

● **N35.811 Other urethral stricture, male, meatal** ♂

● **N35.812 Other urethral bulbous stricture, male** ♂

● N35.813 Other membranous urethral stricture, male ♂

● N35.814 Other anterior urethral stricture, male, anterior ♂

● N35.816 Other urethral stricture, male, overlapping sites ♂

● N35.819 Other urethral stricture, male, unspecified site ♂

● N35.82 Other urethral stricture, female ♀

▲ 5 N35.9 Urethral stricture, unspecified

● 6 N35.91 Urethral stricture, unspecified, male

● N35.911 Unspecified urethral stricture, male, meatal ♂

● N35.912 Unspecified bulbous urethral stricture, male ♂

● N35.913 Unspecified membranous urethral stricture, male ♂

● N35.914 Unspecified anterior urethral stricture, male ♂

● N35.916 Unspecified urethral stricture, male, overlapping sites ♂

● N35.919 Unspecified urethral stricture, male, unspecified site ♂
Pinhole meatus NOS
Urethral stricture NOS

● N35.92 Unspecified urethral stricture, female ♀

4 N36 Other disorders of urethra

N36.0 Urethral fistula
Urethroperineal fistula
Urethrorectal fistula
Urinary fistula NOS

EXCLUDES 1 *urethroscrotal fistula (N50.89)*
urethrovaginal fistula (N82.1)
urethrovesicovaginal fistula (N82.1)

DEFINITION An abnormal passage communicating with the urethra.

N36.1 Urethral diverticulum

DEFINITION Sac-like out-pouching of the urethral wall.

N36.2 Urethral caruncle

DEFINITION A fleshy outgrowth in the urethra that may be normal or abnormal, often growing from mucous membranes.

5 N36.4 Urethral functional and muscular disorders
Use additional code to identify associated urinary stress incontinence (N39.3)

N36.41 Hypermobility of urethra

N36.42 Intrinsic sphincter deficiency (ISD)

N36.43 Combined hypermobility of urethra and intrinsic sphincter deficiency

N36.44 Muscular disorders of urethra
Bladder sphincter dyssynergy

N36.5 Urethral false passage

N36.8 Other specified disorders of urethra

EXCLUDES 1 *congenital urethrocele (Q64.7)*
female urethrocele (N81.0)

N36.9 Urethral disorder, unspecified

N37 *Urethral disorders in diseases classified elsewhere*
Code first:
underlying disease

EXCLUDES 1 *urethritis (in) :*
candidal infection (B37.41)
chlamydial (A56.01)
gonorrhea (A54.01)
syphilis (A52.76)
trichomonal infection (A59.03)
tuberculosis (A18.13)

4 N39 Other disorders of urinary system

EXCLUDES 2 *hematuria NOS (R31.-)*
recurrent or persistent hematuria (N02.-)
recurrent or persistent hematuria with specified morphological lesion (N02.-)
proteinuria NOS (R80.-)

N39.0 Urinary tract infection, site not specified
Use additional code (B95-B97), to identify infectious agent.

EXCLUDES 1 *candidiasis of urinary tract (B37.4-)*
neonatal urinary tract infection (P39.3)
urinary tract infection of specified site, such as:
cystitis (N30.-)
urethritis (N34.-)

CODING TIP ✓ If the urinary tract infection is resolved, or if the patient has recurrent infections, consider the use of Z87.440.

AHA: 4Q 2012, 94
AHA: 1Q 2018, 13

N39.3 Stress incontinence (female) (male)
Code also:
any associated overactive bladder (N32.81)

EXCLUDES 1 *mixed incontinence (N39.46)*

DEFINITION Involuntary loss of bladder control during physical movements, such as coughing, sneezing, or other strenuous activity.

Stress incontinence (female) (male)

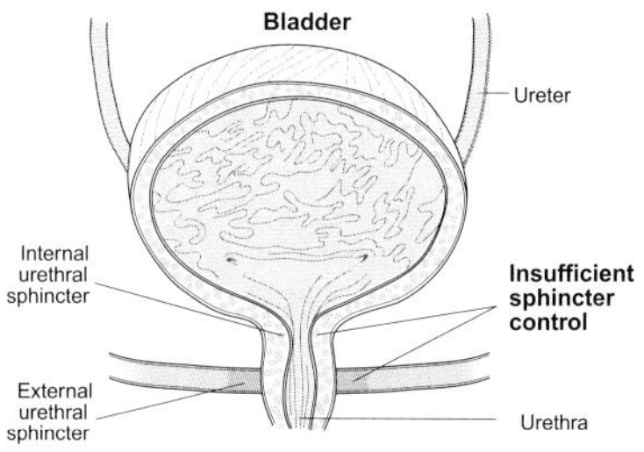

5 N39.4 Other specified urinary incontinence
Code also:
any associated overactive bladder (N32.81)

EXCLUDES 1 *enuresis NOS (R32)*
functional urinary incontinence (R39.81)
urinary incontinence associated with cognitive impairment (R39.81)
urinary incontinence NOS (R32)
urinary incontinence of nonorganic origin (F98.0)

N39.41 Urge incontinence

EXCLUDES 1 *mixed incontinence (N39.46)*

DEFINITION Inability to control urination after the urge to urinate.

N39.42 Incontinence without sensory awareness
Insensible (urinary) incontinence

N39.43 Post-void dribbling

N39.44 Nocturnal enuresis

N39.45 Continuous leakage

N39.46 Mixed incontinence
Urge and stress incontinence

6 N39.49 Other specified urinary incontinence
AHA: 4Q 2016, 44

N39.490 Overflow incontinence

DEFINITION Urinary incontinence due to pressure of retained urine in the bladder, after the bladder has contracted to its limits, with dribbling urine.

N39.491 Coital incontinence

N39.492 Postural (urinary) incontinence

N39.498 Other specified urinary incontinence
Reflex incontinence
Total incontinence

N39.8 Other specified disorders of urinary system

N39.9 Disorder of urinary system, unspecified

Diseases of male genital organs (N40-N53)

4 N40 Benign prostatic hyperplasia

INCLUDES adenofibromatous hypertrophy of prostate
benign hypertrophy of the prostate
benign prostatic hypertrophy
BPH
enlarged prostate
nodular prostate
polyp of prostate

EXCLUDES 1 *benign neoplasms of prostate (adenoma, benign) (fibroadenoma) (fibroma) (myoma) (D29.1)*

EXCLUDES 2 *malignant neoplasm of prostate (C61)*

CODING TIP✓ Although hyperplasia (increase in number of cells) and hypertrophy (increase in size of cells) are not synonymous, benign prostatic hyperplasia and benign prostatic hypertrophy are classified to the same code. When a patient diagnosed with a condition classifiable to N40.- also has lower urinary tract symptoms present – such as obstruction, incontinence, hesitancy, frequency, urgency or other included conditions – assign code N40.1 and the associated symptoms.

N40.0 Benign prostatic hyperplasia without lower urinary tract symptoms ♂ A
Enlarged prostate without LUTS
Enlarged prostate NOS

Enlarged prostate without lower urinary tract symptoms

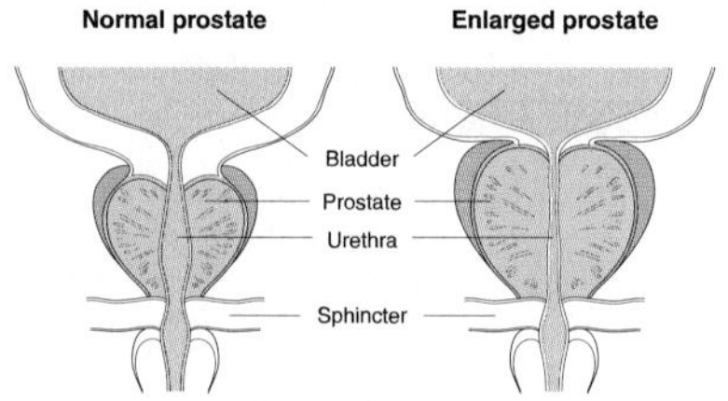

N40.1 Benign prostatic hyperplasia with lower urinary tract symptoms ♂ A
Enlarged prostate with LUTS
Use additional code for associated symptoms, when specified:
incomplete bladder emptying (R39.14)
nocturia (R35.1)
straining on urination (R39.16)
urinary frequency (R35.0)
urinary hesitancy (R39.11)
urinary incontinence (N39.4-)
urinary obstruction (N13.8)
urinary retention (R33.8)
urinary urgency (R39.15)
weak urinary stream (R39.12)

N40.2 Nodular prostate without lower urinary tract symptoms ♂ A
Nodular prostate without LUTS

N40.3 Nodular prostate with lower urinary tract symptoms ♂ A
Use additional code for associated symptoms, when specified:
incomplete bladder emptying (R39.14)
nocturia (R35.1)
straining on urination (R39.16)
urinary frequency (R35.0)
urinary hesitancy (R39.11)
urinary incontinence (N39.4-)
urinary obstruction (N13.8)
urinary retention (R33.8)
urinary urgency (R39.15)
weak urinary stream (R39.12)

4 N41 Inflammatory diseases of prostate

Use additional code (B95-B97), to identify infectious agent.

N41.0 Acute prostatitis ♂ A
N41.1 Chronic prostatitis ♂ A
N41.2 Abscess of prostate ♂ A
N41.3 Prostatocystitis ♂ A
N41.4 Granulomatous prostatitis ♂ A
N41.8 Other inflammatory diseases of prostate ♂ A
N41.9 Inflammatory disease of prostate, unspecified ♂ A
Prostatitis NOS

4 N42 Other and unspecified disorders of prostate

N42.0 Calculus of prostate ♂ A
Prostatic stone

N42.1 Congestion and hemorrhage of prostate ♂ A

EXCLUDES 1 *enlarged prostate (N40.-)*
hematuria (R31.-)
hyperplasia of prostate (N40.-)
inflammatory diseases of prostate (N41.-)

5 N42.3 Dysplasia of prostate
AHA: 4Q 2016, 44

N42.30 Unspecified dysplasia of prostate ♂
N42.31 Prostatic intraepithelial neoplasia ♂
PIN
Prostatic intraepithelial neoplasia I (PIN I)
Prostatic intraepithelial neoplasia II (PIN II)

EXCLUDES 1 *prostatic intraepithelial neoplasia III (PIN III) (D07.5)*

N42.32 Atypical small acinar proliferation of prostate ♂
N42.39 Other dysplasia of prostate ♂

5 N42.8 Other specified disorders of prostate

N42.81 Prostatodynia syndrome ♂ A
Painful prostate syndrome
N42.82 Prostatosis syndrome ♂ A
N42.83 Cyst of prostate ♂ A
N42.89 Other specified disorders of prostate ♂ A

N42.9 Disorder of prostate, unspecified ♂ A

4 N43 Hydrocele and spermatocele

INCLUDES hydrocele of spermatic cord, testis or tunica vaginalis

EXCLUDES 1 *congenital hydrocele (P83.5)*

CODING TIP✓ Conditions classifiable to N43.- indicate cysts of fluid that develop near the head of the epididymis (spermatocele), or surrounding the testicle (hydrocele). They are often painless but may cause discomfort due to pressure on surrounding areas. When a hydrocele is reported as infected, assign N43.1 with an additional code for the causative organism, if known.

Hydrocele

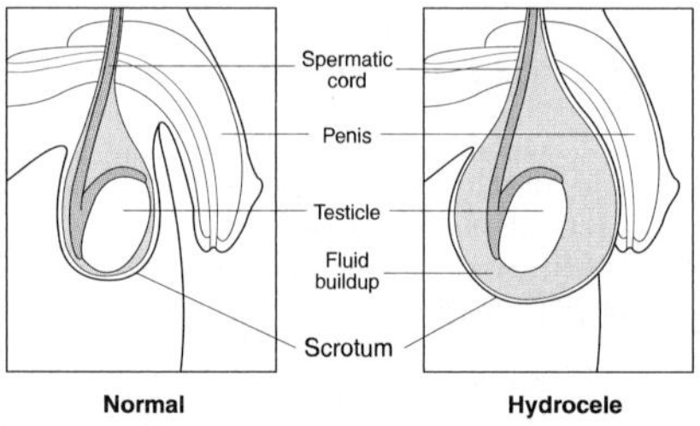

N43.0 Encysted hydrocele ♂
N43.1 Infected hydrocele ♂
Use additional code (B95-B97), to identify infectious agent
N43.2 Other hydrocele ♂
N43.3 Hydrocele, unspecified ♂

DEFINITION Collection of serous fluid on the tunica vaginalis, spermatic cord, or testicle from acute local injury, infection, radiotherapy, or gradual fluid accumulation.

5 N43.4 Spermatocele of epididymis
Spermatic cyst

DEFINITION Cyst on the epididymis containing sperm.

N43.40 Spermatocele of epididymis, unspecified ♂
N43.41 Spermatocele of epididymis, single ♂
N43.42 Spermatocele of epididymis, multiple ♂

4 N44 Noninflammatory disorders of testis

5 N44.0 Torsion of testis

N44.00 Torsion of testis, unspecified ♂

DEFINITION Testicle becomes twisted inside the scrotum, cutting off the blood supply.

N44.01 **Extravaginal torsion of spermatic cord** ♂

N44.02 **Intravaginal torsion of spermatic cord** ♂
Torsion of spermatic cord NOS

N44.03 **Torsion of appendix testis** ♂

N44.04 **Torsion of appendix epididymis** ♂

N44.1 **Cyst of tunica albuginea testis** ♂

N44.2 **Benign cyst of testis** ♂

N44.8 **Other noninflammatory disorders of the testis** ♂

4 N45 Orchitis and epididymitis
Use additional code (B95-B97), to identify infectious agent.

CODING TIP ✓ When coding conditions classifiable to N45.-, review documentation to identify the causative organism(s) if known, and assign an additional code.

N45.1 **Epididymitis** ♂

N45.2 **Orchitis** ♂

N45.3 **Epididymo-orchitis** ♂

N45.4 **Abscess of epididymis or testis** ♂

Abscess of epididymis or testis

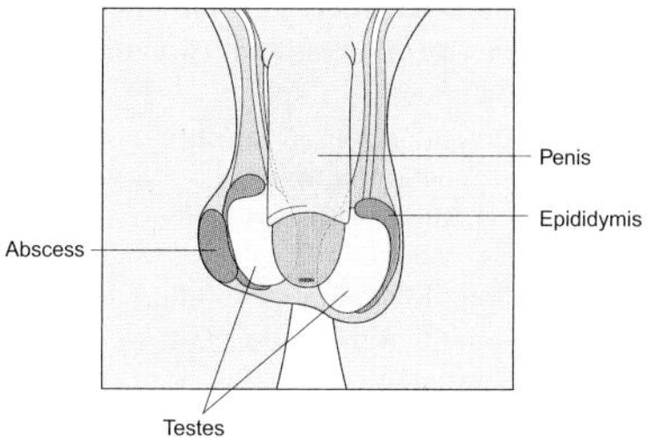

4 N46 Male infertility
EXCLUDES 1 *vasectomy status (Z98.52)*

5 N46.0 **Azoospermia**
Absolute male infertility
Male infertility due to germinal (cell) aplasia
Male infertility due to spermatogenic arrest (complete)

N46.01 **Organic azoospermia** ♂ A
Azoospermia NOS

6 N46.02 **Azoospermia due to extratesticular causes**
Code also:
associated cause

N46.021 **Azoospermia due to drug therapy** ♂ A

N46.022 **Azoospermia due to infection** ♂ A

N46.023 **Azoospermia due to obstruction of efferent ducts** ♂ A

N46.024 **Azoospermia due to radiation** ♂ A

N46.025 **Azoospermia due to systemic disease** ♂ A

N46.029 **Azoospermia due to other extratesticular causes** ♂ A

5 N46.1 **Oligospermia**
Male infertility due to germinal cell desquamation
Male infertility due to hypospermatogenesis
Male infertility due to incomplete spermatogenic arrest

DEFINITION Insufficient spermatozoa in the semen.

N46.11 **Organic oligospermia** ♂ A
Oligospermia NOS

6 N46.12 **Oligospermia due to extratesticular causes**
Code also:
associated cause

N46.121 **Oligospermia due to drug therapy** ♂ A

N46.122 **Oligospermia due to infection** ♂ A

N46.123 **Oligospermia due to obstruction of efferent ducts** ♂ A

N46.124 **Oligospermia due to radiation** ♂ A

N46.125 **Oligospermia due to systemic disease** ♂ A

N46.129 **Oligospermia due to other extratesticular causes** ♂ A

N46.8 **Other male infertility** ♂ A

N46.9 **Male infertility, unspecified** ♂ A

4 N47 Disorders of prepuce

N47.0 **Adherent prepuce, newborn** ♂ N

N47.1 **Phimosis** ♂

N47.2 **Paraphimosis** ♂

N47.3 **Deficient foreskin** ♂

N47.4 **Benign cyst of prepuce** ♂

N47.5 **Adhesions of prepuce and glans penis** ♂

N47.6 **Balanoposthitis** ♂
Use additional code (B95-B97), to identify infectious agent.
EXCLUDES 1 *balanitis (N48.1)*

DEFINITION Inflammation of the head of the penis and foreskin.

N47.7 **Other inflammatory diseases of prepuce** ♂
Use additional code (B95-B97), to identify infectious agent.

N47.8 **Other disorders of prepuce** ♂

4 N48 Other disorders of penis

N48.0 **Leukoplakia of penis** ♂
Balanitis xerotica obliterans
Kraurosis of penis
Lichen sclerosus of external male genital organs
EXCLUDES 1 *carcinoma in situ of penis (D07.4)*

DEFINITION Chronic skin condition of the penis causing atrophic, white, patches on the foreskin and glans with hardened, indurated tissue near the meatus.

N48.1 **Balanitis** ♂
Use additional code (B95-B97), to identify infectious agent
EXCLUDES 1 *amebic balanitis (A06.8)*
balanitis xerotica obliterans (N48.0)
candidal balanitis (B37.42)
gonococcal balanitis (A54.23)
herpesviral [herpes simplex] balanitis (A60.01)

DEFINITION Inflammation of the glans penis (the head of the penis).

5 N48.2 **Other inflammatory disorders of penis**
Use additional code (B95-B97), to identify infectious agent.
EXCLUDES 1 *balanitis (N48.1)*
balanitis xerotica obliterans (N48.0)
balanoposthitis (N47.6)

N48.21 **Abscess of corpus cavernosum and penis** ♂

N48.22 **Cellulitis of corpus cavernosum and penis** ♂

N48.29 **Other inflammatory disorders of penis** ♂

5 N48.3 **Priapism**
Painful erection
Code first:
underlying cause

N48.30 **Priapism, unspecified** ♂

N48.31 **Priapism due to trauma** ♂

N48.32 ***Priapism due to disease classified elsewhere*** ♂

N48.33 **Priapism, drug-induced** ♂

N48.39 **Other priapism** ♂

N48.5 **Ulcer of penis** ♂

N48.6 **Induration penis plastica** ♂
Peyronie's disease
Plastic induration of penis

5 N48.8 **Other specified disorders of penis**

N48.81 **Thrombosis of superficial vein of penis** ♂

N48.82 **Acquired torsion of penis** ♂
Acquired torsion of penis NOS
EXCLUDES 1 *congenital torsion of penis (Q55.63)*

N48.83 **Acquired buried penis** ♂
EXCLUDES 1 *congenital hidden penis (Q55.64)*

N48.89 **Other specified disorders of penis** ♂

N48.9 **Disorder of penis, unspecified** ♂

4 N49 Inflammatory disorders of male genital organs, not elsewhere classified
Use additional code (B95-B97), to identify infectious agent
EXCLUDES 1 *inflammation of penis (N48.1, N48.2-)*
orchitis and epididymitis (N45.-)

N49.0 **Inflammatory disorders of seminal vesicle** ♂
Vesiculitis NOS

Inflammatory disorders of seminal vesicle

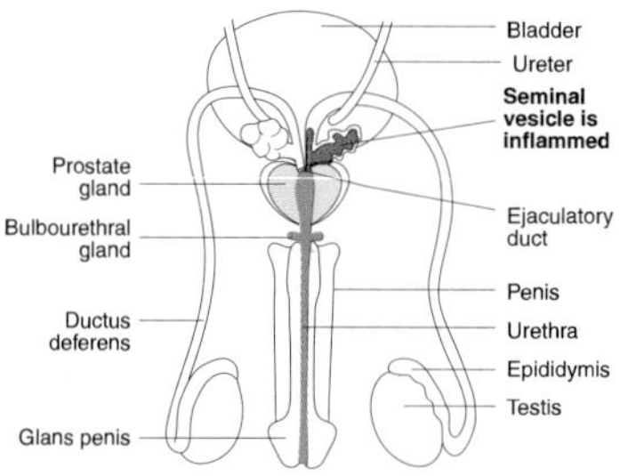

N49.1 **Inflammatory disorders of spermatic cord, tunica vaginalis and vas deferens** ♂
Vasitis

N49.2 **Inflammatory disorders of scrotum** ♂

N49.3 **Fournier gangrene** ♂

CODING TIP ✓ Fournier gangrene is a specific condition typically occurring in males, which includes a necrotizing or gangrenous infection of the perineal region often including a mix of aerobic and anaerobic bacteria. An additional code should be assigned to identify causative organism(s).

DEFINITION Necrosis affecting the perineal, genital, or perianal regions, characterized by black and malodorous tissue decay caused by infection or ischemia.

N49.8 **Inflammatory disorders of other specified male genital organs** ♂
Inflammation of multiple sites in male genital organs

N49.9 **Inflammatory disorder of unspecified male genital organ** ♂
Abscess of unspecified male genital organ
Boil of unspecified male genital organ
Carbuncle of unspecified male genital organ
Cellulitis of unspecified male genital organ

4 **N50** **Other and unspecified disorders of male genital organs**

EXCLUDES 2 *torsion of testis (N44.0-)*

N50.0 **Atrophy of testis** ♂

N50.1 **Vascular disorders of male genital organs** ♂
Hematocele, NOS, of male genital organs
Hemorrhage of male genital organs
Thrombosis of male genital organs

N50.3 **Cyst of epididymis** ♂

5 **N50.8** **Other specified disorders of male genital organs**

DEFINITION Chylocele: A cyst-like lesion resulting from the escape of chyle (milky fluid consisting of lymph and emulsified fat) into the tunica vaginalis of the testes.

AHA: 4Q 2016, 45

6 **N50.81** **Testicular pain**

N50.811 **Right testicular pain** ♂

N50.812 **Left testicular pain** ♂

N50.819 **Testicular pain, unspecified** ♂

N50.82 **Scrotal pain** ♂

N50.89 **Other specified disorders of the male genital organs** ♂
Atrophy of scrotum, seminal vesicle, spermatic cord, tunica vaginalis and vas deferens
Chylocele, tunica vaginalis (nonfilarial) NOS
Edema of scrotum, seminal vesicle, spermatic cord, tunica vaginalis and vas deferens
Hypertrophy of scrotum, seminal vesicle, spermatic cord, tunica vaginalis and vas deferens
Stricture of spermatic cord, tunica vaginalis, and vas deferens
Ulcer of scrotum, seminal vesicle, spermatic cord, testis, tunica vaginalis and vas deferens
Urethroscrotal fistula

N50.9 **Disorder of male genital organs, unspecified** ♂

N51 ***Disorders of male genital organs in diseases classified elsewhere*** ♂
Code first underlying disease, such as:
filariasis (B74.0-B74.9)

EXCLUDES 1 *amebic balanitis (A06.8)*
candidal balanitis (B37.42)
gonococcal balanitis (A54.23)
gonococcal prostatitis (A54.22)
herpesviral [herpes simplex] balanitis (A60.01)
trichomonal prostatitis (A59.02)
tuberculous prostatitis (A18.14)

4 **N52** **Male erectile dysfunction**

EXCLUDES 1 *psychogenic impotence (F52.21)*

5 **N52.0** **Vasculogenic erectile dysfunction**

N52.01 **Erectile dysfunction due to arterial insufficiency** ♂ A

N52.02 **Corporo-venous occlusive erectile dysfunction** ♂ A

N52.03 **Combined arterial insufficiency and corporo-venous occlusive erectile dysfunction** ♂ A

N52.1 ***Erectile dysfunction due to diseases classified elsewhere*** ♂ A
Code first:
underlying disease

N52.2 **Drug-induced erectile dysfunction** ♂ A

5 **N52.3** **Postprocedural erectile dysfunction**
AHA: 4Q 2016, 45

N52.31 **Erectile dysfunction following radical prostatectomy** ♂ A

N52.32 **Erectile dysfunction following radical cystectomy** ♂ A

N52.33 **Erectile dysfunction following urethral surgery** ♂ A

N52.34 **Erectile dysfunction following simple prostatectomy** ♂ A

N52.35 **Erectile dysfunction following radiation therapy** ♂ A

N52.36 **Erectile dysfunction following interstitial seed therapy** ♂ A

N52.37 **Erectile dysfunction following prostate ablative therapy** ♂ A
Erectile dysfunction following cryotherapy
Erectile dysfunction following other prostate ablative therapies
Erectile dysfunction following ultrasound ablative therapies

N52.39 **Other and unspecified postprocedural erectile dysfunction** ♂ A

N52.8 **Other male erectile dysfunction** ♂ A

N52.9 **Male erectile dysfunction, unspecified** ♂ A
Impotence NOS

4 **N53** **Other male sexual dysfunction**

EXCLUDES 1 *psychogenic sexual dysfunction (F52.-)*

5 **N53.1** **Ejaculatory dysfunction**

EXCLUDES 1 *premature ejaculation (F52.4)*

N53.11 **Retarded ejaculation** ♂

N53.12 **Painful ejaculation** ♂

N53.13 **Anejaculatory orgasm** ♂

N53.14 **Retrograde ejaculation** ♂

N53.19 **Other ejaculatory dysfunction** ♂
Ejaculatory dysfunction NOS

N53.8 **Other male sexual dysfunction** ♂

N53.9 **Unspecified male sexual dysfunction** ♂

Disorders of breast (N60-N65)

EXCLUDES 1 *disorders of breast associated with childbirth (O91-O92)*

4 **N60** **Benign mammary dysplasia**

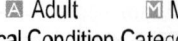

INCLUDES fibrocystic mastopathy

5 **N60.0 Solitary cyst of breast**
Cyst of breast

Solitary cyst of breast

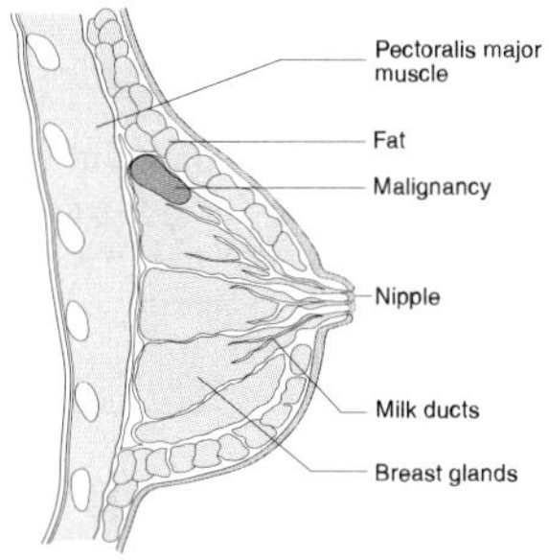

N60.01 Solitary cyst of right breast
N60.02 Solitary cyst of left breast
N60.09 Solitary cyst of unspecified breast

5 **N60.1 Diffuse cystic mastopathy**
Cystic breast
Fibrocystic disease of breast
EXCLUDES 1 *diffuse cystic mastopathy with epithelial proliferation (N60.3-)*
N60.11 Diffuse cystic mastopathy of right breast A
N60.12 Diffuse cystic mastopathy of left breast A
N60.19 Diffuse cystic mastopathy of unspecified breast A

5 **N60.2 Fibroadenosis of breast**
Adenofibrosis of breast
EXCLUDES 2 *fibroadenoma of breast (D24.-)*
N60.21 Fibroadenosis of right breast
N60.22 Fibroadenosis of left breast
N60.29 Fibroadenosis of unspecified breast

5 **N60.3 Fibrosclerosis of breast**
Cystic mastopathy with epithelial proliferation
N60.31 Fibrosclerosis of right breast
N60.32 Fibrosclerosis of left breast
N60.39 Fibrosclerosis of unspecified breast

5 **N60.4 Mammary duct ectasia**
DEFINITION Dilated milk duct filled with fluid; becomes inflamed and clogged with a thick, sticky substance, causing discharge and tenderness.
N60.41 Mammary duct ectasia of right breast
N60.42 Mammary duct ectasia of left breast
N60.49 Mammary duct ectasia of unspecified breast

5 **N60.8 Other benign mammary dysplasias**
N60.81 Other benign mammary dysplasias of right breast
N60.82 Other benign mammary dysplasias of left breast
N60.89 Other benign mammary dysplasias of unspecified breast

5 **N60.9 Unspecified benign mammary dysplasia**
N60.91 Unspecified benign mammary dysplasia of right breast
N60.92 Unspecified benign mammary dysplasia of left breast
N60.99 Unspecified benign mammary dysplasia of unspecified breast

4 **N61 Inflammatory disorders of breast**
EXCLUDES 1 *inflammatory carcinoma of breast (C50.9)*
inflammatory disorder of breast associated with childbirth (O91.-)
neonatal infective mastitis (P39.0)
thrombophlebitis of breast [Mondor's disease] (I80.8)
CODING TIP ✓ Do not assign a code from N61.- for patients who also have breast cancer.

N61.0 Mastitis without abscess
Infective mastitis (acute) (nonpuerperal) (subacute)
Mastitis (acute) (nonpuerperal) (subacute) NOS
Cellulitis (acute) (nonpuerperal) (subacute) of breast NOS
Cellulitis (acute) (nonpuerperal) (subacute) of nipple NOS

N61.1 Abscess of the breast and nipple
Abscess (acute) (chronic) (nonpuerperal) of areola
Abscess (acute) (chronic) (nonpuerperal) of breast
Carbuncle of breast
Mastitis with abscess

N62 Hypertrophy of breast
Gynecomastia
Hypertrophy of breast NOS
Massive pubertal hypertrophy of breast
EXCLUDES 1 *breast engorgement of newborn (P83.4)*
disproportion of reconstructed breast (N65.1)
DEFINITION Abnormal largeness of the breast.

4 **N63 Unspecified lump in breast**
Nodule(s) NOS in breast
N63.0 Unspecified lump in unspecified breast
5 **N63.1 Unspecified lump in the right breast**
AHA: 4Q 2017, 15
N63.10 Unspecified lump in the right breast, unspecified quadrant
N63.11 Unspecified lump in the right breast, upper outer quadrant
N63.12 Unspecified lump in the right breast, upper inner quadrant
N63.13 Unspecified lump in the right breast, lower outer quadrant
N63.14 Unspecified lump in the right breast, lower inner quadrant
5 **N63.2 Unspecified lump in the left breast**
N63.20 Unspecified lump in the left breast, unspecified quadrant
N63.21 Unspecified lump in the left breast, upper outer quadrant
N63.22 Unspecified lump in the left breast, upper inner quadrant
N63.23 Unspecified lump in the left breast, lower outer quadrant
N63.24 Unspecified lump in the left breast, lower inner quadrant
5 **N63.3 Unspecified lump in axillary tail**
N63.31 Unspecified lump in axillary tail of the right breast
N63.32 Unspecified lump in axillary tail of the left breast
5 **N63.4 Unspecified lump in breast, subareolar**
N63.41 Unspecified lump in right breast, subareolar
N63.42 Unspecified lump in left breast, subareolar

4 **N64 Other disorders of breast**
EXCLUDES 2 *mechanical complication of breast prosthesis and implant (T85.4-)*
N64.0 Fissure and fistula of nipple
N64.1 Fat necrosis of breast
Fat necrosis (segmental) of breast
Code first:
breast necrosis due to breast graft (T85.898)
N64.2 Atrophy of breast
N64.3 Galactorrhea not associated with childbirth
DEFINITION Inappropriate discharge of milk from the breast.
N64.4 Mastodynia
5 **N64.5 Other signs and symptoms in breast**
EXCLUDES 2 *abnormal findings on diagnostic imaging of breast (R92.-)*
N64.51 Induration of breast
N64.52 Nipple discharge
EXCLUDES 1 *abnormal findings in nipple discharge (R89.-)*
N64.53 Retraction of nipple
N64.59 Other signs and symptoms in breast
5 **N64.8 Other specified disorders of breast**
N64.81 Ptosis of breast A
EXCLUDES 1 *ptosis of native breast in relation to reconstructed breast (N65.1)*

DEFINITION Falling, drooping, or sagging of the breast tissue which can occur naturally, or following pregnancy or weight gain and loss.

N64.82 **Hypoplasia of breast** A
Micromastia
EXCLUDES 1 *congenital absence of breast (Q83.0)*
hypoplasia of native breast in relation to reconstructed breast (N65.1)

N64.89 **Other specified disorders of breast**
Galactocele
Subinvolution of breast (postlactational)
AHA: 1Q 2018, 3

N64.9 **Disorder of breast, unspecified**

[4] **N65** **Deformity and disproportion of reconstructed breast**

N65.0 **Deformity of reconstructed breast** A
Contour irregularity in reconstructed breast
Excess tissue in reconstructed breast
Misshapen reconstructed breast

N65.1 **Disproportion of reconstructed breast** A
Breast asymmetry between native breast and reconstructed breast
Disproportion between native breast and reconstructed breast

Inflammatory diseases of female pelvic organs (N70-N77)

EXCLUDES 1 *inflammatory diseases of female pelvic organs complicating:*
abortion or ectopic or molar pregnancy (O00-O07, O08.0)
pregnancy, childbirth and the puerperium (O23.-, O75.3, O85, O86.-)

[4] **N70** **Salpingitis and oophoritis**
INCLUDES abscess (of) fallopian tube
abscess (of) ovary
pyosalpinx
salpingo-oophoritis
tubo-ovarian abscess
tubo-ovarian inflammatory disease
Use additional code (B95-B97), to identify infectious agent
EXCLUDES 1 *gonococcal infection (A54.24)*
tuberculous infection (A18.17)

CODING TIP ✓ Conditions classifiable to N70.- should have an additional code assigned to identify the causative organism of infection, when this is known.

[5] **N70.0** **Acute salpingitis and oophoritis**
N70.01 **Acute salpingitis** ♀
N70.02 **Acute oophoritis** ♀
N70.03 **Acute salpingitis and oophoritis** ♀

[5] **N70.1** **Chronic salpingitis and oophoritis**
Hydrosalpinx
N70.11 **Chronic salpingitis** ♀
N70.12 **Chronic oophoritis** ♀
N70.13 **Chronic salpingitis and oophoritis** ♀

[5] **N70.9** **Salpingitis and oophoritis, unspecified**
DEFINITION Inflammation of appendages of the uterus (adnexa uteri).
N70.91 **Salpingitis, unspecified** ♀
N70.92 **Oophoritis, unspecified** ♀
N70.93 **Salpingitis and oophoritis, unspecified** ♀

[4] **N71** **Inflammatory disease of uterus, except cervix**
INCLUDES endo (myo) metritis
metritis
myometritis
pyometra
uterine abscess
Use additional code (B95-B97), to identify infectious agent
EXCLUDES 1 *hyperplastic endometritis (N85.0-)*
infection of uterus following delivery (O85, O86.-)

N71.0 **Acute inflammatory disease of uterus** ♀
N71.1 **Chronic inflammatory disease of uterus** ♀
N71.9 **Inflammatory disease of uterus, unspecified** ♀

N72 **Inflammatory disease of cervix uteri** ♀
INCLUDES cervicitis (with or without erosion or ectropion)
endocervicitis (with or without erosion or ectropion)
exocervicitis (with or without erosion or ectropion)
Use additional code (B95-B97), to identify infectious agent
EXCLUDES 1 *erosion and ectropion of cervix without cervicitis (N86)*

[4] **N73** **Other female pelvic inflammatory diseases**
Use additional code (B95-B97), to identify infectious agent.

N73.0 **Acute parametritis and pelvic cellulitis** ♀
Abscess of broad ligament
Abscess of parametrium
Pelvic cellulitis, female

Acute parametritis and pelvic cellulitis

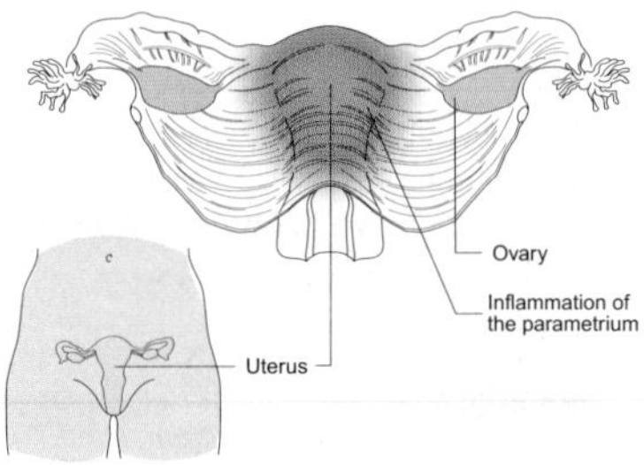

N73.1 **Chronic parametritis and pelvic cellulitis** ♀
Any condition in N73.0 specified as chronic
EXCLUDES 1 *tuberculous parametritis and pelvic cellultis (A18.17)*

N73.2 **Unspecified parametritis and pelvic cellulitis** ♀
Any condition in N73.0 unspecified whether acute or chronic

N73.3 **Female acute pelvic peritonitis** ♀

N73.4 **Female chronic pelvic peritonitis** ♀
EXCLUDES 1 *tuberculous pelvic (female) peritonitis (A18.17)*

N73.5 **Female pelvic peritonitis, unspecified** ♀

N73.6 **Female pelvic peritoneal adhesions (postinfective)** ♀
EXCLUDES 2 *postprocedural pelvic peritoneal adhesions (N99.4)*
AHA: 1Q 2014, 6

N73.8 **Other specified female pelvic inflammatory diseases** ♀

N73.9 **Female pelvic inflammatory disease, unspecified** ♀
Female pelvic infection or inflammation NOS

N74 ***Female pelvic inflammatory disorders in diseases classified elsewhere*** ♀
Code first:
underlying disease
EXCLUDES 1 *chlamydial cervicitis (A56.02)*
chlamydial pelvic inflammatory disease (A56.11)
gonococcal cervicitis (A54.03)
gonococcal pelvic inflammatory disease (A54.24)
herpesviral [herpes simplex] cervicitis (A60.03)
herpesviral [herpes simplex] pelvic inflammatory disease (A60.09)
syphilitic cervicitis (A52.76)
syphilitic pelvic inflammatory disease (A52.76)
trichomonal cervicitis (A59.09)
tuberculous cervicitis (A18.16)
tuberculous pelvic inflammatory disease (A18.17)

[4] **N75** **Diseases of Bartholin's gland**

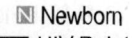

N75.0 Cyst of Bartholin's gland ♀

Cyst of Bartholin's gland

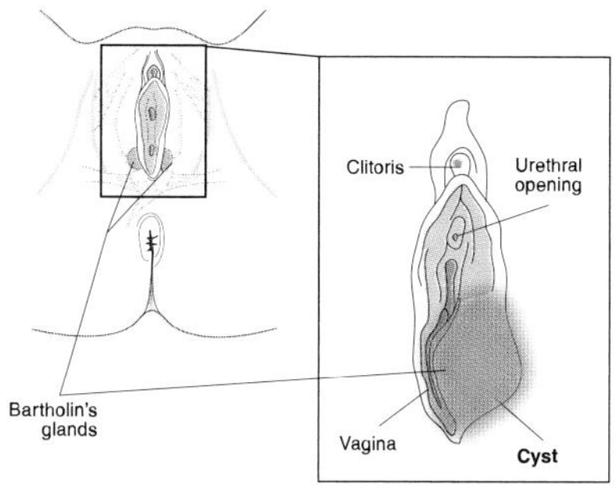

N75.1 Abscess of Bartholin's gland ♀

Abscess of Bartholin's gland

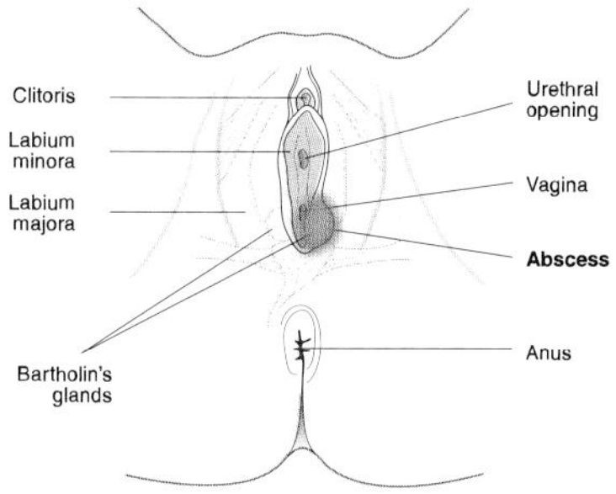

N75.8 Other diseases of Bartholin's gland ♀
Bartholinitis

N75.9 Disease of Bartholin's gland, unspecified ♀

4 N76 Other inflammation of vagina and vulva
Use additional code (B95-B97), to identify infectious agent
EXCLUDES 2 *senile (atrophic) vaginitis (N95.2)*
vulvar vestibulitis (N94.810)

N76.0 Acute vaginitis ♀
Acute vulvovaginitis
Vaginitis NOS
Vulvovaginitis NOS

N76.1 Subacute and chronic vaginitis ♀
Chronic vulvovaginitis
Subacute vulvovaginitis

N76.2 Acute vulvitis ♀
Vulvitis NOS

N76.3 Subacute and chronic vulvitis ♀

N76.4 Abscess of vulva ♀
Furuncle of vulva

N76.5 Ulceration of vagina ♀

N76.6 Ulceration of vulva ♀

5 N76.8 Other specified inflammation of vagina and vulva

N76.81 Mucositis (ulcerative) of vagina and vulva ♀
Code also type of associated therapy, such as:
antineoplastic and immunosuppressive drugs (T45.1X-)
radiological procedure and radiotherapy (Y84.2)
EXCLUDES 2 *gastrointestinal mucositis (ulcerative) (K92.81)*
nasal mucositis (ulcerative) (J34.81)
oral mucositis (ulcerative) (K12.3-)

N76.89 Other specified inflammation of vagina and vulva ♀

4 N77 Vulvovaginal ulceration and inflammation in diseases classified elsewhere

N77.0 *Ulceration of vulva in diseases classified elsewhere* ♀
Code first underlying disease, such as:
Behçet's disease (M35.2)
EXCLUDES 1 *ulceration of vulva in gonococcal infection (A54.02)*
ulceration of vulva in herpesviral [herpes simplex] infection (A60.04)
ulceration of vulva in syphilis (A51.0)
ulceration of vulva in tuberculosis (A18.18)

N77.1 *Vaginitis, vulvitis and vulvovaginitis in diseases classified elsewhere* ♀
Code first underlying disease, such as:
pinworm (B80)
EXCLUDES 1 *candidal vulvovaginitis (B37.3)*
chlamydial vulvovaginitis (A56.02)
gonococcal vulvovaginitis (A54.02)
herpesviral [herpes simplex] vulvovaginitis (A60.04)
trichomonal vulvovaginitis (A59.01)
tuberculous vulvovaginitis (A18.18)
vulvovaginitis in early syphilis (A51.0)
vulvovaginitis in late syphilis (A52.76)

Noninflammatory disorders of female genital tract (N80-N98)

4 N80 Endometriosis

DEFINITION Tissue that lines the uterus growing outside the uterus in the pelvis, abdomen, and on other organs; causes pain and infertility.

N80.0 Endometriosis of uterus ♀
Adenomyosis
EXCLUDES 1 *stromal endometriosis (D39.0)*

N80.1 Endometriosis of ovary ♀

Endometriosis of ovary

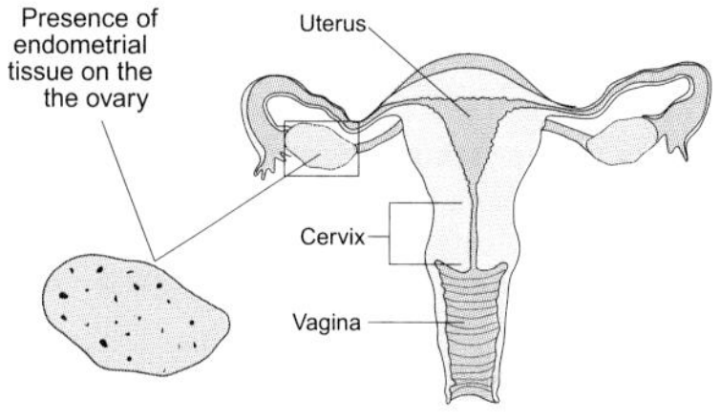

N80.2 Endometriosis of fallopian tube ♀

N80.3 Endometriosis of pelvic peritoneum ♀

N80.4 Endometriosis of rectovaginal septum and vagina ♀

N80.5 Endometriosis of intestine ♀

N80.6 Endometriosis in cutaneous scar ♀

N80.8 Other endometriosis ♀
Endometriosis of thorax

N80.9 Endometriosis, unspecified ♀

4 N81 Female genital prolapse
EXCLUDES 1 *genital prolapse complicating pregnancy, labor or delivery (O34.5-)*
prolapse and hernia of ovary and fallopian tube (N83.4-)
prolapse of vaginal vault after hysterectomy (N99.3)

N81.0 Urethrocele ♀
EXCLUDES 1 *urethrocele with cystocele (N81.1-)*
urethrocele with prolapse of uterus (N81.2-N81.4)

CODING TIP ✓ Urethrocele is identified by prolapse of the urethra into the vaginal canal and may result in urinary disorders, including incontinence.

5 N81.1 Cystocele
Cystocele with urethrocele
Cystourethrocele
EXCLUDES 1 *cystocele with prolapse of uterus (N81.2-N81.4)*

CODING TIP✓ Cystocele is identified by the prolapse of the bladder into the vaginal canal, due to muscle weakening in the pelvic floor, and may result in discomfort and urinary dysfunction, including incontinence.

N81.10 **Cystocele, unspecified** ♀
Prolapse of (anterior) vaginal wall NOS

N81.11 **Cystocele, midline** ♀

N81.12 **Cystocele, lateral** ♀
Paravaginal cystocele

DEFINITION Bladder bulges through the side wall of the vagina.

N81.2 **Incomplete uterovaginal prolapse** ♀
First degree uterine prolapse
Prolapse of cervix NOS
Second degree uterine prolapse
EXCLUDES 1 *cervical stump prolapse (N81.85)*

N81.3 **Complete uterovaginal prolapse** ♀
Procidentia (uteri) NOS
Third degree uterine prolapse

N81.4 **Uterovaginal prolapse, unspecified** ♀
Prolapse of uterus NOS

N81.5 **Vaginal enterocele** ♀
EXCLUDES 1 *enterocele with prolapse of uterus (N81.2-N81.4)*

N81.6 **Rectocele** ♀
Prolapse of posterior vaginal wall
Use additional code for any associated fecal incontinence, if applicable (R15.-)
EXCLUDES 2 *perineocele (N81.81)*
rectal prolapse (K62.3)
rectocele with prolapse of uterus (N81.2-N81.4)

5 **N81.8** **Other female genital prolapse**

N81.81 **Perineocele** ♀

N81.82 **Incompetence or weakening of pubocervical tissue** ♀

N81.83 **Incompetence or weakening of rectovaginal tissue** ♀

N81.84 **Pelvic muscle wasting** ♀
Disuse atrophy of pelvic muscles and anal sphincter

N81.85 **Cervical stump prolapse** ♀

N81.89 **Other female genital prolapse** ♀
Deficient perineum
Old laceration of muscles of pelvic floor

N81.9 **Female genital prolapse, unspecified** ♀

4 **N82** **Fistulae involving female genital tract**
EXCLUDES 1 *vesicointestinal fistulae (N32.1)*

N82.0 **Vesicovaginal fistula** ♀

N82.1 **Other female urinary-genital tract fistulae** ♀
Cervicovesical fistula
Ureterovaginal fistula
Urethrovaginal fistula
Uteroureteric fistula
Uterovesical fistula

N82.2 **Fistula of vagina to small intestine** ♀

N82.3 **Fistula of vagina to large intestine** ♀
Rectovaginal fistula

N82.4 **Other female intestinal-genital tract fistulae** ♀
Intestinouterine fistula

N82.5 **Female genital tract-skin fistulae** ♀
Uterus to abdominal wall fistula
Vaginoperineal fistula

Female genital tract-skin fistula
An abnormal tube-like passage connecting the genital tract to the skin surface

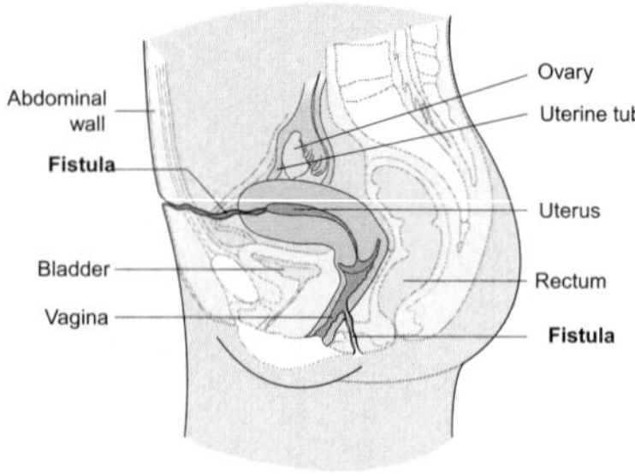

N82.8 **Other female genital tract fistulae** ♀

N82.9 **Female genital tract fistula, unspecified** ♀

4 **N83** **Noninflammatory disorders of ovary, fallopian tube and broad ligament**
EXCLUDES 2 *hydrosalpinx (N70.1-)*
AHA: 4Q 2016, 46

5 **N83.0** **Follicular cyst of ovary**
Cyst of graafian follicle
Hemorrhagic follicular cyst (of ovary)
DEFINITION Fluid-filled sac on the ovary caused by larger than normal growth of a follicle that does not rupture to release the egg.

⊟ **N83.00** **Follicular cyst of ovary, unspecified side** ♀

⊟ **N83.01** **Follicular cyst of right ovary** ♀

⊟ **N83.02** **Follicular cyst of left ovary** ♀

5 **N83.1** **Corpus luteum cyst**
Hemorrhagic corpus luteum cyst

⊟ **N83.10** **Corpus luteum cyst of ovary, unspecified side** ♀

⊟ **N83.11** **Corpus luteum cyst of right ovary** ♀

⊟ **N83.12** **Corpus luteum cyst of left ovary** ♀

5 **N83.2** **Other and unspecified ovarian cysts**
EXCLUDES 1 *developmental ovarian cyst (Q50.1)*
neoplastic ovarian cyst (D27.-)
polycystic ovarian syndrome (E28.2)
Stein-Leventhal syndrome (E28.2)

6 **N83.20** **Unspecified ovarian cysts**

⊟ **N83.201** **Unspecified ovarian cyst, right side** ♀

⊟ **N83.202** **Unspecified ovarian cyst, left side** ♀

⊟ **N83.209** **Unspecified ovarian cyst, unspecified side** ♀
Ovarian cyst, NOS

6 **N83.29** **Other ovarian cysts**
Retention cyst of ovary
Simple cyst of ovary

⊟ **N83.291** **Other ovarian cyst, right side** ♀

⊟ **N83.292** **Other ovarian cyst, left side** ♀

⊟ **N83.299** **Other ovarian cyst, unspecified side** ♀

5 **N83.3** **Acquired atrophy of ovary and fallopian tube**

6 **N83.31** **Acquired atrophy of ovary**

⊟ **N83.311** **Acquired atrophy of right ovary** ♀

⊟ **N83.312** **Acquired atrophy of left ovary** ♀

⊟ **N83.319** **Acquired atrophy of ovary, unspecified side** ♀
Acquired atrophy of ovary, NOS

6 **N83.32** **Acquired atrophy of fallopian tube**

⊟ **N83.321** **Acquired atrophy of right fallopian tube** ♀

⊟ **N83.322** **Acquired atrophy of left fallopian tube** ♀

⊟ **N83.329** **Acquired atrophy of fallopian tube, unspecified side** ♀
Acquired atrophy of fallopian tube, NOS

6 **N83.33** **Acquired atrophy of ovary and fallopian tube**

⊟ **N83.331** **Acquired atrophy of right ovary and fallopian tube** ♀

⊟ **N83.332** **Acquired atrophy of left ovary and fallopian tube** ♀

⊟ **N83.339** **Acquired atrophy of ovary and fallopian tube, unspecified side** ♀
Acquired atrophy of ovary and fallopian tube, NOS

5 **N83.4** **Prolapse and hernia of ovary and fallopian tube**

N83.40 Prolapse and hernia of ovary and fallopian tube, unspecified side ♀
Prolapse and hernia of ovary and fallopian tube, NOS

N83.41 Prolapse and hernia of right ovary and fallopian tube ♀

N83.42 Prolapse and hernia of left ovary and fallopian tube ♀

N83.5 Torsion of ovary, ovarian pedicle and fallopian tube
Torsion of accessory tube

N83.51 Torsion of ovary and ovarian pedicle

N83.511 Torsion of right ovary and ovarian pedicle ♀

N83.512 Torsion of left ovary and ovarian pedicle ♀

N83.519 Torsion of ovary and ovarian pedicle, unspecified side ♀
Torsion of ovary and ovarian pedicle, NOS

N83.52 Torsion of fallopian tube
Torsion of hydatid of Morgagni

N83.521 Torsion of right fallopian tube ♀

N83.522 Torsion of left fallopian tube ♀

N83.529 Torsion of fallopian tube, unspecified side ♀
Torsion of fallopian tube, NOS

N83.53 Torsion of ovary, ovarian pedicle and fallopian tube ♀

N83.6 Hematosalpinx ♀
EXCLUDES 1 *hematosalpinx (with) (in):*
hematocolpos (N89.7)
hematometra (N85.7)
tubal pregnancy (O00.1-)

N83.7 Hematoma of broad ligament ♀

N83.8 Other noninflammatory disorders of ovary, fallopian tube and broad ligament ♀
Broad ligament laceration syndrome [Allen-Masters]

N83.9 Noninflammatory disorder of ovary, fallopian tube and broad ligament, unspecified ♀

N84 Polyp of female genital tract
EXCLUDES 1 *adenomatous polyp (D28.-)*
placental polyp (O90.89)

N84.0 Polyp of corpus uteri ♀
Polyp of endometrium
Polyp of uterus NOS
EXCLUDES 1 *polypoid endometrial hyperplasia (N85.0-)*

N84.1 Polyp of cervix uteri ♀
Mucous polyp of cervix

N84.2 Polyp of vagina ♀

N84.3 Polyp of vulva ♀
Polyp of labia

N84.8 Polyp of other parts of female genital tract ♀

N84.9 Polyp of female genital tract, unspecified ♀

N85 Other noninflammatory disorders of uterus, except cervix
EXCLUDES 1 *endometriosis (N80.-)*
inflammatory diseases of uterus (N71.-)
noninflammatory disorders of cervix, except malposition (N86-N88)
polyp of corpus uteri (N84.0)
uterine prolapse (N81.-)

N85.0 Endometrial hyperplasia
DEFINITION Overgrowth of cells lining the uterus.

Endometrial hyperplasia

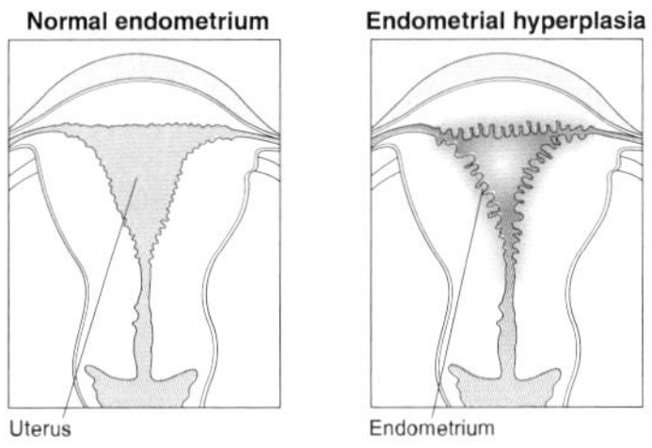

N85.00 Endometrial hyperplasia, unspecified ♀
Hyperplasia (adenomatous) (cystic) (glandular) of endometrium
Hyperplastic endometritis

N85.01 Benign endometrial hyperplasia ♀
Endometrial hyperplasia (complex) (simple) without atypia

N85.02 Endometrial intraepithelial neoplasia [EIN] ♀
Endometrial hyperplasia with atypia
EXCLUDES 1 *malignant neoplasm of endometrium (with endometrial intraepithelial neoplasia [EIN]) (C54.1)*

N85.2 Hypertrophy of uterus ♀
Bulky or enlarged uterus
EXCLUDES 1 *puerperal hypertrophy of uterus (O90.89)*

N85.3 Subinvolution of uterus ♀
EXCLUDES 1 *puerperal subinvolution of uterus (O90.89)*

N85.4 Malposition of uterus ♀
Anteversion of uterus
Retroflexion of uterus
Retroversion of uterus
EXCLUDES 1 *malposition of uterus complicating pregnancy, labor or delivery (O34.5-, O65.5)*

N85.5 Inversion of uterus ♀
EXCLUDES 1 *current obstetric trauma (O71.2)*
postpartum inversion of uterus (O71.2)

N85.6 Intrauterine synechiae ♀

N85.7 Hematometra ♀
Hematosalpinx with hematometra
EXCLUDES 1 *hematometra with hematocolpos (N89.7)*
DEFINITION Blood accumulated in the uterus.

N85.8 Other specified noninflammatory disorders of uterus ♀
Atrophy of uterus, acquired
Fibrosis of uterus NOS

N85.9 Noninflammatory disorder of uterus, unspecified ♀
Disorder of uterus NOS

N86 Erosion and ectropion of cervix uteri ♀
Decubitus (trophic) ulcer of cervix
Eversion of cervix
EXCLUDES 1 *erosion and ectropion of cervix with cervicitis (N72)*

N87 Dysplasia of cervix uteri
EXCLUDES 1 *abnormal results from cervical cytologic examination without histologic confirmation (R87.61-)*
carcinoma in situ of cervix uteri (D06.-)
cervical intraepithelial neoplasia III [CIN III] (D06.-)
HGSIL of cervix (R87.613)
severe dysplasia of cervix uteri (D06.-)

N87.0 Mild cervical dysplasia ♀
Cervical intraepithelial neoplasia I [CIN I]

N87.1 Moderate cervical dysplasia ♀
Cervical intraepithelial neoplasia II [CIN II]

N87.9 Dysplasia of cervix uteri, unspecified ♀
Anaplasia of cervix
Cervical atypism
Cervical dysplasia NOS

N88 Other noninflammatory disorders of cervix uteri
EXCLUDES 2 *inflammatory disease of cervix (N72)*
polyp of cervix (N84.1)

N88.0 Leukoplakia of cervix uteri ♀

N88.1 Old laceration of cervix uteri ♀
Adhesions of cervix
EXCLUDES 1 *current obstetric trauma (O71.3)*

N88.2 Stricture and stenosis of cervix uteri ♀

EXCLUDES 1 *stricture and stenosis of cervix uteri complicating labor (O65.5)*

Stricture and stenosis of cervix uteri

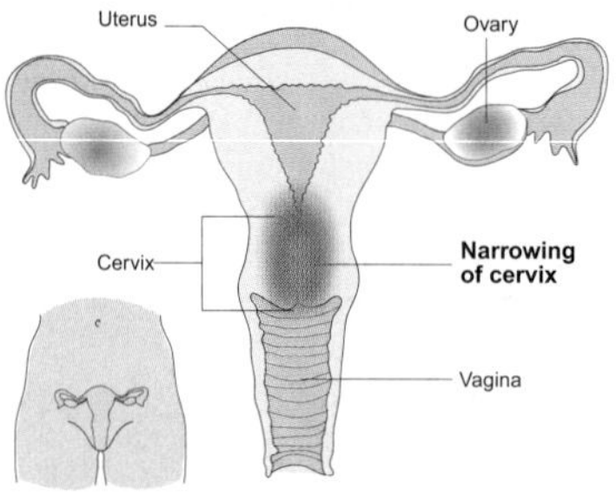

N88.3 Incompetence of cervix uteri ♀

Investigation and management of (suspected) cervical incompetence in a nonpregnant woman

EXCLUDES 1 *cervical incompetence complicating pregnancy (O34.3-)*

N88.4 Hypertrophic elongation of cervix uteri ♀

N88.8 Other specified noninflammatory disorders of cervix uteri ♀

EXCLUDES 1 *current obstetric trauma (O71.3)*

N88.9 Noninflammatory disorder of cervix uteri, unspecified ♀

4 N89 Other noninflammatory disorders of vagina

EXCLUDES 1 *abnormal results from vaginal cytologic examination without histologic confirmation (R87.62-)*
carcinoma in situ of vagina (D07.2)
HGSIL of vagina (R87.623)
inflammation of vagina (N76.-)
senile (atrophic) vaginitis (N95.2)
severe dysplasia of vagina (D07.2)
trichomonal leukorrhea (A59.00)
vaginal intraepithelial neoplasia [VAIN], grade III (D07.2)

N89.0 Mild vaginal dysplasia ♀

Vaginal intraepithelial neoplasia [VAIN], grade I

N89.1 Moderate vaginal dysplasia ♀

Vaginal intraepithelial neoplasia [VAIN], grade II

N89.3 Dysplasia of vagina, unspecified ♀

N89.4 Leukoplakia of vagina ♀

DEFINITION White plaque on the mucosal surface of the vagina that develops into thickened, rough-textured grayish white lesions.

N89.5 Stricture and atresia of vagina ♀

Vaginal adhesions
Vaginal stenosis

EXCLUDES 1 *congenital atresia or stricture (Q52.4)*
postprocedural adhesions of vagina (N99.2)

N89.6 Tight hymenal ring ♀

Rigid hymen
Tight introitus

EXCLUDES 1 *imperforate hymen (Q52.3)*

N89.7 Hematocolpos ♀

Hematocolpos with hematometra or hematosalpinx

N89.8 Other specified noninflammatory disorders of vagina ♀

Leukorrhea NOS
Old vaginal laceration
Pessary ulcer of vagina

EXCLUDES 1 *current obstetric trauma (O70.-, O71.4, O71.7-O71.8)*
old laceration involving muscles of pelvic floor (N81.8)

N89.9 Noninflammatory disorder of vagina, unspecified ♀

4 N90 Other noninflammatory disorders of vulva and perineum

EXCLUDES 1 *anogenital (venereal) warts (A63.0)*
carcinoma in situ of vulva (D07.1)
condyloma acuminatum (A63.0)
current obstetric trauma (O70.-, O71.7-O71.8)
inflammation of vulva (N76.-)
severe dysplasia of vulva (D07.1)
vulvar intraepithelial neoplasm III [VIN III] (D07.1)

N90.0 Mild vulvar dysplasia ♀

Vulvar intraepithelial neoplasia [VIN], grade I

N90.1 Moderate vulvar dysplasia ♀

Vulvar intraepithelial neoplasia [VIN], grade II

N90.3 Dysplasia of vulva, unspecified ♀

N90.4 Leukoplakia of vulva ♀

Dystrophy of vulva
Kraurosis of vulva
Lichen sclerosus of external female genital organs

N90.5 Atrophy of vulva ♀

Stenosis of vulva

5 N90.6 Hypertrophy of vulva

AHA: 4Q 2016, 46

N90.60 Unspecified hypertrophy of vulva ♀

Unspecified hypertrophy of labia

N90.61 Childhood asymmetric labium majus enlargement ♀

CALME

N90.69 Other specified hypertrophy of vulva ♀

Other specified hypertrophy of labia

N90.7 Vulvar cyst ♀

5 N90.8 Other specified noninflammatory disorders of vulva and perineum

6 N90.81 Female genital mutilation status

Female genital cutting status

N90.810 Female genital mutilation status, unspecified ♀

Female genital cutting status, unspecified
Female genital mutilation status NOS

N90.811 Female genital mutilation Type I status ♀

Clitorectomy status
Female genital cutting Type I status

N90.812 Female genital mutilation Type II status ♀

Clitorectomy with excision of labia minora status
Female genital cutting Type II status

N90.813 Female genital mutilation Type III status ♀

Female genital cutting Type III status
Infibulation status

N90.818 Other female genital mutilation status ♀

Female genital cutting Type IV status
Female genital mutilation Type IV status
Other female genital cutting status

N90.89 Other specified noninflammatory disorders of vulva and perineum ♀

Adhesions of vulva
Hypertrophy of clitoris

N90.9 Noninflammatory disorder of vulva and perineum, unspecified ♀

4 N91 Absent, scanty and rare menstruation

EXCLUDES 1 *ovarian dysfunction (E28.-)*

N91.0 Primary amenorrhea ♀

N91.1 Secondary amenorrhea ♀

N91.2 Amenorrhea, unspecified ♀

N91.3 Primary oligomenorrhea ♀

N91.4 Secondary oligomenorrhea ♀

N91.5 Oligomenorrhea, unspecified ♀

Hypomenorrhea NOS

4 N92 Excessive, frequent and irregular menstruation

EXCLUDES 1 *postmenopausal bleeding (N95.0)*
precocious puberty (menstruation) (E30.1)

N92.0 Excessive and frequent menstruation with regular cycle ♀

Heavy periods NOS
Menorrhagia NOS
Polymenorrhea

● New · Manifestation · 4-7 Digit Indicators · Laterality · A Adult · M Maternity · N Newborn · P Pediatric · ♂ Male
▲ Revised · Unspecified · AHA Coding Clinic · HCC Hierarchical Condition Categories · HIV HIV Related Conditions · ♀ Female

N92.1 **Excessive and frequent menstruation with irregular cycle** ♀
Irregular intermenstrual bleeding
Irregular, shortened intervals between menstrual bleeding
Menometrorrhagia
Metrorrhagia

N92.2 **Excessive menstruation at puberty** ♀ P
Excessive bleeding associated with onset of menstrual periods
Pubertal menorrhagia
Puberty bleeding

N92.3 **Ovulation bleeding** ♀
Regular intermenstrual bleeding

N92.4 **Excessive bleeding in the premenopausal period** ♀
Climacteric menorrhagia or metrorrhagia
Menopausal menorrhagia or metrorrhagia
Preclimacteric menorrhagia or metrorrhagia
Premenopausal menorrhagia or metrorrhagia

N92.5 **Other specified irregular menstruation** ♀

N92.6 **Irregular menstruation, unspecified** ♀
Irregular bleeding NOS
Irregular periods NOS
EXCLUDES 1 *irregular menstruation with:*
lengthened intervals or scanty bleeding (N91.3-N91.5)
shortened intervals or excessive bleeding (N92.1)

4 N93 Other abnormal uterine and vaginal bleeding

EXCLUDES 1 *neonatal vaginal hemorrhage (P54.6)*
precocious puberty (menstruation) (E30.1)
pseudomenses (P54.6)

N93.0 **Postcoital and contact bleeding** ♀
DEFINITION Bleeding after sexual intercourse.

N93.1 **Pre-pubertal vaginal bleeding** ♀
AHA: 4Q 2016, 47

N93.8 **Other specified abnormal uterine and vaginal bleeding** ♀
Dysfunctional or functional uterine or vaginal bleeding NOS

N93.9 **Abnormal uterine and vaginal bleeding, unspecified** ♀

4 N94 Pain and other conditions associated with female genital organs and menstrual cycle

N94.0 **Mittelschmerz** ♀
DEFINITION Pain accompanying ovulation, usually occurring midway between menstruation periods.

5 N94.1 **Dyspareunia**
EXCLUDES 1 *psychogenic dyspareunia (F52.6)*
DEFINITION Pain during sexual intercourse.
AHA: 4Q 2016, 47

N94.10 **Unspecified dyspareunia** ♀
N94.11 **Superficial (introital) dyspareunia** ♀
N94.12 **Deep dyspareunia** ♀
N94.19 **Other specified dyspareunia** ♀

N94.2 **Vaginismus** ♀
EXCLUDES 1 *psychogenic vaginismus (F52.5)*
DEFINITION Severe, painful spasms of the vaginal muscles that prevent sexual intercourse.

N94.3 **Premenstrual tension syndrome** ♀
Code also:
associated menstrual migraine (G43.82-, G43.83-)
EXCLUDES 1 *Premenstrual dysphoric disorder (F32.81)*

N94.4 **Primary dysmenorrhea** ♀
N94.5 **Secondary dysmenorrhea** ♀
N94.6 **Dysmenorrhea, unspecified** ♀
EXCLUDES 1 *psychogenic dysmenorrhea (F45.8)*

5 N94.8 **Other specified conditions associated with female genital organs and menstrual cycle**

6 N94.81 **Vulvodynia**

N94.810 **Vulvar vestibulitis** ♀
DEFINITION Pain, tenderness, and redness in the vestibule area of the female external genitalia of unknown cause.

N94.818 **Other vulvodynia** ♀

N94.819 **Vulvodynia, unspecified** ♀
Vulvodynia NOS

N94.89 **Other specified conditions associated with female genital organs and menstrual cycle** ♀

N94.9 **Unspecified condition associated with female genital organs and menstrual cycle** ♀

4 N95 Menopausal and other perimenopausal disorders

Menopausal and other perimenopausal disorders due to naturally occurring (age-related) menopause and perimenopause
EXCLUDES 1 *excessive bleeding in the premenopausal period (N92.4)*
menopausal and perimenopausal disorders due to artificial or premature menopause (E89.4-, E28.31-)
premature menopause (E28.31-)
EXCLUDES 2 *postmenopausal osteoporosis (M81.0-)*
postmenopausal osteoporosis with current pathological fracture (M80.0-)
postmenopausal urethritis (N34.2)

N95.0 **Postmenopausal bleeding** ♀

N95.1 **Menopausal and female climacteric states** ♀
Symptoms such as flushing, sleeplessness, headache, lack of concentration, associated with natural (age-related) menopause
Use additional code for associated symptoms
EXCLUDES 1 *asymptomatic menopausal state (Z78.0)*
symptoms associated with artificial menopause (E89.41)
symptoms associated with premature menopause (E28.310)

N95.2 **Postmenopausal atrophic vaginitis** ♀
Senile (atrophic) vaginitis
DEFINITION Thinning of vaginal epithelium due to decreased estrogen levels.

Postmenopausal atrophic vaginitis

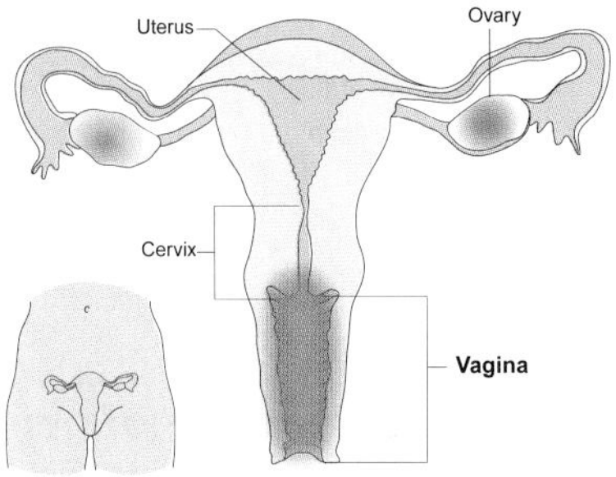

N95.8 **Other specified menopausal and perimenopausal disorders** ♀

N95.9 **Unspecified menopausal and perimenopausal disorder** ♀

N96 Recurrent pregnancy loss ♀

Investigation or care in a nonpregnant woman with history of recurrent pregnancy loss
EXCLUDES 1 *recurrent pregancy loss with current pregnancy (O26.2-)*

4 N97 Female infertility

INCLUDES inability to achieve a pregnancy
sterility, female NOS
EXCLUDES 1 *female infertility associated with:*
hypopituitarism (E23.0)
Stein-Leventhal syndrome (E28.2)
EXCLUDES 2 *incompetence of cervix uteri (N88.3)*

N97.0 **Female infertility associated with anovulation** ♀

N97.1 **Female infertility of tubal origin** ♀
Female infertility associated with congenital anomaly of tube
Female infertility due to tubal block
Female infertility due to tubal occlusion
Female infertility due to tubal stenosis

Female infertility of tubal origin

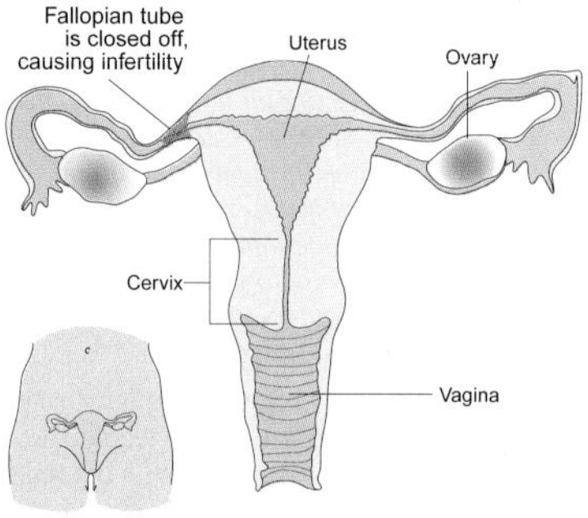

N97.2 **Female infertility of uterine origin** ♀
Female infertility associated with congenital anomaly of uterus
Female infertility due to nonimplantation of ovum

N97.8 **Female infertility of other origin** ♀

N97.9 **Female infertility, unspecified** ♀

4 N98 **Complications associated with artificial fertilization**

N98.0 **Infection associated with artificial insemination** ♀

N98.1 **Hyperstimulation of ovaries** ♀
Hyperstimulation of ovaries NOS
Hyperstimulation of ovaries associated with induced ovulation

N98.2 **Complications of attempted introduction of fertilized ovum following in vitro fertilization** ♀

N98.3 **Complications of attempted introduction of embryo in embryo transfer** ♀

N98.8 **Other complications associated with artificial fertilization** ♀

N98.9 **Complication associated with artificial fertilization, unspecified** ♀

Intraoperative and postprocedural complications and disorders of genitourinary system, not elsewhere classified (N99)

4 N99 **Intraoperative and postprocedural complications and disorders of genitourinary system, not elsewhere classified**

EXCLUDES 2 *irradiation cystitis (N30.4-)*
postoophorectomy osteoporosis with current pathological fracture (M80.8-)
postoophorectomy osteoporosis without current pathological fracture (M81.8)

CODING TIP ✓ **Documentation:** Codes in category N99.- are complication codes and require physician documentation and confirmation of a cause and effect relationship between any specified procedure and the complicated condition.

N99.0 **Postprocedural (acute) (chronic) kidney failure**
Use additional code to type of kidney disease

5 N99.1 **Postprocedural urethral stricture**
Postcatheterization urethral stricture

6 N99.11 **Postprocedural urethral stricture, male**
AHA: 4Q 2016, 47

N99.110 **Postprocedural urethral stricture, male, meatal** ♂

N99.111 **Postprocedural bulbous urethral stricture, male** ♂

N99.112 **Postprocedural membranous urethral stricture, male** ♂

N99.113 **Postprocedural anterior bulbous urethral stricture, male** ♂

N99.114 **Postprocedural urethral stricture, male, unspecified** ♂

N99.115 **Postprocedural fossa navicularis urethral stricture** ♂

● **N99.116** **Postprocedural urethral stricture, male, overlapping sites** ♂

N99.12 **Postprocedural urethral stricture, female** ♀

N99.2 **Postprocedural adhesions of vagina** ♀

N99.3 **Prolapse of vaginal vault after hysterectomy** ♀

N99.4 **Postprocedural pelvic peritoneal adhesions**
EXCLUDES 2 *pelvic peritoneal adhesions NOS (N73.6)*
postinfective pelvic peritoneal adhesions (N73.6)

5 N99.5 **Complications of stoma of urinary tract**
EXCLUDES 2 *mechanical complication of urinary catheter (T83.0-)*

CODING TIP ✓ All cystostomy and other urinary stoma complications (including ileoconduit, urostomy and nephrostomy) are coded to N99.51-N99.53. This includes excoriation and denuding of the skin surrounding the ostomy, infection of the ostomy site, hemorrhage of the ostomy site and other complications. No additional code should be used when coding skin complications unless an infection is present, in which case an additional code should be used to specify the infection. When an ostomy complication is present, do not assign a Z code for the ostomy. Z codes indicate routine ostomy care, which is not appropriate in the case of a complicated ostomy.
AHA: 4Q 2016, 48

6 N99.51 **Complication of cystostomy**

N99.510 **Cystostomy hemorrhage** HCC

N99.511 **Cystostomy infection** HCC

N99.512 **Cystostomy malfunction** HCC

N99.518 **Other cystostomy complication** HCC

6 N99.52 **Complication of incontinent external stoma of urinary tract**

N99.520 **Hemorrhage of incontinent external stoma of urinary tract** HCC

N99.521 **Infection of incontinent external stoma of urinary tract** HCC

N99.522 **Malfunction of incontinent external stoma of urinary tract** HCC

N99.523 **Herniation of incontinent stoma of urinary tract** HCC

N99.524 **Stenosis of incontinent stoma of urinary tract** HCC

N99.528 **Other complication of incontinent external stoma of urinary tract** HCC

6 N99.53 **Complication of continent stoma of urinary tract**

N99.530 **Hemorrhage of continent stoma of urinary tract** HCC

N99.531 **Infection of continent stoma of urinary tract** HCC

N99.532 **Malfunction of continent stoma of urinary tract** HCC

N99.533 **Herniation of continent stoma of urinary tract** HCC

N99.534 **Stenosis of continent stoma of urinary tract** HCC

N99.538 **Other complication of continent stoma of urinary tract** HCC

5 N99.6 **Intraoperative hemorrhage and hematoma of a genitourinary system organ or structure complicating a procedure**
EXCLUDES 1 *intraoperative hemorrhage and hematoma of a genitourinary system organ or structure due to accidental puncture or laceration during a procedure (N99.7-)*

N99.61 **Intraoperative hemorrhage and hematoma of a genitourinary system organ or structure complicating a genitourinary system procedure**

N99.62 **Intraoperative hemorrhage and hematoma of a genitourinary system organ or structure complicating other procedure**

5 N99.7 **Accidental puncture and laceration of a genitourinary system organ or structure during a procedure**

N99.71 **Accidental puncture and laceration of a genitourinary system organ or structure during a genitourinary system procedure**

N99.72 Accidental puncture and laceration of a genitourinary system organ or structure during other procedure

5 N99.8 Other intraoperative and postprocedural complications and disorders of genitourinary system

N99.81 Other intraoperative complications of genitourinary system

6 N99.82 Postprocedural hemorrhage of a genitourinary system organ or structure following a procedure

N99.820 Postprocedural hemorrhage of a genitourinary system organ or structure following a genitourinary system procedure

N99.821 Postprocedural hemorrhage of a genitourinary system organ or structure following other procedure

N99.83 Residual ovary syndrome ♀

6 N99.84 Postprocedural hematoma and seroma of a genitourinary system organ or structure following a procedure

N99.840 Postprocedural hematoma of a genitourinary system organ or structure following a genitourinary system procedure

N99.841 Postprocedural hematoma of a genitourinary system organ or structure following other procedure

N99.842 Postprocedural seroma of a genitourinary system organ or structure following a genitourinary system procedure

N99.843 Postprocedural seroma of a genitourinary system organ or structure following other procedure

N99.89 Other postprocedural complications and disorders of genitourinary system

CHAPTER 15: PREGNANCY, CHILDBIRTH AND THE PUERPERIUM (O00-O9A)

Note: CODES FROM THIS CHAPTER ARE FOR USE ONLY ON MATERNAL RECORDS, NEVER ON NEWBORN RECORDS
Codes from this chapter are for use for conditions related to or aggravated by the pregnancy, childbirth, or by the puerperium (maternal causes or obstetric causes)
Trimesters are counted from the first day of the last menstrual period. They are defined as follows:
1st trimester- less than 14 weeks 0 days
2nd trimester- 14 weeks 0 days to less than 28 weeks 0 days
3rd trimester- 28 weeks 0 days until delivery
Use additional code from category Z3A, Weeks of gestation, to identify the specific week of the pregnancy, if known.

EXCLUDES 1 *supervision of normal pregnancy (Z34.-)*

EXCLUDES 2 *mental and behavioral disorders associated with the puerperium (F53.-)*
obstetrical tetanus (A34)
postpartum necrosis of pituitary gland (E23.0)
puerperal osteomalacia (M83.0)

GUIDELINES **Section I.C.15.a.1)**
Obstetric cases require codes from chapter 15, codes in the range O00-O9A, Pregnancy, Childbirth, and the Puerperium. Chapter 15 codes have sequencing priority over codes from other chapters. Additional codes from other chapters may be used in conjunction with chapter 15 codes to further specify conditions. Should the provider document that the pregnancy is incidental to the encounter, then code Z33.1, Pregnant state, incidental, should be used in place of any chapter 15 codes. It is the provider's responsibility to state that the condition being treated is not affecting the pregnancy.

GUIDELINES **Section I.C.15.a.2)**
Chapter 15 codes are to be used only on the maternal record, never on the record of the newborn.

GUIDELINES **Section I.C.15.c**
When assigning codes from Chapter 15, it is important to assess if a condition was pre-existing prior to pregnancy or developed during or due to the pregnancy in order to assign the correct code. Categories that do not distinguish between pre-existing and pregnancy related conditions may be used for either. It is acceptable to use codes specifically for the puerperium with codes complicating pregnancy and childbirth if a condition arises postpartum during the delivery encounter.

This chapter contains the following blocks:

O00-O08	Pregnancy with abortive outcome
O09	Supervision of high risk pregnancy
O10-O16	Edema, proteinuria and hypertensive disorders in pregnancy, childbirth and the puerperium
O20-O29	Other maternal disorders predominantly related to pregnancy
O30-O48	Maternal care related to the fetus and amniotic cavity and possible delivery problems
O60-O77	Complications of labor and delivery
O80-O82	Encounter for delivery
O85-O92	Complications predominantly related to the puerperium
O94-O9A	Other obstetric conditions, not elsewhere classified

Pregnancy with abortive outcome (O00-O08)

EXCLUDES 1 *continuing pregnancy in multiple gestation after abortion of one fetus or more (O31.1-, O31.3-)*

4 **O00 Ectopic pregnancy**
INCLUDES ruptured ectopic pregnancy
Use additional code from category O08 to identify any associated complication

5 **O00.0 Abdominal pregnancy**
EXCLUDES 1 *maternal care for viable fetus in abdominal pregnancy (O36.7-)*

O00.00 Abdominal pregnancy without intrauterine pregnancy ♀ M
Abdominal pregnancy NOS

O00.01 Abdominal pregnancy with intrauterine pregnancy ♀ M

5 **O00.1 Tubal pregnancy**
Fallopian pregnancy
Rupture of (fallopian) tube due to pregnancy
Tubal abortion

DEFINITION Fertilized egg implants itself within the fallopian tube where the embryo grows and may rupture the tube.
AHA: 4Q 2017, 15

Tubal pregnancy

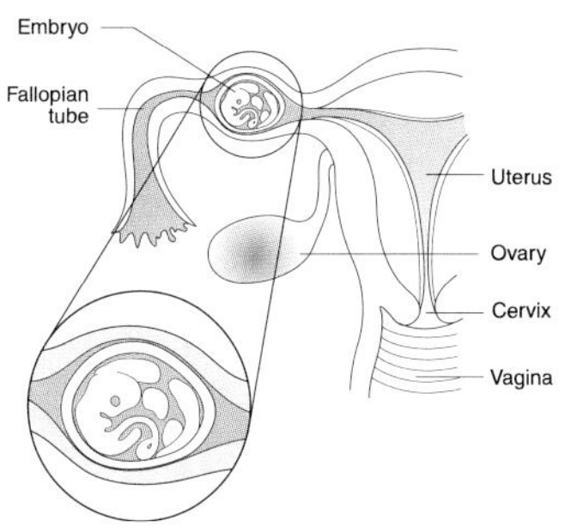

6 **O00.10 Tubal pregnancy without intrauterine pregnancy**
Tubal pregnancy NOS

L **O00.101 Right tubal pregnancy without intrauterine pregnancy** ♀ M

L **O00.102 Left tubal pregnancy without intrauterine pregnancy** ♀ M

L **O00.109 Unspecified tubal pregnancy without intrauterine pregnancy** ♀ M

6 **O00.11 Tubal pregnancy with intrauterine pregnancy**

L **O00.111 Right tubal pregnancy with intrauterine pregnancy** ♀ M

L **O00.112 Left tubal pregnancy with intrauterine pregnancy** ♀ M

L **O00.119 Unspecified tubal pregnancy with intrauterine pregnancy** ♀ M

5 **O00.2 Ovarian pregnancy**
AHA: 4Q 2017, 15

6 **O00.20 Ovarian pregnancy without intrauterine pregnancy**
Ovarian pregnancy NOS

L **O00.201 Right ovarian pregnancy without intrauterine pregnancy** ♀ M

L **O00.202 Left ovarian pregnancy without intrauterine pregnancy** ♀ M

L **O00.209 Unspecified ovarian pregnancy without intrauterine pregnancy** ♀ M

6 **O00.21 Ovarian pregnancy with intrauterine pregnancy**

L **O00.211 Right ovarian pregnancy with intrauterine pregnancy** ♀ M

▲ L **O00.212 Left ovarian pregnancy with intrauterine pregnancy** ♀ M

L **O00.219 Unspecified ovarian pregnancy with intrauterine pregnancy** ♀ M

5 **O00.8 Other ectopic pregnancy**
Cervical pregnancy
Cornual pregnancy
Intraligamentous pregnancy
Mural pregnancy

O00.80 Other ectopic pregnancy without intrauterine pregnancy ♀ M
Other ectopic pregnancy NOS

O00.81 Other ectopic pregnancy with intrauterine pregnancy ♀ M

5 **O00.9 Ectopic pregnancy, unspecified**

O00.90 Unspecified ectopic pregnancy without intrauterine pregnancy ♀ M
Ectopic pregnancy NOS

O00.91 Unspecified ectopic pregnancy with intrauterine pregnancy ♀ M

4 **O01 Hydatidiform mole**
Use additional code from category O08 to identify any associated complication.
EXCLUDES 1 *chorioadenoma (destruens) (D39.2)*
malignant hydatidiform mole (D39.2)

O01.0 Classical hydatidiform mole ♀M
Complete hydatidiform mole

O01.1 Incomplete and partial hydatidiform mole ♀M

O01.9 Hydatidiform mole, unspecified ♀M
Trophoblastic disease NOS
Vesicular mole NOS

4 O02 Other abnormal products of conception
Use additional code from category O08 to identify any associated complication.
EXCLUDES 1 *papyraceous fetus (O31.0-)*

O02.0 Blighted ovum and nonhydatidiform mole ♀M
Carneous mole
Fleshy mole
Intrauterine mole NOS
Molar pregnancy NEC
Pathological ovum

O02.1 Missed abortion ♀M
Early fetal death, before completion of 20 weeks of gestation, with retention of dead fetus
EXCLUDES 1 *failed induced abortion (O07.-)*
fetal death (intrauterine) (late) (O36.4)
missed abortion with blighted ovum (O02.0)
missed abortion with hydatidiform mole (O01.-)
missed abortion with nonhydatidiform (O02.0)
missed abortion with other abnormal products of conception (O02.8-)
missed delivery (O36.4)
stillbirth (P95)

5 O02.8 Other specified abnormal products of conception
EXCLUDES 1 *abnormal products of conception with blighted ovum (O02.0)*
abnormal products of conception with hydatidiform mole (O01.-)
abnormal products of conception with nonhydatidiform mole (O02.0)

O02.81 Inappropriate change in quantitative human chorionic gonadotropin (hCG) in early pregnancy ♀M
Biochemical pregnancy
Chemical pregnancy
Inappropriate level of quantitative human chorionic gonadotropin (hCG) for gestational age in early pregnancy

O02.89 Other abnormal products of conception ♀M

O02.9 Abnormal product of conception, unspecified ♀M

4 O03 Spontaneous abortion
Note: Incomplete abortion includes retained products of conception following spontaneous abortion
INCLUDES miscarriage

O03.0 Genital tract and pelvic infection following incomplete spontaneous abortion ♀M
Endometritis following incomplete spontaneous abortion
Oophoritis following incomplete spontaneous abortion
Parametritis following incomplete spontaneous abortion
Pelvic peritonitis following incomplete spontaneous abortion
Salpingitis following incomplete spontaneous abortion
Salpingo-oophoritis following incomplete spontaneous abortion
EXCLUDES 1 *sepsis following incomplete spontaneous abortion (O03.37)*
urinary tract infection following incomplete spontaneous abortion (O03.38)

O03.1 Delayed or excessive hemorrhage following incomplete spontaneous abortion ♀M
Afibrinogenemia following incomplete spontaneous abortion
Defibrination syndrome following incomplete spontaneous abortion
Hemolysis following incomplete spontaneous abortion
Intravascular coagulation following incomplete spontaneous abortion

O03.2 Embolism following incomplete spontaneous abortion ♀M
Air embolism following incomplete spontaneous abortion
Amniotic fluid embolism following incomplete spontaneous abortion
Blood-clot embolism following incomplete spontaneous abortion
Embolism NOS following incomplete spontaneous abortion
Fat embolism following incomplete spontaneous abortion
Pulmonary embolism following incomplete spontaneous abortion
Pyemic embolism following incomplete spontaneous abortion
Septic or septicopyemic embolism following incomplete spontaneous abortion
Soap embolism following incomplete spontaneous abortion

5 O03.3 Other and unspecified complications following incomplete spontaneous abortion

O03.30 Unspecified complication following incomplete spontaneous abortion ♀M

O03.31 Shock following incomplete spontaneous abortion ♀M
Circulatory collapse following incomplete spontaneous abortion
Shock (postprocedural) following incomplete spontaneous abortion
EXCLUDES 1 *shock due to infection following incomplete spontaneous abortion (O03.37)*

O03.32 Renal failure following incomplete spontaneous abortion ♀M
Kidney failure (acute) following incomplete spontaneous abortion
Oliguria following incomplete spontaneous abortion
Renal shutdown following incomplete spontaneous abortion
Renal tubular necrosis following incomplete spontaneous abortion
Uremia following incomplete spontaneous abortion

O03.33 Metabolic disorder following incomplete spontaneous abortion ♀M

O03.34 Damage to pelvic organs following incomplete spontaneous abortion ♀M
Laceration, perforation, tear or chemical damage of bladder following incomplete spontaneous abortion
Laceration, perforation, tear or chemical damage of bowel following incomplete spontaneous abortion
Laceration, perforation, tear or chemical damage of broad ligament following incomplete spontaneous abortion
Laceration, perforation, tear or chemical damage of cervix following incomplete spontaneous abortion
Laceration, perforation, tear or chemical damage of periurethral tissue following incomplete spontaneous abortion
Laceration, perforation, tear or chemical damage of uterus following incomplete spontaneous abortion
Laceration, perforation, tear or chemical damage of vagina following incomplete spontaneous abortion

O03.35 Other venous complications following incomplete spontaneous abortion ♀M

O03.36 Cardiac arrest following incomplete spontaneous abortion ♀M

O03.37 Sepsis following incomplete spontaneous abortion ♀M
Use additional code to identify infectious agent (B95-B97)
Use additional code to identify severe sepsis, if applicable (R65.2-)
EXCLUDES 1 *septic or septicopyemic embolism following incomplete spontaneous abortion (O03.2)*

O03.38 Urinary tract infection following incomplete spontaneous abortion ♀M
Cystitis following incomplete spontaneous abortion

O03.39 Incomplete spontaneous abortion with other complications ♀M

O03.4 Incomplete spontaneous abortion without complication ♀M

O03.5 Genital tract and pelvic infection following complete or unspecified spontaneous abortion ♀ M

Endometritis following complete or unspecified spontaneous abortion
Oophoritis following complete or unspecified spontaneous abortion
Parametritis following complete or unspecified spontaneous abortion
Pelvic peritonitis following complete or unspecified spontaneous abortion
Salpingitis following complete or unspecified spontaneous abortion
Salpingo-oophoritis following complete or unspecified spontaneous abortion

EXCLUDES 1 *sepsis following complete or unspecified spontaneous abortion (O03.87)*
urinary tract infection following complete or unspecified spontaneous abortion (O03.88)

O03.6 Delayed or excessive hemorrhage following complete or unspecified spontaneous abortion ♀ M

Afibrinogenemia following complete or unspecified spontaneous abortion
Defibrination syndrome following complete or unspecified spontaneous abortion
Hemolysis following complete or unspecified spontaneous abortion
Intravascular coagulation following complete or unspecified spontaneous abortion

O03.7 Embolism following complete or unspecified spontaneous abortion ♀ M

Air embolism following complete or unspecified spontaneous abortion
Amniotic fluid embolism following complete or unspecified spontaneous abortion
Blood-clot embolism following complete or unspecified spontaneous abortion
Embolism NOS following complete or unspecified spontaneous abortion
Fat embolism following complete or unspecified spontaneous abortion
Pulmonary embolism following complete or unspecified spontaneous abortion
Pyemic embolism following complete or unspecified spontaneous abortion
Septic or septicopyemic embolism following complete or unspecified spontaneous abortion
Soap embolism following complete or unspecified spontaneous abortion

5 O03.8 Other and unspecified complications following complete or unspecified spontaneous abortion

O03.80 Unspecified complication following complete or unspecified spontaneous abortion ♀ M

O03.81 Shock following complete or unspecified spontaneous abortion ♀ M

Circulatory collapse following complete or unspecified spontaneous abortion
Shock (postprocedural) following complete or unspecified spontaneous abortion

EXCLUDES 1 *shock due to infection following complete or unspecified spontaneous abortion (O03.87)*

O03.82 Renal failure following complete or unspecified spontaneous abortion ♀ M

Kidney failure (acute) following complete or unspecified spontaneous abortion
Oliguria following complete or unspecified spontaneous abortion
Renal shutdown following complete or unspecified spontaneous abortion
Renal tubular necrosis following complete or unspecified spontaneous abortion
Uremia following complete or unspecified spontaneous abortion

O03.83 Metabolic disorder following complete or unspecified spontaneous abortion ♀ M

O03.84 Damage to pelvic organs following complete or unspecified spontaneous abortion ♀ M

Laceration, perforation, tear or chemical damage of bladder following complete or unspecified spontaneous abortion
Laceration, perforation, tear or chemical damage of bowel following complete or unspecified spontaneous abortion
Laceration, perforation, tear or chemical damage of broad ligament following complete or unspecified spontaneous abortion
Laceration, perforation, tear or chemical damage of cervix following complete or unspecified spontaneous abortion
Laceration, perforation, tear or chemical damage of periurethral tissue following complete or unspecified spontaneous abortion
Laceration, perforation, tear or chemical damage of uterus following complete or unspecified spontaneous abortion
Laceration, perforation, tear or chemical damage of vagina following complete or unspecified spontaneous abortion

O03.85 Other venous complications following complete or unspecified spontaneous abortion ♀ M

O03.86 Cardiac arrest following complete or unspecified spontaneous abortion ♀ M

O03.87 Sepsis following complete or unspecified spontaneous abortion ♀ M

Use additional code to identify infectious agent (B95-B97)
Use additional code to identify severe sepsis, if applicable (R65.2-)

EXCLUDES 1 *septic or septicopyemic embolism following complete or unspecified spontaneous abortion (O03.7)*

O03.88 Urinary tract infection following complete or unspecified spontaneous abortion ♀ M

Cystitis following complete or unspecified spontaneous abortion

O03.89 Complete or unspecified spontaneous abortion with other complications ♀ M

O03.9 Complete or unspecified spontaneous abortion without complication ♀ M

Miscarriage NOS
Spontaneous abortion NOS

4 O04 Complications following (induced) termination of pregnancy

INCLUDES complications following (induced) termination of pregnancy

EXCLUDES 1 *encounter for elective termination of pregnancy, uncomplicated (Z33.2)*
failed attempted termination of pregnancy (O07.-)

O04.5 Genital tract and pelvic infection following (induced) termination of pregnancy ♀ M

Endometritis following (induced) termination of pregnancy
Oophoritis following (induced) termination of pregnancy
Parametritis following (induced) termination of pregnancy
Pelvic peritonitis following (induced) termination of pregnancy
Salpingitis following (induced) termination of pregnancy
Salpingo-oophoritis following (induced) termination of pregnancy

EXCLUDES 1 *sepsis following (induced) termination of pregnancy (O04.87)*
urinary tract infection following (induced) termination of pregnancy (O04.88)

O04.6 Delayed or excessive hemorrhage following (induced) termination of pregnancy ♀ M

Afibrinogenemia following (induced) termination of pregnancy
Defibrination syndrome following (induced) termination of pregnancy
Hemolysis following (induced) termination of pregnancy
Intravascular coagulation following (induced) termination of pregnancy

O04.7 Embolism following (induced) termination of pregnancy ♀ M
Air embolism following (induced) termination of pregnancy
Amniotic fluid embolism following (induced) termination of pregnancy
Blood-clot embolism following (induced) termination of pregnancy
Embolism NOS following (induced) termination of pregnancy
Fat embolism following (induced) termination of pregnancy
Pulmonary embolism following (induced) termination of pregnancy
Pyemic embolism following (induced) termination of pregnancy
Septic or septicopyemic embolism following (induced) termination of pregnancy
Soap embolism following (induced) termination of pregnancy

5 O04.8 (Induced) termination of pregnancy with other and unspecified complications

O04.80 (Induced) termination of pregnancy with unspecified complications ♀ M

O04.81 Shock following (induced) termination of pregnancy ♀ M
Circulatory collapse following (induced) termination of pregnancy
Shock (postprocedural) following (induced) termination of pregnancy
EXCLUDES 1 *shock due to infection following (induced) termination of pregnancy (O04.87)*

O04.82 Renal failure following (induced) termination of pregnancy ♀ M
Kidney failure (acute) following (induced) termination of pregnancy
Oliguria following (induced) termination of pregnancy
Renal shutdown following (induced) termination of pregnancy
Renal tubular necrosis following (induced) termination of pregnancy
Uremia following (induced) termination of pregnancy

O04.83 Metabolic disorder following (induced) termination of pregnancy ♀ M

O04.84 Damage to pelvic organs following (induced) termination of pregnancy ♀ M
Laceration, perforation, tear or chemical damage of bladder following (induced) termination of pregnancy
Laceration, perforation, tear or chemical damage of bowel following (induced) termination of pregnancy
Laceration, perforation, tear or chemical damage of broad ligament following (induced) termination of pregnancy
Laceration, perforation, tear or chemical damage of cervix following (induced) termination of pregnancy
Laceration, perforation, tear or chemical damage of periurethral tissue following (induced) termination of pregnancy
Laceration, perforation, tear or chemical damage of uterus following (induced) termination of pregnancy
Laceration, perforation, tear or chemical damage of vagina following (induced) termination of pregnancy

O04.85 Other venous complications following (induced) termination of pregnancy ♀ M

O04.86 Cardiac arrest following (induced) termination of pregnancy ♀ M

O04.87 Sepsis following (induced) termination of pregnancy ♀ M
Use additional code to identify infectious agent (B95-B97)
Use additional code to identify severe sepsis, if applicable (R65.2-)
EXCLUDES 1 *septic or septicopyemic embolism following (induced) termination of pregnancy (O04.7)*

O04.88 Urinary tract infection following (induced) termination of pregnancy ♀ M
Cystitis following (induced) termination of pregnancy

O04.89 (Induced) termination of pregnancy with other complications ♀ M

4 O07 Failed attempted termination of pregnancy
INCLUDES failure of attempted induction of termination of pregnancy
incomplete elective abortion
EXCLUDES 1 *incomplete spontaneous abortion (O03.0-)*

O07.0 Genital tract and pelvic infection following failed attempted termination of pregnancy ♀ M
Endometritis following failed attempted termination of pregnancy
Oophoritis following failed attempted termination of pregnancy
Parametritis following failed attempted termination of pregnancy
Pelvic peritonitis following failed attempted termination of pregnancy
Salpingitis following failed attempted termination of pregnancy
Salpingo-oophoritis following failed attempted termination of pregnancy
EXCLUDES 1 *sepsis following failed attempted termination of pregnancy (O07.37)*
urinary tract infection following failed attempted termination of pregnancy (O07.38)

O07.1 Delayed or excessive hemorrhage following failed attempted termination of pregnancy ♀ M
Afibrinogenemia following failed attempted termination of pregnancy
Defibrination syndrome following failed attempted termination of pregnancy
Hemolysis following failed attempted termination of pregnancy
Intravascular coagulation following failed attempted termination of pregnancy

O07.2 Embolism following failed attempted termination of pregnancy ♀ M
Air embolism following failed attempted termination of pregnancy
Amniotic fluid embolism following failed attempted termination of pregnancy
Blood-clot embolism following failed attempted termination of pregnancy
Embolism NOS following failed attempted termination of pregnancy
Fat embolism following failed attempted termination of pregnancy
Pulmonary embolism following failed attempted termination of pregnancy
Pyemic embolism following failed attempted termination of pregnancy
Septic or septicopyemic embolism following failed attempted termination of pregnancy
Soap embolism following failed attempted termination of pregnancy

5 O07.3 Failed attempted termination of pregnancy with other and unspecified complications

O07.30 Failed attempted termination of pregnancy with unspecified complications ♀ M

O07.31 Shock following failed attempted termination of pregnancy ♀ M
Circulatory collapse following failed attempted termination of pregnancy
Shock (postprocedural) following failed attempted termination of pregnancy
EXCLUDES 1 *shock due to infection following failed attempted termination of pregnancy (O07.37)*

O07.32 Renal failure following failed attempted termination of pregnancy ♀ M
Kidney failure (acute) following failed attempted termination of pregnancy
Oliguria following failed attempted termination of pregnancy
Renal shutdown following failed attempted termination of pregnancy
Renal tubular necrosis following failed attempted termination of pregnancy
Uremia following failed attempted termination of pregnancy

O07.33 Metabolic disorder following failed attempted termination of pregnancy ♀ M

O07.34 **Damage to pelvic organs following failed attempted termination of pregnancy** ♀M
Laceration, perforation, tear or chemical damage of bladder following failed attempted termination of pregnancy
Laceration, perforation, tear or chemical damage of bowel following failed attempted termination of pregnancy
Laceration, perforation, tear or chemical damage of broad ligament following failed attempted termination of pregnancy
Laceration, perforation, tear or chemical damage of cervix following failed attempted termination of pregnancy
Laceration, perforation, tear or chemical damage of periurethral tissue following failed attempted termination of pregnancy
Laceration, perforation, tear or chemical damage of uterus following failed attempted termination of pregnancy
Laceration, perforation, tear or chemical damage of vagina following failed attempted termination of pregnancy

O07.35 **Other venous complications following failed attempted termination of pregnancy** ♀M

O07.36 **Cardiac arrest following failed attempted termination of pregnancy** ♀M

O07.37 **Sepsis following failed attempted termination of pregnancy** ♀M
Use additional code (B95-B97), to identify infectious agent
Use additional code (R65.2-) to identify severe sepsis, if applicable
EXCLUDES 1 *septic or septicopyemic embolism following failed attempted termination of pregnancy (O07.2)*

O07.38 **Urinary tract infection following failed attempted termination of pregnancy** ♀M
Cystitis following failed attempted termination of pregnancy

O07.39 **Failed attempted termination of pregnancy with other complications** ♀M

O07.4 **Failed attempted termination of pregnancy without complication** ♀M

4 O08 Complications following ectopic and molar pregnancy

This category is for use with categories O00-O02 to identify any associated complications

O08.0 **Genital tract and pelvic infection following ectopic and molar pregnancy** ♀M
Endometritis following ectopic and molar pregnancy
Oophoritis following ectopic and molar pregnancy
Parametritis following ectopic and molar pregnancy
Pelvic peritonitis following ectopic and molar pregnancy
Salpingitis following ectopic and molar pregnancy
Salpingo-oophoritis following ectopic and molar pregnancy
EXCLUDES 1 *sepsis following ectopic and molar pregnancy (O08.82)*
urinary tract infection (O08.83)

O08.1 **Delayed or excessive hemorrhage following ectopic and molar pregnancy** ♀M
Afibrinogenemia following ectopic and molar pregnancy
Defibrination syndrome following ectopic and molar pregnancy
Hemolysis following ectopic and molar pregnancy
Intravascular coagulation following ectopic and molar pregnancy
EXCLUDES 1 *delayed or excessive hemorrhage due to incomplete abortion (O03.1)*

O08.2 **Embolism following ectopic and molar pregnancy** ♀M
Air embolism following ectopic and molar pregnancy
Amniotic fluid embolism following ectopic and molar pregnancy
Blood-clot embolism following ectopic and molar pregnancy
Embolism NOS following ectopic and molar pregnancy
Fat embolism following ectopic and molar pregnancy
Pulmonary embolism following ectopic and molar pregnancy
Pyemic embolism following ectopic and molar pregnancy
Septic or septicopyemic embolism following ectopic and molar pregnancy
Soap embolism following ectopic and molar pregnancy

O08.3 **Shock following ectopic and molar pregnancy** ♀M
Circulatory collapse following ectopic and molar pregnancy
Shock (postprocedural) following ectopic and molar pregnancy
EXCLUDES 1 *shock due to infection following ectopic and molar pregnancy (O08.82)*

O08.4 **Renal failure following ectopic and molar pregnancy** ♀M
Kidney failure (acute) following ectopic and molar pregnancy
Oliguria following ectopic and molar pregnancy
Renal shutdown following ectopic and molar pregnancy
Renal tubular necrosis following ectopic and molar pregnancy
Uremia following ectopic and molar pregnancy

O08.5 **Metabolic disorders following an ectopic and molar pregnancy** ♀M

O08.6 **Damage to pelvic organs and tissues following an ectopic and molar pregnancy** ♀M
Laceration, perforation, tear or chemical damage of bladder following an ectopic and molar pregnancy
Laceration, perforation, tear or chemical damage of bowel following an ectopic and molar pregnancy
Laceration, perforation, tear or chemical damage of broad ligament following an ectopic and molar pregnancy
Laceration, perforation, tear or chemical damage of cervix following an ectopic and molar pregnancy
Laceration, perforation, tear or chemical damage of periurethral tissue following an ectopic and molar pregnancy
Laceration, perforation, tear or chemical damage of uterus following an ectopic and molar pregnancy
Laceration, perforation, tear or chemical damage of vagina following an ectopic and molar pregnancy

O08.7 **Other venous complications following an ectopic and molar pregnancy** ♀M

5 O08.8 **Other complications following an ectopic and molar pregnancy**

O08.81 **Cardiac arrest following an ectopic and molar pregnancy** ♀M

O08.82 **Sepsis following ectopic and molar pregnancy** ♀M
Use additional code (B95-B97), to identify infectious agent
Use additional code (R65.2-) to identify severe sepsis, if applicable
EXCLUDES 1 *septic or septicopyemic embolism following ectopic and molar pregnancy (O08.2)*

O08.83 **Urinary tract infection following an ectopic and molar pregnancy** ♀M
Cystitis following an ectopic and molar pregnancy

O08.89 **Other complications following an ectopic and molar pregnancy** ♀M

O08.9 **Unspecified complication following an ectopic and molar pregnancy** ♀M

Supervision of high risk pregnancy (O09)

4 O09 Supervision of high risk pregnancy

5 O09.0 **Supervision of pregnancy with history of infertility**

O09.00 **Supervision of pregnancy with history of infertility, unspecified trimester** ♀M

O09.01 **Supervision of pregnancy with history of infertility, first trimester** ♀M

O09.02 **Supervision of pregnancy with history of infertility, second trimester** ♀M

O09.03 **Supervision of pregnancy with history of infertility, third trimester** ♀M

5 O09.1 **Supervision of pregnancy with history of ectopic pregnancy**

O09.10 **Supervision of pregnancy with history of ectopic pregnancy, unspecified trimester** ♀M

O09.11 **Supervision of pregnancy with history of ectopic pregnancy, first trimester** ♀M

O09.12 **Supervision of pregnancy with history of ectopic pregnancy, second trimester** ♀M

O09.13 **Supervision of pregnancy with history of ectopic pregnancy, third trimester** ♀M

5 O09.A **Supervision of pregnancy with history of molar pregnancy**

DEFINITION An abnormal product of conception that occurs when the cells proliferate out of control, creating a growth or mass of cell clusters that causes the body to continue producing hormones as if in pregnancy, even though there is no fetus developing. This gives a false positive pregnancy result. Molar pregnancies have the potential of developing into a cancerous growth, called choriocarinoma if left untreated.

O09.A0 **Supervision of pregnancy with history of molar pregnancy, unspecified trimester** ♀

O09.A1 **Supervision of pregnancy with history of molar pregnancy, first trimester** ♀

O09.A2 **Supervision of pregnancy with history of molar pregnancy, second trimester** ♀

O09.A3 **Supervision of pregnancy with history of molar pregnancy, third trimester** ♀

5 **O09.2** **Supervision of pregnancy with other poor reproductive or obstetric history**

EXCLUDES 2 *pregnancy care for patient with history of recurrent pregnancy loss (O26.2-)*

6 **O09.21** **Supervision of pregnancy with history of pre-term labor**

O09.211 **Supervision of pregnancy with history of pre-term labor, first trimester** ♀

O09.212 **Supervision of pregnancy with history of pre-term labor, second trimester** ♀

O09.213 **Supervision of pregnancy with history of pre-term labor, third trimester** ♀

O09.219 **Supervision of pregnancy with history of pre-term labor, unspecified trimester** ♀

6 **O09.29** **Supervision of pregnancy with other poor reproductive or obstetric history**

Supervision of pregnancy with history of neonatal death
Supervision of pregnancy with history of stillbirth

O09.291 **Supervision of pregnancy with other poor reproductive or obstetric history, first trimester** ♀

O09.292 **Supervision of pregnancy with other poor reproductive or obstetric history, second trimester** ♀

O09.293 **Supervision of pregnancy with other poor reproductive or obstetric history, third trimester** ♀

O09.299 **Supervision of pregnancy with other poor reproductive or obstetric history, unspecified trimester** ♀

5 **O09.3** **Supervision of pregnancy with insufficient antenatal care**

Supervision of concealed pregnancy
Supervision of hidden pregnancy

O09.30 **Supervision of pregnancy with insufficient antenatal care, unspecified trimester** ♀

O09.31 **Supervision of pregnancy with insufficient antenatal care, first trimester** ♀

O09.32 **Supervision of pregnancy with insufficient antenatal care, second trimester** ♀

O09.33 **Supervision of pregnancy with insufficient antenatal care, third trimester** ♀

5 **O09.4** **Supervision of pregnancy with grand multiparity**

O09.40 **Supervision of pregnancy with grand multiparity, unspecified trimester** ♀

O09.41 **Supervision of pregnancy with grand multiparity, first trimester** ♀

O09.42 **Supervision of pregnancy with grand multiparity, second trimester** ♀

O09.43 **Supervision of pregnancy with grand multiparity, third trimester** ♀

5 **O09.5** **Supervision of elderly primigravida and multigravida**

Pregnancy for a female 35 years and older at expected date of delivery

6 **O09.51** **Supervision of elderly primigravida**

O09.511 **Supervision of elderly primigravida, first trimester** ♀

O09.512 **Supervision of elderly primigravida, second trimester** ♀

O09.513 **Supervision of elderly primigravida, third trimester** ♀

O09.519 **Supervision of elderly primigravida, unspecified trimester** ♀

6 **O09.52** **Supervision of elderly multigravida**

O09.521 **Supervision of elderly multigravida, first trimester** ♀

O09.522 **Supervision of elderly multigravida, second trimester** ♀

O09.523 **Supervision of elderly multigravida, third trimester** ♀

O09.529 **Supervision of elderly multigravida, unspecified trimester** ♀

5 **O09.6** **Supervision of young primigravida and multigravida**

Supervision of pregnancy for a female less than 16 years old at expected date of delivery

6 **O09.61** **Supervision of young primigravida**

O09.611 **Supervision of young primigravida, first trimester** ♀

O09.612 **Supervision of young primigravida, second trimester** ♀

O09.613 **Supervision of young primigravida, third trimester** ♀

O09.619 **Supervision of young primigravida, unspecified trimester** ♀

6 **O09.62** **Supervision of young multigravida**

O09.621 **Supervision of young multigravida, first trimester** ♀

O09.622 **Supervision of young multigravida, second trimester** ♀

O09.623 **Supervision of young multigravida, third trimester** ♀

O09.629 **Supervision of young multigravida, unspecified trimester** ♀

5 **O09.7** **Supervision of high risk pregnancy due to social problems**

O09.70 **Supervision of high risk pregnancy due to social problems, unspecified trimester** ♀

O09.71 **Supervision of high risk pregnancy due to social problems, first trimester** ♀

O09.72 **Supervision of high risk pregnancy due to social problems, second trimester** ♀

O09.73 **Supervision of high risk pregnancy due to social problems, third trimester** ♀

5 **O09.8** **Supervision of other high risk pregnancies**

6 **O09.81** **Supervision of pregnancy resulting from assisted reproductive technology**

Supervision of pregnancy resulting from in-vitro fertilization

EXCLUDES 2 *gestational carrier status (Z33.3)*

O09.811 **Supervision of pregnancy resulting from assisted reproductive technology, first trimester** ♀

O09.812 **Supervision of pregnancy resulting from assisted reproductive technology, second trimester** ♀

O09.813 **Supervision of pregnancy resulting from assisted reproductive technology, third trimester** ♀

O09.819 **Supervision of pregnancy resulting from assisted reproductive technology, unspecified trimester** ♀

6 **O09.82** **Supervision of pregnancy with history of in utero procedure during previous pregnancy**

O09.821 **Supervision of pregnancy with history of in utero procedure during previous pregnancy, first trimester** ♀

O09.822 **Supervision of pregnancy with history of in utero procedure during previous pregnancy, second trimester** ♀

O09.823 **Supervision of pregnancy with history of in utero procedure during previous pregnancy, third trimester** ♀

O09.829 **Supervision of pregnancy with history of in utero procedure during previous pregnancy, unspecified trimester** ♀

EXCLUDES 1 *supervision of pregnancy affected by in utero procedure during current pregnancy (O35.7)*

6 **O09.89** **Supervision of other high risk pregnancies**

O09.891 Supervision of other high risk pregnancies, first trimester ♀M

O09.892 Supervision of other high risk pregnancies, second trimester ♀M

O09.893 Supervision of other high risk pregnancies, third trimester ♀M

O09.899 Supervision of other high risk pregnancies, unspecified trimester ♀M

5 O09.9 Supervision of high risk pregnancy, unspecified

O09.90 Supervision of high risk pregnancy, unspecified, unspecified trimester ♀M

O09.91 Supervision of high risk pregnancy, unspecified, first trimester ♀M

O09.92 Supervision of high risk pregnancy, unspecified, second trimester ♀M

O09.93 Supervision of high risk pregnancy, unspecified, third trimester ♀M

Edema, proteinuria and hypertensive disorders in pregnancy, childbirth and the puerperium (O10-O16)

4 **O10 Pre-existing hypertension complicating pregnancy, childbirth and the puerperium**

INCLUDES pre-existing hypertension with pre-existing proteinuria complicating pregnancy, childbirth and the puerperium

EXCLUDES 2 *pre-existing hypertension with superimposed pre-eclampsia complicating pregnancy, childbirth and the puerperium (O11.-)*

GUIDELINES Section I.C.15.d

Category O10 includes codes for hypertensive heart and hypertensive chronic kidney disease. When assigning one of the O10 codes that includes hypertensive heart disease or hypertensive chronic kidney disease, it is necessary to add a secondary code from the appropriate hypertension category to specify the type of heart failure or chronic kidney disease.

AHA: 4Q 2016, 50

5 O10.0 Pre-existing essential hypertension complicating pregnancy, childbirth and the puerperium

Any condition in I10 specified as a reason for obstetric care during pregnancy, childbirth or the puerperium

AHA: 4Q 2016, 50

6 O10.01 Pre-existing essential hypertension complicating pregnancy,

AHA: 4Q 2016, 50

O10.011 Pre-existing essential hypertension complicating pregnancy, first trimester ♀M

AHA: 4Q 2016, 50

O10.012 Pre-existing essential hypertension complicating pregnancy, second trimester ♀M

AHA: 4Q 2016, 50

O10.013 Pre-existing essential hypertension complicating pregnancy, third trimester ♀M

AHA: 4Q 2016, 50

O10.019 Pre-existing essential hypertension complicating pregnancy, unspecified trimester ♀M

AHA: 4Q 2016, 50

O10.02 Pre-existing essential hypertension complicating childbirth ♀M

AHA: 4Q 2016, 50

O10.03 Pre-existing essential hypertension complicating the puerperium ♀M

AHA: 4Q 2016, 50

5 O10.1 Pre-existing hypertensive heart disease complicating pregnancy, childbirth and the puerperium

Any condition in I11 specified as a reason for obstetric care during pregnancy, childbirth or the puerperium

Use additional code from I11 to identify the type of hypertensive heart disease

AHA: 4Q 2016, 50

6 O10.11 Pre-existing hypertensive heart disease complicating pregnancy

AHA: 4Q 2016, 50

O10.111 Pre-existing hypertensive heart disease complicating pregnancy, first trimester ♀M

AHA: 4Q 2016, 50

O10.112 Pre-existing hypertensive heart disease complicating pregnancy, second trimester ♀M

AHA: 4Q 2016, 50

O10.113 Pre-existing hypertensive heart disease complicating pregnancy, third trimester ♀M

AHA: 4Q 2016, 50

O10.119 Pre-existing hypertensive heart disease complicating pregnancy, unspecified trimester ♀M

AHA: 4Q 2016, 50

O10.12 Pre-existing hypertensive heart disease complicating childbirth ♀M

AHA: 4Q 2016, 50

O10.13 Pre-existing hypertensive heart disease complicating the puerperium ♀M

AHA: 4Q 2016, 50

5 O10.2 Pre-existing hypertensive chronic kidney disease complicating pregnancy, childbirth and the puerperium

Any condition in I12 specified as a reason for obstetric care during pregnancy, childbirth or the puerperium

Use additional code from I12 to identify the type of hypertensive chronic kidney disease

AHA: 4Q 2016, 50

6 O10.21 Pre-existing hypertensive chronic kidney disease complicating pregnancy

AHA: 4Q 2016, 50

O10.211 Pre-existing hypertensive chronic kidney disease complicating pregnancy, first trimester ♀M

AHA: 4Q 2016, 50

O10.212 Pre-existing hypertensive chronic kidney disease complicating pregnancy, second trimester ♀M

AHA: 4Q 2016, 50

O10.213 Pre-existing hypertensive chronic kidney disease complicating pregnancy, third trimester ♀M

AHA: 4Q 2016, 50

O10.219 Pre-existing hypertensive chronic kidney disease complicating pregnancy, unspecified trimester ♀M

AHA: 4Q 2016, 50

O10.22 Pre-existing hypertensive chronic kidney disease complicating childbirth ♀M

AHA: 4Q 2016, 50

O10.23 Pre-existing hypertensive chronic kidney disease complicating the puerperium ♀M

AHA: 4Q 2016, 50

5 O10.3 Pre-existing hypertensive heart and chronic kidney disease complicating pregnancy, childbirth and the puerperium

Any condition in I13 specified as a reason for obstetric care during pregnancy, childbirth or the puerperium

Use additional code from I13 to identify the type of hypertensive heart and chronic kidney disease

AHA: 4Q 2016, 50

6 O10.31 Pre-existing hypertensive heart and chronic kidney disease complicating pregnancy

AHA: 4Q 2016, 50

O10.311 Pre-existing hypertensive heart and chronic kidney disease complicating pregnancy, first trimester ♀M

AHA: 4Q 2016, 50

O10.312 Pre-existing hypertensive heart and chronic kidney disease complicating pregnancy, second trimester ♀M

AHA: 4Q 2016, 50

O10.313 Pre-existing hypertensive heart and chronic kidney disease complicating pregnancy, third trimester ♀M

AHA: 4Q 2016, 50

O10.319 Pre-existing hypertensive heart and chronic kidney disease complicating pregnancy, unspecified trimester ♀M

AHA: 4Q 2016, 50

O10.32 **Pre-existing hypertensive heart and chronic kidney disease complicating childbirth** ♀M
AHA: 4Q 2016, 50

O10.33 **Pre-existing hypertensive heart and chronic kidney disease complicating the puerperium** ♀M
AHA: 4Q 2016, 50

5 O10.4 **Pre-existing secondary hypertension complicating pregnancy, childbirth and the puerperium**
Any condition in I15 specified as a reason for obstetric care during pregnancy, childbirth or the puerperium
Use additional code from I15 to identify the type of secondary hypertension
AHA: 4Q 2016, 50

6 O10.41 **Pre-existing secondary hypertension complicating pregnancy**
AHA: 4Q 2016, 50

O10.411 **Pre-existing secondary hypertension complicating pregnancy, first trimester** ♀M
AHA: 4Q 2016, 50

O10.412 **Pre-existing secondary hypertension complicating pregnancy, second trimester** ♀M
AHA: 4Q 2016, 50

O10.413 **Pre-existing secondary hypertension complicating pregnancy, third trimester** ♀M
AHA: 4Q 2016, 50

O10.419 **Pre-existing secondary hypertension complicating pregnancy, unspecified trimester** ♀M
AHA: 4Q 2016, 50

O10.42 **Pre-existing secondary hypertension complicating childbirth** ♀M
AHA: 4Q 2016, 50

O10.43 **Pre-existing secondary hypertension complicating the puerperium** ♀M
AHA: 4Q 2016, 50

5 O10.9 **Unspecified pre-existing hypertension complicating pregnancy, childbirth and the puerperium**
AHA: 4Q 2016, 50

6 O10.91 **Unspecified pre-existing hypertension complicating pregnancy**
AHA: 4Q 2016, 50

O10.911 **Unspecified pre-existing hypertension complicating pregnancy, first trimester** ♀M
AHA: 4Q 2016, 50

O10.912 **Unspecified pre-existing hypertension complicating pregnancy, second trimester** ♀M
AHA: 4Q 2016, 50

O10.913 **Unspecified pre-existing hypertension complicating pregnancy, third trimester** ♀M
AHA: 4Q 2016, 50

O10.919 **Unspecified pre-existing hypertension complicating pregnancy, unspecified trimester** ♀M
AHA: 4Q 2016, 50

O10.92 **Unspecified pre-existing hypertension complicating childbirth** ♀M
AHA: 4Q 2016, 50

O10.93 **Unspecified pre-existing hypertension complicating the puerperium** ♀M
AHA: 4Q 2016, 50

4 O11 **Pre-existing hypertension with pre-eclampsia**
INCLUDES conditions in O10 complicated by pre-eclampsia
pre-eclampsia superimposed pre-existing hypertension
Use additional code from O10 to identify the type of hypertension
AHA: 4Q 2016, 50

Pre-existing hypertension with pre-eclampsia

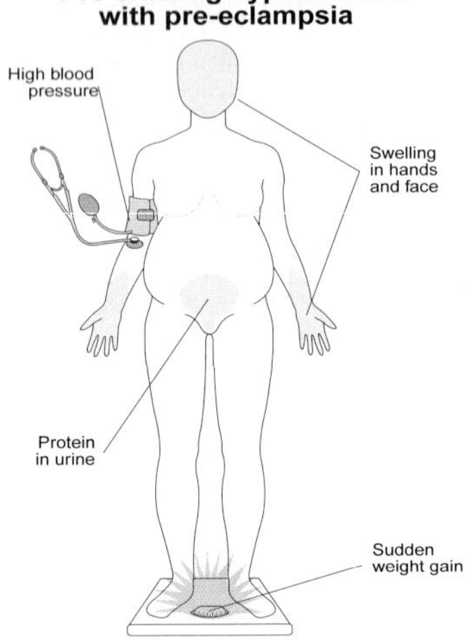

O11.1 **Pre-existing hypertension with pre-eclampsia, first trimester** ♀M
AHA: 4Q 2016, 50

O11.2 **Pre-existing hypertension with pre-eclampsia, second trimester** ♀M
AHA: 4Q 2016, 50

O11.3 **Pre-existing hypertension with pre-eclampsia, third trimester** ♀M
AHA: 4Q 2016, 50

O11.4 **Pre-existing hypertension with pre-eclampsia, complicating childbirth** ♀M
AHA: 4Q 2016, 50

O11.5 **Pre-existing hypertension with pre-eclampsia, complicating the puerperium** ♀M
AHA: 4Q 2016, 50

O11.9 **Pre-existing hypertension with pre-eclampsia, unspecified trimester** ♀M
AHA: 4Q 2016, 50

4 O12 **Gestational [pregnancy-induced] edema and proteinuria without hypertension**
AHA: 4Q 2016, 50

5 O12.0 **Gestational edema**
AHA: 4Q 2016, 50

O12.00 **Gestational edema, unspecified trimester** ♀M
AHA: 4Q 2016, 50

O12.01 **Gestational edema, first trimester** ♀M
AHA: 4Q 2016, 50

O12.02 **Gestational edema, second trimester** ♀M
AHA: 4Q 2016, 50

O12.03 **Gestational edema, third trimester** ♀M
AHA: 4Q 2016, 50

O12.04 **Gestational edema, complicating childbirth** ♀M
AHA: 4Q 2016, 50

O12.05 **Gestational edema, complicating the puerperium** ♀M
AHA: 4Q 2016, 50

5 O12.1 **Gestational proteinuria**
AHA: 4Q 2016, 50

O12.10 **Gestational proteinuria, unspecified trimester** ♀M
AHA: 4Q 2016, 50

O12.11 **Gestational proteinuria, first trimester** ♀M
AHA: 4Q 2016, 50

O12.12 **Gestational proteinuria, second trimester** ♀M
AHA: 4Q 2016, 50

O12.13 **Gestational proteinuria, third trimester** ♀M
AHA: 4Q 2016, 50

O12.14 **Gestational proteinuria, complicating childbirth** ♀M
AHA: 4Q 2016, 50

O12.15 **Gestational proteinuria, complicating the puerperium** ♀M
AHA: 4Q 2016, 50

O12.2 Gestational edema with proteinuria
AHA: 4Q 2016, 50

O12.20 Gestational edema with proteinuria, unspecified trimester ♀ M
AHA: 4Q 2016, 50

O12.21 Gestational edema with proteinuria, first trimester ♀ M
AHA: 4Q 2016, 50

O12.22 Gestational edema with proteinuria, second trimester ♀ M
AHA: 4Q 2016, 50

O12.23 Gestational edema with proteinuria, third trimester ♀ M
AHA: 4Q 2016, 50

O12.24 Gestational edema with proteinuria, complicating childbirth ♀ M
AHA: 4Q 2016, 50

O12.25 Gestational edema with proteinuria, complicating the puerperium ♀ M
AHA: 4Q 2016, 50

O13 Gestational [pregnancy-induced] hypertension without significant proteinuria

INCLUDES gestational hypertension NOS
transient hypertension of pregnancy

GUIDELINES Section I.9.a.7)
Unless patient has an established diagnosis of hypertension, assign code O13.-, Gestational [pregnancy-induced] hypertension without significant proteinuria, or O14.-, Pre-eclampsia, for transient hypertension of pregnancy.
AHA: 4Q 2016, 50

O13.1 Gestational [pregnancy-induced] hypertension without significant proteinuria, first trimester ♀ M
AHA: 4Q 2016, 50

O13.2 Gestational [pregnancy-induced] hypertension without significant proteinuria, second trimester ♀ M
AHA: 4Q 2016, 50

O13.3 Gestational [pregnancy-induced] hypertension without significant proteinuria, third trimester ♀ M
AHA: 4Q 2016, 50

O13.4 Gestational [pregnancy-induced] hypertension without significant proteinuria, complicating childbirth ♀ M
AHA: 4Q 2016, 50

O13.5 Gestational [pregnancy-induced] hypertension without significant proteinuria, complicating the puerperium ♀ M
AHA: 4Q 2016, 50

O13.9 Gestational [pregnancy-induced] hypertension without significant proteinuria, unspecified trimester ♀ M
AHA: 4Q 2016, 50

O14 Pre-eclampsia

EXCLUDES 1 *pre-existing hypertension with pre-eclampsia (O11)*

GUIDELINES Section I.9.a.7)
Unless patient has an established diagnosis of hypertension, assign code O13.-, Gestational [pregnancy-induced] hypertension without significant proteinuria, or O14.-, Pre-eclampsia, for transient hypertension of pregnancy.
AHA: 4Q 2016, 50

O14.0 Mild to moderate pre-eclampsia

DEFINITION Hypertension (BP >140/90 mmHg) after the 20th week of gestation and up to 6 weeks postpartum, with proteinuria.
AHA: 4Q 2016, 50

O14.00 Mild to moderate pre-eclampsia, unspecified trimester ♀ M
AHA: 4Q 2016, 50

O14.02 Mild to moderate pre-eclampsia, second trimester ♀ M
AHA: 4Q 2016, 50

O14.03 Mild to moderate pre-eclampsia, third trimester ♀ M
AHA: 4Q 2016, 50

O14.04 Mild to moderate pre-eclampsia, complicating childbirth ♀ M
AHA: 4Q 2016, 50

O14.05 Mild to moderate pre-eclampsia, complicating the puerperium ♀ M
AHA: 4Q 2016, 50

O14.1 Severe pre-eclampsia

EXCLUDES 1 *HELLP syndrome (O14.2-)*

DEFINITION Severe hypertension (BP >160/110 mmHg) after the 20th week of gestation and up to 6 weeks postpartum, with proteinuria, and additional symptoms such as pulmonary edema, upper abdominal pain, severe headaches, and blurred vision.
AHA: 4Q 2016, 50

O14.10 Severe pre-eclampsia, unspecified trimester ♀ M
AHA: 4Q 2016, 50

O14.12 Severe pre-eclampsia, second trimester ♀ M
AHA: 4Q 2016, 50

O14.13 Severe pre-eclampsia, third trimester ♀ M
AHA: 4Q 2016, 50

O14.14 Severe pre-eclampsia complicating childbirth ♀ M
AHA: 4Q 2016, 50

O14.15 Severe pre-eclampsia, complicating the puerperium ♀ M
AHA: 4Q 2016, 50

O14.2 HELLP syndrome
Severe pre-eclampsia with hemolysis, elevated liver enzymes and low platelet count (HELLP)

DEFINITION Severe pre-eclampsia with hemolysis, elevated liver enzymes and low platelet count (HELLP).
AHA: 4Q 2016, 50

O14.20 HELLP syndrome (HELLP), unspecified trimester ♀ M
AHA: 4Q 2016, 50

O14.22 HELLP syndrome (HELLP), second trimester ♀ M
AHA: 4Q 2016, 50

O14.23 HELLP syndrome (HELLP), third trimester ♀ M
AHA: 4Q 2016, 50

O14.24 HELLP syndrome, complicating childbirth ♀ M
AHA: 4Q 2016, 50

O14.25 HELLP syndrome, complicating the puerperium ♀ M
AHA: 4Q 2016, 50

O14.9 Unspecified pre-eclampsia
AHA: 4Q 2016, 50

O14.90 Unspecified pre-eclampsia, unspecified trimester ♀ M
AHA: 4Q 2016, 50

O14.92 Unspecified pre-eclampsia, second trimester ♀ M
AHA: 4Q 2016, 50

O14.93 Unspecified pre-eclampsia, third trimester ♀ M
AHA: 4Q 2016, 50

O14.94 Unspecified pre-eclampsia, complicating childbirth ♀ M
AHA: 4Q 2016, 50

O14.95 Unspecified pre-eclampsia, complicating the puerperium ♀ M
AHA: 4Q 2016, 50

O15 Eclampsia

INCLUDES convulsions following conditions in O10-O14 and O16
AHA: 4Q 2016, 50

O15.0 Eclampsia complicating pregnancy
AHA: 4Q 2016, 50

O15.00 Eclampsia complicating pregnancy, unspecified trimester ♀ M
AHA: 4Q 2016, 50

O15.02 Eclampsia complicating pregnancy, second trimester ♀ M
AHA: 4Q 2016, 50

O15.03 Eclampsia complicating pregnancy, third trimester ♀ M
AHA: 4Q 2016, 50

O15.1 Eclampsia complicating labor ♀ M

AHA: 4Q 2016, 50

O15.2 Eclampsia complicating the puerperium ♀M
AHA: 4Q 2016, 50

O15.9 Eclampsia, unspecified as to time period ♀M
Eclampsia NOS
AHA: 4Q 2016, 50

4 O16 Unspecified maternal hypertension
AHA: 4Q 2016, 50

O16.1 Unspecified maternal hypertension, first trimester ♀M

O16.2 Unspecified maternal hypertension, second trimester ♀M

O16.3 Unspecified maternal hypertension, third trimester ♀M

O16.4 Unspecified maternal hypertension, complicating childbirth ♀M

O16.5 Unspecified maternal hypertension, complicating the puerperium ♀M

O16.9 Unspecified maternal hypertension, unspecified trimester ♀M

Other maternal disorders predominantly related to pregnancy (O20-O29)

EXCLUDES 2 *maternal care related to the fetus and amniotic cavity and possible delivery problems (O30-O48)*
maternal diseases classifiable elsewhere but complicating pregnancy, labor and delivery, and the puerperium (O98-O99)

4 O20 Hemorrhage in early pregnancy
INCLUDES hemorrhage before completion of 20 weeks gestation
EXCLUDES 1 *pregnancy with abortive outcome (O00-O08)*

O20.0 Threatened abortion ♀M
Hemorrhage specified as due to threatened abortion

O20.8 Other hemorrhage in early pregnancy ♀M

O20.9 Hemorrhage in early pregnancy, unspecified ♀M

4 O21 Excessive vomiting in pregnancy

O21.0 Mild hyperemesis gravidarum ♀M
Hyperemesis gravidarum, mild or unspecified, starting before the end of the 20th week of gestation

O21.1 Hyperemesis gravidarum with metabolic disturbance ♀M
Hyperemesis gravidarum, starting before the end of the 20th week of gestation, with metabolic disturbance such as carbohydrate depletion
Hyperemesis gravidarum, starting before the end of the 20th week of gestation, with metabolic disturbance such as dehydration
Hyperemesis gravidarum, starting before the end of the 20th week of gestation, with metabolic disturbance such as electrolyte imbalance

O21.2 Late vomiting of pregnancy ♀M
Excessive vomiting starting after 20 completed weeks of gestation

O21.8 Other vomiting complicating pregnancy ♀M
Vomiting due to diseases classified elsewhere, complicating pregnancy
Use additional code, to identify cause.

O21.9 Vomiting of pregnancy, unspecified ♀M

4 O22 Venous complications and hemorrhoids in pregnancy
EXCLUDES 1 *venous complications of:*
abortion NOS (O03.9)
ectopic or molar pregnancy (O08.7)
failed attempted abortion (O07.35)
induced abortion (O04.85)
spontaneous abortion (O03.89)
EXCLUDES 2 *obstetric pulmonary embolism (O88.-)*
venous complications and hemorrhoids of childbirth and the puerperium (O87.-)

5 O22.0 Varicose veins of lower extremity in pregnancy
Varicose veins NOS in pregnancy

O22.00 Varicose veins of lower extremity in pregnancy, unspecified trimester ♀M

O22.01 Varicose veins of lower extremity in pregnancy, first trimester ♀M

O22.02 Varicose veins of lower extremity in pregnancy, second trimester ♀M

O22.03 Varicose veins of lower extremity in pregnancy, third trimester ♀M

5 O22.1 Genital varices in pregnancy
Perineal varices in pregnancy
Vaginal varices in pregnancy
Vulval varices in pregnancy

O22.10 Genital varices in pregnancy, unspecified trimester ♀M

O22.11 Genital varices in pregnancy, first trimester ♀M

O22.12 Genital varices in pregnancy, second trimester ♀M

O22.13 Genital varices in pregnancy, third trimester ♀M

5 O22.2 Superficial thrombophlebitis in pregnancy
Phlebitis in pregnancy NOS
Thrombophlebitis of legs in pregnancy
Thrombosis in pregnancy NOS
Use additional code to identify the superficial thrombophlebitis (I80.0-)

O22.20 Superficial thrombophlebitis in pregnancy, unspecified trimester ♀M

O22.21 Superficial thrombophlebitis in pregnancy, first trimester ♀M

O22.22 Superficial thrombophlebitis in pregnancy, second trimester ♀M

O22.23 Superficial thrombophlebitis in pregnancy, third trimester ♀M

5 O22.3 Deep phlebothrombosis in pregnancy
Deep vein thrombosis, antepartum
Use additional code to identify the deep vein thrombosis (I82.4-, I82.5-, I82.62-. I82.72-)
Use additional code, if applicable, for associated long-term (current) use of anticoagulants (Z79.01)

O22.30 Deep phlebothrombosis in pregnancy, unspecified trimester ♀M

O22.31 Deep phlebothrombosis in pregnancy, first trimester ♀M

O22.32 Deep phlebothrombosis in pregnancy, second trimester ♀M

O22.33 Deep phlebothrombosis in pregnancy, third trimester ♀M

5 O22.4 Hemorrhoids in pregnancy

O22.40 Hemorrhoids in pregnancy, unspecified trimester ♀M

O22.41 Hemorrhoids in pregnancy, first trimester ♀M

O22.42 Hemorrhoids in pregnancy, second trimester ♀M

O22.43 Hemorrhoids in pregnancy, third trimester ♀M

5 O22.5 Cerebral venous thrombosis in pregnancy
Cerebrovenous sinus thrombosis in pregnancy

O22.50 Cerebral venous thrombosis in pregnancy, unspecified trimester ♀M

O22.51 Cerebral venous thrombosis in pregnancy, first trimester ♀M

O22.52 Cerebral venous thrombosis in pregnancy, second trimester ♀M

O22.53 Cerebral venous thrombosis in pregnancy, third trimester ♀M

5 O22.8 Other venous complications in pregnancy

6 O22.8X Other venous complications in pregnancy

O22.8X1 Other venous complications in pregnancy, first trimester ♀M

O22.8X2 Other venous complications in pregnancy, second trimester ♀M

O22.8X3 Other venous complications in pregnancy, third trimester ♀M

O22.8X9 Other venous complications in pregnancy, unspecified trimester ♀M

5 O22.9 Venous complication in pregnancy, unspecified
Gestational phlebitis NOS
Gestational phlebopathy NOS
Gestational thrombosis NOS

O22.90 Venous complication in pregnancy, unspecified, unspecified trimester ♀M

O22.91 Venous complication in pregnancy, unspecified, first trimester ♀M

O22.92 Venous complication in pregnancy, unspecified, second trimester ♀M

O22.93 Venous complication in pregnancy, unspecified, third trimester ♀M

O23 Infections of genitourinary tract in pregnancy

Use additional code to identify organism (B95.-, B96.-)

EXCLUDES 2 *gonococcal infections complicating pregnancy, childbirth and the puerperium (O98.2)*
infections with a predominantly sexual mode of transmission NOS complicating pregnancy, childbirth and the puerperium (O98.3)
syphilis complicating pregnancy, childbirth and the puerperium (O98.1)
tuberculosis of genitourinary system complicating pregnancy, childbirth and the puerperium (O98.0)
venereal disease NOS complicating pregnancy, childbirth and the puerperium (O98.3)

O23.0 Infections of kidney in pregnancy
Pyelonephritis in pregnancy

O23.00 Infections of kidney in pregnancy, unspecified trimester ♀
O23.01 Infections of kidney in pregnancy, first trimester ♀
O23.02 Infections of kidney in pregnancy, second trimester ♀
O23.03 Infections of kidney in pregnancy, third trimester ♀

O23.1 Infections of bladder in pregnancy

O23.10 Infections of bladder in pregnancy, unspecified trimester ♀
O23.11 Infections of bladder in pregnancy, first trimester ♀
O23.12 Infections of bladder in pregnancy, second trimester ♀
O23.13 Infections of bladder in pregnancy, third trimester ♀

O23.2 Infections of urethra in pregnancy

O23.20 Infections of urethra in pregnancy, unspecified trimester ♀
O23.21 Infections of urethra in pregnancy, first trimester ♀
O23.22 Infections of urethra in pregnancy, second trimester ♀
O23.23 Infections of urethra in pregnancy, third trimester ♀

O23.3 Infections of other parts of urinary tract in pregnancy

O23.30 Infections of other parts of urinary tract in pregnancy, unspecified trimester ♀
O23.31 Infections of other parts of urinary tract in pregnancy, first trimester ♀
O23.32 Infections of other parts of urinary tract in pregnancy, second trimester ♀
O23.33 Infections of other parts of urinary tract in pregnancy, third trimester ♀

O23.4 Unspecified infection of urinary tract in pregnancy

O23.40 Unspecified infection of urinary tract in pregnancy, unspecified trimester ♀
O23.41 Unspecified infection of urinary tract in pregnancy, first trimester ♀
O23.42 Unspecified infection of urinary tract in pregnancy, second trimester ♀
O23.43 Unspecified infection of urinary tract in pregnancy, third trimester ♀
AHA: 2Q 2018, 15

O23.5 Infections of the genital tract in pregnancy

O23.51 Infection of cervix in pregnancy

O23.511 Infections of cervix in pregnancy, first trimester ♀
O23.512 Infections of cervix in pregnancy, second trimester ♀
O23.513 Infections of cervix in pregnancy, third trimester ♀
O23.519 Infections of cervix in pregnancy, unspecified trimester ♀

O23.52 Salpingo-oophoritis in pregnancy
Oophoritis in pregnancy
Salpingitis in pregnancy

O23.521 Salpingo-oophoritis in pregnancy, first trimester ♀
O23.522 Salpingo-oophoritis in pregnancy, second trimester ♀
O23.523 Salpingo-oophoritis in pregnancy, third trimester ♀
O23.529 Salpingo-oophoritis in pregnancy, unspecified trimester ♀

O23.59 Infection of other part of genital tract in pregnancy

O23.591 Infection of other part of genital tract in pregnancy, first trimester ♀
O23.592 Infection of other part of genital tract in pregnancy, second trimester ♀
O23.593 Infection of other part of genital tract in pregnancy, third trimester ♀
O23.599 Infection of other part of genital tract in pregnancy, unspecified trimester ♀

O23.9 Unspecified genitourinary tract infection in pregnancy
Genitourinary tract infection in pregnancy NOS

O23.90 Unspecified genitourinary tract infection in pregnancy, unspecified trimester ♀
O23.91 Unspecified genitourinary tract infection in pregnancy, first trimester ♀
O23.92 Unspecified genitourinary tract infection in pregnancy, second trimester ♀
O23.93 Unspecified genitourinary tract infection in pregnancy, third trimester ♀

O24 Diabetes mellitus in pregnancy, childbirth, and the puerperium

GUIDELINES **Section I.C.15.g-h**

Diabetes mellitus is a significant complicating factor in pregnancy. Pregnant women who are diabetic should be assigned a code from category O24, Diabetes mellitus in pregnancy, childbirth, and the puerperium, first, followed by the appropriate diabetes code(s) (E08-E13) from Chapter 4. An additional code should be assigned from category Z79 to identify the long-term (current) use of insulin or oral hypoglycemic drugs. If the patient is treated with both oral medications and insulin, only the code for long-term (current) use of insulin should be assigned. Code Z79.4 should not be assigned if insulin is given temporarily to bring a type 2 patient's blood sugar under control during an encounter.

CODING TIP ✓ For an obstetric patient who had pre-existing diabetes before pregnancy, assign the appropriate code from category O24.0, O24.1, O24.3 or O24.8. Use the appropriate code from categories E08-E13 to identify the type and any manifestations.

O24.0 Pre-existing type 1 diabetes mellitus, in pregnancy, childbirth and the puerperium
Juvenile onset diabetes mellitus, in pregnancy, childbirth and the puerperium
Ketosis-prone diabetes mellitus in pregnancy, childbirth and the puerperium
Use additional code from category E10 to further identify any manifestations

O24.01 Pre-existing type 1 diabetes mellitus, in pregnancy

O24.011 Pre-existing type 1 diabetes mellitus, in pregnancy, first trimester ♀
O24.012 Pre-existing type 1 diabetes mellitus, in pregnancy, second trimester ♀
O24.013 Pre-existing type 1 diabetes mellitus, in pregnancy, third trimester ♀
O24.019 Pre-existing type 1 diabetes mellitus, in pregnancy, unspecified trimester ♀

O24.02 Pre-existing type 1 diabetes mellitus, in childbirth ♀
O24.03 Pre-existing type 1 diabetes mellitus, in the puerperium ♀

O24.1 Pre-existing type 2 diabetes mellitus, in pregnancy, childbirth and the puerperium
Insulin-resistant diabetes mellitus in pregnancy, childbirth and the puerperium
Use additional code (for):
from category E11 to further identify any manifestations
long-term (current) use of insulin (Z79.4)

O24.11 Pre-existing type 2 diabetes mellitus, in pregnancy

O24.111 Pre-existing type 2 diabetes mellitus, in pregnancy, first trimester ♀
O24.112 Pre-existing type 2 diabetes mellitus, in pregnancy, second trimester ♀

O24.113 **Pre-existing type 2 diabetes mellitus, in pregnancy, third trimester** ♀M

O24.119 **Pre-existing type 2 diabetes mellitus, in pregnancy, unspecified trimester** ♀M

O24.12 **Pre-existing type 2 diabetes mellitus, in childbirth** ♀M

O24.13 **Pre-existing type 2 diabetes mellitus, in the puerperium** ♀M

5 O24.3 **Unspecified pre-existing diabetes mellitus in pregnancy, childbirth and the puerperium**

Use additional code (for):

from category E11 to further identify any manifestation

long-term (current) use of insulin (Z79.4)

6 O24.31 **Unspecified pre-existing diabetes mellitus in pregnancy**

O24.311 **Unspecified pre-existing diabetes mellitus in pregnancy, first trimester** ♀M

O24.312 **Unspecified pre-existing diabetes mellitus in pregnancy, second trimester** ♀M

O24.313 **Unspecified pre-existing diabetes mellitus in pregnancy, third trimester** ♀M

O24.319 **Unspecified pre-existing diabetes mellitus in pregnancy, unspecified trimester** ♀M

O24.32 **Unspecified pre-existing diabetes mellitus in childbirth** ♀M

O24.33 **Unspecified pre-existing diabetes mellitus in the puerperium** ♀M

5 O24.4 **Gestational diabetes mellitus**

Diabetes mellitus arising in pregnancy

Gestational diabetes mellitus NOS

GUIDELINES **Section I.C.15.i**

Gestational (pregnancy induced) diabetes can occur during the second and third trimester of pregnancy in women who were not diabetic prior to pregnancy. Gestational diabetes can cause complications in the pregnancy similar to those of pre-existing diabetes mellitus. It also puts the woman at greater risk of developing diabetes after the pregnancy. Codes for gestational diabetes are in subcategory O24.4, Gestational diabetes mellitus. No other code from category O24, Diabetes mellitus in pregnancy, childbirth, and the puerperium, should be used with a code from O24.4.

The codes under subcategory O24.4 include diet controlled, insulin controlled, and controlled by oral hypoglycemic drugs. If a patient with gestational diabetes is treated with both diet and insulin, only the code for insulin-controlled is required. If a patient with gestational diabetes is treated with both diet and oral hypoglycemic medications, only the code for "controlled by oral hypoglycemic drugs" is required.

An abnormal glucose tolerance in pregnancy is assigned a code from subcategory O99.81, Abnormal glucose complicating pregnancy, childbirth, and the puerperium.

CODING TIP ✓ Do not use O24.4 if diabetes persists after pregnancy. Use E08 -E13 code.

AHA: 4Q 2016, 50

6 O24.41 **Gestational diabetes mellitus in pregnancy**

O24.410 **Gestational diabetes mellitus in pregnancy, diet controlled** ♀M

O24.414 **Gestational diabetes mellitus in pregnancy, insulin controlled** ♀M

O24.415 **Gestational diabetes mellitus in pregnancy, controlled by oral hypoglycemic drugs** ♀M

Gestational diabetes mellitus in pregnancy, controlled by oral antidiabetic drugs

O24.419 **Gestational diabetes mellitus in pregnancy, unspecified control** ♀M

AHA: 4Q 2015, 34

6 O24.42 **Gestational diabetes mellitus in childbirth**

O24.420 **Gestational diabetes mellitus in childbirth, diet controlled** ♀M

O24.424 **Gestational diabetes mellitus in childbirth, insulin controlled** ♀M

O24.425 **Gestational diabetes mellitus in childbirth, controlled by oral hypoglycemic drugs** ♀M

Gestational diabetes mellitus in childbirth, controlled by oral antidiabetic drugs

O24.429 **Gestational diabetes mellitus in childbirth, unspecified control** ♀M

6 O24.43 **Gestational diabetes mellitus in the puerperium**

O24.430 **Gestational diabetes mellitus in the puerperium, diet controlled** ♀M

O24.434 **Gestational diabetes mellitus in the puerperium, insulin controlled** ♀M

O24.435 **Gestational diabetes mellitus in puerperium, controlled by oral hypoglycemic drugs** ♀M

Gestational diabetes mellitus in puerperium, controlled by oral antidiabetic drugs

O24.439 **Gestational diabetes mellitus in the puerperium, unspecified control** ♀M

5 O24.8 **Other pre-existing diabetes mellitus in pregnancy, childbirth, and the puerperium**

Use additional code (for):

from categories E08, E09 and E13 to further identify any manifestation

long-term (current) use of insulin (Z79.4)

6 O24.81 **Other pre-existing diabetes mellitus in pregnancy**

O24.811 **Other pre-existing diabetes mellitus in pregnancy, first trimester** ♀M

O24.812 **Other pre-existing diabetes mellitus in pregnancy, second trimester** ♀M

O24.813 **Other pre-existing diabetes mellitus in pregnancy, third trimester** ♀M

O24.819 **Other pre-existing diabetes mellitus in pregnancy, unspecified trimester** ♀M

O24.82 **Other pre-existing diabetes mellitus in childbirth** ♀M

O24.83 **Other pre-existing diabetes mellitus in the puerperium** ♀M

5 O24.9 **Unspecified diabetes mellitus in pregnancy, childbirth and the puerperium**

Use additional code for long-term (current) use of insulin (Z79.4)

6 O24.91 **Unspecified diabetes mellitus in pregnancy**

O24.911 **Unspecified diabetes mellitus in pregnancy, first trimester** ♀M

O24.912 **Unspecified diabetes mellitus in pregnancy, second trimester** ♀M

O24.913 **Unspecified diabetes mellitus in pregnancy, third trimester** ♀M

O24.919 **Unspecified diabetes mellitus in pregnancy, unspecified trimester** ♀M

O24.92 **Unspecified diabetes mellitus in childbirth** ♀M

O24.93 **Unspecified diabetes mellitus in the puerperium** ♀M

4 O25 Malnutrition in pregnancy, childbirth and the puerperium

5 O25.1 **Malnutrition in pregnancy**

O25.10 **Malnutrition in pregnancy, unspecified trimester** ♀M

O25.11 **Malnutrition in pregnancy, first trimester** ♀M

O25.12 **Malnutrition in pregnancy, second trimester** ♀M

O25.13 **Malnutrition in pregnancy, third trimester** ♀M

O25.2 **Malnutrition in childbirth** ♀M

O25.3 **Malnutrition in the puerperium** ♀M

4 O26 Maternal care for other conditions predominantly related to pregnancy

5 O26.0 **Excessive weight gain in pregnancy**

EXCLUDES 2 *gestational edema (O12.0, O12.2)*

O26.00 **Excessive weight gain in pregnancy, unspecified trimester** ♀M

O26.01 **Excessive weight gain in pregnancy, first trimester** ♀M

O26.02 **Excessive weight gain in pregnancy, second trimester** ♀M

O26.03 **Excessive weight gain in pregnancy, third trimester** ♀M

5 O26.1 **Low weight gain in pregnancy**

O26.10 **Low weight gain in pregnancy, unspecified trimester** ♀M

O26.11 **Low weight gain in pregnancy, first trimester** ♀M

O26.12 Low weight gain in pregnancy, second trimester ♀M
O26.13 Low weight gain in pregnancy, third trimester ♀M

5 O26.2 Pregnancy care for patient with recurrent pregnancy loss
O26.20 Pregnancy care for patient with recurrent pregnancy loss, unspecified trimester ♀M
O26.21 Pregnancy care for patient with recurrent pregnancy loss, first trimester ♀M
O26.22 Pregnancy care for patient with recurrent pregnancy loss, second trimester ♀M
O26.23 Pregnancy care for patient with recurrent pregnancy loss, third trimester ♀M

5 O26.3 Retained intrauterine contraceptive device in pregnancy
O26.30 Retained intrauterine contraceptive device in pregnancy, unspecified trimester ♀M
O26.31 Retained intrauterine contraceptive device in pregnancy, first trimester ♀M
O26.32 Retained intrauterine contraceptive device in pregnancy, second trimester ♀M
O26.33 Retained intrauterine contraceptive device in pregnancy, third trimester ♀M

5 O26.4 Herpes gestationis
O26.40 Herpes gestationis, unspecified trimester ♀M
O26.41 Herpes gestationis, first trimester ♀M
O26.42 Herpes gestationis, second trimester ♀M
O26.43 Herpes gestationis, third trimester ♀M

5 O26.5 Maternal hypotension syndrome
Supine hypotensive syndrome
O26.50 Maternal hypotension syndrome, unspecified trimester ♀M
O26.51 Maternal hypotension syndrome, first trimester ♀M
O26.52 Maternal hypotension syndrome, second trimester ♀M
O26.53 Maternal hypotension syndrome, third trimester ♀M

5 O26.6 Liver and biliary tract disorders in pregnancy, childbirth and the puerperium
Use additional code to identify the specific disorder
EXCLUDES 2 *hepatorenal syndrome following labor and delivery (O90.4)*

6 O26.61 Liver and biliary tract disorders in pregnancy
O26.611 Liver and biliary tract disorders in pregnancy, first trimester ♀M
O26.612 Liver and biliary tract disorders in pregnancy, second trimester ♀M
O26.613 Liver and biliary tract disorders in pregnancy, third trimester ♀M
O26.619 Liver and biliary tract disorders in pregnancy, unspecified trimester ♀M
O26.62 Liver and biliary tract disorders in childbirth ♀M
O26.63 Liver and biliary tract disorders in the puerperium ♀M

5 O26.7 Subluxation of symphysis (pubis) in pregnancy, childbirth and the puerperium
EXCLUDES 1 *traumatic separation of symphysis (pubis) during childbirth (O71.6)*

6 O26.71 Subluxation of symphysis (pubis) in pregnancy
O26.711 Subluxation of symphysis (pubis) in pregnancy, first trimester ♀M
O26.712 Subluxation of symphysis (pubis) in pregnancy, second trimester ♀M
O26.713 Subluxation of symphysis (pubis) in pregnancy, third trimester ♀M
O26.719 Subluxation of symphysis (pubis) in pregnancy, unspecified trimester ♀M
O26.72 Subluxation of symphysis (pubis) in childbirth ♀M
O26.73 Subluxation of symphysis (pubis) in the puerperium ♀M

5 O26.8 Other specified pregnancy related conditions

6 O26.81 Pregnancy related exhaustion and fatigue
O26.811 Pregnancy related exhaustion and fatigue, first trimester ♀M
O26.812 Pregnancy related exhaustion and fatigue, second trimester ♀M
O26.813 Pregnancy related exhaustion and fatigue, third trimester ♀M
O26.819 Pregnancy related exhaustion and fatigue, unspecified trimester ♀M

6 O26.82 Pregnancy related peripheral neuritis
O26.821 Pregnancy related peripheral neuritis, first trimester ♀M
O26.822 Pregnancy related peripheral neuritis, second trimester ♀M
O26.823 Pregnancy related peripheral neuritis, third trimester ♀M
O26.829 Pregnancy related peripheral neuritis, unspecified trimester ♀M

6 O26.83 Pregnancy related renal disease
Use additional code to identify the specific disorder
O26.831 Pregnancy related renal disease, first trimester ♀M
O26.832 Pregnancy related renal disease, second trimester ♀M
O26.833 Pregnancy related renal disease, third trimester ♀M
O26.839 Pregnancy related renal disease, unspecified trimester ♀M

6 O26.84 Uterine size-date discrepancy complicating pregnancy
EXCLUDES 1 *encounter for suspected problem with fetal growth ruled out (Z03.74)*
O26.841 Uterine size-date discrepancy, first trimester ♀M
O26.842 Uterine size-date discrepancy, second trimester ♀M
O26.843 Uterine size-date discrepancy, third trimester ♀M
O26.849 Uterine size-date discrepancy, unspecified trimester ♀M

6 O26.85 Spotting complicating pregnancy
O26.851 Spotting complicating pregnancy, first trimester ♀M
O26.852 Spotting complicating pregnancy, second trimester ♀M
O26.853 Spotting complicating pregnancy, third trimester ♀M
O26.859 Spotting complicating pregnancy, unspecified trimester ♀M

O26.86 Pruritic urticarial papules and plaques of pregnancy (PUPPP) ♀M
Polymorphic eruption of pregnancy

6 O26.87 Cervical shortening
EXCLUDES 1 *encounter for suspected cervical shortening ruled out (Z03.75)*
O26.872 Cervical shortening, second trimester ♀M
DEFINITION Sonographic evidence of a cervix shortened to 2.5 cm or less in the second trimester; a warning of impending premature birth in women with a prior history of early delivery.
O26.873 Cervical shortening, third trimester ♀M
O26.879 Cervical shortening, unspecified trimester ♀M

6 O26.89 Other specified pregnancy related conditions
O26.891 Other specified pregnancy related conditions, first trimester ♀M
O26.892 Other specified pregnancy related conditions, second trimester ♀M
O26.893 Other specified pregnancy related conditions, third trimester ♀M
AHA: 3Q 2015, 40
O26.899 Other specified pregnancy related conditions, unspecified trimester ♀M

5 O26.9 Pregnancy related conditions, unspecified
O26.90 Pregnancy related conditions, unspecified, unspecified trimester ♀M
O26.91 Pregnancy related conditions, unspecified, first trimester ♀M
O26.92 Pregnancy related conditions, unspecified, second trimester ♀M
O26.93 Pregnancy related conditions, unspecified, third trimester ♀M

4 O28 Abnormal findings on antenatal screening of mother
EXCLUDES 1 *diagnostic findings classified elsewhere - see Alphabetical Index*
O28.0 Abnormal hematological finding on antenatal screening of mother ♀M
O28.1 Abnormal biochemical finding on antenatal screening of mother ♀M

O28.2 Abnormal cytological finding on antenatal screening of mother
O28.3 Abnormal ultrasonic finding on antenatal screening of mother
O28.4 Abnormal radiological finding on antenatal screening of mother
O28.5 Abnormal chromosomal and genetic finding on antenatal screening of mother
O28.8 Other abnormal findings on antenatal screening of mother
O28.9 Unspecified abnormal findings on antenatal screening of mother

O29 Complications of anesthesia during pregnancy

INCLUDES maternal complications arising from the administration of a general, regional or local anesthetic, analgesic or other sedation during pregnancy

Use additional code, if necessary, to identify the complication

EXCLUDES 2 *complications of anesthesia during labor and delivery (O74.-)*
complications of anesthesia during the puerperium (O89.-)

O29.0 Pulmonary complications of anesthesia during pregnancy
O29.01 Aspiration pneumonitis due to anesthesia during pregnancy
Inhalation of stomach contents or secretions NOS due to anesthesia during pregnancy
Mendelson's syndrome due to anesthesia during pregnancy
O29.011 Aspiration pneumonitis due to anesthesia during pregnancy, first trimester
O29.012 Aspiration pneumonitis due to anesthesia during pregnancy, second trimester
O29.013 Aspiration pneumonitis due to anesthesia during pregnancy, third trimester
O29.019 Aspiration pneumonitis due to anesthesia during pregnancy, unspecified trimester
O29.02 Pressure collapse of lung due to anesthesia during pregnancy
O29.021 Pressure collapse of lung due to anesthesia during pregnancy, first trimester
O29.022 Pressure collapse of lung due to anesthesia during pregnancy, second trimester
O29.023 Pressure collapse of lung due to anesthesia during pregnancy, third trimester
O29.029 Pressure collapse of lung due to anesthesia during pregnancy, unspecified trimester
O29.09 Other pulmonary complications of anesthesia during pregnancy
O29.091 Other pulmonary complications of anesthesia during pregnancy, first trimester
O29.092 Other pulmonary complications of anesthesia during pregnancy, second trimester
O29.093 Other pulmonary complications of anesthesia during pregnancy, third trimester
O29.099 Other pulmonary complications of anesthesia during pregnancy, unspecified trimester
O29.1 Cardiac complications of anesthesia during pregnancy
O29.11 Cardiac arrest due to anesthesia during pregnancy
O29.111 Cardiac arrest due to anesthesia during pregnancy, first trimester
O29.112 Cardiac arrest due to anesthesia during pregnancy, second trimester
O29.113 Cardiac arrest due to anesthesia during pregnancy, third trimester
O29.119 Cardiac arrest due to anesthesia during pregnancy, unspecified trimester
O29.12 Cardiac failure due to anesthesia during pregnancy
O29.121 Cardiac failure due to anesthesia during pregnancy, first trimester
O29.122 Cardiac failure due to anesthesia during pregnancy, second trimester
O29.123 Cardiac failure due to anesthesia during pregnancy, third trimester
O29.129 Cardiac failure due to anesthesia during pregnancy, unspecified trimester
O29.19 Other cardiac complications of anesthesia during pregnancy
O29.191 Other cardiac complications of anesthesia during pregnancy, first trimester
O29.192 Other cardiac complications of anesthesia during pregnancy, second trimester
O29.193 Other cardiac complications of anesthesia during pregnancy, third trimester
O29.199 Other cardiac complications of anesthesia during pregnancy, unspecified trimester
O29.2 Central nervous system complications of anesthesia during pregnancy
O29.21 Cerebral anoxia due to anesthesia during pregnancy
O29.211 Cerebral anoxia due to anesthesia during pregnancy, first trimester
O29.212 Cerebral anoxia due to anesthesia during pregnancy, second trimester
O29.213 Cerebral anoxia due to anesthesia during pregnancy, third trimester
O29.219 Cerebral anoxia due to anesthesia during pregnancy, unspecified trimester
O29.29 Other central nervous system complications of anesthesia during pregnancy
O29.291 Other central nervous system complications of anesthesia during pregnancy, first trimester
O29.292 Other central nervous system complications of anesthesia during pregnancy, second trimester
O29.293 Other central nervous system complications of anesthesia during pregnancy, third trimester
O29.299 Other central nervous system complications of anesthesia during pregnancy, unspecified trimester
O29.3 Toxic reaction to local anesthesia during pregnancy
O29.3X Toxic reaction to local anesthesia during pregnancy
O29.3X1 Toxic reaction to local anesthesia during pregnancy, first trimester
O29.3X2 Toxic reaction to local anesthesia during pregnancy, second trimester
O29.3X3 Toxic reaction to local anesthesia during pregnancy, third trimester
O29.3X9 Toxic reaction to local anesthesia during pregnancy, unspecified trimester
O29.4 Spinal and epidural anesthesia induced headache during pregnancy
O29.40 Spinal and epidural anesthesia induced headache during pregnancy, unspecified trimester
O29.41 Spinal and epidural anesthesia induced headache during pregnancy, first trimester
O29.42 Spinal and epidural anesthesia induced headache during pregnancy, second trimester
O29.43 Spinal and epidural anesthesia induced headache during pregnancy, third trimester
O29.5 Other complications of spinal and epidural anesthesia during pregnancy
O29.5X Other complications of spinal and epidural anesthesia during pregnancy
O29.5X1 Other complications of spinal and epidural anesthesia during pregnancy, first trimester
O29.5X2 Other complications of spinal and epidural anesthesia during pregnancy, second trimester
O29.5X3 Other complications of spinal and epidural anesthesia during pregnancy, third trimester
O29.5X9 Other complications of spinal and epidural anesthesia during pregnancy, unspecified trimester
O29.6 Failed or difficult intubation for anesthesia during pregnancy
O29.60 Failed or difficult intubation for anesthesia during pregnancy, unspecified trimester
O29.61 Failed or difficult intubation for anesthesia during pregnancy, first trimester

O29.62 Failed or difficult intubation for anesthesia during pregnancy, second trimester ♀M

O29.63 Failed or difficult intubation for anesthesia during pregnancy, third trimester ♀M

5 O29.8 Other complications of anesthesia during pregnancy

6 O29.8X Other complications of anesthesia during pregnancy

O29.8X1 Other complications of anesthesia during pregnancy, first trimester ♀M

O29.8X2 Other complications of anesthesia during pregnancy, second trimester ♀M

O29.8X3 Other complications of anesthesia during pregnancy, third trimester ♀M

O29.8X9 Other complications of anesthesia during pregnancy, unspecified trimester ♀M

5 O29.9 Unspecified complication of anesthesia during pregnancy

O29.90 Unspecified complication of anesthesia during pregnancy, unspecified trimester ♀M

O29.91 Unspecified complication of anesthesia during pregnancy, first trimester ♀M

O29.92 Unspecified complication of anesthesia during pregnancy, second trimester ♀M

O29.93 Unspecified complication of anesthesia during pregnancy, third trimester ♀M

Maternal care related to the fetus and amniotic cavity and possible delivery problems (O30-O48)

4 O30 Multiple gestation

Code also:
any complications specific to multiple gestation

5 O30.0 Twin pregnancy

6 O30.00 Twin pregnancy, unspecified number of placenta and unspecified number of amniotic sacs

O30.001 Twin pregnancy, unspecified number of placenta and unspecified number of amniotic sacs, first trimester ♀M

O30.002 Twin pregnancy, unspecified number of placenta and unspecified number of amniotic sacs, second trimester ♀M

O30.003 Twin pregnancy, unspecified number of placenta and unspecified number of amniotic sacs, third trimester ♀M

O30.009 Twin pregnancy, unspecified number of placenta and unspecified number of amniotic sacs, unspecified trimester ♀M

6 O30.01 Twin pregnancy, monochorionic/monoamniotic

Twin pregnancy, one placenta, one amniotic sac

EXCLUDES 1 *conjoined twins (O30.02-)*

O30.011 Twin pregnancy, monochorionic/monoamniotic, first trimester ♀M

O30.012 Twin pregnancy, monochorionic/monoamniotic, second trimester ♀M

O30.013 Twin pregnancy, monochorionic/monoamniotic, third trimester ♀M

O30.019 Twin pregnancy, monochorionic/monoamniotic, unspecified trimester ♀M

6 O30.02 Conjoined twin pregnancy

O30.021 Conjoined twin pregnancy, first trimester ♀M

O30.022 Conjoined twin pregnancy, second trimester ♀M

O30.023 Conjoined twin pregnancy, third trimester ♀M

O30.029 Conjoined twin pregnancy, unspecified trimester ♀M

6 O30.03 Twin pregnancy, monochorionic/diamniotic

Twin pregnancy, one placenta, two amniotic sacs

O30.031 Twin pregnancy, monochorionic/diamniotic, first trimester ♀M

O30.032 Twin pregnancy, monochorionic/diamniotic, second trimester ♀M

O30.033 Twin pregnancy, monochorionic/diamniotic, third trimester ♀M

O30.039 Twin pregnancy, monochorionic/diamniotic, unspecified trimester ♀M

6 O30.04 Twin pregnancy, dichorionic/diamniotic

Twin pregnancy, two placentae, two amniotic sacs

O30.041 Twin pregnancy, dichorionic/diamniotic, first trimester ♀M

O30.042 Twin pregnancy, dichorionic/diamniotic, second trimester ♀M

O30.043 Twin pregnancy, dichorionic/diamniotic, third trimester ♀M

O30.049 Twin pregnancy, dichorionic/diamniotic, unspecified trimester ♀M

6 O30.09 Twin pregnancy, unable to determine number of placenta and number of amniotic sacs

O30.091 Twin pregnancy, unable to determine number of placenta and number of amniotic sacs, first trimester ♀M

O30.092 Twin pregnancy, unable to determine number of placenta and number of amniotic sacs, second trimester ♀M

O30.093 Twin pregnancy, unable to determine number of placenta and number of amniotic sacs, third trimester ♀M

O30.099 Twin pregnancy, unable to determine number of placenta and number of amniotic sacs, unspecified trimester ♀M

5 O30.1 Triplet pregnancy

6 O30.10 Triplet pregnancy, unspecified number of placenta and unspecified number of amniotic sacs

O30.101 Triplet pregnancy, unspecified number of placenta and unspecified number of amniotic sacs, first trimester ♀M

O30.102 Triplet pregnancy, unspecified number of placenta and unspecified number of amniotic sacs, second trimester ♀M

O30.103 Triplet pregnancy, unspecified number of placenta and unspecified number of amniotic sacs, third trimester ♀M

AHA: 2Q 2016, 8

O30.109 Triplet pregnancy, unspecified number of placenta and unspecified number of amniotic sacs, unspecified trimester ♀M

6 O30.11 Triplet pregnancy with two or more monochorionic fetuses

O30.111 Triplet pregnancy with two or more monochorionic fetuses, first trimester ♀M

O30.112 Triplet pregnancy with two or more monochorionic fetuses, second trimester ♀M

O30.113 Triplet pregnancy with two or more monochorionic fetuses, third trimester ♀M

O30.119 Triplet pregnancy with two or more monochorionic fetuses, unspecified trimester ♀M

6 O30.12 Triplet pregnancy with two or more monoamniotic fetuses

O30.121 Triplet pregnancy with two or more monoamniotic fetuses, first trimester ♀M

O30.122 Triplet pregnancy with two or more monoamniotic fetuses, second trimester ♀M

O30.123 Triplet pregnancy with two or more monoamniotic fetuses, third trimester ♀M

O30.129 Triplet pregnancy with two or more monoamniotic fetuses, unspecified trimester ♀M

● 6 O30.13 Triplet pregnancy, trichorionic/triamniotic

● O30.131 Triplet pregnancy, trichorionic/triamniotic, first trimester ♀M

● O30.132 Triplet pregnancy, trichorionic/triamniotic, second trimester ♀M

● O30.133 Triplet pregnancy, trichorionic/triamniotic, third trimester ♀M

● O30.139 Triplet pregnancy, trichorionic/triamniotic, unspecified trimester ♀M

6 O30.19 Triplet pregnancy, unable to determine number of placenta and number of amniotic sacs

O30.191 Triplet pregnancy, unable to determine number of placenta and number of amniotic sacs, first trimester ♀M

O30.192 Triplet pregnancy, unable to determine number of placenta and number of amniotic sacs, second trimester ♀M

O30.193 Triplet pregnancy, unable to determine number of placenta and number of amniotic sacs, third trimester ♀M

O30.199 Triplet pregnancy, unable to determine number of placenta and number of amniotic sacs, unspecified trimester ♀M

5 O30.2 Quadruplet pregnancy

6 O30.20 Quadruplet pregnancy, unspecified number of placenta and unspecified number of amniotic sacs

O30.201 Quadruplet pregnancy, unspecified number of placenta and unspecified number of amniotic sacs, first trimester ♀M

O30.202 Quadruplet pregnancy, unspecified number of placenta and unspecified number of amniotic sacs, second trimester ♀M

O30.203 Quadruplet pregnancy, unspecified number of placenta and unspecified number of amniotic sacs, third trimester ♀M

O30.209 Quadruplet pregnancy, unspecified number of placenta and unspecified number of amniotic sacs, unspecified trimester ♀M

6 O30.21 Quadruplet pregnancy with two or more monochorionic fetuses

O30.211 Quadruplet pregnancy with two or more monochorionic fetuses, first trimester ♀M

O30.212 Quadruplet pregnancy with two or more monochorionic fetuses, second trimester ♀M

O30.213 Quadruplet pregnancy with two or more monochorionic fetuses, third trimester ♀M

O30.219 Quadruplet pregnancy with two or more monochorionic fetuses, unspecified trimester ♀M

6 O30.22 Quadruplet pregnancy with two or more monoamniotic fetuses

O30.221 Quadruplet pregnancy with two or more monoamniotic fetuses, first trimester ♀M

O30.222 Quadruplet pregnancy with two or more monoamniotic fetuses, second trimester ♀M

O30.223 Quadruplet pregnancy with two or more monoamniotic fetuses, third trimester ♀M

O30.229 Quadruplet pregnancy with two or more monoamniotic fetuses, unspecified trimester ♀M

● 6 O30.23 Quadruplet pregnancy, quadrachorionic/quadra-amniotic

● O30.231 Quadruplet pregnancy, quadrachorionic/quadra-amniotic, first trimester ♀M

● O30.232 Quadruplet pregnancy, quadrachorionic/quadra-amniotic, second trimester ♀M

● O30.233 Quadruplet pregnancy, quadrachorionic/quadra-amniotic, third trimester ♀M

● O30.239 Quadruplet pregnancy, quadrachorionic/quadra-amniotic, unspecified trimester ♀M

6 O30.29 Quadruplet pregnancy, unable to determine number of placenta and number of amniotic sacs

O30.291 Quadruplet pregnancy, unable to determine number of placenta and number of amniotic sacs, first trimester ♀M

O30.292 Quadruplet pregnancy, unable to determine number of placenta and number of amniotic sacs, second trimester ♀M

O30.293 Quadruplet pregnancy, unable to determine number of placenta and number of amniotic sacs, third trimester ♀M

O30.299 Quadruplet pregnancy, unable to determine number of placenta and number of amniotic sacs, unspecified trimester ♀M

5 O30.8 Other specified multiple gestation

Multiple gestation pregnancy greater then quadruplets

6 O30.80 Other specified multiple gestation, unspecified number of placenta and unspecified number of amniotic sacs

O30.801 Other specified multiple gestation, unspecified number of placenta and unspecified number of amniotic sacs, first trimester ♀M

O30.802 Other specified multiple gestation, unspecified number of placenta and unspecified number of amniotic sacs, second trimester ♀M

O30.803 Other specified multiple gestation, unspecified number of placenta and unspecified number of amniotic sacs, third trimester ♀M

O30.809 Other specified multiple gestation, unspecified number of placenta and unspecified number of amniotic sacs, unspecified trimester ♀M

6 O30.81 Other specified multiple gestation with two or more monochorionic fetuses

O30.811 Other specified multiple gestation with two or more monochorionic fetuses, first trimester ♀M

O30.812 Other specified multiple gestation with two or more monochorionic fetuses, second trimester ♀M

O30.813 Other specified multiple gestation with two or more monochorionic fetuses, third trimester ♀M

O30.819 Other specified multiple gestation with two or more monochorionic fetuses, unspecified trimester ♀M

6 O30.82 Other specified multiple gestation with two or more monoamniotic fetuses

O30.821 Other specified multiple gestation with two or more monoamniotic fetuses, first trimester ♀M

O30.822 Other specified multiple gestation with two or more monoamniotic fetuses, second trimester ♀M

O30.823 Other specified multiple gestation with two or more monoamniotic fetuses, third trimester ♀M

O30.829 Other specified multiple gestation with two or more monoamniotic fetuses, unspecified trimester ♀M

● 6 O30.83 Other specified multiple gestation, number of chorions and amnions are both equal to the number of fetuses

Pentachorionic, penta-amniotic pregnancy (quintuplets)
Hexachorionic, hexa-amniotic pregnancy (sextuplets)
Heptachorionic, hepta-amniotic pregnancy (septuplets)

● O30.831 Other specified multiple gestation, number of chorions and amnions are both equal to the number of fetuses, first trimester ♀M

● O30.832 Other specified multiple gestation, number of chorions and amnions are both equal to the number of fetuses, second trimester ♀M

● O30.833 Other specified multiple gestation, number of chorions and amnions are both equal to the number of fetuses, third trimester ♀M

● O30.839 Other specified multiple gestation, number of chorions and amnions are both equal to the number of fetuses, unspecified trimester ♀M

6 O30.89 Other specified multiple gestation, unable to determine number of placenta and number of amniotic sacs

O30.891 **Other specified multiple gestation, unable to determine number of placenta and number of amniotic sacs, first trimester** ♀M

O30.892 **Other specified multiple gestation, unable to determine number of placenta and number of amniotic sacs, second trimester** ♀M

O30.893 **Other specified multiple gestation, unable to determine number of placenta and number of amniotic sacs, third trimester** ♀M

O30.899 **Other specified multiple gestation, unable to determine number of placenta and number of amniotic sacs, unspecified trimester** ♀M

5 O30.9 **Multiple gestation, unspecified**

Multiple pregnancy NOS

O30.90 **Multiple gestation, unspecified, unspecified trimester** ♀M

O30.91 **Multiple gestation, unspecified, first trimester** ♀M

O30.92 **Multiple gestation, unspecified, second trimester** ♀M

O30.93 **Multiple gestation, unspecified, third trimester** ♀M

4 O31 Complications specific to multiple gestation

EXCLUDES 2 *delayed delivery of second twin, triplet, etc. (O63.2)*
malpresentation of one fetus or more (O32.9)
placental transfusion syndromes (O43.0-)

One of the following 7th characters is to be assigned to each code under category O31. 7th character 0 is for single gestations and multiple gestations where the fetus is unspecified. 7th characters 1 through 9 are for cases of multiple gestations to identify the fetus for which the code applies. The appropriate code from category O30, Multiple gestation, must also be assigned when assigning a code from category O31 that has a 7th character of 1 through 9.

0 not applicable or unspecified
1 fetus 1
2 fetus 2
3 fetus 3
4 fetus 4
5 fetus 5
9 other fetus

AHA: 4Q 2012, 107-108

5 O31.0 **Papyraceous fetus**

Fetus compressus

7 O31.00X- **Papyraceous fetus, unspecified trimester** ♀M

7 O31.01X- **Papyraceous fetus, first trimester** ♀M

7 O31.02X- **Papyraceous fetus, second trimester** ♀M

7 O31.03X- **Papyraceous fetus, third trimester** ♀M

5 O31.1 **Continuing pregnancy after spontaneous abortion of one fetus or more**

7 O31.10X- **Continuing pregnancy after spontaneous abortion of one fetus or more, unspecified trimester** ♀M

7 O31.11X- **Continuing pregnancy after spontaneous abortion of one fetus or more, first trimester** ♀M

7 O31.12X- **Continuing pregnancy after spontaneous abortion of one fetus or more, second trimester** ♀M

7 O31.13X- **Continuing pregnancy after spontaneous abortion of one fetus or more, third trimester** ♀M

5 O31.2 **Continuing pregnancy after intrauterine death of one fetus or more**

7 O31.20X- **Continuing pregnancy after intrauterine death of one fetus or more, unspecified trimester** ♀M

7 O31.21X- **Continuing pregnancy after intrauterine death of one fetus or more, first trimester** ♀M

7 O31.22X- **Continuing pregnancy after intrauterine death of one fetus or more, second trimester** ♀M

7 O31.23X- **Continuing pregnancy after intrauterine death of one fetus or more, third trimester** ♀M

5 O31.3 **Continuing pregnancy after elective fetal reduction of one fetus or more**

Continuing pregnancy after selective termination of one fetus or more

7 O31.30X- **Continuing pregnancy after elective fetal reduction of one fetus or more, unspecified trimester** ♀M

7 O31.31X- **Continuing pregnancy after elective fetal reduction of one fetus or more, first trimester** ♀M

7 O31.32X- **Continuing pregnancy after elective fetal reduction of one fetus or more, second trimester** ♀M

7 O31.33X- **Continuing pregnancy after elective fetal reduction of one fetus or more, third trimester** ♀M

5 O31.8 **Other complications specific to multiple gestation**

6 O31.8X **Other complications specific to multiple gestation**

7 O31.8X1- **Other complications specific to multiple gestation, first trimester** ♀M

7 O31.8X2- **Other complications specific to multiple gestation, second trimester** ♀M

7 O31.8X3- **Other complications specific to multiple gestation, third trimester** ♀M

7 O31.8X9- **Other complications specific to multiple gestation, unspecified trimester** ♀M

4 O32 Maternal care for malpresentation of fetus

INCLUDES the listed conditions as a reason for observation, hospitalization or other obstetric care of the mother, or for cesarean delivery before onset of labor

EXCLUDES 1 *malpresentation of fetus with obstructed labor (O64.-)*

One of the following 7th characters is to be assigned to each code under category O32. 7th character 0 is for single gestations and multiple gestations where the fetus is unspecified. 7th characters 1 through 9 are for cases of multiple gestations to identify the fetus for which the code applies. The appropriate code from category O30, Multiple gestation, must also be assigned when assigning a code from category O32 that has a 7th character of 1 through 9.

0 not applicable or unspecified
1 fetus 1
2 fetus 2
3 fetus 3
4 fetus 4
5 fetus 5
9 other fetus

AHA: 4Q 2012, 107-108

7 O32.0XX- **Maternal care for unstable lie** ♀M

7 O32.1XX- **Maternal care for breech presentation** ♀M

Maternal care for buttocks presentation
Maternal care for complete breech
Maternal care for frank breech

EXCLUDES 1 *footling presentation (O32.8)*
incomplete breech (O32.8)

7 O32.2XX- **Maternal care for transverse and oblique lie** ♀M

Maternal care for oblique presentation
Maternal care for transverse presentation

7 O32.3XX- **Maternal care for face, brow and chin presentation** ♀M

7 O32.4XX- **Maternal care for high head at term** ♀M

Maternal care for failure of head to enter pelvic brim

7 O32.6XX- **Maternal care for compound presentation** ♀M

7 O32.8XX- **Maternal care for other malpresentation of fetus** ♀M

Maternal care for footling presentation
Maternal care for incomplete breech

7 O32.9XX- **Maternal care for malpresentation of fetus, unspecified** ♀M

4 O33 Maternal care for disproportion

INCLUDES the listed conditions as a reason for observation, hospitalization or other obstetric care of the mother, or for cesarean delivery before onset of labor

EXCLUDES 1 *disproportion with obstructed labor (O65-O66)*

O33.0 **Maternal care for disproportion due to deformity of maternal pelvic bones** ♀M

Maternal care for disproportion due to pelvic deformity causing disproportion NOS

O33.1 **Maternal care for disproportion due to generally contracted pelvis** ♀ M
Maternal care for disproportion due to contracted pelvis NOS causing disproportion

O33.2 **Maternal care for disproportion due to inlet contraction of pelvis** ♀ M
Maternal care for disproportion due to inlet contraction (pelvis) causing disproportion

7 **O33.3XX-** **Maternal care for disproportion due to outlet contraction of pelvis** ♀ M
Maternal care for disproportion due to mid-cavity contraction (pelvis)
Maternal care for disproportion due to outlet contraction (pelvis)

One of the following 7th characters is to be assigned to code O33.3. 7th character 0 is for single gestations and multiple gestations where the fetus is unspecified. 7th characters 1 through 9 are for cases of multiple gestations to identify the fetus for which the code applies. The appropriate code from category O30, Multiple gestation, must also be assigned when assigning code O33.3 with a 7th character of 1 through 9.

0 not applicable or unspecified
1 fetus 1
2 fetus 2
3 fetus 3
4 fetus 4
5 fetus 5
9 other fetus

7 **O33.4XX-** **Maternal care for disproportion of mixed maternal and fetal origin** ♀ M

One of the following 7th characters is to be assigned to code O33.4. 7th character 0 is for single gestations and multiple gestations where the fetus is unspecified. 7th characters 1 through 9 are for cases of multiple gestations to identify the fetus for which the code applies. The appropriate code from category O30, Multiple gestation, must also be assigned when assigning code O33.4 with a 7th character of 1 through 9.

0 not applicable or unspecified
1 fetus 1
2 fetus 2
3 fetus 3
4 fetus 4
5 fetus 5
9 other fetus

7 **O33.5XX-** **Maternal care for disproportion due to unusually large fetus** ♀ M
Maternal care for disproportion due to disproportion of fetal origin with normally formed fetus
Maternal care for disproportion due to fetal disproportion NOS

One of the following 7th characters is to be assigned to code O33.5. 7th character 0 is for single gestations and multiple gestations where the fetus is unspecified. 7th characters 1 through 9 are for cases of multiple gestations to identify the fetus for which the code applies. The appropriate code from category O30, Multiple gestation, must also be assigned when assigning code O33.5 with a 7th character of 1 through 9.

0 not applicable or unspecified
1 fetus 1
2 fetus 2
3 fetus 3
4 fetus 4
5 fetus 5
9 other fetus

7 **O33.6XX-** **Maternal care for disproportion due to hydrocephalic fetus** ♀ M

One of the following 7th characters is to be assigned to code O33.6. 7th character 0 is for single gestations and multiple gestations where the fetus is unspecified. 7th characters 1 through 9 are for cases of multiple gestations to identify the fetus for which the code applies. The appropriate code from category O30, Multiple gestation, must also be assigned when assigning code O33.6 with a 7th character of 1 through 9.

0 not applicable or unspecified
1 fetus 1
2 fetus 2
3 fetus 3
4 fetus 4
5 fetus 5
9 other fetus

7 **O33.7XX-** **Maternal care for disproportion due to other fetal deformities** ♀ M
Maternal care for disproportion due to fetal ascites
Maternal care for disproportion due to fetal hydrops
Maternal care for disproportion due to fetal meningomyelocele
Maternal care for disproportion due to fetal sacral teratoma
Maternal care for disproportion due to fetal tumor
EXCLUDES 1 *obstructed labor due to other fetal deformities (O66.3)*

One of the following 7th characters is to be assigned to code O33.7. 7th character 0 is for single gestations and multiple gestations where the fetus is unspecified. 7th characters 1 through 9 are for cases of multiple gestations to identify the fetus for which the code applies. The appropriate code from category O30, Multiple gestation, must also be assigned when assigning code O33.7 with a 7th character of 1 through 9.

0 not applicable or unspecified
1 fetus 1
2 fetus 2
3 fetus 3
4 fetus 4
5 fetus 5
9 other fetus

AHA: 4Q 2016, 51

O33.8 **Maternal care for disproportion of other origin** ♀ M

O33.9 **Maternal care for disproportion, unspecified** ♀ M
Maternal care for disproportion due to cephalopelvic disproportion NOS
Maternal care for disproportion due to fetopelvic disproportion NOS

4 **O34** **Maternal care for abnormality of pelvic organs**
INCLUDES the listed conditions as a reason for hospitalization or other obstetric care of the mother, or for cesarean delivery before onset of labor

Code first:
any associated obstructed labor (O65.5)
Use additional code for specific condition

Maternal care for cervical incompetence

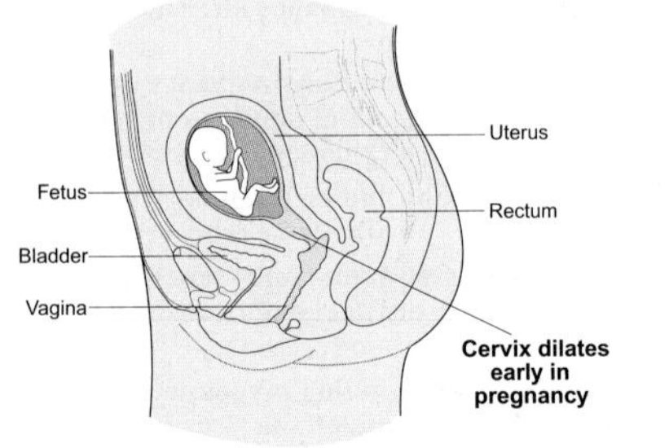

O34.0 Maternal care for congenital malformation of uterus
Maternal care for double uterus
Maternal care for uterus bicornis

- **O34.00** Maternal care for unspecified congenital malformation of uterus, unspecified trimester
- **O34.01** Maternal care for unspecified congenital malformation of uterus, first trimester
- **O34.02** Maternal care for unspecified congenital malformation of uterus, second trimester
- **O34.03** Maternal care for unspecified congenital malformation of uterus, third trimester

O34.1 Maternal care for benign tumor of corpus uteri
EXCLUDES 2 *maternal care for benign tumor of cervix (O34.4-)*
maternal care for malignant neoplasm of uterus (O9A.1-)

- **O34.10** Maternal care for benign tumor of corpus uteri, unspecified trimester
- **O34.11** Maternal care for benign tumor of corpus uteri, first trimester
- **O34.12** Maternal care for benign tumor of corpus uteri, second trimester
- **O34.13** Maternal care for benign tumor of corpus uteri, third trimester

O34.2 Maternal care due to uterine scar from previous surgery

O34.21 Maternal care for scar from previous cesarean delivery

- **O34.211** Maternal care for low transverse scar from previous cesarean delivery
  AHA: 4Q 2016, 51
- **O34.212** Maternal care for vertical scar from previous cesarean delivery
  Maternal care for classical scar from previous cesarean delivery
  AHA: 4Q 2016, 51
- **O34.219** Maternal care for unspecified type scar from previous cesarean delivery
  AHA: 4Q 2016, 51
- **O34.29** Maternal care due to uterine scar from other previous surgery
  Maternal care due to uterine scar from other transmural uterine incision

O34.3 Maternal care for cervical incompetence
Maternal care for cerclage with or without cervical incompetence
Maternal care for Shirodkar suture with or without cervical incompetence

- **O34.30** Maternal care for cervical incompetence, unspecified trimester
- **O34.31** Maternal care for cervical incompetence, first trimester
- **O34.32** Maternal care for cervical incompetence, second trimester
- **O34.33** Maternal care for cervical incompetence, third trimester

O34.4 Maternal care for other abnormalities of cervix

- **O34.40** Maternal care for other abnormalities of cervix, unspecified trimester
- **O34.41** Maternal care for other abnormalities of cervix, first trimester
- **O34.42** Maternal care for other abnormalities of cervix, second trimester
- **O34.43** Maternal care for other abnormalities of cervix, third trimester

O34.5 Maternal care for other abnormalities of gravid uterus

O34.51 Maternal care for incarceration of gravid uterus

- **O34.511** Maternal care for incarceration of gravid uterus, first trimester
- **O34.512** Maternal care for incarceration of gravid uterus, second trimester
- **O34.513** Maternal care for incarceration of gravid uterus, third trimester
- **O34.519** Maternal care for incarceration of gravid uterus, unspecified trimester

O34.52 Maternal care for prolapse of gravid uterus

- **O34.521** Maternal care for prolapse of gravid uterus, first trimester
- **O34.522** Maternal care for prolapse of gravid uterus, second trimester
- **O34.523** Maternal care for prolapse of gravid uterus, third trimester
- **O34.529** Maternal care for prolapse of gravid uterus, unspecified trimester

O34.53 Maternal care for retroversion of gravid uterus

- **O34.531** Maternal care for retroversion of gravid uterus, first trimester
- **O34.532** Maternal care for retroversion of gravid uterus, second trimester
- **O34.533** Maternal care for retroversion of gravid uterus, third trimester
- **O34.539** Maternal care for retroversion of gravid uterus, unspecified trimester

O34.59 Maternal care for other abnormalities of gravid uterus

- **O34.591** Maternal care for other abnormalities of gravid uterus, first trimester
- **O34.592** Maternal care for other abnormalities of gravid uterus, second trimester
- **O34.593** Maternal care for other abnormalities of gravid uterus, third trimester
- **O34.599** Maternal care for other abnormalities of gravid uterus, unspecified trimester

O34.6 Maternal care for abnormality of vagina
EXCLUDES 2 *maternal care for vaginal varices in pregnancy (O22.1-)*

- **O34.60** Maternal care for abnormality of vagina, unspecified trimester
- **O34.61** Maternal care for abnormality of vagina, first trimester
- **O34.62** Maternal care for abnormality of vagina, second trimester
- **O34.63** Maternal care for abnormality of vagina, third trimester

O34.7 Maternal care for abnormality of vulva and perineum
EXCLUDES 2 *maternal care for perineal and vulval varices in pregnancy (O22.1-)*

- **O34.70** Maternal care for abnormality of vulva and perineum, unspecified trimester
- **O34.71** Maternal care for abnormality of vulva and perineum, first trimester
- **O34.72** Maternal care for abnormality of vulva and perineum, second trimester
- **O34.73** Maternal care for abnormality of vulva and perineum, third trimester

O34.8 Maternal care for other abnormalities of pelvic organs

- **O34.80** Maternal care for other abnormalities of pelvic organs, unspecified trimester
- **O34.81** Maternal care for other abnormalities of pelvic organs, first trimester
- **O34.82** Maternal care for other abnormalities of pelvic organs, second trimester
- **O34.83** Maternal care for other abnormalities of pelvic organs, third trimester

O34.9 Maternal care for abnormality of pelvic organ, unspecified

- **O34.90** Maternal care for abnormality of pelvic organ, unspecified, unspecified trimester
- **O34.91** Maternal care for abnormality of pelvic organ, unspecified, first trimester
- **O34.92** Maternal care for abnormality of pelvic organ, unspecified, second trimester
- **O34.93** Maternal care for abnormality of pelvic organ, unspecified, third trimester

O35 Maternal care for known or suspected fetal abnormality and damage

INCLUDES the listed conditions in the fetus as a reason for hospitalization or other obstetric care to the mother, or for termination of pregnancy

Code also:
any associated maternal condition

EXCLUDES 1 *encounter for suspected maternal and fetal conditions ruled out (Z03.7-)*

One of the following 7th characters is to be assigned to each code under category O35. 7th character 0 is for single gestations and multiple gestations where the fetus is unspecified. 7th characters 1 through 9 are for cases of multiple gestations to identify the fetus for which the code applies. The appropriate code from category O30, Multiple gestation, must also be assigned when assigning a code from category O35 that has a 7th character of 1 through 9.

0 not applicable or unspecified
1 fetus 1
2 fetus 2
3 fetus 3
4 fetus 4
5 fetus 5
9 other fetus

O35.0XX- **Maternal care for (suspected) central nervous system malformation in fetus**
Maternal care for fetal anencephaly
Maternal care for fetal hydrocephalus
Maternal care for fetal spina bifida
EXCLUDES 2 *chromosomal abnormality in fetus (O35.1)*

O35.1XX- **Maternal care for (suspected) chromosomal abnormality in fetus**

O35.2XX- **Maternal care for (suspected) hereditary disease in fetus**
EXCLUDES 2 *chromosomal abnormality in fetus (O35.1)*

O35.3XX- **Maternal care for (suspected) damage to fetus from viral disease in mother**
Maternal care for damage to fetus from maternal cytomegalovirus infection
Maternal care for damage to fetus from maternal rubella

O35.4XX- **Maternal care for (suspected) damage to fetus from alcohol**

O35.5XX- **Maternal care for (suspected) damage to fetus by drugs**
Maternal care for damage to fetus from drug addiction

O35.6XX- **Maternal care for (suspected) damage to fetus by radiation**

O35.7XX- **Maternal care for (suspected) damage to fetus by other medical procedures**
Maternal care for damage to fetus by amniocentesis
Maternal care for damage to fetus by biopsy procedures
Maternal care for damage to fetus by hematological investigation
Maternal care for damage to fetus by intrauterine contraceptive device
Maternal care for damage to fetus by intrauterine surgery

O35.8XX- **Maternal care for other (suspected) fetal abnormality and damage**
Maternal care for damage to fetus from maternal listeriosis
Maternal care for damage to fetus from maternal toxoplasmosis

O35.9XX- **Maternal care for (suspected) fetal abnormality and damage, unspecified**

O36 Maternal care for other fetal problems

INCLUDES the listed conditions in the fetus as a reason for hospitalization or other obstetric care of the mother, or for termination of pregnancy

EXCLUDES 1 *encounter for suspected maternal and fetal conditions ruled out (Z03.7-)*
placental transfusion syndromes (O43.0-)

EXCLUDES 2 *labor and delivery complicated by fetal stress (O77.-)*

One of the following 7th characters is to be assigned to each code under category O36. 7th character 0 is for single gestations and multiple gestations where the fetus is unspecified. 7th characters 1 through 9 are for cases of multiple gestations to identify the fetus for which the code applies. The appropriate code from category O30, Multiple gestation, must also be assigned when assigning a code from category O36 that has a 7th character of 1 through 9.

0 not applicable or unspecified
1 fetus 1
2 fetus 2
3 fetus 3
4 fetus 4
5 fetus 5
9 other fetus

CODING TIP ✓ It is common to have abnormalities of the fetal heart rate or rhythm during the antepartum period, including fetal tachycardia, fetal bradycardia, decelerations of the fetal heart rate and loss of variability. Abnormalities during antenatal tests such as non-stress tests (NSTs) and contraction stress tests (CSTs) are also reported.

O36.0 Maternal care for rhesus isoimmunization
Maternal care for Rh incompatibility (with hydrops fetalis)

O36.01 Maternal care for anti-D [Rh] antibodies
AHA: 4Q 2014, 17

O36.011- **Maternal care for anti-D [Rh] antibodies, first trimester**

O36.012- **Maternal care for anti-D [Rh] antibodies, second trimester**

O36.013- **Maternal care for anti-D [Rh] antibodies, third trimester**
AHA: 4Q 2014, 17

O36.019- **Maternal care for anti-D [Rh] antibodies, unspecified trimester**

O36.09 Maternal care for other rhesus isoimmunization

O36.091- **Maternal care for other rhesus isoimmunization, first trimester**

O36.092- **Maternal care for other rhesus isoimmunization, second trimester**

O36.093- **Maternal care for other rhesus isoimmunization, third trimester**
AHA: 3Q 2015, 40

O36.099- **Maternal care for other rhesus isoimmunization, unspecified trimester**

O36.1 Maternal care for other isoimmunization
Maternal care for ABO isoimmunization

O36.11 Maternal care for Anti-A sensitization
Maternal care for isoimmunization NOS (with hydrops fetalis)

O36.111- **Maternal care for Anti-A sensitization, first trimester**

O36.112- **Maternal care for Anti-A sensitization, second trimester**

O36.113- **Maternal care for Anti-A sensitization, third trimester**

O36.119- **Maternal care for Anti-A sensitization, unspecified trimester**

O36.19 Maternal care for other isoimmunization
Maternal care for Anti-B sensitization

O36.191- **Maternal care for other isoimmunization, first trimester**

O36.192- **Maternal care for other isoimmunization, second trimester**

O36.193- **Maternal care for other isoimmunization, third trimester**

O36.199- **Maternal care for other isoimmunization, unspecified trimester**

5 O36.2 **Maternal care for hydrops fetalis**
Maternal care for hydrops fetalis NOS
Maternal care for hydrops fetalis not associated with isoimmunization
EXCLUDES 1 *hydrops fetalis associated with ABO isoimmunization (O36.1-)*
hydrops fetalis associated with rhesus isoimmunization (O36.0-)

7 O36.20X- **Maternal care for hydrops fetalis, unspecified trimester** ♀ M
7 O36.21X- **Maternal care for hydrops fetalis, first trimester** ♀ M
7 O36.22X- **Maternal care for hydrops fetalis, second trimester** ♀ M
7 O36.23X- **Maternal care for hydrops fetalis, third trimester** ♀ M

7 O36.4XX- **Maternal care for intrauterine death** ♀ M
Maternal care for intrauterine fetal death NOS
Maternal care for intrauterine fetal death after completion of 20 weeks of gestation
Maternal care for late fetal death
Maternal care for missed delivery
EXCLUDES 1 *missed abortion (O02.1)*
stillbirth (P95)

5 O36.5 **Maternal care for known or suspected poor fetal growth**
6 O36.51 **Maternal care for known or suspected placental insufficiency**
7 O36.511- **Maternal care for known or suspected placental insufficiency, first trimester** ♀ M
7 O36.512- **Maternal care for known or suspected placental insufficiency, second trimester** ♀ M
7 O36.513- **Maternal care for known or suspected placental insufficiency, third trimester** ♀ M
7 O36.519- **Maternal care for known or suspected placental insufficiency, unspecified trimester** ♀ M

6 O36.59 **Maternal care for other known or suspected poor fetal growth**
Maternal care for known or suspected light-for-dates NOS
Maternal care for known or suspected small-for-dates NOS
7 O36.591- **Maternal care for other known or suspected poor fetal growth, first trimester** ♀ M
7 O36.592- **Maternal care for other known or suspected poor fetal growth, second trimester** ♀ M
7 O36.593- **Maternal care for other known or suspected poor fetal growth, third trimester** ♀ M
7 O36.599- **Maternal care for other known or suspected poor fetal growth, unspecified trimester** ♀ M

5 O36.6 **Maternal care for excessive fetal growth**
Maternal care for known or suspected large-for-dates
7 O36.60X- **Maternal care for excessive fetal growth, unspecified trimester** ♀ M
7 O36.61X- **Maternal care for excessive fetal growth, first trimester** ♀ M
7 O36.62X- **Maternal care for excessive fetal growth, second trimester** ♀ M
7 O36.63X- **Maternal care for excessive fetal growth, third trimester** ♀ M

5 O36.7 **Maternal care for viable fetus in abdominal pregnancy**
7 O36.70X- **Maternal care for viable fetus in abdominal pregnancy, unspecified trimester** ♀ M
7 O36.71X- **Maternal care for viable fetus in abdominal pregnancy, first trimester** ♀ M
7 O36.72X- **Maternal care for viable fetus in abdominal pregnancy, second trimester** ♀ M
7 O36.73X- **Maternal care for viable fetus in abdominal pregnancy, third trimester** ♀ M

5 O36.8 **Maternal care for other specified fetal problems**
7 O36.80X- **Pregnancy with inconclusive fetal viability** ♀ M
Encounter to determine fetal viability of pregnancy
6 O36.81 **Decreased fetal movements**
7 O36.812- **Decreased fetal movements, second trimester** ♀ M
7 O36.813- **Decreased fetal movements, third trimester** ♀ M
7 O36.819- **Decreased fetal movements, unspecified trimester** ♀ M
6 O36.82 **Fetal anemia and thrombocytopenia**
7 O36.821- **Fetal anemia and thrombocytopenia, first trimester** ♀ M
7 O36.822- **Fetal anemia and thrombocytopenia, second trimester** ♀ M
7 O36.823- **Fetal anemia and thrombocytopenia, third trimester** ♀ M
7 O36.829- **Fetal anemia and thrombocytopenia, unspecified trimester** ♀ M
6 O36.83 **Maternal care for abnormalities of the fetal heart rate or rhythm**
AHA: 4Q 2017, 15
7 O36.831- **Maternal care for abnormalities of the fetal heart rate or rhythm, first trimester** ♀ M
7 O36.832- **Maternal care for abnormalities of the fetal heart rate or rhythm, second trimester** ♀ M
7 O36.833- **Maternal care for abnormalities of the fetal heart rate or rhythm, third trimester** ♀ M
7 O36.839- **Maternal care for abnormalities of the fetal heart rate or rhythm, unspecified trimester** ♀ M
6 O36.89 **Maternal care for other specified fetal problems**
7 O36.891- **Maternal care for other specified fetal problems, first trimester** ♀ M
7 O36.892- **Maternal care for other specified fetal problems, second trimester** ♀ M
7 O36.893- **Maternal care for other specified fetal problems, third trimester** ♀ M
7 O36.899- **Maternal care for other specified fetal problems, unspecified trimester** ♀ M

5 O36.9 **Maternal care for fetal problem, unspecified**
7 O36.90X- **Maternal care for fetal problem, unspecified, unspecified trimester** ♀ M
7 O36.91X- **Maternal care for fetal problem, unspecified, first trimester** ♀ M
7 O36.92X- **Maternal care for fetal problem, unspecified, second trimester** ♀ M
7 O36.93X- **Maternal care for fetal problem, unspecified, third trimester** ♀ M

4 O40 Polyhydramnios
INCLUDES hydramnios
EXCLUDES 1 *encounter for suspected maternal and fetal conditions ruled out (Z03.7-)*

One of the following 7th characters is to be assigned to each code under category O40. 7th character 0 is for single gestations and multiple gestations where the fetus is unspecified. 7th characters 1 through 9 are for cases of multiple gestations to identify the fetus for which the code applies. The appropriate code from category O30, Multiple gestation, must also be assigned when assigning a code from category O40 that has a 7th character of 1 through 9.

0 not applicable or unspecified
1 fetus 1
2 fetus 2
3 fetus 3
4 fetus 4
5 fetus 5
9 other fetus

7 O40.1XX- **Polyhydramnios, first trimester** ♀ M
7 O40.2XX- **Polyhydramnios, second trimester** ♀ M
7 O40.3XX- **Polyhydramnios, third trimester** ♀ M
7 O40.9XX- **Polyhydramnios, unspecified trimester** ♀ M

O41 Other disorders of amniotic fluid and membranes

EXCLUDES 1 *encounter for suspected maternal and fetal conditions ruled out (Z03.7-)*

One of the following 7th characters is to be assigned to each code under category O41. 7th character 0 is for single gestations and multiple gestations where the fetus is unspecified. 7th characters 1 through 9 are for cases of multiple gestations to identify the fetus for which the code applies. The appropriate code from category O30, Multiple gestation, must also be assigned when assigning a code from category O41 that has a 7th character of 1 through 9.

- 0 not applicable or unspecified
- 1 fetus 1
- 2 fetus 2
- 3 fetus 3
- 4 fetus 4
- 5 fetus 5
- 9 other fetus

O41.0 Oligohydramnios
Oligohydramnios without rupture of membranes

- **O41.00X- Oligohydramnios, unspecified trimester**
- **O41.01X- Oligohydramnios, first trimester**
- **O41.02X- Oligohydramnios, second trimester**
- **O41.03X- Oligohydramnios, third trimester**

O41.1 Infection of amniotic sac and membranes

O41.10 Infection of amniotic sac and membranes, unspecified

- **O41.101- Infection of amniotic sac and membranes, unspecified, first trimester**
- **O41.102- Infection of amniotic sac and membranes, unspecified, second trimester**
- **O41.103- Infection of amniotic sac and membranes, unspecified, third trimester**
- **O41.109- Infection of amniotic sac and membranes, unspecified, unspecified trimester**

O41.12 Chorioamnionitis

- **O41.121- Chorioamnionitis, first trimester**
- **O41.122- Chorioamnionitis, second trimester**
- **O41.123- Chorioamnionitis, third trimester**
- **O41.129- Chorioamnionitis, unspecified trimester**

O41.14 Placentitis

- **O41.141- Placentitis, first trimester**
- **O41.142- Placentitis, second trimester**
- **O41.143- Placentitis, third trimester**
- **O41.149- Placentitis, unspecified trimester**

O41.8 Other specified disorders of amniotic fluid and membranes

O41.8X Other specified disorders of amniotic fluid and membranes

- **O41.8X1- Other specified disorders of amniotic fluid and membranes, first trimester**
- **O41.8X2- Other specified disorders of amniotic fluid and membranes, second trimester**
- **O41.8X3- Other specified disorders of amniotic fluid and membranes, third trimester**
- **O41.8X9- Other specified disorders of amniotic fluid and membranes, unspecified trimester**

O41.9 Disorder of amniotic fluid and membranes, unspecified

- **O41.90X- Disorder of amniotic fluid and membranes, unspecified, unspecified trimester**
- **O41.91X- Disorder of amniotic fluid and membranes, unspecified, first trimester**
- **O41.92X- Disorder of amniotic fluid and membranes, unspecified, second trimester**
- **O41.93X- Disorder of amniotic fluid and membranes, unspecified, third trimester**

O42 Premature rupture of membranes

O42.0 Premature rupture of membranes, onset of labor within 24 hours of rupture

- **O42.00 Premature rupture of membranes, onset of labor within 24 hours of rupture, unspecified weeks of gestation**

O42.01 Preterm premature rupture of membranes, onset of labor within 24 hours of rupture
Premature rupture of membranes before 37 completed weeks of gestation

- **O42.011 Preterm premature rupture of membranes, onset of labor within 24 hours of rupture, first trimester**
- **O42.012 Preterm premature rupture of membranes, onset of labor within 24 hours of rupture, second trimester**
- **O42.013 Preterm premature rupture of membranes, onset of labor within 24 hours of rupture, third trimester**
- **O42.019 Preterm premature rupture of membranes, onset of labor within 24 hours of rupture, unspecified trimester**

O42.02 Full-term premature rupture of membranes, onset of labor within 24 hours of rupture
Premature rupture of membranes at or after 37 completed weeks of gestation, onset of labor within 24 hours of rupture

O42.1 Premature rupture of membranes, onset of labor more than 24 hours following rupture

- **O42.10 Premature rupture of membranes, onset of labor more than 24 hours following rupture, unspecified weeks of gestation**

O42.11 Preterm premature rupture of membranes, onset of labor more than 24 hours following rupture
Premature rupture of membranes before 37 completed weeks of gestation

- **O42.111 Preterm premature rupture of membranes, onset of labor more than 24 hours following rupture, first trimester**
- **O42.112 Preterm premature rupture of membranes, onset of labor more than 24 hours following rupture, second trimester**
- **O42.113 Preterm premature rupture of membranes, onset of labor more than 24 hours following rupture, third trimester**
- **O42.119 Preterm premature rupture of membranes, onset of labor more than 24 hours following rupture, unspecified trimester**

O42.12 Full-term premature rupture of membranes, onset of labor more than 24 hours following rupture
Premature rupture of membranes at or after 37 completed weeks of gestation, onset of labor more than 24 hours following rupture

O42.9 Premature rupture of membranes, unspecified as to length of time between rupture and onset of labor

- **O42.90 Premature rupture of membranes, unspecified as to length of time between rupture and onset of labor, unspecified weeks of gestation**

O42.91 Preterm premature rupture of membranes, unspecified as to length of time between rupture and onset of labor
Premature rupture of membranes before 37 completed weeks of gestation

- **O42.911 Preterm premature rupture of membranes, unspecified as to length of time between rupture and onset of labor, first trimester**
- **O42.912 Preterm premature rupture of membranes, unspecified as to length of time between rupture and onset of labor, second trimester**
- **O42.913 Preterm premature rupture of membranes, unspecified as to length of time between rupture and onset of labor, third trimester**
- **O42.919 Preterm premature rupture of membranes, unspecified as to length of time between rupture and onset of labor, unspecified trimester**

O42.92 Full-term premature rupture of membranes, unspecified as to length of time between rupture and onset of labor
Premature rupture of membranes at or after 37 completed weeks of gestation, unspecified as to length of time between rupture and onset of labor

4 O43 Placental disorders

EXCLUDES 2 *maternal care for poor fetal growth due to placental insufficiency (O36.5-)*
placenta previa (O44.-)
placental polyp (O90.89)
placentitis (O41.14-)
premature separation of placenta [abruptio placentae] (O45.-)

5 O43.0 Placental transfusion syndromes

6 O43.01 Fetomaternal placental transfusion syndrome
Maternofetal placental transfusion syndrome

- **O43.011** Fetomaternal placental transfusion syndrome, first trimester ♀ M
- **O43.012** Fetomaternal placental transfusion syndrome, second trimester ♀ M
- **O43.013** Fetomaternal placental transfusion syndrome, third trimester ♀ M
- **O43.019** Fetomaternal placental transfusion syndrome, unspecified trimester ♀ M

6 O43.02 Fetus-to-fetus placental transfusion syndrome

- **O43.021** Fetus-to-fetus placental transfusion syndrome, first trimester ♀ M
- **O43.022** Fetus-to-fetus placental transfusion syndrome, second trimester ♀ M
- **O43.023** Fetus-to-fetus placental transfusion syndrome, third trimester ♀ M
- **O43.029** Fetus-to-fetus placental transfusion syndrome, unspecified trimester ♀ M

5 O43.1 Malformation of placenta

6 O43.10 Malformation of placenta, unspecified
Abnormal placenta NOS

- **O43.101** Malformation of placenta, unspecified, first trimester ♀ M
- **O43.102** Malformation of placenta, unspecified, second trimester ♀ M
- **O43.103** Malformation of placenta, unspecified, third trimester ♀ M
- **O43.109** Malformation of placenta, unspecified, unspecified trimester ♀ M

6 O43.11 Circumvallate placenta

- **O43.111** Circumvallate placenta, first trimester ♀ M
- **O43.112** Circumvallate placenta, second trimester ♀ M
- **O43.113** Circumvallate placenta, third trimester ♀ M
- **O43.119** Circumvallate placenta, unspecified trimester ♀ M

6 O43.12 Velamentous insertion of umbilical cord

- **O43.121** Velamentous insertion of umbilical cord, first trimester ♀ M
- **O43.122** Velamentous insertion of umbilical cord, second trimester ♀ M
- **O43.123** Velamentous insertion of umbilical cord, third trimester ♀ M
- **O43.129** Velamentous insertion of umbilical cord, unspecified trimester ♀ M

6 O43.19 Other malformation of placenta

- **O43.191** Other malformation of placenta, first trimester ♀ M
- **O43.192** Other malformation of placenta, second trimester ♀ M
- **O43.193** Other malformation of placenta, third trimester ♀ M
- **O43.199** Other malformation of placenta, unspecified trimester ♀ M

5 O43.2 Morbidly adherent placenta
Code also:
associated third stage postpartum hemorrhage, if applicable (O72.0)

EXCLUDES 1 *retained placenta (O73.-)*

6 O43.21 Placenta accreta

- **O43.211** Placenta accreta, first trimester ♀ M
- **O43.212** Placenta accreta, second trimester ♀ M
- **O43.213** Placenta accreta, third trimester ♀ M
- **O43.219** Placenta accreta, unspecified trimester ♀ M

6 O43.22 Placenta increta

- **O43.221** Placenta increta, first trimester ♀ M
- **O43.222** Placenta increta, second trimester ♀ M
- **O43.223** Placenta increta, third trimester ♀ M
- **O43.229** Placenta increta, unspecified trimester ♀ M

6 O43.23 Placenta percreta

- **O43.231** Placenta percreta, first trimester ♀ M
- **O43.232** Placenta percreta, second trimester ♀ M
- **O43.233** Placenta percreta, third trimester ♀ M
- **O43.239** Placenta percreta, unspecified trimester ♀ M

5 O43.8 Other placental disorders

6 O43.81 Placental infarction

- **O43.811** Placental infarction, first trimester ♀ M
- **O43.812** Placental infarction, second trimester ♀ M
- **O43.813** Placental infarction, third trimester ♀ M
- **O43.819** Placental infarction, unspecified trimester ♀ M

6 O43.89 Other placental disorders
Placental dysfunction

- **O43.891** Other placental disorders, first trimester ♀ M
- **O43.892** Other placental disorders, second trimester ♀ M
- **O43.893** Other placental disorders, third trimester ♀ M
- **O43.899** Other placental disorders, unspecified trimester ♀ M

5 O43.9 Unspecified placental disorder

- **O43.90** Unspecified placental disorder, unspecified trimester ♀ M
- **O43.91** Unspecified placental disorder, first trimester ♀ M
- **O43.92** Unspecified placental disorder, second trimester ♀ M
- **O43.93** Unspecified placental disorder, third trimester ♀ M

4 O44 Placenta previa

Placenta previa

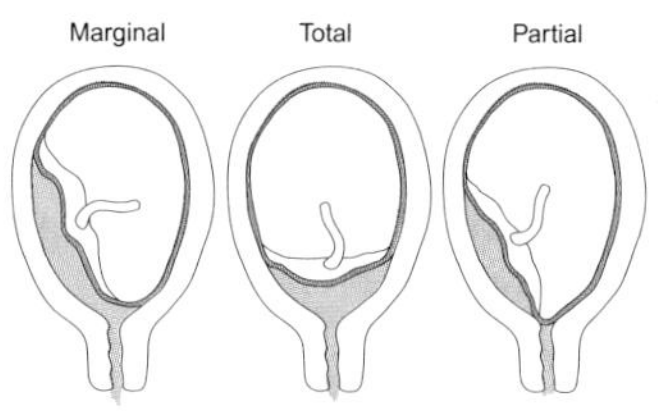

5 O44.0 Complete placenta previa NOS or without hemorrhage
Placenta previa NOS
AHA: 4Q 2016, 52

- **O44.00** Complete placenta previa NOS or without hemorrhage, unspecified trimester ♀ M
  AHA: 4Q 2016, 52
- **O44.01** Complete placenta previa NOS or without hemorrhage, first trimester ♀ M
  AHA: 4Q 2016, 52
- **O44.02** Complete placenta previa NOS or without hemorrhage, second trimester ♀ M
  AHA: 4Q 2016, 52
- **O44.03** Complete placenta previa NOS or without hemorrhage, third trimester ♀ M
  AHA: 4Q 2016, 52

5 O44.1 Complete placenta previa with hemorrhage

EXCLUDES 1 *labor and delivery complicated by hemorrhage from vasa previa (O69.4)*

AHA: 4Q 2016, 52

- **O44.10** Complete placenta previa with hemorrhage, unspecified trimester ♀ M
  AHA: 4Q 2016, 52
- **O44.11** Complete placenta previa with hemorrhage, first trimester ♀ M
  AHA: 4Q 2016, 52
- **O44.12** Complete placenta previa with hemorrhage, second trimester ♀ M
  AHA: 4Q 2016, 52
- **O44.13** Complete placenta previa with hemorrhage, third trimester ♀ M
  AHA: 4Q 2016, 52

5 O44.2 Partial placenta previa without hemorrhage
Marginal placenta previa, NOS or without hemorrhage
AHA: 4Q 2016, 52

O44.20 **Partial placenta previa NOS or without hemorrhage, unspecified trimester** ♀ M
AHA: 4Q 2016, 52

O44.21 **Partial placenta previa NOS or without hemorrhage, first trimester** ♀ M
AHA: 4Q 2016, 52

O44.22 **Partial placenta previa NOS or without hemorrhage, second trimester** ♀ M
AHA: 4Q 2016, 52

O44.23 **Partial placenta previa NOS or without hemorrhage, third trimester** ♀ M
AHA: 4Q 2016, 52

5 O44.3 Partial placenta previa with hemorrhage
Marginal placenta previa with hemorrhage
AHA: 4Q 2016, 52

O44.30 **Partial placenta previa with hemorrhage, unspecified trimester** ♀ M
AHA: 4Q 2016, 52

O44.31 **Partial placenta previa with hemorrhage, first trimester** ♀ M
AHA: 4Q 2016, 52

O44.32 **Partial placenta previa with hemorrhage, second trimester** ♀ M
AHA: 4Q 2016, 52

O44.33 **Partial placenta previa with hemorrhage, third trimester** ♀ M
AHA: 4Q 2016, 52

5 O44.4 Low lying placenta NOS or without hemorrhage
Low implantation of placenta NOS or without hemorrhage
AHA: 4Q 2016, 52

O44.40 **Low lying placenta NOS or without hemorrhage, unspecified trimester** ♀ M
AHA: 4Q 2016, 52

O44.41 **Low lying placenta NOS or without hemorrhage, first trimester** ♀ M
AHA: 4Q 2016, 52

O44.42 **Low lying placenta NOS or without hemorrhage, second trimester** ♀ M
AHA: 4Q 2016, 52

O44.43 **Low lying placenta NOS or without hemorrhage, third trimester** ♀ M
AHA: 4Q 2016, 52

5 O44.5 Low lying placenta with hemorrhage
Low implantation of placenta with hemorrhage
AHA: 4Q 2016, 52

O44.50 **Low lying placenta with hemorrhage, unspecified trimester** ♀ M

O44.51 **Low lying placenta with hemorrhage, first trimester** ♀ M

O44.52 **Low lying placenta with hemorrhage, second trimester** ♀ M

O44.53 **Low lying placenta with hemorrhage, third trimester** ♀ M

4 O45 Premature separation of placenta [abruptio placentae]

5 O45.0 Premature separation of placenta with coagulation defect

6 O45.00 Premature separation of placenta with coagulation defect, unspecified

O45.001 **Premature separation of placenta with coagulation defect, unspecified, first trimester** ♀ M

O45.002 **Premature separation of placenta with coagulation defect, unspecified, second trimester** ♀ M

O45.003 **Premature separation of placenta with coagulation defect, unspecified, third trimester** ♀ M

O45.009 **Premature separation of placenta with coagulation defect, unspecified, unspecified trimester** ♀ M

6 O45.01 Premature separation of placenta with afibrinogenemia
Premature separation of placenta with hypofibrinogenemia

O45.011 **Premature separation of placenta with afibrinogenemia, first trimester** ♀ M

O45.012 **Premature separation of placenta with afibrinogenemia, second trimester** ♀ M

O45.013 **Premature separation of placenta with afibrinogenemia, third trimester** ♀ M

O45.019 **Premature separation of placenta with afibrinogenemia, unspecified trimester** ♀ M

6 O45.02 Premature separation of placenta with disseminated intravascular coagulation

O45.021 **Premature separation of placenta with disseminated intravascular coagulation, first trimester** ♀ M

O45.022 **Premature separation of placenta with disseminated intravascular coagulation, second trimester** ♀ M

O45.023 **Premature separation of placenta with disseminated intravascular coagulation, third trimester** ♀ M

O45.029 **Premature separation of placenta with disseminated intravascular coagulation, unspecified trimester** ♀ M

6 O45.09 Premature separation of placenta with other coagulation defect

O45.091 **Premature separation of placenta with other coagulation defect, first trimester** ♀ M

O45.092 **Premature separation of placenta with other coagulation defect, second trimester** ♀ M

O45.093 **Premature separation of placenta with other coagulation defect, third trimester** ♀ M

O45.099 **Premature separation of placenta with other coagulation defect, unspecified trimester** ♀ M

5 O45.8 Other premature separation of placenta

6 O45.8X Other premature separation of placenta

O45.8X1 **Other premature separation of placenta, first trimester** ♀ M

O45.8X2 **Other premature separation of placenta, second trimester** ♀ M

O45.8X3 **Other premature separation of placenta, third trimester** ♀ M

O45.8X9 **Other premature separation of placenta, unspecified trimester** ♀ M

5 O45.9 Premature separation of placenta, unspecified
Abruptio placentae NOS

O45.90 **Premature separation of placenta, unspecified, unspecified trimester** ♀ M

O45.91 **Premature separation of placenta, unspecified, first trimester** ♀ M

O45.92 **Premature separation of placenta, unspecified, second trimester** ♀ M

O45.93 **Premature separation of placenta, unspecified, third trimester** ♀ M

4 O46 Antepartum hemorrhage, not elsewhere classified

EXCLUDES 1 *hemorrhage in early pregnancy (O20.-)*
intrapartum hemorrhage NEC (O67.-)
placenta previa (O44.-)
premature separation of placenta [abruptio placentae] (O45.-)

5 O46.0 Antepartum hemorrhage with coagulation defect

6 O46.00 Antepartum hemorrhage with coagulation defect, unspecified

O46.001 **Antepartum hemorrhage with coagulation defect, unspecified, first trimester** ♀ M

O46.002 **Antepartum hemorrhage with coagulation defect, unspecified, second trimester** ♀ M

O46.003 **Antepartum hemorrhage with coagulation defect, unspecified, third trimester** ♀ M

O46.009 **Antepartum hemorrhage with coagulation defect, unspecified, unspecified trimester** ♀ M

6 O46.01 Antepartum hemorrhage with afibrinogenemia
Antepartum hemorrhage with hypofibrinogenemia

O46.011 **Antepartum hemorrhage with afibrinogenemia, first trimester** ♀ M

O46.012 **Antepartum hemorrhage with afibrinogenemia, second trimester** ♀ M

O46.013 Antepartum hemorrhage with afibrinogenemia, third trimester ♀M

O46.019 Antepartum hemorrhage with afibrinogenemia, unspecified trimester ♀M

6 O46.02 Antepartum hemorrhage with disseminated intravascular coagulation

O46.021 Antepartum hemorrhage with disseminated intravascular coagulation, first trimester ♀M

O46.022 Antepartum hemorrhage with disseminated intravascular coagulation, second trimester ♀M

O46.023 Antepartum hemorrhage with disseminated intravascular coagulation, third trimester ♀M

O46.029 Antepartum hemorrhage with disseminated intravascular coagulation, unspecified trimester ♀M

6 O46.09 Antepartum hemorrhage with other coagulation defect

O46.091 Antepartum hemorrhage with other coagulation defect, first trimester ♀M

O46.092 Antepartum hemorrhage with other coagulation defect, second trimester ♀M

O46.093 Antepartum hemorrhage with other coagulation defect, third trimester ♀M

O46.099 Antepartum hemorrhage with other coagulation defect, unspecified trimester ♀M

5 O46.8 Other antepartum hemorrhage

6 O46.8X Other antepartum hemorrhage

O46.8X1 Other antepartum hemorrhage, first trimester ♀M

O46.8X2 Other antepartum hemorrhage, second trimester ♀M

O46.8X3 Other antepartum hemorrhage, third trimester ♀M

O46.8X9 Other antepartum hemorrhage, unspecified trimester ♀M

5 O46.9 Antepartum hemorrhage, unspecified

O46.90 Antepartum hemorrhage, unspecified, unspecified trimester ♀M

O46.91 Antepartum hemorrhage, unspecified, first trimester ♀M

O46.92 Antepartum hemorrhage, unspecified, second trimester ♀M

O46.93 Antepartum hemorrhage, unspecified, third trimester ♀M

4 O47 False labor

INCLUDES Braxton Hicks contractions
threatened labor

EXCLUDES 1 *preterm labor (O60.-)*

5 O47.0 False labor before 37 completed weeks of gestation

O47.00 False labor before 37 completed weeks of gestation, unspecified trimester ♀M

O47.02 False labor before 37 completed weeks of gestation, second trimester ♀M

O47.03 False labor before 37 completed weeks of gestation, third trimester ♀M

O47.1 False labor at or after 37 completed weeks of gestation ♀M

O47.9 False labor, unspecified ♀M

4 O48 Late pregnancy

O48.0 Post-term pregnancy ♀M
Pregnancy over 40 completed weeks to 42 completed weeks gestation

O48.1 Prolonged pregnancy ♀M
Pregnancy which has advanced beyond 42 completed weeks gestation

Complications of labor and delivery (O60-O77)

4 O60 Preterm labor

INCLUDES onset (spontaneous) of labor before 37 completed weeks of gestation

EXCLUDES 1 *false labor (O47.0-)*
threatened labor NOS (O47.0-)

5 O60.0 Preterm labor without delivery

O60.00 Preterm labor without delivery, unspecified trimester ♀M

O60.02 Preterm labor without delivery, second trimester ♀M

O60.03 Preterm labor without delivery, third trimester ♀M

5 O60.1 Preterm labor with preterm delivery

One of the following 7th characters is to be assigned to each code under subcategory O60.1. 7th character 0 is for single gestations and multiple gestations where the fetus is unspecified. 7th characters 1 through 9 are for cases of multiple gestations to identify the fetus for which the code applies. The appropriate code from category O30, Multiple gestation, must also be assigned when assigning a code from subcategory O60.1 that has a 7th character of 1 through 9.

0 not applicable or unspecified
1 fetus 1
2 fetus 2
3 fetus 3
4 fetus 4
5 fetus 5
9 other fetus

7 O60.10X- Preterm labor with preterm delivery, unspecified trimester ♀M
Preterm labor with delivery NOS

7 O60.12X- Preterm labor second trimester with preterm delivery second trimester ♀M

7 O60.13X- Preterm labor second trimester with preterm delivery third trimester ♀M

7 O60.14X- Preterm labor third trimester with preterm delivery third trimester ♀M
AHA: (O60.14X0) 2Q 2016, 10
AHA: (O60.14X1) 2Q 2016, 10
AHA: (O60.14X2) 2Q 2016, 10

5 O60.2 Term delivery with preterm labor

One of the following 7th characters is to be assigned to each code under subcategory O60.2. 7th character 0 is for single gestations and multiple gestations where the fetus is unspecified. 7th characters 1 through 9 are for cases of multiple gestations to identify the fetus for which the code applies. The appropriate code from category O30, Multiple gestation, must also be assigned when assigning a code from subcategory O60.2 that has a 7th character of 1 through 9.

0 not applicable or unspecified
1 fetus 1
2 fetus 2
3 fetus 3
4 fetus 4
5 fetus 5
9 other fetus

7 O60.20X- Term delivery with preterm labor, unspecified trimester ♀M

7 O60.22X- Term delivery with preterm labor, second trimester ♀M

7 O60.23X- Term delivery with preterm labor, third trimester ♀M

4 O61 Failed induction of labor

O61.0 Failed medical induction of labor ♀M
Failed induction (of labor) by oxytocin
Failed induction (of labor) by prostaglandins

O61.1 Failed instrumental induction of labor ♀M
Failed mechanical induction (of labor)
Failed surgical induction (of labor)

O61.8 Other failed induction of labor ♀M

O61.9 Failed induction of labor, unspecified ♀M

4 O62 Abnormalities of forces of labor

O62.0 Primary inadequate contractions ♀M
Failure of cervical dilatation
Primary hypotonic uterine dysfunction
Uterine inertia during latent phase of labor

O62.1 Secondary uterine inertia ♀M
Arrested active phase of labor
Secondary hypotonic uterine dysfunction

O62.2 Other uterine inertia
Atony of uterus without hemorrhage
Atony of uterus NOS
Desultory labor
Hypotonic uterine dysfunction NOS
Irregular labor
Poor contractions
Slow slope active phase of labor
Uterine inertia NOS
EXCLUDES 1 *atony of uterus with hemorrhage (postpartum) (O72.1)*
postpartum atony of uterus without hemorrhage (O75.89)

O62.3 Precipitate labor
DEFINITION Labor occurring quickly, with rapid expulsion of the fetus.

O62.4 Hypertonic, incoordinate, and prolonged uterine contractions
Cervical spasm
Contraction ring dystocia
Dyscoordinate labor
Hour-glass contraction of uterus
Hypertonic uterine dysfunction
Incoordinate uterine action
Tetanic contractions
Uterine dystocia NOS
Uterine spasm
EXCLUDES 1 *dystocia (fetal) (maternal) NOS (O66.9)*

O62.8 Other abnormalities of forces of labor

O62.9 Abnormality of forces of labor, unspecified

O63 Long labor

O63.0 Prolonged first stage (of labor)

O63.1 Prolonged second stage (of labor)

O63.2 Delayed delivery of second twin, triplet, etc.

O63.9 Long labor, unspecified
Prolonged labor NOS

O64 Obstructed labor due to malposition and malpresentation of fetus

One of the following 7th characters is to be assigned to each code under category O64. 7th character 0 is for single gestations and multiple gestations where the fetus is unspecified. 7th characters 1 through 9 are for cases of multiple gestations to identify the fetus for which the code applies. The appropriate code from category O30, Multiple gestation, must also be assigned when assigning a code from category O64 that has a 7th character of 1 through 9.

0	not applicable or unspecified
1	fetus 1
2	fetus 2
3	fetus 3
4	fetus 4
5	fetus 5
9	other fetus

O64.0XX- Obstructed labor due to incomplete rotation of fetal head
Deep transverse arrest
Obstructed labor due to persistent occipitoiliac (position)
Obstructed labor due to persistent occipitoposterior (position)
Obstructed labor due to persistent occipitosacral (position)
Obstructed labor due to persistent occipitotransverse (position)

O64.1XX- Obstructed labor due to breech presentation
Obstructed labor due to buttocks presentation
Obstructed labor due to complete breech presentation
Obstructed labor due to frank breech presentation

O64.2XX- Obstructed labor due to face presentation
Obstructed labor due to chin presentation

O64.3XX- Obstructed labor due to brow presentation

O64.4XX- Obstructed labor due to shoulder presentation
Prolapsed arm
EXCLUDES 1 *impacted shoulders (O66.0)*
shoulder dystocia (O66.0)

O64.5XX- Obstructed labor due to compound presentation

O64.8XX- Obstructed labor due to other malposition and malpresentation
Obstructed labor due to footling presentation
Obstructed labor due to incomplete breech presentation

O64.9XX- Obstructed labor due to malposition and malpresentation, unspecified

O65 Obstructed labor due to maternal pelvic abnormality

O65.0 Obstructed labor due to deformed pelvis

O65.1 Obstructed labor due to generally contracted pelvis

O65.2 Obstructed labor due to pelvic inlet contraction

O65.3 Obstructed labor due to pelvic outlet and mid-cavity contraction

O65.4 Obstructed labor due to fetopelvic disproportion, unspecified
EXCLUDES 1 *dystocia due to abnormality of fetus (O66.2-O66.3)*

O65.5 Obstructed labor due to abnormality of maternal pelvic organs
Obstructed labor due to conditions listed in O34.-
Use additional code to identify abnormality of pelvic organs O34.-

O65.8 Obstructed labor due to other maternal pelvic abnormalities

O65.9 Obstructed labor due to maternal pelvic abnormality, unspecified

O66 Other obstructed labor

O66.0 Obstructed labor due to shoulder dystocia
Impacted shoulders
DEFINITION Shoulders of the fetus become caught in the pelvis during delivery.

O66.1 Obstructed labor due to locked twins

O66.2 Obstructed labor due to unusually large fetus

O66.3 Obstructed labor due to other abnormalities of fetus
Dystocia due to fetal ascites
Dystocia due to fetal hydrops
Dystocia due to fetal meningomyelocele
Dystocia due to fetal sacral teratoma
Dystocia due to fetal tumor
Dystocia due to hydrocephalic fetus
Use additional code to identify cause of obstruction

O66.4 Failed trial of labor

O66.40 Failed trial of labor, unspecified

O66.41 Failed attempted vaginal birth after previous cesarean delivery
Code first:
rupture of uterus, if applicable (O71.0-, O71.1)

O66.5 Attempted application of vacuum extractor and forceps
Attempted application of vacuum or forceps, with subsequent delivery by forceps or cesarean delivery

O66.6 Obstructed labor due to other multiple fetuses

O66.8 Other specified obstructed labor
Use additional code to identify cause of obstruction

O66.9 Obstructed labor, unspecified
Dystocia NOS
Fetal dystocia NOS
Maternal dystocia NOS

O67 Labor and delivery complicated by intrapartum hemorrhage, not elsewhere classified

EXCLUDES 1 *antepartum hemorrhage NEC (O46.-)*
placenta previa (O44.-)
premature separation of placenta [abruptio placentae] (O45.-)
EXCLUDES 2 *postpartum hemorrhage (O72.-)*

O67.0 Intrapartum hemorrhage with coagulation defect
Intrapartum hemorrhage (excessive) associated with afibrinogenemia
Intrapartum hemorrhage (excessive) associated with disseminated intravascular coagulation
Intrapartum hemorrhage (excessive) associated with hyperfibrinolysis
Intrapartum hemorrhage (excessive) associated with hypofibrinogenemia

O67.8 Other intrapartum hemorrhage
Excessive intrapartum hemorrhage

O67.9 Intrapartum hemorrhage, unspecified

O68 Labor and delivery complicated by abnormality of fetal acid-base balance

Fetal acidemia complicating labor and delivery
Fetal acidosis complicating labor and delivery
Fetal alkalosis complicating labor and delivery
Fetal metabolic acidemia complicating labor and delivery

EXCLUDES 1 *fetal stress NOS (O77.9)*
labor and delivery complicated by electrocardiographic evidence of fetal stress (O77.8)
labor and delivery complicated by ultrasonic evidence of fetal stress (O77.8)

EXCLUDES 2 *abnormality in fetal heart rate or rhythm (O76)*
labor and delivery complicated by meconium in amniotic fluid (O77.0)

O69 Labor and delivery complicated by umbilical cord complications

One of the following 7th characters is to be assigned to each code under category O69. 7th character 0 is for single gestations and multiple gestations where the fetus is unspecified. 7th characters 1 through 9 are for cases of multiple gestations to identify the fetus for which the code applies. The appropriate code from category O30, Multiple gestation, must also be assigned when assigning a code from category O69 that has a 7th character of 1 through 9.

0	not applicable or unspecified
1	fetus 1
2	fetus 2
3	fetus 3
4	fetus 4
5	fetus 5
9	other fetus

O69.0XX- Labor and delivery complicated by prolapse of cord

O69.1XX- Labor and delivery complicated by cord around neck, with compression

EXCLUDES 1 *labor and delivery complicated by cord around neck, without compression (O69.81)*

O69.2XX- Labor and delivery complicated by other cord entanglement, with compression

Labor and delivery complicated by compression of cord NOS
Labor and delivery complicated by entanglement of cords of twins in monoamniotic sac
Labor and delivery complicated by knot in cord

EXCLUDES 1 *labor and delivery complicated by other cord entanglement, without compression (O69.82)*

O69.3XX- Labor and delivery complicated by short cord

O69.4XX- Labor and delivery complicated by vasa previa

Labor and delivery complicated by hemorrhage from vasa previa

O69.5XX- Labor and delivery complicated by vascular lesion of cord

Labor and delivery complicated by cord bruising
Labor and delivery complicated by cord hematoma
Labor and delivery complicated by thrombosis of umbilical vessels

O69.8 Labor and delivery complicated by other cord complications

O69.81X- Labor and delivery complicated by cord around neck, without compression

O69.82X- Labor and delivery complicated by other cord entanglement, without compression

O69.89X- Labor and delivery complicated by other cord complications

O69.9XX- Labor and delivery complicated by cord complication, unspecified

O70 Perineal laceration during delivery

INCLUDES episiotomy extended by laceration

EXCLUDES 1 *obstetric high vaginal laceration alone (O71.4)*

O70.0 First degree perineal laceration during delivery

Perineal laceration, rupture or tear involving fourchette during delivery
Perineal laceration, rupture or tear involving labia during delivery
Perineal laceration, rupture or tear involving skin during delivery
Perineal laceration, rupture or tear involving vagina during delivery
Perineal laceration, rupture or tear involving vulva during delivery
Slight perineal laceration, rupture or tear during delivery

O70.1 Second degree perineal laceration during delivery

Perineal laceration, rupture or tear during delivery as in O70.0, also involving pelvic floor
Perineal laceration, rupture or tear during delivery as in O70.0, also involving perineal muscles
Perineal laceration, rupture or tear during delivery as in O70.0, also involving vaginal muscles

EXCLUDES 1 *perineal laceration involving anal sphincter (O70.2)*

AHA: 2Q 2016, 34

O70.2 Third degree perineal laceration during delivery

Perineal laceration, rupture or tear during delivery as in O70.1, also involving anal sphincter
Perineal laceration, rupture or tear during delivery as in O70.1, also involving rectovaginal septum
Perineal laceration, rupture or tear during delivery as in O70.1, also involving sphincter NOS

EXCLUDES 1 *anal sphincter tear during delivery without third degree perineal laceration (O70.4)*
perineal laceration involving anal or rectal mucosa (O70.3)

O70.20 Third degree perineal laceration during delivery, unspecified

AHA: 4Q 2016, 53

O70.21 Third degree perineal laceration during delivery, IIIa

Third degree perineal laceration during delivery with less than 50% of external anal sphincter (EAS) thickness torn

AHA: 4Q 2016, 53

O70.22 Third degree perineal laceration during delivery, IIIb

Third degree perineal laceration during delivery with more than 50% external anal sphincter (EAS) thickness torn

AHA: 4Q 2016, 53

O70.23 Third degree perineal laceration during delivery, IIIc

Third degree perineal laceration during delivery with both external anal sphincter (EAS) and internal anal sphincter (IAS) torn

AHA: 4Q 2016, 53

O70.3 Fourth degree perineal laceration during delivery

Perineal laceration, rupture or tear during delivery as in O70.2, also involving anal mucosa
Perineal laceration, rupture or tear during delivery as in O70.2, also involving rectal mucosa

O70.4 Anal sphincter tear complicating delivery, not associated with third degree laceration

EXCLUDES 1 *anal sphincter tear with third degree perineal laceration (O70.2)*

O70.9 Perineal laceration during delivery, unspecified

O71 Other obstetric trauma

INCLUDES obstetric damage from instruments

O71.0 Rupture of uterus (spontaneous) before onset of labor

EXCLUDES 1 *disruption of (current) cesarean delivery wound (O90.0)*
laceration of uterus, NEC (O71.81)

O71.00 Rupture of uterus before onset of labor, unspecified trimester

O71.02 Rupture of uterus before onset of labor, second trimester

O71.03 Rupture of uterus before onset of labor, third trimester

O71.1 Rupture of uterus during labor ♀ M
Rupture of uterus not stated as occurring before onset of labor
EXCLUDES 1 *disruption of cesarean delivery wound (O90.0)*
laceration of uterus, NEC (O71.81)

O71.2 Postpartum inversion of uterus ♀ M

O71.3 Obstetric laceration of cervix ♀ M
Annular detachment of cervix

O71.4 Obstetric high vaginal laceration alone ♀ M
Laceration of vaginal wall without perineal laceration
EXCLUDES 1 *obstetric high vaginal laceration with perineal laceration (O70.-)*

O71.5 Other obstetric injury to pelvic organs ♀ M
Obstetric injury to bladder
Obstetric injury to urethra
EXCLUDES 2 *obstetric periurethral trauma (O71.82)*
AHA: 4Q 2014, 18

O71.6 Obstetric damage to pelvic joints and ligaments ♀ M
Obstetric avulsion of inner symphyseal cartilage
Obstetric damage to coccyx
Obstetric traumatic separation of symphysis (pubis)

O71.7 Obstetric hematoma of pelvis ♀ M
Obstetric hematoma of perineum
Obstetric hematoma of vagina
Obstetric hematoma of vulva

5 **O71.8 Other specified obstetric trauma**

O71.81 Laceration of uterus, not elsewhere classified ♀ M

O71.82 Other specified trauma to perineum and vulva ♀ M
Obstetric periurethral trauma
AHA: 4Q 2014, 18

O71.89 Other specified obstetric trauma ♀ M

O71.9 Obstetric trauma, unspecified ♀ M

4 O72 Postpartum hemorrhage

INCLUDES hemorrhage after delivery of fetus or infant

O72.0 Third-stage hemorrhage ♀ M
Hemorrhage associated with retained, trapped or adherent placenta
Retained placenta NOS
Code also:
type of adherent placenta (O43.2-)

O72.1 Other immediate postpartum hemorrhage ♀ M
Hemorrhage following delivery of placenta
Postpartum hemorrhage (atonic) NOS
Uterine atony with hemorrhage
EXCLUDES 1 *uterine atony NOS (O62.2)*
uterine atony without hemorrhage (O62.2)
postpartum atony of uterus without hemorrhage (O75.89)

O72.2 Delayed and secondary postpartum hemorrhage ♀ M
Hemorrhage associated with retained portions of placenta or membranes after the first 24 hours following delivery of placenta
Retained products of conception NOS, following delivery

O72.3 Postpartum coagulation defects ♀ M
Postpartum afibrinogenemia
Postpartum fibrinolysis

4 O73 Retained placenta and membranes, without hemorrhage

EXCLUDES 1 *placenta accreta (O43.21-)*
placenta increta (O43.22-)
placenta percreta (O43.23-)

O73.0 Retained placenta without hemorrhage ♀ M
Adherent placenta, without hemorrhage
Trapped placenta without hemorrhage

O73.1 Retained portions of placenta and membranes, without hemorrhage ♀ M
Retained products of conception following delivery, without hemorrhage

4 O74 Complications of anesthesia during labor and delivery

INCLUDES maternal complications arising from the administration of a general, regional or local anesthetic, analgesic or other sedation during labor and delivery

Use additional code, if applicable, to identify specific complication

O74.0 Aspiration pneumonitis due to anesthesia during labor and delivery ♀ M
Inhalation of stomach contents or secretions NOS due to anesthesia during labor and delivery
Mendelson's syndrome due to anesthesia during labor and delivery

O74.1 Other pulmonary complications of anesthesia during labor and delivery ♀ M

O74.2 Cardiac complications of anesthesia during labor and delivery ♀ M

O74.3 Central nervous system complications of anesthesia during labor and delivery ♀ M

O74.4 Toxic reaction to local anesthesia during labor and delivery ♀ M

O74.5 Spinal and epidural anesthesia-induced headache during labor and delivery ♀ M

O74.6 Other complications of spinal and epidural anesthesia during labor and delivery ♀ M

O74.7 Failed or difficult intubation for anesthesia during labor and delivery ♀ M

O74.8 Other complications of anesthesia during labor and delivery ♀ M

O74.9 Complication of anesthesia during labor and delivery, unspecified ♀ M

4 O75 Other complications of labor and delivery, not elsewhere classified

EXCLUDES 2 *puerperal (postpartum) infection (O86.-)*
puerperal (postpartum) sepsis (O85)

O75.0 Maternal distress during labor and delivery ♀ M

O75.1 Shock during or following labor and delivery ♀ M
Obstetric shock following labor and delivery

O75.2 Pyrexia during labor, not elsewhere classified ♀ M

O75.3 Other infection during labor ♀ M
Sepsis during labor
Use additional code (B95-B97), to identify infectious agent

▲ **O75.4 Other complications of obstetric surgery and procedures** ♀ M
Cardiac arrest following obstetric surgery or procedures
Cardiac failure following obstetric surgery or procedures
Cerebral anoxia following obstetric surgery or procedures
Pulmonary edema following obstetric surgery or procedures
Use additional code to identify specific complication
EXCLUDES 2 *complications of anesthesia during labor and delivery (O74.-)*
disruption of obstetrical (surgical) wound (O90.0-O90.1)
hematoma of obstetrical (surgical) wound (O90.2)
infection of obstetrical (surgical) wound (O86.0-)

O75.5 Delayed delivery after artificial rupture of membranes ♀ M

5 **O75.8 Other specified complications of labor and delivery**

O75.81 Maternal exhaustion complicating labor and delivery ♀ M

O75.82 Onset (spontaneous) of labor after 37 completed weeks of gestation but before 39 completed weeks gestation, with delivery by (planned) cesarean section ♀ M
Delivery by (planned) cesarean section occurring after 37 completed weeks of gestation but before 39 completed weeks gestation due to (spontaneous) onset of labor
Code first to specify reason for planned cesarean section such as:
cephalopelvic disproportion (normally formed fetus) (O33.9)
previous cesarean delivery (O34.21)

O75.89 Other specified complications of labor and delivery ♀ M

O75.9 Complication of labor and delivery, unspecified ♀ M

O76 Abnormality in fetal heart rate and rhythmcomplicating labor and delivery ♀M

Depressed fetal heart rate tones complicating labor and delivery
Fetal bradycardia complicating labor and delivery
Fetal heart rate decelerations complicating labor and delivery
Fetal heart rate irregularity complicating labor and delivery
Fetal heart rate abnormal variability complicating labor and delivery
Fetal tachycardia complicating labor and delivery
Non-reassuring fetal heart rate or rhythm complicating labor and delivery

EXCLUDES 1 *fetal stress NOS (O77.9)*
labor and delivery complicated by electrocardiographic evidence of fetal stress (O77.8)
labor and delivery complicated by ultrasonic evidence of fetal stress (O77.8)

EXCLUDES 2 *fetal metabolic acidemia (O68)*
other fetal stress (O77.0-O77.1)

AHA: 4Q 2013, 118

4 O77 Other fetal stress complicating labor and delivery

O77.0 Labor and delivery complicated by meconium in amniotic fluid ♀M
AHA: 4Q 2013, 118

O77.1 Fetal stress in labor or delivery due to drug administration ♀M

O77.8 Labor and delivery complicated by other evidence of fetal stress ♀M
Labor and delivery complicated by electrocardiographic evidence of fetal stress
Labor and delivery complicated by ultrasonic evidence of fetal stress

EXCLUDES 1 *abnormality of fetal acid-base balance (O68)*
abnormality in fetal heart rate or rhythm (O76)
fetal metabolic acidemia (O68)

O77.9 Labor and delivery complicated by fetal stress, unspecified ♀M

EXCLUDES 1 *abnormality of fetal acid-base balance (O68)*
abnormality in fetal heart rate or rhythm (O76)
fetal metabolic acidemia (O68)

Encounter for delivery (O80-O82)

O80 Encounter for full-term uncomplicated delivery ♀M
Delivery requiring minimal or no assistance, with or without episiotomy, without fetal manipulation [e.g., rotation version] or instrumentation [forceps] of a spontaneous, cephalic, vaginal, full-term, single, live-born infant. This code is for use as a single diagnosis code and is not to be used with any other code from chapter 15.
Use additional code to indicate outcome of delivery (Z37.0)
AHA: 2Q 2014, 9
AHA: 4Q 2016, 150

O82 Encounter for cesarean delivery without indication ♀M
Use additional code to indicate outcome of delivery (Z37.0)

Complications predominantly related to the puerperium (O85-O92)

EXCLUDES 2 *mental and behavioral disorders associated with the puerperium (F53.-)*
obstetrical tetanus (A34)
puerperal osteomalacia (M83.0)

GUIDELINES **Section I.C.15.a.2)**
Chapter 15 codes are to be used only on the maternal record, never on the record of the newborn.

O85 Puerperal sepsis ♀M
Postpartum sepsis
Puerperal peritonitis
Puerperal pyemia
Use additional code (B95-B97), to identify infectious agent
Use additional code (R65.2-) to identify severe sepsis, if applicable

EXCLUDES 1 *fever of unknown origin following delivery (O86.4)*
genital tract infection following delivery (O86.1-)
obstetric pyemic and septic embolism (O88.3-)
puerperal septic thrombophlebitis (O86.81)
urinary tract infection following delivery (O86.2-)

EXCLUDES 2 *sepsis during labor (O75.3)*

GUIDELINES **Section I.C.15.k**
Code O85, Puerperal sepsis, should be assigned with a secondary code to identify the causal organism (e.g., for a bacterial infection, assign a code from category B95-B96, Bacterial infections in conditions classified elsewhere). A code from category A40, Streptococcal sepsis, or A41, Other sepsis, should not be used for puerperal sepsis. If applicable, use additional codes to identify severe sepsis (R65.2-) and any associated acute organ dysfunction.

4 O86 Other puerperal infections
Use additional code (B95-B97), to identify infectious agent

EXCLUDES 2 *infection during labor (O75.3)*
obstetrical tetanus (A34)

GUIDELINES **Section I.C.1.d.5)(b-c)**
For infections following a procedure, a code from T81.40, to T81.43 Infection following a procedure, or a code from O86.00 to O86.03, Infection of obstetric surgical wound, that identifies the site of the infection should be coded first, if known. Assign an additional code for sepsis following a procedure (T81.44) or sepsis following an obstetrical procedure (O86.04). Use an additional code to identify the infectious agent. If the patient has severe sepsis, the appropriate code from subcategory R65.2 should also be assigned with the additional code(s) for any acute organ dysfunction.

If a postprocedural infection has resulted in postprocedural septic shock, assign the codes indicated above for sepsis due to a postprocedural infection, followed by code T81.12-, Postprocedural septic shock. Do not assign code R65.21, Severe sepsis with septic shock. Additional code(s) should be assigned for any acute organ dysfunction.

▲ 5 **O86.0 Infection of obstetric surgical wound**
Infected cesarean delivery wound following delivery
Infected perineal repair following delivery

EXCLUDES 1 *complications of procedures, not elsewhere classified (T81.4-)*
postprocedural fever NOS (R50.82)
postprocedural retroperitoneal abscess (K68.11)

● **O86.00 Infection of obstetric surgical wound, unspecified** ♀M

● **O86.01 Infection of obstetric surgical wound, superficial incisional site** ♀M
Subcutaneous abscess following an obstetrical procedure
Stitch abscess following an obstetrical procedure

● **O86.02 Infection of obstetric surgical wound, deep incisional site** ♀M
Intramuscular abscess following an obstetrical procedure
Sub-fascial abscess following a procedure

● **O86.03 Infection of obstetric surgical wound, organ and space site** ♀M
Intraabdominal abscess following an obstetrical procedure
Subphrenic abscess following an obstetrical procedure

● **O86.04 Sepsis following an obstetrical procedure** ♀M
Use additional code to identify the sepsis

● **O86.09 Infection of obstetric surgical wound, other surgical site** ♀M

5 **O86.1 Other infection of genital tract following delivery**

O86.11 Cervicitis following delivery ♀M

O86.12 **Endometritis following delivery** ♀
O86.13 **Vaginitis following delivery** ♀
O86.19 **Other infection of genital tract following delivery** ♀
O86.2 **Urinary tract infection following delivery**
O86.20 **Urinary tract infection following delivery, unspecified** ♀
Puerperal urinary tract infection NOS
O86.21 **Infection of kidney following delivery** ♀
O86.22 **Infection of bladder following delivery** ♀
Infection of urethra following delivery
O86.29 **Other urinary tract infection following delivery** ♀
O86.4 **Pyrexia of unknown origin following delivery** ♀
Puerperal infection NOS following delivery
Puerperal pyrexia NOS following delivery
EXCLUDES 2 *pyrexia during labor (O75.2)*
O86.8 **Other specified puerperal infections**
O86.81 **Puerperal septic thrombophlebitis** ♀
O86.89 **Other specified puerperal infections** ♀

O87 Venous complications and hemorrhoids in the puerperium

INCLUDES venous complications in labor, delivery and the puerperium
EXCLUDES 2 *obstetric embolism (O88.-)*
puerperal septic thrombophlebitis (O86.81)
venous complications in pregnancy (O22.-)

O87.0 **Superficial thrombophlebitis in the puerperium** ♀
Puerperal phlebitis NOS
Puerperal thrombosis NOS
O87.1 **Deep phlebothrombosis in the puerperium** ♀
Deep vein thrombosis, postpartum
Pelvic thrombophlebitis, postpartum
Use additional code to identify the deep vein thrombosis (I82.4-, I82.5-, I82.62-, I82.72-)
Use additional code, if applicable, for associated long-term (current) use of anticoagulants (Z79.01)
O87.2 **Hemorrhoids in the puerperium** ♀
O87.3 **Cerebral venous thrombosis in the puerperium** ♀
Cerebrovenous sinus thrombosis in the puerperium
O87.4 **Varicose veins of lower extremity in the puerperium** ♀
O87.8 **Other venous complications in the puerperium** ♀
Genital varices in the puerperium
O87.9 **Venous complication in the puerperium, unspecified** ♀
Puerperal phlebopathy NOS

O88 Obstetric embolism

EXCLUDES 1 *embolism complicating abortion NOS (O03.2)*
embolism complicating ectopic or molar pregnancy (O08.2)
embolism complicating failed attempted abortion (O07.2)
embolism complicating induced abortion (O04.7)
embolism complicating spontaneous abortion (O03.2, O03.7)

O88.0 **Obstetric air embolism**
O88.01 **Obstetric air embolism in pregnancy**
O88.011 **Air embolism in pregnancy, first trimester** ♀
O88.012 **Air embolism in pregnancy, second trimester** ♀
O88.013 **Air embolism in pregnancy, third trimester** ♀
O88.019 **Air embolism in pregnancy, unspecified trimester** ♀
O88.02 **Air embolism in childbirth** ♀
O88.03 **Air embolism in the puerperium** ♀
O88.1 **Amniotic fluid embolism**
Anaphylactoid syndrome in pregnancy
O88.11 **Amniotic fluid embolism in pregnancy**
O88.111 **Amniotic fluid embolism in pregnancy, first trimester** ♀
O88.112 **Amniotic fluid embolism in pregnancy, second trimester** ♀
O88.113 **Amniotic fluid embolism in pregnancy, third trimester** ♀
O88.119 **Amniotic fluid embolism in pregnancy, unspecified trimester** ♀
O88.12 **Amniotic fluid embolism in childbirth** ♀
O88.13 **Amniotic fluid embolism in the puerperium** ♀
O88.2 **Obstetric thromboembolism**
O88.21 **Thromboembolism in pregnancy**
Obstetric (pulmonary) embolism NOS
O88.211 **Thromboembolism in pregnancy, first trimester** ♀
O88.212 **Thromboembolism in pregnancy, second trimester** ♀
O88.213 **Thromboembolism in pregnancy, third trimester** ♀
O88.219 **Thromboembolism in pregnancy, unspecified trimester** ♀
O88.22 **Thromboembolism in childbirth** ♀
O88.23 **Thromboembolism in the puerperium** ♀
Puerperal (pulmonary) embolism NOS
O88.3 **Obstetric pyemic and septic embolism**
O88.31 **Pyemic and septic embolism in pregnancy**
O88.311 **Pyemic and septic embolism in pregnancy, first trimester** ♀
O88.312 **Pyemic and septic embolism in pregnancy, second trimester** ♀
O88.313 **Pyemic and septic embolism in pregnancy, third trimester** ♀
O88.319 **Pyemic and septic embolism in pregnancy, unspecified trimester** ♀
O88.32 **Pyemic and septic embolism in childbirth** ♀
O88.33 **Pyemic and septic embolism in the puerperium** ♀
O88.8 **Other obstetric embolism**
Obstetric fat embolism
O88.81 **Other embolism in pregnancy**
O88.811 **Other embolism in pregnancy, first trimester** ♀
O88.812 **Other embolism in pregnancy, second trimester** ♀
O88.813 **Other embolism in pregnancy, third trimester** ♀
O88.819 **Other embolism in pregnancy, unspecified trimester** ♀
O88.82 **Other embolism in childbirth** ♀
O88.83 **Other embolism in the puerperium** ♀

O89 Complications of anesthesia during the puerperium

INCLUDES maternal complications arising from the administration of a general, regional or local anesthetic, analgesic or other sedation during the puerperium
Use additional code, if applicable, to identify specific complication

O89.0 **Pulmonary complications of anesthesia during the puerperium**
O89.01 **Aspiration pneumonitis due to anesthesia during the puerperium** ♀
Inhalation of stomach contents or secretions NOS due to anesthesia during the puerperium
Mendelson's syndrome due to anesthesia during the puerperium
O89.09 **Other pulmonary complications of anesthesia during the puerperium** ♀
O89.1 **Cardiac complications of anesthesia during the puerperium** ♀
O89.2 **Central nervous system complications of anesthesia during the puerperium** ♀
O89.3 **Toxic reaction to local anesthesia during the puerperium** ♀
O89.4 **Spinal and epidural anesthesia-induced headache during the puerperium** ♀
O89.5 **Other complications of spinal and epidural anesthesia during the puerperium** ♀
O89.6 **Failed or difficult intubation for anesthesia during the puerperium** ♀
O89.8 **Other complications of anesthesia during the puerperium** ♀
O89.9 **Complication of anesthesia during the puerperium, unspecified** ♀

O90 Complications of the puerperium, not elsewhere classified

O90.0 Disruption of cesarean delivery wound
Dehiscence of cesarean delivery wound
EXCLUDES 1 *rupture of uterus (spontaneous) before onset of labor (O71.0-)*
rupture of uterus during labor (O71.1)

O90.1 Disruption of perineal obstetric wound
Disruption of wound of episiotomy
Disruption of wound of perineal laceration
Secondary perineal tear

Disruption of perineal obstetric wound

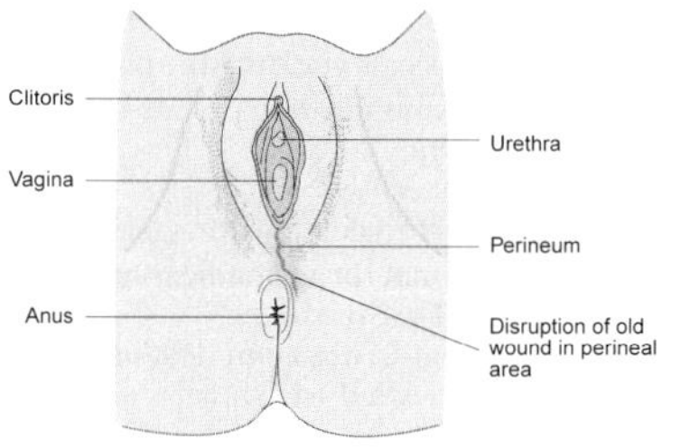

O90.2 Hematoma of obstetric wound

O90.3 Peripartum cardiomyopathy
Conditions in I42.- arising during pregnancy and the puerperium
EXCLUDES 1 *pre-existing heart disease complicating pregnancy and the puerperium (O99.4-)*
GUIDELINES **Section I.C.15.o.5)**
Pregnancy associated cardiomyopathy, code O90.3, is unique in that it may be diagnosed in the third trimester of pregnancy but may continue to progress months after delivery. For this reason, it is referred to as peripartum cardiomyopathy. Code O90.3 is only for use when the cardiomyopathy develops as a result of pregnancy in a woman who did not have pre-existing heart disease.

O90.4 Postpartum acute kidney failure
Hepatorenal syndrome following labor and delivery

O90.5 Postpartum thyroiditis

▲ **O90.6 Postpartum mood disturbance**
Postpartum blues
Postpartum dysphoria
Postpartum sadness
EXCLUDES 1 *postpartum depression (F53.0)*
puerperal psychosis (F53.1)

[5] **O90.8 Other complications of the puerperium, not elsewhere classified**

O90.81 Anemia of the puerperium
Postpartum anemia NOS
EXCLUDES 1 *pre-existing anemia complicating the puerperium (O99.03)*
CODING TIP Use O90.81 for diagnosed anemia complicating the postpartum period. Use O99.01 for anemia complicating pregnancy. Use O99.03 for pre-existing anemia complicating the puerperium.

O90.89 Other complications of the puerperium, not elsewhere classified
Placental polyp

O90.9 Complication of the puerperium, unspecified

[4] **O91 Infections of breast associated with pregnancy, the puerperium and lactation**
Use additional code to identify infection

[5] **O91.0 Infection of nipple associated with pregnancy, the puerperium and lactation**

[6] **O91.01 Infection of nipple associated with pregnancy**
Gestational abscess of nipple

O91.011 Infection of nipple associated with pregnancy, first trimester

O91.012 Infection of nipple associated with pregnancy, second trimester

O91.013 Infection of nipple associated with pregnancy, third trimester

O91.019 Infection of nipple associated with pregnancy, unspecified trimester

O91.02 Infection of nipple associated with the puerperium
Puerperal abscess of nipple

O91.03 Infection of nipple associated with lactation
Abscess of nipple associated with lactation

[5] **O91.1 Abscess of breast associated with pregnancy, the puerperium and lactation**

[6] **O91.11 Abscess of breast associated with pregnancy**
Gestational mammary abscess
Gestational purulent mastitis
Gestational subareolar abscess

O91.111 Abscess of breast associated with pregnancy, first trimester

O91.112 Abscess of breast associated with pregnancy, second trimester

O91.113 Abscess of breast associated with pregnancy, third trimester

O91.119 Abscess of breast associated with pregnancy, unspecified trimester

O91.12 Abscess of breast associated with the puerperium
Puerperal mammary abscess
Puerperal purulent mastitis
Puerperal subareolar abscess

O91.13 Abscess of breast associated with lactation
Mammary abscess associated with lactation
Purulent mastitis associated with lactation
Subareolar abscess associated with lactation

[5] **O91.2 Nonpurulent mastitis associated with pregnancy, the puerperium and lactation**

[6] **O91.21 Nonpurulent mastitis associated with pregnancy**
Gestational interstitial mastitis
Gestational lymphangitis of breast
Gestational mastitis NOS
Gestational parenchymatous mastitis

O91.211 Nonpurulent mastitis associated with pregnancy, first trimester

O91.212 Nonpurulent mastitis associated with pregnancy, second trimester

O91.213 Nonpurulent mastitis associated with pregnancy, third trimester

O91.219 Nonpurulent mastitis associated with pregnancy, unspecified trimester

O91.22 Nonpurulent mastitis associated with the puerperium
Puerperal interstitial mastitis
Puerperal lymphangitis of breast
Puerperal mastitis NOS
Puerperal parenchymatous mastitis

O91.23 Nonpurulent mastitis associated with lactation
Interstitial mastitis associated with lactation
Lymphangitis of breast associated with lactation
Mastitis NOS associated with lactation
Parenchymatous mastitis associated with lactation

[4] **O92 Other disorders of breast and disorders of lactation associated with pregnancy and the puerperium**

[5] **O92.0 Retracted nipple associated with pregnancy, the puerperium, and lactation**

[6] **O92.01 Retracted nipple associated with pregnancy**

O92.011 Retracted nipple associated with pregnancy, first trimester

O92.012 Retracted nipple associated with pregnancy, second trimester

O92.013 Retracted nipple associated with pregnancy, third trimester

O92.019 Retracted nipple associated with pregnancy, unspecified trimester

O92.02 Retracted nipple associated with the puerperium

O92.03 Retracted nipple associated with lactation

[5] **O92.1 Cracked nipple associated with pregnancy, the puerperium, and lactation**
Fissure of nipple, gestational or puerperal

[6] **O92.11 Cracked nipple associated with pregnancy**

O92.111 Cracked nipple associated with pregnancy, first trimester

O92.112 Cracked nipple associated with pregnancy, second trimester

O92.113 Cracked nipple associated with pregnancy, third trimester

O92.119 Cracked nipple associated with pregnancy, unspecified trimester ♀ M

O92.12 Cracked nipple associated with the puerperium ♀ M

O92.13 Cracked nipple associated with lactation ♀ M

5 O92.2 Other and unspecified disorders of breast associated with pregnancy and the puerperium

O92.20 Unspecified disorder of breast associated with pregnancy and the puerperium ♀ M

O92.29 Other disorders of breast associated with pregnancy and the puerperium ♀ M

O92.3 Agalactia ♀ M
Primary agalactia
EXCLUDES 1 *Elective agalactia (O92.5)*
Secondary agalactia (O92.5)
Therapeutic agalactia (O92.5)

O92.4 Hypogalactia ♀ M

O92.5 Suppressed lactation ♀ M
Elective agalactia
Secondary agalactia
Therapeutic agalactia
EXCLUDES 1 *primary agalactia (O92.3)*

O92.6 Galactorrhea ♀ M

5 O92.7 Other and unspecified disorders of lactation

O92.70 Unspecified disorders of lactation ♀ M

O92.79 Other disorders of lactation ♀ M
Puerperal galactocele

Other obstetric conditions, not elsewhere classified (O94-O9A)

O94 Sequelae of complication of pregnancy, childbirth, and the puerperium ♀ M
Note: This category is to be used to indicate conditions in O00-O77.-, O85-O94 and O98-O9A.- as the cause of late effects. The sequelae include conditions specified as such, or as late effects, which may occur at any time after the puerperium
Code first:
condition resulting from (sequela) of complication of pregnancy, childbirth, and the puerperium

GUIDELINES Section I.C.15.p.1)-3)
Code O94 is for use in those cases when an initial complication of a pregnancy develops a sequelae requiring care or treatment at a future date. This code may be used at any time after the initial postpartum period. This code, like all sequela codes, is to be sequenced following the code describing the sequelae of the complication.

4 O98 Maternal infectious and parasitic diseases classifiable elsewhere but complicating pregnancy, childbirth and the puerperium
INCLUDES the listed conditions when complicating the pregnant state, when aggravated by the pregnancy, or as a reason for obstetric care
Use additional code (Chapter 1), to identify specific infectious or parasitic disease
EXCLUDES 2 *herpes gestationis (O26.4-)*
infectious carrier state (O99.82-, O99.83-)
obstetrical tetanus (A34)
puerperal infection (O86.-)
puerperal sepsis (O85)
when the reason for maternal care is that the disease is known or suspected to have affected the fetus (O35-O36)

5 O98.0 Tuberculosis complicating pregnancy, childbirth and the puerperium
Conditions in A15-A19

6 O98.01 Tuberculosis complicating pregnancy

O98.011 Tuberculosis complicating pregnancy, first trimester ♀ M

O98.012 Tuberculosis complicating pregnancy, second trimester ♀ M

O98.013 Tuberculosis complicating pregnancy, third trimester ♀ M

O98.019 Tuberculosis complicating pregnancy, unspecified trimester ♀ M

O98.02 Tuberculosis complicating childbirth ♀ M

O98.03 Tuberculosis complicating the puerperium ♀ M

5 O98.1 Syphilis complicating pregnancy, childbirth and the puerperium
Conditions in A50-A53

6 O98.11 Syphilis complicating pregnancy

O98.111 Syphilis complicating pregnancy, first trimester ♀ M

O98.112 Syphilis complicating pregnancy, second trimester ♀ M

O98.113 Syphilis complicating pregnancy, third trimester ♀ M

O98.119 Syphilis complicating pregnancy, unspecified trimester ♀ M

O98.12 Syphilis complicating childbirth ♀ M

O98.13 Syphilis complicating the puerperium ♀ M

5 O98.2 Gonorrhea complicating pregnancy, childbirth and the puerperium
Conditions in A54.-

6 O98.21 Gonorrhea complicating pregnancy

O98.211 Gonorrhea complicating pregnancy, first trimester ♀ M

O98.212 Gonorrhea complicating pregnancy, second trimester ♀ M

O98.213 Gonorrhea complicating pregnancy, third trimester ♀ M

O98.219 Gonorrhea complicating pregnancy, unspecified trimester ♀ M

O98.22 Gonorrhea complicating childbirth ♀ M

O98.23 Gonorrhea complicating the puerperium ♀ M

5 O98.3 Other infections with a predominantly sexual mode of transmission complicating pregnancy, childbirth and the puerperium
Conditions in A55-A64

6 O98.31 Other infections with a predominantly sexual mode of transmission complicating pregnancy

O98.311 Other infections with a predominantly sexual mode of transmission complicating pregnancy, first trimester ♀ M

O98.312 Other infections with a predominantly sexual mode of transmission complicating pregnancy, second trimester ♀ M

O98.313 Other infections with a predominantly sexual mode of transmission complicating pregnancy, third trimester ♀ M

O98.319 Other infections with a predominantly sexual mode of transmission complicating pregnancy, unspecified trimester ♀ M

O98.32 Other infections with a predominantly sexual mode of transmission complicating childbirth ♀ M

O98.33 Other infections with a predominantly sexual mode of transmission complicating the puerperium ♀ M

5 O98.4 Viral hepatitis complicating pregnancy, childbirth and the puerperium
Conditions in B15-B19

6 O98.41 Viral hepatitis complicating pregnancy

O98.411 Viral hepatitis complicating pregnancy, first trimester ♀ M

O98.412 Viral hepatitis complicating pregnancy, second trimester ♀ M

O98.413 Viral hepatitis complicating pregnancy, third trimester ♀ M

O98.419 Viral hepatitis complicating pregnancy, unspecified trimester ♀ M

O98.42 Viral hepatitis complicating childbirth ♀ M

O98.43 Viral hepatitis complicating the puerperium ♀ M

5 O98.5 Other viral diseases complicating pregnancy, childbirth and the puerperium
Conditions in A80-B09, B25-B34, R87.81-, R87.82-
EXCLUDES 1 *human immunodeficiency virus [HIV] disease complicating pregnancy, childbirth and the puerperium (O98.7-)*

6 O98.51 Other viral diseases complicating pregnancy

O98.511 Other viral diseases complicating pregnancy, first trimester ♀ M

O98.512 Other viral diseases complicating pregnancy, second trimester ♀ M

O98.513 Other viral diseases complicating pregnancy, third trimester ♀ M

O98.519 Other viral diseases complicating pregnancy, unspecified trimester ♀ M

O98.52 **Other viral diseases complicating childbirth** ♀M

O98.53 **Other viral diseases complicating the puerperium** ♀M

5 O98.6 **Protozoal diseases complicating pregnancy, childbirth and the puerperium**

Conditions in B50-B64

6 O98.61 **Protozoal diseases complicating pregnancy**

O98.611 **Protozoal diseases complicating pregnancy, first trimester** ♀M

O98.612 **Protozoal diseases complicating pregnancy, second trimester** ♀M

O98.613 **Protozoal diseases complicating pregnancy, third trimester** ♀M

O98.619 **Protozoal diseases complicating pregnancy, unspecified trimester** ♀M

O98.62 **Protozoal diseases complicating childbirth** ♀M

O98.63 **Protozoal diseases complicating the puerperium** ♀M

5 O98.7 **Human immunodeficiency virus [HIV] disease complicating pregnancy, childbirth and the puerperium**

Use additional code to identify the type of HIV disease:

Acquired immune deficiency syndrome (AIDS) (B20)

Asymptomatic HIV status (Z21)

HIV positive NOS (Z21)

Symptomatic HIV disease (B20)

GUIDELINES **Section I.C.1.a.2)(g)**

During pregnancy, childbirth or the puerperium, a patient admitted (or presenting for a health care encounter) because of an HIV-related illness should receive a principal diagnosis code of O98.7-, followed by B20 and the code(s) for the HIV-related illness(es). Codes from Chapter 15 always take sequencing priority.

Patients with asymptomatic HIV infection status admitted (or presenting for a health care encounter) during pregnancy, childbirth, or the puerperium should receive codes of O98.7- and Z21.

6 O98.71 **Human immunodeficiency virus [HIV] disease complicating pregnancy**

O98.711 **Human immunodeficiency virus [HIV] disease complicating pregnancy, first trimester** ♀M

O98.712 **Human immunodeficiency virus [HIV] disease complicating pregnancy, second trimester** ♀M

O98.713 **Human immunodeficiency virus [HIV] disease complicating pregnancy, third trimester** ♀M

O98.719 **Human immunodeficiency virus [HIV] disease complicating pregnancy, unspecified trimester** ♀M

O98.72 **Human immunodeficiency virus [HIV] disease complicating childbirth** ♀M

O98.73 **Human immunodeficiency virus [HIV] disease complicating the puerperium** ♀M

5 O98.8 **Other maternal infectious and parasitic diseases complicating pregnancy, childbirth and the puerperium**

6 O98.81 **Other maternal infectious and parasitic diseases complicating pregnancy**

O98.811 **Other maternal infectious and parasitic diseases complicating pregnancy, first trimester** ♀M

O98.812 **Other maternal infectious and parasitic diseases complicating pregnancy, second trimester** ♀M

O98.813 **Other maternal infectious and parasitic diseases complicating pregnancy, third trimester** ♀M

O98.819 **Other maternal infectious and parasitic diseases complicating pregnancy, unspecified trimester** ♀M

O98.82 **Other maternal infectious and parasitic diseases complicating childbirth** ♀M

O98.83 **Other maternal infectious and parasitic diseases complicating the puerperium** ♀M

5 O98.9 **Unspecified maternal infectious and parasitic disease complicating pregnancy, childbirth and the puerperium**

6 O98.91 **Unspecified maternal infectious and parasitic disease complicating pregnancy**

O98.911 **Unspecified maternal infectious and parasitic disease complicating pregnancy, first trimester** ♀M

O98.912 **Unspecified maternal infectious and parasitic disease complicating pregnancy, second trimester** ♀M

O98.913 **Unspecified maternal infectious and parasitic disease complicating pregnancy, third trimester** ♀M

O98.919 **Unspecified maternal infectious and parasitic disease complicating pregnancy, unspecified trimester** ♀M

O98.92 **Unspecified maternal infectious and parasitic disease complicating childbirth** ♀M

O98.93 **Unspecified maternal infectious and parasitic disease complicating the puerperium** ♀M

4 O99 **Other maternal diseases classifiable elsewhere but complicating pregnancy, childbirth and the puerperium**

INCLUDES conditions which complicate the pregnant state, are aggravated by the pregnancy or are a main reason for obstetric care

Use additional code to identify specific condition

EXCLUDES 2 *when the reason for maternal care is that the condition is known or suspected to have affected the fetus (O35-O36)*

5 O99.0 **Anemia complicating pregnancy, childbirth and the puerperium**

Conditions in D50-D64

EXCLUDES 1 *anemia arising in the puerperium (O90.81)*
postpartum anemia NOS (O90.81)

6 O99.01 **Anemia complicating pregnancy**

CODING TIP ✓ Use O90.81 for diagnosed anemia complicating the postpartum period. Use O99.01 for anemia complicating pregnancy. Use O99.03 for pre-existing anemia complicating the puerperium.

O99.011 **Anemia complicating pregnancy, first trimester** ♀M

O99.012 **Anemia complicating pregnancy, second trimester** ♀M

O99.013 **Anemia complicating pregnancy, third trimester** ♀M

O99.019 **Anemia complicating pregnancy, unspecified trimester** ♀M

O99.02 **Anemia complicating childbirth** ♀M

O99.03 **Anemia complicating the puerperium** ♀M

EXCLUDES 1 *postpartum anemia not pre-existing prior to delivery (O90.81)*

CODING TIP ✓ Use O90.81 for diagnosed anemia complicating the postpartum period. Use O99.01 for anemia complicating pregnancy. Use O99.03 for pre-existing anemia complicating the puerperium.

5 O99.1 **Other diseases of the blood and blood-forming organs and certain disorders involving the immune mechanism complicating pregnancy, childbirth and the puerperium**

Conditions in D65-D89

EXCLUDES 1 *hemorrhage with coagulation defects (O45.-, O46.0-, O67.0, O72.3)*

6 O99.11 **Other diseases of the blood and blood-forming organs and certain disorders involving the immune mechanism complicating pregnancy**

O99.111 **Other diseases of the blood and blood-forming organs and certain disorders involving the immune mechanism complicating pregnancy, first trimester** ♀M

O99.112 **Other diseases of the blood and blood-forming organs and certain disorders involving the immune mechanism complicating pregnancy, second trimester** ♀M

O99.113 **Other diseases of the blood and blood-forming organs and certain disorders involving the immune mechanism complicating pregnancy, third trimester** ♀M

O99.119 Other diseases of the blood and blood-forming organs and certain disorders involving the immune mechanism complicating pregnancy, unspecified trimester ♀M

O99.12 Other diseases of the blood and blood-forming organs and certain disorders involving the immune mechanism complicating childbirth ♀M

O99.13 Other diseases of the blood and blood-forming organs and certain disorders involving the immune mechanism complicating the puerperium ♀M

5 O99.2 Endocrine, nutritional and metabolic diseases complicating pregnancy, childbirth and the puerperium
Conditions in E00-E88
EXCLUDES 2 *diabetes mellitus (O24.-)*
malnutrition (O25.-)
postpartum thyroiditis (O90.5)

6 O99.21 Obesity complicating pregnancy, childbirth, and the puerperium
Use additional code to identify the type of obesity (E66.-)

O99.210 Obesity complicating pregnancy, unspecified trimester ♀M
O99.211 Obesity complicating pregnancy, first trimester ♀M
O99.212 Obesity complicating pregnancy, second trimester ♀M
O99.213 Obesity complicating pregnancy, third trimester ♀M
O99.214 Obesity complicating childbirth ♀M
O99.215 Obesity complicating the puerperium ♀M

6 O99.28 Other endocrine, nutritional and metabolic diseases complicating pregnancy, childbirth and the puerperium

O99.280 Endocrine, nutritional and metabolic diseases complicating pregnancy, unspecified trimester ♀M
O99.281 Endocrine, nutritional and metabolic diseases complicating pregnancy, first trimester ♀M
O99.282 Endocrine, nutritional and metabolic diseases complicating pregnancy, second trimester ♀M
O99.283 Endocrine, nutritional and metabolic diseases complicating pregnancy, third trimester ♀M
O99.284 Endocrine, nutritional and metabolic diseases complicating childbirth ♀M
O99.285 Endocrine, nutritional and metabolic diseases complicating the puerperium ♀M

5 O99.3 Mental disorders and diseases of the nervous system complicating pregnancy, childbirth and the puerperium

6 O99.31 Alcohol use complicating pregnancy, childbirth, and the puerperium
Use additional code(s) from F10 to identify manifestations of the alcohol use

O99.310 Alcohol use complicating pregnancy, unspecified trimester ♀M
O99.311 Alcohol use complicating pregnancy, first trimester ♀M
O99.312 Alcohol use complicating pregnancy, second trimester ♀M
O99.313 Alcohol use complicating pregnancy, third trimester ♀M
O99.314 Alcohol use complicating childbirth ♀M
O99.315 Alcohol use complicating the puerperium ♀M

6 O99.32 Drug use complicating pregnancy, childbirth, and the puerperium
Use additional code(s) from F11-F16 and F18-F19 to identify manifestations of the drug use
AHA: 2Q 2018, 8

O99.320 Drug use complicating pregnancy, unspecified trimester ♀M
O99.321 Drug use complicating pregnancy, first trimester ♀M
O99.322 Drug use complicating pregnancy, second trimester ♀M
O99.323 Drug use complicating pregnancy, third trimester ♀M
O99.324 Drug use complicating childbirth ♀M
O99.325 Drug use complicating the puerperium ♀M

6 O99.33 Tobacco use disorder complicating pregnancy, childbirth, and the puerperium
Smoking complicating pregnancy, childbirth, and the puerperium
Use additional code from category F17 to identify type of tobacco nicotine dependence

O99.330 Smoking (tobacco) complicating pregnancy, unspecified trimester ♀M
O99.331 Smoking (tobacco) complicating pregnancy, first trimester ♀M
O99.332 Smoking (tobacco) complicating pregnancy, second trimester ♀M
O99.333 Smoking (tobacco) complicating pregnancy, third trimester ♀M
O99.334 Smoking (tobacco) complicating childbirth ♀M
O99.335 Smoking (tobacco) complicating the puerperium ♀M

▲ 6 O99.34 Other mental disorders complicating pregnancy, childbirth, and the puerperium
Conditions in F01-F09 and F20-F99
EXCLUDES 2 *postpartum mood disturbance (O90.6)*
postnatal psychosis (F53.1)
puerperal psychosis (F53.1)

O99.340 Other mental disorders complicating pregnancy, unspecified trimester ♀M
O99.341 Other mental disorders complicating pregnancy, first trimester ♀M
O99.342 Other mental disorders complicating pregnancy, second trimester ♀M
O99.343 Other mental disorders complicating pregnancy, third trimester ♀M
O99.344 Other mental disorders complicating childbirth ♀M
O99.345 Other mental disorders complicating the puerperium ♀M

6 O99.35 Diseases of the nervous system complicating pregnancy, childbirth, and the puerperium
Conditions in G00-G99
EXCLUDES 2 *pregnancy related peripheral neuritis (O26.8-)*

O99.350 Diseases of the nervous system complicating pregnancy, unspecified trimester ♀M
O99.351 Diseases of the nervous system complicating pregnancy, first trimester ♀M
O99.352 Diseases of the nervous system complicating pregnancy, second trimester ♀M
O99.353 Diseases of the nervous system complicating pregnancy, third trimester ♀M
O99.354 Diseases of the nervous system complicating childbirth ♀M
O99.355 Diseases of the nervous system complicating the puerperium ♀M

5 O99.4 Diseases of the circulatory system complicating pregnancy, childbirth and the puerperium
Conditions in I00-I99
EXCLUDES 1 *peripartum cardiomyopathy (O90.3)*
EXCLUDES 2 *hypertensive disorders (O10-O16)*
obstetric embolism (O88.-)
venous complications and cerebrovenous sinus thrombosis in labor, childbirth and the puerperium (O87.-)
venous complications and cerebrovenous sinus thrombosis in pregnancy (O22.-)

6 O99.41 Diseases of the circulatory system complicating pregnancy
AHA: 2Q 2016, 8

O99.411 Diseases of the circulatory system complicating pregnancy, first trimester ♀M
O99.412 Diseases of the circulatory system complicating pregnancy, second trimester ♀M
O99.413 Diseases of the circulatory system complicating pregnancy, third trimester ♀M
O99.419 Diseases of the circulatory system complicating pregnancy, unspecified trimester ♀M

O99.42 Diseases of the circulatory system complicating childbirth ♀M

O99.43 **Diseases of the circulatory system complicating the puerperium** ♀

5 O99.5 **Diseases of the respiratory system complicating pregnancy, childbirth and the puerperium**
Conditions in J00-J99

6 O99.51 **Diseases of the respiratory system complicating pregnancy**

O99.511 **Diseases of the respiratory system complicating pregnancy, first trimester** ♀

O99.512 **Diseases of the respiratory system complicating pregnancy, second trimester** ♀

O99.513 **Diseases of the respiratory system complicating pregnancy, third trimester** ♀

O99.519 **Diseases of the respiratory system complicating pregnancy, unspecified trimester** ♀

O99.52 **Diseases of the respiratory system complicating childbirth** ♀

O99.53 **Diseases of the respiratory system complicating the puerperium** ♀

5 O99.6 **Diseases of the digestive system complicating pregnancy, childbirth and the puerperium**
Conditions in K00-K93
EXCLUDES 2 *hemorrhoids in pregnancy (O22.4-)*
liver and biliary tract disorders in pregnancy, childbirth and the puerperium (O26.6-)

6 O99.61 **Diseases of the digestive system complicating pregnancy**

O99.611 **Diseases of the digestive system complicating pregnancy, first trimester** ♀

O99.612 **Diseases of the digestive system complicating pregnancy, second trimester** ♀

O99.613 **Diseases of the digestive system complicating pregnancy, third trimester** ♀

O99.619 **Diseases of the digestive system complicating pregnancy, unspecified trimester** ♀

O99.62 **Diseases of the digestive system complicating childbirth** ♀

O99.63 **Diseases of the digestive system complicating the puerperium** ♀

5 O99.7 **Diseases of the skin and subcutaneous tissue complicating pregnancy, childbirth and the puerperium**
Conditions in L00-L99
EXCLUDES 2 *herpes gestationis (O26.4)*
pruritic urticarial papules and plaques of pregnancy (PUPPP) (O26.86)

6 O99.71 **Diseases of the skin and subcutaneous tissue complicating pregnancy**

O99.711 **Diseases of the skin and subcutaneous tissue complicating pregnancy, first trimester** ♀

O99.712 **Diseases of the skin and subcutaneous tissue complicating pregnancy, second trimester** ♀

O99.713 **Diseases of the skin and subcutaneous tissue complicating pregnancy, third trimester** ♀

O99.719 **Diseases of the skin and subcutaneous tissue complicating pregnancy, unspecified trimester** ♀

O99.72 **Diseases of the skin and subcutaneous tissue complicating childbirth** ♀

O99.73 **Diseases of the skin and subcutaneous tissue complicating the puerperium** ♀

5 O99.8 **Other specified diseases and conditions complicating pregnancy, childbirth and the puerperium**
Conditions in D00-D48, H00-H95, M00-N99, and Q00-Q99
Use additional code to identify condition
EXCLUDES 2 *genitourinary infections in pregnancy (O23.-)*
infection of genitourinary tract following delivery (O86.1-O86.3)
malignant neoplasm complicating pregnancy, childbirth and the puerperium (O9A.1-)
maternal care for known or suspected abnormality of maternal pelvic organs (O34.-)
postpartum acute kidney failure (O90.4)
traumatic injuries in pregnancy (O9A.2-)

6 O99.81 **Abnormal glucose complicating pregnancy, childbirth and the puerperium**
EXCLUDES 1 *gestational diabetes (O24.4-)*

O99.810 **Abnormal glucose complicating pregnancy** ♀

O99.814 **Abnormal glucose complicating childbirth** ♀

O99.815 **Abnormal glucose complicating the puerperium** ♀

6 O99.82 **Streptococcus B carrier state complicating pregnancy, childbirth and the puerperium**
EXCLUDES 1 *Carrier of streptococcus group B (GBS) in a nonpregnant woman (Z22.330)*

O99.820 **Streptococcus B carrier state complicating pregnancy** ♀

O99.824 **Streptococcus B carrier state complicating childbirth** ♀

O99.825 **Streptococcus B carrier state complicating the puerperium** ♀

6 O99.83 **Other infection carrier state complicating pregnancy, childbirth and the puerperium**
Use additional code to identify the carrier state (Z22.-)

O99.830 **Other infection carrier state complicating pregnancy** ♀

O99.834 **Other infection carrier state complicating childbirth** ♀

O99.835 **Other infection carrier state complicating the puerperium** ♀

6 O99.84 **Bariatric surgery status complicating pregnancy, childbirth and the puerperium**
Gastric banding status complicating pregnancy, childbirth and the puerperium
Gastric bypass status for obesity complicating pregnancy, childbirth and the puerperium
Obesity surgery status complicating pregnancy, childbirth and the puerperium

O99.840 **Bariatric surgery status complicating pregnancy, unspecified trimester** ♀

O99.841 **Bariatric surgery status complicating pregnancy, first trimester** ♀

O99.842 **Bariatric surgery status complicating pregnancy, second trimester** ♀

O99.843 **Bariatric surgery status complicating pregnancy, third trimester** ♀

O99.844 **Bariatric surgery status complicating childbirth** ♀

O99.845 **Bariatric surgery status complicating the puerperium** ♀

O99.89 **Other specified diseases and conditions complicating pregnancy, childbirth and the puerperium** ♀

4 O9A **Maternal malignant neoplasms, traumatic injuries and abuse classifiable elsewhere but complicating pregnancy, childbirth and the puerperium**

5 O9A.1 **Malignant neoplasm complicating pregnancy, childbirth and the puerperium**
Conditions in C00-C96
Use additional code to identify neoplasm
EXCLUDES 2 *maternal care for benign tumor of corpus uteri (O34.1-)*
maternal care for benign tumor of cervix (O34.4-)

6 O9A.11 **Malignant neoplasm complicating pregnancy**

O9A.111 **Malignant neoplasm complicating pregnancy, first trimester** ♀

O9A.112 **Malignant neoplasm complicating pregnancy, second trimester** ♀

O9A.113 **Malignant neoplasm complicating pregnancy, third trimester** ♀

O9A.119 **Malignant neoplasm complicating pregnancy, unspecified trimester** ♀

O9A.12 **Malignant neoplasm complicating childbirth** ♀

O9A.13 **Malignant neoplasm complicating the puerperium** ♀
AHA: 3Q 2015, 19-20

5 O9A.2 Injury, poisoning and certain other consequences of external causes complicating pregnancy, childbirth and the puerperium
Conditions in S00-T88, except T74 and T76
Use additional code(s) to identify the injury or poisoning
EXCLUDES 2 *physical, sexual and psychological abuse complicating pregnancy, childbirth and the puerperium (O9A.3-, O9A.4-, O9A.5-)*

6 O9A.21 Injury, poisoning and certain other consequences of external causes complicating pregnancy

O9A.211 Injury, poisoning and certain other consequences of external causes complicating pregnancy, first trimester ♀M

O9A.212 Injury, poisoning and certain other consequences of external causes complicating pregnancy, second trimester ♀M

O9A.213 Injury, poisoning and certain other consequences of external causes complicating pregnancy, third trimester ♀M

O9A.219 Injury, poisoning and certain other consequences of external causes complicating pregnancy, unspecified trimester ♀M

O9A.22 Injury, poisoning and certain other consequences of external causes complicating childbirth ♀M

O9A.23 Injury, poisoning and certain other consequences of external causes complicating the puerperium ♀M

5 O9A.3 Physical abuse complicating pregnancy, childbirth and the puerperium
Conditions in T74.11 or T76.11
Use additional code (if applicable):
to identify any associated current injury due to physical abuse
to identify the perpetrator of abuse (Y07.-)
EXCLUDES 2 *sexual abuse complicating pregnancy, childbirth and the puerperium (O9A.4)*

GUIDELINES **Section I.C.15.r**
For suspected or confirmed cases of abuse of a pregnant patient, a code(s) from subcategories O9A.3, O9A.4, and O9A.5, should be sequenced first, followed by the appropriate codes (if applicable) to identify any associated current injury due to physical abuse, sexual abuse, and the perpetrator of abuse.

6 O9A.31 Physical abuse complicating pregnancy

O9A.311 Physical abuse complicating pregnancy, first trimester ♀M

O9A.312 Physical abuse complicating pregnancy, second trimester ♀M

O9A.313 Physical abuse complicating pregnancy, third trimester ♀M

O9A.319 Physical abuse complicating pregnancy, unspecified trimester ♀M

O9A.32 Physical abuse complicating childbirth ♀M

O9A.33 Physical abuse complicating the puerperium ♀M

5 O9A.4 Sexual abuse complicating pregnancy, childbirth and the puerperium
Conditions in T74.21 or T76.21
Use additional code (if applicable):
to identify any associated current injury due to sexual abuse
to identify the perpetrator of abuse (Y07.-)

6 O9A.41 Sexual abuse complicating pregnancy

O9A.411 Sexual abuse complicating pregnancy, first trimester ♀M

O9A.412 Sexual abuse complicating pregnancy, second trimester ♀M

O9A.413 Sexual abuse complicating pregnancy, third trimester ♀M

O9A.419 Sexual abuse complicating pregnancy, unspecified trimester ♀M

O9A.42 Sexual abuse complicating childbirth ♀M

O9A.43 Sexual abuse complicating the puerperium ♀M

5 O9A.5 Psychological abuse complicating pregnancy, childbirth and the puerperium
Conditions in T74.31 or T76.31
Use additional code to identify the perpetrator of abuse (Y07.-)

6 O9A.51 Psychological abuse complicating pregnancy

O9A.511 Psychological abuse complicating pregnancy, first trimester ♀M

O9A.512 Psychological abuse complicating pregnancy, second trimester ♀M

O9A.513 Psychological abuse complicating pregnancy, third trimester ♀M

O9A.519 Psychological abuse complicating pregnancy, unspecified trimester ♀M

O9A.52 Psychological abuse complicating childbirth ♀M

O9A.53 Psychological abuse complicating the puerperium ♀M

CHAPTER 16: CERTAIN CONDITIONS ORIGINATING IN THE PERINATAL PERIOD (P00-P96)

Note: Codes from this chapter are for use on newborn records only, never on maternal records

INCLUDES conditions that have their origin in the fetal or perinatal period (before birth through the first 28 days after birth) even if morbidity occurs later

EXCLUDES 2 *congenital malformations, deformations and chromosomal abnormalities (Q00-Q99)*
endocrine, nutritional and metabolic diseases (E00-E88)
injury, poisoning and certain other consequences of external causes (S00-T88)
neoplasms (C00-D49)
tetanus neonatorum (A33)

This chapter contains the following blocks:

P00-P04 Newborn affected by maternal factors and by complications of pregnancy, labor, and delivery
P05-P08 Disorders of newborn related to length of gestation and fetal growth
P09 Abnormal findings on neonatal screening
P10-P15 Birth trauma
P19-P29 Respiratory and cardiovascular disorders specific to the perinatal period
P35-P39 Infections specific to the perinatal period
P50-P61 Hemorrhagic and hematological disorders of newborn
P70-P74 Transitory endocrine and metabolic disorders specific to newborn
P76-P78 Digestive system disorders of newborn
P80-P83 Conditions involving the integument and temperature regulation of newborn
P84 Other problems with newborn
P90-P96 Other disorders originating in the perinatal period

Newborn affected by maternal factors and by complications of pregnancy, labor, and delivery (P00-P04)

Note: These codes are for use when the listed maternal conditions are specified as the cause of confirmed morbidity or potential morbidity which have their origin in the perinatal period (before birth through the first 28 days after birth).

4 **P00 Newborn affected by maternal conditions that may be unrelated to present pregnancy**
Code first:
any current condition in newborn
EXCLUDES 2 *encounter for observation of newborn for suspected diseases and conditions ruled out (Z05.-)*
newborn affected by maternal complications of pregnancy (P01.-)
newborn affected by maternal endocrine and metabolic disorders (P70-P74)
newborn affected by noxious substances transmitted via placenta or breast milk (P04.-)
AHA: 4Q 2016, 54

P00.0 Newborn affected by maternal hypertensive disorders
Newborn affected by maternal conditions classifiable to O10-O11, O13-O16
AHA: 4Q 2016, 54

P00.1 Newborn affected by maternal renal and urinary tract diseases
Newborn affected by maternal conditions classifiable to N00-N39
AHA: 4Q 2016, 54

P00.2 Newborn affected by maternal infectious and parasitic diseases
Newborn affected by maternal infectious disease classifiable to A00-B99, J09 and J10
EXCLUDES 1 *maternal genital tract or other localized infections (P00.8)*
EXCLUDES 2 *infections specific to the perinatal period (P35-P39)*
AHA: 3Q 2015, 20-21
AHA: 4Q 2016, 54

P00.3 Newborn affected by other maternal circulatory and respiratory diseases
Newborn affected by maternal conditions classifiable to I00-I99, J00-J99, Q20-Q34 and not included in P00.0, P00.2
AHA: 4Q 2016, 54

P00.4 Newborn affected by maternal nutritional disorders
Newborn affected by maternal disorders classifiable to E40-E64
Maternal malnutrition NOS
AHA: 4Q 2016, 54

P00.5 Newborn affected by maternal injury
Newborn affected by maternal conditions classifiable to O9A.2-
AHA: 4Q 2016, 54

P00.6 Newborn affected by surgical procedure on mother
Newborn affected by amniocentesis
EXCLUDES 1 *Cesarean delivery for present delivery (P03.4)*
damage to placenta from amniocentesis, Cesarean delivery or surgical induction (P02.1)
previous surgery to uterus or pelvic organs (P03.89)
EXCLUDES 2 *newborn affected by complication of (fetal) intrauterine procedure (P96.5)*
AHA: 4Q 2016, 54

P00.7 Newborn affected by other medical procedures on mother, not elsewhere classified
Newborn affected by radiation to mother
EXCLUDES 1 *damage to placenta from amniocentesis, cesarean delivery or surgical induction (P02.1)*
newborn affected by other complications of labor and delivery (P03.-)
AHA: 4Q 2016, 54

5 **P00.8 Newborn affected by other maternal conditions**
AHA: 4Q 2016, 54

P00.81 Newborn affected by periodontal disease in mother
AHA: 4Q 2016, 54

P00.89 Newborn affected by other maternal conditions
Newborn affected by conditions classifiable to T80-T88
Newborn affected by maternal genital tract or other localized infections
Newborn affected by maternal systemic lupus erythematosus
AHA: 4Q 2016, 54

P00.9 Newborn affected by unspecified maternal condition
AHA: 4Q 2016, 54

4 **P01 Newborn affected by maternal complications of pregnancy**
Code first:
any current condition in newborn
EXCLUDES 2 *encounter for observation of newborn for suspected diseases and conditions ruled out (Z05.-)*
AHA: 4Q 2016, 54

P01.0 Newborn affected by incompetent cervix
AHA: 4Q 2016, 54

P01.1 Newborn affected by premature rupture of membranes
AHA: 4Q 2016, 54

P01.2 Newborn affected by oligohydramnios
EXCLUDES 1 *oligohydramnios due to premature rupture of membranes (P01.1)*
DEFINITION Inadequate amount of amniotic fluid in the womb affecting the fetus.
AHA: 4Q 2016, 54

P01.3 Newborn affected by polyhydramnios
Newborn affected by hydramnios
DEFINITION Excessive amount of amniotic fluid in the womb affecting the fetus.
AHA: 4Q 2016, 54

P01.4 Newborn affected by ectopic pregnancy
Newborn affected by abdominal pregnancy
AHA: 4Q 2016, 54

P01.5 Newborn affected by multiple pregnancy
Newborn affected by triplet (pregnancy)
Newborn affected by twin (pregnancy)

AHA: 4Q 2016, 54

P01.6 **Newborn affected by maternal death**
AHA: 4Q 2016, 54

P01.7 **Newborn affected by malpresentation before labor**
Newborn affected by breech presentation before labor
Newborn affected by external version before labor
Newborn affected by face presentation before labor
Newborn affected by transverse lie before labor
Newborn affected by unstable lie before labor
AHA: 4Q 2016, 54

P01.8 **Newborn affected by other maternal complications of pregnancy**
AHA: 4Q 2016, 54

P01.9 **Newborn affected by maternal complication of pregnancy, unspecified**
AHA: 4Q 2016, 54

4 P02 **Newborn affected by complications of placenta, cord and membranes**
Code first:
any current condition in newborn
EXCLUDES 2 *encounter for observation of newborn for suspected diseases and conditions ruled out (Z05.-)*
AHA: 4Q 2016, 54

P02.0 **Newborn affected by placenta previa**
AHA: 4Q 2016, 54

P02.1 **Newborn affected by other forms of placental separation and hemorrhage**
Newborn affected by abruptio placenta
Newborn affected by accidental hemorrhage
Newborn affected by antepartum hemorrhage
Newborn affected by damage to placenta from amniocentesis, cesarean delivery or surgical induction
Newborn affected by maternal blood loss
Newborn affected by premature separation of placenta
AHA: 4Q 2016, 54

5 P02.2 **Newborn affected by other and unspecified morphological and functional abnormalities of placenta**
AHA: 4Q 2016, 54

P02.20 **Newborn affected by unspecified morphological and functional abnormalities of placenta**
AHA: 4Q 2016, 54

P02.29 **Newborn affected by other morphological and functional abnormalities of placenta**
Newborn affected by placental dysfunction
Newborn affected by placental infarction
Newborn affected by placental insufficiency
AHA: 4Q 2016, 54

P02.3 **Newborn affected by placental transfusion syndromes**
Newborn affected by placental and cord abnormalities resulting in twin-to-twin or other transplacental transfusion
AHA: 4Q 2016, 54

P02.4 **Newborn affected by prolapsed cord**
AHA: 4Q 2016, 54

Prolapsed umbilical cord

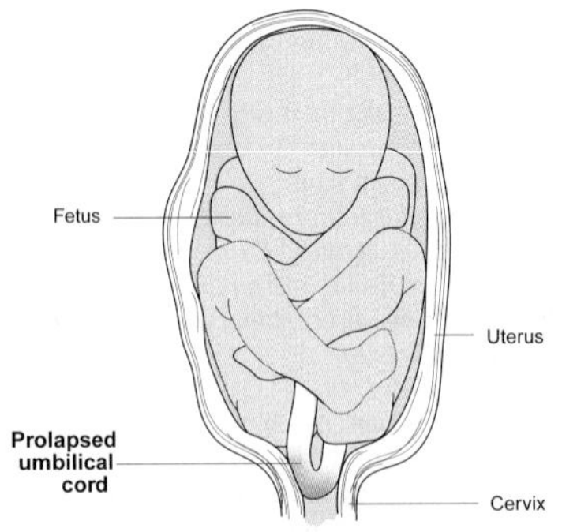

P02.5 **Newborn affected by other compression of umbilical cord**
Newborn affected by umbilical cord (tightly) around neck
Newborn affected by entanglement of umbilical cord
Newborn affected by knot in umbilical cord
AHA: 4Q 2016, 54

5 P02.6 **Newborn affected by other and unspecified conditions of umbilical cord**
AHA: 4Q 2016, 54

P02.60 **Newborn affected by unspecified conditions of umbilical cord**
AHA: 4Q 2016, 54

P02.69 **Newborn affected by other conditions of umbilical cord**
Newborn affected by short umbilical cord
Newborn affected by vasa previa
EXCLUDES 1 *newborn affected by single umbilical artery (Q27.0)*
AHA: 4Q 2016, 54

▲ **5 P02.7** **Newborn affected by chorioamnionitis**
AHA: 4Q 2016, 54

● **P02.70** **Newborn affected by fetal inflammatory response syndrome**
Newborn affected by FIRS
AHA: 4Q 2016, 54

● **P02.78** **Newborn affected by other conditions from chorioamnionitis**
Newborn affected by amnionitis
Newborn affected by membranitis
Newborn affected by placentitis
AHA: 4Q 2016, 54

P02.8 **Newborn affected by other abnormalities of membranes**
AHA: 4Q 2016, 54

P02.9 **Newborn affected by abnormality of membranes, unspecified**
AHA: 4Q 2016, 54

4 P03 **Newborn affected by other complications of labor and delivery**
Code first:
any current condition in newborn
EXCLUDES 2 *encounter for observation of newborn for suspected diseases and conditions ruled out (Z05.-)*
AHA: 4Q 2016, 54

P03.0 **Newborn affected by breech delivery and extraction**
AHA: 4Q 2016, 54

P03.1 **Newborn affected by other malpresentation, malposition and disproportion during labor and delivery**
Newborn affected by contracted pelvis
Newborn affected by conditions classifiable to O64-O66
Newborn affected by persistent occipitoposterior
Newborn affected by transverse lie
AHA: 4Q 2016, 54

P03.2 **Newborn affected by forceps delivery**

AHA: 4Q 2016, 54

P03.3 **Newborn affected by delivery by vacuum extractor [ventouse]**
AHA: 4Q 2016, 54

P03.4 **Newborn affected by Cesarean delivery**
AHA: 4Q 2016, 54

P03.5 **Newborn affected by precipitate delivery**
Newborn affected by rapid second stage
DEFINITION Fetus affected by labor occurring quickly, with rapid expulsion.
AHA: 4Q 2016, 54

P03.6 **Newborn affected by abnormal uterine contractions**
Newborn affected by conditions classifiable to O62.-, except O62.3
Newborn affected by hypertonic labor
Newborn affected by uterine inertia
AHA: 4Q 2016, 54

5 **P03.8** **Newborn affected by other specified complications of labor and delivery**
AHA: 4Q 2016, 54

6 **P03.81** **Newborn affected by abnormality in fetal (intrauterine) heart rate or rhythm**
EXCLUDES 1 *neonatal cardiac dysrhythmia (P29.1-)*
AHA: 4Q 2016, 54

P03.810 **Newborn affected by abnormality in fetal (intrauterine) heart rate or rhythm before the onset of labor**
AHA: 4Q 2016, 54

P03.811 **Newborn affected by abnormality in fetal (intrauterine) heart rate or rhythm during labor**
AHA: 4Q 2016, 54

P03.819 **Newborn affected by abnormality in fetal (intrauterine) heart rate or rhythm, unspecified as to time of onset**
AHA: 4Q 2016, 54

P03.82 **Meconium passage during delivery**
EXCLUDES 1 *meconium aspiration (P24.00, P24.01)*
meconium staining (P96.83)
AHA: 4Q 2016, 54

P03.89 **Newborn affected by other specified complications of labor and delivery**
Newborn affected by abnormality of maternal soft tissues
Newborn affected by conditions classifiable to O60-O75 and by procedures used in labor and delivery not included in P02.- and P03.0-P03.6
Newborn affected by induction of labor
AHA: 4Q 2016, 54

P03.9 **Newborn affected by complication of labor and delivery, unspecified**
AHA: 4Q 2016, 54

4 **P04** **Newborn affected by noxious substances transmitted via placenta or breast milk**
INCLUDES nonteratogenic effects of substances transmitted via placenta
EXCLUDES 2 *congenital malformations (Q00-Q99)*
encounter for observation of newborn for suspected diseases and conditions ruled out (Z05.-)
neonatal jaundice from excessive hemolysis due to drugs or toxins transmitted from mother (P58.4)
newborn in contact with and (suspected) exposures hazardous to health not transmitted via placenta or breast milk (Z77.-)
AHA: 4Q 2016, 54

▲ **P04.0** **Newborn affected by maternal anesthesia and analgesia in pregnancy, labor and delivery**
Newborn affected by reactions and intoxications from maternal opiates and tranquilizers administered for procedures during pregnancy or labor and delivery
EXCLUDES 2 *newborn affected by other maternal medication (P04.1-)*

▲ 5 **P04.1** **Newborn affected by other maternal medication**
Code first:
withdrawal symptoms from maternal use of drugs of addiction, if applicable (P96.1)
EXCLUDES 1 *dysmorphism due to warfarin (Q86.2)*
fetal hydantoin syndrome (Q86.1)
EXCLUDES 2 *maternal anesthesia and analgesia in pregnancy, labor and delivery (P04.0)*
maternal use of drugs of addiction (P04.4-)

● **P04.11** **Newborn affected by maternal antineoplastic chemotherapy**

● **P04.12** **Newborn affected by maternal cytotoxic drugs**

● **P04.13** **Newborn affected by maternal use of anticonvulsants**

● **P04.14** **Newborn affected by maternal use of opiates**

● **P04.15** **Newborn affected by maternal use of antidepressants**

● **P04.16** **Newborn affected by maternal use of amphetamines**

● **P04.17** **Newborn affected by maternal use of sedative-hypnotics**

● **P04.1A** **Newborn affected by maternal use of anxiolytics**

● **P04.18** **Newborn affected by other maternal medication**

● **P04.19** **Newborn affected by maternal use of unspecified medication**

P04.2 **Newborn affected by maternal use of tobacco**
Newborn affected by exposure in utero to tobacco smoke
EXCLUDES 2 *newborn exposure to environmental tobacco smoke (P96.81)*

P04.3 **Newborn affected by maternal use of alcohol**
EXCLUDES 1 *fetal alcohol syndrome (Q86.0)*

5 **P04.4** **Newborn affected by maternal use of drugs of addiction**

● **P04.40** **Newborn affected by maternal use of unspecified drugs of addiction**

P04.41 **Newborn affected by maternal use of cocaine**
'Crack baby'

● **P04.42** **Newborn affected by maternal use of hallucinogens**
EXCLUDES 2 *newborn affected by other maternal medication (P04.1-)*

P04.49 **Newborn affected by maternal use of other drugs of addiction**
EXCLUDES 2 *newborn affected by maternal anesthesia and analgesia (P04.0)*
withdrawal symptoms from maternal use of drugs of addiction (P96.1)

P04.5 **Newborn affected by maternal use of nutritional chemical substances**

P04.6 **Newborn affected by maternal exposure to environmental chemical substances**

▲ 5 **P04.8** **Newborn affected by other maternal noxious substances**

● **P04.81** **Newborn affected by maternal use of cannabis**

● **P04.89** **Newborn affected by other maternal noxious substances**

P04.9 **Newborn affected by maternal noxious substance, unspecified**

Disorders of newborn related to length of gestation and fetal growth (P05-P08)

4 **P05** **Disorders of newborn related to slow fetal growth and fetal malnutrition**

5 **P05.0** **Newborn light for gestational age**
Newborn light-for-dates
Weight below but length above 10th percentile for gestational age

P05.00 **Newborn light for gestational age, unspecified weight**

P05.01 **Newborn light for gestational age, less than 500 grams**

P05.02 **Newborn light for gestational age, 500-749 grams**

P05.03 **Newborn light for gestational age, 750-999 grams**

P05.04 **Newborn light for gestational age, 1000-1249 grams**

P05.05 **Newborn light for gestational age, 1250-1499 grams**

P05.06 **Newborn light for gestational age, 1500-1749 grams**

P05.07 **Newborn light for gestational age, 1750-1999 grams**

P05.08 **Newborn light for gestational age, 2000-2499 grams**

P05.09 **Newborn light for gestational age, 2500 grams and over**
Newborn light for gestational age, other

P05.1 **Newborn small for gestational age**
Newborn small-and-light-for-dates
Newborn small-for-dates
Weight and length below 10th percentile for gestational age

P05.10 **Newborn small for gestational age, unspecified weight**

P05.11 **Newborn small for gestational age, less than 500 grams**

P05.12 **Newborn small for gestational age, 500-749 grams**

P05.13 **Newborn small for gestational age, 750-999 grams**

P05.14 **Newborn small for gestational age, 1000-1249 grams**

P05.15 **Newborn small for gestational age, 1250-1499 grams**

P05.16 **Newborn small for gestational age, 1500-1749 grams**

P05.17 **Newborn small for gestational age, 1750-1999 grams**

P05.18 **Newborn small for gestational age, 2000-2499 grams**

P05.19 **Newborn small for gestational age, other**
Newborn small for gestational age, 2500 grams and over
AHA: 4Q 2016, 55

P05.2 **Newborn affected by fetal (intrauterine) malnutrition not light or small for gestational age**
Infant, not light or small for gestational age, showing signs of fetal malnutrition, such as dry, peeling skin and loss of subcutaneous tissue
EXCLUDES 1 *newborn affected by fetal malnutrition with light for gestational age (P05.0-)*
newborn affected by fetal malnutrition with small for gestational age (P05.1-)

P05.9 **Newborn affected by slow intrauterine growth, unspecified**
Newborn affected by fetal growth retardation NOS

P07 Disorders of newborn related to short gestation and low birth weight, not elsewhere classified

Note: When both birth weight and gestational age of the newborn are available, both should be coded with birth weight sequenced before gestational age
INCLUDES the listed conditions, without further specification, as the cause of morbidity or additional care, in newborn

P07.0 **Extremely low birth weight newborn**
Newborn birth weight 999 g. or less
EXCLUDES 1 *low birth weight due to slow fetal growth and fetal malnutrition (P05.-)*

P07.00 **Extremely low birth weight newborn, unspecified weight**

P07.01 **Extremely low birth weight newborn, less than 500 grams**

P07.02 **Extremely low birth weight newborn, 500-749 grams**

P07.03 **Extremely low birth weight newborn, 750-999 grams**

P07.1 **Other low birth weight newborn**
Newborn birth weight 1000-2499 g.
EXCLUDES 1 *low birth weight due to slow fetal growth and fetal malnutrition (P05.-)*

P07.10 **Other low birth weight newborn, unspecified weight**

P07.14 **Other low birth weight newborn, 1000-1249 grams**

P07.15 **Other low birth weight newborn, 1250-1499 grams**

P07.16 **Other low birth weight newborn, 1500-1749 grams**

P07.17 **Other low birth weight newborn, 1750-1999 grams**

P07.18 **Other low birth weight newborn, 2000-2499 grams**

P07.2 **Extreme immaturity of newborn**
Less than 28 completed weeks (less than 196 completed days) of gestation.

P07.20 **Extreme immaturity of newborn, unspecified weeks of gestation**
Gestational age less than 28 completed weeks NOS

P07.21 **Extreme immaturity of newborn, gestational age less than 23 completed weeks**
Extreme immaturity of newborn, gestational age less than 23 weeks, 0 days

P07.22 **Extreme immaturity of newborn, gestational age 23 completed weeks**
Extreme immaturity of newborn, gestational age 23 weeks, 0 days through 23 weeks, 6 days

P07.23 **Extreme immaturity of newborn, gestational age 24 completed weeks**
Extreme immaturity of newborn, gestational age 24 weeks, 0 days through 24 weeks, 6 days

P07.24 **Extreme immaturity of newborn, gestational age 25 completed weeks**
Extreme immaturity of newborn, gestational age 25 weeks, 0 days through 25 weeks, 6 days

P07.25 **Extreme immaturity of newborn, gestational age 26 completed weeks**
Extreme immaturity of newborn, gestational age 26 weeks, 0 days through 26 weeks, 6 days

P07.26 **Extreme immaturity of newborn, gestational age 27 completed weeks**
Extreme immaturity of newborn, gestational age 27 weeks, 0 days through 27 weeks, 6 days

P07.3 **Preterm [premature] newborn [other]**
28 completed weeks or more but less than 37 completed weeks (196 completed days but less than 259 completed days) of gestation.
Prematurity NOS

P07.30 **Preterm newborn, unspecified weeks of gestation**

P07.31 **Preterm newborn, gestational age 28 completed weeks**
Preterm newborn, gestational age 28 weeks, 0 days through 28 weeks, 6 days

P07.32 **Preterm newborn, gestational age 29 completed weeks**
Preterm newborn, gestational age 29 weeks, 0 days through 29 weeks, 6 days

P07.33 **Preterm newborn, gestational age 30 completed weeks**
Preterm newborn, gestational age 30 weeks, 0 days through 30 weeks, 6 days

P07.34 **Preterm newborn, gestational age 31 completed weeks**
Preterm newborn, gestational age 31 weeks, 0 days through 31 weeks, 6 days

P07.35 **Preterm newborn, gestational age 32 completed weeks**
Preterm newborn, gestational age 32 weeks, 0 days through 32 weeks, 6 days

P07.36 **Preterm newborn, gestational age 33 completed weeks**
Preterm newborn, gestational age 33 weeks, 0 days through 33 weeks, 6 days

P07.37 **Preterm newborn, gestational age 34 completed weeks**
Preterm newborn, gestational age 34 weeks, 0 days through 34 weeks, 6 days

P07.38 **Preterm newborn, gestational age 35 completed weeks**
Preterm newborn, gestational age 35 weeks, 0 days through 35 weeks, 6 days

P07.39 **Preterm newborn, gestational age 36 completed weeks**
Preterm newborn, gestational age 36 weeks, 0 days through 36 weeks, 6 days

P08 Disorders of newborn related to long gestation and high birth weight

Note: When both birth weight and gestational age of the newborn are available, priority of assignment should be given to birth weight
INCLUDES the listed conditions, without further specification, as causes of morbidity or additional care, in newborn

P08.0 **Exceptionally large newborn baby**
Usually implies a birth weight of 4500 g. or more
EXCLUDES 1 *syndrome of infant of diabetic mother (P70.1)*
syndrome of infant of mother with gestational diabetes (P70.0)

P08.1 Other heavy for gestational age newborn
Other newborn heavy- or large-for-dates regardless of period of gestation
Usually implies a birth weight of 4000 g. to 4499 g.
EXCLUDES 1 *newborn with a birth weight of 4500 or more (P08.0)*
syndrome of infant of diabetic mother (P70.1)
syndrome of infant of mother with gestational diabetes (P70.0).

P08.2 Late newborn, not heavy for gestational age
P08.21 Post-term newborn
Newborn with gestation period over 40 completed weeks to 42 completed weeks
AHA: 1Q 2014, 14
P08.22 Prolonged gestation of newborn
Newborn with gestation period over 42 completed weeks (294 days or more), not heavy- or large-for-dates.
Postmaturity NOS
AHA: 1Q 2014, 14

Abnormal findings on neonatal screening (P09)

P09 Abnormal findings on neonatal screening
Use additional code to identify signs, symptoms and conditions associated with the screening
EXCLUDES 2 *nonspecific serologic evidence of human immunodeficiency virus [HIV] (R75)*

Birth trauma (P10-P15)

P10 Intracranial laceration and hemorrhage due to birth injury
EXCLUDES 1 *intracranial hemorrhage of newborn NOS (P52.9)*
intracranial hemorrhage of newborn due to anoxia or hypoxia (P52.-)
nontraumatic intracranial hemorrhage of newborn (P52.-)
P10.0 Subdural hemorrhage due to birth injury
Subdural hematoma (localized) due to birth injury
EXCLUDES 1 *subdural hemorrhage accompanying tentorial tear (P10.4)*
P10.1 Cerebral hemorrhage due to birth injury
P10.2 Intraventricular hemorrhage due to birth injury
P10.3 Subarachnoid hemorrhage due to birth injury
P10.4 Tentorial tear due to birth injury
P10.8 Other intracranial lacerations and hemorrhages due to birth injury
P10.9 Unspecified intracranial laceration and hemorrhage due to birth injury

P11 Other birth injuries to central nervous system
P11.0 Cerebral edema due to birth injury
P11.1 Other specified brain damage due to birth injury
P11.2 Unspecified brain damage due to birth injury
P11.3 Birth injury to facial nerve
Facial palsy due to birth injury
DEFINITION Facial muscle weakness or paralysis resulting from damage or trauma to one of the paired facial nerves.
P11.4 Birth injury to other cranial nerves
P11.5 Birth injury to spine and spinal cord
Fracture of spine due to birth injury
P11.9 Birth injury to central nervous system, unspecified

P12 Birth injury to scalp
P12.0 Cephalhematoma due to birth injury
P12.1 Chignon (from vacuum extraction) due to birth injury
P12.2 Epicranial subaponeurotic hemorrhage due to birth injury
Subgaleal hemorrhage
P12.3 Bruising of scalp due to birth injury
P12.4 Injury of scalp of newborn due to monitoring equipment
Sampling incision of scalp of newborn
Scalp clip (electrode) injury of newborn
P12.8 Other birth injuries to scalp
P12.81 Caput succedaneum
P12.89 Other birth injuries to scalp
P12.9 Birth injury to scalp, unspecified

P13 Birth injury to skeleton
EXCLUDES 2 *birth injury to spine (P11.5)*
P13.0 Fracture of skull due to birth injury
P13.1 Other birth injuries to skull
EXCLUDES 1 *cephalhematoma (P12.0)*
P13.2 Birth injury to femur
P13.3 Birth injury to other long bones
P13.4 Fracture of clavicle due to birth injury
P13.8 Birth injuries to other parts of skeleton
P13.9 Birth injury to skeleton, unspecified

P14 Birth injury to peripheral nervous system
P14.0 Erb's paralysis due to birth injury
P14.1 Klumpke's paralysis due to birth injury
P14.2 Phrenic nerve paralysis due to birth injury
P14.3 Other brachial plexus birth injuries
P14.8 Birth injuries to other parts of peripheral nervous system
P14.9 Birth injury to peripheral nervous system, unspecified

P15 Other birth injuries
P15.0 Birth injury to liver
Rupture of liver due to birth injury
P15.1 Birth injury to spleen
Rupture of spleen due to birth injury
P15.2 Sternomastoid injury due to birth injury
P15.3 Birth injury to eye
Subconjunctival hemorrhage due to birth injury
Traumatic glaucoma due to birth injury
P15.4 Birth injury to face
Facial congestion due to birth injury
P15.5 Birth injury to external genitalia
P15.6 Subcutaneous fat necrosis due to birth injury
P15.8 Other specified birth injuries
P15.9 Birth injury, unspecified

Respiratory and cardiovascular disorders specific to the perinatal period (P19-P29)

P19 Metabolic acidemia in newborn
INCLUDES metabolic acidemia in newborn
P19.0 Metabolic acidemia in newborn first noted before onset of labor
P19.1 Metabolic acidemia in newborn first noted during labor
P19.2 Metabolic acidemia noted at birth
P19.9 Metabolic acidemia, unspecified

P22 Respiratory distress of newborn
EXCLUDES 1 *respiratory arrest of newborn (P28.81)*
respiratory failure of newborn NOS (P28.5)
P22.0 Respiratory distress syndrome of newborn
Cardiorespiratory distress syndrome of newborn
Hyaline membrane disease
Idiopathic respiratory distress syndrome [IRDS or RDS] of newborn
Pulmonary hypoperfusion syndrome
Respiratory distress syndrome, type I
P22.1 Transient tachypnea of newborn
Idiopathic tachypnea of newborn
Respiratory distress syndrome, type II
Wet lung syndrome
DEFINITION Rapid breathing of a newborn.
P22.8 Other respiratory distress of newborn
P22.9 Respiratory distress of newborn, unspecified

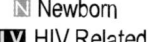

P23 Congenital pneumonia
INCLUDES infective pneumonia acquired in utero or during birth
EXCLUDES 1 *neonatal pneumonia resulting from aspiration (P24.-)*
P23.0 Congenital pneumonia due to viral agent
Use additional code (B97) to identify organism
EXCLUDES 1 *congenital rubella pneumonitis (P35.0)*
P23.1 Congenital pneumonia due to Chlamydia
P23.2 Congenital pneumonia due to staphylococcus

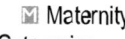

P23.3 **Congenital pneumonia due to streptococcus, group B**
P23.4 **Congenital pneumonia due to Escherichia coli**
P23.5 **Congenital pneumonia due to Pseudomonas**
P23.6 **Congenital pneumonia due to other bacterial agents**
Congenital pneumonia due to Hemophilus influenzae
Congenital pneumonia due to Klebsiella pneumoniae
Congenital pneumonia due to Mycoplasma
Congenital pneumonia due to Streptococcus, except group B
Use additional code (B95-B96) to identify organism
P23.8 **Congenital pneumonia due to other organisms**
P23.9 **Congenital pneumonia, unspecified**

4 P24 **Neonatal aspiration**
INCLUDES aspiration in utero and during delivery

5 P24.0 **Meconium aspiration**
EXCLUDES 1 *meconium passage (without aspiration) during delivery (P03.82)*
meconium staining (P96.83)
P24.00 **Meconium aspiration without respiratory symptoms**
Meconium aspiration NOS
P24.01 **Meconium aspiration with respiratory symptoms**
Meconium aspiration pneumonia
Meconium aspiration pneumonitis
Meconium aspiration syndrome NOS
Use additional code to identify any secondary pulmonary hypertension, if applicable (I27.2-)
5 P24.1 **Neonatal aspiration of (clear) amniotic fluid and mucus**
Neonatal aspiration of liquor (amnii)
P24.10 **Neonatal aspiration of (clear) amniotic fluid and mucus without respiratory symptoms**
Neonatal aspiration of amniotic fluid and mucus NOS
P24.11 **Neonatal aspiration of (clear) amniotic fluid and mucus with respiratory symptoms**
Neonatal aspiration of amniotic fluid and mucus with pneumonia
Neonatal aspiration of amniotic fluid and mucus with pneumonitis
Use additional code to identify any secondary pulmonary hypertension, if applicable (I27.2-)
5 P24.2 **Neonatal aspiration of blood**
P24.20 **Neonatal aspiration of blood without respiratory symptoms**
Neonatal aspiration of blood NOS
P24.21 **Neonatal aspiration of blood with respiratory symptoms**
Neonatal aspiration of blood with pneumonia
Neonatal aspiration of blood with pneumonitis
Use additional code to identify any secondary pulmonary hypertension, if applicable (I27.2-)
5 P24.3 **Neonatal aspiration of milk and regurgitated food**
Neonatal aspiration of stomach contents
P24.30 **Neonatal aspiration of milk and regurgitated food without respiratory symptoms**
Neonatal aspiration of milk and regurgitated food NOS
P24.31 **Neonatal aspiration of milk and regurgitated food with respiratory symptoms**
Neonatal aspiration of milk and regurgitated food with pneumonia
Neonatal aspiration of milk and regurgitated food with pneumonitis
Use additional code to identify any secondary pulmonary hypertension, if applicable (I27.2-)
5 P24.8 **Other neonatal aspiration**
P24.80 **Other neonatal aspiration without respiratory symptoms**
Neonatal aspiration NEC
P24.81 **Other neonatal aspiration with respiratory symptoms**
Neonatal aspiration pneumonia NEC
Neonatal aspiration with pneumonitis NEC
Neonatal aspiration with pneumonia NOS
Neonatal aspiration with pneumonitis NOS
Use additional code to identify any secondary pulmonary hypertension, if applicable (I27.2-)
P24.9 **Neonatal aspiration, unspecified**

4 P25 **Interstitial emphysema and related conditions originating in the perinatal period**
P25.0 **Interstitial emphysema originating in the perinatal period**
P25.1 **Pneumothorax originating in the perinatal period**
P25.2 **Pneumomediastinum originating in the perinatal period**
P25.3 **Pneumopericardium originating in the perinatal period**
P25.8 **Other conditions related to interstitial emphysema originating in the perinatal period**

4 P26 **Pulmonary hemorrhage originating in the perinatal period**
EXCLUDES 1 *acute idiopathic hemorrhage in infants over 28 days old (R04.81)*
P26.0 **Tracheobronchial hemorrhage originating in the perinatal period**
P26.1 **Massive pulmonary hemorrhage originating in the perinatal period**
P26.8 **Other pulmonary hemorrhages originating in the perinatal period**
P26.9 **Unspecified pulmonary hemorrhage originating in the perinatal period**

4 P27 **Chronic respiratory disease originating in the perinatal period**
EXCLUDES 2 *respiratory distress of newborn (P22.0-P22.9)*
P27.0 **Wilson-Mikity syndrome**
Pulmonary dysmaturity
P27.1 **Bronchopulmonary dysplasia originating in the perinatal period**
P27.8 **Other chronic respiratory diseases originating in the perinatal period**
Congenital pulmonary fibrosis
Ventilator lung in newborn
P27.9 **Unspecified chronic respiratory disease originating in the perinatal period**

4 P28 **Other respiratory conditions originating in the perinatal period**
EXCLUDES 1 *congenital malformations of the respiratory system (Q30-Q34)*
P28.0 **Primary atelectasis of newborn**
Primary failure to expand terminal respiratory units
Pulmonary hypoplasia associated with short gestation
Pulmonary immaturity NOS
5 P28.1 **Other and unspecified atelectasis of newborn**
P28.10 **Unspecified atelectasis of newborn**
Atelectasis of newborn NOS
P28.11 **Resorption atelectasis without respiratory distress syndrome**
EXCLUDES 1 *resorption atelectasis with respiratory distress syndrome (P22.0)*
P28.19 **Other atelectasis of newborn**
Partial atelectasis of newborn
Secondary atelectasis of newborn
P28.2 **Cyanotic attacks of newborn**
EXCLUDES 1 *apnea of newborn (P28.3-P28.4)*
DEFINITION A newborn with normal skin tone suddenly turns blue due to a lack of oxygen for a certain period of time before returning to normal color.
P28.3 **Primary sleep apnea of newborn**
Central sleep apnea of newborn
Obstructive sleep apnea of newborn
Sleep apnea of newborn NOS
P28.4 **Other apnea of newborn**
Apnea of prematurity
Obstructive apnea of newborn
EXCLUDES 1 *obstructive sleep apnea of newborn (P28.3)*
P28.5 **Respiratory failure of newborn**
EXCLUDES 1 *respiratory arrest of newborn (P28.81)*
respiratory distress of newborn (P22.0-)
5 P28.8 **Other specified respiratory conditions of newborn**
P28.81 **Respiratory arrest of newborn**
AHA: 2Q 2017, 6
P28.89 **Other specified respiratory conditions of newborn**
Congenital laryngeal stridor
Sniffles in newborn
Snuffles in newborn
EXCLUDES 1 *early congenital syphilitic rhinitis (A50.05)*
P28.9 **Respiratory condition of newborn, unspecified**
Respiratory depression in newborn

4 P29 **Cardiovascular disorders originating in the perinatal period**
EXCLUDES 1 *congenital malformations of the circulatory system (Q20-Q28)*

● New | Manifestation | 4-7 Digit Indicators | Laterality | A Adult | M Maternity | N Newborn | P Pediatric | ♂ Male
▲ Revised | Unspecified | AHA Coding Clinic | HCC Hierarchical Condition Categories | HIV HIV Related Conditions | ♀ Female

P29.0 Neonatal cardiac failure
P29.1 Neonatal cardiac dysrhythmia
P29.11 Neonatal tachycardia
P29.12 Neonatal bradycardia
DEFINITION Abnormally slow newborn heartbeat.
P29.2 Neonatal hypertension
P29.3 Persistent fetal circulation
P29.30 Pulmonary hypertension of newborn
Persistent pulmonary hypertension of newborn
AHA: 4Q 2017, 16
P29.38 Other persistent fetal circulation
Delayed closure of ductus arteriosus
AHA: 4Q 2017, 16
P29.4 Transient myocardial ischemia in newborn
P29.8 Other cardiovascular disorders originating in the perinatal period
P29.81 Cardiac arrest of newborn
P29.89 Other cardiovascular disorders originating in the perinatal period
AHA: 4Q 2014, 23
P29.9 Cardiovascular disorder originating in the perinatal period, unspecified

Infections specific to the perinatal period (P35-P39)

Infections acquired in utero, during birth via the umbilicus, or during the first 28 days after birth

EXCLUDES 2 *asymptomatic human immunodeficiency virus [HIV] infection status (Z21)*
congenital gonococcal infection (A54.-)
congenital pneumonia (P23.-)
congenital syphilis (A50.-)
human immunodeficiency virus [HIV] disease (B20)
infant botulism (A48.51)
infectious diseases not specific to the perinatal period (A00-B99, J09, J10.-)
intestinal infectious disease (A00-A09)
laboratory evidence of human immunodeficiency virus [HIV] (R75)
tetanus neonatorum (A33)

GUIDELINES Section 1.C.16.a.5
If a newborn has a condition that may be either due to the birth process or community acquired and the documentation does not indicate which it is, the default is due to the birth process and the code from Chapter 16 should be used. If the condition is community-acquired, a code from Chapter 16 should not be assigned.

P35 Congenital viral diseases
INCLUDES infections acquired in utero or during birth
P35.0 Congenital rubella syndrome
Congenital rubella pneumonitis
P35.1 Congenital cytomegalovirus infection
P35.2 Congenital herpesviral [herpes simplex] infection
P35.3 Congenital viral hepatitis
● P35.4 Congenital Zika virus disease
Use additional code to identify manifestations of congenital Zika virus disease
P35.8 Other congenital viral diseases
Congenital varicella [chickenpox]
P35.9 Congenital viral disease, unspecified

P36 Bacterial sepsis of newborn
INCLUDES congenital sepsis
Use additional code(s), if applicable, to identify severe sepsis (R65.2-) and associated acute organ dysfunction(s)
P36.0 Sepsis of newborn due to streptococcus, group B HCC
P36.1 Sepsis of newborn due to other and unspecified streptococci
P36.10 Sepsis of newborn due to unspecified streptococci HCC
P36.19 Sepsis of newborn due to other streptococci HCC
P36.2 Sepsis of newborn due to Staphylococcus aureus HCC
P36.3 Sepsis of newborn due to other and unspecified staphylococci
P36.30 Sepsis of newborn due to unspecified staphylococci HCC
P36.39 Sepsis of newborn due to other staphylococci HCC
P36.4 Sepsis of newborn due to Escherichia coli HCC
P36.5 Sepsis of newborn due to anaerobes HCC
P36.8 Other bacterial sepsis of newborn HCC
Use additional code from category B96 to identify organism
P36.9 Bacterial sepsis of newborn, unspecified HCC

P37 Other congenital infectious and parasitic diseases
EXCLUDES 2 *congenital syphilis (A50.-)*
infectious neonatal diarrhea (A00-A09)
necrotizing enterocolitis in newborn (P77.-)
noninfectious neonatal diarrhea (P78.3)
ophthalmia neonatorum due to gonococcus (A54.31)
tetanus neonatorum (A33)
P37.0 Congenital tuberculosis
P37.1 Congenital toxoplasmosis
Hydrocephalus due to congenital toxoplasmosis
P37.2 Neonatal (disseminated) listeriosis
P37.3 Congenital falciparum malaria
P37.4 Other congenital malaria
P37.5 Neonatal candidiasis
P37.8 Other specified congenital infectious and parasitic diseases
P37.9 Congenital infectious or parasitic disease, unspecified

P38 Omphalitis of newborn
EXCLUDES 1 *omphalitis not of newborn (L08.82)*
tetanus omphalitis (A33)
umbilical hemorrhage of newborn (P51.-)
P38.1 Omphalitis with mild hemorrhage
P38.9 Omphalitis without hemorrhage
Omphalitis of newborn NOS

P39 Other infections specific to the perinatal period
Use additional code to identify organism or specific infection
P39.0 Neonatal infective mastitis
EXCLUDES 1 *breast engorgement of newborn (P83.4)*
noninfective mastitis of newborn (P83.4)
DEFINITION Inflammation of the breast in a newborn.
P39.1 Neonatal conjunctivitis and dacryocystitis
Neonatal chlamydial conjunctivitis
Ophthalmia neonatorum NOS
EXCLUDES 1 *gonococcal conjunctivitis (A54.31)*
P39.2 Intra-amniotic infection affecting newborn, not elsewhere classified
P39.3 Neonatal urinary tract infection
P39.4 Neonatal skin infection
Neonatal pyoderma
EXCLUDES 1 *pemphigus neonatorum (L00)*
staphylococcal scalded skin syndrome (L00)
P39.8 Other specified infections specific to the perinatal period
P39.9 Infection specific to the perinatal period, unspecified

Hemorrhagic and hematological disorders of newborn (P50-P61)

EXCLUDES 1 *congenital stenosis and stricture of bile ducts (Q44.3)*
Crigler-Najjar syndrome (E80.5)
Dubin-Johnson syndrome (E80.6)
Gilbert syndrome (E80.4)
hereditary hemolytic anemias (D55-D58)

P50 Newborn affected by intrauterine (fetal) blood loss
EXCLUDES 1 *congenital anemia from intrauterine (fetal) blood loss (P61.3)*
P50.0 Newborn affected by intrauterine (fetal) blood loss from vasa previa
P50.1 Newborn affected by intrauterine (fetal) blood loss from ruptured cord
P50.2 Newborn affected by intrauterine (fetal) blood loss from placenta
P50.3 Newborn affected by hemorrhage into co-twin
P50.4 Newborn affected by hemorrhage into maternal circulation
P50.5 Newborn affected by intrauterine (fetal) blood loss from cut end of co-twin's cord
P50.8 Newborn affected by other intrauterine (fetal) blood loss

P50.9 **Newborn affected by intrauterine (fetal) blood loss, unspecified**
Newborn affected by fetal hemorrhage NOS

P51 **Umbilical hemorrhage of newborn**
EXCLUDES 1 *omphalitis with mild hemorrhage (P38.1)*
umbilical hemorrhage from cut end of co-twins cord (P50.5)

P51.0 **Massive umbilical hemorrhage of newborn**
P51.8 **Other umbilical hemorrhages of newborn**
Slipped umbilical ligature NOS
P51.9 **Umbilical hemorrhage of newborn, unspecified**

P52 **Intracranial nontraumatic hemorrhage of newborn**
INCLUDES intracranial hemorrhage due to anoxia or hypoxia
EXCLUDES 1 *intracranial hemorrhage due to birth injury (P10.-)*
intracranial hemorrhage due to other injury (S06.-)

P52.0 **Intraventricular (nontraumatic) hemorrhage, grade 1, of newborn**
Subependymal hemorrhage (without intraventricular extension)
Bleeding into germinal matrix
P52.1 **Intraventricular (nontraumatic) hemorrhage, grade 2, of newborn**
Subependymal hemorrhage with intraventricular extension
Bleeding into ventricle
P52.2 **Intraventricular (nontraumatic) hemorrhage, grade 3 and grade 4, of newborn**
P52.21 **Intraventricular (nontraumatic) hemorrhage, grade 3, of newborn**
Subependymal hemorrhage with intraventricular extension with enlargement of ventricle
P52.22 **Intraventricular (nontraumatic) hemorrhage, grade 4, of newborn**
Bleeding into cerebral cortex
Subependymal hemorrhage with intracerebral extension
P52.3 **Unspecified intraventricular (nontraumatic) hemorrhage of newborn**
P52.4 **Intracerebral (nontraumatic) hemorrhage of newborn**
P52.5 **Subarachnoid (nontraumatic) hemorrhage of newborn**
P52.6 **Cerebellar (nontraumatic) and posterior fossa hemorrhage of newborn**
P52.8 **Other intracranial (nontraumatic) hemorrhages of newborn**
P52.9 **Intracranial (nontraumatic) hemorrhage of newborn, unspecified**

P53 **Hemorrhagic disease of newborn**
Vitamin K deficiency of newborn

P54 **Other neonatal hemorrhages**
EXCLUDES 1 *newborn affected by (intrauterine) blood loss (P50.-)*
pulmonary hemorrhage originating in the perinatal period (P26.-)

P54.0 **Neonatal hematemesis**
EXCLUDES 1 *neonatal hematemesis due to swallowed maternal blood (P78.2)*
P54.1 **Neonatal melena**
EXCLUDES 1 *neonatal melena due to swallowed maternal blood (P78.2)*
P54.2 **Neonatal rectal hemorrhage**
P54.3 **Other neonatal gastrointestinal hemorrhage**
P54.4 **Neonatal adrenal hemorrhage**
P54.5 **Neonatal cutaneous hemorrhage**
Neonatal bruising
Neonatal ecchymoses
Neonatal petechiae
Neonatal superficial hematomata
EXCLUDES 2 *bruising of scalp due to birth injury (P12.3)*
cephalhematoma due to birth injury (P12.0)
DEFINITION Minute red spots on the surface of the skin, due to escape of a small amount of blood from the vessels.
P54.6 **Neonatal vaginal hemorrhage** ♀
Neonatal pseudomenses
P54.8 **Other specified neonatal hemorrhages**
P54.9 **Neonatal hemorrhage, unspecified**

P55 **Hemolytic disease of newborn**
P55.0 **Rh isoimmunization of newborn**
P55.1 **ABO isoimmunization of newborn**
AHA: 3Q 2015, 20
P55.8 **Other hemolytic diseases of newborn**
P55.9 **Hemolytic disease of newborn, unspecified**

P56 **Hydrops fetalis due to hemolytic disease**
EXCLUDES 1 *hydrops fetalis NOS (P83.2)*

P56.0 **Hydrops fetalis due to isoimmunization**
P56.9 **Hydrops fetalis due to other and unspecified hemolytic disease**
P56.90 **Hydrops fetalis due to unspecified hemolytic disease**
P56.99 **Hydrops fetalis due to other hemolytic disease**

P57 **Kernicterus**
P57.0 **Kernicterus due to isoimmunization**
DEFINITION Encephalopathy due to severe jaundice caused by destruction of the infant's red blood cells by the mother's immune system. Excess bilirubin crosses the blood-brain barrier and accumulates toxically in the brain.
P57.8 **Other specified kernicterus**
EXCLUDES 1 *Crigler-Najjar syndrome (E80.5)*
P57.9 **Kernicterus, unspecified**

P58 **Neonatal jaundice due to other excessive hemolysis**
EXCLUDES 1 *jaundice due to isoimmunization (P55-P57)*

P58.0 **Neonatal jaundice due to bruising**
P58.1 **Neonatal jaundice due to bleeding**
P58.2 **Neonatal jaundice due to infection**
P58.3 **Neonatal jaundice due to polycythemia**
P58.4 **Neonatal jaundice due to drugs or toxins transmitted from mother or given to newborn**
Code first:
poisoning due to drug or toxin, if applicable (T36-T65 with fifth or sixth character 1-4 or 6)
Use additional code for adverse effect, if applicable, to identify drug (T36-T50 with fifth or sixth character 5)
P58.41 **Neonatal jaundice due to drugs or toxins transmitted from mother**
P58.42 **Neonatal jaundice due to drugs or toxins given to newborn**
P58.5 **Neonatal jaundice due to swallowed maternal blood**
P58.8 **Neonatal jaundice due to other specified excessive hemolysis**
P58.9 **Neonatal jaundice due to excessive hemolysis, unspecified**

P59 **Neonatal jaundice from other and unspecified causes**
EXCLUDES 1 *jaundice due to inborn errors of metabolism (E70-E88)*
kernicterus (P57.-)

P59.0 **Neonatal jaundice associated with preterm delivery**
Hyperbilirubinemia of prematurity
Jaundice due to delayed conjugation associated with preterm delivery
P59.1 **Inspissated bile syndrome**
P59.2 **Neonatal jaundice from other and unspecified hepatocellular damage**
EXCLUDES 1 *congenital viral hepatitis (P35.3)*
P59.20 **Neonatal jaundice from unspecified hepatocellular damage**
P59.29 **Neonatal jaundice from other hepatocellular damage**
Neonatal giant cell hepatitis
Neonatal (idiopathic) hepatitis
P59.3 **Neonatal jaundice from breast milk inhibitor**
P59.8 **Neonatal jaundice from other specified causes**
P59.9 **Neonatal jaundice, unspecified**
Neonatal physiological jaundice (intense)(prolonged) NOS
AHA: 3Q 2015, 20

P60 **Disseminated intravascular coagulation of newborn**
Defibrination syndrome of newborn

P61 **Other perinatal hematological disorders**
EXCLUDES 1 *transient hypogammaglobulinemia of infancy (D80.7)*

P61.0 **Transient neonatal thrombocytopenia**
Neonatal thrombocytopenia due to exchange transfusion
Neonatal thrombocytopenia due to idiopathic maternal thrombocytopenia
Neonatal thrombocytopenia due to isoimmunization
P61.1 **Polycythemia neonatorum**

DEFINITION Abnormally increased number of red blood cells in the neonate's bloodstream.

P61.2 **Anemia of prematurity**

P61.3 **Congenital anemia from fetal blood loss**

P61.4 **Other congenital anemias, not elsewhere classified**
Congenital anemia NOS

P61.5 **Transient neonatal neutropenia**
EXCLUDES 1 *congenital neutropenia (nontransient) (D70.0)*

P61.6 **Other transient neonatal disorders of coagulation**

P61.8 **Other specified perinatal hematological disorders**

P61.9 **Perinatal hematological disorder, unspecified**

Transitory endocrine and metabolic disorders specific to newborn (P70-P74)

INCLUDES transitory endocrine and metabolic disturbances caused by the infant's response to maternal endocrine and metabolic factors, or its adjustment to extrauterine environment

4 P70 **Transitory disorders of carbohydrate metabolism specific to newborn**

P70.0 **Syndrome of infant of mother with gestational diabetes**
Newborn (with hypoglycemia) affected by maternal gestational diabetes
EXCLUDES 1 *newborn (with hypoglycemia) affected by maternal (pre-existing) diabetes mellitus (P70.1)*
syndrome of infant of a diabetic mother (P70.1)

P70.1 **Syndrome of infant of a diabetic mother**
Newborn (with hypoglycemia) affected by maternal (pre-existing) diabetes mellitus
EXCLUDES 1 *newborn (with hypoglycemia) affected by maternal gestational diabetes (P70.0)*
syndrome of infant of mother with gestational diabetes (P70.0)

P70.2 **Neonatal diabetes mellitus**

P70.3 **Iatrogenic neonatal hypoglycemia**

P70.4 **Other neonatal hypoglycemia**
Transitory neonatal hypoglycemia

P70.8 **Other transitory disorders of carbohydrate metabolism of newborn**

P70.9 **Transitory disorder of carbohydrate metabolism of newborn, unspecified**

4 P71 **Transitory neonatal disorders of calcium and magnesium metabolism**

P71.0 **Cow's milk hypocalcemia in newborn**

P71.1 **Other neonatal hypocalcemia**
EXCLUDES 1 *neonatal hypoparathyroidism (P71.4)*

P71.2 **Neonatal hypomagnesemia**

P71.3 **Neonatal tetany without calcium or magnesium deficiency**
Neonatal tetany NOS

P71.4 **Transitory neonatal hypoparathyroidism**

P71.8 **Other transitory neonatal disorders of calcium and magnesium metabolism**

P71.9 **Transitory neonatal disorder of calcium and magnesium metabolism, unspecified**

4 P72 **Other transitory neonatal endocrine disorders**
EXCLUDES 1 *congenital hypothyroidism with or without goiter (E03.0-E03.1)*
dyshormogenetic goiter (E07.1)
Pendred's syndrome (E07.1)

P72.0 **Neonatal goiter, not elsewhere classified**
Transitory congenital goiter with normal functioning

P72.1 **Transitory neonatal hyperthyroidism**
Neonatal thyrotoxicosis

DEFINITION Abnormally high levels of thyroid hormone in the neonate.

P72.2 **Other transitory neonatal disorders of thyroid function, not elsewhere classified**
Transitory neonatal hypothyroidism

P72.8 **Other specified transitory neonatal endocrine disorders**

P72.9 **Transitory neonatal endocrine disorder, unspecified**

4 P74 **Other transitory neonatal electrolyte and metabolic disturbances**

P74.0 **Late metabolic acidosis of newborn**
EXCLUDES 1 *(fetal) metabolic acidosis of newborn (P19)*

DEFINITION Imbalance in the acid to alkaline ratio in the blood, most often affecting premature infants in the 2nd and 3rd week of life.

P74.1 **Dehydration of newborn**

▲5 **P74.2** **Disturbances of sodium balance of newborn**
AHA: 2Q 2018, 5

● **P74.21** **Hypernatremia of newborn**

● **P74.22** **Hyponatremia of newborn**

▲5 **P74.3** **Disturbances of potassium balance of newborn**

● **P74.31** **Hyperkalemia of newborn**

● **P74.32** **Hypokalemia of newborn**

▲5 **P74.4** **Other transitory electrolyte disturbances of newborn**

● **P74.41** **Alkalosis of newborn**
Hyperbicarbonatemia

●6 **P74.42** **Disturbances of chlorine balance of newborn**

● **P74.421** **Hyperchloremia of newborn**
Hyperchloremic metabolic acidosis
EXCLUDES 2 *late metabolic acidosis of the newborn (P77.0)*

● **P74.422** **Hypochloremia of newborn**

● **P74.49** **Other transitory electrolyte disturbance of newborn**

P74.5 **Transitory tyrosinemia of newborn**

P74.6 **Transitory hyperammonemia of newborn**

P74.8 **Other transitory metabolic disturbances of newborn**
Amino-acid metabolic disorders described as transitory

P74.9 **Transitory metabolic disturbance of newborn, unspecified**

Digestive system disorders of newborn (P76-P78)

4 P76 **Other intestinal obstruction of newborn**

P76.0 **Meconium plug syndrome**
Meconium ileus NOS
EXCLUDES 1 *meconium ileus in cystic fibrosis (E84.11)*

DEFINITION Dark green feces that normally comprises a newborn's first bowel movement does not pass through the bowel, causing blockage of the intestine.

P76.1 **Transitory ileus of newborn**
EXCLUDES 1 *Hirschsprung's disease (Q43.1)*

P76.2 **Intestinal obstruction due to inspissated milk**

P76.8 **Other specified intestinal obstruction of newborn**
EXCLUDES 1 *intestinal obstruction classifiable to K56.-*

P76.9 **Intestinal obstruction of newborn, unspecified**

4 P77 **Necrotizing enterocolitis of newborn**

P77.1 **Stage 1 necrotizing enterocolitis in newborn**
Necrotizing enterocolitis without pneumatosis, without perforation

P77.2 **Stage 2 necrotizing enterocolitis in newborn**
Necrotizing enterocolitis with pneumatosis, without perforation

P77.3 **Stage 3 necrotizing enterocolitis in newborn**
Necrotizing enterocolitis with perforation
Necrotizing enterocolitis with pneumatosis and perforation

P77.9 **Necrotizing enterocolitis in newborn, unspecified**
Necrotizing enterocolitis in newborn, NOS

4 P78 **Other perinatal digestive system disorders**
EXCLUDES 1 *cystic fibrosis (E84.0-E84.9)*
neonatal gastrointestinal hemorrhages (P54.0-P54.3)

P78.0 **Perinatal intestinal perforation**
Meconium peritonitis

Perinatal intestinal perforation

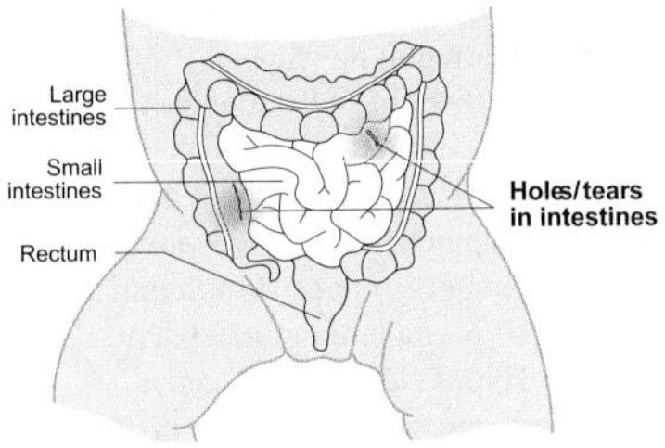

P78.1 **Other neonatal peritonitis**
Neonatal peritonitis NOS

P78.2 **Neonatal hematemesis and melena due to swallowed maternal blood**

P78.3 **Noninfective neonatal diarrhea**
Neonatal diarrhea NOS

5 **P78.8** **Other specified perinatal digestive system disorders**

P78.81 **Congenital cirrhosis (of liver)**

P78.82 **Peptic ulcer of newborn**

P78.83 **Newborn esophageal reflux**
Neonatal esophageal reflux

P78.84 **Gestational alloimmune liver disease**
GALD
Neonatal hemochromatosis
EXCLUDES 1 *hemochromatosis (E83.11-)*
AHA: 4Q 2017, 16

P78.89 **Other specified perinatal digestive system disorders**

P78.9 **Perinatal digestive system disorder, unspecified**

Conditions involving the integument and temperature regulation of newborn (P80-P83)

4 **P80** **Hypothermia of newborn**

P80.0 **Cold injury syndrome**
Severe and usually chronic hypothermia associated with a pink flushed appearance, edema and neurological and biochemical abnormalities.
EXCLUDES 1 *mild hypothermia of newborn (P80.8)*

P80.8 **Other hypothermia of newborn**
Mild hypothermia of newborn

P80.9 **Hypothermia of newborn, unspecified**

4 **P81** **Other disturbances of temperature regulation of newborn**

P81.0 **Environmental hyperthermia of newborn**

P81.8 **Other specified disturbances of temperature regulation of newborn**

P81.9 **Disturbance of temperature regulation of newborn, unspecified**
Fever of newborn NOS

4 **P83** **Other conditions of integument specific to newborn**
EXCLUDES 1 *congenital malformations of skin and integument (Q80-Q84)*
hydrops fetalis due to hemolytic disease (P56.-)
neonatal skin infection (P39.4)
staphylococcal scalded skin syndrome (L00)
EXCLUDES 2 *cradle cap (L21.0)*
diaper [napkin] dermatitis (L22)

P83.0 **Sclerema neonatorum**

P83.1 **Neonatal erythema toxicum**

P83.2 **Hydrops fetalis not due to hemolytic disease**
Hydrops fetalis NOS

5 **P83.3** **Other and unspecified edema specific to newborn**

P83.30 **Unspecified edema specific to newborn**

P83.39 **Other edema specific to newborn**

P83.4 **Breast engorgement of newborn**
Noninfective mastitis of newborn

P83.5 **Congenital hydrocele** ♂

P83.6 **Umbilical polyp of newborn**

5 **P83.8** **Other specified conditions of integument specific to newborn**

P83.81 **Umbilical granuloma**
EXCLUDES 2 *Granulomatous disorder of the skin and subcutaneous tissue, unspecified (L92.9)*
AHA: 4Q 2017, 16

P83.88 **Other specified conditions of integument specific to newborn**
Bronze baby syndrome
Neonatal scleroderma
Urticaria neonatorum
AHA: 4Q 2017, 16

P83.9 **Condition of the integument specific to newborn, unspecified**

Other problems with newborn (P84)

P84 **Other problems with newborn**
Acidemia of newborn
Acidosis of newborn
Anoxia of newborn NOS
Asphyxia of newborn NOS
Hypercapnia of newborn
Hypoxemia of newborn
Hypoxia of newborn NOS
Mixed metabolic and respiratory acidosis of newborn
EXCLUDES 1 *intracranial hemorrhage due to anoxia or hypoxia (P52.-)*
hypoxic ischemic encephalopathy [HIE] (P91.6-)
late metabolic acidosis of newborn (P74.0)

Other disorders originating in the perinatal period (P90-P96)

P90 **Convulsions of newborn**
EXCLUDES 1 *benign myoclonic epilepsy in infancy (G40.3-)*
benign neonatal convulsions (familial) (G40.3-)

4 **P91** **Other disturbances of cerebral status of newborn**

P91.0 **Neonatal cerebral ischemia**

P91.1 **Acquired periventricular cysts of newborn**

P91.2 **Neonatal cerebral leukomalacia**
Periventricular leukomalacia

P91.3 **Neonatal cerebral irritability**

P91.4 **Neonatal cerebral depression**

P91.5 **Neonatal coma**

5 **P91.6** **Hypoxic ischemic encephalopathy [HIE]**
EXCLUDES 1 *Neonatal cerebral depression (P91.4)*
Neonatal cerebral irritability (P91.3)
Neonatal coma (P91.5)

P91.60 **Hypoxic ischemic encephalopathy [HIE], unspecified**

P91.61 **Mild hypoxic ischemic encephalopathy [HIE]**

P91.62 **Moderate hypoxic ischemic encephalopathy [HIE]**

P91.63 **Severe hypoxic ischemic encephalopathy [HIE]**

5 **P91.8** **Other specified disturbances of cerebral status of newborn**

6 **P91.81** **Neonatal encephalopathy**

▲ **P91.811** ***Neonatal encephalopathy in diseases classified elsewhere***
Code first underlying condition, if known, such as:
congenital cirrhosis (of liver) (P78.81)
intracranial nontraumatic hemorrhage of newborn (P52.-)
kernicterus (P57.-)
AHA: 4Q 2017, 17

P91.819 **Neonatal encephalopathy, unspecified**
AHA: 4Q 2017, 17

P91.88 **Other specified disturbances of cerebral status of newborn**

P91.9 **Disturbance of cerebral status of newborn, unspecified**

4 **P92** **Feeding problems of newborn**
EXCLUDES 1 *eating disorders (F50.-)*
feeding problems in child over 28 days old (R63.3)

5 **P92.0** **Vomiting of newborn**
EXCLUDES 1 *vomiting of child over 28 days old (R11.-)*

P92.01 Bilious vomiting of newborn
EXCLUDES 1 *bilious vomiting in child over 28 days old (R11.14)*
P92.09 Other vomiting of newborn
EXCLUDES 1 *regurgitation of food in newborn (P92.1)*
P92.1 Regurgitation and rumination of newborn
P92.2 Slow feeding of newborn
P92.3 Underfeeding of newborn
P92.4 Overfeeding of newborn
P92.5 Neonatal difficulty in feeding at breast
AHA: 3Q 2016, 19
AHA: 1Q 2017, 28
P92.6 Failure to thrive in newborn
EXCLUDES 1 *failure to thrive in child over 28 days old (R62.51)*
P92.8 Other feeding problems of newborn
P92.9 Feeding problem of newborn, unspecified

▲ 4 **P93 Reactions and intoxications due to drugs administered to newborn**
INCLUDES reactions and intoxications due to drugs administered to fetus affecting newborn
EXCLUDES 1 *jaundice due to drugs or toxins transmitted from mother or given to newborn (P58.4-)*
reactions and intoxications from maternal opiates, tranquilizers and other medication (P04.0-P04.1, P04.4-)
withdrawal symptoms from maternal use of drugs of addiction (P96.1)
withdrawal symptoms from therapeutic use of drugs in newborn (P96.2)
P93.0 Grey baby syndrome
Grey syndrome from chloramphenicol administration in newborn
P93.8 Other reactions and intoxications due to drugs administered to newborn
Use additional code for adverse effect, if applicable, to identify drug (T36-T50 with fifth or sixth character 5)

4 **P94 Disorders of muscle tone of newborn**
P94.0 Transient neonatal myasthenia gravis
EXCLUDES 1 *myasthenia gravis (G70.0)*
P94.1 Congenital hypertonia
P94.2 Congenital hypotonia
Floppy baby syndrome, unspecified
P94.8 Other disorders of muscle tone of newborn
P94.9 Disorder of muscle tone of newborn, unspecified

P95 Stillbirth
Deadborn fetus NOS
Fetal death of unspecified cause
Stillbirth NOS
EXCLUDES 1 *maternal care for intrauterine death (O36.4)*
missed abortion (O02.1)
outcome of delivery, stillbirth (Z37.1, Z37.3, Z37.4, Z37.7)

4 **P96 Other conditions originating in the perinatal period**
P96.0 Congenital renal failure
Uremia of newborn
P96.1 Neonatal withdrawal symptoms from maternal use of drugs of addiction
Drug withdrawal syndrome in infant of dependent mother
Neonatal abstinence syndrome
EXCLUDES 1 *reactions and intoxications from maternal opiates and tranquilizers administered during labor and delivery (P04.0)*
P96.2 Withdrawal symptoms from therapeutic use of drugs in newborn
P96.3 Wide cranial sutures of newborn
Neonatal craniotabes
P96.5 Complication to newborn due to (fetal) intrauterine procedure
EXCLUDES 2 *newborn affected by amniocentesis (P00.6)*
5 P96.8 Other specified conditions originating in the perinatal period
P96.81 Exposure to (parental) (environmental) tobacco smoke in the perinatal period
EXCLUDES 2 *newborn affected by in utero exposure to tobacco (P04.2)*
exposure to environmental tobacco smoke after the perinatal period (Z77.22)
P96.82 Delayed separation of umbilical cord
P96.83 Meconium staining
EXCLUDES 1 *meconium aspiration (P24.00, P24.01)*
meconium passage during delivery (P03.82)
P96.89 Other specified conditions originating in the perinatal period
Use additional code to specify condition
P96.9 Condition originating in the perinatal period, unspecified
Congenital debility NOS

CHAPTER 17: CONGENITAL MALFORMATIONS, DEFORMATIONS AND CHROMOSOMAL ABNORMALITIES (Q00-Q99)

Note: Codes from this chapter are not for use on maternal records
EXCLUDES 2 *inborn errors of metabolism (E70-E88)*

GUIDELINES **Section I.C.17**
Codes from Chapter 17 may be used throughout the life of the patient. If a congenital malformation or deformity has been corrected, a personal history code should be used to identify the history of the malformation or deformity. Although present at birth, malformation/deformation/or chromosomal abnormality may not be identified until later in life. Whenever the condition is diagnosed by the physician, it is appropriate to assign a code from codes Q00-Q99. For the birth admission, the appropriate code from category Z38, Liveborn infants, according to place of birth and type of delivery, should be sequenced as the principal diagnosis, followed by any congenital anomaly codes, Q00- Q99.

This chapter contains the following blocks:

Q00-Q07	Congenital malformations of the nervous system
Q10-Q18	Congenital malformations of eye, ear, face and neck
Q20-Q28	Congenital malformations of the circulatory system
Q30-Q34	Congenital malformations of the respiratory system
Q35-Q37	Cleft lip and cleft palate
Q38-Q45	Other congenital malformations of the digestive system
Q50-Q56	Congenital malformations of genital organs
Q60-Q64	Congenital malformations of the urinary system
Q65-Q79	Congenital malformations and deformations of the musculoskeletal system
Q80-Q89	Other congenital malformations
Q90-Q99	Chromosomal abnormalities, not elsewhere classified

Congenital malformations of the nervous system (Q00-Q07)

4 Q00 Anencephaly and similar malformations

Q00.0 Anencephaly HCC
Acephaly
Acrania
Amyelencephaly
Hemianencephaly
Hemicephaly

Q00.1 Craniorachischisis HCC

Q00.2 Iniencephaly HCC

DEFINITION Neural tube birth defect in which the fetal head is severely bent backwards, the neck is usually absent, and other severe birth defects are present.

4 Q01 Encephalocele

INCLUDES Arnold-Chiari syndrome, type III
encephalocystocele
encephalomyelocele
hydroencephalocele
hydromeningocele, cranial
meningocele, cerebral
meningoencephalocele

EXCLUDES 1 *Meckel-Gruber syndrome (Q61.9)*

Q01.0 Frontal encephalocele HCC

Q01.1 Nasofrontal encephalocele HCC

Q01.2 Occipital encephalocele HCC

Q01.8 Encephalocele of other sites HCC

Q01.9 Encephalocele, unspecified HCC

▲ **Q02 Microcephaly** HCC

INCLUDES hydromicrocephaly
micrencephalon

Use additional code, if applicable, to identify congenital Zika virus disease

EXCLUDES 1 *Meckel-Gruber syndrome (Q61.9)*

DEFINITION Abnormal smallness of the head.

4 Q03 Congenital hydrocephalus

INCLUDES hydrocephalus in newborn

EXCLUDES 1 *Arnold-Chiari syndrome, type II (Q07.0-)*
acquired hydrocephalus (G91.-)
hydrocephalus due to congenital toxoplasmosis (P37.1)
hydrocephalus with spina bifida (Q05.0-Q05.4)

CODING TIP✓ Use Z98.2 as a secondary code to indicate a cerebrospinal fluid drainage shunt.

Q03.0 Malformations of aqueduct of Sylvius HCC
Anomaly of aqueduct of Sylvius
Obstruction of aqueduct of Sylvius, congenital
Stenosis of aqueduct of Sylvius

Q03.1 Atresia of foramina of Magendie and Luschka HCC
Dandy-Walker syndrome

Q03.8 Other congenital hydrocephalus HCC

Other congenital hydrocephalus

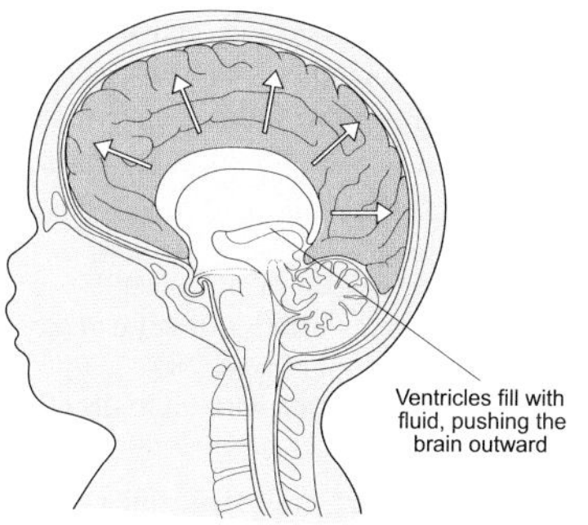
Ventricles fill with fluid, pushing the brain outward

Q03.9 Congenital hydrocephalus, unspecified HCC

4 Q04 Other congenital malformations of brain

EXCLUDES 1 *cyclopia (Q87.0)*
macrocephaly (Q75.3)

Q04.0 Congenital malformations of corpus callosum HCC
Agenesis of corpus callosum

Q04.1 Arhinencephaly HCC

Q04.2 Holoprosencephaly HCC

Q04.3 Other reduction deformities of brain HCC
Absence of part of brain
Agenesis of part of brain
Agyria
Aplasia of part of brain
Hydranencephaly
Hypoplasia of part of brain
Lissencephaly
Microgyria
Pachygyria

EXCLUDES 1 *congenital malformations of corpus callosum (Q04.0)*

Q04.4 Septo-optic dysplasia of brain HCC

Q04.5 Megalencephaly HCC

Q04.6 Congenital cerebral cysts HCC
Porencephaly
Schizencephaly

EXCLUDES 1 *acquired porencephalic cyst (G93.0)*

Q04.8 Other specified congenital malformations of brain HCC
Arnold-Chiari syndrome, type IV
Macrogyria

CODING TIP✓ Chiari malformation, also referred to as Arnold Chiari malformation, is an anomaly where cerebellar tissue extends into the spinal canal. In the rarest form, type IV, the back of the brain fails to develop normally. Type IV is an anomaly where cerebellar hypoplasia is present.

Q04.9 Congenital malformation of brain, unspecified HCC
Congenital anomaly NOS of brain
Congenital deformity NOS of brain
Congenital disease or lesion NOS of brain
Multiple anomalies NOS of brain, congenital

4 Q05 Spina bifida

INCLUDES hydromeningocele (spinal)
meningocele (spinal)
meningomyelocele
myelocele
myelomeningocele
rachischisis
spina bifida (aperta) (cystica)
syringomyelocele

Use additional code for any associated paraplegia (paraparesis) (G82.2-)

EXCLUDES 1 *Arnold-Chiari syndrome, type II (Q07.0-)*
spina bifida occulta (Q76.0)

CODING TIP✓ Use Z98.2 as a secondary code to indicate a cerebrospinal fluid drainage shunt.

Q05.0 Cervical spina bifida with hydrocephalus HCC

Q05.1 Thoracic spina bifida with hydrocephalus HCC
Dorsal spina bifida with hydrocephalus
Thoracolumbar spina bifida with hydrocephalus

Q05.2 Lumbar spina bifida with hydrocephalus HCC
Lumbosacral spina bifida with hydrocephalus

Q05.3 Sacral spina bifida with hydrocephalus HCC

Q05.4 Unspecified spina bifida with hydrocephalus HCC

Q05.5 Cervical spina bifida without hydrocephalus HCC

Q05.6 Thoracic spina bifida without hydrocephalus HCC
Dorsal spina bifida NOS
Thoracolumbar spina bifida NOS

Q05.7 Lumbar spina bifida without hydrocephalus HCC
Lumbosacral spina bifida NOS

Q05.8 Sacral spina bifida without hydrocephalus HCC

Q05.9 Spina bifida, unspecified HCC

4 Q06 Other congenital malformations of spinal cord

Q06.0 Amyelia HCC

Q06.1 Hypoplasia and dysplasia of spinal cord HCC
Atelomyelia
Myelatelia
Myelodysplasia of spinal cord

Q06.2 Diastematomyelia HCC

Q06.3 Other congenital cauda equina malformations HCC

Q06.4 Hydromyelia HCC
Hydrorachis

Q06.8 Other specified congenital malformations of spinal cord HCC

Q06.9 Congenital malformation of spinal cord, unspecified HCC
Congenital anomaly NOS of spinal cord
Congenital deformity NOS of spinal cord
Congenital disease or lesion NOS of spinal cord

4 Q07 Other congenital malformations of nervous system

EXCLUDES 2 *congenital central alveolar hypoventilation syndrome (G47.35)*
familial dysautonomia [Riley-Day] (G90.1)
neurofibromatosis (nonmalignant) (Q85.0-)

5 Q07.0 Arnold-Chiari syndrome
Arnold-Chiari syndrome, type II

EXCLUDES 1 *Arnold-Chiari syndrome, type III (Q01.-)*
Arnold-Chiari syndrome, type IV (Q04.8)

Q07.00 Arnold-Chiari syndrome without spina bifida or hydrocephalus HCC

Q07.01 Arnold-Chiari syndrome with spina bifida HCC

Q07.02 Arnold-Chiari syndrome with hydrocephalus HCC

Q07.03 Arnold-Chiari syndrome with spina bifida and hydrocephalus HCC

Q07.8 Other specified congenital malformations of nervous system HCC
Agenesis of nerve
Displacement of brachial plexus
Jaw-winking syndrome
Marcus Gunn's syndrome

Q07.9 Congenital malformation of nervous system, unspecified HCC
Congenital anomaly NOS of nervous system
Congenital deformity NOS of nervous system
Congenital disease or lesion NOS of nervous system

Congenital malformations of eye, ear, face and neck (Q10-Q18)

EXCLUDES 2 *cleft lip and cleft palate (Q35-Q37)*
congenital malformation of cervical spine (Q05.0, Q05.5, Q67.5, Q76.0-Q76.4)
congenital malformation of larynx (Q31.-)
congenital malformation of lip NEC (Q38.0)
congenital malformation of nose (Q30.-)
congenital malformation of parathyroid gland (Q89.2)
congenital malformation of thyroid gland (Q89.2)

4 Q10 Congenital malformations of eyelid, lacrimal apparatus and orbit

EXCLUDES 1 *cryptophthalmos NOS (Q11.2)*
cryptophthalmos syndrome (Q87.0)

Q10.0 Congenital ptosis

DEFINITION Congenital drooping of the upper eyelid.

Q10.1 Congenital ectropion

Q10.2 Congenital entropion

Q10.3 Other congenital malformations of eyelid
Ablepharon
Blepharophimosis, congenital
Coloboma of eyelid
Congenital absence or agenesis of cilia
Congenital absence or agenesis of eyelid
Congenital accessory eyelid
Congenital accessory eye muscle
Congenital malformation of eyelid NOS

Q10.4 Absence and agenesis of lacrimal apparatus
Congenital absence of punctum lacrimale

Q10.5 Congenital stenosis and stricture of lacrimal duct

Q10.6 Other congenital malformations of lacrimal apparatus
Congenital malformation of lacrimal apparatus NOS

Q10.7 Congenital malformation of orbit

4 Q11 Anophthalmos, microphthalmos and macrophthalmos

Q11.0 Cystic eyeball

Q11.1 Other anophthalmos
Anophthalmos NOS
Agenesis of eye
Aplasia of eye

Q11.2 Microphthalmos
Cryptophthalmos NOS
Dysplasia of eye
Hypoplasia of eye
Rudimentary eye

EXCLUDES 1 *cryptophthalmos syndrome (Q87.0)*

DEFINITION Abnormal smallness in all dimensions of one or both eyes.

Q11.3 Macrophthalmos

EXCLUDES 1 *macrophthalmos in congenital glaucoma (Q15.0)*

4 Q12 Congenital lens malformations

Q12.0 Congenital cataract

Congenital cataract

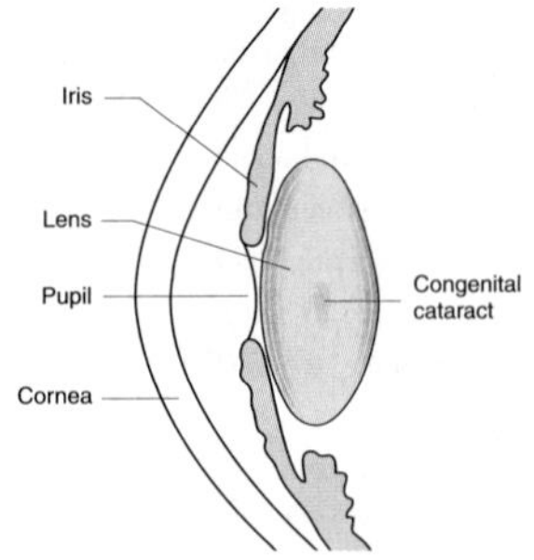

Q12.1 Congenital displaced lens

Q12.2 Coloboma of lens

Q12.3 Congenital aphakia

Q12.4 Spherophakia

Q12.8 **Other congenital lens malformations**
Microphakia
Q12.9 **Congenital lens malformation, unspecified**

Q13 Congenital malformations of anterior segment of eye

Q13.0 **Coloboma of iris**
Coloboma NOS
Q13.1 **Absence of iris**
Aniridia
Use additional code for associated glaucoma (H42)
Q13.2 **Other congenital malformations of iris**
Anisocoria, congenital
Atresia of pupil
Congenital malformation of iris NOS
Corectopia
Q13.3 **Congenital corneal opacity**
Q13.4 **Other congenital corneal malformations**
Congenital malformation of cornea NOS
Microcornea
Peter's anomaly
Q13.5 **Blue sclera**
Q13.8 **Other congenital malformations of anterior segment of eye**
Q13.81 **Rieger's anomaly**
Use additional code for associated glaucoma (H42)
Q13.89 **Other congenital malformations of anterior segment of eye**
Q13.9 **Congenital malformation of anterior segment of eye, unspecified**

Q14 Congenital malformations of posterior segment of eye

EXCLUDES 2 *optic nerve hypoplasia (H47.03-)*

Q14.0 **Congenital malformation of vitreous humor**
Congenital vitreous opacity
Q14.1 **Congenital malformation of retina**
Congenital retinal aneurysm
Q14.2 **Congenital malformation of optic disc**
Coloboma of optic disc
Q14.3 **Congenital malformation of choroid**
Q14.8 **Other congenital malformations of posterior segment of eye**
Coloboma of the fundus
Q14.9 **Congenital malformation of posterior segment of eye, unspecified**

Q15 Other congenital malformations of eye

EXCLUDES 1 *congenital nystagmus (H55.01)*
ocular albinism (E70.31-)
optic nerve hypoplasia (H47.03-)
retinitis pigmentosa (H35.52)

Q15.0 **Congenital glaucoma**
Axenfeld's anomaly
Buphthalmos
Glaucoma of childhood
Glaucoma of newborn
Hydrophthalmos
Keratoglobus, congenital, with glaucoma
Macrocornea with glaucoma
Macrophthalmos in congenital glaucoma
Megalocornea with glaucoma
DEFINITION Disease of infancy, marked by an increase of intraocular fluid, elevated eye pressure, and enlargement of the eyeball.
Q15.8 **Other specified congenital malformations of eye**
Q15.9 **Congenital malformation of eye, unspecified**
Congenital anomaly of eye
Congenital deformity of eye

Q16 Congenital malformations of ear causing impairment of hearing

EXCLUDES 1 *congenital deafness (H90.-)*

Q16.0 **Congenital absence of (ear) auricle**
Q16.1 **Congenital absence, atresia and stricture of auditory canal (external)**
Congenital atresia or stricture of osseous meatus
Q16.2 **Absence of eustachian tube**
Q16.3 **Congenital malformation of ear ossicles**
Congenital fusion of ear ossicles
Q16.4 **Other congenital malformations of middle ear**
Congenital malformation of middle ear NOS
Q16.5 **Congenital malformation of inner ear**
Congenital anomaly of membranous labyrinth
Congenital anomaly of organ of Corti
Q16.9 **Congenital malformation of ear causing impairment of hearing, unspecified**
Congenital absence of ear NOS

Q17 Other congenital malformations of ear

EXCLUDES 1 *congenital malformations of ear with impairment of hearing (Q16.0-Q16.9)*
preauricular sinus (Q18.1)

Q17.0 **Accessory auricle**
Accessory tragus
Polyotia
Preauricular appendage or tag
Supernumerary ear
Supernumerary lobule
Q17.1 **Macrotia**
DEFINITION Excessive enlargement of the auricle (outer portion of ear).
Q17.2 **Microtia**
Q17.3 **Other misshapen ear**
Pointed ear
Q17.4 **Misplaced ear**
Low-set ears
EXCLUDES 1 *cervical auricle (Q18.2)*
Q17.5 **Prominent ear**
Bat ear
Q17.8 **Other specified congenital malformations of ear**
Congenital absence of lobe of ear
Q17.9 **Congenital malformation of ear, unspecified**
Congenital anomaly of ear NOS

Q18 Other congenital malformations of face and neck

EXCLUDES 1 *cleft lip and cleft palate (Q35-Q37)*
conditions classified to Q67.0-Q67.4
congenital malformations of skull and face bones (Q75.-)
cyclopia (Q87.0)
dentofacial anomalies [including malocclusion] (M26.-)
malformation syndromes affecting facial appearance (Q87.0)
persistent thyroglossal duct (Q89.2)

Q18.0 **Sinus, fistula and cyst of branchial cleft**
Branchial vestige
Q18.1 **Preauricular sinus and cyst**
Fistula of auricle, congenital
Cervicoaural fistula
Q18.2 **Other branchial cleft malformations**
Branchial cleft malformation NOS
Cervical auricle
Otocephaly
Q18.3 **Webbing of neck**
Pterygium colli
DEFINITION A thick flap of skin extending from the side of the neck to the shoulder, often in concert with other birth defects.
Q18.4 **Macrostomia**
DEFINITION Abnormally large mouth.
Q18.5 **Microstomia**
DEFINITION Abnormally small mouth.
Q18.6 **Macrocheilia**
Hypertrophy of lip, congenital
DEFINITION Abnormally large lips.
Q18.7 **Microcheilia**
Q18.8 **Other specified congenital malformations of face and neck**
Medial cyst of face and neck
Medial fistula of face and neck
Medial sinus of face and neck
Q18.9 **Congenital malformation of face and neck, unspecified**
Congenital anomaly NOS of face and neck

Congenital malformations of the circulatory system (Q20-Q28)

Q20 Congenital malformations of cardiac chambers and connections

EXCLUDES 1 *dextrocardia with situs inversus (Q89.3)*
mirror-image atrial arrangement with situs inversus (Q89.3)

Q20.0 Common arterial trunk
Persistent truncus arteriosus
EXCLUDES 1 *aortic septal defect (Q21.4)*

DEFINITION Congenital anomaly in which there is abnormal communication between the ascending aorta and pulmonary artery, near the semilunar valve.

Q20.1 Double outlet right ventricle
Taussig-Bing syndrome

Q20.2 Double outlet left ventricle

Q20.3 Discordant ventriculoarterial connection
Dextrotransposition of aorta
Transposition of great vessels (complete)

Q20.4 Double inlet ventricle
Common ventricle
Cor triloculare biatriatum
Single ventricle

DEFINITION No septum or membrane is present dividing the right ventricle from the left ventricle.

Q20.5 Discordant atrioventricular connection
Corrected transposition
Levotransposition
Ventricular inversion

Q20.6 Isomerism of atrial appendages
Isomerism of atrial appendages with asplenia or polysplenia

Q20.8 Other congenital malformations of cardiac chambers and connections
Cor binoculare

Q20.9 Congenital malformation of cardiac chambers and connections, unspecified

Q21 Congenital malformations of cardiac septa

EXCLUDES 1 *acquired cardiac septal defect (I51.0)*

Q21.0 Ventricular septal defect
Roger's disease

Ventricular septal defect

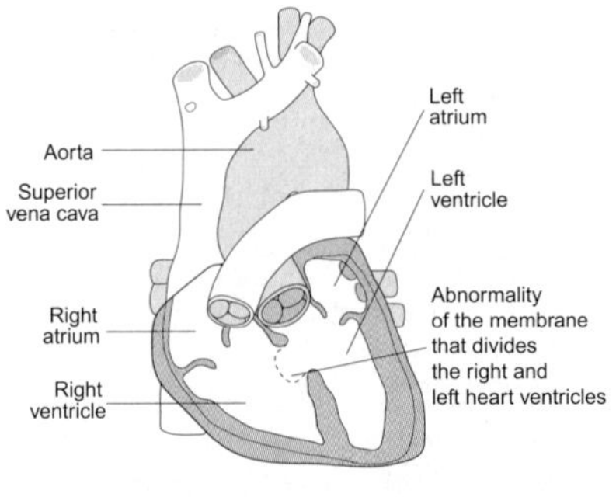

Q21.1 Atrial septal defect
Coronary sinus defect
Patent or persistent foramen ovale
Patent or persistent ostium secundum defect (type II)
Patent or persistent sinus venosus defect

Q21.2 Atrioventricular septal defect
Common atrioventricular canal
Endocardial cushion defect
Ostium primum atrial septal defect (type I)

Q21.3 Tetralogy of Fallot
Ventricular septal defect with pulmonary stenosis or atresia, dextroposition of aorta and hypertrophy of right ventricle.
AHA: 3Q 2014, 17

Tetralogy of Fallot

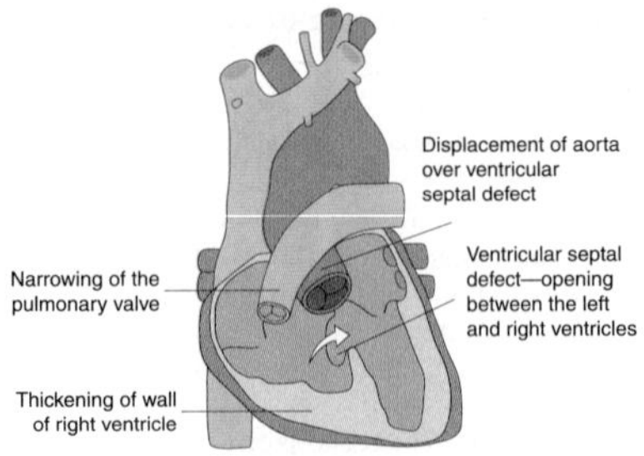

Q21.4 Aortopulmonary septal defect
Aortic septal defect
Aortopulmonary window

Q21.8 Other congenital malformations of cardiac septa
Eisenmenger's defect
Pentalogy of Fallot
Code also if applicable:
Eisenmenger's complex (I27.83)
Eisenmenger's syndrome (I27.83)

Q21.9 Congenital malformation of cardiac septum, unspecified
Septal (heart) defect NOS

Q22 Congenital malformations of pulmonary and tricuspid valves

Q22.0 Pulmonary valve atresia

DEFINITION Congenital absence of a normal valvular opening into the pulmonary artery.

Q22.1 Congenital pulmonary valve stenosis

Q22.2 Congenital pulmonary valve insufficiency
Congenital pulmonary valve regurgitation

Q22.3 Other congenital malformations of pulmonary valve
Congenital malformation of pulmonary valve NOS
Supernumerary cusps of pulmonary valve

Q22.4 Congenital tricuspid stenosis
Congenital tricuspid atresia

DEFINITION Abnormal narrowing of the valve that prevents blood from flowing back into the right atrium from the right ventricle.

Q22.5 Ebstein's anomaly

Q22.6 Hypoplastic right heart syndrome

Q22.8 Other congenital malformations of tricuspid valve

Q22.9 Congenital malformation of tricuspid valve, unspecified

Q23 Congenital malformations of aortic and mitral valves

Q23.0 Congenital stenosis of aortic valve
Congenital aortic atresia
Congenital aortic stenosis NOS
EXCLUDES 1 *congenital stenosis of aortic valve in hypoplastic left heart syndrome (Q23.4)*
congenital subaortic stenosis (Q24.4)
supravalvular aortic stenosis (congenital) (Q25.3)

Q23.1 Congenital insufficiency of aortic valve
Bicuspid aortic valve
Congenital aortic insufficiency

Q23.2 Congenital mitral stenosis
Congenital mitral atresia

Congenital mitral stenosis

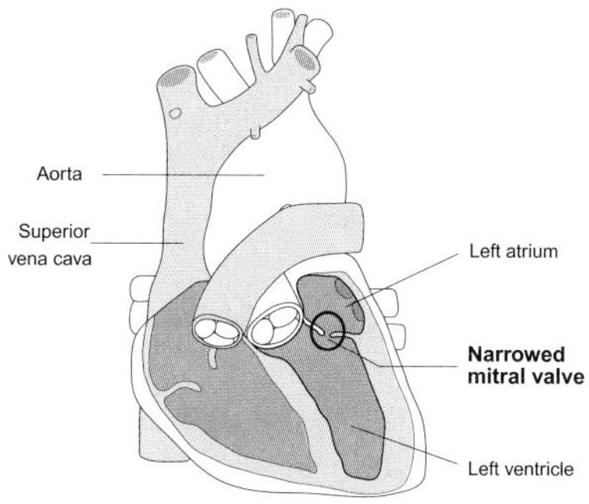

Q23.3 **Congenital mitral insufficiency**
Q23.4 **Hypoplastic left heart syndrome**
Q23.8 **Other congenital malformations of aortic and mitral valves**
Q23.9 **Congenital malformation of aortic and mitral valves, unspecified**

4 Q24 Other congenital malformations of heart

EXCLUDES 1 *endocardial fibroelastosis (I42.4)*

Q24.0 **Dextrocardia**
EXCLUDES 1 *dextrocardia with situs inversus (Q89.3)*
isomerism of atrial appendages (with asplenia or polysplenia) (Q20.6)
mirror-image atrial arrangement with situs inversus (Q89.3)

Q24.1 **Levocardia**
Q24.2 **Cor triatriatum**
DEFINITION The heart has three atrial chambers with the left atrium divided into two segments.

Q24.3 **Pulmonary infundibular stenosis**
Subvalvular pulmonic stenosis
Q24.4 **Congenital subaortic stenosis**
Q24.5 **Malformation of coronary vessels**
Congenital coronary (artery) aneurysm
Q24.6 **Congenital heart block**
Q24.8 **Other specified congenital malformations of heart**
Congenital diverticulum of left ventricle
Congenital malformation of myocardium
Congenital malformation of pericardium
Malposition of heart
Uhl's disease
Q24.9 **Congenital malformation of heart, unspecified**
Congenital anomaly of heart
Congenital disease of heart

4 Q25 Congenital malformations of great arteries

CODING TIP✓ If the condition has been corrected or is no longer a problem, then code Z87.74, Personal history of (corrected) congenital malformations of heart and circulatory system.

Q25.0 **Patent ductus arteriosus**
Patent ductus Botallo
Persistent ductus arteriosus
Q25.1 **Coarctation of aorta**
Coarctation of aorta (preductal) (postductal)
Stenosis of aorta
5 Q25.2 **Atresia of aorta**
Q25.21 **Interruption of aortic arch**
Atresia of aortic arch
AHA: 4Q 2016, 56
Q25.29 **Other atresia of aorta**
Atresia of aorta
AHA: 4Q 2016, 56
Q25.3 **Supravalvular aortic stenosis**
EXCLUDES 1 *congenital aortic stenosis NOS (Q23.0)*
congenital stenosis of aortic valve (Q23.0)
5 Q25.4 **Other congenital malformations of aorta**
EXCLUDES 1 *hypoplasia of aorta in hypoplastic left heart syndrome (Q23.4)*
Q25.40 **Congenital malformation of aorta unspecified**
Q25.41 **Absence and aplasia of aorta**
AHA: 4Q 2016, 57
Q25.42 **Hypoplasia of aorta**
AHA: 4Q 2016, 57
Q25.43 **Congenital aneurysm of aorta**
Congenital aneurysm of aortic root
Congenital aneurysm of aortic sinus
AHA: 4Q 2016, 57
Q25.44 **Congenital dilation of aorta**
AHA: 4Q 2016, 57
Q25.45 **Double aortic arch**
Vascular ring of aorta
AHA: 4Q 2016, 57
Q25.46 **Tortuous aortic arch**
Persistent convolutions of aortic arch
AHA: 4Q 2016, 57
Q25.47 **Right aortic arch**
Persistent right aortic arch
AHA: 4Q 2016, 57
Q25.48 **Anomalous origin of subclavian artery**
AHA: 4Q 2016, 57
Q25.49 **Other congenital malformations of aorta**
Aortic arch
Bovine arch
AHA: 4Q 2016, 57
Q25.5 **Atresia of pulmonary artery**
Q25.6 **Stenosis of pulmonary artery**
Supravalvular pulmonary stenosis
5 Q25.7 **Other congenital malformations of pulmonary artery**
Q25.71 **Coarctation of pulmonary artery**
Q25.72 **Congenital pulmonary arteriovenous malformation**
Congenital pulmonary arteriovenous aneurysm
Q25.79 **Other congenital malformations of pulmonary artery**
Aberrant pulmonary artery
Agenesis of pulmonary artery
Congenital aneurysm of pulmonary artery
Congenital anomaly of pulmonary artery
Hypoplasia of pulmonary artery
Q25.8 **Other congenital malformations of Other great arteries**
Q25.9 **Congenital malformation of great arteries, unspecified**

4 Q26 Congenital malformations of great veins

Q26.0 **Congenital stenosis of vena cava**
Congenital stenosis of vena cava (inferior)(superior)
Q26.1 **Persistent left superior vena cava**
Q26.2 **Total anomalous pulmonary venous connection**
Total anomalous pulmonary venous return [TAPVR], subdiaphragmatic
Total anomalous pulmonary venous return [TAPVR], supradiaphragmatic
Q26.3 **Partial anomalous pulmonary venous connection**
Partial anomalous pulmonary venous return
Q26.4 **Anomalous pulmonary venous connection, unspecified**
Q26.5 **Anomalous portal venous connection**
Q26.6 **Portal vein-hepatic artery fistula**
Q26.8 **Other congenital malformations of great veins**
Absence of vena cava (inferior) (superior)
Azygos continuation of inferior vena cava
Persistent left posterior cardinal vein
Scimitar syndrome
Q26.9 **Congenital malformation of great vein, unspecified**
Congenital anomaly of vena cava (inferior) (superior) NOS

4 Q27 Other congenital malformations of peripheral vascular system

EXCLUDES 2 *anomalies of cerebral and precerebral vessels (Q28.0-Q28.3)*
anomalies of coronary vessels (Q24.5)
anomalies of pulmonary artery (Q25.5-Q25.7)
congenital retinal aneurysm (Q14.1)
hemangioma and lymphangioma (D18.-)

Q27.0 **Congenital absence and hypoplasia of umbilical artery**
Single umbilical artery
Q27.1 **Congenital renal artery stenosis**
Q27.2 **Other congenital malformations of renal artery**
Congenital malformation of renal artery NOS
Multiple renal arteries

Q27.3 Arteriovenous malformation (peripheral)
Arteriovenous aneurysm
EXCLUDES 1 *acquired arteriovenous aneurysm (I77.0)*
EXCLUDES 2 *arteriovenous malformation of cerebral vessels (Q28.2)*
arteriovenous malformation of precerebral vessels (Q28.0)

Q27.30 Arteriovenous malformation, site unspecified
Q27.31 Arteriovenous malformation of vessel of upper limb
Q27.32 Arteriovenous malformation of vessel of lower limb
Q27.33 Arteriovenous malformation of digestive system vessel
Q27.34 Arteriovenous malformation of renal vessel
Q27.39 Arteriovenous malformation, other site

Q27.4 Congenital phlebectasia
Q27.8 Other specified congenital malformations of peripheral vascular system
Absence of peripheral vascular system
Atresia of peripheral vascular system
Congenital aneurysm (peripheral)
Congenital stricture, artery
Congenital varix
EXCLUDES 1 *arteriovenous malformation (Q27.3-)*
Q27.9 Congenital malformation of peripheral vascular system, unspecified
Anomaly of artery or vein NOS

Q28 Other congenital malformations of circulatory system
EXCLUDES 1 *congenital aneurysm NOS (Q27.8)*
congenital coronary aneurysm (Q24.5)
ruptured cerebral arteriovenous malformation (I60.8)
ruptured malformation of precerebral vessels (I72.0)
EXCLUDES 2 *congenital peripheral aneurysm (Q27.8)*
congenital pulmonary aneurysm (Q25.79)
congenital retinal aneurysm (Q14.1)

Q28.0 Arteriovenous malformation of precerebral vessels
Congenital arteriovenous precerebral aneurysm (nonruptured)
Q28.1 Other malformations of precerebral vessels
Congenital malformation of precerebral vessels NOS
Congenital precerebral aneurysm (nonruptured)
Q28.2 Arteriovenous malformation of cerebral vessels
Arteriovenous malformation of brain NOS
Congenital arteriovenous cerebral aneurysm (nonruptured)
Q28.3 Other malformations of cerebral vessels
Congenital cerebral aneurysm (nonruptured)
Congenital malformation of cerebral vessels NOS
Developmental venous anomaly
Q28.8 Other specified congenital malformations of circulatory system
Congenital aneurysm, specified site NEC
Spinal vessel anomaly
Q28.9 Congenital malformation of circulatory system, unspecified

Congenital malformations of the respiratory system (Q30-Q34)

Q30 Congenital malformations of nose
EXCLUDES 1 *congenital deviation of nasal septum (Q67.4)*

Q30.0 Choanal atresia
Atresia of nares (anterior) (posterior)
Congenital stenosis of nares (anterior) (posterior)
DEFINITION Fetal nasal airways are obstructed by membranous or bony tissue; infant is unable to breathe and nurse simultaneously.
Q30.1 Agenesis and underdevelopment of nose
Congenital absent of nose
Q30.2 Fissured, notched and cleft nose
Q30.3 Congenital perforated nasal septum
Q30.8 Other congenital malformations of nose
Accessory nose
Congenital anomaly of nasal sinus wall
Q30.9 Congenital malformation of nose, unspecified

Q31 Congenital malformations of larynx
EXCLUDES 1 *congenital laryngeal stridor NOS (P28.89)*

Q31.0 Web of larynx
Glottic web of larynx
Subglottic web of larynx
Web of larynx NOS
Q31.1 Congenital subglottic stenosis
Q31.2 Laryngeal hypoplasia
Q31.3 Laryngocele
Q31.5 Congenital laryngomalacia
Q31.8 Other congenital malformations of larynx
Absence of larynx
Agenesis of larynx
Atresia of larynx
Congenital cleft thyroid cartilage
Congenital fissure of epiglottis
Congenital stenosis of larynx NEC
Posterior cleft of cricoid cartilage
Q31.9 Congenital malformation of larynx, unspecified

Q32 Congenital malformations of trachea and bronchus
EXCLUDES 1 *congenital bronchiectasis (Q33.4)*

Q32.0 Congenital tracheomalacia
Q32.1 Other congenital malformations of trachea
Atresia of trachea
Congenital anomaly of tracheal cartilage
Congenital dilatation of trachea
Congenital malformation of trachea
Congenital stenosis of trachea
Congenital tracheocele
Q32.2 Congenital bronchomalacia
Q32.3 Congenital stenosis of bronchus
Q32.4 Other congenital malformations of bronchus
Absence of bronchus
Agenesis of bronchus
Atresia of bronchus
Congenital diverticulum of bronchus
Congenital malformation of bronchus NOS

Q33 Congenital malformations of lung
Q33.0 Congenital cystic lung
Congenital cystic lung disease
Congenital honeycomb lung
Congenital polycystic lung disease
EXCLUDES 1 *cystic fibrosis (E84.0)*
cystic lung disease, acquired or unspecified (J98.4)
Q33.1 Accessory lobe of lung
Azygos lobe (fissured), lung
Q33.2 Sequestration of lung
Q33.3 Agenesis of lung
Congenital absence of lung (lobe)
Q33.4 Congenital bronchiectasis
Q33.5 Ectopic tissue in lung
Q33.6 Congenital hypoplasia and dysplasia of lung
EXCLUDES 1 *pulmonary hypoplasia associated with short gestation (P28.0)*
Q33.8 Other congenital malformations of lung
Q33.9 Congenital malformation of lung, unspecified

Q34 Other congenital malformations of respiratory system
EXCLUDES 2 *congenital central alveolar hypoventilation syndrome (G47.35)*

Q34.0 Anomaly of pleura
Q34.1 Congenital cyst of mediastinum
Q34.8 Other specified congenital malformations of respiratory system
Atresia of nasopharynx
Q34.9 Congenital malformation of respiratory system, unspecified
Congenital absence of respiratory system
Congenital anomaly of respiratory system NOS

Cleft lip and cleft palate (Q35-Q37)

Use additional code to identify associated malformation of the nose (Q30.2)
EXCLUDES 1 *Robin's syndrome (Q87.0)*

Q35 Cleft palate
INCLUDES fissure of palate
palatoschisis
EXCLUDES 1 *cleft palate with cleft lip (Q37.-)*

Q35.1 Cleft hard palate
Q35.3 Cleft soft palate

Q35.5 Cleft hard palate with cleft soft palate

Q35.7 Cleft uvula

Q35.9 Cleft palate, unspecified
Cleft palate NOS

DEFINITION A congenital fissure in the roof of the mouth, resulting from incomplete fusion of the palate during embryonic development.

Q36 Cleft lip

INCLUDES cheiloschisis
congenital fissure of lip
harelip
labium leporinum

EXCLUDES 1 *cleft lip with cleft palate (Q37.-)*

CODING TIP ✓ If the cleft palate/cleft lip has been corrected, use Z87.730, Personal history of (corrected) congenital malformations of cleft lip and palate.

Q36.0 Cleft lip, bilateral

Q36.1 Cleft lip, median

Q36.9 Cleft lip, unilateral
Cleft lip NOS

Q37 Cleft palate with cleft lip

INCLUDES cheilopalatoschisis

CODING TIP ✓ If the cleft palate/cleft lip has been corrected, use Z87.730, Personal history of (corrected) congenital malformations of cleft lip and palate.

Q37.0 Cleft hard palate with bilateral cleft lip

Q37.1 Cleft hard palate with unilateral cleft lip
Cleft hard palate with cleft lip NOS

Q37.2 Cleft soft palate with bilateral cleft lip

Q37.3 Cleft soft palate with unilateral cleft lip
Cleft soft palate with cleft lip NOS

Q37.4 Cleft hard and soft palate with bilateral cleft lip

Q37.5 Cleft hard and soft palate with unilateral cleft lip
Cleft hard and soft palate with cleft lip NOS

Cleft hard and soft palate with unilateral cleft lip

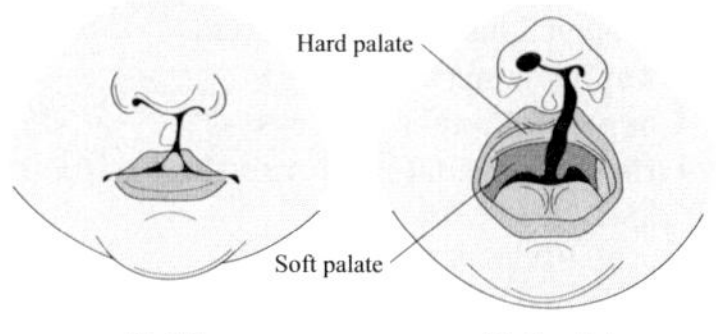

Q37.8 Unspecified cleft palate with bilateral cleft lip

Q37.9 Unspecified cleft palate with unilateral cleft lip
Cleft palate with cleft lip NOS

Other congenital malformations of the digestive system (Q38-Q45)

Q38 Other congenital malformations of tongue, mouth and pharynx

EXCLUDES 1 *dentofacial anomalies (M26.-)*
macrostomia (Q18.4)
microstomia (Q18.5)

Q38.0 Congenital malformations of lips, not elsewhere classified
Congenital fistula of lip
Congenital malformation of lip NOS
Van der Woude's syndrome

EXCLUDES 1 *cleft lip (Q36.-)*
cleft lip with cleft palate (Q37.-)
macrocheilia (Q18.6)
microcheilia (Q18.7)

Q38.1 Ankyloglossia
Tongue tie

Q38.2 Macroglossia
Congenital hypertrophy of tongue

DEFINITION Congenital enlargement of the tongue.

Q38.3 Other congenital malformations of tongue
Aglossia
Bifid tongue
Congenital adhesion of tongue
Congenital fissure of tongue
Congenital malformation of tongue NOS
Double tongue
Hypoglossia
Hypoplasia of tongue
Microglossia

Q38.4 Congenital malformations of salivary glands and ducts
Atresia of salivary glands and ducts
Congenital absence of salivary glands and ducts
Congenital accessory salivary glands and ducts
Congenital fistula of salivary gland

DEFINITION Congenital salivary gland fistula: Abnormal passage communicating with a salivary gland and present at birth.

Q38.5 Congenital malformations of palate, not elsewhere classified
Congenital absence of uvula
Congenital malformation of palate NOS
Congenital high arched palate

EXCLUDES 1 *cleft palate (Q35.-)*
cleft palate with cleft lip (Q37.-)

Q38.6 Other congenital malformations of mouth
Congenital malformation of mouth NOS

Q38.7 Congenital pharyngeal pouch
Congenital diverticulum of pharynx

EXCLUDES 1 *pharyngeal pouch syndrome (D82.1)*

Q38.8 Other congenital malformations of pharynx
Congenital malformation of pharynx NOS
Imperforate pharynx

Q39 Congenital malformations of esophagus

Q39.0 Atresia of esophagus without fistula
Atresia of esophagus NOS

Q39.1 Atresia of esophagus with tracheo-esophageal fistula
Atresia of esophagus with broncho-esophageal fistula

CODING TIP ✓ Code Q39.1 is used for a congenital tracheoesophageal fistula (TE fistula). A fistula as a complication of a tracheostomy is coded J95.04.

Q39.2 Congenital tracheo-esophageal fistula without atresia
Congenital tracheo-esophageal fistula NOS

Q39.3 Congenital stenosis and stricture of esophagus

Q39.4 Esophageal web

Q39.5 Congenital dilatation of esophagus
Congenital cardiospasm

Q39.6 Congenital diverticulum of esophagus
Congenital esophageal pouch

Q39.8 Other congenital malformations of esophagus
Congenital absence of esophagus
Congenital displacement of esophagus
Congenital duplication of esophagus

Q39.9 Congenital malformation of esophagus, unspecified

Q40 Other congenital malformations of upper alimentary tract

Q40.0 Congenital hypertrophic pyloric stenosis
Congenital or infantile constriction
Congenital or infantile hypertrophy
Congenital or infantile spasm
Congenital or infantile stenosis
Congenital or infantile stricture

DEFINITION Congenital narrowing and partial obstruction of the gastric outlet due to muscular hypertrophy and mucosal edema of the ring-like muscle at the lower end of the stomach (pyloric orifice) in newborns.

Q40.1 Congenital hiatus hernia
Congenital displacement of cardia through esophageal hiatus

EXCLUDES 1 *congenital diaphragmatic hernia (Q79.0)*

Q40.2 Other specified congenital malformations of stomach
Congenital displacement of stomach
Congenital diverticulum of stomach
Congenital hourglass stomach
Congenital duplication of stomach
Megalogastria
Microgastria

Q40.3 Congenital malformation of stomach, unspecified

Q40.8 **Other specified congenital malformations of upper alimentary tract**

Q40.9 **Congenital malformation of upper alimentary tract, unspecified**
Congenital anomaly of upper alimentary tract
Congenital deformity of upper alimentary tract

4 Q41 **Congenital absence, atresia and stenosis of small intestine**
INCLUDES congenital obstruction, occlusion or stricture of small intestine or intestine NOS
EXCLUDES 1 *cystic fibrosis with intestinal manifestation (E84.11)*
meconium ileus NOS (without cystic fibrosis) (P76.0)

Q41.0 **Congenital absence, atresia and stenosis of duodenum**

Q41.1 **Congenital absence, atresia and stenosis of jejunum**
Apple peel syndrome
Imperforate jejunum

Q41.2 **Congenital absence, atresia and stenosis of ileum**

Q41.8 **Congenital absence, atresia and stenosis of other specified parts of small intestine**

Q41.9 **Congenital absence, atresia and stenosis of small intestine, part unspecified**
Congenital absence, atresia and stenosis of intestine NOS

4 Q42 **Congenital absence, atresia and stenosis of large intestine**
INCLUDES congenital obstruction, occlusion and stricture of large intestine

Q42.0 **Congenital absence, atresia and stenosis of rectum with fistula**

Q42.1 **Congenital absence, atresia and stenosis of rectum without fistula**
Imperforate rectum

Q42.2 **Congenital absence, atresia and stenosis of anus with fistula**

Q42.3 **Congenital absence, atresia and stenosis of anus without fistula**
Imperforate anus

Q42.8 **Congenital absence, atresia and stenosis of other parts of large intestine**

Q42.9 **Congenital absence, atresia and stenosis of large intestine, part unspecified**

4 Q43 **Other congenital malformations of intestine**

Q43.0 **Meckel's diverticulum (displaced) (hypertrophic)**
Persistent omphalomesenteric duct
Persistent vitelline duct

Q43.1 **Hirschsprung's disease**
Aganglionosis
Congenital (aganglionic) megacolon

Q43.2 **Other congenital functional disorders of colon**
Congenital dilatation of colon

Q43.3 **Congenital malformations of intestinal fixation**
Congenital omental, anomalous adhesions [bands]
Congenital peritoneal adhesions [bands]
Incomplete rotation of cecum and colon
Insufficient rotation of cecum and colon
Jackson's membrane
Malrotation of colon
Rotation failure of cecum and colon
Universal mesentery

Q43.4 **Duplication of intestine**

Q43.5 **Ectopic anus**

Q43.6 **Congenital fistula of rectum and anus**
EXCLUDES 1 *congenital fistula of anus with absence, atresia and stenosis (Q42.2)*
congenital fistula of rectum with absence, atresia and stenosis (Q42.0)
congenital rectovaginal fistula (Q52.2)
congenital urethrorectal fistula (Q64.73)
pilonidal fistula or sinus (L05.-)

Q43.7 **Persistent cloaca**
Cloaca NOS

Q43.8 **Other specified congenital malformations of intestine**
Congenital blind loop syndrome
Congenital diverticulitis, colon
Congenital diverticulum, intestine
Dolichocolon
Megaloappendix
Megaloduodenum
Microcolon
Transposition of appendix
Transposition of colon
Transposition of intestine
AHA: 2Q 2013, 31

Q43.9 **Congenital malformation of intestine, unspecified**

4 Q44 **Congenital malformations of gallbladder, bile ducts and liver**

Q44.0 **Agenesis, aplasia and hypoplasia of gallbladder**
Congenital absence of gallbladder

Q44.1 **Other congenital malformations of gallbladder**
Congenital malformation of gallbladder NOS
Intrahepatic gallbladder

Q44.2 **Atresia of bile ducts**

Q44.3 **Congenital stenosis and stricture of bile ducts**

Q44.4 **Choledochal cyst**

Q44.5 **Other congenital malformations of bile ducts**
Accessory hepatic duct
Biliary duct duplication
Congenital malformation of bile duct NOS
Cystic duct duplication

Q44.6 **Cystic disease of liver**
Fibrocystic disease of liver

Q44.7 **Other congenital malformations of liver**
Accessory liver
Alagille's syndrome
Congenital absence of liver
Congenital hepatomegaly
Congenital malformation of liver NOS

4 Q45 **Other congenital malformations of digestive system**
EXCLUDES 2 *congenital diaphragmatic hernia (Q79.0)*
congenital hiatus hernia (Q40.1)

Q45.0 **Agenesis, aplasia and hypoplasia of pancreas**
Congenital absence of pancreas

Q45.1 **Annular pancreas**

Q45.2 **Congenital pancreatic cyst**

Q45.3 **Other congenital malformations of pancreas and pancreatic duct**
Accessory pancreas
Congenital malformation of pancreas or pancreatic duct NOS
EXCLUDES 1 *congenital diabetes mellitus (E10.-)*
cystic fibrosis (E84.0-E84.9)
fibrocystic disease of pancreas (E84.-)
neonatal diabetes mellitus (P70.2)

Q45.8 **Other specified congenital malformations of digestive system**
Absence (complete) (partial) of alimentary tract NOS
Duplication of digestive system
Malposition, congenital of digestive system

Q45.9 **Congenital malformation of digestive system, unspecified**
Congenital anomaly of digestive system
Congenital deformity of digestive system

Congenital malformations of genital organs (Q50-Q56)

EXCLUDES 1 *androgen insensitivity syndrome (E34.5-)*
syndromes associated with anomalies in the number and form of chromosomes (Q90-Q99)

4 Q50 **Congenital malformations of ovaries, fallopian tubes and broad ligaments**

5 Q50.0 **Congenital absence of ovary**
EXCLUDES 1 *Turner's syndrome (Q96.-)*

Q50.01 **Congenital absence of ovary, unilateral** ♀

Q50.02 **Congenital absence of ovary, bilateral** ♀

Q50.1 **Developmental ovarian cyst** ♀

Q50.2 **Congenital torsion of ovary** ♀

5 Q50.3 **Other congenital malformations of ovary**

Q50.31 **Accessory ovary** ♀

Q50.32 Ovarian streak ♀
46, XX with streak gonads

Q50.39 Other congenital malformation of ovary ♀
Congenital malformation of ovary NOS

Q50.4 Embryonic cyst of fallopian tube ♀
Fimbrial cyst

Q50.5 Embryonic cyst of broad ligament ♀
Epoophoron cyst
Parovarian cyst

Q50.6 Other congenital malformations of fallopian tube and broad ligament ♀
Absence of fallopian tube and broad ligament
Accessory fallopian tube and broad ligament
Atresia of fallopian tube and broad ligament
Congenital malformation of fallopian tube or broad ligament NOS

4 Q51 Congenital malformations of uterus and cervix

Q51.0 Agenesis and aplasia of uterus ♀
Congenital absence of uterus

5 **Q51.1** Doubling of uterus with Doubling of cervix and vagina

Q51.10 Doubling of uterus with doubling of cervix and vagina without obstruction ♀
Doubling of uterus with doubling of cervix and vagina NOS

Q51.11 Doubling of uterus with doubling of cervix and vagina with obstruction ♀

▲ 5 **Q51.2** Other doubling of uterus
Doubling of uterus NOS
Septate uterus

● **Q51.20** Other doubling of uterus, unspecified ♀
Septate uterus, unspecified

● **Q51.21** Other complete doubling of uterus ♀
Complete septate uterus

● **Q51.22** Other partial doubling of uterus ♀
Partial septate uterus

● **Q51.28** Other doubling of uterus, other specified ♀
Septate uterus, other specified

Q51.3 Bicornate uterus ♀
Bicornate uterus, complete or partial

Bicornate uterus

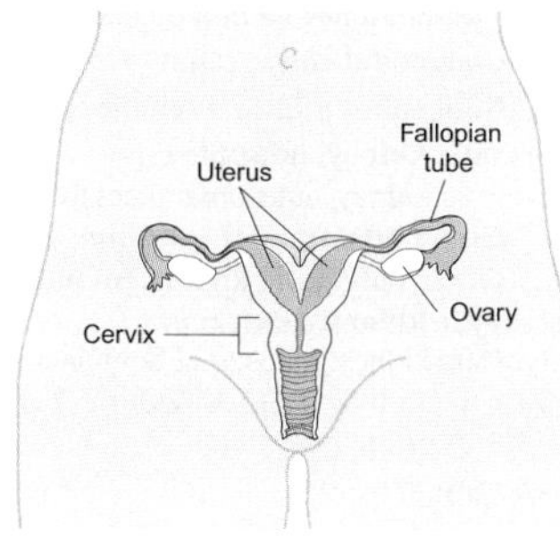

Q51.4 Unicornate uterus ♀
Unicornate uterus with or without a separate uterine horn
Uterus with only one functioning horn

Q51.5 Agenesis and aplasia of cervix ♀
Congenital absence of cervix

Q51.6 Embryonic cyst of cervix ♀

Q51.7 Congenital fistulae between uterus and digestive and urinary tracts ♀

5 **Q51.8** Other congenital malformations of uterus and cervix

6 **Q51.81** Other congenital malformations of uterus

Q51.810 Arcuate uterus ♀
Arcuatus uterus

Q51.811 Hypoplasia of uterus ♀

Q51.818 Other congenital malformations of uterus ♀
Müllerian anomaly of uterus NEC

6 **Q51.82** Other congenital malformations of cervix

Q51.820 Cervical duplication ♀

Q51.821 Hypoplasia of cervix ♀

Q51.828 Other congenital malformations of cervix ♀

Q51.9 Congenital malformation of uterus and cervix, unspecified ♀

4 Q52 Other congenital malformations of female genitalia

Q52.0 Congenital absence of vagina ♀
Vaginal agenesis, total or partial

5 **Q52.1** Doubling of vagina

EXCLUDES 1 *doubling of vagina with doubling of uterus and cervix (Q51.1-)*

Q52.10 Doubling of vagina, unspecified ♀
Septate vagina NOS

Q52.11 Transverse vaginal septum ♀

6 **Q52.12** Longitudinal vaginal septum

Q52.120 Longitudinal vaginal septum, nonobstructing ♀
AHA: 4Q 2016, 58

⊟ **Q52.121** Longitudinal vaginal septum, obstructing, right side ♀
AHA: 4Q 2016, 58

⊟ **Q52.122** Longitudinal vaginal septum, obstructing, left side ♀
AHA: 4Q 2016, 58

⊟ **Q52.123** Longitudinal vaginal septum, microperforate, right side ♀
AHA: 4Q 2016, 58

⊟ **Q52.124** Longitudinal vaginal septum, microperforate, left side ♀
AHA: 4Q 2016, 58

Q52.129 Other and unspecified longitudinal vaginal septum ♀
AHA: 4Q 2016, 58

Q52.2 Congenital rectovaginal fistula ♀

EXCLUDES 1 *cloaca (Q43.7)*

Q52.3 Imperforate hymen ♀

Q52.4 Other congenital malformations of vagina ♀
Canal of Nuck cyst, congenital
Congenital malformation of vagina NOS
Embryonic vaginal cyst
Gartner's duct cyst

Q52.5 Fusion of labia ♀

Q52.6 Congenital malformation of clitoris ♀

5 **Q52.7** Other and unspecified congenital malformations of vulva

Q52.70 Unspecified congenital malformations of vulva ♀
Congenital malformation of vulva NOS

Q52.71 Congenital absence of vulva ♀

Q52.79 Other congenital malformations of vulva ♀
Congenital cyst of vulva

Q52.8 Other specified congenital malformations of female genitalia ♀

Q52.9 Congenital malformation of female genitalia, unspecified ♀

4 Q53 Undescended and ectopic testicle

5 **Q53.0** Ectopic testis

Q53.00 Ectopic testis, unspecified ♂

Q53.01 Ectopic testis, unilateral ♂

Q53.02 Ectopic testes, bilateral ♂

5 **Q53.1** Undescended testicle, unilateral

Q53.10 Unspecified undescended testicle, unilateral ♂

6 **Q53.11** Abdominal testis, unilateral

Q53.111 Unilateral intraabdominal testis ♂
AHA: 4Q 2017, 17

Q53.112 Unilateral inguinal testis ♂
AHA: 4Q 2017, 17

Q53.12 Ectopic perineal testis, unilateral ♂

Q53.13 Unilateral high scrotal testis ♂

5 **Q53.2** Undescended testicle, bilateral

Q53.20 Undescended testicle, unspecified, bilateral ♂

6 **Q53.21** Abdominal testis, bilateral

Q53.211 Bilateral intraabdominal testes ♂
AHA: 4Q 2017, 17

Q53.212 Bilateral inguinal testes ♂
AHA: 4Q 2017, 17

Q53.22 Ectopic perineal testis, bilateral ♂

Q53.23 **Bilateral high scrotal testes** ♂
AHA: 4Q 2017, 17

Q53.9 **Undescended testicle, unspecified** ♂
Cryptorchism NOS

Q54 **Hypospadias**
EXCLUDES 1 *epispadias (Q64.0)*

CODING TIP Use category Q54 when hypospadias is still present. If the condition has been corrected, then code Z87.710, Personal history of hypospadias.

Q54.0 **Hypospadias, balanic** ♂
Hypospadias, coronal
Hypospadias, glandular

Q54.1 **Hypospadias, penile** ♂

Q54.2 **Hypospadias, penoscrotal** ♂

Q54.3 **Hypospadias, perineal** ♂

Q54.4 **Congenital chordee** ♂
Chordee without hypospadias

DEFINITION Abnormal downward or upward bowing of the penis, due to a congenital anomaly.

Q54.8 **Other hypospadias** ♂
Hypospadias with intersex state

Q54.9 **Hypospadias, unspecified** ♂

Q55 **Other congenital malformations of male genital organs**
EXCLUDES 1 *congenital hydrocele (P83.5)*
hypospadias (Q54.-)

Q55.0 **Absence and aplasia of testis** ♂
Monorchism

Q55.1 **Hypoplasia of testis and scrotum** ♂
Fusion of testes

Q55.2 **Other and unspecified congenital malformations of testis and scrotum**

Q55.20 **Unspecified congenital malformations of testis and scrotum** ♂
Congenital malformation of testis or scrotum NOS

Q55.21 **Polyorchism** ♂

Q55.22 **Retractile testis** ♂

Q55.23 **Scrotal transposition** ♂

Q55.29 **Other congenital malformations of testis and scrotum** ♂

Q55.3 **Atresia of vas deferens** ♂
Code first:
any associated cystic fibrosis (E84.-)

Q55.4 **Other congenital malformations of vas deferens, epididymis, seminal vesicles and prostate** ♂
Absence or aplasia of prostate
Absence or aplasia of spermatic cord
Congenital malformation of vas deferens, epididymis, seminal vesicles or prostate NOS

Q55.5 **Congenital absence and aplasia of penis** ♂

Q55.6 **Other congenital malformations of penis**

Q55.61 **Curvature of penis (lateral)** ♂

Q55.62 **Hypoplasia of penis** ♂
Micropenis

Q55.63 **Congenital torsion of penis** ♂
EXCLUDES 1 *acquired torsion of penis (N48.82)*

Q55.64 **Hidden penis** ♂
Buried penis
Concealed penis
EXCLUDES 1 *acquired buried penis (N48.83)*

Q55.69 **Other congenital malformation of penis** ♂
Congenital malformation of penis NOS

Q55.7 **Congenital vasocutaneous fistula** ♂

Q55.8 **Other specified congenital malformations of male genital organs** ♂

Q55.9 **Congenital malformation of male genital organ, unspecified** ♂
Congenital anomaly of male genital organ
Congenital deformity of male genital organ

Q56 **Indeterminate sex and pseudohermaphroditism**
EXCLUDES 1 *46,XX true hermaphrodite (Q99.1)*
androgen insensitivity syndrome (E34.5-)
chimera 46,XX/46,XY true hermaphrodite (Q99.0)
female pseudohermaphroditism with adrenocortical disorder (E25.-)
pseudohermaphroditism with specified chromosomal anomaly (Q96-Q99)
pure gonadal dysgenesis (Q99.1)

Q56.0 **Hermaphroditism, not elsewhere classified**
Ovotestis

Q56.1 **Male pseudohermaphroditism, not elsewhere classified** ♂
46, XY with streak gonads
Male pseudohermaphroditism NOS

Q56.2 **Female pseudohermaphroditism, not elsewhere classified** ♀
Female pseudohermaphroditism NOS

Q56.3 **Pseudohermaphroditism, unspecified**

Q56.4 **Indeterminate sex, unspecified**
Ambiguous genitalia

Congenital malformations of the urinary system (Q60-Q64)

Q60 **Renal agenesis and other reduction defects of kidney**
INCLUDES congenital absence of kidney
congenital atrophy of kidney
infantile atrophy of kidney

Q60.0 **Renal agenesis, unilateral**

Q60.1 **Renal agenesis, bilateral**

Q60.2 **Renal agenesis, unspecified**

Q60.3 **Renal hypoplasia, unilateral**

Q60.4 **Renal hypoplasia, bilateral**

Q60.5 **Renal hypoplasia, unspecified**

Q60.6 **Potter's syndrome**

Q61 **Cystic kidney disease**
EXCLUDES 1 *acquired cyst of kidney (N28.1)*
Potter's syndrome (Q60.6)

Q61.0 **Congenital renal cyst**

Q61.00 **Congenital renal cyst, unspecified**
Cyst of kidney NOS (congenital)

Q61.01 **Congenital single renal cyst**

Q61.02 **Congenital multiple renal cysts**

Q61.1 **Polycystic kidney, infantile type**
Polycystic kidney, autosomal recessive

Q61.11 **Cystic dilatation of collecting ducts**

Q61.19 **Other polycystic kidney, infantile type**

Q61.2 **Polycystic kidney, adult type**
Polycystic kidney, autosomal dominant

Q61.3 **Polycystic kidney, unspecified**
AHA: 3Q 2016, 22
AHA: 3Q 2016, 23

Q61.4 **Renal dysplasia**
Multicystic dysplastic kidney
Multicystic kidney (development)
Multicystic kidney disease
Multicystic renal dysplasia
EXCLUDES 1 *polycystic kidney disease (Q61.11-Q61.3)*

Q61.5 **Medullary cystic kidney**
Nephronopthisis
Sponge kidney NOS

Q61.8 **Other cystic kidney diseases**
Fibrocystic kidney
Fibrocystic renal degeneration or disease

Q61.9 **Cystic kidney disease, unspecified**
Meckel-Gruber syndrome

Q62 **Congenital obstructive defects of renal pelvis and congenital malformations of ureter**

Q62.0 **Congenital hydronephrosis**

Q62.1 **Congenital occlusion of ureter**
Atresia and stenosis of ureter

Q62.10 **Congenital occlusion of ureter, unspecified**

Q62.11 **Congenital occlusion of ureteropelvic junction**

Q62.12 **Congenital occlusion of ureterovesical orifice**

Q62.2 **Congenital megaureter**
Congenital dilatation of ureter
Q62.3 **Other obstructive defects of renal pelvis and ureter**
Q62.31 **Congenital ureterocele, orthotopic**
Q62.32 **Cecoureterocele**
Ectopic ureterocele
Q62.39 **Other obstructive defects of renal pelvis and ureter**
Ureteropelvic junction obstruction NOS
Q62.4 **Agenesis of ureter**
Congenital absence ureter
Q62.5 **Duplication of ureter**
Accessory ureter
Double ureter
Q62.6 **Malposition of ureter**
Q62.60 **Malposition of ureter, unspecified**
Q62.61 **Deviation of ureter**
Q62.62 **Displacement of ureter**
Q62.63 **Anomalous implantation of ureter**
Ectopia of ureter
Ectopic ureter
Q62.69 **Other malposition of ureter**
Q62.7 **Congenital vesico-uretero-renal reflux**
Q62.8 **Other congenital malformations of ureter**
Anomaly of ureter NOS

Q63 **Other congenital malformations of kidney**
EXCLUDES 1 *congenital nephrotic syndrome (N04.-)*
Q63.0 **Accessory kidney**
Q63.1 **Lobulated, fused and horseshoe kidney**
Q63.2 **Ectopic kidney**
Congenital displaced kidney
Malrotation of kidney
Q63.3 **Hyperplastic and giant kidney**
Compensatory hypertrophy of kidney
Q63.8 **Other specified congenital malformations of kidney**
Congenital renal calculi
Q63.9 **Congenital malformation of kidney, unspecified**

Q64 **Other congenital malformations of urinary system**
Q64.0 **Epispadias**
EXCLUDES 1 *hypospadias (Q54.-)*
DEFINITION A rare, congenital defect in which the urethra typically opens on the upper penile surface in boys, although, the urethral opening may also be positioned in the abdomen.
Q64.1 **Exstrophy of urinary bladder**
Q64.10 **Exstrophy of urinary bladder, unspecified**
Ectopia vesicae
Q64.11 **Supravesical fissure of urinary bladder**
Q64.12 **Cloacal exstrophy of urinary bladder**
Q64.19 **Other exstrophy of urinary bladder**
Extroversion of bladder
Q64.2 **Congenital posterior urethral valves**
Q64.3 **Other atresia and stenosis of urethra and bladder neck**
Q64.31 **Congenital bladder neck obstruction**
Congenital obstruction of vesicourethral orifice
Q64.32 **Congenital stricture of urethra**
Q64.33 **Congenital stricture of urinary meatus**
Q64.39 **Other atresia and stenosis of urethra and bladder neck**
Atresia and stenosis of urethra and bladder neck NOS
Q64.4 **Malformation of urachus**
Cyst of urachus
Patent urachus
Prolapse of urachus
Q64.5 **Congenital absence of bladder and urethra**
Q64.6 **Congenital diverticulum of bladder**
Q64.7 **Other and unspecified congenital malformations of bladder and urethra**
EXCLUDES 1 *congenital prolapse of bladder (mucosa) (Q79.4)*
Q64.70 **Unspecified congenital malformation of bladder and urethra**
Malformation of bladder or urethra NOS
Q64.71 **Congenital prolapse of urethra**
Q64.72 **Congenital prolapse of urinary meatus**
Q64.73 **Congenital urethrorectal fistula**
Q64.74 **Double urethra**
Q64.75 **Double urinary meatus**
Q64.79 **Other congenital malformations of bladder and urethra**
Q64.8 **Other specified congenital malformations of urinary system**
Q64.9 **Congenital malformation of urinary system, unspecified**
Congenital anomaly NOS of urinary system
Congenital deformity NOS of urinary system

Congenital malformations and deformations of the musculoskeletal system (Q65-Q79)

Q65 **Congenital deformities of hip**
EXCLUDES 1 *clicking hip (R29.4)*
Q65.0 **Congenital dislocation of hip, unilateral**
Q65.00 **Congenital dislocation of unspecified hip, unilateral**
Q65.01 **Congenital dislocation of right hip, unilateral**
Q65.02 **Congenital dislocation of left hip, unilateral**
Q65.1 **Congenital dislocation of hip, bilateral**
Q65.2 **Congenital dislocation of hip, unspecified**
Q65.3 **Congenital partial dislocation of hip, unilateral**
Q65.30 **Congenital partial dislocation of unspecified hip, unilateral**
Q65.31 **Congenital partial dislocation of right hip, unilateral**
Q65.32 **Congenital partial dislocation of left hip, unilateral**
Q65.4 **Congenital partial dislocation of hip, bilateral**
Q65.5 **Congenital partial dislocation of hip, unspecified**
Q65.6 **Congenital unstable hip**
Congenital dislocatable hip
Q65.8 **Other congenital deformities of hip**
Q65.81 **Congenital coxa valga**
Q65.82 **Congenital coxa vara**
Q65.89 **Other specified congenital deformities of hip**
Anteversion of femoral neck
Congenital acetabular dysplasia
Q65.9 **Congenital deformity of hip, unspecified**

Q66 **Congenital deformities of feet**
EXCLUDES 1 *reduction defects of feet (Q72.-)*
valgus deformities (acquired) (M21.0-)
varus deformities (acquired) (M21.1-)
Q66.0 **Congenital talipes equinovarus**

Congenital talipes equinovarus

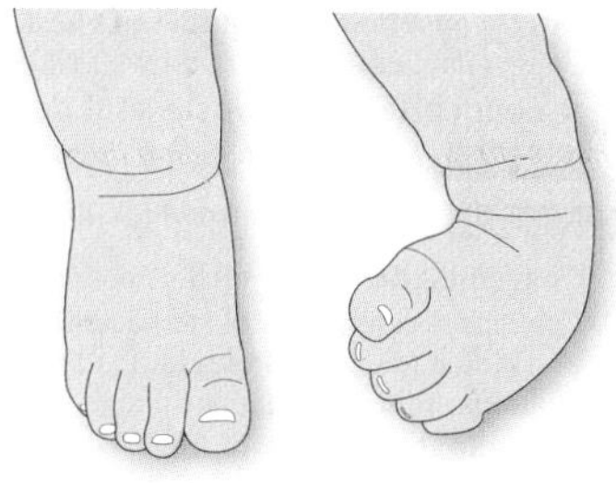

Q66.1 **Congenital talipes calcaneovarus**
Q66.2 **Congenital metatarsus (primus) varus**
Q66.21 **Congenital metatarsus primus varus**
AHA: 4Q 2016, 59
Q66.22 **Congenital metatarsus adductus**
Congenital metatarsus varus
AHA: 4Q 2016, 59
Q66.3 **Other congenital varus deformities of feet**
Hallux varus, congenital
Q66.4 **Congenital talipes calcaneovalgus**
Q66.5 **Congenital pes planus**
Congenital flat foot
Congenital rigid flat foot
Congenital spastic (everted) flat foot
EXCLUDES 1 *pes planus, acquired (M21.4)*
Q66.50 **Congenital pes planus, unspecified foot**
Q66.51 **Congenital pes planus, right foot**

Q66.52 **Congenital pes planus, left foot**

Q66.6 **Other congenital valgus deformities of feet**
Congenital metatarsus valgus

Q66.7 **Congenital pes cavus**

Q66.8 **Other congenital deformities of feet**

Q66.80 **Congenital vertical talus deformity, unspecified foot**

Q66.81 **Congenital vertical talus deformity, right foot**

Q66.82 **Congenital vertical talus deformity, left foot**

Q66.89 **Other specified congenital deformities of feet**
Congenital asymmetric talipes
Congenital clubfoot NOS
Congenital talipes NOS
Congenital tarsal coalition
Hammer toe, congenital

Q66.9 **Congenital deformity of feet, unspecified**

Q67 Congenital musculoskeletal deformities of head, face, spine and chest

EXCLUDES 1 *congenital malformation syndromes classified to Q87.-*
Potter's syndrome (Q60.6)

Q67.0 **Congenital facial asymmetry**

Q67.1 **Congenital compression facies**

Q67.2 **Dolichocephaly**

Q67.3 **Plagiocephaly**

Q67.4 **Other congenital deformities of skull, face and jaw**
Congenital depressions in skull
Congenital hemifacial atrophy or hypertrophy
Deviation of nasal septum, congenital
Squashed or bent nose, congenital

EXCLUDES 1 *dentofacial anomalies [including malocclusion] (M26.-)*
syphilitic saddle nose (A50.5)

Q67.5 **Congenital deformity of spine**
Congenital postural scoliosis
Congenital scoliosis NOS

EXCLUDES 1 *infantile idiopathic scoliosis (M41.0)*
scoliosis due to congenital bony malformation (Q76.3)

AHA: 4Q 2014, 26

Q67.6 **Pectus excavatum**
Congenital funnel chest

Q67.7 **Pectus carinatum**
Congenital pigeon chest

DEFINITION A protrusion deformity of the chest wall in which the sternum and ribs are prominent, due to obstruction of infantile respiration or to rickets.

Q67.8 **Other congenital deformities of chest**
Congenital deformity of chest wall NOS

Q68 Other congenital musculoskeletal deformities

EXCLUDES 1 *reduction defects of limb (s) (Q71-Q73)*

EXCLUDES 2 *congenital myotonic chondrodystrophy (G71.13)*

Q68.0 **Congenital deformity of sternocleidomastoid muscle**
Congenital contracture of sternocleidomastoid (muscle)
Congenital (sternomastoid) torticollis
Sternomastoid tumor (congenital)

Q68.1 **Congenital deformity of finger(s) and hand**
Congenital clubfinger
Spade-like hand (congenital)

Q68.2 **Congenital deformity of knee**
Congenital dislocation of knee
Congenital genu recurvatum

Q68.3 **Congenital bowing of femur**

EXCLUDES 1 *anteversion of femur (neck) (Q65.89)*

Q68.4 **Congenital bowing of tibia and fibula**

Q68.5 **Congenital bowing of long bones of leg, unspecified**

Q68.6 **Discoid meniscus**

Q68.8 **Other specified congenital musculoskeletal deformities**
Congenital deformity of clavicle
Congenital deformity of elbow
Congenital deformity of forearm
Congenital deformity of scapula
Congenital deformity of wrist
Congenital dislocation of elbow
Congenital dislocation of shoulder
Congenital dislocation of wrist

Q69 Polydactyly

Q69.0 **Accessory finger(s)**

Q69.1 **Accessory thumb(s)**

Q69.2 **Accessory toe(s)**
Accessory hallux

Q69.9 **Polydactyly, unspecified**
Supernumerary digit(s) NOS

DEFINITION An extra number of digits on a hand or foot.

Q70 Syndactyly

Q70.0 **Fused fingers**
Complex syndactyly of fingers with synostosis

Q70.00 **Fused fingers, unspecified hand**

Q70.01 **Fused fingers, right hand**

Q70.02 **Fused fingers, left hand**

Q70.03 **Fused fingers, bilateral**

Q70.1 **Webbed fingers**
Simple syndactyly of fingers without synostosis

Q70.10 **Webbed fingers, unspecified hand**

Q70.11 **Webbed fingers, right hand**

Q70.12 **Webbed fingers, left hand**

Q70.13 **Webbed fingers, bilateral**

Q70.2 **Fused toes**
Complex syndactyly of toes with synostosis

Q70.20 **Fused toes, unspecified foot**

Q70.21 **Fused toes, right foot**

Q70.22 **Fused toes, left foot**

Q70.23 **Fused toes, bilateral**

Q70.3 **Webbed toes**
Simple syndactyly of toes without synostosis

Q70.30 **Webbed toes, unspecified foot**

Q70.31 **Webbed toes, right foot**

Q70.32 **Webbed toes, left foot**

Q70.33 **Webbed toes, bilateral**

Q70.4 **Polysyndactyly, unspecified**

EXCLUDES 1 *specified syndactyly of hand and feet - code to specified conditions (Q70.0- -Q70.3-)*

Q70.9 **Syndactyly, unspecified**
Symphalangy NOS

DEFINITION Partial or total webbing connecting two or more fingers or toes; may involve skin/soft tissue only or include fusion of bone.

Q71 Reduction defects of upper limb

Q71.0 **Congenital complete absence of upper limb**

Q71.00 **Congenital complete absence of unspecified upper limb**

Q71.01 **Congenital complete absence of right upper limb**

Q71.02 **Congenital complete absence of left upper limb**

Q71.03 **Congenital complete absence of upper limb, bilateral**

Q71.1 **Congenital absence of upper arm and forearm with hand present**

Q71.10 **Congenital absence of unspecified upper arm and forearm with hand present**

Q71.11 **Congenital absence of right upper arm and forearm with hand present**

Q71.12 **Congenital absence of left upper arm and forearm with hand present**

Q71.13 **Congenital absence of upper arm and forearm with hand present, bilateral**

Q71.2 **Congenital absence of both forearm and hand**

Q71.20 **Congenital absence of both forearm and hand, unspecified upper limb**

Q71.21 **Congenital absence of both forearm and hand, right upper limb**

Q71.22 **Congenital absence of both forearm and hand, left upper limb**

Q71.23 **Congenital absence of both forearm and hand, bilateral**

Q71.3 **Congenital absence of hand and finger**

Q71.30 **Congenital absence of unspecified hand and finger**

Q71.31 **Congenital absence of right hand and finger**

Q71.32 **Congenital absence of left hand and finger**

Q71.33 **Congenital absence of hand and finger, bilateral**

Q71.4 Longitudinal reduction defect of radius
Clubhand (congenital)
Radial clubhand
Q71.40 Longitudinal reduction defect of unspecified radius
Q71.41 Longitudinal reduction defect of right radius
Q71.42 Longitudinal reduction defect of left radius
Q71.43 Longitudinal reduction defect of radius, bilateral
Q71.5 Longitudinal reduction defect of ulna
Q71.50 Longitudinal reduction defect of unspecified ulna
Q71.51 Longitudinal reduction defect of right ulna
Q71.52 Longitudinal reduction defect of left ulna
Q71.53 Longitudinal reduction defect of ulna, bilateral
Q71.6 Lobster-claw hand
Q71.60 Lobster-claw hand, unspecified hand
Q71.61 Lobster-claw right hand
Q71.62 Lobster-claw left hand
Q71.63 Lobster-claw hand, bilateral
Q71.8 Other reduction defects of upper limb
Q71.81 Congenital shortening of upper limb
Q71.811 Congenital shortening of right upper limb
Q71.812 Congenital shortening of left upper limb
Q71.813 Congenital shortening of upper limb, bilateral
Q71.819 Congenital shortening of unspecified upper limb
Q71.89 Other reduction defects of upper limb
Q71.891 Other reduction defects of right upper limb
Q71.892 Other reduction defects of left upper limb
Q71.893 Other reduction defects of upper limb, bilateral
Q71.899 Other reduction defects of unspecified upper limb
Q71.9 Unspecified reduction defect of upper limb
Q71.90 Unspecified reduction defect of unspecified upper limb
Q71.91 Unspecified reduction defect of right upper limb
Q71.92 Unspecified reduction defect of left upper limb
Q71.93 Unspecified reduction defect of upper limb, bilateral

Q72 Reduction defects of lower limb

Q72.0 Congenital complete absence of lower limb
Q72.00 Congenital complete absence of unspecified lower limb
Q72.01 Congenital complete absence of right lower limb
Q72.02 Congenital complete absence of left lower limb
Q72.03 Congenital complete absence of lower limb, bilateral
Q72.1 Congenital absence of thigh and lower leg with foot present
Q72.10 Congenital absence of unspecified thigh and lower leg with foot present
Q72.11 Congenital absence of right thigh and lower leg with foot present
Q72.12 Congenital absence of left thigh and lower leg with foot present
Q72.13 Congenital absence of thigh and lower leg with foot present, bilateral
Q72.2 Congenital absence of both lower leg and foot
Q72.20 Congenital absence of both lower leg and foot, unspecified lower limb
Q72.21 Congenital absence of both lower leg and foot, right lower limb
Q72.22 Congenital absence of both lower leg and foot, left lower limb
Q72.23 Congenital absence of both lower leg and foot, bilateral
Q72.3 Congenital absence of foot and toe(s)
Q72.30 Congenital absence of unspecified foot and toe(s)
Q72.31 Congenital absence of right foot and toe(s)
Q72.32 Congenital absence of left foot and toe(s)
Q72.33 Congenital absence of foot and toe(s), bilateral
Q72.4 Longitudinal reduction defect of femur
Proximal femoral focal deficiency
Q72.40 Longitudinal reduction defect of unspecified femur
Q72.41 Longitudinal reduction defect of right femur
Q72.42 Longitudinal reduction defect of left femur
Q72.43 Longitudinal reduction defect of femur, bilateral
Q72.5 Longitudinal reduction defect of tibia
Q72.50 Longitudinal reduction defect of unspecified tibia
Q72.51 Longitudinal reduction defect of right tibia
Q72.52 Longitudinal reduction defect of left tibia
Q72.53 Longitudinal reduction defect of tibia, bilateral
Q72.6 Longitudinal reduction defect of fibula
Q72.60 Longitudinal reduction defect of unspecified fibula
Q72.61 Longitudinal reduction defect of right fibula
Q72.62 Longitudinal reduction defect of left fibula
Q72.63 Longitudinal reduction defect of fibula, bilateral
Q72.7 Split foot
Q72.70 Split foot, unspecified lower limb
Q72.71 Split foot, right lower limb
Q72.72 Split foot, left lower limb
Q72.73 Split foot, bilateral
Q72.8 Other reduction defects of lower limb
Q72.81 Congenital shortening of lower limb
Q72.811 Congenital shortening of right lower limb
Q72.812 Congenital shortening of left lower limb
Q72.813 Congenital shortening of lower limb, bilateral
Q72.819 Congenital shortening of unspecified lower limb
Q72.89 Other reduction defects of lower limb
Q72.891 Other reduction defects of right lower limb
Q72.892 Other reduction defects of left lower limb
Q72.893 Other reduction defects of lower limb, bilateral
Q72.899 Other reduction defects of unspecified lower limb
Q72.9 Unspecified reduction defect of lower limb
Q72.90 Unspecified reduction defect of unspecified lower limb
Q72.91 Unspecified reduction defect of right lower limb
Q72.92 Unspecified reduction defect of left lower limb
Q72.93 Unspecified reduction defect of lower limb, bilateral

Q73 Reduction defects of unspecified limb

Q73.0 Congenital absence of unspecified limb(s)
Amelia NOS
Q73.1 Phocomelia, unspecified limb(s)
Phocomelia NOS
Q73.8 Other reduction defects of unspecified limb(s)
Longitudinal reduction deformity of unspecified limb(s)
Ectromelia of limb NOS
Hemimelia of limb NOS
Reduction defect of limb NOS

Q74 Other congenital malformations of limb(s)

EXCLUDES 1 *polydactyly (Q69.-)*
reduction defect of limb (Q71-Q73)
syndactyly (Q70.-)

Q74.0 Other congenital malformations of upper limb(s), including shoulder girdle
Accessory carpal bones
Cleidocranial dysostosis
Congenital pseudarthrosis of clavicle
Macrodactylia (fingers)
Madelung's deformity
Radioulnar synostosis
Sprengel's deformity
Triphalangeal thumb
Q74.1 Congenital malformation of knee
Congenital absence of patella
Congenital dislocation of patella
Congenital genu valgum
Congenital genu varum
Rudimentary patella
EXCLUDES 1 *congenital dislocation of knee (Q68.2)*
congenital genu recurvatum (Q68.2)
nail patella syndrome (Q87.2)
Q74.2 Other congenital malformations of lower limb(s), including pelvic girdle
Congenital fusion of sacroiliac joint
Congenital malformation of ankle joint
Congenital malformation of sacroiliac joint
EXCLUDES 1 *anteversion of femur (neck) (Q65.89)*
Q74.3 Arthrogryposis multiplex congenita
Q74.8 Other specified congenital malformations of limb(s)

Q74.9 Unspecified congenital malformation of limb(s)
Congenital anomaly of limb(s) NOS

4 Q75 Other congenital malformations of skull and face bones

EXCLUDES 1 *congenital malformation of face NOS (Q18.-)*
congenital malformation syndromes classified to Q87.-
dentofacial anomalies [including malocclusion] (M26.-)
musculoskeletal deformities of head and face (Q67.0-Q67.4)
skull defects associated with congenital anomalies of brain such as:
anencephaly (Q00.0)
encephalocele (Q01.-)
hydrocephalus (Q03.-)
microcephaly (Q02)

Q75.0 Craniosynostosis
Acrocephaly
Imperfect fusion of skull
Oxycephaly
Trigonocephaly

Q75.1 Craniofacial dysostosis
Crouzon's disease

Q75.2 Hypertelorism

Q75.3 Macrocephaly

Q75.4 Mandibulofacial dysostosis
Franceschetti syndrome
Treacher Collins syndrome

Q75.5 Oculomandibular dysostosis

Q75.8 Other specified congenital malformations of skull and face bones
Absence of skull bone, congenital
Congenital deformity of forehead
Platybasia

Q75.9 Congenital malformation of skull and face bones, unspecified
Congenital anomaly of face bones NOS
Congenital anomaly of skull NOS

4 Q76 Congenital malformations of spine and bony thorax

EXCLUDES 1 *congenital musculoskeletal deformities of spine and chest (Q67.5-Q67.8)*

Q76.0 Spina bifida occulta
EXCLUDES 1 *meningocele (spinal) (Q05.-)*
spina bifida (aperta) (cystica) (Q05.-)

Q76.1 Klippel-Feil syndrome
Cervical fusion syndrome

Q76.2 Congenital spondylolisthesis
Congenital spondylolysis
EXCLUDES 1 *spondylolisthesis (acquired) (M43.1-)*
spondylolysis (acquired) (M43.0-)

Congenital spondylolisthesis

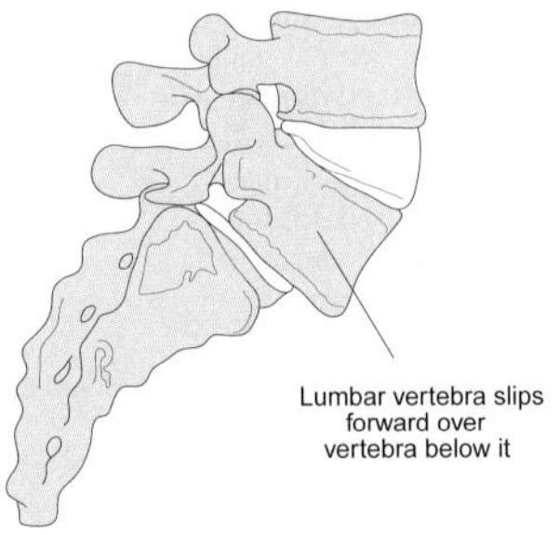
Lumbar vertebra slips forward over vertebra below it

Q76.3 Congenital scoliosis due to congenital bony malformation
Hemivertebra fusion or failure of segmentation with scoliosis

5 Q76.4 Other congenital malformations of spine, not associated with scoliosis

6 Q76.41 Congenital kyphosis

Q76.411 Congenital kyphosis, occipito-atlanto-axial region

Q76.412 Congenital kyphosis, cervical region

Q76.413 Congenital kyphosis, cervicothoracic region

Q76.414 Congenital kyphosis, thoracic region

Q76.415 Congenital kyphosis, thoracolumbar region

Q76.419 Congenital kyphosis, unspecified region

6 Q76.42 Congenital lordosis

Q76.425 Congenital lordosis, thoracolumbar region

Q76.426 Congenital lordosis, lumbar region

Q76.427 Congenital lordosis, lumbosacral region

Q76.428 Congenital lordosis, sacral and sacrococcygeal region

Q76.429 Congenital lordosis, unspecified region

Q76.49 Other congenital malformations of spine, not associated with scoliosis
Congenital absence of vertebra NOS
Congenital fusion of spine NOS
Congenital malformation of lumbosacral (joint) (region) NOS
Congenital malformation of spine NOS
Hemivertebra NOS
Malformation of spine NOS
Platyspondylisis NOS
Supernumerary vertebra NOS

Q76.5 Cervical rib
Supernumerary rib in cervical region

Q76.6 Other congenital malformations of ribs
Accessory rib
Congenital absence of rib
Congenital fusion of ribs
Congenital malformation of ribs NOS
EXCLUDES 1 *short rib syndrome (Q77.2)*

Q76.7 Congenital malformation of sternum
Congenital absence of sternum
Sternum bifidum

Q76.8 Other congenital malformations of bony thorax

Q76.9 Congenital malformation of bony thorax, unspecified

4 Q77 Osteochondrodysplasia with defects of growth of tubular bones and spine

EXCLUDES 1 *mucopolysaccharidosis (E76.0-E76.3)*

EXCLUDES 2 *congenital myotonic chondrodystrophy (G71.13)*

Q77.0 Achondrogenesis
Hypochondrogenesis

Q77.1 Thanatophoric short stature

Q77.2 Short rib syndrome
Asphyxiating thoracic dysplasia [Jeune]

Q77.3 Chondrodysplasia punctata
EXCLUDES 1 *Rhizomelic chondrodysplasia punctata (E71.43)*

Q77.4 Achondroplasia
Hypochondroplasia
Osteosclerosis congenita

Q77.5 Diastrophic dysplasia

Q77.6 Chondroectodermal dysplasia
Ellis-van Creveld syndrome

Q77.7 Spondyloepiphyseal dysplasia

Q77.8 Other osteochondrodysplasia with defects of growth of tubular bones and spine

Q77.9 Osteochondrodysplasia with defects of growth of tubular bones and spine, unspecified

4 Q78 Other osteochondrodysplasias

EXCLUDES 2 *congenital myotonic chondrodystrophy (G71.13)*

Q78.0 Osteogenesis imperfecta
Fragilitas ossium
Osteopsathyrosis

Q78.1 Polyostotic fibrous dysplasia
Albright(-McCune)(-Sternberg) syndrome

DEFINITION Genetic bone disorder causing multiple areas of normal bone to be replaced by bands of abnormal fibrous tissue, causing pain, fractures, and deformity.

Q78.2 Osteopetrosis
Albers-Schönberg syndrome
Osteosclerosis NOS

Q78.3 Progressive diaphyseal dysplasia
Camurati-Engelmann syndrome

Q78.4 Enchondromatosis
Maffucci's syndrome
Ollier's disease

Q78.5 Metaphyseal dysplasia
Pyle's syndrome

Q78.6 **Multiple congenital exostoses**
Diaphyseal aclasis
Q78.8 **Other specified osteochondrodysplasias**
Osteopoikilosis
Q78.9 **Osteochondrodysplasia, unspecified**
Chondrodystrophy NOS
Osteodystrophy NOS

Q79 Congenital malformations of musculoskeletal system, not elsewhere classified
EXCLUDES 2 *congenital (sternomastoid) torticollis (Q68.0)*

Q79.0 **Congenital diaphragmatic hernia**
EXCLUDES 1 *congenital hiatus hernia (Q40.1)*
Q79.1 **Other congenital malformations of diaphragm**
Absence of diaphragm
Congenital malformation of diaphragm NOS
Eventration of diaphragm
Q79.2 **Exomphalos**
Omphalocele
EXCLUDES 1 *umbilical hernia (K42.-)*
Q79.3 **Gastroschisis**
Q79.4 **Prune belly syndrome**
Congenital prolapse of bladder mucosa
Eagle-Barrett syndrome
Q79.5 **Other congenital malformations of abdominal wall**
EXCLUDES 1 *umbilical hernia (K42.-)*
Q79.51 **Congenital hernia of bladder**
Q79.59 **Other congenital malformations of abdominal wall**
Q79.6 **Ehlers-Danlos syndrome**
Q79.8 **Other congenital malformations of musculoskeletal system**
Absence of muscle
Absence of tendon
Accessory muscle
Amyotrophia congenita
Congenital constricting bands
Congenital shortening of tendon
Poland syndrome
Q79.9 **Congenital malformation of musculoskeletal system, unspecified**
Congenital anomaly of musculoskeletal system NOS
Congenital deformity of musculoskeletal system NOS

Other congenital malformations (Q80-Q89)

Q80 Congenital ichthyosis
EXCLUDES 1 *Refsum's disease (G60.1)*

Q80.0 **Ichthyosis vulgaris**
Q80.1 **X-linked ichthyosis**
Q80.2 **Lamellar ichthyosis**
Collodion baby
Q80.3 **Congenital bullous ichthyosiform erythroderma**
Q80.4 **Harlequin fetus**
Q80.8 **Other congenital ichthyosis**
Q80.9 **Congenital ichthyosis, unspecified**

Q81 Epidermolysis bullosa

Q81.0 **Epidermolysis bullosa simplex**
EXCLUDES 1 *Cockayne's syndrome (Q87.1)*
Q81.1 **Epidermolysis bullosa letalis**
Herlitz' syndrome
Q81.2 **Epidermolysis bullosa dystrophica**
Q81.8 **Other epidermolysis bullosa**
Q81.9 **Epidermolysis bullosa, unspecified**

Q82 Other congenital malformations of skin
EXCLUDES 1 *acrodermatitis enteropathica (E83.2)*
congenital erythropoietic porphyria (E80.0)
pilonidal cyst or sinus (L05.-)
Sturge-Weber (-Dimitri) syndrome (Q85.8)

Q82.0 **Hereditary lymphedema**
Q82.1 **Xeroderma pigmentosum**
Q82.2 **Congenital cutaneous mastocytosis**
Congenital diffuse cutaneous mastocytosis
Congenital maculopapular cutaneous mastocytosis
Congenital urticaria pigmentosa
EXCLUDES 1 *cutaneous mastocytosis NOS (D47.01)*
diffuse cutaneous mastocytosis (with onset after newborn period) (D47.01)
malignant mastocytosis (C96.2-)
systemic mastocytosis (D47.02)
urticaria pigmentosa (non-congenital) (with onset after newborn period) (D47.01)
AHA: 4Q 2017, 4
Q82.3 **Incontinentia pigmenti**
Q82.4 **Ectodermal dysplasia (anhidrotic)**
EXCLUDES 1 *Ellis-van Creveld syndrome (Q77.6)*
Q82.5 **Congenital non-neoplastic nevus**
Birthmark NOS
Flammeus Nevus
Portwine Nevus
Sanguineous Nevus
Strawberry Nevus
Vascular Nevus NOS
Verrucous Nevus
EXCLUDES 2 *Café au lait spots (L81.3)*
lentigo (L81.4)
nevus NOS (D22.-)
araneus nevus (I78.1)
melanocytic nevus (D22.-)
pigmented nevus (D22.-)
spider nevus (I78.1)
stellar nevus (I78.1)
Q82.6 **Congenital sacral dimple**
Parasacral dimple
EXCLUDES 2 *pilonidal cyst with abscess (L05.01)*
pilonidal cyst without abscess (L05.91)
AHA: 4Q 2016, 60
Q82.8 **Other specified congenital malformations of skin**
Abnormal palmar creases
Accessory skin tags
Benign familial pemphigus [Hailey-Hailey]
Congenital poikiloderma
Cutis laxa (hyperelastica)
Dermatoglyphic anomalies
Inherited keratosis palmaris et plantaris
Keratosis follicularis [Darier-White]
EXCLUDES 1 *Ehlers-Danlos syndrome (Q79.6)*
AHA: 1Q 2016, 17
Q82.9 **Congenital malformation of skin, unspecified**

Q83 Congenital malformations of breast
EXCLUDES 2 *absence of pectoral muscle (Q79.8)*
hypoplasia of breast (N64.82)
micromastia (N64.82)

Q83.0 **Congenital absence of breast with absent nipple**
Q83.1 **Accessory breast**
Supernumerary breast
Q83.2 **Absent nipple**
Q83.3 **Accessory nipple**
Supernumerary nipple
Q83.8 **Other congenital malformations of breast**
Q83.9 **Congenital malformation of breast, unspecified**

Q84 Other congenital malformations of integument

Q84.0 **Congenital alopecia**
Congenital atrichosis
Q84.1 **Congenital morphological disturbances of hair, not elsewhere classified**
Beaded hair
Monilethrix
Pili annulati
EXCLUDES 1 *Menkes' kinky hair syndrome (E83.0)*
Q84.2 **Other congenital malformations of hair**
Congenital hypertrichosis
Congenital malformation of hair NOS
Persistent lanugo
Q84.3 **Anonychia**
EXCLUDES 1 *nail patella syndrome (Q87.2)*
Q84.4 **Congenital leukonychia**

Q84.5 Enlarged and hypertrophic nails
Congenital onychauxis
Pachyonychia

Q84.6 Other congenital malformations of nails
Congenital clubnail
Congenital koilonychia
Congenital malformation of nail NOS

Q84.8 Other specified congenital malformations of integument
Aplasia cutis congenita

Q84.9 Congenital malformation of integument, unspecified
Congenital anomaly of integument NOS
Congenital deformity of integument NOS

Q85 Phakomatoses, not elsewhere classified

EXCLUDES 1 *ataxia telangiectasia [Louis-Bar] (G11.3)*
familial dysautonomia [Riley-Day] (G90.1)

Q85.0 Neurofibromatosis (nonmalignant)

Q85.00 Neurofibromatosis, unspecified HCC

Q85.01 Neurofibromatosis, type 1 HCC
Von Recklinghausen disease

Q85.02 Neurofibromatosis, type 2 HCC
Acoustic neurofibromatosis

Q85.03 Schwannomatosis HCC

DEFINITION A rare type of neurofibromatosis causing tumors on nerve sheaths of spinal, peripheral, and cranial nerves - except the eighth (vestibular) cranial nerve.

Q85.09 Other neurofibromatosis HCC

Q85.1 Tuberous sclerosis HCC
Bourneville's disease
Epiloia

Q85.8 Other phakomatoses, not elsewhere classified HCC
Peutz-Jeghers Syndrome
Sturge-Weber(-Dimitri) syndrome
von Hippel-Lindau syndrome
EXCLUDES 1 *Meckel-Gruber syndrome (Q61.9)*

Q85.9 Phakomatosis, unspecified HCC
Hamartosis NOS

Q86 Congenital malformation syndromes due to known exogenous causes, not elsewhere classified

EXCLUDES 2 *iodine-deficiency-related hypothyroidism (E00-E02)*
nonteratogenic effects of substances transmitted via placenta or breast milk (P04.-)

Q86.0 Fetal alcohol syndrome (dysmorphic)

Q86.1 Fetal hydantoin syndrome
Meadow's syndrome

Q86.2 Dysmorphism due to warfarin

Q86.8 Other congenital malformation syndromes due to known exogenous causes

Q87 Other specified congenital malformation syndromes affecting multiple systems

Use additional code(s) to identify all associated manifestations

Q87.0 Congenital malformation syndromes predominantly affecting facial appearance
Acrocephalopolysyndactyly
Acrocephalosyndactyly [Apert]
Cryptophthalmos syndrome
Cyclopia
Goldenhar syndrome
Moebius syndrome
Oro-facial-digital syndrome
Robin syndrome
Whistling face

Q87.1 Congenital malformation syndromes predominantly associated with short stature
Aarskog syndrome
Cockayne syndrome
De Lange syndrome
Dubowitz syndrome
Noonan syndrome
Prader-Willi syndrome
Robinow-Silverman-Smith syndrome
Russell-Silver syndrome
Seckel syndrome
EXCLUDES 1 *Ellis-van Creveld syndrome (Q77.6)*
Smith-Lemli-Opitz syndrome (E78.72)

Q87.2 Congenital malformation syndromes predominantly involving limbs
Holt-Oram syndrome
Klippel-Trenaunay-Weber syndrome
Nail patella syndrome
Rubinstein-Taybi syndrome
Sirenomelia syndrome
Thrombocytopenia with absent radius [TAR] syndrome
VATER syndrome

Q87.3 Congenital malformation syndromes involving early overgrowth
Beckwith-Wiedemann syndrome
Sotos syndrome
Weaver syndrome

Q87.4 Marfan's syndrome

Q87.40 Marfan's syndrome, unspecified

Q87.41 Marfan's syndrome with cardiovascular manifestations

Q87.410 Marfan's syndrome with aortic dilation

Q87.418 Marfan's syndrome with other cardiovascular manifestations

Q87.42 Marfan's syndrome with ocular manifestations

Q87.43 Marfan's syndrome with skeletal manifestation

Q87.5 Other congenital malformation syndromes with other skeletal changes

Q87.8 Other specified congenital malformation syndromes, not elsewhere classified
EXCLUDES 1 *Zellweger syndrome (E71.510)*

Q87.81 Alport syndrome
Use additional code to identify stage of chronic kidney disease (N18.1-N18.6)

Q87.82 Arterial tortuosity syndrome
AHA: 4Q 2016, 60

Q87.89 Other specified congenital malformation syndromes, not elsewhere classified
Laurence-Moon (-Bardet)-Biedl syndrome

Q89 Other congenital malformations, not elsewhere classified

Q89.0 Congenital absence and malformations of spleen
EXCLUDES 1 *isomerism of atrial appendages (with asplenia or polysplenia) (Q20.6)*

Q89.01 Asplenia (congenital)

Q89.09 Congenital malformations of spleen
Congenital splenomegaly

Q89.1 Congenital malformations of adrenal gland
EXCLUDES 1 *adrenogenital disorders (E25.-)*
congenital adrenal hyperplasia (E25.0)

Q89.2 Congenital malformations of other endocrine glands
Congenital malformation of parathyroid or thyroid gland
Persistent thyroglossal duct
Thyroglossal cyst
EXCLUDES 1 *congenital goiter (E03.0)*
congenital hypothyroidism (E03.1)

Q89.3 Situs inversus
Dextrocardia with situs inversus
Mirror-image atrial arrangement with situs inversus
Situs inversus or transversus abdominalis
Situs inversus or transversus thoracis
Transposition of abdominal viscera
Transposition of thoracic viscera
EXCLUDES 1 *dextrocardia NOS (Q24.0)*

DEFINITION Congenital disorder in which the position of all major organs in the chest and abdomen are reversed horizontally.

Q89.4 Conjoined twins
Craniopagus
Dicephaly
Pygopagus
Thoracopagus

Q89.7 Multiple congenital malformations, not elsewhere classified
Multiple congenital anomalies NOS
Multiple congenital deformities NOS
EXCLUDES 1 *congenital malformation syndromes affecting multiple systems (Q87.-)*

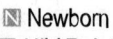

Q89.8 Other specified congenital malformations
Use additional code(s) to identify all associated manifestations

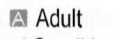

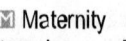

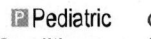

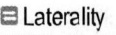

Q89.9 **Congenital malformation, unspecified**
Congenital anomaly NOS
Congenital deformity NOS

Chromosomal abnormalities, not elsewhere classified (Q90-Q99)

EXCLUDES 2 *mitochondrial metabolic disorders (E88.4-)*

Q90 Down syndrome
Use additional code(s) to identify any associated physical conditions and degree of intellectual disabilities (F70-F79)
Q90.0 **Trisomy 21, nonmosaicism (meiotic nondisjunction)**
Q90.1 **Trisomy 21, mosaicism (mitotic nondisjunction)**
Q90.2 **Trisomy 21, translocation**
Q90.9 **Down syndrome, unspecified**
Trisomy 21 NOS

Q91 Trisomy 18 and Trisomy 13
Q91.0 **Trisomy 18, nonmosaicism (meiotic nondisjunction)**
Q91.1 **Trisomy 18, mosaicism (mitotic nondisjunction)**
Q91.2 **Trisomy 18, translocation**
Q91.3 **Trisomy 18, unspecified**
Q91.4 **Trisomy 13, nonmosaicism (meiotic nondisjunction)**
Q91.5 **Trisomy 13, mosaicism (mitotic nondisjunction)**
Q91.6 **Trisomy 13, translocation**
Q91.7 **Trisomy 13, unspecified**

Q92 Other trisomies and partial trisomies of the autosomes, not elsewhere classified
INCLUDES unbalanced translocations and insertions
EXCLUDES 1 *trisomies of chromosomes 13, 18, 21 (Q90-Q91)*
Q92.0 **Whole chromosome trisomy, nonmosaicism (meiotic nondisjunction)**
Q92.1 **Whole chromosome trisomy, mosaicism (mitotic nondisjunction)**
Q92.2 **Partial trisomy**
Less than whole arm duplicated
Whole arm or more duplicated
EXCLUDES 1 *partial trisomy due to unbalanced translocation (Q92.5)*
Q92.5 **Duplications with other complex rearrangements**
Partial trisomy due to unbalanced translocations
Code also:
any associated deletions due to unbalanced translocations, inversions and insertions (Q93.7)
Q92.6 **Marker chromosomes**
Trisomies due to dicentrics
Trisomies due to extra rings
Trisomies due to isochromosomes
Individual with marker heterochromatin
Q92.61 **Marker chromosomes in normal individual**
Q92.62 **Marker chromosomes in abnormal individual**
Q92.7 **Triploidy and polyploidy**
Q92.8 **Other specified trisomies and partial trisomies of autosomes**
Duplications identified by fluorescence in situ hybridization (FISH)
Duplications identified by in situ hybridization (ISH)
Duplications seen only at prometaphase
Q92.9 **Trisomy and partial trisomy of autosomes, unspecified**

Q93 Monosomies and deletions from the autosomes, not elsewhere classified
Q93.0 **Whole chromosome monosomy, nonmosaicism (meiotic nondisjunction)**
Q93.1 **Whole chromosome monosomy, mosaicism (mitotic nondisjunction)**
Q93.2 **Chromosome replaced with ring, dicentric or isochromosome**
Q93.3 **Deletion of short arm of chromosome 4**
Wolff-Hirschorn syndrome
Q93.4 **Deletion of short arm of chromosome 5**
Cri-du-chat syndrome
▲ Q93.5 **Other deletions of part of a chromosome**
● Q93.51 **Angelman syndrome**
● Q93.59 **Other deletions of part of a chromosome**
Q93.7 **Deletions with other complex rearrangements**
Deletions due to unbalanced translocations, inversions and insertions
Code also:
any associated duplications due to unbalanced translocations, inversions and insertions (Q92.5)
Q93.8 **Other deletions from the autosomes**
Q93.81 **Velo-cardio-facial syndrome**
Deletion 22q11.2
● Q93.82 **Williams syndrome**
Q93.88 **Other microdeletions**
Miller-Dieker syndrome
Smith-Magenis syndrome
Q93.89 **Other deletions from the autosomes**
Deletions identified by fluorescence in situ hybridization (FISH)
Deletions identified by in situ hybridization (ISH)
Deletions seen only at prometaphase
Q93.9 **Deletion from autosomes, unspecified**

Q95 Balanced rearrangements and structural markers, not elsewhere classified
INCLUDES Robertsonian and balanced reciprocal translocations and insertions
Q95.0 **Balanced translocation and insertion in normal individual**
Q95.1 **Chromosome inversion in normal individual**
Q95.2 **Balanced autosomal rearrangement in abnormal individual**
Q95.3 **Balanced sex/autosomal rearrangement in abnormal individual**
Q95.5 **Individual with autosomal fragile site**
Q95.8 **Other balanced rearrangements and structural markers**
Q95.9 **Balanced rearrangement and structural marker, unspecified**

Q96 Turner's syndrome
EXCLUDES 1 *Noonan syndrome (Q87.1)*
Q96.0 **Karyotype 45, X** ♀
Q96.1 **Karyotype 46, X iso (Xq)** ♀
Karyotype 46, isochromosome Xq
Q96.2 **Karyotype 46, X with abnormal sex chromosome, except iso (Xq)** ♀
Karyotype 46, X with abnormal sex chromosome, except isochromosome Xq
Q96.3 **Mosaicism, 45, X/46, XX or XY** ♀
Q96.4 **Mosaicism, 45, X/other cell line(s) with abnormal sex chromosome** ♀
Q96.8 **Other variants of Turner's syndrome** ♀
Q96.9 **Turner's syndrome, unspecified** ♀

Q97 Other sex chromosome abnormalities, female phenotype, not elsewhere classified
EXCLUDES 1 *Turner's syndrome (Q96.-)*
Q97.0 **Karyotype 47, XXX** ♀
Q97.1 **Female with more than three X chromosomes** ♀
Q97.2 **Mosaicism, lines with various numbers of X chromosomes** ♀
Q97.3 **Female with 46, XY karyotype** ♀
Q97.8 **Other specified sex chromosome abnormalities, female phenotype** ♀
Q97.9 **Sex chromosome abnormality, female phenotype, unspecified** ♀

Q98 Other sex chromosome abnormalities, male phenotype, not elsewhere classified
Q98.0 **Klinefelter syndrome karyotype 47, XXY** ♂
Q98.1 **Klinefelter syndrome, male with more than two X chromosomes** ♂
Q98.3 **Other male with 46, XX karyotype** ♂
Q98.4 **Klinefelter syndrome, unspecified** ♂
Q98.5 **Karyotype 47, XYY**
Q98.6 **Male with structurally abnormal sex chromosome** ♂
Q98.7 **Male with sex chromosome mosaicism** ♂
Q98.8 **Other specified sex chromosome abnormalities, male phenotype** ♂
Q98.9 **Sex chromosome abnormality, male phenotype, unspecified** ♂

Q99 Other chromosome abnormalities, not elsewhere classified

Q99.0 **Chimera 46, XX/46, XY**
Chimera 46, XX/46, XY true hermaphrodite

Q99.1 **46, XX true hermaphrodite**
46, XX with streak gonads
46, XY with streak gonads
Pure gonadal dysgenesis

Q99.2 **Fragile X chromosome**
Fragile X syndrome

Q99.8 **Other specified chromosome abnormalities**

Q99.9 **Chromosomal abnormality, unspecified**

CHAPTER 18: SYMPTOMS, SIGNS AND ABNORMAL CLINICAL AND LABORATORY FINDINGS, NOT ELSEWHERE CLASSIFIED (R00-R99)

Note: This chapter includes symptoms, signs, abnormal results of clinical or other investigative procedures, and ill-defined conditions regarding which no diagnosis classifiable elsewhere is recorded.
Signs and symptoms that point rather definitely to a given diagnosis have been assigned to a category in other chapters of the classification. In general, categories in this chapter include the less well-defined conditions and symptoms that, without the necessary study of the case to establish a final diagnosis, point perhaps equally to two or more diseases or to two or more systems of the body. Practically all categories in the chapter could be designated 'not otherwise specified', 'unknown etiology' or 'transient'. The Alphabetical Index should be consulted to determine which symptoms and signs are to be allocated here and which to other chapters. The residual subcategories, numbered .8, are generally provided for other relevant symptoms that cannot be allocated elsewhere in the classification.
The conditions and signs or symptoms included in categories R00-R94 consist of:
(a) cases for which no more specific diagnosis can be made even after all the facts bearing on the case have been investigated;
(b) signs or symptoms existing at the time of initial encounter that proved to be transient and whose causes could not be determined;
(c) provisional diagnosis in a patient who failed to return for further investigation or care;
(d) cases referred elsewhere for investigation or treatment before the diagnosis was made;
(e) cases in which a more precise diagnosis was not available for any other reason;
(f) certain symptoms, for which supplementary information is provided, that represent important problems in medical care in their own right.

EXCLUDES 2 *abnormal findings on antenatal screening of mother (O28.-)*
certain conditions originating in the perinatal period (P04-P96)
signs and symptoms classified in the body system chapters
signs and symptoms of breast (N63, N64.5)

GUIDELINES **Section I.C.18.a-c**
Codes that describe symptoms and signs are acceptable for reporting purposes when a related definitive diagnosis has not been established (confirmed) by the provider.

Codes for signs and symptoms may be reported in addition to a related definitive diagnosis when the sign or symptom is not routinely associated with that diagnosis, such as the various signs and symptoms associated with complex syndromes. The definitive diagnosis code should be sequenced before the symptom code. Signs or symptoms that are associated routinely with a disease process should not be assigned as additional codes, unless otherwise instructed by the classification.

ICD-10-CM contains a number of combination codes that identify both the definitive diagnosis and common symptoms of that diagnosis. When using one of these combination codes, an additional code should not be assigned for the symptom.

This chapter contains the following blocks:

R00-R09	Symptoms and signs involving the circulatory and respiratory systems
R10-R19	Symptoms and signs involving the digestive system and abdomen
R20-R23	Symptoms and signs involving the skin and subcutaneous tissue
R25-R29	Symptoms and signs involving the nervous and musculoskeletal systems
R30-R39	Symptoms and signs involving the genitourinary system
R40-R46	Symptoms and signs involving cognition, perception, emotional state and behavior
R47-R49	Symptoms and signs involving speech and voice
R50-R69	General symptoms and signs
R70-R79	Abnormal findings on examination of blood, without diagnosis
R80-R82	Abnormal findings on examination of urine, without diagnosis
R83-R89	Abnormal findings on examination of other body fluids, substances and tissues, without diagnosis
R90-R94	Abnormal findings on diagnostic imaging and in function studies, without diagnosis
R97	Abnormal tumor markers
R99	Ill-defined and unknown cause of mortality

Symptoms and signs involving the circulatory and respiratory systems (R00-R09)

4 R00 Abnormalities of heart beat
EXCLUDES 1 *abnormalities originating in the perinatal period (P29.1-)*
EXCLUDES 2 *specified arrhythmias (I47-I49)*

R00.0 Tachycardia, unspecified
Rapid heart beat
Sinoauricular tachycardia NOS
Sinus [sinusal] tachycardia NOS
EXCLUDES 1 *neonatal tachycardia (P29.11)*
paroxysmal tachycardia (I47.-)
CODING TIP✓ Tachycardia that is not specified as due to a specific arrhythmia or any particular cause is coded here. When the record reports "sinus tachycardia," assign code R00.0. Sinus tachycardia indicates a high heart rate with an impulse that continues to originate from the SA node.

Tachycardia

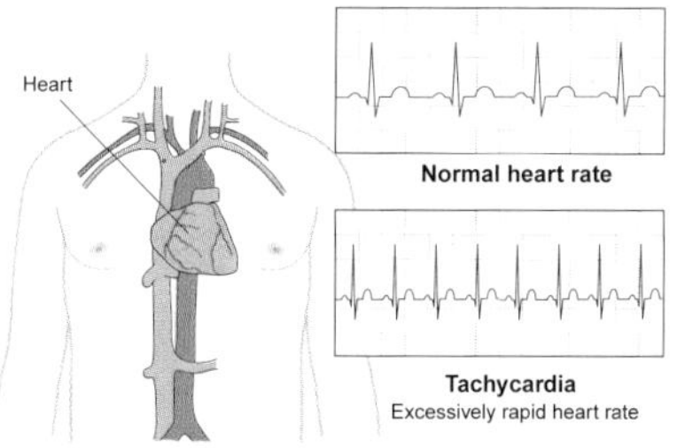

R00.1 Bradycardia, unspecified
Sinoatrial bradycardia
Sinus bradycardia
Slow heart beat
Vagal bradycardia
Use additional code for adverse effect, if applicable, to identify drug (T36-T50 with fifth or sixth character 5)
EXCLUDES 1 *neonatal bradycardia (P29.12)*

R00.2 Palpitations
Awareness of heart beat
DEFINITION Sensation of feeling the heart beat.

R00.8 Other abnormalities of heart beat

R00.9 Unspecified abnormalities of heart beat

4 R01 Cardiac murmurs and other cardiac sounds
EXCLUDES 1 *cardiac murmurs and sounds originating in the perinatal period (P29.8)*

R01.0 Benign and innocent cardiac murmurs
Functional cardiac murmur

R01.1 Cardiac murmur, unspecified
Cardiac bruit NOS
Heart murmur NOS
Systolic murmur NOS

R01.2 Other cardiac sounds
Cardiac dullness, increased or decreased
Precordial friction

4 R03 Abnormal blood-pressure reading, without diagnosis

R03.0 Elevated blood-pressure reading, without diagnosis of hypertension
Note: This category is to be used to record an episode of elevated blood pressure in a patient in whom no formal diagnosis of hypertension has been made, or as an isolated incidental finding.
GUIDELINES **Section I.C.9.a.7)**
Assign code R03.0, Elevated blood pressure reading without diagnosis of hypertension, unless patient has an established diagnosis of hypertension. Assign code O13.-, Gestational [pregnancy-induced] hypertension without significant proteinuria, or O14.-, Pre-eclampsia, for transient hypertension of pregnancy.
CODING TIP✓ Do not assign this code for a patient with a diagnosis of hypertension (I10-I13).

R03.1 **Nonspecific low blood-pressure reading**
EXCLUDES 1 *hypotension (I95.-)*
maternal hypotension syndrome (O26.5-)
neurogenic orthostatic hypotension (G90.3)
CODING TIP ✓ Assign code R03.1 when a patient has a low blood pressure reading but has not been diagnosed with hypotension or orthostasis.

4 R04 Hemorrhage from respiratory passages
CODING TIP ✓ If these bleeds are the result of an adverse effect of anticoagulant, add D68.32 and the T code for anticoagulant from the Table of Drugs and Chemicals.

R04.0 **Epistaxis**
Hemorrhage from nose
Nosebleed

R04.1 **Hemorrhage from throat**
EXCLUDES 2 *hemoptysis (R04.2)*

R04.2 **Hemoptysis**
Blood-stained sputum
Cough with hemorrhage
DEFINITION Coughing up blood or bloody mucous.
AHA: 4Q 2013, 118

5 R04.8 **Hemorrhage from other sites in respiratory passages**

R04.81 **Acute idiopathic pulmonary hemorrhage in infants** P
AIPHI
Acute idiopathic hemorrhage in infants over 28 days old
EXCLUDES 1 *perinatal pulmonary hemorrhage (P26.-)*
von Willebrand's disease (D68.0)

R04.89 **Hemorrhage from other sites in respiratory passages**
Pulmonary hemorrhage NOS

R04.9 **Hemorrhage from respiratory passages, unspecified**

R05 Cough
EXCLUDES 1 *cough with hemorrhage (R04.2)*
smoker's cough (J41.0)
CODING TIP ✓ Do not assign R05 as an additional code when the cough is an integral symptom of another disease process also coded, such as COPD, bronchitis, asthma, or another pulmonary condition known to be the cause of the cough.
AHA: 2Q 2016, 34

4 R06 Abnormalities of breathing
EXCLUDES 1 *acute respiratory distress syndrome (J80)*
respiratory arrest (R09.2)
respiratory arrest of newborn (P28.81)
respiratory distress syndrome of newborn (P22.-)
respiratory failure (J96.-)
respiratory failure of newborn (P28.5)
CODING TIP ✓ Do not assign a code from R06.- as an additional code when the respiratory symptom is routinely associated with another disease process also coded, such as COPD, bronchitis, asthma, or another condition known to be the cause of the presenting symptom. The more specific condition should be coded.

5 R06.0 **Dyspnea**
EXCLUDES 1 *tachypnea NOS (R06.82)*
transient tachypnea of newborn (P22.1)

R06.00 **Dyspnea, unspecified**
AHA: 1Q 2017, 26

R06.01 **Orthopnea**
DEFINITION Difficulty breathing while lying down, necessitating sleeping propped up or in a chair.

R06.02 **Shortness of breath**

R06.03 **Acute respiratory distress**
AHA: 4Q 2017, 18

R06.09 **Other forms of dyspnea**

R06.1 **Stridor**
EXCLUDES 1 *congenital laryngeal stridor (P28.89)*
laryngismus (stridulus) (J38.5)
DEFINITION A whistling sound when breathing, usually heard on inspiration, indicating obstruction of the trachea or larynx.

R06.2 **Wheezing**
EXCLUDES 1 *Asthma (J45.-)*
AHA: 2Q 2016, 34

R06.3 **Periodic breathing**
Cheyne-Stokes breathing

R06.4 **Hyperventilation**
EXCLUDES 1 *psychogenic hyperventilation (F45.8)*

R06.5 **Mouth breathing**
EXCLUDES 2 *dry mouth NOS (R68.2)*

R06.6 **Hiccough**
EXCLUDES 1 *psychogenic hiccough (F45.8)*
DEFINITION Sharp sound of inhalation, with spasm of the glottis and diaphragm.

R06.7 **Sneezing**

5 R06.8 **Other abnormalities of breathing**

R06.81 **Apnea, not elsewhere classified**
Apnea NOS
EXCLUDES 1 *apnea (of) newborn (P28.4)*
sleep apnea (G47.3-)
sleep apnea of newborn (primary) (P28.3)
DEFINITION Temporary cessation of breathing.

R06.82 **Tachypnea, not elsewhere classified**
Tachypnea NOS
EXCLUDES 1 *transitory tachypnea of newborn (P22.1)*
DEFINITION Rapid breathing.

R06.83 **Snoring**

R06.89 **Other abnormalities of breathing**
Breath-holding (spells)
Sighing

R06.9 **Unspecified abnormalities of breathing**

4 R07 Pain in throat and chest
EXCLUDES 1 *epidemic myalgia (B33.0)*
EXCLUDES 2 *jaw pain R68.84*
pain in breast (N64.4)
CODING TIP ✓ Do not assign a code from R07.- for a patient with angina. Chest pain due to angina should be coded to the appropriate I20.- or I25.- code

R07.0 **Pain in throat**
EXCLUDES 1 *chronic sore throat (J31.2)*
sore throat (acute) NOS (J02.9)
EXCLUDES 2 *dysphagia (R13.1-)*
pain in neck (M54.2)

R07.1 **Chest pain on breathing**
Painful respiration

R07.2 **Precordial pain**

5 R07.8 **Other chest pain**

R07.81 **Pleurodynia**
Pleurodynia NOS
EXCLUDES 1 *epidemic pleurodynia (B33.0)*

R07.82 **Intercostal pain**

R07.89 **Other chest pain**
Anterior chest-wall pain NOS

R07.9 **Chest pain, unspecified**

4 R09 Other symptoms and signs involving the circulatory and respiratory system
EXCLUDES 1 *acute respiratory distress syndrome (J80)*
respiratory arrest of newborn (P28.81)
respiratory distress syndrome of newborn (P22.0)
respiratory failure (J96.-)
respiratory failure of newborn (P28.5)

5 R09.0 **Asphyxia and hypoxemia**
EXCLUDES 1 *asphyxia due to carbon monoxide (T58.-)*
asphyxia due to foreign body in respiratory tract (T17.-)
birth (intrauterine) asphyxia (P84)
hyperventilation (R06.4)
traumatic asphyxia (T71.-)
EXCLUDES 2 *hypercapnia (R06.89)*

R09.01 **Asphyxia**

DEFINITION Extreme decrease in the amount of oxygen in the body, accompanied by an increase of carbon dioxide, leading to loss of consciousness or death.

R09.02 Hypoxemia

DEFINITION Abnormally low levels of oxygen in arterial blood.

R09.1 Pleurisy

EXCLUDES 1 *pleurisy with effusion (J90)*

R09.2 Respiratory arrest HCC

Cardiorespiratory failure

EXCLUDES 1 *cardiac arrest (I46.-)*
respiratory arrest of newborn (P28.81)
respiratory distress of newborn (P22.0)
respiratory failure (J96.-)
respiratory failure of newborn (P28.5)
respiratory insufficiency (R06.89)
respiratory insufficiency of newborn (P28.5)

R09.3 Abnormal sputum

Abnormal amount of sputum
Abnormal color of sputum
Abnormal odor of sputum
Excessive sputum

EXCLUDES 1 *blood-stained sputum (R04.2)*

5 **R09.8 Other specified symptoms and signs involving the circulatory and respiratory systems**

R09.81 Nasal congestion

R09.82 Postnasal drip

R09.89 Other specified symptoms and signs involving the circulatory and respiratory systems

Bruit (arterial)
Abnormal chest percussion
Feeling of foreign body in throat
Friction sounds in chest
Chest tympany
Choking sensation
Rales
Weak pulse

EXCLUDES 2 *foreign body in throat (T17.2-)*
wheezing (R06.2)

Symptoms and signs involving the digestive system and abdomen (R10-R19)

EXCLUDES 2 *congenital or infantile pylorospasm (Q40.0)*
gastrointestinal hemorrhage (K92.0-K92.2)
intestinal obstruction (K56.-)
newborn gastrointestinal hemorrhage (P54.0-P54.3)
newborn intestinal obstruction (P76.-)
pylorospasm (K31.3)
signs and symptoms involving the urinary system (R30-R39)
symptoms referable to female genital organs (N94.-)
symptoms referable to male genital organs (N48-N50)

4 **R10 Abdominal and pelvic pain**

EXCLUDES 1 *renal colic (N23)*

EXCLUDES 2 *dorsalgia (M54.-)*
flatulence and related conditions (R14.-)

R10.0 Acute abdomen

Severe abdominal pain (generalized) (with abdominal rigidity)

EXCLUDES 1 *abdominal rigidity NOS (R19.3)*
generalized abdominal pain NOS (R10.84)
localized abdominal pain (R10.1-R10.3-)

5 **R10.1 Pain localized to upper abdomen**

R10.10 Upper abdominal pain, unspecified

⊟ **R10.11 Right upper quadrant pain**

⊟ **R10.12 Left upper quadrant pain**

R10.13 Epigastric pain

Dyspepsia

EXCLUDES 1 *functional dyspepsia (K30)*

R10.2 Pelvic and perineal pain

EXCLUDES 1 *vulvodynia (N94.81)*

5 **R10.3 Pain localized to other parts of lower abdomen**

R10.30 Lower abdominal pain, unspecified

⊟ **R10.31 Right lower quadrant pain**

⊟ **R10.32 Left lower quadrant pain**

R10.33 Periumbilical pain

5 **R10.8 Other abdominal pain**

6 **R10.81 Abdominal tenderness**

Abdominal tenderness NOS

⊟ **R10.811 Right upper quadrant abdominal tenderness**

⊟ **R10.812 Left upper quadrant abdominal tenderness**

⊟ **R10.813 Right lower quadrant abdominal tenderness**

⊟ **R10.814 Left lower quadrant abdominal tenderness**

R10.815 Periumbilic abdominal tenderness

R10.816 Epigastric abdominal tenderness

R10.817 Generalized abdominal tenderness

R10.819 Abdominal tenderness, unspecified site

6 **R10.82 Rebound abdominal tenderness**

⊟ **R10.821 Right upper quadrant rebound abdominal tenderness**

⊟ **R10.822 Left upper quadrant rebound abdominal tenderness**

⊟ **R10.823 Right lower quadrant rebound abdominal tenderness**

⊟ **R10.824 Left lower quadrant rebound abdominal tenderness**

R10.825 Periumbilic rebound abdominal tenderness

R10.826 Epigastric rebound abdominal tenderness

R10.827 Generalized rebound abdominal tenderness

R10.829 Rebound abdominal tenderness, unspecified site

R10.83 Colic P

Colic NOS
Infantile colic

EXCLUDES 1 *colic in adult and child over 12 months old (R10.84)*

R10.84 Generalized abdominal pain

EXCLUDES 1 *generalized abdominal pain associated with acute abdomen (R10.0)*

R10.9 Unspecified abdominal pain

4 **R11 Nausea and vomiting**

EXCLUDES 1 *cyclical vomiting associated with migraine (G43.A-)*
excessive vomiting in pregnancy (O21.-)
hematemesis (K92.0)
neonatal hematemesis (P54.0)
newborn vomiting (P92.0-)
psychogenic vomiting (F50.89)
vomiting associated with bulimia nervosa (F50.2)
vomiting following gastrointestinal surgery (K91.0)

AHA: 1Q 2017, 28

R11.0 Nausea

Nausea NOS
Nausea without vomiting

5 **R11.1 Vomiting**

R11.10 Vomiting, unspecified

Vomiting NOS

R11.11 Vomiting without nausea

R11.12 Projectile vomiting

R11.13 Vomiting of fecal matter

R11.14 Bilious vomiting

Bilious emesis

R11.2 Nausea with vomiting, unspecified

Persistent nausea with vomiting NOS

R12 Heartburn

EXCLUDES 1 *dyspepsia NOS (R10.13)*
functional dyspepsia (K30)

4 **R13 Aphagia and dysphagia**

R13.0 Aphagia

Inability to swallow

EXCLUDES 1 *psychogenic aphagia (F50.9)*

R13.1 Dysphagia
Code first:
, if applicable, dysphagia following cerebrovascular disease (I69. with final characters -91)
EXCLUDES 1 *psychogenic dysphagia (F45.8)*

CODING TIP ✓ Assign a code from R13.1- following a code from I69.- when dysphagia is reported as a sequela of cerebral vascular disease to report the specified level of dysphagia.

DEFINITION Difficulty in swallowing.

R13.10 Dysphagia, unspecified
Difficulty in swallowing NOS
R13.11 Dysphagia, oral phase
R13.12 Dysphagia, oropharyngeal phase
R13.13 Dysphagia, pharyngeal phase
R13.14 Dysphagia, pharyngoesophageal phase
R13.19 Other dysphagia
Cervical dysphagia
Neurogenic dysphagia

R14 Flatulence and related conditions
EXCLUDES 1 *psychogenic aerophagy (F45.8)*
R14.0 Abdominal distension (gaseous)
Bloating
Tympanites (abdominal) (intestinal)
R14.1 Gas pain
R14.2 Eructation
R14.3 Flatulence

R15 Fecal incontinence
INCLUDES encopresis NOS
EXCLUDES 1 *fecal incontinence of nonorganic origin (F98.1)*
R15.0 Incomplete defecation
EXCLUDES 1 *constipation (K59.0-)*
fecal impaction (K56.41)
R15.1 Fecal smearing
Fecal soiling
R15.2 Fecal urgency
R15.9 Full incontinence of feces
Fecal incontinence NOS

R16 Hepatomegaly and splenomegaly, not elsewhere classified
R16.0 Hepatomegaly, not elsewhere classified
Hepatomegaly NOS
R16.1 Splenomegaly, not elsewhere classified
Splenomegaly NOS
R16.2 Hepatomegaly with splenomegaly, not elsewhere classified
Hepatosplenomegaly NOS

R17 Unspecified jaundice
EXCLUDES 1 *neonatal jaundice (P55, P57-P59)*

R18 Ascites
INCLUDES fluid in peritoneal cavity
EXCLUDES 1 *ascites in alcoholic cirrhosis (K70.31)*
ascites in alcoholic hepatitis (K70.11)
ascites in toxic liver disease with chronic active hepatitis (K71.51)
R18.0 Malignant ascites
Code first malignancy, such as:
malignant neoplasm of ovary (C56.-)
secondary malignant neoplasm of retroperitoneum and peritoneum (C78.6)

DEFINITION Abnormal accumulation of fluid containing cancer cells in the peritoneal cavity, usually from metastatic spread of a malignancy.

R18.8 Other ascites
Ascites NOS
Peritoneal effusion (chronic)

R19 Other symptoms and signs involving the digestive system and abdomen
EXCLUDES 1 *acute abdomen (R10.0)*
R19.0 Intra-abdominal and pelvic swelling, mass and lump
EXCLUDES 1 *abdominal distension (gaseous) (R14.-)*
ascites (R18.-)

CODING TIP ✓ A mass should not be coded for an area that has been clearly identified as a neoplasm. If a mass has been biopsied and reported as a neoplasm, code the appropriate neoplasm code.

R19.00 Intra-abdominal and pelvic swelling, mass and lump, unspecified site
R19.01 Right upper quadrant abdominal swelling, mass and lump
R19.02 Left upper quadrant abdominal swelling, mass and lump
R19.03 Right lower quadrant abdominal swelling, mass and lump
R19.04 Left lower quadrant abdominal swelling, mass and lump
R19.05 Periumbilic swelling, mass or lump
Diffuse or generalized umbilical swelling or mass
R19.06 Epigastric swelling, mass or lump
R19.07 Generalized intra-abdominal and pelvic swelling, mass and lump
Diffuse or generalized intra-abdominal swelling or mass NOS
Diffuse or generalized pelvic swelling or mass NOS
R19.09 Other intra-abdominal and pelvic swelling, mass and lump
R19.1 Abnormal bowel sounds
R19.11 Absent bowel sounds
R19.12 Hyperactive bowel sounds
R19.15 Other abnormal bowel sounds
Abnormal bowel sounds NOS
R19.2 Visible peristalsis
Hyperperistalsis
R19.3 Abdominal rigidity
EXCLUDES 1 *abdominal rigidity with severe abdominal pain (R10.0)*
R19.30 Abdominal rigidity, unspecified site
R19.31 Right upper quadrant abdominal rigidity
R19.32 Left upper quadrant abdominal rigidity
R19.33 Right lower quadrant abdominal rigidity
R19.34 Left lower quadrant abdominal rigidity
R19.35 Periumbilic abdominal rigidity
R19.36 Epigastric abdominal rigidity
R19.37 Generalized abdominal rigidity
R19.4 Change in bowel habit
EXCLUDES 1 *constipation (K59.0-)*
functional diarrhea (K59.1)
R19.5 Other fecal abnormalities
Abnormal stool color
Bulky stools
Mucus in stools
Occult blood in feces
Occult blood in stools
EXCLUDES 1 *melena (K92.1)*
neonatal melena (P54.1)
R19.6 Halitosis
R19.7 Diarrhea, unspecified
Diarrhea NOS
EXCLUDES 1 *functional diarrhea (K59.1)*
neonatal diarrhea (P78.3)
psychogenic diarrhea (F45.8)
R19.8 Other specified symptoms and signs involving the digestive system and abdomen

Symptoms and signs involving the skin and subcutaneous tissue (R20-R23)

EXCLUDES 2 *symptoms relating to breast (N64.4-N64.5)*

R20 Disturbances of skin sensation
EXCLUDES 1 *dissociative anesthesia and sensory loss (F44.6)*
psychogenic disturbances (F45.8)
R20.0 Anesthesia of skin
R20.1 Hypoesthesia of skin
R20.2 Paresthesia of skin
Formication
Pins and needles
Tingling skin
EXCLUDES 1 *acroparesthesia (I73.8)*

● New ▲ Revised *Manifestation* Unspecified 4-7 Digit Indicators AHA Coding Clinic Laterality Adult HCC Hierarchical Condition Categories Maternity Newborn HIV HIV Related Conditions Pediatric ♂ Male ♀ Female

R20.3 **Hyperesthesia**
R20.8 Other **disturbances of skin sensation**
R20.9 Unspecified **disturbances of skin sensation**

R21 Rash and other nonspecific skin eruption
INCLUDES rash NOS
EXCLUDES 1 *specified type of rash- code to condition*
vesicular eruption (R23.8)

R22 Localized swelling, mass and lump of skin and subcutaneous tissue
INCLUDES subcutaneous nodules (localized) (superficial)
EXCLUDES 1 *abnormal findings on diagnostic imaging (R90-R93)*
edema (R60.-)
enlarged lymph nodes (R59.-)
localized adiposity (E65)
swelling of joint (M25.4-)

R22.0 **Localized swelling, mass and lump, head**
R22.1 **Localized swelling, mass and lump, neck**
R22.2 **Localized swelling, mass and lump, trunk**
EXCLUDES 1 *intra-abdominal or pelvic mass and lump (R19.0-)*
intra-abdominal or pelvic swelling (R19.0-)
EXCLUDES 2 *breast mass and lump (N63)*
R22.3 **Localized swelling, mass and lump, upper limb**
R22.30 **Localized swelling, mass and lump, unspecified upper limb**
R22.31 **Localized swelling, mass and lump, right upper limb**
R22.32 **Localized swelling, mass and lump, left upper limb**
R22.33 **Localized swelling, mass and lump, upper limb, bilateral**
R22.4 **Localized swelling, mass and lump, lower limb**
R22.40 **Localized swelling, mass and lump, unspecified lower limb**
R22.41 **Localized swelling, mass and lump, right lower limb**
R22.42 **Localized swelling, mass and lump, left lower limb**
R22.43 **Localized swelling, mass and lump, lower limb, bilateral**
R22.9 **Localized swelling, mass and lump, unspecified**

R23 Other skin changes
R23.0 **Cyanosis**
EXCLUDES 1 *acrocyanosis (I73.8)*
cyanotic attacks of newborn (P28.2)
DEFINITION Bluish tint of the skin from lack of oxygen.
R23.1 **Pallor**
Clammy skin
DEFINITION Excessive paleness of the skin, especially the face.
R23.2 **Flushing**
Excessive blushing
Code first:
, if applicable, menopausal and female climacteric states (N95.1)
R23.3 **Spontaneous ecchymoses**
Petechiae
EXCLUDES 1 *ecchymoses of newborn (P54.5)*
purpura (D69.-)
DEFINITION Minute red spots on the skin, due to escape of a small amount of blood from the vessels.
R23.4 **Changes in skin texture**
Desquamation of skin
Induration of skin
Scaling of skin
EXCLUDES 1 *epidermal thickening NOS (L85.9)*
R23.8 **Other skin changes**
CODING TIP✓ When vesicular ulcerations (weeping ulcers) occur to the lower extremities as a result of edema (such as due to CHF or other edema producing conditions), assign R23.8 to indicate the resulting open vesicular (blister) ulceration. Do not assign this code to indicate other ulcerations such as due to friction or unspecified ulcers.
R23.9 **Unspecified skin changes**

Symptoms and signs involving the nervous and musculoskeletal systems (R25-R29)

R25 Abnormal involuntary movements
EXCLUDES 1 *specific movement disorders (G20-G26)*
stereotyped movement disorders (F98.4)
tic disorders (F95.-)
R25.0 **Abnormal head movements**
R25.1 **Tremor, unspecified**
EXCLUDES 1 *chorea NOS (G25.5)*
essential tremor (G25.0)
hysterical tremor (F44.4)
intention tremor (G25.2)
R25.2 **Cramp and spasm**
EXCLUDES 2 *carpopedal spasm (R29.0)*
charley-horse (M62.831)
infantile spasms (G40.4-)
muscle spasm of back (M62.830)
muscle spasm of calf (M62.831)
R25.3 **Fasciculation**
Twitching NOS
R25.8 **Other abnormal involuntary movements**
R25.9 **Unspecified abnormal involuntary movements**

R26 Abnormalities of gait and mobility
EXCLUDES 1 *ataxia NOS (R27.0)*
hereditary ataxia (G11.-)
locomotor (syphilitic) ataxia (A52.11)
immobility syndrome (paraplegic) (M62.3)
R26.0 **Ataxic gait**
Staggering gait
CODING TIP✓ Note the definition of ataxia, a staggering, unsteady gait indicating a lack of muscle coordination.
R26.1 **Paralytic gait**
Spastic gait
R26.2 **Difficulty in walking, not elsewhere classified**
EXCLUDES 1 *falling (R29.6)*
unsteadiness on feet (R26.81)
AHA: 2Q 2016, 7
R26.8 **Other abnormalities of gait and mobility**
R26.81 **Unsteadiness on feet**
R26.89 **Other abnormalities of gait and mobility**
R26.9 **Unspecified abnormalities of gait and mobility**
CODING TIP✓ Keep in mind when assigning R26.9 that if the cause of the gait abnormality is known, the code for the underlying cause of the gait abnormality should be assigned. It is not appropriate to assign the code for a symptom when a more specific condition has been identified.

R27 Other lack of coordination
EXCLUDES 1 *ataxic gait (R26.0)*
hereditary ataxia (G11.-)
vertigo NOS (R42)
R27.0 **Ataxia, unspecified**
EXCLUDES 1 *ataxia following cerebrovascular disease (I69. with final characters -93)*
DEFINITION Distortion or impairment of voluntary movement.
R27.8 **Other lack of coordination**
R27.9 **Unspecified lack of coordination**

R29 Other symptoms and signs involving the nervous and musculoskeletal systems
R29.0 **Tetany**
Carpopedal spasm
EXCLUDES 1 *hysterical tetany (F44.5)*
neonatal tetany (P71.3)
parathyroid tetany (E20.9)
post-thyroidectomy tetany (E89.2)
R29.1 **Meningismus**
R29.2 **Abnormal reflex**
EXCLUDES 2 *abnormal pupillary reflex (H57.0)*
hyperactive gag reflex (J39.2)
vasovagal reaction or syncope (R55)
R29.3 **Abnormal posture**
R29.4 **Clicking hip**
EXCLUDES 1 *congenital deformities of hip (Q65.-)*

R29.5 Transient paralysis
Code first:
any associated spinal cord injury (S14.0, S14.1-, S24.0, S24.1-, S34.0-, S34.1-)
EXCLUDES 1 *transient ischemic attack (G45.9)*

R29.6 Repeated falls
Falling
Tendency to fall
EXCLUDES 2 *at risk for falling (Z91.81)*
history of falling (Z91.81)
GUIDELINES **Section I.C.18.d**
Code R29.6, Repeated falls, is for use for encounters when a patient has recently fallen and the reason for the fall is being investigated. Code Z91.81, History of falling, is for use when a patient has fallen in the past and is at risk for future falls. When appropriate, both codes R29.6 and Z91.81 may be assigned together.
AHA: 2Q 2016, 7

5 **R29.7 National Institutes of Health Stroke Scale (NIHSS) score**
Code first:
the type of cerebral infarction (I63-)
AHA: 4Q 2016, 61

6 **R29.70 NIHSS score 0-9**
R29.700 NIHSS score 0
R29.701 NIHSS score 1
R29.702 NIHSS score 2
R29.703 NIHSS score 3
R29.704 NIHSS score 4
R29.705 NIHSS score 5
R29.706 NIHSS score 6
R29.707 NIHSS score 7
R29.708 NIHSS score 8
R29.709 NIHSS score 9

6 **R29.71 NIHSS score 10-19**
R29.710 NIHSS score 10
R29.711 NIHSS score 11
R29.712 NIHSS score 12
R29.713 NIHSS score 13
R29.714 NIHSS score 14
R29.715 NIHSS score 15
R29.716 NIHSS score 16
R29.717 NIHSS score 17
R29.718 NIHSS score 18
R29.719 NIHSS score 19

6 **R29.72 NIHSS score 20-29**
R29.720 NIHSS score 20
R29.721 NIHSS score 21
R29.722 NIHSS score 22
R29.723 NIHSS score 23
R29.724 NIHSS score 24
R29.725 NIHSS score 25
R29.726 NIHSS score 26
R29.727 NIHSS score 27
R29.728 NIHSS score 28
R29.729 NIHSS score 29

6 **R29.73 NIHSS score 30-39**
R29.730 NIHSS score 30
R29.731 NIHSS score 31
R29.732 NIHSS score 32
R29.733 NIHSS score 33
R29.734 NIHSS score 34
R29.735 NIHSS score 35
R29.736 NIHSS score 36
R29.737 NIHSS score 37
R29.738 NIHSS score 38
R29.739 NIHSS score 39

6 **R29.74 NIHSS score 40-42**
R29.740 NIHSS score 40
R29.741 NIHSS score 41
R29.742 NIHSS score 42

5 **R29.8 Other symptoms and signs involving the nervous and musculoskeletal systems**

6 **R29.81 Other symptoms and signs involving the nervous system**

R29.810 Facial weakness
Facial droop
EXCLUDES 1 *Bell's palsy (G51.0)*
facial weakness following cerebrovascular disease (I69. with final characters -92)

R29.818 Other symptoms and signs involving the nervous system

6 **R29.89 Other symptoms and signs involving the musculoskeletal system**
EXCLUDES 2 *pain in limb (M79.6-)*

R29.890 Loss of height
EXCLUDES 1 *osteoporosis (M80-M81)*

R29.891 Ocular torticollis
EXCLUDES 1 *congenital (sternomastoid) torticollis Q68.0*
psychogenic torticollis (F45.8)
spasmodic torticollis (G24.3)
torticollis due to birth injury (P15.8)
torticollis NOS M43.6

R29.898 Other symptoms and signs involving the musculoskeletal system

5 **R29.9 Unspecified symptoms and signs involving the nervous and musculoskeletal systems**
R29.90 Unspecified symptoms and signs involving the nervous system
R29.91 Unspecified symptoms and signs involving the musculoskeletal system

Symptoms and signs involving the genitourinary system (R30-R39)

4 **R30 Pain associated with micturition**
EXCLUDES 1 *psychogenic pain associated with micturition (F45.8)*

R30.0 Dysuria
Strangury
R30.1 Vesical tenesmus
R30.9 Painful micturition, unspecified
Painful urination NOS

4 **R31 Hematuria**
EXCLUDES 1 *hematuria included with underlying conditions, such as:*
acute cystitis with hematuria (N30.01)
recurrent and persistent hematuria in glomerular diseases (N02.-)

R31.0 Gross hematuria
R31.1 Benign essential microscopic hematuria
5 **R31.2 Other microscopic hematuria**
R31.21 Asymptomatic microscopic hematuria
AMH
AHA: 4Q 2016, 62
R31.29 Other microscopic hematuria
AHA: 4Q 2016, 62
R31.9 Hematuria, unspecified
DEFINITION Presence of blood in the urine.

R32 Unspecified urinary incontinence
Enuresis NOS
EXCLUDES 1 *functional urinary incontinence (R39.81)*
nonorganic enuresis (F98.0)
stress incontinence and other specified urinary incontinence (N39.3-N39.4-)
urinary incontinence associated with cognitive impairment (R39.81)

4 **R33 Retention of urine**
EXCLUDES 1 *psychogenic retention of urine (F45.8)*

R33.0 Drug induced retention of urine
Use additional code for adverse effect, if applicable, to identify drug (T36-T50 with fifth or sixth character 5)
R33.8 Other retention of urine
Code first, if applicable, any causal condition, such as:
enlarged prostate (N40.1)
R33.9 Retention of urine, unspecified

● New | Manifestation | 4-7 Digit Indicators | Laterality | A Adult | M Maternity | N Newborn | P Pediatric | ♂ Male
▲ Revised | Unspecified | AHA Coding Clinic | HCC Hierarchical Condition Categories | HIV HIV Related Conditions | ♀ Female

R34 Anuria and oliguria
EXCLUDES 1 *anuria and oliguria complicating abortion or ectopic or molar pregnancy (O00-O07, O08.4)*
anuria and oliguria complicating pregnancy (O26.83-)
anuria and oliguria complicating the puerperium (O90.4)

4 **R35 Polyuria**
Code first, if applicable, any causal condition, such as:
enlarged prostate (N40.1)
EXCLUDES 1 *psychogenic polyuria (F45.8)*

R35.0 Frequency of micturition
R35.1 Nocturia
R35.8 Other polyuria
Polyuria NOS

4 **R36 Urethral discharge**
R36.0 Urethral discharge without blood
R36.1 Hematospermia ♂
R36.9 Urethral discharge, unspecified
Penile discharge NOS
Urethrorrhea

R37 Sexual dysfunction, unspecified

4 **R39 Other and unspecified symptoms and signs involving the genitourinary system**
R39.0 Extravasation of urine
5 **R39.1 Other difficulties with micturition**
Code first, if applicable, any causal condition, such as:
enlarged prostate (N40.1)
R39.11 Hesitancy of micturition
DEFINITION Difficulty starting urination.
R39.12 Poor urinary stream
Weak urinary steam
R39.13 Splitting of urinary stream
R39.14 Feeling of incomplete bladder emptying
R39.15 Urgency of urination
EXCLUDES 1 *urge incontinence (N39.41, N39.46)*
R39.16 Straining to void
6 **R39.19 Other difficulties with micturition**
R39.191 Need to immediately re-void
AHA: 4Q 2016, 63
R39.192 Position dependent micturition
AHA: 4Q 2016, 63
R39.198 Other difficulties with micturition
AHA: 4Q 2016, 63
R39.2 Extrarenal uremia
Prerenal uremia
EXCLUDES 1 *uremia NOS (N19)*
5 **R39.8 Other symptoms and signs involving the genitourinary system**
R39.81 Functional urinary incontinence
Urinary incontinence due to cognitive impairment, or severe physical disability or immobility
EXCLUDES 1 *stress incontinence and other specified urinary incontinence (N39.3-N39.4-)*
urinary incontinence NOS (R32)
DEFINITION Leaking urine due to cognitive impairment or physical disability leading to the inability for volitional control over bladder function.
R39.82 Chronic bladder pain
AHA: 4Q 2016, 64
R39.83 Unilateral non-palpable testicle ♂
AHA: 4Q 2017, 17
R39.84 Bilateral non-palpable testicles ♂
AHA: 4Q 2017, 17
R39.89 Other symptoms and signs involving the genitourinary system
R39.9 Unspecified symptoms and signs involving the genitourinary system

Symptoms and signs involving cognition, perception, emotional state and behavior (R40-R46)

EXCLUDES 2 *symptoms and signs constituting part of a pattern of mental disorder (F01-F99)*

4 **R40 Somnolence, stupor and coma**
EXCLUDES 1 *neonatal coma (P91.5)*
somnolence, stupor and coma in diabetes (E08-E13)
somnolence, stupor and coma in hepatic failure (K72.-)
somnolence, stupor and coma in hypoglycemia (nondiabetic) (E15)

R40.0 Somnolence
Drowsiness
EXCLUDES 1 *coma (R40.2-)*
R40.1 Stupor
Catatonic stupor
Semicoma
EXCLUDES 1 *catatonic schizophrenia (F20.2)*
coma (R40.2-)
depressive stupor (F31-F33)
dissociative stupor (F44.2)
manic stupor (F30.2)
5 **R40.2 Coma**
Note: One code from each subcategory, R40.21-R40.23, is required to complete the coma scale
Code first any associated:
fracture of skull (S02.-)
intracranial injury (S06.-)

GUIDELINES **Section I.B.14**
For the Body Mass Index (BMI), depth of non-pressure chronic ulcers, pressure ulcer stage, coma scale, and NIH stroke scale (NIHSS) codes, code assignment may be based on medical record documentation from clinicians who are not the patient's provider (i.e., physician or other qualified healthcare practitioner legally accountable for establishing the patient's diagnosis), since this information is typically documented by other clinicians involved in the care of the patient (e.g., a dietitian often documents the BMI, a nurse often documents the pressure ulcer stages, and an emergency medical technician often documents the coma scale). However, the associated diagnosis (such as overweight, obesity, acute stroke, or pressure ulcer) must be documented by the patient's provider.

R40.20 Unspecified coma HCC
Coma NOS
Unconsciousness NOS
6 **R40.21 Coma scale, eyes open**

The following appropriate 7th character is to be added to subcategory R40.21-:
0 unspecified time
1 in the field [EMT or ambulance]
2 at arrival to emergency department
3 at hospital admission
4 24 hours or more after hospital admission

AHA: 2Q 2015, 18

▲ 7 **R40.211- Coma scale, eyes open, never** HCC
Coma scale eye opening score of 1
▲ 7 **R40.212- Coma scale, eyes open, to pain** HCC
Coma scale eye opening score of 2
▲ 7 **R40.213- Coma scale, eyes open, to sound**
Coma scale eye opening score of 3
▲ 7 **R40.214- Coma scale, eyes open, spontaneous**
Coma scale eye opening score of 4

6 **R40.22** **Coma scale, best verbal response**

The following appropriate 7th character is to be added to subcategory R40.22-:
0 unspecified time
1 in the field [EMT or ambulance]
2 at arrival to emergency department
3 at hospital admission
4 24 hours or more after hospital admission

AHA: 2Q 2015, 18
AHA: 4Q 2017, 18

▲ 7 **R40.221-** **Coma scale, best verbal response, none** HCC
Coma scale verbal score of 1

▲ 7 **R40.222-** **Coma scale, best verbal response, incomprehensible words** HCC
Coma scale verbal score of 2
Incomprehensible sounds (2-5 years of age)
Moans/grunts to pain; restless (<2 years old)

▲ 7 **R40.223-** **Coma scale, best verbal response, inappropriate words**
Coma scale verbal score of 3
Inappropriate crying or screaming (< 2 years of age)
Screaming (2-5 years of age)

▲ 7 **R40.224-** **Coma scale, best verbal response, confused conversation**
Coma scale verbal score of 4
Inappropriate words (2-5 years of age)
Irritable cries (< 2 years of age)

▲ 7 **R40.225-** **Coma scale, best verbal response, oriented**
Coma scale verbal score of 5
Cooing or babbling or crying appropriately (< 2 years of age)
Uses appropriate words (2- 5 years of age)

6 **R40.23** **Coma scale, best motor response**

The following appropriate 7th character is to be added to subcategory R40.23-:
0 unspecified time
1 in the field [EMT or ambulance]
2 at arrival to emergency department
3 at hospital admission
4 24 hours or more after hospital admission

AHA: 2Q 2015, 18
AHA: 4Q 2017, 18

▲ 7 **R40.231-** **Coma scale, best motor response, none** HCC
Coma scale motor score of 1

▲ 7 **R40.232-** **Coma scale, best motor response, extension** HCC
Abnormal extensor posturing to pain or noxious stimuli (< 2 years of age)
Coma scale motor score of 2
Extensor posturing to pain or noxious stimuli (2-5 years of age)

▲ 7 **R40.233-** **Coma scale, best motor response, abnormal flexion**
Abnormal flexure posturing to pain or noxious stimuli (2-5 years of age)
Coma scale motor score of 3
Flexion/decorticate posturing (< 2 years of age)

▲ 7 **R40.234-** **Coma scale, best motor response, flexion withdrawal** HCC
Coma scale motor score of 4
Withdraws from pain or noxious stimuli (2-5 years of age)

▲ 7 **R40.235-** **Coma scale, best motor response, localizes pain**
Coma scale motor score of 5
Localizes pain (2-5 years of age)
Withdraws to touch (< 2 years of age)

▲ 7 **R40.236-** **Coma scale, best motor response, obeys commands**
Coma scale motor score of 6
Normal or spontaneous movement (< 2 years of age)
Obeys commands (2-5 years of age)

6 **R40.24** **Glasgow coma scale, total score**
Note: Assign a code from subcategory R40.24, when only the total coma score is documented

The following appropriate 7th character is to be added to subcategory R40.24-:
0 unspecified time
1 in the field [EMT or ambulance]
2 at arrival to emergency department
3 at hospital admission
4 24 hours or more after hospital admission

AHA: 2Q 2015, 18
AHA: 4Q 2016, 64

7 **R40.241-** **Glasgow coma scale score 13-15**
7 **R40.242-** **Glasgow coma scale score 9-12**
7 **R40.243-** **Glasgow coma scale score 3-8** HCC
7 **R40.244-** **Other coma, without documented Glasgow coma scale score, or with partial score reported** HCC

R40.3 **Persistent vegetative state** HCC

CODING TIP ✓ Assign code R40.3 only when the physician has specifically confirmed persistent vegetative state (PVS). Also note that PVS differs from coma.

R40.4 **Transient alteration of awareness**

4 **R41** **Other symptoms and signs involving cognitive functions and awareness**

EXCLUDES 1 *dissociative [conversion] disorders (F44.-)*
mild cognitive impairment, so stated (G31.84)

R41.0 **Disorientation, unspecified**
Confusion NOS
Delirium NOS

R41.1 **Anterograde amnesia**

R41.2 **Retrograde amnesia**

R41.3 **Other amnesia**
Amnesia NOS
Memory loss NOS

EXCLUDES 1 *amnestic disorder due to known physiologic condition (F04)*
amnestic syndrome due to psychoactive substance use (F10-F19 with 5th character .6)
mild memory disturbance due to known physiological condition (F06.8)
transient global amnesia (G45.4)

R41.4 **Neurologic neglect syndrome**
Asomatognosia
Hemi-akinesia
Hemi-inattention
Hemispatial neglect
Left-sided neglect
Sensory neglect
Visuospatial neglect

EXCLUDES 1 *visuospatial deficit (R41.842)*

5 **R41.8** **Other symptoms and signs involving cognitive functions and awareness**

R41.81 **Age-related cognitive decline** A
Senility NOS

R41.82 **Altered mental status, unspecified**
Change in mental status NOS

EXCLUDES 1 *altered level of consciousness (R40.-)*
altered mental status due to known condition - code to condition
delirium NOS (R41.0)

AHA: 4Q 2012, 98

R41.83 **Borderline intellectual functioning**
IQ level 71 to 84

EXCLUDES 1 *intellectual disabilities (F70-F79)*

6 **R41.84** **Other specified cognitive deficit**

EXCLUDES 1 *cognitive deficits as sequelae of cerebrovascular disease (I69.01-, I69.11-, I69.21-, I69.31-, I69.81-, I69.91-)*

R41.840 **Attention and concentration deficit**

EXCLUDES 1 *attention-deficit hyperactivity disorders (F90.-)*

R41.841 **Cognitive communication deficit**

R41.842 Visuospatial deficit
R41.843 Psychomotor deficit
R41.844 Frontal lobe and executive function deficit
R41.89 Other symptoms and signs involving cognitive functions and awareness
Anosognosia
R41.9 Unspecified symptoms and signs involving cognitive functions and awareness
Unspecified neurocognitive disorder

R42 Dizziness and giddiness
Light-headedness
Vertigo NOS
EXCLUDES 1 *vertiginous syndromes (H81.-)*
vertigo from infrasound (T75.23)

R43 Disturbances of smell and taste
R43.0 Anosmia
R43.1 Parosmia
R43.2 Parageusia
R43.8 Other disturbances of smell and taste
Mixed disturbance of smell and taste
R43.9 Unspecified disturbances of smell and taste

R44 Other symptoms and signs involving general sensations and perceptions
EXCLUDES 1 *alcoholic hallucinations (F1.5)*
hallucinations in drug psychosis (F11-F19 with .5)
hallucinations in mood disorders with psychotic symptoms (F30.2, F31.5, F32.3, F33.3)
hallucinations in schizophrenia, schizotypal and delusional disorders (F20-F29)
EXCLUDES 2 *disturbances of skin sensation (R20.-)*
R44.0 Auditory hallucinations
R44.1 Visual hallucinations
R44.2 Other hallucinations
R44.3 Hallucinations, unspecified
R44.8 Other symptoms and signs involving general sensations and perceptions
R44.9 Unspecified symptoms and signs involving general sensations and perceptions

R45 Symptoms and signs involving emotional state
R45.0 Nervousness
Nervous tension
R45.1 Restlessness and agitation
R45.2 Unhappiness
R45.3 Demoralization and apathy
EXCLUDES 1 *anhedonia (R45.84)*
R45.4 Irritability and anger
R45.5 Hostility
R45.6 Violent behavior
R45.7 State of emotional shock and stress, unspecified
R45.8 Other symptoms and signs involving emotional state
R45.81 Low self-esteem
R45.82 Worries
R45.83 Excessive crying of child, adolescent or adult
EXCLUDES 1 *excessive crying of infant (baby) R68.11*
R45.84 Anhedonia
R45.85 Homicidal and suicidal ideations
EXCLUDES 1 *suicide attempt (T14.91)*
R45.850 Homicidal ideations
R45.851 Suicidal ideations
R45.86 Emotional lability
R45.87 Impulsiveness
R45.89 Other symptoms and signs involving emotional state

R46 Symptoms and signs involving appearance and behavior
EXCLUDES 1 *appearance and behavior in schizophrenia, schizotypal and delusional disorders (F20-F29)*
mental and behavioral disorders (F01-F99)
R46.0 Very low level of personal hygiene
R46.1 Bizarre personal appearance
R46.2 Strange and inexplicable behavior
R46.3 Overactivity
R46.4 Slowness and poor responsiveness
EXCLUDES 1 *stupor (R40.1)*
R46.5 Suspiciousness and marked evasiveness
R46.6 Undue concern and preoccupation with stressful events
R46.7 Verbosity and circumstantial detail obscuring reason for contact
R46.8 Other symptoms and signs involving appearance and behavior
R46.81 Obsessive-compulsive behavior
EXCLUDES 1 *obsessive-compulsive disorder (F42-)*
CODING TIP ✓ Do not assign R46.81 for obsessive compulsive disorder, which is a specific syndrome coded to F42. R46.81 indicates the presence of behaviors in the absence of a specific diagnosis.
R46.89 Other symptoms and signs involving appearance and behavior

Symptoms and signs involving speech and voice (R47-R49)

R47 Speech disturbances, not elsewhere classified
EXCLUDES 1 *autism (F84.0)*
cluttering (F80.81)
specific developmental disorders of speech and language (F80.-)
stuttering (F80.81)
R47.0 Dysphasia and aphasia
R47.01 Aphasia
EXCLUDES 1 *aphasia following cerebrovascular disease (I69. with final characters -20)*
progressive isolated aphasia (G31.01)
DEFINITION The inability to speak, write, or understand spoken or written language.
R47.02 Dysphasia
EXCLUDES 1 *dysphasia following cerebrovascular disease (I69. with final characters -21)*
R47.1 Dysarthria and anarthria
EXCLUDES 1 *dysarthria following cerebrovascular disease (I69. with final characters -22)*
R47.8 Other speech disturbances
EXCLUDES 1 *dysarthria following cerebrovascular disease (I69. with final characters -28)*
R47.81 Slurred speech
R47.82 *Fluency disorder in conditions classified elsewhere*
Stuttering in conditions classified elsewhere
Code first underlying disease or condition, such as:
Parkinson's disease (G20)
EXCLUDES 1 *adult onset fluency disorder (F98.5)*
childhood onset fluency disorder (F80.81)
fluency disorder (stuttering) following cerebrovascular disease (I69. with final characters -23)
R47.89 Other speech disturbances
R47.9 Unspecified speech disturbances

R48 Dyslexia and other symbolic dysfunctions, not elsewhere classified
EXCLUDES 1 *specific developmental disorders of scholastic skills (F81.-)*
R48.0 Dyslexia and alexia
R48.1 Agnosia
Astereognosia (astereognosis)
Autotopagnosia
EXCLUDES 1 *visual object agnosia (R48.3)*
R48.2 Apraxia
EXCLUDES 1 *apraxia following cerebrovascular disease (I69. with final characters -90)*
R48.3 Visual agnosia
Prosopagnosia
Simultanagnosia (asimultagnosia)
R48.8 Other symbolic dysfunctions
Acalculia
Agraphia
R48.9 Unspecified symbolic dysfunctions

R49 Voice and resonance disorders

EXCLUDES 1 *psychogenic voice and resonance disorders (F44.4)*

R49.0 Dysphonia
Hoarseness

R49.1 Aphonia
Loss of voice

DEFINITION Inability to produce vocal sounds.

R49.2 Hypernasality and hyponasality

R49.21 Hypernasality

R49.22 Hyponasality

R49.8 Other voice and resonance disorders

R49.9 Unspecified voice and resonance disorder
Change in voice NOS
Resonance disorder NOS

General symptoms and signs (R50-R69)

R50 Fever of other and unknown origin

EXCLUDES 1 *chills without fever (R68.83)*
febrile convulsions (R56.0-)
fever of unknown origin during labor (O75.2)
fever of unknown origin in newborn (P81.9)
hypothermia due to illness (R68.0)
malignant hyperthermia due to anesthesia (T88.3)
puerperal pyrexia NOS (O86.4)

R50.2 Drug induced fever
Use additional code for adverse effect, if applicable, to identify drug (T36-T50 with fifth or sixth character 5)

EXCLUDES 1 *postvaccination (postimmunization) fever (R50.83)*

R50.8 Other specified fever

R50.81 *Fever presenting with conditions classified elsewhere*
Code first underlying condition when associated fever is present, such as with:
leukemia (C91-C95)
neutropenia (D70.-)
sickle-cell disease (D57.-)
AHA: 4Q 2014, 22

R50.82 Postprocedural fever

EXCLUDES 1 *postprocedural infection (T81.4-)*
posttransfusion fever (R50.84)
postvaccination (postimmunization) fever (R50.83)

R50.83 Postvaccination fever
Postimmunization fever

R50.84 Febrile nonhemolytic transfusion reaction
FNHTR
Posttransfusion fever

R50.9 Fever, unspecified
Fever NOS
Fever of unknown origin [FUO]
Fever with chills
Fever with rigors
Hyperpyrexia NOS
Persistent fever
Pyrexia NOS

CODING TIP ✓ When an infection causing a fever has been diagnosed, do not assign R50.9, but instead code the causative infectious disease specifically.

R51 Headache
Facial pain NOS

EXCLUDES 1 *atypical face pain (G50.1)*
migraine and other headache syndromes (G43-G44)
trigeminal neuralgia (G50.0)

R52 Pain, unspecified
Acute pain NOS
Generalized pain NOS
Pain NOS

EXCLUDES 1 *acute and chronic pain, not elsewhere classified (G89.-)*
localized pain, unspecified type - code to pain by site, such as:
abdomen pain (R10.-)
back pain (M54.9)
breast pain (N64.4)
chest pain (R07.1-R07.9)
ear pain (H92.0-)
eye pain (H57.1)
headache (R51)
joint pain (M25.5-)
limb pain (M79.6-)
lumbar region pain (M54.5)
pelvic and perineal pain (R10.2)
shoulder pain (M25.51-)
spine pain (M54.-)
throat pain (R07.0)
tongue pain (K14.6)
tooth pain (K08.8)
renal colic (N23)
pain disorders exclusively related to psychological factors (F45.41)

CODING TIP ✓ R52 should not be coded to identify pain when the underlying cause of pain is known. Code the specific cause of the pain when a diagnosis is present for the cause, such as osteoarthritis. Pay special attention to the Excludes 1 note.

R53 Malaise and fatigue

R53.0 Neoplastic (malignant) related fatigue
Code first:
associated neoplasm

R53.1 Weakness
Asthenia NOS

EXCLUDES 1 *age-related weakness (R54)*
muscle weakness (M62.8-)
sarcopenia (M62.84)
senile asthenia (R54)

CODING TIP ✓ Also known as general weakness. If code R53.1 is used to support therapy, documentation should establish medical necessity. The condition may include excessive tiredness, lacking energy, listlessness, and/or sleepiness. Excludes generalized muscle weakness. Generally used for patients with cardiorespiratory diseases. May be part of many different illnesses, including the flu, pneumonia, congestive heart failure (CHF) and arteriosclerotic heart disease (ASHD).

CODING TIP ✓ Do not assign R53.1 to indicate muscle weakness or weakness resulting as a sequela of a cerebral vascular accident. Muscle weakness is coded to M62.8-.

R53.2 Functional quadriplegia HCC
Complete immobility due to severe physical disability or frailty

EXCLUDES 1 *frailty NOS (R54)*
hysterical paralysis (F44.4)
immobility syndrome (M62.3)
neurologic quadriplegia (G82.5-)
quadriplegia (G82.50)

DEFINITION Inability to move due to non-neurological condition, such as severe spasticity, arthritis, or severe muscle contracture.

AHA: 2Q 2016, 6

R53.8 Other malaise and fatigue

EXCLUDES 1 *combat exhaustion and fatigue (F43.0)*
congenital debility (P96.9)
exhaustion and fatigue due to excessive exertion (T73.3)
exhaustion and fatigue due to exposure (T73.2)
exhaustion and fatigue due to heat (T67.-)
exhaustion and fatigue due to pregnancy (O26.8-)
exhaustion and fatigue due to recurrent depressive episode (F33)
exhaustion and fatigue due to senile debility (R54)

R53.81 Other malaise
Chronic debility
Debility NOS
General physical deterioration
Malaise NOS
Nervous debility
EXCLUDES 1 *age-related physical debility (R54)*

CODING TIP✓ Note that debility is a non-specific condition characterized by weight loss, functional decline, malnutrition and multiple chronic conditions. Coding a non-specific diagnosis such as this should be avoided if possible. If the diagnosis causing the debility is known, code that condition.

R53.82 Chronic fatigue, unspecified
Chronic fatigue syndrome NOS
EXCLUDES 1 *postviral fatigue syndrome (G93.3)*

R53.83 Other fatigue
Fatigue NOS
Lack of energy
Lethargy
Tiredness
EXCLUDES 2 *exhaustion and fatigue due to depressive episode (F32.-)*

R54 Age-related physical debility A
Frailty
Old age
Senescence
Senile asthenia
Senile debility
EXCLUDES 1 *age-related cognitive decline (R41.81)*
sarcopenia (M62.84)
senile psychosis (F03)
senility NOS (R41.81)

CODING TIP✓ Note that debility is a non-specific condition characterized by weight loss, functional decline, malnutrition and multiple chronic conditions. Coding a non-specific diagnosis such as this should be avoided if possible. If the diagnosis causing the debility is known, code that condition.

R55 Syncope and collapse
Blackout
Fainting
Vasovagal attack
EXCLUDES 1 *cardiogenic shock (R57.0)*
carotid sinus syncope (G90.01)
heat syncope (T67.1)
neurocirculatory asthenia (F45.8)
neurogenic orthostatic hypotension (G90.3)
orthostatic hypotension (I95.1)
postprocedural shock (T81.1-)
psychogenic syncope (F48.8)
shock NOS (R57.9)
shock complicating or following abortion or ectopic or molar pregnancy (O00-O07, O08.3)
shock complicating or following labor and delivery (O75.1)
Stokes-Adams attack (I45.9)
unconsciousness NOS (R40.2-)

DEFINITION Fainting and collapse due to a lack of blood flow to the brain.

R56 Convulsions, not elsewhere classified
EXCLUDES 1 *dissociative convulsions and seizures (F44.5)*
epileptic convulsions and seizures (G40.-)
newborn convulsions and seizures (P90)

R56.0 Febrile convulsions

DEFINITION A convulsion accompanying high fever, characterized by loss of consciousness with stiffness and jerking of the limbs. The skin may become pale or turn blue. Once the jerking subsides, the child goes limp and then normal color and consciousness return.

R56.00 Simple febrile convulsions HCC
Febrile convulsion NOS
Febrile seizure NOS

R56.01 Complex febrile convulsions HCC
Atypical febrile seizure
Complex febrile seizure
Complicated febrile seizure
EXCLUDES 1 *status epilepticus (G40.901)*

R56.1 Post traumatic seizures HCC
EXCLUDES 1 *post traumatic epilepsy (G40.-)*

R56.9 Unspecified convulsions HCC
Convulsion disorder
Fit NOS
Recurrent convulsions
Seizure(s) (convulsive) NOS

CODING TIP✓ Do not assign R56.9 when a patient has had recurrent seizures or a seizure disorder. When recurrent seizures or seizure disorder are present, report the appropriate code from category G40.-.

R57 Shock, not elsewhere classified
EXCLUDES 1 *anaphylactic shock NOS (T78.2)*
anaphylactic reaction or shock due to adverse food reaction (T78.0-)
anaphylactic shock due to adverse effect of correct drug or medicament properly administered (T88.6)
anaphylactic shock due to serum (T80.5-)
anesthetic shock (T88.3)
electric shock (T75.4)
obstetric shock (O75.1)
postprocedural shock (T81.1-)
psychic shock (F43.0)
shock complicating or following ectopic or molar pregnancy (O00-O07, O08.3)
shock due to lightning (T75.01)
traumatic shock (T79.4)
toxic shock syndrome (A48.3)

R57.0 Cardiogenic shock HCC
EXCLUDES 2 *septic shock (R65.21)*

R57.1 Hypovolemic shock HCC

R57.8 Other shock HCC

R57.9 Shock, unspecified HCC
Failure of peripheral circulation NOS

R58 Hemorrhage, not elsewhere classified
Hemorrhage NOS
EXCLUDES 1 *hemorrhage included with underlying conditions, such as:*
acute duodenal ulcer with hemorrhage (K26.0)
acute gastritis with bleeding (K29.01)
ulcerative enterocolitis with rectal bleeding (K51.01)

R59 Enlarged lymph nodes
INCLUDES swollen glands
EXCLUDES 1 *lymphadenitis NOS (I88.9)*
acute lymphadenitis (L04.-)
chronic lymphadenitis (I88.1)
mesenteric (acute) (chronic) lymphadenitis (I88.0)

R59.0 Localized enlarged lymph nodes

R59.1 Generalized enlarged lymph nodes
Lymphadenopathy NOS

R59.9 Enlarged lymph nodes, unspecified

[4] **R60 Edema, not elsewhere classified**

EXCLUDES 1 *angioneurotic edema (T78.3)*
ascites (R18.-)
cerebral edema (G93.6)
cerebral edema due to birth injury (P11.0)
edema of larynx (J38.4)
edema of nasopharynx (J39.2)
edema of pharynx (J39.2)
gestational edema (O12.0-)
hereditary edema (Q82.0)
hydrops fetalis NOS (P83.2)
hydrothorax (J94.8)
hydrops fetalis NOS (P83.2)
newborn edema (P83.3)
pulmonary edema (J81.-)

R60.0 Localized edema

CODING TIP ✓ Do not report R60.0 in a patient with heart failure or any other known cause for the edema.

R60.1 Generalized edema

EXCLUDES 2 *nutritional edema (E40-E46)*

Generalized edema

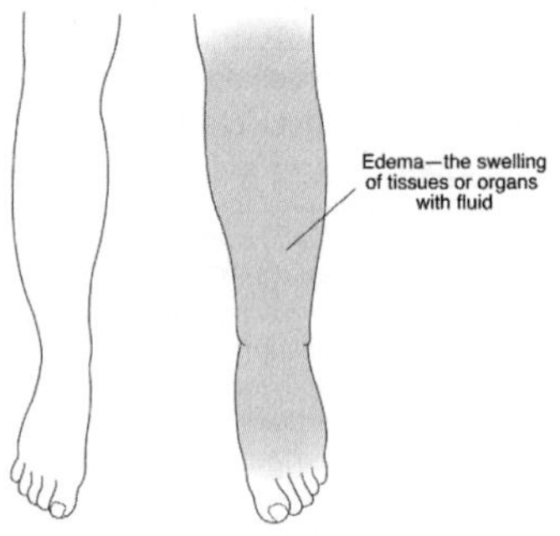
Edema—the swelling of tissues or organs with fluid

R60.9 Edema, unspecified
Fluid retention NOS

R61 Generalized hyperhidrosis
Excessive sweating
Night sweats
Secondary hyperhidrosis
Code first:
, if applicable, menopausal and female climacteric states (N95.1)

EXCLUDES 1 *focal (primary) (secondary) hyperhidrosis (L74.5-)*
Frey's syndrome (L74.52)
localized (primary) (secondary) hyperhidrosis (L74.5-)

[4] **R62 Lack of expected normal physiological development in childhood and adults**

EXCLUDES 1 *delayed puberty (E30.0)*
gonadal dysgenesis (Q99.1)
hypopituitarism (E23.0)

R62.0 Delayed milestone in childhood P
Delayed attainment of expected physiological developmental stage
Late talker
Late walker

[5] **R62.5 Other and unspecified lack of expected normal physiological development in childhood**

EXCLUDES 1 *HIV disease resulting in failure to thrive (B20)*
physical retardation due to malnutrition (E45)

R62.50 Unspecified lack of expected normal physiological development in childhood
Infantilism NOS

R62.51 Failure to thrive (child) P
Failure to gain weight

EXCLUDES 1 *failure to thrive in child under 28 days old (P92.6)*

R62.52 Short stature (child)
Lack of growth
Physical retardation
Short stature NOS

EXCLUDES 1 *short stature due to endocrine disorder (E34.3)*

R62.59 Other lack of expected normal physiological development in childhood

R62.7 Adult failure to thrive A

CODING TIP ✓ When coding failure to thrive, identify the conditions leading to the patient's failure to thrive and code these underlying conditions first.

[4] **R63 Symptoms and signs concerning food and fluid intake**

EXCLUDES 1 *bulimia NOS (F50.2)*
eating disorders of nonorganic origin (F50.-)
malnutrition (E40-E46)

R63.0 Anorexia
Loss of appetite

EXCLUDES 1 *anorexia nervosa (F50.0-)*
loss of appetite of nonorganic origin (F50.89)

CODING TIP ✓ Anorexia indicates a loss of appetite or intake resulting from appetite loss. Note that anorexia nervosa, which is coded to F50.0-, differs from anorexia coded to R63.0 in that anorexia nervosa includes a psychological component of body image disturbance.

R63.1 Polydipsia
Excessive thirst

R63.2 Polyphagia
Excessive eating
Hyperalimentation NOS

R63.3 Feeding difficulties
Feeding problem (elderly) (infant) NOS
Picky eater

EXCLUDES 1 *eating disorders (F50.-)*
feeding problems of newborn (P92.-)
infant feeding disorder of nonorganic origin (F98.2-)

AHA: 3Q 2016, 19
AHA: 1Q 2017, 28

R63.4 Abnormal weight loss

R63.5 Abnormal weight gain

EXCLUDES 1 *excessive weight gain in pregnancy (O26.0-)*
obesity (E66.-)

R63.6 Underweight
Use additional code to identify body mass index (BMI), if known (Z68.-)

EXCLUDES 1 *abnormal weight loss (R63.4)*
anorexia nervosa (F50.0-)
malnutrition (E40-E46)

R63.8 Other symptoms and signs concerning food and fluid intake

R64 Cachexia HCC
Wasting syndrome
Code first:
underlying condition, if known

EXCLUDES 1 *abnormal weight loss (R63.4)*
nutritional marasmus (E41)

AHA: 3Q 2017, 24

[4] **R65 Symptoms and signs specifically associated with systemic inflammation and infection**

GUIDELINES **Section I.C.1.d.6)**
Only one code from category R65, Symptoms and signs specifically associated with systemic inflammation and infection, should be assigned. Therefore, when a non-infectious condition leads to an infection resulting in severe sepsis, assign the appropriate code from subcategory R65.2, Severe sepsis. Do not additionally assign a code from subcategory R65.1, Systemic inflammatory response syndrome (SIRS) of noninfectious origin.

[5] **R65.1 Systemic inflammatory response syndrome (SIRS) of non-infectious origin**
Code first underlying condition, such as:
heatstroke (T67.0)
injury and trauma (S00-T88)

EXCLUDES 1 *sepsis- code to infection*
severe sepsis (R65.2)

CODING TIP✓ Systemic inflammatory response syndrome (SIRS) is defined as two or more of the following: fever <38° C or >36°C, heart rate >90 beats/min, respirations >30/min or PaCO2 < 32mmHg and/or abnormal white blood cell count.

R65.10 **Systemic inflammatory response syndrome (SIRS) of non-infectious origin without acute organ dysfunction** HCC
Systemic inflammatory response syndrome (SIRS) NOS

R65.11 **Systemic inflammatory response syndrome (SIRS) of non-infectious origin with acute organ dysfunction** HCC
Use additional code to identify specific acute organ dysfunction, such as:
acute kidney failure (N17.-)
acute respiratory failure (J96.0-)
critical illness myopathy (G72.81)
critical illness polyneuropathy (G62.81)
disseminated intravascular coagulopathy [DIC] (D65)
encephalopathy (metabolic) (septic) (G93.41)
hepatic failure (K72.0-)

GUIDELINES **Section I.C.18.g**
The systemic inflammatory response syndrome (SIRS) can develop as a result of certain non-infectious disease processes, such as trauma, malignant neoplasm, or pancreatitis. When SIRS is documented with a noninfectious condition, and no subsequent infection is documented, the code for the underlying condition, such as an injury, should be assigned, followed by code R65.10, Systemic inflammatory response syndrome (SIRS) of non-infectious origin without acute organ dysfunction, or code R65.11, Systemic inflammatory response syndrome (SIRS) of non-infectious origin with acute organ dysfunction. If an associated acute organ dysfunction is documented, the appropriate code(s) for the specific type of organ dysfunction(s) should be assigned in addition to code R65.11. If acute organ dysfunction is documented, but it cannot be determined if the acute organ dysfunction is associated with SIRS or due to another condition (e.g., directly due to the trauma), the provider should be queried.

5 **R65.2** **Severe sepsis**
Infection with associated acute organ dysfunction
Sepsis with acute organ dysfunction
Sepsis with multiple organ dysfunction
Systemic inflammatory response syndrome due to infectious process with acute organ dysfunction
Code first underlying infection, such as:
infection following a procedure (T81.4-)
infections following infusion, transfusion and therapeutic injection (T80.2-)
puerperal sepsis (O85)
sepsis following complete or unspecified spontaneous abortion (O03.87)
sepsis following ectopic and molar pregnancy (O08.82)
sepsis following incomplete spontaneous abortion (O03.37)
sepsis following (induced) termination of pregnancy (O04.87)
sepsis NOS (A41.9)
Use additional code to identify specific acute organ dysfunction, such as:
acute kidney failure (N17.-)
acute respiratory failure (J96.0-)
critical illness myopathy (G72.81)
critical illness polyneuropathy (G62.81)
disseminated intravascular coagulopathy [DIC] (D65)
encephalopathy (metabolic) (septic) (G93.41)
hepatic failure (K72.0-)

GUIDELINES **Section I.C.1.d.1)(b)**
The coding of severe sepsis requires a minimum of two codes: first a code for the underlying systemic infection, followed by a code from subcategory R65.2, Severe sepsis. If the causal organism is not documented, assign code A41.9, Sepsis, unspecified organism, for the infection. Additional code(s) for the associated acute organ dysfunction are also required. Due to the complex nature of severe sepsis, some cases may require querying the provider prior to assignment of the codes.

GUIDELINES **Section I.C.1.d.1)(a)(iv)**
If a patient has sepsis and an acute organ dysfunction, but the medical record documentation indicates that the acute organ dysfunction is related to a medical condition other than the sepsis, do not assign a code from subcategory R65.2, Severe sepsis. An acute organ dysfunction must be associated with the sepsis in order to assign the severe sepsis code. If the documentation is not clear as to whether an acute organ dysfunction is related to the sepsis or another medical condition, query the provider.

GUIDELINES **Section I.C.1.d.4)**
If the reason for admission is both sepsis or severe sepsis and a localized infection, such as pneumonia or cellulitis, a code(s) for the underlying systemic infection should be assigned first and the code for the localized infection should be assigned as a secondary diagnosis. If the patient has severe sepsis, a code from subcategory R65.2 should also be assigned as a secondary diagnosis. If the patient is admitted with a localized infection, such as pneumonia, and sepsis/severe sepsis doesn't develop until after admission, the localized infection should be assigned first, followed by the appropriate sepsis/severe sepsis codes.

CODING TIP✓ When severe sepsis is present in a patient (sepsis with the additional presence of organ dysfunction, hypotension, or hypoperfusion), a code from R65.2- must be assigned in addition to the code identifying the underlying infection. An additional code(s) also should be assigned to identify all organ dysfunction present.
AHA: 3Q 2016, 8-9

R65.20 **Severe sepsis without septic shock** HCC
Severe sepsis NOS

GUIDELINES **Section I.C.1.d.5)(b-c)**
For infections following a procedure, a code from T81.40, to T81.43 Infection following a procedure, or a code from O86.00 to O86.03, Infection of obstetric surgical wound, that identifies the site of the infection should be coded first, if known. Assign an additional code for sepsis following a procedure (T81.44) or sepsis following an obstetrical procedure (O86.04). Use an additional code to identify the infectious agent. If the patient has severe sepsis, the appropriate code from subcategory R65.2 should also be assigned with the additional code(s) for any acute organ dysfunction.

If a postprocedural infection has resulted in postprocedural septic shock, assign the codes indicated above for sepsis due to a postprocedural infection, followed by code T81.12-, Postprocedural septic shock. Do not assign code R65.21, Severe sepsis with septic shock. Additional code(s) should be assigned for any acute organ dysfunction.
AHA: 3Q 2016, 14

R65.21 **Severe sepsis with septic shock** HCC

GUIDELINES **Section I.C.1.d.2)(a)**
Septic shock generally refers to circulatory failure associated with severe sepsis, and therefore, it represents a type of acute organ dysfunction. For cases of septic shock, the code for the systemic infection should be sequenced first, followed by code R65.21, Severe sepsis with septic shock or code T81.12, Postprocedural septic shock. Any additional codes for the other acute organ dysfunctions should also be assigned. As noted in the sequencing instructions in the Tabular List, the code for septic shock cannot be assigned as a principal diagnosis.

4 R68 Other general symptoms and signs

R68.0 Hypothermia, not associated with low environmental temperature
EXCLUDES 1 *hypothermia NOS (accidental) (T68)*
hypothermia due to anesthesia (T88.51)
hypothermia due to low environmental temperature (T68)
newborn hypothermia (P80.-)

5 R68.1 Nonspecific symptoms peculiar to infancy
EXCLUDES 1 *colic, infantile (R10.83)*
neonatal cerebral irritability (P91.3)
teething syndrome (K00.7)

R68.11 Excessive crying of infant (baby) P
EXCLUDES 1 *excessive crying of child, adolescent, or adult (R45.83)*

R68.12 Fussy infant (baby) P
Irritable infant

R68.13 Apparent life threatening event in infant (ALTE) P
Apparent life threatening event in newborn
Brief resolved unexplained event (BRUE)
Code first:
confirmed diagnosis, if known
Use additional code(s) for associated signs and symptoms if no confirmed diagnosis established, or if signs and symptoms are not associated routinely with confirmed diagnosis, or provide additional information for cause of ALTE

R68.19 Other nonspecific symptoms peculiar to infancy P

R68.2 Dry mouth, unspecified
EXCLUDES 1 *dry mouth due to dehydration (E86.0)*
dry mouth due to sicca syndrome [Sjögren] (M35.0-)
salivary gland hyposecretion (K11.7)

R68.3 Clubbing of fingers
Clubbing of nails
EXCLUDES 1 *congenital clubfinger (Q68.1)*

5 R68.8 Other general symptoms and signs

R68.81 Early satiety

R68.82 Decreased libido A
Decreased sexual desire

R68.83 Chills (without fever)
Chills NOS
EXCLUDES 1 *chills with fever (R50.9)*

R68.84 Jaw pain
Mandibular pain
Maxilla pain
EXCLUDES 1 *temporomandibular joint arthralgia (M26.62-)*

R68.89 Other general symptoms and signs

R69 Illness, unspecified
Unknown and unspecified cases of morbidity

Abnormal findings on examination of blood, without diagnosis (R70-R79)

EXCLUDES 2 *abnormal findings on antenatal screening of mother (O28.-)*
abnormalities of lipids (E78.-)
abnormalities of platelets and thrombocytes (D69.-)
abnormalities of white blood cells classified elsewhere (D70-D72)
coagulation hemorrhagic disorders (D65-D68)
diagnostic abnormal findings classified elsewhere - see Alphabetical Index
hemorrhagic and hematological disorders of newborn (P50-P61)

4 R70 Elevated erythrocyte sedimentation rate and abnormality of plasma viscosity

R70.0 Elevated erythrocyte sedimentation rate

R70.1 Abnormal plasma viscosity

4 R71 Abnormality of red blood cells
EXCLUDES 1 *anemias (D50-D64)*
anemia of premature infant (P61.2)
benign (familial) polycythemia (D75.0)
congenital anemias (P61.2-P61.4)
newborn anemia due to isoimmunization (P55.-)
polycythemia neonatorum (P61.1)
polycythemia NOS (D75.1)
polycythemia vera (D45)
secondary polycythemia (D75.1)

R71.0 Precipitous drop in hematocrit
Drop (precipitous) in hemoglobin
Drop in hematocrit

R71.8 Other abnormality of red blood cells
Abnormal red-cell morphology NOS
Abnormal red-cell volume NOS
Anisocytosis
Poikilocytosis

4 R73 Elevated blood glucose level
EXCLUDES 1 *diabetes mellitus (E08-E13)*
diabetes mellitus in pregnancy, childbirth and the puerperium (O24.-)
neonatal disorders (P70.0-P70.2)
postsurgical hypoinsulinemia (E89.1)

5 R73.0 Abnormal glucose
EXCLUDES 1 *abnormal glucose in pregnancy (O99.81-)*
diabetes mellitus (E08-E13)
dysmetabolic syndrome X (E88.81)
gestational diabetes (O24.4-)
glycosuria (R81)
hypoglycemia (E16.2)

R73.01 Impaired fasting glucose
Elevated fasting glucose

R73.02 Impaired glucose tolerance (oral)
Elevated glucose tolerance

R73.03 Prediabetes
Latent diabetes
DEFINITION An elevated blood sugar level that is higher than normal, but not high enough to be diagnosed as type 2 diabetes. When left untreated, prediabetes progresses to type 2 diabetes in less than 10 years. For many people, prediabetes has no signs or symptoms.
AHA: 4Q 2016, 65

R73.09 Other abnormal glucose
Abnormal glucose NOS
Abnormal non-fasting glucose tolerance

R73.9 Hyperglycemia, unspecified
CODING TIP ✓ Hyperglycemia should be coded to R73.9 only when not associated with diabetes mellitus or any form of post-procedural hyperinsulinemia. R73.9 indicates hyperglycemia that is of an unspecified origin.

4 R74 Abnormal serum enzyme levels

R74.0 Nonspecific elevation of levels of transaminase and lactic acid dehydrogenase [LDH]

R74.8 Abnormal levels of other serum enzymes
Abnormal level of acid phosphatase
Abnormal level of alkaline phosphatase
Abnormal level of amylase
Abnormal level of lipase [triacylglycerol lipase]

R74.9 Abnormal serum enzyme level, unspecified

R75 Inconclusive laboratory evidence of human immunodeficiency virus [HIV]
Nonconclusive HIV-test finding in infants
EXCLUDES 1 *asymptomatic human immunodeficiency virus [HIV] infection status (Z21)*
human immunodeficiency virus [HIV] disease (B20)

GUIDELINES **Section I.C.1.a.2)(e)**
Patients with inconclusive HIV serology, but no definitive diagnosis or manifestations of the illness, may be assigned code R75, Inconclusive laboratory evidence of human immunodeficiency virus [HIV].

GUIDELINES Section I.C.1.a.2)(f)
Patients previously diagnosed with any HIV illness (B20) should never be assigned to R75 or Z21, Asymptomatic human immunodeficiency virus [HIV] infection status.

4 R76 Other abnormal immunological findings in serum

R76.0 Raised antibody titer
EXCLUDES 1 *isoimmunization in pregnancy (O36.0-O36.1)*
isoimmunization affecting newborn (P55.-)

5 R76.1 Nonspecific reaction to test for tuberculosis

R76.11 Nonspecific reaction to tuberculin skin test without active tuberculosis
Abnormal result of Mantoux test
PPD positive
Tuberculin (skin test) positive
Tuberculin (skin test) reactor
EXCLUDES 1 *nonspecific reaction to cell mediated immunity measurement of gamma interferon antigen response without active tuberculosis (R76.12)*

R76.12 Nonspecific reaction to cell mediated immunity measurement of gamma interferon antigen response without active tuberculosis
Nonspecific reaction to QuantiFERON-TB test (QFT) without active tuberculosis
EXCLUDES 1 *nonspecific reaction to tuberculin skin test without active tuberculosis (R76.11)*
positive tuberculin skin test (R76.11)

R76.8 Other specified abnormal immunological findings in serum
Raised level of immunoglobulins NOS

R76.9 Abnormal immunological finding in serum, unspecified

▲ 4 R77 Other abnormalities of plasma proteins
EXCLUDES 1 *disorders of plasma-protein metabolism (E88.0-)*

R77.0 Abnormality of albumin

R77.1 Abnormality of globulin
Hyperglobulinemia NOS

R77.2 Abnormality of alphafetoprotein

R77.8 Other specified abnormalities of plasma proteins

R77.9 Abnormality of plasma protein, unspecified

4 R78 Findings of drugs and other substances, not normally found in blood
Use additional code to identify the any retained foreign body, if applicable (Z18.-)
EXCLUDES 1 *mental or behavioral disorders due to psychoactive substance use (F10-F19)*

R78.0 Finding of alcohol in blood
Use additional external cause code (Y90.-), for detail regarding alcohol level.

R78.1 Finding of opiate drug in blood

R78.2 Finding of cocaine in blood

R78.3 Finding of hallucinogen in blood

R78.4 Finding of other drugs of addictive potential in blood

R78.5 Finding of other psychotropic drug in blood

R78.6 Finding of steroid agent in blood

5 R78.7 Finding of abnormal level of heavy metals in blood

R78.71 Abnormal lead level in blood
EXCLUDES 1 *lead poisoning (T56.0-)*

R78.79 Finding of abnormal level of heavy metals in blood

5 R78.8 Finding of other specified substances, not normally found in blood

R78.81 Bacteremia
EXCLUDES 1 *sepsis-code to specified infection*

CODING TIP✓ Do not assign code R78.81 to indicate the presence of sepsis. Bacteremia only indicates the presence of bacteria identified in the bloodstream, not the infectious process. Do not assign R78.81 with any code identifying sepsis. Sepsis should be coded to the appropriate code identifying the specific type of sepsis present.

DEFINITION The presence of small numbers of bacteria in the bloodstream, usually as a temporary condition, and without causing symptoms.

R78.89 Finding of other specified substances, not normally found in blood
Finding of abnormal level of lithium in blood

R78.9 Finding of unspecified substance, not normally found in blood

4 R79 Other abnormal findings of blood chemistry
Use additional code to identify any retained foreign body, if applicable (Z18.-)
EXCLUDES 1 *asymptomatic hyperuricemia (E79.0)*
hyperglycemia NOS (R73.9)
hypoglycemia NOS (E16.2)
neonatal hypoglycemia (P70.3-P70.4)
specific findings indicating disorder of amino-acid metabolism (E70-E72)
specific findings indicating disorder of carbohydrate metabolism (E73-E74)
specific findings indicating disorder of lipid metabolism (E75.-)

R79.0 Abnormal level of blood mineral
Abnormal blood level of cobalt
Abnormal blood level of copper
Abnormal blood level of iron
Abnormal blood level of magnesium
Abnormal blood level of mineral NEC
Abnormal blood level of zinc
EXCLUDES 1 *abnormal level of lithium (R78.89)*
disorders of mineral metabolism (E83.-)
neonatal hypomagnesemia (P71.2)
nutritional mineral deficiency (E58-E61)

R79.1 Abnormal coagulation profile
Abnormal or prolonged bleeding time
Abnormal or prolonged coagulation time
Abnormal or prolonged partial thromboplastin time [PTT]
Abnormal or prolonged prothrombin time [PT]
EXCLUDES 1 *coagulation defects (D68.-)*
EXCLUDES 2 *abnormality of fluid, electrolyte or acid-base balance (E86-E87)*

5 R79.8 Other specified abnormal findings of blood chemistry

R79.81 Abnormal blood-gas level
DEFINITION Abnormal oxygen or carbon dioxide level in the blood.

R79.82 Elevated C-reactive protein (CRP)

R79.89 Other specified abnormal findings of blood chemistry

R79.9 Abnormal finding of blood chemistry, unspecified

Abnormal findings on examination of urine, without diagnosis (R80-R82)

EXCLUDES 1 *abnormal findings on antenatal screening of mother (O28.-)*
diagnostic abnormal findings classified elsewhere - see Alphabetical Index
specific findings indicating disorder of amino-acid metabolism (E70-E72)
specific findings indicating disorder of carbohydrate metabolism (E73-E74)

4 R80 Proteinuria
EXCLUDES 1 *gestational proteinuria (O12.1-)*

R80.0 Isolated proteinuria
Idiopathic proteinuria
EXCLUDES 1 *isolated proteinuria with specific morphological lesion (N06.-)*

R80.1 Persistent proteinuria, unspecified

R80.2 Orthostatic proteinuria, unspecified
Postural proteinuria

R80.3 Bence Jones proteinuria

R80.8 Other proteinuria

R80.9 Proteinuria, unspecified
Albuminuria NOS

R81 Glycosuria
EXCLUDES 1 *renal glycosuria (E74.8)*

4 R82 Other and unspecified abnormal findings in urine
INCLUDES chromoabnormalities in urine
Use additional code to identify any retained foreign body, if applicable (Z18.-)
EXCLUDES 2 *hematuria (R31.-)*

R82.0 Chyluria
EXCLUDES 1 *filarial chyluria (B74.-)*

R82.1 Myoglobinuria

R82.2 Biliuria

R82.3 Hemoglobinuria
EXCLUDES 1 *hemoglobinuria due to hemolysis from external causes NEC (D59.6)*
hemoglobinuria due to paroxysmal nocturnal [Marchiafava-Micheli] (D59.5)

R82.4 Acetonuria
Ketonuria

R82.5 Elevated urine levels of drugs, medicaments and biological substances
Elevated urine levels of catecholamines
Elevated urine levels of indoleacetic acid
Elevated urine levels of 17-ketosteroids
Elevated urine levels of steroids

R82.6 Abnormal urine levels of substances chiefly nonmedicinal as to source
Abnormal urine level of heavy metals

5 **R82.7 Abnormal findings on microbiological examination of urine**
EXCLUDES 1 *colonization status (Z22.-)*
AHA: 4Q 2016, 65

R82.71 Bacteriuria
DEFINITION The presence of bacteria identified in the urine. It affects more women than men and commonly occurs asymptomatically.

R82.79 Other abnormal findings on microbiological examination of urine
Positive culture findings of urine

R82.8 Abnormal findings on cytological and histological examination of urine

5 **R82.9 Other and unspecified abnormal findings in urine**

R82.90 Unspecified abnormal findings in urine

R82.91 Other chromoabnormalities of urine
Chromoconversion (dipstick)
Idiopathic dipstick converts positive for blood with no cellular forms in sediment
EXCLUDES 1 *hemoglobinuria (R82.3)*
myoglobinuria (R82.1)

▲ 6 **R82.99 Other abnormal findings in urine**

● **R82.991 Hypocitraturia**

● **R82.992 Hyperoxaluria**
EXCLUDES 1 *Primary hyperoxaluria (E72.53)*

● **R82.993 Hyperuricosuria**

● **R82.994 Hypercalciuria**
Idiopathic hypercalciuria

● **R82.998 Other abnormal findings in urine**
Cells and casts in urine
Crystalluria
Melanuria

Abnormal findings on examination of other body fluids, substances and tissues, without diagnosis (R83-R89)

EXCLUDES 1 *abnormal findings on antenatal screening of mother (O28.-)*
diagnostic abnormal findings classified elsewhere - see Alphabetical Index

EXCLUDES 2 *abnormal findings on examination of blood, without diagnosis (R70-R79)*
abnormal findings on examination of urine, without diagnosis (R80-R82)
abnormal tumor markers (R97.-)

4 **R83 Abnormal findings in cerebrospinal fluid**

R83.0 Abnormal level of enzymes in cerebrospinal fluid

R83.1 Abnormal level of hormones in cerebrospinal fluid

R83.2 Abnormal level of other drugs, medicaments and biological substances in cerebrospinal fluid

R83.3 Abnormal level of substances chiefly nonmedicinal as to source in cerebrospinal fluid

R83.4 Abnormal immunological findings in cerebrospinal fluid

R83.5 Abnormal microbiological findings in cerebrospinal fluid
Positive culture findings in cerebrospinal fluid
EXCLUDES 1 *colonization status (Z22.-)*

R83.6 Abnormal cytological findings in cerebrospinal fluid

R83.8 Other abnormal findings in cerebrospinal fluid
Abnormal chromosomal findings in cerebrospinal fluid

R83.9 Unspecified abnormal finding in cerebrospinal fluid

4 **R84 Abnormal findings in specimens from respiratory organs and thorax**
INCLUDES abnormal findings in bronchial washings
abnormal findings in nasal secretions
abnormal findings in pleural fluid
abnormal findings in sputum
abnormal findings in throat scrapings
EXCLUDES 1 *blood-stained sputum (R04.2)*

R84.0 Abnormal level of enzymes in specimens from respiratory organs and thorax

R84.1 Abnormal level of hormones in specimens from respiratory organs and thorax

R84.2 Abnormal level of other drugs, medicaments and biological substances in specimens from respiratory organs and thorax

R84.3 Abnormal level of substances chiefly nonmedicinal as to source in specimens from respiratory organs and thorax

R84.4 Abnormal immunological findings in specimens from respiratory organs and thorax

R84.5 Abnormal microbiological findings in specimens from respiratory organs and thorax
Positive culture findings in specimens from respiratory organs and thorax
EXCLUDES 1 *colonization status (Z22.-)*

R84.6 Abnormal cytological findings in specimens from respiratory organs and thorax

R84.7 Abnormal histological findings in specimens from respiratory organs and thorax

R84.8 Other abnormal findings in specimens from respiratory organs and thorax
Abnormal chromosomal findings in specimens from respiratory organs and thorax

R84.9 Unspecified abnormal finding in specimens from respiratory organs and thorax

4 **R85 Abnormal findings in specimens from digestive organs and abdominal cavity**
INCLUDES abnormal findings in peritoneal fluid
abnormal findings in saliva
EXCLUDES 1 *cloudy peritoneal dialysis effluent (R88.0)*
fecal abnormalities (R19.5)

R85.0 Abnormal level of enzymes in specimens from digestive organs and abdominal cavity

R85.1 Abnormal level of hormones in specimens from digestive organs and abdominal cavity

R85.2 Abnormal level of other drugs, medicaments and biological substances in specimens from digestive organs and abdominal cavity

R85.3 Abnormal level of substances chiefly nonmedicinal as to source in specimens from digestive organs and abdominal cavity

R85.4 Abnormal immunological findings in specimens from digestive organs and abdominal cavity

R85.5 Abnormal microbiological findings in specimens from digestive organs and abdominal cavity
Positive culture findings in specimens from digestive organs and abdominal cavity
EXCLUDES 1 *colonization status (Z22.-)*

5 **R85.6 Abnormal cytological findings in specimens from digestive organs and abdominal cavity**

6 **R85.61 Abnormal cytologic smear of anus**

EXCLUDES 1 *abnormal cytological findings in specimens from other digestive organs and abdominal cavity (R85.69)*
carcinoma in situ of anus (histologically confirmed) (D01.3)
anal intraepithelial neoplasia I [AIN I] (K62.82)
anal intraepithelial neoplasia II [AIN II] (K62.82)
anal intraepithelial neoplasia III [AIN III] (D01.3)
dysplasia (mild) (moderate) of anus (histologically confirmed) (K62.82)
severe dysplasia of anus (histologically confirmed) (D01.3)

EXCLUDES 2 *anal high risk human papillomavirus (HPV) DNA test positive (R85.81)*
anal low risk human papillomavirus (HPV) DNA test positive (R85.82)

R85.610 Atypical squamous cells of undetermined significance on cytologic smear of anus (ASC-US)

R85.611 Atypical squamous cells cannot exclude high grade squamous intraepithelial lesion on cytologic smear of anus (ASC-H)

R85.612 Low grade squamous intraepithelial lesion on cytologic smear of anus (LGSIL)

R85.613 High grade squamous intraepithelial lesion on cytologic smear of anus (HGSIL)

R85.614 Cytologic evidence of malignancy on smear of anus

R85.615 Unsatisfactory cytologic smear of anus
Inadequate sample of cytologic smear of anus

R85.616 Satisfactory anal smear but lacking transformation zone

R85.618 Other abnormal cytological findings on specimens from anus

R85.619 Unspecified abnormal cytological findings in specimens from anus
Abnormal anal cytology NOS
Atypical glandular cells of anus NOS

R85.69 Abnormal cytological findings in specimens from other digestive organs and abdominal cavity

R85.7 Abnormal histological findings in specimens from digestive organs and abdominal cavity

5 **R85.8 Other abnormal findings in specimens from digestive organs and abdominal cavity**

R85.81 Anal high risk human papillomavirus (HPV) DNA test positive

EXCLUDES 1 *anogenital warts due to human papillomavirus (HPV) (A63.0)*
condyloma acuminatum (A63.0)

R85.82 Anal low risk human papillomavirus (HPV) DNA test positive
Use additional code for associated human papillomavirus (B97.7)

R85.89 Other abnormal findings in specimens from digestive organs and abdominal cavity
Abnormal chromosomal findings in specimens from digestive organs and abdominal cavity

R85.9 Unspecified abnormal finding in specimens from digestive organs and abdominal cavity

4 R86 Abnormal findings in specimens from male genital organs

INCLUDES abnormal findings in prostatic secretions
abnormal findings in semen, seminal fluid
abnormal spermatozoa

EXCLUDES 1 *azoospermia (N46.0-)*
oligospermia (N46.1-)

R86.0 Abnormal level of enzymes in specimens from male genital organs ♂

R86.1 Abnormal level of hormones in specimens from male genital organs ♂

R86.2 Abnormal level of other drugs, medicaments and biological substances in specimens from male genital organs ♂

R86.3 Abnormal level of substances chiefly nonmedicinal as to source in specimens from male genital organs ♂

R86.4 Abnormal immunological findings in specimens from male genital organs ♂

R86.5 Abnormal microbiological findings in specimens from male genital organs ♂
Positive culture findings in specimens from male genital organs

EXCLUDES 1 *colonization status (Z22.-)*

R86.6 Abnormal cytological findings in specimens from male genital organs ♂

R86.7 Abnormal histological findings in specimens from male genital organs ♂

R86.8 Other abnormal findings in specimens from male genital organs ♂
Abnormal chromosomal findings in specimens from male genital organs

R86.9 Unspecified abnormal finding in specimens from male genital organs ♂

4 R87 Abnormal findings in specimens from female genital organs

INCLUDES abnormal findings in secretion and smears from cervix uteri
abnormal findings in secretion and smears from vagina
abnormal findings in secretion and smears from vulva

R87.0 Abnormal level of enzymes in specimens from female genital organs ♀

R87.1 Abnormal level of hormones in specimens from female genital organs ♀

R87.2 Abnormal level of other drugs, medicaments and biological substances in specimens from female genital organs ♀

R87.3 Abnormal level of substances chiefly nonmedicinal as to source in specimens from female genital organs ♀

R87.4 Abnormal immunological findings in specimens from female genital organs ♀

R87.5 Abnormal microbiological findings in specimens from female genital organs ♀
Positive culture findings in specimens from female genital organs

EXCLUDES 1 *colonization status (Z22.-)*

5 **R87.6 Abnormal cytological findings in specimens from female genital organs**

6 **R87.61 Abnormal cytological findings in specimens from cervix uteri**

EXCLUDES 1 *abnormal cytological findings in specimens from other female genital organs (R87.69)*
abnormal cytological findings in specimens from vagina (R87.62-)
carcinoma in situ of cervix uteri (histologically confirmed) (D06.-)
cervical intraepithelial neoplasia I [CIN I] (N87.0)
cervical intraepithelial neoplasia II [CIN II] (N87.1)
cervical intraepithelial neoplasia III [CIN III] (D06.-)
dysplasia (mild) (moderate) of cervix uteri (histologically confirmed) (N87.-)
severe dysplasia of cervix uteri (histologically confirmed) (D06.-)

EXCLUDES 2 *cervical high risk human papillomavirus (HPV) DNA test positive (R87.810)*
cervical low risk human papillomavirus (HPV) DNA test positive (R87.820)

R87.610 Atypical squamous cells of undetermined significance on cytologic smear of cervix (ASC-US) ♀

R87.611 Atypical squamous cells cannot exclude high grade squamous intraepithelial lesion on cytologic smear of cervix (ASC-H) ♀

R87.612 Low grade squamous intraepithelial lesion on cytologic smear of cervix (LGSIL) ♀

R87.613 High grade squamous intraepithelial lesion on cytologic smear of cervix (HGSIL) ♀

R87.614 Cytologic evidence of malignancy on smear of cervix ♀

R87.615 **Unsatisfactory cytologic smear of cervix** ♀
Inadequate sample of cytologic smear of cervix

R87.616 **Satisfactory cervical smear but lacking transformation zone** ♀

R87.618 **Other abnormal cytological findings on specimens from cervix uteri** ♀

R87.619 **Unspecified abnormal cytological findings in specimens from cervix uteri** ♀
Abnormal cervical cytology NOS
Abnormal Papanicolaou smear of cervix NOS
Abnormal thin preparation smear of cervix NOS
Atypical endocervial cells of cervix NOS
Atypical endometrial cells of cervix NOS
Atypical glandular cells of cervix NOS

6 **R87.62** **Abnormal cytological findings in specimens from vagina**
Use additional code to identify acquired absence of uterus and cervix, if applicable (Z90.71-)
EXCLUDES 1 *abnormal cytological findings in specimens from cervix uteri (R87.61-)*
abnormal cytological findings in specimens from other female genital organs (R87.69)
carcinoma in situ of vagina (histologically confirmed) (D07.2)
vaginal intraepithelial neoplasia I [VAIN I] (N89.0)
vaginal intraepithelial neoplasia II [VAIN II] (N89.1)
vaginal intraepithelial neoplasia III [VAIN III] (D07.2)
dysplasia (mild) (moderate) of vagina (histologically confirmed) (N89.-)
severe dysplasia of vagina (histologically confirmed) (D07.2)
EXCLUDES 2 *vaginal high risk human papillomavirus (HPV) DNA test positive (R87.811)*
vaginal low risk human papillomavirus (HPV) DNA test positive (R87.821)

R87.620 **Atypical squamous cells of undetermined significance on cytologic smear of vagina (ASC-US)** ♀

R87.621 **Atypical squamous cells cannot exclude high grade squamous intraepithelial lesion on cytologic smear of vagina (ASC-H)** ♀

R87.622 **Low grade squamous intraepithelial lesion on cytologic smear of vagina (LGSIL)** ♀

R87.623 **High grade squamous intraepithelial lesion on cytologic smear of vagina (HGSIL)** ♀

R87.624 **Cytologic evidence of malignancy on smear of vagina** ♀

R87.625 **Unsatisfactory cytologic smear of vagina** ♀
Inadequate sample of cytologic smear of vagina

R87.628 **Other abnormal cytological findings on specimens from vagina** ♀

R87.629 **Unspecified abnormal cytological findings in specimens from vagina** ♀
Abnormal Papanicolaou smear of vagina NOS
Abnormal thin preparation smear of vagina NOS
Abnormal vaginal cytology NOS
Atypical endocervical cells of vagina NOS
Atypical endometrial cells of vagina NOS
Atypical glandular cells of vagina NOS

R87.69 **Abnormal cytological findings in specimens from other female genital organs** ♀
Abnormal cytological findings in specimens from female genital organs NOS
EXCLUDES 1 *dysplasia of vulva (histologically confirmed) (N90.0-N90.3)*

R87.7 **Abnormal histological findings in specimens from female genital organs** ♀
EXCLUDES 1 *carcinoma in situ (histologically confirmed) of female genital organs (D06-D07.3)*
cervical intraepithelial neoplasia I [CIN I] (N87.0)
cervical intraepithelial neoplasia II [CIN II] (N87.1)
cervical intraepithelial neoplasia III [CIN III] (D06.-)
dysplasia (mild) (moderate) of cervix uteri (histologically confirmed) (N87.-)
dysplasia (mild) (moderate) of vagina (histologically confirmed) (N89.-)
vaginal intraepithelial neoplasia I [VAIN I] (N89.0)
vaginal intraepithelial neoplasia II [VAIN II] (N89.1)
vaginal intraepithelial neoplasia III [VAIN III] (D07.2)
severe dysplasia of cervix uteri (histologically confirmed) (D06.-)
severe dysplasia of vagina (histologically confirmed) (D07.2)

5 **R87.8** **Other abnormal findings in specimens from female genital organs**

6 **R87.81** **High risk human papillomavirus (HPV) DNA test positive from female genital organs**
EXCLUDES 1 *anogenital warts due to human papillomavirus (HPV) (A63.0)*
condyloma acuminatum (A63.0)

R87.810 **Cervical high risk human papillomavirus (HPV) DNA test positive** ♀

R87.811 **Vaginal high risk human papillomavirus (HPV) DNA test positive** ♀

6 **R87.82** **Low risk human papillomavirus (HPV) DNA test positive from female genital organs**
Use additional code for associated human papillomavirus (B97.7)

R87.820 **Cervical low risk human papillomavirus (HPV) DNA test positive** ♀

R87.821 **Vaginal low risk human papillomavirus (HPV) DNA test positive** ♀

R87.89 **Other abnormal findings in specimens from female genital organs** ♀
Abnormal chromosomal findings in specimens from female genital organs

R87.9 **Unspecified abnormal finding in specimens from female genital organs** ♀

4 R88 Abnormal findings in other body fluids and substances

R88.0 **Cloudy (hemodialysis) (peritoneal) dialysis effluent**

R88.8 **Abnormal findings in other body fluids and substances**

4 R89 Abnormal findings in specimens from other organs, systems and tissues

INCLUDES abnormal findings in nipple discharge
abnormal findings in synovial fluid
abnormal findings in wound secretions

R89.0 **Abnormal level of enzymes in specimens from other organs, systems and tissues**

R89.1 **Abnormal level of hormones in specimens from other organs, systems and tissues**

R89.2 **Abnormal level of other drugs, medicaments and biological substances in specimens from other organs, systems and tissues**

R89.3 **Abnormal level of substances chiefly nonmedicinal as to source in specimens from other organs, systems and tissues**

R89.4 **Abnormal immunological findings in specimens from other organs, systems and tissues**

R89.5 **Abnormal microbiological findings in specimens from other organs, systems and tissues**
Positive culture findings in specimens from other organs, systems and tissues
EXCLUDES 1 *colonization status (Z22.-)*

R89.6 **Abnormal cytological findings in specimens from other organs, systems and tissues**

R89.7 **Abnormal histological findings in specimens from other organs, systems and tissues**

R89.8 **Other abnormal findings in specimens from Otherorgans, systems and tissues**
Abnormal chromosomal findings in specimens from other organs, systems and tissues

R89.9 **Unspecified abnormal finding in specimens from other organs, systems and tissues**

Abnormal findings on diagnostic imaging and in function studies, without diagnosis (R90-R94)

INCLUDES nonspecific abnormal findings on diagnostic imaging by computerized axial tomography [CAT scan]
nonspecific abnormal findings on diagnostic imaging by magnetic resonance imaging [MRI][NMR]
nonspecific abnormal findings on diagnostic imaging by positron emission tomography [PET scan]
nonspecific abnormal findings on diagnostic imaging by thermography
nonspecific abnormal findings on diagnostic imaging by ultrasound [echogram]
nonspecific abnormal findings on diagnostic imaging by X-ray examination

EXCLUDES 1 *abnormal findings on antenatal screening of mother (O28.-)*
diagnostic abnormal findings classified elsewhere - see Alphabetical Index

4 R90 **Abnormal findings on diagnostic imaging of central nervous system**

R90.0 **Intracranial space-occupying lesion found on diagnostic imaging of central nervous system**

5 R90.8 **Other abnormal findings on diagnostic imaging of central nervous system**

R90.81 **Abnormal echoencephalogram**

R90.82 **White matter disease, unspecified**

R90.89 **Other abnormal findings on diagnostic imaging of central nervous system**
Other cerebrovascular abnormality found on diagnostic imaging of central nervous system

4 R91 **Abnormal findings on diagnostic imaging of lung**

R91.1 **Solitary pulmonary nodule**
Coin lesion lung
Solitary pulmonary nodule, subsegmental branch of the bronchial tree

R91.8 **Other nonspecific abnormal finding of lung field**
Lung mass NOS found on diagnostic imaging of lung
Pulmonary infiltrate NOS
Shadow, lung

4 R92 **Abnormal and inconclusive findings on diagnostic imaging of breast**

R92.0 **Mammographic microcalcification found on diagnostic imaging of breast**
EXCLUDES 2 *mammographic calcification (calculus) found on diagnostic imaging of breast (R92.1)*

R92.1 **Mammographic calcification found on diagnostic imaging of breast**
Mammographic calculus found on diagnostic imaging of breast

R92.2 **Inconclusive mammogram**
Dense breasts NOS
Inconclusive mammogram NEC
Inconclusive mammography due to dense breasts
Inconclusive mammography NEC
AHA: 1Q 2015, 24

R92.8 **Other abnormal and inconclusive findings on diagnostic imaging of breast**

4 R93 **Abnormal findings on diagnostic imaging of other body structures**

R93.0 **Abnormal findings on diagnostic imaging of skull and head, not elsewhere classified**
EXCLUDES 1 *intracranial space-occupying lesion found on diagnostic imaging (R90.0)*

R93.1 **Abnormal findings on diagnostic imaging of heart and coronary circulation**
Abnormal echocardiogram NOS
Abnormal heart shadow

R93.2 **Abnormal findings on diagnostic imaging of liver and biliary tract**
Nonvisualization of gallbladder

R93.3 **Abnormal findings on diagnostic imaging of other parts of digestive tract**

5 R93.4 **Abnormal findings on diagnostic imaging of urinary organs**
EXCLUDES 2 *hypertrophy of kidney (N28.81)*

R93.41 **Abnormal radiologic findings on diagnostic imaging of renal pelvis, ureter, or bladder**
Filling defect of bladder found on diagnostic imaging
Filling defect of renal pelvis found on diagnostic imaging
Filling defect of ureter found on diagnostic imaging
AHA: 4Q 2016, 66

6 R93.42 **Abnormal radiologic findings on diagnostic imaging of kidney**

R93.421 **Abnormal radiologic findings on diagnostic imaging of right kidney**
AHA: 4Q 2016, 66

R93.422 **Abnormal radiologic findings on diagnostic imaging of left kidney**
AHA: 4Q 2016, 66

R93.429 **Abnormal radiologic findings on diagnostic imaging of unspecified kidney**
AHA: 4Q 2016, 66

R93.49 **Abnormal radiologic findings on diagnostic imaging of other urinary organs**
AHA: 4Q 2016, 66

R93.5 **Abnormal findings on diagnostic imaging of other abdominal regions, including retroperitoneum**

▲ R93.6 **Abnormal findings on diagnostic imaging of limbs**
EXCLUDES 2 *abnormal finding in skin and subcutaneous tissue (R93.8-)*

R93.7 **Abnormal findings on diagnostic imaging of other parts of musculoskeletal system**
EXCLUDES 2 *abnormal findings on diagnostic imaging of skull (R93.0)*

▲5 R93.8 **Abnormal findings on diagnostic imaging of other specified body structures**

● 6 R93.81 **Abnormal radiologic findings on diagnostic imaging of testis**

● R93.811 **Abnormal radiologic findings on diagnostic imaging of right testicle** ♂

● R93.812 **Abnormal radiologic findings on diagnostic imaging of left testicle** ♂

● R93.813 **Abnormal radiologic findings on diagnostic imaging of testicles, bilateral** ♂

● R93.819 **Abnormal radiologic findings on diagnostic imaging of unspecified testicle** ♂

● R93.89 **Abnormal findings on diagnostic imaging of other specified body structures**
Abnormal finding by radioisotope localization of placenta
Abnormal radiological finding in skin and subcutaneous tissue
Mediastinal shift

R93.9 **Diagnostic imaging inconclusive due to excess body fat of patient**

4 R94 **Abnormal results of function studies**
INCLUDES abnormal results of radionuclide [radioisotope] uptake studies
abnormal results of scintigraphy

5 R94.0 **Abnormal results of function studies of central nervous system**

R94.01 **Abnormal electroencephalogram [EEG]**

R94.02 **Abnormal brain scan**

R94.09 **Abnormal results of other function studies of central nervous system**

5 R94.1 **Abnormal results of function studies of peripheral nervous system and special senses**

6 R94.11 **Abnormal results of function studies of eye**

R94.110 **Abnormal electro-oculogram [EOG]**

R94.111 **Abnormal electroretinogram [ERG]**
Abnormal retinal function study

R94.112 **Abnormal visually evoked potential [VEP]**

R94.113 **Abnormal oculomotor study**

R94.118 **Abnormal results of other function studies of eye**

6 R94.12 **Abnormal results of function studies of ear and other special senses**

R94.120 **Abnormal auditory function study**

AHA: 3Q 2016, 17

R94.121 Abnormal vestibular function study

R94.128 Abnormal results of other function studies of ear and other special senses

R94.13 Abnormal results of function studies of peripheral nervous system

R94.130 Abnormal response to nerve stimulation, unspecified

R94.131 Abnormal electromyogram [EMG]

EXCLUDES 1 *electromyogram of eye (R94.113)*

R94.138 Abnormal results of other function studies of peripheral nervous system

R94.2 Abnormal results of pulmonary function studies

Reduced ventilatory capacity

Reduced vital capacity

R94.3 Abnormal results of cardiovascular function studies

R94.30 Abnormal result of cardiovascular function study, unspecified

R94.31 Abnormal electrocardiogram [ECG] [EKG]

EXCLUDES 1 *long QT syndrome (I45.81)*

R94.39 Abnormal result of other cardiovascular function study

Abnormal electrophysiological intracardiac studies

Abnormal phonocardiogram

Abnormal vectorcardiogram

R94.4 Abnormal results of kidney function studies

Abnormal renal function test

R94.5 Abnormal results of liver function studies

R94.6 Abnormal results of thyroid function studies

R94.7 Abnormal results of other endocrine function studies

EXCLUDES 2 *abnormal glucose (R73.0-)*

R94.8 Abnormal results of function studies of other organs and systems

Abnormal basal metabolic rate [BMR]

Abnormal bladder function test

Abnormal splenic function test

Abnormal tumor markers (R97)

R97 Abnormal tumor markers

Elevated tumor associated antigens [TAA]

Elevated tumor specific antigens [TSA]

R97.0 Elevated carcinoembryonic antigen [CEA]

R97.1 Elevated cancer antigen 125 [CA 125]

R97.2 Elevated prostate specific antigen [PSA]

R97.20 Elevated prostate specific antigen [PSA] ♂ A

DEFINITION Elevated levels of prostate specific antigen (PSA) in the bloodstream can indicate prostate cancer, or precursor conditions that can develop into prostate cancer.

AHA: 4Q 2016, 66

R97.21 Rising PSA following treatment for malignant neoplasm of prostate ♂ A

AHA: 4Q 2016, 66

R97.8 Other abnormal tumor markers

Ill-defined and unknown cause of mortality (R99)

R99 Ill-defined and unknown cause of mortality

Death (unexplained) NOS

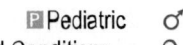

Unspecified cause of mortality

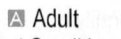

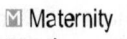

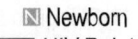

CHAPTER 19: INJURY, POISONING AND CERTAIN OTHER CONSEQUENCES OF EXTERNAL CAUSES (S00-T88)

Note: Use secondary code(s) from Chapter 20, External causes of morbidity, to indicate cause of injury. Codes within the T section that include the external cause do not require an additional external cause code

The chapter uses the S-section for coding different types of injuries related to single body regions and the T-section to cover injuries to unspecified body regions as well as poisoning and certain other consequences of external causes.

Use additional code to identify any retained foreign body, if applicable (Z18.-)

EXCLUDES 1 *birth trauma (P10-P15)*
obstetric trauma (O70-O71)

GUIDELINES **Section I.C.19.a**

Most categories in chapter 19 have a 7th character requirement for each applicable code ... While the patient may be seen by a new or different provider over the course of treatment for an injury, assignment of the 7th character is based on whether the patient is undergoing active treatment and not whether the provider is seeing the patient for the first time ... 7th character "D" subsequent encounter is used for encounters after the patient has completed active treatment of the condition and is receiving routine care for the condition during the healing or recovery phase.

The aftercare Z codes should not be used for aftercare for conditions such as injuries or poisonings, where 7th characters are provided to identify subsequent care. For example, for aftercare of an injury, assign the acute injury code with the 7th character "D" (subsequent encounter).

7th character "S", sequela, is for use for complications or conditions that arise as a direct result of a condition, such as scar formation after a burn. The scars are sequelae of the burn. When using 7th character "S", it is necessary to use both the injury code that precipitated the sequela and the code for the sequela itself. The "S" is added only to the injury code, not the sequela code. The 7th character "S" identifies the injury responsible for the sequela. The specific type of sequela (e.g. scar) is sequenced first, followed by the injury code.

This chapter contains the following blocks:

S00-S09	Injuries to the head
S10-S19	Injuries to the neck
S20-S29	Injuries to the thorax
S30-S39	Injuries to the abdomen, lower back, lumbar spine, pelvis and external genitals
S40-S49	Injuries to the shoulder and upper arm
S50-S59	Injuries to the elbow and forearm
S60-S69	Injuries to the wrist, hand and fingers
S70-S79	Injuries to the hip and thigh
S80-S89	Injuries to the knee and lower leg
S90-S99	Injuries to the ankle and foot
T07	Injuries involving multiple body regions
T14	Injury of unspecified body region
T15-T19	Effects of foreign body entering through natural orifice
T20-T25	Burns and corrosions of external body surface, specified by site
T26-T28	Burns and corrosions confined to eye and internal organs
T30-T32	Burns and corrosions of multiple and unspecified body regions
T33-T34	Frostbite
T36-T50	Poisoning by, adverse effect of and underdosing of drugs, medicaments and biological substances
T51-T65	Toxic effects of substances chiefly nonmedicinal as to source
T66-T78	Other and unspecified effects of external causes
T79	Certain early complications of trauma
T80-T88	Complications of surgical and medical care, not elsewhere classified

Injuries to the head (S00-S09)

INCLUDES injuries of ear
injuries of eye
injuries of face [any part]
injuries of gum
injuries of jaw
injuries of oral cavity
injuries of palate
injuries of periocular area
injuries of scalp
injuries of temporomandibular joint area
injuries of tongue
injuries of tooth

Code also:
for any associated infection

EXCLUDES 2 *burns and corrosions (T20-T32)*
effects of foreign body in ear (T16)
effects of foreign body in larynx (T17.3)
effects of foreign body in mouth NOS (T18.0)
effects of foreign body in nose (T17.0-T17.1)
effects of foreign body in pharynx (T17.2)
effects of foreign body on external eye (T15.-)
frostbite (T33-T34)
insect bite or sting, venomous (T63.4)

GUIDELINES **Section I.C.19.c.2)**

Multiple fractures are sequenced in accordance with the severity of the fracture.

GUIDELINES **Section I.C.19.b.1)-2)**

When coding injuries, assign separate codes for each injury unless a combination code is provided, in which case the combination code is assigned ... Traumatic injury codes (S00-T14.9) are not to be used for normal, healing surgical wounds or to identify complications of surgical wounds. The code for the most serious injury, as determined by the provider and the focus of treatment, is sequenced first.

1) Superficial injuries such as abrasions or contusions are not coded when associated with more severe injuries of the same site.

2) When a primary injury results in minor damage to peripheral nerves or blood vessels, the primary injury is sequenced first with additional code(s) for injuries to nerves and spinal cord (such as category S04), and/or injury to blood vessels (such as category S15). When the primary injury is to the blood vessels or nerves, that injury should be sequenced first.

GUIDELINES **Section I.C.19.c**

Coding of Traumatic Fractures: The principles of multiple coding of injuries should be followed in coding fractures. Fractures of specified sites are coded individually by site in accordance with both the provisions within categories S02, S12, S22, S32, S42, S49, S52, S59, S62, S72, S79, S82, S89, S92 and the level of detail furnished by medical record content. A fracture not indicated as open or closed should be coded to closed. A fracture not indicated whether displaced or not displaced should be coded to displaced.

4 S00 Superficial injury of head

EXCLUDES 1 *diffuse cerebral contusion (S06.2-)*
focal cerebral contusion (S06.3-)
injury of eye and orbit (S05.-)
open wound of head (S01.-)

The appropriate 7th character is to be added to each code from category S00
A initial encounter
D subsequent encounter
S sequela

5 S00.0 Superficial injury of scalp

- **7 S00.00X- Unspecified superficial injury of scalp**
- **7 S00.01X- Abrasion of scalp**
- **7 S00.02X- Blister (nonthermal) of scalp**
- **7 S00.03X- Contusion of scalp**
  Bruise of scalp
  Hematoma of scalp
- **7 S00.04X- External constriction of part of scalp**
- **7 S00.05X- Superficial foreign body of scalp**
  Splinter in the scalp
- **7 S00.06X- Insect bite (nonvenomous) of scalp**

7 S00.07X- Other superficial bite of scalp
EXCLUDES 1 *open bite of scalp (S01.05)*

5 S00.1 Contusion of eyelid and periocular area
Black eye
EXCLUDES 2 *contusion of eyeball and orbital tissues (S05.1)*

7 S00.10X- Contusion of unspecified eyelid and periocular area
7 S00.11X- Contusion of right eyelid and periocular area
7 S00.12X- Contusion of left eyelid and periocular area

5 S00.2 Other and unspecified superficial injuries of eyelid and periocular area
EXCLUDES 2 *superficial injury of conjunctiva and cornea (S05.0-)*

6 S00.20 Unspecified superficial injury of eyelid and periocular area
7 S00.201- Unspecified superficial injury of right eyelid and periocular area
7 S00.202- Unspecified superficial injury of left eyelid and periocular area
7 S00.209- Unspecified superficial injury of unspecified eyelid and periocular area

6 S00.21 Abrasion of eyelid and periocular area
7 S00.211- Abrasion of right eyelid and periocular area
7 S00.212- Abrasion of left eyelid and periocular area
7 S00.219- Abrasion of unspecified eyelid and periocular area

6 S00.22 Blister (nonthermal) of eyelid and periocular area
7 S00.221- Blister (nonthermal) of right eyelid and periocular area
7 S00.222- Blister (nonthermal) of left eyelid and periocular area
7 S00.229- Blister (nonthermal) of unspecified eyelid and periocular area

6 S00.24 External constriction of eyelid and periocular area
7 S00.241- External constriction of right eyelid and periocular area
7 S00.242- External constriction of left eyelid and periocular area
7 S00.249- External constriction of unspecified eyelid and periocular area

6 S00.25 Superficial foreign body of eyelid and periocular area
Splinter of eyelid and periocular area
EXCLUDES 2 *retained foreign body in eyelid (H02.81-)*

7 S00.251- Superficial foreign body of right eyelid and periocular area
7 S00.252- Superficial foreign body of left eyelid and periocular area
7 S00.259- Superficial foreign body of unspecified eyelid and periocular area

6 S00.26 Insect bite (nonvenomous) of eyelid and periocular area
7 S00.261- Insect bite (nonvenomous) of right eyelid and periocular area
7 S00.262- Insect bite (nonvenomous) of left eyelid and periocular area
7 S00.269- Insect bite (nonvenomous) of unspecified eyelid and periocular area

6 S00.27 Other superficial bite of eyelid and periocular area
EXCLUDES 1 *open bite of eyelid and periocular area (S01.15)*

7 S00.271- Other superficial bite of right eyelid and periocular area
7 S00.272- Other superficial bite of left eyelid and periocular area
7 S00.279- Other superficial bite of unspecified eyelid and periocular area

5 S00.3 Superficial injury of nose
7 S00.30X- Unspecified superficial injury of nose
7 S00.31X- Abrasion of nose
7 S00.32X- Blister (nonthermal) of nose
7 S00.33X- Contusion of nose
Bruise of nose
Hematoma of nose
7 S00.34X- External constriction of nose
7 S00.35X- Superficial foreign body of nose
Splinter in the nose
7 S00.36X- Insect bite (nonvenomous) of nose
7 S00.37X- Other superficial bite of nose
EXCLUDES 1 *open bite of nose (S01.25)*

5 S00.4 Superficial injury of ear

6 S00.40 Unspecified superficial injury of ear
7 S00.401- Unspecified superficial injury of right ear
7 S00.402- Unspecified superficial injury of left ear
7 S00.409- Unspecified superficial injury of unspecified ear

6 S00.41 Abrasion of ear
7 S00.411- Abrasion of right ear
7 S00.412- Abrasion of left ear
7 S00.419- Abrasion of unspecified ear

6 S00.42 Blister (nonthermal) of ear
7 S00.421- Blister (nonthermal) of right ear
7 S00.422- Blister (nonthermal) of left ear
7 S00.429- Blister (nonthermal) of unspecified ear

6 S00.43 Contusion of ear
Bruise of ear
Hematoma of ear
7 S00.431- Contusion of right ear
7 S00.432- Contusion of left ear
7 S00.439- Contusion of unspecified ear

6 S00.44 External constriction of ear
7 S00.441- External constriction of right ear
7 S00.442- External constriction of left ear
7 S00.449- External constriction of unspecified ear

6 S00.45 Superficial foreign body of ear
Splinter in the ear
7 S00.451- Superficial foreign body of right ear
7 S00.452- Superficial foreign body of left ear
7 S00.459- Superficial foreign body of unspecified ear

6 S00.46 Insect bite (nonvenomous) of ear
7 S00.461- Insect bite (nonvenomous) of right ear
7 S00.462- Insect bite (nonvenomous) of left ear
7 S00.469- Insect bite (nonvenomous) of unspecified ear

6 S00.47 Other superficial bite of ear
EXCLUDES 1 *open bite of ear (S01.35)*

7 S00.471- Other superficial bite of right ear
7 S00.472- Other superficial bite of left ear
7 S00.479- Other superficial bite of unspecified ear

5 S00.5 Superficial injury of lip and oral cavity

6 S00.50 Unspecified superficial injury of lip and oral cavity
7 S00.501- Unspecified superficial injury of lip
7 S00.502- Unspecified superficial injury of oral cavity

6 S00.51 Abrasion of lip and oral cavity
7 S00.511- Abrasion of lip
7 S00.512- Abrasion of oral cavity

6 S00.52 Blister (nonthermal) of lip and oral cavity
7 S00.521- Blister (nonthermal) of lip
7 S00.522- Blister (nonthermal) of oral cavity

6 S00.53 Contusion of lip and oral cavity
7 S00.531- Contusion of lip
Bruise of lip
Hematoma of lip
7 S00.532- Contusion of oral cavity
Bruise of oral cavity
Hematoma of oral cavity

6 S00.54 External constriction of lip and oral cavity
7 S00.541- External constriction of lip
7 S00.542- External constriction of oral cavity

6 S00.55 **Superficial foreign body of lip and oral cavity**

7 S00.551- **Superficial foreign body of lip**
Splinter of lip and oral cavity

7 S00.552- **Superficial foreign body of oral cavity**
Splinter of lip and oral cavity

6 S00.56 **Insect bite (nonvenomous) of lip and oral cavity**

7 S00.561- **Insect bite (nonvenomous) of lip**

7 S00.562- **Insect bite (nonvenomous) of oral cavity**

6 S00.57 **Other superficial bite of lip and oral cavity**

7 S00.571- **Other superficial bite of lip**
EXCLUDES 1 *open bite of lip (S01.551)*

7 S00.572- **Other superficial bite of oral cavity**
EXCLUDES 1 *open bite of oral cavity (S01.552)*

5 S00.8 **Superficial injury of other parts of head**
Superficial injuries of face [any part]

7 S00.80X- **Unspecified superficial injury of other part of head**

7 S00.81X- **Abrasion of other part of head**

7 S00.82X- **Blister (nonthermal) of other part of head**

7 S00.83X- **Contusion of other part of head**
Bruise of other part of head
Hematoma of other part of head

7 S00.84X- **External constriction of other part of head**

7 S00.85X- **Superficial foreign body of other part of head**
Splinter in other part of head

7 S00.86X- **Insect bite (nonvenomous) of other part of head**

7 S00.87X- **Other superficial bite of other part of head**
EXCLUDES 1 *open bite of other part of head (S01.85)*

5 S00.9 **Superficial injury of unspecified part of head**

7 S00.90X- **Unspecified superficial injury of Unspecified part of head**

7 S00.91X- **Abrasion of unspecified part of head**

7 S00.92X- **Blister (nonthermal) of unspecified part of head**

7 S00.93X- **Contusion of unspecified part of head**
Bruise of head
Hematoma of head

7 S00.94X- **External constriction of unspecified part of head**

7 S00.95X- **Superficial foreign body of unspecified part of head**
Splinter of head

7 S00.96X- **Insect bite (nonvenomous) of unspecified part of head**

7 S00.97X- **Other superficial bite of unspecified part of head**
EXCLUDES 1 *open bite of head (S01.95)*

4 S01 Open wound of head

Code also any associated:
injury of cranial nerve (S04.-)
injury of muscle and tendon of head (S09.1-)
intracranial injury (S06.-)
wound infection

EXCLUDES 1 *open skull fracture (S02.- with 7th character B)*

EXCLUDES 2 *injury of eye and orbit (S05.-)*
traumatic amputation of part of head (S08.-)

The appropriate 7th character is to be added to each code from category S01
A initial encounter
D subsequent encounter
S sequela

CODING TIP Open wound codes are used for wounds caused by trauma. Do not assign a code for "open wound" unless the etiology of the wound is related to trauma. Do not use Z codes for any aspect of care of a trauma wound, e.g. no Z code for dressing changes, drain care, or suture removal. Report instead the appropriate subsequent care 7th character with the injury code.

CODING TIP Open wound codes are used for wounds caused by trauma. Do not assign a code for "open wound" unless the etiology of the wound is related to trauma.

5 S01.0 **Open wound of scalp**
EXCLUDES 1 *avulsion of scalp (S08.0)*

7 S01.00X- **Unspecified open wound of scalp**

7 S01.01X- **Laceration without foreign body of scalp**

7 S01.02X- **Laceration with foreign body of scalp**
AHA: (S01.02XA) 1Q 2015, 5
AHA: (S01.02XD) 1Q 2015, 6, 7

7 S01.03X- **Puncture wound without foreign body of scalp**

7 S01.04X- **Puncture wound with foreign body of scalp**

7 S01.05X- **Open bite of scalp**
Bite of scalp NOS
EXCLUDES 1 *superficial bite of scalp (S00.06, S00.07-)*

5 S01.1 **Open wound of eyelid and periocular area**
Open wound of eyelid and periocular area with or without involvement of lacrimal passages

6 S01.10 **Unspecified open wound of eyelid and periocular area**

7 ⊟ S01.101- **Unspecified open wound of right eyelid and periocular area**

7 ⊟ S01.102- **Unspecified open wound of left eyelid and periocular area**

7 ⊟ S01.109- **Unspecified open wound of unspecified eyelid and periocular area**

6 S01.11 **Laceration without foreign body of eyelid and periocular area**

7 ⊟ S01.111- **Laceration without foreign body of right eyelid and periocular area**

7 ⊟ S01.112- **Laceration without foreign body of left eyelid and periocular area**

7 ⊟ S01.119- **Laceration without foreign body of unspecified eyelid and periocular area**

6 S01.12 **Laceration with foreign body of eyelid and periocular area**

7 ⊟ S01.121- **Laceration with foreign body of right eyelid and periocular area**

7 ⊟ S01.122- **Laceration with foreign body of left eyelid and periocular area**

7 ⊟ S01.129- **Laceration with foreign body of unspecified eyelid and periocular area**

6 S01.13 **Puncture wound without foreign body of eyelid and periocular area**

7 ⊟ S01.131- **Puncture wound without foreign body of right eyelid and periocular area**

7 ⊟ S01.132- **Puncture wound without foreign body of left eyelid and periocular area**

7 ⊟ S01.139- **Puncture wound without foreign body of unspecified eyelid and periocular area**

6 S01.14 **Puncture wound with foreign body of eyelid and periocular area**

7 ⊟ S01.141- **Puncture wound with foreign body of right eyelid and periocular area**

7 ⊟ S01.142- **Puncture wound with foreign body of left eyelid and periocular area**

7 ⊟ S01.149- **Puncture wound with foreign body of unspecified eyelid and periocular area**

6 S01.15 **Open bite of eyelid and periocular area**
Bite of eyelid and periocular area NOS
EXCLUDES 1 *superficial bite of eyelid and periocular area (S00.26, S00.27)*

7 ⊟ S01.151- **Open bite of right eyelid and periocular area**

7 ⊟ S01.152- **Open bite of left eyelid and periocular area**

7 ⊟ S01.159- **Open bite of unspecified eyelid and periocular area**

5 S01.2 **Open wound of nose**

7 S01.20X- **Unspecified open wound of nose**

7 S01.21X- **Laceration without foreign body of nose**
AHA: (S01.21XA) 1Q 2015, 5
AHA: (S01.21XD) 1Q 2015, 6

7 S01.22X- **Laceration with foreign body of nose**

7 S01.23X- **Puncture wound without foreign body of nose**

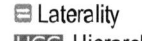

7 S01.24X- **Puncture wound with foreign body of nose**

S01.25X- Open bite of nose
Bite of nose NOS
EXCLUDES 1 *superficial bite of nose (S00.36, S00.37)*

S01.3 Open wound of ear

S01.30 Unspecified open wound of ear
- **S01.301-** Unspecified open wound of right ear
- **S01.302-** Unspecified open wound of left ear
- **S01.309-** Unspecified open wound of unspecified ear

S01.31 Laceration without foreign body of ear
- **S01.311-** Laceration without foreign body of right ear
- **S01.312-** Laceration without foreign body of left ear
- **S01.319-** Laceration without foreign body of unspecified ear

S01.32 Laceration with foreign body of ear
- **S01.321-** Laceration with foreign body of right ear
- **S01.322-** Laceration with foreign body of left ear
- **S01.329-** Laceration with foreign body of unspecified ear

S01.33 Puncture wound without foreign body of ear
- **S01.331-** Puncture wound without foreign body of right ear
- **S01.332-** Puncture wound without foreign body of left ear
- **S01.339-** Puncture wound without foreign body of unspecified ear

S01.34 Puncture wound with foreign body of ear
- **S01.341-** Puncture wound with foreign body of right ear
- **S01.342-** Puncture wound with foreign body of left ear
- **S01.349-** Puncture wound with foreign body of unspecified ear

S01.35 Open bite of ear
Bite of ear NOS
EXCLUDES 1 *superficial bite of ear (S00.46, S00.47)*
- **S01.351-** Open bite of right ear
- **S01.352-** Open bite of left ear
- **S01.359-** Open bite of unspecified ear

S01.4 Open wound of cheek and temporomandibular area

S01.40 Unspecified open wound of cheek and temporomandibular area
- **S01.401-** Unspecified open wound of right cheek and temporomandibular area
- **S01.402-** Unspecified open wound of left cheek and temporomandibular area
- **S01.409-** Unspecified open wound of unspecified cheek and temporomandibular area

S01.41 Laceration without foreign body of cheek and temporomandibular area
- **S01.411-** Laceration without foreign body of right cheek and temporomandibular area
  AHA: (S01.411A) 1Q 2015, 5
  AHA: (S01.411D) 1Q 2015, 6, 7
- **S01.412-** Laceration without foreign body of left cheek and temporomandibular area
- **S01.419-** Laceration without foreign body of unspecified cheek and temporomandibular area

S01.42 Laceration with foreign body of cheek and temporomandibular area
- **S01.421-** Laceration with foreign body of right cheek and temporomandibular area
- **S01.422-** Laceration with foreign body of left cheek and temporomandibular area
- **S01.429-** Laceration with foreign body of unspecified cheek and temporomandibular area

S01.43 Puncture wound without foreign body of cheek and temporomandibular area
- **S01.431-** Puncture wound without foreign body of right cheek and temporomandibular area
- **S01.432-** Puncture wound without foreign body of left cheek and temporomandibular area
- **S01.439-** Puncture wound without foreign body of unspecified cheek and temporomandibular area

S01.44 Puncture wound with foreign body of cheek and temporomandibular area
- **S01.441-** Puncture wound with foreign body of right cheek and temporomandibular area
- **S01.442-** Puncture wound with foreign body of left cheek and temporomandibular area
- **S01.449-** Puncture wound with foreign body of unspecified cheek and temporomandibular area

S01.45 Open bite of cheek and temporomandibular area
Bite of cheek and temporomandibular area NOS
EXCLUDES 2 *superficial bite of cheek and temporomandibular area (S00.86, S00.87)*
- **S01.451-** Open bite of right cheek and temporomandibular area
- **S01.452-** Open bite of left cheek and temporomandibular area
- **S01.459-** Open bite of unspecified cheek and temporomandibular area

S01.5 Open wound of lip and oral cavity
EXCLUDES 2 *tooth dislocation (S03.2)*
tooth fracture (S02.5)

S01.50 Unspecified open wound of lip and oral cavity
- **S01.501-** Unspecified open wound of lip
- **S01.502-** Unspecified open wound of oral cavity

S01.51 Laceration of lip and oral cavity without foreign body
- **S01.511-** Laceration without foreign body of lip
- **S01.512-** Laceration without foreign body of oral cavity

S01.52 Laceration of lip and oral cavity with foreign body
- **S01.521-** Laceration with foreign body of lip
- **S01.522-** Laceration with foreign body of oral cavity

S01.53 Puncture wound of lip and oral cavity without foreign body
- **S01.531-** Puncture wound without foreign body of lip
- **S01.532-** Puncture wound without foreign body of oral cavity

S01.54 Puncture wound of lip and oral cavity with foreign body
- **S01.541-** Puncture wound with foreign body of lip
- **S01.542-** Puncture wound with foreign body of oral cavity

S01.55 Open bite of lip and oral cavity
- **S01.551-** Open bite of lip
  Bite of lip NOS
  EXCLUDES 1 *superficial bite of lip (S00.571)*
- **S01.552-** Open bite of oral cavity
  Bite of oral cavity NOS
  EXCLUDES 1 *superficial bite of oral cavity (S00.572)*

S01.8 Open wound of other parts of head
- **S01.80X-** Unspecified open wound of other part of head
- **S01.81X-** Laceration without foreign body of other part of head
- **S01.82X-** Laceration with foreign body of other part of head
- **S01.83X-** Puncture wound without foreign body of other part of head
- **S01.84X-** Puncture wound with foreign body of other part of head
- **S01.85X-** Open bite of other part of head
  Bite of other part of head NOS
  EXCLUDES 1 *superficial bite of other part of head (S00.87)*

S01.9 Open wound of unspecified part of head
- **S01.90X-** Unspecified open wound of Unspecified part of head
- **S01.91X-** Laceration without foreign body of unspecified part of head

7 **S01.92X-** Laceration with foreign body of unspecified part of head

7 **S01.93X-** Puncture wound without foreign body of unspecified part of head

7 **S01.94X-** Puncture wound with foreign body of unspecified part of head

7 **S01.95X-** Open bite of unspecified part of head
Bite of head NOS
EXCLUDES 1 *superficial bite of head NOS (S00.97)*

4 **S02 Fracture of skull and facial bones**
Note: A fracture not indicated as open or closed should be coded to closed
Code also:
any associated intracranial injury (S06.-)

The appropriate 7th character is to be added to each code from category S02

A	initial encounter for closed fracture
B	initial encounter for open fracture
D	subsequent encounter for fracture with routine healing
G	subsequent encounter for fracture with delayed healing
K	subsequent encounter for fracture with nonunion
S	sequela

CODING TIP ✓ A fracture not indicated as open or closed should be coded to closed.

7 **S02.0XX-** **Fracture of vault of skull** HCC
Fracture of frontal bone
Fracture of parietal bone

5 **S02.1 Fracture of base of skull**
EXCLUDES 1 *orbit NOS (S02.8)*
EXCLUDES 2 *orbital floor (S02.3-)*
AHA: 4Q 2016, 66

6 **S02.10** Unspecified fracture of base of skull
AHA: 4Q 2016, 66

Fracture of base of skull

Exterior view

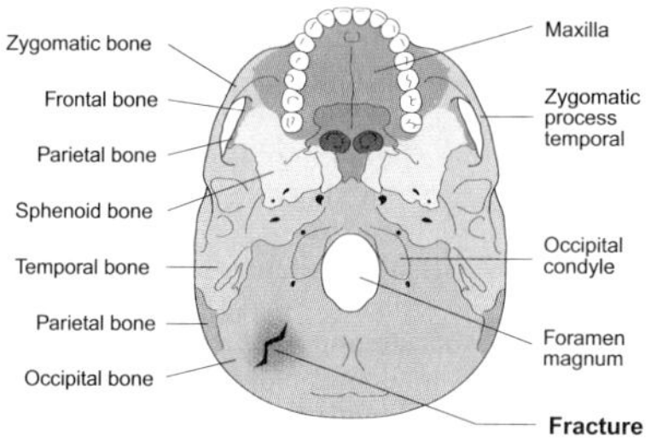

7 ⊟ **S02.101-** **Fracture of base of skull, right side** HCC
AHA: 4Q 2016, 66

7 ⊟ **S02.102-** **Fracture of base of skull, left side** HCC
AHA: 4Q 2016, 66

7 ⊟ **S02.109-** **Fracture of base of skull, unspecified side** HCC
AHA: 4Q 2016, 66

6 **S02.11** **Fracture of occiput**
AHA: 4Q 2016, 66

7 ⊟ **S02.110-** **Type I occipital condyle fracture, unspecified side** HCC
AHA: 4Q 2016, 66

7 ⊟ **S02.111-** **Type II occipital condyle fracture, unspecified side** HCC
AHA: 4Q 2016, 66

7 ⊟ **S02.112-** **Type III occipital condyle fracture, unspecified side** HCC
AHA: 4Q 2016, 66

7 **S02.113-** **Unspecified occipital condyle fracture** HCC
AHA: 4Q 2016, 66

7 ⊟ **S02.118-** **Other fracture of occiput, unspecified side** HCC
AHA: 4Q 2016, 66

7 **S02.119-** **Unspecified fracture of occiput** HCC
AHA: 4Q 2016, 66

7 ⊟ **S02.11A-** **Type I occipital condyle fracture, right side** HCC
AHA: 4Q 2016, 66

7 ⊟ **S02.11B-** **Type I occipital condyle fracture, left side** HCC
AHA: 4Q 2016, 66

7 ⊟ **S02.11C-** **Type II occipital condyle fracture, right side** HCC
AHA: 4Q 2016, 66

7 ⊟ **S02.11D-** **Type II occipital condyle fracture, left side** HCC
AHA: 4Q 2016, 66

7 ⊟ **S02.11E-** **Type III occipital condyle fracture, right side** HCC
AHA: 4Q 2016, 66

7 ⊟ **S02.11F-** **Type III occipital condyle fracture, left side** HCC
AHA: 4Q 2016, 66

7 ⊟ **S02.11G-** **Other fracture of occiput, right side** HCC
AHA: 4Q 2016, 66

7 ⊟ **S02.11H-** **Other fracture of occiput, left side** HCC
AHA: 4Q 2016, 66

7 **S02.19X-** **Other fracture of base of skull** HCC
Fracture of anterior fossa of base of skull
Fracture of ethmoid sinus
Fracture of frontal sinus
Fracture of middle fossa of base of skull
Fracture of orbital roof
Fracture of posterior fossa of base of skull
Fracture of sphenoid
Fracture of temporal bone
AHA: 4Q 2016, 66

7 **S02.2XX-** **Fracture of nasal bones**
AHA: 4Q 2016, 66

5 **S02.3** **Fracture of orbital floor**
EXCLUDES 1 *orbit NOS (S02.8)*
EXCLUDES 2 *orbital roof (S02.1-)*
AHA: 4Q 2016, 66

7 ⊟ **S02.30X-** **Fracture of orbital floor, unspecified side** HCC
AHA: 4Q 2016, 66

7 ⊟ **S02.31X-** **Fracture of orbital floor, right side** HCC
AHA: 4Q 2016, 66

7 ⊟ **S02.32X-** **Fracture of orbital floor, left side** HCC
AHA: 4Q 2016, 66

5 **S02.4** **Fracture of malar, maxillary and zygoma bones**
Fracture of superior maxilla
Fracture of upper jaw (bone)
Fracture of zygomatic process of temporal bone
AHA: 4Q 2016, 66

6 **S02.40** **Fracture of malar, maxillary and zygoma bones, unspecified**
AHA: 4Q 2016, 66

7 ⊟ **S02.400-** **Malar fracture, unspecified side** HCC
AHA: 4Q 2016, 66

7 ⊟ **S02.401-** **Maxillary fracture, unspecified side** HCC
AHA: 4Q 2016, 66

7 ⊟ **S02.402-** **Zygomatic fracture, unspecified side** HCC
AHA: 4Q 2016, 66

7 ⊟ **S02.40A-** **Malar fracture, right side** HCC
AHA: 4Q 2016, 66

7 ⊟ **S02.40B-** **Malar fracture, left side** HCC
AHA: 4Q 2016, 66

7 ⊟ **S02.40C-** **Maxillary fracture, right side** HCC
AHA: 4Q 2016, 66

7 ⊟ **S02.40D-** **Maxillary fracture, left side** HCC
AHA: 4Q 2016, 66

7 ⊟ **S02.40E-** **Zygomatic fracture, right side** HCC
AHA: 4Q 2016, 66

7 ⊟ **S02.40F-** **Zygomatic fracture, left side** HCC
AHA: 4Q 2016, 66

6 **S02.41** **LeFort fracture**
AHA: 4Q 2016, 66

7 **S02.411-** **LeFort I fracture** HCC
AHA: 4Q 2016, 66

7 **S02.412-** **LeFort II fracture** HCC
AHA: 4Q 2016, 66

7 **S02.413-** **LeFort III fracture** HCC
AHA: 4Q 2016, 66

7 **S02.42X-** **Fracture of alveolus of maxilla** HCC
AHA: 4Q 2016, 66

7 **S02.5XX-** **Fracture of tooth (traumatic)**
Broken tooth
EXCLUDES 1 *cracked tooth (nontraumatic) (K03.81)*
AHA: 4Q 2016, 66

5 **S02.6** **Fracture of mandible**
Fracture of lower jaw (bone)
AHA: 4Q 2016, 66

6 **S02.60** **Fracture of mandible, unspecified**
AHA: 4Q 2016, 66

7 ⊟ **S02.600-** **Fracture of unspecified part of body of mandible, unspecified side** HCC
AHA: 4Q 2016, 66

7 ⊟ **S02.601-** **Fracture of unspecified part of body of right mandible** HCC
AHA: 4Q 2016, 66

7 ⊟ **S02.602-** **Fracture of unspecified part of body of left mandible** HCC
AHA: 4Q 2016, 66

7 **S02.609-** **Fracture of mandible, unspecified** HCC
AHA: 4Q 2016, 66

6 **S02.61** **Fracture of condylar process of mandible**
AHA: 4Q 2016, 66

7 ⊟ **S02.610-** **Fracture of condylar process of mandible, unspecified side** HCC
AHA: 4Q 2016, 66

7 ⊟ **S02.611-** **Fracture of condylar process of right mandible** HCC
AHA: 4Q 2016, 66

7 ⊟ **S02.612-** **Fracture of condylar process of left mandible** HCC
AHA: 4Q 2016, 66

6 **S02.62** **Fracture of subcondylar process of mandible**
AHA: 4Q 2016, 66

7 ⊟ **S02.620-** **Fracture of subcondylar process of mandible, unspecified side** HCC
AHA: 4Q 2016, 66

7 ⊟ **S02.621-** **Fracture of subcondylar process of right mandible** HCC
AHA: 4Q 2016, 66

7 ⊟ **S02.622-** **Fracture of subcondylar process of left mandible** HCC
AHA: 4Q 2016, 66

6 **S02.63** **Fracture of coronoid process of mandible**
AHA: 4Q 2016, 66

7 ⊟ **S02.630-** **Fracture of coronoid process of mandible, unspecified side** HCC
AHA: 4Q 2016, 66

7 ⊟ **S02.631-** **Fracture of coronoid process of right mandible** HCC
AHA: 4Q 2016, 66

7 ⊟ **S02.632-** **Fracture of coronoid process of left mandible** HCC
AHA: 4Q 2016, 66

6 **S02.64** **Fracture of ramus of mandible**
AHA: 4Q 2016, 66

7 ⊟ **S02.640-** **Fracture of ramus of mandible, unspecified side** HCC
AHA: 4Q 2016, 66

7 ⊟ **S02.641-** **Fracture of ramus of right mandible** HCC
AHA: 4Q 2016, 66

7 ⊟ **S02.642-** **Fracture of ramus of left mandible** HCC
AHA: 4Q 2016, 66

6 **S02.65** **Fracture of angle of mandible**
AHA: 4Q 2016, 66

7 ⊟ **S02.650-** **Fracture of angle of mandible, unspecified side** HCC
AHA: 4Q 2016, 66

7 ⊟ **S02.651-** **Fracture of angle of right mandible** HCC
AHA: 4Q 2016, 66

7 ⊟ **S02.652-** **Fracture of angle of left mandible** HCC
AHA: 4Q 2016, 66

7 **S02.66X-** **Fracture of symphysis of mandible** HCC
AHA: 4Q 2016, 66

6 **S02.67** **Fracture of alveolus of mandible**
AHA: 4Q 2016, 66

7 ⊟ **S02.670-** **Fracture of alveolus of mandible, unspecified side** HCC
AHA: 4Q 2016, 66

7 ⊟ **S02.671-** **Fracture of alveolus of right mandible** HCC
AHA: 4Q 2016, 66

7 ⊟ **S02.672-** **Fracture of alveolus of left mandible** HCC
AHA: 4Q 2016, 66

7 **S02.69X-** **Fracture of mandible of other specified site** HCC
AHA: 4Q 2016, 66

5 **S02.8** **Fractures of other specified skull and facial bones**
Fracture of orbit NOS
Fracture of palate
EXCLUDES 1 *fracture of orbital floor (S02.3-)*
fracture of orbital roof (S02.1-)
AHA: 4Q 2016, 66

7 ⊟ **S02.80X-** **Fracture of other specified skull and facial bones, unspecified side** HCC

7 ⊟ **S02.81X-** **Fracture of other specified skull and facial bones, right side** HCC

7 ⊟ **S02.82X-** **Fracture of other specified skull and facial bones, left side** HCC

5 **S02.9** **Fracture of unspecified skull and facial bones**

7 **S02.91X-** **Unspecified fracture of skull** HCC

7 **S02.92X-** **Unspecified fracture of facial bones** HCC

4 S03 Dislocation and sprain of joints and ligaments of head

INCLUDES avulsion of joint (capsule) or ligament of head
laceration of cartilage, joint (capsule) or ligament of head
sprain of cartilage, joint (capsule) or ligament of head
traumatic hemarthrosis of joint or ligament of head
traumatic rupture of joint or ligament of head
traumatic subluxation of joint or ligament of head
traumatic tear of joint or ligament of head

Code also:
any associated open wound

EXCLUDES 2 *Strain of muscle or tendon of head (S09.1)*

The appropriate 7th character is to be added to each code from category S03

A	initial encounter
D	subsequent encounter
S	sequela

5 **S03.0** **Dislocation of jaw**
Dislocation of jaw (cartilage) (meniscus)
Dislocation of mandible
Dislocation of temporomandibular (joint)
AHA: 4Q 2016, 67

7 ⊟ **S03.00X-** **Dislocation of jaw, unspecified side**

7 ⊟ **S03.01X-** **Dislocation of jaw, right side**

7 ⊟ **S03.02X-** **Dislocation of jaw, left side**

7 ⊟ **S03.03X-** **Dislocation of jaw, bilateral**

7 **S03.1XX-** **Dislocation of septal cartilage of nose**

7 **S03.2XX-** **Dislocation of tooth**

5 **S03.4** **Sprain of jaw**
Sprain of temporomandibular (joint) (ligament)
AHA: 4Q 2016, 67

7 ⊟ **S03.40X-** **Sprain of jaw, unspecified side**

7 ⊟ S03.41X- **Sprain of jaw, right side**

7 ⊟ S03.42X- **Sprain of jaw, left side**

7 ⊟ S03.43X- **Sprain of jaw, bilateral**

7 S03.8XX- **Sprain of joints and ligaments of other parts of head**

7 S03.9XX- **Sprain of joints and ligaments of unspecified parts of head**

4 S04 **Injury of cranial nerve**

The selection of side should be based on the side of the body being affected

Code first:

any associated intracranial injury (S06.-)

Code also any associated:

open wound of head (S01.-)

skull fracture (S02.-)

The appropriate 7th character is to be added to each code from category S04

A initial encounter

D subsequent encounter

S sequela

CODING TIP ✓ Late effects of injuries are coded with seventh character S (sequela) and are sequenced after the residual condition of the late effect.

5 S04.0 **Injury of optic nerve and pathways**

Use additional code to identify any visual field defect or blindness (H53.4-, H54.-)

6 S04.01 **Injury of optic nerve**

Injury of 2nd cranial nerve

7 ⊟ S04.011- **Injury of optic nerve, right eye**

7 ⊟ S04.012- **Injury of optic nerve, left eye**

7 ⊟ S04.019- **Injury of optic nerve, unspecified eye**

Injury of optic nerve NOS

7 S04.02X- **Injury of optic chiasm**

6 S04.03 **Injury of optic tract and pathways**

Injury of optic radiation

7 ⊟ S04.031- **Injury of optic tract and pathways, right side**

7 ⊟ S04.032- **Injury of optic tract and pathways, left side**

7 ⊟ S04.039- **Injury of optic tract and pathways, unspecified side**

Injury of optic tract and pathways NOS

6 S04.04 **Injury of visual cortex**

7 ⊟ S04.041- **Injury of visual cortex, right side**

7 ⊟ S04.042- **Injury of visual cortex, left side**

7 ⊟ S04.049- **Injury of visual cortex, unspecified side**

Injury of visual cortex NOS

5 S04.1 **Injury of oculomotor nerve**

Injury of 3rd cranial nerve

7 ⊟ S04.10X- **Injury of oculomotor nerve, unspecified side**

7 ⊟ S04.11X- **Injury of oculomotor nerve, right side**

7 ⊟ S04.12X- **Injury of oculomotor nerve, left side**

5 S04.2 **Injury of trochlear nerve**

Injury of 4th cranial nerve

7 ⊟ S04.20X- **Injury of trochlear nerve, unspecified side**

7 ⊟ S04.21X- **Injury of trochlear nerve, right side**

7 ⊟ S04.22X- **Injury of trochlear nerve, left side**

5 S04.3 **Injury of trigeminal nerve**

Injury of 5th cranial nerve

7 ⊟ S04.30X- **Injury of trigeminal nerve, unspecified side**

7 ⊟ S04.31X- **Injury of trigeminal nerve, right side**

7 ⊟ S04.32X- **Injury of trigeminal nerve, left side**

5 S04.4 **Injury of abducent nerve**

Injury of 6th cranial nerve

7 ⊟ S04.40X- **Injury of abducent nerve, unspecified side**

7 ⊟ S04.41X- **Injury of abducent nerve, right side**

7 ⊟ S04.42X- **Injury of abducent nerve, left side**

5 S04.5 **Injury of facial nerve**

Injury of 7th cranial nerve

7 ⊟ S04.50X- **Injury of facial nerve, unspecified side**

7 ⊟ S04.51X- **Injury of facial nerve, right side**

7 ⊟ S04.52X- **Injury of facial nerve, left side**

5 S04.6 **Injury of acoustic nerve**

Injury of auditory nerve

Injury of 8th cranial nerve

7 ⊟ S04.60X- **Injury of acoustic nerve, unspecified side**

7 ⊟ S04.61X- **Injury of acoustic nerve, right side**

7 ⊟ S04.62X- **Injury of acoustic nerve, left side**

5 S04.7 **Injury of accessory nerve**

Injury of 11th cranial nerve

7 ⊟ S04.70X- **Injury of accessory nerve, unspecified side**

7 ⊟ S04.71X- **Injury of accessory nerve, right side**

7 ⊟ S04.72X- **Injury of accessory nerve, left side**

5 S04.8 **Injury of other cranial nerves**

6 S04.81 **Injury of olfactory [1st] nerve**

7 ⊟ S04.811- **Injury of olfactory [1st] nerve, right side**

7 ⊟ S04.812- **Injury of olfactory [1st] nerve, left side**

7 ⊟ S04.819- **Injury of olfactory [1st] nerve, unspecified side**

6 S04.89 **Injury of other cranial nerves**

Injury of vagus [10th] nerve

7 ⊟ S04.891- **Injury of other cranial nerves, right side**

7 ⊟ S04.892- **Injury of other cranial nerves, left side**

7 ⊟ S04.899- **Injury of other cranial nerves, unspecified side**

7 S04.9XX- **Injury of unspecified cranial nerve**

4 S05 **Injury of eye and orbit**

INCLUDES open wound of eye and orbit

EXCLUDES 2 *2nd cranial [optic] nerve injury (S04.0-)*
3rd cranial [oculomotor] nerve injury (S04.1-)
open wound of eyelid and periocular area (S01.1-)
orbital bone fracture (S02.1-, S02.3-, S02.8-)
superficial injury of eyelid (S00.1-S00.2)

The appropriate 7th character is to be added to each code from category S05

A initial encounter

D subsequent encounter

S sequela

5 S05.0 **Injury of conjunctiva and corneal abrasion without foreign body**

EXCLUDES 1 *foreign body in conjunctival sac (T15.1)*
foreign body in cornea (T15.0)

7 ⊟ S05.00X- **Injury of conjunctiva and corneal abrasion without foreign body, unspecified eye**

7 ⊟ S05.01X- **Injury of conjunctiva and corneal abrasion without foreign body, right eye**

7 ⊟ S05.02X- **Injury of conjunctiva and corneal abrasion without foreign body, left eye**

5 S05.1 **Contusion of eyeball and orbital tissues**

Traumatic hyphema

EXCLUDES 2 *black eye NOS (S00.1)*
contusion of eyelid and periocular area (S00.1)

7 ⊟ S05.10X- **Contusion of eyeball and orbital tissues, unspecified eye**

7 ⊟ S05.11X- **Contusion of eyeball and orbital tissues, right eye**

7 ⊟ S05.12X- **Contusion of eyeball and orbital tissues, left eye**

5 S05.2 **Ocular laceration and rupture with prolapse or loss of intraocular tissue**

7 ⊟ S05.20X- **Ocular laceration and rupture with prolapse or loss of intraocular tissue, unspecified eye**

7 ⊟ S05.21X- **Ocular laceration and rupture with prolapse or loss of intraocular tissue, right eye**

7 ⊟ S05.22X- **Ocular laceration and rupture with prolapse or loss of intraocular tissue, left eye**

5 S05.3 **Ocular laceration without prolapse or loss of intraocular tissue**

Laceration of eye NOS

7 ⊟ S05.30X- **Ocular laceration without prolapse or loss of intraocular tissue, unspecified eye**

7 ⊟ S05.31X- **Ocular laceration without prolapse or loss of intraocular tissue, right eye**

7 ⊟ S05.32X- **Ocular laceration without prolapse or loss of intraocular tissue, left eye**

S05.4 Penetrating wound of orbit with or without foreign body

EXCLUDES 2 *retained (old) foreign body following penetrating wound in orbit (H05.5-)*

S05.40X- Penetrating wound of orbit with or without foreign body, unspecified eye

S05.41X- Penetrating wound of orbit with or without foreign body, right eye

S05.42X- Penetrating wound of orbit with or without foreign body, left eye

S05.5 Penetrating wound with foreign body of eyeball

EXCLUDES 2 *retained (old) intraocular foreign body (H44.6-, H44.7)*

S05.50X- Penetrating wound with foreign body of unspecified eyeball

S05.51X- Penetrating wound with foreign body of right eyeball

S05.52X- Penetrating wound with foreign body of left eyeball

S05.6 Penetrating wound without foreign body of eyeball

Ocular penetration NOS

S05.60X- Penetrating wound without foreign body of unspecified eyeball

S05.61X- Penetrating wound without foreign body of right eyeball

S05.62X- Penetrating wound without foreign body of left eyeball

S05.7 Avulsion of eye

Traumatic enucleation

S05.70X- Avulsion of unspecified eye

S05.71X- Avulsion of right eye

S05.72X- Avulsion of left eye

S05.8 Other injuries of eye and orbit

Lacrimal duct injury

S05.8X Other injuries of eye and orbit

S05.8X1- Other injuries of right eye and orbit

S05.8X2- Other injuries of left eye and orbit

S05.8X9- Other injuries of unspecified eye and orbit

S05.9 Unspecified injury of eye and orbit

Injury of eye NOS

S05.90X- Unspecified injury of unspecified eye and orbit

S05.91X- Unspecified injury of right eye and orbit

S05.92X- Unspecified injury of left eye and orbit

S06 Intracranial injury

Note: 7th characters D and S do not apply to codes in category S06 with 6th character 7 - death due to brain injury prior to regaining consciousness, or 8 - death due to other cause prior to regaining consciousness.

INCLUDES traumatic brain injury

Code also any associated:
open wound of head (S01.-)
skull fracture (S02.-)

EXCLUDES 1 *head injury NOS (S09.90)*

The appropriate 7th character is to be added to each code from category S06

A	initial encounter
D	subsequent encounter
S	sequela

CODING TIP ✓ When coding sequelae of a traumatic brain injury, the guideline indicates to first list the residual condition(s), followed by the specific traumatic brain injury diagnosed, using the appropriate code from category S06 with the seventh character "S" to indicate sequelae. In some cases with traumatic brain injury, there is a tabular convention that indicates to code the intracranial injury first and then the residual, e.g. R40.2-. A convention always overrules a conflicting guideline.

AHA: 4Q 2017, 19

S06.0 Concussion

Commotio cerebri

EXCLUDES 1 *concussion with other intracranial injuries classified in subcategories S06.1- to S06.6-, S06.81- and S06.82- code to specified intracranial injury*

AHA: 4Q 2016, 67

S06.0X Concussion

S06.0X0- Concussion without loss of consciousness HCC

S06.0X1- Concussion with loss of consciousness of 30 minutes or less HCC

S06.0X9- Concussion with loss of consciousness of unspecified duration HCC

Concussion NOS

S06.1 Traumatic cerebral edema

Diffuse traumatic cerebral edema
Focal traumatic cerebral edema
AHA: (S06.1X0A) 1Q 2015, 12

S06.1X Traumatic cerebral edema

S06.1X0- Traumatic cerebral edema without loss of consciousness HCC

S06.1X1- Traumatic cerebral edema with loss of consciousness of 30 minutes or less HCC

S06.1X2- Traumatic cerebral edema with loss of consciousness of 31 minutes to 59 minutes HCC

S06.1X3- Traumatic cerebral edema with loss of consciousness of 1 hour to 5 hours 59 minutes HCC

S06.1X4- Traumatic cerebral edema with loss of consciousness of 6 hours to 24 hours HCC

S06.1X5- Traumatic cerebral edema with loss of consciousness greater than 24 hours with return to pre-existing conscious level HCC

S06.1X6- Traumatic cerebral edema with loss of consciousness greater than 24 hours without return to pre-existing conscious level with patient surviving HCC

S06.1X7- Traumatic cerebral edema with loss of consciousness of any duration with death due to brain injury prior to regaining consciousness

S06.1X8- Traumatic cerebral edema with loss of consciousness of any duration with death due to other cause prior to regaining consciousness

S06.1X9- Traumatic cerebral edema with loss of consciousness of unspecified duration HCC

Traumatic cerebral edema NOS

S06.2 Diffuse traumatic brain injury

Diffuse axonal brain injury

EXCLUDES 1 *traumatic diffuse cerebral edema (S06.1X-)*

S06.2X Diffuse traumatic brain injury

S06.2X0- Diffuse traumatic brain injury without loss of consciousness HCC

S06.2X1- Diffuse traumatic brain injury with loss of consciousness of 30 minutes or less HCC

S06.2X2- Diffuse traumatic brain injury with loss of consciousness of 31 minutes to 59 minutes HCC

S06.2X3- Diffuse traumatic brain injury with loss of consciousness of 1 hour to 5 hours 59 minutes HCC

S06.2X4- Diffuse traumatic brain injury with loss of consciousness of 6 hours to 24 hours HCC

S06.2X5- Diffuse traumatic brain injury with loss of consciousness greater than 24 hours with return to pre-existing conscious levels HCC

S06.2X6- Diffuse traumatic brain injury with loss of consciousness greater than 24 hours without return to pre-existing conscious level with patient surviving HCC

S06.2X7- Diffuse traumatic brain injury with loss of consciousness of any duration with death due to brain injury prior to regaining consciousness

S06.2X8- Diffuse traumatic brain injury with loss of consciousness of any duration with death due to other cause prior to regaining consciousness

S06.2X9- Diffuse traumatic brain injury with loss of consciousness of unspecified duration HCC
Diffuse traumatic brain injury NOS

S06.3 Focal traumatic brain injury
EXCLUDES 1 *any condition classifiable to S06.4-S06.6*
focal cerebral edema (S06.1)

S06.30 Unspecified focal traumatic brain injury

S06.300- Unspecified focal traumatic brain injury without loss of consciousness HCC

S06.301- Unspecified focal traumatic brain injury with loss of consciousness of 30 minutes or less HCC

S06.302- Unspecified focal traumatic brain injury with loss of consciousness of 31 minutes to 59 minutes HCC

S06.303- Unspecified focal traumatic brain injury with loss of consciousness of 1 hour to 5 hours 59 minutes HCC

S06.304- Unspecified focal traumatic brain injury with loss of consciousness of 6 hours to 24 hours HCC

S06.305- Unspecified focal traumatic brain injury with loss of consciousness greater than 24 hours with return to pre-existing conscious level HCC

S06.306- Unspecified focal traumatic brain injury with loss of consciousness greater than 24 hours without return to pre-existing conscious level with patient surviving HCC

S06.307- Unspecified focal traumatic brain injury with loss of consciousness of any duration with death due to brain injury prior to regaining consciousness

S06.308- Unspecified focal traumatic brain injury with loss of consciousness of any duration with death due to other cause prior to regaining consciousness

S06.309- Unspecified focal traumatic brain injury with loss of consciousness of unspecified duration HCC
Unspecified focal traumatic brain injury NOS

S06.31 Contusion and laceration of right cerebrum

S06.310- Contusion and laceration of right cerebrum without loss of consciousness HCC

S06.311- Contusion and laceration of right cerebrum with loss of consciousness of 30 minutes or less HCC

S06.312- Contusion and laceration of right cerebrum with loss of consciousness of 31 minutes to 59 minutes HCC

S06.313- Contusion and laceration of right cerebrum with loss of consciousness of 1 hour to 5 hours 59 minutes HCC

S06.314- Contusion and laceration of right cerebrum with loss of consciousness of 6 hours to 24 hours HCC

S06.315- Contusion and laceration of right cerebrum with loss of consciousness greater than 24 hours with return to pre-existing conscious level HCC

S06.316- Contusion and laceration of right cerebrum with loss of consciousness greater than 24 hours without return to pre-existing conscious level with patient surviving HCC

S06.317- Contusion and laceration of right cerebrum with loss of consciousness of any duration with death due to brain injury prior to regaining consciousness

S06.318- Contusion and laceration of right cerebrum with loss of consciousness of any duration with death due to other cause prior to regaining consciousness

S06.319- Contusion and laceration of right cerebrum with loss of consciousness of unspecified duration HCC
Contusion and laceration of right cerebrum NOS

S06.32 Contusion and laceration of left cerebrum

S06.320- Contusion and laceration of left cerebrum without loss of consciousness HCC

S06.321- Contusion and laceration of left cerebrum with loss of consciousness of 30 minutes or less HCC

S06.322- Contusion and laceration of left cerebrum with loss of consciousness of 31 minutes to 59 minutes HCC

S06.323- Contusion and laceration of left cerebrum with loss of consciousness of 1 hour to 5 hours 59 minutes HCC

S06.324- Contusion and laceration of left cerebrum with loss of consciousness of 6 hours to 24 hours HCC

S06.325- Contusion and laceration of left cerebrum with loss of consciousness greater than 24 hours with return to pre-existing conscious level HCC

S06.326- Contusion and laceration of left cerebrum with loss of consciousness greater than 24 hours without return to pre-existing conscious level with patient surviving HCC

S06.327- Contusion and laceration of left cerebrum with loss of consciousness of any duration with death due to brain injury prior to regaining consciousness

S06.328- Contusion and laceration of left cerebrum with loss of consciousness of any duration with death due to other cause prior to regaining consciousness

S06.329- Contusion and laceration of left cerebrum with loss of consciousness of unspecified duration HCC
Contusion and laceration of left cerebrum NOS

S06.33 Contusion and laceration of cerebrum, unspecified

S06.330- Contusion and laceration of cerebrum, unspecified, without loss of consciousness HCC

S06.331- Contusion and laceration of cerebrum, unspecified, with loss of consciousness of 30 minutes or less HCC

S06.332- Contusion and laceration of cerebrum, unspecified, with loss of consciousness of 31 minutes to 59 minutes HCC

S06.333- Contusion and laceration of cerebrum, unspecified, with loss of consciousness of 1 hour to 5 hours 59 minutes HCC

S06.334- Contusion and laceration of cerebrum, unspecified, with loss of consciousness of 6 hours to 24 hours HCC

S06.335- Contusion and laceration of cerebrum, unspecified, with loss of consciousness greater than 24 hours with return to pre-existing conscious level HCC

S06.336- Contusion and laceration of cerebrum, unspecified, with loss of consciousness greater than 24 hours without return to pre-existing conscious level with patient surviving HCC

S06.337- Contusion and laceration of cerebrum, unspecified, with loss of consciousness of any duration with death due to brain injury prior to regaining consciousness

7 S06.338- **Contusion and laceration of cerebrum, unspecified,** with loss of consciousness of any duration with death due to other cause prior to regaining consciousness

7 S06.339- **Contusion and laceration of cerebrum, unspecified,** with loss of consciousness of unspecified duration HCC
Contusion and laceration of cerebrum NOS

6 **S06.34 Traumatic hemorrhage of right cerebrum**
Traumatic intracerebral hemorrhage and hematoma of right cerebrum

7 ⊟ S06.340- **Traumatic hemorrhage of right cerebrum** without loss of consciousness HCC
AHA: (S06.340A) 1Q 2015, 12

7 ⊟ S06.341- **Traumatic hemorrhage of right cerebrum** with loss of consciousness of 30 minutes or less HCC

7 ⊟ S06.342- **Traumatic hemorrhage of right cerebrum** with loss of consciousness of 31 minutes to 59 minutes HCC

7 ⊟ S06.343- **Traumatic hemorrhage of right cerebrum** with loss of consciousness of 1 hours to 5 hours 59 minutes HCC

7 ⊟ S06.344- **Traumatic hemorrhage of right cerebrum** with loss of consciousness of 6 hours to 24 hours HCC

7 ⊟ S06.345- **Traumatic hemorrhage of right cerebrum** with loss of consciousness greater than 24 hours with return to pre-existing conscious level HCC

7 ⊟ S06.346- **Traumatic hemorrhage of right cerebrum** with loss of consciousness greater than 24 hours without return to pre-existing conscious level with patient surviving HCC

7 ⊟ S06.347- **Traumatic hemorrhage of right cerebrum** with loss of consciousness of any duration with death due to brain injury prior to regaining consciousness

7 ⊟ S06.348- **Traumatic hemorrhage of right cerebrum** with loss of consciousness of any duration with death due to other cause prior to regaining consciousness

7 ⊟ S06.349- **Traumatic hemorrhage of right cerebrum** with loss of consciousness of unspecified duration HCC
Traumatic hemorrhage of right cerebrum NOS

6 **S06.35 Traumatic hemorrhage of left cerebrum**
Traumatic intracerebral hemorrhage and hematoma of left cerebrum

7 ⊟ S06.350- **Traumatic hemorrhage of left cerebrum** without loss of consciousness HCC

7 ⊟ S06.351- **Traumatic hemorrhage of left cerebrum** with loss of consciousness of 30 minutes or less HCC

7 ⊟ S06.352- **Traumatic hemorrhage of left cerebrum** with loss of consciousness of 31 minutes to 59 minutes HCC

7 ⊟ S06.353- **Traumatic hemorrhage of left cerebrum** with loss of consciousness of 1 hours to 5 hours 59 minutes HCC

7 ⊟ S06.354- **Traumatic hemorrhage of left cerebrum** with loss of consciousness of 6 hours to 24 hours HCC

7 ⊟ S06.355- **Traumatic hemorrhage of left cerebrum** with loss of consciousness greater than 24 hours with return to pre-existing conscious level HCC

7 ⊟ S06.356- **Traumatic hemorrhage of left cerebrum** with loss of consciousness greater than 24 hours without return to pre-existing conscious level with patient surviving HCC

7 ⊟ S06.357- **Traumatic hemorrhage of left cerebrum** with loss of consciousness of any duration with death due to brain injury prior to regaining consciousness

7 ⊟ S06.358- **Traumatic hemorrhage of left cerebrum** with loss of consciousness of any duration with death due to other cause prior to regaining consciousness

7 ⊟ S06.359- **Traumatic hemorrhage of left cerebrum** with loss of consciousness of unspecified duration HCC
Traumatic hemorrhage of left cerebrum NOS

6 **S06.36 Traumatic hemorrhage of cerebrum, unspecified**
Traumatic intracerebral hemorrhage and hematoma, unspecified

7 S06.360- **Traumatic hemorrhage of cerebrum, unspecified,** without loss of consciousness HCC

7 S06.361- **Traumatic hemorrhage of cerebrum, unspecified,** with loss of consciousness of 30 minutes or less HCC

7 S06.362- **Traumatic hemorrhage of cerebrum, unspecified,** with loss of consciousness of 31 minutes to 59 minutes HCC

7 S06.363- **Traumatic hemorrhage of cerebrum, unspecified,** with loss of consciousness of 1 hours to 5 hours 59 minutes HCC

7 S06.364- **Traumatic hemorrhage of cerebrum, unspecified,** with loss of consciousness of 6 hours to 24 hours HCC

7 S06.365- **Traumatic hemorrhage of cerebrum, unspecified,** with loss of consciousness greater than 24 hours with return to pre-existing conscious level HCC

7 S06.366- **Traumatic hemorrhage of cerebrum, unspecified,** with loss of consciousness greater than 24 hours without return to pre-existing conscious level with patient surviving HCC

7 S06.367- **Traumatic hemorrhage of cerebrum, unspecified,** with loss of consciousness of any duration with death due to brain injury prior to regaining consciousness

7 S06.368- **Traumatic hemorrhage of cerebrum, unspecified,** with loss of consciousness of any duration with death due to other cause prior to regaining consciousness

7 S06.369- **Traumatic hemorrhage of cerebrum, unspecified,** with loss of consciousness of unspecified duration HCC
Traumatic hemorrhage of cerebrum NOS

6 **S06.37 Contusion, laceration, and hemorrhage of cerebellum**

7 S06.370- **Contusion, laceration, and hemorrhage of cerebellum** without loss of consciousness HCC

7 S06.371- **Contusion, laceration, and hemorrhage of cerebellum** with loss of consciousness of 30 minutes or less HCC

7 S06.372- **Contusion, laceration, and hemorrhage of cerebellum** with loss of consciousness of 31 minutes to 59 minutes HCC

7 S06.373- **Contusion, laceration, and hemorrhage of cerebellum** with loss of consciousness of 1 hour to 5 hours 59 minutes HCC

7 S06.374- **Contusion, laceration, and hemorrhage of cerebellum** with loss of consciousness of 6 hours to 24 hours HCC

7 S06.375- **Contusion, laceration, and hemorrhage of cerebellum** with loss of consciousness greater than 24 hours with return to pre-existing conscious level HCC

7 S06.376- **Contusion, laceration, and hemorrhage of cerebellum** with loss of consciousness greater than 24 hours without return to pre-existing conscious level with patient surviving HCC

7 S06.377- **Contusion, laceration, and hemorrhage of cerebellum** with loss of consciousness of any duration with death due to brain injury prior to regaining consciousness

7 S06.378- **Contusion, laceration, and hemorrhage of cerebellum** with loss of consciousness of any duration with death due to other cause prior to regaining consciousness

7 S06.379- **Contusion, laceration, and hemorrhage of cerebellum** with loss of consciousness of unspecified duration HCC
Contusion, laceration, and hemorrhage of cerebellum NOS

6 **S06.38** Contusion, laceration, and hemorrhage **of brainstem**

7 S06.380- **Contusion, laceration, and hemorrhage of brainstem** without loss of consciousness HCC

7 S06.381- **Contusion, laceration, and hemorrhage of brainstem** with loss of consciousness of 30 minutes or less HCC

7 S06.382- **Contusion, laceration, and hemorrhage of brainstem** with loss of consciousness of 31 minutes to 59 minutes HCC

7 S06.383- **Contusion, laceration, and hemorrhage of brainstem** with loss of consciousness of 1 hour to 5 hours 59 minutes HCC

7 S06.384- **Contusion, laceration, and hemorrhage of brainstem** with loss of consciousness of 6 hours to 24 hours HCC

7 S06.385- **Contusion, laceration, and hemorrhage of brainstem** with loss of consciousness greater than 24 hours with return to pre-existing conscious level HCC

7 S06.386- **Contusion, laceration, and hemorrhage of brainstem** with loss of consciousness greater than 24 hours without return to pre-existing conscious level with patient surviving HCC

7 S06.387- **Contusion, laceration, and hemorrhage of brainstem** with loss of consciousness of any duration with death due to brain injury prior to regaining consciousness

7 S06.388- **Contusion, laceration, and hemorrhage of brainstem** with loss of consciousness of any duration with death due to other cause prior to regaining consciousness

7 S06.389- **Contusion, laceration, and hemorrhage of brainstem** with loss of consciousness of unspecified duration HCC
Contusion, laceration, and hemorrhage of brainstem NOS

5 **S06.4 Epidural hemorrhage**
Extradural hemorrhage NOS
Extradural hemorrhage (traumatic)

6 **S06.4X Epidural hemorrhage**

7 S06.4X0- **Epidural hemorrhage** without loss of consciousness HCC

7 S06.4X1- **Epidural hemorrhage** with loss of consciousness of 30 minutes or less HCC

7 S06.4X2- **Epidural hemorrhage** with loss of consciousness of 31 minutes to 59 minutes HCC

7 S06.4X3- **Epidural hemorrhage** with loss of consciousness of 1 hour to 5 hours 59 minutes HCC

7 S06.4X4- **Epidural hemorrhage** with loss of consciousness of 6 hours to 24 hours HCC

7 S06.4X5- **Epidural hemorrhage** with loss of consciousness greater than 24 hours with return to pre-existing conscious level HCC

7 S06.4X6- **Epidural hemorrhage** with loss of consciousness greater than 24 hours without return to pre-existing conscious level with patient surviving HCC

7 S06.4X7- **Epidural hemorrhage** with loss of consciousness of any duration with death due to brain injury prior to regaining consciousness

7 S06.4X8- **Epidural hemorrhage** with loss of consciousness of any duration with death due to other causes prior to regaining consciousness

7 S06.4X9- **Epidural hemorrhage** with loss of consciousness of unspecified duration HCC
Epidural hemorrhage NOS

5 **S06.5 Traumatic subdural hemorrhage**
AHA: (S06.5X0A) 3Q 2015, 37

6 **S06.5X Traumatic subdural hemorrhage**

7 S06.5X0- **Traumatic subdural hemorrhage** without loss of consciousness HCC
AHA: 2Q 2018, 10

7 S06.5X1- **Traumatic subdural hemorrhage** with loss of consciousness of 30 minutes or less HCC

7 S06.5X2- **Traumatic subdural hemorrhage** with loss of consciousness of 31 minutes to 59 minutes HCC

7 S06.5X3- **Traumatic subdural hemorrhage** with loss of consciousness of 1 hour to 5 hours 59 minutes HCC

7 S06.5X4- **Traumatic subdural hemorrhage** with loss of consciousness of 6 hours to 24 hours HCC

7 S06.5X5- **Traumatic subdural hemorrhage** with loss of consciousness greater than 24 hours with return to pre-existing conscious level HCC

7 S06.5X6- **Traumatic subdural hemorrhage** with loss of consciousness greater than 24 hours without return to pre-existing conscious level with patient surviving HCC

7 S06.5X7- **Traumatic subdural hemorrhage** with loss of consciousness of any duration with death due to brain injury before regaining consciousness

7 S06.5X8- **Traumatic subdural hemorrhage** with loss of consciousness of any duration with death due to other cause before regaining consciousness

7 S06.5X9- **Traumatic subdural hemorrhage** with loss of consciousness of unspecified duration HCC
Traumatic subdural hemorrhage NOS

5 **S06.6 Traumatic subarachnoid hemorrhage**
AHA: (S06.6X0A) 3Q 2015, 37

6 **S06.6X Traumatic subarachnoid hemorrhage**

7 S06.6X0- **Traumatic subarachnoid hemorrhage** without loss of consciousness HCC

7 S06.6X1- **Traumatic subarachnoid hemorrhage** with loss of consciousness of 30 minutes or less HCC

7 S06.6X2- **Traumatic subarachnoid hemorrhage** with loss of consciousness of 31 minutes to 59 minutes HCC

7 **S06.6X3-** Traumatic subarachnoid hemorrhage with loss of consciousness of 1 hour to 5 hours 59 minutes HCC

7 **S06.6X4-** Traumatic subarachnoid hemorrhage with loss of consciousness of 6 hours to 24 hours HCC

7 **S06.6X5-** Traumatic subarachnoid hemorrhage with loss of consciousness greater than 24 hours with return to pre-existing conscious level HCC

7 **S06.6X6-** Traumatic subarachnoid hemorrhage with loss of consciousness greater than 24 hours without return to pre-existing conscious level with patient surviving HCC

7 **S06.6X7-** Traumatic subarachnoid hemorrhage with loss of consciousness of any duration with death due to brain injury prior to regaining consciousness

7 **S06.6X8-** Traumatic subarachnoid hemorrhage with loss of consciousness of any duration with death due to other cause prior to regaining consciousness

7 **S06.6X9-** Traumatic subarachnoid hemorrhage with loss of consciousness of unspecified duration HCC

Traumatic subarachnoid hemorrhage NOS

5 **S06.8** Other specified intracranial injuries

6 **S06.81** Injury of right internal carotid artery, intracranial portion, not elsewhere classified

7 ⊟ **S06.810-** Injury of right internal carotid artery, intracranial portion, not elsewhere classified without loss of consciousness HCC

7 ⊟ **S06.811-** Injury of right internal carotid artery, intracranial portion, not elsewhere classified with loss of consciousness of 30 minutes or less HCC

7 ⊟ **S06.812-** Injury of right internal carotid artery, intracranial portion, not elsewhere classified with loss of consciousness of 31 minutes to 59 minutes HCC

7 ⊟ **S06.813-** Injury of right internal carotid artery, intracranial portion, not elsewhere classified with loss of consciousness of 1 hour to 5 hours 59 minutes HCC

7 ⊟ **S06.814-** Injury of right internal carotid artery, intracranial portion, not elsewhere classified with loss of consciousness of 6 hours to 24 hours HCC

7 ⊟ **S06.815-** Injury of right internal carotid artery, intracranial portion, not elsewhere classified with loss of consciousness greater than 24 hours with return to pre-existing conscious level HCC

7 ⊟ **S06.816-** Injury of right internal carotid artery, intracranial portion, not elsewhere classified with loss of consciousness greater than 24 hours without return to pre-existing conscious level with patient surviving HCC

7 ⊟ **S06.817-** Injury of right internal carotid artery, intracranial portion, not elsewhere classified with loss of consciousness of any duration with death due to brain injury prior to regaining consciousness

7 ⊟ **S06.818-** Injury of right internal carotid artery, intracranial portion, not elsewhere classified with loss of consciousness of any duration with death due to other cause prior to regaining consciousness

7 ⊟ **S06.819-** Injury of right internal carotid artery, intracranial portion, not elsewhere classified with loss of consciousness of unspecified duration HCC

Injury of right internal carotid artery, intracranial portion, not elsewhere classified NOS

6 **S06.82** Injury of left internal carotid artery, intracranial portion, not elsewhere classified

7 ⊟ **S06.820-** Injury of left internal carotid artery, intracranial portion, not elsewhere classified without loss of consciousness HCC

7 ⊟ **S06.821-** Injury of left internal carotid artery, intracranial portion, not elsewhere classified with loss of consciousness of 30 minutes or less HCC

7 ⊟ **S06.822-** Injury of left internal carotid artery, intracranial portion, not elsewhere classified with loss of consciousness of 31 minutes to 59 minutes HCC

7 ⊟ **S06.823-** Injury of left internal carotid artery, intracranial portion, not elsewhere classified with loss of consciousness of 1 hour to 5 hours 59 minutes HCC

7 ⊟ **S06.824-** Injury of left internal carotid artery, intracranial portion, not elsewhere classified with loss of consciousness of 6 hours to 24 hours HCC

7 ⊟ **S06.825-** Injury of left internal carotid artery, intracranial portion, not elsewhere classified with loss of consciousness greater than 24 hours with return to pre-existing conscious level HCC

7 ⊟ **S06.826-** Injury of left internal carotid artery, intracranial portion, not elsewhere classified with loss of consciousness greater than 24 hours without return to pre-existing conscious level with patient surviving HCC

7 ⊟ **S06.827-** Injury of left internal carotid artery, intracranial portion, not elsewhere classified with loss of consciousness of any duration with death due to brain injury prior to regaining consciousness

7 ⊟ **S06.828-** Injury of left internal carotid artery, intracranial portion, not elsewhere classified with loss of consciousness of any duration with death due to other cause prior to regaining consciousness

7 ⊟ **S06.829-** Injury of left internal carotid artery, intracranial portion, not elsewhere classified with loss of consciousness of unspecified duration HCC

Injury of left internal carotid artery, intracranial portion, not elsewhere classified NOS

6 **S06.89** Other specified intracranial injury

EXCLUDES 1 *concussion (S06.0X-)*

7 **S06.890-** Other specified intracranial injury without loss of consciousness HCC

7 **S06.891-** Other specified intracranial injury with loss of consciousness of 30 minutes or less HCC

7 **S06.892-** Other specified intracranial injury with loss of consciousness of 31 minutes to 59 minutes HCC

7 **S06.893-** Other specified intracranial injury with loss of consciousness of 1 hour to 5 hours 59 minutes HCC

7 **S06.894-** Other specified intracranial injury with loss of consciousness of 6 hours to 24 hours HCC

7 **S06.895-** Other specified intracranial injury with loss of consciousness greater than 24 hours with return to pre-existing conscious level HCC

7 **S06.896-** Other specified intracranial injury with loss of consciousness greater than 24 hours without return to pre-existing conscious level with patient surviving HCC

7 **S06.897-** **Other specified intracranial injury with loss of consciousness of any duration with death due to brain injury prior to regaining consciousness**

7 **S06.898-** **Other specified intracranial injury with loss of consciousness of any duration with death due to other cause prior to regaining consciousness**

7 **S06.899-** **Other specified intracranial injury with loss of consciousness of unspecified duration** HCC

5 **S06.9** **Unspecified intracranial injury**
Brain injury NOS
Head injury NOS with loss of consciousness
Traumatic brain injury NOS
EXCLUDES 1 *conditions classifiable to S06.0- to S06.8- code to specified intracranial injury*
head injury NOS (S09.90)

6 **S06.9X** **Unspecified intracranial injury**

7 **S06.9X0-** **Unspecified intracranial injury without loss of consciousness** HCC

7 **S06.9X1-** **Unspecified intracranial injury with loss of consciousness of 30 minutes or less** HCC

7 **S06.9X2-** **Unspecified intracranial injury with loss of consciousness of 31 minutes to 59 minutes** HCC

7 **S06.9X3-** **Unspecified intracranial injury with loss of consciousness of 1 hour to 5 hours 59 minutes** HCC

7 **S06.9X4-** **Unspecified intracranial injury with loss of consciousness of 6 hours to 24 hours** HCC

7 **S06.9X5-** **Unspecified intracranial injury with loss of consciousness greater than 24 hours with return to pre-existing conscious level** HCC

7 **S06.9X6-** **Unspecified intracranial injury with loss of consciousness greater than 24 hours without return to pre-existing conscious level with patient surviving** HCC

7 **S06.9X7-** **Unspecified intracranial injury with loss of consciousness of any duration with death due to brain injury prior to regaining consciousness**

7 **S06.9X8-** **Unspecified intracranial injury with loss of consciousness of any duration with death due to other cause prior to regaining consciousness**

7 **S06.9X9-** **Unspecified intracranial injury with loss of consciousness of unspecified duration** HCC

4 S07 Crushing injury of head

Use additional code for all associated injuries, such as:
intracranial injuries (S06.-)
skull fractures (S02.-)

The appropriate 7th character is to be added to each code from category S07
A initial encounter
D subsequent encounter
S sequela

7 **S07.0XX-** **Crushing injury of face**

7 **S07.1XX-** **Crushing injury of skull**

7 **S07.8XX-** **Crushing injury of other parts of head**

7 **S07.9XX-** **Crushing injury of head, part unspecified**

4 S08 Avulsion and traumatic amputation of part of head

An amputation not identified as partial or complete should be coded to complete

The appropriate 7th character is to be added to each code from category S08
A initial encounter
D subsequent encounter
S sequela

7 **S08.0XX-** **Avulsion of scalp**

5 **S08.1** **Traumatic amputation of ear**

6 **S08.11** **Complete traumatic amputation of ear**

7 ⊟ **S08.111-** **Complete traumatic amputation of right ear**

7 ⊟ **S08.112-** **Complete traumatic amputation of left ear**

7 ⊟ **S08.119-** **Complete traumatic amputation of unspecified ear**

6 **S08.12** **Partial traumatic amputation of ear**

7 ⊟ **S08.121-** **Partial traumatic amputation of right ear**

7 ⊟ **S08.122-** **Partial traumatic amputation of left ear**

7 ⊟ **S08.129-** **Partial traumatic amputation of unspecified ear**

5 **S08.8** **Traumatic amputation of other parts of head**

6 **S08.81** **Traumatic amputation of nose**

7 **S08.811-** **Complete traumatic amputation of nose**

7 **S08.812-** **Partial traumatic amputation of nose**

7 **S08.89X-** **Traumatic amputation of other parts of head**

4 S09 Other and unspecified injuries of head

The appropriate 7th character is to be added to each code from category S09
A initial encounter
D subsequent encounter
S sequela

7 **S09.0XX-** **Injury of blood vessels of head, not elsewhere classified**
EXCLUDES 1 *injury of cerebral blood vessels (S06.-)*
injury of precerebral blood vessels (S15.-)

5 **S09.1** **Injury of muscle and tendon of head**
Code also:
any associated open wound (S01.-)
EXCLUDES 2 *sprain to joints and ligament of head (S03.9)*

7 **S09.10X-** **Unspecified injury of muscle and tendon of head**
Injury of muscle and tendon of head NOS

7 **S09.11X-** **Strain of muscle and tendon of head**

7 **S09.12X-** **Laceration of muscle and tendon of head**

7 **S09.19X-** **Other specified injury of muscle and tendon of head**

5 **S09.2** **Traumatic rupture of ear drum**
EXCLUDES 1 *traumatic rupture of ear drum due to blast injury (S09.31-)*

7 ⊟ **S09.20X-** **Traumatic rupture of unspecified ear drum**

7 ⊟ **S09.21X-** **Traumatic rupture of right ear drum**

7 ⊟ **S09.22X-** **Traumatic rupture of left ear drum**

5 **S09.3** **Other specified and unspecified injury of middle and inner ear**
EXCLUDES 1 *injury to ear NOS (S09.91-)*
EXCLUDES 2 *injury to external ear (S00.4-, S01.3-, S08.1-)*

6 **S09.30** **Unspecified injury of middle and inner ear**

7 ⊟ **S09.301-** **Unspecified injury of right middle and inner ear**

7 ⊟ **S09.302-** **Unspecified injury of left middle and inner ear**

7 ⊟ **S09.309-** **Unspecified injury of unspecified middle and inner ear**

6 **S09.31** **Primary blast injury of ear**
Blast injury of ear NOS

7 ⊟ **S09.311-** **Primary blast injury of right ear**

7 ⊟ **S09.312-** **Primary blast injury of left ear**

7 ⊟ **S09.313-** **Primary blast injury of ear, bilateral**

7 ⊟ **S09.319-** **Primary blast injury of unspecified ear**

6 **S09.39** **Other specified injury of middle and inner ear**
Secondary blast injury to ear

7 ⊟ **S09.391-** **Other specified injury of right middle and inner ear**

7 ⊟ **S09.392-** **Other specified injury of left middle and inner ear**

7 ⊟ **S09.399-** **Other specified injury of unspecified middle and inner ear**

7 **S09.8XX-** **Other specified injuries of head**

5 **S09.9** **Unspecified injury of face and head**

7 S09.90X- **Unspecified injury of head**
Head injury NOS
EXCLUDES 1 *brain injury NOS (S06.9-)*
head injury NOS with loss of consciousness (S06.9-)
intracranial injury NOS (S06.9-)

7 S09.91X- **Unspecified injury of ear**
Injury of ear NOS

7 S09.92X- **Unspecified injury of nose**
Injury of nose NOS

7 S09.93X- **Unspecified injury of face**
Injury of face NOS

Injuries to the neck (S10-S19)

INCLUDES injuries of nape
injuries of supraclavicular region
injuries of throat

EXCLUDES 2 *burns and corrosions (T20-T32)*
effects of foreign body in esophagus (T18.1)
effects of foreign body in larynx (T17.3)
effects of foreign body in pharynx (T17.2)
effects of foreign body in trachea (T17.4)
frostbite (T33-T34)
insect bite or sting, venomous (T63.4)

GUIDELINES **Section I.C.19.c.2)**
Multiple fractures are sequenced in accordance with the severity of the fracture.

GUIDELINES **Section I.C.19.b.1)-2)**
When coding injuries, assign separate codes for each injury unless a combination code is provided, in which case the combination code is assigned ... Traumatic injury codes (S00-T14.9) are not to be used for normal, healing surgical wounds or to identify complications of surgical wounds. The code for the most serious injury, as determined by the provider and the focus of treatment, is sequenced first.

1) Superficial injuries such as abrasions or contusions are not coded when associated with more severe injuries of the same site.

2) When a primary injury results in minor damage to peripheral nerves or blood vessels, the primary injury is sequenced first with additional code(s) for injuries to nerves and spinal cord (such as category S04), and/or injury to blood vessels (such as category S15). When the primary injury is to the blood vessels or nerves, that injury should be sequenced first.

GUIDELINES **Section I.C.19.c**
Coding of Traumatic Fractures: The principles of multiple coding of injuries should be followed in coding fractures. Fractures of specified sites are coded individually by site in accordance with both the provisions within categories S02, S12, S22, S32, S42, S49, S52, S59, S62, S72, S79, S82, S89, S92 and the level of detail furnished by medical record content. A fracture not indicated as open or closed should be coded to closed. A fracture not indicated whether displaced or not displaced should be coded to displaced.

4 S10 **Superficial injury of neck**

The appropriate 7th character is to be added to each code from category S10
A initial encounter
D subsequent encounter
S sequela

7 S10.0XX- **Contusion of throat**
Contusion of cervical esophagus
Contusion of larynx
Contusion of pharynx
Contusion of trachea

5 S10.1 **Other and unspecified superficial injuries of throat**
7 S10.10X- **Unspecified superficial injuries of throat**
7 S10.11X- **Abrasion of throat**
7 S10.12X- **Blister (nonthermal) of throat**
7 S10.14X- **External constriction of part of throat**
7 S10.15X- **Superficial foreign body of throat**
Splinter in the throat
7 S10.16X- **Insect bite (nonvenomous) of throat**
7 S10.17X- **Other superficial bite of throat**
EXCLUDES 1 *open bite of throat (S11.85)*

5 S10.8 **Superficial injury of other specified parts of neck**
7 S10.80X- **Unspecified superficial injury of other specified part of neck**
7 S10.81X- **Abrasion of other specified part of neck**
7 S10.82X- **Blister (nonthermal) of other specified part of neck**
7 S10.83X- **Contusion of other specified part of neck**
7 S10.84X- **External constriction of other specified part of neck**
7 S10.85X- **Superficial foreign body of other specified part of neck**
Splinter in other specified part of neck
7 S10.86X- **Insect bite of other specified part of neck**
7 S10.87X- **Other superficial bite of other specified part of neck**
EXCLUDES 1 *open bite of other specified parts of neck (S11.85)*

5 S10.9 **Superficial injury of unspecified part of neck**
7 S10.90X- **Unspecified superficial injury of Unspecified part of neck**
7 S10.91X- **Abrasion of unspecified part of neck**
7 S10.92X- **Blister (nonthermal) of unspecified part of neck**
7 S10.93X- **Contusion of unspecified part of neck**
7 S10.94X- **External constriction of unspecified part of neck**
7 S10.95X- **Superficial foreign body of unspecified part of neck**
7 S10.96X- **Insect bite of unspecified part of neck**
7 S10.97X- **Other superficial bite of unspecified part of neck**

4 S11 **Open wound of neck**
Code also any associated:
spinal cord injury (S14.0, S14.1-)
wound infection
EXCLUDES 2 *open fracture of vertebra (S12.- with 7th character B)*

The appropriate 7th character is to be added to each code from category S11
A initial encounter
D subsequent encounter
S sequela

CODING TIP✓ Open wound codes are used for wounds caused by trauma. Do not assign a code for "open wound" unless the etiology of the wound is related to trauma. Do not use Z codes for any aspect of care of a trauma wound, e.g. no Z code for dressing changes, drain care, or suture removal. Report instead the appropriate subsequent care 7th character with the injury code.

CODING TIP✓ Open wound codes are used for wounds caused by trauma. Do not assign a code for "open wound" unless the etiology of the wound is related to trauma.

5 S11.0 **Open wound of larynx and trachea**
6 S11.01 **Open wound of larynx**
EXCLUDES 2 *open wound of vocal cord (S11.03)*
7 S11.011- **Laceration without foreign body of larynx**
7 S11.012- **Laceration with foreign body of larynx**
7 S11.013- **Puncture wound without foreign body of larynx**
7 S11.014- **Puncture wound with foreign body of larynx**
7 S11.015- **Open bite of larynx**
Bite of larynx NOS
7 S11.019- **Unspecified open wound of larynx**
6 S11.02 **Open wound of trachea**
Open wound of cervical trachea
Open wound of trachea NOS
EXCLUDES 2 *open wound of thoracic trachea (S27.5-)*
7 S11.021- **Laceration without foreign body of trachea**
7 S11.022- **Laceration with foreign body of trachea**
7 S11.023- **Puncture wound without foreign body of trachea**
7 S11.024- **Puncture wound with foreign body of trachea**

7 S11.025- **Open bite of trachea**
Bite of trachea NOS
7 S11.029- **Unspecified open wound of trachea**
6 S11.03 **Open wound of vocal cord**
7 S11.031- **Laceration without foreign body of vocal cord**
7 S11.032- **Laceration with foreign body of vocal cord**
7 S11.033- **Puncture wound without foreign body of vocal cord**
7 S11.034- **Puncture wound with foreign body of vocal cord**
7 S11.035- **Open bite of vocal cord**
Bite of vocal cord NOS
7 S11.039- **Unspecified open wound of vocal cord**
5 S11.1 **Open wound of thyroid gland**
7 S11.10X- **Unspecified open wound of thyroid gland**
7 S11.11X- **Laceration without foreign body of thyroid gland**
7 S11.12X- **Laceration with foreign body of thyroid gland**
7 S11.13X- **Puncture wound without foreign body of thyroid gland**
7 S11.14X- **Puncture wound with foreign body of thyroid gland**
7 S11.15X- **Open bite of thyroid gland**
Bite of thyroid gland NOS
5 S11.2 **Open wound of pharynx and cervical esophagus**
EXCLUDES 1 *open wound of esophagus NOS (S27.8-)*
7 S11.20X- **Unspecified open wound of pharynx and cervical esophagus**
7 S11.21X- **Laceration without foreign body of pharynx and cervical esophagus**
7 S11.22X- **Laceration with foreign body of pharynx and cervical esophagus**
7 S11.23X- **Puncture wound without foreign body of pharynx and cervical esophagus**
7 S11.24X- **Puncture wound with foreign body of pharynx and cervical esophagus**
7 S11.25X- **Open bite of pharynx and cervical esophagus**
Bite of pharynx and cervical esophagus NOS
5 S11.8 **Open wound of other specified parts of neck**
7 S11.80X- **Unspecified open wound of other specified part of neck**
7 S11.81X- **Laceration without foreign body of other specified part of neck**
7 S11.82X- **Laceration with foreign body of other specified part of neck**
7 S11.83X- **Puncture wound without foreign body of other specified part of neck**
7 S11.84X- **Puncture wound with foreign body of other specified part of neck**
7 S11.85X- **Open bite of other specified part of neck**
Bite of other specified part of neck NOS
EXCLUDES 1 *superficial bite of other specified part of neck (S10.87)*
7 S11.89X- **Other open wound of other specified part of neck**
5 S11.9 **Open wound of unspecified part of neck**
7 S11.90X- **Unspecified open wound of Unspecified part of neck**
7 S11.91X- **Laceration without foreign body of unspecified part of neck**
7 S11.92X- **Laceration with foreign body of unspecified part of neck**
7 S11.93X- **Puncture wound without foreign body of unspecified part of neck**
7 S11.94X- **Puncture wound with foreign body of unspecified part of neck**
7 S11.95X- **Open bite of unspecified part of neck**
Bite of neck NOS
EXCLUDES 1 *superficial bite of neck (S10.97)*

4 S12 **Fracture of cervical vertebra and other parts of neck**
Note: A fracture not indicated as displaced or nondisplaced should be coded to displaced
A fracture not indicated as open or closed should be coded to closed
INCLUDES fracture of cervical neural arch
fracture of cervical spine
fracture of cervical spinous process
fracture of cervical transverse process
fracture of cervical vertebral arch
fracture of neck
Code first:
any associated cervical spinal cord injury (S14.0, S14.1-)

The appropriate 7th character is to be added to all codes from subcategories S12.0-S12.6

A	initial encounter for closed fracture
B	initial encounter for open fracture
D	subsequent encounter for fracture with routine healing
G	subsequent encounter for fracture with delayed healing
K	subsequent encounter for fracture with nonunion
S	sequela

CODING TIP ✓ A fracture not indicated as displaced or nondisplaced should be coded to displaced. A fracture not indicated as open or closed should be coded to closed. Query providers on fractures not documented as displaced/nondisplaced; otherwise, a displaced fracture diagnosis could be assigned without a reduction being performed, potentially resulting in claim denials.

5 S12.0 **Fracture of first cervical vertebra**
Atlas
6 S12.00 **Unspecified fracture of first cervical vertebra**
7 S12.000- **Unspecified displaced fracture of first cervical vertebra** HCC
7 S12.001- **Unspecified nondisplaced fracture of first cervical vertebra** HCC
7 S12.01X- **Stable burst fracture of first cervical vertebra** HCC
7 S12.02X- **Unstable burst fracture of first cervical vertebra** HCC
6 S12.03 **Posterior arch fracture of first cervical vertebra**
7 S12.030- **Displaced posterior arch fracture of first cervical vertebra** HCC
7 S12.031- **Nondisplaced posterior arch fracture of first cervical vertebra** HCC
6 S12.04 **Lateral mass fracture of first cervical vertebra**
7 S12.040- **Displaced lateral mass fracture of first cervical vertebra** HCC
7 S12.041- **Nondisplaced lateral mass fracture of first cervical vertebra** HCC
6 S12.09 **Other fracture of first cervical vertebra**
7 S12.090- **Other displaced fracture of first cervical vertebra** HCC
7 S12.091- **Other nondisplaced fracture of first cervical vertebra** HCC
5 S12.1 **Fracture of second cervical vertebra**
Axis
6 S12.10 **Unspecified fracture of second cervical vertebra**
7 S12.100- **Unspecified displaced fracture of second cervical vertebra** HCC
7 S12.101- **Unspecified nondisplaced fracture of second cervical vertebra** HCC
6 S12.11 **Type II dens fracture**
7 S12.110- **Anterior displaced Type II dens fracture** HCC
7 S12.111- **Posterior displaced Type II dens fracture** HCC
7 S12.112- **Nondisplaced Type II dens fracture** HCC
6 S12.12 **Other dens fracture**
7 S12.120- **Other displaced dens fracture** HCC
7 S12.121- **Other nondisplaced dens fracture** HCC
6 S12.13 **Unspecified traumatic spondylolisthesis of second cervical vertebra**
7 S12.130- **Unspecified traumatic displaced spondylolisthesis of second cervical vertebra** HCC

7 S12.131- Unspecified traumatic nondisplacedspondylolisthesis of second cervical vertebra HCC

7 S12.14X- Type III traumatic spondylolisthesis of second cervical vertebra HCC

6 S12.15 Other traumatic spondylolisthesis of second cervical vertebra

7 S12.150- Other traumatic displaced spondylolisthesis of second cervical vertebra HCC

7 S12.151- Other traumatic nondisplaced spondylolisthesis of second cervical vertebra HCC

6 S12.19 Other fracture of second cervical vertebra

7 S12.190- Other displaced fracture of second cervical vertebra HCC

7 S12.191- Other nondisplaced fracture of second cervical vertebra HCC

5 S12.2 Fracture of third cervical vertebra

6 S12.20 Unspecified fracture of third cervical vertebra

7 S12.200- Unspecified displaced fracture of third cervical vertebra HCC

7 S12.201- Unspecified nondisplaced fracture of third cervical vertebra HCC

6 S12.23 Unspecified traumatic spondylolisthesis of third cervical vertebra

7 S12.230- Unspecified traumatic displaced spondylolisthesis of third cervical vertebra HCC

7 S12.231- Unspecified traumatic nondisplaced spondylolisthesis of third cervical vertebra HCC

7 S12.24X- Type III traumatic spondylolisthesis of third cervical vertebra HCC

6 S12.25 Other traumatic spondylolisthesis of third cervical vertebra

7 S12.250- Other traumatic displaced spondylolisthesis of third cervical vertebra HCC

7 S12.251- Other traumatic nondisplaced spondylolisthesis of third cervical vertebra HCC

6 S12.29 Other fracture of third cervical vertebra

7 S12.290- Other displaced fracture of third cervical vertebra HCC

7 S12.291- Other nondisplaced fracture of third cervical vertebra HCC

5 S12.3 Fracture of fourth cervical vertebra

6 S12.30 Unspecified fracture of fourth cervical vertebra

7 S12.300- Unspecified displaced fracture of fourth cervical vertebra HCC

7 S12.301- Unspecified nondisplaced fracture of fourth cervical vertebra HCC

6 S12.33 Unspecified traumatic spondylolisthesis of fourth cervical vertebra

7 S12.330- Unspecified traumatic displaced spondylolisthesis of fourth cervical vertebra HCC

7 S12.331- Unspecified traumatic nondisplaced spondylolisthesis of fourth cervical vertebra HCC

7 S12.34X- Type III traumatic spondylolisthesis of fourth cervical vertebra HCC

6 S12.35 Other traumatic spondylolisthesis of fourth cervical vertebra

7 S12.350- Other traumatic displaced spondylolisthesis of fourth cervical vertebra HCC

7 S12.351- Other traumatic nondisplaced spondylolisthesis of fourth cervical vertebra HCC

6 S12.39 Other fracture of fourth cervical vertebra

7 S12.390- Other displaced fracture of fourth cervical vertebra HCC

7 S12.391- Other nondisplaced fracture of fourth cervical vertebra HCC

5 S12.4 Fracture of fifth cervical vertebra

6 S12.40 Unspecified fracture of fifth cervical vertebra

7 S12.400- Unspecified displaced fracture of fifth cervical vertebra HCC

7 S12.401- Unspecified nondisplaced fracture of fifth cervical vertebra HCC

6 S12.43 Unspecified traumatic spondylolisthesis of fifth cervical vertebra

7 S12.430- Unspecified traumatic displaced spondylolisthesis of fifth cervical vertebra HCC

7 S12.431- Unspecified traumatic nondisplaced spondylolisthesis of fifth cervical vertebra HCC

7 S12.44X- Type III traumatic spondylolisthesis of fifth cervical vertebra HCC

6 S12.45 Other traumatic spondylolisthesis of fifth cervical vertebra

7 S12.450- Other traumatic displaced spondylolisthesis of fifth cervical vertebra HCC

7 S12.451- Other traumatic nondisplaced spondylolisthesis of fifth cervical vertebra HCC

6 S12.49 Other fracture of fifth cervical vertebra

7 S12.490- Other displaced fracture of fifth cervical vertebra HCC

7 S12.491- Other nondisplaced fracture of fifth cervical vertebra HCC

5 S12.5 Fracture of sixth cervical vertebra

6 S12.50 Unspecified fracture of sixth cervical vertebra

7 S12.500- Unspecified displaced fracture of sixth cervical vertebra HCC

7 S12.501- Unspecified nondisplaced fracture of sixth cervical vertebra HCC

6 S12.53 Unspecified traumatic spondylolisthesis of sixth cervical vertebra

7 S12.530- Unspecified traumatic displaced spondylolisthesis of sixth cervical vertebra HCC

7 S12.531- Unspecified traumatic nondisplaced spondylolisthesis of sixth cervical vertebra HCC

7 S12.54X- Type III traumatic spondylolisthesis of sixth cervical vertebra HCC

6 S12.55 Other traumatic spondylolisthesis of sixth cervical vertebra

7 S12.550- Other traumatic displaced spondylolisthesis of sixth cervical vertebra HCC

7 S12.551- Other traumatic nondisplaced spondylolisthesis of sixth cervical vertebra HCC

6 S12.59 Other fracture of sixth cervical vertebra

7 S12.590- Other displaced fracture of sixth cervical vertebra HCC

7 S12.591- Other nondisplaced fracture of sixth cervical vertebra HCC

5 S12.6 Fracture of seventh cervical vertebra

6 S12.60 Unspecified fracture of seventh cervical vertebra

7 S12.600- Unspecified displaced fracture of seventh cervical vertebra HCC

7 S12.601- Unspecified nondisplaced fracture of seventh cervical vertebra HCC

6 S12.63 Unspecified traumatic spondylolisthesis of seventh cervical vertebra

7 S12.630- Unspecified traumatic displaced spondylolisthesis of seventh cervical vertebra HCC

7 S12.631- Unspecified traumatic nondisplaced spondylolisthesis of seventh cervical vertebra HCC

7 S12.64X- Type III traumatic spondylolisthesis of seventh cervical vertebra HCC

6 S12.65 Other traumatic spondylolisthesis of seventh cervical vertebra

7 S12.650- Other traumatic displaced spondylolisthesis of seventh cervical vertebra HCC

7 S12.651- **Other traumatic nondisplaced spondylolisthesis of seventh cervical vertebra** HCC

6 S12.69 **Other fracture of seventh cervical vertebra**

7 S12.690- **Other displaced fracture of seventh cervical vertebra** HCC

7 S12.691- **Other nondisplaced fracture of seventh cervical vertebra** HCC

7 S12.8XX- **Fracture of other parts of neck** HCC
Hyoid bone
Larynx
Thyroid cartilage
Trachea

The appropriate 7th character is to be added to code S12.8
A initial encounter
D subsequent encounter
S sequela

7 S12.9XX- **Fracture of neck, unspecified** HCC
Fracture of neck NOS
Fracture of cervical spine NOS
Fracture of cervical vertebra NOS

The appropriate 7th character is to be added to code S12.9
A initial encounter
D subsequent encounter
S sequela

4 S13 Dislocation and sprain of joints and ligaments at neck level

INCLUDES avulsion of joint or ligament at neck level
laceration of cartilage, joint or ligament at neck level
sprain of cartilage, joint or ligament at neck level
traumatic hemarthrosis of joint or ligament at neck level
traumatic rupture of joint or ligament at neck level
traumatic subluxation of joint or ligament at neck level
traumatic tear of joint or ligament at neck level

Code also:
any associated open wound

EXCLUDES 2 *strain of muscle or tendon at neck level (S16.1)*

The appropriate 7th character is to be added to each code from category S13
A initial encounter
D subsequent encounter
S sequela

CODING TIP✓ There are no codes for open dislocations. When a dislocation is documented as open, assign an additional code for the open wound.

7 S13.0XX- **Traumatic rupture of cervical intervertebral disc**
EXCLUDES 1 *rupture or displacement (nontraumatic) of cervical intervertebral disc NOS (M50.-)*

5 S13.1 **Subluxation and dislocation of cervical vertebrae**
Code also any associated:
open wound of neck (S11.-)
spinal cord injury (S14.1-)
EXCLUDES 2 *fracture of cervical vertebrae (S12.0-S12.3-)*

6 S13.10 **Subluxation and dislocation of unspecified cervical vertebrae**

7 S13.100- **Subluxation of unspecified cervical vertebrae**

7 S13.101- **Dislocation of unspecified cervical vertebrae**

6 S13.11 **Subluxation and dislocation of C0/C1 cervical vertebrae**
Subluxation and dislocation of atlantooccipital joint
Subluxation and dislocation of atloidooccipital joint
Subluxation and dislocation of occipitoatloid joint

7 S13.110- **Subluxation of C0/C1 cervical vertebrae**

7 S13.111- **Dislocation of C0/C1 cervical vertebrae**

6 S13.12 **Subluxation and dislocation of C1/C2 cervical vertebrae**
Subluxation and dislocation of atlantoaxial joint

7 S13.120- **Subluxation of C1/C2 cervical vertebrae**

7 S13.121- **Dislocation of C1/C2 cervical vertebrae**

6 S13.13 **Subluxation and dislocation of C2/C3 cervical vertebrae**

7 S13.130- **Subluxation of C2/C3 cervical vertebrae**

7 S13.131- **Dislocation of C2/C3 cervical vertebrae**

6 S13.14 **Subluxation and dislocation of C3/C4 cervical vertebrae**

7 S13.140- **Subluxation of C3/C4 cervical vertebrae**

7 S13.141- **Dislocation of C3/C4 cervical vertebrae**

6 S13.15 **Subluxation and dislocation of C4/C5 cervical vertebrae**

7 S13.150- **Subluxation of C4/C5 cervical vertebrae**

7 S13.151- **Dislocation of C4/C5 cervical vertebrae**

6 S13.16 **Subluxation and dislocation of C5/C6 cervical vertebrae**

7 S13.160- **Subluxation of C5/C6 cervical vertebrae**

7 S13.161- **Dislocation of C5/C6 cervical vertebrae**

6 S13.17 **Subluxation and dislocation of C6/C7 cervical vertebrae**

7 S13.170- **Subluxation of C6/C7 cervical vertebrae**

7 S13.171- **Dislocation of C6/C7 cervical vertebrae**

6 S13.18 **Subluxation and dislocation of C7/T1 cervical vertebrae**

7 S13.180- **Subluxation of C7/T1 cervical vertebrae**

7 S13.181- **Dislocation of C7/T1 cervical vertebrae**

5 S13.2 **Dislocation of other and unspecified parts of neck**

7 S13.20X- **Dislocation of unspecified parts of neck**

7 S13.29X- **Dislocation of other parts of neck**

7 S13.4XX- **Sprain of ligaments of cervical spine**
Sprain of anterior longitudinal (ligament), cervical
Sprain of atlanto-axial (joints)
Sprain of atlanto-occipital (joints)
Whiplash injury of cervical spine

7 S13.5XX- **Sprain of thyroid region**
Sprain of cricoarytenoid (joint) (ligament)
Sprain of cricothyroid (joint) (ligament)
Sprain of thyroid cartilage

7 S13.8XX- **Sprain of joints and ligaments of other parts of neck**

7 S13.9XX- **Sprain of joints and ligaments of unspecified parts of neck**

4 S14 Injury of nerves and spinal cord at neck level

Note: Code to highest level of cervical cord injury
Code also any associated:
fracture of cervical vertebra (S12.0--S12.6.-)
open wound of neck (S11.-)
transient paralysis (R29.5)

The appropriate 7th character is to be added to each code from category S14
A initial encounter
D subsequent encounter
S sequela

CODING TIP✓ When coding sequelae of a spinal cord injury, first list the residual condition(s), followed by the specific spinal cord injury diagnosed using the appropriate code from this category with the seventh character "S" to indicate sequelae. If there are multiple levels of injury, code only the highest injury.

7 S14.0XX- **Concussion and edema of cervical spinal cord** HCC

5 S14.1 **Other and unspecified injuries of cervical spinal cord**

6 S14.10 **Unspecified injury of cervical spinal cord**

7 S14.101- **Unspecified injury at C1 level of cervical spinal cord** HCC

7 S14.102- **Unspecified injury at C2 level of cervical spinal cord** HCC

7 S14.103- **Unspecified injury at C3 level of cervical spinal cord** HCC

7 S14.104- **Unspecified injury at C4 level of cervical spinal cord** HCC

7 S14.105- **Unspecified injury at C5 level of cervical spinal cord** HCC

7 S14.106- **Unspecified injury at C6 level of cervical spinal cord** HCC

7 S14.107- **Unspecified injury at C7 level of cervical spinal cord** HCC

7 S14.108- Unspecified injury at C8 level of cervical spinal cord HCC

7 S14.109- Unspecified injury at unspecified level of cervical spinal cord HCC
Injury of cervical spinal cord NOS

6 S14.11 Complete lesion of cervical spinal cord

7 S14.111- Complete lesion at C1 level of cervical spinal cord HCC

7 S14.112- Complete lesion at C2 level of cervical spinal cord HCC

7 S14.113- Complete lesion at C3 level of cervical spinal cord HCC

7 S14.114- Complete lesion at C4 level of cervical spinal cord HCC

7 S14.115- Complete lesion at C5 level of cervical spinal cord HCC

7 S14.116- Complete lesion at C6 level of cervical spinal cord HCC

7 S14.117- Complete lesion at C7 level of cervical spinal cord HCC

7 S14.118- Complete lesion at C8 level of cervical spinal cord HCC

7 S14.119- Complete lesion at unspecified level of cervical spinal cord HCC

6 S14.12 Central cord syndrome of cervical spinal cord

7 S14.121- Central cord syndrome at C1 level of cervical spinal cord HCC

7 S14.122- Central cord syndrome at C2 level of cervical spinal cord HCC

7 S14.123- Central cord syndrome at C3 level of cervical spinal cord HCC

7 S14.124- Central cord syndrome at C4 level of cervical spinal cord HCC

7 S14.125- Central cord syndrome at C5 level of cervical spinal cord HCC

7 S14.126- Central cord syndrome at C6 level of cervical spinal cord HCC

7 S14.127- Central cord syndrome at C7 level of cervical spinal cord HCC

7 S14.128- Central cord syndrome at C8 level of cervical spinal cord HCC

7 S14.129- Central cord syndrome at unspecified level of cervical spinal cord HCC

6 S14.13 Anterior cord syndrome of cervical spinal cord

7 S14.131- Anterior cord syndrome at C1 level of cervical spinal cord HCC

7 S14.132- Anterior cord syndrome at C2 level of cervical spinal cord HCC

7 S14.133- Anterior cord syndrome at C3 level of cervical spinal cord HCC

7 S14.134- Anterior cord syndrome at C4 level of cervical spinal cord HCC

7 S14.135- Anterior cord syndrome at C5 level of cervical spinal cord HCC

7 S14.136- Anterior cord syndrome at C6 level of cervical spinal cord HCC

7 S14.137- Anterior cord syndrome at C7 level of cervical spinal cord HCC

7 S14.138- Anterior cord syndrome at C8 level of cervical spinal cord HCC

7 S14.139- Anterior cord syndrome at unspecified level of cervical spinal cord HCC

6 S14.14 Brown-Séquard syndrome of cervical spinal cord

7 S14.141- Brown-Séquard syndrome at C1 level of cervical spinal cord HCC

7 S14.142- Brown-Séquard syndrome at C2 level of cervical spinal cord HCC

7 S14.143- Brown-Séquard syndrome at C3 level of cervical spinal cord HCC

7 S14.144- Brown-Séquard syndrome at C4 level of cervical spinal cord HCC

7 S14.145- Brown-Séquard syndrome at C5 level of cervical spinal cord HCC

7 S14.146- Brown-Séquard syndrome at C6 level of cervical spinal cord HCC

7 S14.147- Brown-Séquard syndrome at C7 level of cervical spinal cord HCC

7 S14.148- Brown-Séquard syndrome at C8 level of cervical spinal cord HCC

7 S14.149- Brown-Séquard syndrome at unspecified level of cervical spinal cord HCC

6 S14.15 Other incomplete lesions of cervical spinal cord
Incomplete lesion of cervical spinal cord NOS
Posterior cord syndrome of cervical spinal cord

7 S14.151- Other incomplete lesion at C1 level of cervical spinal cord HCC

7 S14.152- Other incomplete lesion at C2 level of cervical spinal cord HCC

7 S14.153- Other incomplete lesion at C3 level of cervical spinal cord HCC

7 S14.154- Other incomplete lesion at C4 level of cervical spinal cord HCC

7 S14.155- Other incomplete lesion at C5 level of cervical spinal cord HCC

7 S14.156- Other incomplete lesion at C6 level of cervical spinal cord HCC

7 S14.157- Other incomplete lesion at C7 level of cervical spinal cord HCC

7 S14.158- Other incomplete lesion at C8 level of cervical spinal cord HCC

7 S14.159- Other incomplete lesion at unspecified level of cervical spinal cord HCC

7 S14.2XX- Injury of nerve root of cervical spine

7 S14.3XX- Injury of brachial plexus

7 S14.4XX- Injury of peripheral nerves of neck

7 S14.5XX- Injury of cervical sympathetic nerves

7 S14.8XX- Injury of other specified nerves of neck

7 S14.9XX- Injury of unspecified nerves of neck

4 S15 Injury of blood vessels at neck level

Code also:
any associated open wound (S11.-)

The appropriate 7th character is to be added to each code from category S15
A initial encounter
D subsequent encounter
S sequela

5 S15.0 Injury of carotid artery of neck
Injury of carotid artery (common) (external) (internal, extracranial portion)
Injury of carotid artery NOS
EXCLUDES 1 *injury of internal carotid artery, intracranial portion (S06.8)*

6 S15.00 Unspecified injury of carotid artery

7 ⊟ S15.001- Unspecified injury of right carotid artery

7 ⊟ S15.002- Unspecified injury of left carotid artery

7 ⊟ S15.009- Unspecified injury of unspecified carotid artery

6 S15.01 Minor laceration of carotid artery
Incomplete transection of carotid artery
Laceration of carotid artery NOS
Superficial laceration of carotid artery

7 ⊟ S15.011- Minor laceration of right carotid artery

7 ⊟ S15.012- Minor laceration of left carotid artery

7 ⊟ S15.019- Minor laceration of unspecified carotid artery

6 S15.02 Major laceration of carotid artery
Complete transection of carotid artery
Traumatic rupture of carotid artery

7 ⊟ S15.021- Major laceration of right carotid artery

7 ⊟ S15.022- Major laceration of left carotid artery

7 ⊟ S15.029- Major laceration of unspecified carotid artery

6 S15.09 Other specified injury of carotid artery

7 ⊟ S15.091- Other specified injury of right carotid artery

7 ⊟ S15.092- Other specified injury of left carotid artery

7 ⊟ S15.099- Other specified injury of unspecified carotid artery

5 S15.1 Injury of vertebral artery

6 S15.10 Unspecified injury of vertebral artery

7 ⊟ S15.101- Unspecified injury of right vertebral artery

7 ⊟ S15.102- Unspecified injury of left vertebral artery

7 ⊟ S15.109- Unspecified injury of unspecified vertebral artery

6 S15.11 Minor laceration of vertebral artery
Incomplete transection of vertebral artery
Laceration of vertebral artery NOS
Superficial laceration of vertebral artery
7 S15.111- Minor laceration of right vertebral artery
7 S15.112- Minor laceration of left vertebral artery
7 S15.119- Minor laceration of unspecified vertebral artery
6 S15.12 Major laceration of vertebral artery
Complete transection of vertebral artery
Traumatic rupture of vertebral artery
7 S15.121- Major laceration of right vertebral artery
7 S15.122- Major laceration of left vertebral artery
7 S15.129- Major laceration of unspecified vertebral artery
6 S15.19 Other specified injury of vertebral artery
7 S15.191- Other specified injury of right vertebral artery
7 S15.192- Other specified injury of left vertebral artery
7 S15.199- Other specified injury of unspecified vertebral artery
5 S15.2 Injury of external jugular vein
6 S15.20 Unspecified injury of external jugular vein
7 S15.201- Unspecified injury of right external jugular vein
7 S15.202- Unspecified injury of left external jugular vein
7 S15.209- Unspecified injury of unspecified external jugular vein
6 S15.21 Minor laceration of external jugular vein
Incomplete transection of external jugular vein
Laceration of external jugular vein NOS
Superficial laceration of external jugular vein
7 S15.211- Minor laceration of right external jugular vein
7 S15.212- Minor laceration of left external jugular vein
7 S15.219- Minor laceration of unspecified external jugular vein
6 S15.22 Major laceration of external jugular vein
Complete transection of external jugular vein
Traumatic rupture of external jugular vein
7 S15.221- Major laceration of right external jugular vein
7 S15.222- Major laceration of left external jugular vein
7 S15.229- Major laceration of unspecified external jugular vein
6 S15.29 Other specified injury of external jugular vein
7 S15.291- Other specified injury of right external jugular vein
7 S15.292- Other specified injury of left external jugular vein
7 S15.299- Other specified injury of unspecified external jugular vein
5 S15.3 Injury of internal jugular vein
6 S15.30 Unspecified injury of internal jugular vein
7 S15.301- Unspecified injury of right internal jugular vein
7 S15.302- Unspecified injury of left internal jugular vein
7 S15.309- Unspecified injury of unspecified internal jugular vein
6 S15.31 Minor laceration of internal jugular vein
Incomplete transection of internal jugular vein
Laceration of internal jugular vein NOS
Superficial laceration of internal jugular vein
7 S15.311- Minor laceration of right internal jugular vein
7 S15.312- Minor laceration of left internal jugular vein
7 S15.319- Minor laceration of unspecified internal jugular vein
6 S15.32 Major laceration of internal jugular vein
Complete transection of internal jugular vein
Traumatic rupture of internal jugular vein
7 S15.321- Major laceration of right internal jugular vein
7 S15.322- Major laceration of left internal jugular vein
7 S15.329- Major laceration of unspecified internal jugular vein
6 S15.39 Other specified injury of internal jugular vein
7 S15.391- Other specified injury of right internal jugular vein
7 S15.392- Other specified injury of left internal jugular vein
7 S15.399- Other specified injury of unspecified internal jugular vein
7 S15.8XX- Injury of other specified blood vessels at neck level
7 S15.9XX- Injury of unspecified blood vessel at neck level

4 S16 Injury of muscle, fascia and tendon at neck level
Code also:
any associated open wound (S11.-)
EXCLUDES 2 *sprain of joint or ligament at neck level (S13.9)*

The appropriate 7th character is to be added to each code from category S16
A initial encounter
D subsequent encounter
S sequela

7 S16.1XX- Strain of muscle, fascia and tendon at neck level
7 S16.2XX- Laceration of muscle, fascia and tendon at neck level
7 S16.8XX- Other specified injury of muscle, fascia and tendon at neck level
7 S16.9XX- Unspecified injury of muscle, fascia and tendon at neck level

4 S17 Crushing injury of neck
Use additional code for all associated injuries, such as:
injury of blood vessels (S15.-)
open wound of neck (S11.-)
spinal cord injury (S14.0, S14.1-)
vertebral fracture (S12.0--S12.3-)

The appropriate 7th character is to be added to each code from category S17
A initial encounter
D subsequent encounter
S sequela

7 S17.0XX- Crushing injury of larynx and trachea
7 S17.8XX- Crushing injury of other specified parts of neck
7 S17.9XX- Crushing injury of neck, part unspecified

4 S19 Other specified and unspecified injuries of neck

The appropriate 7th character is to be added to each code from category S19
A initial encounter
D subsequent encounter
S sequela

5 S19.8 Other specified injuries of neck
7 S19.80X- Other specified injuries of unspecified part of neck
7 S19.81X- Other specified injuries of larynx
7 S19.82X- Other specified injuries of cervical trachea
EXCLUDES 2 *other specified injury of thoracic trachea (S27.5-)*
7 S19.83X- Other specified injuries of vocal cord
7 S19.84X- Other specified injuries of thyroid gland
7 S19.85X- Other specified injuries of pharynx and cervical esophagus
7 S19.89X- Other specified injuries of other specified part of neck
7 S19.9XX- Unspecified injury of neck

Injuries to the thorax (S20-S29)

INCLUDES injuries of breast
injuries of chest (wall)
injuries of interscapular area

EXCLUDES 2 *burns and corrosions (T20-T32)*
effects of foreign body in bronchus (T17.5)
effects of foreign body in esophagus (T18.1)
effects of foreign body in lung (T17.8)
effects of foreign body in trachea (T17.4)
frostbite (T33-T34)
injuries of axilla
injuries of clavicle
injuries of scapular region
injuries of shoulder
insect bite or sting, venomous (T63.4)

GUIDELINES **Section I.C.19.c.2)**
Multiple fractures are sequenced in accordance with the severity of the fracture.

GUIDELINES **Section I.C.19.b.1)-2)**
When coding injuries, assign separate codes for each injury unless a combination code is provided, in which case the combination code is assigned ... Traumatic injury codes (S00-T14.9) are not to be used for normal, healing surgical wounds or to identify complications of surgical wounds. The code for the most serious injury, as determined by the provider and the focus of treatment, is sequenced first.

1) Superficial injuries such as abrasions or contusions are not coded when associated with more severe injuries of the same site.

2) When a primary injury results in minor damage to peripheral nerves or blood vessels, the primary injury is sequenced first with additional code(s) for injuries to nerves and spinal cord (such as category S04), and/or injury to blood vessels (such as category S15). When the primary injury is to the blood vessels or nerves, that injury should be sequenced first.

GUIDELINES **Section I.C.19.c**
Coding of Traumatic Fractures: The principles of multiple coding of injuries should be followed in coding fractures. Fractures of specified sites are coded individually by site in accordance with both the provisions within categories S02, S12, S22, S32, S42, S49, S52, S59, S62, S72, S79, S82, S89, S92 and the level of detail furnished by medical record content. A fracture not indicated as open or closed should be coded to closed. A fracture not indicated whether displaced or not displaced should be coded to displaced.

4 S20 Superficial injury of thorax

The appropriate 7th character is to be added to each code from category S20
A initial encounter
D subsequent encounter
S sequela

5 **S20.0** Contusion of breast
7 ⊟ **S20.00X-** Contusion of breast, unspecified breast
7 ⊟ **S20.01X-** Contusion of right breast
7 ⊟ **S20.02X-** Contusion of left breast
5 **S20.1** Other and unspecified superficial injuries of breast
6 **S20.10** Unspecified superficial injuries of breast
7 ⊟ **S20.101-** Unspecified superficial injuries of breast, right breast
7 ⊟ **S20.102-** Unspecified superficial injuries of breast, left breast
7 ⊟ **S20.109-** Unspecified superficial injuries of breast, unspecified breast
6 **S20.11** Abrasion of breast
7 ⊟ **S20.111-** Abrasion of breast, right breast
7 ⊟ **S20.112-** Abrasion of breast, left breast
7 ⊟ **S20.119-** Abrasion of breast, unspecified breast
6 **S20.12** Blister (nonthermal) of breast
7 ⊟ **S20.121-** Blister (nonthermal) of breast, right breast
7 ⊟ **S20.122-** Blister (nonthermal) of breast, left breast
7 ⊟ **S20.129-** Blister (nonthermal) of breast, unspecified breast
6 **S20.14** External constriction of part of breast
7 ⊟ **S20.141-** External constriction of part of breast, right breast
7 ⊟ **S20.142-** External constriction of part of breast, left breast
7 ⊟ **S20.149-** External constriction of part of breast, unspecified breast
6 **S20.15** Superficial foreign body of breast
Splinter in the breast
7 ⊟ **S20.151-** Superficial foreign body of breast, right breast
7 ⊟ **S20.152-** Superficial foreign body of breast, left breast
7 ⊟ **S20.159-** Superficial foreign body of breast, unspecified breast
6 **S20.16** Insect bite (nonvenomous) of breast
7 ⊟ **S20.161-** Insect bite (nonvenomous) of breast, right breast
7 ⊟ **S20.162-** Insect bite (nonvenomous) of breast, left breast
7 ⊟ **S20.169-** Insect bite (nonvenomous) of breast, unspecified breast
6 **S20.17** Other superficial bite of breast
EXCLUDES 1 *open bite of breast (S21.05-)*
7 ⊟ **S20.171-** Other superficial bite of breast, right breast
7 ⊟ **S20.172-** Other superficial bite of breast, left breast
7 ⊟ **S20.179-** Other superficial bite of breast, unspecified breast
5 **S20.2** Contusion of thorax
7 **S20.20X-** Contusion of thorax, unspecified
6 **S20.21** Contusion of front wall of thorax
7 ⊟ **S20.211-** Contusion of right front wall of thorax
7 ⊟ **S20.212-** Contusion of left front wall of thorax
7 ⊟ **S20.219-** Contusion of unspecified front wall of thorax
6 **S20.22** Contusion of back wall of thorax
7 ⊟ **S20.221-** Contusion of right back wall of thorax
7 ⊟ **S20.222-** Contusion of left back wall of thorax
7 ⊟ **S20.229-** Contusion of unspecified back wall of thorax
5 **S20.3** Other and unspecified superficial injuries of front wall of thorax
6 **S20.30** Unspecified superficial injuries of front wall of thorax
7 ⊟ **S20.301-** Unspecified superficial injuries of right front wall of thorax
7 ⊟ **S20.302-** Unspecified superficial injuries of left front wall of thorax
7 ⊟ **S20.309-** Unspecified superficial injuries of unspecified front wall of thorax
6 **S20.31** Abrasion of front wall of thorax
7 ⊟ **S20.311-** Abrasion of right front wall of thorax
7 ⊟ **S20.312-** Abrasion of left front wall of thorax
7 ⊟ **S20.319-** Abrasion of unspecified front wall of thorax
6 **S20.32** Blister (nonthermal) of front wall of thorax
7 ⊟ **S20.321-** Blister (nonthermal) of right front wall of thorax
7 ⊟ **S20.322-** Blister (nonthermal) of left front wall of thorax
7 ⊟ **S20.329-** Blister (nonthermal) of unspecified front wall of thorax
6 **S20.34** External constriction of front wall of thorax
7 ⊟ **S20.341-** External constriction of right front wall of thorax
7 ⊟ **S20.342-** External constriction of left front wall of thorax
7 ⊟ **S20.349-** External constriction of unspecified front wall of thorax
6 **S20.35** Superficial foreign body of front wall of thorax
Splinter in front wall of thorax
7 ⊟ **S20.351-** Superficial foreign body of right front wall of thorax
7 ⊟ **S20.352-** Superficial foreign body of left front wall of thorax
7 ⊟ **S20.359-** Superficial foreign body of unspecified front wall of thorax
6 **S20.36** Insect bite (nonvenomous) of front wall of thorax
7 ⊟ **S20.361-** Insect bite (nonvenomous) of right front wall of thorax
7 ⊟ **S20.362-** Insect bite (nonvenomous) of left front wall of thorax
7 ⊟ **S20.369-** Insect bite (nonvenomous) of unspecified front wall of thorax
6 **S20.37** Other superficial bite of front wall of thorax
EXCLUDES 1 *open bite of front wall of thorax (S21.14)*
7 ⊟ **S20.371-** Other superficial bite of right front wall of thorax
7 ⊟ **S20.372-** Other superficial bite of left front wall of thorax
7 ⊟ **S20.379-** Other superficial bite of unspecified front wall of thorax

5 S20.4 Other and unspecified superficial injuries of back wall of thorax

6 S20.40 Unspecified superficial injuries of back wall of thorax

7 S20.401- Unspecified superficial injuries of right back wall of thorax

7 S20.402- Unspecified superficial injuries of left back wall of thorax

7 S20.409- Unspecified superficial injuries of unspecified back wall of thorax

6 S20.41 Abrasion of back wall of thorax

7 S20.411- Abrasion of right back wall of thorax

7 S20.412- Abrasion of left back wall of thorax

7 S20.419- Abrasion of unspecified back wall of thorax

6 S20.42 Blister (nonthermal) of back wall of thorax

7 S20.421- Blister (nonthermal) of right back wall of thorax

7 S20.422- Blister (nonthermal) of left back wall of thorax

7 S20.429- Blister (nonthermal) of unspecified back wall of thorax

6 S20.44 External constriction of back wall of thorax

7 S20.441- External constriction of right back wall of thorax

7 S20.442- External constriction of left back wall of thorax

7 S20.449- External constriction of unspecified back wall of thorax

6 S20.45 Superficial foreign body of back wall of thorax

Splinter of back wall of thorax

7 S20.451- Superficial foreign body of right back wall of thorax

7 S20.452- Superficial foreign body of left back wall of thorax

7 S20.459- Superficial foreign body of unspecified back wall of thorax

6 S20.46 Insect bite (nonvenomous) of back wall of thorax

7 S20.461- Insect bite (nonvenomous) of right back wall of thorax

7 S20.462- Insect bite (nonvenomous) of left back wall of thorax

7 S20.469- Insect bite (nonvenomous) of unspecified back wall of thorax

6 S20.47 Other superficial bite of back wall of thorax

EXCLUDES 1 *open bite of back wall of thorax (S21.24)*

7 S20.471- Other superficial bite of right back wall of thorax

7 S20.472- Other superficial bite of left back wall of thorax

7 S20.479- Other superficial bite of unspecified back wall of thorax

5 S20.9 Superficial injury of unspecified parts of thorax

EXCLUDES 1 *contusion of thorax NOS (S20.20)*

7 S20.90X- Unspecified superficial injury of Unspecified parts of thorax

Superficial injury of thoracic wall NOS

7 S20.91X- Abrasion of unspecified parts of thorax

7 S20.92X- Blister (nonthermal) of unspecified parts of thorax

7 S20.94X- External constriction of unspecified parts of thorax

7 S20.95X- Superficial foreign body of unspecified parts of thorax

Splinter in thorax NOS

7 S20.96X- Insect bite (nonvenomous) of unspecified parts of thorax

7 S20.97X- Other superficial bite of unspecified parts of thorax

EXCLUDES 1 *open bite of thorax NOS (S21.95)*

4 S21 Open wound of thorax

Code also any associated injury, such as:
- injury of heart (S26.-)
- injury of intrathoracic organs (S27.-)
- rib fracture (S22.3-, S22.4-)
- spinal cord injury (S24.0-, S24.1-)
- traumatic hemopneumothorax (S27.3)
- traumatic hemothorax (S27.1)
- traumatic pneumothorax (S27.0)
- wound infection

EXCLUDES 1 *traumatic amputation (partial) of thorax (S28.1)*

The appropriate 7th character is to be added to each code from category S21

A	initial encounter
D	subsequent encounter
S	sequela

CODING TIP ✓ Open wound codes are used for wounds caused by trauma. Do not assign a code for "open wound" unless the etiology of the wound is related to trauma. Do not use Z codes for any aspect of care of a trauma wound, e.g. no Z code for dressing changes, drain care, or suture removal. Report instead the appropriate subsequent care 7th character with the injury code.

CODING TIP ✓ Open wound codes are used for wounds caused by trauma. Do not assign a code for "open wound" unless the etiology of the wound is related to trauma.

5 S21.0 Open wound of breast

6 S21.00 Unspecified open wound of breast

7 S21.001- Unspecified open wound of right breast

7 S21.002- Unspecified open wound of left breast

7 S21.009- Unspecified open wound of unspecified breast

6 S21.01 Laceration without foreign body of breast

7 S21.011- Laceration without foreign body of right breast

7 S21.012- Laceration without foreign body of left breast

7 S21.019- Laceration without foreign body of unspecified breast

6 S21.02 Laceration with foreign body of breast

7 S21.021- Laceration with foreign body of right breast

7 S21.022- Laceration with foreign body of left breast

7 S21.029- Laceration with foreign body of unspecified breast

6 S21.03 Puncture wound without foreign body of breast

7 S21.031- Puncture wound without foreign body of right breast

7 S21.032- Puncture wound without foreign body of left breast

7 S21.039- Puncture wound without foreign body of unspecified breast

6 S21.04 Puncture wound with foreign body of breast

7 S21.041- Puncture wound with foreign body of right breast

7 S21.042- Puncture wound with foreign body of left breast

7 S21.049- Puncture wound with foreign body of unspecified breast

6 S21.05 Open bite of breast

Bite of breast NOS

EXCLUDES 1 *superficial bite of breast (S20.17)*

7 S21.051- Open bite of right breast

7 S21.052- Open bite of left breast

7 S21.059- Open bite of unspecified breast

5 S21.1 Open wound of front wall of thorax without penetration into thoracic cavity

Open wound of chest without penetration into thoracic cavity

6 S21.10 Unspecified open wound of front wall of thorax without penetration into thoracic cavity

7 S21.101- Unspecified open wound of right front wall of thorax without penetration into thoracic cavity

7 S21.102- Unspecified open wound of left front wall of thorax without penetration into thoracic cavity

7 ⊟ S21.109- Unspecified open wound of unspecified front wall of thorax without penetration into thoracic cavity

6 S21.11 Laceration without foreign body of front wall of thorax without penetration into thoracic cavity

7 ⊟ S21.111- Laceration without foreign body of right front wall of thorax without penetration into thoracic cavity

7 ⊟ S21.112- Laceration without foreign body of left front wall of thorax without penetration into thoracic cavity

7 ⊟ S21.119- Laceration without foreign body of unspecified front wall of thorax without penetration into thoracic cavity

6 S21.12 Laceration with foreign body of front wall of thorax without penetration into thoracic cavity

7 ⊟ S21.121- Laceration with foreign body of right front wall of thorax without penetration into thoracic cavity

7 ⊟ S21.122- Laceration with foreign body of left front wall of thorax without penetration into thoracic cavity

7 ⊟ S21.129- Laceration with foreign body of unspecified front wall of thorax without penetration into thoracic cavity

6 S21.13 Puncture wound without foreign body of front wall of thorax without penetration into thoracic cavity

7 ⊟ S21.131- Puncture wound without foreign body of right front wall of thorax without penetration into thoracic cavity

7 ⊟ S21.132- Puncture wound without foreign body of left front wall of thorax without penetration into thoracic cavity

7 ⊟ S21.139- Puncture wound without foreign body of unspecified front wall of thorax without penetration into thoracic cavity

6 S21.14 Puncture wound with foreign body of front wall of thorax without penetration into thoracic cavity

7 ⊟ S21.141- Puncture wound with foreign body of right front wall of thorax without penetration into thoracic cavity

7 ⊟ S21.142- Puncture wound with foreign body of left front wall of thorax without penetration into thoracic cavity

7 ⊟ S21.149- Puncture wound with foreign body of unspecified front wall of thorax without penetration into thoracic cavity

6 S21.15 Open bite of front wall of thorax without penetration into thoracic cavity

Bite of front wall of thorax NOS

EXCLUDES 1 *superficial bite of front wall of thorax (S20.37)*

7 ⊟ S21.151- Open bite of right front wall of thorax without penetration into thoracic cavity

7 ⊟ S21.152- Open bite of left front wall of thorax without penetration into thoracic cavity

7 ⊟ S21.159- Open bite of unspecified front wall of thorax without penetration into thoracic cavity

5 S21.2 Open wound of back wall of thorax without penetration into thoracic cavity

6 S21.20 Unspecified open wound of back wall of thorax without penetration into thoracic cavity

7 ⊟ S21.201- Unspecified open wound of right back wall of thorax without penetration into thoracic cavity

7 ⊟ S21.202- Unspecified open wound of left back wall of thorax without penetration into thoracic cavity

7 ⊟ S21.209- Unspecified open wound of unspecified back wall of thorax without penetration into thoracic cavity

6 S21.21 Laceration without foreign body of back wall of thorax without penetration into thoracic cavity

7 ⊟ S21.211- Laceration without foreign body of right back wall of thorax without penetration into thoracic cavity

7 ⊟ S21.212- Laceration without foreign body of left back wall of thorax without penetration into thoracic cavity

7 ⊟ S21.219- Laceration without foreign body of unspecified back wall of thorax without penetration into thoracic cavity

6 S21.22 Laceration with foreign body of back wall of thorax without penetration into thoracic cavity

7 ⊟ S21.221- Laceration with foreign body of right back wall of thorax without penetration into thoracic cavity

7 ⊟ S21.222- Laceration with foreign body of left back wall of thorax without penetration into thoracic cavity

7 ⊟ S21.229- Laceration with foreign body of unspecified back wall of thorax without penetration into thoracic cavity

6 S21.23 Puncture wound without foreign body of back wall of thorax without penetration into thoracic cavity

7 ⊟ S21.231- Puncture wound without foreign body of right back wall of thorax without penetration into thoracic cavity

7 ⊟ S21.232- Puncture wound without foreign body of left back wall of thorax without penetration into thoracic cavity

7 ⊟ S21.239- Puncture wound without foreign body of unspecified back wall of thorax without penetration into thoracic cavity

6 S21.24 Puncture wound with foreign body of back wall of thorax without penetration into thoracic cavity

7 ⊟ S21.241- Puncture wound with foreign body of right back wall of thorax without penetration into thoracic cavity

7 ⊟ S21.242- Puncture wound with foreign body of left back wall of thorax without penetration into thoracic cavity

7 ⊟ S21.249- Puncture wound with foreign body of unspecified back wall of thorax without penetration into thoracic cavity

6 S21.25 Open bite of back wall of thorax without penetration into thoracic cavity

Bite of back wall of thorax NOS

EXCLUDES 1 *superficial bite of back wall of thorax (S20.47)*

7 ⊟ S21.251- Open bite of right back wall of thorax without penetration into thoracic cavity

7 ⊟ S21.252- Open bite of left back wall of thorax without penetration into thoracic cavity

7 ⊟ S21.259- Open bite of unspecified back wall of thorax without penetration into thoracic cavity

5 S21.3 Open wound of front wall of thorax with penetration into thoracic cavity

Open wound of chest with penetration into thoracic cavity

6 S21.30 Unspecified open wound of front wall of thorax with penetration into thoracic cavity

7 ⊟ S21.301- Unspecified open wound of right front wall of thorax with penetration into thoracic cavity

7 ⊟ S21.302- Unspecified open wound of left front wall of thorax with penetration into thoracic cavity

7 ⊟ S21.309- Unspecified open wound of unspecified front wall of thorax with penetration into thoracic cavity

6 S21.31 Laceration without foreign body of front wall of thorax with penetration into thoracic cavity

7 ⊟ S21.311- Laceration without foreign body of right front wall of thorax with penetration into thoracic cavity

7 ⊟ S21.312- Laceration without foreign body of left front wall of thorax with penetration into thoracic cavity

7 ⊟ S21.319- Laceration without foreign body of unspecified front wall of thorax with penetration into thoracic cavity

6 S21.32 Laceration with foreign body of front wall of thorax with penetration into thoracic cavity

7 ⊟ S21.321- Laceration with foreign body of right front wall of thorax with penetration into thoracic cavity

7 ⊟ S21.322- Laceration with foreign body of left front wall of thorax with penetration into thoracic cavity

7 ⊟ S21.329- **Laceration with foreign body of unspecifiedfront wall of thorax with penetration into thoracic cavity**

6 S21.33 **Puncture wound without foreign body of front wall of thorax with penetration into thoracic cavity**

7 ⊟ S21.331- **Puncture wound without foreign body of right front wall of thorax with penetration into thoracic cavity**

7 ⊟ S21.332- **Puncture wound without foreign body of left front wall of thorax with penetration into thoracic cavity**

7 ⊟ S21.339- **Puncture wound without foreign body of unspecified front wall of thorax with penetration into thoracic cavity**

6 S21.34 **Puncture wound with foreign body of front wall of thorax with penetration into thoracic cavity**

7 ⊟ S21.341- **Puncture wound with foreign body of right front wall of thorax with penetration into thoracic cavity**

7 ⊟ S21.342- **Puncture wound with foreign body of left front wall of thorax with penetration into thoracic cavity**

7 ⊟ S21.349- **Puncture wound with foreign body of unspecified front wall of thorax with penetration into thoracic cavity**

6 S21.35 **Open bite of front wall of thorax with penetration into thoracic cavity**

EXCLUDES 1 *superficial bite of front wall of thorax (S20.37)*

7 ⊟ S21.351- **Open bite of right front wall of thorax with penetration into thoracic cavity**

7 ⊟ S21.352- **Open bite of left front wall of thorax with penetration into thoracic cavity**

7 ⊟ S21.359- **Open bite of unspecified front wall of thorax with penetration into thoracic cavity**

5 S21.4 **Open wound of back wall of thorax with penetration into thoracic cavity**

6 S21.40 **Unspecified open wound of back wall of thorax with penetration into thoracic cavity**

7 ⊟ S21.401- **Unspecified open wound of right back wall of thorax with penetration into thoracic cavity**

7 ⊟ S21.402- **Unspecified open wound of left back wall of thorax with penetration into thoracic cavity**

7 ⊟ S21.409- **Unspecified open wound of unspecified back wall of thorax with penetration into thoracic cavity**

6 S21.41 **Laceration without foreign body of back wall of thorax with penetration into thoracic cavity**

7 ⊟ S21.411- **Laceration without foreign body of right back wall of thorax with penetration into thoracic cavity**

7 ⊟ S21.412- **Laceration without foreign body of left back wall of thorax with penetration into thoracic cavity**

7 ⊟ S21.419- **Laceration without foreign body of unspecified back wall of thorax with penetration into thoracic cavity**

6 S21.42 **Laceration with foreign body of back wall of thorax with penetration into thoracic cavity**

7 ⊟ S21.421- **Laceration with foreign body of right back wall of thorax with penetration into thoracic cavity**

7 ⊟ S21.422- **Laceration with foreign body of left back wall of thorax with penetration into thoracic cavity**

7 ⊟ S21.429- **Laceration with foreign body of unspecified back wall of thorax with penetration into thoracic cavity**

6 S21.43 **Puncture wound without foreign body of back wall of thorax with penetration into thoracic cavity**

7 ⊟ S21.431- **Puncture wound without foreign body of right back wall of thorax with penetration into thoracic cavity**

7 ⊟ S21.432- **Puncture wound without foreign body of left back wall of thorax with penetration into thoracic cavity**

7 ⊟ S21.439- **Puncture wound without foreign body of unspecified back wall of thorax with penetration into thoracic cavity**

6 S21.44 **Puncture wound with foreign body of back wall of thorax with penetration into thoracic cavity**

7 ⊟ S21.441- **Puncture wound with foreign body of right back wall of thorax with penetration into thoracic cavity**

7 ⊟ S21.442- **Puncture wound with foreign body of left back wall of thorax with penetration into thoracic cavity**

7 ⊟ S21.449- **Puncture wound with foreign body of unspecified back wall of thorax with penetration into thoracic cavity**

6 S21.45 **Open bite of back wall of thorax with penetration into thoracic cavity**

Bite of back wall of thorax NOS

EXCLUDES 1 *superficial bite of back wall of thorax (S20.47)*

7 ⊟ S21.451- **Open bite of right back wall of thorax with penetration into thoracic cavity**

7 ⊟ S21.452- **Open bite of left back wall of thorax with penetration into thoracic cavity**

7 ⊟ S21.459- **Open bite of unspecified back wall of thorax with penetration into thoracic cavity**

5 S21.9 **Open wound of unspecified part of thorax**

Open wound of thoracic wall NOS

7 S21.90X- **Unspecified open wound of Unspecified part of thorax**

7 S21.91X- **Laceration without foreign body of unspecified part of thorax**

7 S21.92X- **Laceration with foreign body of unspecified part of thorax**

7 S21.93X- **Puncture wound without foreign body of unspecified part of thorax**

7 S21.94X- **Puncture wound with foreign body of unspecified part of thorax**

7 S21.95X- **Open bite of unspecified part of thorax**

EXCLUDES 1 *superficial bite of thorax (S20.97)*

4 S22 **Fracture of rib(s), sternum and thoracic spine**

Note: A fracture not indicated as displaced or nondisplaced should be coded to displaced

A fracture not indicated as open or closed should be coded to closed

INCLUDES fracture of thoracic neural arch
fracture of thoracic spinous process
fracture of thoracic transverse process
fracture of thoracic vertebra
fracture of thoracic vertebral arch

Code first any associated:
injury of intrathoracic organ (S27.-)
spinal cord injury (S24.0-, S24.1-)

EXCLUDES 1 *transection of thorax (S28.1)*

EXCLUDES 2 *fracture of clavicle (S42.0-)*
fracture of scapula (S42.1-)

The appropriate 7th character is to be added to each code from category S22

A	initial encounter for closed fracture
B	initial encounter for open fracture
D	subsequent encounter for fracture with routine healing
G	subsequent encounter for fracture with delayed healing
K	subsequent encounter for fracture with nonunion
S	sequela

CODING TIP ✓ A fracture not indicated as displaced or nondisplaced should be coded to displaced. A fracture not indicated as open or closed should be coded to closed. Query providers on fractures not documented as displaced/nondisplaced; otherwise, a displaced fracture diagnosis could be assigned without a reduction being performed, potentially resulting in claim denials.

5 S22.0 **Fracture of thoracic vertebra**

6 S22.00 **Fracture of unspecified thoracic vertebra**

7 S22.000- **Wedge compression fracture of unspecified thoracic vertebra** HCC

7 S22.001- **Stable burst fracture of unspecified thoracic vertebra** HCC

7 S22.002- **Unstable burst fracture of unspecified thoracic vertebra** HCC

7 S22.008- Other fracture of unspecified thoracic vertebra HCC
7 S22.009- Unspecified fracture of Unspecified thoracic vertebra HCC
6 S22.01 Fracture of first thoracic vertebra
7 S22.010- Wedge compression fracture of first thoracic vertebra HCC
7 S22.011- Stable burst fracture of first thoracic vertebra HCC
7 S22.012- Unstable burst fracture of first thoracic vertebra HCC
7 S22.018- Other fracture of first thoracic vertebra HCC
7 S22.019- Unspecified fracture of first thoracic vertebra HCC
6 S22.02 Fracture of second thoracic vertebra
7 S22.020- Wedge compression fracture of second thoracic vertebra HCC
7 S22.021- Stable burst fracture of second thoracic vertebra HCC
7 S22.022- Unstable burst fracture of second thoracic vertebra HCC
7 S22.028- Other fracture of second thoracic vertebra HCC
7 S22.029- Unspecified fracture of second thoracic vertebra HCC
6 S22.03 Fracture of third thoracic vertebra
7 S22.030- Wedge compression fracture of third thoracic vertebra HCC
7 S22.031- Stable burst fracture of third thoracic vertebra HCC
7 S22.032- Unstable burst fracture of third thoracic vertebra HCC
7 S22.038- Other fracture of third thoracic vertebra HCC
7 S22.039- Unspecified fracture of third thoracic vertebra HCC
6 S22.04 Fracture of fourth thoracic vertebra
7 S22.040- Wedge compression fracture of fourth thoracic vertebra HCC
7 S22.041- Stable burst fracture of fourth thoracic vertebra HCC
7 S22.042- Unstable burst fracture of fourth thoracic vertebra HCC
7 S22.048- Other fracture of fourth thoracic vertebra HCC
7 S22.049- Unspecified fracture of fourth thoracic vertebra HCC
6 S22.05 Fracture of T5-T6 vertebra
7 S22.050- Wedge compression fracture of T5-T6 vertebra HCC
7 S22.051- Stable burst fracture of T5-T6 vertebra HCC
7 S22.052- Unstable burst fracture of T5-T6 vertebra HCC
7 S22.058- Other fracture of T5-T6 vertebra HCC
7 S22.059- Unspecified fracture of T5-T6 vertebra HCC
6 S22.06 Fracture of T7-T8 vertebra
7 S22.060- Wedge compression fracture of T7-T8 vertebra HCC
7 S22.061- Stable burst fracture of T7-T8 vertebra HCC
7 S22.062- Unstable burst fracture of T7-T8 vertebra HCC
7 S22.068- Other fracture of T7-T8 thoracic vertebra HCC
7 S22.069- Unspecified fracture of T7-T8 vertebra HCC
6 S22.07 Fracture of T9-T10 vertebra
7 S22.070- Wedge compression fracture of T9-T10 vertebra HCC
7 S22.071- Stable burst fracture of T9-T10 vertebra HCC
7 S22.072- Unstable burst fracture of T9-T10 vertebra HCC
7 S22.078- Other fracture of T9-T10 vertebra HCC
7 S22.079- Unspecified fracture of T9-T10 vertebra HCC
6 S22.08 Fracture of T11-T12 vertebra
7 S22.080- Wedge compression fracture of T11-T12 vertebra HCC
7 S22.081- Stable burst fracture of T11-T12 vertebra HCC
7 S22.082- Unstable burst fracture of T11-T12 vertebra HCC
7 S22.088- Other fracture of T11-T12 vertebra HCC
7 S22.089- Unspecified fracture of T11-T12 vertebra HCC
5 S22.2 Fracture of sternum
7 S22.20X- Unspecified fracture of sternum
7 S22.21X- Fracture of manubrium
7 S22.22X- Fracture of body of sternum
7 S22.23X- Sternal manubrial dissociation
7 S22.24X- Fracture of xiphoid process
5 S22.3 Fracture of one rib
7 ⊟ S22.31X- Fracture of one rib, right side
7 ⊟ S22.32X- Fracture of one rib, left side
7 ⊟ S22.39X- Fracture of one rib, unspecified side
5 S22.4 Multiple fractures of ribs
Fractures of two or more ribs
EXCLUDES 1 *flail chest (S22.5-)*
7 ⊟ S22.41X- Multiple fractures of ribs, right side
7 ⊟ S22.42X- Multiple fractures of ribs, left side
7 ⊟ S22.43X- Multiple fractures of ribs, bilateral
7 ⊟ S22.49X- Multiple fractures of ribs, unspecified side
7 S22.5XX- Flail chest
7 S22.9XX- Fracture of bony thorax, part unspecified

4 S23 Dislocation and sprain of joints and ligaments of thorax

INCLUDES avulsion of joint or ligament of thorax
laceration of cartilage, joint or ligament of thorax
sprain of cartilage, joint or ligament of thorax
traumatic hemarthrosis of joint or ligament of thorax
traumatic rupture of joint or ligament of thorax
traumatic subluxation of joint or ligament of thorax
traumatic tear of joint or ligament of thorax

Code also:
any associated open wound

EXCLUDES 2 *dislocation, sprain of sternoclavicular joint (S43.2, S43.6)*
strain of muscle or tendon of thorax (S29.01-)

The appropriate 7th character is to be added to each code from category S23
A initial encounter
D subsequent encounter
S sequela

CODING TIP ✓ There are no codes for open dislocations. When a dislocation is documented as open, assign an additional code for the open wound.

7 S23.0XX- Traumatic rupture of thoracic intervertebral disc
EXCLUDES 1 *rupture or displacement (nontraumatic) of thoracic intervertebral disc NOS (M51.- with fifth character 4)*
5 S23.1 Subluxation and dislocation of thoracic vertebra
Code also:
any associated
open wound of thorax (S21.-)
spinal cord injury (S24.0-, S24.1-)
EXCLUDES 2 *fracture of thoracic vertebrae (S22.0-)*
6 S23.10 Subluxation and dislocation of unspecified thoracic vertebra
7 S23.100- Subluxation of unspecified thoracic vertebra
7 S23.101- Dislocation of unspecified thoracic vertebra
6 S23.11 Subluxation and dislocation of T1/T2 thoracic vertebra
7 S23.110- Subluxation of T1/T2 thoracic vertebra
7 S23.111- Dislocation of T1/T2 thoracic vertebra
6 S23.12 Subluxation and dislocation of T2/T3-T3/T4 thoracic vertebra
7 S23.120- Subluxation of T2/T3 thoracic vertebra
7 S23.121- Dislocation of T2/T3 thoracic vertebra
7 S23.122- Subluxation of T3/T4 thoracic vertebra
7 S23.123- Dislocation of T3/T4 thoracic vertebra
6 S23.13 Subluxation and dislocation of T4/T5-T5/T6 thoracic vertebra
7 S23.130- Subluxation of T4/T5 thoracic vertebra
7 S23.131- Dislocation of T4/T5 thoracic vertebra

7 S23.132- Subluxation of T5/T6 thoracic vertebra
7 S23.133- Dislocation of T5/T6 thoracic vertebra
6 S23.14 Subluxation and dislocation of T6/T7-T7/T8 thoracic vertebra
7 S23.140- Subluxation of T6/T7 thoracic vertebra
7 S23.141- Dislocation of T6/T7 thoracic vertebra
7 S23.142- Subluxation of T7/T8 thoracic vertebra
7 S23.143- Dislocation of T7/T8 thoracic vertebra
6 S23.15 Subluxation and dislocation of T8/T9-T9/T10 thoracic vertebra
7 S23.150- Subluxation of T8/T9 thoracic vertebra
7 S23.151- Dislocation of T8/T9 thoracic vertebra
7 S23.152- Subluxation of T9/T10 thoracic vertebra
7 S23.153- Dislocation of T9/T10 thoracic vertebra
6 S23.16 Subluxation and dislocation of T10/T11-T11/T12 thoracic vertebra
7 S23.160- Subluxation of T10/T11 thoracic vertebra
7 S23.161- Dislocation of T10/T11 thoracic vertebra
7 S23.162- Subluxation of T11/T12 thoracic vertebra
7 S23.163- Dislocation of T11/T12 thoracic vertebra
6 S23.17 Subluxation and dislocation of T12/L1 thoracic vertebra
7 S23.170- Subluxation of T12/L1 thoracic vertebra
7 S23.171- Dislocation of T12/L1 thoracic vertebra
5 S23.2 Dislocation of other and unspecified parts of thorax
7 S23.20X- Dislocation of unspecified part of thorax
7 S23.29X- Dislocation of other parts of thorax
7 S23.3XX- Sprain of ligaments of thoracic spine
5 S23.4 Sprain of ribs and sternum
7 S23.41X- Sprain of ribs
6 S23.42 Sprain of sternum
7 S23.420- Sprain of sternoclavicular (joint) (ligament)
7 S23.421- Sprain of chondrosternal joint
7 S23.428- Other sprain of sternum
7 S23.429- Unspecified sprain of sternum
7 S23.8XX- Sprain of other specified parts of thorax
7 S23.9XX- Sprain of unspecified parts of thorax

4 S24 Injury of nerves and spinal cord at thorax level

Note: Code to highest level of thoracic spinal cord injury
Injuries to the spinal cord (S24.0 and S24.1) refer to the cord level and not bone level injury, and can affect nerve roots at and below the level given.
Code also any associated:
fracture of thoracic vertebra (S22.0-)
open wound of thorax (S21.-)
transient paralysis (R29.5)

EXCLUDES 2 *injury of brachial plexus (S14.3)*

The appropriate 7th character is to be added to each code from category S24
A initial encounter
D subsequent encounter
S sequela

CODING TIP ✓ When coding sequelae of a spinal cord injury, first list the residual condition(s), followed by the specific spinal cord injury diagnosed using the appropriate code from this category with the seventh character "S" to indicate sequelae. If there are multiple levels of injury, code only the highest injury.

CODING TIP ✓ When coding sequelae of a thoracic spinal cord injury, first list the residual condition(s), followed by the specific spinal cord injury diagnosed using the appropriate code from category S24 with the seventh character "S" to indicate sequelae.

7 S24.0XX- Concussion and edema of thoracic spinal cord HCC
5 S24.1 Other and unspecified injuries of thoracic spinal cord
6 S24.10 Unspecified injury of thoracic spinal cord
7 S24.101- Unspecified injury at T1 level of thoracic spinal cord HCC
7 S24.102- Unspecified injury at T2-T6 level of thoracic spinal cord HCC
7 S24.103- Unspecified injury at T7-T10 level of thoracic spinal cord HCC
7 S24.104- Unspecified injury at T11-T12 level of thoracic spinal cord HCC
7 S24.109- Unspecified injury at unspecified level of thoracic spinal cord HCC
Injury of thoracic spinal cord NOS
6 S24.11 Complete lesion of thoracic spinal cord
7 S24.111- Complete lesion at T1 level of thoracic spinal cord HCC
7 S24.112- Complete lesion at T2-T6 level of thoracic spinal cord HCC
7 S24.113- Complete lesion at T7-T10 level of thoracic spinal cord HCC
7 S24.114- Complete lesion at T11-T12 level of thoracic spinal cord HCC
7 S24.119- Complete lesion at unspecified level of thoracic spinal cord HCC
6 S24.13 Anterior cord syndrome of thoracic spinal cord
7 S24.131- Anterior cord syndrome at T1 level of thoracic spinal cord HCC
7 S24.132- Anterior cord syndrome at T2-T6 level of thoracic spinal cord HCC
7 S24.133- Anterior cord syndrome at T7-T10 level of thoracic spinal cord HCC
7 S24.134- Anterior cord syndrome at T11-T12 level of thoracic spinal cord HCC
7 S24.139- Anterior cord syndrome at unspecified level of thoracic spinal cord HCC
6 S24.14 Brown-Séquard syndrome of thoracic spinal cord
7 S24.141- Brown-Séquard syndrome at T1 level of thoracic spinal cord HCC
7 S24.142- Brown-Séquard syndrome at T2-T6 level of thoracic spinal cord HCC
7 S24.143- Brown-Séquard syndrome at T7-T10 level of thoracic spinal cord HCC
7 S24.144- Brown-Séquard syndrome at T11-T12 level of thoracic spinal cord HCC
7 S24.149- Brown-Séquard syndrome at unspecified level of thoracic spinal cord HCC
6 S24.15 Other incomplete lesions of thoracic spinal cord
Incomplete lesion of thoracic spinal cord NOS
Posterior cord syndrome of thoracic spinal cord
7 S24.151- Other incomplete lesion at T1 level of thoracic spinal cord HCC
7 S24.152- Other incomplete lesion at T2-T6 level of thoracic spinal cord HCC
7 S24.153- Other incomplete lesion at T7-T10 level of thoracic spinal cord HCC
7 S24.154- Other incomplete lesion at T11-T12 level of thoracic spinal cord HCC
7 S24.159- Other incomplete lesion at unspecified level of thoracic spinal cord HCC
7 S24.2XX- Injury of nerve root of thoracic spine
7 S24.3XX- Injury of peripheral nerves of thorax
7 S24.4XX- Injury of thoracic sympathetic nervous system
Injury of cardiac plexus
Injury of esophageal plexus
Injury of pulmonary plexus
Injury of stellate ganglion
Injury of thoracic sympathetic ganglion
7 S24.8XX- Injury of other specified nerves of thorax
7 S24.9XX- Injury of unspecified nerve of thorax

4 S25 Injury of blood vessels of thorax

Code also:
any associated open wound (S21.-)

The appropriate 7th character is to be added to each code from category S25
A initial encounter
D subsequent encounter
S sequela

5 S25.0 Injury of thoracic aorta
Injury of aorta NOS
7 S25.00X- Unspecified injury of thoracic aorta
7 S25.01X- Minor laceration of thoracic aorta
Incomplete transection of thoracic aorta
Laceration of thoracic aorta NOS
Superficial laceration of thoracic aorta

7 S25.02X- **Major laceration of thoracic aorta**
Complete transection of thoracic aorta
Traumatic rupture of thoracic aorta

7 S25.09X- **Other specified injury of thoracic aorta**

5 S25.1 **Injury of innominate or subclavian artery**

6 S25.10 **Unspecified injury of innominate or subclavian artery**

7 ⊟ S25.101- **Unspecified injury of right innominate or subclavian artery**

7 ⊟ S25.102- **Unspecified injury of left innominate or subclavian artery**

7 ⊟ S25.109- **Unspecified injury of unspecified innominate or subclavian artery**

6 S25.11 **Minor laceration of innominate or subclavian artery**
Incomplete transection of innominate or subclavian artery
Laceration of innominate or subclavian artery NOS
Superficial laceration of innominate or subclavian artery

7 ⊟ S25.111- **Minor laceration of right innominate or subclavian artery**

7 ⊟ S25.112- **Minor laceration of left innominate or subclavian artery**

7 ⊟ S25.119- **Minor laceration of unspecified innominate or subclavian artery**

6 S25.12 **Major laceration of innominate or subclavian artery**
Complete transection of innominate or subclavian artery
Traumatic rupture of innominate or subclavian artery

7 ⊟ S25.121- **Major laceration of right innominate or subclavian artery**

7 ⊟ S25.122- **Major laceration of left innominate or subclavian artery**

7 ⊟ S25.129- **Major laceration of unspecified innominate or subclavian artery**

6 S25.19 **Other specified injury of innominate or subclavian artery**

7 ⊟ S25.191- **Other specified injury of right innominate or subclavian artery**

7 ⊟ S25.192- **Other specified injury of left innominate or subclavian artery**

7 ⊟ S25.199- **Other specified injury of unspecified innominate or subclavian artery**

5 S25.2 **Injury of superior vena cava**
Injury of vena cava NOS

7 S25.20X- **Unspecified injury of superior vena cava**

7 S25.21X- **Minor laceration of superior vena cava**
Incomplete transection of superior vena cava
Laceration of superior vena cava NOS
Superficial laceration of superior vena cava

7 S25.22X- **Major laceration of superior vena cava**
Complete transection of superior vena cava
Traumatic rupture of superior vena cava

7 S25.29X- **Other specified injury of superior vena cava**

5 S25.3 **Injury of innominate or subclavian vein**

6 S25.30 **Unspecified injury of innominate or subclavian vein**

7 ⊟ S25.301- **Unspecified injury of right innominate or subclavian vein**

7 ⊟ S25.302- **Unspecified injury of left innominate or subclavian vein**

7 ⊟ S25.309- **Unspecified injury of unspecified innominate or subclavian vein**

6 S25.31 **Minor laceration of innominate or subclavian vein**
Incomplete transection of innominate or subclavian vein
Laceration of innominate or subclavian vein NOS
Superficial laceration of innominate or subclavian vein

7 ⊟ S25.311- **Minor laceration of right innominate or subclavian vein**

7 ⊟ S25.312- **Minor laceration of left innominate or subclavian vein**

7 ⊟ S25.319- **Minor laceration of unspecified innominate or subclavian vein**

6 S25.32 **Major laceration of innominate or subclavian vein**
Complete transection of innominate or subclavian vein
Traumatic rupture of innominate or subclavian vein

7 ⊟ S25.321- **Major laceration of right innominate or subclavian vein**

7 ⊟ S25.322- **Major laceration of left innominate or subclavian vein**

7 ⊟ S25.329- **Major laceration of unspecified innominate or subclavian vein**

6 S25.39 **Other specified injury of innominate or subclavian vein**

7 ⊟ S25.391- **Other specified injury of right innominate or subclavian vein**

7 ⊟ S25.392- **Other specified injury of left innominate or subclavian vein**

7 ⊟ S25.399- **Other specified injury of unspecified innominate or subclavian vein**

5 S25.4 **Injury of pulmonary blood vessels**

6 S25.40 **Unspecified injury of pulmonary blood vessels**

7 ⊟ S25.401- **Unspecified injury of right pulmonary blood vessels**

7 ⊟ S25.402- **Unspecified injury of left pulmonary blood vessels**

7 ⊟ S25.409- **Unspecified injury of unspecified pulmonary blood vessels**

6 S25.41 **Minor laceration of pulmonary blood vessels**
Incomplete transection of pulmonary blood vessels
Laceration of pulmonary blood vessels NOS
Superficial laceration of pulmonary blood vessels

7 ⊟ S25.411- **Minor laceration of right pulmonary blood vessels**

7 ⊟ S25.412- **Minor laceration of left pulmonary blood vessels**

7 ⊟ S25.419- **Minor laceration of unspecified pulmonary blood vessels**

6 S25.42 **Major laceration of pulmonary blood vessels**
Complete transection of pulmonary blood vessels
Traumatic rupture of pulmonary blood vessels

7 ⊟ S25.421- **Major laceration of right pulmonary blood vessels**

7 ⊟ S25.422- **Major laceration of left pulmonary blood vessels**

7 ⊟ S25.429- **Major laceration of unspecified pulmonary blood vessels**

6 S25.49 **Other specified injury of pulmonary blood vessels**

7 ⊟ S25.491- **Other specified injury of right pulmonary blood vessels**

7 ⊟ S25.492- **Other specified injury of left pulmonary blood vessels**

7 ⊟ S25.499- **Other specified injury of unspecified pulmonary blood vessels**

5 S25.5 **Injury of intercostal blood vessels**

6 S25.50 **Unspecified injury of intercostal blood vessels**

7 ⊟ S25.501- **Unspecified injury of intercostal blood vessels, right side**

7 ⊟ S25.502- **Unspecified injury of intercostal blood vessels, left side**

7 ⊟ S25.509- **Unspecified injury of intercostal blood vessels, unspecified side**

6 S25.51 **Laceration of intercostal blood vessels**

7 ⊟ S25.511- **Laceration of intercostal blood vessels, right side**

7 ⊟ S25.512- **Laceration of intercostal blood vessels, left side**

7 ⊟ S25.519- **Laceration of intercostal blood vessels, unspecified side**

6 S25.59 **Other specified injury of intercostal blood vessels**

7 ⊟ S25.591- **Other specified injury of intercostal blood vessels, right side**

7 ⊟ S25.592- **Other specified injury of intercostal blood vessels, left side**

7 ⊟ S25.599- **Other specified injury of intercostal blood vessels, unspecified side**

5 S25.8 **Injury of other blood vessels of thorax**
Injury of azygos vein
Injury of mammary artery or vein

6 S25.80 **Unspecified injury of other blood vessels of thorax**

7 ⊟ S25.801- **Unspecified injury of other blood vessels of thorax, right side**

7 ⊟ S25.802- **Unspecified injury of other blood vessels of thorax, left side**

S25.809- Unspecified injury of other blood vessels of thorax, unspecified side

S25.81 Laceration of other blood vessels of thorax

S25.811- Laceration of other blood vessels of thorax, right side

S25.812- Laceration of other blood vessels of thorax, left side

S25.819- Laceration of other blood vessels of thorax, unspecified side

S25.89 Other specified injury of other blood vessels of thorax

S25.891- Other specified injury of other blood vessels of thorax, right side

S25.892- Other specified injury of other blood vessels of thorax, left side

S25.899- Other specified injury of other blood vessels of thorax, unspecified side

S25.9 Injury of unspecified blood vessel of thorax

S25.90X- Unspecified injury of Unspecified blood vessel of thorax

S25.91X- Laceration of unspecified blood vessel of thorax

S25.99X- Other specified injury of unspecified blood vessel of thorax

S26 Injury of heart

Code also any associated:
open wound of thorax (S21.-)
traumatic hemopneumothorax (S27.2)
traumatic hemothorax (S27.1)
traumatic pneumothorax (S27.0)

The appropriate 7th character is to be added to each code from category S26
A initial encounter
D subsequent encounter
S sequela

S26.0 Injury of heart with hemopericardium

S26.00X- Unspecified injury of heart with hemopericardium

S26.01X- Contusion of heart with hemopericardium

S26.02 Laceration of heart with hemopericardium

S26.020- Mild laceration of heart with hemopericardium
Laceration of heart without penetration of heart chamber

S26.021- Moderate laceration of heart with hemopericardium
Laceration of heart with penetration of heart chamber

S26.022- Major laceration of heart with hemopericardium
Laceration of heart with penetration of multiple heart chambers

S26.09X- Other injury of heart with hemopericardium

S26.1 Injury of heart without hemopericardium

S26.10X- Unspecified injury of heart without hemopericardium

S26.11X- Contusion of heart without hemopericardium

S26.12X- Laceration of heart without hemopericardium

S26.19X- Other injury of heart without hemopericardium

S26.9 Injury of heart, unspecified with or without hemopericardium

S26.90X- Unspecified injury of heart, Unspecified with or without hemopericardium

S26.91X- Contusion of heart, unspecified with or without hemopericardium

S26.92X- Laceration of heart, unspecified with or without hemopericardium
Laceration of heart NOS

S26.99X- Other injury of heart, unspecified with or without hemopericardium

S27 Injury of other and unspecified intrathoracic organs

Code also:
any associated open wound of thorax (S21.-)

EXCLUDES 2 *injury of cervical esophagus (S10-S19)*
injury of trachea (cervical) (S10-S19)

The appropriate 7th character is to be added to each code from category S27
A initial encounter
D subsequent encounter
S sequela

S27.0XX- Traumatic pneumothorax

EXCLUDES 1 *spontaneous pneumothorax (J93.-)*

CODING TIP ✓ Do not assign S27.0- to indicate a pneumothorax that is not specifically identified as due to trauma. Chapter 19 codes are for those diagnoses due to injury and trauma. S27.0- indicates pneumothorax resulting from traumatic origin. Nontraumatic (spontaneous or unspecified pneumothorax) should be coded to J93.-.

S27.1XX- Traumatic hemothorax

S27.2XX- Traumatic hemopneumothorax

S27.3 Other and unspecified injuries of lung

S27.30 Unspecified injury of lung

S27.301- Unspecified injury of lung, unilateral

S27.302- Unspecified injury of lung, bilateral

S27.309- unspecified injury of lung, unspecified

S27.31 Primary blast injury of lung
Blast injury of lung NOS

S27.311- Primary blast injury of lung, unilateral

S27.312- Primary blast injury of lung, bilateral

S27.319- Primary blast injury of lung, unspecified

S27.32 Contusion of lung

S27.321- Contusion of lung, unilateral

S27.322- Contusion of lung, bilateral

S27.329- Contusion of lung, unspecified

S27.33 Laceration of lung

S27.331- Laceration of lung, unilateral

S27.332- Laceration of lung, bilateral

S27.339- Laceration of lung, unspecified

S27.39 Other injuries of lung
Secondary blast injury of lung

S27.391- Other injuries of lung, unilateral

S27.392- Other injuries of lung, bilateral

S27.399- Other injuries of lung, unspecified

S27.4 Injury of bronchus

S27.40 Unspecified injury of bronchus

S27.401- Unspecified injury of bronchus, unilateral

S27.402- Unspecified injury of bronchus, bilateral

S27.409- unspecified injury of bronchus, unspecified

S27.41 Primary blast injury of bronchus
Blast injury of bronchus NOS

S27.411- Primary blast injury of bronchus, unilateral

S27.412- Primary blast injury of bronchus, bilateral

S27.419- Primary blast injury of bronchus, unspecified

S27.42 Contusion of bronchus

S27.421- Contusion of bronchus, unilateral

S27.422- Contusion of bronchus, bilateral

S27.429- Contusion of bronchus, unspecified

S27.43 Laceration of bronchus

S27.431- Laceration of bronchus, unilateral

S27.432- Laceration of bronchus, bilateral

S27.439- Laceration of bronchus, unspecified

S27.49 Other injury of bronchus
Secondary blast injury of bronchus

S27.491- Other injury of bronchus, unilateral

S27.492- Other injury of bronchus, bilateral

S27.499- Other injury of bronchus, unspecified

S27.5 Injury of thoracic trachea

S27.50X- Unspecified injury of thoracic trachea

S27.51X- Primary blast injury of thoracic trachea
Blast injury of thoracic trachea NOS

7 S27.52X- Contusion of thoracic trachea
7 S27.53X- Laceration of thoracic trachea
7 S27.59X- Other injury of thoracic trachea
Secondary blast injury of thoracic trachea
5 S27.6 Injury of pleura
7 S27.60X- Unspecified injury of pleura
7 S27.63X- Laceration of pleura
7 S27.69X- Other injury of pleura
5 S27.8 Injury of other specified intrathoracic organs
6 S27.80 Injury of diaphragm
7 S27.802- Contusion of diaphragm
7 S27.803- Laceration of diaphragm
7 S27.808- Other injury of diaphragm
7 S27.809- Unspecified injury of diaphragm
6 S27.81 Injury of esophagus (thoracic part)
7 S27.812- Contusion of esophagus (thoracic part)
7 S27.813- Laceration of esophagus (thoracic part)
7 S27.818- Other injury of esophagus (thoracic part)
7 S27.819- Unspecified injury of esophagus (thoracic part)
6 S27.89 Injury of other specified intrathoracic organs
Injury of lymphatic thoracic duct
Injury of thymus gland
7 S27.892- Contusion of other specified intrathoracic organs
7 S27.893- Laceration of other specified intrathoracic organs
7 S27.898- Other injury of Other specified intrathoracic organs
7 S27.899- Unspecified injury of other specified intrathoracic organs
7 S27.9XX- Injury of unspecified intrathoracic organ

4 S28 Crushing injury of thorax, and traumatic amputation of part of thorax

The appropriate 7th character is to be added to each code from category S28
A initial encounter
D subsequent encounter
S sequela

7 S28.0XX- Crushed chest
Use additional code for all associated injuries
EXCLUDES 1 *flail chest (S22.5)*
7 S28.1XX- Traumatic amputation (partial) of part of thorax, except breast
5 S28.2 Traumatic amputation of breast
6 S28.21 Complete traumatic amputation of breast
Traumatic amputation of breast NOS
7 ⊟ S28.211- Complete traumatic amputation of right breast
7 ⊟ S28.212- Complete traumatic amputation of left breast
7 ⊟ S28.219- Complete traumatic amputation of unspecified breast
6 S28.22 Partial traumatic amputation of breast
7 ⊟ S28.221- Partial traumatic amputation of right breast
7 ⊟ S28.222- Partial traumatic amputation of left breast
7 ⊟ S28.229- Partial traumatic amputation of unspecified breast

4 S29 Other and unspecified injuries of thorax
Code also:
any associated open wound (S21.-)

The appropriate 7th character is to be added to each code from category S29
A initial encounter
D subsequent encounter
S sequela

5 S29.0 Injury of muscle and tendon at thorax level
6 S29.00 Unspecified injury of muscle and tendon of thorax
7 S29.001- Unspecified injury of muscle and tendon of front wall of thorax
7 S29.002- Unspecified injury of muscle and tendon of back wall of thorax
7 S29.009- Unspecified injury of muscle and tendon of unspecified wall of thorax
6 S29.01 Strain of muscle and tendon of thorax
7 S29.011- Strain of muscle and tendon of front wall of thorax
7 S29.012- Strain of muscle and tendon of back wall of thorax
7 S29.019- Strain of muscle and tendon of unspecified wall of thorax
6 S29.02 Laceration of muscle and tendon of thorax
7 S29.021- Laceration of muscle and tendon of front wall of thorax
7 S29.022- Laceration of muscle and tendon of back wall of thorax
7 S29.029- Laceration of muscle and tendon of unspecified wall of thorax
6 S29.09 Other injury of muscle and tendon of thorax
7 S29.091- Other injury of muscle and tendon of front wall of thorax
7 S29.092- Other injury of muscle and tendon of back wall of thorax
7 S29.099- Other injury of muscle and tendon of unspecified wall of thorax
7 S29.8XX- Other specified injuries of thorax
7 S29.9XX- Unspecified injury of thorax

Injuries to the abdomen, lower back, lumbar spine, pelvis and external genitals (S30-S39)

INCLUDES injuries to the abdominal wall
injuries to the anus
injuries to the buttock
injuries to the external genitalia
injuries to the flank
injuries to the groin

EXCLUDES 2 *burns and corrosions (T20-T32)*
effects of foreign body in anus and rectum (T18.5)
effects of foreign body in genitourinary tract (T19.-)
effects of foreign body in stomach, small intestine and colon (T18.2-T18.4)
frostbite (T33-T34)
insect bite or sting, venomous (T63.4)

GUIDELINES **Section I.C.19.c.2)**
Multiple fractures are sequenced in accordance with the severity of the fracture.

GUIDELINES **Section I.C.19.b.1)-2)**
When coding injuries, assign separate codes for each injury unless a combination code is provided, in which case the combination code is assigned ... Traumatic injury codes (S00-T14.9) are not to be used for normal, healing surgical wounds or to identify complications of surgical wounds. The code for the most serious injury, as determined by the provider and the focus of treatment, is sequenced first.

1) Superficial injuries such as abrasions or contusions are not coded when associated with more severe injuries of the same site.

2) When a primary injury results in minor damage to peripheral nerves or blood vessels, the primary injury is sequenced first with additional code(s) for injuries to nerves and spinal cord (such as category S04), and/or injury to blood vessels (such as category S15). When the primary injury is to the blood vessels or nerves, that injury should be sequenced first.

GUIDELINES **Section I.C.19.c**
Coding of Traumatic Fractures: The principles of multiple coding of injuries should be followed in coding fractures. Fractures of specified sites are coded individually by site in accordance with both the provisions within categories S02, S12, S22, S32, S42, S49, S52, S59, S62, S72, S79, S82, S89, S92 and the level of detail furnished by medical record content. A fracture not indicated as open or closed should be coded to closed. A fracture not indicated whether displaced or not displaced should be coded to displaced.

4 S30 Superficial injury of abdomen, lower back, pelvis and external genitals

EXCLUDES 2 *superficial injury of hip (S70.-)*

The appropriate 7th character is to be added to each code from category S30
A initial encounter
D subsequent encounter
S sequela

7 S30.0XX- Contusion of lower back and pelvis
Contusion of buttock

7 S30.1XX- Contusion of abdominal wall
Contusion of flank
Contusion of groin

5 S30.2 Contusion of external genital organs

6 S30.20 Contusion of unspecified external genital organ

7 S30.201- Contusion of unspecified external genital organ, male ♂

7 S30.202- Contusion of unspecified external genital organ, female ♀

7 S30.21X- Contusion of penis ♂

7 S30.22X- Contusion of scrotum and testes ♂

7 S30.23X- Contusion of vagina and vulva ♀

7 S30.3XX- Contusion of anus

5 S30.8 Other superficial injuries of abdomen, lower back, pelvis and external genitals

6 S30.81 Abrasion of abdomen, lower back, pelvis and external genitals

7 S30.810- Abrasion of lower back and pelvis

7 S30.811- Abrasion of abdominal wall

7 S30.812- Abrasion of penis ♂

7 S30.813- Abrasion of scrotum and testes ♂

7 S30.814- Abrasion of vagina and vulva ♀

7 S30.815- Abrasion of unspecified external genital organs, male ♂

7 S30.816- Abrasion of unspecified external genital organs, female ♀

7 S30.817- Abrasion of anus

6 S30.82 Blister (nonthermal) of abdomen, lower back, pelvis and external genitals

7 S30.820- Blister (nonthermal) of lower back and pelvis

7 S30.821- Blister (nonthermal) of abdominal wall

7 S30.822- Blister (nonthermal) of penis ♂

7 S30.823- Blister (nonthermal) of scrotum and testes ♂

7 S30.824- Blister (nonthermal) of vagina and vulva ♀

7 S30.825- Blister (nonthermal) of unspecified external genital organs, male ♂

7 S30.826- Blister (nonthermal) of unspecified external genital organs, female ♀

7 S30.827- Blister (nonthermal) of anus

6 S30.84 External constriction of abdomen, lower back, pelvis and external genitals

7 S30.840- External constriction of lower back and pelvis

7 S30.841- External constriction of abdominal wall

7 S30.842- External constriction of penis ♂
Hair tourniquet syndrome of penis
Use additional cause code to identify the constricting item (W49.0-)

7 S30.843- External constriction of scrotum and testes ♂

7 S30.844- External constriction of vagina and vulva ♀

7 S30.845- External constriction of unspecified external genital organs, male ♂

7 S30.846- External constriction of unspecified external genital organs, female ♀

6 S30.85 Superficial foreign body of abdomen, lower back, pelvis and external genitals
Splinter in the abdomen, lower back, pelvis and external genitals

7 S30.850- Superficial foreign body of lower back and pelvis

7 S30.851- Superficial foreign body of abdominal wall

7 S30.852- Superficial foreign body of penis ♂

7 S30.853- Superficial foreign body of scrotum and testes ♂

7 S30.854- Superficial foreign body of vagina and vulva ♀

7 S30.855- Superficial foreign body of unspecified external genital organs, male ♂

7 S30.856- Superficial foreign body of unspecified external genital organs, female ♀

7 S30.857- Superficial foreign body of anus

6 S30.86 Insect bite (nonvenomous) of abdomen, lower back, pelvis and external genitals

7 S30.860- Insect bite (nonvenomous) of lower back and pelvis

7 S30.861- Insect bite (nonvenomous) of abdominal wall

7 S30.862- Insect bite (nonvenomous) of penis ♂

7 S30.863- Insect bite (nonvenomous) of scrotum and testes ♂

7 S30.864- Insect bite (nonvenomous) of vagina and vulva ♀

7 S30.865- Insect bite (nonvenomous) of unspecified external genital organs, male ♂

7 S30.866- Insect bite (nonvenomous) of unspecified external genital organs, female ♀

7 S30.867- Insect bite (nonvenomous) of anus

6 S30.87 Other superficial bite of abdomen, lower back, pelvis and external genitals

EXCLUDES 1 *open bite of abdomen, lower back, pelvis and external genitals (S31.05, S31.15, S31.25, S31.35, S31.45, S31.55)*

7 S30.870- Other superficial bite of lower back and pelvis

7 S30.871- Other superficial bite of abdominal wall

7 S30.872- Other superficial bite of penis ♂

7 S30.873- Other superficial bite of scrotum and testes ♂

7 S30.874- Other superficial bite of vagina and vulva ♀

7 S30.875- Other superficial bite of unspecified external genital organs, male ♂

7 S30.876- Other superficial bite of unspecified external genital organs, female ♀

7 S30.877- Other superficial bite of anus

5 S30.9 Unspecified superficial injury of abdomen, lower back, pelvis and external genitals

7 S30.91X- Unspecified superficial injury of lower back and pelvis

7 S30.92X- Unspecified superficial injury of abdominal wall

7 S30.93X- Unspecified superficial injury of penis ♂

7 S30.94X- Unspecified superficial injury of scrotum and testes ♂

7 S30.95X- Unspecified superficial injury of vagina and vulva ♀

7 S30.96X- Unspecified superficial injury of unspecified external genital organs, male ♂

7 S30.97X- Unspecified superficial injury of unspecified external genital organs, female ♀

7 S30.98X- Unspecified superficial injury of anus

4 S31 Open wound of abdomen, lower back, pelvis and external genitals

Code also any associated:
spinal cord injury (S24.0, S24.1-, S34.0-, S34.1-)
wound infection

EXCLUDES 1 *traumatic amputation of part of abdomen, lower back and pelvis (S38.2-, S38.3)*

EXCLUDES 2 *open wound of hip (S71.00-S71.02)*
open fracture of pelvis (S32.1--S32.9 with 7th character B)

The appropriate 7th character is to be added to each code from category S31
A initial encounter
D subsequent encounter
S sequela

CODING TIP ✓ Open wound codes are used for wounds caused by trauma. Do not assign a code for "open wound" unless the etiology of the wound is related to trauma. Do not use Z codes for any aspect of care of a trauma wound, e.g. no Z code for dressing changes, drain care, or suture removal. Report instead the appropriate subsequent care 7th character with the injury code.

CODING TIP ✓ Open wound codes are used for wounds caused by trauma. Do not assign a code for "open wound" unless the etiology of the wound is related to trauma.

5 S31.0 Open wound of lower back and pelvis

6 S31.00 Unspecified open wound of lower back and pelvis

7 S31.000- Unspecified open wound of lower back and pelvis without penetration into retroperitoneum
Unspecified open wound of lower back and pelvis NOS

7 S31.001- Unspecified open wound of lower back and pelvis with penetration into retroperitoneum

6 S31.01 Laceration without foreign body of lower back and pelvis

7 S31.010- Laceration without foreign body of lower back and pelvis without penetration into retroperitoneum
Laceration without foreign body of lower back and pelvis NOS

7 S31.011- Laceration without foreign body of lower back and pelvis with penetration into retroperitoneum

6 S31.02 Laceration with foreign body of lower back and pelvis

7 S31.020- Laceration with foreign body of lower back and pelvis without penetration into retroperitoneum
Laceration with foreign body of lower back and pelvis NOS

7 S31.021- Laceration with foreign body of lower back and pelvis with penetration into retroperitoneum

6 S31.03 Puncture wound without foreign body of lower back and pelvis

7 S31.030- Puncture wound without foreign body of lower back and pelvis without penetration into retroperitoneum
Puncture wound without foreign body of lower back and pelvis NOS

7 S31.031- Puncture wound without foreign body of lower back and pelvis with penetration into retroperitoneum

6 S31.04 Puncture wound with foreign body of lower back and pelvis

7 S31.040- Puncture wound with foreign body of lower back and pelvis without penetration into retroperitoneum
Puncture wound with foreign body of lower back and pelvis NOS

7 S31.041- Puncture wound with foreign body of lower back and pelvis with penetration into retroperitoneum

6 S31.05 Open bite of lower back and pelvis
Bite of lower back and pelvis NOS
EXCLUDES 1 *superficial bite of lower back and pelvis (S30.860, S30.870)*

7 S31.050- Open bite of lower back and pelvis without penetration into retroperitoneum
Open bite of lower back and pelvis NOS

7 S31.051- Open bite of lower back and pelvis with penetration into retroperitoneum

5 S31.1 Open wound of abdominal wall without penetration into peritoneal cavity
Open wound of abdominal wall NOS
EXCLUDES 2 *open wound of abdominal wall with penetration into peritoneal cavity (S31.6-)*

6 S31.10 Unspecified open wound of abdominal wall without penetration into peritoneal cavity

7 ⊟ S31.100- Unspecified open wound of abdominal wall, right upper quadrant without penetration into peritoneal cavity

7 ⊟ S31.101- Unspecified open wound of abdominal wall, left upper quadrant without penetration into peritoneal cavity

7 ⊟ S31.102- Unspecified open wound of abdominal wall, epigastric region without penetration into peritoneal cavity

7 ⊟ S31.103- Unspecified open wound of abdominal wall, right lower quadrant without penetration into peritoneal cavity

7 ⊟ S31.104- Unspecified open wound of abdominal wall, left lower quadrant without penetration into peritoneal cavity

7 ⊟ S31.105- Unspecified open wound of abdominal wall, periumbilic region without penetration into peritoneal cavity

7 ⊟ S31.109- Unspecified open wound of abdominal wall, unspecified quadrant without penetration into peritoneal cavity
Unspecified open wound of abdominal wall NOS

6 S31.11 Laceration without foreign body of abdominal wall without penetration into peritoneal cavity

7 ⊟ S31.110- Laceration without foreign body of abdominal wall, right upper quadrant without penetration into peritoneal cavity

7 ⊟ S31.111- Laceration without foreign body of abdominal wall, left upper quadrant without penetration into peritoneal cavity

7 ⊟ S31.112- Laceration without foreign body of abdominal wall, epigastric region without penetration into peritoneal cavity

7 ⊟ S31.113- Laceration without foreign body of abdominal wall, right lower quadrant without penetration into peritoneal cavity

7 ⊟ S31.114- Laceration without foreign body of abdominal wall, left lower quadrant without penetration into peritoneal cavity

7 ⊟ S31.115- Laceration without foreign body of abdominal wall, periumbilic region without penetration into peritoneal cavity

7 ⊟ S31.119- Laceration without foreign body of abdominal wall, unspecified quadrant without penetration into peritoneal cavity

6 S31.12 Laceration with foreign body of abdominal wall without penetration into peritoneal cavity

7 ⊟ S31.120- Laceration of abdominal wall with foreign body, right upper quadrant without penetration into peritoneal cavity

7 ⊟ S31.121- Laceration of abdominal wall with foreign body, left upper quadrant without penetration into peritoneal cavity

7 ⊟ S31.122- Laceration of abdominal wall with foreign body, epigastric region without penetration into peritoneal cavity

7 ⊟ S31.123- Laceration of abdominal wall with foreign body, right lower quadrant without penetration into peritoneal cavity

7 ⊟ S31.124- Laceration of abdominal wall with foreign body, left lower quadrant without penetration into peritoneal cavity

7 ⊟ S31.125- Laceration of abdominal wall with foreign body, periumbilic region without penetration into peritoneal cavity

7 ⊟ S31.129- Laceration of abdominal wall with foreign body, unspecified quadrant without penetration into peritoneal cavity

6 S31.13 Puncture wound of abdominal wall without foreign body without penetration into peritoneal cavity

7 ⊟ S31.130- Puncture wound of abdominal wall without foreign body, right upper quadrant without penetration into peritoneal cavity

7 ⊟ S31.131- Puncture wound of abdominal wall without foreign body, left upper quadrant without penetration into peritoneal cavity

7 ⊟ S31.132- Puncture wound of abdominal wall without foreign body, epigastric region without penetration into peritoneal cavity

● New | Manifestation | 4-7 Digit Indicators | ⊟ Laterality | A Adult | M Maternity | N Newborn | P Pediatric | ♂ Male
▲ Revised | Unspecified | AHA Coding Clinic | HCC Hierarchical Condition Categories | HIV HIV Related Conditions | ♀ Female

7 ⊟ S31.133- **Puncture wound of abdominal wall without foreign body, right lower quadrant without penetration into peritoneal cavity**

7 ⊟ S31.134- **Puncture wound of abdominal wall without foreign body, left lower quadrant without penetration into peritoneal cavity**

7 ⊟ S31.135- **Puncture wound of abdominal wall without foreign body, periumbilic region without penetration into peritoneal cavity**

7 ⊟ S31.139- **Puncture wound of abdominal wall without foreign body, unspecified quadrant without penetration into peritoneal cavity**

6 S31.14 **Puncture wound of abdominal wall with foreign body without penetration into peritoneal cavity**

7 ⊟ S31.140- **Puncture wound of abdominal wall with foreign body, right upper quadrant without penetration into peritoneal cavity**

7 ⊟ S31.141- **Puncture wound of abdominal wall with foreign body, left upper quadrant without penetration into peritoneal cavity**

7 ⊟ S31.142- **Puncture wound of abdominal wall with foreign body, epigastric region without penetration into peritoneal cavity**

7 ⊟ S31.143- **Puncture wound of abdominal wall with foreign body, right lower quadrant without penetration into peritoneal cavity**

7 ⊟ S31.144- **Puncture wound of abdominal wall with foreign body, left lower quadrant without penetration into peritoneal cavity**

7 ⊟ S31.145- **Puncture wound of abdominal wall with foreign body, periumbilic region without penetration into peritoneal cavity**

7 ⊟ S31.149- **Puncture wound of abdominal wall with foreign body, unspecified quadrant without penetration into peritoneal cavity**

6 S31.15 **Open bite of abdominal wall without penetration into peritoneal cavity**

Bite of abdominal wall NOS

EXCLUDES 1 *superficial bite of abdominal wall (S30.871)*

7 ⊟ S31.150- **Open bite of abdominal wall, right upper quadrant without penetration into peritoneal cavity**

7 ⊟ S31.151- **Open bite of abdominal wall, left upper quadrant without penetration into peritoneal cavity**

7 ⊟ S31.152- **Open bite of abdominal wall, epigastric region without penetration into peritoneal cavity**

7 ⊟ S31.153- **Open bite of abdominal wall, right lower quadrant without penetration into peritoneal cavity**

7 ⊟ S31.154- **Open bite of abdominal wall, left lower quadrant without penetration into peritoneal cavity**

7 ⊟ S31.155- **Open bite of abdominal wall, periumbilic region without penetration into peritoneal cavity**

7 ⊟ S31.159- **Open bite of abdominal wall, unspecified quadrant without penetration into peritoneal cavity**

5 S31.2 **Open wound of penis**

7 S31.20X- **Unspecified open wound of penis** ♂

7 S31.21X- **Laceration without foreign body of penis** ♂

7 S31.22X- **Laceration with foreign body of penis** ♂

7 S31.23X- **Puncture wound without foreign body of penis** ♂

7 S31.24X- **Puncture wound with foreign body of penis** ♂

7 S31.25X- **Open bite of penis** ♂

Bite of penis NOS

EXCLUDES 1 *superficial bite of penis (S30.862, S30.872)*

5 S31.3 **Open wound of scrotum and testes**

7 S31.30X- **Unspecified open wound of scrotum and testes** ♂

7 S31.31X- **Laceration without foreign body of scrotum and testes** ♂

7 S31.32X- **Laceration with foreign body of scrotum and testes** ♂

7 S31.33X- **Puncture wound without foreign body of scrotum and testes** ♂

7 S31.34X- **Puncture wound with foreign body of scrotum and testes** ♂

7 S31.35X- **Open bite of scrotum and testes** ♂

Bite of scrotum and testes NOS

EXCLUDES 1 *superficial bite of scrotum and testes (S30.863, S30.873)*

5 S31.4 **Open wound of vagina and vulva**

EXCLUDES 1 *injury to vagina and vulva during delivery (O70.-, O71.4)*

7 S31.40X- **Unspecified open wound of vagina and vulva** ♀

7 S31.41X- **Laceration without foreign body of vagina and vulva** ♀

7 S31.42X- **Laceration with foreign body of vagina and vulva** ♀

7 S31.43X- **Puncture wound without foreign body of vagina and vulva** ♀

7 S31.44X- **Puncture wound with foreign body of vagina and vulva** ♀

7 S31.45X- **Open bite of vagina and vulva** ♀

Bite of vagina and vulva NOS

EXCLUDES 1 *superficial bite of vagina and vulva (S30.864, S30.874)*

5 S31.5 **Open wound of unspecified external genital organs**

EXCLUDES 1 *traumatic amputation of external genital organs (S38.21, S38.22)*

6 S31.50 **Unspecified open wound of Unspecified external genital organs**

7 S31.501- **Unspecified open wound of unspecified external genital organs, male** ♂

7 S31.502- **Unspecified open wound of unspecified external genital organs, female** ♀

6 S31.51 **Laceration without foreign body of unspecified external genital organs**

7 S31.511- **Laceration without foreign body of unspecified external genital organs, male** ♂

7 S31.512- **Laceration without foreign body of unspecified external genital organs, female** ♀

6 S31.52 **Laceration with foreign body of unspecified external genital organs**

7 S31.521- **Laceration with foreign body of unspecified external genital organs, male** ♂

7 S31.522- **Laceration with foreign body of unspecified external genital organs, female** ♀

6 S31.53 **Puncture wound without foreign body of unspecified external genital organs**

7 S31.531- **Puncture wound without foreign body of unspecified external genital organs, male** ♂

7 S31.532- **Puncture wound without foreign body of unspecified external genital organs, female** ♀

6 S31.54 **Puncture wound with foreign body of unspecified external genital organs**

7 S31.541- **Puncture wound with foreign body of unspecified external genital organs, male** ♂

7 S31.542- **Puncture wound with foreign body of unspecified external genital organs, female** ♀

6 S31.55 **Open bite of unspecified external genital organs**

Bite of unspecified external genital organs NOS

EXCLUDES 1 *superficial bite of unspecified external genital organs (S30.865, S30.866, S30.875, S30.876)*

7 S31.551- **Open bite of unspecified external genital organs, male** ♂

7 S31.552- **Open bite of unspecified external genital organs, female** ♀

5 S31.6 **Open wound of abdominal wall with penetration into peritoneal cavity**

6 S31.60 **Unspecified open wound of abdominal wall with penetration into peritoneal cavity**

7 ⊟ S31.600- **Unspecified open wound of abdominal wall, right upper quadrant with penetration into peritoneal cavity**

7 ⊟ S31.601- **Unspecified open wound of abdominal wall, left upper quadrant with penetration into peritoneal cavity**

S31.602- Unspecified open wound of abdominal wall, epigastric region with penetration into peritoneal cavity

S31.603- Unspecified open wound of abdominal wall, right lower quadrant with penetration into peritoneal cavity

S31.604- Unspecified open wound of abdominal wall, left lower quadrant with penetration into peritoneal cavity

S31.605- Unspecified open wound of abdominal wall, periumbilic region with penetration into peritoneal cavity

S31.609- Unspecified open wound of abdominal wall, unspecified quadrant with penetration into peritoneal cavity

S31.61 Laceration without foreign body of abdominal wall with penetration into peritoneal cavity

S31.610- Laceration without foreign body of abdominal wall, right upper quadrant with penetration into peritoneal cavity

S31.611- Laceration without foreign body of abdominal wall, left upper quadrant with penetration into peritoneal cavity

S31.612- Laceration without foreign body of abdominal wall, epigastric region with penetration into peritoneal cavity

S31.613- Laceration without foreign body of abdominal wall, right lower quadrant with penetration into peritoneal cavity

AHA: (S31.613A) 4Q 2015, 37-38

S31.614- Laceration without foreign body of abdominal wall, left lower quadrant with penetration into peritoneal cavity

S31.615- Laceration without foreign body of abdominal wall, periumbilic region with penetration into peritoneal cavity

S31.619- Laceration without foreign body of abdominal wall, unspecified quadrant with penetration into peritoneal cavity

S31.62 Laceration with foreign body of abdominal wall with penetration into peritoneal cavity

S31.620- Laceration with foreign body of abdominal wall, right upper quadrant with penetration into peritoneal cavity

S31.621- Laceration with foreign body of abdominal wall, left upper quadrant with penetration into peritoneal cavity

S31.622- Laceration with foreign body of abdominal wall, epigastric region with penetration into peritoneal cavity

S31.623- Laceration with foreign body of abdominal wall, right lower quadrant with penetration into peritoneal cavity

S31.624- Laceration with foreign body of abdominal wall, left lower quadrant with penetration into peritoneal cavity

S31.625- Laceration with foreign body of abdominal wall, periumbilic region with penetration into peritoneal cavity

S31.629- Laceration with foreign body of abdominal wall, unspecified quadrant with penetration into peritoneal cavity

S31.63 Puncture wound without foreign body of abdominal wall with penetration into peritoneal cavity

S31.630- Puncture wound without foreign body of abdominal wall, right upper quadrant with penetration into peritoneal cavity

S31.631- Puncture wound without foreign body of abdominal wall, left upper quadrant with penetration into peritoneal cavity

S31.632- Puncture wound without foreign body of abdominal wall, epigastric region with penetration into peritoneal cavity

S31.633- Puncture wound without foreign body of abdominal wall, right lower quadrant with penetration into peritoneal cavity

S31.634- Puncture wound without foreign body of abdominal wall, left lower quadrant with penetration into peritoneal cavity

S31.635- Puncture wound without foreign body of abdominal wall, periumbilic region with penetration into peritoneal cavity

S31.639- Puncture wound without foreign body of abdominal wall, unspecified quadrant with penetration into peritoneal cavity

S31.64 Puncture wound with foreign body of abdominal wall with penetration into peritoneal cavity

S31.640- Puncture wound with foreign body of abdominal wall, right upper quadrant with penetration into peritoneal cavity

S31.641- Puncture wound with foreign body of abdominal wall, left upper quadrant with penetration into peritoneal cavity

S31.642- Puncture wound with foreign body of abdominal wall, epigastric region with penetration into peritoneal cavity

S31.643- Puncture wound with foreign body of abdominal wall, right lower quadrant with penetration into peritoneal cavity

S31.644- Puncture wound with foreign body of abdominal wall, left lower quadrant with penetration into peritoneal cavity

S31.645- Puncture wound with foreign body of abdominal wall, periumbilic region with penetration into peritoneal cavity

S31.649- Puncture wound with foreign body of abdominal wall, unspecified quadrant with penetration into peritoneal cavity

S31.65 Open bite of abdominal wall with penetration into peritoneal cavity

EXCLUDES 1 *superficial bite of abdominal wall (S30.861, S30.871)*

S31.650- Open bite of abdominal wall, right upper quadrant with penetration into peritoneal cavity

S31.651- Open bite of abdominal wall, left upper quadrant with penetration into peritoneal cavity

S31.652- Open bite of abdominal wall, epigastric region with penetration into peritoneal cavity

S31.653- Open bite of abdominal wall, right lower quadrant with penetration into peritoneal cavity

S31.654- Open bite of abdominal wall, left lower quadrant with penetration into peritoneal cavity

S31.655- Open bite of abdominal wall, periumbilic region with penetration into peritoneal cavity

S31.659- Open bite of abdominal wall, unspecified quadrant with penetration into peritoneal cavity

S31.8 Open wound of other parts of abdomen, lower back and pelvis

S31.80 Open wound of unspecified buttock

S31.801- Laceration without foreign body of unspecified buttock

S31.802- Laceration with foreign body of unspecified buttock

S31.803- Puncture wound without foreign body of unspecified buttock

S31.804- Puncture wound with foreign body of unspecified buttock

S31.805- Open bite of unspecified buttock

Bite of buttock NOS

EXCLUDES 1 *superficial bite of buttock (S30.870)*

S31.809- Unspecified open wound of Unspecified buttock

S31.81 Open wound of right buttock

S31.811- Laceration without foreign body of right buttock

S31.812- Laceration with foreign body of right buttock

S31.813- Puncture wound without foreign body of right buttock

S31.814- Puncture wound with foreign body of right buttock

● New ▲ Revised | *Manifestation* Unspecified | 4-7 Digit Indicators | AHA Coding Clinic | Laterality | HCC Hierarchical Condition Categories | A Adult | M Maternity | N Newborn | HIV HIV Related Conditions | P Pediatric | ♂ Male | ♀ Female

7 ⊟ S31.815- **Open bite of right buttock**
Bite of right buttock NOS
EXCLUDES 1 *superficial bite of buttock (S30.870)*

7 ⊟ S31.819- **Unspecified open wound of right buttock**

6 S31.82 **Open wound of left buttock**

7 ⊟ S31.821- **Laceration without foreign body of left buttock**

7 ⊟ S31.822- **Laceration with foreign body of left buttock**

7 ⊟ S31.823- **Puncture wound without foreign body of left buttock**

7 ⊟ S31.824- **Puncture wound with foreign body of left buttock**

7 ⊟ S31.825- **Open bite of left buttock**
Bite of left buttock NOS
EXCLUDES 1 *superficial bite of buttock (S30.870)*

7 ⊟ S31.829- **Unspecified open wound of left buttock**

6 S31.83 **Open wound of anus**

7 S31.831- **Laceration without foreign body of anus**

7 S31.832- **Laceration with foreign body of anus**

7 S31.833- **Puncture wound without foreign body of anus**

7 S31.834- **Puncture wound with foreign body of anus**

7 S31.835- **Open bite of anus**
Bite of anus NOS
EXCLUDES 1 *superficial bite of anus (S30.877)*

7 S31.839- **Unspecified open wound of anus**

4 S32 Fracture of lumbar spine and pelvis

Note: A fracture not indicated as displaced or nondisplaced should be coded to displaced
A fracture not indicated as opened or closed should be coded to closed

INCLUDES fracture of lumbosacral neural arch
fracture of lumbosacral spinous process
fracture of lumbosacral transverse process
fracture of lumbosacral vertebra
fracture of lumbosacral vertebral arch

Code first:
any associated spinal cord and spinal nerve injury (S34.-)

EXCLUDES 1 *transection of abdomen (S38.3)*

EXCLUDES 2 *fracture of hip NOS (S72.0-)*

The appropriate 7th character is to be added to each code from category S32

A	initial encounter for closed fracture
B	initial encounter for open fracture
D	subsequent encounter for fracture with routine healing
G	subsequent encounter for fracture with delayed healing
K	subsequent encounter for fracture with nonunion
S	sequela

CODING TIP ✓ A fracture not indicated as displaced or nondisplaced should be coded to displaced. A fracture not indicated as open or closed should be coded to closed. Query providers on fractures not documented as displaced/nondisplaced; otherwise, a displaced fracture diagnosis could be assigned without a reduction being performed, potentially resulting in claim denials.

5 S32.0 **Fracture of lumbar vertebra**
Fracture of lumbar spine NOS

6 S32.00 **Fracture of unspecified lumbar vertebra**

7 S32.000- **Wedge compression fracture of unspecified lumbar vertebra** HCC

7 S32.001- **Stable burst fracture of unspecified lumbar vertebra** HCC

7 S32.002- **Unstable burst fracture of unspecified lumbar vertebra** HCC

7 S32.008- **Other fracture of unspecified lumbar vertebra** HCC

7 S32.009- **Unspecified fracture of Unspecified lumbar vertebra** HCC

6 S32.01 **Fracture of first lumbar vertebra**

7 S32.010- **Wedge compression fracture of first lumbar vertebra** HCC

7 S32.011- **Stable burst fracture of first lumbar vertebra** HCC

7 S32.012- **Unstable burst fracture of first lumbar vertebra** HCC

7 S32.018- **Other fracture of first lumbar vertebra** HCC

7 S32.019- **Unspecified fracture of first lumbar vertebra** HCC

6 S32.02 **Fracture of second lumbar vertebra**

7 S32.020- **Wedge compression fracture of second lumbar vertebra** HCC

7 S32.021- **Stable burst fracture of second lumbar vertebra** HCC

7 S32.022- **Unstable burst fracture of second lumbar vertebra** HCC

7 S32.028- **Other fracture of second lumbar vertebra** HCC

7 S32.029- **Unspecified fracture of second lumbar vertebra** HCC

6 S32.03 **Fracture of third lumbar vertebra**

7 S32.030- **Wedge compression fracture of third lumbar vertebra** HCC

7 S32.031- **Stable burst fracture of third lumbar vertebra** HCC

7 S32.032- **Unstable burst fracture of third lumbar vertebra** HCC

7 S32.038- **Other fracture of third lumbar vertebra** HCC

7 S32.039- **Unspecified fracture of third lumbar vertebra** HCC

6 S32.04 **Fracture of fourth lumbar vertebra**

7 S32.040- **Wedge compression fracture of fourth lumbar vertebra** HCC

7 S32.041- **Stable burst fracture of fourth lumbar vertebra** HCC

7 S32.042- **Unstable burst fracture of fourth lumbar vertebra** HCC

7 S32.048- **Other fracture of fourth lumbar vertebra** HCC

7 S32.049- **Unspecified fracture of fourth lumbar vertebra** HCC

6 S32.05 **Fracture of fifth lumbar vertebra**

7 S32.050- **Wedge compression fracture of fifth lumbar vertebra** HCC

7 S32.051- **Stable burst fracture of fifth lumbar vertebra** HCC

7 S32.052- **Unstable burst fracture of fifth lumbar vertebra** HCC

7 S32.058- **Other fracture of fifth lumbar vertebra** HCC

7 S32.059- **Unspecified fracture of fifth lumbar vertebra** HCC

5 S32.1 **Fracture of sacrum**
For vertical fractures, code to most medial fracture extension
Use two codes if both a vertical and transverse fracture are present
Code also:
any associated fracture of pelvic ring (S32.8-)

7 S32.10X- **Unspecified fracture of sacrum** HCC

6 S32.11 **Zone I fracture of sacrum**
Vertical sacral ala fracture of sacrum

7 S32.110- **Nondisplaced Zone I fracture of sacrum** HCC

7 S32.111- **Minimally displaced Zone I fracture of sacrum** HCC

7 S32.112- **Severely displaced Zone I fracture of sacrum** HCC

7 S32.119- **Unspecified Zone I fracture of sacrum** HCC

6 S32.12 **Zone II fracture of sacrum**
Vertical foraminal region fracture of sacrum

7 S32.120- **Nondisplaced Zone II fracture of sacrum** HCC

7 S32.121- **Minimally displaced Zone II fracture of sacrum** HCC

7 S32.122- **Severely displaced Zone II fracture of sacrum** HCC

7 S32.129- **Unspecified Zone II fracture of sacrum** HCC

6 S32.13 **Zone III fracture of sacrum**
Vertical fracture into spinal canal region of sacrum

7 S32.130- **Nondisplaced Zone III fracture of sacrum** HCC

7 S32.131- **Minimally displaced Zone III fracture of sacrum** HCC

7 S32.132- **Severely displaced Zone III fracture of sacrum** HCC

7 S32.139- Unspecified Zone III fracture of sacrum HCC
7 S32.14X- Type 1 fracture of sacrum HCC
Transverse flexion fracture of sacrum without displacement
7 S32.15X- Type 2 fracture of sacrum HCC
Transverse flexion fracture of sacrum with posterior displacement
7 S32.16X- Type 3 fracture of sacrum HCC
Transverse extension fracture of sacrum with anterior displacement
7 S32.17X- Type 4 fracture of sacrum HCC
Transverse segmental comminution of upper sacrum
7 S32.19X- Other fracture of sacrum HCC
7 S32.2XX- Fracture of coccyx HCC
5 S32.3 Fracture of ilium
EXCLUDES 1 *fracture of ilium with associated disruption of pelvic ring (S32.8-)*
6 S32.30 Unspecified fracture of ilium
7 ⊟ S32.301- Unspecified fracture of right ilium HCC
7 ⊟ S32.302- Unspecified fracture of left ilium HCC
7 ⊟ S32.309- Unspecified fracture of unspecified ilium HCC
6 S32.31 Avulsion fracture of ilium
7 ⊟ S32.311- Displaced avulsion fracture of right ilium HCC
7 ⊟ S32.312- Displaced avulsion fracture of left ilium HCC
7 ⊟ S32.313- Displaced avulsion fracture of unspecified ilium HCC
7 ⊟ S32.314- Nondisplaced avulsion fracture of right ilium HCC
7 ⊟ S32.315- Nondisplaced avulsion fracture of left ilium HCC
7 ⊟ S32.316- Nondisplaced avulsion fracture of unspecified ilium HCC
6 S32.39 Other fracture of ilium
7 ⊟ S32.391- Other fracture of right ilium HCC
7 ⊟ S32.392- Other fracture of left ilium HCC
7 ⊟ S32.399- Other fracture of unspecified ilium HCC
5 S32.4 Fracture of acetabulum
Code also:
any associated fracture of pelvic ring (S32.8-)
6 S32.40 Unspecified fracture of acetabulum
7 ⊟ S32.401- Unspecified fracture of right acetabulum HCC
7 ⊟ S32.402- Unspecified fracture of left acetabulum HCC
7 ⊟ S32.409- Unspecified fracture of unspecified acetabulum HCC
6 S32.41 Fracture of anterior wall of acetabulum
7 ⊟ S32.411- Displaced fracture of anterior wall of right acetabulum HCC
7 ⊟ S32.412- Displaced fracture of anterior wall of left acetabulum HCC
7 ⊟ S32.413- Displaced fracture of anterior wall of unspecified acetabulum HCC
7 ⊟ S32.414- Nondisplaced fracture of anterior wall of right acetabulum HCC
7 ⊟ S32.415- Nondisplaced fracture of anterior wall of left acetabulum HCC
7 ⊟ S32.416- Nondisplaced fracture of anterior wall of unspecified acetabulum HCC
6 S32.42 Fracture of posterior wall of acetabulum
7 ⊟ S32.421- Displaced fracture of posterior wall of right acetabulum HCC
7 ⊟ S32.422- Displaced fracture of posterior wall of left acetabulum HCC
7 ⊟ S32.423- Displaced fracture of posterior wall of unspecified acetabulum HCC
7 ⊟ S32.424- Nondisplaced fracture of posterior wall of right acetabulum HCC
7 ⊟ S32.425- Nondisplaced fracture of posterior wall of left acetabulum HCC
7 ⊟ S32.426- Nondisplaced fracture of posterior wall of unspecified acetabulum HCC
6 S32.43 Fracture of anterior column [iliopubic] of acetabulum
7 ⊟ S32.431- Displaced fracture of anterior column [iliopubic] of right acetabulum HCC
7 ⊟ S32.432- Displaced fracture of anterior column [iliopubic] of left acetabulum HCC
7 ⊟ S32.433- Displaced fracture of anterior column [iliopubic] of unspecified acetabulum HCC
7 ⊟ S32.434- Nondisplaced fracture of anterior column [iliopubic] of right acetabulum HCC
7 ⊟ S32.435- Nondisplaced fracture of anterior column [iliopubic] of left acetabulum HCC
7 ⊟ S32.436- Nondisplaced fracture of anterior column [iliopubic] of unspecified acetabulum HCC
6 S32.44 Fracture of posterior column [ilioischial] of acetabulum
7 ⊟ S32.441- Displaced fracture of posterior column [ilioischial] of right acetabulum HCC
7 ⊟ S32.442- Displaced fracture of posterior column [ilioischial] of left acetabulum HCC
7 ⊟ S32.443- Displaced fracture of posterior column [ilioischial] of unspecified acetabulum HCC
7 ⊟ S32.444- Nondisplaced fracture of posterior column [ilioischial] of right acetabulum HCC
7 ⊟ S32.445- Nondisplaced fracture of posterior column [ilioischial] of left acetabulum HCC
7 ⊟ S32.446- Nondisplaced fracture of posterior column [ilioischial] of unspecified acetabulum HCC
6 S32.45 Transverse fracture of acetabulum
7 ⊟ S32.451- Displaced transverse fracture of right acetabulum HCC
7 ⊟ S32.452- Displaced transverse fracture of left acetabulum HCC
7 ⊟ S32.453- Displaced transverse fracture of unspecified acetabulum HCC
7 ⊟ S32.454- Nondisplaced transverse fracture of right acetabulum HCC
7 ⊟ S32.455- Nondisplaced transverse fracture of left acetabulum HCC
7 ⊟ S32.456- Nondisplaced transverse fracture of unspecified acetabulum HCC
6 S32.46 Associated transverse-posterior fracture of acetabulum
7 ⊟ S32.461- Displaced associated transverse-posterior fracture of right acetabulum HCC
7 ⊟ S32.462- Displaced associated transverse-posterior fracture of left acetabulum HCC
7 ⊟ S32.463- Displaced associated transverse-posterior fracture of unspecified acetabulum HCC
7 ⊟ S32.464- Nondisplaced associated transverse-posterior fracture of right acetabulum HCC
7 ⊟ S32.465- Nondisplaced associated transverse-posterior fracture of left acetabulum HCC
7 ⊟ S32.466- Nondisplaced associated transverse-posterior fracture of unspecified acetabulum HCC
6 S32.47 Fracture of medial wall of acetabulum
7 ⊟ S32.471- Displaced fracture of medial wall of right acetabulum HCC
7 ⊟ S32.472- Displaced fracture of medial wall of left acetabulum HCC
7 ⊟ S32.473- Displaced fracture of medial wall of unspecified acetabulum HCC
7 ⊟ S32.474- Nondisplaced fracture of medial wall of right acetabulum HCC
7 ⊟ S32.475- Nondisplaced fracture of medial wall of left acetabulum HCC
7 ⊟ S32.476- Nondisplaced fracture of medial wall of unspecified acetabulum HCC
6 S32.48 Dome fracture of acetabulum
7 ⊟ S32.481- Displaced dome fracture of right acetabulum HCC
7 ⊟ S32.482- Displaced dome fracture of left acetabulum HCC
7 ⊟ S32.483- Displaced dome fracture of unspecified acetabulum HCC
7 ⊟ S32.484- Nondisplaced dome fracture of right acetabulum HCC
7 ⊟ S32.485- Nondisplaced dome fracture of left acetabulum HCC
7 ⊟ S32.486- Nondisplaced dome fracture of unspecified acetabulum HCC
6 S32.49 Other specified fracture of acetabulum

7 ⊟ S32.491- Other specified fracture of right acetabulum HCC
7 ⊟ S32.492- Other specified fracture of left acetabulum HCC
7 ⊟ S32.499- Other specified fracture of unspecified acetabulum HCC

5 S32.5 Fracture of pubis
EXCLUDES 1 *fracture of pubis with associated disruption of pelvic ring (S32.8-)*

6 S32.50 Unspecified fracture of pubis
7 ⊟ S32.501- Unspecified fracture of right pubis HCC
7 ⊟ S32.502- Unspecified fracture of left pubis HCC
7 ⊟ S32.509- Unspecified fracture of unspecified pubis HCC

6 S32.51 Fracture of superior rim of pubis
7 ⊟ S32.511- Fracture of superior rim of right pubis HCC
7 ⊟ S32.512- Fracture of superior rim of left pubis HCC
7 ⊟ S32.519- Fracture of superior rim of unspecified pubis HCC

6 S32.59 Other specified fracture of pubis
7 ⊟ S32.591- Other specified fracture of right pubis HCC
7 ⊟ S32.592- Other specified fracture of left pubis HCC
7 ⊟ S32.599- Other specified fracture of unspecified pubis HCC

5 S32.6 Fracture of ischium
EXCLUDES 1 *fracture of ischium with associated disruption of pelvic ring (S32.8-)*

6 S32.60 Unspecified fracture of ischium
7 ⊟ S32.601- Unspecified fracture of right ischium HCC
7 ⊟ S32.602- Unspecified fracture of left ischium HCC
7 ⊟ S32.609- Unspecified fracture of unspecified ischium HCC

6 S32.61 Avulsion fracture of ischium
7 ⊟ S32.611- Displaced avulsion fracture of right ischium HCC
7 ⊟ S32.612- Displaced avulsion fracture of left ischium HCC
7 ⊟ S32.613- Displaced avulsion fracture of unspecified ischium HCC
7 ⊟ S32.614- Nondisplaced avulsion fracture of right ischium HCC
7 ⊟ S32.615- Nondisplaced avulsion fracture of left ischium HCC
7 ⊟ S32.616- Nondisplaced avulsion fracture of unspecified ischium HCC

6 S32.69 Other specified fracture of ischium
7 ⊟ S32.691- Other specified fracture of right ischium HCC
7 ⊟ S32.692- Other specified fracture of left ischium HCC
7 ⊟ S32.699- Other specified fracture of unspecified ischium HCC

5 S32.8 Fracture of other parts of pelvis
Code also any associated:
fracture of acetabulum (S32.4-)
sacral fracture (S32.1-)

6 S32.81 Multiple fractures of pelvis with disruption of pelvic ring
Multiple pelvic fractures with disruption of pelvic circle
7 S32.810- Multiple fractures of pelvis with stable disruption of pelvic ring HCC
7 S32.811 Multiple fractures of pelvis with unstable disruption of pelvic ring HCC

7 S32.82X- Multiple fractures of pelvis without disruption of pelvic ring HCC
Multiple pelvic fractures without disruption of pelvic circle

7 S32.89X- Fracture of other parts of pelvis HCC

7 S32.9XX- Fracture of unspecified parts of lumbosacral spine and pelvis HCC
Fracture of lumbosacral spine NOS
Fracture of pelvis NOS
AHA: (S32.9XXD) 4Q 2012, 93

4 S33 Dislocation and sprain of joints and ligaments of lumbar spine and pelvis
INCLUDES avulsion of joint or ligament of lumbar spine and pelvis
laceration of cartilage, joint or ligament of lumbar spine and pelvis
sprain of cartilage, joint or ligament of lumbar spine and pelvis
traumatic hemarthrosis of joint or ligament of lumbar spine and pelvis
traumatic rupture of joint or ligament of lumbar spine and pelvis
traumatic subluxation of joint or ligament of lumbar spine and pelvis
traumatic tear of joint or ligament of lumbar spine and pelvis

Code also:
any associated open wound

EXCLUDES 1 *nontraumatic rupture or displacement of lumbar intervertebral disc NOS (M51.-)*
obstetric damage to pelvic joints and ligaments (O71.6)

EXCLUDES 2 *dislocation and sprain of joints and ligaments of hip (S73.-)*
strain of muscle of lower back and pelvis (S39.01-)

The appropriate 7th character is to be added to each code from category S33
A initial encounter
D subsequent encounter
S sequela

CODING TIP ✓ There are no codes for open dislocations. When a dislocation is documented as open, assign an additional code for the open wound.

7 S33.0XX- Traumatic rupture of lumbar intervertebral disc
EXCLUDES 1 *rupture or displacement (nontraumatic) of lumbar intervertebral disc NOS (M51.- with fifth character 6)*

5 S33.1 Subluxation and dislocation of lumbar vertebra
Code also any associated:
open wound of abdomen, lower back and pelvis (S31)
spinal cord injury (S24.0, S24.1-, S34.0-, S34.1-)
EXCLUDES 2 *fracture of lumbar vertebrae (S32.0-)*

6 S33.10 Subluxation and dislocation of unspecified lumbar vertebra
7 S33.100- Subluxation of unspecified lumbar vertebra
7 S33.101- Dislocation of unspecified lumbar vertebra

6 S33.11 Subluxation and dislocation of L1/L2 lumbar vertebra
7 S33.110- Subluxation of L1/L2 lumbar vertebra
7 S33.111- Dislocation of L1/L2 lumbar vertebra

6 S33.12 Subluxation and dislocation of L2/L3 lumbar vertebra
7 S33.120- Subluxation of L2/L3 lumbar vertebra
7 S33.121- Dislocation of L2/L3 lumbar vertebra

6 S33.13 Subluxation and dislocation of L3/L4 lumbar vertebra
7 S33.130- Subluxation of L3/L4 lumbar vertebra
7 S33.131- Dislocation of L3/L4 lumbar vertebra

6 S33.14 Subluxation and dislocation of L4/L5 lumbar vertebra
7 S33.140- Subluxation of L4/L5 lumbar vertebra
7 S33.141- Dislocation of L4/L5 lumbar vertebra

7 S33.2XX- Dislocation of sacroiliac and sacrococcygeal joint

5 S33.3 Dislocation of other and unspecified parts of lumbar spine and pelvis
7 S33.30X- Dislocation of unspecified parts of lumbar spine and pelvis
7 S33.39X- Dislocation of other parts of lumbar spine and pelvis

7 S33.4XX- Traumatic rupture of symphysis pubis
7 S33.5XX- Sprain of ligaments of lumbar spine
7 S33.6XX- Sprain of sacroiliac joint
7 S33.8XX- Sprain of other parts of lumbar spine and pelvis

S33.9XX- **Sprain of unspecified parts of lumbar spine and pelvis**

S34 Injury of lumbar and sacral spinal cord and nerves at abdomen, lower back and pelvis level

Note: Code to highest level of lumbar cord injury

Injuries to the spinal cord (S34.0 and S34.1) refer to the cord level and not bone level injury, and can affect nerve roots at and below the level given.

Code also any associated:
- fracture of vertebra (S22.0-, S32.0-)
- open wound of abdomen, lower back and pelvis (S31.-)
- transient paralysis (R29.5)

The appropriate 7th character is to be added to each code from category S34
- A initial encounter
- D subsequent encounter
- S sequela

CODING TIP ✓ When coding sequelae of a spinal cord injury, first list the residual condition(s), followed by the specific spinal cord injury diagnosed using the appropriate code from this category with the seventh character "S" to indicate sequelae. If there are multiple levels of injury, code only the highest injury.

CODING TIP ✓ When coding sequelae of a lumbar and/or sacral spinal cord injury, first list the residual condition(s), followed by the specific spinal cord injury diagnosed using the appropriate code from category S34 with the seventh character "S" to indicate sequelae.

S34.0 **Concussion and edema of lumbar and sacral spinal cord**

S34.01X- **Concussion and edema of lumbar spinal cord** HCC

S34.02X- **Concussion and edema of sacral spinal cord** HCC
Concussion and edema of conus medullaris

S34.1 **Other and unspecified injury of lumbar and sacral spinal cord**

S34.10 **Unspecified injury to lumbar spinal cord**

S34.101- **Unspecified injury to L1 level of lumbar spinal cord** HCC
Unspecified injury to lumbar spinal cord level 1

S34.102- **Unspecified injury to L2 level of lumbar spinal cord** HCC
Unspecified injury to lumbar spinal cord level 2

S34.103- **Unspecified injury to L3 level of lumbar spinal cord** HCC
Unspecified injury to lumbar spinal cord level 3

S34.104- **Unspecified injury to L4 level of lumbar spinal cord** HCC
Unspecified injury to lumbar spinal cord level 4

S34.105- **Unspecified injury to L5 level of lumbar spinal cord** HCC
Unspecified injury to lumbar spinal cord level 5

S34.109- **Unspecified injury to unspecified level of lumbar spinal cord** HCC

S34.11 **Complete lesion of lumbar spinal cord**

S34.111- **Complete lesion of L1 level of lumbar spinal cord** HCC
Complete lesion of lumbar spinal cord level 1

S34.112- **Complete lesion of L2 level of lumbar spinal cord** HCC
Complete lesion of lumbar spinal cord level 2

S34.113- **Complete lesion of L3 level of lumbar spinal cord** HCC
Complete lesion of lumbar spinal cord level 3

S34.114- **Complete lesion of L4 level of lumbar spinal cord** HCC
Complete lesion of lumbar spinal cord level 4

S34.115- **Complete lesion of L5 level of lumbar spinal cord** HCC
Complete lesion of lumbar spinal cord level 5

S34.119- **Complete lesion of unspecified level of lumbar spinal cord** HCC

S34.12 **Incomplete lesion of lumbar spinal cord**

S34.121- **Incomplete lesion of L1 level of lumbar spinal cord** HCC
Incomplete lesion of lumbar spinal cord level 1

S34.122- **Incomplete lesion of L2 level of lumbar spinal cord** HCC
Incomplete lesion of lumbar spinal cord level 2

S34.123- **Incomplete lesion of L3 level of lumbar spinal cord** HCC
Incomplete lesion of lumbar spinal cord level 3

S34.124- **Incomplete lesion of L4 level of lumbar spinal cord** HCC
Incomplete lesion of lumbar spinal cord level 4

S34.125- **Incomplete lesion of L5 level of lumbar spinal cord** HCC
Incomplete lesion of lumbar spinal cord level 5

S34.129- **Incomplete lesion of unspecified level of lumbar spinal cord** HCC

S34.13 **Other and unspecified injury to sacral spinal cord**
Other injury to conus medullaris

S34.131- **Complete lesion of sacral spinal cord** HCC
Complete lesion of conus medullaris

S34.132- **Incomplete lesion of sacral spinal cord** HCC
Incomplete lesion of conus medullaris

S34.139- **Unspecified injury to sacral spinal cord** HCC
Unspecified injury of conus medullaris

S34.2 **Injury of nerve root of lumbar and sacral spine**

S34.21X- **Injury of nerve root of lumbar spine**

S34.22X- **Injury of nerve root of sacral spine**

S34.3XX- **Injury of cauda equina** HCC

S34.4XX- **Injury of lumbosacral plexus**

S34.5XX- **Injury of lumbar, sacral and pelvic sympathetic nerves**
Injury of celiac ganglion or plexus
Injury of hypogastric plexus
Injury of mesenteric plexus (inferior) (superior)
Injury of splanchnic nerve

S34.6XX- **Injury of peripheral nerve(s) at abdomen, lower back and pelvis level**

S34.8XX- **Injury of other nerves at abdomen, lower back and pelvis level**

S34.9XX- **Injury of unspecified nerves at abdomen, lower back and pelvis level**

S35 Injury of blood vessels at abdomen, lower back and pelvis level

Code also:
any associated open wound (S31.-)

The appropriate 7th character is to be added to each code from category S35
- A initial encounter
- D subsequent encounter
- S sequela

S35.0 **Injury of abdominal aorta**
EXCLUDES 1 *injury of aorta NOS (S25.0)*

S35.00X- **Unspecified injury of abdominal aorta**

S35.01X- **Minor laceration of abdominal aorta**
Incomplete transection of abdominal aorta
Laceration of abdominal aorta NOS
Superficial laceration of abdominal aorta

S35.02X- **Major laceration of abdominal aorta**
Complete transection of abdominal aorta
Traumatic rupture of abdominal aorta

S35.09X- **Other injury of abdominal aorta**

S35.1 **Injury of inferior vena cava**
Injury of hepatic vein
EXCLUDES 1 *injury of vena cava NOS (S25.2)*

S35.10X- **Unspecified injury of inferior vena cava**

S35.11X- **Minor laceration of inferior vena cava**
Incomplete transection of inferior vena cava
Laceration of inferior vena cava NOS
Superficial laceration of inferior vena cava

S35.12X- **Major laceration of inferior vena cava**
Complete transection of inferior vena cava
Traumatic rupture of inferior vena cava

S35.19X- **Other injury of inferior vena cava**

S35.2 **Injury of celiac or mesenteric artery and branches**

S35.21 **Injury of celiac artery**

S35.211- **Minor laceration of celiac artery**
Incomplete transection of celiac artery
Laceration of celiac artery NOS
Superficial laceration of celiac artery

7 S35.212- Major laceration of celiac artery
Complete transection of celiac artery
Traumatic rupture of celiac artery
7 S35.218- Other injury of celiac artery
7 S35.219- Unspecified injury of celiac artery
6 S35.22 Injury of superior mesenteric artery
7 S35.221- Minor laceration of superior mesenteric artery
Incomplete transection of superior mesenteric artery
Laceration of superior mesenteric artery NOS
Superficial laceration of superior mesenteric artery
7 S35.222- Major laceration of superior mesenteric artery
Complete transection of superior mesenteric artery
Traumatic rupture of superior mesenteric artery
7 S35.228- Other injury of superior mesenteric artery
7 S35.229- Unspecified injury of superior mesenteric artery
6 S35.23 Injury of inferior mesenteric artery
7 S35.231- Minor laceration of inferior mesenteric artery
Incomplete transection of inferior mesenteric artery
Laceration of inferior mesenteric artery NOS
Superficial laceration of inferior mesenteric artery
7 S35.232- Major laceration of inferior mesenteric artery
Complete transection of inferior mesenteric artery
Traumatic rupture of inferior mesenteric artery
7 S35.238- Other injury of inferior mesenteric artery
7 S35.239- Unspecified injury of inferior mesenteric artery
6 S35.29 Injury of branches of celiac and mesenteric artery
Injury of gastric artery
Injury of gastroduodenal artery
Injury of hepatic artery
Injury of splenic artery
7 S35.291- Minor laceration of branches of celiac and mesenteric artery
Incomplete transection of branches of celiac and mesenteric artery
Laceration of branches of celiac and mesenteric artery NOS
Superficial laceration of branches of celiac and mesenteric artery
7 S35.292- Major laceration of branches of celiac and mesenteric artery
Complete transection of branches of celiac and mesenteric artery
Traumatic rupture of branches of celiac and mesenteric artery
7 S35.298- Other injury of branches of celiac and mesenteric artery
7 S35.299- Unspecified injury of branches of celiac and mesenteric artery
5 S35.3 Injury of portal or splenic vein and branches
6 S35.31 Injury of portal vein
7 S35.311- Laceration of portal vein
7 S35.318- Other specified injury of portal vein
7 S35.319- Unspecified injury of portal vein
6 S35.32 Injury of splenic vein
7 S35.321- Laceration of splenic vein
7 S35.328- Other specified injury of splenic vein
7 S35.329- Unspecified injury of splenic vein
6 S35.33 Injury of superior mesenteric vein
7 S35.331- Laceration of superior mesenteric vein
7 S35.338- Other specified injury of superior mesenteric vein
7 S35.339- Unspecified injury of superior mesenteric vein
6 S35.34 Injury of inferior mesenteric vein
7 S35.341- Laceration of inferior mesenteric vein
7 S35.348- Other specified injury of inferior mesenteric vein
7 S35.349- Unspecified injury of inferior mesenteric vein
5 S35.4 Injury of renal blood vessels
6 S35.40 Unspecified injury of renal blood vessel
7 ⊟ S35.401- Unspecified injury of right renal artery
7 ⊟ S35.402- Unspecified injury of left renal artery
7 ⊟ S35.403- Unspecified injury of unspecified renal artery
7 ⊟ S35.404- Unspecified injury of right renal vein
7 ⊟ S35.405- Unspecified injury of left renal vein
7 ⊟ S35.406- Unspecified injury of unspecified renal vein
6 S35.41 Laceration of renal blood vessel
7 ⊟ S35.411- Laceration of right renal artery
7 ⊟ S35.412- Laceration of left renal artery
7 ⊟ S35.413- Laceration of unspecified renal artery
7 ⊟ S35.414- Laceration of right renal vein
7 ⊟ S35.415- Laceration of left renal vein
7 ⊟ S35.416- Laceration of unspecified renal vein
6 S35.49 Other specified injury of renal blood vessel
7 ⊟ S35.491- Other specified injury of right renal artery
7 ⊟ S35.492- Other specified injury of left renal artery
7 ⊟ S35.493- Other specified injury of unspecified renal artery
7 ⊟ S35.494- Other specified injury of right renal vein
7 ⊟ S35.495- Other specified injury of left renal vein
7 ⊟ S35.496- Other specified injury of unspecified renal vein
5 S35.5 Injury of iliac blood vessels
7 S35.50X- Injury of unspecified iliac blood vessel(s)
6 S35.51 Injury of iliac artery or vein
Injury of hypogastric artery or vein
7 ⊟ S35.511- Injury of right iliac artery
7 ⊟ S35.512- Injury of left iliac artery
7 ⊟ S35.513- Injury of unspecified iliac artery
7 ⊟ S35.514- Injury of right iliac vein
7 ⊟ S35.515- Injury of left iliac vein
7 ⊟ S35.516- Injury of unspecified iliac vein
6 S35.53 Injury of uterine artery or vein
7 ⊟ S35.531- Injury of right uterine artery ♀
7 ⊟ S35.532- Injury of left uterine artery ♀
7 ⊟ S35.533- Injury of unspecified uterine artery ♀
7 ⊟ S35.534- Injury of right uterine vein ♀
7 ⊟ S35.535- Injury of left uterine vein ♀
7 ⊟ S35.536- Injury of unspecified uterine vein ♀
7 S35.59X- Injury of other iliac blood vessels
5 S35.8 Injury of other blood vessels at abdomen, lower back and pelvis level
Injury of ovarian artery or vein
6 S35.8X Injury of other blood vessels at abdomen, lower back and pelvis level
7 S35.8X1- Laceration of other blood vessels at abdomen, lower back and pelvis level
7 S35.8X8- Other specified injury of other blood vessels at abdomen, lower back and pelvis level
7 S35.8X9- Unspecified injury of other blood vessels at abdomen, lower back and pelvis level
5 S35.9 Injury of unspecified blood vessel at abdomen, lower back and pelvis level
7 S35.90X- Unspecified injury of Unspecified blood vessel at abdomen, lower back and pelvis level
7 S35.91X- Laceration of unspecified blood vessel at abdomen, lower back and pelvis level
7 S35.99X- Other specified injury of unspecified blood vessel at abdomen, lower back and pelvis level

4 S36 Injury of intra-abdominal organs
Code also:
any associated open wound (S31.-)

The appropriate 7th character is to be added to each code from category S36
A initial encounter
D subsequent encounter
S sequela

CODING TIP✓ Codes from category S36 do not include injury to intra-abdominal organs resulting from intraoperative complications. When intraoperative complications occur, the appropriate complication code from the disease-specific chapter should be assigned (intraoperative and post-procedural complications), as well as any T codes indicating further information on the complication.

5 S36.0 Injury of spleen

7 S36.00X- **Unspecified injury of spleen**
6 S36.02 **Contusion of spleen**
7 S36.020- **Minor contusion of spleen**
Contusion of spleen less than 2 cm
7 S36.021- **Major contusion of spleen**
Contusion of spleen greater than 2 cm
7 S36.029- **Unspecified contusion of spleen**
AHA: (S36.029A) 1Q 2015, 11
6 S36.03 **Laceration of spleen**
7 S36.030- **Superficial (capsular) laceration of spleen**
Laceration of spleen less than 1 cm
Minor laceration of spleen
7 S36.031- **Moderate laceration of spleen**
Laceration of spleen 1 to 3 cm
AHA: (S36.031A) 1Q 2015, 11
7 S36.032- **Major laceration of spleen**
Avulsion of spleen
Laceration of spleen greater than 3 cm
Massive laceration of spleen
Multiple moderate lacerations of spleen
Stellate laceration of spleen
7 S36.039- **Unspecified laceration of spleen**
7 S36.09X- **Other injury of spleen**
5 S36.1 **Injury of liver and gallbladder and bile duct**
6 S36.11 **Injury of liver**
7 S36.112- **Contusion of liver**
7 S36.113- **Laceration of liver, unspecified degree**
7 S36.114- **Minor laceration of liver**
Laceration involving capsule only, or, without significant involvement of hepatic parenchyma [i.e., less than 1 cm deep]
7 S36.115- **Moderate laceration of liver**
Laceration involving parenchyma but without major disruption of parenchyma [i.e., less than 10 cm long and less than 3 cm deep]
7 S36.116- **Major laceration of liver**
Laceration with significant disruption of hepatic parenchyma [i.e., greater than 10 cm long and 3 cm deep]
Multiple moderate lacerations, with or without hematoma
Stellate laceration of liver
7 S36.118- **Other injury of liver**
7 S36.119- **Unspecified injury of liver**
AHA: 2Q 2015, 17
6 S36.12 **Injury of gallbladder**
7 S36.122- **Contusion of gallbladder**
7 S36.123- **Laceration of gallbladder**
7 S36.128- **Other injury of gallbladder**
7 S36.129- **Unspecified injury of gallbladder**
7 S36.13X- **Injury of bile duct**
5 S36.2 **Injury of pancreas**
6 S36.20 **Unspecified injury of pancreas**
7 S36.200- **Unspecified injury of head of pancreas**
7 S36.201- **Unspecified injury of body of pancreas**
7 S36.202- **Unspecified injury of tail of pancreas**
7 S36.209- **Unspecified injury of unspecified part of pancreas**
6 S36.22 **Contusion of pancreas**
7 S36.220- **Contusion of head of pancreas**
7 S36.221- **Contusion of body of pancreas**
7 S36.222- **Contusion of tail of pancreas**
7 S36.229- **Contusion of unspecified part of pancreas**
6 S36.23 **Laceration of pancreas, unspecified degree**
7 S36.230- **Laceration of head of pancreas, unspecified degree**
7 S36.231- **Laceration of body of pancreas, unspecified degree**
7 S36.232- **Laceration of tail of pancreas, unspecified degree**
7 S36.239- **Laceration of unspecified part of pancreas, unspecified degree**
6 S36.24 **Minor laceration of pancreas**
7 S36.240- **Minor laceration of head of pancreas**
7 S36.241- **Minor laceration of body of pancreas**
7 S36.242- **Minor laceration of tail of pancreas**
7 S36.249- **Minor laceration of unspecified part of pancreas**
6 S36.25 **Moderate laceration of pancreas**
7 S36.250- **Moderate laceration of head of pancreas**
7 S36.251- **Moderate laceration of body of pancreas**
7 S36.252- **Moderate laceration of tail of pancreas**
7 S36.259- **Moderate laceration of unspecified part of pancreas**
6 S36.26 **Major laceration of pancreas**
7 S36.260- **Major laceration of head of pancreas**
7 S36.261- **Major laceration of body of pancreas**
7 S36.262- **Major laceration of tail of pancreas**
7 S36.269- **Major laceration of unspecified part of pancreas**
6 S36.29 **Other injury of pancreas**
7 S36.290- **Other injury of head of pancreas**
7 S36.291- **Other injury of body of pancreas**
7 S36.292- **Other injury of tail of pancreas**
7 S36.299- **Other injury of unspecified part of pancreas**
5 S36.3 **Injury of stomach**
7 S36.30X- **Unspecified injury of stomach**
7 S36.32X- **Contusion of stomach**
7 S36.33X- **Laceration of stomach**
7 S36.39X- **Other injury of stomach**
5 S36.4 **Injury of small intestine**
6 S36.40 **Unspecified injury of small intestine**
7 S36.400- **Unspecified injury of duodenum**
7 S36.408- **Unspecified injury of other part of small intestine**
7 S36.409- **Unspecified injury of unspecified part of small intestine**
6 S36.41 **Primary blast injury of small intestine**
Blast injury of small intestine NOS
7 S36.410- **Primary blast injury of duodenum**
7 S36.418- **Primary blast injury of other part of small intestine**
7 S36.419- **Primary blast injury of unspecified part of small intestine**
6 S36.42 **Contusion of small intestine**
7 S36.420- **Contusion of duodenum**
7 S36.428- **Contusion of other part of small intestine**
7 S36.429- **Contusion of unspecified part of small intestine**
6 S36.43 **Laceration of small intestine**
7 S36.430- **Laceration of duodenum**
7 S36.438- **Laceration of other part of small intestine**
7 S36.439- **Laceration of unspecified part of small intestine**
6 S36.49 **Other injury of small intestine**
7 S36.490- **Other injury of duodenum**
7 S36.498- **Other injury of other part of small intestine**
7 S36.499- **Other injury of unspecified part of small intestine**
5 S36.5 **Injury of colon**
EXCLUDES 2 *injury of rectum (S36.6-)*
6 S36.50 **Unspecified injury of colon**
7 S36.500- **Unspecified injury of ascending [right] colon**
7 S36.501- **Unspecified injury of transverse colon**
7 S36.502- **Unspecified injury of descending [left] colon**
7 S36.503- **Unspecified injury of sigmoid colon**
7 S36.508- **Unspecified injury of other part of colon**
7 S36.509- **Unspecified injury of unspecified part of colon**
6 S36.51 **Primary blast injury of colon**
Blast injury of colon NOS
7 S36.510- **Primary blast injury of ascending [right] colon**
7 S36.511- **Primary blast injury of transverse colon**
7 S36.512- **Primary blast injury of descending [left] colon**
7 S36.513- **Primary blast injury of sigmoid colon**

7 S36.518- **Primary blast injury of other part of colon**
7 S36.519- **Primary blast injury of unspecified part of colon**
6 S36.52 **Contusion of colon**
7 S36.520- **Contusion of ascending [right] colon**
7 S36.521- **Contusion of transverse colon**
7 S36.522- **Contusion of descending [left] colon**
7 S36.523- **Contusion of sigmoid colon**
7 S36.528- **Contusion of other part of colon**
7 S36.529- **Contusion of unspecified part of colon**
6 S36.53 **Laceration of colon**
7 S36.530- **Laceration of ascending [right] colon**
7 S36.531- **Laceration of transverse colon**
7 S36.532- **Laceration of descending [left] colon**
7 S36.533- **Laceration of sigmoid colon**
7 S36.538- **Laceration of other part of colon**
7 S36.539- **Laceration of unspecified part of colon**
6 S36.59 **Other injury of colon**
Secondary blast injury of colon
7 S36.590- **Other injury of ascending [right] colon**
7 S36.591- **Other injury of transverse colon**
7 S36.592- **Other injury of descending [left] colon**
7 S36.593- **Other injury of sigmoid colon**
7 S36.598- **Other injury of other part of colon**
7 S36.599- **Other injury of unspecified part of colon**
5 S36.6 **Injury of rectum**
7 S36.60X- **Unspecified injury of rectum**
7 S36.61X- **Primary blast injury of rectum**
Blast injury of rectum NOS
7 S36.62X- **Contusion of rectum**
7 S36.63X- **Laceration of rectum**
7 S36.69X- **Other injury of rectum**
Secondary blast injury of rectum
5 S36.8 **Injury of other intra-abdominal organs**
7 S36.81X- **Injury of peritoneum**
6 S36.89 **Injury of other intra-abdominal organs**
Injury of retroperitoneum
7 S36.892- **Contusion of other intra-abdominal organs**
7 S36.893- **Laceration of other intra-abdominal organs**
7 S36.898- **Other injury of Other intra-abdominal organs**
7 S36.899- **Unspecified injury of other intra-abdominal organs**
5 S36.9 **Injury of unspecified intra-abdominal organ**
7 S36.90X- **Unspecified injury of Unspecified intra-abdominal organ**
7 S36.92X- **Contusion of unspecified intra-abdominal organ**
7 S36.93X- **Laceration of unspecified intra-abdominal organ**
7 S36.99X- **Other injury of unspecified intra-abdominal organ**

4 S37 **Injury of urinary and pelvic organs**
Code also:
any associated open wound (S31.-)
EXCLUDES 1 *obstetric trauma to pelvic organs (O71.-)*
EXCLUDES 2 *injury of peritoneum (S36.81)*
injury of retroperitoneum (S36.89-)

The appropriate 7th character is to be added to each code from category S37
A initial encounter
D subsequent encounter
S sequela

CODING TIP ✓ Codes from category S37 do not include injury to urinary and pelvic organs resulting from intraoperative complications. When intraoperative complications occur, the appropriate complication code from the disease-specific chapter should be assigned (intraoperative and post-procedural complications), as well as any T codes indicating further information on the complication.

5 S37.0 **Injury of kidney**
EXCLUDES 2 *acute kidney injury (nontraumatic) (N17.9)*
6 S37.00 **Unspecified injury of kidney**
7 ⊟ S37.001- **Unspecified injury of right kidney**
7 ⊟ S37.002- **Unspecified injury of left kidney**
7 ⊟ S37.009- **Unspecified injury of unspecified kidney**
6 S37.01 **Minor contusion of kidney**
Contusion of kidney less than 2 cm
Contusion of kidney NOS
7 ⊟ S37.011- **Minor contusion of right kidney**
7 ⊟ S37.012- **Minor contusion of left kidney**
7 ⊟ S37.019- **Minor contusion of unspecified kidney**
6 S37.02 **Major contusion of kidney**
Contusion of kidney greater than 2 cm
7 ⊟ S37.021- **Major contusion of right kidney**
7 ⊟ S37.022- **Major contusion of left kidney**
7 ⊟ S37.029- **Major contusion of unspecified kidney**
6 S37.03 **Laceration of kidney, unspecified degree**
7 ⊟ S37.031- **Laceration of right kidney, unspecified degree**
7 ⊟ S37.032- **Laceration of left kidney, unspecified degree**
7 ⊟ S37.039- **Laceration of unspecified kidney, unspecified degree**
6 S37.04 **Minor laceration of kidney**
Laceration of kidney less than 1 cm
7 ⊟ S37.041- **Minor laceration of right kidney**
7 ⊟ S37.042- **Minor laceration of left kidney**
7 ⊟ S37.049- **Minor laceration of unspecified kidney**
6 S37.05 **Moderate laceration of kidney**
Laceration of kidney 1 to 3 cm
7 ⊟ S37.051- **Moderate laceration of right kidney**
7 ⊟ S37.052- **Moderate laceration of left kidney**
7 ⊟ S37.059- **Moderate laceration of unspecified kidney**
6 S37.06 **Major laceration of kidney**
Avulsion of kidney
Laceration of kidney greater than 3 cm
Massive laceration of kidney
Multiple moderate lacerations of kidney
Stellate laceration of kidney
7 ⊟ S37.061- **Major laceration of right kidney**
7 ⊟ S37.062- **Major laceration of left kidney**
7 ⊟ S37.069- **Major laceration of unspecified kidney**
6 S37.09 **Other injury of kidney**
7 ⊟ S37.091- **Other injury of right kidney**
7 ⊟ S37.092- **Other injury of left kidney**
7 ⊟ S37.099- **Other injury of unspecified kidney**
5 S37.1 **Injury of ureter**
7 S37.10X- **Unspecified injury of ureter**
7 S37.12X- **Contusion of ureter**
7 S37.13X- **Laceration of ureter**
7 S37.19X- **Other injury of ureter**
5 S37.2 **Injury of bladder**
7 S37.20X- **Unspecified injury of bladder**
7 S37.22X- **Contusion of bladder**
7 S37.23X- **Laceration of bladder**
7 S37.29X- **Other injury of bladder**
5 S37.3 **Injury of urethra**
7 S37.30X- **Unspecified injury of urethra**
7 S37.32X- **Contusion of urethra**
7 S37.33X- **Laceration of urethra**
7 S37.39X- **Other injury of urethra**
5 S37.4 **Injury of ovary**
6 S37.40 **Unspecified injury of ovary**
7 S37.401- **Unspecified injury of ovary, unilateral** ♀
7 S37.402- **Unspecified injury of ovary, bilateral** ♀
7 S37.409- **unspecified injury of ovary, unspecified** ♀
6 S37.42 **Contusion of ovary**
7 S37.421- **Contusion of ovary, unilateral** ♀
7 S37.422- **Contusion of ovary, bilateral** ♀
7 S37.429- **Contusion of ovary, unspecified** ♀
6 S37.43 **Laceration of ovary**
7 S37.431- **Laceration of ovary, unilateral** ♀
7 S37.432- **Laceration of ovary, bilateral** ♀
7 S37.439- **Laceration of ovary, unspecified** ♀

6 S37.49 Other injury of ovary
- 7 S37.491- Other injury of ovary, unilateral ♀
- 7 S37.492- Other injury of ovary, bilateral ♀
- 7 S37.499- Other injury of ovary, unspecified ♀

5 S37.5 Injury of fallopian tube

6 S37.50 Unspecified injury of fallopian tube
- 7 S37.501- Unspecified injury of fallopian tube, unilateral ♀
- 7 S37.502- Unspecified injury of fallopian tube, bilateral ♀
- 7 S37.509- unspecified injury of fallopian tube, unspecified ♀

6 S37.51 Primary blast injury of fallopian tube
Blast injury of fallopian tube NOS
- 7 S37.511- Primary blast injury of fallopian tube, unilateral ♀
- 7 S37.512- Primary blast injury of fallopian tube, bilateral ♀
- 7 S37.519- Primary blast injury of fallopian tube, unspecified ♀

6 S37.52 Contusion of fallopian tube
- 7 S37.521- Contusion of fallopian tube, unilateral ♀
- 7 S37.522- Contusion of fallopian tube, bilateral ♀
- 7 S37.529- Contusion of fallopian tube, unspecified ♀

6 S37.53 Laceration of fallopian tube
- 7 S37.531- Laceration of fallopian tube, unilateral ♀
- 7 S37.532- Laceration of fallopian tube, bilateral ♀
- 7 S37.539- Laceration of fallopian tube, unspecified ♀

6 S37.59 Other injury of fallopian tube
Secondary blast injury of fallopian tube
- 7 S37.591- Other injury of fallopian tube, unilateral ♀
- 7 S37.592- Other injury of fallopian tube, bilateral ♀
- 7 S37.599- Other injury of fallopian tube, unspecified ♀

5 S37.6 Injury of uterus

EXCLUDES 1 *injury to gravid uterus (O9A.2-)*
injury to uterus during delivery (O71.-)

- 7 S37.60X- Unspecified injury of uterus ♀
- 7 S37.62X- Contusion of uterus ♀
- 7 S37.63X- Laceration of uterus ♀
- 7 S37.69X- Other injury of uterus ♀

5 S37.8 Injury of other urinary and pelvic organs

6 S37.81 Injury of adrenal gland
- 7 S37.812- Contusion of adrenal gland
- 7 S37.813- Laceration of adrenal gland
- 7 S37.818- Other injury of adrenal gland
- 7 S37.819- Unspecified injury of adrenal gland

6 S37.82 Injury of prostate
- 7 S37.822- Contusion of prostate ♂
- 7 S37.823- Laceration of prostate ♂
- 7 S37.828- Other injury of prostate ♂
- 7 S37.829- Unspecified injury of prostate ♂

6 S37.89 Injury of other urinary and pelvic organ
- 7 S37.892- Contusion of other urinary and pelvic organ
- 7 S37.893- Laceration of other urinary and pelvic organ
- 7 S37.898- Other injury of Other urinary and pelvic organ
- 7 S37.899- Unspecified injury of other urinary and pelvic organ

5 S37.9 Injury of unspecified urinary and pelvic organ
- 7 S37.90X- Unspecified injury of Unspecified urinary and pelvic organ
- 7 S37.92X- Contusion of unspecified urinary and pelvic organ
- 7 S37.93X- Laceration of unspecified urinary and pelvic organ
- 7 S37.99X- Other injury of unspecified urinary and pelvic organ

4 S38 Crushing injury and traumatic amputation of abdomen, lower back, pelvis and external genitals

An amputation not identified as partial or complete should be coded to complete

The appropriate 7th character is to be added to each code from category S38
- A initial encounter
- D subsequent encounter
- S sequela

CODING TIP✓ Use these codes only when the amputation was due to trauma. There is no need for adding Z89 with traumatic amputations. See Z47.81 for care of amputations not due to trauma.

5 S38.0 Crushing injury of external genital organs
Use additional code for any associated injuries

6 S38.00 Crushing injury of unspecified external genital organs
- 7 S38.001- Crushing injury of unspecified external genital organs, male ♂
- 7 S38.002- Crushing injury of unspecified external genital organs, female ♀

- 7 S38.01X- Crushing injury of penis ♂
- 7 S38.02X- Crushing injury of scrotum and testis ♂
- 7 S38.03X- Crushing injury of vulva ♀

7 S38.1XX- Crushing injury of abdomen, lower back, and pelvis
Use additional code for all associated injuries, such as:
fracture of thoracic or lumbar spine and pelvis (S22.0-, S32.-)
injury to intra-abdominal organs (S36.-)
injury to urinary and pelvic organs (S37.-)
open wound of abdominal wall (S31.-)
spinal cord injury (S34.0, S34.1-)

EXCLUDES 2 *crushing injury of external genital organs (S38.0-)*

5 S38.2 Traumatic amputation of external genital organs

6 S38.21 Traumatic amputation of female external genital organs
Traumatic amputation of clitoris
Traumatic amputation of labium (majus) (minus)
Traumatic amputation of vulva
- 7 S38.211- Complete traumatic amputation of female external genital organs ♀
- 7 S38.212- Partial traumatic amputation of female external genital organs ♀

6 S38.22 Traumatic amputation of penis
- 7 S38.221- Complete traumatic amputation of penis ♂
- 7 S38.222- Partial traumatic amputation of penis ♂

6 S38.23 Traumatic amputation of scrotum and testis
- 7 S38.231- Complete traumatic amputation of scrotum and testis ♂
- 7 S38.232- Partial traumatic amputation of scrotum and testis ♂

7 S38.3XX- Transection (partial) of abdomen

4 S39 Other and unspecified injuries of abdomen, lower back, pelvis and external genitals

Code also:
any associated open wound (S31.-)

EXCLUDES 2 *sprain of joints and ligaments of lumbar spine and pelvis (S33.-)*

The appropriate 7th character is to be added to each code from category S39
- A initial encounter
- D subsequent encounter
- S sequela

5 S39.0 Injury of muscle, fascia and tendon of abdomen, lower back and pelvis

6 S39.00 Unspecified injury of muscle, fascia and tendon of abdomen, lower back and pelvis
- 7 S39.001- Unspecified injury of muscle, fascia and tendon of abdomen
- 7 S39.002- Unspecified injury of muscle, fascia and tendon of lower back
- 7 S39.003- Unspecified injury of muscle, fascia and tendon of pelvis

6 S39.01 Strain of muscle, fascia and tendon of abdomen, lower back and pelvis
7 S39.011- Strain of muscle, fascia and tendon of abdomen
7 S39.012- Strain of muscle, fascia and tendon of lower back
7 S39.013- Strain of muscle, fascia and tendon of pelvis
6 S39.02 Laceration of muscle, fascia and tendon of abdomen, lower back and pelvis
7 S39.021- Laceration of muscle, fascia and tendon of abdomen
7 S39.022- Laceration of muscle, fascia and tendon of lower back
7 S39.023- Laceration of muscle, fascia and tendon of pelvis
6 S39.09 Other injury of muscle, fascia and tendon of abdomen, lower back and pelvis
7 S39.091- Other injury of muscle, fascia and tendon of abdomen
7 S39.092- Other injury of muscle, fascia and tendon of lower back
7 S39.093- Other injury of muscle, fascia and tendon of pelvis
5 S39.8 Other specified injuries of abdomen, lower back, pelvis and external genitals
7 S39.81X- Other specified injuries of abdomen
7 S39.82X- Other specified injuries of lower back
7 S39.83X- Other specified injuries of pelvis
6 S39.84 Other specified injuries of external genitals
7 S39.840- Fracture of corpus cavernosum penis ♂
7 S39.848- Other specified injuries of external genitals
5 S39.9 Unspecified injury of abdomen, lower back, pelvis and external genitals
7 S39.91X- Unspecified injury of abdomen
7 S39.92X- Unspecified injury of lower back
7 S39.93X- Unspecified injury of pelvis
7 S39.94X- Unspecified injury of external genitals

Injuries to the shoulder and upper arm (S40-S49)

INCLUDES injuries of axilla
injuries of scapular region

EXCLUDES 2 *burns and corrosions (T20-T32)*
frostbite (T33-T34)
injuries of elbow (S50-S59)
insect bite or sting, venomous (T63.4)

GUIDELINES Section I.C.19.c.2)

Multiple fractures are sequenced in accordance with the severity of the fracture.

GUIDELINES Section I.C.19.b.1)-2)

When coding injuries, assign separate codes for each injury unless a combination code is provided, in which case the combination code is assigned ... Traumatic injury codes (S00-T14.9) are not to be used for normal, healing surgical wounds or to identify complications of surgical wounds. The code for the most serious injury, as determined by the provider and the focus of treatment, is sequenced first.

1) Superficial injuries such as abrasions or contusions are not coded when associated with more severe injuries of the same site.

2) When a primary injury results in minor damage to peripheral nerves or blood vessels, the primary injury is sequenced first with additional code(s) for injuries to nerves and spinal cord (such as category S04), and/or injury to blood vessels (such as category S15). When the primary injury is to the blood vessels or nerves, that injury should be sequenced first.

GUIDELINES Section I.C.19.c

Coding of Traumatic Fractures: The principles of multiple coding of injuries should be followed in coding fractures. Fractures of specified sites are coded individually by site in accordance with both the provisions within categories S02, S12, S22, S32, S42, S49, S52, S59, S62, S72, S79, S82, S89, S92 and the level of detail furnished by medical record content. A fracture not indicated as open or closed should be coded to closed. A fracture not indicated whether displaced or not displaced should be coded to displaced.

4 S40 Superficial injury of shoulder and upper arm

The appropriate 7th character is to be added to each code from category S40

A initial encounter
D subsequent encounter
S sequela

5 S40.0 Contusion of shoulder and upper arm
6 S40.01 Contusion of shoulder
7 S40.011- Contusion of right shoulder
7 S40.012- Contusion of left shoulder
7 S40.019- Contusion of unspecified shoulder
6 S40.02 Contusion of upper arm
7 S40.021- Contusion of right upper arm
7 S40.022- Contusion of left upper arm
7 S40.029- Contusion of unspecified upper arm
5 S40.2 Other superficial injuries of shoulder
6 S40.21 Abrasion of shoulder
7 S40.211- Abrasion of right shoulder
7 S40.212- Abrasion of left shoulder
7 S40.219- Abrasion of unspecified shoulder
6 S40.22 Blister (nonthermal) of shoulder
7 S40.221- Blister (nonthermal) of right shoulder
7 S40.222- Blister (nonthermal) of left shoulder
7 S40.229- Blister (nonthermal) of unspecified shoulder
6 S40.24 External constriction of shoulder
7 S40.241- External constriction of right shoulder
7 S40.242- External constriction of left shoulder
7 S40.249- External constriction of unspecified shoulder
6 S40.25 Superficial foreign body of shoulder
Splinter in the shoulder
7 S40.251- Superficial foreign body of right shoulder
7 S40.252- Superficial foreign body of left shoulder
7 S40.259- Superficial foreign body of unspecified shoulder
6 S40.26 Insect bite (nonvenomous) of shoulder
7 S40.261- Insect bite (nonvenomous) of right shoulder
7 S40.262- Insect bite (nonvenomous) of left shoulder
7 S40.269- Insect bite (nonvenomous) of unspecified shoulder
6 S40.27 Other superficial bite of shoulder
EXCLUDES 1 *open bite of shoulder (S41.05)*
7 S40.271- Other superficial bite of right shoulder
7 S40.272- Other superficial bite of left shoulder
7 S40.279- Other superficial bite of unspecified shoulder
5 S40.8 Other superficial injuries of upper arm
6 S40.81 Abrasion of upper arm
7 S40.811- Abrasion of right upper arm
7 S40.812- Abrasion of left upper arm
7 S40.819- Abrasion of unspecified upper arm
6 S40.82 Blister (nonthermal) of upper arm
7 S40.821- Blister (nonthermal) of right upper arm
7 S40.822- Blister (nonthermal) of left upper arm
7 S40.829- Blister (nonthermal) of unspecified upper arm
6 S40.84 External constriction of upper arm
7 S40.841- External constriction of right upper arm
7 S40.842- External constriction of left upper arm

7 ⊟ S40.849- **External constriction of unspecified upper arm**

6 S40.85 **Superficial foreign body of upper arm**
Splinter in the upper arm

7 ⊟ S40.851- **Superficial foreign body of right upper arm**
7 ⊟ S40.852- **Superficial foreign body of left upper arm**
7 ⊟ S40.859- **Superficial foreign body of unspecified upper arm**

6 S40.86 **Insect bite (nonvenomous) of upper arm**

7 ⊟ S40.861- **Insect bite (nonvenomous) of right upper arm**
7 ⊟ S40.862- **Insect bite (nonvenomous) of left upper arm**
7 ⊟ S40.869- **Insect bite (nonvenomous) of unspecified upper arm**

6 S40.87 **Other superficial bite of upper arm**

EXCLUDES 1 *open bite of upper arm (S41.14)*

EXCLUDES 2 *other superficial bite of shoulder (S40.27-)*

7 ⊟ S40.871- **Other superficial bite of right upper arm**
7 ⊟ S40.872- **Other superficial bite of left upper arm**
7 ⊟ S40.879- **Other superficial bite of unspecified upper arm**

5 S40.9 **Unspecified superficial injury of shoulder and upper arm**

6 S40.91 **Unspecified superficial injury of shoulder**

7 ⊟ S40.911- **Unspecified superficial injury of right shoulder**
7 ⊟ S40.912- **Unspecified superficial injury of left shoulder**
7 ⊟ S40.919- **Unspecified superficial injury of unspecified shoulder**

6 S40.92 **Unspecified superficial injury of upper arm**

7 ⊟ S40.921- **Unspecified superficial injury of right upper arm**
7 ⊟ S40.922- **Unspecified superficial injury of left upper arm**
7 ⊟ S40.929- **Unspecified superficial injury of unspecified upper arm**

4 S41 Open wound of shoulder and upper arm

Code also:
any associated wound infection

EXCLUDES 1 *traumatic amputation of shoulder and upper arm (S48.-)*

EXCLUDES 2 *open fracture of shoulder and upper arm (S42.- with 7th character B or C)*

The appropriate 7th character is to be added to each code from category S41
A initial encounter
D subsequent encounter
S sequela

CODING TIP ✓ Open wound codes indicate a wound resulting from a traumatic origin. Do not assign a code for "open wound" unless the etiology of the wound is related to trauma.

5 S41.0 **Open wound of shoulder**

6 S41.00 **Unspecified open wound of shoulder**

7 ⊟ S41.001- **Unspecified open wound of right shoulder**
7 ⊟ S41.002- **Unspecified open wound of left shoulder**
7 ⊟ S41.009- **Unspecified open wound of unspecified shoulder**

6 S41.01 **Laceration without foreign body of shoulder**

7 ⊟ S41.011- **Laceration without foreign body of right shoulder**
7 ⊟ S41.012- **Laceration without foreign body of left shoulder**
7 ⊟ S41.019- **Laceration without foreign body of unspecified shoulder**

6 S41.02 **Laceration with foreign body of shoulder**

7 ⊟ S41.021- **Laceration with foreign body of right shoulder**
7 ⊟ S41.022- **Laceration with foreign body of left shoulder**
7 ⊟ S41.029- **Laceration with foreign body of unspecified shoulder**

6 S41.03 **Puncture wound without foreign body of shoulder**

7 ⊟ S41.031- **Puncture wound without foreign body of right shoulder**
7 ⊟ S41.032- **Puncture wound without foreign body of left shoulder**
7 ⊟ S41.039- **Puncture wound without foreign body of unspecified shoulder**

6 S41.04 **Puncture wound with foreign body of shoulder**

7 ⊟ S41.041- **Puncture wound with foreign body of right shoulder**
7 ⊟ S41.042- **Puncture wound with foreign body of left shoulder**
7 ⊟ S41.049- **Puncture wound with foreign body of unspecified shoulder**

6 S41.05 **Open bite of shoulder**
Bite of shoulder NOS

EXCLUDES 1 *superficial bite of shoulder (S40.27)*

7 ⊟ S41.051- **Open bite of right shoulder**
7 ⊟ S41.052- **Open bite of left shoulder**
7 ⊟ S41.059- **Open bite of unspecified shoulder**

5 S41.1 **Open wound of upper arm**

6 S41.10 **Unspecified open wound of upper arm**

7 ⊟ S41.101- **Unspecified open wound of right upper arm**
7 ⊟ S41.102- **Unspecified open wound of left upper arm**
7 ⊟ S41.109- **Unspecified open wound of unspecified upper arm**

6 S41.11 **Laceration without foreign body of upper arm**

7 ⊟ S41.111- **Laceration without foreign body of right upper arm**
7 ⊟ S41.112- **Laceration without foreign body of left upper arm**
7 ⊟ S41.119- **Laceration without foreign body of unspecified upper arm**

6 S41.12 **Laceration with foreign body of upper arm**

7 ⊟ S41.121- **Laceration with foreign body of right upper arm**
7 ⊟ S41.122- **Laceration with foreign body of left upper arm**
7 ⊟ S41.129- **Laceration with foreign body of unspecified upper arm**

6 S41.13 **Puncture wound without foreign body of upper arm**

7 ⊟ S41.131- **Puncture wound without foreign body of right upper arm**
7 ⊟ S41.132- **Puncture wound without foreign body of left upper arm**
7 ⊟ S41.139- **Puncture wound without foreign body of unspecified upper arm**

6 S41.14 **Puncture wound with foreign body of upper arm**

7 ⊟ S41.141- **Puncture wound with foreign body of right upper arm**
7 ⊟ S41.142- **Puncture wound with foreign body of left upper arm**
7 ⊟ S41.149- **Puncture wound with foreign body of unspecified upper arm**

6 S41.15 **Open bite of upper arm**
Bite of upper arm NOS

EXCLUDES 1 *superficial bite of upper arm (S40.87)*

7 ⊟ S41.151- **Open bite of right upper arm**
7 ⊟ S41.152- **Open bite of left upper arm**
7 ⊟ S41.159- **Open bite of unspecified upper arm**

4 S42 Fracture of shoulder and upper arm

Note: A fracture not indicated as displaced or nondisplaced should be coded to displaced
A fracture not indicated as open or closed should be coded to closed

EXCLUDES 1 *traumatic amputation of shoulder and upper arm (S48.-)*

The appropriate 7th character is to be added to all codes from category S42
A initial encounter for closed fracture
B initial encounter for open fracture
D subsequent encounter for fracture with routine healing
G subsequent encounter for fracture with delayed healing
K subsequent encounter for fracture with nonunion
P subsequent encounter for fracture with malunion
S sequela

CODING TIP ✓ A fracture not indicated as displaced or nondisplaced should be coded to displaced. A fracture not indicated as open or closed should be coded to closed. Query providers on fractures not documented as displaced/nondisplaced; otherwise, a displaced fracture diagnosis could be assigned without a reduction being performed, potentially resulting in claim denials.

S42.0 Fracture of clavicle

S42.00 Fracture of unspecified part of clavicle

S42.001- Fracture of unspecified part of right clavicle

S42.002- Fracture of unspecified part of left clavicle

S42.009- Fracture of unspecified part of unspecified clavicle

AHA: (S42.009D) 4Q 2012, 93

S42.01 Fracture of sternal end of clavicle

S42.011- Anterior displaced fracture of sternal end of right clavicle

S42.012- Anterior displaced fracture of sternal end of left clavicle

S42.013- Anterior displaced fracture of sternal end of unspecified clavicle

Displaced fracture of sternal end of clavicle NOS

S42.014- Posterior displaced fracture of sternal end of right clavicle

S42.015- Posterior displaced fracture of sternal end of left clavicle

S42.016- Posterior displaced fracture of sternal end of unspecified clavicle

S42.017- Nondisplaced fracture of sternal end of right clavicle

S42.018- Nondisplaced fracture of sternal end of left clavicle

S42.019- Nondisplaced fracture of sternal end of unspecified clavicle

S42.02 Fracture of shaft of clavicle

S42.021- Displaced fracture of shaft of right clavicle

S42.022- Displaced fracture of shaft of left clavicle

S42.023- Displaced fracture of shaft of unspecified clavicle

S42.024- Nondisplaced fracture of shaft of right clavicle

S42.025- Nondisplaced fracture of shaft of left clavicle

S42.026- Nondisplaced fracture of shaft of unspecified clavicle

S42.03 Fracture of lateral end of clavicle

Fracture of acromial end of clavicle

S42.031- Displaced fracture of lateral end of right clavicle

S42.032- Displaced fracture of lateral end of left clavicle

S42.033- Displaced fracture of lateral end of unspecified clavicle

S42.034- Nondisplaced fracture of lateral end of right clavicle

S42.035- Nondisplaced fracture of lateral end of left clavicle

S42.036- Nondisplaced fracture of lateral end of unspecified clavicle

S42.1 Fracture of scapula

S42.10 Fracture of unspecified part of scapula

S42.101- Fracture of unspecified part of scapula, right shoulder

S42.102- Fracture of unspecified part of scapula, left shoulder

S42.109- Fracture of unspecified part of scapula, unspecified shoulder

S42.11 Fracture of body of scapula

S42.111- Displaced fracture of body of scapula, right shoulder

S42.112- Displaced fracture of body of scapula, left shoulder

S42.113- Displaced fracture of body of scapula, unspecified shoulder

S42.114- Nondisplaced fracture of body of scapula, right shoulder

S42.115- Nondisplaced fracture of body of scapula, left shoulder

S42.116- Nondisplaced fracture of body of scapula, unspecified shoulder

S42.12 Fracture of acromial process

S42.121- Displaced fracture of acromial process, right shoulder

S42.122- Displaced fracture of acromial process, left shoulder

S42.123- Displaced fracture of acromial process, unspecified shoulder

S42.124- Nondisplaced fracture of acromial process, right shoulder

S42.125- Nondisplaced fracture of acromial process, left shoulder

S42.126- Nondisplaced fracture of acromial process, unspecified shoulder

S42.13 Fracture of coracoid process

S42.131- Displaced fracture of coracoid process, right shoulder

S42.132- Displaced fracture of coracoid process, left shoulder

S42.133- Displaced fracture of coracoid process, unspecified shoulder

S42.134- Nondisplaced fracture of coracoid process, right shoulder

S42.135- Nondisplaced fracture of coracoid process, left shoulder

S42.136- Nondisplaced fracture of coracoid process, unspecified shoulder

S42.14 Fracture of glenoid cavity of scapula

S42.141- Displaced fracture of glenoid cavity of scapula, right shoulder

S42.142- Displaced fracture of glenoid cavity of scapula, left shoulder

S42.143- Displaced fracture of glenoid cavity of scapula, unspecified shoulder

S42.144- Nondisplaced fracture of glenoid cavity of scapula, right shoulder

S42.145- Nondisplaced fracture of glenoid cavity of scapula, left shoulder

S42.146- Nondisplaced fracture of glenoid cavity of scapula, unspecified shoulder

S42.15 Fracture of neck of scapula

S42.151- Displaced fracture of neck of scapula, right shoulder

S42.152- Displaced fracture of neck of scapula, left shoulder

S42.153- Displaced fracture of neck of scapula, unspecified shoulder

S42.154- Nondisplaced fracture of neck of scapula, right shoulder

S42.155- Nondisplaced fracture of neck of scapula, left shoulder

S42.156- Nondisplaced fracture of neck of scapula, unspecified shoulder

S42.19 Fracture of other part of scapula

S42.191- Fracture of other part of scapula, right shoulder

S42.192- Fracture of other part of scapula, left shoulder

S42.199- Fracture of other part of scapula, unspecified shoulder

S42.2 Fracture of upper end of humerus

Fracture of proximal end of humerus

EXCLUDES 2 *fracture of shaft of humerus (S42.3-)*
physeal fracture of upper end of humerus (S49.0-)

S42.20 Unspecified fracture of upper end of humerus

S42.201- Unspecified fracture of upper end of right humerus

S42.202- Unspecified fracture of upper end of left humerus

S42.209- Unspecified fracture of upper end of unspecified humerus

S42.21 Unspecified fracture of surgical neck of humerus

Fracture of neck of humerus NOS

7 ⊟ S42.211- **Unspecified displaced fracture of surgical neck of right humerus**

7 ⊟ S42.212- **Unspecified displaced fracture of surgical neck of left humerus**

7 ⊟ S42.213- **Unspecified displaced fracture of surgical neck of unspecified humerus**

7 ⊟ S42.214- **Unspecified nondisplaced fracture of surgical neck of right humerus**

7 ⊟ S42.215- **Unspecified nondisplaced fracture of surgical neck of left humerus**

7 ⊟ S42.216- **Unspecified nondisplaced fracture of surgical neck of unspecified humerus**

6 S42.22 **2-part fracture of surgical neck of humerus**

7 ⊟ S42.221- **2-part displaced fracture of surgical neck of right humerus**

7 ⊟ S42.222- **2-part displaced fracture of surgical neck of left humerus**

7 ⊟ S42.223- **2-part displaced fracture of surgical neck of unspecified humerus**

7 ⊟ S42.224- **2-part nondisplaced fracture of surgical neck of right humerus**

7 ⊟ S42.225- **2-part nondisplaced fracture of surgical neck of left humerus**

7 ⊟ S42.226- **2-part nondisplaced fracture of surgical neck of unspecified humerus**

6 S42.23 **3-part fracture of surgical neck of humerus**

7 ⊟ S42.231- **3-part fracture of surgical neck of right humerus**

3-part fracture of surgical neck of humerus

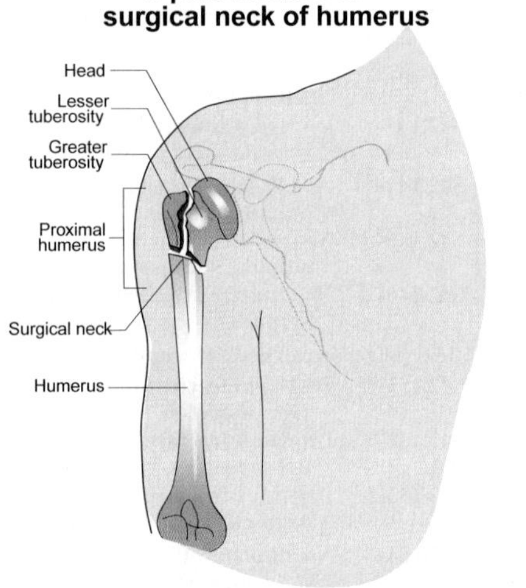

7 ⊟ S42.232- **3-part fracture of surgical neck of left humerus**

7 ⊟ S42.239- **3-part fracture of surgical neck of unspecified humerus**

6 S42.24 **4-part fracture of surgical neck of humerus**

7 ⊟ S42.241- **4-part fracture of surgical neck of right humerus**

4-part fracture of surgical neck of humerus

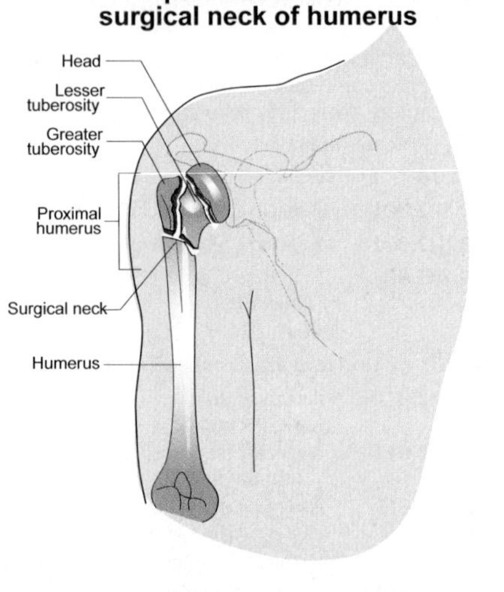

7 ⊟ S42.242- **4-part fracture of surgical neck of left humerus**

7 ⊟ S42.249- **4-part fracture of surgical neck of unspecified humerus**

6 S42.25 **Fracture of greater tuberosity of humerus**

7 ⊟ S42.251- **Displaced fracture of greater tuberosity of right humerus**

7 ⊟ S42.252- **Displaced fracture of greater tuberosity of left humerus**

7 ⊟ S42.253- **Displaced fracture of greater tuberosity of unspecified humerus**

7 ⊟ S42.254- **Nondisplaced fracture of greater tuberosity of right humerus**

7 ⊟ S42.255- **Nondisplaced fracture of greater tuberosity of left humerus**

7 ⊟ S42.256- **Nondisplaced fracture of greater tuberosity of unspecified humerus**

6 S42.26 **Fracture of lesser tuberosity of humerus**

7 ⊟ S42.261- **Displaced fracture of lesser tuberosity of right humerus**

7 ⊟ S42.262- **Displaced fracture of lesser tuberosity of left humerus**

7 ⊟ S42.263- **Displaced fracture of lesser tuberosity of unspecified humerus**

7 ⊟ S42.264- **Nondisplaced fracture of lesser tuberosity of right humerus**

7 ⊟ S42.265- **Nondisplaced fracture of lesser tuberosity of left humerus**

7 ⊟ S42.266- **Nondisplaced fracture of lesser tuberosity of unspecified humerus**

6 S42.27 **Torus fracture of upper end of humerus**

The appropriate 7th character is to be added to all codes in subcategory S42.27

A	initial encounter for closed fracture
D	subsequent encounter for fracture with routine healing
G	subsequent encounter for fracture with delayed healing
K	subsequent encounter for fracture with nonunion
P	subsequent encounter for fracture with malunion
S	sequela

7 ⊟ S42.271- **Torus fracture of upper end of right humerus**

7 ⊟ S42.272- **Torus fracture of upper end of left humerus**

7 ⊟ S42.279- **Torus fracture of upper end of unspecified humerus**

6 S42.29 **Other fracture of upper end of humerus**

Fracture of anatomical neck of humerus
Fracture of articular head of humerus

7 ⊟ S42.291- **Other displaced fracture of upper end of right humerus**

S42.292- Other displaced fracture of upper end of left humerus

S42.293- Other displaced fracture of upper end of unspecified humerus

S42.294- Other nondisplaced fracture of upper end of right humerus

S42.295- Other nondisplaced fracture of upper end of left humerus

S42.296- Other nondisplaced fracture of upper end of unspecified humerus

S42.3 Fracture of shaft of humerus

Fracture of humerus NOS

Fracture of upper arm NOS

EXCLUDES 2 *physeal fractures of upper end of humerus (S49.0-)*
physeal fractures of lower end of humerus (S49.1-)

S42.30 Unspecified fracture of shaft of humerus

S42.301- Unspecified fracture of shaft of humerus, right arm

S42.302- Unspecified fracture of shaft of humerus, left arm

S42.309- Unspecified fracture of shaft of humerus, unspecified arm

S42.31 Greenstick fracture of shaft of humerus

The appropriate 7th character is to be added to all codes in subcategory S42.31

A	initial encounter for closed fracture
D	subsequent encounter for fracture with routine healing
G	subsequent encounter for fracture with delayed healing
K	subsequent encounter for fracture with nonunion
P	subsequent encounter for fracture with malunion
S	sequela

S42.311- Greenstick fracture of shaft of humerus, right arm

S42.312- Greenstick fracture of shaft of humerus, left arm

S42.319- Greenstick fracture of shaft of humerus, unspecified arm

S42.32 Transverse fracture of shaft of humerus

S42.321- Displaced transverse fracture of shaft of humerus, right arm

Displaced transverse fracture, shaft of right humerus

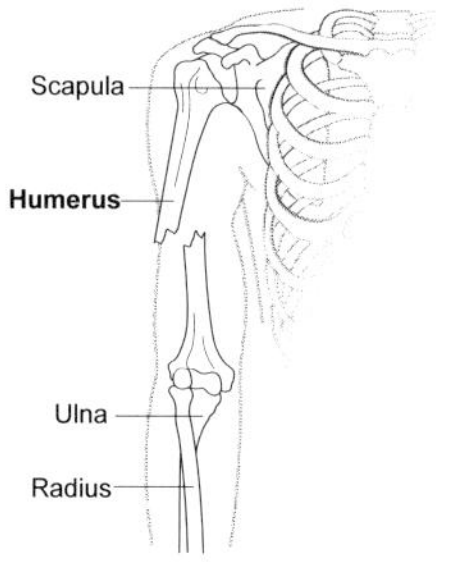

S42.322- Displaced transverse fracture of shaft of humerus, left arm

S42.323- Displaced transverse fracture of shaft of humerus, unspecified arm

S42.324- Nondisplaced transverse fracture of shaft of humerus, right arm

S42.325- Nondisplaced transverse fracture of shaft of humerus, left arm

S42.326- Nondisplaced transverse fracture of shaft of humerus, unspecified arm

S42.33 Oblique fracture of shaft of humerus

S42.331- Displaced oblique fracture of shaft of humerus, right arm

S42.332- Displaced oblique fracture of shaft of humerus, left arm

S42.333- Displaced oblique fracture of shaft of humerus, unspecified arm

S42.334- Nondisplaced oblique fracture of shaft of humerus, right arm

S42.335- Nondisplaced oblique fracture of shaft of humerus, left arm

S42.336- Nondisplaced oblique fracture of shaft of humerus, unspecified arm

S42.34 Spiral fracture of shaft of humerus

S42.341- Displaced spiral fracture of shaft of humerus, right arm

S42.342- Displaced spiral fracture of shaft of humerus, left arm

S42.343- Displaced spiral fracture of shaft of humerus, unspecified arm

S42.344- Nondisplaced spiral fracture of shaft of humerus, right arm

S42.345- Nondisplaced spiral fracture of shaft of humerus, left arm

S42.346- Nondisplaced spiral fracture of shaft of humerus, unspecified arm

S42.35 Comminuted fracture of shaft of humerus

S42.351- Displaced comminuted fracture of shaft of humerus, right arm

S42.352- Displaced comminuted fracture of shaft of humerus, left arm

S42.353- Displaced comminuted fracture of shaft of humerus, unspecified arm

S42.354- Nondisplaced comminuted fracture of shaft of humerus, right arm

S42.355- Nondisplaced comminuted fracture of shaft of humerus, left arm

S42.356- Nondisplaced comminuted fracture of shaft of humerus, unspecified arm

S42.36 Segmental fracture of shaft of humerus

S42.361- Displaced segmental fracture of shaft of humerus, right arm

S42.362- Displaced segmental fracture of shaft of humerus, left arm

S42.363- Displaced segmental fracture of shaft of humerus, unspecified arm

S42.364- Nondisplaced segmental fracture of shaft of humerus, right arm

S42.365- Nondisplaced segmental fracture of shaft of humerus, left arm

S42.366- Nondisplaced segmental fracture of shaft of humerus, unspecified arm

S42.39 Other fracture of shaft of humerus

S42.391- Other fracture of shaft of right humerus

S42.392- Other fracture of shaft of left humerus

S42.399- Other fracture of shaft of unspecified humerus

S42.4 Fracture of lower end of humerus

Fracture of distal end of humerus

EXCLUDES 2 *fracture of shaft of humerus (S42.3-)*
physeal fracture of lower end of humerus (S49.1-)

S42.40 Unspecified fracture of lower end of humerus

Fracture of elbow NOS

S42.401- Unspecified fracture of lower end of right humerus

S42.402- Unspecified fracture of lower end of left humerus

S42.409- Unspecified fracture of lower end of unspecified humerus

S42.41 Simple supracondylar fracture without intercondylar fracture of humerus

S42.411- Displaced simple supracondylar fracture without intercondylar fracture of right humerus

S42.412- Displaced simple supracondylar fracture without intercondylar fracture of left humerus

S42.413- Displaced simple supracondylar fracture without intercondylar fracture of unspecified humerus

S42.414- Nondisplaced simple supracondylar fracture without intercondylar fracture of right humerus
S42.415- Nondisplaced simple supracondylar fracture without intercondylar fracture of left humerus
S42.416- Nondisplaced simple supracondylar fracture without intercondylar fracture of unspecified humerus

S42.42 Comminuted supracondylar fracture without intercondylar fracture of humerus
S42.421- Displaced comminuted supracondylar fracture without intercondylar fracture of right humerus
S42.422- Displaced comminuted supracondylar fracture without intercondylar fracture of left humerus
S42.423- Displaced comminuted supracondylar fracture without intercondylar fracture of unspecified humerus
S42.424- Nondisplaced comminuted supracondylar fracture without intercondylar fracture of right humerus
S42.425- Nondisplaced comminuted supracondylar fracture without intercondylar fracture of left humerus
S42.426- Nondisplaced comminuted supracondylar fracture without intercondylar fracture of unspecified humerus

S42.43 Fracture (avulsion) of lateral epicondyle of humerus
S42.431- Displaced fracture (avulsion) of lateral epicondyle of right humerus
S42.432- Displaced fracture (avulsion) of lateral epicondyle of left humerus
S42.433- Displaced fracture (avulsion) of lateral epicondyle of unspecified humerus
S42.434- Nondisplaced fracture (avulsion) of lateral epicondyle of right humerus
S42.435- Nondisplaced fracture (avulsion) of lateral epicondyle of left humerus
S42.436- Nondisplaced fracture (avulsion) of lateral epicondyle of unspecified humerus

S42.44 Fracture (avulsion) of medial epicondyle of humerus
S42.441- Displaced fracture (avulsion) of medial epicondyle of right humerus
S42.442- Displaced fracture (avulsion) of medial epicondyle of left humerus
S42.443- Displaced fracture (avulsion) of medial epicondyle of unspecified humerus
S42.444- Nondisplaced fracture (avulsion) of medial epicondyle of right humerus
S42.445- Nondisplaced fracture (avulsion) of medial epicondyle of left humerus
S42.446- Nondisplaced fracture (avulsion) of medial epicondyle of unspecified humerus
S42.447- Incarcerated fracture (avulsion) of medial epicondyle of right humerus
S42.448- Incarcerated fracture (avulsion) of medial epicondyle of left humerus
S42.449- Incarcerated fracture (avulsion) of medial epicondyle of unspecified humerus

S42.45 Fracture of lateral condyle of humerus
Fracture of capitellum of humerus
S42.451- Displaced fracture of lateral condyle of right humerus
S42.452- Displaced fracture of lateral condyle of left humerus
S42.453- Displaced fracture of lateral condyle of unspecified humerus
S42.454- Nondisplaced fracture of lateral condyle of right humerus
S42.455- Nondisplaced fracture of lateral condyle of left humerus
S42.456- Nondisplaced fracture of lateral condyle of unspecified humerus

S42.46 Fracture of medial condyle of humerus
Trochlea fracture of humerus
S42.461- Displaced fracture of medial condyle of right humerus
S42.462- Displaced fracture of medial condyle of left humerus
S42.463- Displaced fracture of medial condyle of unspecified humerus
S42.464- Nondisplaced fracture of medial condyle of right humerus
S42.465- Nondisplaced fracture of medial condyle of left humerus
S42.466- Nondisplaced fracture of medial condyle of unspecified humerus

S42.47 Transcondylar fracture of humerus
S42.471- Displaced transcondylar fracture of right humerus
S42.472- Displaced transcondylar fracture of left humerus
S42.473- Displaced transcondylar fracture of unspecified humerus
S42.474- Nondisplaced transcondylar fracture of right humerus
S42.475- Nondisplaced transcondylar fracture of left humerus
S42.476- Nondisplaced transcondylar fracture of unspecified humerus

S42.48 Torus fracture of lower end of humerus

The appropriate 7th character is to be added to all codes in subcategory S42.48

A	initial encounter for closed fracture
D	subsequent encounter for fracture with routine healing
G	subsequent encounter for fracture with delayed healing
K	subsequent encounter for fracture with nonunion
P	subsequent encounter for fracture with malunion
S	sequela

S42.481- Torus fracture of lower end of right humerus
S42.482- Torus fracture of lower end of left humerus
S42.489- Torus fracture of lower end of unspecified humerus

S42.49 Other fracture of lower end of humerus
S42.491- Other displaced fracture of lower end of right humerus
S42.492- Other displaced fracture of lower end of left humerus
S42.493- Other displaced fracture of lower end of unspecified humerus
S42.494- Other nondisplaced fracture of lower end of right humerus
S42.495- Other nondisplaced fracture of lower end of left humerus
S42.496- Other nondisplaced fracture of lower end of unspecified humerus

S42.9 Fracture of shoulder girdle, part unspecified
Fracture of shoulder NOS
S42.90X- Fracture of unspecified shoulder girdle, part unspecified
S42.91X- Fracture of right shoulder girdle, part unspecified
S42.92X- Fracture of left shoulder girdle, part unspecified

S43 Dislocation and sprain of joints and ligaments of shoulder girdle

INCLUDES avulsion of joint or ligament of shoulder girdle
laceration of cartilage, joint or ligament of shoulder girdle
sprain of cartilage, joint or ligament of shoulder girdle
traumatic hemarthrosis of joint or ligament of shoulder girdle
traumatic rupture of joint or ligament of shoulder girdle
traumatic subluxation of joint or ligament of shoulder girdle
traumatic tear of joint or ligament of shoulder girdle

Code also:
any associated open wound

EXCLUDES 2 *strain of muscle, fascia and tendon of shoulder and upper arm (S46.-)*

The appropriate 7th character is to be added to each code from category S43
A initial encounter
D subsequent encounter
S sequela

CODING TIP ✓ There are no codes for open dislocations. When a dislocation is documented as open, assign an additional code for the open wound.

S43.0 Subluxation and dislocation of shoulder joint
Dislocation of glenohumeral joint
Subluxation of glenohumeral joint

S43.00 Unspecified subluxation and dislocation of shoulder joint
Dislocation of humerus NOS
Subluxation of humerus NOS

- **S43.001- Unspecified subluxation of right shoulder joint**
- **S43.002- Unspecified subluxation of left shoulder joint**
- **S43.003- Unspecified subluxation of unspecified shoulder joint**
- **S43.004- Unspecified dislocation of right shoulder joint**
- **S43.005- Unspecified dislocation of left shoulder joint**
- **S43.006- Unspecified dislocation of unspecified shoulder joint**

S43.01 Anterior subluxation and dislocation of humerus
- **S43.011- Anterior subluxation of right humerus**
- **S43.012- Anterior subluxation of left humerus**
- **S43.013- Anterior subluxation of unspecified humerus**
- **S43.014- Anterior dislocation of right humerus**
- **S43.015- Anterior dislocation of left humerus**
- **S43.016- Anterior dislocation of unspecified humerus**

S43.02 Posterior subluxation and dislocation of humerus
- **S43.021- Posterior subluxation of right humerus**
- **S43.022- Posterior subluxation of left humerus**
- **S43.023- Posterior subluxation of unspecified humerus**
- **S43.024- Posterior dislocation of right humerus**
- **S43.025- Posterior dislocation of left humerus**
- **S43.026- Posterior dislocation of unspecified humerus**

S43.03 Inferior subluxation and dislocation of humerus
- **S43.031- Inferior subluxation of right humerus**
- **S43.032- Inferior subluxation of left humerus**
- **S43.033- Inferior subluxation of unspecified humerus**
- **S43.034- Inferior dislocation of right humerus**
- **S43.035- Inferior dislocation of left humerus**
- **S43.036- Inferior dislocation of unspecified humerus**

S43.08 Other subluxation and dislocation of shoulder joint
- **S43.081- Other subluxation of right shoulder joint**
- **S43.082- Other subluxation of left shoulder joint**
- **S43.083- Other subluxation of unspecified shoulder joint**
- **S43.084- Other dislocation of right shoulder joint**
- **S43.085- Other dislocation of left shoulder joint**
- **S43.086- Other dislocation of unspecified shoulder joint**

S43.1 Subluxation and dislocation of acromioclavicular joint

S43.10 Unspecified dislocation of acromioclavicular joint
- **S43.101- Unspecified dislocation of right acromioclavicular joint**
- **S43.102- Unspecified dislocation of left acromioclavicular joint**
- **S43.109- Unspecified dislocation of unspecified acromioclavicular joint**

S43.11 Subluxation of acromioclavicular joint
- **S43.111- Subluxation of right acromioclavicular joint**
- **S43.112- Subluxation of left acromioclavicular joint**
- **S43.119- Subluxation of unspecified acromioclavicular joint**

S43.12 Dislocation of acromioclavicular joint, 100%-200% displacement
- **S43.121- Dislocation of right acromioclavicular joint, 100%-200% displacement**
- **S43.122- Dislocation of left acromioclavicular joint, 100%-200% displacement**
- **S43.129- Dislocation of unspecified acromioclavicular joint, 100%-200% displacement**

S43.13 Dislocation of acromioclavicular joint, greater than 200% displacement
- **S43.131- Dislocation of right acromioclavicular joint, greater than 200% displacement**
- **S43.132- Dislocation of left acromioclavicular joint, greater than 200% displacement**
- **S43.139- Dislocation of unspecified acromioclavicular joint, greater than 200% displacement**

S43.14 Inferior dislocation of acromioclavicular joint
- **S43.141- Inferior dislocation of right acromioclavicular joint**
- **S43.142- Inferior dislocation of left acromioclavicular joint**
- **S43.149- Inferior dislocation of unspecified acromioclavicular joint**

S43.15 Posterior dislocation of acromioclavicular joint
- **S43.151- Posterior dislocation of right acromioclavicular joint**
- **S43.152- Posterior dislocation of left acromioclavicular joint**
- **S43.159- Posterior dislocation of unspecified acromioclavicular joint**

S43.2 Subluxation and dislocation of sternoclavicular joint

S43.20 Unspecified subluxation and dislocation of sternoclavicular joint
- **S43.201- Unspecified subluxation of right sternoclavicular joint**
- **S43.202- Unspecified subluxation of left sternoclavicular joint**
- **S43.203- Unspecified subluxation of unspecified sternoclavicular joint**
- **S43.204- Unspecified dislocation of right sternoclavicular joint**
- **S43.205- Unspecified dislocation of left sternoclavicular joint**
- **S43.206- Unspecified dislocation of unspecified sternoclavicular joint**

S43.21 Anterior subluxation and dislocation of sternoclavicular joint
- **S43.211- Anterior subluxation of right sternoclavicular joint**
- **S43.212- Anterior subluxation of left sternoclavicular joint**
- **S43.213- Anterior subluxation of unspecified sternoclavicular joint**
- **S43.214- Anterior dislocation of right sternoclavicular joint**
- **S43.215- Anterior dislocation of left sternoclavicular joint**
- **S43.216- Anterior dislocation of unspecified sternoclavicular joint**

S43.22 Posterior subluxation and dislocation of sternoclavicular joint

S43.221- Posterior subluxation of right sternoclavicular joint
S43.222- Posterior subluxation of left sternoclavicular joint
S43.223- Posterior subluxation of unspecified sternoclavicular joint
S43.224- Posterior dislocation of right sternoclavicular joint
S43.225- Posterior dislocation of left sternoclavicular joint
S43.226- Posterior dislocation of unspecified sternoclavicular joint

S43.3 Subluxation and dislocation of other and unspecified parts of shoulder girdle

S43.30 Subluxation and dislocation of unspecified parts of shoulder girdle
Dislocation of shoulder girdle NOS
Subluxation of shoulder girdle NOS
S43.301- Subluxation of unspecified parts of right shoulder girdle
S43.302- Subluxation of unspecified parts of left shoulder girdle
S43.303- Subluxation of unspecified parts of unspecified shoulder girdle
S43.304- Dislocation of unspecified parts of right shoulder girdle
S43.305- Dislocation of unspecified parts of left shoulder girdle
S43.306- Dislocation of unspecified parts of unspecified shoulder girdle

S43.31 Subluxation and dislocation of scapula
S43.311- Subluxation of right scapula
S43.312- Subluxation of left scapula
S43.313- Subluxation of unspecified scapula
S43.314- Dislocation of right scapula
S43.315- Dislocation of left scapula
S43.316- Dislocation of unspecified scapula

S43.39 Subluxation and dislocation of other parts of shoulder girdle
S43.391- Subluxation of other parts of right shoulder girdle
S43.392- Subluxation of other parts of left shoulder girdle
S43.393- Subluxation of other parts of unspecified shoulder girdle
S43.394- Dislocation of other parts of right shoulder girdle
S43.395- Dislocation of other parts of left shoulder girdle
S43.396- Dislocation of other parts of unspecified shoulder girdle

S43.4 Sprain of shoulder joint

S43.40 Unspecified sprain of shoulder joint
S43.401- Unspecified sprain of right shoulder joint
S43.402- Unspecified sprain of left shoulder joint
S43.409- Unspecified sprain of unspecified shoulder joint

S43.41 Sprain of coracohumeral (ligament)
S43.411- Sprain of right coracohumeral (ligament)
S43.412- Sprain of left coracohumeral (ligament)
S43.419- Sprain of unspecified coracohumeral (ligament)

S43.42 Sprain of rotator cuff capsule
EXCLUDES 1 *rotator cuff syndrome (complete) (incomplete), not specified as traumatic (M75.1-)*
EXCLUDES 2 *injury of tendon of rotator cuff (S46.0-)*
S43.421- Sprain of right rotator cuff capsule
S43.422- Sprain of left rotator cuff capsule
S43.429- Sprain of unspecified rotator cuff capsule

S43.43 Superior glenoid labrum lesion
SLAP lesion
S43.431- Superior glenoid labrum lesion of right shoulder
S43.432- Superior glenoid labrum lesion of left shoulder
S43.439- Superior glenoid labrum lesion of unspecified shoulder

S43.49 Other sprain of shoulder joint
S43.491- Other sprain of right shoulder joint
S43.492- Other sprain of left shoulder joint
S43.499- Other sprain of unspecified shoulder joint

S43.5 Sprain of acromioclavicular joint
Sprain of acromioclavicular ligament
S43.50X- Sprain of unspecified acromioclavicular joint
S43.51X- Sprain of right acromioclavicular joint
S43.52X- Sprain of left acromioclavicular joint

S43.6 Sprain of sternoclavicular joint
S43.60X- Sprain of unspecified sternoclavicular joint
S43.61X- Sprain of right sternoclavicular joint
S43.62X- Sprain of left sternoclavicular joint

S43.8 Sprain of other specified parts of shoulder girdle
S43.80X- Sprain of other specified parts of unspecified shoulder girdle
S43.81X- Sprain of other specified parts of right shoulder girdle
S43.82X- Sprain of other specified parts of left shoulder girdle

S43.9 Sprain of unspecified parts of shoulder girdle
S43.90X- Sprain of unspecified parts of unspecified shoulder girdle
Sprain of shoulder girdle NOS
S43.91X- Sprain of unspecified parts of right shoulder girdle
S43.92X- Sprain of unspecified parts of left shoulder girdle

S44 Injury of nerves at shoulder and upper arm level

Code also:
any associated open wound (S41.-)
EXCLUDES 2 *injury of brachial plexus (S14.3-)*

The appropriate 7th character is to be added to each code from category S44
A initial encounter
D subsequent encounter
S sequela

CODING TIP ✓ Late effects of injuries are coded with seventh character S (sequela) and are sequenced after the residual condition of the late effect.

S44.0 Injury of ulnar nerve at upper arm level
EXCLUDES 1 *ulnar nerve NOS (S54.0)*
S44.00X- Injury of ulnar nerve at upper arm level, unspecified arm
S44.01X- Injury of ulnar nerve at upper arm level, right arm
S44.02X- Injury of ulnar nerve at upper arm level, left arm

S44.1 Injury of median nerve at upper arm level
EXCLUDES 1 *median nerve NOS (S54.1)*
S44.10X- Injury of median nerve at upper arm level, unspecified arm
S44.11X- Injury of median nerve at upper arm level, right arm
S44.12X- Injury of median nerve at upper arm level, left arm

S44.2 Injury of radial nerve at upper arm level
EXCLUDES 1 *radial nerve NOS (S54.2)*
S44.20X- Injury of radial nerve at upper arm level, unspecified arm
S44.21X- Injury of radial nerve at upper arm level, right arm
S44.22X- Injury of radial nerve at upper arm level, left arm

S44.3 Injury of axillary nerve
S44.30X- Injury of axillary nerve, unspecified arm
S44.31X- Injury of axillary nerve, right arm
S44.32X- Injury of axillary nerve, left arm

S44.4 Injury of musculocutaneous nerve
S44.40X- Injury of musculocutaneous nerve, unspecified arm
S44.41X- Injury of musculocutaneous nerve, right arm

● New ▲ Revised | Manifestation Unspecified | 4-7 Digit Indicators AHA Coding Clinic | Laterality HCC Hierarchical Condition Categories | A Adult | M Maternity | N Newborn | P Pediatric | HIV HIV Related Conditions | ♂ Male ♀ Female

S44.42X- Injury of musculocutaneous nerve, left arm

S44.5 Injury of cutaneous sensory nerve at shoulder and upper arm level

S44.50X- Injury of cutaneous sensory nerve at shoulder and upper arm level, unspecified arm

S44.51X- Injury of cutaneous sensory nerve at shoulder and upper arm level, right arm

S44.52X- Injury of cutaneous sensory nerve at shoulder and upper arm level, left arm

S44.8 Injury of other nerves at shoulder and upper arm level

S44.8X Injury of other nerves at shoulder and upper arm level

S44.8X1- Injury of other nerves at shoulder and upper arm level, right arm

S44.8X2- Injury of other nerves at shoulder and upper arm level, left arm

S44.8X9- Injury of other nerves at shoulder and upper arm level, unspecified arm

S44.9 Injury of unspecified nerve at shoulder and upper arm level

S44.90X- Injury of unspecified nerve at shoulder and upper arm level, unspecified arm

S44.91X- Injury of unspecified nerve at shoulder and upper arm level, right arm

S44.92X- Injury of unspecified nerve at shoulder and upper arm level, left arm

S45 Injury of blood vessels at shoulder and upper arm level

Code also:

any associated open wound (S41.-)

EXCLUDES 2 *injury of subclavian artery (S25.1)*
injury of subclavian vein (S25.3)

The appropriate 7th character is to be added to each code from category S45

A initial encounter

D subsequent encounter

S sequela

S45.0 Injury of axillary artery

S45.00 Unspecified injury of axillary artery

S45.001- Unspecified injury of axillary artery, right side

S45.002- Unspecified injury of axillary artery, left side

S45.009- Unspecified injury of axillary artery, unspecified side

S45.01 Laceration of axillary artery

S45.011- Laceration of axillary artery, right side

S45.012- Laceration of axillary artery, left side

S45.019- Laceration of axillary artery, unspecified side

S45.09 Other specified injury of axillary artery

S45.091- Other specified injury of axillary artery, right side

S45.092- Other specified injury of axillary artery, left side

S45.099- Other specified injury of axillary artery, unspecified side

S45.1 Injury of brachial artery

S45.10 Unspecified injury of brachial artery

S45.101- Unspecified injury of brachial artery, right side

S45.102- Unspecified injury of brachial artery, left side

S45.109- Unspecified injury of brachial artery, unspecified side

S45.11 Laceration of brachial artery

S45.111- Laceration of brachial artery, right side

S45.112- Laceration of brachial artery, left side

S45.119- Laceration of brachial artery, unspecified side

S45.19 Other specified injury of brachial artery

S45.191- Other specified injury of brachial artery, right side

S45.192- Other specified injury of brachial artery, left side

S45.199- Other specified injury of brachial artery, unspecified side

S45.2 Injury of axillary or brachial vein

S45.20 Unspecified injury of axillary or brachial vein

S45.201- Unspecified injury of axillary or brachial vein, right side

S45.202- Unspecified injury of axillary or brachial vein, left side

S45.209- Unspecified injury of axillary or brachial vein, unspecified side

S45.21 Laceration of axillary or brachial vein

S45.211- Laceration of axillary or brachial vein, right side

S45.212- Laceration of axillary or brachial vein, left side

S45.219- Laceration of axillary or brachial vein, unspecified side

S45.29 Other specified injury of axillary or brachial vein

S45.291- Other specified injury of axillary or brachial vein, right side

S45.292- Other specified injury of axillary or brachial vein, left side

S45.299- Other specified injury of axillary or brachial vein, unspecified side

S45.3 Injury of superficial vein at shoulder and upper arm level

S45.30 Unspecified injury of superficial vein at shoulder and upper arm level

S45.301- Unspecified injury of superficial vein at shoulder and upper arm level, right arm

S45.302- Unspecified injury of superficial vein at shoulder and upper arm level, left arm

S45.309- Unspecified injury of superficial vein at shoulder and upper arm level, unspecified arm

S45.31 Laceration of superficial vein at shoulder and upper arm level

S45.311- Laceration of superficial vein at shoulder and upper arm level, right arm

S45.312- Laceration of superficial vein at shoulder and upper arm level, left arm

S45.319- Laceration of superficial vein at shoulder and upper arm level, unspecified arm

S45.39 Other specified injury of superficial vein at shoulder and upper arm level

S45.391- Other specified injury of superficial vein at shoulder and upper arm level, right arm

S45.392- Other specified injury of superficial vein at shoulder and upper arm level, left arm

S45.399- Other specified injury of superficial vein at shoulder and upper arm level, unspecified arm

S45.8 Injury of other specified blood vessels at shoulder and upper arm level

S45.80 Unspecified injury of other specified blood vessels at shoulder and upper arm level

S45.801- Unspecified injury of other specified blood vessels at shoulder and upper arm level, right arm

S45.802- Unspecified injury of other specified blood vessels at shoulder and upper arm level, left arm

S45.809- Unspecified injury of other specified blood vessels at shoulder and upper arm level, unspecified arm

S45.81 Laceration of other specified blood vessels at shoulder and upper arm level

S45.811- Laceration of other specified blood vessels at shoulder and upper arm level, right arm

S45.812- Laceration of other specified blood vessels at shoulder and upper arm level, left arm

S45.819- Laceration of other specified blood vessels at shoulder and upper arm level, unspecified arm

S45.89 Other specified injury of Other specified blood vessels at shoulder and upper arm level

S45.891- Other specified injury of other specified blood vessels at shoulder and upper arm level, right arm

S45.892- Other specified injury of other specified blood vessels at shoulder and upper arm level, left arm

7 ⊟ S45.899- Other specified injury of other specified blood vessels at shoulder and upper arm level, unspecified arm

5 S45.9 Injury of unspecified blood vessel at shoulder and upper arm level

6 S45.90 Unspecified injury of Unspecified blood vessel at shoulder and upper arm level

7 ⊟ S45.901- Unspecified injury of unspecified blood vessel at shoulder and upper arm level, right arm

7 ⊟ S45.902- Unspecified injury of unspecified blood vessel at shoulder and upper arm level, left arm

7 ⊟ S45.909- Unspecified injury of unspecified blood vessel at shoulder and upper arm level, unspecified arm

6 S45.91 Laceration of unspecified blood vessel at shoulder and upper arm level

7 ⊟ S45.911- Laceration of unspecified blood vessel at shoulder and upper arm level, right arm

7 ⊟ S45.912- Laceration of unspecified blood vessel at shoulder and upper arm level, left arm

7 ⊟ S45.919- Laceration of unspecified blood vessel at shoulder and upper arm level, unspecified arm

6 S45.99 Other specified injury of unspecified blood vessel at shoulder and upper arm level

7 ⊟ S45.991- Other specified injury of unspecified blood vessel at shoulder and upper arm level, right arm

7 ⊟ S45.992- Other specified injury of unspecified blood vessel at shoulder and upper arm level, left arm

7 ⊟ S45.999- Other specified injury of unspecified blood vessel at shoulder and upper arm level, unspecified arm

4 S46 Injury of muscle, fascia and tendon at shoulder and upper arm level

Code also:

any associated open wound (S41.-)

EXCLUDES 2 *injury of muscle, fascia and tendon at elbow (S56.-)*

sprain of joints and ligaments of shoulder girdle (S43.9)

The appropriate 7th character is to be added to each code from category S46

A initial encounter

D subsequent encounter

S sequela

5 S46.0 Injury of muscle(s) and tendon(s) of the rotator cuff of shoulder

6 S46.00 Unspecified injury of muscle(s) and tendon(s) of the rotator cuff of shoulder

7 ⊟ S46.001- Unspecified injury of muscle(s) and tendon(s) of the rotator cuff of right shoulder

7 ⊟ S46.002- Unspecified injury of muscle(s) and tendon(s) of the rotator cuff of left shoulder

7 ⊟ S46.009- Unspecified injury of muscle(s) and tendon(s) of the rotator cuff of unspecified shoulder

6 S46.01 Strain of muscle(s) and tendon(s) of the rotator cuff of shoulder

7 ⊟ S46.011- Strain of muscle(s) and tendon(s) of the rotator cuff of right shoulder

7 ⊟ S46.012- Strain of muscle(s) and tendon(s) of the rotator cuff of left shoulder

7 ⊟ S46.019- Strain of muscle(s) and tendon(s) of the rotator cuff of unspecified shoulder

6 S46.02 Laceration of muscle(s) and tendon(s) of the rotator cuff of shoulder

7 ⊟ S46.021- Laceration of muscle(s) and tendon(s) of the rotator cuff of right shoulder

7 ⊟ S46.022- Laceration of muscle(s) and tendon(s) of the rotator cuff of left shoulder

7 ⊟ S46.029- Laceration of muscle(s) and tendon(s) of the rotator cuff of unspecified shoulder

6 S46.09 Other injury of muscle(s) and tendon(s) of the rotator cuff of shoulder

7 ⊟ S46.091- Other injury of muscle(s) and tendon(s) of the rotator cuff of right shoulder

7 ⊟ S46.092- Other injury of muscle(s) and tendon(s) of the rotator cuff of left shoulder

7 ⊟ S46.099- Other injury of muscle(s) and tendon(s) of the rotator cuff of unspecified shoulder

5 S46.1 Injury of muscle, fascia and tendon of long head of biceps

6 S46.10 Unspecified injury of muscle, fascia and tendon of long head of biceps

7 ⊟ S46.101- Unspecified injury of muscle, fascia and tendon of long head of biceps, right arm

7 ⊟ S46.102- Unspecified injury of muscle, fascia and tendon of long head of biceps, left arm

7 ⊟ S46.109- Unspecified injury of muscle, fascia and tendon of long head of biceps, unspecified arm

6 S46.11 Strain of muscle, fascia and tendon of long head of biceps

7 ⊟ S46.111- Strain of muscle, fascia and tendon of long head of biceps, right arm

7 ⊟ S46.112- Strain of muscle, fascia and tendon of long head of biceps, left arm

7 ⊟ S46.119- Strain of muscle, fascia and tendon of long head of biceps, unspecified arm

6 S46.12 Laceration of muscle, fascia and tendon of long head of biceps

7 ⊟ S46.121- Laceration of muscle, fascia and tendon of long head of biceps, right arm

7 ⊟ S46.122- Laceration of muscle, fascia and tendon of long head of biceps, left arm

7 ⊟ S46.129- Laceration of muscle, fascia and tendon of long head of biceps, unspecified arm

6 S46.19 Other injury of muscle, fascia and tendon of long head of biceps

7 ⊟ S46.191- Other injury of muscle, fascia and tendon of long head of biceps, right arm

7 ⊟ S46.192- Other injury of muscle, fascia and tendon of long head of biceps, left arm

7 ⊟ S46.199- Other injury of muscle, fascia and tendon of long head of biceps, unspecified arm

5 S46.2 Injury of muscle, fascia and tendon of other parts of biceps

6 S46.20 Unspecified injury of muscle, fascia and tendon of other parts of biceps

7 ⊟ S46.201- Unspecified injury of muscle, fascia and tendon of other parts of biceps, right arm

7 ⊟ S46.202- Unspecified injury of muscle, fascia and tendon of other parts of biceps, left arm

7 ⊟ S46.209- Unspecified injury of muscle, fascia and tendon of other parts of biceps, unspecified arm

6 S46.21 Strain of muscle, fascia and tendon of other parts of biceps

7 ⊟ S46.211- Strain of muscle, fascia and tendon of other parts of biceps, right arm

7 ⊟ S46.212- Strain of muscle, fascia and tendon of other parts of biceps, left arm

7 ⊟ S46.219- Strain of muscle, fascia and tendon of other parts of biceps, unspecified arm

6 S46.22 Laceration of muscle, fascia and tendon of other parts of biceps

7 ⊟ S46.221- Laceration of muscle, fascia and tendon of other parts of biceps, right arm

7 ⊟ S46.222- Laceration of muscle, fascia and tendon of other parts of biceps, left arm

7 ⊟ S46.229- Laceration of muscle, fascia and tendon of other parts of biceps, unspecified arm

6 S46.29 Other injury of muscle, fascia and tendon of Other parts of biceps

7 ⊟ S46.291- Other injury of muscle, fascia and tendon of other parts of biceps, right arm

7 ⊟ S46.292- Other injury of muscle, fascia and tendon of other parts of biceps, left arm

7 ⊟ S46.299- Other injury of muscle, fascia and tendon of other parts of biceps, unspecified arm

5 S46.3 Injury of muscle, fascia and tendon of triceps

6 S46.30 Unspecified injury of muscle, fascia and tendon of triceps

7 ⊟ S46.301- Unspecified injury of muscle, fascia and tendon of triceps, right arm
7 ⊟ S46.302- Unspecified injury of muscle, fascia and tendon of triceps, left arm
7 ⊟ S46.309- Unspecified injury of muscle, fascia and tendon of triceps, unspecified arm
6 S46.31 Strain of muscle, fascia and tendon of triceps
7 ⊟ S46.311- Strain of muscle, fascia and tendon of triceps, right arm
7 ⊟ S46.312- Strain of muscle, fascia and tendon of triceps, left arm
7 ⊟ S46.319- Strain of muscle, fascia and tendon of triceps, unspecified arm
6 S46.32 Laceration of muscle, fascia and tendon of triceps
7 ⊟ S46.321- Laceration of muscle, fascia and tendon of triceps, right arm
7 ⊟ S46.322- Laceration of muscle, fascia and tendon of triceps, left arm
7 ⊟ S46.329- Laceration of muscle, fascia and tendon of triceps, unspecified arm
6 S46.39 Other injury of muscle, fascia and tendon of triceps
7 ⊟ S46.391- Other injury of muscle, fascia and tendon of triceps, right arm
7 ⊟ S46.392- Other injury of muscle, fascia and tendon of triceps, left arm
7 ⊟ S46.399- Other injury of muscle, fascia and tendon of triceps, unspecified arm
5 S46.8 Injury of other muscles, fascia and tendons at shoulder and upper arm level
6 S46.80 Unspecified injury of other muscles, fascia and tendons at shoulder and upper arm level
7 ⊟ S46.801- Unspecified injury of other muscles, fascia and tendons at shoulder and upper arm level, right arm
7 ⊟ S46.802- Unspecified injury of other muscles, fascia and tendons at shoulder and upper arm level, left arm
7 ⊟ S46.809- Unspecified injury of other muscles, fascia and tendons at shoulder and upper arm level, unspecified arm
6 S46.81 Strain of other muscles, fascia and tendons at shoulder and upper arm level
7 ⊟ S46.811- Strain of other muscles, fascia and tendons at shoulder and upper arm level, right arm
7 ⊟ S46.812- Strain of other muscles, fascia and tendons at shoulder and upper arm level, left arm
7 ⊟ S46.819- Strain of other muscles, fascia and tendons at shoulder and upper arm level, unspecified arm
6 S46.82 Laceration of other muscles, fascia and tendons at shoulder and upper arm level
7 ⊟ S46.821- Laceration of other muscles, fascia and tendons at shoulder and upper arm level, right arm
7 ⊟ S46.822- Laceration of other muscles, fascia and tendons at shoulder and upper arm level, left arm
7 ⊟ S46.829- Laceration of other muscles, fascia and tendons at shoulder and upper arm level, unspecified arm
6 S46.89 Other injury of Other muscles, fascia and tendons at shoulder and upper arm level
7 ⊟ S46.891- Other injury of other muscles, fascia and tendons at shoulder and upper arm level, right arm
7 ⊟ S46.892- Other injury of other muscles, fascia and tendons at shoulder and upper arm level, left arm
7 ⊟ S46.899- Other injury of other muscles, fascia and tendons at shoulder and upper arm level, unspecified arm
5 S46.9 Injury of unspecified muscle, fascia and tendon at shoulder and upper arm level
6 S46.90 Unspecified injury of Unspecified muscle, fascia and tendon at shoulder and upper arm level
7 ⊟ S46.901- Unspecified injury of unspecified muscle, fascia and tendon at shoulder and upper arm level, right arm
7 ⊟ S46.902- Unspecified injury of unspecified muscle, fascia and tendon at shoulder and upper arm level, left arm
7 ⊟ S46.909- Unspecified injury of unspecified muscle, fascia and tendon at shoulder and upper arm level, unspecified arm
6 S46.91 Strain of unspecified muscle, fascia and tendon at shoulder and upper arm level
7 ⊟ S46.911- Strain of unspecified muscle, fascia and tendon at shoulder and upper arm level, right arm
7 ⊟ S46.912- Strain of unspecified muscle, fascia and tendon at shoulder and upper arm level, left arm
7 ⊟ S46.919- Strain of unspecified muscle, fascia and tendon at shoulder and upper arm level, unspecified arm
6 S46.92 Laceration of unspecified muscle, fascia and tendon at shoulder and upper arm level
7 ⊟ S46.921- Laceration of unspecified muscle, fascia and tendon at shoulder and upper arm level, right arm
7 ⊟ S46.922- Laceration of unspecified muscle, fascia and tendon at shoulder and upper arm level, left arm
7 ⊟ S46.929- Laceration of unspecified muscle, fascia and tendon at shoulder and upper arm level, unspecified arm
6 S46.99 Other injury of unspecified muscle, fascia and tendon at shoulder and upper arm level
7 ⊟ S46.991- Other injury of unspecified muscle, fascia and tendon at shoulder and upper arm level, right arm
7 ⊟ S46.992- Other injury of unspecified muscle, fascia and tendon at shoulder and upper arm level, left arm
7 ⊟ S46.999- Other injury of unspecified muscle, fascia and tendon at shoulder and upper arm level, unspecified arm

4 S47 Crushing injury of shoulder and upper arm

Use additional code for all associated injuries

EXCLUDES 2 *crushing injury of elbow (S57.0-)*

The appropriate 7th character is to be added to each code from category S47
A initial encounter
D subsequent encounter
S sequela

7 ⊟ S47.1XX- Crushing injury of right shoulder and upper arm
7 ⊟ S47.2XX- Crushing injury of left shoulder and upper arm
7 ⊟ S47.9XX- Crushing injury of shoulder and upper arm, unspecified arm

4 S48 Traumatic amputation of shoulder and upper arm

An amputation not identified as partial or complete should be coded to complete

EXCLUDES 1 *traumatic amputation at elbow level (S58.0)*

The appropriate 7th character is to be added to each code from category S48
A initial encounter
D subsequent encounter
S sequela

CODING TIP ✓ Use these codes only when the amputation was due to trauma. There is no need for adding Z89 with traumatic amputations. See Z47.81 for care of amputations not due to trauma.

5 S48.0 Traumatic amputation at shoulder joint
6 S48.01 Complete traumatic amputation at shoulder joint
7 ⊟ S48.011- Complete traumatic amputation at right shoulder joint HCC
7 ⊟ S48.012- Complete traumatic amputation at left shoulder joint HCC
7 ⊟ S48.019- Complete traumatic amputation at unspecified shoulder joint HCC
6 S48.02 Partial traumatic amputation at shoulder joint

7 ⊟ S48.021- Partial traumatic amputation at right shoulder joint HCC
7 ⊟ S48.022- Partial traumatic amputation at left shoulder joint HCC
7 ⊟ S48.029- Partial traumatic amputation at unspecified shoulder joint HCC
5 S48.1 Traumatic amputation at level between shoulder and elbow
6 S48.11 Complete traumatic amputation at level between shoulder and elbow
7 ⊟ S48.111- Complete traumatic amputation at level between right shoulder and elbow HCC
7 ⊟ S48.112- Complete traumatic amputation at level between left shoulder and elbow HCC
7 ⊟ S48.119- Complete traumatic amputation at level between unspecified shoulder and elbow HCC
6 S48.12 Partial traumatic amputation at level between shoulder and elbow
7 ⊟ S48.121- Partial traumatic amputation at level between right shoulder and elbow HCC
7 ⊟ S48.122- Partial traumatic amputation at level between left shoulder and elbow HCC
7 ⊟ S48.129- Partial traumatic amputation at level between unspecified shoulder and elbow HCC
5 S48.9 Traumatic amputation of shoulder and upper arm, level unspecified
6 S48.91 Complete traumatic amputation of shoulder and upper arm, level unspecified
7 ⊟ S48.911- Complete traumatic amputation of right shoulder and upper arm, level unspecified HCC
7 ⊟ S48.912- Complete traumatic amputation of left shoulder and upper arm, level unspecified HCC
7 ⊟ S48.919- Complete traumatic amputation of unspecified shoulder and upper arm, level unspecified HCC
6 S48.92 Partial traumatic amputation of shoulder and upper arm, level unspecified
7 ⊟ S48.921- Partial traumatic amputation of right shoulder and upper arm, level unspecified HCC
7 ⊟ S48.922- Partial traumatic amputation of left shoulder and upper arm, level unspecified HCC
7 ⊟ S48.929- Partial traumatic amputation of unspecified shoulder and upper arm, level unspecified HCC

4 S49 Other and unspecified injuries of shoulder and upper arm

The appropriate 7th character is to be added to each code from subcategories S49.0 and S49.1

A	initial encounter for closed fracture
D	subsequent encounter for fracture with routine healing
G	subsequent encounter for fracture with delayed healing
K	subsequent encounter for fracture with nonunion
P	subsequent encounter for fracture with malunion
S	sequela

CODING TIP ✓ A Salter-Harris physeal fracture occurs through the growth plate. Only one code is needed to report a single physeal fracture. Because of the implications for future bone development, coding of a Salter-Harris fracture takes priority over a simple fracture code. Assign the physeal fracture code based on location, type, and laterality. Use a code for "other physeal fracture" for Type V.

5 S49.0 Physeal fracture of upper end of humerus
6 S49.00 Unspecified physeal fracture of upper end of humerus
7 ⊟ S49.001- Unspecified physeal fracture of upper end of humerus, right arm
7 ⊟ S49.002- Unspecified physeal fracture of upper end of humerus, left arm
7 ⊟ S49.009- Unspecified physeal fracture of upper end of humerus, unspecified arm
6 S49.01 Salter-Harris Type I physeal fracture of upper end of humerus
7 ⊟ S49.011- Salter-Harris Type I physeal fracture of upper end of humerus, right arm
7 ⊟ S49.012- Salter-Harris Type I physeal fracture of upper end of humerus, left arm
7 ⊟ S49.019- Salter-Harris Type I physeal fracture of upper end of humerus, unspecified arm
6 S49.02 Salter-Harris Type II physeal fracture of upper end of humerus
7 ⊟ S49.021- Salter-Harris Type II physeal fracture of upper end of humerus, right arm
7 ⊟ S49.022- Salter-Harris Type II physeal fracture of upper end of humerus, left arm
7 ⊟ S49.029- Salter-Harris Type II physeal fracture of upper end of humerus, unspecified arm
6 S49.03 Salter-Harris Type III physeal fracture of upper end of humerus
7 ⊟ S49.031- Salter-Harris Type III physeal fracture of upper end of humerus, right arm
7 ⊟ S49.032- Salter-Harris Type III physeal fracture of upper end of humerus, left arm
7 ⊟ S49.039- Salter-Harris Type III physeal fracture of upper end of humerus, unspecified arm
6 S49.04 Salter-Harris Type IV physeal fracture of upper end of humerus
7 ⊟ S49.041- Salter-Harris Type IV physeal fracture of upper end of humerus, right arm
7 ⊟ S49.042- Salter-Harris Type IV physeal fracture of upper end of humerus, left arm
7 ⊟ S49.049- Salter-Harris Type IV physeal fracture of upper end of humerus, unspecified arm
6 S49.09 Other physeal fracture of upper end of humerus
7 ⊟ S49.091- Other physeal fracture of upper end of humerus, right arm
7 ⊟ S49.092- Other physeal fracture of upper end of humerus, left arm
7 ⊟ S49.099- Other physeal fracture of upper end of humerus, unspecified arm
5 S49.1 Physeal fracture of lower end of humerus
6 S49.10 Unspecified physeal fracture of lower end of humerus
7 ⊟ S49.101- Unspecified physeal fracture of lower end of humerus, right arm
7 ⊟ S49.102- Unspecified physeal fracture of lower end of humerus, left arm
7 ⊟ S49.109- Unspecified physeal fracture of lower end of humerus, unspecified arm
6 S49.11 Salter-Harris Type I physeal fracture of lower end of humerus
7 ⊟ S49.111- Salter-Harris Type I physeal fracture of lower end of humerus, right arm
7 ⊟ S49.112- Salter-Harris Type I physeal fracture of lower end of humerus, left arm
7 ⊟ S49.119- Salter-Harris Type I physeal fracture of lower end of humerus, unspecified arm
6 S49.12 Salter-Harris Type II physeal fracture of lower end of humerus
7 ⊟ S49.121- Salter-Harris Type II physeal fracture of lower end of humerus, right arm
7 ⊟ S49.122- Salter-Harris Type II physeal fracture of lower end of humerus, left arm
7 ⊟ S49.129- Salter-Harris Type II physeal fracture of lower end of humerus, unspecified arm
6 S49.13 Salter-Harris Type III physeal fracture of lower end of humerus
7 ⊟ S49.131- Salter-Harris Type III physeal fracture of lower end of humerus, right arm
7 ⊟ S49.132- Salter-Harris Type III physeal fracture of lower end of humerus, left arm
7 ⊟ S49.139- Salter-Harris Type III physeal fracture of lower end of humerus, unspecified arm
6 S49.14 Salter-Harris Type IV physeal fracture of lower end of humerus
7 ⊟ S49.141- Salter-Harris Type IV physeal fracture of lower end of humerus, right arm

7 ⊟ S49.142- Salter-Harris Type IV physeal fracture of lower end of humerus, left arm

7 ⊟ S49.149- Salter-Harris Type IV physeal fracture of lower end of humerus, unspecified arm

6 S49.19 Other physeal fracture of lower end of humerus

7 ⊟ S49.191- Other physeal fracture of lower end of humerus, right arm

7 ⊟ S49.192- Other physeal fracture of lower end of humerus, left arm

7 ⊟ S49.199- Other physeal fracture of lower end of humerus, unspecified arm

5 S49.8 Other specified injuries of shoulder and upper arm

The appropriate 7th character is to be added to each code in subcategory S49.8
A initial encounter
D subsequent encounter
S sequela

7 ⊟ S49.80X- Other specified injuries of shoulder and upper arm, unspecified arm

7 ⊟ S49.81X- Other specified injuries of right shoulder and upper arm

7 ⊟ S49.82X- Other specified injuries of left shoulder and upper arm

5 S49.9 Unspecified injury of shoulder and upper arm

The appropriate 7th character is to be added to each code in subcategory S49.9
A initial encounter
D subsequent encounter
S sequela

7 ⊟ S49.90X- Unspecified injury of shoulder and upper arm, unspecified arm

7 ⊟ S49.91X- Unspecified injury of right shoulder and upper arm

7 ⊟ S49.92X- Unspecified injury of left shoulder and upper arm

Injuries to the elbow and forearm (S50-S59)

EXCLUDES 2 *burns and corrosions (T20-T32)*
frostbite (T33-T34)
injuries of wrist and hand (S60-S69)
insect bite or sting, venomous (T63.4)

GUIDELINES **Section I.C.19.c.2)**
Multiple fractures are sequenced in accordance with the severity of the fracture.

GUIDELINES **Section I.C.19.b.1)-2)**
When coding injuries, assign separate codes for each injury unless a combination code is provided, in which case the combination code is assigned ... Traumatic injury codes (S00-T14.9) are not to be used for normal, healing surgical wounds or to identify complications of surgical wounds. The code for the most serious injury, as determined by the provider and the focus of treatment, is sequenced first.

1) Superficial injuries such as abrasions or contusions are not coded when associated with more severe injuries of the same site.

2) When a primary injury results in minor damage to peripheral nerves or blood vessels, the primary injury is sequenced first with additional code(s) for injuries to nerves and spinal cord (such as category S04), and/or injury to blood vessels (such as category S15). When the primary injury is to the blood vessels or nerves, that injury should be sequenced first.

GUIDELINES **Section I.C.19.c**
Coding of Traumatic Fractures: The principles of multiple coding of injuries should be followed in coding fractures. Fractures of specified sites are coded individually by site in accordance with both the provisions within categories S02, S12, S22, S32, S42, S49, S52, S59, S62, S72, S79, S82, S89, S92 and the level of detail furnished by medical record content. A fracture not indicated as open or closed should be coded to closed. A fracture not indicated whether displaced or not displaced should be coded to displaced.

4 S50 Superficial injury of elbow and forearm

EXCLUDES 2 *superficial injury of wrist and hand (S60.-)*

The appropriate 7th character is to be added to each code from category S50
A initial encounter
D subsequent encounter
S sequela

5 S50.0 Contusion of elbow

7 ⊟ S50.00X- Contusion of unspecified elbow

7 ⊟ S50.01X- Contusion of right elbow

7 ⊟ S50.02X- Contusion of left elbow

5 S50.1 Contusion of forearm

7 ⊟ S50.10X- Contusion of unspecified forearm

7 ⊟ S50.11X- Contusion of right forearm

7 ⊟ S50.12X- Contusion of left forearm

5 S50.3 Other superficial injuries of elbow

6 S50.31 Abrasion of elbow

7 ⊟ S50.311- Abrasion of right elbow

7 ⊟ S50.312- Abrasion of left elbow

7 ⊟ S50.319- Abrasion of unspecified elbow

6 S50.32 Blister (nonthermal) of elbow

7 ⊟ S50.321- Blister (nonthermal) of right elbow

7 ⊟ S50.322- Blister (nonthermal) of left elbow

7 ⊟ S50.329- Blister (nonthermal) of unspecified elbow

6 S50.34 External constriction of elbow

7 ⊟ S50.341- External constriction of right elbow

7 ⊟ S50.342- External constriction of left elbow

7 ⊟ S50.349- External constriction of unspecified elbow

6 S50.35 Superficial foreign body of elbow
Splinter in the elbow

7 ⊟ S50.351- Superficial foreign body of right elbow

7 ⊟ S50.352- Superficial foreign body of left elbow

7 ⊟ S50.359- Superficial foreign body of unspecified elbow

6 S50.36 Insect bite (nonvenomous) of elbow

7 ⊟ S50.361- Insect bite (nonvenomous) of right elbow

7 ⊟ S50.362- Insect bite (nonvenomous) of left elbow

7 ⊟ S50.369- Insect bite (nonvenomous) of unspecified elbow

6 S50.37 Other superficial bite of elbow

EXCLUDES 1 *open bite of elbow (S51.04)*

7 ⊟ S50.371- Other superficial bite of right elbow

7 ⊟ S50.372- Other superficial bite of left elbow

7 ⊟ S50.379- Other superficial bite of unspecified elbow

5 S50.8 Other superficial injuries of forearm

6 S50.81 Abrasion of forearm

7 ⊟ S50.811- Abrasion of right forearm

7 ⊟ S50.812- Abrasion of left forearm

7 ⊟ S50.819- Abrasion of unspecified forearm

6 S50.82 Blister (nonthermal) of forearm

7 ⊟ S50.821- Blister (nonthermal) of right forearm

7 ⊟ S50.822- Blister (nonthermal) of left forearm

7 ⊟ S50.829- Blister (nonthermal) of unspecified forearm

6 S50.84 External constriction of forearm

7 ⊟ S50.841- External constriction of right forearm

7 ⊟ S50.842- External constriction of left forearm

7 ⊟ S50.849- External constriction of unspecified forearm

6 S50.85 Superficial foreign body of forearm
Splinter in the forearm

7 ⊟ S50.851- Superficial foreign body of right forearm

7 ⊟ S50.852- Superficial foreign body of left forearm

7 ⊟ S50.859- Superficial foreign body of unspecified forearm

6 S50.86 Insect bite (nonvenomous) of forearm

7 ⊟ S50.861- Insect bite (nonvenomous) of right forearm

7 ⊟ S50.862- Insect bite (nonvenomous) of left forearm

S50.869- Insect bite (nonvenomous) of unspecified forearm

S50.87 Other superficial bite of forearm

EXCLUDES 1 *open bite of forearm (S51.84)*

S50.871- Other superficial bite of right forearm

S50.872- Other superficial bite of left forearm

S50.879- Other superficial bite of unspecified forearm

S50.9 Unspecified superficial injury of elbow and forearm

S50.90 Unspecified superficial injury of elbow

S50.901- Unspecified superficial injury of right elbow

S50.902- Unspecified superficial injury of left elbow

S50.909- Unspecified superficial injury of unspecified elbow

S50.91 Unspecified superficial injury of forearm

S50.911- Unspecified superficial injury of right forearm

S50.912- Unspecified superficial injury of left forearm

S50.919- Unspecified superficial injury of unspecified forearm

S51 Open wound of elbow and forearm

Code also:

any associated wound infection

EXCLUDES 1 *open fracture of elbow and forearm (S52.- with open fracture 7th character)*
traumatic amputation of elbow and forearm (S58.-)

EXCLUDES 2 *open wound of wrist and hand (S61.-)*

The appropriate 7th character is to be added to each code from category S51
A initial encounter
D subsequent encounter
S sequela

CODING TIP ✓ Open wound codes indicate a wound resulting from a traumatic origin. Do not assign a code for "open wound" unless the etiology of the wound is related to trauma.

S51.0 Open wound of elbow

S51.00 Unspecified open wound of elbow

S51.001- Unspecified open wound of right elbow
AHA: (S51.001A) 4Q 2012, 108

S51.002- Unspecified open wound of left elbow

S51.009- Unspecified open wound of unspecified elbow
Open wound of elbow NOS

S51.01 Laceration without foreign body of elbow

S51.011- Laceration without foreign body of right elbow

S51.012- Laceration without foreign body of left elbow

S51.019- Laceration without foreign body of unspecified elbow

S51.02 Laceration with foreign body of elbow

S51.021- Laceration with foreign body of right elbow

S51.022- Laceration with foreign body of left elbow

S51.029- Laceration with foreign body of unspecified elbow

S51.03 Puncture wound without foreign body of elbow

S51.031- Puncture wound without foreign body of right elbow

S51.032- Puncture wound without foreign body of left elbow

S51.039- Puncture wound without foreign body of unspecified elbow

S51.04 Puncture wound with foreign body of elbow

S51.041- Puncture wound with foreign body of right elbow

S51.042- Puncture wound with foreign body of left elbow

S51.049- Puncture wound with foreign body of unspecified elbow

S51.05 Open bite of elbow
Bite of elbow NOS

EXCLUDES 1 *superficial bite of elbow (S50.36, S50.37)*

S51.051- Open bite, right elbow

S51.052- Open bite, left elbow

S51.059- Open bite, unspecified elbow

S51.8 Open wound of forearm

EXCLUDES 2 *open wound of elbow (S51.0-)*

S51.80 Unspecified open wound of forearm

S51.801- Unspecified open wound of right forearm

S51.802- Unspecified open wound of left forearm

S51.809- Unspecified open wound of unspecified forearm
Open wound of forearm NOS

S51.81 Laceration without foreign body of forearm

S51.811- Laceration without foreign body of right forearm

S51.812- Laceration without foreign body of left forearm

S51.819- Laceration without foreign body of unspecified forearm

S51.82 Laceration with foreign body of forearm

S51.821- Laceration with foreign body of right forearm

S51.822- Laceration with foreign body of left forearm

S51.829- Laceration with foreign body of unspecified forearm

S51.83 Puncture wound without foreign body of forearm

S51.831- Puncture wound without foreign body of right forearm

S51.832- Puncture wound without foreign body of left forearm

S51.839- Puncture wound without foreign body of unspecified forearm

S51.84 Puncture wound with foreign body of forearm

S51.841- Puncture wound with foreign body of right forearm

S51.842- Puncture wound with foreign body of left forearm

S51.849- Puncture wound with foreign body of unspecified forearm

S51.85 Open bite of forearm
Bite of forearm NOS

EXCLUDES 1 *superficial bite of forearm (S50.86, S50.87)*

S51.851- Open bite of right forearm

S51.852- Open bite of left forearm

S51.859- Open bite of unspecified forearm

4 **S52 Fracture of forearm**

Note: A fracture not indicated as displaced or nondisplaced should be coded to displaced

A fracture not indicated as open or closed should be coded to closed

The open fracture designations are based on the Gustilo open fracture classification

EXCLUDES 1 *traumatic amputation of forearm (S58.-)*

EXCLUDES 2 *fracture at wrist and hand level (S62.-)*

The appropriate 7th character is to be added to all codes from category S52

A	initial encounter for closed fracture
B	initial encounter for open fracture type I or II
C	initial encounter for open fracture type IIIA, IIIB, or IIIC
D	subsequent encounter for closed fracture with routine healing
E	subsequent encounter for open fracture type I or II with routine healing
F	subsequent encounter for open fracture type IIIA, IIIB, or IIIC with routine healing
G	subsequent encounter for closed fracture with delayed healing
H	subsequent encounter for open fracture type I or II with delayed healing
J	subsequent encounter for open fracture type IIIA, IIIB, or IIIC with delayed healing
K	subsequent encounter for closed fracture with nonunion
M	subsequent encounter for open fracture type I or II with nonunion
N	subsequent encounter for open fracture type IIIA, IIIB, or IIIC with nonunion
P	subsequent encounter for closed fracture with malunion
Q	subsequent encounter for open fracture type I or II with malunion
R	subsequent encounter for open fracture type IIIA, IIIB, or IIIC with malunion
S	sequela

CODING TIP✓ A fracture not indicated as displaced or nondisplaced should be coded to displaced. A fracture not indicated as open or closed should be coded to closed. Query providers on fractures not documented as displaced/nondisplaced; otherwise, a displaced fracture diagnosis could be assigned without a reduction being performed, potentially resulting in claim denials.

5 **S52.0 Fracture of upper end of ulna**

Fracture of proximal end of ulna

EXCLUDES 2 *fracture of elbow NOS (S42.40-)*
fractures of shaft of ulna (S52.2-)

6 **S52.00 Unspecified fracture of upper end of ulna**

7 ⊟ **S52.001- Unspecified fracture of upper end of right ulna**

7 ⊟ **S52.002- Unspecified fracture of upper end of left ulna**

7 ⊟ **S52.009- Unspecified fracture of upper end of unspecified ulna**

6 **S52.01 Torus fracture of upper end of ulna**

The appropriate 7th character is to be added to all codes in subcategory S52.01

A	initial encounter for closed fracture
D	subsequent encounter for fracture with routine healing
G	subsequent encounter for fracture with delayed healing
K	subsequent encounter for fracture with nonunion
P	subsequent encounter for fracture with malunion
S	sequela

CODING TIP✓ Open fractures do not occur with torus fractures and greenstick fractures, therefore the 7th characters for open fractures are not available.

7 ⊟ **S52.011- Torus fracture of upper end of right ulna**

7 ⊟ **S52.012- Torus fracture of upper end of left ulna**

7 ⊟ **S52.019- Torus fracture of upper end of unspecified ulna**

6 **S52.02 Fracture of olecranon process without intraarticular extension of ulna**

7 ⊟ **S52.021- Displaced fracture of olecranon process without intraarticular extension of right ulna**

7 ⊟ **S52.022- Displaced fracture of olecranon process without intraarticular extension of left ulna**

7 ⊟ **S52.023- Displaced fracture of olecranon process without intraarticular extension of unspecified ulna**

7 ⊟ **S52.024- Nondisplaced fracture of olecranon process without intraarticular extension of right ulna**

7 ⊟ **S52.025- Nondisplaced fracture of olecranon process without intraarticular extension of left ulna**

7 ⊟ **S52.026- Nondisplaced fracture of olecranon process without intraarticular extension of unspecified ulna**

6 **S52.03 Fracture of olecranon process with intraarticular extension of ulna**

7 ⊟ **S52.031- Displaced fracture of olecranon process with intraarticular extension of right ulna**

7 ⊟ **S52.032- Displaced fracture of olecranon process with intraarticular extension of left ulna**

7 ⊟ **S52.033- Displaced fracture of olecranon process with intraarticular extension of unspecified ulna**

7 ⊟ **S52.034- Nondisplaced fracture of olecranon process with intraarticular extension of right ulna**

7 ⊟ **S52.035- Nondisplaced fracture of olecranon process with intraarticular extension of left ulna**

7 ⊟ **S52.036- Nondisplaced fracture of olecranon process with intraarticular extension of unspecified ulna**

6 **S52.04 Fracture of coronoid process of ulna**

7 ⊟ **S52.041- Displaced fracture of coronoid process of right ulna**

7 ⊟ **S52.042- Displaced fracture of coronoid process of left ulna**

7 ⊟ **S52.043- Displaced fracture of coronoid process of unspecified ulna**

7 ⊟ **S52.044- Nondisplaced fracture of coronoid process of right ulna**

7 ⊟ **S52.045- Nondisplaced fracture of coronoid process of left ulna**

7 ⊟ **S52.046- Nondisplaced fracture of coronoid process of unspecified ulna**

6 **S52.09 Other fracture of upper end of ulna**

7 ⊟ **S52.091- Other fracture of upper end of right ulna**

7 ⊟ **S52.092- Other fracture of upper end of left ulna**

7 ⊟ **S52.099- Other fracture of upper end of unspecified ulna**

5 **S52.1 Fracture of upper end of radius**

Fracture of proximal end of radius

EXCLUDES 2 *physeal fractures of upper end of radius (S59.2-)*
fracture of shaft of radius (S52.3-)

6 **S52.10 Unspecified fracture of upper end of radius**

7 ⊟ **S52.101- Unspecified fracture of upper end of right radius**

7 ⊟ **S52.102- Unspecified fracture of upper end of left radius**

7 ⊟ **S52.109- Unspecified fracture of upper end of unspecified radius**

6 **S52.11 Torus fracture of upper end of radius**

The appropriate 7th character is to be added to all codes in subcategory S52.11

A	initial encounter for closed fracture
D	subsequent encounter for fracture with routine healing
G	subsequent encounter for fracture with delayed healing
K	subsequent encounter for fracture with nonunion
P	subsequent encounter for fracture with malunion
S	sequela

CODING TIP✓ Open fractures do not occur with torus fractures and greenstick fractures, therefore the 7th characters for open fractures are not available.

7 ⊟ S52.111- **Torus fracture of upper end of right radius**
7 ⊟ S52.112- **Torus fracture of upper end of left radius**
7 ⊟ S52.119- **Torus fracture of upper end of unspecified radius**

6 S52.12 **Fracture of head of radius**
7 ⊟ S52.121- **Displaced fracture of head of right radius**
7 ⊟ S52.122- **Displaced fracture of head of left radius**
7 ⊟ S52.123- **Displaced fracture of head of unspecified radius**
7 ⊟ S52.124- **Nondisplaced fracture of head of right radius**
7 ⊟ S52.125- **Nondisplaced fracture of head of left radius**
7 ⊟ S52.126- **Nondisplaced fracture of head of unspecified radius**

6 S52.13 **Fracture of neck of radius**
7 ⊟ S52.131- **Displaced fracture of neck of right radius**
7 ⊟ S52.132- **Displaced fracture of neck of left radius**
7 ⊟ S52.133- **Displaced fracture of neck of unspecified radius**
7 ⊟ S52.134- **Nondisplaced fracture of neck of right radius**
7 ⊟ S52.135- **Nondisplaced fracture of neck of left radius**
7 ⊟ S52.136- **Nondisplaced fracture of neck of unspecified radius**

6 S52.18 **Other fracture of upper end of radius**
7 ⊟ S52.181- **Other fracture of upper end of right radius**
7 ⊟ S52.182- **Other fracture of upper end of left radius**
7 ⊟ S52.189- **Other fracture of upper end of unspecified radius**

5 S52.2 **Fracture of shaft of ulna**

6 S52.20 **Unspecified fracture of shaft of ulna**
Fracture of ulna NOS
7 ⊟ S52.201- **Unspecified fracture of shaft of right ulna**
7 ⊟ S52.202- **Unspecified fracture of shaft of left ulna**
7 ⊟ S52.209- **Unspecified fracture of shaft of unspecified ulna**

Displaced transverse fracture, shafts and radius of ulna

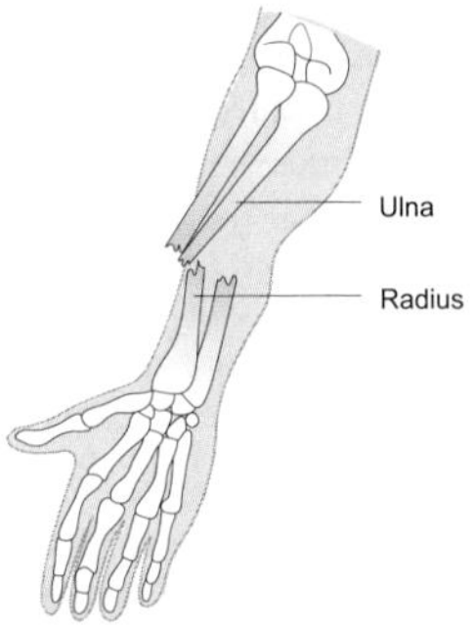

Two codes are required to report fractures of the radius and ulna

6 S52.21 **Greenstick fracture of shaft of ulna**

The appropriate 7th character is to be added to all codes in subcategory S52.21

A	initial encounter for closed fracture
D	subsequent encounter for fracture with routine healing
G	subsequent encounter for fracture with delayed healing
K	subsequent encounter for fracture with nonunion
P	subsequent encounter for fracture with malunion
S	sequela

CODING TIP✓ Open fractures do not occur with torus fractures and greenstick fractures, therefore the 7th characters for open fractures are not available.

7 ⊟ S52.211- **Greenstick fracture of shaft of right ulna**
7 ⊟ S52.212- **Greenstick fracture of shaft of left ulna**
7 ⊟ S52.219- **Greenstick fracture of shaft of unspecified ulna**

6 S52.22 **Transverse fracture of shaft of ulna**
7 ⊟ S52.221- **Displaced transverse fracture of shaft of right ulna**
7 ⊟ S52.222- **Displaced transverse fracture of shaft of left ulna**
7 ⊟ S52.223- **Displaced transverse fracture of shaft of unspecified ulna**
7 ⊟ S52.224- **Nondisplaced transverse fracture of shaft of right ulna**
7 ⊟ S52.225- **Nondisplaced transverse fracture of shaft of left ulna**
7 ⊟ S52.226- **Nondisplaced transverse fracture of shaft of unspecified ulna**

6 S52.23 **Oblique fracture of shaft of ulna**
7 ⊟ S52.231- **Displaced oblique fracture of shaft of right ulna**
7 ⊟ S52.232- **Displaced oblique fracture of shaft of left ulna**
7 ⊟ S52.233- **Displaced oblique fracture of shaft of unspecified ulna**
7 ⊟ S52.234- **Nondisplaced oblique fracture of shaft of right ulna**
7 ⊟ S52.235- **Nondisplaced oblique fracture of shaft of left ulna**
7 ⊟ S52.236- **Nondisplaced oblique fracture of shaft of unspecified ulna**

6 S52.24 **Spiral fracture of shaft of ulna**
7 ⊟ S52.241- **Displaced spiral fracture of shaft of ulna, right arm**
7 ⊟ S52.242- **Displaced spiral fracture of shaft of ulna, left arm**
7 ⊟ S52.243- **Displaced spiral fracture of shaft of ulna, unspecified arm**
7 ⊟ S52.244- **Nondisplaced spiral fracture of shaft of ulna, right arm**
7 ⊟ S52.245- **Nondisplaced spiral fracture of shaft of ulna, left arm**
7 ⊟ S52.246- **Nondisplaced spiral fracture of shaft of ulna, unspecified arm**

6 S52.25 **Comminuted fracture of shaft of ulna**
7 ⊟ S52.251- **Displaced comminuted fracture of shaft of ulna, right arm**
7 ⊟ S52.252- **Displaced comminuted fracture of shaft of ulna, left arm**
7 ⊟ S52.253- **Displaced comminuted fracture of shaft of ulna, unspecified arm**
7 ⊟ S52.254- **Nondisplaced comminuted fracture of shaft of ulna, right arm**
7 ⊟ S52.255- **Nondisplaced comminuted fracture of shaft of ulna, left arm**
7 ⊟ S52.256- **Nondisplaced comminuted fracture of shaft of ulna, unspecified arm**

6 S52.26 **Segmental fracture of shaft of ulna**
7 ⊟ S52.261- **Displaced segmental fracture of shaft of ulna, right arm**
7 ⊟ S52.262- **Displaced segmental fracture of shaft of ulna, left arm**
7 ⊟ S52.263- **Displaced segmental fracture of shaft of ulna, unspecified arm**
7 ⊟ S52.264- **Nondisplaced segmental fracture of shaft of ulna, right arm**
7 ⊟ S52.265- **Nondisplaced segmental fracture of shaft of ulna, left arm**
7 ⊟ S52.266- **Nondisplaced segmental fracture of shaft of ulna, unspecified arm**

6 S52.27 **Monteggia's fracture of ulna**
Fracture of upper shaft of ulna with dislocation of radial head
7 ⊟ S52.271- **Monteggia's fracture of right ulna**
7 ⊟ S52.272- **Monteggia's fracture of left ulna**

7 ⊟ S52.279- **Monteggia's fracture of unspecified ulna**

6 S52.28 **Bent bone of ulna**

7 ⊟ S52.281- **Bent bone of right ulna**

7 ⊟ S52.282- **Bent bone of left ulna**

7 ⊟ S52.283- **Bent bone of unspecified ulna**

6 S52.29 **Other fracture of shaft of ulna**

7 ⊟ S52.291- **Other fracture of shaft of right ulna**

7 ⊟ S52.292- **Other fracture of shaft of left ulna**

7 ⊟ S52.299- **Other fracture of shaft of unspecified ulna**

5 S52.3 **Fracture of shaft of radius**

6 S52.30 **Unspecified fracture of shaft of radius**

7 ⊟ S52.301- **Unspecified fracture of shaft of right radius**

7 ⊟ S52.302- **Unspecified fracture of shaft of left radius**

7 ⊟ S52.309- **Unspecified fracture of shaft of unspecified radius**

6 S52.31 **Greenstick fracture of shaft of radius**

The appropriate 7th character is to be added to all codes in subcategory S52.31

- A initial encounter for closed fracture
- D subsequent encounter for fracture with routine healing
- G subsequent encounter for fracture with delayed healing
- K subsequent encounter for fracture with nonunion
- P subsequent encounter for fracture with malunion
- S sequela

CODING TIP✓ Open fractures do not occur with torus fractures and greenstick fractures, therefore the 7th characters for open fractures are not available.

7 ⊟ S52.311- **Greenstick fracture of shaft of radius, right arm**

7 ⊟ S52.312- **Greenstick fracture of shaft of radius, left arm**

7 ⊟ S52.319- **Greenstick fracture of shaft of radius, unspecified arm**

6 S52.32 **Transverse fracture of shaft of radius**

7 ⊟ S52.321- **Displaced transverse fracture of shaft of right radius**

7 ⊟ S52.322- **Displaced transverse fracture of shaft of left radius**

7 ⊟ S52.323- **Displaced transverse fracture of shaft of unspecified radius**

7 ⊟ S52.324- **Nondisplaced transverse fracture of shaft of right radius**

7 ⊟ S52.325- **Nondisplaced transverse fracture of shaft of left radius**

7 ⊟ S52.326- **Nondisplaced transverse fracture of shaft of unspecified radius**

6 S52.33 **Oblique fracture of shaft of radius**

7 ⊟ S52.331- **Displaced oblique fracture of shaft of right radius**

7 ⊟ S52.332- **Displaced oblique fracture of shaft of left radius**

7 ⊟ S52.333- **Displaced oblique fracture of shaft of unspecified radius**

7 ⊟ S52.334- **Nondisplaced oblique fracture of shaft of right radius**

7 ⊟ S52.335- **Nondisplaced oblique fracture of shaft of left radius**

7 ⊟ S52.336- **Nondisplaced oblique fracture of shaft of unspecified radius**

6 S52.34 **Spiral fracture of shaft of radius**

7 ⊟ S52.341- **Displaced spiral fracture of shaft of radius, right arm**

7 ⊟ S52.342- **Displaced spiral fracture of shaft of radius, left arm**

7 ⊟ S52.343- **Displaced spiral fracture of shaft of radius, unspecified arm**

7 ⊟ S52.344- **Nondisplaced spiral fracture of shaft of radius, right arm**

7 ⊟ S52.345- **Nondisplaced spiral fracture of shaft of radius, left arm**

7 ⊟ S52.346- **Nondisplaced spiral fracture of shaft of radius, unspecified arm**

6 S52.35 **Comminuted fracture of shaft of radius**

7 ⊟ S52.351- **Displaced comminuted fracture of shaft of radius, right arm**

7 ⊟ S52.352- **Displaced comminuted fracture of shaft of radius, left arm**

7 ⊟ S52.353- **Displaced comminuted fracture of shaft of radius, unspecified arm**

7 ⊟ S52.354- **Nondisplaced comminuted fracture of shaft of radius, right arm**

7 ⊟ S52.355- **Nondisplaced comminuted fracture of shaft of radius, left arm**

7 ⊟ S52.356- **Nondisplaced comminuted fracture of shaft of radius, unspecified arm**

6 S52.36 **Segmental fracture of shaft of radius**

7 ⊟ S52.361- **Displaced segmental fracture of shaft of radius, right arm**

7 ⊟ S52.362- **Displaced segmental fracture of shaft of radius, left arm**

7 ⊟ S52.363- **Displaced segmental fracture of shaft of radius, unspecified arm**

7 ⊟ S52.364- **Nondisplaced segmental fracture of shaft of radius, right arm**

7 ⊟ S52.365- **Nondisplaced segmental fracture of shaft of radius, left arm**

7 ⊟ S52.366- **Nondisplaced segmental fracture of shaft of radius, unspecified arm**

6 S52.37 **Galeazzi's fracture**

Fracture of lower shaft of radius with radioulnar joint dislocation

7 ⊟ S52.371- **Galeazzi's fracture of right radius**

7 ⊟ S52.372- **Galeazzi's fracture of left radius**

7 ⊟ S52.379- **Galeazzi's fracture of unspecified radius**

6 S52.38 **Bent bone of radius**

7 ⊟ S52.381- **Bent bone of right radius**

7 ⊟ S52.382- **Bent bone of left radius**

7 ⊟ S52.389- **Bent bone of unspecified radius**

6 S52.39 **Other fracture of shaft of radius**

7 ⊟ S52.391- **Other fracture of shaft of radius, right arm**

7 ⊟ S52.392- **Other fracture of shaft of radius, left arm**

7 ⊟ S52.399- **Other fracture of shaft of radius, unspecified arm**

5 S52.5 **Fracture of lower end of radius**

Fracture of distal end of radius

EXCLUDES 2 *physeal fractures of lower end of radius (S59.2-)*

6 S52.50 **Unspecified fracture of the lower end of radius**

7 ⊟ S52.501- **Unspecified fracture of the lower end of right radius**

7 ⊟ S52.502- **Unspecified fracture of the lower end of left radius**

7 ⊟ S52.509- **Unspecified fracture of the lower end of unspecified radius**

6 S52.51 **Fracture of radial styloid process**

7 ⊟ S52.511- **Displaced fracture of right radial styloid process**

7 ⊟ S52.512- **Displaced fracture of left radial styloid process**

7 ⊟ S52.513- **Displaced fracture of unspecified radial styloid process**

7 ⊟ S52.514- **Nondisplaced fracture of right radial styloid process**

7 ⊟ S52.515- **Nondisplaced fracture of left radial styloid process**

7 ⊟ S52.516- **Nondisplaced fracture of unspecified radial styloid process**

6 S52.52 Torus fracture of lower end of radius

The appropriate 7th character is to be added to all codes in subcategory S52.52
A initial encounter for closed fracture
D subsequent encounter for fracture with routine healing
G subsequent encounter for fracture with delayed healing
K subsequent encounter for fracture with nonunion
P subsequent encounter for fracture with malunion
S sequela

CODING TIP ✓ Open fractures do not occur with torus fractures and greenstick fractures, therefore the 7th characters for open fractures are not available.

- 7 S52.521- **Torus fracture of lower end of right radius**
- 7 S52.522- **Torus fracture of lower end of left radius**
- 7 S52.529- **Torus fracture of lower end of unspecified radius**

6 S52.53 Colles' fracture

DEFINITION Break in the lower end of the radius with posterior displacement of the wrist, often caused by breaking a fall with an extended, outstretched hand.

- 7 S52.531- **Colles' fracture of right radius**
- 7 S52.532- **Colles' fracture of left radius**
  AHA: (S52.532D) 2Q 2016, 5
- 7 S52.539- **Colles' fracture of unspecified radius**

6 S52.54 Smith's fracture

DEFINITION Break in the lower end of the radius with palmar displacement of the wrist; a reverse Colles' fracture.

- 7 S52.541- **Smith's fracture of right radius**
- 7 S52.542- **Smith's fracture of left radius**
- 7 S52.549- **Smith's fracture of unspecified radius**

6 S52.55 Other extraarticular fracture of lower end of radius

- 7 S52.551- **Other extraarticular fracture of lower end of right radius**
- 7 S52.552- **Other extraarticular fracture of lower end of left radius**
- 7 S52.559- **Other extraarticular fracture of lower end of unspecified radius**

6 S52.56 Barton's fracture

- 7 S52.561- **Barton's fracture of right radius**
- 7 S52.562- **Barton's fracture of left radius**
- 7 S52.569- **Barton's fracture of unspecified radius**

6 S52.57 Other intraarticular fracture of lower end of radius

- 7 S52.571- **Other intraarticular fracture of lower end of right radius**
- 7 S52.572- **Other intraarticular fracture of lower end of left radius**
- 7 S52.579- **Other intraarticular fracture of lower end of unspecified radius**

6 S52.59 Other fractures of lower end of radius

- 7 S52.591- **Other fractures of lower end of right radius**
- 7 S52.592- **Other fractures of lower end of left radius**
- 7 S52.599- **Other fractures of lower end of unspecified radius**

5 S52.6 Fracture of lower end of ulna

6 S52.60 Unspecified fracture of lower end of ulna

- 7 S52.601- **Unspecified fracture of lower end of right ulna**
- 7 S52.602- **Unspecified fracture of lower end of left ulna**
- 7 S52.609- **Unspecified fracture of lower end of unspecified ulna**

6 S52.61 Fracture of ulna styloid process

- 7 S52.611- **Displaced fracture of right ulna styloid process**
- 7 S52.612- **Displaced fracture of left ulna styloid process**
- 7 S52.613- **Displaced fracture of unspecified ulna styloid process**
- 7 S52.614- **Nondisplaced fracture of right ulna styloid process**
- 7 S52.615- **Nondisplaced fracture of left ulna styloid process**
- 7 S52.616- **Nondisplaced fracture of unspecified ulna styloid process**

6 S52.62 Torus fracture of lower end of ulna

The appropriate 7th character is to be added to all codes in subcategory S52.62
A initial encounter for closed fracture
D subsequent encounter for fracture with routine healing
G subsequent encounter for fracture with delayed healing
K subsequent encounter for fracture with nonunion
P subsequent encounter for fracture with malunion
S sequela

- 7 S52.621- **Torus fracture of lower end of right ulna**
- 7 S52.622- **Torus fracture of lower end of left ulna**
- 7 S52.629- **Torus fracture of lower end of unspecified ulna**

6 S52.69 Other fracture of lower end of ulna

- 7 S52.691- **Other fracture of lower end of right ulna**
- 7 S52.692- **Other fracture of lower end of left ulna**
- 7 S52.699- **Other fracture of lower end of unspecified ulna**

5 S52.9 Unspecified fracture of forearm

- 7 S52.90X- **Unspecified fracture of unspecified forearm**
- 7 S52.91X- **Unspecified fracture of right forearm**
- 7 S52.92X- **Unspecified fracture of left forearm**

4 S53 Dislocation and sprain of joints and ligaments of elbow

INCLUDES avulsion of joint or ligament of elbow
laceration of cartilage, joint or ligament of elbow
sprain of cartilage, joint or ligament of elbow
traumatic hemarthrosis of joint or ligament of elbow
traumatic rupture of joint or ligament of elbow
traumatic subluxation of joint or ligament of elbow
traumatic tear of joint or ligament of elbow

Code also:
any associated open wound

EXCLUDES 2 *strain of muscle, fascia and tendon at forearm level (S56.-)*

The appropriate 7th character is to be added to each code from category S53
A initial encounter
D subsequent encounter
S sequela

CODING TIP ✓ There are no codes for open dislocations. When a dislocation is documented as open, assign an additional code for the open wound.

5 S53.0 Subluxation and dislocation of radial head

Dislocation of radiohumeral joint
Subluxation of radiohumeral joint

EXCLUDES 1 *Monteggia's fracture-dislocation (S52.27-)*

6 S53.00 Unspecified subluxation and dislocation of radial head

- 7 S53.001- **Unspecified subluxation of right radial head**
- 7 S53.002- **Unspecified subluxation of left radial head**
- 7 S53.003- **Unspecified subluxation of unspecified radial head**
- 7 S53.004- **Unspecified dislocation of right radial head**
- 7 S53.005- **Unspecified dislocation of left radial head**
- 7 S53.006- **Unspecified dislocation of unspecified radial head**

6 S53.01 Anterior subluxation and dislocation of radial head

Anteriomedial subluxation and dislocation of radial head

- 7 S53.011- **Anterior subluxation of right radial head**
- 7 S53.012- **Anterior subluxation of left radial head**
- 7 S53.013- **Anterior subluxation of unspecified radial head**

7 ⊟ S53.014- Anterior dislocation of right radial head
7 ⊟ S53.015- Anterior dislocation of left radial head
7 ⊟ S53.016- Anterior dislocation of unspecified radial head
6 S53.02 Posterior subluxation and dislocation of radial head
Posteriolateral subluxation and dislocation of radial head
7 ⊟ S53.021- Posterior subluxation of right radial head
7 ⊟ S53.022- Posterior subluxation of left radial head
7 ⊟ S53.023- Posterior subluxation of unspecified radial head
7 ⊟ S53.024- Posterior dislocation of right radial head
7 ⊟ S53.025- Posterior dislocation of left radial head
7 ⊟ S53.026- Posterior dislocation of unspecified radial head
6 S53.03 Nursemaid's elbow
7 ⊟ S53.031- Nursemaid's elbow, right elbow
AHA: (S53.031A) 1Q 2015, 7
AHA: (S53.031D) 1Q 2015, 8
7 ⊟ S53.032- Nursemaid's elbow, left elbow
7 ⊟ S53.033- Nursemaid's elbow, unspecified elbow
6 S53.09 Other subluxation and dislocation of radial head
7 ⊟ S53.091- Other subluxation of right radial head
7 ⊟ S53.092- Other subluxation of left radial head
7 ⊟ S53.093- Other subluxation of unspecified radial head
7 ⊟ S53.094- Other dislocation of right radial head
7 ⊟ S53.095- Other dislocation of left radial head
7 ⊟ S53.096- Other dislocation of unspecified radial head
5 S53.1 Subluxation and dislocation of ulnohumeral joint
Subluxation and dislocation of elbow NOS
EXCLUDES 1 *dislocation of radial head alone (S53.0-)*
6 S53.10 Unspecified subluxation and dislocation of ulnohumeral joint
7 ⊟ S53.101- Unspecified subluxation of right ulnohumeral joint
7 ⊟ S53.102- Unspecified subluxation of left ulnohumeral joint
7 ⊟ S53.103- Unspecified subluxation of unspecified ulnohumeral joint
7 ⊟ S53.104- Unspecified dislocation of right ulnohumeral joint
7 ⊟ S53.105- Unspecified dislocation of left ulnohumeral joint
7 ⊟ S53.106- Unspecified dislocation of unspecified ulnohumeral joint
6 S53.11 Anterior subluxation and dislocation of ulnohumeral joint
7 ⊟ S53.111- Anterior subluxation of right ulnohumeral joint
7 ⊟ S53.112- Anterior subluxation of left ulnohumeral joint
7 ⊟ S53.113- Anterior subluxation of unspecified ulnohumeral joint
7 ⊟ S53.114- Anterior dislocation of right ulnohumeral joint
AHA: (S53.114A) 4Q 2012, 108
7 ⊟ S53.115- Anterior dislocation of left ulnohumeral joint
7 ⊟ S53.116- Anterior dislocation of unspecified ulnohumeral joint
6 S53.12 Posterior subluxation and dislocation of ulnohumeral joint
7 ⊟ S53.121- Posterior subluxation of right ulnohumeral joint
7 ⊟ S53.122- Posterior subluxation of left ulnohumeral joint
7 ⊟ S53.123- Posterior subluxation of unspecified ulnohumeral joint
7 ⊟ S53.124- Posterior dislocation of right ulnohumeral joint
7 ⊟ S53.125- Posterior dislocation of left ulnohumeral joint
7 ⊟ S53.126- Posterior dislocation of unspecified ulnohumeral joint
6 S53.13 Medial subluxation and dislocation of ulnohumeral joint
7 ⊟ S53.131- Medial subluxation of right ulnohumeral joint
7 ⊟ S53.132- Medial subluxation of left ulnohumeral joint
7 ⊟ S53.133- Medial subluxation of unspecified ulnohumeral joint
7 ⊟ S53.134- Medial dislocation of right ulnohumeral joint
7 ⊟ S53.135- Medial dislocation of left ulnohumeral joint
7 ⊟ S53.136- Medial dislocation of unspecified ulnohumeral joint
6 S53.14 Lateral subluxation and dislocation of ulnohumeral joint
7 ⊟ S53.141- Lateral subluxation of right ulnohumeral joint
7 ⊟ S53.142- Lateral subluxation of left ulnohumeral joint
7 ⊟ S53.143- Lateral subluxation of unspecified ulnohumeral joint
7 ⊟ S53.144- Lateral dislocation of right ulnohumeral joint
7 ⊟ S53.145- Lateral dislocation of left ulnohumeral joint
7 ⊟ S53.146- Lateral dislocation of unspecified ulnohumeral joint
6 S53.19 Other subluxation and dislocation of ulnohumeral joint
7 ⊟ S53.191- Other subluxation of right ulnohumeral joint
7 ⊟ S53.192- Other subluxation of left ulnohumeral joint
7 ⊟ S53.193- Other subluxation of unspecified ulnohumeral joint
7 ⊟ S53.194- Other dislocation of right ulnohumeral joint
7 ⊟ S53.195- Other dislocation of left ulnohumeral joint
7 ⊟ S53.196- Other dislocation of unspecified ulnohumeral joint
5 S53.2 Traumatic rupture of radial collateral ligament
EXCLUDES 1 *sprain of radial collateral ligament NOS (S53.43-)*
7 ⊟ S53.20X- Traumatic rupture of unspecified radial collateral ligament
7 ⊟ S53.21X- Traumatic rupture of right radial collateral ligament
7 ⊟ S53.22X- Traumatic rupture of left radial collateral ligament
5 S53.3 Traumatic rupture of ulnar collateral ligament
EXCLUDES 1 *sprain of ulnar collateral ligament (S53.44-)*
7 ⊟ S53.30X- Traumatic rupture of unspecified ulnar collateral ligament
7 ⊟ S53.31X- Traumatic rupture of right ulnar collateral ligament
7 ⊟ S53.32X- Traumatic rupture of left ulnar collateral ligament
5 S53.4 Sprain of elbow
EXCLUDES 2 *traumatic rupture of radial collateral ligament (S53.2-)*
traumatic rupture of ulnar collateral ligament (S53.3-)
6 S53.40 Unspecified sprain of elbow
7 ⊟ S53.401- Unspecified sprain of right elbow
7 ⊟ S53.402- Unspecified sprain of left elbow
7 ⊟ S53.409- Unspecified sprain of unspecified elbow
Sprain of elbow NOS
6 S53.41 Radiohumeral (joint) sprain
7 ⊟ S53.411- Radiohumeral (joint) sprain of right elbow
7 ⊟ S53.412- Radiohumeral (joint) sprain of left elbow
7 ⊟ S53.419 Radiohumeral (joint) sprain of unspecified elbow
6 S53.42 Ulnohumeral (joint) sprain
7 ⊟ S53.421- Ulnohumeral (joint) sprain of right elbow
7 ⊟ S53.422- Ulnohumeral (joint) sprain of left elbow
7 ⊟ S53.429- Ulnohumeral (joint) sprain of unspecified elbow
6 S53.43 Radial collateral ligament sprain
7 ⊟ S53.431- Radial collateral ligament sprain of right elbow
7 ⊟ S53.432- Radial collateral ligament sprain of left elbow
7 ⊟ S53.439- Radial collateral ligament sprain of unspecified elbow
6 S53.44 Ulnar collateral ligament sprain
7 ⊟ S53.441- Ulnar collateral ligament sprain of right elbow
7 ⊟ S53.442- Ulnar collateral ligament sprain of left elbow
7 ⊟ S53.449- Ulnar collateral ligament sprain of unspecified elbow

6 S53.49 Other sprain of elbow
7 S53.491- Other sprain of right elbow
7 S53.492- Other sprain of left elbow
7 S53.499- Other sprain of unspecified elbow

4 S54 Injury of nerves at forearm level
Code also:
any associated open wound (S51.-)
EXCLUDES 2 *injury of nerves at wrist and hand level (S64.-)*

The appropriate 7th character is to be added to each code from category S54
A initial encounter
D subsequent encounter
S sequela

CODING TIP✓ Late effects of injuries are coded with seventh character S (sequela) and are sequenced after the residual condition of the late effect.

5 S54.0 Injury of ulnar nerve at forearm level
Injury of ulnar nerve NOS
7 S54.00X- Injury of ulnar nerve at forearm level, unspecified arm
7 S54.01X- Injury of ulnar nerve at forearm level, right arm
7 S54.02X- Injury of ulnar nerve at forearm level, left arm
5 S54.1 Injury of median nerve at forearm level
Injury of median nerve NOS
7 S54.10X- Injury of median nerve at forearm level, unspecified arm
7 S54.11X- Injury of median nerve at forearm level, right arm
7 S54.12X- Injury of median nerve at forearm level, left arm
5 S54.2 Injury of radial nerve at forearm level
Injury of radial nerve NOS
7 S54.20X- Injury of radial nerve at forearm level, unspecified arm
7 S54.21X- Injury of radial nerve at forearm level, right arm
7 S54.22X- Injury of radial nerve at forearm level, left arm
5 S54.3 Injury of cutaneous sensory nerve at forearm level
7 S54.30X- Injury of cutaneous sensory nerve at forearm level, unspecified arm
7 S54.31X- Injury of cutaneous sensory nerve at forearm level, right arm
7 S54.32X- Injury of cutaneous sensory nerve at forearm level, left arm
5 S54.8 Injury of other nerves at forearm level
6 S54.8X Injury of other nerves at forearm level
7 S54.8X1- Injury of other nerves at forearm level, right arm
7 S54.8X2- Injury of other nerves at forearm level, left arm
7 S54.8X9- Injury of other nerves at forearm level, unspecified arm
5 S54.9 Injury of unspecified nerve at forearm level
7 S54.90X- Injury of unspecified nerve at forearm level, unspecified arm
7 S54.91X- Injury of unspecified nerve at forearm level, right arm
7 S54.92X- Injury of unspecified nerve at forearm level, left arm

4 S55 Injury of blood vessels at forearm level
Code also:
any associated open wound (S51.-)
EXCLUDES 2 *injury of blood vessels at wrist and hand level (S65.-)*
injury of brachial vessels (S45.1-S45.2)

The appropriate 7th character is to be added to each code from category S55
A initial encounter
D subsequent encounter
S sequela

5 S55.0 Injury of ulnar artery at forearm level
6 S55.00 Unspecified injury of ulnar artery at forearm level
7 S55.001- Unspecified injury of ulnar artery at forearm level, right arm
7 S55.002- Unspecified injury of ulnar artery at forearm level, left arm
7 S55.009- Unspecified injury of ulnar artery at forearm level, unspecified arm
6 S55.01 Laceration of ulnar artery at forearm level
7 S55.011- Laceration of ulnar artery at forearm level, right arm
7 S55.012- Laceration of ulnar artery at forearm level, left arm
7 S55.019- Laceration of ulnar artery at forearm level, unspecified arm
6 S55.09 Other specified injury of ulnar artery at forearm level
7 S55.091- Other specified injury of ulnar artery at forearm level, right arm
7 S55.092- Other specified injury of ulnar artery at forearm level, left arm
7 S55.099- Other specified injury of ulnar artery at forearm level, unspecified arm
5 S55.1 Injury of radial artery at forearm level
6 S55.10 Unspecified injury of radial artery at forearm level
7 S55.101- Unspecified injury of radial artery at forearm level, right arm
7 S55.102- Unspecified injury of radial artery at forearm level, left arm
7 S55.109- Unspecified injury of radial artery at forearm level, unspecified arm
6 S55.11 Laceration of radial artery at forearm level
7 S55.111- Laceration of radial artery at forearm level, right arm
7 S55.112- Laceration of radial artery at forearm level, left arm
7 S55.119- Laceration of radial artery at forearm level, unspecified arm
6 S55.19 Other specified injury of radial artery at forearm level
7 S55.191- Other specified injury of radial artery at forearm level, right arm
7 S55.192- Other specified injury of radial artery at forearm level, left arm
7 S55.199- Other specified injury of radial artery at forearm level, unspecified arm
5 S55.2 Injury of vein at forearm level
6 S55.20 Unspecified injury of vein at forearm level
7 S55.201- Unspecified injury of vein at forearm level, right arm
7 S55.202- Unspecified injury of vein at forearm level, left arm
7 S55.209- Unspecified injury of vein at forearm level, unspecified arm
6 S55.21 Laceration of vein at forearm level
7 S55.211- Laceration of vein at forearm level, right arm
7 S55.212- Laceration of vein at forearm level, left arm
7 S55.219- Laceration of vein at forearm level, unspecified arm
6 S55.29 Other specified injury of vein at forearm level
7 S55.291- Other specified injury of vein at forearm level, right arm
7 S55.292- Other specified injury of vein at forearm level, left arm
7 S55.299- Other specified injury of vein at forearm level, unspecified arm
5 S55.8 Injury of other blood vessels at forearm level
6 S55.80 Unspecified injury of other blood vessels at forearm level
7 S55.801- Unspecified injury of other blood vessels at forearm level, right arm
7 S55.802- Unspecified injury of other blood vessels at forearm level, left arm
7 S55.809- Unspecified injury of other blood vessels at forearm level, unspecified arm
6 S55.81 Laceration of other blood vessels at forearm level
7 S55.811- Laceration of other blood vessels at forearm level, right arm

7 ⊟ S55.812- Laceration of other blood vessels at forearm level, left arm
7 ⊟ S55.819- Laceration of other blood vessels at forearm level, unspecified arm
6 S55.89 Other specified injury of other blood vessels at forearm level
7 ⊟ S55.891- Other specified injury of other blood vessels at forearm level, right arm
7 ⊟ S55.892- Other specified injury of other blood vessels at forearm level, left arm
7 ⊟ S55.899- Other specified injury of other blood vessels at forearm level, unspecified arm
5 S55.9 Injury of unspecified blood vessel at forearm level
6 S55.90 Unspecified injury of Unspecified blood vessel at forearm level
7 ⊟ S55.901- Unspecified injury of unspecified blood vessel at forearm level, right arm
7 ⊟ S55.902- Unspecified injury of unspecified blood vessel at forearm level, left arm
7 ⊟ S55.909- Unspecified injury of unspecified blood vessel at forearm level, unspecified arm
6 S55.91 Laceration of unspecified blood vessel at forearm level
7 ⊟ S55.911- Laceration of unspecified blood vessel at forearm level, right arm
7 ⊟ S55.912- Laceration of unspecified blood vessel at forearm level, left arm
7 ⊟ S55.919- Laceration of unspecified blood vessel at forearm level, unspecified arm
6 S55.99 Other specified injury of unspecified blood vessel at forearm level
7 ⊟ S55.991- Other specified injury of unspecified blood vessel at forearm level, right arm
7 ⊟ S55.992- Other specified injury of unspecified blood vessel at forearm level, left arm
7 ⊟ S55.999- Other specified injury of unspecified blood vessel at forearm level, unspecified arm

4 S56 Injury of muscle, fascia and tendon at forearm level

Code also:
any associated open wound (S51.-)

EXCLUDES 2 *injury of muscle, fascia and tendon at or below wrist (S66.-)*
sprain of joints and ligaments of elbow (S53.4-)

The appropriate 7th character is to be added to each code from category S56
A initial encounter
D subsequent encounter
S sequela

5 S56.0 Injury of flexor muscle, fascia and tendon of thumb at forearm level
6 S56.00 Unspecified injury of flexor muscle, fascia and tendon of thumb at forearm level
7 ⊟ S56.001- Unspecified injury of flexor muscle, fascia and tendon of right thumb at forearm level
7 ⊟ S56.002- Unspecified injury of flexor muscle, fascia and tendon of left thumb at forearm level
7 ⊟ S56.009- Unspecified injury of flexor muscle, fascia and tendon of unspecified thumb at forearm level
6 S56.01 Strain of flexor muscle, fascia and tendon of thumb at forearm level
7 ⊟ S56.011- Strain of flexor muscle, fascia and tendon of right thumb at forearm level
7 ⊟ S56.012- Strain of flexor muscle, fascia and tendon of left thumb at forearm level
7 ⊟ S56.019- Strain of flexor muscle, fascia and tendon of unspecified thumb at forearm level
6 S56.02 Laceration of flexor muscle, fascia and tendon of thumb at forearm level
7 ⊟ S56.021- Laceration of flexor muscle, fascia and tendon of right thumb at forearm level
7 ⊟ S56.022- Laceration of flexor muscle, fascia and tendon of left thumb at forearm level
7 ⊟ S56.029- Laceration of flexor muscle, fascia and tendon of unspecified thumb at forearm level
6 S56.09 Other injury of flexor muscle, fascia and tendon of thumb at forearm level
7 ⊟ S56.091- Other injury of flexor muscle, fascia and tendon of right thumb at forearm level
7 ⊟ S56.092- Other injury of flexor muscle, fascia and tendon of left thumb at forearm level
7 ⊟ S56.099- Other injury of flexor muscle, fascia and tendon of unspecified thumb at forearm level
5 S56.1 Injury of flexor muscle, fascia and tendon of other and unspecified finger at forearm level
6 S56.10 Unspecified injury of flexor muscle, fascia and tendon of other and Unspecified finger at forearm level
7 ⊟ S56.101- Unspecified injury of flexor muscle, fascia and tendon of right index finger at forearm level
7 ⊟ S56.102- Unspecified injury of flexor muscle, fascia and tendon of left index finger at forearm level
7 ⊟ S56.103- Unspecified injury of flexor muscle, fascia and tendon of right middle finger at forearm level
7 ⊟ S56.104- Unspecified injury of flexor muscle, fascia and tendon of left middle finger at forearm level
7 ⊟ S56.105- Unspecified injury of flexor muscle, fascia and tendon of right ring finger at forearm level
7 ⊟ S56.106- Unspecified injury of flexor muscle, fascia and tendon of left ring finger at forearm level
7 ⊟ S56.107- Unspecified injury of flexor muscle, fascia and tendon of right little finger at forearm level
7 ⊟ S56.108- Unspecified injury of flexor muscle, fascia and tendon of left little finger at forearm level
7 ⊟ S56.109- Unspecified injury of flexor muscle, fascia and tendon of unspecified finger at forearm level
6 S56.11 Strain of flexor muscle, fascia and tendon of other and unspecified finger at forearm level
7 ⊟ S56.111- Strain of flexor muscle, fascia and tendon of right index finger at forearm level
7 ⊟ S56.112- Strain of flexor muscle, fascia and tendon of left index finger at forearm level
7 ⊟ S56.113- Strain of flexor muscle, fascia and tendon of right middle finger at forearm level
7 ⊟ S56.114- Strain of flexor muscle, fascia and tendon of left middle finger at forearm level
7 ⊟ S56.115- Strain of flexor muscle, fascia and tendon of right ring finger at forearm level
7 ⊟ S56.116- Strain of flexor muscle, fascia and tendon of left ring finger at forearm level
7 ⊟ S56.117- Strain of flexor muscle, fascia and tendon of right little finger at forearm level
7 ⊟ S56.118- Strain of flexor muscle, fascia and tendon of left little finger at forearm level
7 ⊟ S56.119- Strain of flexor muscle, fascia and tendon of finger of unspecified finger at forearm level
6 S56.12 Laceration of flexor muscle, fascia and tendon of other and unspecified finger at forearm level
7 ⊟ S56.121- Laceration of flexor muscle, fascia and tendon of right index finger at forearm level
7 ⊟ S56.122- Laceration of flexor muscle, fascia and tendon of left index finger at forearm level
7 ⊟ S56.123- Laceration of flexor muscle, fascia and tendon of right middle finger at forearm level
7 ⊟ S56.124- Laceration of flexor muscle, fascia and tendon of left middle finger at forearm level
7 ⊟ S56.125- Laceration of flexor muscle, fascia and tendon of right ring finger at forearm level
7 ⊟ S56.126- Laceration of flexor muscle, fascia and tendon of left ring finger at forearm level
7 ⊟ S56.127- Laceration of flexor muscle, fascia and tendon of right little finger at forearm level
7 ⊟ S56.128- Laceration of flexor muscle, fascia and tendon of left little finger at forearm level
7 ⊟ S56.129- Laceration of flexor muscle, fascia and tendon of unspecified finger at forearm level
6 S56.19 Other injury of flexor muscle, fascia and tendon of Other and unspecified finger at forearm level
7 ⊟ S56.191- Other injury of flexor muscle, fascia and tendon of right index finger at forearm level

7 ⊟ S56.192- Other injury of flexor muscle, fascia and tendon of left index finger at forearm level
7 ⊟ S56.193- Other injury of flexor muscle, fascia and tendon of right middle finger at forearm level
7 ⊟ S56.194- Other injury of flexor muscle, fascia and tendon of left middle finger at forearm level
7 ⊟ S56.195- Other injury of flexor muscle, fascia and tendon of right ring finger at forearm level
7 ⊟ S56.196- Other injury of flexor muscle, fascia and tendon of left ring finger at forearm level
7 ⊟ S56.197- Other injury of flexor muscle, fascia and tendon of right little finger at forearm level
7 ⊟ S56.198- Other injury of flexor muscle, fascia and tendon of left little finger at forearm level
7 ⊟ S56.199- Other injury of flexor muscle, fascia and tendon of unspecified finger at forearm level

5 S56.2 Injury of other flexor muscle, fascia and tendon at forearm level

6 S56.20 Unspecified injury of other flexor muscle, fascia and tendon at forearm level
7 ⊟ S56.201- Unspecified injury of other flexor muscle, fascia and tendon at forearm level, right arm
7 ⊟ S56.202- Unspecified injury of other flexor muscle, fascia and tendon at forearm level, left arm
7 ⊟ S56.209- Unspecified injury of other flexor muscle, fascia and tendon at forearm level, unspecified arm

6 S56.21 Strain of other flexor muscle, fascia and tendon at forearm level
7 ⊟ S56.211- Strain of other flexor muscle, fascia and tendon at forearm level, right arm
7 ⊟ S56.212- Strain of other flexor muscle, fascia and tendon at forearm level, left arm
7 ⊟ S56.219- Strain of other flexor muscle, fascia and tendon at forearm level, unspecified arm

6 S56.22 Laceration of other flexor muscle, fascia and tendon at forearm level
7 ⊟ S56.221- Laceration of other flexor muscle, fascia and tendon at forearm level, right arm
7 ⊟ S56.222- Laceration of other flexor muscle, fascia and tendon at forearm level, left arm
7 ⊟ S56.229- Laceration of other flexor muscle, fascia and tendon at forearm level, unspecified arm

6 S56.29 Other injury of Other flexor muscle, fascia and tendon at forearm level
7 ⊟ S56.291- Other injury of other flexor muscle, fascia and tendon at forearm level, right arm
7 ⊟ S56.292- Other injury of other flexor muscle, fascia and tendon at forearm level, left arm
7 ⊟ S56.299- Other injury of other flexor muscle, fascia and tendon at forearm level, unspecified arm

5 S56.3 Injury of extensor or abductor muscles, fascia and tendons of thumb at forearm level

6 S56.30 Unspecified injury of extensor or abductor muscles, fascia and tendons of thumb at forearm level
7 ⊟ S56.301- Unspecified injury of extensor or abductor muscles, fascia and tendons of right thumb at forearm level
7 ⊟ S56.302- Unspecified injury of extensor or abductor muscles, fascia and tendons of left thumb at forearm level
7 ⊟ S56.309- Unspecified injury of extensor or abductor muscles, fascia and tendons of unspecified thumb at forearm level

6 S56.31 Strain of extensor or abductor muscles, fascia and tendons of thumb at forearm level
7 ⊟ S56.311- Strain of extensor or abductor muscles, fascia and tendons of right thumb at forearm level
7 ⊟ S56.312- Strain of extensor or abductor muscles, fascia and tendons of left thumb at forearm level
7 ⊟ S56.319- Strain of extensor or abductor muscles, fascia and tendons of unspecified thumb at forearm level

6 S56.32 Laceration of extensor or abductor muscles, fascia and tendons of thumb at forearm level
7 ⊟ S56.321- Laceration of extensor or abductor muscles, fascia and tendons of right thumb at forearm level
7 ⊟ S56.322- Laceration of extensor or abductor muscles, fascia and tendons of left thumb at forearm level
7 ⊟ S56.329- Laceration of extensor or abductor muscles, fascia and tendons of unspecified thumb at forearm level

6 S56.39 Other injury of extensor or abductor muscles, fascia and tendons of thumb at forearm level
7 ⊟ S56.391- Other injury of extensor or abductor muscles, fascia and tendons of right thumb at forearm level
7 ⊟ S56.392- Other injury of extensor or abductor muscles, fascia and tendons of left thumb at forearm level
7 ⊟ S56.399- Other injury of extensor or abductor muscles, fascia and tendons of unspecified thumb at forearm level

5 S56.4 Injury of extensor muscle, fascia and tendon of other and unspecified finger at forearm level

6 S56.40 Unspecified injury of extensor muscle, fascia and tendon of other and Unspecified finger at forearm level
7 ⊟ S56.401- Unspecified injury of extensor muscle, fascia and tendon of right index finger at forearm level
7 ⊟ S56.402- Unspecified injury of extensor muscle, fascia and tendon of left index finger at forearm level
7 ⊟ S56.403- Unspecified injury of extensor muscle, fascia and tendon of right middle finger at forearm level
7 ⊟ S56.404- Unspecified injury of extensor muscle, fascia and tendon of left middle finger at forearm level
7 ⊟ S56.405- Unspecified injury of extensor muscle, fascia and tendon of right ring finger at forearm level
7 ⊟ S56.406- Unspecified injury of extensor muscle, fascia and tendon of left ring finger at forearm level
7 ⊟ S56.407- Unspecified injury of extensor muscle, fascia and tendon of right little finger at forearm level
7 ⊟ S56.408- Unspecified injury of extensor muscle, fascia and tendon of left little finger at forearm level
7 ⊟ S56.409- Unspecified injury of extensor muscle, fascia and tendon of unspecified finger at forearm level

6 S56.41 Strain of extensor muscle, fascia and tendon of other and unspecified finger at forearm level
7 ⊟ S56.411- Strain of extensor muscle, fascia and tendon of right index finger at forearm level
7 ⊟ S56.412- Strain of extensor muscle, fascia and tendon of left index finger at forearm level
7 ⊟ S56.413- Strain of extensor muscle, fascia and tendon of right middle finger at forearm level
7 ⊟ S56.414- Strain of extensor muscle, fascia and tendon of left middle finger at forearm level
7 ⊟ S56.415- Strain of extensor muscle, fascia and tendon of right ring finger at forearm level
7 ⊟ S56.416- Strain of extensor muscle, fascia and tendon of left ring finger at forearm level
7 ⊟ S56.417- Strain of extensor muscle, fascia and tendon of right little finger at forearm level
7 ⊟ S56.418- Strain of extensor muscle, fascia and tendon of left little finger at forearm level
7 ⊟ S56.419- Strain of extensor muscle, fascia and tendon of finger, unspecified finger at forearm level

6 S56.42 Laceration of extensor muscle, fascia and tendon of other and unspecified finger at forearm level
7 ⊟ S56.421- Laceration of extensor muscle, fascia and tendon of right index finger at forearm level
7 ⊟ S56.422- Laceration of extensor muscle, fascia and tendon of left index finger at forearm level

7 ⊟ S56.423- Laceration of extensor muscle, fascia and tendon of right middle finger at forearm level
7 ⊟ S56.424- Laceration of extensor muscle, fascia and tendon of left middle finger at forearm level
7 ⊟ S56.425- Laceration of extensor muscle, fascia and tendon of right ring finger at forearm level
7 ⊟ S56.426- Laceration of extensor muscle, fascia and tendon of left ring finger at forearm level
7 ⊟ S56.427- Laceration of extensor muscle, fascia and tendon of right little finger at forearm level
7 ⊟ S56.428- Laceration of extensor muscle, fascia and tendon of left little finger at forearm level
7 ⊟ S56.429- Laceration of extensor muscle, fascia and tendon of unspecified finger at forearm level

6 S56.49 Other injury of extensor muscle, fascia and tendon of Other and unspecified finger at forearm level
7 ⊟ S56.491- Other injury of extensor muscle, fascia and tendon of right index finger at forearm level
7 ⊟ S56.492- Other injury of extensor muscle, fascia and tendon of left index finger at forearm level
7 ⊟ S56.493- Other injury of extensor muscle, fascia and tendon of right middle finger at forearm level
7 ⊟ S56.494- Other injury of extensor muscle, fascia and tendon of left middle finger at forearm level
7 ⊟ S56.495- Other injury of extensor muscle, fascia and tendon of right ring finger at forearm level
7 ⊟ S56.496- Other injury of extensor muscle, fascia and tendon of left ring finger at forearm level
7 ⊟ S56.497- Other injury of extensor muscle, fascia and tendon of right little finger at forearm level
7 ⊟ S56.498- Other injury of extensor muscle, fascia and tendon of left little finger at forearm level
7 ⊟ S56.499- Other injury of extensor muscle, fascia and tendon of unspecified finger at forearm level

5 S56.5 Injury of other extensor muscle, fascia and tendon at forearm level

6 S56.50 Unspecified injury of other extensor muscle, fascia and tendon at forearm level
7 ⊟ S56.501- Unspecified injury of other extensor muscle, fascia and tendon at forearm level, right arm
7 ⊟ S56.502- Unspecified injury of other extensor muscle, fascia and tendon at forearm level, left arm
7 ⊟ S56.509- Unspecified injury of other extensor muscle, fascia and tendon at forearm level, unspecified arm

6 S56.51 Strain of other extensor muscle, fascia and tendon at forearm level
7 ⊟ S56.511- Strain of other extensor muscle, fascia and tendon at forearm level, right arm
7 ⊟ S56.512- Strain of other extensor muscle, fascia and tendon at forearm level, left arm
7 ⊟ S56.519- Strain of other extensor muscle, fascia and tendon at forearm level, unspecified arm

6 S56.52 Laceration of other extensor muscle, fascia and tendon at forearm level
7 ⊟ S56.521- Laceration of other extensor muscle, fascia and tendon at forearm level, right arm
7 ⊟ S56.522- Laceration of other extensor muscle, fascia and tendon at forearm level, left arm
7 ⊟ S56.529- Laceration of other extensor muscle, fascia and tendon at forearm level, unspecified arm

6 S56.59 Other injury of Other extensor muscle, fascia and tendon at forearm level
7 ⊟ S56.591- Other injury of other extensor muscle, fascia and tendon at forearm level, right arm
7 ⊟ S56.592- Other injury of other extensor muscle, fascia and tendon at forearm level, left arm
7 ⊟ S56.599- Other injury of other extensor muscle, fascia and tendon at forearm level, unspecified arm

5 S56.8 Injury of other muscles, fascia and tendons at forearm level

6 S56.80 Unspecified injury of other muscles, fascia and tendons at forearm level
7 ⊟ S56.801- Unspecified injury of other muscles, fascia and tendons at forearm level, right arm
7 ⊟ S56.802- Unspecified injury of other muscles, fascia and tendons at forearm level, left arm
7 ⊟ S56.809- Unspecified injury of other muscles, fascia and tendons at forearm level, unspecified arm

6 S56.81 Strain of other muscles, fascia and tendons at forearm level
7 ⊟ S56.811- Strain of other muscles, fascia and tendons at forearm level, right arm
7 ⊟ S56.812- Strain of other muscles, fascia and tendons at forearm level, left arm
7 ⊟ S56.819- Strain of other muscles, fascia and tendons at forearm level, unspecified arm

6 S56.82 Laceration of other muscles, fascia and tendons at forearm level
7 ⊟ S56.821- Laceration of other muscles, fascia and tendons at forearm level, right arm
7 ⊟ S56.822- Laceration of other muscles, fascia and tendons at forearm level, left arm
7 ⊟ S56.829- Laceration of other muscles, fascia and tendons at forearm level, unspecified arm

6 S56.89 Other injury of Other muscles, fascia and tendons at forearm level
7 ⊟ S56.891- Other injury of other muscles, fascia and tendons at forearm level, right arm
7 ⊟ S56.892- Other injury of other muscles, fascia and tendons at forearm level, left arm
7 ⊟ S56.899- Other injury of other muscles, fascia and tendons at forearm level, unspecified arm

5 S56.9 Injury of unspecified muscles, fascia and tendons at forearm level

6 S56.90 Unspecified injury of Unspecified muscles, fascia and tendons at forearm level
7 ⊟ S56.901- Unspecified injury of unspecified muscles, fascia and tendons at forearm level, right arm
7 ⊟ S56.902- Unspecified injury of unspecified muscles, fascia and tendons at forearm level, left arm
7 ⊟ S56.909- Unspecified injury of unspecified muscles, fascia and tendons at forearm level, unspecified arm

6 S56.91 Strain of unspecified muscles, fascia and tendons at forearm level
7 ⊟ S56.911- Strain of unspecified muscles, fascia and tendons at forearm level, right arm
7 ⊟ S56.912- Strain of unspecified muscles, fascia and tendons at forearm level, left arm
7 ⊟ S56.919- Strain of unspecified muscles, fascia and tendons at forearm level, unspecified arm

6 S56.92 Laceration of unspecified muscles, fascia and tendons at forearm level
7 ⊟ S56.921- Laceration of unspecified muscles, fascia and tendons at forearm level, right arm
7 ⊟ S56.922- Laceration of unspecified muscles, fascia and tendons at forearm level, left arm
7 ⊟ S56.929- Laceration of unspecified muscles, fascia and tendons at forearm level, unspecified arm

6 S56.99 Other injury of unspecified muscles, fascia and tendons at forearm level
7 ⊟ S56.991- Other injury of unspecified muscles, fascia and tendons at forearm level, right arm
7 ⊟ S56.992- Other injury of unspecified muscles, fascia and tendons at forearm level, left arm
7 ⊟ S56.999- Other injury of unspecified muscles, fascia and tendons at forearm level, unspecified arm

4 S57 Crushing injury of elbow and forearm

Use additional code(s) for all associated injuries

EXCLUDES 2 *crushing injury of wrist and hand (S67.-)*

The appropriate 7th character is to be added to each code from category S57
A initial encounter
D subsequent encounter
S sequela

● New *Manifestation* 4-7 Digit Indicators ⊟ Laterality A Adult M Maternity N Newborn P Pediatric ♂ Male
▲ Revised Unspecified AHA Coding Clinic HCC Hierarchical Condition Categories HIV HIV Related Conditions ♀ Female

S57.0 Crushing injury of elbow
- S57.00X- Crushing injury of unspecified elbow
- S57.01X- Crushing injury of right elbow
- S57.02X- Crushing injury of left elbow

S57.8 Crushing injury of forearm
- S57.80X- Crushing injury of unspecified forearm
- S57.81X- Crushing injury of right forearm
- S57.82X- Crushing injury of left forearm

S58 Traumatic amputation of elbow and forearm

An amputation not identified as partial or complete should be coded to complete

EXCLUDES 1 *traumatic amputation of wrist and hand (S68.-)*

The appropriate 7th character is to be added to each code from category S58
- A initial encounter
- D subsequent encounter
- S sequela

CODING TIP ✓ Use these codes only when the amputation was due to trauma. There is no need for adding Z89 with traumatic amputations. See Z47.81 for care of amputations not due to trauma.

S58.0 Traumatic amputation at elbow level

S58.01 Complete traumatic amputation at elbow level
- S58.011- Complete traumatic amputation at elbow level, right arm HCC
- S58.012- Complete traumatic amputation at elbow level, left arm HCC
- S58.019- Complete traumatic amputation at elbow level, unspecified arm HCC

S58.02 Partial traumatic amputation at elbow level
- S58.021- Partial traumatic amputation at elbow level, right arm HCC
- S58.022- Partial traumatic amputation at elbow level, left arm HCC
- S58.029- Partial traumatic amputation at elbow level, unspecified arm HCC

S58.1 Traumatic amputation at level between elbow and wrist

S58.11 Complete traumatic amputation at level between elbow and wrist
- S58.111- Complete traumatic amputation at level between elbow and wrist, right arm HCC
- S58.112- Complete traumatic amputation at level between elbow and wrist, left arm HCC
- S58.119- Complete traumatic amputation at level between elbow and wrist, unspecified arm HCC

S58.12 Partial traumatic amputation at level between elbow and wrist
- S58.121- Partial traumatic amputation at level between elbow and wrist, right arm HCC
- S58.122- Partial traumatic amputation at level between elbow and wrist, left arm HCC
- S58.129- Partial traumatic amputation at level between elbow and wrist, unspecified arm HCC

S58.9 Traumatic amputation of forearm, level unspecified

EXCLUDES 1 *traumatic amputation of wrist (S68.-)*

S58.91 Complete traumatic amputation of forearm, level unspecified
- S58.911- Complete traumatic amputation of right forearm, level unspecified HCC
- S58.912- Complete traumatic amputation of left forearm, level unspecified HCC
- S58.919- Complete traumatic amputation of unspecified forearm, level unspecified HCC

S58.92 Partial traumatic amputation of forearm, level unspecified
- S58.921- Partial traumatic amputation of right forearm, level unspecified HCC
- S58.922- Partial traumatic amputation of left forearm, level unspecified HCC
- S58.929- Partial traumatic amputation of unspecified forearm, level unspecified HCC

S59 Other and unspecified injuries of elbow and forearm

EXCLUDES 2 *other and unspecified injuries of wrist and hand (S69.-)*

The appropriate 7th character is to be added to each code from subcategories S59.0, S59.1, and S59.2
- A initial encounter for closed fracture
- D subsequent encounter for fracture with routine healing
- G subsequent encounter for fracture with delayed healing
- K subsequent encounter for fracture with nonunion
- P subsequent encounter for fracture with malunion
- S sequela

CODING TIP ✓ A Salter-Harris physeal fracture occurs through the growth plate. Only one code is needed to report a single physeal fracture. Because of the implications for future bone development, coding of a Salter-Harris fracture takes priority over a simple fracture code. Assign the physeal fracture code based on location, type, and laterality. Use a code for "other physeal fracture" for Type V.

S59.0 Physeal fracture of lower end of ulna

S59.00 Unspecified physeal fracture of lower end of ulna
- S59.001- Unspecified physeal fracture of lower end of ulna, right arm
- S59.002- Unspecified physeal fracture of lower end of ulna, left arm
- S59.009- Unspecified physeal fracture of lower end of ulna, unspecified arm

S59.01 Salter-Harris Type I physeal fracture of lower end of ulna
- S59.011- Salter-Harris Type I physeal fracture of lower end of ulna, right arm
- S59.012- Salter-Harris Type I physeal fracture of lower end of ulna, left arm
- S59.019- Salter-Harris Type I physeal fracture of lower end of ulna, unspecified arm

S59.02 Salter-Harris Type II physeal fracture of lower end of ulna
- S59.021- Salter-Harris Type II physeal fracture of lower end of ulna, right arm
- S59.022- Salter-Harris Type II physeal fracture of lower end of ulna, left arm
- S59.029- Salter-Harris Type II physeal fracture of lower end of ulna, unspecified arm

S59.03 Salter-Harris Type III physeal fracture of lower end of ulna
- S59.031- Salter-Harris Type III physeal fracture of lower end of ulna, right arm
- S59.032- Salter-Harris Type III physeal fracture of lower end of ulna, left arm
- S59.039- Salter-Harris Type III physeal fracture of lower end of ulna, unspecified arm

S59.04 Salter-Harris Type IV physeal fracture of lower end of ulna
- S59.041- Salter-Harris Type IV physeal fracture of lower end of ulna, right arm
- S59.042- Salter-Harris Type IV physeal fracture of lower end of ulna, left arm
- S59.049- Salter-Harris Type IV physeal fracture of lower end of ulna, unspecified arm

S59.09 Other physeal fracture of lower end of ulna
- S59.091- Other physeal fracture of lower end of ulna, right arm
- S59.092- Other physeal fracture of lower end of ulna, left arm
- S59.099- Other physeal fracture of lower end of ulna, unspecified arm

S59.1 Physeal fracture of upper end of radius

S59.10 Unspecified physeal fracture of upper end of radius
- S59.101- Unspecified physeal fracture of upper end of radius, right arm
- S59.102- Unspecified physeal fracture of upper end of radius, left arm
- S59.109- Unspecified physeal fracture of upper end of radius, unspecified arm

S59.11 Salter-Harris Type I physeal fracture of upper end of radius

7 ⊟ S59.111- Salter-Harris Type I physeal fracture of upper end of radius, right arm
7 ⊟ S59.112- Salter-Harris Type I physeal fracture of upper end of radius, left arm
7 ⊟ S59.119- Salter-Harris Type I physeal fracture of upper end of radius, unspecified arm
6 S59.12 Salter-Harris Type II physeal fracture of upper end of radius
7 ⊟ S59.121- Salter-Harris Type II physeal fracture of upper end of radius, right arm
7 ⊟ S59.122- Salter-Harris Type II physeal fracture of upper end of radius, left arm
7 ⊟ S59.129- Salter-Harris Type II physeal fracture of upper end of radius, unspecified arm
6 S59.13 Salter-Harris Type III physeal fracture of upper end of radius
7 ⊟ S59.131- Salter-Harris Type III physeal fracture of upper end of radius, right arm
7 ⊟ S59.132- Salter-Harris Type III physeal fracture of upper end of radius, left arm
7 ⊟ S59.139- Salter-Harris Type III physeal fracture of upper end of radius, unspecified arm
6 S59.14 Salter-Harris Type IV physeal fracture of upper end of radius
7 ⊟ S59.141- Salter-Harris Type IV physeal fracture of upper end of radius, right arm
7 ⊟ S59.142- Salter-Harris Type IV physeal fracture of upper end of radius, left arm
7 ⊟ S59.149- Salter-Harris Type IV physeal fracture of upper end of radius, unspecified arm
6 S59.19 Other physeal fracture of upper end of radius
7 ⊟ S59.191- Other physeal fracture of upper end of radius, right arm
7 ⊟ S59.192- Other physeal fracture of upper end of radius, left arm
7 ⊟ S59.199- Other physeal fracture of upper end of radius, unspecified arm
5 S59.2 Physeal fracture of lower end of radius
6 S59.20 Unspecified physeal fracture of lower end of radius
7 ⊟ S59.201- Unspecified physeal fracture of lower end of radius, right arm
7 ⊟ S59.202- Unspecified physeal fracture of lower end of radius, left arm
7 ⊟ S59.209- Unspecified physeal fracture of lower end of radius, unspecified arm
6 S59.21 Salter-Harris Type I physeal fracture of lower end of radius
7 ⊟ S59.211- Salter-Harris Type I physeal fracture of lower end of radius, right arm
7 ⊟ S59.212- Salter-Harris Type I physeal fracture of lower end of radius, left arm
7 ⊟ S59.219- Salter-Harris Type I physeal fracture of lower end of radius, unspecified arm
6 S59.22 Salter-Harris Type II physeal fracture of lower end of radius
7 ⊟ S59.221- Salter-Harris Type II physeal fracture of lower end of radius, right arm
7 ⊟ S59.222- Salter-Harris Type II physeal fracture of lower end of radius, left arm
7 ⊟ S59.229- Salter-Harris Type II physeal fracture of lower end of radius, unspecified arm
6 S59.23 Salter-Harris Type III physeal fracture of lower end of radius
7 ⊟ S59.231- Salter-Harris Type III physeal fracture of lower end of radius, right arm
7 ⊟ S59.232- Salter-Harris Type III physeal fracture of lower end of radius, left arm
7 ⊟ S59.239- Salter-Harris Type III physeal fracture of lower end of radius, unspecified arm
6 S59.24 Salter-Harris Type IV physeal fracture of lower end of radius
7 ⊟ S59.241- Salter-Harris Type IV physeal fracture of lower end of radius, right arm
7 ⊟ S59.242- Salter-Harris Type IV physeal fracture of lower end of radius, left arm
7 ⊟ S59.249- Salter-Harris Type IV physeal fracture of lower end of radius, unspecified arm
6 S59.29 Other physeal fracture of lower end of radius
7 ⊟ S59.291- Other physeal fracture of lower end of radius, right arm
7 ⊟ S59.292- Other physeal fracture of lower end of radius, left arm
7 ⊟ S59.299- Other physeal fracture of lower end of radius, unspecified arm
5 S59.8 Other specified injuries of elbow and forearm

The appropriate 7th character is to be added to each code in subcategory S59.8
A initial encounter
D subsequent encounter
S sequela

6 S59.80 Other specified injuries of elbow
7 ⊟ S59.801- Other specified injuries of right elbow
7 ⊟ S59.802- Other specified injuries of left elbow
7 ⊟ S59.809- Other specified injuries of unspecified elbow
6 S59.81 Other specified injuries of forearm
7 ⊟ S59.811- Other specified injuries right forearm
7 ⊟ S59.812- Other specified injuries left forearm
7 ⊟ S59.819- Other specified injuries unspecified forearm
5 S59.9 Unspecified injury of elbow and forearm

The appropriate 7th character is to be added to each code in subcategory S59.9
A initial encounter
D subsequent encounter
S sequela

6 S59.90 Unspecified injury of elbow
7 ⊟ S59.901- Unspecified injury of right elbow
7 ⊟ S59.902- Unspecified injury of left elbow
7 ⊟ S59.909- Unspecified injury of unspecified elbow
6 S59.91 Unspecified injury of forearm
7 ⊟ S59.911- Unspecified injury of right forearm
7 ⊟ S59.912- Unspecified injury of left forearm
7 ⊟ S59.919- Unspecified injury of unspecified forearm

Injuries to the wrist, hand and fingers (S60-S69)

EXCLUDES 2 *burns and corrosions (T20-T32)*
frostbite (T33-T34)
insect bite or sting, venomous (T63.4)

GUIDELINES **Section I.C.19.c.2)**
Multiple fractures are sequenced in accordance with the severity of the fracture.

GUIDELINES **Section I.C.19.b.1)-2)**
When coding injuries, assign separate codes for each injury unless a combination code is provided, in which case the combination code is assigned ... Traumatic injury codes (S00-T14.9) are not to be used for normal, healing surgical wounds or to identify complications of surgical wounds. The code for the most serious injury, as determined by the provider and the focus of treatment, is sequenced first.

1) Superficial injuries such as abrasions or contusions are not coded when associated with more severe injuries of the same site.

2) When a primary injury results in minor damage to peripheral nerves or blood vessels, the primary injury is sequenced first with additional code(s) for injuries to nerves and spinal cord (such as category S04), and/or injury to blood vessels (such as category S15). When the primary injury is to the blood vessels or nerves, that injury should be sequenced first.

GUIDELINES **Section I.C.19.c**
Coding of Traumatic Fractures: The principles of multiple coding of injuries should be followed in coding fractures. Fractures of specified sites are coded individually by site in accordance with both the provisions within categories S02, S12, S22, S32, S42, S49, S52, S59, S62, S72, S79, S82, S89, S92 and the level of detail furnished by medical record content. A fracture not indicated as open or closed should be coded to closed. A fracture not indicated whether displaced or not displaced should be coded to displaced.

4 S60 Superficial injury of wrist, hand and fingers

The appropriate 7th character is to be added to each code from category S60
A initial encounter
D subsequent encounter
S sequela

5 S60.0 Contusion of finger without damage to nail
EXCLUDES 1 *contusion involving nail (matrix) (S60.1)*

7 S60.00X- Contusion of unspecified finger without damage to nail
Contusion of finger(s) NOS

6 S60.01 Contusion of thumb without damage to nail
- 7 S60.011- Contusion of right thumb without damage to nail
- 7 S60.012- Contusion of left thumb without damage to nail
- 7 S60.019- Contusion of unspecified thumb without damage to nail

6 S60.02 Contusion of index finger without damage to nail
- 7 S60.021- Contusion of right index finger without damage to nail
- 7 S60.022- Contusion of left index finger without damage to nail
- 7 S60.029- Contusion of unspecified index finger without damage to nail

6 S60.03 Contusion of middle finger without damage to nail
- 7 S60.031- Contusion of right middle finger without damage to nail
- 7 S60.032- Contusion of left middle finger without damage to nail
- 7 S60.039- Contusion of unspecified middle finger without damage to nail

6 S60.04 Contusion of ring finger without damage to nail
- 7 S60.041- Contusion of right ring finger without damage to nail
- 7 S60.042- Contusion of left ring finger without damage to nail
- 7 S60.049- Contusion of unspecified ring finger without damage to nail

6 S60.05 Contusion of little finger without damage to nail
- 7 S60.051- Contusion of right little finger without damage to nail
- 7 S60.052- Contusion of left little finger without damage to nail
- 7 S60.059- Contusion of unspecified little finger without damage to nail

5 S60.1 Contusion of finger with damage to nail

7 S60.10X- Contusion of unspecified finger with damage to nail

6 S60.11 Contusion of thumb with damage to nail
- 7 S60.111- Contusion of right thumb with damage to nail
- 7 S60.112- Contusion of left thumb with damage to nail
- 7 S60.119- Contusion of unspecified thumb with damage to nail

6 S60.12 Contusion of index finger with damage to nail
- 7 S60.121- Contusion of right index finger with damage to nail
- 7 S60.122- Contusion of left index finger with damage to nail
- 7 S60.129- Contusion of unspecified index finger with damage to nail

6 S60.13 Contusion of middle finger with damage to nail
- 7 S60.131- Contusion of right middle finger with damage to nail
- 7 S60.132- Contusion of left middle finger with damage to nail
- 7 S60.139- Contusion of unspecified middle finger with damage to nail

6 S60.14 Contusion of ring finger with damage to nail
- 7 S60.141- Contusion of right ring finger with damage to nail
- 7 S60.142- Contusion of left ring finger with damage to nail
- 7 S60.149- Contusion of unspecified ring finger with damage to nail

6 S60.15 Contusion of little finger with damage to nail
- 7 S60.151- Contusion of right little finger with damage to nail
- 7 S60.152- Contusion of left little finger with damage to nail
- 7 S60.159- Contusion of unspecified little finger with damage to nail

5 S60.2 Contusion of wrist and hand
EXCLUDES 2 *contusion of fingers (S60.0-, S60.1-)*

6 S60.21 Contusion of wrist
- 7 S60.211- Contusion of right wrist
- 7 S60.212- Contusion of left wrist
- 7 S60.219- Contusion of unspecified wrist

6 S60.22 Contusion of hand
- 7 S60.221- Contusion of right hand
- 7 S60.222- Contusion of left hand
- 7 S60.229- Contusion of unspecified hand

5 S60.3 Other superficial injuries of thumb

6 S60.31 Abrasion of thumb
- 7 S60.311- Abrasion of right thumb
- 7 S60.312- Abrasion of left thumb
- 7 S60.319- Abrasion of unspecified thumb

6 S60.32 Blister (nonthermal) of thumb
- 7 S60.321- Blister (nonthermal) of right thumb
- 7 S60.322- Blister (nonthermal) of left thumb
- 7 S60.329- Blister (nonthermal) of unspecified thumb

6 S60.34 External constriction of thumb
Hair tourniquet syndrome of thumb
Use additional cause code to identify the constricting item (W49.0-)
- 7 S60.341- External constriction of right thumb
- 7 S60.342- External constriction of left thumb
- 7 S60.349- External constriction of unspecified thumb

6 S60.35 Superficial foreign body of thumb
Splinter in the thumb
- 7 S60.351- Superficial foreign body of right thumb
- 7 S60.352- Superficial foreign body of left thumb
- 7 S60.359- Superficial foreign body of unspecified thumb

6 S60.36 Insect bite (nonvenomous) of thumb
- 7 S60.361- Insect bite (nonvenomous) of right thumb
- 7 S60.362- Insect bite (nonvenomous) of left thumb
- 7 S60.369- Insect bite (nonvenomous) of unspecified thumb

6 S60.37 Other superficial bite of thumb
EXCLUDES 1 *open bite of thumb (S61.05-, S61.15-)*
- 7 S60.371- Other superficial bite of right thumb
- 7 S60.372- Other superficial bite of left thumb
- 7 S60.379- Other superficial bite of unspecified thumb

6 S60.39 Other superficial injuries of thumb
- 7 S60.391- Other superficial injuries of right thumb
- 7 S60.392- Other superficial injuries of left thumb
- 7 S60.399- Other superficial injuries of unspecified thumb

5 S60.4 Other superficial injuries of Other fingers

6 S60.41 Abrasion of fingers
- 7 S60.410- Abrasion of right index finger
- 7 S60.411- Abrasion of left index finger
- 7 S60.412- Abrasion of right middle finger
- 7 S60.413- Abrasion of left middle finger
- 7 S60.414- Abrasion of right ring finger
- 7 S60.415- Abrasion of left ring finger
- 7 S60.416- Abrasion of right little finger
- 7 S60.417- Abrasion of left little finger
- 7 S60.418- Abrasion of other finger
  Abrasion of specified finger with unspecified laterality

7 ⊟ S60.419- **Abrasion of unspecified finger**

6 S60.42 **Blister (nonthermal) of fingers**

7 ⊟ S60.420- Blister (nonthermal) of right index finger
7 ⊟ S60.421- Blister (nonthermal) of left index finger
7 ⊟ S60.422- Blister (nonthermal) of right middle finger
7 ⊟ S60.423- Blister (nonthermal) of left middle finger
7 ⊟ S60.424- Blister (nonthermal) of right ring finger
7 ⊟ S60.425- Blister (nonthermal) of left ring finger
7 ⊟ S60.426- Blister (nonthermal) of right little finger
7 ⊟ S60.427- Blister (nonthermal) of left little finger
7 ⊟ S60.428- Blister (nonthermal) of other finger
Blister (nonthermal) of specified finger with unspecified laterality
7 ⊟ S60.429- **Blister (nonthermal) of unspecified finger**

6 S60.44 **External constriction of fingers**
Hair tourniquet syndrome of finger
Use additional cause code to identify the constricting item (W49.0-)

7 ⊟ S60.440- External constriction of right index finger
7 ⊟ S60.441- External constriction of left index finger
7 ⊟ S60.442- External constriction of right middle finger
7 ⊟ S60.443- External constriction of left middle finger
7 ⊟ S60.444- External constriction of right ring finger
7 ⊟ S60.445- External constriction of left ring finger
7 ⊟ S60.446- External constriction of right little finger
7 ⊟ S60.447- External constriction of left little finger
7 ⊟ S60.448- External constriction of other finger
External constriction of specified finger with unspecified laterality
7 ⊟ S60.449- **External constriction of unspecified finger**

6 S60.45 **Superficial foreign body of fingers**
Splinter in the finger(s)

7 ⊟ S60.450- Superficial foreign body of right index finger
7 ⊟ S60.451- Superficial foreign body of left index finger
7 ⊟ S60.452- Superficial foreign body of right middle finger
7 ⊟ S60.453- Superficial foreign body of left middle finger
7 ⊟ S60.454- Superficial foreign body of right ring finger
7 ⊟ S60.455- Superficial foreign body of left ring finger
7 ⊟ S60.456- Superficial foreign body of right little finger
7 ⊟ S60.457- Superficial foreign body of left little finger
7 ⊟ S60.458- Superficial foreign body of other finger
Superficial foreign body of specified finger with unspecified laterality
7 ⊟ S60.459- **Superficial foreign body of unspecified finger**

6 S60.46 **Insect bite (nonvenomous) of fingers**

7 ⊟ S60.460- Insect bite (nonvenomous) of right index finger
7 ⊟ S60.461- Insect bite (nonvenomous) of left index finger
7 ⊟ S60.462- Insect bite (nonvenomous) of right middle finger
7 ⊟ S60.463- Insect bite (nonvenomous) of left middle finger
7 ⊟ S60.464- Insect bite (nonvenomous) of right ring finger
7 ⊟ S60.465- Insect bite (nonvenomous) of left ring finger
7 ⊟ S60.466- Insect bite (nonvenomous) of right little finger
7 ⊟ S60.467- Insect bite (nonvenomous) of left little finger
7 ⊟ S60.468- Insect bite (nonvenomous) of other finger
Insect bite (nonvenomous) of specified finger with unspecified laterality
7 ⊟ S60.469- **Insect bite (nonvenomous) of unspecified finger**

6 S60.47 **Other superficial bite of fingers**
EXCLUDES 1 *open bite of fingers (S61.25-, S61.35-)*

7 ⊟ S60.470- Other superficial bite of right index finger
7 ⊟ S60.471- Other superficial bite of left index finger
7 ⊟ S60.472- Other superficial bite of right middle finger
7 ⊟ S60.473- Other superficial bite of left middle finger
7 ⊟ S60.474- Other superficial bite of right ring finger
7 ⊟ S60.475- Other superficial bite of left ring finger
7 ⊟ S60.476- Other superficial bite of right little finger
7 ⊟ S60.477- Other superficial bite of left little finger
7 ⊟ S60.478- Other superficial bite of other finger
Other superficial bite of specified finger with unspecified laterality
7 ⊟ S60.479- **Other superficial bite of unspecified finger**

5 S60.5 **Other superficial injuries of hand**
EXCLUDES 2 *superficial injuries of fingers (S60.3-, S60.4-)*

6 S60.51 **Abrasion of hand**

7 ⊟ S60.511- Abrasion of right hand
7 ⊟ S60.512- Abrasion of left hand
7 ⊟ S60.519- **Abrasion of unspecified hand**

6 S60.52 **Blister (nonthermal) of hand**

7 ⊟ S60.521- Blister (nonthermal) of right hand
7 ⊟ S60.522- Blister (nonthermal) of left hand
7 ⊟ S60.529- **Blister (nonthermal) of unspecified hand**

6 S60.54 **External constriction of hand**

7 ⊟ S60.541- External constriction of right hand
7 ⊟ S60.542- External constriction of left hand
7 ⊟ S60.549- **External constriction of unspecified hand**

6 S60.55 **Superficial foreign body of hand**
Splinter in the hand

7 ⊟ S60.551- Superficial foreign body of right hand
7 ⊟ S60.552- Superficial foreign body of left hand
7 ⊟ S60.559- **Superficial foreign body of unspecified hand**

6 S60.56 **Insect bite (nonvenomous) of hand**

7 ⊟ S60.561- Insect bite (nonvenomous) of right hand
7 ⊟ S60.562- Insect bite (nonvenomous) of left hand
7 ⊟ S60.569- **Insect bite (nonvenomous) of unspecified hand**

6 S60.57 **Other superficial bite of hand**
EXCLUDES 1 *open bite of hand (S61.45-)*

7 ⊟ S60.571- Other superficial bite of hand of right hand
7 ⊟ S60.572- Other superficial bite of hand of left hand
7 ⊟ S60.579- **Other superficial bite of hand of unspecified hand**

5 S60.8 **Other superficial injuries of wrist**

6 S60.81 **Abrasion of wrist**

7 ⊟ S60.811- Abrasion of right wrist
7 ⊟ S60.812- Abrasion of left wrist
7 ⊟ S60.819- **Abrasion of unspecified wrist**

6 S60.82 **Blister (nonthermal) of wrist**

7 ⊟ S60.821- Blister (nonthermal) of right wrist
7 ⊟ S60.822- Blister (nonthermal) of left wrist
7 ⊟ S60.829- **Blister (nonthermal) of unspecified wrist**

6 S60.84 **External constriction of wrist**

7 ⊟ S60.841- External constriction of right wrist
7 ⊟ S60.842- External constriction of left wrist
7 ⊟ S60.849- **External constriction of unspecified wrist**

6 S60.85 **Superficial foreign body of wrist**
Splinter in the wrist

7 ⊟ S60.851- Superficial foreign body of right wrist
7 ⊟ S60.852- Superficial foreign body of left wrist
7 ⊟ S60.859- **Superficial foreign body of unspecified wrist**

6 S60.86 **Insect bite (nonvenomous) of wrist**

7 ⊟ S60.861- Insect bite (nonvenomous) of right wrist
7 ⊟ S60.862- Insect bite (nonvenomous) of left wrist
7 ⊟ S60.869- **Insect bite (nonvenomous) of unspecified wrist**

6 S60.87 **Other superficial bite of wrist**
EXCLUDES 1 *open bite of wrist (S61.55)*

7 ⊟ S60.871- Other superficial bite of right wrist
7 ⊟ S60.872- Other superficial bite of left wrist
7 ⊟ S60.879- **Other superficial bite of unspecified wrist**

5 S60.9 **Unspecified superficial injury of wrist, hand and fingers**

6 S60.91 **Unspecified superficial injury of wrist**

7 ⊟ S60.911- **Unspecified superficial injury of right wrist**
7 ⊟ S60.912- **Unspecified superficial injury of left wrist**

7 ⊟ S60.919- **Unspecified superficial injury of unspecified wrist**

6 **S60.92 Unspecified superficial injury of hand**

7 ⊟ S60.921- **Unspecified superficial injury of right hand**

7 ⊟ S60.922- **Unspecified superficial injury of left hand**

7 ⊟ S60.929- **Unspecified superficial injury of unspecified hand**

6 **S60.93 Unspecified superficial injury of thumb**

7 ⊟ S60.931- **Unspecified superficial injury of right thumb**

7 ⊟ S60.932- **Unspecified superficial injury of left thumb**

7 ⊟ S60.939- **Unspecified superficial injury of unspecified thumb**

6 **S60.94 Unspecified superficial injury of other fingers**

7 ⊟ S60.940- **Unspecified superficial injury of right index finger**

7 ⊟ S60.941- **Unspecified superficial injury of left index finger**

7 ⊟ S60.942- **Unspecified superficial injury of right middle finger**

7 ⊟ S60.943- **Unspecified superficial injury of left middle finger**

7 ⊟ S60.944- **Unspecified superficial injury of right ring finger**

7 ⊟ S60.945- **Unspecified superficial injury of left ring finger**

7 ⊟ S60.946- **Unspecified superficial injury of right little finger**

7 ⊟ S60.947- **Unspecified superficial injury of left little finger**

7 ⊟ S60.948- **Unspecified superficial injury of other finger**
Unspecified superficial injury of specified finger with unspecified laterality

7 ⊟ S60.949- **Unspecified superficial injury of unspecified finger**

4 S61 Open wound of wrist, hand and fingers

Code also:
any associated wound infection

EXCLUDES 1 *open fracture of wrist, hand and finger (S62.- with 7th character B)*
traumatic amputation of wrist and hand (S68.-)

The appropriate 7th character is to be added to each code from category S61
A initial encounter
D subsequent encounter
S sequela

CODING TIP ✓ Open wound codes indicate a wound resulting from a traumatic origin. Do not assign a code for "open wound" unless the etiology of the wound is related to trauma.

5 **S61.0 Open wound of thumb without damage to nail**

EXCLUDES 1 *open wound of thumb with damage to nail (S61.1-)*

6 **S61.00 Unspecified open wound of thumb without damage to nail**

7 ⊟ S61.001- **Unspecified open wound of right thumb without damage to nail**

7 ⊟ S61.002- **Unspecified open wound of left thumb without damage to nail**

7 ⊟ S61.009- **Unspecified open wound of unspecified thumb without damage to nail**

6 **S61.01 Laceration without foreign body of thumb without damage to nail**

7 ⊟ S61.011- **Laceration without foreign body of right thumb without damage to nail**

7 ⊟ S61.012- **Laceration without foreign body of left thumb without damage to nail**

7 ⊟ S61.019- **Laceration without foreign body of unspecified thumb without damage to nail**

6 **S61.02 Laceration with foreign body of thumb without damage to nail**

7 ⊟ S61.021- **Laceration with foreign body of right thumb without damage to nail**

7 ⊟ S61.022- **Laceration with foreign body of left thumb without damage to nail**

7 ⊟ S61.029- **Laceration with foreign body of unspecified thumb without damage to nail**

6 **S61.03 Puncture wound without foreign body of thumb without damage to nail**

7 ⊟ S61.031- **Puncture wound without foreign body of right thumb without damage to nail**

7 ⊟ S61.032- **Puncture wound without foreign body of left thumb without damage to nail**

7 ⊟ S61.039- **Puncture wound without foreign body of unspecified thumb without damage to nail**

6 **S61.04 Puncture wound with foreign body of thumb without damage to nail**

7 ⊟ S61.041- **Puncture wound with foreign body of right thumb without damage to nail**

7 ⊟ S61.042- **Puncture wound with foreign body of left thumb without damage to nail**

7 ⊟ S61.049- **Puncture wound with foreign body of unspecified thumb without damage to nail**

6 **S61.05 Open bite of thumb without damage to nail**
Bite of thumb NOS

EXCLUDES 1 *superficial bite of thumb (S60.36-, S60.37-)*

7 ⊟ S61.051- **Open bite of right thumb without damage to nail**

7 ⊟ S61.052- **Open bite of left thumb without damage to nail**

7 ⊟ S61.059- **Open bite of unspecified thumb without damage to nail**

5 **S61.1 Open wound of thumb with damage to nail**

6 **S61.10 Unspecified open wound of thumb with damage to nail**

7 ⊟ S61.101- **Unspecified open wound of right thumb with damage to nail**

7 ⊟ S61.102- **Unspecified open wound of left thumb with damage to nail**

7 ⊟ S61.109- **Unspecified open wound of unspecified thumb with damage to nail**

6 **S61.11 Laceration without foreign body of thumb with damage to nail**

7 ⊟ S61.111- **Laceration without foreign body of right thumb with damage to nail**

7 ⊟ S61.112- **Laceration without foreign body of left thumb with damage to nail**

7 ⊟ S61.119- **Laceration without foreign body of unspecified thumb with damage to nail**

6 **S61.12 Laceration with foreign body of thumb with damage to nail**

7 ⊟ S61.121- **Laceration with foreign body of right thumb with damage to nail**

7 ⊟ S61.122- **Laceration with foreign body of left thumb with damage to nail**

7 ⊟ S61.129- **Laceration with foreign body of unspecified thumb with damage to nail**

6 **S61.13 Puncture wound without foreign body of thumb with damage to nail**

7 ⊟ S61.131- **Puncture wound without foreign body of right thumb with damage to nail**

7 ⊟ S61.132- **Puncture wound without foreign body of left thumb with damage to nail**

7 ⊟ S61.139- **Puncture wound without foreign body of unspecified thumb with damage to nail**

6 **S61.14 Puncture wound with foreign body of thumb with damage to nail**

7 ⊟ S61.141- **Puncture wound with foreign body of right thumb with damage to nail**

7 ⊟ S61.142- **Puncture wound with foreign body of left thumb with damage to nail**

7 ⊟ S61.149- **Puncture wound with foreign body of unspecified thumb with damage to nail**

6 **S61.15 Open bite of thumb with damage to nail**
Bite of thumb with damage to nail NOS

EXCLUDES 1 *superficial bite of thumb (S60.36-, S60.37-)*

7 ⊟ S61.151- **Open bite of right thumb with damage to nail**

7 ⊟ S61.152- **Open bite of left thumb with damage to nail**

7 ⊟ S61.159- **Open bite of unspecified thumb with damage to nail**

5 S61.2 **Open wound of other finger without damage to nail**

EXCLUDES 1 *open wound of finger involving nail (matrix) (S61.3-)*

EXCLUDES 2 *open wound of thumb without damage to nail (S61.0-)*

6 S61.20 **Unspecified open wound of other finger without damage to nail**

7 ⊟ S61.200- **Unspecified open wound of right index finger without damage to nail**

7 ⊟ S61.201- **Unspecified open wound of left index finger without damage to nail**

7 ⊟ S61.202- **Unspecified open wound of right middle finger without damage to nail**

7 ⊟ S61.203- **Unspecified open wound of left middle finger without damage to nail**

7 ⊟ S61.204- **Unspecified open wound of right ring finger without damage to nail**

7 ⊟ S61.205- **Unspecified open wound of left ring finger without damage to nail**

7 ⊟ S61.206- **Unspecified open wound of right little finger without damage to nail**

7 ⊟ S61.207- **Unspecified open wound of left little finger without damage to nail**

7 ⊟ S61.208- **Unspecified open wound of other finger without damage to nail**
Unspecified open wound of specified finger with unspecified laterality without damage to nail

7 ⊟ S61.209- **Unspecified open wound of unspecified finger without damage to nail**

6 S61.21 **Laceration without foreign body of finger without damage to nail**

7 ⊟ S61.210- **Laceration without foreign body of right index finger without damage to nail**

7 ⊟ S61.211- **Laceration without foreign body of left index finger without damage to nail**

7 ⊟ S61.212- **Laceration without foreign body of right middle finger without damage to nail**

7 ⊟ S61.213- **Laceration without foreign body of left middle finger without damage to nail**

7 ⊟ S61.214- **Laceration without foreign body of right ring finger without damage to nail**

7 ⊟ S61.215- **Laceration without foreign body of left ring finger without damage to nail**

7 ⊟ S61.216- **Laceration without foreign body of right little finger without damage to nail**

7 ⊟ S61.217- **Laceration without foreign body of left little finger without damage to nail**

7 ⊟ S61.218- **Laceration without foreign body of other finger without damage to nail**
Laceration without foreign body of specified finger with unspecified laterality without damage to nail

7 ⊟ S61.219- **Laceration without foreign body of unspecified finger without damage to nail**

6 S61.22 **Laceration with foreign body of finger without damage to nail**

7 ⊟ S61.220- **Laceration with foreign body of right index finger without damage to nail**

7 ⊟ S61.221- **Laceration with foreign body of left index finger without damage to nail**

7 ⊟ S61.222- **Laceration with foreign body of right middle finger without damage to nail**

7 ⊟ S61.223- **Laceration with foreign body of left middle finger without damage to nail**

7 ⊟ S61.224- **Laceration with foreign body of right ring finger without damage to nail**

7 ⊟ S61.225- **Laceration with foreign body of left ring finger without damage to nail**

7 ⊟ S61.226- **Laceration with foreign body of right little finger without damage to nail**

7 ⊟ S61.227- **Laceration with foreign body of left little finger without damage to nail**

7 ⊟ S61.228- **Laceration with foreign body of other finger without damage to nail**
Laceration with foreign body of specified finger with unspecified laterality without damage to nail

7 ⊟ S61.229- **Laceration with foreign body of unspecified finger without damage to nail**

6 S61.23 **Puncture wound without foreign body of finger without damage to nail**

7 ⊟ S61.230- **Puncture wound without foreign body of right index finger without damage to nail**

7 ⊟ S61.231- **Puncture wound without foreign body of left index finger without damage to nail**

7 ⊟ S61.232- **Puncture wound without foreign body of right middle finger without damage to nail**

7 ⊟ S61.233- **Puncture wound without foreign body of left middle finger without damage to nail**

7 ⊟ S61.234- **Puncture wound without foreign body of right ring finger without damage to nail**

7 ⊟ S61.235- **Puncture wound without foreign body of left ring finger without damage to nail**

7 ⊟ S61.236- **Puncture wound without foreign body of right little finger without damage to nail**

7 ⊟ S61.237- **Puncture wound without foreign body of left little finger without damage to nail**

7 ⊟ S61.238- **Puncture wound without foreign body of other finger without damage to nail**
Puncture wound without foreign body of specified finger with unspecified laterality without damage to nail

7 ⊟ S61.239- **Puncture wound without foreign body of unspecified finger without damage to nail**

6 S61.24 **Puncture wound with foreign body of finger without damage to nail**

7 ⊟ S61.240- **Puncture wound with foreign body of right index finger without damage to nail**

7 ⊟ S61.241- **Puncture wound with foreign body of left index finger without damage to nail**

7 ⊟ S61.242- **Puncture wound with foreign body of right middle finger without damage to nail**

7 ⊟ S61.243- **Puncture wound with foreign body of left middle finger without damage to nail**

7 ⊟ S61.244- **Puncture wound with foreign body of right ring finger without damage to nail**

7 ⊟ S61.245- **Puncture wound with foreign body of left ring finger without damage to nail**

7 ⊟ S61.246- **Puncture wound with foreign body of right little finger without damage to nail**

7 ⊟ S61.247- **Puncture wound with foreign body of left little finger without damage to nail**

7 ⊟ S61.248- **Puncture wound with foreign body of other finger without damage to nail**
Puncture wound with foreign body of specified finger with unspecified laterality without damage to nail

7 ⊟ S61.249- **Puncture wound with foreign body of unspecified finger without damage to nail**

6 S61.25 **Open bite of finger without damage to nail**
Bite of finger without damage to nail NOS

EXCLUDES 1 *superficial bite of finger (S60.46-, S60.47-)*

7 ⊟ S61.250- **Open bite of right index finger without damage to nail**

7 ⊟ S61.251- **Open bite of left index finger without damage to nail**

7 ⊟ S61.252- **Open bite of right middle finger without damage to nail**

7 ⊟ S61.253- **Open bite of left middle finger without damage to nail**

7 ⊟ S61.254- **Open bite of right ring finger without damage to nail**

7 ⊟ S61.255- **Open bite of left ring finger without damage to nail**

7 ⊟ S61.256- **Open bite of right little finger without damage to nail**

7 ⊟ S61.257- **Open bite of left little finger without damage to nail**

7 ⊟ S61.258- **Open bite of other finger without damage to nail**
Open bite of specified finger with unspecified laterality without damage to nail

S61.259- Open bite of unspecified finger without damage to nail

S61.3 Open wound of other finger with damage to nail

S61.30 Unspecified open wound of finger with damage to nail

S61.300- Unspecified open wound of right index finger with damage to nail

S61.301- Unspecified open wound of left index finger with damage to nail

S61.302- Unspecified open wound of right middle finger with damage to nail

S61.303- Unspecified open wound of left middle finger with damage to nail

S61.304- Unspecified open wound of right ring finger with damage to nail

S61.305- Unspecified open wound of left ring finger with damage to nail

S61.306- Unspecified open wound of right little finger with damage to nail

S61.307- Unspecified open wound of left little finger with damage to nail

S61.308- Unspecified open wound of other finger with damage to nail
Unspecified open wound of specified finger with unspecified laterality with damage to nail

S61.309- Unspecified open wound of unspecified finger with damage to nail

S61.31 Laceration without foreign body of finger with damage to nail

S61.310- Laceration without foreign body of right index finger with damage to nail

S61.311- Laceration without foreign body of left index finger with damage to nail

S61.312- Laceration without foreign body of right middle finger with damage to nail

S61.313- Laceration without foreign body of left middle finger with damage to nail

S61.314- Laceration without foreign body of right ring finger with damage to nail

S61.315- Laceration without foreign body of left ring finger with damage to nail

S61.316- Laceration without foreign body of right little finger with damage to nail

S61.317- Laceration without foreign body of left little finger with damage to nail

S61.318- Laceration without foreign body of other finger with damage to nail
Laceration without foreign body of specified finger with unspecified laterality with damage to nail

S61.319- Laceration without foreign body of unspecified finger with damage to nail

S61.32 Laceration with foreign body of finger with damage to nail

S61.320- Laceration with foreign body of right index finger with damage to nail

S61.321- Laceration with foreign body of left index finger with damage to nail

S61.322- Laceration with foreign body of right middle finger with damage to nail

S61.323- Laceration with foreign body of left middle finger with damage to nail

S61.324- Laceration with foreign body of right ring finger with damage to nail

S61.325- Laceration with foreign body of left ring finger with damage to nail

S61.326- Laceration with foreign body of right little finger with damage to nail

S61.327- Laceration with foreign body of left little finger with damage to nail

S61.328- Laceration with foreign body of other finger with damage to nail
Laceration with foreign body of specified finger with unspecified laterality with damage to nail

S61.329- Laceration with foreign body of unspecified finger with damage to nail

S61.33 Puncture wound without foreign body of finger with damage to nail

S61.330- Puncture wound without foreign body of right index finger with damage to nail

S61.331- Puncture wound without foreign body of left index finger with damage to nail

S61.332- Puncture wound without foreign body of right middle finger with damage to nail

S61.333- Puncture wound without foreign body of left middle finger with damage to nail

S61.334- Puncture wound without foreign body of right ring finger with damage to nail

S61.335- Puncture wound without foreign body of left ring finger with damage to nail

S61.336- Puncture wound without foreign body of right little finger with damage to nail

S61.337- Puncture wound without foreign body of left little finger with damage to nail

S61.338- Puncture wound without foreign body of other finger with damage to nail
Puncture wound without foreign body of specified finger with unspecified laterality with damage to nail

S61.339- Puncture wound without foreign body of unspecified finger with damage to nail

S61.34 Puncture wound with foreign body of finger with damage to nail

S61.340- Puncture wound with foreign body of right index finger with damage to nail

S61.341- Puncture wound with foreign body of left index finger with damage to nail

S61.342- Puncture wound with foreign body of right middle finger with damage to nail

S61.343- Puncture wound with foreign body of left middle finger with damage to nail

S61.344- Puncture wound with foreign body of right ring finger with damage to nail

S61.345- Puncture wound with foreign body of left ring finger with damage to nail

S61.346- Puncture wound with foreign body of right little finger with damage to nail

S61.347- Puncture wound with foreign body of left little finger with damage to nail

S61.348- Puncture wound with foreign body of other finger with damage to nail
Puncture wound with foreign body of specified finger with unspecified laterality with damage to nail

S61.349- Puncture wound with foreign body of unspecified finger with damage to nail

S61.35 Open bite of finger with damage to nail
Bite of finger with damage to nail NOS
EXCLUDES 1 *superficial bite of finger (S60.46-, S60.47-)*

S61.350- Open bite of right index finger with damage to nail

S61.351- Open bite of left index finger with damage to nail

S61.352- Open bite of right middle finger with damage to nail

S61.353- Open bite of left middle finger with damage to nail

S61.354- Open bite of right ring finger with damage to nail

S61.355- Open bite of left ring finger with damage to nail

S61.356- Open bite of right little finger with damage to nail

S61.357- Open bite of left little finger with damage to nail

S61.358- Open bite of other finger with damage to nail
Open bite of specified finger with unspecified laterality with damage to nail

S61.359- Open bite of unspecified finger with damage to nail

S61.4 Open wound of hand

S61.40 Unspecified open wound of hand

S61.401- Unspecified open wound of right hand

S61.402- Unspecified open wound of left hand

S61.409- Unspecified open wound of unspecified hand

S61.41 Laceration without foreign body of hand

7 ⊟ S61.411- Laceration without foreign body of right hand
7 ⊟ S61.412- Laceration without foreign body of left hand
7 ⊟ S61.419- Laceration without foreign body of unspecified hand

6 S61.42 Laceration with foreign body of hand
7 ⊟ S61.421- Laceration with foreign body of right hand
7 ⊟ S61.422- Laceration with foreign body of left hand
7 ⊟ S61.429- Laceration with foreign body of unspecified hand

6 S61.43 Puncture wound without foreign body of hand
7 ⊟ S61.431- Puncture wound without foreign body of right hand
7 ⊟ S61.432- Puncture wound without foreign body of left hand
7 ⊟ S61.439- Puncture wound without foreign body of unspecified hand

6 S61.44 Puncture wound with foreign body of hand
7 ⊟ S61.441- Puncture wound with foreign body of right hand
7 ⊟ S61.442- Puncture wound with foreign body of left hand
7 ⊟ S61.449- Puncture wound with foreign body of unspecified hand

6 S61.45 Open bite of hand
Bite of hand NOS
EXCLUDES 1 *superficial bite of hand (S60.56-, S60.57-)*
7 ⊟ S61.451- Open bite of right hand
7 ⊟ S61.452- Open bite of left hand
7 ⊟ S61.459- Open bite of unspecified hand

5 S61.5 Open wound of wrist

6 S61.50 Unspecified open wound of wrist
7 ⊟ S61.501- Unspecified open wound of right wrist
7 ⊟ S61.502- Unspecified open wound of left wrist
7 ⊟ S61.509- Unspecified open wound of unspecified wrist

6 S61.51 Laceration without foreign body of wrist
7 ⊟ S61.511- Laceration without foreign body of right wrist
7 ⊟ S61.512- Laceration without foreign body of left wrist
7 ⊟ S61.519- Laceration without foreign body of unspecified wrist

6 S61.52 Laceration with foreign body of wrist
7 ⊟ S61.521- Laceration with foreign body of right wrist
7 ⊟ S61.522- Laceration with foreign body of left wrist
7 ⊟ S61.529- Laceration with foreign body of unspecified wrist

6 S61.53 Puncture wound without foreign body of wrist
7 ⊟ S61.531- Puncture wound without foreign body of right wrist
7 ⊟ S61.532- Puncture wound without foreign body of left wrist
7 ⊟ S61.539- Puncture wound without foreign body of unspecified wrist

6 S61.54 Puncture wound with foreign body of wrist
7 ⊟ S61.541- Puncture wound with foreign body of right wrist
7 ⊟ S61.542- Puncture wound with foreign body of left wrist
7 ⊟ S61.549- Puncture wound with foreign body of unspecified wrist

6 S61.55 Open bite of wrist
Bite of wrist NOS
EXCLUDES 1 *superficial bite of wrist (S60.86-, S60.87-)*
7 ⊟ S61.551- Open bite of right wrist
7 ⊟ S61.552- Open bite of left wrist
7 ⊟ S61.559- Open bite of unspecified wrist

4 S62 Fracture at wrist and hand level

Note: A fracture not indicated as displaced or nondisplaced should be coded to displaced
A fracture not indicated as open or closed should be coded to closed

EXCLUDES 1 *traumatic amputation of wrist and hand (S68.-)*
EXCLUDES 2 *fracture of distal parts of ulna and radius (S52.-)*

The appropriate 7th character is to be added to each code from category S62

A	initial encounter for closed fracture
B	initial encounter for open fracture
D	subsequent encounter for fracture with routine healing
G	subsequent encounter for fracture with delayed healing
K	subsequent encounter for fracture with nonunion
P	subsequent encounter for fracture with malunion
S	sequela

CODING TIP ✓ A fracture not indicated as displaced or nondisplaced should be coded to displaced. A fracture not indicated as open or closed should be coded to closed. Query providers on fractures not documented as displaced/nondisplaced; otherwise, a displaced fracture diagnosis could be assigned without a reduction being performed, potentially resulting in claim denials.

5 S62.0 Fracture of navicular [scaphoid] bone of wrist

6 S62.00 Unspecified fracture of navicular [scaphoid] bone of wrist
7 ⊟ S62.001- Unspecified fracture of navicular [scaphoid] bone of right wrist
7 ⊟ S62.002- Unspecified fracture of navicular [scaphoid] bone of left wrist
AHA: (S62.002A) 4Q 2012, 106
7 ⊟ S62.009- Unspecified fracture of navicular [scaphoid] bone of unspecified wrist

6 S62.01 Fracture of distal pole of navicular [scaphoid] bone of wrist
Fracture of volar tuberosity of navicular [scaphoid] bone of wrist
7 ⊟ S62.011- Displaced fracture of distal pole of navicular [scaphoid] bone of right wrist
7 ⊟ S62.012- Displaced fracture of distal pole of navicular [scaphoid] bone of left wrist
7 ⊟ S62.013- Displaced fracture of distal pole of navicular [scaphoid] bone of unspecified wrist
7 ⊟ S62.014- Nondisplaced fracture of distal pole of navicular [scaphoid] bone of right wrist
7 ⊟ S62.015- Nondisplaced fracture of distal pole of navicular [scaphoid] bone of left wrist
7 ⊟ S62.016- Nondisplaced fracture of distal pole of navicular [scaphoid] bone of unspecified wrist

6 S62.02 Fracture of middle third of navicular [scaphoid] bone of wrist
7 ⊟ S62.021- Displaced fracture of middle third of navicular [scaphoid] bone of right wrist
7 ⊟ S62.022- Displaced fracture of middle third of navicular [scaphoid] bone of left wrist
7 ⊟ S62.023- Displaced fracture of middle third of navicular [scaphoid] bone of unspecified wrist
7 ⊟ S62.024- Nondisplaced fracture of middle third of navicular [scaphoid] bone of right wrist
7 ⊟ S62.025- Nondisplaced fracture of middle third of navicular [scaphoid] bone of left wrist
7 ⊟ S62.026- Nondisplaced fracture of middle third of navicular [scaphoid] bone of unspecified wrist

6 S62.03 Fracture of proximal third of navicular [scaphoid] bone of wrist
7 ⊟ S62.031- Displaced fracture of proximal third of navicular [scaphoid] bone of right wrist
7 ⊟ S62.032- Displaced fracture of proximal third of navicular [scaphoid] bone of left wrist
7 ⊟ S62.033- Displaced fracture of proximal third of navicular [scaphoid] bone of unspecified wrist

7 ⊟ **S62.034-** Nondisplaced **fracture of proximal third of navicular [scaphoid] bone of** right **wrist**

7 ⊟ **S62.035-** Nondisplaced **fracture of proximal third of navicular [scaphoid] bone of** left **wrist**

7 ⊟ **S62.036-** Nondisplaced **fracture of proximal third of navicular [scaphoid] bone of** unspecified **wrist**

5 **S62.1** **Fracture of** other and unspecified carpal bone(s)

EXCLUDES 2 *fracture of scaphoid of wrist (S62.0-)*

6 **S62.10** **Fracture of unspecified carpal bone**

Fracture of wrist NOS

7 ⊟ **S62.101-** **Fracture of unspecified carpal bone,** right wrist

7 ⊟ **S62.102-** **Fracture of unspecified carpal bone,** left wrist

AHA: (S62.102D) 4Q 2012, 95

7 ⊟ **S62.109-** **Fracture of unspecified carpal bone,** unspecified wrist

6 **S62.11** **Fracture of** triquetrum [cuneiform] **bone of** wrist

7 ⊟ **S62.111-** Displaced **fracture of triquetrum [cuneiform] bone,** right **wrist**

7 ⊟ **S62.112-** Displaced **fracture of triquetrum [cuneiform] bone,** left **wrist**

7 ⊟ **S62.113-** Displaced **fracture of triquetrum [cuneiform] bone,** unspecified **wrist**

7 ⊟ **S62.114-** Nondisplaced **fracture of triquetrum [cuneiform] bone,** right **wrist**

7 ⊟ **S62.115-** Nondisplaced **fracture of triquetrum [cuneiform] bone,** left **wrist**

7 ⊟ **S62.116-** Nondisplaced **fracture of triquetrum [cuneiform] bone,** unspecified **wrist**

6 **S62.12** **Fracture of** lunate [semilunar]

7 ⊟ **S62.121-** Displaced **fracture of lunate [semilunar],** right wrist

7 ⊟ **S62.122-** Displaced **fracture of lunate [semilunar],** left wrist

7 ⊟ **S62.123-** Displaced **fracture of lunate [semilunar],** unspecified wrist

7 ⊟ **S62.124-** Nondisplaced **fracture of lunate [semilunar],** right wrist

7 ⊟ **S62.125-** Nondisplaced **fracture of lunate [semilunar],** left wrist

7 ⊟ **S62.126-** Nondisplaced **fracture of lunate [semilunar],** unspecified wrist

6 **S62.13** **Fracture of** capitate [os magnum] **bone**

7 ⊟ **S62.131-** Displaced **fracture of capitate [os magnum] bone,** right wrist

7 ⊟ **S62.132-** Displaced **fracture of capitate [os magnum] bone,** left wrist

7 ⊟ **S62.133-** Displaced **fracture of capitate [os magnum] bone,** unspecified wrist

7 ⊟ **S62.134-** Nondisplaced **fracture of capitate [os magnum] bone,** right wrist

7 ⊟ **S62.135-** Nondisplaced **fracture of capitate [os magnum] bone,** left wrist

7 ⊟ **S62.136-** Nondisplaced **fracture of capitate [os magnum] bone,** unspecified wrist

6 **S62.14** **Fracture of** body of hamate [unciform] **bone**

Fracture of hamate [unciform] bone NOS

7 ⊟ **S62.141-** Displaced **fracture of body of hamate [unciform] bone,** right wrist

7 ⊟ **S62.142-** Displaced **fracture of body of hamate [unciform] bone,** left wrist

7 ⊟ **S62.143-** Displaced **fracture of body of hamate [unciform] bone,** unspecified wrist

7 ⊟ **S62.144-** Nondisplaced **fracture of body of hamate [unciform] bone,** right wrist

7 ⊟ **S62.145-** Nondisplaced **fracture of body of hamate [unciform] bone,** left wrist

7 ⊟ **S62.146-** Nondisplaced **fracture of body of hamate [unciform] bone,** unspecified wrist

6 **S62.15** **Fracture of** hook process of hamate [unciform] **bone**

Fracture of unciform process of hamate [unciform] bone

7 ⊟ **S62.151-** Displaced **fracture of hook process of hamate [unciform] bone,** right wrist

7 ⊟ **S62.152-** Displaced **fracture of hook process of hamate [unciform] bone,** left wrist

7 ⊟ **S62.153-** Displaced **fracture of hook process of hamate [unciform] bone,** unspecified wrist

7 ⊟ **S62.154-** Nondisplaced **fracture of hook process of hamate [unciform] bone,** right wrist

7 ⊟ **S62.155-** Nondisplaced **fracture of hook process of hamate [unciform] bone,** left wrist

7 ⊟ **S62.156-** Nondisplaced **fracture of hook process of hamate [unciform] bone,** unspecified wrist

6 **S62.16** **Fracture of** pisiform

7 ⊟ **S62.161-** Displaced **fracture of pisiform,** right wrist

7 ⊟ **S62.162-** Displaced **fracture of pisiform,** left wrist

7 ⊟ **S62.163-** Displaced **fracture of pisiform,** unspecified wrist

7 ⊟ **S62.164-** Nondisplaced **fracture of pisiform,** right wrist

7 ⊟ **S62.165-** Nondisplaced **fracture of pisiform,** left wrist

7 ⊟ **S62.166-** Nondisplaced **fracture of pisiform,** unspecified wrist

6 **S62.17** **Fracture of** trapezium [larger multangular]

7 ⊟ **S62.171-** Displaced **fracture of trapezium [larger multangular],** right wrist

7 ⊟ **S62.172-** Displaced **fracture of trapezium [larger multangular],** left wrist

7 ⊟ **S62.173-** Displaced **fracture of trapezium [larger multangular],** unspecified wrist

7 ⊟ **S62.174-** Nondisplaced **fracture of trapezium [larger multangular],** right wrist

7 ⊟ **S62.175-** Nondisplaced **fracture of trapezium [larger multangular],** left wrist

7 ⊟ **S62.176-** Nondisplaced **fracture of trapezium [larger multangular],** unspecified wrist

6 **S62.18** **Fracture of** trapezoid [smaller multangular]

7 ⊟ **S62.181-** Displaced **fracture of trapezoid [smaller multangular],** right wrist

7 ⊟ **S62.182-** Displaced **fracture of trapezoid [smaller multangular],** left wrist

7 ⊟ **S62.183-** Displaced **fracture of trapezoid [smaller multangular],** unspecified wrist

7 ⊟ **S62.184-** Nondisplaced **fracture of trapezoid [smaller multangular],** right wrist

7 ⊟ **S62.185-** Nondisplaced **fracture of trapezoid [smaller multangular],** left wrist

7 ⊟ **S62.186-** Nondisplaced **fracture of trapezoid [smaller multangular],** unspecified wrist

5 **S62.2** **Fracture of** first metacarpal bone

6 **S62.20** Unspecified **fracture of first metacarpal bone**

7 ⊟ **S62.201-** **Unspecified fracture of first metacarpal bone,** right hand

7 ⊟ **S62.202-** **Unspecified fracture of first metacarpal bone,** left hand

7 ⊟ **S62.209-** **Unspecified fracture of first metacarpal bone,** unspecified hand

6 **S62.21** **Bennett's fracture**

DEFINITION An intra-articular fracture dislocation of the base of the first metacarpal bone (thumb) extending into the carpometacarpal joint.

7 ⊟ **S62.211-** **Bennett's fracture,** right hand

7 ⊟ **S62.212-** **Bennett's fracture,** left hand

7 ⊟ **S62.213-** **Bennett's fracture,** unspecified hand

6 **S62.22** **Rolando's fracture**

7 ⊟ **S62.221-** Displaced **Rolando's fracture,** right hand

7 ⊟ **S62.222-** Displaced **Rolando's fracture,** left hand

7 ⊟ **S62.223-** Displaced **Rolando's fracture,** unspecified hand

7 ⊟ **S62.224-** Nondisplaced **Rolando's fracture,** right hand

7 ⊟ **S62.225-** Nondisplaced **Rolando's fracture,** left hand

7 ⊟ **S62.226-** Nondisplaced **Rolando's fracture,** unspecified hand

6 **S62.23** Other **fracture of** base **of first metacarpal bone**

7 ⊟ **S62.231-** **Other** displaced **fracture of base of first metacarpal bone,** right hand

7 ⊟ **S62.232-** **Other** displaced **fracture of base of first metacarpal bone,** left hand

7 ⊟ **S62.233-** **Other** displaced **fracture of base of first metacarpal bone,** unspecified hand

7 ⊟ **S62.234-** **Other** nondisplaced **fracture of base of first metacarpal bone,** right hand

S62.235- Other nondisplaced fracture of base of first metacarpal bone, left hand
S62.236- Other nondisplaced fracture of base of first metacarpal bone, unspecified hand

S62.24 Fracture of shaft of first metacarpal bone
S62.241- Displaced fracture of shaft of first metacarpal bone, right hand
S62.242- Displaced fracture of shaft of first metacarpal bone, left hand
S62.243- Displaced fracture of shaft of first metacarpal bone, unspecified hand
S62.244- Nondisplaced fracture of shaft of first metacarpal bone, right hand
S62.245- Nondisplaced fracture of shaft of first metacarpal bone, left hand
S62.246- Nondisplaced fracture of shaft of first metacarpal bone, unspecified hand

S62.25 Fracture of neck of first metacarpal bone
S62.251- Displaced fracture of neck of first metacarpal bone, right hand
S62.252- Displaced fracture of neck of first metacarpal bone, left hand
S62.253- Displaced fracture of neck of first metacarpal bone, unspecified hand
S62.254- Nondisplaced fracture of neck of first metacarpal bone, right hand
S62.255- Nondisplaced fracture of neck of first metacarpal bone, left hand
S62.256- Nondisplaced fracture of neck of first metacarpal bone, unspecified hand

S62.29 Other fracture of first metacarpal bone
S62.291- Other fracture of first metacarpal bone, right hand
S62.292- Other fracture of first metacarpal bone, left hand
S62.299- Other fracture of first metacarpal bone, unspecified hand

S62.3 Fracture of other and unspecified metacarpal bone
EXCLUDES 2 *fracture of first metacarpal bone (S62.2-)*

S62.30 Unspecified fracture of other metacarpal bone
S62.300- Unspecified fracture of second metacarpal bone, right hand
S62.301- Unspecified fracture of second metacarpal bone, left hand
S62.302- Unspecified fracture of third metacarpal bone, right hand
S62.303- Unspecified fracture of third metacarpal bone, left hand
S62.304- Unspecified fracture of fourth metacarpal bone, right hand
S62.305- Unspecified fracture of fourth metacarpal bone, left hand
S62.306- Unspecified fracture of fifth metacarpal bone, right hand
S62.307- Unspecified fracture of fifth metacarpal bone, left hand
S62.308- Unspecified fracture of other metacarpal bone
Unspecified fracture of specified metacarpal bone with unspecified laterality
S62.309- Unspecified fracture of unspecified metacarpal bone

S62.31 Displaced fracture of base of other metacarpal bone
S62.310- Displaced fracture of base of second metacarpal bone, right hand
S62.311- Displaced fracture of base of second metacarpal bone, left hand
S62.312- Displaced fracture of base of third metacarpal bone, right hand
S62.313- Displaced fracture of base of third metacarpal bone, left hand
S62.314- Displaced fracture of base of fourth metacarpal bone, right hand
S62.315- Displaced fracture of base of fourth metacarpal bone, left hand
S62.316- Displaced fracture of base of fifth metacarpal bone, right hand
S62.317- Displaced fracture of base of fifth metacarpal bone, left hand
S62.318- Displaced fracture of base of other metacarpal bone
Displaced fracture of base of specified metacarpal bone with unspecified laterality
S62.319- Displaced fracture of base of unspecified metacarpal bone

S62.32 Displaced fracture of shaft of other metacarpal bone
S62.320- Displaced fracture of shaft of second metacarpal bone, right hand
S62.321- Displaced fracture of shaft of second metacarpal bone, left hand
S62.322- Displaced fracture of shaft of third metacarpal bone, right hand
S62.323- Displaced fracture of shaft of third metacarpal bone, left hand
S62.324- Displaced fracture of shaft of fourth metacarpal bone, right hand
S62.325- Displaced fracture of shaft of fourth metacarpal bone, left hand
S62.326- Displaced fracture of shaft of fifth metacarpal bone, right hand
S62.327- Displaced fracture of shaft of fifth metacarpal bone, left hand
S62.328- Displaced fracture of shaft of other metacarpal bone
Displaced fracture of shaft of specified metacarpal bone with unspecified laterality
S62.329- Displaced fracture of shaft of unspecified metacarpal bone

S62.33 Displaced fracture of neck of other metacarpal bone
S62.330- Displaced fracture of neck of second metacarpal bone, right hand
S62.331- Displaced fracture of neck of second metacarpal bone, left hand
S62.332- Displaced fracture of neck of third metacarpal bone, right hand
S62.333- Displaced fracture of neck of third metacarpal bone, left hand
S62.334- Displaced fracture of neck of fourth metacarpal bone, right hand
S62.335- Displaced fracture of neck of fourth metacarpal bone, left hand
S62.336- Displaced fracture of neck of fifth metacarpal bone, right hand
S62.337- Displaced fracture of neck of fifth metacarpal bone, left hand
S62.338- Displaced fracture of neck of other metacarpal bone
Displaced fracture of neck of specified metacarpal bone with unspecified laterality
S62.339- Displaced fracture of neck of unspecified metacarpal bone

S62.34 Nondisplaced fracture of base of other metacarpal bone
S62.340- Nondisplaced fracture of base of second metacarpal bone, right hand
S62.341- Nondisplaced fracture of base of second metacarpal bone, left hand
S62.342- Nondisplaced fracture of base of third metacarpal bone, right hand
S62.343- Nondisplaced fracture of base of third metacarpal bone, left hand
S62.344- Nondisplaced fracture of base of fourth metacarpal bone, right hand
S62.345- Nondisplaced fracture of base of fourth metacarpal bone, left hand
S62.346- Nondisplaced fracture of base of fifth metacarpal bone, right hand
S62.347- Nondisplaced fracture of base of fifth metacarpal bone, left hand
S62.348- Nondisplaced fracture of base of other metacarpal bone
Nondisplaced fracture of base of specified metacarpal bone with unspecified laterality
S62.349- Nondisplaced fracture of base of unspecified metacarpal bone

S62.35 Nondisplaced fracture of shaft of other metacarpal bone

7 ⊟ S62.350- **Nondisplaced fracture of shaft of second metacarpal bone, right hand**
7 ⊟ S62.351- **Nondisplaced fracture of shaft of second metacarpal bone, left hand**
7 ⊟ S62.352- **Nondisplaced fracture of shaft of third metacarpal bone, right hand**
7 ⊟ S62.353- **Nondisplaced fracture of shaft of third metacarpal bone, left hand**
7 ⊟ S62.354- **Nondisplaced fracture of shaft of fourth metacarpal bone, right hand**
7 ⊟ S62.355- **Nondisplaced fracture of shaft of fourth metacarpal bone, left hand**
7 ⊟ S62.356- **Nondisplaced fracture of shaft of fifth metacarpal bone, right hand**
7 ⊟ S62.357- **Nondisplaced fracture of shaft of fifth metacarpal bone, left hand**
7 ⊟ S62.358- **Nondisplaced fracture of shaft of other metacarpal bone**
Nondisplaced fracture of shaft of specified metacarpal bone with unspecified laterality
7 ⊟ S62.359- **Nondisplaced fracture of shaft of unspecified metacarpal bone**

6 S62.36 **Nondisplaced fracture of neck of other metacarpal bone**
7 ⊟ S62.360- **Nondisplaced fracture of neck of second metacarpal bone, right hand**
7 ⊟ S62.361- **Nondisplaced fracture of neck of second metacarpal bone, left hand**
7 ⊟ S62.362- **Nondisplaced fracture of neck of third metacarpal bone, right hand**
7 ⊟ S62.363- **Nondisplaced fracture of neck of third metacarpal bone, left hand**
7 ⊟ S62.364- **Nondisplaced fracture of neck of fourth metacarpal bone, right hand**
7 ⊟ S62.365- **Nondisplaced fracture of neck of fourth metacarpal bone, left hand**
7 ⊟ S62.366- **Nondisplaced fracture of neck of fifth metacarpal bone, right hand**
7 ⊟ S62.367- **Nondisplaced fracture of neck of fifth metacarpal bone, left hand**
7 ⊟ S62.368- **Nondisplaced fracture of neck of other metacarpal bone**
Nondisplaced fracture of neck of specified metacarpal bone with unspecified laterality
7 ⊟ S62.369- **Nondisplaced fracture of neck of unspecified metacarpal bone**

6 S62.39 **Other fracture of other metacarpal bone**
7 ⊟ S62.390- **Other fracture of second metacarpal bone, right hand**
7 ⊟ S62.391- **Other fracture of second metacarpal bone, left hand**
7 ⊟ S62.392- **Other fracture of third metacarpal bone, right hand**
7 ⊟ S62.393- **Other fracture of third metacarpal bone, left hand**
7 ⊟ S62.394- **Other fracture of fourth metacarpal bone, right hand**
7 ⊟ S62.395- **Other fracture of fourth metacarpal bone, left hand**
7 ⊟ S62.396- **Other fracture of fifth metacarpal bone, right hand**
7 ⊟ S62.397- **Other fracture of fifth metacarpal bone, left hand**
7 ⊟ S62.398- **Other fracture of other metacarpal bone**
Other fracture of specified metacarpal bone with unspecified laterality
7 ⊟ S62.399- **Other fracture of unspecified metacarpal bone**

5 S62.5 **Fracture of thumb**

6 S62.50 **Fracture of unspecified phalanx of thumb**
7 ⊟ S62.501- **Fracture of unspecified phalanx of right thumb**
7 ⊟ S62.502- **Fracture of unspecified phalanx of left thumb**
7 ⊟ S62.509- **Fracture of unspecified phalanx of unspecified thumb**

6 S62.51 **Fracture of proximal phalanx of thumb**
7 ⊟ S62.511- **Displaced fracture of proximal phalanx of right thumb**
7 ⊟ S62.512- **Displaced fracture of proximal phalanx of left thumb**
7 ⊟ S62.513- **Displaced fracture of proximal phalanx of unspecified thumb**
7 ⊟ S62.514- **Nondisplaced fracture of proximal phalanx of right thumb**
7 ⊟ S62.515- **Nondisplaced fracture of proximal phalanx of left thumb**
7 ⊟ S62.516- **Nondisplaced fracture of proximal phalanx of unspecified thumb**

6 S62.52 **Fracture of distal phalanx of thumb**
7 ⊟ S62.521- **Displaced fracture of distal phalanx of right thumb**
7 ⊟ S62.522- **Displaced fracture of distal phalanx of left thumb**
7 ⊟ S62.523- **Displaced fracture of distal phalanx of unspecified thumb**
7 ⊟ S62.524- **Nondisplaced fracture of distal phalanx of right thumb**
7 ⊟ S62.525- **Nondisplaced fracture of distal phalanx of left thumb**
7 ⊟ S62.526- **Nondisplaced fracture of distal phalanx of unspecified thumb**

5 S62.6 **Fracture of other and unspecified finger(s)**
EXCLUDES 2 *fracture of thumb (S62.5-)*

6 S62.60 **Fracture of unspecified phalanx of finger**
7 ⊟ S62.600- **Fracture of unspecified phalanx of right index finger**
7 ⊟ S62.601- **Fracture of unspecified phalanx of left index finger**
7 ⊟ S62.602- **Fracture of unspecified phalanx of right middle finger**
7 ⊟ S62.603- **Fracture of unspecified phalanx of left middle finger**
7 ⊟ S62.604- **Fracture of unspecified phalanx of right ring finger**
7 ⊟ S62.605- **Fracture of unspecified phalanx of left ring finger**
7 ⊟ S62.606- **Fracture of unspecified phalanx of right little finger**
7 ⊟ S62.607- **Fracture of unspecified phalanx of left little finger**
7 ⊟ S62.608- **Fracture of unspecified phalanx of other finger**
Fracture of unspecified phalanx of specified finger with unspecified laterality
7 ⊟ S62.609- **Fracture of unspecified phalanx of unspecified finger**

6 S62.61 **Displaced fracture of proximal phalanx of finger**
7 ⊟ S62.610- **Displaced fracture of proximal phalanx of right index finger**
7 ⊟ S62.611- **Displaced fracture of proximal phalanx of left index finger**
7 ⊟ S62.612- **Displaced fracture of proximal phalanx of right middle finger**
7 ⊟ S62.613- **Displaced fracture of proximal phalanx of left middle finger**
7 ⊟ S62.614- **Displaced fracture of proximal phalanx of right ring finger**
7 ⊟ S62.615- **Displaced fracture of proximal phalanx of left ring finger**
7 ⊟ S62.616- **Displaced fracture of proximal phalanx of right little finger**
7 ⊟ S62.617- **Displaced fracture of proximal phalanx of left little finger**
7 ⊟ S62.618- **Displaced fracture of proximal phalanx of other finger**
Displaced fracture of proximal phalanx of specified finger with unspecified laterality
7 ⊟ S62.619- **Displaced fracture of proximal phalanx of unspecified finger**

6 S62.62 **Displaced fracture of middle phalanx of finger**
7 ⊟ S62.620- **Displaced fracture of middle phalanx of right index finger**
7 ⊟ S62.621- **Displaced fracture of middle phalanx of left index finger**
7 ⊟ S62.622- **Displaced fracture of middle phalanx of right middle finger**

7 ⊟ S62.623- **Displaced fracture of middle phalanx of left middle finger**

7 ⊟ S62.624- **Displaced fracture of middle phalanx of right ring finger**

7 ⊟ S62.625- **Displaced fracture of middle phalanx of left ring finger**

▲ 7 ⊟ S62.626- **Displaced fracture of middle phalanx of right little finger**

▲ 7 ⊟ S62.627- **Displaced fracture of middle phalanx of left little finger**

▲ 7 ⊟ S62.628- **Displaced fracture of middle phalanx of other finger**
Displaced fracture of middle phalanx of specified finger with unspecified laterality

▲ 7 ⊟ S62.629- **Displaced fracture of middle phalanx of unspecified finger**

6 S62.63 **Displaced fracture of distal phalanx of finger**

7 ⊟ S62.630- **Displaced fracture of distal phalanx of right index finger**

7 ⊟ S62.631- **Displaced fracture of distal phalanx of left index finger**

7 ⊟ S62.632- **Displaced fracture of distal phalanx of right middle finger**

7 ⊟ S62.633- **Displaced fracture of distal phalanx of left middle finger**

7 ⊟ S62.634- **Displaced fracture of distal phalanx of right ring finger**

7 ⊟ S62.635- **Displaced fracture of distal phalanx of left ring finger**

7 ⊟ S62.636- **Displaced fracture of distal phalanx of right little finger**

7 ⊟ S62.637- **Displaced fracture of distal phalanx of left little finger**

7 ⊟ S62.638- **Displaced fracture of distal phalanx of other finger**
Displaced fracture of distal phalanx of specified finger with unspecified laterality

7 ⊟ S62.639- **Displaced fracture of distal phalanx of unspecified finger**

6 S62.64 **Nondisplaced fracture of proximal phalanx of finger**

7 ⊟ S62.640- **Nondisplaced fracture of proximal phalanx of right index finger**

7 ⊟ S62.641- **Nondisplaced fracture of proximal phalanx of left index finger**

7 ⊟ S62.642- **Nondisplaced fracture of proximal phalanx of right middle finger**

7 ⊟ S62.643- **Nondisplaced fracture of proximal phalanx of left middle finger**

7 ⊟ S62.644- **Nondisplaced fracture of proximal phalanx of right ring finger**

7 ⊟ S62.645- **Nondisplaced fracture of proximal phalanx of left ring finger**

7 ⊟ S62.646- **Nondisplaced fracture of proximal phalanx of right little finger**

7 ⊟ S62.647- **Nondisplaced fracture of proximal phalanx of left little finger**

7 ⊟ S62.648- **Nondisplaced fracture of proximal phalanx of other finger**
Nondisplaced fracture of proximal phalanx of specified finger with unspecified laterality

7 ⊟ S62.649- **Nondisplaced fracture of proximal phalanx of unspecified finger**

6 S62.65 **Nondisplaced fracture of middle phalanx of finger**

7 ⊟ S62.650- **Nondisplaced fracture of middle phalanx of right index finger**

7 ⊟ S62.651- **Nondisplaced fracture of middle phalanx of left index finger**

7 ⊟ S62.652- **Nondisplaced fracture of middle phalanx of right middle finger**

7 ⊟ S62.653- **Nondisplaced fracture of middle phalanx of left middle finger**

▲ 7 ⊟ S62.654- **Nondisplaced fracture of middle phalanx of right ring finger**

▲ 7 ⊟ S62.655- **Nondisplaced fracture of middle phalanx of left ring finger**

▲ 7 ⊟ S62.656- **Nondisplaced fracture of middle phalanx of right little finger**

▲ 7 ⊟ S62.657- **Nondisplaced fracture of middle phalanx of left little finger**

▲ 7 ⊟ S62.658- **Nondisplaced fracture of middle phalanx of other finger**
Nondisplaced fracture of middle phalanx of specified finger with unspecified laterality

▲ 7 ⊟ S62.659- **Nondisplaced fracture of middle phalanx of unspecified finger**

6 S62.66 **Nondisplaced fracture of distal phalanx of finger**

7 ⊟ S62.660- **Nondisplaced fracture of distal phalanx of right index finger**

7 ⊟ S62.661- **Nondisplaced fracture of distal phalanx of left index finger**

7 ⊟ S62.662- **Nondisplaced fracture of distal phalanx of right middle finger**

7 ⊟ S62.663- **Nondisplaced fracture of distal phalanx of left middle finger**

7 ⊟ S62.664- **Nondisplaced fracture of distal phalanx of right ring finger**

7 ⊟ S62.665- **Nondisplaced fracture of distal phalanx of left ring finger**

7 ⊟ S62.666- **Nondisplaced fracture of distal phalanx of right little finger**

7 ⊟ S62.667- **Nondisplaced fracture of distal phalanx of left little finger**

7 ⊟ S62.668- **Nondisplaced fracture of distal phalanx of other finger**
Nondisplaced fracture of distal phalanx of specified finger with unspecified laterality

7 ⊟ S62.669- **Nondisplaced fracture of distal phalanx of unspecified finger**

5 S62.9 **Unspecified fracture of wrist and hand**

7 ⊟ S62.90X- **Unspecified fracture of unspecified wrist and hand**

7 ⊟ S62.91X- **Unspecified fracture of right wrist and hand**

7 ⊟ S62.92X- **Unspecified fracture of left wrist and hand**

4 S63 Dislocation and sprain of joints and ligaments at wrist and hand level

INCLUDES
avulsion of joint or ligament at wrist and hand level
laceration of cartilage, joint or ligament at wrist and hand level
sprain of cartilage, joint or ligament at wrist and hand level
traumatic hemarthrosis of joint or ligament at wrist and hand level
traumatic rupture of joint or ligament at wrist and hand level
traumatic subluxation of joint or ligament at wrist and hand level
traumatic tear of joint or ligament at wrist and hand level

Code also:
any associated open wound

EXCLUDES 2 *strain of muscle, fascia and tendon of wrist and hand (S66.-)*

The appropriate 7th character is to be added to each code from category S63
A initial encounter
D subsequent encounter
S sequela

CODING TIP ✓ There are no codes for open dislocations. When a dislocation is documented as open, assign an additional code for the open wound.

5 S63.0 **Subluxation and dislocation of wrist and hand joints**

6 S63.00 **Unspecified subluxation and dislocation of wrist and hand**
Dislocation of carpal bone NOS
Dislocation of distal end of radius NOS
Subluxation of carpal bone NOS
Subluxation of distal end of radius NOS

7 ⊟ S63.001- **Unspecified subluxation of right wrist and hand**

7 ⊟ S63.002- **Unspecified subluxation of left wrist and hand**

7 ⊟ S63.003- **Unspecified subluxation of unspecified wrist and hand**

7 ⊟ S63.004- **Unspecified dislocation of right wrist and hand**

7 ⊟ S63.005- **Unspecified dislocation of left wrist and hand**

S63.006- Unspecified dislocation of unspecified wrist and hand

S63.01 Subluxation and dislocation of distal radioulnar joint

S63.011- Subluxation of distal radioulnar joint of right wrist

S63.012- Subluxation of distal radioulnar joint of left wrist

S63.013- Subluxation of distal radioulnar joint of unspecified wrist

S63.014- Dislocation of distal radioulnar joint of right wrist

S63.015- Dislocation of distal radioulnar joint of left wrist

S63.016- Dislocation of distal radioulnar joint of unspecified wrist

S63.02 Subluxation and dislocation of radiocarpal joint

S63.021- Subluxation of radiocarpal joint of right wrist

S63.022- Subluxation of radiocarpal joint of left wrist

S63.023- Subluxation of radiocarpal joint of unspecified wrist

S63.024- Dislocation of radiocarpal joint of right wrist

S63.025- Dislocation of radiocarpal joint of left wrist

S63.026- Dislocation of radiocarpal joint of unspecified wrist

S63.03 Subluxation and dislocation of midcarpal joint

S63.031- Subluxation of midcarpal joint of right wrist

S63.032- Subluxation of midcarpal joint of left wrist

S63.033- Subluxation of midcarpal joint of unspecified wrist

S63.034- Dislocation of midcarpal joint of right wrist

S63.035- Dislocation of midcarpal joint of left wrist

S63.036- Dislocation of midcarpal joint of unspecified wrist

S63.04 Subluxation and dislocation of carpometacarpal joint of thumb

EXCLUDES 2 *interphalangeal subluxation and dislocation of thumb (S63.1-)*

S63.041- Subluxation of carpometacarpal joint of right thumb

S63.042- Subluxation of carpometacarpal joint of left thumb

S63.043- Subluxation of carpometacarpal joint of unspecified thumb

S63.044- Dislocation of carpometacarpal joint of right thumb

S63.045- Dislocation of carpometacarpal joint of left thumb

S63.046- Dislocation of carpometacarpal joint of unspecified thumb

S63.05 Subluxation and dislocation of other carpometacarpal joint

EXCLUDES 2 *subluxation and dislocation of carpometacarpal joint of thumb (S63.04-)*

S63.051- Subluxation of other carpometacarpal joint of right hand

S63.052- Subluxation of other carpometacarpal joint of left hand

S63.053- Subluxation of other carpometacarpal joint of unspecified hand

S63.054- Dislocation of other carpometacarpal joint of right hand

S63.055- Dislocation of other carpometacarpal joint of left hand

S63.056- Dislocation of other carpometacarpal joint of unspecified hand

S63.06 Subluxation and dislocation of metacarpal (bone), proximal end

S63.061- Subluxation of metacarpal (bone), proximal end of right hand

S63.062- Subluxation of metacarpal (bone), proximal end of left hand

S63.063- Subluxation of metacarpal (bone), proximal end of unspecified hand

S63.064- Dislocation of metacarpal (bone), proximal end of right hand

S63.065- Dislocation of metacarpal (bone), proximal end of left hand

S63.066- Dislocation of metacarpal (bone), proximal end of unspecified hand

S63.07 Subluxation and dislocation of distal end of ulna

S63.071- Subluxation of distal end of right ulna

S63.072- Subluxation of distal end of left ulna

S63.073- Subluxation of distal end of unspecified ulna

S63.074- Dislocation of distal end of right ulna

S63.075- Dislocation of distal end of left ulna

S63.076- Dislocation of distal end of unspecified ulna

S63.09 Other subluxation and dislocation of wrist and hand

S63.091- Other subluxation of right wrist and hand

S63.092- Other subluxation of left wrist and hand

S63.093- Other subluxation of unspecified wrist and hand

S63.094- Other dislocation of right wrist and hand

S63.095- Other dislocation of left wrist and hand

S63.096- Other dislocation of unspecified wrist and hand

S63.1 Subluxation and dislocation of thumb

S63.10 Unspecified subluxation and dislocation of thumb

S63.101- Unspecified subluxation of right thumb

S63.102- Unspecified subluxation of left thumb

S63.103- Unspecified subluxation of unspecified thumb

S63.104- Unspecified dislocation of right thumb

S63.105- Unspecified dislocation of left thumb

S63.106- Unspecified dislocation of unspecified thumb

S63.11 Subluxation and dislocation of metacarpophalangeal joint of thumb

S63.111- Subluxation of metacarpophalangeal joint of right thumb

S63.112- Subluxation of metacarpophalangeal joint of left thumb

S63.113- Subluxation of metacarpophalangeal joint of unspecified thumb

S63.114- Dislocation of metacarpophalangeal joint of right thumb

S63.115- Dislocation of metacarpophalangeal joint of left thumb

S63.116- Dislocation of metacarpophalangeal joint of unspecified thumb

S63.12 Subluxation and dislocation of interphalangeal joint of thumb

S63.121- Subluxation of interphalangeal joint of right thumb

S63.122- Subluxation of interphalangeal joint of left thumb

S63.123- Subluxation of interphalangeal joint of unspecified thumb

S63.124- Dislocation of interphalangeal joint of right thumb

S63.125- Dislocation of interphalangeal joint of left thumb

S63.126- Dislocation of interphalangeal joint of unspecified thumb

✖ ~~S63.13 Subluxation and dislocation of proximal interphalangeal joint of thumb~~

✖ ~~S63.131- Subluxation of proximal interphalangeal joint of right thumb~~

✖ ~~S63.132- Subluxation of proximal interphalangeal joint of left thumb~~

✖ ~~S63.133- Subluxation of proximal interphalangeal joint of unspecified thumb~~

✖ ~~S63.134- Dislocation of proximal interphalangeal joint of right thumb~~

✖ ~~S63.135- Dislocation of proximal interphalangeal joint of left thumb~~

✖ ~~S63.136- Dislocation of proximal interphalangeal joint of unspecified thumb~~

✖ ~~S63.14 Subluxation and dislocation of distal interphalangeal joint of thumb~~

✖ ~~S63.141-~~ ~~Subluxation of distal interphalangeal joint of right thumb~~

✖ ~~S63.142-~~ ~~Subluxation of distal interphalangeal joint of left thumb~~

✖ ~~S63.143-~~ ~~Subluxation of distal interphalangeal joint of unspecified thumb~~

✖ ~~S63.144-~~ ~~Dislocation of distal interphalangeal joint of right thumb~~

✖ ~~S63.145-~~ ~~Dislocation of distal interphalangeal joint of left thumb~~

✖ ~~S63.146-~~ ~~Dislocation of distal interphalangeal joint of unspecified thumb~~

5 S63.2 Subluxation and dislocation of other finger(s)

EXCLUDES 2 *subluxation and dislocation of thumb (S63.1-)*

6 **S63.20 Unspecified subluxation of other finger**

7 ⊟ **S63.200- Unspecified subluxation of right index finger**

7 ⊟ **S63.201- Unspecified subluxation of left index finger**

7 ⊟ **S63.202- Unspecified subluxation of right middle finger**

7 ⊟ **S63.203- Unspecified subluxation of left middle finger**

7 ⊟ **S63.204- Unspecified subluxation of right ring finger**

7 ⊟ **S63.205- Unspecified subluxation of left ring finger**

7 ⊟ **S63.206- Unspecified subluxation of right little finger**

7 ⊟ **S63.207- Unspecified subluxation of left little finger**

7 ⊟ **S63.208- Unspecified subluxation of other finger**

Unspecified subluxation of specified finger with unspecified laterality

7 ⊟ **S63.209- Unspecified subluxation of unspecified finger**

6 **S63.21 Subluxation of metacarpophalangeal joint of finger**

7 ⊟ **S63.210- Subluxation of metacarpophalangeal joint of right index finger**

7 ⊟ **S63.211- Subluxation of metacarpophalangeal joint of left index finger**

7 ⊟ **S63.212- Subluxation of metacarpophalangeal joint of right middle finger**

7 ⊟ **S63.213- Subluxation of metacarpophalangeal joint of left middle finger**

7 ⊟ **S63.214- Subluxation of metacarpophalangeal joint of right ring finger**

7 ⊟ **S63.215- Subluxation of metacarpophalangeal joint of left ring finger**

7 ⊟ **S63.216- Subluxation of metacarpophalangeal joint of right little finger**

7 ⊟ **S63.217- Subluxation of metacarpophalangeal joint of left little finger**

7 ⊟ **S63.218- Subluxation of metacarpophalangeal joint of other finger**

Subluxation of metacarpophalangeal joint of specified finger with unspecified laterality

7 ⊟ **S63.219- Subluxation of metacarpophalangeal joint of unspecified finger**

6 **S63.22 Subluxation of unspecified interphalangeal joint of finger**

7 ⊟ **S63.220- Subluxation of unspecified interphalangeal joint of right index finger**

7 ⊟ **S63.221- Subluxation of unspecified interphalangeal joint of left index finger**

7 ⊟ **S63.222- Subluxation of unspecified interphalangeal joint of right middle finger**

7 ⊟ **S63.223- Subluxation of unspecified interphalangeal joint of left middle finger**

7 ⊟ **S63.224- Subluxation of unspecified interphalangeal joint of right ring finger**

7 ⊟ **S63.225- Subluxation of unspecified interphalangeal joint of left ring finger**

7 ⊟ **S63.226- Subluxation of unspecified interphalangeal joint of right little finger**

7 ⊟ **S63.227- Subluxation of unspecified interphalangeal joint of left little finger**

7 ⊟ **S63.228- Subluxation of unspecified interphalangeal joint of other finger**

Subluxation of unspecified interphalangeal joint of specified finger with unspecified laterality

7 ⊟ **S63.229- Subluxation of unspecified interphalangeal joint of unspecified finger**

6 **S63.23 Subluxation of proximal interphalangeal joint of finger**

7 ⊟ **S63.230- Subluxation of proximal interphalangeal joint of right index finger**

7 ⊟ **S63.231- Subluxation of proximal interphalangeal joint of left index finger**

7 ⊟ **S63.232- Subluxation of proximal interphalangeal joint of right middle finger**

7 ⊟ **S63.233- Subluxation of proximal interphalangeal joint of left middle finger**

7 ⊟ **S63.234- Subluxation of proximal interphalangeal joint of right ring finger**

7 ⊟ **S63.235- Subluxation of proximal interphalangeal joint of left ring finger**

7 ⊟ **S63.236- Subluxation of proximal interphalangeal joint of right little finger**

7 ⊟ **S63.237- Subluxation of proximal interphalangeal joint of left little finger**

7 ⊟ **S63.238- Subluxation of proximal interphalangeal joint of other finger**

Subluxation of proximal interphalangeal joint of specified finger with unspecified laterality

7 ⊟ **S63.239- Subluxation of proximal interphalangeal joint of unspecified finger**

6 **S63.24 Subluxation of distal interphalangeal joint of finger**

7 ⊟ **S63.240- Subluxation of distal interphalangeal joint of right index finger**

7 ⊟ **S63.241- Subluxation of distal interphalangeal joint of left index finger**

7 ⊟ **S63.242- Subluxation of distal interphalangeal joint of right middle finger**

7 ⊟ **S63.243- Subluxation of distal interphalangeal joint of left middle finger**

7 ⊟ **S63.244- Subluxation of distal interphalangeal joint of right ring finger**

7 ⊟ **S63.245- Subluxation of distal interphalangeal joint of left ring finger**

7 ⊟ **S63.246- Subluxation of distal interphalangeal joint of right little finger**

7 ⊟ **S63.247- Subluxation of distal interphalangeal joint of left little finger**

7 ⊟ **S63.248- Subluxation of distal interphalangeal joint of other finger**

Subluxation of distal interphalangeal joint of specified finger with unspecified laterality

7 ⊟ **S63.249- Subluxation of distal interphalangeal joint of unspecified finger**

6 **S63.25 Unspecified dislocation of other finger**

7 ⊟ **S63.250- Unspecified dislocation of right index finger**

7 ⊟ **S63.251- Unspecified dislocation of left index finger**

7 ⊟ **S63.252- Unspecified dislocation of right middle finger**

7 ⊟ **S63.253- Unspecified dislocation of left middle finger**

7 ⊟ **S63.254- Unspecified dislocation of right ring finger**

7 ⊟ **S63.255- Unspecified dislocation of left ring finger**

7 ⊟ **S63.256- Unspecified dislocation of right little finger**

7 ⊟ **S63.257- Unspecified dislocation of left little finger**

7 ⊟ **S63.258- Unspecified dislocation of other finger**

Unspecified dislocation of specified finger with unspecified laterality

7 ⊟ **S63.259- Unspecified dislocation of unspecified finger**

Unspecified dislocation of unspecified finger with unspecified laterality

6 **S63.26 Dislocation of metacarpophalangeal joint of finger**

7 ⊟ **S63.260- Dislocation of metacarpophalangeal joint of right index finger**

7 ⊟ **S63.261- Dislocation of metacarpophalangeal joint of left index finger**

7 ⊟ **S63.262- Dislocation of metacarpophalangeal joint of right middle finger**

7 ⊟ **S63.263- Dislocation of metacarpophalangeal joint of left middle finger**

7 ⊟ **S63.264- Dislocation of metacarpophalangeal joint of right ring finger**

7 ⊟ **S63.265- Dislocation of metacarpophalangeal joint of left ring finger**

7 ⊟ **S63.266- Dislocation of metacarpophalangeal joint of right little finger**

7 ⊟ S63.267- **Dislocation of metacarpophalangeal joint of left little finger**

7 ⊟ S63.268- **Dislocation of metacarpophalangeal joint of other finger**
Dislocation of metacarpophalangeal joint of specified finger with unspecified laterality

7 ⊟ S63.269- **Dislocation of metacarpophalangeal joint of unspecified finger**

6 S63.27 **Dislocation of unspecified interphalangeal joint of finger**

7 ⊟ S63.270- **Dislocation of unspecified interphalangeal joint of right index finger**

7 ⊟ S63.271- **Dislocation of unspecified interphalangeal joint of left index finger**

7 ⊟ S63.272- **Dislocation of unspecified interphalangeal joint of right middle finger**

7 ⊟ S63.273- **Dislocation of unspecified interphalangeal joint of left middle finger**

7 ⊟ S63.274- **Dislocation of unspecified interphalangeal joint of right ring finger**

7 ⊟ S63.275- **Dislocation of unspecified interphalangeal joint of left ring finger**

7 ⊟ S63.276- **Dislocation of unspecified interphalangeal joint of right little finger**

7 ⊟ S63.277- **Dislocation of unspecified interphalangeal joint of left little finger**

7 ⊟ S63.278- **Dislocation of unspecified interphalangeal joint of other finger**
Dislocation of unspecified interphalangeal joint of specified finger with unspecified laterality

7 ⊟ S63.279- **Dislocation of unspecified interphalangeal joint of unspecified finger**
Dislocation of unspecified interphalangeal joint of unspecified finger without specified laterality

6 S63.28 **Dislocation of proximal interphalangeal joint of finger**

7 ⊟ S63.280- **Dislocation of proximal interphalangeal joint of right index finger**

7 ⊟ S63.281- **Dislocation of proximal interphalangeal joint of left index finger**

7 ⊟ S63.282- **Dislocation of proximal interphalangeal joint of right middle finger**

7 ⊟ S63.283- **Dislocation of proximal interphalangeal joint of left middle finger**

7 ⊟ S63.284- **Dislocation of proximal interphalangeal joint of right ring finger**

7 ⊟ S63.285- **Dislocation of proximal interphalangeal joint of left ring finger**

7 ⊟ S63.286- **Dislocation of proximal interphalangeal joint of right little finger**

7 ⊟ S63.287- **Dislocation of proximal interphalangeal joint of left little finger**

7 ⊟ S63.288- **Dislocation of proximal interphalangeal joint of other finger**
Dislocation of proximal interphalangeal joint of specified finger with unspecified laterality

7 ⊟ S63.289- **Dislocation of proximal interphalangeal joint of unspecified finger**

6 S63.29 **Dislocation of distal interphalangeal joint of finger**

7 ⊟ S63.290- **Dislocation of distal interphalangeal joint of right index finger**

7 ⊟ S63.291- **Dislocation of distal interphalangeal joint of left index finger**

7 ⊟ S63.292- **Dislocation of distal interphalangeal joint of right middle finger**

7 ⊟ S63.293- **Dislocation of distal interphalangeal joint of left middle finger**

7 ⊟ S63.294- **Dislocation of distal interphalangeal joint of right ring finger**

7 ⊟ S63.295- **Dislocation of distal interphalangeal joint of left ring finger**

7 ⊟ S63.296- **Dislocation of distal interphalangeal joint of right little finger**

7 ⊟ S63.297- **Dislocation of distal interphalangeal joint of left little finger**

7 ⊟ S63.298- **Dislocation of distal interphalangeal joint of other finger**
Dislocation of distal interphalangeal joint of specified finger with unspecified laterality

7 ⊟ S63.299- **Dislocation of distal interphalangeal joint of unspecified finger**

5 S63.3 **Traumatic rupture of ligament of wrist**

6 S63.30 **Traumatic rupture of unspecified ligament of wrist**

7 ⊟ S63.301- **Traumatic rupture of unspecified ligament of right wrist**

7 ⊟ S63.302- **Traumatic rupture of unspecified ligament of left wrist**

7 ⊟ S63.309- **Traumatic rupture of unspecified ligament of unspecified wrist**

6 S63.31 **Traumatic rupture of collateral ligament of wrist**

7 ⊟ S63.311- **Traumatic rupture of collateral ligament of right wrist**

7 ⊟ S63.312- **Traumatic rupture of collateral ligament of left wrist**

7 ⊟ S63.319- **Traumatic rupture of collateral ligament of unspecified wrist**

6 S63.32 **Traumatic rupture of radiocarpal ligament**

7 ⊟ S63.321- **Traumatic rupture of right radiocarpal ligament**

7 ⊟ S63.322- **Traumatic rupture of left radiocarpal ligament**

7 ⊟ S63.329- **Traumatic rupture of unspecified radiocarpal ligament**

6 S63.33 **Traumatic rupture of ulnocarpal (palmar) ligament**

7 ⊟ S63.331- **Traumatic rupture of right ulnocarpal (palmar) ligament**

7 ⊟ S63.332- **Traumatic rupture of left ulnocarpal (palmar) ligament**

7 ⊟ S63.339- **Traumatic rupture of unspecified ulnocarpal (palmar) ligament**

6 S63.39 **Traumatic rupture of other ligament of wrist**

7 ⊟ S63.391- **Traumatic rupture of other ligament of right wrist**

7 ⊟ S63.392- **Traumatic rupture of other ligament of left wrist**

7 ⊟ S63.399- **Traumatic rupture of other ligament of unspecified wrist**

5 S63.4 **Traumatic rupture of ligament of finger at metacarpophalangeal and interphalangeal joint(s)**

6 S63.40 **Traumatic rupture of unspecified ligament of finger at metacarpophalangeal and interphalangeal joint**

7 ⊟ S63.400- **Traumatic rupture of unspecified ligament of right index finger at metacarpophalangeal and interphalangeal joint**

7 ⊟ S63.401- **Traumatic rupture of unspecified ligament of left index finger at metacarpophalangeal and interphalangeal joint**

7 ⊟ S63.402- **Traumatic rupture of unspecified ligament of right middle finger at metacarpophalangeal and interphalangeal joint**

7 ⊟ S63.403- **Traumatic rupture of unspecified ligament of left middle finger at metacarpophalangeal and interphalangeal joint**

7 ⊟ S63.404- **Traumatic rupture of unspecified ligament of right ring finger at metacarpophalangeal and interphalangeal joint**

7 ⊟ S63.405- **Traumatic rupture of unspecified ligament of left ring finger at metacarpophalangeal and interphalangeal joint**

7 ⊟ S63.406- **Traumatic rupture of unspecified ligament of right little finger at metacarpophalangeal and interphalangeal joint**

7 ⊟ S63.407- **Traumatic rupture of unspecified ligament of left little finger at metacarpophalangeal and interphalangeal joint**

7 ⊟ S63.408- **Traumatic rupture of unspecified ligament of other finger at metacarpophalangeal and interphalangeal joint**
Traumatic rupture of unspecified ligament of specified finger with unspecified laterality at metacarpophalangeal and interphalangeal joint

S63.409- **Traumatic rupture of unspecified ligament of unspecified finger at metacarpophalangeal and interphalangeal joint**

S63.41 **Traumatic rupture of collateral ligament of finger at metacarpophalangeal and interphalangeal joint**

S63.410- **Traumatic rupture of collateral ligament of right index finger at metacarpophalangeal and interphalangeal joint**

S63.411- **Traumatic rupture of collateral ligament of left index finger at metacarpophalangeal and interphalangeal joint**

S63.412- **Traumatic rupture of collateral ligament of right middle finger at metacarpophalangeal and interphalangeal joint**

S63.413- **Traumatic rupture of collateral ligament of left middle finger at metacarpophalangeal and interphalangeal joint**

S63.414- **Traumatic rupture of collateral ligament of right ring finger at metacarpophalangeal and interphalangeal joint**

S63.415- **Traumatic rupture of collateral ligament of left ring finger at metacarpophalangeal and interphalangeal joint**

S63.416- **Traumatic rupture of collateral ligament of right little finger at metacarpophalangeal and interphalangeal joint**

S63.417- **Traumatic rupture of collateral ligament of left little finger at metacarpophalangeal and interphalangeal joint**

S63.418- **Traumatic rupture of collateral ligament of other finger at metacarpophalangeal and interphalangeal joint**
Traumatic rupture of collateral ligament of specified finger with unspecified laterality at metacarpophalangeal and interphalangeal joint

S63.419- **Traumatic rupture of collateral ligament of unspecified finger at metacarpophalangeal and interphalangeal joint**

S63.42 **Traumatic rupture of palmar ligament of finger at metacarpophalangeal and interphalangeal joint**

S63.420- **Traumatic rupture of palmar ligament of right index finger at metacarpophalangeal and interphalangeal joint**

S63.421- **Traumatic rupture of palmar ligament of left index finger at metacarpophalangeal and interphalangeal joint**

S63.422- **Traumatic rupture of palmar ligament of right middle finger at metacarpophalangeal and interphalangeal joint**

S63.423- **Traumatic rupture of palmar ligament of left middle finger at metacarpophalangeal and interphalangeal joint**

S63.424- **Traumatic rupture of palmar ligament of right ring finger at metacarpophalangeal and interphalangeal joint**

S63.425- **Traumatic rupture of palmar ligament of left ring finger at metacarpophalangeal and interphalangeal joint**

S63.426- **Traumatic rupture of palmar ligament of right little finger at metacarpophalangeal and interphalangeal joint**

S63.427- **Traumatic rupture of palmar ligament of left little finger at metacarpophalangeal and interphalangeal joint**

S63.428- **Traumatic rupture of palmar ligament of other finger at metacarpophalangeal and interphalangeal joint**
Traumatic rupture of palmar ligament of specified finger with unspecified laterality at metacarpophalangeal and interphalangeal joint

S63.429- **Traumatic rupture of palmar ligament of unspecified finger at metacarpophalangeal and interphalangeal joint**

S63.43 **Traumatic rupture of volar plate of finger at metacarpophalangeal and interphalangeal joint**

S63.430- **Traumatic rupture of volar plate of right index finger at metacarpophalangeal and interphalangeal joint**

S63.431- **Traumatic rupture of volar plate of left index finger at metacarpophalangeal and interphalangeal joint**

S63.432- **Traumatic rupture of volar plate of right middle finger at metacarpophalangeal and interphalangeal joint**

S63.433- **Traumatic rupture of volar plate of left middle finger at metacarpophalangeal and interphalangeal joint**

S63.434- **Traumatic rupture of volar plate of right ring finger at metacarpophalangeal and interphalangeal joint**

S63.435- **Traumatic rupture of volar plate of left ring finger at metacarpophalangeal and interphalangeal joint**

S63.436- **Traumatic rupture of volar plate of right little finger at metacarpophalangeal and interphalangeal joint**

S63.437- **Traumatic rupture of volar plate of left little finger at metacarpophalangeal and interphalangeal joint**

S63.438- **Traumatic rupture of volar plate of other finger at metacarpophalangeal and interphalangeal joint**
Traumatic rupture of volar plate of specified finger with unspecified laterality at metacarpophalangeal and interphalangeal joint

S63.439- **Traumatic rupture of volar plate of unspecified finger at metacarpophalangeal and interphalangeal joint**

S63.49 **Traumatic rupture of other ligament of finger at metacarpophalangeal and interphalangeal joint**

S63.490- **Traumatic rupture of other ligament of right index finger at metacarpophalangeal and interphalangeal joint**

S63.491- **Traumatic rupture of other ligament of left index finger at metacarpophalangeal and interphalangeal joint**

S63.492- **Traumatic rupture of other ligament of right middle finger at metacarpophalangeal and interphalangeal joint**

S63.493- **Traumatic rupture of other ligament of left middle finger at metacarpophalangeal and interphalangeal joint**

S63.494- **Traumatic rupture of other ligament of right ring finger at metacarpophalangeal and interphalangeal joint**

S63.495- **Traumatic rupture of other ligament of left ring finger at metacarpophalangeal and interphalangeal joint**

S63.496- **Traumatic rupture of other ligament of right little finger at metacarpophalangeal and interphalangeal joint**

S63.497- **Traumatic rupture of other ligament of left little finger at metacarpophalangeal and interphalangeal joint**

S63.498- **Traumatic rupture of other ligament of other finger at metacarpophalangeal and interphalangeal joint**
Traumatic rupture of ligament of specified finger with unspecified laterality at metacarpophalangeal and interphalangeal joint

S63.499- **Traumatic rupture of other ligament of unspecified finger at metacarpophalangeal and interphalangeal joint**

S63.5 **Other and unspecified sprain of wrist**

S63.50 **Unspecified sprain of wrist**

S63.501- **Unspecified sprain of right wrist**

S63.502- **Unspecified sprain of left wrist**

S63.509- **Unspecified sprain of unspecified wrist**

S63.51 **Sprain of carpal (joint)**

S63.511- **Sprain of carpal joint of right wrist**

S63.512- **Sprain of carpal joint of left wrist**

S63.519- **Sprain of carpal joint of unspecified wrist**

S63.52 **Sprain of radiocarpal joint**

EXCLUDES 1 *traumatic rupture of radiocarpal ligament (S63.32-)*

S63.521- **Sprain of radiocarpal joint of right wrist**

S63.522- **Sprain of radiocarpal joint of left wrist**

S63.529- **Sprain of radiocarpal joint of unspecified wrist**

S63.59 **Other specified sprain of wrist**

7 ⊟ S63.591- Other specified sprain of right wrist
7 ⊟ S63.592- Other specified sprain of left wrist
7 ⊟ S63.599- Other specified sprain of unspecified wrist

5 S63.6 Other and unspecified sprain of finger(s)
EXCLUDES 1 *traumatic rupture of ligament of finger at metacarpophalangeal and interphalangeal joint (s) (S63.4-)*

6 S63.60 Unspecified sprain of thumb
7 ⊟ S63.601- Unspecified sprain of right thumb
7 ⊟ S63.602- Unspecified sprain of left thumb
7 ⊟ S63.609- Unspecified sprain of unspecified thumb

6 S63.61 Unspecified sprain of other and unspecified finger(s)
7 ⊟ S63.610- Unspecified sprain of right index finger
7 ⊟ S63.611- Unspecified sprain of left index finger
7 ⊟ S63.612- Unspecified sprain of right middle finger
7 ⊟ S63.613- Unspecified sprain of left middle finger
7 ⊟ S63.614- Unspecified sprain of right ring finger
7 ⊟ S63.615- Unspecified sprain of left ring finger
7 ⊟ S63.616- Unspecified sprain of right little finger
7 ⊟ S63.617- Unspecified sprain of left little finger
7 ⊟ S63.618- Unspecified sprain of other finger
Unspecified sprain of specified finger with unspecified laterality
7 ⊟ S63.619- Unspecified sprain of unspecified finger

6 S63.62 Sprain of interphalangeal joint of thumb
7 ⊟ S63.621- Sprain of interphalangeal joint of right thumb
7 ⊟ S63.622- Sprain of interphalangeal joint of left thumb
7 ⊟ S63.629- Sprain of interphalangeal joint of unspecified thumb

6 S63.63 Sprain of interphalangeal joint of other and unspecified finger(s)
7 ⊟ S63.630- Sprain of interphalangeal joint of right index finger
7 ⊟ S63.631- Sprain of interphalangeal joint of left index finger
7 ⊟ S63.632- Sprain of interphalangeal joint of right middle finger
7 ⊟ S63.633- Sprain of interphalangeal joint of left middle finger
7 ⊟ S63.634- Sprain of interphalangeal joint of right ring finger
7 ⊟ S63.635- Sprain of interphalangeal joint of left ring finger
7 ⊟ S63.636- Sprain of interphalangeal joint of right little finger
7 ⊟ S63.637- Sprain of interphalangeal joint of left little finger
7 ⊟ S63.638- Sprain of interphalangeal joint of other finger
7 ⊟ S63.639- Sprain of interphalangeal joint of unspecified finger

6 S63.64 Sprain of metacarpophalangeal joint of thumb
7 ⊟ S63.641- Sprain of metacarpophalangeal joint of right thumb
7 ⊟ S63.642- Sprain of metacarpophalangeal joint of left thumb
7 ⊟ S63.649- Sprain of metacarpophalangeal joint of unspecified thumb

6 S63.65 Sprain of metacarpophalangeal joint of other and unspecified finger(s)
7 ⊟ S63.650- Sprain of metacarpophalangeal joint of right index finger
7 ⊟ S63.651- Sprain of metacarpophalangeal joint of left index finger
7 ⊟ S63.652- Sprain of metacarpophalangeal joint of right middle finger
7 ⊟ S63.653- Sprain of metacarpophalangeal joint of left middle finger
7 ⊟ S63.654- Sprain of metacarpophalangeal joint of right ring finger
7 ⊟ S63.655- Sprain of metacarpophalangeal joint of left ring finger
7 ⊟ S63.656- Sprain of metacarpophalangeal joint of right little finger
7 ⊟ S63.657- Sprain of metacarpophalangeal joint of left little finger
7 ⊟ S63.658- Sprain of metacarpophalangeal joint of other finger
Sprain of metacarpophalangeal joint of specified finger with unspecified laterality
7 ⊟ S63.659- Sprain of metacarpophalangeal joint of unspecified finger

6 S63.68 Other sprain of thumb
7 ⊟ S63.681- Other sprain of right thumb
7 ⊟ S63.682- Other sprain of left thumb
7 ⊟ S63.689- Other sprain of unspecified thumb

6 S63.69 Other sprain of other and unspecified finger(s)
7 ⊟ S63.690- Other sprain of right index finger
7 ⊟ S63.691- Other sprain of left index finger
7 ⊟ S63.692- Other sprain of right middle finger
7 ⊟ S63.693- Other sprain of left middle finger
7 ⊟ S63.694- Other sprain of right ring finger
7 ⊟ S63.695- Other sprain of left ring finger
7 ⊟ S63.696- Other sprain of right little finger
7 ⊟ S63.697- Other sprain of left little finger
7 ⊟ S63.698- Other sprain of other finger
Other sprain of specified finger with unspecified laterality
7 ⊟ S63.699- Other sprain of unspecified finger

5 S63.8 Sprain of other part of wrist and hand
6 S63.8X Sprain of other part of wrist and hand
7 ⊟ S63.8X1- Sprain of other part of right wrist and hand
7 ⊟ S63.8X2- Sprain of other part of left wrist and hand
7 ⊟ S63.8X9- Sprain of other part of unspecified wrist and hand

5 S63.9 Sprain of unspecified part of wrist and hand
7 ⊟ S63.90X- Sprain of unspecified part of unspecified wrist and hand
7 ⊟ S63.91X- Sprain of unspecified part of right wrist and hand
7 ⊟ S63.92X- Sprain of unspecified part of left wrist and hand

4 S64 Injury of nerves at wrist and hand level

Code also:
any associated open wound (S61.-)

The appropriate 7th character is to be added to each code from category S64
A initial encounter
D subsequent encounter
S sequela

CODING TIP ✓ Late effects of injuries are coded with seventh character S (sequela) and are sequenced after the residual condition of the late effect.

5 S64.0 Injury of ulnar nerve at wrist and hand level
7 ⊟ S64.00X- Injury of ulnar nerve at wrist and hand level of unspecified arm
7 ⊟ S64.01X- Injury of ulnar nerve at wrist and hand level of right arm
7 ⊟ S64.02X- Injury of ulnar nerve at wrist and hand level of left arm

5 S64.1 Injury of median nerve at wrist and hand level
7 ⊟ S64.10X- Injury of median nerve at wrist and hand level of unspecified arm
7 ⊟ S64.11X- Injury of median nerve at wrist and hand level of right arm
7 ⊟ S64.12X- Injury of median nerve at wrist and hand level of left arm

5 S64.2 Injury of radial nerve at wrist and hand level
7 ⊟ S64.20X- Injury of radial nerve at wrist and hand level of unspecified arm
7 ⊟ S64.21X- Injury of radial nerve at wrist and hand level of right arm
7 ⊟ S64.22X- Injury of radial nerve at wrist and hand level of left arm

5 S64.3 Injury of digital nerve of thumb
7 ⊟ S64.30X- Injury of digital nerve of unspecified thumb
7 ⊟ S64.31X- Injury of digital nerve of right thumb
7 ⊟ S64.32X- Injury of digital nerve of left thumb

5 S64.4 Injury of digital nerve of other and unspecified finger
7 S64.40X- Injury of digital nerve of unspecified finger

6 S64.49 Injury of digital nerve of other finger
- 7 S64.490- Injury of digital nerve of right index finger
- 7 S64.491- Injury of digital nerve of left index finger
- 7 S64.492- Injury of digital nerve of right middle finger
- 7 S64.493- Injury of digital nerve of left middle finger
- 7 S64.494- Injury of digital nerve of right ring finger
- 7 S64.495- Injury of digital nerve of left ring finger
- 7 S64.496- Injury of digital nerve of right little finger
- 7 S64.497- Injury of digital nerve of left little finger
- 7 S64.498- Injury of digital nerve of other finger
  Injury of digital nerve of specified finger with unspecified laterality

5 S64.8 Injury of other nerves at wrist and hand level

6 S64.8X Injury of other nerves at wrist and hand level
- 7 S64.8X1- Injury of other nerves at wrist and hand level of right arm
- 7 S64.8X2- Injury of other nerves at wrist and hand level of left arm
- 7 S64.8X9- Injury of other nerves at wrist and hand level of unspecified arm

5 S64.9 Injury of unspecified nerve at wrist and hand level
- 7 S64.90X- Injury of unspecified nerve at wrist and hand level of unspecified arm
- 7 S64.91X- Injury of unspecified nerve at wrist and hand level of right arm
- 7 S64.92X- Injury of unspecified nerve at wrist and hand level of left arm

4 S65 Injury of blood vessels at wrist and hand level

Code also:
any associated open wound (S61.-)

The appropriate 7th character is to be added to each code from category S65
- A initial encounter
- D subsequent encounter
- S sequela

5 S65.0 Injury of ulnar artery at wrist and hand level

6 S65.00 Unspecified injury of ulnar artery at wrist and hand level
- 7 S65.001- Unspecified injury of ulnar artery at wrist and hand level of right arm
- 7 S65.002- Unspecified injury of ulnar artery at wrist and hand level of left arm
- 7 S65.009- Unspecified injury of ulnar artery at wrist and hand level of unspecified arm

6 S65.01 Laceration of ulnar artery at wrist and hand level
- 7 S65.011- Laceration of ulnar artery at wrist and hand level of right arm
- 7 S65.012- Laceration of ulnar artery at wrist and hand level of left arm
- 7 S65.019- Laceration of ulnar artery at wrist and hand level of unspecified arm

6 S65.09 Other specified injury of ulnar artery at wrist and hand level
- 7 S65.091- Other specified injury of ulnar artery at wrist and hand level of right arm
- 7 S65.092- Other specified injury of ulnar artery at wrist and hand level of left arm
- 7 S65.099- Other specified injury of ulnar artery at wrist and hand level of unspecified arm

5 S65.1 Injury of radial artery at wrist and hand level

6 S65.10 Unspecified injury of radial artery at wrist and hand level
- 7 S65.101- Unspecified injury of radial artery at wrist and hand level of right arm
- 7 S65.102- Unspecified injury of radial artery at wrist and hand level of left arm
- 7 S65.109- Unspecified injury of radial artery at wrist and hand level of unspecified arm

6 S65.11 Laceration of radial artery at wrist and hand level
- 7 S65.111- Laceration of radial artery at wrist and hand level of right arm
- 7 S65.112- Laceration of radial artery at wrist and hand level of left arm
- 7 S65.119 Laceration of radial artery at wrist and hand level of unspecified arm

6 S65.19 Other specified injury of radial artery at wrist and hand level
- 7 S65.191- Other specified injury of radial artery at wrist and hand level of right arm
- 7 S65.192- Other specified injury of radial artery at wrist and hand level of left arm
- 7 S65.199- Other specified injury of radial artery at wrist and hand level of unspecified arm

5 S65.2 Injury of superficial palmar arch

6 S65.20 Unspecified injury of superficial palmar arch
- 7 S65.201- Unspecified injury of superficial palmar arch of right hand
- 7 S65.202- Unspecified injury of superficial palmar arch of left hand
- 7 S65.209- Unspecified injury of superficial palmar arch of unspecified hand

6 S65.21 Laceration of superficial palmar arch
- 7 S65.211- Laceration of superficial palmar arch of right hand
- 7 S65.212- Laceration of superficial palmar arch of left hand
- 7 S65.219- Laceration of superficial palmar arch of unspecified hand

6 S65.29 Other specified injury of superficial palmar arch
- 7 S65.291- Other specified injury of superficial palmar arch of right hand
- 7 S65.292- Other specified injury of superficial palmar arch of left hand
- 7 S65.299- Other specified injury of superficial palmar arch of unspecified hand

5 S65.3 Injury of deep palmar arch

6 S65.30 Unspecified injury of deep palmar arch
- 7 S65.301- Unspecified injury of deep palmar arch of right hand
- 7 S65.302- Unspecified injury of deep palmar arch of left hand
- 7 S65.309- Unspecified injury of deep palmar arch of unspecified hand

6 S65.31 Laceration of deep palmar arch
- 7 S65.311- Laceration of deep palmar arch of right hand
- 7 S65.312- Laceration of deep palmar arch of left hand
- 7 S65.319- Laceration of deep palmar arch of unspecified hand

6 S65.39 Other specified injury of deep palmar arch
- 7 S65.391- Other specified injury of deep palmar arch of right hand
- 7 S65.392- Other specified injury of deep palmar arch of left hand
- 7 S65.399- Other specified injury of deep palmar arch of unspecified hand

5 S65.4 Injury of blood vessel of thumb

6 S65.40 Unspecified injury of blood vessel of thumb
- 7 S65.401- Unspecified injury of blood vessel of right thumb
- 7 S65.402- Unspecified injury of blood vessel of left thumb
- 7 S65.409- Unspecified injury of blood vessel of unspecified thumb

6 S65.41 Laceration of blood vessel of thumb
- 7 S65.411- Laceration of blood vessel of right thumb
- 7 S65.412- Laceration of blood vessel of left thumb
- 7 S65.419- Laceration of blood vessel of unspecified thumb

6 S65.49 Other specified injury of blood vessel of thumb
- 7 S65.491- Other specified injury of blood vessel of right thumb
- 7 S65.492- Other specified injury of blood vessel of left thumb
- 7 S65.499- Other specified injury of blood vessel of unspecified thumb

5 S65.5 Injury of blood vessel of other and unspecified finger

6 S65.50 Unspecified injury of blood vessel of other and Unspecified finger

S65.500- Unspecified injury of blood vessel of right index finger
S65.501- Unspecified injury of blood vessel of left index finger
S65.502- Unspecified injury of blood vessel of right middle finger
S65.503- Unspecified injury of blood vessel of left middle finger
S65.504- Unspecified injury of blood vessel of right ring finger
S65.505- Unspecified injury of blood vessel of left ring finger
S65.506- Unspecified injury of blood vessel of right little finger
S65.507- Unspecified injury of blood vessel of left little finger
S65.508- Unspecified injury of blood vessel of other finger
Unspecified injury of blood vessel of specified finger with unspecified laterality
S65.509- Unspecified injury of blood vessel of unspecified finger

S65.51 Laceration of blood vessel of other and unspecified finger
S65.510- Laceration of blood vessel of right index finger
S65.511- Laceration of blood vessel of left index finger
S65.512- Laceration of blood vessel of right middle finger
S65.513- Laceration of blood vessel of left middle finger
S65.514- Laceration of blood vessel of right ring finger
S65.515- Laceration of blood vessel of left ring finger
S65.516- Laceration of blood vessel of right little finger
S65.517- Laceration of blood vessel of left little finger
S65.518- Laceration of blood vessel of other finger
Laceration of blood vessel of specified finger with unspecified laterality
S65.519- Laceration of blood vessel of unspecified finger

S65.59 Other specified injury of blood vessel of other and unspecified finger
S65.590- Other specified injury of blood vessel of right index finger
S65.591- Other specified injury of blood vessel of left index finger
S65.592- Other specified injury of blood vessel of right middle finger
S65.593- Other specified injury of blood vessel of left middle finger
S65.594- Other specified injury of blood vessel of right ring finger
S65.595- Other specified injury of blood vessel of left ring finger
S65.596- Other specified injury of blood vessel of right little finger
S65.597- Other specified injury of blood vessel of left little finger
S65.598- Other specified injury of blood vessel of other finger
Other specified injury of blood vessel of specified finger with unspecified laterality
S65.599- Other specified injury of blood vessel of unspecified finger

S65.8 Injury of other blood vessels at wrist and hand level

S65.80 Unspecified injury of other blood vessels at wrist and hand level
S65.801- Unspecified injury of other blood vessels at wrist and hand level of right arm
S65.802- Unspecified injury of other blood vessels at wrist and hand level of left arm
S65.809- Unspecified injury of other blood vessels at wrist and hand level of unspecified arm

S65.81 Laceration of other blood vessels at wrist and hand level
S65.811- Laceration of other blood vessels at wrist and hand level of right arm
S65.812- Laceration of other blood vessels at wrist and hand level of left arm
S65.819- Laceration of other blood vessels at wrist and hand level of unspecified arm

S65.89 Other specified injury of other blood vessels at wrist and hand level
S65.891- Other specified injury of other blood vessels at wrist and hand level of right arm
S65.892- Other specified injury of other blood vessels at wrist and hand level of left arm
S65.899- Other specified injury of other blood vessels at wrist and hand level of unspecified arm

S65.9 Injury of unspecified blood vessel at wrist and hand level

S65.90 Unspecified injury of Unspecified blood vessel at wrist and hand level
S65.901- Unspecified injury of unspecified blood vessel at wrist and hand level of right arm
S65.902- Unspecified injury of unspecified blood vessel at wrist and hand level of left arm
S65.909- Unspecified injury of unspecified blood vessel at wrist and hand level of unspecified arm

S65.91 Laceration of unspecified blood vessel at wrist and hand level
S65.911- Laceration of unspecified blood vessel at wrist and hand level of right arm
S65.912- Laceration of unspecified blood vessel at wrist and hand level of left arm
S65.919- Laceration of unspecified blood vessel at wrist and hand level of unspecified arm

S65.99 Other specified injury of unspecified blood vessel at wrist and hand level
S65.991- Other specified injury of unspecified blood vessel at wrist and hand of right arm
S65.992- Other specified injury of unspecified blood vessel at wrist and hand of left arm
S65.999- Other specified injury of unspecified blood vessel at wrist and hand of unspecified arm

S66 Injury of muscle, fascia and tendon at wrist and hand level

Code also:
any associated open wound (S61.-)

EXCLUDES 2 *sprain of joints and ligaments of wrist and hand (S63.-)*

The appropriate 7th character is to be added to each code from category S66
A initial encounter
D subsequent encounter
S sequela

S66.0 Injury of long flexor muscle, fascia and tendon of thumb at wrist and hand level

S66.00 Unspecified injury of long flexor muscle, fascia and tendon of thumb at wrist and hand level
S66.001- Unspecified injury of long flexor muscle, fascia and tendon of right thumb at wrist and hand level
S66.002- Unspecified injury of long flexor muscle, fascia and tendon of left thumb at wrist and hand level
S66.009- Unspecified injury of long flexor muscle, fascia and tendon of unspecified thumb at wrist and hand level

S66.01 Strain of long flexor muscle, fascia and tendon of thumb at wrist and hand level
S66.011- Strain of long flexor muscle, fascia and tendon of right thumb at wrist and hand level
S66.012- Strain of long flexor muscle, fascia and tendon of left thumb at wrist and hand level
S66.019- Strain of long flexor muscle, fascia and tendon of unspecified thumb at wrist and hand level

S66.02 Laceration of long flexor muscle, fascia and tendon of thumb at wrist and hand level
S66.021- Laceration of long flexor muscle, fascia and tendon of right thumb at wrist and hand level

7 ⊟ S66.022- Laceration of long flexor muscle, fascia and tendon of left thumb at wrist and hand level

7 ⊟ S66.029- Laceration of long flexor muscle, fascia and tendon of unspecified thumb at wrist and hand level

6 S66.09 Other specified injury of long flexor muscle, fascia and tendon of thumb at wrist and hand level

7 ⊟ S66.091- Other specified injury of long flexor muscle, fascia and tendon of right thumb at wrist and hand level

7 ⊟ S66.092- Other specified injury of long flexor muscle, fascia and tendon of left thumb at wrist and hand level

7 ⊟ S66.099- Other specified injury of long flexor muscle, fascia and tendon of unspecified thumb at wrist and hand level

5 S66.1 Injury of flexor muscle, fascia and tendon of other and unspecified finger at wrist and hand level

EXCLUDES 2 *Injury of long flexor muscle, fascia and tendon of thumb at wrist and hand level (S66.0-)*

6 S66.10 Unspecified injury of flexor muscle, fascia and tendon of other and Unspecified finger at wrist and hand level

7 ⊟ S66.100- Unspecified injury of flexor muscle, fascia and tendon of right index finger at wrist and hand level

7 ⊟ S66.101- Unspecified injury of flexor muscle, fascia and tendon of left index finger at wrist and hand level

7 ⊟ S66.102- Unspecified injury of flexor muscle, fascia and tendon of right middle finger at wrist and hand level

7 ⊟ S66.103- Unspecified injury of flexor muscle, fascia and tendon of left middle finger at wrist and hand level

7 ⊟ S66.104- Unspecified injury of flexor muscle, fascia and tendon of right ring finger at wrist and hand level

7 ⊟ S66.105- Unspecified injury of flexor muscle, fascia and tendon of left ring finger at wrist and hand level

7 ⊟ S66.106- Unspecified injury of flexor muscle, fascia and tendon of right little finger at wrist and hand level

7 ⊟ S66.107- Unspecified injury of flexor muscle, fascia and tendon of left little finger at wrist and hand level

7 ⊟ S66.108- Unspecified injury of flexor muscle, fascia and tendon of other finger at wrist and hand level

Unspecified injury of flexor muscle, fascia and tendon of specified finger with unspecified laterality at wrist and hand level

7 ⊟ S66.109- Unspecified injury of flexor muscle, fascia and tendon of unspecified finger at wrist and hand level

6 S66.11 Strain of flexor muscle, fascia and tendon of other and unspecified finger at wrist and hand level

7 ⊟ S66.110- Strain of flexor muscle, fascia and tendon of right index finger at wrist and hand level

7 ⊟ S66.111- Strain of flexor muscle, fascia and tendon of left index finger at wrist and hand level

7 ⊟ S66.112- Strain of flexor muscle, fascia and tendon of right middle finger at wrist and hand level

7 ⊟ S66.113- Strain of flexor muscle, fascia and tendon of left middle finger at wrist and hand level

7 ⊟ S66.114- Strain of flexor muscle, fascia and tendon of right ring finger at wrist and hand level

7 ⊟ S66.115- Strain of flexor muscle, fascia and tendon of left ring finger at wrist and hand level

7 ⊟ S66.116- Strain of flexor muscle, fascia and tendon of right little finger at wrist and hand level

7 ⊟ S66.117- Strain of flexor muscle, fascia and tendon of left little finger at wrist and hand level

7 ⊟ S66.118- Strain of flexor muscle, fascia and tendon of other finger at wrist and hand level

Strain of flexor muscle, fascia and tendon of specified finger with unspecified laterality at wrist and hand level

7 ⊟ S66.119- Strain of flexor muscle, fascia and tendon of unspecified finger at wrist and hand level

6 S66.12 Laceration of flexor muscle, fascia and tendon of other and unspecified finger at wrist and hand level

7 ⊟ S66.120- Laceration of flexor muscle, fascia and tendon of right index finger at wrist and hand level

7 ⊟ S66.121- Laceration of flexor muscle, fascia and tendon of left index finger at wrist and hand level

7 ⊟ S66.122- Laceration of flexor muscle, fascia and tendon of right middle finger at wrist and hand level

7 ⊟ S66.123- Laceration of flexor muscle, fascia and tendon of left middle finger at wrist and hand level

7 ⊟ S66.124- Laceration of flexor muscle, fascia and tendon of right ring finger at wrist and hand level

7 ⊟ S66.125- Laceration of flexor muscle, fascia and tendon of left ring finger at wrist and hand level

7 ⊟ S66.126- Laceration of flexor muscle, fascia and tendon of right little finger at wrist and hand level

7 ⊟ S66.127- Laceration of flexor muscle, fascia and tendon of left little finger at wrist and hand level

7 ⊟ S66.128- Laceration of flexor muscle, fascia and tendon of other finger at wrist and hand level

Laceration of flexor muscle, fascia and tendon of specified finger with unspecified laterality at wrist and hand level

7 ⊟ S66.129- Laceration of flexor muscle, fascia and tendon of unspecified finger at wrist and hand level

6 S66.19 Other injury of flexor muscle, fascia and tendon of Other and unspecified finger at wrist and hand level

7 ⊟ S66.190- Other injury of flexor muscle, fascia and tendon of right index finger at wrist and hand level

7 ⊟ S66.191- Other injury of flexor muscle, fascia and tendon of left index finger at wrist and hand level

7 ⊟ S66.192- Other injury of flexor muscle, fascia and tendon of right middle finger at wrist and hand level

7 ⊟ S66.193- Other injury of flexor muscle, fascia and tendon of left middle finger at wrist and hand level

7 ⊟ S66.194- Other injury of flexor muscle, fascia and tendon of right ring finger at wrist and hand level

7 ⊟ S66.195- Other injury of flexor muscle, fascia and tendon of left ring finger at wrist and hand level

7 ⊟ S66.196- Other injury of flexor muscle, fascia and tendon of right little finger at wrist and hand level

7 ⊟ S66.197- Other injury of flexor muscle, fascia and tendon of left little finger at wrist and hand level

7 ⊟ S66.198- Other injury of flexor muscle, fascia and tendon of other finger at wrist and hand level

Other injury of flexor muscle, fascia and tendon of specified finger with unspecified laterality at wrist and hand level

7 ⊟ S66.199- Other injury of flexor muscle, fascia and tendon of unspecified finger at wrist and hand level

5 S66.2 Injury of extensor muscle, fascia and tendon of thumb at wrist and hand level

6 S66.20 Unspecified injury of extensor muscle, fascia and tendon of thumb at wrist and hand level

7 ⊟ S66.201- Unspecified injury of extensor muscle, fascia and tendon of right thumb at wrist and hand level

7 ⊟ S66.202- Unspecified injury of extensor muscle, fascia and tendon of left thumb at wrist and hand level

7 ⊟ S66.209- Unspecified injury of extensor muscle, fascia and tendon of unspecified thumb at wrist and hand level

6 S66.21 Strain of extensor muscle, fascia and tendon of thumb at wrist and hand level

7 ⊟ S66.211- Strain of extensor muscle, fascia and tendon of right thumb at wrist and hand level

7 ⊟ S66.212- Strain of extensor muscle, fascia and tendon of left thumb at wrist and hand level

7 ⊟ S66.219- Strain of extensor muscle, fascia and tendon of unspecified thumb at wrist and hand level

6 S66.22 Laceration of extensor muscle, fascia and tendon of thumb at wrist and hand level

7 ⊟ S66.221- Laceration of extensor muscle, fascia and tendon of right thumb at wrist and hand level

7 ⊟ S66.222- Laceration of extensor muscle, fascia and tendon of left thumb at wrist and hand level

7 ⊟ S66.229- Laceration of extensor muscle, fascia and tendon of unspecified thumb at wrist and hand level

6 S66.29 Other specified injury of extensor muscle, fascia and tendon of thumb at wrist and hand level

7 ⊟ S66.291- Other specified injury of extensor muscle, fascia and tendon of right thumb at wrist and hand level

7 ⊟ S66.292- Other specified injury of extensor muscle, fascia and tendon of left thumb at wrist and hand level

7 ⊟ S66.299- Other specified injury of extensor muscle, fascia and tendon of unspecified thumb at wrist and hand level

5 S66.3 Injury of extensor muscle, fascia and tendon of other and unspecified finger at wrist and hand level

EXCLUDES 2 *Injury of extensor muscle, fascia and tendon of thumb at wrist and hand level (S66.2-)*

6 S66.30 Unspecified injury of extensor muscle, fascia and tendon of other and Unspecified finger at wrist and hand level

7 ⊟ S66.300- Unspecified injury of extensor muscle, fascia and tendon of right index finger at wrist and hand level

7 ⊟ S66.301- Unspecified injury of extensor muscle, fascia and tendon of left index finger at wrist and hand level

7 ⊟ S66.302- Unspecified injury of extensor muscle, fascia and tendon of right middle finger at wrist and hand level

7 ⊟ S66.303- Unspecified injury of extensor muscle, fascia and tendon of left middle finger at wrist and hand level

7 ⊟ S66.304- Unspecified injury of extensor muscle, fascia and tendon of right ring finger at wrist and hand level

7 ⊟ S66.305- Unspecified injury of extensor muscle, fascia and tendon of left ring finger at wrist and hand level

7 ⊟ S66.306- Unspecified injury of extensor muscle, fascia and tendon of right little finger at wrist and hand level

7 ⊟ S66.307- Unspecified injury of extensor muscle, fascia and tendon of left little finger at wrist and hand level

7 ⊟ S66.308- Unspecified injury of extensor muscle, fascia and tendon of other finger at wrist and hand level

Unspecified injury of extensor muscle, fascia and tendon of specified finger with unspecified laterality at wrist and hand level

7 ⊟ S66.309- Unspecified injury of extensor muscle, fascia and tendon of unspecified finger at wrist and hand level

6 S66.31 Strain of extensor muscle, fascia and tendon of other and unspecified finger at wrist and hand level

7 ⊟ S66.310- Strain of extensor muscle, fascia and tendon of right index finger at wrist and hand level

7 ⊟ S66.311- Strain of extensor muscle, fascia and tendon of left index finger at wrist and hand level

7 ⊟ S66.312- Strain of extensor muscle, fascia and tendon of right middle finger at wrist and hand level

7 ⊟ S66.313- Strain of extensor muscle, fascia and tendon of left middle finger at wrist and hand level

7 ⊟ S66.314- Strain of extensor muscle, fascia and tendon of right ring finger at wrist and hand level

7 ⊟ S66.315- Strain of extensor muscle, fascia and tendon of left ring finger at wrist and hand level

7 ⊟ S66.316- Strain of extensor muscle, fascia and tendon of right little finger at wrist and hand level

7 ⊟ S66.317- Strain of extensor muscle, fascia and tendon of left little finger at wrist and hand level

7 ⊟ S66.318- Strain of extensor muscle, fascia and tendon of other finger at wrist and hand level

Strain of extensor muscle, fascia and tendon of specified finger with unspecified laterality at wrist and hand level

7 ⊟ S66.319- Strain of extensor muscle, fascia and tendon of unspecified finger at wrist and hand level

6 S66.32 Laceration of extensor muscle, fascia and tendon of other and unspecified finger at wrist and hand level

7 ⊟ S66.320- Laceration of extensor muscle, fascia and tendon of right index finger at wrist and hand level

7 ⊟ S66.321- Laceration of extensor muscle, fascia and tendon of left index finger at wrist and hand level

7 ⊟ S66.322- Laceration of extensor muscle, fascia and tendon of right middle finger at wrist and hand level

7 ⊟ S66.323- Laceration of extensor muscle, fascia and tendon of left middle finger at wrist and hand level

7 ⊟ S66.324- Laceration of extensor muscle, fascia and tendon of right ring finger at wrist and hand level

7 ⊟ S66.325- Laceration of extensor muscle, fascia and tendon of left ring finger at wrist and hand level

7 ⊟ S66.326- Laceration of extensor muscle, fascia and tendon of right little finger at wrist and hand level

7 ⊟ S66.327- Laceration of extensor muscle, fascia and tendon of left little finger at wrist and hand level

7 ⊟ S66.328- Laceration of extensor muscle, fascia and tendon of other finger at wrist and hand level

Laceration of extensor muscle, fascia and tendon of specified finger with unspecified laterality at wrist and hand level

7 ⊟ S66.329- Laceration of extensor muscle, fascia and tendon of unspecified finger at wrist and hand level

6 S66.39 Other injury of extensor muscle, fascia and tendon of Other and unspecified finger at wrist and hand level

7 ⊟ S66.390- Other injury of extensor muscle, fascia and tendon of right index finger at wrist and hand level

7 ⊟ S66.391- Other injury of extensor muscle, fascia and tendon of left index finger at wrist and hand level

7 ⊟ S66.392- Other injury of extensor muscle, fascia and tendon of right middle finger at wrist and hand level

7 ⊟ S66.393- Other injury of extensor muscle, fascia and tendon of left middle finger at wrist and hand level

7 ⊟ S66.394- Other injury of extensor muscle, fascia and tendon of right ring finger at wrist and hand level

7 ⊟ S66.395- Other injury of extensor muscle, fascia and tendon of left ring finger at wrist and hand level

7 ⊟ S66.396- Other injury of extensor muscle, fascia and tendon of right little finger at wrist and hand level

S66.397- **Other injury of extensor muscle, fascia and tendon of left little finger at wrist and hand level**

S66.398- **Other injury of extensor muscle, fascia and tendon of other finger at wrist and hand level**
Other injury of extensor muscle, fascia and tendon of specified finger with unspecified laterality at wrist and hand level

S66.399- **Other injury of extensor muscle, fascia and tendon of unspecified finger at wrist and hand level**

S66.4 **Injury of intrinsic muscle, fascia and tendon of thumb at wrist and hand level**

S66.40 **Unspecified injury of intrinsic muscle, fascia and tendon of thumb at wrist and hand level**

S66.401- **Unspecified injury of intrinsic muscle, fascia and tendon of right thumb at wrist and hand level**

S66.402- **Unspecified injury of intrinsic muscle, fascia and tendon of left thumb at wrist and hand level**

S66.409- **Unspecified injury of intrinsic muscle, fascia and tendon of unspecified thumb at wrist and hand level**

S66.41 **Strain of intrinsic muscle, fascia and tendon of thumb at wrist and hand level**

S66.411- **Strain of intrinsic muscle, fascia and tendon of right thumb at wrist and hand level**

S66.412- **Strain of intrinsic muscle, fascia and tendon of left thumb at wrist and hand level**

S66.419- **Strain of intrinsic muscle, fascia and tendon of unspecified thumb at wrist and hand level**

S66.42 **Laceration of intrinsic muscle, fascia and tendon of thumb at wrist and hand level**

S66.421- **Laceration of intrinsic muscle, fascia and tendon of right thumb at wrist and hand level**

S66.422- **Laceration of intrinsic muscle, fascia and tendon of left thumb at wrist and hand level**

S66.429- **Laceration of intrinsic muscle, fascia and tendon of unspecified thumb at wrist and hand level**

S66.49 **Other specified injury of intrinsic muscle, fascia and tendon of thumb at wrist and hand level**

S66.491- **Other specified injury of intrinsic muscle, fascia and tendon of right thumb at wrist and hand level**

S66.492- **Other specified injury of intrinsic muscle, fascia and tendon of left thumb at wrist and hand level**

S66.499- **Other specified injury of intrinsic muscle, fascia and tendon of unspecified thumb at wrist and hand level**

S66.5 **Injury of intrinsic muscle, fascia and tendon of other and unspecified finger at wrist and hand level**

EXCLUDES 2 *injury of intrinsic muscle, fascia and tendon of thumb at wrist and hand level (S66.4-)*

S66.50 **Unspecified injury of intrinsic muscle, fascia and tendon of other and Unspecified finger at wrist and hand level**

S66.500- **Unspecified injury of intrinsic muscle, fascia and tendon of right index finger at wrist and hand level**

S66.501- **Unspecified injury of intrinsic muscle, fascia and tendon of left index finger at wrist and hand level**

S66.502- **Unspecified injury of intrinsic muscle, fascia and tendon of right middle finger at wrist and hand level**

S66.503- **Unspecified injury of intrinsic muscle, fascia and tendon of left middle finger at wrist and hand level**

S66.504- **Unspecified injury of intrinsic muscle, fascia and tendon of right ring finger at wrist and hand level**

S66.505- **Unspecified injury of intrinsic muscle, fascia and tendon of left ring finger at wrist and hand level**

S66.506- **Unspecified injury of intrinsic muscle, fascia and tendon of right little finger at wrist and hand level**

S66.507- **Unspecified injury of intrinsic muscle, fascia and tendon of left little finger at wrist and hand level**

S66.508- **Unspecified injury of intrinsic muscle, fascia and tendon of other finger at wrist and hand level**
Unspecified injury of intrinsic muscle, fascia and tendon of specified finger with unspecified laterality at wrist and hand level

S66.509- **Unspecified injury of intrinsic muscle, fascia and tendon of unspecified finger at wrist and hand level**

S66.51 **Strain of intrinsic muscle, fascia and tendon of other and unspecified finger at wrist and hand level**

S66.510- **Strain of intrinsic muscle, fascia and tendon of right index finger at wrist and hand level**

S66.511- **Strain of intrinsic muscle, fascia and tendon of left index finger at wrist and hand level**

S66.512- **Strain of intrinsic muscle, fascia and tendon of right middle finger at wrist and hand level**

S66.513- **Strain of intrinsic muscle, fascia and tendon of left middle finger at wrist and hand level**

S66.514- **Strain of intrinsic muscle, fascia and tendon of right ring finger at wrist and hand level**

S66.515- **Strain of intrinsic muscle, fascia and tendon of left ring finger at wrist and hand level**

S66.516- **Strain of intrinsic muscle, fascia and tendon of right little finger at wrist and hand level**

S66.517- **Strain of intrinsic muscle, fascia and tendon of left little finger at wrist and hand level**

S66.518- **Strain of intrinsic muscle, fascia and tendon of other finger at wrist and hand level**
Strain of intrinsic muscle, fascia and tendon of specified finger with unspecified laterality at wrist and hand level

S66.519- **Strain of intrinsic muscle, fascia and tendon of unspecified finger at wrist and hand level**

S66.52 **Laceration of intrinsic muscle, fascia and tendon of other and unspecified finger at wrist and hand level**

S66.520- **Laceration of intrinsic muscle, fascia and tendon of right index finger at wrist and hand level**

S66.521- **Laceration of intrinsic muscle, fascia and tendon of left index finger at wrist and hand level**

S66.522- **Laceration of intrinsic muscle, fascia and tendon of right middle finger at wrist and hand level**

S66.523- **Laceration of intrinsic muscle, fascia and tendon of left middle finger at wrist and hand level**

S66.524- **Laceration of intrinsic muscle, fascia and tendon of right ring finger at wrist and hand level**

S66.525- **Laceration of intrinsic muscle, fascia and tendon of left ring finger at wrist and hand level**

S66.526- **Laceration of intrinsic muscle, fascia and tendon of right little finger at wrist and hand level**

S66.527- **Laceration of intrinsic muscle, fascia and tendon of left little finger at wrist and hand level**

S66.528- **Laceration of intrinsic muscle, fascia and tendon of other finger at wrist and hand level**
Laceration of intrinsic muscle, fascia and tendon of specified finger with unspecified laterality at wrist and hand level

S66.529- **Laceration of intrinsic muscle, fascia and tendon of unspecified finger at wrist and hand level**

S66.59 **Other injury of intrinsic muscle, fascia and tendon of Other and unspecified finger at wrist and hand level**

S66.590- Other injury of intrinsic muscle, fascia and tendon of right index finger at wrist and hand level
S66.591- Other injury of intrinsic muscle, fascia and tendon of left index finger at wrist and hand level
S66.592- Other injury of intrinsic muscle, fascia and tendon of right middle finger at wrist and hand level
S66.593- Other injury of intrinsic muscle, fascia and tendon of left middle finger at wrist and hand level
S66.594- Other injury of intrinsic muscle, fascia and tendon of right ring finger at wrist and hand level
S66.595- Other injury of intrinsic muscle, fascia and tendon of left ring finger at wrist and hand level
S66.596- Other injury of intrinsic muscle, fascia and tendon of right little finger at wrist and hand level
S66.597- Other injury of intrinsic muscle, fascia and tendon of left little finger at wrist and hand level
S66.598- Other injury of intrinsic muscle, fascia and tendon of other finger at wrist and hand level
Other injury of intrinsic muscle, fascia and tendon of specified finger with unspecified laterality at wrist and hand level
S66.599- Other injury of intrinsic muscle, fascia and tendon of unspecified finger at wrist and hand level

S66.8 Injury of other specified muscles, fascia and tendons at wrist and hand level
S66.80 Unspecified injury of other specified muscles, fascia and tendons at wrist and hand level
S66.801- Unspecified injury of other specified muscles, fascia and tendons at wrist and hand level, right hand
S66.802- Unspecified injury of other specified muscles, fascia and tendons at wrist and hand level, left hand
S66.809- Unspecified injury of other specified muscles, fascia and tendons at wrist and hand level, unspecified hand
S66.81 Strain of other specified muscles, fascia and tendons at wrist and hand level
S66.811- Strain of other specified muscles, fascia and tendons at wrist and hand level, right hand
S66.812- Strain of other specified muscles, fascia and tendons at wrist and hand level, left hand
S66.819- Strain of other specified muscles, fascia and tendons at wrist and hand level, unspecified hand
S66.82 Laceration of other specified muscles, fascia and tendons at wrist and hand level
S66.821- Laceration of other specified muscles, fascia and tendons at wrist and hand level, right hand
S66.822- Laceration of other specified muscles, fascia and tendons at wrist and hand level, left hand
S66.829- Laceration of other specified muscles, fascia and tendons at wrist and hand level, unspecified hand
S66.89 Other injury of Other specified muscles, fascia and tendons at wrist and hand level
S66.891- Other injury of other specified muscles, fascia and tendons at wrist and hand level, right hand
S66.892- Other injury of other specified muscles, fascia and tendons at wrist and hand level, left hand
S66.899- Other injury of other specified muscles, fascia and tendons at wrist and hand level, unspecified hand

S66.9 Injury of unspecified muscle, fascia and tendon at wrist and hand level
S66.90 Unspecified injury of Unspecified muscle, fascia and tendon at wrist and hand level
S66.901- Unspecified injury of unspecified muscle, fascia and tendon at wrist and hand level, right hand
S66.902- Unspecified injury of unspecified muscle, fascia and tendon at wrist and hand level, left hand
S66.909- Unspecified injury of unspecified muscle, fascia and tendon at wrist and hand level, unspecified hand
S66.91 Strain of unspecified muscle, fascia and tendon at wrist and hand level
S66.911- Strain of unspecified muscle, fascia and tendon at wrist and hand level, right hand
S66.912- Strain of unspecified muscle, fascia and tendon at wrist and hand level, left hand
S66.919- Strain of unspecified muscle, fascia and tendon at wrist and hand level, unspecified hand
S66.92 Laceration of unspecified muscle, fascia and tendon at wrist and hand level
S66.921- Laceration of unspecified muscle, fascia and tendon at wrist and hand level, right hand
S66.922- Laceration of unspecified muscle, fascia and tendon at wrist and hand level, left hand
S66.929- Laceration of unspecified muscle, fascia and tendon at wrist and hand level, unspecified hand
S66.99 Other injury of unspecified muscle, fascia and tendon at wrist and hand level
S66.991- Other injury of unspecified muscle, fascia and tendon at wrist and hand level, right hand
S66.992- Other injury of unspecified muscle, fascia and tendon at wrist and hand level, left hand
S66.999- Other injury of unspecified muscle, fascia and tendon at wrist and hand level, unspecified hand

S67 Crushing injury of wrist, hand and fingers

Use additional code for all associated injuries, such as:
fracture of wrist and hand (S62.-)
open wound of wrist and hand (S61.-)

The appropriate 7th character is to be added to each code from category S67
A initial encounter
D subsequent encounter
S sequela

S67.0 Crushing injury of thumb
S67.00X- Crushing injury of unspecified thumb
S67.01X- Crushing injury of right thumb
S67.02X- Crushing injury of left thumb
S67.1 Crushing injury of other and unspecified finger(s)
EXCLUDES 2 *crushing injury of thumb (S67.0-)*
S67.10X- Crushing injury of unspecified finger(s)
S67.19 Crushing injury of other finger(s)
S67.190- Crushing injury of right index finger
S67.191- Crushing injury of left index finger
S67.192- Crushing injury of right middle finger
S67.193- Crushing injury of left middle finger
S67.194- Crushing injury of right ring finger
S67.195- Crushing injury of left ring finger
S67.196- Crushing injury of right little finger
S67.197- Crushing injury of left little finger
S67.198- Crushing injury of other finger
Crushing injury of specified finger with unspecified laterality
S67.2 Crushing injury of hand
EXCLUDES 2 *crushing injury of fingers (S67.1-)*
crushing injury of thumb (S67.0-)
S67.20X- Crushing injury of unspecified hand
S67.21X- Crushing injury of right hand
S67.22X- Crushing injury of left hand
S67.3 Crushing injury of wrist

7 ⊟ S67.30X- **Crushing injury of unspecified wrist**
7 ⊟ S67.31X- **Crushing injury of right wrist**
7 ⊟ S67.32X- **Crushing injury of left wrist**
5 S67.4 **Crushing injury of wrist and hand**
EXCLUDES 1 *crushing injury of hand alone (S67.2-)*
crushing injury of wrist alone (S67.3-)
EXCLUDES 2 *crushing injury of fingers (S67.1-)*
crushing injury of thumb (S67.0-)
7 ⊟ S67.40X- **Crushing injury of unspecified wrist and hand**
7 ⊟ S67.41X- **Crushing injury of right wrist and hand**
7 ⊟ S67.42X- **Crushing injury of left wrist and hand**
5 S67.9 **Crushing injury of unspecified part(s) of wrist, hand and fingers**
7 ⊟ S67.90X- **Crushing injury of unspecified part(s) of unspecified wrist, hand and fingers**
7 ⊟ S67.91X- **Crushing injury of unspecified part(s) of right wrist, hand and fingers**
7 ⊟ S67.92X- **Crushing injury of unspecified part(s) of left wrist, hand and fingers**

4 S68 **Traumatic amputation of wrist, hand and fingers**
An amputation not identified as partial or complete should be coded to complete

The appropriate 7th character is to be added to each code from category S68
A initial encounter
D subsequent encounter
S sequela

CODING TIP✓ Use these codes only when the amputation was due to trauma. There is no need for adding Z89 with traumatic amputations. See Z47.81 for care of amputations not due to trauma.

CODING TIP✓ Assign only if the amputation is due to accident or violence, i.e., trauma.

5 S68.0 **Traumatic metacarpophalangeal amputation of thumb**
Traumatic amputation of thumb NOS
6 S68.01 **Complete traumatic metacarpophalangeal amputation of thumb**
7 ⊟ S68.011- **Complete traumatic metacarpophalangeal amputation of right thumb** HCC
7 ⊟ S68.012- **Complete traumatic metacarpophalangeal amputation of left thumb** HCC
7 ⊟ S68.019- **Complete traumatic metacarpophalangeal amputation of unspecified thumb** HCC
6 S68.02 **Partial traumatic metacarpophalangeal amputation of thumb**
7 ⊟ S68.021- **Partial traumatic metacarpophalangeal amputation of right thumb** HCC
7 ⊟ S68.022- **Partial traumatic metacarpophalangeal amputation of left thumb** HCC
7 ⊟ S68.029- **Partial traumatic metacarpophalangeal amputation of unspecified thumb** HCC
5 S68.1 **Traumatic metacarpophalangeal amputation of other and unspecified finger**
Traumatic amputation of finger NOS
EXCLUDES 2 *traumatic metacarpophalangeal amputation of thumb (S68.0-)*
6 S68.11 **Complete traumatic metacarpophalangeal amputation of other and unspecified finger**
7 ⊟ S68.110- **Complete traumatic metacarpophalangeal amputation of right index finger** HCC
7 ⊟ S68.111- **Complete traumatic metacarpophalangeal amputation of left index finger** HCC
7 ⊟ S68.112- **Complete traumatic metacarpophalangeal amputation of right middle finger** HCC
7 ⊟ S68.113- **Complete traumatic metacarpophalangeal amputation of left middle finger** HCC
7 ⊟ S68.114- **Complete traumatic metacarpophalangeal amputation of right ring finger** HCC
7 ⊟ S68.115- **Complete traumatic metacarpophalangeal amputation of left ring finger** HCC
7 ⊟ S68.116- **Complete traumatic metacarpophalangeal amputation of right little finger** HCC
7 ⊟ S68.117- **Complete traumatic metacarpophalangeal amputation of left little finger** HCC
7 ⊟ S68.118- **Complete traumatic metacarpophalangeal amputation of other finger** HCC
Complete traumatic metacarpophalangeal amputation of specified finger with unspecified laterality
7 ⊟ S68.119- **Complete traumatic metacarpophalangeal amputation of unspecified finger** HCC
6 S68.12 **Partial traumatic metacarpophalangeal amputation of other and unspecified finger**
7 ⊟ S68.120- **Partial traumatic metacarpophalangeal amputation of right index finger** HCC
7 ⊟ S68.121- **Partial traumatic metacarpophalangeal amputation of left index finger** HCC
7 ⊟ S68.122- **Partial traumatic metacarpophalangeal amputation of right middle finger** HCC
7 ⊟ S68.123- **Partial traumatic metacarpophalangeal amputation of left middle finger** HCC
7 ⊟ S68.124- **Partial traumatic metacarpophalangeal amputation of right ring finger** HCC
7 ⊟ S68.125- **Partial traumatic metacarpophalangeal amputation of left ring finger** HCC
7 ⊟ S68.126- **Partial traumatic metacarpophalangeal amputation of right little finger** HCC
7 ⊟ S68.127- **Partial traumatic metacarpophalangeal amputation of left little finger** HCC
7 ⊟ S68.128- **Partial traumatic metacarpophalangeal amputation of other finger** HCC
Partial traumatic metacarpophalangeal amputation of specified finger with unspecified laterality
7 ⊟ S68.129- **Partial traumatic metacarpophalangeal amputation of unspecified finger** HCC
5 S68.4 **Traumatic amputation of hand at wrist level**
Traumatic amputation of hand NOS
Traumatic amputation of wrist
6 S68.41 **Complete traumatic amputation of hand at wrist level**
7 ⊟ S68.411- **Complete traumatic amputation of right hand at wrist level** HCC
7 ⊟ S68.412- **Complete traumatic amputation of left hand at wrist level** HCC
7 ⊟ S68.419- **Complete traumatic amputation of unspecified hand at wrist level** HCC
6 S68.42 **Partial traumatic amputation of hand at wrist level**
7 ⊟ S68.421- **Partial traumatic amputation of right hand at wrist level** HCC
7 ⊟ S68.422- **Partial traumatic amputation of left hand at wrist level** HCC
7 ⊟ S68.429- **Partial traumatic amputation of unspecified hand at wrist level** HCC
5 S68.5 **Traumatic transphalangeal amputation of thumb**
Traumatic interphalangeal joint amputation of thumb
6 S68.51 **Complete traumatic transphalangeal amputation of thumb**
7 ⊟ S68.511- **Complete traumatic transphalangeal amputation of right thumb** HCC
7 ⊟ S68.512- **Complete traumatic transphalangeal amputation of left thumb** HCC
7 ⊟ S68.519- **Complete traumatic transphalangeal amputation of unspecified thumb** HCC
6 S68.52 **Partial traumatic transphalangeal amputation of thumb**
7 ⊟ S68.521- **Partial traumatic transphalangeal amputation of right thumb** HCC
7 ⊟ S68.522- **Partial traumatic transphalangeal amputation of left thumb** HCC
7 ⊟ S68.529- **Partial traumatic transphalangeal amputation of unspecified thumb** HCC
5 S68.6 **Traumatic transphalangeal amputation of other and unspecified finger**
6 S68.61 **Complete traumatic transphalangeal amputation of other and unspecified finger(s)**
7 ⊟ S68.610- **Complete traumatic transphalangeal amputation of right index finger** HCC
7 ⊟ S68.611- **Complete traumatic transphalangeal amputation of left index finger** HCC
7 ⊟ S68.612- **Complete traumatic transphalangeal amputation of right middle finger** HCC

7 ⊟ S68.613- **Complete traumatic transphalangeal amputation of left middle finger** HCC
7 ⊟ S68.614- **Complete traumatic transphalangeal amputation of right ring finger** HCC
7 ⊟ S68.615- **Complete traumatic transphalangeal amputation of left ring finger** HCC
7 ⊟ S68.616- **Complete traumatic transphalangeal amputation of right little finger** HCC
7 ⊟ S68.617- **Complete traumatic transphalangeal amputation of left little finger** HCC
7 ⊟ S68.618- **Complete traumatic transphalangeal amputation of other finger** HCC
Complete traumatic transphalangeal amputation of specified finger with unspecified laterality
7 ⊟ S68.619- **Complete traumatic transphalangeal amputation of unspecified finger** HCC

6 S68.62 **Partial traumatic transphalangeal amputation of other and unspecified finger**
7 ⊟ S68.620- **Partial traumatic transphalangeal amputation of right index finger** HCC
7 ⊟ S68.621- **Partial traumatic transphalangeal amputation of left index finger** HCC
7 ⊟ S68.622- **Partial traumatic transphalangeal amputation of right middle finger** HCC
7 ⊟ S68.623- **Partial traumatic transphalangeal amputation of left middle finger** HCC
7 ⊟ S68.624- **Partial traumatic transphalangeal amputation of right ring finger** HCC
7 ⊟ S68.625- **Partial traumatic transphalangeal amputation of left ring finger** HCC
7 ⊟ S68.626- **Partial traumatic transphalangeal amputation of right little finger** HCC
7 ⊟ S68.627- **Partial traumatic transphalangeal amputation of left little finger** HCC
7 ⊟ S68.628- **Partial traumatic transphalangeal amputation of other finger** HCC
Partial traumatic transphalangeal amputation of specified finger with unspecified laterality
7 ⊟ S68.629- **Partial traumatic transphalangeal amputation of unspecified finger** HCC

5 S68.7 **Traumatic transmetacarpal amputation of hand**
6 S68.71 **Complete traumatic transmetacarpal amputation of hand**
7 ⊟ S68.711- **Complete traumatic transmetacarpal amputation of right hand** HCC
7 ⊟ S68.712- **Complete traumatic transmetacarpal amputation of left hand** HCC
7 ⊟ S68.719- **Complete traumatic transmetacarpal amputation of unspecified hand** HCC
6 S68.72 **Partial traumatic transmetacarpal amputation of hand**
7 ⊟ S68.721- **Partial traumatic transmetacarpal amputation of right hand** HCC
7 ⊟ S68.722- **Partial traumatic transmetacarpal amputation of left hand** HCC
7 ⊟ S68.729- **Partial traumatic transmetacarpal amputation of unspecified hand** HCC

4 S69 **Other and unspecified injuries of wrist, hand and finger(s)**

The appropriate 7th character is to be added to each code from category S69
A initial encounter
D subsequent encounter
S sequela

5 S69.8 **Other specified injuries of wrist, hand and finger(s)**
7 ⊟ S69.80X- **Other specified injuries of unspecified wrist, hand and finger(s)**
7 ⊟ S69.81X- **Other specified injuries of right wrist, hand and finger(s)**
7 ⊟ S69.82X- **Other specified injuries of left wrist, hand and finger(s)**
5 S69.9 **Unspecified injury of wrist, hand and finger(s)**
7 ⊟ S69.90X- **Unspecified injury of unspecified wrist, hand and finger(s)**
7 ⊟ S69.91X- **Unspecified injury of right wrist, hand and finger(s)**
7 ⊟ S69.92X- **Unspecified injury of left wrist, hand and finger(s)**

Injuries to the hip and thigh (S70-S79)

EXCLUDES 2 *burns and corrosions (T20-T32)*
frostbite (T33-T34)
snake bite (T63.0-)
venomous insect bite or sting (T63.4-)

GUIDELINES **Section I.C.19.c.2)**
Multiple fractures are sequenced in accordance with the severity of the fracture.

GUIDELINES **Section I.C.19.b.1)-2)**
When coding injuries, assign separate codes for each injury unless a combination code is provided, in which case the combination code is assigned ... Traumatic injury codes (S00-T14.9) are not to be used for normal, healing surgical wounds or to identify complications of surgical wounds. The code for the most serious injury, as determined by the provider and the focus of treatment, is sequenced first.

1) Superficial injuries such as abrasions or contusions are not coded when associated with more severe injuries of the same site.

2) When a primary injury results in minor damage to peripheral nerves or blood vessels, the primary injury is sequenced first with additional code(s) for injuries to nerves and spinal cord (such as category S04), and/or injury to blood vessels (such as category S15). When the primary injury is to the blood vessels or nerves, that injury should be sequenced first.

GUIDELINES **Section I.C.19.c**
Coding of Traumatic Fractures: The principles of multiple coding of injuries should be followed in coding fractures. Fractures of specified sites are coded individually by site in accordance with both the provisions within categories S02, S12, S22, S32, S42, S49, S52, S59, S62, S72, S79, S82, S89, S92 and the level of detail furnished by medical record content. A fracture not indicated as open or closed should be coded to closed. A fracture not indicated whether displaced or not displaced should be coded to displaced.

4 S70 **Superficial injury of hip and thigh**

The appropriate 7th character is to be added to each code from category S70
A initial encounter
D subsequent encounter
S sequela

5 S70.0 **Contusion of hip**
7 ⊟ S70.00X- **Contusion of unspecified hip**
7 ⊟ S70.01X- **Contusion of right hip**
7 ⊟ S70.02X- **Contusion of left hip**
5 S70.1 **Contusion of thigh**
7 ⊟ S70.10X- **Contusion of unspecified thigh**
7 ⊟ S70.11X- **Contusion of right thigh**
7 ⊟ S70.12X- **Contusion of left thigh**
5 S70.2 **Other superficial injuries of hip**
6 S70.21 **Abrasion of hip**
7 ⊟ S70.211- **Abrasion, right hip**
7 ⊟ S70.212- **Abrasion, left hip**
7 ⊟ S70.219- **Abrasion, unspecified hip**
6 S70.22 **Blister (nonthermal) of hip**
7 ⊟ S70.221- **Blister (nonthermal), right hip**
7 ⊟ S70.222- **Blister (nonthermal), left hip**
7 ⊟ S70.229- **Blister (nonthermal), unspecified hip**
6 S70.24 **External constriction of hip**
7 ⊟ S70.241- **External constriction, right hip**
7 ⊟ S70.242- **External constriction, left hip**
7 ⊟ S70.249- **External constriction, unspecified hip**
6 S70.25 **Superficial foreign body of hip**
Splinter in the hip
7 ⊟ S70.251- **Superficial foreign body, right hip**
7 ⊟ S70.252- **Superficial foreign body, left hip**
7 ⊟ S70.259- **Superficial foreign body, unspecified hip**
6 S70.26 **Insect bite (nonvenomous) of hip**
7 ⊟ S70.261- **Insect bite (nonvenomous), right hip**

● New | Manifestation | 4-7 Digit Indicators | ⊟ Laterality | A Adult | M Maternity | N Newborn | P Pediatric | ♂ Male
▲ Revised | Unspecified | AHA Coding Clinic | HCC Hierarchical Condition Categories | HIV HIV Related Conditions | ♀ Female

- S70.262- Insect bite (nonvenomous), left hip
- S70.269- Insect bite (nonvenomous), unspecified hip

S70.27 Other superficial bite of hip
EXCLUDES 1 *open bite of hip (S71.05-)*

- S70.271- Other superficial bite of hip, right hip
- S70.272- Other superficial bite of hip, left hip
- S70.279- Other superficial bite of hip, unspecified hip

S70.3 Other superficial injuries of thigh

S70.31 Abrasion of thigh
- S70.311- Abrasion, right thigh
- S70.312- Abrasion, left thigh
- S70.319- Abrasion, unspecified thigh

S70.32 Blister (nonthermal) of thigh
- S70.321- Blister (nonthermal), right thigh
- S70.322- Blister (nonthermal), left thigh
- S70.329- Blister (nonthermal), unspecified thigh

S70.34 External constriction of thigh
- S70.341- External constriction, right thigh
- S70.342- External constriction, left thigh
- S70.349- External constriction, unspecified thigh

S70.35 Superficial foreign body of thigh
Splinter in the thigh
- S70.351- Superficial foreign body, right thigh
- S70.352- Superficial foreign body, left thigh
- S70.359- Superficial foreign body, unspecified thigh

S70.36 Insect bite (nonvenomous) of thigh
- S70.361- Insect bite (nonvenomous), right thigh
- S70.362- Insect bite (nonvenomous), left thigh
- S70.369- Insect bite (nonvenomous), unspecified thigh

S70.37 Other superficial bite of thigh
EXCLUDES 1 *open bite of thigh (S71.15)*
- S70.371- Other superficial bite of right thigh
- S70.372- Other superficial bite of left thigh
- S70.379- Other superficial bite of unspecified thigh

S70.9 Unspecified superficial injury of hip and thigh

S70.91 Unspecified superficial injury of hip
- S70.911- Unspecified superficial injury of right hip
- S70.912- Unspecified superficial injury of left hip
- S70.919- Unspecified superficial injury of unspecified hip

S70.92 Unspecified superficial injury of thigh
- S70.921- Unspecified superficial injury of right thigh
- S70.922- Unspecified superficial injury of left thigh
- S70.929- Unspecified superficial injury of unspecified thigh

S71 Open wound of hip and thigh

Code also:
any associated wound infection

EXCLUDES 1 *open fracture of hip and thigh (S72.-)*
traumatic amputation of hip and thigh (S78.-)

EXCLUDES 2 *bite of venomous animal (T63.-)*
open wound of ankle, foot and toes (S91.-)
open wound of knee and lower leg (S81.-)

The appropriate 7th character is to be added to each code from category S71
- A initial encounter
- D subsequent encounter
- S sequela

CODING TIP✓ Open wound codes indicate a wound resulting from a traumatic origin. Do not assign a code for "open wound" unless the etiology of the wound is related to trauma.

S71.0 Open wound of hip

S71.00 Unspecified open wound of hip
- S71.001- Unspecified open wound, right hip
- S71.002- Unspecified open wound, left hip
- S71.009- Unspecified open wound, unspecified hip

S71.01 Laceration without foreign body of hip
- S71.011- Laceration without foreign body, right hip
- S71.012- Laceration without foreign body, left hip
- S71.019- Laceration without foreign body, unspecified hip

S71.02 Laceration with foreign body of hip
- S71.021- Laceration with foreign body, right hip
- S71.022- Laceration with foreign body, left hip
- S71.029- Laceration with foreign body, unspecified hip

S71.03 Puncture wound without foreign body of hip
- S71.031- Puncture wound without foreign body, right hip
- S71.032- Puncture wound without foreign body, left hip
- S71.039- Puncture wound without foreign body, unspecified hip

S71.04 Puncture wound with foreign body of hip
- S71.041- Puncture wound with foreign body, right hip
- S71.042- Puncture wound with foreign body, left hip
- S71.049- Puncture wound with foreign body, unspecified hip

S71.05 Open bite of hip
Bite of hip NOS
EXCLUDES 1 *superficial bite of hip (S70.26, S70.27)*
- S71.051- Open bite, right hip
- S71.052- Open bite, left hip
- S71.059- Open bite, unspecified hip

S71.1 Open wound of thigh

S71.10 Unspecified open wound of thigh
- S71.101- Unspecified open wound, right thigh
- S71.102- Unspecified open wound, left thigh
- S71.109- Unspecified open wound, unspecified thigh

S71.11 Laceration without foreign body of thigh
- S71.111- Laceration without foreign body, right thigh
- S71.112- Laceration without foreign body, left thigh
- S71.119- Laceration without foreign body, unspecified thigh

S71.12 Laceration with foreign body of thigh
- S71.121- Laceration with foreign body, right thigh
- S71.122- Laceration with foreign body, left thigh
- S71.129- Laceration with foreign body, unspecified thigh

S71.13 Puncture wound without foreign body of thigh
- S71.131- Puncture wound without foreign body, right thigh
- S71.132- Puncture wound without foreign body, left thigh
- S71.139- Puncture wound without foreign body, unspecified thigh

S71.14 Puncture wound with foreign body of thigh
- S71.141- Puncture wound with foreign body, right thigh
- S71.142- Puncture wound with foreign body, left thigh
- S71.149- Puncture wound with foreign body, unspecified thigh

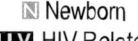

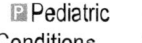

S71.15 Open bite of thigh
Bite of thigh NOS
EXCLUDES 1 *superficial bite of thigh (S70.37-)*
- S71.151- Open bite, right thigh
- S71.152- Open bite, left thigh
- S71.159- Open bite, unspecified thigh

4 S72 Fracture of femur

Note: A fracture not indicated as displaced or nondisplaced should be coded to displaced

A fracture not indicated as open or closed should be coded to closed

The open fracture designations are based on the Gustilo open fracture classification

EXCLUDES 1 *traumatic amputation of hip and thigh (S78.-)*

EXCLUDES 2 *fracture of lower leg and ankle (S82.-)*
fracture of foot (S92.-)
periprosthetic fracture of prosthetic implant of hip (M97.0-)

The appropriate 7th character is to be added to all codes from category S72

A	initial encounter for closed fracture
B	initial encounter for open fracture type I or II
C	initial encounter for open fracture type IIIA, IIIB, or IIIC
D	subsequent encounter for closed fracture with routine healing
E	subsequent encounter for open fracture type I or II with routine healing
F	subsequent encounter for open fracture type IIIA, IIIB, or IIIC with routine healing
G	subsequent encounter for closed fracture with delayed healing
H	subsequent encounter for open fracture type I or II with delayed healing
J	subsequent encounter for open fracture type IIIA, IIIB, or IIIC with delayed healing
K	subsequent encounter for closed fracture with nonunion
M	subsequent encounter for open fracture type I or II with nonunion
N	subsequent encounter for open fracture type IIIA, IIIB, or IIIC with nonunion
P	subsequent encounter for closed fracture with malunion
Q	subsequent encounter for open fracture type I or II with malunion
R	subsequent encounter for open fracture type IIIA, IIIB, or IIIC with malunion
S	sequela

CODING TIP✓ A fracture not indicated as displaced or nondisplaced should be coded to displaced. A fracture not indicated as open or closed should be coded to closed. Query providers on fractures not documented as displaced/nondisplaced; otherwise, a displaced fracture diagnosis could be assigned without a reduction being performed, potentially resulting in claim denials.

5 S72.0 Fracture of head and neck of femur

EXCLUDES 2 *physeal fracture of upper end of femur (S79.0-)*

6 S72.00 Fracture of unspecified part of neck of femur

Fracture of hip NOS
Fracture of neck of femur NOS

CODING TIP✓ A fracture that is only reported as a "hip fracture" should be coded to S72.00- with the appropriate 6th character to indicate laterality, and a 7th character to indicate healing status and episode of care.

7 ⊟ S72.001- **Fracture of unspecified part of neck of right femur** HCC

7 ⊟ S72.002- **Fracture of unspecified part of neck of left femur** HCC
AHA: (S72.002D) 4Q 2015, 36-37
AHA: (S72.002S) 1Q 2015, 17

7 ⊟ S72.009- **Fracture of unspecified part of neck of unspecified femur** HCC

6 S72.01 Unspecified intracapsular fracture of femur

Subcapital fracture of femur

7 ⊟ S72.011- **Unspecified intracapsular fracture of right femur** HCC

7 ⊟ S72.012- **Unspecified intracapsular fracture of left femur** HCC

7 ⊟ S72.019- **Unspecified intracapsular fracture of unspecified femur** HCC

6 S72.02 Fracture of epiphysis (separation) (upper) of femur

Transepiphyseal fracture of femur

EXCLUDES 1 *capital femoral epiphyseal fracture (pediatric) of femur (S79.01-)*
Salter-Harris Type I physeal fracture of upper end of femur (S79.01-)

7 ⊟ S72.021- **Displaced fracture of epiphysis (separation) (upper) of right femur** HCC

7 ⊟ S72.022- **Displaced fracture of epiphysis (separation) (upper) of left femur** HCC

7 ⊟ S72.023- **Displaced fracture of epiphysis (separation) (upper) of unspecified femur** HCC

7 ⊟ S72.024- **Nondisplaced fracture of epiphysis (separation) (upper) of right femur** HCC

7 ⊟ S72.025- **Nondisplaced fracture of epiphysis (separation) (upper) of left femur** HCC

7 ⊟ S72.026- **Nondisplaced fracture of epiphysis (separation) (upper) of unspecified femur** HCC

6 S72.03 Midcervical fracture of femur

Transcervical fracture of femur NOS

7 ⊟ S72.031- **Displaced midcervical fracture of right femur** HCC

7 ⊟ S72.032- **Displaced midcervical fracture of left femur** HCC

7 ⊟ S72.033- **Displaced midcervical fracture of unspecified femur** HCC

7 ⊟ S72.034- **Nondisplaced midcervical fracture of right femur** HCC

7 ⊟ S72.035- **Nondisplaced midcervical fracture of left femur** HCC

7 ⊟ S72.036- **Nondisplaced midcervical fracture of unspecified femur** HCC

6 S72.04 Fracture of base of neck of femur

Cervicotrochanteric fracture of femur

7 ⊟ S72.041- **Displaced fracture of base of neck of right femur** HCC

7 ⊟ S72.042- **Displaced fracture of base of neck of left femur** HCC

7 ⊟ S72.043- **Displaced fracture of base of neck of unspecified femur** HCC

7 ⊟ S72.044- **Nondisplaced fracture of base of neck of right femur** HCC

7 ⊟ S72.045- **Nondisplaced fracture of base of neck of left femur** HCC

7 ⊟ S72.046- **Nondisplaced fracture of base of neck of unspecified femur** HCC

6 S72.05 Unspecified fracture of head of femur

Fracture of head of femur NOS

7 ⊟ S72.051- **Unspecified fracture of head of right femur** HCC

7 ⊟ S72.052- **Unspecified fracture of head of left femur** HCC

7 ⊟ S72.059- **Unspecified fracture of head of unspecified femur** HCC

6 S72.06 Articular fracture of head of femur

7 ⊟ S72.061- **Displaced articular fracture of head of right femur** HCC

7 ⊟ S72.062- **Displaced articular fracture of head of left femur** HCC

7 ⊟ S72.063- **Displaced articular fracture of head of unspecified femur** HCC

7 ⊟ S72.064- **Nondisplaced articular fracture of head of right femur** HCC

7 ⊟ S72.065- **Nondisplaced articular fracture of head of left femur** HCC

7 ⊟ S72.066- **Nondisplaced articular fracture of head of unspecified femur** HCC

6 S72.09 Other fracture of head and neck of femur

7 ⊟ S72.091- **Other fracture of head and neck of right femur** HCC

7 ⊟ S72.092- **Other fracture of head and neck of left femur** HCC

7 ⊟ S72.099- **Other fracture of head and neck of unspecified femur** HCC

5 S72.1 Pertrochanteric fracture

6 S72.10 Unspecified trochanteric fracture of femur
Fracture of trochanter NOS
7 ⊟ S72.101- Unspecified trochanteric fracture of right femur HCC
7 ⊟ S72.102- Unspecified trochanteric fracture of left femur HCC
7 ⊟ S72.109- Unspecified trochanteric fracture of unspecified femur HCC

6 S72.11 Fracture of greater trochanter of femur
7 ⊟ S72.111- Displaced fracture of greater trochanter of right femur HCC
7 ⊟ S72.112- Displaced fracture of greater trochanter of left femur HCC
7 ⊟ S72.113- Displaced fracture of greater trochanter of unspecified femur HCC
7 ⊟ S72.114- Nondisplaced fracture of greater trochanter of right femur HCC
7 ⊟ S72.115- Nondisplaced fracture of greater trochanter of left femur HCC
7 ⊟ S72.116- Nondisplaced fracture of greater trochanter of unspecified femur HCC

6 S72.12 Fracture of lesser trochanter of femur
7 ⊟ S72.121- Displaced fracture of lesser trochanter of right femur HCC
7 ⊟ S72.122- Displaced fracture of lesser trochanter of left femur HCC
7 ⊟ S72.123- Displaced fracture of lesser trochanter of unspecified femur HCC
7 ⊟ S72.124- Nondisplaced fracture of lesser trochanter of right femur HCC
7 ⊟ S72.125- Nondisplaced fracture of lesser trochanter of left femur HCC
7 ⊟ S72.126- Nondisplaced fracture of lesser trochanter of unspecified femur HCC

6 S72.13 Apophyseal fracture of femur
EXCLUDES 1 *chronic (nontraumatic) slipped upper femoral epiphysis (M93.0-)*
7 ⊟ S72.131- Displaced apophyseal fracture of right femur HCC
7 ⊟ S72.132- Displaced apophyseal fracture of left femur HCC
7 ⊟ S72.133- Displaced apophyseal fracture of unspecified femur HCC
7 ⊟ S72.134- Nondisplaced apophyseal fracture of right femur HCC
7 ⊟ S72.135- Nondisplaced apophyseal fracture of left femur HCC
7 ⊟ S72.136- Nondisplaced apophyseal fracture of unspecified femur HCC

6 S72.14 Intertrochanteric fracture of femur
7 ⊟ S72.141- Displaced intertrochanteric fracture of right femur HCC
AHA: 4Q 2013, 129
AHA: 3Q 2016, 16
7 ⊟ S72.142- Displaced intertrochanteric fracture of left femur HCC
7 ⊟ S72.143- Displaced intertrochanteric fracture of unspecified femur HCC
7 ⊟ S72.144- Nondisplaced intertrochanteric fracture of right femur HCC
7 ⊟ S72.145- Nondisplaced intertrochanteric fracture of left femur HCC
7 ⊟ S72.146- Nondisplaced intertrochanteric fracture of unspecified femur HCC

5 S72.2 Subtrochanteric fracture of femur
7 ⊟ S72.21X- Displaced subtrochanteric fracture of right femur HCC
7 ⊟ S72.22X- Displaced subtrochanteric fracture of left femur HCC
7 ⊟ S72.23X- Displaced subtrochanteric fracture of unspecified femur HCC
7 ⊟ S72.24X- Nondisplaced subtrochanteric fracture of right femur HCC
7 ⊟ S72.25X- Nondisplaced subtrochanteric fracture of left femur HCC
7 ⊟ S72.26X- Nondisplaced subtrochanteric fracture of unspecified femur HCC

5 S72.3 Fracture of shaft of femur

6 S72.30 Unspecified fracture of shaft of femur
7 ⊟ S72.301- Unspecified fracture of shaft of right femur HCC
AHA: (S72.301A) 2Q 2018, 9
7 ⊟ S72.302- Unspecified fracture of shaft of left femur HCC
7 ⊟ S72.309- Unspecified fracture of shaft of unspecified femur HCC

6 S72.32 Transverse fracture of shaft of femur
7 ⊟ S72.321- Displaced transverse fracture of shaft of right femur HCC
7 ⊟ S72.322- Displaced transverse fracture of shaft of left femur HCC
7 ⊟ S72.323- Displaced transverse fracture of shaft of unspecified femur HCC
7 ⊟ S72.324- Nondisplaced transverse fracture of shaft of right femur HCC
7 ⊟ S72.325- Nondisplaced transverse fracture of shaft of left femur HCC
7 ⊟ S72.326- Nondisplaced transverse fracture of shaft of unspecified femur HCC

6 S72.33 Oblique fracture of shaft of femur
7 ⊟ S72.331- Displaced oblique fracture of shaft of right femur HCC
7 ⊟ S72.332- Displaced oblique fracture of shaft of left femur HCC
7 ⊟ S72.333- Displaced oblique fracture of shaft of unspecified femur HCC
7 ⊟ S72.334- Nondisplaced oblique fracture of shaft of right femur HCC
7 ⊟ S72.335- Nondisplaced oblique fracture of shaft of left femur HCC
7 ⊟ S72.336- Nondisplaced oblique fracture of shaft of unspecified femur HCC

6 S72.34 Spiral fracture of shaft of femur
7 ⊟ S72.341- Displaced spiral fracture of shaft of right femur HCC
7 ⊟ S72.342- Displaced spiral fracture of shaft of left femur HCC
7 ⊟ S72.343- Displaced spiral fracture of shaft of unspecified femur HCC
7 ⊟ S72.344- Nondisplaced spiral fracture of shaft of right femur HCC
7 ⊟ S72.345- Nondisplaced spiral fracture of shaft of left femur HCC
7 ⊟ S72.346- Nondisplaced spiral fracture of shaft of unspecified femur HCC

6 S72.35 Comminuted fracture of shaft of femur
7 ⊟ S72.351- Displaced comminuted fracture of shaft of right femur HCC
7 ⊟ S72.352- Displaced comminuted fracture of shaft of left femur HCC
7 ⊟ S72.353- Displaced comminuted fracture of shaft of unspecified femur HCC
7 ⊟ S72.354- Nondisplaced comminuted fracture of shaft of right femur HCC
7 ⊟ S72.355- Nondisplaced comminuted fracture of shaft of left femur HCC
7 ⊟ S72.356- Nondisplaced comminuted fracture of shaft of unspecified femur HCC

6 S72.36 Segmental fracture of shaft of femur
7 ⊟ S72.361- Displaced segmental fracture of shaft of right femur HCC
7 ⊟ S72.362- Displaced segmental fracture of shaft of left femur HCC
7 ⊟ S72.363- Displaced segmental fracture of shaft of unspecified femur HCC
7 ⊟ S72.364- Nondisplaced segmental fracture of shaft of right femur HCC
7 ⊟ S72.365- Nondisplaced segmental fracture of shaft of left femur HCC
7 ⊟ S72.366- Nondisplaced segmental fracture of shaft of unspecified femur HCC

6 S72.39 Other fracture of shaft of femur
7 ⊟ S72.391- Other fracture of shaft of right femur HCC
7 ⊟ S72.392- Other fracture of shaft of left femur HCC
7 ⊟ S72.399- Other fracture of shaft of unspecified femur HCC

5 S72.4 Fracture of lower end of femur

Fracture of distal end of femur

EXCLUDES 2 *fracture of shaft of femur (S72.3-)*
physeal fracture of lower end of femur (S79.1-)

6 S72.40 Unspecified fracture of lower end of femur

7 ⊟ S72.401- **Unspecified fracture of lower end of right femur** HCC
AHA: 4Q 2016, 42

7 ⊟ S72.402- **Unspecified fracture of lower end of left femur** HCC

7 ⊟ S72.409- **Unspecified fracture of lower end of unspecified femur** HCC

6 S72.41 Unspecified condyle fracture of lower end of femur

Condyle fracture of femur NOS

7 ⊟ S72.411- **Displaced unspecified condyle fracture of lower end of right femur** HCC

7 ⊟ S72.412- **Displaced unspecified condyle fracture of lower end of left femur** HCC

7 ⊟ S72.413- **Displaced unspecified condyle fracture of lower end of unspecified femur** HCC

7 ⊟ S72.414- **Nondisplaced unspecified condyle fracture of lower end of right femur** HCC

7 ⊟ S72.415- **Nondisplaced unspecified condyle fracture of lower end of left femur** HCC

7 ⊟ S72.416- **Nondisplaced unspecified condyle fracture of lower end of unspecified femur** HCC

6 S72.42 Fracture of lateral condyle of femur

7 ⊟ S72.421- **Displaced fracture of lateral condyle of right femur** HCC

7 ⊟ S72.422- **Displaced fracture of lateral condyle of left femur** HCC

7 ⊟ S72.423- **Displaced fracture of lateral condyle of unspecified femur** HCC

7 ⊟ S72.424- **Nondisplaced fracture of lateral condyle of right femur** HCC

7 ⊟ S72.425- **Nondisplaced fracture of lateral condyle of left femur** HCC

7 ⊟ S72.426- **Nondisplaced fracture of lateral condyle of unspecified femur** HCC

6 S72.43 Fracture of medial condyle of femur

7 ⊟ S72.431- **Displaced fracture of medial condyle of right femur** HCC

7 ⊟ S72.432- **Displaced fracture of medial condyle of left femur** HCC

7 ⊟ S72.433- **Displaced fracture of medial condyle of unspecified femur** HCC

7 ⊟ S72.434- **Nondisplaced fracture of medial condyle of right femur** HCC

7 ⊟ S72.435- **Nondisplaced fracture of medial condyle of left femur** HCC

7 ⊟ S72.436- **Nondisplaced fracture of medial condyle of unspecified femur** HCC

6 S72.44 Fracture of lower epiphysis (separation) of femur

EXCLUDES 1 *Salter-Harris Type I physeal fracture of lower end of femur (S79.11-)*

7 ⊟ S72.441- **Displaced fracture of lower epiphysis (separation) of right femur** HCC

7 ⊟ S72.442- **Displaced fracture of lower epiphysis (separation) of left femur** HCC

7 ⊟ S72.443- **Displaced fracture of lower epiphysis (separation) of unspecified femur** HCC

7 ⊟ S72.444- **Nondisplaced fracture of lower epiphysis (separation) of right femur** HCC

7 ⊟ S72.445- **Nondisplaced fracture of lower epiphysis (separation) of left femur** HCC

7 ⊟ S72.446- **Nondisplaced fracture of lower epiphysis (separation) of unspecified femur** HCC

6 S72.45 Supracondylar fracture without intracondylar extension of lower end of femur

Supracondylar fracture of lower end of femur NOS

EXCLUDES 1 *supracondylar fracture with intracondylar extension of lower end of femur (S72.46-)*

7 ⊟ S72.451- **Displaced supracondylar fracture without intracondylar extension of lower end of right femur** HCC

7 ⊟ S72.452- **Displaced supracondylar fracture without intracondylar extension of lower end of left femur** HCC

7 ⊟ S72.453- **Displaced supracondylar fracture without intracondylar extension of lower end of unspecified femur** HCC

7 ⊟ S72.454- **Nondisplaced supracondylar fracture without intracondylar extension of lower end of right femur** HCC

7 ⊟ S72.455- **Nondisplaced supracondylar fracture without intracondylar extension of lower end of left femur** HCC

7 ⊟ S72.456- **Nondisplaced supracondylar fracture without intracondylar extension of lower end of unspecified femur** HCC

6 S72.46 Supracondylar fracture with intracondylar extension of lower end of femur

EXCLUDES 1 *supracondylar fracture without intracondylar extension of lower end of femur (S72.45-)*

7 ⊟ S72.461- **Displaced supracondylar fracture with intracondylar extension of lower end of right femur** HCC

7 ⊟ S72.462- **Displaced supracondylar fracture with intracondylar extension of lower end of left femur** HCC

7 ⊟ S72.463- **Displaced supracondylar fracture with intracondylar extension of lower end of unspecified femur** HCC

7 ⊟ S72.464- **Nondisplaced supracondylar fracture with intracondylar extension of lower end of right femur** HCC

7 ⊟ S72.465- **Nondisplaced supracondylar fracture with intracondylar extension of lower end of left femur** HCC

7 ⊟ S72.466- **Nondisplaced supracondylar fracture with intracondylar extension of lower end of unspecified femur** HCC

6 S72.47 Torus fracture of lower end of femur

The appropriate 7th character is to be added to all codes in subcategory S72.47

- A initial encounter for closed fracture
- D subsequent encounter for fracture with routine healing
- G subsequent encounter for fracture with delayed healing
- K subsequent encounter for fracture with nonunion
- P subsequent encounter for fracture with malunion
- S sequela

CODING TIP✓ Open fractures do not occur with torus fractures and greenstick fractures, therefore the 7th characters for open fractures are not available.

7 ⊟ S72.471- **Torus fracture of lower end of right femur** HCC

7 ⊟ S72.472- **Torus fracture of lower end of left femur** HCC

7 ⊟ S72.479- **Torus fracture of lower end of unspecified femur** HCC

6 S72.49 Other fracture of lower end of femur

7 ⊟ S72.491- **Other fracture of lower end of right femur** HCC

7 ⊟ S72.492- **Other fracture of lower end of left femur** HCC

7 ⊟ S72.499- **Other fracture of lower end of unspecified femur** HCC

5 S72.8 Other fracture of femur

6 S72.8X Other fracture of femur

7 ⊟ S72.8X1- **Other fracture of right femur** HCC

7 ⊟ S72.8X2- **Other fracture of left femur** HCC

7 ⊟ S72.8X9- **Other fracture of unspecified femur** HCC

5 S72.9 Unspecified fracture of femur

Fracture of thigh NOS
Fracture of upper leg NOS

EXCLUDES 1 *fracture of hip NOS (S72.00-, S72.01-)*

7 ⊟ S72.90X- **Unspecified fracture of unspecified femur** HCC
AHA: (S72.90XD) 4Q 2012, 93-94

7 ⊟ S72.91X- **Unspecified fracture of right femur** HCC

7 ⊟ S72.92X- **Unspecified fracture of left femur** HCC

4 **S73 Dislocation and sprain of joint and ligaments of hip**

INCLUDES avulsion of joint or ligament of hip
laceration of cartilage, joint or ligament of hip
sprain of cartilage, joint or ligament of hip
traumatic hemarthrosis of joint or ligament of hip
traumatic rupture of joint or ligament of hip
traumatic subluxation of joint or ligament of hip
traumatic tear of joint or ligament of hip

Code also:
any associated open wound

EXCLUDES 2 *strain of muscle, fascia and tendon of hip and thigh (S76.-)*

The appropriate 7th character is to be added to each code from category S73
A initial encounter
D subsequent encounter
S sequela

CODING TIP ✓ There are no codes for open dislocations. When a dislocation is documented as open, assign an additional code for the open wound.

5 **S73.0 Subluxation and dislocation of hip**

EXCLUDES 2 *dislocation and subluxation of hip prosthesis (T84.020, T84.021)*

6 **S73.00 Unspecified subluxation and dislocation of hip**
Dislocation of hip NOS
Subluxation of hip NOS

7 ⊟ S73.001- **Unspecified subluxation of right hip** HCC
7 ⊟ S73.002- **Unspecified subluxation of left hip** HCC
7 ⊟ S73.003- **Unspecified subluxation of unspecified hip** HCC
7 ⊟ S73.004- **Unspecified dislocation of right hip** HCC
7 ⊟ S73.005- **Unspecified dislocation of left hip** HCC
7 ⊟ S73.006- **Unspecified dislocation of unspecified hip** HCC

6 **S73.01 Posterior subluxation and dislocation of hip**

7 ⊟ S73.011- **Posterior subluxation of right hip** HCC
7 ⊟ S73.012- **Posterior subluxation of left hip** HCC
7 ⊟ S73.013- **Posterior subluxation of unspecified hip** HCC
7 ⊟ S73.014- **Posterior dislocation of right hip** HCC
7 ⊟ S73.015- **Posterior dislocation of left hip** HCC
7 ⊟ S73.016- **Posterior dislocation of unspecified hip** HCC

6 **S73.02 Obturator subluxation and dislocation of hip**

7 ⊟ S73.021- **Obturator subluxation of right hip** HCC
7 ⊟ S73.022- **Obturator subluxation of left hip** HCC
7 ⊟ S73.023- **Obturator subluxation of unspecified hip** HCC
7 ⊟ S73.024- **Obturator dislocation of right hip** HCC
7 ⊟ S73.025- **Obturator dislocation of left hip** HCC
7 ⊟ S73.026- **Obturator dislocation of unspecified hip** HCC

6 **S73.03 Other anterior subluxation and dislocation of hip**

7 ⊟ S73.031- **Other anterior subluxation of right hip** HCC
7 ⊟ S73.032- **Other anterior subluxation of left hip** HCC
7 ⊟ S73.033- **Other anterior subluxation of unspecified hip** HCC
7 ⊟ S73.034- **Other anterior dislocation of right hip** HCC
7 ⊟ S73.035- **Other anterior dislocation of left hip** HCC
7 ⊟ S73.036- **Other anterior dislocation of unspecified hip** HCC

6 **S73.04 Central subluxation and dislocation of hip**

7 ⊟ S73.041- **Central subluxation of right hip** HCC
7 ⊟ S73.042- **Central subluxation of left hip** HCC
7 ⊟ S73.043- **Central subluxation of unspecified hip** HCC
7 ⊟ S73.044- **Central dislocation of right hip** HCC
7 ⊟ S73.045- **Central dislocation of left hip** HCC
7 ⊟ S73.046- **Central dislocation of unspecified hip** HCC

5 **S73.1 Sprain of hip**
AHA: 4Q 2014, 25

6 **S73.10 Unspecified sprain of hip**

7 ⊟ S73.101- **Unspecified sprain of right hip**
7 ⊟ S73.102- **Unspecified sprain of left hip**
7 ⊟ S73.109- **Unspecified sprain of unspecified hip**

6 **S73.11 Iliofemoral ligament sprain of hip**

7 ⊟ S73.111- **Iliofemoral ligament sprain of right hip**
7 ⊟ S73.112- **Iliofemoral ligament sprain of left hip**
7 ⊟ S73.119- **Iliofemoral ligament sprain of unspecified hip**

6 **S73.12 Ischiocapsular (ligament) sprain of hip**

7 ⊟ S73.121- **Ischiocapsular ligament sprain of right hip**
7 ⊟ S73.122- **Ischiocapsular ligament sprain of left hip**
7 ⊟ S73.129- **Ischiocapsular ligament sprain of unspecified hip**

6 **S73.19 Other sprain of hip**

7 ⊟ S73.191- **Other sprain of right hip**
7 ⊟ S73.192- **Other sprain of left hip**
AHA: (S73.192A) 4Q 2014, 25
7 ⊟ S73.199- **Other sprain of unspecified hip**

4 **S74 Injury of nerves at hip and thigh level**

Code also:
any associated open wound (S71.-)

EXCLUDES 2 *injury of nerves at ankle and foot level (S94.-)*
injury of nerves at lower leg level (S84.-)

The appropriate 7th character is to be added to each code from category S74
A initial encounter
D subsequent encounter
S sequela

CODING TIP ✓ Late effects of injuries are coded with seventh character S (sequela) and are sequenced after the residual condition of the late effect.

5 **S74.0 Injury of sciatic nerve at hip and thigh level**

7 ⊟ S74.00X- **Injury of sciatic nerve at hip and thigh level, unspecified leg**
7 ⊟ S74.01X- **Injury of sciatic nerve at hip and thigh level, right leg**
7 ⊟ S74.02X- **Injury of sciatic nerve at hip and thigh level, left leg**

5 **S74.1 Injury of femoral nerve at hip and thigh level**

7 ⊟ S74.10X- **Injury of femoral nerve at hip and thigh level, unspecified leg**
7 ⊟ S74.11X- **Injury of femoral nerve at hip and thigh level, right leg**
7 ⊟ S74.12X- **Injury of femoral nerve at hip and thigh level, left leg**

5 **S74.2 Injury of cutaneous sensory nerve at hip and thigh level**

7 ⊟ S74.20X- **Injury of cutaneous sensory nerve at hip and thigh level, unspecified leg**
7 ⊟ S74.21X- **Injury of cutaneous sensory nerve at hip and high level, right leg**
7 ⊟ S74.22X- **Injury of cutaneous sensory nerve at hip and thigh level, left leg**

5 **S74.8 Injury of other nerves at hip and thigh level**

6 **S74.8X Injury of other nerves at hip and thigh level**

7 ⊟ S74.8X1- **Injury of other nerves at hip and thigh level, right leg**
7 ⊟ S74.8X2- **Injury of other nerves at hip and thigh level, left leg**
7 ⊟ S74.8X9- **Injury of other nerves at hip and thigh level, unspecified leg**

5 **S74.9 Injury of unspecified nerve at hip and thigh level**

7 ⊟ S74.90X- **Injury of unspecified nerve at hip and thigh level, unspecified leg**
7 ⊟ S74.91X- **Injury of unspecified nerve at hip and thigh level, right leg**
7 ⊟ S74.92X- **Injury of unspecified nerve at hip and thigh level, left leg**

4 **S75 Injury of blood vessels at hip and thigh level**

Code also:
any associated open wound (S71.-)

EXCLUDES 2 *injury of blood vessels at lower leg level (S85.-)*
injury of popliteal artery (S85.0)

The appropriate 7th character is to be added to each code from category S75
A initial encounter
D subsequent encounter
S sequela

S75.0 Injury of femoral artery

S75.00 Unspecified injury of femoral artery

S75.001- Unspecified injury of femoral artery, right leg

S75.002- Unspecified injury of femoral artery, left leg

S75.009- Unspecified injury of femoral artery, unspecified leg

S75.01 Minor laceration of femoral artery
Incomplete transection of femoral artery
Laceration of femoral artery NOS
Superficial laceration of femoral artery

S75.011- Minor laceration of femoral artery, right leg

S75.012- Minor laceration of femoral artery, left leg

S75.019- Minor laceration of femoral artery, unspecified leg

S75.02 Major laceration of femoral artery
Complete transection of femoral artery
Traumatic rupture of femoral artery

S75.021- Major laceration of femoral artery, right leg

S75.022- Major laceration of femoral artery, left leg

S75.029- Major laceration of femoral artery, unspecified leg

S75.09 Other specified injury of femoral artery

S75.091- Other specified injury of femoral artery, right leg

S75.092- Other specified injury of femoral artery, left leg

S75.099- Other specified injury of femoral artery, unspecified leg

S75.1 Injury of femoral vein at hip and thigh level

S75.10 Unspecified injury of femoral vein at hip and thigh level

S75.101- Unspecified injury of femoral vein at hip and thigh level, right leg

S75.102- Unspecified injury of femoral vein at hip and thigh level, left leg

S75.109- Unspecified injury of femoral vein at hip and thigh level, unspecified leg

S75.11 Minor laceration of femoral vein at hip and thigh level
Incomplete transection of femoral vein at hip and thigh level
Laceration of femoral vein at hip and thigh level NOS
Superficial laceration of femoral vein at hip and thigh level

S75.111- Minor laceration of femoral vein at hip and thigh level, right leg

S75.112- Minor laceration of femoral vein at hip and thigh level, left leg

S75.119- Minor laceration of femoral vein at hip and thigh level, unspecified leg

S75.12 Major laceration of femoral vein at hip and thigh level
Complete transection of femoral vein at hip and thigh level
Traumatic rupture of femoral vein at hip and thigh level

S75.121- Major laceration of femoral vein at hip and thigh level, right leg

S75.122- Major laceration of femoral vein at hip and thigh level, left leg

S75.129- Major laceration of femoral vein at hip and thigh level, unspecified leg

S75.19 Other specified injury of femoral vein at hip and thigh level

S75.191- Other specified injury of femoral vein at hip and thigh level, right leg

S75.192- Other specified injury of femoral vein at hip and thigh level, left leg

S75.199- Other specified injury of femoral vein at hip and thigh level, unspecified leg

S75.2 Injury of greater saphenous vein at hip and thigh level
EXCLUDES 1 *greater saphenous vein NOS (S85.3)*

S75.20 Unspecified injury of greater saphenous vein at hip and thigh level

S75.201- Unspecified injury of greater saphenous vein at hip and thigh level, right leg

S75.202- Unspecified injury of greater saphenous vein at hip and thigh level, left leg

S75.209- Unspecified injury of greater saphenous vein at hip and thigh level, unspecified leg

S75.21 Minor laceration of greater saphenous vein at hip and thigh level
Incomplete transection of greater saphenous vein at hip and thigh level
Laceration of greater saphenous vein at hip and thigh level NOS
Superficial laceration of greater saphenous vein at hip and thigh level

S75.211- Minor laceration of greater saphenous vein at hip and thigh level, right leg

S75.212- Minor laceration of greater saphenous vein at hip and thigh level, left leg

S75.219- Minor laceration of greater saphenous vein at hip and thigh level, unspecified leg

S75.22 Major laceration of greater saphenous vein at hip and thigh level
Complete transection of greater saphenous vein at hip and thigh level
Traumatic rupture of greater saphenous vein at hip and thigh level

S75.221- Major laceration of greater saphenous vein at hip and thigh level, right leg

S75.222- Major laceration of greater saphenous vein at hip and thigh level, left leg

S75.229- Major laceration of greater saphenous vein at hip and thigh level, unspecified leg

S75.29 Other specified injury of greater saphenous vein at hip and thigh level

S75.291- Other specified injury of greater saphenous vein at hip and thigh level, right leg

S75.292- Other specified injury of greater saphenous vein at hip and thigh level, left leg

S75.299- Other specified injury of greater saphenous vein at hip and thigh level, unspecified leg

S75.8 Injury of other blood vessels at hip and thigh level

S75.80 Unspecified injury of other blood vessels at hip and thigh level

S75.801- Unspecified injury of other blood vessels at hip and thigh level, right leg

S75.802- Unspecified injury of other blood vessels at hip and thigh level, left leg

S75.809- Unspecified injury of other blood vessels at hip and thigh level, unspecified leg

S75.81 Laceration of other blood vessels at hip and thigh level

S75.811- Laceration of other blood vessels at hip and thigh level, right leg

S75.812- Laceration of other blood vessels at hip and thigh level, left leg

S75.819- Laceration of other blood vessels at hip and thigh level, unspecified leg

S75.89 Other specified injury of other blood vessels at hip and thigh level

S75.891- Other specified injury of other blood vessels at hip and thigh level, right leg

S75.892- Other specified injury of other blood vessels at hip and thigh level, left leg

S75.899- Other specified injury of other blood vessels at hip and thigh level, unspecified leg

S75.9 Injury of unspecified blood vessel at hip and thigh level

S75.90 Unspecified injury of Unspecified blood vessel at hip and thigh level

S75.901- Unspecified injury of unspecified blood vessel at hip and thigh level, right leg

S75.902- Unspecified injury of unspecified blood vessel at hip and thigh level, left leg

S75.909- Unspecified injury of unspecified blood vessel at hip and thigh level, unspecified leg

S75.91 Laceration of unspecified blood vessel at hip and thigh level

S75.911- Laceration of unspecified blood vessel at hip and thigh level, right leg

7 ⊟ S75.912- Laceration of unspecified blood vessel at hip and thigh level, left leg

7 ⊟ S75.919- Laceration of unspecified blood vessel at hip and thigh level, unspecified leg

6 S75.99 Other specified injury of unspecified blood vessel at hip and thigh level

7 ⊟ S75.991- Other specified injury of unspecified blood vessel at hip and thigh level, right leg

7 ⊟ S75.992- Other specified injury of unspecified blood vessel at hip and thigh level, left leg

7 ⊟ S75.999- Other specified injury of unspecified blood vessel at hip and thigh level, unspecified leg

4 S76 Injury of muscle, fascia and tendon at hip and thigh level

Code also:
any associated open wound (S71.-)

EXCLUDES 2 *injury of muscle, fascia and tendon at lower leg level (S86)*
sprain of joint and ligament of hip (S73.1)

The appropriate 7th character is to be added to each code from category S76

A	initial encounter
D	subsequent encounter
S	sequela

5 S76.0 Injury of muscle, fascia and tendon of hip

6 S76.00 Unspecified injury of muscle, fascia and tendon of hip

7 ⊟ S76.001- Unspecified injury of muscle, fascia and tendon of right hip

7 ⊟ S76.002- Unspecified injury of muscle, fascia and tendon of left hip

7 ⊟ S76.009- Unspecified injury of muscle, fascia and tendon of unspecified hip

6 S76.01 Strain of muscle, fascia and tendon of hip

7 ⊟ S76.011- Strain of muscle, fascia and tendon of right hip

7 ⊟ S76.012- Strain of muscle, fascia and tendon of left hip

7 ⊟ S76.019- Strain of muscle, fascia and tendon of unspecified hip

6 S76.02 Laceration of muscle, fascia and tendon of hip

7 ⊟ S76.021- Laceration of muscle, fascia and tendon of right hip

7 ⊟ S76.022- Laceration of muscle, fascia and tendon of left hip

7 ⊟ S76.029- Laceration of muscle, fascia and tendon of unspecified hip

6 S76.09 Other specified injury of muscle, fascia and tendon of hip

7 ⊟ S76.091- Other specified injury of muscle, fascia and tendon of right hip

7 ⊟ S76.092- Other specified injury of muscle, fascia and tendon of left hip

7 ⊟ S76.099- Other specified injury of muscle, fascia and tendon of unspecified hip

5 S76.1 Injury of quadriceps muscle, fascia and tendon
Injury of patellar ligament (tendon)

6 S76.10 Unspecified injury of quadriceps muscle, fascia and tendon

7 ⊟ S76.101- Unspecified injury of right quadriceps muscle, fascia and tendon

7 ⊟ S76.102- Unspecified injury of left quadriceps muscle, fascia and tendon

7 ⊟ S76.109- Unspecified injury of unspecified quadriceps muscle, fascia and tendon

6 S76.11 Strain of quadriceps muscle, fascia and tendon

7 ⊟ S76.111- Strain of right quadriceps muscle, fascia and tendon

7 ⊟ S76.112- Strain of left quadriceps muscle, fascia and tendon

7 ⊟ S76.119- Strain of unspecified quadriceps muscle, fascia and tendon

6 S76.12 Laceration of quadriceps muscle, fascia and tendon

7 ⊟ S76.121- Laceration of right quadriceps muscle, fascia and tendon

7 ⊟ S76.122- Laceration of left quadriceps muscle, fascia and tendon

7 ⊟ S76.129- Laceration of unspecified quadriceps muscle, fascia and tendon

6 S76.19 Other specified injury of quadriceps muscle, fascia and tendon

7 ⊟ S76.191- Other specified injury of right quadriceps muscle, fascia and tendon

7 ⊟ S76.192- Other specified injury of left quadriceps muscle, fascia and tendon

7 ⊟ S76.199- Other specified injury of unspecified quadriceps muscle, fascia and tendon

5 S76.2 Injury of adductor muscle, fascia and tendon of thigh

6 S76.20 Unspecified injury of adductor muscle, fascia and tendon of thigh

7 ⊟ S76.201- Unspecified injury of adductor muscle, fascia and tendon of right thigh

7 ⊟ S76.202- Unspecified injury of adductor muscle, fascia and tendon of left thigh

7 ⊟ S76.209- Unspecified injury of adductor muscle, fascia and tendon of unspecified thigh

6 S76.21 Strain of adductor muscle, fascia and tendon of thigh

7 ⊟ S76.211- Strain of adductor muscle, fascia and tendon of right thigh

7 ⊟ S76.212- Strain of adductor muscle, fascia and tendon of left thigh

7 ⊟ S76.219- Strain of adductor muscle, fascia and tendon of unspecified thigh

6 S76.22 Laceration of adductor muscle, fascia and tendon of thigh

7 ⊟ S76.221- Laceration of adductor muscle, fascia and tendon of right thigh

7 ⊟ S76.222- Laceration of adductor muscle, fascia and tendon of left thigh

7 ⊟ S76.229- Laceration of adductor muscle, fascia and tendon of unspecified thigh

6 S76.29 Other injury of adductor muscle, fascia and tendon of thigh

7 ⊟ S76.291- Other injury of adductor muscle, fascia and tendon of right thigh

7 ⊟ S76.292- Other injury of adductor muscle, fascia and tendon of left thigh

7 ⊟ S76.299- Other injury of adductor muscle, fascia and tendon of unspecified thigh

5 S76.3 Injury of muscle, fascia and tendon of the posterior muscle group at thigh level

6 S76.30 Unspecified injury of muscle, fascia and tendon of the posterior muscle group at thigh level

7 ⊟ S76.301- Unspecified injury of muscle, fascia and tendon of the posterior muscle group at thigh level, right thigh

7 ⊟ S76.302- Unspecified injury of muscle, fascia and tendon of the posterior muscle group at thigh level, left thigh

7 ⊟ S76.309- Unspecified injury of muscle, fascia and tendon of the posterior muscle group at thigh level, unspecified thigh

6 S76.31 Strain of muscle, fascia and tendon of the posterior muscle group at thigh level

7 ⊟ S76.311- Strain of muscle, fascia and tendon of the posterior muscle group at thigh level, right thigh

7 ⊟ S76.312- Strain of muscle, fascia and tendon of the posterior muscle group at thigh level, left thigh

7 ⊟ S76.319- Strain of muscle, fascia and tendon of the posterior muscle group at thigh level, unspecified thigh

6 S76.32 Laceration of muscle, fascia and tendon of the posterior muscle group at thigh level

7 ⊟ S76.321- Laceration of muscle, fascia and tendon of the posterior muscle group at thigh level, right thigh

7 ⊟ S76.322- Laceration of muscle, fascia and tendon of the posterior muscle group at thigh level, left thigh

7 ⊟ S76.329- Laceration of muscle, fascia and tendon of the posterior muscle group at thigh level, unspecified thigh

6 S76.39 Other specified injury of muscle, fascia and tendon of the posterior muscle group at thigh level
7 ⊟ S76.391- Other specified injury of muscle, fascia and tendon of the posterior muscle group at thigh level, right thigh
7 ⊟ S76.392- Other specified injury of muscle, fascia and tendon of the posterior muscle group at thigh level, left thigh
7 ⊟ S76.399- Other specified injury of muscle, fascia and tendon of the posterior muscle group at thigh level, unspecified thigh

5 S76.8 Injury of other specified muscles, fascia and tendons at thigh level
6 S76.80 Unspecified injury of other specified muscles, fascia and tendons at thigh level
7 ⊟ S76.801- Unspecified injury of other specified muscles, fascia and tendons at thigh level, right thigh
7 ⊟ S76.802- Unspecified injury of other specified muscles, fascia and tendons at thigh level, left thigh
7 ⊟ S76.809- Unspecified injury of other specified muscles, fascia and tendons at thigh level, unspecified thigh
6 S76.81 Strain of other specified muscles, fascia and tendons at thigh level
7 ⊟ S76.811- Strain of other specified muscles, fascia and tendons at thigh level, right thigh
7 ⊟ S76.812- Strain of other specified muscles, fascia and tendons at thigh level, left thigh
7 ⊟ S76.819- Strain of other specified muscles, fascia and tendons at thigh level, unspecified thigh
6 S76.82 Laceration of other specified muscles, fascia and tendons at thigh level
7 ⊟ S76.821- Laceration of other specified muscles, fascia and tendons at thigh level, right thigh
7 ⊟ S76.822- Laceration of other specified muscles, fascia and tendons at thigh level, left thigh
7 ⊟ S76.829- Laceration of other specified muscles, fascia and tendons at thigh level, unspecified thigh
6 S76.89 Other injury of Other specified muscles, fascia and tendons at thigh level
7 ⊟ S76.891- Other injury of other specified muscles, fascia and tendons at thigh level, right thigh
7 ⊟ S76.892- Other injury of other specified muscles, fascia and tendons at thigh level, left thigh
7 ⊟ S76.899- Other injury of other specified muscles, fascia and tendons at thigh level, unspecified thigh

5 S76.9 Injury of unspecified muscles, fascia and tendons at thigh level
6 S76.90 Unspecified injury of Unspecified muscles, fascia and tendons at thigh level
7 ⊟ S76.901- Unspecified injury of unspecified muscles, fascia and tendons at thigh level, right thigh
7 ⊟ S76.902- Unspecified injury of unspecified muscles, fascia and tendons at thigh level, left thigh
7 ⊟ S76.909- Unspecified injury of unspecified muscles, fascia and tendons at thigh level, unspecified thigh
6 S76.91 Strain of unspecified muscles, fascia and tendons at thigh level
7 ⊟ S76.911- Strain of unspecified muscles, fascia and tendons at thigh level, right thigh
7 ⊟ S76.912- Strain of unspecified muscles, fascia and tendons at thigh level, left thigh
7 ⊟ S76.919- Strain of unspecified muscles, fascia and tendons at thigh level, unspecified thigh
6 S76.92 Laceration of unspecified muscles, fascia and tendons at thigh level
7 ⊟ S76.921- Laceration of unspecified muscles, fascia and tendons at thigh level, right thigh
7 ⊟ S76.922- Laceration of unspecified muscles, fascia and tendons at thigh level, left thigh
7 ⊟ S76.929- Laceration of unspecified muscles, fascia and tendons at thigh level, unspecified thigh
6 S76.99 Other specified injury of unspecified muscles, fascia and tendons at thigh level
7 ⊟ S76.991- Other specified injury of unspecified muscles, fascia and tendons at thigh level, right thigh
7 ⊟ S76.992- Other specified injury of unspecified muscles, fascia and tendons at thigh level, left thigh
7 ⊟ S76.999- Other specified injury of unspecified muscles, fascia and tendons at thigh level, unspecified thigh

4 S77 Crushing injury of hip and thigh

Use additional code(s) for all associated injuries

EXCLUDES 2 *crushing injury of ankle and foot (S97.-)*
crushing injury of lower leg (S87.-)

The appropriate 7th character is to be added to each code from category S77
A initial encounter
D subsequent encounter
S sequela

5 S77.0 Crushing injury of hip
7 ⊟ S77.00X- Crushing injury of unspecified hip
7 ⊟ S77.01X- Crushing injury of right hip
7 ⊟ S77.02X- Crushing injury of left hip
5 S77.1 Crushing injury of thigh
7 ⊟ S77.10X- Crushing injury of unspecified thigh
7 ⊟ S77.11X- Crushing injury of right thigh
7 ⊟ S77.12X- Crushing injury of left thigh
5 S77.2 Crushing injury of hip with thigh
7 ⊟ S77.20X- Crushing injury of unspecified hip with thigh
7 ⊟ S77.21X- Crushing injury of right hip with thigh
7 ⊟ S77.22X- Crushing injury of left hip with thigh

4 S78 Traumatic amputation of hip and thigh

An amputation not identified as partial or complete should be coded to complete

EXCLUDES 1 *traumatic amputation of knee (S88.0-)*

The appropriate 7th character is to be added to each code from category S78
A initial encounter
D subsequent encounter
S sequela

CODING TIP✓ Use these codes only when the amputation was due to trauma. There is no need for adding Z89 with traumatic amputations. See Z47.81 for care of amputations not due to trauma.

CODING TIP✓ Assign only if the amputation is due to accident or violence, i.e., trauma.

5 S78.0 Traumatic amputation at hip joint
6 S78.01 Complete traumatic amputation at hip joint
7 ⊟ S78.011- Complete traumatic amputation at right hip joint HCC
7 ⊟ S78.012- Complete traumatic amputation at left hip joint HCC
7 ⊟ S78.019- Complete traumatic amputation at unspecified hip joint HCC
6 S78.02 Partial traumatic amputation at hip joint
7 ⊟ S78.021- Partial traumatic amputation at right hip joint HCC
7 ⊟ S78.022- Partial traumatic amputation at left hip joint HCC
7 ⊟ S78.029- Partial traumatic amputation at unspecified hip joint HCC
5 S78.1 Traumatic amputation at level between hip and knee
EXCLUDES 1 *traumatic amputation of knee (S88.0-)*
6 S78.11 Complete traumatic amputation at level between hip and knee
7 ⊟ S78.111- Complete traumatic amputation at level between right hip and knee HCC
7 ⊟ S78.112- Complete traumatic amputation at level between left hip and knee HCC
7 ⊟ S78.119- Complete traumatic amputation at level between unspecified hip and knee HCC
6 S78.12 Partial traumatic amputation at level between hip and knee
7 ⊟ S78.121- Partial traumatic amputation at level between right hip and knee HCC
7 ⊟ S78.122- Partial traumatic amputation at level between left hip and knee HCC

● New *Manifestation* 4-7 Digit Indicators ⊟ Laterality A Adult M Maternity N Newborn P Pediatric ♂ Male
▲ Revised Unspecified AHA Coding Clinic HCC Hierarchical Condition Categories HIV HIV Related Conditions ♀ Female

S78.129- **Partial traumatic amputation at level between unspecified hip and knee** HCC

S78.9 **Traumatic amputation of hip and thigh, level unspecified**

S78.91 **Complete traumatic amputation of hip and thigh, level unspecified**

S78.911- **Complete traumatic amputation of right hip and thigh, level unspecified** HCC

S78.912- **Complete traumatic amputation of left hip and thigh, level unspecified** HCC

S78.919- **Complete traumatic amputation of unspecified hip and thigh, level unspecified** HCC

S78.92 **Partial traumatic amputation of hip and thigh, level unspecified**

S78.921- **Partial traumatic amputation of right hip and thigh, level unspecified** HCC

S78.922- **Partial traumatic amputation of left hip and thigh, level unspecified** HCC

S78.929- **Partial traumatic amputation of unspecified hip and thigh, level unspecified** HCC

S79 Other and unspecified injuries of hip and thigh

Note: A fracture not indicated as open or closed should be coded to closed

The appropriate 7th character is to be added to each code from subcategories S79.0 and S79.1

A	initial encounter for closed fracture
D	subsequent encounter for fracture with routine healing
G	subsequent encounter for fracture with delayed healing
K	subsequent encounter for fracture with nonunion
P	subsequent encounter for fracture with malunion
S	sequela

CODING TIP✓ A Salter-Harris physeal fracture occurs through the growth plate. Only one code is needed to report a single physeal fracture. Because of the implications for future bone development, coding of a Salter-Harris fracture takes priority over a simple fracture code. Assign the physeal fracture code based on location, type, and laterality. Use a code for "other physeal fracture" for Type V.

S79.0 **Physeal fracture of upper end of femur**

EXCLUDES 1 *apophyseal fracture of upper end of femur (S72.13-)*
nontraumatic slipped upper femoral epiphysis (M93.0-)

S79.00 **Unspecified physeal fracture of upper end of femur**

S79.001- **Unspecified physeal fracture of upper end of right femur** HCC

S79.002- **Unspecified physeal fracture of upper end of left femur** HCC

S79.009- **Unspecified physeal fracture of upper end of unspecified femur** HCC

S79.01 **Salter-Harris Type I physeal fracture of upper end of femur**

Acute on chronic slipped capital femoral epiphysis (traumatic)
Acute slipped capital femoral epiphysis (traumatic)
Capital femoral epiphyseal fracture

EXCLUDES 1 *chronic slipped upper femoral epiphysis (nontraumatic) (M93.02-)*

S79.011- **Salter-Harris Type I physeal fracture of upper end of right femur** HCC

Salter-Harris physeal fracture Type 1 upper end of right femur

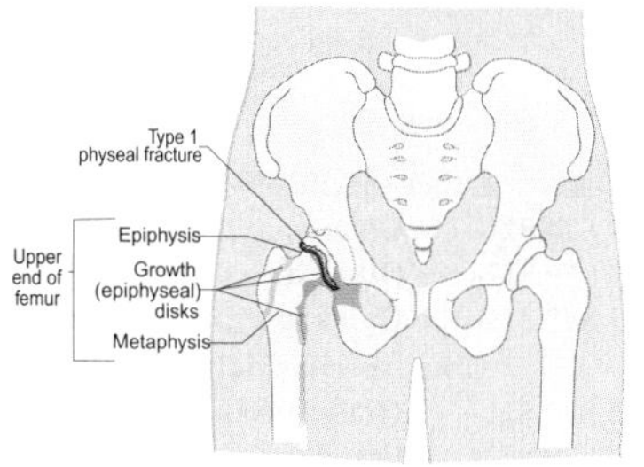

S79.012- **Salter-Harris Type I physeal fracture of upper end of left femur** HCC

S79.019- **Salter-Harris Type I physeal fracture of upper end of unspecified femur** HCC

S79.09 **Other physeal fracture of upper end of femur**

S79.091- **Other physeal fracture of upper end of right femur** HCC

S79.092- **Other physeal fracture of upper end of left femur** HCC

S79.099- **Other physeal fracture of upper end of unspecified femur** HCC

S79.1 **Physeal fracture of lower end of femur**

S79.10 **Unspecified physeal fracture of lower end of femur**

S79.101- **Unspecified physeal fracture of lower end of right femur** HCC

S79.102- **Unspecified physeal fracture of lower end of left femur** HCC

S79.109- **Unspecified physeal fracture of lower end of unspecified femur** HCC

S79.11 **Salter-Harris Type I physeal fracture of lower end of femur**

S79.111- **Salter-Harris Type I physeal fracture of lower end of right femur** HCC

S79.112- **Salter-Harris Type I physeal fracture of lower end of left femur** HCC

S79.119- **Salter-Harris Type I physeal fracture of lower end of unspecified femur** HCC

S79.12 **Salter-Harris Type II physeal fracture of lower end of femur**

S79.121- **Salter-Harris Type II physeal fracture of lower end of right femur** HCC

S79.122- **Salter-Harris Type II physeal fracture of lower end of left femur** HCC

S79.129- **Salter-Harris Type II physeal fracture of lower end of unspecified femur** HCC

S79.13 **Salter-Harris Type III physeal fracture of lower end of femur**

S79.131- **Salter-Harris Type III physeal fracture of lower end of right femur** HCC

S79.132- **Salter-Harris Type III physeal fracture of lower end of left femur** HCC

S79.139- **Salter-Harris Type III physeal fracture of lower end of unspecified femur** HCC

S79.14 **Salter-Harris Type IV physeal fracture of lower end of femur**

S79.141- **Salter-Harris Type IV physeal fracture of lower end of right femur** HCC

S79.142- **Salter-Harris Type IV physeal fracture of lower end of left femur** HCC

S79.149- **Salter-Harris Type IV physeal fracture of lower end of unspecified femur** HCC

S79.19 **Other physeal fracture of lower end of femur**

S79.191- **Other physeal fracture of lower end of right femur** HCC

S79.192- **Other physeal fracture of lower end of left femur** HCC

S79.199- **Other physeal fracture of lower end of unspecified femur** HCC

5 S79.8 Other specified injuries of hip and thigh

The appropriate 7th character is to be added to each code in subcategory S79.8
A initial encounter
D subsequent encounter
S sequela

6 S79.81 Other specified injuries of hip
- 7 S79.811- Other specified injuries of right hip
- 7 S79.812- Other specified injuries of left hip
- 7 S79.819- Other specified injuries of unspecified hip

6 S79.82 Other specified injuries of thigh
- 7 S79.821- Other specified injuries of right thigh
- 7 S79.822- Other specified injuries of left thigh
- 7 S79.829- Other specified injuries of unspecified thigh

5 S79.9 Unspecified injury of hip and thigh

The appropriate 7th character is to be added to each code in subcategory S79.9
A initial encounter
D subsequent encounter
S sequela

6 S79.91 Unspecified injury of hip
- 7 S79.911- Unspecified injury of right hip
- 7 S79.912- Unspecified injury of left hip
- 7 S79.919- Unspecified injury of unspecified hip

6 S79.92 Unspecified injury of thigh
- 7 S79.921- Unspecified injury of right thigh
- 7 S79.922- Unspecified injury of left thigh
- 7 S79.929- Unspecified injury of unspecified thigh

Injuries to the knee and lower leg (S80-S89)

EXCLUDES 2 *burns and corrosions (T20-T32)*
frostbite (T33-T34)
injuries of ankle and foot, except fracture of ankle and malleolus (S90-S99)
insect bite or sting, venomous (T63.4)

GUIDELINES **Section I.C.19.c.2)**
Multiple fractures are sequenced in accordance with the severity of the fracture.

GUIDELINES **Section I.C.19.b.1)-2)**
When coding injuries, assign separate codes for each injury unless a combination code is provided, in which case the combination code is assigned ... Traumatic injury codes (S00-T14.9) are not to be used for normal, healing surgical wounds or to identify complications of surgical wounds. The code for the most serious injury, as determined by the provider and the focus of treatment, is sequenced first.

1) Superficial injuries such as abrasions or contusions are not coded when associated with more severe injuries of the same site.

2) When a primary injury results in minor damage to peripheral nerves or blood vessels, the primary injury is sequenced first with additional code(s) for injuries to nerves and spinal cord (such as category S04), and/or injury to blood vessels (such as category S15). When the primary injury is to the blood vessels or nerves, that injury should be sequenced first.

GUIDELINES **Section I.C.19.c**
Coding of Traumatic Fractures: The principles of multiple coding of injuries should be followed in coding fractures. Fractures of specified sites are coded individually by site in accordance with both the provisions within categories S02, S12, S22, S32, S42, S49, S52, S59, S62, S72, S79, S82, S89, S92 and the level of detail furnished by medical record content. A fracture not indicated as open or closed should be coded to closed. A fracture not indicated whether displaced or not displaced should be coded to displaced.

4 S80 Superficial injury of knee and lower leg

EXCLUDES 2 *superficial injury of ankle and foot (S90.-)*

The appropriate 7th character is to be added to each code from category S80
A initial encounter
D subsequent encounter
S sequela

5 S80.0 Contusion of knee
- 7 S80.00X- Contusion of unspecified knee
- 7 S80.01X- Contusion of right knee
- 7 S80.02X- Contusion of left knee

5 S80.1 Contusion of lower leg
- 7 S80.10X- Contusion of unspecified lower leg
- 7 S80.11X- Contusion of right lower leg
- 7 S80.12X- Contusion of left lower leg

5 S80.2 Other superficial injuries of knee

6 S80.21 Abrasion of knee
- 7 S80.211- Abrasion, right knee
- 7 S80.212- Abrasion, left knee
- 7 S80.219- Abrasion, unspecified knee

6 S80.22 Blister (nonthermal) of knee
- 7 S80.221- Blister (nonthermal), right knee
- 7 S80.222- Blister (nonthermal), left knee
- 7 S80.229- Blister (nonthermal), unspecified knee

6 S80.24 External constriction of knee
- 7 S80.241- External constriction, right knee
- 7 S80.242- External constriction, left knee
- 7 S80.249- External constriction, unspecified knee

6 S80.25 Superficial foreign body of knee
Splinter in the knee
- 7 S80.251- Superficial foreign body, right knee
- 7 S80.252- Superficial foreign body, left knee
- 7 S80.259- Superficial foreign body, unspecified knee

6 S80.26 Insect bite (nonvenomous) of knee
- 7 S80.261- Insect bite (nonvenomous), right knee
- 7 S80.262- Insect bite (nonvenomous), left knee
- 7 S80.269- Insect bite (nonvenomous), unspecified knee

6 S80.27 Other superficial bite of knee
EXCLUDES 1 *open bite of knee (S81.05-)*
- 7 S80.271- Other superficial bite of right knee
- 7 S80.272- Other superficial bite of left knee
- 7 S80.279- Other superficial bite of unspecified knee

5 S80.8 Other superficial injuries of lower leg

6 S80.81 Abrasion of lower leg
- 7 S80.811- Abrasion, right lower leg
- 7 S80.812- Abrasion, left lower leg
- 7 S80.819- Abrasion, unspecified lower leg

6 S80.82 Blister (nonthermal) of lower leg
- 7 S80.821- Blister (nonthermal), right lower leg
- 7 S80.822- Blister (nonthermal), left lower leg
- 7 S80.829- Blister (nonthermal), unspecified lower leg

6 S80.84 External constriction of lower leg
- 7 S80.841- External constriction, right lower leg
- 7 S80.842- External constriction, left lower leg
- 7 S80.849- External constriction, unspecified lower leg

6 S80.85 Superficial foreign body of lower leg
Splinter in the lower leg
- 7 S80.851- Superficial foreign body, right lower leg
- 7 S80.852- Superficial foreign body, left lower leg
- 7 S80.859- Superficial foreign body, unspecified lower leg

6 S80.86 Insect bite (nonvenomous) of lower leg
- 7 S80.861- Insect bite (nonvenomous), right lower leg
- 7 S80.862- Insect bite (nonvenomous), left lower leg
- 7 S80.869- Insect bite (nonvenomous), unspecified lower leg

6 S80.87 Other superficial bite of lower leg
EXCLUDES 1 *open bite of lower leg (S81.85-)*
7 S80.871- Other superficial bite, right lower leg
7 S80.872- Other superficial bite, left lower leg
7 S80.879- Other superficial bite, unspecified lower leg
5 S80.9 Unspecified superficial injury of knee and lower leg
6 S80.91 Unspecified superficial injury of knee
7 S80.911- Unspecified superficial injury of right knee
7 S80.912- Unspecified superficial injury of left knee
7 S80.919- Unspecified superficial injury of unspecified knee
6 S80.92 Unspecified superficial injury of lower leg
7 S80.921- Unspecified superficial injury of right lower leg
7 S80.922- Unspecified superficial injury of left lower leg
7 S80.929- Unspecified superficial injury of unspecified lower leg

4 S81 Open wound of knee and lower leg

Code also:
any associated wound infection
EXCLUDES 1 *open fracture of knee and lower leg (S82.-)*
traumatic amputation of lower leg (S88.-)
EXCLUDES 2 *open wound of ankle and foot (S91.-)*

The appropriate 7th character is to be added to each code from category S81
A initial encounter
D subsequent encounter
S sequela

CODING TIP✓ Open wound codes indicate a wound resulting from a traumatic origin. Do not assign a code for "open wound" unless the etiology of the wound is related to trauma.

5 S81.0 Open wound of knee
6 S81.00 Unspecified open wound of knee
7 S81.001- Unspecified open wound, right knee
7 S81.002- Unspecified open wound, left knee
7 S81.009- Unspecified open wound, unspecified knee
6 S81.01 Laceration without foreign body of knee
7 S81.011- Laceration without foreign body, right knee
7 S81.012- Laceration without foreign body, left knee
7 S81.019- Laceration without foreign body, unspecified knee
6 S81.02 Laceration with foreign body of knee
7 S81.021- Laceration with foreign body, right knee
7 S81.022- Laceration with foreign body, left knee
7 S81.029- Laceration with foreign body, unspecified knee
6 S81.03 Puncture wound without foreign body of knee
7 S81.031- Puncture wound without foreign body, right knee
7 S81.032- Puncture wound without foreign body, left knee
7 S81.039- Puncture wound without foreign body, unspecified knee
6 S81.04 Puncture wound with foreign body of knee
7 S81.041- Puncture wound with foreign body, right knee
7 S81.042- Puncture wound with foreign body, left knee
7 S81.049- Puncture wound with foreign body, unspecified knee
6 S81.05 Open bite of knee
Bite of knee NOS
EXCLUDES 1 *superficial bite of knee (S80.27-)*
7 S81.051- Open bite, right knee
7 S81.052- Open bite, left knee
7 S81.059- Open bite, unspecified knee
5 S81.8 Open wound of lower leg
6 S81.80 Unspecified open wound of lower leg
7 S81.801- Unspecified open wound, right lower leg
7 S81.802- Unspecified open wound, left lower leg
7 S81.809- Unspecified open wound, unspecified lower leg
6 S81.81 Laceration without foreign body of lower leg
7 S81.811- Laceration without foreign body, right lower leg
7 S81.812- Laceration without foreign body, left lower leg
7 S81.819- Laceration without foreign body, unspecified lower leg
6 S81.82 Laceration with foreign body of lower leg
7 S81.821- Laceration with foreign body, right lower leg
7 S81.822- Laceration with foreign body, left lower leg
7 S81.829- Laceration with foreign body, unspecified lower leg
6 S81.83 Puncture wound without foreign body of lower leg
7 S81.831- Puncture wound without foreign body, right lower leg
7 S81.832- Puncture wound without foreign body, left lower leg
7 S81.839- Puncture wound without foreign body, unspecified lower leg
6 S81.84 Puncture wound with foreign body of lower leg
7 S81.841- Puncture wound with foreign body, right lower leg
AHA: 3Q 2016, 23
AHA: 3Q 2016, 24
7 S81.842- Puncture wound with foreign body, left lower leg
7 S81.849- Puncture wound with foreign body, unspecified lower leg
6 S81.85 Open bite of lower leg
Bite of lower leg NOS
EXCLUDES 1 *superficial bite of lower leg (S80.86-, S80.87-)*
7 S81.851- Open bite, right lower leg
7 S81.852- Open bite, left lower leg
7 S81.859- Open bite, unspecified lower leg

4 S82 Fracture of lower leg, including ankle

Note: A fracture not indicated as displaced or nondisplaced should be coded to displaced
A fracture not indicated as open or closed should be coded to closed
The open fracture designations are based on the Gustilo open fracture classification
INCLUDES fracture of malleolus
EXCLUDES 1 *traumatic amputation of lower leg (S88.-)*
EXCLUDES 2 *fracture of foot, except ankle (S92.-)*
periprosthetic fracture of prosthetic implant of knee (M97.0-)

The appropriate 7th character is to be added to all codes from category S82
A initial encounter for closed fracture
B initial encounter for open fracture type I or II
C initial encounter for open fracture type IIIA, IIIB, or IIIC
D subsequent encounter for closed fracture with routine healing
E subsequent encounter for open fracture type I or II with routine healing
F subsequent encounter for open fracture type IIIA, IIIB, or IIIC with routine healing
G subsequent encounter for closed fracture with delayed healing
H subsequent encounter for open fracture type I or II with delayed healing
J subsequent encounter for open fracture type IIIA, IIIB, or IIIC with delayed healing
K subsequent encounter for closed fracture with nonunion
M subsequent encounter for open fracture type I or II with nonunion
N subsequent encounter for open fracture type IIIA, IIIB, or IIIC with nonunion
P subsequent encounter for closed fracture with malunion
Q subsequent encounter for open fracture type I or II with malunion
R subsequent encounter for open fracture type IIIA, IIIB, or IIIC with malunion
S sequela

CODING TIP✓ A fracture not indicated as displaced or nondisplaced should be coded to displaced. A fracture not indicated as open or closed should be coded to closed. Query providers on fractures not documented as displaced/nondisplaced; otherwise, a displaced fracture diagnosis could be assigned without a reduction being performed, potentially resulting in claim denials.

5 **S82.0 Fracture of patella**
Knee cap

6 **S82.00 Unspecified fracture of patella**
- 7 S82.001- Unspecified fracture of right patella
- 7 S82.002- Unspecified fracture of left patella
- 7 S82.009- Unspecified fracture of unspecified patella

6 **S82.01 Osteochondral fracture of patella**
- 7 S82.011- Displaced osteochondral fracture of right patella
- 7 S82.012- Displaced osteochondral fracture of left patella
- 7 S82.013- Displaced osteochondral fracture of unspecified patella
- 7 S82.014- Nondisplaced osteochondral fracture of right patella
- 7 S82.015- Nondisplaced osteochondral fracture of left patella
- 7 S82.016- Nondisplaced osteochondral fracture of unspecified patella

6 **S82.02 Longitudinal fracture of patella**
- 7 S82.021- Displaced longitudinal fracture of right patella
- 7 S82.022- Displaced longitudinal fracture of left patella
- 7 S82.023- Displaced longitudinal fracture of unspecified patella
- 7 S82.024- Nondisplaced longitudinal fracture of right patella
- 7 S82.025- Nondisplaced longitudinal fracture of left patella
- 7 S82.026- Nondisplaced longitudinal fracture of unspecified patella

6 **S82.03 Transverse fracture of patella**
- 7 S82.031- Displaced transverse fracture of right patella
- 7 S82.032- Displaced transverse fracture of left patella
- 7 S82.033- Displaced transverse fracture of unspecified patella
- 7 S82.034- Nondisplaced transverse fracture of right patella
- 7 S82.035- Nondisplaced transverse fracture of left patella
- 7 S82.036- Nondisplaced transverse fracture of unspecified patella

6 **S82.04 Comminuted fracture of patella**
- 7 S82.041- Displaced comminuted fracture of right patella
- 7 S82.042- Displaced comminuted fracture of left patella
- 7 S82.043- Displaced comminuted fracture of unspecified patella
- 7 S82.044- Nondisplaced comminuted fracture of right patella
- 7 S82.045- Nondisplaced comminuted fracture of left patella
- 7 S82.046- Nondisplaced comminuted fracture of unspecified patella

6 **S82.09 Other fracture of patella**
- 7 S82.091- Other fracture of right patella
- 7 S82.092- Other fracture of left patella
- 7 S82.099- Other fracture of unspecified patella

5 **S82.1 Fracture of upper end of tibia**
Fracture of proximal end of tibia

EXCLUDES 2 *fracture of shaft of tibia (S82.2-)*
physeal fracture of upper end of tibia (S89.0-)

6 **S82.10 Unspecified fracture of upper end of tibia**
- 7 S82.101- Unspecified fracture of upper end of right tibia
- 7 S82.102- Unspecified fracture of upper end of left tibia
- 7 S82.109- Unspecified fracture of upper end of unspecified tibia

6 **S82.11 Fracture of tibial spine**
- 7 S82.111- Displaced fracture of right tibial spine
- 7 S82.112- Displaced fracture of left tibial spine
- 7 S82.113- Displaced fracture of unspecified tibial spine
- 7 S82.114- Nondisplaced fracture of right tibial spine
- 7 S82.115- Nondisplaced fracture of left tibial spine
- 7 S82.116- Nondisplaced fracture of unspecified tibial spine

6 **S82.12 Fracture of lateral condyle of tibia**
- 7 S82.121- Displaced fracture of lateral condyle of right tibia
- 7 S82.122- Displaced fracture of lateral condyle of left tibia
- 7 S82.123- Displaced fracture of lateral condyle of unspecified tibia
- 7 S82.124- Nondisplaced fracture of lateral condyle of right tibia
- 7 S82.125- Nondisplaced fracture of lateral condyle of left tibia
- 7 S82.126- Nondisplaced fracture of lateral condyle of unspecified tibia

6 **S82.13 Fracture of medial condyle of tibia**
- 7 S82.131- Displaced fracture of medial condyle of right tibia
- 7 S82.132- Displaced fracture of medial condyle of left tibia
- 7 S82.133- Displaced fracture of medial condyle of unspecified tibia
- 7 S82.134- Nondisplaced fracture of medial condyle of right tibia
- 7 S82.135- Nondisplaced fracture of medial condyle of left tibia
- 7 S82.136- Nondisplaced fracture of medial condyle of unspecified tibia

6 **S82.14 Bicondylar fracture of tibia**
Fracture of tibial plateau NOS
- 7 S82.141- Displaced bicondylar fracture of right tibia
- 7 S82.142- Displaced bicondylar fracture of left tibia
- 7 S82.143- Displaced bicondylar fracture of unspecified tibia
- 7 S82.144- Nondisplaced bicondylar fracture of right tibia
- 7 S82.145- Nondisplaced bicondylar fracture of left tibia
- 7 S82.146- Nondisplaced bicondylar fracture of unspecified tibia

6 **S82.15 Fracture of tibial tuberosity**
- 7 S82.151- Displaced fracture of right tibial tuberosity
- 7 S82.152- Displaced fracture of left tibial tuberosity
- 7 S82.153- Displaced fracture of unspecified tibial tuberosity
- 7 S82.154- Nondisplaced fracture of right tibial tuberosity
- 7 S82.155- Nondisplaced fracture of left tibial tuberosity
- 7 S82.156- Nondisplaced fracture of unspecified tibial tuberosity

6 **S82.16 Torus fracture of upper end of tibia**

The appropriate 7th character is to be added to all codes in subcategory S82.16

A	initial encounter for closed fracture
D	subsequent encounter for fracture with routine healing
G	subsequent encounter for fracture with delayed healing
K	subsequent encounter for fracture with nonunion
P	subsequent encounter for fracture with malunion
S	sequela

CODING TIP✓ Open fractures do not occur with torus fractures and greenstick fractures, therefore the 7th characters for open fractures are not available.

- 7 S82.161- Torus fracture of upper end of right tibia
- 7 S82.162- Torus fracture of upper end of left tibia
- 7 S82.169- Torus fracture of upper end of unspecified tibia

6 **S82.19 Other fracture of upper end of tibia**

7 ⊟ S82.191- Other fracture of upper end of right tibia
7 ⊟ S82.192- Other fracture of upper end of left tibia
7 ⊟ S82.199- Other fracture of upper end of unspecified tibia

5 S82.2 Fracture of shaft of tibia

6 S82.20 Unspecified fracture of shaft of tibia
Fracture of tibia NOS
7 ⊟ S82.201- Unspecified fracture of shaft of right tibia
7 ⊟ S82.202- Unspecified fracture of shaft of left tibia
7 ⊟ S82.209- Unspecified fracture of shaft of unspecified tibia

6 S82.22 Transverse fracture of shaft of tibia
7 ⊟ S82.221- Displaced transverse fracture of shaft of right tibia
7 ⊟ S82.222- Displaced transverse fracture of shaft of left tibia
7 ⊟ S82.223- Displaced transverse fracture of shaft of unspecified tibia
7 ⊟ S82.224- Nondisplaced transverse fracture of shaft of right tibia
7 ⊟ S82.225- Nondisplaced transverse fracture of shaft of left tibia
7 ⊟ S82.226- Nondisplaced transverse fracture of shaft of unspecified tibia

6 S82.23 Oblique fracture of shaft of tibia
7 ⊟ S82.231- Displaced oblique fracture of shaft of right tibia
7 ⊟ S82.232- Displaced oblique fracture of shaft of left tibia
7 ⊟ S82.233- Displaced oblique fracture of shaft of unspecified tibia
7 ⊟ S82.234- Nondisplaced oblique fracture of shaft of right tibia
AHA: (S82.234A) 1Q 2015, 9
AHA: (S82.234D) 1Q 2015, 10
7 ⊟ S82.235- Nondisplaced oblique fracture of shaft of left tibia
7 ⊟ S82.236- Nondisplaced oblique fracture of shaft of unspecified tibia

6 S82.24 Spiral fracture of shaft of tibia
Toddler fracture
7 ⊟ S82.241- Displaced spiral fracture of shaft of right tibia
7 ⊟ S82.242- Displaced spiral fracture of shaft of left tibia
7 ⊟ S82.243- Displaced spiral fracture of shaft of unspecified tibia
7 ⊟ S82.244- Nondisplaced spiral fracture of shaft of right tibia
7 ⊟ S82.245- Nondisplaced spiral fracture of shaft of left tibia
7 ⊟ S82.246- Nondisplaced spiral fracture of shaft of unspecified tibia

6 S82.25 Comminuted fracture of shaft of tibia
7 ⊟ S82.251- Displaced comminuted fracture of shaft of right tibia
AHA: (S82.251D) 2Q 2015, 6
7 ⊟ S82.252- Displaced comminuted fracture of shaft of left tibia
7 ⊟ S82.253- Displaced comminuted fracture of shaft of unspecified tibia
7 ⊟ S82.254- Nondisplaced comminuted fracture of shaft of right tibia
7 ⊟ S82.255- Nondisplaced comminuted fracture of shaft of left tibia
7 ⊟ S82.256- Nondisplaced comminuted fracture of shaft of unspecified tibia

6 S82.26 Segmental fracture of shaft of tibia
7 ⊟ S82.261- Displaced segmental fracture of shaft of right tibia
7 ⊟ S82.262- Displaced segmental fracture of shaft of left tibia
7 ⊟ S82.263- Displaced segmental fracture of shaft of unspecified tibia
7 ⊟ S82.264- Nondisplaced segmental fracture of shaft of right tibia
7 ⊟ S82.265- Nondisplaced segmental fracture of shaft of left tibia
7 ⊟ S82.266- Nondisplaced segmental fracture of shaft of unspecified tibia

6 S82.29 Other fracture of shaft of tibia
7 ⊟ S82.291- Other fracture of shaft of right tibia
7 ⊟ S82.292- Other fracture of shaft of left tibia
7 ⊟ S82.299- Other fracture of shaft of unspecified tibia

5 S82.3 Fracture of lower end of tibia

EXCLUDES 1 *bimalleolar fracture of lower leg (S82.84-)*
fracture of medial malleolus alone (S82.5-)
Maisonneuve's fracture (S82.86-)
pilon fracture of distal tibia (S82.87-)
trimalleolar fractures of lower leg (S82.85-)

6 S82.30 Unspecified fracture of lower end of tibia
7 ⊟ S82.301- Unspecified fracture of lower end of right tibia
7 ⊟ S82.302- Unspecified fracture of lower end of left tibia
7 ⊟ S82.309- Unspecified fracture of lower end of unspecified tibia

6 S82.31 Torus fracture of lower end of tibia

The appropriate 7th character is to be added to all codes in subcategory S82.31
A initial encounter for closed fracture
D subsequent encounter for fracture with routine healing
G subsequent encounter for fracture with delayed healing
K subsequent encounter for fracture with nonunion
P subsequent encounter for fracture with malunion
S sequela

CODING TIP ✓ Open fractures do not occur with torus fractures and greenstick fractures, therefore the 7th characters for open fractures are not available.

7 ⊟ S82.311- Torus fracture of lower end of right tibia
7 ⊟ S82.312- Torus fracture of lower end of left tibia
7 ⊟ S82.319- Torus fracture of lower end of unspecified tibia

6 S82.39 Other fracture of lower end of tibia
7 ⊟ S82.391- Other fracture of lower end of right tibia
7 ⊟ S82.392- Other fracture of lower end of left tibia
AHA: 1Q 2015, 25
7 ⊟ S82.399- Other fracture of lower end of unspecified tibia

5 S82.4 Fracture of shaft of fibula

EXCLUDES 2 *fracture of lateral malleolus alone (S82.6-)*

6 S82.40 Unspecified fracture of shaft of fibula
7 ⊟ S82.401- Unspecified fracture of shaft of right fibula
7 ⊟ S82.402- Unspecified fracture of shaft of left fibula
7 ⊟ S82.409- Unspecified fracture of shaft of unspecified fibula

6 S82.42 Transverse fracture of shaft of fibula
7 ⊟ S82.421- Displaced transverse fracture of shaft of right fibula
7 ⊟ S82.422- Displaced transverse fracture of shaft of left fibula
7 ⊟ S82.423- Displaced transverse fracture of shaft of unspecified fibula
7 ⊟ S82.424- Nondisplaced transverse fracture of shaft of right fibula
7 ⊟ S82.425- Nondisplaced transverse fracture of shaft of left fibula
7 ⊟ S82.426- Nondisplaced transverse fracture of shaft of unspecified fibula

6 S82.43 Oblique fracture of shaft of fibula
7 ⊟ S82.431- Displaced oblique fracture of shaft of right fibula
7 ⊟ S82.432- Displaced oblique fracture of shaft of left fibula
7 ⊟ S82.433- Displaced oblique fracture of shaft of unspecified fibula
7 ⊟ S82.434- Nondisplaced oblique fracture of shaft of right fibula
7 ⊟ S82.435- Nondisplaced oblique fracture of shaft of left fibula

S82.436- Nondisplaced oblique fracture of shaft of unspecified fibula

S82.44 Spiral fracture of shaft of fibula

S82.441- Displaced spiral fracture of shaft of right fibula

S82.442- Displaced spiral fracture of shaft of left fibula

S82.443- Displaced spiral fracture of shaft of unspecified fibula

S82.444- Nondisplaced spiral fracture of shaft of right fibula

S82.445- Nondisplaced spiral fracture of shaft of left fibula

S82.446- Nondisplaced spiral fracture of shaft of unspecified fibula

S82.45 Comminuted fracture of shaft of fibula

S82.451- Displaced comminuted fracture of shaft of right fibula

S82.452- Displaced comminuted fracture of shaft of left fibula

S82.453- Displaced comminuted fracture of shaft of unspecified fibula

S82.454- Nondisplaced comminuted fracture of shaft of right fibula

S82.455- Nondisplaced comminuted fracture of shaft of left fibula

S82.456- Nondisplaced comminuted fracture of shaft of unspecified fibula

S82.46 Segmental fracture of shaft of fibula

S82.461- Displaced segmental fracture of shaft of right fibula

S82.462- Displaced segmental fracture of shaft of left fibula

S82.463- Displaced segmental fracture of shaft of unspecified fibula

S82.464- Nondisplaced segmental fracture of shaft of right fibula

S82.465- Nondisplaced segmental fracture of shaft of left fibula

S82.466- Nondisplaced segmental fracture of shaft of unspecified fibula

S82.49 Other fracture of shaft of fibula

S82.491- Other fracture of shaft of right fibula

S82.492- Other fracture of shaft of left fibula

S82.499- Other fracture of shaft of unspecified fibula

S82.5 Fracture of medial malleolus

EXCLUDES 1 *pilon fracture of distal tibia (S82.87-)*
Salter-Harris type III of lower end of tibia (S89.13-)
Salter-Harris type IV of lower end of tibia (S89.14-)

S82.51X- Displaced fracture of medial malleolus of right tibia

S82.52X- Displaced fracture of medial malleolus of left tibia

S82.53X- Displaced fracture of medial malleolus of unspecified tibia

S82.54X- Nondisplaced fracture of medial malleolus of right tibia

S82.55X- Nondisplaced fracture of medial malleolus of left tibia

S82.56X- Nondisplaced fracture of medial malleolus of unspecified tibia

S82.6 Fracture of lateral malleolus

EXCLUDES 1 *pilon fracture of distal tibia (S82.87-)*

S82.61X- Displaced fracture of lateral malleolus of right fibula

S82.62X- Displaced fracture of lateral malleolus of left fibula

S82.63X- Displaced fracture of lateral malleolus of unspecified fibula

S82.64X- Nondisplaced fracture of lateral malleolus of right fibula

S82.65X- Nondisplaced fracture of lateral malleolus of left fibula

S82.66X- Nondisplaced fracture of lateral malleolus of unspecified fibula

S82.8 Other fractures of lower leg

S82.81 Torus fracture of upper end of fibula

The appropriate 7th character is to be added to all codes in subcategory S82.81

A	initial encounter for closed fracture
D	subsequent encounter for fracture with routine healing
G	subsequent encounter for fracture with delayed healing
K	subsequent encounter for fracture with nonunion
P	subsequent encounter for fracture with malunion
S	sequela

CODING TIP✓ Open fractures do not occur with torus fractures and greenstick fractures, therefore the 7th characters for open fractures are not available.

S82.811- Torus fracture of upper end of right fibula

S82.812- Torus fracture of upper end of left fibula

S82.819- Torus fracture of upper end of unspecified fibula

S82.82 Torus fracture of lower end of fibula

The appropriate 7th character is to be added to all codes in subcategory S82.82

A	initial encounter for closed fracture
D	subsequent encounter for fracture with routine healing
G	subsequent encounter for fracture with delayed healing
K	subsequent encounter for fracture with nonunion
P	subsequent encounter for fracture with malunion
S	sequela

CODING TIP✓ Open fractures do not occur with torus fractures and greenstick fractures, therefore the 7th characters for open fractures are not available.

S82.821- Torus fracture of lower end of right fibula

S82.822- Torus fracture of lower end of left fibula

S82.829- Torus fracture of lower end of unspecified fibula

S82.83 Other fracture of upper and lower end of fibula

S82.831- Other fracture of upper and lower end of right fibula

S82.832- Other fracture of upper and lower end of left fibula
AHA: 1Q 2015, 25

S82.839- Other fracture of upper and lower end of unspecified fibula

S82.84 Bimalleolar fracture of lower leg

S82.841- Displaced bimalleolar fracture of right lower leg

S82.842- Displaced bimalleolar fracture of left lower leg

S82.843- Displaced bimalleolar fracture of unspecified lower leg

S82.844- Nondisplaced bimalleolar fracture of right lower leg

S82.845- Nondisplaced bimalleolar fracture of left lower leg

S82.846- Nondisplaced bimalleolar fracture of unspecified lower leg

S82.85 Trimalleolar fracture of lower leg

S82.851- Displaced trimalleolar fracture of right lower leg

S82.852- Displaced trimalleolar fracture of left lower leg

S82.853- Displaced trimalleolar fracture of unspecified lower leg

S82.854- Nondisplaced trimalleolar fracture of right lower leg

S82.855- Nondisplaced trimalleolar fracture of left lower leg

S82.856- Nondisplaced trimalleolar fracture of unspecified lower leg

S82.86 Maisonneuve's fracture

7 ⊟ S82.861 Displaced Maisonneuve's fracture of right leg
7 ⊟ S82.862- Displaced Maisonneuve's fracture of left leg
7 ⊟ S82.863- Displaced Maisonneuve's fracture of unspecified leg
7 ⊟ S82.864- Nondisplaced Maisonneuve's fracture of right leg
7 ⊟ S82.865- Nondisplaced Maisonneuve's fracture of left leg
7 ⊟ S82.866- Nondisplaced Maisonneuve's fracture of unspecified leg

6 S82.87 Pilon fracture of tibia
7 ⊟ S82.871- Displaced pilon fracture of right tibia
7 ⊟ S82.872- Displaced pilon fracture of left tibia
7 ⊟ S82.873- Displaced pilon fracture of unspecified tibia
7 ⊟ S82.874- Nondisplaced pilon fracture of right tibia
7 ⊟ S82.875- Nondisplaced pilon fracture of left tibia
7 ⊟ S82.876- Nondisplaced pilon fracture of unspecified tibia

6 S82.89 Other fractures of lower leg
Fracture of ankle NOS
7 ⊟ S82.891- Other fracture of right lower leg
7 ⊟ S82.892- Other fracture of left lower leg
7 ⊟ S82.899- Other fracture of unspecified lower leg

5 S82.9 Unspecified fracture of lower leg
7 ⊟ S82.90X- Unspecified fracture of unspecified lower leg
7 ⊟ S82.91X- Unspecified fracture of right lower leg
7 ⊟ S82.92X- Unspecified fracture of left lower leg

4 S83 Dislocation and sprain of joints and ligaments of knee

INCLUDES avulsion of joint or ligament of knee
laceration of cartilage, joint or ligament of knee
sprain of cartilage, joint or ligament of knee
traumatic hemarthrosis of joint or ligament of knee
traumatic rupture of joint or ligament of knee
traumatic subluxation of joint or ligament of knee
traumatic tear of joint or ligament of knee

Code also:
any associated open wound

EXCLUDES 1 *derangement of patella (M22.0-M22.3)*
injury of patellar ligament (tendon) (S76.1-)
internal derangement of knee (M23.-)
old dislocation of knee (M24.36)
pathological dislocation of knee (M24.36)
recurrent dislocation of knee (M22.0)

EXCLUDES 2 *strain of muscle, fascia and tendon of lower leg (S86.-)*

The appropriate 7th character is to be added to each code from category S83
A initial encounter
D subsequent encounter
S sequela

CODING TIP ✓ There are no codes for open dislocations. When a dislocation is documented as open, assign an additional code for the open wound.

5 S83.0 Subluxation and dislocation of patella
6 S83.00 Unspecified subluxation and dislocation of patella
7 ⊟ S83.001- Unspecified subluxation of right patella
7 ⊟ S83.002- Unspecified subluxation of left patella
7 ⊟ S83.003- Unspecified subluxation of unspecified patella
7 ⊟ S83.004- Unspecified dislocation of right patella
7 ⊟ S83.005- Unspecified dislocation of left patella
7 ⊟ S83.006- Unspecified dislocation of unspecified patella

6 S83.01 Lateral subluxation and dislocation of patella
7 ⊟ S83.011- Lateral subluxation of right patella
7 ⊟ S83.012- Lateral subluxation of left patella
7 ⊟ S83.013- Lateral subluxation of unspecified patella
7 ⊟ S83.014- Lateral dislocation of right patella
7 ⊟ S83.015- Lateral dislocation of left patella
7 ⊟ S83.016- Lateral dislocation of unspecified patella

6 S83.09 Other subluxation and dislocation of patella
7 ⊟ S83.091- Other subluxation of right patella
7 ⊟ S83.092- Other subluxation of left patella
7 ⊟ S83.093- Other subluxation of unspecified patella
7 ⊟ S83.094- Other dislocation of right patella
7 ⊟ S83.095- Other dislocation of left patella
7 ⊟ S83.096- Other dislocation of unspecified patella

Dislocation of knee

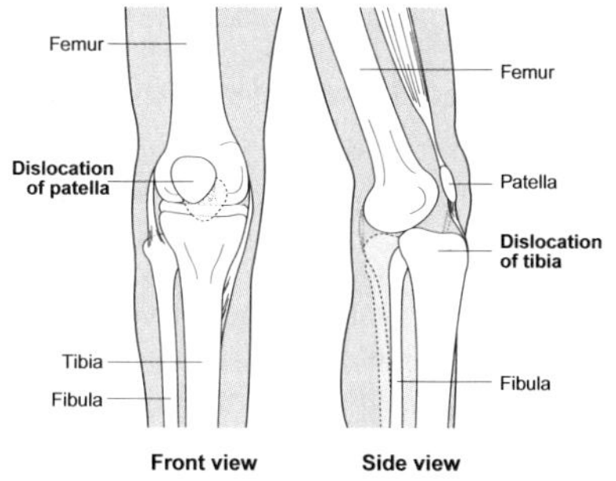

5 S83.1 Subluxation and dislocation of knee
EXCLUDES 2 *instability of knee prosthesis (T84.022, T84.023)*

6 S83.10 Unspecified subluxation and dislocation of knee
7 ⊟ S83.101- Unspecified subluxation of right knee
7 ⊟ S83.102- Unspecified subluxation of left knee
7 ⊟ S83.103- Unspecified subluxation of unspecified knee
7 ⊟ S83.104- Unspecified dislocation of right knee
7 ⊟ S83.105- Unspecified dislocation of left knee
7 ⊟ S83.106- Unspecified dislocation of unspecified knee

6 S83.11 Anterior subluxation and dislocation of proximal end of tibia
Posterior subluxation and dislocation of distal end of femur
7 ⊟ S83.111- Anterior subluxation of proximal end of tibia, right knee
7 ⊟ S83.112- Anterior subluxation of proximal end of tibia, left knee
7 ⊟ S83.113- Anterior subluxation of proximal end of tibia, unspecified knee
7 ⊟ S83.114- Anterior dislocation of proximal end of tibia, right knee
7 ⊟ S83.115- Anterior dislocation of proximal end of tibia, left knee
7 ⊟ S83.116- Anterior dislocation of proximal end of tibia, unspecified knee

6 S83.12 Posterior subluxation and dislocation of proximal end of tibia
Anterior dislocation of distal end of femur
7 ⊟ S83.121- Posterior subluxation of proximal end of tibia, right knee
7 ⊟ S83.122- Posterior subluxation of proximal end of tibia, left knee
7 ⊟ S83.123- Posterior subluxation of proximal end of tibia, unspecified knee
7 ⊟ S83.124- Posterior dislocation of proximal end of tibia, right knee
7 ⊟ S83.125- Posterior dislocation of proximal end of tibia, left knee
7 ⊟ S83.126- Posterior dislocation of proximal end of tibia, unspecified knee

6 S83.13 Medial subluxation and dislocation of proximal end of tibia
7 ⊟ S83.131- Medial subluxation of proximal end of tibia, right knee
7 ⊟ S83.132- Medial subluxation of proximal end of tibia, left knee
7 ⊟ S83.133- Medial subluxation of proximal end of tibia, unspecified knee
7 ⊟ S83.134- Medial dislocation of proximal end of tibia, right knee
7 ⊟ S83.135- Medial dislocation of proximal end of tibia, left knee
7 ⊟ S83.136- Medial dislocation of proximal end of tibia, unspecified knee

6 S83.14 Lateral subluxation and dislocation of proximal end of tibia
- 7 S83.141- Lateral subluxation of proximal end of tibia, right knee
- 7 S83.142- Lateral subluxation of proximal end of tibia, left knee
- 7 S83.143- Lateral subluxation of proximal end of tibia, unspecified knee
- 7 S83.144- Lateral dislocation of proximal end of tibia, right knee
- 7 S83.145- Lateral dislocation of proximal end of tibia, left knee
- 7 S83.146- Lateral dislocation of proximal end of tibia, unspecified knee

6 S83.19 Other subluxation and dislocation of knee
- 7 S83.191- Other subluxation of right knee
- 7 S83.192- Other subluxation of left knee
- 7 S83.193- Other subluxation of unspecified knee
- 7 S83.194- Other dislocation of right knee
- 7 S83.195- Other dislocation of left knee
- 7 S83.196- Other dislocation of unspecified knee

5 S83.2 Tear of meniscus, current injury

EXCLUDES 1 *old bucket-handle tear (M23.2)*

CODING TIP✓ When a meniscus tear is unspecified as to acute or chronic, query the provider. Otherwise, report the default code from S83.2-.

6 S83.20 Tear of unspecified meniscus, current injury

Tear of meniscus of knee NOS
- 7 S83.200- Bucket-handle tear of unspecified meniscus, current injury, right knee
- 7 S83.201- Bucket-handle tear of unspecified meniscus, current injury, left knee
- 7 S83.202- Bucket-handle tear of unspecified meniscus, current injury, unspecified knee
- 7 S83.203- Other tear of unspecified meniscus, current injury, right knee
- 7 S83.204- Other tear of unspecified meniscus, current injury, left knee
- 7 S83.205- Other tear of unspecified meniscus, current injury, unspecified knee
- 7 S83.206- Unspecified tear of Unspecified meniscus, current injury, right knee
- 7 S83.207- Unspecified tear of Unspecified meniscus, current injury, left knee
- 7 S83.209- Unspecified tear of Unspecified meniscus, current injury, Unspecified knee

6 S83.21 Bucket-handle tear of medial meniscus, current injury
- 7 S83.211- Bucket-handle tear of medial meniscus, current injury, right knee
- 7 S83.212- Bucket-handle tear of medial meniscus, current injury, left knee
- 7 S83.219- Bucket-handle tear of medial meniscus, current injury, unspecified knee

6 S83.22 Peripheral tear of medial meniscus, current injury
- 7 S83.221- Peripheral tear of medial meniscus, current injury, right knee
- 7 S83.222- Peripheral tear of medial meniscus, current injury, left knee
- 7 S83.229- Peripheral tear of medial meniscus, current injury, unspecified knee

6 S83.23 Complex tear of medial meniscus, current injury
- 7 S83.231- Complex tear of medial meniscus, current injury, right knee
- 7 S83.232- Complex tear of medial meniscus, current injury, left knee
- 7 S83.239- Complex tear of medial meniscus, current injury, unspecified knee

6 S83.24 Other tear of medial meniscus, current injury
- 7 S83.241- Other tear of medial meniscus, current injury, right knee
- 7 S83.242- Other tear of medial meniscus, current injury, left knee
- 7 S83.249- Other tear of medial meniscus, current injury, unspecified knee

6 S83.25 Bucket-handle tear of lateral meniscus, current injury
- 7 S83.251- Bucket-handle tear of lateral meniscus, current injury, right knee
- 7 S83.252- Bucket-handle tear of lateral meniscus, current injury, left knee
- 7 S83.259- Bucket-handle tear of lateral meniscus, current injury, unspecified knee

6 S83.26 Peripheral tear of lateral meniscus, current injury
- 7 S83.261- Peripheral tear of lateral meniscus, current injury, right knee
- 7 S83.262- Peripheral tear of lateral meniscus, current injury, left knee
- 7 S83.269- Peripheral tear of lateral meniscus, current injury, unspecified knee

6 S83.27 Complex tear of lateral meniscus, current injury
- 7 S83.271- Complex tear of lateral meniscus, current injury, right knee
- 7 S83.272- Complex tear of lateral meniscus, current injury, left knee
- 7 S83.279- Complex tear of lateral meniscus, current injury, unspecified knee

6 S83.28 Other tear of lateral meniscus, current injury
- 7 S83.281- Other tear of lateral meniscus, current injury, right knee
- 7 S83.282- Other tear of lateral meniscus, current injury, left knee
- 7 S83.289- Other tear of lateral meniscus, current injury, unspecified knee

5 S83.3 Tear of articular cartilage of knee, current
- 7 S83.30X- Tear of articular cartilage of unspecified knee, current
- 7 S83.31X- Tear of articular cartilage of right knee, current
- 7 S83.32X- Tear of articular cartilage of left knee, current

5 S83.4 Sprain of collateral ligament of knee

6 S83.40 Sprain of unspecified collateral ligament of knee
- 7 S83.401- Sprain of unspecified collateral ligament of right knee
- 7 S83.402- Sprain of unspecified collateral ligament of left knee
- 7 S83.409- Sprain of unspecified collateral ligament of unspecified knee

6 S83.41 Sprain of medial collateral ligament of knee

Sprain of tibial collateral ligament
- 7 S83.411- Sprain of medial collateral ligament of right knee
- 7 S83.412- Sprain of medial collateral ligament of left knee
- 7 S83.419- Sprain of medial collateral ligament of unspecified knee

6 S83.42 Sprain of lateral collateral ligament of knee

Sprain of fibular collateral ligament
- 7 S83.421- Sprain of lateral collateral ligament of right knee
- 7 S83.422- Sprain of lateral collateral ligament of left knee
- 7 S83.429- Sprain of lateral collateral ligament of unspecified knee

5 S83.5 Sprain of cruciate ligament of knee

6 S83.50 Sprain of unspecified cruciate ligament of knee
- 7 S83.501- Sprain of unspecified cruciate ligament of right knee
- 7 S83.502- Sprain of unspecified cruciate ligament of left knee
- 7 S83.509- Sprain of unspecified cruciate ligament of unspecified knee

6 S83.51 Sprain of anterior cruciate ligament of knee
- 7 S83.511- Sprain of anterior cruciate ligament of right knee
  AHA: (S83.511D) 2Q 2016, 3
- 7 S83.512- Sprain of anterior cruciate ligament of left knee
- 7 S83.519- Sprain of anterior cruciate ligament of unspecified knee

6 S83.52 Sprain of posterior cruciate ligament of knee

- 7 ⊟ S83.521- Sprain of posterior cruciate ligament of right knee
- 7 ⊟ S83.522- Sprain of posterior cruciate ligament of left knee
- 7 ⊟ S83.529- Sprain of posterior cruciate ligament of unspecified knee

5 S83.6 Sprain of the superior tibiofibular joint and ligament
- 7 ⊟ S83.60X- Sprain of the superior tibiofibular joint and ligament, unspecified knee
- 7 ⊟ S83.61X- Sprain of the superior tibiofibular joint and ligament, right knee
- 7 ⊟ S83.62X- Sprain of the superior tibiofibular joint and ligament, left knee

5 S83.8 Sprain of other specified parts of knee

6 S83.8X Sprain of other specified parts of knee
- 7 ⊟ S83.8X1- Sprain of other specified parts of right knee
- 7 ⊟ S83.8X2- Sprain of other specified parts of left knee
- 7 ⊟ S83.8X9- Sprain of other specified parts of unspecified knee

5 S83.9 Sprain of unspecified site of knee
- 7 ⊟ S83.90X- Sprain of unspecified site of unspecified knee
- 7 ⊟ S83.91X- Sprain of unspecified site of right knee
- 7 ⊟ S83.92X- Sprain of unspecified site of left knee

4 S84 Injury of nerves at lower leg level

Code also:

any associated open wound (S81.-)

EXCLUDES 2 *injury of nerves at ankle and foot level (S94.-)*

The appropriate 7th character is to be added to each code from category S84
- A initial encounter
- D subsequent encounter
- S sequela

CODING TIP ✓ Late effects of injuries are coded with seventh character S (sequela) and are sequenced after the residual condition of the late effect.

5 S84.0 Injury of tibial nerve at lower leg level
- 7 ⊟ S84.00X- Injury of tibial nerve at lower leg level, unspecified leg
- 7 ⊟ S84.01X- Injury of tibial nerve at lower leg level, right leg
- 7 ⊟ S84.02X- Injury of tibial nerve at lower leg level, left leg

5 S84.1 Injury of peroneal nerve at lower leg level
- 7 ⊟ S84.10X- Injury of peroneal nerve at lower leg level, unspecified leg
- 7 ⊟ S84.11X- Injury of peroneal nerve at lower leg level, right leg
- 7 ⊟ S84.12X- Injury of peroneal nerve at lower leg level, left leg

5 S84.2 Injury of cutaneous sensory nerve at lower leg level
- 7 ⊟ S84.20X- Injury of cutaneous sensory nerve at lower leg level, unspecified leg
- 7 ⊟ S84.21X- Injury of cutaneous sensory nerve at lower leg level, right leg
- 7 ⊟ S84.22X- Injury of cutaneous sensory nerve at lower leg level, left leg

5 S84.8 Injury of other nerves at lower leg level

6 S84.80 Injury of other nerves at lower leg level
- 7 ⊟ S84.801- Injury of other nerves at lower leg level, right leg
- 7 ⊟ S84.802- Injury of other nerves at lower leg level, left leg
- 7 ⊟ S84.809- Injury of other nerves at lower leg level, unspecified leg

5 S84.9 Injury of unspecified nerve at lower leg level
- 7 ⊟ S84.90X- Injury of unspecified nerve at lower leg level, unspecified leg
- 7 ⊟ S84.91X- Injury of unspecified nerve at lower leg level, right leg
- 7 ⊟ S84.92X- Injury of unspecified nerve at lower leg level, left leg

4 S85 Injury of blood vessels at lower leg level

Code also:

any associated open wound (S81.-)

EXCLUDES 2 *injury of blood vessels at ankle and foot level (S95.-)*

The appropriate 7th character is to be added to each code from category S85
- A initial encounter
- D subsequent encounter
- S sequela

5 S85.0 Injury of popliteal artery

6 S85.00 Unspecified injury of popliteal artery
- 7 ⊟ S85.001- Unspecified injury of popliteal artery, right leg
- 7 ⊟ S85.002- Unspecified injury of popliteal artery, left leg
- 7 ⊟ S85.009- Unspecified injury of popliteal artery, unspecified leg

6 S85.01 Laceration of popliteal artery
- 7 ⊟ S85.011- Laceration of popliteal artery, right leg
- 7 ⊟ S85.012- Laceration of popliteal artery, left leg
- 7 ⊟ S85.019- Laceration of popliteal artery, unspecified leg

6 S85.09 Other specified injury of popliteal artery
- 7 ⊟ S85.091- Other specified injury of popliteal artery, right leg
- 7 ⊟ S85.092- Other specified injury of popliteal artery, left leg
- 7 ⊟ S85.099- Other specified injury of popliteal artery, unspecified leg

5 S85.1 Injury of tibial artery

6 S85.10 Unspecified injury of Unspecified tibial artery

Injury of tibial artery NOS
- 7 ⊟ S85.101- Unspecified injury of unspecified tibial artery, right leg
- 7 ⊟ S85.102- Unspecified injury of unspecified tibial artery, left leg
- 7 ⊟ S85.109- Unspecified injury of unspecified tibial artery, unspecified leg

6 S85.11 Laceration of unspecified tibial artery
- 7 ⊟ S85.111- Laceration of unspecified tibial artery, right leg
- 7 ⊟ S85.112- Laceration of unspecified tibial artery, left leg
- 7 ⊟ S85.119- Laceration of unspecified tibial artery, unspecified leg

6 S85.12 Other specified injury of unspecified tibial artery
- 7 ⊟ S85.121- Other specified injury of unspecified tibial artery, right leg
- 7 ⊟ S85.122- Other specified injury of unspecified tibial artery, left leg
- 7 ⊟ S85.129- Other specified injury of unspecified tibial artery, unspecified leg

6 S85.13 Unspecified injury of anterior tibial artery
- 7 ⊟ S85.131- Unspecified injury of anterior tibial artery, right leg
- 7 ⊟ S85.132- Unspecified injury of anterior tibial artery, left leg
- 7 ⊟ S85.139- Unspecified injury of anterior tibial artery, unspecified leg

6 S85.14 Laceration of anterior tibial artery
- 7 ⊟ S85.141- Laceration of anterior tibial artery, right leg
- 7 ⊟ S85.142- Laceration of anterior tibial artery, left leg
- 7 ⊟ S85.149- Laceration of anterior tibial artery, unspecified leg

6 S85.15 Other specified injury of anterior tibial artery
- 7 ⊟ S85.151- Other specified injury of anterior tibial artery, right leg
- 7 ⊟ S85.152- Other specified injury of anterior tibial artery, left leg
- 7 ⊟ S85.159- Other specified injury of anterior tibial artery, unspecified leg

6 S85.16 Unspecified injury of posterior tibial artery
- 7 ⊟ S85.161- Unspecified injury of posterior tibial artery, right leg
- 7 ⊟ S85.162- Unspecified injury of posterior tibial artery, left leg

7 ⊟ S85.169- Unspecified injury of posterior tibial artery, unspecified leg
6 S85.17 Laceration of posterior tibial artery
7 ⊟ S85.171- Laceration of posterior tibial artery, right leg
7 ⊟ S85.172- Laceration of posterior tibial artery, left leg
7 ⊟ S85.179- Laceration of posterior tibial artery, unspecified leg
6 S85.18 Other specified injury of posterior tibial artery
7 ⊟ S85.181- Other specified injury of posterior tibial artery, right leg
7 ⊟ S85.182- Other specified injury of posterior tibial artery, left leg
7 ⊟ S85.189- Other specified injury of posterior tibial artery, unspecified leg

5 S85.2 Injury of peroneal artery
6 S85.20 Unspecified injury of peroneal artery
7 ⊟ S85.201- Unspecified injury of peroneal artery, right leg
7 ⊟ S85.202- Unspecified injury of peroneal artery, left leg
7 ⊟ S85.209- Unspecified injury of peroneal artery, unspecified leg
6 S85.21 Laceration of peroneal artery
7 ⊟ S85.211- Laceration of peroneal artery, right leg
7 ⊟ S85.212- Laceration of peroneal artery, left leg
7 ⊟ S85.219- Laceration of peroneal artery, unspecified leg
6 S85.29 Other specified injury of peroneal artery
7 ⊟ S85.291- Other specified injury of peroneal artery, right leg
7 ⊟ S85.292- Other specified injury of peroneal artery, left leg
7 ⊟ S85.299- Other specified injury of peroneal artery, unspecified leg

5 S85.3 Injury of greater saphenous vein at lower leg level
Injury of greater saphenous vein NOS
Injury of saphenous vein NOS
6 S85.30 Unspecified injury of greater saphenous vein at lower leg level
7 ⊟ S85.301- Unspecified injury of greater saphenous vein at lower leg level, right leg
7 ⊟ S85.302- Unspecified injury of greater saphenous vein at lower leg level, left leg
7 ⊟ S85.309- Unspecified injury of greater saphenous vein at lower leg level, unspecified leg
6 S85.31 Laceration of greater saphenous vein at lower leg level
7 ⊟ S85.311- Laceration of greater saphenous vein at lower leg level, right leg
7 ⊟ S85.312- Laceration of greater saphenous vein at lower leg level, left leg
7 ⊟ S85.319- Laceration of greater saphenous vein at lower leg level, unspecified leg
6 S85.39 Other specified injury of greater saphenous vein at lower leg level
7 ⊟ S85.391- Other specified injury of greater saphenous vein at lower leg level, right leg
7 ⊟ S85.392- Other specified injury of greater saphenous vein at lower leg level, left leg
7 ⊟ S85.399- Other specified injury of greater saphenous vein at lower leg level, unspecified leg

5 S85.4 Injury of lesser saphenous vein at lower leg level
6 S85.40 Unspecified injury of lesser saphenous vein at lower leg level
7 ⊟ S85.401- Unspecified injury of lesser saphenous vein at lower leg level, right leg
7 ⊟ S85.402- Unspecified injury of lesser saphenous vein at lower leg level, left leg
7 ⊟ S85.409- Unspecified injury of lesser saphenous vein at lower leg level, unspecified leg
6 S85.41 Laceration of lesser saphenous vein at lower leg level
7 ⊟ S85.411- Laceration of lesser saphenous vein at lower leg level, right leg
7 ⊟ S85.412- Laceration of lesser saphenous vein at lower leg level, left leg
7 ⊟ S85.419- Laceration of lesser saphenous vein at lower leg level, unspecified leg
6 S85.49 Other specified injury of lesser saphenous vein at lower leg level
7 ⊟ S85.491- Other specified injury of lesser saphenous vein at lower leg level, right leg
7 ⊟ S85.492- Other specified injury of lesser saphenous vein at lower leg level, left leg
7 ⊟ S85.499- Other specified injury of lesser saphenous vein at lower leg level, unspecified leg

5 S85.5 Injury of popliteal vein
6 S85.50 Unspecified injury of popliteal vein
7 ⊟ S85.501- Unspecified injury of popliteal vein, right leg
7 ⊟ S85.502- Unspecified injury of popliteal vein, left leg
7 ⊟ S85.509- Unspecified injury of popliteal vein, unspecified leg
6 S85.51 Laceration of popliteal vein
7 ⊟ S85.511- Laceration of popliteal vein, right leg
7 ⊟ S85.512- Laceration of popliteal vein, left leg
7 ⊟ S85.519- Laceration of popliteal vein, unspecified leg
6 S85.59 Other specified injury of popliteal vein
7 ⊟ S85.591- Other specified injury of popliteal vein, right leg
7 ⊟ S85.592- Other specified injury of popliteal vein, left leg
7 ⊟ S85.599- Other specified injury of popliteal vein, unspecified leg

5 S85.8 Injury of other blood vessels at lower leg level
6 S85.80 Unspecified injury of other blood vessels at lower leg level
7 ⊟ S85.801- Unspecified injury of other blood vessels at lower leg level, right leg
7 ⊟ S85.802- Unspecified injury of other blood vessels at lower leg level, left leg
7 ⊟ S85.809- Unspecified injury of other blood vessels at lower leg level, unspecified leg
6 S85.81 Laceration of other blood vessels at lower leg level
7 ⊟ S85.811- Laceration of other blood vessels at lower leg level, right leg
7 ⊟ S85.812- Laceration of other blood vessels at lower leg level, left leg
7 ⊟ S85.819- Laceration of other blood vessels at lower leg level, unspecified leg
6 S85.89 Other specified injury of other blood vessels at lower leg level
7 ⊟ S85.891- Other specified injury of other blood vessels at lower leg level, right leg
7 ⊟ S85.892- Other specified injury of other blood vessels at lower leg level, left leg
7 ⊟ S85.899- Other specified injury of other blood vessels at lower leg level, unspecified leg

5 S85.9 Injury of unspecified blood vessel at lower leg level
6 S85.90 Unspecified injury of Unspecified blood vessel at lower leg level
7 ⊟ S85.901- Unspecified injury of unspecified blood vessel at lower leg level, right leg
7 ⊟ S85.902- Unspecified injury of unspecified blood vessel at lower leg level, left leg
7 ⊟ S85.909- Unspecified injury of unspecified blood vessel at lower leg level, unspecified leg
6 S85.91 Laceration of unspecified blood vessel at lower leg level
7 ⊟ S85.911- Laceration of unspecified blood vessel at lower leg level, right leg
7 ⊟ S85.912- Laceration of unspecified blood vessel at lower leg level, left leg
7 ⊟ S85.919- Laceration of unspecified blood vessel at lower leg level, unspecified leg
6 S85.99 Other specified injury of unspecified blood vessel at lower leg level
7 ⊟ S85.991- Other specified injury of unspecified blood vessel at lower leg level, right leg
7 ⊟ S85.992- Other specified injury of unspecified blood vessel at lower leg level, left leg
7 ⊟ S85.999- Other specified injury of unspecified blood vessel at lower leg level, unspecified leg

4 S86 Injury of muscle, fascia and tendon at lower leg level

Code also:
any associated open wound (S81.-)

EXCLUDES 2 *injury of muscle, fascia and tendon at ankle (S96.-)*
injury of patellar ligament (tendon) (S76.1-)
sprain of joints and ligaments of knee (S83.-)

The appropriate 7th character is to be added to each code from category S86

A initial encounter
D subsequent encounter
S sequela

5 S86.0 Injury of Achilles tendon

6 S86.00 Unspecified injury of Achilles tendon

7 S86.001- Unspecified injury of right Achilles tendon

7 S86.002- Unspecified injury of left Achilles tendon

7 S86.009- Unspecified injury of unspecified Achilles tendon

6 S86.01 Strain of Achilles tendon

7 S86.011- Strain of right Achilles tendon

7 S86.012- Strain of left Achilles tendon

7 S86.019- Strain of unspecified Achilles tendon

6 S86.02 Laceration of Achilles tendon

7 S86.021- Laceration of right Achilles tendon

7 S86.022- Laceration of left Achilles tendon

7 S86.029- Laceration of unspecified Achilles tendon

6 S86.09 Other specified injury of Achilles tendon

7 S86.091- Other specified injury of right Achilles tendon

7 S86.092- Other specified injury of left Achilles tendon

7 S86.099- Other specified injury of unspecified Achilles tendon

5 S86.1 Injury of other muscle(s) and tendon(s) of posterior muscle group at lower leg level

6 S86.10 Unspecified injury of other muscle(s) and tendon(s) of posterior muscle group at lower leg level

7 S86.101- Unspecified injury of other muscle(s) and tendon(s) of posterior muscle group at lower leg level, right leg

7 S86.102- Unspecified injury of other muscle(s) and tendon(s) of posterior muscle group at lower leg level, left leg

7 S86.109- Unspecified injury of other muscle(s) and tendon(s) of posterior muscle group at lower leg level, unspecified leg

6 S86.11 Strain of other muscle(s) and tendon(s) of posterior muscle group at lower leg level

7 S86.111- Strain of other muscle(s) and tendon(s) of posterior muscle group at lower leg level, right leg

7 S86.112- Strain of other muscle(s) and tendon(s) of posterior muscle group at lower leg level, left leg

7 S86.119- Strain of other muscle(s) and tendon(s) of posterior muscle group at lower leg level, unspecified leg

6 S86.12 Laceration of other muscle(s) and tendon(s) of posterior muscle group at lower leg level

7 S86.121- Laceration of other muscle(s) and tendon(s) of posterior muscle group at lower leg level, right leg

7 S86.122- Laceration of other muscle(s) and tendon(s) of posterior muscle group at lower leg level, left leg

7 S86.129- Laceration of other muscle(s) and tendon(s) of posterior muscle group at lower leg level, unspecified leg

6 S86.19 Other injury of Other muscle(s) and tendon(s) of posterior muscle group at lower leg level

7 S86.191- Other injury of other muscle(s) and tendon(s) of posterior muscle group at lower leg level, right leg

7 S86.192- Other injury of other muscle(s) and tendon(s) of posterior muscle group at lower leg level, left leg

7 S86.199- Other injury of other muscle(s) and tendon(s) of posterior muscle group at lower leg level, unspecified leg

5 S86.2 Injury of muscle(s) and tendon(s) of anterior muscle group at lower leg level

6 S86.20 Unspecified injury of muscle(s) and tendon(s) of anterior muscle group at lower leg level

7 S86.201- Unspecified injury of muscle(s) and tendon(s) of anterior muscle group at lower leg level, right leg

7 S86.202- Unspecified injury of muscle(s) and tendon(s) of anterior muscle group at lower leg level, left leg

7 S86.209- Unspecified injury of muscle(s) and tendon(s) of anterior muscle group at lower leg level, unspecified leg

6 S86.21 Strain of muscle(s) and tendon(s) of anterior muscle group at lower leg level

7 S86.211- Strain of muscle(s) and tendon(s) of anterior muscle group at lower leg level, right leg

7 S86.212- Strain of muscle(s) and tendon(s) of anterior muscle group at lower leg level, left leg

7 S86.219- Strain of muscle(s) and tendon(s) of anterior muscle group at lower leg level, unspecified leg

6 S86.22 Laceration of muscle(s) and tendon(s) of anterior muscle group at lower leg level

7 S86.221- Laceration of muscle(s) and tendon(s) of anterior muscle group at lower leg level, right leg

7 S86.222- Laceration of muscle(s) and tendon(s) of anterior muscle group at lower leg level, left leg

7 S86.229- Laceration of muscle(s) and tendon(s) of anterior muscle group at lower leg level, unspecified leg

6 S86.29 Other injury of muscle(s) and tendon(s) of anterior muscle group at lower leg level

7 S86.291- Other injury of muscle(s) and tendon(s) of anterior muscle group at lower leg level, right leg

7 S86.292- Other injury of muscle(s) and tendon(s) of anterior muscle group at lower leg level, left leg

7 S86.299- Other injury of muscle(s) and tendon(s) of anterior muscle group at lower leg level, unspecified leg

5 S86.3 Injury of muscle(s) and tendon(s) of peroneal muscle group at lower leg level

6 S86.30 Unspecified injury of muscle(s) and tendon(s) of peroneal muscle group at lower leg level

7 S86.301- Unspecified injury of muscle(s) and tendon(s) of peroneal muscle group at lower leg level, right leg

7 S86.302- Unspecified injury of muscle(s) and tendon(s) of peroneal muscle group at lower leg level, left leg

7 S86.309- Unspecified injury of muscle(s) and tendon(s) of peroneal muscle group at lower leg level, unspecified leg

6 S86.31 Strain of muscle(s) and tendon(s) of peroneal muscle group at lower leg level

7 S86.311- Strain of muscle(s) and tendon(s) of peroneal muscle group at lower leg level, right leg

7 S86.312- Strain of muscle(s) and tendon(s) of peroneal muscle group at lower leg level, left leg

7 S86.319- Strain of muscle(s) and tendon(s) of peroneal muscle group at lower leg level, unspecified leg

6 S86.32 Laceration of muscle(s) and tendon(s) of peroneal muscle group at lower leg level

7 S86.321- Laceration of muscle(s) and tendon(s) of peroneal muscle group at lower leg level, right leg

7 S86.322- Laceration of muscle(s) and tendon(s) of peroneal muscle group at lower leg level, left leg

7 ⊟ S86.329- **Laceration of muscle(s) and tendon(s) of peroneal muscle group at lower leg level, unspecified leg**

6 S86.39 **Other injury of muscle(s) and tendon(s) of peroneal muscle group at lower leg level**

7 ⊟ S86.391- **Other injury of muscle(s) and tendon(s) of peroneal muscle group at lower leg level, right leg**

7 ⊟ S86.392- **Other injury of muscle(s) and tendon(s) of peroneal muscle group at lower leg level, left leg**

7 ⊟ S86.399- **Other injury of muscle(s) and tendon(s) of peroneal muscle group at lower leg level, unspecified leg**

5 S86.8 **Injury of other muscles and tendons at lower leg level**

6 S86.80 **Unspecified injury of other muscles and tendons at lower leg level**

7 ⊟ S86.801- **Unspecified injury of other muscle(s) and tendon(s) at lower leg level, right leg**

7 ⊟ S86.802- **Unspecified injury of other muscle(s) and tendon(s) at lower leg level, left leg**

7 ⊟ S86.809- **Unspecified injury of other muscle(s) and tendon(s) at lower leg level, unspecified leg**

6 S86.81 **Strain of other muscles and tendons at lower leg level**

7 ⊟ S86.811- **Strain of other muscle(s) and tendon(s) at lower leg level, right leg**

7 ⊟ S86.812- **Strain of other muscle(s) and tendon(s) at lower leg level, left leg**

7 ⊟ S86.819- **Strain of other muscle(s) and tendon(s) at lower leg level, unspecified leg**

6 S86.82 **Laceration of other muscles and tendons at lower leg level**

7 ⊟ S86.821- **Laceration of other muscle(s) and tendon(s) at lower leg level, right leg**

7 ⊟ S86.822- **Laceration of other muscle(s) and tendon(s) at lower leg level, left leg**

7 ⊟ S86.829- **Laceration of other muscle(s) and tendon(s) at lower leg level, unspecified leg**

6 S86.89 **Other injury of Other muscles and tendons at lower leg level**

7 ⊟ S86.891- **Other injury of other muscle(s) and tendon(s) at lower leg level, right leg**

7 ⊟ S86.892- **Other injury of other muscle(s) and tendon(s) at lower leg level, left leg**

7 ⊟ S86.899- **Other injury of other muscle(s) and tendon(s) at lower leg level, unspecified leg**

5 S86.9 **Injury of unspecified muscle and tendon at lower leg level**

6 S86.90 **Unspecified injury of Unspecified muscle and tendon at lower leg level**

7 ⊟ S86.901- **Unspecified injury of unspecified muscle(s) and tendon(s) at lower leg level, right leg**

7 ⊟ S86.902- **Unspecified injury of unspecified muscle(s) and tendon(s) at lower leg level, left leg**

7 ⊟ S86.909- **Unspecified injury of unspecified muscle(s) and tendon(s) at lower leg level, unspecified leg**

6 S86.91 **Strain of unspecified muscle and tendon at lower leg level**

7 ⊟ S86.911- **Strain of unspecified muscle(s) and tendon(s) at lower leg level, right leg**

7 ⊟ S86.912- **Strain of unspecified muscle(s) and tendon(s) at lower leg level, left leg**

7 ⊟ S86.919- **Strain of unspecified muscle(s) and tendon(s) at lower leg level, unspecified leg**

6 S86.92 **Laceration of unspecified muscle and tendon at lower leg level**

7 ⊟ S86.921- **Laceration of unspecified muscle(s) and tendon(s) at lower leg level, right leg**

7 ⊟ S86.922- **Laceration of unspecified muscle(s) and tendon(s) at lower leg level, left leg**

7 ⊟ S86.929- **Laceration of unspecified muscle(s) and tendon(s) at lower leg level, unspecified leg**

6 S86.99 **Other injury of unspecified muscle and tendon at lower leg level**

7 ⊟ S86.991- **Other injury of unspecified muscle(s) and tendon(s) at lower leg level, right leg**

7 ⊟ S86.992- **Other injury of unspecified muscle(s) and tendon(s) at lower leg level, left leg**

7 ⊟ S86.999- **Other injury of unspecified muscle(s) and tendon(s) at lower leg level, unspecified leg**

4 S87 Crushing injury of lower leg

Use additional code(s) for all associated injuries

EXCLUDES 2 *crushing injury of ankle and foot (S97.-)*

The appropriate 7th character is to be added to each code from category S87
A initial encounter
D subsequent encounter
S sequela

5 S87.0 **Crushing injury of knee**

7 ⊟ S87.00X- **Crushing injury of unspecified knee**

7 ⊟ S87.01X- **Crushing injury of right knee**

7 ⊟ S87.02X- **Crushing injury of left knee**

5 S87.8 **Crushing injury of lower leg**

7 ⊟ S87.80X- **Crushing injury of unspecified lower leg**

7 ⊟ S87.81X- **Crushing injury of right lower leg**

7 ⊟ S87.82X- **Crushing injury of left lower leg**

4 S88 Traumatic amputation of lower leg

An amputation not identified as partial or complete should be coded to complete

EXCLUDES 1 *traumatic amputation of ankle and foot (S98.-)*

The appropriate 7th character is to be added to each code from category S88
A initial encounter
D subsequent encounter
S sequela

CODING TIP✓ Use these codes only when the amputation was due to trauma. There is no need for adding Z89 with traumatic amputations. See Z47.81 for care of amputations not due to trauma.

CODING TIP✓ Assign only if the amputation is due to accident or violence, i.e., trauma.

5 S88.0 **Traumatic amputation at knee level**

6 S88.01 **Complete traumatic amputation at knee level**

7 ⊟ S88.011- **Complete traumatic amputation at knee level, right lower leg** HCC

7 ⊟ S88.012- **Complete traumatic amputation at knee level, left lower leg** HCC

7 ⊟ S88.019- **Complete traumatic amputation at knee level, unspecified lower leg** HCC

6 S88.02 **Partial traumatic amputation at knee level**

7 ⊟ S88.021- **Partial traumatic amputation at knee level, right lower leg** HCC

7 ⊟ S88.022- **Partial traumatic amputation at knee level, left lower leg** HCC

7 ⊟ S88.029- **Partial traumatic amputation at knee level, unspecified lower leg** HCC

5 S88.1 **Traumatic amputation at level between knee and ankle**

6 S88.11 **Complete traumatic amputation at level between knee and ankle**

7 ⊟ S88.111- **Complete traumatic amputation at level between knee and ankle, right lower leg** HCC

7 ⊟ S88.112- **Complete traumatic amputation at level between knee and ankle, left lower leg** HCC

7 ⊟ S88.119- **Complete traumatic amputation at level between knee and ankle, unspecified lower leg** HCC

6 S88.12 **Partial traumatic amputation at level between knee and ankle**

7 ⊟ S88.121- **Partial traumatic amputation at level between knee and ankle, right lower leg** HCC

7 ⊟ S88.122- **Partial traumatic amputation at level between knee and ankle, left lower leg** HCC

7 ⊟ S88.129- **Partial traumatic amputation at level between knee and ankle, unspecified lower leg** HCC

5 S88.9 **Traumatic amputation of lower leg, level unspecified**

6 S88.91 **Complete traumatic amputation of lower leg, level unspecified**

7 ⊟ S88.911- Complete traumatic amputation of right lower leg, level unspecified HCC

7 ⊟ S88.912- Complete traumatic amputation of left lower leg, level unspecified HCC

7 ⊟ S88.919- Complete traumatic amputation of unspecified lower leg, level unspecified HCC

6 S88.92 Partial traumatic amputation of lower leg, level unspecified

7 ⊟ S88.921- Partial traumatic amputation of right lower leg, level unspecified HCC

7 ⊟ S88.922- Partial traumatic amputation of left lower leg, level unspecified HCC

7 ⊟ S88.929- Partial traumatic amputation of unspecified lower leg, level unspecified HCC

4 S89 Other and unspecified injuries of lower leg

Note: A fracture not indicated as open or closed should be coded to closed

EXCLUDES 2 *other and unspecified injuries of ankle and foot (S99.-)*

The appropriate 7th character is to be added to each code from subcategories S89.0, S89.1, S89.2, and S89.3

A initial encounter for closed fracture
D subsequent encounter for fracture with routine healing
G subsequent encounter for fracture with delayed healing
K subsequent encounter for fracture with nonunion
P subsequent encounter for fracture with malunion
S sequela

CODING TIP✓ A Salter-Harris physeal fracture occurs through the growth plate. Only one code is needed to report a single physeal fracture. Because of the implications for future bone development, coding of a Salter-Harris fracture takes priority over a simple fracture code. Assign the physeal fracture code based on location, type, and laterality. Use a code for "other physeal fracture" for Type V.

CODING TIP✓ A fracture not indicated as open or closed should be coded to closed.

5 S89.0 Physeal fracture of upper end of tibia

6 S89.00 Unspecified physeal fracture of upper end of tibia

7 ⊟ S89.001- Unspecified physeal fracture of upper end of right tibia

7 ⊟ S89.002- Unspecified physeal fracture of upper end of left tibia

7 ⊟ S89.009- Unspecified physeal fracture of upper end of unspecified tibia

6 S89.01 Salter-Harris Type I physeal fracture of upper end of tibia

7 ⊟ S89.011- Salter-Harris Type I physeal fracture of upper end of right tibia

Salter-Harris Type 1 physeal fracture of upper end of right tibia

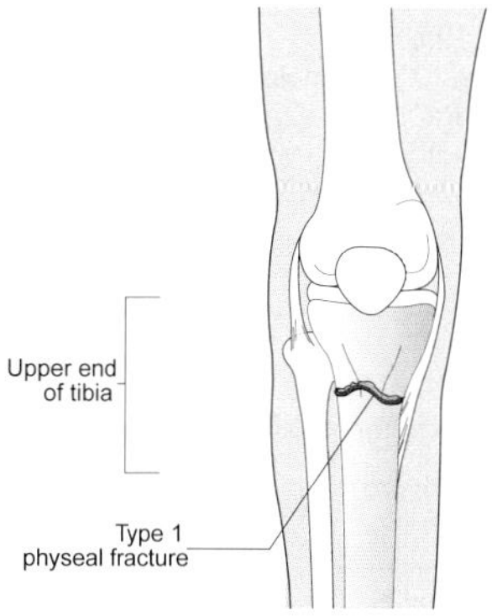

7 ⊟ S89.012- Salter-Harris Type I physeal fracture of upper end of left tibia

7 ⊟ S89.019- Salter-Harris Type I physeal fracture of upper end of unspecified tibia

6 S89.02 Salter-Harris Type II physeal fracture of upper end of tibia

7 ⊟ S89.021- Salter-Harris Type II physeal fracture of upper end of right tibia

7 ⊟ S89.022- Salter-Harris Type II physeal fracture of upper end of left tibia

7 ⊟ S89.029- Salter-Harris Type II physeal fracture of upper end of unspecified tibia

6 S89.03 Salter-Harris Type III physeal fracture of upper end of tibia

7 ⊟ S89.031- Salter-Harris Type III physeal fracture of upper end of right tibia

Salter-Harris Type III physeal fracture of upper end of right tibia

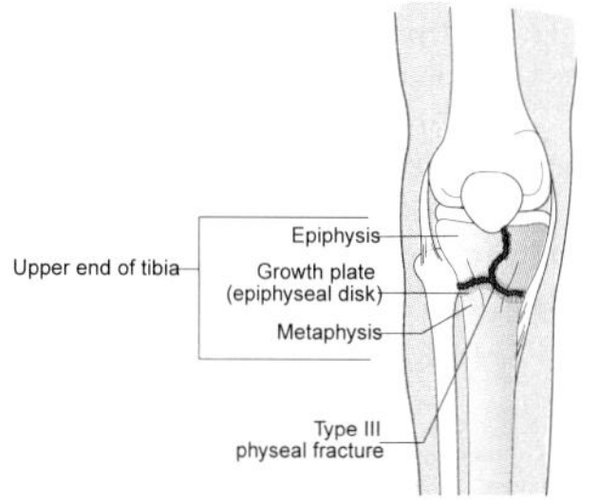

7 ⊟ S89.032- Salter-Harris Type III physeal fracture of upper end of left tibia

7 ⊟ S89.039- Salter-Harris Type III physeal fracture of upper end of unspecified tibia

6 S89.04 Salter-Harris Type IV physeal fracture of upper end of tibia

7 ⊟ S89.041- Salter-Harris Type IV physeal fracture of upper end of right tibia

7 ⊟ S89.042- Salter-Harris Type IV physeal fracture of upper end of left tibia

7 ⊟ S89.049- Salter-Harris Type IV physeal fracture of upper end of unspecified tibia

6 S89.09 Other physeal fracture of upper end of tibia

7 ⊟ S89.091- Other physeal fracture of upper end of right tibia

7 ⊟ S89.092- Other physeal fracture of upper end of left tibia

7 ⊟ S89.099- Other physeal fracture of upper end of unspecified tibia

5 S89.1 Physeal fracture of lower end of tibia

6 S89.10 Unspecified physeal fracture of lower end of tibia

7 ⊟ S89.101- Unspecified physeal fracture of lower end of right tibia

7 ⊟ S89.102- Unspecified physeal fracture of lower end of left tibia

7 ⊟ S89.109- Unspecified physeal fracture of lower end of unspecified tibia

6 S89.11 Salter-Harris Type I physeal fracture of lower end of tibia

7 ⊟ S89.111- Salter-Harris Type I physeal fracture of lower end of right tibia

7 ⊟ S89.112- Salter-Harris Type I physeal fracture of lower end of left tibia

7 ⊟ S89.119- Salter-Harris Type I physeal fracture of lower end of unspecified tibia

6 S89.12 Salter-Harris Type II physeal fracture of lower end of tibia

7 ⊟ S89.121- Salter-Harris Type II physeal fracture of lower end of right tibia

7 ⊟ S89.122- Salter-Harris Type II physeal fracture of lower end of left tibia

7 ⊟ S89.129- Salter-Harris Type II physeal fracture of lower end of unspecified tibia

6 S89.13 Salter-Harris Type III physeal fracture of lower end of tibia

EXCLUDES 1 *fracture of medial malleolus (adult) (S82.5-)*

7 ⊟ S89.131- Salter-Harris Type III physeal fracture of lower end of right tibia

S89.132- Salter-Harris Type III physeal fracture of lower end of left tibia

S89.139- Salter-Harris Type III physeal fracture of lower end of unspecified tibia

S89.14 Salter-Harris Type IV physeal fracture of lower end of tibia

EXCLUDES 1 *fracture of medial malleolus (adult) (S82.5-)*

S89.141- Salter-Harris Type IV physeal fracture of lower end of right tibia

S89.142- Salter-Harris Type IV physeal fracture of lower end of left tibia

S89.149- Salter-Harris Type IV physeal fracture of lower end of unspecified tibia

S89.19 Other physeal fracture of lower end of tibia

S89.191- Other physeal fracture of lower end of right tibia

S89.192- Other physeal fracture of lower end of left tibia

S89.199- Other physeal fracture of lower end of unspecified tibia

S89.2 Physeal fracture of upper end of fibula

S89.20 Unspecified physeal fracture of upper end of fibula

S89.201- Unspecified physeal fracture of upper end of right fibula

S89.202- Unspecified physeal fracture of upper end of left fibula

S89.209- Unspecified physeal fracture of upper end of unspecified fibula

S89.21 Salter-Harris Type I physeal fracture of upper end of fibula

S89.211- Salter-Harris Type I physeal fracture of upper end of right fibula

S89.212- Salter-Harris Type I physeal fracture of upper end of left fibula

S89.219- Salter-Harris Type I physeal fracture of upper end of unspecified fibula

S89.22 Salter-Harris Type II physeal fracture of upper end of fibula

S89.221- Salter-Harris Type II physeal fracture of upper end of right fibula

S89.222- Salter-Harris Type II physeal fracture of upper end of left fibula

S89.229- Salter-Harris Type II physeal fracture of upper end of unspecified fibula

S89.29 Other physeal fracture of upper end of fibula

S89.291- Other physeal fracture of upper end of right fibula

S89.292- Other physeal fracture of upper end of left fibula

S89.299- Other physeal fracture of upper end of unspecified fibula

S89.3 Physeal fracture of lower end of fibula

S89.30 Unspecified physeal fracture of lower end of fibula

S89.301- Unspecified physeal fracture of lower end of right fibula

S89.302- Unspecified physeal fracture of lower end of left fibula

S89.309- Unspecified physeal fracture of lower end of unspecified fibula

S89.31 Salter-Harris Type I physeal fracture of lower end of fibula

S89.311- Salter-Harris Type I physeal fracture of lower end of right fibula

S89.312- Salter-Harris Type I physeal fracture of lower end of left fibula

S89.319- Salter-Harris Type I physeal fracture of lower end of unspecified fibula

S89.32 Salter-Harris Type II physeal fracture of lower end of fibula

S89.321- Salter-Harris Type II physeal fracture of lower end of right fibula

S89.322- Salter-Harris Type II physeal fracture of lower end of left fibula

S89.329- Salter-Harris Type II physeal fracture of lower end of unspecified fibula

S89.39 Other physeal fracture of lower end of fibula

S89.391- Other physeal fracture of lower end of right fibula

S89.392- Other physeal fracture of lower end of left fibula

S89.399- Other physeal fracture of lower end of unspecified fibula

S89.8 Other specified injuries of lower leg

The appropriate 7th character is to be added to each code in subcategory S89.8
A initial encounter
D subsequent encounter
S sequela

S89.80X- Other specified injuries of unspecified lower leg

S89.81X- Other specified injuries of right lower leg

S89.82X- Other specified injuries of left lower leg

S89.9 Unspecified injury of lower leg

The appropriate 7th character is to be added to each code in subcategory S89.9
A initial encounter
D subsequent encounter
S sequela

S89.90X- Unspecified injury of unspecified lower leg

S89.91X- Unspecified injury of right lower leg

S89.92X- Unspecified injury of left lower leg

Injuries to the ankle and foot (S90-S99)

EXCLUDES 2 *burns and corrosions (T20-T32)*
fracture of ankle and malleolus (S82.-)
frostbite (T33-T34)
insect bite or sting, venomous (T63.4)

GUIDELINES **Section I.C.19.c.2)**

Multiple fractures are sequenced in accordance with the severity of the fracture.

GUIDELINES **Section I.C.19.b.1)-2)**

When coding injuries, assign separate codes for each injury unless a combination code is provided, in which case the combination code is assigned ... Traumatic injury codes (S00-T14.9) are not to be used for normal, healing surgical wounds or to identify complications of surgical wounds. The code for the most serious injury, as determined by the provider and the focus of treatment, is sequenced first.

1) Superficial injuries such as abrasions or contusions are not coded when associated with more severe injuries of the same site.

2) When a primary injury results in minor damage to peripheral nerves or blood vessels, the primary injury is sequenced first with additional code(s) for injuries to nerves and spinal cord (such as category S04), and/or injury to blood vessels (such as category S15). When the primary injury is to the blood vessels or nerves, that injury should be sequenced first.

GUIDELINES **Section I.C.19.c**

Coding of Traumatic Fractures: The principles of multiple coding of injuries should be followed in coding fractures. Fractures of specified sites are coded individually by site in accordance with both the provisions within categories S02, S12, S22, S32, S42, S49, S52, S59, S62, S72, S79, S82, S89, S92 and the level of detail furnished by medical record content. A fracture not indicated as open or closed should be coded to closed. A fracture not indicated whether displaced or not displaced should be coded to displaced.

S90 Superficial injury of ankle, foot and toes

The appropriate 7th character is to be added to each code from category S90
A initial encounter
D subsequent encounter
S sequela

S90.0 Contusion of ankle

S90.00X- Contusion of unspecified ankle

S90.01X- Contusion of right ankle

S90.02X- Contusion of left ankle

S90.1 Contusion of toe without damage to nail

6 S90.11 Contusion of great toe without damage to nail
- 7 ⊟ S90.111- Contusion of right great toe without damage to nail
- 7 ⊟ S90.112- Contusion of left great toe without damage to nail
- 7 ⊟ S90.119- Contusion of unspecified great toe without damage to nail

6 S90.12 Contusion of lesser toe without damage to nail
- 7 ⊟ S90.121- Contusion of right lesser toe(s) without damage to nail
- 7 ⊟ S90.122- Contusion of left lesser toe(s) without damage to nail
- 7 ⊟ S90.129- Contusion of unspecified lesser toe(s) without damage to nail
  Contusion of toe NOS

5 S90.2 Contusion of toe with damage to nail

6 S90.21 Contusion of great toe with damage to nail
- 7 ⊟ S90.211- Contusion of right great toe with damage to nail
- 7 ⊟ S90.212- Contusion of left great toe with damage to nail
- 7 ⊟ S90.219- Contusion of unspecified great toe with damage to nail

6 S90.22 Contusion of lesser toe with damage to nail
- 7 ⊟ S90.221- Contusion of right lesser toe(s) with damage to nail
- 7 ⊟ S90.222- Contusion of left lesser toe(s) with damage to nail
- 7 ⊟ S90.229- Contusion of unspecified lesser toe(s) with damage to nail

5 S90.3 Contusion of foot

EXCLUDES 2 *contusion of toes (S90.1-, S90.2-)*

- 7 ⊟ S90.30X- Contusion of unspecified foot
  Contusion of foot NOS
- 7 ⊟ S90.31X- Contusion of right foot
- 7 ⊟ S90.32X- Contusion of left foot

5 S90.4 Other superficial injuries of toe

6 S90.41 Abrasion of toe
- 7 ⊟ S90.411- Abrasion, right great toe
- 7 ⊟ S90.412- Abrasion, left great toe
- 7 ⊟ S90.413- Abrasion, unspecified great toe
- 7 ⊟ S90.414- Abrasion, right lesser toe(s)
- 7 ⊟ S90.415- Abrasion, left lesser toe(s)
- 7 ⊟ S90.416- Abrasion, unspecified lesser toe(s)

6 S90.42 Blister (nonthermal) of toe
- 7 ⊟ S90.421- Blister (nonthermal), right great toe
- 7 ⊟ S90.422- Blister (nonthermal), left great toe
- 7 ⊟ S90.423- Blister (nonthermal), unspecified great toe
- 7 ⊟ S90.424- Blister (nonthermal), right lesser toe(s)
- 7 ⊟ S90.425- Blister (nonthermal), left lesser toe(s)
- 7 ⊟ S90.426- Blister (nonthermal), unspecified lesser toe(s)

6 S90.44 External constriction of toe
  Hair tourniquet syndrome of toe
- 7 ⊟ S90.441- External constriction, right great toe
- 7 ⊟ S90.442- External constriction, left great toe
- 7 ⊟ S90.443- External constriction, unspecified great toe
- 7 ⊟ S90.444- External constriction, right lesser toe(s)
- 7 ⊟ S90.445- External constriction, left lesser toe(s)
- 7 ⊟ S90.446- External constriction, unspecified lesser toe(s)

6 S90.45 Superficial foreign body of toe
  Splinter in the toe
- 7 ⊟ S90.451- Superficial foreign body, right great toe
- 7 ⊟ S90.452- Superficial foreign body, left great toe
- 7 ⊟ S90.453- Superficial foreign body, unspecified great toe
- 7 ⊟ S90.454- Superficial foreign body, right lesser toe(s)
- 7 ⊟ S90.455- Superficial foreign body, left lesser toe(s)
- 7 ⊟ S90.456- Superficial foreign body, unspecified lesser toe(s)

6 S90.46 Insect bite (nonvenomous) of toe
- 7 ⊟ S90.461- Insect bite (nonvenomous), right great toe
- 7 ⊟ S90.462- Insect bite (nonvenomous), left great toe
- 7 ⊟ S90.463- Insect bite (nonvenomous), unspecified great toe
- 7 ⊟ S90.464- Insect bite (nonvenomous), right lesser toe(s)
- 7 ⊟ S90.465- Insect bite (nonvenomous), left lesser toe(s)
- 7 ⊟ S90.466- Insect bite (nonvenomous), unspecified lesser toe(s)

6 S90.47 Other superficial bite of toe

EXCLUDES 1 *open bite of toe (S91.15-, S91.25-)*

- 7 ⊟ S90.471- Other superficial bite of right great toe
- 7 ⊟ S90.472- Other superficial bite of left great toe
- 7 ⊟ S90.473- Other superficial bite of unspecified great toe
- 7 ⊟ S90.474- Other superficial bite of right lesser toe(s)
- 7 ⊟ S90.475- Other superficial bite of left lesser toe(s)
- 7 ⊟ S90.476- Other superficial bite of unspecified lesser toe(s)

5 S90.5 Other superficial injuries of ankle

6 S90.51 Abrasion of ankle
- 7 ⊟ S90.511- Abrasion, right ankle
- 7 ⊟ S90.512- Abrasion, left ankle
- 7 ⊟ S90.519- Abrasion, unspecified ankle

6 S90.52 Blister (nonthermal) of ankle
- 7 ⊟ S90.521- Blister (nonthermal), right ankle
- 7 ⊟ S90.522- Blister (nonthermal), left ankle
- 7 ⊟ S90.529- Blister (nonthermal), unspecified ankle

6 S90.54 External constriction of ankle
- 7 ⊟ S90.541- External constriction, right ankle
- 7 ⊟ S90.542- External constriction, left ankle
- 7 ⊟ S90.549- External constriction, unspecified ankle

6 S90.55 Superficial foreign body of ankle
  Splinter in the ankle
- 7 ⊟ S90.551- Superficial foreign body, right ankle
- 7 ⊟ S90.552- Superficial foreign body, left ankle
- 7 ⊟ S90.559- Superficial foreign body, unspecified ankle

6 S90.56 Insect bite (nonvenomous) of ankle
- 7 ⊟ S90.561- Insect bite (nonvenomous), right ankle
- 7 ⊟ S90.562- Insect bite (nonvenomous), left ankle
- 7 ⊟ S90.569- Insect bite (nonvenomous), unspecified ankle

6 S90.57 Other superficial bite of ankle

EXCLUDES 1 *open bite of ankle (S91.05-)*

- 7 ⊟ S90.571- Other superficial bite of ankle, right ankle
- 7 ⊟ S90.572- Other superficial bite of ankle, left ankle
- 7 ⊟ S90.579- Other superficial bite of ankle, unspecified ankle

5 S90.8 Other superficial injuries of foot

6 S90.81 Abrasion of foot
- 7 ⊟ S90.811- Abrasion, right foot
- 7 ⊟ S90.812- Abrasion, left foot
- 7 ⊟ S90.819- Abrasion, unspecified foot

6 S90.82 Blister (nonthermal) of foot
- 7 ⊟ S90.821- Blister (nonthermal), right foot
- 7 ⊟ S90.822- Blister (nonthermal), left foot
- 7 ⊟ S90.829- Blister (nonthermal), unspecified foot

6 S90.84 External constriction of foot
- 7 ⊟ S90.841- External constriction, right foot
- 7 ⊟ S90.842- External constriction, left foot
- 7 ⊟ S90.849- External constriction, unspecified foot

6 S90.85 Superficial foreign body of foot
  Splinter in the foot
- 7 ⊟ S90.851- Superficial foreign body, right foot
- 7 ⊟ S90.852- Superficial foreign body, left foot
- 7 ⊟ S90.859- Superficial foreign body, unspecified foot

6 S90.86 Insect bite (nonvenomous) of foot
- 7 ⊟ S90.861- Insect bite (nonvenomous), right foot
- 7 ⊟ S90.862- Insect bite (nonvenomous), left foot
- 7 ⊟ S90.869- Insect bite (nonvenomous), unspecified foot

S90.87 Other superficial bite of foot
EXCLUDES 1 *open bite of foot (S91.35-)*
S90.871- Other superficial bite of right foot
S90.872- Other superficial bite of left foot
S90.879- Other superficial bite of unspecified foot
S90.9 Unspecified superficial injury of ankle, foot and toe
S90.91 Unspecified superficial injury of ankle
S90.911- Unspecified superficial injury of right ankle
S90.912- Unspecified superficial injury of left ankle
S90.919- Unspecified superficial injury of unspecified ankle
S90.92 Unspecified superficial injury of foot
S90.921- Unspecified superficial injury of right foot
S90.922- Unspecified superficial injury of left foot
S90.929- Unspecified superficial injury of unspecified foot
S90.93 Unspecified superficial injury of toes
S90.931- Unspecified superficial injury of right great toe
S90.932- Unspecified superficial injury of left great toe
S90.933- Unspecified superficial injury of unspecified great toe
S90.934- Unspecified superficial injury of right lesser toe(s)
S90.935- Unspecified superficial injury of left lesser toe(s)
S90.936- Unspecified superficial injury of unspecified lesser toe(s)

S91 Open wound of ankle, foot and toes

Code also:
any associated wound infection
EXCLUDES 1 *open fracture of ankle, foot and toes (S92.-with 7th character B)*
traumatic amputation of ankle and foot (S98.-)

The appropriate 7th character is to be added to each code from category S91
A initial encounter
D subsequent encounter
S sequela

CODING TIP ✓ Open wound codes indicate a wound resulting from a traumatic origin. Do not assign a code for "open wound" unless the etiology of the wound is related to trauma.

S91.0 Open wound of ankle
S91.00 Unspecified open wound of ankle
S91.001- Unspecified open wound, right ankle
S91.002- Unspecified open wound, left ankle
S91.009- Unspecified open wound, unspecified ankle
S91.01 Laceration without foreign body of ankle
S91.011- Laceration without foreign body, right ankle
S91.012- Laceration without foreign body, left ankle
S91.019- Laceration without foreign body, unspecified ankle
S91.02 Laceration with foreign body of ankle
S91.021- Laceration with foreign body, right ankle
S91.022- Laceration with foreign body, left ankle
S91.029- Laceration with foreign body, unspecified ankle
S91.03 Puncture wound without foreign body of ankle
S91.031- Puncture wound without foreign body, right ankle
S91.032- Puncture wound without foreign body, left ankle
S91.039- Puncture wound without foreign body, unspecified ankle
S91.04 Puncture wound with foreign body of ankle
S91.041- Puncture wound with foreign body, right ankle
S91.042- Puncture wound with foreign body, left ankle
S91.049- Puncture wound with foreign body, unspecified ankle
S91.05 Open bite of ankle
EXCLUDES 1 *superficial bite of ankle (S90.56-, S90.57-)*
S91.051- Open bite, right ankle
S91.052- Open bite, left ankle
S91.059- Open bite, unspecified ankle
S91.1 Open wound of toe without damage to nail
S91.10 Unspecified open wound of toe without damage to nail
S91.101- Unspecified open wound of right great toe without damage to nail
S91.102- Unspecified open wound of left great toe without damage to nail
S91.103- Unspecified open wound of unspecified great toe without damage to nail
S91.104- Unspecified open wound of right lesser toe(s) without damage to nail
S91.105- Unspecified open wound of left lesser toe(s) without damage to nail
S91.106- Unspecified open wound of unspecified lesser toe(s) without damage to nail
S91.109- Unspecified open wound of unspecified toe(s) without damage to nail
S91.11 Laceration without foreign body of toe without damage to nail
S91.111- Laceration without foreign body of right great toe without damage to nail
S91.112- Laceration without foreign body of left great toe without damage to nail
S91.113- Laceration without foreign body of unspecified great toe without damage to nail
S91.114- Laceration without foreign body of right lesser toe(s) without damage to nail
S91.115- Laceration without foreign body of left lesser toe(s) without damage to nail
S91.116- Laceration without foreign body of unspecified lesser toe(s) without damage to nail
S91.119- Laceration without foreign body of unspecified toe without damage to nail
S91.12 Laceration with foreign body of toe without damage to nail
S91.121- Laceration with foreign body of right great toe without damage to nail
S91.122- Laceration with foreign body of left great toe without damage to nail
S91.123- Laceration with foreign body of unspecified great toe without damage to nail
S91.124- Laceration with foreign body of right lesser toe(s) without damage to nail
S91.125- Laceration with foreign body of left lesser toe(s) without damage to nail
S91.126- Laceration with foreign body of unspecified lesser toe(s) without damage to nail
S91.129- Laceration with foreign body of unspecified toe(s) without damage to nail
S91.13 Puncture wound without foreign body of toe without damage to nail
S91.131- Puncture wound without foreign body of right great toe without damage to nail
S91.132- Puncture wound without foreign body of left great toe without damage to nail
S91.133- Puncture wound without foreign body of unspecified great toe without damage to nail
S91.134- Puncture wound without foreign body of right lesser toe(s) without damage to nail
S91.135- Puncture wound without foreign body of left lesser toe(s) without damage to nail
S91.136- Puncture wound without foreign body of unspecified lesser toe(s) without damage to nail
S91.139- Puncture wound without foreign body of unspecified toe(s) without damage to nail
S91.14 Puncture wound with foreign body of toe without damage to nail

7 ⊟ S91.141- Puncture wound with foreign body of right great toe without damage to nail
7 ⊟ S91.142- Puncture wound with foreign body of left great toe without damage to nail
7 ⊟ S91.143- Puncture wound with foreign body of unspecified great toe without damage to nail
7 ⊟ S91.144- Puncture wound with foreign body of right lesser toe(s) without damage to nail
7 ⊟ S91.145- Puncture wound with foreign body of left lesser toe(s) without damage to nail
7 ⊟ S91.146- Puncture wound with foreign body of unspecified lesser toe(s) without damage to nail
7 ⊟ S91.149- Puncture wound with foreign body of unspecified toe(s) without damage to nail

6 S91.15 Open bite of toe without damage to nail
Bite of toe NOS
EXCLUDES 1 *superficial bite of toe (S90.46-, S90.47-)*

7 ⊟ S91.151- Open bite of right great toe without damage to nail
7 ⊟ S91.152- Open bite of left great toe without damage to nail
7 ⊟ S91.153- Open bite of unspecified great toe without damage to nail
7 ⊟ S91.154- Open bite of right lesser toe(s) without damage to nail
7 ⊟ S91.155- Open bite of left lesser toe(s) without damage to nail
7 ⊟ S91.156- Open bite of unspecified lesser toe(s) without damage to nail
7 ⊟ S91.159- Open bite of unspecified toe(s) without damage to nail

5 S91.2 Open wound of toe with damage to nail

6 S91.20 Unspecified open wound of toe with damage to nail
7 ⊟ S91.201- Unspecified open wound of right great toe with damage to nail
7 ⊟ S91.202- Unspecified open wound of left great toe with damage to nail
7 ⊟ S91.203- Unspecified open wound of unspecified great toe with damage to nail
7 ⊟ S91.204- Unspecified open wound of right lesser toe(s) with damage to nail
7 ⊟ S91.205- Unspecified open wound of left lesser toe(s) with damage to nail
7 ⊟ S91.206- Unspecified open wound of unspecified lesser toe(s) with damage to nail
7 ⊟ S91.209- Unspecified open wound of unspecified toe(s) with damage to nail

6 S91.21 Laceration without foreign body of toe with damage to nail
7 ⊟ S91.211- Laceration without foreign body of right great toe with damage to nail
7 ⊟ S91.212- Laceration without foreign body of left great toe with damage to nail
7 ⊟ S91.213- Laceration without foreign body of unspecified great toe with damage to nail
7 ⊟ S91.214- Laceration without foreign body of right lesser toe(s) with damage to nail
7 ⊟ S91.215- Laceration without foreign body of left lesser toe(s) with damage to nail
7 ⊟ S91.216- Laceration without foreign body of unspecified lesser toe(s) with damage to nail
7 ⊟ S91.219- Laceration without foreign body of unspecified toe(s) with damage to nail

6 S91.22 Laceration with foreign body of toe with damage to nail
7 ⊟ S91.221- Laceration with foreign body of right great toe with damage to nail
7 ⊟ S91.222- Laceration with foreign body of left great toe with damage to nail
7 ⊟ S91.223- Laceration with foreign body of unspecified great toe with damage to nail
7 ⊟ S91.224- Laceration with foreign body of right lesser toe(s) with damage to nail
7 ⊟ S91.225- Laceration with foreign body of left lesser toe(s) with damage to nail
7 ⊟ S91.226- Laceration with foreign body of unspecified lesser toe(s) with damage to nail
7 ⊟ S91.229- Laceration with foreign body of unspecified toe(s) with damage to nail

6 S91.23 Puncture wound without foreign body of toe with damage to nail
7 ⊟ S91.231- Puncture wound without foreign body of right great toe with damage to nail
7 ⊟ S91.232- Puncture wound without foreign body of left great toe with damage to nail
7 ⊟ S91.233- Puncture wound without foreign body of unspecified great toe with damage to nail
7 ⊟ S91.234- Puncture wound without foreign body of right lesser toe(s) with damage to nail
7 ⊟ S91.235- Puncture wound without foreign body of left lesser toe(s) with damage to nail
7 ⊟ S91.236- Puncture wound without foreign body of unspecified lesser toe(s) with damage to nail
7 ⊟ S91.239- Puncture wound without foreign body of unspecified toe(s) with damage to nail

6 S91.24 Puncture wound with foreign body of toe with damage to nail
7 ⊟ S91.241- Puncture wound with foreign body of right great toe with damage to nail
7 ⊟ S91.242- Puncture wound with foreign body of left great toe with damage to nail
7 ⊟ S91.243- Puncture wound with foreign body of unspecified great toe with damage to nail
7 ⊟ S91.244- Puncture wound with foreign body of right lesser toe(s) with damage to nail
7 ⊟ S91.245- Puncture wound with foreign body of left lesser toe(s) with damage to nail
7 ⊟ S91.246- Puncture wound with foreign body of unspecified lesser toe(s) with damage to nail
7 ⊟ S91.249- Puncture wound with foreign body of unspecified toe(s) with damage to nail

6 S91.25 Open bite of toe with damage to nail
Bite of toe with damage to nail NOS
EXCLUDES 1 *superficial bite of toe (S90.46-, S90.47-)*

7 ⊟ S91.251- Open bite of right great toe with damage to nail
7 ⊟ S91.252- Open bite of left great toe with damage to nail
7 ⊟ S91.253- Open bite of unspecified great toe with damage to nail
7 ⊟ S91.254- Open bite of right lesser toe(s) with damage to nail
7 ⊟ S91.255- Open bite of left lesser toe(s) with damage to nail
7 ⊟ S91.256- Open bite of unspecified lesser toe(s) with damage to nail
7 ⊟ S91.259- Open bite of unspecified toe(s) with damage to nail

5 S91.3 Open wound of foot

6 S91.30 Unspecified open wound of foot
7 ⊟ S91.301- Unspecified open wound, right foot
7 ⊟ S91.302- Unspecified open wound, left foot
7 ⊟ S91.309- Unspecified open wound, unspecified foot

6 S91.31 Laceration without foreign body of foot
7 ⊟ S91.311- Laceration without foreign body, right foot
7 ⊟ S91.312- Laceration without foreign body, left foot
7 ⊟ S91.319- Laceration without foreign body, unspecified foot

6 S91.32 Laceration with foreign body of foot
7 ⊟ S91.321- Laceration with foreign body, right foot
7 ⊟ S91.322- Laceration with foreign body, left foot
7 ⊟ S91.329- Laceration with foreign body, unspecified foot

6 S91.33 Puncture wound without foreign body of foot
7 ⊟ S91.331- Puncture wound without foreign body, right foot
7 ⊟ S91.332- Puncture wound without foreign body, left foot
7 ⊟ S91.339- Puncture wound without foreign body, unspecified foot

6 S91.34 Puncture wound with foreign body of foot
7 ⊟ S91.341- Puncture wound with foreign body, right foot
7 ⊟ S91.342- Puncture wound with foreign body, left foot

7 ⊟ S91.349- **Puncture wound with foreign body, unspecified foot**

6 S91.35 **Open bite of foot**

EXCLUDES 1 *superficial bite of foot (S90.86-, S90.87-)*

7 ⊟ S91.351- **Open bite, right foot**

7 ⊟ S91.352- **Open bite, left foot**

7 ⊟ S91.359- **Open bite, unspecified foot**

4 S92 **Fracture of foot and toe, except ankle**

Note: A fracture not indicated as displaced or nondisplaced should be coded to displaced

A fracture not indicated as open or closed should be coded to closed

EXCLUDES 1 *traumatic amputation of ankle and foot (S98.-)*

EXCLUDES 2 *fracture of ankle (S82.-)*
fracture of malleolus (S82.-)

The appropriate 7th character is to be added to each code from category S92

A initial encounter for closed fracture
B initial encounter for open fracture
D subsequent encounter for fracture with routine healing
G subsequent encounter for fracture with delayed healing
K subsequent encounter for fracture with nonunion
P subsequent encounter for fracture with malunion
S sequela

CODING TIP ✓ A fracture not indicated as displaced or nondisplaced should be coded to displaced. A fracture not indicated as open or closed should be coded to closed. Query providers on fractures not documented as displaced/nondisplaced; otherwise, a displaced fracture diagnosis could be assigned without a reduction being performed, potentially resulting in claim denials.

5 S92.0 **Fracture of calcaneus**

Heel bone
Os calcis

EXCLUDES 2 *Physeal fracture of calcaneus (S99.0-)*

6 S92.00 **Unspecified fracture of calcaneus**

7 ⊟ S92.001- **Unspecified fracture of right calcaneus**

7 ⊟ S92.002- **Unspecified fracture of left calcaneus**

7 ⊟ S92.009- **Unspecified fracture of unspecified calcaneus**

6 S92.01 **Fracture of body of calcaneus**

7 ⊟ S92.011- **Displaced fracture of body of right calcaneus**

7 ⊟ S92.012- **Displaced fracture of body of left calcaneus**

7 ⊟ S92.013- **Displaced fracture of body of unspecified calcaneus**

7 ⊟ S92.014- **Nondisplaced fracture of body of right calcaneus**

7 ⊟ S92.015- **Nondisplaced fracture of body of left calcaneus**

7 ⊟ S92.016- **Nondisplaced fracture of body of unspecified calcaneus**

6 S92.02 **Fracture of anterior process of calcaneus**

7 ⊟ S92.021- **Displaced fracture of anterior process of right calcaneus**

7 ⊟ S92.022- **Displaced fracture of anterior process of left calcaneus**

7 ⊟ S92.023- **Displaced fracture of anterior process of unspecified calcaneus**

7 ⊟ S92.024- **Nondisplaced fracture of anterior process of right calcaneus**

7 ⊟ S92.025- **Nondisplaced fracture of anterior process of left calcaneus**

7 ⊟ S92.026- **Nondisplaced fracture of anterior process of unspecified calcaneus**

6 S92.03 **Avulsion fracture of tuberosity of calcaneus**

7 ⊟ S92.031- **Displaced avulsion fracture of tuberosity of right calcaneus**

7 ⊟ S92.032- **Displaced avulsion fracture of tuberosity of left calcaneus**

7 ⊟ S92.033- **Displaced avulsion fracture of tuberosity of unspecified calcaneus**

7 ⊟ S92.034- **Nondisplaced avulsion fracture of tuberosity of right calcaneus**

7 ⊟ S92.035- **Nondisplaced avulsion fracture of tuberosity of left calcaneus**

7 ⊟ S92.036- **Nondisplaced avulsion fracture of tuberosity of unspecified calcaneus**

6 S92.04 **Other fracture of tuberosity of calcaneus**

7 ⊟ S92.041- **Displaced other fracture of tuberosity of right calcaneus**

7 ⊟ S92.042- **Displaced other fracture of tuberosity of left calcaneus**

7 ⊟ S92.043- **Displaced other fracture of tuberosity of unspecified calcaneus**

7 ⊟ S92.044- **Nondisplaced other fracture of tuberosity of right calcaneus**

7 ⊟ S92.045- **Nondisplaced other fracture of tuberosity of left calcaneus**

7 ⊟ S92.046- **Nondisplaced other fracture of tuberosity of unspecified calcaneus**

6 S92.05 **Other extraarticular fracture of calcaneus**

7 ⊟ S92.051- **Displaced other extraarticular fracture of right calcaneus**

7 ⊟ S92.052- **Displaced other extraarticular fracture of left calcaneus**

7 ⊟ S92.053- **Displaced other extraarticular fracture of unspecified calcaneus**

7 ⊟ S92.054- **Nondisplaced other extraarticular fracture of right calcaneus**

7 ⊟ S92.055- **Nondisplaced other extraarticular fracture of left calcaneus**

7 ⊟ S92.056- **Nondisplaced other extraarticular fracture of unspecified calcaneus**

6 S92.06 **Intraarticular fracture of calcaneus**

7 ⊟ S92.061- **Displaced intraarticular fracture of right calcaneus**

7 ⊟ S92.062- **Displaced intraarticular fracture of left calcaneus**

7 ⊟ S92.063- **Displaced intraarticular fracture of unspecified calcaneus**

7 ⊟ S92.064- **Nondisplaced intraarticular fracture of right calcaneus**

7 ⊟ S92.065- **Nondisplaced intraarticular fracture of left calcaneus**

7 ⊟ S92.066- **Nondisplaced intraarticular fracture of unspecified calcaneus**

5 S92.1 **Fracture of talus**

Astragalus

6 S92.10 **Unspecified fracture of talus**

7 ⊟ S92.101- **Unspecified fracture of right talus**

7 ⊟ S92.102- **Unspecified fracture of left talus**

7 ⊟ S92.109- **Unspecified fracture of unspecified talus**

6 S92.11 **Fracture of neck of talus**

7 ⊟ S92.111- **Displaced fracture of neck of right talus**

7 ⊟ S92.112- **Displaced fracture of neck of left talus**

7 ⊟ S92.113- **Displaced fracture of neck of unspecified talus**

7 ⊟ S92.114- **Nondisplaced fracture of neck of right talus**

7 ⊟ S92.115- **Nondisplaced fracture of neck of left talus**

7 ⊟ S92.116- **Nondisplaced fracture of neck of unspecified talus**

6 S92.12 **Fracture of body of talus**

7 ⊟ S92.121- **Displaced fracture of body of right talus**

7 ⊟ S92.122- **Displaced fracture of body of left talus**

7 ⊟ S92.123- **Displaced fracture of body of unspecified talus**

7 ⊟ S92.124- **Nondisplaced fracture of body of right talus**

7 ⊟ S92.125- **Nondisplaced fracture of body of left talus**

7 ⊟ S92.126- **Nondisplaced fracture of body of unspecified talus**

6 S92.13 **Fracture of posterior process of talus**

7 ⊟ S92.131- **Displaced fracture of posterior process of right talus**

7 ⊟ S92.132- **Displaced fracture of posterior process of left talus**

7 ⊟ S92.133- **Displaced fracture of posterior process of unspecified talus**

7 ⊟ S92.134- **Nondisplaced fracture of posterior process of right talus**

7 ⊟ S92.135- Nondisplaced fracture of posterior process of left talus
7 ⊟ S92.136- Nondisplaced fracture of posterior process of unspecified talus

6 S92.14 Dome fracture of talus
EXCLUDES 1 *osteochondritis dissecans (M93.2)*
7 ⊟ S92.141- Displaced dome fracture of right talus
7 ⊟ S92.142- Displaced dome fracture of left talus
7 ⊟ S92.143- Displaced dome fracture of unspecified talus
7 ⊟ S92.144- Nondisplaced dome fracture of right talus
7 ⊟ S92.145- Nondisplaced dome fracture of left talus
7 ⊟ S92.146- Nondisplaced dome fracture of unspecified talus

6 S92.15 Avulsion fracture (chip fracture) of talus
7 ⊟ S92.151- Displaced avulsion fracture (chip fracture) of right talus
7 ⊟ S92.152- Displaced avulsion fracture (chip fracture) of left talus
7 ⊟ S92.153- Displaced avulsion fracture (chip fracture) of unspecified talus
7 ⊟ S92.154- Nondisplaced avulsion fracture (chip fracture) of right talus
7 ⊟ S92.155- Nondisplaced avulsion fracture (chip fracture) of left talus
7 ⊟ S92.156- Nondisplaced avulsion fracture (chip fracture) of unspecified talus

6 S92.19 Other fracture of talus
7 ⊟ S92.191- Other fracture of right talus
7 ⊟ S92.192- Other fracture of left talus
7 ⊟ S92.199- Other fracture of unspecified talus

5 S92.2 Fracture of other and unspecified tarsal bone(s)

6 S92.20 Fracture of unspecified tarsal bone(s)
7 ⊟ S92.201- Fracture of unspecified tarsal bone(s) of right foot
7 ⊟ S92.202- Fracture of unspecified tarsal bone(s) of left foot
7 ⊟ S92.209- Fracture of unspecified tarsal bone(s) of unspecified foot

6 S92.21 Fracture of cuboid bone
7 ⊟ S92.211- Displaced fracture of cuboid bone of right foot
7 ⊟ S92.212- Displaced fracture of cuboid bone of left foot
7 ⊟ S92.213- Displaced fracture of cuboid bone of unspecified foot
7 ⊟ S92.214- Nondisplaced fracture of cuboid bone of right foot
7 ⊟ S92.215- Nondisplaced fracture of cuboid bone of left foot
7 ⊟ S92.216- Nondisplaced fracture of cuboid bone of unspecified foot

6 S92.22 Fracture of lateral cuneiform
7 ⊟ S92.221- Displaced fracture of lateral cuneiform of right foot
7 ⊟ S92.222- Displaced fracture of lateral cuneiform of left foot
7 ⊟ S92.223- Displaced fracture of lateral cuneiform of unspecified foot
7 ⊟ S92.224- Nondisplaced fracture of lateral cuneiform of right foot
7 ⊟ S92.225- Nondisplaced fracture of lateral cuneiform of left foot
7 ⊟ S92.226- Nondisplaced fracture of lateral cuneiform of unspecified foot

6 S92.23 Fracture of intermediate cuneiform
7 ⊟ S92.231- Displaced fracture of intermediate cuneiform of right foot
7 ⊟ S92.232- Displaced fracture of intermediate cuneiform of left foot
7 ⊟ S92.233- Displaced fracture of intermediate cuneiform of unspecified foot
7 ⊟ S92.234- Nondisplaced fracture of intermediate cuneiform of right foot
7 ⊟ S92.235- Nondisplaced fracture of intermediate cuneiform of left foot
7 ⊟ S92.236- Nondisplaced fracture of intermediate cuneiform of unspecified foot

6 S92.24 Fracture of medial cuneiform
7 ⊟ S92.241- Displaced fracture of medial cuneiform of right foot
7 ⊟ S92.242- Displaced fracture of medial cuneiform of left foot
7 ⊟ S92.243- Displaced fracture of medial cuneiform of unspecified foot
7 ⊟ S92.244- Nondisplaced fracture of medial cuneiform of right foot
7 ⊟ S92.245- Nondisplaced fracture of medial cuneiform of left foot
7 ⊟ S92.246- Nondisplaced fracture of medial cuneiform of unspecified foot

6 S92.25 Fracture of navicular [scaphoid] of foot
7 ⊟ S92.251- Displaced fracture of navicular [scaphoid] of right foot
7 ⊟ S92.252- Displaced fracture of navicular [scaphoid] of left foot
7 ⊟ S92.253- Displaced fracture of navicular [scaphoid] of unspecified foot
7 ⊟ S92.254- Nondisplaced fracture of navicular [scaphoid] of right foot
7 ⊟ S92.255- Nondisplaced fracture of navicular [scaphoid] of left foot
7 ⊟ S92.256- Nondisplaced fracture of navicular [scaphoid] of unspecified foot

5 S92.3 Fracture of metatarsal bone(s)
EXCLUDES 2 *Physeal fracture of metatarsal (S99.1-)*

6 S92.30 Fracture of unspecified metatarsal bone(s)
7 ⊟ S92.301- Fracture of unspecified metatarsal bone(s), right foot
7 ⊟ S92.302- Fracture of unspecified metatarsal bone(s), left foot
7 ⊟ S92.309- Fracture of unspecified metatarsal bone(s), unspecified foot

6 S92.31 Fracture of first metatarsal bone
7 ⊟ S92.311- Displaced fracture of first metatarsal bone, right foot
7 ⊟ S92.312- Displaced fracture of first metatarsal bone, left foot
7 ⊟ S92.313- Displaced fracture of first metatarsal bone, unspecified foot
7 ⊟ S92.314- Nondisplaced fracture of first metatarsal bone, right foot
7 ⊟ S92.315- Nondisplaced fracture of first metatarsal bone, left foot
7 ⊟ S92.316- Nondisplaced fracture of first metatarsal bone, unspecified foot

6 S92.32 Fracture of second metatarsal bone
7 ⊟ S92.321- Displaced fracture of second metatarsal bone, right foot
7 ⊟ S92.322- Displaced fracture of second metatarsal bone, left foot
7 ⊟ S92.323- Displaced fracture of second metatarsal bone, unspecified foot
7 ⊟ S92.324- Nondisplaced fracture of second metatarsal bone, right foot
7 ⊟ S92.325- Nondisplaced fracture of second metatarsal bone, left foot
7 ⊟ S92.326- Nondisplaced fracture of second metatarsal bone, unspecified foot

6 S92.33 Fracture of third metatarsal bone
7 ⊟ S92.331- Displaced fracture of third metatarsal bone, right foot
7 ⊟ S92.332- Displaced fracture of third metatarsal bone, left foot
7 ⊟ S92.333- Displaced fracture of third metatarsal bone, unspecified foot
7 ⊟ S92.334- Nondisplaced fracture of third metatarsal bone, right foot
7 ⊟ S92.335- Nondisplaced fracture of third metatarsal bone, left foot
7 ⊟ S92.336- Nondisplaced fracture of third metatarsal bone, unspecified foot

6 S92.34 Fracture of fourth metatarsal bone
7 ⊟ S92.341- Displaced fracture of fourth metatarsal bone, right foot

7 ⊟ S92.342- Displaced fracture of fourth metatarsal bone, left foot
7 ⊟ S92.343- Displaced fracture of fourth metatarsal bone, unspecified foot
7 ⊟ S92.344- Nondisplaced fracture of fourth metatarsal bone, right foot
7 ⊟ S92.345- Nondisplaced fracture of fourth metatarsal bone, left foot
7 ⊟ S92.346- Nondisplaced fracture of fourth metatarsal bone, unspecified foot

6 S92.35 Fracture of fifth metatarsal bone
7 ⊟ S92.351- Displaced fracture of fifth metatarsal bone, right foot
7 ⊟ S92.352- Displaced fracture of fifth metatarsal bone, left foot
7 ⊟ S92.353- Displaced fracture of fifth metatarsal bone, unspecified foot
7 ⊟ S92.354- Nondisplaced fracture of fifth metatarsal bone, right foot
7 ⊟ S92.355- Nondisplaced fracture of fifth metatarsal bone, left foot
7 ⊟ S92.356- Nondisplaced fracture of fifth metatarsal bone, unspecified foot

5 S92.4 Fracture of great toe
EXCLUDES 2 *Physeal fracture of phalanx of toe (S99.2-)*

6 S92.40 Unspecified fracture of great toe
7 ⊟ S92.401- Displaced unspecified fracture of right great toe
7 ⊟ S92.402- Displaced unspecified fracture of left great toe
7 ⊟ S92.403- Displaced unspecified fracture of unspecified great toe
7 ⊟ S92.404- Nondisplaced unspecified fracture of right great toe
7 ⊟ S92.405- Nondisplaced unspecified fracture of left great toe
7 ⊟ S92.406- Nondisplaced unspecified fracture of unspecified great toe

6 S92.41 Fracture of proximal phalanx of great toe
7 ⊟ S92.411- Displaced fracture of proximal phalanx of right great toe
7 ⊟ S92.412- Displaced fracture of proximal phalanx of left great toe
7 ⊟ S92.413- Displaced fracture of proximal phalanx of unspecified great toe
7 ⊟ S92.414- Nondisplaced fracture of proximal phalanx of right great toe
7 ⊟ S92.415- Nondisplaced fracture of proximal phalanx of left great toe
7 ⊟ S92.416- Nondisplaced fracture of proximal phalanx of unspecified great toe

6 S92.42 Fracture of distal phalanx of great toe
7 ⊟ S92.421- Displaced fracture of distal phalanx of right great toe
7 ⊟ S92.422- Displaced fracture of distal phalanx of left great toe
7 ⊟ S92.423- Displaced fracture of distal phalanx of unspecified great toe
7 ⊟ S92.424- Nondisplaced fracture of distal phalanx of right great toe
7 ⊟ S92.425- Nondisplaced fracture of distal phalanx of left great toe
7 ⊟ S92.426- Nondisplaced fracture of distal phalanx of unspecified great toe

6 S92.49 Other fracture of great toe
7 ⊟ S92.491- Other fracture of right great toe
7 ⊟ S92.492- Other fracture of left great toe
7 ⊟ S92.499- Other fracture of unspecified great toe

5 S92.5 Fracture of lesser toe(s)
EXCLUDES 2 *Physeal fracture of phalanx of toe (S99.2-)*

6 S92.50 Unspecified fracture of lesser toe(s)
7 ⊟ S92.501- Displaced unspecified fracture of right lesser toe(s)
7 ⊟ S92.502- Displaced unspecified fracture of left lesser toe(s)
7 ⊟ S92.503- Displaced unspecified fracture of unspecified lesser toe(s)
7 ⊟ S92.504- Nondisplaced unspecified fracture of right lesser toe(s)
7 ⊟ S92.505- Nondisplaced unspecified fracture of left lesser toe(s)
7 ⊟ S92.506- Nondisplaced unspecified fracture of unspecified lesser toe(s)

6 S92.51 Fracture of proximal phalanx of lesser toe(s)
7 ⊟ S92.511- Displaced fracture of proximal phalanx of right lesser toe(s)
7 ⊟ S92.512- Displaced fracture of proximal phalanx of left lesser toe(s)
7 ⊟ S92.513- Displaced fracture of proximal phalanx of unspecified lesser toe(s)
7 ⊟ S92.514- Nondisplaced fracture of proximal phalanx of right lesser toe(s)
7 ⊟ S92.515- Nondisplaced fracture of proximal phalanx of left lesser toe(s)
7 ⊟ S92.516- Nondisplaced fracture of proximal phalanx of unspecified lesser toe(s)

6 S92.52 Fracture of middle phalanx of lesser toe(s)
7 ⊟ S92.521- Displaced fracture of middle phalanx of right lesser toe(s)
7 ⊟ S92.522- Displaced fracture of middle phalanx of left lesser toe(s)
7 ⊟ S92.523- Displaced fracture of middle phalanx of unspecified lesser toe(s)
7 ⊟ S92.524- Nondisplaced fracture of middle phalanx of right lesser toe(s)
7 ⊟ S92.525- Nondisplaced fracture of middle phalanx of left lesser toe(s)
7 ⊟ S92.526- Nondisplaced fracture of middle phalanx of unspecified lesser toe(s)

6 S92.53 Fracture of distal phalanx of lesser toe(s)
7 ⊟ S92.531- Displaced fracture of distal phalanx of right lesser toe(s)
7 ⊟ S92.532- Displaced fracture of distal phalanx of left lesser toe(s)
7 ⊟ S92.533- Displaced fracture of distal phalanx of unspecified lesser toe(s)
7 ⊟ S92.534- Nondisplaced fracture of distal phalanx of right lesser toe(s)
7 ⊟ S92.535- Nondisplaced fracture of distal phalanx of left lesser toe(s)
7 ⊟ S92.536- Nondisplaced fracture of distal phalanx of unspecified lesser toe(s)

6 S92.59 Other fracture of lesser toe(s)
7 ⊟ S92.591- Other fracture of right lesser toe(s)
7 ⊟ S92.592- Other fracture of left lesser toe(s)
7 ⊟ S92.599- Other fracture of unspecified lesser toe(s)

5 S92.8 Other fracture of foot, except ankle

6 S92.81 Other fracture of foot
Sesamoid fracture of foot
AHA: 4Q 2016, 68
7 ⊟ S92.811- Other fracture of right foot
7 ⊟ S92.812- Other fracture of left foot
7 ⊟ S92.819- Other fracture of unspecified foot

5 S92.9 Unspecified fracture of foot and toe

6 S92.90 Unspecified fracture of foot
7 ⊟ S92.901- Unspecified fracture of right foot
7 ⊟ S92.902- Unspecified fracture of left foot
7 ⊟ S92.909- Unspecified fracture of unspecified foot

6 S92.91 Unspecified fracture of toe
7 ⊟ S92.911- Unspecified fracture of right toe(s)
7 ⊟ S92.912- Unspecified fracture of left toe(s)
7 ⊟ S92.919- Unspecified fracture of unspecified toe(s)

4 S93 Dislocation and sprain of joints and ligaments at ankle, foot and toe level

INCLUDES avulsion of joint or ligament of ankle, foot and toe
laceration of cartilage, joint or ligament of ankle, foot and toe
sprain of cartilage, joint or ligament of ankle, foot and toe
traumatic hemarthrosis of joint or ligament of ankle, foot and toe
traumatic rupture of joint or ligament of ankle, foot and toe
traumatic subluxation of joint or ligament of ankle, foot and toe
traumatic tear of joint or ligament of ankle, foot and toe

Code also:
any associated open wound

EXCLUDES 2 *strain of muscle and tendon of ankle and foot (S96.-)*

The appropriate 7th character is to be added to each code from category S93
A initial encounter
D subsequent encounter
S sequela

CODING TIP ✓ There are no codes for open dislocations. When a dislocation is documented as open, assign an additional code for the open wound.

5 S93.0 Subluxation and dislocation of ankle joint
Subluxation and dislocation of astragalus
Subluxation and dislocation of fibula, lower end
Subluxation and dislocation of talus
Subluxation and dislocation of tibia, lower end

- 7 S93.01X- **Subluxation of right ankle joint**
- 7 S93.02X- **Subluxation of left ankle joint**
- 7 S93.03X- **Subluxation of unspecified ankle joint**
- 7 S93.04X- **Dislocation of right ankle joint**
- 7 S93.05X- **Dislocation of left ankle joint**
- 7 S93.06X- **Dislocation of unspecified ankle joint**

5 S93.1 Subluxation and dislocation of toe

6 S93.10 Unspecified subluxation and dislocation of toe
Dislocation of toe NOS
Subluxation of toe NOS

- 7 S93.101- **Unspecified subluxation of right toe(s)**
- 7 S93.102- **Unspecified subluxation of left toe(s)**
- 7 S93.103- **Unspecified subluxation of unspecified toe(s)**
- 7 S93.104- **Unspecified dislocation of right toe(s)**
- 7 S93.105- **Unspecified dislocation of left toe(s)**
- 7 S93.106- **Unspecified dislocation of unspecified toe(s)**

6 S93.11 Dislocation of interphalangeal joint

- 7 S93.111- **Dislocation of interphalangeal joint of right great toe**
- 7 S93.112- **Dislocation of interphalangeal joint of left great toe**
- 7 S93.113- **Dislocation of interphalangeal joint of unspecified great toe**
- 7 S93.114- **Dislocation of interphalangeal joint of right lesser toe(s)**
- 7 S93.115- **Dislocation of interphalangeal joint of left lesser toe(s)**
- 7 S93.116- **Dislocation of interphalangeal joint of unspecified lesser toe(s)**
- 7 S93.119- **Dislocation of interphalangeal joint of unspecified toe(s)**

6 S93.12 Dislocation of metatarsophalangeal joint

- 7 S93.121- **Dislocation of metatarsophalangeal joint of right great toe**
- 7 S93.122- **Dislocation of metatarsophalangeal joint of left great toe**
- 7 S93.123- **Dislocation of metatarsophalangeal joint of unspecified great toe**
- 7 S93.124- **Dislocation of metatarsophalangeal joint of right lesser toe(s)**
- 7 S93.125- **Dislocation of metatarsophalangeal joint of left lesser toe(s)**
- 7 S93.126- **Dislocation of metatarsophalangeal joint of unspecified lesser toe(s)**
- 7 S93.129- **Dislocation of metatarsophalangeal joint of unspecified toe(s)**

6 S93.13 Subluxation of interphalangeal joint

- 7 S93.131- **Subluxation of interphalangeal joint of right great toe**
- 7 S93.132- **Subluxation of interphalangeal joint of left great toe**
- 7 S93.133- **Subluxation of interphalangeal joint of unspecified great toe**
- 7 S93.134- **Subluxation of interphalangeal joint of right lesser toe(s)**
- 7 S93.135- **Subluxation of interphalangeal joint of left lesser toe(s)**
- 7 S93.136- **Subluxation of interphalangeal joint of unspecified lesser toe(s)**
- 7 S93.139- **Subluxation of interphalangeal joint of unspecified toe(s)**

6 S93.14 Subluxation of metatarsophalangeal joint

- 7 S93.141- **Subluxation of metatarsophalangeal joint of right great toe**
- 7 S93.142- **Subluxation of metatarsophalangeal joint of left great toe**
- 7 S93.143- **Subluxation of metatarsophalangeal joint of unspecified great toe**
- 7 S93.144- **Subluxation of metatarsophalangeal joint of right lesser toe(s)**
- 7 S93.145- **Subluxation of metatarsophalangeal joint of left lesser toe(s)**
- 7 S93.146- **Subluxation of metatarsophalangeal joint of unspecified lesser toe(s)**
- 7 S93.149- **Subluxation of metatarsophalangeal joint of unspecified toe(s)**

5 S93.3 Subluxation and dislocation of foot

EXCLUDES 2 *dislocation of toe (S93.1-)*

6 S93.30 Unspecified subluxation and dislocation of foot
Dislocation of foot NOS
Subluxation of foot NOS

- 7 S93.301- **Unspecified subluxation of right foot**
- 7 S93.302- **Unspecified subluxation of left foot**
- 7 S93.303- **Unspecified subluxation of unspecified foot**
- 7 S93.304- **Unspecified dislocation of right foot**
- 7 S93.305- **Unspecified dislocation of left foot**
- 7 S93.306- **Unspecified dislocation of unspecified foot**

6 S93.31 Subluxation and dislocation of tarsal joint

- 7 S93.311- **Subluxation of tarsal joint of right foot**
- 7 S93.312- **Subluxation of tarsal joint of left foot**
- 7 S93.313- **Subluxation of tarsal joint of unspecified foot**
- 7 S93.314- **Dislocation of tarsal joint of right foot**
- 7 S93.315- **Dislocation of tarsal joint of left foot**
- 7 S93.316- **Dislocation of tarsal joint of unspecified foot**

6 S93.32 Subluxation and dislocation of tarsometatarsal joint

- 7 S93.321- **Subluxation of tarsometatarsal joint of right foot**
- 7 S93.322- **Subluxation of tarsometatarsal joint of left foot**
- 7 S93.323- **Subluxation of tarsometatarsal joint of unspecified foot**
- 7 S93.324- **Dislocation of tarsometatarsal joint of right foot**
- 7 S93.325- **Dislocation of tarsometatarsal joint of left foot**
- 7 S93.326- **Dislocation of tarsometatarsal joint of unspecified foot**

6 S93.33 Other subluxation and dislocation of foot

- 7 S93.331- **Other subluxation of right foot**
- 7 S93.332- **Other subluxation of left foot**
- 7 S93.333- **Other subluxation of unspecified foot**
- 7 S93.334- **Other dislocation of right foot**
- 7 S93.335- **Other dislocation of left foot**
- 7 S93.336- **Other dislocation of unspecified foot**

5 S93.4 Sprain of ankle

EXCLUDES 2 *injury of Achilles tendon (S86.0-)*

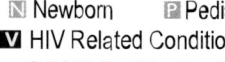

6 S93.40 **Sprain of unspecified ligament of ankle**
Sprain of ankle NOS
Sprained ankle NOS
7 S93.401- **Sprain of unspecified ligament of right ankle**
7 S93.402- **Sprain of unspecified ligament of left ankle**
7 S93.409- **Sprain of unspecified ligament of unspecified ankle**

6 S93.41 **Sprain of calcaneofibular ligament**
7 S93.411- **Sprain of calcaneofibular ligament of right ankle**
7 S93.412- **Sprain of calcaneofibular ligament of left ankle**
7 S93.419- **Sprain of calcaneofibular ligament of unspecified ankle**

6 S93.42 **Sprain of deltoid ligament**
7 S93.421- **Sprain of deltoid ligament of right ankle**
7 S93.422- **Sprain of deltoid ligament of left ankle**
7 S93.429- **Sprain of deltoid ligament of unspecified ankle**

6 S93.43 **Sprain of tibiofibular ligament**
7 S93.431- **Sprain of tibiofibular ligament of right ankle**
7 S93.432- **Sprain of tibiofibular ligament of left ankle**
7 S93.439- **Sprain of tibiofibular ligament of unspecified ankle**

6 S93.49 **Sprain of other ligament of ankle**
Sprain of internal collateral ligament
Sprain of talofibular ligament
7 S93.491- **Sprain of other ligament of right ankle**
7 S93.492- **Sprain of other ligament of left ankle**
7 S93.499- **Sprain of other ligament of unspecified ankle**

5 S93.5 **Sprain of toe**

6 S93.50 **Unspecified sprain of toe**
7 S93.501- **Unspecified sprain of right great toe**
7 S93.502- **Unspecified sprain of left great toe**
7 S93.503- **Unspecified sprain of unspecified great toe**
7 S93.504- **Unspecified sprain of right lesser toe(s)**
7 S93.505- **Unspecified sprain of left lesser toe(s)**
7 S93.506- **Unspecified sprain of unspecified lesser toe(s)**
7 S93.509- **Unspecified sprain of unspecified toe(s)**

6 S93.51 **Sprain of interphalangeal joint of toe**
7 S93.511- **Sprain of interphalangeal joint of right great toe**
7 S93.512- **Sprain of interphalangeal joint of left great toe**
7 S93.513- **Sprain of interphalangeal joint of unspecified great toe**
7 S93.514- **Sprain of interphalangeal joint of right lesser toe(s)**
7 S93.515- **Sprain of interphalangeal joint of left lesser toe(s)**
7 S93.516- **Sprain of interphalangeal joint of unspecified lesser toe(s)**
7 S93.519- **Sprain of interphalangeal joint of unspecified toe(s)**

6 S93.52 **Sprain of metatarsophalangeal joint of toe**
7 S93.521- **Sprain of metatarsophalangeal joint of right great toe**
7 S93.522- **Sprain of metatarsophalangeal joint of left great toe**
7 S93.523- **Sprain of metatarsophalangeal joint of unspecified great toe**
7 S93.524- **Sprain of metatarsophalangeal joint of right lesser toe(s)**
7 S93.525- **Sprain of metatarsophalangeal joint of left lesser toe(s)**
7 S93.526- **Sprain of metatarsophalangeal joint of unspecified lesser toe(s)**
7 S93.529- **Sprain of metatarsophalangeal joint of unspecified toe(s)**

5 S93.6 **Sprain of foot**
EXCLUDES 2 *sprain of metatarsophalangeal joint of toe (S93.52-)*
sprain of toe (S93.5-)

6 S93.60 **Unspecified sprain of foot**
7 S93.601- **Unspecified sprain of right foot**
7 S93.602- **Unspecified sprain of left foot**
7 S93.609- **Unspecified sprain of unspecified foot**

6 S93.61 **Sprain of tarsal ligament of foot**
7 S93.611- **Sprain of tarsal ligament of right foot**
7 S93.612- **Sprain of tarsal ligament of left foot**
7 S93.619- **Sprain of tarsal ligament of unspecified foot**

6 S93.62 **Sprain of tarsometatarsal ligament of foot**
7 S93.621- **Sprain of tarsometatarsal ligament of right foot**
7 S93.622- **Sprain of tarsometatarsal ligament of left foot**
7 S93.629- **Sprain of tarsometatarsal ligament of unspecified foot**

6 S93.69 **Other sprain of foot**
7 S93.691- **Other sprain of right foot**
7 S93.692- **Other sprain of left foot**
7 S93.699- **Other sprain of unspecified foot**

4 S94 Injury of nerves at ankle and foot level

Code also:
any associated open wound (S91.-)

The appropriate 7th character is to be added to each code from category S94
A initial encounter
D subsequent encounter
S sequela

CODING TIP ✓ Late effects of injuries are coded with seventh character S (sequela) and are sequenced after the residual condition of the late effect.

5 S94.0 **Injury of lateral plantar nerve**
7 S94.00X- **Injury of lateral plantar nerve, unspecified leg**
7 S94.01X- **Injury of lateral plantar nerve, right leg**
7 S94.02X- **Injury of lateral plantar nerve, left leg**

5 S94.1 **Injury of medial plantar nerve**
7 S94.10X- **Injury of medial plantar nerve, unspecified leg**
7 S94.11X- **Injury of medial plantar nerve, right leg**
7 S94.12X- **Injury of medial plantar nerve, left leg**

5 S94.2 **Injury of deep peroneal nerve at ankle and foot level**
Injury of terminal, lateral branch of deep peroneal nerve
7 S94.20X- **Injury of deep peroneal nerve at ankle and foot level, unspecified leg**
7 S94.21X- **Injury of deep peroneal nerve at ankle and foot level, right leg**
7 S94.22X- **Injury of deep peroneal nerve at ankle and foot level, left leg**

5 S94.3 **Injury of cutaneous sensory nerve at ankle and foot level**
7 S94.30X- **Injury of cutaneous sensory nerve at ankle and foot level, unspecified leg**
7 S94.31X- **Injury of cutaneous sensory nerve at ankle and foot level, right leg**
7 S94.32X- **Injury of cutaneous sensory nerve at ankle and foot level, left leg**

5 S94.8 **Injury of other nerves at ankle and foot level**
6 S94.8X **Injury of other nerves at ankle and foot level**
7 S94.8X1- **Injury of other nerves at ankle and foot level, right leg**
7 S94.8X2- **Injury of other nerves at ankle and foot level, left leg**
7 S94.8X9- **Injury of other nerves at ankle and foot level, unspecified leg**

5 S94.9 **Injury of unspecified nerve at ankle and foot level**
7 S94.90X- **Injury of unspecified nerve at ankle and foot level, unspecified leg**
7 S94.91X- **Injury of unspecified nerve at ankle and foot level, right leg**
7 S94.92X- **Injury of unspecified nerve at ankle and foot level, left leg**

4 S95 Injury of blood vessels at ankle and foot level

Code also:
any associated open wound (S91.-)

EXCLUDES 2 *injury of posterior tibial artery and vein (S85.1-, S85.8-)*

The appropriate 7th character is to be added to each code from category S95
A initial encounter
D subsequent encounter
S sequela

5 S95.0 Injury of dorsal artery of foot
6 S95.00 Unspecified injury of dorsal artery of foot
7 ⊟ S95.001- Unspecified injury of dorsal artery of right foot
7 ⊟ S95.002- Unspecified injury of dorsal artery of left foot
7 ⊟ S95.009- Unspecified injury of dorsal artery of unspecified foot
6 S95.01 Laceration of dorsal artery of foot
7 ⊟ S95.011- Laceration of dorsal artery of right foot
7 ⊟ S95.012- Laceration of dorsal artery of left foot
7 ⊟ S95.019- Laceration of dorsal artery of unspecified foot
6 S95.09 Other specified injury of dorsal artery of foot
7 ⊟ S95.091- Other specified injury of dorsal artery of right foot
7 ⊟ S95.092- Other specified injury of dorsal artery of left foot
7 ⊟ S95.099- Other specified injury of dorsal artery of unspecified foot
5 S95.1 Injury of plantar artery of foot
6 S95.10 Unspecified injury of plantar artery of foot
7 ⊟ S95.101- Unspecified injury of plantar artery of right foot
7 ⊟ S95.102- Unspecified injury of plantar artery of left foot
7 ⊟ S95.109- Unspecified injury of plantar artery of unspecified foot
6 S95.11 Laceration of plantar artery of foot
7 ⊟ S95.111- Laceration of plantar artery of right foot
7 ⊟ S95.112- Laceration of plantar artery of left foot
7 ⊟ S95.119- Laceration of plantar artery of unspecified foot
6 S95.19 Other specified injury of plantar artery of foot
7 ⊟ S95.191- Other specified injury of plantar artery of right foot
7 ⊟ S95.192- Other specified injury of plantar artery of left foot
7 ⊟ S95.199- Other specified injury of plantar artery of unspecified foot
5 S95.2 Injury of dorsal vein of foot
6 S95.20 Unspecified injury of dorsal vein of foot
7 ⊟ S95.201- Unspecified injury of dorsal vein of right foot
7 ⊟ S95.202- Unspecified injury of dorsal vein of left foot
7 ⊟ S95.209- Unspecified injury of dorsal vein of unspecified foot
6 S95.21 Laceration of dorsal vein of foot
7 ⊟ S95.211- Laceration of dorsal vein of right foot
7 ⊟ S95.212- Laceration of dorsal vein of left foot
7 ⊟ S95.219- Laceration of dorsal vein of unspecified foot
6 S95.29 Other specified injury of dorsal vein of foot
7 ⊟ S95.291- Other specified injury of dorsal vein of right foot
7 ⊟ S95.292- Other specified injury of dorsal vein of left foot
7 ⊟ S95.299- Other specified injury of dorsal vein of unspecified foot
5 S95.8 Injury of other blood vessels at ankle and foot level
6 S95.80 Unspecified injury of other blood vessels at ankle and foot level
7 ⊟ S95.801- Unspecified injury of other blood vessels at ankle and foot level, right leg
7 ⊟ S95.802- Unspecified injury of other blood vessels at ankle and foot level, left leg
7 ⊟ S95.809- Unspecified injury of other blood vessels at ankle and foot level, unspecified leg
6 S95.81 Laceration of other blood vessels at ankle and foot level
7 ⊟ S95.811- Laceration of other blood vessels at ankle and foot level, right leg
7 ⊟ S95.812- Laceration of other blood vessels at ankle and foot level, left leg
7 ⊟ S95.819- Laceration of other blood vessels at ankle and foot level, unspecified leg
6 S95.89 Other specified injury of other blood vessels at ankle and foot level
7 ⊟ S95.891- Other specified injury of other blood vessels at ankle and foot level, right leg
7 ⊟ S95.892- Other specified injury of other blood vessels at ankle and foot level, left leg
7 ⊟ S95.899- Other specified injury of other blood vessels at ankle and foot level, unspecified leg
5 S95.9 Injury of unspecified blood vessel at ankle and foot level
6 S95.90 Unspecified injury of Unspecified blood vessel at ankle and foot level
7 ⊟ S95.901- Unspecified injury of unspecified blood vessel at ankle and foot level, right leg
7 ⊟ S95.902- Unspecified injury of unspecified blood vessel at ankle and foot level, left leg
7 ⊟ S95.909- Unspecified injury of unspecified blood vessel at ankle and foot level, unspecified leg
6 S95.91 Laceration of unspecified blood vessel at ankle and foot level
7 ⊟ S95.911- Laceration of unspecified blood vessel at ankle and foot level, right leg
7 ⊟ S95.912- Laceration of unspecified blood vessel at ankle and foot level, left leg
7 ⊟ S95.919- Laceration of unspecified blood vessel at ankle and foot level, unspecified leg
6 S95.99 Other specified injury of unspecified blood vessel at ankle and foot level
7 ⊟ S95.991- Other specified injury of unspecified blood vessel at ankle and foot level, right leg
7 ⊟ S95.992- Other specified injury of unspecified blood vessel at ankle and foot level, left leg
7 ⊟ S95.999- Other specified injury of unspecified blood vessel at ankle and foot level, unspecified leg

4 S96 Injury of muscle and tendon at ankle and foot level

Code also:
any associated open wound (S91.-)

EXCLUDES 2 *injury of Achilles tendon (S86.0-)*
sprain of joints and ligaments of ankle and foot (S93.-)

The appropriate 7th character is to be added to each code from category S96
A initial encounter
D subsequent encounter
S sequela

5 S96.0 Injury of muscle and tendon of long flexor muscle of toe at ankle and foot level
6 S96.00 Unspecified injury of muscle and tendon of long flexor muscle of toe at ankle and foot level
7 ⊟ S96.001- Unspecified injury of muscle and tendon of long flexor muscle of toe at ankle and foot level, right foot
7 ⊟ S96.002- Unspecified injury of muscle and tendon of long flexor muscle of toe at ankle and foot level, left foot
7 ⊟ S96.009- Unspecified injury of muscle and tendon of long flexor muscle of toe at ankle and foot level, unspecified foot
6 S96.01 Strain of muscle and tendon of long flexor muscle of toe at ankle and foot level
7 ⊟ S96.011- Strain of muscle and tendon of long flexor muscle of toe at ankle and foot level, right foot
7 ⊟ S96.012- Strain of muscle and tendon of long flexor muscle of toe at ankle and foot level, left foot

S96.019- Strain of muscle and tendon of long flexor muscle of toe at ankle and foot level, unspecified foot

S96.02 Laceration of muscle and tendon of long flexor muscle of toe at ankle and foot level

S96.021- Laceration of muscle and tendon of long flexor muscle of toe at ankle and foot level, right foot

S96.022- Laceration of muscle and tendon of long flexor muscle of toe at ankle and foot level, left foot

S96.029- Laceration of muscle and tendon of long flexor muscle of toe at ankle and foot level, unspecified foot

S96.09 Other injury of muscle and tendon of long flexor muscle of toe at ankle and foot level

S96.091- Other injury of muscle and tendon of long flexor muscle of toe at ankle and foot level, right foot

S96.092- Other injury of muscle and tendon of long flexor muscle of toe at ankle and foot level, left foot

S96.099- Other injury of muscle and tendon of long flexor muscle of toe at ankle and foot level, unspecified foot

S96.1 Injury of muscle and tendon of long extensor muscle of toe at ankle and foot level

S96.10 Unspecified injury of muscle and tendon of long extensor muscle of toe at ankle and foot level

S96.101- Unspecified injury of muscle and tendon of long extensor muscle of toe at ankle and foot level, right foot

S96.102- Unspecified injury of muscle and tendon of long extensor muscle of toe at ankle and foot level, left foot

S96.109- Unspecified injury of muscle and tendon of long extensor muscle of toe at ankle and foot level, unspecified foot

S96.11 Strain of muscle and tendon of long extensor muscle of toe at ankle and foot level

S96.111- Strain of muscle and tendon of long extensor muscle of toe at ankle and foot level, right foot

S96.112- Strain of muscle and tendon of long extensor muscle of toe at ankle and foot level, left foot

S96.119- Strain of muscle and tendon of long extensor muscle of toe at ankle and foot level, unspecified foot

S96.12 Laceration of muscle and tendon of long extensor muscle of toe at ankle and foot level

S96.121- Laceration of muscle and tendon of long extensor muscle of toe at ankle and foot level, right foot

S96.122- Laceration of muscle and tendon of long extensor muscle of toe at ankle and foot level, left foot

S96.129- Laceration of muscle and tendon of long extensor muscle of toe at ankle and foot level, unspecified foot

S96.19 Other specified injury of muscle and tendon of long extensor muscle of toe at ankle and foot level

S96.191- Other specified injury of muscle and tendon of long extensor muscle of toe at ankle and foot level, right foot

S96.192- Other specified injury of muscle and tendon of long extensor muscle of toe at ankle and foot level, left foot

S96.199- Other specified injury of muscle and tendon of long extensor muscle of toe at ankle and foot level, unspecified foot

S96.2 Injury of intrinsic muscle and tendon at ankle and foot level

S96.20 Unspecified injury of intrinsic muscle and tendon at ankle and foot level

S96.201- Unspecified injury of intrinsic muscle and tendon at ankle and foot level, right foot

S96.202- Unspecified injury of intrinsic muscle and tendon at ankle and foot level, left foot

S96.209- Unspecified injury of intrinsic muscle and tendon at ankle and foot level, unspecified foot

S96.21 Strain of intrinsic muscle and tendon at ankle and foot level

S96.211- Strain of intrinsic muscle and tendon at ankle and foot level, right foot

S96.212- Strain of intrinsic muscle and tendon at ankle and foot level, left foot

S96.219- Strain of intrinsic muscle and tendon at ankle and foot level, unspecified foot

S96.22 Laceration of intrinsic muscle and tendon at ankle and foot level

S96.221- Laceration of intrinsic muscle and tendon at ankle and foot level, right foot

S96.222- Laceration of intrinsic muscle and tendon at ankle and foot level, left foot

S96.229- Laceration of intrinsic muscle and tendon at ankle and foot level, unspecified foot

S96.29 Other specified injury of intrinsic muscle and tendon at ankle and foot level

S96.291- Other specified injury of intrinsic muscle and tendon at ankle and foot level, right foot

S96.292- Other specified injury of intrinsic muscle and tendon at ankle and foot level, left foot

S96.299- Other specified injury of intrinsic muscle and tendon at ankle and foot level, unspecified foot

S96.8 Injury of other specified muscles and tendons at ankle and foot level

S96.80 Unspecified injury of other specified muscles and tendons at ankle and foot level

S96.801- Unspecified injury of other specified muscles and tendons at ankle and foot level, right foot

S96.802- Unspecified injury of other specified muscles and tendons at ankle and foot level, left foot

S96.809- Unspecified injury of other specified muscles and tendons at ankle and foot level, unspecified foot

S96.81 Strain of other specified muscles and tendons at ankle and foot level

S96.811- Strain of other specified muscles and tendons at ankle and foot level, right foot

S96.812- Strain of other specified muscles and tendons at ankle and foot level, left foot

S96.819- Strain of other specified muscles and tendons at ankle and foot level, unspecified foot

S96.82 Laceration of other specified muscles and tendons at ankle and foot level

S96.821- Laceration of other specified muscles and tendons at ankle and foot level, right foot

S96.822- Laceration of other specified muscles and tendons at ankle and foot level, left foot

S96.829- Laceration of other specified muscles and tendons at ankle and foot level, unspecified foot

S96.89 Other specified injury of Other specified muscles and tendons at ankle and foot level

S96.891- Other specified injury of other specified muscles and tendons at ankle and foot level, right foot

S96.892- Other specified injury of other specified muscles and tendons at ankle and foot level, left foot

S96.899- Other specified injury of other specified muscles and tendons at ankle and foot level, unspecified foot

S96.9 Injury of unspecified muscle and tendon at ankle and foot level

S96.90 Unspecified injury of Unspecified muscle and tendon at ankle and foot level

S96.901- Unspecified injury of unspecified muscle and tendon at ankle and foot level, right foot

S96.902- Unspecified injury of unspecified muscle and tendon at ankle and foot level, left foot

7 ⊟ S96.909- Unspecified injury of unspecified muscle and tendon at ankle and foot level, unspecified foot

6 S96.91 Strain of unspecified muscle and tendon at ankle and foot level

7 ⊟ S96.911- Strain of unspecified muscle and tendon at ankle and foot level, right foot

7 ⊟ S96.912- Strain of unspecified muscle and tendon at ankle and foot level, left foot

7 ⊟ S96.919- Strain of unspecified muscle and tendon at ankle and foot level, unspecified foot

6 S96.92 Laceration of unspecified muscle and tendon at ankle and foot level

7 ⊟ S96.921- Laceration of unspecified muscle and tendon at ankle and foot level, right foot

7 ⊟ S96.922- Laceration of unspecified muscle and tendon at ankle and foot level, left foot

7 ⊟ S96.929- Laceration of unspecified muscle and tendon at ankle and foot level, unspecified foot

6 S96.99 Other specified injury of unspecified muscle and tendon at ankle and foot level

7 ⊟ S96.991- Other specified injury of unspecified muscle and tendon at ankle and foot level, right foot

7 ⊟ S96.992- Other specified injury of unspecified muscle and tendon at ankle and foot level, left foot

7 ⊟ S96.999- Other specified injury of unspecified muscle and tendon at ankle and foot level, unspecified foot

4 S97 Crushing injury of ankle and foot

Use additional code(s) for all associated injuries

The appropriate 7th character is to be added to each code from category S97

A initial encounter

D subsequent encounter

S sequela

5 S97.0 Crushing injury of ankle

7 ⊟ S97.00X- Crushing injury of unspecified ankle

7 ⊟ S97.01X- Crushing injury of right ankle

7 ⊟ S97.02X- Crushing injury of left ankle

5 S97.1 Crushing injury of toe

6 S97.10 Crushing injury of unspecified toe(s)

7 ⊟ S97.101- Crushing injury of unspecified right toe(s)

7 ⊟ S97.102- Crushing injury of unspecified left toe(s)

7 ⊟ S97.109- Crushing injury of unspecified toe(s)

Crushing injury of toe NOS

6 S97.11 Crushing injury of great toe

7 ⊟ S97.111- Crushing injury of right great toe

7 ⊟ S97.112- Crushing injury of left great toe

7 ⊟ S97.119- Crushing injury of unspecified great toe

6 S97.12 Crushing injury of lesser toe(s)

7 ⊟ S97.121- Crushing injury of right lesser toe(s)

7 ⊟ S97.122- Crushing injury of left lesser toe(s)

7 ⊟ S97.129- Crushing injury of unspecified lesser toe(s)

5 S97.8 Crushing injury of foot

7 ⊟ S97.80X- Crushing injury of unspecified foot

Crushing injury of foot NOS

7 ⊟ S97.81X- Crushing injury of right foot

7 ⊟ S97.82X- Crushing injury of left foot

4 S98 Traumatic amputation of ankle and foot

An amputation not identified as partial or complete should be coded to complete

The appropriate 7th character is to be added to each code from category S98

A initial encounter

D subsequent encounter

S sequela

CODING TIP ✓ Use these codes only when the amputation was due to trauma. There is no need for adding Z89 with traumatic amputations. See Z47.81 for care of amputations not due to trauma.

5 S98.0 Traumatic amputation of foot at ankle level

6 S98.01 Complete traumatic amputation of foot at ankle level

7 ⊟ S98.011- Complete traumatic amputation of right foot at ankle level HCC

7 ⊟ S98.012- Complete traumatic amputation of left foot at ankle level HCC

7 ⊟ S98.019- Complete traumatic amputation of unspecified foot at ankle level HCC

6 S98.02 Partial traumatic amputation of foot at ankle level

7 ⊟ S98.021- Partial traumatic amputation of right foot at ankle level HCC

7 ⊟ S98.022- Partial traumatic amputation of left foot at ankle level HCC

7 ⊟ S98.029- Partial traumatic amputation of unspecified foot at ankle level HCC

5 S98.1 Traumatic amputation of one toe

6 S98.11 Complete traumatic amputation of great toe

7 ⊟ S98.111- Complete traumatic amputation of right great toe HCC

7 ⊟ S98.112- Complete traumatic amputation of left great toe HCC

7 ⊟ S98.119- Complete traumatic amputation of unspecified great toe HCC

6 S98.12 Partial traumatic amputation of great toe

7 ⊟ S98.121- Partial traumatic amputation of right great toe HCC

7 ⊟ S98.122- Partial traumatic amputation of left great toe HCC

7 ⊟ S98.129- Partial traumatic amputation of unspecified great toe HCC

6 S98.13 Complete traumatic amputation of one lesser toe

Traumatic amputation of toe NOS

7 ⊟ S98.131- Complete traumatic amputation of one right lesser toe HCC

7 ⊟ S98.132- Complete traumatic amputation of one left lesser toe HCC

7 ⊟ S98.139- Complete traumatic amputation of one unspecified lesser toe HCC

6 S98.14 Partial traumatic amputation of one lesser toe

7 ⊟ S98.141- Partial traumatic amputation of one right lesser toe HCC

7 ⊟ S98.142- Partial traumatic amputation of one left lesser toe HCC

7 ⊟ S98.149- Partial traumatic amputation of one unspecified lesser toe HCC

5 S98.2 Traumatic amputation of two or more lesser toes

6 S98.21 Complete traumatic amputation of two or more lesser toes

7 ⊟ S98.211- Complete traumatic amputation of two or more right lesser toes HCC

7 ⊟ S98.212- Complete traumatic amputation of two or more left lesser toes HCC

7 ⊟ S98.219- Complete traumatic amputation of two or more unspecified lesser toes HCC

6 S98.22 Partial traumatic amputation of two or more lesser toes

7 ⊟ S98.221- Partial traumatic amputation of two or more right lesser toes HCC

7 ⊟ S98.222- Partial traumatic amputation of two or more left lesser toes HCC

7 ⊟ S98.229- Partial traumatic amputation of two or more unspecified lesser toes HCC

5 S98.3 Traumatic amputation of midfoot

6 S98.31 Complete traumatic amputation of midfoot

7 ⊟ S98.311- Complete traumatic amputation of right midfoot HCC

7 ⊟ S98.312- Complete traumatic amputation of left midfoot HCC

7 ⊟ S98.319- Complete traumatic amputation of unspecified midfoot HCC

6 S98.32 Partial traumatic amputation of midfoot

7 ⊟ S98.321- Partial traumatic amputation of right midfoot HCC

7 ⊟ S98.322- Partial traumatic amputation of left midfoot HCC

7 ⊟ S98.329- Partial traumatic amputation of unspecified midfoot HCC

5 S98.9 Traumatic amputation of foot, level unspecified

6 S98.91 Complete traumatic amputation of foot, level unspecified

7 S98.911- Complete traumatic amputation of right foot, level unspecified HCC

7 S98.912- Complete traumatic amputation of left foot, level unspecified HCC

7 S98.919- Complete traumatic amputation of unspecified foot, level unspecified HCC

6 S98.92 Partial traumatic amputation of foot, level unspecified

7 S98.921- Partial traumatic amputation of right foot, level unspecified HCC

7 S98.922- Partial traumatic amputation of left foot, level unspecified HCC

7 S98.929- Partial traumatic amputation of unspecified foot, level unspecified HCC

4 S99 Other and unspecified injuries of ankle and foot

CODING TIP ✓ A Salter-Harris physeal fracture occurs through the growth plate. Only one code is needed to report a single physeal fracture. Because of the implications for future bone development, coding of a Salter-Harris fracture takes priority over a simple fracture code. Assign the physeal fracture code based on location, type, and laterality. Use a code for "other physeal fracture" for Type V.

5 S99.0 Physeal fracture of calcaneus

The appropriate 7th character is to be added to each code from subcategories S99.0

A	initial encounter for closed fracture
B	initial encounter for open fracture
D	subsequent encounter for fracture with routine healing
G	subsequent encounter for fracture with delayed healing
K	subsequent encounter for fracture with nonunion
P	subsequent encounter for fracture with malunion
S	sequela

AHA: 4Q 2016, 68

6 S99.00 Unspecified physeal fracture of calcaneus

7 S99.001- Unspecified physeal fracture of right calcaneus

7 S99.002- Unspecified physeal fracture of left calcaneus

7 S99.009- Unspecified physeal fracture of unspecified calcaneus

6 S99.01 Salter-Harris Type I physeal fracture of calcaneus

7 S99.011- Salter-Harris Type I physeal fracture of right calcaneus

7 S99.012- Salter-Harris Type I physeal fracture of left calcaneus

7 S99.019- Salter-Harris Type I physeal fracture of unspecified calcaneus

6 S99.02 Salter-Harris Type II physeal fracture of calcaneus

7 S99.021- Salter-Harris Type II physeal fracture of right calcaneus

7 S99.022- Salter-Harris Type II physeal fracture of left calcaneus

7 S99.029- Salter-Harris Type II physeal fracture of unspecified calcaneus

6 S99.03 Salter-Harris Type III physeal fracture of calcaneus

7 S99.031- Salter-Harris Type III physeal fracture of right calcaneus

7 S99.032- Salter-Harris Type III physeal fracture of left calcaneus

7 S99.039- Salter-Harris Type III physeal fracture of unspecified calcaneus

6 S99.04 Salter-Harris Type IV physeal fracture of calcaneus

7 S99.041- Salter-Harris Type IV physeal fracture of right calcaneus

7 S99.042- Salter-Harris Type IV physeal fracture of left calcaneus

7 S99.049- Salter-Harris Type IV physeal fracture of unspecified calcaneus

6 S99.09 Other physeal fracture of calcaneus

7 S99.091- Other physeal fracture of right calcaneus

7 S99.092- Other physeal fracture of left calcaneus

7 S99.099- Other physeal fracture of unspecified calcaneus

5 S99.1 Physeal fracture of metatarsal

The appropriate 7th character is to be added to each code from subcategories S99.1

A	initial encounter for closed fracture
B	initial encounter for open fracture
D	subsequent encounter for fracture with routine healing
G	subsequent encounter for fracture with delayed healing
K	subsequent encounter for fracture with nonunion
P	subsequent encounter for fracture with malunion
S	sequela

AHA: 4Q 2016, 68

6 S99.10 Unspecified physeal fracture of metatarsal

7 S99.101- Unspecified physeal fracture of right metatarsal

7 S99.102- Unspecified physeal fracture of left metatarsal

7 S99.109- Unspecified physeal fracture of unspecified metatarsal

6 S99.11 Salter-Harris Type I physeal fracture of metatarsal

7 S99.111- Salter-Harris Type I physeal fracture of right metatarsal

7 S99.112- Salter-Harris Type I physeal fracture of left metatarsal

AHA: 1Q 2018, 3

7 S99.119- Salter-Harris Type I physeal fracture of unspecified metatarsal

6 S99.12 Salter-Harris Type II physeal fracture of metatarsal

7 S99.121- Salter-Harris Type II physeal fracture of right metatarsal

7 S99.122- Salter-Harris Type II physeal fracture of left metatarsal

7 S99.129- Salter-Harris Type II physeal fracture of unspecified metatarsal

6 S99.13 Salter-Harris Type III physeal fracture of metatarsal

7 S99.131- Salter-Harris Type III physeal fracture of right metatarsal

7 S99.132- Salter-Harris Type III physeal fracture of left metatarsal

7 S99.139- Salter-Harris Type III physeal fracture of unspecified metatarsal

6 S99.14 Salter-Harris Type IV physeal fracture of metatarsal

7 S99.141- Salter-Harris Type IV physeal fracture of right metatarsal

7 S99.142- Salter-Harris Type IV physeal fracture of left metatarsal

7 S99.149- Salter-Harris Type IV physeal fracture of unspecified metatarsal

6 S99.19 Other physeal fracture of metatarsal

7 S99.191- Other physeal fracture of right metatarsal

7 S99.192- Other physeal fracture of left metatarsal

7 S99.199- Other physeal fracture of unspecified metatarsal

5 S99.2 Physeal fracture of phalanx of toe

The appropriate 7th character is to be added to each code from subcategories S99.2

A	initial encounter for closed fracture
B	initial encounter for open fracture
D	subsequent encounter for fracture with routine healing
G	subsequent encounter for fracture with delayed healing
K	subsequent encounter for fracture with nonunion
P	subsequent encounter for fracture with malunion
S	sequela

AHA: 4Q 2016, 68

6 S99.20 Unspecified physeal fracture of phalanx of toe

7 S99.201- Unspecified physeal fracture of phalanx of right toe

7 S99.202- Unspecified physeal fracture of phalanx of left toe

7 ⊟ S99.209- **Unspecified physeal fracture of phalanx of unspecified toe**

6 S99.21 **Salter-Harris Type I physeal fracture of phalanx of toe**

7 ⊟ S99.211- Salter-Harris Type I physeal fracture of phalanx of right toe

7 ⊟ S99.212- Salter-Harris Type I physeal fracture of phalanx of left toe

7 ⊟ S99.219- **Salter-Harris Type I physeal fracture of phalanx of unspecified toe**

6 S99.22 **Salter-Harris Type II physeal fracture of phalanx of toe**

7 ⊟ S99.221- Salter-Harris Type II physeal fracture of phalanx of right toe

7 ⊟ S99.222- Salter-Harris Type II physeal fracture of phalanx of left toe

7 ⊟ S99.229- **Salter-Harris Type II physeal fracture of phalanx of unspecified toe**

6 S99.23 **Salter-Harris Type III physeal fracture of phalanx of toe**

7 ⊟ S99.231- Salter-Harris Type III physeal fracture of phalanx of right toe

7 ⊟ S99.232- Salter-Harris Type III physeal fracture of phalanx of left toe

7 ⊟ S99.239- **Salter-Harris Type III physeal fracture of phalanx of unspecified toe**

6 S99.24 **Salter-Harris Type IV physeal fracture of phalanx of toe**

7 ⊟ S99.241- Salter-Harris Type IV physeal fracture of phalanx of right toe

7 ⊟ S99.242- Salter-Harris Type IV physeal fracture of phalanx of left toe

7 ⊟ S99.249- **Salter-Harris Type IV physeal fracture of phalanx of unspecified toe**

6 S99.29 **Other physeal fracture of phalanx of toe**

7 ⊟ S99.291- Other physeal fracture of phalanx of right toe

7 ⊟ S99.292- Other physeal fracture of phalanx of left toe

7 ⊟ S99.299- **Other physeal fracture of phalanx of unspecified toe**

5 S99.8 **Other specified injuries of ankle and foot**

The appropriate 7th character is to be added to each code from subcategory S99.8
A initial encounter
D subsequent encounter
S sequela

6 S99.81 **Other specified injuries of ankle**

7 ⊟ S99.811- Other specified injuries of right ankle

7 ⊟ S99.812- Other specified injuries of left ankle

7 ⊟ S99.819- **Other specified injuries of unspecified ankle**

6 S99.82 **Other specified injuries of foot**

7 ⊟ S99.821- Other specified injuries of right foot

7 ⊟ S99.822- Other specified injuries of left foot

7 ⊟ S99.829- **Other specified injuries of unspecified foot**

5 S99.9 **Unspecified injury of ankle and foot**

The appropriate 7th character is to be added to each code from subcategory S99.9
A initial encounter
D subsequent encounter
S sequela

6 S99.91 **Unspecified injury of ankle**

7 ⊟ S99.911- **Unspecified injury of right ankle**

7 ⊟ S99.912- **Unspecified injury of left ankle**

7 ⊟ S99.919- **Unspecified injury of unspecified ankle**

6 S99.92 **Unspecified injury of foot**

7 ⊟ S99.921- **Unspecified injury of right foot**

7 ⊟ S99.922- **Unspecified injury of left foot**

7 ⊟ S99.929- **Unspecified injury of unspecified foot**

Injury, poisoning and certain other consequences of external causes (T07-T88)

Injuries involving multiple body regions (T07)

EXCLUDES 1 *burns and corrosions (T20-T32)*
frostbite (T33-T34)
insect bite or sting, venomous (T63.4)
sunburn (L55.-)

7 T07.XXX- **Unspecified multiple injuries**

EXCLUDES 1 *injury NOS (T14.90)*

The appropriate 7th character is to be added to code T07
A initial encounter
D subsequent encounter
S sequela

AHA: 4Q 2017, 20

Injury of unspecified body region (T14)

4 T14 **Injury of unspecified body region**

EXCLUDES 1 *multiple unspecified injuries (T07)*

The appropriate 7th character is to be added to each code from category T14
A initial encounter
D subsequent encounter
S sequela

AHA: 4Q 2017, 20

7 T14.8XX- **Other injury of unspecified body region**
Abrasion NOS
Contusion NOS
Crush injury NOS
Fracture NOS
Skin injury NOS
Vascular injury NOS
Wound NOS

5 T14.9 **Unspecified injury**

7 T14.90X- **Injury, unspecified**
Injury NOS

7 T14.91X- **Suicide attempt** HCC
Attempted suicide NOS

Effects of foreign body entering through natural orifice (T15-T19)

EXCLUDES 2 *foreign body accidentally left in operation wound (T81.5-)*
foreign body in penetrating wound - See open wound by body region
residual foreign body in soft tissue (M79.5)
splinter, without open wound - See superficial injury by body region

4 T15 **Foreign body on external eye**

EXCLUDES 2 *foreign body in penetrating wound of orbit and eye ball (S05.4-, S05.5-)*
open wound of eyelid and periocular area (S01.1-)
retained foreign body in eyelid (H02.8-)
retained (old) foreign body in penetrating wound of orbit and eye ball (H05.5-, H44.6-, H44.7-)
superficial foreign body of eyelid and periocular area (S00.25-)

The appropriate 7th character is to be added to each code from category T15
A initial encounter
D subsequent encounter
S sequela

5 T15.0 **Foreign body in cornea**

7 ⊟ T15.00X- **Foreign body in cornea, unspecified eye**

7 ⊟ T15.01X- **Foreign body in cornea, right eye**

7 ⊟ T15.02X- **Foreign body in cornea, left eye**

5 T15.1 **Foreign body in conjunctival sac**

7 ⊟ T15.10X- **Foreign body in conjunctival sac, unspecified eye**

7 ⊟ T15.11X- **Foreign body in conjunctival sac, right eye**
7 ⊟ T15.12X- **Foreign body in conjunctival sac, left eye**
5 T15.8 **Foreign body in other and multiple parts of external eye**
Foreign body in lacrimal punctum
7 ⊟ T15.80X- **Foreign body in other and multiple parts of external eye, unspecified eye**
7 ⊟ T15.81X- **Foreign body in other and multiple parts of external eye, right eye**
7 ⊟ T15.82X- **Foreign body in other and multiple parts of external eye, left eye**
5 T15.9 **Foreign body on external eye, part unspecified**
7 ⊟ T15.90X- **Foreign body on external eye, part unspecified, unspecified eye**
7 ⊟ T15.91X- **Foreign body on external eye, part unspecified, right eye**
7 ⊟ T15.92X- **Foreign body on external eye, part unspecified, left eye**

4 T16 Foreign body in ear

INCLUDES foreign body in auditory canal

The appropriate 7th character is to be added to each code from category T16
A initial encounter
D subsequent encounter
S sequela

7 ⊟ T16.1XX- **Foreign body in right ear**
7 ⊟ T16.2XX- **Foreign body in left ear**
7 ⊟ T16.9XX- **Foreign body in ear, unspecified ear**

4 T17 Foreign body in respiratory tract

The appropriate 7th character is to be added to each code from category T17
A initial encounter
D subsequent encounter
S sequela

7 T17.0XX- **Foreign body in nasal sinus**
7 T17.1XX- **Foreign body in nostril**
Foreign body in nose NOS
5 T17.2 **Foreign body in pharynx**
Foreign body in nasopharynx
Foreign body in throat NOS
6 T17.20 **Unspecified foreign body in pharynx**
7 T17.200- **Unspecified foreign body in pharynx causing asphyxiation**
7 T17.208- **Unspecified foreign body in pharynx causing other injury**
6 T17.21 **Gastric contents in pharynx**
Aspiration of gastric contents into pharynx
Vomitus in pharynx
7 T17.210- **Gastric contents in pharynx causing asphyxiation**
7 T17.218- **Gastric contents in pharynx causing other injury**
6 T17.22 **Food in pharynx**
Bones in pharynx
Seeds in pharynx
7 T17.220- **Food in pharynx causing asphyxiation**
7 T17.228- **Food in pharynx causing other injury**
6 T17.29 **Other foreign object in pharynx**
7 T17.290- **Other foreign object in pharynx causing asphyxiation**
7 T17.298- **Other foreign object in pharynx causing other injury**
5 T17.3 **Foreign body in larynx**
6 T17.30 **Unspecified foreign body in larynx**
7 T17.300- **Unspecified foreign body in larynx causing asphyxiation**
7 T17.308- **Unspecified foreign body in larynx causing other injury**
6 T17.31 **Gastric contents in larynx**
Aspiration of gastric contents into larynx
Vomitus in larynx
7 T17.310- **Gastric contents in larynx causing asphyxiation**
7 T17.318- **Gastric contents in larynx causing other injury**
6 T17.32 **Food in larynx**
Bones in larynx
Seeds in larynx
7 T17.320- **Food in larynx causing asphyxiation**
7 T17.328- **Food in larynx causing other injury**
6 T17.39 **Other foreign object in larynx**
7 T17.390- **Other foreign object in larynx causing asphyxiation**
7 T17.398- **Other foreign object in larynx causing other injury**
5 T17.4 **Foreign body in trachea**
6 T17.40 **Unspecified foreign body in trachea**
7 T17.400- **Unspecified foreign body in trachea causing asphyxiation**
7 T17.408- **Unspecified foreign body in trachea causing other injury**
6 T17.41 **Gastric contents in trachea**
Aspiration of gastric contents into trachea
Vomitus in trachea
7 T17.410- **Gastric contents in trachea causing asphyxiation**
7 T17.418- **Gastric contents in trachea causing other injury**
6 T17.42 **Food in trachea**
Bones in trachea
Seeds in trachea
7 T17.420- **Food in trachea causing asphyxiation**
7 T17.428- **Food in trachea causing other injury**
6 T17.49 **Other foreign object in trachea**
7 T17.490- **Other foreign object in trachea causing asphyxiation**
7 T17.498- **Other foreign object in trachea causing other injury**
5 T17.5 **Foreign body in bronchus**
6 T17.50 **Unspecified foreign body in bronchus**
7 T17.500- **Unspecified foreign body in bronchus causing asphyxiation**
7 T17.508- **Unspecified foreign body in bronchus causing other injury**
6 T17.51 **Gastric contents in bronchus**
Aspiration of gastric contents into bronchus
Vomitus in bronchus
7 T17.510- **Gastric contents in bronchus causing asphyxiation**
7 T17.518- **Gastric contents in bronchus causing other injury**
6 T17.52 **Food in bronchus**
Bones in bronchus
Seeds in bronchus
7 T17.520- **Food in bronchus causing asphyxiation**
7 T17.528- **Food in bronchus causing other injury**
6 T17.59 **Other foreign object in bronchus**
7 T17.590- **Other foreign object in bronchus causing asphyxiation**
7 T17.598- **Other foreign object in bronchus causing other injury**
5 T17.8 **Foreign body in other parts of respiratory tract**
Foreign body in bronchioles
Foreign body in lung
6 T17.80 **Unspecified foreign body in other parts of respiratory tract**
7 T17.800- **Unspecified foreign body in other parts of respiratory tract causing asphyxiation**
7 T17.808- **Unspecified foreign body in other parts of respiratory tract causing other injury**
6 T17.81 **Gastric contents in other parts of respiratory tract**
Aspiration of gastric contents into other parts of respiratory tract
Vomitus in other parts of respiratory tract
7 T17.810- **Gastric contents in other parts of respiratory tract causing asphyxiation**
7 T17.818- **Gastric contents in other parts of respiratory tract causing other injury**
6 T17.82 **Food in other parts of respiratory tract**
Bones in other parts of respiratory tract
Seeds in other parts of respiratory tract

7 T17.820- **Food in other parts of respiratory tract causing asphyxiation**

7 T17.828- **Food in other parts of respiratory tract causing other injury**

6 T17.89 **Other foreign object in other parts of respiratory tract**

7 T17.890- **Other foreign object in other parts of respiratory tract causing asphyxiation**

7 T17.898- **Other foreign object in other parts of respiratory tract causing other injury**

5 T17.9 **Foreign body in respiratory tract, part unspecified**

6 T17.90 **Unspecified foreign body in respiratory tract, part Unspecified**

7 T17.900- **Unspecified foreign body in respiratory tract, part unspecified causing asphyxiation**

7 T17.908- **Unspecified foreign body in respiratory tract, part unspecified causing other injury**

6 T17.91 **Gastric contents in respiratory tract, part unspecified**

Aspiration of gastric contents into respiratory tract, part unspecified

Vomitus in trachea respiratory tract, part unspecified

7 T17.910- **Gastric contents in respiratory tract, part unspecified causing asphyxiation**

7 T17.918- **Gastric contents in respiratory tract, part unspecified causing other injury**

6 T17.92 **Food in respiratory tract, part unspecified**

Bones in respiratory tract, part unspecified

Seeds in respiratory tract, part unspecified

7 T17.920- **Food in respiratory tract, part unspecified causing asphyxiation**

7 T17.928- **Food in respiratory tract, part unspecified causing other injury**

6 T17.99 **Other foreign object in respiratory tract, part unspecified**

7 T17.990- **Other foreign object in respiratory tract, part unspecified in causing asphyxiation**

7 T17.998- **Other foreign object in respiratory tract, part unspecified causing other injury**

4 T18 **Foreign body in alimentary tract**

EXCLUDES 2 *foreign body in pharynx (T17.2-)*

The appropriate 7th character is to be added to each code from category T18

A initial encounter

D subsequent encounter

S sequela

7 T18.0XX- **Foreign body in mouth**

5 T18.1 **Foreign body in esophagus**

EXCLUDES 2 *foreign body in respiratory tract (T17.-)*

6 T18.10 **Unspecified foreign body in esophagus**

7 T18.100- **Unspecified foreign body in esophagus causing compression of trachea**

Unspecified foreign body in esophagus causing obstruction of respiration

7 T18.108- **Unspecified foreign body in esophagus causing other injury**

6 T18.11 **Gastric contents in esophagus**

Vomitus in esophagus

7 T18.110- **Gastric contents in esophagus causing compression of trachea**

Gastric contents in esophagus causing obstruction of respiration

7 T18.118- **Gastric contents in esophagus causing other injury**

6 T18.12 **Food in esophagus**

Bones in esophagus

Seeds in esophagus

7 T18.120- **Food in esophagus causing compression of trachea**

Food in esophagus causing obstruction of respiration

7 T18.128- **Food in esophagus causing other injury**

6 T18.19 **Other foreign object in esophagus**

7 T18.190- **Other foreign object in esophagus causing compression of trachea**

Other foreign body in esophagus causing obstruction of respiration

AHA: 1Q 2015, 24

7 T18.198- **Other foreign object in esophagus causing other injury**

AHA: 1Q 2015, 24

7 T18.2XX- **Foreign body in stomach**

7 T18.3XX- **Foreign body in small intestine**

7 T18.4XX- **Foreign body in colon**

7 T18.5XX- **Foreign body in anus and rectum**

Foreign body in rectosigmoid (junction)

7 T18.8XX- **Foreign body in other parts of alimentary tract**

7 T18.9XX- **Foreign body of alimentary tract, part unspecified**

Foreign body in digestive system NOS

Swallowed foreign body NOS

4 T19 **Foreign body in genitourinary tract**

EXCLUDES 2 *complications due to implanted mesh (T83.7-)*
mechanical complications of contraceptive device (intrauterine) (vaginal) (T83.3-)
presence of contraceptive device (intrauterine) (vaginal) (Z97.5)

The appropriate 7th character is to be added to each code from category T19

A initial encounter

D subsequent encounter

S sequela

7 T19.0XX- **Foreign body in urethra**

7 T19.1XX- **Foreign body in bladder**

7 T19.2XX- **Foreign body in vulva and vagina** ♀

7 T19.3XX- **Foreign body in uterus** ♀

7 T19.4XX- **Foreign body in penis** ♂

7 T19.8XX- **Foreign body in other parts of genitourinary tract**

7 T19.9XX- **Foreign body in genitourinary tract, part unspecified**

Burns and corrosions (T20-T32)

INCLUDES burns (thermal) from electrical heating appliances
burns (thermal) from electricity
burns (thermal) from flame
burns (thermal) from friction
burns (thermal) from hot air and hot gases
burns (thermal) from hot objects
burns (thermal) from lightning
burns (thermal) from radiation
chemical burn [corrosion] (external) (internal)
scalds

EXCLUDES 2 *erythema [dermatitis] ab igne (L59.0)*
radiation-related disorders of the skin and subcutaneous tissue (L55-L59)
sunburn (L55.-)

GUIDELINES Section I.C.19.d.1)-5)

Sequence first the code that reflects the highest degree of burn when more than one burn is present.

a. When the reason for the admission or encounter is for treatment of external multiple burns, sequence first the code that reflects the burn of the highest degree.

b. When a patient has both internal and external burns, the circumstances of admission govern the selection of the principal diagnosis or first-listed diagnosis.

c. When a patient is admitted for burn injuries and other related conditions such as smoke inhalation and/or respiratory failure, the circumstances of admission govern the selection of the principal or first-listed diagnosis.

Classify burns of the same anatomic site and on the same side but of different degrees to the subcategory identifying the highest degree recorded in the diagnosis (e.g., for second and third degree burns of right thigh, assign only code T24.311-).

Non-healing burns are coded as acute burns. Necrosis of burned skin should be coded as a non-healed burn.

For any documented infected burn site, use an additional code for the infection.

When coding burns, assign separate codes for each burn site. Codes for burns of "multiple sites" should only be assigned when the medical record documentation does not specify the individual sites.

GUIDELINES Section I.C.19.d

The ICD-10-CM makes a distinction between burns and corrosions. The burn codes are for thermal burns, except sunburns, that come from a heat source, such as a fire or hot appliance. The burn codes are also for burns resulting from electricity and radiation. Corrosions are burns due to chemicals. The guidelines are the same for burns and corrosions.

CODING TIP ✓ A burn that is referred to as "not healing" should be coded as an acute burn using 7th character "A" or "D" depending upon treatment stage. Sequelae of a burn, such as contracture or keloid scarring, should be coded by first assigning the code for the residual condition, followed by the appropriate code to identify the burn with the 7th character "S" to indicate sequelae.

CODING TIP ✓ When a patient presents with a burn (other than sunburn), an additional code from Chapter 20 (External causes) should be added to indicate the cause (intent) of the burn.

Burns and corrosions of external body surface, specified by site (T20-T25)

INCLUDES burns and corrosions of first degree [erythema]
burns and corrosions of second degree [blisters][epidermal loss]
burns and corrosions of third degree [deep necrosis of underlying tissue] [full- thickness skin loss]

Use additional code from category T31 or T32 to identify extent of body surface involved

GUIDELINES Section I.C.19.d

Current burns (T20-T25) are classified by depth, extent and by agent (X code). Burns are classified by depth as first degree (erythema), second degree (blistering), and third degree (full-thickness involvement). Burns of the eye and internal organs (T26-T28) are classified by site, but not by degree.

4 **T20 Burn and corrosion of head, face, and neck**

EXCLUDES 2 *burn and corrosion of ear drum (T28.41, T28.91)*
burn and corrosion of eye and adnexa (T26.-)
burn and corrosion of mouth and pharynx (T28.0)

The appropriate 7th character is to be added to each code from category T20
A initial encounter
D subsequent encounter
S sequela

5 **T20.0 Burn of unspecified degree of head, face, and neck**
Use additional external cause code to identify the source, place and intent of the burn (X00-X19, X75-X77, X96-X98, Y92)

7 **T20.00X- Burn of unspecified degree of head, face, and neck, unspecified site**

6 **T20.01 Burn of unspecified degree of ear [any part, except ear drum]**
EXCLUDES 2 *burn of ear drum (T28.41-)*

7 ⊟ **T20.011- Burn of unspecified degree of right ear [any part, except ear drum]**

7 ⊟ **T20.012- Burn of unspecified degree of left ear [any part, except ear drum]**

7 ⊟ **T20.019- Burn of unspecified degree of unspecified ear [any part, except ear drum]**

7 **T20.02X- Burn of unspecified degree of lip(s)**

7 **T20.03X- Burn of unspecified degree of chin**

7 **T20.04X- Burn of unspecified degree of nose (septum)**

7 **T20.05X- Burn of unspecified degree of scalp [any part]**

7 **T20.06X- Burn of unspecified degree of forehead and cheek**

7 **T20.07X- Burn of unspecified degree of neck**

7 **T20.09X- Burn of unspecified degree of multiple sites of head, face, and neck**

5 **T20.1 Burn of first degree of head, face, and neck**
Use additional external cause code to identify the source, place and intent of the burn (X00-X19, X75-X77, X96-X98, Y92)

7 **T20.10X- Burn of first degree of head, face, and neck, unspecified site**

6 **T20.11 Burn of first degree of ear [any part, except ear drum]**
EXCLUDES 2 *burn of ear drum (T28.41-)*

7 ⊟ **T20.111- Burn of first degree of right ear [any part, except ear drum]**

7 ⊟ **T20.112- Burn of first degree of left ear [any part, except ear drum]**

7 ⊟ **T20.119- Burn of first degree of unspecified ear [any part, except ear drum]**

7 **T20.12X- Burn of first degree of lip(s)**

7 **T20.13X- Burn of first degree of chin**

7 **T20.14X- Burn of first degree of nose (septum)**

7 **T20.15X- Burn of first degree of scalp [any part]**

7 **T20.16X- Burn of first degree of forehead and cheek**

7 **T20.17X- Burn of first degree of neck**

7 **T20.19X- Burn of first degree of multiple sites of head, face, and neck**

5 **T20.2 Burn of second degree of head, face, and neck**
Use additional external cause code to identify the source, place and intent of the burn (X00-X19, X75-X77, X96-X98, Y92)

7 **T20.20X- Burn of second degree of head, face, and neck, unspecified site**

6 **T20.21 Burn of second degree of ear [any part, except ear drum]**
EXCLUDES 2 *burn of ear drum (T28.41-)*

7 ⊟ **T20.211- Burn of second degree of right ear [any part, except ear drum]**

7 ⊟ **T20.212- Burn of second degree of left ear [any part, except ear drum]**

7 ⊟ **T20.219- Burn of second degree of unspecified ear [any part, except ear drum]**

7 **T20.22X- Burn of second degree of lip(s)**

7 **T20.23X- Burn of second degree of chin**

7 **T20.24X- Burn of second degree of nose (septum)**

7 **T20.25X- Burn of second degree of scalp [any part]**
AHA: (T20.25XS) 1Q 2015, 19

7 **T20.26X- Burn of second degree of forehead and cheek**

7 **T20.27X- Burn of second degree of neck**

7 **T20.29X- Burn of second degree of multiple sites of head, face, and neck**

5 **T20.3 Burn of third degree of head, face, and neck**
Use additional external cause code to identify the source, place and intent of the burn (X00-X19, X75-X77, X96-X98, Y92)

7 **T20.30X- Burn of third degree of head, face, and neck, unspecified site**

6 T20.31 Burn of third degree of ear [any part, except ear drum]
EXCLUDES 2 *burn of ear drum (T28.41-)*

7 T20.311- Burn of third degree of right ear [any part, except ear drum]

7 T20.312- Burn of third degree of left ear [any part, except ear drum]
AHA: (T20.312S) 1Q 2015, 18

7 T20.319- Burn of third degree of unspecified ear [any part, except ear drum]

7 T20.32X- Burn of third degree of lip(s)

7 T20.33X- Burn of third degree of chin

7 T20.34X- Burn of third degree of nose (septum)

7 T20.35X- Burn of third degree of scalp [any part]

7 T20.36X- Burn of third degree of forehead and cheek

7 T20.37X- Burn of third degree of neck

7 T20.39X- Burn of third degree of multiple sites of head, face, and neck

5 T20.4 Corrosion of unspecified degree of head, face, and neck
Code first:
(T51-T65) to identify chemical and intent
Use additional external cause code to identify place (Y92)

7 T20.40X- Corrosion of unspecified degree of head, face, and neck, unspecified site

6 T20.41 Corrosion of unspecified degree of ear [any part, except ear drum]
EXCLUDES 2 *corrosion of ear drum (T28.91-)*

7 T20.411- Corrosion of unspecified degree of right ear [any part, except ear drum]

7 T20.412- Corrosion of unspecified degree of left ear [any part, except ear drum]

7 T20.419- Corrosion of unspecified degree of unspecified ear [any part, except ear drum]

7 T20.42X- Corrosion of unspecified degree of lip(s)

7 T20.43X- Corrosion of unspecified degree of chin

7 T20.44X- Corrosion of unspecified degree of nose (septum)

7 T20.45X- Corrosion of unspecified degree of scalp [any part]

7 T20.46X- Corrosion of unspecified degree of forehead and cheek

7 T20.47X- Corrosion of unspecified degree of neck

7 T20.49X- Corrosion of unspecified degree of multiple sites of head, face, and neck

5 T20.5 Corrosion of first degree of head, face, and neck
Code first:
(T51-T65) to identify chemical and intent
Use additional external cause code to identify place (Y92)

7 T20.50X- Corrosion of first degree of head, face, and neck, unspecified site

6 T20.51 Corrosion of first degree of ear [any part, except ear drum]
EXCLUDES 2 *corrosion of ear drum (T28.91-)*

7 T20.511- Corrosion of first degree of right ear [any part, except ear drum]

7 T20.512- Corrosion of first degree of left ear [any part, except ear drum]

7 T20.519- Corrosion of first degree of unspecified ear [any part, except ear drum]

7 T20.52X- Corrosion of first degree of lip(s)

7 T20.53X- Corrosion of first degree of chin

7 T20.54X- Corrosion of first degree of nose (septum)

7 T20.55X- Corrosion of first degree of scalp [any part]

7 T20.56X- Corrosion of first degree of forehead and cheek

7 T20.57X- Corrosion of first degree of neck

7 T20.59X- Corrosion of first degree of multiple sites of head, face, and neck

5 T20.6 Corrosion of second degree of head, face, and neck
Code first:
(T51-T65) to identify chemical and intent
Use additional external cause code to identify place (Y92)

7 T20.60X- Corrosion of second degree of head, face, and neck, unspecified site

6 T20.61 Corrosion of second degree of ear [any part, except ear drum]
EXCLUDES 2 *corrosion of ear drum (T28.91-)*

7 T20.611- Corrosion of second degree of right ear [any part, except ear drum]

7 T20.612- Corrosion of second degree of left ear [any part, except ear drum]

7 T20.619- Corrosion of second degree of unspecified ear [any part, except ear drum]

7 T20.62X- Corrosion of second degree of lip(s)

7 T20.63X- Corrosion of second degree of chin

7 T20.64X- Corrosion of second degree of nose (septum)

7 T20.65X- Corrosion of second degree of scalp [any part]

7 T20.66X- Corrosion of second degree of forehead and cheek

7 T20.67X- Corrosion of second degree of neck

7 T20.69X- Corrosion of second degree of multiple sites of head, face, and neck

5 T20.7 Corrosion of third degree of head, face, and neck
Code first:
(T51-T65) to identify chemical and intent
Use additional external cause code to identify place (Y92)

7 T20.70X- Corrosion of third degree of head, face, and neck, unspecified site

6 T20.71 Corrosion of third degree of ear [any part, except ear drum]
EXCLUDES 2 *corrosion of ear drum (T28.91-)*

7 T20.711- Corrosion of third degree of right ear [any part, except ear drum]

7 T20.712- Corrosion of third degree of left ear [any part, except ear drum]

7 T20.719- Corrosion of third degree of unspecified ear [any part, except ear drum]

7 T20.72X- Corrosion of third degree of lip(s)

7 T20.73X- Corrosion of third degree of chin

7 T20.74X- Corrosion of third degree of nose (septum)

7 T20.75X- Corrosion of third degree of scalp [any part]

7 T20.76X- Corrosion of third degree of forehead and cheek

7 T20.77X- Corrosion of third degree of neck

7 T20.79X- Corrosion of third degree of multiple sites of head, face, and neck

4 T21 Burn and corrosion of trunk
INCLUDES burns and corrosion of hip region
EXCLUDES 2 *burns and corrosion of axilla (T22.- with fifth character 4)*
burns and corrosion of scapular region (T22.- with fifth character 6)
burns and corrosion of shoulder (T22.- with fifth character 5)

The appropriate 7th character is to be added to each code from category T21
A initial encounter
D subsequent encounter
S sequela

CODING TIP ✓ Do not use Z codes for skin grafts, dressing changes, drains, etc., for traumatic wounds of any type, including burns. Continue to code the burn with the appropriate 7th character.

5 T21.0 Burn of unspecified degree of trunk
Use additional external cause code to identify the source, place and intent of the burn (X00-X19, X75-X77, X96-X98, Y92)

7 T21.00X- Burn of unspecified degree of trunk, unspecified site

▲ 7 T21.01X- Burn of unspecified degree of chest wall
Burn of unspecified degree of breast

7 T21.02X- Burn of unspecified degree of abdominal wall
Burn of unspecified degree of flank
Burn of unspecified degree of groin

7 T21.03X- Burn of unspecified degree of upper back
Burn of unspecified degree of interscapular region

7 T21.04X- Burn of unspecified degree of lower back

7 T21.05X- Burn of unspecified degree of buttock
Burn of unspecified degree of anus

7 T21.06X- Burn of unspecified degree of male genital region ♂
Burn of unspecified degree of penis
Burn of unspecified degree of scrotum
Burn of unspecified degree of testis

7 T21.07X- Burn of unspecified degree of female genital region ♀
Burn of unspecified degree of labium (majus) (minus)
Burn of unspecified degree of perineum
Burn of unspecified degree of vulva
EXCLUDES 2 *burn of vagina (T28.3)*

7 T21.09X- Burn of unspecified degree of other site of trunk

5 T21.1 Burn of first degree of trunk
Use additional external cause code to identify the source, place and intent of the burn (X00-X19, X75-X77, X96-X98, Y92)

7 T21.10X- Burn of first degree of trunk, unspecified site

7 T21.11X- Burn of first degree of chest wall
Burn of first degree of breast

7 T21.12X- Burn of first degree of abdominal wall
Burn of first degree of flank
Burn of first degree of groin

7 T21.13X- Burn of first degree of upper back
Burn of first degree of interscapular region

7 T21.14X- Burn of first degree of lower back

7 T21.15X- Burn of first degree of buttock
Burn of first degree of anus

7 T21.16X- Burn of first degree of male genital region ♂
Burn of first degree of penis
Burn of first degree of scrotum
Burn of first degree of testis

7 T21.17X- Burn of first degree of female genital region ♀
Burn of first degree of labium (majus) (minus)
Burn of first degree of perineum
Burn of first degree of vulva
EXCLUDES 2 *burn of vagina (T28.3)*

7 T21.19X- Burn of first degree of other site of trunk

5 T21.2 Burn of second degree of trunk
Use additional external cause code to identify the source, place and intent of the burn (X00-X19, X75-X77, X96-X98, Y92)

7 T21.20X- Burn of second degree of trunk, unspecified site

7 T21.21X- Burn of second degree of chest wall
Burn of second degree of breast

7 T21.22X- Burn of second degree of abdominal wall
Burn of second degree of flank
Burn of second degree of groin

7 T21.23X- Burn of second degree of upper back
Burn of second degree of interscapular region

7 T21.24X- Burn of second degree of lower back

7 T21.25X- Burn of second degree of buttock
Burn of second degree of anus

7 T21.26X- Burn of second degree of male genital region ♂
Burn of second degree of penis
Burn of second degree of scrotum
Burn of second degree of testis

7 T21.27X- Burn of second degree of female genital region ♀
Burn of second degree of labium (majus) (minus)
Burn of second degree of perineum
Burn of second degree of vulva
EXCLUDES 2 *burn of vagina (T28.3)*

7 T21.29X- Burn of second degree of other site of trunk

5 T21.3 Burn of third degree of trunk
Use additional external cause code to identify the source, place and intent of the burn (X00-X19, X75-X77, X96-X98, Y92)

7 T21.30X- Burn of third degree of trunk, unspecified site

7 T21.31X- Burn of third degree of chest wall
Burn of third degree of breast
AHA: (T21.31XD) 2Q 2016, 6

7 T21.32X- Burn of third degree of abdominal wall
Burn of third degree of flank
Burn of third degree of groin

7 T21.33X- Burn of third degree of upper back
Burn of third degree of interscapular region

7 T21.34X- Burn of third degree of lower back

7 T21.35X- Burn of third degree of buttock
Burn of third degree of anus

7 T21.36X- Burn of third degree of male genital region ♂
Burn of third degree of penis
Burn of third degree of scrotum
Burn of third degree of testis

7 T21.37X- Burn of third degree of female genital region ♀
Burn of third degree of labium (majus) (minus)
Burn of third degree of perineum
Burn of third degree of vulva
EXCLUDES 2 *burn of vagina (T28.3)*

7 T21.39X- Burn of third degree of other site of trunk

5 T21.4 Corrosion of unspecified degree of trunk
Code first:
(T51-T65) to identify chemical and intent
Use additional external cause code to identify place (Y92)

7 T21.40X- Corrosion of unspecified degree of trunk, unspecified site

7 T21.41X- Corrosion of unspecified degree of chest wall
Corrosion of unspecified degree of breast

7 T21.42X- Corrosion of unspecified degree of abdominal wall
Corrosion of unspecified degree of flank
Corrosion of unspecified degree of groin

7 T21.43X- Corrosion of unspecified degree of upper back
Corrosion of unspecified degree of interscapular region

7 T21.44X- Corrosion of unspecified degree of lower back

7 T21.45X- Corrosion of unspecified degree of buttock
Corrosion of unspecified degree of anus

7 T21.46X- Corrosion of unspecified degree of male genital region ♂
Corrosion of unspecified degree of penis
Corrosion of unspecified degree of scrotum
Corrosion of unspecified degree of testis

7 T21.47X- Corrosion of unspecified degree of female genital region ♀
Corrosion of unspecified degree of labium (majus) (minus)
Corrosion of unspecified degree of perineum
Corrosion of unspecified degree of vulva
EXCLUDES 2 *corrosion of vagina (T28.8)*

7 T21.49X- Corrosion of unspecified degree of other site of trunk

5 T21.5 Corrosion of first degree of trunk
Code first:
(T51-T65) to identify chemical and intent
Use additional external cause code to identify place (Y92)

7 T21.50X- Corrosion of first degree of trunk, unspecified site

7 T21.51X- Corrosion of first degree of chest wall
Corrosion of first degree of breast

7 T21.52X- Corrosion of first degree of abdominal wall
Corrosion of first degree of flank
Corrosion of first degree of groin

7 T21.53X- Corrosion of first degree of upper back
Corrosion of first degree of interscapular region

7 T21.54X- Corrosion of first degree of lower back

7 T21.55X- Corrosion of first degree of buttock
Corrosion of first degree of anus

7 T21.56X- Corrosion of first degree of male genital region ♂
Corrosion of first degree of penis
Corrosion of first degree of scrotum
Corrosion of first degree of testis

7 T21.57X- Corrosion of first degree of female genital region ♀
Corrosion of first degree of labium (majus) (minus)
Corrosion of first degree of perineum
Corrosion of first degree of vulva
EXCLUDES 2 *corrosion of vagina (T28.8)*

7 T21.59X- Corrosion of first degree of other site of trunk

5 T21.6 Corrosion of second degree of trunk
Code first:
(T51-T65) to identify chemical and intent
Use additional external cause code to identify place (Y92)

7 T21.60X- **Corrosion of second degree of trunk, unspecified site**

7 T21.61X- **Corrosion of second degree of chest wall**
Corrosion of second degree of breast

7 T21.62X- **Corrosion of second degree of abdominal wall**
Corrosion of second degree of flank
Corrosion of second degree of groin

7 T21.63X- **Corrosion of second degree of upper back**
Corrosion of second degree of interscapular region

7 T21.64X- **Corrosion of second degree of lower back**

7 T21.65X- **Corrosion of second degree of buttock**
Corrosion of second degree of anus

7 T21.66X- **Corrosion of second degree of male genital region** ♂
Corrosion of second degree of penis
Corrosion of second degree of scrotum
Corrosion of second degree of testis

7 T21.67X- **Corrosion of second degree of female genital region** ♀
Corrosion of second degree of labium (majus) (minus)
Corrosion of second degree of perineum
Corrosion of second degree of vulva
EXCLUDES 2 *corrosion of vagina (T28.8)*

7 T21.69X- **Corrosion of second degree of other site of trunk**

5 T21.7 **Corrosion of third degree of trunk**
Code first:
(T51-T65) to identify chemical and intent
Use additional external cause code to identify place (Y92)

7 T21.70X- **Corrosion of third degree of trunk, unspecified site**

7 T21.71X- **Corrosion of third degree of chest wall**
Corrosion of third degree of breast

7 T21.72X- **Corrosion of third degree of abdominal wall**
Corrosion of third degree of flank
Corrosion of third degree of groin

7 T21.73X- **Corrosion of third degree of upper back**
Corrosion of third degree of interscapular region

7 T21.74X- **Corrosion of third degree of lower back**

7 T21.75X- **Corrosion of third degree of buttock**
Corrosion of third degree of anus

7 T21.76X- **Corrosion of third degree of male genital region** ♂
Corrosion of third degree of penis
Corrosion of third degree of scrotum
Corrosion of third degree of testis

7 T21.77X- **Corrosion of third degree of female genital region** ♀
Corrosion of third degree of labium (majus) (minus)
Corrosion of third degree of perineum
Corrosion of third degree of vulva
EXCLUDES 2 *corrosion of vagina (T28.8)*

7 T21.79X- **Corrosion of third degree of other site of trunk**

4 T22 Burn and corrosion of shoulder and upper limb, except wrist and hand

EXCLUDES 2 *burn and corrosion of interscapular region (T21.-)*
burn and corrosion of wrist and hand (T23.-)

The appropriate 7th character is to be added to each code from category T22
A initial encounter
D subsequent encounter
S sequela

CODING TIP ✓ Do not use Z codes for skin grafts, dressing changes, drains, etc., for traumatic wounds of any type, including burns. Continue to code the burn with the appropriate 7th character.

5 T22.0 **Burn of unspecified degree of shoulder and upper limb, except wrist and hand**
Use additional external cause code to identify the source, place and intent of the burn (X00-X19, X75-X77, X96-X98, Y92)

7 T22.00X- **Burn of unspecified degree of shoulder and upper limb, except wrist and hand, unspecified site**

6 T22.01 **Burn of unspecified degree of forearm**

7 ⊟ T22.011- **Burn of unspecified degree of right forearm**

7 ⊟ T22.012- **Burn of unspecified degree of left forearm**

7 ⊟ T22.019- **Burn of unspecified degree of unspecified forearm**

6 T22.02 **Burn of unspecified degree of elbow**

7 ⊟ T22.021- **Burn of unspecified degree of right elbow**

7 ⊟ T22.022- **Burn of unspecified degree of left elbow**

7 ⊟ T22.029- **Burn of unspecified degree of unspecified elbow**

6 T22.03 **Burn of unspecified degree of upper arm**

7 ⊟ T22.031- **Burn of unspecified degree of right upper arm**

7 ⊟ T22.032- **Burn of unspecified degree of left upper arm**

7 ⊟ T22.039- **Burn of unspecified degree of unspecified upper arm**

6 T22.04 **Burn of unspecified degree of axilla**

7 ⊟ T22.041- **Burn of unspecified degree of right axilla**

7 ⊟ T22.042- **Burn of unspecified degree of left axilla**

7 ⊟ T22.049- **Burn of unspecified degree of unspecified axilla**

6 T22.05 **Burn of unspecified degree of shoulder**

7 ⊟ T22.051- **Burn of unspecified degree of right shoulder**

7 ⊟ T22.052- **Burn of unspecified degree of left shoulder**

7 ⊟ T22.059- **Burn of unspecified degree of unspecified shoulder**

6 T22.06 **Burn of unspecified degree of scapular region**

7 ⊟ T22.061- **Burn of unspecified degree of right scapular region**

7 ⊟ T22.062- **Burn of unspecified degree of left scapular region**

7 ⊟ T22.069- **Burn of unspecified degree of unspecified scapular region**

6 T22.09 **Burn of unspecified degree of multiple sites of shoulder and upper limb, except wrist and hand**

7 ⊟ T22.091- **Burn of unspecified degree of multiple sites of right shoulder and upper limb, except wrist and hand**

7 ⊟ T22.092- **Burn of unspecified degree of multiple sites of left shoulder and upper limb, except wrist and hand**

7 ⊟ T22.099- **Burn of unspecified degree of multiple sites of unspecified shoulder and upper limb, except wrist and hand**

5 T22.1 **Burn of first degree of shoulder and upper limb, except wrist and hand**
Use additional external cause code to identify the source, place and intent of the burn (X00-X19, X75-X77, X96-X98, Y92)

7 T22.10X- **Burn of first degree of shoulder and upper limb, except wrist and hand, unspecified site**

6 T22.11 **Burn of first degree of forearm**

7 ⊟ T22.111- **Burn of first degree of right forearm**

7 ⊟ T22.112- **Burn of first degree of left forearm**

7 ⊟ T22.119- **Burn of first degree of unspecified forearm**

6 T22.12 **Burn of first degree of elbow**

7 ⊟ T22.121- **Burn of first degree of right elbow**

7 ⊟ T22.122- **Burn of first degree of left elbow**

7 ⊟ T22.129- **Burn of first degree of unspecified elbow**

6 T22.13 **Burn of first degree of upper arm**

7 ⊟ T22.131- **Burn of first degree of right upper arm**

7 ⊟ T22.132- **Burn of first degree of left upper arm**

7 ⊟ T22.139- **Burn of first degree of unspecified upper arm**

6 T22.14 **Burn of first degree of axilla**

7 ⊟ T22.141- **Burn of first degree of right axilla**

7 ⊟ T22.142- **Burn of first degree of left axilla**

7 ⊟ T22.149- **Burn of first degree of unspecified axilla**

6 T22.15 **Burn of first degree of shoulder**

7 ⊟ T22.151- **Burn of first degree of right shoulder**

7 ⊟ T22.152- **Burn of first degree of left shoulder**

7 ⊟ T22.159- **Burn of first degree of unspecified shoulder**

6 T22.16 **Burn of first degree of scapular region**

7 ⊟ T22.161- **Burn of first degree of right scapular region**

7 ⊟ T22.162- **Burn of first degree of left scapular region**

T22.169- Burn of first degree of unspecified scapular region
T22.19 Burn of first degree of multiple sites of shoulder and upper limb, except wrist and hand
T22.191- Burn of first degree of multiple sites of right shoulder and upper limb, except wrist and hand
T22.192- Burn of first degree of multiple sites of left shoulder and upper limb, except wrist and hand
T22.199- Burn of first degree of multiple sites of unspecified shoulder and upper limb, except wrist and hand
T22.2 Burn of second degree of shoulder and upper limb, except wrist and hand
Use additional external cause code to identify the source, place and intent of the burn (X00-X19, X75-X77, X96-X98, Y92)
T22.20X- Burn of second degree of shoulder and upper limb, except wrist and hand, unspecified site
T22.21 Burn of second degree of forearm
T22.211- Burn of second degree of right forearm
T22.212- Burn of second degree of left forearm
T22.219- Burn of second degree of unspecified forearm
T22.22 Burn of second degree of elbow
T22.221- Burn of second degree of right elbow
T22.222- Burn of second degree of left elbow
T22.229- Burn of second degree of unspecified elbow
T22.23 Burn of second degree of upper arm
T22.231- Burn of second degree of right upper arm
T22.232- Burn of second degree of left upper arm
T22.239- Burn of second degree of unspecified upper arm
T22.24 Burn of second degree of axilla
T22.241- Burn of second degree of right axilla
T22.242- Burn of second degree of left axilla
T22.249- Burn of second degree of unspecified axilla
T22.25 Burn of second degree of shoulder
T22.251- Burn of second degree of right shoulder
T22.252- Burn of second degree of left shoulder
T22.259- Burn of second degree of unspecified shoulder
T22.26 Burn of second degree of scapular region
T22.261- Burn of second degree of right scapular region
T22.262- Burn of second degree of left scapular region
T22.269- Burn of second degree of unspecified scapular region
T22.29 Burn of second degree of multiple sites of shoulder and upper limb, except wrist and hand
T22.291- Burn of second degree of multiple sites of right shoulder and upper limb, except wrist and hand
T22.292- Burn of second degree of multiple sites of left shoulder and upper limb, except wrist and hand
T22.299- Burn of second degree of multiple sites of unspecified shoulder and upper limb, except wrist and hand
T22.3 Burn of third degree of shoulder and upper limb, except wrist and hand
Use additional external cause code to identify the source, place and intent of the burn (X00-X19, X75-X77, X96-X98, Y92)
T22.30X- Burn of third degree of shoulder and upper limb, except wrist and hand, unspecified site
T22.31 Burn of third degree of forearm
T22.311- Burn of third degree of right forearm
T22.312- Burn of third degree of left forearm
T22.319- Burn of third degree of unspecified forearm
T22.32 Burn of third degree of elbow
T22.321- Burn of third degree of right elbow
T22.322- Burn of third degree of left elbow
T22.329- Burn of third degree of unspecified elbow
T22.33 Burn of third degree of upper arm
T22.331- Burn of third degree of right upper arm
T22.332- Burn of third degree of left upper arm
T22.339- Burn of third degree of unspecified upper arm
T22.34 Burn of third degree of axilla
T22.341- Burn of third degree of right axilla
T22.342- Burn of third degree of left axilla
T22.349- Burn of third degree of unspecified axilla
T22.35 Burn of third degree of shoulder
T22.351- Burn of third degree of right shoulder
T22.352- Burn of third degree of left shoulder
T22.359- Burn of third degree of unspecified shoulder
T22.36 Burn of third degree of scapular region
T22.361- Burn of third degree of right scapular region
T22.362- Burn of third degree of left scapular region
T22.369- Burn of third degree of unspecified scapular region
T22.39 Burn of third degree of multiple sites of shoulder and upper limb, except wrist and hand
T22.391- Burn of third degree of multiple sites of right shoulder and upper limb, except wrist and hand
T22.392- Burn of third degree of multiple sites of left shoulder and upper limb, except wrist and hand
T22.399- Burn of third degree of multiple sites of unspecified shoulder and upper limb, except wrist and hand
T22.4 Corrosion of unspecified degree of shoulder and upper limb, except wrist and hand
Code first:
(T51-T65) to identify chemical and intent
Use additional external cause code to identify place (Y92)
T22.40X- Corrosion of unspecified degree of shoulder and upper limb, except wrist and hand, unspecified site
T22.41 Corrosion of unspecified degree of forearm
T22.411- Corrosion of unspecified degree of right forearm
T22.412- Corrosion of unspecified degree of left forearm
T22.419- Corrosion of unspecified degree of unspecified forearm
T22.42 Corrosion of unspecified degree of elbow
T22.421- Corrosion of unspecified degree of right elbow
T22.422- Corrosion of unspecified degree of left elbow
T22.429- Corrosion of unspecified degree of unspecified elbow
T22.43 Corrosion of unspecified degree of upper arm
T22.431- Corrosion of unspecified degree of right upper arm
T22.432- Corrosion of unspecified degree of left upper arm
T22.439- Corrosion of unspecified degree of unspecified upper arm
T22.44 Corrosion of unspecified degree of axilla
T22.441- Corrosion of unspecified degree of right axilla
T22.442- Corrosion of unspecified degree of left axilla
T22.449- Corrosion of unspecified degree of unspecified axilla
T22.45 Corrosion of unspecified degree of shoulder
T22.451- Corrosion of unspecified degree of right shoulder
T22.452- Corrosion of unspecified degree of left shoulder
T22.459- Corrosion of unspecified degree of unspecified shoulder
T22.46 Corrosion of unspecified degree of scapular region
T22.461- Corrosion of unspecified degree of right scapular region
T22.462- Corrosion of unspecified degree of left scapular region
T22.469- Corrosion of unspecified degree of unspecified scapular region
T22.49 Corrosion of unspecified degree of multiple sites of shoulder and upper limb, except wrist and hand

- T22.491- Corrosion of unspecified degree of multiple sites of right shoulder and upper limb, except wrist and hand
- T22.492- Corrosion of unspecified degree of multiple sites of left shoulder and upper limb, except wrist and hand
- T22.499- Corrosion of unspecified degree of multiple sites of unspecified shoulder and upper limb, except wrist and hand

T22.5 Corrosion of first degree of shoulder and upper limb, except wrist and hand
Code first:
(T51-T65) to identify chemical and intent
Use additional external cause code to identify place (Y92)

- T22.50X- Corrosion of first degree of shoulder and upper limb, except wrist and hand unspecified site
- T22.51 Corrosion of first degree of forearm
  - T22.511- Corrosion of first degree of right forearm
  - T22.512- Corrosion of first degree of left forearm
  - T22.519- Corrosion of first degree of unspecified forearm
- T22.52 Corrosion of first degree of elbow
  - T22.521- Corrosion of first degree of right elbow
  - T22.522- Corrosion of first degree of left elbow
  - T22.529- Corrosion of first degree of unspecified elbow
- T22.53 Corrosion of first degree of upper arm
  - T22.531- Corrosion of first degree of right upper arm
  - T22.532- Corrosion of first degree of left upper arm
  - T22.539- Corrosion of first degree of unspecified upper arm
- T22.54 Corrosion of first degree of axilla
  - T22.541- Corrosion of first degree of right axilla
  - T22.542- Corrosion of first degree of left axilla
  - T22.549- Corrosion of first degree of unspecified axilla
- T22.55 Corrosion of first degree of shoulder
  - T22.551- Corrosion of first degree of right shoulder
  - T22.552- Corrosion of first degree of left shoulder
  - T22.559- Corrosion of first degree of unspecified shoulder
- T22.56 Corrosion of first degree of scapular region
  - T22.561- Corrosion of first degree of right scapular region
  - T22.562- Corrosion of first degree of left scapular region
  - T22.569- Corrosion of first degree of unspecified scapular region
- T22.59 Corrosion of first degree of multiple sites of shoulder and upper limb, except wrist and hand
  - T22.591- Corrosion of first degree of multiple sites of right shoulder and upper limb, except wrist and hand
  - T22.592- Corrosion of first degree of multiple sites of left shoulder and upper limb, except wrist and hand
  - T22.599- Corrosion of first degree of multiple sites of unspecified shoulder and upper limb, except wrist and hand

T22.6 Corrosion of second degree of shoulder and upper limb, except wrist and hand
Code first:
(T51-T65) to identify chemical and intent
Use additional external cause code to identify place (Y92)

- T22.60X- Corrosion of second degree of shoulder and upper limb, except wrist and hand, unspecified site
- T22.61 Corrosion of second degree of forearm
  - T22.611- Corrosion of second degree of right forearm
  - T22.612- Corrosion of second degree of left forearm
  - T22.619- Corrosion of second degree of unspecified forearm
- T22.62 Corrosion of second degree of elbow
  - T22.621- Corrosion of second degree of right elbow
  - T22.622- Corrosion of second degree of left elbow
  - T22.629- Corrosion of second degree of unspecified elbow
- T22.63 Corrosion of second degree of upper arm
  - T22.631- Corrosion of second degree of right upper arm
  - T22.632- Corrosion of second degree of left upper arm
  - T22.639- Corrosion of second degree of unspecified upper arm
- T22.64 Corrosion of second degree of axilla
  - T22.641- Corrosion of second degree of right axilla
  - T22.642- Corrosion of second degree of left axilla
  - T22.649- Corrosion of second degree of unspecified axilla
- T22.65 Corrosion of second degree of shoulder
  - T22.651- Corrosion of second degree of right shoulder
  - T22.652- Corrosion of second degree of left shoulder
  - T22.659- Corrosion of second degree of unspecified shoulder
- T22.66 Corrosion of second degree of scapular region
  - T22.661- Corrosion of second degree of right scapular region
  - T22.662- Corrosion of second degree of left scapular region
  - T22.669- Corrosion of second degree of unspecified scapular region
- T22.69 Corrosion of second degree of multiple sites of shoulder and upper limb, except wrist and hand
  - T22.691- Corrosion of second degree of multiple sites of right shoulder and upper limb, except wrist and hand
  - T22.692- Corrosion of second degree of multiple sites of left shoulder and upper limb, except wrist and hand
  - T22.699- Corrosion of second degree of multiple sites of unspecified shoulder and upper limb, except wrist and hand

T22.7 Corrosion of third degree of shoulder and upper limb, except wrist and hand
Code first:
(T51-T65) to identify chemical and intent
Use additional external cause code to identify place (Y92)

- T22.70X- Corrosion of third degree of shoulder and upper limb, except wrist and hand, unspecified site
- T22.71 Corrosion of third degree of forearm
  - T22.711- Corrosion of third degree of right forearm
  - T22.712- Corrosion of third degree of left forearm
  - T22.719- Corrosion of third degree of unspecified forearm
- T22.72 Corrosion of third degree of elbow
  - T22.721- Corrosion of third degree of right elbow
  - T22.722- Corrosion of third degree of left elbow
  - T22.729- Corrosion of third degree of unspecified elbow
- T22.73 Corrosion of third degree of upper arm
  - T22.731- Corrosion of third degree of right upper arm
  - T22.732- Corrosion of third degree of left upper arm
  - T22.739- Corrosion of third degree of unspecified upper arm
- T22.74 Corrosion of third degree of axilla
  - T22.741- Corrosion of third degree of right axilla
  - T22.742- Corrosion of third degree of left axilla
  - T22.749- Corrosion of third degree of unspecified axilla
- T22.75 Corrosion of third degree of shoulder
  - T22.751- Corrosion of third degree of right shoulder
  - T22.752- Corrosion of third degree of left shoulder
  - T22.759- Corrosion of third degree of unspecified shoulder
- T22.76 Corrosion of third degree of scapular region
  - T22.761- Corrosion of third degree of right scapular region
  - T22.762- Corrosion of third degree of left scapular region
  - T22.769- Corrosion of third degree of unspecified scapular region
- T22.79 Corrosion of third degree of multiple sites of shoulder and upper limb, except wrist and hand
  - T22.791- Corrosion of third degree of multiple sites of right shoulder and upper limb, except wrist and hand
  - T22.792- Corrosion of third degree of multiple sites of left shoulder and upper limb, except wrist and hand

T22.799- Corrosion of third degree of multiple sites of unspecified shoulder and upper limb, except wrist and hand

T23 Burn and corrosion of wrist and hand

The appropriate 7th character is to be added to each code from category T23
A initial encounter
D subsequent encounter
S sequela

CODING TIP✓ Do not use Z codes for skin grafts, dressing changes, drains, etc., for traumatic wounds of any type, including burns. Continue to code the burn with the appropriate 7th character.

T23.0 Burn of unspecified degree of wrist and hand
Use additional external cause code to identify the source, place and intent of the burn (X00-X19, X75-X77, X96-X98, Y92)

T23.00 Burn of unspecified degree of hand, unspecified site
T23.001- Burn of unspecified degree of right hand, unspecified site
T23.002- Burn of unspecified degree of left hand, unspecified site
T23.009- Burn of unspecified degree of unspecified hand, unspecified site
T23.01 Burn of unspecified degree of thumb (nail)
T23.011- Burn of unspecified degree of right thumb (nail)
T23.012- Burn of unspecified degree of left thumb (nail)
T23.019- Burn of unspecified degree of unspecified thumb (nail)
T23.02 Burn of unspecified degree of single finger (nail) except thumb
T23.021- Burn of unspecified degree of single right finger (nail) except thumb
T23.022- Burn of unspecified degree of single left finger (nail) except thumb
T23.029- Burn of unspecified degree of unspecified single finger (nail) except thumb
T23.03 Burn of unspecified degree of multiple fingers (nail), not including thumb
T23.031- Burn of unspecified degree of multiple right fingers (nail), not including thumb
T23.032- Burn of unspecified degree of multiple left fingers (nail), not including thumb
T23.039- Burn of unspecified degree of unspecified multiple fingers (nail), not including thumb
T23.04 Burn of unspecified degree of multiple fingers (nail), including thumb
T23.041- Burn of unspecified degree of multiple right fingers (nail), including thumb
T23.042- Burn of unspecified degree of multiple left fingers (nail), including thumb
T23.049- Burn of unspecified degree of unspecified multiple fingers (nail), including thumb
T23.05 Burn of unspecified degree of palm
T23.051- Burn of unspecified degree of right palm
T23.052- Burn of unspecified degree of left palm
T23.059- Burn of unspecified degree of unspecified palm
T23.06 Burn of unspecified degree of back of hand
T23.061- Burn of unspecified degree of back of right hand
T23.062- Burn of unspecified degree of back of left hand
T23.069- Burn of unspecified degree of back of unspecified hand
T23.07 Burn of unspecified degree of wrist
T23.071- Burn of unspecified degree of right wrist
T23.072- Burn of unspecified degree of left wrist
T23.079- Burn of unspecified degree of unspecified wrist
T23.09 Burn of unspecified degree of multiple sites of wrist and hand
T23.091- Burn of unspecified degree of multiple sites of right wrist and hand
T23.092- Burn of unspecified degree of multiple sites of left wrist and hand
T23.099- Burn of unspecified degree of multiple sites of unspecified wrist and hand

T23.1 Burn of first degree of wrist and hand
Use additional external cause code to identify the source, place and intent of the burn (X00-X19, X75-X77, X96-X98, Y92)

T23.10 Burn of first degree of hand, unspecified site
T23.101- Burn of first degree of right hand, unspecified site
T23.102- Burn of first degree of left hand, unspecified site
T23.109- Burn of first degree of unspecified hand, unspecified site
T23.11 Burn of first degree of thumb (nail)
T23.111- Burn of first degree of right thumb (nail)
T23.112- Burn of first degree of left thumb (nail)
T23.119- Burn of first degree of unspecified thumb (nail)
T23.12 Burn of first degree of single finger (nail) except thumb
T23.121- Burn of first degree of single right finger (nail) except thumb
T23.122- Burn of first degree of single left finger (nail) except thumb
T23.129- Burn of first degree of unspecified single finger (nail) except thumb
T23.13 Burn of first degree of multiple fingers (nail), not including thumb
T23.131- Burn of first degree of multiple right fingers (nail), not including thumb
T23.132- Burn of first degree of multiple left fingers (nail), not including thumb
T23.139- Burn of first degree of unspecified multiple fingers (nail), not including thumb
T23.14 Burn of first degree of multiple fingers (nail), including thumb
T23.141- Burn of first degree of multiple right fingers (nail), including thumb
T23.142- Burn of first degree of multiple left fingers (nail), including thumb
T23.149- Burn of first degree of unspecified multiple fingers (nail), including thumb
T23.15 Burn of first degree of palm
T23.151- Burn of first degree of right palm
T23.152- Burn of first degree of left palm
T23.159- Burn of first degree of unspecified palm
T23.16 Burn of first degree of back of hand
T23.161- Burn of first degree of back of right hand
T23.162- Burn of first degree of back of left hand
T23.169- Burn of first degree of back of unspecified hand
T23.17 Burn of first degree of wrist
T23.171- Burn of first degree of right wrist
T23.172- Burn of first degree of left wrist
T23.179- Burn of first degree of unspecified wrist
T23.19 Burn of first degree of multiple sites of wrist and hand
T23.191- Burn of first degree of multiple sites of right wrist and hand
T23.192- Burn of first degree of multiple sites of left wrist and hand
T23.199- Burn of first degree of multiple sites of unspecified wrist and hand

T23.2 Burn of second degree of wrist and hand
Use additional external cause code to identify the source, place and intent of the burn (X00-X19, X75-X77, X96-X98, Y92)

T23.20 Burn of second degree of hand, unspecified site
T23.201- Burn of second degree of right hand, unspecified site

7 T23.202- Burn of second degree of left hand, unspecified site
7 T23.209- Burn of second degree of unspecified hand, unspecified site
6 T23.21 Burn of second degree of thumb (nail)
7 T23.211- Burn of second degree of right thumb (nail)
7 T23.212- Burn of second degree of left thumb (nail)
7 T23.219- Burn of second degree of unspecified thumb (nail)
6 T23.22 Burn of second degree of single finger (nail) except thumb
7 T23.221- Burn of second degree of single right finger (nail) except thumb
7 T23.222- Burn of second degree of single left finger (nail) except thumb
7 T23.229- Burn of second degree of unspecified single finger (nail) except thumb
6 T23.23 Burn of second degree of multiple fingers (nail), not including thumb
7 T23.231- Burn of second degree of multiple right fingers (nail), not including thumb
7 T23.232- Burn of second degree of multiple left fingers (nail), not including thumb
7 T23.239- Burn of second degree of unspecified multiple fingers (nail), not including thumb
6 T23.24 Burn of second degree of multiple fingers (nail), including thumb
7 T23.241- Burn of second degree of multiple right fingers (nail), including thumb
7 T23.242- Burn of second degree of multiple left fingers (nail), including thumb
7 T23.249- Burn of second degree of unspecified multiple fingers (nail), including thumb
6 T23.25 Burn of second degree of palm
7 T23.251- Burn of second degree of right palm
7 T23.252- Burn of second degree of left palm
7 T23.259- Burn of second degree of unspecified palm
6 T23.26 Burn of second degree of back of hand
7 T23.261- Burn of second degree of back of right hand
7 T23.262- Burn of second degree of back of left hand
7 T23.269- Burn of second degree of back of unspecified hand
6 T23.27 Burn of second degree of wrist
7 T23.271- Burn of second degree of right wrist
7 T23.272- Burn of second degree of left wrist
7 T23.279- Burn of second degree of unspecified wrist
6 T23.29 Burn of second degree of multiple sites of wrist and hand
7 T23.291- Burn of second degree of multiple sites of right wrist and hand
7 T23.292- Burn of second degree of multiple sites of left wrist and hand
7 T23.299- Burn of second degree of multiple sites of unspecified wrist and hand
5 T23.3 Burn of third degree of wrist and hand
Use additional external cause code to identify the source, place and intent of the burn (X00-X19, X75-X77, X96-X98, Y92)
6 T23.30 Burn of third degree of hand, unspecified site
7 T23.301- Burn of third degree of right hand, unspecified site
AHA: (T23.301S) 1Q 2015, 19
7 T23.302- Burn of third degree of left hand, unspecified site
AHA: (T23.302S) 2Q 2016, 5
7 T23.309- Burn of third degree of unspecified hand, unspecified site
6 T23.31 Burn of third degree of thumb (nail)
7 T23.311- Burn of third degree of right thumb (nail)
7 T23.312- Burn of third degree of left thumb (nail)
7 T23.319- Burn of third degree of unspecified thumb (nail)
6 T23.32 Burn of third degree of single finger (nail) except thumb
7 T23.321- Burn of third degree of single right finger (nail) except thumb
7 T23.322- Burn of third degree of single left finger (nail) except thumb
7 T23.329- Burn of third degree of unspecified single finger (nail) except thumb
6 T23.33 Burn of third degree of multiple fingers (nail), not including thumb
7 T23.331- Burn of third degree of multiple right fingers (nail), not including thumb
7 T23.332- Burn of third degree of multiple left fingers (nail), not including thumb
7 T23.339- Burn of third degree of unspecified multiple fingers (nail), not including thumb
6 T23.34 Burn of third degree of multiple fingers (nail), including thumb
7 T23.341- Burn of third degree of multiple right fingers (nail), including thumb
7 T23.342- Burn of third degree of multiple left fingers (nail), including thumb
7 T23.349- Burn of third degree of unspecified multiple fingers (nail), including thumb
6 T23.35 Burn of third degree of palm
7 T23.351- Burn of third degree of right palm
7 T23.352- Burn of third degree of left palm
7 T23.359- Burn of third degree of unspecified palm
6 T23.36 Burn of third degree of back of hand
7 T23.361- Burn of third degree of back of right hand
7 T23.362- Burn of third degree of back of left hand
7 T23.369- Burn of third degree of back of unspecified hand
6 T23.37 Burn of third degree of wrist
7 T23.371- Burn of third degree of right wrist
7 T23.372- Burn of third degree of left wrist
7 T23.379- Burn of third degree of unspecified wrist
6 T23.39 Burn of third degree of multiple sites of wrist and hand
7 T23.391- Burn of third degree of multiple sites of right wrist and hand
7 T23.392- Burn of third degree of multiple sites of left wrist and hand
7 T23.399- Burn of third degree of multiple sites of unspecified wrist and hand
5 T23.4 Corrosion of unspecified degree of wrist and hand
Code first:
(T51-T65) to identify chemical and intent
Use additional external cause code to identify place (Y92)
6 T23.40 Corrosion of unspecified degree of hand, unspecified site
7 T23.401- Corrosion of unspecified degree of right hand, unspecified site
7 T23.402- Corrosion of unspecified degree of left hand, unspecified site
7 T23.409- Corrosion of unspecified degree of unspecified hand, unspecified site
6 T23.41 Corrosion of unspecified degree of thumb (nail)
7 T23.411- Corrosion of unspecified degree of right thumb (nail)
7 T23.412- Corrosion of unspecified degree of left thumb (nail)
7 T23.419- Corrosion of unspecified degree of unspecified thumb (nail)
6 T23.42 Corrosion of unspecified degree of single finger (nail) except thumb
7 T23.421- Corrosion of unspecified degree of single right finger (nail) except thumb
7 T23.422- Corrosion of unspecified degree of single left finger (nail) except thumb
7 T23.429- Corrosion of unspecified degree of unspecified single finger (nail) except thumb
6 T23.43 Corrosion of unspecified degree of multiple fingers (nail), not including thumb
7 T23.431- Corrosion of unspecified degree of multiple right fingers (nail), not including thumb
7 T23.432- Corrosion of unspecified degree of multiple left fingers (nail), not including thumb
7 T23.439- Corrosion of unspecified degree of unspecified multiple fingers (nail), not including thumb

6 T23.44 Corrosion of unspecified degree of multiple fingers (nail), including thumb
7 ⊟ T23.441- Corrosion of unspecified degree of multiple right fingers (nail), including thumb
7 ⊟ T23.442- Corrosion of unspecified degree of multiple left fingers (nail), including thumb
7 ⊟ T23.449- Corrosion of unspecified degree of unspecified multiple fingers (nail), including thumb

6 T23.45 Corrosion of unspecified degree of palm
7 ⊟ T23.451- Corrosion of unspecified degree of right palm
7 ⊟ T23.452- Corrosion of unspecified degree of left palm
7 ⊟ T23.459- Corrosion of unspecified degree of unspecified palm

6 T23.46 Corrosion of unspecified degree of back of hand
7 ⊟ T23.461- Corrosion of unspecified degree of back of right hand
7 ⊟ T23.462- Corrosion of unspecified degree of back of left hand
7 ⊟ T23.469- Corrosion of unspecified degree of back of unspecified hand

6 T23.47 Corrosion of unspecified degree of wrist
7 ⊟ T23.471- Corrosion of unspecified degree of right wrist
7 ⊟ T23.472- Corrosion of unspecified degree of left wrist
7 ⊟ T23.479- Corrosion of unspecified degree of unspecified wrist

6 T23.49 Corrosion of unspecified degree of multiple sites of wrist and hand
7 ⊟ T23.491- Corrosion of unspecified degree of multiple sites of right wrist and hand
7 ⊟ T23.492- Corrosion of unspecified degree of multiple sites of left wrist and hand
7 ⊟ T23.499- Corrosion of unspecified degree of multiple sites of unspecified wrist and hand

5 T23.5 Corrosion of first degree of wrist and hand
Code first:
(T51-T65) to identify chemical and intent
Use additional external cause code to identify place (Y92)

6 T23.50 Corrosion of first degree of hand, unspecified site
7 ⊟ T23.501- Corrosion of first degree of right hand, unspecified site
7 ⊟ T23.502- Corrosion of first degree of left hand, unspecified site
7 ⊟ T23.509- Corrosion of first degree of unspecified hand, unspecified site

6 T23.51 Corrosion of first degree of thumb (nail)
7 ⊟ T23.511- Corrosion of first degree of right thumb (nail)
7 ⊟ T23.512- Corrosion of first degree of left thumb (nail)
7 ⊟ T23.519- Corrosion of first degree of unspecified thumb (nail)

6 T23.52 Corrosion of first degree of single finger (nail) except thumb
7 ⊟ T23.521- Corrosion of first degree of single right finger (nail) except thumb
7 ⊟ T23.522- Corrosion of first degree of single left finger (nail) except thumb
7 ⊟ T23.529- Corrosion of first degree of unspecified single finger (nail) except thumb

6 T23.53 Corrosion of first degree of multiple fingers (nail), not including thumb
7 ⊟ T23.531- Corrosion of first degree of multiple right fingers (nail), not including thumb
7 ⊟ T23.532- Corrosion of first degree of multiple left fingers (nail), not including thumb
7 ⊟ T23.539- Corrosion of first degree of unspecified multiple fingers (nail), not including thumb

6 T23.54 Corrosion of first degree of multiple fingers (nail), including thumb
7 ⊟ T23.541- Corrosion of first degree of multiple right fingers (nail), including thumb
7 ⊟ T23.542- Corrosion of first degree of multiple left fingers (nail), including thumb
7 ⊟ T23.549- Corrosion of first degree of unspecified multiple fingers (nail), including thumb

6 T23.55 Corrosion of first degree of palm
7 ⊟ T23.551- Corrosion of first degree of right palm
7 ⊟ T23.552- Corrosion of first degree of left palm
7 ⊟ T23.559- Corrosion of first degree of unspecified palm

6 T23.56 Corrosion of first degree of back of hand
7 ⊟ T23.561- Corrosion of first degree of back of right hand
7 ⊟ T23.562- Corrosion of first degree of back of left hand
7 ⊟ T23.569- Corrosion of first degree of back of unspecified hand

6 T23.57 Corrosion of first degree of wrist
7 ⊟ T23.571- Corrosion of first degree of right wrist
7 ⊟ T23.572- Corrosion of first degree of left wrist
7 ⊟ T23.579- Corrosion of first degree of unspecified wrist

6 T23.59 Corrosion of first degree of multiple sites of wrist and hand
7 ⊟ T23.591- Corrosion of first degree of multiple sites of right wrist and hand
7 ⊟ T23.592- Corrosion of first degree of multiple sites of left wrist and hand
7 ⊟ T23.599- Corrosion of first degree of multiple sites of unspecified wrist and hand

5 T23.6 Corrosion of second degree of wrist and hand
Code first:
(T51-T65) to identify chemical and intent
Use additional external cause code to identify place (Y92)

6 T23.60 Corrosion of second degree of hand, unspecified site
7 ⊟ T23.601- Corrosion of second degree of right hand, unspecified site
7 ⊟ T23.602- Corrosion of second degree of left hand, unspecified site
7 ⊟ T23.609- Corrosion of second degree of unspecified hand, unspecified site

6 T23.61 Corrosion of second degree of thumb (nail)
7 ⊟ T23.611- Corrosion of second degree of right thumb (nail)
7 ⊟ T23.612- Corrosion of second degree of left thumb (nail)
7 ⊟ T23.619- Corrosion of second degree of unspecified thumb (nail)

6 T23.62 Corrosion of second degree of single finger (nail) except thumb
7 ⊟ T23.621- Corrosion of second degree of single right finger (nail) except thumb
7 ⊟ T23.622- Corrosion of second degree of single left finger (nail) except thumb
7 ⊟ T23.629- Corrosion of second degree of unspecified single finger (nail) except thumb

6 T23.63 Corrosion of second degree of multiple fingers (nail), not including thumb
7 ⊟ T23.631- Corrosion of second degree of multiple right fingers (nail), not including thumb
7 ⊟ T23.632- Corrosion of second degree of multiple left fingers (nail), not including thumb
7 ⊟ T23.639- Corrosion of second degree of unspecified multiple fingers (nail), not including thumb

6 T23.64 Corrosion of second degree of multiple fingers (nail), including thumb
7 ⊟ T23.641- Corrosion of second degree of multiple right fingers (nail), including thumb
7 ⊟ T23.642- Corrosion of second degree of multiple left fingers (nail), including thumb
7 ⊟ T23.649- Corrosion of second degree of unspecified multiple fingers (nail), including thumb

6 T23.65 Corrosion of second degree of palm
7 ⊟ T23.651- Corrosion of second degree of right palm
7 ⊟ T23.652- Corrosion of second degree of left palm
7 ⊟ T23.659- Corrosion of second degree of unspecified palm

6 T23.66 Corrosion of second degree of back of hand
7 ⊟ T23.661- Corrosion of second degree back of right hand
7 ⊟ T23.662- Corrosion of second degree back of left hand
7 ⊟ T23.669- Corrosion of second degree back of unspecified hand

6 T23.67 Corrosion of second degree of wrist
7 ⊟ T23.671- Corrosion of second degree of right wrist
7 ⊟ T23.672- Corrosion of second degree of left wrist
7 ⊟ T23.679- Corrosion of second degree of unspecified wrist

6 T23.69 Corrosion of second degree of multiple sites of wrist and hand
7 ⊟ T23.691- Corrosion of second degree of multiple sites of right wrist and hand
7 ⊟ T23.692- Corrosion of second degree of multiple sites of left wrist and hand
7 ⊟ T23.699- Corrosion of second degree of multiple sites of unspecified wrist and hand

5 T23.7 Corrosion of third degree of wrist and hand
Code first:
(T51-T65) to identify chemical and intent
Use additional external cause code to identify place (Y92)

6 T23.70 Corrosion of third degree of hand, unspecified site
7 ⊟ T23.701- Corrosion of third degree of right hand, unspecified site
7 ⊟ T23.702- Corrosion of third degree of left hand, unspecified site
7 ⊟ T23.709- Corrosion of third degree of unspecified hand, unspecified site

6 T23.71 Corrosion of third degree of thumb (nail)
7 ⊟ T23.711- Corrosion of third degree of right thumb (nail)
7 ⊟ T23.712- Corrosion of third degree of left thumb (nail)
7 ⊟ T23.719- Corrosion of third degree of unspecified thumb (nail)

6 T23.72 Corrosion of third degree of single finger (nail) except thumb
7 ⊟ T23.721- Corrosion of third degree of single right finger (nail) except thumb
7 ⊟ T23.722- Corrosion of third degree of single left finger (nail) except thumb
7 ⊟ T23.729- Corrosion of third degree of unspecified single finger (nail) except thumb

6 T23.73 Corrosion of third degree of multiple fingers (nail), not including thumb
7 ⊟ T23.731- Corrosion of third degree of multiple right fingers (nail), not including thumb
7 ⊟ T23.732- Corrosion of third degree of multiple left fingers (nail), not including thumb
7 ⊟ T23.739- Corrosion of third degree of unspecified multiple fingers (nail), not including thumb

6 T23.74 Corrosion of third degree of multiple fingers (nail), including thumb
7 ⊟ T23.741- Corrosion of third degree of multiple right fingers (nail), including thumb
7 ⊟ T23.742- Corrosion of third degree of multiple left fingers (nail), including thumb
7 ⊟ T23.749- Corrosion of third degree of unspecified multiple fingers (nail), including thumb

6 T23.75 Corrosion of third degree of palm
7 ⊟ T23.751- Corrosion of third degree of right palm
7 ⊟ T23.752- Corrosion of third degree of left palm
7 ⊟ T23.759- Corrosion of third degree of unspecified palm

6 T23.76 Corrosion of third degree of back of hand
7 ⊟ T23.761- Corrosion of third degree of back of right hand
7 ⊟ T23.762- Corrosion of third degree of back of left hand
7 ⊟ T23.769- Corrosion of third degree back of unspecified hand

6 T23.77 Corrosion of third degree of wrist
7 ⊟ T23.771- Corrosion of third degree of right wrist
7 ⊟ T23.772- Corrosion of third degree of left wrist
7 ⊟ T23.779- Corrosion of third degree of unspecified wrist

6 T23.79 Corrosion of third degree of multiple sites of wrist and hand
7 ⊟ T23.791- Corrosion of third degree of multiple sites of right wrist and hand
7 ⊟ T23.792- Corrosion of third degree of multiple sites of left wrist and hand
7 ⊟ T23.799- Corrosion of third degree of multiple sites of unspecified wrist and hand

4 T24 Burn and corrosion of lower limb, except ankle and foot

EXCLUDES 2 *burn and corrosion of ankle and foot (T25.-)*
burn and corrosion of hip region (T21.-)

The appropriate 7th character is to be added to each code from category T24
A initial encounter
D subsequent encounter
S sequela

CODING TIP✓ Do not use Z codes for skin grafts, dressing changes, drains, etc., for traumatic wounds of any type, including burns. Continue to code the burn with the appropriate 7th character.

5 T24.0 Burn of unspecified degree of lower limb, except ankle and foot
Use additional external cause code to identify the source, place and intent of the burn (X00-X19, X75-X77, X96-X98, Y92)

6 T24.00 Burn of unspecified degree of unspecified site of lower limb, except ankle and foot
7 ⊟ T24.001- Burn of unspecified degree of unspecified site of right lower limb, except ankle and foot
7 ⊟ T24.002- Burn of unspecified degree of unspecified site of left lower limb, except ankle and foot
7 ⊟ T24.009- Burn of unspecified degree of unspecified site of unspecified lower limb, except ankle and foot

6 T24.01 Burn of unspecified degree of thigh
7 ⊟ T24.011- Burn of unspecified degree of right thigh
7 ⊟ T24.012- Burn of unspecified degree of left thigh
7 ⊟ T24.019- Burn of unspecified degree of unspecified thigh

6 T24.02 Burn of unspecified degree of knee
7 ⊟ T24.021- Burn of unspecified degree of right knee
7 ⊟ T24.022- Burn of unspecified degree of left knee
7 ⊟ T24.029- Burn of unspecified degree of unspecified knee

6 T24.03 Burn of unspecified degree of lower leg
7 ⊟ T24.031- Burn of unspecified degree of right lower leg
7 ⊟ T24.032- Burn of unspecified degree of left lower leg
7 ⊟ T24.039- Burn of unspecified degree of unspecified lower leg

6 T24.09 Burn of unspecified degree of multiple sites of lower limb, except ankle and foot
7 ⊟ T24.091- Burn of unspecified degree of multiple sites of right lower limb, except ankle and foot
7 ⊟ T24.092- Burn of unspecified degree of multiple sites of left lower limb, except ankle and foot
7 ⊟ T24.099- Burn of unspecified degree of multiple sites of unspecified lower limb, except ankle and foot

5 T24.1 Burn of first degree of lower limb, except ankle and foot
Use additional external cause code to identify the source, place and intent of the burn (X00-X19, X75-X77, X96-X98, Y92)

6 T24.10 Burn of first degree of unspecified site of lower limb, except ankle and foot
7 ⊟ T24.101- Burn of first degree of unspecified site of right lower limb, except ankle and foot
7 ⊟ T24.102- Burn of first degree of unspecified site of left lower limb, except ankle and foot
7 ⊟ T24.109- Burn of first degree of unspecified site of unspecified lower limb, except ankle and foot

6 T24.11 Burn of first degree of thigh
7 ⊟ T24.111- Burn of first degree of right thigh
7 ⊟ T24.112- Burn of first degree of left thigh
7 ⊟ T24.119- Burn of first degree of unspecified thigh

6 T24.12 Burn of first degree of knee
7 ⊟ T24.121- Burn of first degree of right knee
7 ⊟ T24.122- Burn of first degree of left knee
7 ⊟ T24.129- Burn of first degree of unspecified knee

6 T24.13 Burn of first degree of lower leg

7 ⊟ T24.131- Burn of first degree of right lower leg
7 ⊟ T24.132- Burn of first degree of left lower leg
7 ⊟ T24.139- Burn of first degree of unspecified lower leg
6 T24.19 Burn of first degree of multiple sites of lower limb, except ankle and foot
7 ⊟ T24.191- Burn of first degree of multiple sites of right lower limb, except ankle and foot
7 ⊟ T24.192- Burn of first degree of multiple sites of left lower limb, except ankle and foot
7 ⊟ T24.199- Burn of first degree of multiple sites of unspecified lower limb, except ankle and foot
5 T24.2 Burn of second degree of lower limb, except ankle and foot
Use additional external cause code to identify the source, place and intent of the burn (X00-X19, X75-X77, X96-X98, Y92)
6 T24.20 Burn of second degree of unspecified site of lower limb, except ankle and foot
7 ⊟ T24.201- Burn of second degree of unspecified site of right lower limb, except ankle and foot
7 ⊟ T24.202- Burn of second degree of unspecified site of left lower limb, except ankle and foot
7 ⊟ T24.209- Burn of second degree of unspecified site of unspecified lower limb, except ankle and foot
6 T24.21 Burn of second degree of thigh
7 ⊟ T24.211- Burn of second degree of right thigh
7 ⊟ T24.212- Burn of second degree of left thigh
7 ⊟ T24.219- Burn of second degree of unspecified thigh
6 T24.22 Burn of second degree of knee
7 ⊟ T24.221- Burn of second degree of right knee
7 ⊟ T24.222- Burn of second degree of left knee
7 ⊟ T24.229- Burn of second degree of unspecified knee
6 T24.23 Burn of second degree of lower leg
7 ⊟ T24.231- Burn of second degree of right lower leg
7 ⊟ T24.232- Burn of second degree of left lower leg
7 ⊟ T24.239- Burn of second degree of unspecified lower leg
6 T24.29 Burn of second degree of multiple sites of lower limb, except ankle and foot
7 ⊟ T24.291- Burn of second degree of multiple sites of right lower limb, except ankle and foot
7 ⊟ T24.292- Burn of second degree of multiple sites of left lower limb, except ankle and foot
7 ⊟ T24.299- Burn of second degree of multiple sites of unspecified lower limb, except ankle and foot
5 T24.3 Burn of third degree of lower limb, except ankle and foot
Use additional external cause code to identify the source, place and intent of the burn (X00-X19, X75-X77, X96-X98, Y92)
6 T24.30 Burn of third degree of unspecified site of lower limb, except ankle and foot
7 ⊟ T24.301- Burn of third degree of unspecified site of right lower limb, except ankle and foot
7 ⊟ T24.302- Burn of third degree of unspecified site of left lower limb, except ankle and foot
7 ⊟ T24.309- Burn of third degree of unspecified site of unspecified lower limb, except ankle and foot
6 T24.31 Burn of third degree of thigh
7 ⊟ T24.311- Burn of third degree of right thigh
7 ⊟ T24.312- Burn of third degree of left thigh
7 ⊟ T24.319- Burn of third degree of unspecified thigh
6 T24.32 Burn of third degree of knee
7 ⊟ T24.321- Burn of third degree of right knee
7 ⊟ T24.322- Burn of third degree of left knee
7 ⊟ T24.329- Burn of third degree of unspecified knee
6 T24.33 Burn of third degree of lower leg
7 ⊟ T24.331- Burn of third degree of right lower leg
7 ⊟ T24.332- Burn of third degree of left lower leg
7 ⊟ T24.339- Burn of third degree of unspecified lower leg
6 T24.39 Burn of third degree of multiple sites of lower limb, except ankle and foot
7 ⊟ T24.391- Burn of third degree of multiple sites of right lower limb, except ankle and foot
AHA: (T24.391A) 2Q 2016, 4
7 ⊟ T24.392- Burn of third degree of multiple sites of left lower limb, except ankle and foot
AHA: (T24.392A) 2Q 2016, 4
7 ⊟ T24.399- Burn of third degree of multiple sites of unspecified lower limb, except ankle and foot
5 T24.4 Corrosion of unspecified degree of lower limb, except ankle and foot
Code first:
(T51-T65) to identify chemical and intent
Use additional external cause code to identify place (Y92)
6 T24.40 Corrosion of unspecified degree of unspecified site of lower limb, except ankle and foot
7 ⊟ T24.401- Corrosion of unspecified degree of unspecified site of right lower limb, except ankle and foot
7 ⊟ T24.402- Corrosion of unspecified degree of unspecified site of left lower limb, except ankle and foot
7 ⊟ T24.409- Corrosion of unspecified degree of unspecified site of unspecified lower limb, except ankle and foot
6 T24.41 Corrosion of unspecified degree of thigh
7 ⊟ T24.411- Corrosion of unspecified degree of right thigh
7 ⊟ T24.412- Corrosion of unspecified degree of left thigh
7 ⊟ T24.419- Corrosion of unspecified degree of unspecified thigh
6 T24.42 Corrosion of unspecified degree of knee
7 ⊟ T24.421- Corrosion of unspecified degree of right knee
7 ⊟ T24.422- Corrosion of unspecified degree of left knee
7 ⊟ T24.429- Corrosion of unspecified degree of unspecified knee
6 T24.43 Corrosion of unspecified degree of lower leg
7 ⊟ T24.431- Corrosion of unspecified degree of right lower leg
7 ⊟ T24.432- Corrosion of unspecified degree of left lower leg
7 ⊟ T24.439- Corrosion of unspecified degree of unspecified lower leg
6 T24.49 Corrosion of unspecified degree of multiple sites of lower limb, except ankle and foot
7 ⊟ T24.491- Corrosion of unspecified degree of multiple sites of right lower limb, except ankle and foot
7 ⊟ T24.492- Corrosion of unspecified degree of multiple sites of left lower limb, except ankle and foot
7 ⊟ T24.499- Corrosion of unspecified degree of multiple sites of unspecified lower limb, except ankle and foot
5 T24.5 Corrosion of first degree of lower limb, except ankle and foot
Code first:
(T51-T65) to identify chemical and intent
Use additional external cause code to identify place (Y92)
6 T24.50 Corrosion of first degree of unspecified site of lower limb, except ankle and foot
7 ⊟ T24.501- Corrosion of first degree of unspecified site of right lower limb, except ankle and foot
7 ⊟ T24.502- Corrosion of first degree of unspecified site of left lower limb, except ankle and foot
7 ⊟ T24.509- Corrosion of first degree of unspecified site of unspecified lower limb, except ankle and foot
6 T24.51 Corrosion of first degree of thigh
7 ⊟ T24.511- Corrosion of first degree of right thigh
7 ⊟ T24.512- Corrosion of first degree of left thigh
7 ⊟ T24.519- Corrosion of first degree of unspecified thigh
6 T24.52 Corrosion of first degree of knee
7 ⊟ T24.521- Corrosion of first degree of right knee
7 ⊟ T24.522- Corrosion of first degree of left knee
7 ⊟ T24.529- Corrosion of first degree of unspecified knee
6 T24.53 Corrosion of first degree of lower leg

7️⃣⊟	T24.531-	Corrosion of first degree of right lower leg
7️⃣⊟	T24.532-	Corrosion of first degree of left lower leg
7️⃣⊟	T24.539-	Corrosion of first degree of unspecified lower leg

6️⃣ **T24.59** Corrosion of first degree of multiple sites of lower limb, except ankle and foot

7️⃣⊟	T24.591-	Corrosion of first degree of multiple sites of right lower limb, except ankle and foot
7️⃣⊟	T24.592-	Corrosion of first degree of multiple sites of left lower limb, except ankle and foot
7️⃣⊟	T24.599-	Corrosion of first degree of multiple sites of unspecified lower limb, except ankle and foot

5️⃣ **T24.6** Corrosion of second degree of lower limb, except ankle and foot
Code first:
(T51-T65) to identify chemical and intent
Use additional external cause code to identify place (Y92)

6️⃣ **T24.60** Corrosion of second degree of unspecified site of lower limb, except ankle and foot

7️⃣⊟	T24.601-	Corrosion of second degree of unspecified site of right lower limb, except ankle and foot
7️⃣⊟	T24.602-	Corrosion of second degree of unspecified site of left lower limb, except ankle and foot
7️⃣⊟	T24.609-	Corrosion of second degree of unspecified site of unspecified lower limb, except ankle and foot

6️⃣ **T24.61** Corrosion of second degree of thigh

7️⃣⊟	T24.611-	Corrosion of second degree of right thigh
7️⃣⊟	T24.612-	Corrosion of second degree of left thigh
7️⃣⊟	T24.619-	Corrosion of second degree of unspecified thigh

6️⃣ **T24.62** Corrosion of second degree of knee

7️⃣⊟	T24.621-	Corrosion of second degree of right knee
7️⃣⊟	T24.622-	Corrosion of second degree of left knee
7️⃣⊟	T24.629-	Corrosion of second degree of unspecified knee

6️⃣ **T24.63** Corrosion of second degree of lower leg

7️⃣⊟	T24.631-	Corrosion of second degree of right lower leg
7️⃣⊟	T24.632-	Corrosion of second degree of left lower leg
7️⃣⊟	T24.639-	Corrosion of second degree of unspecified lower leg

6️⃣ **T24.69** Corrosion of second degree of multiple sites of lower limb, except ankle and foot

7️⃣⊟	T24.691-	Corrosion of second degree of multiple sites of right lower limb, except ankle and foot
7️⃣⊟	T24.692-	Corrosion of second degree of multiple sites of left lower limb, except ankle and foot
7️⃣⊟	T24.699-	Corrosion of second degree of multiple sites of unspecified lower limb, except ankle and foot

5️⃣ **T24.7** Corrosion of third degree of lower limb, except ankle and foot
Code first:
(T51-T65) to identify chemical and intent
Use additional external cause code to identify place (Y92)

6️⃣ **T24.70** Corrosion of third degree of unspecified site of lower limb, except ankle and foot

7️⃣☐	T24.701-	Corrosion of third degree of unspecified site of right lower limb, except ankle and foot
7️⃣⊟	T24.702-	Corrosion of third degree of unspecified site of left lower limb, except ankle and foot
7️⃣⊟	T24.709-	Corrosion of third degree of unspecified site of unspecified lower limb, except ankle and foot

6️⃣ **T24.71** Corrosion of third degree of thigh

7️⃣⊟	T24.711-	Corrosion of third degree of right thigh
7️⃣⊟	T24.712-	Corrosion of third degree of left thigh
7️⃣⊟	T24.719-	Corrosion of third degree of unspecified thigh

6️⃣ **T24.72** Corrosion of third degree of knee

7️⃣⊟	T24.721-	Corrosion of third degree of right knee
7️⃣⊟	T24.722-	Corrosion of third degree of left knee
7️⃣⊟	T24.729-	Corrosion of third degree of unspecified knee

6️⃣ **T24.73** Corrosion of third degree of lower leg

7️⃣⊟	T24.731-	Corrosion of third degree of right lower leg
7️⃣⊟	T24.732-	Corrosion of third degree of left lower leg

7️⃣⊟	T24.739-	Corrosion of third degree of unspecified lower leg

6️⃣ **T24.79** Corrosion of third degree of multiple sites of lower limb, except ankle and foot

7️⃣⊟	T24.791-	Corrosion of third degree of multiple sites of right lower limb, except ankle and foot
7️⃣⊟	T24.792-	Corrosion of third degree of multiple sites of left lower limb, except ankle and foot
7️⃣⊟	T24.799-	Corrosion of third degree of multiple sites of unspecified lower limb, except ankle and foot

4️⃣ **T25** Burn and corrosion of ankle and foot

The appropriate 7th character is to be added to each code from category T25
A   initial encounter
D   subsequent encounter
S   sequela

CODING TIP✓ Do not use Z codes for skin grafts, dressing changes, drains, etc., for traumatic wounds of any type, including burns. Continue to code the burn with the appropriate 7th character.

5️⃣ **T25.0** Burn of unspecified degree of ankle and foot
Use additional external cause code to identify the source, place and intent of the burn (X00-X19, X75-X77, X96-X98, Y92)

6️⃣ **T25.01** Burn of unspecified degree of ankle

7️⃣⊟	T25.011-	Burn of unspecified degree of right ankle
7️⃣⊟	T25.012-	Burn of unspecified degree of left ankle
7️⃣⊟	T25.019-	Burn of unspecified degree of unspecified ankle

6️⃣ **T25.02** Burn of unspecified degree of foot
EXCLUDES 2 *burn of unspecified degree of toe (s) (nail) (T25.03-)*

7️⃣⊟	T25.021-	Burn of unspecified degree of right foot
7️⃣⊟	T25.022-	Burn of unspecified degree of left foot
7️⃣⊟	T25.029-	Burn of unspecified degree of unspecified foot

6️⃣ **T25.03** Burn of unspecified degree of toe(s) (nail)

7️⃣⊟	T25.031-	Burn of unspecified degree of right toe(s) (nail)
7️⃣⊟	T25.032-	Burn of unspecified degree of left toe(s) (nail)
7️⃣⊟	T25.039-	Burn of unspecified degree of unspecified toe(s) (nail)

6️⃣ **T25.09** Burn of unspecified degree of multiple sites of ankle and foot

7️⃣⊟	T25.091-	Burn of unspecified degree of multiple sites of right ankle and foot
7️⃣⊟	T25.092-	Burn of unspecified degree of multiple sites of left ankle and foot
7️⃣⊟	T25.099-	Burn of unspecified degree of multiple sites of unspecified ankle and foot

5️⃣ **T25.1** Burn of first degree of ankle and foot
Use additional external cause code to identify the source, place and intent of the burn (X00-X19, X75-X77, X96-X98, Y92)

6️⃣ **T25.11** Burn of first degree of ankle

7️⃣⊟	T25.111-	Burn of first degree of right ankle
7️⃣⊟	T25.112-	Burn of first degree of left ankle
7️⃣⊟	T25.119-	Burn of first degree of unspecified ankle

6️⃣ **T25.12** Burn of first degree of foot
EXCLUDES 2 *burn of first degree of toe (s) (nail) (T25.13-)*

7️⃣⊟	T25.121-	Burn of first degree of right foot
7️⃣⊟	T25.122-	Burn of first degree of left foot
7️⃣⊟	T25.129-	Burn of first degree of unspecified foot

6️⃣ **T25.13** Burn of first degree of toe(s) (nail)

7️⃣⊟	T25.131-	Burn of first degree of right toe(s) (nail)
7️⃣⊟	T25.132-	Burn of first degree of left toe(s) (nail)
7️⃣⊟	T25.139-	Burn of first degree of unspecified toe(s) (nail)

6️⃣ **T25.19** Burn of first degree of multiple sites of ankle and foot

7️⃣⊟	T25.191-	Burn of first degree of multiple sites of right ankle and foot

T25.192- Burn of first degree of multiple sites of left ankle and foot
T25.199- Burn of first degree of multiple sites of unspecified ankle and foot

T25.2 Burn of second degree of ankle and foot
Use additional external cause code to identify the source, place and intent of the burn (X00-X19, X75-X77, X96-X98, Y92)

T25.21 Burn of second degree of ankle
T25.211- Burn of second degree of right ankle
T25.212- Burn of second degree of left ankle
T25.219- Burn of second degree of unspecified ankle

T25.22 Burn of second degree of foot
EXCLUDES 2 *burn of second degree of toe (s) (nail) (T25.23-)*
T25.221- Burn of second degree of right foot
T25.222- Burn of second degree of left foot
T25.229- Burn of second degree of unspecified foot

T25.23 Burn of second degree of toe(s) (nail)
T25.231- Burn of second degree of right toe(s) (nail)
T25.232- Burn of second degree of left toe(s) (nail)
T25.239- Burn of second degree of unspecified toe(s) (nail)

T25.29 Burn of second degree of multiple sites of ankle and foot
T25.291- Burn of second degree of multiple sites of right ankle and foot
T25.292- Burn of second degree of multiple sites of left ankle and foot
T25.299- Burn of second degree of multiple sites of unspecified ankle and foot

T25.3 Burn of third degree of ankle and foot
Use additional external cause code to identify the source, place and intent of the burn (X00-X19, X75-X77, X96-X98, Y92)

T25.31 Burn of third degree of ankle
T25.311- Burn of third degree of right ankle
T25.312- Burn of third degree of left ankle
T25.319- Burn of third degree of unspecified ankle

T25.32 Burn of third degree of foot
EXCLUDES 2 *burn of third degree of toe (s) (nail) (T25.33-)*
T25.321- Burn of third degree of right foot
T25.322- Burn of third degree of left foot
T25.329- Burn of third degree of unspecified foot

T25.33 Burn of third degree of toe(s) (nail)
T25.331- Burn of third degree of right toe(s) (nail)
T25.332- Burn of third degree of left toe(s) (nail)
T25.339- Burn of third degree of unspecified toe(s) (nail)

T25.39 Burn of third degree of multiple sites of ankle and foot
T25.391- Burn of third degree of multiple sites of right ankle and foot
T25.392- Burn of third degree of multiple sites of left ankle and foot
T25.399- Burn of third degree of multiple sites of unspecified ankle and foot

T25.4 Corrosion of unspecified degree of ankle and foot
Code first:
(T51-T65) to identify chemical and intent
Use additional external cause code to identify place (Y92)

T25.41 Corrosion of unspecified degree of ankle
T25.411- Corrosion of unspecified degree of right ankle
T25.412- Corrosion of unspecified degree of left ankle
T25.419- Corrosion of unspecified degree of unspecified ankle

T25.42 Corrosion of unspecified degree of foot
EXCLUDES 2 *corrosion of unspecified degree of toe (s) (nail) (T25.43-)*
T25.421- Corrosion of unspecified degree of right foot
T25.422- Corrosion of unspecified degree of left foot
T25.429- Corrosion of unspecified degree of unspecified foot

T25.43 Corrosion of unspecified degree of toe(s) (nail)
T25.431- Corrosion of unspecified degree of right toe(s) (nail)
T25.432- Corrosion of unspecified degree of left toe(s) (nail)
T25.439- Corrosion of unspecified degree of unspecified toe(s) (nail)

T25.49 Corrosion of unspecified degree of multiple sites of ankle and foot
T25.491- Corrosion of unspecified degree of multiple sites of right ankle and foot
T25.492- Corrosion of unspecified degree of multiple sites of left ankle and foot
T25.499- Corrosion of unspecified degree of multiple sites of unspecified ankle and foot

T25.5 Corrosion of first degree of ankle and foot
Code first:
(T51-T65) to identify chemical and intent
Use additional external cause code to identify place (Y92)

T25.51 Corrosion of first degree of ankle
T25.511- Corrosion of first degree of right ankle
T25.512- Corrosion of first degree of left ankle
T25.519- Corrosion of first degree of unspecified ankle

T25.52 Corrosion of first degree of foot
EXCLUDES 2 *corrosion of first degree of toe (s) (nail) (T25.53-)*
T25.521- Corrosion of first degree of right foot
T25.522- Corrosion of first degree of left foot
T25.529- Corrosion of first degree of unspecified foot

T25.53 Corrosion of first degree of toe(s) (nail)
T25.531- Corrosion of first degree of right toe(s) (nail)
T25.532- Corrosion of first degree of left toe(s) (nail)
T25.539- Corrosion of first degree of unspecified toe(s) (nail)

T25.59 Corrosion of first degree of multiple sites of ankle and foot
T25.591- Corrosion of first degree of multiple sites of right ankle and foot
T25.592- Corrosion of first degree of multiple sites of left ankle and foot
T25.599- Corrosion of first degree of multiple sites of unspecified ankle and foot

T25.6 Corrosion of second degree of ankle and foot
Code first:
(T51-T65) to identify chemical and intent
Use additional external cause code to identify place (Y92)

T25.61 Corrosion of second degree of ankle
T25.611- Corrosion of second degree of right ankle
T25.612- Corrosion of second degree of left ankle
T25.619- Corrosion of second degree of unspecified ankle

T25.62 Corrosion of second degree of foot
EXCLUDES 2 *corrosion of second degree of toe (s) (nail) (T25.63-)*
T25.621- Corrosion of second degree of right foot
T25.622- Corrosion of second degree of left foot
T25.629- Corrosion of second degree of unspecified foot

T25.63 Corrosion of second degree of toe(s) (nail)
T25.631- Corrosion of second degree of right toe(s) (nail)
T25.632- Corrosion of second degree of left toe(s) (nail)
T25.639- Corrosion of second degree of unspecified toe(s) (nail)

T25.69 Corrosion of second degree of multiple sites of ankle and foot
T25.691- Corrosion of second degree of right ankle and foot
T25.692- Corrosion of second degree of left ankle and foot
T25.699- Corrosion of second degree of unspecified ankle and foot

T25.7 Corrosion of third degree of ankle and foot
Code first:
(T51-T65) to identify chemical and intent
Use additional external cause code to identify place (Y92)

T25.71 Corrosion of third degree of ankle
T25.711- Corrosion of third degree of right ankle

7 ⊟ **T25.712-**   Corrosion of third degree of left ankle

7 ⊟ **T25.719-**   **Corrosion of third degree of unspecified ankle**

6 **T25.72**   **Corrosion of third degree of foot**

   EXCLUDES 2   *corrosion of third degree of toe (s) (nail) (T25.73-)*

7 ⊟ **T25.721-**   Corrosion of third degree of right foot

7 ⊟ **T25.722-**   Corrosion of third degree of left foot

7 ⊟ **T25.729-**   **Corrosion of third degree of unspecified foot**

6 **T25.73**   **Corrosion of third degree of toe(s) (nail)**

7 ⊟ **T25.731-**   Corrosion of third degree of right toe(s) (nail)

7 ⊟ **T25.732-**   Corrosion of third degree of left toe(s) (nail)

7 ⊟ **T25.739-**   **Corrosion of third degree of unspecified toe(s) (nail)**

6 **T25.79**   **Corrosion of third degree of multiple sites of ankle and foot**

7 ⊟ **T25.791-**   Corrosion of third degree of multiple sites of right ankle and foot

7 ⊟ **T25.792-**   Corrosion of third degree of multiple sites of left ankle and foot

7 ⊟ **T25.799-**   **Corrosion of third degree of multiple sites of unspecified ankle and foot**

Burns and corrosions confined to eye and internal organs (T26-T28)

4 **T26**   **Burn and corrosion confined to eye and adnexa**

The appropriate 7th character is to be added to each code from category T26
A   initial encounter
D   subsequent encounter
S   sequela

5 **T26.0**   **Burn of eyelid and periocular area**

Use additional external cause code to identify the source, place and intent of the burn (X00-X19, X75-X77, X96-X98, Y92)

7 ⊟ **T26.00X-**   **Burn of unspecified eyelid and periocular area**

7 ⊟ **T26.01X-**   Burn of right eyelid and periocular area

7 ⊟ **T26.02X-**   Burn of left eyelid and periocular area

5 **T26.1**   **Burn of cornea and conjunctival sac**

Use additional external cause code to identify the source, place and intent of the burn (X00-X19, X75-X77, X96-X98, Y92)

7 ⊟ **T26.10X-**   **Burn of cornea and conjunctival sac, unspecified eye**

7 ⊟ **T26.11X-**   Burn of cornea and conjunctival sac, right eye

7 ⊟ **T26.12X-**   Burn of cornea and conjunctival sac, left eye

5 **T26.2**   **Burn with resulting rupture and destruction of eyeball**

Use additional external cause code to identify the source, place and intent of the burn (X00-X19, X75-X77, X96-X98, Y92)

7 ⊟ **T26.20X-**   **Burn with resulting rupture and destruction of unspecified eyeball**

7 ⊟ **T26.21X-**   Burn with resulting rupture and destruction of right eyeball

7 ⊟ **T26.22X-**   Burn with resulting rupture and destruction of left eyeball

5 **T26.3**   **Burns of other specified parts of eye and adnexa**

Use additional external cause code to identify the source, place and intent of the burn (X00-X19, X75-X77, X96-X98, Y92)

7 ⊟ **T26.30X-**   **Burns of other specified parts of unspecified eye and adnexa**

7 ⊟ **T26.31X-**   Burns of other specified parts of right eye and adnexa

7 ⊟ **T26.32X-**   Burns of other specified parts of left eye and adnexa

5 **T26.4**   **Burn of eye and adnexa, part unspecified**

Use additional external cause code to identify the source, place and intent of the burn (X00-X19, X75-X77, X96-X98, Y92)

7 ⊟ **T26.40X-**   **Burn of unspecified eye and adnexa, part unspecified**

7 ⊟ **T26.41X-**   **Burn of right eye and adnexa, part unspecified**

7 ⊟ **T26.42X-**   **Burn of left eye and adnexa, part unspecified**

5 **T26.5**   **Corrosion of eyelid and periocular area**

Code first:
   (T51-T65) to identify chemical and intent
Use additional external cause code to identify place (Y92)

7 ⊟ **T26.50X-**   **Corrosion of unspecified eyelid and periocular area**

7 ⊟ **T26.51X-**   **Corrosion of right eyelid and periocular area**

7 ⊟ **T26.52X-**   **Corrosion of left eyelid and periocular area**

5 **T26.6**   **Corrosion of cornea and conjunctival sac**

Code first:
   (T51-T65) to identify chemical and intent
Use additional external cause code to identify place (Y92)

7 ⊟ **T26.60X-**   **Corrosion of cornea and conjunctival sac, unspecified eye**

7 ⊟ **T26.61X-**   **Corrosion of cornea and conjunctival sac, right eye**

7 ⊟ **T26.62X-**   **Corrosion of cornea and conjunctival sac, left eye**

5 **T26.7**   **Corrosion with resulting rupture and destruction of eyeball**

Code first:
   (T51-T65) to identify chemical and intent
Use additional external cause code to identify place (Y92)

7 ⊟ **T26.70X-**   **Corrosion with resulting rupture and destruction of unspecified eyeball**

7 ⊟ **T26.71X-**   **Corrosion with resulting rupture and destruction of right eyeball**

7 ⊟ **T26.72X-**   **Corrosion with resulting rupture and destruction of left eyeball**

5 **T26.8**   **Corrosions of other specified parts of eye and adnexa**

Code first:
   (T51-T65) to identify chemical and intent
Use additional external cause code to identify place (Y92)

7 ⊟ **T26.80X-**   **Corrosions of other specified parts of unspecified eye and adnexa**

7 ⊟ **T26.81X-**   **Corrosions of other specified parts of right eye and adnexa**

7 ⊟ **T26.82X-**   **Corrosions of other specified parts of left eye and adnexa**

5 **T26.9**   **Corrosion of eye and adnexa, part unspecified**

Code first:
   (T51-T65) to identify chemical and intent
Use additional external cause code to identify place (Y92)

7 ⊟ **T26.90X-**   **Corrosion of unspecified eye and adnexa, part unspecified**

7 ⊟ **T26.91X-**   **Corrosion of right eye and adnexa, part unspecified**

7 ⊟ **T26.92X-**   **Corrosion of left eye and adnexa, part unspecified**

4 **T27**   **Burn and corrosion of respiratory tract**

Use additional external cause code to identify the source and intent of the burn (X00-X19, X75-X77, X96-X98)
Use additional external cause code to identify place (Y92)

The appropriate 7th character is to be added to each code from category T27
A   initial encounter
D   subsequent encounter
S   sequela

7 **T27.0XX-**   **Burn of larynx and trachea**

7 **T27.1XX-**   **Burn involving larynx and trachea with lung**

7 **T27.2XX-**   **Burn of other parts of respiratory tract**
   Burn of thoracic cavity

7 **T27.3XX-**   **Burn of respiratory tract, part unspecified**

7 **T27.4XX-**   **Corrosion of larynx and trachea**
Code first:
   (T51-T65) to identify chemical and intent

7 **T27.5XX-**   **Corrosion involving larynx and trachea with lung**

7 **T27.6XX-**   **Corrosion of other parts of respiratory tract**
Code first:
   (T51-T65) to identify chemical and intent

7 **T27.7XX-**   **Corrosion of respiratory tract, part unspecified**
Code first:
   (T51-T65) to identify chemical and intent

● New   *Manifestation*   4-7 Digit Indicators   ⊟ Laterality   A Adult   M Maternity   N Newborn   P Pediatric   ♂ Male
▲ Revised   Unspecified   AHA Coding Clinic   HCC Hierarchical Condition Categories   HIV HIV Related Conditions   ♀ Female

2019 ICD-10-CM Experts for Physicians   © 2018 DecisionHealth   1087

Injury, Poisoning and Certain Other Consequences of External Causes   T25.712- — T27.7XX-

4 **T28 Burn and corrosion of other internal organs**

Use additional external cause code to identify the source and intent of the burn (X00-X19, X75-X77, X96-X98)
Use additional external cause code to identify place (Y92)

The appropriate 7th character is to be added to each code from category T28
A initial encounter
D subsequent encounter
S sequela

7 **T28.0XX- Burn of mouth and pharynx**
7 **T28.1XX- Burn of esophagus**
7 **T28.2XX- Burn of other parts of alimentary tract**
7 **T28.3XX- Burn of internal genitourinary organs**
5 **T28.4 Burns of other and unspecified internal organs**
Code first:
(T51-T65) to identify chemical and intent
7 **T28.40X- Burn of unspecified internal organ**
6 **T28.41 Burn of ear drum**
7 ⊟ **T28.411- Burn of right ear drum**
7 ⊟ **T28.412- Burn of left ear drum**
7 ⊟ **T28.419- Burn of unspecified ear drum**
7 **T28.49X- Burn of other internal organ**
7 **T28.5XX- Corrosion of mouth and pharynx**
Code first:
(T51-T65) to identify chemical and intent
7 **T28.6XX- Corrosion of esophagus**
Code first:
(T51-T65) to identify chemical and intent
7 **T28.7XX- Corrosion of other parts of alimentary tract**
Code first:
(T51-T65) to identify chemical and intent
7 **T28.8XX- Corrosion of internal genitourinary organs**
Code first:
(T51-T65) to identify chemical and intent
5 **T28.9 Corrosions of other and unspecified internal organs**
Code first:
(T51-T65) to identify chemical and intent
7 **T28.90X- Corrosions of unspecified internal organs**
6 **T28.91 Corrosions of ear drum**
7 ⊟ **T28.911- Corrosions of right ear drum**
7 ⊟ **T28.912- Corrosions of left ear drum**
7 ⊟ **T28.919- Corrosions of unspecified ear drum**
7 **T28.99X- Corrosions of other internal organs**

Burns and corrosions of multiple and unspecified body regions (T30-T32)

GUIDELINES Section I.C.19.d.6)-9)
Categories T31 and T32 are based on the classic "rule of nines" in estimating body surface involved: head and neck are assigned nine percent, each arm nine percent, each leg 18 percent, the anterior trunk 18 percent, posterior trunk 18 percent, and genitalia one percent. Providers may change these percentage assignments where necessary to accommodate infants and children who have proportionately larger heads than adults, and patients who have large buttocks, thighs, or abdomen that involve burns.

Encounters for the treatment of the late effects of burns or corrosions (i.e., scars or joint contractures) should be coded with a burn or corrosion code with the 7th character "S" for sequela.

When appropriate, both a code for a current burn or corrosion with 7th character "A" or "D" and a burn or corrosion code with 7th character "S" may be assigned on the same record (when both a current burn and sequelae of an old burn exist). Burns and corrosions do not heal at the same rate and a current healing wound may still exist with sequela of a healed burn or corrosion.

An external cause code should be used with burns and corrosions to identify the source and intent of the burn, as well as the place where it occurred.

4 **T30 Burn and corrosion, body region unspecified**

GUIDELINES Section I.C.19.d.5)
Category T30, Burn and corrosion, body region unspecified is extremely vague and should rarely be used.

T30.0 Burn of unspecified body region, unspecified degree
This code is not for inpatient use. Code to specified site and degree of burns
Burn NOS
Multiple burns NOS
T30.4 Corrosion of unspecified body region, unspecified degree
This code is not for inpatient use. Code to specified site and degree of corrosion
Corrosion NOS
Multiple corrosion NOS

4 **T31 Burns classified according to extent of body surface involved**
Note: This category is to be used as the primary code only when the site of the burn is unspecified. It should be used as a supplementary code with categories T20-T25 when the site is specified.

Burns classified according to extent of body surface involved

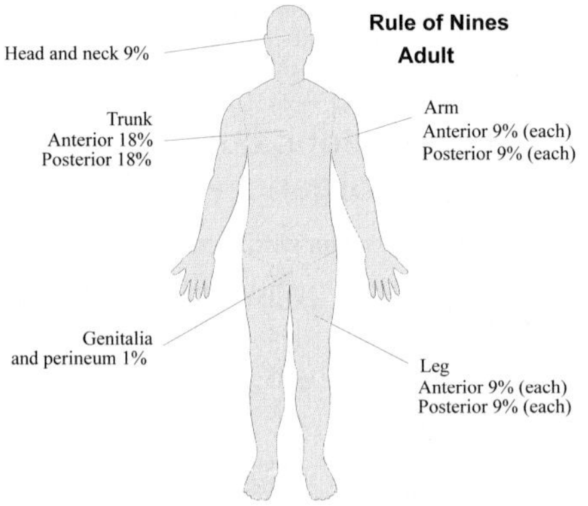

T31.0 Burns involving less than 10% of body surface
5 **T31.1 Burns involving 10-19% of body surface**
T31.10 Burns involving 10-19% of body surface with 0% to 9% third degree burns
Burns involving 10-19% of body surface NOS
T31.11 Burns involving 10-19% of body surface with 10-19% third degree burns HCC
5 **T31.2 Burns involving 20-29% of body surface**
T31.20 Burns involving 20-29% of body surface with 0% to 9% third degree burns
Burns involving 20-29% of body surface NOS
T31.21 Burns involving 20-29% of body surface with 10-19% third degree burns HCC
T31.22 Burns involving 20-29% of body surface with 20-29% third degree burns HCC
5 **T31.3 Burns involving 30-39% of body surface**
T31.30 Burns involving 30-39% of body surface with 0% to 9% third degree burns
Burns involving 30-39% of body surface NOS
T31.31 Burns involving 30-39% of body surface with 10-19% third degree burns HCC
T31.32 Burns involving 30-39% of body surface with 20-29% third degree burns HCC
T31.33 Burns involving 30-39% of body surface with 30-39% third degree burns HCC
5 **T31.4 Burns involving 40-49% of body surface**
T31.40 Burns involving 40-49% of body surface with 0% to 9% third degree burns
Burns involving 40-49% of body surface NOS
T31.41 Burns involving 40-49% of body surface with 10-19% third degree burns HCC
T31.42 Burns involving 40-49% of body surface with 20-29% third degree burns HCC
T31.43 Burns involving 40-49% of body surface with 30-39% third degree burns HCC
T31.44 Burns involving 40-49% of body surface with 40-49% third degree burns HCC
5 **T31.5 Burns involving 50-59% of body surface**
T31.50 Burns involving 50-59% of body surface with 0% to 9% third degree burns
Burns involving 50-59% of body surface NOS
T31.51 Burns involving 50-59% of body surface with 10-19% third degree burns HCC

T31.52 Burns involving 50-59% of body surface with 20-29% third degree burns HCC
T31.53 Burns involving 50-59% of body surface with 30-39% third degree burns HCC
T31.54 Burns involving 50-59% of body surface with 40-49% third degree burns HCC
T31.55 Burns involving 50-59% of body surface with 50-59% third degree burns HCC

5 T31.6 Burns involving 60-69% of body surface
T31.60 Burns involving 60-69% of body surface with 0% to 9% third degree burns
Burns involving 60-69% of body surface NOS
T31.61 Burns involving 60-69% of body surface with 10-19% third degree burns HCC
T31.62 Burns involving 60-69% of body surface with 20-29% third degree burns HCC
T31.63 Burns involving 60-69% of body surface with 30-39% third degree burns HCC
T31.64 Burns involving 60-69% of body surface with 40-49% third degree burns HCC
T31.65 Burns involving 60-69% of body surface with 50-59% third degree burns HCC
T31.66 Burns involving 60-69% of body surface with 60-69% third degree burns HCC

5 T31.7 Burns involving 70-79% of body surface
T31.70 Burns involving 70-79% of body surface with 0% to 9% third degree burns
Burns involving 70-79% of body surface NOS
T31.71 Burns involving 70-79% of body surface with 10-19% third degree burns HCC
T31.72 Burns involving 70-79% of body surface with 20-29% third degree burns HCC
T31.73 Burns involving 70-79% of body surface with 30-39% third degree burns HCC
T31.74 Burns involving 70-79% of body surface with 40-49% third degree burns HCC
T31.75 Burns involving 70-79% of body surface with 50-59% third degree burns HCC
T31.76 Burns involving 70-79% of body surface with 60-69% third degree burns HCC
T31.77 Burns involving 70-79% of body surface with 70-79% third degree burns HCC

5 T31.8 Burns involving 80-89% of body surface
T31.80 Burns involving 80-89% of body surface with 0% to 9% third degree burns
Burns involving 80-89% of body surface NOS
T31.81 Burns involving 80-89% of body surface with 10-19% third degree burns HCC
T31.82 Burns involving 80-89% of body surface with 20-29% third degree burns HCC
T31.83 Burns involving 80-89% of body surface with 30-39% third degree burns HCC
T31.84 Burns involving 80-89% of body surface with 40-49% third degree burns HCC
T31.85 Burns involving 80-89% of body surface with 50-59% third degree burns HCC
T31.86 Burns involving 80-89% of body surface with 60-69% third degree burns HCC
T31.87 Burns involving 80-89% of body surface with 70-79% third degree burns HCC
T31.88 Burns involving 80-89% of body surface with 80-89% third degree burns HCC

5 T31.9 Burns involving 90% or more of body surface
T31.90 Burns involving 90% or more of body surface with 0% to 9% third degree burns
Burns involving 90% or more of body surface NOS
T31.91 Burns involving 90% or more of body surface with 10-19% third degree burns HCC
T31.92 Burns involving 90% or more of body surface with 20-29% third degree burns HCC
T31.93 Burns involving 90% or more of body surface with 30-39% third degree burns HCC
T31.94 Burns involving 90% or more of body surface with 40-49% third degree burns HCC
T31.95 Burns involving 90% or more of body surface with 50-59% third degree burns HCC
T31.96 Burns involving 90% or more of body surface with 60-69% third degree burns HCC
T31.97 Burns involving 90% or more of body surface with 70-79% third degree burns HCC
T31.98 Burns involving 90% or more of body surface with 80-89% third degree burns HCC
T31.99 Burns involving 90% or more of body surface with 90% or more third degree burns HCC

4 T32 Corrosions classified according to extent of body surface involved

Note: This category is to be used as the primary code only when the site of the corrosion is unspecified. It may be used as a supplementary code with categories T20-T25 when the site is specified.

T32.0 Corrosions involving less than 10% of body surface

5 T32.1 Corrosions involving 10-19% of body surface
T32.10 Corrosions involving 10-19% of body surface with 0% to 9% third degree corrosion
Corrosions involving 10-19% of body surface NOS
T32.11 Corrosions involving 10-19% of body surface with 10-19% third degree corrosion HCC

5 T32.2 Corrosions involving 20-29% of body surface
T32.20 Corrosions involving 20-29% of body surface with 0% to 9% third degree corrosion
T32.21 Corrosions involving 20-29% of body surface with 10-19% third degree corrosion HCC
T32.22 Corrosions involving 20-29% of body surface with 20-29% third degree corrosion HCC

5 T32.3 Corrosions involving 30-39% of body surface
T32.30 Corrosions involving 30-39% of body surface with 0% to 9% third degree corrosion
T32.31 Corrosions involving 30-39% of body surface with 10-19% third degree corrosion HCC
T32.32 Corrosions involving 30-39% of body surface with 20-29% third degree corrosion HCC
T32.33 Corrosions involving 30-39% of body surface with 30-39% third degree corrosion HCC

5 T32.4 Corrosions involving 40-49% of body surface
T32.40 Corrosions involving 40-49% of body surface with 0% to 9% third degree corrosion
T32.41 Corrosions involving 40-49% of body surface with 10-19% third degree corrosion HCC
T32.42 Corrosions involving 40-49% of body surface with 20-29% third degree corrosion HCC
T32.43 Corrosions involving 40-49% of body surface with 30-39% third degree corrosion HCC
T32.44 Corrosions involving 40-49% of body surface with 40-49% third degree corrosion HCC

5 T32.5 Corrosions involving 50-59% of body surface
T32.50 Corrosions involving 50-59% of body surface with 0% to 9% third degree corrosion
T32.51 Corrosions involving 50-59% of body surface with 10-19% third degree corrosion HCC
T32.52 Corrosions involving 50-59% of body surface with 20-29% third degree corrosion HCC
T32.53 Corrosions involving 50-59% of body surface with 30-39% third degree corrosion HCC
T32.54 Corrosions involving 50-59% of body surface with 40-49% third degree corrosion HCC
T32.55 Corrosions involving 50-59% of body surface with 50-59% third degree corrosion HCC

5 T32.6 Corrosions involving 60-69% of body surface
T32.60 Corrosions involving 60-69% of body surface with 0% to 9% third degree corrosion
T32.61 Corrosions involving 60-69% of body surface with 10-19% third degree corrosion HCC
T32.62 Corrosions involving 60-69% of body surface with 20-29% third degree corrosion HCC
T32.63 Corrosions involving 60-69% of body surface with 30-39% third degree corrosion HCC
T32.64 Corrosions involving 60-69% of body surface with 40-49% third degree corrosion HCC
T32.65 Corrosions involving 60-69% of body surface with 50-59% third degree corrosion HCC
T32.66 Corrosions involving 60-69% of body surface with 60-69% third degree corrosion HCC

5 T32.7 Corrosions involving 70-79% of body surface
T32.70 Corrosions involving 70-79% of body surface with 0% to 9% third degree corrosion
T32.71 Corrosions involving 70-79% of body surface with 10-19% third degree corrosion HCC
T32.72 Corrosions involving 70-79% of body surface with 20-29% third degree corrosion HCC

T32.73 Corrosions involving 70-79% of body surface with 30-39% third degree corrosion HCC
T32.74 Corrosions involving 70-79% of body surface with 40-49% third degree corrosion HCC
T32.75 Corrosions involving 70-79% of body surface with 50-59% third degree corrosion HCC
T32.76 Corrosions involving 70-79% of body surface with 60-69% third degree corrosion HCC
T32.77 Corrosions involving 70-79% of body surface with 70-79% third degree corrosion HCC

5 T32.8 Corrosions involving 80-89% of body surface
T32.80 Corrosions involving 80-89% of body surface with 0% to 9% third degree corrosion
T32.81 Corrosions involving 80-89% of body surface with 10-19% third degree corrosion HCC
T32.82 Corrosions involving 80-89% of body surface with 20-29% third degree corrosion HCC
T32.83 Corrosions involving 80-89% of body surface with 30-39% third degree corrosion HCC
T32.84 Corrosions involving 80-89% of body surface with 40-49% third degree corrosion HCC
T32.85 Corrosions involving 80-89% of body surface with 50-59% third degree corrosion HCC
T32.86 Corrosions involving 80-89% of body surface with 60-69% third degree corrosion HCC
T32.87 Corrosions involving 80-89% of body surface with 70-79% third degree corrosion HCC
T32.88 Corrosions involving 80-89% of body surface with 80-89% third degree corrosion HCC

5 T32.9 Corrosions involving 90% or more of body surface
T32.90 Corrosions involving 90% or more of body surface with 0% to 9% third degree corrosion
T32.91 Corrosions involving 90% or more of body surface with 10-19% third degree corrosion HCC
T32.92 Corrosions involving 90% or more of body surface with 20-29% third degree corrosion HCC
T32.93 Corrosions involving 90% or more of body surface with 30-39% third degree corrosion HCC
T32.94 Corrosions involving 90% or more of body surface with 40-49% third degree corrosion HCC
T32.95 Corrosions involving 90% or more of body surface with 50-59% third degree corrosion HCC
T32.96 Corrosions involving 90% or more of body surface with 60-69% third degree corrosion HCC
T32.97 Corrosions involving 90% or more of body surface with 70-79% third degree corrosion HCC
T32.98 Corrosions involving 90% or more of body surface with 80-89% third degree corrosion HCC
T32.99 Corrosions involving 90% or more of body surface with 90% or more third degree corrosion HCC

Frostbite (T33-T34)

EXCLUDES 2 *hypothermia and other effects of reduced temperature (T68, T69.-)*

4 **T33 Superficial frostbite**

INCLUDES frostbite with partial thickness skin loss

The appropriate 7th character is to be added to each code from category T33
A initial encounter
D subsequent encounter
S sequela

5 T33.0 Superficial frostbite of head
6 T33.01 Superficial frostbite of ear
7 ⊟ T33.011- Superficial frostbite of right ear
7 ⊟ T33.012- Superficial frostbite of left ear
7 ⊟ T33.019- Superficial frostbite of unspecified ear
7 T33.02X- Superficial frostbite of nose
7 T33.09X- Superficial frostbite of other part of head
7 T33.1XX- Superficial frostbite of neck
7 T33.2XX- Superficial frostbite of thorax
7 T33.3XX- Superficial frostbite of abdominal wall, lower back and pelvis
5 T33.4 Superficial frostbite of arm
EXCLUDES 2 *superficial frostbite of wrist and hand (T33.5-)*
7 ⊟ T33.40X- Superficial frostbite of unspecified arm
7 ⊟ T33.41X- Superficial frostbite of right arm
7 ⊟ T33.42X- Superficial frostbite of left arm
5 T33.5 Superficial frostbite of wrist, hand, and fingers
6 T33.51 Superficial frostbite of wrist
7 ⊟ T33.511- Superficial frostbite of right wrist
7 ⊟ T33.512- Superficial frostbite of left wrist
7 ⊟ T33.519- Superficial frostbite of unspecified wrist
6 T33.52 Superficial frostbite of hand
EXCLUDES 2 *superficial frostbite of fingers (T33.53-)*
7 ⊟ T33.521- Superficial frostbite of right hand
7 ⊟ T33.522- Superficial frostbite of left hand
7 ⊟ T33.529- Superficial frostbite of unspecified hand
6 T33.53 Superficial frostbite of finger(s)
7 ⊟ T33.531- Superficial frostbite of right finger(s)
7 ⊟ T33.532- Superficial frostbite of left finger(s)
7 ⊟ T33.539- Superficial frostbite of unspecified finger(s)
5 T33.6 Superficial frostbite of hip and thigh
7 ⊟ T33.60X- Superficial frostbite of unspecified hip and thigh
7 ⊟ T33.61X- Superficial frostbite of right hip and thigh
7 ⊟ T33.62X- Superficial frostbite of left hip and thigh
5 T33.7 Superficial frostbite of knee and lower leg
EXCLUDES 2 *superficial frostbite of ankle and foot (T33.8-)*
7 ⊟ T33.70X- Superficial frostbite of unspecified knee and lower leg
7 ⊟ T33.71X- Superficial frostbite of right knee and lower leg
7 ⊟ T33.72X- Superficial frostbite of left knee and lower leg
5 T33.8 Superficial frostbite of ankle, foot, and toe(s)
6 T33.81 Superficial frostbite of ankle
7 ⊟ T33.811- Superficial frostbite of right ankle
7 ⊟ T33.812- Superficial frostbite of left ankle
7 ⊟ T33.819- Superficial frostbite of unspecified ankle
6 T33.82 Superficial frostbite of foot
7 ⊟ T33.821- Superficial frostbite of right foot
7 ⊟ T33.822- Superficial frostbite of left foot
7 ⊟ T33.829- Superficial frostbite of unspecified foot
6 T33.83 Superficial frostbite of toe(s)
7 ⊟ T33.831- Superficial frostbite of right toe(s)
7 ⊟ T33.832- Superficial frostbite of left toe(s)
7 ⊟ T33.839- Superficial frostbite of unspecified toe(s)
5 T33.9 Superficial frostbite of other and unspecified sites
7 T33.90X- Superficial frostbite of unspecified sites
Superficial frostbite NOS
7 T33.99X- Superficial frostbite of other sites
Superficial frostbite of leg NOS
Superficial frostbite of trunk NOS

4 **T34 Frostbite with tissue necrosis**

The appropriate 7th character is to be added to each code from category T34
A initial encounter
D subsequent encounter
S sequela

5 T34.0 Frostbite with tissue necrosis of head
6 T34.01 Frostbite with tissue necrosis of ear
7 ⊟ T34.011- Frostbite with tissue necrosis of right ear
7 ⊟ T34.012- Frostbite with tissue necrosis of left ear
7 ⊟ T34.019- Frostbite with tissue necrosis of unspecified ear
7 T34.02X- Frostbite with tissue necrosis of nose
7 T34.09X- Frostbite with tissue necrosis of other part of head
7 T34.1XX- Frostbite with tissue necrosis of neck
7 T34.2XX- Frostbite with tissue necrosis of thorax
7 T34.3XX- Frostbite with tissue necrosis of abdominal wall, lower back and pelvis
5 T34.4 Frostbite with tissue necrosis of arm
EXCLUDES 2 *frostbite with tissue necrosis of wrist and hand (T34.5-)*
7 ⊟ T34.40X- Frostbite with tissue necrosis of unspecified arm
7 ⊟ T34.41X- Frostbite with tissue necrosis of right arm

7 ⊟ T34.42X- **Frostbite with tissue necrosis of left arm**

5 **T34.5 Frostbite with tissue necrosis of wrist, hand, and finger(s)**

6 **T34.51 Frostbite with tissue necrosis of wrist**

7 ⊟ T34.511- **Frostbite with tissue necrosis of right wrist**

7 ⊟ T34.512- **Frostbite with tissue necrosis of left wrist**

7 ⊟ T34.519- **Frostbite with tissue necrosis of unspecified wrist**

6 **T34.52 Frostbite with tissue necrosis of hand**

EXCLUDES 2 *frostbite with tissue necrosis of finger (s) (T34.53-)*

7 ⊟ T34.521- **Frostbite with tissue necrosis of right hand**

7 ⊟ T34.522- **Frostbite with tissue necrosis of left hand**

7 ⊟ T34.529- **Frostbite with tissue necrosis of unspecified hand**

6 **T34.53 Frostbite with tissue necrosis of finger(s)**

7 ⊟ T34.531- **Frostbite with tissue necrosis of right finger(s)**

7 ⊟ T34.532- **Frostbite with tissue necrosis of left finger(s)**

7 ⊟ T34.539- **Frostbite with tissue necrosis of unspecified finger(s)**

5 **T34.6 Frostbite with tissue necrosis of hip and thigh**

7 ⊟ T34.60X- **Frostbite with tissue necrosis of unspecified hip and thigh**

7 ⊟ T34.61X- **Frostbite with tissue necrosis of right hip and thigh**

7 ⊟ T34.62X- **Frostbite with tissue necrosis of left hip and thigh**

5 **T34.7 Frostbite with tissue necrosis of knee and lower leg**

EXCLUDES 2 *frostbite with tissue necrosis of ankle and foot (T34.8-)*

7 ⊟ T34.70X- **Frostbite with tissue necrosis of unspecified knee and lower leg**

7 ⊟ T34.71X- **Frostbite with tissue necrosis of right knee and lower leg**

7 ⊟ T34.72X- **Frostbite with tissue necrosis of left knee and lower leg**

5 **T34.8 Frostbite with tissue necrosis of ankle, foot, and toe(s)**

6 **T34.81 Frostbite with tissue necrosis of ankle**

7 ⊟ T34.811- **Frostbite with tissue necrosis of right ankle**

7 ⊟ T34.812- **Frostbite with tissue necrosis of left ankle**

7 ⊟ T34.819- **Frostbite with tissue necrosis of unspecified ankle**

6 **T34.82 Frostbite with tissue necrosis of foot**

7 ⊟ T34.821- **Frostbite with tissue necrosis of right foot**

7 ⊟ T34.822- **Frostbite with tissue necrosis of left foot**

7 ⊟ T34.829- **Frostbite with tissue necrosis of unspecified foot**

6 **T34.83 Frostbite with tissue necrosis of toe(s)**

7 ⊟ T34.831- **Frostbite with tissue necrosis of right toe(s)**

7 ⊟ T34.832- **Frostbite with tissue necrosis of left toe(s)**

7 ⊟ T34.839- **Frostbite with tissue necrosis of unspecified toe(s)**

5 **T34.9 Frostbite with tissue necrosis of other and unspecified sites**

7 T34.90X- **Frostbite with tissue necrosis of unspecified sites**
Frostbite with tissue necrosis NOS

7 T34.99X- **Frostbite with tissue necrosis of other sites**
Frostbite with tissue necrosis of leg NOS
Frostbite with tissue necrosis of trunk NOS

Poisoning by, adverse effects of and underdosing of drugs, medicaments and biological substances (T36-T50)

Note: The drug giving rise to the adverse effect should be identified by use of codes from categories T36-T50 with fifth or sixth character 5.

INCLUDES adverse effect of correct substance properly administered
poisoning by overdose of substance
poisoning by wrong substance given or taken in error
underdosing by (inadvertently) (deliberately) taking less substance than prescribed or instructed

Code first, for adverse effects, the nature of the adverse effect, such as:
adverse effect NOS (T88.7)
aspirin gastritis (K29.-)
blood disorders (D56-D76)
contact dermatitis (L23-L25)
dermatitis due to substances taken internally (L27.-)
nephropathy (N14.0-N14.2)

Use additional code(s) to specify:
manifestations of poisoning
underdosing or failure in dosage during medical and surgical care (Y63.6, Y63.8-Y63.9)
underdosing of medication regimen (Z91.12-, Z91.13-)

EXCLUDES 1 *toxic reaction to local anesthesia in pregnancy (O29.3-)*

EXCLUDES 2 *abuse and dependence of psychoactive substances (F10-F19)*
abuse of non-dependence-producing substances (F55.-)
drug reaction and poisoning affecting newborn (P00-P96)
pathological drug intoxication (inebriation) (F10-F19)

GUIDELINES **Section I.C.19.e.1)-4)**
Codes in categories T36-T65 are combination codes that include the substance that was taken as well as the intent. No additional external cause code is required for poisonings, toxic effects, adverse effects and underdosing codes.

Do not code directly from the Table of Drugs and Chemicals. Always refer back to the Tabular List. Use as many codes as necessary to describe completely all drugs, medicinal or biological substances. If the same code would describe the causative agent for more than one adverse reaction, poisoning, toxic effect or underdosing, assign the code only once. If two or more drugs, medicinal or biological substances are reported, code each individually unless a combination code is listed in the Table of Drugs and Chemicals.

GUIDELINES **Section I.C.19.e.5)(a)**
When coding an adverse effect of a drug that has been correctly prescribed and properly administered, assign the appropriate code for the nature of the adverse effect followed by the appropriate code for the adverse effect of the drug (T36-T50). The code for the drug should have a 5th or 6th character "5" (for example T36.0X5-). Examples of the nature of an adverse effect are tachycardia, delirium, gastrointestinal hemorrhaging, vomiting, hypokalemia, hepatitis, renal failure, or respiratory failure.

CODING TIP✓ Poisonings are coded as accidental unless there is physician documentation to indicate otherwise. 7th character 'A' means the effect of the drug/chemical requires active treatment. 'D' should be the 7th character if the effect is healing/resolving. 'S' should be used as the 7th character if the condition resulting is still a factor after the medication has long cleared from the body, i.e., glucocorticoids were taken last year resulting in diabetes.

CODING TIP✓ When coding an adverse effect of a drug that has been correctly prescribed and administered, assign "5" as the fifth or sixth character to the appropriate code for the drug.

4 **T36 Poisoning by, adverse effect of and underdosing of systemic antibiotics**

EXCLUDES 1 *antineoplastic antibiotics (T45.1-)*
locally applied antibiotic NEC (T49.0)
topically used antibiotic for ear, nose and throat (T49.6)
topically used antibiotic for eye (T49.5)

The appropriate 7th character is to be added to each code from category T36

A	initial encounter
D	subsequent encounter
S	sequela

GUIDELINES **Section I.C.19.e.5)(c)**
Underdosing refers to taking less of a medication than is prescribed by a provider or a manufacturer's instruction. Discontinuing the use of a prescribed medication on the patient's own initiative (not directed by the patient's provider) is also classified as an underdosing. For underdosing, assign the code from categories T36-T50 (fifth or sixth character "6").

Codes for underdosing should never be assigned as principal or first-listed codes. If a patient has a relapse or exacerbation of the medical condition for which the drug is prescribed because of the reduction in dose, then the medical condition itself should be coded.

Noncompliance (Z91.12-, Z91.13- and Z91.14-) or complication of care (Y63.6-Y63.9) codes are to be used with an underdosing code to indicate intent, if known.

GUIDELINES **Section I.C.19.e.5)(b)**
When coding a poisoning or reaction to the improper use of a medication (e.g., overdose, wrong substance given or taken in error, wrong route of administration), first assign the appropriate code from categories T36-T50. The poisoning codes have an associated intent as their 5th or 6th character (accidental, intentional self harm, assault and undetermined. If the intent of the poisoning is unknown or unspecified, code the intent as accidental intent. The undetermined intent is only for use if the documentation in the record specifies that the intent cannot be determined.

Use additional code(s) for all manifestations of poisonings. If there is also a diagnosis of abuse or dependence of the substance, the abuse or dependence is assigned as an additional code.
See Section I.C.4. if poisoning is the result of insulin pump malfunctions.

5 **T36.0** **Poisoning by, adverse effect of and underdosing of penicillins**
6 **T36.0X** **Poisoning by, adverse effect of and underdosing of penicillins**
7 **T36.0X1-** **Poisoning by penicillins, accidental (unintentional)**
Poisoning by penicillins NOS
7 **T36.0X2-** **Poisoning by penicillins, intentional self-harm** HCC
7 **T36.0X3-** **Poisoning by penicillins, assault**
7 **T36.0X4-** **Poisoning by penicillins, undetermined**
7 **T36.0X5-** **Adverse effect of penicillins**
7 **T36.0X6-** **Underdosing of penicillins**
5 **T36.1** **Poisoning by, adverse effect of and underdosing of cephalosporins and other beta-lactam antibiotics**
6 **T36.1X** **Poisoning by, adverse effect of and underdosing of cephalosporins and other beta-lactam antibiotics**
7 **T36.1X1-** **Poisoning by cephalosporins and other beta-lactam antibiotics, accidental (unintentional)**
Poisoning by cephalosporins and other beta-lactam antibiotics NOS
7 **T36.1X2-** **Poisoning by cephalosporins and other beta-lactam antibiotics, intentional self-harm** HCC
7 **T36.1X3-** **Poisoning by cephalosporins and other beta-lactam antibiotics, assault**
7 **T36.1X4-** **Poisoning by cephalosporins and other beta-lactam antibiotics, undetermined**
7 **T36.1X5-** **Adverse effect of cephalosporins and other beta-lactam antibiotics**
7 **T36.1X6-** **Underdosing of cephalosporins and other beta-lactam antibiotics**
5 **T36.2** **Poisoning by, adverse effect of and underdosing of chloramphenicol group**
6 **T36.2X** **Poisoning by, adverse effect of and underdosing of chloramphenicol group**
7 **T36.2X1-** **Poisoning by chloramphenicol group, accidental (unintentional)**
Poisoning by chloramphenicol group NOS
7 **T36.2X2-** **Poisoning by chloramphenicol group, intentional self-harm** HCC
7 **T36.2X3-** **Poisoning by chloramphenicol group, assault**
7 **T36.2X4-** **Poisoning by chloramphenicol group, undetermined**
7 **T36.2X5-** **Adverse effect of chloramphenicol group**
7 **T36.2X6-** **Underdosing of chloramphenicol group**
5 **T36.3** **Poisoning by, adverse effect of and underdosing of macrolides**
6 **T36.3X** **Poisoning by, adverse effect of and underdosing of macrolides**
7 **T36.3X1-** **Poisoning by macrolides, accidental (unintentional)**
Poisoning by macrolides NOS
7 **T36.3X2-** **Poisoning by macrolides, intentional self-harm** HCC
7 **T36.3X3-** **Poisoning by macrolides, assault**
7 **T36.3X4-** **Poisoning by macrolides, undetermined**
7 **T36.3X5-** **Adverse effect of macrolides**
7 **T36.3X6-** **Underdosing of macrolides**
5 **T36.4** **Poisoning by, adverse effect of and underdosing of tetracyclines**
6 **T36.4X** **Poisoning by, adverse effect of and underdosing of tetracyclines**
7 **T36.4X1-** **Poisoning by tetracyclines, accidental (unintentional)**
Poisoning by tetracyclines NOS
7 **T36.4X2-** **Poisoning by tetracyclines, intentional self-harm** HCC
7 **T36.4X3-** **Poisoning by tetracyclines, assault**
7 **T36.4X4-** **Poisoning by tetracyclines, undetermined**
7 **T36.4X5-** **Adverse effect of tetracyclines**
7 **T36.4X6-** **Underdosing of tetracyclines**
5 **T36.5** **Poisoning by, adverse effect of and underdosing of aminoglycosides**
Poisoning by, adverse effect of and underdosing of streptomycin
6 **T36.5X** **Poisoning by, adverse effect of and underdosing of aminoglycosides**
7 **T36.5X1-** **Poisoning by aminoglycosides, accidental (unintentional)**
Poisoning by aminoglycosides NOS
7 **T36.5X2-** **Poisoning by aminoglycosides, intentional self-harm** HCC
7 **T36.5X3-** **Poisoning by aminoglycosides, assault**
7 **T36.5X4-** **Poisoning by aminoglycosides, undetermined**
7 **T36.5X5-** **Adverse effect of aminoglycosides**
7 **T36.5X6-** **Underdosing of aminoglycosides**
5 **T36.6** **Poisoning by, adverse effect of and underdosing of rifampicins**
6 **T36.6X** **Poisoning by, adverse effect of and underdosing of rifampicins**
7 **T36.6X1-** **Poisoning by rifampicins, accidental (unintentional)**
Poisoning by rifampicins NOS
7 **T36.6X2-** **Poisoning by rifampicins, intentional self-harm** HCC
7 **T36.6X3-** **Poisoning by rifampicins, assault**
7 **T36.6X4-** **Poisoning by rifampicins, undetermined**
7 **T36.6X5-** **Adverse effect of rifampicins**
7 **T36.6X6-** **Underdosing of rifampicins**
5 **T36.7** **Poisoning by, adverse effect of and underdosing of antifungal antibiotics, systemically used**
6 **T36.7X** **Poisoning by, adverse effect of and underdosing of antifungal antibiotics, systemically used**
7 **T36.7X1-** **Poisoning by antifungal antibiotics, systemically used, accidental (unintentional)**
Poisoning by antifungal antibiotics, systemically used NOS
7 **T36.7X2-** **Poisoning by antifungal antibiotics, systemically used, intentional self-harm** HCC
7 **T36.7X3-** **Poisoning by antifungal antibiotics, systemically used, assault**
7 **T36.7X4-** **Poisoning by antifungal antibiotics, systemically used, undetermined**
7 **T36.7X5-** **Adverse effect of antifungal antibiotics, systemically used**
7 **T36.7X6-** **Underdosing of antifungal antibiotics, systemically used**
5 **T36.8** **Poisoning by, adverse effect of and underdosing of other systemic antibiotics**

6 T36.8X Poisoning by, adverse effect of and underdosing of other systemic antibiotics
7 T36.8X1- Poisoning by other systemic antibiotics, accidental (unintentional)
Poisoning by other systemic antibiotics NOS
7 T36.8X2- Poisoning by other systemic antibiotics, intentional self-harm HCC
7 T36.8X3- Poisoning by other systemic antibiotics, assault
7 T36.8X4- Poisoning by other systemic antibiotics, undetermined
7 T36.8X5- Adverse effect of other systemic antibiotics
AHA: 1Q 2017, 39
7 T36.8X6- Underdosing of other systemic antibiotics
5 T36.9 Poisoning by, adverse effect of and underdosing of unspecified systemic antibiotic
7 T36.91X- Poisoning by unspecified systemic antibiotic, accidental (unintentional)
Poisoning by systemic antibiotic NOS
7 T36.92X- Poisoning by unspecified systemic antibiotic, intentional self-harm HCC
7 T36.93X- Poisoning by unspecified systemic antibiotic, assault
7 T36.94X- Poisoning by unspecified systemic antibiotic, undetermined
7 T36.95X- Adverse effect of unspecified systemic antibiotic
7 T36.96X- Underdosing of unspecified systemic antibiotic

4 T37 Poisoning by, adverse effect of and underdosing of other systemic anti-infectives and antiparasitics
EXCLUDES 1 *anti-infectives topically used for ear, nose and throat (T49.6-)*
anti-infectives topically used for eye (T49.5-)
locally applied anti-infectives NEC (T49.0-)

The appropriate 7th character is to be added to each code from category T37
A initial encounter
D subsequent encounter
S sequela

5 T37.0 Poisoning by, adverse effect of and underdosing of sulfonamides
6 T37.0X Poisoning by, adverse effect of and underdosing of sulfonamides
7 T37.0X1- Poisoning by sulfonamides, accidental (unintentional)
Poisoning by sulfonamides NOS
7 T37.0X2- Poisoning by sulfonamides, intentional self-harm HCC
7 T37.0X3- Poisoning by sulfonamides, assault
7 T37.0X4- Poisoning by sulfonamides, undetermined
7 T37.0X5- Adverse effect of sulfonamides
7 T37.0X6- Underdosing of sulfonamides
5 T37.1 Poisoning by, adverse effect of and underdosing of antimycobacterial drugs
EXCLUDES 1 *rifampicins (T36.6-)*
streptomycin (T36.5-)
6 T37.1X Poisoning by, adverse effect of and underdosing of antimycobacterial drugs
7 T37.1X1- Poisoning by antimycobacterial drugs, accidental (unintentional)
Poisoning by antimycobacterial drugs NOS
7 T37.1X2- Poisoning by antimycobacterial drugs, intentional self-harm HCC
7 T37.1X3- Poisoning by antimycobacterial drugs, assault
7 T37.1X4- Poisoning by antimycobacterial drugs, undetermined
7 T37.1X5- Adverse effect of antimycobacterial drugs
7 T37.1X6- Underdosing of antimycobacterial drugs
5 T37.2 Poisoning by, adverse effect of and underdosing of antimalarials and drugs acting on other blood protozoa
EXCLUDES 1 *hydroxyquinoline derivatives (T37.8-)*
6 T37.2X Poisoning by, adverse effect of and underdosing of antimalarials and drugs acting on other blood protozoa
7 T37.2X1- Poisoning by antimalarials and drugs acting on other blood protozoa, accidental (unintentional)
Poisoning by antimalarials and drugs acting on other blood protozoa NOS
7 T37.2X2- Poisoning by antimalarials and drugs acting on other blood protozoa, intentional self-harm HCC
7 T37.2X3- Poisoning by antimalarials and drugs acting on other blood protozoa, assault
7 T37.2X4- Poisoning by antimalarials and drugs acting on other blood protozoa, undetermined
7 T37.2X5- Adverse effect of antimalarials and drugs acting on other blood protozoa
7 T37.2X6- Underdosing of antimalarials and drugs acting on other blood protozoa
5 T37.3 Poisoning by, adverse effect of and underdosing of other antiprotozoal drugs
6 T37.3X Poisoning by, adverse effect of and underdosing of other antiprotozoal drugs
7 T37.3X1- Poisoning by other antiprotozoal drugs, accidental (unintentional)
Poisoning by other antiprotozoal drugs NOS
7 T37.3X2- Poisoning by other antiprotozoal drugs, intentional self-harm HCC
7 T37.3X3- Poisoning by other antiprotozoal drugs, assault
7 T37.3X4- Poisoning by other antiprotozoal drugs, undetermined
7 T37.3X5- Adverse effect of other antiprotozoal drugs
7 T37.3X6- Underdosing of other antiprotozoal drugs
5 T37.4 Poisoning by, adverse effect of and underdosing of anthelminthics
6 T37.4X Poisoning by, adverse effect of and underdosing of anthelminthics
7 T37.4X1- Poisoning by anthelminthics, accidental (unintentional)
Poisoning by anthelminthics NOS
7 T37.4X2- Poisoning by anthelminthics, intentional self-harm HCC
7 T37.4X3- Poisoning by anthelminthics, assault
7 T37.4X4- Poisoning by anthelminthics, undetermined
7 T37.4X5- Adverse effect of anthelminthics
7 T37.4X6- Underdosing of anthelminthics
5 T37.5 Poisoning by, adverse effect of and underdosing of antiviral drugs
EXCLUDES 1 *amantadine (T42.8-)*
cytarabine (T45.1-)
6 T37.5X Poisoning by, adverse effect of and underdosing of antiviral drugs
7 T37.5X1- Poisoning by antiviral drugs, accidental (unintentional)
Poisoning by antiviral drugs NOS
7 T37.5X2- Poisoning by antiviral drugs, intentional self-harm HCC
7 T37.5X3- Poisoning by antiviral drugs, assault
7 T37.5X4- Poisoning by antiviral drugs, undetermined
7 T37.5X5- Adverse effect of antiviral drugs
7 T37.5X6- Underdosing of antiviral drugs
5 T37.8 Poisoning by, adverse effect of and underdosing of other specified systemic anti-infectives and antiparasitics
Poisoning by, adverse effect of and underdosing of hydroxyquinoline derivatives
EXCLUDES 1 *antimalarial drugs (T37.2-)*
6 T37.8X Poisoning by, adverse effect of and underdosing of other specified systemic anti-infectives and antiparasitics
7 T37.8X1- Poisoning by other specified systemic anti-infectives and antiparasitics, accidental (unintentional)
Poisoning by other specified systemic anti-infectives and antiparasitics NOS
7 T37.8X2- Poisoning by other specified systemic anti-infectives and antiparasitics, intentional self-harm HCC
7 T37.8X3- Poisoning by other specified systemic anti-infectives and antiparasitics, assault
7 T37.8X4- Poisoning by other specified systemic anti-infectives and antiparasitics, undetermined
7 T37.8X5- Adverse effect of other specified systemic anti-infectives and antiparasitics
7 T37.8X6- Underdosing of other specified systemic anti-infectives and antiparasitics
5 T37.9 Poisoning by, adverse effect of and underdosing of unspecified systemic anti-infective and antiparasitics

7 T37.91X- **Poisoning by unspecified systemic anti-infective and antiparasitics, accidental (unintentional)**
Poisoning by, adverse effect of and underdosing of systemic anti-infective and antiparasitics NOS

7 T37.92X- **Poisoning by unspecified systemic anti-infective and antiparasitics, intentional self-harm** HCC

7 T37.93X- **Poisoning by unspecified systemic anti-infective and antiparasitics, assault**

7 T37.94X- **Poisoning by unspecified systemic anti-infective and antiparasitics, undetermined**

7 T37.95X- **Adverse effect of unspecified systemic anti-infective and antiparasitic**

7 T37.96X- **Underdosing of unspecified systemic anti-infectives and antiparasitics**

4 T38 **Poisoning by, adverse effect of and underdosing of hormones and their synthetic substitutes and antagonists, not elsewhere classified**

EXCLUDES 1 *mineralocorticoids and their antagonists (T50.0-)*
oxytocic hormones (T48.0-)
parathyroid hormones and derivatives (T50.9-)

The appropriate 7th character is to be added to each code from category T38
A initial encounter
D subsequent encounter
S sequela

5 T38.0 **Poisoning by, adverse effect of and underdosing of glucocorticoids and synthetic analogues**

EXCLUDES 1 *glucocorticoids, topically used (T49.-)*

6 T38.0X **Poisoning by, adverse effect of and underdosing of glucocorticoids and synthetic analogues**

7 T38.0X1- **Poisoning by glucocorticoids and synthetic analogues, accidental (unintentional)**
Poisoning by glucocorticoids and synthetic analogues NOS

7 T38.0X2- **Poisoning by glucocorticoids and synthetic analogues, intentional self-harm** HCC

7 T38.0X3- **Poisoning by glucocorticoids and synthetic analogues, assault**

7 T38.0X4- **Poisoning by glucocorticoids and synthetic analogues, undetermined**

7 T38.0X5- **Adverse effect of glucocorticoids and synthetic analogues**

7 T38.0X6- **Underdosing of glucocorticoids and synthetic analogues**

5 T38.1 **Poisoning by, adverse effect of and underdosing of thyroid hormones and substitutes**

6 T38.1X **Poisoning by, adverse effect of and underdosing of thyroid hormones and substitutes**

7 T38.1X1- **Poisoning by thyroid hormones and substitutes, accidental (unintentional)**
Poisoning by thyroid hormones and substitutes NOS

7 T38.1X2- **Poisoning by thyroid hormones and substitutes, intentional self-harm** HCC

7 T38.1X3- **Poisoning by thyroid hormones and substitutes, assault**

7 T38.1X4- **Poisoning by thyroid hormones and substitutes, undetermined**

7 T38.1X5- **Adverse effect of thyroid hormones and substitutes**

7 T38.1X6- **Underdosing of thyroid hormones and substitutes**

5 T38.2 **Poisoning by, adverse effect of and underdosing of antithyroid drugs**

6 T38.2X **Poisoning by, adverse effect of and underdosing of antithyroid drugs**

7 T38.2X1- **Poisoning by antithyroid drugs, accidental (unintentional)**
Poisoning by antithyroid drugs NOS

7 T38.2X2- **Poisoning by antithyroid drugs, intentional self-harm** HCC

7 T38.2X3- **Poisoning by antithyroid drugs, assault**

7 T38.2X4- **Poisoning by antithyroid drugs, undetermined**

7 T38.2X5- **Adverse effect of antithyroid drugs**

7 T38.2X6- **Underdosing of antithyroid drugs**

5 T38.3 **Poisoning by, adverse effect of and underdosing of insulin and oral hypoglycemic [antidiabetic] drugs**

6 T38.3X **Poisoning by, adverse effect of and underdosing of insulin and oral hypoglycemic [antidiabetic] drugs**

7 T38.3X1- **Poisoning by insulin and oral hypoglycemic [antidiabetic] drugs, accidental (unintentional)**
Poisoning by insulin and oral hypoglycemic [antidiabetic] drugs NOS

GUIDELINES **Section I.C.4.a.5)(b)**
The principal or first-listed code for an encounter due to an insulin pump malfunction resulting in an overdose of insulin, should also be T85.6-, Mechanical complication of other specified internal and external prosthetic devices, implants and grafts, followed by code T38.3x1-.

7 T38.3X2- **Poisoning by insulin and oral hypoglycemic [antidiabetic] drugs, intentional self-harm** HCC

7 T38.3X3- **Poisoning by insulin and oral hypoglycemic [antidiabetic] drugs, assault**

7 T38.3X4- **Poisoning by insulin and oral hypoglycemic [antidiabetic] drugs, undetermined**

7 T38.3X5- **Adverse effect of insulin and oral hypoglycemic [antidiabetic] drugs**

7 T38.3X6- **Underdosing of insulin and oral hypoglycemic [antidiabetic] drugs**

GUIDELINES **Section I.C.4.a.5)(a)**
An underdose of insulin due to an insulin pump failure should be assigned to a code from subcategory T85.6, Mechanical complication of other specified internal and external prosthetic devices, implants and grafts, followed by code T38.3x6-. Additional codes for the type of diabetes mellitus and any associated complications due to the underdosing should also be assigned.

5 T38.4 **Poisoning by, adverse effect of and underdosing of oral contraceptives**
Poisoning by, adverse effect of and underdosing of multiple- and single-ingredient oral contraceptive preparations

6 T38.4X **Poisoning by, adverse effect of and underdosing of oral contraceptives**

7 T38.4X1- **Poisoning by oral contraceptives, accidental (unintentional)**
Poisoning by oral contraceptives NOS

7 T38.4X2- **Poisoning by oral contraceptives, intentional self-harm** HCC

7 T38.4X3- **Poisoning by oral contraceptives, assault**

7 T38.4X4- **Poisoning by oral contraceptives, undetermined**

7 T38.4X5- **Adverse effect of oral contraceptives**

7 T38.4X6- **Underdosing of oral contraceptives**

5 T38.5 **Poisoning by, adverse effect of and underdosing of other estrogens and progestogens**
Poisoning by, adverse effect of and underdosing of estrogens and progestogens mixtures and substitutes

6 T38.5X **Poisoning by, adverse effect of and underdosing of other estrogens and progestogens**

7 T38.5X1- **Poisoning by other estrogens and progestogens, accidental (unintentional)**
Poisoning by other estrogens and progestogens NOS

7 T38.5X2- **Poisoning by other estrogens and progestogens, intentional self-harm** HCC

7 T38.5X3- **Poisoning by other estrogens and progestogens, assault**

7 T38.5X4- **Poisoning by other estrogens and progestogens, undetermined**

7 T38.5X5- **Adverse effect of other estrogens and progestogens**

7 T38.5X6- **Underdosing of other estrogens and progestogens**

5 T38.6 **Poisoning by, adverse effect of and underdosing of antigonadotrophins, antiestrogens, antiandrogens, not elsewhere classified**
Poisoning by, adverse effect of and underdosing of tamoxifen

6 T38.6X **Poisoning by, adverse effect of and underdosing of antigonadotrophins, antiestrogens, antiandrogens, not elsewhere classified**

7 T38.6X1- **Poisoning by antigonadotrophins, antiestrogens, antiandrogens, not elsewhere classified, accidental (unintentional)**
Poisoning by antigonadotrophins, antiestrogens, antiandrogens, not elsewhere classified NOS

7 T38.6X2- **Poisoning by antigonadotrophins, antiestrogens, antiandrogens, not elsewhere classified, intentional self-harm** HCC

7 T38.6X3- **Poisoning by antigonadotrophins, antiestrogens, antiandrogens, not elsewhere classified, assault**

7 T38.6X4- **Poisoning by antigonadotrophins, antiestrogens, antiandrogens, not elsewhere classified, undetermined**

7 T38.6X5- **Adverse effect of antigonadotrophins, antiestrogens, antiandrogens, not elsewhere classified**

7 T38.6X6- **Underdosing of antigonadotrophins, antiestrogens, antiandrogens, not elsewhere classified**

5 T38.7 **Poisoning by, adverse effect of and underdosing of androgens and anabolic congeners**

6 T38.7X **Poisoning by, adverse effect of and underdosing of androgens and anabolic congeners**

7 T38.7X1- **Poisoning by androgens and anabolic congeners, accidental (unintentional)**
Poisoning by androgens and anabolic congeners NOS

7 T38.7X2- **Poisoning by androgens and anabolic congeners, intentional self-harm** HCC

7 T38.7X3- **Poisoning by androgens and anabolic congeners, assault**

7 T38.7X4- **Poisoning by androgens and anabolic congeners, undetermined**

7 T38.7X5- **Adverse effect of androgens and anabolic congeners**

7 T38.7X6- **Underdosing of androgens and anabolic congeners**

5 T38.8 **Poisoning by, adverse effect of and underdosing of other and unspecified hormones and synthetic substitutes**

6 T38.80 **Poisoning by, adverse effect of and underdosing of unspecified hormones and synthetic substitutes**

7 T38.801- **Poisoning by unspecified hormones and synthetic substitutes, accidental (unintentional)**
Poisoning by unspecified hormones and synthetic substitutes NOS

7 T38.802- **Poisoning by unspecified hormones and synthetic substitutes, intentional self-harm** HCC

7 T38.803- **Poisoning by unspecified hormones and synthetic substitutes, assault**

7 T38.804- **Poisoning by unspecified hormones and synthetic substitutes, undetermined**

7 T38.805- **Adverse effect of unspecified hormones and synthetic substitutes**

7 T38.806- **Underdosing of unspecified hormones and synthetic substitutes**

6 T38.81 **Poisoning by, adverse effect of and underdosing of anterior pituitary [adenohypophyseal] hormones**

7 T38.811- **Poisoning by anterior pituitary [adenohypophyseal] hormones, accidental (unintentional)**
Poisoning by anterior pituitary [adenohypophyseal] hormones NOS

7 T38.812- **Poisoning by anterior pituitary [adenohypophyseal] hormones, intentional self-harm** HCC

7 T38.813- **Poisoning by anterior pituitary [adenohypophyseal] hormones, assault**

7 T38.814- **Poisoning by anterior pituitary [adenohypophyseal] hormones, undetermined**

7 T38.815- **Adverse effect of anterior pituitary [adenohypophyseal] hormones**

7 T38.816- **Underdosing of anterior pituitary [adenohypophyseal] hormones**

6 T38.89 **Poisoning by, adverse effect of and underdosing of other hormones and synthetic substitutes**

7 T38.891- **Poisoning by other hormones and synthetic substitutes, accidental (unintentional)**
Poisoning by other hormones and synthetic substitutes NOS

7 T38.892- **Poisoning by other hormones and synthetic substitutes, intentional self-harm** HCC

7 T38.893- **Poisoning by other hormones and synthetic substitutes, assault**

7 T38.894- **Poisoning by other hormones and synthetic substitutes, undetermined**

7 T38.895- **Adverse effect of other hormones and synthetic substitutes**

7 T38.896- **Underdosing of other hormones and synthetic substitutes**

5 T38.9 **Poisoning by, adverse effect of and underdosing of other and unspecified hormone antagonists**

6 T38.90 **Poisoning by, adverse effect of and underdosing of unspecified hormone antagonists**

7 T38.901- **Poisoning by unspecified hormone antagonists, accidental (unintentional)**
Poisoning by unspecified hormone antagonists NOS

7 T38.902- **Poisoning by unspecified hormone antagonists, intentional self-harm** HCC

7 T38.903- **Poisoning by unspecified hormone antagonists, assault**

7 T38.904- **Poisoning by unspecified hormone antagonists, undetermined**

7 T38.905- **Adverse effect of unspecified hormone antagonists**

7 T38.906- **Underdosing of unspecified hormone antagonists**

6 T38.99 **Poisoning by, adverse effect of and underdosing of other hormone antagonists**

7 T38.991- **Poisoning by other hormone antagonists, accidental (unintentional)**
Poisoning by other hormone antagonists NOS

7 T38.992- **Poisoning by other hormone antagonists, intentional self-harm** HCC

7 T38.993- **Poisoning by other hormone antagonists, assault**

7 T38.994- **Poisoning by other hormone antagonists, undetermined**

7 T38.995- **Adverse effect of other hormone antagonists**

7 T38.996- **Underdosing of other hormone antagonists**

4 T39 Poisoning by, adverse effect of and underdosing of nonopioid analgesics, antipyretics and antirheumatics

The appropriate 7th character is to be added to each code from category T39
A initial encounter
D subsequent encounter
S sequela

5 T39.0 **Poisoning by, adverse effect of and underdosing of salicylates**

6 T39.01 **Poisoning by, adverse effect of and underdosing of aspirin**
Poisoning by, adverse effect of and underdosing of acetylsalicylic acid

7 T39.011- **Poisoning by aspirin, accidental (unintentional)**

7 T39.012- **Poisoning by aspirin, intentional self-harm** HCC

7 T39.013- **Poisoning by aspirin, assault**

7 T39.014- **Poisoning by aspirin, undetermined**

7 T39.015- **Adverse effect of aspirin**
AHA: (T39.015A) 1Q 2016, 15

7 T39.016- **Underdosing of aspirin**

6 T39.09 **Poisoning by, adverse effect of and underdosing of other salicylates**

7 **T39.091-** **Poisoning by salicylates, accidental (unintentional)**
Poisoning by salicylates NOS

7 **T39.092-** **Poisoning by salicylates, intentional self-harm** HCC

7 **T39.093-** **Poisoning by salicylates, assault**

7 **T39.094-** **Poisoning by salicylates, undetermined**

7 **T39.095-** **Adverse effect of salicylates**

7 **T39.096-** **Underdosing of salicylates**

5 **T39.1** **Poisoning by, adverse effect of and underdosing of 4-Aminophenol derivatives**

6 **T39.1X** **Poisoning by, adverse effect of and underdosing of 4-Aminophenol derivatives**

7 **T39.1X1-** **Poisoning by 4-Aminophenol derivatives, accidental (unintentional)**
Poisoning by 4-Aminophenol derivatives NOS

7 **T39.1X2-** **Poisoning by 4-Aminophenol derivatives, intentional self-harm** HCC

7 **T39.1X3-** **Poisoning by 4-Aminophenol derivatives, assault**

7 **T39.1X4-** **Poisoning by 4-Aminophenol derivatives, undetermined**

7 **T39.1X5-** **Adverse effect of 4-Aminophenol derivatives**

7 **T39.1X6-** **Underdosing of 4-Aminophenol derivatives**

5 **T39.2** **Poisoning by, adverse effect of and underdosing of pyrazolone derivatives**

6 **T39.2X** **Poisoning by, adverse effect of and underdosing of pyrazolone derivatives**

7 **T39.2X1-** **Poisoning by pyrazolone derivatives, accidental (unintentional)**
Poisoning by pyrazolone derivatives NOS

7 **T39.2X2-** **Poisoning by pyrazolone derivatives, intentional self-harm** HCC

7 **T39.2X3-** **Poisoning by pyrazolone derivatives, assault**

7 **T39.2X4-** **Poisoning by pyrazolone derivatives, undetermined**

7 **T39.2X5-** **Adverse effect of pyrazolone derivatives**

7 **T39.2X6-** **Underdosing of pyrazolone derivatives**

5 **T39.3** **Poisoning by, adverse effect of and underdosing of other nonsteroidal anti-inflammatory drugs [NSAID]**

6 **T39.31** **Poisoning by, adverse effect of and underdosing of propionic acid derivatives**
Poisoning by, adverse effect of and underdosing of fenoprofen
Poisoning by, adverse effect of and underdosing of flurbiprofen
Poisoning by, adverse effect of and underdosing of ibuprofen
Poisoning by, adverse effect of and underdosing of ketoprofen
Poisoning by, adverse effect of and underdosing of naproxen
Poisoning by, adverse effect of and underdosing of oxaprozin

7 **T39.311-** **Poisoning by propionic acid derivatives, accidental (unintentional)**

7 **T39.312-** **Poisoning by propionic acid derivatives, intentional self-harm** HCC

7 **T39.313-** **Poisoning by propionic acid derivatives, assault**

7 **T39.314-** **Poisoning by propionic acid derivatives, undetermined**

7 **T39.315-** **Adverse effect of propionic acid derivatives**

7 **T39.316-** **Underdosing of propionic acid derivatives**

6 **T39.39** **Poisoning by, adverse effect of and underdosing of other nonsteroidal anti-inflammatory drugs [NSAID]**

7 **T39.391-** **Poisoning by other nonsteroidal anti-inflammatory drugs [NSAID], accidental (unintentional)**
Poisoning by other nonsteroidal anti-inflammatory drugs NOS

7 **T39.392-** **Poisoning by other nonsteroidal anti-inflammatory drugs [NSAID], intentional self-harm** HCC

7 **T39.393-** **Poisoning by other nonsteroidal anti-inflammatory drugs [NSAID], assault**

7 **T39.394-** **Poisoning by other nonsteroidal anti-inflammatory drugs [NSAID], undetermined**

7 **T39.395-** **Adverse effect of other nonsteroidal anti-inflammatory drugs [NSAID]**

7 **T39.396-** **Underdosing of other nonsteroidal anti-inflammatory drugs [NSAID]**

5 **T39.4** **Poisoning by, adverse effect of and underdosing of antirheumatics, not elsewhere classified**
EXCLUDES 1 *poisoning by, adverse effect of and underdosing of glucocorticoids (T38.0-)*
poisoning by, adverse effect of and underdosing of salicylates (T39.0-)

6 **T39.4X** **Poisoning by, adverse effect of and underdosing of antirheumatics, not elsewhere classified**

7 **T39.4X1-** **Poisoning by antirheumatics, not elsewhere classified, ~~accidental (unintentional)~~**
Poisoning by antirheumatics, not elsewhere classified NOS

7 **T39.4X2-** **Poisoning by antirheumatics, not elsewhere classified, intentional self-harm** HCC

7 **T39.4X3-** **Poisoning by antirheumatics, not elsewhere classified, assault**

7 **T39.4X4-** **Poisoning by antirheumatics, not elsewhere classified, undetermined**

7 **T39.4X5-** **Adverse effect of antirheumatics, not elsewhere classified**

7 **T39.4X6-** **Underdosing of antirheumatics, not elsewhere classified**

5 **T39.8** **Poisoning by, adverse effect of and underdosing of other nonopioid analgesics and antipyretics, not elsewhere classified**

6 **T39.8X** **Poisoning by, adverse effect of and underdosing of other nonopioid analgesics and antipyretics, not elsewhere classified**

7 **T39.8X1-** **Poisoning by other nonopioid analgesics and antipyretics, not elsewhere classified, accidental (unintentional)**
Poisoning by other nonopioid analgesics and antipyretics, not elsewhere classified NOS

7 **T39.8X2-** **Poisoning by other nonopioid analgesics and antipyretics, not elsewhere classified, intentional self-harm** HCC

7 **T39.8X3-** **Poisoning by other nonopioid analgesics and antipyretics, not elsewhere classified, assault**

7 **T39.8X4-** **Poisoning by other nonopioid analgesics and antipyretics, not elsewhere classified, undetermined**

7 **T39.8X5-** **Adverse effect of other nonopioid analgesics and antipyretics, not elsewhere classified**

7 **T39.8X6-** **Underdosing of other nonopioid analgesics and antipyretics, not elsewhere classified**

5 **T39.9** **Poisoning by, adverse effect of and underdosing of unspecified nonopioid analgesic, antipyretic and antirheumatic**

7 **T39.91X-** **Poisoning by unspecified nonopioid analgesic, antipyretic and antirheumatic, accidental (unintentional)**
Poisoning by nonopioid analgesic, antipyretic and antirheumatic NOS

7 **T39.92X-** **Poisoning by unspecified nonopioid analgesic, antipyretic and antirheumatic, intentional self-harm** HCC

7 **T39.93X-** **Poisoning by unspecified nonopioid analgesic, antipyretic and antirheumatic, assault**

7 **T39.94X-** **Poisoning by unspecified nonopioid analgesic, antipyretic and antirheumatic, undetermined**

7 **T39.95X-** **Adverse effect of unspecified nonopioid analgesic, antipyretic and antirheumatic**

7 **T39.96X-** **Underdosing of unspecified nonopioid analgesic, antipyretic and antirheumatic**

4 **T40** **Poisoning by, adverse effect of and underdosing of narcotics and psychodysleptics [hallucinogens]**
EXCLUDES 2 *drug dependence and related mental and behavioral disorders due to psychoactive substance use (F10.-F19.-)*

The appropriate 7th character is to be added to each code from category T40
A initial encounter
D subsequent encounter
S sequela

5 T40.0 Poisoning by, adverse effect of and underdosing of opium

6 T40.0X Poisoning by, adverse effect of and underdosing of opium

7 T40.0X1- Poisoning by opium, accidental (unintentional) HCC
Poisoning by opium NOS

7 T40.0X2- Poisoning by opium, intentional self-harm HCC

7 T40.0X3- Poisoning by opium, assault

7 T40.0X4- Poisoning by opium, undetermined HCC

7 T40.0X5- Adverse effect of opium

7 T40.0X6- Underdosing of opium

5 T40.1 Poisoning by and adverse effect of heroin

6 T40.1X Poisoning by and adverse effect of heroin

7 T40.1X1- Poisoning by heroin, accidental (unintentional) HCC
Poisoning by heroin NOS

7 T40.1X2- Poisoning by heroin, intentional self-harm HCC

7 T40.1X3- Poisoning by heroin, assault

7 T40.1X4- Poisoning by heroin, undetermined HCC

5 T40.2 Poisoning by, adverse effect of and underdosing of other opioids

6 T40.2X Poisoning by, adverse effect of and underdosing of other opioids

7 T40.2X1- Poisoning by other opioids, accidental (unintentional) HCC
Poisoning by other opioids NOS

7 T40.2X2- Poisoning by other opioids, intentional self-harm HCC

7 T40.2X3- Poisoning by other opioids, assault

7 T40.2X4- Poisoning by other opioids, undetermined HCC

7 T40.2X5- Adverse effect of other opioids

7 T40.2X6- Underdosing of other opioids

5 T40.3 Poisoning by, adverse effect of and underdosing of methadone

6 T40.3X Poisoning by, adverse effect of and underdosing of methadone

7 T40.3X1- Poisoning by methadone, accidental (unintentional) HCC
Poisoning by methadone NOS

7 T40.3X2- Poisoning by methadone, intentional self-harm HCC

7 T40.3X3- Poisoning by methadone, assault

7 T40.3X4- Poisoning by methadone, undetermined HCC

7 T40.3X5- Adverse effect of methadone

7 T40.3X6- Underdosing of methadone

5 T40.4 Poisoning by, adverse effect of and underdosing of other synthetic narcotics

6 T40.4X Poisoning by, adverse effect of and underdosing of other synthetic narcotics

7 T40.4X1- Poisoning by other synthetic narcotics, accidental (unintentional) HCC
Poisoning by other synthetic narcotics NOS

7 T40.4X2- Poisoning by other synthetic narcotics, intentional self-harm HCC

7 T40.4X3- Poisoning by other synthetic narcotics, assault

7 T40.4X4- Poisoning by other synthetic narcotics, undetermined HCC

7 T40.4X5- Adverse effect of other synthetic narcotics

7 T40.4X6- Underdosing of other synthetic narcotics

5 T40.5 Poisoning by, adverse effect of and underdosing of cocaine
AHA: (T40.5X1A) 2Q 2016, 9

6 T40.5X Poisoning by, adverse effect of and underdosing of cocaine

7 T40.5X1- Poisoning by cocaine, accidental (unintentional) HCC
Poisoning by cocaine NOS

7 T40.5X2- Poisoning by cocaine, intentional self-harm HCC

7 T40.5X3- Poisoning by cocaine, assault

7 T40.5X4- Poisoning by cocaine, undetermined HCC

7 T40.5X5- Adverse effect of cocaine

7 T40.5X6- Underdosing of cocaine

5 T40.6 Poisoning by, adverse effect of and underdosing of other and unspecified narcotics

6 T40.60 Poisoning by, adverse effect of and underdosing of unspecified narcotics

7 T40.601- Poisoning by unspecified narcotics, accidental (unintentional) HCC
Poisoning by narcotics NOS

7 T40.602- Poisoning by unspecified narcotics, intentional self-harm HCC

7 T40.603- Poisoning by unspecified narcotics, assault

7 T40.604- Poisoning by unspecified narcotics, undetermined HCC

7 T40.605- Adverse effect of unspecified narcotics

7 T40.606- Underdosing of unspecified narcotics

6 T40.69 Poisoning by, adverse effect of and underdosing of other narcotics

7 T40.691- Poisoning by other narcotics, accidental (unintentional) HCC
Poisoning by other narcotics NOS

7 T40.692- Poisoning by other narcotics, intentional self-harm HCC

7 T40.693- Poisoning by other narcotics, assault

7 T40.694- Poisoning by other narcotics, undetermined HCC

7 T40.695- Adverse effect of other narcotics

7 T40.696- Underdosing of other narcotics

5 T40.7 Poisoning by, adverse effect of and underdosing of cannabis (derivatives)

6 T40.7X Poisoning by, adverse effect of and underdosing of cannabis (derivatives)

7 T40.7X1- Poisoning by cannabis (derivatives), accidental (unintentional)
Poisoning by cannabis NOS

7 T40.7X2- Poisoning by cannabis (derivatives), intentional self-harm HCC

7 T40.7X3- Poisoning by cannabis (derivatives), assault

7 T40.7X4- Poisoning by cannabis (derivatives), undetermined

7 T40.7X5- Adverse effect of cannabis (derivatives)

7 T40.7X6- Underdosing of cannabis (derivatives)

5 T40.8 Poisoning by and adverse effect of lysergide [LSD]

6 T40.8X Poisoning by and adverse effect of lysergide [LSD]

7 T40.8X1- Poisoning by lysergide [LSD], accidental (unintentional) HCC
Poisoning by lysergide [LSD] NOS

7 T40.8X2- Poisoning by lysergide [LSD], intentional self-harm HCC

7 T40.8X3- Poisoning by lysergide [LSD], assault

7 T40.8X4- Poisoning by lysergide [LSD], undetermined HCC

5 T40.9 Poisoning by, adverse effect of and underdosing of other and unspecified psychodysleptics [hallucinogens]

6 T40.90 Poisoning by, adverse effect of and underdosing of unspecified psychodysleptics [hallucinogens]

7 T40.901- Poisoning by unspecified psychodysleptics [hallucinogens], accidental (unintentional) HCC

7 T40.902- Poisoning by unspecified psychodysleptics [hallucinogens], intentional self-harm HCC

7 T40.903- Poisoning by unspecified psychodysleptics [hallucinogens], assault

7 T40.904- Poisoning by unspecified psychodysleptics [hallucinogens], undetermined HCC

7 T40.905- Adverse effect of unspecified psychodysleptics [hallucinogens]

7 T40.906- Underdosing of unspecified psychodysleptics

6 T40.99 Poisoning by, adverse effect of and underdosing of other psychodysleptics [hallucinogens]

7 T40.991- Poisoning by other psychodysleptics [hallucinogens], accidental (unintentional) HCC
Poisoning by other psychodysleptics [hallucinogens] NOS

T40.992- Poisoning by other psychodysleptics [hallucinogens], intentional self-harm HCC
T40.993- Poisoning by other psychodysleptics [hallucinogens], assault
T40.994- Poisoning by other psychodysleptics [hallucinogens], undetermined HCC
T40.995- Adverse effect of other psychodysleptics [hallucinogens]
T40.996- Underdosing of other psychodysleptics

T41 Poisoning by, adverse effect of and underdosing of anesthetics and therapeutic gases

EXCLUDES 1 *benzodiazepines (T42.4-)*
cocaine (T40.5-)
complications of anesthesia during pregnancy (O29.-)
complications of anesthesia during labor and delivery (O74.-)
complications of anesthesia during the puerperium (O89.-)
opioids (T40.0-T40.2-)

The appropriate 7th character is to be added to each code from category T41
A initial encounter
D subsequent encounter
S sequela

T41.0 Poisoning by, adverse effect of and underdosing of inhaled anesthetics
EXCLUDES 1 *oxygen (T41.5-)*
T41.0X Poisoning by, adverse effect of and underdosing of inhaled anesthetics
T41.0X1- Poisoning by inhaled anesthetics, accidental (unintentional)
Poisoning by inhaled anesthetics NOS
T41.0X2- Poisoning by inhaled anesthetics, intentional self-harm HCC
T41.0X3- Poisoning by inhaled anesthetics, assault
T41.0X4- Poisoning by inhaled anesthetics, undetermined
T41.0X5- Adverse effect of inhaled anesthetics
T41.0X6- Underdosing of inhaled anesthetics

T41.1 Poisoning by, adverse effect of and underdosing of intravenous anesthetics
Poisoning by, adverse effect of and underdosing of thiobarbiturates
T41.1X Poisoning by, adverse effect of and underdosing of intravenous anesthetics
T41.1X1- Poisoning by intravenous anesthetics, accidental (unintentional)
Poisoning by intravenous anesthetics NOS
T41.1X2- Poisoning by intravenous anesthetics, intentional self-harm HCC
T41.1X3- Poisoning by intravenous anesthetics, assault
T41.1X4- Poisoning by intravenous anesthetics, undetermined
T41.1X5- Adverse effect of intravenous anesthetics
T41.1X6- Underdosing of intravenous anesthetics

T41.2 Poisoning by, adverse effect of and underdosing of other and unspecified general anesthetics
T41.20 Poisoning by, adverse effect of and underdosing of unspecified general anesthetics
T41.201- Poisoning by unspecified general anesthetics, accidental (unintentional)
Poisoning by general anesthetics NOS
T41.202- Poisoning by unspecified general anesthetics, intentional self-harm HCC
T41.203- Poisoning by unspecified general anesthetics, assault
T41.204- Poisoning by unspecified general anesthetics, undetermined
T41.205- Adverse effect of unspecified general anesthetics
T41.206- Underdosing of unspecified general anesthetics
T41.29 Poisoning by, adverse effect of and underdosing of other general anesthetics
T41.291- Poisoning by other general anesthetics, accidental (unintentional)
Poisoning by other general anesthetics NOS
T41.292- Poisoning by other general anesthetics, intentional self-harm HCC
T41.293- Poisoning by other general anesthetics, assault
T41.294- Poisoning by other general anesthetics, undetermined
T41.295- Adverse effect of other general anesthetics
T41.296- Underdosing of other general anesthetics

T41.3 Poisoning by, adverse effect of and underdosing of local anesthetics
Cocaine (topical)
EXCLUDES 2 *poisoning by cocaine used as a central nervous system stimulant (T40.5X1-T40.5X4)*
T41.3X Poisoning by, adverse effect of and underdosing of local anesthetics
T41.3X1- Poisoning by local anesthetics, accidental (unintentional)
Poisoning by local anesthetics NOS
T41.3X2- Poisoning by local anesthetics, intentional self-harm HCC
T41.3X3- Poisoning by local anesthetics, assault
T41.3X4- Poisoning by local anesthetics, undetermined
T41.3X5- Adverse effect of local anesthetics
T41.3X6- Underdosing of local anesthetics

T41.4 Poisoning by, adverse effect of and underdosing of unspecified anesthetic
T41.41X- Poisoning by unspecified anesthetic, accidental (unintentional)
Poisoning by anesthetic NOS
T41.42X- Poisoning by unspecified anesthetic, intentional self-harm HCC
T41.43X- Poisoning by unspecified anesthetic, assault
T41.44X- Poisoning by unspecified anesthetic, undetermined
T41.45X- Adverse effect of unspecified anesthetic
T41.46X- Underdosing of unspecified anesthetics

T41.5 Poisoning by, adverse effect of and underdosing of therapeutic gases
T41.5X Poisoning by, adverse effect of and underdosing of therapeutic gases
T41.5X1- Poisoning by therapeutic gases, accidental (unintentional)
Poisoning by therapeutic gases NOS
T41.5X2- Poisoning by therapeutic gases, intentional self-harm HCC
T41.5X3- Poisoning by therapeutic gases, assault
T41.5X4- Poisoning by therapeutic gases, undetermined
T41.5X5- Adverse effect of therapeutic gases
T41.5X6- Underdosing of therapeutic gases

T42 Poisoning by, adverse effect of and underdosing of antiepileptic, sedative- hypnotic and antiparkinsonism drugs

EXCLUDES 2 *drug dependence and related mental and behavioral disorders due to psychoactive substance use (F10.--F19.-)*

The appropriate 7th character is to be added to each code from category T42
A initial encounter
D subsequent encounter
S sequela

T42.0 Poisoning by, adverse effect of and underdosing of hydantoin derivatives
T42.0X Poisoning by, adverse effect of and underdosing of hydantoin derivatives
T42.0X1- Poisoning by hydantoin derivatives, accidental (unintentional)
Poisoning by hydantoin derivatives NOS
T42.0X2- Poisoning by hydantoin derivatives, intentional self-harm HCC
T42.0X3- Poisoning by hydantoin derivatives, assault
T42.0X4- Poisoning by hydantoin derivatives, undetermined
T42.0X5- Adverse effect of hydantoin derivatives

7 T42.0X6- **Underdosing of hydantoin derivatives**

5 T42.1 **Poisoning by, adverse effect of and underdosing of iminostilbenes**
Poisoning by, adverse effect of and underdosing of carbamazepine

6 T42.1X **Poisoning by, adverse effect of and underdosing of iminostilbenes**

7 T42.1X1- **Poisoning by iminostilbenes, accidental (unintentional)**
Poisoning by iminostilbenes NOS

7 T42.1X2- **Poisoning by iminostilbenes, intentional self-harm** HCC

7 T42.1X3- **Poisoning by iminostilbenes, assault**

7 T42.1X4- **Poisoning by iminostilbenes, undetermined**

7 T42.1X5- **Adverse effect of iminostilbenes**

7 T42.1X6- **Underdosing of iminostilbenes**

5 T42.2 **Poisoning by, adverse effect of and underdosing of succinimides and oxazolidinediones**

6 T42.2X **Poisoning by, adverse effect of and underdosing of succinimides and oxazolidinediones**

7 T42.2X1- **Poisoning by succinimides and oxazolidinediones, accidental (unintentional)**
Poisoning by succinimides and oxazolidinediones NOS

7 T42.2X2- **Poisoning by succinimides and oxazolidinediones, intentional self-harm** HCC

7 T42.2X3- **Poisoning by succinimides and oxazolidinediones, assault**

7 T42.2X4- **Poisoning by succinimides and oxazolidinediones, undetermined**

7 T42.2X5- **Adverse effect of succinimides and oxazolidinediones**

7 T42.2X6- **Underdosing of succinimides and oxazolidinediones**

5 T42.3 **Poisoning by, adverse effect of and underdosing of barbiturates**

EXCLUDES 1 *poisoning by, adverse effect of and underdosing of thiobarbiturates (T41.1-)*

6 T42.3X **Poisoning by, adverse effect of and underdosing of barbiturates**

7 T42.3X1- **Poisoning by barbiturates, accidental (unintentional)**
Poisoning by barbiturates NOS

7 T42.3X2- **Poisoning by barbiturates, intentional self-harm** HCC

7 T42.3X3- **Poisoning by barbiturates, assault**

7 T42.3X4- **Poisoning by barbiturates, undetermined**

7 T42.3X5- **Adverse effect of barbiturates**

7 T42.3X6- **Underdosing of barbiturates**

5 T42.4 **Poisoning by, adverse effect of and underdosing of benzodiazepines**

6 T42.4X **Poisoning by, adverse effect of and underdosing of benzodiazepines**

7 T42.4X1- **Poisoning by benzodiazepines, accidental (unintentional)**
Poisoning by benzodiazepines NOS

7 T42.4X2- **Poisoning by benzodiazepines, intentional self-harm** HCC

7 T42.4X3- **Poisoning by benzodiazepines, assault**

7 T42.4X4- **Poisoning by benzodiazepines, undetermined**

7 T42.4X5- **Adverse effect of benzodiazepines**

7 T42.4X6- **Underdosing of benzodiazepines**

5 T42.5 **Poisoning by, adverse effect of and underdosing of mixed antiepileptics**

6 T42.5X **Poisoning by, adverse effect of and underdosing of antiepileptics**

7 T42.5X1- **Poisoning by mixed antiepileptics, accidental (unintentional)**
Poisoning by mixed antiepileptics NOS

7 T42.5X2- **Poisoning by mixed antiepileptics, intentional self-harm** HCC

7 T42.5X3- **Poisoning by mixed antiepileptics, assault**

7 T42.5X4- **Poisoning by mixed antiepileptics, undetermined**

7 T42.5X5- **Adverse effect of mixed antiepileptics**

7 T42.5X6- **Underdosing of mixed antiepileptics**

5 T42.6 **Poisoning by, adverse effect of and underdosing of otherantiepileptic and sedative-hypnotic drugs**
Poisoning by, adverse effect of and underdosing of methaqualone
Poisoning by, adverse effect of and underdosing of valproic acid

EXCLUDES 1 *poisoning by, adverse effect of and underdosing of carbamazepine (T42.1-)*

6 T42.6X **Poisoning by, adverse effect of and underdosing of other antiepileptic and sedative-hypnotic drugs**

7 T42.6X1- **Poisoning by other antiepileptic and sedative-hypnotic drugs, accidental (unintentional)**
Poisoning by other antiepileptic and sedative-hypnotic drugs NOS

7 T42.6X2- **Poisoning by other antiepileptic and sedative-hypnotic drugs, intentional self-harm** HCC

7 T42.6X3- **Poisoning by other antiepileptic and sedative-hypnotic drugs, assault**

7 T42.6X4- **Poisoning by other antiepileptic and sedative-hypnotic drugs, undetermined**

7 T42.6X5- **Adverse effect of other antiepileptic and sedative-hypnotic drugs**

7 T42.6X6- **Underdosing of other antiepileptic and sedative-hypnotic drugs**

5 T42.7 **Poisoning by, adverse effect of and underdosing of unspecified antiepileptic and sedative-hypnotic drugs**

7 T42.71X- **Poisoning by unspecified antiepileptic and sedative-hypnotic drugs, accidental (unintentional)**
Poisoning by antiepileptic and sedative-hypnotic drugs NOS

7 T42.72X- **Poisoning by unspecified antiepileptic and sedative-hypnotic drugs, intentional self-harm** HCC

7 T42.73X- **Poisoning by unspecified antiepileptic and sedative-hypnotic drugs, assault**

7 T42.74X- **Poisoning by unspecified antiepileptic and sedative-hypnotic drugs, undetermined**

7 T42.75X- **Adverse effect of unspecified antiepileptic and sedative-hypnotic drugs**

7 T42.76X- **Underdosing of unspecified antiepileptic and sedative-hypnotic drugs**

5 T42.8 **Poisoning by, adverse effect of and underdosing of antiparkinsonism drugs and other central muscle-tone depressants**
Poisoning by, adverse effect of and underdosing of amantadine

6 T42.8X **Poisoning by, adverse effect of and underdosing of antiparkinsonism drugs and other central muscle-tone depressants**

7 T42.8X1- **Poisoning by antiparkinsonism drugs and other central muscle-tone depressants, accidental (unintentional)**
Poisoning by antiparkinsonism drugs and other central muscle-tone depressants NOS

7 T42.8X2- **Poisoning by antiparkinsonism drugs and other central muscle-tone depressants, intentional self-harm** HCC

7 T42.8X3- **Poisoning by antiparkinsonism drugs and other central muscle-tone depressants, assault**

7 T42.8X4- **Poisoning by antiparkinsonism drugs and other central muscle-tone depressants, undetermined**

7 T42.8X5- **Adverse effect of antiparkinsonism drugs and other central muscle-tone depressants**

7 T42.8X6- **Underdosing of antiparkinsonism drugs and other central muscle-tone depressants**

T43 Poisoning by, adverse effect of and underdosing of psychotropic drugs, not elsewhere classified

EXCLUDES 1 *appetite depressants (T50.5-)*
barbiturates (T42.3-)
benzodiazepines (T42.4-)
methaqualone (T42.6-)
psychodysleptics [hallucinogens] (T40.7-T40.9-)

EXCLUDES 2 *drug dependence and related mental and behavioral disorders due to psychoactive substance use (F10.- -F19.-)*

The appropriate 7th character is to be added to each code from category T43
A initial encounter
D subsequent encounter
S sequela

T43.0 Poisoning by, adverse effect of and underdosing of tricyclic and tetracyclic antidepressants

T43.01 Poisoning by, adverse effect of and underdosing of tricyclic antidepressants

T43.011- Poisoning by tricyclic antidepressants, accidental (unintentional)
Poisoning by tricyclic antidepressants NOS

T43.012- Poisoning by tricyclic antidepressants, intentional self-harm HCC

T43.013- Poisoning by tricyclic antidepressants, assault

T43.014- Poisoning by tricyclic antidepressants, undetermined

T43.015- Adverse effect of tricyclic antidepressants

T43.016- Underdosing of tricyclic antidepressants

T43.02 Poisoning by, adverse effect of and underdosing of tetracyclic antidepressants

T43.021- Poisoning by tetracyclic antidepressants, accidental (unintentional)
Poisoning by tetracyclic antidepressants NOS

T43.022- Poisoning by tetracyclic antidepressants, intentional self-harm HCC

T43.023- Poisoning by tetracyclic antidepressants, assault

T43.024- Poisoning by tetracyclic antidepressants, undetermined

T43.025- Adverse effect of tetracyclic antidepressants

T43.026- Underdosing of tetracyclic antidepressants

T43.1 Poisoning by, adverse effect of and underdosing of monoamine-oxidase-inhibitor antidepressants

T43.1X Poisoning by, adverse effect of and underdosing of monoamine-oxidase-inhibitor antidepressants

T43.1X1- Poisoning by monoamine-oxidase-inhibitor antidepressants, accidental (unintentional)
Poisoning by monoamine-oxidase-inhibitor antidepressants NOS

T43.1X2- Poisoning by monoamine-oxidase-inhibitor antidepressants, intentional self-harm HCC

T43.1X3- Poisoning by monoamine-oxidase-inhibitor antidepressants, assault

T43.1X4- Poisoning by monoamine-oxidase-inhibitor antidepressants, undetermined

T43.1X5- Adverse effect of monoamine-oxidase-inhibitor antidepressants

T43.1X6- Underdosing of monoamine-oxidase-inhibitor antidepressants

T43.2 Poisoning by, adverse effect of and underdosing of other and unspecified antidepressants

T43.20 Poisoning by, adverse effect of and underdosing of unspecified antidepressants

T43.201- Poisoning by unspecified antidepressants, accidental (unintentional)
Poisoning by antidepressants NOS

T43.202- Poisoning by unspecified antidepressants, intentional self-harm HCC

T43.203- Poisoning by unspecified antidepressants, assault

T43.204- Poisoning by unspecified antidepressants, undetermined

T43.205- Adverse effect of unspecified antidepressants
Antidepressant discontinuation syndrome

T43.206- Underdosing of unspecified antidepressants

T43.21 Poisoning by, adverse effect of and underdosing of selective serotonin and norepinephrine reuptake inhibitors
Poisoning by, adverse effect of and underdosing of SSNRI antidepressants

T43.211- Poisoning by selective serotonin and norepinephrine reuptake inhibitors, accidental (unintentional)

T43.212- Poisoning by selective serotonin and norepinephrine reuptake inhibitors, intentional self-harm HCC

T43.213- Poisoning by selective serotonin and norepinephrine reuptake inhibitors, assault

T43.214- Poisoning by selective serotonin and norepinephrine reuptake inhibitors, undetermined

T43.215- Adverse effect of selective serotonin and norepinephrine reuptake inhibitors

T43.216- Underdosing of selective serotonin and norepinephrine reuptake inhibitors

T43.22 Poisoning by, adverse effect of and underdosing of selective serotonin reuptake inhibitors
Poisoning by, adverse effect of and underdosing of SSRI antidepressants

T43.221- Poisoning by selective serotonin reuptake inhibitors, accidental (unintentional)

T43.222- Poisoning by selective serotonin reuptake inhibitors, intentional self-harm HCC

T43.223- Poisoning by selective serotonin reuptake inhibitors, assault

T43.224- Poisoning by selective serotonin reuptake inhibitors, undetermined

T43.225- Adverse effect of selective serotonin reuptake inhibitors

T43.226- Underdosing of selective serotonin reuptake inhibitors

T43.29 Poisoning by, adverse effect of and underdosing of other antidepressants

T43.291- Poisoning by other antidepressants, accidental (unintentional)
Poisoning by other antidepressants NOS

T43.292- Poisoning by other antidepressants, intentional self-harm HCC

T43.293- Poisoning by other antidepressants, assault

T43.294- Poisoning by other antidepressants, undetermined

T43.295- Adverse effect of other antidepressants

T43.296- Underdosing of other antidepressants

T43.3 Poisoning by, adverse effect of and underdosing of phenothiazine antipsychotics and neuroleptics

T43.3X Poisoning by, adverse effect of and underdosing of phenothiazine antipsychotics and neuroleptics

T43.3X1- Poisoning by phenothiazine antipsychotics and neuroleptics, accidental (unintentional)
Poisoning by phenothiazine antipsychotics and neuroleptics NOS

T43.3X2- Poisoning by phenothiazine antipsychotics and neuroleptics, intentional self-harm HCC

T43.3X3- Poisoning by phenothiazine antipsychotics and neuroleptics, assault

T43.3X4- Poisoning by phenothiazine antipsychotics and neuroleptics, undetermined

T43.3X5- Adverse effect of phenothiazine antipsychotics and neuroleptics

T43.3X6- Underdosing of phenothiazine antipsychotics and neuroleptics

T43.4 Poisoning by, adverse effect of and underdosing of butyrophenone and thiothixene neuroleptics

T43.4X Poisoning by, adverse effect of and underdosing of butyrophenone and thiothixene neuroleptics

T43.4X1- Poisoning by butyrophenone and thiothixene neuroleptics, accidental (unintentional)
Poisoning by butyrophenone and thiothixene neuroleptics NOS

T43.4X2- Poisoning by butyrophenone and thiothixene neuroleptics, intentional self-harm HCC

T43.4X3- Poisoning by butyrophenone and thiothixene neuroleptics, assault

T43.4X4- Poisoning by butyrophenone and thiothixene neuroleptics, undetermined

T43.4X5- Adverse effect of butyrophenone and thiothixene neuroleptics
T43.4X6- Underdosing of butyrophenone and thiothixene neuroleptics

T43.5 Poisoning by, adverse effect of and underdosing of other and unspecified antipsychotics and neuroleptics
EXCLUDES 1 *poisoning by, adverse effect of and underdosing of rauwolfia (T46.5-)*

T43.50 Poisoning by, adverse effect of and underdosing of unspecified antipsychotics and neuroleptics
T43.501- Poisoning by unspecified antipsychotics and neuroleptics, accidental (unintentional)
Poisoning by antipsychotics and neuroleptics NOS
T43.502- Poisoning by unspecified antipsychotics and neuroleptics, intentional self-harm HCC
T43.503- Poisoning by unspecified antipsychotics and neuroleptics, assault
T43.504- Poisoning by unspecified antipsychotics and neuroleptics, undetermined
T43.505- Adverse effect of unspecified antipsychotics and neuroleptics
T43.506- Underdosing of unspecified antipsychotics and neuroleptics

T43.59 Poisoning by, adverse effect of and underdosing of other antipsychotics and neuroleptics
T43.591- Poisoning by other antipsychotics and neuroleptics, accidental (unintentional)
Poisoning by other antipsychotics and neuroleptics NOS
T43.592- Poisoning by other antipsychotics and neuroleptics, intentional self-harm HCC
AHA: 1Q 2017, 40
T43.593- Poisoning by other antipsychotics and neuroleptics, assault
T43.594- Poisoning by other antipsychotics and neuroleptics, undetermined
T43.595- Adverse effect of other antipsychotics and neuroleptics
T43.596- Underdosing of other antipsychotics and neuroleptics

T43.6 Poisoning by, adverse effect of and underdosing of psychostimulants
EXCLUDES 1 *poisoning by, adverse effect of and underdosing of cocaine (T40.5-)*

T43.60 Poisoning by, adverse effect of and underdosing of unspecified psychostimulant
T43.601- Poisoning by unspecified psychostimulants, accidental (unintentional) HCC
Poisoning by psychostimulants NOS
T43.602- Poisoning by unspecified psychostimulants, intentional self-harm HCC
T43.603- Poisoning by unspecified psychostimulants, assault
T43.604- Poisoning by unspecified psychostimulants, undetermined HCC
T43.605- Adverse effect of unspecified psychostimulants
T43.606- Underdosing of unspecified psychostimulants

T43.61 Poisoning by, adverse effect of and underdosing of caffeine
T43.611- Poisoning by caffeine, accidental (unintentional) HCC
Poisoning by caffeine NOS
T43.612- Poisoning by caffeine, intentional self-harm HCC
T43.613- Poisoning by caffeine, assault
T43.614- Poisoning by caffeine, undetermined HCC
T43.615- Adverse effect of caffeine
T43.616- Underdosing of caffeine

T43.62 Poisoning by, adverse effect of and underdosing of amphetamines
Poisoning by, adverse effect of and underdosing of methamphetamines
T43.621- Poisoning by amphetamines, accidental (unintentional) HCC
Poisoning by amphetamines NOS
T43.622- Poisoning by amphetamines, intentional self-harm HCC
T43.623- Poisoning by amphetamines, assault
T43.624- Poisoning by amphetamines, undetermined HCC
T43.625- Adverse effect of amphetamines
T43.626- Underdosing of amphetamines

T43.63 Poisoning by, adverse effect of and underdosing of methylphenidate
T43.631- Poisoning by methylphenidate, accidental (unintentional) HCC
Poisoning by methylphenidate NOS
T43.632- Poisoning by methylphenidate, intentional self-harm HCC
T43.633- Poisoning by methylphenidate, assault
T43.634- Poisoning by methylphenidate, undetermined HCC
T43.635- Adverse effect of methylphenidate
T43.636- Underdosing of methylphenidate

● T43.64 Poisoning by ecstasy
Poisoning by MDMA
Poisoning by 3,4-methylenedioxymethamphetamine
● T43.641- Poisoning by ecstasy, accidental (unintentional)
Poisoning by ecstasy NOS
● T43.642- Poisoning by ecstasy, intentional self-harm
● T43.643- Poisoning by ecstasy, assault
● T43.644- Poisoning by ecstasy, undetermined

T43.69 Poisoning by, adverse effect of and underdosing of other psychostimulants
T43.691- Poisoning by other psychostimulants, accidental (unintentional) HCC
Poisoning by other psychostimulants NOS
T43.692- Poisoning by other psychostimulants, intentional self-harm HCC
T43.693- Poisoning by other psychostimulants, assault
T43.694- Poisoning by other psychostimulants, undetermined HCC
T43.695- Adverse effect of other psychostimulants
T43.696- Underdosing of other psychostimulants

T43.8 Poisoning by, adverse effect of and underdosing of other psychotropic drugs
T43.8X Poisoning by, adverse effect of and underdosing of other psychotropic drugs
T43.8X1- Poisoning by other psychotropic drugs, accidental (unintentional)
Poisoning by other psychotropic drugs NOS
T43.8X2- Poisoning by other psychotropic drugs, intentional self-harm HCC
T43.8X3- Poisoning by other psychotropic drugs, assault
T43.8X4- Poisoning by other psychotropic drugs, undetermined
T43.8X5- Adverse effect of other psychotropic drugs
T43.8X6- Underdosing of other psychotropic drugs

T43.9 Poisoning by, adverse effect of and underdosing of unspecified psychotropic drug
T43.91X- Poisoning by unspecified psychotropic drug, accidental (unintentional)
Poisoning by psychotropic drug NOS
T43.92X- Poisoning by unspecified psychotropic drug, intentional self-harm HCC
T43.93X- Poisoning by unspecified psychotropic drug, assault
T43.94X- Poisoning by unspecified psychotropic drug, undetermined
T43.95X- Adverse effect of unspecified psychotropic drug
T43.96X- Underdosing of unspecified psychotropic drug

T44 Poisoning by, adverse effect of and underdosing of drugs primarily affecting the autonomic nervous system

The appropriate 7th character is to be added to each code from category T44
A initial encounter
D subsequent encounter
S sequela

T44.0 Poisoning by, adverse effect of and underdosing of anticholinesterase agents

6 T44.0X Poisoning by, adverse effect of and underdosing of anticholinesterase agents
7 T44.0X1- Poisoning by anticholinesterase agents, accidental (unintentional)
Poisoning by anticholinesterase agents NOS
7 T44.0X2- Poisoning by anticholinesterase agents, intentional self-harm HCC
7 T44.0X3- Poisoning by anticholinesterase agents, assault
7 T44.0X4- Poisoning by anticholinesterase agents, undetermined
7 T44.0X5- Adverse effect of anticholinesterase agents
7 T44.0X6- Underdosing of anticholinesterase agents

5 T44.1 Poisoning by, adverse effect of and underdosing of other parasympathomimetics [cholinergics]
6 T44.1X Poisoning by, adverse effect of and underdosing of other parasympathomimetics [cholinergics]
7 T44.1X1- Poisoning by other parasympathomimetics [cholinergics], accidental (unintentional)
Poisoning by other parasympathomimetics [cholinergics] NOS
7 T44.1X2- Poisoning by other parasympathomimetics [cholinergics], intentional self-harm HCC
7 T44.1X3- Poisoning by other parasympathomimetics [cholinergics], assault
7 T44.1X4- Poisoning by other parasympathomimetics [cholinergics], undetermined
7 T44.1X5- Adverse effect of other parasympathomimetics [cholinergics]
7 T44.1X6- Underdosing of other parasympathomimetics

5 T44.2 Poisoning by, adverse effect of and underdosing of ganglionic blocking drugs
6 T44.2X Poisoning by, adverse effect of and underdosing of ganglionic blocking drugs
7 T44.2X1- Poisoning by ganglionic blocking drugs, accidental (unintentional)
Poisoning by ganglionic blocking drugs NOS
7 T44.2X2- Poisoning by ganglionic blocking drugs, intentional self-harm HCC
7 T44.2X3- Poisoning by ganglionic blocking drugs, assault
7 T44.2X4- Poisoning by ganglionic blocking drugs, undetermined
7 T44.2X5- Adverse effect of ganglionic blocking drugs
7 T44.2X6- Underdosing of ganglionic blocking drugs

5 T44.3 Poisoning by, adverse effect of and underdosing of other parasympatholytics [anticholinergics and antimuscarinics] and spasmolytics
Poisoning by, adverse effect of and underdosing of papaverine
6 T44.3X Poisoning by, adverse effect of and underdosing of other parasympatholytics [anticholinergics and antimuscarinics] and spasmolytics
7 T44.3X1- Poisoning by other parasympatholytics [anticholinergics and antimuscarinics] and spasmolytics, accidental (unintentional)
Poisoning by other parasympatholytics [anticholinergics and antimuscarinics] and spasmolytics NOS
7 T44.3X2- Poisoning by other parasympatholytics [anticholinergics and antimuscarinics] and spasmolytics, intentional self-harm HCC
7 T44.3X3- Poisoning by other parasympatholytics [anticholinergics and antimuscarinics] and spasmolytics, assault
7 T44.3X4- Poisoning by other parasympatholytics [anticholinergics and antimuscarinics] and spasmolytics, undetermined
7 T44.3X5- Adverse effect of other parasympatholytics [anticholinergics and antimuscarinics] and spasmolytics
7 T44.3X6- Underdosing of other parasympatholytics [anticholinergics and antimuscarinics] and spasmolytics

5 T44.4 Poisoning by, adverse effect of and underdosing of predominantly alpha-adrenoreceptor agonists
Poisoning by, adverse effect of and underdosing of metaraminol
6 T44.4X Poisoning by, adverse effect of and underdosing of predominantly alpha-adrenoreceptor agonists
7 T44.4X1- Poisoning by predominantly alpha-adrenoreceptor agonists, accidental (unintentional)
Poisoning by predominantly alpha-adrenoreceptor agonists NOS
7 T44.4X2- Poisoning by predominantly alpha-adrenoreceptor agonists, intentional self-harm HCC
7 T44.4X3- Poisoning by predominantly alpha-adrenoreceptor agonists, assault
7 T44.4X4- Poisoning by predominantly alpha-adrenoreceptor agonists, undetermined
7 T44.4X5- Adverse effect of predominantly alpha-adrenoreceptor agonists
7 T44.4X6- Underdosing of predominantly alpha-adrenoreceptor agonists

5 T44.5 Poisoning by, adverse effect of and underdosing of predominantly beta-adrenoreceptor agonists
EXCLUDES 1 *poisoning by, adverse effect of and underdosing of beta-adrenoreceptor agonists used in asthma therapy (T48.6-)*
6 T44.5X Poisoning by, adverse effect of and underdosing of predominantly beta-adrenoreceptor agonists
7 T44.5X1- Poisoning by predominantly beta-adrenoreceptor agonists, accidental (unintentional)
Poisoning by predominantly beta-adrenoreceptor agonists NOS
7 T44.5X2- Poisoning by predominantly beta-adrenoreceptor agonists, intentional self-harm HCC
7 T44.5X3- Poisoning by predominantly beta-adrenoreceptor agonists, assault
7 T44.5X4- Poisoning by predominantly beta-adrenoreceptor agonists, undetermined
7 T44.5X5- Adverse effect of predominantly beta-adrenoreceptor agonists
7 T44.5X6- Underdosing of predominantly beta-adrenoreceptor agonists

5 T44.6 Poisoning by, adverse effect of and underdosing of alpha-adrenoreceptor antagonists
EXCLUDES 1 *poisoning by, adverse effect of and underdosing of ergot alkaloids (T48.0)*
6 T44.6X Poisoning by, adverse effect of and underdosing of alpha-adrenoreceptor antagonists
7 T44.6X1- Poisoning by alpha-adrenoreceptor antagonists, accidental (unintentional)
Poisoning by alpha-adrenoreceptor antagonists NOS
7 T44.6X2- Poisoning by alpha-adrenoreceptor antagonists, intentional self-harm HCC
7 T44.6X3- Poisoning by alpha-adrenoreceptor antagonists, assault
7 T44.6X4- Poisoning by alpha-adrenoreceptor antagonists, undetermined
7 T44.6X5- Adverse effect of alpha-adrenoreceptor antagonists
7 T44.6X6- Underdosing of alpha-adrenoreceptor antagonists

5 T44.7 Poisoning by, adverse effect of and underdosing of beta-adrenoreceptor antagonists
6 T44.7X Poisoning by, adverse effect of and underdosing of beta-adrenoreceptor antagonists
7 T44.7X1- Poisoning by beta-adrenoreceptor antagonists, accidental (unintentional)
Poisoning by beta-adrenoreceptor antagonists NOS
7 T44.7X2- Poisoning by beta-adrenoreceptor antagonists, intentional self-harm HCC
7 T44.7X3- Poisoning by beta-adrenoreceptor antagonists, assault
7 T44.7X4- Poisoning by beta-adrenoreceptor antagonists, undetermined
7 T44.7X5- Adverse effect of beta-adrenoreceptor antagonists
7 T44.7X6- Underdosing of beta-adrenoreceptor antagonists

5 T44.8 **Poisoning by, adverse effect of and underdosing of centrally-acting and adrenergic-neuron- blocking agents**

EXCLUDES 1 *poisoning by, adverse effect of and underdosing of clonidine (T46.5)*
poisoning by, adverse effect of and underdosing of guanethidine (T46.5)

6 T44.8X **Poisoning by, adverse effect of and underdosing of centrally-acting and adrenergic- neuron-blocking agents**

7 T44.8X1- **Poisoning by centrally-acting and adrenergic-neuron-blocking agents, accidental (unintentional)**
Poisoning by centrally-acting and adrenergic-neuron-blocking agents NOS

7 T44.8X2- **Poisoning by centrally-acting and adrenergic-neuron-blocking agents, intentional self-harm** HCC

7 T44.8X3- **Poisoning by centrally-acting and adrenergic-neuron-blocking agents, assault**

7 T44.8X4- **Poisoning by centrally-acting and adrenergic-neuron-blocking agents, undetermined**

7 T44.8X5- **Adverse effect of centrally-acting and adrenergic-neuron-blocking agents**

7 T44.8X6- **Underdosing of centrally-acting and adrenergic-neuron-blocking agents**

5 T44.9 **Poisoning by, adverse effect of and underdosing of other and unspecified drugs primarily affecting the autonomic nervous system**
Poisoning by, adverse effect of and underdosing of drug stimulating both alpha and beta-adrenoreceptors

6 T44.90 **Poisoning by, adverse effect of and underdosing of unspecified drugs primarily affecting the autonomic nervous system**

7 T44.901- **Poisoning by unspecified drugs primarily affecting the autonomic nervous system, accidental (unintentional)**
Poisoning by unspecified drugs primarily affecting the autonomic nervous system NOS

7 T44.902- **Poisoning by unspecified drugs primarily affecting the autonomic nervous system, intentional self-harm** HCC

7 T44.903- **Poisoning by unspecified drugs primarily affecting the autonomic nervous system, assault**

7 T44.904- **Poisoning by unspecified drugs primarily affecting the autonomic nervous system, undetermined**

7 T44.905- **Adverse effect of unspecified drugs primarily affecting the autonomic nervous system**

7 T44.906- **Underdosing of unspecified drugs primarily affecting the autonomic nervous system**

6 T44.99 **Poisoning by, adverse effect of and underdosing of other drugs primarily affecting the autonomic nervous system**

7 T44.991- **Poisoning by other drug primarily affecting the autonomic nervous system, accidental (unintentional)**
Poisoning by other drugs primarily affecting the autonomic nervous system NOS

7 T44.992- **Poisoning by other drug primarily affecting the autonomic nervous system, intentional self-harm** HCC

7 T44.993- **Poisoning by other drug primarily affecting the autonomic nervous system, assault**

7 T44.994- **Poisoning by other drug primarily affecting the autonomic nervous system, undetermined**

7 T44.995- **Adverse effect of other drug primarily affecting the autonomic nervous system**

7 T44.996- **Underdosing of other drug primarily affecting the autonomic nervous system**

4 T45 **Poisoning by, adverse effect of and underdosing of primarily systemic and hematological agents, not elsewhere classified**

The appropriate 7th character is to be added to each code from category T45
A initial encounter
D subsequent encounter
S sequela

5 T45.0 **Poisoning by, adverse effect of and underdosing of antiallergic and antiemetic drugs**

EXCLUDES 1 *poisoning by, adverse effect of and underdosing of phenothiazine-based neuroleptics (T43.3)*

6 T45.0X **Poisoning by, adverse effect of and underdosing of antiallergic and antiemetic drugs**

7 T45.0X1- **Poisoning by antiallergic and antiemetic drugs, accidental (unintentional)**
Poisoning by antiallergic and antiemetic drugs NOS

7 T45.0X2- **Poisoning by antiallergic and antiemetic drugs, intentional self-harm** HCC

7 T45.0X3- **Poisoning by antiallergic and antiemetic drugs, assault**

7 T45.0X4- **Poisoning by antiallergic and antiemetic drugs, undetermined**

7 T45.0X5- **Adverse effect of antiallergic and antiemetic drugs**

7 T45.0X6- **Underdosing of antiallergic and antiemetic drugs**

5 T45.1 **Poisoning by, adverse effect of and underdosing of antineoplastic and immunosuppressive drugs**

EXCLUDES 1 *poisoning by, adverse effect of and underdosing of tamoxifen (T38.6)*

6 T45.1X **Poisoning by, adverse effect of and underdosing of antineoplastic and immunosuppressive drugs**

7 T45.1X1- **Poisoning by antineoplastic and immunosuppressive drugs, accidental (unintentional)**
Poisoning by antineoplastic and immunosuppressive drugs NOS

7 T45.1X2- **Poisoning by antineoplastic and immunosuppressive drugs, intentional self-harm** HCC

7 T45.1X3- **Poisoning by antineoplastic and immunosuppressive drugs, assault**

7 T45.1X4- **Poisoning by antineoplastic and immunosuppressive drugs, undetermined**

7 T45.1X5- **Adverse effect of antineoplastic and immunosuppressive drugs**
AHA: (T45.1X5A) 4Q 2014, 22

7 T45.1X6- **Underdosing of antineoplastic and immunosuppressive drugs**

5 T45.2 **Poisoning by, adverse effect of and underdosing of vitamins**

EXCLUDES 2 *poisoning by, adverse effect of and underdosing of nicotinic acid (derivatives) (T46.7)*
poisoning by, adverse effect of and underdosing of iron (T45.4)
poisoning by, adverse effect of and underdosing of vitamin K (T45.7)

6 T45.2X **Poisoning by, adverse effect of and underdosing of vitamins**

7 T45.2X1- **Poisoning by vitamins, accidental (unintentional)**
Poisoning by vitamins NOS

7 T45.2X2- **Poisoning by vitamins, intentional self-harm** HCC

7 T45.2X3- **Poisoning by vitamins, assault**

7 T45.2X4- **Poisoning by vitamins, undetermined**

7 T45.2X5- **Adverse effect of vitamins**

7 T45.2X6- **Underdosing of vitamins**

EXCLUDES 1 *vitamin deficiencies (E50-E56)*

5 T45.3 **Poisoning by, adverse effect of and underdosing of enzymes**

6 T45.3X **Poisoning by, adverse effect of and underdosing of enzymes**

7 T45.3X1- **Poisoning by enzymes, accidental (unintentional)**
Poisoning by enzymes NOS

7 T45.3X2- **Poisoning by enzymes, intentional self-harm** HCC

7 T45.3X3- **Poisoning by enzymes, assault**

7 T45.3X4- **Poisoning by enzymes, undetermined**

7 T45.3X5- **Adverse effect of enzymes**

7 T45.3X6- **Underdosing of enzymes**

5 T45.4 **Poisoning by, adverse effect of and underdosing of iron and its compounds**

6 T45.4X **Poisoning by, adverse effect of and underdosing of iron and its compounds**

7 T45.4X1- **Poisoning by iron and its compounds, accidental (unintentional)**
Poisoning by iron and its compounds NOS

7 T45.4X2- **Poisoning by iron and its compounds, intentional self-harm** HCC

7 T45.4X3- **Poisoning by iron and its compounds, assault**

7 T45.4X4- **Poisoning by iron and its compounds, undetermined**

7 T45.4X5- **Adverse effect of iron and its compounds**

7 T45.4X6- **Underdosing of iron and its compounds**
EXCLUDES 1 *iron deficiency (E61.1)*

5 T45.5 **Poisoning by, adverse effect of and underdosing of anticoagulants and antithrombotic drugs**

6 T45.51 **Poisoning by, adverse effect of and underdosing of anticoagulants**

7 T45.511- **Poisoning by anticoagulants, accidental (unintentional)**
Poisoning by anticoagulants NOS

7 T45.512- **Poisoning by anticoagulants, intentional self-harm** HCC

7 T45.513- **Poisoning by anticoagulants, assault**

7 T45.514- **Poisoning by anticoagulants, undetermined**

7 T45.515- **Adverse effect of anticoagulants**
AHA: 2Q 2013, 35
AHA: 1Q 2016, 14

7 T45.516- **Underdosing of anticoagulants**

6 T45.52 **Poisoning by, adverse effect of and underdosing of antithrombotic drugs**
Poisoning by, adverse effect of and underdosing of antiplatelet drugs
EXCLUDES 2 *poisoning by, adverse effect of and underdosing of aspirin (T39.01-)*
poisoning by, adverse effect of and underdosing of acetylsalicylic acid (T39.01-)

7 T45.521- **Poisoning by antithrombotic drugs, accidental (unintentional)**
Poisoning by antithrombotic drug NOS

7 T45.522- **Poisoning by antithrombotic drugs, intentional self-harm** HCC

7 T45.523- **Poisoning by antithrombotic drugs, assault**

7 T45.524- **Poisoning by antithrombotic drugs, undetermined**

7 T45.525- **Adverse effect of antithrombotic drugs**
AHA: (T45.525A) 1Q 2016, 15

7 T45.526- **Underdosing of antithrombotic drugs**

5 T45.6 **Poisoning by, adverse effect of and underdosing of fibrinolysis-affecting drugs**

6 T45.60 **Poisoning by, adverse effect of and underdosing of unspecified fibrinolysis-affecting drugs**

7 T45.601- **Poisoning by unspecified fibrinolysis-affecting drugs, accidental (unintentional)**
Poisoning by fibrinolysis-affecting drug NOS

7 T45.602- **Poisoning by unspecified fibrinolysis-affecting drugs, intentional self-harm** HCC

7 T45.603- **Poisoning by unspecified fibrinolysis-affecting drugs, assault**

7 T45.604- **Poisoning by unspecified fibrinolysis-affecting drugs, undetermined**

7 T45.605- **Adverse effect of unspecified fibrinolysis-affecting drugs**

7 T45.606- **Underdosing of unspecified fibrinolysis-affecting drugs**

6 T45.61 **Poisoning by, adverse effect of and underdosing of thrombolytic drugs**

7 T45.611- **Poisoning by thrombolytic drug, accidental (unintentional)**
Poisoning by thrombolytic drug NOS

7 T45.612- **Poisoning by thrombolytic drug, intentional self-harm** HCC

7 T45.613- **Poisoning by thrombolytic drug, assault**

7 T45.614- **Poisoning by thrombolytic drug, undetermined**

7 T45.615- **Adverse effect of thrombolytic drugs**
AHA: 2Q 2017, 9

7 T45.616- **Underdosing of thrombolytic drugs**

6 T45.62 **Poisoning by, adverse effect of and underdosing of hemostatic drugs**

7 T45.621- **Poisoning by hemostatic drug, accidental (unintentional)**
Poisoning by hemostatic drug NOS

7 T45.622- **Poisoning by hemostatic drug, intentional self-harm** HCC

7 T45.623- **Poisoning by hemostatic drug, assault**

7 T45.624- **Poisoning by hemostatic drug, undetermined**

7 T45.625- **Adverse effect of hemostatic drug**

7 T45.626- **Underdosing of hemostatic drugs**

6 T45.69 **Poisoning by, adverse effect of and underdosing of other fibrinolysis-affecting drugs**

7 T45.691- **Poisoning by other fibrinolysis-affecting drugs, accidental (unintentional)**
Poisoning by other fibrinolysis-affecting drug NOS

7 T45.692- **Poisoning by other fibrinolysis-affecting drugs, intentional self-harm** HCC

7 T45.693- **Poisoning by other fibrinolysis-affecting drugs, assault**

7 T45.694- **Poisoning by other fibrinolysis-affecting drugs, undetermined**

7 T45.695- **Adverse effect of other fibrinolysis-affecting drugs**

7 T45.696- **Underdosing of other fibrinolysis-affecting drugs**

5 T45.7 **Poisoning by, adverse effect of and underdosing of anticoagulant antagonists, vitamin K and other coagulants**

6 T45.7X **Poisoning by, adverse effect of and underdosing of anticoagulant antagonists, vitamin K and other coagulants**

7 T45.7X1- **Poisoning by anticoagulant antagonists, vitamin K and other coagulants, accidental (unintentional)**
Poisoning by anticoagulant antagonists, vitamin K and other coagulants NOS

7 T45.7X2- **Poisoning by anticoagulant antagonists, vitamin K and other coagulants, intentional self-harm** HCC

7 T45.7X3- **Poisoning by anticoagulant antagonists, vitamin K and other coagulants, assault**

7 T45.7X4- **Poisoning by anticoagulant antagonists, vitamin K and other coagulants, undetermined**

7 T45.7X5- **Adverse effect of anticoagulant antagonists, vitamin K and other coagulants**

7 T45.7X6- **Underdosing of anticoagulant antagonist, vitamin K and other coagulants**
EXCLUDES 1 *vitamin K deficiency (E56.1)*

5 T45.8 **Poisoning by, adverse effect of and underdosing of other primarily systemic and hematological agents**
Poisoning by, adverse effect of and underdosing of liver preparations and other antianemic agents
Poisoning by, adverse effect of and underdosing of natural blood and blood products
Poisoning by, adverse effect of and underdosing of plasma substitute
EXCLUDES 2 *poisoning by, adverse effect of and underdosing of immunoglobulin (T50.Z1)*
poisoning by, adverse effect of and underdosing of iron (T45.4)
transfusion reactions (T80.-)

6 T45.8X **Poisoning by, adverse effect of and underdosing of other primarily systemic and hematological agents**

7 T45.8X1- **Poisoning by other primarily systemic and hematological agents, accidental (unintentional)**
Poisoning by other primarily systemic and hematological agents NOS

7 T45.8X2- **Poisoning by other primarily systemic and hematological agents, intentional self-harm** HCC

7 T45.8X3- **Poisoning by other primarily systemic and hematological agents, assault**

7 T45.8X4- **Poisoning by other primarily systemic and hematological agents, undetermined**

7 T45.8X5- **Adverse effect of other primarily systemic and hematological agents**

7 T45.8X6- **Underdosing of other primarily systemic and hematological agents**

5 T45.9 **Poisoning by, adverse effect of and underdosing of unspecified primarily systemic and hematological agent**

7 T45.91X- **Poisoning by unspecified primarily systemic and hematological agent, accidental (unintentional)**
Poisoning by primarily systemic and hematological agent NOS

7 T45.92X- **Poisoning by unspecified primarily systemic and hematological agent, intentional self-harm** HCC

7 T45.93X- **Poisoning by unspecified primarily systemic and hematological agent, assault**

7 T45.94X- **Poisoning by unspecified primarily systemic and hematological agent, undetermined**

7 T45.95X- **Adverse effect of unspecified primarily systemic and hematological agent**

7 T45.96X- **Underdosing of unspecified primarily systemic and hematological agent**

4 T46 **Poisoning by, adverse effect of and underdosing of agents primarily affecting the cardiovascular system**

EXCLUDES 1 *poisoning by, adverse effect of and underdosing of metaraminol (T44.4)*

The appropriate 7th character is to be added to each code from category T46
A initial encounter
D subsequent encounter
S sequela

5 T46.0 **Poisoning by, adverse effect of and underdosing of cardiac-stimulant glycosides and drugs of similar action**

6 T46.0X **Poisoning by, adverse effect of and underdosing of cardiac-stimulant glycosides and drugs of similar action**

7 T46.0X1- **Poisoning by cardiac-stimulant glycosides and drugs of similar action, accidental (unintentional)**
Poisoning by cardiac-stimulant glycosides and drugs of similar action NOS

7 T46.0X2- **Poisoning by cardiac-stimulant glycosides and drugs of similar action, intentional self-harm** HCC

7 T46.0X3- **Poisoning by cardiac-stimulant glycosides and drugs of similar action, assault**

7 T46.0X4 **Poisoning by cardiac-stimulant glycosides and drugs of similar action, undetermined**

7 T46.0X5- **Adverse effect of cardiac-stimulant glycosides and drugs of similar action**

7 T46.0X6- **Underdosing of cardiac-stimulant glycosides and drugs of similar action**

5 T46.1 **Poisoning by, adverse effect of and underdosing of calcium-channel blockers**

6 T46.1X **Poisoning by, adverse effect of and underdosing of calcium-channel blockers**

7 T46.1X1- **Poisoning by calcium-channel blockers, accidental (unintentional)**
Poisoning by calcium-channel blockers NOS

7 T46.1X2- **Poisoning by calcium-channel blockers, intentional self-harm** HCC

7 T46.1X3- **Poisoning by calcium-channel blockers, assault**

7 T46.1X4- **Poisoning by calcium-channel blockers, undetermined**

7 T46.1X5- **Adverse effect of calcium-channel blockers**

7 T46.1X6- **Underdosing of calcium-channel blockers**

5 T46.2 **Poisoning by, adverse effect of and underdosing of other antidysrhythmic drugs, not elsewhere classified**

EXCLUDES 1 *poisoning by, adverse effect of and underdosing of beta-adrenoreceptor antagonists (T44.7-)*

6 T46.2X **Poisoning by, adverse effect of and underdosing of other antidysrhythmic drugs**

7 T46.2X1- **Poisoning by other antidysrhythmic drugs, accidental (unintentional)**
Poisoning by other antidysrhythmic drugs NOS

7 T46.2X2- **Poisoning by other antidysrhythmic drugs, intentional self-harm** HCC

7 T46.2X3- **Poisoning by other antidysrhythmic drugs, assault**

7 T46.2X4- **Poisoning by other antidysrhythmic drugs, undetermined**

7 T46.2X5- **Adverse effect of other antidysrhythmic drugs**

7 T46.2X6- **Underdosing of other antidysrhythmic drugs**

5 T46.3 **Poisoning by, adverse effect of and underdosing of coronary vasodilators**
Poisoning by, adverse effect of and underdosing of dipyridamole

EXCLUDES 1 *poisoning by, adverse effect of and underdosing of calcium-channel blockers (T46.1)*

6 T46.3X **Poisoning by, adverse effect of and underdosing of coronary vasodilators**

7 T46.3X1- **Poisoning by coronary vasodilators, accidental (unintentional)**
Poisoning by coronary vasodilators NOS

7 T46.3X2- **Poisoning by coronary vasodilators, intentional self-harm** HCC

7 T46.3X3- **Poisoning by coronary vasodilators, assault**

7 T46.3X4- **Poisoning by coronary vasodilators, undetermined**

7 T46.3X5- **Adverse effect of coronary vasodilators**

7 T46.3X6- **Underdosing of coronary vasodilators**

5 T46.4 **Poisoning by, adverse effect of and underdosing of angiotensin-converting-enzyme inhibitors**

6 T46.4X **Poisoning by, adverse effect of and underdosing of angiotensin-converting-enzyme inhibitors**

7 T46.4X1- **Poisoning by angiotensin-converting-enzyme inhibitors, accidental (unintentional)**
Poisoning by angiotensin-converting-enzyme inhibitors NOS

7 T46.4X2- **Poisoning by angiotensin-converting-enzyme inhibitors, intentional self-harm** HCC

7 T46.4X3- **Poisoning by angiotensin-converting-enzyme inhibitors, assault**

7 T46.4X4- **Poisoning by angiotensin-converting-enzyme inhibitors, undetermined**

7 T46.4X5- **Adverse effect of angiotensin-converting-enzyme inhibitors**

7 T46.4X6- **Underdosing of angiotensin-converting-enzyme inhibitors**

5 T46.5 **Poisoning by, adverse effect of and underdosing of other antihypertensive drugs**

EXCLUDES 2 *poisoning by, adverse effect of and underdosing of beta-adrenoreceptor antagonists (T44.7)*
poisoning by, adverse effect of and underdosing of calcium-channel blockers (T46.1)
poisoning by, adverse effect of and underdosing of diuretics (T50.0-T50.2)

6 T46.5X **Poisoning by, adverse effect of and underdosing of other antihypertensive drugs**

7 T46.5X1- **Poisoning by other antihypertensive drugs, accidental (unintentional)**
Poisoning by other antihypertensive drugs NOS

7 T46.5X2- **Poisoning by other antihypertensive drugs, intentional self-harm** HCC

7 T46.5X3- **Poisoning by other antihypertensive drugs, assault**

7 T46.5X4- **Poisoning by other antihypertensive drugs, undetermined**

7 T46.5X5- **Adverse effect of other antihypertensive drugs**

7 T46.5X6- **Underdosing of other antihypertensive drugs**

5 T46.6 **Poisoning by, adverse effect of and underdosing of antihyperlipidemic and antiarteriosclerotic drugs**

6 T46.6X Poisoning by, adverse effect of and underdosing of antihyperlipidemic and antiarteriosclerotic drugs
7 T46.6X1- Poisoning by antihyperlipidemic and antiarteriosclerotic drugs, accidental (unintentional)
Poisoning by antihyperlipidemic and antiarteriosclerotic drugs NOS
7 T46.6X2- Poisoning by antihyperlipidemic and antiarteriosclerotic drugs, intentional self-harm HCC
7 T46.6X3- Poisoning by antihyperlipidemic and antiarteriosclerotic drugs, assault
7 T46.6X4- Poisoning by antihyperlipidemic and antiarteriosclerotic drugs, undetermined
7 T46.6X5- Adverse effect of antihyperlipidemic and antiarteriosclerotic drugs
7 T46.6X6- Underdosing of antihyperlipidemic and antiarteriosclerotic drugs
5 T46.7 Poisoning by, adverse effect of and underdosing of peripheral vasodilators
Poisoning by, adverse effect of and underdosing of nicotinic acid (derivatives)
EXCLUDES 1 *poisoning by, adverse effect of and underdosing of papaverine (T44.3)*
6 T46.7X Poisoning by, adverse effect of and underdosing of peripheral vasodilators
7 T46.7X1- Poisoning by peripheral vasodilators, accidental (unintentional)
Poisoning by peripheral vasodilators NOS
7 T46.7X2- Poisoning by peripheral vasodilators, intentional self-harm HCC
7 T46.7X3- Poisoning by peripheral vasodilators, assault
7 T46.7X4- Poisoning by peripheral vasodilators, undetermined
7 T46.7X5- Adverse effect of peripheral vasodilators
7 T46.7X6- Underdosing of peripheral vasodilators
5 T46.8 Poisoning by, adverse effect of and underdosing of antivaricose drugs, including sclerosing agents
6 T46.8X Poisoning by, adverse effect of and underdosing of antivaricose drugs, including sclerosing agents
7 T46.8X1- Poisoning by antivaricose drugs, including sclerosing agents, accidental (unintentional)
Poisoning by antivaricose drugs, including sclerosing agents NOS
7 T46.8X2- Poisoning by antivaricose drugs, including sclerosing agents, intentional self-harm HCC
7 T46.8X3- Poisoning by antivaricose drugs, including sclerosing agents, assault
7 T46.8X4- Poisoning by antivaricose drugs, including sclerosing agents, undetermined
7 T46.8X5- Adverse effect of antivaricose drugs, including sclerosing agents
7 T46.8X6- Underdosing of antivaricose drugs, including sclerosing agents
5 T46.9 Poisoning by, adverse effect of and underdosing of other and unspecified agents primarily affecting the cardiovascular system
6 T46.90 Poisoning by, adverse effect of and underdosing of unspecified agents primarily affecting the cardiovascular system
7 T46.901- Poisoning by unspecified agents primarily affecting the cardiovascular system, accidental (unintentional)
7 T46.902- Poisoning by unspecified agents primarily affecting the cardiovascular system, intentional self-harm HCC
7 T46.903- Poisoning by unspecified agents primarily affecting the cardiovascular system, assault
7 T46.904- Poisoning by unspecified agents primarily affecting the cardiovascular system, undetermined
7 T46.905- Adverse effect of unspecified agents primarily affecting the cardiovascular system
7 T46.906- Underdosing of unspecified agents primarily affecting the cardiovascular system
6 T46.99 Poisoning by, adverse effect of and underdosing of other agents primarily affecting the cardiovascular system
7 T46.991- Poisoning by other agents primarily affecting the cardiovascular system, accidental (unintentional)
7 T46.992- Poisoning by other agents primarily affecting the cardiovascular system, intentional self-harm HCC
7 T46.993- Poisoning by other agents primarily affecting the cardiovascular system, assault
7 T46.994- Poisoning by other agents primarily affecting the cardiovascular system, undetermined
7 T46.995- Adverse effect of other agents primarily affecting the cardiovascular system
7 T46.996- Underdosing of other agents primarily affecting the cardiovascular system

4 T47 Poisoning by, adverse effect of and underdosing of agents primarily affecting the gastrointestinal system

The appropriate 7th character is to be added to each code from category T47
A initial encounter
D subsequent encounter
S sequela

5 T47.0 Poisoning by, adverse effect of and underdosing of histamine H2-receptor blockers
6 T47.0X Poisoning by, adverse effect of and underdosing of histamine H2-receptor blockers
7 T47.0X1- Poisoning by histamine H2-receptor blockers, accidental (unintentional)
Poisoning by histamine H2-receptor blockers NOS
7 T47.0X2- Poisoning by histamine H2-receptor blockers, intentional self-harm HCC
7 T47.0X3- Poisoning by histamine H2-receptor blockers, assault
7 T47.0X4- Poisoning by histamine H2-receptor blockers, undetermined
7 T47.0X5- Adverse effect of histamine H2-receptor blockers
7 T47.0X6- Underdosing of histamine H2-receptor blockers
5 T47.1 Poisoning by, adverse effect of and underdosing of other antacids and anti-gastric-secretion drugs
6 T47.1X Poisoning by, adverse effect of and underdosing of other antacids and anti-gastric-secretion drugs
7 T47.1X1- Poisoning by other antacids and anti-gastric-secretion drugs, accidental (unintentional)
Poisoning by other antacids and anti-gastric-secretion drugs NOS
7 T47.1X2- Poisoning by other antacids and anti-gastric-secretion drugs, intentional self-harm HCC
7 T47.1X3- Poisoning by other antacids and anti-gastric-secretion drugs, assault
7 T47.1X4- Poisoning by other antacids and anti-gastric-secretion drugs, undetermined
7 T47.1X5- Adverse effect of other antacids and anti-gastric-secretion drugs
7 T47.1X6- Underdosing of other antacids and anti-gastric-secretion drugs
5 T47.2 Poisoning by, adverse effect of and underdosing of stimulant laxatives
6 T47.2X Poisoning by, adverse effect of and underdosing of stimulant laxatives
7 T47.2X1- Poisoning by stimulant laxatives, accidental (unintentional)
Poisoning by stimulant laxatives NOS
7 T47.2X2- Poisoning by stimulant laxatives, intentional self-harm HCC
7 T47.2X3- Poisoning by stimulant laxatives, assault
7 T47.2X4- Poisoning by stimulant laxatives, undetermined
7 T47.2X5- Adverse effect of stimulant laxatives
7 T47.2X6- Underdosing of stimulant laxatives
5 T47.3 Poisoning by, adverse effect of and underdosing of saline and osmotic laxatives
6 T47.3X Poisoning by and adverse effect of saline and osmotic laxatives
7 T47.3X1- Poisoning by saline and osmotic laxatives, accidental (unintentional)
Poisoning by saline and osmotic laxatives NOS

7 T47.3X2- Poisoning by saline and osmotic laxatives, intentional self-harm HCC

7 T47.3X3- Poisoning by saline and osmotic laxatives, assault

7 T47.3X4- Poisoning by saline and osmotic laxatives, undetermined

7 T47.3X5- Adverse effect of saline and osmotic laxatives

7 T47.3X6- Underdosing of saline and osmotic laxatives

5 T47.4 Poisoning by, adverse effect of and underdosing of other laxatives

6 T47.4X Poisoning by, adverse effect of and underdosing of other laxatives

7 T47.4X1- Poisoning by other laxatives, accidental (unintentional)
Poisoning by other laxatives NOS

7 T47.4X2- Poisoning by other laxatives, intentional self-harm HCC

7 T47.4X3- Poisoning by other laxatives, assault

7 T47.4X4- Poisoning by other laxatives, undetermined

7 T47.4X5- Adverse effect of other laxatives

7 T47.4X6- Underdosing of other laxatives

5 T47.5 Poisoning by, adverse effect of and underdosing of digestants

6 T47.5X Poisoning by, adverse effect of and underdosing of digestants

7 T47.5X1- Poisoning by digestants, accidental (unintentional)
Poisoning by digestants NOS

7 T47.5X2- Poisoning by digestants, intentional self-harm HCC

7 T47.5X3- Poisoning by digestants, assault

7 T47.5X4- Poisoning by digestants, undetermined

7 T47.5X5- Adverse effect of digestants

7 T47.5X6- Underdosing of digestants

5 T47.6 Poisoning by, adverse effect of and underdosing of antidiarrheal drugs

EXCLUDES 2 *poisoning by, adverse effect of and underdosing of systemic antibiotics and other anti-infectives (T36-T37)*

6 T47.6X Poisoning by, adverse effect of and underdosing of antidiarrheal drugs

7 T47.6X1- Poisoning by antidiarrheal drugs, accidental (unintentional)
Poisoning by antidiarrheal drugs NOS

7 T47.6X2- Poisoning by antidiarrheal drugs, intentional self-harm HCC

7 T47.6X3- Poisoning by antidiarrheal drugs, assault

7 T47.6X4- Poisoning by antidiarrheal drugs, undetermined

7 T47.6X5- Adverse effect of antidiarrheal drugs

7 T47.6X6- Underdosing of antidiarrheal drugs

5 T47.7 Poisoning by, adverse effect of and underdosing of emetics

6 T47.7X Poisoning by, adverse effect of and underdosing of emetics

7 T47.7X1- Poisoning by emetics, accidental (unintentional)
Poisoning by emetics NOS

7 T47.7X2- Poisoning by emetics, intentional self-harm HCC

7 T47.7X3- Poisoning by emetics, assault

7 T47.7X4- Poisoning by emetics, undetermined

7 T47.7X5- Adverse effect of emetics

7 T47.7X6- Underdosing of emetics

5 T47.8 Poisoning by, adverse effect of and underdosing of other agents primarily affecting gastrointestinal system

6 T47.8X Poisoning by, adverse effect of and underdosing of other agents primarily affecting gastrointestinal system

7 T47.8X1- Poisoning by other agents primarily affecting gastrointestinal system, accidental (unintentional)
Poisoning by other agents primarily affecting gastrointestinal system NOS

7 T47.8X2- Poisoning by other agents primarily affecting gastrointestinal system, intentional self-harm HCC

7 T47.8X3- Poisoning by other agents primarily affecting gastrointestinal system, assault

7 T47.8X4- Poisoning by other agents primarily affecting gastrointestinal system, undetermined

7 T47.8X5- Adverse effect of other agents primarily affecting gastrointestinal system

7 T47.8X6- Underdosing of other agents primarily affecting gastrointestinal system

5 T47.9 Poisoning by, adverse effect of and underdosing of unspecified agents primarily affecting the gastrointestinal system

7 T47.91X- Poisoning by unspecified agents primarily affecting the gastrointestinal system, accidental (unintentional)
Poisoning by agents primarily affecting the gastrointestinal system NOS

7 T47.92X- Poisoning by unspecified agents primarily affecting the gastrointestinal system, intentional self-harm HCC

7 T47.93X- Poisoning by unspecified agents primarily affecting the gastrointestinal system, assault

7 T47.94X- Poisoning by unspecified agents primarily affecting the gastrointestinal system, undetermined

7 T47.95X- Adverse effect of unspecified agents primarily affecting the gastrointestinal system

7 T47.96X- Underdosing of unspecified agents primarily affecting the gastrointestinal system

4 T48 Poisoning by, adverse effect of and underdosing of agents primarily acting on smooth and skeletal muscles and the respiratory system

The appropriate 7th character is to be added to each code from category T48
A initial encounter
D subsequent encounter
S sequela

5 T48.0 Poisoning by, adverse effect of and underdosing of oxytocic drugs

EXCLUDES 1 *poisoning by, adverse effect of and underdosing of estrogens, progestogens and antagonists (T38.4-T38.6)*

6 T48.0X Poisoning by, adverse effect of and underdosing of oxytocic drugs

7 T48.0X1- Poisoning by oxytocic drugs, accidental (unintentional)
Poisoning by oxytocic drugs NOS

7 T48.0X2- Poisoning by oxytocic drugs, intentional self-harm HCC

7 T48.0X3- Poisoning by oxytocic drugs, assault

7 T48.0X4- Poisoning by oxytocic drugs, undetermined

7 T48.0X5- Adverse effect of oxytocic drugs

7 T48.0X6- Underdosing of oxytocic drugs

5 T48.1 Poisoning by, adverse effect of and underdosing of skeletal muscle relaxants [neuromuscular blocking agents]

6 T48.1X Poisoning by, adverse effect of and underdosing of skeletal muscle relaxants [neuromuscular blocking agents]

7 T48.1X1- Poisoning by skeletal muscle relaxants [neuromuscular blocking agents], accidental (unintentional)
Poisoning by skeletal muscle relaxants [neuromuscular blocking agents] NOS

7 T48.1X2- Poisoning by skeletal muscle relaxants [neuromuscular blocking agents], intentional self-harm HCC

7 T48.1X3- Poisoning by skeletal muscle relaxants [neuromuscular blocking agents], assault

7 T48.1X4- Poisoning by skeletal muscle relaxants [neuromuscular blocking agents], undetermined

7 T48.1X5- Adverse effect of skeletal muscle relaxants [neuromuscular blocking agents]

7 T48.1X6- Underdosing of skeletal muscle relaxants [neuromuscular blocking agents]

5 T48.2 Poisoning by, adverse effect of and underdosing of other and unspecified drugs acting on muscles

6 T48.20 Poisoning by, adverse effect of and underdosing of unspecified drugs acting on muscles

7 **T48.201-** **Poisoning by unspecified drugs acting on muscles, accidental (unintentional)**
Poisoning by unspecified drugs acting on muscles NOS

7 **T48.202-** **Poisoning by unspecified drugs acting on muscles, intentional self-harm** HCC

7 **T48.203-** **Poisoning by unspecified drugs acting on muscles, assault**

7 **T48.204-** **Poisoning by unspecified drugs acting on muscles, undetermined**

7 **T48.205-** **Adverse effect of unspecified drugs acting on muscles**

7 **T48.206-** **Underdosing of unspecified drugs acting on muscles**

6 **T48.29** **Poisoning by, adverse effect of and underdosing of other drugs acting on muscles**

7 **T48.291-** **Poisoning by other drugs acting on muscles, accidental (unintentional)**
Poisoning by other drugs acting on muscles NOS

7 **T48.292-** **Poisoning by other drugs acting on muscles, intentional self-harm** HCC

7 **T48.293-** **Poisoning by other drugs acting on muscles, assault**

7 **T48.294-** **Poisoning by other drugs acting on muscles, undetermined**

7 **T48.295-** **Adverse effect of other drugs acting on muscles**

7 **T48.296-** **Underdosing of other drugs acting on muscles**

5 **T48.3** **Poisoning by, adverse effect of and underdosing of antitussives**

6 **T48.3X** **Poisoning by, adverse effect of and underdosing of antitussives**

7 **T48.3X1-** **Poisoning by antitussives, accidental (unintentional)**
Poisoning by antitussives NOS

7 **T48.3X2-** **Poisoning by antitussives, intentional self-harm** HCC

7 **T48.3X3-** **Poisoning by antitussives, assault**

7 **T48.3X4-** **Poisoning by antitussives, undetermined**

7 **T48.3X5-** **Adverse effect of antitussives**

7 **T48.3X6-** **Underdosing of antitussives**

5 **T48.4** **Poisoning by, adverse effect of and underdosing of expectorants**

6 **T48.4X** **Poisoning by, adverse effect of and underdosing of expectorants**

7 **T48.4X1-** **Poisoning by expectorants, accidental (unintentional)**
Poisoning by expectorants NOS

7 **T48.4X2-** **Poisoning by expectorants, intentional self-harm** HCC

7 **T48.4X3-** **Poisoning by expectorants, assault**

7 **T48.4X4-** **Poisoning by expectorants, undetermined**

7 **T48.4X5-** **Adverse effect of expectorants**

7 **T48.4X6-** **Underdosing of expectorants**

5 **T48.5** **Poisoning by, adverse effect of and underdosing of other anti-common-cold drugs**
Poisoning by, adverse effect of and underdosing of decongestants

EXCLUDES 2 *poisoning by, adverse effect of and underdosing of antipyretics, NEC (T39.9-)*
poisoning by, adverse effect of and underdosing of non-steroidal antiinflammatory drugs (T39.3-)
poisoning by, adverse effect of and underdosing of salicylates (T39.0-)

6 **T48.5X** **Poisoning by, adverse effect of and underdosing of other anti-common-cold drugs**

7 **T48.5X1-** **Poisoning by other anti-common-cold drugs, accidental (unintentional)**
Poisoning by other anti-common-cold drugs NOS

7 **T48.5X2-** **Poisoning by other anti-common-cold drugs, intentional self-harm** HCC

7 **T48.5X3-** **Poisoning by other anti-common-cold drugs, assault**

7 **T48.5X4-** **Poisoning by other anti-common-cold drugs, undetermined**

7 **T48.5X5-** **Adverse effect of other anti-common-cold drugs**

7 **T48.5X6-** **Underdosing of other anti-common-cold drugs**

5 **T48.6** **Poisoning by, adverse effect of and underdosing of antiasthmatics, not elsewhere classified**
Poisoning by, adverse effect of and underdosing of beta-adrenoreceptor agonists used in asthma therapy

EXCLUDES 1 *poisoning by, adverse effect of and underdosing of beta-adrenoreceptor agonists not used in asthma therapy (T44.5)*
poisoning by, adverse effect of and underdosing of anterior pituitary [adenohypophyseal] hormones (T38.8)

6 **T48.6X** **Poisoning by, adverse effect of and underdosing of antiasthmatics**

7 **T48.6X1-** **Poisoning by antiasthmatics, accidental (unintentional)**
Poisoning by antiasthmatics NOS

7 **T48.6X2-** **Poisoning by antiasthmatics, intentional self-harm** HCC

7 **T48.6X3-** **Poisoning by antiasthmatics, assault**

7 **T48.6X4-** **Poisoning by antiasthmatics, undetermined**

7 **T48.6X5-** **Adverse effect of antiasthmatics**

7 **T48.6X6-** **Underdosing of antiasthmatics**

5 **T48.9** **Poisoning by, adverse effect of and underdosing of other and unspecified agents primarily acting on the respiratory system**

6 **T48.90** **Poisoning by, adverse effect of and underdosing of unspecified agents primarily acting on the respiratory system**

7 **T48.901-** **Poisoning by unspecified agents primarily acting on the respiratory system, accidental (unintentional)**

7 **T48.902-** **Poisoning by unspecified agents primarily acting on the respiratory system, intentional self-harm** HCC

7 **T48.903-** **Poisoning by unspecified agents primarily acting on the respiratory system, assault**

7 **T48.904-** **Poisoning by unspecified agents primarily acting on the respiratory system, undetermined**

7 **T48.905-** **Adverse effect of unspecified agents primarily acting on the respiratory system**

7 **T48.906-** **Underdosing of unspecified agents primarily acting on the respiratory system**

6 **T48.99** **Poisoning by, adverse effect of and underdosing of other agents primarily acting on the respiratory system**

7 **T48.991-** **Poisoning by other agents primarily acting on the respiratory system, accidental (unintentional)**

7 **T48.992-** **Poisoning by other agents primarily acting on the respiratory system, intentional self-harm** HCC

7 **T48.993-** **Poisoning by other agents primarily acting on the respiratory system, assault**

7 **T48.994-** **Poisoning by other agents primarily acting on the respiratory system, undetermined**

7 **T48.995-** **Adverse effect of other agents primarily acting on the respiratory system**

7 **T48.996-** **Underdosing of other agents primarily acting on the respiratory system**

4 T49 Poisoning by, adverse effect of and underdosing of topical agents primarily affecting skin and mucous membrane and by ophthalmological, otorhinorlaryngological and dental drugs

INCLUDES poisoning by, adverse effect of and underdosing of glucocorticoids, topically used

The appropriate 7th character is to be added to each code from category T49
A initial encounter
D subsequent encounter
S sequela

5 **T49.0** **Poisoning by, adverse effect of and underdosing of local antifungal, anti-infective and anti-inflammatory drugs**

6 **T49.0X** **Poisoning by, adverse effect of and underdosing of local antifungal, anti-infective and anti-inflammatory drugs**

7 T49.0X1- **Poisoning by local antifungal, anti-infective and anti-inflammatory drugs, accidental (unintentional)**
Poisoning by local antifungal, anti-infective and anti-inflammatory drugs NOS

7 T49.0X2- **Poisoning by local antifungal, anti-infective and anti-inflammatory drugs, intentional self-harm** HCC

7 T49.0X3- **Poisoning by local antifungal, anti-infective and anti-inflammatory drugs, assault**

7 T49.0X4- **Poisoning by local antifungal, anti-infective and anti-inflammatory drugs, undetermined**

7 T49.0X5- **Adverse effect of local antifungal, anti-infective and anti-inflammatory drugs**

7 T49.0X6- **Underdosing of local antifungal, anti-infective and anti-inflammatory drugs**

5 T49.1 **Poisoning by, adverse effect of and underdosing of antipruritics**

6 T49.1X **Poisoning by, adverse effect of and underdosing of antipruritics**

7 T49.1X1- **Poisoning by antipruritics, accidental (unintentional)**
Poisoning by antipruritics NOS

7 T49.1X2- **Poisoning by antipruritics, intentional self-harm** HCC

7 T49.1X3- **Poisoning by antipruritics, assault**

7 T49.1X4- **Poisoning by antipruritics, undetermined**

7 T49.1X5- **Adverse effect of antipruritics**

7 T49.1X6- **Underdosing of antipruritics**

5 T49.2 **Poisoning by, adverse effect of and underdosing of local astringents and local detergents**

6 T49.2X **Poisoning by, adverse effect of and underdosing of local astringents and local detergents**

7 T49.2X1- **Poisoning by local astringents and local detergents, accidental (unintentional)**
Poisoning by local astringents and local detergents NOS

7 T49.2X2- **Poisoning by local astringents and local detergents, intentional self-harm** HCC

7 T49.2X3- **Poisoning by local astringents and local detergents, assault**

7 T49.2X4- **Poisoning by local astringents and local detergents, undetermined**

7 T49.2X5- **Adverse effect of local astringents and local detergents**

7 T49.2X6- **Underdosing of local astringents and local detergents**

5 T49.3 **Poisoning by, adverse effect of and underdosing of emollients, demulcents and protectants**

6 T49.3X **Poisoning by, adverse effect of and underdosing of emollients, demulcents and protectants**

7 T49.3X1- **Poisoning by emollients, demulcents and protectants, accidental (unintentional)**
Poisoning by emollients, demulcents and protectants NOS

7 T49.3X2- **Poisoning by emollients, demulcents and protectants, intentional self-harm** HCC

7 T49.3X3- **Poisoning by emollients, demulcents and protectants, assault**

7 T49.3X4- **Poisoning by emollients, demulcents and protectants, undetermined**

7 T49.3X5- **Adverse effect of emollients, demulcents and protectants**

7 T49.3X6- **Underdosing of emollients, demulcents and protectants**

5 T49.4 **Poisoning by, adverse effect of and underdosing of keratolytics, keratoplastics, and other hair treatment drugs and preparations**

6 T49.4X **Poisoning by, adverse effect of and underdosing of keratolytics, keratoplastics, and other hair treatment drugs and preparations**

7 T49.4X1- **Poisoning by keratolytics, keratoplastics, and other hair treatment drugs and preparations, accidental (unintentional)**
Poisoning by keratolytics, keratoplastics, and other hair treatment drugs and preparations NOS

7 T49.4X2- **Poisoning by keratolytics, keratoplastics, and other hair treatment drugs and preparations, intentional self-harm** HCC

7 T49.4X3- **Poisoning by keratolytics, keratoplastics, and other hair treatment drugs and preparations, assault**

7 T49.4X4- **Poisoning by keratolytics, keratoplastics, and other hair treatment drugs and preparations, undetermined**

7 T49.4X5- **Adverse effect of keratolytics, keratoplastics, and other hair treatment drugs and preparations**

7 T49.4X6- **Underdosing of keratolytics, keratoplastics, and other hair treatment drugs and preparations**

5 T49.5 **Poisoning by, adverse effect of and underdosing of ophthalmological drugs and preparations**

6 T49.5X **Poisoning by, adverse effect of and underdosing of ophthalmological drugs and preparations**

7 T49.5X1- **Poisoning by ophthalmological drugs and preparations, accidental (unintentional)**
Poisoning by ophthalmological drugs and preparations NOS

7 T49.5X2- **Poisoning by ophthalmological drugs and preparations, intentional self-harm** HCC

7 T49.5X3- **Poisoning by ophthalmological drugs and preparations, assault**

7 T49.5X4- **Poisoning by ophthalmological drugs and preparations, undetermined**

7 T49.5X5- **Adverse effect of ophthalmological drugs and preparations**

7 T49.5X6- **Underdosing of ophthalmological drugs and preparations**

5 T49.6 **Poisoning by, adverse effect of and underdosing of otorhinolaryngological drugs and preparations**

6 T49.6X **Poisoning by, adverse effect of and underdosing of otorhinolaryngological drugs and preparations**

7 T49.6X1- **Poisoning by otorhinolaryngological drugs and preparations, accidental (unintentional)**
Poisoning by otorhinolaryngological drugs and preparations NOS

7 T49.6X2- **Poisoning by otorhinolaryngological drugs and preparations, intentional self-harm** HCC

7 T49.6X3- **Poisoning by otorhinolaryngological drugs and preparations, assault**

7 T49.6X4- **Poisoning by otorhinolaryngological drugs and preparations, undetermined**

7 T49.6X5- **Adverse effect of otorhinolaryngological drugs and preparations**

7 T49.6X6- **Underdosing of otorhinolaryngological drugs and preparations**

5 T49.7 **Poisoning by, adverse effect of and underdosing of dental drugs, topically applied**

6 T49.7X **Poisoning by, adverse effect of and underdosing of dental drugs, topically applied**

7 T49.7X1- **Poisoning by dental drugs, topically applied, accidental (unintentional)**
Poisoning by dental drugs, topically applied NOS

7 T49.7X2- **Poisoning by dental drugs, topically applied, intentional self-harm** HCC

7 T49.7X3- **Poisoning by dental drugs, topically applied, assault**

7 T49.7X4- **Poisoning by dental drugs, topically applied, undetermined**

7 T49.7X5- **Adverse effect of dental drugs, topically applied**

7 T49.7X6- **Underdosing of dental drugs, topically applied**

5 T49.8 **Poisoning by, adverse effect of and underdosing of other topical agents**
Poisoning by, adverse effect of and underdosing of spermicides

6 T49.8X **Poisoning by, adverse effect of and underdosing of other topical agents**

7 T49.8X1- **Poisoning by other topical agents, accidental (unintentional)**
Poisoning by other topical agents NOS

7 T49.8X2- **Poisoning by other topical agents, intentional self-harm** HCC

7 T49.8X3- **Poisoning by other topical agents, assault**

7 T49.8X4- **Poisoning by other topical agents, undetermined**

7 T49.8X5- **Adverse effect of other topical agents**

7 T49.8X6- **Underdosing of other topical agents**

5 T49.9 **Poisoning by, adverse effect of and underdosing of unspecified topical agent**

7 T49.91X- **Poisoning by unspecified topical agent, accidental (unintentional)**

7 T49.92X- **Poisoning by unspecified topical agent, intentional self-harm** HCC

7 T49.93X- **Poisoning by unspecified topical agent, assault**

7 T49.94X- **Poisoning by unspecified topical agent, undetermined**

7 T49.95X- **Adverse effect of unspecified topical agent**

7 T49.96X- **Underdosing of unspecified topical agent**

4 T50 **Poisoning by, adverse effect of and underdosing of diuretics and other and unspecified drugs, medicaments and biological substances**

The appropriate 7th character is to be added to each code from category T50
A initial encounter
D subsequent encounter
S sequela

5 T50.0 **Poisoning by, adverse effect of and underdosing of mineralocorticoids and their antagonists**

6 T50.0X **Poisoning by, adverse effect of and underdosing of mineralocorticoids and their antagonists**

7 T50.0X1- **Poisoning by mineralocorticoids and their antagonists, accidental (unintentional)**
Poisoning by mineralocorticoids and their antagonists NOS

7 T50.0X2- **Poisoning by mineralocorticoids and their antagonists, intentional self-harm** HCC

7 T50.0X3- **Poisoning by mineralocorticoids and their antagonists, assault**

7 T50.0X4- **Poisoning by mineralocorticoids and their antagonists, undetermined**

7 T50.0X5- **Adverse effect of mineralocorticoids and their antagonists**

7 T50.0X6- **Underdosing of mineralocorticoids and their antagonists**

5 T50.1 **Poisoning by, adverse effect of and underdosing of loop [high-ceiling] diuretics**

6 T50.1X **Poisoning by, adverse effect of and underdosing of loop [high-ceiling] diuretics**

7 T50.1X1- **Poisoning by loop [high-ceiling] diuretics, accidental (unintentional)**
Poisoning by loop [high-ceiling] diuretics NOS

7 T50.1X2- **Poisoning by loop [high-ceiling] diuretics, intentional self-harm** HCC

7 T50.1X3- **Poisoning by loop [high-ceiling] diuretics, assault**

7 T50.1X4- **Poisoning by loop [high-ceiling] diuretics, undetermined**

7 T50.1X5- **Adverse effect of loop [high-ceiling] diuretics**

7 T50.1X6- **Underdosing of loop [high-ceiling] diuretics**

5 T50.2 **Poisoning by, adverse effect of and underdosing of carbonic-anhydrase inhibitors, benzothiadiazides and other diuretics**
Poisoning by, adverse effect of and underdosing of acetazolamide

6 T50.2X **Poisoning by, adverse effect of and underdosing of carbonic-anhydrase inhibitors, benzothiadiazides and other diuretics**

7 T50.2X1- **Poisoning by carbonic-anhydrase inhibitors, benzothiadiazides and other diuretics, accidental (unintentional)**
Poisoning by carbonic-anhydrase inhibitors, benzothiadiazides and other diuretics NOS

7 T50.2X2- **Poisoning by carbonic-anhydrase inhibitors, benzothiadiazides and other diuretics, intentional self-harm** HCC

7 T50.2X3- **Poisoning by carbonic-anhydrase inhibitors, benzothiadiazides and other diuretics, assault**

7 T50.2X4- **Poisoning by carbonic-anhydrase inhibitors, benzothiadiazides and other diuretics, undetermined**

7 T50.2X5- **Adverse effect of carbonic-anhydrase inhibitors, benzothiadiazides and other diuretics**

7 T50.2X6- **Underdosing of carbonic-anhydrase inhibitors, benzothiadiazides and other diuretics**

5 T50.3 **Poisoning by, adverse effect of and underdosing of electrolytic, caloric and water-balance agents**
Poisoning by, adverse effect of and underdosing of oral rehydration salts

6 T50.3X **Poisoning by, adverse effect of and underdosing of electrolytic, caloric and water-balance agents**

7 T50.3X1- **Poisoning by electrolytic, caloric and water-balance agents, accidental (unintentional)**
Poisoning by electrolytic, caloric and water-balance agents NOS

7 T50.3X2- **Poisoning by electrolytic, caloric and water-balance agents, intentional self-harm** HCC

7 T50.3X3- **Poisoning by electrolytic, caloric and water-balance agents, assault**

7 T50.3X4- **Poisoning by electrolytic, caloric and water-balance agents, undetermined**

7 T50.3X5- **Adverse effect of electrolytic, caloric and water-balance agents**

7 T50.3X6- **Underdosing of electrolytic, caloric and water-balance agents**

5 T50.4 **Poisoning by, adverse effect of and underdosing of drugs affecting uric acid metabolism**

6 T50.4X **Poisoning by, adverse effect of and underdosing of drugs affecting uric acid metabolism**

7 T50.4X1- **Poisoning by drugs affecting uric acid metabolism, accidental (unintentional)**
Poisoning by drugs affecting uric acid metabolism NOS

7 T50.4X2- **Poisoning by drugs affecting uric acid metabolism, intentional self-harm** HCC

7 T50.4X3- **Poisoning by drugs affecting uric acid metabolism, assault**

7 T50.4X4- **Poisoning by drugs affecting uric acid metabolism, undetermined**

7 T50.4X5- **Adverse effect of drugs affecting uric acid metabolism**

7 T50.4X6- **Underdosing of drugs affecting uric acid metabolism**

5 T50.5 **Poisoning by, adverse effect of and underdosing of appetite depressants**

6 T50.5X **Poisoning by, adverse effect of and underdosing of appetite depressants**

7 T50.5X1- **Poisoning by appetite depressants, accidental (unintentional)**
Poisoning by appetite depressants NOS

7 T50.5X2- **Poisoning by appetite depressants, intentional self-harm** HCC

7 T50.5X3- **Poisoning by appetite depressants, assault**

7 T50.5X4- **Poisoning by appetite depressants, undetermined**

7 T50.5X5- **Adverse effect of appetite depressants**

7 T50.5X6- **Underdosing of appetite depressants**

5 T50.6 **Poisoning by, adverse effect of and underdosing of antidotes and chelating agents**
Poisoning by, adverse effect of and underdosing of alcohol deterrents

6 T50.6X **Poisoning by, adverse effect of and underdosing of antidotes and chelating agents**

7 T50.6X1- **Poisoning by antidotes and chelating agents, accidental (unintentional)**
Poisoning by antidotes and chelating agents NOS

7 T50.6X2- **Poisoning by antidotes and chelating agents, intentional self-harm** HCC

7 T50.6X3- **Poisoning by antidotes and chelating agents, assault**

7 T50.6X4- **Poisoning by antidotes and chelating agents, undetermined**

7 T50.6X5- **Adverse effect of antidotes and chelating agents**

7 T50.6X6- **Underdosing of antidotes and chelating agents**

5 T50.7 **Poisoning by, adverse effect of and underdosing of analeptics and opioid receptor antagonists**

6 T50.7X **Poisoning by, adverse effect of and underdosing of analeptics and opioid receptor antagonists**

7 T50.7X1- Poisoning by analeptics and opioid receptor antagonists, accidental (unintentional)
Poisoning by analeptics and opioid receptor antagonists NOS

7 T50.7X2- Poisoning by analeptics and opioid receptor antagonists, intentional self-harm HCC

7 T50.7X3- Poisoning by analeptics and opioid receptor antagonists, assault

7 T50.7X4- Poisoning by analeptics and opioid receptor antagonists, undetermined

7 T50.7X5- Adverse effect of analeptics and opioid receptor antagonists

7 T50.7X6- Underdosing of analeptics and opioid receptor antagonists

5 T50.8 Poisoning by, adverse effect of and underdosing of diagnostic agents

6 T50.8X Poisoning by, adverse effect of and underdosing of diagnostic agents

7 T50.8X1- Poisoning by diagnostic agents, accidental (unintentional)
Poisoning by diagnostic agents NOS

7 T50.8X2- Poisoning by diagnostic agents, intentional self-harm HCC

7 T50.8X3- Poisoning by diagnostic agents, assault

7 T50.8X4- Poisoning by diagnostic agents, undetermined

7 T50.8X5- Adverse effect of diagnostic agents

7 T50.8X6- Underdosing of diagnostic agents

5 T50.A Poisoning by, adverse effect of and underdosing of bacterial vaccines

6 T50.A1 Poisoning by, adverse effect of and underdosing of pertussis vaccine, including combinations with a pertussis component

7 T50.A11- Poisoning by pertussis vaccine, including combinations with a pertussis component, accidental (unintentional)

7 T50.A12- Poisoning by pertussis vaccine, including combinations with a pertussis component, intentional self-harm HCC

7 T50.A13- Poisoning by pertussis vaccine, including combinations with a pertussis component, assault

7 T50.A14- Poisoning by pertussis vaccine, including combinations with a pertussis component, undetermined

7 T50.A15- Adverse effect of pertussis vaccine, including combinations with a pertussis component

7 T50.A16- Underdosing of pertussis vaccine, including combinations with a pertussis component

6 T50.A2 Poisoning by, adverse effect of and underdosing of mixed bacterial vaccines without a pertussis component

7 T50.A21- Poisoning by mixed bacterial vaccines without a pertussis component, accidental (unintentional)

7 T50.A22- Poisoning by mixed bacterial vaccines without a pertussis component, intentional self-harm HCC

7 T50.A23- Poisoning by mixed bacterial vaccines without a pertussis component, assault

7 T50.A24- Poisoning by mixed bacterial vaccines without a pertussis component, undetermined

7 T50.A25- Adverse effect of mixed bacterial vaccines without a pertussis component

7 T50.A26- Underdosing of mixed bacterial vaccines without a pertussis component

6 T50.A9 Poisoning by, adverse effect of and underdosing of other bacterial vaccines

7 T50.A91- Poisoning by other bacterial vaccines, accidental (unintentional)

7 T50.A92- Poisoning by other bacterial vaccines, intentional self-harm HCC

7 T50.A93- Poisoning by other bacterial vaccines, assault

7 T50.A94- Poisoning by other bacterial vaccines, undetermined

7 T50.A95- Adverse effect of other bacterial vaccines

7 T50.A96- Underdosing of other bacterial vaccines

5 T50.B Poisoning by, adverse effect of and underdosing of viral vaccines

6 T50.B1 Poisoning by, adverse effect of and underdosing of smallpox vaccines

7 T50.B11- Poisoning by smallpox vaccines, accidental (unintentional)

7 T50.B12- Poisoning by smallpox vaccines, intentional self-harm HCC

7 T50.B13- Poisoning by smallpox vaccines, assault

7 T50.B14- Poisoning by smallpox vaccines, undetermined

7 T50.B15- Adverse effect of smallpox vaccines

7 T50.B16- Underdosing of smallpox vaccines

6 T50.B9 Poisoning by, adverse effect of and underdosing of other viral vaccines

7 T50.B91- Poisoning by other viral vaccines, accidental (unintentional)

7 T50.B92- Poisoning by other viral vaccines, intentional self-harm HCC

7 T50.B93- Poisoning by other viral vaccines, assault

7 T50.B94- Poisoning by other viral vaccines, undetermined

7 T50.B95- Adverse effect of other viral vaccines

7 T50.B96- Underdosing of other viral vaccines

5 T50.Z Poisoning by, adverse effect of and underdosing of other vaccines and biological substances

6 T50.Z1 Poisoning by, adverse effect of and underdosing of immunoglobulin

7 T50.Z11- Poisoning by immunoglobulin, accidental (unintentional)

7 T50.Z12- Poisoning by immunoglobulin, intentional self-harm HCC

7 T50.Z13- Poisoning by immunoglobulin, assault

7 T50.Z14- Poisoning by immunoglobulin, undetermined

7 T50.Z15- Adverse effect of immunoglobulin

7 T50.Z16- Underdosing of immunoglobulin

6 T50.Z9 Poisoning by, adverse effect of and underdosing of other vaccines and biological substances

7 T50.Z91- Poisoning by other vaccines and biological substances, accidental (unintentional)

7 T50.Z92- Poisoning by other vaccines and biological substances, intentional self-harm HCC

7 T50.Z93- Poisoning by other vaccines and biological substances, assault

7 T50.Z94- Poisoning by other vaccines and biological substances, undetermined

7 T50.Z95- Adverse effect of other vaccines and biological substances

7 T50.Z96- Underdosing of other vaccines and biological substances

5 T50.9 Poisoning by, adverse effect of and underdosing of other and unspecified drugs, medicaments and biological substances

6 T50.90 Poisoning by, adverse effect of and underdosing of unspecified drugs, medicaments and biological substances

7 T50.901- Poisoning by unspecified drugs, medicaments and biological substances, accidental (unintentional)
AHA: (T50.901S) 1Q 2015, 21

7 T50.902- Poisoning by unspecified drugs, medicaments and biological substances, intentional self-harm HCC

7 T50.903- Poisoning by unspecified drugs, medicaments and biological substances, assault

7 T50.904- Poisoning by unspecified drugs, medicaments and biological substances, undetermined

7 T50.905- Adverse effect of unspecified drugs, medicaments and biological substances

7 T50.906- Underdosing of unspecified drugs, medicaments and biological substances

6 T50.99 Poisoning by, adverse effect of and underdosing of other drugs, medicaments and biological substances

7 T50.991- Poisoning by other drugs, medicaments and biological substances, accidental (unintentional)

T50.992- Poisoning by other drugs, medicaments and biological substances, intentional self-harm HCC

T50.993- Poisoning by other drugs, medicaments and biological substances, assault

T50.994- Poisoning by other drugs, medicaments and biological substances, undetermined

T50.995- Adverse effect of other drugs, medicaments and biological substances

T50.996- Underdosing of other drugs, medicaments and biological substances

Toxic effects of substances chiefly nonmedicinal as to source (T51-T65)

Note: When no intent is indicated code to accidental. Undetermined intent is only for use when there is specific documentation in the record that the intent of the toxic effect cannot be determined.

Use additional code(s):

for all associated manifestations of toxic effect, such as: respiratory conditions due to external agents (J60-J70)

personal history of foreign body fully removed (Z87.821)

to identify any retained foreign body, if applicable (Z18.-)

EXCLUDES 1 *contact with and (suspected) exposure to toxic substances (Z77.-)*

GUIDELINES Section I.C.19.e.1)-4)

Codes in categories T36-T65 are combination codes that include the substance that was taken as well as the intent. No additional external cause code is required for poisonings, toxic effects, adverse effects and underdosing codes.

Do not code directly from the Table of Drugs and Chemicals. Always refer back to the Tabular List. Use as many codes as necessary to describe completely all drugs, medicinal or biological substances. If the same code would describe the causative agent for more than one adverse reaction, poisoning, toxic effect or underdosing, assign the code only once. If two or more drugs, medicinal or biological substances are reported, code each individually unless a combination code is listed in the Table of Drugs and Chemicals.

GUIDELINES Section I.C.19.e.5)(d)

When a harmful substance is ingested or comes in contact with a person, this is classified as a toxic effect. The toxic effect codes are in categories T51-T65. Toxic effect codes have an associated intent: accidental, intentional self-harm, assault and undetermined.

CODING TIP When coding toxic effects, first assign the code from T51-T65 to identify the substance and intent, followed by an additional code to identify the manifestations of the toxic substance that resulted in the effect(s). If the intent is not documented, accidental intent should be coded. Undetermined intent should only be coded when documentation specifically indicates that the intent cannot be determined.

CODING TIP Note there are only codes for poisonings or toxic effects. There are no therapeutic uses for the following substances, therefore there are no codes for adverse effects or underdosing.

T51 Toxic effect of alcohol

The appropriate 7th character is to be added to each code from category T51

A initial encounter

D subsequent encounter

S sequela

T51.0 Toxic effect of ethanol

Toxic effect of ethyl alcohol

EXCLUDES 2 *acute alcohol intoxication or 'hangover' effects (F10.129, F10.229, F10.929)*
drunkenness (F10.129, F10.229, F10.929)
pathological alcohol intoxication (F10.129, F10.229, F10.929)

T51.0X Toxic effect of ethanol

T51.0X1- Toxic effect of ethanol, accidental (unintentional) HCC
Toxic effect of ethanol NOS

T51.0X2- Toxic effect of ethanol, intentional self-harm HCC

T51.0X3- Toxic effect of ethanol, assault

T51.0X4- Toxic effect of ethanol, undetermined HCC

T51.1 Toxic effect of methanol

Toxic effect of methyl alcohol

T51.1X Toxic effect of methanol

T51.1X1- Toxic effect of methanol, accidental (unintentional)
Toxic effect of methanol NOS

T51.1X2- Toxic effect of methanol, intentional self-harm HCC

T51.1X3- Toxic effect of methanol, assault

T51.1X4- Toxic effect of methanol, undetermined

T51.2 Toxic effect of 2-Propanol

Toxic effect of isopropyl alcohol

T51.2X Toxic effect of 2-Propanol

T51.2X1- Toxic effect of 2-Propanol, accidental (unintentional)
Toxic effect of 2-Propanol NOS

T51.2X2- Toxic effect of 2-Propanol, intentional self-harm HCC

T51.2X3- Toxic effect of 2-Propanol, assault

T51.2X4- Toxic effect of 2-Propanol, undetermined

T51.3 Toxic effect of fusel oil

Toxic effect of amyl alcohol
Toxic effect of butyl [1-butanol] alcohol
Toxic effect of propyl [1-propanol] alcohol

T51.3X Toxic effect of fusel oil

T51.3X1- Toxic effect of fusel oil, accidental (unintentional)
Toxic effect of fusel oil NOS

T51.3X2- Toxic effect of fusel oil, intentional self-harm HCC

T51.3X3- Toxic effect of fusel oil, assault

T51.3X4- Toxic effect of fusel oil, undetermined

T51.8 Toxic effect of other alcohols

T51.8X Toxic effect of other alcohols

T51.8X1- Toxic effect of other alcohols, accidental (unintentional)
Toxic effect of other alcohols NOS

T51.8X2- Toxic effect of other alcohols, intentional self-harm HCC

T51.8X3- Toxic effect of other alcohols, assault

T51.8X4- Toxic effect of other alcohols, undetermined

T51.9 Toxic effect of unspecified alcohol

T51.91X- Toxic effect of unspecified alcohol, accidental (unintentional)

T51.92X- Toxic effect of unspecified alcohol, intentional self-harm HCC

T51.93X- Toxic effect of unspecified alcohol, assault

T51.94X- Toxic effect of unspecified alcohol, undetermined

T52 Toxic effect of organic solvents

EXCLUDES 1 *halogen derivatives of aliphatic and aromatic hydrocarbons (T53.-)*

The appropriate 7th character is to be added to each code from category T52

A initial encounter

D subsequent encounter

S sequela

T52.0 Toxic effects of petroleum products

Toxic effects of gasoline [petrol]
Toxic effects of kerosene [paraffin oil]
Toxic effects of paraffin wax
Toxic effects of ether petroleum
Toxic effects of naphtha petroleum
Toxic effects of spirit petroleum

T52.0X Toxic effects of petroleum products

T52.0X1- Toxic effect of petroleum products, accidental (unintentional)
Toxic effects of petroleum products NOS

T52.0X2- Toxic effect of petroleum products, intentional self-harm HCC

T52.0X3- Toxic effect of petroleum products, assault

T52.0X4- Toxic effect of petroleum products, undetermined

T52.1 Toxic effects of benzene

EXCLUDES 1 *homologues of benzene (T52.2)*
nitroderivatives and aminoderivatives of benzene and its homologues (T65.3)

T52.1X Toxic effects of benzene

T52.1X1- Toxic effect of benzene, accidental (unintentional)
Toxic effects of benzene NOS

7 T52.1X2- **Toxic effect of benzene, intentional self-harm** HCC

7 T52.1X3- **Toxic effect of benzene, assault**

7 T52.1X4- **Toxic effect of benzene, undetermined**

5 T52.2 **Toxic effects of homologues of benzene**
Toxic effects of toluene [methylbenzene]
Toxic effects of xylene [dimethylbenzene]

6 T52.2X **Toxic effects of homologues of benzene**

7 T52.2X1- **Toxic effect of homologues of benzene, accidental (unintentional)**
Toxic effects of homologues of benzene NOS

7 T52.2X2- **Toxic effect of homologues of benzene, intentional self-harm** HCC

7 T52.2X3- **Toxic effect of homologues of benzene, assault**

7 T52.2X4- **Toxic effect of homologues of benzene, undetermined**

5 T52.3 **Toxic effects of glycols**

6 T52.3X **Toxic effects of glycols**

7 T52.3X1- **Toxic effect of glycols, accidental (unintentional)**
Toxic effects of glycols NOS

7 T52.3X2- **Toxic effect of glycols, intentional self-harm** HCC

7 T52.3X3- **Toxic effect of glycols, assault**

7 T52.3X4- **Toxic effect of glycols, undetermined**

5 T52.4 **Toxic effects of ketones**

6 T52.4X **Toxic effects of ketones**

7 T52.4X1- **Toxic effect of ketones, accidental (unintentional)**
Toxic effects of ketones NOS

7 T52.4X2- **Toxic effect of ketones, intentional self-harm** HCC

7 T52.4X3- **Toxic effect of ketones, assault**

7 T52.4X4- **Toxic effect of ketones, undetermined**

5 T52.8 **Toxic effects of other organic solvents**

6 T52.8X **Toxic effects of other organic solvents**

7 T52.8X1- **Toxic effect of other organic solvents, accidental (unintentional)**
Toxic effects of other organic solvents NOS

7 T52.8X2- **Toxic effect of other organic solvents, intentional self-harm** HCC

7 T52.8X3- **Toxic effect of other organic solvents, assault**

7 T52.8X4- **Toxic effect of other organic solvents, undetermined**

5 T52.9 **Toxic effects of unspecified organic solvent**

7 T52.91X- **Toxic effect of unspecified organic solvent, accidental (unintentional)**

7 T52.92X- **Toxic effect of unspecified organic solvent, intentional self-harm** HCC

7 T52.93X- **Toxic effect of unspecified organic solvent, assault**

7 T52.94X- **Toxic effect of unspecified organic solvent, undetermined**

4 T53 Toxic effect of halogen derivatives of aliphatic and aromatic hydrocarbons

The appropriate 7th character is to be added to each code from category T53
A initial encounter
D subsequent encounter
S sequela

5 T53.0 **Toxic effects of carbon tetrachloride**
Toxic effects of tetrachloromethane

6 T53.0X **Toxic effects of carbon tetrachloride**

7 T53.0X1- **Toxic effect of carbon tetrachloride, accidental (unintentional)**
Toxic effects of carbon tetrachloride NOS

7 T53.0X2- **Toxic effect of carbon tetrachloride, intentional self-harm** HCC

7 T53.0X3- **Toxic effect of carbon tetrachloride, assault**

7 T53.0X4- **Toxic effect of carbon tetrachloride, undetermined**

5 T53.1 **Toxic effects of chloroform**
Toxic effects of trichloromethane

6 T53.1X **Toxic effects of chloroform**

7 T53.1X1- **Toxic effect of chloroform, accidental (unintentional)**
Toxic effects of chloroform NOS

7 T53.1X2- **Toxic effect of chloroform, intentional self-harm** HCC

7 T53.1X3- **Toxic effect of chloroform, assault**

7 T53.1X4- **Toxic effect of chloroform, undetermined**

5 T53.2 **Toxic effects of trichloroethylene**
Toxic effects of trichloroethene

6 T53.2X **Toxic effects of trichloroethylene**

7 T53.2X1- **Toxic effect of trichloroethylene, accidental (unintentional)**
Toxic effects of trichloroethylene NOS

7 T53.2X2- **Toxic effect of trichloroethylene, intentional self-harm** HCC

7 T53.2X3- **Toxic effect of trichloroethylene, assault**

7 T53.2X4- **Toxic effect of trichloroethylene, undetermined**

5 T53.3 **Toxic effects of tetrachloroethylene**
Toxic effects of perchloroethylene
Toxic effect of tetrachloroethene

6 T53.3X **Toxic effects of tetrachloroethylene**

7 T53.3X1- **Toxic effect of tetrachloroethylene, accidental (unintentional)**
Toxic effects of tetrachloroethylene NOS

7 T53.3X2- **Toxic effect of tetrachloroethylene, intentional self-harm** HCC

7 T53.3X3- **Toxic effect of tetrachloroethylene, assault**

7 T53.3X4- **Toxic effect of tetrachloroethylene, undetermined**

5 T53.4 **Toxic effects of dichloromethane**
Toxic effects of methylene chloride

6 T53.4X **Toxic effects of dichloromethane**

7 T53.4X1- **Toxic effect of dichloromethane, accidental (unintentional)**
Toxic effects of dichloromethane NOS

7 T53.4X2- **Toxic effect of dichloromethane, intentional self-harm** HCC

7 T53.4X3- **Toxic effect of dichloromethane, assault**

7 T53.4X4- **Toxic effect of dichloromethane, undetermined**

5 T53.5 **Toxic effects of chlorofluorocarbons**

6 T53.5X **Toxic effects of chlorofluorocarbons**

7 T53.5X1- **Toxic effect of chlorofluorocarbons, accidental (unintentional)**
Toxic effects of chlorofluorocarbons NOS

7 T53.5X2- **Toxic effect of chlorofluorocarbons, intentional self-harm** HCC

7 T53.5X3- **Toxic effect of chlorofluorocarbons, assault**

7 T53.5X4- **Toxic effect of chlorofluorocarbons, undetermined**

5 T53.6 **Toxic effects of other halogen derivatives of aliphatic hydrocarbons**

6 T53.6X **Toxic effects of other halogen derivatives of aliphatic hydrocarbons**

7 T53.6X1- **Toxic effect of other halogen derivatives of aliphatic hydrocarbons, accidental (unintentional)**
Toxic effects of other halogen derivatives of aliphatic hydrocarbons NOS

7 T53.6X2- **Toxic effect of other halogen derivatives of aliphatic hydrocarbons, intentional self-harm** HCC

7 T53.6X3- **Toxic effect of other halogen derivatives of aliphatic hydrocarbons, assault**

7 T53.6X4- **Toxic effect of other halogen derivatives of aliphatic hydrocarbons, undetermined**

5 T53.7 **Toxic effects of other halogen derivatives of aromatic hydrocarbons**

6 T53.7X **Toxic effects of other halogen derivatives of aromatic hydrocarbons**

7 T53.7X1- **Toxic effect of other halogen derivatives of aromatic hydrocarbons, accidental (unintentional)**
Toxic effects of other halogen derivatives of aromatic hydrocarbons NOS

7 T53.7X2- **Toxic effect of other halogen derivatives of aromatic hydrocarbons, intentional self-harm** HCC

7 T53.7X3- **Toxic effect of other halogen derivatives of aromatic hydrocarbons, assault**

7 T53.7X4- **Toxic effect of other halogen derivatives of aromatic hydrocarbons, undetermined**

5 T53.9 **Toxic effects of unspecified halogen derivatives of aliphatic and aromatic hydrocarbons**

T53.91X- Toxic effect of unspecified halogen derivatives of aliphatic and aromatic hydrocarbons, accidental (unintentional)

T53.92X- Toxic effect of unspecified halogen derivatives of aliphatic and aromatic hydrocarbons, intentional self-harm HCC

T53.93X- Toxic effect of unspecified halogen derivatives of aliphatic and aromatic hydrocarbons, assault

T53.94X- Toxic effect of unspecified halogen derivatives of aliphatic and aromatic hydrocarbons, undetermined

T54 Toxic effect of corrosive substances

The appropriate 7th character is to be added to each code from category T54
A initial encounter
D subsequent encounter
S sequela

T54.0 Toxic effects of phenol and phenol homologues

T54.0X Toxic effects of phenol and phenol homologues

T54.0X1- Toxic effect of phenol and phenol homologues, accidental (unintentional)
Toxic effects of phenol and phenol homologues NOS

T54.0X2- Toxic effect of phenol and phenol homologues, intentional self-harm HCC

T54.0X3- Toxic effect of phenol and phenol homologues, assault

T54.0X4- Toxic effect of phenol and phenol homologues, undetermined

T54.1 Toxic effects of other corrosive organic compounds

T54.1X Toxic effects of other corrosive organic compounds

T54.1X1- Toxic effect of other corrosive organic compounds, accidental (unintentional)
Toxic effects of other corrosive organic compounds NOS

T54.1X2- Toxic effect of other corrosive organic compounds, intentional self-harm HCC

T54.1X3- Toxic effect of other corrosive organic compounds, assault

T54.1X4- Toxic effect of other corrosive organic compounds, undetermined

T54.2 Toxic effects of corrosive acids and acid-like substances
Toxic effects of hydrochloric acid
Toxic effects of sulfuric acid

T54.2X Toxic effects of corrosive acids and acid-like substances

T54.2X1- Toxic effect of corrosive acids and acid-like substances, accidental (unintentional)
Toxic effects of corrosive acids and acid-like substances NOS

T54.2X2- Toxic effect of corrosive acids and acid-like substances, intentional self-harm HCC

T54.2X3- Toxic effect of corrosive acids and acid-like substances, assault

T54.2X4- Toxic effect of corrosive acids and acid-like substances, undetermined

T54.3 Toxic effects of corrosive alkalis and alkali-like substances
Toxic effects of potassium hydroxide
Toxic effects of sodium hydroxide

T54.3X Toxic effects of corrosive alkalis and alkali-like substances

T54.3X1- Toxic effect of corrosive alkalis and alkali-like substances, accidental (unintentional)
Toxic effects of corrosive alkalis and alkali-like substances NOS

T54.3X2- Toxic effect of corrosive alkalis and alkali-like substances, intentional self-harm HCC

T54.3X3- Toxic effect of corrosive alkalis and alkali-like substances, assault

T54.3X4- Toxic effect of corrosive alkalis and alkali-like substances, undetermined

T54.9 Toxic effects of unspecified corrosive substance

T54.91X- Toxic effect of unspecified corrosive substance, accidental (unintentional)

T54.92X- Toxic effect of unspecified corrosive substance, intentional self-harm HCC

T54.93X- Toxic effect of unspecified corrosive substance, assault

T54.94X- Toxic effect of unspecified corrosive substance, undetermined

T55 Toxic effect of soaps and detergents

The appropriate 7th character is to be added to each code from category T55
A initial encounter
D subsequent encounter
S sequela

T55.0 Toxic effect of soaps

T55.0X Toxic effect of soaps

T55.0X1- Toxic effect of soaps, accidental (unintentional)
Toxic effect of soaps NOS

T55.0X2- Toxic effect of soaps, intentional self-harm HCC

T55.0X3- Toxic effect of soaps, assault

T55.0X4- Toxic effect of soaps, undetermined

T55.1 Toxic effect of detergents

T55.1X Toxic effect of detergents

T55.1X1- Toxic effect of detergents, accidental (unintentional)
Toxic effect of detergents NOS

T55.1X2- Toxic effect of detergents, intentional self-harm HCC

T55.1X3- Toxic effect of detergents, assault

T55.1X4- Toxic effect of detergents, undetermined

T56 Toxic effect of metals

INCLUDES toxic effects of fumes and vapors of metals
toxic effects of metals from all sources, except medicinal substances

Use additional code to identify any retained metal foreign body, if applicable (Z18.0-, T18.1-)

EXCLUDES 1 *arsenic and its compounds (T57.0)*
manganese and its compounds (T57.2)

The appropriate 7th character is to be added to each code from category T56
A initial encounter
D subsequent encounter
S sequela

T56.0 Toxic effects of lead and its compounds

T56.0X Toxic effects of lead and its compounds

T56.0X1- Toxic effect of lead and its compounds, accidental (unintentional)
Toxic effects of lead and its compounds NOS

T56.0X2- Toxic effect of lead and its compounds, intentional self-harm HCC

T56.0X3- Toxic effect of lead and its compounds, assault

T56.0X4- Toxic effect of lead and its compounds, undetermined

T56.1 Toxic effects of mercury and its compounds

T56.1X Toxic effects of mercury and its compounds

T56.1X1- Toxic effect of mercury and its compounds, accidental (unintentional)
Toxic effects of mercury and its compounds NOS

T56.1X2- Toxic effect of mercury and its compounds, intentional self-harm HCC

T56.1X3- Toxic effect of mercury and its compounds, assault

T56.1X4- Toxic effect of mercury and its compounds, undetermined

T56.2 Toxic effects of chromium and its compounds

T56.2X Toxic effects of chromium and its compounds

T56.2X1- Toxic effect of chromium and its compounds, accidental (unintentional)
Toxic effects of chromium and its compounds NOS

T56.2X2- Toxic effect of chromium and its compounds, intentional self-harm HCC

T56.2X3- Toxic effect of chromium and its compounds, assault

T56.2X4- Toxic effect of chromium and its compounds, undetermined

T56.3 Toxic effects of cadmium and its compounds

T56.3X Toxic effects of cadmium and its compounds

- 7 T56.3X1- **Toxic effect of cadmium and its compounds, accidental (unintentional)**
  Toxic effects of cadmium and its compounds NOS
- 7 T56.3X2- **Toxic effect of cadmium and its compounds, intentional self-harm** HCC
- 7 T56.3X3- **Toxic effect of cadmium and its compounds, assault**
- 7 T56.3X4- **Toxic effect of cadmium and its compounds, undetermined**

5 T56.4 **Toxic effects of copper and its compounds**

6 T56.4X **Toxic effects of copper and its compounds**
- 7 T56.4X1- **Toxic effect of copper and its compounds, accidental (unintentional)**
  Toxic effects of copper and its compounds NOS
- 7 T56.4X2- **Toxic effect of copper and its compounds, intentional self-harm** HCC
- 7 T56.4X3- **Toxic effect of copper and its compounds, assault**
- 7 T56.4X4- **Toxic effect of copper and its compounds, undetermined**

5 T56.5 **Toxic effects of zinc and its compounds**

6 T56.5X **Toxic effects of zinc and its compounds**
- 7 T56.5X1- **Toxic effect of zinc and its compounds, accidental (unintentional)**
  Toxic effects of zinc and its compounds NOS
- 7 T56.5X2- **Toxic effect of zinc and its compounds, intentional self-harm** HCC
- 7 T56.5X3- **Toxic effect of zinc and its compounds, assault**
- 7 T56.5X4- **Toxic effect of zinc and its compounds, undetermined**

5 T56.6 **Toxic effects of tin and its compounds**

6 T56.6X **Toxic effects of tin and its compounds**
- 7 T56.6X1- **Toxic effect of tin and its compounds, accidental (unintentional)**
  Toxic effects of tin and its compounds NOS
- 7 T56.6X2- **Toxic effect of tin and its compounds, intentional self-harm** HCC
- 7 T56.6X3- **Toxic effect of tin and its compounds, assault**
- 7 T56.6X4- **Toxic effect of tin and its compounds, undetermined**

5 T56.7 **Toxic effects of beryllium and its compounds**

6 T56.7X **Toxic effects of beryllium and its compounds**
- 7 T56.7X1- **Toxic effect of beryllium and its compounds, accidental (unintentional)**
  Toxic effects of beryllium and its compounds NOS
- 7 T56.7X2- **Toxic effect of beryllium and its compounds, intentional self-harm** HCC
- 7 T56.7X3- **Toxic effect of beryllium and its compounds, assault**
- 7 T56.7X4- **Toxic effect of beryllium and its compounds, undetermined**

5 T56.8 **Toxic effects of other metals**

6 T56.81 **Toxic effect of thallium**
- 7 T56.811- **Toxic effect of thallium, accidental (unintentional)**
  Toxic effect of thallium NOS
- 7 T56.812- **Toxic effect of thallium, intentional self-harm** HCC
- 7 T56.813- **Toxic effect of thallium, assault**
- 7 T56.814- **Toxic effect of thallium, undetermined**

6 T56.89 **Toxic effects of other metals**
- 7 T56.891- **Toxic effect of other metals, accidental (unintentional)**
  Toxic effects of other metals NOS
- 7 T56.892- **Toxic effect of other metals, intentional self-harm** HCC
- 7 T56.893- **Toxic effect of other metals, assault**
- 7 T56.894- **Toxic effect of other metals, undetermined**

5 T56.9 **Toxic effects of unspecified metal**
- 7 T56.91X- **Toxic effect of unspecified metal, accidental (unintentional)**
- 7 T56.92X- **Toxic effect of unspecified metal, intentional self-harm** HCC
- 7 T56.93X- **Toxic effect of unspecified metal, assault**
- 7 T56.94X- **Toxic effect of unspecified metal, undetermined**

4 T57 Toxic effect of other inorganic substances

The appropriate 7th character is to be added to each code from category T57
- A initial encounter
- D subsequent encounter
- S sequela

5 T57.0 **Toxic effect of arsenic and its compounds**

6 T57.0X **Toxic effect of arsenic and its compounds**
- 7 T57.0X1- **Toxic effect of arsenic and its compounds, accidental (unintentional)**
  Toxic effect of arsenic and its compounds NOS
- 7 T57.0X2- **Toxic effect of arsenic and its compounds, intentional self-harm** HCC
- 7 T57.0X3- **Toxic effect of arsenic and its compounds, assault**
- 7 T57.0X4- **Toxic effect of arsenic and its compounds, undetermined**

5 T57.1 **Toxic effect of phosphorus and its compounds**

EXCLUDES 1 *organophosphate insecticides (T60.0)*

6 T57.1X **Toxic effect of phosphorus and its compounds**
- 7 T57.1X1- **Toxic effect of phosphorus and its compounds, accidental (unintentional)**
  Toxic effect of phosphorus and its compounds NOS
- 7 T57.1X2- **Toxic effect of phosphorus and its compounds, intentional self-harm** HCC
- 7 T57.1X3- **Toxic effect of phosphorus and its compounds, assault**
- 7 T57.1X4- **Toxic effect of phosphorus and its compounds, undetermined**

5 T57.2 **Toxic effect of manganese and its compounds**

6 T57.2X **Toxic effect of manganese and its compounds**
- 7 T57.2X1- **Toxic effect of manganese and its compounds, accidental (unintentional)**
  Toxic effect of manganese and its compounds NOS
- 7 T57.2X2- **Toxic effect of manganese and its compounds, intentional self-harm** HCC
- 7 T57.2X3- **Toxic effect of manganese and its compounds, assault**
- 7 T57.2X4- **Toxic effect of manganese and its compounds, undetermined**

5 T57.3 **Toxic effect of hydrogen cyanide**

6 T57.3X **Toxic effect of hydrogen cyanide**
- 7 T57.3X1- **Toxic effect of hydrogen cyanide, accidental (unintentional)**
  Toxic effect of hydrogen cyanide NOS
- 7 T57.3X2- **Toxic effect of hydrogen cyanide, intentional self-harm** HCC
- 7 T57.3X3- **Toxic effect of hydrogen cyanide, assault**
- 7 T57.3X4- **Toxic effect of hydrogen cyanide, undetermined**

5 T57.8 **Toxic effect of other specified inorganic substances**

6 T57.8X **Toxic effect of other specified inorganic substances**
- 7 T57.8X1- **Toxic effect of other specified inorganic substances, accidental (unintentional)**
  Toxic effect of other specified inorganic substances NOS
- 7 T57.8X2- **Toxic effect of other specified inorganic substances, intentional self-harm** HCC
- 7 T57.8X3- **Toxic effect of other specified inorganic substances, assault**
- 7 T57.8X4- **Toxic effect of other specified inorganic substances, undetermined**

5 T57.9 **Toxic effect of unspecified inorganic substance**
- 7 T57.91X- **Toxic effect of unspecified inorganic substance, accidental (unintentional)**
- 7 T57.92X- **Toxic effect of unspecified inorganic substance, intentional self-harm** HCC
- 7 T57.93X- **Toxic effect of unspecified inorganic substance, assault**
- 7 T57.94X- **Toxic effect of unspecified inorganic substance, undetermined**

T58 Toxic effect of carbon monoxide

INCLUDES asphyxiation from carbon monoxide
toxic effect of carbon monoxide from all sources

The appropriate 7th character is to be added to each code from category T58
A initial encounter
D subsequent encounter
S sequela

T58.0 Toxic effect of carbon monoxide from motor vehicle exhaust
Toxic effect of exhaust gas from gas engine
Toxic effect of exhaust gas from motor pump

T58.01X- Toxic effect of carbon monoxide from motor vehicle exhaust, accidental (unintentional)
T58.02X- Toxic effect of carbon monoxide from motor vehicle exhaust, intentional self-harm HCC
T58.03X- Toxic effect of carbon monoxide from motor vehicle exhaust, assault
T58.04X- Toxic effect of carbon monoxide from motor vehicle exhaust, undetermined

T58.1 Toxic effect of carbon monoxide from utility gas
Toxic effect of acetylene
Toxic effect of gas NOS used for lighting, heating, cooking
Toxic effect of water gas

T58.11X- Toxic effect of carbon monoxide from utility gas, accidental (unintentional)
T58.12X- Toxic effect of carbon monoxide from utility gas, intentional self-harm HCC
T58.13X- Toxic effect of carbon monoxide from utility gas, assault
T58.14X- Toxic effect of carbon monoxide from utility gas, undetermined

T58.2 Toxic effect of carbon monoxide from incomplete combustion of other domestic fuels
Toxic effect of carbon monoxide from incomplete combustion of coal, coke, kerosene, wood

T58.2X Toxic effect of carbon monoxide from incomplete combustion of other domestic fuels
T58.2X1- Toxic effect of carbon monoxide from incomplete combustion of other domestic fuels, accidental (unintentional)
T58.2X2- Toxic effect of carbon monoxide from incomplete combustion of other domestic fuels, intentional self-harm HCC
T58.2X3- Toxic effect of carbon monoxide from incomplete combustion of other domestic fuels, assault
T58.2X4- Toxic effect of carbon monoxide from incomplete combustion of other domestic fuels, undetermined

T58.8 Toxic effect of carbon monoxide from other source
Toxic effect of carbon monoxide from blast furnace gas
Toxic effect of carbon monoxide from fuels in industrial use
Toxic effect of carbon monoxide from kiln vapor

T58.8X Toxic effect of carbon monoxide from other source
T58.8X1- Toxic effect of carbon monoxide from other source, accidental (unintentional)
T58.8X2- Toxic effect of carbon monoxide from other source, intentional self-harm HCC
T58.8X3- Toxic effect of carbon monoxide from other source, assault
T58.8X4- Toxic effect of carbon monoxide from other source, undetermined

T58.9 Toxic effect of carbon monoxide from unspecified source
T58.91X- Toxic effect of carbon monoxide from unspecified source, accidental (unintentional)
T58.92X- Toxic effect of carbon monoxide from unspecified source, intentional self-harm HCC
T58.93X- Toxic effect of carbon monoxide from unspecified source, assault
T58.94X- Toxic effect of carbon monoxide from unspecified source, undetermined

T59 Toxic effect of other gases, fumes and vapors

INCLUDES aerosol propellants

EXCLUDES 1 *chlorofluorocarbons (T53.5)*

The appropriate 7th character is to be added to each code from category T59
A initial encounter
D subsequent encounter
S sequela

T59.0 Toxic effect of nitrogen oxides
T59.0X Toxic effect of nitrogen oxides
T59.0X1- Toxic effect of nitrogen oxides, accidental (unintentional)
Toxic effect of nitrogen oxides NOS
T59.0X2- Toxic effect of nitrogen oxides, intentional self-harm HCC
T59.0X3- Toxic effect of nitrogen oxides, assault
T59.0X4- Toxic effect of nitrogen oxides, undetermined

T59.1 Toxic effect of sulfur dioxide
T59.1X Toxic effect of sulfur dioxide
T59.1X1- Toxic effect of sulfur dioxide, accidental (unintentional)
Toxic effect of sulfur dioxide NOS
T59.1X2- Toxic effect of sulfur dioxide, intentional self-harm HCC
T59.1X3- Toxic effect of sulfur dioxide, assault
T59.1X4- Toxic effect of sulfur dioxide, undetermined

T59.2 Toxic effect of formaldehyde
T59.2X Toxic effect of formaldehyde
T59.2X1- Toxic effect of formaldehyde, accidental (unintentional)
Toxic effect of formaldehyde NOS
T59.2X2- Toxic effect of formaldehyde, intentional self-harm HCC
T59.2X3- Toxic effect of formaldehyde, assault
T59.2X4- Toxic effect of formaldehyde, undetermined

T59.3 Toxic effect of lacrimogenic gas
Toxic effect of tear gas
T59.3X Toxic effect of lacrimogenic gas
T59.3X1- Toxic effect of lacrimogenic gas, accidental (unintentional)
Toxic effect of lacrimogenic gas NOS
T59.3X2- Toxic effect of lacrimogenic gas, intentional self-harm HCC
T59.3X3- Toxic effect of lacrimogenic gas, assault
T59.3X4- Toxic effect of lacrimogenic gas, undetermined

T59.4 Toxic effect of chlorine gas
T59.4X Toxic effect of chlorine gas
T59.4X1- Toxic effect of chlorine gas, accidental (unintentional)
Toxic effect of chlorine gas NOS
T59.4X2- Toxic effect of chlorine gas, intentional self-harm HCC
T59.4X3- Toxic effect of chlorine gas, assault
T59.4X4- Toxic effect of chlorine gas, undetermined

T59.5 Toxic effect of fluorine gas and hydrogen fluoride
T59.5X Toxic effect of fluorine gas and hydrogen fluoride
T59.5X1- Toxic effect of fluorine gas and hydrogen fluoride, accidental (unintentional)
Toxic effect of fluorine gas and hydrogen fluoride NOS
T59.5X2- Toxic effect of fluorine gas and hydrogen fluoride, intentional self-harm HCC
T59.5X3- Toxic effect of fluorine gas and hydrogen fluoride, assault
T59.5X4- Toxic effect of fluorine gas and hydrogen fluoride, undetermined

T59.6 Toxic effect of hydrogen sulfide
T59.6X Toxic effect of hydrogen sulfide
T59.6X1- Toxic effect of hydrogen sulfide, accidental (unintentional)
Toxic effect of hydrogen sulfide NOS
T59.6X2- Toxic effect of hydrogen sulfide, intentional self-harm HCC
T59.6X3- Toxic effect of hydrogen sulfide, assault
T59.6X4- Toxic effect of hydrogen sulfide, undetermined

T59.7 Toxic effect of carbon dioxide

T59.7X Toxic effect of carbon dioxide

T59.7X1- Toxic effect of carbon dioxide, accidental (unintentional)
Toxic effect of carbon dioxide NOS

T59.7X2- Toxic effect of carbon dioxide, intentional self-harm HCC

T59.7X3- Toxic effect of carbon dioxide, assault

T59.7X4- Toxic effect of carbon dioxide, undetermined

T59.8 Toxic effect of other specified gases, fumes and vapors

T59.81 Toxic effect of smoke
Smoke inhalation
EXCLUDES 2 *toxic effect of cigarette (tobacco) smoke (T65.22-)*

T59.811- Toxic effect of smoke, accidental (unintentional)
Toxic effect of smoke NOS
AHA: 4Q 2013, 121

T59.812- Toxic effect of smoke, intentional self-harm HCC

T59.813- Toxic effect of smoke, assault

T59.814- Toxic effect of smoke, undetermined

T59.89 Toxic effect of other specified gases, fumes and vapors

T59.891- Toxic effect of other specified gases, fumes and vapors, accidental (unintentional)

T59.892- Toxic effect of other specified gases, fumes and vapors, intentional self-harm HCC

T59.893- Toxic effect of other specified gases, fumes and vapors, assault

T59.894- Toxic effect of other specified gases, fumes and vapors, undetermined

T59.9 Toxic effect of unspecified gases, fumes and vapors

T59.91X- Toxic effect of unspecified gases, fumes and vapors, accidental (unintentional)

T59.92X- Toxic effect of unspecified gases, fumes and vapors, intentional self-harm HCC

T59.93X- Toxic effect of unspecified gases, fumes and vapors, assault

T59.94X- Toxic effect of unspecified gases, fumes and vapors, undetermined

T60 Toxic effect of pesticides

INCLUDES toxic effect of wood preservatives

The appropriate 7th character is to be added to each code from category T60
A initial encounter
D subsequent encounter
S sequela

T60.0 Toxic effect of organophosphate and carbamate insecticides

T60.0X Toxic effect of organophosphate and carbamate insecticides

T60.0X1- Toxic effect of organophosphate and carbamate insecticides, accidental (unintentional)
Toxic effect of organophosphate and carbamate insecticides NOS

T60.0X2- Toxic effect of organophosphate and carbamate insecticides, intentional self-harm HCC

T60.0X3- Toxic effect of organophosphate and carbamate insecticides, assault

T60.0X4- Toxic effect of organophosphate and carbamate insecticides, undetermined

T60.1 Toxic effect of halogenated insecticides
EXCLUDES 1 *chlorinated hydrocarbon (T53.-)*

T60.1X Toxic effect of halogenated insecticides

T60.1X1- Toxic effect of halogenated insecticides, accidental (unintentional)
Toxic effect of halogenated insecticides NOS

T60.1X2- Toxic effect of halogenated insecticides, intentional self-harm HCC

T60.1X3- Toxic effect of halogenated insecticides, assault

T60.1X4- Toxic effect of halogenated insecticides, undetermined

T60.2 Toxic effect of other insecticides

T60.2X Toxic effect of other insecticides

T60.2X1- Toxic effect of other insecticides, accidental (unintentional)
Toxic effect of other insecticides NOS

T60.2X2- Toxic effect of other insecticides, intentional self-harm HCC

T60.2X3- Toxic effect of other insecticides, assault

T60.2X4- Toxic effect of other insecticides, undetermined

T60.3 Toxic effect of herbicides and fungicides

T60.3X Toxic effect of herbicides and fungicides

T60.3X1- Toxic effect of herbicides and fungicides, accidental (unintentional)
Toxic effect of herbicides and fungicides NOS

T60.3X2- Toxic effect of herbicides and fungicides, intentional self-harm HCC

T60.3X3- Toxic effect of herbicides and fungicides, assault

T60.3X4- Toxic effect of herbicides and fungicides, undetermined

T60.4 Toxic effect of rodenticides
EXCLUDES 1 *strychnine and its salts (T65.1)*
thallium (T56.81-)

T60.4X Toxic effect of rodenticides

T60.4X1- Toxic effect of rodenticides, accidental (unintentional)
Toxic effect of rodenticides NOS

T60.4X2- Toxic effect of rodenticides, intentional self-harm HCC

T60.4X3- Toxic effect of rodenticides, assault

T60.4X4- Toxic effect of rodenticides, undetermined

T60.8 Toxic effect of other pesticides

T60.8X Toxic effect of other pesticides

T60.8X1- Toxic effect of other pesticides, accidental (unintentional)
Toxic effect of other pesticides NOS

T60.8X2- Toxic effect of other pesticides, intentional self-harm HCC

T60.8X3- Toxic effect of other pesticides, assault

T60.8X4- Toxic effect of other pesticides, undetermined

T60.9 Toxic effect of unspecified pesticide

T60.91X- Toxic effect of unspecified pesticide, accidental (unintentional)

T60.92X- Toxic effect of unspecified pesticide, intentional self-harm HCC

T60.93X- Toxic effect of unspecified pesticide, assault

T60.94X- Toxic effect of unspecified pesticide, undetermined

T61 Toxic effect of noxious substances eaten as seafood

EXCLUDES 1 *allergic reaction to food, such as:*
anaphylactic reaction or shock due to adverse food reaction (T78.0-)
bacterial foodborne intoxications (A05.-)
dermatitis (L23.6, L25.4, L27.2)
food protein-induced enterocolitis syndrome (K52.21)
food protein induced enteropathy (K52.22)
gastroenteritis (noninfective) (K52.29)
toxic effect of aflatoxin and other mycotoxins (T64)
toxic effect of cyanides (T65.0-)
toxic effect of harmful algae bloom (T65.82-)
toxic effect of hydrogen cyanide (T57.3-)
toxic effect of mercury (T56.1-)
toxic effect of red tide (T65.82-)

The appropriate 7th character is to be added to each code from category T61
A initial encounter
D subsequent encounter
S sequela

T61.0 Ciguatera fish poisoning

T61.01X- Ciguatera fish poisoning, accidental (unintentional)

T61.02X- Ciguatera fish poisoning, intentional self-harm HCC

T61.03X- Ciguatera fish poisoning, assault

7 T61.04X- Ciguatera fish poisoning, undetermined

5 T61.1 Scombroid fish poisoning
Histamine-like syndrome

7 T61.11X- Scombroid fish poisoning, accidental (unintentional)
7 T61.12X- Scombroid fish poisoning, intentional self-harm HCC
7 T61.13X- Scombroid fish poisoning, assault
7 T61.14X- Scombroid fish poisoning, undetermined

5 T61.7 Other fish and shellfish poisoning
6 T61.77 Other fish poisoning
7 T61.771- Other fish poisoning, accidental (unintentional)
7 T61.772- Other fish poisoning, intentional self-harm HCC
7 T61.773- Other fish poisoning, assault
7 T61.774- Other fish poisoning, undetermined
6 T61.78 Other shellfish poisoning
7 T61.781- Other shellfish poisoning, accidental (unintentional)
7 T61.782- Other shellfish poisoning, intentional self-harm HCC
7 T61.783- Other shellfish poisoning, assault
7 T61.784- Other shellfish poisoning, undetermined

5 T61.8 Toxic effect of other seafood
6 T61.8X Toxic effect of other seafood
7 T61.8X1- Toxic effect of other seafood, accidental (unintentional)
7 T61.8X2- Toxic effect of other seafood, intentional self-harm HCC
7 T61.8X3- Toxic effect of other seafood, assault
7 T61.8X4- Toxic effect of other seafood, undetermined

5 T61.9 Toxic effect of unspecified seafood
7 T61.91X- Toxic effect of unspecified seafood, accidental (unintentional)
7 T61.92X- Toxic effect of unspecified seafood, intentional self-harm HCC
7 T61.93X- Toxic effect of unspecified seafood, assault
7 T61.94X- Toxic effect of unspecified seafood, undetermined

4 T62 Toxic effect of other noxious substances eaten as food

EXCLUDES 1 *allergic reaction to food, such as:*
anaphylactic shock (reaction) due to adverse food reaction (T78.0-)
bacterial food borne intoxications (A05.-)
dermatitis (L23.6, L25.4, L27.2)
food protein-induced enterocolitis syndrome (K52.21)
food protein-induced enteropathy (K52.22)
gastroenteritis (noninfective) (K52.29)
toxic effect of aflatoxin and other mycotoxins (T64)
toxic effect of cyanides (T65.0-)
toxic effect of hydrogen cyanide (T57.3-)
toxic effect of mercury (T56.1-)

The appropriate 7th character is to be added to each code from category T62
A initial encounter
D subsequent encounter
S sequela

5 T62.0 Toxic effect of ingested mushrooms
6 T62.0X Toxic effect of ingested mushrooms
7 T62.0X1- Toxic effect of ingested mushrooms, accidental (unintentional)
Toxic effect of ingested mushrooms NOS
7 T62.0X2- Toxic effect of ingested mushrooms, intentional self-harm HCC
7 T62.0X3- Toxic effect of ingested mushrooms, assault
7 T62.0X4- Toxic effect of ingested mushrooms, undetermined

5 T62.1 Toxic effect of ingested berries
6 T62.1X Toxic effect of ingested berries
7 T62.1X1- Toxic effect of ingested berries, accidental (unintentional)
Toxic effect of ingested berries NOS
7 T62.1X2- Toxic effect of ingested berries, intentional self-harm HCC
7 T62.1X3- Toxic effect of ingested berries, assault
7 T62.1X4- Toxic effect of ingested berries, undetermined

5 T62.2 Toxic effect of other ingested (parts of) plant(s)
6 T62.2X Toxic effect of other ingested (parts of) plant(s)
7 T62.2X1- Toxic effect of other ingested (parts of) plant(s), accidental (unintentional)
Toxic effect of other ingested (parts of) plant(s) NOS
7 T62.2X2- Toxic effect of other ingested (parts of) plant(s), intentional self-harm HCC
7 T62.2X3- Toxic effect of other ingested (parts of) plant(s), assault
7 T62.2X4- Toxic effect of other ingested (parts of) plant(s), undetermined

5 T62.8 Toxic effect of other specified noxious substances eaten as food
6 T62.8X Toxic effect of other specified noxious substances eaten as food
7 T62.8X1- Toxic effect of other specified noxious substances eaten as food, accidental (unintentional)
Toxic effect of other specified noxious substances eaten as food NOS
7 T62.8X2- Toxic effect of other specified noxious substances eaten as food, intentional self-harm HCC
7 T62.8X3- Toxic effect of other specified noxious substances eaten as food, assault
7 T62.8X4- Toxic effect of other specified noxious substances eaten as food, undetermined

5 T62.9 Toxic effect of unspecified noxious substance eaten as food
7 T62.91X- Toxic effect of unspecified noxious substance eaten as food, accidental (unintentional)
Toxic effect of unspecified noxious substance eaten as food NOS
7 T62.92X- Toxic effect of unspecified noxious substance eaten as food, intentional self-harm HCC
7 T62.93X- Toxic effect of unspecified noxious substance eaten as food, assault
7 T62.94X- Toxic effect of unspecified noxious substance eaten as food, undetermined

4 T63 Toxic effect of contact with venomous animals and plants

INCLUDES bite or touch of venomous animal
pricked or stuck by thorn or leaf
EXCLUDES 2 *ingestion of toxic animal or plant (T61.-, T62.-)*

The appropriate 7th character is to be added to each code from category T63
A initial encounter
D subsequent encounter
S sequela

5 T63.0 Toxic effect of snake venom
6 T63.00 Toxic effect of unspecified snake venom
7 T63.001- Toxic effect of unspecified snake venom, accidental (unintentional)
Toxic effect of unspecified snake venom NOS
7 T63.002- Toxic effect of unspecified snake venom, intentional self-harm HCC
7 T63.003- Toxic effect of unspecified snake venom, assault
7 T63.004- Toxic effect of unspecified snake venom, undetermined
6 T63.01 Toxic effect of rattlesnake venom
7 T63.011- Toxic effect of rattlesnake venom, accidental (unintentional)
Toxic effect of rattlesnake venom NOS
7 T63.012- Toxic effect of rattlesnake venom, intentional self-harm HCC
7 T63.013- Toxic effect of rattlesnake venom, assault
7 T63.014- Toxic effect of rattlesnake venom, undetermined
6 T63.02 Toxic effect of coral snake venom
7 T63.021- Toxic effect of coral snake venom, accidental (unintentional)
Toxic effect of coral snake venom NOS

7 T63.022- Toxic effect of coral snake venom, intentional self-harm HCC
7 T63.023- Toxic effect of coral snake venom, assault
7 T63.024- Toxic effect of coral snake venom, undetermined
6 T63.03 Toxic effect of taipan venom
7 T63.031- Toxic effect of taipan venom, accidental (unintentional)
Toxic effect of taipan venom NOS
7 T63.032- Toxic effect of taipan venom, intentional self-harm HCC
7 T63.033- Toxic effect of taipan venom, assault
7 T63.034- Toxic effect of taipan venom, undetermined
6 T63.04 Toxic effect of cobra venom
7 T63.041- Toxic effect of cobra venom, accidental (unintentional)
Toxic effect of cobra venom NOS
7 T63.042- Toxic effect of cobra venom, intentional self-harm HCC
7 T63.043- Toxic effect of cobra venom, assault
7 T63.044- Toxic effect of cobra venom, undetermined
6 T63.06 Toxic effect of venom of other North and South American snake
7 T63.061- Toxic effect of venom of other North and South American snake, accidental (unintentional)
Toxic effect of venom of other North and South American snake NOS
7 T63.062- Toxic effect of venom of other North and South American snake, intentional self-harm HCC
7 T63.063- Toxic effect of venom of other North and South American snake, assault
7 T63.064- Toxic effect of venom of other North and South American snake, undetermined
6 T63.07 Toxic effect of venom of other Australian snake
7 T63.071- Toxic effect of venom of other Australian snake, accidental (unintentional)
Toxic effect of venom of other Australian snake NOS
7 T63.072- Toxic effect of venom of other Australian snake, intentional self-harm HCC
7 T63.073- Toxic effect of venom of other Australian snake, assault
7 T63.074- Toxic effect of venom of other Australian snake, undetermined
6 T63.08 Toxic effect of venom of other African and Asian snake
7 T63.081- Toxic effect of venom of other African and Asian snake, accidental (unintentional)
Toxic effect of venom of other African and Asian snake NOS
7 T63.082- Toxic effect of venom of other African and Asian snake, intentional self-harm HCC
7 T63.083- Toxic effect of venom of other African and Asian snake, assault
7 T63.084- Toxic effect of venom of other African and Asian snake, undetermined
6 T63.09 Toxic effect of venom of other snake
7 T63.091- Toxic effect of venom of other snake, accidental (unintentional)
Toxic effect of venom of other snake NOS
7 T63.092- Toxic effect of venom of other snake, intentional self-harm HCC
7 T63.093- Toxic effect of venom of other snake, assault
7 T63.094- Toxic effect of venom of other snake, undetermined
5 T63.1 Toxic effect of venom of other reptiles
6 T63.11 Toxic effect of venom of gila monster
7 T63.111- Toxic effect of venom of gila monster, accidental (unintentional)
Toxic effect of venom of gila monster NOS
7 T63.112- Toxic effect of venom of gila monster, intentional self-harm HCC
7 T63.113- Toxic effect of venom of gila monster, assault
7 T63.114- Toxic effect of venom of gila monster, undetermined
6 T63.12 Toxic effect of venom of other venomous lizard
7 T63.121- Toxic effect of venom of other venomous lizard, accidental (unintentional)
Toxic effect of venom of other venomous lizard NOS
7 T63.122- Toxic effect of venom of other venomous lizard, intentional self-harm HCC
7 T63.123- Toxic effect of venom of other venomous lizard, assault
7 T63.124- Toxic effect of venom of other venomous lizard, undetermined
6 T63.19 Toxic effect of venom of other reptiles
7 T63.191- Toxic effect of venom of other reptiles, accidental (unintentional)
Toxic effect of venom of other reptiles NOS
7 T63.192- Toxic effect of venom of other reptiles, intentional self-harm HCC
7 T63.193- Toxic effect of venom of other reptiles, assault
7 T63.194- Toxic effect of venom of other reptiles, undetermined
5 T63.2 Toxic effect of venom of scorpion
6 T63.2X Toxic effect of venom of scorpion
7 T63.2X1- Toxic effect of venom of scorpion, accidental (unintentional)
Toxic effect of venom of scorpion NOS
7 T63.2X2- Toxic effect of venom of scorpion, intentional self-harm HCC
7 T63.2X3- Toxic effect of venom of scorpion, assault
7 T63.2X4- Toxic effect of venom of scorpion, undetermined
5 T63.3 Toxic effect of venom of spider
6 T63.30 Toxic effect of unspecified spider venom
7 T63.301- Toxic effect of unspecified spider venom, accidental (unintentional)
7 T63.302- Toxic effect of unspecified spider venom, intentional self-harm HCC
7 T63.303- Toxic effect of unspecified spider venom, assault
7 T63.304- Toxic effect of unspecified spider venom, undetermined
6 T63.31 Toxic effect of venom of black widow spider
7 T63.311- Toxic effect of venom of black widow spider, accidental (unintentional)
7 T63.312- Toxic effect of venom of black widow spider, intentional self-harm HCC
7 T63.313- Toxic effect of venom of black widow spider, assault
7 T63.314- Toxic effect of venom of black widow spider, undetermined
6 T63.32 Toxic effect of venom of tarantula
7 T63.321- Toxic effect of venom of tarantula, accidental (unintentional)
7 T63.322- Toxic effect of venom of tarantula, intentional self-harm HCC
7 T63.323- Toxic effect of venom of tarantula, assault
7 T63.324- Toxic effect of venom of tarantula, undetermined
6 T63.33 Toxic effect of venom of brown recluse spider
7 T63.331- Toxic effect of venom of brown recluse spider, accidental (unintentional)
7 T63.332- Toxic effect of venom of brown recluse spider, intentional self-harm HCC
7 T63.333- Toxic effect of venom of brown recluse spider, assault
7 T63.334- Toxic effect of venom of brown recluse spider, undetermined
6 T63.39 Toxic effect of venom of other spider
7 T63.391- Toxic effect of venom of other spider, accidental (unintentional)
7 T63.392- Toxic effect of venom of other spider, intentional self-harm HCC
7 T63.393- Toxic effect of venom of other spider, assault
7 T63.394- Toxic effect of venom of other spider, undetermined
5 T63.4 Toxic effect of venom of other arthropods
6 T63.41 Toxic effect of venom of centipedes and venomous millipedes
7 T63.411- Toxic effect of venom of centipedes and venomous millipedes, accidental (unintentional)

7 T63.412- Toxic effect of venom of centipedes and venomous millipedes, intentional self-harm HCC
7 T63.413- Toxic effect of venom of centipedes and venomous millipedes, assault
7 T63.414- Toxic effect of venom of centipedes and venomous millipedes, undetermined
6 T63.42 Toxic effect of venom of ants
7 T63.421- Toxic effect of venom of ants, accidental (unintentional)
7 T63.422- Toxic effect of venom of ants, intentional self-harm HCC
7 T63.423- Toxic effect of venom of ants, assault
7 T63.424- Toxic effect of venom of ants, undetermined
6 T63.43 Toxic effect of venom of caterpillars
7 T63.431- Toxic effect of venom of caterpillars, accidental (unintentional)
7 T63.432- Toxic effect of venom of caterpillars, intentional self-harm HCC
7 T63.433- Toxic effect of venom of caterpillars, assault
7 T63.434- Toxic effect of venom of caterpillars, undetermined
6 T63.44 Toxic effect of venom of bees
7 T63.441- Toxic effect of venom of bees, accidental (unintentional)
7 T63.442- Toxic effect of venom of bees, intentional self-harm HCC
7 T63.443- Toxic effect of venom of bees, assault
7 T63.444- Toxic effect of venom of bees, undetermined
6 T63.45 Toxic effect of venom of hornets
7 T63.451- Toxic effect of venom of hornets, accidental (unintentional)
7 T63.452- Toxic effect of venom of hornets, intentional self-harm HCC
7 T63.453- Toxic effect of venom of hornets, assault
7 T63.454- Toxic effect of venom of hornets, undetermined
6 T63.46 Toxic effect of venom of wasps
Toxic effect of yellow jacket
7 T63.461- Toxic effect of venom of wasps, accidental (unintentional)
7 T63.462- Toxic effect of venom of wasps, intentional self-harm HCC
7 T63.463- Toxic effect of venom of wasps, assault
7 T63.464- Toxic effect of venom of wasps, undetermined
6 T63.48 Toxic effect of venom of other arthropod
7 T63.481- Toxic effect of venom of other arthropod, accidental (unintentional)
7 T63.482- Toxic effect of venom of other arthropod, intentional self-harm HCC
7 T63.483- Toxic effect of venom of other arthropod, assault
7 T63.484- Toxic effect of venom of other arthropod, undetermined
5 T63.5 Toxic effect of contact with venomous fish
EXCLUDES 2 *poisoning by ingestion of fish (T61.-)*
6 T63.51 Toxic effect of contact with stingray
7 T63.511- Toxic effect of contact with stingray, accidental (unintentional)
7 T63.512- Toxic effect of contact with stingray, intentional self-harm HCC
7 T63.513- Toxic effect of contact with stingray, assault
7 T63.514- Toxic effect of contact with stingray, undetermined
6 T63.59 Toxic effect of contact with other venomous fish
7 T63.591- Toxic effect of contact with other venomous fish, accidental (unintentional)
7 T63.592- Toxic effect of contact with other venomous fish, intentional self-harm HCC
7 T63.593- Toxic effect of contact with other venomous fish, assault
7 T63.594- Toxic effect of contact with other venomous fish, undetermined
5 T63.6 Toxic effect of contact with other venomous marine animals
EXCLUDES 1 *sea-snake venom (T63.09)*
EXCLUDES 2 *poisoning by ingestion of shellfish (T61.78-)*
6 T63.61 Toxic effect of contact with Portugese Man-o-war
Toxic effect of contact with bluebottle
7 T63.611- Toxic effect of contact with Portugese Man-o-war, accidental (unintentional)
7 T63.612- Toxic effect of contact with Portugese Man-o-war, intentional self-harm HCC
7 T63.613- Toxic effect of contact with Portugese Man-o-war, assault
7 T63.614- Toxic effect of contact with Portugese Man-o-war, undetermined
6 T63.62 Toxic effect of contact with other jellyfish
7 T63.621- Toxic effect of contact with other jellyfish, accidental (unintentional)
7 T63.622- Toxic effect of contact with other jellyfish, intentional self-harm HCC
7 T63.623- Toxic effect of contact with other jellyfish, assault
7 T63.624- Toxic effect of contact with other jellyfish, undetermined
6 T63.63 Toxic effect of contact with sea anemone
7 T63.631- Toxic effect of contact with sea anemone, accidental (unintentional)
7 T63.632- Toxic effect of contact with sea anemone, intentional self-harm HCC
7 T63.633- Toxic effect of contact with sea anemone, assault
7 T63.634- Toxic effect of contact with sea anemone, undetermined
6 T63.69 Toxic effect of contact with other venomous marine animals
7 T63.691- Toxic effect of contact with other venomous marine animals, accidental (unintentional)
7 T63.692- Toxic effect of contact with other venomous marine animals, intentional self-harm HCC
7 T63.693- Toxic effect of contact with other venomous marine animals, assault
7 T63.694- Toxic effect of contact with other venomous marine animals, undetermined
5 T63.7 Toxic effect of contact with venomous plant
6 T63.71 Toxic effect of contact with venomous marine plant
7 T63.711- Toxic effect of contact with venomous marine plant, accidental (unintentional)
7 T63.712- Toxic effect of contact with venomous marine plant, intentional self-harm HCC
7 T63.713- Toxic effect of contact with venomous marine plant, assault
7 T63.714- Toxic effect of contact with venomous marine plant, undetermined
6 T63.79 Toxic effect of contact with other venomous plant
7 T63.791- Toxic effect of contact with other venomous plant, accidental (unintentional)
7 T63.792- Toxic effect of contact with other venomous plant, intentional self-harm HCC
7 T63.793- Toxic effect of contact with other venomous plant, assault
7 T63.794- Toxic effect of contact with other venomous plant, undetermined
5 T63.8 Toxic effect of contact with other venomous animals
6 T63.81 Toxic effect of contact with venomous frog
EXCLUDES 1 *contact with nonvenomous frog (W62.0)*
7 T63.811- Toxic effect of contact with venomous frog, accidental (unintentional)
7 T63.812- Toxic effect of contact with venomous frog, intentional self-harm HCC
7 T63.813- Toxic effect of contact with venomous frog, assault
7 T63.814- Toxic effect of contact with venomous frog, undetermined
6 T63.82 Toxic effect of contact with venomous toad
EXCLUDES 1 *contact with nonvenomous toad (W62.1)*
7 T63.821- Toxic effect of contact with venomous toad, accidental (unintentional)
7 T63.822- Toxic effect of contact with venomous toad, intentional self-harm HCC
7 T63.823- Toxic effect of contact with venomous toad, assault
7 T63.824- Toxic effect of contact with venomous toad, undetermined

6 T63.83 Toxic effect of contact with other venomous amphibian
EXCLUDES 1 *contact with nonvenomous amphibian (W62.9)*
7 T63.831- Toxic effect of contact with other venomous amphibian, accidental (unintentional)
7 T63.832- Toxic effect of contact with other venomous amphibian, intentional self-harm HCC
7 T63.833- Toxic effect of contact with other venomous amphibian, assault
7 T63.834- Toxic effect of contact with other venomous amphibian, undetermined
6 T63.89 Toxic effect of contact with other venomous animals
7 T63.891- Toxic effect of contact with other venomous animals, accidental (unintentional)
7 T63.892- Toxic effect of contact with other venomous animals, intentional self-harm HCC
7 T63.893- Toxic effect of contact with other venomous animals, assault
7 T63.894- Toxic effect of contact with other venomous animals, undetermined
5 T63.9 Toxic effect of contact with unspecified venomous animal
7 T63.91X- Toxic effect of contact with unspecified venomous animal, accidental (unintentional)
7 T63.92X- Toxic effect of contact with unspecified venomous animal, intentional self-harm HCC
7 T63.93X- Toxic effect of contact with unspecified venomous animal, assault
7 T63.94X- Toxic effect of contact with unspecified venomous animal, undetermined

4 T64 Toxic effect of aflatoxin and other mycotoxin food contaminants

The appropriate 7th character is to be added to each code from category T64
A initial encounter
D subsequent encounter
S sequela

5 T64.0 Toxic effect of aflatoxin
7 T64.01X- Toxic effect of aflatoxin, accidental (unintentional)
7 T64.02X- Toxic effect of aflatoxin, intentional self-harm HCC
7 T64.03X- Toxic effect of aflatoxin, assault
7 T64.04X- Toxic effect of aflatoxin, undetermined
5 T64.8 Toxic effect of other mycotoxin food contaminants
7 T64.81X- Toxic effect of other mycotoxin food contaminants, accidental (unintentional)
7 T64.82X- Toxic effect of other mycotoxin food contaminants, intentional self-harm HCC
7 T64.83X- Toxic effect of other mycotoxin food contaminants, assault
7 T64.84X- Toxic effect of other mycotoxin food contaminants, undetermined

4 T65 Toxic effect of other and unspecified substances

The appropriate 7th character is to be added to each code from category T65
A initial encounter
D subsequent encounter
S sequela

5 T65.0 Toxic effect of cyanides
EXCLUDES 1 *hydrogen cyanide (T57.3-)*
6 T65.0X Toxic effect of cyanides
7 T65.0X1- Toxic effect of cyanides, accidental (unintentional)
Toxic effect of cyanides NOS
7 T65.0X2- Toxic effect of cyanides, intentional self-harm HCC
7 T65.0X3- Toxic effect of cyanides, assault
7 T65.0X4- Toxic effect of cyanides, undetermined
5 T65.1 Toxic effect of strychnine and its salts
6 T65.1X Toxic effect of strychnine and its salts
7 T65.1X1- Toxic effect of strychnine and its salts, accidental (unintentional)
Toxic effect of strychnine and its salts NOS
7 T65.1X2- Toxic effect of strychnine and its salts, intentional self-harm HCC
7 T65.1X3- Toxic effect of strychnine and its salts, assault
7 T65.1X4- Toxic effect of strychnine and its salts, undetermined
5 T65.2 Toxic effect of tobacco and nicotine
EXCLUDES 2 *nicotine dependence (F17.-)*
6 T65.21 Toxic effect of chewing tobacco
7 T65.211- Toxic effect of chewing tobacco, accidental (unintentional)
Toxic effect of chewing tobacco NOS
7 T65.212- Toxic effect of chewing tobacco, intentional self-harm HCC
7 T65.213- Toxic effect of chewing tobacco, assault
7 T65.214- Toxic effect of chewing tobacco, undetermined
6 T65.22 Toxic effect of tobacco cigarettes
Toxic effect of tobacco smoke
Use additional code for exposure to second hand tobacco smoke (Z57.31, Z77.22)
7 T65.221- Toxic effect of tobacco cigarettes, accidental (unintentional)
Toxic effect of tobacco cigarettes NOS
7 T65.222- Toxic effect of tobacco cigarettes, intentional self-harm HCC
7 T65.223- Toxic effect of tobacco cigarettes, assault
7 T65.224- Toxic effect of tobacco cigarettes, undetermined
6 T65.29 Toxic effect of other tobacco and nicotine
7 T65.291- Toxic effect of other tobacco and nicotine, accidental (unintentional)
Toxic effect of other tobacco and nicotine NOS
7 T65.292- Toxic effect of other tobacco and nicotine, intentional self-harm HCC
7 T65.293- Toxic effect of other tobacco and nicotine, assault
7 T65.294- Toxic effect of other tobacco and nicotine, undetermined
5 T65.3 Toxic effect of nitroderivatives and aminoderivatives of benzene and its homologues
Toxic effect of anilin [benzenamine]
Toxic effect of nitrobenzene
Toxic effect of trinitrotoluene
6 T65.3X Toxic effect of nitroderivatives and aminoderivatives of benzene and its homologues
7 T65.3X1- Toxic effect of nitroderivatives and aminoderivatives of benzene and its homologues, accidental (unintentional)
Toxic effect of nitroderivatives and aminoderivatives of benzene and its homologues NOS
7 T65.3X2- Toxic effect of nitroderivatives and aminoderivatives of benzene and its homologues, intentional self-harm HCC
7 T65.3X3- Toxic effect of nitroderivatives and aminoderivatives of benzene and its homologues, assault
7 T65.3X4- Toxic effect of nitroderivatives and aminoderivatives of benzene and its homologues, undetermined
5 T65.4 Toxic effect of carbon disulfide
6 T65.4X Toxic effect of carbon disulfide
7 T65.4X1- Toxic effect of carbon disulfide, accidental (unintentional)
Toxic effect of carbon disulfide NOS
7 T65.4X2- Toxic effect of carbon disulfide, intentional self-harm HCC
7 T65.4X3- Toxic effect of carbon disulfide, assault
7 T65.4X4- Toxic effect of carbon disulfide, undetermined
5 T65.5 Toxic effect of nitroglycerin and other nitric acids and esters
Toxic effect of 1,2,3-Propanetriol trinitrate
6 T65.5X Toxic effect of nitroglycerin and other nitric acids and esters
7 T65.5X1- Toxic effect of nitroglycerin and other nitric acids and esters, accidental (unintentional)
Toxic effect of nitroglycerin and other nitric acids and esters NOS

7 T65.5X2- **Toxic effect of nitroglycerin and other nitric acids and esters, intentional self-harm** HCC

7 T65.5X3- **Toxic effect of nitroglycerin and other nitric acids and esters, assault**

7 T65.5X4- **Toxic effect of nitroglycerin and other nitric acids and esters, undetermined**

5 T65.6 **Toxic effect of paints and dyes, not elsewhere classified**

6 T65.6X **Toxic effect of paints and dyes, not elsewhere classified**

7 T65.6X1- **Toxic effect of paints and dyes, not elsewhere classified, accidental (unintentional)**
Toxic effect of paints and dyes NOS

7 T65.6X2- **Toxic effect of paints and dyes, not elsewhere classified, intentional self-harm** HCC

7 T65.6X3- **Toxic effect of paints and dyes, not elsewhere classified, assault**

7 T65.6X4- **Toxic effect of paints and dyes, not elsewhere classified, undetermined**

5 T65.8 **Toxic effect of other specified substances**

6 T65.81 **Toxic effect of latex**

7 T65.811- **Toxic effect of latex, accidental (unintentional)**
Toxic effect of latex NOS

7 T65.812- **Toxic effect of latex, intentional self-harm** HCC

7 T65.813- **Toxic effect of latex, assault**

7 T65.814- **Toxic effect of latex, undetermined**

6 T65.82 **Toxic effect of harmful algae and algae toxins**
Toxic effect of (harmful) algae bloom NOS
Toxic effect of blue-green algae bloom
Toxic effect of brown tide
Toxic effect of cyanobacteria bloom
Toxic effect of Florida red tide
Toxic effect of pfiesteria piscicida
Toxic effect of red tide

7 T65.821- **Toxic effect of harmful algae and algae toxins, accidental (unintentional)**
Toxic effect of harmful algae and algae toxins NOS

7 T65.822- **Toxic effect of harmful algae and algae toxins, intentional self-harm** HCC

7 T65.823- **Toxic effect of harmful algae and algae toxins, assault**

7 T65.824- **Toxic effect of harmful algae and algae toxins, undetermined**

6 T65.83 **Toxic effect of fiberglass**

7 T65.831- **Toxic effect of fiberglass, accidental (unintentional)**
Toxic effect of fiberglass NOS

7 T65.832- **Toxic effect of fiberglass, intentional self-harm** HCC

7 T65.833- **Toxic effect of fiberglass, assault**

7 T65.834- **Toxic effect of fiberglass, undetermined**

6 T65.89 **Toxic effect of other specified substances**

7 T65.891- **Toxic effect of other specified substances, accidental (unintentional)**
Toxic effect of other specified substances NOS

7 T65.892- **Toxic effect of other specified substances, intentional self-harm** HCC

7 T65.893- **Toxic effect of other specified substances, assault**

7 T65.894- **Toxic effect of other specified substances, undetermined**

5 T65.9 **Toxic effect of unspecified substance**

7 T65.91X- **Toxic effect of unspecified substance, accidental (unintentional)**
Poisoning NOS

7 T65.92X- **Toxic effect of unspecified substance, intentional self-harm** HCC

7 T65.93X- **Toxic effect of unspecified substance, assault**

7 T65.94X- **Toxic effect of unspecified substance, undetermined**

Other and unspecified effects of external causes (T66-T78)

7 T66.XXX- **Radiation sickness, unspecified**

EXCLUDES 1 *specified adverse effects of radiation, such as:*
burns (T20-T31)
leukemia (C91-C95)
radiation gastroenteritis and colitis (K52.0)
radiation pneumonitis (J70.0)
radiation related disorders of the skin and subcutaneous tissue (L55-L59)
sunburn (L55.-)

The appropriate 7th character is to be added to code T66
A initial encounter
D subsequent encounter
S sequela

4 T67 **Effects of heat and light**

EXCLUDES 1 *erythema [dermatitis] ab igne (L59.0)*
malignant hyperpyrexia due to anesthesia (T88.3)
radiation-related disorders of the skin and subcutaneous tissue (L55-L59)

EXCLUDES 2 *burns (T20-T31)*
sunburn (L55.-)
sweat disorder due to heat (L74-L75)

The appropriate 7th character is to be added to each code from category T67
A initial encounter
D subsequent encounter
S sequela

7 T67.0XX- **Heatstroke and sunstroke**
Heat apoplexy
Heat pyrexia
Siriasis
Thermoplegia
Use additional code(s) to identify any associated complications of heatstroke, such as:
coma and stupor (R40.-)
systemic inflammatory response syndrome (R65.1-)

7 T67.1XX- **Heat syncope**
Heat collapse

7 T67.2XX- **Heat cramp**

7 T67.3XX- **Heat exhaustion, anhydrotic**
Heat prostration due to water depletion
EXCLUDES 1 *heat exhaustion due to salt depletion (T67.4)*

7 T67.4XX- **Heat exhaustion due to salt depletion**
Heat prostration due to salt (and water) depletion

7 T67.5XX- **Heat exhaustion, unspecified**
Heat prostration NOS

7 T67.6XX- **Heat fatigue, transient**

7 T67.7XX- **Heat edema**

7 T67.8XX- **Other effects of heat and light**

7 T67.9XX- **Effect of heat and light, unspecified**

7 T68.XXX- **Hypothermia**
Accidental hypothermia
Hypothermia NOS
Use additional code to identify source of exposure:
Exposure to excessive cold of man-made origin (W93)
Exposure to excessive cold of natural origin (X31)

EXCLUDES 1 *hypothermia following anesthesia (T88.51)*
hypothermia not associated with low environmental temperature (R68.0)
hypothermia of newborn (P80.-)

EXCLUDES 2 *frostbite (T33-T34)*

The appropriate 7th character is to be added to code T68
A initial encounter
D subsequent encounter
S sequela

T69 Other effects of reduced temperature

Use additional code to identify source of exposure:
Exposure to excessive cold of man-made origin (W93)
Exposure to excessive cold of natural origin (X31)

EXCLUDES 2 *frostbite (T33-T34)*

The appropriate 7th character is to be added to each code from category T69
A initial encounter
D subsequent encounter
S sequela

T69.0 Immersion hand and foot

T69.01 Immersion hand

T69.011- Immersion hand, right hand

T69.012- Immersion hand, left hand

T69.019- Immersion hand, unspecified hand

T69.02 Immersion foot
Trench foot

T69.021- Immersion foot, right foot

T69.022- Immersion foot, left foot

T69.029- Immersion foot, unspecified foot

T69.1XX- Chilblains

T69.8XX- Other specified effects of reduced temperature

T69.9XX- Effect of reduced temperature, unspecified

T70 Effects of air pressure and water pressure

The appropriate 7th character is to be added to each code from category T70
A initial encounter
D subsequent encounter
S sequela

T70.0XX- Otitic barotrauma
Aero-otitis media
Effects of change in ambient atmospheric pressure or water pressure on ears

T70.1XX- Sinus barotrauma
Aerosinusitis
Effects of change in ambient atmospheric pressure on sinuses

T70.2 Other and unspecified effects of high altitude

EXCLUDES 2 *polycythemia due to high altitude (D75.1)*

T70.20X- Unspecified effects of high altitude

T70.29X- Other effects of high altitude
Alpine sickness
Anoxia due to high altitude
Barotrauma NOS
Hypobaropathy
Mountain sickness

T70.3XX- Caisson disease [decompression sickness]
Compressed-air disease
Diver's palsy or paralysis

T70.4XX- Effects of high-pressure fluids
Hydraulic jet injection (industrial)
Pneumatic jet injection (industrial)
Traumatic jet injection (industrial)

T70.8XX- Other effects of air pressure and water pressure

T70.9XX- Effect of air pressure and water pressure, unspecified

T71 Asphyxiation
Mechanical suffocation
Traumatic suffocation

EXCLUDES 1 *acute respiratory distress (syndrome) (J80)*
anoxia due to high altitude (T70.2)
asphyxia NOS (R09.01)
asphyxia from carbon monoxide (T58.-)
asphyxia from inhalation of food or foreign body (T17.-)
asphyxia from other gases, fumes and vapors (T59.-)
respiratory distress (syndrome) in newborn (P22.-)

The appropriate 7th character is to be added to each code from category T71
A initial encounter
D subsequent encounter
S sequela

T71.1 Asphyxiation due to mechanical threat to breathing
Suffocation due to mechanical threat to breathing

T71.11 Asphyxiation due to smothering under pillow

T71.111- Asphyxiation due to smothering under pillow, accidental
Asphyxiation due to smothering under pillow NOS

T71.112- Asphyxiation due to smothering under pillow, intentional self-harm HCC

T71.113- Asphyxiation due to smothering under pillow, assault

T71.114- Asphyxiation due to smothering under pillow, undetermined

T71.12 Asphyxiation due to plastic bag

T71.121- Asphyxiation due to plastic bag, accidental
Asphyxiation due to plastic bag NOS

T71.122- Asphyxiation due to plastic bag, intentional self-harm HCC

T71.123- Asphyxiation due to plastic bag, assault

T71.124- Asphyxiation due to plastic bag, undetermined

T71.13 Asphyxiation due to being trapped in bed linens

T71.131- Asphyxiation due to being trapped in bed linens, accidental
Asphyxiation due to being trapped in bed linens NOS

T71.132- Asphyxiation due to being trapped in bed linens, intentional self-harm HCC

T71.133- Asphyxiation due to being trapped in bed linens, assault

T71.134- Asphyxiation due to being trapped in bed linens, undetermined

T71.14 Asphyxiation due to smothering under another person's body (in bed)

T71.141- Asphyxiation due to smothering under another person's body (in bed), accidental
Asphyxiation due to smothering under another person's body (in bed) NOS

T71.143- Asphyxiation due to smothering under another person's body (in bed), assault

T71.144- Asphyxiation due to smothering under another person's body (in bed), undetermined

T71.15 Asphyxiation due to smothering in furniture

T71.151- Asphyxiation due to smothering in furniture, accidental
Asphyxiation due to smothering in furniture NOS

T71.152- Asphyxiation due to smothering in furniture, intentional self-harm HCC

T71.153- Asphyxiation due to smothering in furniture, assault

T71.154- Asphyxiation due to smothering in furniture, undetermined

T71.16 Asphyxiation due to hanging
Hanging by window shade cord
Use additional code for any associated injuries, such as:
crushing injury of neck (S17.-)
fracture of cervical vertebrae (S12.0-S12.2-)
open wound of neck (S11.-)

T71.161- Asphyxiation due to hanging, accidental
Asphyxiation due to hanging NOS
Hanging NOS

T71.162- **Asphyxiation due to hanging, intentional self-harm** HCC

T71.163- **Asphyxiation due to hanging, assault**

T71.164- **Asphyxiation due to hanging, undetermined**

T71.19 **Asphyxiation due to mechanical threat to breathing due to other causes**

T71.191- **Asphyxiation due to mechanical threat to breathing due to other causes, accidental**
Asphyxiation due to other causes NOS

T71.192- **Asphyxiation due to mechanical threat to breathing due to other causes, intentional self-harm** HCC

T71.193- **Asphyxiation due to mechanical threat to breathing due to other causes, assault**

T71.194- **Asphyxiation due to mechanical threat to breathing due to other causes, undetermined**

T71.2 **Asphyxiation due to systemic oxygen deficiency due to low oxygen content in ambient air**
Suffocation due to systemic oxygen deficiency due to low oxygen content in ambient air

T71.20X- **Asphyxiation due to systemic oxygen deficiency due to low oxygen content in ambient air due to unspecified cause**

T71.21X- **Asphyxiation due to cave-in or falling earth**
Use additional code for any associated cataclysm (X34-X38)

T71.22 **Asphyxiation due to being trapped in a car trunk**

T71.221- **Asphyxiation due to being trapped in a car trunk, accidental**

T71.222- **Asphyxiation due to being trapped in a car trunk, intentional self-harm** HCC

T71.223- **Asphyxiation due to being trapped in a car trunk, assault**

T71.224- **Asphyxiation due to being trapped in a car trunk, undetermined**

T71.23 **Asphyxiation due to being trapped in a (discarded) refrigerator**

T71.231- **Asphyxiation due to being trapped in a (discarded) refrigerator, accidental**

T71.232- **Asphyxiation due to being trapped in a (discarded) refrigerator, intentional self-harm** HCC

T71.233- **Asphyxiation due to being trapped in a (discarded) refrigerator, assault**

T71.234- **Asphyxiation due to being trapped in a (discarded) refrigerator, undetermined**

T71.29X- **Asphyxiation due to being trapped in other low oxygen environment**

T71.9XX- **Asphyxiation due to unspecified cause**
Suffocation (by strangulation) due to unspecified cause
Suffocation NOS
Systemic oxygen deficiency due to low oxygen content in ambient air due to unspecified cause
Systemic oxygen deficiency due to mechanical threat to breathing due to unspecified cause
Traumatic asphyxia NOS

T73 Effects of other deprivation

The appropriate 7th character is to be added to each code from category T73

A	initial encounter
D	subsequent encounter
S	sequela

T73.0XX- **Starvation**
Deprivation of food

T73.1XX- **Deprivation of water**

T73.2XX- **Exhaustion due to exposure**

T73.3XX- **Exhaustion due to excessive exertion**
Exhaustion due to overexertion

T73.8XX- **Other effects of deprivation**

T73.9XX- **Effect of deprivation, unspecified**

T74 Adult and child abuse, neglect and other maltreatment, confirmed

Use additional code, if applicable, to identify any associated current injury
Use additional external cause code to identify perpetrator, if known (Y07.-)

EXCLUDES 1 *abuse and maltreatment in pregnancy (O9A.3-, O9A.4-, O9A.5-)*
adult and child maltreatment, suspected (T76.-)

The appropriate 7th character is to be added to each code from category T74

A	initial encounter
D	subsequent encounter
S	sequela

GUIDELINES **Section I.C.19.f**
Sequence first the appropriate code from categories T74.- (Adult and child abuse, neglect and other maltreatment, confirmed) or T76.- (Adult and child abuse, neglect and other maltreatment, suspected) for abuse, neglect and other maltreatment, followed by any accompanying mental health or injury code(s). If the documentation in the medical record states abuse or neglect it is coded as confirmed (T74.-). It is coded as suspected if it is documented as suspected (T76.-).

For cases of confirmed abuse or neglect an external cause code from the assault section (X92-Y09) should be added to identify the cause of any physical injuries. A perpetrator code (Y07) should be added when the perpetrator of the abuse is known. For suspected cases of abuse or neglect, do not report external cause or perpetrator code. If a suspected case of abuse, neglect or mistreatment is ruled out during an encounter code Z04.71, Encounter for examination and observation following alleged physical adult abuse, ruled out, or code Z04.72, Encounter for examination and observation following alleged child physical abuse, ruled out, should be used, not a code from T76.

T74.0 **Neglect or abandonment, confirmed**

T74.01X- **Adult neglect or abandonment, confirmed** A

T74.02X- **Child neglect or abandonment, confirmed** P

T74.1 **Physical abuse, confirmed**
EXCLUDES 2 *sexual abuse (T74.2-)*

T74.11X- **Adult physical abuse, confirmed** A

T74.12X- **Child physical abuse, confirmed** P
EXCLUDES 2 *shaken infant syndrome (T74.4)*

T74.2 **Sexual abuse, confirmed**
Rape, confirmed
Sexual assault, confirmed

T74.21X- **Adult sexual abuse, confirmed** A

T74.22X- **Child sexual abuse, confirmed** P

▲ **T74.3** **Psychological abuse, confirmed**
Bullying and intimidation, confirmed
Intimidation through social media, confirmed

T74.31X- **Adult psychological abuse, confirmed** A

T74.32X- **Child psychological abuse, confirmed** P

T74.4XX- **Shaken infant syndrome** P

● **T74.5** **Forced sexual exploitation, confirmed**

● **T74.51X-** **Adult forced sexual exploitation, confirmed** A

● **T74.52X-** **Child sexual exploitation, confirmed** P

● **T74.6** **Forced labor exploitation, confirmed**

● **T74.61X-** **Adult forced labor exploitation, confirmed** A

● **T74.62X-** **Child forced labor exploitation, confirmed** P

T74.9 **Unspecified maltreatment, confirmed**

T74.91X- **Unspecified adult maltreatment, confirmed** A

T74.92X- **Unspecified child maltreatment, confirmed** P

T75 Other and unspecified effects of other external causes

EXCLUDES 1 *adverse effects NEC (T78.-)*

EXCLUDES 2 *burns (electric) (T20-T31)*

The appropriate 7th character is to be added to each code from category T75

A	initial encounter
D	subsequent encounter
S	sequela

T75.0 Effects of lightning
Struck by lightning

T75.00X- Unspecified effects of lightning
Struck by lightning NOS

T75.01X- Shock due to being struck by lightning

T75.09X- Other effects of lightning
Use additional code for other effects of lightning

T75.1XX- Unspecified effects of drowning and nonfatal submersion
Immersion
EXCLUDES 1 *specified effects of drowning- code to effects*

T75.2 Effects of vibration

T75.20X- Unspecified effects of vibration

T75.21X- Pneumatic hammer syndrome

T75.22X- Traumatic vasospastic syndrome

T75.23X- Vertigo from infrasound
EXCLUDES 1 *vertigo NOS (R42)*

T75.29X- Other effects of vibration

T75.3XX- Motion sickness
Airsickness
Seasickness
Travel sickness
Use additional external cause code to identify vehicle or type of motion (Y92.81-, Y93.5-)

T75.4XX- Electrocution
Shock from electric current
Shock from electroshock gun (taser)

T75.8 Other specified effects of external causes

T75.81X- Effects of abnormal gravitation [G] forces

T75.82X- Effects of weightlessness

T75.89X- Other specified effects of external causes

T76 Adult and child abuse, neglect and other maltreatment, suspected

Use additional code, if applicable, to identify any associated current injury

EXCLUDES 1 *adult and child maltreatment, confirmed (T74.-)*
suspected abuse and maltreatment in pregnancy (O9A.3-, O9A.4-, O9A.5-)
suspected adult physical abuse, ruled out (Z04.71)
suspected adult sexual abuse, ruled out (Z04.41)
suspected child physical abuse, ruled out (Z04.72)
suspected child sexual abuse, ruled out (Z04.42)

The appropriate 7th character is to be added to each code from category T76
A initial encounter
D subsequent encounter
S sequela

GUIDELINES **Section I.C.19.f**
Sequence first the appropriate code from categories T74.- (Adult and child abuse, neglect and other maltreatment, confirmed) or T76.- (Adult and child abuse, neglect and other maltreatment, suspected) for abuse, neglect and other maltreatment, followed by any accompanying mental health or injury code(s). If the documentation in the medical record states abuse or neglect it is coded as confirmed (T74 -) It is coded as suspected if it is documented as suspected (T76.-).

For cases of confirmed abuse or neglect an external cause code from the assault section (X92-Y09) should be added to identify the cause of any physical injuries. A perpetrator code (Y07) should be added when the perpetrator of the abuse is known. For suspected cases of abuse or neglect, do not report external cause or perpetrator code. If a suspected case of abuse, neglect or mistreatment is ruled out during an encounter code Z04.71, Encounter for examination and observation following alleged physical adult abuse, ruled out, or code Z04.72, Encounter for examination and observation following alleged child physical abuse, ruled out, should be used, not a code from T76.

T76.0 Neglect or abandonment, suspected

T76.01X- Adult neglect or abandonment, suspected A

T76.02X- Child neglect or abandonment, suspected P

T76.1 Physical abuse, suspected

T76.11X- Adult physical abuse, suspected A

T76.12X- Child physical abuse, suspected P

T76.2 Sexual abuse, suspected
Rape, suspected
EXCLUDES 1 *alleged abuse, ruled out (Z04.7)*

T76.21X- Adult sexual abuse, suspected A

T76.22X- Child sexual abuse, suspected P

▲ **T76.3 Psychological abuse, suspected**
Bullying and intimidation, suspected
Intimidation through social media, suspected

T76.31X- Adult psychological abuse, suspected A

T76.32X- Child psychological abuse, suspected P

● **T76.5 Forced sexual exploitation, suspected**

● **T76.51X- Adult forced sexual exploitation, suspected** A

● **T76.52X- Child sexual exploitation, suspected** P

● **T76.6 Forced labor exploitation, suspected**

● **T76.61X- Adult forced labor exploitation, suspected** A

● **T76.62X- Child forced labor exploitation, suspected** P

T76.9 Unspecified maltreatment, suspected

T76.91X- Unspecified adult maltreatment, suspected A

T76.92X- Unspecified child maltreatment, suspected P

T78 Adverse effects, not elsewhere classified

EXCLUDES 2 *complications of surgical and medical care NEC (T80-T88)*

The appropriate 7th character is to be added to each code from category T78
A initial encounter
D subsequent encounter
S sequela

T78.0 Anaphylactic reaction due to food
Anaphylactic reaction due to adverse food reaction
Anaphylactic shock or reaction due to nonpoisonous foods
Anaphylactoid reaction due to food

T78.00X- Anaphylactic reaction due to unspecified food

T78.01X- Anaphylactic reaction due to peanuts

T78.02X- Anaphylactic reaction due to shellfish (crustaceans)

T78.03X- Anaphylactic reaction due to other fish

T78.04X- Anaphylactic reaction due to fruits and vegetables

T78.05X- Anaphylactic reaction due to tree nuts and seeds
EXCLUDES 2 *anaphylactic reaction due to peanuts (T78.01)*

T78.06X- Anaphylactic reaction due to food additives

T78.07X- Anaphylactic reaction due to milk and dairy products

T78.08X- Anaphylactic reaction due to eggs

T78.09X- Anaphylactic reaction due to other food products

T78.1XX- Other adverse food reactions, not elsewhere classified
Use additional code to identify the type of reaction, if applicable
EXCLUDES 1 *anaphylactic reaction or shock due to adverse food reaction (T78.0-)*
anaphylactic reaction due to food (T78.0-)
bacterial food borne intoxications (A05.-)
EXCLUDES 2 *allergic and dietetic gastroenteritis and colitis (K52.29)*
allergic rhinitis due to food (J30.5)
dermatitis due to food in contact with skin (L23.6, L24.6, L25.4)
dermatitis due to ingested food (L27.2)
food protein-induced enterocolitis syndrome (K52.21)
food protein-induced enteropathy (K52.22)

7 T78.2XX- Anaphylactic shock, unspecified
Allergic shock
Anaphylactic reaction
Anaphylaxis
EXCLUDES 1 *anaphylactic reaction or shock due to adverse effect of correct medicinal substance properly administered (T88.6)*
anaphylactic reaction or shock due to adverse food reaction (T78.0-)
anaphylactic reaction or shock due to serum (T80.5-)

7 T78.3XX- Angioneurotic edema
Allergic angioedema
Giant urticaria
Quincke's edema
EXCLUDES 1 *serum urticaria (T80.6-)*
urticaria (L50.-)

5 T78.4 Other and unspecified allergy
EXCLUDES 1 *specified types of allergic reaction such as:*
allergic diarrhea (K52.29)
allergic gastroenteritis and colitis (K52.29)
dermatitis (L23-L25, L27.-)
food protein-induced enterocolitis syndrome (K52.21)
food protein-induced enteropathy (K52.22)
hay fever (J30.1)

7 T78.40X- Allergy, unspecified
Allergic reaction NOS
Hypersensitivity NOS

7 T78.41X- Arthus phenomenon
Arthus reaction

7 T78.49X- Other allergy

7 T78.8XX- Other adverse effects, not elsewhere classified

Certain early complications of trauma (T79)

4 T79 Certain early complications of trauma, not elsewhere classified
EXCLUDES 2 *acute respiratory distress syndrome (J80)*
complications occurring during or following medical procedures (T80-T88)
complications of surgical and medical care NEC (T80-T88)
newborn respiratory distress syndrome (P22.0)

The appropriate 7th character is to be added to each code from category T79
A initial encounter
D subsequent encounter
S sequela

7 T79.0XX- Air embolism (traumatic) HCC
EXCLUDES 1 *air embolism complicating abortion or ectopic or molar pregnancy (O00-O07, O08.2)*
air embolism complicating pregnancy, childbirth and the puerperium (O88.0)
air embolism following infusion, transfusion, and therapeutic injection (T80.0)
air embolism following procedure NEC (T81.7-)

CODING TIP ✓ Code T79.0- should not be assigned for an air embolus that is not specified as due to a traumatic cause.

7 T79.1XX- Fat embolism (traumatic) HCC
EXCLUDES 1 *fat embolism complicating:*
abortion or ectopic or molar pregnancy (O00-O07, O08.2)
pregnancy, childbirth and the puerperium (O88.8)

7 T79.2XX- Traumatic secondary and recurrent hemorrhage and seroma HCC

7 T79.4XX- Traumatic shock HCC
Shock (immediate) (delayed) following injury
EXCLUDES 1 *anaphylactic shock due to adverse food reaction (T78.0-)*
anaphylactic shock due to correct medicinal substance properly administered (T88.6)
anaphylactic shock due to serum (T80.5-)
anaphylactic shock NOS (T78.2)
anesthetic shock (T88.2)
electric shock (T75.4)
nontraumatic shock NEC (R57.-)
obstetric shock (O75.1)
postprocedural shock (T81.1-)
septic shock (R65.21)
shock complicating abortion or ectopic or molar pregnancy (O00-O07, O08.3)
shock due to lightning (T75.01)
shock NOS (R57.9)

7 T79.5XX- Traumatic anuria HCC
Crush syndrome
Renal failure following crushing

7 T79.6XX- Traumatic ischemia of muscle HCC
Traumatic rhabdomyolysis
Volkmann's ischemic contracture
EXCLUDES 2 *anterior tibial syndrome (M76.8)*
compartment syndrome (traumatic) (T79.A-)
nontraumatic ischemia of muscle (M62.2-)

7 T79.7XX- Traumatic subcutaneous emphysema HCC
EXCLUDES 1 *emphysema NOS (J43)*
emphysema (subcutaneous) resulting from a procedure (T81.82)

5 T79.A Traumatic compartment syndrome
EXCLUDES 1 *fibromyalgia (M79.7)*
nontraumatic compartment syndrome (M79.A-)
traumatic ischemic infarction of muscle (T79.6)

CODING TIP ✓ Do not assign any code from subcategory T79.A- to indicate compartment syndrome that is not specifically stated as due to a traumatic cause. Non-traumatic compartment syndrome is coded to M79.A-.

CODING TIP ✓ Compartment syndrome occurs when increased pressure in an enclosed tissue space leads to decreased blood flow and possibly tissue necrosis. The necrosis may become an ulcer. This usually occurs within part of an extremity, but may occur in the abdomen or other sites. Possible causes include external compression or soft tissue swelling (edema, hematoma). For example, trauma such as snake bite, burns, frostbite or falls (e.g., hematoma due to a fall in a patient on anticoagulant therapy) may cause this syndrome.

7 T79.A0X- Compartment syndrome, unspecified HCC
Compartment syndrome NOS

6 T79.A1 Traumatic compartment syndrome of upper extremity
Traumatic compartment syndrome of shoulder, arm, forearm, wrist, hand, and fingers

7 ⊟ T79.A11- Traumatic compartment syndrome of right upper extremity HCC

7 ⊟ T79.A12- Traumatic compartment syndrome of left upper extremity HCC

7 ⊟ T79.A19- Traumatic compartment syndrome of unspecified upper extremity HCC

6 T79.A2 Traumatic compartment syndrome of lower extremity
Traumatic compartment syndrome of hip, buttock, thigh, leg, foot, and toes

7 ⊟ T79.A21- Traumatic compartment syndrome of right lower extremity HCC

7 ⊟ T79.A22- Traumatic compartment syndrome of left lower extremity HCC

7 ⊟ T79.A29- Traumatic compartment syndrome of unspecified lower extremity HCC

7 T79.A3X- **Traumatic compartment syndrome of abdomen** HCC

7 T79.A9X- **Traumatic compartment syndrome of other sites** HCC

7 T79.8XX- **Other early complications of trauma** HCC

7 T79.9XX- **Unspecified early complication of trauma** HCC

Complications of surgical and medical care, not elsewhere classified (T80-T88)

Use additional code for adverse effect, if applicable, to identify drug (T36-T50 with fifth or sixth character 5)

Use additional code(s) to identify the specified condition resulting from the complication

Use additional code to identify devices involved and details of circumstances (Y62-Y82)

EXCLUDES 2 *any encounters with medical care for postprocedural conditions in which no complications are present, such as:*
artificial opening status (Z93.-)
closure of external stoma (Z43.-)
fitting and adjustment of external prosthetic device (Z44.-)
burns and corrosions from local applications and irradiation (T20-T32)
complications of surgical procedures during pregnancy, childbirth and the puerperium (O00-O9A)
mechanical complication of respirator [ventilator] (J95.850)
poisoning and toxic effects of drugs and chemicals (T36-T65 with fifth or sixth character 1-4 or 6)
postprocedural fever (R50.82)
specified complications classified elsewhere, such as:
cerebrospinal fluid leak from spinal puncture (G97.0)
colostomy malfunction (K94.0-)
disorders of fluid and electrolyte imbalance (E86-E87)
functional disturbances following cardiac surgery (I97.0-I97.1)
intraoperative and postprocedural complications of specified body systems (D78.-, E36.-, E89.-, G97.3-, G97.4, H59.3-, H59.-, H95.2-, H95.3, I97.4-, I97.5, J95.6-, J95.7, K91.6-, L76.-, M96.-, N99.-)
ostomy complications (J95.0-, K94.-, N99.5-)
postgastric surgery syndromes (K91.1)
postlaminectomy syndrome NEC (M96.1)
postmastectomy lymphedema syndrome (I97.2)
postsurgical blind-loop syndrome (K91.2)
ventilator associated pneumonia (J95.851)

GUIDELINES **Section I.B.16**

Documentation of Complication of Care: Code assignment is based on the provider's documentation of the relationship between the condition and the care or procedure. The guideline extends to any complications of care, regardless of the chapter the code is located in. It is important to note that not all conditions that occur during or following medical care or surgery are classified as complications. There must be a cause-and-effect relationship between the care provided and the condition, and an indication in the documentation that it is a complication. Query the provider for clarification, if the complication is not clearly documented.

GUIDELINES **Section I.C.19.g.5)**

Intraoperative and postprocedural complication codes are found within the body system chapters with codes specific to the organs and structures of that body system. These codes should be sequenced first, followed by a code(s) for the specific complication, if applicable.

CODING TIP✓ Conditions classifiable to T80-T88 are classifiable as complications of surgical and medical care. These conditions should only be assigned when diagnostic statements clearly indicate that the condition is a complication. Additional codes may be assigned to fully describe the complication.

4 **T80 Complications following infusion, transfusion and therapeutic injection**

INCLUDES complications following perfusion

EXCLUDES 2 *bone marrow transplant rejection (T86.01)*
febrile nonhemolytic transfusion reaction (R50.84)
fluid overload due to transfusion (E87.71)
posttransfusion purpura (D69.51)
transfusion associated circulatory overload (TACO) (E87.71)
transfusion (red blood cell) associated hemochromatosis (E83.111)
transfusion related acute lung injury (TRALI) (J95.84)

The appropriate 7th character is to be added to each code from category T80
A initial encounter
D subsequent encounter
S sequela

7 T80.0XX- **Air embolism following infusion, transfusion and therapeutic injection**

7 T80.1XX- **Vascular complications following infusion, transfusion and therapeutic injection**
Use additional code to identify the vascular complication
EXCLUDES 2 *extravasation of vesicant agent (T80.81-)*
infiltration of vesicant agent (T80.81-)
vascular complications specified as due to prosthetic devices, implants and grafts (T82.8-, T83.8-, T84.8-, T85.8-)
postprocedural vascular complications (T81.7-)

5 T80.2 **Infections following infusion, transfusion and therapeutic injection**
Use additional code to identify the specific infection, such as: sepsis (A41.9)
Use additional code (R65.2-) to identify severe sepsis, if applicable
EXCLUDES 2 *infections specified as due to prosthetic devices, implants and grafts (T82.6-T82.7, T83.5-T83.6, T84.5-T84.7, T85.7)*
postprocedural infections (T81.4-)

6 T80.21 **Infection due to central venous catheter**
Infection due to pulmonary artery catheter (Swan-Ganz catheter)

7 T80.211- **Bloodstream infection due to central venous catheter**
Catheter-related bloodstream infection (CRBSI) NOS
Central line-associated bloodstream infection (CLABSI)
Bloodstream infection due to Hickman catheter
Bloodstream infection due to peripherally inserted central catheter (PICC)
Bloodstream infection due to portacath (port-a-cath)
Bloodstream infection due to pulmonary artery catheter
Bloodstream infection due to triple lumen catheter
Bloodstream infection due to umbilical venous catheter

7 T80.212- **Local infection due to central venous catheter**
Exit or insertion site infection
Local infection due to Hickman catheter
Local infection due to peripherally inserted central catheter (PICC)
Local infection due to portacath (port-a-cath)
Local infection due to pulmonary artery catheter
Local infection due to triple lumen catheter
Local infection due to umbilical venous catheter
Port or reservoir infection
Tunnel infection

7 **T80.218-** **Other infection due to central venous catheter**
Other central line-associated infection
Other infection due to Hickman catheter
Other infection due to peripherally inserted central catheter (PICC)
Other infection due to portacath (port-a-cath)
Other infection due to pulmonary artery catheter
Other infection due to triple lumen catheter
Other infection due to umbilical venous catheter

7 **T80.219-** **Unspecified infection due to central venous catheter**
Central line-associated infection NOS
Unspecified infection due to Hickman catheter
Unspecified infection due to peripherally inserted central catheter (PICC)
Unspecified infection due to portacath (port-a-cath)
Unspecified infection due to pulmonary artery catheter
Unspecified infection due to triple lumen catheter
Unspecified infection due to umbilical venous catheter

7 **T80.22X-** **Acute infection following transfusion, infusion, or injection of blood and blood products**

7 **T80.29X-** **Infection following other infusion, transfusion and therapeutic injection**

▲ 5 **T80.3** **ABO incompatibility reaction due to transfusion of blood or blood products**
EXCLUDES 1 *minor blood group antigens reactions (Duffy) (E) (K) (Kell) (Kidd) (Lewis) (M) (N) (P) (S) (T80.A-)*

7 **T80.30X-** **ABO incompatibility reaction due to transfusion of blood or blood products, unspecified**
ABO incompatibility blood transfusion NOS
Reaction to ABO incompatibility from transfusion NOS

6 **T80.31** **ABO incompatibility with hemolytic transfusion reaction**

7 **T80.310-** **ABO incompatibility with acute hemolytic transfusion reaction**
ABO incompatibility with hemolytic transfusion reaction less than 24 hours after transfusion
Acute hemolytic transfusion reaction (AHTR) due to ABO incompatibility

7 **T80.311-** **ABO incompatibility with delayed hemolytic transfusion reaction**
ABO incompatibility with hemolytic transfusion reaction 24 hours or more after transfusion
Delayed hemolytic transfusion reaction (DHTR) due to ABO incompatibility

7 **T80.319-** **ABO incompatibility with hemolytic transfusion reaction, unspecified**
ABO incompatibility with hemolytic transfusion reaction at unspecified time after transfusion
Hemolytic transfusion reaction (HTR) due to ABO incompatibility NOS

7 **T80.39X-** **Other ABO incompatibility reaction due to transfusion of blood or blood products**
Delayed serologic transfusion reaction (DSTR) from ABO incompatibility
Other ABO incompatible blood transfusion
Other reaction to ABO incompatible blood transfusion

5 **T80.4** **Rh incompatibility reaction due to transfusion of blood or blood products**
Reaction due to incompatibility of Rh antigens (C) (c) (D) (E) (e)

7 **T80.40X-** **Rh incompatibility reaction due to transfusion of blood or blood products, unspecified**
Reaction due to Rh factor in transfusion NOS
Rh incompatible blood transfusion NOS

6 **T80.41** **Rh incompatibility with hemolytic transfusion reaction**

7 **T80.410-** **Rh incompatibility with acute hemolytic transfusion reaction**
Acute hemolytic transfusion reaction (AHTR) due to Rh incompatibility
Rh incompatibility with hemolytic transfusion reaction less than 24 hours after transfusion

7 **T80.411-** **Rh incompatibility with delayed hemolytic transfusion reaction**
Delayed hemolytic transfusion reaction (DHTR) due to Rh incompatibility
Rh incompatibility with hemolytic transfusion reaction 24 hours or more after transfusion

7 **T80.419-** **Rh incompatibility with hemolytic transfusion reaction, unspecified**
Rh incompatibility with hemolytic transfusion reaction at unspecified time after transfusion
Hemolytic transfusion reaction (HTR) due to Rh incompatibility NOS

7 **T80.49X-** **Other Rh incompatibility reaction due to transfusion of blood or blood products**
Delayed serologic transfusion reaction (DSTR) from Rh incompatibility
Other reaction to Rh incompatible blood transfusion

5 **T80.A** **Non-ABO incompatibility reaction due to transfusion of blood or blood products**
Reaction due to incompatibility of minor antigens (Duffy) (Kell) (Kidd) (Lewis) (M) (N) (P) (S)

7 **T80.A0X-** **Non-ABO incompatibility reaction due to transfusion of blood or blood products, unspecified**
Non-ABO antigen incompatibility reaction from transfusion NOS

6 **T80.A1** **Non-ABO incompatibility with hemolytic transfusion reaction**

7 **T80.A10-** **Non-ABO incompatibility with acute hemolytic transfusion reaction**
Acute hemolytic transfusion reaction (AHTR) due to non-ABO incompatibility
Non-ABO incompatibility with hemolytic transfusion reaction less than 24 hours after transfusion

7 **T80.A11-** **Non-ABO incompatibility with delayed hemolytic transfusion reaction**
Delayed hemolytic transfusion reaction (DHTR) due to non-ABO incompatibility
Non-ABO incompatibility with hemolytic transfusion reaction 24 or more hours after transfusion

7 **T80.A19-** **Non-ABO incompatibility with hemolytic transfusion reaction, unspecified**
Hemolytic transfusion reaction (HTR) due to non-ABO incompatibility NOS
Non-ABO incompatibility with hemolytic transfusion reaction at unspecified time after transfusion

7 **T80.A9X-** **Other non-ABO incompatibility reaction due to transfusion of blood or blood products**
Delayed serologic transfusion reaction (DSTR) from non-ABO incompatibility
Other reaction to non-ABO incompatible blood transfusion

5 **T80.5** **Anaphylactic reaction due to serum**
Allergic shock due to serum
Anaphylactic shock due to serum
Anaphylactoid reaction due to serum
Anaphylaxis due to serum
EXCLUDES 1 *ABO incompatibility reaction due to transfusion of blood or blood products (T80.3-)*
allergic reaction or shock NOS (T78.2)
anaphylactic reaction or shock NOS (T78.2)
anaphylactic reaction or shock due to adverse effect of correct medicinal substance properly administered (T88.6)
other serum reaction (T80.6-)

7 **T80.51X-** **Anaphylactic reaction due to administration of blood and blood products**

7 **T80.52X-** **Anaphylactic reaction due to vaccination**

7 **T80.59X-** **Anaphylactic reaction due to other serum**

5 **T80.6** **Other serum reactions**
Intoxication by serum
Protein sickness
Serum rash
Serum sickness
Serum urticaria
EXCLUDES 2 *serum hepatitis (B16-B19)*

7 T80.61X- Other serum reaction due to administration of blood and blood products

7 T80.62X- Other serum reaction due to vaccination

7 T80.69X- Other serum reaction due to other serum
Code also:
, if applicable, arthropathy in hypersensitivity reactions classified elsewhere (M36.4)

5 T80.8 Other complications following infusion, transfusion and therapeutic injection

6 T80.81 Extravasation of vesicant agent
Infiltration of vesicant agent

7 T80.810- Extravasation of vesicant antineoplastic chemotherapy
Infiltration of vesicant antineoplastic chemotherapy

7 T80.818- Extravasation of other vesicant agent
Infiltration of other vesicant agent

7 T80.89X- Other complications following infusion, transfusion and therapeutic injection
Delayed serologic transfusion reaction (DSTR), unspecified incompatibility
Use additional code to identify graft-versus-host reaction, if applicable, (D89.81-)

5 T80.9 Unspecified complication following infusion, transfusion and therapeutic injection

7 T80.90X- Unspecified complication following infusion and therapeutic injection

6 T80.91 Hemolytic transfusion reaction, unspecified incompatibility
EXCLUDES 1 *ABO incompatibility with hemolytic transfusion reaction (T80.31-)*
Non-ABO incompatibility with hemolytic transfusion reaction (T80.A1-)
Rh incompatibility with hemolytic transfusion reaction (T80.41-)

7 T80.910- Acute hemolytic transfusion reaction, unspecified incompatibility

7 T80.911- Delayed hemolytic transfusion reaction, unspecified incompatibility

7 T80.919- Hemolytic transfusion reaction, unspecified incompatibility, unspecified as acute or delayed
Hemolytic transfusion reaction NOS

7 T80.92X- Unspecified transfusion reaction
Transfusion reaction NOS

4 T81 Complications of procedures, not elsewhere classified
Use additional code for adverse effect, if applicable, to identify drug (T36-T50 with fifth or sixth character 5)
EXCLUDES 2 *complications following immunization (T88.0-T88.1)*
complications following infusion, transfusion and therapeutic injection (T80.-)
complications of transplanted organs and tissue (T86.-)
specified complications classified elsewhere, such as:
complication of prosthetic devices, implants and grafts (T82-T85)
dermatitis due to drugs and medicaments (L23.3, L24.4, L25.1, L27.0-L27.1)
endosseous dental implant failure (M27.6-)
floppy iris syndrome (IFIS) (intraoperative) H21.81
intraoperative and postprocedural complications of specific body system (D78.-, E36.-, E89.-, G97.3-, G97.4, H59.3-, H59.-, H95.2-, H95.3, I97.4-, I97.5, J95, K91.-, L76.-, M96.-, N99.-)
ostomy complications (J95.0-, K94.-, N99.5-)
plateau iris syndrome (post-iridectomy) (postprocedural) H21.82
poisoning and toxic effects of drugs and chemicals (T36-T65 with fifth or sixth character 1-4 or 6)

The appropriate 7th character is to be added to each code from category T81
A initial encounter
D subsequent encounter
S sequela

5 T81.1 Postprocedural shock
Shock during or resulting from a procedure, not elsewhere classified
EXCLUDES 1 *anaphylactic shock NOS (T78.2)*
anaphylactic shock due to correct substance properly administered (T88.6)
anaphylactic shock due to serum (T80.5-)
anesthetic shock (T88.2)
electric shock (T75.4)
obstetric shock (O75.1)
septic shock (R65.21)
shock following abortion or ectopic or molar pregnancy (O00-O07, O08.3)
traumatic shock (T79.4)

7 T81.10X- Postprocedural shock unspecified
Collapse NOS during or resulting from a procedure, not elsewhere classified
Postprocedural failure of peripheral circulation
Postprocedural shock NOS

7 T81.11X- Postprocedural cardiogenic shock HCC

7 T81.12X- Postprocedural septic shock HCC
Postprocedural endotoxic shock resulting from a procedure, not elsewhere classified
Postprocedural gram-negative shock resulting from a procedure, not elsewhere classified
Code first:
underlying infection
Use additional code, to identify any associated acute organ dysfunction, if applicable

Injury, Poisoning and Certain Other Consequences of External Causes
T80.61X— T81.12X-

GUIDELINES **Section I.C.1.d.5)(b-c)**
For infections following a procedure, a code from T81.40, to T81.43 Infection following a procedure, or a code from O86.00 to O86.03, Infection of obstetric surgical wound, that identifies the site of the infection should be coded first, if known. Assign an additional code for sepsis following a procedure (T81.44) or sepsis following an obstetrical procedure (O86.04). Use an additional code to identify the infectious agent. If the patient has severe sepsis, the appropriate code from subcategory R65.2 should also be assigned with the additional code(s) for any acute organ dysfunction.

If a postprocedural infection has resulted in postprocedural septic shock, assign the codes indicated above for sepsis due to a postprocedural infection, followed by code T81.12-, Postprocedural septic shock. Do not assign code R65.21, Severe sepsis with septic shock. Additional code(s) should be assigned for any acute organ dysfunction.

CODING TIP✓ **Documentation:** Only assign T81.12- when the provider diagnostic statements clearly indicate septic shock as a postprocedural complication.

7 **T81.19X-** **Other postprocedural shock**
Postprocedural hypovolemic shock

5 **T81.3** **Disruption of wound, not elsewhere classified**
Disruption of any suture materials or other closure methods
EXCLUDES 1 *breakdown (mechanical) of permanent sutures (T85.612)*
displacement of permanent sutures (T85.622)
disruption of cesarean delivery wound (O90.0)
disruption of perineal obstetric wound (O90.1)
mechanical complication of permanent sutures NEC (T85.692)
AHA: 1Q 2014, 23

7 **T81.30X-** **Disruption of wound, unspecified**
Disruption of wound NOS

7 **T81.31X-** **Disruption of external operation (surgical) wound, not elsewhere classified**
Dehiscence of operation wound NOS
Disruption of operation wound NOS
Disruption or dehiscence of closure of cornea
Disruption or dehiscence of closure of mucosa
Disruption or dehiscence of closure of skin and subcutaneous tissue
Full-thickness skin disruption or dehiscence
Superficial disruption or dehiscence of operation wound
EXCLUDES 1 *dehiscence of amputation stump (T87.81)*
CODING TIP✓ Assign T81.31- for an unspecified dehiscence of a surgical wound.
AHA: (T81.31XA) 1Q 2015, 20

7 **T81.32X-** **Disruption of internal operation (surgical) wound, not elsewhere classified**
Deep disruption or dehiscence of operation wound NOS
Disruption or dehiscence of closure of internal organ or other internal tissue
Disruption or dehiscence of closure of muscle or muscle flap
Disruption or dehiscence of closure of ribs or rib cage
Disruption or dehiscence of closure of skull or craniotomy
Disruption or dehiscence of closure of sternum or sternotomy
Disruption or dehiscence of closure of tendon or ligament
Disruption or dehiscence of closure of superficial or muscular fascia

7 **T81.33X-** **Disruption of traumatic injury wound repair**
Disruption or dehiscence of closure of traumatic laceration (external) (internal)
CODING TIP✓ Assign code T81.33- for a repaired (sutured) traumatic laceration, which has dehisced. This code should not be used for surgically created wounds.

▲ 5 **T81.4** **Infection following a procedure**
Wound abscess following a procedure
Use additional code to identify infection
Use additional code (R65.2-) to identify severe sepsis, if applicable
EXCLUDES 2 *bleb associated endophthalmitis (H59.4-)*
infection due to infusion, transfusion and therapeutic injection (T80.2-)
infection due to prosthetic devices, implants and grafts (T82.6-T82.7, T83.5-T83.6, T84.5-T84.7, T85.7)
obstetric surgical wound infection (O86.0-)
postprocedural fever NOS (R50.82)
postprocedural retroperitoneal abscess (K68.11)

GUIDELINES **Section I.C.1.d.5)(b-c)**
For infections following a procedure, a code from T81.40, to T81.43 Infection following a procedure, or a code from O86.00 to O86.03, Infection of obstetric surgical wound, that identifies the site of the infection should be coded first, if known. Assign an additional code for sepsis following a procedure (T81.44) or sepsis following an obstetrical procedure (O86.04). Use an additional code to identify the infectious agent. If the patient has severe sepsis, the appropriate code from subcategory R65.2 should also be assigned with the additional code(s) for any acute organ dysfunction.

If a postprocedural infection has resulted in postprocedural septic shock, assign the codes indicated above for sepsis due to a postprocedural infection, followed by code T81.12-, Postprocedural septic shock. Do not assign code R65.21, Severe sepsis with septic shock. Additional code(s) should be assigned for any acute organ dysfunction.

CODING TIP✓ Assign a code from T81.4- to indicate the presence of a post-operative infection. Codes are reported based on the depth of the infection: At the skin or subcutaneous level (T81.41-), the intramuscular level (T81.42-), in the organ or space of the surgical site (T81.42-) or when sepsis has developed following the procedure (T81.44-).
AHA: (T81.4XXD) 4Q 2015, 37
AHA: 1Q 2014, 23

● 7 **T81.40X-** **Infection following a procedure, unspecified**

● 7 **T81.41X-** **Infection following a procedure, superficial incisional surgical site**
Subcutaneous abscess following a procedure
Stitch abscess following a procedure
CODING TIP✓ A superficial incisional infection involves only the skin and subcutaneous tissue and may be indicated by localized signs such as redness, pain, heat or swelling at the site of the incision or by the drainage of pus.

● 7 **T81.42X-** **Infection following a procedure, deep incisional surgical site**
Intra-muscular abscess following a procedure
CODING TIP✓ A deep incisional infection involves deep tissues, such as fascial and muscle layers, and may be indicated by the presence of pus or an abscess, fever with tenderness of the wound, or separation of incision edges exposing deeper tissues.

● 7 **T81.43X-** **Infection following a procedure, organ and space surgical site**
Intra-abdominal abscess following a procedure
Subphrenic abscess following a procedure

CODING TIP✓ An organ and space infection involves any part of the anatomy in organs and spaces other than the incision, which was opened or manipulated during operation, such as the joint or the peritoneum, and may be indicated by the drainage of pus or the formation of an abscess detected by histopathological or radiological examination or during re-operation; does not include organ infection.

● 7 T81.44X- **Sepsis following a procedure**
Use additional code to identify the sepsis

● 7 T81.49X- **Infection following a procedure, other surgical site**

5 T81.5 **Complications of foreign body accidentally left in body following procedure**

6 T81.50 **Unspecified complication of foreign body accidentally left in body following procedure**

7 ⊟ T81.500- **Unspecified complication of foreign body accidentally left in body following surgical operation**

7 ⊟ T81.501- **Unspecified complication of foreign body accidentally left in body following infusion or transfusion**

7 ⊟ T81.502- **Unspecified complication of foreign body accidentally left in body following kidney dialysis** HCC

7 ⊟ T81.503- **Unspecified complication of foreign body accidentally left in body following injection or immunization**

7 ⊟ T81.504- **Unspecified complication of foreign body accidentally left in body following endoscopic examination**

7 ⊟ T81.505- **Unspecified complication of foreign body accidentally left in body following heart catheterization**

7 ⊟ T81.506- **Unspecified complication of foreign body accidentally left in body following aspiration, puncture or other catheterization**

7 ⊟ T81.507- **Unspecified complication of foreign body accidentally left in body following removal of catheter or packing**

7 ⊟ T81.508- **Unspecified complication of foreign body accidentally left in body following other procedure**

7 ⊟ T81.509- **Unspecified complication of foreign body accidentally left in body following unspecified procedure**

6 T81.51 **Adhesions due to foreign body accidentally left in body following procedure**

7 ⊟ T81.510- **Adhesions due to foreign body accidentally left in body following surgical operation**

7 ⊟ T81.511- **Adhesions due to foreign body accidentally left in body following infusion or transfusion**

7 ⊟ T81.512- **Adhesions due to foreign body accidentally left in body following kidney dialysis** HCC

7 ⊟ T81.513- **Adhesions due to foreign body accidentally left in body following injection or immunization**

7 ⊟ T81.514- **Adhesions due to foreign body accidentally left in body following endoscopic examination**

7 ⊟ T81.515- **Adhesions due to foreign body accidentally left in body following heart catheterization**

7 ⊟ T81.516- **Adhesions due to foreign body accidentally left in body following aspiration, puncture or other catheterization**

7 ⊟ T81.517- **Adhesions due to foreign body accidentally left in body following removal of catheter or packing**

7 ⊟ T81.518- **Adhesions due to foreign body accidentally left in body following other procedure**

7 ⊟ T81.519- **Adhesions due to foreign body accidentally left in body following unspecified procedure**

6 T81.52 **Obstruction due to foreign body accidentally left in body following procedure**

7 ⊟ T81.520- **Obstruction due to foreign body accidentally left in body following surgical operation**

7 ⊟ T81.521- **Obstruction due to foreign body accidentally left in body following infusion or transfusion**

7 ⊟ T81.522- **Obstruction due to foreign body accidentally left in body following kidney dialysis** HCC

7 ⊟ T81.523- **Obstruction due to foreign body accidentally left in body following injection or immunization**

7 ⊟ T81.524- **Obstruction due to foreign body accidentally left in body following endoscopic examination**

7 ⊟ T81.525- **Obstruction due to foreign body accidentally left in body following heart catheterization**

7 ⊟ T81.526- **Obstruction due to foreign body accidentally left in body following aspiration, puncture or other catheterization**

7 ⊟ T81.527- **Obstruction due to foreign body accidentally left in body following removal of catheter or packing**

7 ⊟ T81.528- **Obstruction due to foreign body accidentally left in body following other procedure**

7 ⊟ T81.529- **Obstruction due to foreign body accidentally left in body following unspecified procedure**

6 T81.53 **Perforation due to foreign body accidentally left in body following procedure**

7 ⊟ T81.530- **Perforation due to foreign body accidentally left in body following surgical operation**

7 ⊟ T81.531- **Perforation due to foreign body accidentally left in body following infusion or transfusion**

7 ⊟ T81.532- **Perforation due to foreign body accidentally left in body following kidney dialysis** HCC

7 ⊟ T81.533- **Perforation due to foreign body accidentally left in body following injection or immunization**

7 ⊟ T81.534- **Perforation due to foreign body accidentally left in body following endoscopic examination**

7 ⊟ T81.535- **Perforation due to foreign body accidentally left in body following heart catheterization**

7 ⊟ T81.536- **Perforation due to foreign body accidentally left in body following aspiration, puncture or other catheterization**

7 ⊟ T81.537- **Perforation due to foreign body accidentally left in body following removal of catheter or packing**

7 ⊟ T81.538- **Perforation due to foreign body accidentally left in body following other procedure**

7 ⊟ T81.539- **Perforation due to foreign body accidentally left in body following unspecified procedure**

6 T81.59 **Other complications of foreign body accidentally left in body following procedure**

EXCLUDES 2 *obstruction or perforation due to prosthetic devices and implants intentionally left in body (T82.0-T82.5, T83.0-T83.4, T83.7, T84.0-T84.4, T85.0-T85.6)*

7 ⊟ T81.590- **Other complications of foreign body accidentally left in body following surgical operation**
AHA: (T81.590A) 4Q 2014, 24

7 ⊟ T81.591- **Other complications of foreign body accidentally left in body following infusion or transfusion**

7 ⊟ T81.592- **Other complications of foreign body accidentally left in body following kidney dialysis** HCC

7 ⊟ T81.593- **Other complications of foreign body accidentally left in body following injection or immunization**

7 ⊟ T81.594- **Other complications of foreign body accidentally left in body following endoscopic examination**

7 ⊟ T81.595- **Other complications of foreign body accidentally left in body following heart catheterization**

7 ⊟ T81.596- **Other complications of foreign body accidentally left in body following aspiration , puncture or other catheterization**

7 ⊟ T81.597- **Other complications of foreign body accidentally left in body following removal of catheter or packing**

7 ⊟ T81.598- **Other complications of foreign body accidentally left in body following other procedure**

7 ⊟ T81.599- **Other complications of foreign body accidentally left in body following unspecified procedure**

5 T81.6 **Acute reaction to foreign substance accidentally left during a procedure**

EXCLUDES 2 *complications of foreign body accidentally left in body cavity or operation wound following procedure (T81.5-)*

7 T81.60X- **Unspecified acute reaction to foreign substance accidentally left during a procedure**

7 T81.61X- **Aseptic peritonitis due to foreign substance accidentally left during a procedure**
Chemical peritonitis

7 T81.69X- **Other acute reaction to foreign substance accidentally left during a procedure**

5 T81.7 **Vascular complications following a procedure, not elsewhere classified**
Air embolism following procedure NEC
Phlebitis or thrombophlebitis resulting from a procedure

EXCLUDES 1 *embolism complicating abortion or ectopic or molar pregnancy (O00-O07, O08.2)*
embolism complicating pregnancy, childbirth and the puerperium (O88.-)
traumatic embolism (T79.0)

EXCLUDES 2 *embolism due to prosthetic devices, implants and grafts (T82.8-, T83.81, T84.8-, T85.81-)*
embolism following infusion, transfusion and therapeutic injection (T80.0)

6 T81.71 **Complication of artery following a procedure, not elsewhere classified**

7 T81.710- **Complication of mesenteric artery following a procedure, not elsewhere classified**

7 T81.711- **Complication of renal artery following a procedure, not elsewhere classified**

7 T81.718- **Complication of other artery following a procedure, not elsewhere classified**

7 T81.719- **Complication of unspecified artery following a procedure, not elsewhere classified**

7 T81.72X- **Complication of vein following a procedure, not elsewhere classified**

5 T81.8 **Other complications of procedures, not elsewhere classified**

EXCLUDES 2 *hypothermia following anesthesia (T88.51)*
malignant hyperpyrexia due to anesthesia (T88.3)

7 T81.81X- **Complication of inhalation therapy**

7 T81.82X- **Emphysema (subcutaneous) resulting from a procedure**

7 T81.83X- **Persistent postprocedural fistula**
AHA: 3Q 2017, 3
AHA: 3Q 2017, 4

7 T81.89X- **Other complications of procedures, not elsewhere classified**
Use additional code to specify complication, such as: postprocedural delirium (F05)
AHA: (T81.89X) 1Q 2014, 23

7 ⊟ T81.9XX- **Unspecified complication of procedure**

4 T82 **Complications of cardiac and vascular prosthetic devices, implants and grafts**

EXCLUDES 2 *failure and rejection of transplanted organs and tissue (T86.-)*

The appropriate 7th character is to be added to each code from category T82
A initial encounter
D subsequent encounter
S sequela

5 T82.0 **Mechanical complication of heart valve prosthesis**
Mechanical complication of artificial heart valve

EXCLUDES 1 *mechanical complication of biological heart valve graft (T82.22-)*

CODING TIP ✓ Do not use Z95.2 when the heart valve is complicated.

7 T82.01X- **Breakdown (mechanical) of heart valve prosthesis**

7 T82.02X- **Displacement of heart valve prosthesis**
Malposition of heart valve prosthesis

7 T82.03X- **Leakage of heart valve prosthesis**

7 T82.09X- **Other mechanical complication of heart valve prosthesis**
Obstruction (mechanical) of heart valve prosthesis
Perforation of heart valve prosthesis
Protrusion of heart valve prosthesis

5 T82.1 **Mechanical complication of cardiac electronic device**

6 T82.11 **Breakdown (mechanical) of cardiac electronic device**

7 T82.110- **Breakdown (mechanical) of cardiac electrode**

7 T82.111- **Breakdown (mechanical) of cardiac pulse generator (battery)**

7 T82.118- **Breakdown (mechanical) of other cardiac electronic device**

7 T82.119- **Breakdown (mechanical) of unspecified cardiac electronic device**

6 T82.12 **Displacement of cardiac electronic device**
Malposition of cardiac electronic device

7 T82.120- **Displacement of cardiac electrode**

7 T82.121- **Displacement of cardiac pulse generator (battery)**

7 T82.128- **Displacement of other cardiac electronic device**

7 T82.129- **Displacement of unspecified cardiac electronic device**

6 T82.19 **Other mechanical complication of cardiac electronic device**
Leakage of cardiac electronic device
Obstruction of cardiac electronic device
Perforation of cardiac electronic device
Protrusion of cardiac electronic device

7 T82.190- **Other mechanical complication of cardiac electrode**

7 T82.191- **Other mechanical complication of cardiac pulse generator (battery)**

7 T82.198- **Other mechanical complication of other cardiac electronic device**

7 T82.199- **Other mechanical complication of unspecified cardiac device**

5 T82.2 **Mechanical complication of coronary artery bypass graft and biological heart valve graft**

EXCLUDES 1 *mechanical complication of artificial heart valve prosthesis (T82.0-)*

CODING TIP ✓ Do not use Z95.5 when the bypass graft is complicated.

6 T82.21 **Mechanical complication of coronary artery bypass graft**

7 T82.211- **Breakdown (mechanical) of coronary artery bypass graft**

7 T82.212- **Displacement of coronary artery bypass graft**
Malposition of coronary artery bypass graft

7 T82.213- **Leakage of coronary artery bypass graft**

7 T82.218- **Other mechanical complication of coronary artery bypass graft**
Obstruction, mechanical of coronary artery bypass graft
Perforation of coronary artery bypass graft
Protrusion of coronary artery bypass graft

6 T82.22 **Mechanical complication of biological heart valve graft**

7 T82.221- **Breakdown (mechanical) of biological heart valve graft**

7 T82.222- **Displacement of biological heart valve graft**
Malposition of biological heart valve graft

7 T82.223- **Leakage of biological heart valve graft**

7 T82.228- **Other mechanical complication of biological heart valve graft**
Obstruction of biological heart valve graft
Perforation of biological heart valve graft
Protrusion of biological heart valve graft

5 T82.3 **Mechanical complication of other vascular grafts**

6 T82.31 **Breakdown (mechanical) of other vascular grafts**

7 T82.310- **Breakdown (mechanical) of aortic (bifurcation) graft (replacement)** HCC

7 T82.311- **Breakdown (mechanical) of carotid arterial graft (bypass)** HCC

7 T82.312- **Breakdown (mechanical) of femoral arterial graft (bypass)** HCC

7 T82.318- Breakdown (mechanical) of other vascular grafts HCC
7 T82.319- Breakdown (mechanical) of unspecified vascular grafts HCC

6 T82.32 Displacement of other vascular grafts
Malposition of other vascular grafts
7 T82.320- Displacement of aortic (bifurcation) graft (replacement) HCC
7 T82.321- Displacement of carotid arterial graft (bypass) HCC
7 T82.322- Displacement of femoral arterial graft (bypass) HCC
7 T82.328- Displacement of other vascular grafts HCC
7 T82.329- Displacement of unspecified vascular grafts HCC

6 T82.33 Leakage of other vascular grafts
7 T82.330- Leakage of aortic (bifurcation) graft (replacement) HCC
7 T82.331- Leakage of carotid arterial graft (bypass) HCC
7 T82.332- Leakage of femoral arterial graft (bypass) HCC
7 T82.338- Leakage of other vascular grafts HCC
7 T82.339- Leakage of unspecified vascular graft HCC

6 T82.39 Other mechanical complication of Other vascular grafts
Obstruction (mechanical) of other vascular grafts
Perforation of other vascular grafts
Protrusion of other vascular grafts
7 T82.390- Other mechanical complication of aortic (bifurcation) graft (replacement) HCC
7 T82.391- Other mechanical complication of carotid arterial graft (bypass) HCC
7 T82.392- Other mechanical complication of femoral arterial graft (bypass) HCC
7 T82.398- Other mechanical complication of other vascular grafts HCC
7 T82.399- Other mechanical complication of unspecified vascular grafts HCC

5 T82.4 Mechanical complication of vascular dialysis catheter
Mechanical complication of hemodialysis catheter
EXCLUDES 1 *mechanical complication of intraperitoneal dialysis catheter (T85.62)*
7 T82.41X- Breakdown (mechanical) of vascular dialysis catheter HCC
7 T82.42X- Displacement of vascular dialysis catheter HCC
Malposition of vascular dialysis catheter
7 T82.43X- Leakage of vascular dialysis catheter HCC
7 T82.49X- Other complication of vascular dialysis catheter HCC
Obstruction (mechanical) of vascular dialysis catheter
Perforation of vascular dialysis catheter
Protrusion of vascular dialysis catheter

5 T82.5 Mechanical complication of other cardiac and vascular devices and implants
EXCLUDES 2 *mechanical complication of epidural and subdural infusion catheter (T85.61)*

6 T82.51 Breakdown (mechanical) of other cardiac and vascular devices and implants
7 T82.510- Breakdown (mechanical) of surgically created arteriovenous fistula HCC
7 T82.511- Breakdown (mechanical) of surgically created arteriovenous shunt HCC
7 T82.512- Breakdown (mechanical) of artificial heart
7 T82.513- Breakdown (mechanical) of balloon (counterpulsation) device HCC
7 T82.514- Breakdown (mechanical) of infusion catheter HCC
7 T82.515- Breakdown (mechanical) of umbrella device HCC
7 T82.518- Breakdown (mechanical) of other cardiac and vascular devices and implants HCC
7 T82.519- Breakdown (mechanical) of unspecified cardiac and vascular devices and implants

6 T82.52 Displacement of other cardiac and vascular devices and implants
Malposition of other cardiac and vascular devices and implants
7 T82.520- Displacement of surgically created arteriovenous fistula HCC
7 T82.521- Displacement of surgically created arteriovenous shunt HCC
7 T82.522- Displacement of artificial heart
7 T82.523- Displacement of balloon (counterpulsation) device HCC
7 T82.524- Displacement of infusion catheter HCC
7 T82.525- Displacement of umbrella device HCC
7 T82.528- Displacement of other cardiac and vascular devices and implants HCC
7 T82.529- Displacement of unspecified cardiac and vascular devices and implants

6 T82.53 Leakage of other cardiac and vascular devices and implants
7 T82.530- Leakage of surgically created arteriovenous fistula HCC
7 T82.531- Leakage of surgically created arteriovenous shunt HCC
7 T82.532- Leakage of artificial heart
7 T82.533- Leakage of balloon (counterpulsation) device HCC
7 T82.534- Leakage of infusion catheter HCC
7 T82.535- Leakage of umbrella device HCC
7 T82.538- Leakage of other cardiac and vascular devices and implants HCC
7 T82.539- Leakage of unspecified cardiac and vascular devices and implants

6 T82.59 Other mechanical complication of Other cardiac and vascular devices and implants
Obstruction (mechanical) of other cardiac and vascular devices and implants
Perforation of other cardiac and vascular devices and implants
Protrusion of other cardiac and vascular devices and implants
7 T82.590- Other mechanical complication of surgically created arteriovenous fistula HCC
7 T82.591- Other mechanical complication of surgically created arteriovenous shunt HCC
7 T82.592- Other mechanical complication of artificial heart
7 T82.593- Other mechanical complication of balloon (counterpulsation) device HCC
7 T82.594- Other mechanical complication of infusion catheter HCC
7 T82.595- Other mechanical complication of umbrella device HCC
7 T82.598- Other mechanical complication of other cardiac and vascular devices and implants HCC
7 T82.599- Other mechanical complication of unspecified cardiac and vascular devices and implants

7 T82.6XX- Infection and inflammatory reaction due to cardiac valve prosthesis HCC
Use additional code to identify infection

7 T82.7XX- Infection and inflammatory reaction due to other cardiac and vascular devices, implants and grafts HCC
Use additional code to identify infection
AHA: (T82.7XXA) 1Q 2015, 20

5 T82.8 Other specified complications of cardiac and vascular prosthetic devices, implants and grafts

6 T82.81 Embolism due to cardiac and vascular prosthetic devices, implants and grafts
7 T82.817- Embolism due to cardiac prosthetic devices, implants and grafts
7 T82.818- Embolism due to vascular prosthetic devices, implants and grafts HCC

6 T82.82 Fibrosis due to cardiac and vascular prosthetic devices, implants and grafts
7 T82.827- Fibrosis due to cardiac prosthetic devices, implants and grafts
7 T82.828- Fibrosis due to vascular prosthetic devices, implants and grafts HCC

6 T82.83 Hemorrhage due to cardiac and vascular prosthetic devices, implants and grafts
7 T82.837- Hemorrhage due to cardiac prosthetic devices, implants and grafts
7 T82.838- Hemorrhage due to vascular prosthetic devices, implants and grafts HCC

6 T82.84 Pain due to cardiac and vascular prosthetic devices, implants and grafts
7 T82.847- Pain due to cardiac prosthetic devices, implants and grafts
7 T82.848- Pain due to vascular prosthetic devices, implants and grafts HCC
6 T82.85 Stenosis due to cardiac and vascular prosthetic devices, implants and grafts
7 T82.855- Stenosis of coronary artery stent
In-stent stenosis (restenosis) of coronary artery stent
Restenosis of coronary artery stent
AHA: 4Q 2016, 70
7 T82.856- Stenosis of peripheral vascular stent HCC
In-stent stenosis (restenosis) of peripheral vascular stent
Restenosis of peripheral vascular stent
AHA: 4Q 2016, 70
7 T82.857- Stenosis of other cardiac prosthetic devices, implants and grafts
7 T82.858- Stenosis of other vascular prosthetic devices, implants and grafts HCC
6 T82.86 Thrombosis of cardiac and vascular prosthetic devices, implants and grafts
7 T82.867- Thrombosis due to cardiac prosthetic devices, implants and grafts
7 T82.868- Thrombosis due to vascular prosthetic devices, implants and grafts HCC
6 T82.89 Other specified complication of cardiac and vascular prosthetic devices, implants and grafts
7 T82.897- Other specified complication of cardiac prosthetic devices, implants and grafts
7 T82.898- Other specified complication of vascular prosthetic devices, implants and grafts HCC
7 T82.9XX- Unspecified complication of cardiac and vascular prosthetic device, implant and graft

4 T83 Complications of genitourinary prosthetic devices, implants and grafts

EXCLUDES 2 *failure and rejection of transplanted organs and tissue (T86.-)*

The appropriate 7th character is to be added to each code from category T83
A initial encounter
D subsequent encounter
S sequela

5 T83.0 Mechanical complication of urinary catheter
EXCLUDES 2 *complications of stoma of urinary tract (N99.5-)*
6 T83.01 Breakdown (mechanical) of urinary catheter
7 T83.010- Breakdown (mechanical) of cystostomy catheter HCC
7 T83.011- Breakdown (mechanical) of indwelling urethral catheter HCC
7 T83.012- Breakdown (mechanical) of nephrostomy catheter HCC
7 T83.018- Breakdown (mechanical) of other urinary catheter HCC
Breakdown (mechanical) of Hopkins catheter
Breakdown (mechanical) of ileostomy catheter
Breakdown (mechanical) urostomy catheter
6 T83.02 Displacement of urinary catheter
Malposition of urinary catheter
7 T83.020- Displacement of cystostomy catheter HCC
7 T83.021- Displacement of indwelling urethral catheter HCC
7 T83.022- Displacement of nephrostomy catheter HCC
7 T83.028- Displacement of other urinary catheter HCC
Displacement of Hopkins catheter
Displacement of ileostomy catheter
Displacement of urostomy catheter
6 T83.03 Leakage of urinary catheter
7 T83.030- Leakage of cystostomy catheter HCC
7 T83.031- Leakage of indwelling urethral catheter HCC
7 T83.032- Leakage of nephrostomy catheter HCC
7 T83.038- Leakage of other urinary catheter HCC
Leakage of Hopkins catheter
Leakage of ileostomy catheter
Leakage of urostomy catheter
6 T83.09 Other mechanical complication of urinary catheter
Obstruction (mechanical) of urinary catheter
Perforation of urinary catheter
Protrusion of urinary catheter
7 T83.090- Other mechanical complication of cystostomy catheter HCC
7 T83.091- Other mechanical complication of indwelling urethral catheter HCC
7 T83.092- Other mechanical complication of nephrostomy catheter HCC
7 T83.098- Other mechanical complication of other urinary catheter HCC
Other mechanical complication of Hopkins catheter
Other mechanical complication of ileostomy catheter
Other mechanical complication of urostomy catheter
5 T83.1 Mechanical complication of other urinary devices and implants
6 T83.11 Breakdown (mechanical) of other urinary devices and implants
7 T83.110- Breakdown (mechanical) of urinary electronic stimulator device HCC
EXCLUDES 2 *Breakdown (mechanical) of electrode (lead) for sacral nerve neurostimulator (T85.111)*
Breakdown (mechanical) of implanted electronic sacral neurostimulator, pulse generator or receiver (T85.113)
7 T83.111- Breakdown (mechanical) of implanted urinary sphincter HCC
7 T83.112- Breakdown (mechanical) of indwelling ureteral stent HCC
7 T83.113- Breakdown (mechanical) of other urinary stents HCC
Breakdown (mechanical) of ileal conduit stent
Breakdown (mechanical) of nephroureteral stent
7 T83.118- Breakdown (mechanical) of other urinary devices and implants HCC
6 T83.12 Displacement of other urinary devices and implants
Malposition of other urinary devices and implants
7 T83.120- Displacement of urinary electronic stimulator device HCC
EXCLUDES 2 *Displacement of electrode (lead) for sacral nerve neurostimulator (T85.121)*
Displacement of implanted electronic sacral neurostimulator, pulse generator or receiver (T85.123)
7 T83.121- Displacement of implanted urinary sphincter HCC
7 T83.122- Displacement of indwelling ureteral stent HCC
7 T83.123- Displacement of other urinary stents HCC
Displacement of ileal conduit stent
Displacement of nephroureteral stent
7 T83.128- Displacement of other urinary devices and implants HCC
6 T83.19 Other mechanical complication of Other urinary devices and implants
Leakage of other urinary devices and implants
Obstruction (mechanical) of other urinary devices and implants
Perforation of other urinary devices and implants
Protrusion of other urinary devices and implants

7 **T83.190- Other mechanical complication of urinary electronic stimulator device** HCC

EXCLUDES 2 *Other mechanical complication of electrode (lead) for sacral nerve neurostimulator (T85.191)*
Other mechanical complication of implanted electronic sacral neurostimulator, pulse generator or receiver (T85.193)

7 **T83.191- Other mechanical complication of implanted urinary sphincter** HCC

7 **T83.192- Other mechanical complication of indwelling ureteral stent** HCC

7 **T83.193- Other mechanical complication of other urinary stent** HCC
Other mechanical complication of ileal conduit stent
Other mechanical complication of nephroureteral stent

7 **T83.198- Other mechanical complication of other urinary devices and implants** HCC

5 **T83.2 Mechanical complication of graft of urinary organ**
AHA: 4Q 2016, 70

7 **T83.21X- Breakdown (mechanical) of graft of urinary organ** HCC

7 **T83.22X- Displacement of graft of urinary organ** HCC
Malposition of graft of urinary organ

7 **T83.23X- Leakage of graft of urinary organ** HCC

7 **T83.24X- Erosion of graft of urinary organ** HCC

7 **T83.25X- Exposure of graft of urinary organ** HCC

7 **T83.29X- Other mechanical complication of graft of urinary organ** HCC
Obstruction (mechanical) of graft of urinary organ
Perforation of graft of urinary organ
Protrusion of graft of urinary organ

5 **T83.3 Mechanical complication of intrauterine contraceptive device**

7 **T83.31X- Breakdown (mechanical) of intrauterine contraceptive device** ♀

7 **T83.32X- Displacement of intrauterine contraceptive device** ♀
Malposition of intrauterine contraceptive device
Missing string of intrauterine contraceptive device

7 **T83.39X- Other mechanical complication of intrauterine contraceptive device** ♀
Leakage of intrauterine contraceptive device
Obstruction (mechanical) of intrauterine contraceptive device
Perforation of intrauterine contraceptive device
Protrusion of intrauterine contraceptive device

5 **T83.4 Mechanical complication of other prosthetic devices, implants and grafts of genital tract**

6 **T83.41 Breakdown (mechanical) of other prosthetic devices, implants and grafts of genital tract**

7 **T83.410- Breakdown (mechanical) of implanted penile prosthesis** ♂ HCC
Breakdown (mechanical) of penile prosthesis cylinder
Breakdown (mechanical) of penile prosthesis pump
Breakdown (mechanical) of penile prosthesis reservoir

7 **T83.411- Breakdown (mechanical) of implanted testicular prosthesis** HCC

7 **T83.418- Breakdown (mechanical) of other prosthetic devices, implants and grafts of genital tract** HCC

6 **T83.42 Displacement of other prosthetic devices, implants and grafts of genital tract**
Malposition of other prosthetic devices, implants and grafts of genital tract

7 **T83.420- Displacement of implanted penile prosthesis** ♂ HCC
Displacement of penile prosthesis cylinder
Displacement of penile prosthesis pump
Displacement of penile prosthesis reservoir

7 **T83.421- Displacement of implanted testicular prosthesis** HCC

7 **T83.428- Displacement of other prosthetic devices, implants and grafts of genital tract** HCC
AHA: (T83.428A) 1Q 2018, 5

6 **T83.49 Other mechanical complication of Other prosthetic devices, implants and grafts of genital tract**
Leakage of other prosthetic devices, implants and grafts of genital tract
Obstruction, mechanical of other prosthetic devices, implants and grafts of genital tract
Perforation of other prosthetic devices, implants and grafts of genital tract
Protrusion of other prosthetic devices, implants and grafts of genital tract

7 **T83.490- Other mechanical complication of implanted penile prosthesis** ♂ HCC
Other mechanical complication of penile prosthesis cylinder
Other mechanical complication of penile prosthesis pump
Other mechanical complication of penile prosthesis reservoir

7 **T83.491- Other mechanical complication of implanted testicular prosthesis** HCC

7 **T83.498- Other mechanical complication of other prosthetic devices, implants and grafts of genital tract** HCC

5 **T83.5 Infection and inflammatory reaction due to prosthetic device, implant and graft in urinary system**
Use additional code to identify infection

CODING TIP✓ Do not use Z43 or Z93 codes for routine care when a complication is documented.

6 **T83.51 Infection and inflammatory reaction due to urinary catheter**

EXCLUDES 2 *complications of stoma of urinary tract (N99.5-)*

7 **T83.510- Infection and inflammatory reaction due to cystostomy catheter** HCC

7 **T83.511- Infection and inflammatory reaction due to indwelling urethral catheter** HCC

7 **T83.512- Infection and inflammatory reaction due to nephrostomy catheter** HCC

7 **T83.518- Infection and inflammatory reaction due to other urinary catheter** HCC
Infection and inflammatory reaction due to Hopkins catheter
Infection and inflammatory reaction due to ileostomy catheter
Infection and inflammatory reaction due to urostomy catheter

6 **T83.59 Infection and inflammatory reaction due to prosthetic device, implant and graft in urinary system**

7 **T83.590- Infection and inflammatory reaction due to implanted urinary neurostimulation device** HCC

EXCLUDES 2 *Infection and inflammatory reaction due to electrode lead of sacral nerve neurostimulator (T85.732)*
Infection and inflammatory reaction due to pulse generator or receiver of sacral nerve neurostimulator (T85.734)

7 **T83.591- Infection and inflammatory reaction due to implanted urinary sphincter** HCC

7 **T83.592- Infection and inflammatory reaction due to indwelling ureteral stent** HCC

7 **T83.593- Infection and inflammatory reaction due to other urinary stents** HCC
Infection and inflammatory reaction due to ileal conduit stents
Infection and inflammatory reaction due to nephroureteral stent

7 **T83.598- Infection and inflammatory reaction due to other prosthetic device, implant and graft in urinary system** HCC

5 **T83.6 Infection and inflammatory reaction due to prosthetic device, implant and graft in genital tract**
Use additional code to identify infection

7 T83.61X- **Infection and inflammatory reaction due to implanted penile prosthesis** HCC
Infection and inflammatory reaction due to penile prosthesis cylinder
Infection and inflammatory reaction due to penile prosthesis pump
Infection and inflammatory reaction due to penile prosthesis reservoir
7 T83.62X- **Infection and inflammatory reaction due to implanted testicular prosthesis** HCC
7 T83.69X- **Infection and inflammatory reaction due to other prosthetic device, implant and graft in genital tract** HCC

5 T83.7 **Complications due to implanted mesh and other prosthetic materials**
6 T83.71 **Erosion of implanted mesh and other prosthetic materials to surrounding organ or tissue**
7 T83.711- **Erosion of implanted vaginal mesh to surrounding organ or tissue** ♀ HCC
Erosion of implanted vaginal mesh into pelvic floor muscles
7 T83.712- **Erosion of implanted urethral mesh to surrounding organ or tissue** HCC
Erosion of implanted female urethral sling
Erosion of implanted male urethral sling
Erosion of implanted urethral mesh into pelvic floor muscles
7 T83.713- **Erosion of implanted urethral bulking agent to surrounding organ or tissue** HCC
7 T83.714- **Erosion of implanted ureteral bulking agent to surrounding organ or tissue** HCC
7 T83.718- **Erosion of other implanted mesh to organ or tissue** HCC
7 T83.719- **Erosion of other prosthetic materials to surrounding organ or tissue** HCC
6 T83.72 **Exposure of implanted mesh and other prosthetic materials into surrounding organ or tissue**
Extrusion of implanted mesh
7 T83.721- **Exposure of implanted vaginal mesh into vagina** ♀ HCC
Exposure of implanted vaginal mesh through vaginal wall
7 T83.722- **Exposure of implanted urethral mesh into urethra** HCC
Exposure of implanted female urethral sling
Exposure of implanted male urethral sling
Exposure of implanted urethral mesh through urethral wall
7 T83.723- **Exposure of implanted urethral bulking agent into urethra** HCC
7 T83.724- **Exposure of implanted ureteral bulking agent into ureter** HCC
7 T83.728- **Exposure of other implanted mesh into organ or tissue** HCC
7 T83.729- **Exposure of other prosthetic materials into organ or tissue** HCC
7 T83.79X- **Other specified complications due to other genitourinary prosthetic materials** HCC

5 T83.8 **Other specified complications of genitourinary prosthetic devices, implants and grafts**
7 T83.81X- **Embolism due to genitourinary prosthetic devices, implants and grafts** HCC
7 T83.82X- **Fibrosis due to genitourinary prosthetic devices, implants and grafts** HCC
7 T83.83X- **Hemorrhage due to genitourinary prosthetic devices, implants and grafts** HCC
7 T83.84X- **Pain due to genitourinary prosthetic devices, implants and grafts** HCC
7 T83.85X- **Stenosis due to genitourinary prosthetic devices, implants and grafts** HCC
7 T83.86X- **Thrombosis due to genitourinary prosthetic devices, implants and grafts** HCC
7 T83.89X- **Other specified complication of genitourinary prosthetic devices, implants and grafts** HCC
7 T83.9XX- **Unspecified complication of genitourinary prosthetic device, implant and graft** HCC

4 T84 **Complications of internal orthopedic prosthetic devices, implants and grafts**
EXCLUDES 2 *failure and rejection of transplanted organs and tissues (T86.-)*
fracture of bone following insertion of orthopedic implant, joint prosthesis or bone plate (M96.6)

The appropriate 7th character is to be added to each code from category T84
A initial encounter
D subsequent encounter
S sequela

5 T84.0 **Mechanical complication of internal joint prosthesis**
CODING TIP ✓ Site and laterality should be documented. Sixth character 8 is used for shoulder, elbow, wrist, hand, ankle, foot and spine prostheses.
CODING TIP ✓ Subcategory T84.0 is for mechanical complications of joint replacements. If the complication is an infection, see T84.5. If the joint prosthesis has been removed, use the appropriate code for the removed prosthesis and use of spacer.
6 T84.01 **Broken internal joint prosthesis**
Breakage (fracture) of prosthetic joint
Broken prosthetic joint implant
EXCLUDES 1 *periprosthetic joint implant fracture (M97-)*
7 ⊟ T84.010- **Broken internal right hip prosthesis** HCC
7 ⊟ T84.011- **Broken internal left hip prosthesis** HCC
7 ⊟ T84.012- **Broken internal right knee prosthesis** HCC
7 ⊟ T84.013- **Broken internal left knee prosthesis** HCC
7 ⊟ T84.018- **Broken internal joint prosthesis, other site** HCC
Use additional code to identify the joint (Z96.6-)
7 ⊟ T84.019- **Broken internal joint prosthesis, unspecified site** HCC
6 T84.02 **Dislocation of internal joint prosthesis**
Instability of internal joint prosthesis
Subluxation of internal joint prosthesis
7 ⊟ T84.020- **Dislocation of internal right hip prosthesis** HCC
7 ⊟ T84.021- **Dislocation of internal left hip prosthesis** HCC
7 ⊟ T84.022- **Instability of internal right knee prosthesis** HCC
7 ⊟ T84.023- **Instability of internal left knee prosthesis** HCC
7 ⊟ T84.028- **Dislocation of other internal joint prosthesis** HCC
Use additional code to identify the joint (Z96.6-)
7 ⊟ T84.029- **Dislocation of unspecified internal joint prosthesis** HCC
6 T84.03 **Mechanical loosening of internal prosthetic joint**
Aseptic loosening of prosthetic joint
7 ⊟ T84.030- **Mechanical loosening of internal right hip prosthetic joint** HCC
7 ⊟ T84.031- **Mechanical loosening of internal left hip prosthetic joint** HCC
7 ⊟ T84.032- **Mechanical loosening of internal right knee prosthetic joint** HCC
7 ⊟ T84.033- **Mechanical loosening of internal left knee prosthetic joint** HCC
7 ⊟ T84.038- **Mechanical loosening of other internal prosthetic joint** HCC
Use additional code to identify the joint (Z96.6-)
7 ⊟ T84.039- **Mechanical loosening of unspecified internal prosthetic joint** HCC
6 T84.05 **Periprosthetic osteolysis of internal prosthetic joint**
Use additional code to identify major osseous defect, if applicable (M89.7-)
7 ⊟ T84.050- **Periprosthetic osteolysis of internal prosthetic right hip joint** HCC
7 ⊟ T84.051- **Periprosthetic osteolysis of internal prosthetic left hip joint** HCC
7 ⊟ T84.052- **Periprosthetic osteolysis of internal prosthetic right knee joint** HCC
7 ⊟ T84.053- **Periprosthetic osteolysis of internal prosthetic left knee joint** HCC
7 ⊟ T84.058- **Periprosthetic osteolysis of other internal prosthetic joint** HCC
Use additional code to identify the joint (Z96.6-)

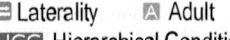

7 ⊟ T84.059- Periprosthetic osteolysis of unspecified internal prosthetic joint HCC

6 T84.06 Wear of articular bearing surface of internal prosthetic joint

7 ⊟ T84.060- Wear of articular bearing surface of internal prosthetic right hip joint HCC

7 ⊟ T84.061- Wear of articular bearing surface of internal prosthetic left hip joint HCC

7 ⊟ T84.062- Wear of articular bearing surface of internal prosthetic right knee joint HCC

7 ⊟ T84.063- Wear of articular bearing surface of internal prosthetic left knee joint HCC

7 ⊟ T84.068- Wear of articular bearing surface of other internal prosthetic joint HCC
Use additional code to identify the joint (Z96.6-)

7 ⊟ T84.069- Wear of articular bearing surface of unspecified internal prosthetic joint HCC

6 T84.09 Other mechanical complication of internal joint prosthesis
Prosthetic joint implant failure NOS

7 ⊟ T84.090- Other mechanical complication of internal right hip prosthesis HCC

7 ⊟ T84.091- Other mechanical complication of internal left hip prosthesis HCC

7 ⊟ T84.092- Other mechanical complication of internal right knee prosthesis HCC

7 ⊟ T84.093- Other mechanical complication of internal left knee prosthesis HCC

7 ⊟ T84.098- Other mechanical complication of other internal joint prosthesis HCC
Use additional code to identify the joint (Z96.6-)

7 ⊟ T84.099- Other mechanical complication of unspecified internal joint prosthesis HCC

5 T84.1 Mechanical complication of internal fixation device of bones of limb

EXCLUDES 2 *mechanical complication of internal fixation device of bones of feet (T84.2-)*
mechanical complication of internal fixation device of bones of fingers (T84.2-)
mechanical complication of internal fixation device of bones of hands (T84.2-)
mechanical complication of internal fixation device of bones of toes (T84.2-)

6 T84.11 Breakdown (mechanical) of internal fixation device of bones of limb

7 ⊟ T84.110- Breakdown (mechanical) of internal fixation device of right humerus HCC

7 ⊟ T84.111- Breakdown (mechanical) of internal fixation device of left humerus HCC

7 ⊟ T84.112- Breakdown (mechanical) of internal fixation device of bone of right forearm HCC

7 ⊟ T84.113- Breakdown (mechanical) of internal fixation device of bone of left forearm HCC

7 ⊟ T84.114- Breakdown (mechanical) of internal fixation device of right femur HCC

7 ⊟ T84.115- Breakdown (mechanical) of internal fixation device of left femur HCC

7 ⊟ T84.116- Breakdown (mechanical) of internal fixation device of bone of right lower leg HCC

7 ⊟ T84.117- Breakdown (mechanical) of internal fixation device of bone of left lower leg HCC

7 ⊟ T84.119- Breakdown (mechanical) of internal fixation device of unspecified bone of limb HCC

6 T84.12 Displacement of internal fixation device of bones of limb
Malposition of internal fixation device of bones of limb

7 ⊟ T84.120- Displacement of internal fixation device of right humerus HCC

7 ⊟ T84.121- Displacement of internal fixation device of left humerus HCC

7 ⊟ T84.122- Displacement of internal fixation device of bone of right forearm HCC

7 ⊟ T84.123- Displacement of internal fixation device of bone of left forearm HCC

7 ⊟ T84.124- Displacement of internal fixation device of right femur HCC

7 ⊟ T84.125- Displacement of internal fixation device of left femur HCC

7 ⊟ T84.126- Displacement of internal fixation device of bone of right lower leg HCC

7 ⊟ T84.127- Displacement of internal fixation device of bone of left lower leg HCC

7 ⊟ T84.129- Displacement of internal fixation device of unspecified bone of limb HCC

6 T84.19 Other mechanical complication of internal fixation device of bones of limb
Obstruction (mechanical) of internal fixation device of bones of limb
Perforation of internal fixation device of bones of limb
Protrusion of internal fixation device of bones of limb

7 ⊟ T84.190- Other mechanical complication of internal fixation device of right humerus HCC

7 ⊟ T84.191- Other mechanical complication of internal fixation device of left humerus HCC

7 ⊟ T84.192- Other mechanical complication of internal fixation device of bone of right forearm HCC

7 ⊟ T84.193- Other mechanical complication of internal fixation device of bone of left forearm HCC

7 ⊟ T84.194- Other mechanical complication of internal fixation device of right femur HCC

7 ⊟ T84.195- Other mechanical complication of internal fixation device of left femur HCC

7 ⊟ T84.196- Other mechanical complication of internal fixation device of bone of right lower leg HCC

7 ⊟ T84.197- Other mechanical complication of internal fixation device of bone of left lower leg HCC

7 ⊟ T84.199- Other mechanical complication of internal fixation device of unspecified bone of limb HCC

5 T84.2 Mechanical complication of internal fixation device of other bones

6 T84.21 Breakdown (mechanical) of internal fixation device of other bones

7 T84.210- Breakdown (mechanical) of internal fixation device of bones of hand and fingers HCC

7 T84.213- Breakdown (mechanical) of internal fixation device of bones of foot and toes HCC

7 T84.216- Breakdown (mechanical) of internal fixation device of vertebrae HCC

7 T84.218- Breakdown (mechanical) of internal fixation device of other bones HCC

6 T84.22 Displacement of internal fixation device of other bones
Malposition of internal fixation device of other bones

7 T84.220- Displacement of internal fixation device of bones of hand and fingers HCC

7 T84.223- Displacement of internal fixation device of bones of foot and toes HCC

7 T84.226- Displacement of internal fixation device of vertebrae HCC

7 T84.228- Displacement of internal fixation device of other bones HCC

6 T84.29 Other mechanical complication of internal fixation device of other bones
Obstruction (mechanical) of internal fixation device of other bones
Perforation of internal fixation device of other bones
Protrusion of internal fixation device of other bones

7 T84.290- Other mechanical complication of internal fixation device of bones of hand and fingers HCC

7 T84.293- Other mechanical complication of internal fixation device of bones of foot and toes HCC

7 T84.296- Other mechanical complication of internal fixation device of vertebrae HCC

7 T84.298- Other mechanical complication of internal fixation device of other bones HCC

5 T84.3 Mechanical complication of other bone devices, implants and grafts

EXCLUDES 2 *other complications of bone graft (T86.83-)*

6 T84.31 Breakdown (mechanical) of other bone devices, implants and grafts

T84.310- **Breakdown (mechanical) of electronic bone stimulator** HCC

T84.318- **Breakdown (mechanical) of other bone devices, implants and grafts** HCC

T84.32 **Displacement of other bone devices, implants and grafts**
Malposition of other bone devices, implants and grafts

T84.320- **Displacement of electronic bone stimulator** HCC

T84.328- **Displacement of other bone devices, implants and grafts** HCC
AHA: (T84.328A) 4Q 2014, 29

T84.39 **Other mechanical complication of Other bone devices, implants and grafts**
Obstruction (mechanical) of other bone devices, implants and grafts
Perforation of other bone devices, implants and grafts
Protrusion of other bone devices, implants and grafts

T84.390- **Other mechanical complication of electronic bone stimulator** HCC

T84.398- **Other mechanical complication of other bone devices, implants and grafts** HCC

T84.4 **Mechanical complication of other internal orthopedic devices, implants and grafts**

CODING TIP✓ Use subcategory T84.4 for disruptions of tendon grafts such as ACL. Do not use a current sprain/strain series code.

T84.41 **Breakdown (mechanical) of other internal orthopedic devices, implants and grafts**

T84.410- **Breakdown (mechanical) of muscle and tendon graft** HCC

T84.418- **Breakdown (mechanical) of other internal orthopedic devices, implants and grafts** HCC

T84.42 **Displacement of other internal orthopedic devices, implants and grafts**
Malposition of other internal orthopedic devices, implants and grafts

T84.420- **Displacement of muscle and tendon graft** HCC

T84.428- **Displacement of other internal orthopedic devices, implants and grafts** HCC

T84.49 **Other mechanical complication of Other internal orthopedic devices, implants and grafts**
Mechanical complication of other internal orthopedic devices, implants and grafts NOS
Obstruction (mechanical) of other internal orthopedic devices, implants and grafts
Perforation of other internal orthopedic devices, implants and grafts
Protrusion of other internal orthopedic devices, implants and grafts

T84.490- **Other mechanical complication of muscle and tendon graft** HCC

T84.498- **Other mechanical complication of other internal orthopedic devices, implants and grafts** HCC

T84.5 **Infection and inflammatory reaction due to internal joint prosthesis**
Use additional code to identify infection

CODING TIP✓ If the infection is superficial, query the physician before using T84.5-. If the joint prosthesis has been removed, use appropriate Z codes for the removed prosthesis and use of spacer.

CODING TIP✓ Use a code from T84.5 for the initial admission to remove an infected joint prosthesis. Code also the affected prosthetic joint with a code from Z96.64-. For aftercare following explantation or for staged reimplantation, use the Z47.3- subcategory of codes along with Z96.64- for the type of prosthesis.
AHA: 1Q 2015, 16

T84.50X- **Infection and inflammatory reaction due to unspecified internal joint prosthesis** HCC

T84.51X- **Infection and inflammatory reaction due to internal right hip prosthesis** HCC
AHA: (T84.51XA) 4Q 2015, 36

T84.52X- **Infection and inflammatory reaction due to internal left hip prosthesis** HCC
AHA: (T84.52X-) 1Q 2015, 17
AHA: (T84.52XA) 1Q 2015, 16

T84.53X- **Infection and inflammatory reaction due to internal right knee prosthesis** HCC

T84.54X- **Infection and inflammatory reaction due to internal left knee prosthesis** HCC

T84.59X- **Infection and inflammatory reaction due to other internal joint prosthesis** HCC

T84.6 **Infection and inflammatory reaction due to internal fixation device**
Use additional code to identify infection

T84.60X- **Infection and inflammatory reaction due to internal fixation device of unspecified site** HCC

T84.61 **Infection and inflammatory reaction due to internal fixation device of arm**

T84.610- **Infection and inflammatory reaction due to internal fixation device of right humerus** HCC

T84.611- **Infection and inflammatory reaction due to internal fixation device of left humerus** HCC

T84.612- **Infection and inflammatory reaction due to internal fixation device of right radius** HCC

T84.613- **Infection and inflammatory reaction due to internal fixation device of left radius** HCC

T84.614- **Infection and inflammatory reaction due to internal fixation device of right ulna** HCC

T84.615- **Infection and inflammatory reaction due to internal fixation device of left ulna** HCC

T84.619- **Infection and inflammatory reaction due to internal fixation device of unspecified bone of arm** HCC

T84.62 **Infection and inflammatory reaction due to internal fixation device of leg**

T84.620- **Infection and inflammatory reaction due to internal fixation device of right femur** HCC

T84.621- **Infection and inflammatory reaction due to internal fixation device of left femur** HCC

T84.622- **Infection and inflammatory reaction due to internal fixation device of right tibia** HCC

T84.623- **Infection and inflammatory reaction due to internal fixation device of left tibia** HCC

T84.624- **Infection and inflammatory reaction due to internal fixation device of right fibula** HCC

T84.625- **Infection and inflammatory reaction due to internal fixation device of left fibula** HCC

T84.629- **Infection and inflammatory reaction due to internal fixation device of unspecified bone of leg** HCC

T84.63X- **Infection and inflammatory reaction due to internal fixation device of spine** HCC

T84.69X- **Infection and inflammatory reaction due to internal fixation device of other site** HCC

T84.7XX- **Infection and inflammatory reaction due to other internal orthopedic prosthetic devices, implants and grafts** HCC
Use additional code to identify infection

T84.8 **Other specified complications of internal orthopedic prosthetic devices, implants and grafts**

T84.81X- **Embolism due to internal orthopedic prosthetic devices, implants and grafts** HCC

T84.82X- **Fibrosis due to internal orthopedic prosthetic devices, implants and grafts** HCC

T84.83X- **Hemorrhage due to internal orthopedic prosthetic devices, implants and grafts** HCC

T84.84X- **Pain due to internal orthopedic prosthetic devices, implants and grafts** HCC

CODING TIP✓ A G89.- code may be added to indicate the nature of the pain, e.g. post surgical vs traumatic, and acute vs chronic.

T84.85X- **Stenosis due to internal orthopedic prosthetic devices, implants and grafts** HCC

T84.86X- **Thrombosis due to internal orthopedic prosthetic devices, implants and grafts** HCC

T84.89X- **Other specified complication of internal orthopedic prosthetic devices, implants and grafts** HCC

T84.9XX- **Unspecified complication of internal orthopedic prosthetic device, implant and graft** HCC

T85 Complications of other internal prosthetic devices, implants and grafts

EXCLUDES 2 *failure and rejection of transplanted organs and tissue (T86.-)*

The appropriate 7th character is to be added to each code from category T85
A initial encounter
D subsequent encounter
S sequela

AHA: 4Q 2016, 71

T85.0 Mechanical complication of ventricular intracranial (communicating) shunt

CODING TIP Do not use Z98.2 if the ventricular shunt is complicated.

T85.01X- Breakdown (mechanical) of ventricular intracranial (communicating) shunt HCC

T85.02X- Displacement of ventricular intracranial (communicating) shunt HCC
Malposition of ventricular intracranial (communicating) shunt

T85.03X- Leakage of ventricular intracranial (communicating) shunt HCC

T85.09X- Other mechanical complication of ventricular intracranial (communicating) shunt HCC
Obstruction (mechanical) of ventricular intracranial (communicating) shunt
Perforation of ventricular intracranial (communicating) shunt
Protrusion of ventricular intracranial (communicating) shunt

T85.1 Mechanical complication of implanted electronic stimulator of nervous system

T85.11 Breakdown (mechanical) of implanted electronic stimulator of nervous system

T85.110- Breakdown (mechanical) of implanted electronic neurostimulator of brain electrode (lead) HCC

T85.111- Breakdown (mechanical) of implanted electronic neurostimulator of peripheral nerve electrode (lead) HCC
Breakdown of electrode (lead) for cranial nerve neurostimulators
Breakdown of electrode (lead) for gastric neurostimulator
Breakdown of electrode (lead) for sacral nerve neurostimulator
Breakdown of electrode (lead) for vagal nerve neurostimulators

T85.112- Breakdown (mechanical) of implanted electronic neurostimulator of spinal cord electrode (lead) HCC

▲ **T85.113- Breakdown (mechanical) of implanted electronic neurostimulator, generator** HCC
Breakdown (mechanical) of implanted electronic neurostimulator generator, brain, peripheral, gastric, spinal
Breakdown (mechanical) of implanted electronic sacral neurostimulator, pulse generator or receiver

T85.118- Breakdown (mechanical) of other implanted electronic stimulator of nervous system HCC

T85.12 Displacement of implanted electronic stimulator of nervous system
Malposition of implanted electronic stimulator of nervous system

T85.120- Displacement of implanted electronic neurostimulator of brain electrode (lead) HCC

T85.121- Displacement of implanted electronic neurostimulator of peripheral nerve electrode (lead) HCC
Displacement of electrode (lead) for cranial nerve neurostimulators
Displacement of electrode (lead) for gastric neurostimulator
Displacement of electrode (lead) for sacral nerve neurostimulator
Displacement of electrode (lead) for vagal nerve neurostimulators

T85.122- Displacement of implanted electronic neurostimulator of spinal cord electrode (lead) HCC

T85.123- Displacement of implanted electronic neurostimulator, generator HCC
Displacement of implanted electronic neurostimulator generator, brain, peripheral, gastric, spinal
Displacement of implanted electronic sacral neurostimulator, pulse generator or receiver

T85.128- Displacement of other implanted electronic stimulator of nervous system HCC

T85.19 Other mechanical complication of implanted electronic stimulator of nervous system
Leakage of implanted electronic stimulator of nervous system
Obstruction (mechanical) of implanted electronic stimulator of nervous system
Perforation of implanted electronic stimulator of nervous system
Protrusion of implanted electronic stimulator of nervous system

T85.190- Other mechanical complication of implanted electronic neurostimulator of brain electrode (lead) HCC

T85.191- Other mechanical complication of implanted electronic neurostimulator of peripheral nerve electrode (lead) HCC
Other mechanical complication of electrode (lead) for cranial nerve neurostimulators
Other mechanical complication of electrode (lead) for gastric neurostimulator
Other mechanical complication of electrode (lead) for sacral nerve neurostimulator
Other mechanical complication of electrode (lead) for vagal nerve neurostimulators

T85.192- Other mechanical complication of implanted electronic neurostimulator of spinal cord electrode (lead) HCC

T85.193- Other mechanical complication of implanted electronic neurostimulator, generator HCC
Other mechanical complication of implanted electronic neurostimulator generator, brain, peripheral, gastric, spinal
Other mechanical complication of implanted electronic sacral neurostimulator, pulse generator or receiver

T85.199- Other mechanical complication of other implanted electronic stimulator of nervous system HCC

T85.2 Mechanical complication of intraocular lens

T85.21X- Breakdown (mechanical) of intraocular lens

T85.22X- Displacement of intraocular lens
Malposition of intraocular lens

T85.29X- Other mechanical complication of intraocular lens
Obstruction (mechanical) of intraocular lens
Perforation of intraocular lens
Protrusion of intraocular lens

T85.3 Mechanical complication of other ocular prosthetic devices, implants and grafts

EXCLUDES 2 *other complications of corneal graft (T86.84-)*

T85.31 Breakdown (mechanical) of other ocular prosthetic devices, implants and grafts

T85.310- Breakdown (mechanical) of prosthetic orbit of right eye

T85.311- Breakdown (mechanical) of prosthetic orbit of left eye

7 T85.318- Breakdown (mechanical) of other ocular prosthetic devices, implants and grafts

6 T85.32 Displacement of other ocular prosthetic devices, implants and grafts
Malposition of other ocular prosthetic devices, implants and grafts

7 T85.320- Displacement of prosthetic orbit of right eye

7 T85.321- Displacement of prosthetic orbit of left eye

7 T85.328- Displacement of other ocular prosthetic devices, implants and grafts

6 T85.39 Other mechanical complication of Other ocular prosthetic devices, implants and grafts
Obstruction (mechanical) of other ocular prosthetic devices, implants and grafts
Perforation of other ocular prosthetic devices, implants and grafts
Protrusion of other ocular prosthetic devices, implants and grafts

7 T85.390- Other mechanical complication of prosthetic orbit of right eye

7 T85.391- Other mechanical complication of prosthetic orbit of left eye

7 T85.398- Other mechanical complication of other ocular prosthetic devices, implants and grafts

5 T85.4 Mechanical complication of breast prosthesis and implant

7 T85.41X- Breakdown (mechanical) of breast prosthesis and implant

7 T85.42X- Displacement of breast prosthesis and implant
Malposition of breast prosthesis and implant

7 T85.43X- Leakage of breast prosthesis and implant

7 T85.44X- Capsular contracture of breast implant

7 T85.49X- Other mechanical complication of breast prosthesis and implant
Obstruction (mechanical) of breast prosthesis and implant
Perforation of breast prosthesis and implant
Protrusion of breast prosthesis and implant

5 T85.5 Mechanical complication of gastrointestinal prosthetic devices, implants and grafts

6 T85.51 Breakdown (mechanical) of gastrointestinal prosthetic devices, implants and grafts

7 T85.510- Breakdown (mechanical) of bile duct prosthesis

7 T85.511- Breakdown (mechanical) of esophageal anti-reflux device

7 T85.518- Breakdown (mechanical) of other gastrointestinal prosthetic devices, implants and grafts

6 T85.52 Displacement of gastrointestinal prosthetic devices, implants and grafts
Malposition of gastrointestinal prosthetic devices, implants and grafts

7 T85.520- Displacement of bile duct prosthesis

7 T85.521- Displacement of esophageal anti-reflux device

7 T85.528- Displacement of other gastrointestinal prosthetic devices, implants and grafts

6 T85.59 Other mechanical complication of gastrointestinal prosthetic devices, implants and
Obstruction, mechanical of gastrointestinal prosthetic devices, implants and grafts
Perforation of gastrointestinal prosthetic devices, implants and grafts
Protrusion of gastrointestinal prosthetic devices, implants and grafts

7 T85.590- Other mechanical complication of bile duct prosthesis

7 T85.591- Other mechanical complication of esophageal anti-reflux device

7 T85.598- Other mechanical complication of other gastrointestinal prosthetic devices, implants and grafts

5 T85.6 Mechanical complication of other specified internal and external prosthetic devices, implants and grafts

GUIDELINES **Section I.C.4.a.5)(a)-(b)**
An underdose of insulin due to an insulin pump failure should be assigned to a code from subcategory T85.6 followed by code T38.3x6-, Underdosing of insulin and oral hypoglycemic [antidiabetic] drugs. Additional codes for the type of diabetes mellitus and any associated complications due to the underdosing should also be assigned.

The principal or first-listed code for an encounter due to an insulin pump malfunction resulting in an overdose of insulin, should also be T85.6- followed by code T38.3x1-, Poisoning by insulin and oral hypoglycemic [antidiabetic] drugs, accidental (unintentional).

6 T85.61 Breakdown (mechanical) of other specified internal prosthetic devices, implants and grafts

7 T85.610- Breakdown (mechanical) of cranial or spinal infusion catheter
Breakdown (mechanical) of epidural infusion catheter
Breakdown (mechanical) of intrathecal infusion catheter
Breakdown (mechanical) of subarachnoid infusion catheter
Breakdown (mechanical) of subdural infusion catheter

7 T85.611- Breakdown (mechanical) of intraperitoneal dialysis catheter HCC
EXCLUDES 1 *mechanical complication of vascular dialysis catheter (T82.4-)*

7 T85.612- Breakdown (mechanical) of permanent sutures
EXCLUDES 1 *mechanical complication of permanent (wire) suture used in bone repair (T84.1-T84.2)*

7 T85.613- Breakdown (mechanical) of artificial skin graft and decellularized allodermis
Failure of artificial skin graft and decellularized allodermis
Non-adherence of artificial skin graft and decellularized allodermis
Poor incorporation of artificial skin graft and decellularized allodermis
Shearing of artificial skin graft and decellularized allodermis

7 T85.614- Breakdown (mechanical) of insulin pump

7 T85.615- Breakdown (mechanical) of other nervous system device, implant or graft HCC
Breakdown (mechanical) of intrathecal infusion pump

7 T85.618- Breakdown (mechanical) of other specified internal prosthetic devices, implants and grafts

6 T85.62 Displacement of other specified internal prosthetic devices, implants and grafts
Malposition of other specified internal prosthetic devices, implants and grafts

7 T85.620- Displacement of cranial or spinal infusion catheter
Displacement of epidural infusion catheter
Displacement of intrathecal infusion catheter
Displacement of subarachnoid infusion catheter
Displacement of subdural infusion catheter

7 T85.621- Displacement of intraperitoneal dialysis catheter HCC
EXCLUDES 1 *mechanical complication of vascular dialysis catheter (T82.4-)*

7 T85.622- Displacement of permanent sutures
EXCLUDES 1 *mechanical complication of permanent (wire) suture used in bone repair (T84.1-T84.2)*

7 T85.623- Displacement of artificial skin graft and decellularized allodermis
Dislodgement of artificial skin graft and decellularized allodermis

7 T85.624- Displacement of insulin pump

7 T85.625- Displacement of other nervous system device, implant or graft HCC
Displacement of intrathecal infusion pump

7 **T85.628- Displacement of other specified internal prosthetic devices, implants and grafts**
AHA: (T85.628A) 1Q 2015, 15

6 **T85.63 Leakage of other specified internal prosthetic devices, implants and grafts**

7 **T85.630- Leakage of cranial or spinal infusion catheter**
Leakage of epidural infusion catheter
Leakage of intrathecal infusion catheter infusion catheter
Leakage of subdural infusion catheter
Leakage of subarachnoid infusion catheter

7 **T85.631- Leakage of intraperitoneal dialysis catheter** HCC
EXCLUDES 1 *mechanical complication of vascular dialysis catheter (T82.4)*

7 **T85.633- Leakage of insulin pump**

7 **T85.635- Leakage of other nervous system device, implant or graft** HCC
Leakage of intrathecal infusion pump

7 **T85.638- Leakage of other specified internal prosthetic devices, implants and grafts**

6 **T85.69 Other mechanical complication of other specified internal prosthetic devices, implants and grafts**
Obstruction, mechanical of other specified internal prosthetic devices, implants and grafts
Perforation of other specified internal prosthetic devices, implants and grafts
Protrusion of other specified internal prosthetic devices, implants and grafts

7 **T85.690- Other mechanical complication of cranial or spinal infusion catheter**
Other mechanical complication of epidural infusion catheter
Other mechanical complication of intrathecal infusion catheter
Other mechanical complication of subarachnoid infusion catheter
Other mechanical complication of subdural infusion catheter

7 **T85.691- Other mechanical complication of intraperitoneal dialysis catheter** HCC
EXCLUDES 1 *mechanical complication of vascular dialysis catheter (T82.4)*

7 **T85.692- Other mechanical complication of permanent sutures**
EXCLUDES 1 *mechanical complication of permanent (wire) suture used in bone repair (T84.1-T84.2)*

7 **T85.693- Other mechanical complication of artificial skin graft and decellularized allodermis**

7 **T85.694- Other mechanical complication of insulin pump**

7 **T85.695- Other mechanical complication of other nervous system device, implant or graft** HCC
Other mechanical complication of intrathecal infusion pump

7 **T85.698- Other mechanical complication of other specified internal prosthetic devices, implants and grafts**
Mechanical complication of nonabsorbable surgical material NOS

5 **T85.7 Infection and inflammatory reaction due to other internal prosthetic devices, implants and grafts**
Use additional code to identify infection

7 **T85.71X- Infection and inflammatory reaction due to peritoneal dialysis catheter** HCC

7 **T85.72X- Infection and inflammatory reaction due to insulin pump** HCC

6 **T85.73 Infection and inflammatory reaction due to nervous system devices, implants and graft**

7 **T85.730- Infection and inflammatory reaction due to ventricular intracranial (communicating) shunt** HCC

7 **T85.731- Infection and inflammatory reaction due to implanted electronic neurostimulator of brain, electrode (lead)** HCC

7 **T85.732- Infection and inflammatory reaction due to implanted electronic neurostimulator of peripheral nerve, electrode (lead)** HCC
Infection and inflammatory reaction due to electrode (lead) for cranial nerve neurostimulators
Infection and inflammatory reaction due to electrode (lead) for gastric neurostimulator
Infection and inflammatory reaction due to electrode (lead) for sacral nerve neurostimulator
Infection and inflammatory reaction due to electrode (lead) for vagal nerve neurostimulators

7 **T85.733- Infection and inflammatory reaction due to implanted electronic neurostimulator of spinal cord, electrode (lead)** HCC

7 **T85.734- Infection and inflammatory reaction due to implanted electronic neurostimulator , generator** HCC
Generator pocket infection

7 **T85.735- Infection and inflammatory reaction due to cranial or spinal infusion catheter** HCC
Infection and inflammatory reaction due to epidural catheter
Infection and inflammatory reaction due to intrathecal infusion catheter
Infection and inflammatory reaction due to subarachnoid catheter
Infection and inflammatory reaction due to subdural catheter

7 **T85.738- Infection and inflammatory reaction due to other nervous system device, implant or graft** HCC
Infection and inflammatory reaction due to intrathecal infusion pump

7 **T85.79X- Infection and inflammatory reaction due to other internal prosthetic devices, implants and grafts** HCC

5 **T85.8 Other specified complications of internal prosthetic devices, implants and grafts, not elsewhere classified**

6 **T85.81 Embolism due to internal prosthetic devices, implants and grafts, not elsewhere classified**

7 **T85.810- Embolism due to nervous system prosthetic devices, implants and grafts** HCC

7 **T85.818- Embolism due to other internal prosthetic devices, implants and grafts**

6 **T85.82 Fibrosis due to internal prosthetic devices, implants and grafts, not elsewhere classified**

7 **T85.820- Fibrosis due to nervous system prosthetic devices, implants and grafts** HCC

7 **T85.828- Fibrosis due to other internal prosthetic devices, implants and grafts**

6 **T85.83 Hemorrhage due to internal prosthetic devices, implants and grafts, not elsewhere classified**

7 **T85.830- Hemorrhage due to nervous system prosthetic devices, implants and grafts** HCC

7 **T85.838- Hemorrhage due to other internal prosthetic devices, implants and grafts**

6 **T85.84 Pain due to internal prosthetic devices, implants and grafts, not elsewhere classified**

7 **T85.840- Pain due to nervous system prosthetic devices, implants and grafts** HCC

7 **T85.848- Pain due to other internal prosthetic devices, implants and grafts**

6 **T85.85 Stenosis due to internal prosthetic devices, implants and grafts, not elsewhere classified**

7 **T85.850- Stenosis due to nervous system prosthetic devices, implants and grafts** HCC

7 **T85.858- Stenosis due to other internal prosthetic devices, implants and grafts**

6 **T85.86 Thrombosis due to internal prosthetic devices, implants and grafts, not elsewhere classified**

7 **T85.860- Thrombosis due to nervous system prosthetic devices, implants and grafts** HCC

7 **T85.868- Thrombosis due to other internal prosthetic devices, implants and grafts**

6 **T85.89 Other specified complication of internal prosthetic devices, implants and grafts, not elsewhere classified**
Erosion or breakdown of subcutaneous device pocket

7 T85.890- Other specified complication of nervous system prosthetic devices, implants and grafts HCC
7 T85.898- Other specified complication of other internal prosthetic devices, implants and grafts
7 T85.9XX- Unspecified complication of internal prosthetic device, implant and graft
Complication of internal prosthetic device, implant and graft NOS

4 **T86 Complications of transplanted organs and tissue**
Use additional code to identify other transplant complications, such as:
graft-versus-host disease (D89.81-)
malignancy associated with organ transplant (C80.2)
post-transplant lymphoproliferative disorders (PTLD) (D47.Z1)

GUIDELINES Section I.C.2.r
A malignant neoplasm of a transplanted organ should be coded as a transplant complication. Assign first the appropriate code from category T86.-, Complications of transplanted organs and tissue, followed by code C80.2. Use an additional code for the specific malignancy.

GUIDELINES Section I.C.19.g.3)(a)
Codes under category T86, Complications of transplanted organs and tissues, are for use for both complications and rejection of transplanted organs. A transplant complication code is only assigned if the complication affects the function of the transplanted organ. Two codes are required to fully describe a transplant complication: the appropriate code from category T86 and a secondary code that identifies the complication.

Pre-existing conditions or conditions that develop after the transplant are not coded as complications unless they affect the function of the transplanted organs.

CODING TIP✓ Do not assume dysfunction in a transplanted organ to be a complication of a transplanted organ unless specifically stated by a provider diagnostic statement. The only exception to this is a malignant neoplasm of a transplanted organ. A neoplasm associated with a transplant is coded as an "other complication of transplant" unless specified by the physician as a failure or rejection.

5 **T86.0 Complications of bone marrow transplant**
T86.00 Unspecified complication of bone marrow transplant HCC
T86.01 Bone marrow transplant rejection HCC
T86.02 Bone marrow transplant failure HCC
T86.03 Bone marrow transplant infection HCC
T86.09 Other complications of bone marrow transplant HCC

5 **T86.1 Complications of kidney transplant**

GUIDELINES Section I.C.19.g.3)(b)
Patients who have undergone kidney transplant may still have some form of chronic kidney disease (CKD) because the kidney transplant may not fully restore kidney function ... Code T86.1- should not be assigned for post kidney transplant patients who have CKD unless a transplant complication such as transplant failure or rejection is documented. If the documentation is unclear as to whether the patient has a complication of the transplant, query the provider.

Conditions that affect the function of the transplanted kidney, other than CKD, should be assigned a code from subcategory T86.1 and a secondary code that identifies the complication. For patients with CKD following a kidney transplant, but who do not have a complication such as failure or rejection
, see section I.C.14. Chronic kidney disease and kidney transplant status.

T86.10 Unspecified complication of kidney transplant
T86.11 Kidney transplant rejection
T86.12 Kidney transplant failure
AHA: 1Q 2013, 24
T86.13 Kidney transplant infection
Use additional code to specify infection
T86.19 Other complication of kidney transplant

5 **T86.2 Complications of heart transplant**
EXCLUDES 1 *complication of:*
artificial heart device (T82.5)
heart-lung transplant (T86.3)
T86.20 Unspecified complication of heart transplant HCC
T86.21 Heart transplant rejection HCC
T86.22 Heart transplant failure HCC
T86.23 Heart transplant infection HCC
Use additional code to specify infection
6 T86.29 Other complications of heart transplant
T86.290 Cardiac allograft vasculopathy HCC
EXCLUDES 1 *atherosclerosis of coronary arteries (I25.75-, I25.76-, I25.81-)*
T86.298 Other complications of heart transplant HCC

5 **T86.3 Complications of heart-lung transplant**
T86.30 Unspecified complication of heart-lung transplant HCC
T86.31 Heart-lung transplant rejection HCC
T86.32 Heart-lung transplant failure HCC
T86.33 Heart-lung transplant infection HCC
Use additional code to specify infection
T86.39 Other complications of heart-lung transplant HCC

5 **T86.4 Complications of liver transplant**
T86.40 Unspecified complication of liver transplant HCC
T86.41 Liver transplant rejection HCC
T86.42 Liver transplant failure HCC
T86.43 Liver transplant infection HCC
Use additional code to identify infection, such as: Cytomegalovirus (CMV) infection (B25.-)
T86.49 Other complications of liver transplant HCC

T86.5 Complications of stem cell transplant HCC
Complications from stem cells from peripheral blood
Complications from stem cells from umbilical cord

5 **T86.8 Complications of other transplanted organs and tissues**
6 T86.81 Complications of lung transplant
EXCLUDES 1 *complication of heart-lung transplant (T86.3-)*
T86.810 Lung transplant rejection HCC
T86.811 Lung transplant failure HCC
T86.812 Lung transplant infection HCC
Use additional code to specify infection
T86.818 Other complications of lung transplant HCC
T86.819 Unspecified complication of lung transplant HCC

6 T86.82 Complications of skin graft (allograft) (autograft)
EXCLUDES 2 *complication of artificial skin graft (T85.693)*
CODING TIP✓ Use code T86.82- when a skin graft fails. Use T85.693- if the skin graft is artificial.
T86.820 Skin graft (allograft) rejection
T86.821 Skin graft (allograft) (autograft) failure
T86.822 Skin graft (allograft) (autograft) infection
Use additional code to specify infection
T86.828 Other complications of skin graft (allograft) (autograft)
T86.829 Unspecified complication of skin graft (allograft) (autograft)

6 T86.83 Complications of bone graft
EXCLUDES 2 *mechanical complications of bone graft (T84.3-)*
T86.830 Bone graft rejection
T86.831 Bone graft failure
T86.832 Bone graft infection
Use additional code to specify infection
T86.838 Other complications of bone graft
T86.839 Unspecified complication of bone graft

6 T86.84 Complications of corneal transplant
EXCLUDES 2 *mechanical complications of corneal graft (T85.3-)*
T86.840 Corneal transplant rejection
T86.841 Corneal transplant failure
T86.842 Corneal transplant infection HCC
Use additional code to specify infection
T86.848 Other complications of corneal transplant

T86.849 Unspecified complication of corneal transplant

T86.85 Complication of intestine transplant

T86.850 Intestine transplant rejection HCC

T86.851 Intestine transplant failure HCC

T86.852 Intestine transplant infection HCC

Use additional code to specify infection

T86.858 Other complications of intestine transplant HCC

T86.859 Unspecified complication of intestine transplant HCC

T86.89 Complications of other transplanted tissue

Transplant failure or rejection of pancreas

T86.890 Other transplanted tissue rejection

T86.891 Other transplanted tissue failure

T86.892 Other transplanted tissue infection

Use additional code to specify infection

T86.898 Other complications of Other transplanted tissue

T86.899 Unspecified complication of other transplanted tissue

T86.9 Complication of unspecified transplanted organ and tissue

T86.90 Unspecified complication of Unspecified transplanted organ and tissue

T86.91 Unspecified transplanted organ and tissue rejection

T86.92 Unspecified transplanted organ and tissue failure

T86.93 Unspecified transplanted organ and tissue infection

Use additional code to specify infection

T86.99 Other complications of unspecified transplanted organ and tissue

T87 Complications peculiar to reattachment and amputation

T87.0 Complications of reattached (part of) upper extremity

T87.0X Complications of reattached (part of) upper extremity

T87.0X1 Complications of reattached (part of) right upper extremity HCC

T87.0X2 Complications of reattached (part of) left upper extremity HCC

T87.0X9 Complications of reattached (part of) unspecified upper extremity HCC

T87.1 Complications of reattached (part of) lower extremity

T87.1X Complications of reattached (part of) lower extremity

T87.1X1 Complications of reattached (part of) right lower extremity HCC

T87.1X2 Complications of reattached (part of) left lower extremity HCC

T87.1X9 Complications of reattached (part of) unspecified lower extremity HCC

T87.2 Complications of other reattached body part HCC

T87.3 Neuroma of amputation stump

CODING TIP ✓ Use T87.3-T87.89 to report a complication of a surgical stump amputation. The complication may or may not be chronic. Do not report a code from T87 when the encounter is related to treatment of a traumatic amputation.

T87.30 Neuroma of amputation stump, unspecified extremity HCC

T87.31 Neuroma of amputation stump, right upper extremity HCC

T87.32 Neuroma of amputation stump, left upper extremity HCC

T87.33 Neuroma of amputation stump, right lower extremity HCC

T87.34 Neuroma of amputation stump, left lower extremity HCC

T87.4 Infection of amputation stump

T87.40 Infection of amputation stump, unspecified extremity HCC

T87.41 Infection of amputation stump, right upper extremity HCC

T87.42 Infection of amputation stump, left upper extremity HCC

T87.43 Infection of amputation stump, right lower extremity HCC

T87.44 Infection of amputation stump, left lower extremity HCC

T87.5 Necrosis of amputation stump

T87.50 Necrosis of amputation stump, unspecified extremity HCC

T87.51 Necrosis of amputation stump, right upper extremity HCC

T87.52 Necrosis of amputation stump, left upper extremity HCC

T87.53 Necrosis of amputation stump, right lower extremity HCC

T87.54 Necrosis of amputation stump, left lower extremity HCC

T87.8 Other complications of amputation stump

T87.81 Dehiscence of amputation stump HCC

CODING TIP ✓ When a patient presents with a dehiscence of an amputation stump wound, assign code T87.81. When both dehiscence and infection are present, code the dehiscence first (T87.81), followed by infection. Use an additional code to specify the infection.

CODING TIP ✓ Disruption of the operative wound for an amputation is coded here and not with T81.31-.

T87.89 Other complications of amputation stump HCC

Amputation stump contracture

Amputation stump contracture of next proximal joint

Amputation stump flexion

Amputation stump edema

Amputation stump hematoma

EXCLUDES 2 *phantom limb syndrome (G54.6-G54.7)*

CODING TIP ✓ Do not assign a code for complication of an amputation stump for an ulcer (due to pressure, diabetic ulcer, arterial, trauma, stasis, or other) of the amputation stump. Ulcers of the amputation stump are not considered amputation stump complications. Use the L89 codes for pressure ulcer/injury and the staging system to stage.

T87.9 Unspecified complications of amputation stump HCC

T88 Other complications of surgical and medical care, not elsewhere classified

EXCLUDES 2
complication following infusion, transfusion and therapeutic injection (T80.-)
complication following procedure NEC (T81.-)
complications of anesthesia in labor and delivery (O74.-)
complications of anesthesia in pregnancy (O29.-)
complications of anesthesia in puerperium (O89.-)
complications of devices, implants and grafts (T82-T85)
complications of obstetric surgery and procedure (O75.4)
dermatitis due to drugs and medicaments (L23.3, L24.4, L25.1, L27.0-L27.1)
poisoning and toxic effects of drugs and chemicals (T36-T65 with fifth or sixth character 1-4 or 6)
specified complications classified elsewhere

The appropriate 7th character is to be added to each code from category T88
A initial encounter
D subsequent encounter
S sequela

T88.0XX- Infection following immunization

Sepsis following immunization

7 T88.1XX- **Other complications following immunization, not elsewhere classified**
Generalized vaccinia
Rash following immunization
EXCLUDES 1 *vaccinia not from vaccine (B08.011)*
EXCLUDES 2 *anaphylactic shock due to serum (T80.5-)*
other serum reactions (T80.6-)
postimmunization arthropathy (M02.2)
postimmunization encephalitis (G04.02)
postimmunization fever (R50.83)

7 T88.2XX- **Shock due to anesthesia**
Use additional code for adverse effect, if applicable, to identify drug (T41.- with fifth or sixth character 5)
EXCLUDES 1 *complications of anesthesia (in) :*
labor and delivery (O74.-)
pregnancy (O29.-)
puerperium (O89.-)
postprocedural shock NOS (T81.1-)

7 T88.3XX- **Malignant hyperthermia due to anesthesia**
Use additional code for adverse effect, if applicable, to identify drug (T41.- with fifth or sixth character 5)

7 T88.4XX- **Failed or difficult intubation**

5 T88.5 **Other complications of anesthesia**
Use additional code for adverse effect, if applicable, to identify drug (T41.- with fifth or sixth character 5)

7 T88.51X- **Hypothermia following anesthesia**

7 T88.52X- **Failed moderate sedation during procedure**
Failed conscious sedation during procedure
EXCLUDES 2 *personal history of failed moderate sedation (Z92.83)*

7 T88.53X- **Unintended awareness under general anesthesia during procedure**
EXCLUDES 2 *personal history of unintended awareness under general anesthesia (Z92.84)*
AHA: 4Q 2016, 72

7 T88.59X- **Other complications of anesthesia**

7 T88.6XX- **Anaphylactic reaction due to adverse effect of correct drug or medicament properly administered**
Anaphylactic shock due to adverse effect of correct drug or medicament properly administered
Anaphylactoid reaction NOS
Use additional code for adverse effect, if applicable, to identify drug (T36-T50 with fifth or sixth character 5)
EXCLUDES 1 *anaphylactic reaction due to serum (T80.5-)*
anaphylactic shock or reaction due to adverse food reaction (T78.0-)

7 T88.7XX- **Unspecified adverse effect of drug or medicament**
Drug hypersensitivity NOS
Drug reaction NOS
Use additional code for adverse effect, if applicable, to identify drug (T36-T50 with fifth or sixth character 5)
EXCLUDES 1 *specified adverse effects of drugs and medicaments (A00-R94 and T80-T88.6, T88.8)*

7 T88.8XX- **Other specified complications of surgical and medical care, not elsewhere classified**
Use additional code to identify the complication

7 T88.9XX- **Complication of surgical and medical care, unspecified**

CHAPTER 20: EXTERNAL CAUSES OF MORBIDITY (V00-Y99)

Note: This chapter permits the classification of environmental events and circumstances as the cause of injury, and other adverse effects. Where a code from this section is applicable, it is intended that it shall be used secondary to a code from another chapter of the Classification indicating the nature of the condition. Most often, the condition will be classifiable to Chapter 19, Injury, poisoning and certain other consequences of external causes (S00-T88). Other conditions that may be stated to be due to external causes are classified in Chapters I to XVIII. For these conditions, codes from Chapter 20 should be used to provide additional information as to the cause of the condition.

GUIDELINES **Section I.C.20**

The external causes of morbidity codes should never be sequenced as the first-listed or principal diagnosis. External cause codes are intended to provide data for injury research and evaluation of injury prevention strategies. These codes capture how the injury or health condition happened (cause), the intent (unintentional or accidental; or intentional, such as suicide or assault), the place where the event occurred the activity of the patient at the time of the event, and the person's status (e.g., civilian, military).

There is no national requirement for mandatory ICD-10-CM external cause code reporting. Unless a provider is subject to a state-based external cause code reporting mandate or these codes are required by a particular payer, reporting of ICD-10-CM codes in Chapter 20, External Causes of Morbidity, is not required. In the absence of a mandatory reporting requirement, providers are encouraged to voluntarily report external cause codes, as they provide valuable data for injury research and evaluation of injury prevention strategies.

GUIDELINES **Section I.C.20.a.2)**

Most categories in chapter 20 have a 7th character requirement for each applicable code. ... While the patient may be seen by a new or different provider over the course of treatment for an injury or condition, assignment of the 7th character for external cause should match the 7th character of the code assigned for the associated injury or condition for the encounter.

This chapter contains the following blocks:

V00-X58	Accidents
V00-V99	Transport accidents
V00-V09	Pedestrian injured in transport accident
V10-V19	Pedal cycle rider injured in transport accident
V20-V29	Motorcycle rider injured in transport accident
V30-V39	Occupant of three-wheeled motor vehicle injured in transport accident
V40-V49	Car occupant injured in transport accident
V50-V59	Occupant of pick-up truck or van injured in transport accident
V60-V69	Occupant of heavy transport vehicle injured in transport accident
V70-V79	Bus occupant injured in transport accident
V80-V89	Other land transport accidents
V90-V94	Water transport accidents
V95-V97	Air and space transport accidents
V98-V99	Other and unspecified transport accidents
W00-X58	Other external causes of accidental injury
W00-W19	Slipping, tripping, stumbling and falls
W20-W49	Exposure to inanimate mechanical forces
W50-W64	Exposure to animate mechanical forces
W65-W74	Accidental non-transport drowning and submersion
W85-W99	Exposure to electric current, radiation and extreme ambient air temperature and pressure
X00-X08	Exposure to smoke, fire and flames
X10-X19	Contact with heat and hot substances
X30-X39	Exposure to forces of nature
X50	Overexertion and strenuous or repetitive movements
X52-X58	Accidental exposure to other specified factors
X71-X83	Intentional self-harm
X92-Y09	Assault
Y21-Y33	Event of undetermined intent
Y35-Y38	Legal intervention, operations of war, military operations, and terrorism
Y62-Y84	Complications of medical and surgical care
Y62-Y69	Misadventures to patients during surgical and medical care
Y70-Y82	Medical devices associated with adverse incidents in diagnostic and therapeutic use
Y83-Y84	Surgical and other medical procedures as the cause of abnormal reaction of the patient, or of later complication, without mention of misadventure at the time of the procedure
Y90-Y99	Supplementary factors related to causes of morbidity classified elsewhere

Accidents (V00-X58)

Transport accidents (V00-V99)

Note: This section is structured in 12 groups. Those relating to land transport accidents (V00-V89) reflect the victim's mode of transport and are subdivided to identify the victim's 'counterpart' or the type of event. The vehicle of which the injured person is an occupant is identified in the first two characters since it is seen as the most important factor to identify for prevention purposes. A transport accident is one in which the vehicle involved must be moving or running or in use for transport purposes at the time of the accident.

Definitions related to transport accidents:

(a) A transport accident (V00-V99) is any accident involving a device designed primarily for, or used at the time primarily for, conveying persons or good from one place to another.

(b) A public highway [trafficway] or street is the entire width between property lines (or other boundary lines) of land open to the public as a matter of right or custom for purposes of moving persons or property from one place to another. A roadway is that part of the public highway designed, improved and customarily used for vehicular traffic.

(c) A traffic accident is any vehicle accident occurring on the public highway [i.e. originating on, terminating on, or involving a vehicle partially on the highway]. A vehicle accident is assumed to have occurred on the public highway unless another place is specified, except in the case of accidents involving only off-road motor vehicles, which are classified as nontraffic accidents unless the contrary is stated.

(d) A nontraffic accident is any vehicle accident that occurs entirely in any place other than a public highway.

(e) A pedestrian is any person involved in an accident who was not at the time of the accident riding in or on a motor vehicle, railway train, streetcar or animal-drawn or other vehicle, or on a pedal cycle or animal. This includes, a person changing a tire, working on a parked car, or a person on foot. It also includes the user of a pedestrian conveyance such as a baby stroller, ice-skates, skis, sled, roller skates, a skateboard, nonmotorized or motorized wheelchair, motorized mobility scooter, or nonmotorized scooter.

(f) A driver is an occupant of a transport vehicle who is operating or intending to operate it.

(g) A passenger is any occupant of a transport vehicle other than the driver, except a person traveling on the outside of the vehicle.

(h) A person on the outside of a vehicle is any person being transported by a vehicle but not occupying the space normally reserved for the driver or passengers, or the space intended for the transport of property. This includes a person travelling on the bodywork, bumper, fender, roof, running board or step of a vehicle, as well as, hanging on the outside of the vehicle.

(i) A pedal cycle is any land transport vehicle operated solely by nonmotorized pedals including a bicycle or tricycle.

(j) A pedal cyclist is any person riding a pedal cycle or in a sidecar or trailer attached to a pedal cycle.

(k) A motorcycle is a two-wheeled motor vehicle with one or two riding saddles and sometimes with a third wheel for the support of a sidecar. The sidecar is considered part of the motorcycle. This includes a moped, motor scooter, or motorized bicycle.

(l) A motorcycle rider is any person riding a motorcycle or in a sidecar or trailer attached to the motorcycle.

(m) A three-wheeled motor vehicle is a motorized tricycle designed primarily for on-road use. This includes a motor-driven tricycle, a motorized rickshaw, or a three-wheeled motor car.

(n) A car [automobile] is a four-wheeled motor vehicle designed primarily for carrying up to 7 persons. A trailer being towed by the car is considered part of the car. It does not include a van or minivan - see definition (o)

(o) A pick-up truck or van is a four or six-wheeled motor vehicle designed for carrying passengers as well as property or cargo weighing less than the local limit for classification as a heavy goods vehicle, and not requiring a special driver's license. This includes a minivan and a sport-utility vehicle (SUV).

(p) A heavy transport vehicle is a motor vehicle designed primarily for carrying property, meeting local criteria for classification as a heavy goods vehicle in terms of weight and requiring a special driver's license.

(q) A bus (coach) is a motor vehicle designed or adapted primarily for carrying more than 10 passengers, and requiring a special driver's license.

(r) A railway train or railway vehicle is any device, with or without freight or passenger cars couple to it, designed for traffic on a railway track. This includes subterranean (subways) or elevated trains.

(s) A streetcar, is a device designed and used primarily for transporting passengers within a municipality, running on rails, usually subject to normal traffic control signals, and operated principally on a right-of-way that forms part of the roadway. This includes a tram or trolley that runs on rails. A trailer being towed by a streetcar is considered part of the streetcar.

(t) A special vehicle mainly used on industrial premises is a motor vehicle designed primarily for use within the buildings and premises of industrial or commercial establishments. This includes battery-powered airport passenger vehicles or baggage/mail trucks, forklifts, coal-cars in a coal mine, logging cars and trucks used in mines or quarries.

(u) A special vehicle mainly used in agriculture is a motor vehicle designed specifically for use in farming and agriculture (horticulture), to work the land, tend and harvest crops and transport materials on the farm. This includes harvesters, farm machinery and tractor and trailers.

(v) A special construction vehicle is a motor vehicle designed specifically for use on construction and demolition sites. This includes bulldozers, diggers, earth levellers, dump trucks. backhoes, front-end loaders, pavers, and mechanical shovels.

(w) A special all-terrain vehicle is a motor vehicle of special design to enable it to negotiate over rough or soft terrain, snow or sand. Examples of special design are high construction, special wheels and tires, tracks, and support on a cushion of air. This includes snow mobiles, All-terrain vehicles (ATV), and dune buggies. It does not include passenger vehicle designated as Sport Utility Vehicles. (SUV)

(x) A watercraft is any device designed for transporting passengers or goods on water. This includes motor or sail boats, ships, and hovercraft.

(y) An aircraft is any device for transporting passengers or goods in the air. This includes hot-air balloons, gliders, helicopters and airplanes.

(z) A military vehicle is any motorized vehicle operating on a public roadway owned by the military and being operated by a member of the military.

Use additional code to identify:
Airbag injury (W22.1)
Type of street or road (Y92.4-)
Use of cellular telephone and other electronic equipment at the time of the transport accident (Y93.C-)

EXCLUDES 1 *agricultural vehicles in stationary use or maintenance (W31.-)*
assault by crashing of motor vehicle (Y03.-)
automobile or motor cycle in stationary use or maintenance- code to type of accident
crashing of motor vehicle, undetermined intent (Y32)
intentional self-harm by crashing of motor vehicle (X82)

EXCLUDES 2 *transport accidents due to cataclysm (X34-X38)*

Pedestrian injured in transport accident (V00-V09)

INCLUDES person changing tire on transport vehicle
person examining engine of vehicle broken down in (on side of) road

EXCLUDES 1 *fall due to non-transport collision with other person (W03)*
pedestrian on foot falling (slipping) on ice and snow (W00.-)
struck or bumped by another person (W51)

4 V00 Pedestrian conveyance accident
Use additional place of occurrence and activity external cause codes, if known (Y92.-, Y93.-)

EXCLUDES 1 *collision with another person without fall (W51)*
fall due to person on foot colliding with another person on foot (W03)
fall from non-moving wheelchair, nonmotorized scooter and motorized mobility scooter without collision (W05.-)
pedestrian (conveyance) collision with other land transport vehicle (V01-V09)
pedestrian on foot falling (slipping) on ice and snow (W00.-)

The appropriate 7th character is to be added to each code from category V00
A initial encounter
D subsequent encounter
S sequela

5 V00.0 Pedestrian on foot injured in collision with pedestrian conveyance

7 V00.01X- Pedestrian on foot injured in collision with roller-skater

7 V00.02X- Pedestrian on foot injured in collision with skateboarder

7 V00.09X- Pedestrian on foot injured in collision with other pedestrian conveyance

▲ **5 V00.1 Rolling-type pedestrian conveyance accident**

EXCLUDES 1 *accident with baby stroller (V00.82-)*
accident with wheelchair (powered) (V00.81-)
accident with motorized mobility scooter (V00.83-)

6 V00.11 In-line roller-skate accident

7 V00.111- Fall from in-line roller-skates

7 V00.112- In-line roller-skater colliding with stationary object
7 V00.118- Other in-line roller-skate accident
EXCLUDES 1 *roller-skater collision with other land transport vehicle (V01-V09 with 5th character 1)*
6 V00.12 Non-in- line roller-skate accident
7 V00.121- Fall from non-in-line roller-skates
7 V00.122- Non-in-line roller-skater colliding with stationary object
7 V00.128- Other non-in-line roller-skating accident
EXCLUDES 1 *roller-skater collision with other land transport vehicle (V01-V09 with 5th character 1)*
6 V00.13 Skateboard accident
7 V00.131- Fall from skateboard
7 V00.132- Skateboarder colliding with stationary object
7 V00.138- Other skateboard accident
EXCLUDES 1 *skateboarder collision with other land transport vehicle (V01-V09 with 5th character 2)*
▲ 6 V00.14 Scooter (nonmotorized) accident
EXCLUDES 1 *motor scooter accident (V20-V29)*
7 V00.141- Fall from scooter (nonmotorized)
7 V00.142- Scooter (nonmotorized) colliding with stationary object
7 V00.148- Other scooter (nonmotorized) accident
EXCLUDES 1 *scooter (nonmotorized) collision with other land transport vehicle (V01-V09 with fifth character 9)*
6 V00.15 Heelies accident
Rolling shoe
Wheeled shoe
Wheelies accident
7 V00.151- Fall from heelies
7 V00.152- Heelies colliding with stationary object
7 V00.158- Other heelies accident
6 V00.18 Accident on other rolling-type pedestrian conveyance
7 V00.181- Fall from other rolling-type pedestrian conveyance
7 V00.182- Pedestrian on other rolling-type pedestrian conveyance colliding with stationary object
7 V00.188- Other accident on Other rolling-type pedestrian conveyance
5 V00.2 Gliding-type pedestrian conveyance accident
6 V00.21 Ice-skates accident
7 V00.211- Fall from ice-skates
7 V00.212- Ice-skater colliding with stationary object
▲ 7 V00.218- Other ice-skates accident
EXCLUDES 1 *ice-skater collision with other land transport vehicle (V01-V09 with 5th character 9)*
6 V00.22 Sled accident
7 V00.221- Fall from sled
7 V00.222- Sledder colliding with stationary object
▲ 7 V00.228- Other sled accident
EXCLUDES 1 *sled collision with other land transport vehicle (V01-V09 with 5th character 9)*
6 V00.28 Other gliding-type pedestrian conveyance accident
7 V00.281- Fall from other gliding-type pedestrian conveyance
7 V00.282- Pedestrian on other gliding-type pedestrian conveyance colliding with stationary object
▲ 7 V00.288- Other accident on other gliding-type pedestrian conveyance
EXCLUDES 1 *gliding-type pedestrian conveyance collision with other land transport vehicle (V01-V09 with 5th character 9)*
5 V00.3 Flat-bottomed pedestrian conveyance accident
6 V00.31 Snowboard accident
7 V00.311- Fall from snowboard
7 V00.312- Snowboarder colliding with stationary object
▲ 7 V00.318- Other snowboard accident
EXCLUDES 1 *snowboarder collision with other land transport vehicle (V01-V09 with 5th character 9)*
6 V00.32 Snow-ski accident
7 V00.321- Fall from snow-skis
AHA: (V00.321A) 1Q 2015, 12
7 V00.322- Snow-skier colliding with stationary object
▲ 7 V00.328- Other snow-ski accident
EXCLUDES 1 *snow-skier collision with other land transport vehicle (V01-V09 with 5th character 9)*
6 V00.38 Other flat-bottomed pedestrian conveyance accident
7 V00.381- Fall from other flat-bottomed pedestrian conveyance
7 V00.382- Pedestrian on other flat-bottomed pedestrian conveyance colliding with stationary object
7 V00.388- Other accident on other flat-bottomed pedestrian conveyance
5 V00.8 Accident on other pedestrian conveyance
6 V00.81 Accident with wheelchair (powered)
7 V00.811- Fall from moving wheelchair (powered)
EXCLUDES 1 *fall from non-moving wheelchair (W05.0)*
7 V00.812- Wheelchair (powered) colliding with stationary object
7 V00.818- Other accident with wheelchair (powered)
▲ 6 V00.82 Accident with baby stroller
▲ 7 V00.821- Fall from baby stroller
▲ 7 V00.822- Baby stroller colliding with stationary object
▲ 7 V00.828- Other accident with baby stroller
6 V00.83 Accident with motorized mobility scooter
7 V00.831- Fall from motorized mobility scooter
EXCLUDES 1 *fall from non-moving motorized mobility scooter (W05.2)*
7 V00.832- Motorized mobility scooter colliding with stationary object
7 V00.838- Other accident with motorized mobility scooter
6 V00.89 Accident on other pedestrian conveyance
7 V00.891- Fall from other pedestrian conveyance
7 V00.892- Pedestrian on other pedestrian conveyance colliding with stationary object
▲ 7 V00.898- Other accident on Other pedestrian conveyance
EXCLUDES 1 *other pedestrian (conveyance) collision with other land transport vehicle (V01-V09 with 5th character 9)*

4 V01 Pedestrian injured in collision with pedal cycle

The appropriate 7th character is to be added to each code from category V01
A initial encounter
D subsequent encounter
S sequela

5 V01.0 Pedestrian injured in collision with pedal cycle in nontraffic accident
7 V01.00X- Pedestrian on foot injured in collision with pedal cycle in nontraffic accident
Pedestrian NOS injured in collision with pedal cycle in nontraffic accident

7 **V01.01X- Pedestrian on roller-skates injured in collision with pedal cycle in nontraffic accident**

7 **V01.02X- Pedestrian on skateboard injured in collision with pedal cycle in nontraffic accident**

▲ 7 **V01.09X- Pedestrian with other conveyance injured in collision with pedal cycle in nontraffic accident**
Pedestrian with baby stroller injured in collision with pedal cycle in nontraffic accident
Pedestrian on ice-skates injured in collision with pedal cycle in nontraffic accident
Pedestrian on nonmotorized scooter injured in collision with pedal cycle in nontraffic accident
Pedestrian on sled injured in collision with pedal cycle in nontraffic accident
Pedestrian on snowboard injured in collision with pedal cycle in nontraffic accident
Pedestrian on snow-skis injured in collision with pedal cycle in nontraffic accident
Pedestrian in wheelchair (powered) injured in collision with pedal cycle in nontraffic accident
Pedestrian in motorized mobility scooter injured in collision with pedal cycle in nontraffic accident

5 **V01.1 Pedestrian injured in collision with pedal cycle in traffic accident**

7 **V01.10X- Pedestrian on foot injured in collision with pedal cycle in traffic accident**
Pedestrian NOS injured in collision with pedal cycle in traffic accident

7 **V01.11X- Pedestrian on roller-skates injured in collision with pedal cycle in traffic accident**

7 **V01.12X- Pedestrian on skateboard injured in collision with pedal cycle in traffic accident**

▲ 7 **V01.19X- Pedestrian with other conveyance injured in collision with pedal cycle in traffic accident**
Pedestrian with baby stroller injured in collision with pedal cycle in traffic accident
Pedestrian on ice-skates injured in collision with pedal cycle in traffic accident
Pedestrian on nonmotorized scooter injured in collision with pedal cycle in traffic accident
Pedestrian on sled injured in collision with pedal cycle in traffic accident
Pedestrian on snowboard injured in collision with pedal cycle in traffic accident
Pedestrian on snow-skis injured in collision with pedal cycle in traffic accident
Pedestrian in wheelchair (powered) injured in collision with pedal cycle in traffic accident
Pedestrian in motorized mobility scooter injured in collision with pedal cycle in traffic accident

5 **V01.9 Pedestrian injured in collision with pedal cycle, unspecified whether traffic or nontraffic accident**

7 **V01.90X- Pedestrian on foot injured in collision with pedal cycle, unspecified whether traffic or nontraffic accident**
Pedestrian NOS injured in collision with pedal cycle, unspecified whether traffic or nontraffic accident

7 **V01.91X- Pedestrian on roller-skates injured in collision with pedal cycle, unspecified whether traffic or nontraffic accident**

7 **V01.92X- Pedestrian on skateboard injured in collision with pedal cycle, unspecified whether traffic or nontraffic accident**

▲ 7 **V01.99X- Pedestrian with other conveyance injured in collision with pedal cycle, unspecified whether traffic or nontraffic accident**
Pedestrian with baby stroller injured in collision with pedal cycle, unspecified whether traffic or nontraffic accident
Pedestrian on ice-skates injured in collision with pedal cycle unspecified, whether traffic or nontraffic accident
Pedestrian on nonmotorized scooter injured in collision with pedal cycle, unspecified whether traffic or nontraffic accident
Pedestrian on sled injured in collision with pedal cycle unspecified, whether traffic or nontraffic accident
Pedestrian on snowboard injured in collision with pedal cycle, unspecified whether traffic or nontraffic accident
Pedestrian on snow-skis injured in collision with pedal cycle, unspecified whether traffic or nontraffic accident
Pedestrian in wheelchair (powered) injured in collision with pedal cycle, unspecified whether traffic or nontraffic accident
Pedestrian in motorized mobility scooter injured in collision with pedal cycle, unspecified whether traffic or nontraffic accident

4 V02 Pedestrian injured in collision with two- or three-wheeled motor vehicle

The appropriate 7th character is to be added to each code from category V02

A	initial encounter
D	subsequent encounter
S	sequela

5 **V02.0 Pedestrian injured in collision with two- or three-wheeled motor vehicle in nontraffic accident**

7 **V02.00X- Pedestrian on foot injured in collision with two- or three-wheeled motor vehicle in nontraffic accident**
Pedestrian NOS injured in collision with two- or three-wheeled motor vehicle in nontraffic accident

7 **V02.01X- Pedestrian on roller-skates injured in collision with two- or three-wheeled motor vehicle in nontraffic accident**

7 **V02.02X- Pedestrian on skateboard injured in collision with two- or three-wheeled motor vehicle in nontraffic accident**

▲ 7 **V02.09X- Pedestrian with other conveyance injured in collision with two- or three-wheeled motor vehicle in nontraffic accident**
Pedestrian with baby stroller injured in collision with two- or three-wheeled motor vehicle in nontraffic accident
Pedestrian on ice-skates injured in collision with two- or three-wheeled motor vehicle in nontraffic accident
Pedestrian on nonmotorized scooter injured in collision with two- or three-wheeled motor vehicle in nontraffic accident
Pedestrian on sled injured in collision with two- or three-wheeled motor vehicle in nontraffic accident
Pedestrian on snowboard injured in collision with two- or three-wheeled motor vehicle in nontraffic accident
Pedestrian on snow-skis injured in collision with two- or three-wheeled motor vehicle in nontraffic accident
Pedestrian in wheelchair (powered) injured in collision with two- or three-wheeled motor vehicle in nontraffic accident
Pedestrian in motorized mobility scooter injured in collision with two- or three-wheeled motor vehicle in nontraffic accident

5 **V02.1 Pedestrian injured in collision with two- or three-wheeled motor vehicle in traffic accident**

7 **V02.10X- Pedestrian on foot injured in collision with two- or three-wheeled motor vehicle in traffic accident**
Pedestrian NOS injured in collision with two- or three-wheeled motor vehicle in traffic accident

7 V02.11X- **Pedestrian on roller-skates injured in collision with two- or three-wheeled motor vehicle in traffic accident**

7 V02.12X- **Pedestrian on skateboard injured in collision with two- or three-wheeled motor vehicle in traffic accident**

▲ 7 V02.19X- **Pedestrian with other conveyance injured in collision with two- or three-wheeled motor vehicle in traffic accident**
Pedestrian with baby stroller injured in collision with two- or three-wheeled motor vehicle in traffic accident
Pedestrian on ice-skates injured in collision with two- or three-wheeled motor vehicle in traffic accident
Pedestrian on nonmotorized scooter injured in collision with two- or three-wheeled motor vehicle in traffic accident
Pedestrian on sled injured in collision with two- or three-wheeled motor vehicle in traffic accident
Pedestrian on snowboard injured in collision with two- or three-wheeled motor vehicle in traffic accident
Pedestrian on snow-skis injured in collision with two- or three-wheeled motor vehicle in traffic accident
Pedestrian in wheelchair (powered) injured in collision with two- or three-wheeled motor vehicle in traffic accident
Pedestrian in motorized mobility scooter injured in collision with two- or three-wheeled motor vehicle in traffic accident

5 V02.9 **Pedestrian injured in collision with two- or three-wheeled motor vehicle, unspecified whether traffic or nontraffic accident**

7 V02.90X- **Pedestrian on foot injured in collision with two- or three-wheeled motor vehicle, unspecified whether traffic or nontraffic accident**
Pedestrian NOS injured in collision with two- or three-wheeled motor vehicle, unspecified whether traffic or nontraffic accident

7 V02.91X- **Pedestrian on roller-skates injured in collision with two- or three-wheeled motor vehicle, unspecified whether traffic or nontraffic accident**

7 V02.92X- **Pedestrian on skateboard injured in collision with two- or three-wheeled motor vehicle, unspecified whether traffic or nontraffic accident**

▲ 7 V02.99X- **Pedestrian with other conveyance injured in collision with two- or three-wheeled motor vehicle, unspecified whether traffic or nontraffic accident**
Pedestrian with baby stroller injured in collision with two- or three-wheeled motor vehicle, unspecified whether traffic or nontraffic accident
Pedestrian on ice-skates injured in collision with two- or three-wheeled motor vehicle, unspecified whether traffic or nontraffic accident
Pedestrian on nonmotorized scooter injured in collision with two- or three-wheeled motor vehicle, unspecified whether traffic or nontraffic accident
Pedestrian on sled injured in collision with two- or three-wheeled motor vehicle, unspecified whether traffic or nontraffic accident
Pedestrian on snowboard injured in collision with two- or three-wheeled motor vehicle, unspecified whether traffic or nontraffic accident
Pedestrian on snow-skis injured in collision with two- or three-wheeled motor vehicle, unspecified whether traffic or nontraffic accident
Pedestrian in wheelchair (powered) injured in collision with two- or three-wheeled motor vehicle, unspecified whether traffic or nontraffic accident
Pedestrian in motorized mobility scooter injured in collision with two- or three-wheeled motor vehicle, unspecified whether traffic or nontraffic accident

4 V03 Pedestrian injured in collision with car, pick-up truck or van

The appropriate 7th character is to be added to each code from category V03
A initial encounter
D subsequent encounter
S sequela

5 V03.0 **Pedestrian injured in collision with car, pick-up truck or van in nontraffic accident**

7 V03.00X- **Pedestrian on foot injured in collision with car, pick-up truck or van in nontraffic accident**
Pedestrian NOS injured in collision with car, pick-up truck or van in nontraffic accident

7 V03.01X- **Pedestrian on roller-skates injured in collision with car, pick-up truck or van in nontraffic accident**

7 V03.02X- **Pedestrian on skateboard injured in collision with car, pick-up truck or van in nontraffic accident**

▲ 7 V03.09X- **Pedestrian with other conveyance injured in collision with car, pick-up truck or van in nontraffic accident**
Pedestrian with baby stroller injured in collision with car, pick-up truck or van in nontraffic accident
Pedestrian on ice-skates injured in collision with car, pick-up truck or van in nontraffic accident
Pedestrian on nonmotorized scooter injured in collision with car, pick-up truck or van in nontraffic accident
Pedestrian on sled injured in collision with car, pick-up truck or van in nontraffic accident
Pedestrian on snowboard injured in collision with car, pick-up truck or van in nontraffic accident
Pedestrian on snow-skis injured in collision with car, pick-up truck or van in nontraffic accident
Pedestrian in wheelchair (powered) injured in collision with car, pick-up truck or van in nontraffic accident
Pedestrian in motorized mobility scooter injured in collision with car, pick-up truck or van in nontraffic accident

5 V03.1 **Pedestrian injured in collision with car, pick-up truck or van in traffic accident**

7 V03.10X- **Pedestrian on foot injured in collision with car, pick-up truck or van in traffic accident**
Pedestrian NOS injured in collision with car, pick-up truck or van in traffic accident

7 V03.11X- **Pedestrian on roller-skates injured in collision with car, pick-up truck or van in traffic accident**

7 V03.12X- **Pedestrian on skateboard injured in collision with car, pick-up truck or van in traffic accident**

▲ 7 V03.19X- **Pedestrian with other conveyance injured in collision with car, pick-up truck or van in traffic accident**
Pedestrian with baby stroller injured in collision with car, pick-up truck or van in traffic accident
Pedestrian on ice-skates injured in collision with car, pick-up truck or van in traffic accident
Pedestrian on nonmotorized scooter injured in collision with car, pick-up truck or van in traffic accident
Pedestrian on sled injured in collision with car, pick-up truck or van in traffic accident
Pedestrian on snowboard injured in collision with car, pick-up truck or van in traffic accident
Pedestrian on snow-skis injured in collision with car, pick-up truck or van in traffic accident
Pedestrian in wheelchair (powered) injured in collision with car, pick-up truck or van in traffic accident
Pedestrian in motorized mobility scooter injured in collision with car, pick-up truck or van in traffic accident

5 V03.9 **Pedestrian injured in collision with car, pick-up truck or van, unspecified whether traffic or nontraffic accident**

7 V03.90X- **Pedestrian on foot injured in collision with car, pick-up truck or van, unspecified whether traffic or nontraffic accident**
Pedestrian NOS injured in collision with car, pick-up truck or van, unspecified whether traffic or nontraffic accident

7 V03.91X- **Pedestrian on roller-skates injured in collision with car, pick-up truck or van, unspecified whether traffic or nontraffic accident**

7 V03.92X- **Pedestrian on skateboard injured in collision with car, pick-up truck or van, unspecified whether traffic or nontraffic accident**

▲ 7 V03.99X- **Pedestrian with other conveyance injured in collision with car, pick-up truck or van, unspecified whether traffic or nontraffic accident**
Pedestrian with baby stroller injured in collision with car, pick-up truck or van, unspecified whether traffic or nontraffic accident
Pedestrian on ice-skates injured in collision with car, pick-up truck or van, unspecified whether traffic or nontraffic accident
Pedestrian on nonmotorized scooter injured in collision with car, pick-up truck or van, unspecified whether traffic or nontraffic accident
Pedestrian on sled injured in collision with car, pick-up truck or van in nontraffic accident
Pedestrian on snowboard injured in collision with car, pick-up truck or van, unspecified whether traffic or nontraffic accident
Pedestrian on snow-skis injured in collision with car, pick-up truck or van, unspecified whether traffic or nontraffic accident
Pedestrian in wheelchair (powered) injured in collision with car, pick-up truck or van, unspecified whether traffic or nontraffic accident
Pedestrian in motorized mobility scooter injured in collision with car, pick-up truck or van, unspecified whether traffic or nontraffic accident

4 V04 Pedestrian injured in collision with heavy transport vehicle or bus

EXCLUDES 1 *pedestrian injured in collision with military vehicle (V09.01, V09.21)*

The appropriate 7th character is to be added to each code from category V04
A initial encounter
D subsequent encounter
S sequela

5 V04.0 **Pedestrian injured in collision with heavy transport vehicle or bus in nontraffic accident**

7 V04.00X- **Pedestrian on foot injured in collision with heavy transport vehicle or bus in nontraffic accident**
Pedestrian NOS injured in collision with heavy transport vehicle or bus in nontraffic accident

7 V04.01X- **Pedestrian on roller-skates injured in collision with heavy transport vehicle or bus in nontraffic accident**

7 V04.02X- **Pedestrian on skateboard injured in collision with heavy transport vehicle or bus in nontraffic accident**

▲ 7 V04.09X- **Pedestrian with other conveyance injured in collision with heavy transport vehicle or bus in nontraffic accident**
Pedestrian with baby stroller injured in collision with heavy transport vehicle or bus in nontraffic accident
Pedestrian on ice-skates injured in collision with heavy transport vehicle or bus in nontraffic accident
Pedestrian on nonmotorized scooter injured in collision with heavy transport vehicle or bus in nontraffic accident
Pedestrian on sled injured in collision with heavy transport vehicle or bus in nontraffic accident
Pedestrian on snowboard injured in collision with heavy transport vehicle or bus in nontraffic accident
Pedestrian on snow-skis injured in collision with heavy transport vehicle or bus in nontraffic accident
Pedestrian in wheelchair (powered) injured in collision with heavy transport vehicle or bus in nontraffic accident
Pedestrian in motorized mobility scooter injured in collision with heavy transport vehicle or bus in nontraffic accident

5 V04.1 **Pedestrian injured in collision with heavy transport vehicle or bus in traffic accident**

7 V04.10X- **Pedestrian on foot injured in collision with heavy transport vehicle or bus in traffic accident**
Pedestrian NOS injured in collision with heavy transport vehicle or bus in traffic accident

7 V04.11X- **Pedestrian on roller-skates injured in collision with heavy transport vehicle or bus in traffic accident**

7 V04.12X- **Pedestrian on skateboard injured in collision with heavy transport vehicle or bus in traffic accident**

▲ 7 V04.19X- **Pedestrian with other conveyance injured in collision with heavy transport vehicle or bus in traffic accident**
Pedestrian with baby stroller injured in collision with heavy transport vehicle or bus in traffic accident
Pedestrian on ice-skates injured in collision with heavy transport vehicle or bus in traffic accident
Pedestrian on nonmotorized scooter injured in collision with heavy transport vehicle or bus in traffic accident
Pedestrian on sled injured in collision with heavy transport vehicle or bus in traffic accident
Pedestrian on snowboard injured in collision with heavy transport vehicle or bus in traffic accident
Pedestrian on snow-skis injured in collision with heavy transport vehicle or bus in traffic accident
Pedestrian in wheelchair (powered) injured in collision with heavy transport vehicle or bus in traffic accident
Pedestrian in motorized mobility scooter injured in collision with heavy transport vehicle or bus in traffic accident

5 V04.9 **Pedestrian injured in collision with heavy transport vehicle or bus, unspecified whether traffic or nontraffic accident**

7 V04.90X- **Pedestrian on foot injured in collision with heavy transport vehicle or bus, unspecified whether traffic or nontraffic accident**
Pedestrian NOS injured in collision with heavy transport vehicle or bus, unspecified whether traffic or nontraffic accident

7 V04.91X- **Pedestrian on roller-skates injured in collision with heavy transport vehicle or bus, unspecified whether traffic or nontraffic accident**

7 V04.92X- **Pedestrian on skateboard injured in collision with heavy transport vehicle or bus, unspecified whether traffic or nontraffic accident**

▲ 7 **V04.99X- Pedestrian with other conveyance injured in collision with heavy transport vehicle or bus, unspecified whether traffic or nontraffic accident**

Pedestrian with baby stroller injured in collision with heavy transport vehicle or bus, unspecified whether traffic or nontraffic accident
Pedestrian on ice-skates injured in collision with heavy transport vehicle or bus, unspecified whether traffic or nontraffic accident
Pedestrian on nonmotorized scooter injured in collision with heavy transport vehicle or bus, unspecified whether traffic or nontraffic accident
Pedestrian on sled injured in collision with heavy transport vehicle or bus, unspecified whether traffic or nontraffic accident
Pedestrian on snowboard injured in collision with heavy transport vehicle or bus, unspecified whether traffic or nontraffic accident
Pedestrian on snow-skis injured in collision with heavy transport vehicle or bus, unspecified whether traffic or nontraffic accident
Pedestrian in wheelchair (powered) injured in collision with heavy transport vehicle or bus, unspecified whether traffic or nontraffic accident
Pedestrian in motorized mobility scooter injured in collision with heavy transport vehicle or bus, unspecified whether traffic or nontraffic accident

4 **V05 Pedestrian injured in collision with railway train or railway vehicle**

The appropriate 7th character is to be added to each code from category V05
A initial encounter
D subsequent encounter
S sequela

5 **V05.0 Pedestrian injured in collision with railway train or railway vehicle in nontraffic accident**

7 **V05.00X- Pedestrian on foot injured in collision with railway train or railway vehicle in nontraffic accident**

Pedestrian NOS injured in collision with railway train or railway vehicle in nontraffic accident

7 **V05.01X- Pedestrian on roller-skates injured in collision with railway train or railway vehicle in nontraffic accident**

7 **V05.02X- Pedestrian on skateboard injured in collision with railway train or railway vehicle in nontraffic accident**

▲ 7 **V05.09X- Pedestrian with other conveyance injured in collision with railway train or railway vehicle in nontraffic accident**

Pedestrian with baby stroller injured in collision with railway train or railway vehicle in nontraffic accident
Pedestrian on ice-skates injured in collision with railway train or railway vehicle in nontraffic accident
Pedestrian on nonmotorized scooter injured in collision with railway train or railway vehicle in nontraffic accident
Pedestrian on sled injured in collision with railway train or railway vehicle in nontraffic accident
Pedestrian on snowboard injured in collision with railway train or railway vehicle in nontraffic accident
Pedestrian on snow-skis injured in collision with railway train or railway vehicle in nontraffic accident
Pedestrian in wheelchair (powered) injured in collision with railway train or railway vehicle in nontraffic accident
Pedestrian in motorized mobility scooter injured in collision with railway train or railway vehicle in nontraffic accident

5 **V05.1 Pedestrian injured in collision with railway train or railway vehicle in traffic accident**

7 **V05.10X- Pedestrian on foot injured in collision with railway train or railway vehicle in traffic accident**

Pedestrian NOS injured in collision with railway train or railway vehicle in traffic accident

7 **V05.11X- Pedestrian on roller-skates injured in collision with railway train or railway vehicle in traffic accident**

7 **V05.12X- Pedestrian on skateboard injured in collision with railway train or railway vehicle in traffic accident**

▲ 7 **V05.19X- Pedestrian with other conveyance injured in collision with railway train or railway vehicle in traffic accident**

Pedestrian with baby stroller injured in collision with railway train or railway vehicle in traffic accident
Pedestrian on ice-skates injured in collision with railway train or railway vehicle in traffic accident
Pedestrian on nonmotorized scooter injured in collision with railway train or railway vehicle in traffic accident
Pedestrian on sled injured in collision with railway train or railway vehicle in traffic accident
Pedestrian on snowboard injured in collision with railway train or railway vehicle in traffic accident
Pedestrian on snow-skis injured in collision with railway train or railway vehicle in traffic accident
Pedestrian in wheelchair (powered) injured in collision with railway train or railway vehicle in traffic accident
Pedestrian in motorized mobility scooter injured in collision with railway train or railway vehicle in traffic accident

5 **V05.9 Pedestrian injured in collision with railway train or railway vehicle, unspecified whether traffic or nontraffic accident**

7 **V05.90X- Pedestrian on foot injured in collision with railway train or railway vehicle, unspecified whether traffic or nontraffic accident**

Pedestrian NOS injured in collision with railway train or railway vehicle, unspecified whether traffic or nontraffic accident

7 **V05.91X- Pedestrian on roller-skates injured in collision with railway train or railway vehicle, unspecified whether traffic or nontraffic accident**

7 **V05.92X- Pedestrian on skateboard injured in collision with railway train or railway vehicle, unspecified whether traffic or nontraffic accident**

▲ 7 **V05.99X- Pedestrian with other conveyance injured in collision with railway train or railway vehicle, unspecified whether traffic or nontraffic accident**

Pedestrian with baby stroller injured in collision with railway train or railway vehicle, unspecified whether traffic or nontraffic
Pedestrian on ice-skates injured in collision with railway train or railway vehicle, unspecified whether traffic or nontraffic
Pedestrian on nonmotorized scooter injured in collision with railway train or railway vehicle, unspecified whether traffic or nontraffic
Pedestrian on sled injured in collision with railway train or railway vehicle, unspecified whether traffic or nontraffic
Pedestrian on snowboard injured in collision with railway train or railway vehicle, unspecified whether traffic or nontraffic
Pedestrian on snow-skis injured in collision with railway train or railway vehicle, unspecified whether traffic or nontraffic
Pedestrian in wheelchair (powered) injured in collision with railway train or railway vehicle, unspecified whether traffic or nontraffic
Pedestrian in motorized mobility scooter injured in collision with railway train or railway vehicle, unspecified whether traffic or nontraffic

4 V06 Pedestrian injured in collision with other nonmotor vehicle

INCLUDES collision with animal-drawn vehicle, animal being ridden, nonpowered streetcar

EXCLUDES 1 *pedestrian injured in collision with pedestrian conveyance (V00.0-)*

The appropriate 7th character is to be added to each code from category V06
A initial encounter
D subsequent encounter
S sequela

5 V06.0 Pedestrian injured in collision with other nonmotor vehicle in nontraffic accident

7 V06.00X- Pedestrian on foot injured in collision with other nonmotor vehicle in nontraffic accident
Pedestrian NOS injured in collision with other nonmotor vehicle in nontraffic accident

7 V06.01X- Pedestrian on roller-skates injured in collision with other nonmotor vehicle in nontraffic accident

7 V06.02X- Pedestrian on skateboard injured in collision with other nonmotor vehicle in nontraffic accident

▲ 7 V06.09X- Pedestrian with other conveyance injured in collision with other nonmotor vehicle in nontraffic accident
Pedestrian with baby stroller injured in collision with other nonmotor vehicle in nontraffic accident
Pedestrian on ice-skates injured in collision with other nonmotor vehicle in nontraffic accident
Pedestrian on nonmotorized scooter injured in collision with other nonmotor vehicle in nontraffic accident
Pedestrian on sled injured in collision with other nonmotor vehicle in nontraffic accident
Pedestrian on snowboard injured in collision with other nonmotor vehicle in nontraffic accident
Pedestrian on snow-skis injured in collision with other nonmotor vehicle in nontraffic accident
Pedestrian in wheelchair (powered) injured in collision with other nonmotor vehicle in nontraffic accident
Pedestrian in motorized mobility scooter injured in collision with other nonmotor vehicle in nontraffic accident

5 V06.1 Pedestrian injured in collision with other nonmotor vehicle in traffic accident

7 V06.10X- Pedestrian on foot injured in collision with other nonmotor vehicle in traffic accident
Pedestrian NOS injured in collision with other nonmotor vehicle in traffic accident

7 V06.11X- Pedestrian on roller-skates injured in collision with other nonmotor vehicle in traffic accident

7 V06.12X- Pedestrian on skateboard injured in collision with other nonmotor vehicle in traffic accident

▲ 7 V06.19X- Pedestrian with other conveyance injured in collision with other nonmotor vehicle in traffic accident
Pedestrian with baby stroller injured in collision with other nonmotor vehicle in nontraffic accident
Pedestrian on ice-skates injured in collision with other nonmotor vehicle in traffic accident
Pedestrian on nonmotorized scooter injured in collision with other nonmotor vehicle in traffic accident
Pedestrian on sled injured in collision with other nonmotor vehicle in traffic accident
Pedestrian on snowboard injured in collision with other nonmotor vehicle in traffic accident
Pedestrian on snow-skis injured in collision with other nonmotor vehicle in traffic accident
Pedestrian in wheelchair (powered) injured in collision with other nonmotor vehicle in traffic accident
Pedestrian in motorized mobility scooter injured in collision with other nonmotor vehicle in traffic accident

5 V06.9 Pedestrian injured in collision with other nonmotor vehicle, unspecified whether traffic or nontraffic accident

7 V06.90X- Pedestrian on foot injured in collision with other nonmotor vehicle, unspecified whether traffic or nontraffic accident
Pedestrian NOS injured in collision with other nonmotor vehicle, unspecified whether traffic or nontraffic accident

7 V06.91X- Pedestrian on roller-skates injured in collision with other nonmotor vehicle, unspecified whether traffic or nontraffic accident

7 V06.92X- Pedestrian on skateboard injured in collision with other nonmotor vehicle, unspecified whether traffic or nontraffic accident

▲ 7 V06.99X- Pedestrian with other conveyance injured in collision with other nonmotor vehicle, unspecified whether traffic or nontraffic accident
Pedestrian with baby stroller injured in collision with other nonmotor vehicle, unspecified whether traffic or nontraffic accident
Pedestrian on ice-skates injured in collision with other nonmotor vehicle, unspecified whether traffic or nontraffic accident
Pedestrian on nonmotorized scooter injured in collision with other nonmotor vehicle, unspecified whether traffic or nontraffic accident
Pedestrian on sled injured in collision with other nonmotor vehicle, unspecified whether traffic or nontraffic accident
Pedestrian on snowboard injured in collision with other nonmotor vehicle, unspecified whether traffic or nontraffic accident
Pedestrian on snow-skis injured in collision with other nonmotor vehicle, unspecified whether traffic or nontraffic accident
Pedestrian in wheelchair (powered) injured in collision with other nonmotor vehicle, unspecified whether traffic or nontraffic accident
Pedestrian in motorized mobility scooter injured in collision with other nonmotor vehicle, unspecified whether traffic or nontraffic accident

4 V09 Pedestrian injured in other and unspecified transport accidents

The appropriate 7th character is to be added to each code from category V09
A initial encounter
D subsequent encounter
S sequela

5 V09.0 Pedestrian injured in nontraffic accident involving other and unspecified motor vehicles

7 V09.00X- Pedestrian injured in nontraffic accident involving unspecified motor vehicles

7 V09.01X- Pedestrian injured in nontraffic accident involving military vehicle

7 V09.09X- Pedestrian injured in nontraffic accident involving other motor vehicles
Pedestrian injured in nontraffic accident by special vehicle

7 V09.1XX- Pedestrian injured in unspecified nontraffic accident

5 V09.2 Pedestrian injured in traffic accident involving other and unspecified motor vehicles

7 V09.20X- Pedestrian injured in traffic accident involving unspecified motor vehicles

7 V09.21X- Pedestrian injured in traffic accident involving military vehicle

7 V09.29X- Pedestrian injured in traffic accident involving other motor vehicles

7 V09.3XX- Pedestrian injured in unspecified traffic accident

7 V09.9XX- Pedestrian injured in unspecified transport accident

Pedal cycle rider injured in transport accident (V10-V19)

INCLUDES any non-motorized vehicle, excluding an animal-drawn vehicle, or a sidecar or trailer attached to the pedal cycle

EXCLUDES 2 *rupture of pedal cycle tire (W37.0)*

V10 Pedal cycle rider injured in collision with pedestrian or animal

EXCLUDES 1 *pedal cycle rider collision with animal-drawn vehicle or animal being ridden (V16.-)*

The appropriate 7th character is to be added to each code from category V10
A initial encounter
D subsequent encounter
S sequela

V10.0XX- **Pedal cycle driver injured in collision with pedestrian or animal in nontraffic accident**
V10.1XX- **Pedal cycle passenger injured in collision with pedestrian or animal in nontraffic accident**
V10.2XX- **Unspecified pedal cyclist injured in collision with pedestrian or animal in nontraffic accident**
V10.3XX- **Person boarding or alighting a pedal cycle injured in collision with pedestrian or animal**
V10.4XX- **Pedal cycle driver injured in collision with pedestrian or animal in traffic accident**
V10.5XX- **Pedal cycle passenger injured in collision with pedestrian or animal in traffic accident**
V10.9XX- **Unspecified pedal cyclist injured in collision with pedestrian or animal in traffic accident**

V11 Pedal cycle rider injured in collision with other pedal cycle

The appropriate 7th character is to be added to each code from category V11
A initial encounter
D subsequent encounter
S sequela

V11.0XX- **Pedal cycle driver injured in collision with other pedal cycle in nontraffic accident**
V11.1XX- **Pedal cycle passenger injured in collision with other pedal cycle in nontraffic accident**
V11.2XX- **Unspecified pedal cyclist injured in collision with other pedal cycle in nontraffic accident**
V11.3XX- **Person boarding or alighting a pedal cycle injured in collision with other pedal cycle**
V11.4XX- **Pedal cycle driver injured in collision with other pedal cycle in traffic accident**
V11.5XX- **Pedal cycle passenger injured in collision with other pedal cycle in traffic accident**
V11.9XX- **Unspecified pedal cyclist injured in collision with other pedal cycle in traffic accident**

V12 Pedal cycle rider injured in collision with two- or three-wheeled motor vehicle

The appropriate 7th character is to be added to each code from category V12
A initial encounter
D subsequent encounter
S sequela

V12.0XX- **Pedal cycle driver injured in collision with two- or three-wheeled motor vehicle in nontraffic accident**
V12.1XX- **Pedal cycle passenger injured in collision with two- or three-wheeled motor vehicle in nontraffic accident**
V12.2XX- **Unspecified pedal cyclist injured in collision with two- or three-wheeled motor vehicle in nontraffic accident**
V12.3XX- **Person boarding or alighting a pedal cycle injured in collision with two- or three-wheeled motor vehicle**
V12.4XX- **Pedal cycle driver injured in collision with two- or three-wheeled motor vehicle in traffic accident**
V12.5XX- **Pedal cycle passenger injured in collision with two- or three-wheeled motor vehicle in traffic accident**
V12.9XX- **Unspecified pedal cyclist injured in collision with two- or three-wheeled motor vehicle in traffic accident**

V13 Pedal cycle rider injured in collision with car, pick-up truck or van

The appropriate 7th character is to be added to each code from category V13
A initial encounter
D subsequent encounter
S sequela

V13.0XX- **Pedal cycle driver injured in collision with car, pick-up truck or van in nontraffic accident**
V13.1XX- **Pedal cycle passenger injured in collision with car, pick-up truck or van in nontraffic accident**
V13.2XX- **Unspecified pedal cyclist injured in collision with car, pick-up truck or van in nontraffic accident**
V13.3XX- **Person boarding or alighting a pedal cycle injured in collision with car, pick-up truck or van**
V13.4XX- **Pedal cycle driver injured in collision with car, pick-up truck or van in traffic accident**
V13.5XX- **Pedal cycle passenger injured in collision with car, pick-up truck or van in traffic accident**
V13.9XX- **Unspecified pedal cyclist injured in collision with car, pick-up truck or van in traffic accident**

V14 Pedal cycle rider injured in collision with heavy transport vehicle or bus

EXCLUDES 1 *pedal cycle rider injured in collision with military vehicle (V19.81)*

The appropriate 7th character is to be added to each code from category V14
A initial encounter
D subsequent encounter
S sequela

V14.0XX- **Pedal cycle driver injured in collision with heavy transport vehicle or bus in nontraffic accident**
V14.1XX- **Pedal cycle passenger injured in collision with heavy transport vehicle or bus in nontraffic accident**
V14.2XX- **Unspecified pedal cyclist injured in collision with heavy transport vehicle or bus in nontraffic accident**
V14.3XX- **Person boarding or alighting a pedal cycle injured in collision with heavy transport vehicle or bus**
V14.4XX- **Pedal cycle driver injured in collision with heavy transport vehicle or bus in traffic accident**
V14.5XX- **Pedal cycle passenger injured in collision with heavy transport vehicle or bus in traffic accident**
V14.9XX- **Unspecified pedal cyclist injured in collision with heavy transport vehicle or bus in traffic accident**

V15 Pedal cycle rider injured in collision with railway train or railway vehicle

The appropriate 7th character is to be added to each code from category V15
A initial encounter
D subsequent encounter
S sequela

V15.0XX- **Pedal cycle driver injured in collision with railway train or railway vehicle in nontraffic accident**
V15.1XX- **Pedal cycle passenger injured in collision with railway train or railway vehicle in nontraffic accident**
V15.2XX- **Unspecified pedal cyclist injured in collision with railway train or railway vehicle in nontraffic accident**
V15.3XX- **Person boarding or alighting a pedal cycle injured in collision with railway train or railway vehicle**
V15.4XX- **Pedal cycle driver injured in collision with railway train or railway vehicle in traffic accident**
V15.5XX- **Pedal cycle passenger injured in collision with railway train or railway vehicle in traffic accident**
V15.9XX- **Unspecified pedal cyclist injured in collision with railway train or railway vehicle in traffic accident**

V16 Pedal cycle rider injured in collision with other nonmotor vehicle

INCLUDES collision with animal-drawn vehicle, animal being ridden, streetcar

The appropriate 7th character is to be added to each code from category V16
A initial encounter
D subsequent encounter
S sequela

- V16.0XX- **Pedal cycle driver injured in collision with other nonmotor vehicle in nontraffic accident**
- V16.1XX- **Pedal cycle passenger injured in collision with other nonmotor vehicle in nontraffic accident**
- V16.2XX- **Unspecified pedal cyclist injured in collision with other nonmotor vehicle in nontraffic accident**
- V16.3XX- **Person boarding or alighting a pedal cycle injured in collision with other nonmotor vehicle in nontraffic accident**
- V16.4XX- **Pedal cycle driver injured in collision with other nonmotor vehicle in traffic accident**
- V16.5XX- **Pedal cycle passenger injured in collision with other nonmotor vehicle in traffic accident**
- V16.9XX- **Unspecified pedal cyclist injured in collision with other nonmotor vehicle in traffic accident**

V17 Pedal cycle rider injured in collision with fixed or stationary object

The appropriate 7th character is to be added to each code from category V17
A initial encounter
D subsequent encounter
S sequela

- V17.0XX- **Pedal cycle driver injured in collision with fixed or stationary object in nontraffic accident**
- V17.1XX- **Pedal cycle passenger injured in collision with fixed or stationary object in nontraffic accident**
- V17.2XX- **Unspecified pedal cyclist injured in collision with fixed or stationary object in nontraffic accident**
- V17.3XX- **Person boarding or alighting a pedal cycle injured in collision with fixed or stationary object**
- V17.4XX- **Pedal cycle driver injured in collision with fixed or stationary object in traffic accident**
- V17.5XX- **Pedal cycle passenger injured in collision with fixed or stationary object in traffic accident**
- V17.9XX- **Unspecified pedal cyclist injured in collision with fixed or stationary object in traffic accident**

V18 Pedal cycle rider injured in noncollision transport accident

INCLUDES fall or thrown from pedal cycle (without antecedent collision)
overturning pedal cycle NOS
overturning pedal cycle without collision

The appropriate 7th character is to be added to each code from category V18
A initial encounter
D subsequent encounter
S sequela

- V18.0XX- **Pedal cycle driver injured in noncollision transport accident in nontraffic accident**
- V18.1XX- **Pedal cycle passenger injured in noncollision transport accident in nontraffic accident**
- V18.2XX- **Unspecified pedal cyclist injured in noncollision transport accident in nontraffic accident**
- V18.3XX- **Person boarding or alighting a pedal cycle injured in noncollision transport accident**
- V18.4XX- **Pedal cycle driver injured in noncollision transport accident in traffic accident**
- V18.5XX- **Pedal cycle passenger injured in noncollision transport accident in traffic accident**
- V18.9XX- **Unspecified pedal cyclist injured in noncollision transport accident in traffic accident**

V19 Pedal cycle rider injured in other and unspecifiedtransport accidents

The appropriate 7th character is to be added to each code from category V19
A initial encounter
D subsequent encounter
S sequela

- V19.0 **Pedal cycle driver injured in collision with other and unspecified motor vehicles in nontraffic accident**
  - V19.00X- **Pedal cycle driver injured in collision with unspecified motor vehicles in nontraffic accident**
  - V19.09X- **Pedal cycle driver injured in collision with other motor vehicles in nontraffic accident**
- V19.1 **Pedal cycle passenger injured in collision with other and unspecified motor vehicles in nontraffic accident**
  - V19.10X- **Pedal cycle passenger injured in collision with unspecified motor vehicles in nontraffic accident**
  - V19.19X- **Pedal cycle passenger injured in collision with other motor vehicles in nontraffic accident**
- V19.2 **Unspecified pedal cyclist injured in collision with other and unspecified motor vehicles in nontraffic accident**
  - V19.20X- **Unspecified pedal cyclist injured in collision with unspecified motor vehicles in nontraffic accident**
    Pedal cycle collision NOS, nontraffic
  - V19.29X- **Unspecified pedal cyclist injured in collision with other motor vehicles in nontraffic accident**
- V19.3XX- **Pedal cyclist (driver) (passenger) injured in unspecified nontraffic accident**
  Pedal cycle accident NOS, nontraffic
  Pedal cyclist injured in nontraffic accident NOS
- V19.4 **Pedal cycle driver injured in collision with other and unspecified motor vehicles in traffic accident**
  - V19.40X- **Pedal cycle driver injured in collision with unspecified motor vehicles in traffic accident**
  - V19.49X- **Pedal cycle driver injured in collision with other motor vehicles in traffic accident**
- V19.5 **Pedal cycle passenger injured in collision with other and unspecified motor vehicles in traffic accident**
  - V19.50X- **Pedal cycle passenger injured in collision with unspecified motor vehicles in traffic accident**
  - V19.59X- **Pedal cycle passenger injured in collision with other motor vehicles in traffic accident**
- V19.6 **Unspecified pedal cyclist injured in collision with other and unspecified motor vehicles in traffic accident**
  - V19.60X- **Unspecified pedal cyclist injured in collision with unspecified motor vehicles in traffic accident**
    Pedal cycle collision NOS (traffic)
  - V19.69X- **Unspecified pedal cyclist injured in collision with other motor vehicles in traffic accident**
- V19.8 **Pedal cyclist (driver) (passenger) injured in other specified transport accidents**
  - V19.81X- **Pedal cyclist (driver) (passenger) injured in transport accident with military vehicle**
  - V19.88X- **Pedal cyclist (driver) (passenger) injured in other specified transport accidents**
- V19.9XX- **Pedal cyclist (driver) (passenger) injured in unspecified traffic accident**
  Pedal cycle accident NOS

Motorcycle rider injured in transport accident (V20-V29)

INCLUDES moped
motorcycle with sidecar
motorized bicycle
motor scooter

EXCLUDES 1 *three-wheeled motor vehicle (V30-V39)*

V20 Motorcycle rider injured in collision with pedestrian or animal

EXCLUDES 1 *motorcycle rider collision with animal-drawn vehicle or animal being ridden (V26.-)*

The appropriate 7th character is to be added to each code from category V20
A initial encounter
D subsequent encounter
S sequela

- **V20.0XX-** Motorcycle driver injured in collision with pedestrian or animal in nontraffic accident
- **V20.1XX-** Motorcycle passenger injured in collision with pedestrian or animal in nontraffic accident
- **V20.2XX-** Unspecified motorcycle rider injured in collision with pedestrian or animal in nontraffic accident
- **V20.3XX-** Person boarding or alighting a motorcycle injured in collision with pedestrian or animal
- **V20.4XX-** Motorcycle driver injured in collision with pedestrian or animal in traffic accident
- **V20.5XX-** Motorcycle passenger injured in collision with pedestrian or animal in traffic accident
- **V20.9XX-** Unspecified motorcycle rider injured in collision with pedestrian or animal in traffic accident

V21 Motorcycle rider injured in collision with pedal cycle

The appropriate 7th character is to be added to each code from category V21
A initial encounter
D subsequent encounter
S sequela

- **V21.0XX-** Motorcycle driver injured in collision with pedal cycle in nontraffic accident
- **V21.1XX-** Motorcycle passenger injured in collision with pedal cycle in nontraffic accident
- **V21.2XX-** Unspecified motorcycle rider injured in collision with pedal cycle in nontraffic accident
- **V21.3XX-** Person boarding or alighting a motorcycle injured in collision with pedal cycle
- **V21.4XX-** Motorcycle driver injured in collision with pedal cycle in traffic accident
- **V21.5XX-** Motorcycle passenger injured in collision with pedal cycle in traffic accident
- **V21.9XX-** Unspecified motorcycle rider injured in collision with pedal cycle in traffic accident

V22 Motorcycle rider injured in collision with two- or three-wheeled motor vehicle

The appropriate 7th character is to be added to each code from category V22
A initial encounter
D subsequent encounter
S sequela

- **V22.0XX-** Motorcycle driver injured in collision with two- or three-wheeled motor vehicle in nontraffic accident
- **V22.1XX-** Motorcycle passenger injured in collision with two- or three-wheeled motor vehicle in nontraffic accident
- **V22.2XX** Unspecified motorcycle rider injured in collision with two- or three-wheeled motor vehicle in nontraffic accident
- **V22.3XX-** Person boarding or alighting a motorcycle injured in collision with two- or three-wheeled motor vehicle
- **V22.4XX-** Motorcycle driver injured in collision with two- or three-wheeled motor vehicle in traffic accident
- **V22.5XX-** Motorcycle passenger injured in collision with two- or three-wheeled motor vehicle in traffic accident
- **V22.9XX-** Unspecified motorcycle rider injured in collision with two- or three-wheeled motor vehicle in traffic accident

V23 Motorcycle rider injured in collision with car, pick-up truck or van

The appropriate 7th character is to be added to each code from category V23
A initial encounter
D subsequent encounter
S sequela

- **V23.0XX-** Motorcycle driver injured in collision with car, pick-up truck or van in nontraffic accident
- **V23.1XX-** Motorcycle passenger injured in collision with car, pick-up truck or van in nontraffic accident
- **V23.2XX-** Unspecified motorcycle rider injured in collision with car, pick-up truck or van in nontraffic accident
- **V23.3XX-** Person boarding or alighting a motorcycle injured in collision with car, pick-up truck or van
- **V23.4XX-** Motorcycle driver injured in collision with car, pick-up truck or van in traffic accident
- **V23.5XX-** Motorcycle passenger injured in collision with car, pick-up truck or van in traffic accident
- **V23.9XX-** Unspecified motorcycle rider injured in collision with car, pick-up truck or van in traffic accident

V24 Motorcycle rider injured in collision with heavy transport vehicle or bus

EXCLUDES 1 *motorcycle rider injured in collision with military vehicle (V29.81)*

The appropriate 7th character is to be added to each code from category V24
A initial encounter
D subsequent encounter
S sequela

- **V24.0XX-** Motorcycle driver injured in collision with heavy transport vehicle or bus in nontraffic accident
- **V24.1XX-** Motorcycle passenger injured in collision with heavy transport vehicle or bus in nontraffic accident
- **V24.2XX-** Unspecified motorcycle rider injured in collision with heavy transport vehicle or bus in nontraffic accident
- **V24.3XX-** Person boarding or alighting a motorcycle injured in collision with heavy transport vehicle or bus
- **V24.4XX-** Motorcycle driver injured in collision with heavy transport vehicle or bus in traffic accident
- **V24.5XX-** Motorcycle passenger injured in collision with heavy transport vehicle or bus in traffic accident
- **V24.9XX-** Unspecified motorcycle rider injured in collision with heavy transport vehicle or bus in traffic accident

V25 Motorcycle rider injured in collision with railway train or railway vehicle

The appropriate 7th character is to be added to each code from category V25
A initial encounter
D subsequent encounter
S sequela

- **V25.0XX-** Motorcycle driver injured in collision with railway train or railway vehicle in nontraffic accident
- **V25.1XX-** Motorcycle passenger injured in collision with railway train or railway vehicle in nontraffic accident
- **V25.2XX-** Unspecified motorcycle rider injured in collision with railway train or railway vehicle in nontraffic accident
- **V25.3XX-** Person boarding or alighting a motorcycle injured in collision with railway train or railway vehicle
- **V25.4XX-** Motorcycle driver injured in collision with railway train or railway vehicle in traffic accident
- **V25.5XX-** Motorcycle passenger injured in collision with railway train or railway vehicle in traffic accident
- **V25.9XX-** Unspecified motorcycle rider injured in collision with railway train or railway vehicle in traffic accident

V26 Motorcycle rider injured in collision with other nonmotor vehicle

INCLUDES collision with animal-drawn vehicle, animal being ridden, streetcar

The appropriate 7th character is to be added to each code from category V26
A initial encounter
D subsequent encounter
S sequela

- **V26.0XX-** Motorcycle driver injured in collision with other nonmotor vehicle in nontraffic accident
- **V26.1XX-** Motorcycle passenger injured in collision with other nonmotor vehicle in nontraffic accident

7 V26.2XX- Unspecified motorcycle rider injured in collision with other nonmotor vehicle in nontraffic accident

7 V26.3XX- Person boarding or alighting a motorcycle injured in collision with other nonmotor vehicle

7 V26.4XX- Motorcycle driver injured in collision with other nonmotor vehicle in traffic accident

7 V26.5XX- Motorcycle passenger injured in collision with other nonmotor vehicle in traffic accident

7 V26.9XX- Unspecified motorcycle rider injured in collision with other nonmotor vehicle in traffic accident

4 V27 Motorcycle rider injured in collision with fixed or stationary object

The appropriate 7th character is to be added to each code from category V27
A initial encounter
D subsequent encounter
S sequela

7 V27.0XX- Motorcycle driver injured in collision with fixed or stationary object in nontraffic accident

7 V27.1XX- Motorcycle passenger injured in collision with fixed or stationary object in nontraffic accident

7 V27.2XX- Unspecified motorcycle rider injured in collision with fixed or stationary object in nontraffic accident

7 V27.3XX- Person boarding or alighting a motorcycle injured in collision with fixed or stationary object

7 V27.4XX- Motorcycle driver injured in collision with fixed or stationary object in traffic accident

7 V27.5XX- Motorcycle passenger injured in collision with fixed or stationary object in traffic accident

7 V27.9XX- Unspecified motorcycle rider injured in collision with fixed or stationary object in traffic accident

4 V28 Motorcycle rider injured in noncollision transport accident

INCLUDES fall or thrown from motorcycle (without antecedent collision)
overturning motorcycle NOS
overturning motorcycle without collision

The appropriate 7th character is to be added to each code from category V28
A initial encounter
D subsequent encounter
S sequela

7 V28.0XX- Motorcycle driver injured in noncollision transport accident in nontraffic accident

7 V28.1XX- Motorcycle passenger injured in noncollision transport accident in nontraffic accident

7 V28.2XX- Unspecified motorcycle rider injured in noncollision transport accident in nontraffic accident

7 V28.3XX- Person boarding or alighting a motorcycle injured in noncollision transport accident

7 V28.4XX- Motorcycle driver injured in noncollision transport accident in traffic accident

7 V28.5XX- Motorcycle passenger injured in noncollision transport accident in traffic accident

7 V28.9XX- Unspecified motorcycle rider injured in noncollision transport accident in traffic accident

4 V29 Motorcycle rider injured in other and unspecified transport accidents

The appropriate 7th character is to be added to each code from category V29
A initial encounter
D subsequent encounter
S sequela

5 V29.0 Motorcycle driver injured in collision with other and unspecified motor vehicles in nontraffic accident

7 V29.00X- Motorcycle driver injured in collision with unspecified motor vehicles in nontraffic accident

7 V29.09X- Motorcycle driver injured in collision with other motor vehicles in nontraffic accident

5 V29.1 Motorcycle passenger injured in collision with other and unspecified motor vehicles in nontraffic accident

7 V29.10X- Motorcycle passenger injured in collision with unspecified motor vehicles in nontraffic accident

7 V29.19X- Motorcycle passenger injured in collision with other motor vehicles in nontraffic accident

5 V29.2 Unspecified motorcycle rider injured in collision with other and unspecified motor vehicles in nontraffic accident

7 V29.20X- Unspecified motorcycle rider injured in collision with unspecified motor vehicles in nontraffic accident
Motorcycle collision NOS, nontraffic

7 V29.29X- Unspecified motorcycle rider injured in collision with other motor vehicles in nontraffic accident

7 V29.3XX- Motorcycle rider (driver) (passenger) injured in unspecified nontraffic accident
Motorcycle accident NOS, nontraffic
Motorcycle rider injured in nontraffic accident NOS

5 V29.4 Motorcycle driver injured in collision with other and unspecified motor vehicles in traffic accident

7 V29.40X- Motorcycle driver injured in collision with unspecified motor vehicles in traffic accident

7 V29.49X- Motorcycle driver injured in collision with other motor vehicles in traffic accident

5 V29.5 Motorcycle passenger injured in collision with other and unspecified motor vehicles in traffic accident

7 V29.50X- Motorcycle passenger injured in collision with unspecified motor vehicles in traffic accident

7 V29.59X- Motorcycle passenger injured in collision with other motor vehicles in traffic accident

5 V29.6 Unspecified motorcycle rider injured in collision with other and unspecified motor vehicles in traffic accident

7 V29.60X- Unspecified motorcycle rider injured in collision with unspecified motor vehicles in traffic accident
Motorcycle collision NOS (traffic)

7 V29.69X- Unspecified motorcycle rider injured in collision with other motor vehicles in traffic accident

5 V29.8 Motorcycle rider (driver) (passenger) injured in other specified transport accidents

7 V29.81X- Motorcycle rider (driver) (passenger) injured in transport accident with military vehicle

7 V29.88X- Motorcycle rider (driver) (passenger) injured in other specified transport accidents

7 V29.9XX- Motorcycle rider (driver) (passenger) injured in unspecified traffic accident
Motorcycle accident NOS

Occupant of three-wheeled motor vehicle injured in transport accident (V30-V39)

INCLUDES motorized tricycle
motorized rickshaw
three-wheeled motor car

EXCLUDES 1 *all-terrain vehicles (V86.-)*
motorcycle with sidecar (V20-V29)
vehicle designed primarily for off-road use (V86.-)

4 V30 Occupant of three-wheeled motor vehicle injured in collision with pedestrian or animal

EXCLUDES 1 *three-wheeled motor vehicle collision with animal-drawn vehicle or animal being ridden (V36.-)*

The appropriate 7th character is to be added to each code from category V30
A initial encounter
D subsequent encounter
S sequela

7 V30.0XX- Driver of three-wheeled motor vehicle injured in collision with pedestrian or animal in nontraffic accident

7 V30.1XX- Passenger in three-wheeled motor vehicle injured in collision with pedestrian or animal in nontraffic accident

7 V30.2XX- Person on outside of three-wheeled motor vehicle injured in collision with pedestrian or animal in nontraffic accident

V30.3XX- Unspecified occupant of three-wheeled motor vehicle injured in collision with pedestrian or animal in nontraffic accident

V30.4XX- Person boarding or alighting a three-wheeled motor vehicle injured in collision with pedestrian or animal

V30.5XX- Driver of three-wheeled motor vehicle injured in collision with pedestrian or animal in traffic accident

V30.6XX- Passenger in three-wheeled motor vehicle injured in collision with pedestrian or animal in traffic accident

V30.7XX- Person on outside of three-wheeled motor vehicle injured in collision with pedestrian or animal in traffic accident

V30.9XX- Unspecified occupant of three-wheeled motor vehicle injured in collision with pedestrian or animal in traffic accident

V31 Occupant of three-wheeled motor vehicle injured in collision with pedal cycle

The appropriate 7th character is to be added to each code from category V31

A initial encounter
D subsequent encounter
S sequela

V31.0XX- Driver of three-wheeled motor vehicle injured in collision with pedal cycle in nontraffic accident

V31.1XX- Passenger in three-wheeled motor vehicle injured in collision with pedal cycle in nontraffic accident

V31.2XX- Person on outside of three-wheeled motor vehicle injured in collision with pedal cycle in nontraffic accident

V31.3XX- Unspecified occupant of three-wheeled motor vehicle injured in collision with pedal cycle in nontraffic accident

V31.4XX- Person boarding or alighting a three-wheeled motor vehicle injured in collision with pedal cycle

V31.5XX- Driver of three-wheeled motor vehicle injured in collision with pedal cycle in traffic accident

V31.6XX- Passenger in three-wheeled motor vehicle injured in collision with pedal cycle in traffic accident

V31.7XX- Person on outside of three-wheeled motor vehicle injured in collision with pedal cycle in traffic accident

V31.9XX- Unspecified occupant of three-wheeled motor vehicle injured in collision with pedal cycle in traffic accident

V32 Occupant of three-wheeled motor vehicle injured in collision with two- or three-wheeled motor vehicle

The appropriate 7th character is to be added to each code from category V32

A initial encounter
D subsequent encounter
S sequela

V32.0XX- Driver of three-wheeled motor vehicle injured in collision with two- or three-wheeled motor vehicle in nontraffic accident

V32.1XX- Passenger in three-wheeled motor vehicle injured in collision with two- or three-wheeled motor vehicle in nontraffic accident

V32.2XX- Person on outside of three-wheeled motor vehicle injured in collision with two- or three-wheeled motor vehicle in nontraffic accident

V32.3XX- Unspecified occupant of three-wheeled motor vehicle injured in collision with two- or three-wheeled motor vehicle in nontraffic accident

V32.4XX- Person boarding or alighting a three-wheeled motor vehicle injured in collision with two- or three-wheeled motor vehicle

V32.5XX- Driver of three-wheeled motor vehicle injured in collision with two- or three-wheeled motor vehicle in traffic accident

V32.6XX- Passenger in three-wheeled motor vehicle injured in collision with two- or three-wheeled motor vehicle in traffic accident

V32.7XX- Person on outside of three-wheeled motor vehicle injured in collision with two- or three-wheeled motor vehicle in traffic accident

V32.9XX- Unspecified occupant of three-wheeled motor vehicle injured in collision with two- or three-wheeled motor vehicle in traffic accident

V33 Occupant of three-wheeled motor vehicle injured in collision with car, pick-up truck or van

The appropriate 7th character is to be added to each code from category V33

A initial encounter
D subsequent encounter
S sequela

V33.0XX- Driver of three-wheeled motor vehicle injured in collision with car, pick-up truck or van in nontraffic accident

V33.1XX- Passenger in three-wheeled motor vehicle injured in collision with car, pick-up truck or van in nontraffic accident

V33.2XX- Person on outside of three-wheeled motor vehicle injured in collision with car, pick-up truck or van in nontraffic accident

V33.3XX- Unspecified occupant of three-wheeled motor vehicle injured in collision with car, pick-up truck or van in nontraffic accident

V33.4XX- Person boarding or alighting a three-wheeled motor vehicle injured in collision with car, pick-up truck or van

V33.5XX- Driver of three-wheeled motor vehicle injured in collision with car, pick-up truck or van in traffic accident

V33.6XX- Passenger in three-wheeled motor vehicle injured in collision with car, pick-up truck or van in traffic accident

V33.7XX- Person on outside of three-wheeled motor vehicle injured in collision with car, pick-up truck or van in traffic accident

V33.9XX- Unspecified occupant of three-wheeled motor vehicle injured in collision with car, pick-up truck or van in traffic accident

V34 Occupant of three-wheeled motor vehicle injured in collision with heavy transport vehicle or bus

EXCLUDES 1 *occupant of three-wheeled motor vehicle injured in collision with military vehicle (V39.81)*

The appropriate 7th character is to be added to each code from category V34

A initial encounter
D subsequent encounter
S sequela

V34.0XX- Driver of three-wheeled motor vehicle injured in collision with heavy transport vehicle or bus in nontraffic accident

V34.1XX- Passenger in three-wheeled motor vehicle injured in collision with heavy transport vehicle or bus in nontraffic accident

V34.2XX- Person on outside of three-wheeled motor vehicle injured in collision with heavy transport vehicle or bus in nontraffic accident

V34.3XX- Unspecified occupant of three-wheeled motor vehicle injured in collision with heavy transport vehicle or bus in nontraffic accident

V34.4XX- Person boarding or alighting a three-wheeled motor vehicle injured in collision with heavy transport vehicle or bus

V34.5XX- Driver of three-wheeled motor vehicle injured in collision with heavy transport vehicle or bus in traffic accident

V34.6XX- Passenger in three-wheeled motor vehicle injured in collision with heavy transport vehicle or bus in traffic accident

V34.7XX- Person on outside of three-wheeled motor vehicle injured in collision with heavy transport vehicle or bus in traffic accident

V34.9XX- Unspecified occupant of three-wheeled motor vehicle injured in collision with heavy transport vehicle or bus in traffic accident

V35 Occupant of three-wheeled motor vehicle injured in collision with railway train or railway vehicle

The appropriate 7th character is to be added to each code from category V35
A initial encounter
D subsequent encounter
S sequela

V35.0XX- **Driver of three-wheeled motor vehicle injured in collision with railway train or railway vehicle in nontraffic accident**

V35.1XX- **Passenger in three-wheeled motor vehicle injured in collision with railway train or railway vehicle in nontraffic accident**

V35.2XX- **Person on outside of three-wheeled motor vehicle injured in collision with railway train or railway vehicle in nontraffic accident**

V35.3XX- **Unspecified occupant of three-wheeled motor vehicle injured in collision with railway train or railway vehicle in nontraffic accident**

V35.4XX- **Person boarding or alighting a three-wheeled motor vehicle injured in collision with railway train or railway vehicle**

V35.5XX- **Driver of three-wheeled motor vehicle injured in collision with railway train or railway vehicle in traffic accident**

V35.6XX- **Passenger in three-wheeled motor vehicle injured in collision with railway train or railway vehicle in traffic accident**

V35.7XX- **Person on outside of three-wheeled motor vehicle injured in collision with railway train or railway vehicle in traffic accident**

V35.9XX- **Unspecified occupant of three-wheeled motor vehicle injured in collision with railway train or railway vehicle in traffic accident**

V36 Occupant of three-wheeled motor vehicle injured in collision with other nonmotor vehicle

INCLUDES collision with animal-drawn vehicle, animal being ridden, streetcar

The appropriate 7th character is to be added to each code from category V36
A initial encounter
D subsequent encounter
S sequela

V36.0XX- **Driver of three-wheeled motor vehicle injured in collision with other nonmotor vehicle in nontraffic accident**

V36.1XX- **Passenger in three-wheeled motor vehicle injured in collision with other nonmotor vehicle in nontraffic accident**

V36.2XX- **Person on outside of three-wheeled motor vehicle injured in collision with other nonmotor vehicle in nontraffic accident**

V36.3XX- **Unspecified occupant of three-wheeled motor vehicle injured in collision with other nonmotor vehicle in nontraffic accident**

V36.4XX- **Person boarding or alighting a three-wheeled motor vehicle injured in collision with other nonmotor vehicle**

V36.5XX- **Driver of three-wheeled motor vehicle injured in collision with other nonmotor vehicle in traffic accident**

V36.6XX- **Passenger in three-wheeled motor vehicle injured in collision with other nonmotor vehicle in traffic accident**

V36.7XX- **Person on outside of three-wheeled motor vehicle injured in collision with other nonmotor vehicle in traffic accident**

V36.9XX- **Unspecified occupant of three-wheeled motor vehicle injured in collision with other nonmotor vehicle in traffic accident**

V37 Occupant of three-wheeled motor vehicle injured in collision with fixed or stationary object

The appropriate 7th character is to be added to each code from category V37
A initial encounter
D subsequent encounter
S sequela

V37.0XX- **Driver of three-wheeled motor vehicle injured in collision with fixed or stationary object in nontraffic accident**

V37.1XX- **Passenger in three-wheeled motor vehicle injured in collision with fixed or stationary object in nontraffic accident**

V37.2XX- **Person on outside of three-wheeled motor vehicle injured in collision with fixed or stationary object in nontraffic accident**

V37.3XX- **Unspecified occupant of three-wheeled motor vehicle injured in collision with fixed or stationary object in nontraffic accident**

V37.4XX- **Person boarding or alighting a three-wheeled motor vehicle injured in collision with fixed or stationary object**

V37.5XX- **Driver of three-wheeled motor vehicle injured in collision with fixed or stationary object in traffic accident**

V37.6XX- **Passenger in three-wheeled motor vehicle injured in collision with fixed or stationary object in traffic accident**

V37.7XX- **Person on outside of three-wheeled motor vehicle injured in collision with fixed or stationary object in traffic accident**

V37.9XX- **Unspecified occupant of three-wheeled motor vehicle injured in collision with fixed or stationary object in traffic accident**

V38 Occupant of three-wheeled motor vehicle injured in noncollision transport accident

INCLUDES fall or thrown from three-wheeled motor vehicle
overturning of three-wheeled motor vehicle NOS
overturning of three-wheeled motor vehicle without collision

The appropriate 7th character is to be added to each code from category V38
A initial encounter
D subsequent encounter
S sequela

V38.0XX- **Driver of three-wheeled motor vehicle injured in noncollision transport accident in nontraffic accident**

V38.1XX- **Passenger in three-wheeled motor vehicle injured in noncollision transport accident in nontraffic accident**

V38.2XX- **Person on outside of three-wheeled motor vehicle injured in noncollision transport accident in nontraffic accident**

V38.3XX- **Unspecified occupant of three-wheeled motor vehicle injured in noncollision transport accident in nontraffic accident**

V38.4XX- **Person boarding or alighting a three-wheeled motor vehicle injured in noncollision transport accident**

V38.5XX- **Driver of three-wheeled motor vehicle injured in noncollision transport accident in traffic accident**

V38.6XX- **Passenger in three-wheeled motor vehicle injured in noncollision transport accident in traffic accident**

V38.7XX- **Person on outside of three-wheeled motor vehicle injured in noncollision transport accident in traffic accident**

V38.9XX- **Unspecified occupant of three-wheeled motor vehicle injured in noncollision transport accident in traffic accident**

V39 Occupant of three-wheeled motor vehicle injured in other and unspecified transport accidents

The appropriate 7th character is to be added to each code from category V39
A initial encounter
D subsequent encounter
S sequela

V39.0 **Driver of three-wheeled motor vehicle injured in collision with other and unspecified motor vehicles in nontraffic accident**

V39.00X- **Driver of three-wheeled motor vehicle injured in collision with unspecified motor vehicles in nontraffic accident**

V39.09X- **Driver of three-wheeled motor vehicle injured in collision with other motor vehicles in nontraffic accident**

5 V39.1 **Passenger in three-wheeled motor vehicle injured in collision with other and unspecified motor vehicles in nontraffic accident**

7 V39.10X- **Passenger in three-wheeled motor vehicle injured in collision with unspecified motor vehicles in nontraffic accident**

7 V39.19X- **Passenger in three-wheeled motor vehicle injured in collision with other motor vehicles in nontraffic accident**

5 V39.2 **Unspecified occupant of three-wheeled motor vehicle injured in collision with other and unspecified motor vehicles in nontraffic accident**

7 V39.20X- **Unspecified occupant of three-wheeled motor vehicle injured in collision with unspecified motor vehicles in nontraffic accident**

Collision NOS involving three-wheeled motor vehicle, nontraffic

7 V39.29X- **Unspecified occupant of three-wheeled motor vehicle injured in collision with other motor vehicles in nontraffic accident**

7 V39.3XX- **Occupant (driver) (passenger) of three-wheeled motor vehicle injured in unspecified nontraffic accident**

Accident NOS involving three-wheeled motor vehicle, nontraffic

Occupant of three-wheeled motor vehicle injured in nontraffic accident NOS

5 V39.4 **Driver of three-wheeled motor vehicle injured in collision with other and unspecified motor vehicles in traffic accident**

7 V39.40X- **Driver of three-wheeled motor vehicle injured in collision with unspecified motor vehicles in traffic accident**

7 V39.49X- **Driver of three-wheeled motor vehicle injured in collision with other motor vehicles in traffic accident**

5 V39.5 **Passenger in three-wheeled motor vehicle injured in collision with other and unspecified motor vehicles in traffic accident**

7 V39.50X- **Passenger in three-wheeled motor vehicle injured in collision with unspecified motor vehicles in traffic accident**

7 V39.59X- **Passenger in three-wheeled motor vehicle injured in collision with other motor vehicles in traffic accident**

5 V39.6 **Unspecified occupant of three-wheeled motor vehicle injured in collision with other and unspecified motor vehicles in traffic accident**

7 V39.60X- **Unspecified occupant of three-wheeled motor vehicle injured in collision with unspecified motor vehicles in traffic accident**

Collision NOS involving three-wheeled motor vehicle (traffic)

7 V39.69X- **Unspecified occupant of three-wheeled motor vehicle injured in collision with other motor vehicles in traffic accident**

5 V39.8 **Occupant (driver) (passenger) of three-wheeled motor vehicle injured in other specified transport accidents**

7 V39.81X- **Occupant (driver) (passenger) of three-wheeled motor vehicle injured in transport accident with military vehicle**

7 V39.89X- **Occupant (driver) (passenger) of three-wheeled motor vehicle injured in other specified transport accidents**

7 V39.9XX- **Occupant (driver) (passenger) of three-wheeled motor vehicle injured in unspecified traffic accident**

Accident NOS involving three-wheeled motor vehicle

Car occupant injured in transport accident (V40-V49)

INCLUDES a four-wheeled motor vehicle designed primarily for carrying passengers
automobile (pulling a trailer or camper)

EXCLUDES 1 *bus (V50-V59)*
minibus (V50-V59)
minivan (V50-V59)
motorcoach (V70-V79)
pick-up truck (V50-V59)
sport utility vehicle (SUV) (V50-V59)

4 V40 **Car occupant injured in collision with pedestrian or animal**

EXCLUDES 1 *car collision with animal-drawn vehicle or animal being ridden (V46.-)*

The appropriate 7th character is to be added to each code from category V40
A initial encounter
D subsequent encounter
S sequela

7 V40.0XX- **Car driver injured in collision with pedestrian or animal in nontraffic accident**

7 V40.1XX- **Car passenger injured in collision with pedestrian or animal in nontraffic accident**

7 V40.2XX- **Person on outside of car injured in collision with pedestrian or animal in nontraffic accident**

7 V40.3XX- **Unspecified car occupant injured in collision with pedestrian or animal in nontraffic accident**

7 V40.4XX- **Person boarding or alighting a car injured in collision with pedestrian or animal**

7 V40.5XX- **Car driver injured in collision with pedestrian or animal in traffic accident**

7 V40.6XX- **Car passenger injured in collision with pedestrian or animal in traffic accident**

7 V40.7XX- **Person on outside of car injured in collision with pedestrian or animal in traffic accident**

7 V40.9XX- **Unspecified car occupant injured in collision with pedestrian or animal in traffic accident**

4 V41 **Car occupant injured in collision with pedal cycle**

The appropriate 7th character is to be added to each code from category V41
A initial encounter
D subsequent encounter
S sequela

7 V41.0XX- **Car driver injured in collision with pedal cycle in nontraffic accident**

7 V41.1XX- **Car passenger injured in collision with pedal cycle in nontraffic accident**

7 V41.2XX- **Person on outside of car injured in collision with pedal cycle in nontraffic accident**

7 V41.3XX- **Unspecified car occupant injured in collision with pedal cycle in nontraffic accident**

7 V41.4XX- **Person boarding or alighting a car injured in collision with pedal cycle**

7 V41.5XX- **Car driver injured in collision with pedal cycle in traffic accident**

7 V41.6XX- **Car passenger injured in collision with pedal cycle in traffic accident**

7 V41.7XX- **Person on outside of car injured in collision with pedal cycle in traffic accident**

7 V41.9XX- **Unspecified car occupant injured in collision with pedal cycle in traffic accident**

4 V42 **Car occupant injured in collision with two- or three-wheeled motor vehicle**

The appropriate 7th character is to be added to each code from category V42
A initial encounter
D subsequent encounter
S sequela

7 V42.0XX- **Car driver injured in collision with two- or three-wheeled motor vehicle in nontraffic accident**

7 V42.1XX- **Car passenger injured in collision with two- or three-wheeled motor vehicle in nontraffic accident**

7 V42.2XX- Person on outside of car injured in collision with two- or three-wheeled motor vehicle in nontraffic accident

7 V42.3XX- Unspecified car occupant injured in collision with two- or three-wheeled motor vehicle in nontraffic accident

7 V42.4XX- Person boarding or alighting a car injured in collision with two- or three-wheeled motor vehicle

7 V42.5XX- Car driver injured in collision with two- or three-wheeled motor vehicle in traffic accident

7 V42.6XX- Car passenger injured in collision with two- or three-wheeled motor vehicle in traffic accident

7 V42.7XX- Person on outside of car injured in collision with two- or three-wheeled motor vehicle in traffic accident

7 V42.9XX- Unspecified car occupant injured in collision with two- or three-wheeled motor vehicle in traffic accident

4 V43 Car occupant injured in collision with car, pick-up truck or van

The appropriate 7th character is to be added to each code from category V43
A initial encounter
D subsequent encounter
S sequela

5 V43.0 Car driver injured in collision with car, pick-up truck or van in nontraffic accident

7 V43.01X- Car driver injured in collision with sport utility vehicle in nontraffic accident

7 V43.02X- Car driver injured in collision with other type car in nontraffic accident

7 V43.03X- Car driver injured in collision with pick-up truck in nontraffic accident

7 V43.04X- Car driver injured in collision with van in nontraffic accident

5 V43.1 Car passenger injured in collision with car, pick-up truck or van in nontraffic accident

7 V43.11X- Car passenger injured in collision with sport utility vehicle in nontraffic accident

7 V43.12X- Car passenger injured in collision with other type car in nontraffic accident

7 V43.13X- Car passenger injured in collision with pick-up in nontraffic accident

7 V43.14X- Car passenger injured in collision with van in nontraffic accident

5 V43.2 Person on outside of car injured in collision with car, pick-up truck or van in nontraffic accident

7 V43.21X- Person on outside of car injured in collision with sport utility vehicle in nontraffic accident

7 V43.22X- Person on outside of car injured in collision with other type car in nontraffic accident

7 V43.23X- Person on outside of car injured in collision with pick-up truck in nontraffic accident

7 V43.24X- Person on outside of car injured in collision with van in nontraffic accident

5 V43.3 Unspecified car occupant injured in collision with car, pick-up truck or van in nontraffic accident

7 V43.31X- Unspecified car occupant injured in collision with sport utility vehicle in nontraffic accident

7 V43.32X- Unspecified car occupant injured in collision with other type car in nontraffic accident

7 V43.33X- Unspecified car occupant injured in collision with pick-up truck in nontraffic accident

7 V43.34X- Unspecified car occupant injured in collision with van in nontraffic accident

5 V43.4 Person boarding or alighting a car injured in collision with car, pick-up truck or van

7 V43.41X- Person boarding or alighting a car injured in collision with sport utility vehicle

7 V43.42X- Person boarding or alighting a car injured in collision with other type car

7 V43.43X- Person boarding or alighting a car injured in collision with pick-up truck

7 V43.44X- Person boarding or alighting a car injured in collision with van

5 V43.5 Car driver injured in collision with car, pick-up truck or van in traffic accident

7 V43.51X- Car driver injured in collision with sport utility vehicle in traffic accident

7 V43.52X- Car driver injured in collision with other type car in traffic accident

7 V43.53X- Car driver injured in collision with pick-up truck in traffic accident

7 V43.54X- Car driver injured in collision with van in traffic accident

5 V43.6 Car passenger injured in collision with car, pick-up truck or van in traffic accident

7 V43.61X- Car passenger injured in collision with sport utility vehicle in traffic accident
AHA: (V43.61XA) 1Q 2015, 5
AHA: (V43.61XD) 1Q 2015, 5, 7

7 V43.62X- Car passenger injured in collision with other type car in traffic accident

7 V43.63X- Car passenger injured in collision with pick-up truck in traffic accident

7 V43.64X- Car passenger injured in collision with van in traffic accident

5 V43.7 Person on outside of car injured in collision with car, pick-up truck or van in traffic accident

7 V43.71X- Person on outside of car injured in collision with sport utility vehicle in traffic accident

7 V43.72X- Person on outside of car injured in collision with other type car in traffic accident

7 V43.73X- Person on outside of car injured in collision with pick-up truck in traffic accident

7 V43.74X- Person on outside of car injured in collision with van in traffic accident

5 V43.9 Unspecified car occupant injured in collision with car, pick-up truck or van in traffic accident

7 V43.91X- Unspecified car occupant injured in collision with sport utility vehicle in traffic accident

7 V43.92X- Unspecified car occupant injured in collision with other type car in traffic accident

7 V43.93X- Unspecified car occupant injured in collision with pick-up truck in traffic accident

7 V43.94X- Unspecified car occupant injured in collision with van in traffic accident

4 V44 Car occupant injured in collision with heavy transport vehicle or bus

EXCLUDES 1 *car occupant injured in collision with military vehicle (V49.81)*

The appropriate 7th character is to be added to each code from category V44
A initial encounter
D subsequent encounter
S sequela

7 V44.0XX- Car driver injured in collision with heavy transport vehicle or bus in nontraffic accident

7 V44.1XX- Car passenger injured in collision with heavy transport vehicle or bus in nontraffic accident

7 V44.2XX- Person on outside of car injured in collision with heavy transport vehicle or bus in nontraffic accident

7 V44.3XX- Unspecified car occupant injured in collision with heavy transport vehicle or bus in nontraffic accident

7 V44.4XX- Person boarding or alighting a car injured in collision with heavy transport vehicle or bus

7 V44.5XX- Car driver injured in collision with heavy transport vehicle or bus in traffic accident

7 V44.6XX- Car passenger injured in collision with heavy transport vehicle or bus in traffic accident

7 V44.7XX- Person on outside of car injured in collision with heavy transport vehicle or bus in traffic accident

7 V44.9XX- Unspecified car occupant injured in collision with heavy transport vehicle or bus in traffic accident

4 V45 Car occupant injured in collision with railway train or railway vehicle

The appropriate 7th character is to be added to each code from category V45
A initial encounter
D subsequent encounter
S sequela

7 V45.0XX- Car driver injured in collision with railway train or railway vehicle in nontraffic accident

V45.1XX- **Car passenger injured in collision with railway train or railway vehicle in nontraffic accident**

V45.2XX- **Person on outside of car injured in collision with railway train or railway vehicle in nontraffic accident**

V45.3XX- **Unspecified car occupant injured in collision with railway train or railway vehicle in nontraffic accident**

V45.4XX- **Person boarding or alighting a car injured in collision with railway train or railway vehicle**

V45.5XX- **Car driver injured in collision with railway train or railway vehicle in traffic accident**

V45.6XX- **Car passenger injured in collision with railway train or railway vehicle in traffic accident**

V45.7XX- **Person on outside of car injured in collision with railway train or railway vehicle in traffic accident**

V45.9XX- **Unspecified car occupant injured in collision with railway train or railway vehicle in traffic accident**

V46 Car occupant injured in collision with other nonmotor vehicle

INCLUDES collision with animal-drawn vehicle, animal being ridden, streetcar

The appropriate 7th character is to be added to each code from category V46
A initial encounter
D subsequent encounter
S sequela

V46.0XX- **Car driver injured in collision with other nonmotor vehicle in nontraffic accident**

V46.1XX- **Car passenger injured in collision with other nonmotor vehicle in nontraffic accident**

V46.2XX- **Person on outside of car injured in collision with other nonmotor vehicle in nontraffic accident**

V46.3XX- **Unspecified car occupant injured in collision with other nonmotor vehicle in nontraffic accident**

V46.4XX- **Person boarding or alighting a car injured in collision with other nonmotor vehicle**

V46.5XX- **Car driver injured in collision with other nonmotor vehicle in traffic accident**

V46.6XX- **Car passenger injured in collision with other nonmotor vehicle in traffic accident**

V46.7XX- **Person on outside of car injured in collision with other nonmotor vehicle in traffic accident**

V46.9XX- **Unspecified car occupant injured in collision with other nonmotor vehicle in traffic accident**

V47 Car occupant injured in collision with fixed or stationary object

The appropriate 7th character is to be added to each code from category V47
A initial encounter
D subsequent encounter
S sequela

AHA: 4Q 2016, 73

V47.0XX- **Car driver injured in collision with fixed or stationary object in nontraffic accident**

V47.1XX- **Car passenger injured in collision with fixed or stationary object in nontraffic accident**

V47.2XX- **Person on outside of car injured in collision with fixed or stationary object in nontraffic accident**

V47.3XX- **Unspecified car occupant injured in collision with fixed or stationary object in nontraffic accident**

V47.4XX- **Person boarding or alighting a car injured in collision with fixed or stationary object**

V47.5XX- **Car driver injured in collision with fixed or stationary object in traffic accident**

V47.6XX- **Car passenger injured in collision with fixed or stationary object in traffic accident**

V47.7XX- **Person on outside of car injured in collision with fixed or stationary object in traffic accident**

V47.9XX- **Unspecified car occupant injured in collision with fixed or stationary object in traffic accident**

V48 Car occupant injured in noncollision transport accident

INCLUDES overturning car NOS
overturning car without collision

The appropriate 7th character is to be added to each code from category V48
A initial encounter
D subsequent encounter
S sequela

V48.0XX- **Car driver injured in noncollision transport accident in nontraffic accident**

V48.1XX- **Car passenger injured in noncollision transport accident in nontraffic accident**

V48.2XX- **Person on outside of car injured in noncollision transport accident in nontraffic accident**

V48.3XX- **Unspecified car occupant injured in noncollision transport accident in nontraffic accident**

V48.4XX- **Person boarding or alighting a car injured in noncollision transport accident**

V48.5XX- **Car driver injured in noncollision transport accident in traffic accident**

V48.6XX- **Car passenger injured in noncollision transport accident in traffic accident**

V48.7XX- **Person on outside of car injured in noncollision transport accident in traffic accident**

V48.9XX- **Unspecified car occupant injured in noncollision transport accident in traffic accident**

V49 Car occupant injured in other and unspecified transport accidents

The appropriate 7th character is to be added to each code from category V49
A initial encounter
D subsequent encounter
S sequela

V49.0 **Driver injured in collision with other and unspecified motor vehicles in nontraffic accident**

V49.00X- **Driver injured in collision with unspecified motor vehicles in nontraffic accident**

V49.09X- **Driver injured in collision with other motor vehicles in nontraffic accident**

V49.1 **Passenger injured in collision with other and unspecified motor vehicles in nontraffic accident**

V49.10X- **Passenger injured in collision with unspecified motor vehicles in nontraffic accident**

V49.19X- **Passenger injured in collision with other motor vehicles in nontraffic accident**

V49.2 **Unspecified car occupant injured in collision with other and unspecified motor vehicles in nontraffic accident**

V49.20X- **Unspecified car occupant injured in collision with unspecified motor vehicles in nontraffic accident**
Car collision NOS, nontraffic

V49.29X- **Unspecified car occupant injured in collision with other motor vehicles in nontraffic accident**

V49.3XX- **Car occupant (driver) (passenger) injured in unspecified nontraffic accident**
Car accident NOS, nontraffic
Car occupant injured in nontraffic accident NOS

V49.4 **Driver injured in collision with other and unspecified motor vehicles in traffic accident**

V49.40X- **Driver injured in collision with unspecified motor vehicles in traffic accident**

V49.49X- **Driver injured in collision with other motor vehicles in traffic accident**

V49.5 **Passenger injured in collision with other and unspecified motor vehicles in traffic accident**

V49.50X- **Passenger injured in collision with unspecified motor vehicles in traffic accident**

V49.59X- **Passenger injured in collision with other motor vehicles in traffic accident**

V49.6 **Unspecified car occupant injured in collision with other and unspecified motor vehicles in traffic accident**

V49.60X- **Unspecified car occupant injured in collision with unspecified motor vehicles in traffic accident**
Car collision NOS (traffic)

7 V49.69X- **Unspecified car occupant injured in collision with other motor vehicles in traffic accident**

5 V49.8 **Car occupant (driver) (passenger) injured in other specified transport accidents**

7 V49.81X- **Car occupant (driver) (passenger) injured in transport accident with military vehicle**

7 V49.88X- **Car occupant (driver) (passenger) injured in other specified transport accidents**

7 V49.9XX- **Car occupant (driver) (passenger) injured in unspecified traffic accident**

Car accident NOS
AHA: (V49.9XXA) 1Q 2015, 11

Occupant of pick-up truck or van injured in transport accident (V50-V59)

INCLUDES a four or six wheel motor vehicle designed primarily for carrying passengers and property but weighing less than the local limit for classification as a heavy goods vehicle
minibus
minivan
sport utility vehicle (SUV)
truck
van

EXCLUDES 1 *heavy transport vehicle (V60-V69)*

4 V50 **Occupant of pick-up truck or van injured in collision with pedestrian or animal**

EXCLUDES 1 *pick-up truck or van collision with animal-drawn vehicle or animal being ridden (V56.-)*

The appropriate 7th character is to be added to each code from category V50
A initial encounter
D subsequent encounter
S sequela

7 V50.0XX- **Driver of pick-up truck or van injured in collision with pedestrian or animal in nontraffic accident**

7 V50.1XX- **Passenger in pick-up truck or van injured in collision with pedestrian or animal in nontraffic accident**

7 V50.2XX- **Person on outside of pick-up truck or van injured in collision with pedestrian or animal in nontraffic accident**

7 V50.3XX- **Unspecified occupant of pick-up truck or van injured in collision with pedestrian or animal in nontraffic accident**

7 V50.4XX- **Person boarding or alighting a pick-up truck or van injured in collision with pedestrian or animal**

7 V50.5XX- **Driver of pick-up truck or van injured in collision with pedestrian or animal in traffic accident**

7 V50.6XX- **Passenger in pick-up truck or van injured in collision with pedestrian or animal in traffic accident**

7 V50.7XX- **Person on outside of pick-up truck or van injured in collision with pedestrian or animal in traffic accident**

7 V50.9XX- **Unspecified occupant of pick-up truck or van injured in collision with pedestrian or animal in traffic accident**

4 V51 **Occupant of pick-up truck or van injured in collision with pedal cycle**

The appropriate 7th character is to be added to each code from category V51
A initial encounter
D subsequent encounter
S sequela

7 V51.0XX- **Driver of pick-up truck or van injured in collision with pedal cycle in nontraffic accident**

7 V51.1XX- **Passenger in pick-up truck or van injured in collision with pedal cycle in nontraffic accident**

7 V51.2XX- **Person on outside of pick-up truck or van injured in collision with pedal cycle in nontraffic accident**

7 V51.3XX- **Unspecified occupant of pick-up truck or van injured in collision with pedal cycle in nontraffic accident**

7 V51.4XX- **Person boarding or alighting a pick-up truck or van injured in collision with pedal cycle**

7 V51.5XX- **Driver of pick-up truck or van injured in collision with pedal cycle in traffic accident**

7 V51.6XX- **Passenger in pick-up truck or van injured in collision with pedal cycle in traffic accident**

7 V51.7XX- **Person on outside of pick-up truck or van injured in collision with pedal cycle in traffic accident**

7 V51.9XX- **Unspecified occupant of pick-up truck or van injured in collision with pedal cycle in traffic accident**

4 V52 **Occupant of pick-up truck or van injured in collision with two- or three-wheeled motor vehicle**

The appropriate 7th character is to be added to each code from category V52
A initial encounter
D subsequent encounter
S sequela

7 V52.0XX- **Driver of pick-up truck or van injured in collision with two- or three-wheeled motor vehicle in nontraffic accident**

7 V52.1XX- **Passenger in pick-up truck or van injured in collision with two- or three-wheeled motor vehicle in nontraffic accident**

7 V52.2XX- **Person on outside of pick-up truck or van injured in collision with two- or three-wheeled motor vehicle in nontraffic accident**

7 V52.3XX- **Unspecified occupant of pick-up truck or van injured in collision with two- or three-wheeled motor vehicle in nontraffic accident**

7 V52.4XX- **Person boarding or alighting a pick-up truck or van injured in collision with two- or three-wheeled motor vehicle**

7 V52.5XX- **Driver of pick-up truck or van injured in collision with two- or three-wheeled motor vehicle in traffic accident**

7 V52.6XX- **Passenger in pick-up truck or van injured in collision with two- or three-wheeled motor vehicle in traffic accident**

7 V52.7XX- **Person on outside of pick-up truck or van injured in collision with two- or three-wheeled motor vehicle in traffic accident**

7 V52.9XX- **Unspecified occupant of pick-up truck or van injured in collision with two- or three-wheeled motor vehicle in traffic accident**

4 V53 **Occupant of pick-up truck or van injured in collision with car, pick-up truck or van**

The appropriate 7th character is to be added to each code from category V53
A initial encounter
D subsequent encounter
S sequela

7 V53.0XX- **Driver of pick-up truck or van injured in collision with car, pick-up truck or van in nontraffic accident**

7 V53.1XX- **Passenger in pick-up truck or van injured in collision with car, pick-up truck or van in nontraffic accident**

7 V53.2XX- **Person on outside of pick-up truck or van injured in collision with car, pick-up truck or van in nontraffic accident**

7 V53.3XX- **Unspecified occupant of pick-up truck or van injured in collision with car, pick-up truck or van in nontraffic accident**

7 V53.4XX- **Person boarding or alighting a pick-up truck or van injured in collision with car, pick-up truck or van**

7 V53.5XX- **Driver of pick-up truck or van injured in collision with car, pick-up truck or van in traffic accident**

7 V53.6XX- **Passenger in pick-up truck or van injured in collision with car, pick-up truck or van in traffic accident**

7 V53.7XX- **Person on outside of pick-up truck or van injured in collision with car, pick-up truck or van in traffic accident**

7 V53.9XX- **Unspecified occupant of pick-up truck or van injured in collision with car, pick-up truck or van in traffic accident**

V54 Occupant of pick-up truck or van injured in collisionwith heavy transport vehicle or bus

EXCLUDES 1 *occupant of pick-up truck or van injured in collision with military vehicle (V59.81)*

The appropriate 7th character is to be added to each code from category V54
A initial encounter
D subsequent encounter
S sequela

- V54.0XX- **Driver of pick-up truck or van injured in collision with heavy transport vehicle or bus in nontraffic accident**
- V54.1XX- **Passenger in pick-up truck or van injured in collision with heavy transport vehicle or bus in nontraffic accident**
- V54.2XX- **Person on outside of pick-up truck or van injured in collision with heavy transport vehicle or bus in nontraffic accident**
- V54.3XX- **Unspecified occupant of pick-up truck or van injured in collision with heavy transport vehicle or bus in nontraffic accident**
- V54.4XX- **Person boarding or alighting a pick-up truck or van injured in collision with heavy transport vehicle or bus**
- V54.5XX- **Driver of pick-up truck or van injured in collision with heavy transport vehicle or bus in traffic accident**
- V54.6XX- **Passenger in pick-up truck or van injured in collision with heavy transport vehicle or bus in traffic accident**
- V54.7XX- **Person on outside of pick-up truck or van injured in collision with heavy transport vehicle or bus in traffic accident**
- V54.9XX- **Unspecified occupant of pick-up truck or van injured in collision with heavy transport vehicle or bus in traffic accident**

V55 Occupant of pick-up truck or van injured in collision with railway train or railway vehicle

The appropriate 7th character is to be added to each code from category V55
A initial encounter
D subsequent encounter
S sequela

- V55.0XX- **Driver of pick-up truck or van injured in collision with railway train or railway vehicle in nontraffic accident**
- V55.1XX- **Passenger in pick-up truck or van injured in collision with railway train or railway vehicle in nontraffic accident**
- V55.2XX- **Person on outside of pick-up truck or van injured in collision with railway train or railway vehicle in nontraffic accident**
- V55.3XX- **Unspecified occupant of pick-up truck or van injured in collision with railway train or railway vehicle in nontraffic accident**
- V55.4XX- **Person boarding or alighting a pick-up truck or van injured in collision with railway train or railway vehicle**
- V55.5XX- **Driver of pick-up truck or van injured in collision with railway train or railway vehicle in traffic accident**
- V55.6XX- **Passenger in pick-up truck or van injured in collision with railway train or railway vehicle in traffic accident**
- V55.7XX- **Person on outside of pick-up truck or van injured in collision with railway train or railway vehicle in traffic accident**
- V55.9XX- **Unspecified occupant of pick-up truck or van injured in collision with railway train or railway vehicle in traffic accident**

V56 Occupant of pick-up truck or van injured in collisionwith other nonmotor vehicle

INCLUDES collision with animal-drawn vehicle, animal being ridden, streetcar

The appropriate 7th character is to be added to each code from category V56
A initial encounter
D subsequent encounter
S sequela

- V56.0XX- **Driver of pick-up truck or van injured in collision with other nonmotor vehicle in nontraffic accident**
- V56.1XX- **Passenger in pick-up truck or van injured in collision with other nonmotor vehicle in nontraffic accident**
- V56.2XX- **Person on outside of pick-up truck or van injured in collision with other nonmotor vehicle in nontraffic accident**
- V56.3XX- **Unspecified occupant of pick-up truck or van injured in collision with other nonmotor vehicle in nontraffic accident**
- V56.4XX- **Person boarding or alighting a pick-up truck or van injured in collision with other nonmotor vehicle**
- V56.5XX- **Driver of pick-up truck or van injured in collision with other nonmotor vehicle in traffic accident**
- V56.6XX- **Passenger in pick-up truck or van injured in collision with other nonmotor vehicle in traffic accident**
- V56.7XX- **Person on outside of pick-up truck or van injured in collision with other nonmotor vehicle in traffic accident**
- V56.9XX- **Unspecified occupant of pick-up truck or van injured in collision with other nonmotor vehicle in traffic accident**

V57 Occupant of pick-up truck or van injured in collision with fixed or stationary object

The appropriate 7th character is to be added to each code from category V57
A initial encounter
D subsequent encounter
S sequela

- V57.0XX- **Driver of pick-up truck or van injured in collision with fixed or stationary object in nontraffic accident**
- V57.1XX- **Passenger in pick-up truck or van injured in collision with fixed or stationary object in nontraffic accident**
- V57.2XX- **Person on outside of pick-up truck or van injured in collision with fixed or stationary object in nontraffic accident**
- V57.3XX- **Unspecified occupant of pick-up truck or van injured in collision with fixed or stationary object in nontraffic accident**
- V57.4XX- **Person boarding or alighting a pick-up truck or van injured in collision with fixed or stationary object**
- V57.5XX- **Driver of pick-up truck or van injured in collision with fixed or stationary object in traffic accident**
- V57.6XX- **Passenger in pick-up truck or van injured in collision with fixed or stationary object in traffic accident**
- V57.7XX- **Person on outside of pick-up truck or van injured in collision with fixed or stationary object in traffic accident**
- V57.9XX- **Unspecified occupant of pick-up truck or van injured in collision with fixed or stationary object in traffic accident**

V58 Occupant of pick-up truck or van injured in noncollision transport accident

INCLUDES overturning pick-up truck or van NOS
overturning pick-up truck or van without collision

The appropriate 7th character is to be added to each code from category V58
A initial encounter
D subsequent encounter
S sequela

7 V58.0XX- Driver of pick-up truck or van injured in noncollision transport accident in nontraffic accident

7 V58.1XX- Passenger in pick-up truck or van injured in noncollision transport accident in nontraffic accident

7 V58.2XX- Person on outside of pick-up truck or van injured in noncollision transport accident in nontraffic accident

7 V58.3XX- Unspecified occupant of pick-up truck or van injured in noncollision transport accident in nontraffic accident

7 V58.4XX- Person boarding or alighting a pick-up truck or van injured in noncollision transport accident

7 V58.5XX- Driver of pick-up truck or van injured in noncollision transport accident in traffic accident

7 V58.6XX- Passenger in pick-up truck or van injured in noncollision transport accident in traffic accident

7 V58.7XX- Person on outside of pick-up truck or van injured in noncollision transport accident in traffic accident

7 V58.9XX- Unspecified occupant of pick-up truck or van injured in noncollision transport accident in traffic accident

4 V59 **Occupant of pick-up truck or van injured in other and unspecified transport accidents**

The appropriate 7th character is to be added to each code from category V59
A initial encounter
D subsequent encounter
S sequela

5 V59.0 Driver of pick-up truck or van injured in collision with other and unspecified motor vehicles in nontraffic accident

7 V59.00X- Driver of pick-up truck or van injured in collision with unspecified motor vehicles in nontraffic accident

7 V59.09X- Driver of pick-up truck or van injured in collision with other motor vehicles in nontraffic accident

5 V59.1 Passenger in pick-up truck or van injured in collision with other and unspecified motor vehicles in nontraffic accident

7 V59.10X- Passenger in pick-up truck or van injured in collision with unspecified motor vehicles in nontraffic accident

7 V59.19X- Passenger in pick-up truck or van injured in collision with other motor vehicles in nontraffic accident

5 V59.2 Unspecified occupant of pick-up truck or van injured in collision with other and unspecified motor vehicles in nontraffic accident

7 V59.20X- Unspecified occupant of pick-up truck or van injured in collision with unspecified motor vehicles in nontraffic accident

Collision NOS involving pick-up truck or van, nontraffic

7 V59.29X- Unspecified occupant of pick-up truck or van injured in collision with other motor vehicles in nontraffic accident

7 V59.3XX- Occupant (driver) (passenger) of pick-up truck or van injured in unspecified nontraffic accident

Accident NOS involving pick-up truck or van, nontraffic

Occupant of pick-up truck or van injured in nontraffic accident NOS

5 V59.4 Driver of pick-up truck or van injured in collision with other and unspecified motor vehicles in traffic accident

7 V59.40X- Driver of pick-up truck or van injured in collision with unspecified motor vehicles in traffic accident

7 V59.49X- Driver of pick-up truck or van injured in collision with other motor vehicles in traffic accident

5 V59.5 Passenger in pick-up truck or van injured in collision with other and unspecified motor vehicles in traffic accident

7 V59.50X- Passenger in pick-up truck or van injured in collision with unspecified motor vehicles in traffic accident

7 V59.59X- Passenger in pick-up truck or van injured in collision with other motor vehicles in traffic accident

5 V59.6 Unspecified occupant of pick-up truck or van injured in collision with other and unspecified motor vehicles in traffic accident

7 V59.60X- Unspecified occupant of pick-up truck or van injured in collision with unspecified motor vehicles in traffic accident

Collision NOS involving pick-up truck or van (traffic)

7 V59.69X- Unspecified occupant of pick-up truck or van injured in collision with other motor vehicles in traffic accident

5 V59.8 Occupant (driver) (passenger) of pick-up truck or van injured in other specified transport accidents

7 V59.81X- Occupant (driver) (passenger) of pick-up truck or van injured in transport accident with military vehicle

7 V59.88X- Occupant (driver) (passenger) of pick-up truck or van injured in other specified transport accidents

7 V59.9XX- Occupant (driver) (passenger) of pick-up truck or van injured in unspecified traffic accident

Accident NOS involving pick-up truck or van

Occupant of heavy transport vehicle injured in transport accident (V60-V69)

INCLUDES 18 wheeler
armored car
panel truck

EXCLUDES 1 *bus*
motorcoach

4 V60 **Occupant of heavy transport vehicle injured in collision with pedestrian or animal**

EXCLUDES 1 *heavy transport vehicle collision with animal-drawn vehicle or animal being ridden (V66.-)*

The appropriate 7th character is to be added to each code from category V60
A initial encounter
D subsequent encounter
S sequela

7 V60.0XX- Driver of heavy transport vehicle injured in collision with pedestrian or animal in nontraffic accident

7 V60.1XX- Passenger in heavy transport vehicle injured in collision with pedestrian or animal in nontraffic accident

7 V60.2XX- Person on outside of heavy transport vehicle injured in collision with pedestrian or animal in nontraffic accident

7 V60.3XX- Unspecified occupant of heavy transport vehicle injured in collision with pedestrian or animal in nontraffic accident

7 V60.4XX- Person boarding or alighting a heavy transport vehicle injured in collision with pedestrian or animal

7 V60.5XX- Driver of heavy transport vehicle injured in collision with pedestrian or animal in traffic accident

7 V60.6XX- Passenger in heavy transport vehicle injured in collision with pedestrian or animal in traffic accident

7 V60.7XX- Person on outside of heavy transport vehicle injured in collision with pedestrian or animal in traffic accident

7 V60.9XX- Unspecified occupant of heavy transport vehicle injured in collision with pedestrian or animal in traffic accident

4 V61 **Occupant of heavy transport vehicle injured in collision with pedal cycle**

The appropriate 7th character is to be added to each code from category V61
A initial encounter
D subsequent encounter
S sequela

7 V61.0XX- Driver of heavy transport vehicle injured in collision with pedal cycle in nontraffic accident

V61.1XX- Passenger in heavy transport vehicle injured in collision with pedal cycle in nontraffic accident

V61.2XX- Person on outside of heavy transport vehicle injured in collision with pedal cycle in nontraffic accident

V61.3XX- Unspecified occupant of heavy transport vehicle injured in collision with pedal cycle in nontraffic accident

V61.4XX- Person boarding or alighting a heavy transport vehicle injured in collision with pedal cycle while boarding or alighting

V61.5XX- Driver of heavy transport vehicle injured in collision with pedal cycle in traffic accident

V61.6XX- Passenger in heavy transport vehicle injured in collision with pedal cycle in traffic accident

V61.7XX- Person on outside of heavy transport vehicle injured in collision with pedal cycle in traffic accident

V61.9XX- Unspecified occupant of heavy transport vehicle injured in collision with pedal cycle in traffic accident

V62 Occupant of heavy transport vehicle injured in collision with two- or three-wheeled motor vehicle

The appropriate 7th character is to be added to each code from category V62
A initial encounter
D subsequent encounter
S sequela

V62.0XX- Driver of heavy transport vehicle injured in collision with two- or three-wheeled motor vehicle in nontraffic accident

V62.1XX- Passenger in heavy transport vehicle injured in collision with two- or three-wheeled motor vehicle in nontraffic accident

V62.2XX- Person on outside of heavy transport vehicle injured in collision with two- or three-wheeled motor vehicle in nontraffic accident

V62.3XX- Unspecified occupant of heavy transport vehicle injured in collision with two- or three-wheeled motor vehicle in nontraffic accident

V62.4XX- Person boarding or alighting a heavy transport vehicle injured in collision with two- or three-wheeled motor vehicle

V62.5XX- Driver of heavy transport vehicle injured in collision with two- or three-wheeled motor vehicle in traffic accident

V62.6XX- Passenger in heavy transport vehicle injured in collision with two- or three-wheeled motor vehicle in traffic accident

V62.7XX- Person on outside of heavy transport vehicle injured in collision with two- or three-wheeled motor vehicle in traffic accident

V62.9XX- Unspecified occupant of heavy transport vehicle injured in collision with two- or three-wheeled motor vehicle in traffic accident

V63 Occupant of heavy transport vehicle injured in collision with car, pick-up truck or van

The appropriate 7th character is to be added to each code from category V63
A initial encounter
D subsequent encounter
S sequela

V63.0XX- Driver of heavy transport vehicle injured in collision with car, pick-up truck or van in nontraffic accident

V63.1XX- Passenger in heavy transport vehicle injured in collision with car, pick-up truck or van in nontraffic accident

V63.2XX- Person on outside of heavy transport vehicle injured in collision with car, pick-up truck or van in nontraffic accident

V63.3XX- Unspecified occupant of heavy transport vehicle injured in collision with car, pick-up truck or van in nontraffic accident

V63.4XX- Person boarding or alighting a heavy transport vehicle injured in collision with car, pick-up truck or van

V63.5XX- Driver of heavy transport vehicle injured in collision with car, pick-up truck or van in traffic accident

V63.6XX- Passenger in heavy transport vehicle injured in collision with car, pick-up truck or van in traffic accident

V63.7XX- Person on outside of heavy transport vehicle injured in collision with car, pick-up truck or van in traffic accident

V63.9XX- Unspecified occupant of heavy transport vehicle injured in collision with car, pick-up truck or van in traffic accident

V64 Occupant of heavy transport vehicle injured in collision with heavy transport vehicle or bus

EXCLUDES 1 *occupant of heavy transport vehicle injured in collision with military vehicle (V69.81)*

The appropriate 7th character is to be added to each code from category V64
A initial encounter
D subsequent encounter
S sequela

V64.0XX- Driver of heavy transport vehicle injured in collision with heavy transport vehicle or bus in nontraffic accident

V64.1XX- Passenger in heavy transport vehicle injured in collision with heavy transport vehicle or bus in nontraffic accident

V64.2XX- Person on outside of heavy transport vehicle injured in collision with heavy transport vehicle or bus in nontraffic accident

V64.3XX- Unspecified occupant of heavy transport vehicle injured in collision with heavy transport vehicle or bus in nontraffic accident

V64.4XX- Person boarding or alighting a heavy transport vehicle injured in collision with heavy transport vehicle or bus while boarding or alighting

V64.5XX- Driver of heavy transport vehicle injured in collision with heavy transport vehicle or bus in traffic accident

V64.6XX- Passenger in heavy transport vehicle injured in collision with heavy transport vehicle or bus in traffic accident

V64.7XX- Person on outside of heavy transport vehicle injured in collision with heavy transport vehicle or bus in traffic accident

V64.9XX- Unspecified occupant of heavy transport vehicle injured in collision with heavy transport vehicle or bus in traffic accident

V65 Occupant of heavy transport vehicle injured in collision with railway train or railway vehicle

The appropriate 7th character is to be added to each code from category V65
A initial encounter
D subsequent encounter
S sequela

V65.0XX- Driver of heavy transport vehicle injured in collision with railway train or railway vehicle in nontraffic accident

V65.1XX- Passenger in heavy transport vehicle injured in collision with railway train or railway vehicle in nontraffic accident

V65.2XX- Person on outside of heavy transport vehicle injured in collision with railway train or railway vehicle in nontraffic accident

V65.3XX- Unspecified occupant of heavy transport vehicle injured in collision with railway train or railway vehicle in nontraffic accident

V65.4XX- Person boarding or alighting a heavy transport vehicle injured in collision with railway train or railway vehicle

V65.5XX- Driver of heavy transport vehicle injured in collision with railway train or railway vehicle in traffic accident

V65.6XX- Passenger in heavy transport vehicle injured in collision with railway train or railway vehicle in traffic accident

V65.7XX- Person on outside of heavy transport vehicle injured in collision with railway train or railway vehicle in traffic accident

V65.9XX- Unspecified occupant of heavy transport vehicle injured in collision with railway train or railway vehicle in traffic accident

4 V66 Occupant of heavy transport vehicle injured in collision with other nonmotor vehicle

INCLUDES collision with animal-drawn vehicle, animal being ridden, streetcar

The appropriate 7th character is to be added to each code from category V66
A initial encounter
D subsequent encounter
S sequela

7 V66.0XX- **Driver of heavy transport vehicle injured in collision with other nonmotor vehicle in nontraffic accident**

7 V66.1XX- **Passenger in heavy transport vehicle injured in collision with other nonmotor vehicle in nontraffic accident**

7 V66.2XX- **Person on outside of heavy transport vehicle injured in collision with other nonmotor vehicle in nontraffic accident**

7 V66.3XX- **Unspecified occupant of heavy transport vehicle injured in collision with other nonmotor vehicle in nontraffic accident**

7 V66.4XX- **Person boarding or alighting a heavy transport vehicle injured in collision with other nonmotor vehicle**

7 V66.5XX- **Driver of heavy transport vehicle injured in collision with other nonmotor vehicle in traffic accident**

7 V66.6XX- **Passenger in heavy transport vehicle injured in collision with other nonmotor vehicle in traffic accident**

7 V66.7XX- **Person on outside of heavy transport vehicle injured in collision with other nonmotor vehicle in traffic accident**

7 V66.9XX- **Unspecified occupant of heavy transport vehicle injured in collision with other nonmotor vehicle in traffic accident**

4 V67 Occupant of heavy transport vehicle injured in collision with fixed or stationary object

The appropriate 7th character is to be added to each code from category V67
A initial encounter
D subsequent encounter
S sequela

7 V67.0XX- **Driver of heavy transport vehicle injured in collision with fixed or stationary object in nontraffic accident**

7 V67.1XX- **Passenger in heavy transport vehicle injured in collision with fixed or stationary object in nontraffic accident**

7 V67.2XX- **Person on outside of heavy transport vehicle injured in collision with fixed or stationary object in nontraffic accident**

7 V67.3XX- **Unspecified occupant of heavy transport vehicle injured in collision with fixed or stationary object in nontraffic accident**

7 V67.4XX- **Person boarding or alighting a heavy transport vehicle injured in collision with fixed or stationary object**

7 V67.5XX- **Driver of heavy transport vehicle injured in collision with fixed or stationary object in traffic accident**

7 V67.6XX- **Passenger in heavy transport vehicle injured in collision with fixed or stationary object in traffic accident**

7 V67.7XX- **Person on outside of heavy transport vehicle injured in collision with fixed or stationary object in traffic accident**

7 V67.9XX- **Unspecified occupant of heavy transport vehicle injured in collision with fixed or stationary object in traffic accident**

4 V68 Occupant of heavy transport vehicle injured in noncollision transport accident

INCLUDES overturning heavy transport vehicle NOS
overturning heavy transport vehicle without collision

The appropriate 7th character is to be added to each code from category V68
A initial encounter
D subsequent encounter
S sequela

7 V68.0XX- **Driver of heavy transport vehicle injured in noncollision transport accident in nontraffic accident**

7 V68.1XX- **Passenger in heavy transport vehicle injured in noncollision transport accident in nontraffic accident**

7 V68.2XX- **Person on outside of heavy transport vehicle injured in noncollision transport accident in nontraffic accident**

7 V68.3XX- **Unspecified occupant of heavy transport vehicle injured in noncollision transport accident in nontraffic accident**

7 V68.4XX- **Person boarding or alighting a heavy transport vehicle injured in noncollision transport accident**

7 V68.5XX- **Driver of heavy transport vehicle injured in noncollision transport accident in traffic accident**

7 V68.6XX- **Passenger in heavy transport vehicle injured in noncollision transport accident in traffic accident**

7 V68.7XX- **Person on outside of heavy transport vehicle injured in noncollision transport accident in traffic accident**

7 V68.9XX- **Unspecified occupant of heavy transport vehicle injured in noncollision transport accident in traffic accident**

4 V69 Occupant of heavy transport vehicle injured in other and unspecified transport accidents

The appropriate 7th character is to be added to each code from category V69
A initial encounter
D subsequent encounter
S sequela

5 V69.0 **Driver of heavy transport vehicle injured in collision with other and unspecified motor vehicles in nontraffic accident**

7 V69.00X- **Driver of heavy transport vehicle injured in collision with unspecified motor vehicles in nontraffic accident**

7 V69.09X- **Driver of heavy transport vehicle injured in collision with other motor vehicles in nontraffic accident**

5 V69.1 **Passenger in heavy transport vehicle injured in collision with other and unspecified motor vehicles in nontraffic accident**

7 V69.10X- **Passenger in heavy transport vehicle injured in collision with unspecified motor vehicles in nontraffic accident**

7 V69.19X- **Passenger in heavy transport vehicle injured in collision with other motor vehicles in nontraffic accident**

5 V69.2 **Unspecified occupant of heavy transport vehicle injured in collision with other and unspecified motor vehicles in nontraffic accident**

7 V69.20X- **Unspecified occupant of heavy transport vehicle injured in collision with unspecified motor vehicles in nontraffic accident**

Collision NOS involving heavy transport vehicle, nontraffic

7 V69.29X- **Unspecified occupant of heavy transport vehicle injured in collision with other motor vehicles in nontraffic accident**

7 V69.3XX- **Occupant (driver) (passenger) of heavy transport vehicle injured in unspecified nontraffic accident**

Accident NOS involving heavy transport vehicle, nontraffic
Occupant of heavy transport vehicle injured in nontraffic accident NOS

5 V69.4 **Driver of heavy transport vehicle injured in collision with other and unspecified motor vehicles in traffic accident**

7 V69.40X- **Driver of heavy transport vehicle injured in collision with unspecified motor vehicles in traffic accident**

7 V69.49X- **Driver of heavy transport vehicle injured in collision with other motor vehicles in traffic accident**

5 V69.5 **Passenger in heavy transport vehicle injured in collision with other and unspecified motor vehicles in traffic accident**

7 V69.50X- **Passenger in heavy transport vehicle injured in collision with unspecified motor vehicles in traffic accident**

7 V69.59X- **Passenger in heavy transport vehicle injured in collision with other motor vehicles in traffic accident**

5 V69.6 **Unspecified occupant of heavy transport vehicle injured in collision with other and unspecified motor vehicles in traffic accident**

7 V69.60X- **Unspecified occupant of heavy transport vehicle injured in collision with unspecified motor vehicles in traffic accident**

Collision NOS involving heavy transport vehicle (traffic)

7 V69.69X- **Unspecified occupant of heavy transport vehicle injured in collision with other motor vehicles in traffic accident**

5 V69.8 **Occupant (driver) (passenger) of heavy transport vehicle injured in other specified transport accidents**

7 V69.81X- **Occupant (driver) (passenger) of heavy transport vehicle injured in transport accidents with military vehicle**

7 V69.88X- **Occupant (driver) (passenger) of heavy transport vehicle injured in other specified transport accidents**

7 V69.9XX- **Occupant (driver) (passenger) of heavy transport vehicle injured in unspecified traffic accident**

Accident NOS involving heavy transport vehicle

Bus occupant injured in transport accident (V70-V79)

INCLUDES motorcoach

EXCLUDES 1 *minibus (V50-V59)*

4 V70 **Bus occupant injured in collision with pedestrian or animal**

EXCLUDES 1 *bus collision with animal-drawn vehicle or animal being ridden (V76.-)*

The appropriate 7th character is to be added to each code from category V70

A initial encounter
D subsequent encounter
S sequela

7 V70.0XX- **Driver of bus injured in collision with pedestrian or animal in nontraffic accident**

7 V70.1XX- **Passenger on bus injured in collision with pedestrian or animal in nontraffic accident**

7 V70.2XX- **Person on outside of bus injured in collision with pedestrian or animal in nontraffic accident**

7 V70.3XX- **Unspecified occupant of bus injured in collision with pedestrian or animal in nontraffic accident**

7 V70.4XX- **Person boarding or alighting from bus injured in collision with pedestrian or animal**

7 V70.5XX- **Driver of bus injured in collision with pedestrian or animal in traffic accident**

7 V70.6XX- **Passenger on bus injured in collision with pedestrian or animal in traffic accident**

7 V70.7XX- **Person on outside of bus injured in collision with pedestrian or animal in traffic accident**

7 V70.9XX- **Unspecified occupant of bus injured in collision with pedestrian or animal in traffic accident**

4 V71 **Bus occupant injured in collision with pedal cycle**

The appropriate 7th character is to be added to each code from category V71

A initial encounter
D subsequent encounter
S sequela

7 V71.0XX- **Driver of bus injured in collision with pedal cycle in nontraffic accident**

7 V71.1XX- **Passenger on bus injured in collision with pedal cycle in nontraffic accident**

7 V71.2XX- **Person on outside of bus injured in collision with pedal cycle in nontraffic accident**

7 V71.3XX- **Unspecified occupant of bus injured in collision with pedal cycle in nontraffic accident**

7 V71.4XX- **Person boarding or alighting from bus injured in collision with pedal cycle**

7 V71.5XX- **Driver of bus injured in collision with pedal cycle in traffic accident**

7 V71.6XX- **Passenger on bus injured in collision with pedal cycle in traffic accident**

7 V71.7XX- **Person on outside of bus injured in collision with pedal cycle in traffic accident**

7 V71.9XX- **Unspecified occupant of bus injured in collision with pedal cycle in traffic accident**

4 V72 **Bus occupant injured in collision with two- or three-wheeled motor vehicle**

The appropriate 7th character is to be added to each code from category V72

A initial encounter
D subsequent encounter
S sequela

7 V72.0XX- **Driver of bus injured in collision with two- or three-wheeled motor vehicle in nontraffic accident**

7 V72.1XX- **Passenger on bus injured in collision with two- or three-wheeled motor vehicle in nontraffic accident**

7 V72.2XX- **Person on outside of bus injured in collision with two- or three-wheeled motor vehicle in nontraffic accident**

7 V72.3XX- **Unspecified occupant of bus injured in collision with two- or three-wheeled motor vehicle in nontraffic accident**

7 V72.4XX- **Person boarding or alighting from bus injured in collision with two- or three-wheeled motor vehicle**

7 V72.5XX- **Driver of bus injured in collision with two- or three-wheeled motor vehicle in traffic accident**

7 V72.6XX- **Passenger on bus injured in collision with two- or three-wheeled motor vehicle in traffic accident**

7 V72.7XX- **Person on outside of bus injured in collision with two- or three-wheeled motor vehicle in traffic accident**

7 V72.9XX- **Unspecified occupant of bus injured in collision with two- or three-wheeled motor vehicle in traffic accident**

4 V73 **Bus occupant injured in collision with car, pick-up truck or van**

The appropriate 7th character is to be added to each code from category V73

A initial encounter
D subsequent encounter
S sequela

7 V73.0XX- **Driver of bus injured in collision with car, pick-up truck or van in nontraffic accident**

7 V73.1XX- **Passenger on bus injured in collision with car, pick-up truck or van in nontraffic accident**

7 V73.2XX- **Person on outside of bus injured in collision with car, pick-up truck or van in nontraffic accident**

7 V73.3XX- **Unspecified occupant of bus injured in collision with car, pick-up truck or van in nontraffic accident**

7 V73.4XX- **Person boarding or alighting from bus injured in collision with car, pick-up truck or van**

7 V73.5XX- **Driver of bus injured in collision with car, pick-up truck or van in traffic accident**

7 V73.6XX- **Passenger on bus injured in collision with car, pick-up truck or van in traffic accident**

7 V73.7XX- **Person on outside of bus injured in collision with car, pick-up truck or van in traffic accident**

7 V73.9XX- **Unspecified occupant of bus injured in collision with car, pick-up truck or van in traffic accident**

4 V74 **Bus occupant injured in collision with heavy transport vehicle or bus**

EXCLUDES 1 *bus occupant injured in collision with military vehicle (V79.81)*

The appropriate 7th character is to be added to each code from category V74

A initial encounter
D subsequent encounter
S sequela

7 V74.0XX- **Driver of bus injured in collision with heavy transport vehicle or bus in nontraffic accident**

- 7 V74.1XX- Passenger on bus injured in collision with heavy transport vehicle or bus in nontraffic accident
- 7 V74.2XX- Person on outside of bus injured in collision with heavy transport vehicle or bus in nontraffic accident
- 7 V74.3XX- Unspecified occupant of bus injured in collision with heavy transport vehicle or bus in nontraffic accident
- 7 V74.4XX- Person boarding or alighting from bus injured in collision with heavy transport vehicle or bus
- 7 V74.5XX- Driver of bus injured in collision with heavy transport vehicle or bus in traffic accident
- 7 V74.6XX- Passenger on bus injured in collision with heavy transport vehicle or bus in traffic accident
- 7 V74.7XX- Person on outside of bus injured in collision with heavy transport vehicle or bus in traffic accident
- 7 V74.9XX- Unspecified occupant of bus injured in collision with heavy transport vehicle or bus in traffic accident

4 V75 Bus occupant injured in collision with railway train or railway vehicle

The appropriate 7th character is to be added to each code from category V75
A initial encounter
D subsequent encounter
S sequela

- 7 V75.0XX- Driver of bus injured in collision with railway train or railway vehicle in nontraffic accident
- 7 V75.1XX- Passenger on bus injured in collision with railway train or railway vehicle in nontraffic accident
- 7 V75.2XX- Person on outside of bus injured in collision with railway train or railway vehicle in nontraffic accident
- 7 V75.3XX- Unspecified occupant of bus injured in collision with railway train or railway vehicle in nontraffic accident
- 7 V75.4XX- Person boarding or alighting from bus injured in collision with railway train or railway vehicle
- 7 V75.5XX- Driver of bus injured in collision with railway train or railway vehicle in traffic accident
- 7 V75.6XX- Passenger on bus injured in collision with railway train or railway vehicle in traffic accident
- 7 V75.7XX- Person on outside of bus injured in collision with railway train or railway vehicle in traffic accident
- 7 V75.9XX- Unspecified occupant of bus injured in collision with railway train or railway vehicle in traffic accident

4 V76 Bus occupant injured in collision with other nonmotor vehicle

INCLUDES collision with animal-drawn vehicle, animal being ridden, streetcar

The appropriate 7th character is to be added to each code from category V76
A initial encounter
D subsequent encounter
S sequela

- 7 V76.0XX- Driver of bus injured in collision with other nonmotor vehicle in nontraffic accident
- 7 V76.1XX- Passenger on bus injured in collision with other nonmotor vehicle in nontraffic accident
- 7 V76.2XX- Person on outside of bus injured in collision with other nonmotor vehicle in nontraffic accident
- 7 V76.3XX- Unspecified occupant of bus injured in collision with other nonmotor vehicle in nontraffic accident
- 7 V76.4XX- Person boarding or alighting from bus injured in collision with other nonmotor vehicle
- 7 V76.5XX- Driver of bus injured in collision with other nonmotor vehicle in traffic accident
- 7 V76.6XX- Passenger on bus injured in collision with other nonmotor vehicle in traffic accident
- 7 V76.7XX- Person on outside of bus injured in collision with other nonmotor vehicle in traffic accident
- 7 V76.9XX- Unspecified occupant of bus injured in collision with other nonmotor vehicle in traffic accident

4 V77 Bus occupant injured in collision with fixed or stationary object

The appropriate 7th character is to be added to each code from category V77
A initial encounter
D subsequent encounter
S sequela

- 7 V77.0XX- Driver of bus injured in collision with fixed or stationary object in nontraffic accident
- 7 V77.1XX- Passenger on bus injured in collision with fixed or stationary object in nontraffic accident
- 7 V77.2XX- Person on outside of bus injured in collision with fixed or stationary object in nontraffic accident
- 7 V77.3XX- Unspecified occupant of bus injured in collision with fixed or stationary object in nontraffic accident
- 7 V77.4XX- Person boarding or alighting from bus injured in collision with fixed or stationary object
- 7 V77.5XX- Driver of bus injured in collision with fixed or stationary object in traffic accident
- 7 V77.6XX- Passenger on bus injured in collision with fixed or stationary object in traffic accident
- 7 V77.7XX- Person on outside of bus injured in collision with fixed or stationary object in traffic accident
- 7 V77.9XX- Unspecified occupant of bus injured in collision with fixed or stationary object in traffic accident

4 V78 Bus occupant injured in noncollision transport accident

INCLUDES overturning bus NOS
overturning bus without collision

The appropriate 7th character is to be added to each code from category V78
A initial encounter
D subsequent encounter
S sequela

- 7 V78.0XX- Driver of bus injured in noncollision transport accident in nontraffic accident
- 7 V78.1XX- Passenger on bus injured in noncollision transport accident in nontraffic accident
- 7 V78.2XX- Person on outside of bus injured in noncollision transport accident in nontraffic accident
- 7 V78.3XX- Unspecified occupant of bus injured in noncollision transport accident in nontraffic accident
- 7 V78.4XX- Person boarding or alighting from bus injured in noncollision transport accident
- 7 V78.5XX- Driver of bus injured in noncollision transport accident in traffic accident
- 7 V78.6XX- Passenger on bus injured in noncollision transport accident in traffic accident
- 7 V78.7XX- Person on outside of bus injured in noncollision transport accident in traffic accident
- 7 V78.9XX- Unspecified occupant of bus injured in noncollision transport accident in traffic accident

4 V79 Bus occupant injured in other and unspecified transport accidents

The appropriate 7th character is to be added to each code from category V79
A initial encounter
D subsequent encounter
S sequela

- 5 V79.0 Driver of bus injured in collision with other and unspecified motor vehicles in nontraffic accident
  - 7 V79.00X- Driver of bus injured in collision with unspecified motor vehicles in nontraffic accident
  - 7 V79.09X- Driver of bus injured in collision with other motor vehicles in nontraffic accident
- 5 V79.1 Passenger on bus injured in collision with other and unspecified motor vehicles in nontraffic accident
  - 7 V79.10X- Passenger on bus injured in collision with unspecified motor vehicles in nontraffic accident
  - 7 V79.19X- Passenger on bus injured in collision with other motor vehicles in nontraffic accident
- 5 V79.2 Unspecified bus occupant injured in collision with other and unspecified motor vehicles in nontraffic accident

● New Manifestation 4-7 Digit Indicators Laterality A Adult M Maternity N Newborn P Pediatric ♂ Male
▲ Revised Unspecified AHA Coding Clinic HCC Hierarchical Condition Categories HIV HIV Related Conditions ♀ Female

V79.20X- Unspecified bus occupant injured in collision with unspecified motor vehicles in nontraffic accident
Bus collision NOS, nontraffic

V79.29X- Unspecified bus occupant injured in collision with other motor vehicles in nontraffic accident

V79.3XX- Bus occupant (driver) (passenger) injured in unspecified nontraffic accident
Bus accident NOS, nontraffic
Bus occupant injured in nontraffic accident NOS

V79.4 Driver of bus injured in collision with other and unspecified motor vehicles in traffic accident

V79.40X- Driver of bus injured in collision with unspecified motor vehicles in traffic accident

V79.49X- Driver of bus injured in collision with other motor vehicles in traffic accident

V79.5 Passenger on bus injured in collision with other and unspecified motor vehicles in traffic accident

V79.50X- Passenger on bus injured in collision with unspecified motor vehicles in traffic accident

V79.59X- Passenger on bus injured in collision with other motor vehicles in traffic accident

V79.6 Unspecified bus occupant injured in collision with other and unspecified motor vehicles in traffic accident

V79.60X- Unspecified bus occupant injured in collision with unspecified motor vehicles in traffic accident
Bus collision NOS (traffic)

V79.69X- Unspecified bus occupant injured in collision with other motor vehicles in traffic accident

V79.8 Bus occupant (driver) (passenger) injured in other specified transport accidents

V79.81X- Bus occupant (driver) (passenger) injured in transport accidents with military vehicle

V79.88X- Bus occupant (driver) (passenger) injured in other specified transport accidents

V79.9XX- Bus occupant (driver) (passenger) injured in unspecified traffic accident
Bus accident NOS

Other land transport accidents (V80-V89)

V80 Animal-rider or occupant of animal-drawn vehicle injured in transport accident

The appropriate 7th character is to be added to each code from category V80
A initial encounter
D subsequent encounter
S sequela

V80.0 Animal-rider or occupant of animal drawn vehicle injured by fall from or being thrown from animal or animal-drawn vehicle in noncollision accident

V80.01 Animal-rider injured by fall from or being thrown from animal in noncollision accident

V80.010- Animal-rider injured by fall from or being thrown from horse in noncollision accident

V80.018- Animal-rider injured by fall from or being thrown from other animal in noncollision accident

V80.02X- Occupant of animal-drawn vehicle injured by fall from or being thrown from animal-drawn vehicle in noncollision accident
Overturning animal-drawn vehicle NOS
Overturning animal-drawn vehicle without collision

V80.1 Animal-rider or occupant of animal-drawn vehicle injured in collision with pedestrian or animal
EXCLUDES 1 *animal-rider or animal-drawn vehicle collision with animal-drawn vehicle or animal being ridden (V80.7)*

V80.11X- Animal-rider injured in collision with pedestrian or animal

V80.12X- Occupant of animal-drawn vehicle injured in collision with pedestrian or animal

V80.2 Animal-rider or occupant of animal-drawn vehicle injured in collision with pedal cycle

V80.21X- Animal-rider injured in collision with pedal cycle

V80.22X- Occupant of animal-drawn vehicle injured in collision with pedal cycle

V80.3 Animal-rider or occupant of animal-drawn vehicle injured in collision with two- or three-wheeled motor vehicle

V80.31X- Animal-rider injured in collision with two- or three-wheeled motor vehicle

V80.32X- Occupant of animal-drawn vehicle injured in collision with two- or three-wheeled motor vehicle

V80.4 Animal-rider or occupant of animal-drawn vehicle injured in collision with car, pick-up truck, van, heavy transport vehicle or bus
EXCLUDES 1 *animal-rider injured in collision with military vehicle (V80.910)*
occupant of animal-drawn vehicle injured in collision with military vehicle (V80.920)

V80.41X- Animal-rider injured in collision with car, pick-up truck, van, heavy transport vehicle or bus

V80.42X- Occupant of animal-drawn vehicle injured in collision with car, pick-up truck, van, heavy transport vehicle or bus

V80.5 Animal-rider or occupant of animal-drawn vehicle injured in collision with other specified motor vehicle

V80.51X- Animal-rider injured in collision with other specified motor vehicle

V80.52X- Occupant of animal-drawn vehicle injured in collision with other specified motor vehicle

V80.6 Animal-rider or occupant of animal-drawn vehicle injured in collision with railway train or railway vehicle

V80.61X- Animal-rider injured in collision with railway train or railway vehicle

V80.62X- Occupant of animal-drawn vehicle injured in collision with railway train or railway vehicle

V80.7 Animal-rider or occupant of animal-drawn vehicle injured in collision with other nonmotor vehicles

V80.71 Animal-rider or occupant of animal-drawn vehicle injured in collision with animal being ridden

V80.710- Animal-rider injured in collision with other animal being ridden

V80.711- Occupant of animal-drawn vehicle injured in collision with animal being ridden

V80.72 Animal-rider or occupant of animal-drawn vehicle injured in collision with other animal-drawn vehicle

V80.720- Animal-rider injured in collision with animal-drawn vehicle

V80.721- Occupant of animal-drawn vehicle injured in collision with other animal-drawn vehicle

V80.73 Animal-rider or occupant of animal-drawn vehicle injured in collision with streetcar

V80.730- Animal-rider injured in collision with streetcar

V80.731- Occupant of animal-drawn vehicle injured in collision with streetcar

V80.79 Animal-rider or occupant of animal-drawn vehicle injured in collision with other nonmotor vehicles

V80.790- Animal-rider injured in collision with other nonmotor vehicles

V80.791- Occupant of animal-drawn vehicle injured in collision with other nonmotor vehicles

V80.8 Animal-rider or occupant of animal-drawn vehicle injured in collision with fixed or stationary object

V80.81X- Animal-rider injured in collision with fixed or stationary object

V80.82X- Occupant of animal-drawn vehicle injured in collision with fixed or stationary object

V80.9 Animal-rider or occupant of animal-drawn vehicle injured in other and unspecified transport accidents

V80.91 Animal-rider injured in other and unspecified transport accidents

V80.910- Animal-rider injured in transport accident with military vehicle

V80.918- Animal-rider injured in other transport accident

V80.919- Animal-rider injured in unspecified transport accident
Animal rider accident NOS

V80.92 Occupant of animal-drawn vehicle injured in other and unspecified transport accidents

7 V80.920- **Occupant of animal-drawn vehicle injured in transport accident with military vehicle**

7 V80.928- **Occupant of animal-drawn vehicle injured in other transport accident**

7 V80.929- **Occupant of animal-drawn vehicle injured in unspecified transport accident**
Animal-drawn vehicle accident NOS

4 V81 **Occupant of railway train or railway vehicle injured in transport accident**
INCLUDES derailment of railway train or railway vehicle
person on outside of train
EXCLUDES 1 *streetcar (V82.-)*

The appropriate 7th character is to be added to each code from category V81
A initial encounter
D subsequent encounter
S sequela

7 V81.0XX- **Occupant of railway train or railway vehicle injured in collision with motor vehicle in nontraffic accident**
EXCLUDES 1 *Occupant of railway train or railway vehicle injured due to collision with military vehicle (V81.83)*

7 V81.1XX- **Occupant of railway train or railway vehicle injured in collision with motor vehicle in traffic accident**
EXCLUDES 1 *Occupant of railway train or railway vehicle injured due to collision with military vehicle (V81.83)*

7 V81.2XX- **Occupant of railway train or railway vehicle injured in collision with or hit by rolling stock**

7 V81.3XX- **Occupant of railway train or railway vehicle injured in collision with other object**
Railway collision NOS

7 V81.4XX- **Person injured while boarding or alighting from railway train or railway vehicle**

7 V81.5XX- **Occupant of railway train or railway vehicle injured by fall in railway train or railway vehicle**

7 V81.6XX- **Occupant of railway train or railway vehicle injured by fall from railway train or railway vehicle**

7 V81.7XX- **Occupant of railway train or railway vehicle injured in derailment without antecedent collision**

5 V81.8 **Occupant of railway train or railway vehicle injured in other specified railway accidents**

7 V81.81X- **Occupant of railway train or railway vehicle injured due to explosion or fire on train**

7 V81.82X- **Occupant of railway train or railway vehicle injured due to object falling onto train**
Occupant of railway train or railway vehicle injured due to falling earth onto train
Occupant of railway train or railway vehicle injured due to falling rocks onto train
Occupant of railway train or railway vehicle injured due to falling snow onto train
Occupant of railway train or railway vehicle injured due to falling trees onto train

7 V81.83X- **Occupant of railway train or railway vehicle injured due to collision with military vehicle**

7 V81.89X- **Occupant of railway train or railway vehicle injured due to other specified railway accident**

7 V81.9XX- **Occupant of railway train or railway vehicle injured in unspecified railway accident**
Railway accident NOS

4 V82 **Occupant of powered streetcar injured in transport accident**
INCLUDES interurban electric car
person on outside of streetcar
tram (car)
trolley (car)
EXCLUDES 1 *bus (V70-V79)*
motorcoach (V70-V79)
nonpowered streetcar (V76.-)
train (V81.-)

The appropriate 7th character is to be added to each code from category V82
A initial encounter
D subsequent encounter
S sequela

7 V82.0XX- **Occupant of streetcar injured in collision with motor vehicle in nontraffic accident**

7 V82.1XX- **Occupant of streetcar injured in collision with motor vehicle in traffic accident**

7 V82.2XX- **Occupant of streetcar injured in collision with or hit by rolling stock**

7 V82.3XX- **Occupant of streetcar injured in collision with other object**
EXCLUDES 1 *collision with animal-drawn vehicle or animal being ridden (V82.8)*

7 V82.4XX- **Person injured while boarding or alighting from streetcar**

7 V82.5XX- **Occupant of streetcar injured by fall in streetcar**
EXCLUDES 1 *fall in streetcar:*
while boarding or alighting (V82.4)
with antecedent collision (V82.0-V82.3)

7 V82.6XX- **Occupant of streetcar injured by fall from streetcar**
EXCLUDES 1 *fall from streetcar:*
while boarding or alighting (V82.4)
with antecedent collision (V82.0-V82.3)

7 V82.7XX- **Occupant of streetcar injured in derailment without antecedent collision**
EXCLUDES 1 *occupant of streetcar injured in derailment with antecedent collision (V82.0-V82.3)*

7 V82.8XX- **Occupant of streetcar injured in other specified transport accidents**
Streetcar collision with military vehicle
Streetcar collision with train or nonmotor vehicles

7 V82.9XX- **Occupant of streetcar injured in unspecified traffic accident**
Streetcar accident NOS

4 V83 **Occupant of special vehicle mainly used on industrial premises injured in transport accident**
INCLUDES battery-powered airport passenger vehicle
battery-powered truck (baggage) (mail)
coal-car in mine
forklift (truck)
logging car
self-propelled industrial truck
station baggage truck (powered)
tram, truck, or tub (powered) in mine or quarry
EXCLUDES 1 *special construction vehicles (V85.-)*
special industrial vehicle in stationary use or maintenance (W31.-)

The appropriate 7th character is to be added to each code from category V83
A initial encounter
D subsequent encounter
S sequela

7 V83.0XX- **Driver of special industrial vehicle injured in traffic accident**

7 V83.1XX- **Passenger of special industrial vehicle injured in traffic accident**

7 V83.2XX- **Person on outside of special industrial vehicle injured in traffic accident**

7 V83.3XX- **Unspecified occupant of special industrial vehicle injured in traffic accident**

7 V83.4XX- **Person injured while boarding or alighting from special industrial vehicle**

7 V83.5XX- **Driver of special industrial vehicle injured in nontraffic accident**

7 V83.6XX- **Passenger of special industrial vehicle injured in nontraffic accident**

7 V83.7XX- **Person on outside of special industrial vehicle injured in nontraffic accident**

7 V83.9XX- **Unspecified occupant of special industrial vehicle injured in nontraffic accident**
Special-industrial-vehicle accident NOS

4 V84 Occupant of special vehicle mainly used in agriculture injured in transport accident

INCLUDES self-propelled farm machinery
tractor (and trailer)

EXCLUDES 1 *animal-powered farm machinery accident (W30.8-)*
contact with combine harvester (W30.0)
special agricultural vehicle in stationary use or maintenance (W30.-)

The appropriate 7th character is to be added to each code from category V84
A initial encounter
D subsequent encounter
S sequela

7 V84.0XX- **Driver of special agricultural vehicle injured in traffic accident**

7 V84.1XX- **Passenger of special agricultural vehicle injured in traffic accident**

7 V84.2XX- **Person on outside of special agricultural vehicle injured in traffic accident**

7 V84.3XX- **Unspecified occupant of special agricultural vehicle injured in traffic accident**

7 V84.4XX- **Person injured while boarding or alighting from special agricultural vehicle**

7 V84.5XX- **Driver of special agricultural vehicle injured in nontraffic accident**

7 V84.6XX- **Passenger of special agricultural vehicle injured in nontraffic accident**

7 V84.7XX- **Person on outside of special agricultural vehicle injured in nontraffic accident**

7 V84.9XX- **Unspecified occupant of special agricultural vehicle injured in nontraffic accident**
Special-agricultural vehicle accident NOS

4 V85 Occupant of special construction vehicle injured in transport accident

INCLUDES bulldozer
digger
dump truck
earth-leveller
mechanical shovel
road-roller

EXCLUDES 1 *special industrial vehicle (V83.-)*
special construction vehicle in stationary use or maintenance (W31.-)

The appropriate 7th character is to be added to each code from category V85
A initial encounter
D subsequent encounter
S sequela

7 V85.0XX- **Driver of special construction vehicle injured in traffic accident**

7 V85.1XX- **Passenger of special construction vehicle injured in traffic accident**

7 V85.2XX- **Person on outside of special construction vehicle injured in traffic accident**

7 V85.3XX- **Unspecified occupant of special construction vehicle injured in traffic accident**

7 V85.4XX- **Person injured while boarding or alighting from special construction vehicle**

7 V85.5XX- **Driver of special construction vehicle injured in nontraffic accident**

7 V85.6XX- **Passenger of special construction vehicle injured in nontraffic accident**

7 V85.7XX- **Person on outside of special construction vehicle injured in nontraffic accident**

7 V85.9XX- **Unspecified occupant of special construction vehicle injured in nontraffic accident**
Special-construction-vehicle accident NOS

4 V86 Occupant of special all-terrain or other off-road motor vehicle, injured in transport accident

EXCLUDES 1 *special all-terrain vehicle in stationary use or maintenance (W31.-)*
sport-utility vehicle (V50-V59)
three-wheeled motor vehicle designed for on-road use (V30-V39)

The appropriate 7th character is to be added to each code from category V86
A initial encounter
D subsequent encounter
S sequela

AHA: 4Q 2017, 20

5 V86.0 **Driver of special all-terrain or other off-road motor vehicle injured in traffic accident**

7 V86.01X- **Driver of ambulance or fire engine injured in traffic accident**

7 V86.02X- **Driver of snowmobile injured in traffic accident**

7 V86.03X- **Driver of dune buggy injured in traffic accident**

7 V86.04X- **Driver of military vehicle injured in traffic accident**

7 V86.05X- **Driver of 3- or 4- wheeled all-terrain vehicle (ATV) injured in traffic accident**

7 V86.06X- **Driver of dirt bike or motor/cross bike injured in traffic accident**

7 V86.09X- **Driver of other special all-terrain or other off-road motor vehicle injured in traffic accident**
Driver of dirt bike injured in traffic accident
Driver of go cart injured in traffic accident
Driver of golf cart injured in traffic accident

5 V86.1 **Passenger of special all-terrain or other off-road motor vehicle injured in traffic accident**

7 V86.11X- **Passenger of ambulance or fire engine injured in traffic accident**

7 V86.12X- **Passenger of snowmobile injured in traffic accident**

7 V86.13X- **Passenger of dune buggy injured in traffic accident**

7 V86.14X- **Passenger of military vehicle injured in traffic accident**

7 V86.15X- **Passenger of 3- or 4- wheeled all-terrain vehicle (ATV) injured in traffic accident**

7 V86.16X- **Passenger of dirt bike or motor/cross bike injured in traffic accident**

7 V86.19X- **Passenger of other special all-terrain or other off-road motor vehicle injured in traffic accident**
Passenger of dirt bike injured in traffic accident
Passenger of go cart injured in traffic accident
Passenger of golf cart injured in traffic accident

5 V86.2 **Person on outside of special all-terrain or other off-road motor vehicle injured in traffic accident**

7 V86.21X- **Person on outside of ambulance or fire engine injured in traffic accident**

7 V86.22X- **Person on outside of snowmobile injured in traffic accident**

7 V86.23X- **Person on outside of dune buggy injured in traffic accident**

7 V86.24X- **Person on outside of military vehicle injured in traffic accident**

7 V86.25X- **Person on outside of 3- or 4- wheeled all-terrain vehicle (ATV) injured in traffic accident**

7 V86.26X- **Person on outside of dirt bike or motor/cross bike injured in traffic accident**

7 V86.29X- **Person on outside of other special all-terrain or other off-road motor vehicle injured in traffic accident**
Person on outside of dirt bike injured in traffic accident
Person on outside of go cart in traffic accident
Person on outside of golf cart injured in traffic accident

5 V86.3 **Unspecified occupant of special all-terrain or other off-road motor vehicle injured in traffic accident**

7 V86.31X- **Unspecified occupant of ambulance or fire engine injured in traffic accident**

7 V86.32X- **Unspecified occupant of snowmobile injured in traffic accident**

7 V86.33X- **Unspecified occupant of dune buggy injured in traffic accident**

V86.34X- **Unspecified occupant of military vehicle injured in traffic accident**

V86.35X- **Unspecified occupant of 3- or 4- wheeled all-terrain vehicle (ATV) injured in traffic accident**

V86.36X- **Unspecified occupant of dirt bike or motor/cross bike injured in traffic accident**

V86.39X- **Unspecified occupant of other special all-terrain or other off-road motor vehicle injured in traffic accident**
Unspecified occupant of dirt bike injured in traffic accident
Unspecified occupant of go cart injured in traffic accident
Unspecified occupant of golf cart injured in traffic accident

V86.4 **Person injured while boarding or alighting from special all-terrain or other off-road motor vehicle**

V86.41X- **Person injured while boarding or alighting from ambulance or fire engine**

V86.42X- **Person injured while boarding or alighting from snowmobile**

V86.43X- **Person injured while boarding or alighting from dune buggy**

V86.44X- **Person injured while boarding or alighting from military vehicle**

V86.45X- **Person injured while boarding or alighting from a 3- or 4- wheeled all-terrain vehicle (ATV)**

V86.46X- **Person injured while boarding or alighting from a dirt bike or motor/cross bike**

V86.49X- **Person injured while boarding or alighting from other special all-terrain or other off-road motor vehicle**
Person injured while boarding or alighting from dirt bike
Person injured while boarding or alighting from go cart
Person injured while boarding or alighting from golf cart

V86.5 **Driver of special all-terrain or other off-road motor vehicle injured in nontraffic accident**

V86.51X- **Driver of ambulance or fire engine injured in nontraffic accident**

V86.52X- **Driver of snowmobile injured in nontraffic accident**

V86.53X- **Driver of dune buggy injured in nontraffic accident**

V86.54X- **Driver of military vehicle injured in nontraffic accident**

V86.55X- **Driver of 3- or 4- wheeled all-terrain vehicle (ATV) injured in nontraffic accident**

V86.56X- **Driver of dirt bike or motor/cross bike injured in nontraffic accident**

V86.59X- **Driver of other special all-terrain or other off-road motor vehicle injured in nontraffic accident**
Driver of dirt bike injured in nontraffic accident
Driver of go cart injured in nontraffic accident
Driver of golf cart injured in nontraffic accident

V86.6 **Passenger of special all-terrain or other off-road motor vehicle injured in nontraffic accident**

V86.61X- **Passenger of ambulance or fire engine injured in nontraffic accident**

V86.62X- **Passenger of snowmobile injured in nontraffic accident**

V86.63X- **Passenger of dune buggy injured in nontraffic accident**

V86.64X- **Passenger of military vehicle injured in nontraffic accident**

V86.65X- **Passenger of 3- or 4- wheeled all-terrain vehicle (ATV) injured in nontraffic accident**

V86.66X- **Passenger of dirt bike or motor/cross bike injured in nontraffic accident**

V86.69X- **Passenger of other special all-terrain or other off-road motor vehicle injured in nontraffic accident**
Passenger of dirt bike injured in nontraffic accident
Passenger of go cart injured in nontraffic accident
Passenger of golf cart injured in nontraffic accident

V86.7 **Person on outside of special all-terrain or other off-road motor vehicle injured in nontraffic accident**

V86.71X- **Person on outside of ambulance or fire engine injured in nontraffic accident**

V86.72X- **Person on outside of snowmobile injured in nontraffic accident**

V86.73X- **Person on outside of dune buggy injured in nontraffic accident**

V86.74X- **Person on outside of military vehicle injured in nontraffic accident**

V86.75X- **Person on outside of 3- or 4- wheeled all-terrain vehicle (ATV) injured in nontraffic accident**

V86.76X- **Person on outside of dirt bike or motor/cross bike injured in nontraffic accident**

V86.79X- **Person on outside of other special all-terrain or other off-road motor vehicles injured in nontraffic accident**
Person on outside of dirt bike injured in nontraffic accident
Person on outside of go cart injured in nontraffic accident
Person on outside of golf cart injured in nontraffic accident

V86.9 **Unspecified occupant of special all-terrain or other off-road motor vehicle injured in nontraffic accident**

V86.91X- **Unspecified occupant of ambulance or fire engine injured in nontraffic accident**

V86.92X- **Unspecified occupant of snowmobile injured in nontraffic accident**

V86.93X- **Unspecified occupant of dune buggy injured in nontraffic accident**

V86.94X- **Unspecified occupant of military vehicle injured in nontraffic accident**

V86.95X- **Unspecified occupant of 3- or 4- wheeled all-terrain vehicle (ATV) injured in nontraffic accident**

V86.96X- **Unspecified occupant of dirt bike or motor/cross bike injured in nontraffic accident**

V86.99X- **Unspecified occupant of other special all-terrain or other off-road motor vehicle injured in nontraffic accident**
Off-road motor-vehicle accident NOS
Other motor-vehicle accident NOS
Unspecified occupant of go cart injured in nontraffic accident
Unspecified occupant of golf cart injured in nontraffic accident

V87 Traffic accident of specified type but victim's mode of transport unknown

EXCLUDES 1 *collision involving:*
pedal cycle (V10-V19)
pedestrian (V01-V09)

The appropriate 7th character is to be added to each code from category V87
A initial encounter
D subsequent encounter
S sequela

V87.0XX- **Person injured in collision between car and two- or three-wheeled powered vehicle (traffic)**

V87.1XX- **Person injured in collision between other motor vehicle and two- or three-wheeled motor vehicle (traffic)**

V87.2XX- **Person injured in collision between car and pick-up truck or van (traffic)**

V87.3XX- **Person injured in collision between car and bus (traffic)**

V87.4XX- **Person injured in collision between car and heavy transport vehicle (traffic)**

V87.5XX- **Person injured in collision between heavy transport vehicle and bus (traffic)**

V87.6XX- **Person injured in collision between railway train or railway vehicle and car (traffic)**

V87.7XX- **Person injured in collision between other specified motor vehicles (traffic)**

V87.8XX- **Person injured in other specified noncollision transport accidents involving motor vehicle (traffic)**

V87.9XX- **Person injured in other specified (collision)(noncollision) transport accidents involving nonmotor vehicle (traffic)**

V88 Nontraffic accident of specified type but victim's mode of transport unknown

EXCLUDES 1 *collision involving:*
pedal cycle (V10-V19)
pedestrian (V01-V09)

The appropriate 7th character is to be added to each code from category V88
A initial encounter
D subsequent encounter
S sequela

V88.0XX- **Person injured in collision between car and two- or three-wheeled motor vehicle, nontraffic**

V88.1XX- **Person injured in collision between other motor vehicle and two- or three-wheeled motor vehicle, nontraffic**

V88.2XX- **Person injured in collision between car and pick-up truck or van, nontraffic**

V88.3XX- **Person injured in collision between car and bus, nontraffic**

V88.4XX- **Person injured in collision between car and heavy transport vehicle, nontraffic**

V88.5XX- **Person injured in collision between heavy transport vehicle and bus, nontraffic**

V88.6XX- **Person injured in collision between railway train or railway vehicle and car, nontraffic**

V88.7XX- **Person injured in collision between other specified motor vehicle, nontraffic**

V88.8XX- **Person injured in other specified noncollision transport accidents involving motor vehicle, nontraffic**

V88.9XX- **Person injured in other specified (collision)(noncollision) transport accidents involving nonmotor vehicle, nontraffic**

V89 Motor- or nonmotor- accident, type of vehicle unspecified

The appropriate 7th character is to be added to each code from category V89
A initial encounter
D subsequent encounter
S sequela

V89.0XX- **Person injured in unspecified motor-vehicle accident, nontraffic**
Motor-vehicle accident NOS, nontraffic

V89.1XX- **Person injured in unspecified nonmotor-vehicle accident, nontraffic**
Nonmotor-vehicle accident NOS (nontraffic)

V89.2XX- **Person injured in unspecified motor-vehicle accident, traffic**
Motor-vehicle accident [MVA] NOS
Road (traffic) accident [RTA] NOS

V89.3XX- **Person injured in unspecified nonmotor-vehicle accident, traffic**
Nonmotor-vehicle traffic accident NOS

V89.9XX- **Person injured in unspecified vehicle accident**
Collision NOS

Water transport accidents (V90-V94)

V90 Drowning and submersion due to accident to watercraft

EXCLUDES 1 *civilian water transport accident involving military watercraft (V94.81-)*
fall into water not from watercraft (W16.-)
military watercraft accident in military or war operations (Y36.0-, Y37.0-)
water-transport-related drowning or submersion without accident to watercraft (V92.-)

The appropriate 7th character is to be added to each code from category V90
A initial encounter
D subsequent encounter
S sequela

V90.0 Drowning and submersion due to watercraft overturning

V90.00X- **Drowning and submersion due to merchant ship overturning**

V90.01X- **Drowning and submersion due to passenger ship overturning**
Drowning and submersion due to Ferry-boat overturning
Drowning and submersion due to Liner overturning

V90.02X- **Drowning and submersion due to fishing boat overturning**

V90.03X- **Drowning and submersion due to other powered watercraft overturning**
Drowning and submersion due to Hovercraft (on open water) overturning
Drowning and submersion due to Jet ski overturning

V90.04X- **Drowning and submersion due to sailboat overturning**

V90.05X- **Drowning and submersion due to canoe or kayak overturning**

V90.06X- **Drowning and submersion due to (nonpowered) inflatable craft overturning**

V90.08X- **Drowning and submersion due to other unpowered watercraft overturning**
Drowning and submersion due to windsurfer overturning

V90.09X- **Drowning and submersion due to unspecified watercraft overturning**
Drowning and submersion due to boat NOS overturning
Drowning and submersion due to ship NOS overturning
Drowning and submersion due to watercraft NOS overturning

V90.1 Drowning and submersion due to watercraft sinking

V90.10X- **Drowning and submersion due to merchant ship sinking**

V90.11X- **Drowning and submersion due to passenger ship sinking**
Drowning and submersion due to Ferry-boat sinking
Drowning and submersion due to Liner sinking

V90.12X- **Drowning and submersion due to fishing boat sinking**

V90.13X- **Drowning and submersion due to other powered watercraft sinking**
Drowning and submersion due to Hovercraft (on open water) sinking
Drowning and submersion due to Jet ski sinking

V90.14X- **Drowning and submersion due to sailboat sinking**

V90.15X- **Drowning and submersion due to canoe or kayak sinking**

V90.16X- **Drowning and submersion due to (nonpowered) inflatable craft sinking**

V90.18X- **Drowning and submersion due to other unpowered watercraft sinking**

V90.19X- **Drowning and submersion due to unspecified watercraft sinking**
Drowning and submersion due to boat NOS sinking
Drowning and submersion due to ship NOS sinking
Drowning and submersion due to watercraft NOS sinking

V90.2 Drowning and submersion due to falling or jumping from burning watercraft

V90.20X- **Drowning and submersion due to falling or jumping from burning merchant ship**

V90.21X- **Drowning and submersion due to falling or jumping from burning passenger ship**
Drowning and submersion due to falling or jumping from burning Ferry-boat
Drowning and submersion due to falling or jumping from burning Liner

V90.22X- **Drowning and submersion due to falling or jumping from burning fishing boat**

V90.23X- **Drowning and submersion due to falling or jumping from other burning powered watercraft**
Drowning and submersion due to falling and jumping from burning Hovercraft (on open water)
Drowning and submersion due to falling and jumping from burning Jet ski

V90.24X- **Drowning and submersion due to falling or jumping from burning sailboat**

V90.25X- **Drowning and submersion due to falling or jumping from burning canoe or kayak**

V90.26X- **Drowning and submersion due to falling or jumping from burning (nonpowered) inflatable craft**

V90.27X- **Drowning and submersion due to falling or jumping from burning water-skis**

V90.28X- **Drowning and submersion due to falling or jumping from other burning unpowered watercraft**
Drowning and submersion due to falling and jumping from burning surf-board
Drowning and submersion due to falling and jumping from burning windsurfer

V90.29X- **Drowning and submersion due to falling or jumping from unspecified burning watercraft**
Drowning and submersion due to falling or jumping from burning boat NOS
Drowning and submersion due to falling or jumping from burning ship NOS
Drowning and submersion due to falling or jumping from burning watercraft NOS

V90.3 **Drowning and submersion due to falling or jumping from crushed watercraft**

V90.30X- **Drowning and submersion due to falling or jumping from crushed merchant ship**

V90.31X- **Drowning and submersion due to falling or jumping from crushed passenger ship**
Drowning and submersion due to falling and jumping from crushed Ferry boat
Drowning and submersion due to falling and jumping from crushed Liner

V90.32X- **Drowning and submersion due to falling or jumping from crushed fishing boat**

V90.33X- **Drowning and submersion due to falling or jumping from other crushed powered watercraft**
Drowning and submersion due to falling and jumping from crushed Hovercraft
Drowning and submersion due to falling and jumping from crushed Jet ski

V90.34X- **Drowning and submersion due to falling or jumping from crushed sailboat**

V90.35X- **Drowning and submersion due to falling or jumping from crushed canoe or kayak**

V90.36X- **Drowning and submersion due to falling or jumping from crushed (nonpowered) inflatable craft**

V90.37X- **Drowning and submersion due to falling or jumping from crushed water-skis**

V90.38X- **Drowning and submersion due to falling or jumping from other crushed unpowered watercraft**
Drowning and submersion due to falling and jumping from crushed surf-board
Drowning and submersion due to falling and jumping from crushed windsurfer

V90.39X- **Drowning and submersion due to falling or jumping from crushed unspecified watercraft**
Drowning and submersion due to falling and jumping from crushed boat NOS
Drowning and submersion due to falling and jumping from crushed ship NOS
Drowning and submersion due to falling and jumping from crushed watercraft NOS

V90.8 **Drowning and submersion due to other accident to watercraft**

V90.80X- **Drowning and submersion due to other accident to merchant ship**

V90.81X- **Drowning and submersion due to other accident to passenger ship**
Drowning and submersion due to other accident to Ferry-boat
Drowning and submersion due to other accident to Liner

V90.82X- **Drowning and submersion due to other accident to fishing boat**

V90.83X- **Drowning and submersion due to other accident to other powered watercraft**
Drowning and submersion due to other accident to Hovercraft (on open water)
Drowning and submersion due to other accident to Jet ski

V90.84X- **Drowning and submersion due to other accident to sailboat**

V90.85X- **Drowning and submersion due to other accident to canoe or kayak**

V90.86X- **Drowning and submersion due to other accident to (nonpowered) inflatable craft**

V90.87X- **Drowning and submersion due to other accident to water-skis**

V90.88X- **Drowning and submersion due to other accident to other unpowered watercraft**
Drowning and submersion due to other accident to surf-board
Drowning and submersion due to other accident to windsurfer

V90.89X- **Drowning and submersion due to other accident to unspecified watercraft**
Drowning and submersion due to other accident to boat NOS
Drowning and submersion due to other accident to ship NOS
Drowning and submersion due to other accident to watercraft NOS

V91 Other injury due to accident to watercraft

INCLUDES any injury except drowning and submersion as a result of an accident to watercraft

EXCLUDES 1 *civilian water transport accident involving military watercraft (V94.81-)*
military watercraft accident in military or war operations (Y36, Y37.-)

EXCLUDES 2 *drowning and submersion due to accident to watercraft (V90.-)*

The appropriate 7th character is to be added to each code from category V91
A initial encounter
D subsequent encounter
S sequela

V91.0 **Burn due to watercraft on fire**

EXCLUDES 1 *burn from localized fire or explosion on board ship without accident to watercraft (V93.-)*

V91.00X- **Burn due to merchant ship on fire**

V91.01X- **Burn due to passenger ship on fire**
Burn due to Ferry-boat on fire
Burn due to Liner on fire

V91.02X- **Burn due to fishing boat on fire**

V91.03X- **Burn due to other powered watercraft on fire**
Burn due to Hovercraft (on open water) on fire
Burn due to Jet ski on fire

V91.04X- **Burn due to sailboat on fire**

V91.05X- **Burn due to canoe or kayak on fire**

V91.06X- **Burn due to (nonpowered) inflatable craft on fire**

V91.07X- **Burn due to water-skis on fire**

V91.08X- **Burn due to other unpowered watercraft on fire**

V91.09X- **Burn due to unspecified watercraft on fire**
Burn due to boat NOS on fire
Burn due to ship NOS on fire
Burn due to watercraft NOS on fire

V91.1 **Crushed between watercraft and other watercraft or other object due to collision**
Crushed by lifeboat after abandoning ship in a collision
Note: select the specified type of watercraft that the victim was on at the time of the collision

V91.10X- **Crushed between merchant ship and other watercraft or other object due to collision**

V91.11X- **Crushed between passenger ship and other watercraft or other object due to collision**
Crushed between Ferry-boat and other watercraft or other object due to collision
Crushed between Liner and other watercraft or other object due to collision

V91.12X- **Crushed between fishing boat and other watercraft or other object due to collision**

V91.13X- **Crushed between other powered watercraft and other watercraft or other object due to collision**
Crushed between Hovercraft (on open water) and other watercraft or other object due to collision
Crushed between Jet ski and other watercraft or other object due to collision

7 V91.14X- **Crushed between sailboat and other watercraft or other object due to collision**

7 V91.15X- **Crushed between canoe or kayak and other watercraft or other object due to collision**

7 V91.16X- **Crushed between (nonpowered) inflatable craft and other watercraft or other object due to collision**

7 V91.18X- **Crushed between other unpowered watercraft and other watercraft or other object due to collision**
Crushed between surfboard and other watercraft or other object due to collision
Crushed between windsurfer and other watercraft or other object due to collision

7 V91.19X- **Crushed between unspecified watercraft and other watercraft or other object due to collision**
Crushed between boat NOS and other watercraft or other object due to collision
Crushed between ship NOS and other watercraft or other object due to collision
Crushed between watercraft NOS and other watercraft or other object due to collision

5 V91.2 **Fall due to collision between watercraft and other watercraft or other object**
Fall while remaining on watercraft after collision
Note: select the specified type of watercraft that the victim was on at the time of the collision
EXCLUDES 1 *crushed between watercraft and other watercraft and other object due to collision (V91.1-)*
drowning and submersion due to falling from crushed watercraft (V90.3-)

7 V91.20X- **Fall due to collision between merchant ship and other watercraft or other object**

7 V91.21X- **Fall due to collision between passenger ship and other watercraft or other object**
Fall due to collision between Ferry-boat and other watercraft or other object
Fall due to collision between Liner and other watercraft or other object

7 V91.22X- **Fall due to collision between fishing boat and other watercraft or other object**

7 V91.23X- **Fall due to collision between other powered watercraft and other watercraft or other object**
Fall due to collision between Hovercraft (on open water) and other watercraft or other object
Fall due to collision between Jet ski and other watercraft or other object

7 V91.24X- **Fall due to collision between sailboat and other watercraft or other object**

7 V91.25X- **Fall due to collision between canoe or kayak and other watercraft or other object**

7 V91.26X- **Fall due to collision between (nonpowered) inflatable craft and other watercraft or other object**

7 V91.29X- **Fall due to collision between unspecified watercraft and other watercraft or other object**
Fall due to collision between boat NOS and other watercraft or other object
Fall due to collision between ship NOS and other watercraft or other object
Fall due to collision between watercraft NOS and other watercraft or other object

5 V91.3 **Hit or struck by falling object due to accident to watercraft**
Hit or struck by falling object (part of damaged watercraft or other object) after falling or jumping from damaged watercraft
EXCLUDES 2 *drowning or submersion due to fall or jumping from damaged watercraft (V90.2-, V90.3-)*

7 V91.30X- **Hit or struck by falling object due to accident to merchant ship**

7 V91.31X- **Hit or struck by falling object due to accident to passenger ship**
Hit or struck by falling object due to accident to Ferry-boat
Hit or struck by falling object due to accident to Liner

7 V91.32X- **Hit or struck by falling object due to accident to fishing boat**

7 V91.33X- **Hit or struck by falling object due to accident to other powered watercraft**
Hit or struck by falling object due to accident to Hovercraft (on open water)
Hit or struck by falling object due to accident to Jet ski

7 V91.34X- **Hit or struck by falling object due to accident to sailboat**

7 V91.35X- **Hit or struck by falling object due to accident to canoe or kayak**

7 V91.36X- **Hit or struck by falling object due to accident to (nonpowered) inflatable craft**

7 V91.37X- **Hit or struck by falling object due to accident to water-skis**
Hit by water-skis after jumping off of waterskis

7 V91.38X- **Hit or struck by falling object due to accident to other unpowered watercraft**
Hit or struck by surf-board after falling off damaged surf-board
Hit or struck by object after falling off damaged windsurfer

7 V91.39X- **Hit or struck by falling object due to accident to unspecified watercraft**
Hit or struck by falling object due to accident to boat NOS
Hit or struck by falling object due to accident to ship NOS
Hit or struck by falling object due to accident to watercraft NOS

5 V91.8 **Other injury due to other accident to watercraft**

7 V91.80X- **Other injury due to other accident to merchant ship**

7 V91.81X- **Other injury due to other accident to passenger ship**
Other injury due to other accident to Ferry-boat
Other injury due to other accident to Liner

7 V91.82X- **Other injury due to other accident to fishing boat**

7 V91.83X- **Other injury due to other accident to other powered watercraft**
Other injury due to other accident to Hovercraft (on open water)
Other injury due to other accident to Jet ski

7 V91.84X- **Other injury due to other accident to sailboat**

7 V91.85X- **Other injury due to other accident to canoe or kayak**

7 V91.86X- **Other injury due to other accident to (nonpowered) inflatable craft**

7 V91.87X- **Other injury due to other accident to water-skis**

7 V91.88X- **Other injury due to other accident to other unpowered watercraft**
Other injury due to other accident to surf-board
Other injury due to other accident to windsurfer

7 V91.89X- **Other injury due to other accident to unspecified watercraft**
Other injury due to other accident to boat NOS
Other injury due to other accident to ship NOS
Other injury due to other accident to watercraft NOS

4 V92 **Drowning and submersion due to accident on board watercraft, without accident to watercraft**
EXCLUDES 1 *civilian water transport accident involving military watercraft (V94.81-)*
drowning or submersion due to accident to watercraft (V90-V91)
drowning or submersion of diver who voluntarily jumps from boat not involved in an accident (W16.711, W16.721)
fall into water without watercraft (W16.-)
military watercraft accident in military or war operations (Y36, Y37)

The appropriate 7th character is to be added to each code from category V92
A initial encounter
D subsequent encounter
S sequela

5 V92.0 **Drowning and submersion due to fall off watercraft**
Drowning and submersion due to fall from gangplank of watercraft
Drowning and submersion due to fall overboard watercraft
EXCLUDES 2 *hitting head on object or bottom of body of water due to fall from watercraft (V94.0-)*

7 **V92.00X- Drowning and submersion due to fall off merchant ship**

7 **V92.01X- Drowning and submersion due to fall off passenger ship**
Drowning and submersion due to fall off Ferry-boat
Drowning and submersion due to fall off Liner

7 **V92.02X- Drowning and submersion due to fall off fishing boat**

7 **V92.03X- Drowning and submersion due to fall off other powered watercraft**
Drowning and submersion due to fall off Hovercraft (on open water)
Drowning and submersion due to fall off Jet ski

7 **V92.04X- Drowning and submersion due to fall off sailboat**

7 **V92.05X- Drowning and submersion due to fall off canoe or kayak**

7 **V92.06X- Drowning and submersion due to fall off (nonpowered) inflatable craft**

7 **V92.07X- Drowning and submersion due to fall off water-skis**
EXCLUDES 1 *drowning and submersion due to falling off burning water-skis (V90.27)*
drowning and submersion due to falling off crushed water-skis (V90.37)
hit by boat while water-skiing NOS (V94.X)

7 **V92.08X- Drowning and submersion due to fall off other unpowered watercraft**
Drowning and submersion due to fall off surf-board
Drowning and submersion due to fall off windsurfer
EXCLUDES 1 *drowning and submersion due to fall off burning unpowered watercraft (V90.28)*
drowning and submersion due to fall off crushed unpowered watercraft (V90.38)
drowning and submersion due to fall off damaged unpowered watercraft (V90.88)
drowning and submersion due to rider of nonpowered watercraft being hit by other watercraft (V94.-)
other injury due to rider of nonpowered watercraft being hit by other watercraft (V94.-)

7 **V92.09X- Drowning and submersion due to fall off unspecified watercraft**
Drowning and submersion due to fall off boat NOS
Drowning and submersion due to fall off ship
Drowning and submersion due to fall off watercraft NOS

5 **V92.1 Drowning and submersion due to being thrown overboard by motion of watercraft**
EXCLUDES 1 *drowning and submersion due to fall off surf-board (V92.08)*
drowning and submersion due to fall off water-skis (V92.07)
drowning and submersion due to fall off windsurfer (V92.08)

7 **V92.10X- Drowning and submersion due to being thrown overboard by motion of merchant ship**

7 **V92.11X- Drowning and submersion due to being thrown overboard by motion of passenger ship**
Drowning and submersion due to being thrown overboard by motion of Ferry-boat
Drowning and submersion due to being thrown overboard by motion of Liner

7 **V92.12X- Drowning and submersion due to being thrown overboard by motion of fishing boat**

7 **V92.13X- Drowning and submersion due to being thrown overboard by motion of other powered watercraft**
Drowning and submersion due to being thrown overboard by motion of Hovercraft

7 **V92.14X- Drowning and submersion due to being thrown overboard by motion of sailboat**

7 **V92.15X- Drowning and submersion due to being thrown overboard by motion of canoe or kayak**

7 **V92.16X- Drowning and submersion due to being thrown overboard by motion of (nonpowered) inflatable craft**

7 **V92.19X- Drowning and submersion due to being thrown overboard by motion of unspecified watercraft**
Drowning and submersion due to being thrown overboard by motion of boat NOS
Drowning and submersion due to being thrown overboard by motion of ship NOS
Drowning and submersion due to being thrown overboard by motion of watercraft NOS

5 **V92.2 Drowning and submersion due to being washed overboard from watercraft**
Code first:
any associated cataclysm (X37.0-)

7 **V92.20X- Drowning and submersion due to being washed overboard from merchant ship**

7 **V92.21X- Drowning and submersion due to being washed overboard from passenger ship**
Drowning and submersion due to being washed overboard from Ferry-boat
Drowning and submersion due to being washed overboard from Liner

7 **V92.22X- Drowning and submersion due to being washed overboard from fishing boat**

7 **V92.23X- Drowning and submersion due to being washed overboard from other powered watercraft**
Drowning and submersion due to being washed overboard from Hovercraft (on open water)
Drowning and submersion due to being washed overboard from Jet ski

7 **V92.24X- Drowning and submersion due to being washed overboard from sailboat**

7 **V92.25X- Drowning and submersion due to being washed overboard from canoe or kayak**

7 **V92.26X- Drowning and submersion due to being washed overboard from (nonpowered) inflatable craft**

7 **V92.27X- Drowning and submersion due to being washed overboard from water-skis**
EXCLUDES 1 *drowning and submersion due to fall off water-skis (V92.07)*

7 **V92.28X- Drowning and submersion due to being washed overboard from other unpowered watercraft**
Drowning and submersion due to being washed overboard from surf-board
Drowning and submersion due to being washed overboard from windsurfer

7 **V92.29X- Drowning and submersion due to being washed overboard from unspecified watercraft**
Drowning and submersion due to being washed overboard from boat NOS
Drowning and submersion due to being washed overboard from ship NOS
Drowning and submersion due to being washed overboard from watercraft NOS

4 **V93 Other injury due to accident on board watercraft, without accident to watercraft**
EXCLUDES 1 *civilian water transport accident involving military watercraft (V94.81-)*
other injury due to accident to watercraft (V91.-)
military watercraft accident in military or war operations (Y36, Y37.-)
EXCLUDES 2 *drowning and submersion due to accident on board watercraft, without accident to watercraft (V92.-)*

The appropriate 7th character is to be added to each code from category V93
A initial encounter
D subsequent encounter
S sequela

5 **V93.0 Burn due to localized fire on board watercraft**
EXCLUDES 1 *burn due to watercraft on fire (V91.0-)*

7 **V93.00X- Burn due to localized fire on board merchant vessel**

7 **V93.01X- Burn due to localized fire on board passenger vessel**
Burn due to localized fire on board Ferry-boat
Burn due to localized fire on board Liner

7 **V93.02X- Burn due to localized fire on board fishing boat**

7 **V93.03X-** **Burn due to localized fire on board other powered watercraft**
Burn due to localized fire on board Hovercraft
Burn due to localized fire on board Jet ski

7 **V93.04X-** **Burn due to localized fire on board sailboat**

7 **V93.09X-** **Burn due to localized fire on board unspecified watercraft**
Burn due to localized fire on board boat NOS
Burn due to localized fire on board ship NOS
Burn due to localized fire on board watercraft NOS

5 **V93.1** **Other burn on board watercraft**
Burn due to source other than fire on board watercraft
EXCLUDES 1 *burn due to watercraft on fire (V91.0-)*

7 **V93.10X-** **Other burn on board merchant vessel**

7 **V93.11X-** **Other burn on board passenger vessel**
Other burn on board Ferry-boat
Other burn on board Liner

7 **V93.12X-** **Other burn on board fishing boat**

7 **V93.13X-** **Other burn on board other powered watercraft**
Other burn on board Hovercraft
Other burn on board Jet ski

7 **V93.14X-** **Other burn on board sailboat**

7 **V93.19X-** **Other burn on board unspecified watercraft**
Other burn on board boat NOS
Other burn on board ship NOS
Other burn on board watercraft NOS

5 **V93.2** **Heat exposure on board watercraft**
EXCLUDES 1 *exposure to man-made heat not aboard watercraft (W92)*
exposure to natural heat while on board watercraft (X30)
exposure to sunlight while on board watercraft (X32)
EXCLUDES 2 *burn due to fire on board watercraft (V93.0-)*

7 **V93.20X-** **Heat exposure on board merchant ship**

7 **V93.21X-** **Heat exposure on board passenger ship**
Heat exposure on board Ferry-boat
Heat exposure on board Liner

7 **V93.22X-** **Heat exposure on board fishing boat**

7 **V93.23X-** **Heat exposure on board other powered watercraft**
Heat exposure on board hovercraft

7 **V93.24X-** **Heat exposure on board sailboat**

7 **V93.29X-** **Heat exposure on board unspecified watercraft**
Heat exposure on board boat NOS
Heat exposure on board ship NOS
Heat exposure on board watercraft NOS

5 **V93.3** **Fall on board watercraft**
EXCLUDES 1 *fall due to collision of watercraft (V91.2-)*

7 **V93.30X-** **Fall on board merchant ship**

7 **V93.31X-** **Fall on board passenger ship**
Fall on board Ferry-boat
Fall on board Liner

7 **V93.32X-** **Fall on board fishing boat**

7 **V93.33X-** **Fall on board other powered watercraft**
Fall on board Hovercraft (on open water)
Fall on board Jet ski

7 **V93.34X-** **Fall on board sailboat**

7 **V93.35X-** **Fall on board canoe or kayak**

7 **V93.36X-** **Fall on board (nonpowered) inflatable craft**

7 **V93.38X-** **Fall on board other unpowered watercraft**

7 **V93.39X-** **Fall on board unspecified watercraft**
Fall on board boat NOS
Fall on board ship NOS
Fall on board watercraft NOS

5 **V93.4** **Struck by falling object on board watercraft**
Hit by falling object on board watercraft
EXCLUDES 1 *struck by falling object due to accident to watercraft (V91.3)*

7 **V93.40X-** **Struck by falling object on merchant ship**

7 **V93.41X-** **Struck by falling object on passenger ship**
Struck by falling object on Ferry-boat
Struck by falling object on Liner

7 **V93.42X-** **Struck by falling object on fishing boat**

7 **V93.43X-** **Struck by falling object on other powered watercraft**
Struck by falling object on Hovercraft

7 **V93.44X-** **Struck by falling object on sailboat**

7 **V93.48X-** **Struck by falling object on other unpowered watercraft**

7 **V93.49X-** **Struck by falling object on unspecified watercraft**

5 **V93.5** **Explosion on board watercraft**
Boiler explosion on steamship
EXCLUDES 2 *fire on board watercraft (V93.0-)*

7 **V93.50X-** **Explosion on board merchant ship**

7 **V93.51X-** **Explosion on board passenger ship**
Explosion on board Ferry-boat
Explosion on board Liner

7 **V93.52X-** **Explosion on board fishing boat**

7 **V93.53X-** **Explosion on board other powered watercraft**
Explosion on board Hovercraft
Explosion on board Jet ski

7 **V93.54X-** **Explosion on board sailboat**

7 **V93.59X-** **Explosion on board unspecified watercraft**
Explosion on board boat NOS
Explosion on board ship NOS
Explosion on board watercraft NOS

5 **V93.6** **Machinery accident on board watercraft**
EXCLUDES 1 *machinery explosion on board watercraft (V93.4-)*
machinery fire on board watercraft (V93.0-)

7 **V93.60X-** **Machinery accident on board merchant ship**

7 **V93.61X-** **Machinery accident on board passenger ship**
Machinery accident on board Ferry-boat
Machinery accident on board Liner

7 **V93.62X-** **Machinery accident on board fishing boat**

7 **V93.63X-** **Machinery accident on board other powered watercraft**
Machinery accident on board Hovercraft

7 **V93.64X-** **Machinery accident on board sailboat**

7 **V93.69X-** **Machinery accident on board unspecified watercraft**
Machinery accident on board boat NOS
Machinery accident on board ship NOS
Machinery accident on board watercraft NOS

5 **V93.8** **Other injury due to other accident on board watercraft**
Accidental poisoning by gases or fumes on watercraft

7 **V93.80X-** **Other injury due to other accident on board merchant ship**

7 **V93.81X-** **Other injury due to other accident on board passenger ship**
Other injury due to other accident on board Ferry-boat
Other injury due to other accident on board Liner

7 **V93.82X-** **Other injury due to other accident on board fishing boat**

7 **V93.83X-** **Other injury due to other accident on board other powered watercraft**
Other injury due to other accident on board Hovercraft
Other injury due to other accident on board Jet ski

7 **V93.84X-** **Other injury due to other accident on board sailboat**

7 **V93.85X-** **Other injury due to other accident on board canoe or kayak**

7 **V93.86X-** **Other injury due to other accident on board (nonpowered) inflatable craft**

7 **V93.87X-** **Other injury due to other accident on board water-skis**
Hit or struck by object while waterskiing

7 **V93.88X-** **Other injury due to other accident on board other unpowered watercraft**
Hit or struck by object while surfing
Hit or struck by object while on board windsurfer

7 **V93.89X-** **Other injury due to other accident on board unspecified watercraft**
Other injury due to other accident on board boat NOS
Other injury due to other accident on board ship NOS
Other injury due to other accident on board watercraft NOS

4 V94 Other and unspecified water transport accidents

EXCLUDES 1 *military watercraft accidents in military or war operations (Y36, Y37)*

The appropriate 7th character is to be added to each code from category V94
A initial encounter
D subsequent encounter
S sequela

7 V94.0XX- Hitting object or bottom of body of water due to fall from watercraft
EXCLUDES 2 *drowning and submersion due to fall from watercraft (V92.0-)*

5 V94.1 Bather struck by watercraft
Swimmer hit by watercraft

7 V94.11X- Bather struck by powered watercraft

7 V94.12X- Bather struck by nonpowered watercraft

5 V94.2 Rider of nonpowered watercraft struck by other watercraft

7 V94.21X- Rider of nonpowered watercraft struck by other nonpowered watercraft
Canoer hit by other nonpowered watercraft
Surfer hit by other nonpowered watercraft
Windsurfer hit by other nonpowered watercraft

7 V94.22X- Rider of nonpowered watercraft struck by powered watercraft
Canoer hit by motorboat
Surfer hit by motorboat
Windsurfer hit by motorboat

5 V94.3 Injury to rider of (inflatable) watercraft being pulled behind other watercraft

7 V94.31X- Injury to rider of (inflatable) recreational watercraft being pulled behind other watercraft
Injury to rider of inner-tube pulled behind motor boat

7 V94.32X- Injury to rider of non-recreational watercraft being pulled behind other watercraft
Injury to occupant of dingy being pulled behind boat or ship
Injury to occupant of life-raft being pulled behind boat or ship

7 V94.4XX- Injury to barefoot water-skier
Injury to person being pulled behind boat or ship

5 V94.8 Other water transport accident

6 V94.81 Water transport accident involving military watercraft

7 V94.810- Civilian watercraft involved in water transport accident with military watercraft
Passenger on civilian watercraft injured due to accident with military watercraft

7 V94.811- Civilian in water injured by military watercraft

7 V94.818- Other water transport accident involving military watercraft

7 V94.89X- Other water transport accident

7 V94.9XX- Unspecified water transport accident
Water transport accident NOS

Air and space transport accidents (V95-V97)

EXCLUDES 1 *military aircraft accidents in military or war operations (Y36, Y37)*

4 V95 Accident to powered aircraft causing injury to occupant

The appropriate 7th character is to be added to each code from category V95
A initial encounter
D subsequent encounter
S sequela

5 V95.0 Helicopter accident injuring occupant

7 V95.00X- Unspecified helicopter accident injuring occupant

7 V95.01X- Helicopter crash injuring occupant

7 V95.02X- Forced landing of helicopter injuring occupant

7 V95.03X- Helicopter collision injuring occupant
Helicopter collision with any object, fixed, movable or moving

7 V95.04X- Helicopter fire injuring occupant

7 V95.05X- Helicopter explosion injuring occupant

7 V95.09X- Other helicopter accident injuring occupant

5 V95.1 Ultralight, microlight or powered-glider accident injuring occupant

7 V95.10X- Unspecified ultralight, microlight or powered-glider accident injuring occupant

7 V95.11X- Ultralight, microlight or powered-glider crash injuring occupant

7 V95.12X- Forced landing of ultralight, microlight or powered-glider injuring occupant

7 V95.13X- Ultralight, microlight or powered-glider collision injuring occupant
Ultralight, microlight or powered-glider collision with any object, fixed, movable or moving

7 V95.14X- Ultralight, microlight or powered-glider fire injuring occupant

7 V95.15X- Ultralight, microlight or powered-glider explosion injuring occupant

7 V95.19X- Other ultralight, microlight or powered-glider accident injuring occupant

5 V95.2 Other private fixed-wing aircraft accident injuring occupant

7 V95.20X- Unspecified accident to other private fixed-wing aircraft, injuring occupant

7 V95.21X- Other private fixed-wing aircraft crash injuring occupant

7 V95.22X- Forced landing of other private fixed-wing aircraft injuring occupant

7 V95.23X- Other private fixed-wing aircraft collision injuring occupant
Other private fixed-wing aircraft collision with any object, fixed, movable or moving

7 V95.24X- Other private fixed-wing aircraft fire injuring occupant

7 V95.25X- Other private fixed-wing aircraft explosion injuring occupant

7 V95.29X- Other accident to other private fixed-wing aircraft injuring occupant

5 V95.3 Commercial fixed-wing aircraft accident injuring occupant

7 V95.30X- Unspecified accident to commercial fixed-wing aircraft injuring occupant

7 V95.31X- Commercial fixed-wing aircraft crash injuring occupant

7 V95.32X- Forced landing of commercial fixed-wing aircraft injuring occupant

7 V95.33X- Commercial fixed-wing aircraft collision injuring occupant
Commercial fixed-wing aircraft collision with any object, fixed, movable or moving

7 V95.34X- Commercial fixed-wing aircraft fire injuring occupant

7 V95.35X- Commercial fixed-wing aircraft explosion injuring occupant

7 V95.39X- Other accident to commercial fixed-wing aircraft injuring occupant

5 V95.4 Spacecraft accident injuring occupant

7 V95.40X- Unspecified spacecraft accident injuring occupant

7 V95.41X- Spacecraft crash injuring occupant

7 V95.42X- Forced landing of spacecraft injuring occupant

7 V95.43X- Spacecraft collision injuring occupant
Spacecraft collision with any object, fixed, moveable or moving

7 V95.44X- Spacecraft fire injuring occupant

7 V95.45X- Spacecraft explosion injuring occupant

7 V95.49X- Other spacecraft accident injuring occupant

7 V95.8XX- Other powered aircraft accidents injuring occupant

7 V95.9XX- Unspecified aircraft accident injuring occupant
Aircraft accident NOS
Air transport accident NOS

4 V96 Accident to nonpowered aircraft causing injury to occupant

The appropriate 7th character is to be added to each code from category V96
A initial encounter
D subsequent encounter
S sequela

5 V96.0 Balloon accident injuring occupant

7 V96.00X- Unspecified **balloon accident injuring occupant**

7 V96.01X- **Balloon** crash **injuring occupant**

7 V96.02X- Forced landing **of balloon injuring occupant**

7 V96.03X- **Balloon** collision **injuring occupant**

Balloon collision with any object, fixed, moveable or moving

7 V96.04X- **Balloon** fire **injuring occupant**

7 V96.05X- **Balloon** explosion **injuring occupant**

7 V96.09X- Other **balloon accident injuring occupant**

5 V96.1 Hang-glider **accident injuring occupant**

7 V96.10X- Unspecified **hang-glider accident injuring occupant**

7 V96.11X- **Hang-glider** crash **injuring occupant**

7 V96.12X- Forced landing **of hang-glider injuring occupant**

7 V96.13X- **Hang-glider** collision **injuring occupant**

Hang-glider collision with any object, fixed, moveable or moving

7 V96.14X- **Hang-glider** fire **injuring occupant**

7 V96.15X- **Hang-glider** explosion **injuring occupant**

7 V96.19X- Other **hang-glider accident injuring occupant**

5 V96.2 Glider (nonpowered) **accident injuring occupant**

7 V96.20X- Unspecified **glider (nonpowered) accident injuring occupant**

7 V96.21X- **Glider (nonpowered)** crash **injuring occupant**

7 V96.22X- Forced landing **of glider (nonpowered) injuring occupant**

7 V96.23X- **Glider (nonpowered)** collision **injuring occupant**

Glider (nonpowered) collision with any object, fixed, moveable or moving

7 V96.24X- **Glider (nonpowered)** fire **injuring occupant**

7 V96.25X- **Glider (nonpowered)** explosion **injuring occupant**

7 V96.29X- Other **glider (nonpowered) accident injuring occupant**

7 V96.8XX- Other **nonpowered-aircraft accidents injuring occupant**

Kite carrying a person accident injuring occupant

7 V96.9XX- Unspecified **nonpowered-aircraft accident injuring occupant**

Nonpowered-aircraft accident NOS

4 V97 Other specified **air transport accidents**

The appropriate 7th character is to be added to each code from category V97
A initial encounter
D subsequent encounter
S sequela

7 V97.0XX- Occupant of aircraft injured in **other specified air transport accidents**

Fall in, on or from aircraft in air transport accident

EXCLUDES 1 *accident while boarding or alighting aircraft (V97.1)*

7 V97.1XX- **Person injured while boarding or alighting from aircraft**

5 V97.2 Parachutist **accident**

7 V97.21X- **Parachutist** entangled in object

Parachutist landing in tree

7 V97.22X- **Parachutist** injured on landing

7 V97.29X- Other **parachutist accident**

5 V97.3 Person on ground injured **in air transport accident**

7 V97.31X- **Hit by object falling from aircraft**

Hit by crashing aircraft
Injured by aircraft hitting house
Injured by aircraft hitting car

7 V97.32X- **Injured by** rotating propeller

7 V97.33X- **Sucked into jet engine**

7 V97.39X- Other **injury to person on ground due to air transport accident**

5 V97.8 **Other air transport accidents,** not elsewhere classified

EXCLUDES 1 *aircraft accident NOS (V95.9)*
exposure to changes in air pressure during ascent or descent (W94.-)

6 V97.81 **Air transport accident** involving military aircraft

7 V97.810- Civilian **aircraft involved in air transport accident with military aircraft**

Passenger in civilian aircraft injured due to accident with military aircraft

7 V97.811- Civilian injured **by military aircraft**

7 V97.818- Other **air transport accident involving military aircraft**

7 V97.89X- **Other air transport accidents, not elsewhere classified**

Injury from machinery on aircraft

Other and unspecified transport accidents (V98-V99)

EXCLUDES 1 *vehicle accident, type of vehicle unspecified (V89.-)*

4 V98 **Other** specified **transport accidents**

The appropriate 7th character is to be added to each code from category V98
A initial encounter
D subsequent encounter
S sequela

7 V98.0XX- **Accident to,** on or involving **cable-car,** not on rails

Caught or dragged by cable-car, not on rails
Fall or jump from cable-car, not on rails
Object thrown from or in cable-car, not on rails

7 V98.1XX- **Accident to,** on or involving **land-yacht**

7 V98.2XX- **Accident to,** on or involving **ice yacht**

7 V98.3XX- **Accident to,** on or involving **ski lift**

Accident to, on or involving ski chair-lift
Accident to, on or involving ski-lift with gondola

7 V98.8XX- **Other specified transport accidents**

7 V99.XXX- **Unspecified transport accident**

The appropriate 7th character is to be added to code V99
A initial encounter
D subsequent encounter
S sequela

Other external causes of accidental injury (W00-X58)

Slipping, tripping, stumbling and falls (W00-W19)

EXCLUDES 1 *assault involving a fall (Y01-Y02)*
fall from animal (V80.-)
fall (in) (from) machinery (in operation) (W28-W31)
fall (in) (from) transport vehicle (V01-V99)
intentional self-harm involving a fall (X80-X81)

EXCLUDES 2 *at risk for fall (history of fall) Z91.81*
fall (in) (from) burning building (X00.-)
fall into fire (X00-X04, X08)

4 W00 **Fall due to** ice and snow

INCLUDES pedestrian on foot falling (slipping) on ice and snow

EXCLUDES 1 *fall on (from) ice and snow involving pedestrian conveyance (V00.-)*
fall from stairs and steps not due to ice and snow (W10.-)

The appropriate 7th character is to be added to each code from category W00
A initial encounter
D subsequent encounter
S sequela

7 W00.0XX- **Fall** on same level **due to ice and snow**

AHA: (W00.0XXD) 2Q 2016, 5

7 W00.1XX- **Fall from** stairs and steps **due to ice and snow**

7 W00.2XX- Other **fall from** one level to another **due to ice and snow**

7 W00.9XX- Unspecified **fall due to ice and snow**

W01 Fall on same level from slipping, tripping and stumbling

INCLUDES fall on moving sidewalk

EXCLUDES 1 *fall due to bumping (striking) against object (W18.0-)*
fall in shower or bathtub (W18.2-)
fall on same level NOS (W18.30)
fall on same level from slipping, tripping and stumbling due to ice or snow (W00.0)
fall off or from toilet (W18.1-)
slipping, tripping and stumbling NOS (W18.40)
slipping, tripping and stumbling without falling (W18.4-)

The appropriate 7th character is to be added to each code from category W01
A initial encounter
D subsequent encounter
S sequela

W01.0XX- Fall on same level from slipping, tripping and stumbling without subsequent striking against object
Falling over animal

W01.1 Fall on same level from slipping, tripping and stumbling with subsequent striking against object

W01.10X- Fall on same level from slipping, tripping and stumbling with subsequent striking against unspecified object

W01.11 Fall on same level from slipping, tripping and stumbling with subsequent striking against sharp object

W01.110- Fall on same level from slipping, tripping and stumbling with subsequent striking against sharp glass

W01.111- Fall on same level from slipping, tripping and stumbling with subsequent striking against power tool or machine

W01.118- Fall on same level from slipping, tripping and stumbling with subsequent striking against other sharp object

W01.119- Fall on same level from slipping, tripping and stumbling with subsequent striking against unspecified sharp object

W01.19 Fall on same level from slipping, tripping and stumbling with subsequent striking against other object

W01.190- Fall on same level from slipping, tripping and stumbling with subsequent striking against furniture

W01.198- Fall on same level from slipping, tripping and stumbling with subsequent striking against other object

W03.XXX- Other fall on same level due to collision with another person
Fall due to non-transport collision with other person

EXCLUDES 1 *collision with another person without fall (W51)*
crushed or pushed by a crowd or human stampede (W52)
fall involving pedestrian conveyance (V00-V09)
fall due to ice or snow (W00)
fall on same level NOS (W18.30)

The appropriate 7th character is to be added to code W03
A initial encounter
D subsequent encounter
S sequela

AHA: (W03.xxxD) 1Q 2015, 10
AHA: (WO3.xxxA) 1Q 2015, 9
AHA: (WO3.xxxA) 4Q 2012, 108

W04.XXX- Fall while being carried or supported by other persons
Accidentally dropped while being carried

The appropriate 7th character is to be added to code W04
A initial encounter
D subsequent encounter
S sequela

W05 Fall from non-moving wheelchair, nonmotorized scooter and motorized mobility scooter

EXCLUDES 1 *fall from moving wheelchair (powered) (V00.811)*
fall from moving motorized mobility scooter (V00.831)
fall from nonmotorized scooter (V00.141)

The appropriate 7th character is to be added to each code from category W05
A initial encounter
D subsequent encounter
S sequela

W05.0XX- Fall from non-moving wheelchair

W05.1XX- Fall from non-moving nonmotorized scooter

W05.2XX- Fall from non-moving motorized mobility scooter

W06.XXX- Fall from bed

The appropriate 7th character is to be added to code W06
A initial encounter
D subsequent encounter
S sequela

W07.XXX- Fall from chair

The appropriate 7th character is to be added to code W07
A initial encounter
D subsequent encounter
S sequela

W08.XXX- Fall from other furniture

The appropriate 7th character is to be added to code W08
A initial encounter
D subsequent encounter
S sequela

W09 Fall on and from playground equipment

EXCLUDES 1 *fall involving recreational machinery (W31)*

The appropriate 7th character is to be added to each code from category W09
A initial encounter
D subsequent encounter
S sequela

W09.0XX- Fall on or from playground slide

W09.1XX- Fall from playground swing

W09.2XX- Fall on or from jungle gym

W09.8XX- Fall on or from other playground equipment

W10 Fall on and from stairs and steps

EXCLUDES 1 *Fall from stairs and steps due to ice and snow (W00.1)*

The appropriate 7th character is to be added to each code from category W10
A initial encounter
D subsequent encounter
S sequela

W10.0XX- Fall (on)(from) escalator

W10.1XX- Fall (on)(from) sidewalk curb

W10.2XX- Fall (on)(from) incline
Fall (on) (from) ramp

W10.8XX- Fall (on) (from) other stairs and steps

W10.9XX- Fall (on) (from) unspecified stairs and steps

W11.XXX- Fall on and from ladder

The appropriate 7th character is to be added to code W11
A initial encounter
D subsequent encounter
S sequela

W12.XXX- Fall on and from scaffolding

The appropriate 7th character is to be added to code W12
A initial encounter
D subsequent encounter
S sequela

4 W13 Fall from, out of or through building or structure

The appropriate 7th character is to be added to each code from category W13
A initial encounter
D subsequent encounter
S sequela

7 W13.0XX- Fall from, out of or through balcony
Fall from, out of or through railing
7 W13.1XX- Fall from, out of or through bridge
7 W13.2XX- Fall from, out of or through roof
7 W13.3XX- Fall through floor
7 W13.4XX- Fall from, out of or through window
EXCLUDES 2 *fall with subsequent striking against sharp glass (W01.110)*
7 W13.8XX- Fall from, out of or through other building or structure
Fall from, out of or through viaduct
Fall from, out of or through wall
Fall from, out of or through flag-pole
7 W13.9XX- Fall from, out of or through building, not otherwise specified
EXCLUDES 1 *collapse of a building or structure (W20.-)*
fall or jump from burning building or structure (X00.-)

7 W14.XXX- Fall from tree

The appropriate 7th character is to be added to code W14
A initial encounter
D subsequent encounter
S sequela

7 W15.XXX- Fall from cliff

The appropriate 7th character is to be added to code W15
A initial encounter
D subsequent encounter
S sequela

4 W16 Fall, jump or diving into water
EXCLUDES 1 *accidental non-watercraft drowning and submersion not involving fall (W65-W74)*
effects of air pressure from diving (W94.-)
fall into water from watercraft (V90-V94)
hitting an object or against bottom when falling from watercraft (V94.0)
EXCLUDES 2 *striking or hitting diving board (W21.4)*

The appropriate 7th character is to be added to each code from category W16
A initial encounter
D subsequent encounter
S sequela

5 W16.0 Fall into swimming pool
Fall into swimming pool NOS
EXCLUDES 1 *fall into empty swimming pool (W17.3)*
6 W16.01 Fall into swimming pool striking water surface
7 W16.011- Fall into swimming pool striking water surface causing drowning and submersion
EXCLUDES 1 *drowning and submersion while in swimming pool without fall (W67)*
7 W16.012- Fall into swimming pool striking water surface causing other injury
6 W16.02 Fall into swimming pool striking bottom
7 W16.021- Fall into swimming pool striking bottom causing drowning and submersion
EXCLUDES 1 *drowning and submersion while in swimming pool without fall (W67)*
7 W16.022- Fall into swimming pool striking bottom causing other injury
6 W16.03 Fall into swimming pool striking wall
7 W16.031- Fall into swimming pool striking wall causing drowning and submersion
EXCLUDES 1 *drowning and submersion while in swimming pool without fall (W67)*
7 W16.032- Fall into swimming pool striking wall causing other injury

5 W16.1 Fall into natural body of water
Fall into lake
Fall into open sea
Fall into river
Fall into stream
6 W16.11 Fall into natural body of water striking water surface
7 W16.111- Fall into natural body of water striking water surface causing drowning and submersion
EXCLUDES 1 *drowning and submersion while in natural body of water without fall (W69)*
7 W16.112- Fall into natural body of water striking water surface causing other injury
6 W16.12 Fall into natural body of water striking bottom
7 W16.121- Fall into natural body of water striking bottom causing drowning and submersion
EXCLUDES 1 *drowning and submersion while in natural body of water without fall (W69)*
7 W16.122- Fall into natural body of water striking bottom causing other injury
6 W16.13 Fall into natural body of water striking side
7 W16.131- Fall into natural body of water striking side causing drowning and submersion
EXCLUDES 1 *drowning and submersion while in natural body of water without fall (W69)*
7 W16.132- Fall into natural body of water striking side causing other injury

5 W16.2 Fall in (into) filled bathtub or bucket of water
6 W16.21 Fall in (into) filled bathtub
EXCLUDES 1 *fall into empty bathtub (W18.2)*
7 W16.211- Fall in (into) filled bathtub causing drowning and submersion
EXCLUDES 1 *drowning and submersion while in filled bathtub without fall (W65)*
7 W16.212- Fall in (into) filled bathtub causing other injury
6 W16.22 Fall in (into) bucket of water
7 W16.221- Fall in (into) bucket of water causing drowning and submersion
7 W16.222- Fall in (into) bucket of water causing other injury

5 W16.3 Fall into other water
Fall into fountain
Fall into reservoir
6 W16.31 Fall into other water striking water surface
7 W16.311- Fall into other water striking water surface causing drowning and submersion
EXCLUDES 1 *drowning and submersion while in other water without fall (W73)*
7 W16.312- Fall into other water striking water surface causing other injury
6 W16.32 Fall into other water striking bottom
7 W16.321- Fall into other water striking bottom causing drowning and submersion
EXCLUDES 1 *drowning and submersion while in other water without fall (W73)*
7 W16.322- Fall into other water striking bottom causing other injury
6 W16.33 Fall into other water striking wall
7 W16.331- Fall into other water striking wall causing drowning and submersion
EXCLUDES 1 *drowning and submersion while in other water without fall (W73)*
7 W16.332- Fall into other water striking wall causing other injury

5 W16.4 Fall into unspecified water
7 W16.41X- Fall into unspecified water causing drowning and submersion
7 W16.42X- Fall into unspecified water causing other injury

5 W16.5 Jumping or diving into swimming pool

6 W16.51 Jumping or diving into swimming pool striking water surface
7 W16.511- Jumping or diving into swimming pool striking water surface causing drowning and submersion
EXCLUDES 1 *drowning and submersion while in swimming pool without jumping or diving (W67)*
7 W16.512- Jumping or diving into swimming pool striking water surface causing other injury
6 W16.52 Jumping or diving into swimming pool striking bottom
7 W16.521- Jumping or diving into swimming pool striking bottom causing drowning and submersion
EXCLUDES 1 *drowning and submersion while in swimming pool without jumping or diving (W67)*
7 W16.522- Jumping or diving into swimming pool striking bottom causing other injury
6 W16.53 Jumping or diving into swimming pool striking wall
7 W16.531- Jumping or diving into swimming pool striking wall causing drowning and submersion
EXCLUDES 1 *drowning and submersion while in swimming pool without jumping or diving (W67)*
7 W16.532- Jumping or diving into swimming pool striking wall causing other injury
5 W16.6 Jumping or diving into natural body of water
Jumping or diving into lake
Jumping or diving into open sea
Jumping or diving into river
Jumping or diving into stream
6 W16.61 Jumping or diving into natural body of water striking water surface
7 W16.611- Jumping or diving into natural body of water striking water surface causing drowning and submersion
EXCLUDES 1 *drowning and submersion while in natural body of water without jumping or diving (W69)*
7 W16.612- Jumping or diving into natural body of water striking water surface causing other injury
6 W16.62 Jumping or diving into natural body of water striking bottom
7 W16.621- Jumping or diving into natural body of water striking bottom causing drowning and submersion
EXCLUDES 1 *drowning and submersion while in natural body of water without jumping or diving (W69)*
7 W16.622- Jumping or diving into natural body of water striking bottom causing other injury
5 W16.7 Jumping or diving from boat
EXCLUDES 1 *Fall from boat into water -see watercraft accident (V90-V94)*
6 W16.71 Jumping or diving from boat striking water surface
7 W16.711- Jumping or diving from boat striking water surface causing drowning and submersion
7 W16.712- Jumping or diving from boat striking water surface causing other injury
6 W16.72 Jumping or diving from boat striking bottom
7 W16.721- Jumping or diving from boat striking bottom causing drowning and submersion
7 W16.722- Jumping or diving from boat striking bottom causing other injury
5 W16.8 Jumping or diving into other water
Jumping or diving into fountain
Jumping or diving into reservoir
6 W16.81 Jumping or diving into other water striking water surface
7 W16.811- Jumping or diving into other water striking water surface causing drowning and submersion
EXCLUDES 1 *drowning and submersion while in other water without jumping or diving (W73)*
7 W16.812- Jumping or diving into other water striking water surface causing other injury
6 W16.82 Jumping or diving into other water striking bottom
7 W16.821- Jumping or diving into other water striking bottom causing drowning and submersion
EXCLUDES 1 *drowning and submersion while in other water without jumping or diving (W73)*
7 W16.822- Jumping or diving into other water striking bottom causing other injury
6 W16.83 Jumping or diving into other water striking wall
7 W16.831- Jumping or diving into other water striking wall causing drowning and submersion
EXCLUDES 1 *drowning and submersion while in other water without jumping or diving (W73)*
7 W16.832- Jumping or diving into other water striking wall causing other injury
5 W16.9 Jumping or diving into unspecified water
7 W16.91X- Jumping or diving into unspecified water causing drowning and submersion
7 W16.92X- Jumping or diving into unspecified water causing other injury

4 W17 Other fall from one level to another

The appropriate 7th character is to be added to each code from category W17
A initial encounter
D subsequent encounter
S sequela

7 W17.0XX- Fall into well
7 W17.1XX- Fall into storm drain or manhole
7 W17.2XX- Fall into hole
Fall into pit
7 W17.3XX- Fall into empty swimming pool
EXCLUDES 1 *fall into filled swimming pool (W16.0-)*
7 W17.4XX- Fall from dock
5 W17.8 Other fall from one level to another
7 W17.81X- Fall down embankment (hill)
7 W17.82X- Fall from (out of) grocery cart
Fall due to grocery cart tipping over
7 W17.89X- Other fall from one level to another
Fall from cherry picker
Fall from lifting device
Fall from mobile elevated work platform [MEWP]
Fall from sky lift
AHA: (W17.89XD) 2Q 2015, 6

4 W18 Other slipping, tripping and stumbling and falls

The appropriate 7th character is to be added to each code from category W18
A initial encounter
D subsequent encounter
S sequela

5 W18.0 Fall due to bumping against object
Striking against object with subsequent fall
EXCLUDES 1 *fall on same level due to slipping, tripping, or stumbling with subsequent striking against object (W01.1-)*
7 W18.00X- Striking against unspecified object with subsequent fall
7 W18.01X- Striking against sports equipment with subsequent fall
7 W18.02X- Striking against glass with subsequent fall
7 W18.09X- Striking against other object with subsequent fall
5 W18.1 Fall from or off toilet
7 W18.11X- Fall from or off toilet without subsequent striking against object
Fall from (off) toilet NOS
7 W18.12X- Fall from or off toilet with subsequent striking against object
7 W18.2XX- Fall in (into) shower or empty bathtub
EXCLUDES 1 *fall in full bathtub causing drowning or submersion (W16.21-)*
5 W18.3 Other and unspecified fall on same level
7 W18.30X- Fall on same level, unspecified

W18.31X- **Fall on same level due to stepping on an object**
Fall on same level due to stepping on an animal
EXCLUDES 1 *slipping, tripping and stumbling without fall due to stepping on animal (W18.41)*

W18.39X- **Other fall on same level**

W18.4 **Slipping, tripping and stumbling without falling**
EXCLUDES 1 *collision with another person without fall (W51)*

W18.40X- **Slipping, tripping and stumbling without falling, unspecified**

W18.41X- **Slipping, tripping and stumbling without falling due to stepping on object**
Slipping, tripping and stumbling without falling due to stepping on animal
EXCLUDES 1 *slipping, tripping and stumbling with fall due to stepping on animal (W18.31)*

W18.42X- **Slipping, tripping and stumbling without falling due to stepping into hole or opening**

W18.43X- **Slipping, tripping and stumbling without falling due to stepping from one level to another**

W18.49X- **Other slipping, tripping and stumbling without falling**

W19.XXX- **Unspecified fall**
Accidental fall NOS
The appropriate 7th character is to be added to code W19
A initial encounter
D subsequent encounter
S sequela
AHA: (W19.XXXD) 4Q 2012, 95

Exposure to inanimate mechanical forces (W20-W49)

EXCLUDES 1 *assault (X92-Y09)*
contact or collision with animals or persons (W50-W64)
exposure to inanimate mechanical forces involving military or war operations (Y36.-, Y37.-)
intentional self-harm (X71-X83)

W20 **Struck by thrown, projected or falling object**
Code first any associated:
cataclysm (X34-X39)
lightning strike (T75.00)
EXCLUDES 1 *falling object in machinery accident (W24, W28-W31)*
falling object in transport accident (V01-V99)
object set in motion by explosion (W35-W40)
object set in motion by firearm (W32-W34)
struck by thrown sports equipment (W21.-)

The appropriate 7th character is to be added to each code from category W20
A initial encounter
D subsequent encounter
S sequela

W20.0XX- **Struck by falling object in cave-in**
EXCLUDES 2 *asphyxiation due to cave-in (T71.21)*

W20.1XX- **Struck by object due to collapse of building**
EXCLUDES 1 *struck by object due to collapse of burning building (X00.2, X02.2)*

W20.8XX- **Other cause of strike by thrown, projected or falling object**
EXCLUDES 1 *struck by thrown sports equipment (W21.-)*

W21 **Striking against or struck by sports equipment**
EXCLUDES 1 *assault with sports equipment (Y08.0-)*
striking against or struck by sports equipment with subsequent fall (W18.01)

The appropriate 7th character is to be added to each code from category W21
A initial encounter
D subsequent encounter
S sequela

W21.0 **Struck by hit or thrown ball**

W21.00X- **Struck by hit or thrown ball, unspecified type**

W21.01X- **Struck by football**

W21.02X- **Struck by soccer ball**

W21.03X- **Struck by baseball**

W21.04X- **Struck by golf ball**

W21.05X- **Struck by basketball**

W21.06X- **Struck by volleyball**

W21.07X- **Struck by softball**

W21.09X- **Struck by other hit or thrown ball**

W21.1 **Struck by bat, racquet or club**

W21.11X- **Struck by baseball bat**

W21.12X- **Struck by tennis racquet**

W21.13X- **Struck by golf club**

W21.19X- **Struck by other bat, racquet or club**

W21.2 **Struck by hockey stick or puck**

W21.21 **Struck by hockey stick**

W21.210- **Struck by ice hockey stick**

W21.211- **Struck by field hockey stick**

W21.22 **Struck by hockey puck**

W21.220- **Struck by ice hockey puck**

W21.221- **Struck by field hockey puck**

W21.3 **Struck by sports foot wear**

W21.31X- **Struck by shoe cleats**
Stepped on by shoe cleats

W21.32X- **Struck by skate blades**
Skated over by skate blades

W21.39X- **Struck by other sports foot wear**

W21.4XX- **Striking against diving board**
Use additional code for subsequent falling into water, if applicable (W16.-)

W21.8 **Striking against or struck by other sports equipment**

W21.81X- **Striking against or struck by football helmet**

W21.89X- **Striking against or struck by other sports equipment**

W21.9XX- **Striking against or struck by unspecified sports equipment**

W22 **Striking against or struck by other objects**
EXCLUDES 1 *striking against or struck by object with subsequent fall (W18.09)*

The appropriate 7th character is to be added to each code from category W22
A initial encounter
D subsequent encounter
S sequela

W22.0 **Striking against stationary object**
EXCLUDES 1 *striking against stationary sports equipment (W21.8)*

W22.01X- **Walked into wall**

W22.02X- **Walked into lamppost**

W22.03X- **Walked into furniture**

W22.04 **Striking against wall of swimming pool**

W22.041- **Striking against wall of swimming pool causing drowning and submersion**
EXCLUDES 1 *drowning and submersion while swimming without striking against wall (W67)*

W22.042- **Striking against wall of swimming pool causing other injury**

W22.09X- **Striking against other stationary object**

W22.1 **Striking against or struck by automobile airbag**

W22.10X- **Striking against or struck by unspecified automobile airbag**

W22.11X- **Striking against or struck by driver side automobile airbag**

W22.12X- **Striking against or struck by front passenger side automobile airbag**

W22.19X- **Striking against or struck by other automobile airbag**

W22.8XX- **Striking against or struck by other objects**
Striking against or struck by object NOS
EXCLUDES 1 *struck by thrown, projected or falling object (W20.-)*

W23 Caught, crushed, jammed or pinched in or between objects

EXCLUDES 1 *injury caused by cutting or piercing instruments (W25-W27)*
injury caused by firearms malfunction (W32.1, W33.1-, W34.1-)
injury caused by lifting and transmission devices (W24.-)
injury caused by machinery (W28-W31)
injury caused by nonpowered hand tools (W27.-)
injury caused by transport vehicle being used as a means of transportation (V01-V99)
injury caused by struck by thrown, projected or falling object (W20.-)

The appropriate 7th character is to be added to each code from category W23
A initial encounter
D subsequent encounter
S sequela

W23.0XX- Caught, crushed, jammed, or pinched between moving objects

W23.1XX- Caught, crushed, jammed, or pinched between stationary objects

W24 Contact with lifting and transmission devices, not elsewhere classified

EXCLUDES 1 *transport accidents (V01-V99)*

The appropriate 7th character is to be added to each code from category W24
A initial encounter
D subsequent encounter
S sequela

W24.0XX- Contact with lifting devices, not elsewhere classified
Contact with chain hoist
Contact with drive belt
Contact with pulley (block)

W24.1XX- Contact with transmission devices, not elsewhere classified
Contact with transmission belt or cable

W25.XXX- Contact with sharp glass
Code first any associated:
injury due to flying glass from explosion or firearm discharge (W32-W40)
transport accident (V00-V99)

EXCLUDES 1 *fall on same level due to slipping, tripping and stumbling with subsequent striking against sharp glass (W01.10)*
striking against sharp glass with subsequent fall (W18.02)

EXCLUDES 2 *glass embedded in skin (W45)*

The appropriate 7th character is to be added to code W25
A initial encounter
D subsequent encounter
S sequela

W26 Contact with other sharp objects

EXCLUDES 2 *sharp object (s) embedded in skin (W45)*

The appropriate 7th character is to be added to each code from category W26
A initial encounter
D subsequent encounter
S sequela

AHA: 4Q 2016, 73

W26.0XX- Contact with knife
EXCLUDES 1 *contact with electric knife (W29.1)*

W26.1XX- Contact with sword or dagger

W26.2XX- Contact with edge of stiff paper
Paper cut

W26.8XX- Contact with other sharp object(s), not elsewhere classified
Contact with tin can lid

W26.9XX- Contact with unspecified sharp object(s)

W27 Contact with nonpowered hand tool

The appropriate 7th character is to be added to each code from category W27
A initial encounter
D subsequent encounter
S sequela

W27.0XX- Contact with workbench tool
Contact with auger
Contact with axe
Contact with chisel
Contact with handsaw
Contact with screwdriver

W27.1XX- Contact with garden tool
Contact with hoe
Contact with nonpowered lawn mower
Contact with pitchfork
Contact with rake

W27.2XX- Contact with scissors

W27.3XX- Contact with needle (sewing)
EXCLUDES 1 *contact with hypodermic needle (W46.-)*

W27.4XX- Contact with kitchen utensil
Contact with fork
Contact with ice-pick
Contact with can-opener NOS

W27.5XX- Contact with paper-cutter

W27.8XX- Contact with other nonpowered hand tool
Contact with nonpowered sewing machine
Contact with shovel

W28.XXX- Contact with powered lawn mower
Powered lawn mower (commercial) (residential)

EXCLUDES 1 *contact with nonpowered lawn mower (W27.1)*

EXCLUDES 2 *exposure to electric current (W86.-)*

The appropriate 7th character is to be added to code W28
A initial encounter
D subsequent encounter
S sequela

W29 Contact with other powered hand tools and household machinery

EXCLUDES 1 *contact with commercial machinery (W31.82)*
contact with hot household appliance (X15)
contact with nonpowered hand tool (W27.-)
exposure to electric current (W86)

The appropriate 7th character is to be added to each code from category W29
A initial encounter
D subsequent encounter
S sequela

W29.0XX- Contact with powered kitchen appliance
Contact with blender
Contact with can-opener
Contact with garbage disposal
Contact with mixer

W29.1XX- Contact with electric knife

W29.2XX- Contact with other powered household machinery
Contact with electric fan
Contact with powered dryer (clothes) (powered) (spin)
Contact with washing-machine
Contact with sewing machine

W29.3XX- Contact with powered garden and outdoor hand tools and machinery
Contact with chainsaw
Contact with edger
Contact with garden cultivator (tiller)
Contact with hedge trimmer
Contact with other powered garden tool

EXCLUDES 1 *contact with powered lawn mower (W28)*

W29.4XX- Contact with nail gun

W29.8XX- Contact with other powered hand tools and household machinery
Contact with do-it-yourself tool NOS

W30 Contact with agricultural machinery

INCLUDES animal-powered farm machine

EXCLUDES 1 *agricultural transport vehicle accident (V01-V99)*
explosion of grain store (W40.8)
exposure to electric current (W86.-)

The appropriate 7th character is to be added to each code from category W30
A initial encounter
D subsequent encounter
S sequela

W30.0XX- Contact with combine harvester
Contact with reaper
Contact with thresher

W30.1XX- Contact with power take-off devices (PTO)

W30.2XX- Contact with hay derrick

W30.3XX- Contact with grain storage elevator
EXCLUDES 1 *explosion of grain store (W40.8)*

W30.8 Contact with other specified agricultural machinery

W30.81X- Contact with agricultural transport vehicle in stationary use
Contact with agricultural transport vehicle under repair, not on public roadway
EXCLUDES 1 *agricultural transport vehicle accident (V01-V99)*

W30.89X- Contact with other specified agricultural machinery

W30.9XX- Contact with unspecified agricultural machinery
Contact with farm machinery NOS

W31 Contact with other and unspecified machinery

EXCLUDES 1 *contact with agricultural machinery (W30.-)*
contact with machinery in transport under own power or being towed by a vehicle (V01-V99)
exposure to electric current (W86)

The appropriate 7th character is to be added to each code from category W31
A initial encounter
D subsequent encounter
S sequela

W31.0XX- Contact with mining and earth-drilling machinery
Contact with bore or drill (land) (seabed)
Contact with shaft hoist
Contact with shaft lift
Contact with undercutter

W31.1XX- Contact with metalworking machines
Contact with abrasive wheel
Contact with forging machine
Contact with lathe
Contact with mechanical shears
Contact with metal drilling machine
Contact with milling machine
Contact with power press
Contact with rolling-mill
Contact with metal sawing machine

W31.2XX- Contact with powered woodworking and forming machines
Contact with band saw
Contact with bench saw
Contact with circular saw
Contact with molding machine
Contact with overhead plane
Contact with powered saw
Contact with radial saw
Contact with sander
EXCLUDES 1 *nonpowered woodworking tools (W27.0)*

W31.3XX- Contact with prime movers
Contact with gas turbine
Contact with internal combustion engine
Contact with steam engine
Contact with water driven turbine

W31.8 Contact with other specified machinery

W31.81X- Contact with recreational machinery
Contact with roller coaster

W31.82X- Contact with other commercial machinery
Contact with commercial electric fan
Contact with commercial kitchen appliances
Contact with commercial powered dryer (clothes) (powered) (spin)
Contact with commercial washing-machine
Contact with commercial sewing machine
EXCLUDES 1 *contact with household machinery (W29.-)*
contact with powered lawn mower (W28)

W31.83X- Contact with special construction vehicle in stationary use
Contact with special construction vehicle under repair, not on public roadway
EXCLUDES 1 *special construction vehicle accident (V01-V99)*

W31.89X- Contact with other specified machinery

W31.9XX- Contact with unspecified machinery
Contact with machinery NOS

W32 Accidental handgun discharge and malfunction

INCLUDES accidental discharge and malfunction of gun for single hand use
accidental discharge and malfunction of pistol
accidental discharge and malfunction of revolver
Handgun discharge and malfunction NOS

EXCLUDES 1 *accidental airgun discharge and malfunction (W34.010, W34.110)*
accidental BB gun discharge and malfunction (W34.010, W34.110)
accidental pellet gun discharge and malfunction (W34.010, W34.110)
accidental shotgun discharge and malfunction (W33.01, W33.11)
assault by handgun discharge (X93)
handgun discharge involving legal intervention (Y35.0-)
handgun discharge involving military or war operations (Y36.4-)
intentional self-harm by handgun discharge (X72)
Very pistol discharge and malfunction (W34.09, W34.19)

The appropriate 7th character is to be added to each code from category W32
A initial encounter
D subsequent encounter
S sequela

W32.0XX- Accidental handgun discharge

W32.1XX- Accidental handgun malfunction
Injury due to explosion of handgun (parts)
Injury due to malfunction of mechanism or component of handgun
Injury due to recoil of handgun
Powder burn from handgun

4 W33 Accidental rifle, shotgun and larger firearm discharge and malfunction

INCLUDES rifle, shotgun and larger firearm discharge and malfunction NOS

EXCLUDES 1 *accidental airgun discharge and malfunction (W34.010, W34.110)*
accidental BB gun discharge and malfunction (W34.010, W34.110)
accidental handgun discharge and malfunction (W32.-)
accidental pellet gun discharge and malfunction (W34.010, W34.110)
assault by rifle, shotgun and larger firearm discharge (X94)
firearm discharge involving legal intervention (Y35.0-)
firearm discharge involving military or war operations (Y36.4-)
intentional self-harm by rifle, shotgun and larger firearm discharge (X73)

The appropriate 7th character is to be added to each code from category W33
A initial encounter
D subsequent encounter
S sequela

5 W33.0 Accidental rifle, shotgun and larger firearm discharge

7 W33.00X- Accidental discharge of unspecified larger firearm
Discharge of unspecified larger firearm NOS

7 W33.01X- Accidental discharge of shotgun
Discharge of shotgun NOS

7 W33.02X- Accidental discharge of hunting rifle
Discharge of hunting rifle NOS

7 W33.03X- Accidental discharge of machine gun
Discharge of machine gun NOS

7 W33.09X- Accidental discharge of other larger firearm
Discharge of other larger firearm NOS

5 W33.1 Accidental rifle, shotgun and larger firearm malfunction
Injury due to explosion of rifle, shotgun and larger firearm (parts)
Injury due to malfunction of mechanism or component of rifle, shotgun and larger firearm
Injury due to piercing, cutting, crushing or pinching due to (by) slide trigger mechanism, scope or other gun part
Injury due to recoil of rifle, shotgun and larger firearm
Powder burn from rifle, shotgun and larger firearm

7 W33.10X- Accidental malfunction of unspecified larger firearm
Malfunction of unspecified larger firearm NOS

7 W33.11X- Accidental malfunction of shotgun
Malfunction of shotgun NOS

7 W33.12X- Accidental malfunction of hunting rifle
Malfunction of hunting rifle NOS

7 W33.13X- Accidental malfunction of machine gun
Malfunction of machine gun NOS

7 W33.19X- Accidental malfunction of other larger firearm
Malfunction of other larger firearm NOS

4 W34 Accidental discharge and malfunction from other and unspecified firearms and guns

The appropriate 7th character is to be added to each code from category W34
A initial encounter
D subsequent encounter
S sequela

5 W34.0 Accidental discharge from other and unspecified firearms and guns

7 W34.00X- Accidental discharge from unspecified firearms or gun
Discharge from firearm NOS
Gunshot wound NOS
Shot NOS
AHA: (W34.00XS) 1Q 2015, 17

6 W34.01 Accidental discharge of gas, air or spring-operated guns

7 W34.010- Accidental discharge of airgun
Accidental discharge of BB gun
Accidental discharge of pellet gun

7 W34.011- Accidental discharge of paintball gun
Accidental injury due to paintball discharge

7 W34.018- Accidental discharge of other gas, air or spring-operated gun

7 W34.09X- Accidental discharge from other specified firearms
Accidental discharge from Very pistol [flare]

5 W34.1 Accidental malfunction from other and unspecified firearms and guns

7 W34.10X- Accidental malfunction from unspecified firearms or gun
Firearm malfunction NOS

6 W34.11 Accidental malfunction of gas, air or spring-operated guns

7 W34.110- Accidental malfunction of airgun
Accidental malfunction of BB gun
Accidental malfunction of pellet gun

7 W34.111- Accidental malfunction of paintball gun
Accidental injury due to paintball gun malfunction

7 W34.118- Accidental malfunction of other gas, air or spring-operated gun

7 W34.19X- Accidental malfunction from other specified firearms
Accidental malfunction from Very pistol [flare]

7 W35.XXX- Explosion and rupture of boiler

EXCLUDES 1 *explosion and rupture of boiler on watercraft (V93.4)*

The appropriate 7th character is to be added to code W35
A initial encounter
D subsequent encounter
S sequela

4 W36 Explosion and rupture of gas cylinder

The appropriate 7th character is to be added to each code from category W36
A initial encounter
D subsequent encounter
S sequela

7 W36.1XX- Explosion and rupture of aerosol can
7 W36.2XX- Explosion and rupture of air tank
7 W36.3XX- Explosion and rupture of pressurized-gas tank
7 W36.8XX- Explosion and rupture of other gas cylinder
7 W36.9XX- Explosion and rupture of unspecified gas cylinder

4 W37 Explosion and rupture of pressurized tire, pipe or hose

The appropriate 7th character is to be added to each code from category W37
A initial encounter
D subsequent encounter
S sequela

7 W37.0XX- Explosion of bicycle tire
7 W37.8XX- Explosion and rupture of other pressurized tire, pipe or hose

7 W38.XXX- Explosion and rupture of other specified pressurized devices

The appropriate 7th character is to be added to code W38
A initial encounter
D subsequent encounter
S sequela

7 W39.XXX- Discharge of firework

The appropriate 7th character is to be added to code W39
A initial encounter
D subsequent encounter
S sequela

W40 Explosion of other materials

EXCLUDES 1 *assault by explosive material (X96)*
explosion involving legal intervention (Y35.1-)
explosion involving military or war operations (Y36.0-, Y36.2-)
intentional self-harm by explosive material (X75)

The appropriate 7th character is to be added to each code from category W40
A initial encounter
D subsequent encounter
S sequela

W40.0XX- Explosion of blasting material
Explosion of blasting cap
Explosion of detonator
Explosion of dynamite
Explosion of explosive (any) used in blasting operations

W40.1XX- Explosion of explosive gases
Explosion of acetylene
Explosion of butane
Explosion of coal gas
Explosion in mine NOS
Explosion of explosive gas
Explosion of fire damp
Explosion of gasoline fumes
Explosion of methane
Explosion of propane

W40.8XX- Explosion of other specified explosive materials
Explosion in dump NOS
Explosion in factory NOS
Explosion in grain store
Explosion in munitions
EXCLUDES 1 *explosion involving legal intervention (Y35.1-)*
explosion involving military or war operations (Y36.0-, Y36.2-)

W40.9XX- Explosion of unspecified explosive materials
Explosion NOS

W42 Exposure to noise

The appropriate 7th character is to be added to each code from category W42
A initial encounter
D subsequent encounter
S sequela

W42.0XX- Exposure to supersonic waves
W42.9XX- Exposure to other noise
Exposure to sound waves NOS

W45 Foreign body or object entering through skin

INCLUDES foreign body or object embedded in skin
nail embedded in skin
EXCLUDES 2 *contact with hand tools (nonpowered) (powered) (W27-W29)*
contact with other sharp object (s) (W26.-)
contact with sharp glass (W25.-)
struck by objects (W20-W22)

The appropriate 7th character is to be added to each code from category W45
A initial encounter
D subsequent encounter
S sequela

W45.0XX- Nail entering through skin
W45.8XX- Other foreign body or object entering through skin
Splinter in skin NOS

W46 Contact with hypodermic needle

The appropriate 7th character is to be added to each code from category W46
A initial encounter
D subsequent encounter
S sequela

W46.0XX- Contact with hypodermic needle
Hypodermic needle stick NOS
W46.1XX- Contact with contaminated hypodermic needle

W49 Exposure to other inanimate mechanical forces

INCLUDES exposure to abnormal gravitational [G] forces
exposure to inanimate mechanical forces NEC
EXCLUDES 1 *exposure to inanimate mechanical forces involving military or war operations (Y36.-, Y37.-)*

The appropriate 7th character is to be added to each code from category W49
A initial encounter
D subsequent encounter
S sequela

W49.0 Item causing external constriction
W49.01X- Hair causing external constriction
W49.02X- String or thread causing external constriction
W49.03X- Rubber band causing external constriction
W49.04X- Ring or other jewelry causing external constriction
W49.09X- Other specified item causing external constriction
W49.9XX- Exposure to other inanimate mechanical forces

Exposure to animate mechanical forces (W50-W64)

EXCLUDES 1 *Toxic effect of contact with venomous animals and plants (T63.-)*

W50 Accidental hit, strike, kick, twist, bite or scratch by another person

INCLUDES hit, strike, kick, twist, bite, or scratch by another person NOS
EXCLUDES 1 *assault by bodily force (Y04)*
struck by objects (W20-W22)

The appropriate 7th character is to be added to each code from category W50
A initial encounter
D subsequent encounter
S sequela

W50.0XX- Accidental hit or strike by another person
Hit or strike by another person NOS
W50.1XX- Accidental kick by another person
Kick by another person NOS
W50.2XX- Accidental twist by another person
Twist by another person NOS
AHA: (W50.2XXA) 1Q 2015, 8
AHA: (W50.2XXD) 1Q 2015, 8
W50.3XX- Accidental bite by another person
Human bite
Bite by another person NOS
W50.4XX- Accidental scratch by another person
Scratch by another person NOS

W51.XXX- Accidental striking against or bumped into by another person
EXCLUDES 1 *assault by striking against or bumping into by another person (Y04.2)*
fall due to collision with another person (W03)

The appropriate 7th character is to be added to code W51
A initial encounter
D subsequent encounter
S sequela

W52.XXX- Crushed, pushed or stepped on by crowd or human stampede
Crushed, pushed or stepped on by crowd or human stampede with or without fall

The appropriate 7th character is to be added to code W52
A initial encounter
D subsequent encounter
S sequela

W53 Contact with rodent

INCLUDES contact with saliva, feces or urine of rodent

The appropriate 7th character is to be added to each code from category W53
A initial encounter
D subsequent encounter
S sequela

W53.0 Contact with mouse
- W53.01X- Bitten by mouse
- W53.09X- Other contact with mouse

W53.1 Contact with rat
- W53.11X- Bitten by rat
- W53.19X- Other contact with rat

W53.2 Contact with squirrel
- W53.21X- Bitten by squirrel
- W53.29X- Other contact with squirrel

W53.8 Contact with other rodent
- W53.81X- Bitten by other rodent
- W53.89X- Other contact with Other rodent

W54 Contact with dog

INCLUDES contact with saliva, feces or urine of dog

The appropriate 7th character is to be added to each code from category W54
A initial encounter
D subsequent encounter
S sequela

- W54.0XX- Bitten by dog
- W54.1XX- Struck by dog
  Knocked over by dog
- W54.8XX- Other contact with dog

W55 Contact with other mammals

INCLUDES contact with saliva, feces or urine of mammal

EXCLUDES 1 *animal being ridden- see transport accidents*
bitten or struck by dog (W54)
bitten or struck by rodent (W53.-)
contact with marine mammals (W56.-)

The appropriate 7th character is to be added to each code from category W55
A initial encounter
D subsequent encounter
S sequela

W55.0 Contact with cat
- W55.01X- Bitten by cat
- W55.03X- Scratched by cat
- W55.09X- Other contact with cat

W55.1 Contact with horse
- W55.11X- Bitten by horse
- W55.12X- Struck by horse
- W55.19X- Other contact with horse

W55.2 Contact with cow
Contact with bull
- W55.21X- Bitten by cow
- W55.22X- Struck by cow
  Gored by bull
- W55.29X- Other contact with cow

W55.3 Contact with other hoof stock
Contact with goats
Contact with sheep
- W55.31X- Bitten by other hoof stock
- W55.32X- Struck by other hoof stock
  Gored by goat
  Gored by ram
- W55.39X- Other contact with Other hoof stock

W55.4 Contact with pig
- W55.41X- Bitten by pig
- W55.42X- Struck by pig
- W55.49X- Other contact with pig

W55.5 Contact with raccoon
- W55.51X- Bitten by raccoon
- W55.52X- Struck by raccoon
- W55.59X- Other contact with raccoon

W55.8 Contact with other mammals
- W55.81X- Bitten by other mammals
- W55.82X- Struck by other mammals
- W55.89X- Other contact with Other mammals

W56 Contact with nonvenomous marine animal

EXCLUDES 1 *contact with venomous marine animal (T63.-)*

The appropriate 7th character is to be added to each code from category W56
A initial encounter
D subsequent encounter
S sequela

W56.0 Contact with dolphin
- W56.01X- Bitten by dolphin
- W56.02X- Struck by dolphin
- W56.09X- Other contact with dolphin

W56.1 Contact with sea lion
- W56.11X- Bitten by sea lion
- W56.12X- Struck by sea lion
- W56.19X- Other contact with sea lion

W56.2 Contact with orca
Contact with killer whale
- W56.21X- Bitten by orca
- W56.22X- Struck by orca
- W56.29X- Other contact with orca

W56.3 Contact with other marine mammals
- W56.31X- Bitten by other marine mammals
- W56.32X- Struck by other marine mammals
- W56.39X- Other contact with Other marine mammals

W56.4 Contact with shark
- W56.41X- Bitten by shark
- W56.42X- Struck by shark
- W56.49X- Other contact with shark

W56.5 Contact with other fish
- W56.51X- Bitten by other fish
- W56.52X- Struck by other fish
- W56.59X- Other contact with Other fish

W56.8 Contact with other nonvenomous marine animals
- W56.81X- Bitten by other nonvenomous marine animals
- W56.82X- Struck by other nonvenomous marine animals
- W56.89X- Other contact with Other nonvenomous marine animals

W57.XXX- Bitten or stung by nonvenomous insect and other nonvenomous arthropods

EXCLUDES 1 *contact with venomous insects and arthropods (T63.2-, T63.3-, T63.4-)*

The appropriate 7th character is to be added to code W57
A initial encounter
D subsequent encounter
S sequela

W58 Contact with crocodile or alligator

The appropriate 7th character is to be added to each code from category W58
A initial encounter
D subsequent encounter
S sequela

W58.0 Contact with alligator
- W58.01X- Bitten by alligator
- W58.02X- Struck by alligator
- W58.03X- Crushed by alligator
- W58.09X- Other contact with alligator

W58.1 Contact with crocodile
- W58.11X- Bitten by crocodile
- W58.12X- Struck by crocodile
- W58.13X- Crushed by crocodile
- W58.19X- Other contact with crocodile

4 W59 Contact with other nonvenomous reptiles
EXCLUDES 1 *contact with venomous reptile (T63.0-, T63.1-)*

The appropriate 7th character is to be added to each code from category W59
A initial encounter
D subsequent encounter
S sequela

5 W59.0 Contact with nonvenomous lizards
7 W59.01X- Bitten by nonvenomous lizards
7 W59.02X- Struck by nonvenomous lizards
7 W59.09X- Other contact with nonvenomous lizards
Exposure to nonvenomous lizards
5 W59.1 Contact with nonvenomous snakes
7 W59.11X- Bitten by nonvenomous snake
7 W59.12X- Struck by nonvenomous snake
7 W59.13X- Crushed by nonvenomous snake
7 W59.19X- Other contact with nonvenomous snake
5 W59.2 Contact with turtles
EXCLUDES 1 *contact with tortoises (W59.8-)*
7 W59.21X- Bitten by turtle
7 W59.22X- Struck by turtle
7 W59.29X- Other contact with turtle
Exposure to turtles
5 W59.8 Contact with other nonvenomous reptiles
7 W59.81X- Bitten by other nonvenomous reptiles
7 W59.82X- Struck by other nonvenomous reptiles
7 W59.83X- Crushed by other nonvenomous reptiles
7 W59.89X- Other contact with Other nonvenomous reptiles

7 W60.XXX- Contact with nonvenomous plant thorns and spines and sharp leaves
EXCLUDES 1 *Contact with venomous plants (T63.7-)*

The appropriate 7th character is to be added to code W60
A initial encounter
D subsequent encounter
S sequela

4 W61 Contact with birds (domestic) (wild)
INCLUDES contact with excreta of birds

The appropriate 7th character is to be added to each code from category W61
A initial encounter
D subsequent encounter
S sequela

5 W61.0 Contact with parrot
7 W61.01X- Bitten by parrot
7 W61.02X- Struck by parrot
7 W61.09X- Other contact with parrot
Exposure to parrots
5 W61.1 Contact with macaw
7 W61.11X- Bitten by macaw
7 W61.12X- Struck by macaw
7 W61.19X- Other contact with macaw
Exposure to macaws
5 W61.2 Contact with other psittacines
7 W61.21X- Bitten by other psittacines
7 W61.22X- Struck by other psittacines
7 W61.29X- Other contact with Other psittacines
Exposure to other psittacines
5 W61.3 Contact with chicken
7 W61.32X- Struck by chicken
7 W61.33X- Pecked by chicken
7 W61.39X- Other contact with chicken
Exposure to chickens
5 W61.4 Contact with turkey
7 W61.42X- Struck by turkey
7 W61.43X- Pecked by turkey
7 W61.49X- Other contact with turkey
5 W61.5 Contact with goose
7 W61.51X- Bitten by goose
7 W61.52X- Struck by goose
7 W61.59X- Other contact with goose
5 W61.6 Contact with duck
7 W61.61X- Bitten by duck
7 W61.62X- Struck by duck
7 W61.69X- Other contact with duck
5 W61.9 Contact with other birds
7 W61.91X- Bitten by other birds
7 W61.92X- Struck by other birds
7 W61.99X- Other contact with Other birds
Contact with bird NOS

4 W62 Contact with nonvenomous amphibians
EXCLUDES 1 *contact with venomous amphibians (T63.81-R63.83)*

The appropriate 7th character is to be added to each code from category W62
A initial encounter
D subsequent encounter
S sequela

7 W62.0XX- Contact with nonvenomous frogs
7 W62.1XX- Contact with nonvenomous toads
7 W62.9XX- Contact with other nonvenomous amphibians

7 W64.XXX- Exposure to other animate mechanical forces
INCLUDES exposure to nonvenomous animal NOS
EXCLUDES 1 *contact with venomous animal (T63.-)*

The appropriate 7th character is to be added to code W64
A initial encounter
D subsequent encounter
S sequela

Accidental non-transport drowning and submersion (W65-W74)

EXCLUDES 1 *accidental drowning and submersion due to fall into water (W16.-)*
accidental drowning and submersion due to water transport accident (V90.-, V92.-)
EXCLUDES 2 *accidental drowning and submersion due to cataclysm (X34-X39)*

7 W65.XXX- Accidental drowning and submersion while in bath-tub
EXCLUDES 1 *accidental drowning and submersion due to fall in (into) bathtub (W16.211)*

The appropriate 7th character is to be added to code W65
A initial encounter
D subsequent encounter
S sequela

7 W67.XXX- Accidental drowning and submersion while in swimming-pool
EXCLUDES 1 *accidental drowning and submersion due to fall into swimming pool (W16.011, W16.021, W16.031)*
accidental drowning and submersion due to striking into wall of swimming pool (W22.041)

The appropriate 7th character is to be added to code W67
A initial encounter
D subsequent encounter
S sequela

7 W69.XXX- Accidental drowning and submersion while in natural water
Accidental drowning and submersion while in lake
Accidental drowning and submersion while in open sea
Accidental drowning and submersion while in river
Accidental drowning and submersion while in stream
EXCLUDES 1 *accidental drowning and submersion due to fall into natural body of water (W16.111, W16.121, W16.131)*

The appropriate 7th character is to be added to code W69
A initial encounter
D subsequent encounter
S sequela

W73.XXX- Other specified cause of accidental non-transport drowning and submersion
Accidental drowning and submersion while in quenching tank
Accidental drowning and submersion while in reservoir
EXCLUDES 1 *accidental drowning and submersion due to fall into other water (W16.311, W16.321, W16.331)*

The appropriate 7th character is to be added to code W73
A initial encounter
D subsequent encounter
S sequela

W74.XXX- Unspecified cause of accidental drowning and submersion
Drowning NOS

The appropriate 7th character is to be added to code W74
A initial encounter
D subsequent encounter
S sequela

Exposure to electric current, radiation and extreme ambient air temperature and pressure (W85-W99)

EXCLUDES 1 *exposure to:*
failure in dosage of radiation or temperature during surgical and medical care (Y63.2-Y63.5)
lightning (T75.0-)
natural cold (X31)
natural heat (X30)
natural radiation NOS (X39)
radiological procedure and radiotherapy (Y84.2)
sunlight (X32)

W85.XXX- Exposure to electric transmission lines
Broken power line

The appropriate 7th character is to be added to code W85
A initial encounter
D subsequent encounter
S sequela

W86 Exposure to other specified electric current

The appropriate 7th character is to be added to each code from category W86
A initial encounter
D subsequent encounter
S sequela

W86.0XX- Exposure to domestic wiring and appliances
W86.1XX- Exposure to industrial wiring, appliances and electrical machinery
Exposure to conductors
Exposure to control apparatus
Exposure to electrical equipment and machinery
Exposure to transformers
W86.8XX- Exposure to other electric current
Exposure to wiring and appliances in or on farm (not farmhouse)
Exposure to wiring and appliances outdoors
Exposure to wiring and appliances in or on public building
Exposure to wiring and appliances in or on residential institutions
Exposure to wiring and appliances in or on schools

W88 Exposure to ionizing radiation
EXCLUDES 1 *exposure to sunlight (X32)*

The appropriate 7th character is to be added to each code from category W88
A initial encounter
D subsequent encounter
S sequela

W88.0XX- Exposure to X-rays
W88.1XX- Exposure to radioactive isotopes
W88.8XX- Exposure to other ionizing radiation

W89 Exposure to man-made visible and ultraviolet light
INCLUDES exposure to welding light (arc)
EXCLUDES 1 *exposure to sunlight (X32)*

The appropriate 7th character is to be added to each code from category W89
A initial encounter
D subsequent encounter
S sequela

W89.0XX- Exposure to welding light (arc)
W89.1XX- Exposure to tanning bed
W89.8XX- Exposure to other man-made visible and ultraviolet light
W89.9XX- Exposure to unspecified man-made visible and ultraviolet light

W90 Exposure to other nonionizing radiation
EXCLUDES 1 *exposure to sunlight (X32)*

The appropriate 7th character is to be added to each code from category W90
A initial encounter
D subsequent encounter
S sequela

W90.0XX- Exposure to radiofrequency
W90.1XX- Exposure to infrared radiation
W90.2XX- Exposure to laser radiation
W90.8XX- Exposure to other nonionizing radiation

W92.XXX- Exposure to excessive heat of man-made origin

The appropriate 7th character is to be added to code W92
A initial encounter
D subsequent encounter
S sequela

W93 Exposure to excessive cold of man-made origin

The appropriate 7th character is to be added to each code from category W93
A initial encounter
D subsequent encounter
S sequela

W93.0 Contact with or inhalation of dry ice
W93.01X- Contact with dry ice
W93.02X- Inhalation of dry ice
W93.1 Contact with or inhalation of liquid air
W93.11X- Contact with liquid air
Contact with liquid hydrogen
Contact with liquid nitrogen
W93.12X- Inhalation of liquid air
Inhalation of liquid hydrogen
Inhalation of liquid nitrogen
W93.2XX- Prolonged exposure in deep freeze unit or refrigerator
W93.8XX- Exposure to other excessive cold of man-made origin

W94 Exposure to high and low air pressure and changes in air pressure

The appropriate 7th character is to be added to each code from category W94
A initial encounter
D subsequent encounter
S sequela

W94.0XX- Exposure to prolonged high air pressure
W94.1 Exposure to prolonged low air pressure
W94.11X- Exposure to residence or prolonged visit at high altitude
W94.12X- Exposure to other prolonged low air pressure
W94.2 Exposure to rapid changes in air pressure during ascent
W94.21X- Exposure to reduction in atmospheric pressure while surfacing from deep-water diving
W94.22X- Exposure to reduction in atmospheric pressure while surfacing from underground
W94.23X- Exposure to sudden change in air pressure in aircraft during ascent

W94.29X- **Exposure to other rapid changes in air pressure during ascent**

W94.3 **Exposure to rapid changes in air pressure during descent**

W94.31X- **Exposure to sudden change in air pressure in aircraft during descent**

W94.32X- **Exposure to high air pressure from rapid descent in water**

W94.39X- **Exposure to other rapid changes in air pressure during descent**

W99.XXX- **Exposure to other man-made environmental factors**

The appropriate 7th character is to be added to code W99
A initial encounter
D subsequent encounter
S sequela

Exposure to smoke, fire and flames (X00-X08)

EXCLUDES 1 *arson (X97)*

EXCLUDES 2 *explosions (W35-W40)*
lightning (T75.0-)
transport accident (V01-V99)

X00 **Exposure to uncontrolled fire in building or structure**

INCLUDES conflagration in building or structure

Code first:
any associated cataclysm

EXCLUDES 2 *Exposure to ignition or melting of nightwear (X05)*
Exposure to ignition or melting of other clothing and apparel (X06.-)
Exposure to other specified smoke, fire and flames (X08.-)

The appropriate 7th character is to be added to each code from category X00
A initial encounter
D subsequent encounter
S sequela

X00.0XX- **Exposure to flames in uncontrolled fire in building or structure**
AHA: (X00.0XXD) 2Q 2016, 6
AHA: (X00.0XXS) 2Q 2016, 5; 1Q 2015, 19

X00.1XX- **Exposure to smoke in uncontrolled fire in building or structure**

X00.2XX- **Injury due to collapse of burning building or structure in uncontrolled fire**
EXCLUDES 1 *injury due to collapse of building not on fire (W20.1)*

X00.3XX- **Fall from burning building or structure in uncontrolled fire**

X00.4XX- **Hit by object from burning building or structure in uncontrolled fire**

X00.5XX- **Jump from burning building or structure in uncontrolled fire**

X00.8XX- **Other exposure to uncontrolled fire in building or structure**

X01 **Exposure to uncontrolled fire, not in building or structure**

INCLUDES exposure to forest fire

The appropriate 7th character is to be added to each code from category X01
A initial encounter
D subsequent encounter
S sequela

X01.0XX- **Exposure to flames in uncontrolled fire, not in building or structure**

X01.1XX- **Exposure to smoke in uncontrolled fire, not in building or structure**

X01.3XX- **Fall due to uncontrolled fire, not in building or structure**

X01.4XX- **Hit by object due to uncontrolled fire, not in building or structure**

X01.8XX- **Other exposure to uncontrolled fire, not in building or structure**

X02 **Exposure to controlled fire in building or structure**

INCLUDES exposure to fire in fireplace
exposure to fire in stove

The appropriate 7th character is to be added to each code from category X02
A initial encounter
D subsequent encounter
S sequela

X02.0XX- **Exposure to flames in controlled fire in building or structure**

X02.1XX- **Exposure to smoke in controlled fire in building or structure**

X02.2XX- **Injury due to collapse of burning building or structure in controlled fire**
EXCLUDES 1 *injury due to collapse of building not on fire (W20.1)*

X02.3XX- **Fall from burning building or structure in controlled fire**

X02.4XX- **Hit by object from burning building or structure in controlled fire**

X02.5XX- **Jump from burning building or structure in controlled fire**

X02.8XX- **Other exposure to controlled fire in building or structure**

X03 **Exposure to controlled fire, not in building or structure**

INCLUDES exposure to bon fire
exposure to camp-fire
exposure to trash fire

The appropriate 7th character is to be added to each code from category X03
A initial encounter
D subsequent encounter
S sequela

X03.0XX- **Exposure to flames in controlled fire, not in building or structure**
AHA: (X03.0XXS) 1Q 2015, 19

X03.1XX- **Exposure to smoke in controlled fire, not in building or structure**

X03.3XX- **Fall due to controlled fire, not in building or structure**

X03.4XX- **Hit by object due to controlled fire, not in building or structure**

X03.8XX- **Other exposure to controlled fire, not in building or structure**

X04.XXX- **Exposure to ignition of highly flammable material**
Exposure to ignition of gasoline
Exposure to ignition of kerosene
Exposure to ignition of petrol

EXCLUDES 2 *exposure to ignition or melting of nightwear (X05)*
exposure to ignition or melting of other clothing and apparel (X06)

The appropriate 7th character is to be added to code X04
A initial encounter
D subsequent encounter
S sequela

AHA: (X04.xxxA) 2Q 2017, 30
AHA: (X04.XXA) 2Q 2016, 4

X05.XXX- **Exposure to ignition or melting of nightwear**

EXCLUDES 2 *exposure to uncontrolled fire in building or structure (X00.-)*
exposure to uncontrolled fire, not in building or structure (X01.-)
exposure to controlled fire in building or structure (X02.-)
exposure to controlled fire, not in building or structure (X03.-)
exposure to ignition of highly flammable materials (X04.-)

The appropriate 7th character is to be added to code X05
A initial encounter
D subsequent encounter
S sequela

4 X06 Exposure to ignition or melting of other clothing and apparel

EXCLUDES 2 *exposure to uncontrolled fire in building or structure (X00.-)*
exposure to uncontrolled fire, not in building or structure (X01.-)
exposure to controlled fire in building or structure (X02.-)
exposure to controlled fire, not in building or structure (X03.-)
exposure to ignition of highly flammable materials (X04.-)

The appropriate 7th character is to be added to each code from category X06
A initial encounter
D subsequent encounter
S sequela

7 X06.0XX- Exposure to ignition of plastic jewelry
7 X06.1XX- Exposure to melting of plastic jewelry
7 X06.2XX- Exposure to ignition of other clothing and apparel
7 X06.3XX- Exposure to melting of other clothing and apparel

4 X08 Exposure to other specified smoke, fire and flames

The appropriate 7th character is to be added to each code from category X08
A initial encounter
D subsequent encounter
S sequela

5 X08.0 Exposure to bed fire
Exposure to mattress fire

7 X08.00X- Exposure to bed fire due to unspecified burning material
7 X08.01X- Exposure to bed fire due to burning cigarette
AHA: (X08.01XS) 1Q 2015, 19
7 X08.09X- Exposure to bed fire due to other burning material

5 X08.1 Exposure to sofa fire
7 X08.10X- Exposure to sofa fire due to unspecified burning material
7 X08.11X- Exposure to sofa fire due to burning cigarette
7 X08.19X- Exposure to sofa fire due to other burning material

5 X08.2 Exposure to other furniture fire
7 X08.20X- Exposure to other furniture fire due to unspecified burning material
7 X08.21X- Exposure to other furniture fire due to burning cigarette
7 X08.29X- Exposure to other furniture fire due to other burning material

7 X08.8XX- Exposure to other specified smoke, fire and flames

Contact with heat and hot substances (X10-X19)

EXCLUDES 1 *exposure to excessive natural heat (X30)*
exposure to fire and flames (X00-X08)

4 X10 Contact with hot drinks, food, fats and cooking oils

The appropriate 7th character is to be added to each code from category X10
A initial encounter
D subsequent encounter
S sequela

7 X10.0XX- Contact with hot drinks
7 X10.1XX- Contact with hot food
7 X10.2XX- Contact with fats and cooking oils

4 X11 Contact with hot tap-water

INCLUDES contact with boiling tap-water
contact with boiling water NOS

EXCLUDES 1 *contact with water heated on stove (X12)*

The appropriate 7th character is to be added to each code from category X11
A initial encounter
D subsequent encounter
S sequela

7 X11.0XX- Contact with hot water in bath or tub
EXCLUDES 1 *contact with running hot water in bath or tub (X11.1)*
7 X11.1XX- Contact with running hot water
Contact with hot water running out of hose
Contact with hot water running out of tap
7 X11.8XX- Contact with other hot tap-water
Contact with hot water in bucket
Contact with hot tap-water NOS

7 X12.XXX- Contact with other hot fluids
Contact with water heated on stove
EXCLUDES 1 *hot (liquid) metals (X18)*

The appropriate 7th character is to be added to code X12
A initial encounter
D subsequent encounter
S sequela

4 X13 Contact with steam and other hot vapors

The appropriate 7th character is to be added to each code from category X13
A initial encounter
D subsequent encounter
S sequela

7 X13.0XX- Inhalation of steam and other hot vapors
7 X13.1XX- Other contact with steam and Other hot vapors

4 X14 Contact with hot air and other hot gases

The appropriate 7th character is to be added to each code from category X14
A initial encounter
D subsequent encounter
S sequela

7 X14.0XX- Inhalation of hot air and gases
7 X14.1XX- Other contact with hot air and Other hot gases

4 X15 Contact with hot household appliances

EXCLUDES 1 *contact with heating appliances (X16)*
contact with powered household appliances (W29.-)
exposure to controlled fire in building or structure due to household appliance (X02.8)
exposure to household appliances electrical current (W86.0)

The appropriate 7th character is to be added to each code from category X15
A initial encounter
D subsequent encounter
S sequela

7 X15.0XX- Contact with hot stove (kitchen)
7 X15.1XX- Contact with hot toaster
7 X15.2XX- Contact with hotplate
7 X15.3XX- Contact with hot saucepan or skillet
7 X15.8XX- Contact with other hot household appliances
Contact with cooker
Contact with kettle
Contact with light bulbs

X16.XXX- Contact with hot heating appliances, radiatorsand pipes

EXCLUDES 1 *contact with powered appliances (W29.-)*
exposure to controlled fire in building or structure due to appliance (X02.8)
exposure to industrial appliances electrical current (W86.1)

The appropriate 7th character is to be added to code X16
A initial encounter
D subsequent encounter
S sequela

X17.XXX- Contact with hot engines, machinery and tools

EXCLUDES 1 *contact with hot heating appliances, radiators and pipes (X16)*
contact with hot household appliances (X15)

The appropriate 7th character is to be added to code X17
A initial encounter
D subsequent encounter
S sequela

X18.XXX- Contact with other hot metals
Contact with liquid metal

The appropriate 7th character is to be added to code X18
A initial encounter
D subsequent encounter
S sequela

X19.XXX- Contact with other heat and hot substances

EXCLUDES 1 *objects that are not normally hot, e.g., an object made hot by a house fire (X00-X08)*

The appropriate 7th character is to be added to code X19
A initial encounter
D subsequent encounter
S sequela

Exposure to forces of nature (X30-X39)

X30.XXX- Exposure to excessive natural heat
Exposure to excessive heat as the cause of sunstroke
Exposure to heat NOS

EXCLUDES 1 *excessive heat of man-made origin (W92)*
exposure to man-made radiation (W89)
exposure to sunlight (X32)
exposure to tanning bed (W89)

The appropriate 7th character is to be added to code X30
A initial encounter
D subsequent encounter
S sequela

X31.XXX- Exposure to excessive natural cold
Excessive cold as the cause of chilblains NOS
Excessive cold as the cause of immersion foot or hand
Exposure to cold NOS
Exposure to weather conditions

EXCLUDES 1 *cold of man-made origin (W93.-)*
contact with or inhalation of dry ice (W93.-)
contact with or inhalation of liquefied gas (W93.-)

The appropriate 7th character is to be added to code X31
A initial encounter
D subsequent encounter
S sequela

X32.XXX- Exposure to sunlight

EXCLUDES 1 *man-made radiation (tanning bed) (W89)*

EXCLUDES 2 *radiation-related disorders of the skin and subcutaneous tissue (L55-L59)*

The appropriate 7th character is to be added to code X32
A initial encounter
D subsequent encounter
S sequela

X34.XXX- Earthquake

EXCLUDES 2 *tidal wave (tsunami) due to earthquake (X37.41)*

The appropriate 7th character is to be added to code X34
A initial encounter
D subsequent encounter
S sequela

X35.XXX- Volcanic eruption

EXCLUDES 2 *tidal wave (tsunami) due to volcanic eruption (X37.41)*

The appropriate 7th character is to be added to code X35
A initial encounter
D subsequent encounter
S sequela

X36 Avalanche, landslide and other earth movements

INCLUDES victim of mudslide of cataclysmic nature

EXCLUDES 1 *earthquake (X34)*

EXCLUDES 2 *transport accident involving collision with avalanche or landslide not in motion (V01-V99)*

The appropriate 7th character is to be added to each code from category X36
A initial encounter
D subsequent encounter
S sequela

X36.0XX- Collapse of dam or man-made structure causing earth movement

X36.1XX- Avalanche, landslide, or mudslide

X37 Cataclysmic storm

The appropriate 7th character is to be added to each code from category X37
A initial encounter
D subsequent encounter
S sequela

X37.0XX- Hurricane
Storm surge
Typhoon
AHA: 4Q 2017, 88

X37.1XX- Tornado
Cyclone
Twister

X37.2XX- Blizzard (snow)(ice)

X37.3XX- Dust storm

X37.4 Tidalwave

X37.41X- Tidal wave due to earthquake or volcanic eruption
Tidal wave NOS
Tsunami

X37.42X- Tidal wave due to storm

X37.43X- Tidal wave due to landslide

X37.8XX- Other cataclysmic storms
Cloudburst
Torrential rain

EXCLUDES 2 *flood (X38)*

▲ **X37.9XX- Unspecified cataclysmic storm**
Storm NOS

EXCLUDES 1 *collapse of dam or man-made structure causing earth movement (X36.0)*

▲ **X38.XXX- Flood**
Flood arising from remote storm
Flood of cataclysmic nature arising from melting snow
Flood resulting directly from storm

EXCLUDES 1 *collapse of dam or man-made structure causing earth movement (X36.0)*
tidal wave NOS (X37.41)
tidal wave caused by storm (X37.42)

The appropriate 7th character is to be added to code X38
A initial encounter
D subsequent encounter
S sequela

4 X39 Exposure to other forces of nature

The appropriate 7th character is to be added to each code from category X39
A initial encounter
D subsequent encounter
S sequela

▲ 5 **X39.0 Exposure to natural radiation**

EXCLUDES 1 *contact with and (suspected) exposure to radon and other naturally occurring radiation (Z77.123)*
exposure to man-made radiation (W88-W90)
exposure to sunlight (X32)

7 **X39.01X- Exposure to radon**

7 **X39.08X- Exposure to other natural radiation**

7 **X39.8XX- Other exposure to forces of nature**

Overexertion and strenuous or repetitive movements (X50)

4 X50 Overexertion and strenuous or repetitive movements

The appropriate 7th character is to be added to each code from category X50
A initial encounter
D subsequent encounter
S sequela

AHA: 4Q 2016, 73

7 **X50.0XX- Overexertion from strenuous movement or load**
Lifting heavy objects
Lifting weights

7 **X50.1XX- Overexertion from prolonged static or awkward postures**
Prolonged bending
Prolonged kneeling
Prolonged reaching
Prolonged sitting
Prolonged standing
Prolonged twisting
Static bending
Static kneeling
Static reaching
Static sitting
Static standing
Static twisting

7 **X50.3XX- Overexertion from repetitive movements**
Use of hand as hammer
EXCLUDES 2 *Overuse from prolonged static or awkward postures (X50.1)*

7 **X50.9XX- Other and unspecified overexertion or strenuous movements or postures**
Contact pressure
Contact stress

Accidental exposure to other specified factors (X52-X58)

7 **X52.XXX- Prolonged stay in weightless environment**
Weightlessness in spacecraft (simulator)

The appropriate 7th character is to be added to code X52
A initial encounter
D subsequent encounter
S sequela

7 **X58.XXX- Exposure to other specified factors**
Accident NOS
Exposure NOS

The appropriate 7th character is to be added to code X58
A initial encounter
D subsequent encounter
S sequela

Intentional self-harm (X71-X83)

Purposely self-inflicted injury
Suicide (attempted)

4 X71 Intentional self-harm by drowning and submersion

The appropriate 7th character is to be added to each code from category X71
A initial encounter
D subsequent encounter
S sequela

7 **X71.0XX- Intentional self-harm by drowning and submersion while in bathtub** HCC

7 **X71.1XX- Intentional self-harm by drowning and submersion while in swimming pool** HCC

7 **X71.2XX- Intentional self-harm by drowning and submersion after jump into swimming pool** HCC

7 **X71.3XX- Intentional self-harm by drowning and submersion in natural water** HCC

7 **X71.8XX- Other intentional self-harm by drowning and submersion** HCC

7 **X71.9XX- Intentional self-harm by drowning and submersion, unspecified** HCC

7 **X72.XXX- Intentional self-harm by handgun discharge** HCC
Intentional self-harm by gun for single hand use
Intentional self-harm by pistol
Intentional self-harm by revolver
EXCLUDES 1 *Very pistol (X74.8)*

The appropriate 7th character is to be added to code X72
A initial encounter
D subsequent encounter
S sequela

4 X73 Intentional self-harm by rifle, shotgun and larger firearm discharge
EXCLUDES 1 *airgun (X74.01)*

The appropriate 7th character is to be added to each code from category X73
A initial encounter
D subsequent encounter
S sequela

7 **X73.0XX- Intentional self-harm by shotgun discharge** HCC

7 **X73.1XX- Intentional self-harm by hunting rifle discharge** HCC

7 **X73.2XX- Intentional self-harm by machine gun discharge** HCC

7 **X73.8XX- Intentional self-harm by other larger firearm discharge** HCC

7 **X73.9XX- Intentional self-harm by unspecified larger firearm discharge** HCC

4 X74 Intentional self-harm by other and unspecified firearm and gun discharge

The appropriate 7th character is to be added to each code from category X74
A initial encounter
D subsequent encounter
S sequela

5 **X74.0 Intentional self-harm by gas, air or spring-operated guns**

7 **X74.01X- Intentional self-harm by airgun** HCC
Intentional self-harm by BB gun discharge
Intentional self-harm by pellet gun discharge

7 **X74.02X- Intentional self-harm by paintball gun** HCC

7 **X74.09X- Intentional self-harm by other gas, air or spring-operated gun** HCC

7 **X74.8XX- Intentional self-harm by other firearm discharge** HCC
Intentional self-harm by Very pistol [flare] discharge

7 **X74.9XX- Intentional self-harm by unspecified firearm discharge** HCC

7 **X75.XXX- Intentional self-harm by explosive material** HCC

The appropriate 7th character is to be added to code X75
A initial encounter
D subsequent encounter
S sequela

7 X76.XXX- Intentional self-harm by smoke, fire and flames HCC

The appropriate 7th character is to be added to code X76
A initial encounter
D subsequent encounter
S sequela

4 X77 Intentional self-harm by steam, hot vapors and hot objects

The appropriate 7th character is to be added to each code from category X77
A initial encounter
D subsequent encounter
S sequela

7 X77.0XX- Intentional self-harm by steam or hot vapors HCC
7 X77.1XX- Intentional self-harm by hot tap water HCC
7 X77.2XX- Intentional self-harm by other hot fluids HCC
7 X77.3XX- Intentional self-harm by hot household appliances HCC
7 X77.8XX- Intentional self-harm by other hot objects HCC
7 X77.9XX- Intentional self-harm by unspecified hot objects HCC

4 X78 Intentional self-harm by sharp object

The appropriate 7th character is to be added to each code from category X78
A initial encounter
D subsequent encounter
S sequela

7 X78.0XX- Intentional self-harm by sharp glass HCC
7 X78.1XX- Intentional self-harm by knife HCC
7 X78.2XX- Intentional self-harm by sword or dagger HCC
7 X78.8XX- Intentional self-harm by other sharp object HCC
7 X78.9XX- Intentional self-harm by unspecified sharp object HCC

7 X79.XXX- Intentional self-harm by blunt object HCC

The appropriate 7th character is to be added to code X79
A initial encounter
D subsequent encounter
S sequela

7 X80.XXX- Intentional self-harm by jumping from a high place HCC
Intentional fall from one level to another

The appropriate 7th character is to be added to code X80
A initial encounter
D subsequent encounter
S sequela

4 X81 Intentional self-harm by jumping or lying in front of moving object

The appropriate 7th character is to be added to each code from category X81
A initial encounter
D subsequent encounter
S sequela

7 X81.0XX- Intentional self-harm by jumping or lying in front of motor vehicle HCC
7 X81.1XX- Intentional self-harm by jumping or lying in front of (subway) train HCC
7 X81.8XX- Intentional self-harm by jumping or lying in front of other moving object HCC

4 X82 Intentional self-harm by crashing of motor vehicle

The appropriate 7th character is to be added to each code from category X82
A initial encounter
D subsequent encounter
S sequela

7 X82.0XX- Intentional collision of motor vehicle with other motor vehicle HCC
7 X82.1XX- Intentional collision of motor vehicle with train HCC
7 X82.2XX- Intentional collision of motor vehicle with tree HCC
7 X82.8XX- Other intentional self-harm by crashing of motor vehicle HCC

4 X83 Intentional self-harm by other specified means
EXCLUDES 1 *intentional self-harm by poisoning or contact with toxic substance- See Table of Drugs and Chemicals*

The appropriate 7th character is to be added to each code from category X83
A initial encounter
D subsequent encounter
S sequela

7 X83.0XX- Intentional self-harm by crashing of aircraft HCC
7 X83.1XX- Intentional self-harm by electrocution HCC
7 X83.2XX- Intentional self-harm by exposure to extremes of cold HCC
7 X83.8XX- Intentional self-harm by other specified means HCC

Assault (X92-Y09)

INCLUDES homicide
injuries inflicted by another person with intent to injure or kill, by any means

EXCLUDES 1 *injuries due to legal intervention (Y35.-)*
injuries due to operations of war (Y36.-)
injuries due to terrorism (Y38.-)

4 X92 Assault by drowning and submersion

The appropriate 7th character is to be added to each code from category X92
A initial encounter
D subsequent encounter
S sequela

7 X92.0XX- Assault by drowning and submersion while in bathtub
7 X92.1XX- Assault by drowning and submersion while in swimming pool
7 X92.2XX- Assault by drowning and submersion after push into swimming pool
7 X92.3XX- Assault by drowning and submersion in natural water
7 X92.8XX- Other assault by drowning and submersion
7 X92.9XX- Assault by drowning and submersion, unspecified

7 X93.XXX- Assault by handgun discharge
Assault by discharge of gun for single hand use
Assault by discharge of pistol
Assault by discharge of revolver
EXCLUDES 1 *Very pistol (X95.8)*

The appropriate 7th character is to be added to code X93
A initial encounter
D subsequent encounter
S sequela

4 X94 Assault by rifle, shotgun and larger firearm discharge
EXCLUDES 1 *airgun (X95.01)*

The appropriate 7th character is to be added to each code from category X94
A initial encounter
D subsequent encounter
S sequela

7 X94.0XX- Assault by shotgun
7 X94.1XX- Assault by hunting rifle
7 X94.2XX- Assault by machine gun
7 X94.8XX- Assault by other larger firearm discharge
7 X94.9XX- Assault by unspecified larger firearm discharge

4 X95 Assault by other and unspecified firearm and gun discharge

The appropriate 7th character is to be added to each code from category X95
A initial encounter
D subsequent encounter
S sequela

5 X95.0 Assault by gas, air or spring-operated guns

7 X95.01X- Assault by airgun discharge
Assault by BB gun discharge
Assault by pellet gun discharge

7 X95.02X- **Assault by paintball gun discharge**

7 X95.09X- **Assault by other gas, air or spring-operated gun**

7 X95.8XX- **Assault by other firearm discharge**
Assault by very pistol [flare] discharge

7 X95.9XX- **Assault by unspecified firearm discharge**
AHA: 3Q 2016, 23
AHA: 3Q 2016, 24

4 **X96 Assault by explosive material**
EXCLUDES 1 *incendiary device (X97)*
terrorism involving explosive material (Y38.2-)

The appropriate 7th character is to be added to each code from category X96
A initial encounter
D subsequent encounter
S sequela

7 X96.0XX- **Assault by antipersonnel bomb**
EXCLUDES 1 *antipersonnel bomb use in military or war (Y36.2-)*

7 X96.1XX- **Assault by gasoline bomb**

7 X96.2XX- **Assault by letter bomb**

7 X96.3XX- **Assault by fertilizer bomb**

7 X96.4XX- **Assault by pipe bomb**

7 X96.8XX- **Assault by other specified explosive**

7 X96.9XX- **Assault by unspecified explosive**

7 **X97.XXX- Assault by smoke, fire and flames**
Assault by arson
Assault by cigarettes
Assault by incendiary device

The appropriate 7th character is to be added to code X97
A initial encounter
D subsequent encounter
S sequela

4 **X98 Assault by steam, hot vapors and hot objects**

The appropriate 7th character is to be added to each code from category X98
A initial encounter
D subsequent encounter
S sequela

7 X98.0XX- **Assault by steam or hot vapors**

7 X98.1XX- **Assault by hot tap water**

7 X98.2XX- **Assault by hot fluids**

7 X98.3XX- **Assault by hot household appliances**

7 X98.8XX- **Assault by other hot objects**

7 X98.9XX- **Assault by unspecified hot objects**

4 **X99 Assault by sharp object**
EXCLUDES 1 *assault by strike by sports equipment (Y08.0-)*

The appropriate 7th character is to be added to each code from category X99
A initial encounter
D subsequent encounter
S sequela

7 X99.0XX- **Assault by sharp glass**

7 X99.1XX- **Assault by knife**

7 X99.2XX- **Assault by sword or dagger**

7 X99.8XX- **Assault by other sharp object**

7 X99.9XX- **Assault by unspecified sharp object**
Assault by stabbing NOS

7 **Y00.XXX- Assault by blunt object**
EXCLUDES 1 *assault by strike by sports equipment (Y08.0-)*

The appropriate 7th character is to be added to code Y00
A initial encounter
D subsequent encounter
S sequela

7 **Y01.XXX- Assault by pushing from high place**

The appropriate 7th character is to be added to code Y01
A initial encounter
D subsequent encounter
S sequela

4 **Y02 Assault by pushing or placing victim in front of moving object**

The appropriate 7th character is to be added to each code from category Y02
A initial encounter
D subsequent encounter
S sequela

7 Y02.0XX- **Assault by pushing or placing victim in front of motor vehicle**

7 Y02.1XX- **Assault by pushing or placing victim in front of (subway) train**

7 Y02.8XX- **Assault by pushing or placing victim in front of other moving object**

4 **Y03 Assault by crashing of motor vehicle**

The appropriate 7th character is to be added to each code from category Y03
A initial encounter
D subsequent encounter
S sequela

7 Y03.0XX- **Assault by being hit or run over by motor vehicle**

7 Y03.8XX- **Other assault by crashing of motor vehicle**

4 **Y04 Assault by bodily force**
EXCLUDES 1 *assault by:*
submersion (X92.-)
use of weapon (X93-X95, X99, Y00)

The appropriate 7th character is to be added to each code from category Y04
A initial encounter
D subsequent encounter
S sequela

7 Y04.0XX- **Assault by unarmed brawl or fight**

7 Y04.1XX- **Assault by human bite**

7 Y04.2XX- **Assault by strike against or bumped into by another person**

7 Y04.8XX- **Assault by other bodily force**
Assault by bodily force NOS

4 **Y07 Perpetrator of assault, maltreatment and neglect**
Note: Codes from this category are for use only in cases of confirmed abuse (T74.-)
Selection of the correct perpetrator code is based on the relationship between the perpetrator and the victim
INCLUDES perpetrator of abandonment
perpetrator of emotional neglect
perpetrator of mental cruelty
perpetrator of physical abuse
perpetrator of physical neglect
perpetrator of sexual abuse
perpetrator of torture

5 Y07.0 **Spouse or partner, perpetrator of maltreatment and neglect**
Spouse or partner, perpetrator of maltreatment and neglect against spouse or partner

Y07.01 **Husband, perpetrator of maltreatment and neglect**

Y07.02 **Wife, perpetrator of maltreatment and neglect**

Y07.03 **Male partner, perpetrator of maltreatment and neglect**

Y07.04 **Female partner, perpetrator of maltreatment and neglect**

5 Y07.1 **Parent (adoptive) (biological), perpetrator of maltreatment and neglect**

Y07.11 **Biological father, perpetrator of maltreatment and neglect**

Y07.12 **Biological mother, perpetrator of maltreatment and neglect**

Y07.13 **Adoptive father, perpetrator of maltreatment and neglect**

Y07.14 **Adoptive mother, perpetrator of maltreatment and neglect**

5 Y07.4 **Other family member, perpetrator of maltreatment and neglect**

6 Y07.41 **Sibling, perpetrator of maltreatment and neglect**
EXCLUDES 1 *stepsibling, perpetrator of maltreatment and neglect (Y07.435, Y07.436)*

Y07.410 Brother, perpetrator of maltreatment and neglect

Y07.411 Sister, perpetrator of maltreatment and neglect

6 Y07.42 Foster parent, perpetrator of maltreatment and neglect

Y07.420 Foster father, perpetrator of maltreatment and neglect

Y07.421 Foster mother, perpetrator of maltreatment and neglect

6 Y07.43 Stepparent or stepsibling, perpetrator of maltreatment and neglect

Y07.430 Stepfather, perpetrator of maltreatment and neglect

Y07.432 Male friend of parent (co-residing in household), perpetrator of maltreatment and neglect

Y07.433 Stepmother, perpetrator of maltreatment and neglect

Y07.434 Female friend of parent (co-residing in household), perpetrator of maltreatment and neglect

Y07.435 Stepbrother, perpetrator or maltreatment and neglect

Y07.436 Stepsister, perpetrator of maltreatment and neglect

6 Y07.49 Other family member, perpetrator of maltreatment and neglect

Y07.490 Male cousin, perpetrator of maltreatment and neglect

Y07.491 Female cousin, perpetrator of maltreatment and neglect

Y07.499 Other family member, perpetrator of maltreatment and neglect

5 Y07.5 Non-family member, perpetrator of maltreatment and neglect

Y07.50 Unspecified non-family member, perpetrator of maltreatment and neglect

6 Y07.51 Daycare provider, perpetrator of maltreatment and neglect

Y07.510 At-home childcare provider, perpetrator of maltreatment and neglect

Y07.511 Daycare center childcare provider, perpetrator of maltreatment and neglect

Y07.512 At-home adultcare provider, perpetrator of maltreatment and neglect

Y07.513 Adultcare center provider, perpetrator of maltreatment and neglect

Y07.519 Unspecified daycare provider, perpetrator of maltreatment and neglect

6 Y07.52 Healthcare provider, perpetrator of maltreatment and neglect

Y07.521 Mental health provider, perpetrator of maltreatment and neglect

Y07.528 Other therapist or healthcare provider, perpetrator of maltreatment and neglect

Nurse perpetrator of maltreatment and neglect
Occupational therapist perpetrator of maltreatment and neglect
Physical therapist perpetrator of maltreatment and neglect
Speech therapist perpetrator of maltreatment and neglect

Y07.529 Unspecified healthcare provider, perpetrator of maltreatment and neglect

Y07.53 Teacher or instructor, perpetrator of maltreatment and neglect

Coach, perpetrator of maltreatment and neglect

Y07.59 Other non-family member, perpetrator of maltreatment and neglect

● **Y07.6 Multiple perpetrators of maltreatment and neglect**

Y07.9 Unspecified perpetrator of maltreatment and neglect

4 Y08 Assault by other specified means

The appropriate 7th character is to be added to each code from category Y08
A initial encounter
D subsequent encounter
S sequela

5 Y08.0 Assault by strike by sport equipment

7 Y08.01X- Assault by strike by hockey stick

7 Y08.02X- Assault by strike by baseball bat

7 Y08.09X- Assault by strike by other specified type of sport equipment

5 Y08.8 Assault by other specified means

7 Y08.81X- Assault by crashing of aircraft

7 Y08.89X- Assault by other specified means

Y09 Assault by unspecified means

Assassination (attempted) NOS
Homicide (attempted) NOS
Manslaughter (attempted) NOS
Murder (attempted) NOS

Event of undetermined intent (Y21-Y33)

Undetermined intent is only for use when there is specific documentation in the record that the intent of the injury cannot be determined. If no such documentation is present, code to accidental (unintentional)

4 Y21 Drowning and submersion, undetermined intent

The appropriate 7th character is to be added to each code from category Y21
A initial encounter
D subsequent encounter
S sequela

7 Y21.0XX- Drowning and submersion while in bathtub, undetermined intent

7 Y21.1XX- Drowning and submersion after fall into bathtub, undetermined intent

7 Y21.2XX- Drowning and submersion while in swimming pool, undetermined intent

7 Y21.3XX- Drowning and submersion after fall into swimming pool, undetermined intent

7 Y21.4XX- Drowning and submersion in natural water, undetermined intent

7 Y21.8XX- Other drowning and submersion, undetermined intent

7 Y21.9XX- Unspecified drowning and submersion, undetermined intent

7 Y22.XXX- Handgun discharge, undetermined intent

Discharge of gun for single hand use, undetermined intent
Discharge of pistol, undetermined intent
Discharge of revolver, undetermined intent

EXCLUDES 2 *very pistol (Y24.8)*

The appropriate 7th character is to be added to code Y22
A initial encounter
D subsequent encounter
S sequela

4 Y23 Rifle, shotgun and larger firearm discharge, undetermined intent

EXCLUDES 2 *airgun (Y24.0)*

The appropriate 7th character is to be added to each code from category Y23
A initial encounter
D subsequent encounter
S sequela

7 Y23.0XX- Shotgun discharge, undetermined intent

7 Y23.1XX- Hunting rifle discharge, undetermined intent

7 Y23.2XX- Military firearm discharge, undetermined intent

7 Y23.3XX- Machine gun discharge, undetermined intent

7 Y23.8XX- Other larger firearm discharge, undetermined intent

7 Y23.9XX- Unspecified larger firearm discharge, undetermined intent

4 Y24 Other and unspecified firearm discharge, undetermined intent

The appropriate 7th character is to be added to each code from category Y24
A initial encounter
D subsequent encounter
S sequela

Y24.0XX- **Airgun discharge, undetermined intent**
BB gun discharge, undetermined intent
Pellet gun discharge, undetermined intent

Y24.8XX- **Other firearm discharge, undetermined intent**
Paintball gun discharge, undetermined intent
Very pistol [flare] discharge, undetermined intent

Y24.9XX- **Unspecified firearm discharge, undetermined intent**

Y25.XXX- **Contact with explosive material, undetermined intent**

The appropriate 7th character is to be added to code Y25
A initial encounter
D subsequent encounter
S sequela

Y26.XXX- **Exposure to smoke, fire and flames, undetermined intent**

The appropriate 7th character is to be added to code Y26
A initial encounter
D subsequent encounter
S sequela

Y27 **Contact with steam, hot vapors and hot objects, undetermined intent**

The appropriate 7th character is to be added to each code from category Y27
A initial encounter
D subsequent encounter
S sequela

Y27.0XX- **Contact with steam and hot vapors, undetermined intent**

Y27.1XX- **Contact with hot tap water, undetermined intent**

Y27.2XX- **Contact with hot fluids, undetermined intent**

Y27.3XX- **Contact with hot household appliance, undetermined intent**

Y27.8XX- **Contact with other hot objects, undetermined intent**

Y27.9XX- **Contact with unspecified hot objects, undetermined intent**

Y28 **Contact with sharp object, undetermined intent**

The appropriate 7th character is to be added to each code from category Y28
A initial encounter
D subsequent encounter
S sequela

Y28.0XX- **Contact with sharp glass, undetermined intent**

Y28.1XX- **Contact with knife, undetermined intent**

Y28.2XX- **Contact with sword or dagger, undetermined intent**

Y28.8XX- **Contact with other sharp object, undetermined intent**

Y28.9XX- **Contact with unspecified sharp object, undetermined intent**

Y29.XXX- **Contact with blunt object, undetermined intent**

The appropriate 7th character is to be added to code Y29
A initial encounter
D subsequent encounter
S sequela

Y30.XXX- **Falling, jumping or pushed from a high place, undetermined intent**
Victim falling from one level to another, undetermined intent

The appropriate 7th character is to be added to code Y30
A initial encounter
D subsequent encounter
S sequela

Y31.XXX- **Falling, lying or running before or into moving object, undetermined intent**

The appropriate 7th character is to be added to code Y31
A initial encounter
D subsequent encounter
S sequela

Y32.XXX- **Crashing of motor vehicle, undetermined intent**

The appropriate 7th character is to be added to code Y32
A initial encounter
D subsequent encounter
S sequela

Y33.XXX- **Other specified events, undetermined intent**

The appropriate 7th character is to be added to code Y33
A initial encounter
D subsequent encounter
S sequela

Legal intervention, operations of war, military operations, and terrorism (Y35-Y38)

Y35 **Legal intervention**

INCLUDES any injury sustained as a result of an encounter with any law enforcement official, serving in any capacity at the time of the encounter, whether on-duty or off-duty. Includes: injury to law enforcement official, suspect and bystander

The appropriate 7th character is to be added to each code from category Y35
A initial encounter
D subsequent encounter
S sequela

Y35.0 **Legal intervention involving firearm discharge**

Y35.00 **Legal intervention involving unspecified firearm discharge**
Legal intervention involving gunshot wound
Legal intervention involving shot NOS

Y35.001- **Legal intervention involving unspecified firearm discharge, law enforcement official injured**

Y35.002- **Legal intervention involving unspecified firearm discharge, bystander injured**

Y35.003- **Legal intervention involving unspecified firearm discharge, suspect injured**

Y35.01 **Legal intervention involving injury by machine gun**

Y35.011- **Legal intervention involving injury by machine gun, law enforcement official injured**

Y35.012- **Legal intervention involving injury by machine gun, bystander injured**

Y35.013- **Legal intervention involving injury by machine gun, suspect injured**

Y35.02 **Legal intervention involving injury by handgun**

Y35.021- **Legal intervention involving injury by handgun, law enforcement official injured**

Y35.022- **Legal intervention involving injury by handgun, bystander injured**

Y35.023- **Legal intervention involving injury by handgun, suspect injured**

Y35.03 **Legal intervention involving injury by rifle pellet**

Y35.031- **Legal intervention involving injury by rifle pellet, law enforcement official injured**

Y35.032- **Legal intervention involving injury by rifle pellet, bystander injured**

Y35.033- **Legal intervention involving injury by rifle pellet, suspect injured**

Y35.04 **Legal intervention involving injury by rubber bullet**

Y35.041- **Legal intervention involving injury by rubber bullet, law enforcement official injured**

Y35.042- **Legal intervention involving injury by rubber bullet, bystander injured**

Y35.043- **Legal intervention involving injury by rubber bullet, suspect injured**

Y35.09 **Legal intervention involving other firearm discharge**

Y35.091- **Legal intervention involving other firearm discharge, law enforcement official injured**

Y35.092- **Legal intervention involving other firearm discharge, bystander injured**

Y35.093- **Legal intervention involving other firearm discharge, suspect injured**

Y35.1 **Legal intervention involving explosives**

6 Y35.10 **Legal intervention involving unspecified explosives**
- 7 Y35.101- **Legal intervention involving unspecified explosives, law enforcement official injured**
- 7 Y35.102- **Legal intervention involving unspecified explosives, bystander injured**
- 7 Y35.103- **Legal intervention involving unspecified explosives, suspect injured**

6 Y35.11 **Legal intervention involving injury by dynamite**
- 7 Y35.111- **Legal intervention involving injury by dynamite, law enforcement official injured**
- 7 Y35.112- **Legal intervention involving injury by dynamite, bystander injured**
- 7 Y35.113- **Legal intervention involving injury by dynamite, suspect injured**

6 Y35.12 **Legal intervention involving injury by explosive shell**
- 7 Y35.121- **Legal intervention involving injury by explosive shell, law enforcement official injured**
- 7 Y35.122- **Legal intervention involving injury by explosive shell, bystander injured**
- 7 Y35.123- **Legal intervention involving injury by explosive shell, suspect injured**

6 Y35.19 **Legal intervention involving other explosives**
Legal intervention involving injury by grenade
Legal intervention involving injury by mortar bomb
- 7 Y35.191- **Legal intervention involving other explosives, law enforcement official injured**
- 7 Y35.192- **Legal intervention involving other explosives, bystander injured**
- 7 Y35.193- **Legal intervention involving other explosives, suspect injured**

5 Y35.2 **Legal intervention involving gas**
Legal intervention involving asphyxiation by gas
Legal intervention involving poisoning by gas

6 Y35.20 **Legal intervention involving unspecified gas**
- 7 Y35.201- **Legal intervention involving unspecified gas, law enforcement official injured**
- 7 Y35.202- **Legal intervention involving unspecified gas, bystander injured**
- 7 Y35.203- **Legal intervention involving unspecified gas, suspect injured**

6 Y35.21 **Legal intervention involving injury by tear gas**
- 7 Y35.211- **Legal intervention involving injury by tear gas, law enforcement official injured**
- 7 Y35.212- **Legal intervention involving injury by tear gas, bystander injured**
- 7 Y35.213- **Legal intervention involving injury by tear gas, suspect injured**

6 Y35.29 **Legal intervention involving other gas**
- 7 Y35.291- **Legal intervention involving other gas, law enforcement official injured**
- 7 Y35.292- **Legal intervention involving other gas, bystander injured**
- 7 Y35.293- **Legal intervention involving other gas, suspect injured**

5 Y35.3 **Legal intervention involving blunt objects**
Legal intervention involving being hit or struck by blunt object

6 Y35.30 **Legal intervention involving unspecified blunt objects**
- 7 Y35.301- **Legal intervention involving unspecified blunt objects, law enforcement official injured**
- 7 Y35.302- **Legal intervention involving unspecified blunt objects, bystander injured**
- 7 Y35.303- **Legal intervention involving unspecified blunt objects, suspect injured**

6 Y35.31 **Legal intervention involving baton**
- 7 Y35.311- **Legal intervention involving baton, law enforcement official injured**
- 7 Y35.312- **Legal intervention involving baton, bystander injured**
- 7 Y35.313- **Legal intervention involving baton, suspect injured**

6 Y35.39 **Legal intervention involving other blunt objects**
- 7 Y35.391- **Legal intervention involving other blunt objects, law enforcement official injured**
- 7 Y35.392- **Legal intervention involving other blunt objects, bystander injured**
- 7 Y35.393- **Legal intervention involving other blunt objects, suspect injured**

5 Y35.4 **Legal intervention involving sharp objects**
Legal intervention involving being cut by sharp objects
Legal intervention involving being stabbed by sharp objects

6 Y35.40 **Legal intervention involving unspecified sharp objects**
- 7 Y35.401- **Legal intervention involving unspecified sharp objects, law enforcement official injured**
- 7 Y35.402- **Legal intervention involving unspecified sharp objects, bystander injured**
- 7 Y35.403- **Legal intervention involving unspecified sharp objects, suspect injured**

6 Y35.41 **Legal intervention involving bayonet**
- 7 Y35.411- **Legal intervention involving bayonet, law enforcement official injured**
- 7 Y35.412- **Legal intervention involving bayonet, bystander injured**
- 7 Y35.413- **Legal intervention involving bayonet, suspect injured**

6 Y35.49 **Legal intervention involving other sharp objects**
- 7 Y35.491- **Legal intervention involving other sharp objects, law enforcement official injured**
- 7 Y35.492- **Legal intervention involving other sharp objects, bystander injured**
- 7 Y35.493- **Legal intervention involving other sharp objects, suspect injured**

5 Y35.8 **Legal intervention involving other specified means**

6 Y35.81 **Legal intervention involving manhandling**
- 7 Y35.811- **Legal intervention involving manhandling, law enforcement official injured**
- 7 Y35.812- **Legal intervention involving manhandling, bystander injured**
- 7 Y35.813- **Legal intervention involving manhandling, suspect injured**

6 Y35.89 **Legal intervention involving other specified means**
- 7 Y35.891- **Legal intervention involving other specified means, law enforcement official injured**
- 7 Y35.892- **Legal intervention involving other specified means, bystander injured**
- 7 Y35.893- **Legal intervention involving other specified means, suspect injured**

5 Y35.9 **Legal intervention, means unspecified**
- 7 Y35.91X- **Legal intervention, means unspecified, law enforcement official injured**
- 7 Y35.92X- **Legal intervention, means unspecified, bystander injured**
- 7 Y35.93X- **Legal intervention, means unspecified, suspect injured**

4 Y36 Operations of war

INCLUDES injuries to military personnel and civilians caused by war, civil insurrection, and peacekeeping missions

EXCLUDES 1 *injury to military personnel occurring during peacetime military operations (Y37.-)*
military vehicles involved in transport accidents with non-military vehicle during peacetime (V09.01, V09.21, V19.81, V29.81, V39.81, V49.81, V59.81, V69.81, V79.81)

The appropriate 7th character is to be added to each code from category Y36
- A initial encounter
- D subsequent encounter
- S sequela

AHA: 3Q 2014, 5

5 Y36.0 **War operations involving explosion of marine weapons**

6 Y36.00 **War operations involving explosion of unspecified marine weapon**
War operations involving underwater blast NOS
- 7 Y36.000- **War operations involving explosion of unspecified marine weapon, military personnel**
- 7 Y36.001- **War operations involving explosion of unspecified marine weapon, civilian**

6 Y36.01 **War operations involving explosion of depth-charge**

7 Y36.010- **War operations involving explosion of depth-charge, military personnel**

7 Y36.011- **War operations involving explosion of depth-charge, civilian**

6 Y36.02 **War operations involving explosion of marine mine**

War operations involving explosion of marine mine, at sea or in harbor

7 Y36.020- **War operations involving explosion of marine mine, military personnel**

7 Y36.021- **War operations involving explosion of marine mine, civilian**

6 Y36.03 **War operations involving explosion of sea-based artillery shell**

7 Y36.030- **War operations involving explosion of sea-based artillery shell, military personnel**

7 Y36.031- **War operations involving explosion of sea-based artillery shell, civilian**

6 Y36.04 **War operations involving explosion of torpedo**

7 Y36.040- **War operations involving explosion of torpedo, military personnel**

7 Y36.041- **War operations involving explosion of torpedo, civilian**

6 Y36.05 **War operations involving accidental detonation of onboard marine weapons**

7 Y36.050- **War operations involving accidental detonation of onboard marine weapons, military personnel**

7 Y36.051- **War operations involving accidental detonation of onboard marine weapons, civilian**

6 Y36.09 **War operations involving explosion of other marine weapons**

7 Y36.090- **War operations involving explosion of other marine weapons, military personnel**

7 Y36.091- **War operations involving explosion of other marine weapons, civilian**

5 Y36.1 **War operations involving destruction of aircraft**

6 Y36.10 **War operations involving unspecified destruction of aircraft**

7 Y36.100- **War operations involving unspecified destruction of aircraft, military personnel**

7 Y36.101- **War operations involving unspecified destruction of aircraft, civilian**

6 Y36.11 **War operations involving destruction of aircraft due to enemy fire or explosives**

War operations involving destruction of aircraft due to air to air missile

War operations involving destruction of aircraft due to explosive placed on aircraft

War operations involving destruction of aircraft due to rocket propelled grenade [RPG]

War operations involving destruction of aircraft due to small arms fire

War operations involving destruction of aircraft due to surface to air missile

7 Y36.110- **War operations involving destruction of aircraft due to enemy fire or explosives, military personnel**

7 Y36.111- **War operations involving destruction of aircraft due to enemy fire or explosives, civilian**

6 Y36.12 **War operations involving destruction of aircraft due to collision with other aircraft**

7 Y36.120- **War operations involving destruction of aircraft due to collision with other aircraft, military personnel**

7 Y36.121- **War operations involving destruction of aircraft due to collision with other aircraft, civilian**

6 Y36.13 **War operations involving destruction of aircraft due to onboard fire**

7 Y36.130- **War operations involving destruction of aircraft due to onboard fire, military personnel**

7 Y36.131- **War operations involving destruction of aircraft due to onboard fire, civilian**

6 Y36.14 **War operations involving destruction of aircraft due to accidental detonation of onboard munitions and explosives**

7 Y36.140- **War operations involving destruction of aircraft due to accidental detonation of onboard munitions and explosives, military personnel**

7 Y36.141- **War operations involving destruction of aircraft due to accidental detonation of onboard munitions and explosives, civilian**

6 Y36.19 **War operations involving other destruction of aircraft**

7 Y36.190- **War operations involving other destruction of aircraft, military personnel**

7 Y36.191- **War operations involving other destruction of aircraft, civilian**

5 Y36.2 **War operations involving other explosions and fragments**

EXCLUDES 1 *war operations involving explosion of aircraft (Y36.1-)*
war operations involving explosion of marine weapons (Y36.0-)
war operations involving explosion of nuclear weapons (Y36.5-)
war operations involving explosion occurring after cessation of hostilities (Y36.8-)

6 Y36.20 **War operations involving unspecified explosion and fragments**

War operations involving air blast NOS
War operations involving blast NOS
War operations involving blast fragments NOS
War operations involving blast wave NOS
War operations involving blast wind NOS
War operations involving explosion NOS
War operations involving explosion of bomb NOS

7 Y36.200- **War operations involving unspecified explosion and fragments, military personnel**

7 Y36.201- **War operations involving unspecified explosion and fragments, civilian**

6 Y36.21 **War operations involving explosion of aerial bomb**

7 Y36.210- **War operations involving explosion of aerial bomb, military personnel**

7 Y36.211- **War operations involving explosion of aerial bomb, civilian**

6 Y36.22 **War operations involving explosion of guided missile**

7 Y36.220- **War operations involving explosion of guided missile, military personnel**

7 Y36.221- **War operations involving explosion of guided missile, civilian**

6 Y36.23 **War operations involving explosion of improvised explosive device [IED]**

War operations involving explosion of person-borne improvised explosive device [IED]

War operations involving explosion of vehicle-borne improvised explosive device [IED]

War operations involving explosion of roadside improvised explosive device [IED]

7 Y36.230- **War operations involving explosion of improvised explosive device [IED], military personnel**

7 Y36.231- **War operations involving explosion of improvised explosive device [IED], civilian**

6 Y36.24 **War operations involving explosion due to accidental detonation and discharge of own munitions or munitions launch device**

7 Y36.240- **War operations involving explosion due to accidental detonation and discharge of own munitions or munitions launch device, military personnel**

7 Y36.241- **War operations involving explosion due to accidental detonation and discharge of own munitions or munitions launch device, civilian**

6 Y36.25 **War operations involving fragments from munitions**

7 Y36.250- **War operations involving fragments from munitions, military personnel**

7 Y36.251- **War operations involving fragments from munitions, civilian**

6 Y36.26 **War operations involving fragments of improvisedexplosive device [IED]**
War operations involving fragments of person-borne improvised explosive device [IED]
War operations involving fragments of vehicle-borne improvised explosive device [IED]
War operations involving fragments of roadside improvised explosive device [IED]

7 Y36.260- **War operations involving fragments of improvised explosive device [IED], military personnel**

7 Y36.261- **War operations involving fragments of improvised explosive device [IED], civilian**

6 Y36.27 **War operations involving fragments from weapons**

7 Y36.270- **War operations involving fragments from weapons, military personnel**

7 Y36.271- **War operations involving fragments from weapons, civilian**

6 Y36.29 **War operations involving other explosions and fragments**
War operations involving explosion of grenade
War operations involving explosions of land mine
War operations involving shrapnel NOS

7 Y36.290- **War operations involving other explosions and fragments, military personnel**

7 Y36.291- **War operations involving other explosions and fragments, civilian**

5 Y36.3 **War operations involving fires, conflagrations and hot substances**
War operations involving smoke, fumes, and heat from fires, conflagrations and hot substances
EXCLUDES 1 *war operations involving fires and conflagrations aboard military aircraft (Y36.1-)*
war operations involving fires and conflagrations aboard military watercraft (Y36.0-)
war operations involving fires and conflagrations caused indirectly by conventional weapons (Y36.2-)
war operations involving fires and thermal effects of nuclear weapons (Y36.53-)

6 Y36.30 **War operations involving unspecified fire, conflagration and hot substance**

7 Y36.300- **War operations involving unspecified fire, conflagration and hot substance, military personnel**

7 Y36.301- **War operations involving unspecified fire, conflagration and hot substance, civilian**

6 Y36.31 **War operations involving gasoline bomb**
War operations involving incendiary bomb
War operations involving petrol bomb

7 Y36.310- **War operations involving gasoline bomb, military personnel**

7 Y36.311- **War operations involving gasoline bomb, civilian**

6 Y36.32 **War operations involving incendiary bullet**

7 Y36.320- **War operations involving incendiary bullet, military personnel**

7 Y36.321- **War operations involving incendiary bullet, civilian**

6 Y36.33 **War operations involving flamethrower**

7 Y36.330- **War operations involving flamethrower, military personnel**

7 Y36.331- **War operations involving flamethrower, civilian**

6 Y36.39 **War operations involving other fires, conflagrations and hot substances**

7 Y36.390- **War operations involving other fires, conflagrations and hot substances, military personnel**

7 Y36.391- **War operations involving other fires, conflagrations and hot substances, civilian**

5 Y36.4 **War operations involving firearm discharge and other forms of conventional warfare**

6 Y36.41 **War operations involving rubber bullets**

7 Y36.410- **War operations involving rubber bullets, military personnel**

7 Y36.411- **War operations involving rubber bullets, civilian**

6 Y36.42 **War operations involving firearms pellets**

7 Y36.420- **War operations involving firearms pellets, military personnel**

7 Y36.421- **War operations involving firearms pellets, civilian**

6 Y36.43 **War operations involving other firearms discharge**
War operations involving bullets NOS
EXCLUDES 1 *war operations involving munitions fragments (Y36.25-)*
war operations involving incendiary bullets (Y36.32-)

7 Y36.430- **War operations involving other firearms discharge, military personnel**

7 Y36.431- **War operations involving other firearms discharge, civilian**

6 Y36.44 **War operations involving unarmed hand to hand combat**
EXCLUDES 1 *war operations involving combat using blunt or piercing object (Y36.45-)*
war operations involving intentional restriction of air and airway (Y36.46-)
war operations involving unintentional restriction of air and airway (Y36.47-)

7 Y36.440- **War operations involving unarmed hand to hand combat, military personnel**

7 Y36.441- **War operations involving unarmed hand to hand combat, civilian**

6 Y36.45 **War operations involving combat using blunt or piercing object**

7 Y36.450- **War operations involving combat using blunt or piercing object, military personnel**

7 Y36.451- **War operations involving combat using blunt or piercing object, civilian**

6 Y36.46 **War operations involving intentional restriction of air and airway**

7 Y36.460- **War operations involving intentional restriction of air and airway, military personnel**

7 Y36.461- **War operations involving intentional restriction of air and airway, civilian**

6 Y36.47 **War operations involving unintentional restriction of air and airway**

7 Y36.470- **War operations involving unintentional restriction of air and airway, military personnel**

7 Y36.471- **War operations involving unintentional restriction of air and airway, civilian**

6 Y36.49 **War operations involving other forms of conventional warfare**

7 Y36.490- **War operations involving other forms of conventional warfare, military personnel**

7 Y36.491- **War operations involving other forms of conventional warfare, civilian**

5 Y36.5 **War operations involving nuclear weapons**
War operations involving dirty bomb NOS

6 Y36.50 **War operations involving unspecified effect of nuclear weapon**

7 Y36.500- **War operations involving unspecified effect of nuclear weapon, military personnel**

7 Y36.501- **War operations involving unspecified effect of nuclear weapon, civilian**

6 Y36.51 **War operations involving direct blast effect of nuclear weapon**
War operations involving blast pressure of nuclear weapon

7 Y36.510- **War operations involving direct blast effect of nuclear weapon, military personnel**

7 Y36.511- **War operations involving direct blast effect of nuclear weapon, civilian**

6 Y36.52 **War operations involving indirect blast effect of nuclear weapon**
War operations involving being thrown by blast of nuclear weapon
War operations involving being struck or crushed by blast debris of nuclear weapon

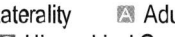

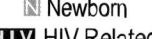

7 Y36.520- **War operations involving indirect blast effect of nuclear weapon, military personnel**

7 Y36.521- War operations involving indirect blast effect of nuclear weapon, civilian

6 Y36.53 War operations involving thermal radiation effect of nuclear weapon
War operations involving direct heat from nuclear weapon
War operation involving fireball effects from nuclear weapon

7 Y36.530- War operations involving thermal radiation effect of nuclear weapon, military personnel

7 Y36.531- War operations involving thermal radiation effect of nuclear weapon, civilian

6 Y36.54 War operation involving nuclear radiation effects of nuclear weapon
War operation involving acute radiation exposure from nuclear weapon
War operation involving exposure to immediate ionizing radiation from nuclear weapon
War operation involving fallout exposure from nuclear weapon
War operation involving secondary effects of nuclear weapons

7 Y36.540- War operation involving nuclear radiation effects of nuclear weapon, military personnel

7 Y36.541- War operation involving nuclear radiation effects of nuclear weapon, civilian

6 Y36.59 War operation involving other effects of nuclear weapons

7 Y36.590- War operation involving other effects of nuclear weapons, military personnel

7 Y36.591- War operation involving other effects of nuclear weapons, civilian

5 Y36.6 War operations involving biological weapons

6 Y36.6X War operations involving biological weapons

7 Y36.6X0- War operations involving biological weapons, military personnel

7 Y36.6X1- War operations involving biological weapons, civilian

5 Y36.7 War operations involving chemical weapons and other forms of unconventional warfare

EXCLUDES 1 *war operations involving incendiary devices (Y36.3-, Y36.5-)*

6 Y36.7X War operations involving chemical weapons and other forms of unconventional warfare

7 Y36.7X0- War operations involving chemical weapons and other forms of unconventional warfare, military personnel

7 Y36.7X1- War operations involving chemical weapons and other forms of unconventional warfare, civilian

5 Y36.8 War operations occurring after cessation of hostilities
War operations classifiable to categories Y36.0-Y36.8 but occurring after cessation of hostilities

6 Y36.81 Explosion of mine placed during war operations but exploding after cessation of hostilities

7 Y36.810- Explosion of mine placed during war operations but exploding after cessation of hostilities, military personnel

7 Y36.811- Explosion of mine placed during war operations but exploding after cessation of hostilities, civilian

6 Y36.82 Explosion of bomb placed during war operations but exploding after cessation of hostilities

7 Y36.820- Explosion of bomb placed during war operations but exploding after cessation of hostilities, military personnel

7 Y36.821- Explosion of bomb placed during war operations but exploding after cessation of hostilities, civilian

6 Y36.88 Other war operations occurring after cessation of hostilities

7 Y36.880- Other war operations occurring after cessation of hostilities, military personnel

7 Y36.881- Other war operations occurring after cessation of hostilities, civilian

6 Y36.89 Unspecified war operations occurring after cessation of hostilities

7 Y36.890- Unspecified war operations occurring after cessation of hostilities, military personnel

7 Y36.891- Unspecified war operations occurring after cessation of hostilities, civilian

5 Y36.9 Other and unspecified war operations

7 Y36.90X- War operations, unspecified

7 Y36.91X- War operations involving unspecified weapon of mass destruction [WMD]

7 Y36.92X- War operations involving friendly fire

4 Y37 Military operations

INCLUDES injuries to military personnel and civilians occurring during peacetime on military property and during routine military exercises and operations

EXCLUDES 1 *military aircraft involved in aircraft accident with civilian aircraft (V97.81-)*
military vehicles involved in transport accident with civilian vehicle (V09.01, V09.21, V19.81, V29.81, V39.81, V49.81, V59.81, V69.81, V79.81)
military watercraft involved in water transport accident with civilian watercraft (V94.81-)
war operations (Y36.-)

The appropriate 7th character is to be added to each code from category Y37

A	initial encounter
D	subsequent encounter
S	sequela

5 Y37.0 Military operations involving explosion of marine weapons

6 Y37.00 Military operations involving explosion of unspecified marine weapon
Military operations involving underwater blast NOS

7 Y37.000- Military operations involving explosion of unspecified marine weapon, military personnel

7 Y37.001- Military operations involving explosion of unspecified marine weapon, civilian

6 Y37.01 Military operations involving explosion of depth-charge

7 Y37.010- Military operations involving explosion of depth-charge, military personnel

7 Y37.011- Military operations involving explosion of depth-charge, civilian

6 Y37.02 Military operations involving explosion of marine mine
Military operations involving explosion of marine mine, at sea or in harbor

7 Y37.020- Military operations involving explosion of marine mine, military personnel

7 Y37.021- Military operations involving explosion of marine mine, civilian

6 Y37.03 Military operations involving explosion of sea-based artillery shell

7 Y37.030- Military operations involving explosion of sea-based artillery shell, military personnel

7 Y37.031- Military operations involving explosion of sea-based artillery shell, civilian

6 Y37.04 Military operations involving explosion of torpedo

7 Y37.040- Military operations involving explosion of torpedo, military personnel

7 Y37.041- Military operations involving explosion of torpedo, civilian

6 Y37.05 Military operations involving accidental detonation of onboard marine weapons

7 Y37.050- Military operations involving accidental detonation of onboard marine weapons, military personnel

7 Y37.051- Military operations involving accidental detonation of onboard marine weapons, civilian

6 Y37.09 Military operations involving explosion of other marine weapons

7 Y37.090- Military operations involving explosion of other marine weapons, military personnel

7 Y37.091- Military operations involving explosion of other marine weapons, civilian

5 Y37.1 Military operations involving destruction of aircraft

6 Y37.10 **Military operations involving unspecified destruction of aircraft**

7 Y37.100- **Military operations involving unspecified destruction of aircraft, military personnel**

7 Y37.101- **Military operations involving unspecified destruction of aircraft, civilian**

6 Y37.11 **Military operations involving destruction of aircraft due to enemy fire or explosives**
Military operations involving destruction of aircraft due to air to air missile
Military operations involving destruction of aircraft due to explosive placed on aircraft
Military operations involving destruction of aircraft due to rocket propelled grenade [RPG]
Military operations involving destruction of aircraft due to small arms fire
Military operations involving destruction of aircraft due to surface to air missile

7 Y37.110- **Military operations involving destruction of aircraft due to enemy fire or explosives, military personnel**

7 Y37.111- **Military operations involving destruction of aircraft due to enemy fire or explosives, civilian**

6 Y37.12 **Military operations involving destruction of aircraft due to collision with other aircraft**

7 Y37.120- **Military operations involving destruction of aircraft due to collision with other aircraft, military personnel**

7 Y37.121- **Military operations involving destruction of aircraft due to collision with other aircraft, civilian**

6 Y37.13 **Military operations involving destruction of aircraft due to onboard fire**

7 Y37.130- **Military operations involving destruction of aircraft due to onboard fire, military personnel**

7 Y37.131- **Military operations involving destruction of aircraft due to onboard fire, civilian**

6 Y37.14 **Military operations involving destruction of aircraft due to accidental detonation of onboard munitions and explosives**

7 Y37.140- **Military operations involving destruction of aircraft due to accidental detonation of onboard munitions and explosives, military personnel**

7 Y37.141- **Military operations involving destruction of aircraft due to accidental detonation of onboard munitions and explosives, civilian**

6 Y37.19 **Military operations involving other destruction of aircraft**

7 Y37.190- **Military operations involving other destruction of aircraft, military personnel**

7 Y37.191- **Military operations involving other destruction of aircraft, civilian**

5 Y37.2 **Military operations involving other explosions and fragments**

EXCLUDES 1 *military operations involving explosion of aircraft (Y37.1-)*
military operations involving explosion of marine weapons (Y37.0-)
military operations involving explosion of nuclear weapons (Y37.5-)

6 Y37.20 **Military operations involving unspecified explosion and fragments**
Military operations involving air blast NOS
Military operations involving blast NOS
Military operations involving blast fragments NOS
Military operations involving blast wave NOS
Military operations involving blast wind NOS
Military operations involving explosion NOS
Military operations involving explosion of bomb NOS

7 Y37.200- **Military operations involving unspecified explosion and fragments, military personnel**

7 Y37.201- **Military operations involving unspecified explosion and fragments, civilian**

6 Y37.21 **Military operations involving explosion of aerial bomb**

7 Y37.210- **Military operations involving explosion of aerial bomb, military personnel**

7 Y37.211- **Military operations involving explosion of aerial bomb, civilian**

6 Y37.22 **Military operations involving explosion of guided missile**

7 Y37.220- **Military operations involving explosion of guided missile, military personnel**

7 Y37.221- **Military operations involving explosion of guided missile, civilian**

6 Y37.23 **Military operations involving explosion of improvised explosive device [IED]**
Military operations involving explosion of person-borne improvised explosive device [IED]
Military operations involving explosion of vehicle-borne improvised explosive device [IED]
Military operations involving explosion of roadside improvised explosive device [IED]

7 Y37.230- **Military operations involving explosion of improvised explosive device [IED], military personnel**

7 Y37.231- **Military operations involving explosion of improvised explosive device [IED], civilian**

6 Y37.24 **Military operations involving explosion due to accidental detonation and discharge of own munitions or munitions launch device**

7 Y37.240- **Military operations involving explosion due to accidental detonation and discharge of own munitions or munitions launch device, military personnel**

7 Y37.241- **Military operations involving explosion due to accidental detonation and discharge of own munitions or munitions launch device, civilian**

6 Y37.25 **Military operations involving fragments from munitions**

7 Y37.250- **Military operations involving fragments from munitions, military personnel**

7 Y37.251- **Military operations involving fragments from munitions, civilian**

6 Y37.26 **Military operations involving fragments of improvised explosive device [IED]**
Military operations involving fragments of person-borne improvised explosive device [IED]
Military operations involving fragments of vehicle-borne improvised explosive device [IED]
Military operations involving fragments of roadside improvised explosive device [IED]

7 Y37.260- **Military operations involving fragments of improvised explosive device [IED], military personnel**

7 Y37.261- **Military operations involving fragments of improvised explosive device [IED], civilian**

6 Y37.27 **Military operations involving fragments from weapons**

7 Y37.270- **Military operations involving fragments from weapons, military personnel**

7 Y37.271- **Military operations involving fragments from weapons, civilian**

6 Y37.29 **Military operations involving other explosions and fragments**
Military operations involving explosion of grenade
Military operations involving explosions of land mine
Military operations involving shrapnel NOS

7 Y37.290- **Military operations involving other explosions and fragments, military personnel**

7 Y37.291- **Military operations involving other explosions and fragments, civilian**

5 Y37.3 **Military operations involving fires, conflagrations and hot substances**
Military operations involving smoke, fumes, and heat from fires, conflagrations and hot substances

EXCLUDES 1 *military operations involving fires and conflagrations aboard military aircraft (Y37.1-)*
military operations involving fires and conflagrations aboard military watercraft (Y37.0-)
military operations involving fires and conflagrations caused indirectly by conventional weapons (Y37.2-)
military operations involving fires and thermal effects of nuclear weapons (Y36.53-)

6 Y37.30 Military operations involving unspecified fire, conflagration and hot substance
7 Y37.300- Military operations involving unspecified fire, conflagration and hot substance, military personnel
7 Y37.301- Military operations involving unspecified fire, conflagration and hot substance, civilian
6 Y37.31 Military operations involving gasoline bomb
Military operations involving incendiary bomb
Military operations involving petrol bomb
7 Y37.310- Military operations involving gasoline bomb, military personnel
7 Y37.311- Military operations involving gasoline bomb, civilian
6 Y37.32 Military operations involving incendiary bullet
7 Y37.320- Military operations involving incendiary bullet, military personnel
7 Y37.321- Military operations involving incendiary bullet, civilian
6 Y37.33 Military operations involving flamethrower
7 Y37.330- Military operations involving flamethrower, military personnel
7 Y37.331- Military operations involving flamethrower, civilian
6 Y37.39 Military operations involving other fires, conflagrations and hot substances
7 Y37.390- Military operations involving other fires, conflagrations and hot substances, military personnel
7 Y37.391- Military operations involving other fires, conflagrations and hot substances, civilian
5 Y37.4 Military operations involving firearm discharge and other forms of conventional warfare
6 Y37.41 Military operations involving rubber bullets
7 Y37.410- Military operations involving rubber bullets, military personnel
7 Y37.411- Military operations involving rubber bullets, civilian
6 Y37.42 Military operations involving firearms pellets
7 Y37.420- Military operations involving firearms pellets, military personnel
7 Y37.421- Military operations involving firearms pellets, civilian
6 Y37.43 Military operations involving other firearms discharge
Military operations involving bullets NOS
EXCLUDES 1 *military operations involving munitions fragments (Y37.25-)*
military operations involving incendiary bullets (Y37.32-)
7 Y37.430- Military operations involving other firearms discharge, military personnel
7 Y37.431- Military operations involving other firearms discharge, civilian
6 Y37.44 Military operations involving unarmed hand to hand combat
EXCLUDES 1 *military operations involving combat using blunt or piercing object (Y37.45-)*
military operations involving intentional restriction of air and airway (Y37.46-)
military operations involving unintentional restriction of air and airway (Y37.47-)
7 Y37.440- Military operations involving unarmed hand to hand combat, military personnel
7 Y37.441- Military operations involving unarmed hand to hand combat, civilian
6 Y37.45 Military operations involving combat using blunt or piercing object
7 Y37.450- Military operations involving combat using blunt or piercing object, military personnel
7 Y37.451- Military operations involving combat using blunt or piercing object, civilian
6 Y37.46 Military operations involving intentional restriction of air and airway
7 Y37.460- Military operations involving intentional restriction of air and airway, military personnel
7 Y37.461- Military operations involving intentional restriction of air and airway, civilian
6 Y37.47 Military operations involving unintentional restriction of air and airway
7 Y37.470- Military operations involving unintentional restriction of air and airway, military personnel
7 Y37.471- Military operations involving unintentional restriction of air and airway, civilian
6 Y37.49 Military operations involving other forms of conventional warfare
7 Y37.490- Military operations involving other forms of conventional warfare, military personnel
7 Y37.491- Military operations involving other forms of conventional warfare, civilian
5 Y37.5 Military operations involving nuclear weapons
Military operation involving dirty bomb NOS
6 Y37.50 Military operations involving unspecified effect of nuclear weapon
7 Y37.500- Military operations involving unspecified effect of nuclear weapon, military personnel
7 Y37.501- Military operations involving unspecified effect of nuclear weapon, civilian
6 Y37.51 Military operations involving direct blast effect of nuclear weapon
Military operations involving blast pressure of nuclear weapon
7 Y37.510- Military operations involving direct blast effect of nuclear weapon, military personnel
7 Y37.511- Military operations involving direct blast effect of nuclear weapon, civilian
6 Y37.52 Military operations involving indirect blast effect of nuclear weapon
Military operations involving being thrown by blast of nuclear weapon
Military operations involving being struck or crushed by blast debris of nuclear weapon
7 Y37.520- Military operations involving indirect blast effect of nuclear weapon, military personnel
7 Y37.521- Military operations involving indirect blast effect of nuclear weapon, civilian
6 Y37.53 Military operations involving thermal radiation effect of nuclear weapon
Military operations involving direct heat from nuclear weapon
Military operation involving fireball effects from nuclear weapon
7 Y37.530- Military operations involving thermal radiation effect of nuclear weapon, military personnel
7 Y37.531- Military operations involving thermal radiation effect of nuclear weapon, civilian
6 Y37.54 Military operation involving nuclear radiation effects of nuclear weapon
Military operation involving acute radiation exposure from nuclear weapon
Military operation involving exposure to immediate ionizing radiation from nuclear weapon
Military operation involving fallout exposure from nuclear weapon
Military operation involving secondary effects of nuclear weapons
7 Y37.540- Military operation involving nuclear radiation effects of nuclear weapon, military personnel
7 Y37.541- Military operation involving nuclear radiation effects of nuclear weapon, civilian
6 Y37.59 Military operation involving other effects of nuclear weapons
7 Y37.590- Military operation involving other effects of nuclear weapons, military personnel
7 Y37.591- Military operation involving other effects of nuclear weapons, civilian
5 Y37.6 Military operations involving biological weapons
6 Y37.6X Military operations involving biological weapons
7 Y37.6X0- Military operations involving biological weapons, military personnel

7 Y37.6X1- **Military operations involving biological weapons, civilian**

5 Y37.7 **Military operations involving chemical weapons and other forms of unconventional warfare**

EXCLUDES 1 *military operations involving incendiary devices (Y36.3-, Y36.5-)*

6 Y37.7X **Military operations involving chemical weapons and other forms of unconventional warfare**

7 Y37.7X0- **Military operations involving chemical weapons and other forms of unconventional warfare, military personnel**

7 Y37.7X1- **Military operations involving chemical weapons and other forms of unconventional warfare, civilian**

5 Y37.9 **Other and unspecified military operations**

7 Y37.90X- **Military operations, unspecified**

7 Y37.91X- **Military operations involving unspecified weapon of mass destruction [WMD]**

7 Y37.92X- **Military operations involving friendly fire**

4 Y38 Terrorism

These codes are for use to identify injuries resulting from the unlawful use of force or violence against persons or property to intimidate or coerce a Government, the civilian population, or any segment thereof, in furtherance of political or social objective

Use additional code for place of occurrence (Y92.-)

The appropriate 7th character is to be added to each code from category Y38

A	initial encounter
D	subsequent encounter
S	sequela

5 Y38.0 **Terrorism involving explosion of marine weapons**

Terrorism involving depth-charge
Terrorism involving marine mine
Terrorism involving mine NOS, at sea or in harbor
Terrorism involving sea-based artillery shell
Terrorism involving torpedo
Terrorism involving underwater blast

6 Y38.0X **Terrorism involving explosion of marine weapons**

7 Y38.0X1- **Terrorism involving explosion of marine weapons, public safety official injured**

7 Y38.0X2- **Terrorism involving explosion of marine weapons, civilian injured**

7 Y38.0X3- **Terrorism involving explosion of marine weapons, terrorist injured**

5 Y38.1 **Terrorism involving destruction of aircraft**

Terrorism involving aircraft burned
Terrorism involving aircraft exploded
Terrorism involving aircraft being shot down
Terrorism involving aircraft used as a weapon

6 Y38.1X **Terrorism involving destruction of aircraft**

7 Y38.1X1- **Terrorism involving destruction of aircraft, public safety official injured**

7 Y38.1X2- **Terrorism involving destruction of aircraft, civilian injured**

7 Y38.1X3- **Terrorism involving destruction of aircraft, terrorist injured**

5 Y38.2 **Terrorism involving other explosions and fragments**

Terrorism involving antipersonnel (fragments) bomb
Terrorism involving blast NOS
Terrorism involving explosion NOS
Terrorism involving explosion of breech block
Terrorism involving explosion of cannon block
Terrorism involving explosion (fragments) of artillery shell
Terrorism involving explosion (fragments) of bomb
Terrorism involving explosion (fragments) of grenade
Terrorism involving explosion (fragments) of guided missile
Terrorism involving explosion (fragments) of land mine
Terrorism involving explosion of mortar bomb
Terrorism involving explosion of munitions
Terrorism involving explosion (fragments) of rocket
Terrorism involving explosion (fragments) of shell
Terrorism involving shrapnel
Terrorism involving mine NOS, on land

EXCLUDES 1 *terrorism involving explosion of nuclear weapon (Y38.5)*
terrorism involving suicide bomber (Y38.81)

6 Y38.2X **Terrorism involving other explosions and fragments**

7 Y38.2X1- **Terrorism involving other explosions and fragments, public safety official injured**

7 Y38.2X2- **Terrorism involving other explosions and fragments, civilian injured**

7 Y38.2X3- **Terrorism involving other explosions and fragments, terrorist injured**

5 Y38.3 **Terrorism involving fires, conflagration and hot substances**

Terrorism involving conflagration NOS
Terrorism involving fire NOS
Terrorism involving petrol bomb

EXCLUDES 1 *terrorism involving fire or heat of nuclear weapon (Y38.5)*

6 Y38.3X **Terrorism involving fires, conflagration and hot substances**

7 Y38.3X1- **Terrorism involving fires, conflagration and hot substances, public safety official injured**

7 Y38.3X2- **Terrorism involving fires, conflagration and hot substances, civilian injured**

7 Y38.3X3- **Terrorism involving fires, conflagration and hot substances, terrorist injured**

5 Y38.4 **Terrorism involving firearms**

Terrorism involving carbine bullet
Terrorism involving machine gun bullet
Terrorism involving pellets (shotgun)
Terrorism involving pistol bullet
Terrorism involving rifle bullet
Terrorism involving rubber (rifle) bullet

6 Y38.4X **Terrorism involving firearms**

7 Y38.4X1- **Terrorism involving firearms, public safety official injured**

7 Y38.4X2- **Terrorism involving firearms, civilian injured**

7 Y38.4X3- **Terrorism involving firearms, terrorist injured**

5 Y38.5 **Terrorism involving nuclear weapons**

Terrorism involving blast effects of nuclear weapon
Terrorism involving exposure to ionizing radiation from nuclear weapon
Terrorism involving fireball effect of nuclear weapon
Terrorism involving heat from nuclear weapon

6 Y38.5X **Terrorism involving nuclear weapons**

7 Y38.5X1- **Terrorism involving nuclear weapons, public safety official injured**

7 Y38.5X2- **Terrorism involving nuclear weapons, civilian injured**

7 Y38.5X3- **Terrorism involving nuclear weapons, terrorist injured**

5 Y38.6 **Terrorism involving biological weapons**

Terrorism involving anthrax
Terrorism involving cholera
Terrorism involving smallpox

6 Y38.6X **Terrorism involving biological weapons**

7 Y38.6X1- **Terrorism involving biological weapons, public safety official injured**

7 Y38.6X2- **Terrorism involving biological weapons, civilian injured**

7 Y38.6X3- **Terrorism involving biological weapons, terrorist injured**

5 Y38.7 **Terrorism involving chemical weapons**

Terrorism involving gases, fumes, chemicals
Terrorism involving hydrogen cyanide
Terrorism involving phosgene
Terrorism involving sarin

6 Y38.7X **Terrorism involving chemical weapons**

7 Y38.7X1- **Terrorism involving chemical weapons, public safety official injured**

7 Y38.7X2- **Terrorism involving chemical weapons, civilian injured**

7 Y38.7X3- **Terrorism involving chemical weapons, terrorist injured**

5 Y38.8 **Terrorism involving other and unspecified means**

7 Y38.80X- **Terrorism involving unspecified means**

Terrorism NOS

6 Y38.81 **Terrorism involving suicide bomber**

7 Y38.811- **Terrorism involving suicide bomber, public safety official injured**

7 Y38.812- **Terrorism involving suicide bomber, civilian injured**

6 **Y38.89 Terrorism involving other means**

Terrorism involving drowning and submersion

Terrorism involving lasers

Terrorism involving piercing or stabbing instruments

7 **Y38.891- Terrorism involving other means, public safety official injured**

7 **Y38.892- Terrorism involving other means, civilian injured**

7 **Y38.893- Terrorism involving other means, terrorist injured**

5 **Y38.9 Terrorism, secondary effects**

Note: This code is for use to identify conditions occurring subsequent to a terrorist attack not those that are due to the initial terrorist attack

6 **Y38.9X Terrorism, secondary effects**

7 **Y38.9X1- Terrorism, secondary effects, public safety official injured**

7 **Y38.9X2- Terrorism, secondary effects, civilian injured**

Complications of medical and surgical care (Y62-Y84)

INCLUDES complications of medical devices

surgical and medical procedures as the cause of abnormal reaction of the patient, or of later complication, without mention of misadventure at the time of the procedure

Misadventures to patients during surgical and medical care (Y62-Y69)

EXCLUDES 1 *surgical and medical procedures as the cause of abnormal reaction of the patient, without mention of misadventure at the time of the procedure (Y83-Y84)*

EXCLUDES 2 *breakdown or malfunctioning of medical device (during procedure) (after implantation) (ongoing use) (Y70-Y82)*

4 **Y62 Failure of sterile precautions during surgical and medical care**

Y62.0 Failure of sterile precautions during surgical operation

Y62.1 Failure of sterile precautions during infusion or transfusion

Y62.2 Failure of sterile precautions during kidney dialysis and other perfusion HCC

Y62.3 Failure of sterile precautions during injection or immunization

Y62.4 Failure of sterile precautions during endoscopic examination

Y62.5 Failure of sterile precautions during heart catheterization

Y62.6 Failure of sterile precautions during aspiration, puncture and other catheterization

Y62.8 Failure of sterile precautions during other surgical and medical care

Y62.9 Failure of sterile precautions during unspecified surgical and medical care

4 **Y63 Failure in dosage during surgical and medical care**

EXCLUDES 2 *accidental overdose of drug or wrong drug given in error (T36-T50)*

Y63.0 Excessive amount of blood or other fluid given during transfusion or infusion

Y63.1 Incorrect dilution of fluid used during infusion

Y63.2 Overdose of radiation given during therapy

Y63.3 Inadvertent exposure of patient to radiation during medical care

Y63.4 Failure in dosage in electroshock or insulin-shock therapy

Y63.5 Inappropriate temperature in local application and packing

Y63.6 Underdosing and nonadministration of necessary drug, medicament or biological substance

GUIDELINES Section I.C.19.e.5)(c)

Noncompliance (Z91.12-, Z91.13- and Z91.14-) or complication of care (Y63.6-Y63.9) codes are to be used with an underdosing code to indicate intent, if known.

Y63.8 Failure in dosage during other surgical and medical care

GUIDELINES Section I.C.19.e.5)(c)

Noncompliance (Z91.12-, Z91.13- and Z91.14-) or complication of care (Y63.6-Y63.9) codes are to be used with an underdosing code to indicate intent, if known.

Y63.9 Failure in dosage during unspecified surgical and medical care

GUIDELINES Section I.C.19.e.5)(c)

Noncompliance (Z91.12-, Z91.13- and Z91.14-) or complication of care (Y63.6-Y63.9) codes are to be used with an underdosing code to indicate intent, if known.

4 **Y64 Contaminated medical or biological substances**

Y64.0 Contaminated medical or biological substance, transfused or infused

Y64.1 Contaminated medical or biological substance, injected or used for immunization

Y64.8 Contaminated medical or biological substance administered by other means

Y64.9 Contaminated medical or biological substance administered by unspecified means

Administered contaminated medical or biological substance NOS

4 **Y65 Other misadventures during surgical and medical care**

Y65.0 Mismatched blood in transfusion

Y65.1 Wrong fluid used in infusion

Y65.2 Failure in suture or ligature during surgical operation

Y65.3 Endotracheal tube wrongly placed during anesthetic procedure

Y65.4 Failure to introduce or to remove other tube or instrument

5 **Y65.5 Performance of wrong procedure (operation)**

Y65.51 Performance of wrong procedure (operation) on correct patient

Wrong device implanted into correct surgical site

EXCLUDES 1 *performance of correct procedure (operation) on wrong side or body part (Y65.53)*

Y65.52 Performance of procedure (operation) on patient not scheduled for surgery

Performance of procedure (operation) intended for another patient

Performance of procedure (operation) on wrong patient

Y65.53 Performance of correct procedure (operation) on wrong side or body part

Performance of correct procedure (operation) on wrong side

Performance of correct procedure (operation) on wrong site

Y65.8 Other specified misadventures during surgical and medical care

Y66 Nonadministration of surgical and medical care

Premature cessation of surgical and medical care

EXCLUDES 1 *DNR status (Z66)*

palliative care (Z51.5)

Y69 Unspecified misadventure during surgical and medical care

Medical devices associated with adverse incidents in diagnostic and therapeutic use (Y70-Y82)

INCLUDES breakdown or malfunction of medical devices (during use) (after implantation) (ongoing use)

EXCLUDES 2 *later complications following use of medical devices without breakdown or malfunctioning of device (Y83-Y84)*

misadventure to patients during surgical and medical care, classifiable to (Y62-Y69)

surgical and other medical procedures as the cause of abnormal reaction of the patient, or of later complication, without mention of misadventure at the time of the procedure (Y83-Y84)

4 **Y70 Anesthesiology devices associated with adverse incidents**

Y70.0 Diagnostic and monitoring anesthesiology devices associated with adverse incidents

Y70.1 Therapeutic (nonsurgical) and rehabilitative anesthesiology devices associated with adverse incidents
Y70.2 Prosthetic and other implants, materials and accessory anesthesiology devices associated with adverse incidents
Y70.3 Surgical instruments, materials and anesthesiology devices (including sutures) associated with adverse incidents
Y70.8 Miscellaneous anesthesiology devices associated with adverse incidents, not elsewhere classified

Y71 Cardiovascular devices associated with adverse incidents
Y71.0 Diagnostic and monitoring cardiovascular devices associated with adverse incidents
Y71.1 Therapeutic (nonsurgical) and rehabilitative cardiovascular devices associated with adverse incidents
Y71.2 Prosthetic and other implants, materials and accessory cardiovascular devices associated with adverse incidents
Y71.3 Surgical instruments, materials and cardiovascular devices (including sutures) associated with adverse incidents
Y71.8 Miscellaneous cardiovascular devices associated with adverse incidents, not elsewhere classified

Y72 Otorhinolaryngological devices associated with adverse incidents
Y72.0 Diagnostic and monitoring otorhinolaryngological devices associated with adverse incidents
Y72.1 Therapeutic (nonsurgical) and rehabilitative otorhinolaryngological devices associated with adverse incidents
Y72.2 Prosthetic and other implants, materials and accessory otorhinolaryngological devices associated with adverse incidents
Y72.3 Surgical instruments, materials and otorhinolaryngological devices (including sutures) associated with adverse incidents
Y72.8 Miscellaneous otorhinolaryngological devices associated with adverse incidents, not elsewhere classified

Y73 Gastroenterology and urology devices associated with adverse incidents
Y73.0 Diagnostic and monitoring gastroenterology and urology devices associated with adverse incidents
Y73.1 Therapeutic (nonsurgical) and rehabilitative gastroenterology and urology devices associated with adverse incidents
Y73.2 Prosthetic and other implants, materials and accessory gastroenterology and urology devices associated with adverse incidents
Y73.3 Surgical instruments, materials and gastroenterology and urology devices (including sutures) associated with adverse incidents
Y73.8 Miscellaneous gastroenterology and urology devices associated with adverse incidents, not elsewhere classified

Y74 General hospital and personal-use devices associated with adverse incidents
Y74.0 Diagnostic and monitoring general hospital and personal-use devices associated with adverse incidents
Y74.1 Therapeutic (nonsurgical) and rehabilitative general hospital and personal-use devices associated with adverse incidents
Y74.2 Prosthetic and other implants, materials and accessory general hospital and personal-use devices associated with adverse incidents
Y74.3 Surgical instruments, materials and general hospital and personal-use devices (including sutures) associated with adverse incidents
Y74.8 Miscellaneous general hospital and personal-use devices associated with adverse incidents, not elsewhere classified

Y75 Neurological devices associated with adverse incidents
Y75.0 Diagnostic and monitoring neurological devices associated with adverse incidents
Y75.1 Therapeutic (nonsurgical) and rehabilitative neurological devices associated with adverse incidents
Y75.2 Prosthetic and other implants, materials and neurological devices associated with adverse incidents
Y75.3 Surgical instruments, materials and neurological devices (including sutures) associated with adverse incidents
Y75.8 Miscellaneous neurological devices associated with adverse incidents, not elsewhere classified

Y76 Obstetric and gynecological devices associated with adverse incidents
Y76.0 Diagnostic and monitoring obstetric and gynecological devices associated with adverse incidents ♀
Y76.1 Therapeutic (nonsurgical) and rehabilitative obstetric and gynecological devices associated with adverse incidents ♀
Y76.2 Prosthetic and other implants, materials and accessory obstetric and gynecological devices associated with adverse incidents ♀
Y76.3 Surgical instruments, materials and obstetric and gynecological devices (including sutures) associated with adverse incidents ♀
Y76.8 Miscellaneous obstetric and gynecological devices associated with adverse incidents, not elsewhere classified ♀

Y77 Ophthalmic devices associated with adverse incidents
Y77.0 Diagnostic and monitoring ophthalmic devices associated with adverse incidents
Y77.1 Therapeutic (nonsurgical) and rehabilitative ophthalmic devices associated with adverse incidents
Y77.2 Prosthetic and other implants, materials and accessory ophthalmic devices associated with adverse incidents
Y77.3 Surgical instruments, materials and ophthalmic devices (including sutures) associated with adverse incidents
Y77.8 Miscellaneous ophthalmic devices associated with adverse incidents, not elsewhere classified

Y78 Radiological devices associated with adverse incidents
Y78.0 Diagnostic and monitoring radiological devices associated with adverse incidents
Y78.1 Therapeutic (nonsurgical) and rehabilitative radiological devices associated with adverse incidents
Y78.2 Prosthetic and other implants, materials and accessory radiological devices associated with adverse incidents
Y78.3 Surgical instruments, materials and radiological devices (including sutures) associated with adverse incidents
Y78.8 Miscellaneous radiological devices associated with adverse incidents, not elsewhere classified

Y79 Orthopedic devices associated with adverse incidents
Y79.0 Diagnostic and monitoring orthopedic devices associated with adverse incidents
Y79.1 Therapeutic (nonsurgical) and rehabilitative orthopedic devices associated with adverse incidents
Y79.2 Prosthetic and other implants, materials and accessory orthopedic devices associated with adverse incidents
Y79.3 Surgical instruments, materials and orthopedic devices (including sutures) associated with adverse incidents
Y79.8 Miscellaneous orthopedic devices associated with adverse incidents, not elsewhere classified

Y80 Physical medicine devices associated with adverse incidents
Y80.0 Diagnostic and monitoring physical medicine devices associated with adverse incidents
Y80.1 Therapeutic (nonsurgical) and rehabilitative physical medicine devices associated with adverse incidents
Y80.2 Prosthetic and other implants, materials and accessory physical medicine devices associated with adverse incidents
Y80.3 Surgical instruments, materials and physical medicine devices (including sutures) associated with adverse incidents
Y80.8 Miscellaneous physical medicine devices associated with adverse incidents, not elsewhere classified

Y81 General- and plastic-surgery devices associated with adverse incidents
Y81.0 Diagnostic and monitoring general- and plastic-surgery devices associated with adverse incidents
Y81.1 Therapeutic (nonsurgical) and rehabilitative general- and plastic-surgery devices associated with adverse incidents
Y81.2 Prosthetic and other implants, materials and accessory general- and plastic-surgery devices associated with adverse incidents
Y81.3 Surgical instruments, materials and general- and plastic-surgery devices (including sutures) associated with adverse incidents

Y81.8 Miscellaneous general- and plastic-surgery devices associated with adverse incidents, not elsewhere classified

4 **Y82 Other and unspecified medical devices associated with adverse incidents**

Y82.8 Other medical devices associated with adverse incidents

Y82.9 Unspecified medical devices associated with adverse incidents

Surgical and other medical procedures as the cause of abnormal reaction of the patient, or of later complication, without mention of misadventure at the time of the procedure (Y83-Y84)

EXCLUDES 1 *misadventures to patients during surgical and medical care, classifiable to (Y62-Y69)*

EXCLUDES 2 *breakdown or malfunctioning of medical device (after implantation) (during procedure) (ongoing use) (Y70-Y82)*

4 **Y83 Surgical operation and other surgical procedures as the cause of abnormal reaction of the patient, or of later complication, without mention of misadventure at the time of the procedure**

Y83.0 Surgical operation with transplant of whole organ as the cause of abnormal reaction of the patient, or of later complication, without mention of misadventure at the time of the procedure

Y83.1 Surgical operation with implant of artificial internal device as the cause of abnormal reaction of the patient, or of later complication, without mention of misadventure at the time of the procedure

Y83.2 Surgical operation with anastomosis, bypass or graft as the cause of abnormal reaction of the patient, or of later complication, without mention of misadventure at the time of the procedure

Y83.3 Surgical operation with formation of external stoma as the cause of abnormal reaction of the patient, or of later complication, without mention of misadventure at the time of the procedure

Y83.4 Other reconstructive surgery as the cause of abnormal reaction of the patient, or of later complication, without mention of misadventure at the time of the procedure

Y83.5 Amputation of limb(s) as the cause of abnormal reaction of the patient, or of later complication, without mention of misadventure at the time of the procedure

Y83.6 Removal of other organ (partial) (total) as the cause of abnormal reaction of the patient, or of later complication, without mention of misadventure at the time of the procedure

Y83.8 Other surgical procedures as the cause of abnormal reaction of the patient, or of later complication, without mention of misadventure at the time of the procedure

Y83.9 Surgical procedure, unspecified as the cause of abnormal reaction of the patient, or of later complication, without mention of misadventure at the time of the procedure

4 **Y84 Other medical procedures as the cause of abnormal reaction of the patient, or of later complication, without mention of misadventure at the time of the procedure**

Y84.0 Cardiac catheterization as the cause of abnormal reaction of the patient, or of later complication, without mention of misadventure at the time of the procedure

Y84.1 Kidney dialysis as the cause of abnormal reaction of the patient, or of later complication, without mention of misadventure at the time of the procedure

Y84.2 Radiological procedure and radiotherapy as the cause of abnormal reaction of the patient, or of later complication, without mention of misadventure at the time of the procedure
AHA: 1Q 2017, 33

Y84.3 Shock therapy as the cause of abnormal reaction of the patient, or of later complication, without mention of misadventure at the time of the procedure

Y84.4 Aspiration of fluid as the cause of abnormal reaction of the patient, or of later complication, without mention of misadventure at the time of the procedure

Y84.5 Insertion of gastric or duodenal sound as the cause of abnormal reaction of the patient, or of later complication, without mention of misadventure at the time of the procedure

Y84.6 Urinary catheterization as the cause of abnormal reaction of the patient, or of later complication, without mention of misadventure at the time of the procedure

Y84.7 Blood-sampling as the cause of abnormal reaction of the patient, or of later complication, without mention of misadventure at the time of the procedure

Y84.8 Other medical procedures as the cause of abnormal reaction of the patient, or of later complication, without mention of misadventure at the time of the procedure
AHA: 4Q 2014, 24

Y84.9 Medical procedure, unspecified as the cause of abnormal reaction of the patient, or of later complication, without mention of misadventure at the time of the procedure

Supplementary factors related to causes of morbidity classified elsewhere (Y90-Y99)

Note: These categories may be used to provide supplementary information concerning causes of morbidity. They are not to be used for single-condition coding.

4 **Y90 Evidence of alcohol involvement determined by blood alcohol level**

Code first:
any associated alcohol related disorders (F10)

Y90.0 Blood alcohol level of less than 20 mg/100 ml

Y90.1 Blood alcohol level of 20-39 mg/100 ml

Y90.2 Blood alcohol level of 40-59 mg/100 ml

Y90.3 Blood alcohol level of 60-79 mg/100 ml

Y90.4 Blood alcohol level of 80-99 mg/100 ml

Y90.5 Blood alcohol level of 100-119 mg/100 ml

Y90.6 Blood alcohol level of 120-199 mg/100 ml

Y90.7 Blood alcohol level of 200-239 mg/100 ml

Y90.8 Blood alcohol level of 240 mg/100 ml or more

Y90.9 Presence of alcohol in blood, level not specified

4 **Y92 Place of occurrence of the external cause**

The following category is for use, when relevant, to identify the place of occurrence of the external cause. Use in conjunction with an activity code.

Place of occurrence should be recorded only at the initial encounter for treatment

5 Y92.0 Non-institutional (private) residence as the place of occurrence of the external cause

EXCLUDES 1 *abandoned or derelict house (Y92.89)*
home under construction but not yet occupied (Y92.6-)
institutional place of residence (Y92.1-)

6 Y92.00 Unspecified non-institutional (private) residence as the place of occurrence of the external cause

Y92.000 Kitchen of unspecified non-institutional (private) residence as the place of occurrence of the external cause

Y92.001 Dining room of unspecified non-institutional (private) residence as the place of occurrence of the external cause

Y92.002 Bathroom of unspecified non-institutional (private) residence single-family (private) house as the place of occurrence of the external cause

Y92.003 Bedroom of unspecified non-institutional (private) residence as the place of occurrence of the external cause

Y92.007 Garden or yard of unspecified non-institutional (private) residence as the place of occurrence of the external cause

Y92.008 Other place in unspecified non-institutional (private) residence as the place of occurrence of the external cause

Y92.009 Unspecified place in unspecified non-institutional (private) residence as the place of occurrence of the external cause
Home (NOS) as the place of occurrence of the external cause

6 **Y92.01** Single-family **non-institutional (private)** house **as the place of occurrence of the external cause**
Farmhouse as the place of occurrence of the external cause
EXCLUDES 1 *barn (Y92.71)*
chicken coop or hen house (Y92.72)
farm field (Y92.73)
orchard (Y92.74)
single family mobile home or trailer (Y92.02-)
slaughter house (Y92.86)

Y92.010 Kitchen **of single-family (private) house as the place of occurrence of the external cause**
Y92.011 Dining room **of single-family (private) house as the place of occurrence of the external cause**
Y92.012 Bathroom **of single-family (private) house as the place of occurrence of the external cause**
Y92.013 Bedroom **of single-family (private) house as the place of occurrence of the external cause**
Y92.014 Private driveway **to single-family (private) house as the place of occurrence of the external cause**
Y92.015 Private garage **of single-family (private) house as the place of occurrence of the external cause**
Y92.016 Swimming-pool **in single-family (private) house or** garden **as the place of occurrence of the external cause**
Y92.017 Garden or yard **in single-family (private) house as the place of occurrence of the external cause**
Y92.018 Other **place in single-family (private) house as the place of occurrence of the external cause**
Y92.019 Unspecified **place in single-family (private) house as the place of occurrence of the external cause**

6 **Y92.02** Mobile home **as the place of occurrence of the external cause**
Y92.020 Kitchen in **mobile home as the place of occurrence of the external cause**
Y92.021 Dining room in **mobile home as the place of occurrence of the external cause**
Y92.022 Bathroom in **mobile home as the place of occurrence of the external cause**
Y92.023 Bedroom in **mobile home as the place of occurrence of the external cause**
Y92.024 Driveway of **mobile home as the place of occurrence of the external cause**
Y92.025 Garage of **mobile home as the place of occurrence of the external cause**
Y92.026 Swimming-pool of **mobile home as the place of occurrence of the external cause**
Y92.027 Garden or yard of **mobile home as the place of occurrence of the external cause**
Y92.028 Other place in **mobile home as the place of occurrence of the external cause**
Y92.029 Unspecified place in **mobile home as the place of occurrence of the external cause**

6 **Y92.03** Apartment **as the place of occurrence of the external cause**
Condominium as the place of occurrence of the external cause
Co-op apartment as the place of occurrence of the external cause
Y92.030 Kitchen in **apartment as the place of occurrence of the external cause**
Y92.031 Bathroom in **apartment as the place of occurrence of the external cause**
Y92.032 Bedroom in **apartment as the place of occurrence of the external cause**
Y92.038 Other place in **apartment as the place of occurrence of the external cause**
Y92.039 Unspecified place in **apartment as the place of occurrence of the external cause**

6 **Y92.04** Boarding-house **as the place of occurrence of the external cause**
Y92.040 Kitchen in **boarding-house as the place of occurrence of the external cause**
Y92.041 Bathroom in **boarding-house as the place of occurrence of the external cause**
Y92.042 Bedroom in **boarding-house as the place of occurrence of the external cause**
Y92.043 Driveway of **boarding-house as the place of occurrence of the external cause**
Y92.044 Garage of **boarding-house as the place of occurrence of the external cause**
Y92.045 Swimming-pool of **boarding-house as the place of occurrence of the external cause**
Y92.046 Garden or yard of **boarding-house as the place of occurrence of the external cause**
Y92.048 Other place in **boarding-house as the place of occurrence of the external cause**
Y92.049 Unspecified place in **boarding-house as the place of occurrence of the external cause**

6 **Y92.09** Other **non-institutional residence as the place of occurrence of the external cause**
Y92.090 Kitchen in **other non-institutional residence as the place of occurrence of the external cause**
Y92.091 Bathroom in **other non-institutional residence as the place of occurrence of the external cause**
Y92.092 Bedroom in **other non-institutional residence as the place of occurrence of the external cause**
Y92.093 Driveway of **other non-institutional residence as the place of occurrence of the external cause**
Y92.094 Garage of **other non-institutional residence as the place of occurrence of the external cause**
Y92.095 Swimming-pool of **other non-institutional residence as the place of occurrence of the external cause**
Y92.096 Garden or yard of **other non-institutional residence as the place of occurrence of the external cause**
Y92.098 Other place in **other non-institutional residence as the place of occurrence of the external cause**
CODING TIP✓ Assign Y92.098, Other place in other noninstitutional residence, as the place of occurrence of the external cause, for an assisted living facility.
AHA: 2Q 2017, 10
Y92.099 Unspecified place in **other non-institutional residence as the place of occurrence of the external cause**

5 **Y92.1** Institutional (nonprivate) residence as the **place of occurrence of the external cause**
Y92.10 Unspecified **residential institution as the place of occurrence of the external cause**

6 **Y92.11** Children's home and orphanage **as the place of occurrence of the external cause**
Y92.110 Kitchen in **children's home and orphanage as the place of occurrence of the external cause**
Y92.111 Bathroom in **children's home and orphanage as the place of occurrence of the external cause**
Y92.112 Bedroom in **children's home and orphanage as the place of occurrence of the external cause**
Y92.113 Driveway of **children's home and orphanage as the place of occurrence of the external cause**
Y92.114 Garage of **children's home and orphanage as the place of occurrence of the external cause**
Y92.115 Swimming-pool of **children's home and orphanage as the place of occurrence of the external cause**
Y92.116 Garden or yard of **children's home and orphanage as the place of occurrence of the external cause**
Y92.118 Other place in **children's home and orphanage as the place of occurrence of the external cause**
Y92.119 Unspecified place in **children's home and orphanage as the place of occurrence of the external cause**

6 **Y92.12** Nursing home **as the place of occurrence of the external cause**
Home for the sick as the place of occurrence of the external cause
Hospice as the place of occurrence of the external cause

Y92.120 Kitchen in nursing home as the place of occurrence of the external cause
Y92.121 Bathroom in nursing home as the place of occurrence of the external cause
Y92.122 Bedroom in nursing home as the place of occurrence of the external cause
Y92.123 Driveway of nursing home as the place of occurrence of the external cause
Y92.124 Garage of nursing home as the place of occurrence of the external cause
Y92.125 Swimming-pool of nursing home as the place of occurrence of the external cause
Y92.126 Garden or yard of nursing home as the place of occurrence of the external cause
Y92.128 Other place in nursing home as the place of occurrence of the external cause
Y92.129 Unspecified place in nursing home as the place of occurrence of the external cause

6 Y92.13 Military base as the place of occurrence of the external cause
EXCLUDES 1 *military training grounds (Y92.83)*

Y92.130 Kitchen on military base as the place of occurrence of the external cause
Y92.131 Mess hall on military base as the place of occurrence of the external cause
Y92.133 Barracks on military base as the place of occurrence of the external cause
Y92.135 Garage on military base as the place of occurrence of the external cause
Y92.136 Swimming-pool on military base as the place of occurrence of the external cause
Y92.137 Garden or yard on military base as the place of occurrence of the external cause
Y92.138 Other place on military base as the place of occurrence of the external cause
Y92.139 Unspecified place military base as the place of occurrence of the external cause

6 Y92.14 Prison as the place of occurrence of the external cause

Y92.140 Kitchen in prison as the place of occurrence of the external cause
Y92.141 Dining room in prison as the place of occurrence of the external cause
Y92.142 Bathroom in prison as the place of occurrence of the external cause
Y92.143 Cell of prison as the place of occurrence of the external cause
Y92.146 Swimming-pool of prison as the place of occurrence of the external cause
Y92.147 Courtyard of prison as the place of occurrence of the external cause
Y92.148 Other place in prison as the place of occurrence of the external cause
Y92.149 Unspecified place in prison as the place of occurrence of the external cause

6 Y92.15 Reform school as the place of occurrence of the external cause

Y92.150 Kitchen in reform school as the place of occurrence of the external cause
Y92.151 Dining room in reform school as the place of occurrence of the external cause
Y92.152 Bathroom in reform school as the place of occurrence of the external cause
Y92.153 Bedroom in reform school as the place of occurrence of the external cause
Y92.154 Driveway of reform school as the place of occurrence of the external cause
Y92.155 Garage of reform school as the place of occurrence of the external cause
Y92.156 Swimming-pool of reform school as the place of occurrence of the external cause
Y92.157 Garden or yard of reform school as the place of occurrence of the external cause
Y92.158 Other place in reform school as the place of occurrence of the external cause
Y92.159 Unspecified place in reform school as the place of occurrence of the external cause

6 Y92.16 School dormitory as the place of occurrence of the external cause
EXCLUDES 1 *reform school as the place of occurrence of the external cause (Y92.15-)*
school buildings and grounds as the place of occurrence of the external cause (Y92.2-)
school sports and athletic areas as the place of occurrence of the external cause (Y92.3-)

Y92.160 Kitchen in school dormitory as the place of occurrence of the external cause
Y92.161 Dining room in school dormitory as the place of occurrence of the external cause
Y92.162 Bathroom in school dormitory as the place of occurrence of the external cause
Y92.163 Bedroom in school dormitory as the place of occurrence of the external cause
Y92.168 Other place in school dormitory as the place of occurrence of the external cause
Y92.169 Unspecified place in school dormitory as the place of occurrence of the external cause

6 Y92.19 Other specified residential institution as the place of occurrence of the external cause

Y92.190 Kitchen in other specified residential institution as the place of occurrence of the external cause
Y92.191 Dining room in other specified residential institution as the place of occurrence of the external cause
Y92.192 Bathroom in other specified residential institution as the place of occurrence of the external cause
Y92.193 Bedroom in other specified residential institution as the place of occurrence of the external cause
Y92.194 Driveway of other specified residential institution as the place of occurrence of the external cause
Y92.195 Garage of other specified residential institution as the place of occurrence of the external cause
Y92.196 Pool of other specified residential institution as the place of occurrence of the external cause
Y92.197 Garden or yard of other specified residential institution as the place of occurrence of the external cause
Y92.198 Other place in other specified residential institution as the place of occurrence of the external cause
Y92.199 Unspecified place in other specified residential institution as the place of occurrence of the external cause

5 Y92.2 School, other institution and public administrative area as the place of occurrence of the external cause
Building and adjacent grounds used by the general public or by a particular group of the public
EXCLUDES 1 *building under construction as the place of occurrence of the external cause (Y92.6)*
residential institution as the place of occurrence of the external cause (Y92.1)
school dormitory as the place of occurrence of the external cause (Y92.16-)
sports and athletics area of schools as the place of occurrence of the external cause (Y92.3-)

6 Y92.21 School (private) (public) (state) as the place of occurrence of the external cause

Y92.210 Daycare center as the place of occurrence of the external cause
Y92.211 Elementary school as the place of occurrence of the external cause
Kindergarten as the place of occurrence of the external cause
Y92.212 Middle school as the place of occurrence of the external cause
Y92.213 High school as the place of occurrence of the external cause
AHA: 4Q 2012, 108

Y92.214 **College as the place of occurrence of the external cause**
University as the place of occurrence of the external cause

Y92.215 **Trade school as the place of occurrence of the external cause**

Y92.218 **Other school as the place of occurrence of the external cause**

Y92.219 **Unspecified school as the place of occurrence of the external cause**

Y92.22 **Religious institution as the place of occurrence of the external cause**
Church as the place of occurrence of the external cause
Mosque as the place of occurrence of the external cause
Synagogue as the place of occurrence of the external cause

6 Y92.23 **Hospital as the place of occurrence of the external cause**

EXCLUDES 1 *ambulatory (outpatient) health services establishments (Y92.53-)*
home for the sick as the place of occurrence of the external cause (Y92.12-)
hospice as the place of occurrence of the external cause (Y92.12-)
nursing home as the place of occurrence of the external cause (Y92.12-)

Y92.230 **Patient room in hospital as the place of occurrence of the external cause**

Y92.231 **Patient bathroom in hospital as the place of occurrence of the external cause**

Y92.232 **Corridor of hospital as the place of occurrence of the external cause**

Y92.233 **Cafeteria of hospital as the place of occurrence of the external cause**

Y92.234 **Operating room of hospital as the place of occurrence of the external cause**

Y92.238 **Other place in hospital as the place of occurrence of the external cause**

Y92.239 **Unspecified place in hospital as the place of occurrence of the external cause**

6 Y92.24 **Public administrative building as the place of occurrence of the external cause**

Y92.240 **Courthouse as the place of occurrence of the external cause**

Y92.241 **Library as the place of occurrence of the external cause**

Y92.242 **Post office as the place of occurrence of the external cause**

Y92.243 **City hall as the place of occurrence of the external cause**

Y92.248 **Other public administrative building as the place of occurrence of the external cause**

6 Y92.25 **Cultural building as the place of occurrence of the external cause**

Y92.250 **Art Gallery as the place of occurrence of the external cause**

Y92.251 **Museum as the place of occurrence of the external cause**

Y92.252 **Music hall as the place of occurrence of the external cause**

Y92.253 **Opera house as the place of occurrence of the external cause**

Y92.254 **Theater (live) as the place of occurrence of the external cause**

Y92.258 **Other cultural public building as the place of occurrence of the external cause**

Y92.26 **Movie house or cinema as the place of occurrence of the external cause**

Y92.29 **Other specified public building as the place of occurrence of the external cause**
Assembly hall as the place of occurrence of the external cause
Clubhouse as the place of occurrence of the external cause

5 Y92.3 **Sports and athletics area as the place of occurrence of the external cause**

6 Y92.31 **Athletic court as the place of occurrence of the external cause**

EXCLUDES 1 *tennis court in private home or garden (Y92.09)*

Y92.310 **Basketball court as the place of occurrence of the external cause**

Y92.311 **Squash court as the place of occurrence of the external cause**

Y92.312 **Tennis court as the place of occurrence of the external cause**

Y92.318 **Other athletic court as the place of occurrence of the external cause**

6 Y92.32 **Athletic field as the place of occurrence of the external cause**

Y92.320 **Baseball field as the place of occurrence of the external cause**

Y92.321 **Football field as the place of occurrence of the external cause**

Y92.322 **Soccer field as the place of occurrence of the external cause**

Y92.328 **Other athletic field as the place of occurrence of the external cause**
Cricket field as the place of occurrence of the external cause
Hockey field as the place of occurrence of the external cause

6 Y92.33 **Skating rink as the place of occurrence of the external cause**

Y92.330 **Ice skating rink (indoor) (outdoor) as the place of occurrence of the external cause**

Y92.331 **Roller skating rink as the place of occurrence of the external cause**

Y92.34 **Swimming pool (public) as the place of occurrence of the external cause**

EXCLUDES 1 *swimming pool in private home or garden (Y92.016)*

Y92.39 **Other specified sports and athletic area as the place of occurrence of the external cause**
Golf-course as the place of occurrence of the external cause
Gymnasium as the place of occurrence of the external cause
Riding-school as the place of occurrence of the external cause
Stadium as the place of occurrence of the external cause

5 Y92.4 **Street, highway and other paved roadways as the place of occurrence of the external cause**

EXCLUDES 1 *private driveway of residence (Y92.014, Y92.024, Y92.043, Y92.093, Y92.113, Y92.123, Y92.154, Y92.194)*

6 Y92.41 **Street and highway as the place of occurrence of the external cause**

Y92.410 **Unspecified street and highway as the place of occurrence of the external cause**
Road NOS as the place of occurrence of the external cause

Y92.411 **Interstate highway as the place of occurrence of the external cause**
Freeway as the place of occurrence of the external cause
Motorway as the place of occurrence of the external cause

Y92.412 **Parkway as the place of occurrence of the external cause**

Y92.413 **State road as the place of occurrence of the external cause**

Y92.414 **Local residential or business street as the place of occurrence of the external cause**

Y92.415 **Exit ramp or entrance ramp of street or highway as the place of occurrence of the external cause**

6 Y92.48 **Other paved roadways as the place of occurrence of the external cause**

Y92.480 **Sidewalk as the place of occurrence of the external cause**

Y92.481 **Parking lot as the place of occurrence of the external cause**

Y92.482 **Bike path as the place of occurrence of the external cause**

Y92.488 **Other paved roadways as the place of occurrence of the external cause**

5 **Y92.5** **Trade and service area as the place of occurrence of the external cause**
EXCLUDES 1 *garage in private home (Y92.015)*
schools and other public administration buildings (Y92.2-)

6 **Y92.51** **Private commercial establishments as the place of occurrence of the external cause**

Y92.510 **Bank as the place of occurrence of the external cause**

Y92.511 **Restaurant or café as the place of occurrence of the external cause**

Y92.512 **Supermarket, store or market as the place of occurrence of the external cause**

Y92.513 **Shop (commercial) as the place of occurrence of the external cause**

6 **Y92.52** **Service areas as the place of occurrence of the external cause**

Y92.520 **Airport as the place of occurrence of the external cause**

Y92.521 **Bus station as the place of occurrence of the external cause**

Y92.522 **Railway station as the place of occurrence of the external cause**

Y92.523 **Highway rest stop as the place of occurrence of the external cause**

Y92.524 **Gas station as the place of occurrence of the external cause**
Petroleum station as the place of occurrence of the external cause
Service station as the place of occurrence of the external cause

6 **Y92.53** **Ambulatory health services establishments as the place of occurrence of the external cause**

Y92.530 **Ambulatory surgery center as the place of occurrence of the external cause**
Outpatient surgery center, including that connected with a hospital as the place of occurrence of the external cause
Same day surgery center, including that connected with a hospital as the place of occurrence of the external cause

Y92.531 **Health care provider office as the place of occurrence of the external cause**
Physician office as the place of occurrence of the external cause

Y92.532 **Urgent care center as the place of occurrence of the external cause**

Y92.538 **Other ambulatory health services establishments as the place of occurrence of the external cause**

Y92.59 **Other trade areas as the place of occurrence of the external cause**
Office building as the place of occurrence of the external cause
Casino as the place of occurrence of the external cause
Garage (commercial) as the place of occurrence of the external cause
Hotel as the place of occurrence of the external cause
Radio or television station as the place of occurrence of the external cause
Shopping mall as the place of occurrence of the external cause
Warehouse as the place of occurrence of the external cause

5 **Y92.6** **Industrial and construction area as the place of occurrence of the external cause**

Y92.61 **Building [any] under construction as the place of occurrence of the external cause**

Y92.62 **Dock or shipyard as the place of occurrence of the external cause**
Dockyard as the place of occurrence of the external cause
Dry dock as the place of occurrence of the external cause
Shipyard as the place of occurrence of the external cause

Y92.63 **Factory as the place of occurrence of the external cause**
Factory building as the place of occurrence of the external cause
Factory premises as the place of occurrence of the external cause
Industrial yard as the place of occurrence of the external cause

Y92.64 **Mine or pit as the place of occurrence of the external cause**
Mine as the place of occurrence of the external cause

Y92.65 **Oil rig as the place of occurrence of the external cause**
Pit (coal) (gravel) (sand) as the place of occurrence of the external cause

Y92.69 **Other specified industrial and construction area as the place of occurrence of the external cause**
Gasworks as the place of occurrence of the external cause
Power-station (coal) (nuclear) (oil) as the place of occurrence of the external cause
Tunnel under construction as the place of occurrence of the external cause
Workshop as the place of occurrence of the external cause

5 **Y92.7** **Farm as the place of occurrence of the external cause**
Ranch as the place of occurrence of the external cause
EXCLUDES 1 *farmhouse and home premises of farm (Y92.01-)*

Y92.71 **Barn as the place of occurrence of the external cause**

Y92.72 **Chicken coop as the place of occurrence of the external cause**
Hen house as the place of occurrence of the external cause

Y92.73 **Farm field as the place of occurrence of the external cause**

Y92.74 **Orchard as the place of occurrence of the external cause**

Y92.79 **Other farm location as the place of occurrence of the external cause**

5 **Y92.8** **Other places as the place of occurrence of the external cause**

6 **Y92.81** **Transport vehicle as the place of occurrence of the external cause**
EXCLUDES 1 *transport accidents (V00-V99)*

Y92.810 **Car as the place of occurrence of the external cause**

Y92.811 **Bus as the place of occurrence of the external cause**

Y92.812 **Truck as the place of occurrence of the external cause**

Y92.813 **Airplane as the place of occurrence of the external cause**

Y92.814 **Boat as the place of occurrence of the external cause**

Y92.815 **Train as the place of occurrence of the external cause**

Y92.816 **Subway car as the place of occurrence of the external cause**

Y92.818 **Other transport vehicle as the place of occurrence of the external cause**

6 **Y92.82** **Wilderness area**

Y92.820 **Desert as the place of occurrence of the external cause**

Y92.821 **Forest as the place of occurrence of the external cause**

Y92.828 **Other wilderness area as the place of occurrence of the external cause**
Swamp as the place of occurrence of the external cause
Mountain as the place of occurrence of the external cause
Marsh as the place of occurrence of the external cause
Prairie as the place of occurrence of the external cause

6 **Y92.83** **Recreation area as the place of occurrence of the external cause**

Y92.830 **Public park as the place of occurrence of the external cause**

Y92.831 **Amusement park as the place of occurrence of the external cause**

Y92.832 **Beach as the place of occurrence of the external cause**
Seashore as the place of occurrence of the external cause

Y92.833 **Campsite as the place of occurrence of the external cause**

Y92.834 **Zoological garden (Zoo) as the place of occurrence of the external cause**

Y92.838 **Other recreation area as the place of occurrence of the external cause**

Y92.84 **Military training ground as the place of occurrence of the external cause**

Y92.85 **Railroad track as the place of occurrence of the external cause**

Y92.86 **Slaughter house as the place of occurrence of the external cause**

Y92.89 **Other specified places as the place of occurrence of the external cause**
Derelict house as the place of occurrence of the external cause

Y92.9 **Unspecified place or not applicable**

Y93 Activity codes

Note: Category Y93 is provided for use to indicate the activity of the person seeking healthcare for an injury or health condition, such as a heart attack while shoveling snow, which resulted from, or was contributed to, by the activity. These codes are appropriate for use for both acute injuries, such as those from chapter 19, and conditions that are due to the long-term, cumulative effects of an activity, such as those from chapter 13. They are also appropriate for use with external cause codes for cause and intent if identifying the activity provides additional information on the event. These codes should be used in conjunction with codes for external cause status (Y99) and place of occurrence (Y92).

This section contains the following broad activity categories:
Y93.0 Activities involving walking and running
Y93.1 Activities involving water and water craft
Y93.2 Activities involving ice and snow
Y93.3 Activities involving climbing, rappelling, and jumping off
Y93.4 Activities involving dancing and other rhythmic movement
Y93.5 Activities involving other sports and athletics played individually
Y93.6 Activities involving other sports and athletics played as a team or group
Y93.7 Activities involving other specified sports and athletics
Y93.A Activities involving other cardiorespiratory exercise
Y93.B Activities involving other muscle strengthening exercises
Y93.C Activities involving computer technology and electronic devices
Y93.D Activities involving arts and handcrafts
Y93.E Activities involving personal hygiene and interior property and clothing maintenance
Y93.F Activities involving caregiving
Y93.G Activities involving food preparation, cooking and grilling
Y93.H Activities involving exterior property and land maintenance, building and construction
Y93.I Activities involving roller coasters and other types of external motion
Y93.J Activities involving playing musical instrument
Y93.K Activities involving animal care
Y93.8 Activities, other specified
Y93.9 Activity, unspecified

Y93.0 **Activities involving walking and running**
EXCLUDES 1 *activity, walking an animal (Y93.K1)*
activity, walking or running on a treadmill (Y93.A1)

Y93.01 **Activity, walking, marching and hiking**
Activity, walking, marching and hiking on level or elevated terrain
EXCLUDES 1 *activity, mountain climbing (Y93.31)*

Y93.02 **Activity, running**

Y93.1 **Activities involving water and water craft**
EXCLUDES 1 *activities involving ice (Y93.2-)*

Y93.11 **Activity, swimming**

Y93.12 **Activity, springboard and platform diving**

Y93.13 **Activity, water polo**

Y93.14 **Activity, water aerobics and water exercise**

Y93.15 **Activity, underwater diving and snorkeling**
Activity, SCUBA diving

Y93.16 **Activity, rowing, canoeing, kayaking, rafting and tubing**
Activity, canoeing, kayaking, rafting and tubing in calm and turbulent water

Y93.17 **Activity, water skiing and wake boarding**

Y93.18 **Activity, surfing, windsurfing and boogie boarding**
Activity, water sliding

Y93.19 **Activity, other involving water and watercraft**
Activity involving water NOS
Activity, parasailing
Activity, water survival training and testing

Y93.2 **Activities involving ice and snow**
EXCLUDES 1 *activity, shoveling ice and snow (Y93.H1)*

Y93.21 **Activity, ice skating**
Activity, figure skating (singles) (pairs)
Activity, ice dancing
EXCLUDES 1 *activity, ice hockey (Y93.22)*

Y93.22 **Activity, ice hockey**

▲ Y93.23 **Activity, snow (alpine) (downhill) skiing, snowboarding, sledding, tobogganing and snow tubing**
EXCLUDES 1 *activity, cross country skiing (Y93.24)*

Y93.24 **Activity, cross country skiing**
Activity, nordic skiing

Y93.29 **Activity, other involving ice and snow**
Activity involving ice and snow NOS

Y93.3 **Activities involving climbing, rappelling and jumping off**
EXCLUDES 1 *activity, hiking on level or elevated terrain (Y93.01)*
activity, jumping rope (Y93.56)
activity, trampoline jumping (Y93.44)

Y93.31 **Activity, mountain climbing, rock climbing and wall climbing**

Y93.32 **Activity, rappelling**

Y93.33 **Activity, BASE jumping**
Activity, Building, Antenna, Span, Earth jumping

Y93.34 **Activity, bungee jumping**

Y93.35 **Activity, hang gliding**

Y93.39 **Activity, other involving climbing, rappelling and jumping off**

Y93.4 **Activities involving dancing and other rhythmic movement**
EXCLUDES 1 *activity, martial arts (Y93.75)*

Y93.41 **Activity, dancing**
AHA: 4Q 2012, 108

Y93.42 **Activity, yoga**

Y93.43 **Activity, gymnastics**
Activity, rhythmic gymnastics
EXCLUDES 1 *activity, trampolining (Y93.44)*

Y93.44 **Activity, trampolining**

Y93.45 **Activity, cheerleading**

Y93.49 **Activity, other involving dancing and other rhythmic movements**

Y93.5 **Activities involving other sports and athletics played individually**
EXCLUDES 1 *activity, dancing (Y93.41)*
activity, gymnastic (Y93.43)
activity, trampolining (Y93.44)
activity, yoga (Y93.42)

Y93.51 **Activity, roller skating (inline) and skateboarding**

Y93.52 **Activity, horseback riding**

Y93.53 **Activity, golf**

Y93.54 **Activity, bowling**

Y93.55 **Activity, bike riding**

Y93.56 **Activity, jumping rope**

Y93.57 **Activity, non-running track and field events**
EXCLUDES 1 *activity, running (any form) (Y93.02)*

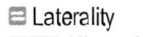

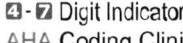

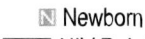

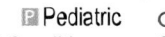

Y93.59 **Activity, other involving other sports and athletics played individually**
EXCLUDES 1 *activities involving climbing, rappelling, and jumping (Y93.3-)*
activities involving ice and snow (Y93.2-)
activities involving walking and running (Y93.0-)
activities involving water and watercraft (Y93.1-)

5 **Y93.6** **Activities involving other sports and athletics played as a team or group**
EXCLUDES 1 *activity, ice hockey (Y93.22)*
activity, water polo (Y93.13)

Y93.61 **Activity, american tackle football**
Activity, football NOS

Y93.62 **Activity, american flag or touch football**

Y93.63 **Activity, rugby**

Y93.64 **Activity, baseball**
Activity, softball

Y93.65 **Activity, lacrosse and field hockey**
AHA: 1Q 2015, 9

Y93.66 **Activity, soccer**

Y93.67 **Activity, basketball**

Y93.68 **Activity, volleyball (beach) (court)**

Y93.6A **Activity, physical games generally associated with school recess, summer camp and children**
Activity, capture the flag
Activity, dodge ball
Activity, four square
Activity, kickball

Y93.69 **Activity, other involving other sports and athletics played as a team or group**
Activity, cricket

5 **Y93.7** **Activities involving other specified sports and athletics**

Y93.71 **Activity, boxing**

Y93.72 **Activity, wrestling**

Y93.73 **Activity, racquet and hand sports**
Activity, handball
Activity, racquetball
Activity, squash
Activity, tennis

Y93.74 **Activity, frisbee**
Activity, ultimate frisbee

Y93.75 **Activity, martial arts**
Activity, combatives

Y93.79 **Activity, other specified sports and athletics**
EXCLUDES 1 *sports and athletics activities specified in categories Y93.0-Y93.6*

5 **Y93.A** **Activities involving other cardiorespiratory exercise**
Activities involving physical training

Y93.A1 **Activity, exercise machines primarily for cardiorespiratory conditioning**
Activity, elliptical and stepper machines
Activity, stationary bike
Activity, treadmill

Y93.A2 **Activity, calisthenics**
Activity, jumping jacks
Activity, warm up and cool down

Y93.A3 **Activity, aerobic and step exercise**

Y93.A4 **Activity, circuit training**

Y93.A5 **Activity, obstacle course**
Activity, challenge course
Activity, confidence course

Y93.A6 **Activity, grass drills**
Activity, guerilla drills

Y93.A9 **Activity, other involving cardiorespiratory exercise**
EXCLUDES 1 *activities involving cardiorespiratory exercise specified in categories Y93.0-Y93.7*

5 **Y93.B** **Activities involving other muscle strengthening exercises**

Y93.B1 **Activity, exercise machines primarily for muscle strengthening**

Y93.B2 **Activity, push-ups, pull-ups, sit-ups**

Y93.B3 **Activity, free weights**
Activity, barbells
Activity, dumbbells

Y93.B4 **Activity, pilates**

Y93.B9 **Activity, other involving muscle strengthening exercises**
EXCLUDES 1 *activities involving muscle strengthening specified in categories Y93.0-Y93.A*

5 **Y93.C** **Activities involving computer technology and electronic devices**
EXCLUDES 1 *activity, electronic musical keyboard or instruments (Y93.J-)*

Y93.C1 **Activity, computer keyboarding**
Activity, electronic game playing using keyboard or other stationary device

Y93.C2 **Activity, hand held interactive electronic device**
Activity, cellular telephone and communication device
Activity, electronic game playing using interactive device
EXCLUDES 1 *activity, electronic game playing using keyboard or other stationary device (Y93.C1)*

Y93.C9 **Activity, other involving computer technology and electronic devices**

5 **Y93.D** **Activities involving arts and handcrafts**
EXCLUDES 1 *activities involving playing musical instrument (Y93.J-)*

Y93.D1 **Activity, knitting and crocheting**

Y93.D2 **Activity, sewing**

Y93.D3 **Activity, furniture building and finishing**
Activity, furniture repair

Y93.D9 **Activity, other involving arts and handcrafts**

5 **Y93.E** **Activities involving personal hygiene and interior property and clothing maintenance**
EXCLUDES 1 *activities involving cooking and grilling (Y93.G-)*
activities involving exterior property and land maintenance, building and construction (Y93.H-)
activities involving caregiving (Y93.F-)
activity, dishwashing (Y93.G1)
activity, food preparation (Y93.G1)
activity, gardening (Y93.H2)

Y93.E1 **Activity, personal bathing and showering**

Y93.E2 **Activity, laundry**

Y93.E3 **Activity, vacuuming**

Y93.E4 **Activity, ironing**

Y93.E5 **Activity, floor mopping and cleaning**

Y93.E6 **Activity, residential relocation**
Activity, packing up and unpacking involved in moving to a new residence

Y93.E8 **Activity, other personal hygiene**

Y93.E9 **Activity, other interior property and clothing maintenance**

5 **Y93.F** **Activities involving caregiving**
Activity involving the provider of caregiving

Y93.F1 **Activity, caregiving, bathing**

Y93.F2 **Activity, caregiving, lifting**

Y93.F9 **Activity, other caregiving**

5 **Y93.G** **Activities involving food preparation, cooking and grilling**

Y93.G1 **Activity, food preparation and clean up**
Activity, dishwashing

Y93.G2 **Activity, grilling and smoking food**

Y93.G3 **Activity, cooking and baking**
Activity, use of stove, oven and microwave oven

Y93.G9 **Activity, other involving cooking and grilling**

5 **Y93.H** **Activities involving exterior property and land maintenance, building and construction**

Y93.H1 **Activity, digging, shoveling and raking**
Activity, dirt digging
Activity, raking leaves
Activity, snow shoveling

Y93.H2 **Activity, gardening and landscaping**
Activity, pruning, trimming shrubs, weeding

Y93.H3 **Activity, building and construction**

Y93.H9 **Activity, other involving exterior property and land maintenance, building and construction**

5 **Y93.I** **Activities involving roller coasters and other types of external motion**

Y93.I1 **Activity, roller coaster riding**

Y93.I9 **Activity, other involving external motion**

5 **Y93.J** **Activities involving playing musical instrument**
Activity involving playing electric musical instrument

Y93.J1 **Activity, piano playing**
Activity, musical keyboard (electronic) playing
Y93.J2 **Activity, drum and other percussion instrument playing**
Y93.J3 **Activity, string instrument playing**
Y93.J4 **Activity, winds and brass instrument playing**
Y93.K **Activities involving animal care**
EXCLUDES 1 *activity, horseback riding (Y93.52)*
Y93.K1 **Activity, walking an animal**
Y93.K2 **Activity, milking an animal**
Y93.K3 **Activity, grooming and shearing an animal**
Y93.K9 **Activity, other involving animal care**
Y93.8 **Activities, other specified**
Y93.81 **Activity, refereeing a sports activity**
Y93.82 **Activity, spectator at an event**
Y93.83 **Activity, rough housing and horseplay**
AHA: 1Q 2015, 8
Y93.84 **Activity, sleeping**
Y93.85 **Activity, choking game**
Activity, blackout game
Activity, fainting game
Activity, pass out game
AHA: 4Q 2016, 74
Y93.89 **Activity, other specified**
Y93.9 **Activity, unspecified**

Y95 Nosocomial condition
AHA: 4Q 2013, 119

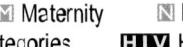

Y99 External cause status
Note: A single code from category Y99 should be used in conjunction with the external cause code(s) assigned to a record to indicate the status of the person at the time the event occurred.
Y99.0 **Civilian activity done for income or pay**
Civilian activity done for financial or other compensation
EXCLUDES 1 *military activity (Y99.1)*
volunteer activity (Y99.2)
Y99.1 **Military activity**
EXCLUDES 1 *activity of off duty military personnel (Y99.8)*
Y99.2 **Volunteer activity**
EXCLUDES 1 *activity of child or other family member assisting in compensated work of other family member (Y99.8)*
Y99.8 **Other external cause status**
Activity NEC
Activity of child or other family member assisting in compensated work of other family member
Hobby not done for income
Leisure activity
Off-duty activity of military personnel
Recreation or sport not for income or while a student
Student activity
EXCLUDES 1 *civilian activity done for income or compensation (Y99.0)*
military activity (Y99.1)
AHA: 4Q 2012, 108
Y99.9 **Unspecified external cause status**

CHAPTER 21: FACTORS INFLUENCING HEALTH STATUS AND CONTACT WITH HEALTH SERVICES (Z00-Z99)

Note: Z codes represent reasons for encounters. A corresponding procedure code must accompany a Z code if a procedure is performed. Categories Z00-Z99 are provided for occasions when circumstances other than a disease, injury or external cause classifiable to categories A00-Y89 are recorded as 'diagnoses' or 'problems'. This can arise in two main ways:
(a) When a person who may or may not be sick encounters the health services for some specific purpose, such as to receive limited care or service for a current condition, to donate an organ or tissue, to receive prophylactic vaccination (immunization), or to discuss a problem which is in itself not a disease or injury.
(b) When some circumstance or problem is present which influences the person's health status but is not in itself a current illness or injury.

GUIDELINES **Section I.C.21.a**
Z codes are for use in any healthcare setting. Z codes may be used as either a first-listed (principal diagnosis code in the inpatient setting) or secondary code, depending on the circumstances of the encounter. Certain Z codes may only be used as first-listed or principal diagnosis.

CODING TIP✓ Aftercare Z codes should not be used for aftercare of injuries. For aftercare of an injury, assign the injury code with the appropriate 7th character, usually "D" if the condition meets the definition of aftercare (patient requires continued care during the healing or recovery phase or long term consequences of the disease/Injury).

This chapter contains the following blocks:

Z00-Z13	Persons encountering health services for examinations
Z14-Z15	Genetic carrier and genetic susceptibility to disease
Z16	Resistance to antimicrobial drugs
Z17	Estrogen receptor status
Z18	Retained foreign body fragments
Z19	Hormone sensitivity malignancy status
Z20-Z29	Persons with potential health hazards related to communicable diseases
Z30-Z39	Persons encountering health services in circumstances related to reproduction
Z40-Z53	Encounters for other specific health care
Z55-Z65	Persons with potential health hazards related to socioeconomic and psychosocial circumstances
Z66	Do not resuscitate status
Z67	Blood type
Z68	Body mass index (BMI)
Z69-Z76	Persons encountering health services in other circumstances
Z77-Z99	Persons with potential health hazards related to family and personal history and certain conditions influencing health status

Persons encountering health services for examinations (Z00-Z13)

Note: Nonspecific abnormal findings disclosed at the time of these examinations are classified to categories R70-R94.

EXCLUDES 1 *examinations related to pregnancy and reproduction (Z30-Z36, Z39.-)*

④ Z00 Encounter for general examination without complaint, suspected or reported diagnosis

EXCLUDES 1 *encounter for examination for administrative purposes (Z02.-)*

EXCLUDES 2 *encounter for pre-procedural examinations (Z01.81-)*
special screening examinations (Z11-Z13)

⑤ Z00.0 Encounter for general adult medical examination
Encounter for adult periodic examination (annual) (physical) and any associated laboratory and radiologic examinations

EXCLUDES 1 *encounter for examination of sign or symptom- code to sign or symptom*
general health check-up of infant or child (Z00.12.-)

Z00.00 Encounter for general adult medical examination without abnormal findings Ⓐ
Encounter for adult health check-up NOS
AHA: 1Q 2016, 36-37

Z00.01 Encounter for general adult medical examination with abnormal findings Ⓐ
Use additional code to identify abnormal findings
AHA: 1Q 2016, 35, 36

⑤ Z00.1 Encounter for newborn, infant and child health examinations

⑥ Z00.11 Newborn health examination
Health check for child under 29 days old
Use additional code to identify any abnormal findings

EXCLUDES 1 *health check for child over 28 days old (Z00.12-)*

Z00.110 Health examination for newborn under 8 days old Ⓝ
Health check for newborn under 8 days old

Z00.111 Health examination for newborn 8 to 28 days old Ⓝ
Health check for newborn 8 to 28 days old
Newborn weight check

▲⑥ Z00.12 Encounter for routine child health examination
Health check (routine) for child over 28 days old
Immunizations appropriate for age
Routine developmental screening of infant or child
Routine vision and hearing testing

EXCLUDES 1 *health check for child under 29 days old (Z00.11-)*
health supervision of foundling or other healthy infant or child (Z76.1-Z76.2)
newborn health examination (Z00.11-)

Z00.121 Encounter for routine child health examination with abnormal findings Ⓟ
Use additional code to identify abnormal findings
AHA: 1Q 2016, 34, 35

Z00.129 Encounter for routine child health examination without abnormal findings Ⓟ
Encounter for routine child health examination NOS
AHA: 1Q 2016, 34-35

Z00.2 Encounter for examination for period of rapid growth in childhood Ⓟ

Z00.3 Encounter for examination for adolescent development state Ⓟ
Encounter for puberty development state

Z00.5 Encounter for examination of potential donor of organ and tissue

Z00.6 Encounter for examination for normal comparison and control in clinical research program
Examination of participant or control in clinical research program

⑤ Z00.7 Encounter for examination for period of delayed growth in childhood

Z00.70 Encounter for examination for period of delayed growth in childhood without abnormal findings Ⓟ

Z00.71 Encounter for examination for period of delayed growth in childhood with abnormal findings Ⓟ
Use additional code to identify abnormal findings

Z00.8 Encounter for other general examination
Encounter for health examination in population surveys

④ Z01 Encounter for other special examination without complaint, suspected or reported diagnosis
Note: Codes from category Z01 represent the reason for the encounter. A separate procedure code is required to identify any examinations or procedures performed

INCLUDES routine examination of specific system

EXCLUDES 1 *encounter for examination for administrative purposes (Z02.)*
encounter for examination for suspected conditions, proven not to exist (Z03.-)
encounter for laboratory and radiologic examinations as a component of general medical examinations (Z00.0-)
encounter for laboratory, radiologic and imaging examinations for sign (s) and symptom(s) - code to the sign(s) or symptom(s)

EXCLUDES 2 *screening examinations (Z11-Z13)*

⑤ Z01.0 Encounter for examination of eyes and vision

EXCLUDES 1 *examination for driving license (Z02.4)*

Z01.00 Encounter for examination of eyes and vision without abnormal findings
Encounter for examination of eyes and vision NOS

Z01.01 Encounter for examination of eyes and vision with abnormal findings
Use additional code to identify abnormal findings

⑤ Z01.1 Encounter for examination of ears and hearing

Z01.10 Encounter for examination of ears and hearing without abnormal findings
Encounter for examination of ears and hearing NOS

6 **Z01.11 Encounter for examination of ears and hearing with abnormal findings**

Z01.110 Encounter for hearing examination following failed hearing screening
AHA: 3Q 2016, 17
AHA: 3Q 2016, 18

Z01.118 Encounter for examination of ears and hearing with other abnormal findings
Use additional code to identify abnormal findings
AHA: 3Q 2016, 17

Z01.12 Encounter for hearing conservation and treatment

5 **Z01.2 Encounter for dental examination and cleaning**

Z01.20 Encounter for dental examination and cleaning without abnormal findings
Encounter for dental examination and cleaning NOS

Z01.21 Encounter for dental examination and cleaning with abnormal findings
Use additional code to identify abnormal findings

5 **Z01.3 Encounter for examination of blood pressure**

Z01.30 Encounter for examination of blood pressure without abnormal findings
Encounter for examination of blood pressure NOS

Z01.31 Encounter for examination of blood pressure with abnormal findings
Use additional code to identify abnormal findings

5 **Z01.4 Encounter for gynecological examination**
EXCLUDES 2 *pregnancy examination or test (Z32.0-)*
routine examination for contraceptive maintenance (Z30.4-)

6 **Z01.41 Encounter for routine gynecological examination**
Encounter for general gynecological examination with or without cervical smear
Encounter for gynecological examination (general) (routine) NOS
Encounter for pelvic examination (annual) (periodic)
Use additional code:
for screening for human papillomavirus, if applicable, (Z11.51)
for screening vaginal pap smear, if applicable (Z12.72)
to identify acquired absence of uterus, if applicable (Z90.71-)
EXCLUDES 1 *gynecologic examination status-post hysterectomy for malignant condition (Z08)*
screening cervical pap smear not a part of a routine gynecological examination (Z12.4)

Z01.411 Encounter for gynecological examination (general) (routine) with abnormal findings ♀
Use additional code to identify abnormal findings

Z01.419 Encounter for gynecological examination (general) (routine) without abnormal findings ♀

Z01.42 Encounter for cervical smear to confirm findings of recent normal smear following initial abnormal smear ♀

5 **Z01.8 Encounter for other specified special examinations**

6 **Z01.81 Encounter for preprocedural examinations**
Encounter for preoperative examinations
Encounter for radiological and imaging examinations as part of preprocedural examination

Z01.810 Encounter for preprocedural cardiovascular examination

Z01.811 Encounter for preprocedural respiratory examination

Z01.812 Encounter for preprocedural laboratory examination
Blood and urine tests prior to treatment or procedure

Z01.818 Encounter for other preprocedural examination
Encounter for preprocedural examination NOS
Encounter for examinations prior to antineoplastic chemotherapy

Z01.82 Encounter for allergy testing
EXCLUDES 1 *encounter for antibody response examination (Z01.84)*

Z01.83 Encounter for blood typing
Encounter for Rh typing

Z01.84 Encounter for antibody response examination
Encounter for immunity status testing
EXCLUDES 1 *encounter for allergy testing (Z01.82)*

Z01.89 Encounter for other specified special examinations

4 **Z02 Encounter for administrative examination**

Z02.0 Encounter for examination for admission to educational institution
Encounter for examination for admission to preschool (education)
Encounter for examination for re-admission to school following illness or medical treatment

Z02.1 Encounter for pre-employment examination

Z02.2 Encounter for examination for admission to residential institution
EXCLUDES 1 *examination for admission to prison (Z02.89)*

Z02.3 Encounter for examination for recruitment to armed forces

Z02.4 Encounter for examination for driving license

Z02.5 Encounter for examination for participation in sport
EXCLUDES 1 *blood-alcohol and blood-drug test (Z02.83)*

Z02.6 Encounter for examination for insurance purposes

▲ 5 **Z02.7 Encounter for issue of medical certificate**
EXCLUDES 1 *encounter for general medical examination (Z00-Z01, Z02.0-Z02.6, Z02.8-Z02.9)*

Z02.71 Encounter for disability determination
Encounter for issue of medical certificate of incapacity
Encounter for issue of medical certificate of invalidity

Z02.79 Encounter for issue of other medical certificate

5 **Z02.8 Encounter for other administrative examinations**

Z02.81 Encounter for paternity testing

Z02.82 Encounter for adoption services

Z02.83 Encounter for blood-alcohol and blood-drug test
Use additional code for findings of alcohol or drugs in blood (R78.-)

Z02.89 Encounter for other administrative examinations
Encounter for examination for admission to prison
Encounter for examination for admission to summer camp
Encounter for immigration examination
Encounter for naturalization examination
Encounter for premarital examination
EXCLUDES 1 *health supervision of foundling or other healthy infant or child (Z76.1-Z76.2)*

Z02.9 Encounter for administrative examinations, unspecified

▲ 4 **Z03 Encounter for medical observation for suspected diseases and conditions ruled out**
This category is to be used when a person without a diagnosis is suspected of having an abnormal condition, without signs or symptoms, which requires study, but after examination and observation, is ruled out. This category is also for use for administrative and legal observation status.
EXCLUDES 1 *contact with and (suspected) exposures hazardous to health (Z77.-)*
encounter for observation and evaluation of newborn for suspected diseases and conditions ruled out (Z05.-)
person with feared complaint in whom no diagnosis is made (Z71.1)
signs or symptoms under study- code to signs or symptoms
AHA: 4Q 2017, 20

Z03.6 Encounter for observation for suspected toxic effect from ingested substance ruled out
Encounter for observation for suspected adverse effect from drug
Encounter for observation for suspected poisoning

Z03.7 **Encounter for suspected maternal and fetal conditions ruled out**
Encounter for suspected maternal and fetal conditions not found
EXCLUDES 1 *known or suspected fetal anomalies affecting management of mother, not ruled out (O26.-, O35.-, O36.-, O40.-, O41.-)*

Z03.71 **Encounter for suspected problem with amniotic cavity and membrane ruled out** ♀ M
Encounter for suspected oligohydramnios ruled out
Encounter for suspected polyhydramnios ruled out

Z03.72 **Encounter for suspected placental problem ruled out** ♀ M

Z03.73 **Encounter for suspected fetal anomaly ruled out** ♀ M

Z03.74 **Encounter for suspected problem with fetal growth ruled out** ♀ M

Z03.75 **Encounter for suspected cervical shortening ruled out** ♀ M

Z03.79 **Encounter for other suspected maternal and fetal conditions ruled out** ♀ M

Z03.8 **Encounter for observation for other suspected diseases and conditions ruled out**

Z03.81 **Encounter for observation for suspected exposure to biological agents ruled out**

Z03.810 **Encounter for observation for suspected exposure to anthrax ruled out**

Z03.818 **Encounter for observation for suspected exposure to other biological agents ruled out**

Z03.89 **Encounter for observation for other suspected diseases and conditions ruled out**

Z04 Encounter for examination and observation for other reasons

INCLUDES encounter for examination for medicolegal reasons
This category is to be used when a person without a diagnosis is suspected of having an abnormal condition, without signs or symptoms, which requires study, but after examination and observation, is ruled-out. This category is also for use for administrative and legal observation status.

Z04.1 **Encounter for examination and observation following transport accident**
EXCLUDES 1 *encounter for examination and observation following work accident (Z04.2)*
AHA: 2Q 2018, 6

Z04.2 **Encounter for examination and observation following work accident**

Z04.3 **Encounter for examination and observation following other accident**
AHA: 2Q 2018, 6

Z04.4 **Encounter for examination and observation following alleged rape**
Encounter for examination and observation of victim following alleged rape
Encounter for examination and observation of victim following alleged sexual abuse

Z04.41 **Encounter for examination and observation following alleged adult rape** A
Suspected adult rape, ruled out
Suspected adult sexual abuse, ruled out

Z04.42 **Encounter for examination and observation following alleged child rape** P
Suspected child rape, ruled out
Suspected child sexual abuse, ruled out

Z04.6 **Encounter for general psychiatric examination, requested by authority**

Z04.7 **Encounter for examination and observation following alleged physical abuse**

Z04.71 **Encounter for examination and observation following alleged adult physical abuse** A
Suspected adult physical abuse, ruled out
EXCLUDES 1 *confirmed case of adult physical abuse (T74.-)*
encounter for examination and observation following alleged adult sexual abuse (Z04.41)
suspected case of adult physical abuse, not ruled out (T76.-)

Z04.72 **Encounter for examination and observation following alleged child physical abuse** P
Suspected child physical abuse, ruled out
EXCLUDES 1 *confirmed case of child physical abuse (T74.-)*
encounter for examination and observation following alleged child sexual abuse (Z04.42)
suspected case of child physical abuse, not ruled out (T76.-)

▲ Z04.8 **Encounter for examination and observation for other specified reasons**
Encounter for examination and observation for request for expert evidence

● Z04.81 **Encounter for examination and observation of victim following forced sexual exploitation**

● Z04.82 **Encounter for examination and observation of victim following forced labor exploitation**

● Z04.89 **Encounter for examination and observation for other specified reasons**

Z04.9 **Encounter for examination and observation for unspecified reason**
Encounter for observation NOS

Z05 Encounter for observation and evaluation of newborn for suspected diseases and conditions ruled out

This category is to be used for newborns, within the neonatal period (the first 28 days of life), who are suspected of having an abnormal condition, but without signs or symptoms, and which, after examination and observation, is ruled out.

Z05.0 **Observation and evaluation of newborn for suspected cardiac condition ruled out** N

Z05.1 **Observation and evaluation of newborn for suspected infectious condition ruled out** N

Z05.2 **Observation and evaluation of newborn for suspected neurological condition ruled out** N

Z05.3 **Observation and evaluation of newborn for suspected respiratory condition ruled out** N

Z05.4 **Observation and evaluation of newborn for suspected genetic, metabolic or immunologic condition ruled out**

Z05.41 **Observation and evaluation of newborn for suspected genetic condition ruled out** N

Z05.42 **Observation and evaluation of newborn for suspected metabolic condition ruled out** N

Z05.43 **Observation and evaluation of newborn for suspected immunologic condition ruled out** N

Z05.5 **Observation and evaluation of newborn for suspected gastrointestinal condition ruled out** N

Z05.6 **Observation and evaluation of newborn for suspected genitourinary condition ruled out** N

Z05.7 **Observation and evaluation of newborn for suspected skin, subcutaneous, musculoskeletal and connective tissue condition ruled out**

Z05.71 **Observation and evaluation of newborn for suspected skin and subcutaneous tissue condition ruled out** N

Z05.72 **Observation and evaluation of newborn for suspected musculoskeletal condition ruled out** N

Z05.73 **Observation and evaluation of newborn for suspected connective tissue condition ruled out** N

Z05.8 **Observation and evaluation of newborn for other specified suspected condition ruled out** N

Z05.9 **Observation and evaluation of newborn for unspecified suspected condition ruled out** N

Z08 Encounter for follow-up examination after completed treatment for malignant neoplasm

Medical surveillance following completed treatment
Use additional code to identify any acquired absence of organs (Z90.-)
Use additional code to identify the personal history of malignant neoplasm (Z85.-)
EXCLUDES 1 *aftercare following medical care (Z43-Z49, Z51)*

Z09 Encounter for follow-up examination after completed treatment for conditions other than malignant neoplasm

Medical surveillance following completed treatment

Use additional code to identify any applicable history of disease code (Z86.-, Z87.-)

EXCLUDES 1 *aftercare following medical care (Z43-Z49, Z51)*
surveillance of contraception (Z30.4-)
surveillance of prosthetic and other medical devices (Z44-Z46)

GUIDELINES **Section 1.C.21.c.8**

The follow-up codes are used to explain continuing surveillance following completed treatment of a disease, condition, or injury. They imply that the condition has been fully treated and no longer exists. They should not be confused with aftercare codes, or injury codes with a 7th character for subsequent encounter, that explain ongoing care of a healing condition or its sequelae. Follow-up codes may be used in conjunction with history codes to provide the full picture of the healed condition and its treatment. The follow-up code is sequenced first, followed by the history code.

AHA: 1Q 2015, 8
AHA: 1Q 2017, 8

4 **Z11 Encounter for screening for infectious and parasitic diseases**

Screening is the testing for disease or disease precursors in asymptomatic individuals so that early detection and treatment can be provided for those who test positive for the disease.

EXCLUDES 1 *encounter for diagnostic examination-code to sign or symptom*

Z11.0 Encounter for screening for intestinal infectious diseases

Z11.1 Encounter for screening for respiratory tuberculosis

Z11.2 Encounter for screening for other bacterial diseases

Z11.3 Encounter for screening for infections with a predominantly sexual mode of transmission

EXCLUDES 2 *encounter for screening for human immunodeficiency virus [HIV] (Z11.4)*
encounter for screening for human papillomavirus (Z11.51)

Z11.4 Encounter for screening for human immunodeficiency virus [HIV]

5 **Z11.5 Encounter for screening for other viral diseases**

EXCLUDES 2 *encounter for screening for viral intestinal disease (Z11.0)*

Z11.51 Encounter for screening for human papillomavirus (HPV)

Z11.59 Encounter for screening for other viral diseases

Z11.6 Encounter for screening for other protozoal diseases and helminthiases

EXCLUDES 2 *encounter for screening for protozoal intestinal disease (Z11.0)*

Z11.8 Encounter for screening for other infectious and parasitic diseases

Encounter for screening for chlamydia
Encounter for screening for rickettsial
Encounter for screening for spirochetal
Encounter for screening for mycoses

Z11.9 Encounter for screening for infectious and parasitic diseases, unspecified

4 **Z12 Encounter for screening for malignant neoplasms**

Screening is the testing for disease or disease precursors in asymptomatic individuals so that early detection and treatment can be provided for those who test positive for the disease.

Use additional code to identify any family history of malignant neoplasm (Z80.-)

EXCLUDES 1 *encounter for diagnostic examination-code to sign or symptom*

Z12.0 Encounter for screening for malignant neoplasm of stomach

5 **Z12.1 Encounter for screening for malignant neoplasm of intestinal tract**

Z12.10 Encounter for screening for malignant neoplasm of intestinal tract, unspecified

Z12.11 Encounter for screening for malignant neoplasm of colon

Encounter for screening colonoscopy NOS

AHA: 1Q 2017, 8

Z12.12 Encounter for screening for malignant neoplasm of rectum

Z12.13 Encounter for screening for malignant neoplasm of small intestine

Z12.2 Encounter for screening for malignant neoplasm of respiratory organs

5 **Z12.3 Encounter for screening for malignant neoplasm of breast**

Z12.31 Encounter for screening mammogram for malignant neoplasm of breast

EXCLUDES 1 *inconclusive mammogram (R92.2)*

AHA: 1Q 2015, 24

Z12.39 Encounter for other screening for malignant neoplasm of breast

Z12.4 Encounter for screening for malignant neoplasm of cervix ♀

Encounter for screening pap smear for malignant neoplasm of cervix

EXCLUDES 1 *when screening is part of general gynecological examination (Z01.4-)*

EXCLUDES 2 *encounter for screening for human papillomavirus (Z11.51)*

Z12.5 Encounter for screening for malignant neoplasm of prostate ♂

Z12.6 Encounter for screening for malignant neoplasm of bladder

5 **Z12.7 Encounter for screening for malignant neoplasm of other genitourinary organs**

Z12.71 Encounter for screening for malignant neoplasm of testis ♂

Z12.72 Encounter for screening for malignant neoplasm of vagina ♀

Vaginal pap smear status-post hysterectomy for non-malignant condition

Use additional code to identify acquired absence of uterus (Z90.71-)

EXCLUDES 1 *vaginal pap smear status-post hysterectomy for malignant conditions (Z08)*

Z12.73 Encounter for screening for malignant neoplasm of ovary ♀

Z12.79 Encounter for screening for malignant neoplasm of other genitourinary organs

5 **Z12.8 Encounter for screening for malignant neoplasm of other sites**

Z12.81 Encounter for screening for malignant neoplasm of oral cavity

Z12.82 Encounter for screening for malignant neoplasm of nervous system

Z12.83 Encounter for screening for malignant neoplasm of skin

Z12.89 Encounter for screening for malignant neoplasm of other sites

Z12.9 Encounter for screening for malignant neoplasm, site unspecified

4 **Z13 Encounter for screening for other diseases and disorders**

Screening is the testing for disease or disease precursors in asymptomatic individuals so that early detection and treatment can be provided for those who test positive for the disease.

EXCLUDES 1 *encounter for diagnostic examination-code to sign or symptom*

Z13.0 Encounter for screening for diseases of the blood and blood-forming organs and certain disorders involving the immune mechanism

Z13.1 Encounter for screening for diabetes mellitus

5 **Z13.2 Encounter for screening for nutritional, metabolic and other endocrine disorders**

Z13.21 Encounter for screening for nutritional disorder

6 **Z13.22 Encounter for screening for metabolic disorder**

Z13.220 Encounter for screening for lipoid disorders

Encounter for screening for cholesterol level
Encounter for screening for hypercholesterolemia
Encounter for screening for hyperlipidemia

Z13.228 Encounter for screening for other metabolic disorders

Z13.29 Encounter for screening for other suspected endocrine disorder

EXCLUDES 1 *encounter for screening for diabetes mellitus (Z13.1)*

● 5 **Z13.3 Encounter for screening examination for mental health and behavioral disorders**

● **Z13.30 Encounter for screening examination for mental health and behavioral disorders, unspecified**

● **Z13.31 Encounter for screening for depression**
Encounter for screening for depression, adult
Encounter for screening for depression for child or adolescent

● **Z13.32 Encounter for screening for maternal depression** ♀
Encounter for screening for perinatal depression

● **Z13.39 Encounter for screening examination for other mental health and behavioral disorders**
Encounter for screening for alcoholism
Encounter for screening for intellectual disabilities

▲ 5 **Z13.4 Encounter for screening for certain developmental disorders in childhood**
Encounter for development testing of infant or child
Encounter for screening for developmental handicaps in early childhood
EXCLUDES 2 *encounter for routine child health examination (Z00.12-)*

● **Z13.40 Encounter for screening for unspecified developmental delays**

● **Z13.41 Encounter for autism screening**

● **Z13.42 Encounter for screening for global developmental delays (milestones)**
Encounter for screening for developmental handicaps in early childhood

● **Z13.49 Encounter for screening for other developmental delays**

Z13.5 Encounter for screening for eye and ear disorders
EXCLUDES 2 *encounter for general hearing examination (Z01.1-)*
encounter for general vision examination (Z01.0-)
AHA: 3Q 2016, 17
AHA: 3Q 2016, 17
AHA: 3Q 2016, 18

Z13.6 Encounter for screening for cardiovascular disorders

5 **Z13.7 Encounter for screening for genetic and chromosomal anomalies**
EXCLUDES 1 *genetic testing for procreative management (Z31.4-)*

Z13.71 Encounter for nonprocreative screening for genetic disease carrier status

Z13.79 Encounter for other screening for genetic and chromosomal anomalies

5 **Z13.8 Encounter for screening for other specified diseases and disorders**
EXCLUDES 2 *screening for malignant neoplasms (Z12.-)*

6 **Z13.81 Encounter for screening for digestive system disorders**

Z13.810 Encounter for screening for upper gastrointestinal disorder

Z13.811 Encounter for screening for lower gastrointestinal disorder
EXCLUDES 1 *encounter for screening for intestinal infectious disease (Z11.0)*

Z13.818 Encounter for screening for other digestive system disorders

6 **Z13.82 Encounter for screening for musculoskeletal disorder**

Z13.820 Encounter for screening for osteoporosis

Z13.828 Encounter for screening for other musculoskeletal disorder

Z13.83 Encounter for screening for respiratory disorder NEC
EXCLUDES 1 *encounter for screening for respiratory tuberculosis (Z11.1)*

Z13.84 Encounter for screening for dental disorders

6 **Z13.85 Encounter for screening for nervous system disorders**

Z13.850 Encounter for screening for traumatic brain injury

Z13.858 Encounter for screening for other nervous system disorders

Z13.88 Encounter for screening for disorder due to exposure to contaminants
EXCLUDES 1 *those exposed to contaminants without suspected disorders (Z57.-, Z77.-)*

Z13.89 Encounter for screening for other disorder
Encounter for screening for genitourinary disorders

Z13.9 Encounter for screening, unspecified

Genetic carrier and genetic susceptibility to disease (Z14-Z15)

4 **Z14 Genetic carrier**

5 **Z14.0 Hemophilia A carrier**

Z14.01 Asymptomatic hemophilia A carrier

Z14.02 Symptomatic hemophilia A carrier

Z14.1 Cystic fibrosis carrier

Z14.8 Genetic carrier of other disease

4 **Z15 Genetic susceptibility to disease**
INCLUDES confirmed abnormal gene
Use additional code, if applicable, for any associated family history of the disease (Z80-Z84)
EXCLUDES 1 *chromosomal anomalies (Q90-Q99)*

GUIDELINES Section I.C.21.c.3)
Codes from category Z15 should not be used as principal or first-listed codes. If the patient has the condition to which he/she is susceptible, and that condition is the reason for the encounter, the code for the current condition should be sequenced first.

5 **Z15.0 Genetic susceptibility to malignant neoplasm**
Code first:
, if applicable, any current malignant neoplasm (C00-C75, C81-C96)
Use additional code, if applicable, for any personal history of malignant neoplasm (Z85.-)

Z15.01 Genetic susceptibility to malignant neoplasm of breast
CODING TIP✓ Assign Z15.01 for a patient who has prophylactic breast removal due to genetic susceptibility to breast cancer.

Z15.02 Genetic susceptibility to malignant neoplasm of ovary ♀

Z15.03 Genetic susceptibility to malignant neoplasm of prostate ♂

Z15.04 Genetic susceptibility to malignant neoplasm of endometrium ♀

Z15.09 Genetic susceptibility to other malignant neoplasm

5 **Z15.8 Genetic susceptibility to other disease**

Z15.81 Genetic susceptibility to multiple endocrine neoplasia [MEN]
EXCLUDES 1 *multiple endocrine neoplasia [MEN] syndromes (E31.2-)*

Z15.89 Genetic susceptibility to other disease

Resistance to antimicrobial drugs (Z16)

4 **Z16 Resistance to antimicrobial drugs**
Note: The codes in this category are provided for use as additional codes to identify the resistance and non-responsiveness of a condition to antimicrobial drugs.
Code first:
the infection
EXCLUDES 1 *Methicillin resistant Staphylococcus aureus infection (A49.02)*
Methicillin resistant Staphylococcus aureus pneumonia (J15.212)
Sepsis due to Methicillin resistant Staphylococcus aureus (A41.02)

GUIDELINES Section I.C.1.c
Many bacterial infections are resistant to current antibiotics. It is necessary to identify all infections documented as antibiotic resistant. Assign a code from category Z16, Resistance to antimicrobial drugs, following the infection code only if the infection code does not identify drug resistance.

5 **Z16.1 Resistance to beta lactam antibiotics**

Z16.10 Resistance to unspecified beta lactam antibiotics

Z16.11 **Resistance to penicillins**
Resistance to amoxicillin
Resistance to ampicillin

GUIDELINES **Section I.C.e.1)(a)**
When a patient is diagnosed with an infection that is due to methicillin resistant Staphylococcus aureus (MRSA), and that infection has a combination code that includes the causal organism (e.g., sepsis, pneumonia) assign the appropriate combination code for the condition.

Do not assign code B95.62, MRSA infection as the cause of diseases classified elsewhere, as an additional code, because the combination code includes the type of infection and the MRSA organism. Do not assign a code from subcategory Z16.11, Resistance to penicillins, as an additional diagnosis.

Z16.12 **Extended spectrum beta lactamase (ESBL) resistance**
EXCLUDES 2 *Methicillin resistant Staphylococcus aureus infection in diseases classified elsewhere (B95.62)*

Z16.19 **Resistance to other specified beta lactam antibiotics**
Resistance to cephalosporins

5 **Z16.2** **Resistance to other antibiotics**

Z16.20 **Resistance to unspecified antibiotic**
Resistance to antibiotics NOS

Z16.21 **Resistance to vancomycin**

Z16.22 **Resistance to vancomycin related antibiotics**

Z16.23 **Resistance to quinolones and fluoroquinolones**

Z16.24 **Resistance to multiple antibiotics**

Z16.29 **Resistance to other single specified antibiotic**
Resistance to aminoglycosides
Resistance to macrolides
Resistance to sulfonamides
Resistance to tetracyclines

5 **Z16.3** **Resistance to other antimicrobial drugs**
EXCLUDES 1 *resistance to antibiotics (Z16.1-, Z16.2-)*

Z16.30 **Resistance to unspecified antimicrobial drugs**
Drug resistance NOS

Z16.31 **Resistance to antiparasitic drug(s)**
Resistance to quinine and related compounds

Z16.32 **Resistance to antifungal drug(s)**

Z16.33 **Resistance to antiviral drug(s)**

6 **Z16.34** **Resistance to antimycobacterial drug(s)**
Resistance to tuberculostatics

Z16.341 **Resistance to single antimycobacterial drug**
Resistance to antimycobacterial drug NOS

Z16.342 **Resistance to multiple antimycobacterial drugs**

Z16.35 **Resistance to multiple antimicrobial drugs**
EXCLUDES 1 *Resistance to multiple antibiotics only (Z16.24)*

Z16.39 **Resistance to other specified antimicrobial drug**

Estrogen receptor status (Z17)

4 **Z17** **Estrogen receptor status**
Code first:
malignant neoplasm of breast (C50.-)

CODING TIP✓ When a patient has breast cancer and the estrogen receptor status is specified, the appropriate code from category Z17 should be assigned to indicate the ER positive or negative status. Breast cancers that are ER+ may be treated with selective estrogen receptor modulators (SERMs). When SERM therapy is also present in an ER+ breast cancer patient, an additional Z code may be assigned to identify SERM therapy (Z79.810).

Z17.0 **Estrogen receptor positive status [ER+]**

Z17.1 **Estrogen receptor negative status [ER-]**

Retained foreign body fragments (Z18)

4 **Z18** **Retained foreign body fragments**
INCLUDES embedded fragment (status)
embedded splinter (status)
retained foreign body status
EXCLUDES 1 *artificial joint prosthesis status (Z96.6-)*
foreign body accidentally left during a procedure (T81.5-)
foreign body entering through orifice (T15-T19)
in situ cardiac device (Z95.-)
organ or tissue replaced by means other than transplant (Z96.-, Z97.-)
organ or tissue replaced by transplant (Z94.-)
personal history of retained foreign body fully removed Z87.821
superficial foreign body (non-embedded splinter) - code to superficial foreign body, by site

5 **Z18.0** **Retained radioactive fragments**

Z18.01 **Retained depleted uranium fragments**

Z18.09 **Other retained radioactive fragments**
Other retained depleted isotope fragments
Retained nontherapeutic radioactive fragments

5 **Z18.1** **Retained metal fragments**
EXCLUDES 1 *retained radioactive metal fragments (Z18.01-Z18.09)*

Z18.10 **Retained metal fragments, unspecified**
Retained metal fragment NOS

Z18.11 **Retained magnetic metal fragments**

Z18.12 **Retained nonmagnetic metal fragments**

▲ **Z18.2** **Retained plastic fragments**
Acrylics fragments
Diethylhexyl phthalates fragments
Isocyanate fragments

5 **Z18.3** **Retained organic fragments**

Z18.31 **Retained animal quills or spines**

Z18.32 **Retained tooth**

Z18.33 **Retained wood fragments**

Z18.39 **Other retained organic fragments**

5 **Z18.8** **Other specified retained foreign body**

Z18.81 **Retained glass fragments**

Z18.83 **Retained stone or crystalline fragments**
Retained concrete or cement fragments

Z18.89 **Other specified retained foreign body fragments**
AHA: 3Q 2016, 23
AHA: 3Q 2016, 24

Z18.9 **Retained foreign body fragments, unspecified material**

Hormone sensitivity malignancy status (Z19)

4 **Z19** **Hormone sensitivity malignancy status**
Code first:
malignant neoplasm - see Table of Neoplasms, by site, malignant

Z19.1 **Hormone sensitive malignancy status**
DEFINITION Identifies cancers that are known to be hormone dependent and for which the use of hormone therapy drugs in treatment is effective.

Z19.2 **Hormone resistant malignancy status**
Castrate resistant prostate malignancy status

Persons with potential health hazards related to communicable diseases (Z20-Z29)

4 **Z20** **Contact with and (suspected) exposure to communicable diseases**
EXCLUDES 1 *carrier of infectious disease (Z22.-)*
diagnosed current infectious or parasitic disease -see Alphabetic Index
EXCLUDES 2 *personal history of infectious and parasitic diseases (Z86.1-)*

GUIDELINES Section I.C.21.c.1)
Category Z20 indicates contact with, and suspected exposure to, communicable diseases. These codes are for patients who do not show any sign or symptom of a disease but are suspected to have been exposed to it by close personal contact with an infected individual or are in an area where a disease is epidemic. Category Z77 indicates contact with and suspected exposures hazardous to health.

Contact/exposure codes may be used as a first-listed code to explain an encounter for testing, or, more commonly, as a secondary code to identify a potential risk.

5 **Z20.0 Contact with and (suspected) exposure to intestinal infectious diseases**

Z20.01 Contact with and (suspected) exposure to intestinal infectious diseases due to Escherichia coli (E. coli)

Z20.09 Contact with and (suspected) exposure to other intestinal infectious diseases

Z20.1 Contact with and (suspected) exposure to tuberculosis

Z20.2 Contact with and (suspected) exposure to infections with a predominantly sexual mode of transmission

Z20.3 Contact with and (suspected) exposure to rabies

Z20.4 Contact with and (suspected) exposure to rubella

Z20.5 Contact with and (suspected) exposure to viral hepatitis

Z20.6 Contact with and (suspected) exposure to human immunodeficiency virus [HIV]

EXCLUDES 1 *asymptomatic human immunodeficiency virus [HIV]*
HIV infection status (Z21)

Z20.7 Contact with and (suspected) exposure to pediculosis, acariasis and other infestations

5 **Z20.8 Contact with and (suspected) exposure to other communicable diseases**

6 **Z20.81 Contact with and (suspected) exposure to other bacterial communicable diseases**

Z20.810 Contact with and (suspected) exposure to anthrax

Z20.811 Contact with and (suspected) exposure to meningococcus

Z20.818 Contact with and (suspected) exposure to other bacterial communicable diseases

6 **Z20.82 Contact with and (suspected) exposure to other viral communicable diseases**

Z20.820 Contact with and (suspected) exposure to varicella

● **Z20.821 Contact with and (suspected) exposure to Zika virus**

Z20.828 Contact with and (suspected) exposure to other viral communicable diseases

Z20.89 Contact with and (suspected) exposure to other communicable diseases

Z20.9 Contact with and (suspected) exposure to unspecified communicable disease

Z21 Asymptomatic human immunodeficiency virus [HIV] infection status HCC

HIV positive NOS

Code first:

Human immunodeficiency virus [HIV] disease complicating pregnancy, childbirth and the puerperium, if applicable (O98.7-)

EXCLUDES 1 *acquired immunodeficiency syndrome (B20)*
contact with human immunodeficiency virus [HIV] (Z20.6)
exposure to human immunodeficiency virus [HIV] (Z20.6)
human immunodeficiency virus [HIV] disease (B20)
inconclusive laboratory evidence of human immunodeficiency virus [HIV] (R75)

GUIDELINES Section I.C.1.a.2)(f)
Patients previously diagnosed with any HIV illness (B20) should never be assigned to R75 or Z21, Asymptomatic human immunodeficiency virus [HIV] infection status.

GUIDELINES Section I.C.1.a.2)(d)
Z21, Asymptomatic human immunodeficiency virus [HIV] infection status, is to be applied when the patient without any documentation of symptoms is listed as being "HIV positive," "known HIV," "HIV test positive," or similar terminology. Do not use this code if the term "AIDS" is used or if the patient is treated for any HIV-related illness or is described as having any condition(s) resulting from his/her HIV positive status; use B20 in these cases.

4 Z22 Carrier of infectious disease

INCLUDES colonization status
suspected carrier

EXCLUDES 2 *carrier of viral hepatitis (B18.-)*

Z22.0 Carrier of typhoid

Z22.1 Carrier of other intestinal infectious diseases

Z22.2 Carrier of diphtheria

5 **Z22.3 Carrier of other specified bacterial diseases**

Z22.31 Carrier of bacterial disease due to meningococci

6 **Z22.32 Carrier of bacterial disease due to staphylococci**

GUIDELINES Section I.C.1.e.1)(c)
Assign code Z22.322 for patients documented as having MRSA colonization. Assign code Z22.321 for patient documented as having MSSA colonization. Colonization is not necessarily indicative of a disease process or as the cause of a specific condition the patient may have unless documented as such by the provider.

Z22.321 Carrier or suspected carrier of Methicillin susceptible Staphylococcus aureus
MSSA colonization

Z22.322 Carrier or suspected carrier of Methicillin resistant Staphylococcus aureus
MRSA colonization

GUIDELINES Section I.C.1.e.1)(d)
If a patient is documented as having both MRSA colonization and infection during a hospital admission, code Z22.322 and a code for the MRSA infection may both be assigned.

6 **Z22.33 Carrier of bacterial disease due to streptococci**

Z22.330 Carrier of Group B streptococcus

EXCLUDES 1 *Carrier of streptococcus group B (GBS) complicating pregnancy, childbirth and the puerperium (O99.82-)*

Z22.338 Carrier of other streptococcus

Z22.39 Carrier of other specified bacterial diseases

Z22.4 Carrier of infections with a predominantly sexual mode of transmission

Z22.6 Carrier of human T-lymphotropic virus type-1 [HTLV-1] infection

Z22.8 Carrier of other infectious diseases

Z22.9 Carrier of infectious disease, unspecified

Z23 Encounter for immunization

Note: procedure codes are required to identify the types of immunizations given

Code first:

any routine childhood examination

GUIDELINES Section I.C.21.c.2)
Code Z23 is for encounters for inoculations and vaccinations. It indicates that a patient is being seen to receive a prophylactic inoculation against a disease. Procedure codes are required to identify the actual administration of the injection and the type(s) of immunizations given. Code Z23 may be used as a secondary code if the inoculation is given as a routine part of preventive health care, such as a well-baby visit.

4 Z28 Immunization not carried out and underimmunization status

INCLUDES vaccination not carried out

5 **Z28.0 Immunization not carried out because of contraindication**

Z28.01 Immunization not carried out because of acute illness of patient

Z28.02 Immunization not carried out because of chronic illness or condition of patient

Z28.03 Immunization not carried out because of immune compromised state of patient

Z28.04 **Immunization not carried out because of patient allergy to vaccine or component**

Z28.09 **Immunization not carried out because of other contraindication**

Z28.1 **Immunization not carried out because of patient decision for reasons of belief or group pressure**
Immunization not carried out because of religious belief

5 Z28.2 **Immunization not carried out because of patient decision for other and unspecified reason**

Z28.20 **Immunization not carried out because of patient decision for unspecified reason**

Z28.21 **Immunization not carried out because of patient refusal**

Z28.29 **Immunization not carried out because of patient decision for other reason**

Z28.3 **Underimmunization status**
Delinquent immunization status
Lapsed immunization schedule status

5 Z28.8 **Immunization not carried out for other reason**

Z28.81 **Immunization not carried out due to patient having had the disease**

Z28.82 **Immunization not carried out because of caregiver refusal**
Immunization not carried out because of guardian refusal
Immunization not carried out because of parent refusal
EXCLUDES 1 *immunization not carried out because of caregiver refusal because of religious belief (Z28.1)*

● Z28.83 **Immunization not carried out due to unavailability of vaccine**
Delay in delivery of vaccine
Lack of availability of vaccine
Manufacturer delay of vaccine

Z28.89 **Immunization not carried out for other reason**

Z28.9 **Immunization not carried out for unspecified reason**

4 Z29 **Encounter for other prophylactic measures**
EXCLUDES 1 *desensitization to allergens (Z51.6)*
prophylactic surgery (Z40.-)

5 Z29.1 **Encounter for prophylactic immunotherapy**
Encounter for administration of immunoglobulin

Z29.11 **Encounter for prophylactic immunotherapy for respiratory syncytial virus (RSV)**

Z29.12 **Encounter for prophylactic antivenin**

Z29.13 **Encounter for prophylactic Rho(D) immune globulin**

Z29.14 **Encounter for prophylactic rabies immune globin**

Z29.3 **Encounter for prophylactic fluoride administration**

Z29.8 **Encounter for other specified prophylactic measures**

Z29.9 **Encounter for prophylactic measures, unspecified**

Persons encountering health services in circumstances related to reproduction (Z30-Z39)

4 Z30 **Encounter for contraceptive management**

5 Z30.0 **Encounter for general counseling and advice on contraception**

6 Z30.01 **Encounter for initial prescription of contraceptives**
EXCLUDES 1 *encounter for surveillance of contraceptives (Z30.4-)*

Z30.011 **Encounter for initial prescription of contraceptive pills** ♀

Z30.012 **Encounter for prescription of emergency contraception** ♀
Encounter for postcoital contraception

Z30.013 **Encounter for initial prescription of injectable contraceptive** ♀

Z30.014 **Encounter for initial prescription of intrauterine contraceptive device** ♀
EXCLUDES 1 *encounter for insertion of intrauterine contraceptive device (Z30.430, Z30.432)*

Z30.015 **Encounter for initial prescription of vaginal ring hormonal contraceptive** ♀

Z30.016 **Encounter for initial prescription of transdermal patch hormonal contraceptive device**

Z30.017 **Encounter for initial prescription of implantable subdermal contraceptive**

Z30.018 **Encounter for initial prescription of other contraceptives** ♀
Encounter for initial prescription of barrier contraception
Encounter for initial prescription of diaphragm

Z30.019 **Encounter for initial prescription of contraceptives, unspecified** ♀

Z30.02 **Counseling and instruction in natural family planning to avoid pregnancy**

Z30.09 **Encounter for other general counseling and advice on contraception**
Encounter for family planning advice NOS

Z30.2 **Encounter for sterilization**

5 Z30.4 **Encounter for surveillance of contraceptives**

Z30.40 **Encounter for surveillance of contraceptives, unspecified**

Z30.41 **Encounter for surveillance of contraceptive pills** ♀
Encounter for repeat prescription for contraceptive pill

Z30.42 **Encounter for surveillance of injectable contraceptive** ♀

6 Z30.43 **Encounter for surveillance of intrauterine contraceptive device**

Z30.430 **Encounter for insertion of intrauterine contraceptive device** ♀

Z30.431 **Encounter for routine checking of intrauterine contraceptive device** ♀

Z30.432 **Encounter for removal of intrauterine contraceptive device** ♀

Z30.433 **Encounter for removal and reinsertion of intrauterine contraceptive device** ♀
Encounter for replacement of intrauterine contraceptive device

Z30.44 **Encounter for surveillance of vaginal ring hormonal contraceptive device** ♀

Z30.45 **Encounter for surveillance of transdermal patch hormonal contraceptive device** ♀

Z30.46 **Encounter for surveillance of implantable subdermal contraceptive** ♀
Encounter for checking, reinsertion or removal of implantable subdermal contraceptive

Z30.49 **Encounter for surveillance of other contraceptives** ♀
Encounter for surveillance of barrier contraception
Encounter for surveillance of diaphragm

Z30.8 **Encounter for other contraceptive management**
Encounter for postvasectomy sperm count
Encounter for routine examination for contraceptive maintenance
EXCLUDES 1 *sperm count following sterilization reversal (Z31.42)*
sperm count for fertility testing (Z31.41)

Z30.9 **Encounter for contraceptive management, unspecified**

4 Z31 **Encounter for procreative management**
EXCLUDES 1 *complications associated with artificial fertilization (N98.-)*
female infertility (N97.-)
male infertility (N46.-)

Z31.0 **Encounter for reversal of previous sterilization**

5 Z31.4 **Encounter for procreative investigation and testing**
EXCLUDES 1 *postvasectomy sperm count (Z30.8)*

Z31.41 **Encounter for fertility testing**
Encounter for fallopian tube patency testing
Encounter for sperm count for fertility testing

Z31.42 **Aftercare following sterilization reversal**
Sperm count following sterilization reversal

6 Z31.43 **Encounter for genetic testing of female for procreative management**
Use additional code for recurrent pregnancy loss, if applicable (N96, O26.2-)
EXCLUDES 1 *nonprocreative genetic testing (Z13.7-)*

Z31.430 **Encounter of female for testing for genetic disease carrier status for procreative management** ♀

Z31.438 **Encounter for other genetic testing of female for procreative management** ♀

6 Z31.44 **Encounter for genetic testing of male for procreative management**
EXCLUDES 1 *nonprocreative genetic testing (Z13.7-)*
Z31.440 **Encounter of male for testing for genetic disease carrier status for procreative management** ♂
Z31.441 **Encounter for testing of male partner of patient with recurrent pregnancy loss** ♂ A
Z31.448 **Encounter for other genetic testing of male for procreative management** ♂ A
Z31.49 **Encounter for other procreative investigation and testing**
Z31.5 **Encounter for procreative genetic counseling**
AHA: 4Q 2017, 21
5 Z31.6 **Encounter for general counseling and advice on procreation**
Z31.61 **Procreative counseling and advice using natural family planning**
Z31.62 **Encounter for fertility preservation counseling**
Encounter for fertility preservation counseling prior to cancer therapy
Encounter for fertility preservation counseling prior to surgical removal of gonads
Z31.69 **Encounter for other general counseling and advice on procreation**
Z31.7 **Encounter for procreative management and counseling for gestational carrier** ♀
EXCLUDES 1 *pregnant state, gestational carrier (Z33.3)*
5 Z31.8 **Encounter for other procreative management**
Z31.81 **Encounter for male factor infertility in female patient** ♀
Z31.82 **Encounter for Rh incompatibility status** ♀
AHA: 4Q 2014, 17
AHA: 3Q 2015, 40
Z31.83 **Encounter for assisted reproductive fertility procedure cycle** ♀
Patient undergoing in vitro fertilization cycle
Use additional code to identify the type of infertility
EXCLUDES 1 *pre-cycle diagnosis and testing - code to reason for encounter*
Z31.84 **Encounter for fertility preservation procedure**
Encounter for fertility preservation procedure prior to cancer therapy
Encounter for fertility preservation procedure prior to surgical removal of gonads
Z31.89 **Encounter for other procreative management**
Z31.9 **Encounter for procreative management, unspecified**

4 Z32 **Encounter for pregnancy test and childbirth and childcare instruction**
5 Z32.0 **Encounter for pregnancy test**
Z32.00 **Encounter for pregnancy test, result unknown** ♀
Encounter for pregnancy test NOS
Z32.01 **Encounter for pregnancy test, result positive** ♀ M
Z32.02 **Encounter for pregnancy test, result negative** ♀
Z32.2 **Encounter for childbirth instruction**
Z32.3 **Encounter for childcare instruction**
Encounter for prenatal or postpartum childcare instruction

4 Z33 **Pregnant state**
Z33.1 **Pregnant state, incidental** ♀ M
Pregnant state NOS
EXCLUDES 1 *complications of pregnancy (O00-O9A)*
pregnant state, gestational carrier (Z33.3)
GUIDELINES **Section I.C.15.a.1)**
Should the provider document that the pregnancy is incidental to the encounter, then code Z33.1 should be used in place of any chapter 15 codes. It is the provider's responsibility to state that the condition being treated is not affecting the pregnancy.
Z33.2 **Encounter for elective termination of pregnancy** ♀ M
EXCLUDES 1 *early fetal death with retention of dead fetus (O02.1)*
late fetal death (O36.4)
spontaneous abortion (O03)
Z33.3 **Pregnant state, gestational carrier** ♀ M
EXCLUDES 1 *encounter for procreative management and counseling for gestational carrier (Z31.7)*

4 Z34 **Encounter for supervision of normal pregnancy**
EXCLUDES 1 *any complication of pregnancy (O00-O9A)*
encounter for pregnancy test (Z32.0-)
encounter for supervision of high risk pregnancy (O09.-)
5 Z34.0 **Encounter for supervision of normal first pregnancy**
Z34.00 **Encounter for supervision of normal first pregnancy, unspecified trimester** ♀ M
Z34.01 **Encounter for supervision of normal first pregnancy, first trimester** ♀ M
Z34.02 **Encounter for supervision of normal first pregnancy, second trimester** ♀ M
Z34.03 **Encounter for supervision of normal first pregnancy, third trimester** ♀ M
5 Z34.8 **Encounter for supervision of other normal pregnancy**
Z34.80 **Encounter for supervision of other normal pregnancy, unspecified trimester** ♀ M
Z34.81 **Encounter for supervision of other normal pregnancy, first trimester** ♀ M
Z34.82 **Encounter for supervision of other normal pregnancy, second trimester** ♀ M
Z34.83 **Encounter for supervision of other normal pregnancy, third trimester** ♀ M
AHA: 4Q 2014, 17
5 Z34.9 **Encounter for supervision of normal pregnancy, unspecified**
Z34.90 **Encounter for supervision of normal pregnancy, unspecified, unspecified trimester** ♀ M
Z34.91 **Encounter for supervision of normal pregnancy, unspecified, first trimester** ♀ M
Z34.92 **Encounter for supervision of normal pregnancy, unspecified, second trimester** ♀ M
Z34.93 **Encounter for supervision of normal pregnancy, unspecified, third trimester** ♀ M

4 Z36 **Encounter for antenatal screening of mother**
INCLUDES Encounter for placental sample (taken vaginally)
Screening is the testing for disease or disease precursors in asymptomatic individuals so that early detection and treatment can be provided for those who test positive for the disease.
EXCLUDES 1 *diagnostic examination- code to sign or symptom*
encounter for suspected maternal and fetal conditions ruled out (Z03.7-)
suspected fetal condition affecting management of pregnancy - code to condition in Chapter 15
EXCLUDES 2 *abnormal findings on antenatal screening of mother (O28.-)*
genetic counseling and testing (Z31.43-, Z31.5)
routine prenatal care (Z34)
Z36.0 **Encounter for antenatal screening for chromosomal anomalies** ♀ M
AHA: 4Q 2017, 21
Z36.1 **Encounter for antenatal screening for raised alphafetoprotein level** ♀ M
Encounter for antenatal screening for elevated maternal serum alphafetoprotein level
AHA: 4Q 2017, 21
Z36.2 **Encounter for other antenatal screening follow-up** ♀ M
Non-visualized anatomy on a previous scan
AHA: 4Q 2017, 21
Z36.3 **Encounter for antenatal screening for malformations** ♀ M
Screening for a suspected anomaly
AHA: 4Q 2017, 21
Z36.4 **Encounter for antenatal screening for fetal growth retardation** ♀ M
Intrauterine growth restriction (IUGR)/small-for-dates
AHA: 4Q 2017, 21
Z36.5 **Encounter for antenatal screening for isoimmunization** ♀ M
AHA: 4Q 2017, 21
5 Z36.8 **Encounter for other antenatal screening**
Z36.81 **Encounter for antenatal screening for hydrops fetalis** ♀ M
AHA: 4Q 2017, 21
Z36.82 **Encounter for antenatal screening for nuchal translucency** ♀ M
AHA: 4Q 2017, 21

Z36.83 **Encounter for fetal screening for congenital cardiac abnormalities** ♀ M
AHA: 4Q 2017, 21

Z36.84 **Encounter for antenatal screening for fetal lung maturity** ♀ M
AHA: 4Q 2017, 21

Z36.85 **Encounter for antenatal screening for Streptococcus B** ♀ M
AHA: 4Q 2017, 21

Z36.86 **Encounter for antenatal screening for cervical length** ♀ M
Screening for risk of pre-term labor
AHA: 4Q 2017, 21

Z36.87 **Encounter for antenatal screening for uncertain dates** ♀ M
AHA: 4Q 2017, 21

Z36.88 **Encounter for antenatal screening for fetal macrosomia** ♀ M
Screening for large-for-dates
AHA: 4Q 2017, 21

Z36.89 **Encounter for other specified antenatal screening** ♀ M
AHA: 4Q 2017, 21

Z36.8A **Encounter for antenatal screening for other genetic defects** ♀ M
AHA: 4Q 2017, 21

Z36.9 **Encounter for antenatal screening, unspecified** ♀ M
AHA: 4Q 2017, 21

4 Z3A Weeks of gestation

Note: Codes from category Z3A are for use, only on the maternal record, to indicate the weeks of gestation of the pregnancy, if known.
Code first:
complications of pregnancy, childbirth and the puerperium (O09-O9A)
AHA: 2Q 2013, 33

5 Z3A.0 **Weeks of gestation of pregnancy, unspecified or less than 10 weeks**

Z3A.00 **Weeks of gestation of pregnancy not specified** ♀ M
AHA: 3Q 2014, 18

Z3A.01 **Less than 8 weeks gestation of pregnancy** ♀ M

Z3A.08 **8 weeks gestation of pregnancy** ♀ M

Z3A.09 **9 weeks gestation of pregnancy** ♀ M

5 Z3A.1 **Weeks of gestation of pregnancy, weeks 10-19**

Z3A.10 **10 weeks gestation of pregnancy** ♀ M
Z3A.11 **11 weeks gestation of pregnancy** ♀ M
Z3A.12 **12 weeks gestation of pregnancy** ♀ M
Z3A.13 **13 weeks gestation of pregnancy** ♀ M
Z3A.14 **14 weeks gestation of pregnancy** ♀ M
Z3A.15 **15 weeks gestation of pregnancy** ♀ M
Z3A.16 **16 weeks gestation of pregnancy** ♀ M
Z3A.17 **17 weeks gestation of pregnancy** ♀ M
Z3A.18 **18 weeks gestation of pregnancy** ♀ M
Z3A.19 **19 weeks gestation of pregnancy** ♀ M

5 Z3A.2 **Weeks of gestation of pregnancy, weeks 20-29**

Z3A.20 **20 weeks gestation of pregnancy** ♀ M
Z3A.21 **21 weeks gestation of pregnancy** ♀ M
Z3A.22 **22 weeks gestation of pregnancy** ♀ M
Z3A.23 **23 weeks gestation of pregnancy** ♀ M
Z3A.24 **24 weeks gestation of pregnancy** ♀ M
Z3A.25 **25 weeks gestation of pregnancy** ♀ M
Z3A.26 **26 weeks gestation of pregnancy** ♀ M
Z3A.27 **27 weeks gestation of pregnancy** ♀ M
Z3A.28 **28 weeks gestation of pregnancy** ♀ M
AHA: 4Q 2014, 17
Z3A.29 **29 weeks gestation of pregnancy** ♀ M

5 Z3A.3 **Weeks of gestation of pregnancy, weeks 30-39**

Z3A.30 **30 weeks gestation of pregnancy** ♀ M
Z3A.31 **31 weeks gestation of pregnancy** ♀ M
Z3A.32 **32 weeks gestation of pregnancy** ♀ M
Z3A.33 **33 weeks gestation of pregnancy** ♀ M
Z3A.34 **34 weeks gestation of pregnancy** ♀ M
Z3A.35 **35 weeks gestation of pregnancy** ♀ M
Z3A.36 **36 weeks gestation of pregnancy** ♀ M
Z3A.37 **37 weeks gestation of pregnancy** ♀ M
AHA: 4Q 2014, 18
Z3A.38 **38 weeks gestation of pregnancy** ♀ M
AHA: 2Q 2016, 34
Z3A.39 **39 weeks gestation of pregnancy** ♀ M

5 Z3A.4 **Weeks of gestation of pregnancy, weeks 40 or greater**

Z3A.40 **40 weeks gestation of pregnancy** ♀ M
AHA: 2Q 2014, 9
Z3A.41 **41 weeks gestation of pregnancy** ♀ M
Z3A.42 **42 weeks gestation of pregnancy** ♀ M
AHA: 4Q 2014, 23
Z3A.49 **Greater than 42 weeks gestation of pregnancy** ♀ M
AHA: 4Q 2014, 23

4 Z37 Outcome of delivery

This category is intended for use as an additional code to identify the outcome of delivery on the mother's record. It is not for use on the newborn record.
EXCLUDES 1 *stillbirth (P95)*

Z37.0 **Single live birth** ♀ M
AHA: 2Q 2014, 9
AHA: 4Q 2014, 18
AHA: 2Q 2016, 34
Z37.1 **Single stillbirth** ♀ M
Z37.2 **Twins, both liveborn** ♀ M
Z37.3 **Twins, one liveborn and one stillborn** ♀ M
Z37.4 **Twins, both stillborn** ♀ M

5 Z37.5 **Other multiple births, all liveborn**

Z37.50 **Multiple births, unspecified, all liveborn** ♀ M
Z37.51 **Triplets, all liveborn** ♀ M
Z37.52 **Quadruplets, all liveborn** ♀ M
Z37.53 **Quintuplets, all liveborn** ♀ M
Z37.54 **Sextuplets, all liveborn** ♀ M
Z37.59 **Other multiple births, all liveborn** ♀ M

5 Z37.6 **Other multiple births, some liveborn**

Z37.60 **Multiple births, unspecified, some liveborn** ♀ M
Z37.61 **Triplets, some liveborn** ♀ M
Z37.62 **Quadruplets, some liveborn** ♀ M
Z37.63 **Quintuplets, some liveborn** ♀ M
Z37.64 **Sextuplets, some liveborn** ♀ M
Z37.69 **Other multiple births, some liveborn** ♀ M

Z37.7 **Other multiple births, all stillborn** ♀ M
Z37.9 **Outcome of delivery, unspecified** ♀ M
Multiple birth NOS
Single birth NOS

4 Z38 Liveborn infants according to place of birth and type of delivery

This category is for use as the principal code on the initial record of a newborn baby. It is to be used for the initial birth record only. It is not to be used on the mother's record.
AHA: 2Q 2015, 15
AHA: 2Q 2017, 7

5 Z38.0 **Single liveborn infant, born in hospital**
Single liveborn infant, born in birthing center or other health care facility
AHA: 2Q 2017, 5
AHA: 2Q 2017, 6

Z38.00 **Single liveborn infant, delivered vaginally** N
Z38.01 **Single liveborn infant, delivered by cesarean** N
AHA: 3Q 2016, 17
AHA: 3Q 2016, 18

Z38.1 **Single liveborn infant, born outside hospital** N
Z38.2 **Single liveborn infant, unspecified as to place of birth** N
Single liveborn infant NOS

5 Z38.3 **Twin liveborn infant, born in hospital**

Z38.30 **Twin liveborn infant, delivered vaginally** N
Z38.31 **Twin liveborn infant, delivered by cesarean** N

Z38.4 **Twin liveborn infant, born outside hospital** N
Z38.5 **Twin liveborn infant, unspecified as to place of birth** N

5 Z38.6 **Other multiple liveborn infant, born in hospital**

Z38.61 **Triplet liveborn infant, delivered vaginally** N
Z38.62 **Triplet liveborn infant, delivered by cesarean** N
Z38.63 **Quadruplet liveborn infant, delivered vaginally** N

Z38.64 **Quadruplet liveborn infant, delivered by cesarean** N
Z38.65 **Quintuplet liveborn infant, delivered vaginally** N
Z38.66 **Quintuplet liveborn infant, delivered by cesarean** N
Z38.68 **Other multiple liveborn infant, delivered vaginally** N
Z38.69 **Other multiple liveborn infant, delivered by cesarean** N
Z38.7 **Other multiple liveborn infant, born outside hospital** N
Z38.8 **Other multiple liveborn infant, unspecified as to place of birth** N

4 Z39 **Encounter for maternal postpartum care and examination**

Z39.0 **Encounter for care and examination of mother immediately after delivery** ♀M
Care and observation in uncomplicated cases when the delivery occurs outside a healthcare facility
EXCLUDES 1 *care for postpartum complication- see Alphabetic index*

Z39.1 **Encounter for care and examination of lactating mother** ♀M
Encounter for supervision of lactation
EXCLUDES 1 *disorders of lactation (O92.-)*

Z39.2 **Encounter for routine postpartum follow-up** ♀M

Encounters for other specific health care (Z40-Z53)

Categories Z40-Z53 are intended for use to indicate a reason for care. They may be used for patients who have already been treated for a disease or injury, but who are receiving aftercare or prophylactic care, or care to consolidate the treatment, or to deal with a residual state

EXCLUDES 2 *follow-up examination for medical surveillance after treatment (Z08-Z09)*

4 Z40 **Encounter for prophylactic surgery**
EXCLUDES 1 *organ donations (Z52.-)*
therapeutic organ removal-code to condition

5 Z40.0 **Encounter for prophylactic surgery for risk factors related to malignant neoplasms**
Admission for prophylactic organ removal
Use additional code to identify risk factor

Z40.00 **Encounter for prophylactic removal of unspecified organ**
Z40.01 **Encounter for prophylactic removal of breast**
Z40.02 **Encounter for prophylactic removal of ovary(s)** ♀
Encounter for prophylactic removal of ovary(s) and fallopian tube(s)
Z40.03 **Encounter for prophylactic removal of fallopian tube(s)** ♀
AHA: 4Q 2017, 22
Z40.09 **Encounter for prophylactic removal of other organ**

Z40.8 **Encounter for other prophylactic surgery**
Z40.9 **Encounter for prophylactic surgery, unspecified**

4 Z41 **Encounter for procedures for purposes other than remedying health state**

Z41.1 **Encounter for cosmetic surgery**
Encounter for cosmetic breast implant
Encounter for cosmetic procedure
EXCLUDES 1 *encounter for plastic and reconstructive surgery following medical procedure or healed injury (Z42.-)*
encounter for post-mastectomy breast implantation (Z42.1)

Z41.2 **Encounter for routine and ritual male circumcision** ♂
Z41.3 **Encounter for ear piercing**
Z41.8 **Encounter for other procedures for purposes other than remedying health state**
Z41.9 **Encounter for procedure for purposes other than remedying health state, unspecified**

4 Z42 **Encounter for plastic and reconstructive surgery following medical procedure or healed injury**
EXCLUDES 1 *encounter for cosmetic plastic surgery (Z41.1)*
encounter for plastic surgery for treatment of current injury - code to relevent injury

Z42.1 **Encounter for breast reconstruction following mastectomy** A
EXCLUDES 1 *deformity and disproportion of reconstructed breast (N65.1-)*

Z42.8 **Encounter for other plastic and reconstructive surgery following medical procedure or healed injury**
AHA: 1Q 2017, 42

4 Z43 **Encounter for attention to artificial openings**
INCLUDES closure of artificial openings
passage of sounds or bougies through artificial openings
reforming artificial openings
removal of catheter from artificial openings
toilet or cleansing of artificial openings
EXCLUDES 1 *complications of external stoma (J95.0-, K94.-, N99.5-)*
EXCLUDES 2 *fitting and adjustment of prosthetic and other devices (Z44-Z46)*

CODING TIP✓ When assigning a code from Z43 for an encounter for attention to artificial openings, such as a tracheostomy or cystostomy, the plan of care should include interventions for the treatment of the artificial opening.

CODING TIP✓ Assign codes from category Z43 when reason for encounter is to provide active care/intervention to the artificial opening. Do not use codes in the Z43 category with status ostomy codes (Z93) or when there is a complication with the ostomy.

Z43.0 **Encounter for attention to tracheostomy** HCC
Z43.1 **Encounter for attention to gastrostomy** HCC
EXCLUDES 2 *artificial opening status only, without need for care (Z93.-)*
Z43.2 **Encounter for attention to ileostomy** HCC
AHA: Q3 2016, 5
Z43.3 **Encounter for attention to colostomy** HCC
Z43.4 **Encounter for attention to other artificial openings of digestive tract** HCC
Z43.5 **Encounter for attention to cystostomy** HCC
Z43.6 **Encounter for attention to other artificial openings of urinary tract** HCC
Encounter for attention to nephrostomy
Encounter for attention to ureterostomy
Encounter for attention to urethrostomy
Z43.7 **Encounter for attention to artificial vagina**
Z43.8 **Encounter for attention to other artificial openings** HCC
Z43.9 **Encounter for attention to unspecified artificial opening** HCC

4 Z44 **Encounter for fitting and adjustment of external prosthetic device**
INCLUDES removal or replacement of external prosthetic device
EXCLUDES 1 *malfunction or other complications of device - see Alphabetical Index*
presence of prosthetic device (Z97.-)

5 Z44.0 **Encounter for fitting and adjustment of artificial arm**
6 Z44.00 **Encounter for fitting and adjustment of unspecified artificial arm**
⊟ Z44.001 **Encounter for fitting and adjustment of unspecified right artificial arm**
⊟ Z44.002 **Encounter for fitting and adjustment of unspecified left artificial arm**
⊟ Z44.009 **Encounter for fitting and adjustment of unspecified artificial arm, unspecified arm**
6 Z44.01 **Encounter for fitting and adjustment of complete artificial arm**
⊟ Z44.011 **Encounter for fitting and adjustment of complete right artificial arm**
⊟ Z44.012 **Encounter for fitting and adjustment of complete left artificial arm**
⊟ Z44.019 **Encounter for fitting and adjustment of complete artificial arm, unspecified arm**
6 Z44.02 **Encounter for fitting and adjustment of partial artificial arm**
⊟ Z44.021 **Encounter for fitting and adjustment of partial artificial right arm**
⊟ Z44.022 **Encounter for fitting and adjustment of partial artificial left arm**
⊟ Z44.029 **Encounter for fitting and adjustment of partial artificial arm, unspecified arm**
5 Z44.1 **Encounter for fitting and adjustment of artificial leg**
6 Z44.10 **Encounter for fitting and adjustment of unspecified artificial leg**

Z44.101 **Encounter for fitting and adjustment of unspecified right artificial leg** HCC

Z44.102 **Encounter for fitting and adjustment of unspecified left artificial leg** HCC

Z44.109 **Encounter for fitting and adjustment of unspecified artificial leg, unspecified leg** HCC

Z44.11 **Encounter for fitting and adjustment of complete artificial leg**

Z44.111 **Encounter for fitting and adjustment of complete right artificial leg** HCC

Z44.112 **Encounter for fitting and adjustment of complete left artificial leg** HCC

Z44.119 **Encounter for fitting and adjustment of complete artificial leg, unspecified leg** HCC

Z44.12 **Encounter for fitting and adjustment of partial artificial leg**

Z44.121 **Encounter for fitting and adjustment of partial artificial right leg** HCC

Z44.122 **Encounter for fitting and adjustment of partial artificial left leg** HCC

Z44.129 **Encounter for fitting and adjustment of partial artificial leg, unspecified leg** HCC

Z44.2 **Encounter for fitting and adjustment of artificial eye**

EXCLUDES 1 *mechanical complication of ocular prosthesis (T85.3)*

Z44.20 **Encounter for fitting and adjustment of artificial eye, unspecified**

Z44.21 **Encounter for fitting and adjustment of artificial right eye**

Z44.22 **Encounter for fitting and adjustment of artificial left eye**

Z44.3 **Encounter for fitting and adjustment of external breast prosthesis**

EXCLUDES 1 *complications of breast implant (T85.4-)*
encounter for adjustment or removal of breast implant (Z45.81-)
encounter for initial breast implant insertion for cosmetic breast augmentation (Z41.1)
encounter for breast reconstruction following mastectomy (Z42.1)

Z44.30 **Encounter for fitting and adjustment of external breast prosthesis, unspecified breast**

Z44.31 **Encounter for fitting and adjustment of external right breast prosthesis**

Z44.32 **Encounter for fitting and adjustment of external left breast prosthesis**

Z44.8 **Encounter for fitting and adjustment of other external prosthetic devices**

Z44.9 **Encounter for fitting and adjustment of unspecified external prosthetic device**

Z45 Encounter for adjustment and management of implanted device

INCLUDES removal or replacement of implanted device

EXCLUDES 1 *malfunction or other complications of device - see Alphabetical Index*

EXCLUDES 2 *encounter for fitting and adjustment of non-implanted device (Z46.-)*

Z45.0 **Encounter for adjustment and management of cardiac device**

Z45.01 **Encounter for adjustment and management of cardiac pacemaker**
Encounter for adjustment and management of cardiac resynchronization therapy pacemaker (CRT-P)

EXCLUDES 1 *encounter for adjustment and management of automatic implantable cardiac defibrillator with synchronous cardiac pacemaker (Z45.02)*

Z45.010 **Encounter for checking and testing of cardiac pacemaker pulse generator [battery]**
Encounter for replacing cardiac pacemaker pulse generator [battery]

Z45.018 **Encounter for adjustment and management of other part of cardiac pacemaker**

EXCLUDES 2 *presence of prosthetic and other devices (Z95-Z97)*

Z45.02 **Encounter for adjustment and management of automatic implantable cardiac defibrillator**
Encounter for adjustment and management of automatic implantable cardiac defibrillator with synchronous cardiac pacemaker
Encounter for adjustment and management of cardiac resynchronization therapy defibrillator (CRT-D)

Z45.09 **Encounter for adjustment and management of other cardiac device**

Z45.1 **Encounter for adjustment and management of infusion pump**

Z45.2 **Encounter for adjustment and management of vascular access device**
Encounter for adjustment and management of vascular catheters

EXCLUDES 1 *encounter for adjustment and management of renal dialysis catheter (Z49.01)*

CODING TIP ✓ This code is used for routine care of vascular access devices, including peripheral, PICC and central lines. Do not use this code if the line is complicated. See T80 for complications.

Z45.3 **Encounter for adjustment and management of implanted devices of the special senses**

Z45.31 **Encounter for adjustment and management of implanted visual substitution device**

Z45.32 **Encounter for adjustment and management of implanted hearing device**

EXCLUDES 1 *Encounter for fitting and adjustment of hearing aide (Z46.1)*

Z45.320 **Encounter for adjustment and management of bone conduction device**

Z45.321 **Encounter for adjustment and management of cochlear device**

Z45.328 **Encounter for adjustment and management of other implanted hearing device**

Z45.4 **Encounter for adjustment and management of implanted nervous system device**

Z45.41 **Encounter for adjustment and management of cerebrospinal fluid drainage device**
Encounter for adjustment and management of cerebral ventricular (communicating) shunt

Z45.42 **Encounter for adjustment and management of neuropacemaker (brain) (peripheral nerve) (spinal cord)**

Z45.49 **Encounter for adjustment and management of other implanted nervous system device**
AHA: 3Q 2014, 20

Z45.8 **Encounter for adjustment and management of other implanted devices**

Z45.81 **Encounter for adjustment or removal of breast implant**
Encounter for elective implant exchange (different material) (different size)
Encounter removal of tissue expander without synchronous insertion of permanent implant

EXCLUDES 1 *complications of breast implant (T85.4-)*
encounter for initial breast implant insertion for cosmetic breast augmentation (Z41.1)
encounter for breast reconstruction following mastectomy (Z42.1)

Z45.811 **Encounter for adjustment or removal of right breast implant**

Z45.812 **Encounter for adjustment or removal of left breast implant**

Z45.819 **Encounter for adjustment or removal of unspecified breast implant**

Z45.82 **Encounter for adjustment or removal of myringotomy device (stent) (tube)**

Z45.89 **Encounter for adjustment and management of other implanted devices**
AHA: 4Q 2014, 27, 28

Z45.9 **Encounter for adjustment and management of unspecified implanted device**

4 Z46 Encounter for fitting and adjustment of other devices

INCLUDES removal or replacement of other device

EXCLUDES 1 *malfunction or other complications of device - see Alphabetical Index*

EXCLUDES 2 *encounter for fitting and management of implanted devices (Z45.-)*
issue of repeat prescription only (Z76.0)
presence of prosthetic and other devices (Z95-Z97)

Z46.0 Encounter for fitting and adjustment of spectacles and contact lenses

Z46.1 Encounter for fitting and adjustment of hearing aid

EXCLUDES 1 *encounter for adjustment and management of implanted hearing device (Z45.32-)*

Z46.2 Encounter for fitting and adjustment of other devices related to nervous system and special senses

EXCLUDES 2 *encounter for adjustment and management of implanted nervous system device (Z45.4-)*
encounter for adjustment and management of implanted visual substitution device (Z45.31)

Z46.3 Encounter for fitting and adjustment of dental prosthetic device
Encounter for fitting and adjustment of dentures

Z46.4 Encounter for fitting and adjustment of orthodontic device

5 Z46.5 Encounter for fitting and adjustment of other gastrointestinal appliance and device

EXCLUDES 1 *encounter for attention to artificial openings of digestive tract (Z43.1-Z43.4)*

Z46.51 Encounter for fitting and adjustment of gastric lap band

Z46.59 Encounter for fitting and adjustment of other gastrointestinal appliance and device

Z46.6 Encounter for fitting and adjustment of urinary device

EXCLUDES 2 *attention to artificial openings of urinary tract (Z43.5, Z43.6)*

CODING TIP✓ Code Z46.6 includes removal and intermittent catheterization as well as indwelling catheter care. Do not use this code for complications of urinary catheters; instead, code to complications, such as T83.0.

CODING TIP✓ Code Z46.6 includes removal and intermittent catheterization as well as indwelling catheter care.

5 Z46.8 Encounter for fitting and adjustment of other specified devices

Z46.81 Encounter for fitting and adjustment of insulin pump
Encounter for insulin pump instruction and training
Encounter for insulin pump titration

Z46.82 Encounter for fitting and adjustment of non-vascular catheter

Z46.89 Encounter for fitting and adjustment of other specified devices
Encounter for fitting and adjustment of wheelchair

Z46.9 Encounter for fitting and adjustment of unspecified device

4 Z47 Orthopedic aftercare

EXCLUDES 1 *aftercare for healing fracture-code to fracture with 7th character D*

Z47.1 Aftercare following joint replacement surgery
Use additional code to identify the joint (Z96.6-)

CODING TIP✓ The use of Z47.1 for aftercare for joint replacement when the joint replacement was for treatment of a fracture is inappropriate. Code the fracture with the appropriate 7th character followed by a Z96.6 code to indicate the joint prosthesis.

Z47.2 Encounter for removal of internal fixation device

EXCLUDES 1 *encounter for adjustment of internal fixation device for fracture treatment- code to fracture with appropriate 7th character*
encounter for removal of external fixation device- code to fracture with 7th character D
infection or inflammatory reaction to internal fixation device (T84.6-)
mechanical complication of internal fixation device (T84.1-)

5 Z47.3 Aftercare following explantation of joint prosthesis
Aftercare following explantation of joint prosthesis, staged procedure
Encounter for joint prosthesis insertion following prior explantation of joint prosthesis
AHA: 1Q 2015, 17

Z47.31 Aftercare following explantation of shoulder joint prosthesis

EXCLUDES 1 *acquired absence of shoulder joint following prior explantation of shoulder joint prosthesis (Z89.23-)*
shoulder joint prosthesis explantation status (Z89.23-)

Z47.32 Aftercare following explantation of hip joint prosthesis

EXCLUDES 1 *acquired absence of hip joint following prior explantation of hip joint prosthesis (Z89.62-)*
hip joint prosthesis explantation status (Z89.62-)

AHA: 1Q 2015, 17

Z47.33 Aftercare following explantation of knee joint prosthesis

EXCLUDES 1 *acquired absence of knee joint following prior explantation of knee prosthesis ()*
knee joint prosthesis explantation status (Z89.52-)

5 Z47.8 Encounter for other orthopedic aftercare

Z47.81 Encounter for orthopedic aftercare following surgical amputation
Use additional code to identify the limb amputated (Z89.-)

CODING TIP✓ This code is only used for planned amputations. Do not assign Z47.81 for care following a traumatic amputation or when a surgical amputation is complicated by infection, dehiscence, or other complication.

Z47.82 Encounter for orthopedic aftercare following scoliosis surgery

CODING TIP✓ If the condition treated by surgery is coded with a M41 code, this aftercare code is correct.

Z47.89 Encounter for other orthopedic aftercare
AHA: 1Q 2015, 8

4 Z48 Encounter for other postprocedural aftercare

EXCLUDES 1 *encounter for follow-up examination after completed treatment (Z08-Z09)*
encounter for aftercare following injury - code to Injury, by site, with appropriate 7th character for subsequent encounter

EXCLUDES 2 *encounter for attention to artificial openings (Z43.-)*
encounter for fitting and adjustment of prosthetic and other devices (Z44-Z46)

5 Z48.0 Encounter for attention to dressings, sutures and drains

EXCLUDES 1 *encounter for planned postprocedural wound closure (Z48.1)*

Z48.00 Encounter for change or removal of nonsurgical wound dressing
Encounter for change or removal of wound dressing NOS

Z48.01 Encounter for change or removal of surgical wound dressing
AHA: 4Q 2015, 38

Z48.02 Encounter for removal of sutures
Encounter for removal of staples
AHA: 1Q 2015, 6

Z48.03 Encounter for change or removal of drains

Z48.1 Encounter for planned postprocedural wound closure

EXCLUDES 1 *encounter for attention to dressings and sutures (Z48.0-)*

5 Z48.2 Encounter for aftercare following organ transplant

Z48.21 Encounter for aftercare following heart transplant HCC

Z48.22 Encounter for aftercare following kidney transplant

Z48.23 Encounter for aftercare following liver transplant HCC

Z48.24 **Encounter for aftercare following lung transplant** HCC

6 Z48.28 **Encounter for aftercare following multiple organ transplant**

Z48.280 **Encounter for aftercare following heart-lung transplant** HCC

Z48.288 **Encounter for aftercare following multiple organ transplant**

6 Z48.29 **Encounter for aftercare following other organ transplant**

Z48.290 **Encounter for aftercare following bone marrow transplant** HCC

Z48.298 **Encounter for aftercare following other organ transplant**

Z48.3 **Aftercare following surgery for neoplasm**
Use additional code to identify the neoplasm

CODING TIP ✓ When coding Z48.3, an additional code should be assigned to identify the neoplasm. If it is unclear if the neoplasm has been eradicated or if there are plans to continue treatment for the neoplastic disease, assign the appropriate code from Chapter 2 to indicate the neoplasm. If documentation clearly indicates that the neoplasm has been eradicated, assign the appropriate Z85 code to report personal history of neoplasm.

5 Z48.8 **Encounter for other specified postprocedural aftercare**

6 Z48.81 **Encounter for surgical aftercare following surgery on specified body systems**
These codes identify the body system requiring aftercare. They are for use in conjunction with other aftercare codes to fully explain the aftercare encounter. The condition treated should also be coded if still present.

EXCLUDES 1 *aftercare for injury- code the injury with 7th character D*
aftercare following surgery for neoplasm (Z48.3)

EXCLUDES 2 *aftercare following organ transplant (Z48.2-)*
orthopedic aftercare (Z47.-)

Z48.810 **Encounter for surgical aftercare following surgery on the sense organs**

CODING TIP ✓ Use this aftercare code for pre-operative conditions coded with H codes.

Z48.811 **Encounter for surgical aftercare following surgery on the nervous system**

EXCLUDES 2 *encounter for surgical aftercare following surgery on the sense organs (Z48.810)*

CODING TIP ✓ Use this aftercare code for pre-operative conditions coded with G codes.

Z48.812 **Encounter for surgical aftercare following surgery on the circulatory system**

CODING TIP ✓ Use this aftercare code for pre-operative conditions coded with I codes.
AHA: 4Q 2012, 96-97

Z48.813 **Encounter for surgical aftercare following surgery on the respiratory system**

CODING TIP ✓ Use this aftercare code for pre-operative conditions coded with J codes.

Z48.814 **Encounter for surgical aftercare following surgery on the teeth or oral cavity**

Z48.815 **Encounter for surgical aftercare following surgery on the digestive system**

CODING TIP ✓ Use this aftercare code for pre-operative conditions coded with K codes.
AHA: 4Q 2015, 38

Z48.816 **Encounter for surgical aftercare following surgery on the genitourinary system**

EXCLUDES 1 *encounter for aftercare following sterilization reversal (Z31.42)*

CODING TIP ✓ Use this aftercare code for pre-operative conditions coded with N codes.

Z48.817 **Encounter for surgical aftercare following surgery on the skin and subcutaneous tissue**

CODING TIP ✓ Use this aftercare code for pre-operative conditions coded with L codes.
AHA: 1Q 2015, 6

Z48.89 **Encounter for other specified surgical aftercare**

4 Z49 **Encounter for care involving renal dialysis**
Code also:
associated end stage renal disease (N18.6)

5 Z49.0 **Preparatory care for renal dialysis**
Encounter for dialysis instruction and training

Z49.01 **Encounter for fitting and adjustment of extracorporeal dialysis catheter** HCC
Removal or replacement of renal dialysis catheter
Toilet or cleansing of renal dialysis catheter

Z49.02 **Encounter for fitting and adjustment of peritoneal dialysis catheter** HCC

5 Z49.3 **Encounter for adequacy testing for dialysis**

Z49.31 **Encounter for adequacy testing for hemodialysis** HCC

Z49.32 **Encounter for adequacy testing for peritoneal dialysis** HCC
Encounter for peritoneal equilibration test

4 Z51 **Encounter for other aftercare and medical care**
Code also:
condition requiring care

EXCLUDES 1 *follow-up examination after treatment (Z08-Z09)*

GUIDELINES **Section I.C.2.e.2)**
If a patient admission/encounter is solely for the administration of chemotherapy, immunotherapy or external beam radiation therapy, assign code Z51.0, Encounter for antineoplastic radiation therapy, or Z51.11, Encounter for antineoplastic chemotherapy, or Z51.12, Encounter for antineoplastic immunotherapy as the first-listed or principal diagnosis.

The malignancy for which the therapy is being administered should be assigned as a secondary diagnosis.

If a patient admission/encounter is for the insertion or implantation of radioactive elements (e.g., brachytherapy) the appropriate code for the malignancy is sequenced as the principal or first-listed diagnosis. Code Z51.0 should not be assigned.

CODING TIP ✓ Only the provider administering the radiation, chemotherapy or immunotherapy may assign a code from category Z51 to report encounter for radiation, chemotherapy, or immunotherapy.

Z51.0 **Encounter for antineoplastic radiation therapy**

GUIDELINES **Section I.C.2.e.3)**
When a patient is admitted for the purpose of external beam radiotherapy, immunotherapy or chemotherapy and develops complications such as uncontrolled nausea and vomiting or dehydration, the principal or first-listed diagnosis is Z51.0 or Z51.11 or Z51.12, followed by any codes for the complications.

5 Z51.1 **Encounter for antineoplastic chemotherapy and immunotherapy**

EXCLUDES 2 *encounter for chemotherapy and immunotherapy for nonneoplastic condition - code to condition*

Z51.11 **Encounter for antineoplastic chemotherapy**
AHA: 3Q 2015, 19

Z51.12 **Encounter for antineoplastic immunotherapy**

Z51.5 **Encounter for palliative care**
AHA: 1Q 2017, 48

Z51.6 **Encounter for desensitization to allergens**

5 Z51.8 **Encounter for other specified aftercare**

EXCLUDES 1 *holiday relief care (Z75.5)*

AHA: 4Q 2012, 96, 97

Z51.81 **Encounter for therapeutic drug level monitoring**
Code also:
any long-term (current) drug therapy (Z79.-)

EXCLUDES 1 *encounter for blood-drug test for administrative or medicolegal reasons (Z02.83)*

Z51.89 **Encounter for other specified aftercare**

4 Z52 **Donors of organs and tissues**

INCLUDES autologous and other living donors

EXCLUDES 1 *cadaveric donor - omit code*
examination of potential donor (Z00.5)

AHA: 4Q 2012, 99-100

5 Z52.0 Blood donor
6 Z52.00 Unspecified blood donor
Z52.000 Unspecified donor, whole blood
Z52.001 Unspecified donor, stem cells
Z52.008 Unspecified donor, other blood
6 Z52.01 Autologous blood donor
Z52.010 Autologous donor, whole blood
Z52.011 Autologous donor, stem cells
Z52.018 Autologous donor, other blood
6 Z52.09 Other blood donor
Volunteer donor
Z52.090 Other blood donor, whole blood
Z52.091 Other blood donor, stem cells
Z52.098 other blood donor, other blood
5 Z52.1 Skin donor
Z52.10 Skin donor, unspecified
Z52.11 Skin donor, autologous
Z52.19 Skin donor, other
5 Z52.2 Bone donor
Z52.20 Bone donor, unspecified
Z52.21 Bone donor, autologous
Z52.29 Bone donor, other
Z52.3 Bone marrow donor
Z52.4 Kidney donor
Z52.5 Cornea donor
Z52.6 Liver donor
AHA: 4Q 2012, 99-100
5 Z52.8 Donor of other specified organs or tissues
6 Z52.81 Egg (Oocyte) donor
Z52.810 Egg (Oocyte) donor under age 35, anonymous recipient ♀
Egg donor under age 35 NOS
Z52.811 Egg (Oocyte) donor under age 35, designated recipient ♀
Z52.812 Egg (Oocyte) donor age 35 and over, anonymous recipient ♀
Egg donor age 35 and over NOS
Z52.813 Egg (Oocyte) donor age 35 and over, designated recipient ♀
Z52.819 Egg (Oocyte) donor, unspecified ♀
Z52.89 Donor of other specified organs or tissues
Z52.9 Donor of unspecified organ or tissue
Donor NOS

4 Z53 Persons encountering health services for specific procedures and treatment, not carried out
5 Z53.0 Procedure and treatment not carried out because of contraindication
Z53.01 Procedure and treatment not carried out due to patient smoking
Z53.09 Procedure and treatment not carried out because of other contraindication
Z53.1 Procedure and treatment not carried out because of patient's decision for reasons of belief and group pressure
5 Z53.2 Procedure and treatment not carried out because of patient's decision for other and unspecified reasons
Z53.20 Procedure and treatment not carried out because of patient's decision for unspecified reasons
Z53.21 Procedure and treatment not carried out due to patient leaving prior to being seen by health care provider
Z53.29 Procedure and treatment not carried out because of patient's decision for other reasons
5 Z53.3 Procedure converted to open procedure
Z53.31 Laparoscopic surgical procedure converted to open procedure
Z53.32 Thoracoscopic surgical procedure converted to open procedure
Z53.33 Arthroscopic surgical procedure converted to open procedure
Z53.39 Other specified procedure converted to open procedure
Z53.8 Procedure and treatment not carried out for other reasons
Z53.9 Procedure and treatment not carried out, unspecified reason

Persons with potential health hazards related to socioeconomic and psychosocial circumstances (Z55-Z65)

4 Z55 Problems related to education and literacy
EXCLUDES 1 *disorders of psychological development (F80-F89)*
AHA: 1Q 2018, 14
Z55.0 Illiteracy and low-level literacy
AHA: 1Q 2018, 14
Z55.1 Schooling unavailable and unattainable
AHA: 1Q 2018, 14
Z55.2 Failed school examinations
AHA: 1Q 2018, 14
Z55.3 Underachievement in school
AHA: 1Q 2018, 14
Z55.4 Educational maladjustment and discord with teachers and classmates
AHA: 1Q 2018, 14
Z55.8 Other problems related to education and literacy
Problems related to inadequate teaching
AHA: 1Q 2018, 14
Z55.9 Problems related to education and literacy, unspecified
Academic problems NOS
AHA: 1Q 2018, 14

4 Z56 Problems related to employment and unemployment
EXCLUDES 2 *occupational exposure to risk factors (Z57.-)*
problems related to housing and economic circumstances (Z59.-)
AHA: 1Q 2018, 14
Z56.0 Unemployment, unspecified
AHA: 1Q 2018, 14
Z56.1 Change of job A
AHA: 1Q 2018, 14
Z56.2 Threat of job loss
AHA: 1Q 2018, 14
Z56.3 Stressful work schedule
AHA: 1Q 2018, 14
Z56.4 Discord with boss and workmates
AHA: 1Q 2018, 14
Z56.5 Uncongenial work environment
Difficult conditions at work
AHA: 1Q 2018, 14
Z56.6 Other physical and mental strain related to work
AHA: 1Q 2018, 14
5 Z56.8 Other problems related to employment
AHA: 1Q 2018, 14
Z56.81 Sexual harassment on the job
AHA: 1Q 2018, 14
Z56.82 Military deployment status
Individual (civilian or military) currently deployed in theater or in support of military war, peacekeeping and humanitarian operations
AHA: 1Q 2018, 14
Z56.89 Other problems related to employment
AHA: 1Q 2018, 14
Z56.9 Unspecified problems related to employment
Occupational problems NOS
AHA: 1Q 2018, 14

4 Z57 Occupational exposure to risk factors
AHA: 1Q 2018, 14
Z57.0 Occupational exposure to noise
AHA: 1Q 2018, 14
Z57.1 Occupational exposure to radiation
AHA: 1Q 2018, 14
Z57.2 Occupational exposure to dust
AHA: 1Q 2018, 14
5 Z57.3 Occupational exposure to other air contaminants
AHA: 1Q 2018, 14

Z57.31 Occupational exposure to environmental tobacco smoke
EXCLUDES 2 *exposure to environmental tobacco smoke (Z77.22)*
AHA: 1Q 2018, 14

Z57.39 Occupational exposure to other air contaminants
AHA: 1Q 2018, 14

Z57.4 Occupational exposure to toxic agents in agriculture
Occupational exposure to solids, liquids, gases or vapors in agriculture
AHA: 1Q 2018, 14

Z57.5 Occupational exposure to toxic agents in other industries
Occupational exposure to solids, liquids, gases or vapors in other industries
AHA: 1Q 2018, 14

Z57.6 Occupational exposure to extreme temperature
AHA: 1Q 2018, 14

Z57.7 Occupational exposure to vibration
AHA: 1Q 2018, 14

Z57.8 Occupational exposure to other risk factors
AHA: 1Q 2018, 14

Z57.9 Occupational exposure to unspecified risk factor
AHA: 1Q 2018, 14

4 Z59 Problems related to housing and economic circumstances
EXCLUDES 2 *problems related to upbringing (Z62.-)*
AHA: 1Q 2018, 14

Z59.0 Homelessness
AHA: 1Q 2018, 14

Z59.1 Inadequate housing
Lack of heating
Restriction of space
Technical defects in home preventing adequate care
Unsatisfactory surroundings
EXCLUDES 1 *problems related to the natural and physical environment (Z77.1-)*
AHA: 1Q 2018, 14

Z59.2 Discord with neighbors, lodgers and landlord
AHA: 1Q 2018, 14

Z59.3 Problems related to living in residential institution
Boarding-school resident
EXCLUDES 1 *institutional upbringing (Z62.2)*
AHA: 1Q 2018, 14

Z59.4 Lack of adequate food and safe drinking water
Inadequate drinking water supply
EXCLUDES 1 *effects of hunger (T73.0)*
inappropriate diet or eating habits (Z72.4)
malnutrition (E40-E46)
AHA: 1Q 2018, 14

Z59.5 Extreme poverty
AHA: 1Q 2018, 14

Z59.6 Low income
AHA: 1Q 2018, 14

Z59.7 Insufficient social insurance and welfare support
AHA: 1Q 2018, 14

Z59.8 Other problems related to housing and economic circumstances
Foreclosure on loan
Isolated dwelling
Problems with creditors
AHA: 1Q 2018, 14

Z59.9 Problem related to housing and economic circumstances, unspecified
AHA: 1Q 2018, 14

4 Z60 Problems related to social environment
AHA: 1Q 2018, 14

Z60.0 Problems of adjustment to life-cycle transitions
Empty nest syndrome
Phase of life problem
Problem with adjustment to retirement [pension]
AHA: 1Q 2018, 14

Z60.2 Problems related to living alone
AHA: 1Q 2018, 14

Z60.3 Acculturation difficulty
Problem with migration
Problem with social transplantation
AHA: 1Q 2018, 14

Z60.4 Social exclusion and rejection
Exclusion and rejection on the basis of personal characteristics, such as unusual physical appearance, illness or behavior.
EXCLUDES 1 *target of adverse discrimination such as for racial or religious reasons (Z60.5)*
AHA: 1Q 2018, 14

Z60.5 Target of (perceived) adverse discrimination and persecution
EXCLUDES 1 *social exclusion and rejection (Z60.4)*
AHA: 1Q 2018, 14

Z60.8 Other problems related to social environment
AHA: 1Q 2018, 14

Z60.9 Problem related to social environment, unspecified
AHA: 1Q 2018, 14

4 Z62 Problems related to upbringing
INCLUDES current and past negative life events in childhood
current and past problems of a child related to upbringing
EXCLUDES 2 *maltreatment syndrome (T74.-)*
problems related to housing and economic circumstances (Z59.-)
AHA: 1Q 2018, 14

Z62.0 Inadequate parental supervision and control
AHA: 1Q 2018, 14

Z62.1 Parental overprotection
AHA: 1Q 2018, 14

5 Z62.2 Upbringing away from parents
EXCLUDES 1 *problems with boarding school (Z59.3)*
AHA: 1Q 2018, 14

Z62.21 Child in welfare custody P
Child in care of non-parental family member
Child in foster care
EXCLUDES 2 *problem for parent due to child in welfare custody (Z63.5)*
AHA: 1Q 2018, 14

Z62.22 Institutional upbringing
Child living in orphanage or group home
AHA: 1Q 2018, 14

Z62.29 Other upbringing away from parents
AHA: 1Q 2018, 14

Z62.3 Hostility towards and scapegoating of child P
AHA: 1Q 2018, 14

Z62.6 Inappropriate (excessive) parental pressure
AHA: 1Q 2018, 14

5 Z62.8 Other specified problems related to upbringing
AHA: 1Q 2018, 14

6 Z62.81 Personal history of abuse in childhood
AHA: 1Q 2018, 14

Z62.810 Personal history of physical and sexual abuse in childhood
EXCLUDES 1 *current child physical abuse (T74.12, T76.12)*
current child sexual abuse (T74.22, T76.22)
AHA: 1Q 2018, 14

Z62.811 Personal history of psychological abuse in childhood
EXCLUDES 1 *current child psychological abuse (T74.32, T76.32)*
AHA: 1Q 2018, 14

Z62.812 Personal history of neglect in childhood
EXCLUDES 1 *current child neglect (T74.02, T76.02)*
AHA: 1Q 2018, 14

● **Z62.813 Personal history of forced labor or sexual exploitation in childhood**
AHA: 1Q 2018, 14

Z62.819 Personal history of unspecified abuse in childhood
EXCLUDES 1 *current child abuse NOS (T74.92, T76.92)*
AHA: 1Q 2018, 14

6 Z62.82 Parent-child conflict
AHA: 1Q 2018, 14

Z62.820 Parent-biological child conflict
Parent-child problem NOS
AHA: 1Q 2018, 14

Z62.821 Parent-adopted child conflict
AHA: 1Q 2018, 14

Z62.822 Parent-foster child conflict
AHA: 1Q 2018, 14

6 **Z62.89 Other specified problems related to upbringing**
AHA: 1Q 2018, 14

Z62.890 Parent-child estrangement NEC
AHA: 1Q 2018, 14

Z62.891 Sibling rivalry
AHA: 1Q 2018, 14

Z62.898 Other specified problems related to upbringing
AHA: 1Q 2018, 14

Z62.9 Problem related to upbringing, unspecified
AHA: 1Q 2018, 14

4 **Z63 Other problems related to primary support group, including family circumstances**
EXCLUDES 2 *maltreatment syndrome (T74.-, T76)*
parent-child problems (Z62.-)
problems related to negative life events in childhood (Z62.-)
problems related to upbringing (Z62.-)
AHA: 1Q 2018, 14

Z63.0 Problems in relationship with spouse or partner
Relationship distress with spouse or intimate partner
EXCLUDES 1 *counseling for spousal or partner abuse problems (Z69.1)*
counseling related to sexual attitude, behavior, and orientation (Z70.-)
AHA: 1Q 2018, 14

Z63.1 Problems in relationship with in-laws
AHA: 1Q 2018, 14

5 **Z63.3 Absence of family member**
EXCLUDES 1 *absence of family member due to disappearance and death (Z63.4)*
absence of family member due to separation and divorce (Z63.5)
AHA: 1Q 2018, 14

Z63.31 Absence of family member due to military deployment
Individual or family affected by other family member being on military deployment
EXCLUDES 1 *family disruption due to return of family member from military deployment (Z63.71)*
AHA: 1Q 2018, 14

Z63.32 Other absence of family member
AHA: 1Q 2018, 14

Z63.4 Disappearance and death of family member
Assumed death of family member
Bereavement
AHA: 1Q 2014, 25
AHA: 1Q 2018, 14

Z63.5 Disruption of family by separation and divorce
Marital estrangement
AHA: 1Q 2018, 14

Z63.6 Dependent relative needing care at home
AHA: 1Q 2018, 14

5 **Z63.7 Other stressful life events affecting family and household**
AHA: 1Q 2018, 14

Z63.71 Stress on family due to return of family member from military deployment
Individual or family affected by family member having returned from military deployment (current or past conflict)
AHA: 1Q 2018, 14

Z63.72 Alcoholism and drug addiction in family
AHA: 1Q 2018, 14

Z63.79 Other stressful life events affecting family and household
Anxiety (normal) about sick person in family
Health problems within family
Ill or disturbed family member
Isolated family
AHA: 1Q 2018, 14

Z63.8 Other specified problems related to primary support group
Family discord NOS
Family estrangement NOS
High expressed emotional level within family
Inadequate family support NOS
Inadequate or distorted communication within family
AHA: 1Q 2018, 14

Z63.9 Problem related to primary support group, unspecified
Relationship disorder NOS
AHA: 1Q 2018, 14

4 **Z64 Problems related to certain psychosocial circumstances**
AHA: 1Q 2018, 14

Z64.0 Problems related to unwanted pregnancy ♀
AHA: 1Q 2018, 14

Z64.1 Problems related to multiparity ♀
AHA: 1Q 2018, 14

Z64.4 Discord with counselors
Discord with probation officer
Discord with social worker
AHA: 1Q 2018, 14

4 **Z65 Problems related to other psychosocial circumstances**
AHA: 1Q 2018, 14

Z65.0 Conviction in civil and criminal proceedings without imprisonment

Z65.1 Imprisonment and other incarceration

Z65.2 Problems related to release from prison

Z65.3 Problems related to other legal circumstances
Arrest
Child custody or support proceedings
Litigation
Prosecution

Z65.4 Victim of crime and terrorism
Victim of torture

Z65.5 Exposure to disaster, war and other hostilities
EXCLUDES 1 *target of perceived discrimination or persecution (Z60.5)*

Z65.8 Other specified problems related to psychosocial circumstances
Religious or spiritual problem

Z65.9 Problem related to unspecified psychosocial circumstances

Do not resuscitate status (Z66)

Z66 Do not resuscitate
DNR status

Blood type (Z67)

4 **Z67 Blood type**

5 **Z67.1 Type A blood**

Z67.10 Type A blood, Rh positive

Z67.11 Type A blood, Rh negative

5 **Z67.2 Type B blood**

Z67.20 Type B blood, Rh positive

Z67.21 Type B blood, Rh negative

5 **Z67.3 Type AB blood**

Z67.30 Type AB blood, Rh positive

Z67.31 Type AB blood, Rh negative

5 **Z67.4 Type O blood**

Z67.40 Type O blood, Rh positive

Z67.41 Type O blood, Rh negative

5 **Z67.9 Unspecified blood type**

Z67.90 Unspecified blood type, Rh positive

Z67.91 Unspecified blood type, Rh negative
AHA: 3Q 2015, 40

Body mass index [BMI] (Z68)

Z68 Body mass index [BMI]
Kilograms per meters squared
Note: BMI adult codes are for use for persons 21 years of age or older
BMI pediatric codes are for use for persons 2-20 years of age. These percentiles are based on the growth charts published by the Centers for Disease Control and Prevention (CDC)

CODING TIP✓ BMI adult codes are for use in persons 21 years of age or older. Pediatric BMI codes (Z69.5-) are for use in persons aged 2-20 years of age. Percentiles are based on growth charts published by the CDC. BMI code assignment may be based on documentation from clinicians other than the physician.

CODING TIP✓ When coding weight loss, obesity, overweight or morbid obesity, it is recommended to calculate and code the associated BMI. BMI may be calculated and coded based upon documentation from clinicians other than the physician.

Z68.1 Body mass index (BMI) 19.9 or less, adult A
AHA: 1Q 2017, 39

Z68.2 Body mass index (BMI) 20-29, adult
- **Z68.20 Body mass index (BMI) 20.0-20.9, adult** A
- **Z68.21 Body mass index (BMI) 21.0-21.9, adult** A
- **Z68.22 Body mass index (BMI) 22.0-22.9, adult** A
- **Z68.23 Body mass index (BMI) 23.0-23.9, adult** A
- **Z68.24 Body mass index (BMI) 24.0-24.9, adult** A
- **Z68.25 Body mass index (BMI) 25.0-25.9, adult** A
- **Z68.26 Body mass index (BMI) 26.0-26.9, adult** A
- **Z68.27 Body mass index (BMI) 27.0-27.9, adult** A
- **Z68.28 Body mass index (BMI) 28.0-28.9, adult** A
- **Z68.29 Body mass index (BMI) 29.0-29.9, adult** A

Z68.3 Body mass index (BMI) 30-39, adult
- **Z68.30 Body mass index (BMI) 30.0-30.9, adult** A
- **Z68.31 Body mass index (BMI) 31.0-31.9, adult** A
- **Z68.32 Body mass index (BMI) 32.0-32.9, adult** A
- **Z68.33 Body mass index (BMI) 33.0-33.9, adult** A
- **Z68.34 Body mass index (BMI) 34.0-34.9, adult** A
- **Z68.35 Body mass index (BMI) 35.0-35.9, adult** A
- **Z68.36 Body mass index (BMI) 36.0-36.9, adult** A
- **Z68.37 Body mass index (BMI) 37.0-37.9, adult** A
- **Z68.38 Body mass index (BMI) 38.0-38.9, adult** A
- **Z68.39 Body mass index (BMI) 39.0-39.9, adult** A

Z68.4 Body mass index (BMI) 40 or greater, adult
- **Z68.41 Body mass index (BMI) 40.0-44.9, adult** A HCC
- **Z68.42 Body mass index (BMI) 45.0-49.9, adult** A HCC
- **Z68.43 Body mass index (BMI) 50-59.9, adult** A HCC
- **Z68.44 Body mass index (BMI) 60.0-69.9, adult** A HCC
- **Z68.45 Body mass index (BMI) 70 or greater, adult** A HCC

Z68.5 Body mass index (BMI) pediatric
- **Z68.51 Body mass index (BMI) pediatric, less than 5th percentile for age**
- **Z68.52 Body mass index (BMI) pediatric, 5th percentile to less than 85th percentile for age**
- **Z68.53 Body mass index (BMI) pediatric, 85th percentile to less than 95th percentile for age**
- **Z68.54 Body mass index (BMI) pediatric, greater than or equal to 95th percentile for age**

Persons encountering health services in other circumstances (Z69-Z76)

Z69 Encounter for mental health services for victim and perpetrator of abuse
INCLUDES counseling for victims and perpetrators of abuse

Z69.0 Encounter for mental health services for child abuse problems

Z69.01 Encounter for mental health services for parental child abuse

Z69.010 Encounter for mental health services for victim of parental child abuse P
Encounter for mental health services for victim of child abuse by parent
Encounter for mental health services for victim of child neglect by parent
Encounter for mental health services for victim of child psychological abuse by parent
Encounter for mental health services for victim of child sexual abuse by parent

Z69.011 Encounter for mental health services for perpetrator of parental child abuse
Encounter for mental health services for perpetrator of parental child neglect
Encounter for mental health services for perpetrator of parental child psychological abuse
Encounter for mental health services for perpetrator of parental child sexual abuse
EXCLUDES 1 *encounter for mental health services for non-parental child abuse (Z69.02-)*

Z69.02 Encounter for mental health services for non-parental child abuse

Z69.020 Encounter for mental health services for victim of non-parental child abuse P
Encounter for mental health services for victim of non-parental child neglect
Encounter for mental health services for victim of non-parental child psychological abuse
Encounter for mental health services for victim of non-parental child sexual abuse

Z69.021 Encounter for mental health services for perpetrator of non-parental child abuse
Encounter for mental health services for perpetrator of non-parental child neglect
Encounter for mental health services for perpetrator of non-parental child psychological abuse
Encounter for mental health services for perpetrator of non-parental child sexual abuse

Z69.1 Encounter for mental health services for spousal or partner abuse problems

Z69.11 Encounter for mental health services for victim of spousal or partner abuse
Encounter for mental health services for victim of spouse or partner neglect
Encounter for mental health services for victim of spouse or partner psychological abuse
Encounter for mental health services for victim of spouse or partner violence, physical

Z69.12 Encounter for mental health services for perpetrator of spousal or partner abuse
Encounter for mental health services for perpetrator of spouse or partner neglect
Encounter for mental health services for perpetrator of spouse or partner psychological abuse
Encounter for mental health services for perpetrator of spouse or partner violence, physical
Encounter for mental health services for perpetrator of spouse or partner violence, sexual

Z69.8 Encounter for mental health services for victim or perpetrator of other abuse

Z69.81 Encounter for mental health services for victim of other abuse
Encounter for mental health services for perpetrator of non-spousal adult abuse
Encounter for mental health services for victim of non-spousal adult abuse
Encounter for mental health services for victim of spouse or partner violence, sexual
Encounter for rape victim counseling

Z69.82 Encounter for mental health services for perpetrator of other abuse

Z70 Counseling related to sexual attitude, behavior and orientation
INCLUDES encounter for mental health services for sexual attitude, behavior and orientation
EXCLUDES 2 *contraceptive or procreative counseling (Z30-Z31)*

Z70.0 Counseling related to sexual attitude

Z70.1 Counseling related to patient's sexual behavior and orientation
Patient concerned regarding impotence
Patient concerned regarding non-responsiveness
Patient concerned regarding promiscuity
Patient concerned regarding sexual orientation

Z70.2 Counseling related to sexual behavior and orientation of third party
Advice sought regarding sexual behavior and orientation of child
Advice sought regarding sexual behavior and orientation of partner
Advice sought regarding sexual behavior and orientation of spouse

Z70.3 Counseling related to combined concerns regarding sexual attitude, behavior and orientation

Z70.8 Other sex counseling
Encounter for sex education

Z70.9 Sex counseling, unspecified

4 Z71 Persons encountering health services for other counseling and medical advice, not elsewhere classified

EXCLUDES 2 *contraceptive or procreation counseling (Z30-Z31)*
sex counseling (Z70.-)

Z71.0 Person encountering health services to consult on behalf of another person
Person encountering health services to seek advice or treatment for non-attending third party
EXCLUDES 2 *anxiety (normal) about sick person in family (Z63.7)*
expectant (adoptive) parent(s) pre-birth pediatrician visit (Z76.81)

Z71.1 Person with feared health complaint in whom no diagnosis is made
Person encountering health services with feared condition which was not demonstrated
Person encountering health services in which problem was normal state
'Worried well'
EXCLUDES 1 *medical observation for suspected diseases and conditions proven not to exist (Z03.-)*

Z71.2 Person consulting for explanation of examination or test findings

Z71.3 Dietary counseling and surveillance
Use additional code for any associated underlying medical condition
Use additional code to identify body mass index (BMI), if known (Z68.-)

5 Z71.4 Alcohol abuse counseling and surveillance
Use additional code for alcohol abuse or dependence (F10.-)

Z71.41 Alcohol abuse counseling and surveillance of alcoholic

Z71.42 Counseling for family member of alcoholic
Counseling for significant other, partner, or friend of alcoholic

5 Z71.5 Drug abuse counseling and surveillance
Use additional code for drug abuse or dependence (F11-F16, F18-F19)

Z71.51 Drug abuse counseling and surveillance of drug abuser

Z71.52 Counseling for family member of drug abuser
Counseling for significant other, partner, or friend of drug abuser

Z71.6 Tobacco abuse counseling
Use additional code for nicotine dependence (F17.-)

Z71.7 Human immunodeficiency virus [HIV] counseling

5 Z71.8 Other specified counseling
EXCLUDES 2 *counseling for contraception (Z30.0-)*

Z71.81 Spiritual or religious counseling

Z71.82 Exercise counseling
AHA: 4Q 2017, 21

Z71.83 Encounter for nonprocreative genetic counseling
EXCLUDES 1 *counseling for procreative genetics (Z31.5)*
counseling for procreative management (Z31.6)
AHA: 4Q 2017, 21

Z71.89 Other specified counseling

Z71.9 Counseling, unspecified
Encounter for medical advice NOS

4 Z72 Problems related to lifestyle

EXCLUDES 2 *problems related to life-management difficulty (Z73.-)*
problems related to socioeconomic and psychosocial circumstances (Z55-Z65)

CODING TIP ✓ These codes should be assigned only when the documentation specifies that the patient has an associated problem.

Z72.0 Tobacco use
Tobacco use NOS
EXCLUDES 1 *history of tobacco dependence (Z87.891)*
nicotine dependence (F17.2-)
tobacco dependence (F17.2-)
tobacco use during pregnancy (O99.33-)

Z72.3 Lack of physical exercise

Z72.4 Inappropriate diet and eating habits
EXCLUDES 1 *behavioral eating disorders of infancy or childhood (F98.2.-F98.3)*
eating disorders (F50.-)
lack of adequate food (Z59.4)
malnutrition and other nutritional deficiencies (E40-E64)

5 Z72.5 High risk sexual behavior
Promiscuity
EXCLUDES 1 *paraphilias (F65)*

Z72.51 High risk heterosexual behavior

Z72.52 High risk homosexual behavior

Z72.53 High risk bisexual behavior

Z72.6 Gambling and betting
EXCLUDES 1 *compulsive or pathological gambling (F63.0)*

5 Z72.8 Other problems related to lifestyle

6 Z72.81 Antisocial behavior
EXCLUDES 1 *conduct disorders (F91.-)*

Z72.810 Child and adolescent antisocial behavior P
Antisocial behavior (child) (adolescent) without manifest psychiatric disorder
Delinquency NOS
Group delinquency
Offenses in the context of gang membership
Stealing in company with others
Truancy from school

Z72.811 Adult antisocial behavior A
Adult antisocial behavior without manifest psychiatric disorder

6 Z72.82 Problems related to sleep

Z72.820 Sleep deprivation
Lack of adequate sleep
EXCLUDES 1 *insomnia (G47.0-)*

Z72.821 Inadequate sleep hygiene
Bad sleep habits
Irregular sleep habits
Unhealthy sleep wake schedule
EXCLUDES 1 *insomnia (F51.0-, G47.0-)*

Z72.89 Other problems related to lifestyle
Self damaging behavior

Z72.9 Problem related to lifestyle, unspecified

4 Z73 Problems related to life management difficulty

EXCLUDES 2 *problems related to socioeconomic and psychosocial circumstances (Z55-Z65)*

Z73.0 Burn-out

Z73.1 Type A behavior pattern

Z73.2 Lack of relaxation and leisure

Z73.3 Stress, not elsewhere classified
Physical and mental strain NOS
EXCLUDES 1 *stress related to employment or unemployment (Z56.-)*

Z73.4 Inadequate social skills, not elsewhere classified

Z73.5 Social role conflict, not elsewhere classified

Z73.6 Limitation of activities due to disability
EXCLUDES 1 *care-provider dependency (Z74.-)*

5 Z73.8 Other problems related to life management difficulty

6 Z73.81 Behavioral insomnia of childhood

Z73.810 **Behavioral insomnia of childhood, sleep-onset association type** P
Z73.811 **Behavioral insomnia of childhood, limit setting type** P
Z73.812 **Behavioral insomnia of childhood, combined type** P
Z73.819 **Behavioral insomnia of childhood, unspecified type** P
Z73.82 **Dual sensory impairment**
Z73.89 **Other problems related to life management difficulty**
Z73.9 **Problem related to life management difficulty, unspecified**

4 Z74 **Problems related to care provider dependency**
EXCLUDES 2 *dependence on enabling machines or devices NEC (Z99.-)*

5 Z74.0 **Reduced mobility**
Z74.01 **Bed confinement status**
Bedridden
Z74.09 **Other reduced mobility**
Chairridden
Reduced mobility NOS
EXCLUDES 2 *wheelchair dependence (Z99.3)*

Z74.1 **Need for assistance with personal care**
Z74.2 **Need for assistance at home and no other household member able to render care**
Z74.3 **Need for continuous supervision**
Z74.8 **Other problems related to care provider dependency**
Z74.9 **Problem related to care provider dependency, unspecified**

4 Z75 **Problems related to medical facilities and other health care**
Z75.0 **Medical services not available in home**
EXCLUDES 1 *no other household member able to render care (Z74.2)*
Z75.1 **Person awaiting admission to adequate facility elsewhere**
Z75.2 **Other waiting period for investigation and treatment**
Z75.3 **Unavailability and inaccessibility of health-care facilities**
EXCLUDES 1 *bed unavailable (Z75.1)*
Z75.4 **Unavailability and inaccessibility of other helping agencies**
Z75.5 **Holiday relief care**
Z75.8 **Other problems related to medical facilities and Other health care**
Z75.9 **Unspecified problem related to medical facilities and other health care**

4 Z76 **Persons encountering health services in other circumstances**
Z76.0 **Encounter for issue of repeat prescription**
Encounter for issue of repeat prescription for appliance
Encounter for issue of repeat prescription for medicaments
Encounter for issue of repeat prescription for spectacles
EXCLUDES 2 *issue of medical certificate (Z02.7)*
repeat prescription for contraceptive (Z30.4-)
Z76.1 **Encounter for health supervision and care of foundling**
Z76.2 **Encounter for health supervision and care of other healthy infant and child** P
Encounter for medical or nursing care or supervision of healthy infant under circumstances such as adverse socioeconomic conditions at home
Encounter for medical or nursing care or supervision of healthy infant under circumstances such as awaiting foster or adoptive placement
Encounter for medical or nursing care or supervision of healthy infant under circumstances such as maternal illness
Encounter for medical or nursing care or supervision of healthy infant under circumstances such as number of children at home preventing or interfering with normal care
Z76.3 **Healthy person accompanying sick person**
Z76.4 **Other boarder to healthcare facility**
EXCLUDES 1 *homelessness (Z59.0)*
▲ Z76.5 **Malingerer [conscious simulation]**
Person feigning illness (with obvious motivation)
EXCLUDES 1 *factitious disorder (F68.1-, F68.A)*
peregrinating patient (F68.1-)
5 Z76.8 **Persons encountering health services in other specified circumstances**
Z76.81 **Expectant parent(s) prebirth pediatrician visit**
Pre-adoption pediatrician visit for adoptive parent(s)
Z76.82 **Awaiting organ transplant status**
Patient waiting for organ availability
Z76.89 **Persons encountering health services in other specified circumstances**
Persons encountering health services NOS
AHA: 2Q 2014, 10

Persons with potential health hazards related to family and personal history and certain conditions influencing health status (Z77-Z99)

Code also:
any follow-up examination (Z08-Z09)

4 Z77 **Other contact with and (suspected) exposures hazardous to health**
INCLUDES contact with and (suspected) exposures to potential hazards to health
EXCLUDES 2 *contact with and (suspected) exposure to communicable diseases (Z20.-)*
exposure to (parental) (environmental) tobacco smoke in the perinatal period (P96.81)
newborn affected by noxious substances transmitted via placenta or breast milk (P04.-)
occupational exposure to risk factors (Z57.-)
retained foreign body (Z18.-)
retained foreign body fully removed (Z87.821)
toxic effects of substances chiefly nonmedicinal as to source (T51-T65)

GUIDELINES **Section I.C.21.c.1)**
Category Z20 indicates contact with, and suspected exposure to, communicable diseases. These codes are for patients who do not show any sign or symptom of a disease but are suspected to have been exposed to it by close personal contact with an infected individual or are in an area where a disease is epidemic. Category Z77 indicates contact with and suspected exposures hazardous to health.

Contact/exposure codes may be used as a first-listed code to explain an encounter for testing, or, more commonly, as a secondary code to identify a potential risk.

5 Z77.0 **Contact with and (suspected) exposure to hazardous, chiefly nonmedicinal, chemicals**
6 Z77.01 **Contact with and (suspected) exposure to hazardous metals**
Z77.010 **Contact with and (suspected) exposure to arsenic**
Z77.011 **Contact with and (suspected) exposure to lead**
Z77.012 **Contact with and (suspected) exposure to uranium**
EXCLUDES 1 *retained depleted uranium fragments (Z18.01)*
Z77.018 **Contact with and (suspected) exposure to other hazardous metals**
Contact with and (suspected) exposure to chromium compounds
Contact with and (suspected) exposure to nickel dust
6 Z77.02 **Contact with and (suspected) exposure to hazardous aromatic compounds**
Z77.020 **Contact with and (suspected) exposure to aromatic amines**
Z77.021 **Contact with and (suspected) exposure to benzene**
Z77.028 **Contact with and (suspected) exposure to other hazardous aromatic compounds**
Aromatic dyes NOS
Polycyclic aromatic hydrocarbons
6 Z77.09 **Contact with and (suspected) exposure to other hazardous, chiefly nonmedicinal, chemicals**
Z77.090 **Contact with and (suspected) exposure to asbestos**
Z77.098 **Contact with and (suspected) exposure to other hazardous, chiefly nonmedicinal, chemicals**
Dyes NOS
5 Z77.1 **Contact with and (suspected) exposure to environmental pollution and hazards in the physical environment**

6 **Z77.11 Contact with and (suspected) exposure to environmental pollution**

Z77.110 Contact with and (suspected) exposure to air pollution

Z77.111 Contact with and (suspected) exposure to water pollution

Z77.112 Contact with and (suspected) exposure to soil pollution

Z77.118 Contact with and (suspected) exposure to other environmental pollution

6 **Z77.12 Contact with and (suspected) exposure to hazards in the physical environment**

Z77.120 Contact with and (suspected) exposure to mold (toxic)

Z77.121 Contact with and (suspected) exposure to harmful algae and algae toxins

Contact with and (suspected) exposure to (harmful) algae bloom NOS

Contact with and (suspected) exposure to blue-green algae bloom

Contact with and (suspected) exposure to brown tide

Contact with and (suspected) exposure to cyanobacteria bloom

Contact with and (suspected) exposure to Florida red tide

Contact with and (suspected) exposure to pfiesteria piscicida

Contact with and (suspected) exposure to red tide

Z77.122 Contact with and (suspected) exposure to noise

▲ **Z77.123 Contact with and (suspected) exposure to radon and other naturally occurring radiation**

EXCLUDES 2 *radiation exposure as the cause of a confirmed condition (W88-W90, X39.0-)*
radiation sickness NOS (T66)

Z77.128 Contact with and (suspected) exposure to other hazards in the physical environment

5 **Z77.2 Contact with and (suspected) exposure to other hazardous substances**

Z77.21 Contact with and (suspected) exposure to potentially hazardous body fluids

Z77.22 Contact with and (suspected) exposure to environmental tobacco smoke (acute) (chronic)

Exposure to second hand tobacco smoke (acute) (chronic)

Passive smoking (acute) (chronic)

EXCLUDES 1 *nicotine dependence (F17.-)*
tobacco use (Z72.0)

EXCLUDES 2 *occupational exposure to environmental tobacco smoke (Z57.31)*

Z77.29 Contact with and (suspected) exposure to other hazardous substances

CODING TIP✓ This code may be used to indicate passive exposure to e-cigarettes or vaping.

AHA: 2Q 2016, 34

Z77.9 Other contact with and (suspected) exposures hazardous to health

4 **Z78 Other specified health status**

EXCLUDES 2 *asymptomatic human immunodeficiency virus [HIV] infection status (Z21)*
postprocedural status (Z93-Z99)
sex reassignment status (Z87.890)

Z78.0 Asymptomatic menopausal state ♀A

Menopausal state NOS

Postmenopausal status NOS

EXCLUDES 2 *symptomatic menopausal state (N95.1)*

Z78.1 Physical restraint status

EXCLUDES 1 *physical restraint due to a procedure - omit code*

Z78.9 Other specified health status

4 **Z79 Long term (current) drug therapy**

INCLUDES long term (current) drug use for prophylactic purposes

Code also:

any therapeutic drug level monitoring (Z51.81)

EXCLUDES 2 *drug abuse and dependence (F11-F19)*
drug use complicating pregnancy, childbirth, and the puerperium (O99.32-)
long term (current) use of oral antidiabetic drugs (Z79.84)
long term (current) use of oral hypoglycemic drugs (Z79.84)

GUIDELINES **Section I.C.21.c.3)**

Codes from this category [Z79] indicate a patient's continuous use of a prescribed drug (including such things as aspirin therapy) for the long-term treatment of a condition or for prophylactic use. It is not for use for patients who have addictions to drugs. This subcategory is not for use of medications for detoxification or maintenance programs to prevent withdrawal symptoms in patients with drug dependence (e.g., methadone maintenance for opiate dependence). Assign the appropriate code for the drug dependence instead.

Assign a code from Z79 if the patient is receiving a medication for an extended period as a prophylactic measure (such as for the prevention of deep vein thrombosis) or as treatment of a chronic condition (such as arthritis) or a disease requiring a lengthy course of treatment (such as cancer). Do not assign a code from category Z79 for medication being administered for a brief period of time to treat an acute illness or injury (such as a course of antibiotics to treat acute bronchitis).

CODING TIP✓ Codes classifiable to category Z79 should not be assigned as primary diagnoses. When the management of any of these medications is integral to the plan of care, consider the confirmed diagnosis for which the patient is under treatment with the medication. This diagnosis should be coded, with a code from Z79 as an additional diagnosis.

5 **Z79.0 Long term (current) use of anticoagulants and antithrombotics/antiplatelets**

EXCLUDES 2 *long term (current) use of aspirin (Z79.82)*

Z79.01 Long term (current) use of anticoagulants

Z79.02 Long term (current) use of antithrombotics/antiplatelets

Z79.1 Long term (current) use of non-steroidal anti-inflammatories (NSAID)

EXCLUDES 2 *long term (current) use of aspirin (Z79.82)*

Z79.2 Long term (current) use of antibiotics

Z79.3 Long term (current) use of hormonal contraceptives

Long term (current) use of birth control pill or patch

Z79.4 Long term (current) use of insulin HCC

GUIDELINES **Section I.C.4.a.3)**

If the documentation in a medical record does not indicate the type of diabetes but does indicate that the patient uses insulin, code E11, Type 2 diabetes mellitus, should be assigned. An additional code should be assigned from category Z79 to identify the long-term (current) use of insulin or oral hypoglycemic drugs. If the patient is treated with both oral medications and insulin, only the code for long-term (current) use of insulin should be assigned if insulin is given temporarily to bring a type 2 patient's blood sugar under control during an encounter.

GUIDELINES **Section I.C.15.i**

Code Z79.4, Long-term (current) use of insulin or code Z79.84, Long-term (current) use of oral hypoglycemic drugs, should not be assigned with codes from subcategory O24.4.

5 **Z79.5 Long term (current) use of steroids**

Z79.51 Long term (current) use of inhaled steroids

Z79.52 Long term (current) use of systemic steroids

5 **Z79.8 Other long term (current) drug therapy**

Z79.81 Long term (current) use of agents affecting estrogen receptors and estrogen levels

Code first, if applicable:
- malignant neoplasm of breast (C50.-)
- malignant neoplasm of prostate (C61)

Use additional code, if applicable, to identify:
- *estrogen receptor positive status (Z17.0)*
- *family history of breast cancer (Z80.3)*
- *genetic susceptibility to malignant neoplasm (cancer) (Z15.0-)*
- *personal history of breast cancer (Z85.3)*
- *personal history of prostate cancer (Z85.46)*
- *postmenopausal status (Z78.0)*

EXCLUDES 1 *hormone replacement therapy (Z79.890)*

Z79.810 Long term (current) use of selective estrogen receptor modulators (SERMs)
- Long term (current) use of raloxifene (Evista)
- Long term (current) use of tamoxifen (Nolvadex)
- Long term (current) use of toremifene (Fareston)

Z79.811 Long term (current) use of aromatase inhibitors
- Long term (current) use of anastrozole (Arimidex)
- Long term (current) use of exemestane (Aromasin)
- Long term (current) use of letrozole (Femara)

Z79.818 Long term (current) use of other agents affecting estrogen receptors and estrogen levels
- Long term (current) use of estrogen receptor downregulators
- Long term (current) use of fulvestrant (Faslodex)
- Long term (current) use of gonadotropin-releasing hormone (GnRH) agonist
- Long term (current) use of goserelin acetate (Zoladex)
- Long term (current) use of leuprolide acetate (leuprorelin) (Lupron)
- Long term (current) use of megestrol acetate (Megace)

Z79.82 Long term (current) use of aspirin

Z79.83 Long term (current) use of bisphosphonates

Z79.84 Long term (current) use of oral hypoglycemic drugs
- Long term (current) use of oral antidiabetic drugs

EXCLUDES 2 *long term (current) use of insulin (Z79.4)*

Z79.89 Other long term (current) drug therapy

Z79.890 Hormone replacement therapy

Z79.891 Long term (current) use of opiate analgesic
- Long term (current) use of methadone for pain management

EXCLUDES 1 *methodone use NOS (F11.9-)*
use of methodone for treatment of heroin addiction (F11.2-)

Z79.899 Other long term (current) drug therapy

AHA: 3Q 2015, 21-22

AHA: 4Q 2015, 34

Z80 Family history of primary malignant neoplasm

GUIDELINES **Section I.C.21.c.4)**

There are two types of history Z codes, personal and family. Personal history codes explain a patient's past medical condition that no longer exists and is not receiving any treatment, but that has the potential for recurrence, and therefore may require continued monitoring.

Family history codes are for use when a patient has a family member(s) who has had a particular disease that causes the patient to be at higher risk of also contracting the disease. Personal history codes may be used in conjunction with follow-up codes and family history codes may be used in conjunction with screening codes to explain the need for a test or procedure. History codes are also acceptable on any medical record regardless of the reason for visit. A history of an illness, even if no longer present, is important information that may alter the type of treatment ordered.

Z80.0 Family history of malignant neoplasm of digestive organs
Conditions classifiable to C15-C26

Z80.1 Family history of malignant neoplasm of trachea, bronchus and lung
Conditions classifiable to C33-C34

Z80.2 Family history of malignant neoplasm of other respiratory and intrathoracic organs
Conditions classifiable to C30-C32, C37-C39

Z80.3 Family history of malignant neoplasm of breast
Conditions classifiable to C50.-

Z80.4 Family history of malignant neoplasm of genital organs
Conditions classifiable to C51-C63

Z80.41 Family history of malignant neoplasm of ovary

Z80.42 Family history of malignant neoplasm of prostate

Z80.43 Family history of malignant neoplasm of testis

Z80.49 Family history of malignant neoplasm of other genital organs

Z80.5 Family history of malignant neoplasm of urinary tract
Conditions classifiable to C64-C68

Z80.51 Family history of malignant neoplasm of kidney

Z80.52 Family history of malignant neoplasm of bladder

Z80.59 Family history of malignant neoplasm of other urinary tract organ

Z80.6 Family history of leukemia
Conditions classifiable to C91-C95

Z80.7 Family history of other malignant neoplasms of lymphoid, hematopoietic and related tissues
Conditions classifiable to C81-C90, C96.-

Z80.8 Family history of malignant neoplasm of other organs or systems
Conditions classifiable to C00-C14, C40-C49, C69-C79

Z80.9 Family history of malignant neoplasm, unspecified
Conditions classifiable to C80.1

Z81 Family history of mental and behavioral disorders

GUIDELINES **Section I.C.21.c.4)**

There are two types of history Z codes, personal and family. Personal history codes explain a patient's past medical condition that no longer exists and is not receiving any treatment, but that has the potential for recurrence, and therefore may require continued monitoring.

Family history codes are for use when a patient has a family member(s) who has had a particular disease that causes the patient to be at higher risk of also contracting the disease. Personal history codes may be used in conjunction with follow-up codes and family history codes may be used in conjunction with screening codes to explain the need for a test or procedure. History codes are also acceptable on any medical record regardless of the reason for visit. A history of an illness, even if no longer present, is important information that may alter the type of treatment ordered.

Z81.0 Family history of intellectual disabilities
Conditions classifiable to F70-F79

Z81.1 Family history of alcohol abuse and dependence
Conditions classifiable to F10.-

Z81.2 Family history of tobacco abuse and dependence
Conditions classifiable to F17.-

Z81.3 Family history of other psychoactive substance abuse and dependence
Conditions classifiable to F11-F16, F18-F19

Z81.4 Family history of other substance abuse and dependence
Conditions classifiable to F55

Z81.8 Family history of other mental and behavioral disorders
Conditions classifiable elsewhere in F01-F99

Z82 Family history of certain disabilities and chronic diseases (leading to disablement)

GUIDELINES Section I.C.21.c.4)

There are two types of history Z codes, personal and family. Personal history codes explain a patient's past medical condition that no longer exists and is not receiving any treatment, but that has the potential for recurrence, and therefore may require continued monitoring.

Family history codes are for use when a patient has a family member(s) who has had a particular disease that causes the patient to be at higher risk of also contracting the disease. Personal history codes may be used in conjunction with follow-up codes and family history codes may be used in conjunction with screening codes to explain the need for a test or procedure. History codes are also acceptable on any medical record regardless of the reason for visit. A history of an illness, even if no longer present, is important information that may alter the type of treatment ordered.

Z82.0 **Family history of epilepsy and other diseases of the nervous system**
Conditions classifiable to G00-G99

Z82.1 **Family history of blindness and visual loss**
Conditions classifiable to H54.-

Z82.2 **Family history of deafness and hearing loss**
Conditions classifiable to H90-H91

Z82.3 **Family history of stroke**
Conditions classifiable to I60-I64

5 **Z82.4** **Family history of ischemic heart disease and other diseases of the circulatory system**
Conditions classifiable to I00-I52, I65-I99

Z82.41 **Family history of sudden cardiac death**

Z82.49 **Family history of ischemic heart disease and other diseases of the circulatory system**

Z82.5 **Family history of asthma and other chronic lower respiratory diseases**
Conditions classifiable to J40-J47

EXCLUDES 2 *family history of other diseases of the respiratory system (Z83.6)*

5 **Z82.6** **Family history of arthritis and other diseases of the musculoskeletal system and connective tissue**
Conditions classifiable to M00-M99

Z82.61 **Family history of arthritis**

Z82.62 **Family history of osteoporosis**

Z82.69 **Family history of other diseases of the musculoskeletal system and connective tissue**

5 **Z82.7** **Family history of congenital malformations, deformations and chromosomal abnormalities**
Conditions classifiable to Q00-Q99

Z82.71 **Family history of polycystic kidney**

Z82.79 **Family history of other congenital malformations, deformations and chromosomal abnormalities**

Z82.8 **Family history of other disabilities and chronic diseases leading to disablement, not elsewhere classified**

4 **Z83** **Family history of other specific disorders**

EXCLUDES 2 *contact with and (suspected) exposure to communicable disease in the family (Z20.-)*

GUIDELINES Section I.C.21.c.4)

There are two types of history Z codes, personal and family. Personal history codes explain a patient's past medical condition that no longer exists and is not receiving any treatment, but that has the potential for recurrence, and therefore may require continued monitoring.

Family history codes are for use when a patient has a family member(s) who has had a particular disease that causes the patient to be at higher risk of also contracting the disease. Personal history codes may be used in conjunction with follow-up codes and family history codes may be used in conjunction with screening codes to explain the need for a test or procedure. History codes are also acceptable on any medical record regardless of the reason for visit. A history of an illness, even if no longer present, is important information that may alter the type of treatment ordered.

Z83.0 **Family history of human immunodeficiency virus [HIV] disease**
Conditions classifiable to B20

Z83.1 **Family history of other infectious and parasitic diseases**
Conditions classifiable to A00-B19, B25-B94, B99

Z83.2 **Family history of diseases of the blood and blood-forming organs and certain disorders involving the immune mechanism**
Conditions classifiable to D50-D89

Z83.3 **Family history of diabetes mellitus**
Conditions classifiable to E08-E13

5 **Z83.4** **Family history of other endocrine, nutritional and metabolic diseases**
Conditions classifiable to E00-E07, E15-E88

Z83.41 **Family history of multiple endocrine neoplasia [MEN] syndrome**

Z83.42 **Family history of familial hypercholesterolemia**

● 6 **Z83.43** **Family history of other disorder of lipoprotein metabolism and other lipidemias**

● **Z83.430** **Family history of elevated lipoprotein(a)**
Family history of elevated Lp(a)

● **Z83.438** **Family history of other disorder of lipoprotein metabolism and other lipidemia**
Family history of familial combined hyperlipidemia

Z83.49 **Family history of other endocrine, nutritional and metabolic diseases**

5 **Z83.5** **Family history of eye and ear disorders**

6 **Z83.51** **Family history of eye disorders**
Conditions classifiable to H00-H53, H55-H59

EXCLUDES 2 *family history of blindness and visual loss (Z82.1)*

Z83.511 **Family history of glaucoma**

Z83.518 **Family history of other specified eye disorder**

Z83.52 **Family history of ear disorders**
Conditions classifiable to H60-H83, H92-H95

EXCLUDES 2 *family history of deafness and hearing loss (Z82.2)*

Z83.6 **Family history of other diseases of the respiratory system**
Conditions classifiable to J00-J39, J60-J99

EXCLUDES 2 *family history of asthma and other chronic lower respiratory diseases (Z82.5)*

5 **Z83.7** **Family history of diseases of the digestive system**
Conditions classifiable to K00-K93

Z83.71 **Family history of colonic polyps**

EXCLUDES 2 *family history of malignant neoplasm of digestive organs (Z80.0)*

Z83.79 **Family history of other diseases of the digestive system**

4 **Z84** **Family history of other conditions**

GUIDELINES Section I.C.21.c.4)

There are two types of history Z codes, personal and family. Personal history codes explain a patient's past medical condition that no longer exists and is not receiving any treatment, but that has the potential for recurrence, and therefore may require continued monitoring.

Family history codes are for use when a patient has a family member(s) who has had a particular disease that causes the patient to be at higher risk of also contracting the disease. Personal history codes may be used in conjunction with follow-up codes and family history codes may be used in conjunction with screening codes to explain the need for a test or procedure. History codes are also acceptable on any medical record regardless of the reason for visit. A history of an illness, even if no longer present, is important information that may alter the type of treatment ordered.

Z84.0 **Family history of diseases of the skin and subcutaneous tissue**
Conditions classifiable to L00-L99

Z84.1 **Family history of disorders of kidney and ureter**
Conditions classifiable to N00-N29

Z84.2 **Family history of other diseases of the genitourinary system**
Conditions classifiable to N30-N99

Z84.3 **Family history of consanguinity**

5 **Z84.8** **Family history of other specified conditions**

Z84.81 **Family history of carrier of genetic disease**

Z84.82 **Family history of sudden infant death syndrome**
Family history of SIDS

Z84.89 **Family history of other specified conditions**

4 Z85 Personal history of malignant neoplasm

Code first:
any follow-up examination after treatment of malignant neoplasm (Z08)

Use additional code to identify:
alcohol use and dependence (F10.-)
exposure to environmental tobacco smoke (Z77.22)
history of tobacco dependence (Z87.891)
occupational exposure to environmental tobacco smoke (Z57.31)
tobacco dependence (F17.-)
tobacco use (Z72.0)

EXCLUDES 2 *personal history of benign neoplasm (Z86.01-)*
personal history of carcinoma-in-situ (Z86.00-)

GUIDELINES **Section I.C.2.m**

When a primary malignancy has been excised but further treatment, such as an additional surgery for the malignancy, radiation therapy or chemotherapy is directed to that site, the primary malignancy code should be used until treatment is completed.

When a primary malignancy has been previously excised or eradicated from its site, there is no further treatment (of the malignancy) directed at that site, and there is no evidence of any existing primary malignancy, a code from category Z85 should be used to indicate the former site of the malignancy.

Subcategories Z85.0 – Z85.7 should only be assigned for the former site of a primary malignancy, not the site of a secondary malignancy. Codes from subcategory Z85.8-, may be assigned for the former site(s) of either a primary or secondary malignancy included in this subcategory.

GUIDELINES **Section I.C.21.c.4)**

There are two types of history Z codes, personal and family. Personal history codes explain a patient's past medical condition that no longer exists and is not receiving any treatment, but that has the potential for recurrence, and therefore may require continued monitoring.

Family history codes are for use when a patient has a family member(s) who has had a particular disease that causes the patient to be at higher risk of also contracting the disease. Personal history codes may be used in conjunction with follow-up codes and family history codes may be used in conjunction with screening codes to explain the need for a test or procedure. History codes are also acceptable on any medical record regardless of the reason for visit. A history of an illness, even if no longer present, is important information that may alter the type of treatment ordered.

CODING TIP✓ The codes in this section are commonly referred to as the "history of cancer" codes. "History" in this case means the cancer has been eradicated from its primary site. It does not necessarily mean the patient no longer has cancer. The cancer may have already metastasized to other sites.

5 Z85.0 Personal history of malignant neoplasm of digestive organs

Z85.00 Personal history of malignant neoplasm of unspecified digestive organ

Z85.01 Personal history of malignant neoplasm of esophagus
Conditions classifiable to C15

6 Z85.02 Personal history of malignant neoplasm of stomach

Z85.020 Personal history of malignant carcinoid tumor of stomach
Conditions classifiable to C7A.092

Z85.028 Personal history of other malignant neoplasm of stomach
Conditions classifiable to C16

6 Z85.03 Personal history of malignant neoplasm of large intestine

Z85.030 Personal history of malignant carcinoid tumor of large intestine
Conditions classifiable to C7A.022-C7A.025, C7A.029

Z85.038 Personal history of other malignant neoplasm of large intestine
Conditions classifiable to C18

6 Z85.04 Personal history of malignant neoplasm of rectum, rectosigmoid junction, and anus

Z85.040 Personal history of malignant carcinoid tumor of rectum
Conditions classifiable to C7A.026

Z85.048 Personal history of other malignant neoplasm of rectum, rectosigmoid junction, and anus
Conditions classifiable to C19-C21

Z85.05 Personal history of malignant neoplasm of liver
Conditions classifiable to C22

6 Z85.06 Personal history of malignant neoplasm of small intestine

Z85.060 Personal history of malignant carcinoid tumor of small intestine
Conditions classifiable to C7A.01-

Z85.068 Personal history of other malignant neoplasm of small intestine
Conditions classifiable to C17

Z85.07 Personal history of malignant neoplasm of pancreas
Conditions classifiable to C25

Z85.09 Personal history of malignant neoplasm of other digestive organs

5 Z85.1 Personal history of malignant neoplasm of trachea, bronchus and lung

6 Z85.11 Personal history of malignant neoplasm of bronchus and lung

Z85.110 Personal history of malignant carcinoid tumor of bronchus and lung
Conditions classifiable to C7A.090

Z85.118 Personal history of other malignant neoplasm of bronchus and lung
Conditions classifiable to C34

Z85.12 Personal history of malignant neoplasm of trachea
Conditions classifiable to C33

5 Z85.2 Personal history of malignant neoplasm of other respiratory and intrathoracic organs

Z85.20 Personal history of malignant neoplasm of unspecified respiratory organ

Z85.21 Personal history of malignant neoplasm of larynx
Conditions classifiable to C32

Z85.22 Personal history of malignant neoplasm of nasal cavities, middle ear, and accessory sinuses
Conditions classifiable to C30-C31

6 Z85.23 Personal history of malignant neoplasm of thymus

Z85.230 Personal history of malignant carcinoid tumor of thymus
Conditions classifiable to C7A.091

Z85.238 Personal history of other malignant neoplasm of thymus
Conditions classifiable to C37

Z85.29 Personal history of malignant neoplasm of other respiratory and intrathoracic organs

Z85.3 Personal history of malignant neoplasm of breast
Conditions classifiable to C50.-

5 Z85.4 Personal history of malignant neoplasm of genital organs
Conditions classifiable to C51-C63

Z85.40 Personal history of malignant neoplasm of unspecified female genital organ ♀

Z85.41 Personal history of malignant neoplasm of cervix uteri ♀

Z85.42 Personal history of malignant neoplasm of other parts of uterus ♀

Z85.43 Personal history of malignant neoplasm of ovary ♀

Z85.44 Personal history of malignant neoplasm of other female genital organs ♀

Z85.45 Personal history of malignant neoplasm of unspecified male genital organ ♂

Z85.46 Personal history of malignant neoplasm of prostate ♂

Z85.47 Personal history of malignant neoplasm of testis ♂

Z85.48 Personal history of malignant neoplasm of epididymis ♂

Z85.49 Personal history of malignant neoplasm of other male genital organs ♂

5 Z85.5 Personal history of malignant neoplasm of urinary tract
Conditions classifiable to C64-C68

Z85.50 Personal history of malignant neoplasm of unspecified urinary tract organ

Z85.51 Personal history of malignant neoplasm of bladder

6 **Z85.52 Personal history of malignant neoplasm of kidney**
EXCLUDES 1 *personal history of malignant neoplasm of renal pelvis (Z85.53)*
Z85.520 Personal history of malignant carcinoid tumor of kidney
Conditions classifiable to C7A.093
Z85.528 Personal history of other malignant neoplasm of kidney
Conditions classifiable to C64
Z85.53 Personal history of malignant neoplasm of renal pelvis
Z85.54 Personal history of malignant neoplasm of ureter
Z85.59 Personal history of malignant neoplasm of other urinary tract organ
Z85.6 Personal history of leukemia
Conditions classifiable to C91-C95
EXCLUDES 1 *leukemia in remission C91.0-C95.9 with 5th character 1*
5 **Z85.7 Personal history of other malignant neoplasms of lymphoid, hematopoietic and related tissues**
Z85.71 Personal history of Hodgkin lymphoma
Conditions classifiable to C81
Z85.72 Personal history of non-Hodgkin lymphomas
Conditions classifiable to C82-C85
Z85.79 Personal history of other malignant neoplasms of lymphoid, hematopoietic and related tissues
Conditions classifiable to C88-C90, C96
EXCLUDES 1 *multiple myeloma in remission (C90.01)*
plasma cell leukemia in remission (C90.11)
plasmacytoma in remission (C90.21)
GUIDELINES **Section I.C.2.n**
The categories for leukemia, and category C90, Multiple myeloma and malignant plasma cell neoplasms, have codes indicating whether or not the leukemia has achieved remission. There are also codes Z85.6, Personal history of leukemia, and Z85.79, Personal history of other malignant neoplasms of lymphoid, hematopoietic and related tissues. If the documentation is unclear, as to whether the leukemia has achieved remission, the provider should be queried.
5 **Z85.8 Personal history of malignant neoplasms of other organs and systems**
Conditions classifiable to C00-C14, C40-C49, C69-C75, C7A.098, C76-C79
6 **Z85.81 Personal history of malignant neoplasm of lip, oral cavity, and pharynx**
Z85.810 Personal history of malignant neoplasm of tongue
Z85.818 Personal history of malignant neoplasm of other sites of lip, oral cavity, and pharynx
Z85.819 Personal history of malignant neoplasm of unspecified site of lip, oral cavity, and pharynx
6 **Z85.82 Personal history of malignant neoplasm of skin**
Z85.820 Personal history of malignant melanoma of skin
Conditions classifiable to C43
Z85.821 Personal history of Merkel cell carcinoma
Conditions classifiable to C4A
Z85.828 Personal history of other malignant neoplasm of skin
Conditions classifiable to C44
6 **Z85.83 Personal history of malignant neoplasm of bone and soft tissue**
Z85.830 Personal history of malignant neoplasm of bone
Z85.831 Personal history of malignant neoplasm of soft tissue
EXCLUDES 2 *personal history of malignant neoplasm of skin (Z85.82-)*
6 **Z85.84 Personal history of malignant neoplasm of eye and nervous tissue**
Z85.840 Personal history of malignant neoplasm of eye
Z85.841 Personal history of malignant neoplasm of brain
Z85.848 Personal history of malignant neoplasm of other parts of nervous tissue
6 **Z85.85 Personal history of malignant neoplasm of endocrine glands**
Z85.850 Personal history of malignant neoplasm of thyroid
Z85.858 Personal history of malignant neoplasm of other endocrine glands
Z85.89 Personal history of malignant neoplasm of other organs and systems
Z85.9 Personal history of malignant neoplasm, unspecified
Conditions classifiable to C7A.00, C80.1

4 **Z86 Personal history of certain other diseases**
Code first:
any follow-up examination after treatment (Z09)
GUIDELINES **Section I.C.21.c.4)**
There are two types of history Z codes, personal and family. Personal history codes explain a patient's past medical condition that no longer exists and is not receiving any treatment, but that has the potential for recurrence, and therefore may require continued monitoring.

Family history codes are for use when a patient has a family member(s) who has had a particular disease that causes the patient to be at higher risk of also contracting the disease. Personal history codes may be used in conjunction with follow-up codes and family history codes may be used in conjunction with screening codes to explain the need for a test or procedure. History codes are also acceptable on any medical record regardless of the reason for visit. A history of an illness, even if no longer present, is important information that may alter the type of treatment ordered.
5 **Z86.0 Personal history of in-situ and benign neoplasms and neoplasms of uncertain behavior**
EXCLUDES 2 *personal history of malignant neoplasms (Z85.-)*
6 **Z86.00 Personal history of in-situ neoplasm**
Conditions classifiable to D00-D09
Z86.000 Personal history of in-situ neoplasm of breast
Z86.001 Personal history of in-situ neoplasm of cervix uteri ♀
Personal history of cervical intraepithelial neoplasia III [CIN III]
Z86.008 Personal history of in-situ neoplasm of other site
Personal history of vaginal intraepithelial neoplasia III [VAIN III]
Personal history of vulvar intraepithelial neoplasia III [VIN III]
6 **Z86.01 Personal history of benign neoplasm**
AHA: 1Q 2017, 14
Z86.010 Personal history of colonic polyps
AHA: 1Q 2017, 8
Z86.011 Personal history of benign neoplasm of the brain
Z86.012 Personal history of benign carcinoid tumor
Z86.018 Personal history of other benign neoplasm
Z86.03 Personal history of neoplasm of uncertain behavior
5 **Z86.1 Personal history of infectious and parasitic diseases**
Conditions classifiable to A00-B89, B99
EXCLUDES 1 *personal history of infectious diseases specific to a body system*
sequelae of infectious and parasitic diseases (B90-B94)
Z86.11 Personal history of tuberculosis
Z86.12 Personal history of poliomyelitis
Z86.13 Personal history of malaria
Z86.14 Personal history of Methicillin resistant Staphylococcus aureus infection
Personal history of MRSA infection
Z86.19 Personal history of other infectious and parasitic diseases
Z86.2 Personal history of diseases of the blood and blood-forming organs and certain disorders involving the immune mechanism
Conditions classifiable to D50-D89
5 **Z86.3 Personal history of endocrine, nutritional and metabolic diseases**
Conditions classifiable to E00-E88
Z86.31 Personal history of diabetic foot ulcer
EXCLUDES 2 *current diabetic foot ulcer (E08.621, E09.621, E10.621, E11.621, E13.621)*

Z86.32 Personal history of gestational diabetes ♀
Personal history of conditions classifiable to O24.4-
EXCLUDES 1 *gestational diabetes mellitus in current pregnancy (O24.4-)*

Z86.39 Personal history of other endocrine, nutritional and metabolic disease

Z86.5 Personal history of mental and behavioral disorders
Conditions classifiable to F40-F59

Z86.51 Personal history of combat and operational stress reaction A

Z86.59 Personal history of other mental and behavioral disorders

Z86.6 Personal history of diseases of the nervous system and sense organs
Conditions classifiable to G00-G99, H00-H95

Z86.61 Personal history of infections of the central nervous system
Personal history of encephalitis
Personal history of meningitis

Z86.69 Personal history of other diseases of the nervous system and sense organs

Z86.7 Personal history of diseases of the circulatory system
Conditions classifiable to I00-I99
EXCLUDES 2 *old myocardial infarction (I25.2)*
personal history of anaphylactic shock (Z87.892)
postmyocardial infarction syndrome (I24.1)

Z86.71 Personal history of venous thrombosis and embolism

Z86.711 Personal history of pulmonary embolism

Z86.718 Personal history of other venous thrombosis and embolism

Z86.72 Personal history of thrombophlebitis

Z86.73 Personal history of transient ischemic attack (TIA), and cerebral infarction without residual deficits
Personal history of prolonged reversible ischemic neurological deficit (PRIND)
Personal history of stroke NOS without residual deficits
EXCLUDES 1 *personal history of traumatic brain injury (Z87.820)*
sequelae of cerebrovascular disease (I69.-)

GUIDELINES **Section I.C.9.d.3)**
Codes from category I69, Sequela of cerebrovascular disease, should not be assigned if the patient does not have neurologic deficits. Assign Z86.73, Personal history of transient ischemic attack (TIA) and cerebral infarction
AHA: 4Q 2012, 92-93

Z86.74 Personal history of sudden cardiac arrest
Personal history of sudden cardiac death successfully resuscitated

Z86.79 Personal history of other diseases of the circulatory system

Z87 Personal history of other diseases and conditions

Code first:
any follow-up examination after treatment (Z09)

GUIDELINES **Section I.C.21.c.4)**
There are two types of history Z codes, personal and family. Personal history codes explain a patient's past medical condition that no longer exists and is not receiving any treatment, but that has the potential for recurrence, and therefore may require continued monitoring.

Family history codes are for use when a patient has a family member(s) who has had a particular disease that causes the patient to be at higher risk of also contracting the disease. Personal history codes may be used in conjunction with follow-up codes and family history codes may be used in conjunction with screening codes to explain the need for a test or procedure. History codes are also acceptable on any medical record regardless of the reason for visit. A history of an illness, even if no longer present, is important information that may alter the type of treatment ordered.

Z87.0 Personal history of diseases of the respiratory system
Conditions classifiable to J00-J99

Z87.01 Personal history of pneumonia (recurrent)

Z87.09 Personal history of other diseases of the respiratory system

Z87.1 Personal history of diseases of the digestive system
Conditions classifiable to K00-K93

Z87.11 Personal history of peptic ulcer disease

Z87.19 Personal history of other diseases of the digestive system
AHA: 1Q 2017, 14

Z87.2 Personal history of diseases of the skin and subcutaneous tissue
Conditions classifiable to L00-L99
EXCLUDES 2 *personal history of diabetic foot ulcer (Z86.31)*

Z87.3 Personal history of diseases of the musculoskeletal system and connective tissue
Conditions classifiable to M00-M99
EXCLUDES 2 *personal history of (healed) traumatic fracture (Z87.81)*

Z87.31 Personal history of (healed) nontraumatic fracture

Z87.310 Personal history of (healed) osteoporosis fracture
Personal history of (healed) fragility fracture
Personal history of (healed) collapsed vertebra due to osteoporosis

GUIDELINES **Section I.C.13.d.1)**
Category M81, Osteoporosis without current pathological fracture, is for use for patients with osteoporosis who do not currently have a pathologic fracture due to the osteoporosis, even if they have had a fracture in the past. For patients with a history of osteoporosis fractures, status code Z87.310, Personal history of (healed) osteoporosis fracture, should follow the code from M81.

Z87.311 Personal history of (healed) other pathological fracture
Personal history of (healed) collapsed vertebra NOS
EXCLUDES 2 *personal history of osteoporosis fracture (Z87.310)*

Z87.312 Personal history of (healed) stress fracture
Personal history of (healed) fatigue fracture

Z87.39 Personal history of other diseases of the musculoskeletal system and connective tissue

Z87.4 Personal history of diseases of genitourinary system
Conditions classifiable to N00-N99

Z87.41 Personal history of dysplasia of the female genital tract
EXCLUDES 1 *personal history of intraepithelial neoplasia III of female genital tract (Z86.001, Z86.008)*
personal history of malignant neoplasm of female genital tract (Z85.40-Z85.44)

Z87.410 Personal history of cervical dysplasia ♀

Z87.411 Personal history of vaginal dysplasia ♀

Z87.412 Personal history of vulvar dysplasia ♀

Z87.42 Personal history of other diseases of the female genital tract ♀

Z87.43 Personal history of diseases of male genital organs

Z87.430 Personal history of prostatic dysplasia ♂
EXCLUDES 1 *personal history of malignant neoplasm of prostate (Z85.46)*

Z87.438 Personal history of other diseases of male genital organs ♂

Z87.44 Personal history of diseases of urinary system
EXCLUDES 1 *personal history of malignant neoplasm of cervix uteri (Z85.41)*

Z87.440 Personal history of urinary (tract) infections

Z87.441 Personal history of nephrotic syndrome

Z87.442 Personal history of urinary calculi
Personal history of kidney stones

Z87.448 Personal history of other diseases of urinary system

Z87.5 Personal history of complications of pregnancy, childbirth and the puerperium
Conditions classifiable to O00-O9A
EXCLUDES 2 *recurrent pregnancy loss (N96)*

Z87.51 Personal history of pre-term labor ♀
EXCLUDES 1 *current pregnancy with history of pre-term labor (O09.21-)*

Z87.59 **Personal history of other complications of pregnancy, childbirth and the puerperium** ♀
Personal history of trophoblastic disease

5 Z87.7 **Personal history of (corrected) congenital malformations**
Conditions classifiable to Q00-Q89 that have been repaired or corrected
EXCLUDES 1 *congenital malformations that have been partially corrected or repair but which still require medical treatment - code to condition*
EXCLUDES 2 *other postprocedural states (Z98.-)*
personal history of medical treatment (Z92.-)
presence of cardiac and vascular implants and grafts (Z95.-)
presence of other devices (Z97.-)
presence of other functional implants (Z96.-)
transplanted organ and tissue status (Z94.-)

6 Z87.71 **Personal history of (corrected) congenital malformations of genitourinary system**
Z87.710 **Personal history of (corrected) hypospadias** ♂
Z87.718 **Personal history of other specified (corrected) congenital malformations of genitourinary system**

6 Z87.72 **Personal history of (corrected) congenital malformations of nervous system and sense organs**
Z87.720 **Personal history of (corrected) congenital malformations of eye**
Z87.721 **Personal history of (corrected) congenital malformations of ear**
Z87.728 **Personal history of other specified (corrected) congenital malformations of nervous system and sense organs**

6 Z87.73 **Personal history of (corrected) congenital malformations of digestive system**
Z87.730 **Personal history of (corrected) cleft lip and palate**
Z87.738 **Personal history of other specified (corrected) congenital malformations of digestive system**

Z87.74 **Personal history of (corrected) congenital malformations of heart and circulatory system**
Z87.75 **Personal history of (corrected) congenital malformations of respiratory system**
Z87.76 **Personal history of (corrected) congenital malformations of integument, limbs and musculoskeletal system**

6 Z87.79 **Personal history of other (corrected) congenital malformations**
Z87.790 **Personal history of (corrected) congenital malformations of face and neck**
Z87.798 **Personal history of other (corrected) congenital malformations**

5 Z87.8 **Personal history of other specified conditions**
EXCLUDES 2 *personal history of self harm (Z91.5)*

Z87.81 **Personal history of (healed) traumatic fracture**
EXCLUDES 2 *personal history of (healed) nontraumatic fracture (Z87.31-)*

6 Z87.82 **Personal history of other (healed) physical injury and trauma**
Conditions classifiable to S00-T88, except traumatic fractures
Z87.820 **Personal history of traumatic brain injury**
EXCLUDES 1 *personal history of transient ischemic attack (TIA), and cerebral infarction without residual deficits (Z86.73)*
Z87.821 **Personal history of retained foreign body fully removed**
Z87.828 **Personal history of other (healed) physical injury and trauma**

6 Z87.89 **Personal history of other specified conditions**
Z87.890 **Personal history of sex reassignment**
Z87.891 **Personal history of nicotine dependence**
EXCLUDES 1 *current nicotine dependence (F17.2-)*
CODING TIP ✓ Use this code if the physician uses the term "history." Remission is coded to F17.2 codes.
AHA: 2Q 2017, 27
Z87.892 **Personal history of anaphylaxis**
Code also allergy status such as:
allergy status to drugs, medicaments and biological substances (Z88.-)
allergy status, other than to drugs and biological substances (Z91.0-)
Z87.898 **Personal history of other specified conditions**
AHA: 1Q 2013, 21

4 Z88 **Allergy status to drugs, medicaments and biological substances**
EXCLUDES 2 *Allergy status, other than to drugs and biological substances (Z91.0-)*

Z88.0 **Allergy status to penicillin**
Z88.1 **Allergy status to other antibiotic agents status**
Z88.2 **Allergy status to sulfonamides status**
AHA: 3Q 2015, 23
Z88.3 **Allergy status to other anti-infective agents status**
Z88.4 **Allergy status to anesthetic agent status**
Z88.5 **Allergy status to narcotic agent status**
Z88.6 **Allergy status to analgesic agent status**
Z88.7 **Allergy status to serum and vaccine status**
Z88.8 **Allergy status to other drugs, medicaments and biological substances status**
Z88.9 **Allergy status to unspecified drugs, medicaments and biological substances status**

4 Z89 **Acquired absence of limb**
INCLUDES amputation status
postprocedural loss of limb
post-traumatic loss of limb
EXCLUDES 1 *acquired deformities of limbs (M20-M21)*
congenital absence of limbs (Q71-Q73)

5 Z89.0 **Acquired absence of thumb and other finger(s)**
6 Z89.01 **Acquired absence of thumb**
⊟ Z89.011 **Acquired absence of right thumb**
⊟ Z89.012 **Acquired absence of left thumb**
⊟ Z89.019 **Acquired absence of unspecified thumb**
6 Z89.02 **Acquired absence of other finger(s)**
EXCLUDES 2 *acquired absence of thumb (Z89.01-)*
⊟ Z89.021 **Acquired absence of right finger(s)**
⊟ Z89.022 **Acquired absence of left finger(s)**
⊟ Z89.029 **Acquired absence of unspecified finger(s)**

5 Z89.1 **Acquired absence of hand and wrist**
6 Z89.11 **Acquired absence of hand**
⊟ Z89.111 **Acquired absence of right hand**
⊟ Z89.112 **Acquired absence of left hand**
⊟ Z89.119 **Acquired absence of unspecified hand**
6 Z89.12 **Acquired absence of wrist**
Disarticulation at wrist
⊟ Z89.121 **Acquired absence of right wrist**
⊟ Z89.122 **Acquired absence of left wrist**
⊟ Z89.129 **Acquired absence of unspecified wrist**

5 Z89.2 **Acquired absence of upper limb above wrist**
6 Z89.20 **Acquired absence of upper limb, unspecified level**
⊟ Z89.201 **Acquired absence of right upper limb, unspecified level**
⊟ Z89.202 **Acquired absence of left upper limb, unspecified level**
⊟ Z89.209 **Acquired absence of unspecified upper limb, unspecified level**
Acquired absence of arm NOS
6 Z89.21 **Acquired absence of upper limb below elbow**
⊟ Z89.211 **Acquired absence of right upper limb below elbow**
⊟ Z89.212 **Acquired absence of left upper limb below elbow**
⊟ Z89.219 **Acquired absence of unspecified upper limb below elbow**
6 Z89.22 **Acquired absence of upper limb above elbow**
Disarticulation at elbow

Z89.221 **Acquired absence of right upper limb above elbow**

Z89.222 **Acquired absence of left upper limb above elbow**

Z89.229 **Acquired absence of unspecified upper limb above elbow**

Z89.23 **Acquired absence of shoulder**

Acquired absence of shoulder joint following explantation of shoulder joint prosthesis, with or without presence of antibiotic-impregnated cement spacer

Z89.231 **Acquired absence of right shoulder**

Z89.232 **Acquired absence of left shoulder**

Z89.239 **Acquired absence of unspecified shoulder**

Z89.4 **Acquired absence of toe(s), foot, and ankle**

Z89.41 **Acquired absence of great toe**

Z89.411 **Acquired absence of right great toe** HCC

Z89.412 **Acquired absence of left great toe** HCC

Z89.419 **Acquired absence of unspecified great toe** HCC

Z89.42 **Acquired absence of other toe(s)**

EXCLUDES 2 *acquired absence of great toe (Z89.41-)*

Z89.421 **Acquired absence of other right toe(s)** HCC

Z89.422 **Acquired absence of other left toe(s)** HCC

Z89.429 **Acquired absence of other toe(s), unspecified side** HCC

Z89.43 **Acquired absence of foot**

Z89.431 **Acquired absence of right foot** HCC

Z89.432 **Acquired absence of left foot** HCC

Z89.439 **Acquired absence of unspecified foot** HCC

Z89.44 **Acquired absence of ankle**

Disarticulation of ankle

Z89.441 **Acquired absence of right ankle** HCC

Z89.442 **Acquired absence of left ankle** HCC

Z89.449 **Acquired absence of unspecified ankle** HCC

Z89.5 **Acquired absence of leg below knee**

Z89.51 **Acquired absence of leg below knee**

Z89.511 **Acquired absence of right leg below knee** HCC

Z89.512 **Acquired absence of left leg below knee** HCC

Z89.519 **Acquired absence of unspecified leg below knee** HCC

Z89.52 **Acquired absence of knee**

Acquired absence of knee joint following explantation of knee joint prosthesis, with or without presence of antibiotic-impregnated cement spacer

Z89.521 **Acquired absence of right knee**

Z89.522 **Acquired absence of left knee**

Z89.529 **Acquired absence of unspecified knee**

Z89.6 **Acquired absence of leg above knee**

Z89.61 **Acquired absence of leg above knee**

Acquired absence of leg NOS

Disarticulation at knee

Z89.611 **Acquired absence of right leg above knee** HCC

Z89.612 **Acquired absence of left leg above knee** HCC

Z89.619 **Acquired absence of unspecified leg above knee** HCC

Z89.62 **Acquired absence of hip**

Acquired absence of hip joint following explantation of hip joint prosthesis, with or without presence of antibiotic-impregnated cement spacer

Disarticulation at hip

Z89.621 **Acquired absence of right hip joint**

Z89.622 **Acquired absence of left hip joint**

Z89.629 **Acquired absence of unspecified hip joint**

Z89.9 **Acquired absence of limb, unspecified**

Z90 Acquired absence of organs, not elsewhere classified

INCLUDES postprocedural or post-traumatic loss of body part NEC

EXCLUDES 1 *congenital absence - see Alphabetical Index*

EXCLUDES 2 *postprocedural absence of endocrine glands (E89.-)*

Z90.0 **Acquired absence of part of head and neck**

Z90.01 **Acquired absence of eye**

Z90.02 **Acquired absence of larynx**

Z90.09 **Acquired absence of other part of head and neck**

Acquired absence of nose

EXCLUDES 2 *teeth (K08.1)*

Z90.1 **Acquired absence of breast and nipple**

Z90.10 **Acquired absence of unspecified breast and nipple**

Z90.11 **Acquired absence of right breast and nipple**

Z90.12 **Acquired absence of left breast and nipple**

Z90.13 **Acquired absence of bilateral breasts and nipples**

Z90.2 **Acquired absence of lung [part of]**

Z90.3 **Acquired absence of stomach [part of]**

Z90.4 **Acquired absence of other specified parts of digestive tract**

Z90.41 **Acquired absence of pancreas**

Code also:

exocrine pancreatic insufficiency (K86.81)

Use additional code to identify any associated:

insulin use (Z79.4)

diabetes mellitus, postpancreatectomy (E13.-)

GUIDELINES **Section I.C.4.a.6)(b)(i)**

For postpancreatectomy diabetes mellitus (lack of insulin due to the surgical removal of all or part of the pancreas), assign code E89.1, Postprocedural hypoinsulinemia. Assign a code from category E13 and a code from subcategory Z90.41-, Acquired absence of pancreas, as additional codes.

Z90.410 **Acquired total absence of pancreas**

Acquired absence of pancreas NOS

Z90.411 **Acquired partial absence of pancreas**

Z90.49 **Acquired absence of other specified parts of digestive tract**

Z90.5 **Acquired absence of kidney**

Z90.6 **Acquired absence of other parts of urinary tract**

Acquired absence of bladder

Z90.7 **Acquired absence of genital organ(s)**

EXCLUDES 1 *personal history of sex reassignment (Z87.890)*

EXCLUDES 2 *female genital mutilation status (N90.81-)*

Z90.71 **Acquired absence of cervix and uterus**

Z90.710 **Acquired absence of both cervix and uterus** ♀

Acquired absence of uterus NOS

Status post total hysterectomy

Z90.711 **Acquired absence of uterus with remaining cervical stump** ♀

Status post partial hysterectomy with remaining cervical stump

Z90.712 **Acquired absence of cervix with remaining uterus** ♀

Z90.72 **Acquired absence of ovaries**

Z90.721 **Acquired absence of ovaries, unilateral** ♀

Z90.722 **Acquired absence of ovaries, bilateral** ♀

Z90.79 **Acquired absence of other genital organ(s)**

Z90.8 **Acquired absence of other organs**

Z90.81 **Acquired absence of spleen**

Z90.89 **Acquired absence of other organs**

Z91 Personal risk factors, not elsewhere classified

EXCLUDES 2 *contact with and (suspected) exposures hazardous to health (Z77.-)*

exposure to pollution and other problems related to physical environment (Z77.1-)

female genital mutilation status (N90.81-)

personal history of physical injury and trauma (Z87.81, Z87.82-)

occupational exposure to risk factors (Z57.-)

Z91.0 **Allergy status, other than to drugs and biological substances**

EXCLUDES 2 *Allergy status to drugs, medicaments, and biological substances (Z88.-)*

Z91.01 **Food allergy status**

EXCLUDES 2 *food additives allergy status (Z91.02)*

Z91.010 **Allergy to peanuts**

Z91.011 **Allergy to milk products**

EXCLUDES 1 *lactose intolerance (E73.-)*

Z91.012 **Allergy to eggs**

Z91.013 **Allergy to seafood**
Allergy to shellfish
Allergy to octopus or squid ink

Z91.018 **Allergy to other foods**
Allergy to nuts other than peanuts

Z91.02 **Food additives allergy status**

6 Z91.03 **Insect allergy status**

Z91.030 **Bee allergy status**

Z91.038 **Other insect allergy status**

6 Z91.04 **Nonmedicinal substance allergy status**

Z91.040 **Latex allergy status**
Latex sensitivity status

Z91.041 **Radiographic dye allergy status**
Allergy status to contrast media used for diagnostic X-ray procedure

Z91.048 **Other nonmedicinal substance allergy status**

Z91.09 **Other allergy status, Other than to drugs and biological substances**

5 Z91.1 **Patient's noncompliance with medical treatment and regimen**

Z91.11 **Patient's noncompliance with dietary regimen**

6 Z91.12 **Patient's intentional underdosing of medication regimen**
Code first:
underdosing of medication (T36-T50) with fifth or sixth character 6

EXCLUDES 1 *adverse effect of prescribed drug taken as directed- code to adverse effect*
poisoning (overdose) -code to poisoning

GUIDELINES Section I.C.19.e.5)(c)
Noncompliance (Z91.12-, Z91.13- and Z91.14-) or complication of care (Y63.6-Y63.9) codes are to be used with an underdosing code to indicate intent, if known.

CODING TIP✓ A code from Z91.12- or Z91.13- should be assigned when underdosing has been identified and coded in the plan of care/medical record.

Z91.120 **Patient's intentional underdosing of medication regimen due to financial hardship**

Z91.128 **Patient's intentional underdosing of medication regimen for other reason**

6 Z91.13 **Patient's unintentional underdosing of medication regimen**
Code first:
underdosing of medication (T36-T50) with fifth or sixth character 6

EXCLUDES 1 *adverse effect of prescribed drug taken as directed- code to adverse effect*
poisoning (overdose) -code to poisoning

GUIDELINES Section I.C.19.e.5)(c)
Noncompliance (Z91.12-, Z91.13- and Z91.14-) or complication of care (Y63.6-Y63.9) codes are to be used with an underdosing code to indicate intent, if known.

CODING TIP✓ A code from Z91.12- or Z91.13- should be assigned when underdosing has been identified and coded in the plan of care/medical record.

Z91.130 **Patient's unintentional underdosing of medication regimen due to age-related debility**

Z91.138 **Patient's unintentional underdosing of medication regimen for other reason**

Z91.14 **Patient's other noncompliance with medication regimen**
Patient's underdosing of medication NOS

GUIDELINES Section I.C.19.e.5)(c)
Noncompliance (Z91.12-, Z91.13- and Z91.14-) or complication of care (Y63.6-Y63.9) codes are to be used with an underdosing code to indicate intent, if known.

Z91.15 **Patient's noncompliance with renal dialysis** HCC

Z91.19 **Patient's noncompliance with other medical treatment and regimen**
Nonadherence to medical treatment

5 Z91.4 **Personal history of psychological trauma, not elsewhere classified**

GUIDELINES Section I.C.21.c.4)
There are two types of history Z codes, personal and family. Personal history codes explain a patient's past medical condition that no longer exists and is not receiving any treatment, but that has the potential for recurrence, and therefore may require continued monitoring.

Family history codes are for use when a patient has a family member(s) who has had a particular disease that causes the patient to be at higher risk of also contracting the disease. Personal history codes may be used in conjunction with follow-up codes and family history codes may be used in conjunction with screening codes to explain the need for a test or procedure. History codes are also acceptable on any medical record regardless of the reason for visit. A history of an illness, even if no longer present, is important information that may alter the type of treatment ordered.

6 Z91.41 **Personal history of adult abuse**

EXCLUDES 2 *personal history of abuse in childhood (Z62.81-)*

Z91.410 **Personal history of adult physical and sexual abuse** A

EXCLUDES 1 *current adult physical abuse (T74.11, T76.11)*
current adult sexual abuse (T74.21, T76.11)

Z91.411 **Personal history of adult psychological abuse** A

Z91.412 **Personal history of adult neglect** A

EXCLUDES 1 *current adult neglect (T74.01, T76.01)*

Z91.419 **Personal history of unspecified adult abuse** A

● Z91.42 **Personal history of forced labor or sexual exploitation**

Z91.49 **Other personal history of psychological trauma, not elsewhere classified**

Z91.5 **Personal history of self-harm**
Personal history of parasuicide
Personal history of self-poisoning
Personal history of suicide attempt

GUIDELINES Section I.C.21.c.4)
There are two types of history Z codes, personal and family. Personal history codes explain a patient's past medical condition that no longer exists and is not receiving any treatment, but that has the potential for recurrence, and therefore may require continued monitoring.

Family history codes are for use when a patient has a family member(s) who has had a particular disease that causes the patient to be at higher risk of also contracting the disease. Personal history codes may be used in conjunction with follow-up codes and family history codes may be used in conjunction with screening codes to explain the need for a test or procedure. History codes are also acceptable on any medical record regardless of the reason for visit. A history of an illness, even if no longer present, is important information that may alter the type of treatment ordered.

5 Z91.8 **Other specified personal risk factors, not elsewhere classified**

GUIDELINES **Section I.C.21.c.4)**
There are two types of history Z codes, personal and family. Personal history codes explain a patient's past medical condition that no longer exists and is not receiving any treatment, but that has the potential for recurrence, and therefore may require continued monitoring.

Family history codes are for use when a patient has a family member(s) who has had a particular disease that causes the patient to be at higher risk of also contracting the disease. Personal history codes may be used in conjunction with follow-up codes and family history codes may be used in conjunction with screening codes to explain the need for a test or procedure. History codes are also acceptable on any medical record regardless of the reason for visit. A history of an illness, even if no longer present, is important information that may alter the type of treatment ordered.

Z91.81 History of falling
At risk for falling

GUIDELINES **Section I.C.21.c.4)**
There are two types of history Z codes, personal and family. Personal history codes explain a patient's past medical condition that no longer exists and is not receiving any treatment, but that has the potential for recurrence, and therefore may require continued monitoring.

Family history codes are for use when a patient has a family member(s) who has had a particular disease that causes the patient to be at higher risk of also contracting the disease. Personal history codes may be used in conjunction with follow-up codes and family history codes may be used in conjunction with screening codes to explain the need for a test or procedure. History codes are also acceptable on any medical record regardless of the reason for visit. A history of an illness, even if no longer present, is important information that may alter the type of treatment ordered.

GUIDELINES **Section I.C.18.d**
Code R29.6, Repeated falls, is for use for encounters when a patient has recently fallen and the reason for the fall is being investigated. Code Z91.81, History of falling, is for use when a patient has fallen in the past and is at risk for future falls. When appropriate, both codes R29.6 and Z91.81 may be assigned together.

CODING TIP✓ Use this code when a patient has fallen in the past and is at risk for future falls. In some cases, it may be appropriate to assign R29.6, Repeated falls, on the same claim with Z91.81 if the patient is experiencing current, repeated falls and the intent of the episode is to investigate and treat the falls. Z91.81 may not be first listed on hospital claims.

CODING TIP✓ Code Z91.81 may be listed primary or secondary. Use this code when a patient has fallen in the past and is at risk for future falls.

Z91.82 Personal history of military deployment A
Individual (civilian or military) with past history of military war, peacekeeping and humanitarian deployment (current or past conflict)
Returned from military deployment

Z91.83 *Wandering in diseases classified elsewhere*
Code first underlying disorder such as:
Alzheimer's disease (G30.-)
autism or pervasive developmental disorder (F84.-)
intellectual disabilities (F70-F79)
unspecified dementia with behavioral disturbance (F03.9-)

6 **Z91.84 Oral health risk factors**
Z91.841 Risk for dental caries, low
Z91.842 Risk for dental caries, moderate
Z91.843 Risk for dental caries, high
Z91.849 Unspecified risk for dental caries

Z91.89 Other specified personal risk factors, not elsewhere classified
AHA: 1Q 2017, 45

4 **Z92 Personal history of medical treatment**
EXCLUDES 2 *postprocedural states (Z98.-)*

Z92.0 Personal history of contraception
EXCLUDES 1 *counseling or management of current contraceptive practices (Z30.-)*
long term (current) use of contraception (Z79.3)
presence of (intrauterine) contraceptive device (Z97.5)

5 **Z92.2 Personal history of drug therapy**
EXCLUDES 2 *long term (current) drug therapy (Z79.-)*

Z92.21 Personal history of antineoplastic chemotherapy
Z92.22 Personal history of monoclonal drug therapy
Z92.23 Personal history of estrogen therapy
6 **Z92.24 Personal history of steroid therapy**
Z92.240 Personal history of inhaled steroid therapy
Z92.241 Personal history of systemic steroid therapy
Personal history of steroid therapy NOS
Z92.25 Personal history of immunosupression therapy
EXCLUDES 2 *personal history of steroid therapy (Z92.24)*
Z92.29 Personal history of other drug therapy

Z92.3 Personal history of irradiation
Personal history of exposure to therapeutic radiation
EXCLUDES 1 *exposure to radiation in the physical environment (Z77.12)*
occupational exposure to radiation (Z57.1)

5 **Z92.8 Personal history of other medical treatment**
Z92.81 Personal history of extracorporeal membrane oxygenation (ECMO)
Z92.82 Status post administration of tPA (rtPA) in a different facility within the last 24 hours prior to admission to current facility
Code first condition requiring tPA administration, such as:
acute cerebral infarction (I63.-)
acute myocardial infarction (I21.-, I22.-)
AHA: 4Q 2013, 124
Z92.83 Personal history of failed moderate sedation
Personal history of failed conscious sedation
EXCLUDES 2 *failed moderate sedation during procedure (T88.52)*
Z92.84 Personal history of unintended awareness under general anesthesia
EXCLUDES 2 *unintended awareness under general anesthesia during procedure (T88.53)*
AHA: 4Q 2016, 72
Z92.89 Personal history of other medical treatment

4 **Z93 Artificial opening status**
EXCLUDES 1 *artificial openings requiring attention or management (Z43.-)*
complications of external stoma (J95.0-, K94.-, N99.5-)

CODING TIP✓ Assign codes from category Z93 to indicate artificial openings which are present but do not require intervention or management by the agency. Do not use codes in the Z93 category with attention to artificial opening codes (Z43) codes for the same ostomy or when the ostomy is complicated.

Z93.0 Tracheostomy status HCC
AHA: 4Q 2013, 129
Z93.1 Gastrostomy status HCC
Z93.2 Ileostomy status HCC
Z93.3 Colostomy status HCC
Z93.4 Other artificial openings of gastrointestinal tract status HCC
5 **Z93.5 Cystostomy status**
Z93.50 Unspecified cystostomy status HCC
Z93.51 Cutaneous-vesicostomy status HCC
Z93.52 Appendico-vesicostomy status HCC
Z93.59 Other cystostomy status HCC

Z93.6 **Other artificial openings of urinary tract status** HCC
Nephrostomy status
Ureterostomy status
Urethrostomy status
Z93.8 **Other artificial opening status** HCC
Z93.9 **Artificial opening status, unspecified** HCC

Z94 Transplanted organ and tissue status
INCLUDES organ or tissue replaced by heterogenous or homogenous transplant
EXCLUDES 1 *complications of transplanted organ or tissue - see Alphabetical Index*
EXCLUDES 2 *presence of vascular grafts (Z95.-)*
CODING TIP These are status codes and are used to 1) indicate that a transplant has occurred in the past; and 2) to provide more information as to type of transplant, **if needed**, in the case of aftercare (Z48.2) or transplant complications (T86).

Z94.0 **Kidney transplant status**
GUIDELINES **Section I.C.14.a.2)**
Patients who have undergone kidney transplant may still have some form of chronic kidney disease (CKD) because the kidney transplant may not fully restore kidney function. Therefore, the presence of CKD alone does not constitute a transplant complication. Assign the appropriate N18 code for the patient's stage of CKD and code Z94.0, Kidney transplant status. If a transplant complication such as failure or rejection or other transplant complication is documented, see section I.C.19.g for information on coding complications of a kidney transplant. If the documentation is unclear as to whether the patient has a complication of the transplant, query the provider.
Z94.1 **Heart transplant status** HCC
EXCLUDES 1 *artificial heart status (Z95.812)*
heart-valve replacement status (Z95.2-Z95.4)
Z94.2 **Lung transplant status** HCC
Z94.3 **Heart and lungs transplant status** HCC
Z94.4 **Liver transplant status** HCC
Z94.5 **Skin transplant status**
Autogenous skin transplant status
Z94.6 **Bone transplant status**
Z94.7 **Corneal transplant status**
Z94.8 **Other transplanted organ and tissue status**
Z94.81 **Bone marrow transplant status** HCC
Z94.82 **Intestine transplant status** HCC
Z94.83 **Pancreas transplant status** HCC
Z94.84 **Stem cells transplant status** HCC
Z94.89 **Other transplanted organ and tissue status**
Z94.9 **Transplanted organ and tissue status, unspecified**

Z95 Presence of cardiac and vascular implants and grafts
EXCLUDES 2 *complications of cardiac and vascular devices, implants and grafts (T82.-)*
Z95.0 **Presence of cardiac pacemaker**
Presence of cardiac resynchronization therapy (CRT-P) pacemaker
EXCLUDES 1 *adjustment or management of cardiac device (Z45.0-)*
adjustment or management of cardiac pacemaker (Z45.0)
presence of automatic (implantable) cardiac defibrillator with synchronous cardiac pacemaker (Z95.810)
Z95.1 **Presence of aortocoronary bypass graft**
Presence of coronary artery bypass graft
CODING TIP Z95.1 and Z95.5 are used to indicate the presence of a coronary bypass grafts and implants without complications. If complications are documented, see T82.2-.
Z95.2 **Presence of prosthetic heart valve**
Presence of heart valve NOS
CODING TIP Code Z95.2 is used to indicate the presence of a heart valve prosthesis without complications. If complications are documented, see T82.0-.
Z95.3 **Presence of xenogenic heart valve**
Z95.4 **Presence of other heart-valve replacement**
Z95.5 **Presence of coronary angioplasty implant and graft**
EXCLUDES 1 *coronary angioplasty status without implant and graft (Z98.61)*
CODING TIP Z95.1 and Z95.5 are used to indicate the presence of a coronary bypass grafts and implants without complications. If complications are documented, see T82.2-.
Z95.8 **Presence of other cardiac and vascular implants and grafts**
Z95.81 **Presence of other cardiac implants and grafts**
CODING TIP Do not use these codes if the condition is complicated, unless the status code provides information about the specific type of device. See T82 for complications.
▲ Z95.810 **Presence of automatic (implantable) cardiac defibrillator**
Presence of automatic (implantable) cardiac defibrillator with synchronous cardiac pacemaker
Presence of cardiac resynchronization therapy defibrillator (CRT-D)
Presence of cardioverter-defibrillator (ICD)
Z95.811 **Presence of heart assist device** HCC
Z95.812 **Presence of fully implantable artificial heart** HCC
Z95.818 **Presence of other cardiac implants and grafts**
Z95.82 **Presence of other vascular implants and grafts**
Z95.820 **Peripheral vascular angioplasty status with implants and grafts**
EXCLUDES 1 *peripheral vascular angioplasty without implant and graft (Z98.62)*
Z95.828 **Presence of other vascular implants and grafts**
Presence of intravascular prosthesis NEC
Z95.9 **Presence of cardiac and vascular implant and graft, unspecified**

Z96 Presence of other functional implants
EXCLUDES 2 *complications of internal prosthetic devices, implants and grafts (T82-T85)*
fitting and adjustment of prosthetic and other devices (Z44-Z46)
Z96.0 **Presence of urogenital implants**
Z96.1 **Presence of intraocular lens**
Presence of pseudophakia
Z96.2 **Presence of otological and audiological implants**
Z96.20 **Presence of otological and audiological implant, unspecified**
Z96.21 **Cochlear implant status**
Z96.22 **Myringotomy tube(s) status**
Z96.29 **Presence of other otological and audiological implants**
Presence of bone-conduction hearing device
Presence of eustachian tube stent
Stapes replacement
Z96.3 **Presence of artificial larynx**
Z96.4 **Presence of endocrine implants**
Z96.41 **Presence of insulin pump (external) (internal)**
CODING TIP If the patient uses an insulin pump, use Z96.41 as an secondary code. If there is a complication involving the insulin pump, use a code from T85.6- or T85.7- instead of the Z code.
Z96.49 **Presence of other endocrine implants**
Z96.5 **Presence of tooth-root and mandibular implants**
Z96.6 **Presence of orthopedic joint implants**
Z96.60 **Presence of unspecified orthopedic joint implant**
Z96.61 **Presence of artificial shoulder joint**
Z96.611 **Presence of right artificial shoulder joint**
Z96.612 **Presence of left artificial shoulder joint**
Z96.619 **Presence of unspecified artificial shoulder joint**
Z96.62 **Presence of artificial elbow joint**
Z96.621 **Presence of right artificial elbow joint**
Z96.622 **Presence of left artificial elbow joint**
Z96.629 **Presence of unspecified artificial elbow joint**
Z96.63 **Presence of artificial wrist joint**
Z96.631 **Presence of right artificial wrist joint**
Z96.632 **Presence of left artificial wrist joint**

Z96.639 Presence of unspecified artificial wrist joint

Z96.64 Presence of artificial hip joint
Hip-joint replacement (partial) (total)

Z96.641 Presence of right artificial hip joint
AHA: 3Q 2016, 16

Z96.642 Presence of left artificial hip joint
AHA: 1Q 2015, 16

Z96.643 Presence of artificial hip joint, bilateral

Z96.649 Presence of unspecified artificial hip joint

Z96.65 Presence of artificial knee joint

Z96.651 Presence of right artificial knee joint

Z96.652 Presence of left artificial knee joint

Z96.653 Presence of artificial knee joint, bilateral

Z96.659 Presence of unspecified artificial knee joint

Z96.66 Presence of artificial ankle joint

Z96.661 Presence of right artificial ankle joint

Z96.662 Presence of left artificial ankle joint

Z96.669 Presence of unspecified artificial ankle joint

Z96.69 Presence of other orthopedic joint implants

Z96.691 Finger-joint replacement of right hand

Z96.692 Finger-joint replacement of left hand

Z96.693 Finger-joint replacement, bilateral

Z96.698 Presence of other orthopedic joint implants

Z96.7 Presence of other bone and tendon implants
Presence of skull plate

Z96.8 Presence of other specified functional implants

Z96.81 Presence of artificial skin

Z96.89 Presence of other specified functional implants

Z96.9 Presence of functional implant, unspecified

Z97 Presence of other devices

EXCLUDES 1 *complications of internal prosthetic devices, implants and grafts (T82-T85)*
fitting and adjustment of prosthetic and other devices (Z44-Z46)

EXCLUDES 2 *presence of cerebrospinal fluid drainage device (Z98.2)*

Z97.0 Presence of artificial eye

Z97.1 Presence of artificial limb (complete) (partial)

Z97.10 Presence of artificial limb (complete) (partial), unspecified

Z97.11 Presence of artificial right arm (complete) (partial)

Z97.12 Presence of artificial left arm (complete) (partial)

Z97.13 Presence of artificial right leg (complete) (partial)

Z97.14 Presence of artificial left leg (complete) (partial)

Z97.15 Presence of artificial arms, bilateral (complete) (partial)

Z97.16 Presence of artificial legs, bilateral (complete) (partial)

Z97.2 Presence of dental prosthetic device (complete) (partial)
Presence of dentures (complete) (partial)

Z97.3 Presence of spectacles and contact lenses

Z97.4 Presence of external hearing-aid

Z97.5 Presence of (intrauterine) contraceptive device ♀

EXCLUDES 1 *checking, reinsertion or removal of implantable subdermal contraceptive (Z30.46)*
checking, reinsertion or removal of intrauterine contraceptive device (Z30.43-)

Z97.8 Presence of other specified devices

Z98 Other postprocedural states

EXCLUDES 2 *aftercare (Z43-Z49, Z51)*
follow-up medical care (Z08-Z09)
postprocedural complication - see Alphabetical Index

Z98.0 Intestinal bypass and anastomosis status

EXCLUDES 2 *bariatric surgery status (Z98.84)*
gastric bypass status (Z98.84)
obesity surgery status (Z98.84)

Z98.1 Arthrodesis status

CODING TIP✓ This is a status code and should not be used for joint ankylosis or nonsurgical joint fusion.

Z98.2 Presence of cerebrospinal fluid drainage device
Presence of CSF shunt

CODING TIP✓ Do not use this code for complications of a CSF shunt/drainage device. See T85.0.-

Z98.3 Post therapeutic collapse of lung status
Code first:
underlying disease

Z98.4 Cataract extraction status
Use additional code to identify intraocular lens implant status (Z96.1)

EXCLUDES 1 *aphakia (H27.0)*

Z98.41 Cataract extraction status, right eye

Z98.42 Cataract extraction status, left eye

Z98.49 Cataract extraction status, unspecified eye

Z98.5 Sterilization status

EXCLUDES 1 *female infertility (N97.-)*
male infertility (N46.-)

Z98.51 Tubal ligation status ♀

Z98.52 Vasectomy status ♂ A

Z98.6 Angioplasty status

Z98.61 Coronary angioplasty status

EXCLUDES 1 *coronary angioplasty status with implant and graft (Z95.5)*

Z98.62 Peripheral vascular angioplasty status

EXCLUDES 1 *peripheral vascular angioplasty status with implant and graft (Z95.820)*

Z98.8 Other specified postprocedural states

Z98.81 Dental procedure status

Z98.810 Dental sealant status

Z98.811 Dental restoration status
Dental crown status
Dental fillings status

Z98.818 Other dental procedure status

Z98.82 Breast implant status

EXCLUDES 1 *breast implant removal status (Z98.86)*

Z98.83 Filtering (vitreous) bleb after glaucoma surgery status

EXCLUDES 1 *Inflammation (infection) of postprocedural bleb (H59.4-)*

Z98.84 Bariatric surgery status
Gastric banding status
Gastric bypass status for obesity
Obesity surgery status

EXCLUDES 1 *bariatric surgery status complicating pregnancy, childbirth, or the puerperium (O99.84)*

EXCLUDES 2 *intestinal bypass and anastomosis status (Z98.0)*

CODING TIP✓ Do not use this code for complications related to bariatric surgery. Use a code from K95 instead.

Z98.85 Transplanted organ removal status
Transplanted organ previously removed due to complication, failure, rejection or infection

EXCLUDES 1 *encounter for removal of transplanted organ -code to complication of transplanted organ (T86.-)*

GUIDELINES **Section I.C.21.c.3)**
Assign code Z98.85, Transplanted organ removal status, to indicate that a transplanted organ has been previously removed. This code should not be assigned for the encounter in which the transplanted organ is removed. The complication necessitating removal of the transplant organ should be assigned for that encounter.

Z98.86 Personal history of breast implant removal

Z98.87 Personal history of in utero procedure

Z98.870 Personal history of in utero procedure during pregnancy ♀

EXCLUDES 2 *complications from in utero procedure for current pregnancy (O35.7)*
supervision of current pregnancy with history of in utero procedure during previous pregnancy (O09.82-)

Z98.871 Personal history of in utero procedure while a fetus

Z98.89 Other specified postprocedural states

Z98.890 Other specified postprocedural states
Personal history of surgery, not elsewhere classified

Z98.891 History of uterine scar from previous surgery ♀
EXCLUDES 1 *Maternal care due to uterine scar from previous surgery (O34.2-)*

Z99 Dependence on enabling machines and devices, not elsewhere classified
EXCLUDES 1 *cardiac pacemaker status (Z95.0)*

Z99.0 Dependence on aspirator

Z99.1 Dependence on respirator
Dependence on ventilator

Z99.11 Dependence on respirator [ventilator] status HCC
AHA: 1Q 2015, 21
AHA: 1Q 2018, 11

Z99.12 Encounter for respirator [ventilator] dependence during power failure HCC
EXCLUDES 1 *mechanical complication of respirator [ventilator] (J95.850)*

Z99.2 Dependence on renal dialysis HCC
Hemodialysis status
Peritoneal dialysis status
Presence of arteriovenous shunt for dialysis
Renal dialysis status NOS
EXCLUDES 1 *encounter for fitting and adjustment of dialysis catheter (Z49.0-)*
EXCLUDES 2 *noncompliance with renal dialysis (Z91.15)*
AHA: 1Q 2016, 12-13

▲ **Z99.3 Dependence on wheelchair**
Wheelchair confinement status
Code first cause of dependence, such as:
muscular dystrophy (G71.0-)
obesity (E66.-)

Z99.8 Dependence on other enabling machines and devices

Z99.81 Dependence on supplemental oxygen
Dependence on long-term oxygen
AHA: 4Q 2013, 129

Z99.89 Dependence on other enabling machines and devices
Dependence on machine or device NOS

Male Figure
(Anterior View)

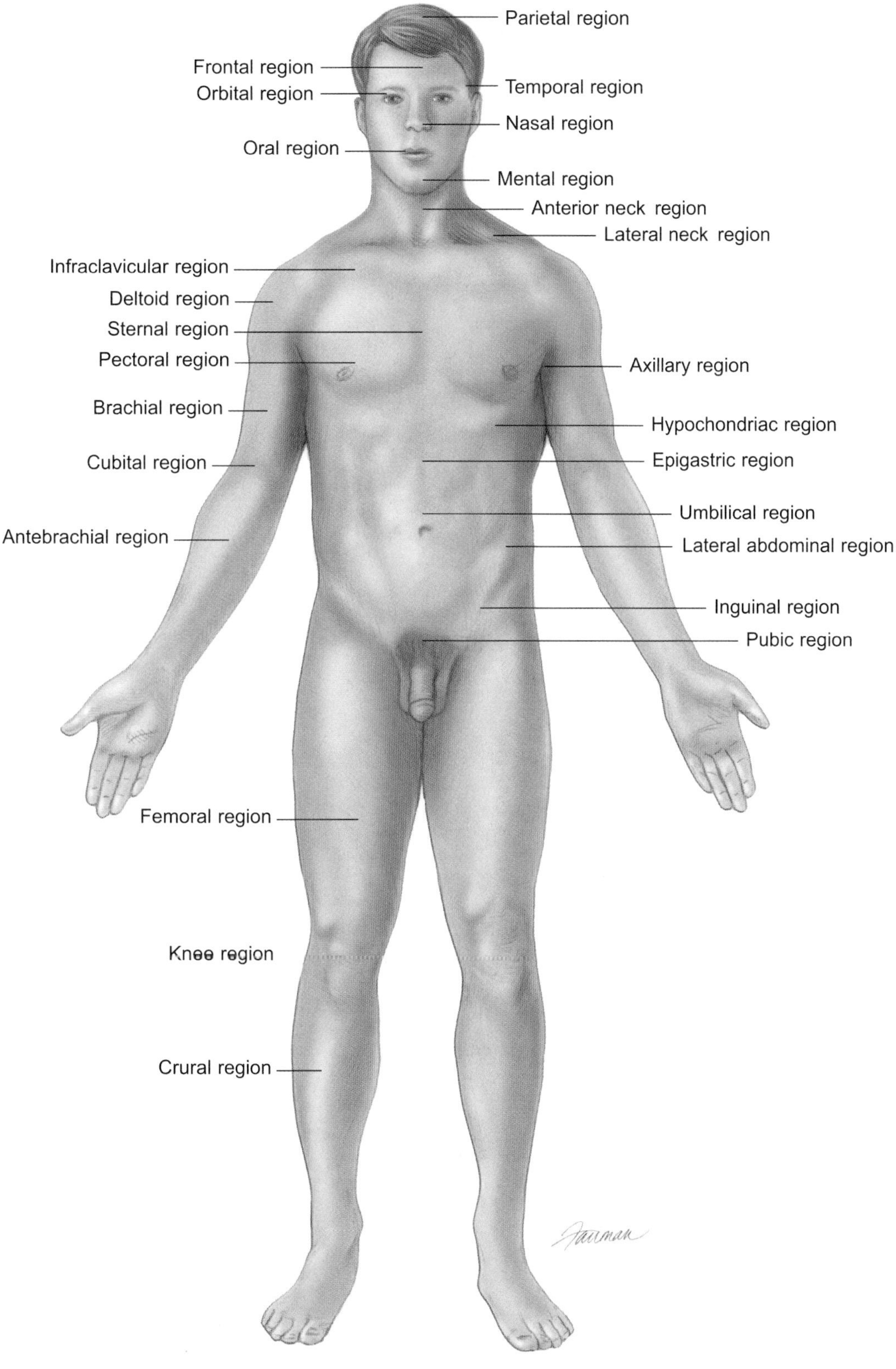
Parietal region
Frontal region
Orbital region
Temporal region
Nasal region
Oral region
Mental region
Anterior neck region
Lateral neck region
Infraclavicular region
Deltoid region
Sternal region
Pectoral region
Axillary region
Brachial region
Hypochondriac region
Cubital region
Epigastric region
Umbilical region
Antebrachial region
Lateral abdominal region
Inguinal region
Pubic region
Femoral region
Knee region
Crural region

Female Figure
(Anterior View)

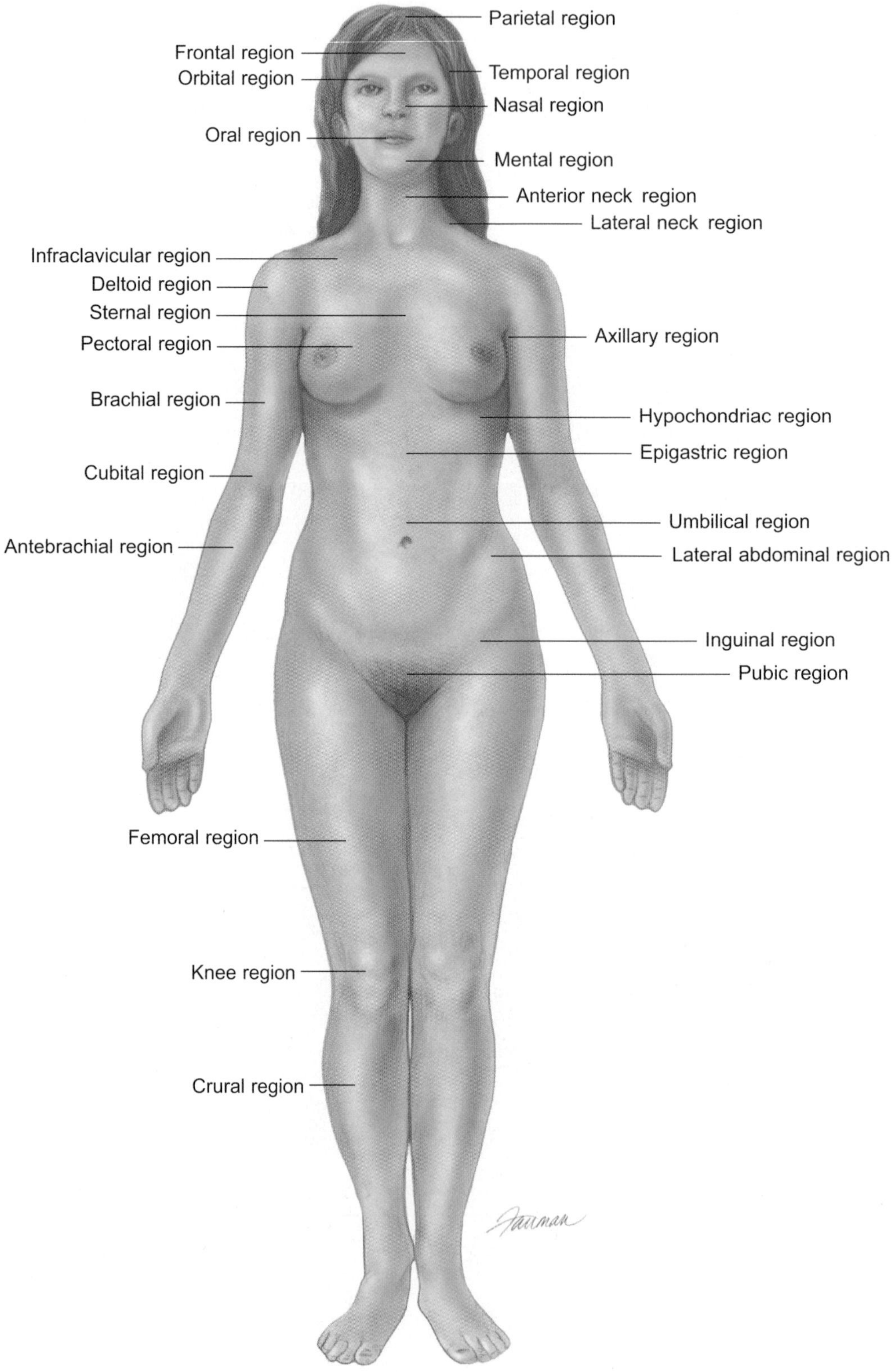
Parietal region
Frontal region
Orbital region
Temporal region
Nasal region
Oral region
Mental region
Anterior neck region
Lateral neck region
Infraclavicular region
Deltoid region
Sternal region
Pectoral region
Axillary region
Brachial region
Hypochondriac region
Epigastric region
Cubital region
Umbilical region
Antebrachial region
Lateral abdominal region
Inguinal region
Pubic region
Femoral region
Knee region
Crural region
Fairman

Female Breast

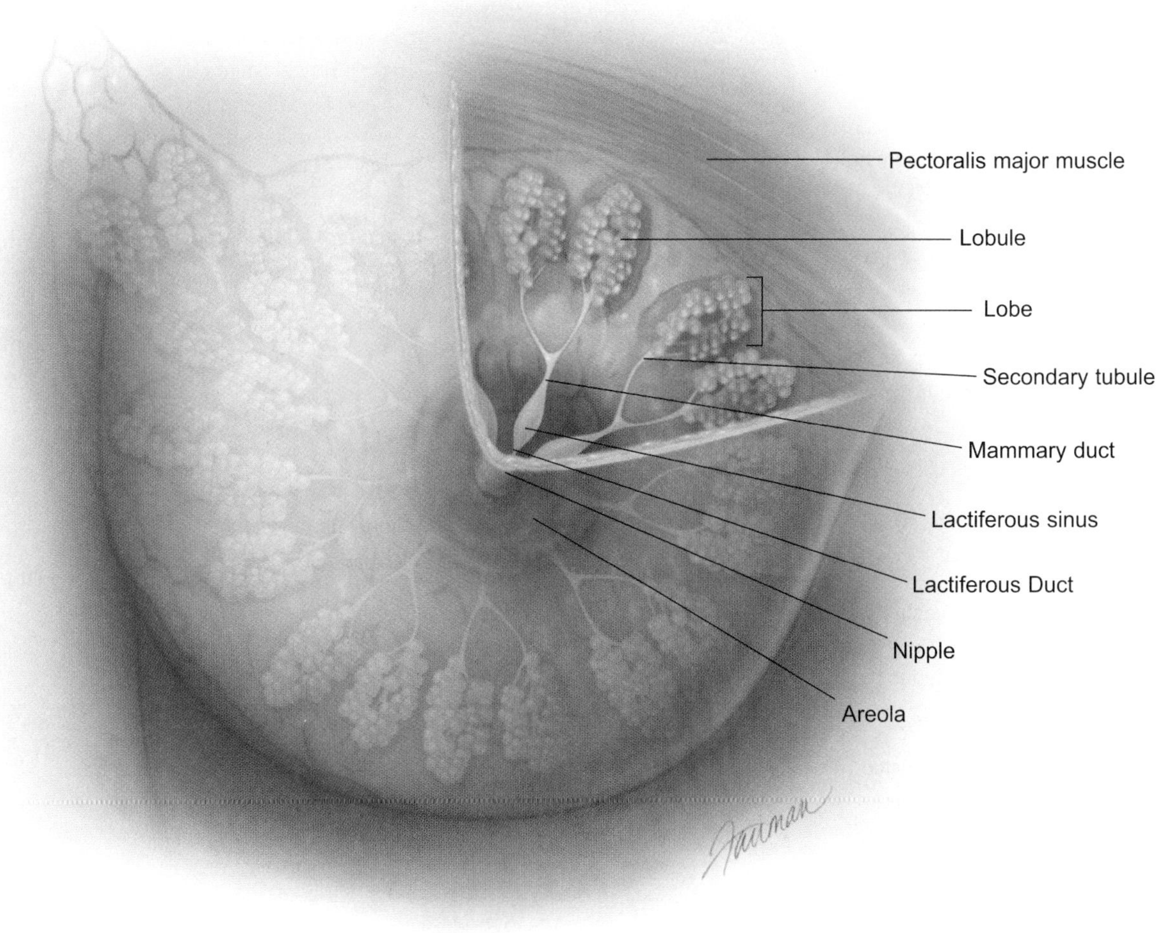

Muscular System
(Anterior View)

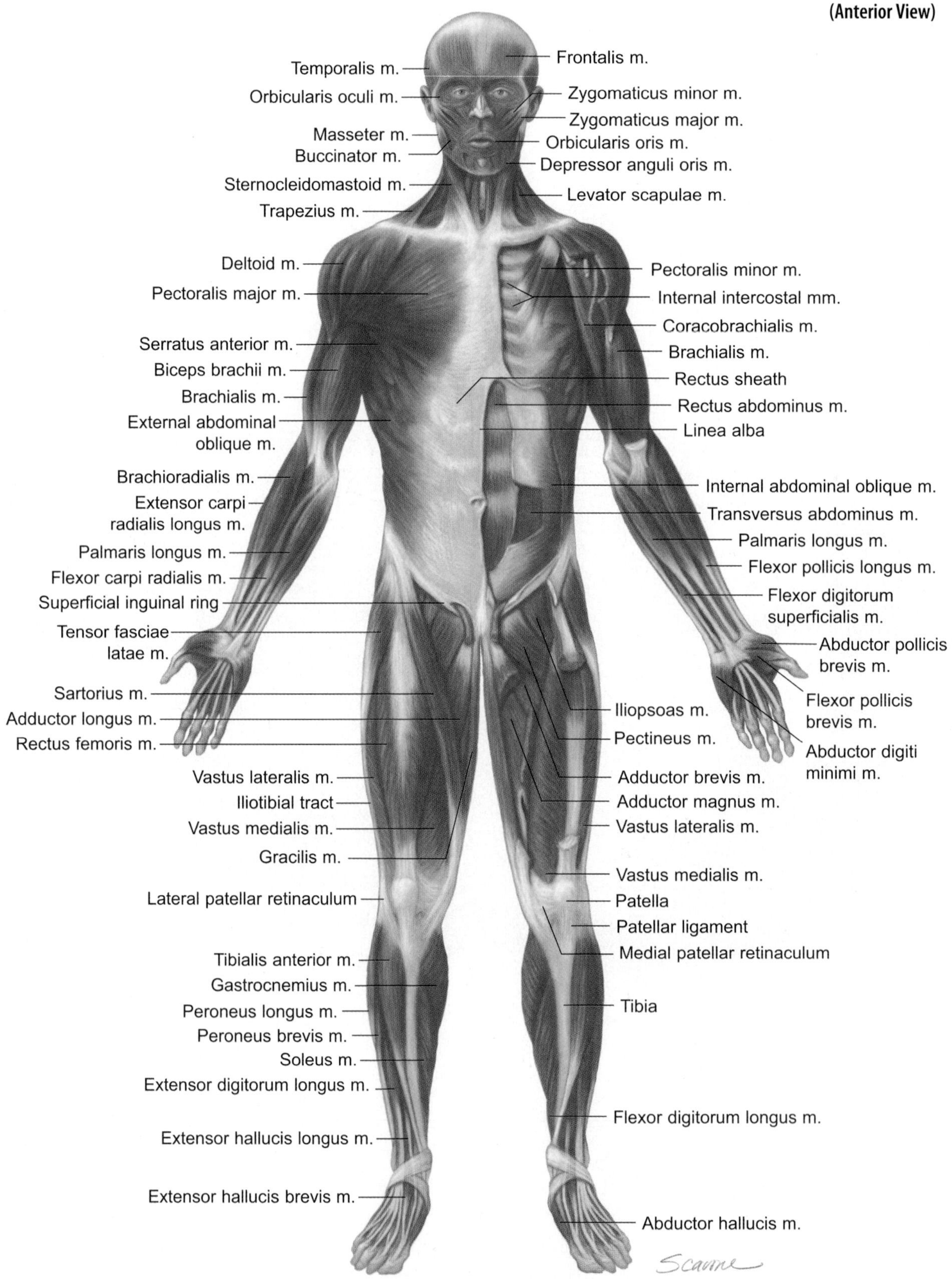

Frontalis m.
Temporalis m.
Orbicularis oculi m.
Zygomaticus minor m.
Zygomaticus major m.
Masseter m.
Orbicularis oris m.
Buccinator m.
Depressor anguli oris m.
Sternocleidomastoid m.
Levator scapulae m.
Trapezius m.
Deltoid m.
Pectoralis minor m.
Pectoralis major m.
Internal intercostal mm.
Coracobrachialis m.
Serratus anterior m.
Brachialis m.
Biceps brachii m.
Rectus sheath
Brachialis m.
Rectus abdominus m.
External abdominal oblique m.
Linea alba
Brachioradialis m.
Internal abdominal oblique m.
Extensor carpi radialis longus m.
Transversus abdominus m.
Palmaris longus m.
Palmaris longus m.
Flexor pollicis longus m.
Flexor carpi radialis m.
Flexor digitorum superficialis m.
Superficial inguinal ring
Tensor fasciae latae m.
Abductor pollicis brevis m.
Flexor pollicis brevis m.
Sartorius m.
Iliopsoas m.
Adductor longus m.
Rectus femoris m.
Pectineus m.
Abductor digiti minimi m.
Vastus lateralis m.
Adductor brevis m.
Iliotibial tract
Adductor magnus m.
Vastus medialis m.
Vastus lateralis m.
Gracilis m.
Vastus medialis m.
Lateral patellar retinaculum
Patella
Patellar ligament
Medial patellar retinaculum
Tibialis anterior m.
Gastrocnemius m.
Tibia
Peroneus longus m.
Peroneus brevis m.
Soleus m.
Extensor digitorum longus m.
Flexor digitorum longus m.
Extensor hallucis longus m.
Extensor hallucis brevis m.
Abductor hallucis m.
Scavone

Muscular System
(Posterior View)

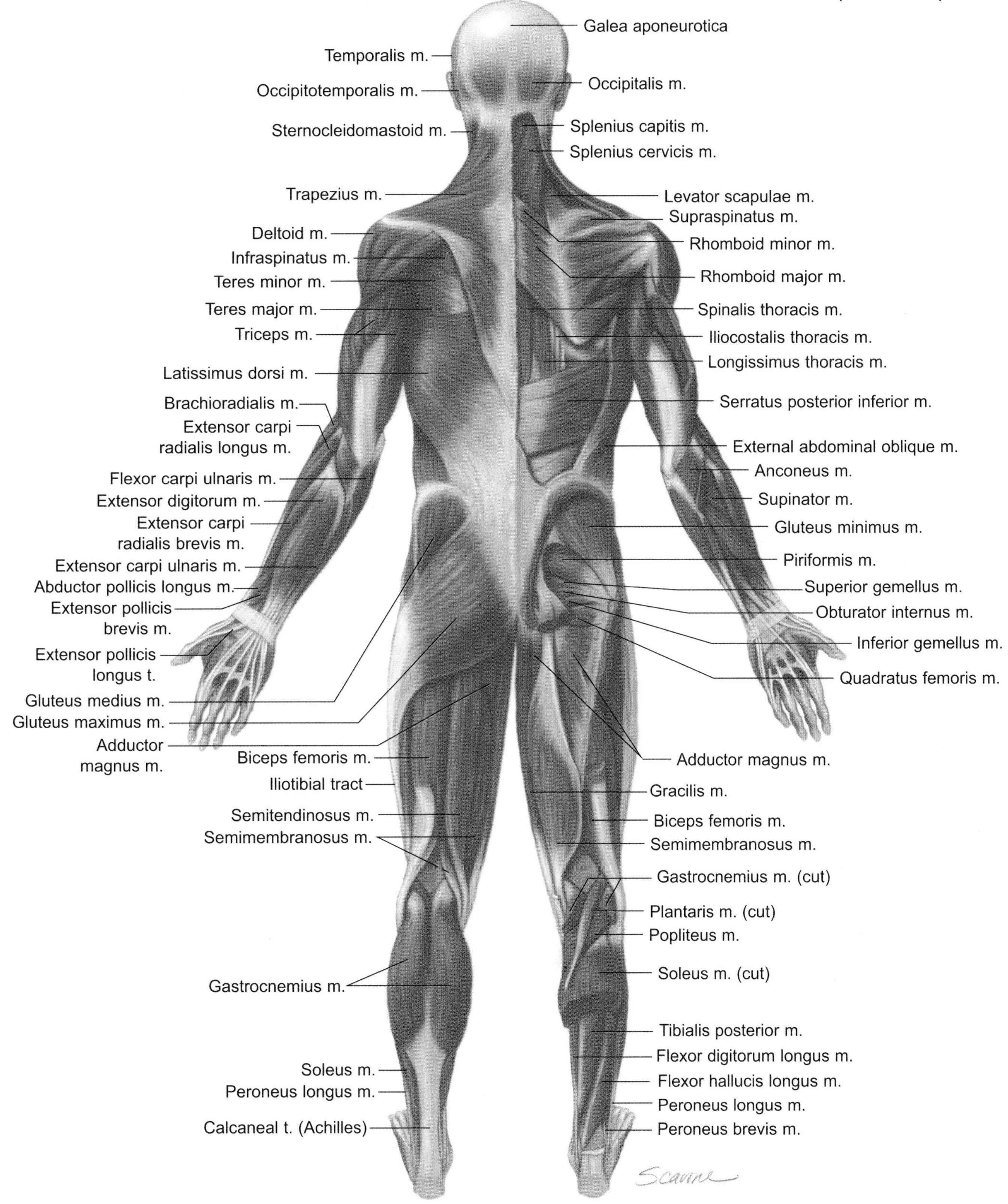
Galea aponeurotica
Temporalis m.
Occipitotemporalis m.
Occipitalis m.
Sternocleidomastoid m.
Splenius capitis m.
Splenius cervicis m.
Trapezius m.
Levator scapulae m.
Supraspinatus m.
Deltoid m.
Rhomboid minor m.
Infraspinatus m.
Rhomboid major m.
Teres minor m.
Teres major m.
Spinalis thoracis m.
Triceps m.
Iliocostalis thoracis m.
Longissimus thoracis m.
Latissimus dorsi m.
Brachioradialis m.
Serratus posterior inferior m.
Extensor carpi radialis longus m.
External abdominal oblique m.
Flexor carpi ulnaris m.
Anconeus m.
Extensor digitorum m.
Supinator m.
Extensor carpi radialis brevis m.
Gluteus minimus m.
Piriformis m.
Extensor carpi ulnaris m.
Abductor pollicis longus m.
Superior gemellus m.
Extensor pollicis brevis m.
Obturator internus m.
Inferior gemellus m.
Extensor pollicis longus t.
Quadratus femoris m.
Gluteus medius m.
Gluteus maximus m.
Adductor magnus m.
Adductor magnus m.
Biceps femoris m.
Iliotibial tract
Gracilis m.
Semitendinosus m.
Biceps femoris m.
Semimembranosus m.
Semimembranosus m.
Gastrocnemius m. (cut)
Plantaris m. (cut)
Popliteus m.
Gastrocnemius m.
Soleus m. (cut)
Tibialis posterior m.
Flexor digitorum longus m.
Soleus m.
Flexor hallucis longus m.
Peroneus longus m.
Peroneus longus m.
Calcaneal t. (Achilles)
Peroneus brevis m.
Scanne

Skeletal System
(Anterior View)

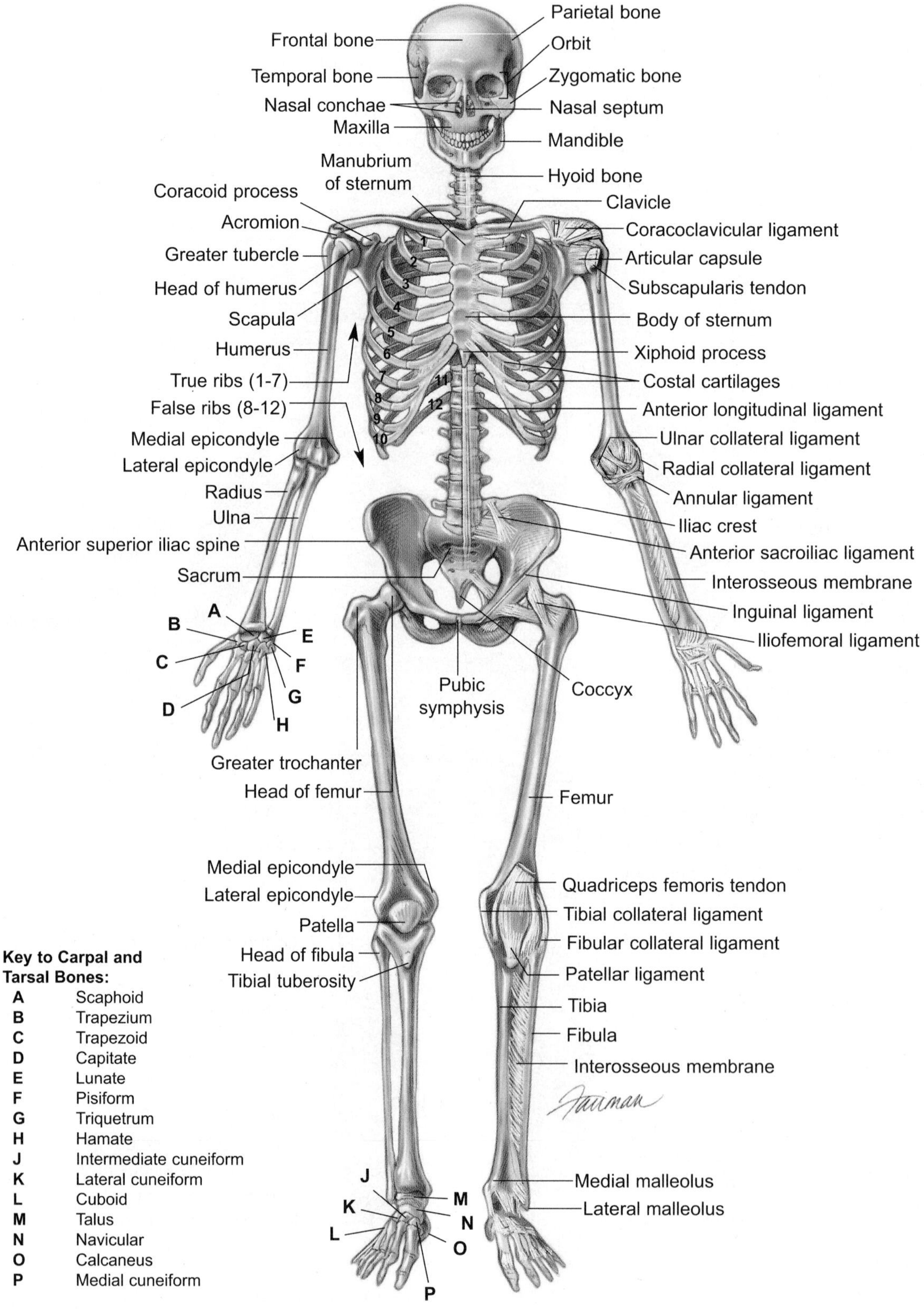

Key to Carpal and Tarsal Bones:

A Scaphoid
B Trapezium
C Trapezoid
D Capitate
E Lunate
F Pisiform
G Triquetrum
H Hamate
J Intermediate cuneiform
K Lateral cuneiform
L Cuboid
M Talus
N Navicular
O Calcaneus
P Medial cuneiform

Skeletal System
(Posterior View)

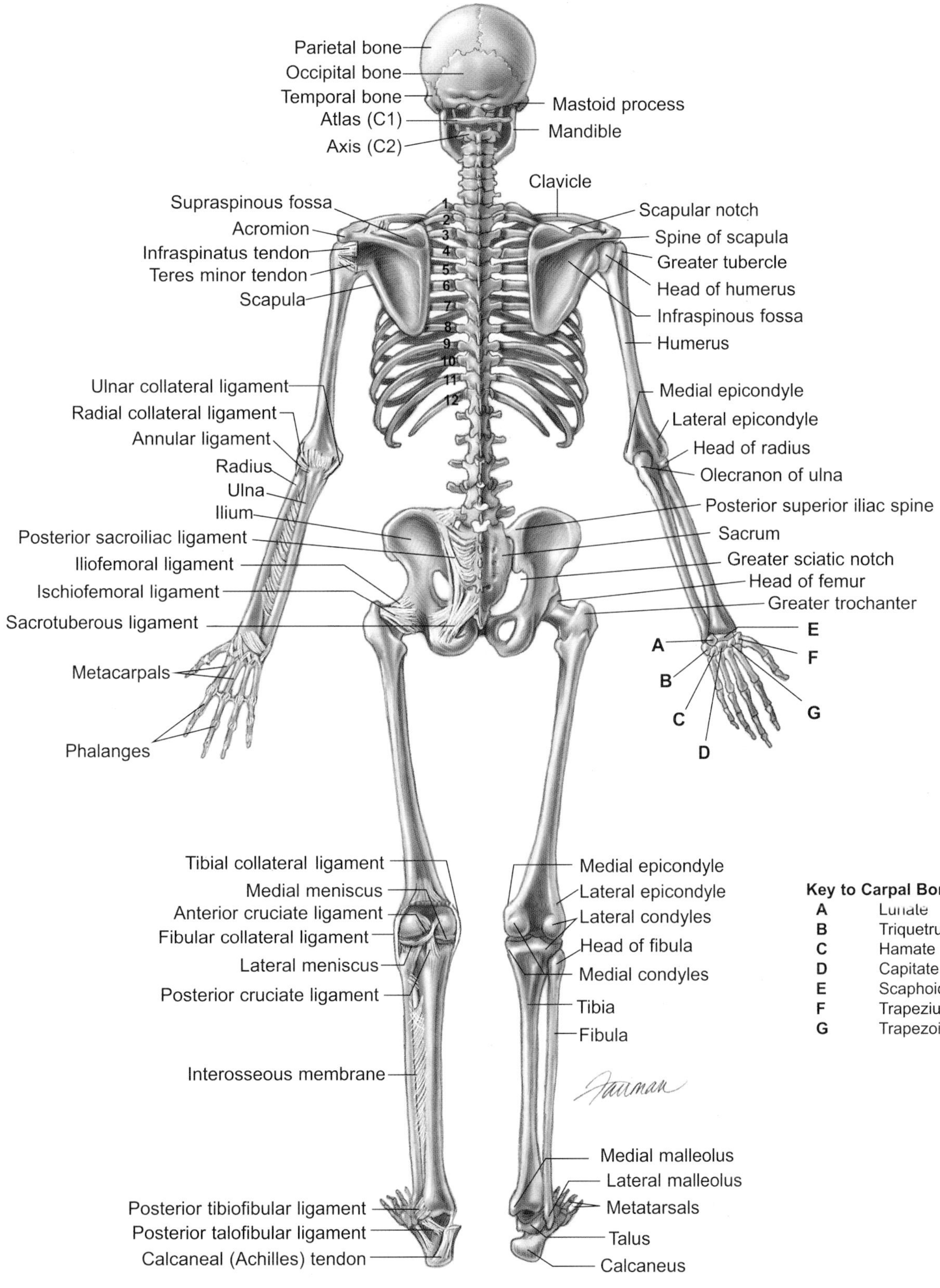

Key to Carpal Bones:

A	Lunate
B	Triquetrum
C	Hamate
D	Capitate
E	Scaphoid
F	Trapezium
G	Trapezoid

Skeletal System

(Vertebral Column – Left Lateral View)

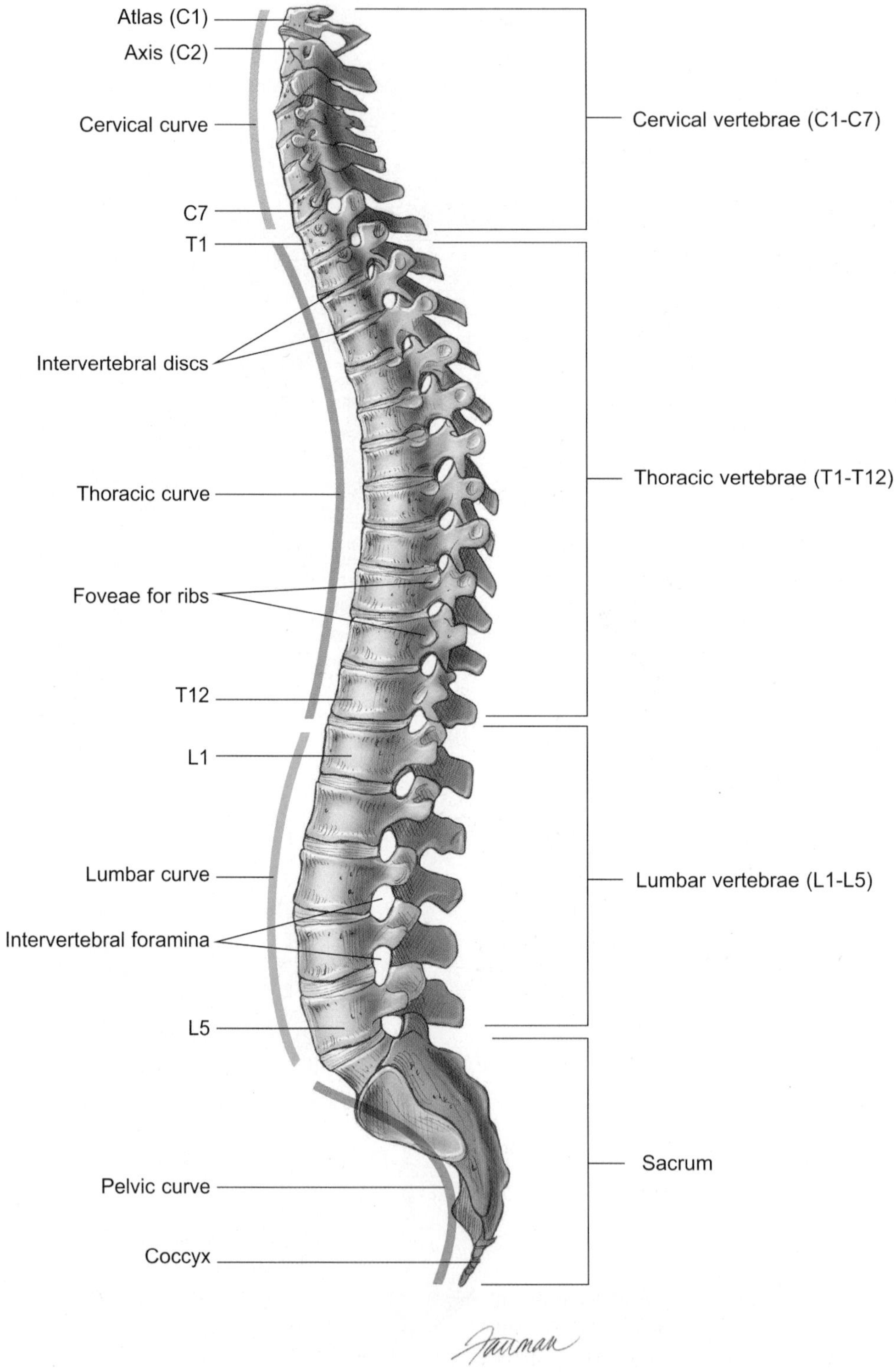

Shoulder and Elbow

(Anterior View)

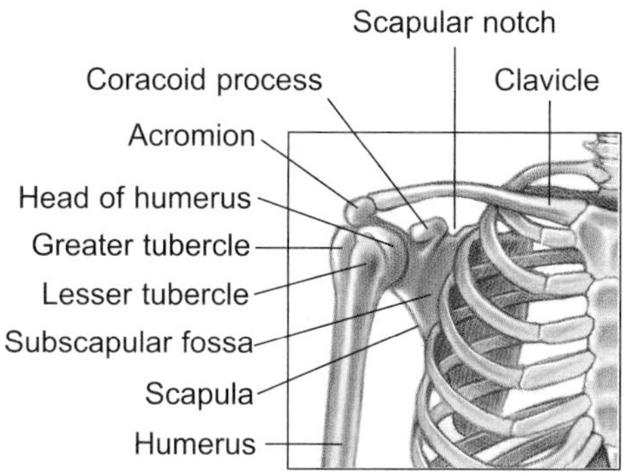

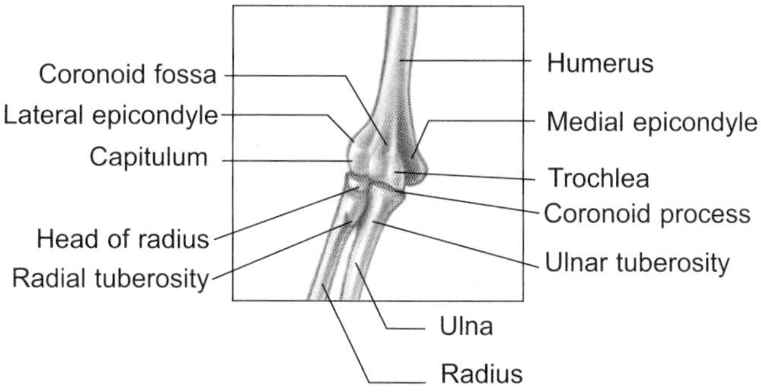

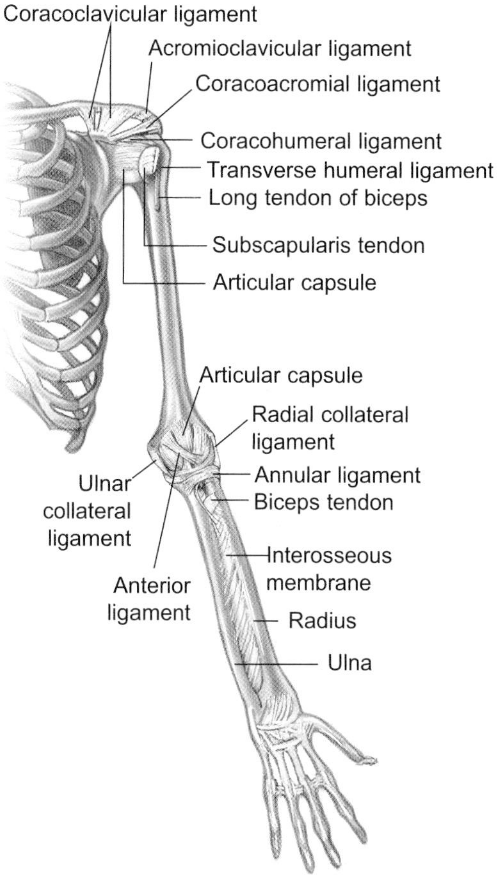

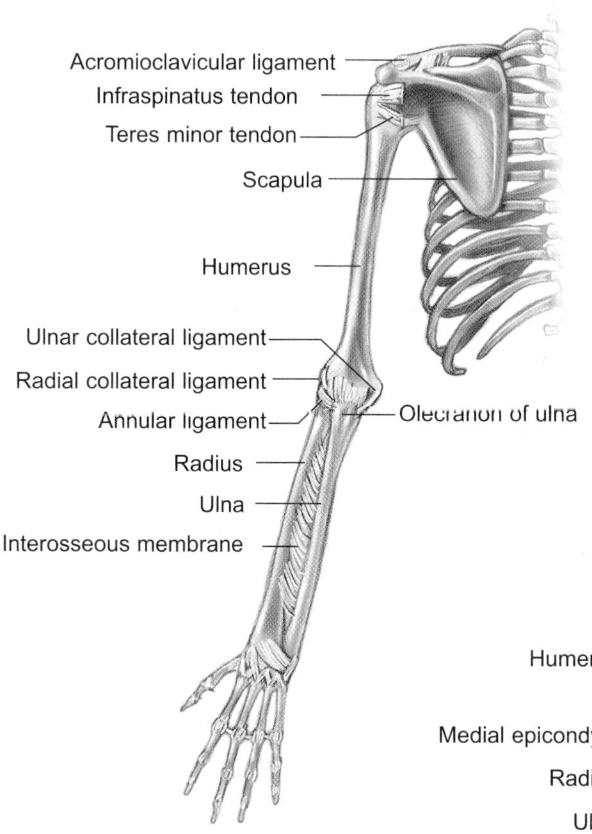

(Posterior View)

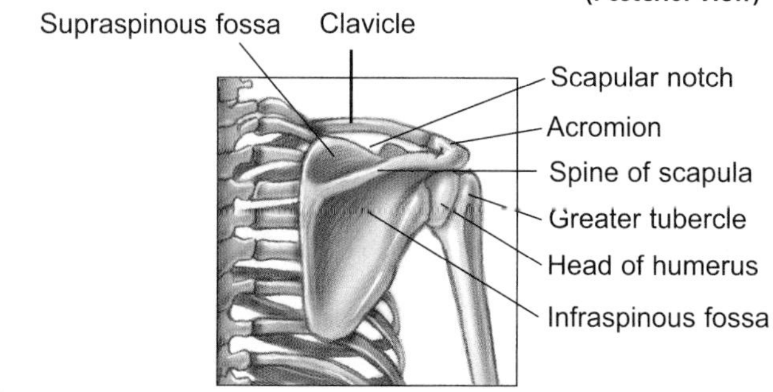

Fairman

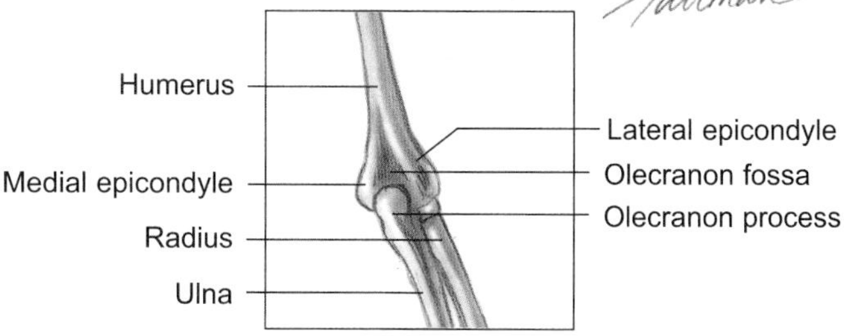

Anatomy Illustrations/Muscle & Tendon Table

Anatomy Illustrations/Muscle & Tendon Table

Musculoskeletal System – Hand and Wrist

(Dorsal and Palmar Views)

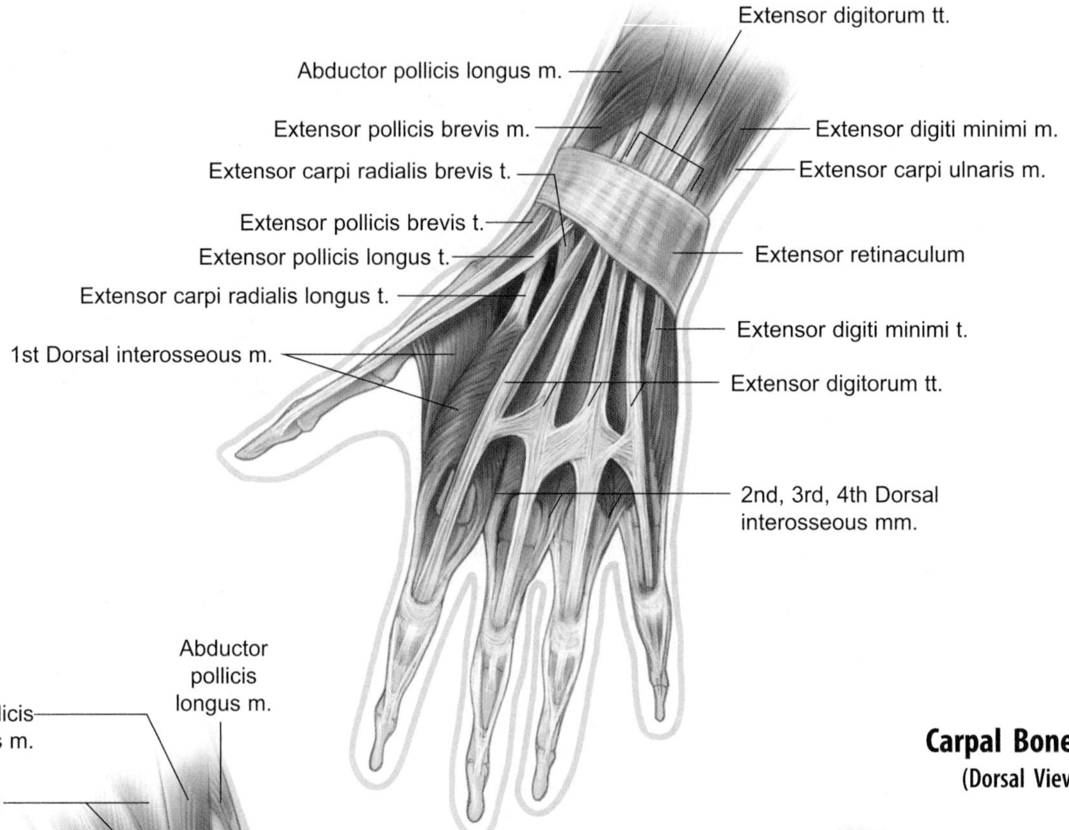

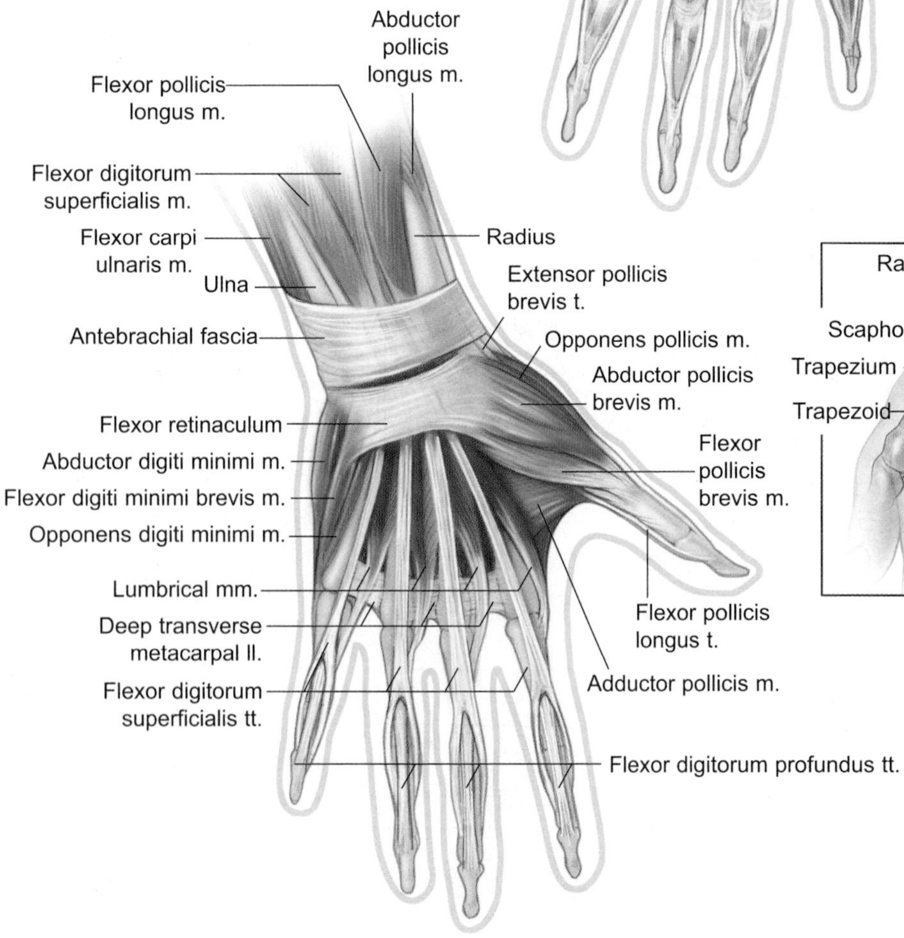

Carpal Bones

(Dorsal View)

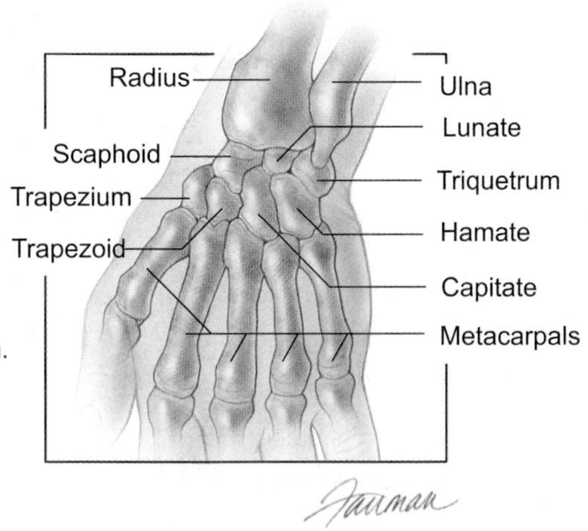

Musculoskeletal System – Hip and Knee

(Anterior and Posterior Views)

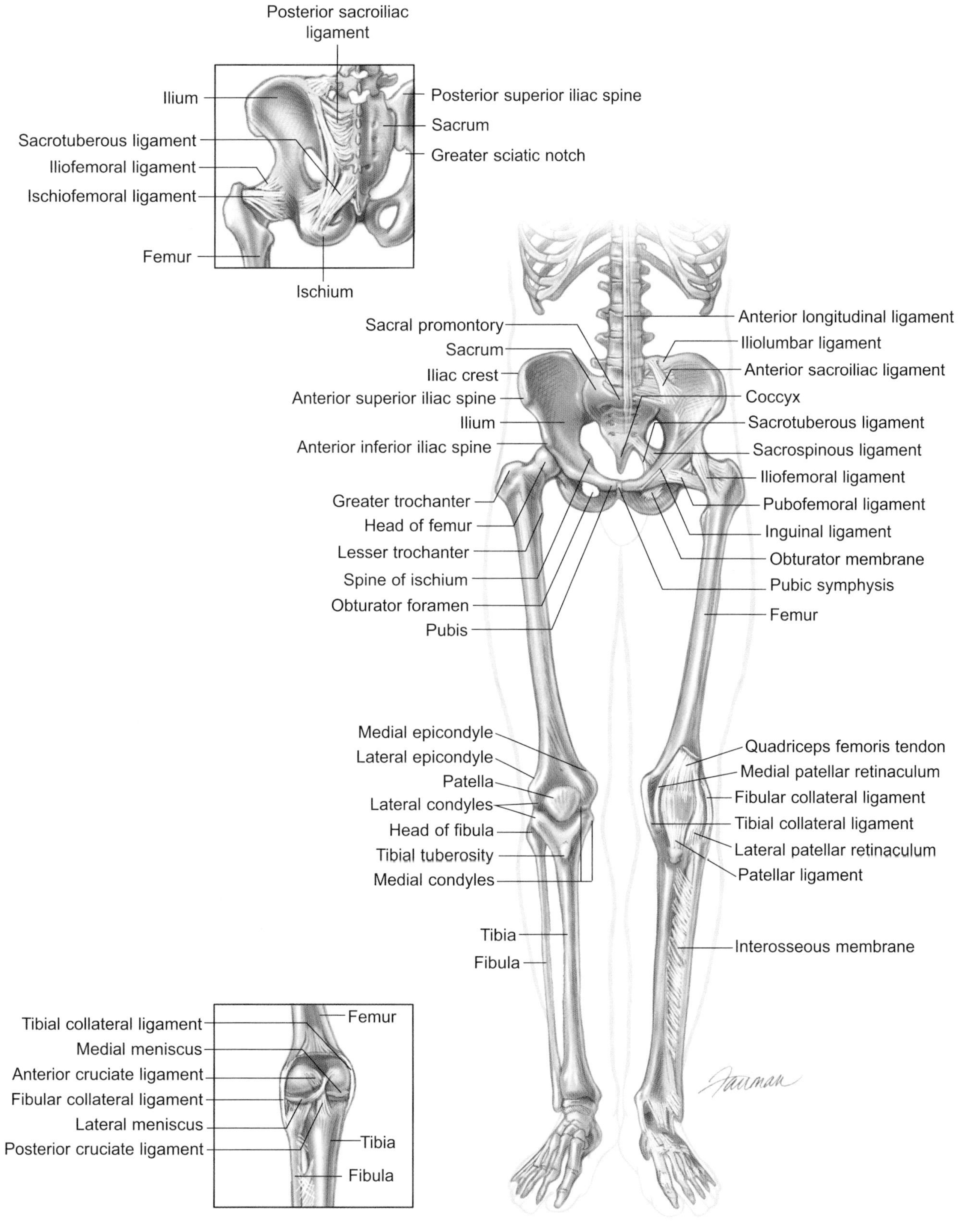
Posterior sacroiliac ligament
Ilium
Sacrotuberous ligament
Iliofemoral ligament
Ischiofemoral ligament
Femur
Ischium
Posterior superior iliac spine
Sacrum
Greater sciatic notch
Sacral promontory
Sacrum
Iliac crest
Anterior superior iliac spine
Ilium
Anterior inferior iliac spine
Greater trochanter
Head of femur
Lesser trochanter
Spine of ischium
Obturator foramen
Pubis
Anterior longitudinal ligament
Iliolumbar ligament
Anterior sacroiliac ligament
Coccyx
Sacrotuberous ligament
Sacrospinous ligament
Iliofemoral ligament
Pubofemoral ligament
Inguinal ligament
Obturator membrane
Pubic symphysis
Femur
Medial epicondyle
Lateral epicondyle
Patella
Lateral condyles
Head of fibula
Tibial tuberosity
Medial condyles
Tibia
Fibula
Quadriceps femoris tendon
Medial patellar retinaculum
Fibular collateral ligament
Tibial collateral ligament
Lateral patellar retinaculum
Patellar ligament
Interosseous membrane
Fairman
Tibial collateral ligament
Medial meniscus
Anterior cruciate ligament
Fibular collateral ligament
Lateral meniscus
Posterior cruciate ligament
Femur
Tibia
Fibula

Anatomy Illustrations/Muscle & Tendon Table

Musculoskeletal System – Foot and Ankle

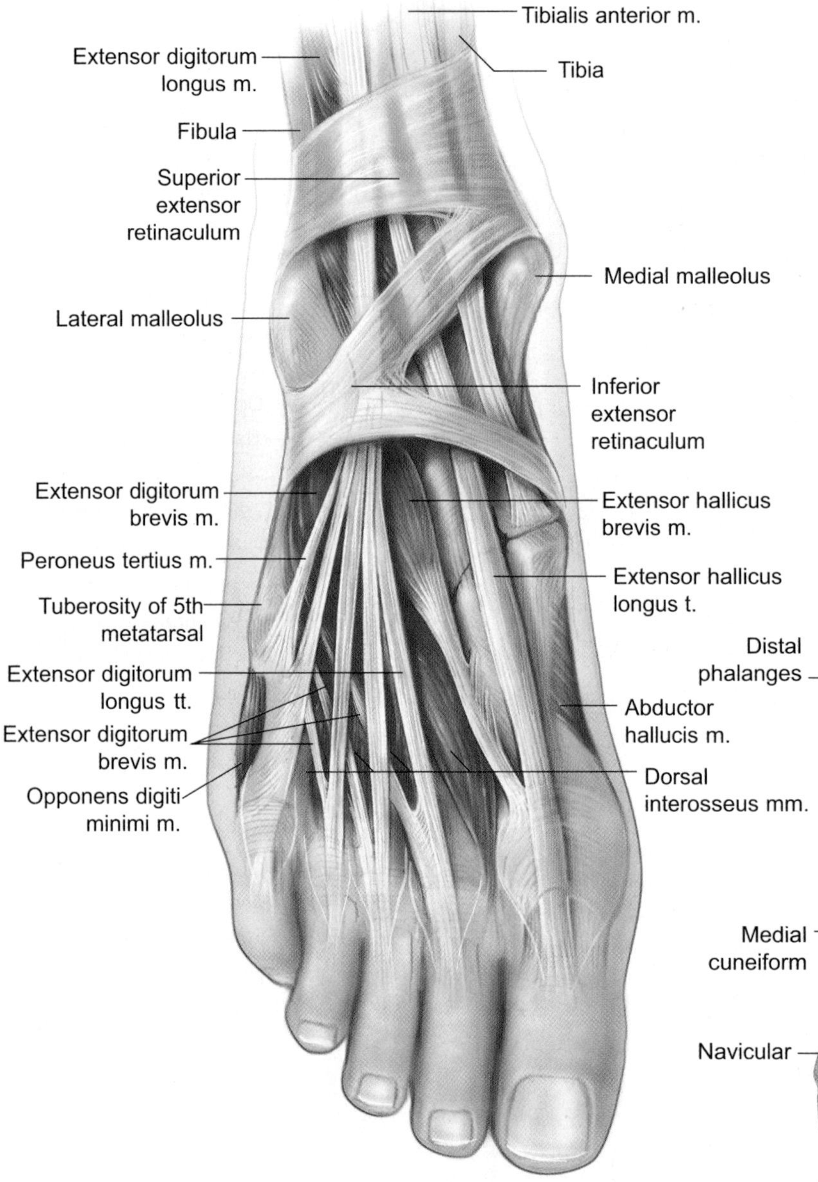
Tibialis anterior m.
Extensor digitorum longus m.
Tibia
Fibula
Superior extensor retinaculum
Medial malleolus
Lateral malleolus
Inferior extensor retinaculum
Extensor digitorum brevis m.
Extensor hallicus brevis m.
Peroneus tertius m.
Extensor hallicus longus t.
Tuberosity of 5th metatarsal
Extensor digitorum longus tt.
Abductor hallucis m.
Extensor digitorum brevis m.
Dorsal interosseus mm.
Opponens digiti minimi m.

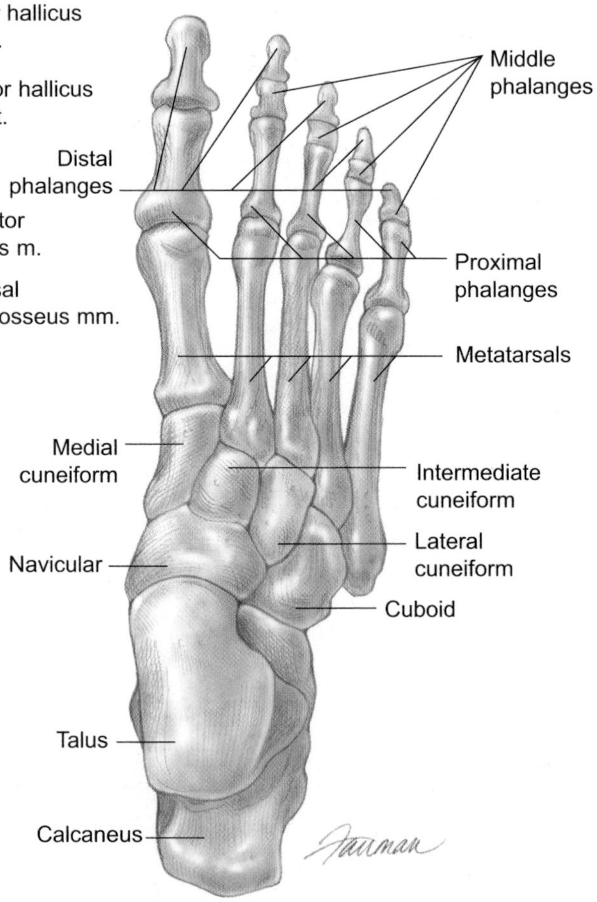
Middle phalanges
Distal phalanges
Proximal phalanges
Metatarsals
Medial cuneiform
Intermediate cuneiform
Lateral cuneiform
Navicular
Cuboid
Talus
Calcaneus
Fairman

Vascular System

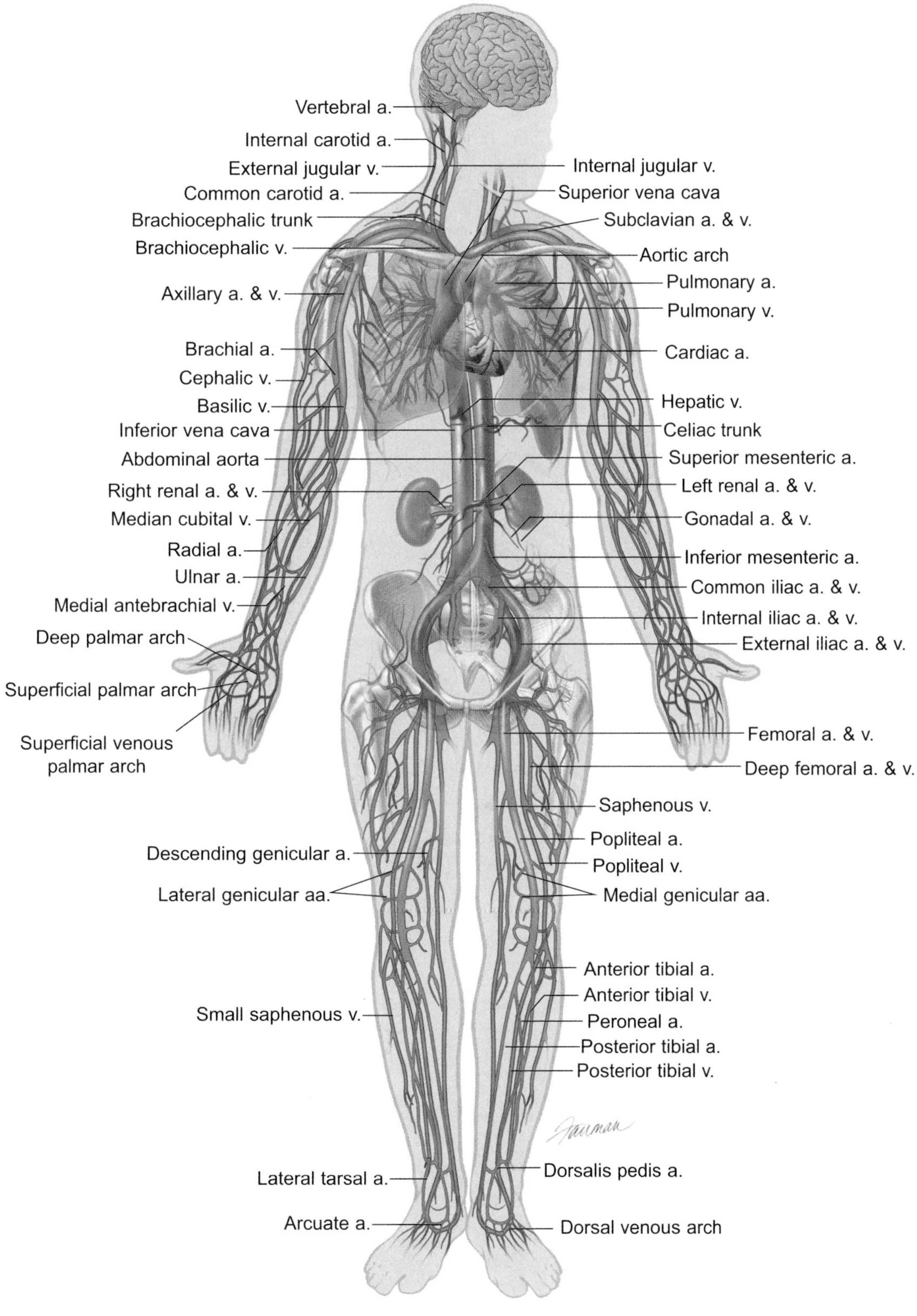

Vertebral a.
Internal carotid a.
External jugular v.
Common carotid a.
Brachiocephalic trunk
Brachiocephalic v.
Axillary a. & v.
Brachial a.
Cephalic v.
Basilic v.
Inferior vena cava
Abdominal aorta
Right renal a. & v.
Median cubital v.
Radial a.
Ulnar a.
Medial antebrachial v.
Deep palmar arch
Superficial palmar arch
Superficial venous palmar arch
Internal jugular v.
Superior vena cava
Subclavian a. & v.
Aortic arch
Pulmonary a.
Pulmonary v.
Cardiac a.
Hepatic v.
Celiac trunk
Superior mesenteric a.
Left renal a. & v.
Gonadal a. & v.
Inferior mesenteric a.
Common iliac a. & v.
Internal iliac a. & v.
External iliac a. & v.
Femoral a. & v.
Deep femoral a. & v.
Saphenous v.
Popliteal a.
Popliteal v.
Medial genicular aa.
Descending genicular a.
Lateral genicular aa.
Anterior tibial a.
Anterior tibial v.
Peroneal a.
Posterior tibial a.
Posterior tibial v.
Small saphenous v.
Fairman
Lateral tarsal a.
Dorsalis pedis a.
Arcuate a.
Dorsal venous arch

Heart
(External View)

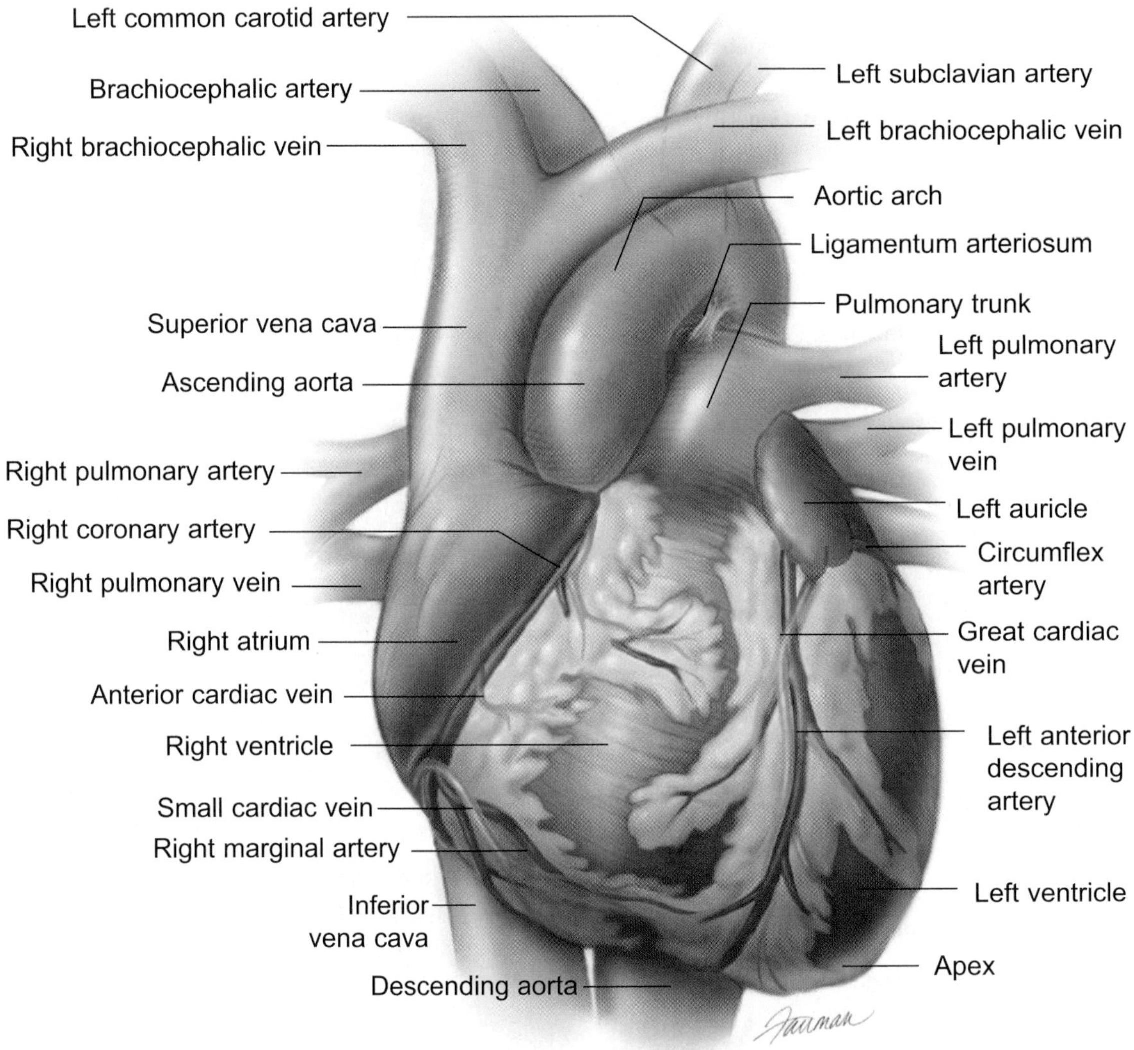

Left common carotid artery
Brachiocephalic artery
Right brachiocephalic vein
Superior vena cava
Ascending aorta
Right pulmonary artery
Right coronary artery
Right pulmonary vein
Right atrium
Anterior cardiac vein
Right ventricle
Small cardiac vein
Right marginal artery
Inferior vena cava
Descending aorta
Left subclavian artery
Left brachiocephalic vein
Aortic arch
Ligamentum arteriosum
Pulmonary trunk
Left pulmonary artery
Left pulmonary vein
Left auricle
Circumflex artery
Great cardiac vein
Left anterior descending artery
Left ventricle
Apex
Fairman

Heart
(Internal View)

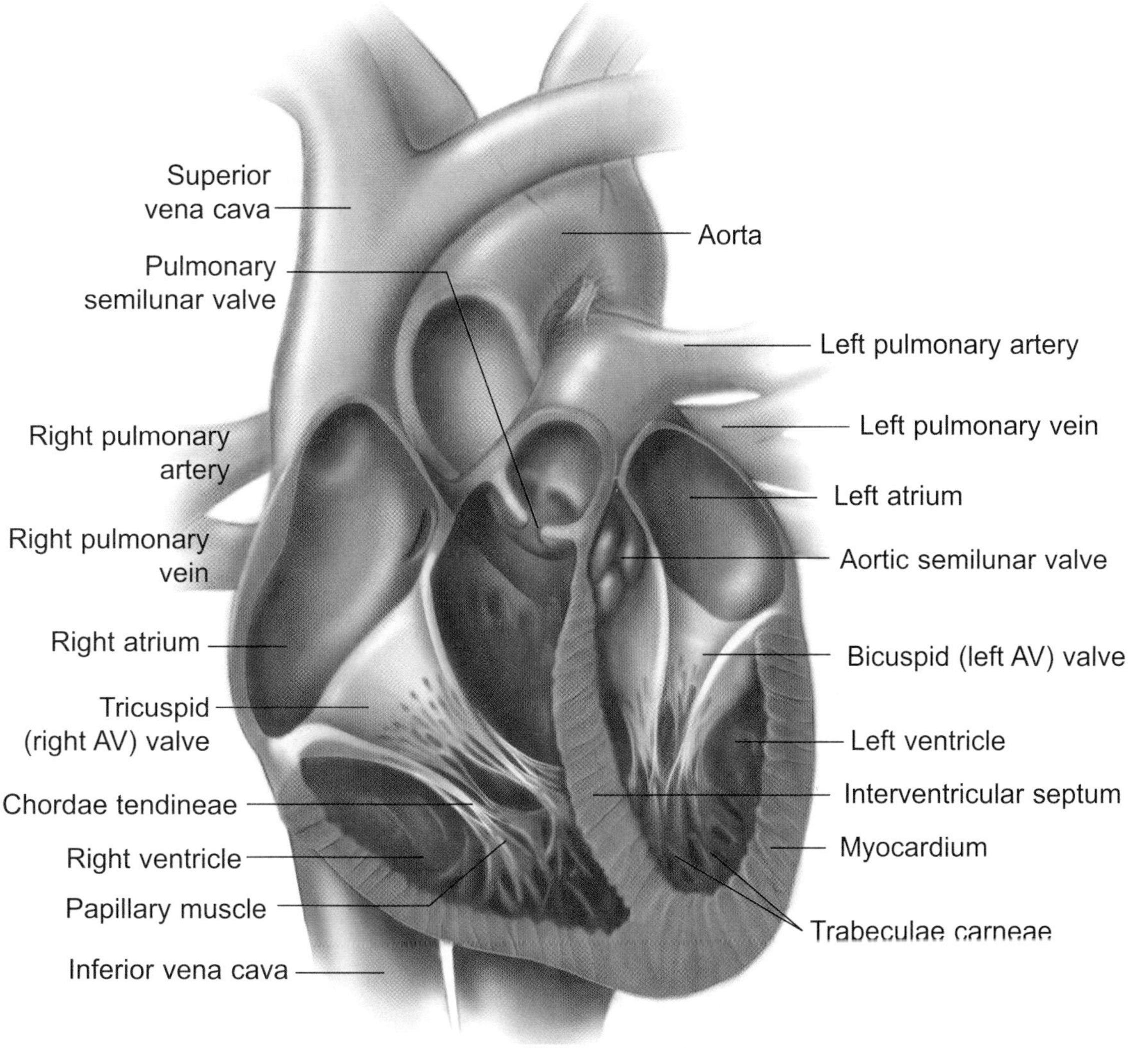
Superior vena cava
Aorta
Pulmonary semilunar valve
Left pulmonary artery
Left pulmonary vein
Right pulmonary artery
Left atrium
Right pulmonary vein
Aortic semilunar valve
Right atrium
Bicuspid (left AV) valve
Tricuspid (right AV) valve
Left ventricle
Interventricular septum
Chordae tendineae
Myocardium
Right ventricle
Papillary muscle
Trabeculae carneae
Inferior vena cava

Respiratory System

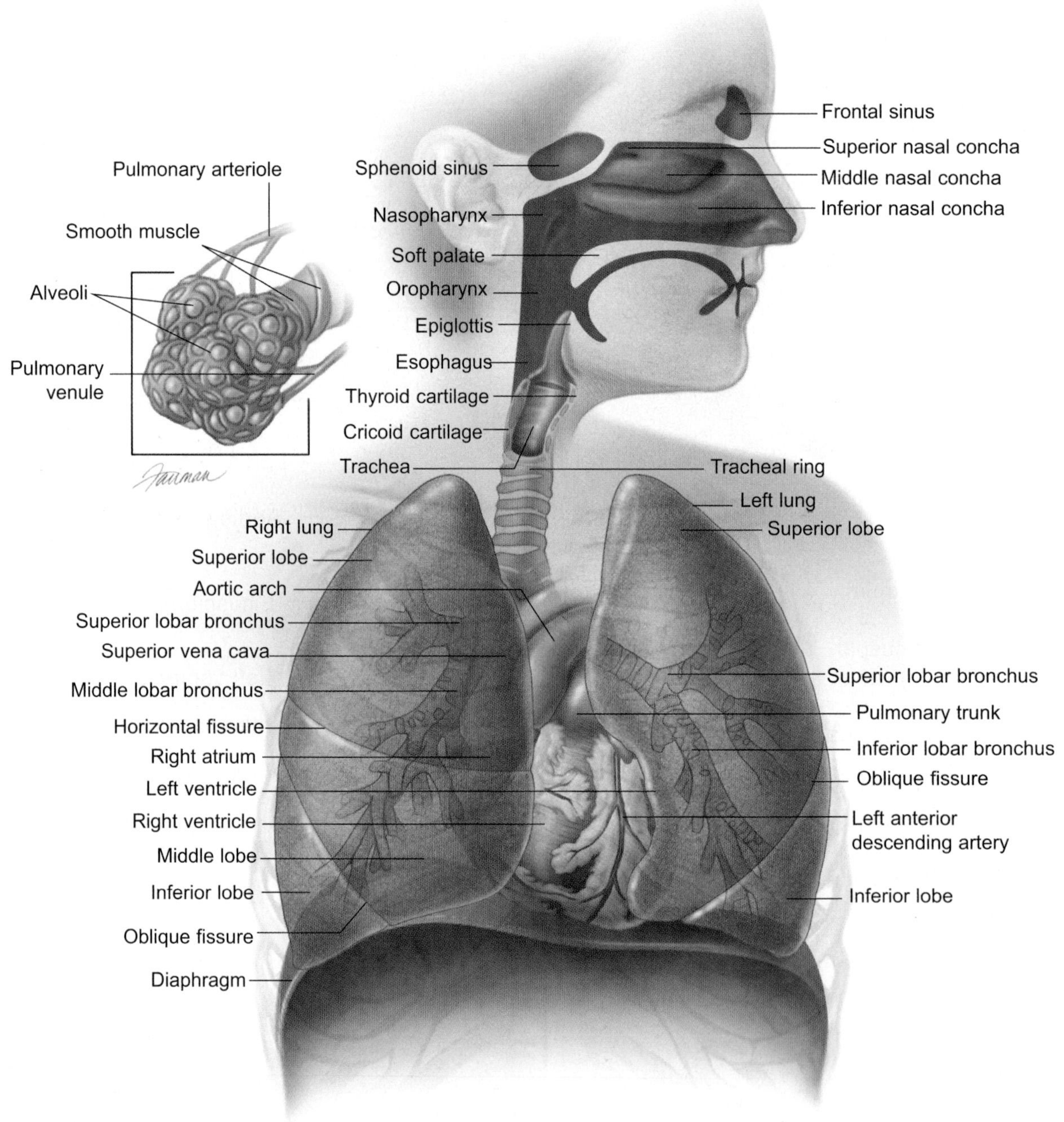
Pulmonary arteriole
Smooth muscle
Alveoli
Pulmonary venule
Frontal sinus
Superior nasal concha
Middle nasal concha
Inferior nasal concha
Sphenoid sinus
Nasopharynx
Soft palate
Oropharynx
Epiglottis
Esophagus
Thyroid cartilage
Cricoid cartilage
Trachea
Tracheal ring
Left lung
Superior lobe
Right lung
Superior lobe
Aortic arch
Superior lobar bronchus
Superior vena cava
Middle lobar bronchus
Horizontal fissure
Right atrium
Left ventricle
Right ventricle
Middle lobe
Inferior lobe
Oblique fissure
Diaphragm
Superior lobar bronchus
Pulmonary trunk
Inferior lobar bronchus
Oblique fissure
Left anterior descending artery
Inferior lobe

Digestive System

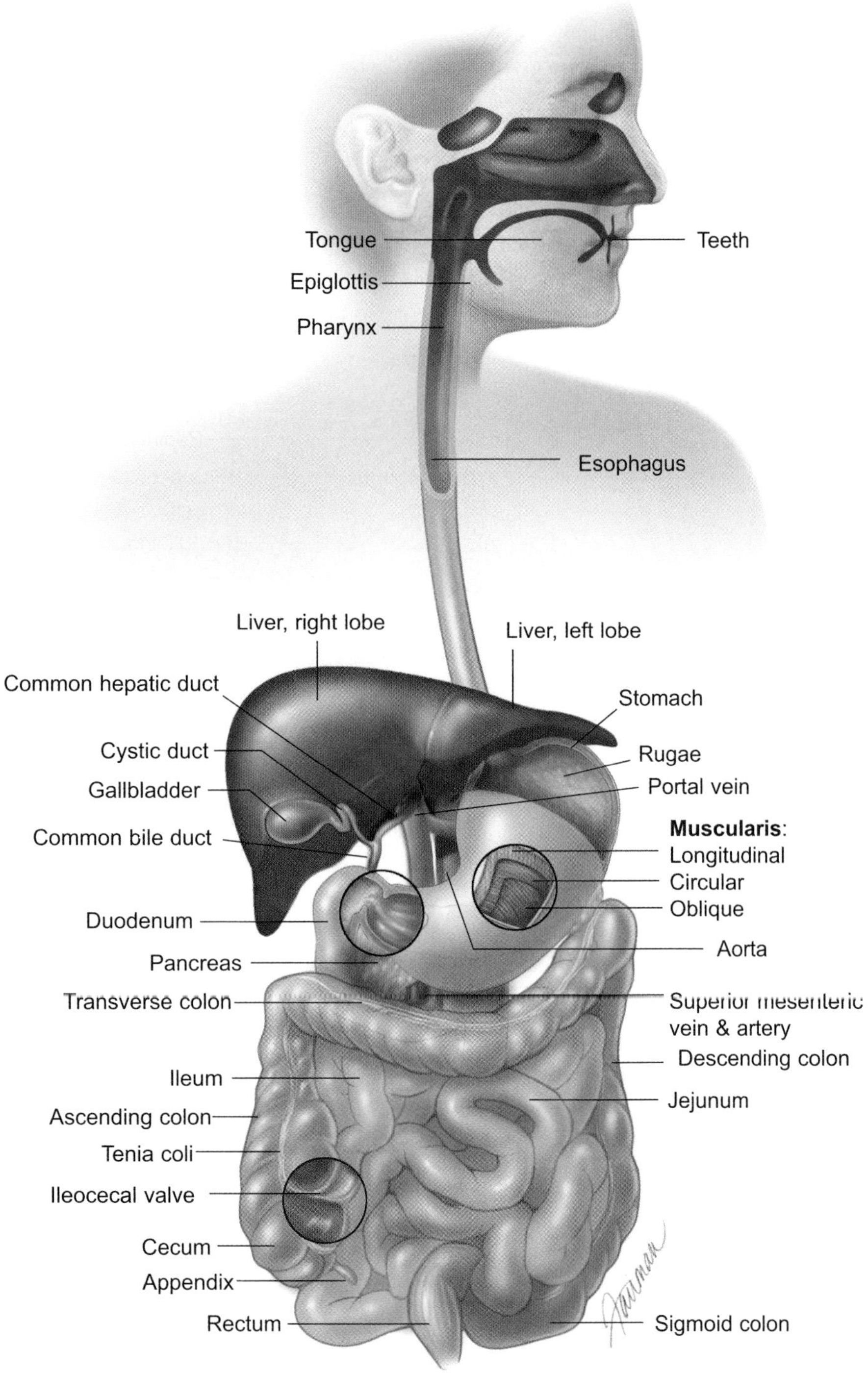
Tongue
Teeth
Epiglottis
Pharynx
Esophagus
Liver, right lobe
Liver, left lobe
Common hepatic duct
Stomach
Cystic duct
Rugae
Gallbladder
Portal vein
Common bile duct
Muscularis:
Longitudinal
Circular
Oblique
Duodenum
Aorta
Pancreas
Transverse colon
Superior mesenteric vein & artery
Descending colon
Ileum
Jejunum
Ascending colon
Tenia coli
Ileocecal valve
Cecum
Appendix
Rectum
Sigmoid colon

Nervous System

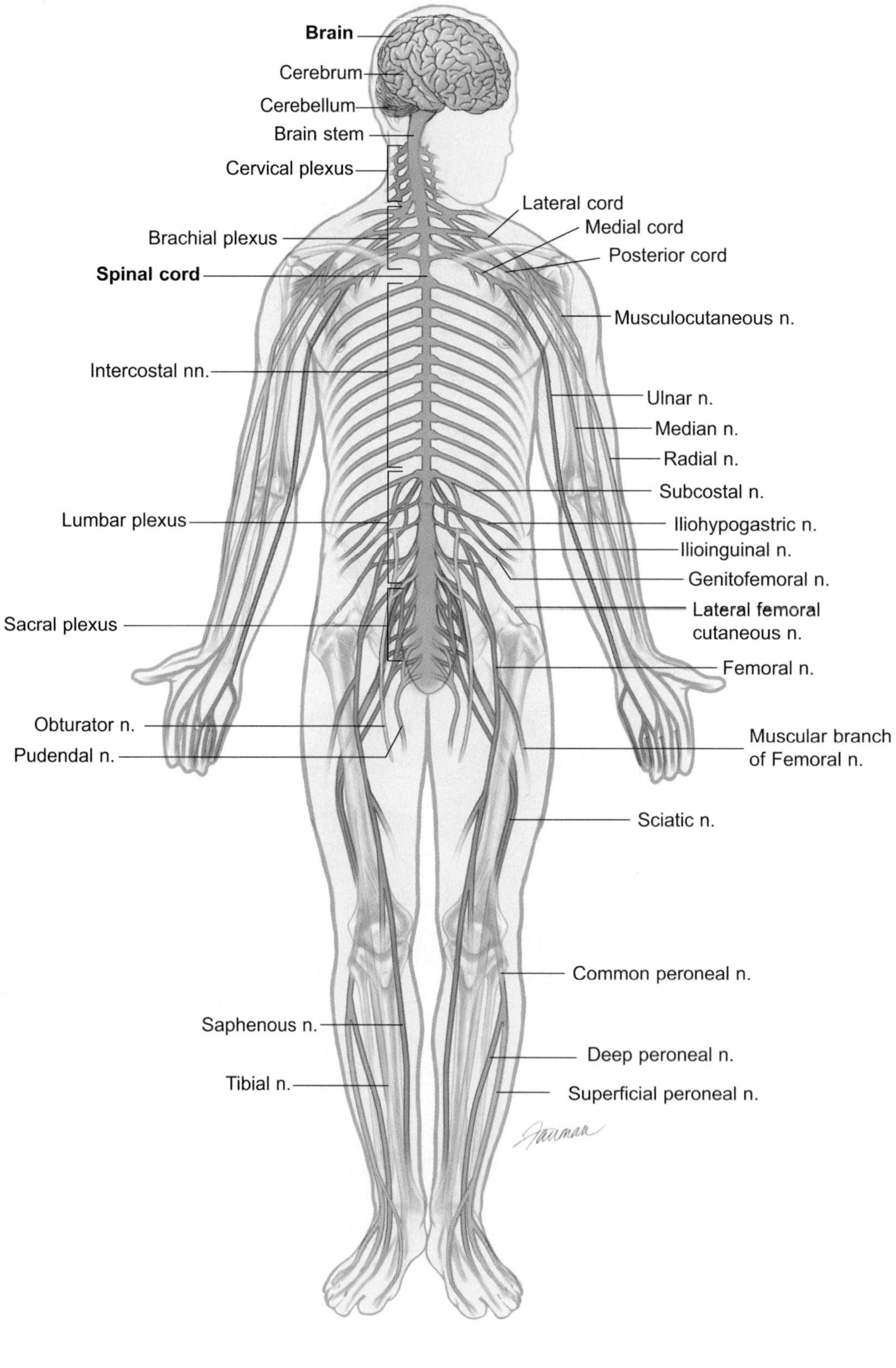
Brain
Cerebrum
Cerebellum
Brain stem
Cervical plexus
Brachial plexus
Spinal cord
Intercostal nn.
Lumbar plexus
Sacral plexus
Obturator n.
Pudendal n.
Saphenous n.
Tibial n.
Lateral cord
Medial cord
Posterior cord
Musculocutaneous n.
Ulnar n.
Median n.
Radial n.
Subcostal n.
Iliohypogastric n.
Ilioinguinal n.
Genitofemoral n.
Lateral femoral cutaneous n.
Femoral n.
Muscular branch of Femoral n.
Sciatic n.
Common peroneal n.
Deep peroneal n.
Superficial peroneal n.

Brain
(Inferior View)

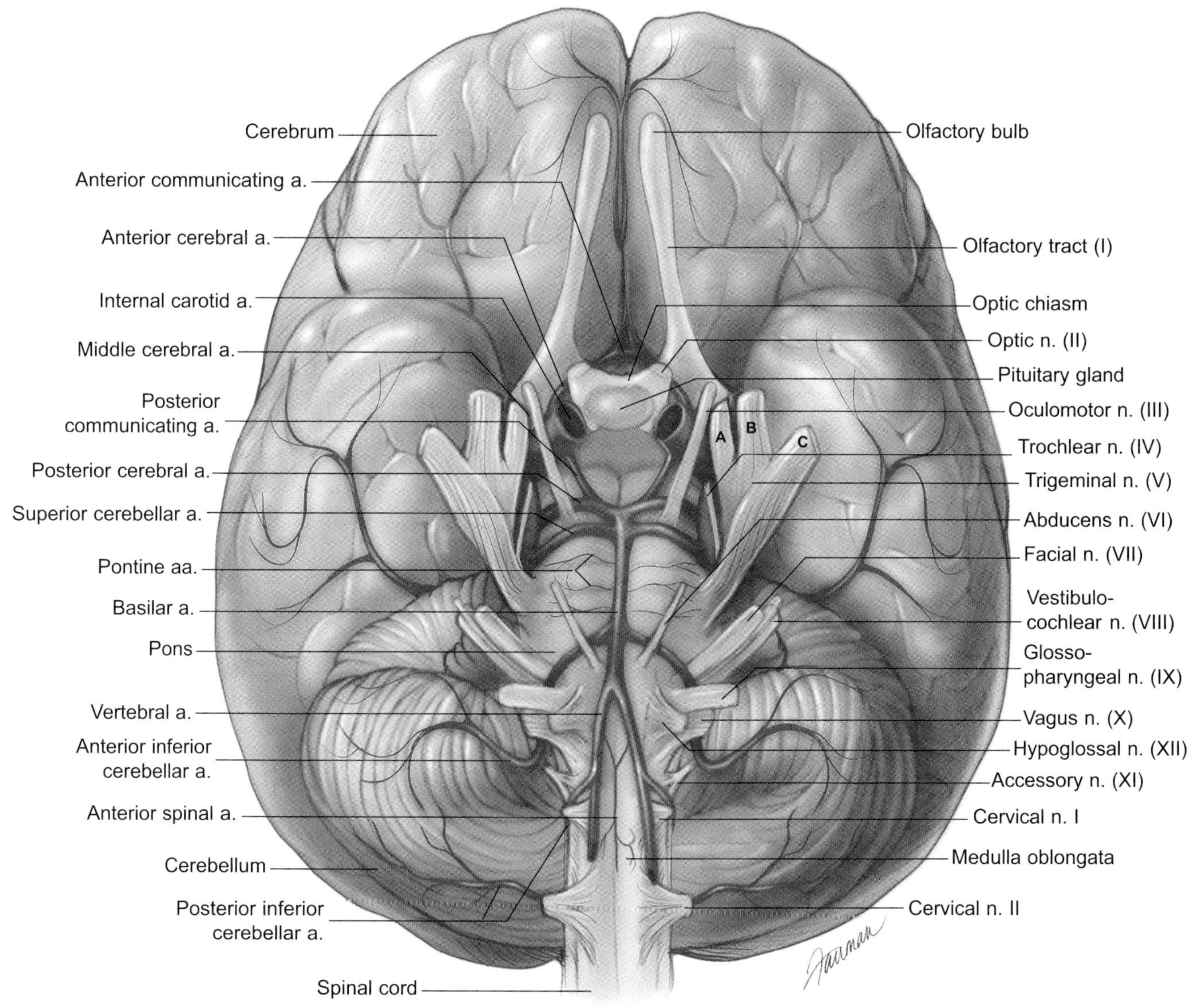

Trigeminal nerve (V) branches:

A	Ophthalmic branch
B	Maxillary branch
C	Mandibular branch

The Right Eye
(Transverse Section)

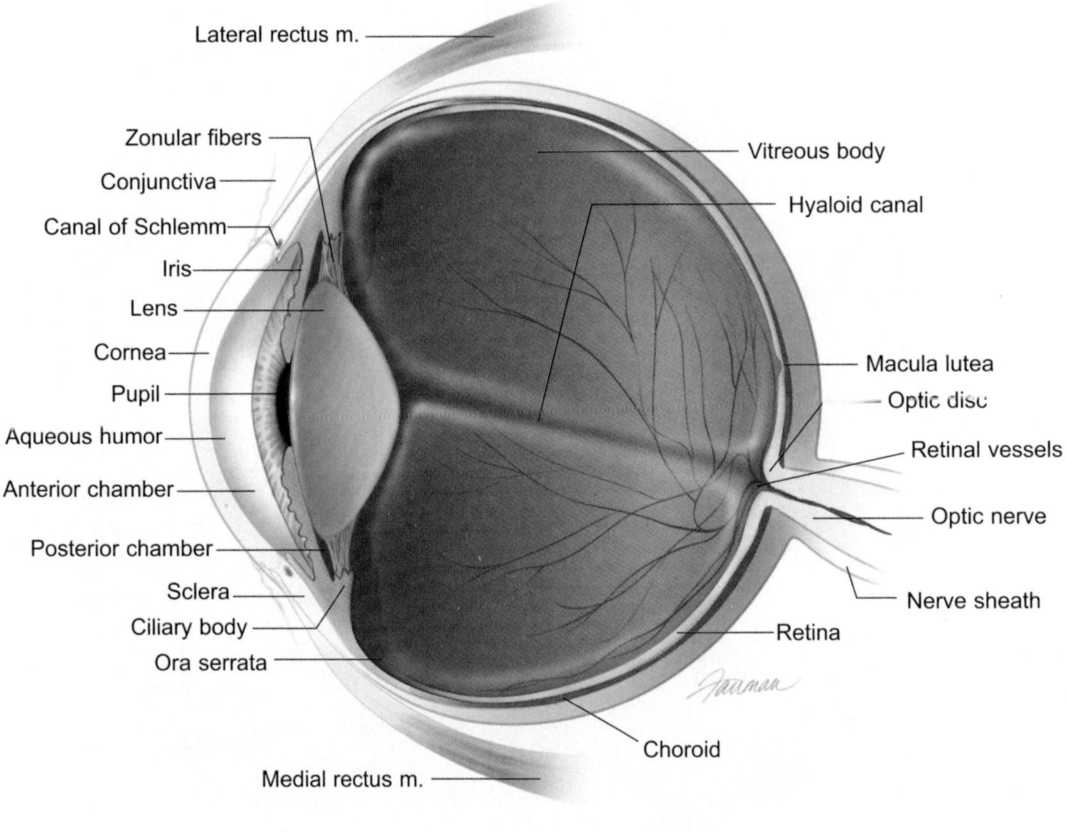

The Right Ear

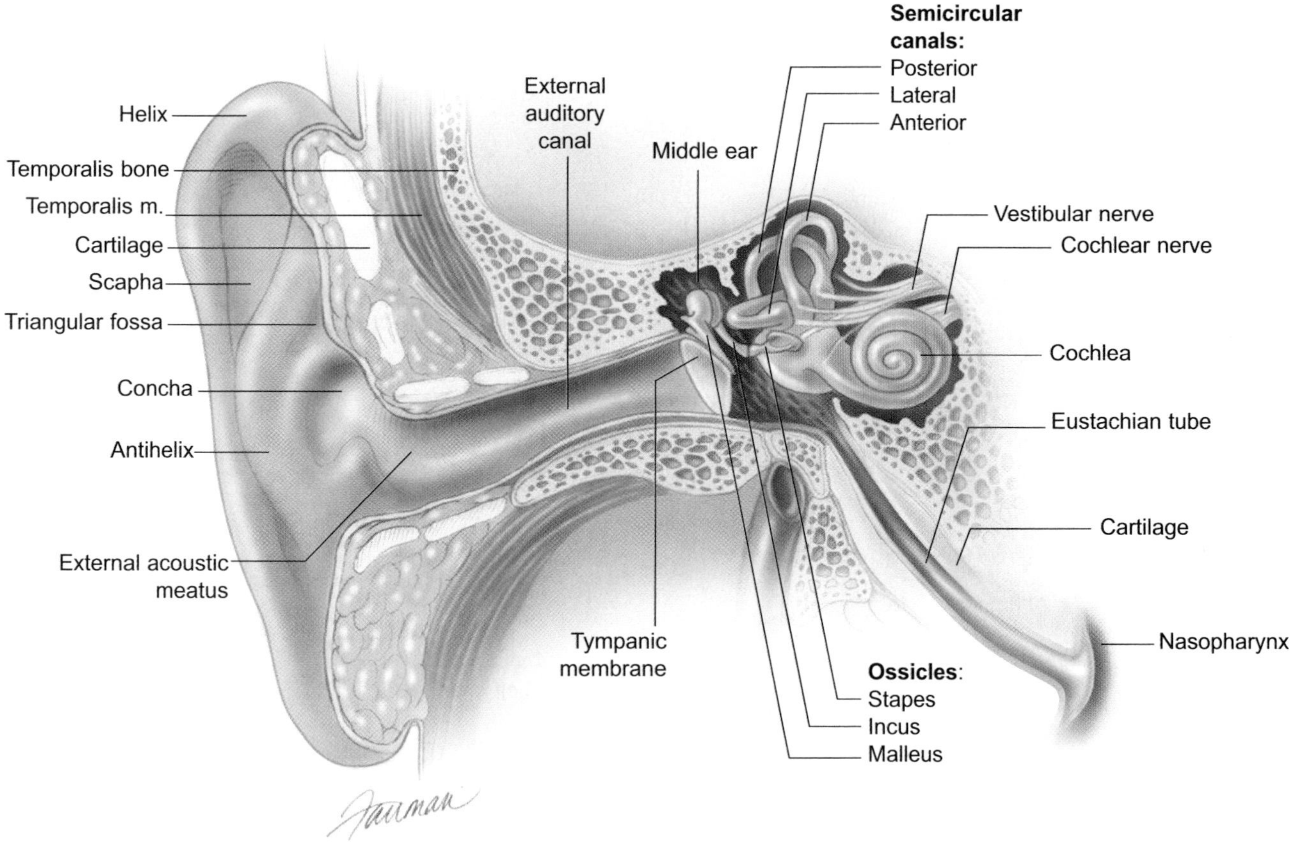
Semicircular canals:
Posterior
Lateral
Anterior
External auditory canal
Middle ear
Helix
Temporalis bone
Temporalis m.
Cartilage
Scapha
Triangular fossa
Concha
Antihelix
External acoustic meatus
Vestibular nerve
Cochlear nerve
Cochlea
Eustachian tube
Cartilage
Nasopharynx
Tympanic membrane
Ossicles:
Stapes
Incus
Malleus
Fairman

Urinary System

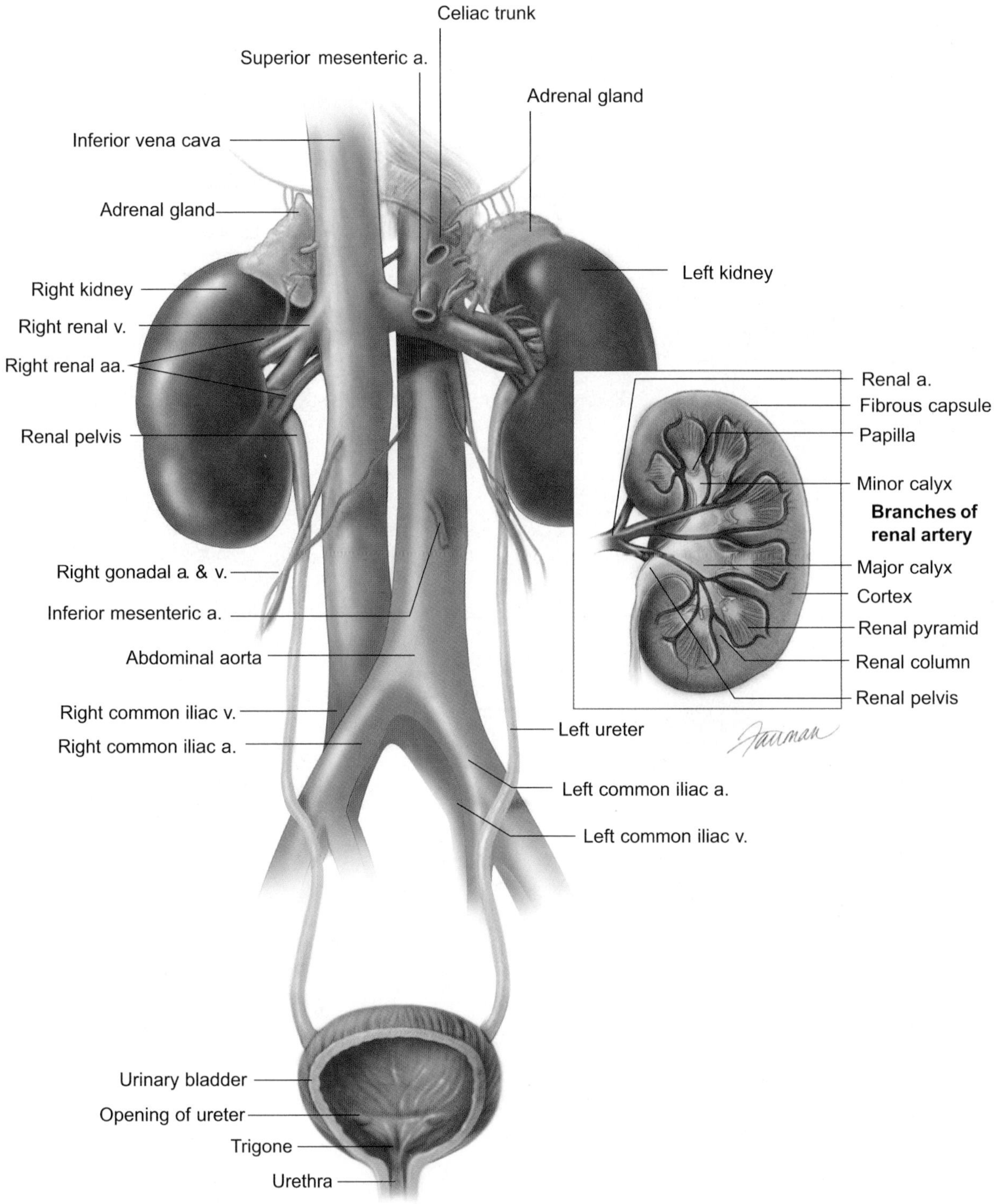
Celiac trunk
Superior mesenteric a.
Adrenal gland
Inferior vena cava
Adrenal gland
Left kidney
Right kidney
Right renal v.
Right renal aa.
Renal a.
Fibrous capsule
Papilla
Renal pelvis
Minor calyx
Branches of renal artery
Major calyx
Cortex
Renal pyramid
Renal column
Renal pelvis
Right gonadal a. & v.
Inferior mesenteric a.
Abdominal aorta
Right common iliac v.
Left ureter
Right common iliac a.
Left common iliac a.
Left common iliac v.
Urinary bladder
Opening of ureter
Trigone
Urethra

Male Genital System

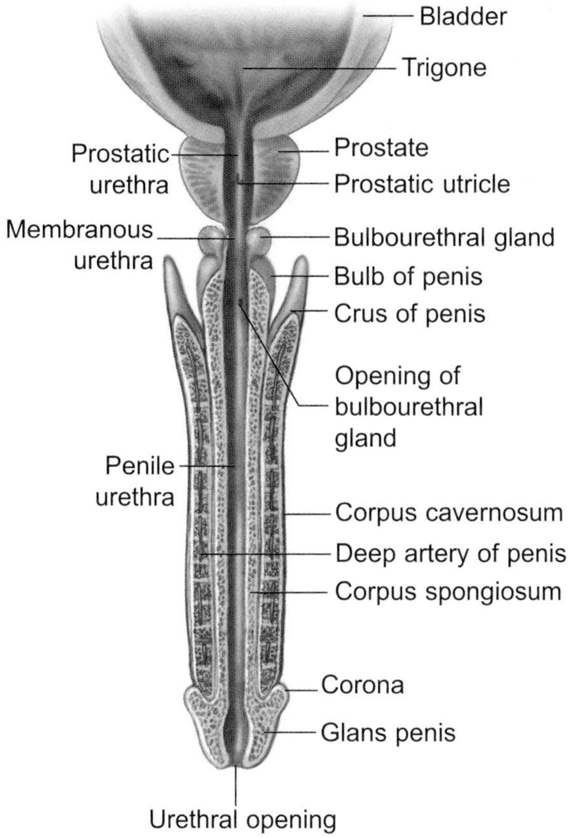
Bladder
Trigone
Prostatic urethra
Prostate
Prostatic utricle
Membranous urethra
Bulbourethral gland
Bulb of penis
Crus of penis
Opening of bulbourethral gland
Penile urethra
Corpus cavernosum
Deep artery of penis
Corpus spongiosum
Corona
Glans penis
Urethral opening

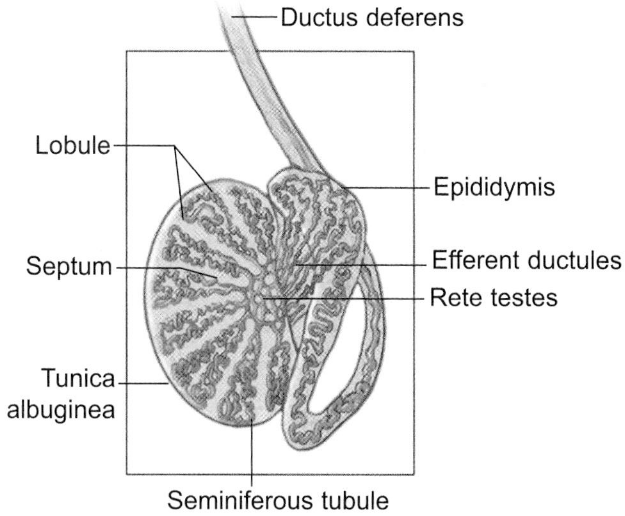
Ductus deferens
Lobule
Epididymis
Septum
Efferent ductules
Rete testes
Tunica albuginea
Seminiferous tubule

Male Genital System

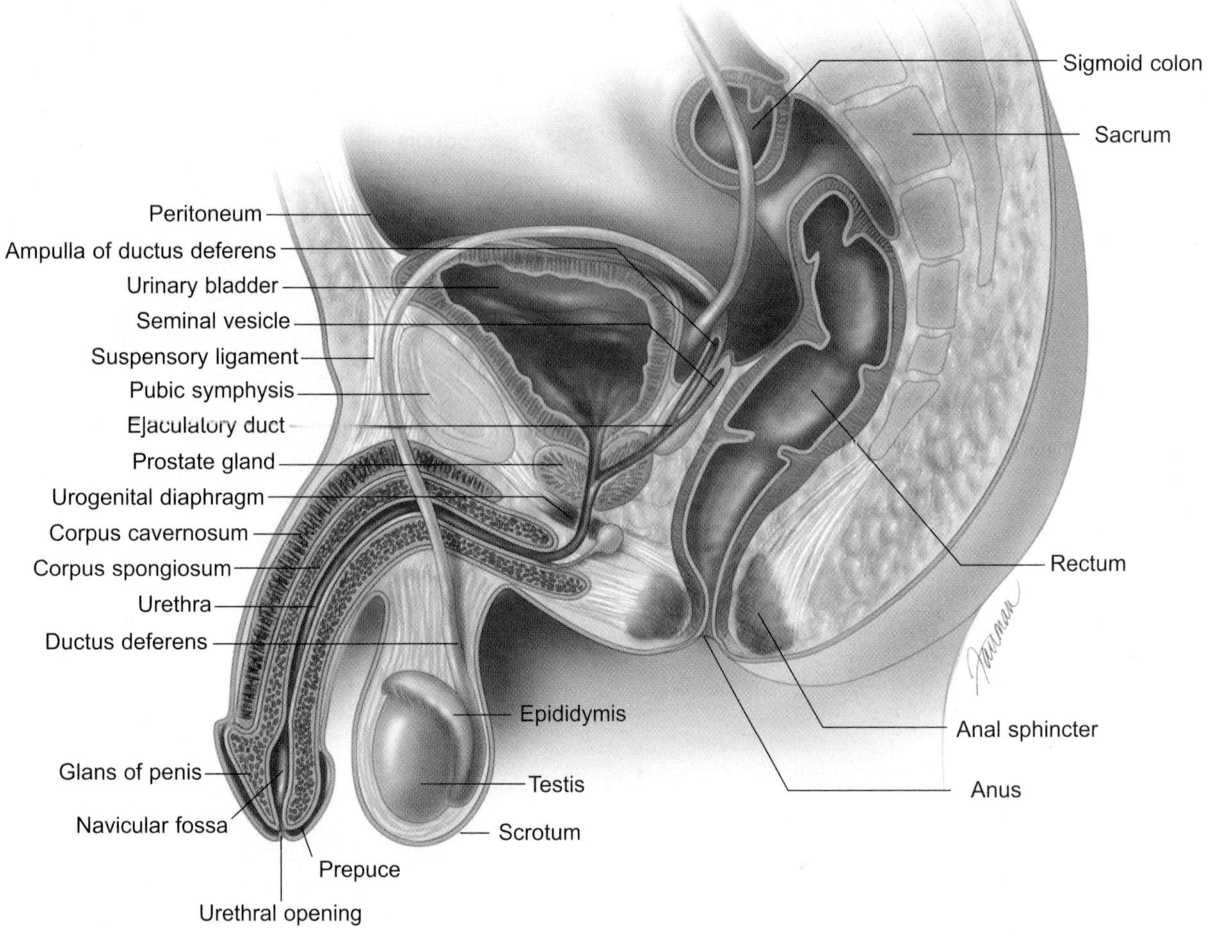
Sigmoid colon
Sacrum
Peritoneum
Ampulla of ductus deferens
Urinary bladder
Seminal vesicle
Suspensory ligament
Pubic symphysis
Ejaculatory duct
Prostate gland
Urogenital diaphragm
Corpus cavernosum
Corpus spongiosum
Urethra
Ductus deferens
Rectum
Epididymis
Anal sphincter
Glans of penis
Testis
Anus
Navicular fossa
Scrotum
Prepuce
Urethral opening

Female Genital System

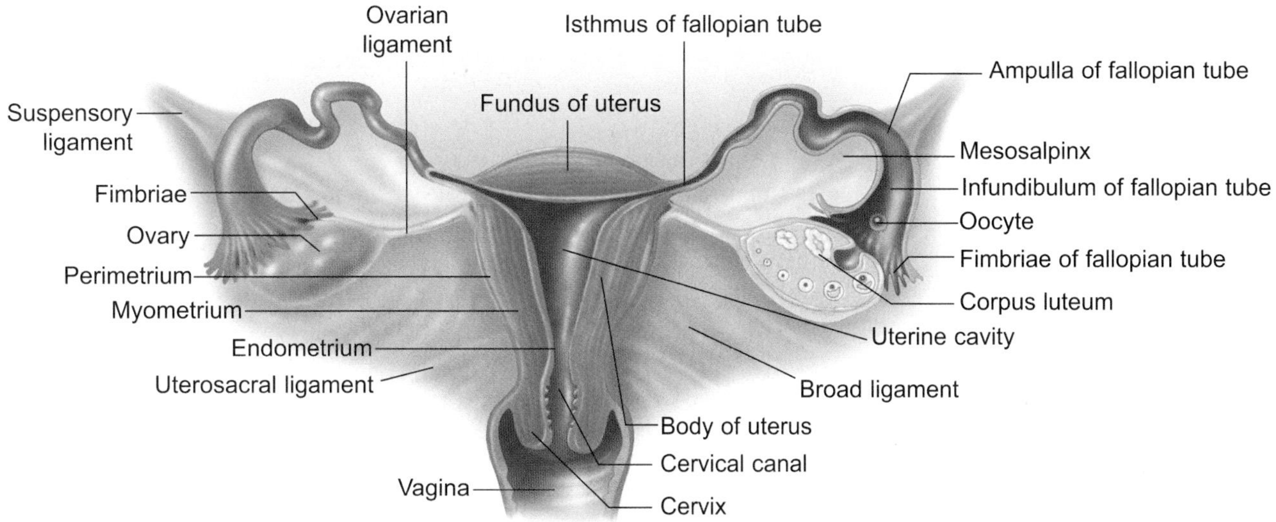

Female Genital System

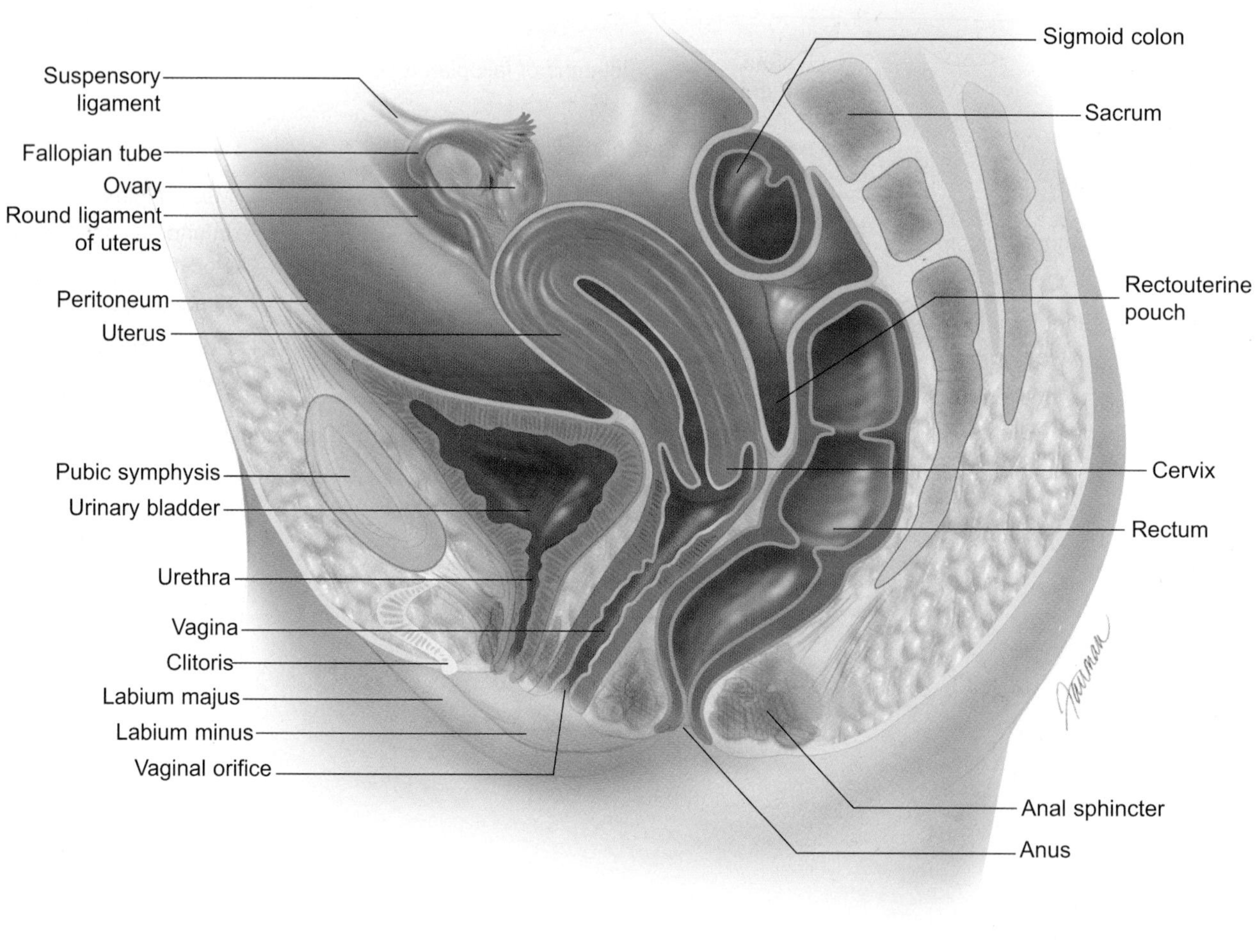
Suspensory ligament
Fallopian tube
Ovary
Round ligament of uterus
Peritoneum
Uterus
Pubic symphysis
Urinary bladder
Urethra
Vagina
Clitoris
Labium majus
Labium minus
Vaginal orifice
Sigmoid colon
Sacrum
Rectouterine pouch
Cervix
Rectum
Anal sphincter
Anus

Female Reproductive System – Pregnancy
(Lateral View)

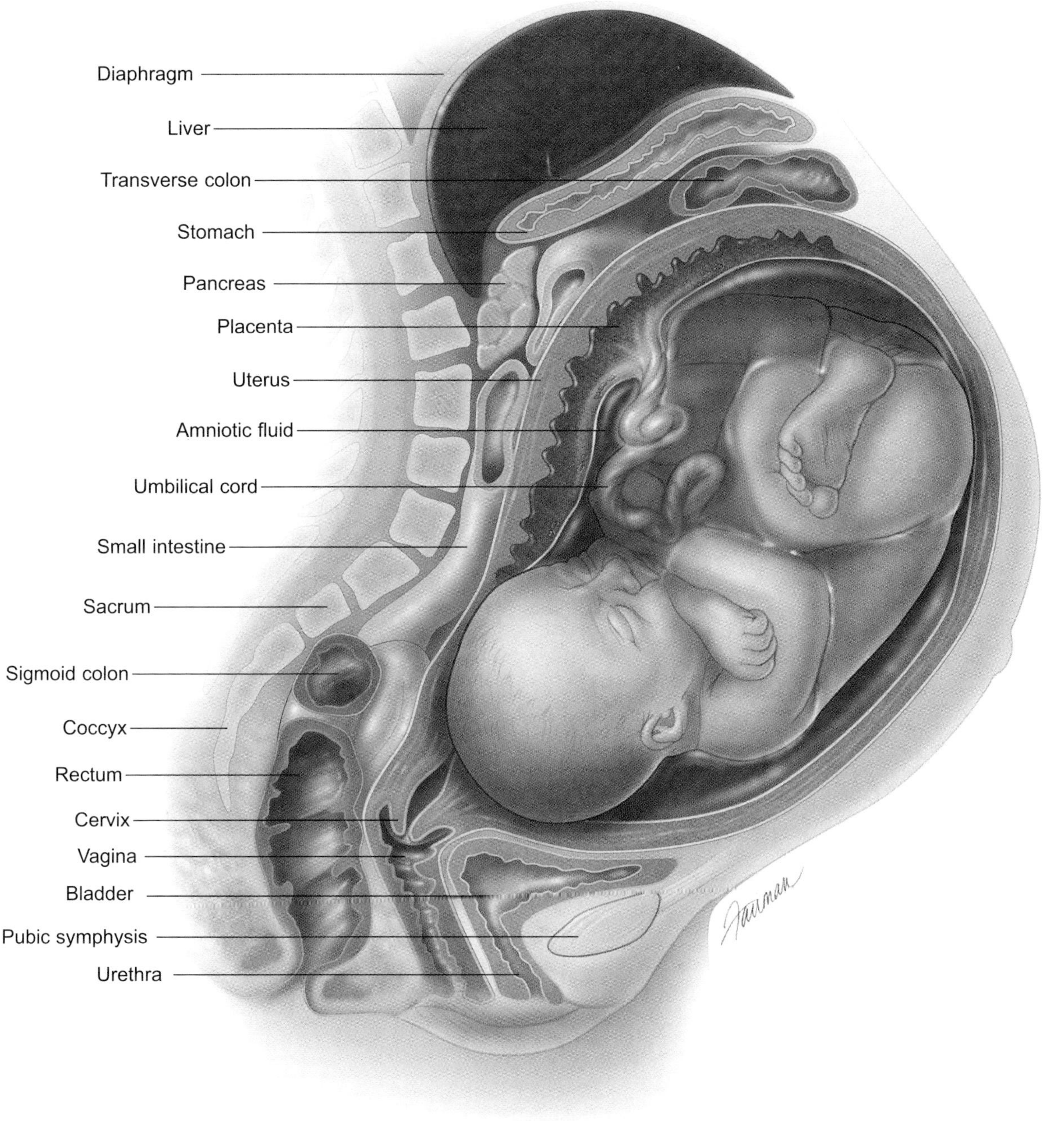

Cerebral Vasculature

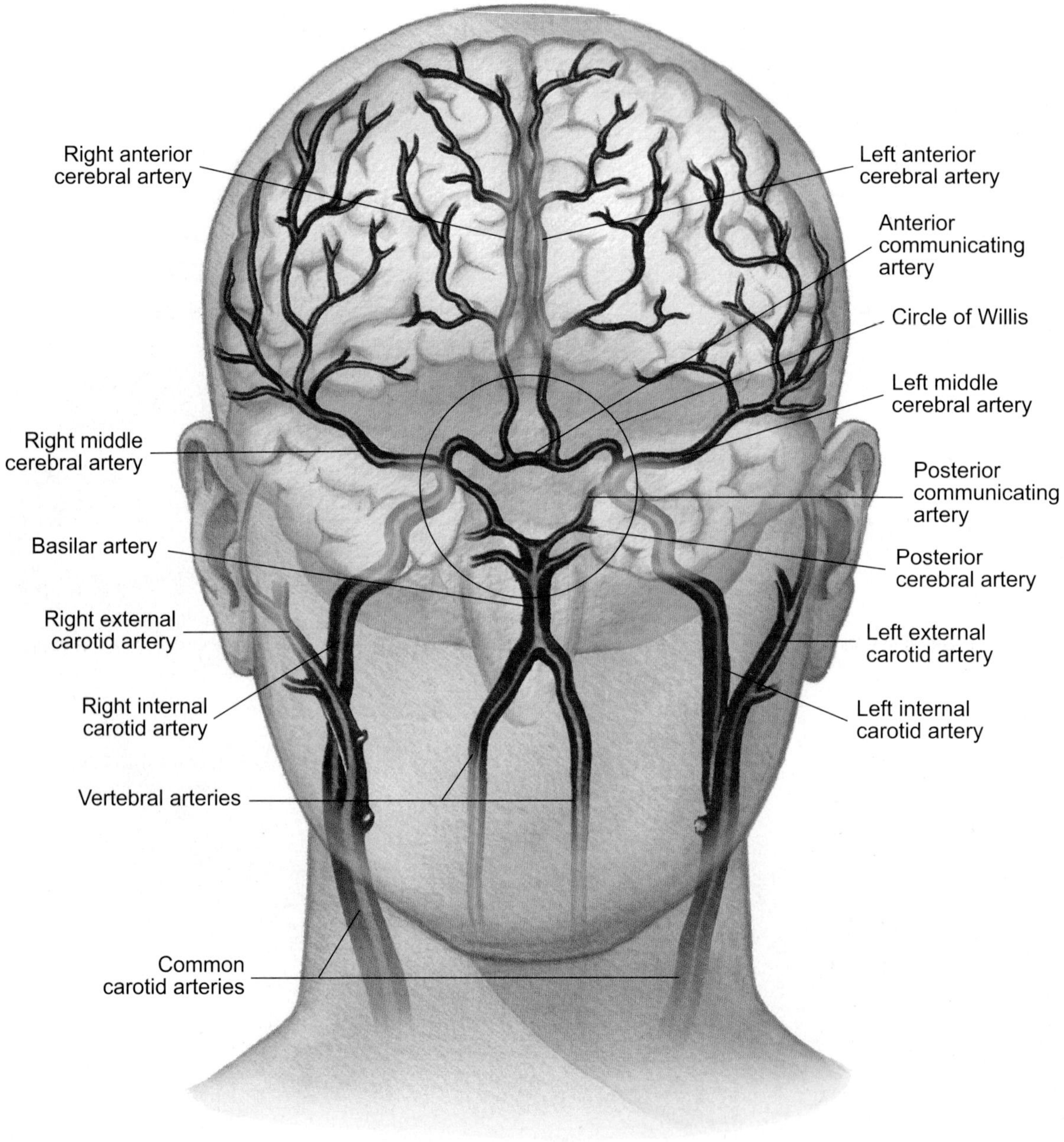
Right anterior cerebral artery
Left anterior cerebral artery
Anterior communicating artery
Circle of Willis
Left middle cerebral artery
Right middle cerebral artery
Posterior communicating artery
Basilar artery
Posterior cerebral artery
Right external carotid artery
Left external carotid artery
Right internal carotid artery
Left internal carotid artery
Vertebral arteries
Common carotid arteries

Muscle & Tendon Table

Muscle/Tendon	Location	Origin (O)/Insertion (I)	Action
Abductor pollicis brevis	Wrist/Hand/Thumb	O: Transverse carpal ligament and the tubercle of the scaphoid bone or (occasionally) the tubercle of the trapezium I: Base of the proximal phalanx of the thumb	Abducts the thumb and with muscles of the thenar eminence, acts to oppose the thumb
Abductor pollicis longus (APL)	Forearm/Thumb/Hand/Wrist	O: Posterior radius, posterior ulna and interosseous membrane I: Base 1st metacarpal Combined with the extensor pollicis brevis makes the anatomic snuff box.	Abducts and extends thumb at CMC joint; assists wrist abduction (radial deviation)
Achilles tendon	Lower Leg	O: Joins the gastrocnemius and soleus muscles I: Calcaneus	Flexor tendon – plantar flexes foot
Anconeus	Elbow	O: Lateral epicondyle humerus I: Posterior olecranon	Extends forearm
Brachialis	Elbow	O: Distal ½ anterior humeral shaft I: Coronoid process and ulnar tuberosity	Flexes forearm
Biceps brachii	Shoulder/Upper Arm	Long Head: O: Supraglenoid tubercle of the scapula to join the biceps tendon, short head in the middle of the humerus forming the biceps muscle belly Short Head: O: Coracoid process at the top of the scapula I: Radial tuberosity Long head and short head join in the middle of the humerus forming the biceps muscle belly	Flexes elbow Supinates forearm Weakly assists shoulder with forward flexion (long head) Short head provides horizontal adduction to stabilize shoulder joint and resist dislocation. With elbow flexed becomes a powerful supinator
Common flexor tendon 1. Pronator teres 2. Flexor carpi radialis (FCR) 3. Palmaris longus 4. Flexor digitorum superficialis (sublimis) (FDS) 5. Flexor carpi ulnaris (FCU)	Forearm/Hand	Common flexor tendon formed by 5 muscles of the forearm. There are slight variations in the site of origin and insertion 1. O: Medial epicondyle humerus and coronoid process of the ulna. I: Mid-lateral surface radial shaft 2. O: Medial epicondyle humerus. I: Base of 2nd and 3rd metacarpal 3. O: Medial epicondyle humerus. I: Palmar aponeurosis and flexor retinaculum 4. O: Medial epicondyle humerus, coronoid process ulna and anterior oblique line of radius. I: shaft middle phalanx digits 2-5 5. O: Medial epicondyle of the humerus, olecranon and posterior border ulna I: Pisiform, hook of hamate and 5th metacarpal.	1. Pronator Teres-pronation of forearm; assists elbow flexion 2. FCR- flexion and abduction of wrist (radial deviation) 3. Palmaris longus-assists wrist flexion 4. FDS- flexion middle phalanx PIP joint digits 2-4; assists wrist flexion 5. FCU- flexes and adducts hand at the wrist
Coracobrachialis	Shoulder/Upper Arm	O: Coracoid process I: Midshaft of humerus	Adducts & flexes shoulder
Deltoid	Shoulder/Upper Arm	O: Lateral 1/3 of clavicle, acromion and spine of scapula I: Deltoid tuberosity of humerus Large triangular shaped muscle composed of three parts	Anterior-Flex & medially rotate shoulder; Middle-assist w/abduction of humerus at shoulder; Posterior-extend & laterally rotate humerus
Extensor carpi radialis longus (ECRL)	Forearm/Hand	O: Lateral epicondyle humerus I: Dorsal surface 2nd metacarpal	Extends and abducts wrist; active during fist clenching
Extensor (digitorum) communis (EDC)	Forearm/Wrist/Hand/Finger	O: Lateral epicondyle humerus terminates into 4 tendons in the hand I: On the lateral and dorsal surfaces of digits 2-5 (fingers)	Extends the metacarpophalangeal (MCP), proximal interphalangeal (PIP) and distal interphalangeal (DIP) joints of 2nd-5th fingers and wrist
Extensor digitorum longus (EDL)	Lower Leg/Ankle/Foot	O: Lateral condyle tibia, proximal 2/3 anterior fibula shaft and interosseous membrane I: Middle and distal phalanx toes 2-5	Extension lateral 4 digits at metatarsophalangeal joint; assists dorsiflexion of foot at ankle
Extensor hallicus longus (EHL)	Lower Leg/Ankle/Foot	O: Middle part anterior surface fibula and interosseous membrane I: Dorsal aspect base distal phalanx great toe	Extends great toe; assists dorsiflexion of foot at ankle; weak invertor

Muscle/Tendon	Location	Origin (O)/Insertion (I)	Action
Extensor pollicis brevis (EPB)	Wrist/Hand/Thumb	O: Distal radius (dorsal surface) and interosseous membrane I: Base proximal phalanx thumb Combined with the abductor pollicis longus makes the anatomic snuff box	Extends the thumb at metacarpophalangeal joint (MCPJ)
Extensor pollicis longus (EPL)	Wrist/Hand/Thumb	O: Dorsal surface of the ulna and interosseous membrane I: Base distal phalanx thumb	Extends distal phalanx thumb at IP joint; assists wrist abduction
Flexor digitorum longus (FDL)	Lower Leg/Ankle/Foot	O: Medial posterior tibia shaft I: Base distal phalanx digits 2-5	Flexes digits 2-5; plantar flex ankle; supports longitudinal arch of foot
Flexor digitorum profundus (FDP)	Forearm/Wrist/Hand	O: Proximal 1/3 anterior-medial surface ulna and interosseous membrane; in the hand splits into 4 tendons I: Base of the distal phalanx, digits 2-5 (fingers)	Flexes the distal phalanx, digits 2-5 (fingers)
Flexor hallucis longus (FHL)	Lower Leg/Ankle/Foot	O: Inferior 2/3 posterior fibula; inferior interosseous membrane I: Base distal phalanx great toe (hallux)	Flexes great toe at all joints; weakly plantar flexes ankle; supports medial longitudinal arches of foot
Flexor pollicis brevis (FPB)	Wrist/Hand/Thumb	O: Distal edge of the transverse carpal ligament and the tubercle of the trapezium I: Proximal phalanx of the thumb	Flexes the thumb at the metacarpophalangeal (MCPJ) and carpometacarpal (CMC) joint
Flexor pollicis longus (FPL)	Forearm/Wrist/Hand/ Thumb	O: Below the radial tuberosity on the anterior surface of the radius and interosseous membrane I: Base distal phalanx thumb	Flexes the thumb at the metacarpophalangeal (MCPJ) and interphalangeal (IPJ) joint
Hamstring	Upper Leg/Knee	Composed of three muscles 1. Semitendinosus O: Ischial tuberosity I: Anterior proximal tibial shaft Semimembranosus O: Ischial tuberosity I: Posterior medial tibial condyle 2. Biceps femoris O: Long head ischial tuberosity; short head linea aspera femoral shaft and lateral supracondylar line I: Head of fibula	1. Semitendinosus and Semimembranosus-Flexes leg at knee, when knee flexed medially rotates tibia; thigh extensor at hip joint; when hip & knee both flexed, extends trunk 2. Biceps femoris-Flexes leg and rotates laterally when knee flexed; extends thigh
Intrinsics of hand hypothenar 1. Abductor digiti minimi 2. Flexor digiti minimi brevis 3. Opponens digiti minimi	Wrist/Hand/Finger	1. O: Pisiform I: Medial side of base proximal phalanx 5th finger 2. O: Hook of hamate & flexor retinaculum I: Medial side of base proximal phalanx 5th finger 3. O: Hook of hamate and transverse carpal ligament I: Uulnar aspect shaft 5th metacarpal	1. Abducts 5th finger; assists flexion proximal phalanx 2. Flexes proximal phalanx 5th finger 3. Rotates the 5th metacarpal bone forward
Intrinsics of hand short 1. Dorsal interossei 1-4 2. Dorsal interossei 1-3 3. Lumbricals 1st & 2nd 4. Lumbricals 3rd & 4th	Wrist/Hand	1. O: Adjacent sides of 2 MC I: Bases of proximal phalanges; extensor expansions of 2-4 fingers 2. O: Palmar surface 2nd, 4th & 5th MC I: Bases of proximal phalanges; extensor expansions of 2nd, 4th & 5th fingers 3. O: Lateral two tendons of FDP I: Lateral sides of extensor expansion of 2nd-5th 4. O: Medial 3 tendons of FDP I: Lateral sides of extensor expansion of 2nd-5th	1. Abduct 2-4 fingers from axial line; acts w/ lumbricals to flex MCP jt and extend IP jt 2. Adduct 2nd, 4th, 5th fingers from axial line; assist lumbricals to flex MCP jt and extend IP jt; extensor expansions of 2nd-4th fingers 3. Flex MCP jt; extend IP joint 2-5 4. Flex MCP jt; extend IP joint 2-5

Muscle/Tendon	Location	Origin (O)/Insertion (I)	Action
Intrinsics of hand thenar 1. Abductor pollicis brevis 2. Adductor pollicis 3. Flexor pollicis brevis 4. Opponens pollicis	Wrist/Hand/Thumb	1. O: Flexor retinaculum & tubercle scaphoid & trapezium I: :Lateral side of base of proximal phalanx thumb 2. O: Oblique head base 2nd & 3rd MC, capitate, adjacent carpals and transverse head anterior surface shaft 3rd MC I: Medial side base of proximal phalanx thumb 3. O: Flexor retinaculum & tubercle scaphoid & trapezium I: Lateral side of base of proximal phalanx thumb 4. O: Transverse carpal ligament and the tubercle of the trapezium I: Lateral border shaft 1st metacarpal	1. Abducts thumb; helps w/opposition 2. Adducts thumb toward lateral border of palm 3. Flexes thumb 4. Rotates the thumb in opposition with fingers
Lumbricals (foot)	Foot	O: Lumbricals-flexor digitorum longus tendon I: Medial side base proximal phalanges 2-5	Assist in joint movement between metatarsals
Patellar tendon	Knee/Lower Leg	Connects the bottom of the patella to the top of the tibia The tendon is actually a ligament because it joins bone to bone	Works with the quadriceps tendon to bend and straighten the knee
Pectoralis major	Chest/Upper Arm	O: Clavicle, sternum, ribs 2-6 I: Upper shaft of humerus	Adducts, flexes, medially rotates humerus
Peroneus (fibularis) brevis	Lower Leg/Ankle/Foot	O: Distal 2/3 lateral shaft fibula I: Becomes a tendon midcalf that runs behind the lateral malleolus inserts on tuberosity base 5th metatarsal	Eversion of foot; assists with plantar flexion of foot at ankle
Peroneus (fibularis) longus	Lower Leg/Ankle/Foot	O: Head and upper 2/3 lateral surface fibula I: Becomes a long tendon midcalf that runs behind the lateral malleolus and crosses obliquely on plantar surface of foot inserts on base 1st metatarsal and medial cuneiform	Eversion of foot; weak plantar flexion foot at ankle
Peroneus (fibularis) tertius	Lower Leg/Ankle/Foot	O: Inferior 1/3 anterior surface fibula and interosseous membrane I: Dorsum base 5th metatarsal	Dorsiflexes ankle and aids inversion of foot
Quadratus plantae	Foot	O: Calcaneus I: Flexor digitorum tendons	Assists flexor muscles
Quadriceps femoris	Upper Leg/Knee	Composed of four muscles: Rectus femoris O: Anterior inferior iliac spine and ilium superior to acetabulum I: Combines to form quadriceps tendon; inserts base of patella and tibial tuberosity via patellar ligament Vastus lateralis O: Greater trochanter and lateral aspect femoral shaft I: Lateral patella and tendon of rectus femoris Vastus medialis O: Intertrochanteric line and medial aspect femoral shaft I: Medial border of quadriceps tendon and medial aspect of patella; tibial tuberosity via patellar ligament Vastus intermedius: O: Anterior and lateral surface femoral shaft I: Posterior surface upper border of patella; tibial tuberosity via patellar ligament	Extends leg at knee joint; rectus femoris with iliopsoas helps flex thigh and stabilized hip joint
Quadriceps tendon	Upper Leg/Knee	Fibrous band of tissue that connects the quadriceps muscle of the anterior thigh to the patella (kneecap)	Holds the patella (kneecap) in the patellofemoral groove of the femur enabling it to act as a fulcrum and provide power to bend and straighten the knee

Muscle/Tendon	Location	Origin (O)/Insertion (I)	Action
Rotator cuff tendons: 1. Supraspinatus 2. Infraspinatus 3. Teres minor 4. Subscapularis	Shoulder/Upper Arm	Rotator cuff tendons are formed by 4 muscles of the shoulder/upper arm. They all originate from the scapula and insert (terminate) on the humerus: 1. O: Supraspinous fossa of scapula. I: Superior facet greater tuberosity humerus. 2. O: Infraspinous fossa of scapula. I: Middle facet greater tuberosity humerus. 3. O: Middle half of the lateral border of the scapula. I: Inferior facet greater tuberosity humerus 4. O: Subscapular fossa of scapula. I: Either the lesser tuberosity humerus or the humeral neck.	1. Initiates abduction of shoulder joint (completed by deltoid) 2. Externally rotates the arm; helps hold humeral head in glenoid cavity 3. Externally rotates the arm; helps hold humeral head in glenoid cavity 4. Internally rotates and adducts the humerus; helps hold humeral head in glenoid cavity
Tibialis anterior	Lower Leg/Ankle/Foot	O: Lateral condyle and superior half lateral tibia I: Base 1st metatarsal, plantar surface medial cuneiform	Dorsiflexion ankle, foot inversion at subtalar and midtarsal joints
Tibialis posterior	Lower Leg/Ankle/Foot	O: Interosseus membrane; posterior surface of tibia and fibula I: Tuberosity of tarsal navicula, cuneiform and cuboid and bases of 2nd, 3rd and 4th metatarsals	Plantar flexes ankle; inverts foot
Triceps	Shoulder/Upper Arm	Long head: O: Infraglenoid tubercle of scapula; Lateral head: O: Upper half of posterior surface shaft of humerus Medial head O: Lower half of posterior surface shaft of humerus I: Olecranon process Only muscle on the back of the arm	Extends elbow joint; long head can adduct humerus and extend it from flexed position; stabilizes shoulder joint

